Principles
and Practice
of Mechanical
Ventilation

Principles

and Practice

of Mechanical

Ventilation

Second Edition

Editor

Martin J. Tobin, MD

Professor of Medicine and Anesthesiology
Director, Division of Pulmonary and Critical Care Medicine
Loyola University of Chicago Stritch School of Medicine and
Edward Hines, Jr., Veterans Administration Hospital
Attending Physician, RML Specialty Hospital
Maywood, Illinois

McGraw-Hill

Medical Publishing Division

New York   Chicago   San Francisco   Lisbon   London   Madrid   Mexico City   Milan
New Delhi   San Juan   Seoul   Singapore   Sydney   Toronto

1234567890 CCI/CCI 09876

ISBN 0-07-144767-9

This book was set in Palatino by TechBooks, Inc.
The editors were Martin J. Wonsiewicz, Christie Naglieri, and Penny Linskey
The production supervisor was Sherri Souffrance
The index was prepared by Pat Perrier
The cover designer was Mary McKeon
The book was printed at Courier Kendallville

Library of Congress Cataloging-in-Publication Data

Principles and practice of mechanical ventilation / editor, Martin J. Tobin.—2nd ed.
    p. ;   cm.
    Includes bibliographical references and index.
    ISBN 0-07-144767-9 (hardcover)
    1. Respiratory therapy.   2. Respirators (Medical equipment)   3. Artificial respiration.
  I. Tobin, Martin J.
    [DNLM: 1. Respiration, Artificial—methods.   2. Respiratory Therapy—methods.
  3. Ventilators, Mechanical. WF 145 P957 2006]
  RC735.I5P75 2006
  615.8′36—dc22

                  2005054371

To Sareen, Damien, Kate, and Kieran

CONTENTS

CONTRIBUTORS

Charles G. Alex, MD
Professor of Medicine, Division of Pulmonary and Critical Care Medicine, Loyola University of Chicago, Stritch School of Medicine and Edward Hines Jr. Veterans Administration Hospital, Hines, Illinois
Chapter 53: Fighting the Ventilator

Marcelo B.P. Amato, MD, PhD
Laboratory of Medical Investigation (LIM-09) and Respiratory ICU–Hospital das Clínicas Pulmonary Division–University of São Paulo Medical School, São Paulo, SP, Brazil
Chapter 10: Pressure-Controlled and Inverse-Ratio Ventilation

Lorenzo Appendini, MD
Fondazione Salvatore Maugeri, IRCCS, Scientific Institute of Veruno, Pulmonary Division, Veruno (NO), Italy
Chapter 31: Mechanical Ventilation in Chronic Obstructive Pulmonary Disease

Elie Azoulay, MD, PhD
Service de Réanimation Médicale, Hôpital Saint-Louis et Université Paris 7
Chapter 66: The Ethics of Withholding and Withdrawing Mechanical Ventilation

Steven M. Banks, PhD
Mathematical Statistician, Critical Care Medicine Department, Clinical Center, National Institutes of Health, Bethesda, Maryland
Chapter 67: Interpreting Clinical Trials of Mechanical Ventilation: The Importance of Routine Care

Robert B. Banzett, PhD
Associate Professor, Physiology Program, Department of Environmental Health, Harvard School of Public Health & Beth Israel Deaconess Medical Center, Harvard Medical School, Boston, Massachusetts
Chapter 55: Addressing Respiratory Discomfort in the Ventilated Patient
Chapter 56: Ventilator-Supported Speech

Robert Bartlett, MD, FACS
Professor, General and Thoracic Surgery, The University of Michigan Health System, Ann Arbor, Michigan
Chapter 21: Extracorporeal Membrane Oxygenation and Extracorporal Life Support

Jason H.T. Bates, PhD, DSc
Research Professor, Vermont Lung Center, University of Vermont College of Medicine Burlington, Vermont
Chapter 14: Closed-Loop Ventilation

Ahmet Baydur, MD, FACP, FCCP
Professor of Clinical Medicine, Division of Pulmonary and Critical Care Medicine, Department of Medicine, Keck School of Medicine, University of Southern California, Los Angeles, California
Chapter 32: Mechanical Ventilation in Neuromuscular Disease

Andrew D. Bersten, MB, BS, MD, FJFICM
Professor, Department of Critical Care Medicine, Flinders Medical Centre and School of Medicine, Flinders University, Adelaide, South Australia
Chapter 65: Fluid Management in the Ventilated Patient

Michael J. Bishop, MD
Professor of Anesthesiology and Medicine (Adjunct, Pulmonary and Critical Care), Veterans Affairs Puget Sound Health Care System, University of Washington, Seattle, Washington
Chapter 38: Airway Management

Lluís Blanch, MD, PhD
Critical Care Center, Hospital de Sabadell, Corporació Parc Taulí, Institut Universitari Fundació Parc Taulí Universitat Autónoma de Barcelona Sabadell, Spain
Chapter 24: Transtracheal Gas Insufflation

Michela Bombino, MD
Staff, Department of Perioperative Medicine and Intensive Care, A.O. Ospedale S. Gerardo, Monza, Italy
Chapter 22: Extracorporeal Carbon Dioxide Removal

Richard D. Branson, MS, RRT
Associate Professor of Surgery, University of Cincinnati
Medical Center, Cincinnati, Ohio
Chapter 16: Feedback Enhancements on Ventilator Breaths
Chapter 28: Transport of the Ventilator Supported Patient

Laurent Brochard, MD
Réanimation Médicale, Assistance Publique-Hôpitaux de
Paris, Hôpital Henri Mondor, Université Paris 12, and
INSERM U 615, Créteil, France
Chapter 9: Pressure Support Ventilation

Robert Brown, MD
Director, Respiratory Acute Care Unit; Director, Pulmonary
Function Laboratory; Associate Professor of Medicine,
Pulmonary and Critical Care Medicine Unit, Department of
Medicine, Massachusetts General Hospital, Harvard
Medical School, Boston, MA.
*Chapter 55: Addressing Respiratory Discomfort in the Ventilated
Patient*
Chapter 56: Ventilator-Supported Speech

Shannon S. Carson, MD
Assistant Professor, Division of Pulmonary and Critical Care
Medicine, University of North Carolina School of Medicine,
Chapel Hill, North Carolina
Chapter 68: Economics of Ventilator Care

Jean Chastre, MD
Service de Réanimation Médicale, Institut de Cardiologie,
Groupe Hospitalier Pitié, Paris, France
Chapter 46: Pneumonia in the Ventilator-Dependent Patient

Robert L. Chatburn, BS, RRT-NPS, FAARC
Director, Respiratory Care Department, University
Hospitals of Cleveland; Associate Professor, Department of
Pediatrics, Case Western Reserve University,
Cleveland, Ohio
Chapter 2: Classification of Mechanical Ventilators

Daniel W. Chipman, BS, RRT
Assistant Director, Department of Respiratory Care,
Massachusetts General Hospital, Boston, Massachusetts
Chapter 3: Basic Principles of Ventilator Machinery

Gene L. Colice, MD
Professor of Medicine, The George Washington University
School of Medicine; Director, Pulmonary, Critical Care and
Respiratory Services, Washington Hospital Center,
Washington, DC
*Chapter 1: Historical Perspective on the Development of
Mechanical Ventilation*

Antonio Corrado, MD
Unità di Terapia Intensiva Respiratoria-Fisiopatologia
Toracica, Azienda Ospedaliera-Universitaria Careggi,
Firenze, Italy
Chapter 17: Negative Pressure Ventilation

Gerard J. Criner, MD
Professor of Medicine and Director, Pulmonary and Critical
Care Medicine, Temple University School of Medicine and
Temple Lung Center, Philadelphia, Pennsylvania
Chapter 54: Psychological Problems in the Ventilated Patient

Xizhong Cui, MD, PhD
Senior Research Specialist, Critical Care Medicine
Department, Clinical Center, National Institutes
of Health, Bethesda, Maryland
*Chapter 67: Interpreting Clinical Trials of Mechanical Ventilation:
The Importance of Routine Care*

J. Randall Curtis, MD, MPH
Professor of Medicine, Division of Pulmonary and Critical
Care Medicine, and Director, Harborview/University of
Washington End-of-life Care Research Program, University
of Washington, Harborview Medical Center, Seattle,
Washington
Chapter 70: Long-Term Outcomes After Mechanical Ventilation

Katherine J. Deans, MD
Research Fellow, Critical Care Medicine Department,
Clinical Center, National Institutes of Health, Bethesda,
Maryland; Department of Surgery, Massachusetts General
Hospital, Boston, Massachusetts
*Chapter 67: Interpreting Clinical Trials of Mechanical Ventilation:
The Importance of Routine Care*

Steven Deem, MD
Associate Professor of Anesthesiology and Medicine
(Adjunct, Pulmonary and Critical Care), University of
Washington, Harborview Medical Center, Seattle,
Washington
Chapter 38: Airway Management

Rajiv Dhand, MD, FCCP
Professor of Medicine and Director, Division of Pulmonary,
Critical Care, and Environmental Medicine, Department of
Internal Medicine, University of Missouri- Columbia; Staff
Physician, Harry S. Truman VA Hospital, Columbia,
Missouri
Chapter 63: Bronchodilator Therapy

Anthony F. DiMarco, MD
Professor of Medicine, Physiology and Biophysics, Case
Western Reserve University, Cleveland, Ohio; Director,
Department of Respiratory Therapy and Chief, Department
of Medicine, University Hospitals Health System, Geauga
Regional Hospital
Chapter 62: Diaphragmatic Pacing

Didier Dreyfuss, MD
Professor of Critical Care Medicine, Faculté Denis Diderot,
Paris; Chairman of Critical Care Department, Hôpital
Louis-Mourier, Colombes, (Assistance Publique- Hôpitaux
de Paris); and Institut National de la Santé et de la Récherche
Médicale, Faculté Denis Diderot, Université Paris VII, France
Chapter 42: Ventilator-Induced Lung Injury

Peter Q. Eichacker, MD
Senior Investigator, Head Critical Care Section, Critical Care Medicine Department, Clinical Center, National Institutes of Health, Bethesda, MD
Chapter 67: Interpreting Clinical Trials of Mechanical Ventilation: The Importance of Routine Care

Mark Elliott, MD, FRCP
Department of Respiratory Medicine, St James's University Hospital, Beckett Street, Leeds, England
Chapter 34: Non Invasive Ventilation on a General Ward

Scott K. Epstein, MD
Vice Chair, Department of Medicine, Caritas-St. Elizabeth's Medical Center; Professor of Medicine, Department of Medicine, Tufts University School of Medicine Boston, Massachusetts
Chapter 41: Complications Associated with Mechanical Ventilation

Jean-Yves Fagon, MD, PhD
Service de Réanimation Médicale, Hôpital Européen Georges-Pompidou, Assistance Publique-Hôpitaux de Paris, Université René Descartes-Paris 5, Paris, France
Chapter 46: Pneumonia in the Ventilator-Dependent Patient

Patrick J. Fahey, MD, FACP
The John W. Clarke Professor and Chairman, Department of Medicine, Loyola University Medical Center, Maywood
Chapter 53: Fighting the Ventilator

Antoni Ferrer, MD
Servei de Pneumologia, Hospital de Sabadell, Corporació Parc Taulí, Institut Universitari Fundació Parc Taulí, Universitat Autònoma de Barcelona, Sabadell, Spain
Chapter 37: Effect of Mechanical Ventilation on Gas Exchange

James B. Fink, MS, RRT, FAARC
Fellow, Respiratory Science, Nektar Therapeutics, Mountain View, California
Chapter 69: Purchasing a Ventilator

Alison B. Froese, MD, FRCPC
Professor of Anesthesiology, Physiology and Pediatrics, Queen's University; Staff Anesthesiologist, Department of Anesthesiology, Kingston General Hospital, Kingston, Ontario, Canada
Chapter 20: High Frequency Ventilation

Luciano Gattinoni, MD, FRCP
Professor of Anesthesia and Intensive Care, University of Milan, Istituto di Anestesia e Rianimazione, Fondazione IRCCS, Ospedale Maggiore Policlinico, Mangiagalli e Regina Elena, Milano, Italy
Chapter 22: Extracorporeal Carbon Dioxide Removal
Chapter 50: Prone Positioning in Acute Respiratory Failure

Dimitris Georgopoulos, MD, PhD
Professor of Medicine and Director of Intensive Care Medicine Department, University Hospital of Heraklion, University of Crete, Heraklion, Crete, Greece
Chapter 35: Effects of Mechanical Ventilation on Control of Breathing

Achim von Goedecke, MD
Associate Professor of Anesthesiology and Critical Care Medicine, Department of Anesthesiology and Critical Care Medicine, Innsbruck Medical University, Innsbruck, Austria
Chapter 27: Mechanical Ventilation During Resuscitation

Ivan Goldstein, MD, PhD
Réanimation Chirugicale Polyvalente Pierre Viars, Hôpital Pitié-Salpêtrière, Assistance Publique Hôpitaux de Paris, Université Pierre et Marie Curie, Paris, France
Chapter 64: Inhaled Antibiotic Therapy

Lawrence R. Goodman, MD
Professor, Diagnostic Radiology & Pulmonary Medicine, Medical College of Wisconsin, Milwaukee, Wisconsin
Chapter 48: Imaging of the Mechanically Ventilated Patient

Massimo Gorini, MD
Unità di Terapia Intensiva Respiratoria-Fisiopatologia Toracica, Azienda Ospedaliera-Universitaria Careggi, Firenze, Italy
Chapter 17: Negative Pressure Ventilation

Jesse B. Hall, MD
Professor of Medicine, Section Chief Pulmonary and Critical Care Medicine, Department of Medicine, Section of Pulmonary and Critical Care University of Chicago, Chicago, Illinois
Chapter 51: Pain Control, Sedation, and Neuromuscular Blockade

Juerg Hammer, MD
Professor of Pediatrics, Head, Division of Intensive Care and Pulmonology, University Children's Hospital Basel, Basel, Switzerland
Chapter 25: Mechanical Ventilation in the Neonatal and Pediatric Setting

Patrick J. Hanly, MD, MRCPI, FRCPC, ABSM
Professor of Medicine, University of Calgary, Alberta, Canada; Director, Lung Association Sleep Centre, Foothills Medical Centre, Calgary, Alberta, Canada
Chapter 57: Sleep in the Ventilated Patient

John E. Heffner, MD
Professor of Medicine and Executive Medical Director, Medical University of South Carolina, Charleston, South Carolina
Chapter 40: Care of the Mechanically-Ventilated Patient with a Tracheostomy

Nicholas S. Hill, MD
Chief, Division of Pulmonary, Critical Care and Sleep
Medicine, Tufts-New England Medical Center; Professor of
Medicine, Tufts University School of Medicine, Boston,
Massachusetts
*Chapter 18: Noninvasive Respiratory Aids: Rocking Bed,
Pneumobelt, and Glossopharyngeal Breathing*
Chapter 19: Noninvasive Positive-Pressure Ventilation

Ronald B. Hirschl, MD
Professor of Surgery and Section Head, Department of
Pediatric Surgery, C.S. Mott Children's Hospital and
The University of Michigan Health System,
Ann Arbor, Michigan
Chapter 23: Liquid Ventilation

Jeannette D. Hoit, PhD, CCC-SLP
Professor, Department of Speech, Language, and Hearing
Sciences, University of Arizona, Tucson, AZ
Chapter 56: Ventilator-Supported Speech

Steven R. Holets, RRT
Anesthesia Clinical Research Unit, Department of
Anesthesiology, Division of Intensive Care and Respiratory
Care, Mayo Clinic College of Medicine, Rochester,
Minnesota
Chapter 6: Setting the Ventilator

Catherine Lee Hough, MD, MSc
Assistant Professor of Medicine, Division of Pulmonary and
Critical Care Medicine, Department of Medicine, University
of Washington, Harborview Medical Center, Seattle,
Washington
Chapter 70: Long-Term Outcomes After Mechanical Ventilation

Rolf D. Hubmayr, MD
Professor of Medicine and Physiology, Mayo Clinic College
of Medicine, Rochester, Minnesota
Chapter 6: Setting the Ventilator

Jay A. Johannigman, MD, Col USAFR
Associate Professor of Surgery, Director Division of Trauma
and Critical Care, University of Cincinnati Medical Center,
Cincinnati, Ohio
Chapter 28: Transport of the Ventilator Supported Patient

Amal Jubran, MD
Professor of Medicine, Division of Pulmonary and Critical
Care Medicine, Loyola University of Chicago, Stritch School
of Medicine; Section Chief, Edward Hines Jr. Veterans
Administration Hospital, Hines, Illinois
Chapter 49: Monitoring During Mechanical Ventilation
Chapter 58: Weaning from Mechanical Ventilation

Robert M. Kacmarek, PhD, RRT
Professor, Department of Anesthesia, Harvard Medical
School; Director, Respiratory Care Services, Massachusetts
General Hospital, Boston, Massachusetts
Chapter 3: Basic Principles of Ventilator Machinery
Chapter 4: Equipment Required for Home Mechanical Ventilation

Brian P. Kavanagh, MB BSc MRCP(I) FRCP(C)
Dr. Geoffrey Barker Chair in Critical Care Medicine
Professor of Anesthesia, Medicine & Physiology, University
of Toronto Staff Physician & Director of Research,
Department of Critical Care Medicine,
Hospital for Sick Children, Toronto, Canada
Chapter 15: Permissive Hypercapnia

Sonia Khirani
Recipient of a European Respiratory Society Fellowship
(Number 174), U.S.C. Pneumologia, A.O. Ospedali Riuniti,
Bergamo, Italy
*Chapter 31: Mechanical Ventilation in Chronic Obstructive
Pulmonary Disease*

Theodor Kolobow, MD
Chief, Section on Pulmonary and Cardiac Assist Devices,
Pulmonary and Critical Care Medicine Branch, National
Heart, Lung and Blood Institute, National Institutes of
Health, Bethesda, Maryland
*Chapter 21: Extracorporeal Membrane Oxygenation and
Extracorporal Life Support*

John P. Kress, MD
Assistant Professor of Medicine, Department of Medicine,
Section of Pulmonary and Critical Care, University of
Chicago, Chicago, Illinois
*Chapter 51: Pain Control, Sedation, and
Neuromuscular Blockade*

John G. Laffey, MD, BSc, MA
Consultant and Clinical Lecturer, Department of Anesthesia
and Intensive Care, Galway University Hospitals and
National University of Ireland,
Galway, Ireland
Chapter 15: Permissive Hypercapnia

Franco Laghi, MD
Associate Professor of Medicine, Division of Pulmonary and
Critical Care Medicine, Loyola University of Chicago Stritch
School of Medicine and Edward Hines Jr. Veterans
Administration Hospital, Hines, Illinois
Chapter 5: Indications for Mechanical Ventilation
Chapter 59: Extubation

James W. Leatherman, MD
Associate Professor of Medicine, Pulmonary and Critical
Care Medicine, University of Minnesota, Hennepin County
Medical Center, Minneapolis, Minnesota
Chapter 30: Mechanical Ventilation for Severe Asthma

François Lellouche, MD
Réanimation Médicale, Assistance Publique-Hôpitaux de
Paris, Hôpital Henri Mondor, Université Paris 12,
Créteil, France
Chapter 9: Pressure Support Ventilation

Klaus Lewandowski, Prof. Dr. med.
Direktor der Klinik für Anästhesiologie, Intensivmedizin
und Schmerztherapie, Elisabeth-Krankenhaus Essen,
Akademisches Lehrkrankenhaus der Universität
Duisburg-Essen, Germany
Chapter 61: Inhaled Nitric Oxide

James F. Lewis, MD, FRCPC
Professor of Medicine/Physiology/Pharmacology,
St. Joseph's Health Centre University of Western Ontario,
London, Ontario Canada
Chapter 60: Surfactant

Robert F. Lodato, MD, PhD
Associate Professor of Medicine, Division of Pulmonary and
Critical Care Medicine, University of Texas Health Science
Center at Houston, Houston, Texas
Chapter 45: Oxygen Toxicity

Qin Lu, MD, PhD
Réanimation Chirurgicale Polyvalente, Research
Coordinator, Hôpital Pitié- Salpêtrière, Faculté de Médecine
Pierre et Marie Curie, Paris, France
Chapter 47: Sinus Infections in the Ventilated Patient
Chapter 64: Inhaled Antibiotic Therapy

Neil MacIntyre, MD
Professor of Medicine, Division of Pulmonary and Critical
Care Medicine, and Medical Director of Respiratory Care
Service, Duke University Medical Center, Durham,
North Carolina
Chapter 16: Feedback Enhancements on Ventilator Breaths

Salvatore Maurizio Maggiore, MD, PhD
Department of Anesthesiology and Intensive Care, Agostino
Gemelli University Hospital Università Cattolica del Sacro
Cuore, Rome, Italy
Chapter 11: Positive End-Expiratory Pressure

Atul Malhotra, MD
Staff, Department of Pathology, Massachusetts General
Hospital, Boston, Massachusetts
Chapter 4: Equipment Required for Home Mechanical Ventilation

Jordi Mancebo, MD
Unit Director, Servei de Medicina Intensiva, Hospital de
Sant Pau, Barcelona, Spain Associate Professor of Medicine,
Universitat Autònoma de Barcelona,
Barcelona, Spain
Chapter 7: Assist-Control Ventilation

John J. Marini, MD
Professor of Medicine, University of Minnesota,
Minneapolis/St. Paul; Director of Physiological and
Translational Research, Regions Hospital,
St. Paul, Minnesota
Chapter 10: Pressure-Controlled and Inverse-Ratio Ventilation
*Chapter 29: Mechanical Ventilation in the Acute Respiratory
Distress Syndrome*

Ubaldo Martin, MD
Assistant Professor of Medicine, Division of Pulmonary and
Critical Care Medicine, Temple University School of
Medicine, Temple Lung Center, Temple University Hospital,
Philadelphia, Pennsylvania
*Chapter 54: Psychological Problems in the
Ventilated Patient*

Bonnie Martin-Harris, PhD, CCC-SLP
Associate Professor, Otolaryngology-Head and Neck
Surgery and College of Health Professions, College of
Dental Medicine; Director, MUSC Evelyn Trammell Institute
for Voice and Swallowing, Medical University of South
Carolina, Charleston; Consultant, Evelyn Trammell Voice &
Swallowing Center, Saint Joseph's Hospital of Atlanta,
Atlanta, Georgia
*Chapter 40: Care of the Mechanically-Ventilated Patient
with a Tracheostomy*

Daniele Mascheroni, MD
Ospedale Policlinico, Servizio di Anesthesia e Rianimazione,
Milano, Italy
Chapter 50: Prone Positioning in Acute Respiratory Failure

Peter C. Minneci, MD
Research Fellow, Critical Care Medicine Department,
Clinical Center, National Institutes of Health, Bethesda,
Maryland; Department of Surgery, Massachusetts
General Hospital, Boston, Massachusetts
*Chapter 67: Interpreting Clinical Trials of Mechanical Ventilation:
The Importance of Routine Care*

Avi Nahum, MD, PhD
Section Head, Department of Pulmonary and Critical Care
Medicine, Regions Hospital, St Paul, Minnesota; Associate
Professor of Medicine, University of Minnesota.
Chapter 24: Transtracheal Gas Insufflation

Charles Natanson, MD
Senior Investigator, Critical Care Medicine Department,
Clinical Center, National Institutes of Health,
Bethesda, Maryland
*Chapter 67: Interpreting Clinical Trials of Mechanical Ventilation:
The Importance of Routine Care*

Stefano Nava, MD
Respiratory Intensive Care Unit, Fondazione S. Maugeri,
Istituto Scientifico di Pavia, Pavia, Italy
Chapter 33: Chronic Ventilator Facilities

Paolo Navalesi, MD
Respiratory Intensive Care Unit,
Fondazione S. Maugeri-IRCCS, Pavia, Italy
Chapter 11: Positive End-Expiratory Pressure

Paolo Pelosi, MD
Ospedale Policlinico, Servizio di Anesthesia e Rianimazione,
Milano, Italy
Chapter 50: Prone Positioning in Acute Respiratory Failure

Antonio Pesenti, MD
Professor of Anesthesia and Intensive Care, University of
Milan-Bicocca; Director, Department of Perioperative
Medicine and Intensive Care, A.O. Ospedale S. Gerardo,
Monza, Italy
Chapter 22: Extracorporeal Carbon Dioxide Removal

David J. Pierson, MD
Medical Director, Respiratory Care, Harborview Medical
Center; Professor of Medicine, Division of Pulmonary and
Critical Care Medicine, University of Washington,
Seattle, Washington.
Chapter 44: Barotrauma and Bronchopleural Fistula

Michael R. Pinsky, MD, CM, Dr hc, FCCP, FCCM
Professor of Critical Care Medicine, Bioengineering and
Anesthesiology, University of Pittsburgh,
Pittsburgh, Pennsylvania
*Chapter 36: Effect of Mechanical Ventilation on
Heart-Lung Interactions*

Guido Polese, MD
U.S.C. Pneumologia, A.O. Ospedali Riuniti, Bergamo, Italy
*Chapter 31: Mechanical Ventilation in Chronic Obstructive
Pulmonary Disease*

Christian Putensen, MD
Professor of Intensive Care Medicine, Division of Intensive
Care Medicine, Department of Anesthesiology and
Intensive Care Medicine, University of Bonn,
Bonn, Germany
Chapter 12: Airway Pressure Release Ventilation

Jean-Damien Ricard, MD, PhD
Associate Professor of Intensive Care Medicine, Denis
Diderot Medical School, Paris VII University, Paris and
Service de Réanimation Médicale, Hôpital Louis-Mourier,
Assistance Publique – Hôpitaux de Paris, Colombes, France.
Chapter 42: Ventilator-Induced Lung Injury
Chapter 52: Humidification

Peter C. Rimensberger, MD
Associate Professor of Intensive Care Medicine, Pediatric
and Neonatal Intensive Care, Children's Hospital,
University Hospitals of Geneva, Geneva, Switzerland
*Chapter 25: Mechanical Ventilation in the Neonatal and Pediatric
Setting*

Robert Rodriguez-Roison, MD, FRCPE
Professor of Medicine, Chair, Servei de Pneumologia,
Hospital Clínic, Institut d'Investigacions Biomédiques
August Pi i Sunyer (IDIBAPS), Departament de Medicina,
Universitat de Barcelona, Barcelona, Spain
*Chapter 37: Effect of Mechanical Ventilation on
Gas Exchange*

Andrea Rossi, MD
Director U.S.C. Pneumologia, A.O. Ospedali Riuniti,
Bergamo, Italia
*Chapter 31: Mechanical Ventilation in Chronic Obstructive
Pulmonary Disease*

Jean-Jacques Rouby, MD, PhD
Professor of Anesthesiology and Critical Care Medicine,
Director, Réanimation Chirurgicale Polyvalente, Hôpital
Pitié-Salpêtrière, Faculté de Médecine Pierre et Marie Curie,
Paris, France
Chapter 47: Sinus Infections in the Ventilated Patient
Chapter 64: Inhaled Antibiotic Therapy

Catherine S.H. Sassoon, MD
Professor of Medicine, Pulmonary and Critical Care Section,
University of California, Irvine and
Veterans Affairs Long Beach Healthcare System,
Long Beach, California
Chapter 8: Intermittent Mandatory Ventilation

Georges Saumon, MD
Institut National de la Santé et de la Recherche Médicale,
Faculté Xavier Bichat, Paris, France
Chapter 42: Ventilator-Induced Lung Injury

Rupa Seetharamaiah, MD
Research Fellow, Section of Pediatric Surgery, C.S. Mott
Children's Hospital and The University of Michigan Health
System, Ann Arbor, Michigan
Chapter 23: Liquid Ventilation

John L. Stauffer, MD
Clinical Professor of Medicine, Division of Pulmonary,
Allergy, and Critical Care Medicine, The Pennsylvania State
University College of Medicine, The Milton S. Hershey
Medical Center, Hershey, Pennsylvania; Senior Director,
Respiratory Medicine Development Center,
GlaxoSmithKline, Research Triangle Park, North Carolina
Chapter 39: Complications of Translaryngeal Intubation

Martin J. Tobin, MD
Professor of Medicine and Anesthesiology; Director,
Division of Pulmonary and Critical Care Medicine, Loyola
University of Chicago Stritch School of Medicine and
Edward Hines, Jr., Veterans Administration Hospital;
Attending Physician, RML Specialty Hospital,
Maywood, Illinois
Chapter 5: Indications for Mechanical Ventilation
Chapter 49: Monitoring During Mechanical Ventilation
Chapter 53: Fighting the Ventilator
Chapter 58: Weaning from Mechanical Ventilation
Chapter 59: Extubation

Stefano Tredici, MD
Research Fellow, Department of General Surgery,
C.S. Mott Children's Hospital and The University of
Michigan Health System, Ann Arbor, Michigan
Chapter 23: Liquid Ventilation

David V. Tuxen, MB, BS, FRACP, Dip DHM, MD, FJFICM
Assoc Professor, Senior Intensivist, Department of Intensive Care Unit and Hyperbaric Medicine, The Alfred, Prahran, Victoria, Australia
Chapter 26: Independent Lung Ventilation

Franco Valenza, MD
Assistant Professor, Università degli Studi di Milano, Department of Anesthesia and Intensive Care, Ospedale Maggiore Policlinico, Mangiagalli e Regina Elena, Servizio di Anestesia e Rianimazione, Milano, Italy
Chapter 50: Prone Positioning in Acute Respiratory Failure

Theodoros Vassilakopoulos, MD
Assistant Professor, Department of Pulmonary and Critical Care Medicine, National and Kapodistrian University of Athens Medical School, Athens, Greece
Chapter 43: Ventilator-Induced Diaphragm Dysfunction

Michele Vitacca, MD
Pulmonary Rehabilitation and Weaning Center, Fondazione S. Maugeri IRCCS, Gussago/ Lumezzane (BS) Italy
Chapter 33: Chronic Ventilator Facilities

Volker Wenzel, MD
Associate Professor of Anesthesiology and Critical Care Medicine; Head, Experimental Anesthesiology, Department of Anesthesiology and Critical Care Medicine, Innsbruck Medical University, Innsbruck, Austria
Chapter 27: Mechanical Ventilation During Resuscitation

Hermann Wrigge, MD
Associate Professor of Anesthesiology, Department of Anesthesiology and Intensive Care Medicine, University of Bonn, Bonn, Germany
Chapter 12: Airway Pressure Release Ventilation

Magdy Younes, MD
Departments of Medicine, St. Michael's Hospital and the University of Toronto, Toronto, Ontario, Canada
Chapter 13: Proportional Assist Ventilation

PREFACE

The second edition of a textbook is typically a cosmetic job. A snip here. A tuck there. And correction of major howlers. New editions usually arrive within three or four years of their predecessor. This short interval decreases the incentive of contributing authors to make substantial changes to their chapters. As such, content changes much less than might be expected. Twelve years have passed before bringing out a new edition of *Principles and Practice of Mechanical Ventilation*. Thus, this volume is more representative of a fourth than of a second edition. Rather than confess to laziness, I would like readers to believe that I did not wish to burden them with the usual second and third editions.

The goal of the book is unchanged: to provide a comprehensive and contemporary discussion of mechanical ventilation based on the application of knowledge gained through research. By providing a single resource where clinicians can find answers to all their questions about mechanical ventilation, I hope the contained information will improve the care of ventilated-supported patients.

The content of the book, however, is drastically changed. The new edition contains twenty-four completely new chapters. Subjects include dyspnea in the ventilated patient, diaphragmatic pacing, inhaled antibiotic therapy, liquid ventilation, inhaled nitric oxide, ventilator-induced diaphragmatic damage, and speech and sleep in the ventilated patient. Other new chapters cover additional exciting developments since the early 1990s. Integrated accounts of ventilator strategies in major disease states, such as the acute respiratory distress syndrome, asthma and chronic obstructive pulmonary disease, are presented in new chapters. Today, mechanical ventilation is used increasingly outside the intensive care unit; several new chapters distill the expertise that has been garnered at these locations. For seventeen of previously included chapters, new authors provide completely fresh accounts. To make way for all this new material, several chapters (in the previous edition) have been deleted. All in all, the content bears little resemblance to that of the first edition, with the exception of the historical perspective chapter.

Editing this book has been a tremendous educational experience. It is fascinating to see how mechanical ventilation has changed over the past twelve years. When engaged in day-to-day practice of a discipline, we underestimate how much it changes from year to year. Leafing through the two editions of this book makes it clear that few areas of medicine have undergone so much change as mechanical ventilation. I hope that future developments will be stimulated by the new edition, through its shining a spotlight on hidden recesses of ignorance and areas of controversy.

In the Internet age, readers have questioned the usefulness of textbooks. Today's physicians can access the latest research across a wide spectrum of journals. By design, however, the information is fragmented, and little effort is made to fit new research into the mosaic of existing knowledge. A state-of-the-art review article can provide comprehensive discussion of a subject. The authors of such an article, however, cannot achieve substantial depth unless they focus on a narrow area. A detailed discussion of all the nuances of positive end-expiratory pressure requires much more space than a journal editor would be willing to allow. Thus, physicians wishing to gain expertise across a broad field are left with many gaps–especially of subjects that journal editors deem unfashionable. For trainees struggling to acquire expertise in a field, new understanding necessarily depends on the epistemic ideals they set for themselves, the path they choose for gaining knowledge. One vital epistemic ideal is coherence: that beliefs within a field not only make sense individually but they also hang together in a coherent pattern. From the Middle Ages onwards, *Summa* accounts that collate, synthesize and integrate all known information in a field have been sought after by scholars and professionals. For this task, the textbook has no competitor.

Book chapters can vary enormously in organization, presentation, and readability. To minimize such variation, authors of the new edition of *Principles and Practice of Mechanical Ventilation* were given detailed guidance on the structure of their chapter and also the expected content of every other chapter. This planned structure should make it easier for readers to contrast the advantages and disadvantages of various ventilator techniques. To enhance clarity and readability and to achieve a relatively uniform style throughout the book, I personally copy-edited each manuscript. Some chapters underwent several revisions after their first submission.

The dread of every textbook editor is the delay between arrival of the first and last chapter. A year or more may elapse, making chapters of punctual contributors appear dated by the time a book is published. Every effort was made to avoid this problem, and chapters arrived within four months of their due date. (A couple of authors who could not meet an extension of the deadline were dropped.) McGraw-Hill placed the book on a rapid production track. As such, the book achieves a freshness attained by few medical journals.

A multi-authored text can only be as good as its authors. For each chapter, I selected the scientists and clinicians at the forefront of research in that area. Such authors are attuned to evolving developments in a field, thus guarding against early obsolescence of covered material. A striking feature is the geographical diversity of the authors, reflecting the international base of advances in this field.

The corpus of knowledge required for the practice of a medical subspecialty is generated by researchers who typically devote their professional life to that field. Virtually all patients admitted to an intensive care unit can be classified under one or two headings: admission for the delivery of mechanical ventilation or for detailed monitoring of vital organ function. Thus, the unique corpus of knowledge required for expert practice of intensive care medicine is provided by *Principles and Practice of Mechanical Ventilation* and its companion text, *Principles and Practice of Intensive Care Monitoring*. Outside these two areas, intensive care physicians who seek the most authoritative writing on a subject must turn to articles and texts published by non-intensivists.

This book would not have been possible without the help of several people, and to them I am extremely grateful. First are the more than one hundred authors, whose knowledge, commitment and wisdom form the core of the book. I am grateful to Jane LaMarre, Lynnel Hodge, and Karen Janata for invaluable assistance at several stages of the project. I thank Patrick J Fahey, MD, Chairman of Medicine at Loyola and Brian Schmitt, MD Chairman of Medicine at Hines for their support of scholarly activity. The faculty and fellows in the Division of Pulmonary and Critical Care Medicine at Loyola-Hines provided stimulation and insight. Penelope Linskey, Christie Naglieri, and Karen Edmonson at McGraw-Hill guided the book through its production. Finally, I thank my family for their forbearance.

Kilkenny, 2006

Principles
and Practice
of Mechanical
Ventilation

PART I
HISTORICAL BACKGROUND

Chapter 1

HISTORICAL PERSPECTIVE ON THE DEVELOPMENT OF MECHANICAL VENTILATION

GENE L. COLICE

Breathing is both fundamentally obvious and essential to life. From ancient times, humankind has attributed to air and the inhalation of air unique and almost mystical properties. Chinese philosophers as far back as 2000 BC described *lien ch'i* as the process of transmitting the inspired breath into the "soul substance." Anaximenes of Miltus, a Greek physician born around 570 BC, stated that *pneuma*, or breath, was the essence of all things and recognized it as essential to life. He noted that "as our soul, being air, sustains us, so *pneuma* and air pervade the whole world." Biblical references similarly emphasize the importance of breathing: "then the Lord God formed man of dust from the ground and breathed into his nostrils the breath of life and man became a living being" (Genesis 2:7); "when thou takest away their breath, they die and return to their dust"(Psalms 104:29). Understanding why breathing is essential to life, that is, the physiologic role of ventilation, however, was not intuitively apparent. It has taken millennia and a circuitous route encompassing advances in widely disparate fields before humankind has developed clear insights into the purpose of ventilation.

The history of understanding ventilation is intimately intertwined with the history of anatomy, chemistry, and physiology; exploration under water and in the air; and of course, modern medicine. Anatomists from the early Greek physician-scholars to Malpighi described the structural connections of the lungs to the heart and vasculature and developed the earliest insights into the functional relationships of these organs. They emphasized the role of the lungs in bringing air into the body and probably expelling waste products but showed little understanding of how air was used by the body. Chemists defined the constituents of air and explained the metabolic processes by which the cells used oxygen and produced carbon dioxide. Physiologists complemented these studies by exploring the relationships between levels of oxygen and carbon dioxide in the blood and ventilation. Explorers tested the true limits of physiology. Travel in the air and underwater exposed humans to extremes in ventilatory demands and prompted the development of mechanical adjuncts to ventilation. Following the various historical threads provided by the anatomists, chemists, physiologists, and explorers will provide a useful perspective on the tapestry of a technique modern physicians accept casually: mechanical ventilation.

Anatomists: Of the Heart and Lungs

EARLY GREEKS

The Chinese and Egyptian civilizations apparently developed practical and reliable medical treatments millennia before the birth of Christ but left little evidence of an interest in either anatomy or physiology. During the Greco-Roman period, study in many aspects of biology flourished. Beginning with Anaximenes around 550 BC and ending with Galen about AD 160, the Greeks showed great interest in the structure and function of the human body. Early Greek physicians endorsed Empedocles' view that all matter was composed of four essential elements: earth, air, fire, and water. Each of these elements had primary qualities of heat and cold, moisture and dryness.[1] Empedocles applied this global philosophic view to the human body by stating that "innate heat," or the soul, was distributed from the heart via the blood to various parts of the body.

This concept of the heart as a source and distributor of an innate heat played an important role in how these early physicians viewed the relationship among the lungs, heart, and blood. The Hippocratic corpus, for instance, stated that the purpose of respiration was to cool the heart. Air was thought to be pumped by the atria from the lungs to the right ventricle via the pulmonary artery and to the left ventricle through the pulmonary vein.[2] Aristotle performed vivisections and dissections on hundreds of species but did little to clarify how the heart and lungs cooperated. He believed that blood was an indispensable part of animals but that blood was found only in veins. Arteries, in contrast, contained only air. This conclusion probably was based on his methods of sacrificing animals. The animals were starved, to better define their vessels, and then they were strangled. During the strangulation, blood probably pooled in the right side of the heart and venous circulation, leaving the left side of the heart and arteries empty.[2] Aristotle described a three-chamber heart connected with passages leading in the direction of the lung, but these connections were minute and indiscernible.[3] Presumably, the lungs cooled the blood and somehow supplied it with air.[4]

Erasistratus (born around 300 BC) took significant steps forward from Aristotle's views. He believed that air taken in by the lungs was transferred via the pulmonary artery to the left ventricle. Within the left ventricle, air was transformed into *pneuma zotikon*, or the "vital spirit," and was distributed through air-filled arteries to various parts of the body. The *pneuma zotikon* carried to the brain was secondarily changed to the *pneuma psychikon* ("animal spirit"). This animal spirit was transmitted to the muscles by the hollow nerves. Apparently, Erasistratus understood that the right ventricle facilitated venous return to the heart by suction during diastole and also that venous valves allowed only one-way flow of blood. These concepts would become instrumental in leading to understanding the true nature of circulation.[1]

As Greek civilization waned and the Roman Empire flourished, medicine became more pragmatic, with one outstanding exception. The Greek physician Claudius Galen established a practice in Rome in AD 161 and soon became recognized as the most influential physician in the world. Galen's insights, based on extensive vivisection and physiologic studies, are well worth examining. He demonstrated that arteries contain blood by inserting a tube into the femoral artery of a dog.[5,6] Blood flow through the tube could be controlled by adjusting tension on a ligature placed around the proximal portion of the artery. He described a four-chamber heart with auricles distinct from the right and left ventricles. Galen also believed that the "power of pulsation has its origin in the heart itself" and that the "power [to contract and dilate] belongs by nature to the heart and is infused into the arteries from it."[5,6] He described valves in the heart in detail and, as did Erasistratus, recognized their essential importance in preventing the backward discharge of blood from the heart. He alluded several times to blood flowing, for example, from the body through the vena cava into the right ventricle and even made the remarkable statement that "in the entire body the arteries come together with the veins and exchange air and blood through extremely fine invisible orifices."[6] Furthermore, Galen believed that "fuliginous wastes" were somehow discharged from the blood through the lung.[6] This appreciation that the lungs served both to supply some property of air to the body and to discharge a waste product from the blood was the first true insight into the lung's role in ventilation. Ap-

parently, however, he did not understand the true circular nature of blood flow. Galen also failed in two critical ways to appreciate the true interaction of the heart and lungs. First, he believed, as did Aristotle and other earlier Greeks, that the left ventricle is the source of the innate heat that vitalizes the animal. Respiration in animals exists for the sake of the heart, which requires the substance of air to cool it. Expansion of the lung caused the lightest substance, that is, the outside air, to rush in and fill the bronchi. Galen provided no insight, though, into how air, or *pneuma*, might be drawn out from the bronchi and lungs into the heart. Second, he did not clearly describe blood flow from the right ventricle through the lungs and into the left ventricle. Indeed, his writings left the serious misconception that blood was somehow transported directly from the right to the left ventricle through the interventricular septum.[1,5,6]

RENAISSANCE PHYSICIANS

Galen's influence was pervasive for hundreds of years, in large part because the Romans did little to encourage experimentation in anatomy, and feudal lords and barbarians disparaged all science during the Dark Ages. Fortunately, Byzantine and Arab scholars maintained Galen's legacy and provided a foundation for the rebirth of science during the Renaissance.[1,6,7] A renewed interest in anatomy was triggered in the 1400s and 1500s by artists such as Leonardo da Vinci, who strove for an accurate and natural representation of the human form. For the first time in over a millennium, there was a surge of interest, primarily by Italian physicians, in dissection. Around 1550, Vesalius, the foremost anatomist of his time, corrected many inaccuracies in Galen's work and even questioned Galen's concept of blood flow from the right ventricle to the left ventricle. He specifically was skeptical about the flow of blood through the interventricular pores Galen described.[1,6,8] Vesalius's ideas may have been the critical catalyst for subsequent work leading to a true understanding of the circulation.

Servetus, a fellow student of Vesalius in Paris, suggested that the vital spirit is elaborated both by the force of heat from the left ventricle and by a change in color of the blood to reddish yellow. This change in color "is generated in the lungs from a mixture of inspired air with elaborated subtle blood which the right ventricle of the heart communicates to the left. However, this communication is made not through the middle wall of the heart, as is commonly believed, but by a very ingenious arrangement: the subtle blood courses through the lungs from the pulmonary artery to pulmonary vein, where it changes color. During this passage the blood is mixed with inspired air and through expiration it is cleansed of its sooty vapors. This mixture, suitably prepared for the production of the vital spirit, is drawn onward to the left ventricle of the heart by diastole."[6,9] Although Servetus' views proved ultimately to be correct, they were considered heretical at the time, and he was subsequently burned at the stake, along with most copies of his book, in 1553.

Fortunately, religious fervor did not dissuade Columbus, a dissectionist to Vesalius at Padua, from continuing the line of reasoning advanced by Servetus. In 1559 he cited evidence supporting the view that blood travels to the lungs via the pulmonary artery and then, along with air, is taken to the left ventricle through the pulmonary vein. He further advanced the concept of circulation by noting that the left ventricle distributes blood to the body through the aorta, blood returns to the right ventricle in the vena cava, and venous valves in the heart allow only one-way flow.[1,6,10]

These views clearly influenced William Harvey, who studied anatomy with Fabricius in Padua from 1600 to 1602. Harvey set out to investigate the "true movement, pulse, action, use and usefulness of the heart and arteries." He questioned why the left ventricle and right ventricle traditionally were felt to play such fundamentally different roles. If the right ventricle existed simply to nourish the lungs, why was its structure so similar to that of the left ventricle? Furthermore, when one directly observed the beating heart in animals, it was clear that the function of both right and left ventricles also was similar. In both cases, when the ventricle contracted, it expelled blood, and when it relaxed, it received blood. Cardiac systole coincided with arterial pulsations. The motion of the auricles preceded that of the ventricles. Indeed, the motions are consecutive with a rhythm about them, the auricles contracting and forcing blood into the ventricles and the ventricles, in turn, contracting and forcing blood into the arteries. "Since blood is constantly sent from the right ventricle into the lungs through the pulmonary artery and likewise constantly is drawn the left ventricle from the lungs . . . it cannot do otherwise than flow through continuously. This flow must occur by way of tiny pores and vascular openings through the lungs. Thus, the right ventricle may be said to be made for the sake of transmitting blood through the lungs, not for nourishing them."[6,11]

Harvey described blood flow through the body as being circular. This was easily understood if one just considered the quantity of blood pumped by the heart. If the heart pumped 1 to 2 drachms of blood per beat and beat 1000 times per half-hour, it put out almost 2000 drachms in this short time. This was more blood than was contained in the whole body. Clearly, the body could not produce amounts of blood fast enough to supply these needs. Where else could all the blood go but around and around "like a stage army in an opera." If this theory were correct, Harvey went on to say, then blood must be only a carrier of critical nutrients for the body. Presumably, the problem of the elimination of waste vapors from the lungs also was explained by the idea of blood as the carrier.[1,6,11]

With Harvey's remarkable insights, the relationship between the lungs and the heart and the role of blood were finally understood. Only two steps remained for the anatomists to resolve. First, the nature of the tiny pores and vascular openings through the lungs had to be explained. About 1650, Malpighi provided such an explanation through his work with early microscopes. He found that air passes via the trachea and bronchi into and out of microscopic saccules with no clear connection to the bloodstream. He further described capillaries: ". . . and such is the wandering about of these vessels as they proceed on this side from the vein and on the other side from the artery, that the vessels no longer maintain a straight direction, but there appears a network made up of the articulations of the two vessels. . . . blood flowed away along [these] tortuous vessels . . . always contained within tubules."[1,6] Second, Borelli, a mathematician in Pisa and a friend of Malpighi, first suggested the concept of diffusion. Air dissolved in liquids could pass through membranes without the existence of pores. Air and blood finally had been linked in a plausible manner.[1]

Chemists and Physiologists: Of the Air and Blood

UNDERSTANDING GASES

The anatomists had identified an entirely new set of problems for chemists and physiologists to consider. The concept of blood circulation had been well developed. It was accepted that the right ventricle pumped blood through the pulmonary artery to the lungs. In the lungs the blood took up some substance. This was evidenced by the change in color observed as blood passes through the pulmonary circulation. It also was presumed that the blood released "fuliginous wastes" into the lung. The site of this exchange was thought to be at the alveolar-capillary interface, and it probably occurred by the process of diffusion. What were the substances exchanged between blood and air in the lung? What changed the color of blood and was essential for the production of the "innate heat"? What was the process by which "innate heat" was produced, and where did this combustion occur, in the left ventricle as supposed from the earliest Greek physician-philosophers or elsewhere? Where were the "fuliginous wastes" produced, and were they in any way related to the production of "innate heat"? If the blood was a carrier, pumped by the left ventricle to the body, what was it carrying to the tissues and then again back to the heart?

Von Helmont provided a new approach to these problems by performing experiments with gases. In about 1620 he added acid to limestone and potash and collected the "air" liberated by the chemical reaction. This "air" extinguished a flame and seemed to be similar to the gas produced by fermentation. This "air" also appeared to be the same gas as that found in the Grotto del Cane. This grotto was notorious for containing air that would kill dogs but spare their taller masters.[1] The gas, of course, was carbon dioxide, but von Helmont's studies were not appreciated for well over a hundred years. What was appreciated, however, was that air was a complex substance. In the late seventeenth century, Boyle described this new insight well. He considered the constitution of air, which he called "atmospherical air," a confused aggregate of effluviums. For example, he recognized that sulfur particles could impregnate the air. This was apparent by the odor. Furthermore, there is some substance in air that is necessary to keep a flame burning and an animal alive. Place a flame in a bell jar, and the flame eventually will go out. Place an animal in such a chamber, and the animal eventually will die. If another animal is placed in that same chamber soon thereafter, it will die suddenly. This concept was nicely supported by Mayow's simple experiments around 1670. Enclosing a mouse in a bell jar resulted eventually in the mouse's death. If the bell jar was covered by a moistened bladder, the bladder bulged inward when the mouse died. Obviously, the animals needed something in air for survival. Mayow called this the "nitro-aereal spirit," and when it was depleted, the animals died.[1,12] It was well recognized that air had at least four qualities: heat, cold, dryness, and moisture. Philosophers and chemists recognized that air also had gravity, springiness, and the power to refract light. Boyle's suspicions, however, that air had other qualities primarily owing to its ingredients seemed well founded.[13,14]

In a remarkable and probably entirely intuitive insight, Mayow suggested that the ingredient essential for life, the "nitro-aereal spirit," was taken up by the blood and formed the basis of muscular contraction. Evidence supporting this concept came indirectly. The concept of air pressure apparently had just been appreciated by Galileo in the early 1600s. Torricelli found in 1644 that a column of mercury 30 inches high could be supported in a glass tube with its lower end in a base of mercury. He postulated that the weight of air supported this column of mercury. Pascal realized that if air did have weight, air pressure should vary with altitude. This hypothesis was confirmed when the height of a column of mercury was measured simultaneously by Pascal's brother-in-law Perier in the Puy-de-Dôme mountains and at sea level in 1648.

The ability to study the effects of changes in air pressure became possible when von Guericke invented the pneumatic machine, a device that reduced air pressure.[1,15] Robert Boyle was stimulated by Harvey's work on circulation to ask what part did air and respiration play. He saw the pneumatic pump as an ideal way to answer this question, and he commissioned Robert Hooke and the instrument maker Ralph Greatorex to design and build a closed vessel from which air could be extracted using a pumping mechanism to produce something approaching a vacuum (Fig. 1-1). Hooke, being an impatient and demanding type, soon dropped Greatorex from the endeavor and developed the pump himself. He also was the only one who could consistently operate the tempermental device. Boyle and Hooke used this pneumatic engine to study animals under low-pressure conditions. Apparently Hooke favored dramatic experiments, and he often demonstrated in front of crowds that small animals died after air was evacuated from the chamber. Hooke actually built a human-sized chamber in 1671 and volunteered to enter it. Fortunately, the pump effectively removed only about a quarter of the air, and Hooke survived.[16] Boyle believed that the difficulty encountered in breathing under these conditions was caused solely by the loss of elasticity in the air. He also went on to observe, however, that animal blood bubbled when placed in a vacuum. This observation clearly showed that blood contained a gas of some type.[13,14] In 1727 Hales introduced the pneumatic trough (Fig. 1-2). With this device he was able to distinguish between free gas and gas no longer in its elastic state but combined with a liquid.[1] The basis for blood gas machines had been invented.

The first constituent of air to be truly recognized was carbon dioxide. Joseph Black (around 1754) probably was

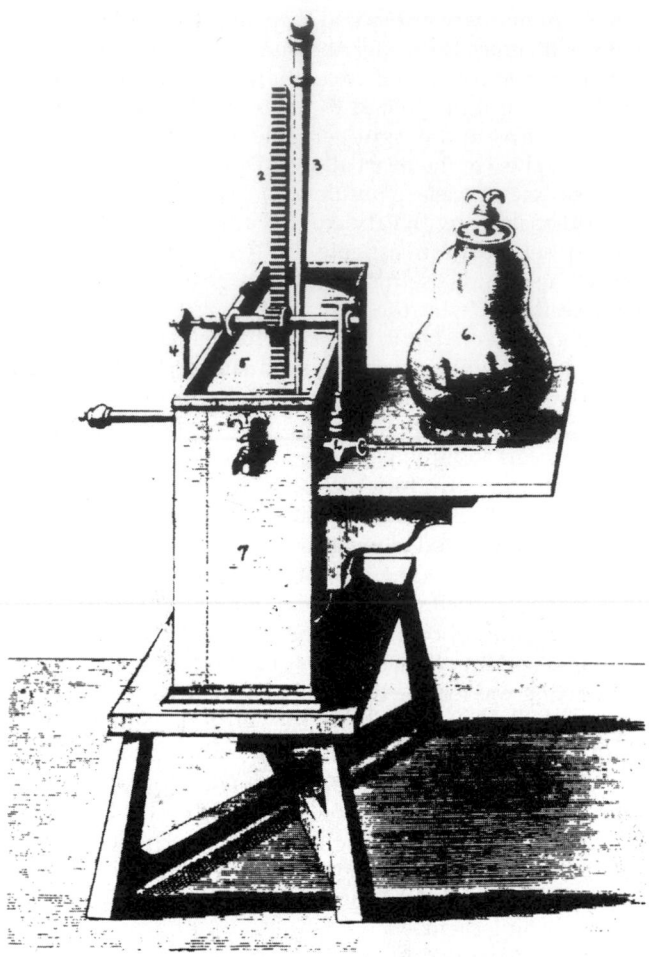

FIGURE 1-1 A pneumatical engine, or vacuum pump, devised by Hooke in collaboration with Boyle around 1660. The jar (6) contains an animal in this illustration. Pressure is lowered in the jar by raising the tightly fitting slide (5) with the crank (4). (*Used, with permission, from Graubard.*[6])

working on a cure for kidney stones when he found that limestone was transformed into caustic lime and lost weight on being heated. The weight loss occurred because a gas was liberated during the heating process. The same results occurred when the carbonates of alkali metals were treated with an acid such as hydrochloric acid. He called the liberated gas "fixed air" and found that it would react with lime water to form a white insoluble precipitate of chalk. This reaction became an invaluable marker for the presence of "fixed air." Black subsequently found that "fixed air" was produced by burning charcoal and fermenting beer. In a remarkable experiment he showed that "fixed air" was given off by respiration. In a Scottish church where a large congregation gathered for religious devotions, he allowed limewater to drip over rags in the air ducts. After the service, which lasted about 10 hours, he found a precipitate of crystalline lime ($CaCO_3$) in the rags, proof that "fixed air" was produced during the services. Black recognized that "fixed air" was the same gas described by von Helmont and would extinguish flame and life.[1,4,14]

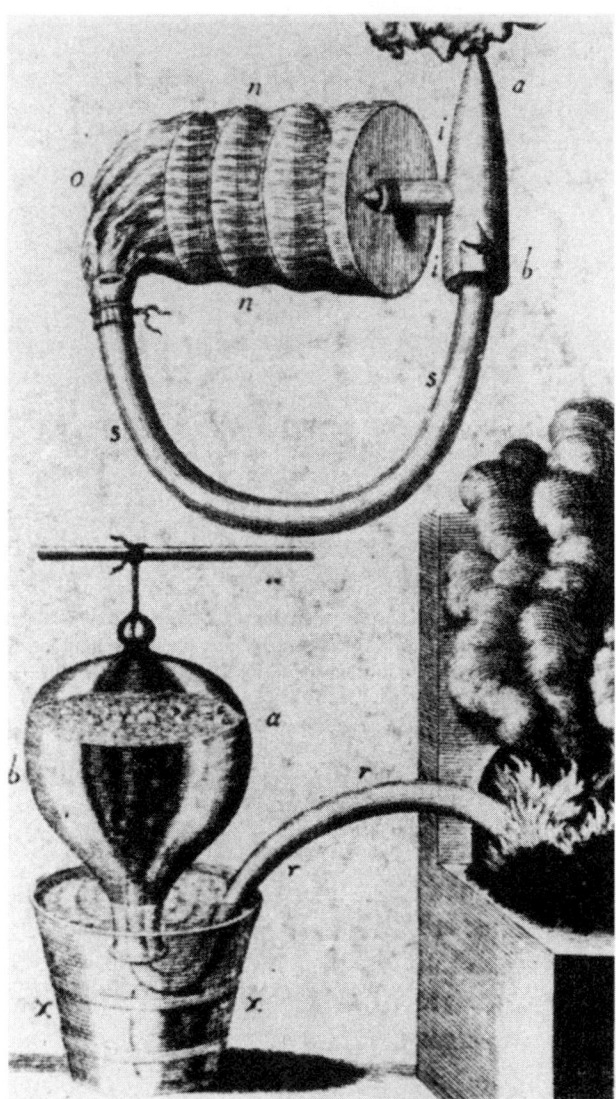

FIGURE 1-2 In 1727, Hales developed the pneumatic trough, shown on the bottom of this illustration. This device enabled him to collect gases produced by heating. On the top is a closed-circuit respiratory apparatus for inhaling the collected gases. (*Used, with permission, from Perkins.*[1])

In the early 1770s, Priestley and Scheele, working independently of each other but using similar methods, both produced and isolated "pure air." Priestley used a 12-inch lens to heat mercuric oxide. The gas released in this process passed through the long neck of a flask and was isolated over mercury. This gas allowed a flame to burn brighter and a mouse to live longer than in ordinary air.[1,4,15] Scheele also heated chemicals such as mercuric oxide and isolated the gases produced. He collected the gases in ox or hog bladders. Like Priestley, Scheele found that the gas isolated made a flame burn brighter. Neither Priestley nor Scheele understood the real significance of their findings. They attempted to explain their findings by the phlogiston theory of Stahl. Stahl felt that all material contained variable amounts of a substance called *phlogiston*, which could transform itself into fire on heating. The residual material, or ash, left after heat-

ing was *nonphlogiston*.[1,4] Remarkably, both men described their observations to Antoine Lavoisier, who would go on to discredit the phlogiston theory. Lavoisier was a successful businessman but enjoyed dabbling in science on an intermittent basis. His research proved to have a profound influence on chemistry. He repeated Priestley's experiments and found that if mercuric oxide was heated in the presence of charcoal, Black's "fixed air" would be produced. Further work led Lavoisier to the conclusion that ordinary air must have at least two separate components. One part was respirable, combined with metals during heating, and supported combustion. The other part was nonrespirable. In 1779 Lavoisier called the respirable component of air "oxygen." He also concluded from his experiments that "fixed air" was a combination of coal and the respirable portion of air. It was apparent to Lavoisier that oxygen, not phlogiston, was the explanation for combustion.[1,4,17]

METABOLISM

Political upheavals kept Lavoisier from his scientific work for several years, but later in the 1780s he performed a brilliant series of studies with the French mathematician Laplace on the use of oxygen by animals. Lavoisier knew that oxygen was essential for combustion and necessary for life. Furthermore, he was well aware of the Greek concept of internal heat presumably produced by the left ventricle. The obvious question was whether animals used oxygen for some type of internal combustion. Would this internal combustion be similar to that readily perceived by the burning of coal? To answer this question, the two great scientists built an ice calorimeter (Fig. 1-3). This device could do two things. Because the melting of ice was a heat-consuming process, the rate at which ice melted in the calorimeter could be used as a quantitative measure of heat production within the calorimeter. In addition, the consumption of oxygen could be measured. It then was a relatively simple task to put an animal inside the calorimeter and carefully measure heat production and oxygen consumption. As Lavoisier suspected, the amount of heat generated by the animal was similar to that produced by burning coal for the quantity of oxygen consumed.[1,4]

Despite Lavoisier's prodigious achievements in identifying the respirable portion of atmospheric air and in defining the chemical processes involved in the production of "innate heat," his political and business activities were caught up in the vortex of the French Revolution. In May 1794 the Father of Modern Chemistry was guillotined.[17] Fortunately, Lavoisier's findings and opinions were distributed widely and believed. More important, they stimulated intensive research in two areas: metabolism and the role of oxygen and carbon dioxide in ventilation.

It was not clear from Lavoisier's work where in the body internal combustion actually took place. The Greeks suspected that the left ventricle produced innate heat, and Lavoisier himself may have thought that internal combustion occurred in the lungs.[4] Spallanzani redirected attention to the tissue level. He took a variety of tissues from freshly killed animals and found that they took up oxygen

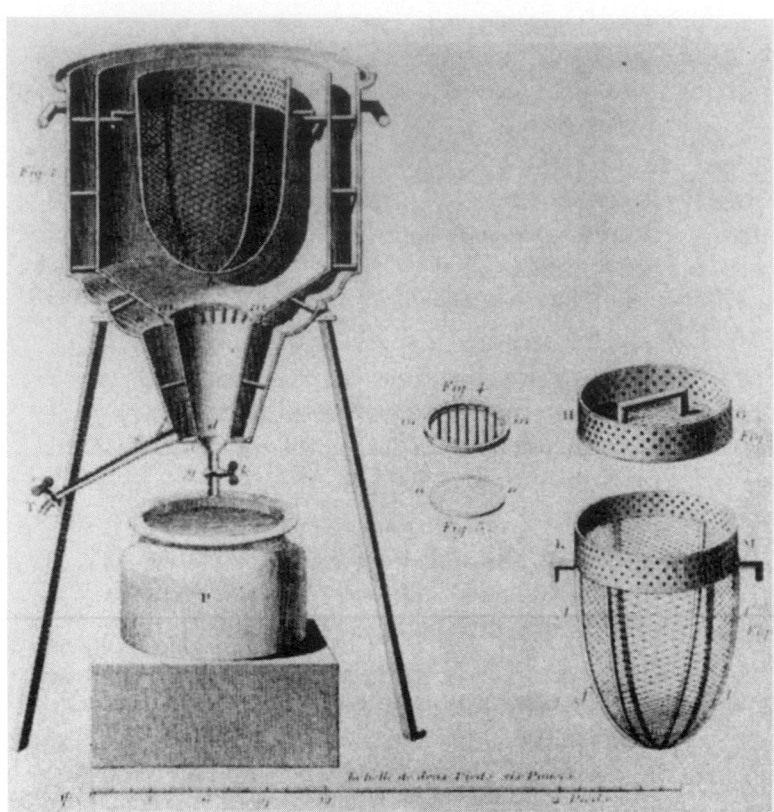

FIGURE 1-3 The ice calorimeter, designed by Lavoisier and Laplace, allowed these French scientists to measure the oxygen consumed by an animal and the heat produced by that same animal. With careful measurements, the internal combustion of animals was found to be similar, in terms of oxygen consumption and heat production, to open fires. (*Used, with permission, from Perkins.*[1])

and released carbon dioxide.[1] Magnus, relying on improved methods of analyzing the gas content of blood, found higher oxygen levels in arterial blood than in venous blood but higher carbon dioxide levels in venous blood than in arterial blood. He believed that inhaled oxygen was absorbed into the blood, transported throughout the body, given off at the capillary level to the tissues, and there formed the basis for the formation of carbon dioxide.[18] Many other scientists pursued this area of research and built elaborate devices to study metabolism and respiration. In 1849 Regnault and Reiset perfected a closed-circuit metabolic chamber with devices for circulating air, absorbing carbon dioxide, and periodically adding oxygen (Fig. 1-4). Pettenkofer built a closed-circuit metabolic chamber large enough for a man and a bicycle ergometer (Fig. 1-5).[19] This device relied on a steam engine to pump air, gas meters to measure air volumes, and barium hydroxide to collect carbon dioxide. Although these devices were intended to examine the relationship between inhaled oxygen and exhaled carbon dioxide, they also could be viewed as among some of the earliest methods of controlled ventilation. These efforts were essential in leading chemists to study cellular metabolism.

BLOOD GASES AND VENTILATION

Lavoisier's work also provided the critical pieces of data necessary for an explosion of knowledge on the role of gases in ventilation. From ancient times it was understood that some element in air was necessary for life and, furthermore, that "fuliginous wastes" were released from the lung. In separate experiments, the British scientist Lower and the Irish scientist Boyle provided the first evidence that uptake of gases in the lungs was related to gas content in the blood. In 1669 Lower placed a cork in the trachea of an animal and found that arterial blood took on a venous appearance. Removing the cork and ventilating the lungs with a bellows made the arterial blood bright red again. Lower felt that the blood must take in air during its course through the lungs and therefore owed its bright color entirely to an admixture of air. Moreover, after the air had in large measure left the blood again in the viscera, the venous blood became dark red.[20] A year later Boyle showed with his vacuum pump that blood contained gas. Following Lavoisier's studies, scientists knew that oxygen was the component of air essential for life and that carbon dioxide was the "fuliginous waste." The next step, understanding how oxygen and carbon dioxide were related to ventilation, required valid methods of measuring the content of these gases in blood.

In about 1797 Davey was the first actually to measure the amount of oxygen and carbon dioxide extracted from blood by an air pump.[4] The significance of this finding was not appreciated at the time. Magnus in 1837, however, successfully built a device for quantitative analysis of blood oxygen and carbon dioxide content.[18] This was a mercurial blood pump. Blood was enclosed in a glass tube in continuity with a vacuum pump. Carbon dioxide extracted by means of the vacuum was quantified by the change in weight of carbon dioxide–absorbent caustic potash. Oxygen content was determined by detonating the gas in hydrogen.[15] A limiting

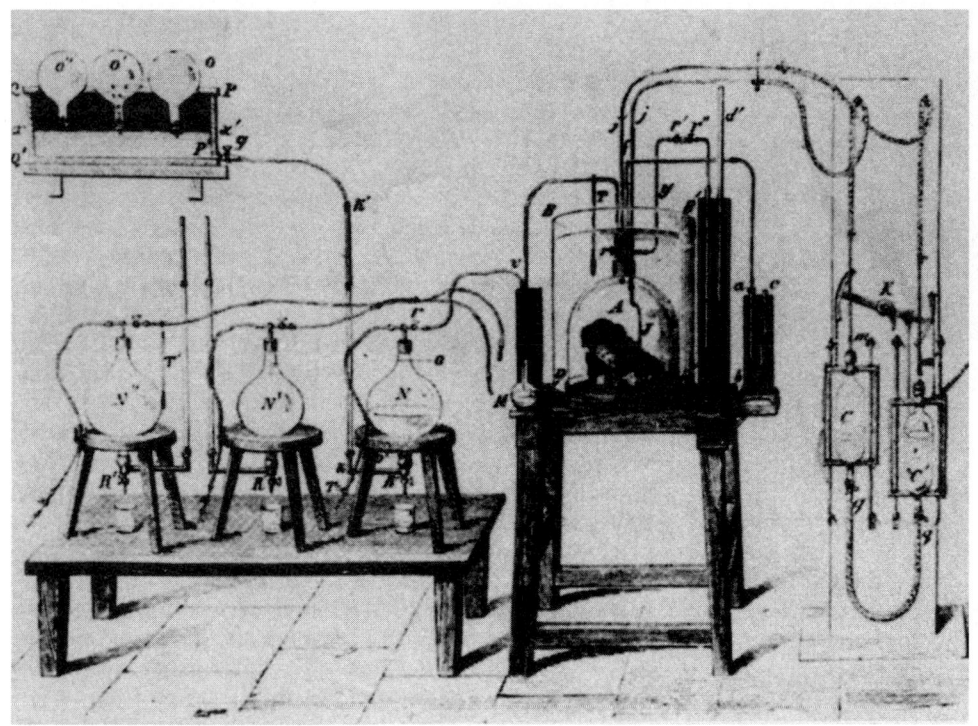

FIGURE 1-4 Regnault and Reiset developed a closed-circuit metabolic chamber in 1849 for studying oxygen consumption and carbon dioxide production in animals. (*Used, with permission, from Perkins.*[1])

factor in Magnus's work was the assumption that the quantity of oxygen and carbon dioxide in blood simply depended on absorption. Hence the variables determining gas content in blood were presumed to be the absorption coefficients and partial pressures of the gases. In the 1860s, working in concert, Meyer and Fernet showed that the gas content of blood was determined by more than just simple physical properties. Meyer found that the oxygen content of blood remained relatively stable despite large fluctuations in its partial pressure.[21] Fernet showed that blood absorbed more oxygen than did saline solution at a given partial pressure.[15]

Paul Bert was trained originally in law but later turned to medicine and studied under Claude Bernard in Paris in the 1860s. He became interested in altitude physiology through a close friendship with Jourdanet, a wealthy patron who had developed mountain sickness during a trip to Mexico. Jourdanet was willing to support many of Bert's experiments financially; through this work, Bert made a series of extremely important contributions to this field. For instance, he felt that it was intuitively obvious that oxygen consumption could not be strictly dependent on the physical properties of oxygen dissolving under pressure in the blood. As an example, he posed the problem of a bird in flight changing altitude abruptly. Oxygen consumption could be maintained with the sudden changes in pressure only if chemical reactions contributed to the oxygen-carrying capacity of blood.[15] In 1878 Bert went on to describe the first air curvilinear oxygen dissociation curves relating oxygen content of the blood to its pressure. Hoppe-Seyler was instrumental in attributing the oxygen-carrying capacity of the blood to hemoglobin.[22]

Remarkable insights into the relationship among ventilation and blood oxygen and carbon dioxide contents were achieved during the latter half of the nineteenth century. Besides his extensive experiments with animals in either high- or low-pressure chambers, Bert also examined the effect of ventilation on blood gas levels. Using a bellows to artificially ventilate animals through a tracheostomy, he found that increasing ventilation would increase oxygen content in blood and decrease the carbon dioxide content. Decreasing ventilation had the opposite effect.[15] Dohman, in Pflüger's laboratory, showed that both carbon dioxide excess and lack of oxygen would stimulate ventilation.[23] Miescher-Rusch demonstrated in 1885 that carbon dioxide excess was the more potent stimulus for ventilation.[1] Haldane and Priestley, building on this work, made great strides in analyzing the chemical control of ventilation. They developed a device for sampling end-tidal, or alveolar exhaled, gas (Fig. 1-6). Even small changes in alveolar carbon dioxide fraction greatly increased minute ventilation, but hypoxia did not increase minute ventilation until the alveolar oxygen fraction fell to 12–13%.[24]

Early measurements of arterial oxygen and carbon dioxide tensions led to widely divergent results. In Ludwig's laboratory the arterial partial pressure of oxygen was thought to be about 20 mmHg. The partial pressure of carbon dioxide reportedly was much higher than currently believed. These results could not entirely support the concept of passive gas movement between lung blood and tissues based on pressure gradients. Ludwig and others began to suspect that an active secretory process was involved in gas transport.[4] This hypothesis was suggested in part by the French biologist Biot, who observed that some deep-water fish had extremely large swim bladders. Of immense interest was the fact that the composition of the gas in those swim bladders seemed to be different than that of atmospheric

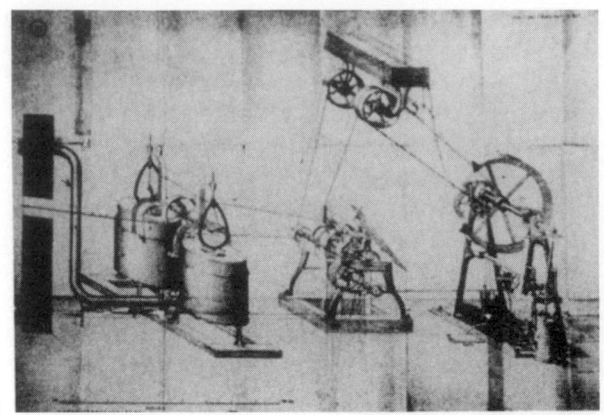

A

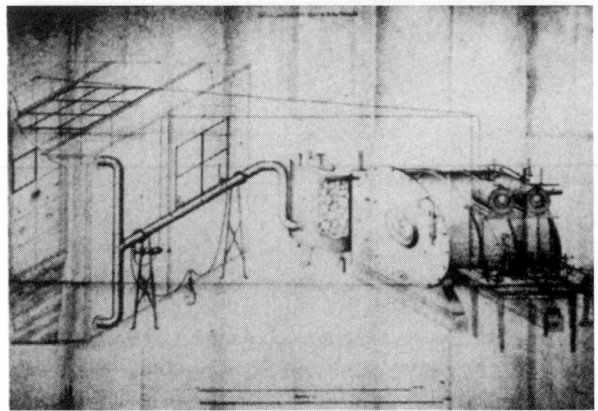

B

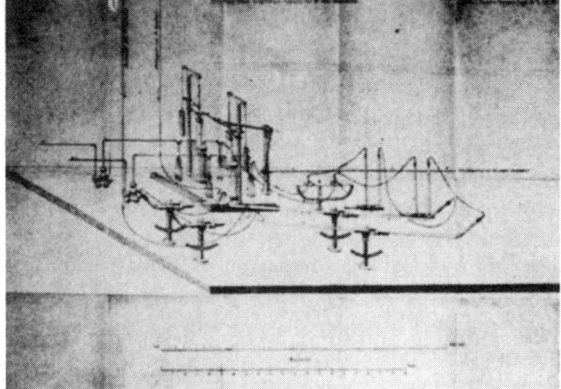

C

FIGURE 1-5 *A.* This huge device, constructed by Pettenkoffer, was large enough for a person. *B.* The actual chamber. The gas meters used to measure gas volumes are shown next to the chamber. The steam engine and gasometers for circulating air are labeled *A*. *C.* A close-up view of the gas-absorbing device adjacent to the gas meter in *B*. With this device Pettenkoffer and Voit studied the effect of diet on the respiratory quotient. (*Used, with permission, from Perkins.[1]*)

air. Biot concluded that gas was actively secreted into these bladders.[4,15,24,25] Pflüger and his coworkers developed the aerotonometer, a far more accurate device for measuring gas tensions than that used by Ludwig. When they obstructed a bronchus, they found no difference in the gas composition of air distal to the bronchial obstruction and that of pulmonary venous blood draining the area. They concluded that the

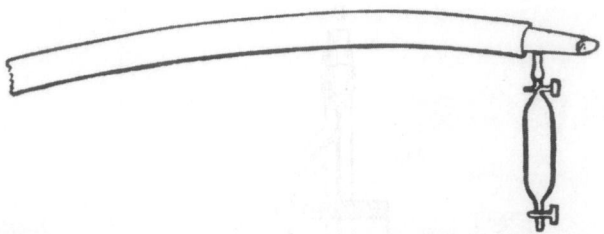

FIGURE 1-6 This relatively simple device enabled Haldane and Priestley to collect end-tidal expired air, which they felt approximated alveolar air. The subject exhaled through the mouthpiece at the right. At the end of expiration, the stopcock on the accessory collecting bag was opened, and a small aliquot of air was trapped in this device. (*Used, with permission, from Best et al: Physiological basis of medical practice. Baltimore: Williams & Wilkins, 1939: 509.*)

lung did not rely on active processes for transporting oxygen and carbon dioxide; passive diffusion was a sufficient explanation.[26]

Although Pflüger's findings were fairly convincing at the time, Bohr resurrected this controversy.[27] He found greater variability in blood and air carbon dioxide and oxygen tensions than previously reported by Pflüger and suspected that under some circumstances secretion of gases might occur. In response to this suspicion, Krogh, a student of Bohr's, developed an improved blood gas-measuring technique relying on the microaerotonometer (Fig. 1-7). With his wife, Krogh convincingly showed that alveolar air oxygen tension was higher than blood oxygen tension and vice versa for carbon dioxide tensions, even when the composition of inspired air was varied.[28] Douglas and Haldane confirmed Krogh's findings but wondered whether they were applicable only to people at rest. Perhaps during the stress of either exercise or high-altitude exposure, passive diffusion might not be sufficient. Indeed, the ability to secrete oxygen might explain the tolerance to high altitude developed by repeated or chronic exposures. Possibly carbon dioxide excretion might occur with increased carbon dioxide levels.[26] In a classic series of experiments, Marie Krogh showed that diffusion increased with exercise secondary to the concomitant increase in cardiac output.[29] Barcroft put to rest the diffusion-versus-secretion controversy with his "glass chamber" experiment. For 6 days he remained in a closed chamber subjected to hypoxia similar to that found on Pike's Peak. Oxygen saturation of radial artery blood was always less than that of blood exposed to simultaneously obtained alveolar gas, even during exercise. These were expected findings for gas transport based simply on passive diffusion.[30]

With this body of work, the chemists and physiologists had provided the fundamental knowledge necessary for the development of mechanical ventilation. Oxygen was the component of atmospheric gas understood to be essential for life. Carbon dioxide was the "fuliginous waste" gas released from the lungs. The exchange of oxygen and carbon dioxide between air and blood was determined by the tensions of these gases and simple passive diffusion. Blood was a carrier of these two gases, as Harvey first suggested. Oxygen was carried in two ways, both dissolved in plasma

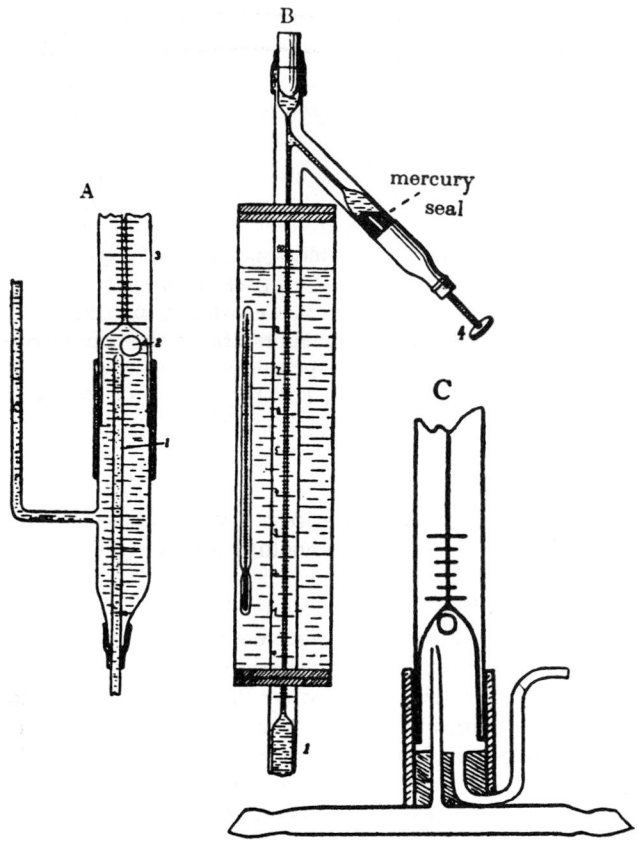

FIGURE 1-7   Krogh's microaerotonometer. *A.* **An enlarged view of the lower part of** *B.* **Through the bottom of the narrow tube (1) in** *A,* **blood is introduced. The blood leaves the upper end of the narrow tube (1) in a fine jet and plays on the air bubble (2). Once equilibrium is reached between the air bubble and blood, the air bubble is drawn by the screw plunger (4) into the graduated capillary tube shown in** *B.* **The volume of the air bubble is measured before and after treatment with KOH to absorb** CO_2 **and potassium pyrogallate to absorb** O_2. **The changes in volume of the bubble reflect blood** CO_2 **and** O_2 **content.** *C.* **A model of** *A* **designed for direct connection to a blood vessel. (***Used, with permission, from Best et al: Physiological basis of medical practice. Baltimore: Williams & Wilkins, 1939: 521.***)**

The concept of blood acid-base activity was just beginning to be examined in the early 1900s. By the 1930s, a practical electrode became available for determining anaerobic blood pH,[33] but pH was not thought to be useful clinically until the 1950s. In 1952, during the polio epidemic in Copenhagen, Ibsen suggested that hypoventilation, hypercapnia, and respiratory acidosis caused the high mortality rate in polio patients with respiratory paralysis. Clinicians disagreed because a high level of "bicarbonate" in the blood of these patients indicated an alkalosis of uncertain origin. By measuring pH, Ibsen was proved correct, and clinicians soon became acutely aware of the importance of determining both carbon dioxide levels and pH.[4] Numerous workers looked carefully at such factors as base excess, duration of hypercapnia, and renal buffering activity before Siggaard-Anderson published a pH/log P_{CO_2} acid-base chart in 1971.[34] This chart proved to be an invaluable basis for evaluating acute and chronic respiratory and metabolic acid-base disturbances. The development of practical blood gas machines suitable for use in clinical medicine did not occur until electrodes became available for measuring oxygen and carbon dioxide tensions in liquid solutions. Stow built the first electrode capable of measuring blood P_{CO_2}. As the basis for this device, he used a glass pH electrode with a coaxial central calomel electrode opening at its tip. A unique adaptation, however, was the use of a rubber finger cot to wrap the electrode. This wrap trapped a film of distilled water over the electrode. The finger cot then acted as a semipermeable membrane to separate the measuring electrode from the sample.[35] Clark used a similar idea in the development of an oxygen measuring device. Platinum electrodes were used as the measuring device, and polyethylene served as the semipermeable membrane.[36] By 1973, Radiometer was able to commercially produce the first automated blood gas analyzer, the ABL, capable of measuring P_{O_2}, P_{CO_2}, and pH in blood.[4]

Explorers and Working Men: Of Submarines and Balloons

Travel in the deep sea and flight have intrigued humankind for centuries. Achieving these goals has followed a typical pattern. First, individual explorers tested the limits of human endurance. As mechanical devices were developed to extend those limits, the deep sea and the air became accessible to commercial and military exploration. These forces further intensified the need for safe and efficient underwater and high-altitude travel. Unfortunately, the development of vehicles to carry humans aloft and under water proceeded faster than the appreciation of the physiologic risks. Calamitous events ensued, with serious injury and death often a consequence. Only a clear understanding of the ventilatory problems associated with flight and deep-sea travel has enabled human beings to reach outer space and the depths of the ocean floor. Appreciation of the requirements for mechanical ventilation in submarines and planes has provided valuable insights into methods of providing mechanical ventilation in disease.

and chemically combined with hemoglobin. Blood carried oxygen to the tissues, where oxygen was used in cellular metabolism, that is, the production of the body's "innate heat." Carbon dioxide was the waste product of this reaction. Oxygen and carbon dioxide tensions in the blood were related to ventilation in two critical ways. Increasing ventilation would secondarily increase oxygen tensions and decrease carbon dioxide levels. Decreasing ventilation would have the opposite effect. Because blood levels of oxygen and carbon dioxide could be measured, physiologists now had a means of assessing the adequacy of ventilation. Decreased oxygen tensions and increased carbon dioxide tensions played a critical role in the chemical control of ventilation.

Of course, much work remained. How carbon dioxide was carried by the blood was not entirely understood until experiments were performed by Bohr[31] and Haldane.[32]

EXPLORATION UNDER WATER

Diving bells undoubtedly were derived from ancient humans' inverting a clay pot over their heads and breathing the trapped air while under water. These devices were used in various forms by Alexander the Great at the siege of Tyre in 332 BC, the Romans in numerous naval battles, and pirates in the Black Sea.[37,38] In the 1500s, Sturmius constructed a heavy bell that, even though full of air, sank of its own weight. When the bell was positioned at the bottom of fairly shallow bodies of water, workers were able to enter and work within the protected area. Unfortunately, these bells had to be raised periodically to the surface to refresh the air. Although the nature of the foul air was not understood, an important principle of underwater work, the absolute need for adequate ventilation, was appreciated.[15]

Halley devised the first modern version of the diving bell in 1690 (Fig. 1-8). To drive out the air accumulated in the bell and "made foul" by the workers' respiration, small barrels of air were let down periodically from the surface and opened within the bell. Old air was released through the top of the bell by a valve. In 1691, Papin developed a technique for constantly injecting fresh air from the surface directly into the bell by means of a strong leather bellows. In 1788, Smeaton replaced the bellows with a pump for supplying fresh air to the submerged bell.[15,37,38]

Techniques used to make diving bells practical also were applied to divers. Naked divers have been described since the beginnings of recorded history. Xerxes used them to recover sunken treasure.[39] Sponge divers in the Mediterranean in the 1860s could stay submerged for 2 to 4 minutes and reach depths of 45 to 55 m.[40] *Amas*, female Japanese divers using only goggles and a weight to facilitate rapid descent, made up to 60 to 90 dives a day to similar depths.[41] Despite the remarkable adaptations of breath-holding measures developed by these naked divers,[42] the commercial and military use of naked divers was limited. In AD 77, Pliny described divers breathing through tubes while submerged and engaged in warfare. More sophisticated diving suits were described by Leonardo da Vinci in 1500 and Renatus in 1511. These suits also relied on tubes connected to the surface for ventilation. Although these breathing tubes prolonged underwater activities, they did not enable divers to reach even moderate depths.[15] Borelli described a complete diving dress with tubes in the helmet for recirculating and purifying air in 1680. Whether this actually was useful is unclear (Fig. 1-9).[37]

Klingert described the first modern diving suit in 1797.[37] It consisted of a large helmet connected by twin breathing pipes to an air reservoir that was large enough to have an associated platform. The diver stood on the platform and inhaled from the air reservoir through an intake pipe on the top of the reservoir and exhaled through a tube connected to the bottom of the reservoir. Siebe made substantial

FIGURE 1-8 Halley's version of the diving bell. Small barrels of fresh air were lowered periodically to the bell, and the worker inside the bell released the air. "Foul air" often was released by way of a valve at the top of the bell. Workers could exit the bell for short periods. (*Used, with permission, from Hill.*[38])

FIGURE 1-9 A fanciful diving suit designed by Borelli in 1680. (*Used, with permission, from Hill.*[38])

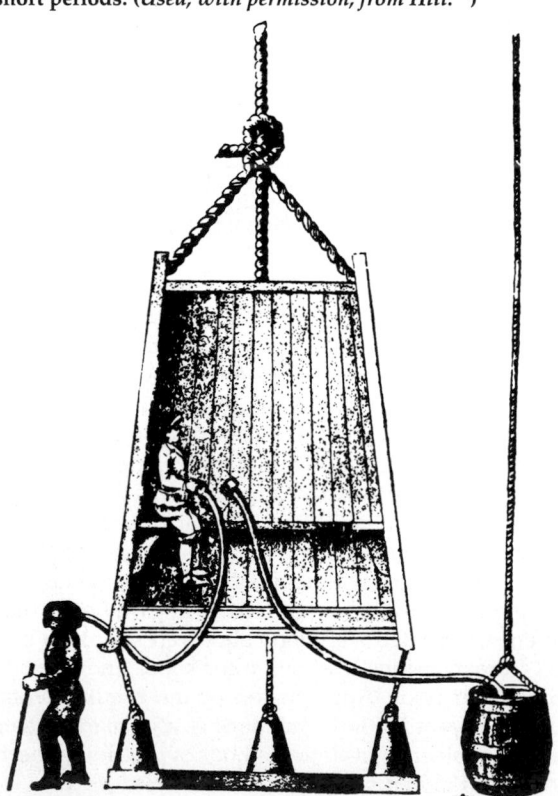

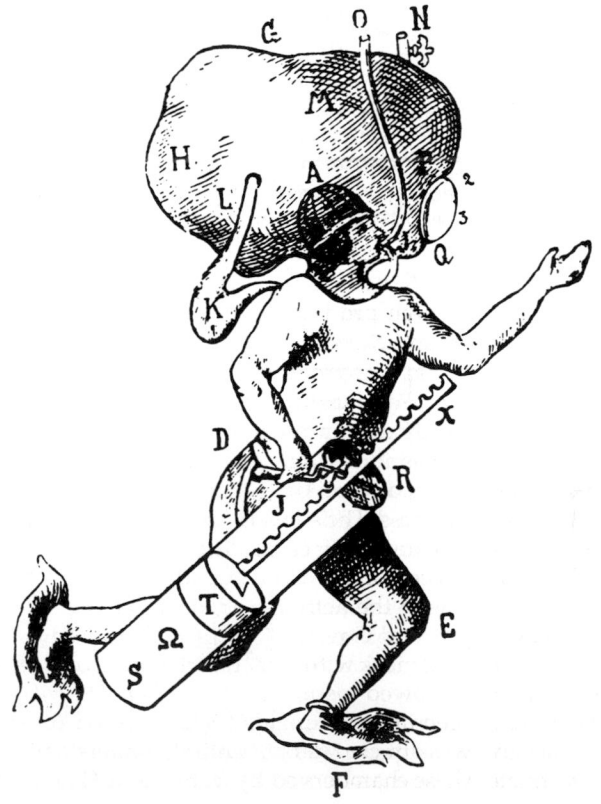

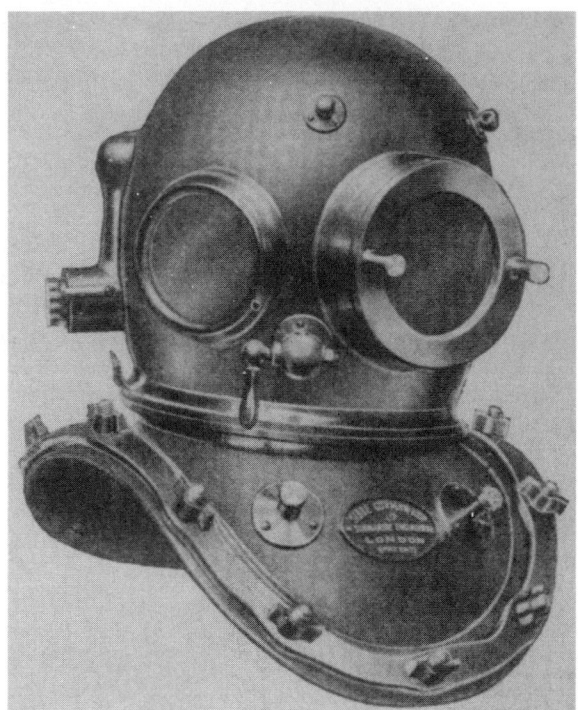
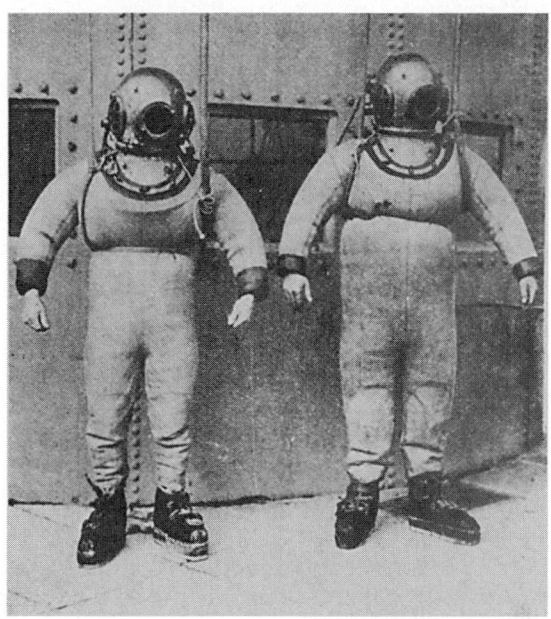

A   B

FIGURE 1-10   *A.*The metal helmet devised by Siebe is still used today. *B.* The complete diving suit produced by Siebe, Gorman, and Company in the nineteenth century included the metal helmet, a diving dress sealed at the wrists and ankles, and weighted shoes. (*Used, with permission, from Hill.*[38])

revisions in this diving suit and constructed the first commercially viable diving dress. The diver wore a metal helmet riveted to a flexible waterproof jacket. This jacket extended to the diver's waist but was not sealed. Air under pressure was pumped from the surface into the diver's helmet and escaped through the lower end of the jacket. In 1837, Siebe modified this diving dress by extending the jacket to cover the whole body. The suit was watertight at the wrists and ankles. Air under pressure entered the suit through a one-way valve at the back of the helmet and was released from the suit by an adjustable valve at the side of the helmet. Variations of this diving suit are still in use (Fig. 1-10).[37]

Siebe, Gorman, and Company became the world-recognized leaders in producing diving suits in the nineteenth century. Modifications of Siebe's original design were encouraged by this company. In 1866, Denayouze incorporated a metal air reservoir on the back of the diver's suit. Air was pumped directly into the reservoir, and escape of air from the suit was adjusted by the diver.[15] In 1878, Siebe, Gorman, and Company produced the first practical self-contained diving dress. The suit had a copper chamber containing potash for absorbing carbon dioxide and a cylinder of oxygen under pressure.[37] Fleuss cleverly revised this diving suit in 1879 with the help of Davis, managing director of Siebe, Gorman, and Company. The Fleuss appliance included an oronasal mask with an inlet and an exhaust valve. The inlet valve allowed inspiration from a metal chamber containing oxygen under pressure. Expiration through the exhaust valve was directed into metal chambers underlying a breastplate. These chambers contained carbon dioxide ab-

sorbents. Construction of this appliance was so precise that Fleuss used it not only to stay underwater for hours but also to enter chambers containing only noxious gases. The Fleuss appliance was adapted rapidly and successfully to mine rescue work, where explosions and toxic gases previously had prevented such efforts.[43]

As Siebe, Gorman, and Company successfully marketed diving suits, commercial divers began to dive deeper and longer. Unfortunately, complications developed for two separate reasons. Decompression illness was recognized first. In 1830, Lord Cochrane took out a patent in England for "an apparatus for compressing atmospheric air within the interior capacity of subterraneous excavations [to] . . . counteract the tendency of superincumbent water to flow by gravitation into such excavations . . . and which apparatus at the same time is adapted to allowing workmen to carry out their ordinary operations of excavating, sinking, and mining."[38] In 1841, Triger described the first practically applied caisson for penetrating the quicksands of the Loire River (Fig. 1-11).[44] This caisson, or hollow iron tube, was sunk to a depth of 20 m. The air within the caisson was compressed by a pump at the surface. The high air pressure within the caisson was sufficient to keep water out of the tube and allow workers to excavate the bottom. Once the excavation reached the prescribed depth, the caisson was filled with cement, providing a firm foundation. During the excavation process, workers entered and exited the caisson through an airlock. During this work, Triger described the first cases of "caisson disease," or decompression illness, in workers after they had left the pressurized caisson.

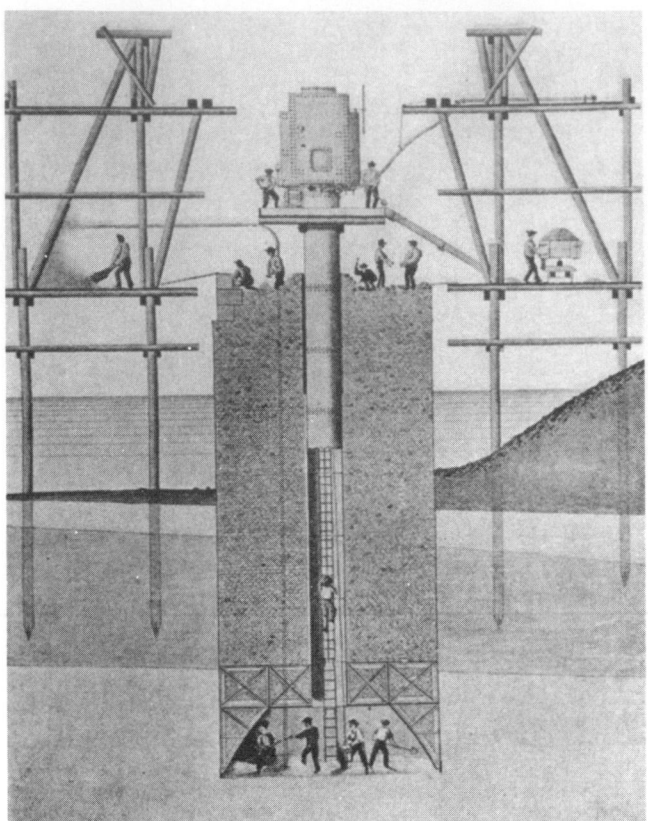

FIGURE 1-11 The caisson is a complex device enabling workers to function in dry conditions under shallow bodies of water or in other potentially flooded circumstances. A tube composed of concentric rings opens at the bottom to a widened chamber, where workers can be seen. At the top of the tube is a blowing chamber for maintaining air pressure and dry conditions within the tube. Workers enter at the top through an air lock and gain access to the working area via a ladder through the middle of the tube. (*Used, with permission, from Hill.*[38])

As this new technology was applied increasingly in shaft and tunnel work (e.g., the Douchy mines in France in 1846; bridges across the Midway and Tamar rivers in England in 1851 and 1855, respectively; and the Brooklyn Bridge, constructed between 1870 and 1873), caisson disease was recognized more frequently. Bert was especially instrumental in pointing out the dangers of high pressure.[15] Denayouze supervised many commercial divers and probably was among the first to recognize that decompression caused illness in these divers.[15] In the early 1900s, Haldane developed safe and acceptable techniques for staged decompression based on physiologic principles.[38]

Haldane also played a critical role in examining how well Siebe's closed diving suit supplied the ventilation needs of divers. This work may have been prompted by Bert's studies with animals placed in high-pressure chambers. Bert found that death invariably occurred when inspired carbon dioxide levels reached a certain threshold. Carbon dioxide absorbents placed in the high-pressure chamber prevented deaths.[15] Haldane's studies in this area were encouraged by a British Admiralty committee studying the risks of deep

diving in 1906. Haldane understood that minute ventilation varied directly with alveolar carbon dioxide levels. It appeared reasonable that the same minute ventilation needed to maintain an appropriate Pa_{CO_2} at sea level would be needed to maintain a similar Pa_{CO_2} under water. What was not appreciated initially was that as the diver descended and pressure increased, pump ventilation at the surface necessarily also would have to increase to maintain minute ventilation. Haldane realized that at 2 atm, or 33 ft under water, pump ventilation would have to double to ensure appropriate ventilation. This does not take into account muscular effort, which would further increase ventilatory demands. Unfortunately, early divers did not appreciate the need to adjust ventilation to the diving suit. Furthermore, air pumps often leaked or were maintained inadequately. Haldane demonstrated the relationship between divers' symptoms and hypercapnia by collecting exhaled gas from divers at various depths. The fraction of carbon dioxide in the divers' helmets ranged from 0.0018 to 0.10 atm.[26,38] The investigations of Bert and Haldane finally clarified the nature of "foul air" in diving bells and suits and the role of adequate ventilation in protecting underwater workers from hypercapnia. Besides his work with divers, Haldane also demonstrated that the "black damp" found in mines actually was a dangerously toxic blend of 10% CO_2 and 1.45% O_2.[45] He developed a self-contained rescue apparatus for use in mine accidents that apparently was more successful than the Fleuss appliance.[46]

Diving boats were fancifully described by Marsenius in 1638 and others. Only the boat designed by Debrell in 1648 appeared plausible because "besides the mechanical contrivances of his boat, he had a chemical liquor, the fumes of which, when the vessel containing it was unstopped, would speedily restore to the air, fouled by the respiration, such a portion of vital spirits as would make it again fit for that office." Although the liquor was never identified, it undoubtedly was an alkali for absorbing carbon dioxide.[38] More successful submarine boats were built in the nineteenth century. Fulton demonstrated such a vessel in the Seine. Payerne built a submarine for underwater excavation in 1844. Since 1850, the modern submarine has been developed primarily for military actions at sea.

As naval warfare became more sophisticated, submarines were seen as an invaluable asset for preying on shipping. They also could be viewed as an intriguing physiologic experiment in simultaneously ventilating many subjects. Ventilation under these conditions became more complex because it involved not only oxygen and carbon dioxide levels but also heat, humidity, and body odors. Early work in submarines documented substantial increases in temperature, humidity, and carbon dioxide levels.[47] Mechanical devices for absorption of carbon dioxide and air renewal were developed quickly,[48] and by 1928, Du Bois felt that submarines could remain submerged safely for up to 96 hours.[49] With the available carbon dioxide absorbents, such as caustic soda, caustic potash, and soda lime, carbon dioxide levels could be kept within relatively safe levels of less than 3%. Supplemental oxygen could be carried by the submarine and used to maintain a preferred fractional inspired oxygen concentration (FI_{O_2}) of above 17%.[39,50–52]

EXPLORATION IN THE AIR

In 1782, the Montgolfier brothers astounded the world by constructing a linen balloon about 18 m in diameter, filling it with hot air, and letting it rise about 2000 m into the air. Soon after, a larger balloon was constructed and carried a sheep, a cock, and a duck to a great height above the palace square at Versailles. After a series of experiments with tethered balloons, two Frenchmen, de Rozier and the Marquis d'Arlandes, had the honor of being the first humans to fly in a Montgolfier balloon on November 21, 1783.[53] Within a few years, Jeffreys and Blanchard had crossed the English Channel in a balloon, and Charles had reached the astonishing height of 13,000 ft in a hydrogen-filled balloon. As with diving, however, the machines that carried them aloft brought human passengers past the limits of their physiologic endurance. By 1804, balloonists were reaching heights of over 20,000 ft but were greatly affected. Glaisher and Coxwell reached possibly 29,000 ft in a memorable flight in 1862 and suffered temporary paralysis and loss of consciousness. Only heroic efforts by Coxwell enabled them to survive.[4,26,54]

The French physiologist Bert was greatly intrigued by the risks of high-altitude flight. He was very much aware of the symptoms described by climbers at high altitude. Acoste's description in 1573 of vomiting, disequilibrium, fatigue, and distressing grief as he traversed the Escaleras (Stairs) de Pariacaca, between Cuzco and Lima, Peru ("one of the highest places in the universe"), was widely known in Europe.[55] In 1804, von Humboldt attributed the symptoms he felt at high altitude to a lack of oxygen. Surprisingly, however, he found that the fraction of inspired oxygen in high-altitude air was similar to that found in sea-level air. He actually suggested that respiratory air might be used to prevent mountain sickness.[56] Longet expanded on this idea in 1857 by suggesting that the blood of high-altitude dwellers should have a lower oxygen content than that of sea-level natives. In a remarkable series of observations during the 1860s, Coindet described respiratory patterns of French people living at high altitude in Mexico City. Compared with sea-level values, respirations were deeper and more frequent, and the quantity of air expired in 1 minute was somewhat increased. He felt that "this is logical since the air of altitudes contains in a given volume less oxygen at a lower barometric pressure . . . [and therefore] a greater quantity of this air must be absorbed to compensate for the difference."[15] Although these conclusions might seem reasonable now, physiologists of the time also considered decreased air elasticity, wind currents, exhalations from harmful plants, expansion of intestinal gas, and lack of support in blood vessels as other possible explanations for the breathing problems experienced at high altitude. Bert, the father of aviation medicine, was instrumental in clarifying the interrelationship among barometric pressure, oxygen tension, and symptoms. He performed a series of experiments on animals exposed to low-pressure conditions in chambers (Fig. 1-12). Carbonic acid levels increased within the chamber, but carbon dioxide absorbents did not prevent death. Supplying supplemental oxygen to the animals, however, protected them from dying under simulated high-altitude conditions (Fig. 1-13). More important, he recognized a critical physiologic concept. Death occurred as a result of the interaction of both the fraction of inspired oxygen and barometric pressure. When a multiple of these two variables—that is, the partial pressure of oxygen—reached a critical threshold, death ensued.[15,39]

Croce-Spinelli, Sivel, and Tissandier were adventurous French balloonists eager to reach the record height of 8000 m. At Bert's urging, they experimented with the use of oxygen tanks in preliminary balloon flights and even in Bert's decompression chamber. In 1875, they began their historic attempt to set an altitude record supplied with oxygen cylinders (Fig. 1-14). Unfortunately, at 24,600 ft they released too much ballast, and their balloon ascended so rapidly that they were stricken unconscious before they could use the oxygen. When the balloon eventually returned to earth, only Tissandier remained alive.[4,54] This tragedy shook France.

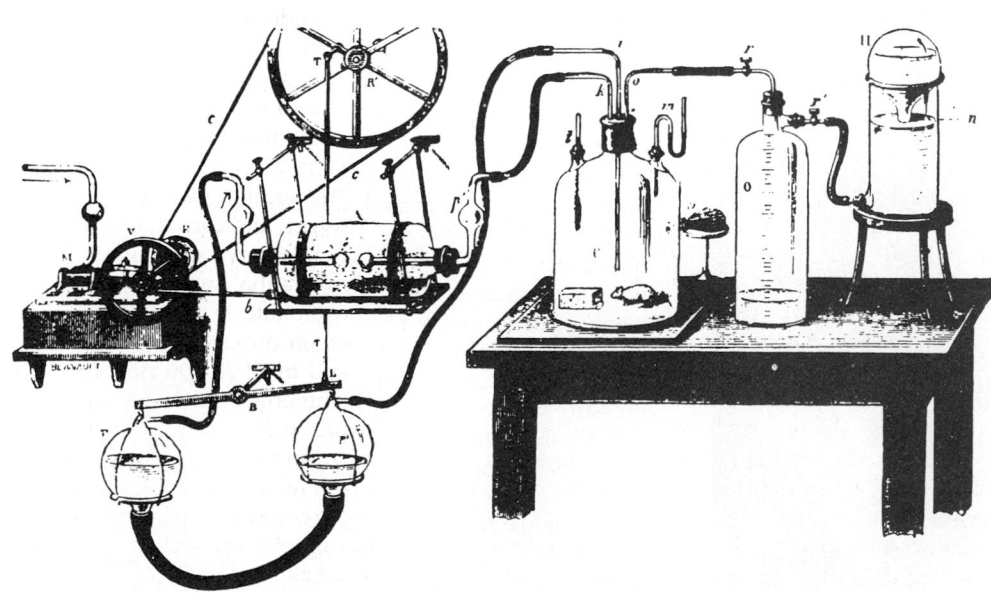

FIGURE 1-12 A typical device used by Bert to study animals under low-pressure conditions. (*Used, with permission, from Bert.*[15])

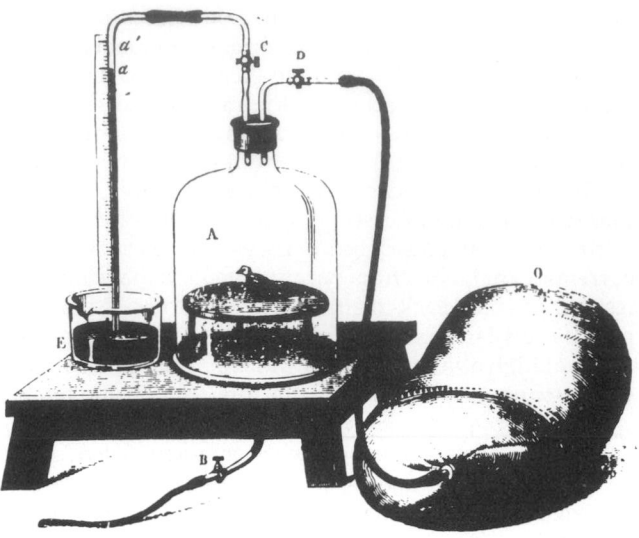

FIGURE 1-13 A bird placed in a low-pressure bell jar can supplement the enclosed atmospheric air with oxygen inspired from the bag labeled *O*. Supplemental oxygen prolonged survival in these experiments. (*Used, with permission, from Bert.*[15])

FIGURE 1-14 The adventurous French balloonists Croce-Spinelli, Sivel, and Tissandier begin their attempt at a record ascent. The balloonist at the right can be seen inhaling from an oxygen tank. Unfortunately, the supplemental oxygen did not prevent tragic results from a too rapid ascent. (*Used, with permission, from Armstrong: Principles and practice of aviation medicine. Baltimore: Williams & Wilkins, 1939: 4.*)

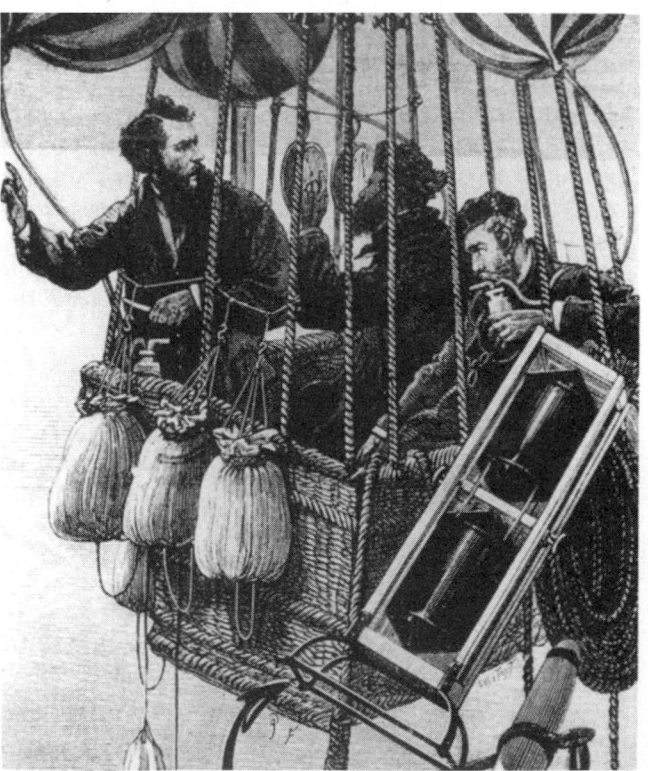

The idea that two men had died in the air was especially disquieting.[53] Unfortunately, the reasons for the deaths of Croce-Spinelli and Sivel were not clearly attributed to hypoxia. Von Schrotter, an Austrian physiologist, believed Bert's position regarding oxygen deficit as the lethal threat and encouraged Berson to attempt further high-altitude balloon flights. He originally devised a system for supplying oxygen from a steel cylinder with tubing leading to the balloonists. Later, von Schrotter conceived the idea of a face mask to supply oxygen more easily and also began to use liquid oxygen. With these devices, Berson reached 36,000 ft in 1901.[4,54]

The Wright brothers' historic flight at Kitty Hawk in 1903 substantially changed the nature of flight. The military value of airplanes soon was appreciated and applied during World War I. The Germans were especially interested in increasing the altitude limits for their pilots. They applied the concepts advocated by von Schrotter and provided liquid oxygen supplies for high-altitude bombing flights. Interest in airplane flights for commercial and military uses was especially high following Lindbergh's solo flight across the Atlantic in 1927. Much work was done on valves and oxygen gas regulators in the hope of further improving altitude tolerance. A series of high-altitude airplane flights using simple face masks and supplemental oxygen culminated in Donati's reaching an altitude of 47,358 ft in 1934. This was clearly the limit for human endurance using this technology.[4,54]

Somewhat before Donati's record, a breakthrough in flight was achieved by Piccard, who enclosed an aeronaut in a spherical metal chamber sealed with an ambient barometric pressure equivalent to that of sea level. The aeronaut easily exceeded what soon would be Donati's record and reached 55,000 ft. This work recapitulated the important physiologic concept, gained from Bert's earlier experimental work in high-altitude chambers, that oxygen availability is a function of both fractional inspired oxygen and barometric pressure. Piccard's work stimulated two separate investigators to adapt pressurized diving suits for high-altitude flying. In 1933, Post devised a rubberized, hermetically sealed silk suit. In the same year, Ridge worked with Siebe, Gorman, and Company to modify a self-contained diving dress for flight. This suit provided oxygen under pressure and an air circulator with a soda lime canister for carbon dioxide removal. These suits proved quite successful, and soon pilots were exceeding heights of 50,000 ft. Parallel work with sealed gondolas attached to huge balloons led to ascents over 70,000 ft. In 1938, Lockheed produced the XC-35, which was the first successful airplane with a pressurized cabin (Fig. 1-15).[4,54] These advances were applied quickly to military aviation in World War II. The German Air Ministry was particularly interested in developing oxygen regulators and valves and positive-pressure face masks for facilitating high-altitude flying.[57]

Work throughout World War II had defined certain limits for technological support of high-altitude flight. Pilots could reach up to 10,000 to 12,000 ft safely without oxygen supplements. Above this limit, oxygen-enriched air was essential. With flights going above 25,000 ft, oxygen supplementation alone usually was not sufficient, and some type of

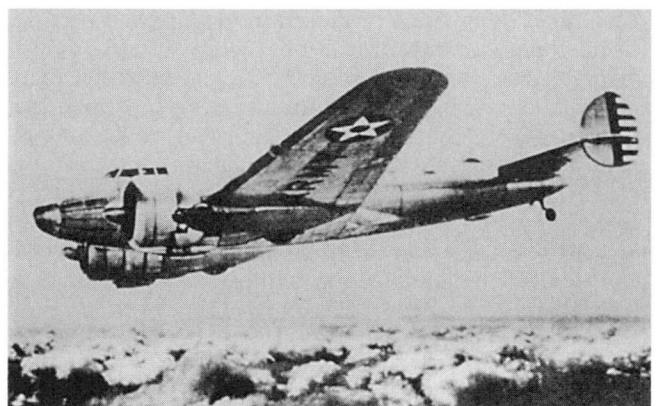

FIGURE 1-15 Lockheed produced the XC-35 in 1938. This was the first plane to have a pressurized cabin. (*Used, with permission, Armstrong: Principles and practice of aviation medicine. Baltimore: Williams & Wilkins, 1939: 337.*)

pressurized system—cabin, suit, or mask—was needed. Pressurization as an adjunct, however, reached its limit of usefulness at about 80,000 ft. At this altitude, air compressors became too leaky and inefficient to maintain adequate pressurization. A completely sealed cabin was essential to protect passengers adequately from the rarefied atmosphere outside. An altitude of 80,000 ft thus became a functional definition of space because at this height complete control of the atmosphere in the plane (i.e., the supply of oxygen, a means of removing carbon dioxide, and adequate control of temperature and humidity) was required.[58,59] Advances in submarine ventilatory physiology were adapted easily to the space program. In 1947, the American Air Force began the XI program, which culminated in the production in 1952 of the X15 aircraft. This plane reached a top speed of 4159 mi/h at an altitude of 314,750 ft. More important, the technology developed for this plane was a prelude to manned satellite programs. The United States Mercury and the Russian Vostok programs both relied on rockets to boost small, one-person capsules into space orbit. The Mercury capsule had a pure oxygen atmosphere at a reduced cabin pressure. In addition, the pilot wore a pressurized suit with an independent, closed oxygen supply. In April 1961, Gagarin was the first person to be launched into space. Shepard followed soon after, in May 1961, and reached an altitude of 116 miles. More sophisticated space flight—in the Gemini, Apollo, and space station programs—was based on similar ventilation systems and principles.[60]

Mechanical Ventilation: Of Resuscitation and Anesthesia

VIVISECTION

Galen is the first to have described ventilating an animal: "If you take a dead animal and blow air through its larynx [through a reed], you will fill its bronchi and watch its lungs attain the greatest distention."[61] He was fascinated by the question of how air could be drawn into the heart. Unfortunately for Galen, this was a question that could not be solved before the development of the microscope and the concept of diffusion. Also unfortunate for Galen was his failure to appreciate how ventilating the lungs could help him in his vivisection work. Galen operated on many living animals, but his studies on the function of the heart were limited by the risk of pneumothorax. Opening the thoracic cavity almost certainly resulted in death of the animal.[1,6] It was over a thousand years later that Vesalius realized that ventilation could protect animals from pneumothorax.[62,63] The beating heart would almost stop when Vesalius opened the chest cavity, and the lungs would collapse but could be restarted by inflating the lungs through a reed tied into the trachea. It is unclear whether Vesalius learned this procedure from others or developed the idea directly from Galen's work. A fascinating coincidence is that Paracelsus, a contemporary of Vesalius, is reported to have used a similar technique around 1530 in attempting to resuscitate a human. Did Paracelsus adapt Vesalius's research efforts, or vice versa?[63] It is also unclear whether Vesalius himself tried artificial ventilation during the dissection of a Spanish nobleman. Legend has it that when the nobleman's heart began to beat once more, Vesalius's medical associates were so outraged that they reported him to the religious authorities. Vesalius only avoided being burned at the stake by embarking on a pilgrimage to the Holy Land, but he died during the voyage.[64]

It is probably reasonable to assume that Vesalius's technique for ventilation during open-chest procedures remained well known in Padua. Presumably, Harvey, during his studies in Padua, became familiar with this technique because he mentions artificial ventilation in his work later in England.[63] Other English scientists soon after began to mention artificial ventilation in their own studies.[65] In 1664, Hooke dramatically described dissecting a dog, placing a pipe into the windpipe of the animal, and using a pair of bellows to ventilate the dog (and keep the heart beating) for well over an hour.[63] Lower, an associate of Hooke, later showed that artificial respiration kept the color of blood red during dissection.[63]

RESUSCITATING THE APPARENTLY DROWNED

Artificial respiration with a bellows and tracheal tube remained popular for vivisection work but was applied to humans only after a curious turn of events. Attempts to resuscitate apparently dead people were first recorded in the mid-eighteenth century. The origins of this movement are not entirely clear. Indeed, there were strong reasons for people to fear the dead. The risk of contagious disease was well known—memories of the plague were still fresh—and religious beliefs dissuaded many from believing in the wisdom of resuscitation. Despite these disincentives, sporadic attempts were made at organized resuscitation. In 1740, the Académie des Sciences in Paris issued an *avis* strongly advising mouth-to-mouth respiration for resuscitating the apparently drowned.[63] In 1744, Tossach may have been the first to use this technique successfully in saving a life.[66]

Fothergill soon after provided an excellent description of the mouth-to-mouth resuscitation technique, including the use of bellows if the "blast of a man's mouth" were not sufficient.[63,64,67,68] In 1760, Buchan went on to advise creating "an opening in the windpipe" when air cannot be forced into the chest through the mouth or nose.[69] Societal pressures led to widespread dissemination of knowledge about resuscitation techniques. In response to citizens' concerns about the large number of lives lost in canals, a group of influential laymen in Amsterdam formed the Society for the Rescue of Drowned Persons (*Maatschappy tot Redding von Dreykhingen*) in 1767.[63,64,67] The express purpose of this society was to publicize the need for and the techniques of resuscitation. Similar societies soon were formed in other maritime cities, such as Venice and Milan in 1768, Paris in 1771, London in 1774, and Philadelphia in 1780.

The Dutch method emphasized five steps: keeping the patient warm, artificial respiration through the mouth, fumigation with tobacco smoke through the rectum (Fig. 1-16), stimulants placed orally or rectally, and bleeding. Cogan, an English physician with a Dutch wife, translated a pamphlet describing the Dutch method into English. Hawes, an apothecary, read the pamphlet and led a concerted effort to introduce this technique into England. In encouraging this work, Hawes' activities led directly to the formation of the Royal Humane Society in 1774.[67] Through this society, many physicians were encouraged to develop techniques for resuscitating the apparently drowned. In 1776, Hunter advocated the use of a double bellows for artificial ventilation. The first stroke blew fresh air into the lung, and the second stroke sucked out stale air. He had perfected this technique during physiologic studies with dogs. Almost certainly this physiologic work was influenced by the earlier studies of Hooke and Lower. Hunter also advised the use of Priestley's pure air (oxygen) for resuscitation, but it is unclear whether this advice was ever followed.[64,67,70] Also in 1776, Cullen suggested relying on tracheal intubation and bellows ventilation for reviving the apparently dead.[71] In 1791, Curry developed an intralaryngeal cannula for this purpose, as

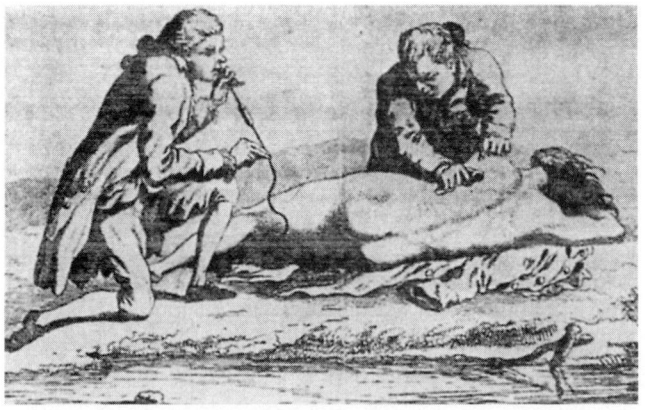

FIGURE 1-16 An attempt at resuscitating an apparently drowned person using the modified Dutch method. One resuscitator is assisting respiration by massaging the chest. The fumigator is instilling tobacco smoke through the rectum. (*Used, with permission, from Morch.*[64])

did Fine in 1800. These cannulas could be placed through the nose, mouth, or trachea.

Many other physicians were encouraged to develop ingenious devices as resuscitation aids by the Royal Humane Society (Fig. 1-17). This society held competitions and offered prizes and medals for the best work in this area.[63,64,67,72] As an alternative to tracheal intubation, Chaussier constructed a simple bag and face mask for artificial ventilation in 1780 (Fig. 1-18). He felt that this device would protect the rescuer from the deleterious effects of exhaled air. Chaussier devised accessory tubing for the face mask to allow the use of supplemental oxygen.[73] Kite, Curry, and Chaussier also developed devices to assist the operator in cannulating the trachea through the mouth.[73,74]

As these techniques for resuscitation were gaining widespread acceptance, concerns were being raised about the effectiveness of bellows ventilation. Leroy confirmed these doubts in a dramatic series of studies in 1827 and 1828. By subjecting an animal to overzealous bellows inflation, he caused fatal pneumothorax.[75,76] Although only later would it be realized that the pressures reached in this demonstration were unlikely to be achieved in clinical practice,[63] the French Academy quickly condemned the technique. Despite adaptations of bellows to limit the ventilatory volumes,[77] the Royal Humane Society also abandoned the use of tracheal intubation and bellows ventilation for resuscitation.[63] Consequently, positive-pressure ventilation was banned from medical practice early in its infancy, not to be routinely relied on for patient care until well into the twentieth century.

NEGATIVE-PRESSURE VENTILATORS

As an alternative to positive-pressure ventilation, physicians began to develop machines for negative-pressure ventilation. The first tank respirator was produced by Dalziel, of Scotland, in 1832. It was an airtight box in which the patient sat enclosed up to the neck. Negative pressure was created by bellows placed within the box but operated from the outside by a piston rod and one-way valve.[78,79] Jones, of Kentucky, patented the first tank respirator in America in 1864. The design appears similar to that of Dalziel's apparatus (Fig. 1-19).[78,80] Although Jones used this device to treat asthma and bronchitis, he also claimed cures for paralysis, neuralgia, rheumatism, seminal weakness, and dyspepsia.[80] Von Hauke designed a series of cuirass and tank respirators in the 1870s that were intended specifically to treat patients with respiratory diseases, but he showed little insight into the physiologic basis for how this type of respirator might be of benefit in lung disease. Woillez presented his version of a tank respirator to the French Academy of Medicine in 1876 (Fig. 1-20). It was basically a hollow cylinder of metal with a rigid lower end and an upper end enclosing a neck made of a rubber diaphragm seal. Air was evacuated from the cylinder by a bellows. Woillez understood the physiologic basis of ventilation and incorporated a bar placed on the patient's sternum to measure tidal excursions and adequacy of ventilation. Unfortunately, this device seemed to have been used only for resuscitating the apparently drowned and with little success.[78,81]

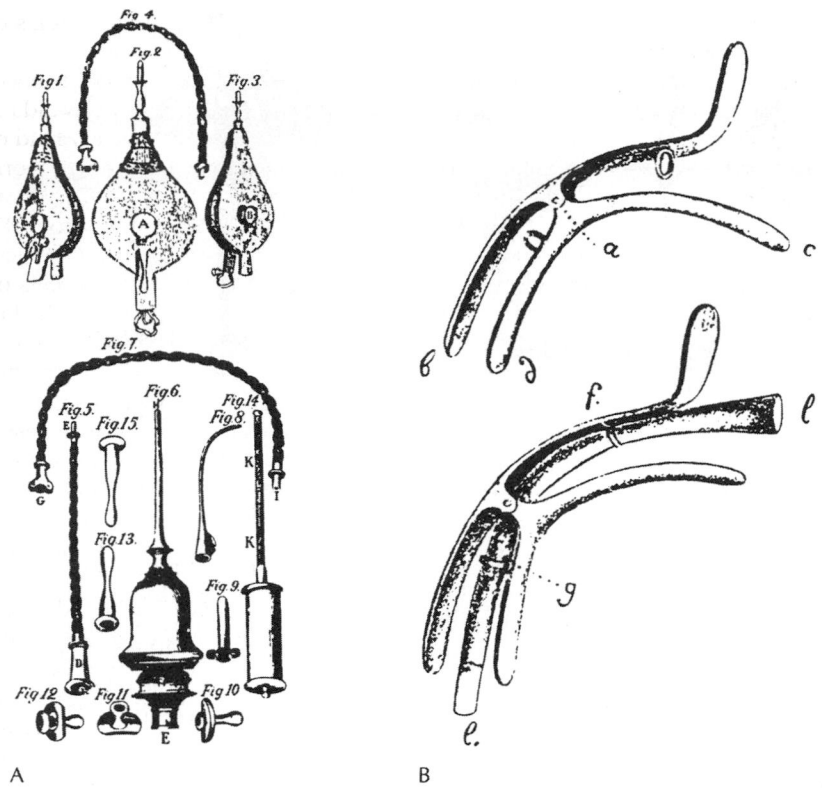

A

B

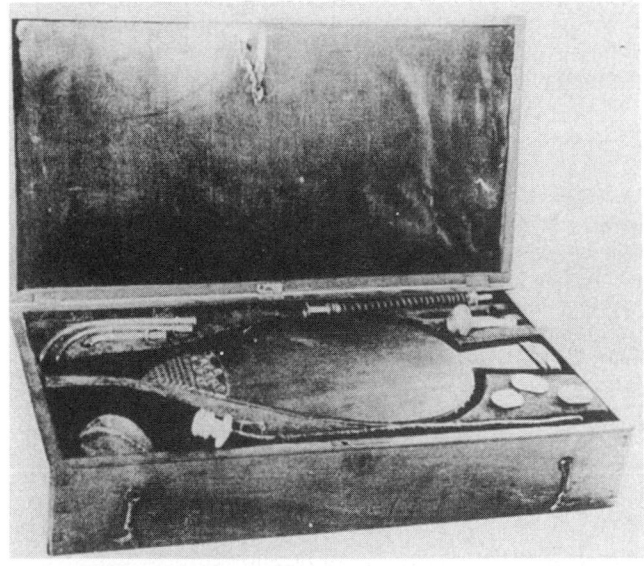

C

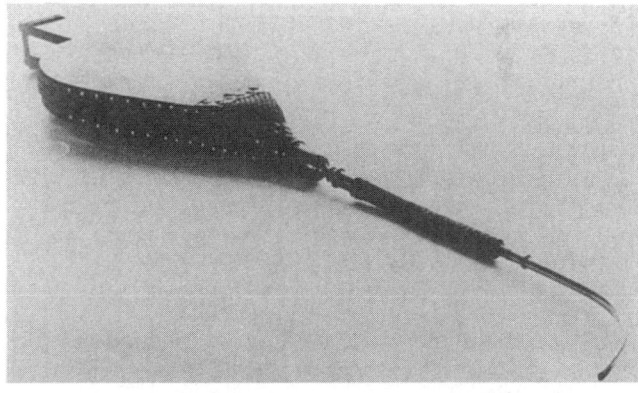

D

FIGURE 1-17 *A.* Examples of some of the devices included in the Royal Humane Society's compendium of resuscitation techniques in 1806. Figures 1, 2, and 3 are bellows of different sizes. Figure 6 is a brass box for holding a stimulating substance. Various connecting tubes and nozzles are also enclosed. (*Used, with permission, from Mushin et al: The principles and practice of thoracic anesthesia. Oxford, England: Blackwell Scientific Publications, 1953:32.*) *B.* A two-bladed intubating spatula was developed to hold the mouth open and allow passage of the tracheal tube through the larynx. (*Used, with permission, from Mushin et al: The principles and practice of thoracic anesthesia. Oxford, England: Blackwell Scientific Publications, 1953:36.*) *C.* The Royal Humane Society approved this type of box of intubation equipment with a bellows ventilator for distribution in 1806. (*Used, with permission, from McClellan: Anaesthesia 36:308, 1981.*) *D.* The bellows is shown connected to the otolaryngeal cannula and ready for use. (*Used with permission. McClellan: Anaesthesia 36:308, 1981.*)

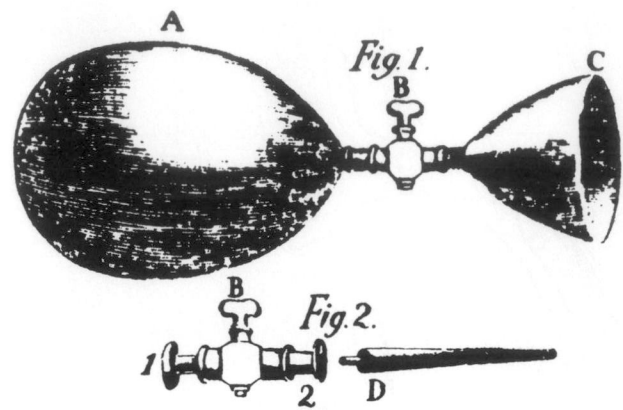

FIGURE 1-18 Chaussier developed this face mask and bag for artificial ventilation in 1780. (*Used, with permission, from Mushin et al: The principles and practice of thoracic anesthesia. Oxford, England: Blackwell Scientific Publications, 1953:39.*)

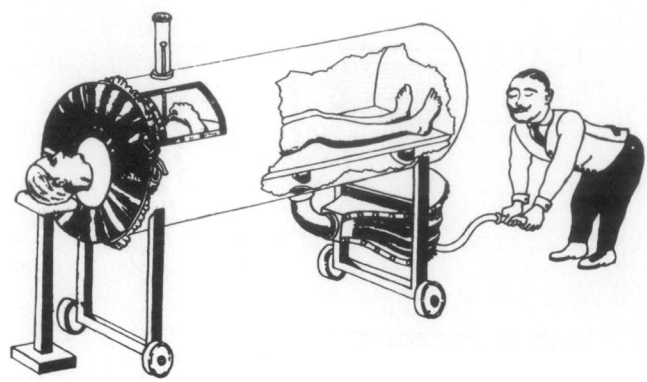

FIGURE 1-20 The spirophore produced by Woillez in 1876 had a rod placed on the patient's sternum to indicate the adequacy of tidal excursions. (*Used, with permission, from Emerson: Evolution of iron lungs. JH Emerson Co., 1978: fig. 2.*)

Many other ingenious devices were invented for negative-pressure ventilation over the next 50 years. Breuillard, of Paris, patented a tank respirator operated by a steam boiler.[78,80] Bell devised a vacuum jacket for newborns with neonatal respiratory distress. It is unlikely that this was ever used clinically, but a resuscitation box developed by Braun reportedly was quite useful for children with respiratory distress (Fig. 1-21).[78,80,82] Eisenmenger designed several respirators that, like Bell's, did not cover the entire body. His first prototype extended from the upper part of the sternum to the pubis (Fig. 1-22*A*). A more sophisticated device covered the chest and only a portion of the abdomen (Fig. 1-22*B*). These devices allowed positive-pressure compression of the chest to assist exhalation and negative-pressure suction to facilitate inhalation.[78,80,83] A later device, called the *Eisenmenger biomotor,* was patented in 1927 and had only

an abdominal cuirass shell.[84] An important advantage of these devices was the access they allowed to the patient for nursing care. This consideration prompted Lord, of Worcester, to build a respirator room (Fig. 1-23). Huge pistons in the ceiling created the pressure changes but required heavy equipment.[78,80] Severy in 1916 and Schwake in 1926 built negative-pressure ventilators that required the patient to stand (Fig. 1-24). Although they incorporated ingenious mechanical elements, their practicality for severely ill patients was limited.[80]

The first negative-pressure ventilator to be used successfully in clinical practice on a widespread basis was the Drinker-Shaw "iron lung" developed in 1928 (Fig. 1-25).[80,84–86] With this device, the body was enclosed entirely

FIGURE 1-21 In Egon Braun's resuscitation box, children were seated in a plaster mold with their noses and mouths protruding through a rubber diaphragm. The operator blew through the tube on the right first, compressing the chest. Then suction was applied to the tube expanding the chest. (*Used, with permission, from Emerson: Evolution of iron lungs. Cambridge, MA: JH Emerson Co., 1978: fig. 4.*)

FIGURE 1-19 The body-enclosing tank respirator constructed by Jones in 1864. The large syringe was used to create negative pressure. (*Used, with permission, from Emerson: Evolution of iron lungs. Cambridge, MA: JH Emerson Co., 1978: fig. 1.*)

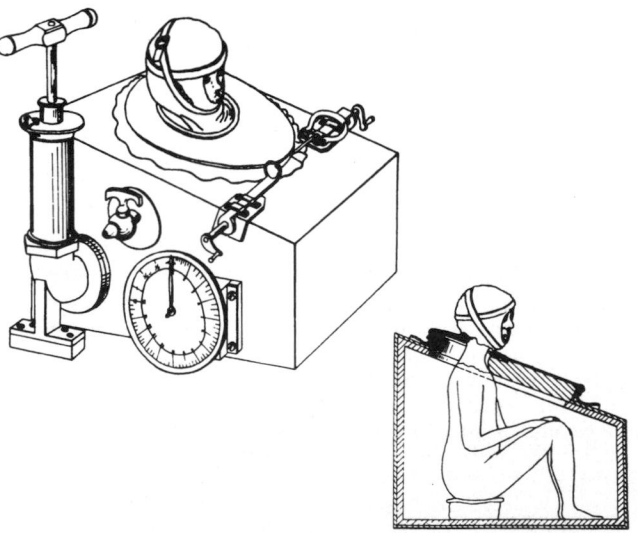

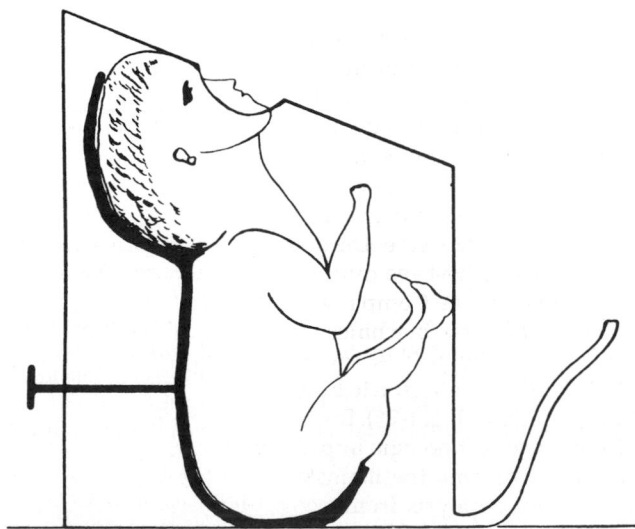

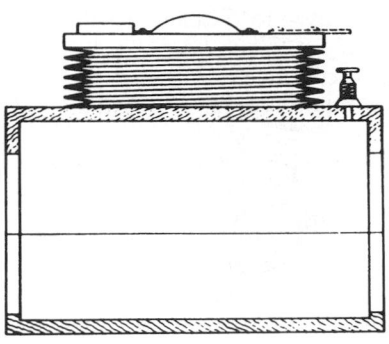
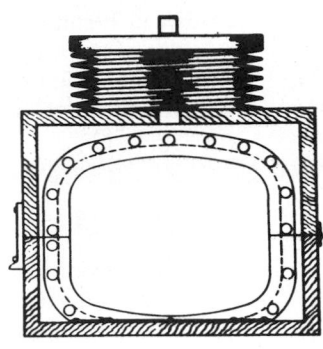

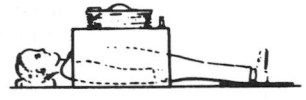

A

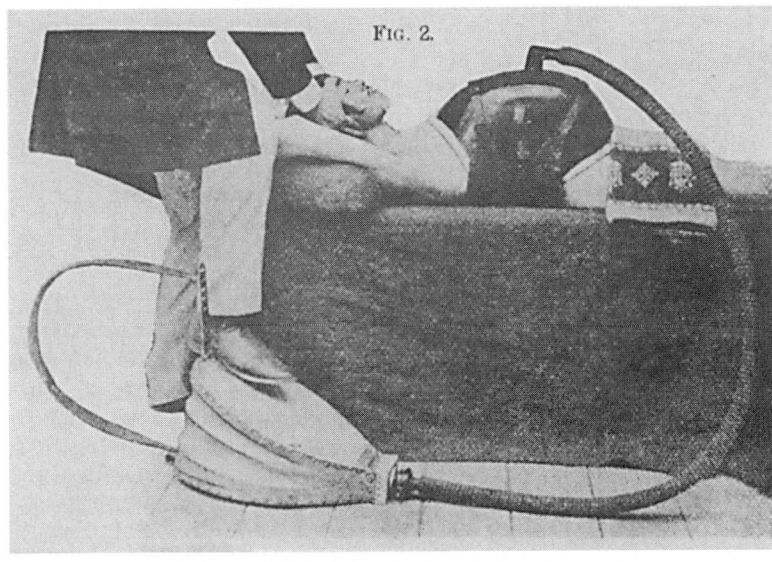

B

FIGURE 1-22 *A.* Eisenmenger's earlier version of his cuirass shell. (*Used, with permission, from Emerson: Evolution of iron lungs. Cambridge, MA: JH Emerson Co., 1978: fig. 5.*) *B.* The more sophisticated version described in 1904. A foot bellows allows positive and negative pressure to assist expiration and inspiration, respectively. This device is quite similar to chest shells still in use today. (*Used, with permission, from Eisenmenger: Lancet, ii:515, 1904.*)

within a cylindrical sheet-metal tank sealed at the lower end. The patient's head protruded out the upper end through a close-fitting rubber collar. Pressure within the chamber could be either increased or decreased by air blowers. This design is remarkably similar to the spirophore first built by Woillez in 1876. Unfortunately, it suffered from several of the same disadvantages, being cumbersome and inconvenient for patient care. Despite these limitations, this iron lung saved many lives during polio epidemics. When the Consolidated Gas Company of New York paid for large numbers of these machines to be built, their use spread quickly worldwide.[80] A severe poliomyelitis epidemic in 1931 prompted Emerson to build a simplified and improved tank respirator (Fig. 1-26). Because of its low cost, ease of operation, and technologic improvements, the Emerson tank respirator became the mainstay in treating patients with respiratory paralysis from polio[80] until reintroduction of positive-pressure ventilation in the 1950s.

POSITIVE-PRESSURE VENTILATION

IN THE PHYSIOLOGY LABORATORY

Following the admonitions against bellows ventilation, the use of positive-pressure ventilation was disavowed by clinicians but flourished in the physiology laboratory. Throughout the middle to late 1800s, physiologists were becoming more sophisticated in their investigative techniques and were relying increasingly on positive-pressure ventilation in animal experiments. Hering and Breuer used this technique to examine how alterations in lung volume influenced the vagi in 1868.[87] Bert, in his studies on blood oxygen and carbon dioxide content, wrote of giving animals sufficient curare to induce total paralysis and of providing artificial ventilation through a tracheostomy tube in 1878. A bellows with a graduated handle for controlling tidal volume proved to be quite effective in these experiments (Fig. 1-27).[15] Pflüger[26] and Head[88] described complex experiments

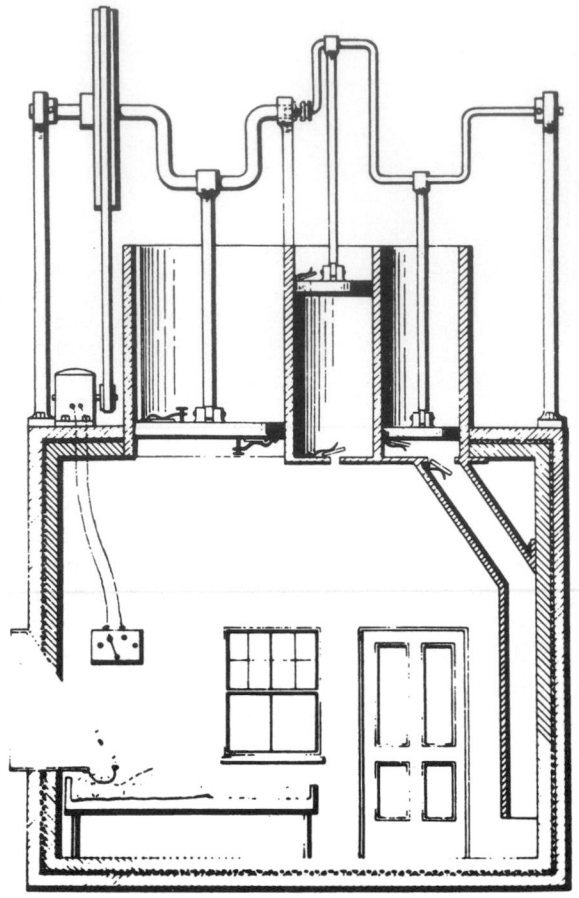

FIGURE 1-23 A negative-pressure respirator room, patented by Lord in 1908, provided optimal access to the patient for the nursing staff. (*Used, with permission, from Emerson: Evolution of iron lungs. Cambridge, MA: JH Emerson Co., 1978: fig. 8.*)

FIGURE 1-24 Severy's negative-pressure ventilator obliged the patient to stand but had a remarkable set of eletromagnetic controls and pulleys for adjusting pressure changes within the box. (*Used, with permission, from Emerson: Evolution of iron lungs. Cambridge, MA: JH Emerson Co., 1978: fig. 9.*)

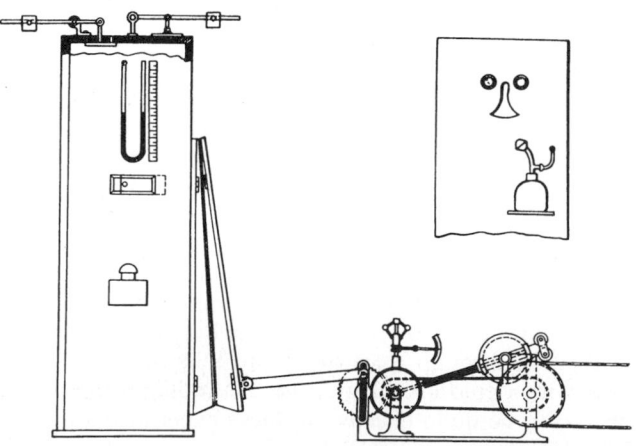

in which cuffed tubes were used to ventilate isolated portions of the lung. Bowditch wrote of a simple but reliable volume-cycled ventilator used for animal studies as a standard piece of laboratory equipment at Harvard in 1879 (Fig. 1-28).[89]

IN THE OPERATING ROOM

The reintroduction of positive-pressure ventilation into clinical medicine occurred in two distinctly different stages. The initial stage began around the turn of the twentieth century and involved the use of this technique in the operating room. Only after positive-pressure ventilation had become a well-established technique during surgery was it applied to nonoperative patients, beginning in the 1950s. There was a clear and pressing need for positive-pressure ventilation to facilitate thoracic surgery. From the time of Galen, it was appreciated that opening the thorax invariably caused fatal pneumothorax. Vesalius had shown that positive-pressure ventilation could keep an animal's lungs inflated and the animal alive during these operations, but this lesson seems to have been forgotten. Consequently, lung surgery in the nineteenth century was limited to rare cases of draining lung abscesses and bronchiectatic or tuberculous cavities. Although pneumonectomy had been performed successfully in animals by 1881,[90,91] between 1880 and 1920 the mortality rate for thoracic surgery remained high, and these procedures were performed infrequently.[90,92] By 1896, Quénu and Longuet realized that to have success in thoracic operations, one had "to maintain a difference in pressure between the intra-alveolar air and the surrounding air." The surgeon could choose either to "lower the extra thoracic pressure, the intrapulmonary tension remaining the same, making it necessary . . . to operate in a relative vacuum, or to increase the intrabronchial pressure."[93] Over the ensuing 10 to 15 years, ingenious methods were devised to achieve both these ventilatory end points.

Tracheal Intubation

Intuitively, the obvious way to increase intrabronchial pressure would be to follow Vesalius's example by placing a tube in the trachea and inflating the lungs with a bellows. Positive-pressure ventilation had been well standardized in the physiology laboratory. Although techniques to cannulate the trachea had been developed in the late eighteenth century, translaryngeal intubation still was viewed skeptically by many physicians until the early 1900s.[94] Physicians only became reassured about the usefulness of translaryngeal intubation through work on controlling the airway. The most compelling reason for airway control always had been upper-airway obstruction. Tracheostomy historically was a well-known method of gaining access to the airway in such situations. Indirect references to this technique can be found in such ancient texts as the Rig Veda, written between 2000 and 1000 BC, and Eber's Papyrus, from about 1550 BC. Alexander the Great reputedly performed a tracheostomy with his sword in 400 BC on a soldier who was choking on a bone.[95] According to Frost[96] and McClelland,[97] Asclepiades of Bithynia was the first surgeon to perform

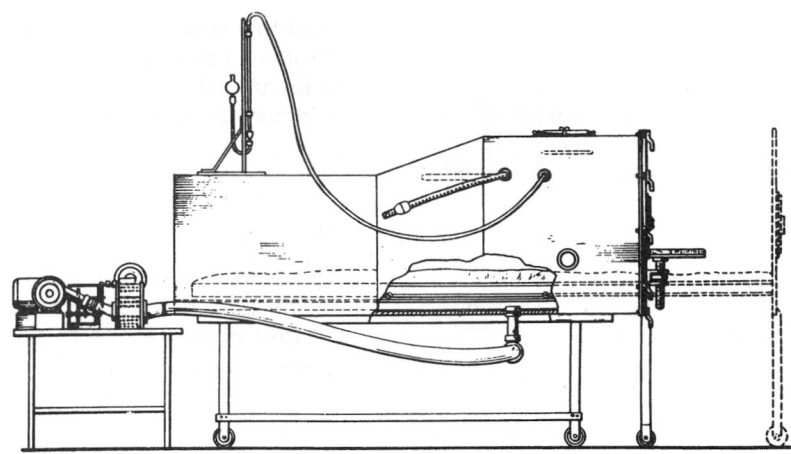

FIGURE 1-25 The Drinker-Shaw iron lung developed in 1928 had a sliding bed and a close-fitting rubber collar for sealing the patient's neck. The patient's head protruded from the device at the right and rested on a flat support. (*Used, with permission, from Emerson: Evolution of iron lungs. Cambridge, MA: JH Emerson Co., 1978: fig. 13.*)

tracheostomy routinely, around 100 BC. The Roman Antyllos also was noted for his skill in this procedure in AD 340.[96] Although few surgeons were reported to have performed this procedure during the Dark Ages, Brasavola reintroduced the technique to the medical community in 1546. In 1833, Trousseau clearly demonstrated the lifesaving value of tracheostomy for managing upper-airway obstruction with his report on 200 of these operations for diphtheria.[96,97]

With the development of techniques and devices to cannulate the trachea through either the nose or the mouth (translaryngeal intubation) in the late eighteenth century, physicians had a practical alternative to tracheostomy for managing upper-airway obstruction. Depaul, who succeeded Chaussier at the maternity hospital in Paris, believed

FIGURE 1-26 The Emerson tank respirator build in 1931 used a bellows device to change pressure (hand pumps also were available in case of electricity failure), was less cumbersome and expensive than the Drinker-Shaw iron lung, and was easily opened and closed for nursing care. (*Used, with permission, from Emerson: Evolution of iron lungs. Cambridge, MA: JH Emerson Co., 1978: fig. 15.*)

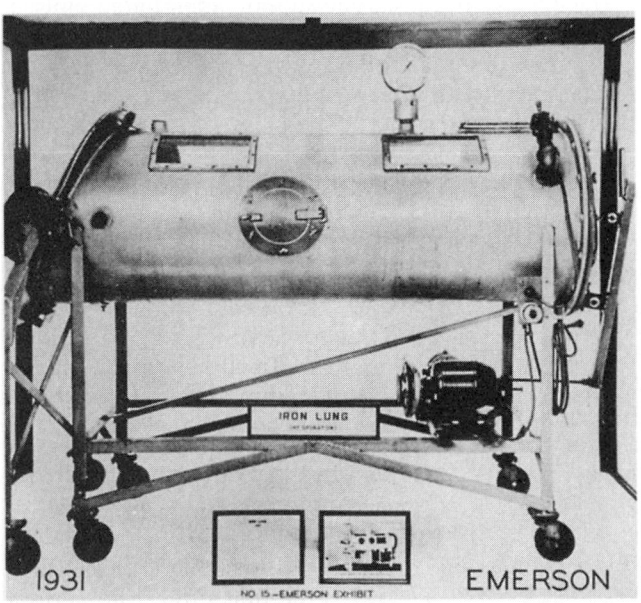

Chaussier's tubes to be useful in managing neonatal respiratory distress. He devised and successfully used modifications of Chaussier's tubes for this purpose.[73] Apparently, Bouchut unsuccessfully attempted translaryngeal intubation to relieve diphtheritic croup in 1848.[73] Later, MacEwen of Glasgow in 1880[98] and O'Dwyer of New York in 1887 [99–101] would be recognized as the first physicians to use translaryngeal intubation successfully for managing upper-airway obstruction.

Tracheal Anesthesia

As clinicians began to appreciate the value of translaryngeal intubation for managing upper-airway obstruction, anesthetists slowly began to grasp how useful this technique might be for administering anesthesia in the operating room. Ether anesthesia had first been used during an operation by Morton in 1846.[102] Snow recognized the potential value of such anesthesia and developed various ways of administering inhalational agents. One novel method he described in 1858 was to give rabbits chloroform vapor through a tracheostomy tube.[103] Trendelenberg apparently adapted this method for use in patients during operations on the mouth and larynx. A practical problem limiting these operations at the time was aspiration of blood into the lungs during the procedure. Trendelenberg solved this problem by devising a cuffed tracheostomy tube for sealing the airway in 1869 (Fig. 1-29).[73,104] With this cuffed tube in place, inhalational anesthesia could only be given

FIGURE 1-27 A bellows with graduated handle for controlling tidal volume was used by Bert to ventilate paralyzed animals in 1878. (*Used, with permission, from Bert.[15]*)

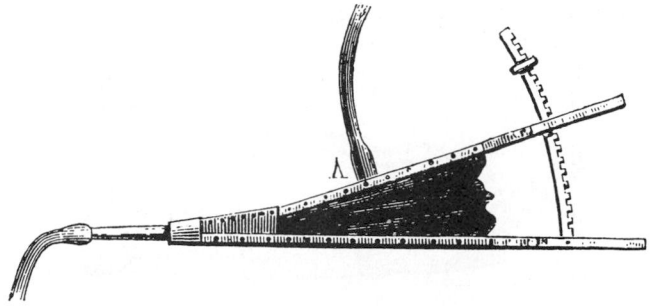

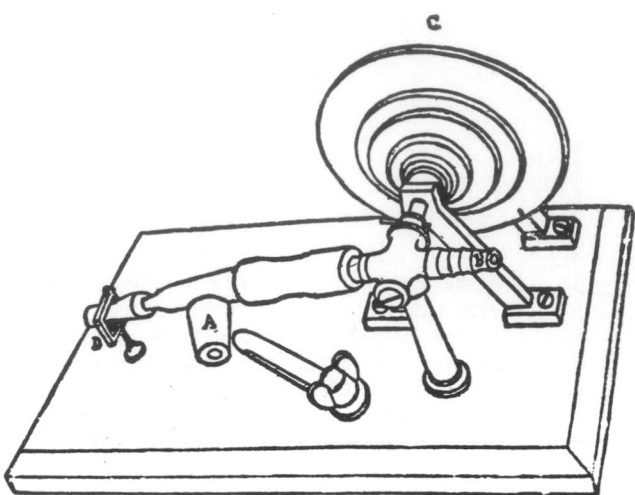

FIGURE 1-28 The volume-cycled ventilator used in the Harvard Physiology Department in 1870s. Air from a bellows or tromp enters *A* and passes to the animal through *B*. The respiratory rate is determined by adjusting the driving band on cone *C*. The amount of air entering the animal is determined by screw clamp *D*, which permits air to escape. (*Used, with permission, from Bowditch: J Physiol 2:202, 1879–1880.*)

practically through the tube itself. MacEwen's original work on translaryngeal intubation for upper-airway obstruction included one case in which successful anesthesia given through the tube allowed surgical removal of a pharyngeal tumor.[98] Maydl of Prague and Eisenmenger of Vienna both described cases of upper-airway surgery in 1893 using endotracheal anesthesia.[104]

Matas is recognized as playing a pivotal role in introducing positive-pressure ventilation into the operating room, but he clearly credited others with inspiring him. Tuffier and Hallion in 1896 described the efficacy of artificial ventilation of the lungs through a translaryngeal tube in preventing lung collapse during surgery in animals.[105] Doyen improved their techniques.[106] At about the same time, Fell devised a bellows for positive-pressure ventilation of patients with respiratory paralysis from opiate overdose.[107] This bellows could be connected to either a face mask or a tracheotomy tube. O'Dwyer modified Fell's device so that it could be attached to a translaryngeal tube, and soon the Fell-O'Dwyer apparatus for mechanical ventilation was marketed. Matas realized that if anesthesia could be ad-

FIGURE 1-29 Trendelenberg first used this type of tracheostomy tube with inflatable cuff to prevent aspiration during operations on the mouth and larynx in 1780. (*Used, with permission, from Lomholt: Acta Anaesthesiol Scand 11:312, 1967.*)

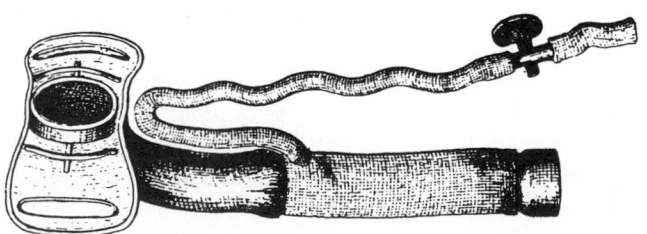

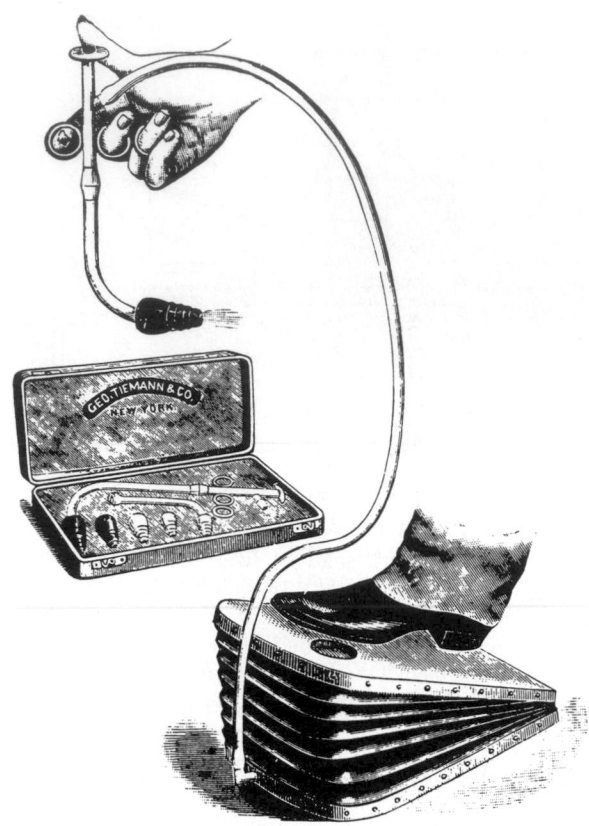

FIGURE 1-30 The Fell-O'Dwyer apparatus with modifications by Matas for delivering anaesthesia. (*Used, with permission, from Matas: JAMA 34:1468–73, 1900.*)

ministered readily through the apparatus, the Fell-O'Dwyer ventilator would be well suited for managing intrathoracic surgery. Matas modified this ventilator successfully and indicated that the new machine indeed was effective (Fig. 1-30).[106,108]

The interest in translaryngeal intubation for administering anesthesia and facilitating positive-pressure ventilation was stuttering at first. Kuhn apparently used this technique regularly and with great success. He experimented extensively with both the size and position of the tracheal tube, even using separate tubes for inhalation and exhalation.[109] In 1909, Meltzer and Auer presented a modified approach to this technique. Instead of using a tracheal tube that nearly approximated the diameter of the trachea and allowing the patients to inhale and exhale through that same tube, these physiologists used a narrow-bore tube. Air was blown into the lung through the tube and allowed to escape from the lung between the external wall of the tube and the trachea. This technique was referred to as *endotracheal insufflation*.[110] Ellsberg was the first to use endotracheal insufflation on a patient,[111] but others criticized the technique. Meyer disparagingly called Meltzer's insufflation method the "blowpipe apparatus." Meyer cited numerous concerns (i.e., risks of aspiration through the tube; incomplete control of airway pressure, especially when closing the chest; unreliable administration of anesthesia; and difficulties placing the

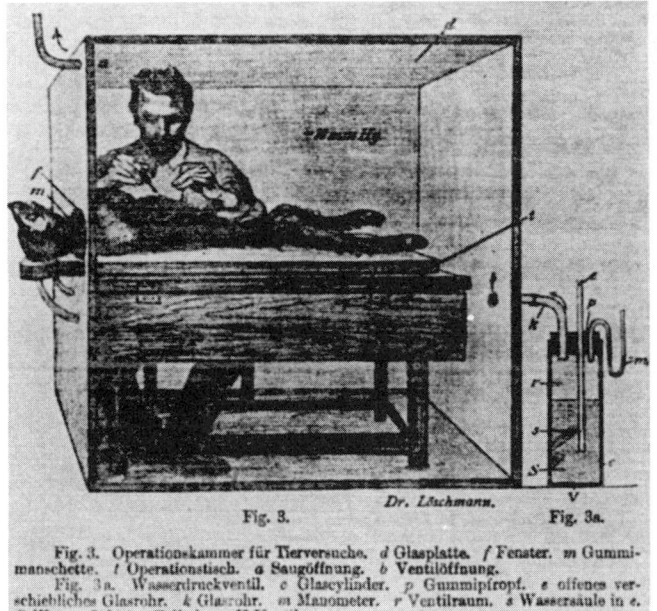

Fig. 3. Operationskammer für Tierversuche. *d* Glasplatte. *f* Fenster. *m* Gummimanschette. *t* Operationstisch. *a* Saugöffnung. *b* Ventilöffnung.

Fig. 3a. Wasserdruckventil. *c* Glascylinder. *p* Gummipfropf. *e* offenes verschiebliches Glasrohr. *k* Glasrohr. *m* Manometer. *r* Ventilraum. *s* Wassersäule in *e*. *S* Wassersäule im Cylinder. *V* Ventil.

FIGURE 1-31 The differential-pressure cabinet, developed by Sauerbruch, had the surgeon placed inside a small chamber. Suction was applied to this chamber. With the animal's (in this case) or patient's head outside the chamber, the intrabronchial pressure remained at effective sea level. This differential pressure maintained lung inflation when the thorax was open. (*Used, with permission, from Morch.*[64])

tracheal tube correctly) and concluded that endotracheal insufflation was not suitable for thoracic surgery.[94]

Differential Pressure

Meyer advocated the use of a differential-pressure apparatus for open-chest procedures. Around 1904, Sauerbruch devised a working model of a cabinet that generated negative pressure around the lung. Sauerbruch built a small airtight operating room with the patient's body and the surgeon inside. The patient's head extended out of the room. By applying suction to this room, differential pressure was created across the pleural surface, atmospheric pressure within the bronchial tree, and negative pressure outside the lung (Fig. 1-31).[64] Meyer built a much larger version of a negative-pressure apparatus. The entire operating room was subjected to suction, and a small chamber was built within the operating room to enclose the patient's head and the anesthetist. This chamber either could be kept at atmospheric pressure or could subjected to positive pressure (Fig. 1-32).[112]

Surgeons also had the option of using devices that employed positive pressure without intubation to inflate the lungs. Brauer generally is credited as devising the first positive-pressure cabinet in 1904. This apparatus apparently was large enough for the patient's head to fit inside. Positive pressure in the cabinet would be transmitted to the lungs during the patient's respiratory efforts.[64,113–115] Modifications of the positive-pressure cabinet were put forth by Murphy,[113] Green,[114] and Green and Janeway (Fig. 1-33).[115] As an alternative to cabinets, other surgeons used

face masks and helmets to supply positive-pressure ventilation (Fig. 1-34).[116–118]

Several factors favored the endotracheal insufflation method for both anesthesia and lung inflation during thoracic operations. The differential-pressure chambers were either large and cumbersome or small and confining, and all were expensive. A device for endotracheal insufflation, which was portable and easy to use, was built in 1910 by Elsberg for less than $100,[119] although more complex devices also were built (Fig. 1-35). The positive-pressure cabinets limited access to the patient's head during the procedure. Positive-pressure masks were not reliable in maintaining lung inflation. Techniques and devices for facilitating translaryngeal intubation were being developed quickly. Dorrance,[120] for example, described a simple endotracheal tube made of flexible rubber with an inflatable cuff at its distal end. Janeway developed the first modem laryngoscope, an invaluable aid for translaryngeal intubation.[64] Jackson was instrumental in providing clear guidelines for performing translaryngeal intubation.[121] With these developments, endotracheal insufflation became firmly established, and new devices for anesthesia and ventilation by insufflation were developed quickly.[122,123] Many other devices for positive-pressure ventilation, including the "pulmotor" portable resuscitator, were devised in the early 1900s.[64]

Translaryngeal Intubation

By World War I, endotracheal intubation had become an invaluable method, especially for extensive plastic facial reconstructions. However, anesthetists began to express dissatisfaction with the insufflation technique for anesthesia and ventilation. Insufflation did not protect from aspiration, especially during upper-airway operations. In these procedures, pharyngeal packing to prevent aspiration required placement of two tubes, one for insufflation and the other for exhalation. Placement of two tubes was technically difficult. Anesthetists would much prefer to use a cuffed tracheal tube, which, of course, was not feasible with insufflation. Anesthetists were finding that nitrous oxide was a better anesthetic agent than chloroform or ether, but it was very expensive to administer by insufflation. Periodic deflations of the lung usually were required, with insufflation to ensure adequate carbon dioxide removal. As a consequence of these problems with insufflation, Magill and Rowbotham returned to Matas's old "inhalation" method. They used a tracheal tube large enough to allow both inhalation and exhalation. A balloon cuff could be attached to the outer distal end of the tube to prevent aspiration.[104,124,125] Rowbotham also was instrumental in popularizing nasotracheal intubation.[126] A number of cleverly designed machines were produced before World War II that could be used to administer anesthesia and artificial ventilation via positive-pressure rhythmic "insufflation" (ventilation) through these large-diameter tubes.[64,127,128] By 1934, Guedel and Treweek described apneic anesthesia, or purposely giving enough anesthesia to cause complete respiratory paralysis. Artificial respiration by rhythmic bag ventilation adequately supported the patient during apnea. This technique provided the "quiet" field necessary for abdominal and thoracic surgery.[129]

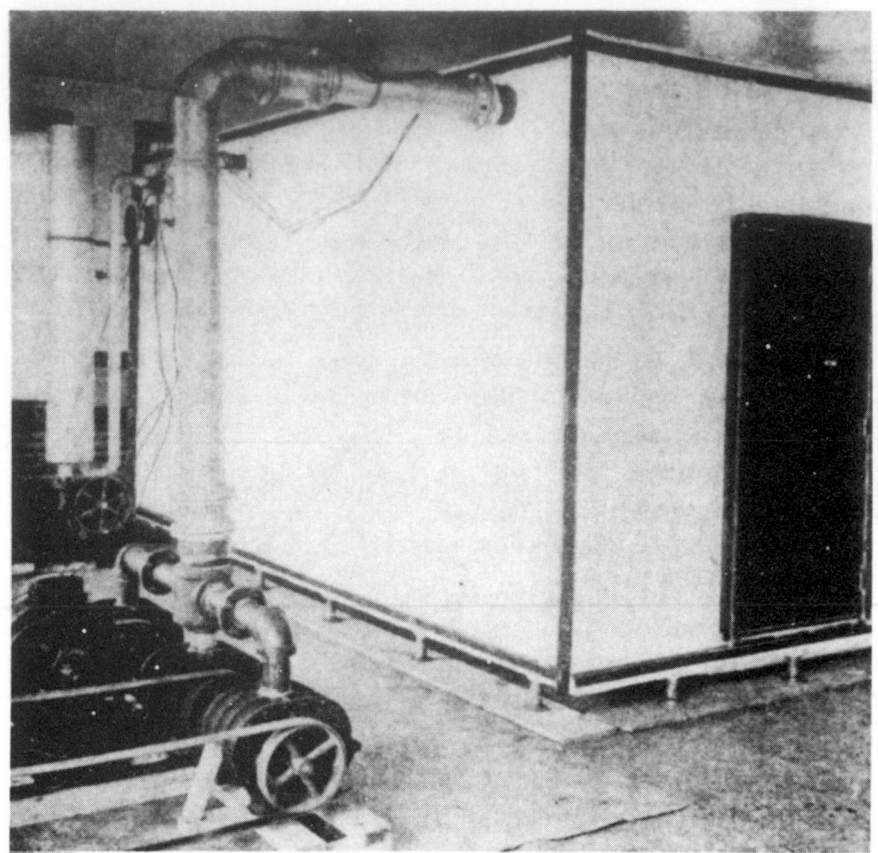

A

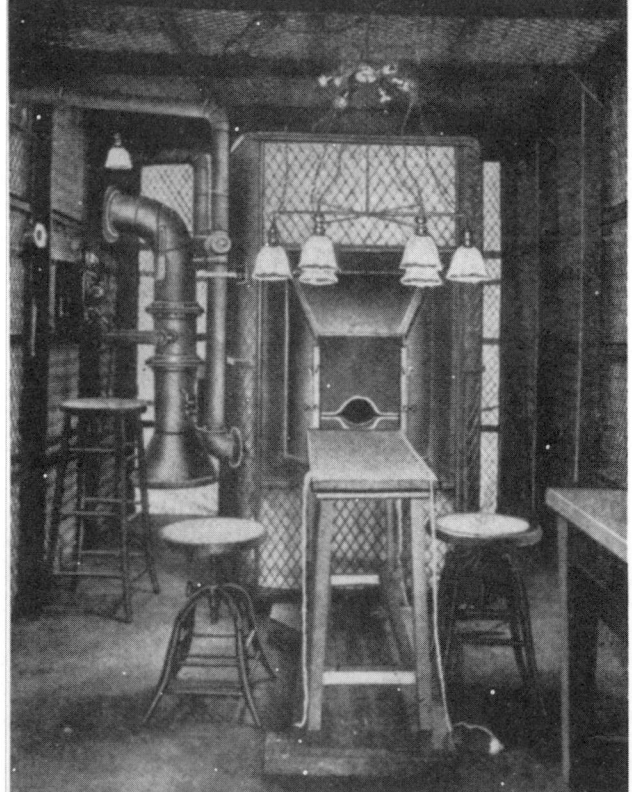

B

FIGURE 1-32 A larger version of the differential-pressure cabinet was constructed by Meyer. *A.* The large chamber, shown from an outside view on the left, has suction applied to it. Inside this chamber, the patient is placed on a table with the patient's head inserted into a smaller chamber. Within this smaller chamber (*B*), kept at positive pressure, resides the anesthetist. (*Used, with permission, from Meyer: JAMA 77:1984, 1909.*)

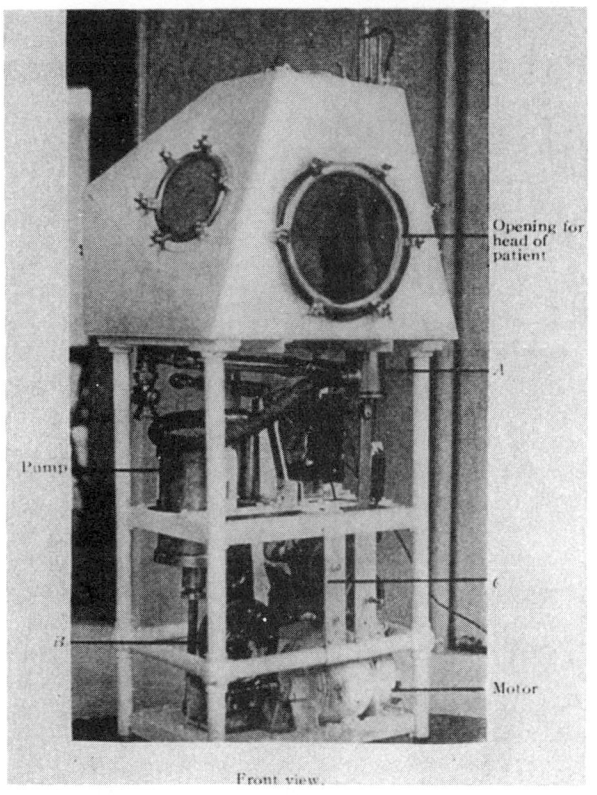

A

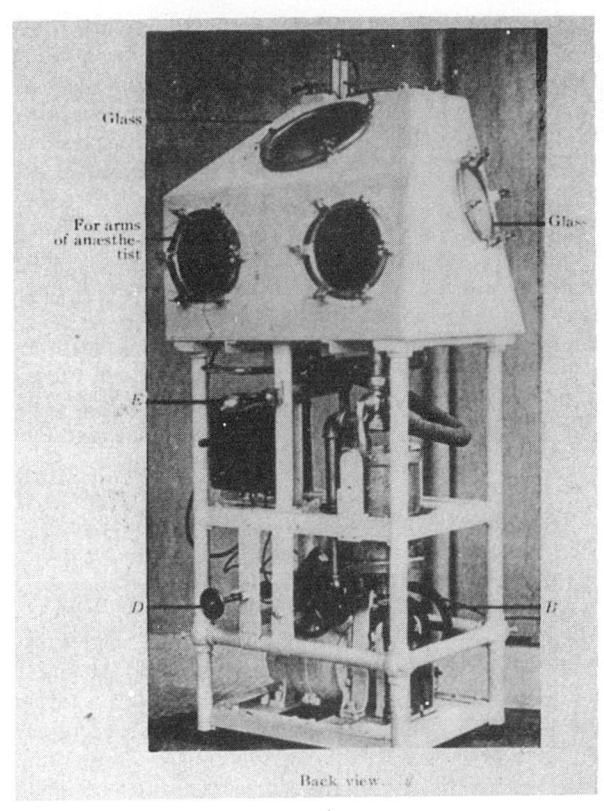

B

FIGURE 1-33 Green and Janeway proposed this positive-pressure chamber in 1910. The patient's head is inserted into the chamber (*A*). The anesthetist's arms also can reach into the chamber (*B*). (*Used, with permission, from Green: Ann Surg 52:58–66, 1910.*)

FIGURE 1-34 A positive-pressure mask used by Bunnell in 1912. (*Used, with permission, from Bunnell: JAMA 58:836, 1912.*)

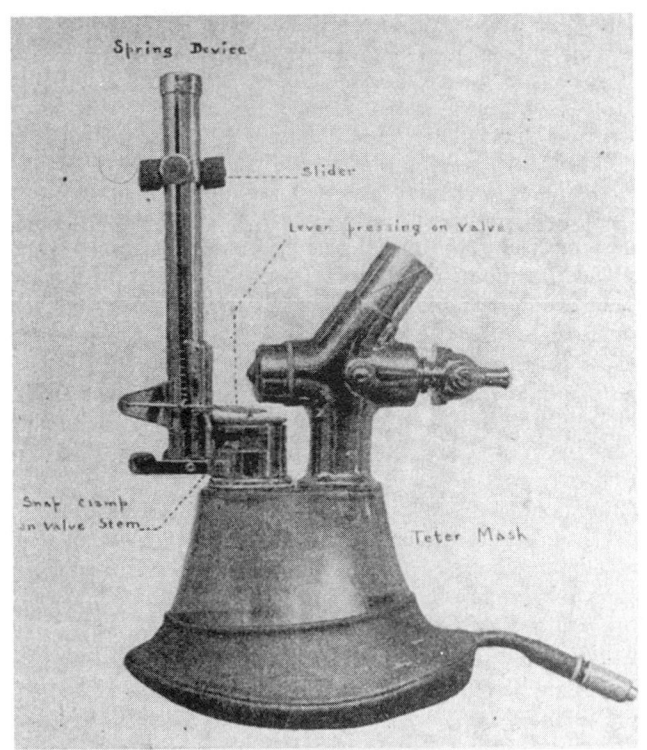

Further favoring the use of translaryngeal intubation was recognition of retained pulmonary secretions as a cause of postoperative morbidity and mortality. As pointed out by Jackson in 1911, "when tracheal and bronchial secretions are in excess of the amount required properly to moisten the inspired air, they become a menace to life unless removed."[130] Postoperative atelectasis, attributed to retention of thick bronchial secretions and inhibition of coughing, was first

FIGURE 1-35 A sophisticated and complex ventilator built by Janeway in 1912. (*Used, with permission, from Janeway: Ann Surg 56:328–30, 1912.*)

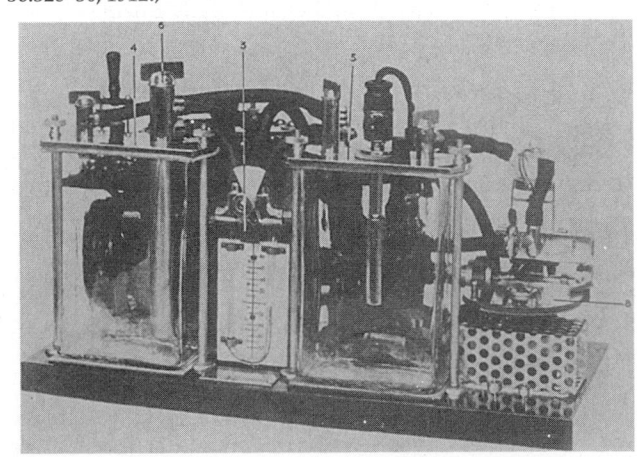

described in 1928.[131] Bronchoscopy and intratracheal suctioning were the earliest techniques advised for removing secretions,[130,132,133] but it became apparent that easy access to the tracheobronchial tree for repeated suctioning might be necessary in difficult cases. Tracheostomy was recommended as early as 1932 specifically for this problem in polio patients[134,135] and later for patients with a variety of surgical problems.[136–139] Physicians soon realized that suctioning through a large tube placed translaryngeally might be just as effective as through a tracheotomy tube. In the 1940s, case reports began to appear describing the successful and prolonged use of translaryngeal intubation for tracheobronchial toilet.[140–142] Modification of tracheal tubes to include "Murphy eyes" at the tips probably has reduced the likelihood that these tubes would become occluded by mucus.[143]

FOR THE NONOPERATIVE PATIENT

The second stage of the reintroduction of positive-pressure ventilation into clinical practice involved nonoperative patients and occurred dramatically in the 1950s. There had been isolated reports of physicians' using positive-pressure ventilation for purely mechanical problems before this time. Bert describes a positive-pressure chamber built by Jourdanet in the 1870s (Fig. 1-36) and used for a variety of mechanical problems.[15] Williams wrote of treating pulmonary disease with a pneumatic differentiation chamber in 1885. The patients were placed within a cabinet, and the air in this cabinet was exhausted by suction. Simultaneously, "antiseptic air charged with remedial agents" was administered to the patient's mouth. The reduced pressure around the thorax and atmospheric pressure applied to the lungs were thought to dilate the lungs beneficially. Remarkable improvements were described for a wide variety of lung disorders with this device.[144] Fell used a bellows ventilator to manage respiratory depression secondary to opiate overdose in the late 1880s.[107] A remarkable series of studies described the use of positive-pressure respiration for the treatment of pulmonary edema.[145–147] The emphasis of these studies was not to assist respiration—forced respiration by intubation was felt to be unjustifiable[145]—but to use positive pressure to counterbalance the backward pressure on the pulmonary capillaries.[147] The widespread use of positive-pressure ventilation did not begin, however, until its value was demonstrated dramatically during a polio epidemic in Copenhagen in 1952.

Paralytic Polio

A series of polio epidemics had swept across Europe and the United States in the 1930s and 1940s. Respiratory paralysis secondary to poliomyelitis was an infrequent but feared complication. Even with the best management techniques using iron lungs and cuirass ventilators (Fig. 1-37), the mortality rate for polio-induced respiratory paralysis probably was about 85 percent.[64] In the late summer of 1952, an epidemic struck Copenhagen. Of the first 31 patients admitted to Blegdamshospital, Copenhagen's hospital for communicable diseases, during this epidemic with respiratory paralysis, 27 died within 3 days. Out of desperation, Henry Lassen, the chief physician and epidemiologist, called the

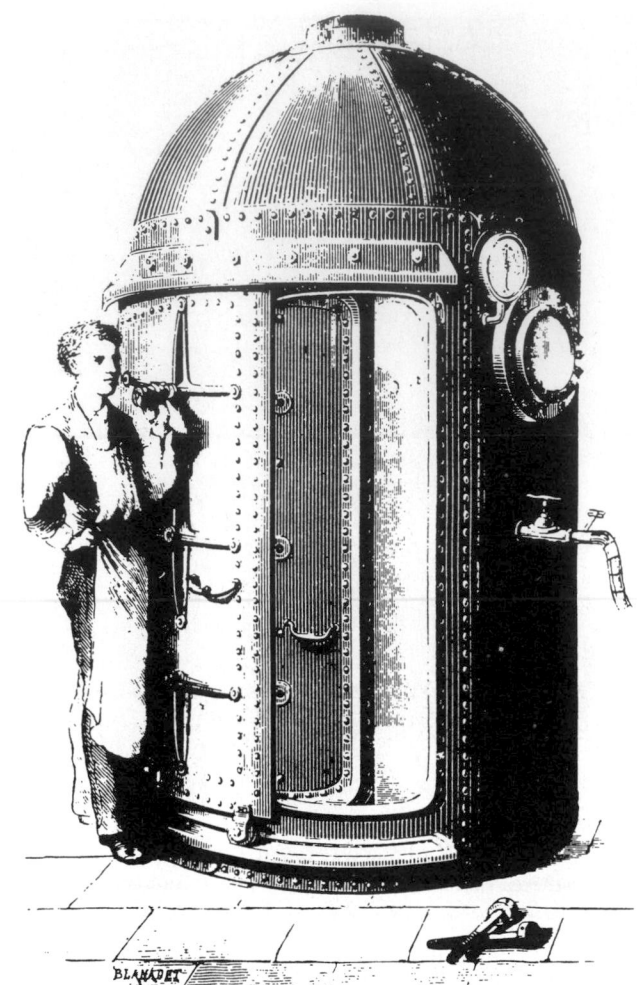

FIGURE 1-36 Jourdanet used this positive-pressure chamber to treat patients with a wide variety of disorders in the 1870s. (*Used, with permission, from Bert.*[15])

freelance anesthetist Bjorn Ibsen for consultative advice. After reviewing the medical records and autopsy results, Ibsen made two startling conclusions. First, he felt that in the fatal cases there was not sufficient atelectasis within the lungs to make adequate ventilation impossible. Second, he suggested that the increased blood levels of total CO_2 did not reflect metabolic alkalosis, as was generally believed, but rather acute respiratory acidosis. Ibsen's observations about respiratory acidosis were derived directly from work he had performed measuring exhaled carbon dioxide levels in the operating theater. Ibsen, as the anesthetist, had noted that exhaled carbon dioxide levels fluctuated during the course of surgery and could be compensated by more vigorous bag ventilation. Most important, when exhaled carbon dioxide levels increased, the patients in the operating theater had developed clammy skin and high blood pressure, similar signs to those found in the paralytic polio patients just before death. Based on these observations, Ibsen suggested inadequate ventilation as the cause of death and advised tracheostomy to allow the operative techniques of positive-pressure ventilation. Lassen was not convinced; the iron lung and cuirass respirators had reliably provided adequate

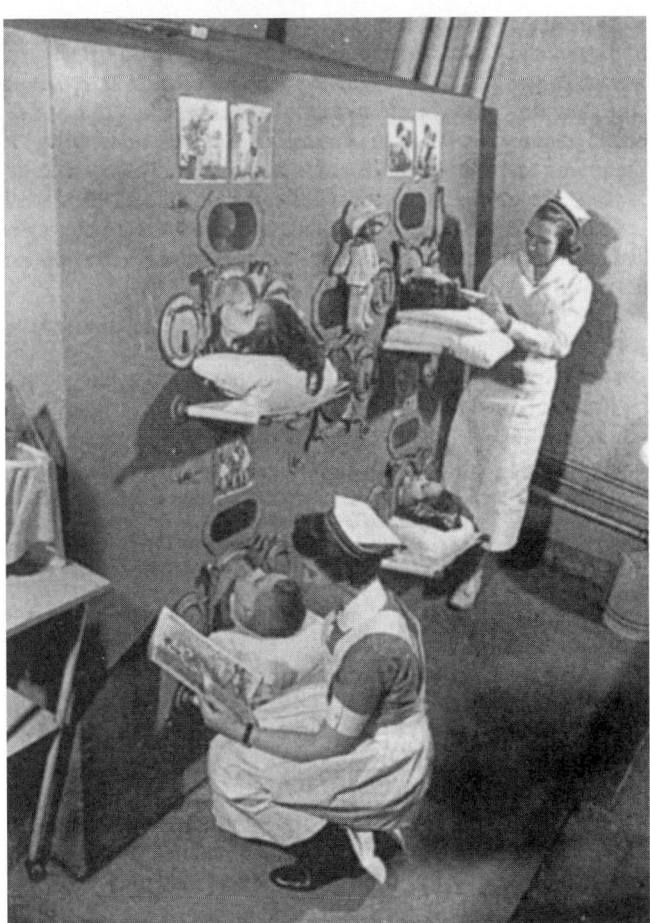

FIGURE 1-37 Young patients with respiratory paralysis from polio being treated in an "iron lung."(*Used, with permission, from Hansel Mieth, Time Life Pictures, Getty Images, 1938.*)

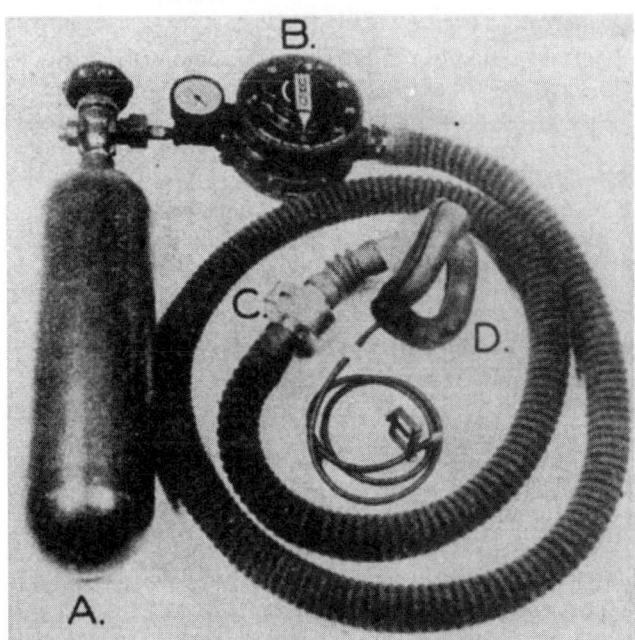

FIGURE 1-38 A prototype intermittent positive-pressure breathing device used by Motley in 1948. (*Used, with permission, Motley et al: JAMA 137:371, 1948.*)

ventilation in the past. Lassen argued that it was unlikely that positive-pressure ventilation would save paralytic polio patients if the underlying disease process actually included extensive brain-stem involvement.[148]

As a counterargument, Ibsen cited recent experience from the United States with a positive-pressure valve capable of providing mechanical positive-pressure ventilation to polio patients. These valves were developed as a result of intense interest by the U.S. Air Force during World War II in using positive pressure to increase altitude tolerance in pilots.[149,150] The unique attribute of these valves, such as the pneumatic balance respirator (PBR) and the Bennett clinical research model, was their ability to convert a continuous positive pressure into intermittent positive pressure. It was believed to be important that positive pressure only assist inspiration, allowing expiration to be passive. Intermittent positive-pressure breathing was applied in the late 1940s to a variety of medical problems and found to be effective in providing artificial ventilation to an apneic person[151–153]; in managing acute pulmonary edema, acute asthma, and postoperative patients with poor respiratory excursion[152]; possibly in improving oxygenation in various lung diseases[154]; and in administering medications by nebulization[155] (Fig. 1-38). The Bennett valve was adapted as a positive-pressure

respirator attachment for the standard tank respirator during the 1948 Los Angeles poliomyelitis epidemic (Fig. 1-39). This device was installed easily and supplied intermittent positive-pressure breaths in synchrony with the tank respirator's inspiratory negative-pressure phase.[156]

Lassen eventually agreed to a trial of Ibsen's theory. The thirty-second patient with respiratory paralysis admitted to Blegdamshospital was the poignant case of a 12-year-old girl. When her condition deteriorated, Ibsen asked a surgeon to perform a tracheostomy, and a cuffed tracheal tube was introduced. During the procedure, the girl became comatose. Ibsen initially was unable to ventilate her effectively. He assumed that retained secretions were the problem, and he suctioned her. Her condition deteriorated further, and many physicians observing the trial began to leave, assuming that the outcome would be fatal. In this desperate situation, Ibsen decided to paralyze the girl. She collapsed immediately, and Ibsen finally was able to ventilate her adequately. Her condition improved immediately.[148] Eventually, arterial blood-gas levels confirmed Ibsen's suspicions about respiratory acidosis as the cause of death in the previous patients, and positive-pressure ventilation proved successful in substantially reducing the mortality rates from paralytic polio. The only drawback was the equipment available (Fig. 1-40). Only bag ventilation was possible. During the remainder of the epidemic, it is estimated that 1500 medical and dental students worked around the clock providing bag ventilation by hand to help support these patients.[157,158]

The Copenhagen experience provided the impetus for a revolution in the medical care of patients with respiratory failure. First, it confirmed the value of positive-pressure ventilation and demonstrated the need for practical mechanical ventilators. Second, by encouraging the grouping

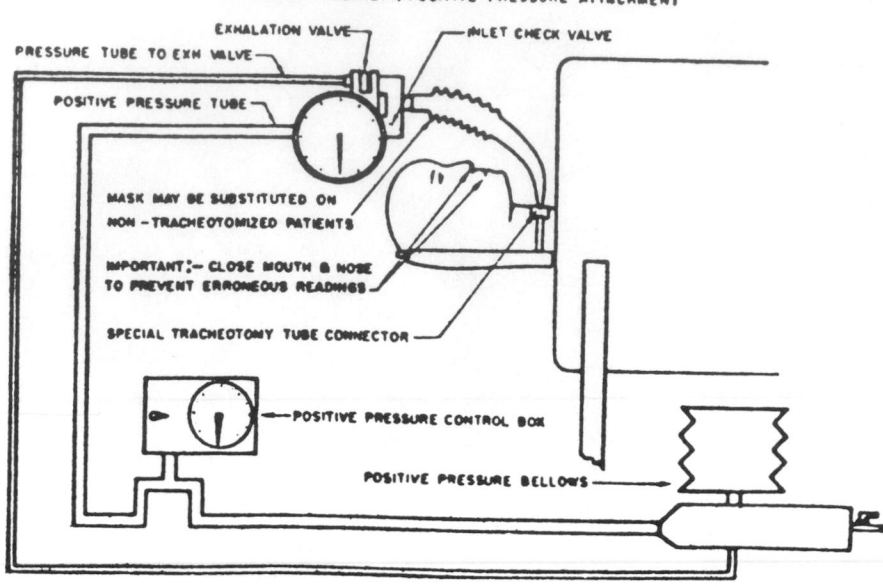

FIGURE 1-39 A schematic of the Bennett positive-pressure valve used via a tracheostomy tube in a patient in an iron lung. (*Used, with permission, from Bower et al: Ann West Med Surg 4:567, 1950.*)

of acutely ill patients in certain sections of the hospital and the organization of intensive care for these patients, it led the way for the later development of intensive-care units.[157,158] Third, Ibsen realized that provisions had to be made for resuscitating acutely ill patients in small outlying towns and transporting them to specialized centers.[159] Accordingly, mobile teams were formed with expertise in performing translaryngeal intubation and tracheotomy. After intubation and stabilization, patients could be transferred secondarily. This was obviously the precursor of our present emergency medical system.

Other Diseases with Inadequate Ventilation
Although the results using positive-pressure ventilation for the respiratory paralytic form of polio were remark-

FIGURE 1-40 This hand ventilator was used in the Copenhagen polio epidemic of 1952 by hundreds of "ventilators"(i.e., medical students, technicians, volunteers, and others) to save many lives. (*Used, with permission, from Lassen: Lancet i:38, 1953.*)

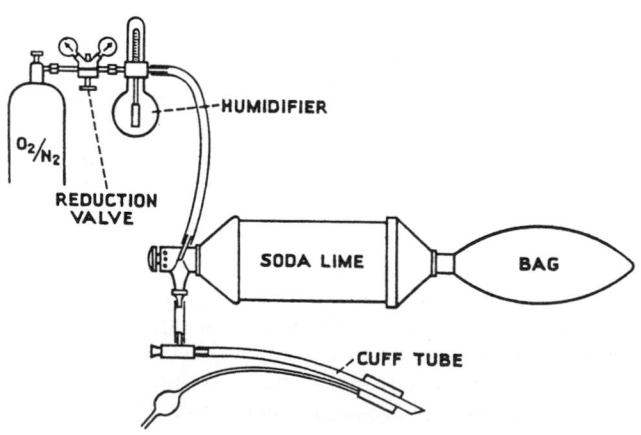

able, application of this technique to other medical problems was slow. Again, the Scandinavians took the lead in applying positive-pressure ventilation to other conditions characterized by inadequate ventilation. Extensive work in pulmonary emphysema and chronic bronchitis had confirmed that in severe cases ventilatory failure was accompanied by high carbon dioxide levels and low oxygen levels. Supplemental oxygen alone seemed to worsen the situation.[160] Sporadic reports described the use of mechanical ventilation for treating this problem. Usually used were body respirators,[160–164] but occasionally either intermittent positive-pressure breathing via a pneumatic balance respirator[161] or hand ventilation[163,164] was used transiently. By 1961, Munck had collected a total of 42 case reports describing some form of mechanical ventilation for exacerbations of chronic obstructive pulmonary disease (COPD) with successful outcomes in 31.[165] Munck's group was the first to rely strictly on positive-pressure ventilation through a tracheotomy tube to treat patients with COPD in acute respiratory crises. Their methods emphasized reliance on monitoring arterial blood oxygen, carbon dioxide, and pH levels. The average duration of treatment in their series was 24 days. They emphasized that mechanical ventilation provides a fair chance of "tiding patients with diffuse chronic lung disease over an episode of life-threatening respiratory failure—and of obtaining a reasonable recovery," provided there is some historical evidence of pulmonary reserve.[165]

Many other groups throughout the 1960s and early 1970s found that positive-pressure ventilation through either a translaryngeal tube or tracheostomy was an effective method of managing acute exacerbations of COPD.[166–175] Conservative treatment, including the use of controlled levels of supplemental oxygen, antibiotics, bronchodilators, and respiratory stimulants, was useful for treating some patients with acute ventilatory failure complicating chronic lung disease,[176,177] but it soon became clearly recognized that in severe cases with either coma or deteriorating arterial blood-gas values, endotracheal intubation and mechanical ventilation provided the most appropriate alternative.[178]

The Scandinavians also adapted these techniques to other medical problems. As early as 1951, Nilsson recognized the value of translaryngeal intubation for controlling the airway in patients with barbiturate poisoning.[179] He later emphasized that artificial respiration via a mechanical ventilator is essential when barbiturate poisoning causes apnea or respiratory insufficiency.[180] Avoiding the potentially stigmatizing tracheotomy scar also was an important consideration in patients prone to depression. Bjork pioneered the use of positive-pressure respirator treatment in postoperative thoracic surgery patients. Initially, he was conservative in his approach and postponed tracheotomy until the patient was in severe respiratory failure. By the late 1950s, however, he was performing elective tracheotomy after pulmonary resections and cardiovascular surgery and providing "prophylactic" positive-pressure ventilation to prevent atelectasis and to minimize "heavy respiratory work." He believed that any patient with a small cardiopulmonary reserve, who could become exhausted rapidly following major surgery, would benefit from this approach.[181–184] As these principles were established in thoracic surgery, the Scandinavians also began to apply them to patients with crush injury of the chest, pulmonary edema, renal failure, tetanus, pneumonia, peritonitis, and so on. The best results were obtained when respirator treatment was initiated early in the acute illness and not when chances for recovery were nil.[185]

Modern Respirators

Providing mechanical ventilation on a widespread basis could only be achieved with reliable respirators, and again, it was the Scandinavians who led the way in developing these machines. Morch built the first clinically proven volume ventilator during World War II in Denmark for use in the operating room. Because of the war, pistons and cylinders for this ventilator were made from discarded sewer pipes.[64] As a direct result of the 1952 polio epidemic in Denmark, Bang constructed a mechanical respirator. Manual ventilation of patients with respiratory paralysis was possible in Copenhagen because of the availability of medical students. In Skive, where Bang practiced, medical students were not available, and Bang's respirator was a practical necessity. Fortunately, it worked.[186,187] The Engstrom respirator, built for the same reasons, proved to be hugely successful for managing poliomyelitis patients.[188] This volume-cycled respirator also was used by Bjork in his outstanding work in postoperative respiratory care. By 1954, a number of modern automatic respirators had been developed in Europe.[189] Morch was instrumental in bringing the concept of positive-pressure ventilation across the Atlantic to America.[64,190] The incorporation of this technique into standard medical practice apparently was slower in the United States than in Scandinavia.[64] Tank respirators still were used routinely in the United States until the 1960s,[191,192] although the benefits of endotracheal intubation and positive-pressure ventilation were slowly being appreciated.[191,193] Since the 1950s, an enormous number of

TABLE 1-1   Mechanical Ventilation

Year of Introduction	Brand
1948	Bennett TV-2P
1950	Engstrom 150
1954	Drager Poliomat
1954	Thompson Portable Respirator
1955	Morch "Piston"
1955	Bird Mark 7
1955	Emerson High-Frequency Ventilator
1958	Emerson Assistor/Controller
1963	Air-Shields 1000
1963	Puritan Bennett PR-2
1964	Emerson "Post-Op" 3-PV
1964	Bourns LS-104-150
1967	Puritan Bennett MA-1
1968	Ohio/Monaghan 560
1968	Drager Spiromat
1968	Loos Co. Amsterdam
1968	Engstrom 300
1970	Veriflo CV 2000
1970	Hamilton Standard PAD 1
1972	Monaghan 225, 225-SIMV
1972	Bird-Baby Bird
1972	Bird-IMV Bird
1972	Siemens Servo 900/900B
1973	Chemtron Gill 1
1974	Emerson IMV
1974	Searle VVA
1974	Ohio 550
1975	Bourns Bear 1
1976	Forreger 210
1978	Puritan Bennett MA-II.2-2
1980	Engstrom Erica
1982	Siemens Servo 900C
1983	Biomed IC-5
1984	Puritan Bennett 7200
1984	Sechrist Adult 2200B
1985	Bear Medical Bear 5
1985	Ohmeda CPU
1986	Hamilton Veolar
1986	Bird 6400 ST
1986	Infrasonics Infant Star
1988	Bear 3
1988	Hamilton Amadeus
1988	Siemens E
1988	Bird 8400ST
1989	Bunnell Life Pulse
1989	PPG (Drager)IRISA
1989	Bird VIP
1989	Infrasonics Adult Star
1991	Siemens Servo 300
1993	Bear 1000

SOURCE: Adapted, with permission from, Masferrer et al: History of the respiratory care profession. In: Respiratory Care. Philadelphia: Lippincott, 1991:12.

practical ventilators have been introduced for everyday use (Table 1-1). This was paralleled by a significant increase in the number of patients receiving mechanical ventilation in American hospitals throughout the 1960s. Pontoppidan found a fivefold increase in artificial respiration cases at the Massachusetts General Hospital between 1960 and 1968.[194]

Intesive Care

Incorporating positive-pressure ventilation into the standard clinical practice of medical patients was not easy. Many practical problems had to be overcome. Organizing the "intensive care" that patients with ventilatory failure required was a substantial logistical problem. The Danes had answered this problem by congregating respiratory patients in special units. In the United States and elsewhere in the world, intensive-care units similarly were developed. By the middle to late 1960s, widespread experience had been accumulated with intensive-care units specifically designed for managing patients requiring sophisticated respiratory care and mechanical ventilation.[195–199] By the 1970s, several centers reported impressive reductions in mortality rate through reliance on the intensive-care-unit approach.[200–202] At present, intensive-care units are accepted as a standard and essential part of any modem acute-care hospital.

Adequacy of Ventilation

Assessing the adequacy of positive-pressure ventilation was critically important. Until arterial blood-gas machines became available commercially, physicians had to rely on laborious and exacting methods of measuring blood oxygen and carbon dioxide levels. Astrup and others emphasized that measuring Pao_2, $Paco_2$, and pH should be the ultimate goal for determining how well the respirator actually was ventilating the patient.[203,204] By 1957 it was realized that intermittent positive-pressure breathing was not always effective in reducing hypercapnia in emphysema. In fact, the more severe the obstructive lung disease, the less effective pressure-cycled respirators seemed to be in producing hyperventilation.[205] Conversely, pressure-cycled respirators easily could overventilate a patient and convert a dangerous acidosis into an equally dangerous alkalosis.[206] The issue of pulmonary encephalopathy secondary to hypercapnia was of serious concern to physicians,[207] as was the realization that mechanical ventilation could be followed by paradoxical central nervous system acidosis.[208,209]

Adequacy of ventilation also was determined by oxygenation. Supplemental oxygen had been used to treat numerous medical ailments since Priestley and Scheele had identified "pure air" in the 1770s. By the beginning of the twentieth century, the physiologic benefits of oxygen therapy were better understood, and physicians became more interested in using oxygen specifically to treat respiratory disorders. The intravenous injection of oxygen was advocated by Tunnicliffe and Stebbing in 1916[210] but attracted little interest from others. Haldane devised an apparatus for supplying controlled amounts of oxygen[211] that was used on soldiers exposed to suffocating gases during World War I. Building on the observation that patients with pneumonia had low blood oxygen levels, Meakins used the Haldane apparatus to treat hypoxic patients with pneumonia.[212] Stadie constructed and used an oxygen chamber for treating pneumonia in 1922.[213,214] Barach described the introduction of other methods of oxygen administration, including the oxygen tent, nasal catheter, and mouth funnel in 1926.[215] Physicians believed that oxygen was useful in reducing the mortality rate in pneumonia but did not understand why it was effective.[216,217] The belief that oxygen

treatment was beneficial unfortunately led to its indiscriminant use. It was not appreciated that supplemental oxygen given to a patient with COPD who had an acute ventilatory crisis with hypercapnia could result in paradoxic hypoventilation and worsened respiratory acidosis. Campbell played a leading role in recognizing this problem and devising a device, the venturi mask, for administering oxygen in a controlled fashion with a reduced risk of carbon dioxide retention.[218–220]

Just as oxygen use generally was believed to be beneficial for treating respiratory disorders, the use of oxygen was incorporated routinely into many early mechanical ventilators. This approach was justified in some cases because oxygen requirements to achieve adequate arterial oxygenation often were surprisingly high.[221] Mean inspired oxygen levels in the early respirators, however, could not be regulated accurately. Substantial and occasionally dangerous variations in inspired oxygen levels were found when ventilators were compared directly.[222–224] Nash and coworkers pointed out the potential gravity of this problem when they linked, for the first time in humans, diffuse alveolar damage (or the *respirator lung syndrome*) with the prolonged use of ventilators delivering a high inspired oxygen concentration.[225]

As an interesting aside to the issue of inspired oxygen variability among various ventilators, Frumin and coworkers found that insertion of an expiratory resistance increased arterial oxygen levels in anesthetized, paralyzed, artificially ventilated humans.[226] Manipulation of airway pressure by immersion of the exhalation limb from a tracheotomy tube 1 to 4 cm under water had been shown previously to improve ventilation in patients with multiple rib fractures.[227] These simple measures for increasing airway pressure, termed variously the *positive expiratory pressure plateau,*[228] *continuous positive airway pressure,*[229,230] and later, *positive end-expiratory pressure,* were to prove enormously successful in improving oxygenation in patients with both adult and infant respiratory distress syndromes.

Quality Control of Ventilators

The variability in oxygen concentrations found among various respirators reflected a more serious underlying problem. As the need for ventilators, gas cylinders, connectors, oxygen-delivery masks, and myriad other types of respiratory equipment increased, the number of manufacturers producing this equipment proliferated. Quality control among manufacturers varied. More important, manufacturers tended to produce equipment of various size specifications, often making integration of breathing circuits impossible. Anesthesiologists were particularly concerned with these problems because of the difficulties they had encountered in establishing universal color codes for anesthetic gas cylinders during World War II. For example, carbon dioxide cylinders in Britain were painted green, but U.S. oxygen cylinders also were painted green. Inevitably, when U.S. and British anesthesiologists worked together, cylinders were filled with the wrong gas, and deaths occurred.[231–233]

The American Society for Anesthetists (ASA) performed a critically important service by organizing a Committee on Standardization of Anesthetic and Resuscitating Equipment, charged with forging a consensus on manufacturing standards for this type of equipment. In 1955, the committee met with representatives of anesthesia equipment manufacturers and the American Standards Association (later the American National Standards Institute, or ANSI). Following this meeting, the ASA approved financial support for the American National Standards Committee Z79 on Anesthesia and Respiratory Equipment to operate under the umbrella of ANSI. Members of this committee included representatives of various medical specialties and principal manufacturers of anesthesia and respiratory equipment.

Committee Z79 tried to obtain consensus on equipment production both within the United States and internationally. Initially, it worked closely with the British Standards Committee SGC 15. In 1967, the International Standards Organization (ISO) convened its own technical committee in this field, for which the British Standards Committee acted as secretariat. Committee Z79 was extraordinarily effective in developing standards for a wide range of respiratory equipment. Under the Medical Device Amendments of 1976, the Food and Drug Administration (FDA) was charged with regulatory responsibility for the safety and efficacy of medical devices. The FDA had a significant impact on refining the standards established by Committee Z79. In 1983, the relationship between ANSI and Committee Z79 was terminated for financial and liability reasons. At that time, the ASA agreed to transfer this committee's sponsorship to the American Society for Testing Materials (ASTM). The committee's name was then changed to F29. American medicine indeed has been quite fortunate in having ongoing committees to gain consensus effectively and voluntarily on manufacturing and performance standards for ventilators (ASTM F1100-90, for standard specifications for ventilators intended for use in critical care), tracheal tubes (ASTM F1242-89, standard specifications for cuffed and uncuffed tracheal tubes), and many other standard pieces of respiratory equipment.[233]

Numerous other problems were encountered with the regular and prolonged use of positive-pressure ventilation. There was serious concern about accidental disconnections from the ventilator. Appropriate safeguards and alarm systems were incorporated gradually into respirator systems to reassure the nursing staff, respiratory therapists, and physicians that such disconnections would be recognized promptly. Adequate humidification of the ventilator air supply had to be ensured.[190] The risks of nosocomial pneumonia were not understood initially. Vigilant attention to sterilization of respiratory equipment, proper suctioning technique, and minimization of stagnant water in tubing and humidification sources was advised to reduce the risk of "ventilator lung."[196] There was considerable debate for decades over whether translaryngeal intubation was preferred over tracheotomy for patients requiring prolonged mechanical ventilation. Although this subject is still controversial, a consensus conference in 1986 reached agreement that translaryngeal intubation is the preferred initial choice for obtaining airway control in most patients needing artificial respiration. A secondary tracheotomy can be deferred for up to 20 days or longer depending on the individual situation.[234]

Weaning

An intriguing problem developed as the use of positive-pressure ventilation became more widespread. Once patients were placed on a mechanical ventilator, how were they to be "weaned" eventually from such respiratory support? This question actually had two components: How could the physician determine when a patient was ready to be weaned? What methods could be used to facilitate the weaning process? Numerous criteria have been advocated as reasonable indicators that patients are weaning candidates, but none has yet proved infallible.[194,235–237] Similarly, numerous techniques have been proposed as useful modalities for maximizing the chances for a successful weaning process. Modifications of ventilator technology in the 1970s led to the proposal of such methods as intermittent mandatory ventilation (IMV)[238,239] and mandatory minute volume[240] as alternatives to the standard T-piece method of weaning.[241–243] Although many physicians expressed strong preferences for one weaning modality over another,[244] it has never been shown clearly that modalities such as IMV hasten the weaning process.[245,246] Whether more recently introduced technological advances in ventilator techniques, such as pressure-support and pressure-control ventilation, will improve clinicians' ability to wean patients is still unclear.

Conclusion

In this historical review of the development of mechanical ventilation, a rich and complex weave of discoveries in many different scientific and technical areas has brought us to the early 1990s, a time during which physicians have been trained to rely routinely on mechanical ventilation for managing all manner of acute, serious illnesses. It is remarkable that only 40 years ago, cadres of medical and dental students were needed to manually ventilate polio patients with respiratory paralysis, and at the turn of the century, a foot-operated bellows for mechanical ventilation was a remarkable innovation. In the late eighteenth century, the concept of using a bellows and translaryngeal tube for resuscitating the apparently drowned was just being introduced, and in the sixteenth century, Vesalius was forced to make a pilgrimage to the Holy Land to atone for the sin of restarting a Spanish nobleman's heart by inflating his lungs. The debt we owe to the many pioneers who have contributed to the advances in the field of mechanical ventilation is humbling, just as the hope for future unforeseeable developments in this field is enthralling.

References

1. Perkins JF. Historical development of respiratory physiology. In: Fenn WO, Rahn H, editors. Handbook of physiology. Washington: American Physiological Society, 1964: 1–62.
2. Wilson LG. Erasistratus, Galen and the pneuma. Bull Hist Med 1959; 33:293–314.

3. Aristotle. Historia animalium. Thompson DW, translator. London: Oxford University Press, 1910.

4. Astrup P, Severinghaus JW. The history of blood gases, acids and bases. Copenhagen: Munksgaard, 1986.

5. Galen C. On anatomical procedures. Singer C, translator. London: Oxford University Press, 1956.

6. Graubard M. Circulation and respiration. New York: Harcourt, Brace & World, 1964.

7. Haddad SI, Khalrallah AA. A forgotten chapter in the history of the circulation of the blood. Ann Surg 1936; 104:1–8.

8. Vesalius A. The epitome. Lind LR, translator. New York: Macmillan, 1949.

9. Servetus M. The restoration of christianity. O'Malley CD, translator. Philadelphia: American Philosophical Society, 1953.

10. Columbus R. Of things anatomical. DeWitt NJ, translator. Venice, 1559.

11. Harvey W. Anatomical studies on the motion of the heart and blood in animals. Leake CD, translator. Springfield, IL: Charles C Thomas, 1941.

12. Mayow J. Medico-physical works. English translation. Edinburgh: Alembic Club, 1907.

13. Boyle R. The philosophical works of the honorable Robert Boyle. Shaw P, Innys W, Innys J, editors. London, 1725.

14. Boyle R. New pneumatical experiments about respiration. Philos Trans R Soc London 1670; 5:2011–58.

15. Bert P. Barometric pressure (1878). Hitchcock MA, Hitchcock FA, translators. Columbus, OH: College Book, 1943.

16. Jardine L. Ingenious pursuits. New York: Doubleday, 1999.

17. McKie D. Antoine Lavoisier: Scientist, economist and social reformer. New York: Schuman, 1952.

18. Magnus HG. De la presence de l'oxigéne, de l'azote et de acide carbonique dans la théorie de la respiration. Ann Sci Nat Zool 1837; 8:79–96.

19. Pettenkofer M. Ueber die respiration. Ann Chern U Pharm Suppl 1862; 2:1–52.

20. Lower R. On the movement and color of the blood from early science in Oxford. Gunther RT, editor. London: Oxford University Press, 1932.

21. Meyer L. Die Gase des Blutes. Gottingen, Germany, 1857.

22. Hoppe-Seyler F. Über die Oxidation im lebenden Blute. Medicinisch-chemischie Untersuchungen 1866–1871; 132:1–4.

23. Dohmen W. Untersuchungen über den Einfluss, den die Blutgase in Uutersuchungen aus dein physiologischen Laboratorium 20. Bonn: Relin F Fruegen, 1865: 83.

24. Haldane JS, Priestley JG. The regulation of lung ventilation. J Physiol 1905; 32:225–66.

25. Biot JB. Sür la nature de l'air contenu dans la vessie natatoire des poissons. Mem d' Arcueil 1809; 2:405.

26. Haldane JS, Priestly JG. Respiration. New Haven: Yale University Press, 1935.

27. Bohr C. On the specific activity of the lung in respiratory gas uptake and its relation to the gas diffusions occurring across the alveolar wall. Scand Arch Physiol 1907; 22:221–80.

28. Krogh A, Krogh M. On the tensions of gases in the arterial blood. Scand Arch Physiol 1910; 23:179–96.

29. Krogh M. The diffusion of gases through the lungs of man. J Physiol 1915; 49:271–300.

30. Barcroft J, Cooke A, Hartridge H, et al. The flow of oxygen through the pulmonary epithelium. J Physiol 1920; 53:450–72.

31. Bohr C, Hasselbalch KA, Krogh A. Ueber einen in biologisches beziehung wichtigen ein fluss, den die kohlensaine spannung des blutes auf dessen sauerstoffburdung ubt. Scand Arch Physiol 1904; 16:402–12.

32. Christiansen J, Douglas CG, Haldane JS. The absorption and dissociation of carbon dioxide by blood. J Physiol 1914; 48:244–71.

33. Mcinnes DA, Belcher D. A durable glass electrode. Ind Eng Chem Anal Ed 1933; 5:199–200.

34. Siggaard-Anderson O. An acid-base chart for arterial blood with normal and pathophysiological reference areas. Scand J Clin Lab Invest 1971; 27:239–45.

35. Stow RW, Randall BF. Electrical measurement of the P_{CO_2} in blood. Am J Physiol 1954; 179:678.

36. Clark LC Jr. Monitoring and control of blood and tissue O_2 tensions. Trans Am Soc Artif Intern Organs 1956; 2:41–57.

37. Hoff EC. A bibliographical sourcebook of compressed air, diving and submarine medicine. Washington: US Government Printing Office, 1948.

38. Hill L. Caisson sickness. New York: Longmans, Green, 1912.

39. Davis RH. Deep sea diving and underwater rescue. J R Soc Arts 1934; 82:1032–47, 1049–65, 1069–80.

40. Méricourt L. Considerations sûr l'hygiene des pecheurs d'éponges. Ann Hyg Publique Paris 1869; 31:274–86.

41. Teruoka G. Die Ama und ihre Arbeit. Arbeitsphysiologie 1931–1932; 5:239–51.

42. Thooris A. Contribution à l'étude biologique des plongeurs. C R Acad Sci Paris 1921; 172:1529–32.

43. Foregger R. Development of mine rescue and underwater breathing apparatus: Appliances of Henry Fleuss. J Hist Med 1974; 29:317–30.

44. Triger. Mémoire sûr un appareil à qui comprimé, pour Ie percement des pants de mines et autres travaux, sous les eaux et dans les sables submergés. C R Acad Sci Paris 1841; 13:884–96.

45. Haldane JS, Atkinson WN. Investigations on the composition, occurrence and properties of black damp. Trans Inst Miner Eng Lond 1895; 8:549–62.

46. Haldane JS. Self-contained rescue apparatus for use in irrespirable atmosphere. Trans Inst Miner Eng Lond 1914; 47:725–6.

47. Belli CM. Les alterations de l'air dans les sousmarins. Int Congr Hyg 1907; 14:718–9.

48. Marantonio R. Mechanical devices for ventilation and air renewal on the submarine "Ballila." Nav Med Bull Wash 1917; 11:156–75.

49. Du Bois EF. Physiology of respiration in relationship to the problems of naval medicine: III. Submarine ventilation. Nav Med Bull Wash 1928; 26:515–52.

50. Carpenter DN. Habitability of submarines. Nav Med Bull Wash 1928; 26:31–40.

51. Dudley SF. Some atmospheric hazards encountered in naval life. Proc R Soc Med 1934–1935; 28:1282–92.

52. Johnson LW. Medical problems of diving and submarines. NY State J Med 1940; 40:1065–74.

53. Gibson WC. Medical pioneers in aviation. J Hist Med 1962; 17:83–93.

54. Armstrong HG. Principles and practice of aviation medicine. Baltimore: Williams & Wilkins, 1939.

55. Gilbert DL. The first documented report of mountain sickness: The Andean or Pariacaca story. Respir Physiol 1983; 52:327–47.

56. Ruff S, Strughold H. Compendium of aviation medicine. Washington: National Research Council, 1942.

57. Department of the Air Force. German aviation medicine: World War II. Washington: US Government Printing Office, 1951.

58. Clamann HG. The engineered environment of the space vehicle. In: Sells SB, Berry CA, editors. Human factors in jet and space travel. New York: Ronald Press, 1961: 330–4.

59. Welds BE. Ecological systems. In: Brown JHU, editor. Physiology of man in space. New York: Academic Press, 1963: 310–35.

60. Kuettner JP, Ordway FI. The development of manned space vehicles. In: Bourne GH, editor. Medical and biological problems of space flight. New York: Academic Press, 1963: 1–4.

61. Galen C. On the functions of parts of the human body. Daremberg C, translator. Paris: JB Bailliére, 1954.

62. Vesalius A. De humani corporis fabrica. Basel: Oporinus, 1543.

63. Baker AB. Artificial respiration, the history of an idea. Med Hist 1971; 15:336–51.

64. Morch ET. History of mechanical ventilation. In: Kirby RR, Smith RA, Desautels DA, editors. Mechanical ventilation. New York: Churchill Livingstone, 1985; 1–58.

65. Highmore N. Corporis humani disquisitio anatomica. The Hague: Comitis S Broun, 1651.

66. Tossach W. A man dead in appearance recovered by distending the lungs with air. Medical Essays and Observations 1744; 5:605.

67. Lee RV. Cardiopulmonary resuscitation in the eighteenth century. J Hist Med 1972; 27:418–33.

68. Fothergill J. Observations on a case published in the last volume of Medical Essays. Philos Trans R Soc London 1745; 43:378.

69. Buchan W. Domestic medicine. London: W Strahan, 1760.

70. Hunter J. Proposals for the recovery of persons apparently drowned. Philos Trans R Soc London 1775; 66:412–25.

71. Cullen W. A letter to Lord Cathcart: Concerning the recovery of persons drowned and seemingly dead. Edinburgh, 1776: 1–41.

72. McClellan I. Nineteenth century resuscitation apparatus. Anaesthesia 1981; 36:307–11.

73. Mushin M, Rendell-Baker L. The principles and practices of thoracic anesthesia. Oxford: Blackwell, 1953.

74. Kite C. An essay on the recovery of the apparently drowned. London, 1788.

75. Leroy J. Recherches sûr l'asphyxie. J Physiol Exp Pathol 1827; 7:45.

76. Leroy J. Second mémoire sûr l'asphyxie. J Physiol Exp Pathol 1828; 8:97.

77. Price JL. The evolution of breathing machines. Med Hist 1962; 6:67–72.

78. Woollam CHM. The development of apparatus for intermittent negative pressure respiration 1832–1918. Anaesthesia 1976; 31:537–47.

79. Dalziel J. On sleep and an apparatus for promoting artificial respiration. Br Assoc Adv Sci 1838; 2:127.

80. Emerson JH. The evolution of iron lungs. Cambridge: JH Emerson, 1978.

81. Woillez EJ. Du spirophore, apparell de sauvatage pour Ie traitment de l'asphyxie, et princepalement de l'asphyxie des noyes et des noureauvés. Bull Acad Med 1876; 5:611.

82. Doe OW. Apparatus for resuscitating asphyxiated children. Boston Med Surg J 1889; 120:9–11.

83. Eisenmenger R. Apparatus for maintaining artificial respiration. Lancet 1904; 1:515.

84. Woollam CHM. The development of apparatus for intermittent negative pressure respiration 1919–1976. Anaesthesia 1976; 31:666–85.

85. Drinker P, Shaw LA. An apparatus for the prolonged administration of artificial respiration. J Clin Invest 1929; 7:229–47.

86. Drinker P, McKhann CF. The use of a new apparatus for the prolonged administration of artificial respiration. JAMA 1929; 92:1658–60.

87. Hering E, Breuer J. Die Selbsteurung den Athmung derch den Nervus vagus. Sitzungsber Akad Wiss Wien 1868; 57:672–7.

88. Head H. On the regulation of respiration. J Physiol 1889; 10:1–55.

89. Bowditch HP. Physiological apparatus in use at the Harvard Medical School. J Physiol 1879–1880; 2:202–5.

90. Herbsman H. Early history of pulmonary surgery. J Hist Med 1958; 13:329–48.

91. Marcus S. Recherches relatives aux consequences de l'extirpation experimentale des poumons. Gaz Med Paris 1881; 52:695.

92. Heuer GJ. The development of lobectomy and pneumonectomy in man. J Thorac Surg 1934; 3:560–72.

93. Quenu, Longuet. Note sûr quelques recherches experimentales concernant la chirurgie thoracique. C R Soc Biol Paris 1896; 48:1007–8.

94. Meyer W. Avoidance of apparatus complicating the operation. Med Rec 1910; 77:483–90.

95. Colice GL. Prolonged intubation versus tracheostomy in the adult. J Intens Care Med 1987; 2:85–102.

96. Frost E. Tracing the tracheostomy. Ann Otol 1976; 85:618–24.

97. McClelland RMA. Tracheostomy: Its management and alternatives. Proc R Soc Med 1972; 65:401–4.

98. MacEwen W. Clinical observations on the introduction of tracheal tubes by the mouth instead of performing tracheostomy or laryngotomy. Br Med J 1880; 2:122–4, 163–5.

99. O'Dwyer J. Fifty cases of croup in private practice treated by intubation of the larynx with a description of the method and of the dangers incident thereto. Med Rec 1887; 32:497–502.

100. O'Dwyer J. Intubation of the larynx. NY Med J 1885; 42:145.

101. O'Dwyer J. Intubation in the treatment of chronic stenosis of the larynx. Br Med J 1894; 2:1478–81.

102. Warren JC. Inhalation of ethereal vapor for the prevention of pain in surgical operations. Boston Med Surg J 1846; 35:375–9.

103. Snow J. On chloroform and other anesthetics: Their action and administration. London: Churchill, 1858.

104. Gillespie NA. The evolution of endotracheal anesthesia. J Hist Med 1946; 1:583–94.

105. Tuffier, Hallion. Opérations intrathoraciques avec respiration artificielle par insufflation. C R Soc Biol Paris 1896; 48:951–3.

106. Matas R. Intralaryngeal insufflation. JAMA 1900; 34:1468–73.

107. Fell GE. Forced respiration. JAMA 1891; 16:325–30.

108. Matas R. Artificial respiration by direct intralaryngeal intubation with a modified O'Dwyer tube and a new graduated air pump, in its applications to medical and surgical practice. Am Med 1902; 3:97–103.

109. Kuhn F. Die perorale Intubation. Berlin, 1911.

110. Meltzer SJ, Auer J. Continuous respiration without respiratory movements. J Exp Med 1909; 11:622–5.

111. Elsberg CA. Clinical experiences with intratracheal insufflation (Meltzer) with remarks upon the value of the method for thoracic surgery. Ann Surg 1910; 52:23–9.

112. Meyer W. Pneumectomy with the aid of differential air pressure. JAMA 1909; 53:1978–87.

113. Murphy FT. A suggestion for a practical apparatus for use in intrathoracic operations. Boston Med Surg J 1905; 152:428–31.

114. Green NW. The positive-pressure method of artificial respiration. Surg Gynecol Obstet 1906; 2:512–37.

115. Green NW, Janeway HH. Artificial respiration and intrathoracic esophageal surgery. Ann Surg 1910; 52:58–66.

116. Robinson S. Experimental surgery of the lungs. Ann Surg 1908; 47:182–221.

117. Robinson S. Artificial intrapulmonary positive pressure. JAMA 1908; 51:803–5.

118. Bunnell S. The use of nitrous oxide and oxygen to maintain anesthesia and positive pressure for thoracic surgery. JAMA 1912; 58:835–8.

119. Elsberg CA. The value of continuous intratracheal insufflation of air (Meltzer) in thoracic surgery. Med Rec 1910; 77:493–5.

120. Dorrance GM. On the treatment of traumatic injuries of the lungs and pleura. Surg Gynecol Obstet 1910; 11:160–73.

121. Jackson C. The technique of insertion of intratracheal insufflation tubes. Surg Gynecol Obstet 1913; 17:507–9.

122. Janeway HH. An apparatus for the intratracheal insufflation. Ann Surg 1912; 56:328–30.

123. Kelly RE. Anesthesia by the intratracheal insufflation of ether. Br Med J 1912; 2:112–3.

124. Magill IW. Endotracheal anesthesia. Proc R Soc Med 1928; 22:83–8.

125. Magill IW. Technique in endotracheal anesthesia. Br Med J 1930; 2:817–9.

126. Rowbotham S. Intratracheal anaesthesia by the nasal route for operations on the mouth and lips. Br Med J 1920; 1:590–1.

127. Jackson DE. A universal artificial respiration and closed anesthesia machine. J Lab Clin Med 1927; 12:998–1002.

128. Starling EH. An improved method of artificial respiration. Proc Physiol Soc 1926; 61:14–5.

129. Guedel AE, Treweek DN. Ether apneas. Anesth Analg 1934; 13:263–4.

130. Jackson C. The drowning of the patient in his own secretion. Laryngoscope 1911; 21:1183–5.

131. Lee WE, Tucker G, Clerf L. Post-operative pulmonary atelectasis. Ann Surg 1928; 88:6–14.

132. Haight C. Intratracheal suction in the management of postoperative pulmonary complications. Ann Surg 1938; 107:218–28.

133. Cardon L. Tracheobronchial aspiration with a urethral catheter. JAMA 1950; 142:1039–44.

134. Wilson JL. Acute anterior poliomyelitis. New Engl J Med 1932; 206:887–93.

135. Galloway TC. Tracheotomy in bulbar poliomyelitis. JAMA 1943; 123:1096–7.

136. Reynolds JT, Holinger TH, Andrews AH, et al. Role of tracheotomy in the postoperative care of patients subjected to esophagectomy. Arch Surg 1950; 61:211–28.

137. Echols DH, Llewellyn R, Kirgis HD, et al. Tracheotomy in the management of severe head injuries. Surgery 1950; 28: 801–11.

138. Carter N, Giuseffi J. Tracheotomy, a useful procedure in thoracic surgery. J Thorac Cardiovasc Surg 1951; 21:495–505.

139. Taylor GW, Austin GM. Treatment of pulmonary complications in neurosurgical patients by tracheotomy. Arch Otolaryngol 1951; 53:386–92.

140. Gillespie NA. Prolonged use of an endotracheal tube. Anesthesiology 1942; 3:217–8.

141. Foregger R. Use of endotracheal tube in therapy of posttraumatic pulmonary secretions. Anesthesiology 1946; 7:285–9.

142. Briggs BD. Prolonged endotracheal intubation. Anesthesiology 1950; 11:129–31.

143. Murphy FJ. Two improved intratracheal catheters. Anesth Analg 1941; 27:102–5. 144.

144. Williams HF. Antiseptic treatment of pulmonary disease by means of pneumatic differentiation. Med Rec 1885; 27:57–62.

145. Emerson H. Artificial respiration in the treatment of edema of the lungs. Arch Intern Med 1909; 3:368–71.

146. Poulton EP. Left-sided heart failure with pulmonary edema. Lancet 1936; 2:981–3.

147. Barach AL, Martin J, Eckman M. Positive pressure respiration and its application to the treatment of acute pulmonary edema. Ann Intern Med 1938; 17:754–95.

148. Wackers GL. Modern anaesthesiological principles for bulbar polio: Manual IPPR in the 1952 polio-epidemic in Copenhagen. Acta Anaesthesiol Scand 1994; 38:420–31.

149. Eckman M, Barach B, Fox C, et al. An appraisal of intermittent pressure breathing as a method of increasing altitude tolerance. J Aviat Med 1947; 18:565–74.

150. Barach AL, Fenn WO, Ferris EB, Schmidt CP. The physiology of pressure breathing. J Aviat Med 1947; 18:73–86.

151. Motley HL, Coumand A, Eckman M, Richards DW. Physiological studies on man with the pneumatic balance resuscitator, "Bums model." J Aviat Med 1946; 17:431–61.

152. Motley HL, Werko L, Coumand A, Richards DW. Observations on the clinical use of intermittent positive pressure. J Aviat Med 1947; 18:417–35.

153. Motley HL, Coumand A, Werko L, et al. Intermittent positive pressure breathing. JAMA 1948; 137:370–82.

154. Motley HL, Lang LP, Gordon B. Effect of intermittent positive pressure breathing on respiratory gas exchange. J Aviat Med 1950; 21:14–27.

155. Motley HL, Lang LP, Gordon B. Use of intermittent positive pressure breathing combined with nebulization in pulmonary disease. Am J Med 1948; 5:853–5.

156. Bower AG, Bennett VR, Dillon JB, Axelrod B. Investigation on the case and treatment of poliomyelitis patients. Ann West Med Surg 1950; 4:561–715.

157. Lassen HCA. A preliminary report on the 1952 epidemic of poliomyelitis in Copenhagen with special reference to the treatment of acute respiratory insufficiency. Lancet 1953; i:37–40.

158. Ibsen B. The anaesthetist's viewpoint on the treatment of respiratory complications in poliomyelitis during the epidemic in Copenhagen, 1952. Proc R Soc Med 1954; 47:72–4.

159. Andersen EW, Ibsen B. The anaesthetic management of patients with poliomyelitis and respiratory paralysis. Br Med J 1954; 1:786–8.

160. Boutourline-Young HJ, Whittenberger JL. The use of artificial respiration in pulmonary emphysema accompanied by high carbon dioxide levels. J Clin Invest 1951; 30:838–47.

161. Stone DJ, Schwartz A, Newman W, et al. Precipitation by pulmonary infection of acute anoxia, cardiac failure and respiratory acidosis in chronic pulmonary disease. Am J Med 1953; 14:14–22.

162. Lovejoy FW, Yu PNG, Nye R, et al. Pulmonary hypertension. Am J Med 1954; 16:4–11.

163. Bjorneboe M, Astrup P, Harvald B, et al. Active ventilation in treatment of respiratory acidosis in chronic diseases of the lungs. Lancet 1955; ii:901–3.

164. Lindsay A, Davidson G. Tracheotomy in acute respiratory disease. Lancet 1959; 2:597–600.

165. Munck O, Kristensen HS, Lassen HCA. Mechanical ventilation for acute respiratory failure in diffuse chronic lung disease. Lancet 1961; i:66–7.

166. Billingham M, Eldridge F. Use of a pressure-cycled respirator (Bird) in respiratory failure due to severe obstructive pulmonary disease. Ann Intern Med 1969; 70:1121–33.

167. Weill H, George R, Munsakul N, et al. Management of acute respiratory failure in chronic obstructive pulmonary disease. South Med J 1970; 63:90–5.

168. Kettel LJ, Diener CF, Morse JO, et al. Treatment of acute respiratory acidosis in chronic obstructive lung disease. JAMA 1971; 217:1503–8.

169. Sluiter HI, Blokzijl EJ, van Dijl W, et al. Conservative and respirator treatment of acute respiratory insufficiency in patients with chronic obstructive lung disease. Am Rev Respir Dis 1972; 103:932–43.

170. Bradley RD, Spencer GT, Semple SJG. Tracheostomy and artificial ventilation in the treatment of acute exacerbations of chronic lung disease. Lancet 1964; i:854–9.

171. Ebert RV, Pierce JA. The results of intensive treatment of patients with chronic bronchitis and pulmonary emphysema. Trans Am Assoc Climatol 1965; 77:183–7.

172. Williams MH. Ventilatory failure. Medicine 1966; 45:317–30.

173. Jessen O, Kristensen HS, Rasmussen K. Tracheostomy and artificial ventilation in chronic lung disease. Lancet 1967; ii:9–12.

174. Weg JG. Prolonged endotracheal intubation in respiratory failure. Arch Intern Med 1967; 120:679–86.

175. Smith JP, Stone RW, Muschenheim C. Acute respiratory failure in chronic lung disease. Am Rev Respir Dis 1968; 97:791–803.

176. Canter HG, Luchsinger PC. The treatment of respiratory failure without mechanical assistance. Am J Med Sci 1964; 248:206–10.

177. Vandenbergh E, van de Woestijne KP, Gyselen A. Conservative treatment of acute respiratory failure in patients with chronic obstructive lung disease. Am Rev Respir Dis 1968; 98: 60–9.

178. Warren PM, Flenley DC, Millar JS, Avery A. Respiratory failure revisited: Acute exacerbations of chronic bronchitis between 1961–68 and 1970–76. Lancet 1980; i:467–70.

179. Nilsson E. Frequency and occurrence of barbiturate poisoning. Acta Med Scand 1951; S253:9–98.

180. Clemmesen C, Nilsson E. Therapeutic trends in the treatment of barbiturate poisoning. Clin Pharm Ther 1960; 2:220–9.

181. Bjork VO, Engstom CG. The treatment of ventilatory insufficiency after pulmonary resection with tracheostomy and prolonged artificial ventilation. J Thoracic Surg 1955; 30:356–67.

182. Bjork VO, Engstrom CG, Friberg O, et al. Ventilatory problems in thoracic anesthesia. J Thoracic Surg 1956; 31:117–23.

183. Bjork VO, Engstrom CG. The treatment of ventilatory insufficiency by tracheostomy and artificial ventilation. J Thoracic Surg 1957; 34:228–41.

184. Bjork VO, Holmdahl MH. Respirator treatment for hypoventilation following thoracic surgery. Ann NY Acad Sci 1963; 110:920–5.

185. Norlander OP, Bjork VO, Crafoord C, et al. Controlled ventilation in medical practice. Anaesthesia 1961; 16:285–307.

186. Bang C. A new respirator. Lancet 1953; i:723–6.

187. Kristensen LK, Lunding M. Early Danish respirators designed for prolonged artificial ventilation. Acta Anesth 1978; S67:96–105.

188. Engstrom CG. Treatment of severe cases of respiratory paralysis by the Engstrom universal respirator. Br Med J 1954; 2:666–9.

189. Mushin W, Rendell-Baker L. Modem automatic respirators. Br J Anaesth 1954; 26:131–47.

190. Morch ET, Saxton GA, Gish G. Artificial respiration via the uncuffed tracheostomy tube. JAMA 1956; 160:864–7.

191. Safar P, Berman B, Diamond E, et al. Cuffed tracheotomy tube vs tank respirator for prolonged artificial ventilation. Arch Phys Med Rehabil 1962; 43:487–93.

192. McClement JH, Christianson LC, Hubaytar RT, Simpson DG. The body-type respirator in the treatment of chronic obstructive pulmonary disease. Ann NY Acad Sci 1964–1965; 121:746–9.

193. Block AJ, Ball WC. Acute respiratory failure: Observations on the use of the Morch piston respirator. Ann Intern Med 1966; 65:957–75.

194. Pontoppidan H, Laver M, Geffin B. Acute respiratory failure in the surgical patient. Adv Surg 1970; 4:163–254.

195. Bates DV, Klassen GA, Broadhurst CA, et al. Management of respiratory failure. Ann NY Acad Sci 1965; 121:781–6.

196. Linton RC, Walker FW, Spoerel WE. Respirator care in a general hospital: A five-year survey. Can Anaesth Soc J 1965;12:450–7.

197. Bigelow DB, Petty TL, Ashbaugh DG, et al. Acute respiratory failure: Experiences of a respiratory care unit. Med Clin North Am 1967; 51:323–39.

198. Noehren TH, Friedman I. A ventilation unit for special intensive care of patients with respiratory failure. JAMA 1968; 203:125–7.

199. Holmdahl MH. The respiratory care unit. Anesthesiology 1962; 23:559–67.

200. O'Donohue WI, Baker JP, Bell GM, et al. The management of acute respiratory failure in a respiratory intensive care unit. Chest 1970; 58:603–10.

201. Rogers RM, Weiler C, Ruppenthal B. Impact of the respiratory intensive care unit on survival of patients with acute respiratory failure. Chest 1972; 62:94–7.

202. Snell JD. Treatment of acute respiratory failure in chronic obstructive pulmonary disease: Results without a special respiratory care unit. South Med J 1973; 66:153–8.

203. Astrup P, Gotzche H, Neukirch F. Laboratory investigations during treatment of patients with poliomyelitis and respiratory paralysis. Br Med J 1954; 1:780–6.

204. Radford EP, Ferris BG, Kriete BC. Clinical use of a nomogram to estimate proper ventilation during artificial respiration. New Engl J Med 1954; 251:879–83.

205. Fraimow W, Cathcart RT, Goodman E. The use of intermittent positive pressure breathing in the prevention of the carbon dioxide narcosis associated with oxygen therapy. Am Rev Respir Dis 1960; 81:815–21.

206. Herzog H. Pressure-cycled ventilators. Ann NY Acad Sci 1964–1968; 121:751–65.

207. Austin FK, Carmichael MW, Adams RD. Neurologic manifestations of chronic pulmonary insufficiency. New Engl J Med 1957; 257:579–89.

208. Kilburn KH. Shock, seizures, and coma with alkalosis during mechanical ventilation. Ann Intern Med 1966; 65:977–983.

209. Bulger RJ, Schrier RW, Arend WP, Swanson AG. Spinal-fluid acidosis and the diagnosis of pulmonary encephalopathy. New Engl J Med 1966; 274:433–7.

210. Tunnidiffe FW, Stebbing GF. The intravenous injection of oxygen gas as a therapeutic measure. Lancet 1916; ii:321–32.

211. Haldane JS. The therapeutic administration of oxygen. Br Med J 1917; 1:181–3.

212. Meakins J. Observations on the gases in human arterial blood in certain pathological pulmonary conditions, and their treatment with oxygen. J Pathol Bacteriol 1921; 24:79–90.

213. Stadie WC. Construction of an oxygen chamber for the treatment of pneumonia. J Exp Med 1922; 35:323–35.

214. Stadie WC. The treatment of anoxemia in pneumonia in an oxygen chamber. J Exp Med 1922; 35:337–60.

215. Barach AL. Methods and results of oxygen treatment in pneumonia. Arch Intern Med 1926; 37:186–211.

216. Binger CAL. Anoxemia in pneumonia and its relief by oxygen inhalation. J Clin Invest 1928–1929; 6:203–19.

217. Boothby WM, Haines SF. Oxygen therapy. JAMA 1928; 90:372–5.

218. Campbell EJM. A method of controlled oxygen administration which reduces the risk of carbon-dioxide retention. Lancet 1960; ii:12–4.

219. Campbell EJM. Respiratory failure 30 years ago. Br Med J 1979; 2:657–8.

220. Campbell EJM. The management of acute respiratory failure in chronic bronchitis and emphysema. Am Rev Respir Dis 1967; 96:626–39.

221. Pontoppidan H, Hedley-White J, Bendixen HH, et al. Ventilation and oxygen requirements during prolonged artificial ventilation in patients with respiratory failure. New Engl J Med 1965; 273:401–9.

222. Fairley HB, Britt BA. The adequacy of the air-mix control in ventilators operated from an oxygen source. Can Med Assoc J 1964; 90:1394–6.

223. Fairley HB, Hunter DD. The performance of respirators used in the treatment of respiratory insufficiency. Can Med Assoc J 1964; 90:1397–1406.

224. Pontoppidan H, Berry PR. Regulation of the inspired oxygen concentration during artificial ventilation. JAMA 1967; 201:89–92.

225. Nash G, Blennerhassett JB, Pontoppidan H. Pulmonary lesions associated with oxygen therapy and artificial ventilation. New Engl J Med 1967; 276:368–73.

226. Frumin MJ, Bergman NA, Holaday DA, et al. Alveolar-arterial O_2 difference during artificial respiration in man. J Appl Physiol 1959; 14:694–700.

227. Jensen NK. Recovery of pulmonary function after crushing injuries of the chest. Dis Chest 1952; 22:319–43.

228. McIntyre RW. Laws AK, Ramachandran PR. Positive expiratory pressure plateau: Improved gas exchange during mechanical ventilation. Can Anaesth Soc J 1969; 16:477–86.

229. Ashbaugh DG, Petty TL, Bigelow DB, Harris TM. Continuous positive-pressure breathing (CPPB) in adult respiratory distress syndrome. J Thorac Cardiovasc Surg 1969; 57:31–41.

230. Gregory GA, Kitterman JA, Phibbs RH, et al. Treatment of the idiopathic respiratory-distress syndrome with continuous positive airway pressure. New Engl J Med 1971; 284:1333–9.

231. Rendell-Baker L. Standards for anesthesia. In: Brown BR, Clakins JM, Saunders RJ, editors. The issues in future anesthesia delivery systems. Philadelphia: FA Davis, 1984: 59–86.

232. Rendell-Baker L. Standards for anesthetic and ventilatory equipment: Problems with anesthetic and respiratory therapy equipment. Int Anesth Clin 1950; 2:171–90.

233. Colice GL. Technical standards for tracheal tubes. Clin Chest Med 1991; 12:433–48.

234. Gracey D, Plummer A. Consensus conference on artificial airways in patients receiving mechanical ventilation. Chest 1989; 96:178–84.

235. Skillman J, Malhotra IV, Pallotta JA, Bushnell LS. Determinants of weaning from controlled ventilation. Surg Forum 1971; 22:198–200.

236. Sahn SA, Lakshminarayan S. Bedside criteria for discontinuation of mechanical ventilation. Chest 1973; 63:1002–5.

237. Yang KL, Tobin MJ. A prospective study of indexes predicting the outcome of trials of weaning from mechanical ventilation. New Engl J Med 1991; 324:1445–50.

238. Downs JB, Block AJ, Vennum KB. Intermittent mandatory ventilation in the treatment of patients with chronic obstructive pulmonary disease. Anesth Analg 1974; 53:437–42.

239. Downs JB, Perkins HM, Modell JH. Intermittent mandatory ventilation. Arch Surg 1974; 109:519–23.

240. Hewlett AM, Platt AS, Terry VG. Mandatory minute volume. Anaesthesia 1977; 32:163–9.

241. Hodgkin JE, Bowser MA, Burton GG. Respirator weaning. Crit Care Med 1974; 2:96–102.

242. Feeley TW, Hedley-White J. Weaning from controlled ventilation and supplemental oxygen. New Engl J Med 1975; 292:903–6.

243. Sahn SA, Lakshminarayan S, Petty TL. Weaning from mechanical ventilation. JAMA 1976; 235:2208–12.

244. Petty TL. IMV vs IMC. Chest 1975; 67:630–1.

245. Tomlinson JR, Miller KS, Lorch DG, et al. A prospective comparison of IMV and T-piece weaning from mechanical ventilation. Chest 1989; 96:348–52.

246. Schachter EN, Tucker D, Beck GJ. Does intermittent mandatory ventilation accelerate weaning? JAMA 1981; 246:1210–4.

PART II
PHYSICAL BASIS OF MECHANICAL VENTILATION

Chapter 2
CLASSIFICATION OF MECHANICAL VENTILATORS

ROBERT L. CHATBURN

CONTROL SCHEME
    Models of Patient-Ventilator Interaction
    Control Variables
    Phase Variables
OUTPUT WAVEFORMS
    Idealized Pressure, Volume, and Flow Waveforms
    Effects of the Patient Circuit
MODES OF VENTILATION
    Breathing Pattern
    Control Type
    Control Strategy
VENTILATOR ALARM SYSTEMS
THE FUTURE
SUMMARY AND CONCLUSION

A good ventilator classification scheme describes how ventilators work in general terms, but with enough detail so that one particular model can be distinguished from others. It facilitates description by focusing on key attributes in a logical and consistent manner. A clear description allows us to quickly assess new facts in relation to our previous knowledge. Learning the operation of a new ventilator or describing it to others then becomes much easier. Understanding how the ventilator operates, we can then anticipate appropriate ventilator management strategies for particular clinical situations. The classification system described in this chapter is based on previously published work.[1-7]

A ventilator is simply a machine, a system of related elements designed to alter, transmit, and direct energy in a predetermined manner to perform useful work. We put energy into the ventilator in the form of electricity (energy = volts × amps × time) or compressed gas (energy = pressure × volume). That energy is transmitted or transformed (by the ventilator's drive mechanism) in a predetermined manner (by the control circuit) to augment or replace the patient's muscles in performing the work of breathing. Therefore, to understand mechanical ventilators in general, we must first understand their basic functions: (1) power input, (2) power transmission or conversion, (3) control scheme, and (4) output. This simple format can be expanded to add as much detail as desired (Table 2-1).

A discussion of input power sources and power conversion/transmission is beyond the scope of this chapter, and these topics have been treated elsewhere.[7,8] I will, however, explore in detail control schemes and ventilator output because these directly affect patient management.

Control Scheme

MODELS OF PATIENT-VENTILATOR INTERACTION

To understand how a machine can be controlled to replace or supplement the natural function of breathing, we need to first understand something about the mechanics of breathing itself. The study of mechanics deals with forces, displacements, and the rate of change of displacement. In physiology, force is measured as pressure (pressure = force/area), displacement as volume (volume = area × displacement), and the relevant rate of change as flow (average flow = Δvolume/Δtime; instantaneous flow ($\dot{V}$) = dv/dt, the derivative of volume with respect to time). Specifically, we are interested in the *pressure* necessary to cause a *flow* of gas to enter the airway and increase the *volume* of the lungs.

The study of respiratory mechanics is essentially the search for simple but useful models of respiratory system mechanical behavior. Figure 2-1 illustrates the process by which the respiratory system is represented first by a graphical model, and then by a mathematical model based on the graphical model. Pressure, volume, and flow are measurable variables in the mathematical model that change with time over the course of one inspiration and expiration. The relation among them is described by the *equation of motion for the respiratory system*.[9] The derivation of this equation stems from a force-balance equation that is an expression of Newton's third law of motion (for every action, there is an equal and opposite reaction):

$$P_{TR} = P_E + P_R \qquad (1)$$

where P_{TR} is the transrespiratory pressure (i.e., pressure at the airway opening minus pressure at the body surface), P_E is the pressure secondary to elastic recoil (elastic load), and P_R is the pressure secondary to flow resistance (resistive load).

Transrespiratory pressure can have two components, one secondary to the ventilator (Pvent) and one secondary to the respiratory muscles (Pmusc). Elastic recoil pressure is the product of elastance (E = Δpressure/Δvolume) and volume. Resistive pressure is the product of resistance (R = Δpressure/Δflow) and flow. Thus Eq. (1) can be expanded to yield the following equation for inspiration:

$$P_{vent} + P_{musc} = EV + R\dot{V} \qquad (2)$$

TABLE 2-1 Outline of Ventilator Classification System

I. Input
  A. Pneumatic
  B. Electric
    1. AC
    2. DC (battery)
II. Power conversion and
  transmission
  A. External compressor
  B. Internal compressor
  C. Output control valves
III. Control scheme
  A. Control circuit
    1. Mechanical
    2. Pneumatic
    3. Fluidic
    4. Electric
    5. Electronic
  B. Control variables
    1. Pressure
    2. Volume
    3. Flow
    4. Time
  C. Phase variables
    1. Trigger
    2. Limit
    3. Cycle
    4. Baseline
  D. Conditional variables
  E. Modes of ventilation
    1. Breathing pattern
    2. Control type
    3. Specific control
      strategy
	IV. Output
	  A. Pressure waveforms
	    1. Rectangular
	    2. Exponential
	    3. Sinusoidal
	    4. Oscillating
	  B. Volume waveforms
	    1. Ascending ramp
	    2. Sinusoidal
	  C. Flow waveforms
	    1. Rectangular
	    2. Ascending ramp
	    3. Descending ramp
	    4. Sinusoidal
	V. Alarms
	  A. Input power alarms
	    1. Loss of electric power
	    2. Loss of pneumatic power
	  B. Control circuit alarms
	    1. General systems failure
	    2. Incompatible ventilator
	      settings
	    3. Warnings (e.g., inverse
	      I:E ratio)
	  C. Output alarms (high/low
	    conditions)
	    1. Pressure
	    2. Volume
	    3. Flow
	    4. Time
	      a. Frequency
	      b. Inspiratory time
	      c. Expiratory time
	    5. Inspired gas
	      a. Temperature
	      b. $F_{I_{O_2}}$

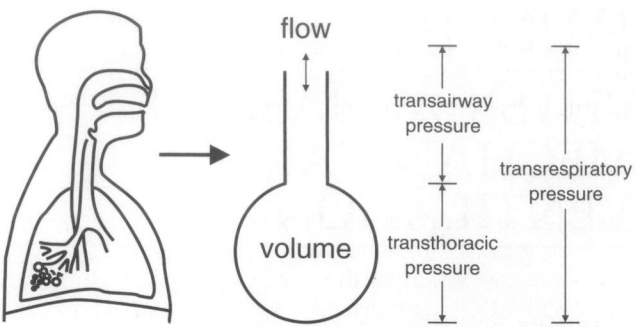

FIGURE 2-1 The respiratory system is often modeled as a single flow resistance (representing the endotracheal tube and the airways) connected to an elastic chamber (representing the lungs and chest wall). Flow through the airways is generated by transairway pressure (pressure at the airway opening minus pressure in the lungs). Expansion of the elastic chamber is generated by transthoracic pressure (pressure in the lungs minus pressure on the body surface). Transrespiratory pressure (pressure at the airway opening minus pressure on the body surface) is the sum of these two pressures and is the total pressure required to generate inspiration. The "airway-pressure" gauge on a positive-pressure ventilator displays transrespiratory pressure.

spontaneous breathing (i.e., vent pressure = 0). Between those two extremes, an infinite number of combinations of muscle pressure (i.e., patient effort) and ventilator pressure are possible under the general heading of "partial ventilator support." The equation of motion also gives the basis for defining an *assisted* breath as one for which ventilator pressure rises above baseline during inspiration or falls below baseline during expiration.

The combined ventilator and muscle pressure causes volume and flow to be delivered to the patient. (Of course, muscle pressure may subtract rather than add to ventilator pressure in the case of patient-ventilator dyssynchrony, in which case both volume and flow delivery are reduced.) Pressure, volume, and flow are functions of time and are called *variables*. They are all measured relative to their values at end expiration. Elastance and resistance are assumed to remain constant and are called *parameters*.

For passive expiration, both ventilator and muscle pressure are absent, so Eq. (2) becomes

$$-R\dot{V} = EV \qquad (3)$$

The negative sign on the left side of the equation indicates flow in the expiratory direction. This equation also shows that passive expiratory flow is generated by the energy stored in the elastic compartment (i.e., lungs and chest wall) during inspiration.

Equation (2) shows that if the patient's respiratory muscles are not functioning, muscle pressure is zero, and the ventilator must generate all the pressure for inspiration. On the other hand, a ventilator is not needed for normal

CONTROL VARIABLES

In the equation of motion, the mathematical form of any of the three variables (i.e., pressure, volume, or flow as functions of time) can be predetermined, making it the independent variable and making the other two the dependent variables. We now have a theoretical basis for classifying ventilators as pressure, volume, or flow controllers. Thus, during pressure-controlled ventilation, pressure is the independent variable and may take the form of, say, a step function (i.e., a rectangular pressure waveform). The shapes of the volume and flow waveforms then will depend on the shape of the pressure waveform as well as the parameters of resistance and compliance. On the other hand, during volume-controlled ventilation, we can specify the shape of the volume waveform making flow- and pressure-dependent variables. The same reasoning applies to a flow controller. Very crude ventilators, such as the early jet ventilators, controlled only the duration of inspiration and expiration, making them what we could call "time controllers."

It follows from the preceding discussion that any conceivable ventilator can control only one variable at a time: pressure, volume, or flow. Therefore, pressure, volume, and flow are referred to in this context as *control variables*. I will discuss later in the section on modes of ventilation exactly how ventilator control systems work. We will see that it is possible for a ventilator to switch quickly from one control variable to another, not only from breath to breath but even during a single inspiration.

PHASE VARIABLES

Because breathing is a periodic event, the ventilator must be able to control a number of variables during the respiratory cycle (i.e., the time from the beginning of one breath to the beginning of the next). Mapelson[10] proposed that this time span be divided into four phases: the change from expiration to inspiration, inspiration, the change from inspiration to expiration, and expiration. This convention is useful for examining how a ventilator starts, sustains, and stops an inspiration and what it does between inspirations. A particular variable is measured and used to start, sustain, and end each phase. In this context, pressure, volume, flow, and time are referred to as *phase variables*.[11] The criteria for determining phase variables are shown in Fig. 2-2.

TRIGGER VARIABLE

All ventilators measure one or more variables associated with the equation of motion (i.e., pressure, volume, flow, or time). Inspiration is started when one of these variables reaches a preset value. Thus the variable of interest is considered an initiating, or *trigger,* variable. Time is a trigger variable when the ventilator starts a breath according to a set frequency independent of the patient's spontaneous efforts. Pressure is the trigger variable when the ventilator senses a drop in baseline pressure caused by the patient's inspiratory effort and begins a breath independent of the set frequency. Flow or volume are the trigger variables when the ventilator senses the patient's inspiratory effort in the form of either flow of volume into the lungs.

Flow triggering has been shown to reduce the work the patient must perform to start inspiration.[12] This is so because work is proportional to the volume the patient inspires times the change in baseline pressure necessary to trigger. Pressure triggering requires some pressure change and hence an irreducible amount of work to trigger. With flow or volume triggering, however, baseline pressure need not change, and theoretically, the patient need do no work on the ventilator to trigger.

The patient effort required to trigger inspiration is determined by the ventilator's *sensitivity* setting. Some ventilators indicate sensitivity qualitatively ("min" or "max"). Alternatively, a ventilator may specify a trigger threshold quantitatively (e.g., 5 cmH$_2$O below baseline). Once the trigger variable signals the start of inspiration, there is always a short delay before flow to the patient starts. This delay is called the *response time* and is secondary to the signal-processing time and the mechanical inertia of the drive mechanisms. It is important for the ventilator to have a short response time to maintain optimal synchrony with patient inspiratory effort.

FIGURE 2-2   Criteria for determining the phase variables during a ventilator-assisted breath.

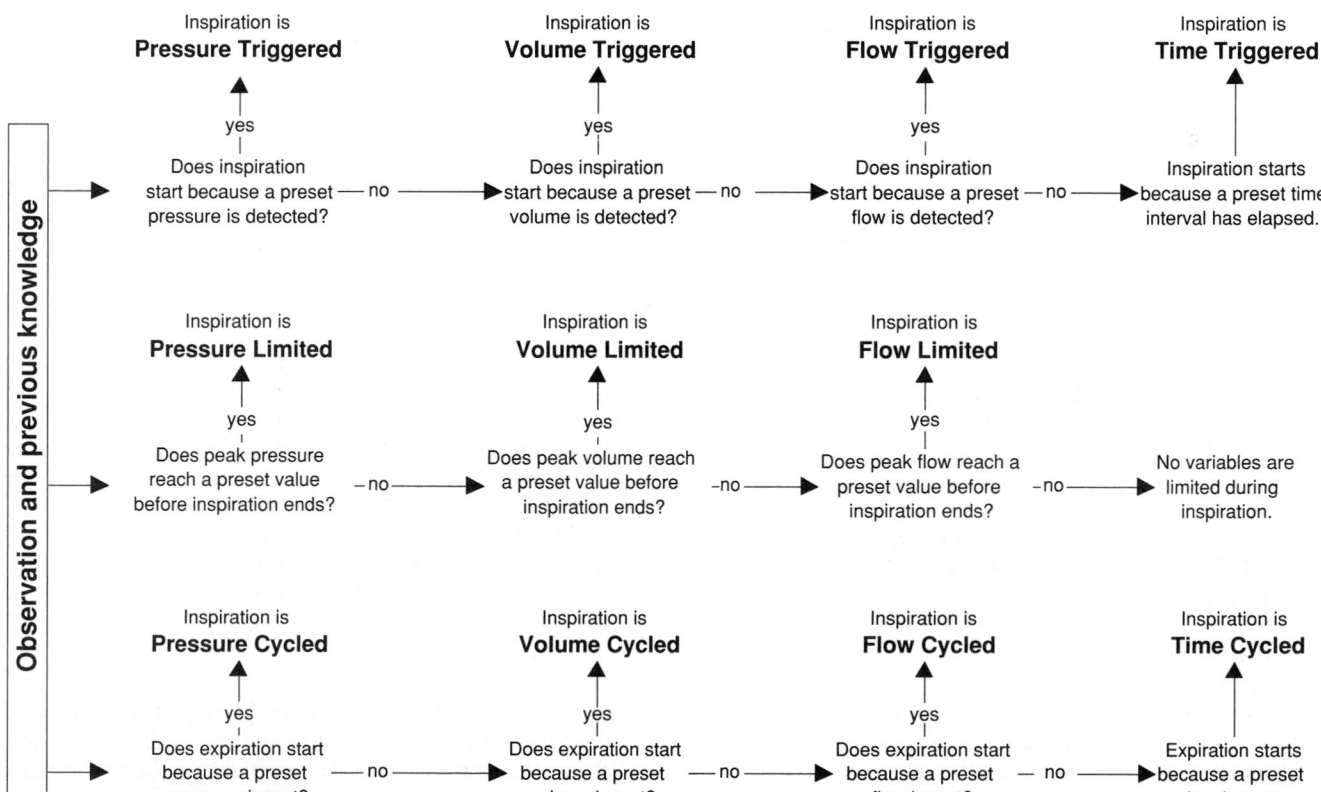

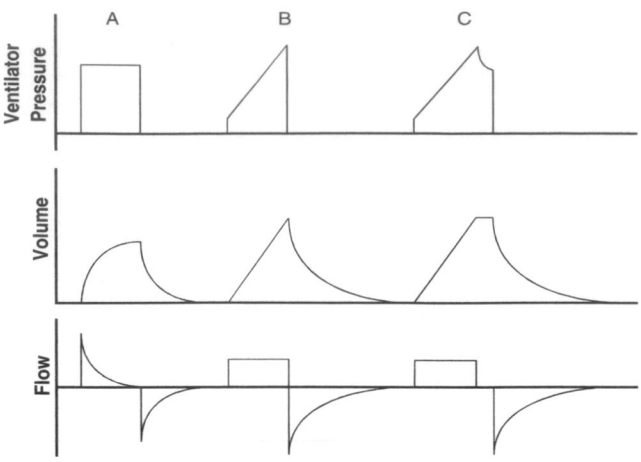

FIGURE 2-3 This figure illustrates the distinction between the terms *limit* and *cycle*. **A.** Inspiration is pressure-limited and time-cycled. **B.** Flow is limited, but volume is not, and inspiration is volume-cycled. **C.** Both volume and flow are limited, and inspiration is time-cycled. (*Reproduced, with permission, from Chatburn Fundamentals of Mechanical Ventilation.*)[6]

LIMIT VARIABLE

Here, *limit* means restricting the magnitude of a variable during inspiration. A *limit variable* is one that can reach and maintain a preset level *before* inspiration ends (i.e., it does not end inspiration). Pressure, flow, or volume can be limit variables and actually all can be active for a single breath (e.g., using the Pmax feature on a Dräger ventilator). Note that time cannot be a limit variable because limiting inspiratory time would cause inspiration to end, violating the preceding definition.

Clinicians often confuse limit variables with cycle variables. To *cycle* means "to end inspiration." A cycle variable always ends inspiration. A limit variable does not terminate inspiration; it only sets an upper bound for pressure, volume, or flow (see Fig. 2-3). The confusion over limit and cycle variables is caused, in part, by the nomenclature used by many ventilator manufacturers. They often use the term *limit* to describe what happens when a pressure or time alarm threshold is met (i.e., inspiration is terminated, and an alarm is activated). To be consistent with accepted nomenclature, it is best to refer to these alarm thresholds as *backup cycling mechanisms* rather than limits.

CYCLE VARIABLE

The inspiratory phase always ends when some variable reaches a preset value. The variable that is measured and used to end inspiration is called the *cycle variable*. The cycle variable can be pressure, volume, flow, or time. Manual cycling is also available on some ventilators.

When a ventilator is set to pressure cycle, it delivers flow until a preset pressure is reached, at which time inspiratory flow stops and expiratory flow begins. The most common application of pressure cycling is for alarm settings.

When a ventilator is set to volume cycle, it delivers flow until a preset volume has passed through the control valve. By definition, as soon as the set volume is met, inspiratory

flow stops and expiratory flow begins. If expiration does not begin immediately after inspiratory flow stops, then an inspiratory hold has been set, and the ventilator is, by definition, time cycled (see Fig. 2-3). Note that the volume that passes through the ventilator's output control valve is never exactly equal to the volume delivered to the patient because of the volume compressed in the patient circuit. Some ventilators use a sensor at the Y-connector (such as the Dräger Evita 4 with the neonatal circuit) for more accurate tidal volume measurement. Others measure volume at some point inside the ventilator, and the operator must know whether the ventilator compensates for compressed gas in its tidal volume readout.

When a ventilator is set to flow cycle, it delivers flow until a preset level is met. Flow then stops, and expiration begins. The most frequent application of flow cycling is in the pressure-support mode. In this mode, the control variable is pressure, and the ventilator provides the flow necessary to meet the inspiratory pressure limit. In doing so, flow starts out at a relatively high value and decays exponentially (assuming that the patient's respiratory muscles are inactive). Once flow has decreased to a relatively low value (such as 25% of peak flow, typically preset by the manufacturer), inspiration is cycled off. Manufactures often set the cycle threshold slightly above zero flow to prevent inspiratory times from getting so long that patient synchrony is degraded. On some ventilators, the flow-cycle threshold may be adjusted by the operator to improve patient synchrony.

Time cycling means that expiratory flow starts because a preset inspiratory time interval has elapsed.

BASELINE VARIABLE

The baseline variable is the parameter controlled during expiration. Although pressure, volume, or flow could serve as the baseline variable, pressure control is the most practical and is implemented by all modern ventilators. Baseline or expiratory pressure is always measured and set relative to atmospheric pressure. Thus, when we want baseline pressure to equal atmospheric pressure, we set it to zero. When we want baseline pressure to exceed atmospheric pressure, we set a positive value, called *positive end-expiratory pressure* (PEEP).

Output Waveforms

Just as the study of cardiology involves the use of electrocardiograms and blood pressure waveforms, the study of mechanical ventilation requires an understanding of output waveforms. The waveforms of interest are, of course, the pressure, volume, and flow waveforms.

IDEALIZED PRESSURE, VOLUME, AND FLOW WAVEFORMS

Output waveforms are conveniently graphed in groups of three. The horizontal axis of all three graphs is the same and has the units of time. The vertical axes are in units of pressure, volume, and flow. For the purpose of identifying

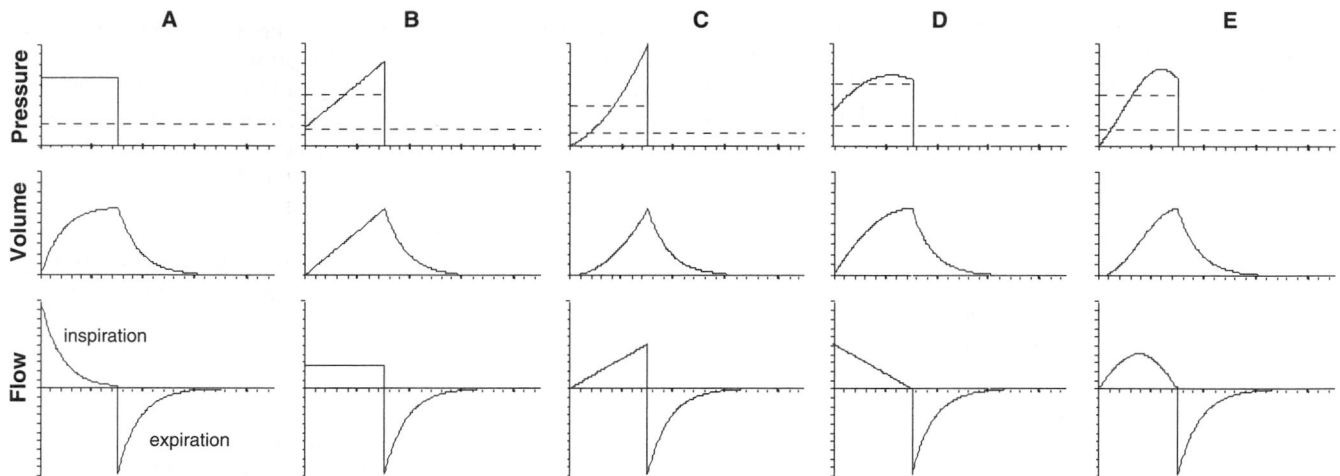

FIGURE 2-4 Idealized ventilator output waveforms. *A*. Pressure-controlled inspiration with a rectangular pressure waveform. Note that this is identical to flow-controlled inspiration with an exponential-decay flow waveform. *B*. Flow-controlled inspiration with a rectangular flow waveform. Note that this is identical to volume-controlled inspiration with an ascending-ramp volume waveform. *C*. Flow-controlled inspiration with an ascending-ramp flow waveform. *D*. Flow-controlled inspiration with a descending-ramp flow waveform. *E*. Flow-controlled inspiration with a sinusoidal flow waveform. The short dashed lines represent mean inspiratory pressure, and the long dashed lines represent mean pressure for the complete respiratory cycle (i.e., mean airway pressure). Note that mean inspiratory pressure is the same as the pressure limit in A. These waveforms were created as follows: (1) defining the control waveform using a mathematical equation (e.g., an ascending-ramp flow waveform is specified as flow = constant × time), (2) specifying the tidal volume for flow- and volume-control waveforms, (3) specifying the resistance and compliance, (4) substituting the preceding information into the equation of motion for the respiratory system, and (5) using a computer to solve the equation for the unknown variables and plotting the results against time. (*Reproduced, with permission, from Chatburn.*)

characteristic waveform shapes, the specific baseline values are irrelevant. What is important is the relative magnitudes of each of the variables and how the value of one affects or is affected by the value of the others.

Typical waveforms available on modern ventilators are illustrated in Fig. 2-4. These waveforms are idealized. That is, they are precisely defined by mathematical equations and are meant to characterize the operation of the ventilator's control system. As such, they do not show the minor deviations, or "noise," often seen in waveforms recorded during actual ventilator use. This noise can be caused by a variety of extraneous factors such as vibration and flow turbulence. Of course, scaling of the horizontal and vertical axes can affect the appearance of actual waveforms considerably. Finally, the waveforms in Fig. 2-4 do not show the effects of the resistance and compliance of the patient circuit.

No ventilator is an ideal pressure, volume, or flow controller, and ventilators are designed to only approximate a particular waveform. Idealized waveforms as shown in Fig. 2-4 are nevertheless helpful because they are used commonly in other fields (e.g., electrical engineering), which makes it possible to use mathematical procedures and terminology that have already been established. For example, a standard mathematical equation is used to describe the most common ventilator waveforms for each control variable. This known equation may be substituted into the equation of motion, which is then solved to get the equations for the other two variables. Once the equations for pressure, volume, and flow are known, they are easily graphed. This is the procedure used to generate the graphs in Fig. 2-4.

EFFECTS OF THE PATIENT CIRCUIT

The pressure, volume, and flow the patient actually receives are never precisely the same as what the clinician sets on the ventilator. Sometimes these differences are caused by instrument inaccuracies or calibration error. More commonly, the patient delivery circuit contributes to discrepancies between the desired and actual patient values. This is so because the patient circuit has its own compliance and resistance. Thus the pressure measured inside a ventilator upstream of the patient always will be higher than the pressure at the airway opening because of patient circuit resistance. In addition, the volume and flow coming out of the ventilator's exhalation manifold will exceed those delivered to the patient because of the compliance of the patient circuit.

Exactly how the mechanical properties of the patient circuit affect ventilator performance depends on whether they are connected in series or in parallel with the patient. It turns out that the resistance of the patient circuit is connected in series while the compliance is modeled as a parallel connection. To understand this, we first make the simplifying assumption that we can examine the patient circuit's resistance separate from its compliance. It is intuitively obvious that the same flow of gas that comes from the ventilator travels through the circuit tubing as through the patient's airway opening. We also can see that the pressure drop across the patient circuit will be different from that across the respiratory system because they have different resistances. By a definition we borrow from electronics, when two circuit components share the same flow but have different pressure drops, they are connected in series. This means that the patient circuit resistance, however small, adds to the total resistive load seen by the ventilator. Thus, in a volume-controlled breath, the peak inspiratory pressure is higher, and in a pressure-controlled breath, the tidal volume and peak flow are lower. In practice, the effect of patient circuit resistance is usually ignored because it is so much lower than the resistance of the respiratory system.

Now consider the patient circuit compliance.[*] As the ventilator delivers the breath to the patient, pressure at the airway opening rises relative to atmospheric pressure, which is the driving force for flow into the lungs. The patient circuit is connected between the ventilator and the airway, so the pressure it experiences across its walls is the same as that experienced by the respiratory system (remember, we are ignoring its resistance now, so we can ignore any pressure drop between the ventilator outlet and the airway opening). The volume change of the patient circuit tubing will be different from that of the respiratory system because the compliance of the circuit is different. Because the patient circuit and the respiratory system fill with different volumes during the same inspiratory time, the flows they experience are different (remember that flow = volume ÷ time). Again borrowing a definition from electronics, if two circuit components share the same pressure drop but different flows, they are connected in parallel. Because they are in parallel, the two compliances are additive, so the total compliance is greater than either component.

Patient circuit compliance sometimes can be greater than respiratory system compliance and thus can have a large effect on ventilation. It must be accounted for either automatically by the ventilator or manually by increasing the tidal volume. For example, when ventilating neonates, patient circuit compliance can be as much as three times that of the respiratory system, even with small-bore tubing and a small-volume humidifier. Thus, when trying to deliver a preset tidal volume during volume-controlled ventilation, as little as 25% of the set volume will be delivered to the patient, with 75% compressed in the patient circuit. The compliance of the patient circuit can be determined by occluding the tubing at the patient Y, delivering a small volume under flow control (using zero PEEP), and noting the resulting pressure. Using a short inspiratory hold will make it easier to read the pressure. Then compliance is calculated as before by dividing the volume by the pressure. Once the patient circuit compliance is known, the set tidal volume can be corrected using the following equation:

$$V_{delivered} = \frac{V_{set}}{1 + (C_{PC}/C_{RS})} \quad (4)$$

where $V_{delivered}$ is the tidal volume delivered to the patient, V_{set} is the tidal volume setting on the ventilator, C_{PC} is the patient circuit compliance, and C_{RS} is the respiratory system compliance. We can get a more intuitive understanding of this equation if we put in some values. Suppose, for example, that we use the perfect patient circuit that has zero

[*] The effective compliance of the patient circuit is a combination of the tubing compliance and the compressibility of the gas inside it.

compliance. Substituting zero for C_{PC}, we get

$$V_{delivered} = \frac{V_{set}}{1 + (C_{PC}/C_{RS})} = \frac{V_{set}}{1 + (0/C_{RS})}$$
$$= \frac{V_{set}}{1 + 0} = \frac{V_{set}}{1} = V_{set} \quad (5)$$

which shows that there is no effect on the delivered tidal volume. Suppose now that C_{PC} is as large as C_{RS} (i.e., $C_{PC} = C_{RS}$). Now we have

$$V_{delivered} = \frac{V_{set}}{1 + (C_{PC}/C_{RS})} = \frac{V_{set}}{1 + 1} = \frac{V_{set}}{2} \quad (6)$$

in which case, half the volume from the ventilator goes to the patient, and the other half is compressed in the patient circuit.

The effect of the patient circuit is more troublesome during volume-controlled modes than during pressure-controlled modes. This is so because during volume control, the ventilator meters out a specific volume of gas, and unless it measures flow at the airway opening, it has no way of knowing how much goes to the patient and how much goes to the patient circuit. In contrast, during pressure-controlled modes, the ventilator simply meters out a set pressure change no matter where the gas goes. Because the respiratory system and the patient circuit compliance are in parallel, they both experience the same driving pressure (peak inspiratory pressure minus end-expiratory pressure), so tidal volume delivery is affected very little. The only effect might be that the patient circuit compliance may tend to increase the pressure rise time, which would tend to decrease peak flow and tidal volume slightly.

Another area where patient circuit compliance causes trouble is in the determination of auto-PEEP. There are several methods for determining auto-PEEP. One method to determine auto-PEEP during mechanical ventilation is to create an expiratory hold manually (i.e., delay the next inspiration) until static conditions prevail throughout the lungs (i.e., no flow anywhere in the lungs). The pressure at this time (total PEEP) minus the applied PEEP is an estimation of global auto-PEEP. Note that auto-PEEP may vary throughout the lungs depending on the distribution of lung disease and may not reflect pressure behind collapsed areas in patients with severe flow limitation. Auto-PEEP ($PEEP_A$) is an index of the gas trapped in the system at end expiration secondary to an insufficient expiratory time:

$$\text{Measured } PEEP_A = \frac{V_{trapped}}{C_{total}} \quad (7)$$

where $PEEP_A$ is auto-PEEP, $V_{trapped}$ is the volume of gas trapped in the patient and the patient circuit at end expiration (above that associated with applied PEEP), and C_{total} is the total compliance of the respiratory system and the patient circuit. The problem is that we want auto-PEEP to reflect the gas trapped in the patient, not in the circuit. If we know the compliances of the patient circuit and the respiratory system, we can correct the measured auto-PEEP as follows:

$$\text{True PEEP}_A = \frac{C_{RS} + C_{PC}}{C_{RS}} \times \text{measured PEEP}_A \qquad (8)$$

where true PEEP_A is the auto-PEEP in the lungs, measured PEEP_A is the auto-PEEP in the lungs and patient circuit, C_{RS} is the respiratory system compliance, and C_{PC} is the patient circuit compliance. If the ventilator displays auto-PEEP on its monitor, check the ventilator's operating's manual to see whether or not the auto-PEEP calculation is corrected for patient circuit compliance. The larger C_{PC} is relative to C_{RS}, the larger will be the error. Again, the error will be most noticeable in pediatric and neonatal patients.

Modes of Ventilation

The objectives of mechanical ventilation are to ensure that the patient receives the minute volume of appropriate gases required to satisfy physiologic needs while not damaging the lungs, impairing circulatory function, or increasing patient discomfort. The manner in which a ventilator achieves these objectives is referred to as a *mode* of ventilation. Specifically, a mode can be identified and/or classified by specifying the

1. Breathing pattern in terms of the primary breath control variable and the breath sequence
2. Control type used to manipulate the primary control variable during inspiration
3. Control strategy, including phase variables and operational logic used to generate the breathing pattern

BREATHING PATTERN

The simplest way to identify a mode is in terms of the inspiratory control variable and the breath sequence. I have already mentioned that pressure, volume, or flow can be controlled during inspiration. When discussing modes rather than specific ventilator design characteristics, it is more convenient simply to refer to inspiration as being pressure-controlled or volume-controlled. We can justify ignoring flow control because when the ventilator controls volume directly (i.e., using a volume-feedback signal), flow is controlled indirectly, and vice versa (i.e., mathematically, volume is the integral of flow, and flow is the derivative of volume).

There are clinical advantages and disadvantages to volume and pressure control. To keep within the scope of this chapter, we can just say that volume control results in a more stable minute ventilation (and hence more stable blood gases) than pressure control if lung mechanics are unstable. On the other hand, pressure control allows better synchronization with the patient because inspiratory flow is not limited to a preset value. While the ventilator must control only one variable at a time during inspiration, it is possible to begin a breath in pressure control and (if certain criteria are met) switch to volume control or vice versa. In addition, it is possible to pressure-control inspiration but to

automatically adjust the pressure limit from breath to breath in an attempt to achieve a preset tidal volume target. To accommodate these situations in which both pressure and volume signals are used to control the size of the breath, we invoke the intuitively satisfying term *dual control*.[2]

The *breath sequence* is the pattern of mandatory or spontaneous breaths that the mode delivers. A *breath* is a positive airway flow (inspiration) relative to baseline, and it is paired with a negative airway flow (expiration), both associated with ventilation of the lungs. This definition excludes flow changes associated with hiccups or cardiogenic oscillations. A *spontaneous breath*, in the context of mechanical ventilation, is a breath for which the patient determines both the timing and the size. That is, the patient both triggers and cycles the breath. On some ventilators, the patient may make a short spontaneous effort during a longer mandatory breath, as in the case of *airway pressure-release ventilation*. It is important to make a distinction between spontaneous breaths and assisted breaths. An *assisted breath* is one for which the ventilator does some work on the patient, as indicated by an increase in airway pressure (i.e., P_{vent}) above baseline during inspiration or below baseline during expiration. For example, in the *pressure-support mode*, each breath is assisted because airway pressures rises to the *pressure-support* setting above PEEP (i.e., $P_{vent} > 0$). Each breath is also spontaneous because the patient both triggers and cycles the breath. The patient may cycle the breath in the *pressure-support* mode by actively exhaling, but even if the patient is passive at end inspiration, his or her resistance and compliance determine the cycle point and thus the size of the breath for a given *pressure-support* setting. In contrast, for a patient on continuous positive airway pressure (CPAP), each breath is spontaneous but unassisted. Breaths are spontaneous because the patient determines the timing and size of the breaths without any interference by the ventilator. Breaths during CPAP are not assisted because airway pressure is controlled by the ventilator to be as constant as possible (i.e., $P_{vent} = 0$). Understanding the difference between assisted and unassisted spontaneous breaths is very important clinically. For example, when making measurements of tidal volume and respiratory rate for calculation of the rapid-shallow breathing index, the breaths must be *spontaneous* and *unassisted*. If they are assisted (e.g., with pressure support), an error of 25–50% may be introduced. A *mandatory breath* is any breath that does not meet the criteria of a spontaneous breath. That is, the machine triggers and/or cycles the breath. It is possible to superimpose a short mandatory breath on top of a longer spontaneous breath, as in the case of high-frequency oscillatory ventilation.

Having defined spontaneous and mandatory breaths, there are three possible breath sequences, designated as follows:

• *Continuous mandatory ventilation (CMV)*. All breaths are mandatory unless the ventilator permits spontaneous breaths during mandatory breaths; spontaneous breaths are not permitted between mandatory breaths. The newer ventilators with the "active" exhalation valves actually will allow a patient to inhale and exhale spontaneously during the mandatory inspiratory time as opposed to older devices that only let a patient inhale. This may be easier to appreciate if you consider an old-fashioned infant ventilator, wherein the mandatory breaths were essentially a transitory high CPAP level, and infants breathed quite freely during both set inspiratory and expiratory times. This is how the "new" *airway pressure-release ventilation* modes work on ventilators such as the Draeger Evita 4.

- *Continuous spontaneous ventilation (CSV).* All breaths are spontaneous.
- *Intermittent mandatory ventilation (IMV).* Spontaneous breaths are permitted between mandatory breaths. When the mandatory breath is triggered by the patient, it is commonly referred to as *synchronized IMV* (SIMV). Because the trigger variable can be specified in the description of phase variables, however, I will use IMV instead of SIMV to designate general breath sequences.

CMV originally meant that every breath was mandatory. The recent development of the "active exhalation valve," however, made it possible for the patient to breathe spontaneously during a mandatory pressure-controlled breath on some ventilators. In fact, it was always possible for the patient to breath spontaneously during pressure-controlled mandatory breaths on infant ventilators. *The key distinction between CMV and IMV is that with CMV, the ventilator attempts to deliver a mandatory breath every time the patient makes an inspiratory effort* (unless a mandatory breath is already in progress). This means that during CMV, if the operator decreases the ventilator rate, the level of ventilator support is unaffected so long as the patient continues making inspiratory efforts. With IMV, the rate setting directly affects the number of mandatory breaths and hence the level of ventilator support. Thus CMV is normally used as a method of full ventilator support, whereas IMV is usually viewed as a method of partial ventilator support.

Given the three ways to control inspiration (i.e., pressure, volume, or dual) and the three breath sequences (i.e., CMV, IMV, or CSV), there are eight possible breathing patterns (Table 2-2).

CONTROL TYPE[13]

OPEN-LOOP CONTROL
The simplest type of control is called *open loop*. Its advantage is low cost. Its weakness is that it is unable to cope with

TABLE 2-2 The Breathing Patterns

Breath-Control Variable	Breath Sequence	Abbreviation
Volume	Continuous mandatory ventilation	VC-CMV
	Intermittent mandatory ventilation	VC-IMV
Pressure	Continuous mandatory ventilation	PC-CMV
	Intermittent mandatory ventilation	PC-IMV
	Continuous spontaneous ventilation	PC-CSV
Dual	Continuous mandatory ventilation	DC-CMV
	Intermittent mandatory ventilation	DC-IMV
	Continuous spontaneous ventilation	DC-CSV

disturbances in the system. Figure 2-5*A* is a diagram of an open-loop system. Shown are three subsystems connected in series: a controller, an effector, and a plant.

The plant is the subsystem being controlled. Its output is the *controlled*, or *output, variable*. The effector is the mechanism that drives the plant to respond in a given way. Its output is the variable that is manipulated to control the behavior of the controlled system. We will refer to it as the *manipulated variable* (we have called it the *control variable* in relation to mechanical ventilators). The effector, typically, is the prime mover or the device that drives or powers the controlled system. In a ventilator, the effector might be a piston pump or an electronic flow-control valve.

The control circuit or controller contains the logic used to interpret or translate the input signal into a signal to which the effector responds. Figure 2-5*B* shows the controller and effector together within the ventilator. One of the few examples of open-loop control of mechanical ventilation is the type of jet ventilator used experimentally in the early 1980s.[14,15] The operator could set a driving pressure, and the controller would turn a valve on and off at a set frequency and inspiration-expiration (I:E) ratio. Gas was metered to the patient, but the actual pressure and volume delivered were dependent on the moment-to-moment changes in the patient's respiratory system impedance.

Thus an open-loop control system cannot correct for disturbances in the conditions affecting the controlled plant. It goes on its merry way oblivious of its surroundings. Disturbances are influences on the system that make the output unpredictable. During mechanical ventilation, the major disturbances are changes in the patient's respiratory drive, respiratory system mechanics, and leaks.

CLOSED-LOOP CONTROL
All modern ventilators use closed-loop control to maintain consistent pressure and flow waveforms in the face of changing environmental conditions. Closed-loop control is accomplished by using the output as a feedback signal that is compared with the operator-set input. The difference between the two is used to drive the system toward the desired output. For example, pressure-controlled modes use airway pressure as the feedback signal to control gas flow from the ventilator. Manufacturers typically do not use flow at the airway opening as a feedback signal because they do not trust the flow sensors available for that purpose. Instead, they would rather measure flow inside the ventilator near the main flow-control valve.

Closed-loop control (also called *feedback control*) uses a sensor to measure the output of the effector. This signal is passed to a comparator (represented by the circles in Fig. 2-6) that essentially applies a simple equation: error = input − output. If the error in the effector output is large enough, an error signal is sent to the controller. The controller then adjusts the effector so that its output is closer to the desired input (i.e., the error is smaller). The advantage of closed-loop control is that the output is adjusted continuously and automatically so that disturbances are not a

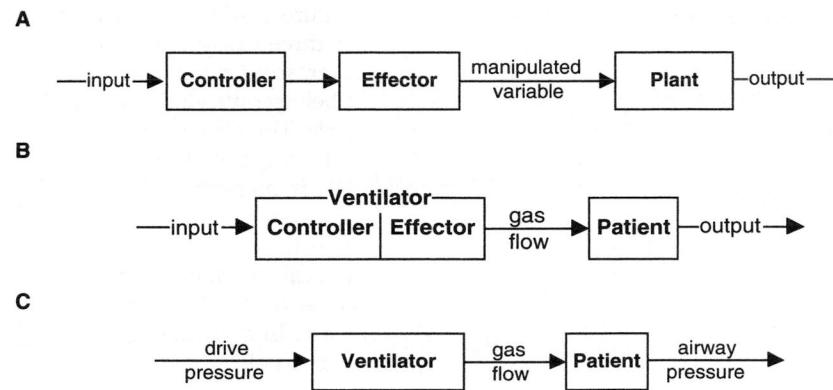

FIGURE 2-5 Schematic diagrams of open-loop control systems: (*A*) basic control circuit; (*B*) open-loop control circuit diagram for a ventilator; (*C*) example of open-loop control of a jet ventilator. (*Reproduced, with permission, from Chatburn: Respir Care 49:507–15, 2004.*)

problem. Of course, the higher complexity of the system makes it more expensive to build and maintain.

Note that a feedback signal may be electrical (e.g., from an electronic pressure transducer) or mechanical (e.g., pressure regulators and CPAP valves). In mechanical devices, a spring provides the input setting, and the position of the diaphragm (a measure of the gas pressure) is the feedback signal. When the force caused by the pressure exceeds the spring load, the diaphragm deflects and vents gas to the atmosphere to relieve the pressure.

THE HIERARCHY OF VENTILATOR CONTROL SYSTEMS

The basic concept of closed-loop control has evolved into at least seven different ventilator control systems (setpoint, auto-setpoint, servo, adaptive, optimal, knowledge-based, and neural-net control). These control types are the foundation that makes possible several dozen apparently different modes of ventilation. Once we understand how these control types work, many of the apparent differences are seen to be similarities. We then avoid a lot of the confusion

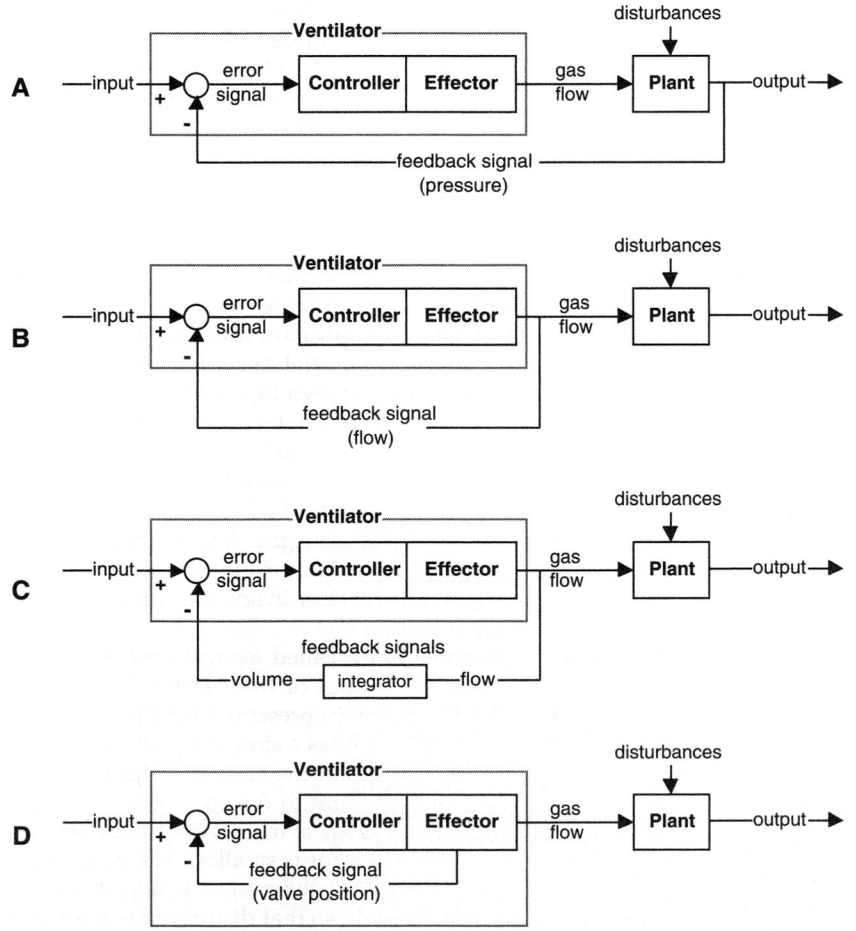

FIGURE 2-6 Schematic diagrams of closed-loop control of mechanical ventilators: (*A*) pressure control; (*B*) flow control; (*C*) the flow signal is integrated to provide a signal for volume control; (*D*) flow/volume control using a calibrated gas-control valve instead of an actual flow sensor. (*Reproduced, with permission, from Chatburn: Respir Care 49:507–15, 2004.*)

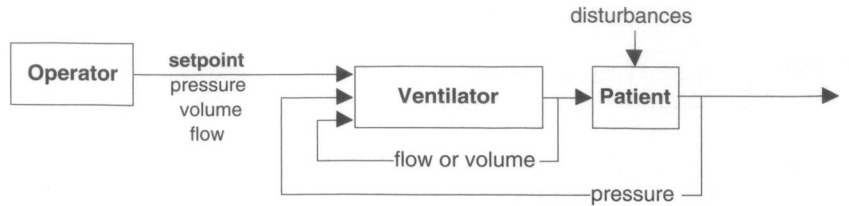

FIGURE 2-7 Setpoint control. (*Reproduced, with permission, from Chatburn: Respir Care 49:507–15, 2004.*)

surrounding ventilator marketing hype and begin to appreciate the true clinical capabilities of different ventilators.

Setpoint Control

All ventilators use at least setpoint control (Fig. 2-7). In setpoint control, the output is constrained to match a constant input (i.e., a set maximum pressure or flow value). This allows the typical ventilator to generate pressure- or flow-controlled inspiration. The operator sets either a fixed pressure or flow limit, and the ventilator then maintains a consistent pressure or flow waveform output. (Recall that the term *limit* means that a control variable reaches a preset maximum value before inspiration ends). This type of control is similar to "cruise control" on an automobile.

Auto-Setpoint Control

Auto-setpoint control is a more advanced version of setpoint control. It gives the ventilator the decision of whether the breath will be pressure- or flow-controlled according to the operator-set priorities. The breath may start out in pressure control and automatically switch to flow, as in the Bird volume-assured pressure-control support (VAPS) mode,[16] or the reverse, as in the Drager P_{max} mode.

Servo Control

While setpoint control attempts to maintain a constant output to match a constant input, servo control is designed to track a moving input, much like power steering on an automobile. Servo control was developed during World War II to aim ship's guns and radar equipment. Servo control makes the proportional-assist mode possible.[17] In this mode, the ventilator's output follows and amplifies the patient's own flow pattern. The ventilator thus can support the abnormal load imposed by disease while the patient's own muscles handle a normal load secondary to natural resistance and compliance of the respiratory system (Fig. 2-8). Recall from Eqs. (1) and (2) that the "load" experienced by the ventilator or the patient has an elastic component (elastance times volume) and a resistive component (resistance times flow).

Adaptive Control

Adaptive control means automatic adjustment of one setpoint to maintain a different operator-selected setpoint (Fig. 2-9). One of the first examples of a mode using adaptive control was *pressure-regulated volume control* on the Siemens Servo ventilator. Adaptive control is an evolutionary step because it gives the ventilator the capability to determine a setpoint level independent of the operator. While setpoint control occurs within breaths, adaptive control introduces another feedback loop that occurs between breaths. The breath-by-breath feedback of exhaled volume, along with calculation of compliance, allows the ventilator to adapt to changes in the patient's lung mechanics (e.g., if compliance decreases, the pressure limit is increased). Despite having various names for the specific modes it allows, adaptive control to date has been implemented as a way for the ventilator to automatically adjust the pressure limit of a breath to meet an operator-set volume target over several breaths. Notice that the operator's influence has subtly moved away, in a sense, from direct control of the breath.

Optimal Control

Optimal control takes adaptive control a step further by allowing the ventilator to determine its own setpoints (Fig. 2-10). Optimal control takes its name from the fact that a mathematical model is used to find the best (e.g., minimum)

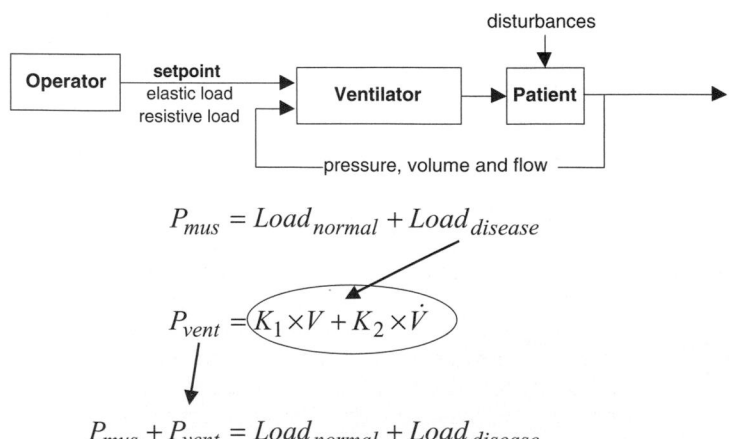

$$P_{mus} = Load_{normal} + Load_{disease}$$

$$P_{vent} = K_1 \times V + K_2 \times \dot{V}$$

$$P_{mus} + P_{vent} = Load_{normal} + Load_{disease}$$

FIGURE 2-8 Servo control is the basis for the proportional-assist mode. In this mode, the operator sets targets for elastic and resistive unloading. The ventilator then delivers airway pressure in proportion to the patient's own inspiratory volume and flow. When the patient's muscles have to contend with an abnormal load secondary to disease, proportional assist allows the operator to set amplification factors (K_1 and K_2) on the feedback volume and flow signals. By amplifying volume and flow, the ventilator generates a pressure that supports the abnormal load, freeing the respiratory muscles to support only the normal load caused by the natural elastance and resistance of the respiratory system. (*Reproduced, with permission, from Chatburn: Respir Care 49:507–15, 2004.*)

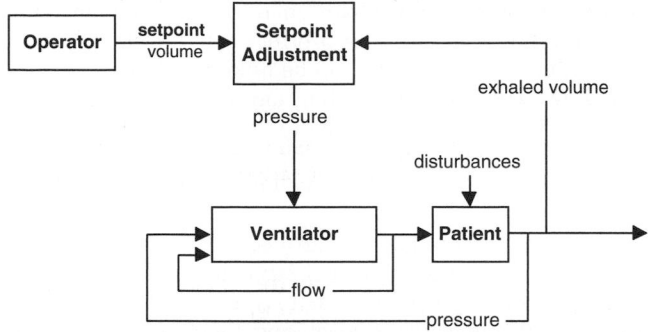

FIGURE 2-9 **Adaptive control. Notice that the operator has stepped back from direct control of the within-breath parameters of pressure and flow. Examples of adaptive control are pressure-regulated volume control (PRVC) on the Siemens ventilator and Autoflow on the Drager Evita 4 ventiltaor.** (*Reproduced, with permission, from Chatburn: Respir Care 49: 507–15, 2004.*)

value of some performance function. For example, once the operator enters the patient's ideal body weight, the ventilator selects the tidal volume and frequency that both meets the patient's minute volume need and minimizes the work of breathing. The Hamilton Galileo is currently the only ventilator with this feature, and it allows the ventilator to make all subsequent adjustments to tidal volume and frequency based on continuous monitoring of exhaled volume and lung mechanics. Again, the operator is moved another step away from direct control of the breath.

An experimental form of optimal control gives the ventilator even more authority.[18] Feedback of the exhaled carbon dioxide signal allows the ventilator to estimate the patient's minute ventilation needs (Fig. 2-11). Now the operator has stepped completely out of the picture. Of course, we are only talking about eliminating the operator in the sense of establishing the level of ventilatory support. Operator input

FIGURE 2-10 **Optimal control. A static mathematical model is used to optimize some performance parameter, such as work of breathing. The only commercially available form of optimal control is the adaptive-support ventilation (ASV) mode on the Hamilton Galileo ventilator.** (*Reproduced, with permission, from Chatburn: Respir Care 49: 507–15, 2004.*)

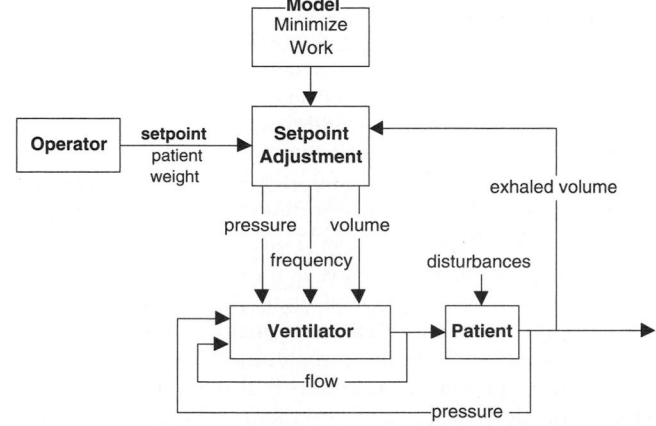

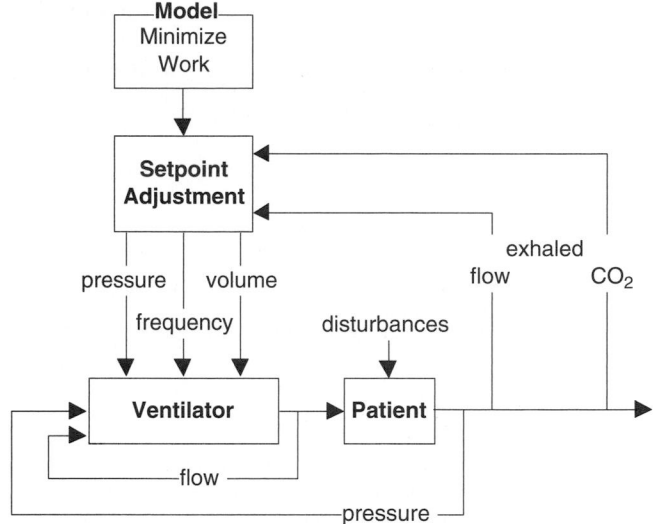

FIGURE 2-11 **An experimental form of optimal control allows the ventilator to estimate the patient's minute ventilation needs by feedback of the exhaled carbon dioxide signal. This eliminates the need for the operator to set any of the major breath parameters. Setpoints, however, for FI_{O_2} and PEEP are still required.** (*Reproduced, with permission, from Chatburn: Respir Care 49:507–15, 2004.*)

is still required for all the other parameters, such a PEEP, fractional inspired oxygen concentration (FI_{O_2}), and alarm settings.

Knowledge-Based Control

Knowledge-based control is yet a further evolutionary step because it gives the ventilator more knowledge than what may be contained in a simple, static, mathematical model. In fact, knowledge-based control attempts to capture the experience of any number of human experts and thus expand the scope of control to potentially all parameters of the ventilator mode. An experimental application of this type of control has been described for automatic adjustment of pressure support.[19] An even more sophisticated approach coupled a knowledge base with fuzzy logic (Fig. 2-12).[20] In this case, the ventilator used both instantaneous measurements of physiologic values, such as respiratory rate and oxygen saturation, and their rates of change. Fuzzy logic[21] was used as a way to integrate the measurements with predefined ranges of values representing the patient status. Once the patient's status was determined, appropriate expert rules were selected from a lookup table and used to adjust the ventilator. While this was a limited application, it proved the concept.

The most convincing proof of the concept was presented by East et al.[22] They used a rule-based expert system for ventilator management in a large, multicenter, prospective, randomized trial. While survival and length of stay were not different between human and computer management, computer control resulted in a significant reduction in multiorgan dysfunction and a lower incidence and severity of lung overdistension injury. The most important finding, however, was that *expert knowledge can be encoded and shared*

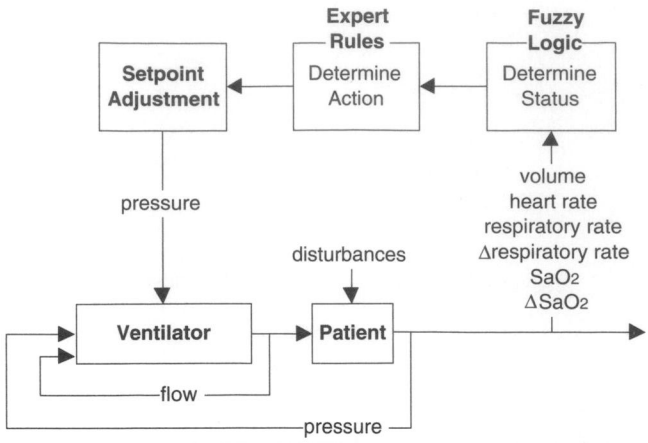

FIGURE 2-12 A knowledge-based control system for automatically adjusting pressure support levels. (*Reproduced, with permission, from Chatburn: Respir Care 49:507–15, 2004.*)

successfully with institutions that had no input into the model. Note that the expert system did not control the ventilator directly but rather made suggestions for the human operator. In theory, of course, the operator could be eliminated.

Artificial Neural-Net Control

The ultimate in ventilator control to date is the artificial neural network (Fig. 2-13).[23] Again, this experimental system did not control the ventilator directly but acted as a decision-support system. What is most interesting is that *the neural network was capable of learning,* which offers significant advantages over static mathematical models and even expert rule-based systems.

Neural nets are essentially data-modeling tools used to capture and represent complex input-output relationships. A neural net learns by experience the same way a human brain does, by storing knowledge in the strengths of internode connections. As data-modeling tools, they have been used in many business and medical applications for both diagnosis and forecasting.[24] A neural network, like an animal brain, is made up of individual neurons. Signals (action potentials) appear at the unit's inputs (synapses). The effect of each signal may be approximated by multiplying the signal by some number or weight to indicate the strength of the signal. The weighted signals then are summed to

produce an overall unit activation. If this activation exceeds a certain threshold, the unit produces an output response. Large numbers of neurons can be linked together in layers (Fig. 2-14). The nodes in the diagram represent the summation and transfer processes. Note that each node contains information from all neurons. As the network learns, the weights change, and thus the values at the nodes change, affecting the final output.

In summary, ventilator control schemes display a definite hierarchy of evolutionary complexity. At the most basic level, control is focused on what happens within a breath. We can call this *tactical control,* and there is a very direct need for operator input of static setpoints. The next level up is what we can call *strategic control.* Here, setpoints are dynamic in that they may be adjusted automatically over time by the ventilator according to some model of desired performance. The operator is somewhat removed in that inputs are entered at the level of the model and take effect over several breaths instead of at the level of individual breath control. Finally, the highest level so far is what might be considered *intelligent control.* Here, the operator can be eliminated altogether. Not only dynamic setpoints but also dynamic models of desired performance are permitted. There is the possibility of the system learning from experience so that the control actually spans between patients instead of just between breaths (Fig. 2-15).

CONTROL STRATEGY

Finally, we can fully characterize a mode by adding the specific strategy it employs. This begins with the naming of the phase variables, followed by detailing the operational logic and, if necessary, giving the parameter values used in the conditional statements. *The specification of the breathing pattern that the mode can produce, the type of control, and the specific strategy it uses, for both mandatory and spontaneous breaths, comprise a complete classification for any mode of ventilation* (Fig. 2-16). This system helps us to distinguish modes that appear similar (i.e., look the same on graphics monitors) and suggests what the operator must do to set the controls. For example, pressure support (any ventilator) is PC-CSV, for which the operator sets the sensitivity and pressure limit. In contrast, volume assist (Siemens 300) is DC-CSV and looks similar to pressure support on the graphics monitor, but the operator must set a tidal volume in addition to sensitivity and pressure limit.

Ventilator Alarm Systems

As with other components of ventilation systems, ventilator alarms have increased in number and complexity. Fortunately, the classification system I have been describing can be expanded to include alarms as well (see Table 2-1).

MacIntyre[25] has suggested that alarms also be categorized by the events that they are designed to detect. Level 1 events include life-threatening situations, such as loss of input power or ventilator malfunction (e.g., excessive or no flow of gas to the patient). The alarms in this

FIGURE 2-13 Artificial neural network control. (*Reproduced, with permission, from Chatburn: Respir Care 49:507–15, 2004.*)

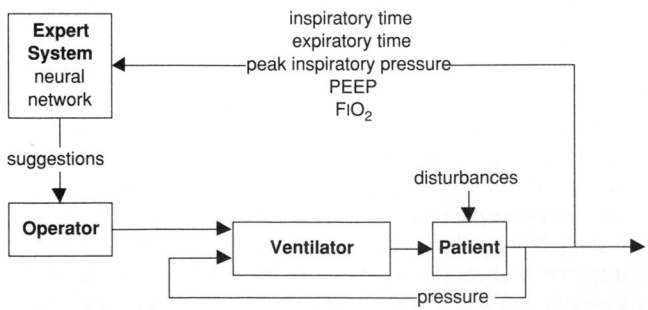

Single Neuron

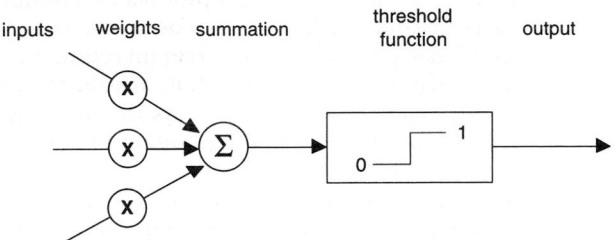

Neural Network

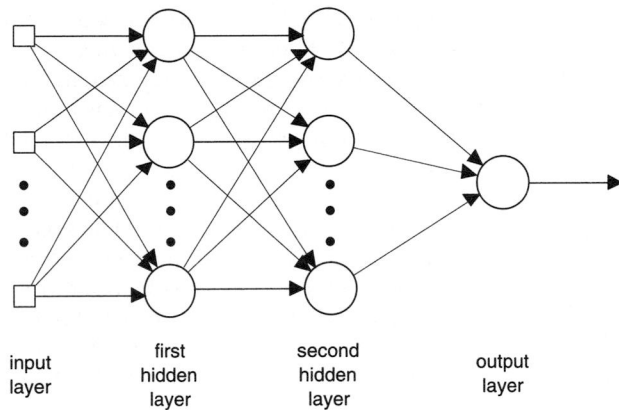

FIGURE 2-14 Neural network structure. A single neuron accepts inputs of any value and weights them to indicate the strength of the synapse. The weighted signals are summed to produce an overall unit activation. If this activation exceeds a certain threshold, the unit produces an output response. A network is made up of layers of individual neurons. (*Reproduced, with permission, from Chatburn: Respir Care 49:507–15, 2004.*)

category should be mandatory (i.e., not subject to operator choice), redundant (i.e., multiple sensors and circuits), and noncanceling (i.e., alarm continues to be activated, even if the event is corrected, and must be reset manually). Level 2 events can lead to life-threatening situations if not corrected in a timely fashion. These events include such things as blender failure, high or low airway pressure, autotriggering, and partial patient circuit occlusion. They also may include suspicious ventilator settings such as an I:E ratio greater than 1:1. Alarms for level 2 events may not be redundant and may be self-canceling (i.e., alarm inactivated if event ceases to occur). Level 3

Tactical Control (within breaths)
Static set points
- set point
- auto set point
- servo

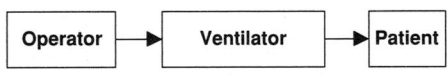

FIGURE 2-15 Summary of control-system hierarchy. (*Reproduced, with permission, from Chatburn: Respir Care 49:507–15, 2004.*)

Strategic Control (between breaths)
Dynamic set points
Static models
- adaptive
- optimal

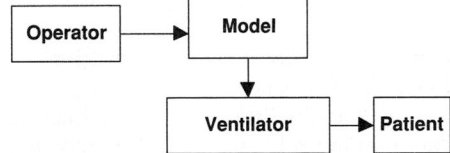

Intelligent Control (between patients)
Dynamic set points
Dynamic models
Ability to learn from experience
- knowledge based
- artificial neural networks

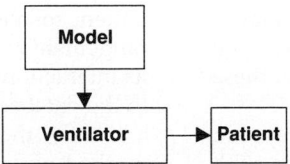

Ventilator Name: Bear 1000
Manufacturer's Mode Name: SIMV/CPAP (PSV)
Breathing Pattern: VC-IMV
Control Type: Setpoint
Control Strategy:

Phase Variables for Mandatory Breaths

Trigger: Pressure (sensitivity adjustable from 0.2 to 5.0 cm H₂O)
time (rate adjustable from 0 to 120 cycles/minute)
Limit: Flow (10 to 150 liters/minute)
volume (whenever the inspiratory pause time is set >0)
Cycle: Volume (tidal volume adjustable from 100 to 2,000 mL)
time (whenever the inspiratory pause time is set >0)
pressure (when inspiratory pressure violates alarm setting)
Baseline: PEEP/CPAP level adjustable from 0 to 50 cm H₂O

Phase Variables for Spontaneous Breaths

Trigger: Pressure (sensitivity adjustable from 0.2 to 5.0 cm H₂O)
Limit: Pressure (0 to 65 cm H₂O above baseline)
Cycle: Flow (when inspiratory flow decays to 30% of peak flow);
time (when inspiration exceeds preset threshold)
Baseline: PEEP/CPAP level adjustable from 0 to 50 cm H₂O

Operational Logic

If the patient triggers a breath after the start of a ventilatory period (the time equal to the reciprocal of the set ventilatory rate) then a mandatory breath is delivered. If subsequent breathing efforts are detected during the same period, then spontaneous breaths are delivered. If a breathing effort is not detected during a given ventilatory period, then a mandatory breath is time triggered at the beginning of the next period and time triggered mandatory breaths will continue at the set rate until a breathing effort is detected and the sequence repeats.

FIGURE 2-16 An example of how a ventilator mode can be completely specified. SIMV, synchronized intermittent mandatory ventilation; VC-IMV, volume-controlled intermittent mandatory ventilation; CPAP, continuous positive airway pressure; PEEP, positive end-expiratory pressure. (*Reproduced, with permission, from Chatburn et al: Respir Care 46:604–21, 2001.*)

events are those that affect the patient-ventilator interface and may influence the level of support provided. Examples of such events are changes in patient compliance and resistance, changes in patient respiratory drive, and auto-PEEP. Alarm function at this level is similar to that of level 2 alarms. Level 4 events reflect the patient condition alone rather than ventilator function. As such, these events usually are detected by stand-alone monitors, such as oximeters, cardiac monitors, and blood gas analyzers. Some ventilators, however, are able to incorporate the readings of a capnograph in their displays and alarm systems.

The Future

There are three directions to go to improve ventilators in the future. First, just like computer games, ventilators need to improve the operator interface constantly. Yet very little, if any, research has been done to call attention to problems with current displays. We have come a long way from using a crank to adjust the stroke of a ventilator's piston to set tidal volume. The operator interface must provide for three basic functions: to allow input of control and alarm parameters, to monitor the ventilator's status, and to monitor the ventilator-patient interaction status. We have a long way to go before the user interface provides an ideal experience with these functions.

Second, the weak link in the patient-ventilator system is the patient circuit. We buy a $30,000 ventilator with state-of-the-art computer control, and then we connect it to the patient with a $1.98 piece of plastic tubing that is subject to filling with condensate from a heated humidifier whose design has not changed appreciably in 20 years. The resistance and compliance of the delivery circuit make flow control and volume delivery more difficult (as discussed earlier). It's like buying a Ferrari and putting wooden wheels on it. In the future, water vapor should be treated like any other gas constituent (e.g., air, oxygen, or nitric oxide) and metered from within the ventilator. The inspiratory part of the patient circuit should be a sterile, insulated, permanent part of the ventilator right up to the patient connection, which can be a disposable tip for cleaning purposes. The gas should be delivered under high pressure as a jet to provide not only conventional pressure, volume, and flow waveforms but also high-frequency ventilation. The jet also can be used to provide a counterflow PEEP effect, eliminating any need for an exhalation-valve system. The disposable tip could be designed to house disposable sensors and would be the only part of the circuit to be exposed to the patient's exhaled gas. If ventilator manufacturers saw themselves as providers of the entire system, instead of letting thirdparties deal in plastic connecting tubing, then I think we would see a huge evolutionary step in ventilator performance, better patient outcomes, and potential savings in labor costs for providers.

Third, the most exciting area for development probably will be in the intelligence built into ventilator control circuits of the future. The real challenge in closed-loop control of ventilation is defining, measuring, and interpreting the appropriate feedback signals. If we stop to consider all the variables a human operator assesses, the problem looks insurmountable. Not only does a human consider a wide range of individual physiologic variables, but there are the more abstract evaluations of such things as metabolic, cardiovascular, and psychological states. Add to this the various environmental factors that may affect operator judgment, and we get a truly complex control problem (Fig. 2-17).

I would like to speculate now about a response to this challenge. The ideal control strategy would have to start out with basic tactical control of the individual breath. Next, we add longer-term strategic control that adapts to changing load characteristics. Mathematical models could provide the basic parameters of the mode, whereas expert rules would place limits to ensure lung protection.

Next, we sample various physiologic parameters and use fuzzy logic to establish the patient's immediate condition. This information is passed on to a neural network, which would then select the best response to the patient's condition.

The neural network ideally would have access to a huge database comprised of both human expert rules and actual patient responses to various ventilator strategies. This arrangement would allow the ventilator not only to learn from its interaction with the current patient but also to contribute to the database.

Finally, the database and this ventilator could be networked with other intelligent ventilators to multiply the

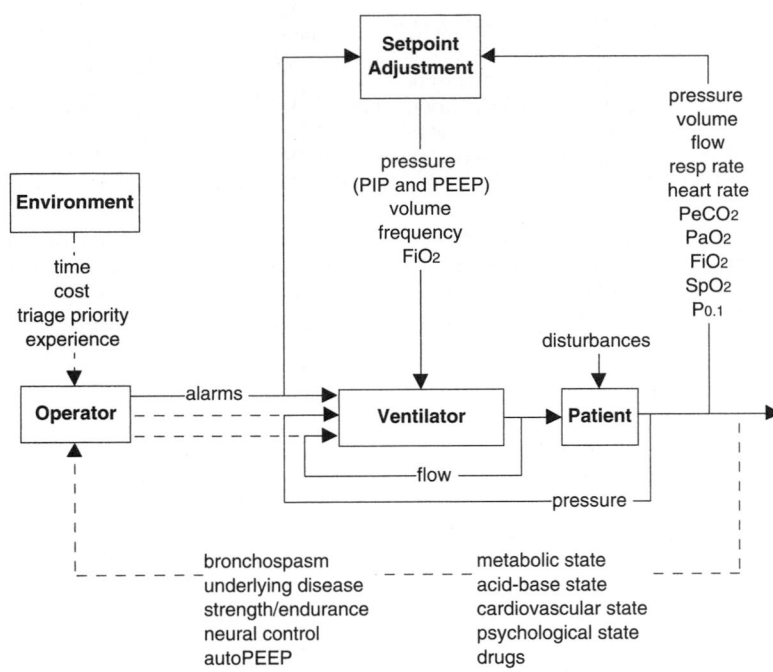

FIGURE 2-17 The challenge of total computer control of mechanical ventilation. Solid arrows depict signals that have been used at least experimentally. Dotted arrows represent potential feedback signals. (*Reproduced, with permission, from Chatburn: Respir Care* 49:507–15, 2004.)

learning capacity exponentially (Fig. 2-18). Whatever the future brings, it seems clear that ventilators will have more intelligence built in to increase patient safety and decrease the time required to provide care.

Summary and Conclusion

Mechanical ventilators have become so complex that a system of classification is necessary to communicate intelligently about them. The theoretical basis for this classification system is a mathematical model of patient-ventilator interaction known as the *equation of motion for the respiratory*

system. From this model we deduce that as far as an individual inspiration is concerned, any conceivable ventilator can be classified as either a pressure, volume, or flow controller (and in rare cases, simply an inspiratory-expiratory time controller). An individual breath is shaped by the phase variables that determine how the breath is triggered (started), limited (sustained), and cycled (stopped). Idealized pressure, volume, and flow waveforms of individual breaths can be identified and named according to conventions in electrical engineering. Individual breaths can be classified as being either mandatory or spontaneous, the definitions of which are very specific and form the basis for characterizing modes.

FIGURE 2-18 A potential approach to the challenge of fully automated control of mechanical ventilation. (*Reproduced, with permission, from Chatburn: Respir Care* 49:507–15, 2004.)

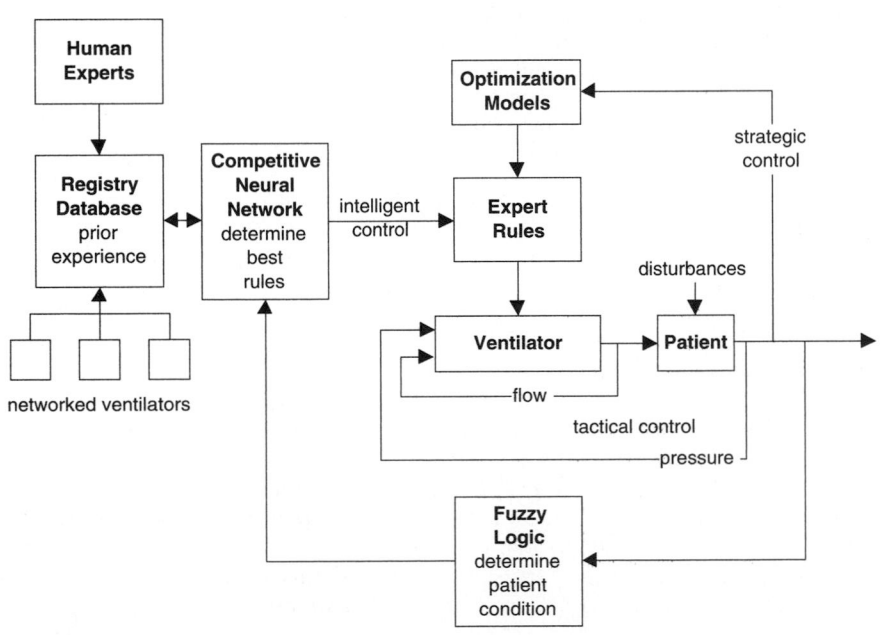

A *mode* of ventilation can be characterized simply as a particular pattern of mandatory and spontaneous breaths that are either volume-controlled, pressure-controlled, or have elements of both (dual-controlled). More detail (enough to distinguish any mode) can be added by describing the control scheme, the phase variables, and the operational logic used in the control circuit.

The trend in ventilator control schemes has been from basic tactical control (within-breath control requiring operator input of static setpoints), to more advanced strategic control (between-breath control of setpoints that are adjusted automatically by the ventilator with minimal operator input), to the highest level of intelligent control (in which the operator theoretically may be eliminated altogether in favor of artificial intelligence systems capable of learning).

References

1. Chatburn RL. A new system for understanding mechanical ventilators. Respir Care 1991; 36:1123–55.
2. Chatburn RL. Classification of mechanical ventilators. Respir Care 1992; 37:1009–25.
3. Chatburn RL, Volsko TA. Mechanical ventilators. In: Wilkins RL, Stoller JK, Scanlan CL, editors. Egan's fundamentals of respiratory care. 8th ed. St. Louis: Mosby, 2003: 929–62.
4. Chatburn RL. Mechanical ventilators: Classification and principles of operation. In: Hess DR, MacIntyre NR, Mishoe SC, et al, editors Respiratory care: Principles and practice. Philadelphia: Saunders, 2002: 757–809.
5. Chatburn RL, Primiano FP Jr. A new system for understanding modes of mechanical ventilation. Respir Care 2001; 46:604–21.
6. Chatburn RL. Fundamentals of mechanical ventilation. Cleveland Heights, OH: Mandu Press, 2003.
7. Branson RD, Hess DR, Chatburn RL. Respiratory care equipment. 2nd ed. Philadelphia: Lippincott Williams & Wilkins, 1999.
8. Cairo JM, Pilbeam SP. Mosby's respiratory care equipment. 7th ed. St. Louis: Mosby; 2004.
9. Rodarte JR, Rehder K. Dynamics of respiration. In: Macklem PT, Mead J, editors. Handbook of physiology. Section 3: The respiratory system. Volume. III: Mechanics of breathing. Part 1. Bethesda, MD: American Physiological Society, 1986.
10. Mushin WW, Rendell-Baker L, Thompson PW, Mapelson WW. Automatic ventilation of the lungs. 3rd ed. Oxford, England: Blackwell Scientific, 1980: 62–131.
11. Desautels DA. Ventilator performance. In: Kirby RR, Smith RA, Desautels DA, editors. Mechanical ventilation. New York: Churchill Livingstone, 1985: 120.
12. Sassoon CSH, Girion AE, Ely EA, Light RW. Inspiratory work of breathing on flow-by and demand flow continuous positive airway pressure. Crit Care Med 1989; 17:1108–14.
13. Chatburn RL. Computer control of mechanical ventilation. Respir Care 2004; 49:507–15.
14. Carlo WA, Chatburn RL, Martin RJ, Lough MD, et al. Decrease in airway pressure during high-frequency jet ventilation in infants with respiratory distress syndrome. J Pediatr 1984; 104:101–7.
15. Branson RD, Hurst JM, DeHaven CB. Use of high frequency jet ventilation during mechanical hyperventilation for control of elevated intracranial pressure: A case report. Respir Care 1984; 29:1121–4.
16. Amato MB, Barbas CS, Bonassa J, Saldiva PH, et al. Volume-assured pressure support ventilation (VAPS): A new approach for reducing muscle workload during acute respiratory failure. Chest 1992; 102:1225–34.
17. Younes M. Proportional assist ventilation, a new approach to ventilator support: I. Theory. Am Rev Respir Dis 1992; 145: 114–20.
18. Laubscher TP, Frutiger A, Fanconi S, Brunner JX. The automatic selection of ventilation parameters during the initial phase of mechanical ventilation. Intensive Care Med 1996; 22: 199–207.
19. Dojat M, Harf A, Touchard D, et al. Clinical evaluation of a computer-controlled pressure support mode. Am J Respir Crit Care Med 2000; 161:1161–6.
20. Nemoto T, Hatzakis G, Thorpe CW, et al. Automatic control of pressure support ventilation using fuzzy logic. Am J Respir Crit Care Med 1999; 160:550–6.
21. Bates JHT, Hatzakis GE, Olivenstein R. Fuzzy logic and mechanical ventilation. In: Iotti GA, ed. Respiratory Care Clinics of North America 2001; 7(3):363–377.
22. East TD, Heermann LK, Bradshaw RL, et al. Efficacy of computerized decision support for mechanical ventilation: Results of a prospective multicenter randomized trial. Proc AMIA Symp 1999; 251–255.
23. Snowden S, Brownlee KG, Smye SW, Dear PR. An advisory system for artificial ventilation of the newborn utilizing a neural network. Med Inform (Lond) 1993; 18:367–76.
24. Gottschalk A, Hyzer MC, Greet RT. A comparison of human and machine-based predictions of successful weaning from mechanical ventilation. Med Decis Making 2000; 20:243–4.
25. MacIntyre NR. Ventilator monitors, displays, and alarms. In: MacIntyre NR, Branson RD, editors. Mechanical ventilation. Philadelphia: Saunders, 2001: 131–44.

Chapter 3

BASIC PRINCIPLES OF VENTILATOR MACHINERY

ROBERT M. KACMAREK
DANIEL CHIPMAN

The newest generation of mechanical ventilators has obtained a level of sophistication unparalleled in previous generations (Fig. 3-1). Most of these units incorporate multiple microprocessors to control the flow of gas precisely, to allow for the provision of ventilator support by multiple modes, and to allow for the monitoring and alarming of virtually every aspect of the ventilator and patient-ventilator interface. The rationale for the development of these highly sophisticated units was to provide a safer, more flexible machine that would ensure a less stressful patient-ventilator interface, as well as a ventilator capable of meeting the needs of an increasingly varied group of critically ill patients. In addition, because of the microprocessor design, these ventilators can be upgraded and updated easily with new modes or monitoring systems without the need to purchase new hardware.

The primary purpose of this chapter is not to compare and contrast individual mechanical ventilator brands (Fig. 3-2) but to provide a detailed discussion of the individual components and operational algorithms of the newest generation of mechanical ventilators (Fig. 3-3). We will begin with the user interface and then proceed with tracing gas flow from its entrance into the ventilator to its exit via the exhalation valve, as well as the various approaches used to monitor and alarm patient-ventilator functions, along with the modes used to provide ventilator support. This chapter provides a detailed description of the technical complexities of gas delivery during ventilator support.

The User Interface

The user interface is the interaction between clinician and ventilator. In first-generation ventilators, this consisted of electrical switches and mechanical adjustments

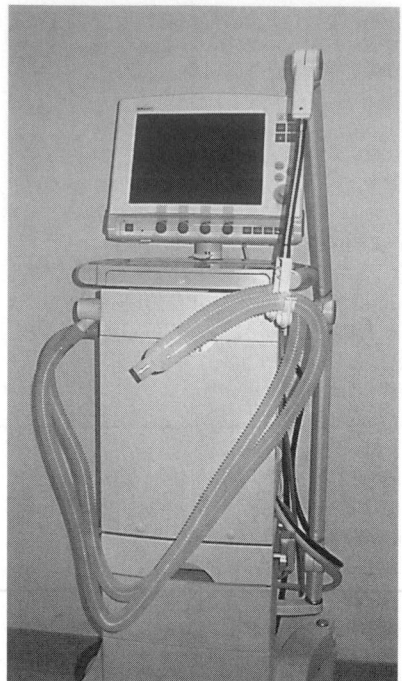

FIGURE 3-1 Maquet Servo I ventilator.

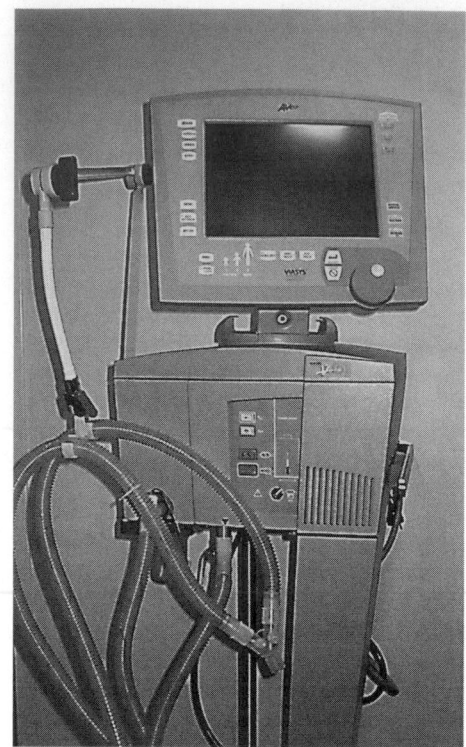

FIGURE 3-3 Viaysis Avea ventilator.

(e.g., Emerson). As the control of ventilators became more electronic and less mechanical, the user interface evolved into an array of rotary knobs that adjusted gas delivery and associated alarms. With the current generation of microprocessor-controlled ventilators, the user inter-

FIGURE 3-2 Puritan-Bennett 840 ventilator.

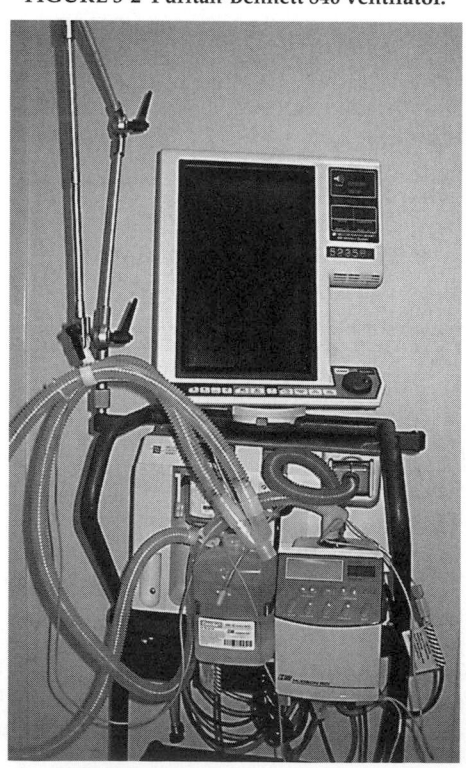

face is commonly a touch pad and/or rotary encoder. Most ventilators incorporate a layering of Windows-type screens displaying the variables that can be adjusted or monitored. Some incorporate touch-screen control of the various parameters. All, however, incorporate a two-step process of changing a particular setting: first selecting the setting and then accepting it with an encorder. The user interface not only allows the clinician to control ventilator settings but also displays information related to ventilator function and patient status. All the current generation of intensive-care unit (ICU) ventilators also have the capability of displaying waveforms of pressure, flow, and volume, as well as pressure-volume and flow-volume loops. Ideally, the user interface should be simple to use, logical in format, and difficult to adjust accidentally.

Unfortunately, there is no consistency among manufacturers in terms of the names and functions of ventilator controls. This is particularly true regarding modes of ventilation and has led to confusion and potentially dangerous situations, especially in hospitals where several ventilator brands are used. Especially confusing are single controls on a ventilator that have multiple functions that depend on the settings of other controls on the ventilator. Most of the newest generation of ventilators have eliminated this problem, although some of the older units still in use do have these multiple variable controls. Because of the multiple interactions that can occur between ventilator settings, adjustments of mechanical ventilators should be restricted to persons with specialized expertise in the technical aspects of mechanical ventilation.

Pneumatic Systems

The primary system that defines the operational capabilities of every ventilator is the pneumatic system, which consists of the mechanical components that physically control gas delivery. All pneumatic systems begin with a gas source, have a means of blending gas to establish specific oxygen concentrations, and include a precision flow-control mechanism capable of regulating and manipulating delivered flow and volume (Fig. 3-4).

GAS SOURCE

A pressurized gas source is needed to power the pneumatics of all ventilator gas-delivery systems. In critical-care applications, this consists of air and oxygen delivered at 50 lb/in² from a bulk-gas-delivery system. Alternatively, the ventilator can be powered by an internal compressor system, with oxygen added to provide the desired oxygen concentration. In some ventilators, air and oxygen are needed only for gas delivery to the patient. In other ventilators, gas is also consumed to power the control functions of the ventilator. This occurs most commonly in ventilators that are driven pneumatically (i.e., require no electricity), such as portable transport ventilators. In these ventilators, the gas flow required and consumed by the unit is greater than the minute ventilation of the patient. Knowledge of this volume is critical

FIGURE 3-4 Primary pneumatic system for the Puritan-Bennett 840 ventilator. Compressed gases enter at the far left of the "inspiratory module"(*center*) **below PS1 and PS2. The lower part of the figure depicts the function of the optional air compressor unit. The top of the figure indicates the expiratory module. (***Used, with permission, from Puritan Bennett 840 Ventilator System Operators Guide 4-075609-00 Rev C (01/99), p. C1.***)**

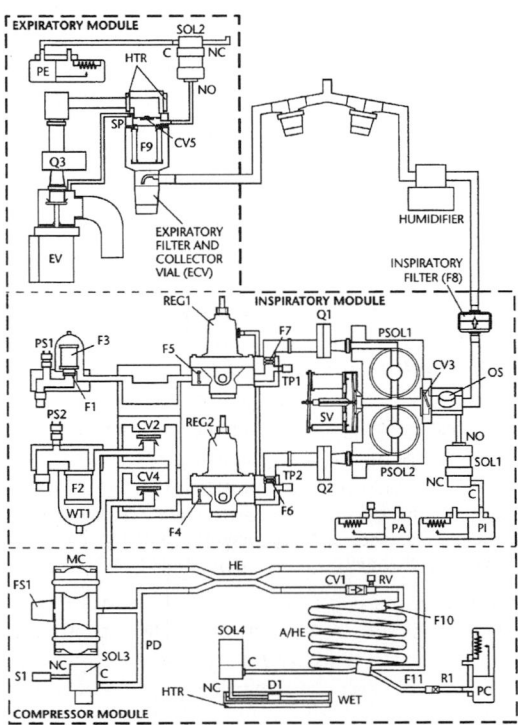

when patients are being transported and pressurized gas is being provided by cylinders.

PRESSURE REDUCTION

Although gases typically enter the ventilator at 50 lb/in², the working pressure usually is reduced immediately to 20 lb/in² or less. Ideally, the working pressure should be as low as possible for safety purposes and to lessen wear on components. If the working pressure is too low, however, flow and volume delivery are affected. Consider the case in which the working pressure is 80 cmH₂O and the patient's peak airway pressure is 40 cmH₂O. During inspiration, the pressure gradient decreases from 80 to 40 cmH₂O, causing the flow to taper to 50% of the initial flow, resulting in decreased volume delivery for a fixed inspiratory time. Working pressure usually is preset, but it has been adjustable in some older-generation ventilators not currently manufactured (e.g., Siemens Servo 900 series). In the Servo 900 series ventilators, marked alterations in peak inspiratory flow are observed as working (driving) pressure is altered. In other old ventilators (e.g., Bear 2), the inspiratory-flow waveform was controlled by adjusting the driving pressure. Fortunately, none of the current generation of ICU ventilators suffers from this deficiency.

Historically, ventilators have been described as single- or double-circuit designs. With the single-circuit design, the gas that enters the pneumatic system is delivered to the patient. In the double-circuit design, the gas that powers the pneumatic system is separate from that delivered to the patient (e.g., Enstrom 300, Puritan-Bennett MA-1). All new-generation ventilators are single-circuit design.

GAS BLENDING

All critical-care ventilators have some mechanism for mixing air and oxygen to achieve oxygen delivery in the range of 21–100%. In first-generation volume ventilators, such as the Emerson postoperative ventilator, oxygen flow was titrated into a reservoir from which the piston drew gas for delivery to the patient. All current-generation critical-care ventilators use either an internal or an external blender. These blenders use a precision metering device called a *proportioning valve*. By altering the opening through which air and oxygen are passed, different oxygen concentrations are delivered. These often work in such a manner that when the oxygen port is opened, the air port is proportionally closed, and vice versa. For these blenders to deliver an accurate oxygen concentration, the gas pressure entering the proportioning valve must be stable and equal. In some of the newest-generation microprocessor ventilators (e.g., Puritan Bennett 840, Respironics Espirit), air and oxygen are mixed by use of proportional solenoid valves (as discussed later). It is important that the ventilator does not allow backflow of oxygen into the compressed-air delivery system and vice versa. Most accomplish this by one-way check valves placed in the individual gas-pressure-reduction mechanisms. This is critical because most institutional compressed-gas systems are not maintained at the same exact pressure. If the oxygen system is at 49 lb/in² and the compressed-air system

TABLE 3-1 Characteristics of 100% Oxygen Suction Feature Available on Adult ICU Ventilators

Ventilator	Activation	Duration	Manual Termination	Alarms
Puritan-Bennett 860	Touchkey entry	2 minutes	Yes	Active
Drager Evita 4	Touchkey entry	Up to 3 minutes	Yes	Active/inactive[b]
Servo i	Touchkey entry	1 minute	Yes	Active
Viasys Avea[a]	Touchkey entry	2 minutes	Yes	Active
Hamilton Galileo	Touchkey entry	2 minutes	Yes	Active
e-Vent Inspiration LS	Touchkey entry	5 minutes	Yes	Active
Datex-Ohmed Engstrom Carestation	Touchkey entry	2 minutes	Yes	Active

[a] The increase in F_{IO_2} can be adjusted with the Avea.
[b] Alarms are inactive on ventilator disconnection.

at 51 lb/in², the accuracy of gas mixing would be altered without check valves.

In some ventilators, the delivered oxygen concentration is not constant throughout inspiration. Although small fluctuations (±1–2%) in delivered oxygen concentrations may not be important clinically, this can be problematic during indirect calorimetry measurements. The delivered oxygen concentration can be stabilized by adding a secondary external blender to ensure gas mixing before entering the ventilator or using a precision gas mixture during these measurements.[1]

A control that is available on most ventilators is 100% oxygen suction. Activation of this control provides 100% oxygen for a defined period of time (e.g., 2 minutes), primarily for hyperoxygenation immediately before and after endotracheal suctioning.[2] This feature also can be used for procedures other than suctioning that may be associated with desaturation (e.g., line insertion and postural drainage). The 100% oxygen suction feature is available on most current-generation ICU ventilators,[2] and characteristics of some of these ventilators are described in Table 3-1.

In all ventilators, except the Siemens Servo 300, Maquet Servo-i, and Viaysis Avea, blending of only oxygen and room air is possible. With these ventilators, a third gas may be blended with oxygen and air. The two gases commonly added to these systems are helium and nitric oxide.

ACCUMULATOR

In some ventilators, gases are stored in an accumulator before delivery to the patient. With the Servo 900 series ventilators, gas accumulates in a 0.9-liter bellows. The pressure in this bellows can be adjusted and serves as the working (driving) pressure during inspiration. Gas accumulates in a 1.1-liter reservoir in the Bird 6400ST, in an 8-liter reservoir in the Hamilton Veolar, and in a 3.4-liter reservoir in the Bear 1000. The accumulator acts as a mixing chamber for blended gases, which increases the stability of the delivered oxygen concentrations. It also allows high peak flows (>200 liters/min), even when gas enters the ventilator at low flows (<80 liters/min). None of the newest-generation ventilators, however, incorporate accumulators. They have been replaced with more efficient gas mixing and delivery systems.

FLOW AND PRESSURE REGULATION

A ventilator can be classified as a pressure, volume, flow, or time controller (Fig. 3-5).[3] If the pressure waveform does not change with changes in patient resistance and compliance, then the ventilator is considered a pressure controller. If the delivered volume is measured directly, then the ventilator is considered a volume controller. If the delivered volume is determined by a flow transducer, then the ventilator is

FIGURE 3-5 Criteria for determining the control variable during a ventilator-assisted inspiration. (*Used, with permission, from Chatburn: Respir Care 37:1009–25, 1992.*)

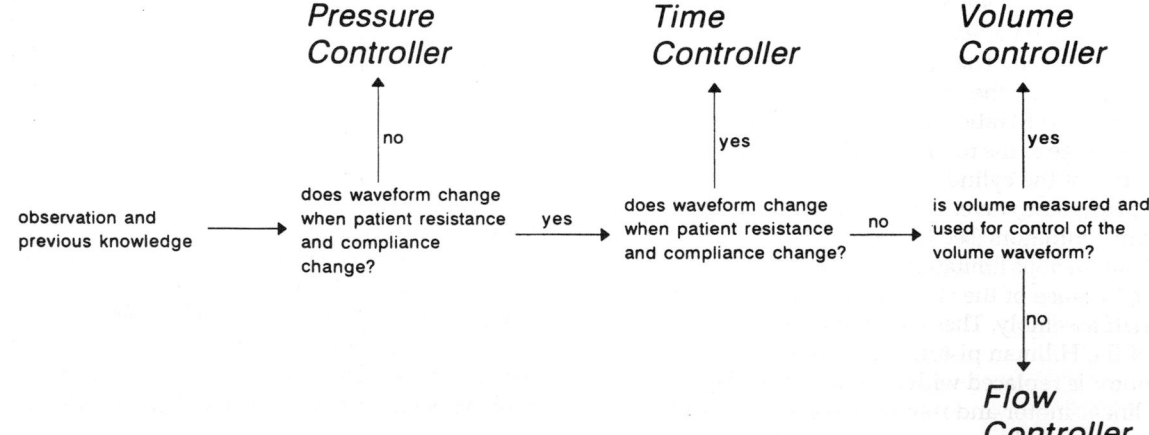

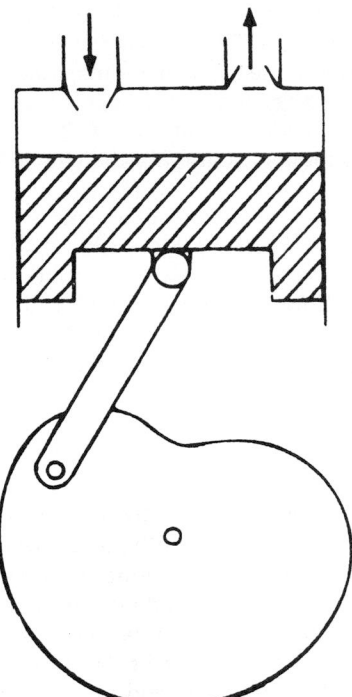

FIGURE 3-6 A rotary, motor-driven piston pneumatic system as used with the Emerson postoperative and IMV ventilators (see text for details). (*Used, with permission, from Sanborn: Respir Care 38:72–109, 1993.*)

a flow controller. If both pressure and volume waveforms change with changes in patient resistance and compliance, then the ventilator is considered a time controller. Most commercially available mechanical ventilators are either pressure, volume, or flow controllers.

A number of methods are and have been used historically on commercially available ventilators to regulate inspiratory flow and manipulate the inspiratory flow pattern. These include the use of a piston, a compressor-bellows, a variable restriction, a stepper motor with a scissors valve, a proportional solenoid, and a proportional manifold with digital valves.[4]

- *Piston.* With this design (Fig. 3-6), a piston draws gas into a cylinder during its downstroke (or return stroke). On its upstroke (or forward stroke), the piston moves gas out of the cylinder to the patient. A motor turns a rotary wheel at a constant speed. The speed of the motor can be adjusted to determine the respiratory rate and inspiratory-expiratory time (I:E) ratio. Because the piston rod connects to the outer edge of the rotary wheel, the movement of gas into and out of the cylinder is not constant and approximates that of a sine wave. This design is still used in many home-care ventilators (see Chap. 4) available throughout world. It has serious limitations in critical-care ventilators, however, because of the slow response of the motor and crank-shaft assembly. These limitations can be overcome by use of the Hillman piston and motor, in which the rotating motor is replaced with a linear motor (Fig. 3-7). By using a linear motor and rolling-seal piston, greater flexibility and responsiveness are achieved. This design was

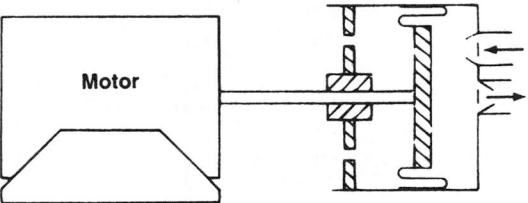

FIGURE 3-7 A linearly accelerating rolling-seal piston pneumatic system, as seen with the Bournes LS-104 ventilator (see text for details). (*Used, with permission, from Sanborn: Respir Care 38:72–109, 1993.*)

used in the original proportional-assist ventilator (Winnipeg ventilator)[5,6] and is used currently on the Puritan Bennett 700 series ventilators. Piston ventilators normally are volume controllers because the volume delivered is determined by the displacement of the piston, and pressure varies secondarily.

- *Compressor-bellows.* With this design (Fig. 3-8), the gas to be delivered is contained in a bellows. Gas is moved to the patient by pressurizing the chamber surrounding the bellows. This method is no longer used in current-generation critical-care ventilators. Most anesthesia ventilators, however, use this design because it separates the breathing gas from any possible mechanical contamination and increases safety with flammable gases. Compressor-bellows ventilators are volume controllers because the volume delivered is measured directly, as determined by the degree of bellows compression. The rate of compression of the bellows determines the rate of gas flow to the patient. A relatively low driving pressure (e.g., 1.8 lb/in^2 or 125 cmH$_2$O) is controlled

FIGURE 3-8 Compressor bellows or a bag within a chamber-type pneumatic system, as used with the Bennett MA-1 and MA-2 and Monaghan 225 ventilators (see text for details). (*Used, with permission, from Sanborn: Respir Care 38:72–109, 1993.*)

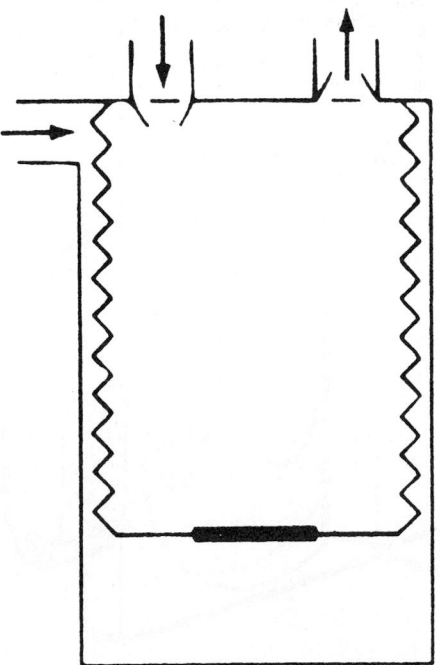

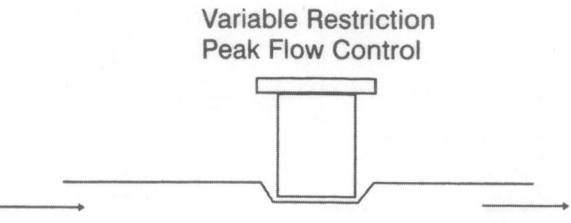

**Variable Restriction
Peak Flow Control**

FIGURE 3-9 A variable-restriction flow-controller pneumatic system as used with the Sechrist infant ventilator (see text for details).

by a variable-orifice peak-flow controller. The peak-flow control determines the flow at the initiation of inspiration. Flow decelerates as airway pressure increases, however, because of the decreasing gradient between the driving pressure and the downstream airway pressure.

- *Variable restriction.* In this design (Fig. 3-9), the flow control is a variable restriction that limits gas flow. In some neonatal ventilators, this is simply a Thorpe-tube flowmeter. In more sophisticated applications of this design, the inspiratory waveform is varied by an adjustable pressure-reducing valve. When a decelerating waveform is selected, the working pressure is reduced (e.g., from 3–1.8 lb/in^2). This decreases the gradient between driving pressure and airway pressure, with a resulting decrease in gas flow. The peak-flow control distal to the pressure-

reducing valve is a variable restriction that limits the maximum flow. This mechanism is a flow controller, and tidal volume is determined by a preset inspiratory time relative to the flow setting.

- *Stepper motor with a scissors valve.* This device meters flow by a stepper motor attached to a scissors valve that pinches a silicon tube (Fig. 3-10). The peak inspiratory flow is determined by the pressure entering the scissors valve (e.g., 120 cmH$_2$O). A stepper motor controls the scissors valve to allow an increase or decrease in flow of approximately 10% increments or decrements, respectively, as required to maintain the selected tidal volume or airway pressure.[7] If tidal volume is determined by a flow transducer, this design is a flow controller. If inspiratory pressure is controlled by a pressure transducer, this design is considered a pressure controller.

- *Proportional solenoid.* With this design, gas flow during inspiration is controlled by either one or two proportional solenoids (one for air and one for oxygen or a single solenoid after gas blending) or flow-control valves. Traditionally, a solenoid has operated in one of two positions, on or off. Proportional solenoids, however, open and close proportionally to control flow. In the case of the Puritan-Bennett 7200, each solenoid has 4095 stops in an operating distance of 762 μm. In some cases the flowmetering orifice of the proportional solenoid is actuated directly by an armature moving linearly in a magnetic field (Fig. 3-11). Alternative designs include the use of a stepper motor coupled directly to the flowmetering orifice or a stepper motor–driven cam (Fig. 3-12). With each of these

FIGURE 3-10 A stepper motor with scissors-valve pneumatic system from the Siemens Servo 900C ventilator (see text for details). (*Used, with permission, from Siemens product literature.*)

FIGURE 3-11 An electromagnetic proportional-solenoid pneumatic system as used with the Puritan-Bennett 7200, the Hamilton Veolar and Amadeus, the Drager Evita, and the Siemens Servo 300 ventilators (see text for details). (*Used, with permission, from Sanborn: Respir Care 38:72–109, 1993.*)

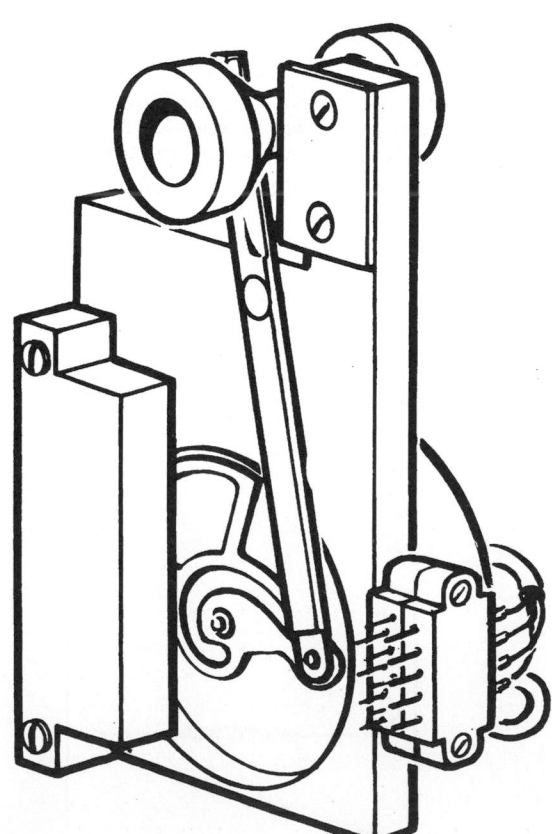

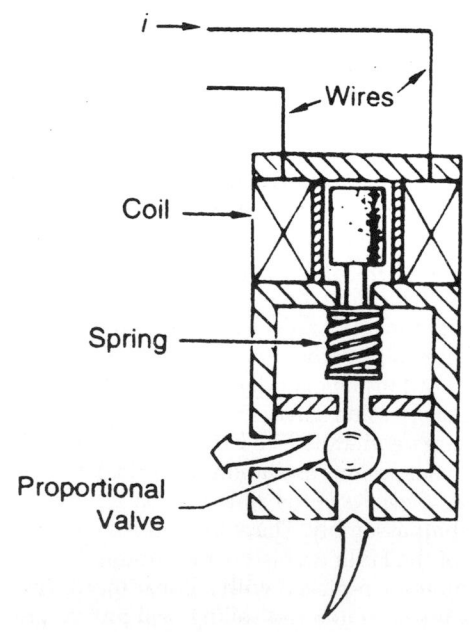

i →

Wires

Coil

Spring

Proportional
Valve

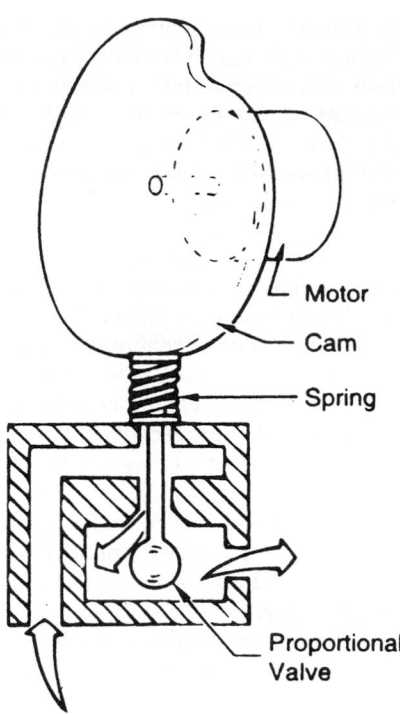

FIGURE 3-12 A step motor–driven cam proportional-solenoid system as used with the Bear 5 and 1000 and the Bird 6400ST and 8400ST ventilators (see text for details). (*Used, with permission, from Sanborn: Respir Care 38:72–109, 1993.*)

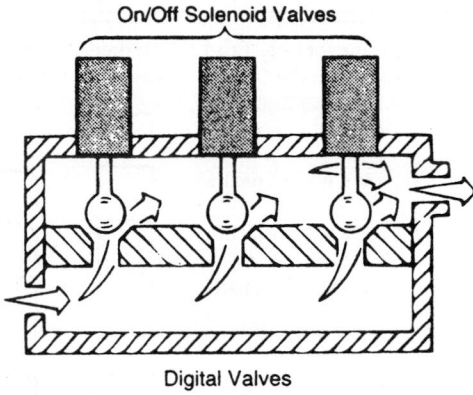

FIGURE 3-13 A proportional manifold with digital valve pneumatic system as used with the Infrasonics Infant Star ventilator (see text for details). (*Used, with permission, from Sanborn: Respir Care 38:72–109, 1993.*)

designs, the position of the solenoid determines peak flow and flow waveform. When proportional solenoids are used for both air and oxygen, the delivered oxygen concentration is also controlled. A proportional solenoid can function as either a flow controller or a pressure controller.

- *Proportional manifold with digital valves.* This design uses digital solenoid valves in which each valve is either open or closed (Fig. 3-13). When open, each valve produces only one calibrated flow. The number of discrete flow steps (including zero) is 2^n, where n is the number of valves. For example, a nine-valve design with 0.5 liter/min increments between valves yields a flow range of 0–255 liters/min at a

resolution of 0.5 liter/min. With this design, flow accuracy from each valve and reliability of the individual components are important. If problems of reliability and accuracy can be solved, the digital valve design is attractive because each valve can be considerably less sophisticated than a full-range proportional valve.[4] This design can serve as either a flow controller or a pressure controller.

INSPIRATORY-FLOW WAVEFORMS

For each control variable (pressure, volume, and flow), a limited number of waveforms can be developed. These can be grouped into four categories: rectangular, exponential, ramp, and sinusoidal (Fig. 3-14).[3] With ventilators that are pressure controllers, rectangular and exponentially increasing waveforms are available. For volume controllers, increasing ramp and sinusoidal waveforms are available. The greatest number of waveforms are possible for flow controllers: rectangular, sinusoidal, ramp (ascending and descending), and exponential decay.

With pressure and flow controllers, the delivered waveform is a function of both ventilator settings and respiratory system impedance (Fig. 3-15).[8] With increased impedance,

FIGURE 3-14 During inspiration, the ventilator is only able to control one of three variables (pressure, volume, or flow) during a given breath. Possible waveforms associated with each control variable are illustrated. (*Used, with permission, from Chatburn: Respir Care 36:1123–55, 1991.*)

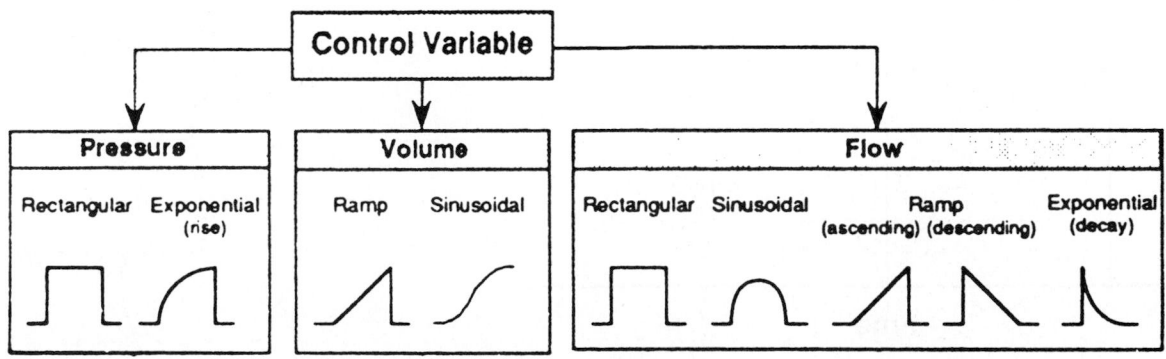

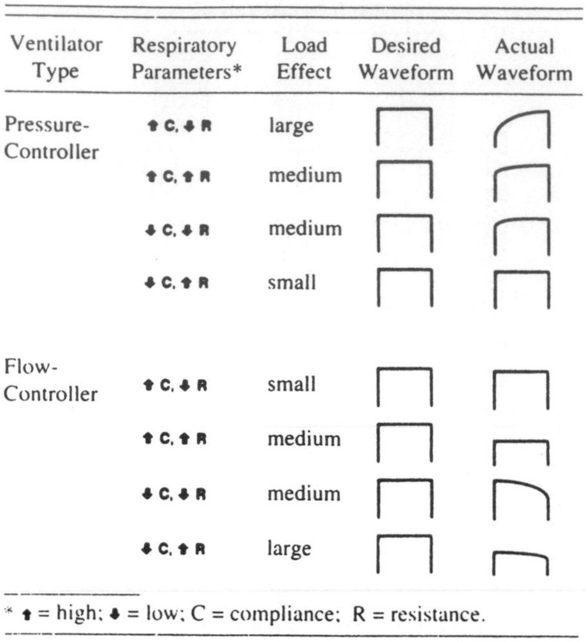

Ventilator Type	Respiratory Parameters*	Load Effect	Desired Waveform	Actual Waveform
Pressure-Controller	↑C, ↓R	large		
	↑C, ↑R	medium		
	↓C, ↓R	medium		
	↓C, ↑R	small		
Flow-Controller	↑C, ↓R	small		
	↑C, ↑R	medium		
	↓C, ↓R	medium		
	↓C, ↑R	large		

* ↑ = high; ↓ = low; C = compliance; R = resistance.

FIGURE 3-15 Idealized effects of increasing impedance on pressure and flow controllers. (*Used, with permission, from Chatburn: Respir Care 36:1123–55, 1991.*)

the desired waveform may differ considerably from the actual delivered waveform. When an inspiratory waveform other than constant flow is chosen, the ventilator must adjust either the peak flow or inspiratory time to maintain a constant delivered tidal volume (Fig. 3-16).

The clinical usefulness of inspiratory waveform manipulations is somewhat unclear.[9] Over the past 40 years, there have been a number of studies that have evaluated inspiratory flow patterns and their effects on system pressures, gas exchange, and other variables (Table 3-2).[10–22] The following conclusions[9] can be drawn from these studies:

• Mean airway pressure is higher with decelerating flow patterns and lower with accelerating flow patterns.

• Peak airway pressure is lower with decelerating flow patterns and higher with accelerating flow patterns.
• Gas distribution is improved with decelerating flow patterns. The result of this improved gas distribution is a decrease in pulmonary shunt and dead space.
• Mean airway pressure is further increased by use of an end-inspiratory breath hold.

A decelerating flow pattern can be produced using either a pressure controller or a flow controller.[23]

Because variation in flow waveform is technically feasible, the spectrum defined earlier has been included on many ventilators despite no clearly established benefit of one over the other. The only exception to this is the decelerating and exponential-decay waveforms, which result in the lowest peak airway pressure. On current-generation ICU ventilators, only three waveforms are available: rectangular, descending ramp, and exponential decay. Rectangular and descending-ramp waveforms are available with volume-targeted modes, and exponential-decay waveforms are available with pressure-targeted modes.

SIGH VOLUME

The sigh breath is a deliberate increase in tidal volume for one or more breaths at regular intervals.[24] Much debate over the use of sigh breaths has occurred over the last 40 years.[25–34] The lack of demonstrated benefit has resulted in none of the current-generation ICU ventilators providing a sigh function. Two recent clinical studies,[35–36] however, have demonstrated improved oxygenation with the use of periodic sighs over the short term. With the current concern over ventilator-induced lung injury, though, it is doubtful that the sigh function will be reintroduced into the current generation of ICU ventilators. No data are available to determine whether the application of peak alveolar pressures of 40 cmH2O and tidal volumes of 12 ml/kg of ideal body weight once every minute or two over days will result in the same level of injury that the application of these volumes and pressures cause when applied continuously.[37]

FIGURE 3-16 When the inspiratory waveform is changed from a square to a decelerating waveform, either peak inspiratory flow or inspiratory time must be increased to maintain constant delivery of tidal volume.

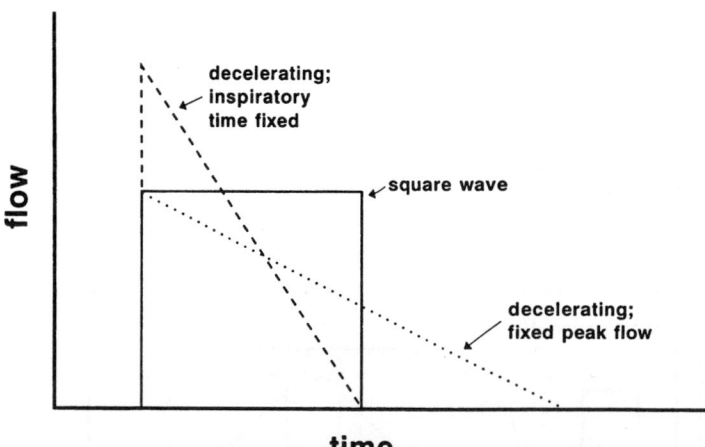

TABLE 3-2   Studies of Inspiratory Flow Patterns and Their Effect on Pressures and Other Variables

Investigator(s)	Model and Flow Generator	Mean Airway Pressure	Peak Airway Pressure	Gas Distribution	Pa_{O_2}	Other
Lyager[10]	Lung model; Engstrom, Bird Mark 8, Bennett PR-2	—	—	Poorest with ascending	—	—
Adams et al[11]	Canine model; experimental flow generator	Highest with sine, descending; lower with ascending square	—	—	—	—
Jansson and Jonson[12]	Computer simulation	Higher with descending; lower with ascending and square	Lower with descending; higher with ascending and square	—	—	—
Johansson and Lofstrom[13]	Human subjects; Servo 900	Highest with ascending	Lowest to highest: descending, square, ascending	—	—	—
Baker et al[14]	Canine model; experimental flow generator	Highest to lowest: descending, square, sine, ascending	—	—	Most favorable with descending	V_D/V_T, C, Pa_{CO_2}, CO most favorable with descending
Damann[15]	Human subjects; Servo 900B	Highest with sine wave	—	Sine better than square	—	—
Modell and Cheney[16]	Canine lung injury; Emerson 3PV	—	—	—	10% increase in Pa_{O_2} with descending vs. ascending and sine wave	—
Baker et al[17,18]	Canine pulmonary edema and emphysema; experimental flow generator	Highest to lowest: descending, square	—	—	—	Lowest Pa_{CO_2} with descending
Banner et al[19]	Lung model of uneven ventilation; Hamilton Veolar (4 waveforms)	—	Lowest with descending, highest with ascending	Improved with descending	—	Lowest Pa_{CO_2} with descending; decrease in Pet_{CO_2} with descending and increasing inspiratory time
Branson and Hurst[20]	Human subjects; Hamilton Veolar (4 waveforms)	Highest with descending and square	Lowest to highest: sine, square, descending, ascending	—	—	—
Smith and Venus[21]	Pigs with high R_{aw}; Hamilton Veolar (4 waveforms)	Higher with ascending than with square, sine, or descending	—	—	—	No differences in gas exchange or hemodynamic values
Rau and Shelledy[22]	Lung model; Hamilton Veolar (7 waveforms) baseline and low compliance	Highest with full descending; lowest with full ascending	Lowest to highest: descending; modified sine, sine, partial descending, square, partial ascending, and full ascending	—	—	—

ABBREVIATIONS: V_DV_T, dead space-to-tidal volume ratio; C, compliance; CO, cardiac output; Pa_{CO_2}, arterial carbon dioxide tension; Pa_{O_2}, arterial oxygen tension; Pet_{CO_2}, end-tidal carbon dioxide tension; R_{aw}, airway resistance.
SOURCE: Used, with permission, from Rau.[9]

NEBULIZER

Some ventilators are capable of powering a nebulizer. When activated, part of the delivered tidal volume is diverted through an auxiliary line to power the nebulizer. Normally, the nebulizer is activated only during the inspiratory phase without affecting the delivered F_{IO_2}. Some ventilators, however, do use either compressed air or 100% oxygen to power the nebulizer (thus affecting F_{IO_2}). This feature of mechanical ventilators has become less useful in recent years in various parts of the world for the delivery of aerosolized bronchodilators because of increased use of metered-dose inhalers during mechanical ventilation. The increasing use of drugs not available as metered-dose inhalers, especially antibiotics, has caused many manufacturers to rethink the addition of the nebulizer feature. Some manufactures (e.g., Maquet Servo-i) have developed ultrasonic nebulizers specific for their ventilators; these offer an increased capacity to deliver a large volume of aerosol in the therapeutic range. With the ongoing development of new nebulizers and continued research on drug delivery by the aerosol route, we expect this to be an area of continued development in ventilator design.[38]

A word of caution about the use of aerosolized medication is in order. Because many ventilators now incorporate highly developed flow-measuring capabilities, the aerosolization of drugs within the ventilator circuit can cause malfunction of the expiratory-flow transducer. Many manufacturers now recommend the inclusion of a filter in the expiratory limb just before gas enters the exhalation manifold. These filters, however, must be removed and discarded after treatment to avoid the buildup of inadvertent positive end-expiratory pressure (PEEP) because of clogging of the filter with drugs and water.

Ventilator Safety Issues

Because mechanical ventilators are life-support devices, it is imperative that they respond in a safe manner if there is a pneumatic or electrical failure. An antiasphyxia valve should be present on the inspiratory limb of the ventilator. In the event of a pneumatic failure, this valve opens to allow the patient to breathe room air. Some ventilators, in the event of an electrical or pneumatic failure, open both the inspiratory and expiratory valves to allow continuous gas flow through the circuit from which the patient may breathe spontaneously.[39,40] All new-generation ventilators incorporate an apnea backup ventilation system that activates if the ventilation rate falls below a clinician-selected level. In most current-generation ventilators, a high continuous gas flow is produced with disconnection in an attempt to compensate for the leak. This can result in aerosolization of tubing condensate into the room, which is potentially hazardous to clinicians at the bedside. When a patient is purposefully disconnected from the ventilator, the Y-piece of the circuit should be capped. Other ventilators (e.g., Puritan-Bennett 840) are able to differentiate between a leak and disconnection and will stop all gas delivery if an actual disconnection occurs.

Modes of Mechanical Ventilation

The relationships between the various possible breath types and inspiratory-phase variables are referred to as the *modes of ventilation*.[41,42] Three phase variables define inspiration: the trigger variable, the limit variable, and the cycle variable (Fig. 3-17).[3,43] The trigger variable begins inspiration and is discussed later in this chapter. The limit variable is the pressure, flow, or volume target that cannot be exceeded during inspiration. The cycle variable ends inspiration. Five control variables describe gas delivery: pressure control, volume control, flow control, time control, and dual control (normally pressure and volume). Finally, two general terms can be applied to the actual breath type: *mandatory breath* (inspiration is triggered and/or cycled by the machine) and *spontaneous breath* (inspiration is triggered and cycled by the patient). A classification of common ventilator modes is summarized in Table 3-3. Some modes must stand alone, based on their function, whereas others can be

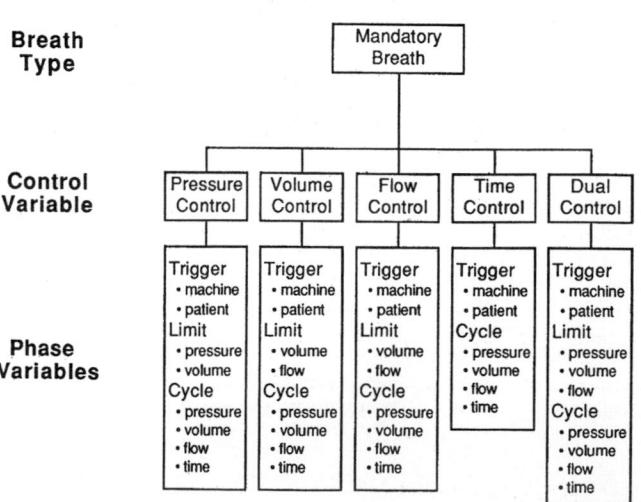

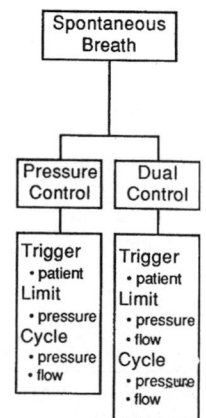

FIGURE 3-17 Classification of control and phase variables for the two basic breath types: mandatory and spontaneous. (*Used, with permission, from Branson et al.[43]*)

TABLE 3-3 Expanded Classification of Modes of Ventilator Operation

Mode	MANDATORY BREATH Control	Trigger	Limit	Cycle	SPONTANEOUS BREATH Control	Trigger	Limit	Cycle
CMV	Pressure, volume, or flow	Time	Pressure, volume, or flow	Time, pressure, volume or flow	—	—	—	—
PCV	Pressure	Time	Pressure	Time	—	—	—	—
V-ACV	Pressure, volume, or flow	Pressure, volume, or flow	Pressure, volume, or flow	Time, pressure, volume, or flow	—	—	—	—
P-ACV	Pressure	Pressure, volume, or flow	Pressure	Time	—	—	—	—
AMV	Pressure, volume, or flow	Pressure, volume, or flow	Pressure, volume, or flow	Time, pressure, volume, or flow	—	—	—	—
VC-IMV	Pressure, volume, or flow	Time	Pressure, volume, or flow	Time, pressure, volume, or flow	Pressure	Pressure, volume, or flow	Pressure	Pressure
VC-SIMV	Pressure, volume, or flow	Time, pressure, volume, or flow	Pressure, volume, or flow	Time, pressure, volume, or flow	Pressure	Pressure, volume, or flow	Pressure	Pressure or flow
CPAP	—	—	—	—	Pressure	Pressure, volume, or flow	Pressure	Pressure or flow
PC-IMV	Pressure	Time	Pressure	Time	Pressure	Pressure, volume, or flow	Pressure	Pressure
PC-SIMV	Pressure	Time, pressure, volume, or flow	Pressure	Time	Pressure	Pressure, volume, or flow	Pressure	Pressure
PCIRV	Pressure	Time	Pressure	Time	—	—	—	—
APRV	Pressure	Time or pressure	Pressure	Time	Pressure	Pressure, volume, or flow	Pressure	Pressure
Bilevel	Pressure	Time, pressure, or flow	Pressure	Time	Pressure	Pressure, volume, or flow	Pressure	Pressure
PSV	—	—	—	—	Pressure	Pressure, volume, or flow	Pressure	Flow
MMV	Volume or flow	Time	Volume or flow	Time, volume, or flow	Pressure	Pressure, volume, or flow	Pressure	Pressure or volume
VAPS	—	—	—	—	Pressure, volume, or flow	Pressure, volume, or flow	Pressure	Pressure, volume, or flow
BiPAP	Pressure	Time	Pressure	Time	Pressure	Flow	Pressure	Flow
VS	—	—	—	—	Pressure	Pressure, volume, or flow	Pressure	Flow
ASV	Pressure	Time, pressure, volume, or flow	Pressure	Time	Pressure	Pressure, volume, or flow	Pressure	Flow
ATC	—	—	—	—	—	Pressure, volume, or flow	Pressure	Flow
PAV	—	—	—	—	—	Pressure, volume, or flow	Pressure	Flow

ABBREVIATIONS: CMV, volume-controlled mechanical ventilation; V-ACV, volume assist-control ventilation, P-ACV, pressure assist-control ventilation; AMV, assisted mechanical ventilation; VC-IMV, volume-controlled intermittent mandatory ventilation; VC-SIMV, volume-controlled synchronized intermittent mandatory ventilation; CPAP, continuous positive airway pressure; PCV, pressure-controlled ventilation; PC-IMV, pressure-controlled IMV; PC-SIMV, pressure-controlled SIMV; PCIRV, pressure-controlled inverse-ratio ventilation; APRV airway pressure release ventilation; Bilevel, bilevel pressure ventilation; MMV, mandatory minute ventilation; VAPS, volume-assured pressure support; BiPAP, bilevel positive airway pressure; VS volume support; ASV, adaptive-support ventilation; ATC, automatic tube compensation; PAV, proportional assist ventilation.
SOURCE: Modified and used, with permission, from Chatburn.[3]

TABLE 3-4 Pressure versus Volume Targeting Modes

	Pressure	Volume
Tidal volume	Variable	Preset
Peak airway pressure	Preset	Variable
Peak alveolar pressure	Preset	Variable
Flow waveform	Preset but variable	Preset
Peak flow	Variable	Preset
Inspiratory time	Preset	Preset
Sensitivity	Preset	Preset
FI_{O_2}	Preset	Preset
PEEP	Preset	Preset
I:E ratio	Preset or variable	Preset or variable

ABBREVIATIONS: FI_{O_2}, fractional inspired oxygen concentration; PEEP, positive end-expiratory pressure; I:E ratio, inspiratory time-to-expiratory time ratio.

TABLE 3-5 New Modes of Ventilation That Vary Gas Delivery within a Breath or between Breaths

Within-Breath Variability	Between-Breath Variability
Proportional-assist ventilation (PAV)	Pressure-regulated volume control (PRVC)
Automatic tube compensation (ATC)	Volume support (VS)
Volume-assured pressure support (VAPS)	Adaptive-support ventilation (ASV)

combined.[42–45] Finally, most modes of ventilation associated with actual gas delivery to the patient can be grouped by their primary gas-delivery target—pressure, volume, or both—although two modes, proportional-assist ventilation (PAV) and automatic tube compensation (ATC), target neither pressure nor volume.

Pressure-targeted modes all set a peak inspiratory pressure that is targeted during inspiration; that is, initial gas flow is delivered rapidly to achieve the pressure target. After the target is reached, flow usually decelerates in an exponentially decaying manner to maintain pressure at the target until the inspiratory phase is complete. If the patient should inspire more forcefully in the middle of the breath, flow accelerates to maintain the target pressure. Because of this gas-delivery format, tidal volume is variable on a breath-to-breath basis. Other aspects of gas delivery, however, are set the same as with volume-targeted modes (Table 3-4).

With volume-targeted modes, the primary gas-delivery target is tidal volume. Normally, all aspects of the inspiratory phase are selected by the clinician with volume-targeted modes. Specifically, tidal volume, flow waveform, peak inspiratory flow, and inspiratory time are set. This contrasts with pressure-targeted modes, where the pressure limit and the inspiratory time are the only variables set. With volume targeting, peak inspiratory pressure may vary on a breath-to-breath basis.

With dual modes, the gas-delivery pattern can vary in two ways. First, each breath can be delivered as a pressure-targeted breath but with a tidal volume target. As a result, to ensure the tidal volume target, pressure may need to vary on a breath-to-breath basis. With this approach, tidal volume on the current breath is compared with the target, and pressure level on the subsequent breath is adjusted if the tidal volume is off target. Second, gas can be delivered as a volume-targeted breath with a set minimum tidal volume and peak flow. On any breath, however, peak flow and, as a result, tidal volume can be exceeded if the patient's ventilatory demand increases. This is accomplished by allowing the patient access to a demand flow any time during the breath. With this approach, the volume-targeted breath can be converted to a pressure-supported breath.

Two modes of ventilation target proportional unloading of patient effort (PAV or ATC). That is, the ventilation target is the percentage of the tidal effort that is unloaded either to minimize overall patient effort (PAV) or to maintain tracheal pressure constant (ATC). As a result, both tidal volume and airway pressure can vary considerably on a breath-to-breath basis from near zero to excessive.

For these more sophisticated or so-called new modes of ventilation, gas delivery can be adjusted either within each breath or between breaths (Table 3-5). That is, pressure or volume vary within a given breath based on patient demand or on the subsequent breath based on the current breath demand to establish a new target level. Modes of ventilation available on select ventilators are listed in Table 3-6.

CONTROLLED MECHANICAL VENTILATION (CMV)

With CMV, all breaths are totally controlled by the ventilator, and patient triggering is not possible (Fig. 3-18). CMV is also called *volume-controlled ventilation* or *pressure-controlled ventilation* (Fig. 3-19). In some ventilators, the only difference between CMV and assist-control ventilation is the sensitivity setting. In reality, assist-control or intermittent mandatory ventilation modes can provide controlled mechanical ventilation if the patient is sedated and/or paralyzed. With volume-targeted CMV, the clinician sets the rate, tidal volume (in some machines, a minute volume is set), flow waveform, peak inspiratory flow or inspiratory time, and I:E ratio. With pressure-targeted CMV, the clinician sets the rate, pressure level, inspiratory time, or I:E ratio.

ASSIST-CONTROL VENTILATION (ACV)

ACV may be either pressure- or volume-targeted. With ACV, a minimal rate and tidal volume (or inspiratory pressure) are set by the clinician. The patient may trigger the ventilator at a more rapid rate, but the clinician-determined tidal volume (or inspiratory pressure) is delivered with each breath (Figs. 3-20 and 3-21). Assisted breaths may be either pressure- or flow-triggered (see discussion related to triggering later in this chapter).

ASSISTED MECHANICAL VENTILATION (AMV)

With this mode of ventilation, all breaths are triggered by the patient (no set backup rate) (Fig. 3-22), and each breath is delivered at the ventilator's set tidal volume (or pressure).

TABLE 3-6 Modes of Ventilation Available on Selected Mechanical Ventilators

	CPAP	C, ACV	SIMV	MMV	APRV	Bilevel	PS	Apnea Vent.	PRVC	VS	ATC	ASV	VAPS
Bear 5	+	V	V	+			+						
Bird 6400ST	+	V	V				+						
Bird 8400ST	+	V	V				+						+
Hamilton Veolar	+	V, P	V, P	+			+	+					
Hamilton Amadeus	+	V	V				+	+					
Infrasonics Adult Star	+	V	V				+						
Ohmeda Advent	+	V, P	V, P	+			+	+					
Orager IRISA	+	V, P	V, P	+			+	+					
Puritan-Bennett													
7200a	+	V, P	V, P				+	+					
7200ae	+	V, P	V, P				+	+					
7200sp	+	V, P	V, P				+	+					
Siemens Servo 900E	+	V	V				+						
Siemens Servo 900C	+	V, P	V, P				+						
Maquet Servo i	+	V, P	V, P			+	+	+	+	+			
Puritan-Bennett 840	+	V, P	V, P			+	+	+			+		
Hamilton Gallileo	+	V, P	V, P				+	+				+	
Viasys Avea	+	V, P	V, P			+	+	+	+	+			
Orager Evita 4	+	V, P	V, P	+	+		+	+	+		+		
e-Vent Inspiration LS	+	V, P	V, P			+	+	+	+	+			
Datex-Ohmeda	+	V, P	V, P			+	+	+	+				

ABBREVIATIONS: V, volume; P, pressure; CPAP, continuous positive airway pressure; ACV, assist-control ventilation; C, control; SIMV, synchronized intermittent mandatory ventilation; MMV, mandatory minute ventilation; APRV, airway pressure-release ventilation; Bilevel, bilevel airway pressure ventilation; apnea vent. backup, apnea ventilation; PRVC, pressure-regulated volume control; VS, volume support; ATC, automatic tube compensation; ASV, adaptive-support ventilation; VAPS, volume-assured pressure support.

FIGURE 3-18 Volume-controlled ventilation (CMV), decelerating ramp flow.

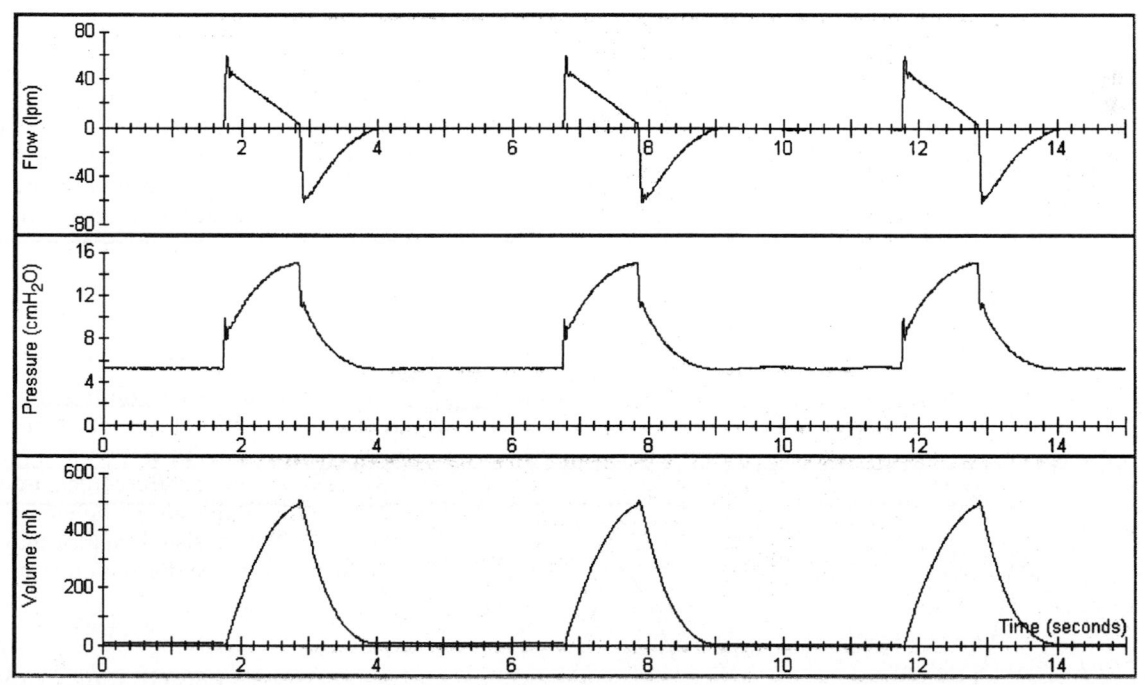

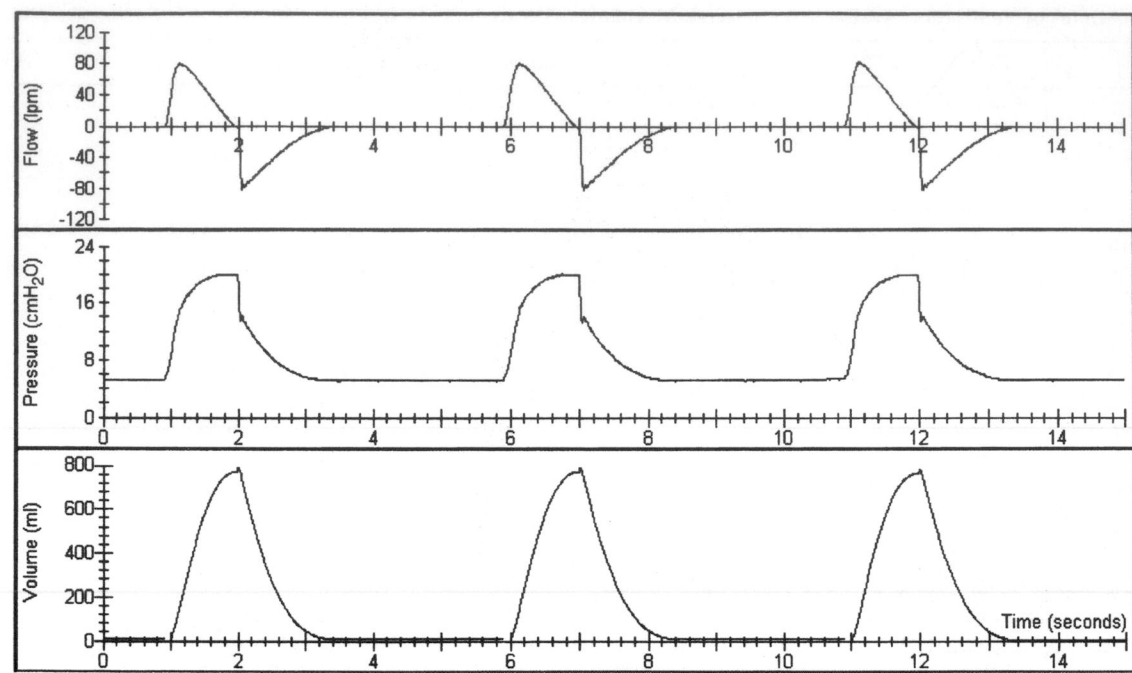

FIGURE 3-19 Pressure-controlled ventilation (CMV).

FIGURE 3-20 Volume assist-control ventilation (V-ACV), decelerating ramp flow.

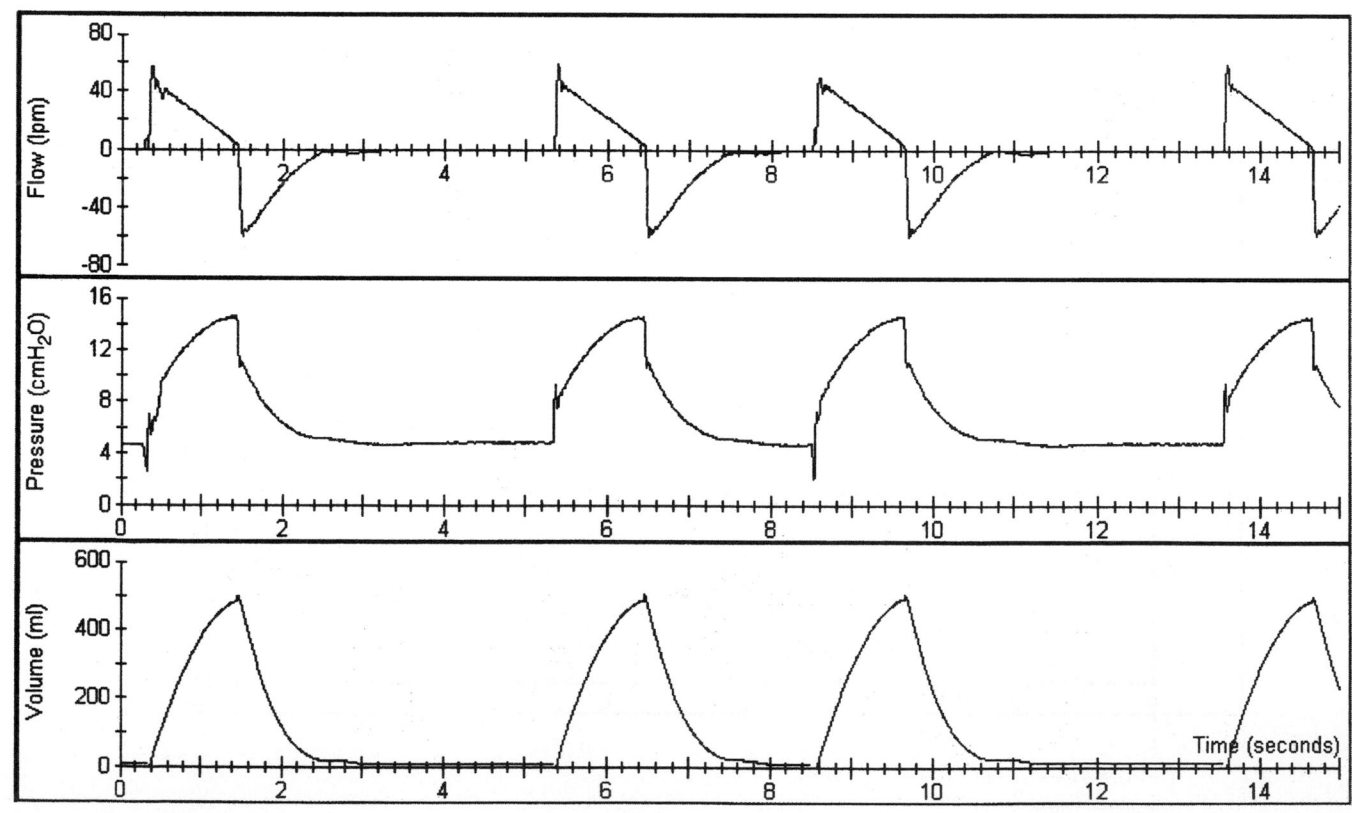

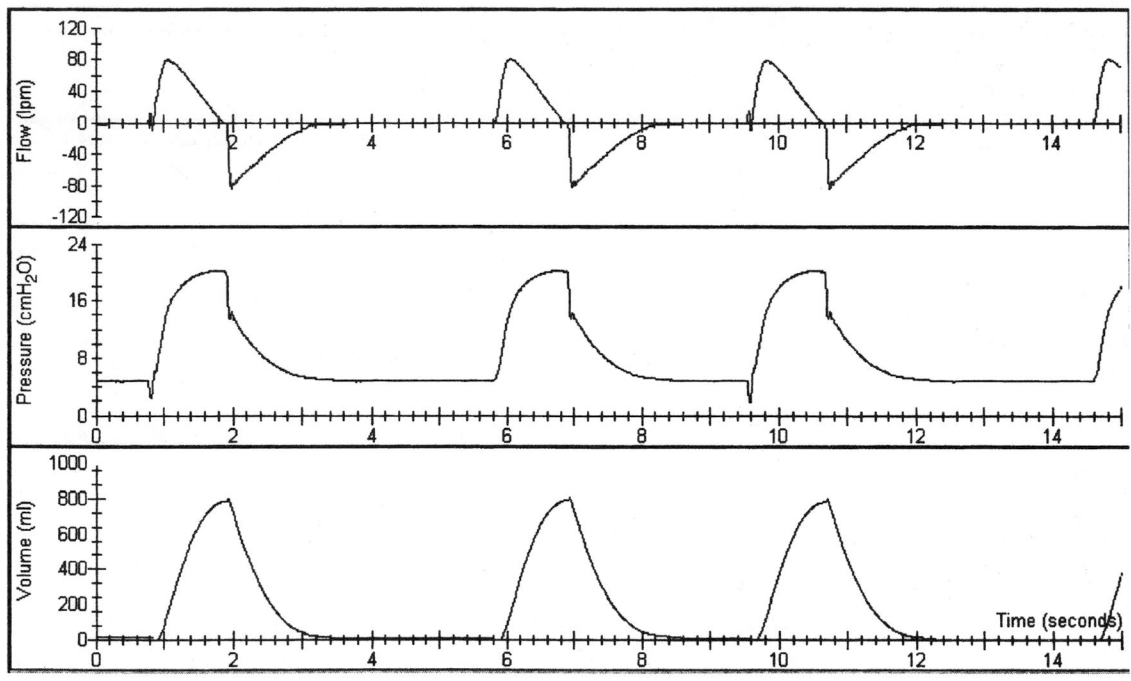

FIGURE 3-21 Pressure assist-control ventilation (P-ACV).

This can be achieved on some ventilators in which the ACM rate can be set to zero. This mode is normally referred to as *pressure support* (see later section).

INTERMITTENT MANDATORY VENTILATION (IMV)

IMV may be pressure- or volume-targeted. With this mode, CMV breaths are delivered at a set rate and volume (or pressure).[40–46] In between the machine-delivered breaths, the patient is allowed to breathe spontaneously from either a demand valve or a continuous flow of gas (Figs. 3-23 and 3-24). The first applications of IMV were achieved by setting the ventilator in the control mode and incorporating a one-way valve into the inspiratory limb of the circuit to allow the patient to breathe spontaneously from atmosphere or from a secondary continuous-flow system between mandatory breaths.[47,48] These early systems essentially coupled a parallel gas-flow system with

FIGURE 3-22 Volume-assisted ventilation (VAV), decelerating ramp flow.

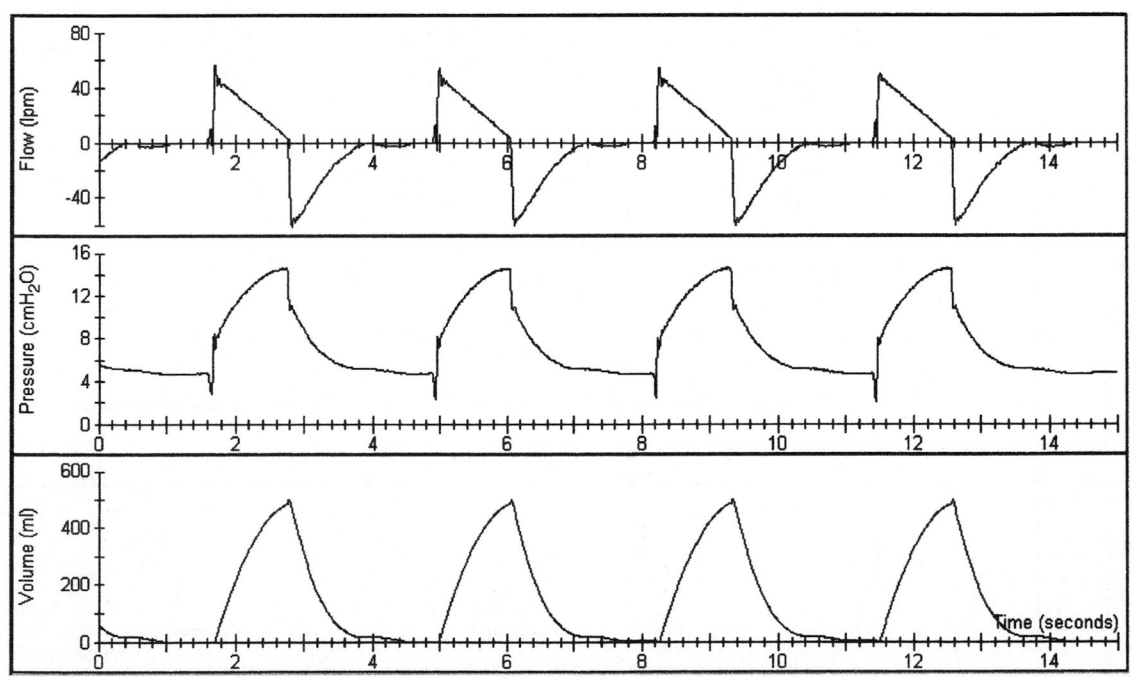

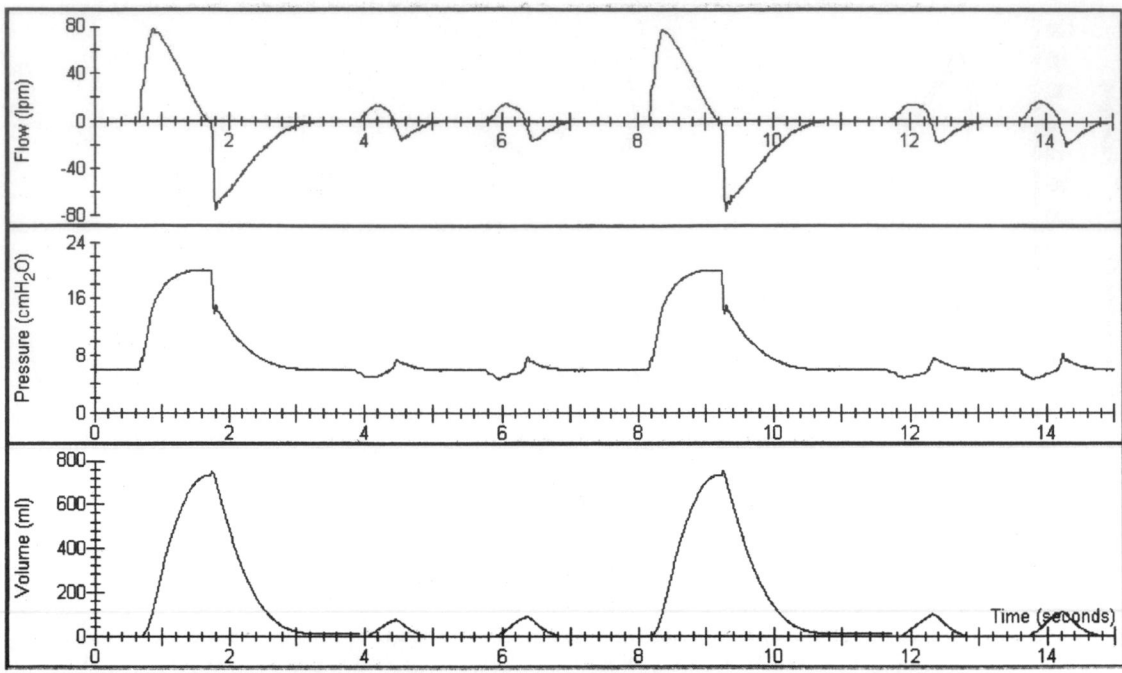

FIGURE 3-23 Pressure-controlled intermittent mandatory ventilation (PC-IMV).

the inspiratory limb of the ventilator circuit via a one-way valve in such a manner that gas did not flow continuously through the circuit.[49–51] Such systems allow accurate measurements of exhaled tidal volumes. They are associated with a high inspiratory work of breathing, however, particularly if PEEP is in use.[47] IMV is available on older-generation ventilators that are still in use but not manufactured any longer. It has been replaced on newer-generation ventilators by synchronized intermittent mandatory ventilation (SIMV) (see next section). The lack of coordina-

tion with the patient's inspiratory effort during IMV results in increased work of breathing and hemodynamic compromise.[52,53]

SYNCHRONIZED INTERMITTENT MANDATORY VENTILATION (SIMV)

This mode of ventilation is similar to IMV and available with pressure (Fig. 3-25) and volume (Fig. 3-26) targeting, except that the ventilator delivers the mandatory breaths in

FIGURE 3-24 Volume-controlled intermittent mandatory ventilation (VC-IMV), decelerating ramp flow.

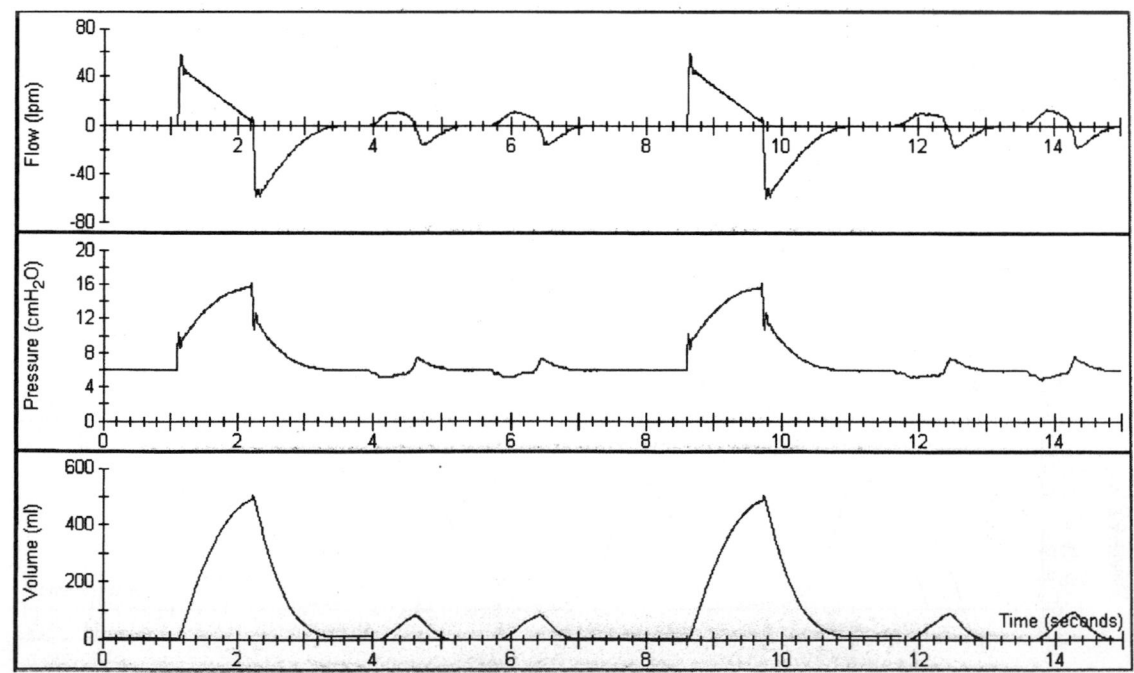

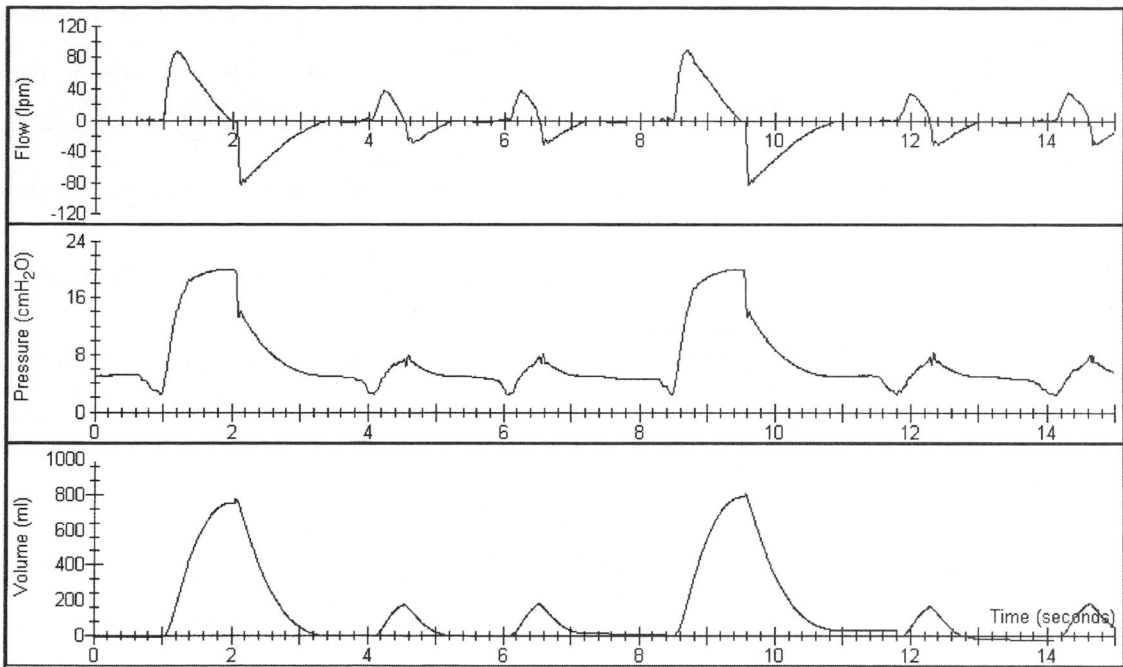

FIGURE 3-25 Pressure-controlled synchronized intermittent mandatory ventilation (PC-SIMV).

synchrony with the patient's inspiratory efforts, and gas is supplied by a patient-triggered demand system during spontaneous breaths.[54,55] In essence, the unit functions in the assist-control mode only during "windows" of time established by the manufacturer (Fig. 3-27). The time available within each window for patient triggering varies among manufacturers but is usually a function of the set respiratory rate. As a result, the mandatory rate may vary from its set rate depending on when triggering occurs in a series of windows. If a patient's inspiratory effort is detected while the window is open, a synchronized breath is delivered. If no patient effort is detected at the time the window closes, the ventilator delivers a mandatory breath. This avoids the stacking of mandatory breaths on top of spontaneous

FIGURE 3-26 Volume-controlled synchronized intermittent mandatory ventilation (VC-SIMV), decelerating ramp flow.

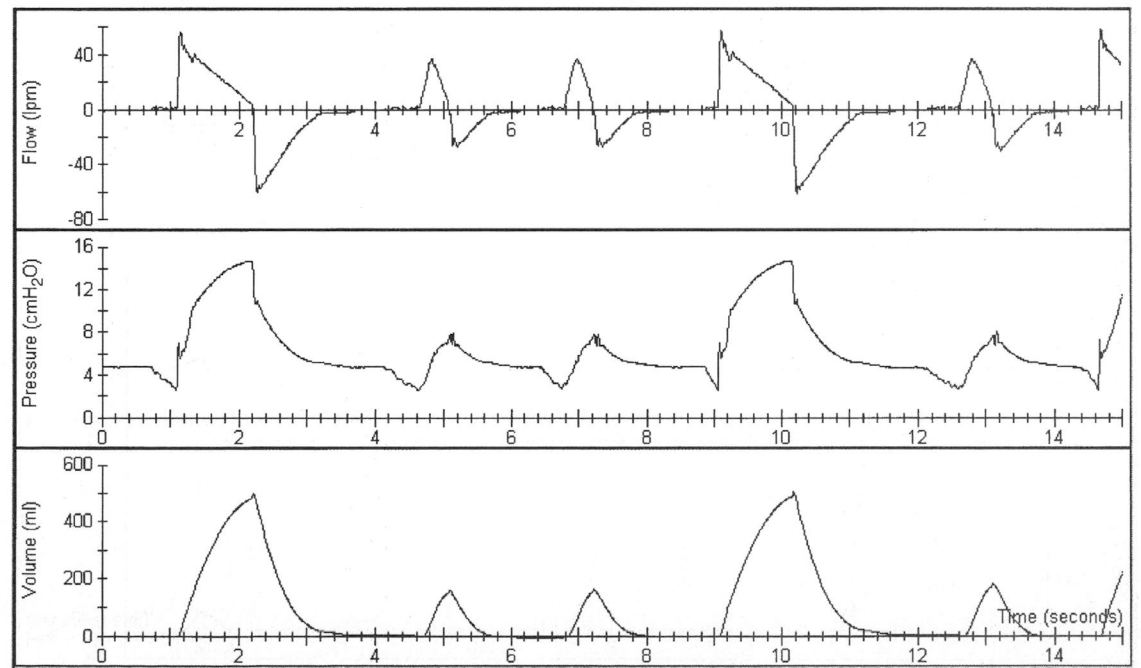

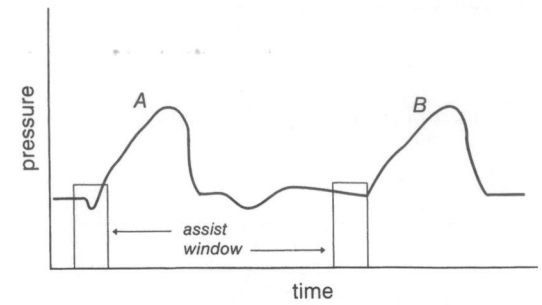

FIGURE 3-27 Depiction of the SIMV assist window. In assisted breaths (*A*), the ventilator senses the patient's inspiratory effort and triggers the breath in synchrony with the patient's desires. In contrast, if patient effort is not sensed by the end of the assist time window (*B*), a controlled positive-pressure breath is delivered.

breaths or machine inspiration or expiration being delivered out of phase with the patient's desired phase of ventilation. In addition, pressure support can be provided during spontaneous breathing with either pressure- or volume-targeted SIMV.

CONTINUOUS POSITIVE AIRWAY PRESSURE (CPAP)

This is a spontaneous breathing mode (Fig. 3-28); no mechanical positive-pressure breaths are delivered. The only variables set by the clinician are the level of CPAP and the sensitivity of the demand system. As noted in Fig. 3-29, differences do exist among ventilators with regard to patient effort during CPAP,[56] although the problems observed with earlier systems and high levels of work of breathing imposed have been eliminated.[57,58] In fact, the use of CPAP via a mechanical ventilator has been advocated in recent weaning guidelines.[59] CPAP often is confused with PEEP.

CPAP is a specific mode on mechanical ventilators, whereas PEEP is the elevation of baseline system pressure during other positive-pressure modes of ventilation. Both establish an elevated system baseline pressure by manipulating operation of the ventilator's exhalation valve (see the section Exhalation Valves below for details), although the CPAP mode can be used without an elevation of baseline pressure (0 cmH$_2$O CPAP).

PRESSURE-CONTROLLED INVERSE-RATIO VENTILATION (PCIRV)

PCIRV is a variation of PCV in which inspiration is longer than expiration.[60-68] PCIRV typically is initiated by selecting PCV and adjusting settings to provide the desired I:E ratio or inspiratory time (Fig. 3-30). In some ventilators, the I:E ratio is set and does not vary when the respiratory rate is changed (e.g., Servo 300). In other ventilators, the inspiratory time is set and does not vary when the rate setting is changed (e.g., Puritan-Bennett 840), whereas others allow the user to select either inspiratory time or I:E ratio as the constant when respiratory rate is changed (e.g., Puritan-Bennett 7200).

AIRWAY PRESSURE-RELEASE VENTILATION (APRV)

APRV is described as two levels of CPAP (high and low) that are applied for defined periods of time where spontaneous breathing is allowed at both levels (Fig. 3-31).[69-73] Normally, inspiratory time is longer than expiratory time. The clinician sets the two levels of CPAP and the amount of time spent at each level. APRV is similar to pressure-controlled SIMV, pressure-controlled ventilation (PCV), or PCIRV. If the patient is not breathing spontaneously, PCIRV and PCV are indistinguishable from APRV. In the initial application of

FIGURE 3-28 Continuous positive airway pressure (CPAP).

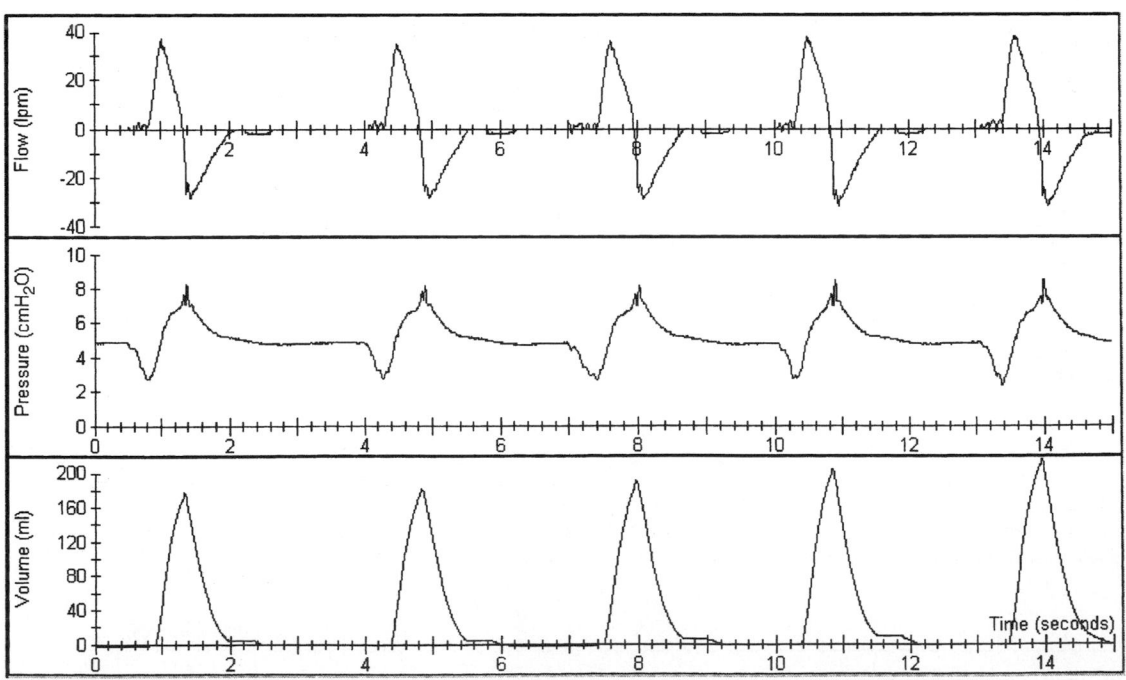

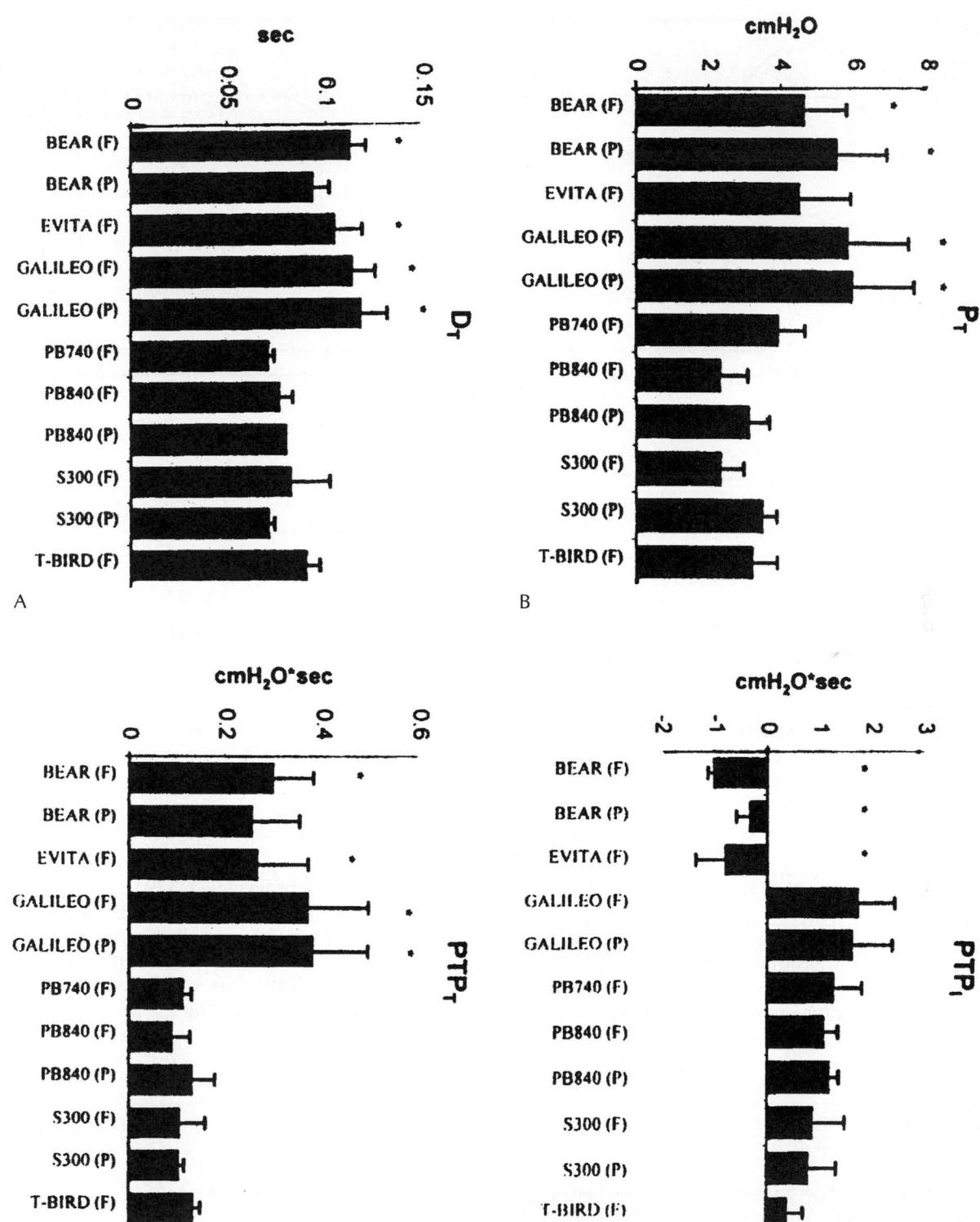

FIGURE 3-29 Inspiratory-phase variables evaluated during CPAP on a number of current-generation ICU ventilators: (*A*) inspiratory trigger delay time (D_T); (*B*) inspiratory trigger pressure (P_T); (*C*) triggering pressure-time product (PTP_I); (*D*) inspiratory pressure-time product (PTP_T). Mean ± SD of all inspiratory peak flows. F, flow triggering; P, pressure triggering; Bear, Bear 1000; Evita, Drager Evita; Galileo, Hamilton Galileo; PB 740, Puritan-Bennett 740; 840, Puritan Bennett 840; S300, Maquet Servo 300; T-Bird, Viasys T-Bird. *$P < 0.05$ versus flow-triggered S300. (*Used, with permission, from Takeuchi et al: Anesthesiology 96:162–72, 2002.*)

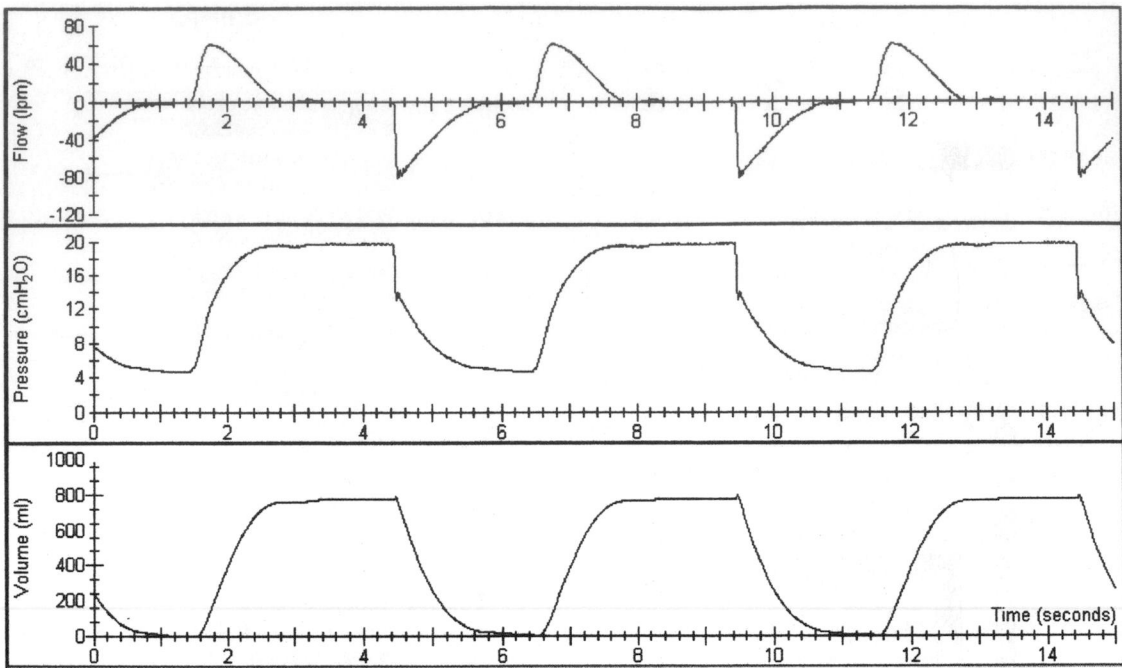

FIGURE 3-30 Pressure-controlled inverse-ratio ventilation (PC-IRV).

APRV, it was assembled using a modified continuous-flow CPAP system (Fig. 3-32). In essence, this system requires a high-flow gas delivery, a rapid-response solenoid valve, and two independent PEEP valves. The solenoid valve switches gas flow in the expiratory limb of the system from one PEEP valve to the other to achieve the two different levels of CPAP. APRV is now available commercially on new-generation mechanical ventilators (i.e., Drager Evita).

BILEVEL AIRWAY PRESSURE VENTILATION (BILEVEL)

Bilevel is a modification of APRV similar to the improvement seen when SIMV was introduced to replace IMV. During bilevel ventilation, the patient's spontaneous breathing efforts and the change from one CPAP level to the other are coordinated. As a result, breath stacking is avoided. In addition, pressure support can be added to the spontaneous breaths at either or both levels of CPAP (Fig. 3-33).

PRESSURE-SUPPORT VENTILATION (PSV)

This is a pressure-targeted mode where the patient's inspiratory effort is supported by the ventilator at a preset level of inspiratory pressure.[74-77] Inspiration is initiated by patient effort and terminated primarily when inspiratory flow falls to a ventilator-specific level (Fig. 3-34). During PSV, the patient determines the respiratory rate, inspiratory time, and tidal volume; the ventilator only controls the inspiratory pressure level. PSV can be combined with SIMV (Figs. 3-35 and 3-36) and applied to the spontaneous breaths during bilevel pressure ventilation (Fig. 3-37).

FIGURE 3-31 Airway pressure-release ventilation (APRV).

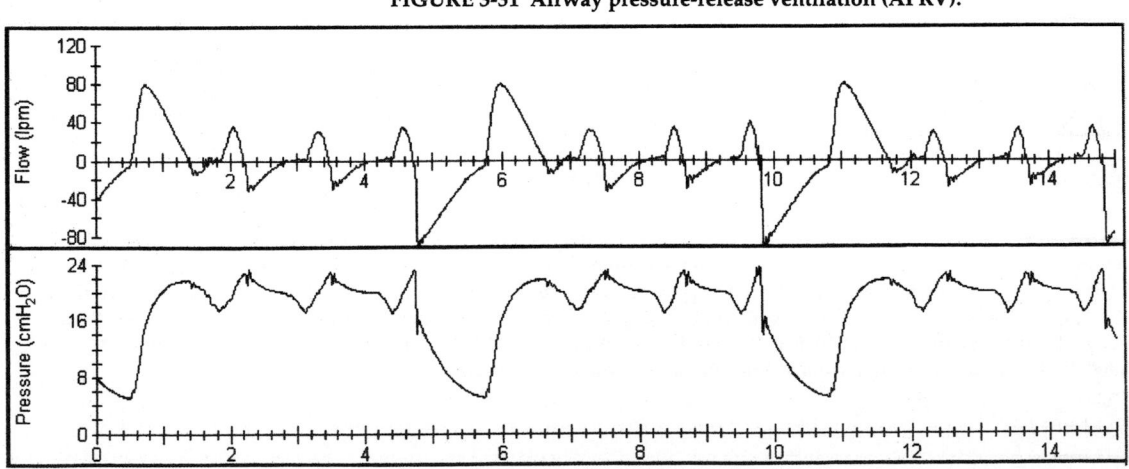

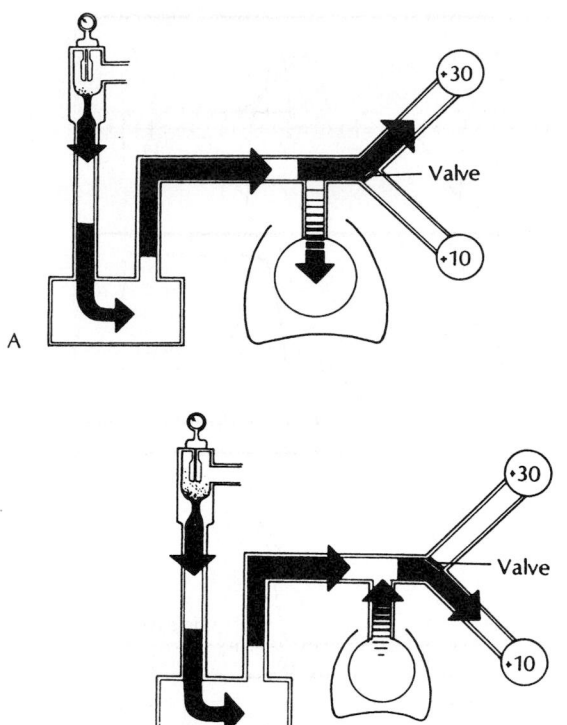

FIGURE 3-32 Schematic presentation of APRV with an inspiratory CPAP level set at 30 cmH$_2$O and an expiratory CPAP level set at 10 cmH$_2$O. Flow is produced by a high-flow generator, and a solenoid valve is used to move gas flow to one of the PEEP valves (+30 and +10). *A.* High CPAP period. *B.* Low CPAP period. (*Used, with permission, from Cane et al: Chest 200:460–3, 1991.*)

PSV is triggered only by the patient; when the pressure-support breath is triggered, the ventilator delivers sufficient flow to rapidly achieve the set pressure level. After the pressure is established, flow must decrease rapidly to ensure that the pressure does not exceed the set level. When the flow decreases to the target cycling level (normally 25% of peak flow), ventilator inspiration is terminated.[78] The breath also may be terminated if pressure, after a manufacturer's spe-

cific period of inspiratory time, exceeds the set level by a specific pressure (e.g., +3 cmH$_2$O).[79] In addition, if inspiratory time exceeds a manufacturer's specific time period (e.g., 3 seconds), inspiration will end (Table 3-7).[79]

Patient-ventilator dyssynchrony can occur during pressure-support ventilation. The three primarily reasons for dyssynchrony are an inappropriate pressure level, an inappropriate initial flow delivery, and an inappropriate cycling criterion (terminal flow).[80] Pressure level can be corrected easily by increasing or decreasing the pressure setting. It should be remembered that setting too high a pressure level can force too large a tidal volume and increase the likelihood of air trapping and auto-PEEP.[81] Frequently, the correct pressure adjustment is a decrease in pressure level to allow a tidal volume consistent with the patient's desired tidal volume.

Dyssynchrony at the onset and termination of a pressure-support breath can be corrected by varying the rate of gas delivery at the onset of inspiration or varying the percent of the peak-flow decrease required to cycle the breath to exhalation. The addition of rise time and inspiratory termination criteria as adjuncts to pressure-targeted breaths can improve synchrony at these two points of the breath.

RISE TIME

As illustrated in Fig. 3-38, the rise-time control on ventilators alters the slope of the rise in flow (to its peak level) at the onset of a pressure-targeted breath.[81] Rise time on most ventilators is active during all pressure-targeted modes of ventilation. A change in rise time from rapid to slow has three potential effects during pressure support. First, the time to peak airway pressure (and flow) is increased. Second, the actual peak flow obtained is decreased. Third, the inspiratory time may be increased to maintain the same tidal volume. As shown in Figs. 3-38 and 3-39, too rapid a rise time causes airway pressure to overshoot the peak level at the onset of the breath. In this situation, the rise time should be slowed.[82] As illustrated in Fig. 3-39, however, too slow a rise time also results in air hunger and a convex initial airway pressure curve.[82] In this situation, rise time should be increased.

FIGURE 3-33 Bilevel airway pressure ventilation (bilevel) with pressure support at the low CPAP level.

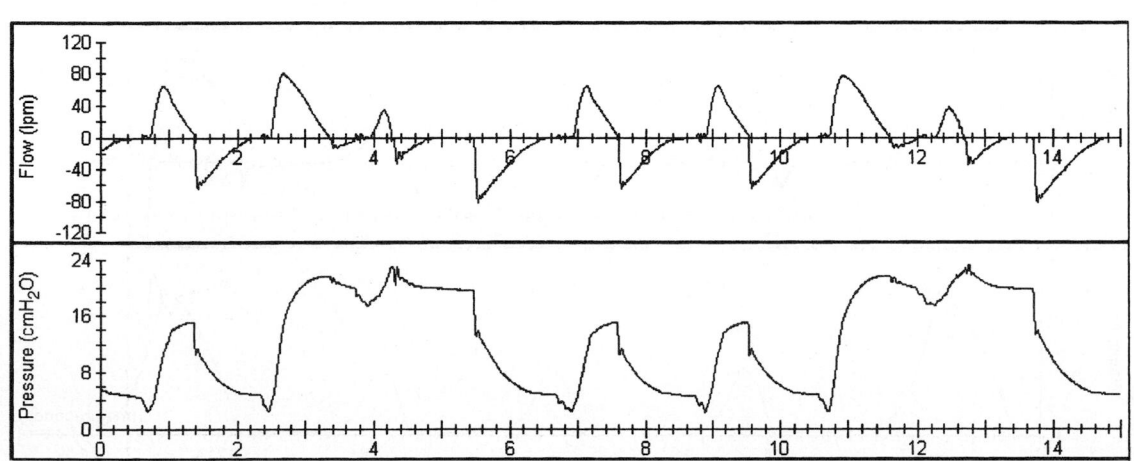

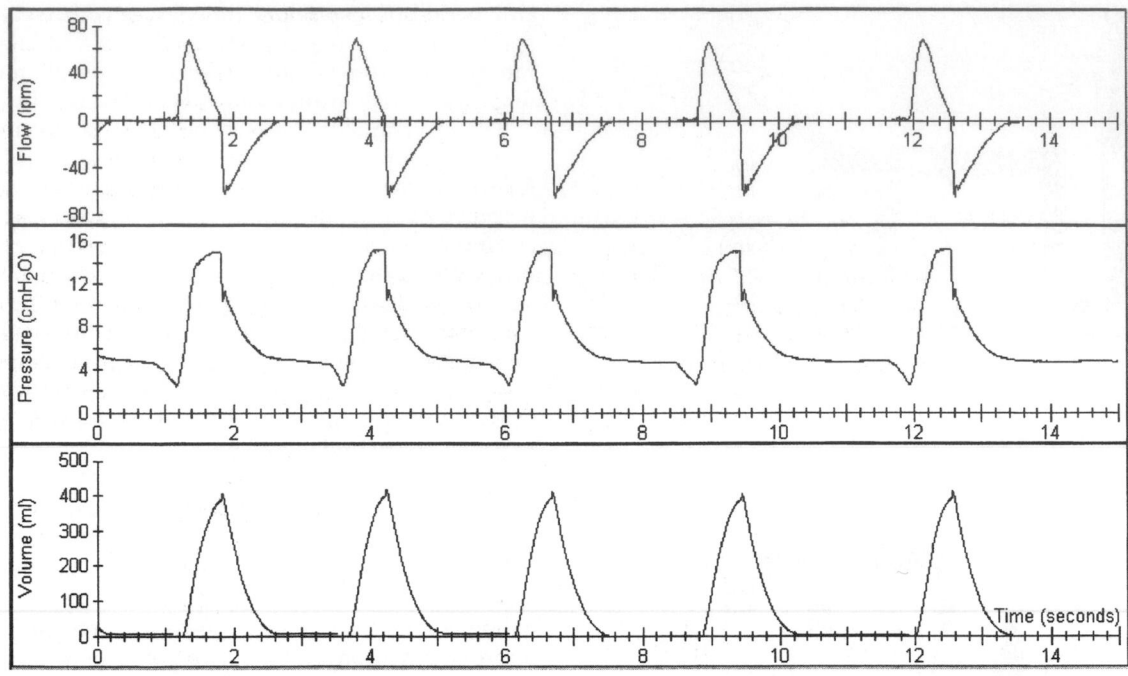

FIGURE 3-34 Pressure-support ventilation (PSV).

INSPIRATORY TERMINATION CRITERIA

This control is effective only in pressure support. It adjusts the percent of peak flow terminating the pressure-support breath. If the airway pressure increases above the set level at the end of a pressure-support breath, the patient is activating the expiratory muscles to achieve exhalation before the ventilator is ready to permit exhalation (Fig. 3-40).[83,84] In this situation, the flow setting for terminating the inspiration (as a percent of peak flow) is too low. The problem is corrected by increasing the latter setting until the spike in airway pressure at the end of the breath disappears. The opposite problem also can occur, as illustrated in Fig. 3-41, where machine inspiration ends before the patient is ready to exhale.[85] In this case, both airway pressure and flow tracing appear as

FIGURE 3-35 Volume-controlled synchronized intermittent mandatory ventilation (VC-SIMV) with pressure-support ventilation, decelerating ramp flow.

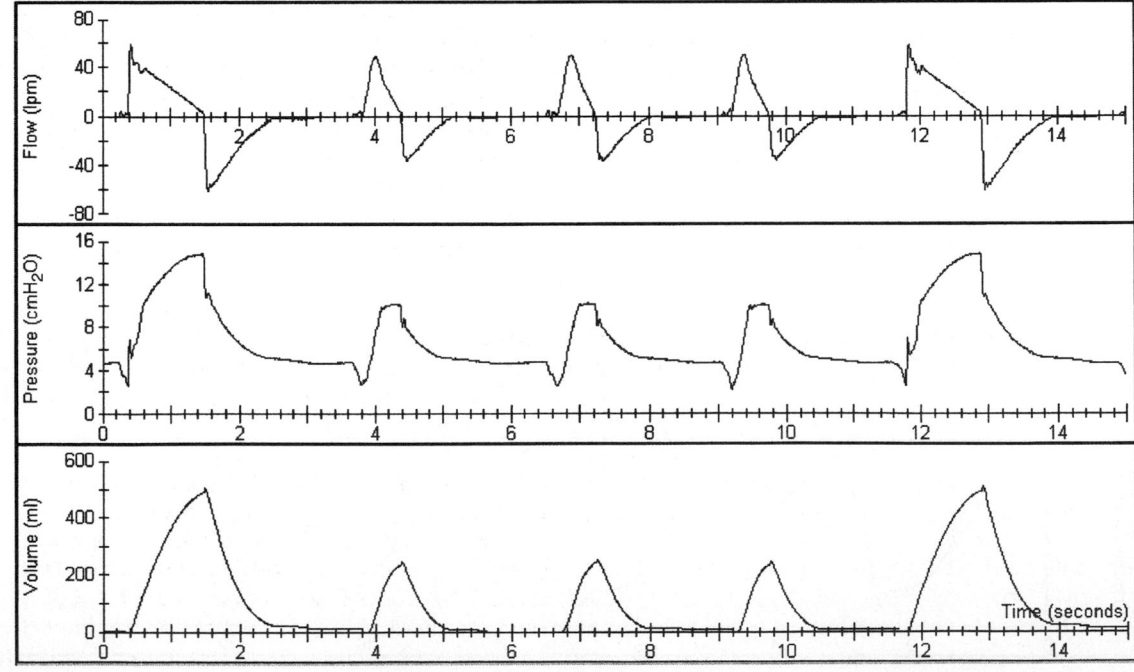

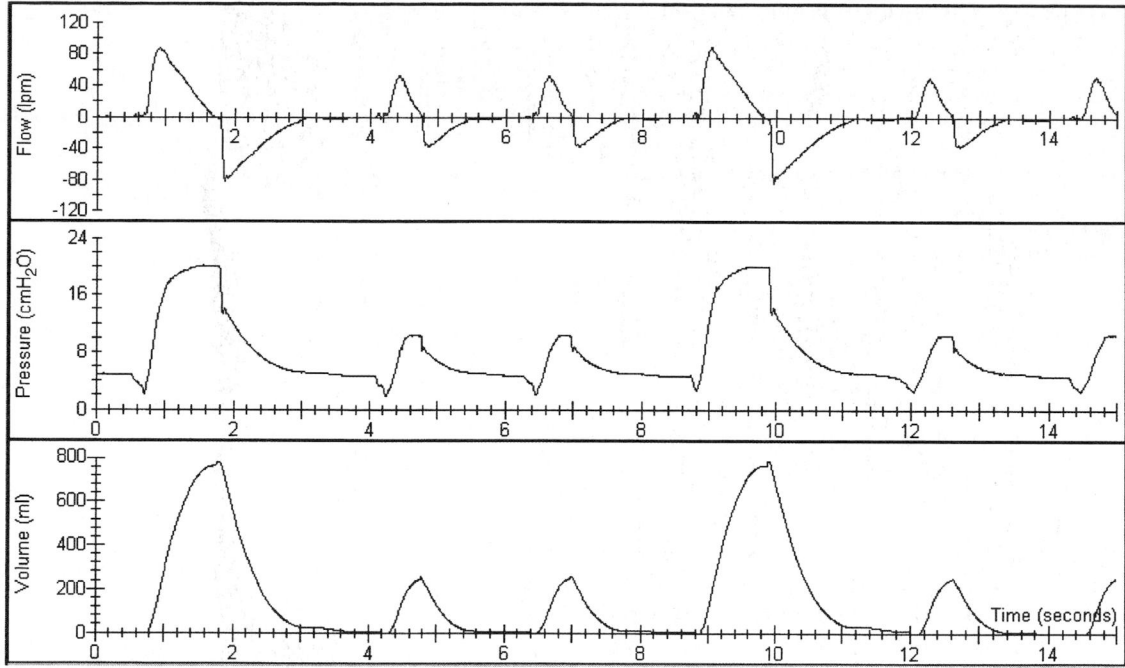

FIGURE 3-36 Pressure-controlled synchronized intermittent mandatory ventilation (PC-SIMV) with pressure-support ventilation.

if a secondary small breath is provided immediately after the end of the normal breath. The problem is corrected by decreasing the flow setting for terminating inspiration (percent of the peak flow) until the abnormality is eliminated.

PROPORTIONAL-ASSIST VENTILATION (PAV)

This mode permits free flow of gas to the patient in response to patient-generated effort (Fig. 3-42).[5,6] The difference between pressure at the patient's proximal airway and pressure in the piston chamber of the device creates flow and volume signals that can be amplified by the device. The airway pressure produced by the device to support the patient's inspiratory effort is determined by patient-generated inspiratory flow ($\dot{V}$) and volume (V) and clinician-determined amplification of these variables. Thus

$$Paw = f_1 V + f_2 \dot{V}$$

where f_1 and f_2 are the amplification factors. In practical application, f_1 and f_2 become volume (elastic) and flow (resistive) assist settings, respectively. Theoretically, this should produce an ideal relationship between inspiratory effort and gas delivery from the ventilator. When adjusting the volume and flow amplification controls, the clinician is determining the level of unloading regardless of patient volume or flow requirements. That is, if the ventilator is set to unload patient effort at the 50% level, all breaths are unloaded at this level regardless of volume or inspiratory flow rate. This mode is equivalent to PSV in a number of settings[86–89] and can support patients during exercise.

FIGURE 3-37 Bilevel pressure ventilation with pressure support applied to breaths at both the high and low CPAP levels.

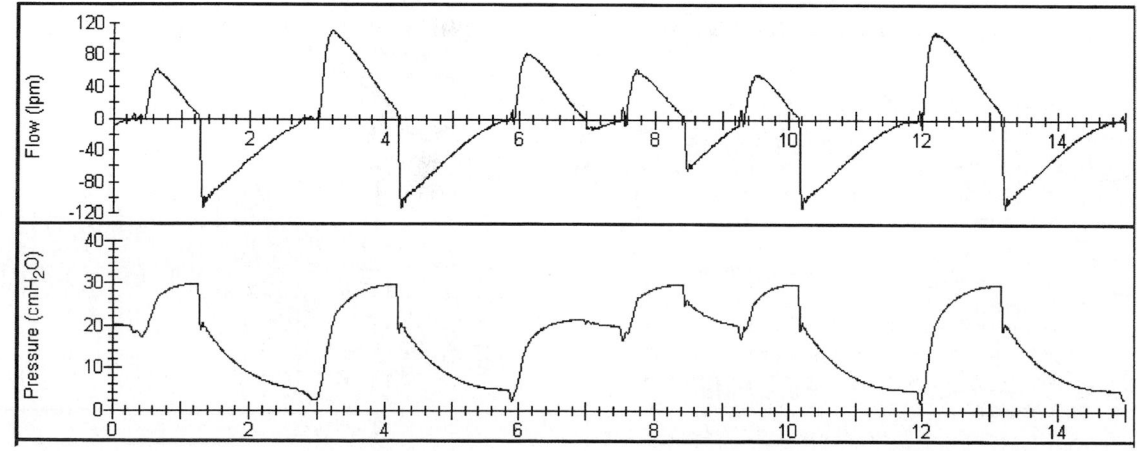

TABLE 3-7 Mechanisms Cycling Pressure Support in All Ventilators

- Primary cycling mechanism: a decrease in inspiratory flow to a specific percentage of peak flow, usually 25%. This is adjustable on some ventilators.
- Secondary cycling mechanism: pressure exceeding target by a specific level (i.e., 3 cmH$_2$O) after inspiratory time has exceeded a manufacturer-specific period.
- Tertiary cycling mechanism: inspiratory time exceeding a manufacturer-specific period, usually about 2–3 seconds.

BiPAP

BiPAP is a manufacturer-established term (Respironics) defining the noninvasive application of positive-pressure ventilation.[90] This mode is designed specifically to provide partial ventilator support. It is the same as PSV with PEEP or PCV with PEEP.[91] This mode is available on specific ventilators designed to provide noninvasive ventilation. A pressure-controlling valve maintains pressure at one of two levels, PEEP (the expiratory positive airway pressure, EPAP) and pressure support (the inspiratory positive airway pressure level, IPAP). These devices and this mode have been used extensively to manage various pathophysiologies with positive pressure noninvasively (see Chap. 4 for details).[91–96]

MANDATORY MINUTE VENTILATION (MMV)

This was the first mode of ventilation in which the ventilator changed gas delivery based on patient response or the first mode considered to constitute computerized control of ventilation. Patients were allowed to breathe spontaneously, but the ventilator ensured a minimum level of

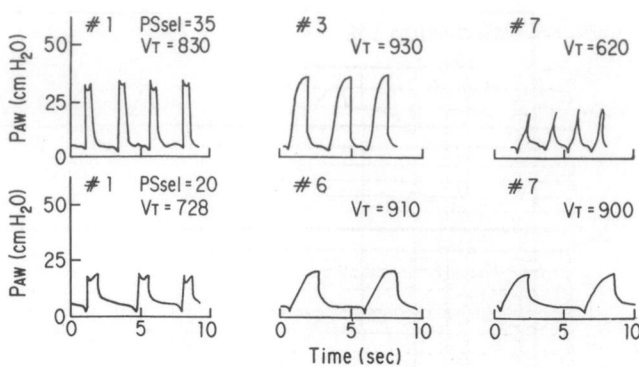

FIGURE 3-39 Examples of airway pressure tracings in two patients with different initial peak flows during pressure support (PS). Initial PS flows are expressed as one of seven discrete settings ranging from maximal (1) to minimal (7). For these two patients, maximal, optimal, and minimal initial PS flow settings are depicted. In the top panels, the optimal initial PS flow setting for this patient was the third fastest (3). Note that the attained pressure and tidal volume (V$_T$) appeared highest and the inspiratory time (T$_I$) longest at the optimal initial PS flow setting. In the bottom panels, the optimal initial PS flow setting for this patient was the second slowest (6). Again note that the attained pressure and V$_T$ appeared highest and the T$_I$ longest at the optimal initial PS flow setting. (*Used, with permission, from MacIntyre et al: Chest 99:134–8, 1991.*)

FIGURE 3-40 Recordings of flow, airway pressure (Paw), and transversus abdominis EMG in a critically ill patient with COPD receiving pressure support of 20 cmH$_2$O. The onset of expiratory muscle activity (*vertical dotted line*) occurred when mechanical inflation was only partly completed. Note the spike in airway pressure at the end of the breath coinciding with the activation of the transversus abdominis muscle. (*Used, with permission, from Parathasarathy et al: Am J Respir Crit Care Med 158:1471–8, 1998.*)

FIGURE 3-38 Effect of changing inspiratory rise time in a patient preferring a midrange flow. *A.* Flow is in excess of patient demand, and a pressure spike is seen. *B.* As flow rate is decreased, inspiratory time (T$_I$) lengthens, and the pressure spike is absent. Machine output matches patient demand. *C.* When flow rate is further reduced patient demand exceeds machine flow rate, and T$_I$ falls. Deformation of the pressure waveform during the rise to the set PSV level is also seen in *C.* (*Used, with permission, from Campbell et al: Respir Care 38:526–37, 1993.*)

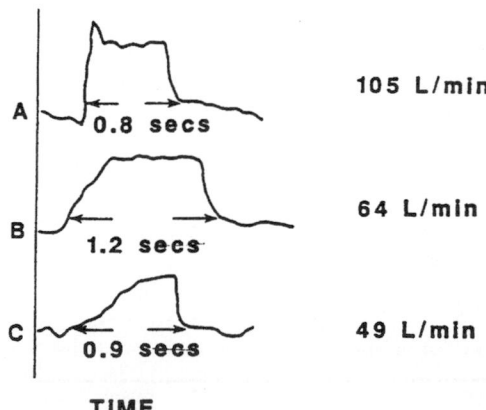

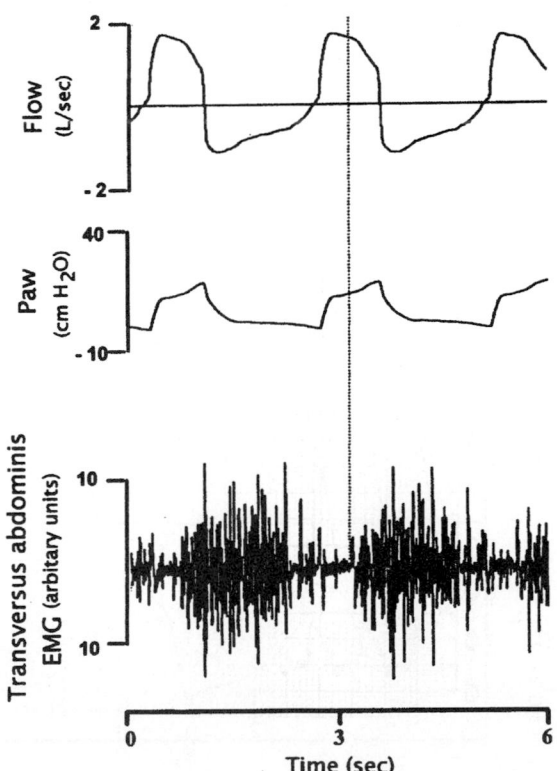

Termination Criterion 5%

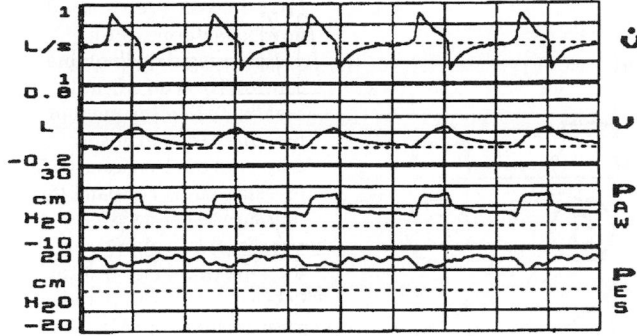

Termination Criterion 45%

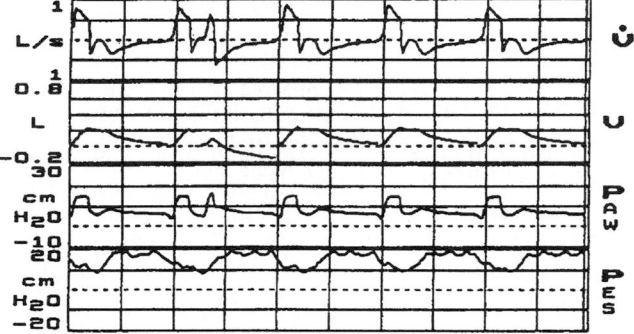

FIGURE 3-41 Flow ($\dot{V}$), volume (V), airway pressure (Paw), and esophageal pressure (Pes) curves with termination criterion (TC) 5% and 45% during 10 cmH$_2$O of pressure-support ventilation. With TC 5%, inspiratory flow terminated simultaneously with the cessation of the patient's inspiratory effort estimated by Pes. In contrast, premature termination with double breathing occurred with TC 45%. Work of breathing also increased from 0.42 J/liter with TC 5% to 0.64 J/liter with TC 45%. (*Used, with permission, from Tokiaka et al: Anesth Analg 92:161–5, 2001.*)

clinician-determined ventilation.[97–100] With MMV, the ventilator monitors the patient's minute ventilation, and the amount of ventilator support provided is adjusted automatically to compensate for fluctuations in the level of spontaneous breathing. The assurance of a preset level of ventilation can be achieved either by increasing the tidal volume or by increasing the frequency of mandatory breath delivery. That is, the ventilator is allowed to alter gas delivery based on feedback from the patient. Although many of the models used to achieve MMV were crude, they opened the door to more sophisticated approaches to closed-loop ventilation. The major problem with MMV was that the ventilator made adjustments based only on minute ventilation. In other words, the ventilator did not distinguish between a tidal volume of 0.6 liter with a rate of 10 breaths per minute and a tidal volume of 0.15 liter and a rate of 40 breaths per minute. The Drager Evita 4 is the only current-generation ventilator that includes this mode.

PRESSURE-REGULATED VOLUME CONTROL (PRVC)

This mode is a form of closed-loop ventilation that has combined the features of volume and pressure ventilation (Fig. 3-43). In essence, the clinician sets a target tidal volume and maximum pressure level. The ventilator attempts to achieve the volume target using a pressure-control gas-delivery format at the lowest possible airway pressure.[101] When activated, the first delivered breath is a test breath at some minimal pressure level (5–10 cmH$_2$O), which is used to calculate patient compliance. The next few breaths may be delivered at a pressure below the calculated pressure needed to deliver the target tidal volume as a further test. After this, the calculated pressure is applied. If the target volume is exceeded, the pressure limit is decreased by 1–3 cmH$_2$O on each breath until the target tidal volume is reached. Similarly, if the volume is low, pressure is increased by 1–3 cmH$_2$O on each breath until the target is met. Of concern with this approach is the potential for an inappropriate decrease in delivered airway pressure when the patient's inspiratory demand is increased as a result of increased

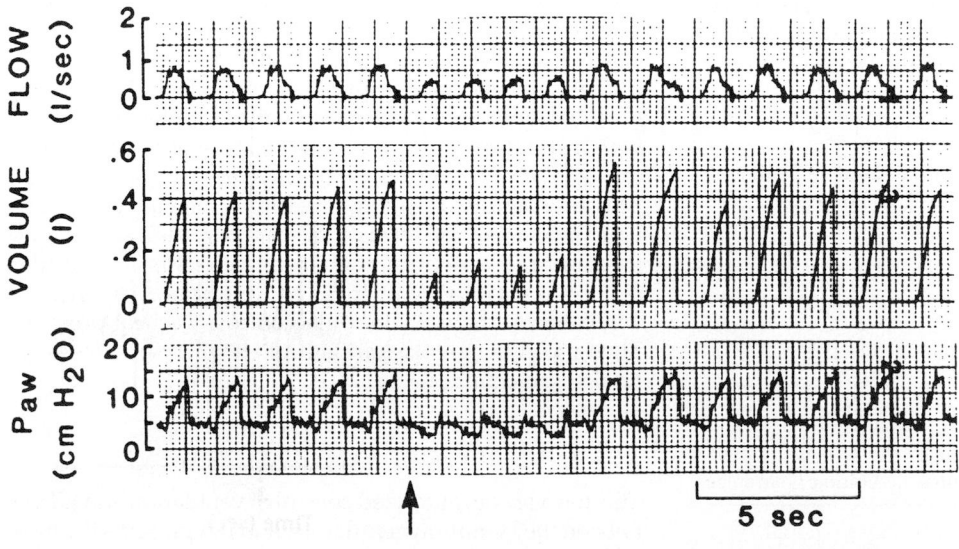

FIGURE 3-42 Airway pressure (Paw), volume, and flow during proportional-assist ventilation and during spontaneous breathing (*arrow*). Note the variation in both pressure and volume on a breath-to-breath basis. (*Used, with permission, from Younes et al: Am Rev Respir Dis 145:114–20, 1992.*)

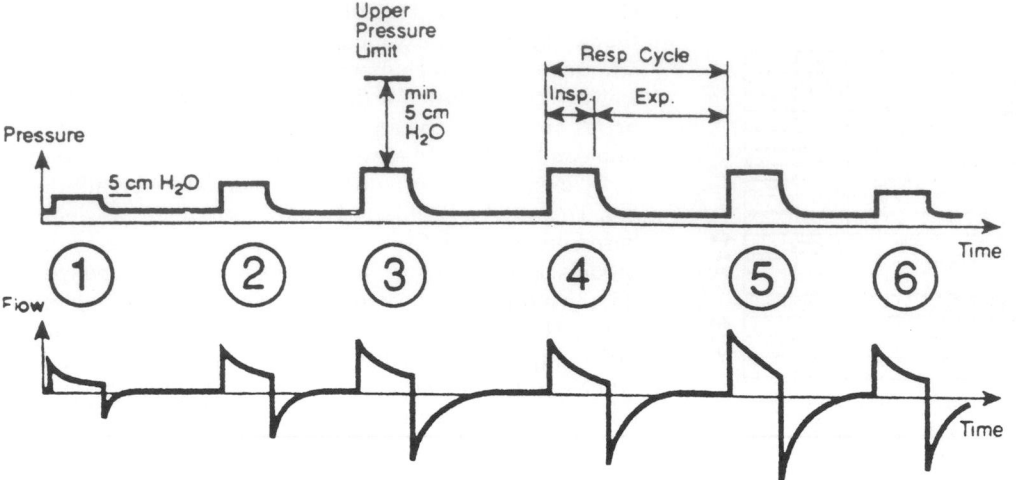

FIGURE 3-43 Pressure and flow waveforms during pressure-regulated volume control: (1) 5 cmH$_2$O test breath; (2, 3) adjustment of pressure target to ensure delivered tidal volume; (4, 5) pressure target constant; (6) pressure target decreased because tidal volume is higher than the target (see text for details). Used with permision: Product literature Maquet Servo I Ventilator, users manual US version No. 66-00-261-E313E Solna, Sweden 2004.)

stress (e.g., hypoxemia, increased temperature, pain, anxiety). That is, ventilator support can be decreased inappropriately in the presence of an increase in ventilatory demand if the increased demand increases tidal volume. This mode is currently available on numerous ventilators by different names (Table 3-8).

VOLUME SUPPORT (VS)

This mode of ventilation is similar to PRVC. It combines volume-targeted ventilation with pressure support in spontaneously breathing patients (Fig. 3-44). Similar to PRVC, it performs an initial test breath (low pressure) to calculate compliance and then administers additional test breaths at a higher pressure before going to the calculated pressure.[101] The inspiratory pressure is controlled automatically between PEEP and the set upper pressure limit. The patient has control of the inspiratory phase as in pressure support, whereas with PRVC, inspiratory time, I:E ratio, and rate are set. If a patient's rate drops below the apneic alarm threshold during volume support, some ventilators switch automatically to PRVC ventilation. Similar concerns as with PRVC regarding patients with strong ventilatory drives and large tidal volume should be exercised. See Table 3-8 for select ventilators in which this mode is available.

TABLE 3-8 Terms Used by Various Manufacturers to Define Pressure-Regulated Volume Control (PRVC) or Volume-Support Modes (VS)

Ventilator	PRVC	VS
Servo 300	PRVC	VS
Servo I	PRVC	VS
Drager Evita	Autoflow	NA[a]
Viasys Vvea	PRVC	NA
e-Vent	PRVC	VS
Datex-Ohmeda	Volume Guarantee	NA
Drager Badylog	Volume Guarantee	Volume Guarantee

[a]NA, not available.

VOLUME-ASSURED PRESSURE SUPPORT (VAPS)

VAPS also combines the benefits of pressure and volume ventilation.[102,103] The clinician sets a pressure-support level, a peak flow, and a tidal volume. If patient demand is high relative to the peak flow and tidal volume settings, VAPS functions similar to PSV but guarantees a minimum tidal volume delivery (Fig. 3-45).[104] If patient demand is low, however, gas is delivered as a typical ACV breath. This approach to closed-loop ventilation was available on the Bird 8400 and Bear 1000 ventilators but is not available on any of the newest-generation ventilators.

AUTOMATIC TUBE COMPENSATION (ATC)

This mode of ventilation is similar to the flow assist of PAV except that it is designed to maintain tracheal pressure at baseline (PEEP level) during both inspiration and expiration. Data from Guttman et al[105] demonstrated that if the resistance properties of the artificial airway were programmed into a ventilator, the ventilator would be able to calculate tracheal pressure if flow could be measured continuously (which is done by all ventilators) (Fig. 3-46). With activation of this mode, the type and size of the airway must be programmed into the ventilator, as well as the percent of ATC to be applied (100% versus lower percentages). In addition, some ventilators apply ATC only during inspiration (i.e., Puritan-Bennett 840); others allow application during both inspiration and expiration (i.e., Drager Evita). Expiratory ATC is of concern because it applies a negative airway pressure, rapidly dropping pressure in the lung and potentially increasing the level of air trapping. ATC seems most useful in the patient with a strong ventilatory drive (Fig. 3-47).[106] As with PAV, there is no control over any normal ventilatory variable. ATC only controls tracheal pressure. Thus patients may assume a rapid-shallow or slow-large tidal volume pattern.

ADAPTIVE-SUPPORT VENTILATION (ASV)

This form of computerized control of ventilation is available only on the Hamilton ventilators, and it represents the most

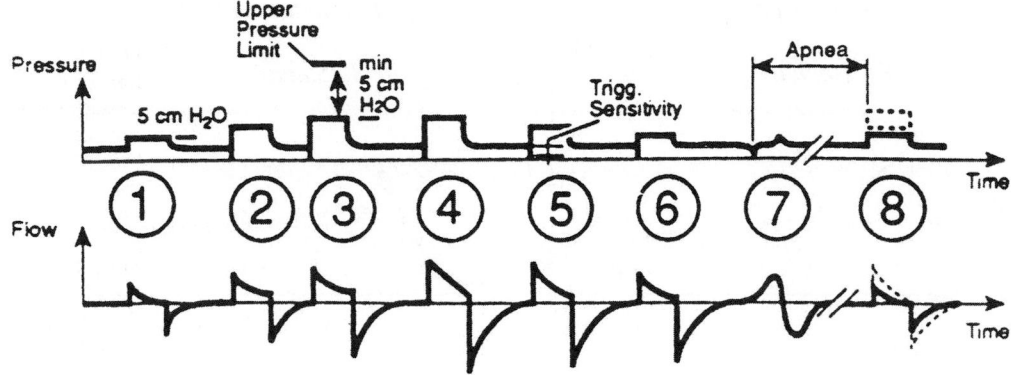

FIGURE 3-44 Pressure and flow waveforms during volume support: (1) test breath; (2–5) adjustment of pressure target to ensure delivered tidal volume; (5, 6) pressure limit decreased to maintain tidal volume at target level; (7) period of apneic ventilation; (8) ventilator switches to pressure-regulated control mode. Used with permision: Product literature Maquet Servo I Ventilator, users manual US version No. 66-00-261-E313E Solna, Sweden 2004.

sophisticated form of computerized control of ventilation available. This mode is designed to establish a ventilatory pattern that results in the least work of breathing based on the original data of Otis,[107] where work of breathing is related to compliance and resistance. That is, if compliance is decreased, a rapid-shallow pattern results in the least work of breathing. Conversely, if resistance is increased, a slow rate with a large tidal volume results in the least work of breathing. The patient's weight and the percent of ideal tidal volume (25–350%) to be delivered must be programmed. The ventilator uses these data as well as measure-

ment of the patient's dynamic compliance and expiratory time constant to determine the ideal ventilatory pattern. A tidal volume versus rate curve for the minute volume selected is determined, as well as high and low limits on the rate and tidal volume. In addition, a target zone of rate and tidal volume is established (Fig. 3-48). If the patient moves outside the defined zone, specific adjustments of airway pressure and rate are established to force the ventilatory pattern into the target zone (Fig. 3-49). As with many of these new modes, gas delivery is based on a pressure-target delivery pattern. Depending on the relationship between a patient's actual rate and the ideal ventilatory rate, ventilation can change between assisted and controlled ventilation. ASV also can be active in SIMV. Currently, ASV is not available in the United States. It is called *adaptive tidal volume ventilation*, where the ventilator provides the clinician with the adjustments needed, but the clinician must make

FIGURE 3-45 The possible breath types during volume-assured pressure support (VAPS). In breath *A*, the set tidal volume and delivered tidal volume are equal. This is a pressure-support breath (patient triggered, pressure limited, and flow cycled). Breath *B* represents a reduction in patient effort. As flow decelerates, the ventilator determines that delivered tidal volume will be less than the minimum set volume. At the shaded portion of the graph, the breath changes from a pressure- to a volume-limited (constant-flow) breath. Breath *C* demonstrates a worsening of compliance and the possibility of extending inspiratory time to ensure the minimum tidal volume delivery. Breath *D* represents a pressure-support breath in which the tidal volume is greater than the set tidal volume. This kind of breath allowed during VAPS may aid in reducing work of breathing and dyspnea. (*Used, with permission, from Branson et al: Respir Clin North Am 7:397–408, 2001.*)

FIGURE 3-46 Volume-pressure diagram in a tracheally intubated patient during spontaneous breathing with inspiratory pressure support (PEEP = 5 cmH$_2$O, pressure support = 5 cmH$_2$O). The pressure drop across the endotracheal tube (ETT) (ΔP_{ETT}) is indicated during both inspiration and expiration by a broken arrow. The direction of the arrow points from airway pressure to tracheal pressure. (*Used, with permission, Guttman et al: Anes 79:503–13, 1993.*)

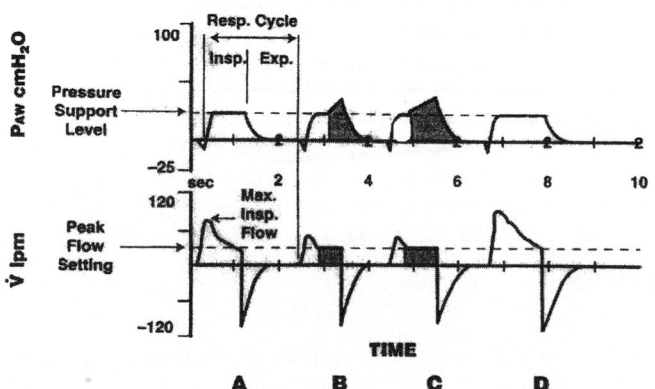

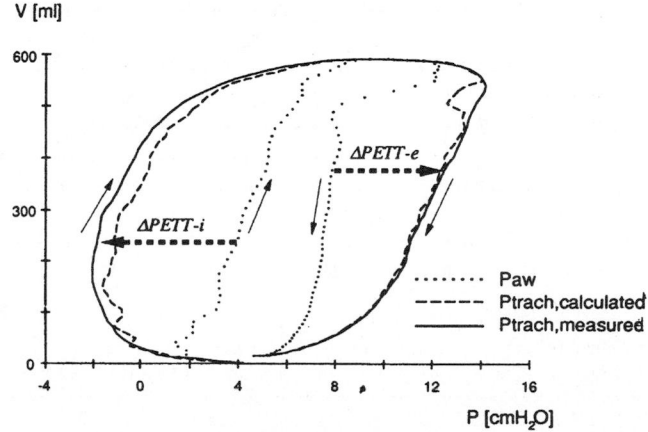

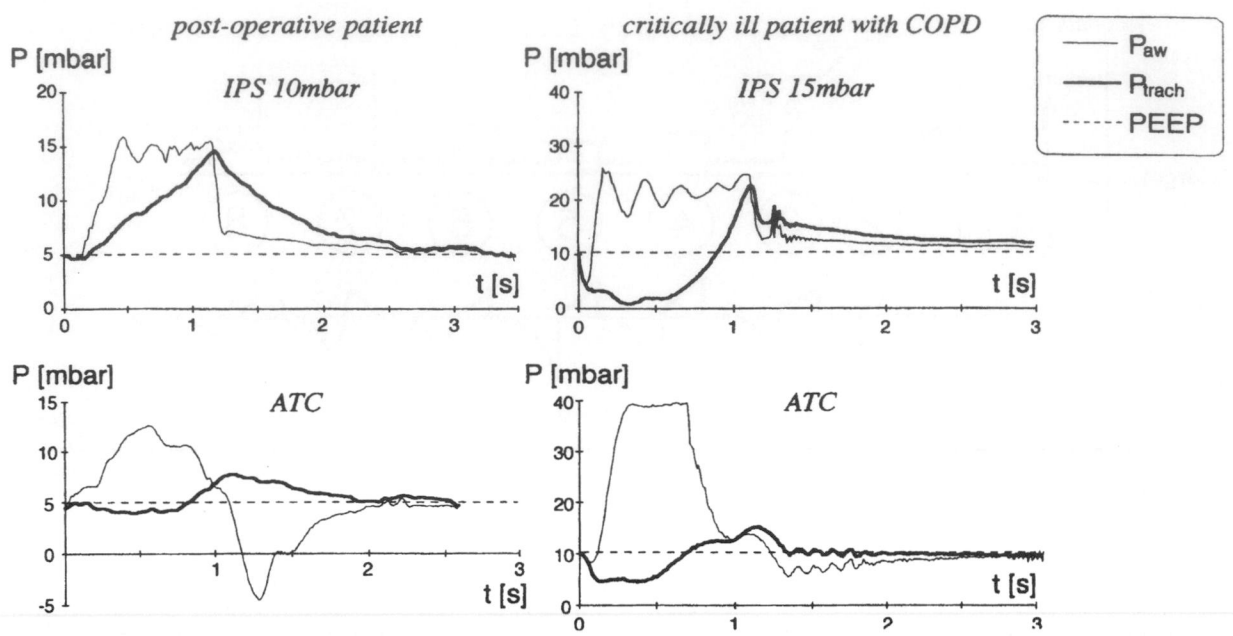

FIGURE 3-47 Airway pressure and tracheal pressure curves during pressure support (IPS) (*top*) and automatic tube compensation (ATC) (*bottom*) in a patient after open-heart surgery (*left*) and a critically ill patient with chronic obstructive pulmonary disease COPD (*right*). Note that although the ventilator lowers Paw during expiration to subatmospheric pressure (*bottom left*), controlling the expiratory valve ensures that Ptrach is above or equal to PEEP. The patient with acute respiratory insufficiency during ATC generates an inspiratory gas flow of greater than 2 liters/s (*bottom right*), which accounts for part of the deviation between P_{trach} and PEEP. (*Used, with permission, from Fabry et al: Intensive Care Med 23:545–52, 1997.*)

FIGURE 3-48 Graphic depicting target ventilatory pattern during adaptive-support ventilation (15 breaths per minute with a 535-ml tidal volume). In addition, the respiratory rate versus tidal volume curve for the specific minute ventilation chosen is illustrated. The dotted-line box indicates the limits of rate and tidal volume. (*Used, with permission, from Campbell et al: Respir Clin North Am 9:425–40, 2001.*)

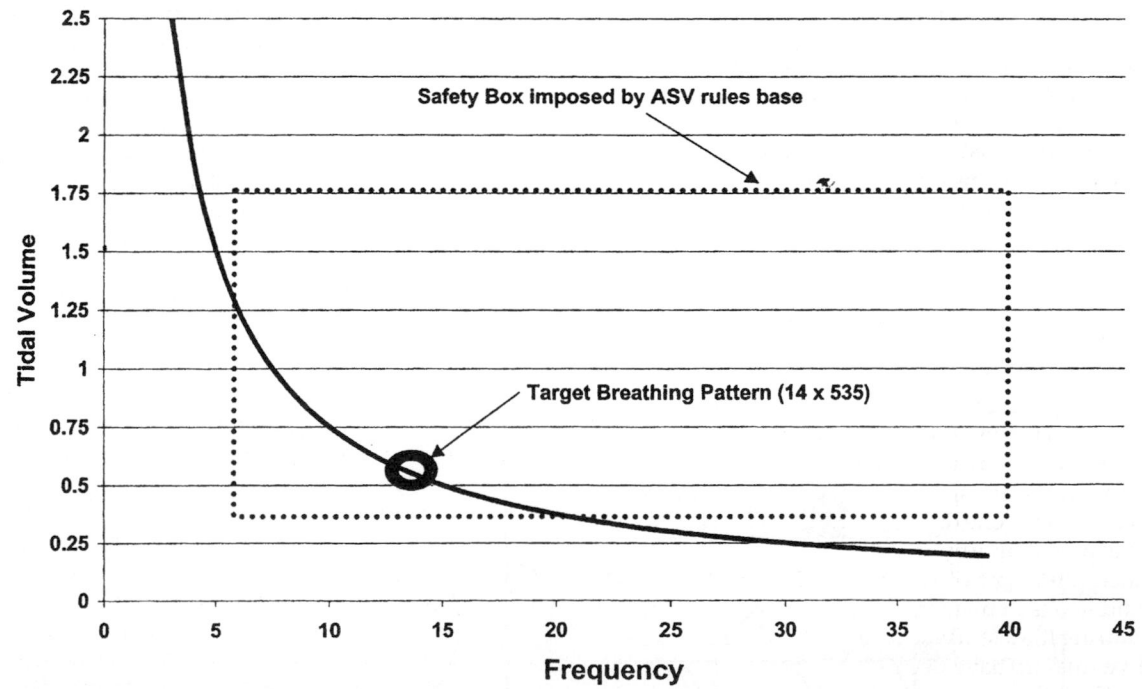

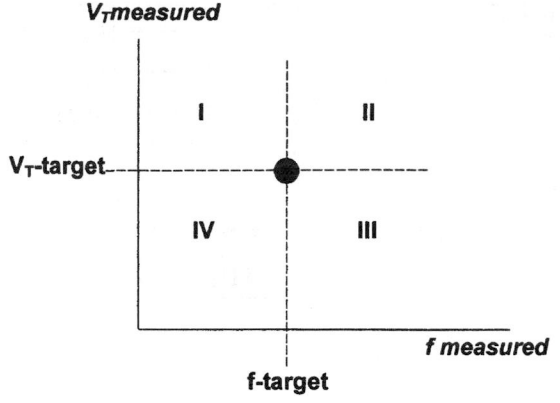

Quadr.	P$_{Insp}$	mand.rate
I	−	+
II	−	−
III	+	−
IV	+	+

FIGURE 3-49 Algorithm used to dictate adaptive-support ventilation response to changing patient effort and lung mechanics in order to maintain the target breathing pattern. (*Used, with permission, from Campbell et al: Respir Clin North Am 9:425–40, 2001.*)

the adjustment himself or herself. Limited data are available defining the efficacy of this mode of ventilation.[108,109]

NONINVASIVE VENTILATION (NIV)

A number of ICU ventilators designed essentially to provide invasive ventilation (via an artificial airway) also include modes that make noninvasive ventilation via a facemask easier. The primary adjustment made automatically by the ventilator is leak compensation. In addition, a number of alarm functions (i.e., low tidal volume) are modified to reduce the number of false-positive alarms.

Adults, Pediatric Patients, and Neonates

An increasing number of the newest-generation ICU ventilators are being designed for use across all age groups: adults, pediatric patients, and neonates. That is, as a result of microprocessor design, ranges and delivery rates can be altered to accommodate specific-sized patients. The same ventilator can be used one day on an adult and the next day on a 500-g neonate simply by selecting the correct size range. With the increasing cost of ICU ventilators and the small pediatric and neonatal market, one can expect this trend to continue. During the last 10 years, more than 10 adult or all-age-range ventilators have been introduced to the market worldwide. Over the same period, no new neonatal ventilator entered the market.

Patient Management Assistance Algorithms

A number of companies have included slow-flow pressure-volume (P-V) curve algorithms that identify the upper and lower inflection points. One company (Hamilton) also allows construction of the deflation limb of the P-V curve. The open-lung approach algorithm on the Maquet Servo i assists the clinician in performing lung recruitment maneuvers and the performance of a decremental PEEP trial. Volume and pressure changes during these procedures are identified carefully for the clinician. It is expected that such algorithms will be more widely available on ventilators as the ability to define precise ventilator management improves in the future.

Ventilator Triggering

The interaction of a patient with a ventilator occurs essentially under two settings: The ventilator delivers a controlled breath, regardless of the patient's desire; or delivery of ventilator support can be coordinated with patient effort. Over the last 25 years, increasing emphasis has been placed on ensuring patient synchrony with the ventilator. If the ventilator is to function in synchrony with the patient, it must respond rapidly to patient inspiratory effort without imposing considerable work or effort.

SITE OF TRIGGER

With perfect patient-ventilator interaction, the ventilator would trigger in synchrony with electrical impulses originating in the central nervous system. Work is currently being done experimentally to evaluate the feasibility of neurally adjusted ventilatory assist (NAVA).[110,111] Ventilator triggering from diaphragmatic electromyographic (EMG) signals, however, is not currently available clinically. The greater the distance from the diaphragm that the ventilator senses patient inspiratory effort, the greater is the potential for dyssynchrony or an increase in patient effort necessary to trigger the ventilator.

The next logical site for ventilator triggering is the trachea. Pressure changes in the trachea are more directly reflective of intrapleural pressure changes than pressures measured in the ventilator circuit; triggering based on tracheal pressure results in marked decreases in imposed work of breathing when compared with triggering from pressure changes within the ventilator circuit.[112–114] The primary reason for these differences is the resistance to gas flow caused by the endotracheal tube.[115–117] The endotracheal tube is a nonlinear resistor. Thus the decrease in work produced by ventilator triggering via sensors located in the trachea versus in the ventilator circuit is magnified by a decrease in the size of the endotracheal tube and an increase in ventilator drive.[117]

Banner et al,[112] using a lung model, clearly demonstrated the beneficial effects of ventilator triggering from the

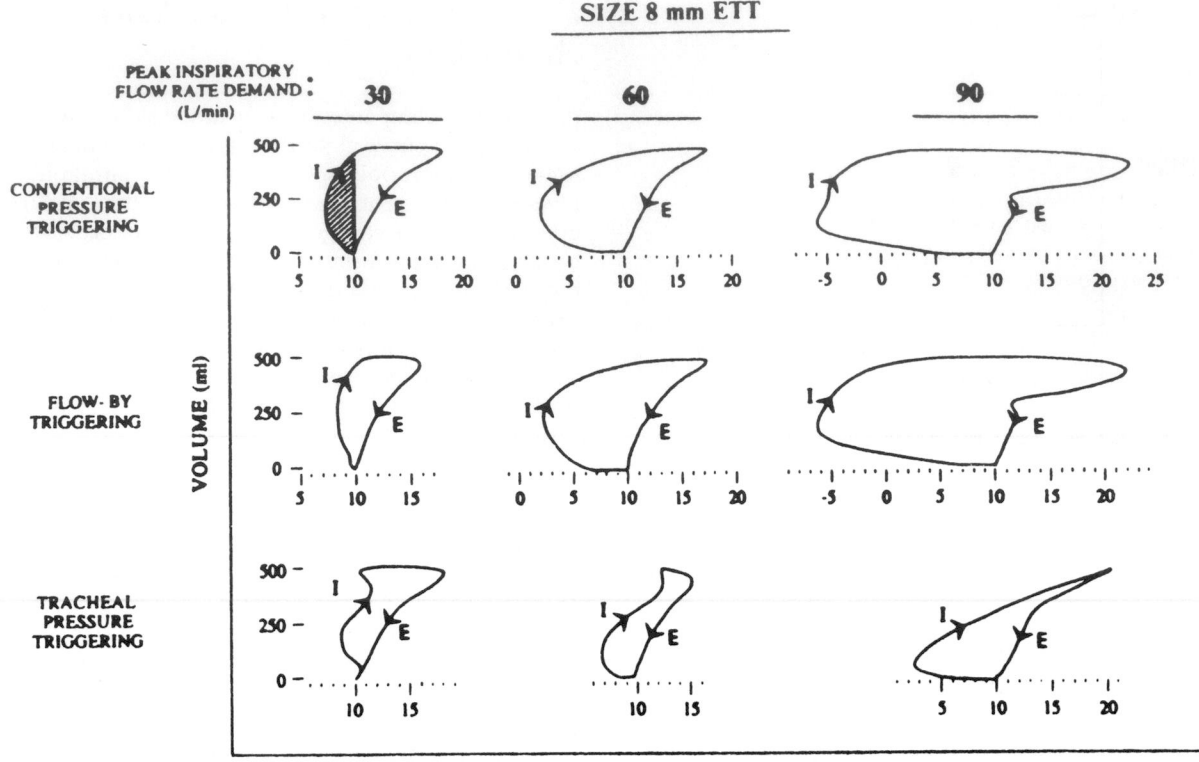

FIGURE 3-50 Pressure-volume (imposed work) loops during spontaneous inhalation (I) and exhalation (E) with continuous positive airway pressure (10 cmH$_2$O) via an 8-mm internal-diameter endotracheal tube (ETT) at peak inspiratory flow rates of 30, 60, and 90 liters/min during conventional pressure triggering, flow (flow-by) triggering, and tracheal triggering. The shaded area circumscribed within the inspiratory portion of the loops is the inspiratory imposed work of breathing. Note that imposed work increased with peak inspiratory flow and always was least with tracheal triggering. (*Used, with permission, from Banner et al: Crit Care Med 21:183–90, 1993.*)

tracheal site. They compared imposed work of breathing calculated from pressures measured within the trachea during conventional pressure triggering, flow triggering, and triggering from pressure measured in the trachea. The effects of endotracheal tube sizes of 6, 7, 8, and 9 mm, as well as flows of 30, 60, and 90 liters/min, were evaluated. As expected, imposed work with all methods of triggering increased with increased peak inspiratory flow and narrower endotracheal tubes but always was lowest with tracheal triggering (Fig. 3-50).

Although the trachea appears to be the optional site for the trigger signal in lung models, practical problems have prevented ventilator manufacturers from using this site. Tracheal pressure triggering or pressure monitoring is unlikely to become an everyday clinical reality until a highly durable and inexpensive means of measuring signals at this site is developed.

Presently, all mechanical ventilators trigger from signals measured within the ventilator circuit. The particular point of measurement, however, as well as the precise signal, varies. The trigger signal can be sensed at the proximal endotracheal tube, in the inspiratory limb, and in the expiratory limb of the circuit, and the signal can be either pressure or flow (Table 3-9).[118] The ventilator must be able to appropriately sense patient effort yet not trigger in response to artifact (autocycling).

Both magnitude of pressure change and delay in trigger activation are important in relation to triggering. *Magnitude* is the amount of patient effort required and should be as small as possible. *Delay* is the time between the initiation of patient effort and the beginning of flow from the ventilator and should be as short as possible. Trigger delay is also related to the pneumatics and electronics of the ventilator system.

PRESSURE TRIGGERING

All ventilators in use today that trigger inspiration from a pressure signal do so from a signal measured within the ventilator circuit. The exact point of measurement may be the patient Y (proximal endotracheal tube) or internal to the ventilator on either the inspiratory or expiratory side of the circuit. Measurement of airway pressure at the proximal airway differs from pressure measured inside the ventilator because of resistance to gas flow created by the ventilator circuit, humidifier, and exhalation valve.[113]

The primary technical concern with triggering from a pressure signal at the circuit Y is water accumulation in the pressure-sensing line. This dampens the pressure signal and results in increased patient effort to trigger. Even if filters and water traps are placed in the pressure-sensing line,

TABLE 3-9 Advantages and Disadvantages of the Different Circuit Pressure-Sensing Sites

Advantages	Disadvantages
A. Exhalation port: Well protected from mechanical abuse. During mechanical inhalation, accurately reads pressure at the Y. During inhalation, increases in inspiratory or expiratory circuit resistance do not compromise inspiratory flow output, except for many-fold increases.	Requires protection from moisture of exhaled gas. During spontaneous inspiration, underestimates pressure generated at the Y to trigger the ventilator. During exhalation, underestimates pressure at the Y. During exhalation, increases in expiratory circuit resistance compromise expiratory flow. Hence system requires well-maintained expiratory filter to ensure that expiratory circuit resistance remains low.
B. Inhalation port: Well protected from mechanical abuse. Does not require protection from moisture or additional filters. During exhalation, accurately reads pressure at the Y as long as the inspiratory circuit remains patient. During inhalation, increases in expiratory circuit resistance do not compromise inspiratory-flow output.	During mechanical inhalation, overestimates pressure at the Y. During spontaneous inspiration, underestimates pressure generated at the Y to trigger the ventilator. During inhalation, increases in inspiratory circuit resistance compromise inspiratory flow output. For example, factors such as selection of humidifier and type of patient circuit yield varying patient inspiratory efforts for fixed ventilator settings.
C. Patient Y: During inhalation and exhalation, accurately reads both inspiratory and expiratory pressures. Pressure readings reflect relative condition of inspiratory and expiratory circuits.	Susceptible to mechanical abuse. Requires a separate pressure-sensing tube, which is prone to occlusion, blockage, and disconnection, all of which prevent sensing of patient effort.

SOURCE: Modified, with permission, from Sassoon. [118]

as they fill with water, patient effort is increased. Pressure sensing internal to the ventilator, on either the inspiratory or expiratory side, is also affected by accumulation of water in the ventilator tubing. This either dampens the signal or results in premature cycling. Stationary water that partially occludes the circuit increases patient effort to trigger. If, however, the water is moving to and fro in the circuit because of high system flow, subbaseline pressure can be developed, causing self-cycling. If the pressure signal is sensed internally on the inspiratory side of the circuit, a bubble-through humidifier should not be used because the patient is required to create a pressure gradient across the water to trigger the ventilator.

As described by Sassoon,[119] a number of factors affect the delay time during pressure triggering. These include errors caused by the speed of the pressure signal, errors caused by digital sampling of the transducer, errors in the pressure-transducing circuit, discrepancies in the set and actual PEEP, and circuit noise.

FLOW TRIGGERING

Most ventilators now allow triggering from a flow signal. Based on imposed work of breathing data, it appears that flow triggering is slightly more efficient than pressure triggering,[56,120] although this does not appear to be a clinical concern if the pressure trigger is set appropriately.[120]

Two technical approaches to flow triggering have emerged. In one, a bias flow is established during the ex-

piratory phase, with triggering occurring when the difference between flow entering and exiting the circuit equals the trigger sensitivity. The other approach is the measurement of flow at the airway by use of a pneumotachometer or hot-wire anemometer.

The major problem with the measurement of flow at the airway and use of this signal for triggering is the accumulation of water and debris on the flow-measuring device. Flow-measuring devices kept at the airway must be changed or cleaned frequently to ensure their optimal function. A potential problem with all flow-triggering mechanisms is system leaks, which are recognized as patient effort. Another potential problem with flow and pressure triggering occurs when uncuffed airways are used. With both flow and pressure triggering, the ventilator should be set at the most sensitive level that avoids self-triggering.

Exhalation Valves

Gas exiting the patient's airway normally travels past the Y connector of the system through a length (about 60 in) of large-bore tubing (22-mm internal diameter), past a filter (in some ventilators), through a flow sensor and a check valve (in some ventilators), and then through the exhalation valve itself. All these components of the expiratory system affect the ability of the system to operate appropriately in accomplishing the following goals: (1) sealing the circuit during inspiration, (2) cycling to exhalation, (3) maintaining the desired PEEP/CPAP level, and (4) minimizing the imposed work of breathing.[4]

A number of different physical designs have been used in the expiratory valving mechanism. The most common of these have been the mushroom and diaphragm types of valves. All disposable exhalation valves used on home care and transport ventilators, as well as some ICU ventilators, are either mushroom or diaphragm valves. In addition, many of the newest ICU ventilators still use these valves. The newest-generation ventilators, however, frequently locate the valve internally within a heated compartment, eliminating the need for changing the valve between patients and enhancing microprocessor control of the valve. In addition, scissors valves and electromagnetic and electronic valves are used as exhalation valves.

MUSHROOM/DIAPHRAGM VALVES

These two types of valves, although slightly different, function physically in a very similar manner. A typical mushroom-type exhalation valve is depicted in Fig. 3-51. In most ventilators, gas is either diverted from the inspiratory limb internal to the ventilator or from a secondary gas-control module to the exhalation valve to inflate the mushroom-shaped balloon and occlude the exhalation port during the inspiratory phase.[121] Because these exhalation valve charging lines are internal to the ventilator and before the system humidifier, the pressure affecting the exha-

lation valve is always higher than the pressure exerted on the airway. Thus leaks through the exhalation valve are very uncommon.

In earlier ventilators, inflation and deflation of the balloon were controlled simply by changes in system pressure. With current-generation ventilators, however, the pressure inflating or deflating the valve is under microprocessor control. In most mechanical ventilators, a pressure transducer is placed just before the exhalation valve to provide feedback via the microprocessor to the inspiratory flow control to maintain sufficient flow to establish the set PEEP. If the PEEP level should fall, this feedback loop increases system flow. As noted in Fig. 3-51, the expiratory gas flow route through many of these valves is rather tortuous, and as a result, expiratory flow is retarded. That is, because of the resistance to gas flow through the valving device and the expiratory circuit, system pressure does not drop to baseline immediately when the expiratory phase begins but requires time to return to baseline.[122–125] With most of the newest ventilator systems, it takes about 0.3–0.5 second for complete passive decompression of the ventilator circuit.[4] If expiratory gas flow is high, or if the patient coughs, high system pressures may be developed.[122,125]

Diaphragm-type exhalation valves (Fig. 3-52) function in exactly the same manner as mushroom-type valves.[126] Gas from the inspiratory limb compresses the diaphragm and closes the valve during inspiration. The valve opens when the inspiratory phase ends and the recoil pressure of the patient-ventilator system exceeds that of the valve. The opening of both mushroom and diaphragm valves is also delayed by the time necessary for gas pressurizing the valve to be evacuated.

SCISSORS VALVES

The prototype for this expiratory valve is the Servo ventilators (e.g., 900 and 300 series). As crudely illustrated in Fig. 3-53, these valves function by compression and

FIGURE 3-51 Schematic representation of balloon-type exhalation valves under varying conditions of pressure. *A.* Inspiration. *B.* Exhalation without PEEP. *C.* End of exhalation with 10 cmH$_2$O of PEEP. *D.* Active exhalation with 10 cmH$_2$O of PEEP. Restriction to flow is greater with the application of PEEP than if end-expiratory pressure is zero. (*Used, with permission, from Shapiro et al.*[121])

FIGURE 3-52 Diaphragm-type exhalation valve with 10 cmH$_2$O of PEEP. This valve is partially closed during the expiratory phase because of the PEEP. As a result, resistance to gas flow is increased compared with zero end-expiratory pressure. (*Used, with permission, from Kacmarek et al: Anesthesiol Clin North Am 5:757–76, 1987.*)

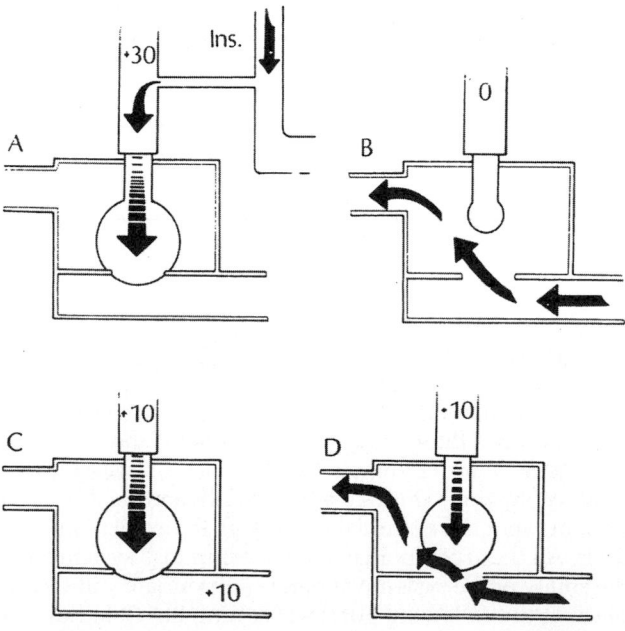

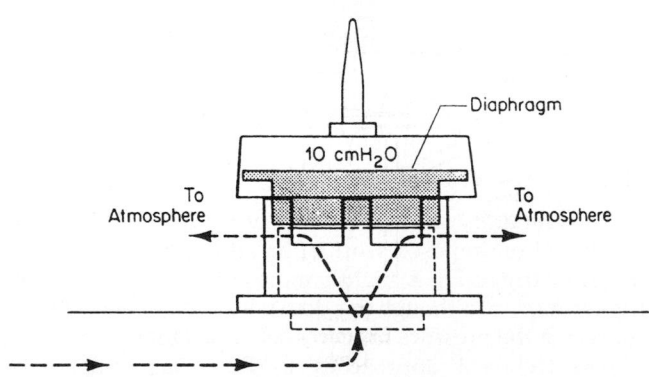

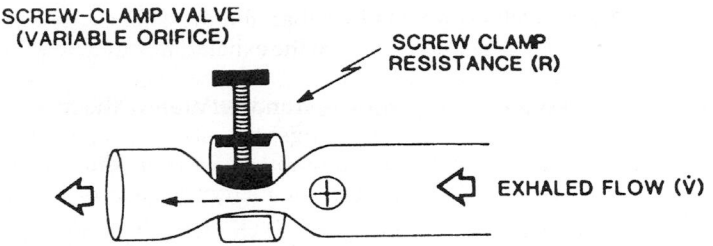

SCREW-CLAMP VALVE
(VARIABLE ORIFICE)

SCREW CLAMP
RESISTANCE (R)

EXHALED FLOW (V̇)

FIGURE 3-53 Crude representation of a scissors-type exhalation/PEEP valve. Because this valve is a variable-orifice flow resistor, resistance to exhalation, as well as the level of PEEP established, depends on the patient's expiratory flow rate. The greater the gas flow, the greater is the retard of exhalation and the greater is the PEEP. (*Used, with permission, from Banner et al: Chest 90:212–7, 1986.*)

relaxation of a silicone tube. Generally, the level of constriction is controlled by a stepper motor.

ELECTROMAGNETIC VALVES

Figure 3-54 depicts the Hamilton exhalation valve, which operates by the electromagnetic positioning of a large-surface-area diaphragm by an actuating shaft. This type of exhalation valve requires microprocessor control. As a result, the resistance to gas flow across this valve is very low even when PEEP/CPAP is applied.[127,128]

ELECTRONIC VALVES

These valves appear and operate in a manner similar to electromagnetic valves (Fig. 3-55). Opening the closure of the valve generally is controlled by a stepper motor under microprocessor control. Thus, as with electromagnetic valves, as long as the surface area across which exhalation occurs is large, resistance to gas flow should be minimized.

MICROPROCESSOR CONTROL

Early exhalation valves functioned in a simple pneumatic manner. When the mechanical inspiratory phase ended,

pressure in the inspiratory limb began to drop, while the recoil of the patient-ventilator system moved gas into the expiratory limb of the circuit. The combined effect of these two phenomena allowed the exhalation valve charging-line pressure to decompress and the valve to open.

Microprocessor control greatly enhances the efficiency of this process by being able to identify precisely when the inspiratory process ends and expiration begins. This is performed easily during all control or assisted breaths in which airway pressure is elevated and where a precise definition of the end of inspiration can be made. Spontaneous unassisted breathing (CPAP) or pressure support are more challenging transitions for the microprocessor to control. In these modes, exhalation becomes a patient-controlled, instead of a ventilator-controlled, event. The microprocessor must identify an elevation of system pressure, a decrease in inspiratory flow demand, or an increase in expiratory flow to establish the onset of expiration. In this setting, microprocessor control is essential.

With most microprocessor-controlled ventilators, there is an intimate linking of the inspiratory and expiratory control systems to ensure that undesirable alterations in system pressure, as during a patient cough, can be controlled.[4] As a result, the valving mechanism for inspiration and expiration can be said to operate in harmony to maximize the reproducibility of the inspiratory and expiratory events. That is, during the inspiratory phase, the exhalation valve is opening and closing to maximize conformance of the inspiratory phase with that programmed. The same process is

FIGURE 3-54 Hamilton ventilator electromagnetic exhalation valve/PEEP device. The exhalation diaphragm is positioned electromagnetically by the actuating shaft. (*Used, with permission, from Kacmarek et al: Anesthesiol Clin North Am 5:757–76, 1987.*)

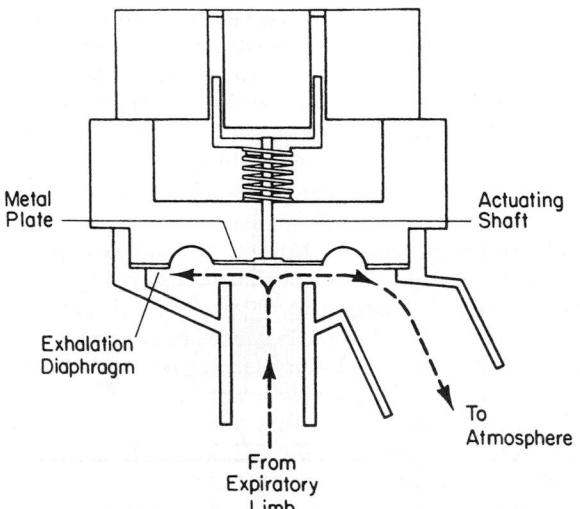

Metal Plate

Actuating Shaft

Exhalation Diaphragm

To Atmosphere

From Expiratory Limb

FIGURE 3-55 The electromechanical exhalation valve of the Bird 8400ST. *A.* The electromechanical driver moves the plunger, seating the exhalation diaphragm. *B.* Gas entry into the valve. *C.* Gas exiting the valve.

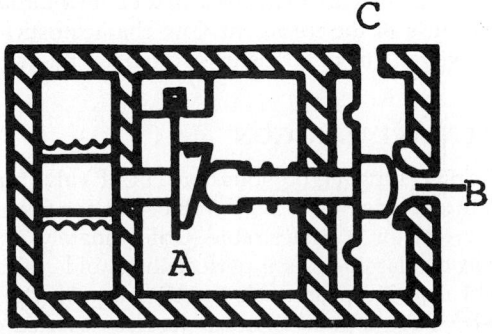

occurring during exhalation to better ensure that the expiratory pressure baseline is maintained.

Establishment of PEEP/CPAP

Since the first description of the use of PEEP in the management of the acute respiratory distress syndrome was published by Ashbaugh and Petty[129] in 1967, numerous approaches have been described for the application of PEEP/CPAP to mechanically ventilated patients, as well as spontaneously breathing patients.[127–130] In general, PEEP devices have been classified historically as one of two types, threshold resistors and orificial (or flow) resistors, based on the mechanisms used to establish PEEP and their effects on resistance to flow.[130]

THRESHOLD RESISTORS

The ideal PEEP valve is a pure threshold resistor, a device that exerts a predictable, quantifiable, and constant force at the expiratory limb outlet of the ventilator or CPAP system.[130] The PEEP level established is proportional to the force (F) applied over the specific surface area (SA):

$$P \propto \frac{F}{SA}$$

That is, a force exceeding the threshold pressure must be developed for gas to flow through the device. Ideally, a threshold resistor maintains a constant force on the system regardless of the gas flow through the device. In fact, PEEP is independent of flow, and no flow is necessary to maintain the PEEP level.

FLOW RESISTORS

The PEEP level established with a flow resistor depends on the flow of gas ($\dot{V}$) through the system and the physical characteristics of the device (resistance R) that affect gas flow. That is, the PEEP level is governed by the law of flow (Ohm's law):

$$P \propto R\dot{V}$$

where P is the expiratory pressure established. For a given R, PEEP increases with an increase in total flow through the valve. Because of the turbulent flow characteristics of the valve, however, this relationship is often not linear.

ACTUAL VALVE FUNCTION

From the preceding it is obvious that a PEEP valve functioning as a threshold resistor is desirable, and one functioning as a flow resistor is undesirable. Unfortunately, no PEEP valve can be classified as a perfect threshold resistor. All threshold resistors possess flow-resistant properties. Banner et al[127] have argued that the pressure exerted during exhalation by any threshold resistor is represented more

appropriately by the following equation:

$$\text{Expiratory pressure} \propto \frac{F}{SA} + R(\dot{V}exh + \dot{V}sys)$$

where SA is surface area, $\dot{V}exh$ is patient-exhaled flow rate, and $\dot{V}sys$ is system flow during exhalation. Based on the evaluation of numerous PEEP devices,[122–128] the preceding relationship more closely predicts the PEEP/CPAP level established by a threshold resistor than the simple F/SA relationship.

PEEP/CPAP IN MICROPROCESSOR SYSTEMS

In all the newest-generation ventilators, PEEP/CPAP is established via the exhalation valve. When baseline pressure is increased, however, the efficiency of exhalation-valve function decreases,[127–128] resulting in greater retardation of exhalation and a prolonged period between peak inspiratory pressure and return to baseline pressure. This inefficiency can be modified by referencing the pressure in the exhalation valve to atmosphere early in the expiratory phase and then gradually referencing it back to the PEEP/CPAP level as expiration continues and system pressure approaches the baseline PEEP/CPAP level.[4] That is, the function of the exhalation valve is under active microprocessor control throughout the entire expiratory period. This active control of exhalation is provided by one of two schemes in all new-generation ventilators (Fig. 3-56): (1) adjustment of the pressure in the air chamber (active pneumatic control) behind the diaphragm (or within the mushroom valve) or (2) manipulation of the diaphragm by a proportional linear solenoid linked either directly or indirectly to the diaphragm.[4]

INTERCHANGEABLE PEEP/CPAP VALVES

In addition to the integrated PEEP systems via the exhalation valves of microprocessor ventilators, numerous disposable/interchangeable PEEP/CPAP devices are available for use on older-generation ICU ventilators, as well as home care, transport, and manual ventilators and free-standing CPAP systems. Most of these devices are either spring-loaded (Fig. 3-57) or magnetic valves (Fig. 3-58). All these devices function as combined threshold/flow resistors, exhibiting greater or lesser flow-resistant properties.[131] As a result, expiratory pressure during CPAP can be expected to increase 2–3 cmH$_2$O,[131] and the time for return of peak inspiratory pressure to baseline during mechanical ventilation is also lengthened. In addition, because of mass production of these devices and their flow-resistant properties, indicated and actual PEEP/CPAP levels established may differ by 3–4 cmH$_2$O.[131] Thus it is necessary to measure actual system PEEP level during the use of these devices. Finally, as a result of the marked flow-resistant properties of these valves, they impose not only additional expiratory but also additional inspiratory work of breathing.[131]

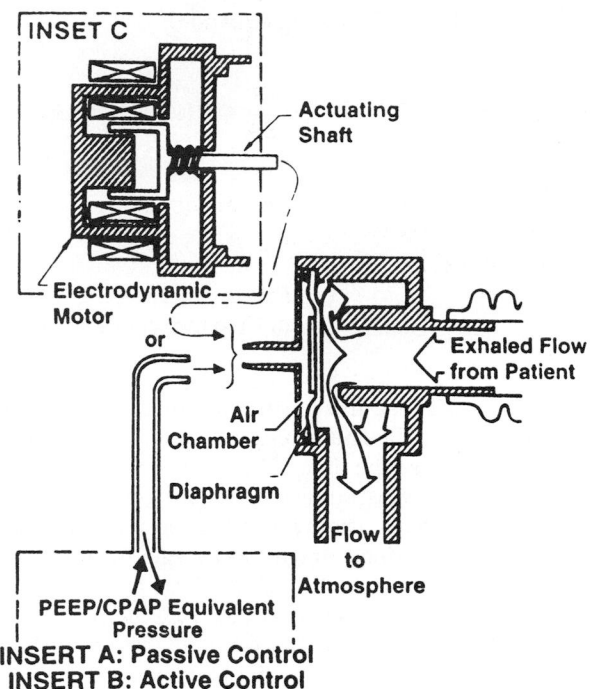

FIGURE 3-56 An illustration of a diaphragm-type expiratory valve. Diaphragm positioning generally follows one of three strategies: (1) maintenance of a specified PEEP/CPAP-equivalent pressure in the air chamber (passive pneumatic control), (2) algorithmic modulation of the chamber pressure between the PEEP/CPAP-equivalent value and a lesser value, thereby improving expiratory efficiency when PEEP/CPAP is finite (active pneumatic control), and (3) algorithmic positioning of the diaphragm via an electrodynamic motor (active direct control). If the electrodynamic motor and the diaphragm are coupled directly (in contrast to physically uncoupled), all positions of the diaphragm must be specified by the control algorithm. In the uncoupled design, the force of exhalation opens the valve, but closure is controlled by the electrodynamic motor. (*Used, with permission, from Sanborn: Respir Care 37:1009–25, 1992.*)

Imposed Work of Breathing

Whenever instrumentation is affixed to the airway, work of breathing is imposed. Artificial airways are responsible in large part for most of the work imposed,[132,133] but a close second is the ventilator itself. Numerous authors have documented the impact of ventilators on imposed work of breathing.[134–138] Ventilator-imposed work historically has been most pronounced (and has had the greatest clinical impact) during CPAP, where the patient is expected to perform all the effort required to ventilate. More recent data on the newest generation of mechanical ventilators, however, indicate that imposed work, when sensitivity is set properly, is minimal and of limited clinical concern.[56,124,139]

Alarms

Today's ventilators, because of their microprocessor control, are capable of monitoring and alarming an indefinite

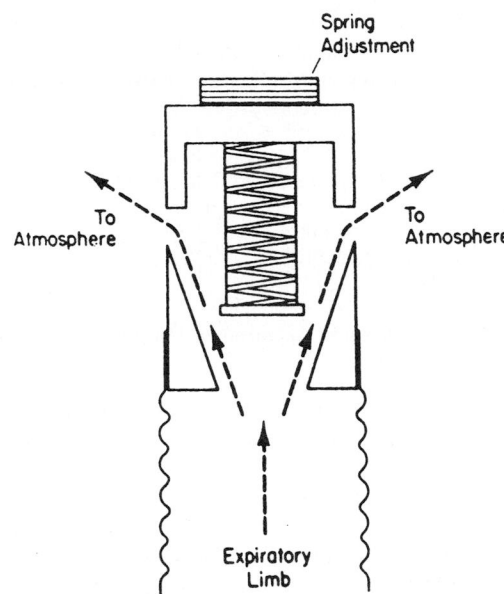

FIGURE 3-57 Spring-loaded interchangeable PEEP valve. As PEEP is increased by adjustment of the spring and diaphragm, the area available for expiratory flow to pass decreases, increasing the flow-resistant properties of the valve. (*Used, with permission, from Kacmarek et al: Anesthesiol Clin North Am 5:757–76, 1987.*)

number of events associated with either the ventilator itself, the patient-ventilator interface, or the patient.[140,142,144] The question that has not been answered clearly, however, is this: Is it necessary to alarm all the events that can be monitored." A secondary and equally important question is: What should the alarm threshold be for a given event?

Ventilator alarms, as designed today, greatly contribute to noise pollution in the ICU and, based on our observation of clinician activities, actually encourage practitioners to ignore them because of the high frequency of false alarms.[140,143,144] Because manufacturers have tried to

FIGURE 3-58 Magnetic PEEP valve. Adjustment of the distance between the two magnets determines the PEEP level established. (*Used, with permission, from Kacmarek et al: Anesthesiol Clin North Am 5:757–76, 1987.*)

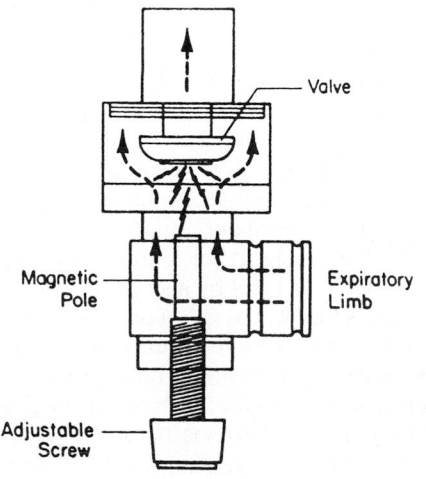

TABLE 3-10 Priorities for Mechanical Ventilator Alarms

Priority	Life-Threatening	Immediate Response Required	Redundant	Alarm Type
Level 1	Yes, immediately	Yes	Yes	Loud audible and visual
Level 2	Yes, potentially	Yes	No	Softly audible and visual
Level 3	No	No	No	Visual

SOURCE: Used, with permission from American Association for Respiratory Care.[147]

maximize the sensitivity of alarms (the percentage of true events that are detected), and because of the type of alarm algorithms currently used, specificity (the percentage of false events that are ignored) of these alarms is frequently low.[140] This is especially true when evaluating the number of false-positive alarms in the area of patient or patient-ventilator interface variables.[144] Even if the false-positive rate is low (5%), however, but there are 20 alarms that all function at this false-positive rate, there is a 64% probability that any given alarm will be false-positive alarm.[126] Such a frequency of false-positive alarms clearly prevents practitioners from taking alarms seriously.

HIERARCHY OF PATIENT-VENTILATOR ALARMS

A few groups, including the International Organization for Standardization and the American Society for Testing and Materials,[145,146] have defined limited specific standards for ventilator alarm systems. The group that has most specifically defined guidelines for ventilator alarms, however, is the American Association for Respiratory Care.[147] This group has recommended classifying ventilator alarms in three levels of priority, with level 1 indicating an immediate life-threatening situation and level 3 indicating no threat to life (Table 3-10). Also recommended was the need for an immediate response to level 1 priority alarms and a distinction between the audio and visual response of the ventilator to each alarm priority level. Table 3-11 lists events that should be monitored and the possible sites for monitoring of each event at all three levels of priority. In general, it is recommended that all ventilators include alarms for all level 1 and level 2 events.[147] Generally, level 3 alarms, although useful in certain settings, are not necessary.[147]

"SMART" ALARMS

Alarm-activation algorithms used historically on most ventilators for patient-ventilator interface events were relatively simplistic in design.[4] For example, when the high inspiratory pressure was met by a single breath violation, an alarm was activated that must be reset by the practitioner. Because the event may have occurred on only one breath as the patient changed position, however, when the practitioner arrived at the bedside, the peak inspiratory pressure had returned to the level before the incident. Such

a scenario may cause the practitioner to disregard future high-pressure events. This is also true of many volume and rate alarms because the time interval over which the monitored variable is integrated is so small with some ventilators (5–10 seconds). That is, a change in tidal volume or rate outside the defined range for a single breath or over

TABLE 3-11 Events and Monitoring Sites for Ventilator Alarms

Event	Possible Monitoring Site
Level 1	
Power failure (including when battery in use)	Electrical control system
Absence of gas delivery (apnea)	Circuit pressures, circuit flows, timing monitor, CO_2 analysis
Loss of gas source	Pneumatic control system
Excessive gas delivery	Circuit pressures, circuit flow, timing monitor
Exhalation value failure	Circuit pressures, circuit flows, timing monitor
Time failure	Circuit pressures, circuit flows, timing monitor
Level 2	
Battery power loss (not in use)	Electrical control system
Circuit leak	Circuit pressures, circuit flows
Blender failure	F_{IO_2} sensor
Circuit partially occluded	Circuit pressures, circuit flows
Heater/humidifier failure	Temperature probe in circuit
Loss of/or excessive PEEP	Circuit pressures
Autocycling	Circuit pressures, circuit flows
Other electrical or preventative subsystem out of limits without immediate overt gas delivery effects	Electrical and pneumatic systems monitor
Level 3	
Change in central nervous system drive	Circuit pressures, circuit flows, timing monitor
Change in impedances	Circuit pressures, circuit flows, timing monitor
Intrinsic (auto) PEEP > 5 cmH_2O	Circuit pressures, circuit flow

SOURCE: Used, with permission, from American Association for Respiratory Care.[147]

a short time but rapidly corrected by itself resulted in a sustained alarm. Many of the newest generation of ventilators, however, reset alarms if the event occurs only for one breath or corrects itself in a short period of time. Other alarms, once activated but self-corrected, provide a visual but not audio indication of the event. Much of the problem with false-positive alarms is a result of the algorithms designed to activate the alarms. More and more emphasis, however, currently is being placed on the development of "smart" alarms, that is, alarms that use up/down counting sequences, time delays, or other software filtering mechanisms that reduce the frequency of false-positive alarms.[141,148]

In addition, designing the alarm audiovisual response in the form of a hierarchy, which increases in urgency as an alarm condition continues, helps to decrease the frequency of false-positive alarms. These types of "smart" alarm systems are being used more frequently on the newest generation of ventilators.

Monitoring

Today's ventilators are capable of alarming various patient and patient-ventilator interface variables as a result of their ability to monitor pressure and flow. Numerous techniques are used to monitor flow, and both flow and pressure are monitored in various locations within the ventilator circuit.[141,149] Ideally, pressure should be measured within the lung.[112,113] As discussed earlier, however, this is rarely done for clinical purposes. As a result, pressure is monitored either at the ventilator circuit Y or internal to the ventilator, on either the inspiratory or expiratory side. The major concern with measurement internal to the ventilator is that airway pressure changes during spontaneous breathing are dampened.

Flow can also be measured at the airway or internal to the ventilator. If measurements are made internal to the ventilator, the volume measured may reflect not only volume delivered to the patient's lung but also volume compressed in the ventilator tubing (compressible volume is generally 2–3 ml/cmH$_2$O). Many of the new-generation ventilators compensate for this volume.[141,142] When flow-measuring devices are located at the airway, only gas entering or leaving the patient is monitored.

The advent of microprocessor control has led to an increase in the development of inexpensive sensors that can be incorporated into ventilators. It is important to realize that the accuracy of these sensors is considerably less than that of laboratory-grade sensors.[141] That is, displayed pressure measurements range between ±3% and ±5% of actual pressure, and displayed flow measurements range between ±6% and ±10% of the actual flow.[141]

PRESSURE MONITORING

Historically, pressure during mechanical ventilation was measured and displayed by aneroid manometers. Today, most microprocessor-based ventilators employ solid-state

integrated silicon-wafer pressure transducers, which are inexpensive and have an accuracy that is a clinically acceptable estimate of the actual value (±0.1 cmH$_2$O ± 3% of reading and can target pressure with an accuracy of ±2 cmH$_2$O ± 3% of reading).[149] The format used to display pressure varies considerably from ventilator to ventilator. Few ventilators still employ analog scales. Most ventilators convert the pressure signal to a digital format and display it either as a moving or expanding bar on a liquid-crystal display or, more commonly, as a digitally displayed value.

FLOW MONITORING

Monitoring flow is considerably more difficult than monitoring pressure. In general, flow is not measured directly but rather is calculated from change in pressure or temperature or the development vortices as gas flows past a partial obstruction.[141] Flow then is converted to volume at body temperature and pressure saturated. All these factors decrease the accuracy of the flow and volume measurements displayed by even the newest of mechanical ventilators.[142] The most common flow sensors used in current mechanical ventilators are (1) pressure-gradient measuring devices (i.e., pneumotachometers, variable orifices or venturis), (2) vane-displacement devices, (3) thermal-cooling sensors, (4) vortex-shedding sensors, and (5) ultrasonic sensors.[141]

Numerous variations of the standard pneumotachometer (Fig. 3-59) are used to measure flow during mechanical ventilation. The Servo 300 and i series ventilators use screened pneumotachometers placed proximal to the exhalation valve and distal to the inspiratory-flow valve. Advantages of these pneumotachometers are decreased dead space, better frequency response, and ease of disassembly for cleaning.[149–151] Moisture, however, significantly alters their accuracy. This is particularly true if aerosolized pharmacologic agents are allowed to contaminate the device. As a result, it is advisable to place filters in the expiratory limb during aerosol therapy.

FIGURE 3-59 Schematic representation of Fleisch pneumotachograph with a differential pressure transducer. (*Used, with permission, from Sullivan et al: Respir Care 29:736–49, 1984.*)

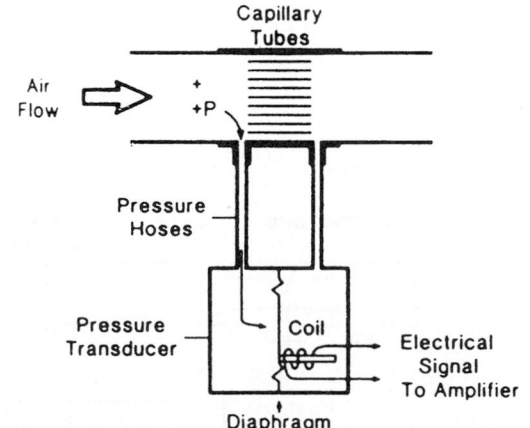

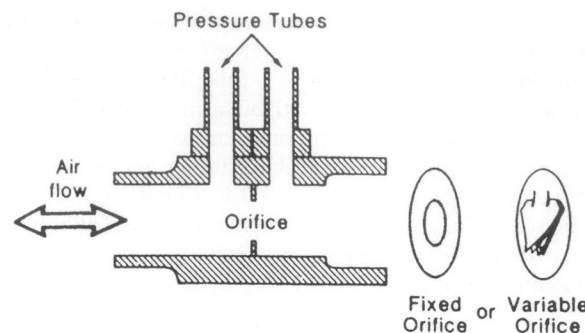

FIGURE 3-60 Schematic representation of an orifice pneumotachograph. (*Used, with permission, from Sullivan et al: Respir Care 29:736–49, 1984.*)

Another popular device used by both the Bird and Hamilton ventilators is the orifice pneumotachometer (Fig. 3-60). This device was designed to circumvent the moisture problems seen with both the Fleisch and screen pneumotachometers. Generally, the orifice is large enough to allow the free passage of water, and the device itself is coated with a water-resistant substance. This device is produced in two designs: one with a large orifice, creating turbulent flow and requiring a linearizing electronic circuit, and the other using an elastic flap in the middle of the orifice, which produces mechanical linearization of flow.[152,153]

A hot-wire pneumotachometer (or anemometer) (Fig 3-61) is used in the Puritan-Bennett 7200 and 840 ventilators. This type of pneumotachometer consists of a heated platinum wire positioned in the middle of a tube.[154,155] As gases pass through the tube, the wire rapidly loses heat. Cooling is offset by an electronic circuit that adds additional current to maintain a constant temperature. The gas flow rate is proportional to the added current.

The old Bear ventilators use a vortex-shedding pneumotachometer. As illustrated in Fig. 3-62, a partial obstruction (strut) is placed in the center of the device, causing turbulence and the formation of vortices as gas flows through the pneumotachometer. The level of turbulence is detected by an ultrasonic beam located downstream from the strut. The degree of turbulence is proportional to the flow rate.[156]

With all the newest-generation ventilators, volume is determined by integrating flow over time. None of these units measures volume displacement directly, as was done with

FIGURE 3-61 Schematic representation of a hot-wire pneumotachograph. (*Used, with permission, from Sullivan et al: Respir Care 29:736–49, 1984.*)

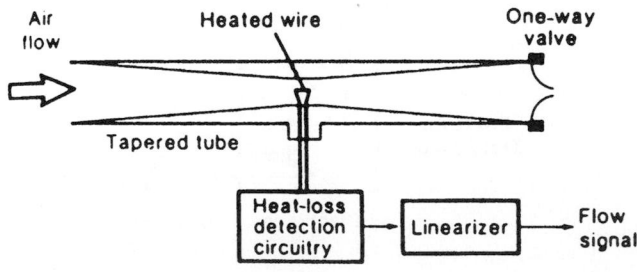

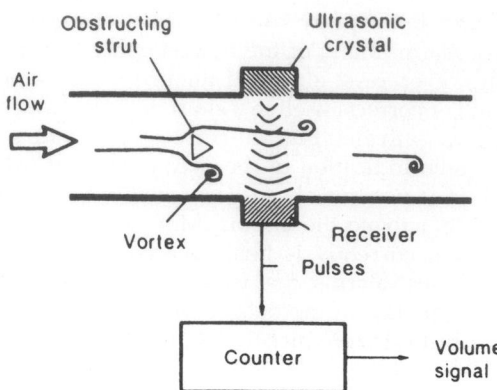

FIGURE 3-62 Schematic representation of a vortex pneumotachograph. (*Used, with permission, from Sullivan et al: Respir Care 29:736–49, 1984.*)

the old MA-1 ventilator. The accuracy of the volume displayed varies considerably from that actually measured at the ventilator circuit Y,[141,149,157,158] and the discrepancy increases with increased tidal volume. Ventilators that actually measure flow at the circuit Y (Hamilton ventilators) display the most accurate tidal volume.[158] A major reason for this difference is compressible volume. Many of the newer-generation ventilators, however, attempt to correct for compressible volume.

WAVEFORMS AND LOOPS

All current-generation ICU ventilators display waveforms of airway pressure, flow, and volume. These waveforms have been invaluable in monitoring overall patient-ventilator interaction,[159] the setting of various modes of ventilation,[160] and the management of patients with specific conditions,[161–165] as well as the identification of auto-PEEP.[165] In addition, many ventilators also display pressure-volume and flow-volume loops. Information regarding patient effort, patient-ventilator synchrony, auto-PEEP, response to bronchodilators, and work performed by the ventilator can be gained from the analysis of waveforms and loops, even if they are measured internal to the ventilator. Specific information regarding waveforms and loops is available elsewhere in this book (See Chapters 49 and 53), as well as in other publications.[159–167]

DERIVED VARIABLES

Because the newest-generation ventilators are microprocessor controlled and monitor airway pressure and flow throughout both the inspiratory and expiratory phases, numerous variables related to pulmonary mechanics can be derived. Of major concern with many of these mechanics packages is that the formula used to calculate a particular variable may not be the most accurate formula. In addition, few data evaluating the accuracy of these packages are available.[168,169]

EFFECTIVE COMPLIANCE

As has been pointed out by Marini[170] and others,[152,168,171] the measurement of compliance in passively ventilated patients requires that total PEEP (auto-PEEP plus applied PEEP) and ventilator tubing compliance be considered when effective static compliance (Ces) is determined:

$$Ces = \frac{V_T - (Pplat - PEEP_{TOT})(\text{compressible volume factor})}{Pplat - PEEP_{TOT}}$$

where Pplat is the plateau (end-inspiratory hold) pressure, $PEEP_{TOT}$ is total PEEP, and the compressible volume factor is the volume compressed in the ventilator circuit per centimeter of water pressure. The algorithms used by specific manufactures should be evaluated carefully to ensure they conform to this equation.

RESISTANCE TO FLOW

Concerns regarding the calculation of either inspiratory or expiratory resistance also exist. Of all the variables calculated by ventilators, however, the estimate of inspiratory resistance is probably the most accurate. This calculation requires gas to be delivered in a square-waveflow pattern. Only peak airway pressure, plateau pressure, and inspiratory flow are required for the calculation. Expiratory resistance also requires the determination of total PEEP for accurate calculation.

AUTO (INTRINSIC) PEEP

Since the original description of auto-PEEP by Pepe and Marini,[172] its importance in the management of patients requiring ventilatory assistance has been increasingly obvious.[173,174] As discussed elsewhere in this book, auto-PEEP usually is identified by the establishment of an end-expiratory hold during passive ventilation. This approach provides an estimate of the mean level of auto-PEEP. Currently, all new-generation ventilators allow for the measurement of auto-PEEP provided that a static end-expiratory pause can be established.

TRENDING OF DATA

Most new-generation ventilators provide some trending of data. This includes monitored patient/ventilator data as well as alarm events. As a result, the specific set of circumstances that produced a particular event in the past frequently can be inferred. What is lacking in most ventilators, however, is an integration of these data in a manner that can be interpreted easily by clinicians.

DIGITAL ELECTRONIC COMMUNICATIONS

Today's ventilator is a highly sophisticated microprocessor-controlled machine. As such, it is capable of interfacing with other microprocessor-controlled systems. Specifically, most of the newest ventilators can be attached to printers, other computers for recording and documentation of all events related to mechanical ventilation, and to the cardiac monitors for display of variables and annunciation of alarms.[175] That is, the exact time and specific changes made can be displayed, as also can all alarm conditions and events leading to the condition.

Airway pressure, flow, and volume waveforms also can be displayed on separate computers or on the cardiac bedside monitor. This transfer of online data to systems capable of manipulating and filtering the data and subsequently packaging them with other data associated with the patient's physiologic status opens the door for an integrated approach to the monitoring of the whole patient-ventilator system.[176] Ventilator data also can be transferred by the institution's Ethernet system to remote locations for assessment or be interfaced directly with nurse call systems. It is anticipated that highly sophisticated interactions of ventilators and other monitors will be available in the near future.

The Future

Today's generation of ICU mechanical ventilators is much more sophisticated than those manufactured in the 1980s or 1990s. This trend toward increasing sophistication, greater versatility, and enhanced capability is expected to continue. From an engineering perspective, essentially anything is feasible. The factors limiting ventilator development today are time and money, not engineering capability.

We still believe that there are areas of ventilator performance where significant improvement is needed and would expect that the mechanical ventilators of the future will incorporate the following and more: (1) Alarms on all patient and patient-ventilator interface variables should be "smart," that is, capable by more appropriate activation algorithms of greatly reducing the number of false-positive alarms; (2) monitoring, not the addition of more monitored variables but a better organization of trended data, should result in a list of the potential problems identified; and (3) more carefully designed approaches to closed-loop ventilation should become standard features of mechanical ventilators. With the introduction of more accurate and continuous monitors, closed-loop ventilation algorithms based on multiple patient physiologic variables should be possible.

References

1. Ritz R, Cunningham J. Indirect calorimetry. In: Kacmarek RM, Hess D, Stoller JK, editors. Monitoring in respiratory care. Chicago: Mosby-Year Book, 1993.
2. Campbell RS, Branson RD. How ventilators provide temporary O_2 enrichment: What happens when you press the 100% suction button? Respir Care 1992; 37:933–7.
3. Chatburn RL. Classification of mechanical ventilators. Respir Care 1992; 37:1009–25.
4. Sanborn WG. Microprocessor-based mechanical ventilation. Respir Care 1993; 38:72–109.
5. Younes M. Proportional assist ventilation, a new approach to ventilatory support. Am Rev Respir Dis 1992; 145:114–20.

6. Younes M, Puddy A, Roberts D, et al. Proportional assist ventilation: Results of an initial clinical trial. Am Rev Respir Dis 1992; 145:121–9.

7. Product literature, Siemens Servo 900C Operating Manual No. 9383011E313E, Solna, Sweden, 1989.

8. Chatburn RL. A new system for understanding mechanical ventilators. Respir Care 1991; 36:1123–55.

9. Rau JL Jr. Inspiratory flow patterns: The shape of ventilation. Respir Care 1993; 38:132–40.

10. Lyager S. Influence of flow pattern on the distribution of respiratory air during intermittent positive pressure ventilation. Acta Anaesthesiol Scand 1968; 12:191–211.

11. Adams AP, Economides AP, Finlay WEI, Sykes MK. The effect of variations of inspiratory flow waveform on cardiorespiratory function during controlled ventilation in normo-, hypo-, and hypervolemic dogs. Br J Anaesth 1970; 42:818–25.

12. Jansson L, Jonson B. A theoretical study on flow patterns of ventilators. Scand J Respir Dis 1972; 53:237–46.

13. Johansson H, Lofstrom JB. Effects on breathing mechanics and gas exchange of different inspiratory gas flow patterns during aesthesia. Acta Anaesthesiol Scand 1975; 19:8–18.

14. Baker AB, Colliss JE, Cowie RW. Effects of varying inspiratory flow waveform and time in intermittent positive pressure ventilation: II. Various physiological variables. Br J Anaesth 1977; 49:1221–34.

15. Dammann JF, McAslan TC, Maffeo CJ. Optimal flow pattern for mechanical ventilation of the lungs: 2. The effect of a sine versus square wave flow pattern with and without an end-inspiratory pause on patients. Crit Care Med 1978; 6:293–310.

16. Modell HI, Cheney FW. Effects of inspiratory flow pattern on gas exchange in normal and abnormal lungs. J Appl Physiol 1979; 46:1103–7.

17. Baker AB, Thompson JB, Turner J, Hansen P. Effects of varying inspiratory flow waveform and time intermittent positive pressure ventilation: Pulmonary oedema. Br J Anaesth 1982; 54:539–46.

18. Baker AB, Restall R, Clark BW. Effects of varying inspiratory flow waveform and time in intermittent positive pressure ventilation: Emphysema. Br J Anaesth 1982; 54:547–54.

19. Banner MJ, Boysen PG, Lampotang S, Jaeger MJ. End-tidal CO_2 affected by inspiratory time and flow waveform-time for a change (abstract). Crit Care Med 1986; 14:374.

20. Branson RD, Hurst JM. Effects of inspiratory flow pattern on airway pressure, ventilation, and hemodynamics (abstract). Respir Care 1987; 32:913.

21. Smith RA, Venus B. Cardiopulmonary effect of various inspiratory flow profiles during controlled mechanical ventilation in a porcine lung model. Crit Care Med 1988; 16:769–72.

22. Rau JL Jr, Shelledy DC. The effect of varying inspiratory flow waveforms on peak and mean airway pressures with a time-cycled volume ventilator: A bench study. Respir Care 1991; 36:347–56.

23. Ravenscraft SA, Burke WC, Marini JJ. Volume-cycled decelerating flow: An alternative form of mechanical ventilation. Chest 1992; 101:1342–51.

24. Branson RD, Campbell RS. Sighs: Wasted breath or breath of fresh air? Respir Care 1992; 37:462–8.

25. Ferris BG, Pollard DS. Effect of deep and quiet breathing on pulmonary compliance in man. J Clin Invest 1960; 39:143–9.

26. Mead J, Collier C. Relation of volume history of lungs to respiratory mechanics in anesthetized dogs. J Appl Physiol 1959; 14:669–78.

27. Bendixen HH, Hedley-Whyte J, Laver MB. Impaired oxygenation in surgical patients during general anesthesia with controlled ventilation. New Engl J Med 1963; 269:991–6.

28. Bendixen HH, Smith G, Mead J. Pattern of ventilation in young adults. J Appl Physiol 1963; 19:195–8.

29. Laver MB, Morgan J, Bendixen HH, Radford EP. Lung volume, compliance and arterial oxygen tension during controlled ventilation. J Appl Physiol 1964; 19:725–33.

30. Fletcher G, Barber JL. Lung mechanics and physiologic shunt during spontaneous breathing in normal subjects. Anesthesiology 1966; 27:638–47.

31. Housley E, Louzda N, Becklake MR. To sigh or not to sigh. Am Rev Respir Dis 1970; 101:611–4.

32. Levine M, Gilbert R, Auchincloss JH. A comparison of the effects of sighs, large tidal volumes, and positive end-expiratory pressure in assisted ventilation. Scand J Respir Dis 1972; 53: 101–8.

33. Balsys AJ, Jones RL, Man SFP, Wells A. Effects of sighs and different tidal volumes on compliance, functional residual capacity and arterial oxygen tension in normal and hypoxemic dogs. Crit Care Med 1980; 8:641–5.

34. Fairley HB. The mechanical ventilation sigh is a dodo. Respir Care 1976; 21:1127–30.

35. Pelosi P, Cadringher P, Bottino N, et al. Sigh in acute respiratory distress syndrome. Am J Respir Crit Care Med 1999; 159: 872–80.

36. Patroniti N, Foti G, Cortinovis B, et al. Sigh improves gas exchange and lung volume in patients with acute respiratory distress syndrome undergoing pressure support ventilation. Anesthesiology 2002; 96:788–94.

37. Dreyfuss D, Saumon G. Ventilator-induced lung injury: Lessons from experimental studies. Am J Respir Crit Care Med 1998; 157:294–323.

38. Rau JL. The inhalation of drugs: Advantages and problems. Respir Care 2005; 50:367–82.

39. Branson RD. Ventilators and loss of electrical power: Response and responsibility (editorial). Respir Care 1988; 33: 177–8.

40. Algren JT, Polston ST. Effect on airway pressure when electrical power to the Servo ventilator is interrupted. Respir Care 1987; 32:1141–4.

41. AARC. Consensus statement on the essentials of mechanical ventilators—1992. Respir Care 1992; 37:1000–8.

42. Branson RD, Chatburn RL. Technical description and classification of modes of ventilator operation. Respir Care 1992; 37: 1026–44.

43. Branson RD, Hess DR, Chatburn RL. Respiratory care equipment, 2nd ed. Philadelphia: Lippincott Williams & Wilkins, 1999.

44. Sassoon CSH. Positive pressure ventilation: Alternate modes. Chest 1991; 100:1421–9.

45. Sassoon CSH, Mahutte CK, Light RW. Ventilator modes: Old and new. Crit Care Clin 1990; 6:605–34.

46. Luce JM, Pierson DJ, Hudson LD. Intermittent mandatory ventilation. Chest 1981; 79:678–85.

47. Weisman 1M, Rinaldo JE, Rogers RM, Sanders MH. Intermittent mandatory ventilation. Am Rev Respir Dis 1983; 127: 641–7.

48. Downs JB, Stock MC, Tabeling B. Intermittent mandatory ventilation (IMV): A primary ventilatory support mode. Ann Chir Gynaecol 1982; 196(suppl):57–63.

49. Downs JB, Block AJ, Vennum KB. Intermittent mandatory ventilation in the treatment of patients with chronic obstructive pulmonary disease. Anesth Analg 1974; 53:437–43.

50. Downs JB, Douglas ME, Sanfelippo PM, et al. Ventilatory pattern, intrapleural pressure and cardiac output. Anesth Analg 1977; 56:88–96.

51. Downs JB, Klein EF Jr, Desautels D, et al. Intermittent mandatory ventilation: A new approach to weaning patients from mechanical ventilators. Chest 1973; 64:331–5.

52. Gibney RTN, Wilson RS, Pontoppidan H. Comparison of work of breathing on high gas flow and demand valve continue positive airway pressure systems. Chest 1982; 82:692–5.

53. Kacmarek RM, Wilson RS. IMV systems: Do they make a difference? Chest 1985; 87:557.

54. Kacmarek RM, Dimas S, Reynolds J, Shapiro BA. Technical aspects of positive end expiratory pressure: II. PEEP with positive pressure ventilation. Respir Care 1982; 27:1490–1504.

55. Shapiro BA, Harrison RA, Walton JR, Davison R. Intermittent demand ventilation: A new technique for supporting ventilation in critically ill patients. Respir Care 1976; 21: 521–5.

56. Takeuchi M, Williams P, Hess D, Kacmarek RM. Continuous positive airway pressure in new-generation mechanical ventilators. Anesthesiology 2002; 96:162–72.

57. Henry WC, West GA, Wilson RS. A comparison of the oxygen cost of breathing between a continuous-flow CPAP system and a demand-flow CPAP system. Respir Care 1983; 28: 1273–81.

58. Cox D, Niblett DJ. Studies on continuous positive airway pressure breathing systems. Br J Anaesth 1984; 56:905–11.

59. ACCP-SCCM-AARC. Evidence-based guidelines for weaning/discontinuation. Chest 2001; S375–484.

60. Abraham E, Yoshihara G. Cardiorespiratory effects of pressure control ventilation in severe respiratory failure. Chest 1990; 98:1445–9.

61. Marini JJ, Crooke PS III, Tmwit JD. Determinants and limits of pressure-preset ventilation: A mathematical model of pressure control. J Appl Physiol 1989; 67:1081–92.

62. East TD, Bohm SH, Wallace CJ, et al. A successful computerized protocol for clinical management of pressure control inverse ratio ventilation in ARDS patients. Chest 1992; 101:697–710.

63. Walley KR, Schmidt GA. Therapeutic use of intrinsic end expiratory pressure. Crit Care Med 1990; 18:336–7.

64. Gurevitch MJ, Van Dyke J, Young ES, Jackson K. Improved oxygenation and lower peak airway pressure in severe adult respiratory distress syndrome: Treatment with inverse ratio ventilation. Chest 1986; 89:211–3.

65. Abraham E, Yoshihara G. Cardiorespiratory effects of pressure controlled inverse ratio ventilation in severe respiratory failure. Chest 1989; 96:1356–9.

66. Lain DC, DiBeneaetto R, Morris SL, et al. Pressure control inverse ratio ventilation as a method to reduce peak inspiratory pressure and provide adequate ventilation and oxygenation. Chest 1989; 95:1081–8.

67. Tharratt RS, Allen RP, Albertson TE. Pressure controlled inverse ratio ventilation in severe adult respiratory failure. Chest 1988; 94:755–62.

68. Kacmarek RM, Hess D. Pressure-controlled inverse-ratio ventilation: Panacea or auto-PEEP (editorial). Respir Care 1990; 35:945–8.

69. Stock MC, Downs JB. Airway pressure release ventilation: A new approach to ventilation support during acute lung injury. Respir Care 1987; 32:517–24.

70. Stock MC, Downs JB, Frolicher DA. Airway pressure release ventilation. Crit Care Med 1987; 15:462–6.

71. Downs JB, Stock MC. Airway pressure release ventilation: A new concept in ventilatory support. Crit Care Med 1987; 15:459–61.

72. Rasanen J, Downs JB, Stock MC. Cardiovascular effect of conventional positive pressure ventilation and airway pressure release ventilation. Chest 1988; 93:911–5.

73. Cane RD, Peruzzi WT, Shapiro BA. Airway pressure release ventilation in severe respiratory failure. Chest 1991; 200:460–3.

74. MacIntyre NR. Respiratory function during pressure support ventilation. Chest 1986; 89:677–83.

75. Murphy DF, Dobb GD. Effect of pressure support of spontaneous breathing during intermittent mandatory ventilation. Crit Care Med 1987; 15:612–3.

76. Macintyre NR. Weaning from mechanical ventilatory support: Volume assisting intermittent breaths versus pressure-assisting every breath. Respir Care 1988; 33:121–5.

77. Kacmarek RM. The role of pressure support ventilation in reducing work of breathing. Respir Care 1988; 33:99–120.

78. Hess DR, Branson RD. Mechanical ventilation. In: Hess DR et al, editors. Respiratory care principles and practice. Philadelphia: Saunders, 2002: 782–809.

79. Chatburn RL, Volsko TA. Mechanical ventilators. In: Wilkens RL et al, editors. Egan's fundamentals of respiratory care, 8th ed. St. Louis: Mosby, 2003: 929–62.

80. MacIntyre N, Nishimura M, Usada Y, et al. The Nagoya conference on system design and patient-ventilator interactions during pressure support ventilation. Chest 1990; 97:1463–6.

81. Campbell RS, Branson RD. Ventilatory support for the 90s: Pressure support ventilation. Respir Care 1993; 38:526–37.

82. MacIntyre NR, Ho L. Effects of initial flow rate and breath termination criteria on pressure support ventilation. Chest 1991; 99:134–8.

83. Jubran A, Van de Graff WB, Tobin MJ. Variability of patient-ventilator interaction with pressure support ventilation in patients with chronic obstructive pulmonary disease. Am J Respir Crit Care Med 1995; 152:129–36.

84. Parathasarathy S, Jubran A, Tobin MJ. Cycling of inspiratory and expiratory muscle groups with the ventilator in airflow limitation. Am J Respir Crit Care Med 1998; 158:1471–8.

85. Tokioka H, Tanaka T, Ishizu T, et al. The effect of breath termination criterion on breathing patterns and the work of breathing during pressure support ventilation. Anesth Analg 2001; 92:161–5.

86. Hart N, Hunt A, Polkey MI, et al. Comparison of proportional assist ventilation and pressure support ventilation in chronic respiratory failure due to neuromuscular and chest wall deformity. Thorax 2002; 57:979–81.

87. Ranieri VM, Giuliani R, Mascia L, et al. Patient-ventilator interaction during acute hypercapnia pressure-support vs proportional-assist ventilation. J Appl Physiol 1996; 81:426–36.

88. Serra A, Polese G, Braggion C, Rossi A. Non-invasive proportional assist and pressure support ventilation in patients with cystic fibrosis and chronic respiratory failure. Thorax 2002; 57:50–4.

89. Polese G, Vitacca M, Bianchi L, et al. Nasal proportional assist ventilation unloads the inspiratory muscles of stable patients with hypercapnia due to COPD. Eur Respir J 2000; 16:491–8.

90. Pennock BE, Kaplan P, Carlin BW, et al. Pressure support ventilation with a simplified ventilatory support system administered with a nasal mask in patients with respiratory failure. Chest 1991;100:1371–6.

91. Hess DR, Kacmarek RM. Essentials of mechanical ventilation, 2nd ed. New York: McGraw-Hill, 2003.

92. Brochard L, Mancebo J, Wysocki M, et al. Noninvasive ventilation for acute exacerbations of chronic obstructive pulmonary disease. New Engl J Med 1995; 333:817–22.

93. Plant PK, Owen JL, Parrott S, Elliott MW. Cost-effectiveness of ward-based non-invasive ventilation for acute exacerbations of chronic obstructive pulmonary disease: Economic analysis of randomized, controlled trial. Br Med J 2003; 326:956.

94. Pank M, Sangean M, Volpe M, et al. Randomized, prospective trial of oxygen, continuous positive airway pressure, and bilevel positive airway pressure by face mask in acute cardiogenic pulmonary edema. Crit Care Med 2004; 32:2407–15.

95. Hilbert F, Gruson D, Vargas F, et al. Noninvasive ventilation in immunosuppressed patients with pulmonary infiltrates, fever, and acute respiratory failure. New Engl J Med 2001; 344:481–7.

96. Ferrer M, Esquinas A, Leon AM, et al. Noninvasive ventilation in severe hypoxemic respiratory failure. Am J Respir Crit Care Med 2003; 168:1438–44.

97. Hewlett AM, Platt AS, Terry VG. Mandatory minute volume. Anesthesia 1977; 32:163–9.

98. East ill, Elkhuizean PHM, Pace CL. Pressure support in mandatory minute ventilation supplied by the Ohmeda CPU-I prevents alveolar hypoventilation due to respiratory depression in a canine model. Respir Care 1989; 34:795–800.

99. Ravenscroft PS. Simple mandatory minute volume. Anesthesia 1978; 33:246–9.

100. Quan SF, Parides GC, Knoper SR. Mandatory minute volume (MVV) ventilation: An overview. Respir Care 1990; 35:898–905.

101. Product literature, Maquet Servo i Ventilator, User's Manual, US Version No. 66–00-261-E313E, Solna, Sweden, 2004.

102. Product literature, Bear 1000 Ventilator Manual, Bear Medical Systems, Inc., Riverside, California, 1992: 4-20–4-27.

103. Amato MBP, Barbas CSV, Bonassa J, et al. Volume-assured pressure support ventilation (VAPSV): A new approach for reducing muscle workload during acute respiratory failure. Chest 1992; 102:1225–34.

104. Branson RD, David K. Dual control modes: Combining volume and pressure breaths. Respir Care Clin North Am 2001; 7:397–408.

105. Guttman J, Eberhard L, Fabry B, et al. Continuous calculation of intratracheal pressure in tracheally intubated patients. Anes 1993; 79:503–13.

106. Fabry B, Haberthur C, Zappe D, et al. Breathing pattern and additional work of breathing in spontaneously breathing patients with different ventilatory demands during inspiratory pressure support and automatic tube compensation. Intensive Care Med 1997; 23:545–52.

107. Otis AB, Fenn WO, Rahn H. Mechanics of breathing in man. J Appl Physiol 1950; 2:592–607.

108. Campbell RS, Branson RD, Johannigman JA. Adaptive support ventilation. Respir Care Clin North Am 2001; 9:425–40.

109. Laubscher TP, Frutiger A, Fanconi S. The automatic selection of ventilation parameters during the initial phase of mechanical ventilation. Intensive Care Med 1996; 22:199–207.

110. Sinderby C, Navalesi P, Beck J, et al. Neutral control of mechanical ventilation in respiratory failure. Nature Med 1999; 5:1433–6.

111. Sharshar T, Desmarais G, Louis B, et al. Transdiaphragmatic pressure control of airway pressure support in healthy subjects. Am J Respir Crit Care Med 2003; 168:760–9.

112. Banner MJ, Blanch PB, Kirby RR. Imposed work of breathing and methods of triggering a demand-flow, continuous positive airway pressure system. Crit Care Med 1993; 21: 183–90.

113. Kacmarek RM, Shimada Y, Ohmura A, et al. The second Nagoya conference: Triggering and optimizing mechanical ventilatory assist. Respir Care 1991; 36:45–51.

114. Banner MJ, Kirby RR, Blanch PB. Site of pressure measurement during spontaneous breathing with continuous positive airway pressure: Effect of calculating imposed work of breathing. Crit Care Med 1992; 20:528–33.

115. Bersten AD, Rutten AJ, Vedig AE, et al. Additional work of breathing imposed by endotracheal tubes, breathing circuits and intensive care ventilators. Crit Care Med 1989; 17:671–7.

116. Bolder PM, Healy EJ, Bolder AR, et al. The extra work of breathing through adult endotracheal tubes. Anesth Analg 1986; 65:853–9.

117. Shapiro M, Wilson RK, Casar G, et al. Work of breathing through different sized endotracheal tubes. Crit Care Med 1986; 14:1028–31.

118. Sassoon CSH. Mechanical ventilator design and function: The trigger variable. Respir Care 1992; 37:1056–69.

119. Sassoon CSH, Giron AE, Ely EA, Light RW. Inspiratory work of breathing on flow-by and demand-flow continuous airway pressure. Crit Care Med 1989; 17:1108–114.

120. Goulet R, Hess DR, Kacmarek RM. Pressure vs flow triggering during pressure support ventilation. Chest 1997; 111:1649–54.

121. Shapiro BA, Kacmarek RM, Cane RD, et al. Clinical applications of respiratory care, 4th ed. Chicago: Mosby–Year Book 1991: 323–34.

122. Marini JJ, Culver BH, Kirk W. Flow resistance of exhalation valves and positive end expiratory pressure devices used in mechanical ventilation. Am Rev Respir Dis 1985; 131:850–4.

123. Pinsky RA, Hrehocik D, Culpepper J, Snyder JV. Flow resistance of expiratory positive pressure systems. Chest 1988; 94:788–91.

124. Williams P, Muelver M, Kratohvil J, et al. Pressure support and pressure assist/control: Are their differences? An evaluation of the newest intensive care ventilators. Respir Care 2000; 45:1169–81.

125. Kayaleh RA, Wilson AF. Mechanisms of expiratory valve resistance. Am Rev Respir Dis 1988; 137:1390–4.

126. Kacmarek RM, Goulet RL. PEEP devices. Anesthesiol Clin North Am 1987; 5:757–76.

127. Banner MJ, Lampotang S, Boysen PG, et al. Flow resistance of expiratory positive pressure valve systems. Chest 1986; 90:212–7.

128. Banner MJ, Downs JB, Kirby RR, et al. Effects of expiratory flow resistance on inspiratory work of breathing. Chest 1988; 93:795–9.

129. Ashbaugh DG, Bigelow DB, Petty TL, Leyine BE. Acute respiratory distress in adults. Lancet 1967; 2:319–23.

130. Kacmarek RM, Dimas S, Reynolds J, Shapiro BA. Technical aspects of positive end-expiratory pressure (PEEP): 1. Physics of PEEP devices. Respir Care 1982; 27:1478–89.

131. Kacmarek RM, Mang H, Barker N, Cycyk-Chapman C. The effects of disposable/interchangeable PEEP valves on work of breathing during CPAP. Crit Care Med 1994; 22:1219–26.

132. Shapiro W, Wilson RK, Casar G, et al. Work of breathing through different sized endotracheal tubes. Crit Care Med 1986; 14:1028–31.

133. Bersten AD, Rutten AJ, Vedig AE, Showronski GA. Additional work of breathing imposed by endotracheal tubes, breathing circuits, and intensive care ventilators. Crit Care Med 1989; 17:671–7.

134. Viale JP, Annat G, Bertrand O. Additional inspiratory work in intubated patients breathing with continuous positive airway pressure systems. Anesthesiology 1985; 63:536–9.

135. Katz JA, Kraemer RW, Gjerde GE. Inspiratory work and airway pressure with continuous positive airway pressure delivery systems. Chest 1985; 88:519–26.

136. Capps JS, Ritz R, Pierson DJ. An evaluation in four ventilators of characteristics that affect work of breathing. Respir Care 1987; 32:1017–24.

137. Samodelov Lf, Falke KJ. Total inspiratory work with modem demand valve devices compared to continuous flow CPAP. Intensive Care Med 1988; 14:632–9.

138. Beydon L, Chasse M, Harf A, Lemaire F. Inspiratory work of breathing during spontaneous ventilation, using demand valve and continuous flow systems Am Rev Respir Dis 1988; 138:300–4.

139. Chatmongkolchart S, Williams P, Hess DR, Kacmarek RM. Evaluation of inspiratory rise time and inspiratory termination criteria in new generation mechanical ventilators: A lung model study. Respir Care 2001; 46:874–96.

140. Macintyre NR, Day S. Essentials for ventilator-alarm systems. Respir Care 1992; 37:1108–12.

141. Sanborn WG. Monitoring respiratory mechanics during mechanical ventilation: Where do the signals come from? Respir Care 2005; 50:28–52.

142. Lucangelo U, Bernabe F, Blanch L. Respiratory mechanics derived from signals in the ventilatory circuit. Respir Care 2005; 50:55–65.

143. Hess D. Noninvasive monitoring in respiratory care—Present, past and future: An overview. Respir Care 1990; 35:482–99.

144. Kacmarek RM. Noninvasive monitoring in respiratory care: Conference summary. Respir Care 1990; 35:740–6.

145. American Society for Testing and Materials, ASTM Committee F-29.03.0. Standard specification for ventilators intended for use in critical care; F1100-90. In: Annual book for ASTM standards. Philadelphia: American Society for Testing and Materials, 1990.

146. International Organization for Standardization, Technical Committee ISO/TC121. Breathing machines for medical use—Lung ventilators, Vol. ISO5369:1987E. Switzerland: International Organization for Standardization, 1987: 1–18.

147. American Association for Respiratory Care. Consensus statement on the essentials of mechanical ventilators—1992. Respir Care 1992; 37:1000–8.

148. Kacmarek RM, Meklaus GT. The new generation of mechanical ventilators. Crit Care Clin 1990; 6:551–78.

149. Tobin MJ. Monitoring of pressure, flow, and volume during mechanical ventilation. Respir Care 1992; 37:1081–96.

150. Wilkens K, Hicks GH. Gas volume, flow, pressure, and temperature monitoring. Probl Respir Care 1984; 29:736–49.

151. Sullivan WJ, Peters GM, Enright PL. Pneumotachography: Theory and clinical application. Respir Care 1984; 29: 736–49.

152. Elliot SE, Shore JH, Barnes CW, et al. Turbulent airflow meter for long-term monitoring in patient-ventilator circuits. J Appl Physiol 1977; 42:456–60.

153. Osborn JJ. A flowmeter for respiratory monitoring. Crit Care Med 1978; 6:349–51.

154. Yoshiya I, Shimada Y, Tanaka K. Evaluation of a hot wire respiratory flowmeter for clinical applicability. J Appl Physiol 1979; 47:1131–5.

155. Fitzgerald MX, Smith AA, Gaensler EA. Evaluation of "electronic" spirometers. New Engl J Med 1973; 289:1283–8.

156. Westenskow DR, Tucker SM. Evaluation of a ventilation monitor. Crit Care Med 1981; 9:64–6.

157. Branson RD, Campbell RS, Srivastava P, et al. Volume monitoring accuracy of four ventilators and the Bicore CP-100 monitor (abstract). Respir Care 1991; 36:1303.

158. Gammage GW, Banner MJ, Blanch PB, Kirby RR. Ventilator displayed tidal volume: What you see may not be what you get (abstract). Crit Care Med 1988; 16:454.

159. Nilsestuen JO, Hargett KD. Using ventilator graphics to identify patient-ventilator asynchrony. Respir Care 2005; 50:202–32.

160. Branson RD, Johannigman JA. The role of ventilator graphics when setting dual-control modes. Respir Care 2005; 50: 187–201.

161. Bigatello LM, Davignon KR, Stelfox HF. Respiratory mechanics and ventilator waveforms in the patient with acute lung injury. Respir Care 2005; 50:235–44.

162. Dhand R. Ventilator graphics and respiratory mechanics in the patient with obstructive lung disease. Respir Care 2005; 50: 246–59.

163. Macintyre NR. Respiratory mechanics in the patient who is weaning from the ventilator. Respir Care 2005; 50:275–84.

164. Murphy BA, Durbin CG. Using ventilator and cardiovascular graphics in the patient who is hemodynamically unstable. Respir Care 2005; 50:262–73.

165. Blanch L, Bernabe F, Lucangelo U. Measurement of air trapping, intrinsic positive end-expiratory pressure, and dynamic hyperinflation in mechanically ventilated patients. Respir Care 2005; 50:110–123.

166. Kacmarek RM. Management of the patient mechanical ventilator system. In: Pierson DJ, Kacmarek RM, editors. Foundations in respiratory care. New York: Churchill Livingstone, 1992: 973–99.

167. Kacmarek RM, Hess D. Monitoring of airway pressure, flow and volume waveforms and pressure-volume and flow-volume loops. In: Kacmarek RM, Hess D, Stoller J, editors. Monitoring in respiratory care. Chicago: Mosby–Year Book, 1993: 497–544.

168. Korst R, Orlando R, Yeaton N, et al. Validation of respiratory mechanics software microprocessor-controlled ventilators. Chest 1989; 96:255S.

169. Branson RD, Hurst JM, Davis K, Campbell R. Measurement of maximal inspiratory pressure: A comparison of three methods. Respir Care 1989; 34:789–94.

170. Marini JJ. Lung mechanics in the adult respiratory distress syndrome. Clin Chest Med 1990; 11:673–90.

171. Rossi A, Gottfried SB, Xocchi L, et al. Measurement of static compliance of the total respiratory system in patients with acute respiratory failure during mechanical ventilation: The effect of intrinsic positive end expiratory pressure. Am Rev Respir Dis 1985; 131:672–7.

172. Pepe PE, Marini JJ. Occult positive end-expiratory pressure in mechanically ventilated patients with airflow obstruction: The auto-PEEP effect. Am Rev Respir Dis 1982; 126:166–70.

173. Smith TC, Marini JJ. Impact of PEEP on lung mechanics and work of breathing in severe airflow obstruction. J Appl Physiol 1988; 65:1488–99.

174. Petrof BJ, Legare M, Goldberg P, et al. Continuous positive airway pressure reduces work of breathing and dyspnea during weaning from mechanical ventilation in severe COPD. Am Rev Respir Dis 1990; 141:281–9.

175. East TD, Young WH, Gardner RM. Digital electronic communication between ICU ventilators and computers and printers. Respir Care 1992; 37:1113–23.

176. Brunner J, Thompson JD. Computerized ventilation monitoring. Respir Care 1993; 38:110–24.

Chapter 4

EQUIPMENT REQUIRED FOR HOME MECHANICAL VENTILATION

ROBERT M. KACMAREK
ATUL MALHOTRA

Long-term home mechanical ventilation has been used worldwide for over 70 years to manage chronic ventilatory failure.[1,2] In the United States, long-term mechanical ventilation via the iron lung was first used with polio victims, although negative-pressure ventilators in Europe trace their history to the mid-nineteenth century.[3,4] In 1952, the use of intermittent positive-pressure ventilation via tracheostomy was introduced,[5] whereas the use of mouthpiece intermittent positive-pressure ventilation began in the late 1950s.[6] All the various approaches to ventilator support have been used successfully for long-term maintenance of patients with respiratory failure secondary to either neuromuscular and primary pulmonary diseases.[7-10]

Over the past 25 years, the number of patients receiving home mechanical ventilator assistance in the form of continuous positive airway pressure (CPAP) and ventilation provided both invasively and noninvasively has increased markedly.[11-18] As a result, there has been a resurgence of interest in the use of all approaches to chronic ventilator support. These include invasive and noninvasive positive- and negative-pressure techniques and the use of CPAP to manage sleep apnea. The concept of long-term mechanical ventilation has been approached from two distinct clinical perspectives: mandatory, for use during true life support, and elective, for managing chronic ventilatory failure and sleep apnea.[6,19,20] In most patients requiring ventilator support on a mandatory basis, invasive approaches have been most common. Many patients in this category, however, are being maintained with noninvasive methods.[21,22] In patients with slowly progressive chronic ventilatory failure who can sustain spontaneous breathing for lengthy periods, noninvasive methods are the primary approach.[8] This is especially true for patients with chronic neuromuscular or neurologic diseases.[17,18]

If one were to gather every possible positive-pressure ventilator produced for home use over the last 40 years, dozens of units would be listed.[23-26] Most of the older units, however, have fallen into disuse, and many are not presently manufactured. Only units currently marketed and those no longer manufactured but still with large numbers in use are presented herein. Detailed discussions of each of these units are presented as well as critical analyses. Following the individual unit discussions, topics applicable to all positive-pressure home-care ventilators are discussed. We begin with a description of all volume-targeted ventilators, followed by the pressure-targeted or bilevel-pressure units.

Invasive Positive-Pressure Ventilators

All the ventilators discussed in this section are designed for use via an artificial airway. That is, all include monitoring and alarms required when providing a patient with ventilator support 24 hours per day. In addition, each of these ventilators includes an internal battery that will maintain

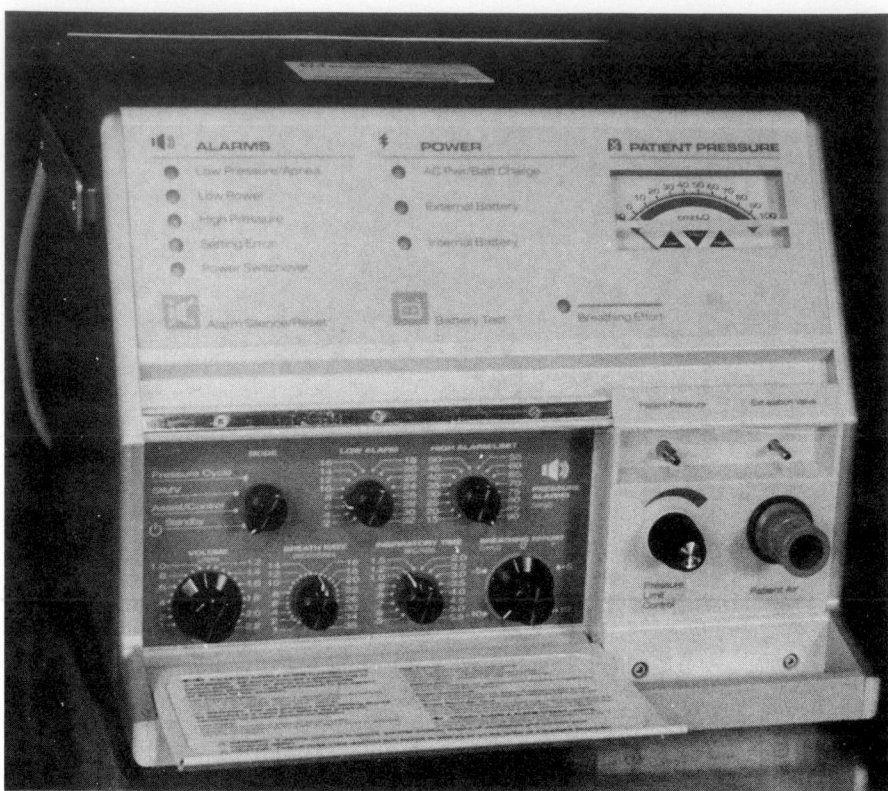

FIGURE 4-1 The Puritan-Bennett LP-10 Ventilator.

ventilation for at least 1 hour. These ventilators may be used for noninvasive ventilator support. They are not designed for this purpose, however, and do not do as good a job as the bilevel-pressure ventilators specifically designed for noninvasive ventilation.

NELCOR PURITAN-BENNETT LP-10

The LP-10[27] (Fig. 4-1) is a compact ($9^3/3$ in high × $14^1/2$ in wide × $13^1/4$ in in diameter), lightweight (weighs 34 lb) microprocessor-based ventilator. The internal gas-flow pathway in this unit is similar to that of the all early-generation positive-pressure home-care ventilators (Fig. 4-2). Gas enters the unit from atmosphere or via a reservoir-bag assembly attached to the gas inlet port on the back panel of the machine. From here, via a one-way valve (see Fig. 4-2A), gas enters the piston chamber; gas exits the piston chamber at a second one-way valve (see Fig. 4-2B), from which it proceeds into the inspiratory circuit. Within the internal inspiratory circuit, a gas tap supplying flow to the exhalation valve is configured. Additionally, a manufacturer-set nonadjustable pressure pop-off valve is located internally on the inspiratory limb. A proximal pressure tap leads from the patient's airways to the ventilator front panel and on to the microprocessor. The system's pressure gauge attaches to this line. The high-pressure limit is identified by the microprocessor that, when reached, alarms and terminates the inspiratory phase.

Parameters set on the control panel are relayed to the piston motor via the microprocessor. Patient effort during assisted ventilation is sensed via the proximal pressure tap. The one-way gas inlet valve (located at C in Fig. 4-2) is not included in the LP-10 gas-flow path. The oxygen-accumulating apparatus used on the LP-10 is depicted in Fig. 4-3. To the gas inlet port on the back of the machine, a 30 × 22 mm adapter is used to attach a large-bore connecting tube that affixes to a specifically designed T piece attached to the unit's accessory side rail on the right side panel of the unit. This T piece is configured with an O_2 tap and a reservoir bag. A detailed discussion of O_2 delivery is provided later in this chapter.

CLASSIFICATION

The LP-10 is a microprocessor-controlled, electrically powered, rotary-piston-driven positive-pressure home-care ventilator. As a result of the piston-driving mechanism, the unit is classified as a non-constant-flow generator that produces a sigmoidal pressure pattern (Fig. 4-4). Inspiration is triggered by either time or pressure based on the patient's inspiratory efforts, and expiration is cycled based on either volume or pressure: volume cycled under normal operating conditions and pressure cycled if the pressure-limited mode is chosen or if the unit's high-pressure alarm/limit is reached. Assist-control ventilation (ACV), synchronized intermittent mandatory ventilation (SIMV), and pressure-limited ventilation modes can be programmed. In addition, apnea ventilation is available. No inspiratory sigh or expiratory maneuvers are included.

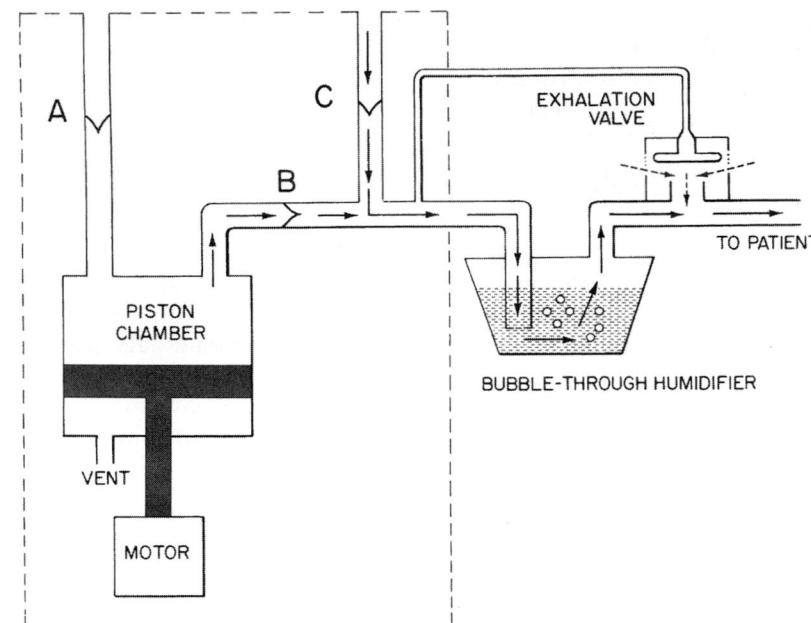

FIGURE 4-2 Diagram showing generalized gas-flow routes through a typical home-care ventilator. *A.* One-way check valve allows gas entry into the piston chamber during the piston backstroke. *B.* One-way check valve prevents subatmospheric pressure from developing in the ventilator circuit during the backstroke of the piston. *C.* One-way check valve (antisuffocation valve) allows patient to inspire spontaneously during closure of *B* when piston backstroke is in progress. Some gas may enter system at the exhalation valve during spontaneous breathing. Arrows depict gas flow possible during spontaneous inspiration. (*Used, with permission, from Kacmarek et al: Respir Care 35:405–14, 1990.*)

MODES

ACV, SIMV, and pressure cycle and pressure limit are the modes available with the LP-10. In the ACV mode, the operator sets a control breath rate, the tidal volume, the inspiratory time, and breathing-effort control (patient-triggered sensitivity). If the breath rate is set at 6 breaths per minute or less and the patient becomes apneic, the apnea alarms sounds.

During SIMV, the operator also must set breath rate, tidal volume, inspiratory time, and breathing effort. Between SIMV positive-pressure breaths, the patient may breathe spontaneously, drawing gas from the piston chamber or through the exhalation valve. As with other piston ventilators, the LP-10 does not have a demand system, nor is it normally configured with a continuous-flow system. If the patient fails to create sufficient inspiratory force to be sensed by the ventilator for a 20-second period, the unit goes into backup ventilation at a rate of 10 breaths per minute, delivering the preset tidal volume. If the SIMV breath rate is set at 6 breaths per minute or greater, the apnea alarm will sound, but the machine will not revert to backup ventilation.

The pressure-cycle mode functions exactly the same as the ACV mode, except that inspiration is terminated when the set high pressure is reached. This mode does not result in

FIGURE 4-3 Schematic of the oxygen accumulator used on the LP series ventilators. See text for discussion. (*Used, with permission, from Puritan-Bennett.*[27])

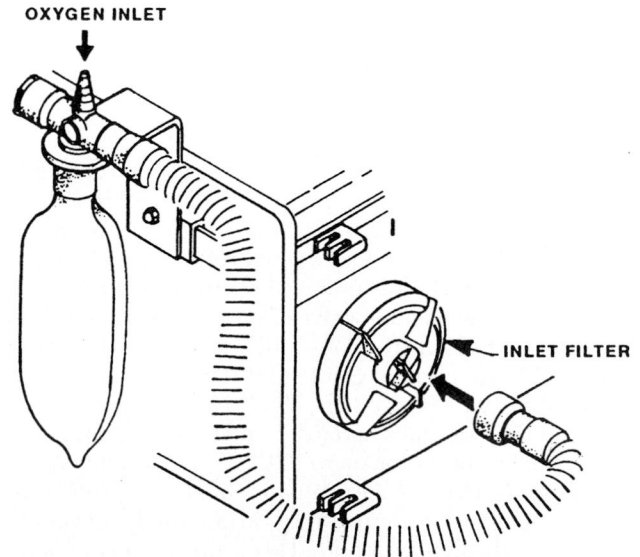

OXYGEN INLET

INLET FILTER

FIGURE 4-4 *A.* Sine-wave flow pattern established by older home-care ventilators during volume-limited ventilation. *B.* Corresponding sigmoidal pressure curve established during inspiration. (*Used, with permission, from Kacmarek et al: J Neuro Rehab 6:103–12, 1992.*)

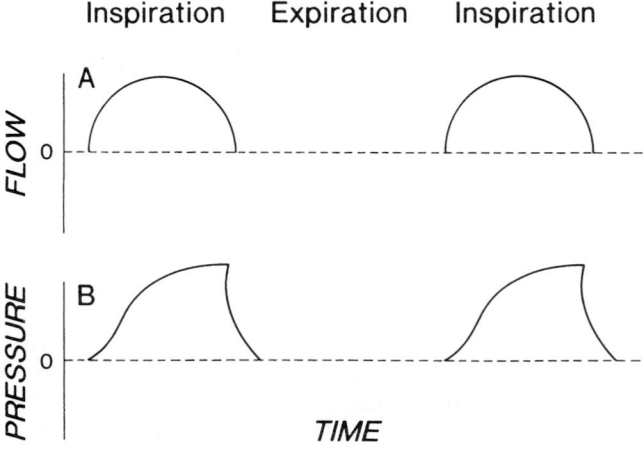

a pressure plateau. Thus the inspiratory time setting in conjunction with the tidal volume determines peak inspiratory flow. As in all pressure-cycled approaches to ventilation, actual tidal volume delivered depends on ventilator settings and the patient's airway resistance and compliance. When this mode is used, the high-pressure alarm is inactivated. Thus any acute change in system compliance or airways resistance may go unnoticed because no method of monitoring tidal volume or minute ventilation is available on this unit.

The LP-10 also has a pressure-limit control. That is, during either SIMV or ACV, a large tidal volume can be set in association with a specific pressure limit. During inspiration, the ventilator delivers the complete tidal volume. Pressure will not be allowed, however, to exceed the pressure limit (volume delivered after the limit has been reached is dumped to the atmosphere). In addition, the high-pressure alarm limit is not affected by the pressure-limit control. If the high-pressure alarm limit is reached, the ventilator alarms and dumps additional volume to the atmosphere without altering inspiratory time. Table 4-1 lists the ranges for gas-delivery variables.

ALARMS

The number of specific alarm conditions identifiable with the LP-10 is 23. These conditions are categorized under five major alarm conditions: high pressure, low pressure/apnea, low power, power switchover, and setting error. Audio and visual indicators are available for these five major categories. No other information except these five indicators is available to the practitioner unless the optional printer is set up and active during ventilation. When the printer is in use, a specific description of the alarm, along with an indication of why the alarm occurred, is provided.

There are six individual alarm specifications in the category low pressure/apnea: low pressure (system pressure below limit for two consecutive breaths), valley alarm (system pressure does not drop below the pressure setting for two consecutive breaths), exhale fail (system pressure is above the low-pressure alarm setting at the beginning of a breath), apnea (10 seconds or greater), stall (failure to complete a breathing cycle in 14 seconds), and failure of system leak self-test.

The power-failure alarm results from two distinct conditions: internal battery voltage below 11.6 V and failure of the battery charger. The power-switchover alarm is activated when the internal dc battery is the primary power source and its voltage is low. Under the high-pressure alarm, three situations are identified: System pressure is above set level, system pressure exceeds set level by 10 cmH_2O, and failure of overpressure-relief valve during self-test. With the setting-error alarm, a total of 11 different user or machine operational errors are identified. See Table 4-2 for details on alarm systems.

POWER SOURCE

The LP-10 can be operated by ac, external dc, and internal dc current. The unit always selects the highest power source available, ac, then external dc, and then internal dc. When the unit is connected to an electrical outlet, the internal dc battery is charged automatically unless the unit is turned off. It takes 2 to 3 hours to recharge a discharged internal battery. The internal battery can operate the LP-10 for up to 1 hour, depending on the actual ventilator setup. The unit converts automatically from ac to dc sources if required. The power-switchover alarm is activated when switchover occurs.

MISCELLANEOUS

The unit has a remote alarm access port and a communications port for an optional printer. If the communications port is used, access to detailed monitoring data is available based on alarm activation (i.e., each alarm condition is categorized, a description of the alarm condition is provided, and an indication of why the condition occurred is detailed).

CRITICAL ANALYSIS

Minimal tidal volume is 100 ml, and possible changes are only in 100-ml increments. This limits the unit's use in pediatric settings. Addition of the pressure-limit control does offset the preceding concern in certain settings; because no volume monitoring is provided, however, extreme care must be exercised whenever the pressure-limit control is used. This includes proper setting of the high- and low-pressure alarms. Another concern with the pressure-limit control is the absence of calibration. The chance of an inadvertent parameter change is decreased (except for the pressure-limit control) by the design of the unit (the recession of the control panel and its door). The design of the control panel is simple and straightforward, improving user-friendliness. The communications port greatly enhances the monitoring of and appropriate response to alarm conditions.

NELLCOR PURITAN-BENNETT LP-6 PLUS

The LP-6 Plus[27] (Fig. 4-5) is exactly the same as the LP-10, except that the pressure-limit control is not included.

PURITAN-BENNETT ACHIEVA[28]

The Achieva is very similar in design to the LP6 plus and LP-10 (Fig. 4-6). It weights 32 lb and is $10^3/_4$ in high, $13^1/_4$ in deep, and $15^1/_2$ in wide. The overall gas-delivery pattern is essentially the same as that illustrated in Fig. 4-2. The piston, however, is accelerated linearly and controlled by a microprocessor; as a result, gas-delivery pattern in volume ventilation is not a sine wave. In addition, pressure-support ventilation (PSV) and pressure assist-control ventilation (P-ACV) are available. This unit also controls the pressure in the mushroom exhalation valve electronically, allowing the setting of up to 20 cmH_2O of positive end-expiratory pressure (PEEP). An internal O_2 blender is included on the upgraded Achieva PSO$_2$. When a 50 lb/in^2 gas source is attached to the external standard-diameter index safety system (DISS) O_2 connector, up to 100% O_2 can be delivered. A flow sensor (internal to the ventilator) allows precise control of the gas-delivery pattern during various modes of ventilation. A specific circuit is required to ensure proper operation

TABLE 4-1 Setting Ranges for Volume-Targeted Home-Care Positive-Pressure Ventilation

	Modes	Tidal Volume, ml	Rate, per minute	Peak Flow Rate, liters/min	Inspiratory Time, seconds	Sensitivity, cmH_2O	Sigh Volume, ml	Sigh Rate	I:E Ratio	PEEP
PB LP-10	ACV, SIMV, pressure-limited, Pressure-limited, plateau	100–2200	1–38	—	0.5–5.5	–10 to +10	—	—	—	—
PB LP-6 Plus	ACV, SIMV, pressure-limited	100–2200	1–38	—	0.5–5.5	–10 to +10	—	—	—	—
Lifecare PLV-100	C, A, SIMV	50–3000	2–40	10–120	—	–6 to +3	—	—	—	—
Lifecare PLV-102	C, C + sign, ACV, ACV + sign, SIMV	50–1800	2–40	10–120	—	–5 to +18	1.5 times set V_T	1 every 100 breaths	—	—
PB Achieva	C, ACV both press. and Vol., SIMV vol, CPAP, PS, apnea	50–2200	1–80	Up to 180	0.2–5.0	3–25 liters/min or 1–15 cmH_2O	—	—	—	Up to 20 cmH_2O
Respironics PLV Continuum	C, ACV, SIMV press. and Vol., PS, apnea	50–2500	1–80	3–120	0.2–5.0	–4 to 18 cmH_2O	150% of set V_T	1 every 100 breaths	—	—
Pulmonetic LTV	C, ACV, SIMV press. and vol., PS, CPAP, apnea, NPPV	50–2000	0–80	Up to 160	0.3–9.9	1 to 9 liters/min and –3 cmH_2O	—	—	—	Up to 20 cmH_2O external
Versa Med iVent$_{201}$	C, ACV, SIMV press. and Vol., PS, CPAP, apnea, NPPV	100–2000	1–50	Up to180	0.3–3.0	1–20 liters/min, –0.5 to –20 cmH_2O	150% of set V_T	1 every 25 to 1 every 150 breaths	—	Up to 20 cmH_2O
Newport HT50	C, ACV, SIMV press. and vol., PS, CPAP	100–2200	1–99	6–100	0.1–3.0	–9.9 to 0 cmH_2O	—	—	—	Up to 30 cmH_2O

NOTE: C, control; ACV, assist-control ventilation; SIMV, synchronized intermittent mandatory ventilation; A, assist; I:E ratio, inspiration/expiration ratio; PEEP, positive end-expiratory pressure; V_T, tidal volume; PB, Puritan-Bennett.

TABLE 4-2 Alarm Systems of Volume-Targeted Home-Care Positive-Pressure Ventilations

	High Inspiratory Pressure Alarm, cmH$_2$O	Low Inspiratory Pressure, cmH$_2$O	Apnea	Low Battery	Inverse I/E Ratio	Ventilator Malfunction	Low Inspiratory Flow	Reverse External Battery Connections	Microprocessor Failure	Switch to Battery	Power Failure	Oxygen	Minimum Minute Volume
PB LP-10	25–100	2–50	Yes	Yes	Yes[a]	Yes	Yes[a]	No	Yes	Yes	Yes	No	No
PB LP-6 Plus	25–100	2–50	Yes	Yes	Yes[a]	Yes	Yes[a]	No	Yes	Yes	Yes	No	No
Lifecare PLV-100	5–95	2–50[c]	Yes[b]	Yes[b]	Yes	Yes	Yes	Yes	Yes	Yes	Yes	No	No
Lifecare PLV-102	5–95	2–50[c]	Yes[b]	Yes[b]	Yes	Yes	Yes	Yes	Yes	Yes	Yes	Yes	No
PB Achieva	2–80	1–59	Yes	Yes	Yes	Yes	No	No	Yes	Yes	Yes	Yes	No
Respironics PLV Continuum	10–80	3–50	Yes	Yes	Yes	Yes	No	Yes	Yes	Yes	Yes	No	No
Pulmonetic LTV	5–100	1–60	Yes	Yes	Yes	No	No	No	Yes	Yes	Yes	Yes	Yes
Versa Med iVent$_{201}$	3–80	1–77	Yes	Yes	Yes	No	No	Yes	Yes	Yes	Yes	Yes	Yes
Newport HT50	4–99	3–98	Yes	Yes	No	Yes	No	No	Yes	Yes	Yes	No	Yes

[a] Actually referred to as setting error; controls are set outside machine limits.
[b] Low inspiratory pressure and apnea alarms are actually combined.
[c] Have separate alarm for low internal and low external battery.

102

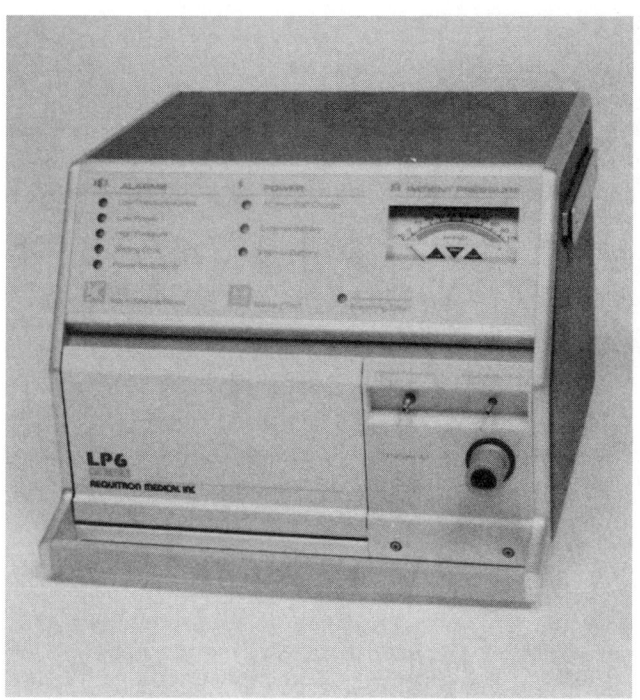

FIGURE 4-5 The Puritan-Bennett LP-6 Plus Ventilator.

of the PEEP control and to ensure that a gas-collection head is available to allow monitoring of exhaled gas.

CLASSIFICATION

The Achieva is an electrically powered, linear-piston-driven, microprocessor-controlled ventilator. It incorporates a single gas-flow system and produces multiple gas-flow patterns. Inspiration is triggered by either time or pressure, whereas exhalation may be cycled based on volume, time, or flow.

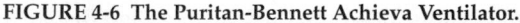

FIGURE 4-6 The Puritan-Bennett Achieva Ventilator.

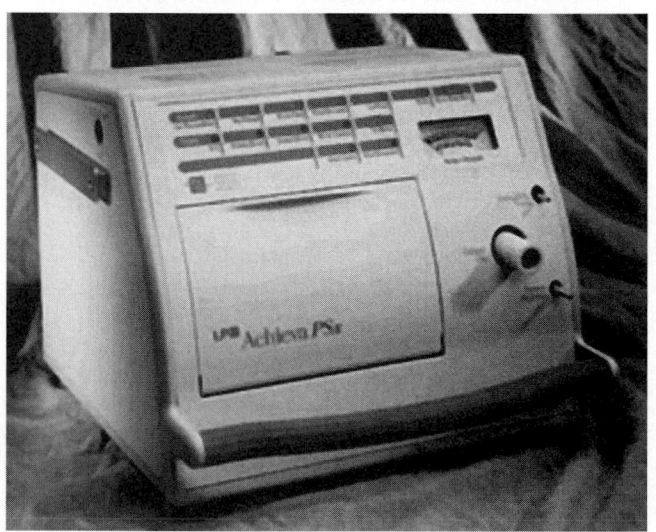

MODES

Both volume and pressure assist-control modes are available. In these modes, the ventilator is set as in most other ventilators. Trigger sensitivity is either via pressure or flow. Flow sensitivity ranges between 3 and 25 liters/min, and pressure sensitivity ranges between off and 1–15 cmH$_2$O. PEEP up to 20 cmH$_2$O can be applied to all modes of ventilation, and CPAP to 20 cmH$_2$O also can be set. During CPAP, as well as during the spontaneous breaths with SIMV, gas delivery is based on patient demand up to 180 liters/min. Only volume-targeted SIMV is available, and PSV can be used as an independent mode or in conjunction with SIMV. Table 4-1 lists ranges for gas-delivery variables.

ALARMS

The Achieva incorporates low- and high-pressure alarms, an apnea alarm, an equipment-failure alarm, a low-power alarm, an O$_2$ fail alarm, a setting-error alarm, a microprocessor-error alarm, and a power-switchover indicator. Alarms activate at different levels to indicate the severity of the alarm activated. Repeating bursts of five alarm pulses occur when low pressure or apnea is identified, the ventilator has detected an equipment error, and the internal battery is depleted. Repeated bursts of three pulses occur when the internal battery is low (10 minutes of power remaining), high pressure has developed, or the O$_2$ system fails. A single beep repeated every 5 minutes indicates inappropriate inspiratory-expiratory time (I:E) ratio, 45 minutes of dc power, or a minor equipment fault. Setting errors are also identified by single beeps. Activation of the apnea alarm results in ventilation being provided at a rate of 10 breaths per minute. See Table 4-2 for details on alarm systems.

POWER SOURCE

As with all ventilators of this class, the Achieva operates via three distinct power sources: ac, external dc, and internal dc. On change of power source, both visual and audio alarms are activated. The internal dc battery lasts from 1 to 4 hours depending on ventilator settings.

MISCELLANEOUS

During machine power-up, a complete unit diagnostic check of all systems occurs. Activation and setting of variables are menu-driven. The ventilator can be connected to a telephone by its internal modem using a standard R11 phone connector; in addition, the ventilator contains an RS-232 port. A remote-alarm connector and nurse-call connection are also available.

CRITICAL ANALYSIS

The overall design of the ventilator interface is somewhat busy and requires knowledge of computer-driven systems. The design, however, prevents inadvertent changing of parameters. The ability of this ventilator to provide pressure-targeted ventilation or demand flow has not been evaluated.

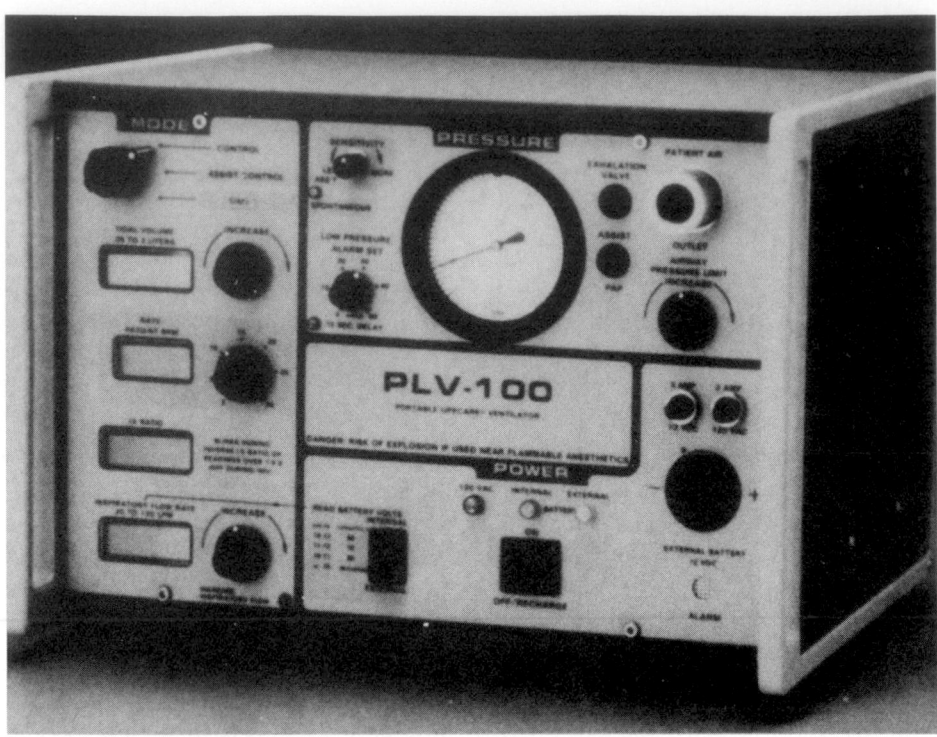

FIGURE 4-7 The Lifecare PLV-100 Ventilator.

LIFECARE PLV-100[29]

The Lifecare PLV-100 (now owned by Respironics) weighs 28.2 lb and has the following overall physical dimensions: 9 in high × 12.5 in wide × 12.25 in deep (Fig. 4-7). It is a compact and highly portable microprocessor-based home-care ventilator. It is not currently manufactured, although a large number of units are still in clinical use. The basic gas-flow pattern for the PLV-100 is illustrated in Fig. 4-2, with two major exceptions. First, no O_2 accumulator is available for attachment to the unit's gas entry port (*A*). Second, the one-way valve at *C*, which allows gas inflow during spontaneous breathing when the piston is in its backstroke, is not present. Essentially, gas enters the piston chamber at *A* and is moved from the chamber into the internal gas-delivery system at *B*. A pressure pop-off valve is also located inside the piston chamber. From *B*, gas proceeds past an inspiratory pressure-limit valve, out of the ventilator, through the inspiratory circuitry, and to the patient. The exhalation-valve line originates from the internal ventilator circuitry. A proximal airway-pressure line provides input to the microprocessor (the system manometer is tapped off this line). O_2 is administered via an adapter interfaced with the unit between the external circuitry and the unit itself. An increase in delivered tidal volume, as well as $F_{I_{O_2}}$, results.

CLASSIFICATION

The PLV-100 home-care positive-pressure ventilator is rotary-piston-driven via an electric motor and under the control of a microprocessor. It incorporates a single gas-flow system, and the rotary-piston design produces a sine-wave gas-flow pattern with a sigmoidal pressure curve.

It is classified as a non-constant-flow generator. Inspiration is triggered by either time (control mode) or pressure (ACV, SIMV), whereas exhalation is always cycled based on volume. System pressure, however, is limited by the high-airway-pressure alarm. This level, once reached, dumps the remaining gas in the piston chamber to the atmosphere but does not alter inspiratory time.

MODES

Control, ACV, and SIMV modes are available on the PLV-100. In the control mode, the practitioner sets ventilator rate, tidal volume, and inspiratory-flow rate. The unit determines inspiratory time based on these settings and displays an I:E ratio. In the control mode, the patient is unable to activate a positive-pressure breath but can breathe spontaneously via the piston chamber or the exhalation valve. In the ACV mode, all settings are identical to the control mode, with the addition of sensitivity setting. Inspiratory time remains constant with each positive-pressure breath, but the I:E ratio display indicates a varied ratio depending on the rate that the patient is assisting. In the SIMV mode, the machine setup is identical to the ACV mode. Because of the patient's spontaneous breathing efforts, however, the I:E ratio display is inactivated. A 6-second window is available for patient triggering of the SIMV mandatory breath; as a result of this large window, delivered positive-pressure rate may vary. The PLV-100 does not contain a demand system. Thus, unless the unit is configured with a continuous-flow system, the patient must draw air during spontaneous ventilation either from the piston chamber or via the exhalation valve. Table 4-1 lists ranges for gas-delivery variables.

ALARMS

The PLV-100 incorporates 11 system alarms: low pressure/apnea, high pressure, inverse I:E ratio, increase inspiratory flow, low internal battery, low external battery, reverse external-battery connection, switch to battery, power failure, microprocessor failure, and ventilator malfunction. The low-pressure audio alarm is activated if the set low airway pressure is not exceeded within a 15-second period. A front-panel light-emitting diode (LED) flashes with each breath as pressure passes the set level. In SIMV, the low-pressure alarm also acts as an apnea alarm. The patient's spontaneous inspiratory efforts are sensed by the low-pressure mechanism, and the 15-second delay is reset. Thus, if either the machine does not sense a spontaneous breath or the positive-pressure level does not exceed the set mark within a 15-second period, the alarm is activated.

The high-airway-pressure alarm (audio only) is activated each time the patient's peak airway pressure exceeds the alarm setting. When this occurs, tidal volume remaining in the piston chamber is dumped to the atmosphere while the piston continues its forward motion. As a result, inspiratory time remains unaltered. The alarm resets automatically after each breath.

The inverse I:E ratio alarm is a visual flashing alarm that is activated whenever the inspiratory time exceeds the expiratory time. No action on the part of the practitioner is indicated if an inverse I:E ratio is desired.

The increase-inspiratory-flow alarm is a visual alarm activated if inspiratory flow is insufficient to meet other set parameters. When activated, the inspiratory-flow display will flash "Increase Inspiratory Flow" while the inspiratory flow is increased automatically. Inspiratory flow, however, will not increase to a level to prevent an inverse I:E ratio.

The low-internal-battery alarm is both an audio and visual alarm, activated if the internal battery falls below 9.5 V. The external-battery alarm functions in precisely the same manner. If an attempt is made to reverse the external-battery connection, an alarm sounds until the connection is corrected.

Whenever the power source switches from ac to either external dc or internal ac, a 3-second audible alarm sounds. Additionally, if the power switch is in the "on" position and no power is applied to the unit, an audible alarm is activated.

If the microprocessor fails to pass its diagnostic self-test, an audio alarm is activated, and the piston motor locks, preventing uncontrolled function. In addition, if the unit's pressure transducer fails or the piston system fails to cycle properly, a "fast beep" audible alarm is continuously activated if attempts are made to use the unit. See Table 4-2 for a comparison of ventilator alarm functions.

POWER SOURCE

As with all the ventilators in this class, the PLV-100 is operational via three distinct power sources: ac, external dc, and internal dc. This unit always selects ac power if the powering mechanism is available. If the unit must switch to either dc source, a 3-second alarm is activated. When functioning on a dc source, the voltage level of the source can be evaluated rapidly by the "Read Battery Volts" indicator on the front panel. The internal battery is capable of providing up to 60 minutes of power, depending on the actual ventilator settings. The higher the demand, the shorter is the time period. The internal battery is charging whenever the unit is plugged into an ac outlet, regardless of activation.

MISCELLANEOUS

During machine power-up, a complete unit diagnostics check of all systems occurs. This lasts about 5 seconds, during which LEDs are active and alarms sound. Digital readouts of tidal volume, rate, I:E ratio, and inspiratory-flow rate are provided. In addition, a front-panel cover is available as an accessory.

CRITICAL ANALYSIS

The overall physical layout of the control panel is very busy, making the machine appear intimidating and increasing the difficulty in teaching its operation initially. The sensitivity and high-airway-pressure-limit control knobs are not calibrated, making them difficult to set. To determine the high-airway-pressure-limit setting, the patient must be removed from the ventilator. It is possible to provide inverse-ratio ventilation, an approach that is not indicated in the home. The attachments for the exhalation-valve line and the proximal-airway-pressure line are of different sizes to avoid inadvertent misconnection.

LIFECARE PLV-102

The PLV-102[30] (Fig. 4-8) is essentially an update of the PLV-100. This ventilator, as with the PLV 100, is not currently manufactured, but a large number of these units are still in clinical use. The internal gas-flow path is the same as with the PLV-100 with the addition of an O_2 proportioning valve and a 50 lb/in^2 gauge O_2 attachment. A DISS O_2 connector exists on the back of the ventilator; from here, O_2 enters a proportional valve, from which it proceeds to a flow sensor and then into the internal inspiratory circuit, bypassing the piston chamber, thus allowing a delivered F_{O_2} of up to 0.90. In ACV and control modes, F_{O_2} is simply set on the front panel. The accuracy of O_2 delivery, however, decreases at low tidal volume settings less than 300 ml and high F_{O_2} settings of greater than 0.40. During SIMV, the manufacturer recommends using the unit's O_2 sensor. The sensor cable originates on the front of the machine and is interfaced between the humidifier and the ventilator at least 18 in proximal to any H valve or to the unit itself. The sensor is necessary to ensure consistent F_{O_2} during spontaneous ventilation. If the sensor is not present during SIMV, room air is inspired during spontaneous unassisted ventilation.

CLASSIFICATION

The PLV-102 is classified in the same manner as the PLV-100.

MODES

In addition to the control, ACV, and SIMV modes, the PLV-102 incorporates control + sigh and ACV + sigh modes. During both these modes, the ventilator automatically delivers a sigh breath at 150% of the set tidal volume once

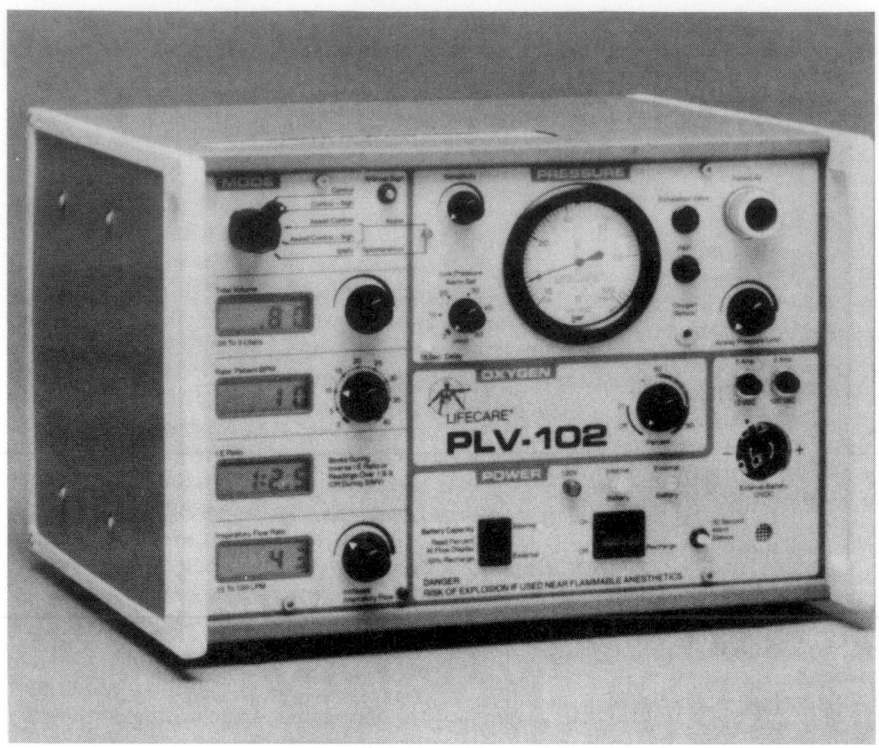

FIGURE 4-8 The Lifecare PLV-102 Ventilator.

every 100 breaths. Table 4-1 lists the ranges for gas-delivery variables.

ALARMS

The PLV-102 incorporates the 11 alarms included on the PLV-100, with the addition of an O_2 alarm that is activated if (1) O_2 source pressure is less than 45 lb/in^2, (2) O_2 source pressure is greater than 55 lb/in^2, (3) the ventilator O_2 valve is stuck open, (4) the O_2 sensor is defective, and (5) the ventilator demand exceeds O_2 valve capability (>90 liters/min). In addition, the PLV-102 displays alarm codes in the peak-flow digital readout window. A decal with code definitions is attached to the machine. A 30-second alarm silence also has been included. See Table 4-2 for a comparison of ventilator alarm conditions.

POWER SOURCE

The power-source data are identical to those of the PLV-100.

MISCELLANEOUS

The PLV-102 has two options not available on the PLV-100: a remote alarm and a printer hookup. In addition, a manual-sigh button allows for sighs on user discretion.

CRITICAL ANALYSIS

The PLV-102 is even more complex than the PLV-100 and less user-friendly. In addition, the 50 lb/in^2 O_2 attachment and F_{IO_2} delivery system make it even less practical for home use. This add-on, however, makes the unit very attractive for use in long-term-care facilities or hospitals. The sensitivity and high-pressure-limit control knobs are not calibrated,

and inverse I:E ratio ventilation is also feasible, as in the PLV-100.

RESPIRONICS PLV CONTINUUM[31]

The PLV Continuum is a highly versatile, compact (10 in wide × 12 in deep × 5.5 in high), lightweight (23 lb), microprocessor-controlled portable home-care ventilator (Fig. 4-9). This unit is turbine-driven; as a result, gas delivery is highly programmable. ACV (pressure or volume), SIMV (pressure or volume), PSV, CPAP, and apnea modes are available. In addition, a sigh can be delivered during

FIGURE 4-9 The Respironics PLV Continuum Ventilator: (1) power on/off, (2) system power indicators, (3) alarm reset button, (4) alarm silence button, (5) status indicators, (6) display control buttons, (7) patient pressure port, (8) exhalation valve port, (9) gas outlet port, and (10) display panel. (*Used, with permission, from Respironics.*[31])

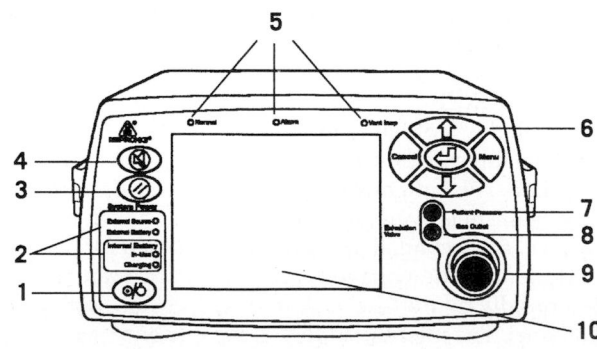

volume ACV. As with other ventilators in this class, it operates from multiple power sources, including an internal battery. Both flow and pressure are monitored during gas delivery; thus tidal volume is displayed. The ventilator can be operated with or without supplemental O_2 entrained, although precise O_2 delivery is not possible.

CLASSIFICATION
The PLV Continuum is an electrically powered, turbine-driven, microprocessor-controlled home-care ventilator. It is single-circuited, with inspiration activated by time or pressure, and expiration cycled based on time, volume, pressure, or flow.

MODES
The ACV and SIMV modes operate like any other demand-flow ventilator. Both modes can be set as volume- or pressure-targeted ventilation. In addition, PSV is available. During PSV, pressure ACV, and pressure SIMV, rise time is active. PSV is terminated by flow decreasing to 25% of peak or by pressure increasing above the set level at the end of a breath by 5 cmH_2O or 10% of the set pressure + 2.5 cmH_2O. Both square and decelerating ramp flows are available during volume breaths. Apnea ventilation at a rate of 12 breaths per minute is also activated after a 20-second apnea period. PEEP is not available. Table 4-1 lists ranges of gas-delivery variables.

ALARMS
A total of 14 ventilator alarms and alerts and 7 patient alarms and alerts are present. From the patient perspective, apnea, high-inflation pressure (two consecutive breaths), excessive inspiratory time, low pressure, and system occlusion/disconnect are alarmed. In addition, patient visual alerts are activated if airway pressure is high for a single breath or if an inverse I:E ratio is established. Machine alarms include alarm failure, barometer failure, depleted external battery, depleted internal battery, external battery connection, high gas temperature, indicator failure, low internal battery, primary alarm failure, using default settings, and ventilator inoperable. Ventilator alerts are activated visually if indicators fail, the external battery power is low, and the ventilator is running on the internal battery. See Table 4-2 for a comparison of ventilator alarm conditions.

POWER SOURCE
Operation is possible by ac, internal dc, and external dc power. The internal battery lasts 15 minutes to 1 hour depending on ventilator settings. When the internal battery is running, a visual alert is provided, as well as when the internal battery charge is low. The internal battery charges whenever the unit is plugged into ac current.

MISCELLANEOUS
The ventilator is set using a series of four screens in a menu format. A group of five control buttons on the front upper-right side control screen and setting selection. Multiple entries are required to make a setting change. With startup, a self-check is performed, and the startup screen indicates the last patient's settings. A settings screen controls settings and modes, and an alarm screen provides control of alarm settings. The final screen is a preference screen, directing the clinician to other screens and functions. The ventilator can download data via an RS-232 port or upload revisions of software via a PC connection port. A remote-alarm attachment is also present. A proximal pressure line is used to monitor pressure and enhance triggering to inspiration.

CRITICAL ANALYSIS
This is a very versatile home-care ventilator, usable in pediatric to adult patients requiring any of the standard modes of ventilation. Its major drawback is the lack of PEEP. Inadvertent parameter change is almost impossible; the use of the system requires knowledge and comfort with computer systems. The function of this ventilator has never been compared with that of other similar units.

PULMONETIC SYSTEMS LTV[32,33]

This is one of the most compact of all volume mechanical ventilators. It is 10 in wide, 12 in deep, and 3 in high, weighting only 12.6 lb (Fig. 4-10). Because of its turbine design, it is able to operate without an external gas source. Because of its microprocessor control, it is able to provide a variety of both pressure and volume modes of ventilation. This ventilator also incorporates leak compensation to coordinate patient triggering more effectively. Depending on the particular model, precise F_{IO_2} delivery to 100% via a high-pressure gas source is available. Despite its small size, an internal battery is included. Patient triggering is primarily by flow

FIGURE 4-10 The Pulmonetic System LTV-1000 Ventilator.

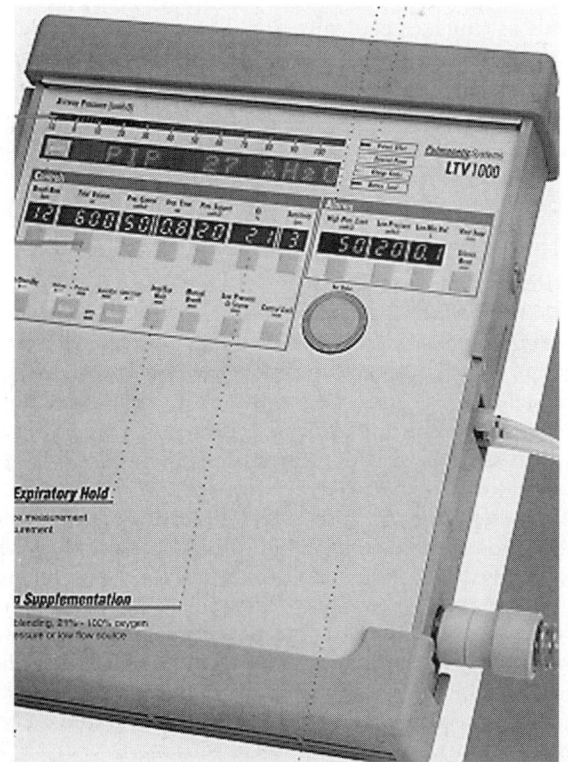

(1–9 liters/min)—diverting flow from the fixed-bias flow of 10 liters/min established during the expiratory phase. A secondary pressure trigger is active when airway pressure falls to –3 cmH_2O. The displayed leak measurement is useful in setting the flow sensitivity.

CLASSIFICATION

The LTV ventilators are electrically powered, turbine-driven, microprocessor-controlled home-care ventilators. This unit is single-circuited, with inspiration triggered by time, flow, or pressure and expiration initiated by time, pressure, volume, or flow.

MODES

ACV and SIMV modes are available in both pressure and volume ventilation. In addition, PS and CPAP are available. During SIMV, PSV can be applied to the spontaneous breaths. During pressure ACV breaths, rise time can be adjusted. During PSV, the terminating flow can be adjusted from 10–40% of peak flow. Pressure ACV breaths also can be terminated by flow if desired. That is, either flow or time can end the breath, whichever is met first. The same can occur in PSV by setting the variable time limit or if inspiratory time exceeds two breath periods. Apnea backup ventilation is present in all modes at a rate equal to the set rate if the set rate is greater than 12 breaths per minute and at a rate of 12 breaths per minute if the set rate is less than 12 breaths per minute. A noninvasive ventilation mode is also included (NPPV). Activation of this mode can occur only in conjunction with the other primary modes of ventilation. When activated, the NPPV LED is lit, and only the following alarms are active: high pressure, apnea, external power lost, internal battery low, ventilator inoperable, and default settings. Specifically, the low-minute-volume and low-peak-pressure alarms are inactive. PEEP is not an integrated microprocessor-controlled function with this ventilator. PEEP is established by addition of a spring-loaded PEEP valve on the expiratory limb. A specific ventilator circuit is required with this ventilator. Table 4-1 lists ranges for gas-delivery variables.

ALARMS

A total of 12 alarms are included on the LTV: apnea, battery depleted, low battery, defaults settings activated, pressure-sensing-line disconnect/malfunction, high O_2 pressure, high airway pressure, hardware faults, ventilator inoperative, low minute ventilation, low O_2 pressure, and low airway pressure. In addition, a number of patient variables are monitored and displayed. In order to measure many of these variables, the inspiratory-hold or expiratory-hold control must be activated periodically. The inspiratory hold, however, is only active in volume ventilation, and the expiratory hold requires passive exhalation. The specific monitored variables are peak inspiratory pressure, mean airway pressure, PEEP, frequency, exhaled tidal volume, minute ventilation, I:E ratio, calculated peak flow, plateau pressure, quasi-static compliance, and auto-PEEP. See Table 4-2 for a comparison of ventilator alarm conditions.

POWER SOURCE

Ac, dc internal, and external dc power are available. The internal battery lasts a maximum 1 hour and 37 minutes depending on ventilator settings. When the internal battery is operational, an alert is activated.

MISCELLANEOUS

On activation, the ventilator performs a power-on self-test that ventilates with the last set parameters. Mode selection is made by pressing the mode-select button twice, and the use of pressure or volume ventilation is determined the pressing these controls twice. In addition, the user may set any of the following extended-feature options by entering a separate field: alarm volume, low-pressure alarm, variable inspiratory time termination, apnea interval, pressure-control flow termination, NPPV mode, high-pressure alarm delay, and variable flow termination. A manual-breath control is also provided. A specific ventilator circuit is required with a proximal pressure-sensing line to monitor pressure and improve triggering.

CRITICAL ANALYSIS

This is a very sophisticated home-care ventilator offering many modes and adjuncts to modes. Its biggest limitation is the lack of electronic integration of the PEEP control. It is also not a user-friendly ventilator. Actual setting of variables is confusing. It has a user-lockout feature, however, preventing inadvertent parameter adjustment.

VERSAMED iVENT$_{201}$[34]

The iVent$_{201}$ is a turbine-driven home-care/subacute-care ventilator incorporating most of the features of an intensive-care-unit (ICU) ventilator. It is the only ventilator of this class that provides continuous waveforms of pressure, flow, and volume. The ventilator is portable and compact (13 in high × 9.5 in wide × 10.3 in deep), weighting only 22 lb (Fig. 4-11). With startup, the ventilator goes through a ventilator verification test to ensure proper function. In addition, an operational verification test requiring attachment of the circuit to a test lung should be preformed with every circuit change. In addition to multiple modes and monitoring and alarm functions, PEEP is an integrated aspect of the function of this ventilator. Ventilator triggering to inspiration can be by either time, pressure, or flow, and cycling to exhalation can be based on time, volume, pressure, or flow. A high-pressure DISS O_2 connection is available providing precise F_{IO_2}, or the unit may be run by entraining room air and titrating O_2 into the system gas inlet.

CLASSIFICATION

The iVent$_{201}$ is an electrically powered, turbine-driven, single-circuited microprocessor-controlled ventilator.

MODES

ACV and SIMV pressure- or volume-targeted ventilation is available. In addition, PSV, CPAP, and bilevel ventilation are included. Sigh breaths during volume ventilation can be provided. Rise-time variability is available for

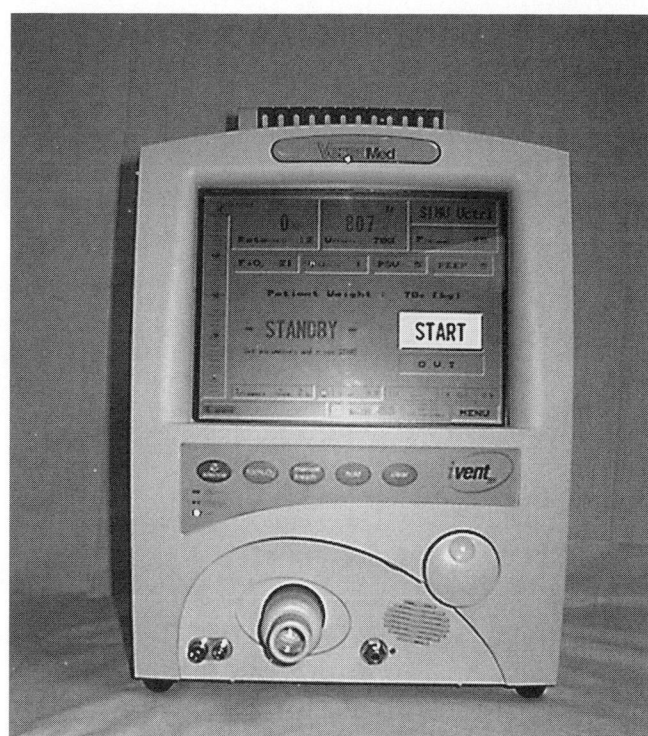

FIGURE 4-11 The VersaMed iVent$_{201}$ Ventilator.

pressure-targeted breaths. Easy exhale is an adjustment recommended for use during bilevel. When activated, this feature momentarily relieves the exhalation-valve diaphragm of pressure immediately at end inspiration. The ventilator also includes two unique mode adjuncts: adaptive peak flow and adaptive time. Adaptive peak flow allows the ventilator to determine the inspiratory peak flow required to meet the set tidal volume while maintaining an I:E ratio of 1:2. Adaptive time allows the ventilator to determine the inspiratory time (in pressure ventilation) to maintain a 1:2 I:E ratio. Bilevel is similar to airway pressure-release ventilation (APRV), where the patient can breathe spontaneously at two levels of CPAP or during SIMV. I:E ratio in this mode can be inverted. Table 4-1 lists ranges of gas-delivery variables.

ALARMS

This ventilator has 26 alarms arranged by priority: high, middle, and low level. High-priority alarms are apnea, battery empty, excessive leak, high F_{IO_2}, high minute volume, high airway pressure, low battery, low breath rate, low F_{IO_2}, low minute volume, low O_2 pressure, needs service, high internal ventilator temperature, patient disconnect, proximal-pressure-sensor disconnect, tubing disconnect, and high PEEP. Middle-priority alarms are ac power disconnect, high breath rate, low airway pressure, needs calibration, low tidal volume, and volume limit reached in pressure ventilation. Inverse I:E ratio is a low-priority alarm. In addition, a number of patient variables are monitored and displayed: exhaled tidal volume, rate, I:E ratio, inspiratory time, and peak inspiratory pressure. Waveforms for pressure, volume, and flow are also displayed continually. In addition, pressure-

volume, flow-volume, and pressure-flow loops can be displayed. A lung mechanics package (compliance, resistance, and mean airway pressure) is also available. Trends of monitored data also can be displayed. See Table 4-2 for a comparison of ventilator alarm conditions.

POWER SOURCE

The iVent$_{201}$ can be operated on ac, dc internal, or dc external current. On switchover to internal dc, indicators are activated. The internal battery may last up to 2 hours depending on ventilator settings.

MISCELLANEOUS

The ventilator operates via a rotating control knob requiring a push to enter a charge and a series of touch pad keys located on the ventilator front panel. Data and options are presented in a series of menus accessible by the rotator controler. The ventilator has an RS-232 port, and an Sp_{O_2} probe can be connected to the ventilator. A specific circuit is required with a proximal pressure-sensing line for monitoring of pressure and to improve triggering.

CRITICAL ANALYSIS

The only major concern with this ventilator is that it may be too much of a ventilator for use in the home. It clearly contains modes and monitoring capabilities more useful in the ICU than in the home. It is very busy and somewhat intimidating to the uneducated user. For home-care use, the airway pressure, flow, and volume waveforms may be too much.

NEWPORT HT50[35]

This ventilator is also a very compact (10.24 in high × 10.63 in wide × 7.87 in deep) and lightweight (15 lb), portable, microprocessor-controlled home-care ventilator (Fig. 4-12). The unit is turbine-driven and has an attachment for the addition of low-flow (1–10 liters/min) O_2. At high minute volumes, however, high F_{IO_2} is not attainable. A specifically designed circuit is required. A proximal-airway-pressure line is included in the circuit for monitoring and triggering. A number of modes of ventilation are offered, and sensitivity is via pressure triggering.

CLASSIFICATION

This is an electrically powered, turbine-driven, microprocessor-controlled single-circuit ventilator producing a variety of gas-flow patterns. Inspiration is triggered by either time or pressure, and expiration is cycled based on either time, volume, flow, or pressure.

MODES

The HT50 provides ACV and SIMV in both pressure and volume ventilation. In addition, CPAP and PSV are available. PSV may be added to the spontaneous breaths during SIMV, and PEEP can be applied with any mode. During PSV, the breath is terminated when the peak flow decreases to 25%, the peak pressure exceeds 3 cmH$_2$O above the set level, or inspiration time equals 3 seconds. Backup ventilation is available in all modes at a frequency of 1.5 times

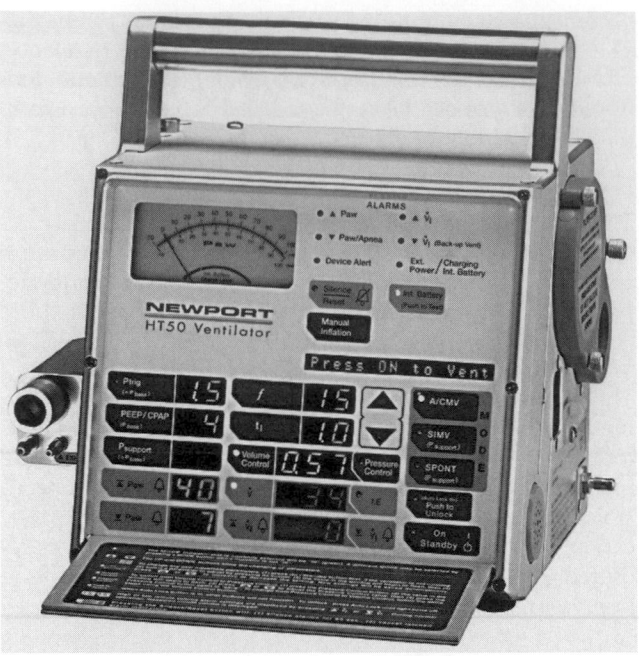

FIGURE 4-12 The Newport HT50 Ventilator.

the frequency setting with a minimum of 15 breaths per minute during ACV and SIMV. During CPAP and PSV, the mode changes to pressure control at a rate of 15 breaths per minute, peak pressure 15 cmH$_2$O, and inspiratory time of 1.0 second. Table 4-1 lists ranges for gas-delivery variables.

ALARMS
A total of 16 alarms are included on the HT50: high and low airway pressure, high and low baseline (PEEP) pressure, high and low minute volume, circuit occlusion, device occlusion, apnea, check proximal pressure line, set pressure not reached (pressure control), low battery, empty battery, power switchover, device alert, and device shut down. The ventilator includes a message window where tidal volume, peak pressure, PEEP, frequency, mean airway pressure, and minute volumes are displayed. In addition, an airway-pressure meter and battery charge indicator are located on the front panel.

POWER SOURCE
As with all these ventilators, the HT50 can be operated by ac, internal dc, and external dc current. Power switchover is indicated on the front panel, as well as internal battery charge level. Low- and empty-battery alarms also are included. The internal battery lasts up to 8 hours when fully charged depending on actual ventilator settings. See Table 4-2 for a comparison of ventilator alarm functions.

MISCELLANEOUS
This ventilator is set by touchpad key entry of all parameters. Individual touchpads for each variable are located on the front panel. An optional humidifier is available, and its operation is monitored on the front panel. A manual inflation control is also on the front panel. Depression of the touchpad delivers a mechanical breath at the set pressure

or volume for up to 3.0 seconds with continued touchpad depression. The panel is locked automatically 20 second after the last adjustment. The unlock-panel touchpad must be depressed for at least 1.0 second to unlock the control panel. An RS-232 port is also included.

CRITICAL ANALYSIS
This is the easiest to operate of all the newest ventilators of this group. The control panel is very user-friendly, and the automatic lockout feature makes undesired changes unlikely. PEEP is an integrated function of the ventilator, making the unit much more useful in a variety of clinical settings. O$_2$ delivery is the one concern. O$_2$ must be titrated into the external gas entrainment port, and the capability of delivering high F$_{IO_2}$ is questionable. The unit's gas-delivery functions have not been compared with those of other ventilators in this class.

Noninvasive Positive-Pressure Ventilators

This group of positive-pressure ventilators only provides pressure ventilation, either pressure ACV or PSV, and generally, they are designed exclusively for noninvasive use. The primary reason for avoidance of invasive application is the inability to provide a high F$_{IO_2}$, inadequate monitoring of patients status, and inadequate alarms. These units have a distinct advantage over ventilators designed for invasive use because they compensate for leaks.[23,24,36,37] In addition, they are highly responsive to patient inspiratory effort, responding at least as well as ICU ventilators.[24,36,37] Each of these ventilators includes some or all of the following modes: control, ACV, PSV, and CPAP. See Table 4-3 for modes offered by specific ventilators.

In addition to the lack of monitoring and alarms, there are two other major issues with these devices: delivery of an increased F$_{IO_2}$ and the "potential" for CO$_2$ rebreathing. As with all ventilators, O$_2$ can be titrated into the inspiratory circuit. With these units (Fig. 4-13),[38] O$_2$ can be titrated into the mask or the circuit at the attachment to the ventilator. The actual F$_{IO_2}$ delivered depends on a number of factors. The first factor is the location of the expiratory port. As noted in Fig. 4-13, the circuit is a single-limb circuit without an exhalation valve. Exhalation occurs through a small orifice either in the mask itself or in the circuit near the mask. A secondary isolation valve can be added to the circuit distal to the expiratory port. Thus the circuit is open. Ventilation is accomplished because these units rapidly compensate for leaks and have a high enough flow to maintain system pressure despite the leaks. The second factor that affects F$_{IO_2}$ is pressure settings: The higher the settings, the lower is the F$_{IO_2}$ because higher settings translate into greater flow compared with the fixed flow of O$_2$ into the circuit. Schwartz et al,[38] using a lung model (see Fig. 4-13), recently demonstrated the large variability in F$_{IO_2}$ at 5 and 10 liters/min O$_2$ flow into the circuit. At high ventilator settings with the leak port in the mask and O$_2$ titrated into the mask itself, only 22–25% delivered O$_2$ could be achieved at O$_2$ flows of 5 and 10 liters/min. With the leak port in the circuit,

TABLE 4-3 Specifications of Bilevel Pressure Noninvasive Ventilators

	Respironics BiPAP S/T	Respironics BiPAP S/T-D 30	Respironics Vision	Respironics BiPAP Pro 2	Respironics BiPAP Plus	Respironics Synchrony	Res Med VPAP III	Res Med VPAP III ST	Res Med VPAP ST-A	Puritan Bennett Knight Star 335	Puritan Bennett Knight Star 330
Modes	C, ACV, A CPAP	C, ACV, A CPAP	C, ACV, CPAP	A	A	C, ACV, A CPAP	A, CPAP CPAP	C, ACV, A	C, ACV, A CPAP	C, ACV, CPAP	A, ACV, CPAP
Inspiratory pressure, cmH_2O	4–20	4–30	4–40	4–25	4–20	4–30	4–25	4–25	3–30	3–35	3–30
Expiratory pressure, cmH_2O	4–20	4–30	4–40	4–25	4–20	4–20	4–25	4–25	3–25	3–20	3–20
Rate, per Min	4–30	4–30	4–40	—	—	4–30	—	5–30	3–30	3–30	3–30
Inspiratory time, %	10–90	10–90	—	—	—	—	—	—	—	—	—
Maximum flow, bites/min	120	120	180	120	120	120	130	130	130	120	120
Inspiratory time, s	—	—	0.5–3.0	—	—	0.5–3.0	—	0.1–4.0	0.1–4.0	—	—
Oxygen concentration	—	—	21–100%	—	—	—	—	—	—	—	—
I:E ratio	—	—	—	—	—	—	—	—	—	1:1 to 1:4	1:1 to 1:4

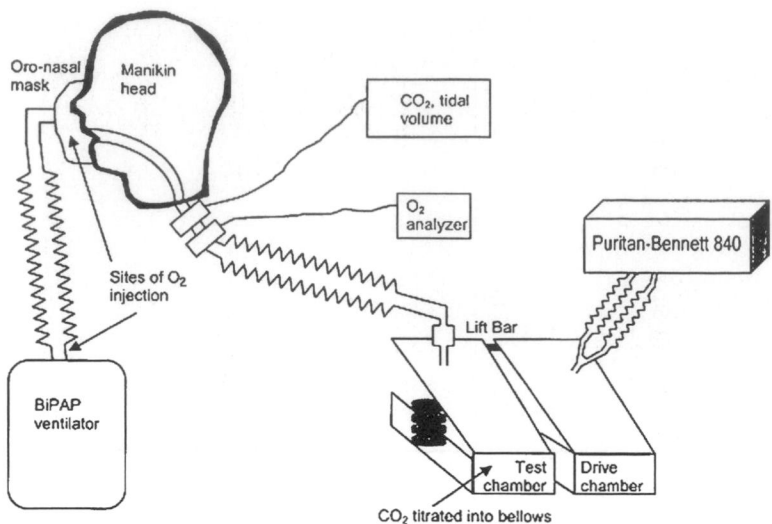

FIGURE 4-13 Illustration of O_2 addition to a bilevel ventilator circuit in a lung model. (*Used, with permission, from Schwartz et al: Respir Care 49:270–5, 1997.*)

however, and O_2 titrated into the mask at 10 liters/min and low ventilator pressures, over 60% O_2 could be delivered. This point is important: It is impossible to predict or measure delivered F_{IO_2} with most of these systems. As a result, very careful monitoring of patient response is required whenever supplemental O_2 is needed. Very high flows of O_2, up to 75 liters/min, can be titrated into some of these units, establishing greater than 90% O_2.[39] These high O_2 flows, however, increases PEEP above the set level and peak airway pressure by as much as 7 cmH_2O.[39] As a result, the addition of high-flow O_2 into the circuit is not recommended.

As discussed earlier, the ventilator circuit is single-limbed without a true exhalation valve. This, coupled with the fact that these ventilators have low internal resistance, increases the possibility of inadvertent CO_2 rebreathing. As noted in Fig. 4-14, when PEEP or end-expiratory airway pressure (EPAP) is set at zero or at a low level, exhaled gas can move retrograde through the ventilator circuit all the way back through the ventilator, causing CO_2 rebreathing.[40] The setting of PEEP, however, ensures flow from the ventilator toward the patient during exhalation, preventing CO_2 rebreathing. CO_2 rebreathing also can be prevented by the use of an isolation valve or a standard exhalation valve. All newer bilevel ventilators maintain a minimum PEEP (2–4 cmH_2O) even when PEEP is turned off to minimize CO_2 rebreathing. The lower the PEEP level, however, the greater is the likelihood of CO_2 rebreathing.

The original bilevel ventilator is the Respironics B_IPAP S/T ventilator[41] (Fig. 4-15). Although these units are no longer manufactured, many of them are still in general use. The unit provides pressure-limited, time- or flow-cycled ventilator assistance via a mask. The B_IPAP S/T is operated by a turbine blower and is designed to provide a continuous flow of gas. It is $7^3/4$ in high, 9 in wide, and 12 3/16 in in diameter and weighs 9.5 lb. Gas is drawn into the unit from the filtered back panel and then passes through an electromagnetically operated solenoid valve (Fig. 4-16) that

controls flow, pressure level, and inspiratory and expiratory cycling times via a microprocessor. Before gas leaves the unit, it passes a flow transducer that provides feedback via the microprocessor to the control solenoid valve.

The unit includes five separate controls: mode selector inspiratory positive airway pressure (IPAP) level; peak inspiratory pressure setting; and EPAP (PEEP) or CPAP level, rate, and inspiratory time percent. Even when the EPAP control is set at minimum, a low level of CPAP/PEEP

FIGURE 4-14 Volume of CO_2 inhaled from the ventilator tubing at various IPAP and EPAP settings during B_IPAP ventilatory assistance in normal subjects (*top*) and patients (*bottom*).
***p < 0.05 compared with other devices at similar B_IPAP settings. (*Used, with permission, from Ferguson et al: Am J Respir Crit Care Med 151:1126–35, 1995.*)**

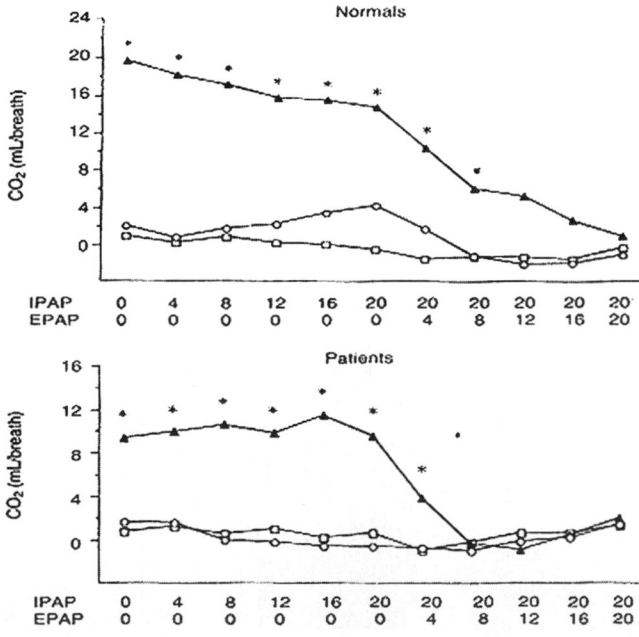

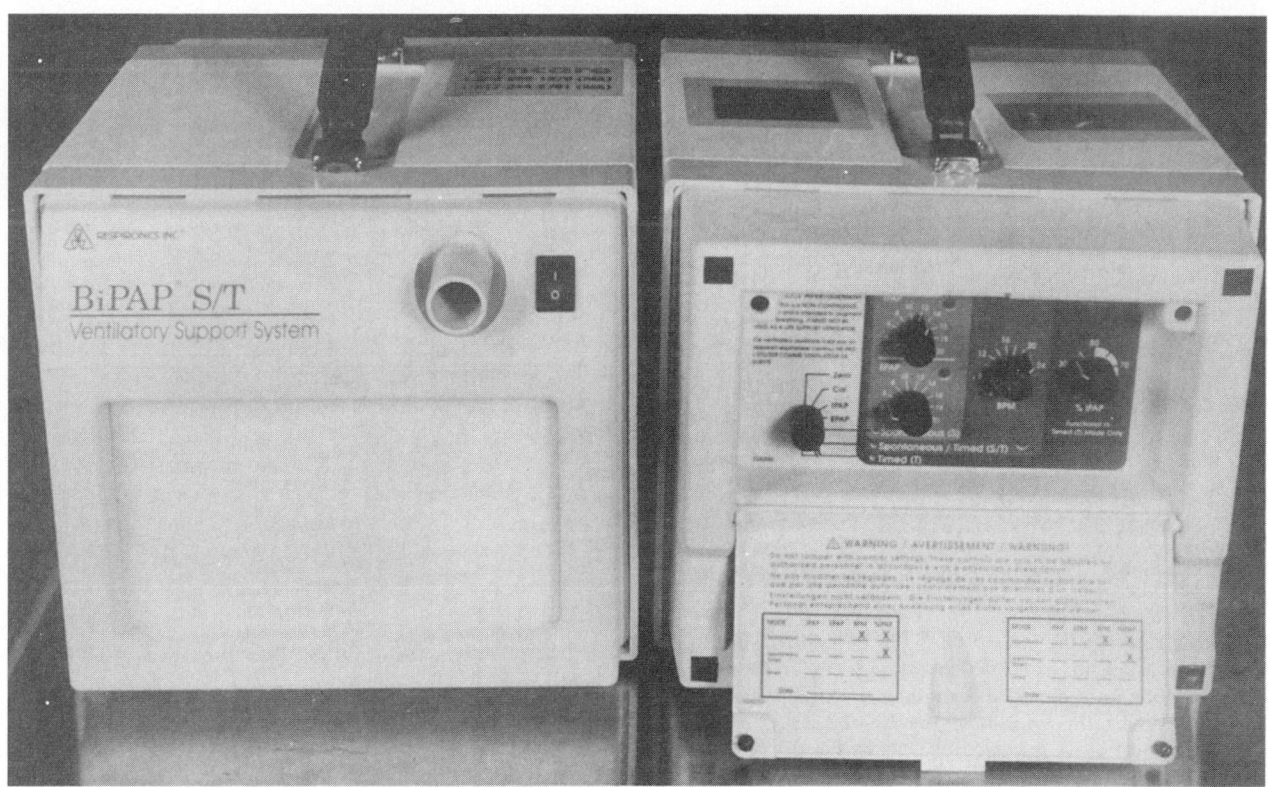

FIGURE 4-15 The Respironics B₁PAP S/T Ventilator.

(2 cmH₂O) is maintained in the system. The B₁PAP S/T ventilator does not incorporate any alarms. The unit only operates via ac current. It does not have an internal battery, although it may be attached to an external dc battery. All other ventilators in this class essentially operate in the same manner. Each has a flow-regulating valve (see Fig. 4-16) as the basis of its operation. This valve allows for easy triggering, cycling, and leak compensation. The electric current in the coil, in combination with a magnetic field, produces a force on the valve disk that must equal the force created by the air pressure in order to maintain a stable pressure level. As changes from the preset pressure are sensed, the electric current adjusts the disk automatically to increase or decrease the amount of air vented from the pressurized valve chamber.

RESPIRONICS BILEVEL VENTILATORS

S/T-D30

This ventilator is lightweight (17.6 lb) and relatively small (7.75 in high × 9 in wide × 15.25 in deep). It offers the same modes as the S/T. It also has an optional alarm package, with high and low pressure monitored. It appearance is essentially the same as the S/T (see Fig. 4-15). The system used to track leaks is "auto-track sensitivity." The ventilator incorporates a process known as "shape signal" to effectively trigger and cycle during spontaneous breathing (Fig. 4-17). The patient's inspiratory and expiratory flow is monitored continuously. The shape signal appears as a shadow image of the patient's actual flow, establishing a sensitivity threshold for inspiration and expiration. When the patient's actual flow crosses the shape signal, the unit changes

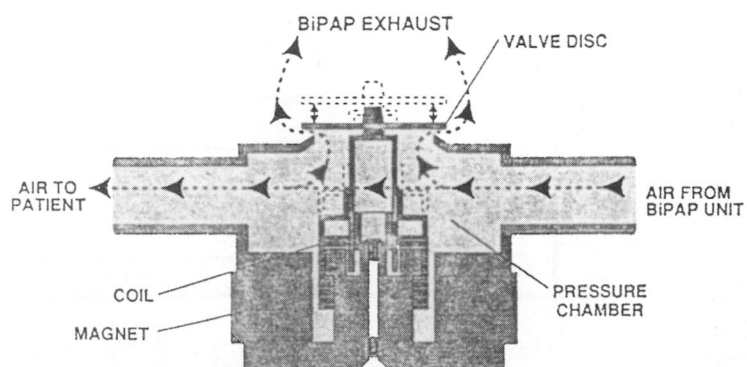

FIGURE 4-16 Schematic of the B₁PAP pressure-flow control valve. The electrical coil and magnet cyclically apply a force to the valve disk that is equal to the IPAP and EPAP settings. Excess pressure is vented to the room, allowing for maintenance of stable pressures despite changes in flow rate. (*Used, with permission, from Respironics.*[41])

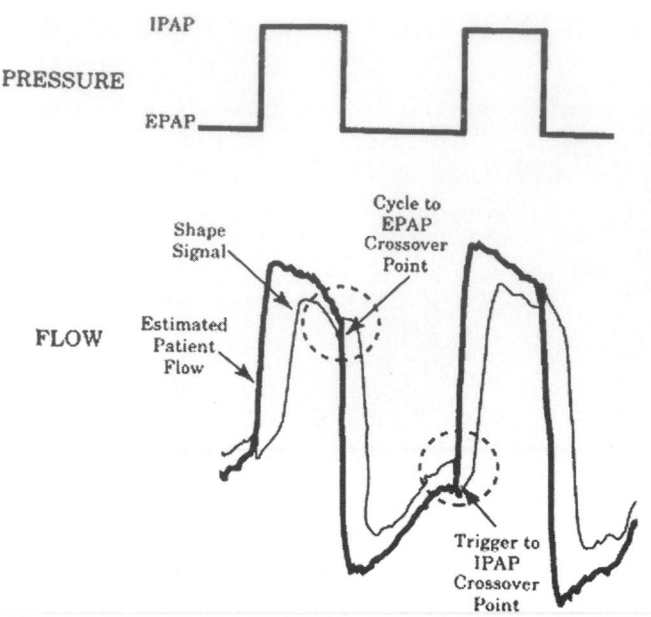

FIGURE 4-17 Tracking the patient's flow pattern with a shape signal provides a sensitive mechanism to trigger inspiration or to cycle to expiration in response to changing breathing patterns and circuit leaks. (*Used, with permission, from Respironics.*[42])

pressure level. The control panel of the S/T-D30 is the same as the S/T, and no internal battery is included.

VISION
This is the only bilevel pressure noninvasive ventilator designed for use in the ICU[43] (Fig. 4-18). Because of size (16 in deep × 14⅜ in wide × 10⅝ in high), weight (34 lb), and cost, it is unlikely that it would be used in the home. This ventilator has the same modes as the S/T-D30 and the same enhanced ability to trigger and cycle. In addition, it monitors and alarms high and low pressure, the delay in establishing low pressure, apnea, low minute ventilation, and high and low rate. The ventilator can be attached to a high-pressure O_2 source and can provide 90% or greater F_{IO_2}. Waveforms

FIGURE 4-18 The Respironics Vision Ventilator.

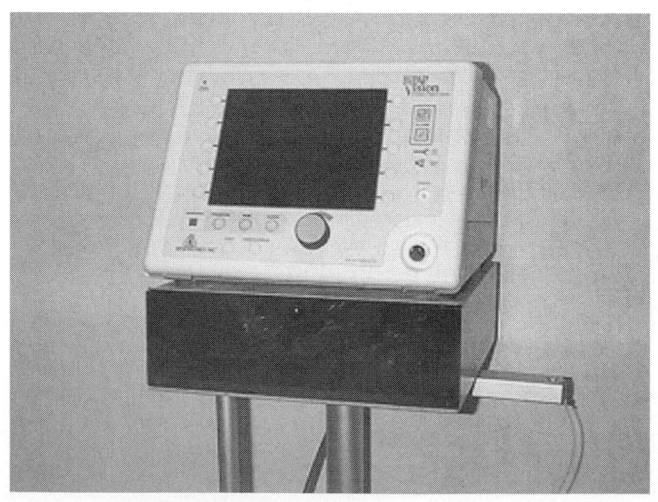

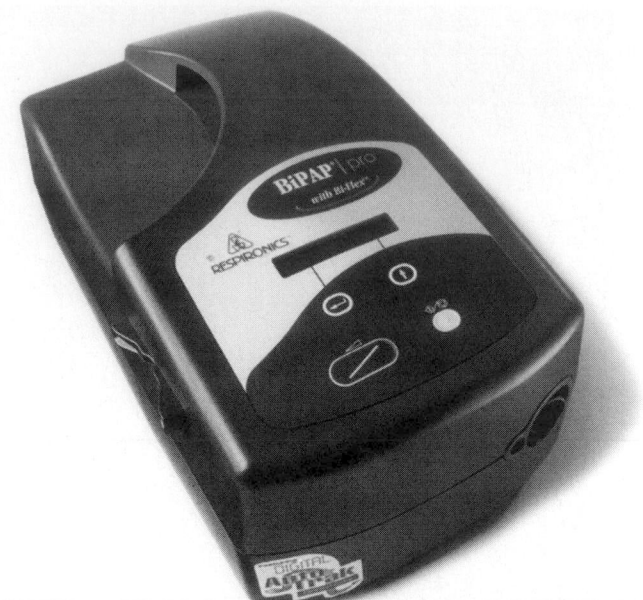

FIGURE 4-19 The Respironics B_IPAP Pro 2 or B_IPAP Plus Ventilators.

for pressure, flow, and volume are provided, and the ventilator displays monitored pressures, volumes, rate, and F_{IO_2}. As with all other ventilators in this group, the Vision does not include an internal battery.

B_IPAP PRO 2 AND B_IPAP PLUS
These two ventilators appears exactly alike except that the Pro 2 has the ability to accept a "Smart Card" for recording of health-status data, and the Plus has a communications connection port[44] (Fig. 4-19). In addition, the Pro 2 allows the activation of the "Bi-Flex" option[45] (Fig. 4-20). This

FIGURE 4-20 Illustration of the function of the Bi-Flex adjunct on the Respironics B_IPAP Pro-2. Adjustment of Bi-Flex allows rapid decompression of the ventilator circuit, making exhalation easier. Three levels can be set. (*Used, with permission, from Hess et al: Chest 124:227S, 2003.*)

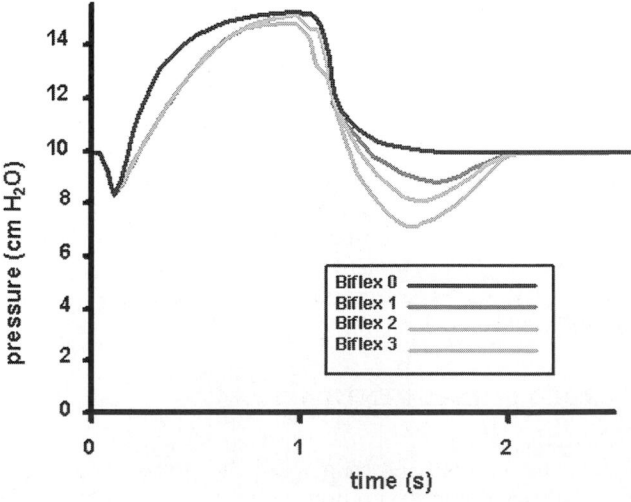

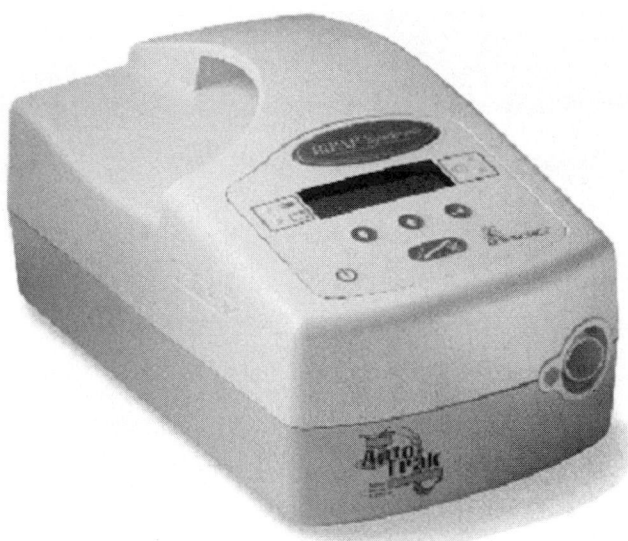

FIGURE 4-21 The Respironics Synchrony Ventilator.

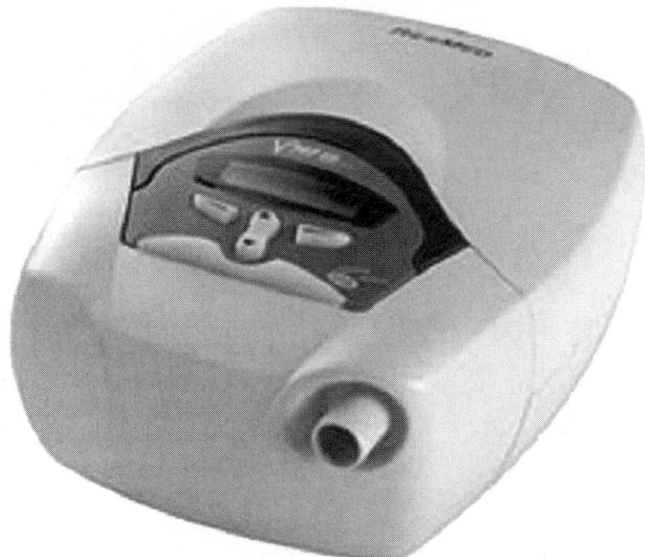

FIGURE 4-22 The ResMed VPAP III or VPAP III ST Ventilators.

control causes a rapid decrease in airway pressure at the start of exhalation that can be set at three levels and is designed to make exhalation easier. Both these ventilators provide only PSV. In addition, each includes a rise-time adjustment. Also, included is an automatic off/on option. This feature allows the unit to turn off automatically when the mask is disconnected and to turn automatically on when the patient begins inhaling (three consecutive breaths). A ramp function slowly increases pressure as assistance is started to make it easier for the patient to accept the ventilator. A dual-time meter is provided to track the time the unit is plugged in versus the time it is operational. In addition, the unit provide alerts to the patient: system error and patient disconnect.

B$_I$PAP SYNCHRONY

The Synchrony, similar to the Pro 2 or Plus, is a small (12 in long × 7 in wide × 6 in high) and lightweight (6 lb) ventilator. Unlike the Pro 2 and Plus, however, all modes are available: control, ACV, PSV, and CPAP. It also includes a ramp to set pressure and a rise-time adjustment. This ventilator incorporates a large number of alarms: high priority (power failure, apnea, low pressure, high pressure, low minute volume, patient disconnect, ventilator inoperative, external dc battery failure), medium priority (low battery), and low priority (battery in use, call for service, and power failure). This unit is designed to allow attachment to an external dc power source but has no internal battery. An integral modem is included to allow for monitoring at a distance via the telephone. An RS-232 communications port is also included. An optional O$_2$ supplement port is provided, which allows automatic shutoff and turn on when the ventilator is turned off and on.

RESMED B$_I$LEVEL VENTILATORS

VPAP III[47]

This is a small (10.6 in long × 9.1 in wide × 5.6 in high) and lightweight (5 lb) noninvasive ventilator that provide

PSV or CPAP (Fig. 4-22). It allows rise-time control over 100–900 ms. A unique feature is T$_I$ control or control over minimal and maximal inspiratory time; that is, a minimal inspiratory and maximal inspiratory time can be set (Fig. 4-23). This unit also evaluates mask fit by measuring the extent of the leak with the particular mask. A "Smart Start" opinion is available, starting and stopping the machine as the patient begins and ends breathing through the ventilator. An additional unique and useful feature is the data-management option. This feature allows the clinician to monitor and compare trends in leak volume, tidal volume, respiratory rate, minute volume, apneas, and hypopneas. Data can be stored for up to 365 sessions of ventilator support. A 9-pin communications port and a 15-pin auxiliary port are included.

FIGURE 4-23 ResMed T$_I$ control. With this option, minimal and maximal inspiratory times during pressure support can be set. (*Used, with permission, from ResMed.*[47])

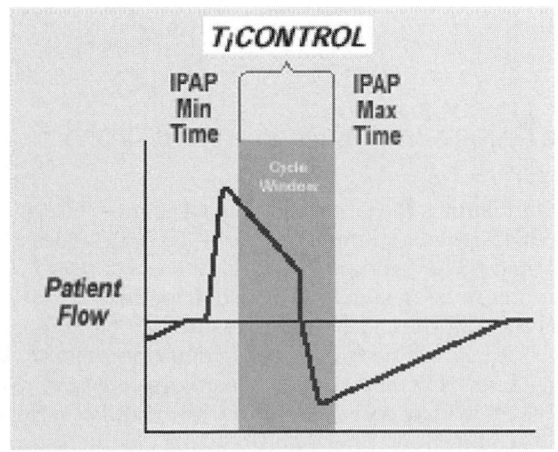

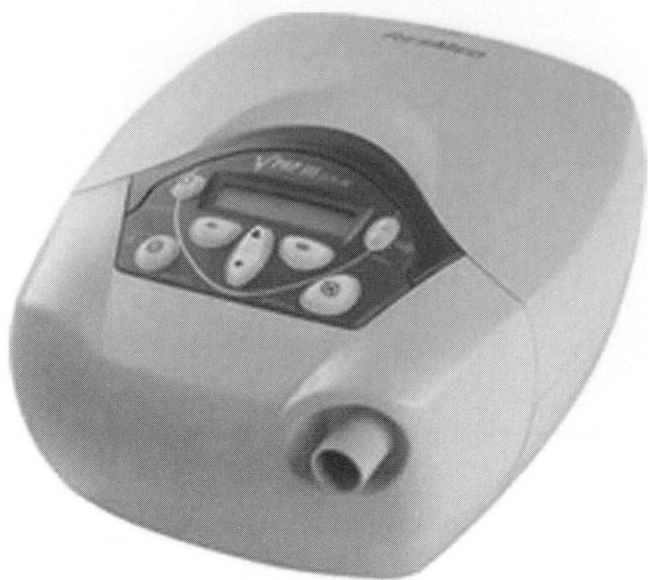

FIGURE 4-24 The ResMed VPAP III ST-A Ventilator.

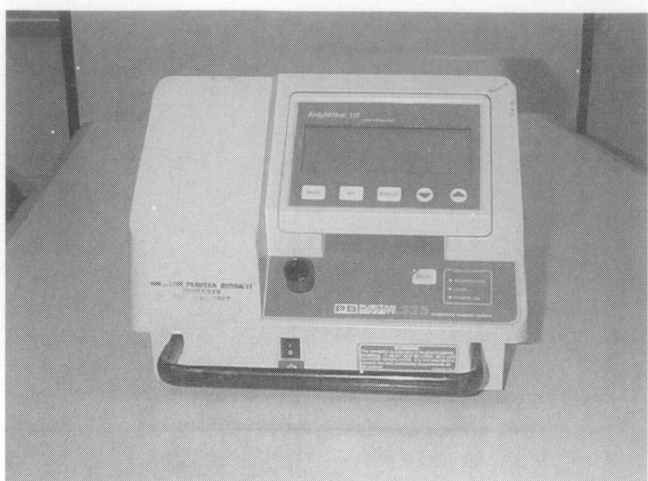

FIGURE 4-25 Puritan-Bennett Knight Star 335 Ventilator.

VPAP III ST

This ventilator looks and operates exactly the same as the VPAP III except that it also includes the ability to deliver ACV and control mode ventilation.

VPAP III ST-A

This ventilator has all the features of the VPAP III ST with the addition of a number of new features[48] (Fig. 4-24). A new leak management system referred to as "Vsync" has been added. This ensures better and faster recognition of system leaks and adjustment of triggering and cycling levels. Both triggering sensitivity and cycling sensitivity are now adjustable. An upgraded data-management system referred to as "Smart Data" is included. This system monitors a number of patient parameters and allows for comparison to trended data. Specifically, hours of use, mask leak, tidal volume, respiratory rate, minute volume, percent spontaneous triggered breaths, percent spontaneous cycled breaths, and pressures are monitored and displayed. A series of adjustable and nonadjustable alarms is included. Adjustable alarms include mask leak, low pressure, high pressure, low minute volume, and nonvented. Preset alarms include power fail, excessive pressure above set level, and system fault/failure.

PURITAN-BENNETT BILEVEL VENTILATORS

KNIGHT STAR 335

This ventilator is the largest and heaviest of the bilevel ventilators designed for home use (Fig. 4-25). It provides assist, ACV, and CPAP modes.[49] During all modes, pressure application can be delayed for a specific period of time after application of the mask, and pressure can be ramped up slowly thereafter in steps of 1–3 cmH$_2$O per minute. Both trigger sensitivity and cycling sensitivity can be adjusted. The machine incorporates basic alarms: ventilator inoperative, disconnect, and power failure. Tidal volume, estimated

peak inspiratory flow, leak volume, respiratory rate, and I:E ratio are monitored and displayed. A unique aspect is the ability to remove the control module after setting the ventilator or using the module at a distance of up to 100 ft to monitor patient response and adjunct settings.

KNIGHT STAR 330

This is the featured ventilator from Puritan-Bennett (Fig. 4-26). It is very small (3.75 in high × 8.25 in deep × 5.62 in wide) and lightweight (2.7 lb), with features similar to the 335. Assist, ACV, and CPAP modes are present, with both delay in starting ventilation and ramp of setting over time. Rise time can be set during assist and ACV. A number of conditions are alarmed: high pressure, low pressure, system leak, ventilator malfunction, apnea, power loss, and pressure above 40 cmH$_2$O. In addition, respiratory rate, pressure, tidal volume, leak, peak flow, and I:E ratio are monitored and displayed. The ventilator can be powered by an external battery or ac current and has an RS-232 port for remote communications.

Common Features of All Positive-Pressure Ventilators

DELIVERY OF INCREASED F$_{IO_2}$

The typical home ventilator is not designed to provide a precise, constant F$_{IO_2}$. These machines have evolved in this manner because many patients receiving home ventilation do not require a precise or high F$_{IO_2}$. Typically, an F$_{IO_2}$ of 0.25–0.35 is needed, and a ±0.05 variation in F$_{IO_2}$ is usually clinically acceptable in these patients.

Of the ventilators presented, only the PLV-102, LTV, iVent$_{201}$, and Vision are capable of setting and maintaining a relatively precise and high F$_{IO_2}$. Each of the other units increases the F$_{IO_2}$ by attachment of an O$_2$ accumulator to the gas entry port (see Fig. 4-3) or titration of O$_2$ into the inspiratory limb between the ventilator and humidifier (Fig. 4-27). The exception to this may occur during noninvasive mask ventilation. In this setting, O$_2$ may be delivered directly into

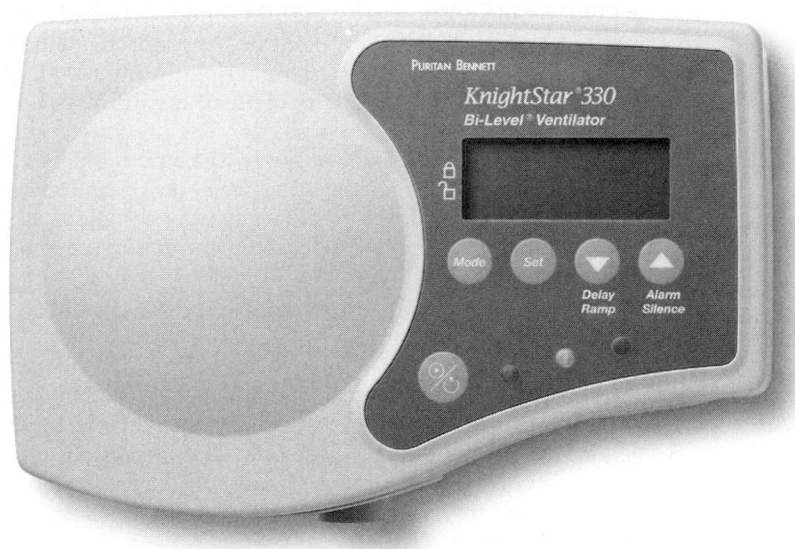

FIGURE 4-26 Puritan-Bennett Knight Star 330 Ventilator.

some masks that include pressure monitoring and O_2 delivery ports. With all noninvasive ventilators, however, it is difficult to approximate and impossible to measure F_{IO_2}, as discussed earlier.

Normally, O_2 is bled into the accumulator while room air is drawn into the accumulator during the backstroke of the piston. Although all manufacturers provide elaborate formulas with which to calculate F_{IO_2} delivered in this way, the formulas hold true only if the patient is ventilated in the volume-control mode. Variation in the ventilator rate, tidal volume, inspiratory flow rate, O_2 flow, and level of spontaneous breathing all affect the breath-by-breath F_{IO_2} delivered.

SIMV/IMV AND WORK OF BREATHING

Most of the new volume-targeted home-care ventilators incorporate a demand system, which allows SIMV to be de-

FIGURE 4-27 Oxygen delivery elbow used on LP series ventilators, although this type of adaptor may be used on any of the home care ventilators. Oxygen is titrated directly into the inspiratory limb, bypassing the piston chamber. (*Used, with permission, from Puritan-Bennett.*[27])

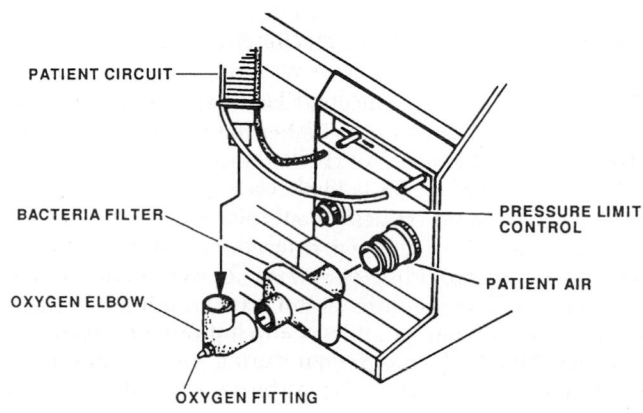

livered in a manner similar to that of ICU ventilators. None of the older units still in use, however, incorporates a demand valve. Thus, during the spontaneous breathing phase of SIMV with these older units, the patient must draw gas from the piston chamber, from a piston chamber bypass valve, or through the exhalation valve. As a result, even with the use of an optimal humidifying system (e.g., a passover humidifier), a large amount of work is imposed by the ventilator system.[26,51] This work increases as patient peak spontaneous inspiratory flow rate increases and with use of a bubble-through humidifier.

Whenever SIMV is used on these older ventilators (e.g., LP-10, LP-6 Plus, PLV-100, PLV-102, or any other older ventilators), the following are highly recommended: the use of a passover humidifier and incorporation of a one-way H-valve between the ventilator and the humidifier (Fig. 4-28). This configuration significantly reduces inspiratory work imposed during the spontaneous phase of SIMV.[26] If an increased F_{IO_2} is required, a reservoir bag, with or without a venturi to provide high flow (see Fig. 4-28), may be used. The addition of a one-way H-valve, particularly if an increased F_{IO_2} is desired, significantly complicates the ventilator setup, limits portability, and wastes O_2 if an elevated F_{IO_2} is needed. For this reason and because of increased workload, use of SIMV on these older ventilators should be avoided.

HUMIDIFICATION

In general, two basic humidification systems are available for home use: heated passover humidifiers and heat and moisture exchangers (HMEs). HMEs, while not recommended on a continuous basis, are very useful during transport and periods of time away from home. Use of these devices greatly simplifies the ventilator setup on a wheelchair or in a car. Once the patient returns home, however, reattachment to a passover humidifier is recommended. It should be remembered that the respiratory resistance of artificial noses increases over time and varies

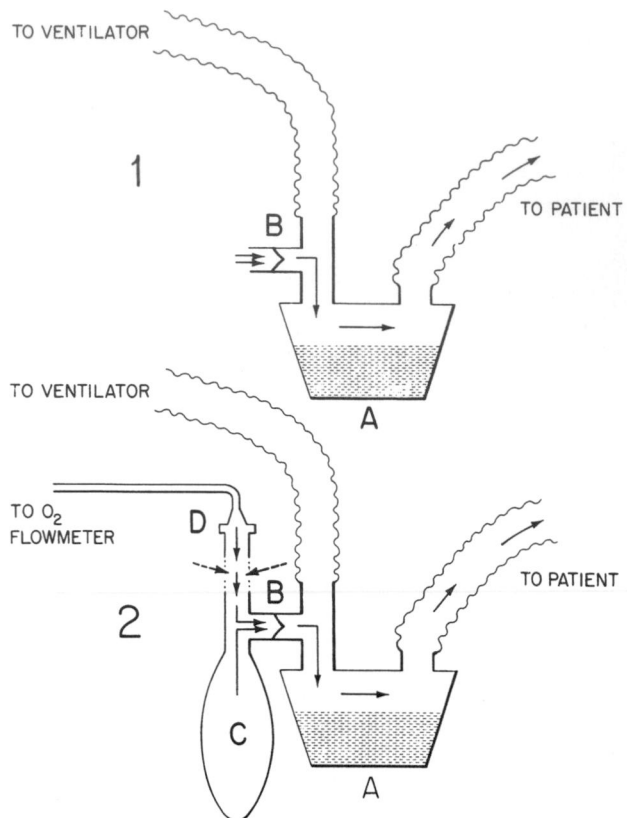

FIGURE 4-28 Diagram of one-way H-valve systems: **(1)** valve open to atmosphere, **(2)** valve with 3-liter reservoir bag attached to 28% oxygen air-entrainment device powered by 4 liter/min oxygen, **(A)** passover humidifier, **(B)** one-way valve, **(C)** reservoir, **(D)** 28% oxygen air-entrainment valve. Arrows indicate gas flow during spontaneous inspiration. Setup **(1)** is used if no supplemental oxygen is required. Setup **(2)** allows for the titration of oxygen into the system. (*Used, with permission, from Kacmarek et al: Respir Care 35:405–14, 1990.*)

from one unit to another.[52] To our knowledge, there are no published data to support the use of artificial noses as the sole source of humidity for ventilated patients in the home.

APPLICATION OF PEEP

Few volume-targeted ventilators available for home ventilation are designed for the application of PEEP. The exceptions are the Achieva, iVent$_{201}$, and Newport HT50. A PEEP device can be affixed easily to the ventilator circuit of any unit, however, work of breathing is increased if ventilation is patient triggered because none of these units automatically compensates for PEEP. With these units in PSV, ACV, or CPAP modes, sensitivity must be adjusted to decrease the pressure gradient necessary to trigger the unit; if 5 cmH$_2$O of PEEP is applied, sensitivity must be set to about +4 cmH$_2$O (1 cmH$_2$O below baseline required to trigger inspiration). Many patients at home do not maintain a tight seal at the tracheostomy cuff, however, which increases the likelihood of self-cycling. Table 4-1 lists the limits of the sensitivity settings of all units discussed. As noted, a significant variation in the range of sensitivities exists.

PEEP should not be used in the SIMV mode on ventilators without an integrated PEEP control. Appropriate setting of the sensitivity may allow for triggering during positive-pressure breaths, although work of breathing during spontaneous breaths is increased markedly. The pressure gradient required to inspire is increased by the amount of PEEP applied. If indications for the use of PEEP arise, use of the ACV mode with an appropriate sensitivity setting is recommended. All the pressure-targeted ventilators have an integrated PEEP function.

PEDIATRIC VENTILATION

The ventilation of pediatric patients, whether they are 8 weeks or 8 months of age, is a challenge with the older generation of home-care ventilators. The introduction of the newer volume ventilators with pressure-targeted modes makes is easy to ventilate children in a manner similar to that used in the ICU. Pediatric ventilation can be accomplished easily with the LTV, iVent$_{201}$, and Newport HT50 ventilators.

THE IDEAL HOME POSITIVE-PRESSURE VENTILATOR

Whether there is such a thing as an ideal home mechanical ventilator is questionable. We will, however, present our perspective on such a unit for use with adults. This description is based on the assumption that adult home mechanical ventilator patients are stable and not weanable. The two key words that describe such a unit are *simplicity* and *reliability*. Because operation of such a unit is primarily by non-health care workers, its design must be straightforward and its operation user-friendly. It should only incorporate modes commonly used in the ICU. It should be alarmed with the following: high pressure, low pressure/apnea, ventilator failure, power switchover, low minute ventilation, and disconnect. In addition, a simple method of increasing the F$_{IO_2}$ to 0.40 should be included. In addition, PEEP should be an integrated function to allow use without imposing work. Many of the newest generation of volume home-care ventilators fulfill this recommendation.

Clinical Application of Positive-Pressure Ventilators

The choice of a specific mechanical ventilator and method of application depends on whether the application is elective or required because of chronic ventilatory failure and whether the application is invasive (via tracheostomy) or noninvasive. Based on design and overall features, all the units discussed, except the pressure-targeted bilevel units, are capable of providing ventilator support under all circumstances. The pressure-targeted bilevel units, because of their lack of alarms and their inability to monitor gas delivery, should be used only for elective, noninvasive applications.

ELECTIVE POSITIVE-PRESSURE VENTILATION

The type of patient who benefits from the elective, non-invasive application of positive-pressure ventilation is still controversial (see Chapter 19). It is our opinion and that of others[53-56] that elective support benefits any patient in whom the progression of ventilatory dysfunction has resulted in retained CO_2, disturbed sleep, loss of energy, and an inability to perform functions of daily diving. This is particularly true if the process is irreversible and progressive.[56]

The goal of elective ventilator support is unloading of the respiratory muscles for about 6–12 hours per day. It is hoped that this rest allows muscles to recover from incipient fatigue and results in normalized sleep, increased energy, and frequently, an improvement in baseline P_{CO_2} during spontaneous breathing.[57-60] To achieve these goals, care must be taken that the application of positive pressure is comfortable, that it is capable of meeting the patient's ventilatory demands, and that it is set to unload effort during sleep.[54,56]

Bilevel positive-pressure ventilators are ideal for this purpose. A major problem with patient acceptance is the periodic blast of air through the nose (or nose and mouth) during inspiration. Because pressure-targeted ventilators maintain a continuous gas flow, it is our experience that the change from expiration to inspiration is not as dramatic with these units and is better tolerated than with volume-targeted ventilators. When setting bilevel pressure, the primary goal is patient comfort. The selection of both inspiratory pressure and PEEP must be acceptable to the patient to ensure compliance. The PEEP level selected depends on the need to (1) establish functional residual capacity, (2) overcome upper airway obstruction, and (3) decrease the work of breathing associated with the presence of air trapping and auto-PEEP. We have found that in the vast majority of patients, a PEEP of minimal (2 cmH_2O) to about 6 cmH_2O is sufficient to accomplish these goals. Higher levels usually result in overdistension and patient discomfort. The inspiratory pressure level is set to ensure an adequate tidal volume and reasonable respiratory rate. With some bilevel pressure units it is impossible to determine tidal volume delivery, and other units have optional monitoring modules available that can estimate tidal volume. We normally base the inspiratory pressure setting on patient comfort, chest expansion, use of accessory muscles, chest auscultation, respiratory rate and pattern, and arterial blood-gas results. Most patients require a peak airway pressure of about 12–16 cmH_2O or a ventilatory pressure of 6–12 cmH_2O.

ELECTIVE VENTILATION VIA TRACHEOSTOMY

Provision of elective ventilation via a tracheostomy is rare. Nevertheless, there are individuals who require a tracheostomy for upper airway disorders who also benefit from elective support. In this setting, a volume ventilator always should be selected because of its monitoring and alarm capabilities in the face of a closed ventilatory system. The setup of the ventilator is the same as that described for noninvasive ventilation, with the actual delivered tidal volume generally in the 6–10 ml/kg range depending on patient tolerance and comfort.

TABLE 4-4   Guidelines for the Use of Elective NPPV

Primary ventilator	Remote alarm
Backup ventilator	Battery
System humidifier	Battery charger
Ventilator circuits	Manual ventilator
Oxygen source	Compressor for aerosol medication
Suction apparatus	Small volume nebulizer[a] (or metered dose inhaler)
Suction catheters	
Spare tracheostomy tube	Electric generator[b]

[a]Only necessary if aerosol medication required.
[b]Only necessary if greater than 16 hours a day ventilator support required or located more than 4 hours from a hospital.

INVASIVE NONELECTIVE VENTILATOR SUPPORT

As indicated earlier, only volume ventilators capable of monitoring patient status with appropriate alarms should be used during invasive ventilator support. The primary controversy in this area is the mode of ventilation. Generally, no attempt is made to wean adult home-care patients. The overriding goal is to maximize ventilator independence for short periods of time, which is the same goal as with elective ventilation. We believe that this can be accomplished best with the ACV mode of pressure or volume ventilation or PSV by maximizing respiratory muscle rest during periods of ventilation to ensure maximum capability during periods of ventilator independence.

Many patients requiring home ventilator support require a secondary backup ventilator. Generally, we recommend a backup ventilator if the patient requires 16 hours or more of ventilatory support per day or if he or she resides more than 4 hours from a hospital. Additional equipment frequently needed by these patients is listed in Table 4-4.

NONINVASIVE NONELECTIVE VENTILATOR SUPPORT

The provision of noninvasive positive-pressure ventilator support to patients requiring home ventilation demands careful monitoring of both the patient and the status of the equipment. Most clinicians prefer to provide ventilator support invasively in these settings. Others,[61-64] however, have demonstrated the effective use of both noninvasive positive-pressure[61,62] and non-positive-pressure techniques[65,66] in large numbers of patients requiring ventilator support. In this setting, a mouthpiece and lip seal, a nasal mask, or an oral-nasal mask have been used to interface the patient with the ventilator. The actual setup of the ventilator is consistent with that of elective, noninvasive ventilator support.

Facial Appliances for Noninvasive Positive-Pressure Ventilation (NPPV)

The most difficult aspect of establishing NPPV is finding a properly fitting facial appliance. Six different approaches are currently in use: (1) total face mask, (2) oral-nasal mask,

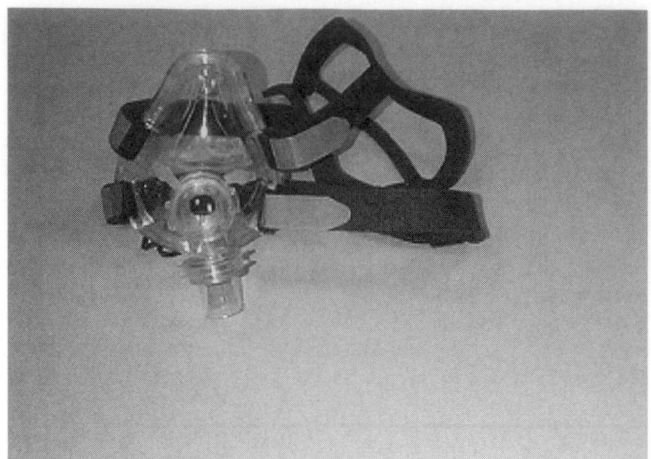

FIGURE 4-29 A *ResMed*. Oral-Nasal Mask.

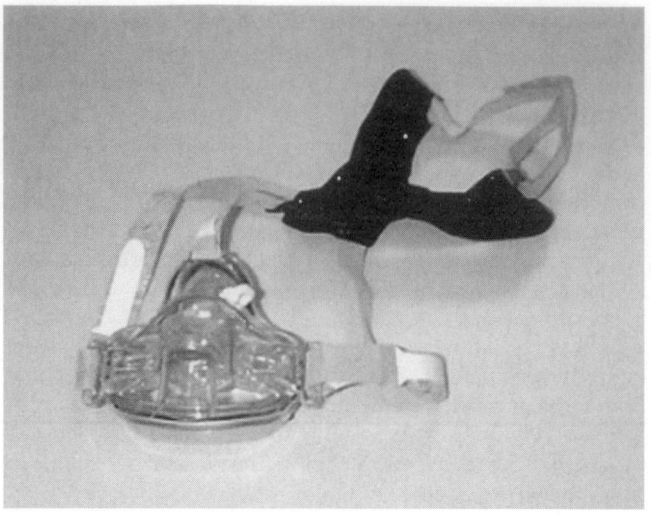

FIGURE 4-30 A nasal mask.

(3) nasal mask, (4) Adams circuit, (5) head hood, and (6) mouthpieces. All approaches should be considered with every patient, although there are different problems with each appliance.

ORAL-NASAL MASKS

For many practitioners,[67–69] an oral-nasal mask has been the appliance of choice for the delivery of NPPV in the emergency room and in the ICU, whereas others[54,59,61,66] have used oral-nasal masks successfully in patients requiring long-term ventilator support (Fig. 4-29). Many oral-nasal masks are available currently; we find that most work well, provided that a proper fit is achieved. The ideal face mask for long-term ventilation (1) is made of clear plastic to allow visual assessment of secretions, (2) has a soft contour that conforms to the anatomy of the patient's face, (3) is deformed easily from its factory shape as needed to fit the patient, and (4) has "memory" so that it maintains its deformed shape when it is removed. Ideally, a number of different masks of varying sizes should be available when attempting to fit a particular patient.

Proper fit is the essential feature in mask selection. Leaks at the bridge of the nose, causing air to blow into the patient's eyes, will result in NPPV failure because of patient intolerance. The mask should fit comfortably from just below the lower lip to about two-thirds of the way up the bridge of the nose. The exact fit is depends on the patient. Patient comfort is essential: The patient is *always* the final judge of proper fit.

The most common error in securing the mask is exerting excessive pressure. With NPPV, low peak airway pressures (generally 12–16 cmH$_2$O) usually are used. Because some leak is expected, masks do not need to be secured so tightly that pressure sores develop. Firm but even pressure distributed over the entire mask usually is sufficient to make a seal. Remember, if a patient cannot tolerate the facial pressure, the whole process may fail. Most mask have inner lips that seal tighter during inspirations.

NASAL MASKS

The most popular approach to the application of NPPV for home use is the nasal mask. Numerous commercial nasal masks are available that work well on most patients (Fig. 4-30). Most, similar to today's oral-nasal masks, have an inner lip of $1/4–1/2$ in that forms an open space between the inner and outer walls of the mask. As a result, when positive pressure is applied, force is exerted between the inner and outer folds, creating a better seal. Because of this, only low to moderate pressure is needed to secure the mask. As with the oral-nasal mask, pressure must be applied equally at all points of connection to the headgear: at the bridge of the nose and at each side of the mask. If a properly fitting mask is chosen, and moderate but equal pressure is applied at each connection, a very comfortable fit can be achieved.

Choosing the proper size mask is critical. As a general rule, the smaller the mask, the better is the fit. There are many types and sizes of masks available, although we would estimate that nearly all patients are fitted with the smaller sizes. The ideal mask fits closely to the lateral contour of the nose, extending from just under the external nares to two-thirds of the way up the bridge of the nose.

Chinstraps are available to reduce mouth leak. Although we frequently try them, they infrequently reduce mouth leak. If patients are actively opposing nasal NPPV, nothing eliminates mouth leak. In many patients, the extent of the mouth leak decreases as they acclimate to ventilation. Also, many patients who have a large leak while awake demonstrate little or no leak while sleeping, or vice versa. Because peak pressures are usually 12–16 cmH$_2$O, during sleep the soft palate and the base of the tongue are elevated sufficiently to prevent excessive leak in many patients.

ADAMS CIRCUIT

A variation on the application of nasal ventilation, the Adams circuit (Fig. 4-31) is available from several manufacturers. Individual "nasal pillows" fit into a manifold that is attached over the top of the patient's head. Some patients prefer this approach to the nasal mask. Others who are more

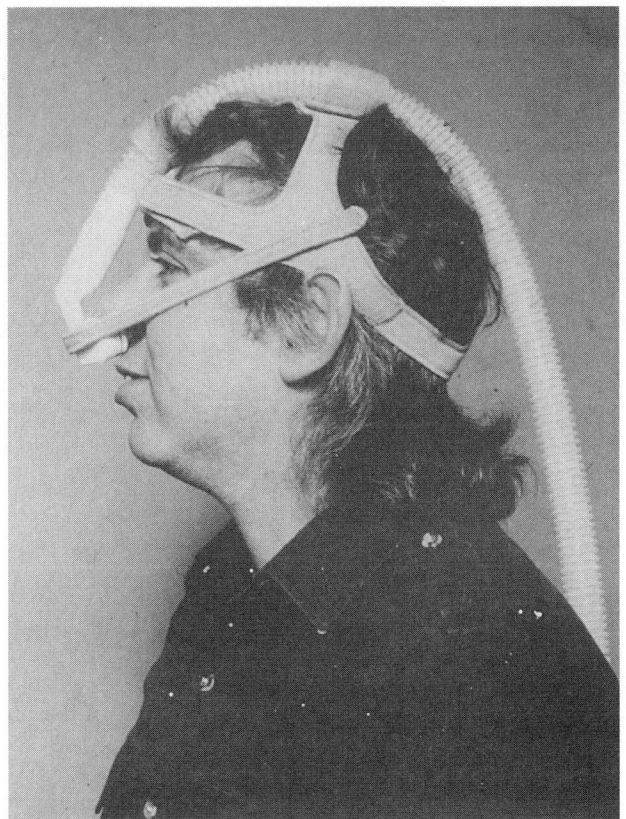

FIGURE 4-31 Adams circuit. (*Courtesy of Puritan-Bennett.*)

sensitive to pressure use both nasal masks and nasal pillows, switching back and forth as irritation develops. Because of differences in design, the points of pressure differ greatly between the two approaches. Multiple sizes of pillows are available, corresponding to the size of an individual's external nares.

MOUTHPIECES

Many patients who use negative-pressure ventilation at night use periodic positive-pressure ventilation during the day. In others, mouthpiece positive-pressure ventilation has been applied 24 hours per day.[70] This requires more than the use of a standard mouthpiece. Many mouthpieces with inner flanges are available commercially (Fig. 4-32). Some patients do best when a customized mouthpiece is made from an impression of the patient's mouth. With a customized mouthpiece, many patients are capable of comfortably maintaining ventilation for indefinite periods. Many do not experience significant nasal leaks during sleep, whereas others also require nasal plugs or nose clips. With this approach, the gumline should be monitored for sores.

TOTAL FACE MASK

One company makes a full face mask (Fig. 4-33). This mask fits over the whole face, including the eyes. Despite its size, it is very comfortable. The primary concern with this mask is deadspace and thus a decreased ability to eliminate CO_2.[71] This interface normally is used for the acute application of NPPV; it is not used commonly in the home.

HEAD HOOD

Figure 4-34 illustrates the newest facial appliance for the application of noninvasive positive pressure. The head hood has been used successfully by a number of European groups[18,72,73] but is not currently available in the United States. Despite its appearance, it is very comfortable. Again, the biggest concern with the device is deadspace and CO_2 rebreathing.[72,74] It appears to be best suited for the application of CPAP using a high-continuous-flow approach to clear CO_2 continually from the hood. The head hood should be reserved for acute application of positive pressure in the ICU.

Non-Positive-Pressure Approaches to Ventilator Support

Three basic approaches are used to provide ventilator support without the application of positive pressure to the airway: (1) negative-pressure ventilation, (2) pneumobelts, and (3) rocking beds.

FIGURE 4-32 A mouthpiece for NPPV application.

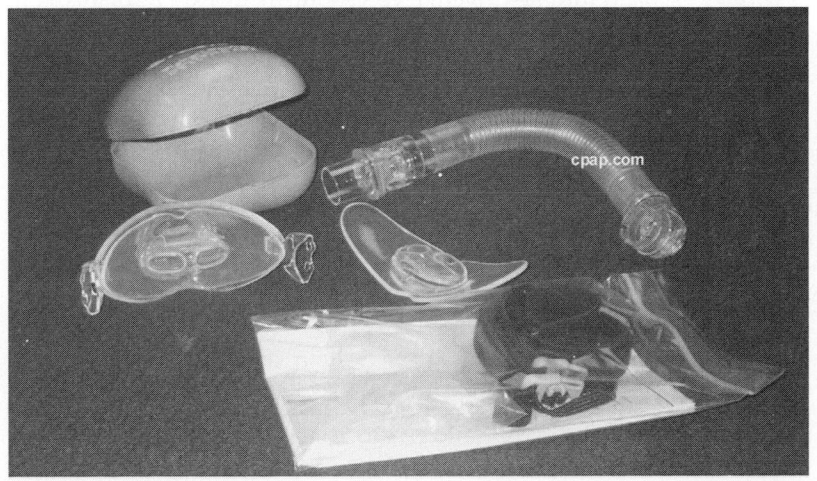

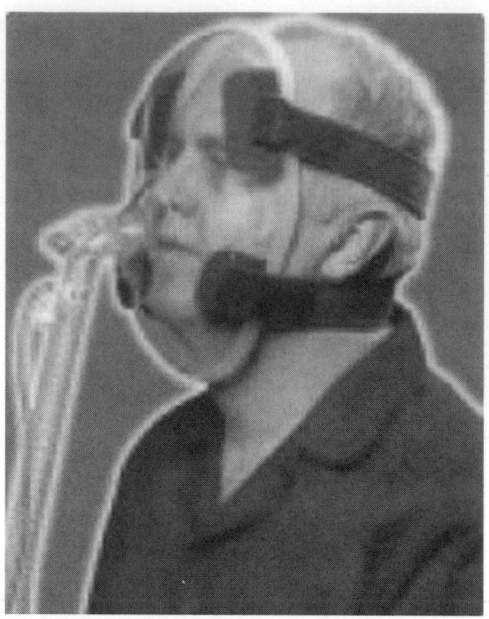

FIGURE 4-33 The Respironics Total Face Mask. (*Used with permission.*)

NEGATIVE-PRESSURE GENERATORS

There is only one commercially available negative-pressure generator in the United States. Iron lungs still exist in many centers and are used by some neuromuscular diseased patients in the home.

EMERSON IRON LUNG

The oldest of all mechanical ventilators still available commercially for use in the United States is the Emerson Iron Lung[75] (Fig. 4-35). Jack Emerson manufactured his first iron lung in 1931.[76] The unit consists of a large, relatively airtight chamber in which the patient's body is placed. The patient's head is exposed to the atmosphere, whereas on the opposite end a flexible diaphragm is attached by a series of arms and gears to an electric motor. The motor drives a variable-sized

FIGURE 4-34 Head hood currently available only in Europe.

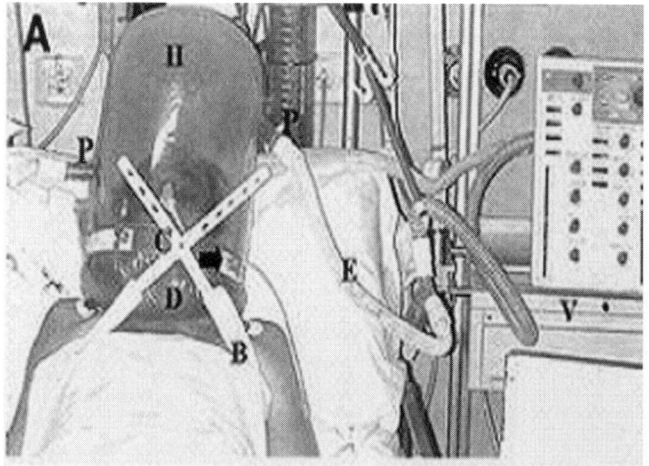

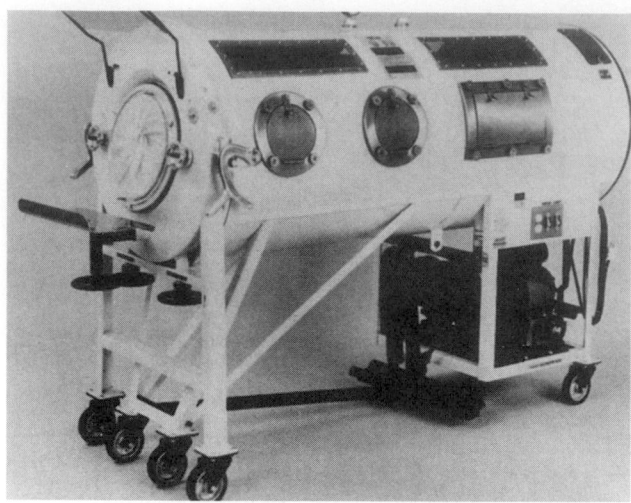

FIGURE 4-35 Emerson Iron Lung.

wheel (the actual diameter of the wheel varies from one end to the other) via a fan belt. The wheel is connected to a cam by a transfer case that translates the motion of the wheel to the cam. The cam is connected by a series of linkages and arms to the movable leather/rubber diaphragm at the rear of the iron lung. The level of negative pressure created is controlled by the size of an adjustable leak. In the event of a power failure, the machine may be cycled manually. The unit functions at a fixed I:E ratio of 1:1, with rates available from about 10–30 breaths per minute in the adult unit. Adolescent and pediatric units are available that provide even greater rates. Pressures up to –60 cmH$_2$O are obtainable. A pressure manometer is affixed to the top of the unit for monitoring. A number of locking ports located on each side of the unit allow access to the patient, and glass panels are configured across the top of the unit. A seal at the patient's neck is achieved with an adjustable plastic ring.

LIFECARE NEV-100

The NEV-100 ventilator (Fig. 4-36) is the most technically sophisticated of the negative-pressure ventilators currently available.[77] It is light (31 lb), compact (21 in high × 12 in wide × 12 in diameter), and portable but is incapable of being operated by battery. It is microprocessor-controlled and turbine-driven. Five specific modes are available: control, control with sigh, ACV, ACV with sigh, and continuous negative extrathoracic pressure (CNEP). In all but the CNEP mode, a negative or positive base pressure (expiratory pressure) can be set. The front panel has three buttons [manual sigh, alarm silence (30 seconds), and panel lock/unlock], a computer screen menu display, and a single rotary parameter controller. All setting adjustments are made with the rotary controller, which must be unlocked before use (it locks automatically 30 seconds after last use).

Three different menus are available on the computer screen. With the first menu, the following parameters are displayed and can be set: mode, negative inspiratory pressure (–5 to –100 cmH$_2$O), base pressure (–30 to +30 cmH$_2$O), rate (4–60 breaths per minute), inspiratory time (0.5–5.0 s), I:E ratio (1:3 to 2:1), sigh pressure (–5 to –100

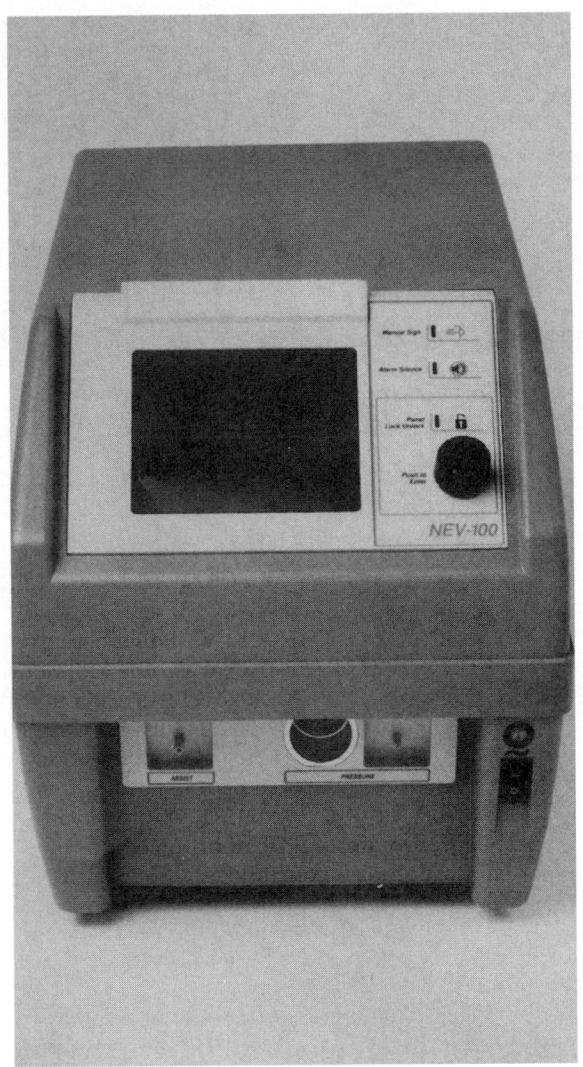

FIGURE 4-36 Lifecare NEV-100 Negative-Pressure Ventilator.

cmH_2O), sigh multiple breaths (one, two, or three, sigh frequency (1–20 per hour), and low-pressure alarm setting.

The second menu indicates frequency of output to a printer, units of pressure displayed (cmH_2O, kPa, mbar), and alarm history. In addition, screen brightness, date and time, alarm volume, assist sensitivity (levels 1–10, no pressure units indicated), alarm pitch, and remote alarm status all can be controlled and adjusted from this screen.

The final menu is for the setting of CNEP levels. Only two variables are set in this menu: base pressure and low-pressure alarm.

In the four ventilation modes, the clinician must set the rate, negative inspiratory pressure, base pressure, inspiratory time, and I:E ratio. Sigh pressure, multiples and frequency, and sensitivity are also set. Although I:E ratio can be set, it depends on rate and inspiratory time and will default to the ratio indicated by the combination of these variables.

Unlike older negative-pressure ventilators, this unit is highly alarmed. It incorporates 13 specific alarms, although only one is set by the clinician: the low-pressure alarm. It can be set from –1 cmH_2O below to +1 cmH_2O above the base pressure setting. If system pressure is below this level for a 20-second period, audio and visual alarms are activated. Both are activated if excessive negative pressure or base pressure develops or if the inspiratory CNEP or base pressure is out of range. Internal system failure, constant pressure failure, missing parameter, and high or low internal temperature alarms are also present. A continuous audio alarm sounds if a power failure occurs, and an information message is displayed if an inverse ratio is set.

This unit has a remote alarm and an hour clock and is capable of being attached to a recorder for the display of alarms and ventilation variables, as well as diagnostic information.

CRITICAL ANALYSIS OF NEGATIVE-PRESSURE GENERATORS

The iron lung is still the standard in the area of negative-pressure ventilation, although it is no longer manufactured. It is the most reliable and effective method of providing negative-pressure ventilation. The rapid development of noninvasive positive-pressure techniques since 1995 has all but eliminated the use of negative pressure. As discussed earlier, only one company in the United States currently makes a negative-pressure generator.

NEGATIVE-PRESSURE CHAMBERS

Negative pressure can be applied to the thorax using a full-body chamber, chest cuirass, or Nu-Mo suit.

FULL-BODY CHAMBERS

The Portal-Lung (Fig. 4-37) is a full-body chamber without a negative-pressure generator. It is available from Respironics, is lightweight and easy to use, and can be driven by any negative-pressure generator. It is presently available in child and adolescent sizes. Its major drawback is the requirement of an assistant to operate. The present model must be secured from the outside.

FIGURE 4-37 The Porta-Lung with the Respironics NEV-100. (*Courtesy of Respironics.*)

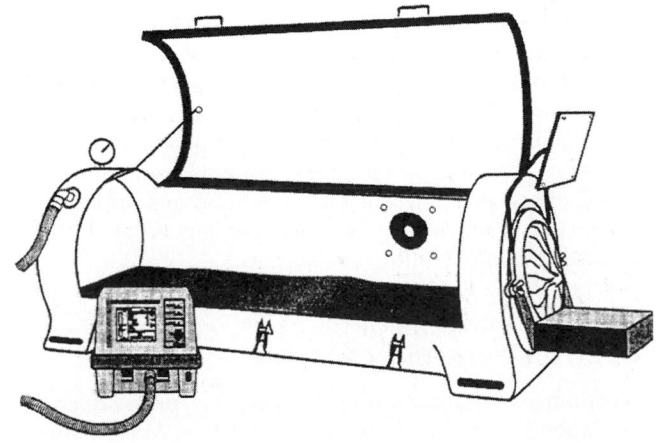

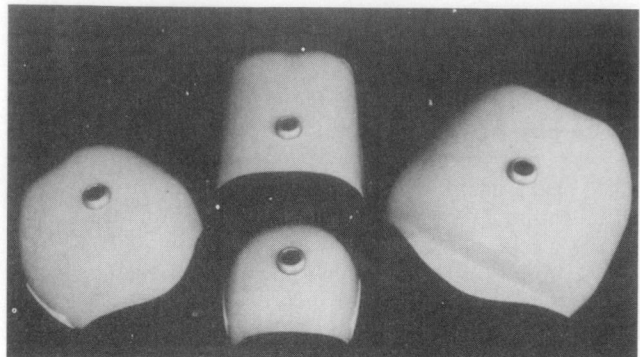

FIGURE 4-38 Commercially available chest cuirass.

CHEST CUIRASS

Figure 4-38 depicts a commercially available chest cuirass. They are designed to be placed over the patient's thorax and abdomen and are secured in place with wide straps. A negative-pressure generator is attached at the opening on the top of the shell. Each shell is designed with a cushion of 2–3 in of air between the patient's maximum chest rise and shell to ensure that the chest wall of the patient does not come directly in contact with the top of the shell, which would negate further thoracic expansion. Most patients find the shell reasonably comfortable. The major problem with commercial shells, however, is fit. In many cases, towels must be stuffed between the shell and the patient to ensure a seal, or foam rubber must be added. Leaks normally occur at the neck and pelvis. For these reasons, it is best to have a shell customized to the patient. Figure 4-39 shows a cast of a patient's chest and abdomen from which a customized shell is designed. Customized shells are particularly important in patients with thoracic deformities. To fit well, the shell should extend from the clavicle to the pelvic arch and along the sides of the chest wall. Ideally, when attached, the shell should not rest on the bed but should extend about halfway down the chest wall. Of all the negative-pressure chambers available, the chest cuirass is the easiest for patients to use independently.

NU-MO SUIT

The Nu-Mo Suit is depicted in Fig. 4-40. This device is actually a modified poncho that is fit over a grid. The grid is necessary to prevent the negative-pressure attachment from being affixed directly to the thorax. It maintains a 2–3-in cushion of air that can be decompressed during inspiration. When applied, the Nu-Mo Suit is secured at the neck with a tie string and at the arms and hips with Velcro straps. It is available in three sizes. The primary problem with this chamber is leakage. In fact, most patients complain about being cold when using the Nu-Mo Suit because of room air drawn into it when negative pressure is generated. Leaks are most prevalent at the hips and neck.

CRITICAL ANALYSIS OF NEGATIVE-PRESSURE CHAMBERS

Acceptance and acclimation to a negative-pressure chamber depend primarily on patient preference. Many patients

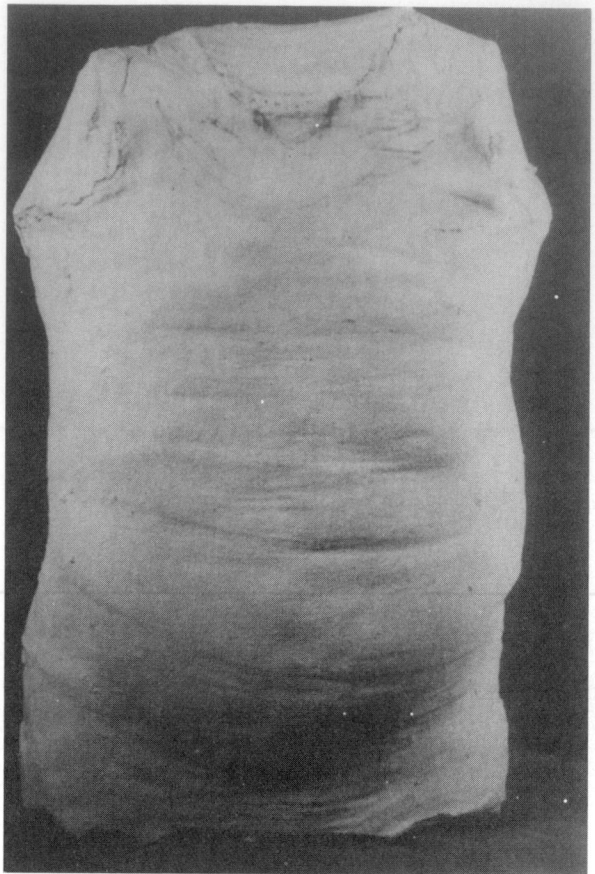

FIGURE 4-39 Cast of the thorax used to make a customized chest cuirass.

simply prefer one chamber to another. In general, the chest cuirass is best tolerated, particularly if the patient is claustrophobic. A customized cuirass is preferable in most situations. The full-body chamber seems to work best with children and adolescents, although many adult polio victims and kyphoscoliosis patients still use iron lungs or portalungs. The Nu-Mo Suit is cumbersome for patients to use, and many become claustrophobic in them. All approaches should be considered and tried clinically before deciding on one method in a given patient.

PNEUMOBELT

The pneumobelt (Fig. 4-41) is actually an adjustable corset that contains an inflatable bladder. It functions by exerting a positive pressure on the abdomen, forcing the abdomen cephalad and thus assisting with exhalation[3,78](Fig. 4-42). Inspiration proceeds under the patient's own efforts. It is hoped, however, that with proper application of the pneumobelt, functional residual capacity is reduced slightly. Thus, on release, elastic recoil leads to an increase in tidal volume.

For proper function, an appropriately sized pneumobelt should be selected and fitted tightly over the abdomen from the xiphoid process to just about the pelvic arch.[79] Fit is important to prevent paradoxical movement of the rib

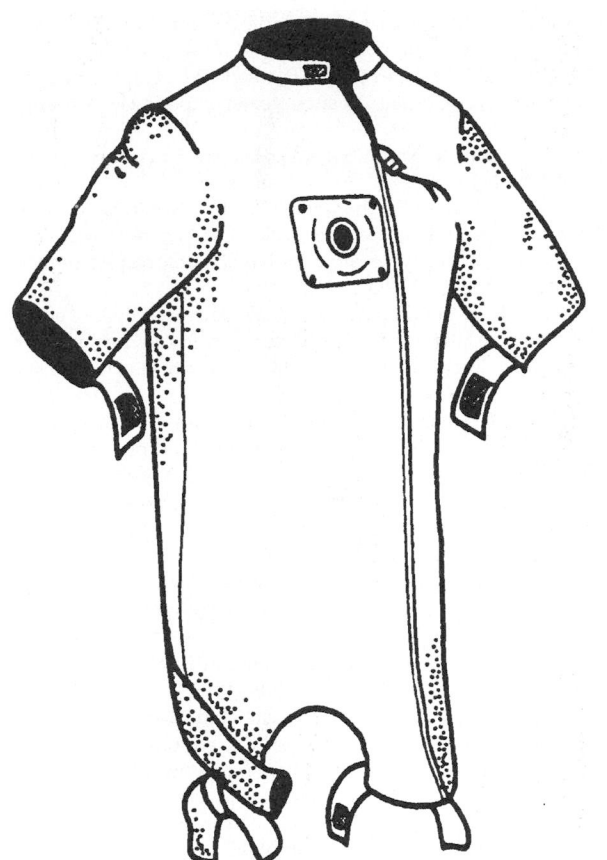

FIGURE 4-40 The Respironics Nu-Mo Suit. (*Courtesy of Respironics.*)

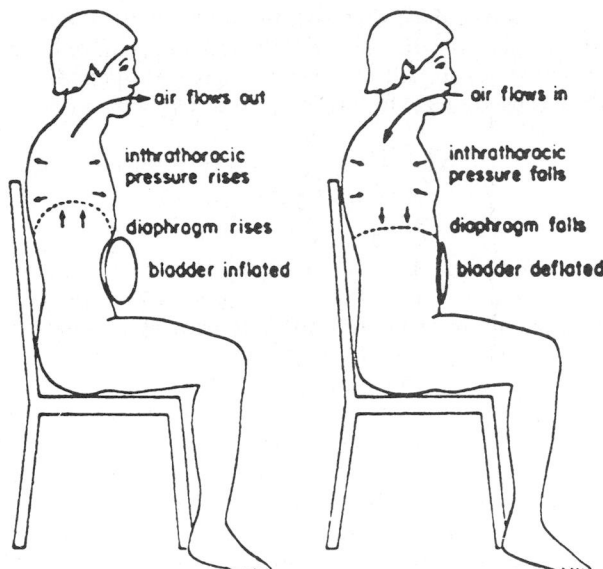

FIGURE 4-42 Illustration of the function of the pneumobelt. The pneumobelt functions by exerting pressure on the abdominal contents by inflation of a rubber bladder, forcing the diaphragm upward and assisting exhalation (*left*). When the bladder deflates, gravity pulls the diaphragm back down, assisting inhalation (*right*). (*Used, with permission, from* ref. 79).

ROCKING BED

Operation of the rocking bed (Fig. 4-43) is based on the effect gravity has on the abdominal contents.[3] That is, as the bed rocks, the abdominal contents assist the movement of the diaphragm. When the bed tilts head down, exhalation is assisted. When the head tilts up, inspiration is assisted.

The rocking bed can move through a total arc of up to 60°: a maximum of 30° head down and 30° head up. Generally, a 15° head-down with a 30° head-up tilt is sufficient for most patients.[3] In addition to the size of the arc, the rate can be adjusted from 8–34 tilts per minute, and a break at the knee

cage during exhalation. Depending on the patient, between 30 and 50 cmH₂O must be applied to the bladder, and patients ideally should be seated at a 75° angle.[78] As the angle from supine decreases, the effectiveness of the belt also decreases. The pneumobelt may be powered by any positive-pressure generator. Although effective in some patients, this device is used rarely today.

FIGURE 4-41 Pneumobelt with its internal inflatable bladder.

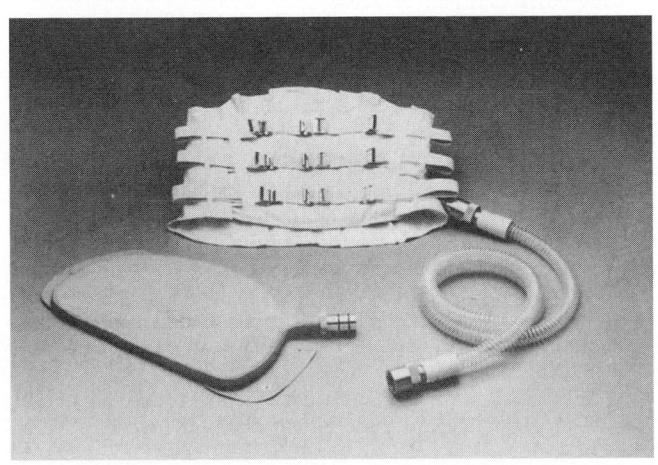

FIGURE 4-43 The Emerson Rocking Bed.

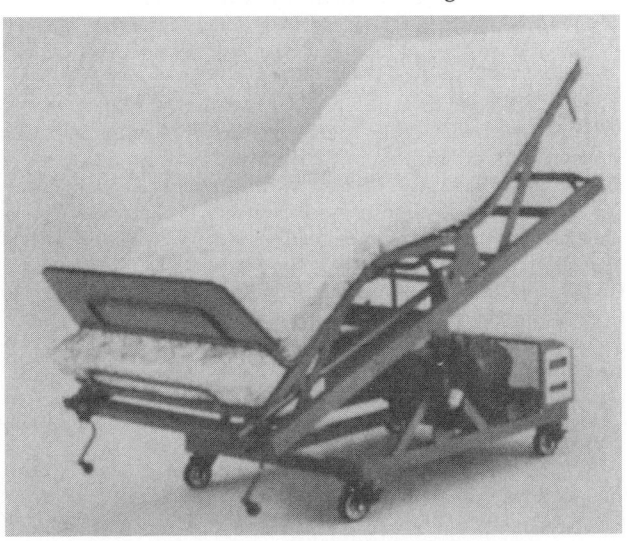

can be established to prevent sliding. Some patients develop motion sickness with the rocking bed and require appropriate medication.[3] Although effective in some patients, this device is used rarely today.

CRITICAL ANALYSIS OF PNEUMOBELT AND ROCKING BED

The pneumobelt and the rocking bed, both noninvasive approaches to ventilatory support, have limited application but may be extremely beneficial in select patients. Neither functions well in patients with chronic lung disease, although patients with primary pneumomuscular/neurologic disorders often benefit from their use. The pneumobelt is used primarily for daytime assistance in patients requiring other forms of support during the night. The same is true with the rocking bed. Some patients, however, can tolerate the motion and sleep comfortably in the rocking bed. Because the pneumobelt requires a sitting position, it is used rarely at night. It must be remembered that both units function as controllers. Patients who are anxious and frequently change their respiratory rate rarely tolerate either.

References

1. Drinker PA, Shaw LA. An apparatus for the prolonged administration of artificial ventilation. J Clin Invest 1929; 7:229–7.
2. Drinker PA, McKhann CF. The iron lung, first practical means of respiratory support. JAMA 1986; 255:1476–80.
3. Hill NS. Clinical application of body ventilators. Chest 1986; 90:897–905.
4. Emerson JH, Loynes JA. The evolution of iron lungs. Cambridge, MA: Emerson, 1958: 1–16.
5. Lassen HCA. The epidemic of poliomyelitus in Copenhagen 1952. Proc R Soc Med 1953; 47:67–71.
6. Kacmarek RM. The practical application of home mechanical ventilatory equipment. J Neuro Rehab 1992; 6:103–12.
7. Yang GW, Alba A, Lee M. Pneumobelt for sleep in the ventilator user: Clinical experience. Arch Phys Med Rehabil 1989; 20:707–11.
8. Farrero E, Prats E, Povedano M, et al. Survival in amyotrophic lateral sclerosis with home mechanical ventilation. Chest 2005; 127:2132–8.
9. Lloyd-Owen SJ, Donaldson SC, Ambrosino N, et al. Patterns of home mechanical ventilation use in Europe: Results from the Eurovent survey. Eur Respir J 2005; 25:1025–31.
10. Cropp A, DiMarco AF. Effects of intermittent negative-pressure ventilation on respiratory muscle function in patients with severe chronic obstructive pulmonary disease. Am Rev Respir Dis 1987; 135:1056–61.
11. Cazzolli P, Oppenheimer EA. Home mechanical ventilation for amyotrophic lateral sclerosis: Nasal compared to tracheostomy-intermittent positive-pressure ventilation. J Neurol Sci 1996; 139:123–8.
12. Kleopa KA, Sherman M, Neal B, et al. Bipap improves survival and rate of pulmonary function decline in patients with ALS. J Neurol Sci 1999; 164:82–8.
13. Bourke SC, Bullock RE, Williams TL, et al. Noninvasive ventilation in ALS: Indications and effect on quality of life. Neurology 2002; 61:171–7.
14. Snider GL. Thirty years of mechanical ventilation: Changing implications. Arch Intern Med 1983; 143:745–9.
15. Splaingard ML, Frates RC Jr, Harrison GM, et al. Home positive-pressure ventilation: Twenty years' experience. Chest 1983; 84:376–82.
16. Metha S, Hill N. Noninvasive ventilation. Am J Respir Crit Care Med 2001; 163:540–77.
17. Meduri G, Turner R, Abou-Shala N, et al. Noninvasive positive-pressure ventilation via face mask: First-line intervention in patients with acute hypercapnic and hypoxemic respiratory failure. Chest 1996; 109:179–93.
18. Antonelli M, Conti G, Pelosi P, et al. New treatment of acute hypoxemic respiratory failure: Noninvasive pressure support ventilation delivered by a helmet—A pilot controlled trial. Crit Care Med 2002; 30:602–8.
19. Pierson DJ, Kacmarek RM. Home ventilator care. In: Casaburi R, Petty T, editors. Principles and practice of pulmonary rehabilitation, 2nd ed. Philadelphia: Saunders, 1993: 274–88.
20. Gilmartin ME. Long-term mechanical ventilation outside the hospital. In: Pierson DJ, Kacmarek RM, editors. Foundations of respiratory care. New York: Churchill Livingstone, 1992: 1185–205.
21. Bach JR, Alba AS. Non-invasive options for ventilatory support of the traumatic high-level quadraplegic patient. Chest 1990; 98:613–9.
22. Back JA, Alba AS. Management of chronic alveolar hypoventilation by nasal ventilation. Chest 1990; 97:52–7.
23. Kacmarek RM. Home mechanical ventilation equipment. In: Branson RD, Hess DR, Chatburn RL, editors. Respiratory care equipment, 2nd ed, Philadelphia: Lippincott, 1995.
24. Hess DR, Kacmarek RM. Noninvasive ventilation. In: Branson RD, Hess DR, Chatburn RL, editors. Respiratory care equipment, 2nd ed Philadelphia: Lippincott, 1995.
25. Battisti A, Tassaux D, Janssens J-P, et al. Performance characteristics of 10 home mechanical ventilators in pressure-support mode: A comparative bench study. Chest 2005; 127:1784–92.
26. Kacmarek RM, Stanek KS, McMahon KM, Wilson RS. Imposed work of breathing during synchronized intermittent mandatory ventilation: Provided by five home care ventilators. Respir Care 1990; 35:405–14.
27. Nellcor Puritan-Bennett LP-6 Plus and LP-10 Volume Ventilators, Clinical manual, no Y-004129–03A, rev 8, The Netherlands, 1999.
28. Puritan-Bennett Achieva, Clinician manual, no 066478B-0603, Pleasanton, CA, 2003.
29. Lifecare PLV-100, Operating manual, Lafayette, CO, 1986.
30. Lifecare PLV-102, Operating manual, form 37-500E, Lafayette, CO, 1991.
31. Respironics PLV Continuum Ventilator, Provider's manual, ref 1009561A, Carlsbad, CA, 2004.
32. Pulmonetic Systems LTV Series, Ventilator operators manual, no P/N 10664, rev J, Colton, CA, May 2001.
33. Wilkens RL, Stoller JK, Scanlan CL. Egan's fundamentals of respiratory care, 8th ed. St Louis: Mosby, 2003.
34. VersaMed iVent$_{201}$, Operator's manual, no OM-01-04, Pearl River, NY, 2003.
35. Newport HT50 Ventilator, Operating manual, no OPRHT50-1, rev B, Newport Beach, CA, 2001.
36. Bundurophong T, Imanaka H, Nishimura M, et al. Performance characteristics of bilevel pressure ventilators: A lung model study. Chest 1997; 111:1050–60.
37. Kacmarek RM. Characteristics of pressure-targeted ventilators used for noninvasive positive-pressure ventilation. Respir Care 1997; 42:380–8.
38. Schwartz AR, Kacmarek RM, Hess DR. Factors affecting oxygen delivery with bilevel positive airway pressure. Respir Care 2004; 49:270–5.

39. Sollars MJ, Hess DR. Effect of oxygen flow on performance of a B$_I$PAP ventilator. Respir Care 2003; 48:1099.

40. Ferguson G, Gilmartin M. CO$_2$ rebreathing during B$_I$PAP ventilatory assistance. Am J Respir Crit Care Med 1995; 151: 1126–35.

41. B$_I$PAP ventilatory support system clinical manual for models S/T and S/T-D, form no 336051, Murrysville, PA, Respironics, 1989.

42. Respironics B$_I$PAP S/T-D30, Clinical manual, no. 556065, Murrysville, PA, 1997.

43. Respironics Vision, Clinical manual, no 1009071, Murryville, PA, 1998.

44. Respironics B$_I$PAP Pro 2 and B$_I$PAP Plus, User manual, no 1018989, Murrysville, PA, 2003.

45. Hess DR, Hardy WH. Laboratory evaluation of Bi-Flex mode of the Respironics Pro bilevel system. Chest 2003; 124:227S.

46. Respironics Synchrony, User guide. no 1003121, Murrysville, PA, 2000.

47. ResMed VPAP III and III ST, Clinician manual, no 24808/3-04-04, Waterloo, Australia, 2004.

48. ResMed VPAP III ST-A, Clinician manual, no 24851/1-04-07, Bella Vista, Australia, 2004.

49. Puritan-Bennett Knight Star 335 Ventilator, Clinical guide, no Y-7999-20-00, rev A, Pleasanton, CA.

50. Puritan-Bennett Knight Star 330 Ventilator, Clinician's manual, no Y-500008-00, rev H, Pleasanton, CA, 2003.

51. Robert P, Hirsch C, Barker S, Kacmarek RM. Work of breathing imposed during spontaneous breathing in the SIMV mode of the newest home care ventilators (abstract). Respir Care 1992; 37:1358.

52. Ploysongsang Y, Branson RD, Rashkin MC, Hurst JM. Effect of flow rate and duration of use on the pressure drop across six artificial noses. Respir Care 1989; 34:902–7.

53. O'Donohue WI, Giovannoni RM, Goldberg AL, et al. Long-term mechanical ventilation: Guidelines for management in the home and at alternate community sites (consensus report). Chest 1986; 90(suppl):ls–37s.

54. Goldstein RS, Avendano MA. Long-term mechanical ventilation as elective therapy: Clinical status and future prospects. Respir Care 1991; 36:297–304.

55. Strumpf DA, Millman RP, Hill NS. The management of chronic hypoventilation. Chest 1990; 98:474–80.

56. American Thoracic Society and European Respiratory Society: International consensus conference in intensive care medicine: Noninvasive positive-pressure ventilation in acute respiratory failure. Am J Respir Crit Care Med 2001; 163:283–91.

57. Stoller JK. Physiologic rationale for resting the ventilatory muscles. Respir Care 1991; 36:290–6.

58. Goldstein RS, DeRosie JA, Avendano MA, Donnage M. Influence of noninvasive positive-pressure ventilation on inspiratory muscles. Chest 1991; 99:408–15.

59. Braun NMT, Marino WD. Effects of daily intermittent rest on respiratory muscles in patients with severe chronic airflow limitation (abstract). Chest 1984; 85:595.

60. Branthwaite MA. Noninvasive and domiciliary ventilation: Positive-pressure techniques. Thorax 1991; 46:208–12.

61. Back JR, O'Brien J, Krotenberg R, Alba A. Management of end-stage respiratory failure in Duchenne muscular dystrophy. Muscle Nerve 1987; 10:177–82.

62. Alexander MA, Johnson EW, Petty J, Stauch D. Mechanical ventilation of patients with late-stage Duchenne muscular dystrophy: Management in the home. Arch Phys Med Rehabil 1979; 60: 289–92.

63. Curren FJ, Golbert AP. Ventilatory management in Duchenne muscular dystrophy and post-poliomyelitis syndrome: Twelve years' experience. Arch Phys Med Rehabib 1989; 70:180–5.

64. Goldstein RS, Molotiu N, Skrastins R. Reversal of sleep-induced hypoventilation in chronic respiratory failure by nocturnal negative-pressure ventilation in patients with restrictive ventilatory impairment. Am Rev Respir Dis, 1987; 135:1049–55.

65. Back JR, Alba AS. Intermittent abdominal pressure ventilation in a regimen of noninvasive ventilatory support. Chest 1991; 99:630–6.

66. Back JR, Alba AS. Noninvasive options for ventilatory support of the traumatic high-level quadriplegic patient. Chest 1990; 98:613–9.

67. Brochard L, Isabey D, Piquet J, et al. Reversal of acute exacerbations of chronic obstructive lung disease by inspiratory assistance with a face mask. New Engl J Med 1990; 323:1523–9.

68. Meduri GU, Abou-Shala N, Fox RC, et al. Noninvasive face mask mechanical ventilation in patients with acute hypercapnia. Chest 1991; 100:445–54.

69. Meduri GU, Conoscenti CC, Menashe PH, Nair S. Noninvasive face mask ventilation in patients with acute respiratory failure. Chest 1989; 95:865–70.

70. Back JR, Alba A, Saporito LR. Intermittent positive-pressure ventilation via the mouth as an alternative to tracheostomy for 257 ventilator users. Chest 1993; 103:174–82.

71. Schettino GPP, Chatmongkolchart S, Hess DR, Kacmarek RM. Position of exhalation port and mask design affect CO$_2$ rebreathing during noninvasive positive pressure ventilation. Crit Care Med 2003; 31:2178–82.

72. Antonelli M, Pennisi MA, Pelosi P, et al. Noninvasive positive-pressure ventilation using a helmet in patients with acute exacerbation of chronic obstructive pulmonary disease. Anesthesiology 2004; 100:16–24.

73. Patroniti N, Foti G, Manfio A. Head helmet versus face mask for non-invasive continuous positive airway pressure: A physiological study. Intensive Care Med 2003; 29:1680–87.

74. Taccoone P, Hess D, Caironi P, Bigatello LM. Continuous positive airway pressure delivered with a "helmet": Effects on carbon dioxide rebreathing. Crit Care Med 2004; 32:2090–6.

75. Emerson Respiratory Instruction, Iron lung accessories, Cambridge, MA, JH Emerson, 1982.

76. Kirby R, Banner M, Desautels D, Downs J. Clinical application of ventilator care, 2nd ed. New York: Churchill Livingstone, 1991.

77. Respironics NEV-100, Operating manual, no 12533, Murrysville, PA, 2000.

78. Adamson JP, Lewis L, Stern JD. Application of abdominal pressure for artificial respiration. JAMA 1959; 169:1613–7.

PART III
INDICATIONS

Chapter 5

INDICATIONS FOR MECHANICAL VENTILATION

FRANCO LAGHI
MARTIN J. TOBIN

In this chapter we discuss the indications for mechanical ventilation in adult patients. We focus on patients who are already in the intensive care unit (ICU) or who are considered for transfer to the ICU, that is, patients with new onset of signs and symptoms over minutes or hours. We do not deal with the indications for mechan-ical ventilation for chronic respiratory failure or in pedi-atric patients; these subjects are covered in Chapters 19, 25, and 32.

There is a paucity of research—and no clinical trials—on the indications for mechanical ventilation. This situation contrasts with the growing amount of research on the dis-continuation of mechanical ventilation. While it is tempting to apply indices used for predicting the outcome of weaning trials as indices to identify patients who require mechanical ventilation, such an approach has not been tested. It is also probably unwise.

Two factors account for the limited research on indica-tions for mechanical ventilation. First, such patients are extremely ill. Any intervention—such as careful collec-tion of physiologic measurements—that delays institution of ventilation might be viewed as unethical. Second, the nosology of respiratory failure is unsatisfactory (see be-low). In everyday practice, clinicians do not decide to institute mechanical ventilation because a patient meets cer-tain diagnostic criteria. Instead, clinicians typically decide to institute ventilation based on their assessment of a pa-tient's signs and symptoms. This decision is also grounded on a foundation of solid biomedical theory, specifically principles of pulmonary pathophysiology. Accordingly, we develop our discussion of ventilator indications along these two lines: physical examination and pathophysiologic principles.

Overall Assessment

Clinical presentations that cause a physician to institute me-chanical ventilation are protean. They range from patients presenting with frank apnea to patients with clinical signs of increased work of breathing with or without laboratory evidence of impaired gas exchange.

APNEA

Apneic patients, such as those who have suffered catas-trophic central nervous system (CNS) damage, need im-mediate institution of mechanical ventilation. To advocate controlled trials to determine the need for mechanical ven-tilations in apneic patients is unethical.

CLINICAL SIGNS OF INCREASED WORK OF BREATHING

Asthma, chronic obstructive pulmonary disease (COPD), pneumonia, cardiogenic pulmonary edema, and acute res-piratory distress syndrome (ARDS) are just a few of the many conditions that cause an increase in work of breathing and, with it, increased energy expenditure by the respira-tory muscles.

The energy expenditure of the respiratory muscles can be quantified in terms of pressure-time product[1]—the time integral of the difference between the esophageal pressure tracing and the estimated recoil pressure of the chest wall[2,3] (Fig. 5-1). The pressure-time product of patients in acute

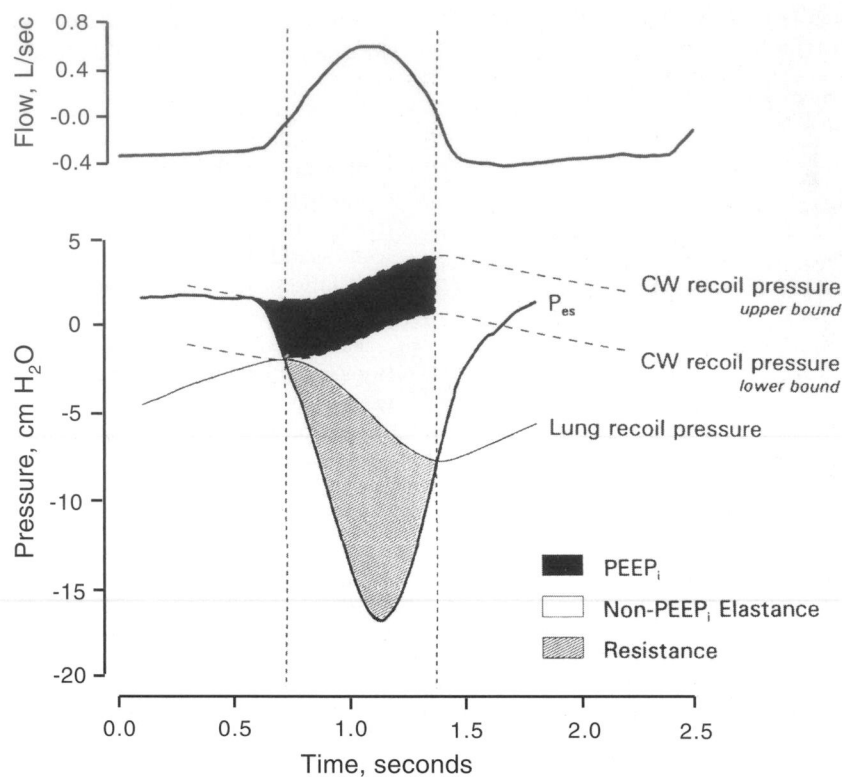

FIGURE 5-1 Flow (*inspiration upward*) and pressure tracings during spontaneous breathing. Recoil pressures of the chest wall (CW) and lung are calculated from dynamic elastances of the chest wall and lung, respectively, and lung volume. Inspiratory pressure-time product (PTP) is calculated using the integral of the difference between esophageal pressure (P_{es}) and CW recoil pressure from the onset of the rapid decrease in P_{es} to the transition from inspiratory to expiratory flow (upper-bound PTP). The component of PTP caused by intrinsic positive end-expiratory pressure ($PEEP_i$) is computed using the integral of the difference between the upper-bound PTP and CW recoil pressure from the onset of rapid decrease in P_{es} to the transition from inspiratory to expiratory flow (lower-bound PTP). The component of PTP caused by non-$PEEP_i$ elastance is computed using the integral of the difference between lung recoil pressure and lower-bound CW recoil pressure from the onset of inspiratory flow to the moment of transition from inspiratory to expiratory flow. The resistive fraction of PTP is computed using the integral of the difference between P_{es} and lung recoil pressure. The vertical interrupted lines represent points for zero flow. (*Used, with permission, from Jubran et al: Pathophysiologic basis of acute respiratory distress in patients who fail a trial of weaning from mechanical ventilation. Am J Respir Crit Care Med 155:906–15, 1997.*)

respiratory failure is about four times[4–6] the normal value (100 cmH$_2$O · s/min), and it can be increased sixfold in individual patients.[4,5] The inspiratory pressure-time product can be partitioned into resistive, elastic, and intrinsic positive end-expiratory pressure (PEEP) components[5] (see Fig. 5-1). Patients in respiratory distress typically have a 30–50% greater inspiratory resistance,[5] 100% greater dynamic elastance,[5] and 100–200% greater intrinsic PEEP[4,5] than do similar patients who are not in acute respiratory failure. Inspiratory effort is almost equally divided in offsetting intrinsic PEEP, elastic recoil, and inspiratory resistance.[5] The increase in respiratory effort means that the respiratory muscles account for a much larger fraction of the body's oxygen (O$_2$) consumption. In healthy subjects, this fraction is only 1–3% of total O$_2$ consumption. In patients with acute hypoxemic respiratory failure and shock who are undergoing cardiopulmonary resuscitation, the respiratory muscles account for about 20% of total O$_2$ consumption.[7]

Increased work by the respiratory muscles causes respiratory distress. Clinical manifestations of respiratory distress include nasal flaring, retraction of the eyelids, accessory muscle recruitment, expiratory muscle recruitment, tracheal tug, intercostal recession, tachypnea, tachycardia, hypertension or hypotension, diaphoresis, and changes in mental status.

FACIAL SIGNS OF RESPIRATORY DISTRESS

Many intensivists often decide to institute mechanical ventilation based on a patient's facial appearance.[8] Gilston has provided an insightful description of many signs that go unstated in reviews on mechanical ventilation.[8] Take, for example, the mouth. At an early stage of respiratory distress, the mouth opens slightly and to a variable extent during inhalation (Fig. 5-2). At a later stage, the mouth opens throughout the respiratory cycle. Patients may switch to mouth breathing perhaps to decrease respiratory work[8,9] and physiologic dead-space ventilation.[8] An open mouth is sometimes seen in patients with a tracheostomy (Fig. 5-3) and in patients receiving ventilator support.[8] The tongue may be seen to jerk in unison with inspiratory efforts.[8]

Some distressed patients also exhibit pursed-lip breathing during exhalation.[8] In stable ambulatory patients with

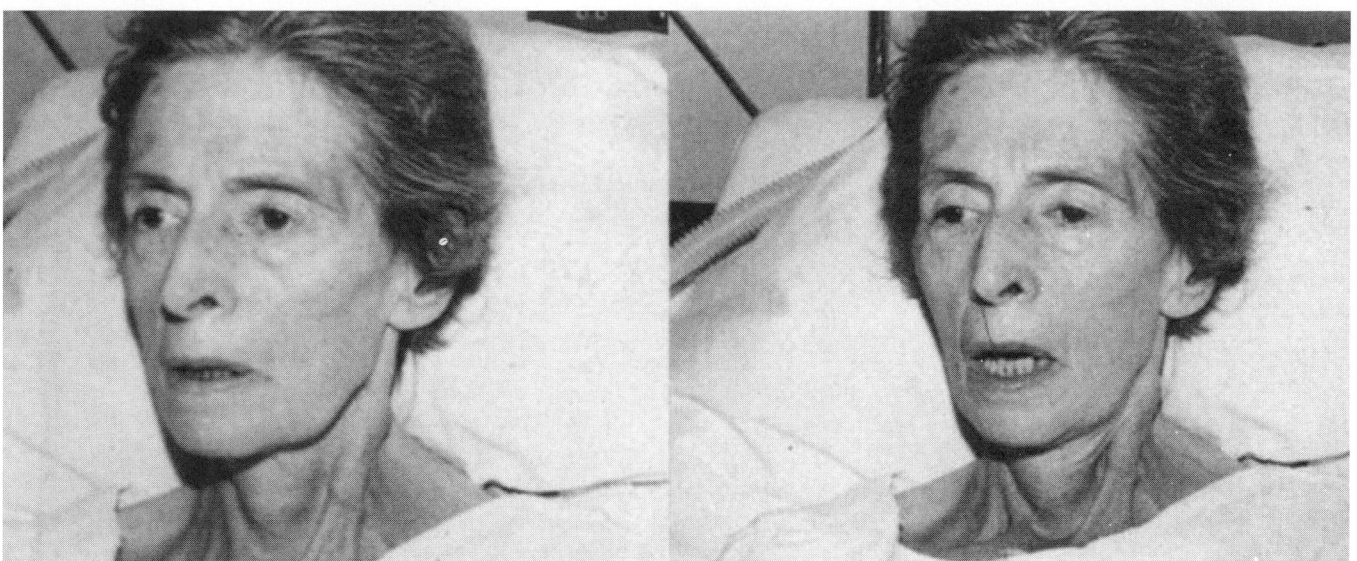

FIGURE 5-2 Mouth opening during respiratory distress. (*Left*) A patient developed respiratory distress precipitated by right-middle- and right-lower-lobe atelectasis 1 week after mitral valve replacement. The patient is moderately dyspneic, especially on talking; the mouth is slightly open; the sternomastoids are prominent; and there is some retraction of the eyelids. She is anxious. (*Right*) Twenty-four hours later the patient is complaining of severe dyspnea. The mouth is now more open, and contraction of the sternomastoids is such that the head is raised off the pillow. The patient is drowsy, and lid retraction has decreased. Also visible is thrombosis of the left external jugular vein. Despite a Pa_{O_2} of 60 mmHg, the patient was intubated and mechanically ventilated (*not shown*). (*Used, with permission, from Gilston: Anesthesia 31:385–97, 1976.*)

COPD, pursed-lip breathing is associated with an increase in tidal volume and a decrease in respiratory rate.[10] Pursed-lip breathing can improve the arterial tensions of both carbon dioxide (Pa_{CO_2}) and oxygen (Pa_{O_2}), whereas oxygen uptake ($\dot{V}_{O_2}$) remains unchanged.[10] The latter finding suggests that pursed-lip breathing may allow a decrease in cardiac output without changing tissue oxygenation.[10] Alternatively, if cardiac output does not decrease, pursed-lip breathing may increase mixed venous oxygen saturation,

resulting in better tissue oxygenation.[10] Pursed-lip breathing is thought to improve gas exchange by preventing airway collapse. As a result, gas trapping is decreased, resulting in an increase in tidal volume.[10]

A few patients in respiratory distress moan during exhalation. Such moans have been compared with the grunting that is typical of neonates with the respiratory distress syndrome.[8] Grunting results from glottic closure and expiratory muscle recruitment during early exhalation.[11]

FIGURE 5-3 Alterations in the configuration of the mouth in a patient with a tracheostomy. (*Left*) The patient is sleeping while respiration is fully supported by mechanical ventilation. The mouth is closed. (*Center*) Eight minutes after being disconnected from the ventilator, the patient has developed dyspnea with nasal flaring, restlessness, and anxiety. The mouth is open. (*Right*) Eleven days later, the patient has recovered and is breathing comfortably without ventilator assistance. Her mouth is open but conveys a smile. (*Used, with permission, from Gilston: Anesthesia 31:385–97, 1976.*)

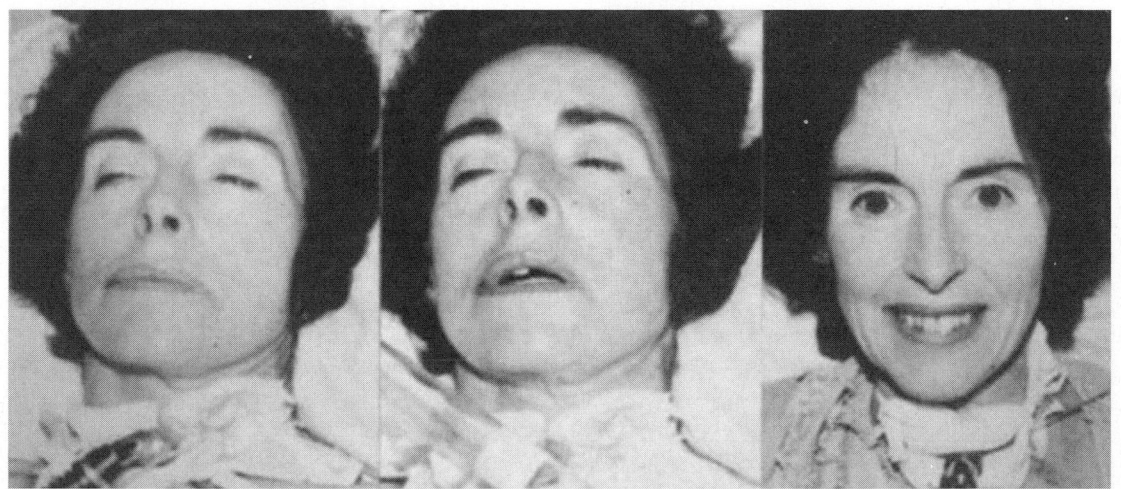

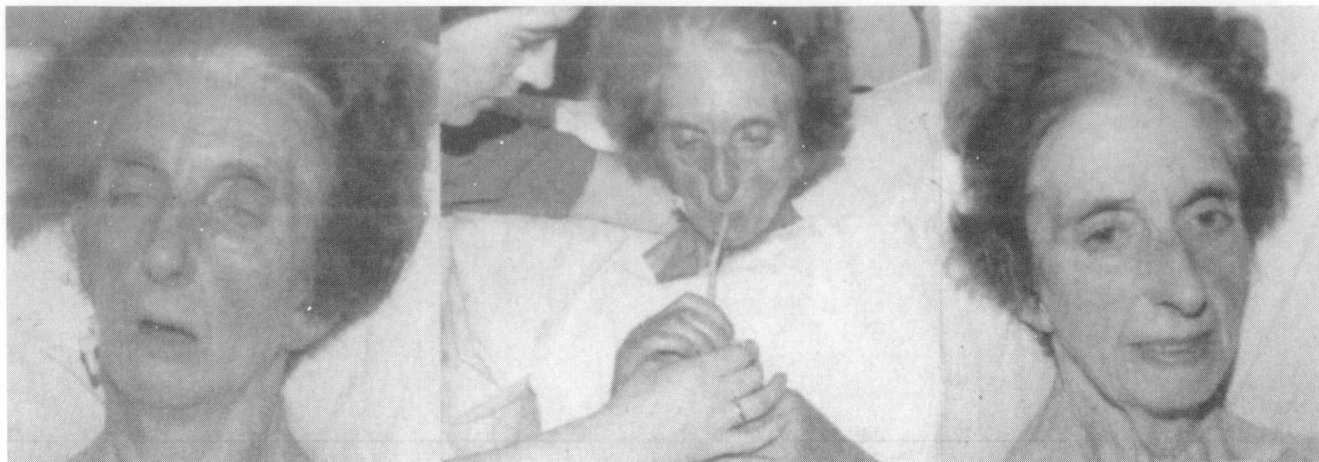

FIGURE 5-4 Drooping of the eyelids accompanying deterioration of mental status during an episode of respiratory distress. (*Left*) A patient developed respiratory distress 3 days after aortic- and mitral-valve replacement. The patient is drowsy and moderately dyspneic. The mouth is open, and she is moaning during exhalation. The eyelids are drooping. Her hemodynamic status was maintained satisfactorily with medical therapy. (*Center*) Despite respiratory distress, the patient is able to drink. (*Right*) After 2 days of medical therapy, which did not include mechanical ventilation, dyspnea has resolved, and the patient is alert, cheerful, and talkative. Her expression is relaxed. (*Used, with permission, from Gilston: Anesthesia 31:385–97, 1976.*)

It is associated with a rise in transpulmonary pressure and oxygenation.[11] If grunting is prevented by tracheal intubation, oxygenation deteriorates.[11] Use of continuous positive airway pressure (CPAP) improves oxygenation and eliminates grunting.[12] The improvement in oxygenation may result from grunting acting as a natural form of PEEP that recruits collapsed alveoli and partially overcomes inequalities in gas distribution caused by differing time constants. Of course, grunting also can arise with disease outside the thorax, such as with an acute abdomen.[13]

Nasal flaring, another facial sign of respiratory distress, is caused by contraction of the alae nasi, the dilator muscle of the external nares.[9] In adults, nasal flaring reduces nasal resistance by about 40–50% and total airway resistance by about 10–30%.[9] Factors regulating alae nasi activity include chemical stimuli that cause hyperpnea (hypoxia and hypercapnia),[9,14,15] inspiratory resistive loading,[15] and local stimuli (negative intraluminal nasal pressure).[14] The proportion of patients in respiratory distress who present with nasal flaring is unknown, as is the level of interobserver agreement in detecting flaring. Ventilator support reduces or eliminates alae nasi activity.[16,17]

Diaphoresis, often best detected on the forehead,[8] accompanies respiratory distress in some patients. Among 49 patients admitted to the emergency ward for acute bronchial asthma, Brenner et al[18] found that 9 patients had profuse sweating. This subgroup displayed greater abnormalities in peak expiratory flow rate and Pa_{CO_2}. In patients with respiratory distress, diaphoresis may result from increased work of breathing,[19] sympathetic stimulation,[19,20] and hypercapnia-associated cutaneous vasodilation.[19,21] In contrast, diaphoresis in patients with heart failure often is associated with hypoperfusion of the skin, vasoconstriction, and cold extremities.[19]

Mentation can be evaluated by inspection of the face and by simple questioning. With early respiratory distress, nearly all patients are anxious, and their eyelids are retracted. As distress increases, the level of consciousness often decreases, and the lids tend to fall (Fig. 5-4). Instead of remaining alert to their surroundings, patients gaze vacantly ahead.[8] If respiratory failure is left untreated, apathy leads to drowsiness and then coma. These changes in mentation arise because of the underlying cause of respiratory failure (decreased cardiac output in cases of shock, impaired neurologic function in sepsis), acute hypercapnia,[22] or to a lesser extent, hypoxemia.[22,23] In a classic description, Campbell noted that most (nonhypotensive) patients with an exacerbation of COPD have preserved consciousness on arrival to the emergency room despite Pa_{O_2} being as low as 20–40 mmHg.[23] While extremely useful in overall patient assessment, facial signs of respiratory distress do not necessarily translate into an automatic decision to intubate a patient (see Fig. 5-4).

ACCESSORY AND EXPIRATORY MUSCLE RECRUITMENT

Increased respiratory loads in healthy subjects[24,25] and in ambulatory patients with COPD[26] are met with a proportionately greater use of the rib-cage muscles than of the diaphragm.[24–26] As the load increases, the expiratory muscles are recruited.[24,25,27] In addition to increased activity of rib-cage and abdominal muscles, the respiratory centers may increase activity of the accessory muscles, especially the sternomastoids.[28,29] The sternomastoids have been shown to be activated in patients with respiratory compromise[28] and in healthy subjects breathing with a high level of inspiratory effort. The threshold for sternomastoid activation, however, is lower in patients.[29] In patients with respiratory distress,[4,30] sternomastoid recruitment can be phasic (during inhalation) or tonic.[27] Some patients hold their head off the pillow to enhance sternomastoid action[8] (see Fig. 5-2).

TACHYPNEA, PARADOX, TRACHEAL TUG, INTERCOSTAL RECESSIONS

Changes in respiratory rate are one of the most useful signs in evaluating the need for mechanical ventilation. Tachypnea is a near-universal sign accompanying respiratory distress.

Obtaining reliable measurements of respiratory rate and interpreting the values are not straightforward. First bedside assessment often is inaccurate. In one study, 40% of nurses' estimations of respiratory frequencies deviated by more than 20% from the true value.[31] Agreement as to the presence of tachypnea among physicians, expressed as a κ value (κ of 0 indicates that agreement is no better than chance; κ of 1 indicates complete agreement), was only 0.25.[32] Second, the within-day (within an individual) coefficient of variation in respiratory rate among young healthy adults is $21 \pm 12\%$; in old healthy adults, it is $29 \pm 11\%$.[33] Thus accurate quantification of respiratory rate requires counting more breaths than contained in the usual 15-second sample.[33,34] Third, the day-to-day coefficient of variation of respiratory rate is $7 \pm 2\%$ in healthy individuals,[33] the value in patients with pulmonary diseases is unknown. Fourth, the typical respiratory rate in patients with different disease states varies from one state to the next[34] (Table 5-1); a rate that is judged high in a previously healthy subject may arouse no concern in a patient with restrictive disease. The upper limit of normal (mean + two standard deviations) in health is 22 breaths per minute.[34] The equivalent value for stable patients with COPD is 30 breaths per minute and for patients with restrictive lung disease 44 breaths per minute.[34]

Despite limitations in its measurement, tachypnea is an important clinical sign. In a retrospective case-controlled study of patients discharged from an ICU, the only continuous variables that predicted readmission to the ICU were higher respiratory rate (24 versus 21 breaths per minute) and lower hematocrit.[35] Readmitted patients had a much higher mortality than the control patients, 42% and 7%,

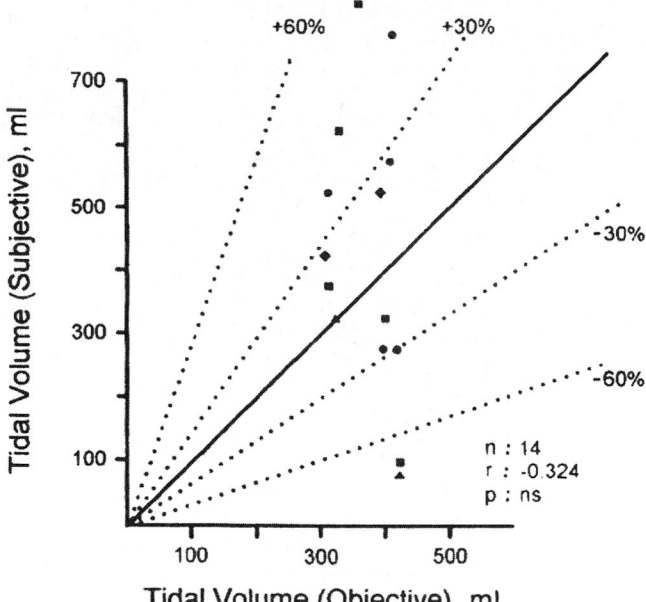

FIGURE 5-5 Subjective estimates by 14 observers of tidal volume in one critically ill patient breathing spontaneously compared with objective measurements at that time. The diamonds signify attending physicians, triangles signify fellows, squares signify respiratory therapists, and circles signify critical-care nurses. The correlation between subjective estimates and objective measurements was not significant. (*Used, with permission, from Semmes et al: Subjective and objective measurement of tidal volume in critically ill patients. Chest 87:577–9, 1985.*).

respectively, and respiratory problems accounted for more than half the readmissions. Of 18 patients who where discharged from the ICU with a respiratory rate of more than 30 breaths per minute, 12 required readmission. In a study of patients who had experienced a cardiopulmonary arrest, 53% had documented deterioration in respiratory function in the 8 hours preceding the arrest.[36] Of interest, respiratory rate was elevated in most patients [mean 29 ± 1 (standard error) breaths per minute], whereas other routine laboratory tests showed no consistent abnormalities. That detection of tachypnea did not lead to a change in patient management (in an effort to prevent the arrest) led the authors to surmise that physicians do not fully appreciate its clinical importance.

Shallow respiration (when measured with instrumentation) is common in patients with acute respiratory distress.[37] Judging tidal volume as shallow based on physical examination is very unreliable[38,39] (Fig. 5-5). Clinical skill in this task is not improved by years of experience.[39]

Patients in distress commonly display abnormal chest-wall movements.[40,41] Abnormal movements can be separated into three categories. One, asynchrony, consists of a difference in the rate of motion of the rib cage and abdomen. Two, paradox, consists of one compartment moving in the opposite direction to tidal volume. The third abnormality is greater than normal breath-to-breath variation in the relative contribution of the rib cage and abdomen to tidal volume; this pattern, termed *respiratory alternans*, represents

TABLE 5-1   Respiratory Rates in Health and Disease

Condition	Number of Subjects	Mean (breaths/min)	SD	Mean + 2 SD
Healthy nonsmoker	65	16.6	2.8	22.2
Healthy smoker	22	18.3	3.0	24.3
Asthma	17	16.6	3.4	23.4
COPD, eucapnia	16	20.4	4.1	28.6
COPD, hypercapnia	12	23.3	3.3	29.9
Restrictive lung disease	14	27.9	7.9	43.7
Pulmonary hypertension	7	25.1	6.4	37.9
Chronic anxiety	13	18.3	2.8	23.9

SD, standard deviation.
SOURCE: Data from Tobin et al: Chest 84:286–94,1983.

recruitment and derecruitment of the accessory intercostal muscles and the diaphragm. In the past it was thought that these three abnormalities of motion represented respiratory muscle fatigue.[42] It is now known that they represent signs of increased load and occur in the absence of fatigue.[43] These abnormalities are seen not only in patients with respiratory distress[44] but also in some ambulatory patients[34,44] or during sleep (sleep apnea syndrome).[45]

Increased tidal swings in intrathoracic pressure are axiomatic to increases in the work of breathing. The greater downward movement of the diaphragm tends to pull down the trachea (just as a sexton ringing a bell) with each inspiration,[46] producing a sign termed *tracheal tug*. Tracheal tug correlates closely with severity of airway obstruction.[47]

The intercostal spaces normally bulge inward during inhalation and outward during exhalation.[13] Inspiratory retraction of the intercostal space—serving as a window into the pleural space—is increased in patients with respiratory disease. The suprasternal fossa also moves inward in direct proportion to swings in pleural pressure.[48,49] Focal exaggerated retraction of the intercostal space can occur with a flail chest. Focal expiratory bulging may be seen on the side of a tension pneumothorax or over the area of a flail chest.[13] As with other physical signs, studies often reveal poor agreement among physicians.[32,50] For example, Godfrey et al[50] found agreement among 11 relatively experienced chest physicians in identifying tracheal tug to be midway between chance and maximum possible agreement. Spiteri et al[32] found poor agreement among experienced physicians for detecting reduced chest movements (κ = 0.38) and cricosternal distance (κ = 0.28)[32] (Fig. 5-6); they did not address tracheal tug or inspiratory retractions.

The interpretation of data generated by studies that quantify physical signs is hazardous. The entity that researchers are quantifying can be very different from the skill involved in the physician's actions. Physical examination is an art—learned through apprenticeship, not out of a book. Thus we should bear in mind Braque's caution about art appreciation: "The only thing that matters in art can't be explained." Likewise, the essence of physical examination is its tacit

coefficient; the explicit, measurable components may be the least relevant. Another problem with research on physical signs is test-referral bias. For example, the studies of Godfrey et al[50] and Spiteri et al[32] were confined to patients with respiratory diseases; a more appropriate design also would have included healthy subjects and patients with diseases not affecting the lungs. These flaws in the methodology of such studies markedly overestimate the diagnostic power of physical examination.

CARDIOVASCULAR SIGNS OF RESPIRATORY DISTRESS

Respiratory distress frequently is associated with tachycardia and hypertension. Tachycardia and hypertension likely are caused by increased sympathetic discharge.[51] In some patients, such as those with sepsis, cardiac impairment, or severe hypoxemia, respiratory distress is associated with hypotension and not hypertension.

Pulsus paradoxus is defined as an inspiratory fall in the systolic pressure of greater than 10 mmHg.[13] Pulsus paradoxus is very common in patients with an exacerbation of asthma but also in patients with COPD, shock, and pericardial tamponade[13,18] (see Chapter 36).

NONUNIFORM PRESENTATION

Patients with impending respiratory failure do not have a uniform presentation. The spectrum ranges from a patient complaining of dyspnea to a patient with impending respiratory arrest. Several factors are responsible. Patients differ in the balance between work of breathing and the capacity of the respiratory muscles to generate pressure. They also differ in the central processing of neural afferents. For instance, patients with a history of near-fatal asthma have a blunted perception of dyspnea,[52] reduced sensitivity to added inspiratory resistive loads,[53] and a reduced chemosensitivity to hypoxia.[52] In addition, hypoxia, and possibly hypercapnia, can impair sensations of respiratory load.[54]

IMPENDING RESPIRATORY FAILURE

A commonly listed indication for mechanical ventilation is development of impending respiratory failure.[55] But impending respiratory failure has no clear definition. Some clinicians use the term to mean development of severe tachypnea, diaphoresis, and use of accessory muscles of respiration. Others use it to mean agonal breathing.

In some circumstances, physicians do not institute mechanical ventilation until they obtain results of diagnostic testing, such as chest radiographs, electrocardiograms, or arterial blood-gas analyses. Even in this situation, clinicians commonly do not change their mind when the test results

FIGURE 5-6 Cricosternal distance. The physician notes the distance in finger breaths between the lower border of the cricoid cartilage and the suprasternal notch. The normal distance is three or four finger breaths. A decrease in this distance is a sign of hyperinflation. (*Used, with permission, from Flenley: Concise medical textbooks: Respiratory medicine. London: Bailliere Tindall, 45, 1981.*)

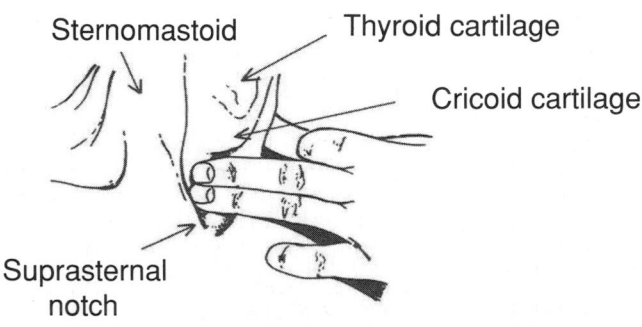

Sternomastoid

Thyroid cartilage

Cricoid cartilage

Suprasternal notch

TABLE 5-2 Common Causes of Hypoxemic Respiratory Failure

Pneumonia
Cardiogenic pulmonary edema
Acute respiratory distress syndrome
Aspiration pneumonia
Multiple trauma
Immunocompromised host with pulmonary infiltrates
Pulmonary embolism

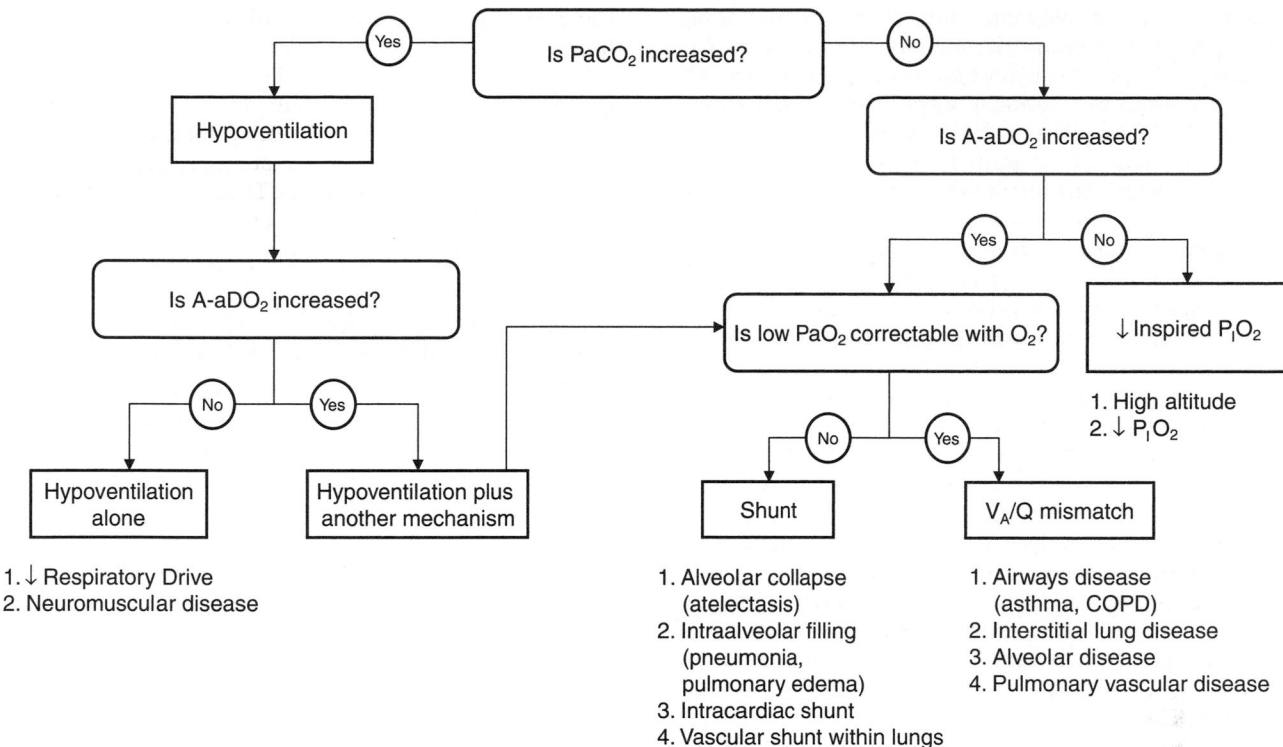

FIGURE 5-7 The diagnostic approach to a patient with hypoxemia or hypercapnia. The alveolar-arterial O₂ gradient (A-aDO₂) is usually less than 10 mmHg for subjects 30 years of age and younger and is increased by ~3 mmHg per decade after age 30. V_A/Q̇, ventilation-perfusion ratio; COPD, chronic obstructive pulmonary disease. Not included are conditions where a decrease in mixed venous O₂ content in the presence of increased A-aDO₂ contributes to hypoxemia. (*Modified, with permission, from Weinberger et al: In: Kasper et al, editors. Harrison's principles of internal medicine. New York: McGraw-Hill, 1498–1505, 2005.*)

are different from those expected. In most circumstances, a patient's clinical presentation is so dramatic that mechanical ventilation is instituted without performing arterial blood-gas analysis. If arterial blood-gas results are not available before connecting a patient to a ventilator, they are almost invariably available shortly after. Arterial blood-gas analysis is helpful in choosing the type of support best suited to a patient's needs. Analysis also serves to classify patients into two broad groups: hypoxemic respiratory failure (Table 5-2) and hypercapnic respiratory failure; some patients display features of both.[56]

HYPOXEMIC RESPIRATORY FAILURE

PATHOPHYSIOLOGY

The pathophysiologic mechanisms responsible for hypoxemia can be grouped into two broad categories depending on whether there is (or is not) an increased alveolar-arterial O₂ gradient (A-aDO₂)* (Fig. 5-7). An increased A-aDO₂ results

from either ventilation-perfusion (V_A/Q̇) abnormalities or excessive right-to-left shunt. (Diffusion impairment, a third cause of increased A-aDO₂, plays only a marginal role in the development of hypoxemia.) Patients with hypoxemic respiratory failure and a normal A-aDO₂ typically have alveolar hypoventilation or inadequate inspiratory partial pressure of O₂. Hypoxemia results from a low inspired P_O₂ or when the fractional concentration of inspired O₂ (FiO₂) is less than 0.21, such as at high altitude or when O₂ is consumed from ambient gas secondary to a fire. A low FiO₂ also can arise during anesthesia if a low-O₂ gas mixture is administered inadvertently. Hypoxemic respiratory failure also can be caused by the combination of a decreased mixed venous O₂ content and impaired gas exchange, such as in patients with heart failure and concurrent V_A/Q̇ derangements or increased shunt.

Right-To-Left Shunt

A right-to-left shunt is present when venous blood returning from the tissues passes to the systemic arterial

*A-aDo₂ is calculated as $P_{AO_2} - P_{aO_2}$, where P_{aO_2} (alveolar O₂ tension) can be estimated according to the simplified alveolar gas equation:

$$P_{AO_2} = F_{IO_2} \times (P_B - P_{H_2O}) - P_{aCO_2}/R$$

where F_{IO_2} is fractional concentration of inspired O₂ (about 0.21 when breathing room air), P_B is barometric pressure (about 760 mmHg at sea level), P_{H_2O} is water vapor pressure (usually taken as 47 mmHg

at 37°C), and R is respiratory exchange ratio of the whole lung. The respiratory exchange ratio (R) = CO₂ production/O₂ consumption ($\dot{V}_{CO_2}/\dot{V}_{O_2}$) is normally about 0.8. In steady state, R is determined by the relative proportions of free fatty acids, protein, and carbohydrate consumed by the tissues. In this equation it is assumed that alveolar P_{CO_2} and P_{aCO_2} are the same (usually they nearly are). In healthy young subjects (≤30 years old) breathing air at sea level, A-aDO₂ is usually less than 10mm Hg, but it increases to as much as 28 mmHg in some healthy 60-year-old subjects.

circulation without coming into contact with gas-containing alveoli. A small degree of shunting (about 2–3% of cardiac output) is caused by the bronchial veins entering the pulmonary veins and the thebesian veins of the myocardium, which empty directly into the left-ventricular cavity.[57] Shunting also may occur through abnormal intracardiac or intrapulmonary anatomic pathways: atrial or ventricular septal defects, patent ductus ateriosus, and pulmonary arteriovenous fistulas. Shunt is the major mechanism of abnormal gas exchange in patients with pulmonary edema, ARDS, pneumonia, and atelectasis. In all the latter instances, the shunt results from the perfusion of alveoli that are unventilated because they are filled with fluid or collapsed.

A characteristics feature of a shunt is the failure of Pa_{O_2} to increase to the expected level when a patient breathes 100% O_2 (Fig. 5-8). This occurs because the shunted blood does not make contact with ventilated alveoli and thus is not exposed to the higher Pa_{O_2}. The addition of well-oxygenated blood of nonshunted areas to the poorly oxygenated blood from the shunted areas is not sufficient to increase the Pa_{O_2}.

Although the shunted blood is rich in CO_2, a patient with an increased shunt typically does not have a raised Pa_{CO_2} because any elevation of Pa_{CO_2} causes chemoreceptor stimulation and an increase in ventilation. Thus P_{CO_2} in the nonshunted blood is lowered such that Pa_{CO_2} returns to normal. In patients with a large shunt (cyanotic congenital heart disease), Pa_{CO_2} may be low because the low Pa_{O_2} stimulates respiratory drive and minute ventilation (V_E).[58] A shunt typically produces more severe hypoxemia than does $V_A/\dot{Q}$ inequality.

Ventilation-Perfusion Inequality

Optimal uptake of O_2 depends on proper matching of ventilation and perfusion within the lung. The lung consists of about 300 million alveoli,[59] each with its own share of ventilation and perfusion. In semirecumbent young healthy subjects breathing room air, the range (or dispersion) of $V_A/\dot{Q}$ ratios is quite small: More than 95% of both ventilation and perfusion is limited between $V_A/\dot{Q}$ ratios of 0.3 and 2.1.[60] The dispersion increases with age.[60] With pulmonary disease, the range of $V_A/\dot{Q}$ ratios widens,[61] varying from 0 (perfused but unventilated, i.e., shunt) to infinity (ventilated by unperfused, i.e., alveolar dead space). In other words, $V_A/\dot{Q}$ inequality does not refer to alterations in the ratio of total ventilation to total perfusion, which constitute global hyper- or hypoventilation. (One lung could receive all ventilation and the other all perfusion for an overall $V_A/\dot{Q}$ ratio of 1.0).[62] $V_A/\dot{Q}$ inequality refers to regional mismatching of ventilation to perfusion. $V_A/\dot{Q}$ inequality, no matter what its mechanism, interferes with overall efficiency of the lung for exchanging all gases, including O_2, CO_2, CO, and anesthetic gases.[58]

$V_A/\dot{Q}$ mismatch is the most common cause of hypoxemia. Most diseases affecting either the airways or lung parenchyma are distributed unevenly. Thus they variably affect ventilation and perfusion. Some lung regions may have good perfusion and poor ventilation, whereas other regions may have poor ventilation but good perfusion.

When $V_A/\dot{Q}$ inequality consists mainly of low $V_A/\dot{Q}$ areas secondary to inadequate ventilation (e.g., COPD when severe bronchitis predominates) or increased perfusion of normally ventilated units (e.g., diversion of blood flow following pulmonary embolism), the effects on gas exchange are more marked for P_{O_2} than for P_{CO_2}.[63] In the low $V_A/\dot{Q}$ units, alveolar O_2 is taken up by the perfusing blood at a high enough rate and is refreshed by ventilation at a slow enough rate to maintain an abnormally low Pa_{O_2}.[64] The result is a shuntlike mixing of poorly oxygenated blood from the low $V_A/\dot{Q}$ units with well-oxygenated blood from the high $V_A/\dot{Q}$ units. The well-oxygenated blood cannot fully compensate for the poorly oxygenated blood for the same reason that supplemental O_2 does not correct the hypoxemia of right-to-left shunt.

When $V_A/\dot{Q}$ inequality consists mainly of high $V_A/\dot{Q}$ areas, such as decreased perfusion of a compartment (severe emphysema where many capillaries are destroyed), decreases in Pa_{O_2} can be accompanied by rises in Pa_{CO_2} because high $V_A/\dot{Q}$ units are inefficient at eliminating CO_2.[58,63] Units such as these constitute part of alveolar (and physiologic) dead space.[58,62]

Compensatory mechanisms tend to minimize the effects of these abnormal $V_A/\dot{Q}$ ratios. The low Pa_{O_2} associated with a low $V_A/\dot{Q}$ ratio causes pulmonary vasoconstriction. The low Pa_{CO_2} associated with a high $V_A/\dot{Q}$ ratio causes hypocapnic bronchoconstriction[65] (e.g., pulmonary embolism). These responses, however, only achieve partial

FIGURE 5-8 Relationship between arterial P_{O_2} (Pa_{O_2}) and increases in inhaled O_2 concentrations for different levels of shunt. When the shunt fraction is 30% or more of cardiac output, Pa_{O_2} increases little despite marked increases in inspired O_2 concentration. The plot is a simplification that ignores factors such as cardiac output and O_2 uptake, which influence the location of the lines. (*Used, with permission, from West: Pulmonary pathophysiology: The essentials, 6th ed. Philadelphia: Lippincott Williams & Wilkins, 163, 2003.*)

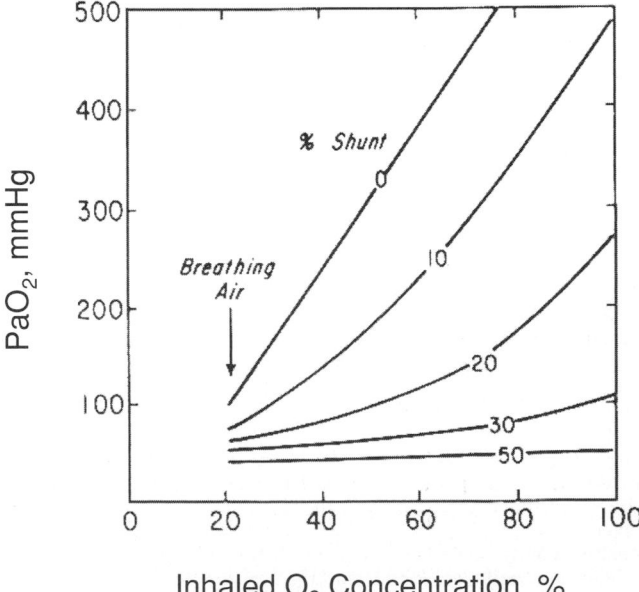

compensation. As $V_A/\dot{Q}$ inequality increases in the presence of a constant $\dot{V}_{O_2}$ and $\dot{V}_{CO_2}$, there is an immediate and marked fall in Pa_{O_2} and a slower increase in Pa_{CO_2}. The increase in Pa_{CO_2} and, to a lesser extent, the fall in Pa_{O_2} stimulates the chemoreceptors and lead to an increase in $\dot{V}_E$. In patients without a significant reduction in ventilatory capacity, the increase in ventilation is sufficient to bring Pa_{CO_2} back to normal, although it has only a small effect on the fall in Pa_{O_2} (Fig. 5-9). Thus most patients with $V_A/\dot{Q}$ inequalities have a low Pa_{O_2} but normal Pa_{CO_2}.[66] Ventilation in excess of normal alveolar requirement is termed *wasted ventilation*.[58] All normocapnic patients with COPD have increased ventilation of their alveoli, as do most hypercapnic patients.[58]

FIGURE 5-9 Effect of increasing overall ventilation on Pa_{O_2} and Pa_{CO_2} (lung model) as a function of different degrees of $V_A/\dot{Q}$ mismatching, represented in terms of dispersion or standard deviations (SD) of the lognormal distribution of ventilation and perfusion. (Dispersion of 0.30–0.05 = normal $V_A/\dot{Q}$ mismatch; 1.0 = moderate $V_A/\dot{Q}$ mismatch; 2.0 = severe $V_A/\dot{Q}$ mismatch.) Increases in overall ventilation have a powerful effect on Pa_{O_2} and Pa_{CO_2} when $V_A/\dot{Q}$ dispersion is small. Abnormal $V_A/\dot{Q}$ dispersion does not cause an increase in Pa_{CO_2} as long as patients are able to increase minute ventilation sufficiently. Pa_{O_2} also increase with increases in overall ventilation, although when $V_A/\dot{Q}$ dispersions are (very) altered, normal Pa_{O_2} cannot be reached very easily, and further effects on ventilation have little effect on Pa_{O_2}. In the patients who cannot maintain a high rate of ventilation owing to the increased work of breathing and in those whose respiratory drive increases only slightly when Pa_{CO_2} is high, hypercapnia can ensue. (Used, with permission, from West: *Am Rev Respir Dis* 116:919–43,1977.)

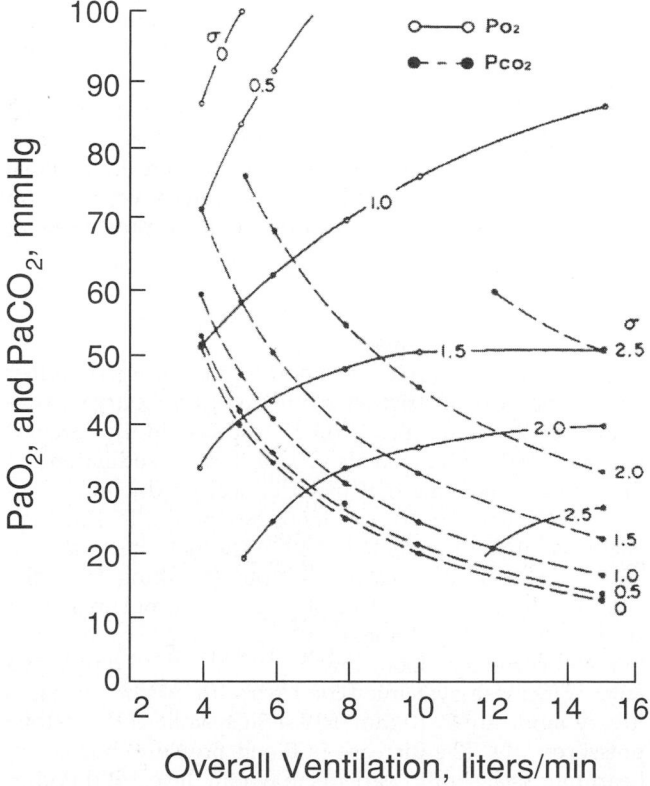

The different responses of Pa_{O_2} and Pa_{CO_2} to an increase in the level of ventilation is caused by the different shapes of the oxyhemoglobin and CO_2 dissociation curves (Fig. 5-10). The oxyhemoglobin dissociation curve is flat in the normal range. Thus only units with moderately low $V_A/\dot{Q}$ ratios benefit appreciably from the increased ventilation. Lung units that are positioned on the upper portion of the dissociation curve (high $V_A/\dot{Q}$ ratio) develop little increase in the O_2 concentration of their effluent blood. The net result is that with increasing V_E, the mixed Pa_{O_2} rises only modestly, and some hypoxemia always remains.[58] By contrast, the CO_2 dissociation curve is almost linear in the physiologic range. Thus an increase in V_E raises CO_2 output of lung units with both high and low $V_A/\dot{Q}$ ratios.[58] The different shapes of the two dissociations curves are the main reason that patients with parenchymal lung disease have greater hypoxemia relative to hypercapnia. One final compensatory adjustment is possible: increase in cardiac output.[63] Adrenergic stimulation by arterial hypoxemia can raise cardiac output by 50% or more; this improves arterial blood gases by raising mixed venous O_2 and by lowering mixed venous CO_2.[63]

Administration of supplemental O_2 in patients with $V_A/\dot{Q}$ inequality will cause arterial hypoxemia to reverse impressively because Pa_{O_2} of even poorly ventilated units increases sufficiently to achieve saturation (Fig. 5-11). Unless Fi_{O_2} is 1.0, it is impossible to determine the relative contribution of right-to-left shunt versus $V_A/\dot{Q}$ inequality to an increase in A-aD_{O_2}.[57] After breathing 100% O_2 for a sufficient time, only units that are totally or almost totally unventilated (shunt, true shunt, or anatomic shunt) will contribute to hypoxemia.[57]

PHYSIOLOGIC EFFECTS OF HYPOXIA

Although the physiologic effects of hypoxia are graded, the damaging effects are sudden.[67] A remarkable degree of arterial hypoxemia is required to cause tissue hypoxia.[23] In clinical practice, Campbell[23] observed that the lowest Pa_{O_2} compatible with life is 20 mmHg [equivalent to an arterial O_2 saturation (Sa_{O_2}) of 30–40%]. Evidence of end-organ damage is difficult to demonstrate in patients with a Pa_{O_2} above 40 mmHg (equivalent to an Sa_{O_2} of about 70%).[23] Obviously, the duration of hypoxemia and the state of circulation (O_2 delivery) play major roles in determining the minimum Pa_{O_2} that does not cause end-organ damage or death.

The threshold Pa_{O_2} commonly used to diagnose hypoxemic respiratory failure is 60 mmHg, which corresponds to an Sa_{O_2} of 90% (hypoxic hypoxia). Pa_{O_2} values below 60 mmHg fall on the steep portion of the oxyhemoglobin dissociation curve, and decreases below that value are associated with precipitous falls in Sa_{O_2} (see Fig. 5-10). Although physiologically reasonable, for self-evident ethical reasons, the 60 mmHg (Pa_{O_2}) threshold cannot be validated experimentally.

The main concern with hypoxemia is impaired tissue oxygenation, especially of the heart and brain. The factors determining O_2 supply to the tissues include hemoglobin (Hb) concentration, Sa_{O_2}, the affinity of Hb for O_2 (P_{50}), cardiac output, regional O_2 consumption-to-perfusion relationships, and the diffusion of O_2 from the capillary to

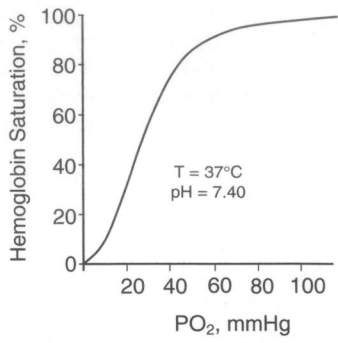 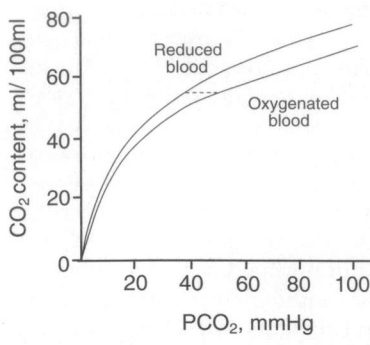

FIGURE 5-10 (*Left*) Normal oxyhemoglobin dissociation curve. The curve has a sigmoid shape because when one subunit of the normal tetrameric form of normal adult hemoglobin becomes oxygenated, it induces a configuration (or structural) arrangement change in the whole complex. As a result, the three other subunits gain a greater affinity for oxygen until four molecules of O_2 are combined with hemoglobin. (*Right*) The CO_2 dissociation curve for oxygenated and reduced blood. The relationship is steeper and more linear than the oxyhemoglobin dissociation curve. Oxygenation of blood causes the curve to shift in a rightward direction (Haldane effect). Thus, for a given CO_2 content, oxygenated blood has a higher P_{CO_2} than reduced blood; this factor is one of the reasons for an increase in P_{CO_2} when breathing supplemental O_2.

intracellular sites. The amount of O_2 delivered to the tissues is calculated as

$$O_2 \text{ delivery} = Ca_{O_2} \times \text{cardiac output}$$

where arterial O_2 content (Ca_{O_2}) is calculated as

$$Ca_{O_2} = (Hb \times 1.34 \times Sa_{O_2}/100) + (0.003 \times Pa_{O_2})$$

Even with a satisfactory Pa_{O_2}, tissue hypoxia may arise because of decreased Ca_{O_2} (e.g., decreased Hb concentration or decreased Hb function, such as in carbon monoxide poisoning or anemic hypoxia), decreased O_2 delivery (e.g., cardiogenic shock or stagnant hypoxia), and decreased capacity of the tissues to use O_2 (e.g., sepsis, cyanide intoxication, or histotoxic hypoxia). Otherwise stated, tissue hypoxia can be present despite adequate Pa_{O_2}, or it can be absent despite an abnormally low Pa_{O_2}.[55]

Respiratory Responses
Peripheral chemoreceptors (carotid and aortic bodies) detect changes in arterial O_2. Within seconds after the onset of hypoxia, they initiate reflexes that are important for maintaining homeostasis.[68–70] The aortic bodies play a minor role in modulating spontaneous respiratory activity, although they have a discernible effect when their gain is increased by hypercapnia.[71]

Although hypoxia augments sensory discharge of both carotid and aortic bodies, it has been proposed that aortic chemoreceptors sense O_2 delivery, whereas carotid bodies sense P_{O_2}.[72] These notions are based on the finding that carboxyhemoglobinemia causes marked stimulation of aortic bodies, whereas it has no effect on the carotid body sensory activity.[72]

Hypoxia augments sensory discharge from the peripheral chemoreceptors, which, in turn, send neural impulses to the respiratory centers (inspiratory neurons of the dorsal respiratory group and ventral respiratory group[73]), causing an increase in the V_E.[68,69,74,75] Hyperpnea, in turn, activates pulmonary afferents, thereby buffering the sympathetic response to hypoxemia.[76]

The ventilatory response to progressive hypoxia is curvilinear[68] and increases in the presence of concurrent hypercapnia[71] (Fig. 5-12). It decreases with age,[77] Chronic hypoxia may induce a reduced ventilatory response to hypoxia in patients with COPD,[71] although the role of airway narrowing in producing this effect cannot be excluded.[71]

The ventilatory response to hypoxemia is attenuated or abolished in patients who have undergone surgical excision of the carotid bodies.[69,70,75,78] The increase in ventilation in response to hypoxemia probably contributes to coronary vasodilation.[79] Stimulation of the carotid bodies with nicotine under normoxic conditions causes an increase in ventilation and coronary vasodilation.[79] Coronary vasodilation does not occur if the increase in ventilation is prevented by general anesthesia.[79]

Cardiovascular Responses
Hypoxic stimulation of chemoreceptors triggers reflex adrenergic vasoconstriction in muscle and coronary vasodilation but does not elicit a reflex response in the cerebral vessels.[70,76,79,80] Hypoxia also causes local vasodilation[68,76] through mechanisms that include local production of nitric oxide, activation of adenosine- and ATP-sensitive channels, and other metabolites.[81] The net effects are increases in heart rate, cardiac output (resulting from the positive chronotropic effect of hypoxemia, not increased stroke volume[82]), pulmonary artery resistance,[83] and cerebral and coronary blood flow[70,76,77,79,80,82,84,85] Hypoxemia fails to increase systemic blood pressure[82,85] or increases it very modestly (<10 mmHg rise in systolic and diastolic pressures[74,84]). The increase in blood pressure, but not in heart rate, is absent in patients in whom the carotid bodies

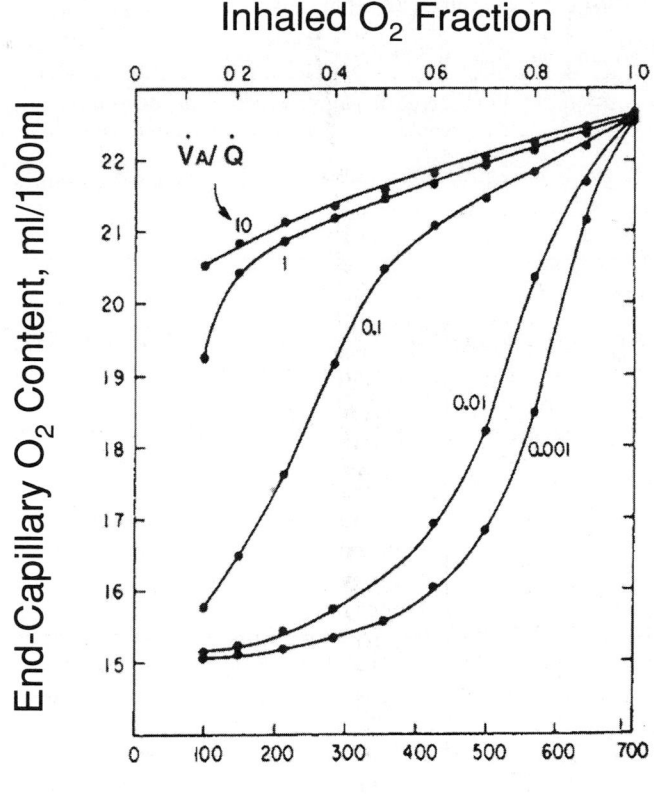

FIGURE 5-11 The effect of alterations in inhaled partial pressure of O_2 on O_2 content of end-capillary blood of a lung unit. Each line depicts a different ventilation-perfusion ratio ($V_A/\dot{Q}$). With mild to moderate degrees of $V_A/\dot{Q}$ inequality ($V_A/\dot{Q}$ down to 0.1), end-capillary O_2 content increases as inspired O_2 is increased. With severe $V_A/\dot{Q}$ inequality ($V_A/\dot{Q}$ below 0.1), the increase in end-capillary O_2 content with an increase in inspired O_2 is much slower; only when inspired P_{O_2} is more than 400–500 mmHg does end-capillary O_2 content of the lung unit reach values equivalent to those seen with mild to moderate degrees of $V_A/\dot{Q}$ inequality. (*Used, with permission, from West: Am Rev Respir Dis 116:919–43, 1977.*)

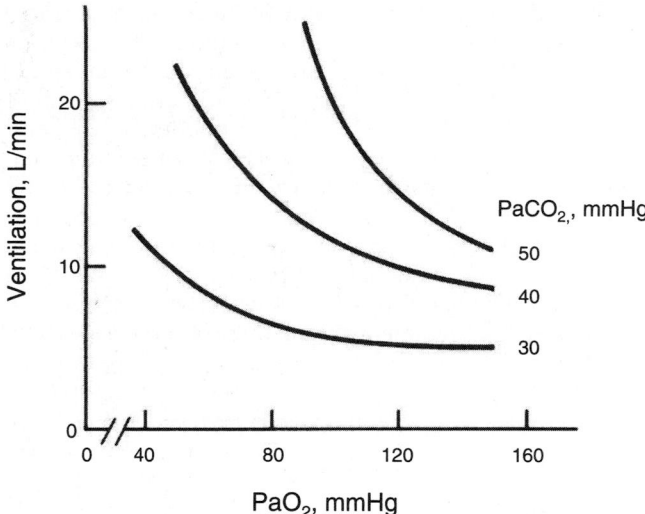

FIGURE 5-12 The curvilinear relationship between ventilation and Pa_{O_2} at various levels of Pa_{CO_2}. When Pa_{CO_2} is 40 mmHg, ventilation increases precipitously as Pa_{O_2} falls below 60 mmHg. When Pa_{CO_2} is elevated, ventilation increases abruptly at a higher Pa_{O_2}. When Pa_{CO_2} is lower, the ventilatory response to hypoxia is less steep. (*Used, with permission, from Grippi et al: In: Fishman, editor. Fishman's pulmonary diseases and disorders, 3rd ed. New York: McGraw-Hill, Chap. 36, 563, 1998.*)

are inactivated.[70,74] Persistent tachycardic response to hypoxemia in patients with bilateral carotid body ablation likely is mediated by the effect of hypoxemia on the aortic bodies.[68]

Tachycardia caused by hypoxemia is mediated by multiple factors, including CNS-mediated sympathetic discharge, effect of P_{O_2} on the cardiac pacemaker, and concomitant hyperpnea.[74] These mechanisms presumably override the cardioinhibitory signals (bradycardic effect) from the carotid body.[74] The importance of hyperpnea in overriding the bradycardic effect is supported by the observation that hypoxemia combined with cessation of lung inflation (sleep apnea,[86] breath holding,[87] or neuromuscular blockade during intubation[88]) or diminution of lung inflation (such as when hyperpnea is prevented by controlled ventilation[89,90]) is more apt to produce bradycardia than tachycardia.[68,86] Bradycardia results from the concurrent activation of the

carotid bodies by hypoxia and increased cardiac vagal activity induced by apnea.[76,80] [The increased vagal activity (induced by apnea) can be so intense as to induce bradycardia in the absence of coexisting hypoxemia; this response has been described in patients with spinal cord injury within seconds of discontinuation from a ventilator.[91]] Simultaneously with the increase in cardiac vagal activity, diminution of lung inflation causes marked potentiation of the sympathetic vasoconstrictor response to hypoxemia (secondary to the lack of inhibitory influence of the pulmonary stretch receptors).[80,92] (This combination of sympathetic vasoconstriction and vagal bradycardia constitutes part of the diving reflex.[80])

Severe hypoxemia is not tolerated by the CNS because it has a high rate of O_2 consumption and lacks alternative energy reserves.[93] Therefore, severe hypoxemia causes cerebral depression.[69,84] Patients with cerebral hypoxia develop bradycardia, hypotension,[88] and hypoventilation,[84] which further worsens hypoxia and induces a potentially lethal viscous cycle.

CLINICAL PRESENTATION OF HYPOXEMIA

Cyanosis

Physicians commonly view cyanosis as the hallmark of hypoxemia.[68] Cyanosis is recognized as a blueness of the capillary blood visible through the mucous membranes or skin, where capillaries are numerous and close together and the tissues over them are thin and transparent, such as the lips (central cyanosis) and nail beds.[68]

Central cyanosis is believed to depend on the presence of at least 5 g/dl of deoxygenated hemoglobin in the blood of the capillaries[94] and of the subpapillary venous plexus.[95]

With mild anemia (hemoglobin of 10 g/dl), hypoxemia should be severe enough (O_2 saturation 50%, capillary P_{O_2} about 24 mmHg) to produce cyanosis.[64] Conversely, with polycythemia (hemoglobin 20 g/dl), cyanosis should be present when hypoxemia is only moderate (O_2 saturation 75%, capillary P_{O_2} 40 mmHg).[64] The dictum that cyanosis requires 5 g/dl of reduced hemoglobin is difficult to substantiate.[96,97] Cyanosis depends not only on variables such as thickness and opacity of the skin and perfusion status but also on the visual skills of the observer.[95,97] In 72 patients who had Sa_{O_2} values ranging between less than 75% and 100%, agreement among three observers was only 69% when inspecting the tongue, 61% when inspecting the lips, and 53% when inspecting the nail bed.[95] In that study,[95] cyanosis of the tongue and lips was recorded in 40–45% of patients with normal Sa_{O_2} values. Rather than a blue or pink color, pallor is seen with both anemia and shock. Thus severe or fatal tissue hypoxia may occur without cyanosis.[68] The skin and arterial blood may be normal in color or even bright red in two other types of tissue hypoxia: cyanide poisoning, where the tissues are unable to use blood O_2 despite its abundance, and carbon monoxide poisoning, where blood contains a bright-red pigment, carboxyhemoglobin,[68] that decreases the oxygen-carrying capacity of the blood and shifts the oxyhemoglobin dissociation curve to the left. Both these changes—together with inhibition of the mitochondrial respiratory chain at the cytochrome C by carbon monoxide[98]—limit the uptake and use of O_2 by peripheral tissues.

Cardiopulmonary Manifestations

Acute hypoxemia increases respiratory frequency, tidal volume, and V_E in almost all subjects.[68] Increases in V_E, however, are an unreliable guide because the interindividual response to hypoxemia is considerable.[97] The standard deviation for the within-subject variability in day-to-day hypoxic ventilatory response is about 22%.[99] The respiratory response to mild or moderate hypoxemia may be barely measurable or absent.[68,92] An increase in heart rate is equally of limited value because many other factors, such as fever, low blood pressure, pain, apprehension, and drugs, can cause it to rise.[68] Moreover, under specific circumstances (see above), hypoxemia causes bradycardia rather than tachycardia. Hypoxemia tends to increase systolic blood pressure in some subjects; the wide variations in response[74] renders arterial pressure of little value in the diagnosis of hypoxemia.[68]

Neurologic Manifestations

The metabolic needs of the brain largely depend on oxidation of glucose to CO_2 and water.[93] The brain cannot store O_2. It survives only for minutes after the supply is reduced to critical levels.[93] In acute anoxia, consciousness is lost within 15 seconds. The electroencephalogram slows with a Pa_{O_2} of less than 35 mmHg or with blood flow of less than 40% of normal.[93] Loss of the electroencephalogram tracing occurs when cerebral P_{O_2} reaches 20 mmHg or following 20 seconds of complete anoxia.[93]

TABLE 5-3 Neurologic Signs and Symptoms of Hypoxia

Pa_{O_2}, mmHg	Signs and Symptoms of Hypoxia
35–50	Loss of critical judgment, confusion, delirium (resembling alcohol intoxication), tremors, asterixis
25–35	Somenolence, obtundation, myoclonic jerks, seizures
20–25	Loss of consciousness
<20	Death

In the absence of defects of cerebral blood flow, Pa_{O_2} below 40 mmHg is required to produce prominent symptoms[22,100,101] (Table 5-3). Confusion and delirium (resembling alcohol intoxication) appear at Pa_{O_2} values of 35–50 mmHg.[62] Tremors and asterixis (flapping tremor elicited by dorsiflexing the wrists with the arms outstretched and caused by a momentary interruption of normal continuous action potentials to both flexor and extensor muscles) are infrequent even when the Pa_{O_2} is less than 40 mmHg.[22,23] Somnolence and obtundation occur at Pa_{O_2} values of 25–35 mmHg. Some patients develop myoclonic jerks (bursts of excitation to resting muscles) and seizures.[22] At about 25 mmHg, consciousness is lost,[62] and death often ensues.

When considering the neurologic manifestations of hypoxemia, Pa_{O_2} is only a small part of a complex situation. A decrease in Pa_{O_2} may be well tolerated if O_2 delivery is maintained by the combination of increased cardiac output and systemic vasoconstriction.[102] These compensatory mechanisms, however, can be overwhelmed by anemia or carbon monoxide poisoning, which decrease oxygen-carrying capacity (anemic hypoxia), or by atherosclerosis or other causes of vascular occlusion (ischemic hypoxia) in which the increased cardiac output does not suffice to prevent tissue damage.

HYPERCAPNIC RESPIRATORY FAILURE

PATHOPHYSIOLOGY

Hypercapnic respiratory failure is a state in which ventilation is insufficient to maintain a normal Pa_{CO_2} for the level of metabolic activity (measured by CO_2 production, $\dot{V}_{CO_2}$). Common causes include COPD, severe asthma, conditions where respiratory drive is decreased (e.g., neoplasm and infections of the CNS, medications, and drugs), neuromuscular-skeletal diseases (e.g., myasthenia gravis, Guillain-Barré syndrome, and trauma), and upper airway obstruction.

Under steady-state conditions, the relationship between Pa_{CO_2}, alveolar ventilation (V_A), and $\dot{V}_{CO_2}$ is given by the equation

$$Pa_{CO_2} = (\dot{V}_{CO_2}/V_A) \times K$$

The constant K is usually stated as 0.863; it converts measurements of $\dot{V}_{CO_2}$ from standard conditions to body-temperature conditions. The term V_A represents the portion of V_E that reaches the terminal gas-exchange units and is calculated as

$$V_A = V_E - V_D$$

where V_D equals dead-space ventilation. A reduction in V_A may result from an inadequate V_E or an increase in V_D (resulting from an increase in true V_D or a functional increase in V_D secondary to lung regions with high $V_A/\dot{Q}$ relationships).

The mechanisms responsible for hypercapnia can be grouped into two categories depending on whether there is (or is not) an increased A-aD_{O_2} (see Fig. 5-7). In pure alveolar hypoventilation (e.g., neuromuscular diseases, drug overdoses, and CNS pathologies), A-aD_{O_2} is usually normal (unless lung abnormalities are present). In disorders associated with $V_A/\dot{Q}$ inequality (e.g., COPD and ARDS), A-aD_{O_2} is increased.

Pa_{CO_2} in excess of 90 mmHg is unlikely in patients breathing room air because the concomitant degree of hypoxia is incompatible with survival.[23] Such Pa_{CO_2} values can occur if a patient is breathing O_2-enriched air.[103]

PHYSIOLOGIC EFFECTS OF HYPERCAPNIA

Hypercapnia elicits autonomic and ventilatory responses primarily through central chemoreceptors located in the rostral ventrolateral medulla.[70] These respond to changes in hydrogen ion concentration.[70] Hypercapnia, probably via a reduction in pH, also stimulates peripheral arterial chemoreceptors located in the carotid bodies, aortic bodies, and abdomen.[104,105] Only 15–30% of the ventilatory response to hypercapnia results from peripheral chemoreceptor stimulation.[106,107] Not surprisingly, the Pa_{CO_2} of patients with bilateral resection of the carotid bodies is higher [by 4.6 ± 1.3 (standard deviation) mmHg] than in healthy subjects.[78]

Respiratory Responses

Hypercapnia causes an increase in V_E; stimulation peaks with an inhaled CO_2 of 10%.[108] In contrast to the curvilinear response to progressive hypoxemia (see Fig. 5-12), the hypercapnic ventilatory response is linear.[68] (Fig. 5-13). The ventilatory response to CO_2 increases when concurrent hypoxemia is present[109] and decreases with age.[77]

Hypercapnia and hypoxia induce different patterns of neuromuscular activation as V_E rises—even when the respiratory components of tidal breathing (tidal volume and inspiratory and expiratory times) are similar.[73] First, hypercapnia is a more potent stimulus for expiratory muscle recruitment than is hypoxemia—one-third of subjects do not recruit their expiratory muscles during hypoxemia.[73] Second, activation of the diaphragm is greater during hypoxemia that during hypercapnia.[73] (The lack of expiratory recruitment during hypoxemia may increase end-expiratory lung volume, which increases O_2 reserves.[73])

The interindividual variation in respiratory response to hypercapnia is large. In 31 healthy subjects inhaling 10.4% CO_2 in O_2, average maximum V_E rose to 76 liters/min, with a range of 40–130 liters/min.[110]

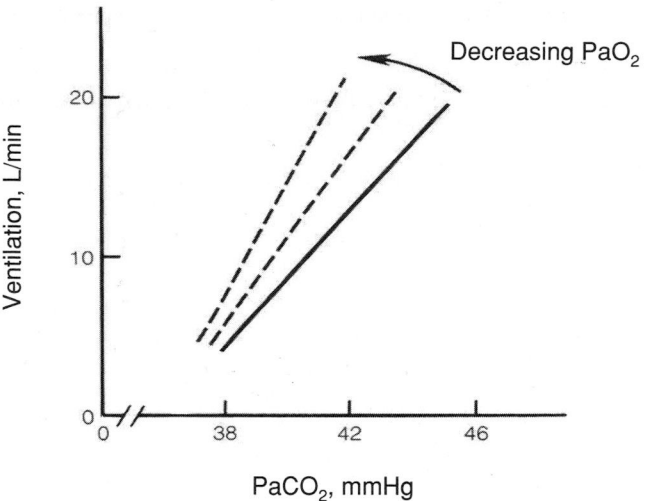

FIGURE 5-13 Ventilatory response to progressive hypercapnia. Ventilation increases linearly with increase in Pa_{CO_2}. Decreases in Pa_{O_2} produce more steep ventilatory response to progressive hypercapnia. (*Used, with permission, from Grippi et al: In: Fishman, editor. Fishman's pulmonary diseases and disorders, 3rd ed. New York: McGraw-Hill, Chap. 36, 561, 1998.*)

Cardiovascular Responses

Hypercapnia causes greater increases in sympathetic activity[92,105,111] (Fig. 5-14) and (usually) greater increases in systemic blood pressure (about 30 mmHg rise in systolic pressure and about 25 mmHg rise in diastolic pressure[110]) than does hypoxemia.[85,105] Acting via baroreflexes, this greater hypertensive response may be partly responsible for the more limited rise in heart rate during hypercapnia than during hypoxemia.[85,105] The tachycardic (and hyperpneic) response to hypercapnia is blunted in the elderly.[77] Apnea increases the sympathetic nerve activity elicited by hypercapnia.[105] This increase, however, is less than the increase during hypoxemia[105] (see Fig. 5-14).

Combined hypoxia and hypercapnia have a synergistic effect on sympathetic nerve activity[105] (see Fig. 5-14) and hyperpnea (see Fig. 5-13). This potentiation may arise because hypercapnia sensitizes the response of peripheral chemoreceptor afferents to hypoxia.[105] Another possibility is that both peripheral and central chemoreceptors synapse on common nuclei in the brain stem.[105]

Hypercapnia not only has a sympathetic vasoconstrictor effect (secondary to chemoreceptor activation) but also has a direct vasodilator effect on systemic arterioles[21,68]; dilatation of conjuntival and superficial facial vessels may be noted. The first action, however, is predominant in conscious persons, and blood pressure and heart rate increase. If the vasomotor center cannot respond (e.g., secondary to brain damage, severe ischemia or hypoxia, or deep anesthesia) or is disconnected from peripheral parts of the sympathetic nervous system (e.g., secondary to spinal cord damage or blocking drug or spinal anesthesia), direct vasodilation becomes the sole or dominant effect, and blood pressure falls.[21,68,112]

Hypercapnia increases cerebral blood flow.[113] Cerebrovascular reactivity to CO_2 depends on age (i.e., there

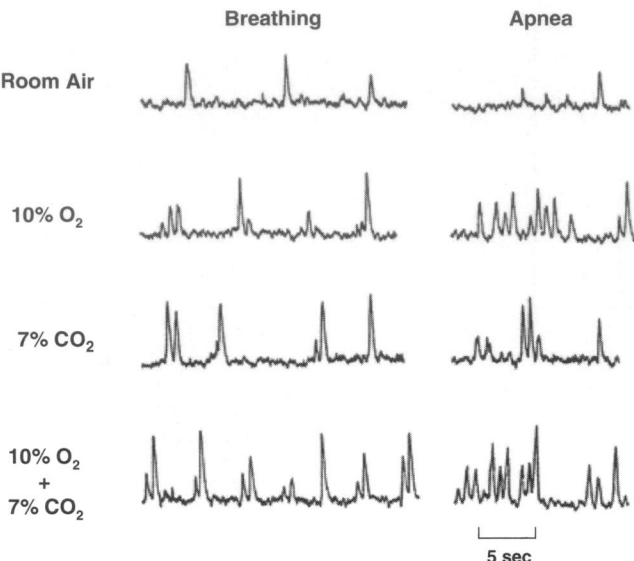

FIGURE 5-14 Direct intraneural recordings of sympathetic nerve activity in during exposure to room air, isocapnic hypoxia (10% O_2, 90% N_2, and titrated CO_2), hyperoxic hypercapnia (7% CO_2, 93% O_2), and hypoxic hypercapnia (10% O_2, 7% CO_2, and 83% N_2) during spontaneous breathing (*left*) and during end-expiratory apnea (*right*). Sympathetic activity is a function of both burst frequency and burst amplitude. Three points can be made. First, sympathetic activity during breathing increased more during hypercapnia (7% CO_2) than during hypoxia (10% O_2). Second, apnea caused greater enhancement of sympathetic nerve activity during hypoxia (10% O_2) than during hypercapnia (7% CO_2). Third, hypoxia and hypercapnia had a synergistic effect on sympathetic nerve activity. (*Used, with permission, from Somers et al: J Appl Physiol 67:2101–6, 1989.*)

is reduced cerebral perfusion reserve in the elderly)[114] and state (i.e., there is a 70% reduction in cerebrovascular reactivity to CO_2 during non–rapid eye movement sleep).[81] Hypercapnic cerebrovascular reactivity also is reduced in patients with preexisting cerebrovascular diseases.[115]

Neurologic Responses

Hypercapnia decreases cerebral metabolic rate for glucose and interferes with cerebral energy production.[116] The cerebral metabolic rate for O_2 is maintained, or slightly increased, provided that Pa_{CO_2} is less than 90–100 mmHg.[116] For higher values of Pa_{CO_2}, cerebral metabolic rate for O_2 decreases.[116] Hypercapnia has a dual effect on neuron excitability: stimulatory at low concentrations and inhibitory at high concentrations.[68] In humans, very high concentrations (30%) can produce surgical anesthesia, which can be associated with seizures.[68,103,108]

CLINICAL PRESENTATION OF HYPERCAPNIA

The clinical manifestations of hypercapnia result from a complex interaction of several factors, including severity of hypercapnia, comorbidities, and the speed at which the increase in CO_2 has occurred. For example, patients receiving chronic O_2 therapy have been reported to function sat-

isfactorily with Pa_{CO} values of greater than 100 mmHg.[68] Therefore, there is no single threshold of Pa_{CO_2} above which mechanical ventilation is mandatory.

Cardiopulmonary Manifestations

Most signs and symptoms of acute hypercapnic respiratory failure, including hyperpnea, dyspnea, tachycardia and hypertension, and diaphoresis, are similar to those of hypoxemia. Some consider it a waste of effort to try to separate which manifestations are related to hypoxemia and which to hypercapnia.[117]

Neurologic Manifestations

The major clinical features of hypercapnia are those affecting the CNS. One difference between acute hypoxemic and acute hypercapnic respiratory failure is the greater incidence of neurologic manifestations with the latter. Acute hypercapnia can cause fine tremors (of the outstretched hands, head, or legs), asterixis, myoclonic jerks, sustained myoclonus, and seizures.[22,108] It also can cause cognitive disorders, hostility, irritability, paranoid behavior, somnolence, stupor, and coma.[22] In a study of 32 episodes of acute respiratory failure, Kilburn[22] reported that the severity of cognitive disorders, asterixis, and somnolence and the presence of stupor and coma were closely related to the severity of respiratory acidosis—and not to the severity of hypoxemia.

Some patients with severe hypercapnia have papilledema and elevated cerebrospinal fluid pressure probably because of the increase in blood volume within the near-rigid cranial cavity.[68,84,113] Under conditions of prolonged hypercapnia (several hours), cortical blood flow may return toward baseline over time.[118] The latter is probably mediated by a buildup of brain extracellular bicarbonate and an increase in pH.[118]

Some patients with combined hypoxemic and hypercapnic respiratory failure become more comatose when treated with O_2 (CO_2 narcosis). The mechanisms responsible for O_2-induced hypercapnia are complex and probably include reduction in ventilation, increased wasted ventilation (alveolar dead space),[119] and the Haldane effect (Pa_{CO_2} increases because of net release of CO_2 from erythrocytes when Sa_{O_2} is increased)[120] (see Fig. 5-10).

POSTOPERATIVE RESPIRATORY FAILURE

Postoperative respiratory failure can be defined as the need for intubation and mechanical ventilation in the 48 hours after surgery.[121] Among more than 180,000 patients undergoing major noncardiac surgery, postoperative respiratory failure occurred in 3%.[121] This exceeds the incidence of myocardial infarction after surgery (0.4–0.7%).[121,122] Among 1055 patients, most of whom underwent lower abdominal/inguinal hernia repair or orthopedic limb surgery, 0.1% required intubation within 7 days of surgery.[123]

Pulmonary complications are estimated to account for nearly 25% of deaths within 6 days of surgery.[124] This figure may be an underestimate; many patients with respiratory failure can be kept alive by ventilator support, only to die from nonrespiratory complications (e.g., sepsis and

TABLE 5-4 Causes of Postoperative Respiratory Failure

Intrapulmonary causes
  Atelectasis
  Aspiration
  Pneumonia
  Acute respiratory distress sysdrome/acute lung injury
  Volume overload/congestive heart failure
  Pulmonary embolism (thrombus, air, fat)
  Bronchoconstriction (asthma/COPD)
  Pneumothorax
Extrapulmonary causes
  Shock
  Decreased respiratory drive
  Phrenic nerve injury
  Diaphragmatic dysfunction
  Upper airway obstruction
  Obstructive sleep apnea

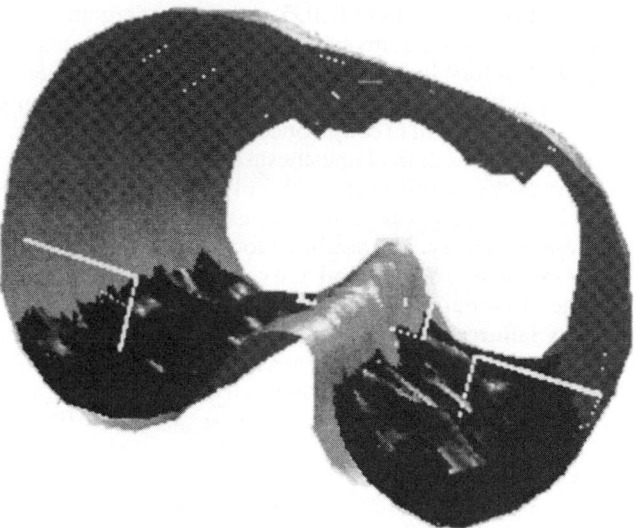

FIGURE 5-15 Three-dimensional reconstruction of atelectasis (in dependent lung regions) and the chest wall in an anesthetized and paralyzed patient before the start of surgery. The chest wall has a gray appearance; the anterior part is directed upward, and the dorsal border is directed downward. The dorsal ridge indicates the spine. The caudal region of the chest wall is closest to the viewer, who is looking into the thorax from the position of the diaphragm. The black regions correspond to the atelectasis. The size of the atelectasis decreases toward the apex, and its surface is coarse. (Used, with permission, from Hedenstierna: Clin Physiol Funct Imaging 23:123–9, 2003.)

multiorgan failure).[125] Among patients who undergo major noncardiac surgery, mortality is 27–42% for those with postoperative respiratory failure versus 1–6% for those without postoperative respiratory failure.[121,126] Respiratory failure is the most important determinant of postoperative mortality in 40–100% of thoracic surgery patients.[127]

A common cause of postoperative respiratory failure is the development of atelectasis.[125,127,128] Atelectasis is the most frequent pulmonary complication after general surgery (particularly thoracic and upper abdominal surgery)[125] (Table 5-4). Atelectasis occurs in about 90% of patients during anesthesia.[129] During uneventful anesthesia, before any surgery is begun, 15–20% of the lung base is collapsed[130] (Fig. 5-15). With thoracic surgery and cardiopulmonary bypass, more than 50% of the lung can be collapsed several hours after surgery.[131] After abdominal surgery, atelectasis can persist for several days.[132]

One mechanism for the development of atelectasis during general anesthesia is decreased respiratory muscle tone, which is accompanied by a cephalad displacing of the diaphragm, 20% reduction in functional residual capacity (60% reduction in obesity), and compression of lung tissue.[125,133] Two other purported mechanisms are impaired function of surfactant and resorption of gas behind occluded airways (particularly with high F_{IO_2}).[130]

Persistent or new atelectasis after anesthesia can be caused by several mechanisms. First, patients undergoing abdominal or thoracic surgery experience a marked reduction in vital capacity and a smaller but clinically important decrease in functional residual capacity.[133] These changes are ascribed to postoperative pain and diaphragmatic dysfunction.[133,134] Abnormal abdominal mechanics reduce end-expiratory lung volume below (the increased) closing volume, leading to absorption of gas from poorly ventilated lung units.[128] Second, the weakened diaphragm no longer acts as a rigid wall between the thoracic and abdominal space.[134] The positive abdominal pressure transmitted to the thoracic cavity increases pleural pressure and causes compression atelectasis—particularly in the dependent thorax.[130,135] Third, mucociliary clearance is impaired.[136,137] Fourth, narcotics[138] and pain[122] suppress

periodic deep breaths. Lack of intermittent deep breaths favors alveolar collapse by precluding alveolar recruitment and decreasing active forms of alveolar surfactant.[139] Fifth, narcotics[138] and pain[122] also suppress cough and interfere with the ability to clear secretions.[140] In a prospective study of 361 patients undergoing elective lung surgery (including pneumonectomy, lobectomy, wedge and segmental resection, and bullectomy), Bonde et al[140] reported that complications related to retention of secretions (i.e., atelectasis, pneumonia, and respiratory failure) occurred in 30% of patients. On multivariate analysis, being a current smoker, having ischemic heart disease, and the absence of regional analgesia or failure of regional analgesia (thoracic epidural or extrapleural intercostal nerve infusion block) increased the risk of secretion retention.[140] Of 12 in-hospital deaths, 10 were considered complications of secretion retention. Sixth, risk of atelectasis is increased with routine use of nasogastric tubes.[123,141,142] Seventh, preexisting pulmonary disease[143] and current smoking[144]—associated with increased postoperative secretions[140]—increase the risk of atelectasis. The end result of atelectasis can be hypoxemic respiratory failure, hypercapnic respiratory failure, or both and pneumonia and sepsis.[128,145]

Preoperative assessment is useful in identifying patients at increased risk after thoracic and nonthoracic surgery.[121,123,146] In a prospective study of 272 patients undergoing nonthoracic surgery, McAlister et al[146] identified three independent risk factors for postoperative complications: age of 65 years or more, smoking of 40 pack-years or more, and maximum laryngeal height of 4 cm or less.

In a subsequent study of 1055 patients undergoing non-thoracic surgery, these investigators reported four independent risk factors for postoperative complications: age of 65 years or more, positive cough test (recurrent coughing after asking a patient to cough once), perioperative nasogastric tube, and duration of anesthesia of 2.5 hours or more.[123] In a prospective study of more than 180,000 patients undergoing major noncardiac surgery, Arozullah et al[121] reported that type of surgery, albumin and blood urea nitrogen levels, functional status, COPD, and age could be used to generate an index to identify patients at risk for postoperative respiratory failure. Solid data on the usefulness of respiratory physiotherapy, including incentive spirometry and noninvasive ventilation to *prevent* pulmonary complications, after cardiac or upper abdominal surgery are lacking.[147,148]

CARDIAC SURGERY

Cardiac surgery requires prolonged anesthesia and often hypothermia.[149,150] Patients also often require therapy for hypotension or hypertension, as well as fluid resuscitation (including blood transfusions).[149,150] Cardiac surgery can temporarily increase respiratory load.[151–153] At the end of coronary bypass surgery, lung compliance is less and lung resistance greater after chest closure than before surgery.[151] An increase in lung water after cardiopulmonary bypass, especially if the lungs remain collapsed during surgery, contributes to the worsening mechanics. In eight patients undergoing valvular surgery, compliances of the chest wall and lung were less at 4 hours after surgery that before surgery.[152] By 7 hours, chest-wall compliance was back to baseline, and lung compliance was higher than before surgery.[152] The investigators speculated that the initial decrease in lung compliance is caused by interstitial fluid secondary to increased vascular permeability.[152] The subsequent increase in lung compliance may result from mobilization of fluid that had accumulated before surgery (as a consequence of valvular disease) and as a result of extracorporeal circulation (increased permeability). Severe restrictive pulmonary defect is the rule,[154,155] and venous admixture (or sum of true shunt and $V_A/\dot{Q}$ mismatch) is increased.[155] At the end of surgery, many patients are transferred to the ICU while fully ventilated. Patients then are given the time to rewarm, to metabolize the medications received during anesthesia, and to receive therapy for any hemodynamic derangements that are present.

From the 1960s to 1990s, prolonged controlled mechanical ventilation was the standard of care following cardiac surgery.[156–158] This strategy was justified by the use of high-dose narcotic anesthesia and concerns about myocardial ischemia in the early postoperative period.[158–160] Since the early 1990s, under pressure of cost containment and improved resource utilization,[161] early extubation strategies have been implemented successfully in uncomplicated cardiac surgery cases.[149,150,162] Early extubation is achieved by modifying intraoperative anesthetic techniques (e.g., usually a decrease in total opioid administration, use of ultra-short-acting opiates, and use of inhaled techniques[150,163,164]), minimizing sedation during the postoperative ICU stay,[150] and improving postoperative pain

control.[165] Recovery to spontaneous respiration and extubation is shorter with rapid tracheal extubation strategies than with conventional strategies—median time of about 4 and 7 hours, respectively.[149,150] About 20–30% of patients, however, do not tolerate (or are not candidates for) rapid tracheal extubation strategies because of postoperative complications (e.g., bleeding, myocardial ischemia, myocardial infarction, refractory hypoxemia, or neurologic complications).[149,150] Early extubation may improve cardiac output[166] and renal perfusion[159,167] and reduce cardiopulmonary morbidity[168] and decrease hospital stay without adverse outcome.[162,163]

In addition to early extubation (extubation achieved in less than 6 hours after surgery[162]), immediate extubation in the operating room has been reported after coronary bypass grafting with or without valve replacement,[158,164,169,170] single-lung transplantation,[171] and two-stage esophagectomy.[172] Recently, coronary bypass grafting with high thoracic epidural anesthesia in the awake and spontaneously breathing patient has been achieved successfully.[173–175] This latter strategy remains highly controversial.[176]

SHOCK

DEFINITION AND CLASSIFICATION

Shock can be defined as a "state in which a profound and widespread reduction of effective tissue perfusion leads to reversible, and, if prolonged, irreversible cellular injury."[177] Based on hemodynamic profile, shock is classified into four categories: cardiogenic, hypovolemic, extracardiac obstructive, and distributive[177] (Fig. 5-16).

PHYSIOLOGIC EFFECTS OF SHOCK

All forms of shock exhibit common cellular metabolic processes that typically lead to cell injury, organ failure, and eventually, death.[177,178] These processes are caused by multiple interrelated factors, including cellular ischemia, circulating or local inflammatory mediators, and free-radical injury.[177,178]

Respiratory Responses

Shock elicits at least three respiratory responses: increase in dead-space ventilation, respiratory muscle dysfunction, and pulmonary inflammation. The increase in dead-space ventilation is an early accompaniment of shock.[179–181] It results from a fall in pulmonary perfusion.[177]* V_E increases to achieve normocapnia.[181,182] V_E also may further increase through other mechanisms. First, baroreflex deactivation (secondary to hypotension) amplifies the ventilatory response to stimulation of the peripheral chemoreceptors.[183] Second, direct stimulation of the aortic chemoreceptors occurs as a result of decreased O_2 delivery.[72] (This point, though clearly

---

*Terminology of dead space is confusing. *Anatomic dead space* is made up of the conducting airways (nose, mouth, pharynx, larynx, trachea, bronchi, and bronchioles). *Alveolar dead space* is made up of alveoli that receive some or no blood flow, which does not match ventilation (units with very high $V_A/\dot{Q}$ ratio). *Physiologic dead space* is the sum of anatomic dead space and alveolar dead space.

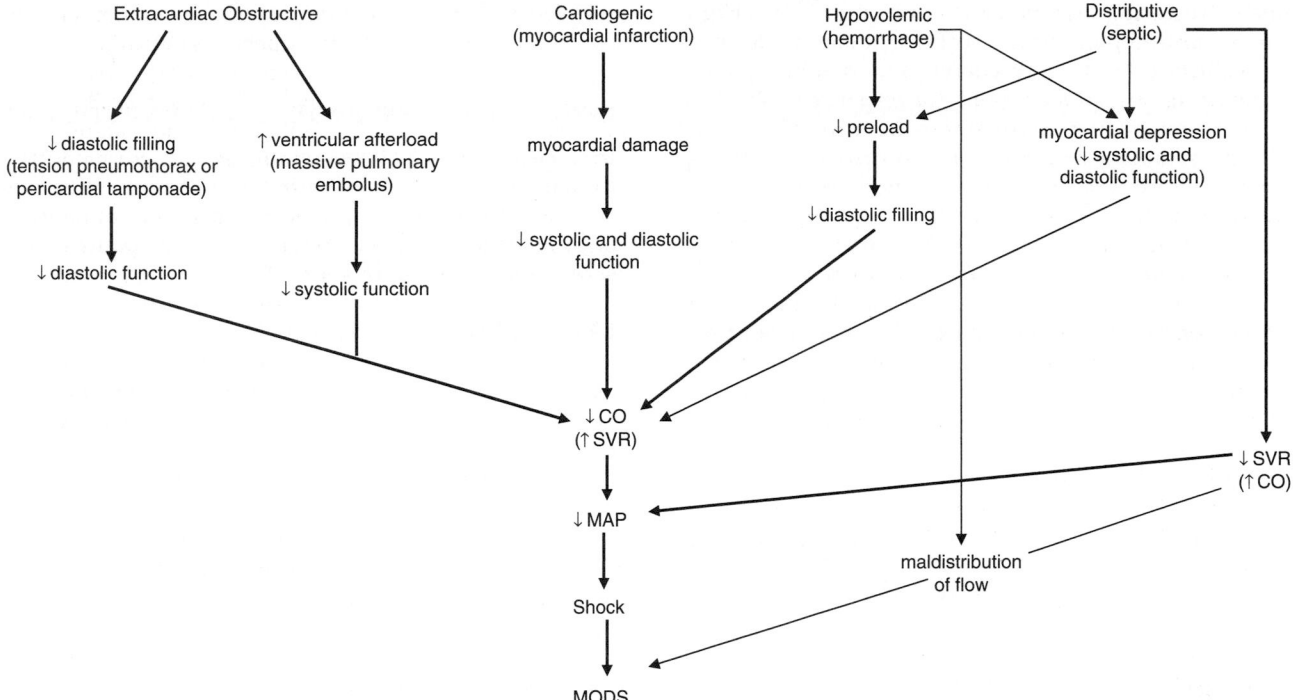

FIGURE 5-16 The hemodynamic profiles of four categories of shock. With extracardiac obstructive, cardiogenic, and hypovolemic shock, hypotension is caused primarily by a decrease in cardiac output (CO), and systemic vascular resistance (SVR) increases secondarily. With distributive shock, hypotension is caused primarily by a decrease in systemic vascular resistance with a secondary increase in cardiac output. In 10% or fewer of patients with distributive shock, cardiac output is decreased. The dominant pathologic pathways are indicated by heavier lines. MAP, mean arterial pressure; MODS, multiple organ dysfunction syndrome. (*Used, with permission, from Kumar et al: In: Parrillo et al, editors. Critical care medicine: Principles of diagnosis and management in the adult. St. Louis: Mosby, 372–420, 2001.*)

demonstrated in the cat,[72] remains controversial in humans.[71]) Third, cerebral hypoperfusion causes intracellular hypercapnia and acidosis[68] and, in turn, induces further hyperventilation unless the neurons are depressed (e.g., by hypoxia, lack of substrates, or excessive accumulation of metabolic products).[68] Fourth, increased respiratory drive occurs as a result of peripheral stimulation of pulmonary J receptors.[177] Fifth, increased respiratory drive results from vestibular activation during orthostasis (vestibulorespiratory reflex).[184] Sixth, V_E increases to compensate for lactic acidosis[185] resulting in part from the overworked and underperfused respiratory muscles.[181,186,187] The increase in V_E accompanying these responses may enhance venous return (through the respiratory pump) and vasoconstriction (through reduced Pa_{CO_2}), helping the cardiovascular system to cope with hypovolemia.[188]

Respiratory muscle dysfunction is one result of the associated cellular dysfunction and injury.[134,189] Many mechanisms contribute to this dysfunction in septic shock, including failure of neuromuscular transmission (because of elevated of muscle membrane potential and failure of excitation-contraction coupling[190–193]), the cytotoxic effect of nitric oxide and its metabolites,[189,194,195] free radicals,[196–198] ubiquitin-proteasome proteolysis,[193,199–202] and possibly, a decrease in nicotinic acetylcholine receptors.[203] Local dysregulation of the circulation and of the Krebs cycle also may contribute.[193] Many pathways purported to be responsible

for respiratory muscle dysfunction in sepsis are also activated in cardiogenic and hemorrhagic shock.[204–209]

Laboratory animals with cardiogenic[210] and septic shock[193,211] die of respiratory failure. Death is not caused by pulmonary disease per se but by an inability of the respiratory muscles to maintain adequate ventilation. In dogs with cardiogenic shock, institution of mechanical ventilation decreases the metabolic needs and thus the blood flow to the respiratory muscles (from 21–3% of the total cardiac output).[212] A nonrandomized study by Kontoyannis et al[213] in 28 patients with cardiogenic shock provides support for the view that hemodynamic instability is an indication for mechanical ventilation. Compared with nonventilated patients, ventilated patients were weaned from an intra-aortic balloon pump more often, and their survival was greater.[213]

The failure to reverse shock and treat the underlying cause promptly predisposes to ARDS (see Chapter 29). ARDS causes hypoxemia because of $V_A/\dot{Q}$ mismatch and shunt. Pulmonary vascular resistance increases during shock, including septic shock (in which peripheral vascular resistance is usually decreased).[214]

Cardiovascular Responses
Hypovolemic, distributive and extracardiac obstructive shock result in decreased diastolic filling. Low-pressure stretch receptors located in right atrium and pulmonary artery consequently signal the medullary vasomotor

centers, triggering sympathetic discharge.[177,215] High-pressure baroreceptors in the aortic arch contribute (negative feedback to the tonic discharge of the medullary vasoconstrictor centers) to the vasomotor response of shock as long as the mean arterial pressure is no lower than 80–90 mmHg.[216] When mean pressure is less than 80–90 mmHg, the aortic baroreceptor response is eliminated (baroreceptor deactivation).[177,216] Likewise, the carotid baroreceptors contribute (negative feedback) to the vasomotor response as long as the mean pressure is no lower than 60 mmHg.[216] When mean pressure is less than 60 mmHg, the carotid baroreceptor response is eliminated.[216] When mean pressure is less than 50–60 mm Hg, the peripheral chemoreceptors (sensitive to Pa_{O_2}, Pa_{CO_2}, and pH) dominate.[177] The most powerful stimulus to sympathetic tone during severe shock, however, is the ischemic response of the CNS.[216] When mean pressure falls below 50–60 mmHg, the medullary chemoreceptors become active.[216] Maximal sympathetic stimulation is induced by these receptors when mean pressure is 15–20 mmHg, resulting in maximal cardiovascular stimulation.[216] The Cushing response to increased intracranial pressure is an example of this reflex operating in a different setting.[177] Increased sympathetic outflow from the CNS is aimed at supporting O_2 delivery to vital organs. Other compensatory responses include releases of adrenocorticotropic hormone, antidiuretic hormone, and aldosterone, which contribute to sodium retention and maintenance of cardiovascular catecholamine responsiveness.[177,178,217]

CLINICAL PRESENTATION OF SHOCK

Cardiopulmonary Manifestations

Patients in shock or in the process of developing it may report dyspnea. Patients are usually tachypneic and tachycardic; they have primary respiratory alkalosis or a metabolic acidosis with some degree of respiratory compensation. Tachypnea, combined with low tidal volume, worsens dead-space ventilation. The skin of patients in septic shock is initially warm and dry. It is typically cold and clammy when cardiac output is low (see Fig. 5-16). Shock is usually not an all-or-none phenomenon that occurs abruptly after injury or infection. Instead, homeostatic compensatory mechanisms are engaged.[177,178] Early in the course, subtle signs of hemodynamic stress include tachycardia and decreased urine output. During early shock, assessment based on vital signs, central venous pressure, and urinary output may fail to detect global tissue hypoxia.[218] If the precipitating insult is too great or progresses quickly, compensatory mechanisms fail, and overt shock follows.[177]

Neurologic Manifestations

Compensatory mechanisms tend to protect the CNS from the ill effects of decreased cerebral perfusion. In the absence of cerebrovascular compromise, ischemic injury is unusual if mean arterial pressure is 50–60 mmHg or higher.[177] Before ischemic injury, consciousness may become altered, depending on perfusion deficit. Contributory factors include electrolyte disturbances, hypoxemia, and hypercapnia.[177] Sepsis-related encephalopathy can occur at higher arterial pressures (secondary to inflammatory mediators); it is as-

sociated with increased mortality.[219] Altered consciousness by itself may be an indication for intubation.

INTUBATION VERSUS MECHANICAL VENTILATION

In some instances, patients require endotracheal intubation to maintain airway patency because of upper airway obstruction, an inability to protect the airway from aspiration, or to manage secretions. Not all intubated patients necessarily require ventilator support.

UPPER AIRWAY OBSTRUCTION

Upper airway obstruction is one of the most urgent and potentially lethal medical emergencies. Complete airway obstruction lasting for as little as 4–6 minutes can cause irreversible brain damage.[220] The upper airway, which encompasses the passage between the nares and carina,[221] can be obstructed for functional or anatomic reasons. Among the first are vocal cord paralysis and laryngospasm.[221–223] Among the second are trauma, burn, infections, foreign bodies, and tumors.[220,221] Functional and anatomic obstruction can occur postoperatively in patients with redundant pharyngeal soft tissue (sleep apnea) and loss of muscle tone related to postanesthetic state.[221–223]

The first warning of airway obstruction in an unconscious patient may be failure of a jaw-thrust maneuver to open the airway or an inability to ventilate with a bag valve.[220] In a conscious patient, respiratory distress, stridor, altered voice (aphonia or dysphonia), snoring, dysphagia, odynophagia, prominence of neck veins, and neck and facial swelling all may indicate impending airway obstruction.[220,221] Patients may bring their hands to their neck, a sign of choking.[221] Other signs include suprasternal and intercostal indrawing and reduced or absent air movement on auscultation. Wheezing may be present (or absent). Thoracoabdominal paradox may be prominent. Sympathetic discharge is high. Patients are diaphoretic, tachycardic, and hypertensive. As asphyxia progresses, bradycardia, hypotension, and death ensue.[221]

Upper airway obstruction can be complicated by pulmonary edema[221,222]—incidence of 11% in one adult series[224]—or pulmonary hemorrhage.[223] Increased venous return (more negative intrathoracic pressure and catecholamine-induced venoconstriction) contributes to pulmonary edema, but it cannot be the sole mechanism[225]; as intrathoracic pressure becomes more negative, venous return to the right ventricle becomes flow-limited.[226] Other factors contributing to pulmonary edema include decreased left-ventricular preload (leftward shift of interventricular septum), increased left-ventricular afterload (increased negative intrathoracic pressure and catecholamine-induced elevation of systemic vascular resistance), pulmonary vasoconstriction (hypoxemia and acidosis), and possibly, stress failure of the alveolar-capillary membrane[223,227] (Fig. 5-17).

Whether pulmonary edema develops during (or after) relief of upper airway obstruction may depend on whether the obstruction is fixed or variable.[222] Fixed upper airway obstruction results in vigorous inspiratory efforts (Mueller maneuver) followed by vigorous expiratory efforts (Valsalva maneuver).[222,224] Exhalation against an obstructed airway

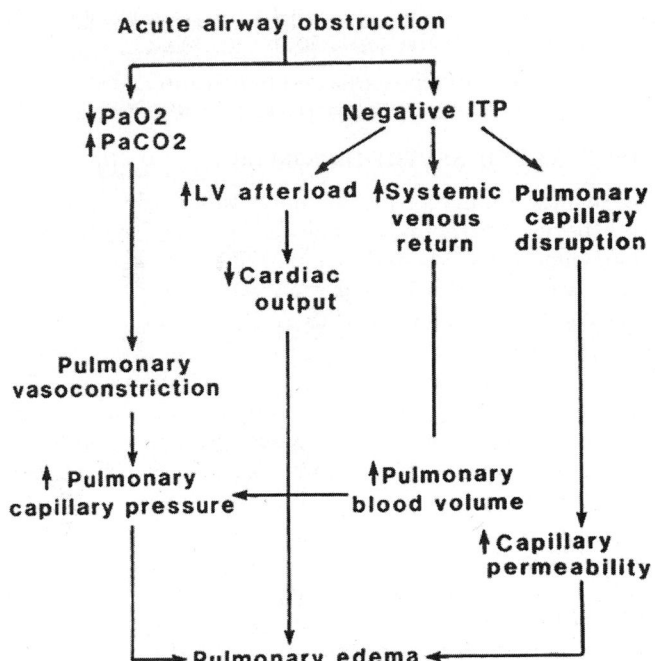

FIGURE 5-17 Mechanisms responsible for the development of pulmonary edema formation during acute airway obstruction. ITP, intrathoracic pressure; LV, left ventricle. (*Used, with permission, from Miro et al: In: Tobin, editor. Principles and practice of mechanical ventilation. New York: McGraw-Hill, 664, 1994.*)

raises intrathoracic and alveolar pressures. The positive expiratory pressure decreases pulmonary vascular filling and opposes the hydrostatic forces that favor transudation of fluid into the alveoli during inhalation.[224] With a sudden relief of obstruction, positive expiratory pressure is lost; consequently, there is a massive transudation of fluid from the pulmonary interstitium into the alveoli (pulmonary edema) over minutes to hours. In contrast to fixed obstruction, variable extrathoracic upper airway obstruction hinders inhalation. Exhalation usually is unaffected. In this situation, the hydrostatic forces, which favor transudation of fluid into the alveoli during inhalation, are unopposed, leading to edema before relief of the obstruction.[222]

Upper airway obstruction may worsen suddenly because resistance varies with the fourth power of the radius. A slight change in airway anatomy may increase resistive load dramatically.[221] For example, manipulation of the upper airway by an inexperienced clinician may induce edema, which can increase airway resistance markedly and induce asphyxia.

An initial assessment is undertaken to determine severity of airway compromise. If compromise is judged severe, the airway should be secured immediately. If ventilation is adequate, more detailed assessment is wise.[220] Arterial blood gases are not particularly helpful because they are not specific to airway patency.[220] They may show little change until a patient is in extremis.[220]

Steps to relieve airway obstruction include use of pharyngeal airways, endotracheal intubation, cricothyrotomy, tracheotomy, endoscopy, intubation over a fiberoptic bronchoscope, and medications (e.g., epinephrine, norepinephrine, antihistamines, steroids, and antibiotics).[221] In general, pharmacotherapy cannot reverse mechanical obstruction. Use of helium-O_2 mixtures should not engender a false sense of security.[221]

The nature of respiratory noises helps to localize lesions.[220] Stridor is an inspiratory sound typically caused by a lesion above the thoracic inlet (usually glottic or supraglottic). Wheezing is generated below this level.[220] Snoring, a feature of obstructive sleep apnea, can be life-threatening. A patient with an obstructed airway should not be sedated until the airway has been secured; minimal sedation may precipitate acute respiratory failure.

Cricothyrotomy and tracheotomy can be performed at the bedside or in the operating room. If time permits and the patient is conscious and moving sufficient air to speak, it may be best to transport the patient to the operating room.[220] Although percutaneous tracheotomy is gaining in popularity, it is best performed in an already intubated patient and not as an emergency procedure.[220]

INABILITY TO PROTECT THE AIRWAY FROM ASPIRATION

Patients with severe bulbar weakness or decreased consciousness may be unable to protect the airway against aspiration.[228,229] The lack of a gag reflex or cough on suctioning suggests impaired protective reflexes.[230] If the cervical spine is stable, the head should be flexed while checking for airway obstruction. Inability to maintain a patent airway is an indication for elective intubation.[230]

Patients who require an oral airway or special appliances may require prophylactic intubation; such patients are unstable and can asphyxiate or vomit and aspirate suddenly.[230] Ideally, patients with depressed consciousness should be assessed while asleep, a time during which they are at greatest risk of obstruction.[230]

Severe head injury is a condition requiring intubation for airway protection. In the past, controlled hyperventilation (Pa_{CO_2} of 25–35 mmHg) was delivered in these patients with the goal of reducing intracranial pressure. Such a strategy, however, has proven harmful[231] and is no longer recommended.[232] It is unknown whether the use of short periods of hyperventilation to suddenly lower intracranial pressure are harmful or not.[55]

SECRETIONS

Occasionally, endotracheal intubation or tracheostomy may be required to manage large amount of secretions or to remove secretions in severely debilitated patients who themselves cannot clear them.[55,140]

Many patients with the preceding conditions are capable of maintaining adequate gas exchange following endotracheal intubation. Yet most intensivists still connect such patients to a ventilator. This decision commonly is taken independently of any consideration about the work of breathing imposed by an endotracheal tube.[233]

Goals of Mechanical Ventilation

The fundamental goal of mechanical ventilation is to keep a patient alive and free from iatrogenic complications so that the catastrophic precipitating event(s) may resolve. Attention should be directed to the primary disorder.

REVERSAL OF APNEA

The goal of mechanical ventilation in the apneic patient is to restore ventilation.

REVERSAL OF RESPIRATORY DISTRESS

For obvious ethical reasons, no human studies have addressed the natural course of acute respiratory failure in the presence of increased work of breathing or, for that matter, with any other type of respiratory failure. Animal data indicate that increased loads can cause respiratory muscle damage,[234,235] CO_2 retention,[236] and as a terminal event respiratory muscle fatigue.[236] Increased load may be responsible for respiratory muscle damage in patients with COPD[237] and in patients dying while supported by mechanical ventilation.[238] In sepsis, increased respiratory efforts are particularly damaging to the respiratory muscles.[239]

Despite intense research, the role of contractile fatigue in the development of respiratory failure in patients is unknown.[134] Diaphragmatic contractility has been quantified objectively (phrenic nerve stimulation) in only one study where patients developed acute respiratory distress (during weaning from mechanical ventilation).[4] No change in diaphragmatic contractility was documented.[4] It is not known if the latter observation applies to patients in respiratory distress who have yet to undergo mechanical ventilation.

It seems self-evident that connecting a patient to a ventilator and providing ventilator assistance should unload the respiratory muscles and, possibly, reduce muscle stress. To date, however, we do not know the desirable level of unloading (and for how long) for a specific patient. Insufficient unloading can be dangerous to the respiratory muscles,[237,238,240] as can excessive unloading[241-246] (see Chapter 43).

Although most patients in acute respiratory failure have increased work of breathing, this may not be the sole problem. Most patients also have abnormal gas exchange, impaired muscle perfusion, and sepsis-induced muscle dysfunction.[5,247,248] In patients with increased work of breathing, unloading by the ventilator may appreciably reduce $\dot{V}_{O_2}$ and $\dot{V}_{CO_2}$.[7,51] These reductions, in turn, may improve concurrent hypoxemia and hypercapnia.

REVERSAL OF SEVERE HYPOXEMIA

Mechanical ventilation is commonly commenced with 100% O_2. The response helps to define the underlying pathophysiology and thus aids in differential diagnosis and therapy (see Figs. 5-8 and 5-11). For example, if 100% O_2 fails to increase Pa_{O_2} in a patient with an exacerbation of COPD, the underlying problem is not pure $V_A/\dot{Q}$ mismatch (as is typical with acute bronchitis); instead, the patient has coexisting shunt. Common causes of shunt include pneumonia, congestive heart failure, lobar atelectasis, and pulmonary embolism. (For a discussion of O_2 toxicity, see Chapter 45.)

SHUNT

Patients with increased shunt commonly exhibit considerable improvement in oxygenation with application of PEEP. The improvement results from a decrease in shunt[249] secondary to recruitment of previously atelectatic areas and redistribution of extravascular lung water from alveoli to peribronchial and perivascular spaces.[250] If cardiac output decreases (with PEEP), this can contribute to the decrease in shunt.[249,251]

PEEP causes an increase in dead space through several mechanisms. First, an increase in lung volume exerts radial traction on the airways, increasing their volume with a consequent increase in *anatomic dead space*. Second, increased airway pressure tends to divert blood flow from ventilated lung units by compressing capillaries. The consequent development of areas of high $V_A/\dot{Q}$ ratio (or even unperfused areas) produces an increase in *alveolar dead space*. Such dead space is especially common in the uppermost lung units, where pulmonary artery pressure is relatively low because of the hydrostatic effect.[252,253] If the capillary pressure falls below airway pressure, the capillaries may collapse completely and the lung units become unperfused[253] (Fig. 5-18). Two factors encourage collapse: very high airway pressure and low venous return.

Dantzker et al[249] showed that increasing levels of PEEP can induce two distinct patterns of $V_A/\dot{Q}$ distribution. Some patients experienced no change in the pattern of $V_A/\dot{Q}$ relationships (Fig. 5-19). Other patients experienced

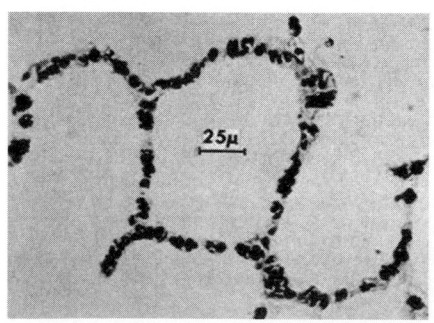
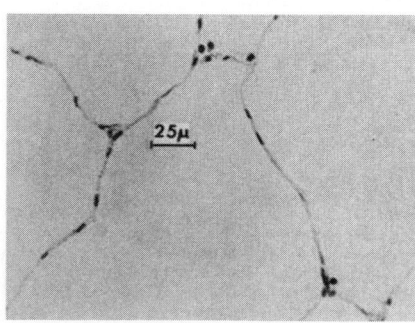

FIGURE 5-18 Effect of an elevated airway pressure on the structure of pulmonary capillaries. (*Left*) Normal appearance. (*Right*) An increase in alveolar pressure above capillary pressure produces capillary collapse. (*Used, with permission, from Glazier et al: J Appl Physiol 26:65–76, 1969.*)

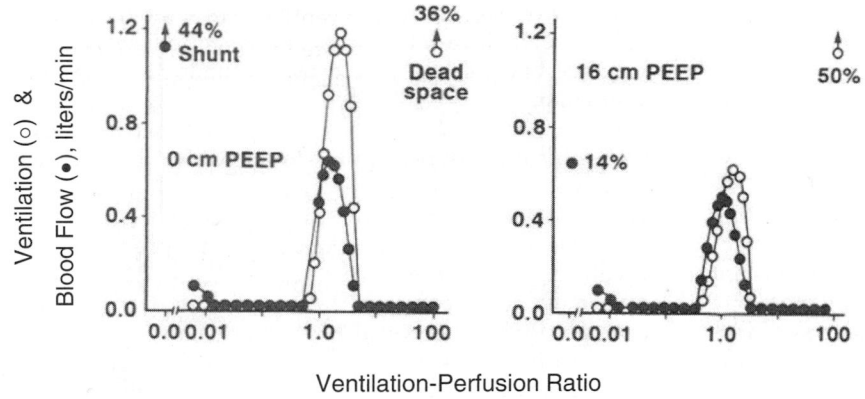

FIGURE 5-19 Effect of PEEP on shunt and dead space in a patient with ARDS. A progressive increase in PEEP from 0 to 16 cmH$_2$O caused a decrease in shunt from 44 to 14% of the cardiac output and an increase in dead space from 36 to 50% of the tidal volume. The shape of the distribution of ventilation and perfusion did not change. (*Used, with permission, from Dantzker et al: Am Rev Respir Dis 120:1039–52, 1979.*)

broadening of the ventilation dispersion—increases of areas with high V$_A$/Q̇ ratios and alveolar dead space (Fig. 5-20). The improvement in gas exchange with PEEP is even greater when pressors are used to prevent the expected decrease in cardiac output during PEEP.[254]

In some patients, PEEP causes no improvement or even a decrease in Pa$_{O_2}$. This effect is the result of increased dead-space ventilation, diversion of blood flow from well-ventilated to unventilated regions, and decreased cardiac output (especially if circulating blood volume is depleted).[252] Lack of improvement in oxygenation with PEEP also may result from a patent foramen ovale because PEEP can increases the right-to-left shunt.[255]

Because PEEP can decrease cardiac output,[249,256] its net effect should be judged in terms of O$_2$ delivery. Mixed venous P$_{O_2}$ has been used as a surrogate for O$_2$ delivery.[218,256] Other potential hazards of PEEP include reduced splachnic and renal blood flow, barotrauma, and ventilator-induced lung injury (see Chapter 11).

In addition to mechanical ventilation, patients with hypoxemic respiratory failure may require other therapies, such as antibiotics (pneumonia), diuretics, and inotropic support (heart failure). Ancillary strategies to reverse hypoxemia include exogenous surfactant,[257] nitric oxide supplementation,[258] prone position,[259,260] and anti-inflammatory agents.[261,262] These strategies can increase oxygenation in patients with ARDS, but none has improved patient outcome.

VENTILATION-PERFUSION INEQUALITY

Theoretically, patients with hypoxemia secondary to V$_A$/Q̇ mismatch can be managed by increasing F$_{IO_2}$ without mechanical ventilation (see Fig. 5-11). In reality, such patients always have increased ventilatory requirements (see Fig. 5-9), which may demand ventilator support. Many patients with V$_A$/Q̇ inequality requiring mechanical ventilation are hyperinflated (e.g., COPD or status asthmaticus). Hyperinflation decreases the efficiency of the respiratory muscles in generating pressure, which contributes to the respiratory distress.[134]

In a study of seven patients with exacerbations of COPD, mechanical ventilation improved V$_A$/Q̇ mismatch by redistributing blood flow away from low V$_A$/Q̇ areas.[263] Dispersion of the distribution of ventilation also improved. Dead space or ventilation of high V$_A$/Q̇ units did not change.[263] Patients with increased V$_A$/Q̇ mismatch associated with COPD or ARDS may benefit from careful application of PEEP (see Chapter 11). Use of PEEP in patients with status asthmaticus is fraught with danger (see Chapter 30).

REVERSAL OF SEVERE HYPERCAPNIA

Severe hypercapnia depresses the CNS and decreases respiratory motor output.[264] A viscous cycle can arise: Hypercapnia depresses drive leading to more hypercapnia.[265,266] Hypercapnia can decrease diaphragmatic contractility,[267,268]

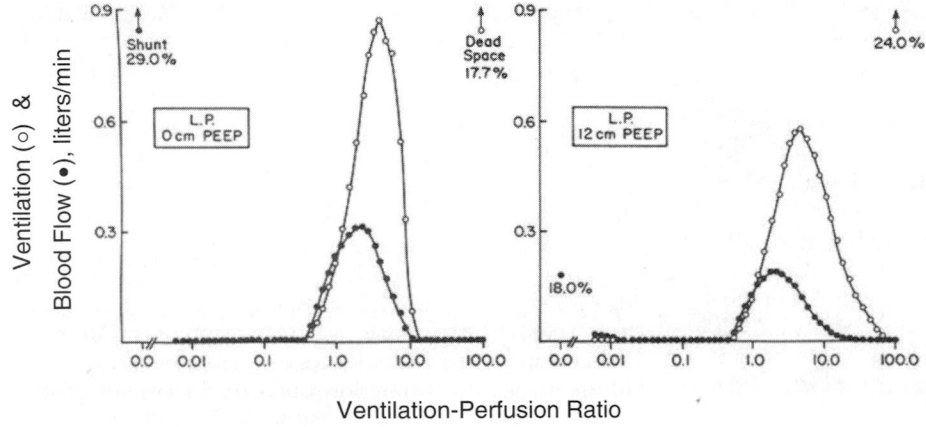

FIGURE 5-20 Effect of PEEP on shunt and dead space in a patient with ARDS. An increase in PEEP from 0 to 12 cmH$_2$O produced a decrease in shunt (from 29 to 18%) and increase in dead space (from 17.7 to 24.0%). Also apparent is a widening of the dispersion in ventilation with the development of units with very high V$_A$/Q̇; these may have resulted from diversion of blood flow or increased ventilation of these areas of the lung. (*Used, with permission, from Dantzker et al: Am Rev Respir Dis 120:1039–52, 1979.*)

although not consistently.[236,269] Acidosis may be more important than hypercapnia in depressing respiratory muscle contractility.[270,271]

The goal of mechanical ventilation in patients with hypercapnic respiratory failure is to improve V_A. Ventilator strategies need to be tailored to the specific setting. In hypercapnic patients with status asthmaticus or COPD, the prolonged respiratory time constant poses a significant challenge. If the ventilator is set to deliver small tidal volumes at high respiratory frequencies, the prolonged time constant may interfere with lung empting, and hyperinflation may ensue. Moreover, small tidal volumes may not achieve adequate alveolar ventilation because physiologic dead space is increased. Larger tidal volumes may achieve adequate alveolar ventilation but require longer expiratory times than do smaller tidal volumes. A common strategy to ensure sufficient time for exhalation is to increase inspiratory flow. The increase in flow decreases the time of mechanical inflation and, if respiratory rate remains constant, prolongs time available for exhalation. An increase in inspiratory flow, however, is commonly associated with an increase in respiratory rate.[272,273] Yet, despite the reduction in the respiratory cycle, the decrease in inspiratory time is accompanied by an increase in time available for exhalation—and a decrease in inspiratory effort.[273]

Neuromuscular disorders such as Guillain-Barré syndrome, myasthenia gravis, and spinal cord injury[134] can cause hypercapnic respiratory failure. These patients usually have normal lung mechanics, unlike patients with COPD or asthma. The normal time constant allows for greater flexibility in the setting of the ventilator.

Overzealous ventilation can cause serious complications, including life-threatening alkalosis, decreased cerebral perfusion, and cardiovascular instability. Patients previously hypercapnic are especially vulnerable to these complications. When severe, alkalosis is occasionally associated with coronary artery spasm,[274] confusion, myoclonus, asterixis, and seizures.[275]

Respiratory alkalosis reduces ionized calcium. For each 0.1-unit rise in pH, ionized calcium falls by 0.05 mmol/liter.[276] These changes are too modest and inconsistent[277] to account for the increased central and peripheral excitability associated with alkalosis. Paresthesias, carpal-pedal spasm, and tetany, seen in acute hyperventilation, are caused by the direct effects of respiratory alkalosis on neurons.[278] Other effects of alkalosis include increase in hemoglobin affinity for O_2 and, in the presence of increased shunt, a possible worsening of $V_A/\dot{Q}$ relationship (secondary to a decrease in hypoxic pulmonary vasoconstriction).[279] Precipitous decrease in Pa_{CO_2} reduces blood flow to the CNS,[280] which may contribute to confusion and loss of consciousness in patients with hyperventilation.[275]

The most common hemodynamic instability associated with overzealous ventilator management of the hypercapnic patient (prolonged time constant) is hypotension. Hypotension often results from an increase in intrinsic PEEP after intubation—although a decrease in sympathetic tone caused by the decrease in Pa_{CO_2} and administration of seda-

tion may be contributory factors. In this setting, the circulation usually is restored promptly by stopping ventilation for 30 seconds (or more) and then resuming less vigorous ventilation.

In the 1940s and 1950s it was reported that rapid CO_2 washout after hypercapnia could cause hypotension (removal of cyclopropane anesthesia in humans)[281,282] and life-threatening ventricular arrhythmias (dog experiments).[283,284] Hyperkalemia appeared to be involved.[283,284] More recent series in patients, however, have not substantiated the earlier studies.[103,285] For example, Prys-Roberts et al[103,285] reported no electrocardiographic alterations when Pa_{CO_2} was reduced from about 80 to less than 20 mmHg over 5 minutes in anesthetized patients. Some practitioners suggest that supraventricular and ventricular arrhythmias associated with alkalemia[286] may occur only in patients with ischemic heart disease.[287] Whether reductions in ionized magnesium could contribute to cardiac irritability remains unclear.[277]

Excessive ventilation, over time, causes bicarbonate wasting by the kidney. In patients who retain CO_2 when clinically stable, this renal wasting (of bicarbonate) will increase ventilatory demands during weaning.

GOALS OF MECHANICAL VENTILATION IN POSTORERATIVE RESPIRATORY FAILURE AND TAUMA

Patients developing postoperative hypoxemia usually are treated with supplemental O_2 and chest physical therapy (including incentive spirometry).[128,155,288–290] In about 10% of patients undergoing major elective abdominal surgery, however, supplemental O_2 and chest physical therapy do not prevent respiratory failure.[291] Squadrone et al[291] recently undertook a randomized study in more than 200 patients who had undergone major elective abdominal surgery and who developed hypoxemia within 1 hour of the operation. They compared the incidence of intubation in patients receiving standard treatment (50% O_2 and chest physical therapy) and patients who also received 7.5 cmH$_2$O CPAP (delivered noninvasively with a helmet). Compared with the control group, patients receiving CPAP had lower rates of intubation (1% versus 10%) and complications (e.g., pneumonia, infection, and sepsis). The CPAP group spent fewer days in the ICU. Exclusion criteria included history of COPD, asthma, sleep apnea, heart failure, hypercapnia, and respiratory acidosis. Thus these results[291] may not apply to patients at greatest risk of postoperative atelectasis.

Bonde et al[145] undertook a prospective, randomized study in 102 patients undergoing elective lung surgery who were considered at high risk for retention of secretions.[140] Minitracheotomy (4-mm percutaneous cricothyroidotomy device) was performed at the conclusion of surgery in one group. Sputum retention was 30% in a conventionally treated group and 2% in the minitracheotomy group ($p < 0.005$).[145] Atelectasis was less common in the minitracheostomy group. Incidences of pneumonia, respiratory failure, myocardial infarction, and death were not affected by minitracheotomy.[145] Significant complications of minitracheostomy have been reported, however.[292,293] Therefore, its routine use, even in patients at risk of secretion retention, needs to be considered on a case-by-case basis.

Some patients with multiple trauma present with a flail chest. Many such patients may have respiratory failure secondary to underlying lung damage or other pathophysiology and may require mechanical ventilation. Flail chest on its own, however, is not an indication for mechanical ventilation.[294] In one randomized study of patients with flail chest who were hypoxemic and in respiratory distress, noninvasive CPAP decreased mortality and nosocomial infection as compared with patients who underwent endotracheal intubation and ventilation.[295]

GOALS OF MECHANICAL VENTILATION IN SHOCK

In hemodynamically unstable patients, tissue perfusion, including that of the CNS, is compromised.[178,218] Two main goals are to establish an adequate airway and reduce $\dot{V}_{O_2}$.[177] By resting the respiratory muscles and allowing for sedation, mechanical ventilation can reduce $\dot{V}_{O_2}$[7,296,297] and decrease sympathetic tone.[51] These effects may improve tissue perfusion,[212,298] which may explain why ventilator support improves outcome in animals[210] and patients in shock.[213] It is important to achieve good patient-ventilator synchronization[299,300]; otherwise, work of breathing increases, which diverts blood to the respiratory muscles and away from other vulnerable tissue beds.

Delivery of Mechanical Ventilation: Invasive versus Noninvasive Mechanical Ventilation

Solid experimental data support the use of noninvasive ventilation in patients with acute respiratory failure caused by severe exacerbations of COPD (limited to patients deemed not to require immediate intubation).[301–305] Noninvasive ventilation is probably superior to invasive ventilation in patients with cardiogenic pulmonary edema complicated with hypercapnia[306] and in immunocompromised patients with early hypoxemic respiratory failure.[307,308] The role of noninvasive ventilation in difficult-to-wean patients is discussed in Chapter 58.

Sinuff et al[309] studied the use of a practice guideline for noninvasive ventilation in patients admitted to hospital for an exacerbation of COPD or congestive heart failure. The developers of the guideline pointed out that data from randomized trials do not support use of noninvasive ventilation in other disease states. Before introduction of the guideline, 65% of patients with diseases other than COPD or cardiogenic pulmonary edema were managed without endotracheal intubation. After introduction of the guideline, 100% of these patients were intubated; mortality also tended to

increase (from 20.5 to 34.3%). This study raises the possibility that introduction of a practice guideline may cause an increase in morbidity and mortality.[309,310] A practice guideline could discourage physicians from the use of noninvasive ventilation in subgroups of patients who are likely to benefit from its use simply because benefit has not yet been demonstrated in a randomized trial and thus has not been incorporated into the practice guideline. In an accompanying editorial, Hill[310] commented: "The concern is that by classifying a sizable category of patients as 'not meeting noninvasive positive pressure ventilation criteria,' the authors could have unintentionally encouraged endotracheal intubation in this subgroup, possibly contributing to morbidity and mortality."

Detailed discussion of noninvasive ventilation is provided in Chapter 19, as well as in Chapters 9 and 31–34.

Indications for Mechanical Ventilation and Nosology

INDICATIONS: TRUE VERUS STATED

In publications on mechanical ventilation, listed indications commonly include acute respiratory failure, exacerbation of chronic respiratory failure (secondary to infection, bronchoconstriction, heart failure), coma, and neuromuscular disease. Many patients, however, have these same conditions but do not require ventilator assistance. Take COPD, one of the most common indications for mechanical ventilation. At any point in time, much, much less than 1% of patients with COPD are receiving mechanical ventilation. This small subset is commonly identified as those with acute respiratory failure. But the definition of acute respiratory failure is vague and the criteria loose. The usual defining criterion is a Pa_{O_2} of less than 60 mmHg (sometimes combined with a Pa_{CO_2} of greater than 50 mmHg). It is patently absurd to suggest, however, that all patients with a Pa_{O_2} of 59 mmHg (or lower) need ventilator assistance and that all patients with a Pa_{O_2} of 61 mmHg (or higher) can be managed without it.

As such, the usually stated indications for mechanical ventilation are elastic, lacking meaningful boundaries. What, then, is the real reason to institute it? We believe that the most honest description of a physician's judgment at this juncture is "The patient looks like he (or she) needs to be placed on the ventilator." That is, a physician institutes mechanical ventilation based on his or her gestalt of disease severity as opposed to slotting a patient into a particular diagnostic pigeonhole.

At first blush, this admission makes the undertaking of mechanical ventilation appear less scientific than other areas of medicine. Students of medicine are taught to make a diagnosis before initiating treatment. The usual teaching is that an accurate diagnosis will make the appropriate treatment relatively obvious. But this medical model is plausible only for diseases where the precise etiology is known (such as a microbial agent). The medical model is also more ideal than real. To understand the limitations of this model—and the apparent lack of science concerning ventilator indications—the reader needs to grapple with nosology, the discipline that names and classifies diseases.* Just as Moliere's "Bourgeois Gentilhomme" was delighted to learn that he had been speaking prose all his life without knowing it, we were astonished to discover (while writing this chapter) that we have been thinking nosologically every day unawares.

NOSOLOGY

The first attempt to introduce a systematic and consistent nomenclature for diagnostic terms was made in the mid-nineteenth century.[311] Diseases were no longer viewed in terms of a Galenic humoral disequilibrium. Instead, they were regarded as discrete entities—real things. This ontologic model grew out of the increasing use of autopsy, which was seen to uncover the true reasons for the corporeal changes induced by disease.[312] Ideally, each disease category would be identified through elicitation of pathognomonic signs on physical examination and the finding of a defining lesion on autopsy. This thinking is conveyed in the quip circulated by nineteenth-century physicians: If you were suffering from some mysterious illness, the best thing to do was go to Vienna (then the Mecca of medical science)[313] and be diagnosed by Skoda and autopsied by Rokitansky.

DISEASE DEFINITION AND CHARACTERISTICS

How is disease defined? A *disease* is "the sum of abnormal phenomena displayed by a group of patients in association with a specified common characteristic (or set of characteristics) by which these patients differ from the norm (of healthy people) in such a way as to place them at a biological disadvantage."[314]

There are four main classes of characteristics by which diseases can be defined:

1. *Syndrome.* Historically, diseases are defined initially by way of a description of symptoms and signs; when these constitute a recognizable pattern, they are referred to as a *syndrome* (e.g., ARDS).
2. *Disorders of structure (morbid anatomy).* When a specifiable disorder is found to be associated constantly with a morbid-anatomic change, it tends to be named in these terms (e.g., the switch from jaundice to hepatitis).
3. *Disorders of function (pathophysiology).* When a disorder is found to be associated constantly with a specific abnormality of function, the abnormality may be used to name the disorder (e.g., hypothyroidism).

---

*The late Guy Scadding has written more lucidly on nosology than most; he made explicit the factual implications of medical usage of disease names. This account borrows extensively from his writings.

4. *Causation (etiology).* When the cause of a disease is discovered, the disease generally is redefined in causal terms (Legionnaire's disease). Scadding[314] refers to another category, "clinical entity," that always needs an ad hoc explanation; he says, "It often seems to be the refuge of one who has not succeeded in clarifying his or her thoughts, but is nevertheless determined to put them into words."

In general, the direction of scientific advance follows the preceding sequence, although many conditions are never described in etiologic terms. The primary purpose of applying a name to a disorder is to provide a brief statement of the medical understanding of its nature (from syndrome to etiologic mechanism) and to serve as a verbal device for ease of communication. The American-European consensus definition of ARDS,[315] for example, has served as the basis of patient recruitment for most of the recent trials of mechanical ventilation in ARDS. Yet, as discussed in detail by Marini (see Chapter 29), this definition lacks scientific rigor. Nevertheless, in everyday practice, the term *ARDS* helps a clinician to predict prognosis and prescribe treatment. Moreover, in emergency settings (such as the ICU), problems are discussed and major decisions often are made without making any explicit diagnosis. Indeed, this is the rule rather than the exception when instituting mechanical ventilation. An experienced critical-care physician can identify a patient who will die if left untreated but who might live if managed by mechanical ventilation—even though the physician is unable to identify the etiology of that patient's illness. Nevertheless, in such situations where physicians cannot put forward a defensible diagnosis, they still apply descriptors (at Scadding's level of "clinical entity"), such as "the patient is tiring out," to justify their judgment that mechanical ventilation is indicated.

DEFINITIONS: ESSENTIALIST AND NOMINALIST

What are the factual implications of the naming of a disease? Diseases are defined in essentialist or nominalist terms. An *essentialist definition* tries to describe the true essence of an entity: the essential quality (invariable and fixed properties) that makes a given entity the type of thing it is—the "whatness" of an entity. (The study of the essence of things is called *ontology*.[316]) Essentialist ideas about diseases are implicit in everyday speech.[317] For example, a patient presents with a cough and mucoid sputum. The doctor makes a diagnosis of chronic bronchitis. The patient then thinks that chronic bronchitis is causing his or her cough. Given that chronic bronchitis is defined as a productive cough, the patient's reasoning is circular.

Such usage lays a linguistic trap: Many laypeople and some doctors think that the names of diseases refer to active agents that cause the illness. To talk of diseases as if they existed as real entities is plausible (at first sight) only in relation to diseases that are defined in etiologic terms.[318] Even then we must not confuse an etiologic agent with the disease itself. The disease is the effect on the affected person;

diseases have no existence apart from patients. We treat patients, not diseases. When we speak of treatment of a disease, we are employing an ellipsis for treatment of patients with that disease.[314] All this brings to mind Osler's admonition: "It is much more important to know what sort of patient has the disease than to know what sort of disease the patient has."[312]

A *nominalist definition* recognizes that the task of revealing the essence of the *definiendum* is impossible.[319,320] Instead, it simply uses words to state the set of characteristics that are used to identify a member of a class (make a diagnosis). Such a definition makes it possible to determine whether a particular example (clinical picture) falls into a category to which a name (a disease) is applied.[321] A nominalist definition avoids the essentialist fallacy of regarding diseases as causes of illness; instead, it is simply naming a class of entities or events.

The nominalist-essentialist distinction becomes clearer if we consider the definition of acute respiratory failure. Karl Popper, who condemned essentialist definitions, observed that a good definition in science should be read from right to left, not left to right.[322] Take the sentence, "Acute respiratory failure is the presence of a Pa_{O_2} of less than 60 mmHg, with or without a Pa_{CO_2} of greater than 50 mmHg, together with physical findings indicative of increased work of breathing." Reading from right to left, the sentence provides a "nominalist" answer to the clinician's question, "What shall we call the presence of a Pa_{O_2} of less than 60 mmHg, with or without a Pa_{CO_2} of greater than 50 mmHg, together with physical findings indicative of increased work of breathing?" rather than providing an "essentialist" answer to the question, "What is acute respiratory failure?" That is, the term *acute respiratory failure* is handy shorthand for the longer, more cumbersome description. Nothing more. The term *acute respiratory failure* contains no information about medicine, and nothing is to be gained from analyzing it.

DIAGNOSTIC PROCESS, TREATMENT, AND VALUE JUDGMENT

The process of making a diagnosis goes through two broad steps. First, the physician undertakes an initial review of the clinical features, looking for a pattern that suggests one or more disease. For example, a clinician notes eyelid retraction, tracheal tug, sternomastoid contraction, tachypnea, and monosyllabic speech. He or she concludes that the patient is in acute respiratory distress (an "entity" rather than a disease). Second, the physician undertakes a directed search for the defining characteristics (pathognomonic findings) of each of a number of suspected diseases.[323] Let us consider a patient who exhibits all the above-listed features of acute respiratory distress. On learning that the patient had been extubated a half hour previously, the physician suspects laryngeal edema and carefully listens for stridor. In a second patient, a physician's initial assessment again may reveal the general features of acute respiratory distress. On learning that this patient also has fever, chills, and rust-colored sputum, the physician suspects pneumonic consolidation. He

or she then undertakes careful palpation (for tactile vocal fremitus), percussion (for dullness), and auscultation (for whispering pectoriloquy, egophony, and bronchial breathing).

The clinical diagnostic criteria are the descriptive features that best discriminate between one disease and other diseases with which it might be confused. In the best-case scenario, the clinical diagnostic criteria are made up largely of defining characteristics. None of the features is conclusive, but together they produce a degree of probability that justifies a diagnosis on which practical management may be based.[321] It is possible to state defining characteristics in objective, demonstrable terms when a disease is defined etiologically or as a disorder of structure or function.[314] The same is also possible for a disease defined syndromically if the description of the syndrome includes objectively demonstrable elements. For example, as entry criteria for a research study, respiratory distress might be defined (arbitrarily) as meeting three of the following four elements; respiratory rate greater than 33 breaths per minute, Pa_{O_2}/F_{IO_2} ratio of less than 300, phasic sternomastoid contraction, and nasal flaring. That is, in the context of this study, respiratory distress can be defined without making subjective value judgments.

When making decisions about the treatment of an individual patient, however, it is not possible to avoid subjective value judgments (things being assessed on a scale of goodness or badness). Ultimately, the decision of whether to institute mechanical ventilation (or not) boils down to a value judgment by the patient's physician. In some instances this decision will be preceded by a physician's making of a diagnosis. In many cases, however, physicians institute mechanical ventilation without having formulated a precise diagnosis. Along the same lines, Gross[324] has argued that it is unlikely that management of asthma would be improved were it possible to articulate a more widely accepted definition of this disease.

FACTUAL IMPLICATIONS OF DISEASE TERMINOLOGY

Nosology is rarely discussed at medical conferences.[311] Questions on terminology are regarded as recondite and pedantic, eliciting yawns from the audience. When a speaker is asked to define the clinical entity about which he or she is speaking, he or she may appear puzzled—feeling that everyone surely knows what the term means. The audience becomes restless, seeing the question as a philosophical diversion that distracts from the hard scientific facts that the speaker is trying to discuss. Yet it makes little sense for a speaker to present detailed data analysis on a condition that he or she cannot define. Likewise, readers should treat with a jaundiced eye statistics in surveys that list precise diagnoses for which mechanical ventilation was used. The ghost of such unrealistic (and unattainable) precision also hovers over lists of reasons for why patients were intubated in reports on controlled trials of noninvasive ventilation versus conventional therapy.

The application of precise mathematical methods to vague and ill-defined concepts gives them a false air of respectability that cloaks ignorance and perpetuates confusion.[318] It is unfortunate that the more fundamental the concept to which a word refers, the less careful we tend to be about the use of a clear definition.[325]

Contraindications to Mechanical Ventilation

Complications associated with mechanical ventilation can be lethal (see Chapters 41, 44, 46, and 47). Thus mechanical ventilation should be used only when it is clearly needed. Intubation is not the first approach for most patients with an exacerbation of COPD; instead, noninvasive ventilation is the first choice. The same sequence probably holds for selected patients with congestive heart failure or immunocompromise. Mechanical ventilation should not be instituted when a mentally competent patient or a surrogate designated to make decisions on behalf of a noncompetent patient refuses it. If time permits, the patient and family should be instructed about the likely impact of mechanical ventilation on prognosis. For instance, hospital mortality of patients with idiopathic pulmonary fibrosis requiring mechanical ventilation is 68%[326] to 100%,[327] and 92% of the survivors are dead within 2 months of hospital discharge.[326]

Conclusion

When we started to write this chapter, we expected to end it by formulating a set of concrete recommendations as to when mechanical ventilation should be instituted. Readers willingly wade their way through complex pathophysiologic concepts if they believe the material enhances their understanding of a clinical topic. At the end, however, they expect to see the complexity reduced to a set of concrete recommendations, preferably conveyed as a list of entities with numerical values attached. That final step is not possible with this chapter. More than is the case for any other chapter in this book, it is not possible to articulate the indications for mechanical ventilation in the form of a list of items.

Thus, if it is not possible to formulate a list, then what? When you, dear reader, are in severe respiratory distress and a physician is standing at your bedside deciding whether or not to ventilate (and possibly intubate) you, what type of physician are you hoping will make this decision? We can speak only for ourselves. The physician we want is a person deeply versed in pathophysiologic concepts, skilled in the art of physical examination, with extensive experience of cases similar to our own illness, and blessed with good clinical judgment. We expect that physician to base the decision (on which our life depends) on his or her clinical gestalt. And we recognize that the physician may not be able to articulate the precise reasons behind this decision in the form of words.

Why can't our ideal physician express these thoughts in explicit terms? A wise physician standing at a patient's bedside senses a great deal of worthwhile information—much more than can be expressed in words. In short, there is a very large tacit coefficient to clinical knowledge—physicians *know* much more than they can communicate verbally.[328] There is an enormous difference between the assessment made by an experienced physician standing at a bedside and the assessment the same physician makes on hearing information (about the same patient) relayed over the telephone by a junior resident. An experienced and wise physician employs intuition rather than explicit rules in deciding what is best for a particular patient in a particular setting. A physician who regards such intuition as unscientific betrays a fundamental misunderstanding of the epistemology of science.[320]

Our failure to formulate a list of indications does not mean that we advocate a laissez-faire approach to instituting mechanical ventilation. Earlier we mentioned the absurdity of saying that mechanical ventilation is always indicated for acute respiratory failure, defined as a Pa_{O_2} of less than 60 mmHg. This does not mean that we consider Pa_{O_2} unimportant. A physician, on learning that a patient has a sustained Pa_{O_2} of 40 mmHg, will take immediate steps to institute assisted ventilation. But it is not possible to pick a Pa_{O_2} breakpoint (between of 40 and 60 mmHg) below which the benefits of mechanical ventilation decidedly outweigh its hazards. It is futile to imagine that decision making about instituting mechanical ventilation can be condensed into an algorithm with numbers at each nodal point. In sum, an algorithm cannot replace the presence of a physician well skilled in the art of clinical evaluation who has a deep understanding of pathophysiologic principles.

Acknowledgment

This work was supported by grants from the Veterans Administration Research Service.

References

1. Field S, Sanci S, Grassino A. Respiratory muscle oxygen consumption estimated by the diaphragm pressure-time index. J Appl Physiol 1984; 57:44–51.

2. Jubran A, Van de Graaff WB, Tobin MJ. Variability of patient-ventilator interaction with pressure support ventilation in patients with chronic obstructive pulmonary disease. Am J Respir Crit Care Med 1995; 152:129–36.

3. Laghi F, Jubran A, Topeli A, et al. Effect of lung volume reduction surgery on diaphragmatic neuromechanical coupling at 2 years. Chest 2004; 125:2188–95.

4. Laghi F, Cattapan SE, Jubran A, et al. Is weaning failure caused by low-frequency fatigue of the diaphragm? Am J Respir Crit Care Med 2003; 167:120–7.

5. Jubran A, Tobin MJ. Pathophysiologic basis of acute respiratory distress in patients who fail a trial of weaning from mechanical ventilation. Am J Respir Crit Care Med 1997; 155:906–15.

6. Appendini L, Purro A, Gudjonsdottir M, et al. Physiologic response of ventilator-dependent patients with chronic obstructive pulmonary disease to proportional assist ventilation and

continuous positive airway pressure. Am J Respir Crit Care Med 1999; 159:1510–7.

7. Manthous CA, Hall JB, Kushner R, et al. The effect of mechanical ventilation on oxygen consumption in critically ill patients. Am J Respir Crit Care Med 1995; 151:210–4.

8. Gilston A. Facial signs of respiratory distress after cardiac surgery: A plea for the clinical approach to mechanical ventilation. Anaesthesia 1976; 31:385–97.

9. Strohl KP, O'Cain CF, Slutsky AS. Alae nasi activation and nasal resistance in healthy subjects. J Appl Physiol 1982; 52:1432–7.

10. Mueller RE, Petty TL, Filley GF. Ventilation and arterial blood gas changes induced by pursed lips breathing. J Appl Physiol 1970; 28:784–9.

11. Harrison VC, Heese H, V, Klein M. The significance of grunting in hyaline membrane disease. Pediatrics 1968; 41:549–59.

12. Speidel BD, Dunn PM. Effect of continuous positive airway pressure on breathing pattern of infants with respiratory-distress syndrome. Lancet 1975; 1:302–4.

13. Sapira JD. The art and science of bedside diagnosis. Baltimore: Urban & Schwarzenberg, 1990.

14. Mezzanotte WS, Tangel DJ, White DP. Mechanisms of control of alae nasi muscle activity. J Appl Physiol 1992; 72:925–33.

15. Redline S, Strohl KP. Influence of upper airway sensory receptors on respiratory muscle activation in humans. J Appl Physiol 1987; 63:368–74.

16. Abdel-Hady H, Mohareb S, Khashaba M, et al. Randomized, controlled trial of discontinuation of nasal-CPAP in stable preterm infants breathing room air. Acta Paediatr 1998; 87:82–7.

17. Strohl KP, Redline S. Nasal CPAP therapy, upper airway muscle activation, and obstructive sleep apnea. Am Rev Respir Dis 1986; 134:555–8.

18. Brenner BE, Abraham E, Simon RR. Position and diaphoresis in acute asthma. Am J Med 1983; 74:1005–9.

19. Brochard L. Profuse diaphoresis as an important sign for the differential diagnosis of acute respiratory distress. Intensive Care Med 1992; 18:445.

20. Timmers HJ, Wieling W, Karemaker JM, Lenders JW. Cardiovascular responses to stress after carotid baroreceptor denervation in humans. Ann NY Acad Sci 2004; 1018:515–9.

21. Wendling MG, Eckstein JW, Abboud FM. Cardiovascular responses to carbon dioxide before and after beta-adrenergic blockade. J Appl Physiol 1967; 22:223–6.

22. Kilburn KH. Neurologic manifestations of respiratotry failure. Arch Intern Med 1965; 116:409–15.

23. Campbell EJ. The J Burns Amberson Lecture: The management of acute respiratory failure in chronic bronchitis and emphysema. Am Rev Respir Dis 1967; 96:626–39.

24. Yan S, Lichros I, Zakynthinos S, Macklem PT. Effect of diaphragmatic fatigue on control of respiratory muscles and ventilation during CO2 rebreathing. J Appl Physiol 1993; 75:1364–70.

25. Laghi F, Topeli A, Tobin MJ. Does resistive loading decrease diaphragmatic contractility before task failure? J Appl Physiol 1998; 85:1103–12.

26. Yan S, Kaminski D, Sliwinski P. Inspiratory muscle mechanics of patients with chronic obstructive pulmonary disease during incremental exercise. Am J Respir Crit Care Med 1997; 156:807–13.

27. Martin J, Powell E, Shore S, et al. The role of respiratory muscles in the hyperinflation of bronchial asthma. Am Rev Respir Dis 1980; 121:441–7.

28. Brochard L, Harf A, Lorino H, Lemaire F. Inspiratory pressure support prevents diaphragmatic fatigue during weaning from mechanical ventilation. Am Rev Respir Dis 1989; 139:513–21.

29. Skarvan K, Mikulenka V. The ventilatory function of sternomastoid and scalene muscles in patients with pulmonary emphysema. Respiration 1970; 27:480–92.

30. Perrigault PF, Pouzeratte YH, Jaber S, et al. Changes in occlusion pressure (P0.1) and breathing pattern during pressure support ventilation. Thorax 1999; 54:119–23.

31. Krieger B, Feinerman D, Zaron A, Bizousky F. Continuous noninvasive monitoring of respiratory rate in critically ill patients. Chest 1986; 90:632–4.

32. Spiteri MA, Cook DG, Clarke SW. Reliability of eliciting physical signs in examination of the chest. Lancet 1988; 1:873–5.

33. Tobin MJ, Mador MJ, Guenther SM, et al. Variability of resting respiratory drive and timing in healthy subjects. J Appl Physiol 1988; 65:309–17.

34. Tobin MJ, Chadha TS, Jenouri G, et al. Breathing patterns: 2. Diseased subjects. Chest 1983; 84:286–94.

35. Durbin CG Jr, Kopel RF. A case-control study of patients readmitted to the intensive care unit. Crit Care Med 1993; 21:1547–53.

36. Schein RM, Hazday N, Pena M, et al. Clinical antecedents to in-hospital cardiopulmonary arrest. Chest 1990; 98:1388–92.

37. Tobin MJ, Perez W, Guenther SM, et al. The pattern of breathing during successful and unsuccessful trials of weaning from mechanical ventilation. Am Rev Respir Dis 1986; 134:1111–8.

38. Semmes BJ, Tobin MJ, Snyder JV, Grenvik A. Subjective and objective measurement of tidal volume in critically ill patients. Chest 1985; 87:577–9.

39. Mithoefer JC, Bossman OG, Thibeault DW, Mead GD. The clinical estimation of alveolar ventilation. Am Rev Respir Dis 1968; 98:868–71.

40. Gilbert R, Ashutosh K, Auchincloss JH Jr, et al. Prospective study of controlled oxygen therapy: Poor prognosis of patients with asynchronous breathing. Chest 1977; 71:456–62.

41. Tobin MJ, Guenther SM, Perez W, et al. Konno-Mead analysis of ribcage-abdominal motion during successful and unsuccessful trials of weaning from mechanical ventilation. Am Rev Respir Dis 1987; 135:1320–8.

42. Cohen CA, Zagelbaum G, Gross D, et al. Clinical manifestations of inspiratory muscle fatigue. Am J Med 1982; 73:308–16.

43. Tobin MJ, Perez W, Guenther SM, et al. Does rib cage–abdominal paradox signify respiratory muscle fatigue? J Appl Physiol 1987; 63:851–60.

44. Ashutosh K, Gilbert R, Auchincloss JH Jr, Peppi D. Asynchronous breathing movements in patients with chronic obstructive pulmonary disease. Chest 1975; 67:553–7.

45. Tobin MJ, Cohn MA, Sackner MA. Breathing abnormalities during sleep. Arch Intern Med 1983; 143:1221–8.

46. Campbell EJ. Physical signs of diffuse airways obstruction and lung distension. Thorax 1969; 24:1–3.

47. Godfrey S, Edwards RH, Campbell EJ, Newton-Howes J. Clinical and physiological associations of some physical signs observed in patients with chronic airways obstruction. Thorax 1970; 25:285–7.

48. Tobin MJ, Jenouri GA, Watson H, Sackner MA. Noninvasive measurement of pleural pressure by surface inductive plethysmography. J Appl Physiol 1983; 55:267–75.

49. Tobin MJ. Noninvasive monitoring of ventilation. In: Tobin MJ, editor. Principles and practice of intensive care monitoring. New York: NcGraw-Hill, 1998: 465–95.

50. Godfrey S, Edwards RH, Campbell EJ, et al. Repeatability of physical signs in airways obstruction. Thorax 1969; 24:4–9.

51. Oh TE, Bhatt S, Lin ES, et al. Plasma catecholamines and oxygen consumption during weaning from mechanical ventilation. Intensive Care Med 1991; 17:199–203.

52. Kikuchi Y, Okabe S, Tamura G, et al. Chemosensitivity and perception of dyspnea in patients with a history of near-fatal asthma. New Engl J Med 1994; 330:1329–34.

53. Kifle Y, Seng V, Davenport PW. Magnitude estimation of inspiratory resistive loads in children with life-threatening asthma. Am J Respir Crit Care Med 1997; 156:1530–5.

54. Eckert DJ, Catcheside PG, Smith JH, et al. Hypoxia suppresses symptom perception in asthma. Am J Respir Crit Care Med 2004; 169:1224–30.

55. Pierson DJ. Indications for mechanical ventilation in adults with acute respiratory failure. Respir Care 2002; 47:249–62.

56. Grippi MA. Respiratory failure: An overview. In: Fishman AP, Elias JA, Fishman JA, et al, editors. Fishman's Pulmonary Diseases and Disorders. New York: McGraw-Hill, 1998: 2525–48.

57. Murray JF. The normal lung, 2nd ed. Philadelphia: Saunders, 1986.

58. West JB, Wagner PD. Respiratory physiology. In: Murray JF, Nadel JA, Mason RJ, Boushey HA, editors. Textbook of respiratory medicine. Philadelphia: Saunders, 2000: 55–89.

59. Dunnill MS. Postnatal growth of the lung. Thorax 1962; 17: 329–33.

60. Wagner PD, Laravuso RB, Uhl RR, West JB. Continuous distributions of ventilation-perfusion ratios in normal subjects breathing air and 100 percent O_2. J Clin Invest 1974; 54:54–68.

61. West JB. State of the art: Ventilation-perfusion relationships. Am Rev Respir Dis 1977; 116:919–43.

62. Marini JJ. Respiratory medicine, 2nd ed. Baltimore: Williams & Wilkins, 1987.

63. Wagner PD. Ventilation, pulmonary blood flow, and ventilation-perfusion relationships. In: Fishman AP, Elias JA, Fishman JA, et al, editors. Fishman's pulmonary diseases and disorders. New York: McGraw-Hill, 1998: 177–92.

64. Aldrich TK, Prezant DJ. Indications for mechanical ventilation. In: Tobin MJ, editor. Principles and practice of mechanical ventilation. New York: McGraw-Hill, 1994: 155–89.

65. Newhouse MT, Becklake MR, Macklem PT, MacGregor M. Effect of alterations in end-tidal CO_2 tension in flow resistance. J Appl Physiol 1964; 19:745–9.

66. West JB. Ventilation-perfusion inequality and overall gas exchange in computer models of the lung. Respir Physiol 1969; 7:88–110.

67. Campbell EJ. Methods of oxygen administration in respiratory failure. Ann NY Acad Sci 1965; 121:861–70.

68. Comroe JH. Physiology of respiration, 2nd ed. Chicago: Year Book Medical Publishers, 1974.

69. Prabhakar NR, Peng YJ. Peripheral chemoreceptors in health and disease. J Appl Physiol 2004; 96:359–66.

70. Timmers HJ, Wieling W, Karemaker JM, Lenders JW. Denervation of carotid baro- and chemoreceptors in humans. J Physiol 2003; 553:3–11.

71. Whipp BJ. Carotid bodies and breathing in humans. Thorax 1994; 49:1081–4.

72. Lahiri S, Mulligan E, Nishino T, et al. Relative responses of aortic body and carotid body chemoreceptors to carboxyhemoglobinemia. J Appl Physiol 1981; 50:580–6.

73. Takasaki Y, Orr D, Popkin J, et al. Effect of hypercapnia and hypoxia on respiratory muscle activation in humans. J Appl Physiol 1989; 67:1776–84.

74. Lugliani R, Whipp BJ, Wasserman K. A role for the carotid body in cardiovascular control in man. Chest 1973; 63:744–50.

75. Lugliani R, Whipp BJ, Seard C, Wasserman K. Effect of bilateral carotid-body resection on ventilatory control at rest and during exercise in man. New Engl J Med 1971; 285:1105–11.

76. Somers VK, Mark AL, Zavala DC, Abboud FM. Influence of ventilation and hypocapnia on sympathetic nerve responses to hypoxia in normal humans. J Appl Physiol 1989; 67:2095–2100.

77. Kronenberg RS, Drage CW. Attenuation of the ventilatory and heart rate responses to hypoxia and hypercapnia with aging in normal men. J Clin Invest 1973; 52:1812–9.

78. Fatemian M, Nieuwenhuijs DJ, Teppema LJ, et al. The respiratory response to carbon dioxide in humans with unilateral and bilateral resections of the carotid bodies. J Physiol 2003; 549:965–73.

79. Vatner SF, McRitchie RJ. Interaction of the chemoreflex and the pulmonary inflation reflex in the regulation of coronary circulation in conscious dogs. Circ Res 1975; 37:664–73.

80. Shamsuzzaman AS, Somers VK. Cardiorespiratory interactions in neural circulatory control in humans. Ann NY Acad Sci 2001; 940:488–99.

81. Meadows GE, O'Driscoll DM, Simonds AK, et al. Cerebral blood flow response to isocapnic hypoxia during slow-wave sleep and wakefulness. J Appl Physiol 2004; 97:1343–8.

82. Cargill RI, Kiely DG, Lipworth BJ. Left ventricular systolic performance during acute hypoxemia. Chest 1995; 108: 899–902.

83. Cargill RI, Lipworth BJ. Lisinopril attenuates acute hypoxic pulmonary vasoconstriction in humans. Chest 1996; 109:424–9.

84. Bernardi L, Hilz M, Stemper B, et al. Respiratory and cerebrovascular responses to hypoxia and hypercapnia in familial dysautonomia. Am J Respir Crit Care Med 2003; 167:141–9.

85. Somers VK, Mark AL, Abboud FM. Interaction of baroreceptor and chemoreceptor reflex control of sympathetic nerve activity in normal humans. J Clin Invest 1991; 87:1953–7.

86. Zwillich C, Devlin T, White D, et al. Bradycardia during sleep apnea: Characteristics and mechanism. J Clin Invest 1982; 69:1286–92.

87. Lin YC, Shida KK, Hong SK. Effects of hypercapnia, hypoxia, and rebreathing on heart rate response during apnea. J Appl Physiol 1983; 54:166–71.

88. Dunford JV, Davis DP, Ochs M, et al. Incidence of transient hypoxia and pulse rate reactivity during paramedic rapid sequence intubation. Ann Emerg Med 2003; 42:721–8.

89. De Daly MB, Scott MJ. The effects of stimulation of the carotid body chemoreceptors on heart rate in the dog. J Physiol 1958; 144:148–66.

90. Kontos HA, Mauck HP Jr, Richardson DW, Patterson JL Jr. Mechanisms of circulatory responses to systemic hypoxia in the anesthetized dog. Am J Physiol 1965; 209:397–403.

91. Berk JL, Levy MN. Profound reflex bradycardia produced by transient hypoxia or hypercapnia in man. Eur Surg Res 1977; 9:75–84.

92. Trzebski A, Smith ML, Beightol LA, et al. Modulation of human sympathetic periodicity by mild, brief hypoxia and hypercapnia. J Physiol Pharmacol 1995; 46:17–35.

93. Maiese K, Caronna JJ. Coma. In: Parrillo JE, Bone RB, editors. Critical care medicine: Principles of diagnosis and management. St. Louis: Mosby, 1995: 1157–76.

94. Lundsgaard C, Van Slyke DD. Cyanosis. Medicine 1923; 2:1–76.

95. Medd WE, French EB, McA.Wyllie V. Cyanosis as a guide to arterial oxygen desaturation. Thorax 1959; 14:247–50.

96. Fleming PR. Cyanosis. In: Hart DF, editor. French's index of differential diagnosis. Bristol, England: John Wright & Sons, 1979: 194–9.

97. Comroe JH, Botelho S. The unreliability of cyanosis in the recognition of arterial anoxemia. Am J Med Sci 1947; 214:1–6.

98. Alonso JR, Cardellach F, Lopez S, et al. Carbon monoxide specifically inhibits cytochrome C oxidase of human mitochondrial respiratory chain. Pharmacol Toxicol 2003; 93: 142–6.

99. Crosby A, Talbot NP, Balanos GM, et al. Respiratory effects in humans of a 5-day elevation of end-tidal P_{CO_2} by 8 torr. J Appl Physiol 2003; 95:1947–54.

100. Naik-Tolani S, Oropello JM, Benjamin E. Neurologic complications in the intensive care unit. Clin Chest Med 1999; 20:423–34.

101. Siesjo BK. Brain dysfunction in cerebral hypoxia and ischemia. In: Plum F, editor. Brain dysfunction in metabolic disorders. New York: Raven Press, 1974: 75–112.

102. West JB, Hackett PH, Maret KH, et al. Pulmonary gas exchange on the summit of Mount Everest. J Appl Physiol 1983; 55:678–87.

103. Prys-Roberts C, Smith WD, Nunn JF. Accidental severe hypercapnia during anaesthesia: A case report and review of some physiological effects. Br J Anaesth 1967; 39:257–67.

104. Henry RA, Lu IL, Beightol LA, Eckberg DL. Interactions between CO_2 chemoreflexes and arterial baroreflexes. Am J Physiol 1998; 274:H2177–87.

105. Somers VK, Mark AL, Zavala DC, Abboud FM. Contrasting effects of hypoxia and hypercapnia on ventilation and sympathetic activity in humans. J Appl Physiol 1989; 67:2101–6.

106. Gelfand R, Lambertsen CJ. Dynamic respiratory response to abrupt change of inspired CO_2 at normal and high P_{O_2}. J Appl Physiol 1973; 35:903–13.

107. Bellville JW, Whipp BJ, Kaufman RD, et al. Central and peripheral chemoreflex loop gain in normal and carotid body-resected subjects. J Appl Physiol 1979; 46:843–53.

108. Seevers MH. The narcotic properties of carbon dioxide. NY State J Med 1944; 44:597–602.

109. Nielsen M, Smith H. Studies on the regulation of respiration in acute hypoxia; with a appendix on respiratory control during prolonged hypoxia. Acta Physiol Scand 1952; 24:293–313.

110. Dripps RD, Comroe JH. The respiratory and circulatory response of normal man to inhalation of 7.6 and 10.4 percent CO_2 with a comparison of the maximal ventilation produced by severe muscular exercise, inhalation of CO_2 and maximal coluntary hyperventilation. Am J Physiol 1947; 149:43–51.

111. McArdle L, Roddie IC, Shepherd JT, Whelan RF. The effect of inhalation of 30% carbon dioxide on the peripheral circulation of the human subject. Br J Pharmacol 1957; 12:293–6.

112. Morisaki H, Serita R, Innami Y, et al. Permissive hypercapnia during thoracic anaesthesia. Acta Anaesthesiol Scand 1999; 43:845–9.

113. Ito H, Ibaraki M, Kanno I, et al. Changes in the arterial fraction of human cerebral blood volume during hypercapnia and hypocapnia measured by positron emission tomography. J Cerebrvasc Blood Flow Metab 2005; 25:852–7.

114. Ito H, Kanno I, Ibaraki M, Hatazawa J. Effect of aging on cerebral vascular response to Pa_{CO_2} changes in humans as measured by positron emission tomography. J Cerebrovasc Blood Flow Metab 2002; 22:997–1003.

115. Marshall RS, Rundek T, Sproule DM, et al. Monitoring of cerebral vasodilatory capacity with transcranial Doppler carbon dioxide inhalation in patients with severe carotid artery disease. Stroke 2003; 34:945–9.

116. Siesjo BK, Ingvar M. Ventilation and brain metabolism. In: Fishman AP, Cherniack NS, Widdicombe JG, Geiger SR, editors. Handbook of physiology: The respiratory system, Vol II. Bethesda, MD: American Physiological Society, 1986: 141–61.

117. Hudson LD. Evaluation of the patient with acute respiratory failure. Respir Care 1983; 28:542–52.

118. Warner DS, Turner DM, Kassell NF. Time-dependent effects of prolonged hypercapnia on cerebrovascular parameters in dogs: Acid-base chemistry. Stroke 1987; 18:142–9.

119. Robinson TD, Freiberg DB, Regnis JA, Young IH. The role of hypoventilation and ventilation-perfusion redistribution in oxygen-induced hypercapnia during acute exacerbations of chronic obstructive pulmonary disease. Am J Respir Crit Care Med 2000; 161:1524–9.

120. Tobin MJ, Jubran A. Oxygen takes the breath away: Old sting, new setting. Mayo Clin Proc 1995; 70:403–4.

121. Arozullah AM, Daley J, Henderson WG, Khuri SF. Multifactorial risk index for predicting postoperative respiratory failure in men after major noncardiac surgery. The National Veterans Administration Surgical Quality Improvement Program. Ann Surg 2000; 232:242–53.

122. Arozullah AM, Khuri SF, Henderson WG, Daley J. Development and validation of a multifactorial risk index for predicting postoperative pneumonia after major noncardiac surgery. Ann Intern Med 2001; 135:847–57.

123. McAlister FA, Bertsch K, Man J, et al. Incidence of and risk factors for pulmonary complications after nonthoracic surgery. Am J Respir Crit Care Med 2005; 171:514–7.

124. Brooks-Brunn JA. Postoperative atelectasis and pneumonia. Heart Lung 1995; 24:94–115.

125. Kotloff RM. Acute respiratory failure in the surgical patient. In: Fishman AP, Elias JA, Fishman JA, et al, editors. Fishman's pulmonary diseases and disorders. New York: McGraw-Hill, 1998: 2589–2604.

126. Money SR, Rice K, Crockett D, et al. Risk of respiratory failure after repair of thoracoabdominal aortic aneurysms. Am J Surg 1994; 168:152–5.

127. Pezzella AT, Adebonojo SA, Hooker SG, et al. Complications of general thoracic surgery. Curr Probl Surg 2000; 37:733–858.

128. Wood LDH, Schmidt GA, Hall JB. Principles of critical care of respiratory failure. In: Murray JF, Nadel JA, Mason RJ, Boushey HA, editors. Textbook of respiratory medicine. Philadelphia: Saunders, 2000: 2377–2411.

129. Gunnarsson L, Tokics L, Gustavsson H, Hedenstierna G. Influence of age on atelectasis formation and gas exchange impairment during general anaesthesia. Br J Anaesth 1991; 66: 423–32.

130. Hedenstierna G. Alveolar collapse and closure of airways: Regular effects of anaesthesia. Clin Physiol Funct Imaging 2003; 23:123–9.

131. Tenling A, Hachenberg T, Tyden H, et al. Atelectasis and gas exchange after cardiac surgery. Anesthesiology 1998; 89: 371–8.

132. Lindberg P, Gunnarsson L, Tokics L, et al. Atelectasis and lung function in the postoperative period. Acta Anaesthesiol Scand 1992; 36:546–53.

133. Schwartz DE, Katz JE. Delivery of mechanical ventilation during general anesthesia. In: Tobin MJ, editor. Principles and practice of mechanical ventilation. New York: McGraw-Hill, 1994: 529–70.

134. Laghi F, Tobin MJ. Disorders of the respiratory muscles. Am J Respir Crit Care Med 2003; 168:10–48.

135. Hedenstierna G, Tokics L, Lundquist H, et al. Phrenic nerve stimulation during halothane anesthesia: Effects of atelectasis. Anesthesiology 1994; 80:751–60.

136. Forbes AR. Halothane depresses mucociliary flow in the trachea. Anesthesiology 1976; 45:59–63.

137. Forbes AR, Horrigan RW. Mucociliary flow in the trachea during anesthesia with enflurane, ether, nitrous oxide, and morphine. Anesthesiology 1977; 46:319–21.

138. Pierce AK, Robertson J. Pulmonary complications of general surgery. Annu Rev Med 1977; 28:211–21.

139. Otis DR Jr, Johnson M, Pedley TJ, Kamm RD. Role of pulmonary surfactant in airway closure: A computational study. J Appl Physiol 1993; 75:1323–33.

140. Bonde P, McManus K, McAnespie M, McGuigan J. Lung surgery: Identifying the subgroup at risk for sputum retention. Eur J Cardiothorac Surg 2002; 22:18–22.

141. Cheatham ML, Chapman WC, Key SP, Sawyers JL. A meta-analysis of selective versus routine nasogastric decompression after elective laparotomy. Ann Surg 1995; 221: 469–76.

142. Keenan SP, Heyland DK, Jacka MJ, et al. Ventilator-associated pneumonia: Prevention, diagnosis, and therapy. Crit Care Clin 2002; 18:107–25.

143. Sekine Y, Behnia M, Fujisawa T. Impact of COPD on pulmonary complications and on long-term survival of patients undergoing surgery for NSCLC. Lung Cancer 2002; 37:95–101.

144. Ashraf MN, Mortasawi A, Grayson AD, Oo AY. Effect of smoking status on mortality and morbidity following coronary artery bypass surgery. Thorac Cardiovasc Surg 2004; 52:268–73.

145. Bonde P, Papachristos I, McCraith A, et al. Sputum retention after lung operation: Prospective, randomized trial shows superiority of prophylactic minitracheostomy in high-risk patients. Ann Thorac Surg 2002; 74:196–202.

146. McAlister FA, Khan NA, Straus SE, et al. Accuracy of the preoperative assessment in predicting pulmonary risk after nonthoracic surgery. Am J Respir Crit Care Med 2003; 167:741–4.

147. Pasquina P, Tramer MR, Walder B. Prophylactic respiratory physiotherapy after cardiac surgery: Systematic review. Br Med J 2003; 327:1379.

148. Overend TJ, Anderson CM, Lucy SD, et al. The effect of incentive spirometry on postoperative pulmonary complications: A systematic review. Chest 2001; 120:971–8.

149. Sulzer CF, Chiolero R, Chassot PG, et al. Adaptive support ventilation for fast tracheal extubation after cardiac surgery: A randomized, controlled study. Anesthesiology 2001; 95:1339–45.

150. Silbert BS, Santamaria JD, O'Brien JL, et al. Early extubation following coronary artery bypass surgery: A prospective, randomized, controlled trial. The Fast Track Cardiac Care Team. Chest 1998; 113:1481–8.

151. Barnas GM, Watson RJ, Green MD, et al. Lung and chest wall mechanical properties before and after cardiac surgery with cardiopulmonary bypass. J Appl Physiol 1994; 76:166–75.

152. Ranieri VM, Vitale N, Grasso S, et al. Time course of impairment of respiratory mechanics after cardiac surgery and cardiopulmonary bypass. Crit Care Med 1999; 27:1454–60.

153. Roosens C, Heerman J, De Somer F, et al. Effects of off-pump coronary surgery on the mechanics of the respiratory system, lung, and chest wall: Comparison with extracorporeal circulation. Crit Care Med 2002; 30:2430–7.

154. Nicholson DJ, Kowalski SE, Hamilton GA, et al. Postoperative pulmonary function in coronary artery bypass graft surgery patients undergoing early tracheal extubation: A comparison between short-term mechanical ventilation and early extubation. J Cardiothorac Vasc Anesth 2002; 16:27–31.

155. Matte P, Jacquet L, Van Dyck M, Goenen M. Effects of conventional physiotherapy, continuous positive airway pressure and non-invasive ventilatory support with bilevel positive airway pressure after coronary artery bypass grafting. Acta Anaesthesiol Scand 2000; 44:75–81.

156. Lefemine AA, Harken DE. Postoperative care following open-heart operations: Routine use of controlled ventilation. J Thorac Cardiovasc Surg 1966; 52:207–16.

157. Cooperman LH, Mann PE. Postoperative respiratory care: A review of 65 consecutive cases of open-heart surgery on the mitral valve. J Thorac Cardiovasc Surg 1967; 53:504–7.

158. Royse CF, Royse AG, Soeding PF. Routine immediate extubation after cardiac operation: A review of our first 100 patients. Ann Thorac Surg 1999; 68:1326–9.

159. Koning HM, Leusink JA, Nas AA, et al. Renal function following open heart surgery: The influence of postoperative artificial ventilation. Thorac Cardiovasc Surg 1988; 36:1–4.

160. Mangano DT, Siliciano D, Hollenberg M, et al. Postoperative myocardial ischemia: Therapeutic trials using intensive analgesia following surgery. The Study of Perioperative Ischemia (SPI) Research Group. Anesthesiology 1992; 76:342–53.

161. Cheng DC, Karski J, Peniston C, et al. Early tracheal extubation after coronary artery bypass graft surgery reduces costs and improves resource use: A prospective, randomized, controlled trial. Anesthesiology 1996; 85:1300–10.

162. Guller U, Anstrom KJ, Holman WL, et al. Outcomes of early extubation after bypass surgery in the elderly. Ann Thorac Surg 2004; 77:781–8.

163. Myles PS, McIlroy D. Fast-track cardiac anesthesia: Choice of anesthetic agents and techniques. Semin Cardiothorac Vasc Anesth 2005; 9:5–16.

164. Straka Z, Brucek P, Vanek T, et al. Routine immediate extubation for off-pump coronary artery bypass grafting without thoracic epidural analgesia. Ann Thorac Surg 2002; 74:1544–7.

165. Tenling A, Joachimsson P-O, Tyden H, Hedenstierna G. Thoracic epidural analgesia as an adjunct to general anaesthesia for cardiac surgery: Effects on pulmonary mechanics. Acta Anaesthesiol Scand 2000; 44:1071–6.

166. Higgins TL. Pro: Early endotracheal extubation is preferable to late extubation in patients following coronary artery surgery. J Cardiothorac Vasc Anesth 1992; 6:488–93.

167. Kuiper JW, Groeneveld AB, Slutsky AS, Plotz FB. Mechanical ventilation and acute renal failure. Crit Care Med 2005; 33: 1408–15.

168. Quasha AL, Loeber N, Feeley TW, et al. Postoperative respiratory care: A controlled trial of early and late extubation following coronary-artery bypass grafting. Anesthesiology 1980; 52:135–41.

169. Hemmerling TM, Le N, Olivier JF, et al. Immediate extubation after aortic valve surgery using high thoracic epidural analgesia or opioid-based analgesia. J Cardiothorac Vasc Anesth 2005; 19:176–81.

170. Oxelbark S, Bengtsson L, Eggersen M, et al. Fast track as a routine for open heart surgery. Eur J Cardiothorac Surg 2001; 19:460–3.

171. Hansen LN, Ravn JB, Yndgaard S. Early extubation after single-lung transplantation: Analysis of the first 106 cases. J Cardiothorac Vasc Anesth 2003; 17:36–9.

172. Chandrashekar MV, Irving M, Wayman J, et al. Immediate extubation and epidural analgesia allow safe management in a high-dependency unit after two-stage oesophagectomy: Results of eight years of experience in a specialized upper gastrointestinal unit in a district general hospital. Br J Anaesth 2003; 90: 474–9.

173. Karagoz HY, Sonmez B, Bakkaloglu B, et al. Coronary artery bypass grafting in the conscious patient without endotracheal general anesthesia. Ann Thorac Surg 2000; 70:91–6.

174. Aybek T, Kessler P, Khan MF, et al. Operative techniques in awake coronary artery bypass grafting. J Thorac Cardiovasc Surg 2003; 125:1394–1400.

175. Karagoz HY, Kurtoglu M, Bakkaloglu B, et al. Coronary artery bypass grafting in the awake patient: Three years' experience in 137 patients. J Thorac Cardiovasc Surg 2003; 125:1401–4.

176. Mangano CT. Risky business. J Thorac Cardiovasc Surg 2003; 125:1204–7.

177. Kumar A, Parrillo JE. Shock: Classification, pathophysiology, and approach to management. In: Parrillo JE, Dellinger RP, editors. Critical care medicine: Principles of diagnosis and management in the adult. St. Louis: Mosby, 2001: 371–420.

178. Annane D, Bellissant E, Cavaillon JM. Septic shock. Lancet 2005; 365:63–78.

179. Jardin F, Eveleigh MC, Gurdjian F, et al. Venous admixture in human septic shock: Comparative effects of blood volume expansion, dopamine infusion and isoproterenol infusion on mismatching of ventilation and pulmonary blood flow in peritonitis. Circulation 1979; 60:155–9.

180. Kamal GD, Symreng T, Tatman DJ, Jebson PJ. Reduced venous admixture in hemorrhagic hypovolemia: Maintenance of

arterial oxygenation by selective pulmonary vascular collapse. Crit Care Med 1990; 18:208–12.

181. Steenblock U, Mannhart H, Wolff G. Effect of hemorrhagic shock on intrapulmonary right-to-left shunt ($\dot{Q}_S/\dot{Q}_T$) and dead space ($\dot{V}_D/\dot{V}_T$). Respiration 1976; 33:133–42.

182. Groeneveld ABJ. Hypovolemic shock. In: Parrillo JE, Dellinger RP, editors. Critical care medicine: Principles of diagnosis and management in the adult. St.Louis: Mosby, 2001: 465–500.

183. Heistad D, Abboud FM, Mark AL, Schmid PG. Effect of baroreceptor activity on ventilatory response to chemoreceptor stimulation. J Appl Physiol 1975; 39:411–6.

184. Monahan KD, Sharpe MK, Drury D, et al. Influence of vestibular activation on respiration in humans. Am J Physiol Regul Integr Comp Physiol 2002; 282:R689–94.

185. Mizock BA, Falk JL. Lactic acidosis in critical illness. Crit Care Med 1992; 20:80–93.

186. Aubier M, Viires N, Syllie G, et al. Respiratory muscle contribution to lactic acidosis in low cardiac output. Am Rev Respir Dis 1982; 126:648–52.

187. Adrogue HJ, Rashad MN, Gorin AB, et al. Arteriovenous acid-base disparity in circulatory failure: Studies on mechanism. Am J Physiol 1989; 257:F1087–93.

188. Hildebrandt W, Ottenbacher A, Schuster M, et al. Increased hypoxic ventilatory response during hypovolemic stress imposed through head-up-tilt and lower-body negative pressure. Eur J Appl Physiol 2000; 81:470–8.

189. Lanone S, Mebazaa A, Heymes C, et al. Muscular contractile failure in septic patients: Role of the inducible nitric oxide synthase pathway. Am J Respir Crit Care Med 2000; 162:2308–15.

190. Leon A, Boczkowski J, Dureuil B, et al. Effects of endotoxic shock on diaphragmatic function in mechanically ventilated rats. J Appl Physiol 1992; 72:1466–72.

191. Lin MC, Ebihara S, El Dwairi Q, et al. Diaphragm sarcolemmal injury is induced by sepsis and alleviated by nitric oxide synthase inhibition. Am J Respir Crit Care Med 1998; 158:1656–63.

192. Callahan LA, Nethery D, Stofan D, et al. Free radical-induced contractile protein dysfunction in endotoxin-induced sepsis. Am J Respir Cell Mol Biol 2001; 24:210–7.

193. Hussain SN. Respiratory muscle dysfunction in sepsis. Mol Cell Biochem 1998; 179:125–34.

194. Boczkowski J, Lisdero CL, Lanone S, et al. Endogenous peroxynitrite mediates mitochondrial dysfunction in rat diaphragm during endotoxemia. FASEB J 1999; 13:1637–46.

195. El Dwairi Q, Comtois A, Guo Y, Hussain SN. Endotoxin-induced skeletal muscle contractile dysfunction: Contribution of nitric oxide synthases. Am J Physiol 1998; 274:C770–9.

196. Taille C, Foresti R, Lanone S, et al. Protective role of heme oxygenases against endotoxin-induced diaphragmatic dysfunction in rats. Am J Respir Crit Care Med 2001; 163:753–61.

197. Javesghani D, Magder SA, Barreiro E, et al. Molecular characterization of a superoxide-generating NAD(P)H oxidase in the ventilatory muscles. Am J Respir Crit Care Med 2002; 165:412–8.

198. Fujimura N, Sumita S, Aimono M, et al. Effect of free radical scavengers on diaphragmatic contractility in septic peritonitis. Am J Respir Crit Care Med 2000; 162:2159–65.

199. Tiao G, Fagan J, Roegner V, et al. Energy-ubiquitin-dependent muscle proteolysis during sepsis in rats is regulated by glucocorticoids. J Clin Invest 1996; 97:339–48.

200. Mitch WE, Goldberg AL. Mechanisms of muscle wasting: The role of the ubiquitin-proteasome pathway. New Engl J Med 1996; 335:1897–1905.

201. Laghi F. Curing the septic diaphragm with the ventilator. Am J Respir Crit Care Med 2002; 165:145–6.

202. Tawa NE Jr, Odessey R, Goldberg AL. Inhibitors of the proteasome reduce the accelerated proteolysis in atrophying rat skeletal muscles. J Clin Invest 1997; 100:197–203.

203. Tsukagoshi H, Morita T, Takahashi K, et al. Cecal ligation and puncture peritonitis model shows decreased nicotinic acetylcholine receptor numbers in rat muscle: Immunopathologic mechanisms? Anesthesiology 1999; 91:448–60.

204. Md S, Moochhala SM, Siew Yang KL, et al. The role of selective nitric oxide synthase inhibitor on nitric oxide and PGE2 levels in refractory hemorrhagic-shocked rats. J Surg Res 2005; 123:206–14.

205. Vallejo JG, Nemoto S, Ishiyama M, et al. Functional significance of inflammatory mediators in a murine model of resuscitated hemorrhagic shock. Am J Physiol Heart Circ Physiol 2005; 288:H1272–7.

206. Liu LM, Dubick MA. Hemorrhagic shock-induced vascular hyporeactivity in the rat: Relationship to gene expression of nitric oxide synthase, endothelin-1, and select cytokines in corresponding organs. J Surg Res 2005; 125:128–36.

207. Appoloni O, Dupont E, Vandercruys M, et al. Association between the TNF-2 allele and a better survival in cardiogenic shock. Chest 2004; 125:2232–7.

208. Cotter G, Kaluski E, Blatt A, et al. L-NMMA (a nitric oxide synthase inhibitor) is effective in the treatment of cardiogenic shock. Circulation 2000; 101:1358–61.

209. Kiang JG. Inducible heat shock protein 70 kD and inducible nitric oxide synthase in hemorrhage/resuscitation-induced injury. Cell Res 2004; 14:450–9.

210. Aubier M, Trippenbach T, Roussos C. Respiratory muscle fatigue during cardiogenic shock. J Appl Physiol 1981; 51:499–508.

211. Hussain SN, Simkus G, Roussos C. Respiratory muscle fatigue: A cause of ventilatory failure in septic shock. J Appl Physiol 1985; 58:2033–40.

212. Viires N, Sillye G, Aubier M, et al. Regional blood flow distribution in dog during induced hypotension and low cardiac output: Spontaneous breathing versus artificial ventilation. J Clin Invest 1983; 72:935–47.

213. Kontoyannis DA, Nanas JN, Kontoyannis SA, et al. Mechanical ventilation in conjunction with the intra-aortic balloon pump improves the outcome of patients in profound cardiogenic shock. Intensive Care Med 1999; 25:835–8.

214. Maier RV. Approach to the patient with shock. In: Kasper DL, Braunwald E, Fauci AS, et al, editors. *Harrison's principles of internal medicine.* New York: McGraw-Hill, 2005: 1600–6.

215. Dodt C, Gunnarsson T, Elam M, et al. Central blood volume influences sympathetic sudomotor nerve traffic in warm humans. Acta Physiol Scand 1995; 155:41–51.

216. Guyton AC, Hall JE. Textbook of medical physiology, 11th ed. Philadelphia: Saunders, 2000.

217. Hamrahian AH, Oseni TS, Arafah BM. Measurements of serum free cortisol in critically ill patients. New Engl J Med 2004; 350:1629–38.

218. Rivers E, Nguyen B, Havstad S, et al. Early goal-directed therapy in the treatment of severe sepsis and septic shock. New Engl J Med 2001; 345:1368–77.

219. Eidelman LA, Putterman D, Putterman C, Sprung CL. The spectrum of septic encephalopathy: Definitions, etiologies, and mortalities. JAMA 1996; 275:470–3.

220. Khosh MM, Lebovics RS. Upper airway obstruction. In: Parrillo JE, Dellinger RP, editors. Critical care medicine. Principles of diagnosis and management in the adult. St. Louis: Mosby, 2001: 808–25.

221. King EG, Sheehan GJ, McDonnell TJ. Upper airway obstruction. In: Hall JB, Schmidt GA, Wood LDH, editors. Principles of critical care. New York: McGraw-Hill, 1992: 1710–8.

222. Deepika K, Kenaan CA, Barrocas AM, et al. Negative pressure pulmonary edema after acute upper airway obstruction. J Clin Anesth 1997; 9:403–8.

223. Schwartz DR, Maroo A, Malhotra A, Kesselman H. Negative pressure pulmonary hemorrhage. Chest 1999; 115:1194–7.

224. Tami TA, Chu F, Wildes TO, Kaplan M. Pulmonary edema and acute upper airway obstruction. Laryngoscope 1986; 96: 506–9.

225. Miro AM, Pinsky MR. Heart-lung interactions. In: Tobin MJ, editor. Principles and practice of mechanical ventilation. New York: McGraw-Hill, 1994: 647–71.

226. Guyton AC, Lindsey AW, Albernathy B, Richardson T. Venous retoun at various right atrial pressures and the normal venous return curve. Am J Physiol 1957; 189:609–15.

227. West JB, Tsukimoto K, Mathieu-Costello O, Prediletto R. Stress failure in pulmonary capillaries. J Appl Physiol 1991; 70: 1731–42.

228. Berrouschot J, Rossler A, Koster J, Schneider D. Mechanical ventilation in patients with hemispheric ischemic stroke. Crit Care Med 2000; 28:2956–61.

229. Shaker R. Airway protective mechanisms: Current concepts. Dysphagia 1995; 10:216–27.

230. Keamy M. Airway management and intubation. In: Hall JB, Schmidt GA, Wood LDH, editors. Principles of critical care. New York: McGraw-Hill, 1992: 123–34.

231. Muizelaar JP, Marmarou A, Ward JD, et al. Adverse effects of prolonged hyperventilation in patients with severe head injury: A randomized clinical trial. J Neurosurg 1991; 75:731–9.

232. The use of hyperventilation in the acute management of severe traumatic brain injury. Brain Trauma Foundation. J Neurotrauma 1996; 13:699–703.

233. Shapiro M, Wilson RK, Casar G, et al. Work of breathing through different sized endotracheal tubes. Crit Care Med 1986; 14: 1028–31.

234. Zhu E, Petrof BJ, Gea J, et al. Diaphragm muscle fiber injury after inspiratory resistive breathing. Am J Respir Crit Care Med 1997; 155:1110–6.

235. Jiang TX, Reid WD, Road JD. Free radical scavengers and diaphragm injury following inspiratory resistive loading. Am J Respir Crit Care Med 2001; 164:1288–94.

236. Sassoon CS, Gruer SE, Sieck GC. Temporal relationships of ventilatory failure, pump failure, and diaphragm fatigue. J Appl Physiol 1996; 81:238–45.

237. Orozco-Levi M, Lloreta J, Minguella J, et al. Injury of the human diaphragm associated with exertion and chronic obstructive pulmonary disease. Am J Respir Crit Care Med 2001; 164: 1734–1739.

238. Silver MM, Smith CR. Diaphragmatic contraction band necrosis in a perinatal and infantile autopsy population. Hum Pathol 1992; 23:817–27.

239. Ebihara S, Hussain SN, Danialou G, et al. Mechanical ventilation protects against diaphragm injury in sepsis: Interaction of oxidative and mechanical stresses. Am J Respir Crit Care Med 2002; 165:221–8.

240. Douglass JA, Tuxen DV, Horne M, et al. Myopathy in severe asthma. Am Rev Respir Dis 1992; 146:517–9.

241. Sassoon CS, Caiozzo VJ, Manka A, Sieck GC. Altered diaphragm contractile properties with controlled mechanical ventilation. J Appl Physiol 2002; 92:2585–95.

242. Sassoon CS, Zhu E, Caiozzo VJ. Assist-control mechanical ventilation attenuates ventilator-induced diaphragmatic dysfunction. Am J Respir Crit Care Med 2004; 170:626–32.

243. Vassilakopoulos T, Petrof BJ. Ventilator-induced diaphragmatic dysfunction. Am J Respir Crit Care Med 2004; 169:336–41.

244. Deruisseau KC, Kavazis AN, Deering MA, et al. Mechanical ventilation induces alterations of the ubiquitin-proteasome pathway in the diaphragm. J Appl Physiol 2005; 98: 1314–21.

245. Shanely RA, Van Gammeren D, Deruisseau KC, et al. Mechanical ventilation depresses protein synthesis in the rat diaphragm. Am J Respir Crit Care Med 2004; 170:994–9.

246. Betters JL, Criswell DS, Shanely RA, et al. Trolox attenuates mechanical ventilation-induced diaphragmatic dysfunction and proteolysis. Am J Respir Crit Care Med 2004; 170:1179–84.

247. Nava S, Rubini F. Lung and chest wall mechanics in ventilated patients with end-stage idiopathic pulmonary fibrosis. Thorax 1999; 54:390–5.

248. Pelosi P, Bottino N, Chiumello D, et al. Sigh in supine and prone position during acute respiratory distress syndrome. Am J Respir Crit Care Med 2003; 167:521–7.

249. Dantzker DR, Brook CJ, Dehart P, et al. Ventilation-perfusion distributions in the adult respiratory distress syndrome. Am Rev Respir Dis 1979; 120:1039–52.

250. Pare PD, Warriner B, Baile EM, Hogg JC. Redistribution of pulmonary extravascular water with positive end-expiratory pressure in canine pulmonary edema. Am Rev Respir Dis 1983; 127:590–3.

251. Dantzker DR, Lynch JP, Weg JG. Depression of cardiac output is a mechanism of shunt reduction in the therapy of acute respiratory failure. Chest 1980; 77:636–42.

252. West JB. Pulmonary pathophysiology: The essentials, 6th ed. Philadelphia: Lippincott Williams & Wilkins, 2003.

253. Glazier JB, Hughes JM, Maloney JE, West JB. Measurements of capillary dimensions and blood volume in rapidly frozen lungs. J Appl Physiol 1969; 26:65–76.

254. Matamis D, Lemaire F, Harf A, et al. Redistribution of pulmonary blood flow induced by positive end-expiratory pressure and dopamine infusion in acute respiratory failure. Am Rev Respir Dis 1984; 129:39–44.

255. Cujec B, Polasek P, Mayers I, Johnson D. Positive end-expiratory pressure increases the right-to-left shunt in mechanically ventilated patients with patent foramen ovale. Ann Intern Med 1993; 119:887–94.

256. Berendes E, Lippert G, Loick HM, Brussel T. Effects of positive end-expiratory pressure ventilation on splanchnic oxygenation in humans. J Cardiothorac Vasc Anesth 1996; 10:598–602.

257. Spragg RG, Lewis JF, Walmrath HD, et al. Effect of recombinant surfactant protein C–based surfactant on the acute respiratory distress syndrome. New Engl J Med 2004; 351:884–92.

258. Taylor RW, Zimmerman JL, Dellinger RP, et al. Low-dose inhaled nitric oxide in patients with acute lung injury: A randomized, controlled trial. JAMA 2004; 291:1603–9.

259. Gattinoni L, Tognoni G, Pesenti A, et al. Effect of prone positioning on the survival of patients with acute respiratory failure. New Engl J Med 2001; 345:568–73.

260. Guerin C, Gaillard S, Lemasson S, et al. Effects of systematic prone positioning in hypoxemic acute respiratory failure: A randomized, controlled trial. JAMA 2004; 292:2379–87.

261. Ketoconazole for early treatment of acute lung injury and acute respiratory distress syndrome: A randomized, controlled trial. The ARDS Network. JAMA 2000; 283:1995–2002.

262. Zeiher BG, Artigas A, Vincent JL, et al. Neutrophil elastase inhibition in acute lung injury: Results of the STRIVE study. Crit Care Med 2004; 32:1695–1702.

263. Torres A, Reyes A, Roca J, et al. Ventilation-perfusion mismatching in chronic obstructive pulmonary disease during ventilator weaning. Am Rev Respir Dis 1989; 140:1246–50.

264. Kellog RH. Central chemical regulation of respiration. In: Fenn WO, Rahn H, editors. Handbook of physiology. Washington: American Physiological Society, 1964: 513.

265. Costello R, Deegan P, Fitzpatrick M, McNicholas WT. Reversible hypercapnia in chronic obstructive pulmonary disease: A distinct pattern of respiratory failure with a favorable prognosis. Am J Med 1997; 102:239–44.

266. Moser KM, Luchsinger PC, Adamson JS, et al. Respiratory stimulation with intravenous doxapram in respiratory failure: A double-blind co-operative study. New Engl J Med 1973; 288:427–31.

267. Rafferty GF, Lou HM, Polkey MI, et al. Effect of hypercapnia on maximal voluntary ventilation and diaphragm fatigue in normal humans. Am J Respir Crit Care Med 1999; 160:1567–71.

268. Juan G, Calverley P, Talamo C, et al. Effect of carbon dioxide on diaphragmatic function in human beings. New Engl J Med 1984; 310:874–9.

269. Mador MJ, Wendel T, Kufel TJ. Effect of acute hypercapnia on diaphragmatic and limb muscle contractility. Am J Respir Crit Care Med 1997; 155:1590–5.

270. Jeffrey AA, Warren PM, Flenley DC. Acute hypercapnic respiratory failure in patients with chronic obstructive lung disease: Risk factors and use of guidelines for management. Thorax 1992; 47:34–40.

271. Plant PK, Owen JL, Elliott MW. Early use of non-invasive ventilation for acute exacerbations of chronic obstructive pulmonary disease on general respiratory wards: A multicentre randomised, controlled trial. Lancet 2000; 355:1931–5.

272. Laghi F, Karamchandani K, Tobin MJ. Influence of ventilator settings in determining respiratory frequency during mechanical ventilation. Am J Respir Crit Care Med 1999; 160:1766–70.

273. Laghi F, Segal J, Choe WK, Tobin MJ. Effect of imposed inflation time on respiratory frequency and hyperinflation in patients with chronic obstructive pulmonary disease. Am J Respir Crit Care Med 2001; 163:1365–70.

274. Ardissino D, De Servi S, Falcone C, et al. Role of hypocapnic alkalosis in hyperventilation-induced coronary artery spasm in variant angina. Am J Cardiol 1987; 59:707–9.

275. Rotheram EBJr, Safar P, Robin E. CNS disorder during mechanical ventilation in chronic pulmonary disease. JAMA 1964; 189:993–6.

276. Seamonds B, Towfighi J, Arvan DA. Determination of ionized calcium in serum by use of an Ion-selective electrode: I. Determination of normal values under physiologic conditions, with comments on the effects of food ingestion and hyperventilation. Clin Chem 1972; 18:155–60.

277. Hafen G, Laux-End R, Truttmann AC, et al. Plasma ionized magnesium during acute hyperventilation in humans. Clin Sci (Lond) 1996; 91:347–51.

278. Somjen GG, Allen BW, Balestrino M, Aitken PG. Pathophysiology of pH and Ca^{2+} in bloodstream and brain. Can J Physiol Pharmacol 1987; 65:1078–85.

279. Brimioulle S, Kahn RJ. Effects of metabolic alkalosis on pulmonary gas exchange. Am Rev Respir Dis 1990; 141:1185–9.

280. Halpern P, Neufeld MY, Sade K, et al. Middle cerebral artery flow velocity decreases and electroencephalogram (EEG) changes occur as acute hypercapnia reverses. Intensive Care Med 2003; 29:1650–5.

281. Dripps RD. The immediate decrease in blood pressure seen at the conclusion of cyclopropane anesthesia: "Cyclopropane shock." Anesthesiology 1947; 8:35.

282. Buckley JJ, Van Bergen FH, Dobkin AB, et al. Postanesthetic hypotension following cyclopropane: Its relationship to hypercapnia. Anesthesiology 1954; 14:226–37.

283. Brown EB, Miller FA. Ventricular fibrillation following a rapid fall in alveolar carbon dioxide concentration. Am J Physiol 1952; 169:56–60.

284. Sealy WC, Young WG, Harris JS. Studies on cardiac arrest: the relationship of hypercapnia to ventricular fibrillation. J Thorac Surg 1954; 28:447–62.

285. Prys-Roberts C, Kelman GR, Nunn JF. Determination of the in vivo carbon dioxide titration curve of anaesthetized man. Br J Anaesth 1966; 38:500–9.

286. Ayres SM, Grace WJ. Inappropriate ventilation and hypoxemia as causes of cardiac arrhythmias: The control of arrhythmias without antiarrhythmic drugs. Am J Med 1969; 46:495–505.

287. Hamm LL, Dubose TD. Acid-base and electrolyte disorders: A companion to Brenner & Rector's the kidney. Philadelphia: Saunders, 2002.

288. O'Donohue WJ Jr. National survey of the usage of lung expansion modalities for the prevention and treatment of postoperative atelectasis following abdominal and thoracic surgery. Chest 1985; 87:76–80.

289. Gosselink R, Schrever K, Cops P, et al. Incentive spirometry does not enhance recovery after thoracic surgery. Crit Care Med 2000; 28:679–83.

290. Celli BR, Rodriguez KS, Snider GL. A controlled trial of intermittent positive pressure breathing, incentive spirometry, and deep breathing exercises in preventing pulmonary complications after abdominal surgery. Am Rev Respir Dis 1984; 130:12–5.

291. Squadrone V, Coha M, Cerutti E, et al. Continuous positive airway pressure for treatment of postoperative hypoxemia: A randomized, controlled trial. JAMA 2005; 293:589–95.

292. Claffey LP, Phelan DM. A complication of cricothyroid "minitracheostomy"—Oesophageal perforation. Intensive Care Med 1989; 15:140–1.

293. Charnley RM, Verma R. Inhalation of a minitracheotomy tube. Intensive Care Med 1986; 12:108–9.

294. Shackford SR, Virgilio RW, Peters RM. Selective use of ventilator therapy in flail chest injury. J Thorac Cardiovasc Surg 1981; 81:194–201.

295. Gunduz M, Unlugenc H, Ozalevli M, et al. A comparative study of continuous positive airway pressure (CPAP) and intermittent positive pressure ventilation (IPPV) in patients with flail chest. Emerg Med J 2005; 22:325–9.

296. Jubran A, Mathru M, Dries D, Tobin MJ. Continuous recordings of mixed venous oxygen saturation during weaning from mechanical ventilation and the ramifications thereof. Am J Respir Crit Care Med 1998; 158:1763–9.

297. Pohman A, O'Connor M, Olson DLA, et al. Sedation with propofol lowers $\dot{V}_{O_2}$ in critically ill patients. Am J Respir Crit Care Med 1995;151:A325

298. Marik PE, Kaufman D. The effects of neuromuscular paralysis on systemic and splanchnic oxygen utilization in mechanically ventilated patients. Chest 1996; 109:1038–42.

299. Leung P, Jubran A, Tobin MJ. Comparison of assisted ventilator modes on triggering, patient effort, and dyspnea. Am J Respir Crit Care Med 1997; 155:1940–8.

300. Laghi F. Assessment of respiratory output in mechanically ventilated patients. Respir Care Clin North Am 2005; 11:173–99.

301. Keenan SP, Sinuff T, Cook DJ, Hill NS. Which patients with acute exacerbation of chronic obstructive pulmonary disease benefit from noninvasive positive-pressure ventilation? A systematic review of the literature. Ann Intern Med 2003; 138:861–70.

302. Brochard L, Mancebo J, Wysocki M, et al. Noninvasive ventilation for acute exacerbations of chronic obstructive pulmonary disease. New Engl J Med 1995; 333:817–22.

303. Kramer N, Meyer TJ, Meharg J, et al. Randomized, prospective trial of noninvasive positive pressure ventilation in acute respiratory failure. Am J Respir Crit Care Med 1995; 151:1799–1806.

304. Martin TJ, Hovis JD, Costantino JP, et al. A randomized, prospective evaluation of noninvasive ventilation for acute respiratory failure. Am J Respir Crit Care Med 2000; 161:807–13.

305. Girou E, Brun-Buisson C, Taille S, et al. Secular trends in nosocomial infections and mortality associated with noninvasive ventilation in patients with exacerbation of COPD and pulmonary edema. JAMA 2003; 290:2985–91.

306. Nava S, Carbone G, DiBattista N, et al. Noninvasive ventilation in cardiogenic pulmonary edema: A multicenter randomized trial. Am J Respir Crit Care Med 2003; 168:1432–7.

307. Hilbert G, Gruson D, Vargas F, et al. Noninvasive ventilation in immunosuppressed patients with pulmonary infiltrates, fever, and acute respiratory failure. New Engl J Med 2001; 344:481–7.

308. Antonelli M, Conti G, Bufi M, et al. Noninvasive ventilation for treatment of acute respiratory failure in patients undergoing solid organ transplantation: A randomized trial. JAMA 2000; 283:235–41.

309. Sinuff T, Cook DJ, Randall J, Allen CJ. Evaluation of a practice guideline for noninvasive positive-pressure ventilation for acute respiratory failure. Chest 2003; 123:2062–73.

310. Hill NS. Practice guidelines for noninvasive positive-pressure ventilation: Help or hindrance? Chest 2003; 123:1784–6.

311. Feinstein AR. The blame-X syndrome: Problems and lessons in nosology, spectrum, and etiology. J Clin Epidemiol 2001; 54: 433–9.

312. Porter R. The greatest benefit to mankind: A medical history of humanity. New York: Norton, 1998.

313. Tobin MJ. ATS centenary: Four-century prologue to a century of progress. Am J Respir Crit Care Med 2004; 169:891–3.

314. Scadding JG. Health and disease: What can medicine do for philosophy? J Med Ethics 1988; 14:118–24.

315. Bernard GR, Artigas A, Brigham KL, et al. The American-European Consensus Conference on ARDS: Definitions, mechanisms, relevant outcomes, and clinical trial coordination. Am J Respir Crit Care Med 1994; 149:818–24.

316. Magee B. The story of philosophy. London: Dorling Kindersley, 1998.

317. Scadding JG. Essentialism and nominalism in medicine: Logic of diagnosis in disease terminology. Lancet 1996; 348:594–6.

318. Scadding JG. The semantics of medical diagnosis. Int J Biomed Comput 1972; 3:83–90.

319. Popper KR. The open society and its enemies. London: Routledge & Kegan Paul, 1945.

320. Popper KR. The logic of scientific discovery. New York: Harper and Row, 1959.

321. Scadding JG. Principles of definition in medicine with special reference to chronic bronchitis and emphysema. Lancet 1959; 1:323–5.

322. Magee B. The criterion of demarcation between what is and what is not science. Glasgow: Popper, Fontana/Collins, 1973: 35–55.

323. Scadding JG. Diagnosis: The clinician and the computer. Lancet 1967; 2:877–82.

324. Gross NJ. What is this thing called love?—Or, defining asthma. Am Rev Respir Dis 1980; 121:203–4.

325. Scadding JG. Meaning of diagnostic terms in bronchopulmonary disease. Br Med J 1963; 5370:1425–30.

326. Saydain G, Islam A, Afessa B, et al. Outcome of patients with idiopathic pulmonary fibrosis admitted to the intensive care unit. Am J Respir Crit Care Med 2002; 166:839–42.

327. Fumeaux T, Rothmeier C, Jolliet P. Outcome of mechanical ventilation for acute respiratory failure in patients with pulmonary fibrosis. Intensive Care Med 2001; 27: 1868–74.

328. Polanyi M. Personal knowledge: Towards a post-critical philosophy. Chicago: University of Chicago Press, 1958.

PART IV
CONVENTIONAL METHODS OF VENTILATORY SUPPORT

Chapter 6
SETTING THE VENTILATOR

STEVE HOLETS
ROLF D. HUBMAYR

The choice of ventilator settings should be guided by clearly defined therapeutic end points. In most instances, the primary goal of mechanical ventilation is to correct abnormalities in arterial blood-gas tensions. In most patients, this is ac-complished easily by adjusting the minute volume to correct hypercapnia and by treating hypoxemia with oxygen (O_2) supplementation. Because the volume, frequency, and timing of gas delivered to the lungs have important disease-specific effects on cardiovascular and respiratory systems functions, however, the physician must avoid simply managing the blood-gas tensions of the ventilator-dependent patient. After a brief review of the capabilities of modern ventilators, this chapter discusses the mechanical determinants of patient-ventilator interactions and defines therapeutic end points in common respiratory failure syndromes. These sections provide background for the major thrust of the chapter, which is to detail the physiologic consequences of positive-pressure ventilation and to develop recommendations for ventilator settings in various disease states based on this knowledge.

Capabilities of Modern Ventilators

The incorporation of microprocessors into ventilator technology has made it possible to program ventilators to deliver gas with virtually any pressure or flow profile. Significant advances have been made in producing machines that are more responsive to changes in patient ventilatory demands, and most full-service mechanical ventilators display diagnostic information contained in airway pressure (Paw), volume (V), and flow ($\dot{V}$) waveforms. Because of these added capabilities, the practitioner is being challenged with a staggering array of descriptive acronyms for so-called new modes of ventilation. To avoid unnecessary confusion, it is useful not to focus on specific modes for the moment but rather to consider three general aspects of ventilator management: (1) the choice of inspired-gas composition, (2) the means to ensure the machine's sensing of the patient's demand, and (3) the definition of the machine's mechanical output.

CHOICE OF INSPIRED-GAS COMPOSITION

Practically speaking, decisions regarding the composition of inspired gas concern only the O_2 concentration (see Hypoxic Respiratory Failure below). While there may be occasions in which the care provider considers supplementing the inspired gas with nitric oxide, the efficacy of nitric oxide therapy for most forms of hypoxic respiratory failure remains to be established. There has been growing interest in the biologic effects of hypercapnia on gas exchange, vascular barrier properties, and innate immunity.[1-9] Therapeutic hypercapnia, that is, the deliberate supplementation of inspired gas with carbon dioxide (CO_2), however, cannot be recommended at this point in time. On extremely rare occasions, it may be appropriate to use a helium-oxygen mixture[10,11] in an attempt to lower the flow resistance across a lesion in the distal trachea or main-stem bronchi, and there has been some interest in the use of helium in asthma. Currently, these approaches must be considered experimental.

MACHINE'S SENSING OF PATIENT'S DEMAND (VENTILATOR TRIGGERING)

Ideally, a mechanical ventilator should adjust not only its rate but also its instantaneous mechanical output in response to changing patient demands. Conventional modes of ventilation cannot do so but rather execute a predefined pressure or flow program after an effort has been sensed.

Controlled mechanical ventilation refers to a mode during which rate, tidal volume (V_T), inspiratory-to-expiratory timing (I:E ratio), and inspiratory flow profile are determined entirely by machine settings and can be altered by neither the rate nor the amplitude of the patient's effort. Occasionally, investigators refer to ventilation as "controlled" when spontaneous respiratory muscle activity has been abolished by mechanical hyperventilation or by pharmacological means (e.g., sedation and neuromuscular blockade).

Assist-control ventilation (ACV) gives the patient the option of initiating additional machine breaths when the rate, set by the physician, is insufficient to meet the patient's rate demand. ACV differs from intermittent mandatory ventilation (IMV) in that all delivered breaths are either volume- or pressure-preset depending on the choice of primary mode. The ACV feature has lured many physicians into the erroneous assumption that the primary machine rate setting is unimportant (see Hypoxic Respiratory Failure: Respiratory Rate, below).

Traditionally, machine algorithms for detecting patient effort have keyed on the airway pressure signal.[12] Because the inspiratory port of ventilators is closed during machine expiration, any inspiratory effort that is initiated near relaxation volume (Vrel) causes a fall in Paw. When Paw reaches a predefined trigger threshold (usually set 1–2 cmH$_2$O below the end-expiratory pressure setting), the machine switches from expiration to inspiration. In the presence of dynamic hyperinflation, the inspiratory muscles must generate considerably more pressure than the set airway trigger pressure before a machine breath is delivered[13] (see Obstructive Lung Diseases, below).

Particularly in older ventilator models and in less sophisticated portable machines intended for home use, it used to be common to find delays of up to 0.5 second between the onset of inspiratory muscle activity and machine response. In most ventilators used nowadays, such delays are less than 100 ms.[14] Sensing delays are common when the Paw is monitored in the machine rather than near the patient-ventilator interphase. In the former case, the ventilator tubing acts as a capacitor, delaying the transmission of pressure from the intrathoracic airway to the pressure transducer. Additional delays can be attributed to dynamic hyperinflation and physical constraints on the opening and closing of demands valves. Considering that most ventilator-dependent patients generate between 4 and 8 cmH$_2$O pressure in 100 ms,[12,15] delays can cause significant effort expenditure and discomfort. More important, patients may terminate seemingly ineffective inspiratory efforts prematurely only to initiate another effort of greater amplitude shortly thereafter. This leads to discrepancies between patient and machine rate.[16] Discrepancies are seen often in weak or heavily sedated patients with severe hyperinflation and high intrinsic respiratory rates.[16,17]

Flow-triggering algorithms are alternatives or adjuncts to Paw-based triggering. During "flow triggering," a base flow of gas is being delivered to the patient during the expiratory as well as the inspiratory phases of the machine cycle.[12] Unless the patient makes an inspiratory effort, gas bypasses the endotracheal tube and is discarded through the expiratory machine port. In the absence of patient effort, expiratory flow is equal to inspiratory base flow. In the presence of an inspiratory effort, gas enters the patient's lungs and is thereby diverted from the expiratory machine port. A discrepancy between inspiratory and expiratory base flow is sensed, and the ventilator switches phase. Because "flow triggering" alleviates the need to rarefy gas against an occluded demand valve, initially it was considered superior to pressure-based trigger algorithms.[12,18] Since many new-generation ventilators have combined pressure and flow sensing capabilities, these distinctions may no longer apply.

OPTIONS FOR DEFINING THE MACHINE'S MECHANICAL OUTPUT

The mode of mechanical ventilation often refers to the shape of the inspiratory pressure or flow profile and determines whether a patient can augment V_T or rate through his or her own efforts.

VOLUME-PRESET MODE

In conventional volume-preset mode, each machine breath is delivered with the same predefined inspiratory flow-time profile. Because the area under a flow-time curve defines volume, V_T remains fixed and is uninfluenced by the patient's effort. Volume-preset ventilation with constant (squarewave) or decelerating inspiratory flow is the most widely used breath-delivery mode. Breath delivery with flows that decrease with increasing lung volume are effective in reducing peak Paw. It is not clear, however, whether they protect the lungs from overdistension injury any more than squarewave flow profiles.

The mechanical output of a ventilator operating in the volume-preset mode is uniquely defined by four settings: (1) the shape of the inspiratory flow profile, (2) V_T, (3) machine rate, and (4) a timing variable in the form of either the I:E ratio, the duty cycle (T_I/T_{TOT}), or the inspiratory time (T_I). In some ventilators, timing is set indirectly through the choice of peak or mean inspiratory flow (V_T/T_I). Figure 6-1 illustrates the relationships among these and other breathing-pattern parameters of significance.

PRESSURE-PRESET MODE

During pressure-preset ventilation, the ventilator applies a predefined target pressure to the endotracheal tube during inspiration. The resulting V_T and inspiratory flow profile varies with the impedance of the respiratory system and with the strength and duration of the patient's inspiratory efforts. Therefore, when the lungs or chest wall become stiff, airway resistance increases, the patient's own inspiratory

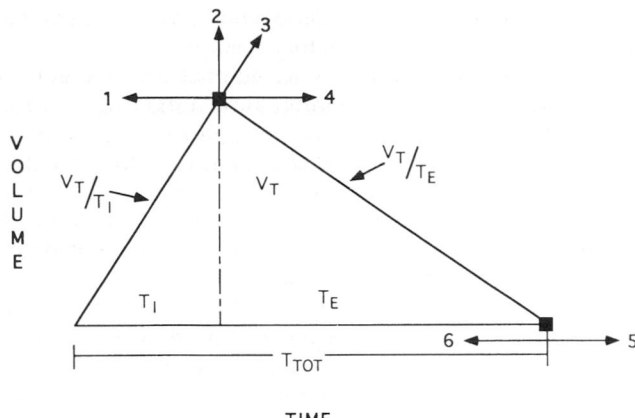

TIME

FIGURE 6-1 Idealized spirogram of a breath delivered during volume-preset mechanical ventilation. Examples 1 through 6 indicate specific changes in ventilator settings and illustrate the consequences on flow and timing variable. (For abbreviations, see Table 6-1.) (1) Increasing mean inspiratory flow (V_T/T_I) at a constant machine rate setting results in a reduced I:E ratio and vice versa. T_I, T_I/T_{TOT}, and mean expiratory flow (V_T/T_E) decline. (2) Increasing V_T at constant T_I/T_{TOT} or I:E setting increases mean inspiratory flow and requires an increase in mean expiratory flow. Remember that mean inspiratory flow equals peak inspiratory flow when delivery modes with constant squarewave flow profiles are used. (3) Increasing V_T at a constant mean inspiratory flow setting increases T_I, T_I/T_{TOT}, I:E ratio, and mean expiratory flow. (4) Decreasing mean inspiratory flow at a constant machine rate setting results in an increase in the I:E ratio and vice versa. T_I, T_I/T_{TOT}), and mean expiratory flow rise. (5) Reducing the machine backup rate (f_M) at a fixed I:E ratio or T_I/T_{TOT} setting always prolongs T_I and lowers mean inspiratory flow. The timing effects of reducing f_M at a fixed inspiratory-flow setting cannot be predicted without knowledge of the patient's actual trigger rate. (6) Increasing f_M at a fixed I:E ratio or T_I/T_{TOT} setting always raises inspiratory flow. The timing effects of increasing f_M at a fixed inspiratory-flow setting cannot be predicted without knowledge of the patient's actual trigger rate.

TABLE 6-1 List of Abbreviations

τ	Time constant
AC	Assist-control mode
ARDS	Adult respiratory distress syndrome
CMV	Controlled mechanical ventilation
CPAP	Continuous positive airway pressure
Ers	Elastance of the respiratory system
Edi	Electromyographic tracing of the diaphragm
F	Force
f_A	Actual breathing rate
FEF_{25-75}	Forced expiratory flow in the mid vital capacity range
FI_{O_2}	Fractional inspired oxygen concentration
f_M	Machine backup rate
I:E ratio	Inspiratory-to-expiratory time ratio
IMV	Intermittent mandatory ventilation
MMV	Mandatory minute ventilation
Pa_{CO_2}	Arterial CO_2 tension
Pa_{O_2}	Arterial O_2 tension
Paw	Airway pressure
PCV	Pressure-controlled ventilation
PEEP	Positive end-expiratory pressure
$PEEP_E$	Extrinsic positive end-expiratory pressure
$PEEP_I$	Intrinsic positive end-expiratory pressure
Pel	Elastic recoil pressure
P_L	Transpulmonary pressure
Pmus	Inflation pressure exerted by inspiratory muscles
Pres	Resistive pressure
Prs	Recoil of respiratory system
PSV	Pressure support ventilation
SIMV	Synchronized intermittent mandatory ventilation
T_E	Expiratory time
T_I	Inspiratory time
T_I/T_{TOT}	Duty cycle
T_{TOT}	Total cycle time
TLC	Total lung capacity
$\dot{V}$	Flow
$\dot{V}/\dot{Q}$	Ventilation-perfusion ratio
$\dot{V}_{CO_2}$	Volume of CO_2 produced in liters per minute
$\dot{V}_E$	Minute ventilation
$\dot{V}_I$	Mean inspiratory flow
V(t)	Instantaneous lung volume
$\dot{V}_E/V_T$	Dead-space-to-tidal-volume ratio
Vee	Volume of lungs at end expiration
Vrel	Relaxation volume
V_T/T_E	Mean expiratory flow
V_T/T_I	Mean inspiratory flow
V_T	Tidal volume
Vtrapped	Volume of gas remaining in the elastic element at the beginning of a new machine inflation
Wel	Elastic work

efforts decline, or T_I decreases, V_T decreases. An increase in respiratory system impedance can lead to a dangerous fall in minute ventilation ($\dot{V}_E$), hypoxemia, and CO_2 retention, but in contrast to volume-preset modes, it does not predispose the patient to an increased risk of barotrauma. On the other hand, pressure-preset modes are no safeguard against ventilator-induced lung injury because large fluctuations in respiratory impedance or patient effort would result in large V_T fluctuations directly undermining the primary objective of lung-protective mechanical ventilation (see discussion of ventilator management in hypoxic respiratory failure).

Pressure-support ventilation (PSV) and pressure-controlled ventilation (PCV) are the most widely used forms of pressure-preset ventilation. In contrast to PCV, PSV requires the patient's effort before a machine breath is delivered. PSV therefore is not suitable for the management of patients with central apneas. During PCV, the physician sets the machine rate, the T_I, and thus the I:E ratio. In PSV, phase switching is linked to inspiratory flow, which, in turn, depends on the impedance of the respiratory system,

as well as on the timing and magnitude of inspiratory muscle pressure output.[14,19]

PSV is a popular weaning mode for adults. Its popularity is based on the premise that weaning from mechanical ventilation should be a gradual process and that the work of unassisted breathing through an endotracheal tube is unreasonably high and could lead to respiratory muscle failure in susceptible patients. Actual measurements of pulmonary resistance and work of breathing before and after extubation do not support this reasoning,[20,21] and several large clinical trials have established equivalence between PSV and T-piece weaning (unassisted breathing from a bias-flow circuit).[22–24] In the PSV mode, a target pressure is applied to the endotracheal tube, which augments the inflation pressure exerted by the inspiratory muscles (Pmus) on the respiratory system. When inspiratory muscles cease to contract and Pmus falls, inspiratory flow (a ventilator-sensed variable) declines, and the machine switches to expiration. Early PSV modules were designed to generate pressure ramps (squarewave inflation pressure) and had relatively rigid flow-based, off-switch criteria. More recent versions of PSV afford control over the rate of rise in inspiratory pressure and the flow threshold at which inspiration is teminated.[14,19,25]

SYNCHRONIZED INTERMITTENT MANDATORY VENTILATION (SIMV)

During SIMV, a specified number of usually volume-preset breaths are delivered every minute. In addition, the patient is free to breathe spontaneously between machine breaths from a reservoir or to take breaths augmented with PSV. Some ventilators allow the operator to choose between volume- and pressure-preset mandatory breaths. Unless the patient fails to breathe spontaneously, machine breaths are delivered only after the ventilator has recognized the patient's effort; that is, ventilator and respiratory muscle activities are "synchronized." Because nowadays all IMV circuits are synchronized, the terms *IMV* and *SIMV* are used interchangeably. Although SIMV remains a viable and popular mode of mechanical ventilation, compared with the alternatives, PSV and T piece, it has clearly proven inferior as a weaning modality.[22,23,26,27] Moreover, the care provider needs to be aware of certain pitfalls when using IMV. Even a small number of volume-preset IMV breaths per minute may make the blood-gas tensions look acceptable in patients who otherwise meet criteria for respiratory failure. One should suspect this in patients with small spontaneous V_T (≤ 3 ml/kg of body weight), in those with 30 or more inspiratory efforts per minute regardless of whether they trigger a machine breath, and when dyspnea and thoracoabdominal paradox indicate a heightened respiratory effort. One reason that IMV remains popular is because it silences apnea alarms by masking PSV-induced respiratory dysrythmias, which are common in sleeping and obtunded patients.[28,29]

DUAL-CONTROL AND ADVANCED CLOSED-LOOP MODES

Many new-generation mechanical ventilators feature modes with closed-loop feedback control of both pressure and volume.[30,31] While a detailed description of the operating principles of every new mode is beyond the scope of this chapter, it is important to understand the rationale behind dual-control modes and some of their general operating characteristics. The idea behind dual-control modes is the meeting of a ventilation target while maintaining low inflation pressures. To this end, ventilator output is adjusted based on volume, flow, and pressure feedback. This may occur within each machine cycle or gradually from one cycle to the next. Modes that adjust output within each cycle execute a predetermined pressure-time program as long as the desired V_T is reached. When the V_T target is not reached, inspiration continues at a preselected inspiratory flow rate (volume-limited) until the target volume is attained. *Volume-assured pressure support* and *pressure augmentation* are examples of such modes.[32] Breath-to-breath dual-control modes are pressure-limited and time- or flow-cycled. Ventilator output is derived from the pressure-volume relationship of the preceding breath and is adjusted within predefined pressure limits to maintain the target V_T. *Pressure-regulated volume control* (PRVC), *volume control+*, *auto-flow*, *adaptive pressure ventilation*, *volume support*, and *variable pressure support* are examples of breath-to-breath control modes. There is no evidence that the use of dual-control modes improves patient outcomes.[33] Moreover, there is a conceptual problem insofar as less complex modes already safeguard against hypoventilation, whereas dual-control modes do little to protect the patient from a potentially harmful increase in the regulated variable, that is, large V_T–mediated lung injury.[34,35]

Neurally adjusted ventilatory assistance (NAVA) and *proportional-assist ventilation* (PAV)[36–38] are the most complex and arguably the most promising closed-loop ventilation modes. At the time of this writing, neither mode is available in the United States. During NAVA, the diaphragm's electrical activity is recorded with an esophageal probe, and the signal is conditioned and transposed into a positive airway pressure output. NAVA is undergoing early clinical testing at this time and must be considered experimental. PAV, on the other hand, is available commercially in Canada and Europe, but it has not achieved mainstream status.[36,37] During PAV, the ventilator derives its mechanical output from continuously monitored Paw, V, and V̇ information, which, in turn, reflects Pmus. The operating principles of PAV will be easier to understand after a review of patient-ventilator interactions (see below).

The Mechanical Determinants of Patient-Ventilator Interactions

INSPIRATORY MECHANICS

It is useful to think of patient-ventilator interactions in terms of a mechanical or electrical analog system consisting of a resistive element (resistor) and an elastic element (capacitor) in series. The forcing function is defined by the pressure or flow "program" that is executed by the mechanical ventilator.

In Fig. 6-2, a piston pump (the mechanical ventilator) is attached to a rigid tube (the resistive element) and a balloon (the elastic element). An in-series mechanical arrangement means that at any time t, the pressure that is applied to the tube inlet Pi(t) (near the attachment to the ventilator) is equal to the sum of two pressures, an elastic pressure Pel(t) and a resistive pressure Pres(t):

$$Pi(t) = Pel(t) + Pres(t) \qquad (1)$$

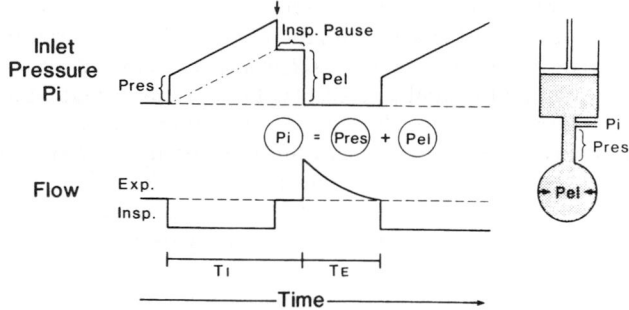

FIGURE 6-2 Components of inlet pressure. The model of the respiratory system at right consists of a resistive element (straight tube) and an elastic element (balloon) connected to a ventilator (piston). During inflation of the model with constant flow (*lower panel*), there is a stepwise increase inlet pressure (Pi) that equals the loss of pressure across the resistive element (Pres) (*upper panel*). Thereafter, Pi increases linearly and reflects the mechanical properties of the elastic element (Pell). Pi is the sum of Pres and Pel. At end inspiration, when flow has ceased (Insp. Pause), Pi decreases by an amount equal to Pres; Pi equals Pel during Insp. Pause. T_I, inspiratory time; T_E, expiratory time. (*Used, with permission, from Hubmayr et al: Crit Care Med 18:103–13, 1990.*)

The tube outlet pressure at the junction with the balloon is equal to the pressure inside the balloon, that is, Pel. Pres is the difference in pressure between the tube inlet and the tube outlet. Assuming linear-system behavior, the inlet pressure-time profile can be computed for any piston stroke volume (Vstroke) and flow ($\dot{V}$) setting, provided the resistive properties of the tube (R) and the elastic properties of the balloon (E) are known:

$$Pi(t) = EV(t) + R\dot{V}(t) \tag{2}$$

The elastance (E) is a measure of balloon stiffness and is equal to the ratio of Pel and Vstroke (assuming 0 volume and pressure at the beginning of balloon inflation). Therefore, Pel(t) in Eq. (1) can be replaced with EV(t) in Eq. (2). Because Ohm's law states that the tube resistance (R) is equal to the ratio of Pres and $\dot{V}$, Pres(t) in Eq. (1) can be replaced with the product $R\dot{V}(t)$ in Eq. (2).

Equations (1) and (2) are based on the equation of motion,[39] which describes the force (F) that must be applied to a mass (M) in order to move it a certain distance (d) at a rate dd/dt against a spring (elastic) load:

$$F(t) = kd(t) + k'(dd/dt)(t) + k''[d(dd/dt)/dt](t) \tag{3}$$

where   k = stiffness of the spring (analogous to E)
        k' = frictional resistance between mass and supporting surface (analogous to R)
        k'' = inertance, which is proportional to mass

The first and second derivatives of *d* (analogous to volume) represent the velocity (dd/dt, analogous to flow) and the acceleration [$d(dd/dt)/dt$] of the mass at time *t*, respectively. As long as the mass of the moving parts in the model of Fig. 6-2[40] is small, any inertive-pressure component that

is dissipated during the acceleration of gas at the beginning of the pump instroke can be ignored. Therefore, the respiratory analog of the equation of motion [Eqs. (1) and (2)] considers only elastic and resistive pressures.

Consider the Pi-time profile of a tube-balloon system with resistance of 10 cmH$_2$O × liter/s and an elastance of 10 cmH$_2$O when the piston pump is programmed to deliver a volume of 0.5 liter with a constant (squarewave) flow of 0.5 liter/s. Because flow and R remain constant throughout inflation, Pres is constant at 5 cmH$_2$O and accounts for the initial step change in inlet pressure at the beginning of inflation. As gas enters the balloon, Pi increases further and reaches a value of 10 cmH$_2$O at end inflation. At that instant, the tube is occluded (end-inflation hold), causing Pi to drop by an amount equal to Pres (as flow returns to 0). The end-inflation hold pressure is equal to Pel at that volume. Its value of 5 cmH$_2$O is equal to the product of piston stroke volume (0.5 liter) and elastance (10 cmH$_2$O/liter), as follows from Eqs. (1) and (2). Subtracting Pres from Pi(*t*) yields the Pel per time course during inflation. Pel increases linearly with time and volume. Its rate of rise ($dPel/dt$) parallels that of Pi and is determined by E and the flow setting of the piston[41]:

$$E \times \dot{V} = (dp/dV) \times (dV/dt) = dP/dt \tag{4}$$

While changes in inspiratory flow result in proportional changes in $dPel/dt$, flow has no effect on peak Pel, provided that stroke volume and thus peak lung volume are held constant. This is in contrast to peak Pi, which reflects flow-dependent changes in Pres, as well as change in Pel, at end inflation. The relevance of this important property of linear single-compartment systems will become apparent later when the relationships between ventilator settings and barotrauma (balloon yield stress) are discussed (see Hypoxic Respiratory Failure, below).

EXPIRATORY MECHANICS

In mechanically ventilated subjects, expiration is usually a passive process that is driven by the elastic recoil (Pel) of the respiratory system. Assuming linear pressure-volume and pressure-flow relationships, the instantaneous expiratory flow [$\dot{V}exp(t)$] is given by

$$\dot{V}exp(t) = Pel(t)/R \tag{5}$$

Because Pel(*t*) is a function of E and of the instantaneous lung volume [V(*t*)], Eq. (5) can be rewritten as

$$\dot{V}exp(t) = E \times V(t)/R = V(t)/R \times C \tag{6}$$

where C (the compliance of the respiratory system) is simply the inverse of the elastance (E). The product of R and C characterizes the time constant (τ) of single-compartment linear systems. The time constant defines the time at which approximately two-thirds of the volume above Vrel has emptied passively. From this it should be clear that patients with increased respiratory system resistances and compliances (e.g., patients with emphysema) are prone to dynamic hyperinflation even if one ignores nonlinear system behavior, such as flow limitation, for the moment.

The volume of gas remaining in the elastic element at the beginning of a new machine inflation (Vtrapped) can be calculated as follows:

$$\text{Vtrapped} = V_T/(e^{TE/\tau} - 1) \qquad (7)$$

In other words, the degree of dynamic hyperinflation is determined by the choice of ventilator settings, specifically mean expiratory flow (V_T/V_E) and the time constant of the respiratory system, which reflects its mechanical constants R and C.[42] These important concepts are expanded on under Obstructive Lung Diseases, below.

LIMITATIONS OF LINEAR SINGLE-COMPARTMENT MODELS

Before linear model principles are applied to the ventilator management of patients, one must be cognizant of the model's limitations. The limitations fall into two general categories: those related to nonlinear respiratory system characteristics and those related to respiratory muscle activation during mechanical ventilation. Sources of nonlinear system behavior include inhomogeneities within the numerous bronchoalveolar compartments (particularly when the lungs are diseased),[43] respiratory system hysteresis from recruitment of alveolar units and time-dependent surface tension phenomena,[44] and phenomena related to dynamic airway collapse and expiratory flow limitation.[45] Coactivation of the respiratory muscles during mechanical ventilation invalidates Eqs. (1) through (7) insofar as they alter the impedance of the respiratory system and change the driving pressure for expiratory flow. If one assumes that the respiratory muscles and the ventilator are arranged in series, then the monitoring of pressure, volume, and flow at the airway opening offers the opportunity to define the magnitude, rate, and duration of respiratory muscle output in mechanically ventilated subjects.[46,47]

Defining Therapeutic Endpoints in Common Respiratory Failure Syndromes

Numerous diseases of cardiopulmonary systems can cause respiratory failure. From a ventilator management perspective, it is useful to group them into those that cause lung failure and those that cause ventilatory pump failure.

The hallmark of lung failure is hypoxemia, which is usually the result of severe ventilation-perfusion mismatch. The hallmark of ventilatory pump failure is hypercapnia. Ventilatory pump failure may be caused by disorders of the central nervous system (CNS), peripheral nerves, or respiratory muscles. It also may accompany diseases of the lungs, such as emphysema, once the ventilatory pump fails to compensate for inefficiencies in pulmonary CO_2 elimination. Two classic examples of hypoxic and hypercapnic

ventilatory failure that require fundamentally different approaches to mechanical ventilation are the acute respiratory distress syndrome (ARDS) and chronic airflow obstruction. The therapeutic goal in ARDS is to raise lung volume in an attempt to reduce shunt by reexpanding collapsed and flooded alveolar units. In contrast, the therapeutic goal in a patient with hypercapnic ventilatory failure from exacerbation of airways obstruction is to reduce dynamic hyperinflation and to protect the respiratory muscles from overuse.

Acute Lung Injury and Hypoxic Respiratory Failure

Acute lung injury (ALI) is a syndrome associated with bilateral pulmonary infiltrates and a gas-exchange impairment severe enough to lower the arterial oxygen tension-to-fractional inspired oxygen concentration ratio (Pa_{O_2}/FI_{O_2}) below 300.[48,49] Heart failure and moderate to severe pre-existing chronic lung disease must be absent. ALI and its more severe form, ARDS, are often complications of systemic illnesses such as sepsis.[50] The impairment on pulmonary gas exchange therefore is accompanied frequently by microcirculatory failure. The general management goal in these disorders is to augment systemic oxygen delivery until the metabolic demands of the organism can be met. This goal requires an integrated approach between cardiovascular and ventilator support.[51]

Ventilator support is often difficult because exceedingly high ventilatory requirements challenge the performance capacity of mechanical ventilators; render patients at risk for barotrauma, ventilator-induced lung injury, and cardiovascular collapse; and often are accompanied by excessive respiratory muscle activity ("fighting the ventilator"). All these conditions on occasion can necessitate heavy sedation and neuromuscular blockade.

FRACTIONAL INSPIRED OXYGEN CONCENTRATION (FI_{O_2})

The two principal means by which the physician can increase Pa_{O_2} in ARDS are to raise the FI_{O_2} and to elevate the volume about which the lungs are being ventilated. The danger inherent in raising FI_{O_2} is oxygen toxicity,[52] whereas manipulating lung and/or V_T may result in ventilator-induced lung injury[53,54] and/or barotrauma.[55] Presented with the choice between two different kinds of adverse reactions, physicians currently tend to be more fearful of mechanical lung injury than of oxygen toxicity. Unfortunately, there are no clinical outcome studies that shed light on the interactions between these two iatrogenic insults. It is common practice to initiate ventilator support with an FI_{O_2} of 1.0 and to ignore the potential for oxygen toxicity during the first few hours of ventilator management. While, generally speaking, the relative and combined risks of oxygen toxicity and overdistension injury of the lungs remain poorly defined, there are instances in which it seems wise to minimize FI_{O_2}, namely, in patients who have received drugs

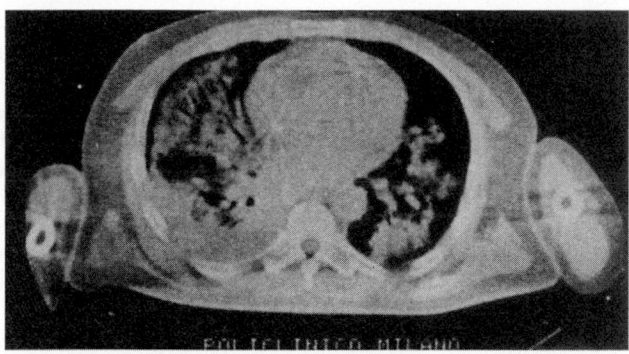

FIGURE 6-3 Computed tomographic (CT) scan of a patient with acute respiratory failure in the supine position. Note the patchy, nonuniform distribution of alveolar edema. (*Used, with permission, from Gattinoni et al: Am Rev Respir Dis 135:730–6, 1987.*)

such as bleomycin or amiodarone, which make the lungs susceptible to reactive O_2 species–mediated injury.[56]

MANIPULATING END-EXPIRATORY LUNG VOLUME

The insults to the lungs of patients with hypoxic respiratory failure are often patchy and result in flooding and closure of dependent airspaces[57,58] (Fig. 6-3). Paraspinal regions of the lung appear most susceptible to atelectasis (lack of aeration) because, in the supine posture, they normally empty close to their residual volume and they receive most of the pulmonary blood flow.[59,60] Therefore, insults to their capillary integrity are most likely to promote alveolar flooding, closure of airspaces by liquid plugs, surfactant inactivation, and gas-absorption atelectasis.[61] The accumulation of airway liquid and foam also generates interfacial forces that are large enough to abrade the epithelial lining of small airways during breathing, causing further injury.[62,63] Ventilator management therefore must be directed toward preventing the repeated opening and closing of unstable lung units, which means reestablishing aeration and ventilation of the flooded lung as much as possible[64] (Fig. 6-4).

There are several ways to achieve this objective: (1) by raising overall lung volume through the judicious use of extrinsic positive end-expiratory pressure (PEEP), (2) by raising lung volume dynamically through "intentional gas trapping," (3) by increasing V_T, and (4) by taking advantage of the local distending forces generated by an actively contracting diaphragm. Any one of these approaches may be combined with so-called recruitment maneuvers, which consist of sustained (up to 40 seconds) inflations of the lungs to high volumes and pressures.[65–69] The preferred and time-tested approach is the judicious use of extrinsic PEEP. All the other means of raising lung volume are comparatively untested, and in the case of V_T, manipulations can be outright harmful.[34–35–70] While there is a strong physiologic rationale to condition (i.e., "open") the lungs with recruitment maneuvers before a PEEP adjustment, most experimental and clinical data indicate that conditioning effects are short-lived.[71–74] Because it is common for patients with ALI to have an increased respiratory rate, a component of dynamic hyperinflation often is present.[75] Despite the short time constant for lung emptying, the use of extrinsic PEEP valves, which in older-generation ventilators represent resistive as well as threshold loads, and ventilator settings that require large mean expiratory flows (V_T/T_E; see Mean Expiratory Flow: The Hidden Variable, below) contribute to dynamic hyperinflation.

Although the experimental evidence in support of PEEP therapy in injured lungs is overwhelming, its specific application to clinical practice remains controversial.[76–79] There is general agreement among experts that patients with injured lungs should be ventilated with PEEP settings greater than 5 cm H_2O.[80] There is no consensus, however, as to whether PEEP should be set arbitrarily to 10, 15, or 20 cm H_2O, whether it should be targeted to specific physiologic endpoints, and if so, what those endpoints and their target thresholds should be. This uncertainty was only amplified by a recent large randomized clinical trial that failed to show an outcome benefit for patients managed with a high-PEEP strategy (mean value 13 cmH_2O) as opposed to a low-PEEP strategy (mean value 8 cmH_2O).[81] While at least one prior clinical trial had demonstrated an impressive survival benefit in patients managed with high PEEP,[34] there were too many covariates, most notably the choice of V_T, to attribute benefit uniquely to the choice of PEEP.

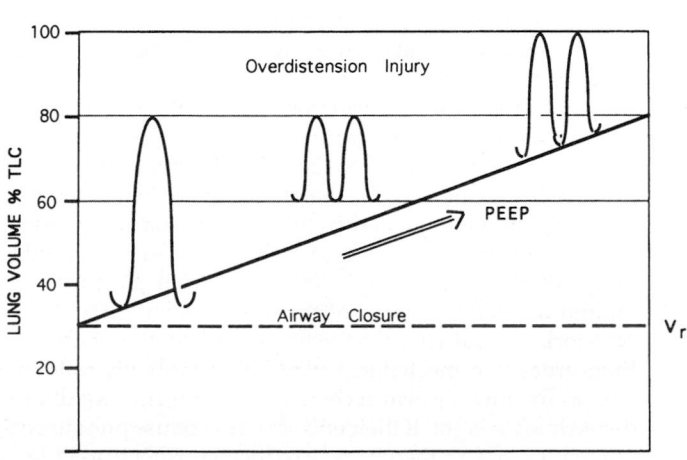

FIGURE 6-4 Schematic representation of the therapeutic endpoints of ventilator management in ARDS. Raising peak lung volume toward TLC increases the risk of barotrauma. Keeping the minimal volume near relaxation volume (Vrel) raises the likelihood of alveolar derecruitment at end expiration and the need to apply large opening pressures in order to recruit collapsed and flooded lung regions during the subsequent breath.

In light of this dilemma in 2005, it seems reasonable to target the initial PEEP settings to a default value of 10 cmH$_2$O. PEEP may be and probably should be increased further if there is evidence of additional lung recruitment at higher PEEP settings. Most physicians assess this by monitoring arterial O$_2$ saturation during step changes in PEEP. A very large step change amounts to a recruitment maneuver. Alternative tools for assessing recruitment responses include (1) measures of regional lung aeration with computed tomography or electrical impedance imaging of the chest,[82–84] (2) measurement of the respiratory system pressure-volume relationships,[85–87] and (3) assessment of within-breath oscillations in arterial O$_2$ tension with indwelling arterial O$_2$ sensors with fast response times.[88] Patients who are likely to recruit in response to PEEP and who may indeed benefit from raising PEEP above 10 cmH$_2$O at the outset are patients with a reduced chest-wall/abdominal compliance[89–91] and patients whose airway and alveolar edema can be redistributed easily.[92] In critically ill patients, the most common conditions associated with reduced chest-wall compliance are obesity, ileus, and ascites.[93,94] The ability to influence the distribution of edema within and between lung regions is greatest in the early stages of inflammation. In the later stages of ARDS, when the inflammatory exudate turns from liquid to a gel, it becomes much harder to "open" a closed airspace. The likelihood of high PEEP causing recruitment is even less once organizing pneumonia, alveolar remodeling, and fibrosis dominate the pathology.[95] One attempt to identify groups of patients who are more or less likely to respond to PEEP has been to classify their insults as indirect versus direct.[89] Indirect insults such as abdominal sepsis are associated with a favorable PEEP response (possibly because their chest-wall compliance is low and their alveolar exudate is liquid), whereas a direct insult, from a microbial lung infection, for example, tends to be PEEP-resistant (airway secretions tend to be viscous, and the alveolar exudate has the consistency of a gel).

To the extent to which many clinicians rely on acute changes in Pa$_{O_2}$ as surrogate endpoints of PEEP management, certain caveats are in order. In critically ill patients with injured lungs, Pa$_{O_2}$ is sensitive to changes in metabolic rate and cardiac output.[96–97] Because patients with injured lungs have $\dot{V}/\dot{Q}$ mismatch as well as shunt, changes in mixed venous oxygen tension, which result from changes in metabolic rate and cardiac output, must influence arterial P$_{O_2}$. Therefore, the P$_{O_2}$ response to step changes in PEEP (and/or recruitment maneuvers) is determined by a net balance between positive and negative effects. Positive effects include (1) reductions in the number of lung units with low $\dot{V}/\dot{Q}$ and shunt as a result of their recruitment, (2) increases in cardiac output driven by the sympathomimetic effects of CO$_2$ retention (the latter invariably accompanies recruitment maneuvers), (3) a fall in oxygen uptake associated with respiratory acidosis.[98,99] Negative effects include (1) increases in low $\dot{V}/\dot{Q}$ and shunt in patients who are PEEP-resistant and in whom the increased alveolar pressure diverts blood away from normal lung toward diseased lung,[100] (2) a fall in cardiac output resulting from volume- and pressure-mediated decreases in venous return,[68] (3) a fall in cardiac output resulting from

volume- and pressure-mediated increases in pulmonary artery pressure and right-ventricular afterload,[101] and (4) increases in systemic oxygen consumption as a behavioral response to increased lung expansion and CO$_2$ retention. The cardiovascular and metabolic confounders of the recruitment response may be deduced from pulse and blood-pressure responses. Alternatively, lung recruitment ought to result in a change in respiratory system mechanics. The clinician, however, should be under no illusion that such change will be large and easy to discern from peak and plateau pressure measurements.[102] This is so because comparisons between states require careful attention to muscle relaxation and the matching of volume and time histories.[103] Finally, because clinicians generally must rely on pulse oximetry as opposed to online P$_{O_2}$ measurements, they must consider the time delays secondary to circulation time and signal processing when assessing the recruitment response.[104]

CHOOSING THE APPROPRIATE TIDAL VOLUME

The choice of V$_T$ is arguably the most important decision a care provider makes when initiating mechanical ventilation. For many years, physicians have chosen ventilator V$_T$ between 10 and 15 cm^3/kg of actual body weight. This recommendation can be traced back to the early days of positive-pressure ventilation, when this therapy was reserved for patients with neuromuscular diseases, such as poliomyelitis. Patients with near-normal lungs feel more comfortable when they are ventilated with two to three times normal V$_T$. In patients with injured lungs, however, a V$_T$ of as little as 10 cm^3/kg of actual body weight can have devastating effects on lung structure, function, and ultimately, outcome.[34,35,105]

To fully appreciate the importance of V$_T$ settings, it is useful to consider distinct physical lung-injury mechanisms: (1) regional overinflation, caused by the application of a local stress or pressure that forces cells and tissues to assume shapes and dimensions that exceed those experienced during even the most strenuous exercise,[54,106] (2) so-called low-volume injury associated with the repeated opening and closure of unstable lung units,[62,63] (3) inactivation of surfactant, on account of large alveolar surface-area oscillations,[107,108] and (4) interdependence mechanisms that raise cell and tissue shear stress between neighboring structures with differing mechanical properties.[109]

The injured lung is particularly susceptible to physical damage because its inspiratory capacity is reduced and its dorsal units tend to get obstructed with liquid plugs.[110] As a result, the greater the V$_T$, the greater is the likelihood that the lung will be damaged by both high- and low-volume injury mechanisms. One approach that requires no judgment whatsoever is simply to adopt in all patients with injured lungs the settings of the low-V$_T$ arm of the ARDS Network clinical trial,[35] which established the efficacy of lung-protective mechanical ventilation. Patients randomized to the low-V$_T$ arm received a V$_T$ of 6 cm^3/kg of predicted body weight. If their end-inflation pause pressure exceeded 30 cmH$_2$O, then V$_T$ was reduced further to as little as

4 cm³/kg of predicted body weight. In patients in whom 6 cm³/kg of predicted body weight resulted in breath stacking, effectively doubling their V_T, and in whom stacking could not be abolished with sedation, V_T was increased up to 8 cm³/kg of predicted body weight. This approach was associated with a 23% reduction in all-cause mortality compared with a high-V_T strategy.[35]

One important lesson from the ARDS Network trial is the scaling of V_T to predicted or ideal as opposed to actual body weight. To the extent to which the treatment objective of lung-protective mechanical ventilation is to minimize lung stretch, one would want to scale V_T to the volume of recruitable lung.[111] Because determining recruitable lung volume requires imaging or more sophisticated respiratory mechanics measurement techniques, estimating the size and volume of the lung before injury is the next best alternative. Epidemiologic studies have established height and gender as opposed to actual body weight as the best predictors of absolute lung volume, including total lung capacity (TLC).[112,113] The ARDS Network investigators predicted ideal body weight from an equation based on height and gender. A graphic comparison of the two predictive equations (Fig. 6-5) shows that 1 cm³/kg of predicted body weight corresponds to 1% predicted TLC. Therefore, the recommendation to restrict V_T of patients with injured lungs to 6 cm³/kg of predicted body weight amounts to restricting V_T during mechanical ventilation to no more than 6% of preinjury TLC. The right-hand side of the figure shows that there is no correlation between predicted TLC and actual body weight in a population of patients who were ventilated at the Mayo Clinic in 2001.[105] Because both reasoning and clinical outcome data are compelling, the practice of scaling V_T to actual body weight should be abandoned.[35,105]

The results of the ARDS Network trial generated a heated debate as to whether outcome differences reflected the obsolete management of the high-V_T group or improved management of the low-V_T group.[114] Be this as it may, the debate produced some important questions: (1) Is the choice of V_T also important in patients who are ventilated with what generally are considered "safe" inflation pressures? (2) Are ventilator modes in which diaphragmatic activity is preserved superior to the low-V_T approach used in the ARDS Network trial? (3) Should one care about V_T restrictions in patients with lung diseases other than ALI?

1. *Is the choice of V_T also important in patients who are ventilated with what generally are considered "safe" inflation pressures?* Inflating the lungs beyond TLC greatly increases the risk for barotrauma. Barotrauma is characterized by extra-alveolar air and is an entity distinct from ventilator-induced lung injury.[53,55] The transpulmonary and alveolar pressures at TLC approximate 25 and 35 cmH₂O, respectively.[115] During mechanical ventilation, peak alveolar pressure can be approximated from pressure at the airway opening after occluding the endotracheal tube at end inflation (hold or plateau pressure). Measurement of the transpulmonary pressure requires placement of an esophageal catheter and thus is invasive. Furthermore, use of esophageal pressure tends to result in overestimation of mean lung surface pressure in the supine position.[116]

There is an ongoing debate as to whether mechanical ventilation with plateau pressures of less than 30 cmH₂O is safe irrespective of the choice of V_T. None of the available clinical and experimental studies is sufficiently convincing to base general management recommendations on. In the absence of convincing data, one should exercise extreme caution when departing from low-V_T guidelines in patients with ALI. Indeed, circumstantial evidence and reasoning favor strict adherence to low-V_T guidelines in patients with ALI because (a) spontaneous hyperventilation, which by definition never exceeds TLC, has been implicated as a cause of surfactant dysfunction and

FIGURE 6-5 Predicted or ideal (*left panel*) and actual body weights (*right panel*) of 332 mechanically ventilated patients have been plotted against their predicted normal total lung capacity (%TLC). The predictive equations for ideal body weight and TLC are based on height and gender. Not surprisingly, then, the correlation between predicted body weight and predicted TLC is excellent. Also note, however, that the correlation between actual body weight and percent TLC is extremely poor. The source data are from patients included in a report by Gajic et al.[105]

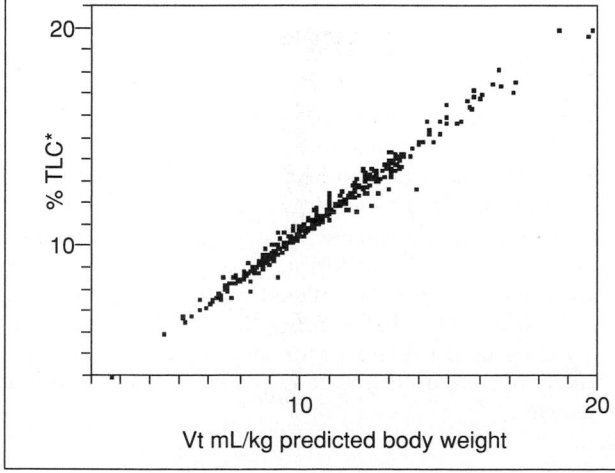
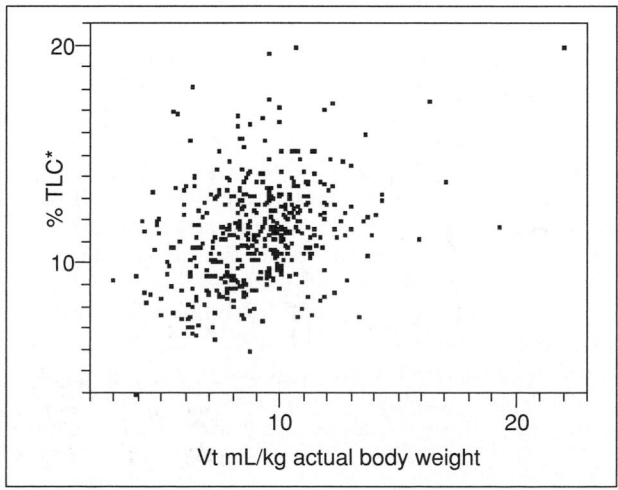

noncardiogenic pulmonary edema,[117] (b) repeated inflations of the respiratory system to pressures and volumes below TLC but above the upper inflection point of the inflation P-V curve have been associated with lung injury,[87] and (c) a post-hoc analysis of ARDS Network data suggested that patients in all plateau pressure quartiles derived benefit from V_T reductions (R. Brower, personal communication).

2. *Are ventilator modes in which diaphragmatic activity is preserved superior to the low-V_T approach used in the ARDS Network trial?* Patient-assisted breathing modes, such as PSV, bilevel pressure ventilation, and airway pressure-release ventilation (APRV), have been touted as modes of choice in the management of patients with ALI.[118,119] The evidence in support of this recommendation is not as strong as that in support of the low-V_T strategy employed in the ARDS Network trial.[35] The rationale for partial support centers on the increased regional ventilation and reduced incidence of atelectasis in dorsal lung regions when diaphragmatic activity is preserved.[120,121] Whether this observation has bearing on patient survival, however, is currently unclear. It should be noted that, on general principles, V_T-related effects on lung structure and function, including injury mechanisms, are not specific to ventilator mode.

3. *Should V_T be restricted in patients with respiratory failure from conditions other than ALI?* To the extent to which alveolar overdistension is a prevailing injury mechanism, lungs with relatively preserved inspiratory capacity ought to be less susceptible to deformation injury. Consistent with this reasoning, ventilator management of patients undergoing major surgery had no apparent effect on pulmonary immune responses.[122] On the other hand, the postoperative use of continuous positive airway pressure (CPAP) was shown recently to reduce the need for reintubation in such patients.[94] Moreover, a retrospective cohort study of patients who were mechanically ventilated for more than 48 hours and who did not have ALI from the outset identified V_T as a major risk factor for the subsequent development of noncardiogenic pulmonary edema.[105] Because there is no compelling reason why any patient with normal or near-normal lungs would benefit from or need a V_T of greater than 10 cm³/kg of predicted body weight, V_T settings above this threshold should be used with caution.

RESPIRATORY RATE

Having settled on a V_T and an end-expiratory volume, adjustments in the machine backup rate (f_M) should be made considering (1) the patient's actual rate demand, (2) the patient's anticipated ventilatory requirement, and (3) the impact of the rate setting on breath timing (see Fig. 6-1). Virtually all patients with hypoxic respiratory failure are tachypneic and usually require f_M settings of between 20 and 30 breaths per minute. Unless the patient has been paralyzed or has been so heavily sedated that spontaneous inspiratory triggering efforts are not sensed, f_M settings of 20 breaths per minute or lower are poorly tolerated be-

cause (1) neurohumoral feedback from lung edema and inflammation induces rapid shallow breathing independent of chemoreceptive and mechanoreceptive effects on central pattern generation, (2) in the presence of a severe gas-exchange impairment, low rates and minute volumes would cause CO_2 retention, which, in turn, elicits its own disease state–independent effects on respiratory rate and drive, and (3) discrepancies between actual (triggered) and set machine (backup) rate promote breathing patterns with inverse inspiratory-to-expiratory timing ratios and double triggering. Inverse breathing-pattern ratios are not compatible with normal phase-switching mechanisms in the presence of respiratory distress. Conventional ventilator modes are not capable of varying T_I or inspiratory flow with the actual machine rate. For example, at an f_M setting of 10 breaths per minute, the total cycle time (T_{TOT}) is 6 seconds. If the I:E ratio is set at 1:2, or if V_T and flow have been set to 0.5 and 0.25 liter/s, respectively, then T_I is fixed at 2 seconds, and expiratory time (T_E) will be 4 seconds. If the patient actually triggers at 20 breaths per minute, then T_{TOT} declines to 3 seconds. T_I remains fixed at 2 seconds because it is determined by the preset machine (backup) rate, the I:E ratio, or the inspiratory-flow setting. T_E now must decrease from 4 seconds to 1 second, and the actual I:E ratio will increase from 1:2 to 2:1. At a rate of 30 breaths per minute (T_{TOT}) = 2 seconds), T_E becomes 0, and "fighting the ventilator" must result. For these reasons, the f_M always should be set close to the patient's actual rate. If the actual rate is so high that effective ventilation cannot be achieved, then the patient needs additional sedation and possibly neuromuscular blockade.

TIMING VARIABLES

I:E RATIO

The setting of timing variables in conjunction with V_T and extrinsic PEEP determines the volume range over which lungs are cycled during ventilation. A long T_I, a high T_I/T_{TOT}), and a low mean inspiratory flow all promote ventilation with an inverse I:E ratio. Despite the considerable number of endorsements of inverse-ratio ventilation in ARDS, the beneficial effects of increasing I:E beyond 1:1 on pulmonary gas exchange tends to be marginal, provided that V_T and end-expiratory volumes are held constant.[123] All ventilators provide the option of maintaining lung volume at end inflation through the use of an inspiratory-hold time or pause time that usually is expressed as a percentage of the total cycle time (%T_{TOT}). For the purpose of defining the I:E ratio, the pause time is considered part of the inspiratory machine cycle. Long pause times favor the recruitment of previously collapsed or flooded alveoli and offer a means of shortening expiration independent of rate and mean inspiratory flow ($\dot{V}_I$). Although alveolar recruitment is a desired therapeutic endpoint in the treatment of patients with edematous lungs, one should at least consider that keeping the lungs expanded at high volumes (and pressures) for some time may damage relatively normal units and may cause adverse hemodynamic effects.

INSPIRATORY FLOW

Most ventilators require that mean $\dot{V}_I$ and its profile be specified. Mean $\dot{V}_I$ is equal to the ratio of V_T and T_I. Therefore, one cannot change flow without affecting at least one of the other timing variables (see Fig. 6-1). It is also important to consider that changing the flow profile from a squarewave to a decelerating or sine-wave pattern prolongs T_I in ventilators that require a peak-flow setting. This is so because nonsquarewave profiles have a higher peak-to-mean flow ratio; that is, it takes longer to deliver the predefined V_T than in squarewave flow delivery modes. Unless the patient is struggling, mean $\dot{V}_I$ usually is set to no more than 1 liter/s during volume-preset ventilation. In patients in whom lung recruitment and oxygenation are the primary therapeutic endpoints, setting flow (and rate) so that the T_I/T_{TOT}) approximates 0.5 (I:E = 1) tends to achieve the goal. Increasing flow always will raise peak airway pressure, but this need not be of concern if most of the added pressure is dissipated across the endotracheal tube. On the other hand, there is experimental evidence that the rate of lung expansion is a V_T-independent risk factor for lung deformation injury. Although $\dot{V}_I$ is one of the factors that determine the regional distribution of inspired gas,[43] the lung volume–independent effects of flow on pulmonary gas exchange are too unpredictable to warrant general guidelines. Much more important is the realization that the combined effects of flow, volume, and time settings influence the functional residual capacity and the degree of dynamic hyperinflation.[42,124,125]

MEAN EXPIRATORY FLOW: THE HIDDEN VARIABLE

Mean expiratory flow is defined by the ratio of V_T and T_E. $T_E = T_{TOT}) - T_I$. $T_{TOT}) = 60/f$ (per minute). Because the f_M and the actual f may differ from each other in the assist-control mode, the assumed and the actual T_{TOT} also may differ. Recall from the discussion on rate and timing that T_I is defined by both the set f_M and the set I:E ratio and that T_I remains constant irrespective of the actual rate. In contrast, T_E is affected by the actual breathing rate (f_A): $T_E = 60/f_A - T_I$. Therefore, the choice of volume and timing settings, together with the patient's trigger rate, determine mean expiratory flow. V_T/T_E is the principal ventilator setting–related determinant of dynamic hyperinflation. A patient with airway obstruction and a maximal forced expiratory flow of 0.2 liter/s in the mid–vital capacity range obviously cannot accommodate a V_T/T_E of 0.5 liter/s without an increase in end-expiratory lung volume (see Obstructive Lung Diseases, below).

MINUTE VENTILATION ($\dot{V}_E$)

With the exception of some older-generation Siemens series ventilators, $\dot{V}_E$ is not a variable that is set directly by the operator, but it is consequence of the V_T and rate settings. $\dot{V}_E$ is an important determinant of the body's CO_2 stores

and consequently of the arterial CO_2 tension (Pa_{CO_2}):

$$Pa_{CO_2} = \frac{\dot{V}_{CO_2} \times k}{\dot{V}_E(1 - V_D/V_T)} \qquad (8)$$

where

$\dot{V}_{CO_2}$ = volume of CO_2 produced in liters per minute

V_D/V_T = dead-space-to-tidal-volume ratio, a variable with which the efficiency of the lung as a CO_2 eliminator can be approximated

k = 0.863 and is a constant that scales $\dot{V}_{CO_2}$ and $\dot{V}_E$ to the same temperature and humidity

If the main goal of mechanical ventilation were to normalize Pa_{CO_2}, then $\dot{V}_E$ would be the most important machine setting. Although a "normal" Pa_{CO_2} is one of the therapeutic endpoints of mechanical ventilation, at times, normocapnia can be achieved only with high lung inflation volumes and pressures. This is particularly true in patients with ALI because they are often hypermetabolic (high $\dot{V}_{CO_2}$ and in addition suffer from $\dot{V}/\dot{Q}$ mismatch (high V_D/V_T). For these reasons, it is not unusual to encounter patients with ALI whose $\dot{V}_E$ requirements exceed 20 liters. In the past, concerns about acid-base status dominated the choice of ventilator settings. In recent years, however, the focus on mechanical lung injury has resulted in a reappraisal of therapeutic priorities that now places the prevention of lung injury above the goal to normalize CO_2 tensions and acid-base status. The corresponding ventilation strategy has been termed *permissive hypercapnia*.[126,127] Permissive hypercapnia means that the physician accepts a Pa_{CO_2} outside the expected or "normal' range in order to minimize the potential for ventilator-induced lung injury. Because such a ventilation strategy runs contrary to the limits set by the chemoresponses of neural ventilatory control mechanisms, permissive hypercapnia usually requires heavy sedation and at times paralysis of the patient.

There is a great deal of interest in the consequences of hypercapnia on pulmonary vascular barrier function, signaling mediated by reactive oxygen and nitrogen species, innate immunity, and ultimately, patient survival.[1–9] The science is fascinating, but it is not sufficiently advanced to derive clinical management decisions. That said, most experts probably would agree that (1) there is no universal pH or P_{CO_2} threshold that mandates a corrective action, (2) the use of bicarbonate buffers to correct respiratory acidemia is unproven, and (3) tracheal gas insufflation generally is effective in reducing Pa_{CO_2} by 10 mmHg or less.[128–130]

Obstructive Lung Diseases

In patients with obstructive lung diseases, there is a reduced capacity for generating expiratory flow. When obstruction is severe enough to cause ventilatory failure, dynamic airway collapse is virtually always present during the expiratory phase of the ventilatory cycle.[13,131] This means that the passive elastic recoil forces of the relaxed respiratory system are large enough to produce maximal expiratory flows in the tidal breathing range. Such patients are prone to dynamic hyperinflation, which may adversely affect circulation,[132] may increase the risk of barotrauma,[133] and can place the diaphragm and inspiratory muscles at a mechanical disadvantage.[134–136] The primary therapeutic goal of mechanical ventilation in obstructive lung disease therefore is to minimize the thoracic volume about which the lungs are ventilated. Additional goals vary with the context in which airflow obstruction is observed. Patients with long-standing obstruction from emphysema or chronic bronchitis (unless they are "fighting the ventilator") usually are easy to ventilate and simply may need respiratory muscle rest and a resetting of the CO_2-response threshold to more normal values. These secondary therapeutic objectives are highly controversial. In contrast, patients with acute severe asthma often "fight the ventilator" and therefore often require sedation, neuromuscular blockade, and ventilation with permissive hypercapnia.[126,133] Such patients are prone to neuromuscular insults from glucocorticoids and paralytic agents and may require prolonged mechanical ventilation for weakness long after lung mechanics normalize.[137]

MINIMIZING DYNAMIC HYPERINFLATION

The ventilator management of patients who are prone to dynamic hyperinflation is best understood after a review of the expiratory mechanics of the relaxed respiratory system (see The Mechanical Determinants of Patient-Ventilator Interactions, above). The key determinants of end-expiratory lung volume in a ventilated patient are the time constant of the respiratory system (R × C) and the V_T/T_E that has been imposed by the ventilator settings.[42] Figure 6-6 underscores these concepts, which are fundamental to formulating a meaningful management plan. If it is assumed that a mechanical inflation of 1 liter is initiated from Vrel at a rate of 20 breaths per minute and an I:E ratio of 1:2, the patient has 2 seconds to exhale. In the example in Fig. 6-6, the maximal mean passive expiratory flow that can be achieved in this volume range (between Vrel and Vrel + 1 liter) is given by the expiratory flow-volume curve. In this example, the maximal mean flow is only 0.25 liter/s. Hence, in the 2 seconds available for expiration, the patient can exhale only half the inspired volume (0.5 liter) before the next inflation is initiated by the machine. The second breath therefore is begun at a lung volume of Vrel + 0.5 liter. Maximal mean expiratory flow over the new volume range (Vrel + 0.5 liter and Vrel + 1.5 liters) is 0.3 liter/s. This flow is still insufficient for adequate lung emptying. A new steady state will be achieved only when the increase in lung volume results in a maximal mean expiratory flow of 0.5 liter/s, which is equal to the obligatory mean expiratory flow imposed by the ventilator settings.

Dynamic hyperinflation is associated with an increase in alveolar pressure at end expiration. This pressure, also called *intrinsic positive end-expiratory pressure* (PEEP$_I$), is the pressure of the respiratory system at end expiration plus

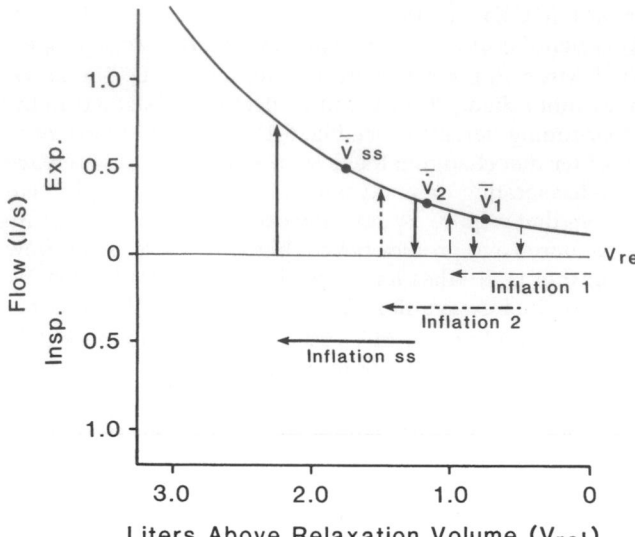

FIGURE 6-6 Diagrammatic demonstration of how insufficient expiratory flow produces dynamic hyperinflation. The broken horizontal arrow shows the first breath of 1 liter initiated from relaxation volume (Vrel) at a rate of 20 breaths per minute and a T_I/T_{TOT}) of 0.33 (inflation 1). The solid curved line shows the maximal expiratory flow that can be produced during passive exhalation by the elastic recoil pressure of the system. In the 2 seconds available from expiration, the maximum mean expiratory flow of the first breath ($\bar{V}_1$) is only 0.25 liter/s. Therefore, only 0.5 liter can be exhaled in the 2 seconds before the next inhalation of 1 liter is initiated (inflation 2). According to the flow-volume relationship, a maximal mean expiratory flow of 0.3 liter/s ($\bar{V}_1$) can be achieved over this volume range. A steady state, during which inspiratory and expiratory volumes are matched, will be reached only when the maximal mean expiratory flow ($\bar{V}_{SS}$) equals 0.5 liter/s. (*Used, with permission, from Hubmayr et al: Crit Care Med 18:103–13, 1990.*)

any pressure generated by respiratory muscles.[13,138] In the absence of muscle activity, the degree of dynamic hyperinflation can be inferred from the end-expiratory airway occlusion pressure (PEEP$_I$) and the elastance of the relaxed respiratory system (Ers):

$$Vee - Vrel = Ers/PEEP_I \qquad (9)$$

where Vee is the volume of the lungs at end expiration.

In the presence of muscle activity from active expiration or inspiratory triggering efforts, PEEP$_I$ is a meaningless measurement. This limitation also applies to some extent to esophageal pressure-derived estimates of PEEP$_I$. In some ventilators, PEEP$_I$ can be estimated at the "press of a button"—by pressing an end-expiratory hold button and waiting until airway opening pressure reaches a steady value. In ventilators in which the timing of end-expiratory occlusions is not automated, the measurement of PEEP$_I$ is considerably more difficult.

As illustrated in Fig. 6-6, ventilator adjustments designed to minimize dynamic hyperinflation should be geared toward lowering mean expiratory flow (V_T/T_E). In a paralyzed patient with asthma, V_T can be reduced to as little as about 4 cm³/kg of predicted body weight, whereas T_E is prolonged through increases in mean inspiratory flow (1–1.5 liters/s), adjustments in the I:E ratio (1:4–1:5), and reductions in f_M (~10 breaths per minute). As discussed earlier, such a strategy is likely to produce hypercapnia, but even severe acidemia is usually well tolerated in paralyzed subjects.[139] High inspiratory-flow settings, which are required to prolong T_E, are bound to increase peak Paw and may raise concerns about barotrauma. It must be emphasized, however, that much of this added "resistive pressure" is dissipated along the endotracheal tube and proximal airways and that, on balance, increasing the rate of lung inflation seems less damaging than ventilating asthmatic lungs near TLC. Consistent with this hypothesis, the incidence of barotrauma can be reduced significantly in patients with status asthmaticus when ventilator settings are chosen to maintain peak lung volume within 1.4 liters of Vrel.[133,140,141]

Permissive hypercapnia and neuromuscular blockade are rarely required in patients with ventilatory failure from exacerbations of chronic obstructive lung diseases. Nevertheless, many such patients have respiratory rates in the high teens and low twenties, making it difficult to prolong T_E beyond about 2 seconds. This makes it virtually impossible to ventilate these patients near Vrel. Recall that patients with end-stage obstruction may have maximal expiratory flows of 0.2 liter/s or less up to volumes near TLC.[131] In the nonparalyzed patient, hypercapnia sets limits to the reductions in V_T; therefore, attempts must be made to reduce the patient's respiratory rate. Sometimes the only way to minimize hyperinflation without having to resort to neuromuscular blockade is through the judicious use of sedatives with the intent of reducing inspiratory efforts until they fail to initiate a machine breath (see Asynchrony between the Patient's Effort and Machine-Delivered Breaths, below).

USE OF CONTINUOUS POSITIVE AIRWAY PRESSURE (CPAP)

In patients with hypoxic respiratory failure, CPAP is used to raise lung volume to recruit closed and flooded alveoli and to improve oxygenation. In contrast, the goal of CPAP therapy in patients with obstruction is to minimize inspiratory work.[142] Potential mechanisms of action of CPAP in obstructed patients are shown schematically in Fig. 6-7A. The figure shows the pressure-volume relationships of the relaxed respiratory system and depicts the elastic work

FIGURE 6-7A. Effect of dynamic hyperinflation of elastic inspiratory work. The solid curve shows the relationship between the volume above Vrel and the recoil of the respiratory system (Prs). Dynamic hyperinflation exists. Inspiration is now initiated from a volume above Vrel. The increase in lung volume necessitates an increase in the elastic inspiratory work, which may be considered to have two components: work to halt expiratory flow (*darker-shaded area*) and work required to inflate the respiratory system (*lighter-shaded area*). B. Effect of CPAP on respiratory work. The solid curve is the pressure-volume curve of the respiratory system. With CPAP, a new Vrel is achieved. To conserve inspiratory elastic work, the patient recruits expiratory muscles and exhales below the new Vrel. The elastic work performed by the expiratory muscles is represented by the darker shaded area. Relaxation of the expiratory muscles inflates the lungs back to the new Vrel without inspiratory effort. The inspiratory muscles then increase lung volume further, performing elastic inspiratory work (*lighter-shaded area*). Hence CPAP reduced the work of the inspiratory muscles by letting the expiratory muscles do part of the inspiratory work. (*Used with permission. From Hubmayr et al: Crit Care Med 18:103–13, 1990.*)

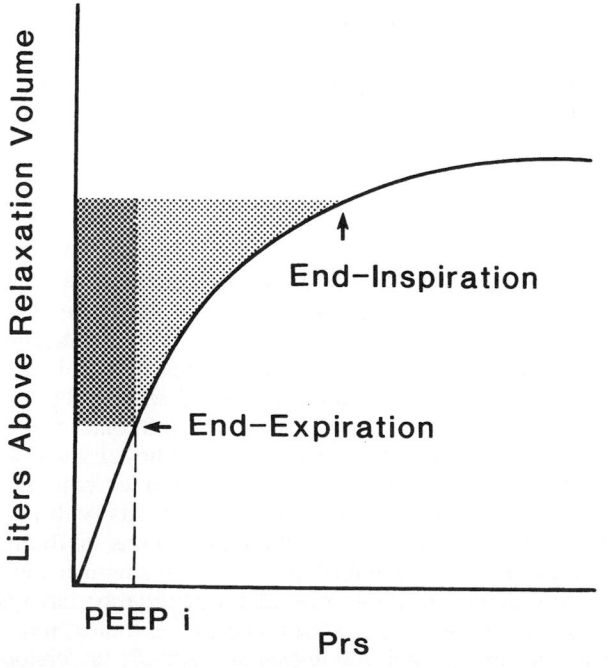

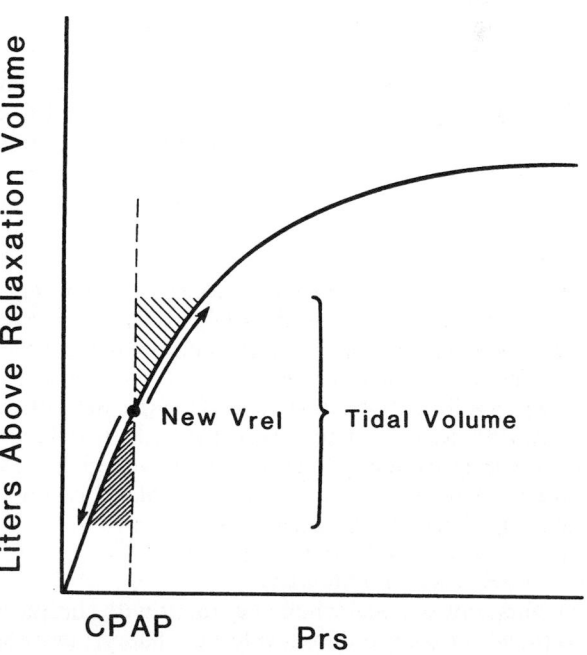

A

B

(Wel) needed to raise lung volume from end expiration to end inspiration (shaded area) in the presence of dynamic hyperinflation. Wel has two components: (1) work required to halt expiratory flow by counterbalancing respiratory system recoil at end expiration (W related to $PEEP_I$) and (2) work expended during inflation of the lungs and thorax. In theory, the inspiratory work related to $PEEP_I$ (darker shaded area) can be provided externally with CPAP equal to $PEEP_I$. As CPAP approaches $PEEP_I$, however, additional hyperinflation may occur.[143] To guard against CPAP-induced worsening of hyperinflation, the physician can monitor peak or end-inflation hold pressure as an indicator of peak lung volume.

An alternative mechanism by which CPAP may reduce inspiratory elastic work is shown in Fig. 6-7B. CPAP may result in exhalation below the new Vrel through the recruitment of expiratory muscles.[138,144] Subsequent relaxation of the expiratory muscle inflates the lungs passively back to the new Vrel. Inspiratory muscles are unloaded because the expiratory muscles do part of the inspiratory work. This is depicted by the lighter-shaded area in Fig. 67B. This mechanism is of limited value in patients with severe obstruction, however, because low maximal flows prevent significant reductions in lung volume below Vrel.

VENTILATORY PUMP FAILURE AND CHRONIC CO₂ RETENTION

RESTING THE RESPIRATORY MUSCLES

In the 1970s and 1980s, much emphasis was placed on respiratory muscle fatigue as a common cause of ventilatory failure.[145] Experimental evidence, however, that this truly occurs in a clinical setting remains elusive.[146] Without addressing all the pros and cons of minimizing the patient's contribution to inspiratory work, evidence is mounting that mechanical ventilation inhibits respiratory motor output primarily through mechanoreceptive pathways. Studies on volunteers and patients have shown that depending on state and ventilator settings, spontaneous respiratory muscle activity can be abolished, reduced, or entrained to the ventilator.[147–149] Two respiratory control aspects of patient-ventilator interactions deserve particular emphasis. First, volume-preset mechanical ventilation at settings that normalize blood gas tensions provides no safeguard against excessive respiratory work.[46] This means that ventilating patients in a volume-preset assist-control mode offers no universal guarantee for sufficient respiratory muscle rest. Second, sleeping and obtunded patients are susceptible to PSV setting–induced central apneas.[28,29] This can lead to problems if a clinician feels compelled to increase ventilator support without a mandatory backup in order to reduce the work of breathing at night. If this is done through low IMV backup rates, then apneas may trigger ventilator alarms and cause arousal and sleep fragmentation.[150]

RESETTING THE CHEMOSTAT

It remains controversial whether patients with chronic hypercapnia and complicating acute ventilatory pump failure should be "mechanically" hyperventilated to normocapnia in an attempt to restore normal chemoresponsiveness.

Proponents of such a ventilator strategy may argue that CO_2 has negative inotropic effects on respiratory muscles[151] and that experience with nocturnal ventilator assistance suggests that resetting CO_2 responsiveness is feasible in some instances.[152] Opponents argue that maintenance of normocapnia in the presence of lung disease requires a high minute volume, which could represent a fatiguing load on the respiratory muscles. As a general rule, at the time weaning is contemplated, sustainable CO_2 tensions should range between 40 and 50 mmHg. Patients who are being weaned with CO_2 tensions in the sixties tend not to do well and are severely limited.

Approaches to Common Potentially Adverse Patient-Ventilator Interactions

RESPIRATORY ALKALOSIS

In spontaneously breathing normal subjects, $\dot{V}_E$ is closely coupled to Pa_{CO_2} and reflects both rate and V_T responses of the ventilatory control system. In mechanically ventilated subjects, V_T is often preset, thereby uncoupling ventilation from respiratory drive and confining the influence of neural control on the regulation of breathing to machine trigger rate. Consequently, ventilated patients with high intrinsic respiratory rates can have CO_2 tensions significantly below normal. Because associated alkalemia may contribute to arrhythmias and cardiovascular instability,[153] patients often are sedated, and the ventilator settings are adjusted with the goal of raising Pa_{CO_2}. In most instances of ventilator-induced hypocapnia, tachypnea is unrelated to hypoxemia or increased CO_2 drive per se. The causes of tachypnea may be behavioral in origin, as with pain and anxiety syndromes, or neurohumoral in origin, as with circulatory failure or in conjunction with lung and airway inflammation. Because tachypnea and increased ventilatory drive rarely are caused by CO_2 itself, any means of reducing ventilator-delivered volumes is effective in raising Pa_{CO_2}.

ASYNCHRONY BETWEEN THE PATIENT'S EFFORT AND MACHINE-DELIVERED BREATHS

Asynchrony between vigorous spontaneous efforts and machine-delivered breaths is often referred to as "fighting the ventilator." Because inspiratory efforts often are followed by active expiration in patients with increased drive, discrepancies between machine and patient T_I cause peak Paw to exceed the alarm (safety) limit (usually set to 45 cmH₂O), resulting in premature termination of inspiratory flow and insufficient ventilation. Although the initial management should be to raise the f_M and increase inspiratory flow up to 1.5 liters/s, many patients with asynchrony require sedation and, on rare occasions, neuromuscular blockade. It is of note that the mechanisms of action by which sedatives facilitate mechanical ventilation have not been fully detailed. When "fighting the ventilator" reflects pain and anxiety, their mode of action is easily understood. Not all manifestations of respiratory distress, however, are

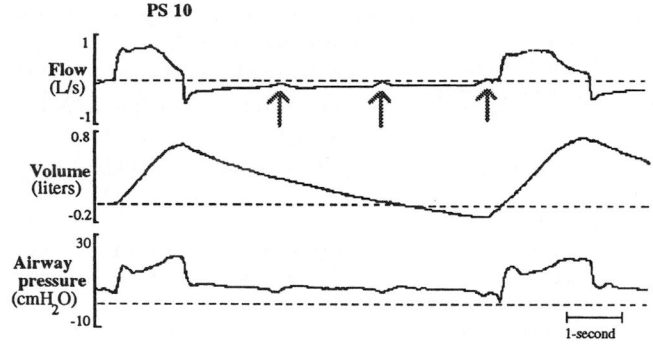

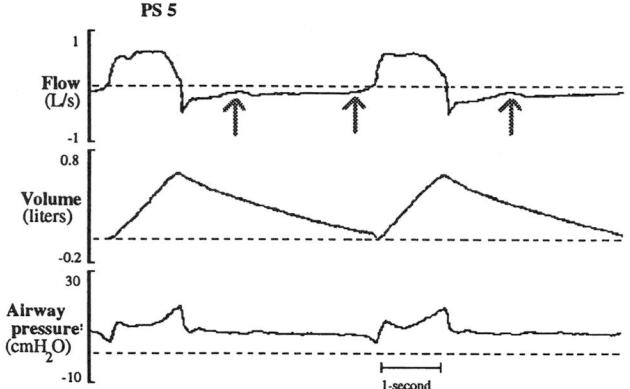

FIGURE 6-8 Flow, volume, and pressure tracings of a patient recorded during PSV with 10 cmH$_2$O (*upper panel*) and 5 cmH$_2$O (*lower panel*). Each arrow indicates an inspiratory effort. See the text for a further explanation. (*Used, with permission, from Hubmayr.*[154])

machine inflation after the cessation of inspiratory effort, and the presence of airways obstruction, with its propensity for dynamic hyperinflation, all contribute to machine trigger failure. Note that the reduction in PSV from 10–5 cmH$_2$O and the lower peak volume account for the reduced number of wasted inspiratory efforts. An awareness of this problem is important because the physician otherwise may attribute an increase in machine rate following reductions in PSV to impending failure or a fatiguing load response.

Because asynchrony between the patient and machine is common, its diagnostic and prognostic significance remains uncertain. When asynchrony impairs ventilator assistance or causes patient discomfort, treatment is required in the form of sedation and adjustments in CPAP, rate, flow, or trigger mode. When "wasted" inspiratory efforts are not perceived as uncomfortable, however, it is not clear that adjustments in ventilator settings are warranted. After all, increases in machine rate to match the rate of patient efforts may cause worsening dynamic hyperinflation and may compromise circulation.

References

1. Shibata K, Cregg N, Engelberts D, et al. Hypercapnic acidosis may attenuate acute lung injury by inhibition of endogenous xanthine oxidase. Am J Respir Crit Care Med 1999; 158:1578–84.
2. Broccard AF, Hotchkiss JR, Vannay C, et al. Protective effects of hypercapnic acidosis on ventilator-induced lung injury. Am J Respir Crit Care Med 2001; 164:802–6.
3. Laffey JG, Tanaka M, Engelberts D, et al. Therapeutic hypercapnia reduces pulmonary and systemic injury following in vivo lung reperfusion. Am J Respir Crit Care Med 2000; 162:2287–94.
4. Sinclair SE, Kregenow DA, Lamm WJ, et al. Hypercapnic acidosis is protective in an in vivo model of ventilator-induced lung injury. Am J Respir Crit Care Med 2002; 166: 403–8.
5. Strand M, Ikegami M, Jobe AH. Effects of high P$_{CO_2}$ on ventilated preterm lamb lungs. Pediatr Res 2003; 53:468–72.
6. Laffey JG, Honan D, Hopkins N, et al. Hypercapnic acidosis attenuates endotoxin-induced acute lung injury. Am J Respir Crit Care Med 2004; 169:46–56.
7. Lang JD Jr, Chumley P, Eiserich JP, et al. Hypercapnia induces injury to alveolar epithelial cells via a nitric oxide-dependent pathway. Am J Physiol Lung Cell Mol Physiol 2000; 279:L994–1002.
8. Lang JD, Figueroa M, Sanders KD, et al. Hypercapnia via reduced rate and tidal volume contributes to lipopolysaccharide-induced lung injury. Am J Respir Crit Care Med 2005; 171:147–57.
9. Doerr CH, Gajic O, Berrios JC, et al. Hypercapnic acidosis impairs plasma membrane wound resealing in ventilator injured lungs. Am J Respir Crit Care Med 2005; 171:1371–7.
10. Jolliet P, Tassaux D, Roeseler J, et al. Helium-oxygen versus air-oxygen noninvasive pressure support in decompensated chronic obstructive disease: A prospective, multicenter study. Crit Care Med 2003; 31:878–84.
11. Jolliet P, Tassaux D. Usefulness of helium-oxygen mixtures in the treatment of mechanically ventilated patients. Curr Opin Crit Care 2003; 9:45–50.
12. Sasson CS. Mechanical ventilation design and function: The trigger variable. Respir Care 1992; 37:1056–69.

behavioral in origin. It is not known to what extent various sedatives reduce the magnitude of inspiratory efforts (drive), slow respiratory rate, or facilitate the entrainment of medullary inspiratory pattern generation to the ventilator.

Asynchrony between patient and machine breaths is very common. This is particularly true for patients with high intrinsic respiratory rates, for patients with reduced inspiratory pressure output from low drive or respiratory muscle weakness, for patients with airways obstruction, and when ventilator support results in greater than normal V$_T$.[16,17,19,138] For example, Fig. 6-8 shows pressure and flow tracings of a patient with airways obstruction and hypercapnic ventilatory failure during PSV of 10 and 5 cmH$_2$O. Arterial O$_2$ and CO$_2$ tensions were normal at both settings, and the patient did not appear to be in distress. The small deflections in expiratory flow marked by arrows represent inspiratory efforts (I) during the expiratory phase of the machine cycle. In the presence of dynamic hyperinflation, Pmus must counterbalance the expiratory recoil forces (Pel) before a new machine breath can be triggered. If ΔPmus is less than Pel minus the machine trigger sensitivity, then the inspiratory effort is wasted and does not result in a machine breath. At the PSV setting of 10 cmH$_2$O in this example, only every third inspiratory effort results in a machine breath (3:1 coupling). The low ΔPmus, the persistence of

13. Rossi A, Gottfried SB, Zocchi L, et al. Measurement of static compliance of the total respiratory system in patients with acute respiratory failure during mechanical ventilation: The effect of intrinsic positive end-expiratory pressure. Am Rev Respir Dis 1985; 131:672–7.

14. Chatmongkolchart S, Williams P, Hess DR, Kacmarek RM. Evaluation of inspiratory rise time and inspiration termination criteria in new-generation mechanical ventilators: A lung model study. Respir Care 2001; 46:666–77.

15. Murciano D, Boczkowski J, Lecocguic Y, et al. Tracheal occlusion pressure: A simple index to monitor respiratory failure in patients with chronic obstructive pulmonary disease. Ann Intern Med 1988; 108:800–5.

16. Tobin MJ, Jubran A, Laghi F. Patient-ventilator interaction. Am J Respir Crit Care Med 2001; 163:1059–63.

17. Sassoon CS, Foster GT. Patient-ventilator asynchrony. Curr Opin Crit Care 2001; 7:28–33.

18. Aslanian P, El Atrous S, Isabey D, et al. Effects of flow triggering on breathing effort during partial ventilatory support. Am J Respir Crit Care Med 1998; 157:135–43.

19. Yamada Y, Du HL. Analysis of the mechanisms of expiratory asynchrony in pressure support ventilation: A mathematical approach. J Appl Physiol 2000; 88:2143–50.

20. Ishaaya AM, Nathan SD, Belman MJ. Work of breathing after extubation. Chest 1995; 107:204–9.

21. Straus C, Louis B, Isabey D, et al. Contribution of the endotracheal tube and the upper airway to breathing workload. Am J Respir Crit Care Med 1998; 157:23–30.

22. Esteban A, Frutos F, Tobin MJ, et al. A comparison of four methods of weaning patients from mechanical ventilation. Spanish Lung Failure Collaborative Group. New Engl J Med 1995; 332: 345–50.

23. Esteban A, Alía I, Gordo F, et al. Extubation outcome after spontaneous breathing trials with T-tube or pressure support ventilation. The Spanish Lung Failure Collaborative Group. Am J Respir Crit Care Med 1997; 156:459–65.

24. Butler R, Keenan SP, Inman, KJ, et al. Is there a preferred technique for weaning the difficult-to-wean patient? A systematic review of the literature. Crit Care Med 1999; 27:2331–6.

25. Bonmarchand G, Chevron V, Menard JF, et al. Effects of pressure ramp slope values on the work of breathing during pressure support ventilation in restrictive patients. Crit Care Med 1999; 27:715–22.

26. Brochard L, Rauss A, Benito S, et al. Comparison of three methods of gradual withdrawal from ventilatory support during weaning from mechanical ventilation. Am J Respir Crit Care Med 1994; 150:896–903.

27. MacIntyre NR, Cook DJ, Ely EW Jr, et al. Evidence-based guidelines for weaning and discontinuing ventilatory support: A collective task force facilitated by the American College of Chest Physicians, the American Association for Respiratory Care, and the American College of Critical Care Medicine. Chest 2001; 120:375S–95S.

28. Morrell MJ, Shea SA, Adams L, Guz A. Effects of inspiratory support upon breathing in humans during wakefulness and sleep. Respir Physiol 1993; 93:57–70.

29. Tobert DG, Simon PM, Stroetz RW, Hubmayr RD. The determinants of respiratory rate during mechanical ventilation. Am J Respir Crit Care Med 1997; 155:485–92.

30. Branson RD, Johannigman JA, Campbell RS, Davis K Jr. Closed loop ventilation. Respir Care 2002; 47:427–51.

31. Brunner JX. Principles and history of closed-loop controlled ventilation. Respir Care Clin North Am 2001; 7:341–62.

32. Sinha SK, Donn SM. Volume-controlled ventilation: Variations on a theme. Clin Perinatol 2001; 28:547–60.

33. Branson RD, Johannigman JA. What is the evidence base for the newer ventilation modes? Respir Care 2004; 49:742–60.

34. Amato MB, Barbas CS, Medeiros DM, et al. Effect of a protective-ventilation strategy on mortality in the acute respiratory distress syndrome. New Engl J Med 1998; 338:347–54.

35. ARDS Network. Ventilation with lower tidal volumes as compared with traditional tidal volumes for acute lung injury and the acute respiratory distress syndrome. New Engl J Med 2000; 342:1301–8.

36. Ambrosino N, Rossi A. Proportional assist ventilation (PAV): A significant advance or a futile struggle between logic and practice? Thorax 2002; 57:272–6.

37. Navalesi P, Costa R. New modes of mechanical ventilation: Proportional assist ventilation, neurally adjusted ventilatory assist, and fractal ventilation. Curr Opin Crit Care 2003; 9:51–8.

38. Sinderby C, Navalesi P, Beck J, et al. Neural control of mechanical ventilation in respiratory failure. Nature Med 1999; 5:1433–6.

39. Rodarte JR, Rehder K. Dynamics of respiration. In: Handbook of physiology, Vol 3. Baltimore: Waverly Press, 1986; 131–44.

40. Hubmayr RD, Abel MD, Rehder K. Physiologic approach to mechanical ventilation. Crit Care Med 1990; 18:103–13.

41. Lavietes MH, Rochester DF. Assessment of airway function during assisted ventilation. Lung 1981; 159:219–29.

42. Gay PC, Rodarte JR, Tayyab M, Hubmayr RD. The evaluation of bronchodilator responsiveness in mechanically ventilated patients. Am Rev Respir Dis 1987; 136:880–5.

43. Otis AB, Mckerrow CB, Barlett RA, et al. Mechanical factors in distribution of pulmonary ventilation. J Appl Physiol 1956; 8:427–43.

44. Fredberg JJ, Stamenovic D. On the imperfect elasticity of lung tissue. J Appl Physiol 1989; 67: 2408–19.

45. Wilson TA, Fredberg JJ, Rodarte JR, Hyatt RE. Interdependence of regional expiratory flow. J Appl Physiol 1985; 59: 1924–8.

46. Marini JJ, Rodriguez RM, Lamb V. The inspiratory workload of patient-initiated mechanical ventilation. Am Rev Respir Dis 1986; 134:902–9.

47. Prechter GC, Nelson SB, Hubmayr RD. The ventilatory recruitment threshold for carbon dioxide. Am Rev Respir Dis 1990; 141:758–64.

48. Bernard GR, Artigas A, Brigham KL, et al. The American-European Consensus Conference on ARDS: Definitions, mechanisms, relevant outcomes, and clinical trial coordination. Am J Respir Crit Care Med 1994; 149:818–24.

49. Artigas A, Bernard GR, Carlet J, et al. The American-European Consensus Conference on ARDS: 2. Ventilatory, pharmacologic, supportive therapy, study design strategies, and issues related to recovery and remodeling: Acute respiratory distress syndrome. Am J Respir Crit Care Med 1998; 157:1332–47.

50. Levy MM, Fink MP, Marshall JC, et al. 2001 SCCM/ESICM/ACCP/ATS/SIS International Sepsis Definitions Conference. Crit Care Med 2003; 31:1250–6.

51. Wood LD, Prewitt RM. Cardiovascular management in acute hypoxemic respiratory failure. Am J Cardiol 1981; 47:963–72.

52. Martindale JL, Holbrook NJ. Cellular response to oxidative stress: Signaling for suicide and survival. J Cell Physiol 2002; 192:1–15.

53. Dreyfuss D, Saumon G. Ventilator-induced lung injury: Lessons from experimental studies. Am J Respir Crit Care Med 1998; 157:294–323.

54. Vlahakis NE, Hubmayr RD. Cellular stress failure in ventilator injured lungs. Am J Respir Cri. Care Med 2005; 171:1328–42.

55. Macklin MT, Macklin CC. Malignant interstitial emphysema of the lungs and mediastinum as an important occult complication in many respiratory diseases and other conditions: An

interpretation of the clinical literature in the light of laboratory experiment. Medicine 1944; 23:281–358.

56. Ryrfeldt A. Drug-induced inflammatory responses to the lung. Toxicol Lett 2000; 112–3:171–6.

57. Maunder RJ, Shuman WP, McHugh JW, et al. Preservation of normal lung regions in the adult respiratory distress syndrome: Analysis by computed tomography. JAMA 1986; 255:2463–5.

58. Gattinoni L, Pesenti A, Avalli L, et al. Pressure-volume curve of total respiratory system in acute respiratory failure: Computed tomographic scan study. Am Rev Respir Dis 1987; 136:730–6.

59. Rodarte JR, Fung YC. Distribution of stresses within the lung. In: Fishman AP, editor. Handbook of physiology, Sec 3: Respiratory system, Vol III: Mechanics of breathing, Part I. Baltimore: Williams & Wilkins, 1986: 233–46.

60. Jones AT, Hansell DM, Evans TW. Pulmonary perfusion in supine and prone positions: An electron-beam computed tomography study. J Appl Physiol 2001; 90:1342–8.

61. Hubmayr RD. Perspective on lung injury and recruitment: A skeptical look at the opening and collapse story. Am J Respir Crit Care Med 2002; 165:1647–53.

62. Bilek AM, Dee KC, Gaver DP 3d. Mechanisms of surface-tension-induced epithelial cell damage in a model of pulmonary airway reopening. J Appl Physiol 2003; 94:770–83.

63. Muscedere JG, Mullen JB, Gan K, Slutsky AS. Tidal ventilation at low airway pressures can augment lung injury. Am J Respir Crit Care Med 1994; 149:1327–34.

64. Lachmann B. Open lung in ARDS. Minerva Anestesiol 2002; 68:637–42.

65. Barbas CS, de Matos GF, Pincelli MP, e al. Mechanical ventilation in acute respiratory failure: Recruitment and high positive end-expiratory pressure are necessary. Curr Opin Crit Care 2005; 11:18–28.

66. Richard JC, Maggiore SM, Jonson B, et al. Influence of tidal volume on alveolar recruitment: Respective role of PEEP and a recruitment maneuver. Am J Respir Crit Care Med 2001; 163:1609–13.

67. Malbouisson LM, Muller JC, Constantin JM, et al. Computed tomography assessment of positive end-expiratory pressure-induced alveolar recruitment in patients with acute respiratory distress syndrome. Am J Respir Crit Care Med 2001; 163:1444–50.

68. Lim SC, Adams AB, Simonson DA, et al. Transient hemodynamic effects of recruitment maneuvers in three experimental models of acute lung injury. Crit Care Med 2004; 32:2378–84.

69. Lim SC, Adams AB, Simonson DA, et al. Intercomparison of recruitment maneuver efficacy in three models of acute lung injury. Crit Care Med 2004; 32:2371–7.

70. Dreyfuss D, Soler P, Basset G, Saumon G. High inflation pressure pulmonary edema: Respective effects of high airway pressure, high tidal volume, and positive end-expiratory pressure. Am Rev Respir Dis 1988; 137:1159–64.

71. Brower RG, Morris A. MacIntyre N, et al. Effects of recruitment maneuvers in patients with acute lung injury and acute respiratory distress syndrome ventilated with high positive end-expiratory pressure. Crit Care Med 2003; 31:2592–7.

72. Oczenski W, Hormann C, Keller C, et al. Recruitment maneuvers after a positive end-expiratory pressure trial do not induce sustained effects in early adult respiratory distress syndrome. Anesthesiology 2004; 101:620–5.

73. Pelosi P, Cadringher P, Bottino N, et al. Sigh in acute respiratory distress syndrome. Am J Respir Crit Care Med 1999; 159:872–80.

74. Villagra A, Ochagavia A, Vatua S, et al. Recruitment maneuvers during lung protective ventilation in acute respiratory distress syndrome. Am J Respir Crit Care Med 2002; 165:165–70.

75. Broseghinin C, Brandolese R, Poggi R, et al. Respiratory resistance and intrinsic positive end-expiratory pressure ($PEEP_i$) in patients with adult respiratory distress syndrome (ARDS). Eur Respir J 1988; 1:726–31.

76. Eisner MD, Thompson BT, Schoenfeld D, et al and Acute Respiratory Distress Syndrome Network. Airway pressures and early barotrauma in patients with acute lung injury and acute respiratory distress syndrome. Am J Respir Crit Care Med 2002; 165:978–82.

77. Esteban A, Anzueto A, Frutos F, et al. Characteristics and outcomes in adult patients receiving mechanical ventilation: A 28-day international study. JAMA. 2002; 287:345–55.

78. Ware LB, Matthay MA. The acute respiratory distress syndrome. New Engl J Med 2000; 342:1334–49.

79. Ferguson ND, Frutos-Vivar F, Esteban A, et al. Airway pressures, tidal volumes, and mortality in patients with acute respiratory distress syndrome. Crit Care Med. 2005; 33:21–30.

80. Tobin MJ. Advances in mechanical ventilation. New Engl J Med 2001; 344:1986–96.

81. Perren A. High versus low PEEP in ARDS. New Engl J Med 2004; 351:2128–9.

82. Albaiceta GM, Taboada F, Parra D, et al. Tomographic study of the inflection points of the pressure volume curve in acute lung injury. Am J Respir Crit Care Med 2004; 170:1066–72.

83. Rouby JJ, Puybasset L, Nieszkowska A, Lu Q. Acute respiratory distress syndrome: Lessons from computed tomography of the whole lung. Crit Care Med 2003; 31:S285–95.

84. Victorino JA, Borges JB, Okamoto VN, et al. Imbalances in regional lung ventilation: A validation study on electrical impedance tomography. Am J Respir Crit Care Med 2004; 169:791–800.

85. Jonson B, Richard JC, Straus C, et al. Pressure-volume curves and compliance in acute lung injury: Evidence of recruitment above the lower inflection point. Am J Respir Crit Care Med 1999; 159:1172–8.

86. Maggiore SM, Jonson B, Richard JC, et al. Alveolar derecruitment at decremental positive end-expiratory pressure levels in acute lung injury: Comparison with the lower inflection point, oxygenation, and compliance. Am J Respir Crit Care Med 2001; 164:759–801.

87. Grasso S, Terragni P, Mascia L, et al. Airway pressure-time curve profile (stress index) detects tidal recruitment/hyperinflation in experimental acute lung injury. Crit Care Med 2004; 32:1018–27.

88. Baumgardner JE, Markstaller K, Pfeiffer B, et al. Effects of respiratory rate, plateau pressure, and positive end-expiratory pressure on Pa_{CO_2} oscillations after saline lavage. Am J Respir Crit Care Med 2002; 166:1556–62.

89. Gattinoni L, Pelosi P, Suter PM, et al. Acute respiratory distress syndrome caused by pulmonary and extrapulmonary disease: Different syndromes? Am J Respir Crit Care Med 1998; 158:3–11.

90. Malbrain ML: Abdominal pressure in the critically ill: Measurement and clinical relevance. Intensive Care Med 1999; 25:1453–8.

91. Pelosi P, Croci M, Ravagnan I, et al. The effects of body mass on lung volumes, respiratory mechanics, and gas exchange during general anesthesia. Anesth Analg 1998; 87:654–60.

92. Malo J, Ali J, Wood LD. How does positive end-expiratory pressure reduce intrapulmonary shunt in canine pulmonary edema? J Appl Physiol 1984; 57:1002–10.

93. Malbrain MLNG, Chiumello D, Pelosi P, et al. Incidence and prognosis of intraabdominal hypertension in a mixed population of critically ill patients: A multiple-center epidemiological study. Crit Care Med 2005; 33:315–22.

94. Squadrone V, Coha M, Cerutti E, et al. Continuous positive airway pressure for treatment of postoperative hypoxemia: A randomized, controlled trial. JAMA 2005; 293:589–95.

95. Rouby JJ, Lu Q, Goldstein I. Selecting the right level of positive end-expiratory pressure in patients with acute respiratory distress syndrome. Am J Respir Crit Care Med 2002; 165:1182–6.

96. Rivers EP, Ander DS, Powell D. Central venous oxygen saturation monitoring in the critically ill patient. Curr Opin Crit Care 2001; 7:204–11.

97. Cain SM. Oxygen supply dependency in the critically ill: A continuing conundrum. Adv Exp Med Biol 1992; 317:35–45.

98. Hood VL, Tannen RL. Protection of acid-base balance by pH regulation of acid production (review). New Engl J Med 1998; 339:81–6.

99. Hickling KG, Joyce C. Permissive hypercapnia in ARDS and its effect on tissue oxygenation. Acta Anaesthesiol Scand Suppl 1995; 107:201–8.

100. Beydon L, Uttman L, Rawal R, Jonson B. Effects of positive end-expiratory pressure on dead space and its partitions in acute lung injury. Intensive Care Med 2002; 28:1239–45.

101. Pinsky MR. Recent advances in the clinical application of heart-lung interactions. Curr Opin Crit Care. 2002; 8:26–31.

102. Jonson B, Richard JC, Straus C, et al. Pressure-volume curves and compliance in acute lung injury: Evidence of recruitment above the lower inflection point. Am J Respir Crit Care Med 1999; 159:1172–8.

103. Horie T, Hildebrandt J. Volume history, static equilibrium, and dynamic compliance of excised cat lung. J Appl Physiol 1972; 33:105–12.

104. Caples SM, Hubmayr RD. Respiratory monitoring tools in the intensive care unit. Curr Opin Crit Care 2003; 9:230–5.

105. Gajic O, Dara SI, Mendez JL, et al. Ventilator-associated lung injury in patients without acute lung injury at the onset of mechanical ventilation. Crit Care Med 2004; 32:1817–24.

106. Nieszkowska A, Lu Q, Vieira S, et al. Incidence and regional distribution of lung overinflation during mechanical ventilation with positive end-expiratory pressure. Crit Care Med 2004; 7:1496–503.

107. Veldhuizen RA, Welk B, Harbottle R, et al. Mechanical ventilation of isolated rat lungs changes the structure and biophysical properties of surfactant. J Appl Physiol 2002; 92:1169–75.

108. Veldhuizen RA, Yao LJ, Lewis JF. An examination of the different variables affecting surfactant aggregate conversion in vitro. Exp Lung Res 1999; 25:127–41.

109. Mead J, Takishima T, Leith D. Stress distribution in lungs: A model of pulmonary elasticity. J Appl Physiol 1970; 28:596–608.

110. Martynowicz MA, Minor TA, Walters BJ, Hubmayr RD. Regional expansion of oleic acid-injured lungs. Am J Respir Crit Care Med 1999; 160:250–8.

111. Gattinoni L, Carlesso E, Valenza F, et al. Acute respiratory distress syndrome, the critical care paradigm: What we learned and what we forgot. Curr Opin Crit Care 2004; 10:272–8.

112. Crapo RO, Morris AH, Clayton PD, Nixon CR. Lung volumes in healthy nonsmoking adults. Bull Eur Physiopathol Respir. 1982; 18:419–25.

113. Standardized lung function testing: Official statement of the European Respiratory Society. Eur Respir J Suppl 1993; 16:1–100.

114. Eichacker PQ, Gerstenberger EP, Banks SM, et al. Meta-analysis of acute lung injury and acute respiratory distress syndrome trials testing low tidal volumes. Am J Respir Crit Care Med 2002; 166:1510–4.

115. Agostoni E, Hyatt RE. Static behavior of the respiratory system. In: Macklem PT, Mead J, editors. Handbook of physiology, Vol 3. Baltimore: Waverly Press, 1986: 113–30.

116. Mead J, Gaensler EA. Esophageal and pleural pressures in man upright and supine. J Appl Physiol 1959; 14:81–3.

117. Mascheroni D, Kolobow T, Fumagalli R, et al. Acute respiratory failure following pharmacologically induced hyperventilation: An experimental animal study. Intensive Care Med 1988; 15:8–14.

118. Putensen C, Mutz NJ, Putensen-Himmer G, Zinserling J. Spontaneous breathing during ventilatory support improves ventilation-perfusion distributions in patients with acute respiratory distress syndrome. Am J Respir Crit Care Med 1999; 159:1241–8.

119. Putensen C, Hering R, Muders T, Wrigge H. Assisted breathing is better in acute respiratory failure. Curr Opin Crit Care. 2005; 11:63–8.

120. Hubmayr RD, Rodarte JR, Walters BJ, Tonelli FM. Regional ventilation during spontaneous breathing and mechanical ventilation in anesthetized dogs. J Appl Physiol 1987; 63:2467–75.

121. Reber A, Nylund U, Hedenstierna G. Position and shape of the diaphragm: Implications for atelectasis formation. Anaesthesia 1998; 53:1054–61.

122. Wrigge H, Uhlig U, Zinserling J, et al. The effects of different ventilatory settings on pulmonary and systemic inflammatory responses during major surgery. Anesth Analg 2004; 98:775–81.

123. Cole AG, Weller SF, Sykes MK. Inverse ratio ventilation compared with PEEP in adult respiratory failure. Intensive Care Med 1984; 10:227–32.

124. Yang SC, Yang SP. Effects of inspiratory flow waveforms on lung mechanics, gas exchange, and respiratory metabolism in COPD patients during mechanical ventilation. Chest 2002; 122:2096–104.

125. Laghi F, Segal J, Choe WK, Tobin MJ. Effect of imposed inflation time on respiratory frequency and hyperinflation in patients with chronic obstructive pulmonary disease. Am J Respir Crit Care Med 2001; 163:1365–70.

126. Darioli R, Peret C. Mechanical controlled hypoventilation in status asthmaticus. Am Rev Respir Dis 1984; 129:385–7.

127. Hickling KG, Henderson SJ, Jackson R. Low mortality associated with low volume pressure limited ventilation with permissive hypercapnia in severe adult respiratory distress syndrome. Intensive Care Med 1990; 16:372–7.

128. Rossi N, Musch G, Sangalli F, et al. Reverse-thrust ventilation in hypercapnic patients with acute respiratory distress syndrome: Acute physiological effects. Am J Respir Crit Care Med 2000; 162:363–8.

129. Richecoeur J, Lu Q, Vieira SR, et al. Expiratory washout versus optimization of mechanical ventilation during permissive hypercapnia in patients with severe acute respiratory distress syndrome. Am J Respir Crit Care Med 1999; 160:77–85.

130. Carter C, Adams AB, Stone M, et al. Tracheal gas insufflation during late exhalation efficiently reduces Pa_{O_2} in experimental acute lung injury. Intensive Care Med 2000; 28:504–8.

131. Reinoso MA, Gracey DR, Hubmayr RD. Interrupter mechanics of patients admitted to a chronic ventilator dependency unit. Am Rev Respir Dis 1993; 148:127–31.

132. Pepe PE, Marini JJ. Occult positive end-expiratory pressure in mechanically ventilated patients with airflow obstruction: The auto-PEEP effect. Am Rev Respir Dis 1982; 126:166–70.

133. Williams TJ, Tuxen DV, Scheinkestel CD, et al. Risk factors for morbidity in mechanically ventilated patients with acute severe asthma. Am Rev Respir Dis 1992; 146:607–15.

134. Sinderby C, Spahija J, Beck J, et al. Diaphragm activation during exercise in chronic obstructive pulmonary disease. Am J Respir Crit Care Med 2001; 163:1637–41.

135. Cassart M, Pettiaux N, Gevenois PA, et al. Effect of chronic hyperinflation on diaphragm length and surface area. Am J Respir Crit Care Med 1997; 156:504–8.

136. Cassart M, Hamacher J, Verbandt Y, et al. Effects of lung volume reduction surgery for emphysema on diaphragm dimensions and configuration. Am J Respir Crit Care Med 2001; 163:1171–5.
137. Rhoney DH, Murry KR. National survey of the use of sedating drugs, neuromuscular blocking agents, and reversal agents in the intensive care unit. J Intensive Care Med 2003; 18:139–45.
138. Parthasarathy S, Jubran A, Tobin MJ. Cycling of inspiratory and expiratory muscle groups with the ventilator in airflow limitation. Am J Respir Crit Care Med 1998; 158:1471–8.
139. Weber T, Tschernich H, Sitzwohl C, et al. Tromethamine buffer modifies the depressant effect of permissive hypercapnia on myocardial contractility in patients with acute respiratory distress syndrome. Am J Respir Crit Care Med 2000; 162:1361–5.
140. Tuxen DV, Lane S. The effects of ventilatory pattern on hyperinflation, airway pressures, and circulation in mechanical ventilation of patients with severe airflow obstruction. Am Rev Respir Dis 1987; 136:872–9.
141. Tuxen DV, Williams TJ, Scheinkestel CD, et al. Use of a measurement of pulmonary hyperinflation to control the level of mechanical ventilation in patients with acute severe asthma. Am Rev Respir Dis 1992; 146:1136–42.
142. Petrof BJ, Legare M, Goldberg P, et al. Continuous positive airway pressure reduced work of breathing and dyspnea during weaning from mechanical ventilation in severe chronic obstructive pulmonary disease. Am Rev Respir Dis 1990; 141:281–9.
143. Gay PC, Rodarte JR, Hubmayr RD. The effects of positive expiratory pressure on isovolume flow and dynamic hyperinflation in patients receiving mechanical ventilation. Am Rev Respir Dis 1989; 139:621–6.
144. Martin JG, Shore S, Engel LA. Effect of continuous positive airway pressure on respiratory mechanics and pattern of breathing in induced asthma. Am Rev Respir Dis 1982; 126:812–7.
145. Roussos C, Macklem PT. The respiratory muscles. New Engl J Med 1982; 307:786–97.
146. Laghi F, Cattapan SE, Jubran A, et al. Is weaning failure caused by low-frequency fatigue of the diaphragm? Am J Respir Crit Care Med 2003; 167:120–7.
147. Gaves C, Glass L, Laporta D, et al. Respiratory phase locking during mechanical ventilation in anesthetized human subjects. Am J Physiol 1986; 250:R902–9.
148. Ingrassia TS 3d, Nelson SB, Harris CD, Hubmayr RD. Influence of sleep state on CO_2 responsiveness: A study of the unloaded respiratory pump in humans. Am Rev Respir Dis 1991; 144:1125–9.
149. Simon PM, Zurob AS, Wies WM, et al. Entrainment of respiration in humans by periodic lung inflations: Effect of state and CO_2. Am J Respir Crit Care Med 1999; 160: 950–60.
150. Parthasarathy S, Tobin MJ. Effect of ventilator mode on sleep quality in critically ill patients. Am J Respir Crit Care Med 2002; 166:1423–9.
151. Juan G, Calverley P, Talamo C, et al. Effect of carbon dioxide on diaphragmatic function in human beings. New Engl J Med 1984; 310:874–9.
152. Nava S, Fanfulla F, Frigerio P, Navalesi P. Physiologic evaluation of 4 weeks of nocturnal nasal positive pressure ventilation in stable hypercapnic patients with chronic obstructive pulmonary disease. Respiration 2001; 68:573–83.
153. Laffey JG, Kavanagh BP. Hypocapnia. New Engl J Med 2002; 347:43–53.
154. Hubmayr RD. Coordinación de la musculatura respiratoria durante la desconexión de la ventilación mecánica en pacientes con enfermedades neurológicas [Respiratory muscle coordination during the weaning of patients with neurological diseases]. In: Net A, Mancebo J, Benito S, editors. Retirada de la ventilación mecánica. Barcelona: Springer-Verlag Ibérica, 1995: 164–81.

ASSIST-CONTROL VENTILATION

JORDI MANCEBO

Volume assist-control ventilation (ACV) is a ventilator mode in which the machine always delivers the same tidal volume during every inspiration, whether initiated by the ventilator or by the patient. This occurs regardless of the mechanical load on the respiratory system and no matter how strenuous or feeble the inspiratory muscle effort. Although it is one of the oldest ventilator modes, current data indicate that ACV is still the most frequently used mode in intensive-care units (ICUs).[1] The main reason for patients being admitted to an ICU is the need for mechanical ventilation,[2] and the most common reason to initiate mechanical ventilation is acute respiratory failure.[1]

About 60% of intubated, ventilated patients receive ACV and continue mainly with this mode throughout the course of mechanical ventilation, at least within the first 4 weeks of its initiation.[3] This percentage is similar for patients ventilated for acute respiratory distress syndrome (ARDS) or for decompensated chronic obstructive pulmonary disease (COPD).[3] An international survey revealed that ACV was the preferred mode for 62% of physicians.[1]

Basic Principles

In ACV, mechanical breaths can be triggered by the ventilator or the patient. With the former, triggering occurs when a certain time has elapsed after the previous inspiration if the patient fails to make a new inspiratory muscle effort (Fig. 7-1). The frequency at which time triggering takes place is determined by the backup rate set on the ventilator. When patients trigger a mechanical breath, their spontaneous inspiratory effort is sensed by the machine, usually as a change in airway pressure or airflow (Fig. 7-2). When such a change crosses the trigger-sensitivity threshold, the ventilator delivers the preset tidal volume. Most machines delivering ACV are flow controllers because they measure and control flow and calculate volume by appropriate flow transducers. Special valves, run by microprocessors or by analog electronics, control flow delivery. Their performance is similar, although it has been claimed that using microprocessors provides increased flexibility[4] because they are run by software programs. Such valves open and close proportionally by different motor mechanisms: solenoids (a current generates a magnetic field), motor-driven cams, or digital on-off solenoid systems. In some ventilators, volume is measured directly by volumetric displacement via a built-in linear motor and a rolling-seal piston. Apart from delivering gas to the patient, the ventilators control exhalation with appropriate valves. Expiratory valves are closed during inspiration and open during exhalation. Importantly, they should provide minimal airflow resistance, which depends on their physical design, and maintain the desired levels of positive end-expiratory pressure (PEEP) throughout exhalation. This can be achieved with microprocessor active control mechanisms, with inflatable diaphragms, or by pinching silicon tubes.[4]

Mechanical breaths have precise mechanisms for being initiated (trigger variable), sustained (limit variable), and stopped (cycle variable). These are known as *phase variables*.[5] In ACV, the mechanical breaths are limited by volume and/or flow and cycled by volume or time. The limit variable is that which increases to a preset value before inspiration ends. The cycle variable is that used to declare the end of inspiration. The inspiratory flow-shape delivery is usually a square (constant) during ACV, although some ventilators also permit sinusoidal and/or ramp (ascending or descending) gas flows.

Physiologic Effects

Mechanical ventilation is a lifesaving supportive treatment that improves gas exchange and decreases the mechanical workload of the respiratory muscles while buying time for the patient to recover. The way mechanical ventilation is used is central to its short- and long-term effects. Ventilator settings are a major determinant of the physiologic and clinical effects of ACV. The physiologic effects of ACV on gas exchange and cardiovascular function are dealt with in Chapters 38 and 39.

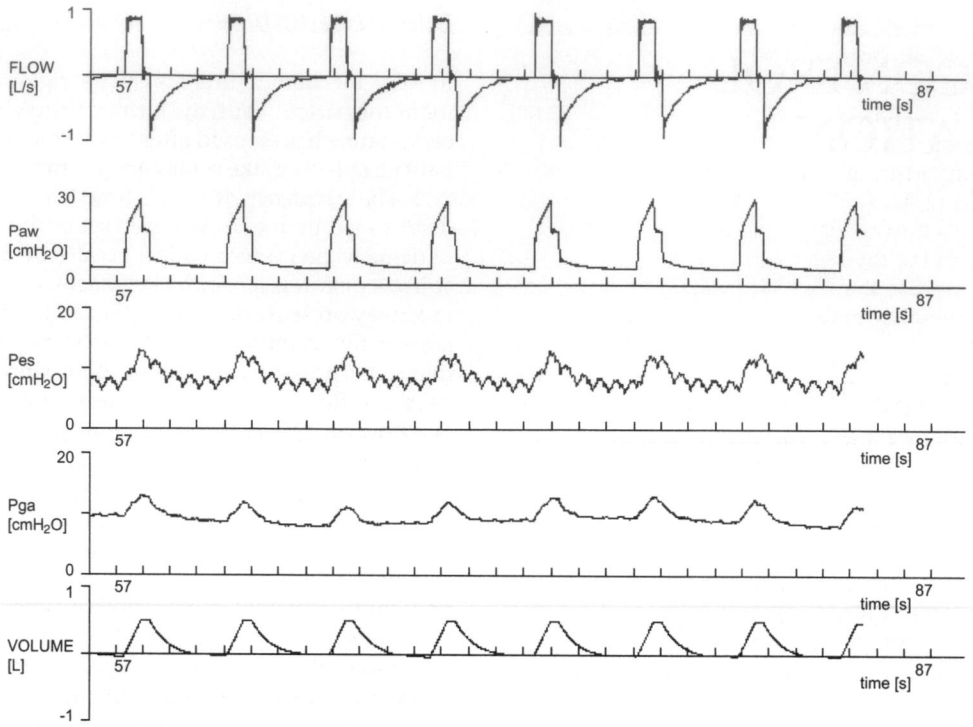

FIGURE 7-1 (*From top to bottom*) Tracings of airflow (flow), airway pressure (Paw), esophageal pressure (Pes), gastric pressure (Pga), and tidal volume (volume). Each mark on the time axis denotes 1 second. These recordings were obtained in a passively ventilated patient. Each breath is time-triggered.

FIGURE 7-2 (*From top to bottom*) tracings of airflow (flow), airway pressure (Paw), esophageal pressure (Pes), gastric pressure (Pga), and tidal volume (volume). Each mark on the time axis denotes 1 second. These recordings were obtained during patient-triggered assist-control ventilation (ACV). Every spontaneous inspiratory muscle effort is followed by a mechanically delivered breath. Note the delay between the beginning of inspiratory effort (Pes tracings) and the beginning of the mechanical breath (Paw tracings). The presence of intrinsic PEEP and the demand-valve sensitivity setting account for this delay.

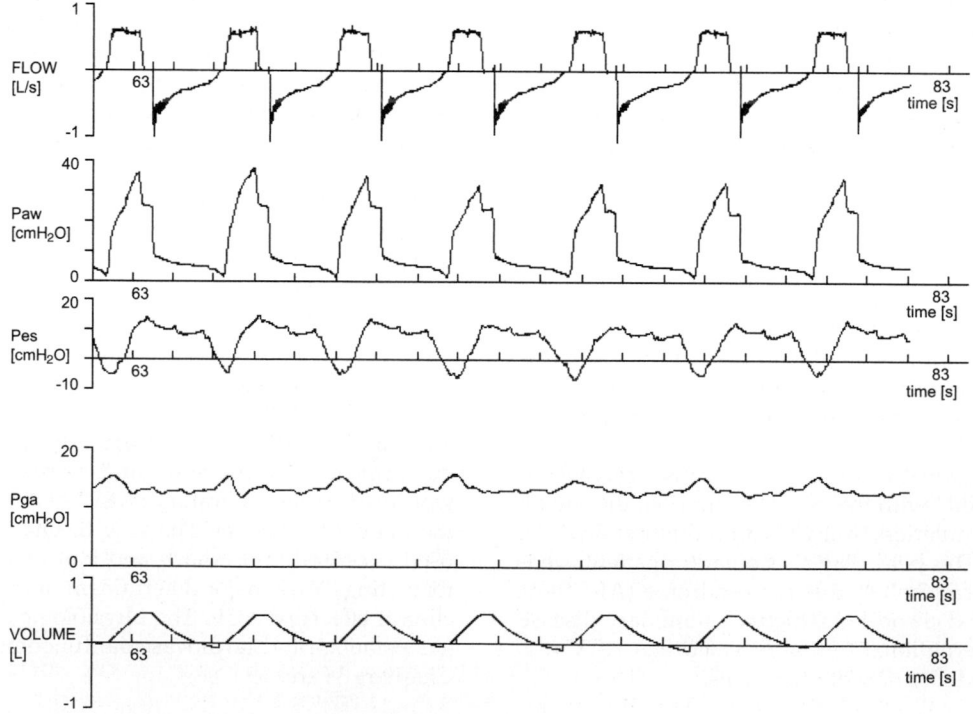

In every assisted mode, the ventilator responds to a patient's inspiratory effort. Both pressure- and flow-triggering systems of modern ventilators offer high performance, and the differences are small in terms of added work of breathing. Flow triggering, however, seems slightly superior to pressure triggering during pressure-support ventilation (PSV) but not during ACV. This is probably true because of the relatively small effort needed to open the demand valves in comparison with the total effort made during the whole inspiration and because the fixed inspiratory flow during ACV does not necessarily match the patient's demand.[6]

INSPIRATORY MUSCLE EFFORT

Marini et al[7] reported that decreases in trigger sensitivity increased work of breathing. Although decreasing the inspiratory flow rate from 100 to 80 liters/min did not affect the effort to breathe at a moderate minute ventilation (12 liters/min), it increased the work expenditure significantly when the minute ventilation was doubled.[7] When inspiratory flow was reduced to 40 liters/min and thus did not match the subject's demand, the work of breathing increased by 50%. Marini et al[8] later analyzed the inspiratory work at two inspiratory flow settings, 60 and 100 liters/min, in 20 patients. Tidal volume was unchanged. Such airflow rates generally exceeded those measured during unassisted breathing. The patients' work per liter of ventilation at both ACV inspiratory flow settings represented around 60% of the work dissipated during spontaneous breathing. In comparison with the nonsedated state, sedation and curarization did not modify the work to inflate the respiratory system. Dead space was added in half the patients and led to marked increases in muscle effort. Patients' work of breathing did not correlate with minute ventilation, although it was highly correlated with respiratory drive and muscle strength. A decrease in inspiratory flow to 40 liters/min (in five patients) led not only to an increase in effort but also to premature expiratory efforts, encroaching on the ventilator's inspiratory time. In total, these data demonstrated that inspiratory muscle effort persists throughout the inflation and that a substantial amount of muscle work is dissipated during ACV.

Ward et al[9] analyzed the inspiratory muscle effort at several inspiratory flow rates between 25 and 65 liters/min and two trigger-sensitivity settings, -2 and -5 cmH_2O. Tidal volume was constant, and no PEEP was used. As expected, the less sensitive the trigger sensitivity, the more work the patients performed. As inspiratory flow rate increased, inspiratory muscle effort decreased. During time-triggered ACV, in particular at inspiratory flow rates of 45 liters/min or lower, the muscles contracted after the onset of inspiratory flow.[9] The authors suggested that the stimulus for muscle contraction, rather than arising from a generalized increase in respiratory drive, arises within the breath in response to an abnormal imposed flow pattern. Flick et al[10] analyzed the duration of the diaphragmatic contraction at different ACV settings by using electromyography. They found that the diaphragmatic activity persisted well after triggering. Cinella et al[11] analyzed the effects of different tidal volumes (12 and 8 ml/kg) with an unchanged inspiratory time

(1 second without end-inspiratory pause), as well as different inspiratory time settings (0.6 and 1 second), with the same tidal volume (8 ml/kg). When inspiratory flow was reduced either by reducing tidal volume or by lengthening inspiratory time, work of breathing was increased consistently. The duration of diaphragmatic contraction was unaffected by the ventilator settings and always was shorter than 1 second.[11] Thus it appears that the effects of high airflow settings on muscle unloading are mainly exerted at the very beginning of inspiratory efforts.

Compared with spontaneous breathing, Leung et al[12] reported a fivefold reduction in inspiratory effort during ACV adjusted to deliver a tidal volume of 10 ml/kg and an inspiratory flow of 60 liters/min. Although such settings induced a major decrease in the sensation of dyspnea, they also were accompanied by the highest number of inspiratory efforts failing to trigger the machine. The patients, who mostly had obstructive airway disease, were ventilated without PEEP.

INSPIRATORY FLOW SETTINGS AND BREATHING PATTERN

A number of authors have shown that patients[11,13–15] and healthy individuals[16,17] react to an increase in inspiratory flow with an increase in respiratory rate when tidal volume is kept constant. In these circumstances, the imposed ventilator inspiratory time shortens as flow increases. This leads to a decrease in neural inspiratory time. When tidal volume is increased by lengthening the duration of inspiratory flow, neural expiratory time increases, and respiratory rate tends to decrease. These changes have opposite effects on respiratory rate. The mechanisms explaining these responses are complex and include the Hering-Breuer reflex (inhibits inspiration and prolongs expiration), reflexes mediated by vagal mechanoreceptors, and perhaps consciousness-mediated reflexes.[18–20] A study in nonintubated normal subjects who were ventilated with ACV[21] also reported the greatest breathing discomfort when inspiratory flow rates were at the extremes of those tested: 25 and 93 liters/min. Discomfort was minimal when flow rates were set at 34 and 63 liters/min.

Airflow-induced changes in breathing pattern carry important clinical implications, especially in patients with dynamic hyperinflation. Because inspiratory time is made up of the time of flow delivery and inspiratory pause, Laghi et al[14] hypothesized that a decrease in ventilator inflation time would cause an increase in rate. In 10 noninvasively ventilated stable patients with an obstructive airway disease, the authors increased flow at constant tidal volume and decreased the inspiratory pause, keeping inspiratory flow and tidal volume constant. Decreasing inspiratory time by increasing flow from 30–90 liters/min increased both respiratory rate and expiratory time significantly. Intrinsic PEEP diminished significantly despite the increase in respiratory rate. When inspiratory time was decreased by shortening the inspiratory pause, both respiratory frequency and expiratory time increased significantly. Again, this decreased intrinsic PEEP significantly. Additionally, the higher inspiratory flow rates also decreased respiratory drive and inspiratory effort. These results suggest that imposed ventilator inspiratory time duration determines the respiratory rate and that the strategies that reduce ventilator inspiratory time, although accompanied by tachypnea, also prolong the time for exhalation, thus decreasing intrinsic PEEP.

INVERSE INSPIRATORY-TO-EXPIRATORY RATIO

ACV has been used with inverse inspiratory-to-expiratory (I:E) ratio (i.e., >1:1). The rationale is that a lower inspiratory flow may improve intrapulmonary distribution of gas (via a better mixing of gas or by improving the efficacy of collateral ventilation), reduce dead space, improve the ventilation-to-perfusion relationships, and enhance alveolar recruitment.[22,23]

In an experimental study of oleic acid–induced lung injury,[24] the short-term effects of ACV with PEEP were compared with those of inverse-ratio ACV at the same total PEEP. The authors found no differences in lung mechanics, hemodynamics, gas exchange, or computed tomographic lung densities. In sheep with bronchoalveolar lavage–induced acute lung injury, Mang et al[25] analyzed the effects of ACV and PCV (both with PEEP) at different I:E ratios while maintaining the mean airway pressure constant. No differences were found in gas exchange or hemodynamics, most probably because mean airway pressure did not change.

In a study that compared ACV with inverse-ratio ACV, no differences in gas exchange were reported in patients with acute respiratory failure.[26] Mercat et al[27] compared ACV with and without inverse-ratio ACV (I:E ratio 2:1 versus 1:2) at unchanged total PEEP, respiratory rate, and tidal volume in patients with ARDS. No advantages in terms of arterial oxygen tension (Pa_{O_2}) were seen. In the first hour of the study, cardiac index, oxygen delivery, and Pa_{CO_2} were lower with inverse-ratio ACV, but differences disappeared over time.

RESPIRATORY MUSCLES

Mechanical ventilation per se can induce respiratory muscle damage,[28–30] and patients appear to exhibit diaphragmatic weakness after a period of mechanical ventilation.[31] Le Bourdellès et al[32] showed that anesthetized, passively ventilated rats had lower diaphragmatic weight and a reduction in their force-generating capacity in comparison with spontaneously breathing control animals. The force-generating capacity was not reduced in peripheral muscles, and the authors suggested that this might be secondary to the prior history of muscle activation. Anzueto et al[33] studied sedated, paralyzed baboons under ACV for 11 days. Endurance time decreased over this period, and transdiaphragmatic pressure diminished by 25%, suggesting that the duration of passive ACV is also a relevant factor.

Sassoon et al[34] showed that 3 days of passive ventilation in rabbits led to a progressive decrease in the force-generating capacity of the diaphragm in comparison with control animals who received the same total amounts of sedatives but were breathing spontaneously. They also showed that

significant diaphragmatic myofibril damage had occurred. This investigation supports the notion that a decrease in diaphragmatic force-generating capacity depends on time and that muscle inactivity is associated with injury. Similar data have been reported by others studying the same animal species.[35] Yang et al[36] reported structural remodeling of the diaphragm in rats under passive ACV for 4 days. They also found a decreased diaphragm-to-body-weight ratio and a decrease in the maximal force generated by the diaphragm as compared with spontaneously breathing controls. Several investigators[37–39] have begun to elucidate the complex cellular and molecular mechanisms underlying passive ventilation-induced respiratory muscle damage.

Recent findings by Sassoon et al[40] carry important clinical implications. The authors found that ACV, as compared with passive ACV, can attenuate markedly the decrease in diaphragmatic force induced by total inactivity in rabbits. Another investigation with clinical ramifications has shown that passive ACV improves diaphragmatic force production in rats challenged with intravascular endotoxin as compared with equally challenged spontaneously breathing animals.[41]

If passive ventilation is one extreme, the other is a fatiguing loading. Both extremes are harmful to the respiratory muscles. Normal subjects submitted to inspiratory resistive loading up to a fatiguing threshold showed a decrease in diaphragmatic contractility lasting for at least 24 hours.[42] Jiang et al[43] showed diaphragmatic injury and inflammation at 3 days after a 90-minute period of acute moderate and high inspiratory resistive loading in rabbits. The same group[44] subsequently reported a marked decrease in the force production of the diaphragm at 3 days after high inspiratory resistive loading over the same time. Such stress also induces selective upregulation of a number of cytokines in the diaphragmatic fibers and eventually may lead to systemic effects.[45,46]

SLEEP

Sleep is new area of investigation in patients admitted to an ICU. Studies using appropriate tools reveal that patients have major sleep disturbances in terms of quantity and quality.[47] The acuity of illness, the use of medications (such as sedatives or opioids), the caregivers' interventions, and the environmental elements are contributing factors. Gabor et al[48] indicated that only 30% of sleep disruption in ventilated patients was attributable to elements of the ICU environment. A large proportion of sleep disruption was unexplained, and—quoting preliminary work by Parthasarathy et al—the authors suggested the mode of ventilation and patient-ventilator dyssynchrony as plausible explanations.[48]

Parthasarathy and Tobin[49] sought to determine if sleep quality was influenced by the mode of ventilation. They hypothesized that sleep is more fragmented during PSV as compared to ACV because of the development of central apneas. Eleven patients were ventilated with ACV at tidal volumes of 8 ml/kg, inspiratory flow rate 1 liter/s, and a backup rate of four breaths below the total assisted rate. PSV was set to deliver the same tidal volume. Patients also received PSV with 100 ml of added dead space. During wakefulness, respiratory rate was similar with the two modes. During sleep, minute ventilation fell more during PSV than with ACV. Sleep fragmentation, measured as the number of arousals and awakenings, was significantly greater during PSV than during ACV (79 versus 54 events per hour). Six patients had apneas while receiving PSV and none while receiving ACV. The percentage of patients who had congestive heart failure was significantly higher among patients exhibiting apneas than among patients free of apneas (83% versus 20%). Minute ventilation during sleep was greater in patients who did not develop apneas, suggesting that increased drive protects against the development of apneas. The addition of dead space reduced the number of apneas markedly: from 54 to 4 apneas per hour. Whether or not similar results would be obtained with PSV titrated at lower levels of assist is unknown.

Rationale, Advantages, and Limitations

The main reasons for using ACV are to unload the inspiratory muscles and to improve gas exchange. ACV permits complete respiratory muscle rest, which is usually the case when patients do not trigger the machine, and a variable degree of respiratory muscle work. ACV commonly achieves an improvement in gas exchange, and only a minority of ventilated patients die because of refractory hypoxemia.

During passive ventilation with ACV at a constant inspiratory flow, fundamental variables related to respiratory system mechanics, such as tidal volume, inspiratory flow, peak airway pressure, end-inspiratory plateau airway pressure, and total PEEP (the sum of external PEEP and intrinsic PEEP, if any), are measured easily (Fig. 7-3). These variables allow calculation of resistance, compliance, and the time constant of the respiratory system.

If airway pressure tracings are obtained during passive ACV as well as during patient-triggered ACV at the same settings, we can estimate a patient's work of breathing simply by superimposing the two tracings (Fig. 7-4). When patients are triggering the breaths, the end-inspiratory plateau pressure also can be influenced by the amount and duration of inspiratory muscle effort (Fig. 7-5). When mechanical breaths are triggered by the patient, the scooping on the airway pressure profile allows indirect evaluation of patient-ventilator interaction (Fig. 7-6). Such capabilities are unique to ACV. These capabilities represent a major advantage because they enable one to properly understand respiratory system mechanics and patient-ventilator interactions.

A major limitation of ACV is that it imposes a number of constraints on the variability of the patient's breathing pattern: inspiratory flow, inspiratory time, and backup rate. Adjusting ACV settings may be more complex than with pressure-limited modes. One reason is that manufacturers employ different algorithms for implementing the delivery of a tidal breath. The other reason is that during ACV it is difficult to pinpoint the inspiratory flow rate and tidal volume settings that are optimal for an individual patient (Fig. 7-7).

Some settings are almost impossible to achieve with ACV. For instance, the simultaneous adjustment of a moderate tidal volume at a high inspiratory flow rate will produce a short machine inspiratory time, which under certain circumstances may not match the patient's neural inspiratory time properly. In addition, the patient's varying ventilatory needs and the change in the mechanical properties of the respiratory system over the course of ventilation imply that periods of underassist are likely to be interspersed with periods of overassist. These problems, however, are common to virtually all ventilator modes.

Indications and Contraindications

ACV is indicated when a life-threatening physiologic derangement in gas exchange or cardiovascular dynamics has not been corrected by other means. Clinical manifestations of severely increased work of breathing or impending respiratory arrest are indications for instituting ACV.[50] Although there appear to be no absolute contraindications to ACV, some of its shortcomings may prompt physicians to use other modes.

Comparison with Other Modes

The main difference between ACV and PCV is that with the latter the ventilator functions as a pressure controller, and it is a pressure-limited and time-cycled mode. The trigger variable is identical to ACV. With the PCV mode, delivery of airflow and tidal volume changes according to the mechanical impedance of the respiratory system and patient inspiratory muscle effort. This mechanism implies that every increase in transpulmonary pressure is accompanied by an increase in tidal volume.

PRESSURE-CONTROLLED VENTILATION IN ANIMAL STUDIES

In rabbits with oleic acid–induced lung injury, Ludwigs et al[51] compared ACV with PEEP and inverse-ratio PCV at equal total PEEP and found that arterial oxygenation and a radionuclide index of lung epithelial permeability both worsened during inverse-ratio PCV. Recently, Maeda et al[52] compared ACV at I:E ratios of 1:4 and 1:1 with pressure-regulated volume control ventilation at an I:E ratio of 1:4 in healthy animals. After 6 hours, the animals ventilated with pressure-regulated volume control, which delivered a high peak inspiratory flow, exhibited a greater decrease in Pa_{O_2} and respiratory system compliance and more macroscopic and microscopic lung injury in comparison with animals undergoing the other two modes.

PRESSURE-CONTROLLED VENTILATION IN ACUTE RESPIRATORY FAILURE PATIENTS

Numerous studies[53–61] have compared the effects of PCV and ACV. These are summarized in the Table 7-1. They are

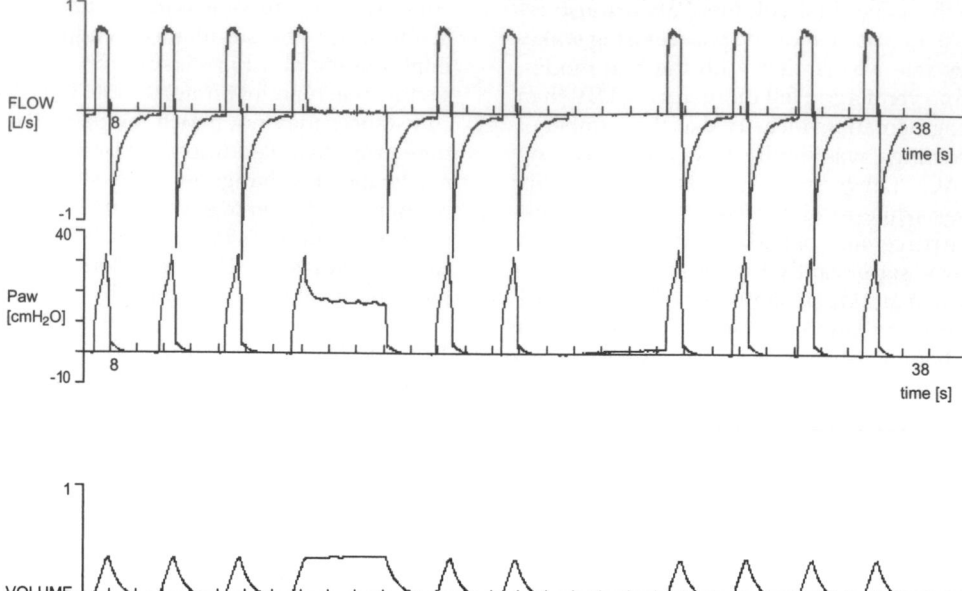

FIGURE 7-3 (*From top to bottom*) Tracings of airflow (flow), airway pressure (Paw), and tidal volume (volume). Each mark on the time axis denotes 1 second. Note that expiratory flow is interrupted by the beginning of each breath, thus heralding dynamic hyperinflation. A prolonged end-inspiratory occlusion (fourth breath from the left) enables measurement of the static recoil pressure of the respiratory system. A prolonged end-expiratory occlusion (sixth breath from the left) illustrates the presence of intrinsic PEEP (3 cmH_2O). These values, together with peak airway pressure, inspiratory flow rate, and tidal volume, enable the calculation of resistance, compliance, and respiratory system time constant in passively ventilated patients.

all short-term studies with a limited number of patients. Different adjustments were used. Taken together, no major differences in terms of gas exchange seem to emerge between ACV and PCV.

A randomized monocenter trial performed with a small number of patients[62] showed an early trend toward respiratory system compliance improvement during PCV compared with ACV. Differences in gas exchange between the two modes were minimal. In a randomized multicenter study,[63] PCV and ACV were compared. End-inspiratory plateau airway pressure was kept at a maximum of 35 cmH_2O during both modes, and I:E ratio adjustment was at the discretion of the physicians. This resulted in a similar inverse I:E ratio in the two groups, about 2:1. Arterial oxygenation did not differ between the modes. ICU mortality was 69% (29 of 42 patients) in the ACV group and 49% (18 of 37 patients) in the PCV group; the difference was not significant. A multivariate analysis did not find ventilator mode to be independently associated with increased mortality. Although difficult to interpret, this study cast doubts on the usefulness of inverse-ratio ACV in patients with ARDS.

PRESSURE-CONTROLLED VENTILATION AND INSPIRATORY MUSCLE EFFORT

Cinella et al[11] compared ACV and assist PCV and used two tidal volume settings (12 and 8 ml/kg) with an inspiratory time of 1 second and no end-inspiratory pause. At high tidal volumes, no differences were observed between the two modes in terms of breathing pattern or indexes of inspiratory muscle effort. When a tidal volume of 8 ml/kg was used (and thus inspiratory flow decreased with ACV), differences arose. Respiratory rate and occlusion pressure (a measure of respiratory drive) tended to be higher with ACV, and indexes of inspiratory muscle effort showed a marked increase as compared with PCV.

In a second part of this study[11] the authors compared the effects of ACV and assist PCV using a fixed tidal volume (8 ml/kg) and two different settings for inspiratory time: 1 second and 0.6 second with no pause. With the longer inspiratory time, the differences were the same as stated previously. When inspiratory time was reduced and thus inspiratory flow increased during ACV, however, the differences between the modes virtually vanished. The study showed that both modes unloaded the respiratory muscles equally, provided that the inspiratory flow rate was set appropriately during ACV. These data confirm the importance of maintaining an inspiratory flow rate high enough to unload the respiratory muscles adequately and also point out that moderate- to low-tidal-volume ventilation using high flow rates results in a short inspiratory time, which may not be optimal for some patients. Similar results were obtained by McIntyre et al[64] comparing ACV with a pressure-limited volume-guaranteed dual mode. These authors, however, suggested that the pressure-limited breaths could reduce

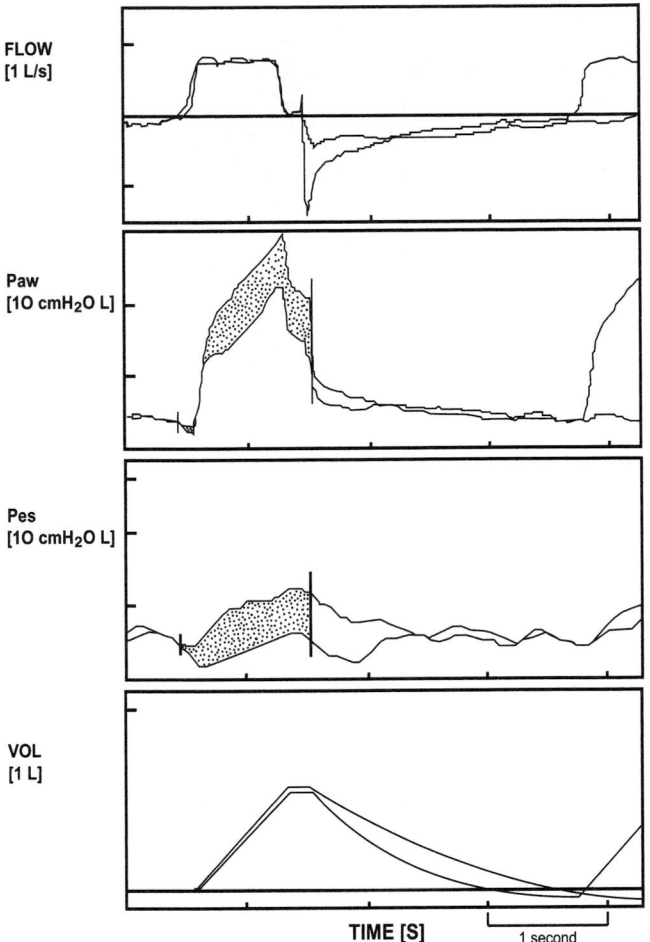

FLOW
[1 L/s]

Paw
[10 cmH₂O L]

Pes
[10 cmH₂O L]

VOL
[1 L]

TIME [S] 1 second

FIGURE 7-4 (*From top to bottom*) Tracings of airflow (flow), airway pressure (Paw), esophageal pressure (Pes), and tidal volume (volume). Each mark on the time axis denotes 1 second. The tracings in each panel were obtained from the same individual at two different times. They were then superimposed. Ventilator settings were identical. The vertical line on the airflow, airway pressure, and esophageal pressure tracings indicates the end of ventilator's total inspiratory time. The dotted areas within the airway pressure and esophageal pressure tracings are identical. The dotted areas denote the amount of inspiratory muscle effort that the patient made during the assisted breath.

patient-ventilator flow dyssynchrony, although total inspiratory effort was similar between the modes, and tidal volume was significantly higher with the pressure-limiting strategy.

INTERMITTENT MANDATORY VENTILATION

Early studies compared ACV with intermittent mandatory ventilation (IMV). In a study by Hudson et al,[65] the mandatory rates were 50% and 25% of the ACV rate. In a study by Groeger et al,[66] the mandatory rates were 50% of the ACV rate, and patients always remained normocapnic. Patients in the study of Hudson et al were markedly hypocapnic and alkalotic during ACV, and a slight increase in Pa_{CO_2} was observed during IMV. This change was attributed to

an increased CO_2 production, presumably caused by an increase in work of breathing.

Marini et al[67] compared ACV (100% IMV) with IMV to provide 80%, 60%, 40%, 20%, and 0% of the ventilation observed during ACV. Tidal volume and flow settings during ACV were 10 ml/kg and 1 liter/s, respectively, and average respiratory rate was 23 breaths per minute. The total breathing frequency and spontaneous tidal volume increased as far as IMV assistance was decreased. Duration of inspiratory effort during assisted breaths was similar across the different IMV levels. At all levels of support, patients performed a substantial effort during the machine-assisted breaths that increased progressively as IMV assistance was withdrawn. These data emphasize several points. Machine assistance does not suppress patient effort. There is a poor adaptation to ventilator assistance on a breath-by-breath basis, suggesting that the intensity of muscle effort is fixed before cycle initiation. Off-switching of inspiratory muscle contraction is independent of volume and flow ventilator settings.

Leung et al[12] compared ACV, IMV (80%, 60%, 40%, and 20% levels of assist), pressure support (100%, 80%, 60%, 40%, and 20% levels of assist) and a combination of IMV with a pressure support of 10 cmH₂O. No PEEP was used. Average tidal volume and respiratory rate during ACV were 600 ml and 17 breaths per minute, respectively. The observed rate during ACV was considered equivalent to IMV 100%. Pressure support 100% (average 17 cmH₂O) was the level of assistance that resulted in the same tidal volume as during ACV; this led to a respiratory rate of 16 breaths per minute. Nontriggering attempts occurred with every mode and were most numerous at the highest levels of assistance. At 100% levels of assistance, the inspiratory effort and dyspnea sensation were similar among the modes, and both increased progressively when assistance was decreased. When the total inspiratory effort was partitioned between its triggering and posttriggering components, the former was unchanged despite varying levels of ventilator assistance. The posttriggering effort, however, was highly correlated with the respiratory drive at the beginning of the breath.

PRESSURE-SUPPORT VENTILATION

Tokioka et al[68] compared ACV with pressure-support ventilation (PSV) set to achieve the same value of peak airway pressure as during ACV. This resulted in PSV levels of 27 cmH₂O above a PEEP of 12 cmH₂O. With these settings, tidal volume was significantly higher and machine respiratory rate significantly lower during pressure support. These data indicate that peak airway pressure during ACV is an inappropriate surrogate variable to adjust pressure support to get similar levels of assistance. Tejeda et al[69] compared ACV with PSV in patients with respiratory failure of assorted etiologies. PSV was adjusted to deliver the same tidal volume as with ACV, although it actually resulted in significantly higher tidal volumes. The authors found a slightly better Pa_{O_2} only in a subgroup of patients with restrictive disorders. Surprisingly, the calculated shunt in these

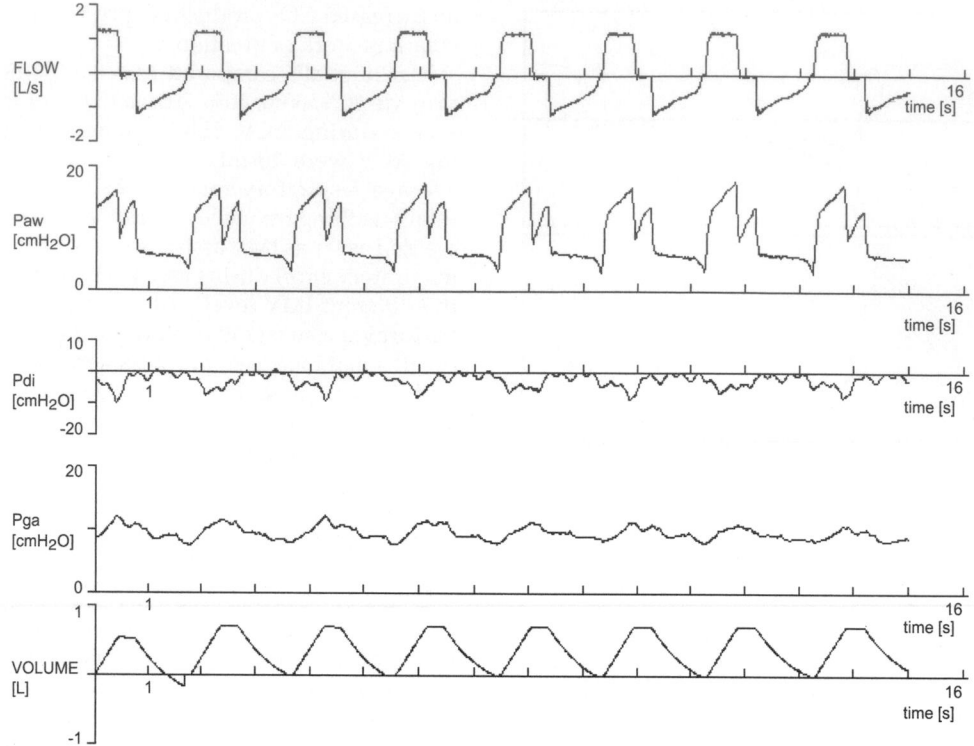

FIGURE 7-5 (*From top to bottom*) Tracings of airflow (flow), airway pressure (Paw), transdiaphragmatic pressure (Pes), gastric pressure (Pga), and tidal volume (volume). Each mark on the time axis denotes 1 second. The time of inspiratory flow is shorter than the duration of diaphragmatic contraction. This patient did not exhibit expiratory muscle recruitment, as indicated by the gastric pressure recording. Inspiratory muscles relax at the end of the inspiratory pause time, thus explaining the "M"wave shape on the airway pressure recording.

patients (18–20%) was lower than in patients with COPD (26–29%). A significantly higher dead-space-to-tidal-volume ratio also was observed during PSV (24%) than during ACV (18%). These are extremely low values for patients with respiratory failure. For these reasons, the overall clinical significance of these findings is difficult to judge.

Kreit et al[70] analyzed work of breathing during ACV and PSV in 11 patients. During ACV, tidal volume was 10–12 ml/kg, and inspiratory flow 75–80 liters/min. PSV was increased progressively to reach the same tidal volume as during ACV. This strategy resulted in an average pressure support of about 19 cmH$_2$O. The authors confirmed previous studies indicating that both work of breathing and respiratory rate vary inversely with the PSV level. With such adjustments, the patient's work of breathing and minute ventilation were almost identical between the modes.

In a study not specifically designed to compare ACV with PSV, Aslanian et al[6] used the average tidal volume measured during clinician-titrated PSV for later adjustments of ACV. PSV levels were set at a target respiratory rate of between 15 and 30 breaths per minute, which resulted in an average pressure support of 16 cmH$_2$O and an average tidal volume of 500 ml. Settings during ACV were tidal volume 500 ml with an inspiratory flow rate at 50 liters/min. With such adjustments, respiratory rate, minute ventilation,

breathing pattern, and several indexes of inspiratory muscle effort were similar between the modes.

Chiumello et al[71] compared the effects of PSV at 5, 15, and 25 cmH$_2$O with assist PCV at the same levels of pressure and inspiratory time as during PSV and ACV. ACV was delivered with a square and decelerating flow pattern, both matched for the same tidal volume and peak inspiratory flow as during PSV. No differences among the modes were observed. The authors also compared clinician-titrated PSV (average 10 cmH$_2$O) with two ACV modes (square and decelerating flow), both at two flow settings (high and low). Tidal volume was always the same. The peak inspiratory flow obtained during PSV (0.78 liter/s) was the high-flow setting for both ACV types. When high-flow settings were used, no differences were observed. The low-flow setting, about 0.64 liter/s, induced a significant increase in work of breathing without differences in respiratory rate or gas exchange.

In a very selected population of patients with acute lung injury, Cereda et al[72] studied the physiologic changes that appeared during the 48 hours after the transition from ACV to PSV. Hemodynamics and oxygenation were similar. An increase in minute ventilation and a lower Pa$_{CO_2}$ were observed during PSV. Of 48 patients, 10 did not tolerate PSV. These patients had a lower static compliance and a higher dead-space-to-tidal-volume ratio when compared with patients who succeeded. These data suggest that PSV might

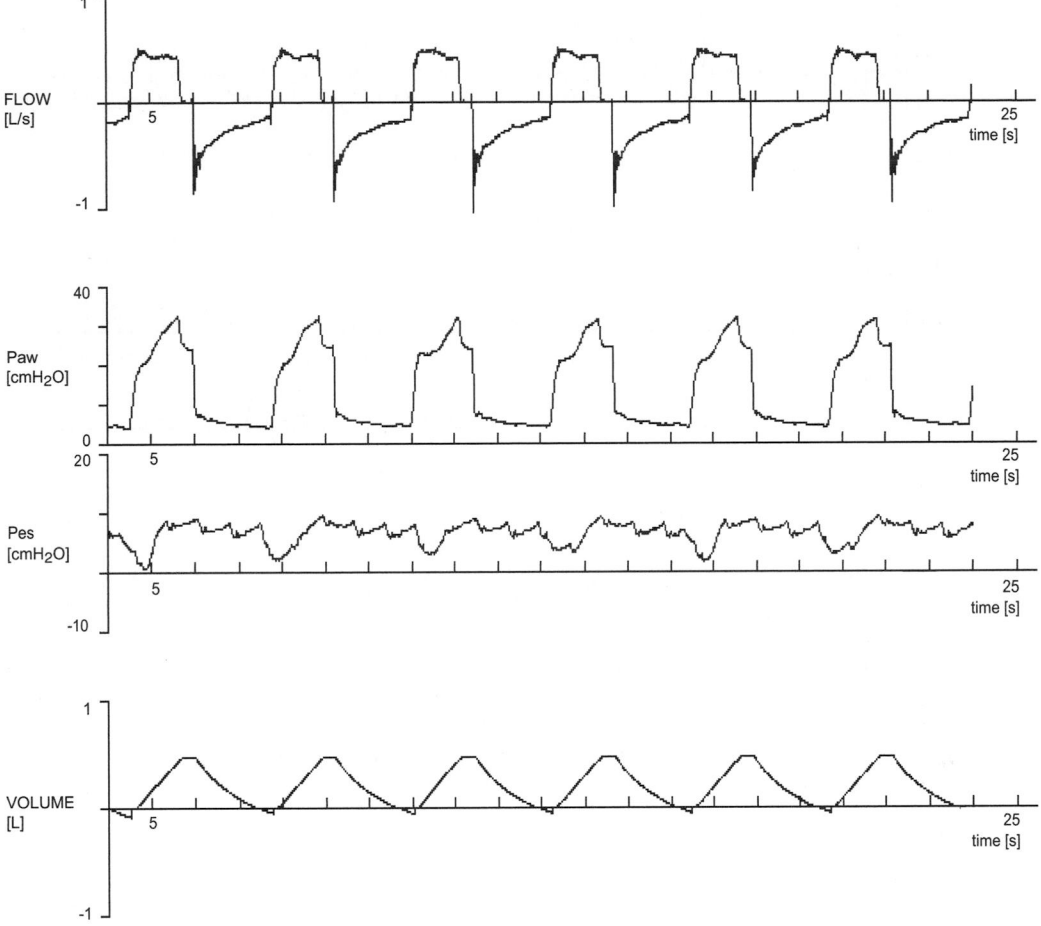

FIGURE 7-6 (*From top to bottom*) Tracings of airflow (flow), airway pressure (Paw), esophageal pressure (Pes), and tidal volume (volume). Each mark on the time axis denotes 1 second. The scooping on the airway pressure recording immediately after peak inspiratory flow delivery is apparent on all these assisted breaths.

be an alternative to ACV in carefully selected patients with acute lung injury.

BIOLOGICALLY VARIABLE VENTILATION

Tidal volume during ACV is, by design, delivered in a monotonous manner. To recreate the spontaneous variability of physiologic rhythms, mechanical ventilation using computer-generated biologic variability in respiratory rate and tidal volume has been used. The goal of this approach is to improve gas exchange and respiratory system mechanics and minimize ventilator-induced lung injury. Data comparing ACV with ventilation achieved with randomly variable tidal volumes and respiratory rates have been obtained in several experimental models of acute lung injury.[73–77] Models include different animal species (e.g., rodents, pigs, and dogs), different type of insults (e.g., chemical, mechanical, and biological), and different ventilator settings (e.g., PEEP or no PEEP). In these short-term experiments, variable ventilation was matched to ACV in terms of minute ventilation.

The study by Nam et al[74] in a canine oleic acid–induced lung-injury model showed no benefits of one mode over the other. Other studies[73,75–77] reported benefits of variable ventilation over ACV in terms of arterial oxygenation, lung mechanics, degree of lung edema, proinflammatory cytokine production, or combinations of these. Variable ventilation may induce a better distribution of tidal volume—thereby matching ventilation to perfusion—better recruitment, and increased surfactant production. Whether these putative benefits are attributable directly to the ventilator mode per se, the type of injury, the animal species, the ventilator settings (degree of variability, PEEP levels), or the respiratory system mechanical characteristics is unclear. The physiologic effects of this new mode in patients with acute lung injury are unknown.

Variation in Delivery among Ventilator Brands

This section does not pretend to explain exhaustively the working principles of the dozens of different mechanical ventilators available on the market. It only explains some major differences in the way ACV settings are to be adjusted.

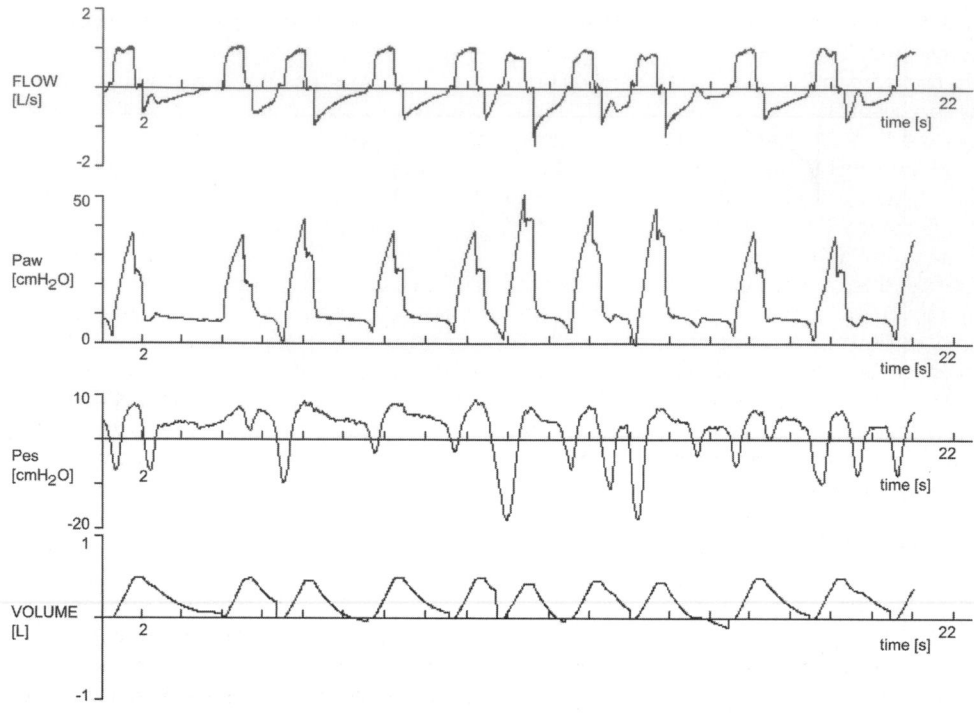

FIGURE 7-7 (*From top to bottom*) Tracings of airflow (flow), airway pressure (Paw), esophageal pressure (Pes), and tidal volume (volume). Each mark on the time axis denotes 1 second. Note the marked breath-by-breath variability in inspiratory muscle effort (esophageal pressure swings) and airway pressure profile. There is profound patient-ventilator dyssynchrony, and numerous inspiratory attempts fail to trigger the ventilator. It is also remarkable how difficult it can be to estimate the end-inspiratory plateau airway pressure in such circumstances.

TABLE 7-1   Comparison of ACV and PCV in Acute Respiratory Failure

Author, Year (Reference)	Modes	Matching	Measurements	Main Findings
Abraham, 1990 (53)	ACV, PCV	Same total PEEP	Gas exchange, hemodynamics	Gas exchange improved with PCV
Muñoz, 1993 (54)	ACV decelerated flow, PCV, no PEEP	Same intrinsic PEEP	Gas exchange, mechanics	Compliance higher with PCV
Mercat, 1993 (55)	ACV, PCV, PCV-IR	Same total PEEP	Gas exchange, hemodynamics	Pa_{CO_2}, cardiac index, and O_2 delivery lower with PCV-IR
Lessard, 1994 (56)	ACV, PCV, PCV-IR	Same total PEEP	Gas exchange, hemodynamics, mechanics	Pa_{O_2} and systemic blood pressure lower and mean airway pressure higher with PCV-IR
Mancebo, 1994 (57)	ACV, PCV-IR	Same total PEEP, respiratory rate, and tidal volume	Gas exchange, hemodynamics, mechanics	Mean airway pressure higher with PCV-IR
Davis, 1996 (58)	ACV, ACV decelerated flow, PCV; all with PEEP	Same setting as ACV	Gas exchange and hemodynamics	Lower Pa_{O_2} and mean airway pressure with ACV
Zavala, 1998 (59)	ACV no PEEP, ACV, ACV-IR, PCV-IR	ACV, ACV-IR, and PCV-IR; all with same PEEP	Gas exchange and multiple inert-gas elimination technique	Pa_{CO_2} improved and shunt decreased with ACV Pa_{CO_2} and dead space decreased with PCV-IR
Prella, 2002 (60)	ACV, PCV	Patients' needs	Gas exchange and gas distribution by computed tomography	Better gas distribution at end expiration during PCV
Edibam, 2003 (61)	ACV, PCV, PCV-IR	Same total PEEP, respiratory rate, and tidal volume	Gas exchange, hemodynamics, mechanics, and gas distribution by computed tomography	More overinflated units at end inspiration during PCV-IR, suggesting further stretch

ABBREVIATIONS: PCV, pressure-controlled ventilation; PCV-IR, inverse-ratio, pressure-controlled ventilation; ACV-IR, inverse-ratio, assist-control ventilation.

The decision to stick with one style or another depends solely on the manufacturer. The fundamental settings during ACV are respiratory rate, tidal volume, and inspiratory flow rate. The backup respiratory rate determines the total breath duration, and both tidal volume and inspiratory flow rate determine the duration of mechanical inflation within a breath. The inspiratory pause, if used, appears immediately after the machine's flow delivery has ceased and thus increases the inspiratory time. The expiratory time is the only part of the breathing cycle that is allowed to vary when a patient triggers an ACV breath. For this reason, we consider machines that require I:E ratio adjustment during ACV to be totally counterintuitive.

The Puritan-Bennett 7200,[78] 740, 760,[79] and 840[80] ventilators allow direct setting of respiratory rate, tidal volume, inspiratory flow rate, and inspiratory pause time. In my opinion, this is the most comprehensive approach because the time for flow delivery depends on the tidal volume and inspiratory flow rate. The I:E ratio thus is a consequence of those settings.

The Dräger Evita 2 ventilator[81] allows direct settings for respiratory rate, tidal volume, inspiratory flow rate, and I:E ratio. This kind of configuration mandates that the inspiratory pause time will vary depending on those settings. With this particular ventilator, the airway pressure alarm (Pmax) limits the peak airway pressure in a way that flow decelerates when the Pmax threshold is reached, and then airway pressure flattens. Flow decelerates throughout the remaining total inspiratory time in an attempt to deliver the preset tidal volume, but the common peak airway pressure alarm (which is configurated automatically at 10 cmH2O above Pmax) does not sound. In these circumstances, the only high-priority alarm that alerts caregivers is the minute-ventilation alarm. This may occur when tidal volume is extremely low. This kind of setting may be dangerous and can lead to life-threatening situations, such as in the case of an endotracheal tube obstruction.

In the Dräger Evita 4 ventilator,[82] the settings to be adjusted during ACV are similar to those of the Evita 2, with the exception that instead of adjusting the I:E ratio, it is necessary to adjust the total inspiratory time. There is no independent adjustment of inspiratory pause time. With the Evita 4 machine, there are two airway pressure alarms. That which appears together with the other adjustable settings in ACV, Pmax, limits airway pressure in the same way as with the Evita 2. There is another airway pressure alarm that is to be adjusted in the main alarm settings screen, and it appears in a different ventilator window. The latter is a true alarm in the sense that when the preset pressure threshold is reached, the alarm sounds, and the machine cycles off. In consequence, it is highly advisable to set the Pmax value (which limits pressure) above the level of the true airway pressure alarm so as to inhibit Pmax from working.

The Hamilton Galileo ventilator[83] is user-configurable in three different ways. One is inspiratory flow rate and inspiratory pause time. The second is I:E ratio and inspiratory pause time. The third allows adjustment of inspiratory time as a percentage of the total cycle duration 60 divided by backup respiratory rate [60: backup rate]. Example: if rate is 15, the total cycle duration is 4(60/15 = 4 seconds), and

inspiratory pause time. Respiratory rate and tidal volume are mandatory for all three.

With the Siemens Servo 300,[84] the required adjustments are tidal volume, respiratory rate, inspiratory time (from 10–80% of total cycle duration), and inspiratory pause time (from 0–30% of total cycle duration). The maximal I:E ratio is 4:1. The Maquet Servo^i ventilator[85] allows a choice of internal configurations, either tidal volume and respiratory rate or minute ventilation and respiratory rate. Each one of these is also internally configurable, either inspiratory time or I:E ratio. The inspiratory pause time is adjustable from 0–30% of total cycle duration and is independent of the preselected internal configuration. This machine has a particular feature during ACV: If airway pressure drops more than 3 cmH2O during the inspiratory time window, for instance, because of a huge inspiratory muscle effort, the ventilator delivers more flow. The machine does so in a similar way to PSV and switches off when flow reaches the preset ACV flow value. This is obviously a hybrid ACV, and the clinical consequences of the machine reacting to this change in airway pressure are unknown. We can speculate what might happen, however, when ventilating patients with ARDS. When they are receiving ACV and make an inspiratory effort that it is not well matched with the preset machine settings, the ventilator will deliver more flow and volume when faced with an increase in muscle effort. Of course, this scenario (i.e., an increase in volume and transpulmonary pressure) is extremely harmful for these patients. A similar extra flow delivery occurs with the Servo 300. With this machine, however, extra flow is delivered when the airway pressure decreases 2 cmH2O below the preset PEEP level.

Finally, the Servo 300 and the Servo^i have an adjustable inspiratory pressure rise time (from 0–20% of the total cycle duration). When set at 0%, the flow delivery is completely squared. At the 20% extreme setting, the peak flow arrives at the very end of the inspiratory flow delivery time, and because the volume is controlled, the peak flow increases.

Adjustments at the Bedside

Settings to be adjusted in ACV are inspired oxygen concentration (FI_{O_2}), trigger sensitivity (to be set above the threshold of auto-triggering), backup rate, tidal volume, inspiratory flow rate (or inspiratory time), and end-inspiratory pause and external PEEP, if any. When ACV is instituted after tracheal intubation, patients usually are sedated and passively ventilated. Proper calculations of compliance and airflow resistance may help in adjusting the ventilator's backup breathing pattern. The time constant of the respiratory system determines the rate of passive lung emptying. The product of three time constants is the time needed to passively exhale 95% of the inspired volume.[86,87] If expiratory time is insufficient to allow for passive emptying, this will generate hyperinflation.

Mechanical ventilation in specific scenarios, for example, patients with obstructive disease, ARDS, and neuromuscular disorders, are dealt with in Chapters 31, 33, and 34. Some general principles, however, are worth recalling.

The goals of mechanical ventilation, in particular during ACV, have changed profoundly in the last decade.

Nowadays, moderate tidal volumes are customary, and achieving normocapnia is no longer required per se. This is the case for virtually all mechanically ventilated patients. One exception, however, is patients with brain injury and relatively normal lungs, in whom a tight Pa_{CO_2} control is required to avoid undesirable episodes of brain ischemia or hyperemia.

In patients with COPD, Tuxen and Lane[88] showed that at constant minute ventilation, the lowest degree of dynamic hyperinflation was obtained when ventilation was performed at a high inspiratory airflow and long expiratory time.[88] These data indicate that the quotient between tidal volume and expiratory time—mean expiratory flow—is the principal ventilator setting influencing the degree of dynamic hyperinflation.[87,88] Connors et al[89] showed improvements in gas exchange using high inspiratory airflows and suggested that they produced a more even distribution of ventilation. At the present time, a physiologically sound recommendation can be made when initiating ACV in these patients. A moderate F_{IO_2}, usually 0.4, suffices to improve hypoxemia; an arterial oxygen saturation of about 90% is acceptable. Initiate ventilation with a respiratory rate of 12 breaths per minute, tidal volume of about 8 ml/kg, and a constant inspiratory flow rate of between 60 and 90 liters/min. These settings need to be readjusted, as needed, once basic respiratory system mechanics and arterial blood gases have been measured. In these patients, the goal is to keep a balance between minimizing dynamic hyperinflation and providing sufficient alveolar ventilation to maintain arterial pH near the low-normal limit, not a normal Pa_{CO_2}. When patients are receiving ACV and mechanical breaths are triggered by the patient, external PEEP counterbalances the elastic mechanical load induced by intrinsic PEEP secondary to expiratory flow limitation and decreases the breathing workload markedly.[90] It is important to remember that external PEEP does not decrease the degree of dynamic hyperinflation either in passively ventilated patients or in patients with spontaneous inspiratory efforts. During ACV, when a patient triggers a mechanical breath, the expiratory time is no longer constant. Exhaled volume therefore might change on a cycle-to-cycle basis and modify the degree of dynamic hyperinflation. This may alter patient-ventilator synchrony and cause subsequent wasted inspiratory efforts, as is seen in patients with low inspiratory drive (i.e., sedated) and those with prolonged time constants.

Data[91–97] indicate consistently that the ventilator strategy in acute asthma should favor moderate tidal volumes, high inspiratory flow rates, and a long expiratory time. These settings avoid large end-inspiratory lung volumes, thus decreasing the risks of barotrauma and hypotension. The main goal in asthma is to avoid these complications rather than to achieve normocapnia. A reasonable recommendation from physiologic and clinical viewpoints when initiating ACV is to provide an inspiratory flow of 80 to 100 liters/min and a tidal volume of about 8 ml/kg and to avoid end-inspiratory plateau airway pressures higher than 30 cmH_2O. The respiratory rate should be adjusted to relatively low frequencies (about 10–12 cycles/min) so as to minimize hyperinflation. These settings are accompanied most often by hypercapnia and respiratory acidosis and require adequate sedation and even neuromuscular blockade in some patients. Current knowledge, however, indicates that this is probably the less dangerous approach in patients with asthma.[91,93,96,98] Ventilator settings should be readjusted in accordance with the time course of changes in gas exchange and respiratory system mechanics.

Most patients with ARDS require mechanical ventilation during their illness. In this setting, mechanical ventilation is harmful when delivering high tidal volumes.[99,100] There is general agreement that end-inspiratory plateau airway pressure should be kept at values no higher than 30–35 cmH_2O. End-inspiratory plateau airway pressure, however, is a function of tidal volume, total PEEP level, and elastance of both the lung and chest wall. Importantly, patients with ARDS have small lungs with different mechanical characteristics of the lungs and chest wall,[101,102] and recommending a single combination of tidal volume and PEEP for all patients is not sound. Patients with more compliant lungs possibly can receive somewhat higher tidal volumes than those delivered to patients with poorly compliant lungs. As in any other disease state, individual titration of tidal volume and PEEP according to underlying physiologic abnormalities and to the time course of the disease seems the most reasonable. Besides, such an approach serves as a control for comparison purposes.

Once the precipitating cause of the acute respiratory failure is partially or totally reversed, a patient's ability to tolerate ACV discontinuation should be evaluated, at least on a daily basis. This is best done carrying out a spontaneous breathing trial using a T tube or low PSV levels for 30 to 120 minutes. This simple approach is successful in the vast majority (~70%) of intubated ventilated patients, although it may be particularly difficult when COPD is present[103–107] and in patients in whom cardiovascular function is not well preserved.[108–116]

Troubleshooting

Solving problems related to mechanical equipment requires special skills and intuition. Some troubles are intrinsically related to machines and their own working principles/algorithms but can be minimized if manufacturers' recommendations are followed. It should be unnecessary to emphasize that thorough reading of the operator's manual is mandatory. One study showed that hospital environment (e.g., electric power supply) affects ventilator reliability.[117] Overall, and according to a retrospective survey,[118] the frequency of ventilator malfunctions is very low, about 176 mechanical failures and 106 operator-related errors from over 2 million hours of ventilator running time. This author also reported that ventilator reliability improves in direct relationship to its utilization.[117]

Important Unknowns and the Future

Mechanical ventilation is instituted mainly to improve gas exchange and to decrease respiratory muscle workload. The clinical response to this lifesaving treatment in terms of gas

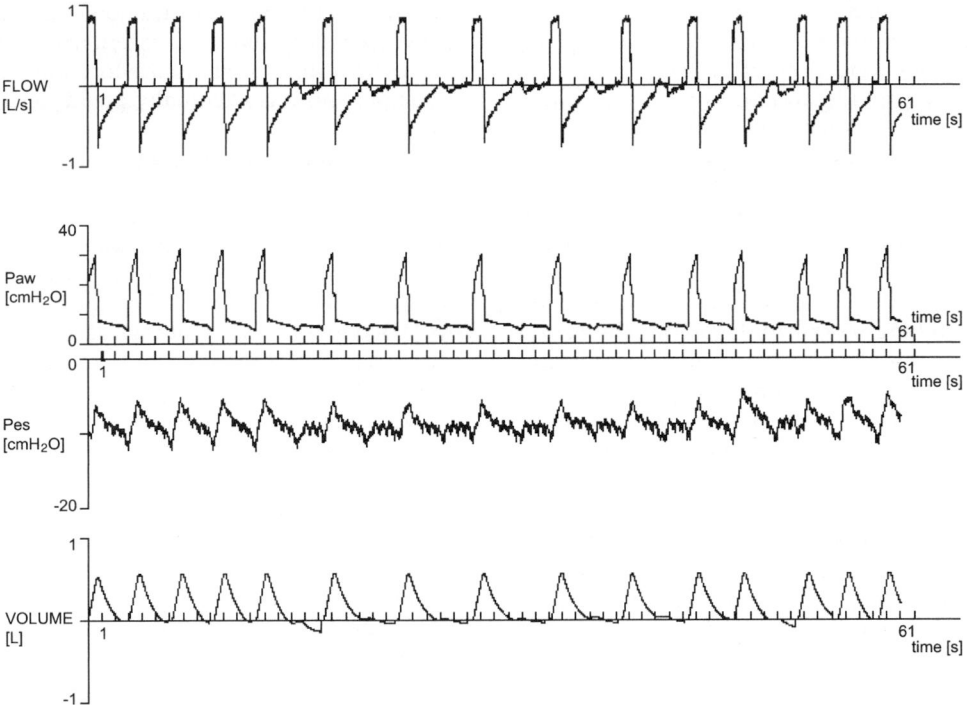

FIGURE 7-8 (*From top to bottom*) Tracings of airflow (flow), airway pressure (Paw), esophageal pressure (Pes), and tidal volume (volume). Each mark on the time axis denotes 1 second. As can be seen from the esophageal pressure recordings, this patient was markedly unloaded and exhibited a feeble respiratory drive. As a result, multiple wasted inspiratory efforts are interspersed between the patient-triggered breaths.

FIGURE 7-9 (*From top to bottom*) Tracings of airflow (flow), airway pressure (Paw), esophageal pressure (Pes), and tidal volume (volume). Each mark on the time axis denotes 1 second. These recordings and those in Fig. 7-6 were obtained in the same patient. As seen easily on the esophageal pressure tracing, there is a highly variable inspiratory muscle effort over time, thus inducing permanent scooping on the airway pressure recording.

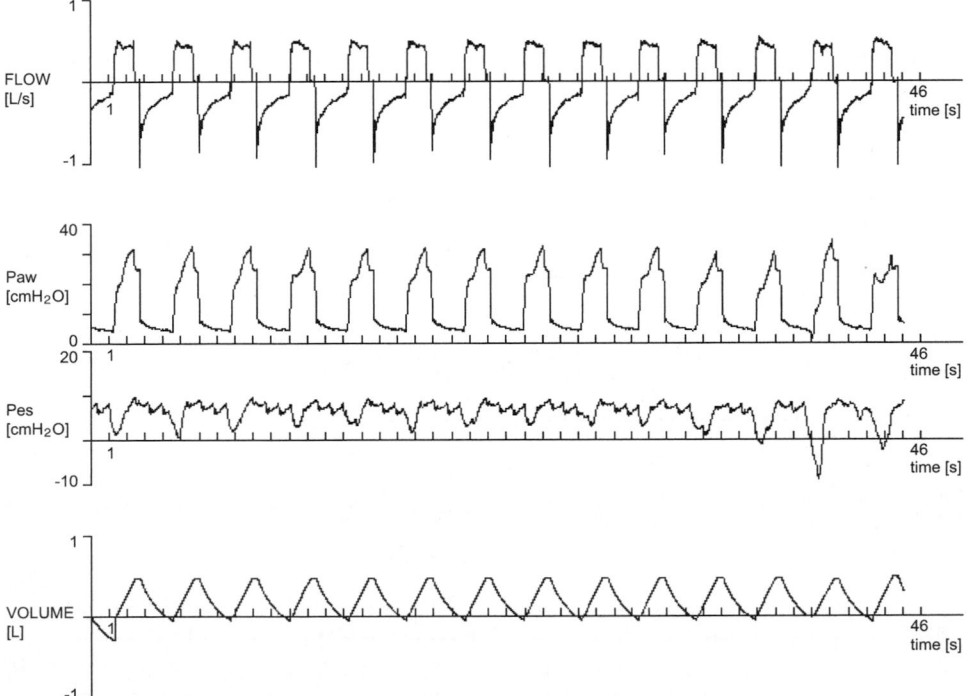

exchange is usually evaluated by means of intermittent arterial blood gas measurements, continuous pulse oximetry monitoring, and less often, monitoring end-tidal CO_2. These measurements provide an objective way to titrate therapy. Although gas exchange is the main function of the lungs, the respiratory system also has a muscular pump that is central to its main purposes. The way we evaluate the function of the respiratory muscles clinically during the course of ACV and patient-ventilator interactions is rudimentary.

When ACV is first initiated, the ventilator usually overcomes the total breathing workload. How long the period of respiratory muscle inactivity is to be maintained is unknown. This is relevant because it may induce muscle atrophy and eventually may jeopardize withdrawal from the ventilator. When ACV is triggered by the patient, multiple factors interplay between the patient and the ventilator. Although high levels of assistance decrease the sensation of dyspnea, they also increase the likelihood of wasted inspiratory efforts (Fig. 7-8). The clinical relevance of such abnormal patient-ventilator interactions has not been elucidated. How ACV is adjusted, in particular concerning inspiratory flow rate and tidal volume settings, is a major determinant of its physiologic effects. Knowing how much effort a particular patient is making and how much unloading is to be provided is very difficult to ascertain on clinical grounds. An excessive respiratory muscle effort may induce muscle dysfunction, and this eventually could delay ventilator withdrawal.

Clinicians sometimes judge tolerance to ACV from the respiratory-rate readings, but this can be very misleading when spontaneous inspiratory efforts do not trigger mechanical breaths. During the course of ACV, it is also difficult to know how many efforts are triggered by the patient and how many are triggered by time. In addition, tolerance to ACV depends on the settings. If selected inappropriately, these may lead the physician to erroneously interpret that the problem lies with the patient and perhaps administer a sedative agent when, in reality, the patient is simply reacting against improper adjustment of the machine.

When patients are receiving ACV, they are at risk of undergoing periods of underassistance alternating with periods of overassistance. This is so because of the varying ventilatory demands (Fig. 7-9) and because the mechanical characteristics of the respiratory system also change over time. The frequency of such phenomena and their clinical consequences are unknown. The effects of permanent monotonous tidal volume delivery, as well as whether or

FIGURE 7-10 (*From top to bottom*) Tracings of airflow (flow), airway pressure (Paw), esophageal pressure (Pes), gastric pressure (Pga) and tidal volume (volume). Each mark on the time axis denotes one second. These tracings were obtained in the same patient as in Figure 7-1. The calculated compliance was 0.049 L/cmH$_2$O, airflow resistance was 14.8 cmH$_2$O/L/s, and total PEEP was 6 cmH$_2$O. There are two superimposed airway pressure tracings: the spontaneous tracing generated by the patient and the tracing calculated by applying the equation of motion (Paw + Pmus = [tidal volume/compliance] + [airflow × resistance] + total PEEP). Pmus denotes the pressure developed by the inspiratory muscles. In this case, Pmus is zero because the patient was relaxed. As predicted, the two tracings are virtually identical. The tracing obtained by applying the equation of motion is the one that shows the expiratory airway pressure trajectory below the recorded waveform from the patient. This is explained by the fact that the equation of motion assumed identical compliance and resistance during both inspiration and expiration.

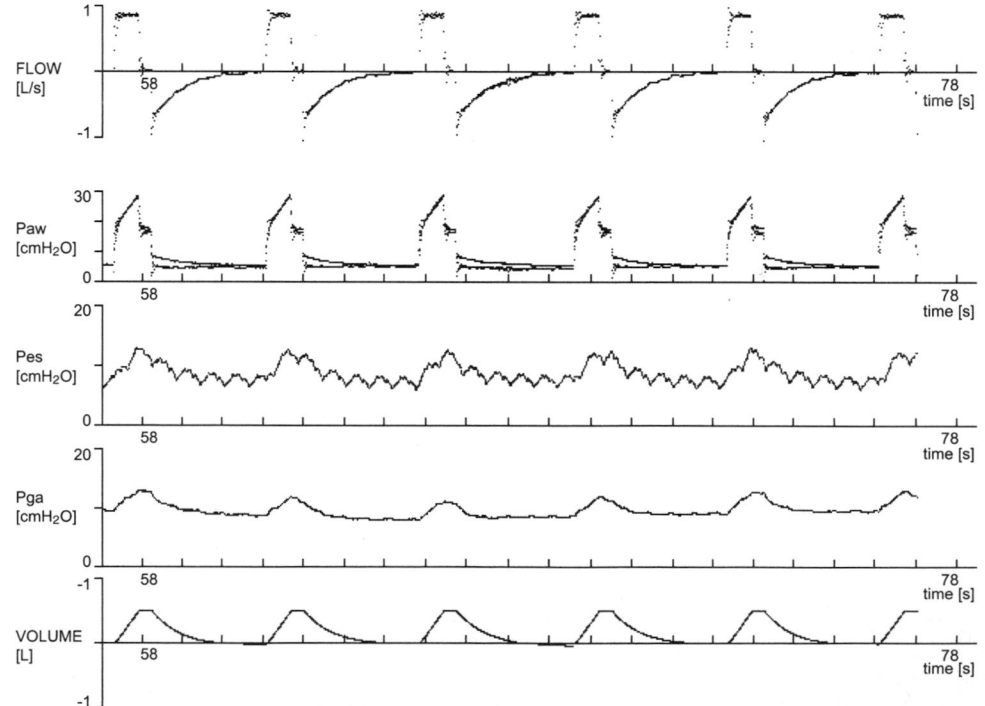

not sighs are to be used in this setting, also remain to be elucidated.

The only way to interpret clinically whether the patient is doing well or not during ACV is to evaluate respiratory rate and the airway pressure trajectory over time. The latter can be monitored on the ventilator simply by applying the equation of motion (Fig. 7-10). During patient-triggered ACV, muscle effort can be estimated by superimposing the current and the passive airway pressure trajectories. Airway occlusion pressure is an important component of the airway pressure trajectory during patient-triggered breaths. This variable is a good estimate of the central respiratory drive and is highly correlated with the inspiratory muscle effort. Pressure-triggered demand-valve ventilators are well suited to make precise measurements of airway pressure decay during the first 100 ms of an occluded inspiration on a breath-by-breath basis. Such measurements would allow clinicians to analyze trends and estimate patient-ventilator interactions objectively. It is indeed surprising that such sound noninvasive monitoring possibilities have yet to be implemented. And it is ironic to realize how many new ventilator modes are introduced without having passed rigorous physiologic and clinical evaluations.

Summary and Conclusions

The most widely used ventilator mode in mechanically ventilated patients is ACV. Many of its physiologic effects have been well characterized, and it is conceivable that, in the main, its purposes are met. ACV is also very versatile because it offers ventilator support throughout the entire period of mechanical ventilation. As with any other mode, the effects depend on the way ACV is implemented. The necessity to impose a number of fixed settings, in essence, tidal volume and inspiratory flow rate, implies that the respiratory pump may be unloaded suboptimally and contracts out of synchrony with the ventilator. The real magnitude and the clinical consequences of these phenomena is unknown.

Since its introduction, ACV implementation has undergone considerable changes, and it is presently applied less aggressively than in the past. Thanks to an enormous amount of physiologic and clinically oriented research, we have learned that ACV can be harmful to patients, injuring both the lungs and the respiratory muscles. Future research should help us to deliver ACV in such a manner that a patient's clinical needs are served more optimally.

References

1. Esteban A, Anzueto A, Alia I, et al. How is mechanical ventilation employed in the intensive care unit? An international utilization review. Am J Respir Crit Care Med 2000; 161:1450–8.
2. Tobin MJ. Advances in mechanical ventilation. New Engl J Med 2001; 344:1986–96.
3. Esteban A, Anzueto A, Frutos F, et al. Characteristics and outcomes in adult patients receiving mechanical ventilation: A 28-day international study. JAMA 2002; 287:345–55.
4. Sanborn WG. Microprocessor-based mechanical ventilation. Respir Care 1993; 38:72–109.
5. Chatburn RL. Classification of mechanical ventilators. In: Tobin MJ, editor. Principles and practice of mechanical ventilation. New York; McGraw-Hill, 1994: 37–64.
6. Aslanian P, El Atrous S, Isabey D, et al. Effects of flow triggering on breathing effort during partial ventilatory support. Am J Respir Crit Care Med 1998; 157:135–43.
7. Marini JJ, Capps JS, Culver BH. The inspiratory work of breathing during assisted mechanical ventilation. Chest 1985; 87:612–8.
8. Marini JJ, Rodriguez RM, Lamb V. The inspiratory workload of patient-initiated mechanical ventilation. Am Rev Respir Dis 1986; 134:902–9.
9. Ward ME, Corbeil C, Gibbons W, et al. Optimization of respiratory muscle relaxation during mechanical ventilation. Anesthesiology 1988; 69:29–35.
10. Flick GR, Bellamy PE, Simmons DH. Diaphragmatic contraction during assisted mechanical ventilation. Chest 1989; 96:130–5.
11. Cinnella G, Conti G, Lofaso F, et al. Effects of assisted ventilation on the work of breathing: Volume-controlled versus pressure-controlled ventilation. Am J Respir Crit Care Med 1996; 153:1025–33.
12. Leung P, Jubran A, Tobin M. Comparison of assisted ventilator modes on triggering, patient effort and dyspnea. Am J Respir Crit Care Med 1997; 155:1940–8.
13. Corne S, Gillespie D, Roberts D, Younes M. Effect of inspiratory flow rate on respiratory rate in intubated ventilated patients. Am J Respir Crit Care Med 1997; 156:304–8.
14. Laghi F, Segal J, Choe WK, Tobin MJ. Effect of imposed inflation time on respiratory frequency and hyperinflation in patients with chronic obstructive pulmonary disease. Am J Respir Crit Care Med 2001; 163:1365–70.
15. Kondili E, Prinianakis G, Anastasaki M, Georgopoulos D. Acute effects of ventilator settings on respiratory motor output in patients with acute lung injury. Intensive Care Med 2001; 27:1147–57.
16. Laghi F, Karamchandani K, Tobin MJ. Influence of ventilator settings in determining respiratory frequency during mechanical ventilation. Am J Respir Crit Care Med 1999; 160:1766–70.
17. Fernández R, Méndez M, Yones M. Effect of ventilator flow rate on respiratory timing in normal humans. Am J Respir Crit Care Med 1999; 159:710–9.
18. Younes M, Georgopoulos D. Control of breathing relevant to mechanical ventilation. In: Marini JJ, Slutsky AS, editors. Physiological basis of ventilatory support: Lung biology in health and disease, Vol 118. New York: Marcel Dekker, 1998:1–73.
19. Laghi F. Effect of inspiratory time and flow settings during assist-control ventilation. Curr Opin Crit Care 2003; 9:39–44.
20. Younes M. Control of breathing during mechanical ventilation. In: Slutsky AS, Brochard L, editors. Mechanical ventilation: Update in intensive care and emergency medicine, Vol 40. Berlin: Springer-Verlag, 2004: 63–82.
21. Manning HL, Molinary EJ, Leiter JC. Effect of inspiratory flow rate on respiratory sensation and pattern of breathing. Am J Respir Crit Care Med 1995; 151:751–7.
22. Marcy TW, Marini JJ. Inverse ratio ventilation in ARDS: Rationale and implementation. Chest 1991; 100:494–504.
23. Shanholtz C, Brower R. Should inverse ratio ventilation be used in adult respiratory distress syndrome? Am J Respir Crit Care Med 1994; 149:1354–8.
24. Ludwigs U, Klingstedt C, Baehrendtz S, et al. Volume-controlled inverse ratio ventilation in oleic acid–induced lung injury: Effects on gas exchange, hemodynamics, and computed tomographic lung density. Chest 1995; 108:804–9.

25. Mang H, Kacmarek RM, Ritz R, et al. Cardiorespiratory effects of volume and pressure-controlled ventilation at various I:E ratios in an acute lung injury model. Am J Respir Crit Care Med 1995; 151:731–6.

26. Cole AGH, Weller SF, Sykes MK. Inverse ratio ventilation compared with PEEP in adult respiratory failure. Intensive Care Med 1984; 10:227–32.

27. Mercat A, Titiriga M, Anguel N, et al. Inverse ratio ventilation (I:E = 2:1) in acute respiratory distress syndrome: A six-hour controlled study. Am J Respir Crit Care Med 1997; 155: 1637–42.

28. Gayan-Ramirez G, Decramer M. Effects of mechanical ventilation on diaphragm function and biology. Eur Respir J 2002; 20:1579–86.

29. Laghi F, Tobin MJ. Disorders of the respiratory muscles. Am J Respir Crit Care Med 2003; 168:10–48.

30. Vassilakopoulos T, Petrof BJ. Ventilator-induced diaphragmatic dysfunction. Am J Respir Crit Care Med 2004; 169:336–41.

31. Laghi F, Cattapan SE, Jubran A, et al. Is weaning failure caused by low-frequency fatigue of the diaphragm? Am J Respir Crit Care Med 2003; 167:120–7.

32. Le Bourdellès G, Viires N, Boczkowski J, et al. Effects of mechanical ventilation on diaphragmatic contractile properties in rats. Am J Respir Crit Care Med 1994; 149:1539–44.

33. Anzueto A, Peters JI, Tobin MJ, et al. Effects of prolonged controlled mechanical ventilation on diaphragmatic function in healthy adult baboons. Crit Care Med 1997; 25:1187–90.

34. Sassoon CSH. Ventilator-associated diaphragmatic dysfunction. Am J Respir Crit Care Med 2002; 166:1017–8.

35. Capdevila X, Lopez S, Bernard N, et al. Effects of controlled mechanical ventilation on respiratory muscle contractile properties in rabbits. Intensive Care Med 2003; 29:103–10.

36. Yang L, Luo J, Bourdon J, et al. Controlled mechanical ventilation leads to remodeling of the rat diaphragm. Am J Respir Crit Care Med 2002; 166:1135–40.

37. Rácz GZ, Gayan-Ramirez G, Testelmans D, et al. Early changes in rat diaphragm biology with mechanical ventilation. Am J Respir Crit Care Med 2003; 168:297–304.

38. Shanely RA, Zergeroglu MA, Lennon SL, et al. Mechanical ventilation-induced diaphragmatic atrophy is associated with oxidative injury and increased proteolytic activity. Am J Respir Crit Care Med 2002; 166:1369–74.

39. Shanely RA, Van Gammeren D, DeRuisseau KC, et al. Mechanical ventilation depresses protein synthesis in the rat diaphragm. Am J Respir Crit Care Med 2004; 170:994–9.

40. Sassoon CSH, Zhu E, Caiozzo VJ. Assist-control mechanical ventilation attenuates ventilator-induced diaphragmatic dysfunction. Am J Respir Crit Care Med 2004; 170:626–32.

41. Ebihara S, Hussain SNA, Danialou G, et al. Mechanical ventilation protects against diaphragm injury in sepsis: Interaction of oxidative and mechanical stresses. Am J Respir Crit Care Med 2002; 165:221–8.

42. Laghi F, D'Alfonso N, Tobin MJ. Pattern of recovery from diaphragmatic fatigue over 24 hours. J Appl Physiol 1995; 79:539–46.

43. Jiang T-X, Reid WD, Belcastro A, Road JD. Load dependence of secondary diaphragm inflammation and injury after acute inspiratory loading. Am J Respir Crit Care Med 1998; 157:230–6.

44. Jiang T-X, Reid WD, Road JD. Delayed diaphragm injury and diaphragm force production. Am J Respir Crit Care Med 1998; 157:736–42.

45. Vassilakopoulos T, Divangahi M, Rallis G, et al. Differential cytokine gene expression in the diaphragm in response to strenuous resistive breathing. Am J Respir Crit Care Med 2004; 170:154–61.

46. Vassilakopoulos T, Roussos C, Zakynthinos S. The immune response to resistive breathing. Eur Respir J 2004; 24:1033–43.

47. Parthasarathy S, Tobin MJ. Sleep in the intensive care unit. Intensive Care Med 2004; 30:197–206.

48. Gabor JY, Cooper AB, Crombach SA, et al. Contribution of the intensive care unit environment to sleep disruption in mechanically ventilated patients and healthy subjects. Am J Respir Crit Care Med 2003; 167:708–15.

49. Parthasarathy S, Tobin MJ. Effect of ventilator mode on sleep quality in critically ill patients. Am J Respir Crit Care Med 2002; 166:1423–9.

50. Mador JF. Assist-control ventilation. In: Tobin MJ, editor. Principles and practice of mechanical ventilation. New York: McGraw-Hill, 1994: 207–19.

51. Ludwigs U, Philip A. Pulmonary epithelial permeability and gas exchange: A comparison of inverse ratio ventilation and conventional mechanical ventilation in oleic acid–induced lung injury in rabbits. Chest 1998; 113:459–66.

52. Maeda Y, Fujino Y, Uchiyama A, et al. Effects of peak inspiratory flow on development of ventilator-induced lung injury in rabbits. Anesthesiology 2004; 101:722–8.

53. Abraham E, Yoshihara G. Cardiorespiratory effects of pressure controlled ventilation in severe respiratory failure. Chest 1990; 98:1445–9.

54. Muñoz J, Guerrero JE, Escalante JL, et al. Pressure-controlled ventilation versus controlled mechanical ventilation with decelerating inspiratory flow. Crit Care Med 1993; 21:1143–8.

55. Mercat A, Graini L, Teboul JL, et al. Cardiorespiratory effects of pressure controlled ventilation with and without inverse ratio in the adult respiratory distress syndrome. Chest 1993; 104: 871–5.

56. Lessard MR, Guerot E, Lorino H, et al. Effects of pressure-controlled with different I:E ratios versus volume-controlled ventilation on respiratory mechanics, gas exchange, and hemodynamics in patients with adult respiratory distress syndrome. Anesthesiology 1994; 80:983–91.

57. Mancebo J, Vallverdu I, Bak E, et al. Volume-controlled ventilation and pressure-controlled inverse ratio ventilation: A comparison of their effects in ARDS patients. Monaldi Arch Chest Dis 1994; 49:201–7.

58. Davis KJ, Branson RD, Campbell RS, Porembka DT. Comparison of volume control and pressure control ventilation: Is flow waveform the difference? J Trauma 1996; 41:808–14.

59. Zavala E, Ferrer M, Polese G, et al. Effect of inverse I:E ratio ventilation on pulmonary gas exchange in acute respiratory distress syndrome. Anesthesiology 1998; 88:35–42.

60. Prella M, Feihl F, Domenighetti G. Effects of short-term pressure-controlled ventilation on gas exchange, airway pressures, and gas distribution in patients with acute lung injury/ARDS: Comparison with volume-controlled ventilation. Chest 2002; 122:1382–8.

61. Edibam C, Rutten AJ, Collins DV, Bersten AD. Effect of inspiratory flow pattern and inspiratory to expiratory ratio on nonlinear elastic behavior in patients with acute lung injury. Am J Respir Crit Care Med 2003; 167:702–7.

62. Rappaport SH, Shpiner R, Yoshihara G, et al. Randomized, prospective trial of pressure-limited versus volume-controlled ventilation in severe respiratory failure. Crit Care Med 1994; 22:22–32.

63. Esteban A, Alía I, Gordo F, et al. Prospective, randomized trial comparing pressure-controlled ventilation and volume-controlled ventilation in ARDS. Chest 2000; 117:1690–6.

64. MacIntyre NR, McConnell R, Cheng K-CG, Sane A. Patient-ventilator flow dyssynchrony: Flow-limited versus pressure-limited breaths. Crit Care Med 1997; 25:1671–7.

65. Hudson LD, Hurlow RS, Craig KC, Pierson DJ. Does intermittent mandatory ventilation correct respiratory alkalosis in patients receiving assisted mechanical ventilation? Am Rev Respir Dis 1985; 132:1071–4.

66. Groeger JS, Levinson MR, Carlon GC. Assist control versus synchronized intermittent mandatory ventilation during acute respiratory failure. Crit Care Med 1989; 17:607–12.

67. Marini JJ, Smith TC, Lamb VT. External work output and force generation during synchronized intermittent mechanical ventilation: Effect of machine assistance on breathing effort. Am Rev Respir Dis 1988; 138:1169–79.

68. Tokioka H, Saito S, Kosaka F. Comparison of pressure support ventilation and assist control ventilation in patients with acute respiratory failure. Intensive Care Med 1989; 15:364–7.

69. Tejeda M, Boix JH, Alvarez F, et al. Comparison of pressure support ventilation and assist-control ventilation in the treatment of respiratory failure. Chest 1997; 111:1322–5.

70. Kreit J, Capper M, Eschenbacher W. Patient work of breathing during pressure support and volume-cycled mechanical ventilation. Am J Respir Crit Care Med 1994; 149:1085–91.

71. Chiumello D, Pelosi P, Calvi E, et al. Different modes of assisted ventilation in patients with acute respiratory failure. Eur Respir J 2002; 20:925–33.

72. Cereda M, Foti G, Marcora B, et al. Pressure support ventilation in patients with acute lung injury. Crit Care Med 2000; 28: 1269–75.

73. Lefevre G, Kowalski S, Girling L, et al. Improved arterial oxygenation after oleic acid lung injury in the pig using a computer-controlled mechanical ventilator. Am J Respir Crit Care Med 1996; 154:1567–72.

74. Nam AJ, Brower RG, Fessler HE, Simon BA. Biologic variability in mechanical ventilation rate and tidal volume does not improve oxygenation or lung mechanics in canine oleic acid lung injury. Am J Respir Crit Care Med 2000; 161:1797–804.

75. Mutch WAC, Harms S, Graham MR, et al. Biologically variable or naturally noisy mechanical ventilation recruits atelectatic lung. Am J Respir Crit Care Med 2000; 162:319–23.

76. Arold SP, Mora R, Lutchen KR, et al. Variable tidal volume ventilation improves lung mechanics and gas exchange in a rodent model of acute lung injury. Am J Respir Crit Care Med 2002; 165:366–71.

77. Boker A, Graham MR, Walley KR, et al. Improved arterial oxygenation with biologically variable or fractal ventilation using low tidal volumes in a porcine model of acute respiratory distress syndrome. Am J Respir Crit Care Med 2002; 165: 456–62.

78. Puritan-Bennett Corporation. 7200 series microprocessor ventilator: Operator's manual. Carslbad, CA, 1988.

79. Nellcor Puritan-Bennett. Sistema de ventilador serie 700: Manual del usuario. Pleasanton, CA, 1998.

80. Nellcor Puritan-Bennett. Sistema ventilador 840: Manual del operador y referencia técnica. Pleasanton, CA, 1997.

81. Drägerwerk AG. Evita 2 Ventilador para cuidados intensivos: Instrucciones de uso, software 1.n. Lübeck, Germany, 1993.

82. Dräger Medizintechnik GmbH. Evita 4 intensive care ventilator: Instructions for use, software 2.n. Lübeck, Germany, 1997.

83. Hamilton Medical AG. Ventilador de cuidados intensivos Galileo: Manual del operador, versión del software 3. Rhäzüns, Switzerland, 2002.

84. Siemens-Elema AB. Servo ventilator 300/300A: Manual de instrucciones 8.0/9.0. Solna, Sweden, 1996.

85. Maquet Critical Care AB. Servo-i ventilator system V. 2.0: Manual del usuario. Solna, Sweden, 2004.

86. Hubmayr RD, Abel MD, Rehder K. Physiologic approach to mechanical ventilation. Crit Care Med 1990; 18:103–13.

87. Hubmayr RD. Setting the ventilator. In: Tobin MJ, editor. Principles and practice of mechanical ventilation. New York: McGraw-Hill, 1994: 191–206.

88. Tuxen D, Lane S. The effects of ventilatory pattern on hyperinflation, airway pressures, and circulation in mechanical ventilation of patients with severe airflow obstruction. Am Rev Respir Dis 1987; 136:872–9.

89. Connors AF, McCaffree DR, Gray BA. Effect of inspiratory flow rate on gas exchange during mechanical ventilation. Am Rev Respir Dis 1981; 124:537–43.

90. Smith TC, Marini JJ. Impact of PEEP on lung mechanics and work of breathing in severe airflow obstruction. J Appl Physiol 1988; 65:1488–99.

91. Darioli R, Perret C. Mechanical controlled hypoventilation in status asthmaticus. Am Rev Respir Dis 1984; 129:385–7.

92. Williams TJ, Tuxen DV, Scheinkestel CD, et al. Risk factors for morbidity in mechanically ventilated patients with acute severe asthma. Am Rev Respir Dis 1992; 146:607–15.

93. Tuxen DV. Permissive hypercapnia. In: Tobin MJ, editor. Principles and practice of mechanical ventilation. New York: McGraw-Hill, 1994: 371–92.

94. Manthous CA. Management of severe exacerbations of asthma. Am J Med 1995; 151:298–308.

95. Corbridge TC, Hall JB. The assessment and management of adults with status asthmaticus. Am J Respir Crit Care Med 1995; 151:1296–316.

96. Leatherman JW. Mechanical ventilation in severe asthma. In: Marini JJ, Slutsky AS, editors. Physiological basis of ventilatory support. New York: Marcel Dekker, 1998: 1155–85.

97. Leatherman JW, McArthur C, Shapiro RS. Effect of prolongation of expiratory time on dynamic hyperinflation in mechanically ventilated patients with severe asthma. Crit Care Med 2004; 32:1542–5.

98. Feihl F, Perret C. Permissive hypercapnia: How permissive should we be? Am J Respir Crit Care Med 1994; 150: 1722–37.

99. Amato MBP, Barbas CSV, Medeiros DM, et al. Effect of a protective-ventilation strategy on mortality in the acute respiratory distress syndrome. New Engl J Med 1998; 338:347–54.

100. The Acute Respiratory Distress Syndrome Network. Ventilation with lower tidal volumes as compared with traditional tidal volumes for acute lung injury and the acute respiratory distress syndrome. New Engl J Med 2000; 342:1301–8.

101. Gattinoni L, Carlesso E, Cadringher P, et al. Physical and biological triggers of ventilator-induced lung injury and its prevention. Eur Respir J 2003; 22(suppl 47):15–25s.

102. Gattinoni L, Pesenti A. The concept of "baby lung." Intensive Care Med 2005; in press 2005; 31:776–84.

103. Brochard L, Rauss A, Benito S, et al. Comparison of three methods of gradual withdrawal from ventilatory support during weaning from mechanical ventilation. Am J Respir Crit Care Med 1994; 150:896–903.

104. Jubran A, Tobin MJ. Pathophysiologic basis of acute respiratory distress in patients who fail a trial of weaning from mechanical ventilation. Am J Respir Crit Care Med 1997; 155:906–15.

105. Esteban A, Alia I, Gordo F, et al. Extubation outcome after spontaneous breathing trials with T-tube or pressure support ventilation. Am J Respir Crit Care Med 1997; 156:459–65.

106. Vallverdú I, Calaf N, Subirana M, et al. Clinical characteristics, respiratory functional parameters, and outcome of a two-hour T-piece trial in patients weaning from mechanical ventilation. Am J Respir Crit Care Med 1998; 158:1855–62.

107. Esteban A, Alia I, Tobin MJ, et al. Effect of spontaneous breathing trial duration on outcome of attempts to discontinue mechanical ventilation. Am J Respir Crit Care Med 1999; 159:512–8.

108. Derenne J, Fleury B, Pariente R. Acute respiratory failure of chronic obstructive pulmonary disease. Am Rev Respir Dis 1988; 138:1006–33.

109. Lemaire F, Teboul JL, Cinotti L, et al. Acute left ventricular dysfunction during unsuccessful weaning from mechanical ventilation. Anesthesiology 1988; 69:171–9.

110. Richard C, Teboul JL, Archambaud F, et al. Left ventricular function during weaning of patients with chronic obstructive pulmonary disease. Intensive Care Med 1994; 20:181–6.

111. Chatila W, Ani S, Guaglianone D, et al. Cardiac ischemia during weaning from mechanical ventilation. Chest 1996; 109:1577–83.

112. Jubran A, Mathru M, Dries D, Tobin MJ. Continuous recordings of mixed venous oxygen saturation during weaning from mechanical ventilation and the ramifications thereof. Am J Respir Crit Care Med 1998; 158:1763–9.

113. Jones NL, Killian KJ. Exercise limitation in health and disease. New Engl J Med 2000; 343:632–41.

114. O'Donnell DE, Revill SM, Webb KA. Dynamic hyperinflation and exercise intolerance in chronic obstructive pulmonary disease. Am J Respir Crit Care Med 2001; 164: 770–7.

115. O'Donnell DE, D'Arsigny C, Fitzpatrick M, Webb KA. Exercise hypercapnia in advanced chronic obstructive pulmonary disease: The role of lung hyperinflation. Am J Respir Crit Care Med 2002; 166:663–8.

116. Scharf SM, Iqbal M, Keller C, et al. Hemodynamic characterization of patients with severe emphysema. Am J Respir Crit Care Med 2002; 166:314–22.

117. Blanch PB. An evaluation of ventilator reliability: A multivariate, failure time analysis of 5 common ventilator brands. Respir Care 2001; 46:789–97.

118. Blanch PB. Mechanical ventilator malfunctions: A descriptive and comparative study of 6 common ventilator brands. Respir Care 1999; 44:1183–92.

Chapter 8

INTERMITTENT MANDATORY VENTILATION

CATHERINE S. H. SASSOON

Intermittent mandatory ventilation (IMV) allows the patient to breathe spontaneously between machine-cycled or mandatory breaths. This concept originated in 1955 with an unnamed ventilator designed by Engstrom.[1,2] In the early 1970s, Kirby et al[3,4] introduced IMV as a means of ventilator support of infants with respiratory distress syndrome. In 1973, Downs et al[5] were the first to propose IMV as a method to facilitate discontinuation from mechanical ventilation in adults. Those investigators[6,7] also pioneered IMV use as a primary means of ventilator support during acute respiratory failure. Subsequently, breath-delivery design has been modified. Mandatory breaths initially delivered regardless of respiratory timing are synchronized with the patient's inspiratory effort.[8,9] This mode of ventilation has been termed *intermittent demand ventilation,*[8] *intermittent assisted ventilation,*[9] and *synchronous intermittent mandatory ventilation* (SIMV); the latter designation is now standard. Currently, SIMV is an established partial mechanical ventilation mode in critically ill patients, both adults[10] and neonates.[11] This chapter will use the terms *IMV* and *SIMV* interchangeably unless specifically indicated for clarification.

Basic Principles

DESCRIPTION

IMV is a means of ventilator support in which a preset number of positive-pressure (mandatory) breaths are delivered while the patient breathes spontaneously between the mandatory breaths. The mandatory breaths can be in the form of a preset volume (flow-limited, volume-cycled, or time-cycled), pressure (pressure-limited, time-cycled),[12] or a combination of pressure and volume (dual control).[13] In principle, IMV is similar to controlled mechanical ventilation (CMV), in which the patient receives a predetermined number of mandatory machine-triggered breaths independent of spontaneous breathing effort. Likewise, SIMV is similar to assist-control ventilation (ACV), in which mandatory breaths are triggered by the patient. In contrast to CMV and ACV, however, in both IMV and SIMV the patient is allowed to breathe spontaneously between the mandatory breaths. In addition, with IMV/SIMV, the clinician can vary the ventilator support level according to the set IMV rate. At a high IMV rate, in which the patient's spontaneous effort is suppressed, IMV provides full ventilator support. At a zero IMV rate, it provides no support, and all breaths are spontaneous. Between these extremes, IMV provides partial ventilator support.

SYSTEM DESIGN

Three types of IMV systems are described: continuous-flow IMV and pressure-triggered and flow-triggered SIMV systems.

CONTINUOUS-FLOW IMV

The original IMV design uses a continuous-flow system.[3] Two parallel circuits—one for the patient's spontaneous breaths and the other for the mechanical breaths—are connected through a sidearm and a one-way valve and share a common oxygen and air source. The continuous-flow IMV setup can be either an open or a closed system.[14] The open system employs a reservoir tube that has a capacity of at least 1.5 times the patient's tidal volume (V_T) and is open to the atmosphere (Fig. 8-1). For this reason, continuous positive airway pressure (CPAP) cannot be applied during the spontaneous breathing cycles. To reduce inspiratory resistance, the side port of the spontaneous breathing circuit is placed between the patient Y and the humidifier. The continuous flow of fresh gas is humidified using a venturi nebulizer. The reservoir tubing's considerable length and the inability to maintain a CPAP level make this open system cumbersome.

The closed system employs a reservoir bag (Fig. 8-2) that minimizes airway pressure fluctuations because the inspired gas flow rate may be limited by the maximum flow generated by the hospital's compressed air and oxygen source. In addition, constant positive airway pressure can be maintained during both the mandatory [i.e., positive

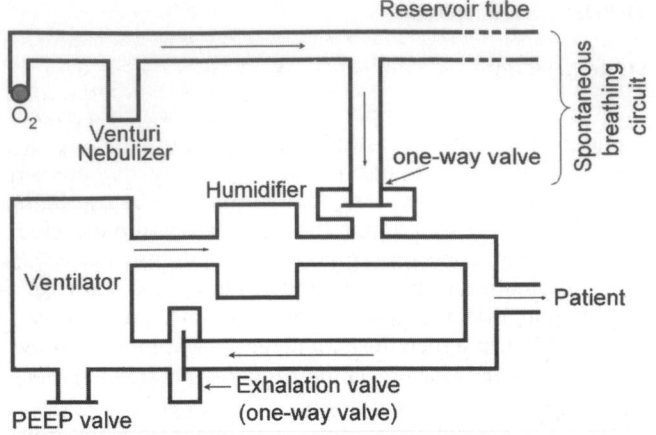

FIGURE 8-1 Continuous-flow intermittent mandatory ventilation setup with a reservoir tube. The sidearm of the spontaneous breathing circuit is connected through a one-way valve to the inspiratory limb of the ventilator circuit. The sidearm is placed between the humidifier and the patient Y. See text for further explanation.

end-expiratory airway pressure (PEEP)] and spontaneous breaths (i.e., CPAP). During spontaneous breathing, the patient breathes from the reservoir bag via the one-way valve. When the ventilator cycles, the one-way valve closes, and a positive-pressure breath is delivered to the patient. During the mechanical breath, excess gas in the reservoir bag is vented through a relief valve. Exhalation occurs through the ventilator's exhalation circuit, which is supplied with a PEEP valve.

In a continuous-flow IMV system, the inspired gas flow rate within the spontaneous breathing circuit must exceed the patient's peak inspiratory flow rate to minimize airway pressure fluctuations and hence the patient's inspiratory work. When set appropriately, spontaneous breathing in

FIGURE 8-2 Continuous-flow intermittent mandatory ventilation setup with a reservoir bag. The sidearm for the spontaneous breathing circuit is connected through a one-way valve to the inspiratory limb of the ventilator circuit. The sidearm is placed proximal to the humidifier. See text for further explanation.

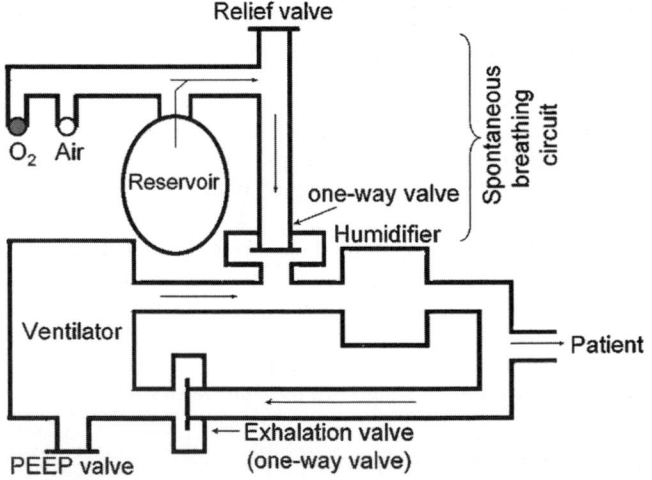

continuous-flow IMV should resemble breathing from the atmosphere.

Continuous-flow IMV has several disadvantages. First, the high flow rate of fresh gas results in gas wastage, although it can be minimized by applying a weighted or high-compliance reservoir bag.[15,16] Second, measurement of exhaled volume is inaccurate because the continuous flow of fresh gas contaminates the exhaled gas within the expiratory circuit, making monitoring of V_T difficult.[17] Third, IMV requires extra circuitry,[18] with the risk of tubing disconnection,[19] incompetence,[20] and incorrect assembly of the one-way valve, as well as added cost. Fourth, patient-ventilator asynchrony potentially can occur because mandatory breaths are not delivered in concert with the patient's inspiratory effort (Fig. 8-3A). Whereas asynchrony has no significant effect in adults,[21] in neonates, asynchrony associated with continuous-flow IMV resulted in large

FIGURE 8-3 A. Continuous-flow intermittent mandatory ventilation (IMV). Airway pressure (Paw) and flow tracings ($\dot{V}$). The dashed line indicates the onset of inspiratory flow. Minimal fluctuations of Paw are due to circuit resistance. Large fluctuations of Paw occur when inspiratory flow rates are insufficient and a reservoir bag is not used. PEEP, positive end-expiratory airway pressure. B. Pressure-triggered synchronous intermittent mandatory ventilation (SIMV). A period of zero flow before the onset of flow (indicated by the dashed line) can be detected on the flow tracing. Zero flow coincides with patient triggering to open the proportional valve. During the unassisted breathing after flow onset, Paw continues to drop during inspiration because of inadequate flow delivery. C. Flow-triggered synchronous intermittent mandatory ventilation (SIMV). Triggering phase is significantly shorter than with pressure-triggered SIMV. During the unassisted breathing following patient triggering, Paw is maintained at or slightly above the PEEP level, suggesting adequate flow delivery during inspiration.

A. Continuous-flow IMV

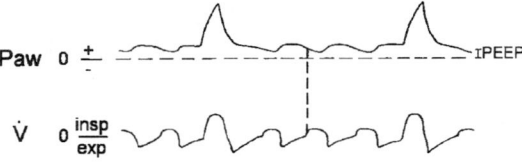
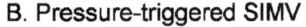

B. Pressure-triggered SIMV

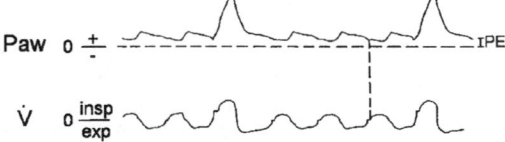

C. Flow-triggered SIMV

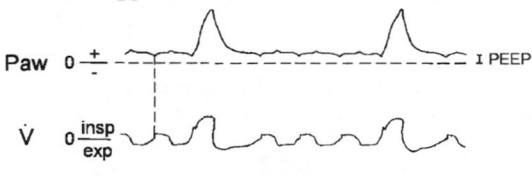

Time

fluctuations of V_T[22] and lower Pa_{O_2}[23] than with SIMV. The effect of IMV on Pa_{O_2} was confirmed in a large randomized multicenter trial.[24] Low Pa_{O_2} was postulated to result from active exhalation because muscle relaxant improves oxygenation.[25,26]

A technologically advanced continuous-flow IMV machine is the flow-regulated IMV/CPAP machine described by Akashi et al.[27] Flow within the circuit is polled, for example, every 20 minutes and used as a feedback signal to increase the basal flow to match the patient's ventilatory demand during inspiration and subtract it during exhalation. Flow-regulated CPAP eliminates airway fluctuations and decreases imposed work during both inspiration and exhalation. Using a mechanical lung model with flow-regulated CPAP of 5 cmH_2O, the total imposed work was 3.4 mJ/breath versus 43.5 mJ/breath with a continuous-flow CPAP device and an added 20-liter reservoir bag.[27]

PRESSURE- AND FLOW-TRIGGERED SIMV
SIMV is currently the standard for clinical use.[10,11] SIMV incorporates a demand valve that is triggered by the patient with each spontaneous breath and delivers a mandatory breath in concert with the patient's inspiratory effort. If the patient ceases to trigger the ventilator, mandatory breaths will be triggered by the machine and delivered according to the preset rate. The demand valve is triggered by either a fall in pressure (pressure-triggered) or a change in flow (flow-triggered). In pressure-triggered (or *demand-flow*) SIMV, a preset pressure sensitivity must be achieved before the ventilator delivers fresh gas into the inspiratory circuit.[28,29] A noticeable delay in opening the demand valve occurs between onset of inspiratory effort and flow delivery (see Fig. 8-3*B*). Flow-triggered (or *flow-by*) SIMV uses a preset flow sensitivity as the trigger mechanism.[28,29] The terms *pressure-triggered SIMV* and *flow-triggered SIMV* are preferred over demand-flow SIMV and flow-by SIMV, respectively, because with both demand-flow and flow-by SIMV systems, flow delivery is essentially "on demand." In addition, the term *flow-by* signifies continuous flow rather than flow sensitivity.

The pressure- and flow-triggering characteristics of the spontaneous breaths (CPAP) are an important component of the imposed work of an SIMV system (see Chapter 3).[30,31] This situation arises because there is little adaptation to the mandatory breaths' ventilatory assistance unless the system is set at a substantial assistance level.[32] Fortunately, most modern microprocessor-based ventilators employ a remarkably responsive proportional solenoid valve such that the work imposed during the trigger phase (the interval from onset of patient effort to valve opening or flow delivery) is a small percentage of the total inspiratory work of breathing (<10% with pressure-triggered SIMV).[33] Nevertheless, flow triggering has become the preferred triggering method not only for SIMV but also for various other ventilation modes because of its faster response time and therefore shorter triggering phase compared with pressure triggering (see Fig. 8-3*C*).[34] In the posttrigger phase (the interval from onset of flow delivery to the end of inspiration), flow delivery

with pressure triggering may not be adequate during the spontaneous breaths.[28] The feedback signal for flow delivery is the gradient between a manufacturer-determined target pressure and circuit pressure. As the pressure gradient increases, flow delivery increases. This pressure gradient can be enhanced by adding pressure support (PS) or sensing the circuit pressure at the distal end of the endotracheal tube.[35,36] From a practical standpoint, adding PS is preferable. Alternatively, flow delivery during the spontaneous breaths may be augmented by using changes in flow instead of pressure as a feedback signal for adding and subtracting flow from the base flow during inspiration and exhalation, respectively.[27]

Augmenting flow delivery during the mandatory breaths can be accomplished by setting the pressure-attack rate sufficiently high when pressure-limited mandatory breaths are employed.[37,38] To maintain a constant V_T with pressure-limited mandatory breaths, both pressure- and volume-limited breaths can be combined in the form of dual control within breaths[39] or breath-to-breath ventilation (see Chapter 16).[40] Several microprocessor-based ventilators are equipped with dual-control breath-to-breath ventilation that can be applied in the SIMV mode.[41] In essence, this form of mandatory breath is a pressure-limited, time-cycled breath that uses V_T as feedback control for continuously adjusting the pressure limit to attain the set V_T. The volume signal used as feedback to the ventilator controller is the volume exiting the ventilator and not the exhaled V_T. This step prevents runaway of airway pressure that could occur if a leak in the circuit caused inaccurate measurement of exhaled volume. With dual-control mandatory breaths, a "test breath" is delivered, and the dynamic compliance of the respiratory system is calculated. The next three breaths are delivered at a pressure limit of 75% of that necessary to achieve the desired V_T. The ensuing breaths will increase or decrease the pressure limit at less than 3 cmH_2O per breath in an attempt to achieve a relatively smooth transition from the initial V_T to the target volume. The pressure limit will fluctuate between 5 cmH_2O above the PEEP level and 5 cmH_2O below the upper pressure alarm setting.[41] As a safety feature, if the volume exiting the ventilator exceeds 150% of the set V_T, then the ventilator exhalation valve opens, ending the mechanical inspiration. Thus, with SIMV, most microprocessor-based ventilators are able to apply PS and dual-control breathing to the spontaneous and mandatory breaths, respectively, to improve flow delivery and maintain a set V_T during pressure-limited mandatory breaths. In preterm infants, because changes in respiratory system mechanics occur frequently, the set V_T of the mandatory dual-control breaths not only provides a guaranteed volume when respiratory system compliance decreases but also prevents overinflation when compliance improves.[42,43]

Physiologic Effects

The physiologic effects of IMV not listed in this section are discussed in comparison with other ventilation modes.

CONTROL OF BREATHING AND BREATHING PATTERNS

In early IMV development, it was thought that inspiratory muscle activity is downregulated during the mandatory breaths and that IMV therefore allows a combination of unassisted breathing with respiratory muscle rest to promote weaning.[5,44] By adjusting mandatory breath frequency, inspiratory effort could be modified until the patient resumed complete control of spontaneous breathing. Several studies, however, disproved this hypothesis.[32,45–47] Imsand et al[45] studied the neuromuscular output of patients recovering from acute exacerbation of chronic obstructive pulmonary disease (COPD) who were receiving pressure-triggered SIMV. The mandatory-breath V_T was set at 10–12 ml/kg. Neuromuscular output was estimated from the amplitude of the integrated diaphragmatic electrical activity (EMGd), measured using bipolar esophageal electrodes. Sternocleidomastoid muscle electrical activity (EMGscm) was recorded using surface electrodes. Neuromuscular output, occlusion esophageal pressure (Pes$_{0.1}$, another index of neuromuscular output), and neural inspiratory time (T_I) were measured at three ventilator support levels: >60%, 50–20%, and 0% of total support. Total support was defined as the support at which EMGd was suppressed completely. Only at the highest machine assistance rate did EMGd decrease significantly, whereas EMGscm did not (Fig. 8-4). Moreover, across all levels of ventilator support, both EMGd (Fig. 8-5) and Pes$_{0.1}$ of the unassisted and machine breaths were similar. Pes$_{0.1}$, however, tended to increase with

FIGURE 8-4 Peak inspiratory amplitude of integrated electrical activity of the diaphragm (EMGd) and sternocleidomastoid muscles (EMGscm) at three levels of machine assistance during SIMV, expressed as a percentage of mean value of 0% of or minimal (4 breaths per minute) machine assistance. Values are mean ± SE. *$P < 0.01$ compared with 0% of machine assistance. †$P < 0.05$ compared with spontaneous cycles at 50–20% of assistance. Assist, machine-assisted breaths; spont, intervening spontaneous breaths. (*Adapted, with permission, from Imsand et al: Anesthesiology 80:13–22, 1994.*)

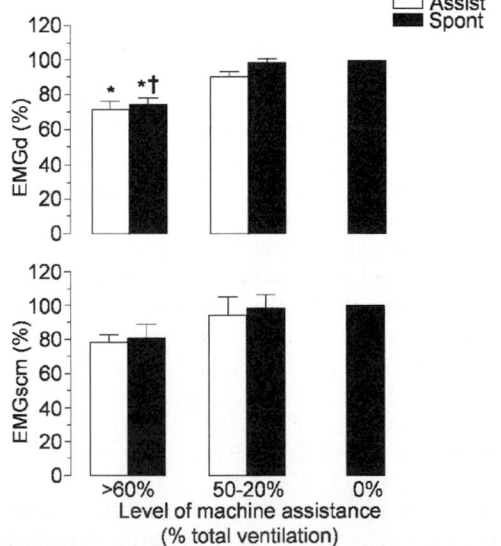

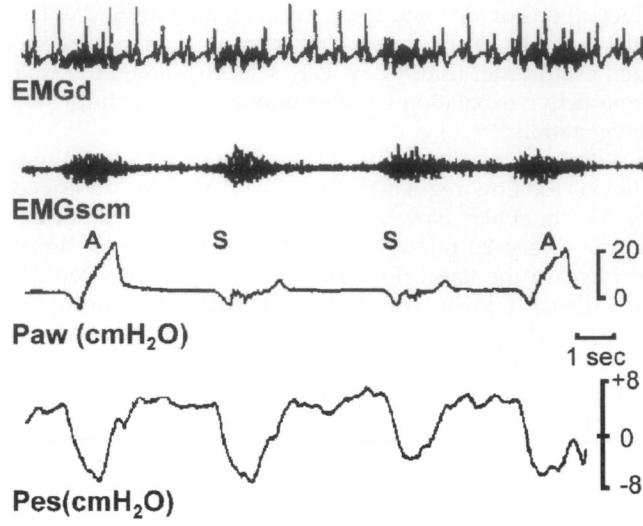

FIGURE 8-5 Electrical activity of the diaphragm (EMGd) and sternocleidomastoid muscles (EMGscm) in a patient receiving SIMV. Intensity and duration of electrical activity in successive assisted (A) and intervening spontaneous (S) breaths are similar. The regular spikes in the EMGd tracing are the QRS complex of the electrocardiogram signal. Paw, airway pressure; Pes, esophageal pressure. (*Adapted, with permission, from Imsand et al: Anesthesiology 80:13–22, 1994.*)

decreasing machine assistance. Likewise, neural T_I, defined as the interval from onset to peak EMGd, was equivalent for unassisted and machine breaths.

In another study, Uchiyama et al[46] applied continuous-flow IMV in anesthetized rabbits and measured EMGd with implanted electrodes into the diaphragm. The IMV rate was set at 0, 5, 10, 15, and 20 breaths per minute, at which EMGd was suppressed completely. EMGd was expressed as percent of EMGd at zero IMV rate per minute. Compared with spontaneous breathing, EMGd decreased significantly only at an IMV rate of 15 breaths per minute (75% of total support). In contrast with the study of Imsand et al,[45] at an IMV rate of 10 and 15 breaths per minute, EMGd of the mandatory breaths was absent. The difference in neuromuscular output response during mandatory breaths in the study of Uchiyama et al[46] may be related to the effect of anesthesia and the large V_T applied (15 ml/kg), causing vagally mediated inspiratory inhibition.[48] It appears that in anesthetized animals at ventilator support of 50% or greater, breath-by-breath adaptation to ventilator assistance occurred, but it was not observed in conscious humans.

In unsedated preterm infants with acute respiratory failure receiving flow-triggered SIMV, Beck et al[47] measured EMGd and neural timing of mandatory breaths and the unassisted breaths immediately preceding and following the mandatory breaths using miniaturized electrodes mounted on a feeding tube. The set SIMV rate ranged from 5–25 breaths per minute. Both EMGd and neural T_I amplitude were similar for the mandatory and unassisted breaths (Fig. 8-6). In contrast to improved triggering in adults,[45] during the mandatory breaths, a substantial delay was observed from onset of EMGd to flow delivery, an average of 95 ms (range 5–110 ms).

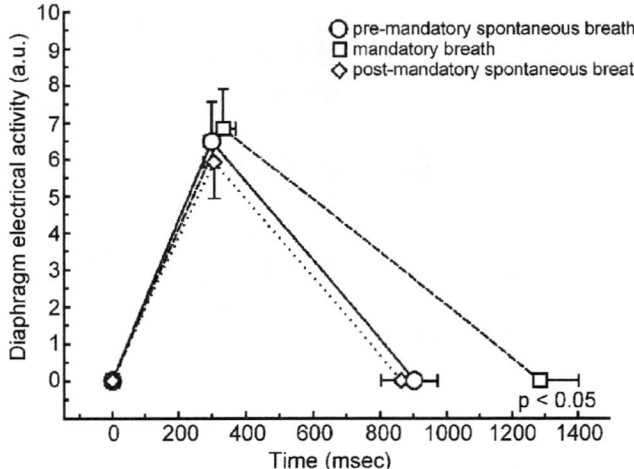

FIGURE 8-6 Diaphragmatic electrical activity (EMGd) time profile for group mean data. No significant difference exists between peak EMGd amplitude and neural timing on inspiration for the premandatory spontaneous breaths (*solid line*), mandatory breaths (*dashed line*), or after mandatory spontaneous breaths (*dotted line*). Neural expiratory time was prolonged significantly for the mandatory breaths (*dashed line*). The plot does not represent the shape of the EMGd recruitment pattern but simply represents three points: the onset of EMGd, peak of EMGd, and onset of EMGd of subsequent breath. Values are mean ± SE. (*Adapted, with permission, from Beck et al: Pediatr Res 55:747–54, 2004.*)

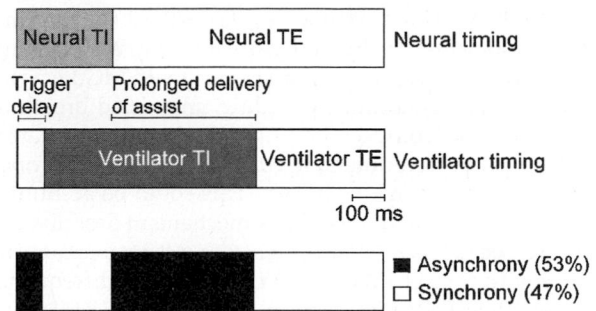

FIGURE 8-7 Inspiratory and expiratory asynchrony during mandatory breaths. Schematic representation of patient neural timing (*upper bar*) and ventilator timing (*middle bar*) during mandatory breaths. Upper bar shows the neural inspiratory time (T_I) (*light-gray area*) and neural expiratory time (T_E) (*white area*). Middle bar shows periods of ventilator timing, including trigger delay, ventilator T_I (*dark-gray area*), and ventilator T_E. Bottom bar shows periods of infant-ventilator synchrony (*white area*) and asynchrony (*black area*). (*Adapted, with permission, from Beck et al: Pediatr Res 55: 747–54, 2004.*)

Because most of the infants had bronchiolitis and likely were hyperinflated, the authors attributed the trigger delay or inspiratory asynchrony to neuroventilatory uncoupling (a delay from onset of diaphragmatic activation to flow generation)[49] rather than to the ventilator triggering system. Neural expiratory time (T_E) of the mandatory breath, defined as the interval from peak to EMGd onset of the subsequent breath, was prolonged. The relative increase in neural T_E during the mandatory breaths was related to the time the ventilator continued to inflate beyond the end of neural T_I ($R^2 = 0.66$; $P = 0.01$). This extended time was consistent with a vagally mediated reflex when pulse inflation was delivered into early expiration.[50,51] Both inspiratory asynchrony and expiratory asynchrony were present during every mandatory breath and constituted, on average, 53% of the total breath duration (Fig. 8-7). Expiratory asynchrony may result in increased peak airway pressure as the subject attempts to terminate inspiration by recruiting the expiratory muscles.[52] It also may result in increased work of breathing and discomfort and manifest as a patient "fighting the ventilator,"[53] potentially dictating sedation.

Using airway occlusion pressure ($P_{0.1}$) and mean inspiratory flow rate (V_T/T_I) as indices of neuromuscular output, Weiss et al[54] examined the effect of IMV on respiratory drive in stable ventilator-dependent patients who received mechanical ventilation for 12–24 hours each day. The IMV rate was initially set at 10 breaths per minute and reduced gradually to 6, 3, 2, and 1 breath per minute, and each level was maintained for 10 minutes. The V_T of the mandatory breaths was set at 8–12 ml/kg. End tidal P_{CO_2} and arterial oxygen saturation did not change as the IMV rate was reduced.

In the presence of stable chemical input, $P_{0.1}$ and V_T/T_I measured during spontaneous breathing varied inversely with IMV rate. Increases in V_T/T_I with IMV rate reduction primarily were the result of progressive V_T augmentation because inspiratory time (T_I) and the duty cycle (T_I/T_{TOT}) remained unchanged at all IMV support levels. This V_T response probably was related to changes in CO_2 production that stimulated chemoreceptors. In acutely ill patients,[32] the effect of IMV on $P_{0.1}$, measured during spontaneous breathing, is similar to that in stable patients.[54] Using another index of neuromuscular output, dP/dt of esophageal pressure at the onset of ventilator triggering, Leung et al[33] also demonstrated an inverse relationship between dP/dt and machine assistance level.

As with neuromuscular output, IMV's effects on breathing patterns are determined by assistance level. Both V_T and unassisted breath frequency increase progressively with a decreasing IMV rate.[32,33,45,55] Because V_T of the unassisted breaths is relatively small compared with the mandatory breaths, dead-space-to-tidal-volume ratio inevitably increases. Consequently, spontaneous breathing frequency increases to maintain constant alveolar ventilation. Indeed, Pa_{CO_2} remained constant at all machine assistance levels.[55]

The sensation of dyspnea during SIMV depends on assistance level when applied without pressure-support ventilation (PSV) but was independent of assistance level when 10 cmH$_2$O of PS was added to the unassisted breaths.[33] During low assistance levels, dyspnea probably is secondary to increased inspiratory effort, whereas the high rate of nontriggering efforts may be responsible for the dyspnea at higher assistance levels. Knebel et al[56] also demonstrated that during the weaning trial on SIMV, the sensation of dyspnea and patient anxiety were independent of support level. In that study,[56] a PEEP of 5 cmH$_2$O was maintained, which might have offset the increased inspiratory muscle work with a decreasing IMV rate.[57,58]

In summary, with IMV, the neuromuscular output of both the mandatory and unassisted breaths is downregulated only at high machine assistance levels (~75–80% of total machine assistance).[45,46] Breath-by-breath adaptation to machine assistance does not occur. The fact that EMGd was the same during assisted and preceding unassisted breathing suggests that neuromuscular output during the mandatory breaths must be determined at least in part by factors operating during the previous breath. This could be accounted for by the central neural feedback mechanism described by Eldridge (see below).[59] Neuromuscular output increases inversely with the set IMV rate. Whereas V_T and frequency increase when IMV rate decreases, neural inspiratory timing of the mandatory and unassisted breaths is of the same duration across all levels of machine assistance. Neural expiratory timing of the mandatory breaths is prolonged secondary to mechanical T_I encroaching into neural T_E, causing expiratory asynchrony. Respiratory timing asynchrony, however, potentially can be abolished by using inspiratory and expiratory neural triggering with a neurally adjusted ventilatory assist (NAVA).[49]

WORK OF BREATHING AND INSPIRATORY EFFORT

The effect of IMV on inspiratory muscle work and inspiratory effort is, as expected, determined by the level of machine assistance, and the response is similar in adults[32,33,45] and neonates.[55] A higher number of mandatory breaths reduces total workload and inspiratory effort in patients during acute respiratory failure[32] or recovery.[33,60,61] Marini et al[32] measured work of breathing (WOB) per liter of ventilation (joules per liter) and pressure-time product (PTP) per breath (PTPb) during ACV and at SIMV support levels of 80%, 60%, 40%, 20%, and 0% of the ACV rate. When the SIMV support level was less than 80% of the ACV rate, the patient's total workload was increased markedly compared with that during ACV. Moreover, at all SIMV levels, the patient expended a similar effort during both the mandatory and spontaneous breaths, as gauged by PTPb, which reflects the energy consumed by contracting respiratory muscles (patient effort). The patient does not vary effort on a breath-by-breath basis in response to machine unloading, as confirmed by others on the basis of EMGd recording.[45,47] It appears that during SIMV the heightened respiratory activity during the spontaneous breath is carried over to the subsequent mandatory breath in the manner of an "afterdischarge" or "memory" phenomenon.[59] In fact, when 10 cmH_2O of PS was applied during the intervening spontaneous breaths, inspiratory muscle effort decreased not only during the intervening breaths but also during the mandatory breaths (Fig. 8-8).[33] This afterdischarge phenomenon is central in origin and unrelated to chemoreceptor or mechanoreceptor feedback or the state of sleep/wakefulness.[59,62]

The patient workload during IMV is determined not only by machine assistance level but also by the IMV system employed.[60,61] Patient workload or inspiratory effort during spontaneous breathing cycles with flow-triggered SIMV was significantly less than with a pressure-triggered SIMV system,[60,61] particularly at a relatively low SIMV rate.[61] The effect, however, of the triggering system on patient mandatory breath workload is conflicting. Sassoon et al[61] demon-

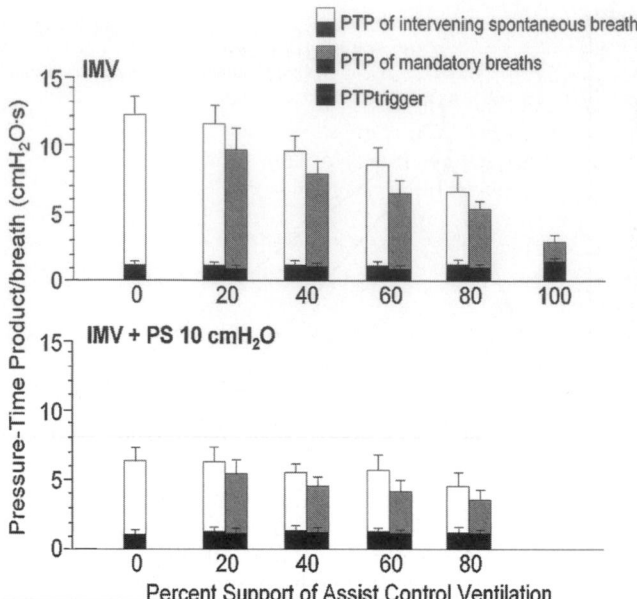

FIGURE 8-8 Pressure-time product (PTP) per breath during synchronous intermittent mandatory ventilation (IMV) in the presence and absence of pressure support (PS). The addition of 10 cmH_2O PS to the intervening spontaneous breaths decreased the overall PTP per breath. PTP per breath, however, did not differ between the mandatory and intervening spontaneous IMV breaths at each level of machine assistance, irrespective of whether PS was present or absent. (*Adapted, with permission, from Leung et al: Am J Respir Crit Care Med 155:1940–8, 1997.*)

strated that the triggering system had no effect on patient mandatory-breath workload. In contrast, Giuliani et al[60] found that patient mandatory-breath workload was significantly less with flow-triggered than with pressure-triggered SIMV irrespective of the mandatory-breath type (whether SIMV was flow- or pressure-limited). Moreover, patient workload with combined flow-triggered and pressure-limited mandatory breaths was lower than the other combinations of triggering and mandatory-breath types (flow-triggered flow limit and pressure-triggered flow and pressure limit).[60] The decrease was so substantial that the PTPb of the mandatory breath was significantly less than that of the intervening spontaneous breaths. It is not clear as to why the data of Giuliani et al[60] differed from the data of others[32,33,45,47] who demonstrated the lack of breath-by-breath adaptation to machine unloading.

In summary, during acute respiratory failure or recovery, patient workload during SIMV remains substantial unless the SIMV support is equivalent to or greater than 80% of the support during ACV.[32,33] IMV often allows adequate gas exchange at lower support levels[63] (see below) but at the expense of increased patient workload.[32,33,45]

Rationale, Advantages, and Limitations

IMV was developed as an alternative to CMV and ACV. The rationale for developing IMV was based on the premise that by maintaining spontaneous breathing amid the mechanical breaths, (1) machine breaths can be titrated to adjust alveolar ventilation, thereby decreasing the incidence of respiratory alkalemia,[64] (2) distribution of inspired gas and ventilation-perfusion to the lung base improve, and physiologic dead space decreases,[65] (3) mean airway pressure and pulmonary vascular resistance decrease, allowing PEEP titration and therefore more effective treatment of hypoxemia,[66] and (4) pleural pressure decreases, resulting in better venous return and cardiac output.[65] Unfortunately, subsequent clinical trials did not support some of the rationales (see below).

IMV's flexibility in providing a range of support levels makes it advantageous for use as a primary means of ventilator support[67] and as a method for discontinuing mechanical ventilation.[5] An inherent limitation of IMV is the fixed rate of machine breaths. When set at a very high rate, IMV functions as CMV and potentially may lead to diaphragmatic muscle atrophy.[68–70] During weaning from mechanical ventilation, the pace of decreasing the IMV rate potentially can prolong weaning when it is inappropriately slow.

Indications and Contraindications

IMV has been used as a primary means of ventilator support in postoperative patients[71] and during acute respiratory failure of various etiologies.[6,7,72–76] For treatment of acute respiratory failure, North Americans apply SIMV, with and without PS, more frequently than ACV (40% versus 34%, respectively).[10] The level of machine assistance must be tailored to the patient's ventilatory requirement. The optimal mandatory-breath settings are similar in principle to those for ACV.[77–79] A low IMV setting is contraindicated when the patient's ventilatory demand is high; likewise, the setting should not be left high after the patient's ventilatory requirement has decreased. A gradual decrease in the IMV rate is unwarranted when discontinuation from mechanical ventilation is imminent.

Comparison with Other Modes

IMV AS A PRIMARY MEANS OF VENTILATOR SUPPORT

IMV AND CMV

Unlike IMV, CMV imposes a fixed breathing pattern. Hence, to some extent, a comparison favors IMV, which has been claimed to be superior to CMV for the following reasons: (1) it prevents the patient from "fighting the ventilator," reducing the need for sedation and paralysis, (2) it prevents respiratory alkalosis, (3) it improves intrapulmonary gas distribution, (4) it lowers mean airway pressure, benefiting cardiac output and preventing barotrauma, (5) it decreases oxygen consumption ($\dot{V}_{O_2}$), (6) it prevents muscle atrophy and discoordination, and (7) it improves renal function.

1. *IMV prevents the patient from "fighting the ventilator," reducing the need for sedation and paralysis.* Because the patient has no autonomy to alter breathing pattern with CMV, the patient will increase inspiratory effort, which is manifested as "fighting the ventilator" when ventilatory demand rises. No studies, however, have compared the respective sedative doses used during CMV and IMV.

2. *IMV prevents respiratory alkalosis.* In a prospective study comparing IMV and CMV in patients with acute respiratory failure, CMV resulted in a mean pH of 7.49 and a Pa_{CO_2} of 32.3 mmHg, whereas IMV resulted in a mean pH of 7.44 and a Pa_{CO_2} of 39.9 mmHg.[7] The CMV rate, however, was set to suppress spontaneous respiratory effort, whereas, during IMV, the rate was adjusted downward continuously as long as pH remained greater than 7.30. Hence the result in favor of IMV is to be expected. When a normal pH is achieved at a low IMV rate, subsequent data suggested that it was at the expense of increased work of breathing.[32,60] Moreover, some patients on mechanical ventilation who are allowed to set their own Pa_{CO_2} do not always choose a normal level (e.g., patients with brain injury). These patients will have persistent respiratory alkalosis regardless of ventilation mode.[63,80]

3. *IMV improves intrapulmonary gas distribution.* This hypothesis is based on the premise that in the supine position, spontaneous breathing causes inspired gas to be distributed preferentially to dependent lung regions because the dependent diaphragm, which is displaced cephalad, operates at an improved mechanical advantage.[81] Conversely, during mechanical ventilation, ventilation is distributed preferentially to nondependent lung regions because the diaphragm is not used, and the nondependent lung and chest wall are more compliant.[82] Therefore, IMV's combination of spontaneous and mechanical breaths theoretically should result in a better matching of ventilation and perfusion.[83] A comparison study evaluating IMV and CMV ventilation-perfusion distribution with the inert-gas elimination technique[84] was performed in stable patients recovering from major abdominal aortic surgery.[85] During CMV, V_T was set at 14–16 ml/kg with a set rate of 8–10 breaths per minute. During SIMV, the rate was set at 50% of the CMV rate (4–5 breaths per minute); a PS of 5–8 cmH$_2$O was added to the intervening spontaneous breaths to overcome the ventilator circuit and endotracheal tube resistance.[86] Each ventilator mode was maintained for 45 minutes. Compared with CMV, physiologic dead space increased with SIMV (22.0% versus 26.8 %, respectively; $p < 0.05$) and was associated with a significant increase in $\dot{V}_E$, resulting in a similar Pa_{CO_2}. The SIMV perfusion distributions remained unaltered. This study, using the inert-gas elimination technique, shows that IMV does not improve ventilation-perfusion distributions.

4. *IMV lowers mean airway pressure, benefiting cardiac output and preventing barotrauma.* Since IMV intersperses spontaneous breaths between mechanical breaths, mean airway pressure averaged over time is lower than with CMV. The lower mean airway pressure results in maintenance of cardiac output. Several studies have shown a higher cardiac output with IMV than with CMV.[75,76,87] The interactions between intrathoracic pressure associated with mechanical ventilation and cardiac performance, however, are quite complex.[88] Right- and left-ventricular interaction,

direct pressure on the heart, and changes in systemic and pulmonary venous return all play a role. The net effect of this interaction depends on left-ventricular filling pressure and reserve. Mathru et al[89] compared the effect of CMV, IMV with 5 cmH$_2$O PEEP (IMV–5PEEP), and IMV with 0 cmH$_2$O PEEP (IMV–0PEEP) in two groups of patients following aortocoronary bypass surgery. V$_T$ and ventilator rate were adjusted to achieve a Pa$_{CO_2}$ of between 35 and 40 mmHg. One group had normal left-ventricular function. The second group had decreased left-ventricular reserve: left-ventricular diastolic pressure of greater than 16 mmHg and ejection fraction of less than 0.6. In the first group, IMV–0PEEP resulted in an increase in cardiac output of 27% compared with CMV. In the second group, however, IMV resulted in a significant decrease in cardiac output (19%) compared with CMV. IMV–5PEEP affected cardiac output similarly to CMV. These data indicate that when compared with CMV, IMV improves cardiac output in patients with normal left-ventricular function or hypovolemia, but it may be harmful in patients with poor left-ventricular reserve.

The frequency of barotrauma with IMV and CMV was compared in a retrospective study of 292 postoperative and nonsurgical patients who received mechanical ventilation for 24 hours or more.[90] The ventilator V$_T$ was set at 12–15 ml/kg. The IMV rate was set at 6 breaths per minute or lower, provided that normocapnia was maintained. If hypercapnia developed, it was treated by increasing V$_T$ to 15 ml/kg and, if necessary, by increasing the IMV rate to 8 breaths per minute. No sedation or muscle relaxants were used. In the CMV group, the rate was set at 12 breaths per minute. Hypercapnia was corrected by increasing V$_T$. The patients were sedated and paralyzed. Compared with the CMV group, patients receiving IMV had a significantly higher peak airway pressure (34 versus 51 cmH$_2$O, respectively) and PEEP/CPAP (15 versus 27 cmH$_2$O, respectively). Yet the barotrauma was 22% in the CMV group compared with 7% in the IMV group. The authors speculated that the less frequent barotrauma with IMV was related to the smaller number of mechanical breaths with large V$_T$. Mean transpulmonary pressure, which may be responsible for the barotrauma, was not measured in either group.

5. *IMV decreases oxygen consumption.* Downs et al[7] found that $\dot{V}_{O_2}$ was lower both during mechanical ventilation and 15 minutes after its discontinuation in patients ventilated with IMV versus CMV. The authors speculated that the higher $\dot{V}_{O_2}$ on CMV could be ascribed to respiratory alkalosis[91,92] and abrupt withdrawal from mechanical ventilation rather than reflecting metabolic work of breathing. In contrast, Wolff et al[87] showed that CO$_2$ production ($\dot{V}_{CO_2}$) tended to be lower with CMV than with IMV. Because the respiratory quotient was similar with both ventilation modes, it is reasonable to assume that $\dot{V}_{O_2}$ during CMV was lower than that during IMV. In this study, Pa$_{CO_2}$ was 39 and 44 mmHg on CMV and IMV, respectively, suggesting that pH was within the normal range. This observation suggests that, in the absence of alkalemia, $\dot{V}_{O_2}$ is lower on CMV than on IMV.

6. *IMV prevents muscle atrophy and discoordination.* Maintaining spontaneous breathing activity during IMV has been proposed to achieve respiratory muscle conditioning and preserve respiratory muscle function.[5] The periodic hyperinflation also may reinforce coordinated breathing.[5,93] During CMV, muscle atrophy[70,94,95,96] and myofibrillar damage[69,98,99] that account for ventilator-induced diaphragmatic dysfunction have been demonstrated in experimental animals. Conversely, maintaining diaphragmatic activation with ACV attenuates expression of the gene responsible for developing muscle atrophy: the *muscle atrophy F-box* (see Chapter 46).[70] The extent to which respiratory muscle atrophy develops during prolonged CMV in humans is unknown. With IMV, diaphragmatic electrical activity of both mandatory and spontaneous breaths persists. Thus it is possible that IMV prevents respiratory muscle atrophy. This hypothesis remains to be investigated.

Respiratory muscle discoordination with IMV and CMV has not been compared. IMV's efficacy in counteracting respiratory muscle discoordination was demonstrated by Andersen et al[93] in a study of 28 patients during discontinuation of mechanical ventilation. The mandatory breaths were increased gradually to 75% of the patient's $\dot{V}_E$. In contrast, Gibbons et al[100] failed to show similar results when IMV was applied to six patients receiving prolonged mechanical ventilation. The lowest spontaneous breathing rate was 29 breaths per minute at the lowest IMV rate of 10 breaths per minute. Gas exchange was adequate. Five of the six patients manifested breathing discoordination in the form of either rib-cage or abdominal paradox. In the patients whose diaphragmatic electrical activity was measured, an electromyographic fatigue pattern also was observed. In this study, IMV was insufficient to reduce respiratory muscle workload, as reflected by the relatively high spontaneous breathing rate. IMV's efficacy in counteracting respiratory muscle discoordination appears to depend primarily on the extent of respiratory muscle unloading.

7. *IMV improves renal function.* Steinhoff et al[101] studied the effect of CMV and IMV on renal function in patients with acute respiratory failure. With CMV, the ventilator rate was set to suppress inspiratory efforts, which averaged 10–16 breaths per minute. IMV was set at 4–10 breaths per minute. PEEP was maintained constant during both CMV and IMV. With CMV, urinary flow and creatinine and osmolal clearance decreased, with a net effect of water retention, in comparison with IMV. Impaired renal function during CMV was attributed to the increased intrathoracic pressure, which caused stimulation of atrial stretch receptors and release of antidiuretic hormone. A more important factor may be that increased intrathoracic pressure during CMV decreases venous return, and the consequent decrease in cardiac output produces a decrease in renal plasma flow. Hence the effects of CMV and IMV on renal function are related directly to their respective effects on cardiac function.

IMV AND ACV

Comparison of IMV with ACV is more appropriate than comparison of IMV with CMV because both IMV and ACV provide partial ventilator support. Few studies have compared IMV with ACV. As discussed below, these studies primarily concern effects on cardiac output,[102,103] $\dot{V}_{O_2}$,[102–104] and respiratory alkalosis.[63,102,105] (Since IMV's effects on work of breathing were discussed extensively earlier, comparison of IMV with ACV will be limited to its application in the neonate.[106,107])

1. *Effect on cardiac output.* Groeger et al[102] studied the effect of SIMV and ACV in 40 patients with acute respiratory failure of various etiologies other than COPD. SIMV, at a set V_T of 10–15 ml/kg, was the initial ventilation mode in all patients, and the mandatory rate was adjusted to the minimum required to maintain a normal pH and Pa_{CO2}. When the combined mandatory and spontaneous breathing rates were greater than 35 breaths per minute, the IMV rate was increased to ensure patient comfort. The ventilator mode was then switched to ACV, and V_T, PEEP, inspiratory flow rate, and inspired oxygen fraction (F_{IO_2}) were held constant. After 30 minutes on SIMV or ACV, hemodynamic variables were measured. At this point, mean IMV rate was 7 breaths per minute, with a total rate of 34 breaths per minute, whereas the ACV rate was 15 breaths per minute. Cardiac output, measured by thermodilution, was 6% higher with SIMV than with ACV. Likewise, studying 12 patients recovering from acute respiratory failure of various etiologies, Sternberg and Sahebjami[103] demonstrated that cardiac index was significantly higher with SIMV than with ACV (3.6 versus 3.3 liters/min/m²). (The investigators also compared SIMV with PSV, which will be discussed below.) The average V_T with ACV was 715 ml, whereas with SIMV it was 491 ml. The SIMV mandatory breaths were set at 75% of the ACV rate. Although the cardiac output with SIMV was significantly higher than with ACV, the changes fall within the variability of the thermodilution technique.[108] Despite the limited differences in cardiac output with IMV and ACV, IMV may be helpful in patients who demonstrate significant hemodynamic deterioration during ACV. In the original description of intrinsic PEEP ($PEEP_I$),[109] two patients with COPD developed hemodynamic compromise secondary to significant $PEEP_I$ while receiving ACV. The institution of IMV and fluid repletion produced an improvement,

although cardiac output was not measured directly during either IMV or ACV. The conflicting data concerning the effects of ACV and IMV on cardiac output underscore the complex interaction between intrathoracic pressure and cardiac function.

2. *Effect on oxygen consumption.* In the above-mentioned study by Groeger et al,[102] $\dot{V}_{O_2}$ was comparable for both pressure-triggered SIMV and ACV. When the patients were grouped according to the ratio between $\dot{V}_E$ achieved by the mandatory breaths and total $\dot{V}_E$, however, the mean $\dot{V}_{O_2}$ for patients with a ratio of less than 0.5 was significantly higher during SIMV than during ACV (320 versus 296 ml/min/m², respectively; $p \leq 0.05$). Conversely, in the study of Sternberg and Sebahjami,[103] when the mandatory breaths during SIMV were set at 75% of the ACV rate, $\dot{V}_{O_2}$ was unaltered during SIMV despite total frequency being higher with SIMV than with ACV (20 breaths per minute versus 12 breaths per minute). In healthy subjects breathing via a mouthpiece on SIMV or ACV, $\dot{V}_{O_2}$ (measured with a metabolic cart) also was similar with the two modes.[104] With SIMV, both the V_T and mandatory-breath rate were equivalent to those of the ACV: 10 ml/kg and 12 breaths per minute, respectively, with a total rate of 15 breaths per minute. These studies[102–104] demonstrate that compared with ACV, the degree of machine assistance during IMV determines $\dot{V}_{O_2}$.

3. *Effect on respiratory alkalosis.* Three prospective studies[63,102,105] comparing IMV and ACV showed a significantly lower pH and higher Pa_{CO_2} during IMV than during ACV (Table 8-1). Groeger et al[102] suggested that the higher Pa_{CO_2} during IMV was related to an increased dead-space-to-tidal-volume ratio (V_D/V_T), because $\dot{V}_{CO_2}$ and $\dot{V}_E$ were similar for both IMV and ACV. Conversely, Hudson et al[63] showed that the higher Pa_{CO_2} during IMV came at the expense of a high patient workload given elevated CO_2 and an unchanged alveolar ventilation level. Regardless of the mechanisms of the elevated Pa_{CO_2} during IMV, all three groups of investigators concluded that the

TABLE 8-1   Effect of IMV versus ACV on pH and Pa_{CO_2}

Reference No.	pH		Pa_{CO_2} (mmHg)		RATE (BREATHS PER MINUTE)		
	IMV	ACV	IMV	ACV	IMV	ACV	*n*
63	7.41 ± 0.06[a]	7.45 ± 0.06	43.0 ± 6.3[a]	38.0 ± 6.3	7.1 (33.6)	15.1	40
102	7.48 ± 0.05[b]	7.51 ± 0.04	29.7 ± 6.1	28.6 ± 4.9	1/2 ACV rate	NA	26
105	7.42 ± 0.08[a]	7.45 ± 0.04	40.7 ± 7.6[a]	37.9 ± 6.7	4 (21)	15.0	18
PATIENTS WITH PREEXISTING RESPIRATORY ALKALOSIS							
63	7.49 ± 0.03	7.49 ± 0.03	27.4 ± 6.3	29.1 ± 4.7			17
105	7.46 ± 0.07[b]	7.49 ± 0.03	37.8 ± 7.4	35.7 ± 6.7			12

[a]$p < 0.01$.
[b]$p < 0.05$.
NOTE: Values are mean ± SD; only mean rate is shown. Number in parenthesis denotes total mandatory and spontaneous breath rates. Tidal volume was maintained the same for the mandatory breath with both IMV and ACV.
ABBREVIATIONS: IMV, intermittent mandatory ventilation; ACV, assist-control ventilation; NA, not available.
SOURCES: Adapted, with permission, from Hudson et al,[63] Groeger et al,[102] and Culpepper et al.[105]

decrease in pH and increase in Pa_{CO_2} were minimal and of questionable clinical significance. Furthermore, in studies where IMV was compared with ACV in a subgroup of patients with preexisting respiratory alkalosis, respiratory alkalosis persisted during IMV (Table 8-1).[63,105]

4. *Effects on work of breathing in the neonate.* Kapasi et al[107] undertook a comparison of the effects of pressure-limited ACV, SIMV, and IMV on WOB and inspiratory effort of clinically stable neonates with respiratory distress syndrome. The mandatory breath rate with both SIMV and IMV was set the same as that of the ACV (range 14–25 breaths per minute). Average total respiratory rate was not significantly different among the modes (IMV, 56.3 breaths per minute; SIMV, 58.3 breaths per minute; ACV, 58.8 breaths per minute). The WOB was estimated using the esophageal pressure, calculated using the Campbell diagram.[110,111] Both WOB and inspiratory effort were least with ACV and highest with IMV; SIMV had values between ACV and IMV. Patient-ventilator asynchrony occurred only with IMV. Jarreau et al[106] reported a similar result when comparing IMV, ACV with inspiratory pressure set at 10–15 cmH_2O, and spontaneous breathing on CPAP. WOB with IMV was similar to that with CPAP: 0.81 versus 0.90 J/liter. WOB fell significantly only during ACV to 0.48–0.47 J/liter at inspiratory pressures of 10 and 15 cmH_2O, respectively. Thus, in neonates, patient-triggered ACV provides better patient-ventilator synchrony and unloading of workload than continuous-flow IMV does.

In summary, the limited number of studies suggests minimal differences between the effects of high levels of IMV and ACV on cardiac output, $\dot{V}_{O_2}$, and respiratory alkalosis. Because of lower mean airway and intrapleural pressures, IMV should help to improve cardiovascular function in patients who exhibit hemodynamic compromise during ACV. In neonates, ACV is more effective in unloading the WOB and providing synchrony than IMV.

IMV AND PSV

As with IMV, PSV provides the patient with some autonomy to alter breathing patterns in response to ventilatory demand. PSV is a form of ventilatory support in which the patient's inspiratory effort is assisted by the ventilator up to a preset inspiratory pressure level and remains at that level until the ventilator cycle-off algorithm is activated.[112,114] Unlike IMV, in which the number of mandatory breaths is fixed, PSV assists every breath, and the ventilator contribution to total workload is variable. Because the set inspiratory pressure is fixed with PSV, when patient ventilatory demand increases, inspiratory effort may exceed the ventilator contribution to total workload (see Chapter 9).[115] PSV can be added to IMV to unload inspiratory muscle work during the spontaneous breathing cycles. The addition of a small amount of PSV (5 cmH_2O) to pressure-triggered SIMV is adequate to overcome the lack of flow delivery observed with some pressure-triggered SIMV systems.[31] Higher levels of PSV not only help in overcoming the ventilator circuit and endotracheal tube resistance[116,117] but also augment V_T and unload the elastic work of the spontaneous breaths.[118,119] In

one study of a small number of patients with acute respiratory failure,[120] PSV application at levels of up to 30 cmH_2O during SIMV (IMV rate of 6–10 breaths per minute) and PEEP of 3–13 cmH_2O did not result in cardiovascular compromise. Comparison between IMV and PSV will be discussed pertaining to cardiac output,[103] ventilation-perfusion distribution,[121] and unloading of patient effort.[33]

1. *Effects on cardiac output.* Hemodynamics during SIMV and PSV were studied in critically ill patients by initially applying ACV to the patients.[103] The V_T of the mandatory breaths with SIMV then was set the same as that of ACV, at a rate of 75% of the ACV rate. With PSV, the inspiratory pressure was set to produce a V_T similar to that of ACV (average pressure of 21 cmH_2O). Cardiac output (measured by thermodilution), oxygen transport, and $\dot{V}_{O_2}$ were the same for both ventilation modes. As a primary means of ventilatory support, both SIMV and PSV have comparable effects on hemodynamics.

2. *Effects on ventilation-perfusion.* Valentine et al[121] studied the effect of SIMV, PSV, and airway pressure-release ventilation (see below) on ventilation-perfusion distribution in post–cardiac surgery patients who were ready to be weaned; this section will discuss only the comparison between SIMV and PSV. SIMV was the initial ventilatory support mode. The IMV rate was adjusted to maintain a pH of greater than 7.35. With PSV, pressure was titrated to achieve a mean end-tidal P_{CO_2} of 40 mmHg. Ventilation-perfusion distribution was assessed using the inert-gas elimination technique.[84] The dispersion of ventilation-perfusion ratios, calculated as the logarithmic standard deviation of perfusion (log SD$\dot{Q}$) and ventilation (log SD$\dot{V}$), was similar for SIMV and PSV. Right-to-left intrapulmonary shunt and fractional dead-space ventilation did not differ significantly. Table 8-2 shows the effects on arterial blood gases, respiratory mechanics, and $\dot{V}_{O_2}$. Differences in arterial blood gases were of questionable clinical significance. Peak airway pressure was significantly higher with SIMV, but mean transpulmonary pressure was comparable. As sole ventilator support, SIMV and PSV provide comparable and adequate gas exchange in postoperative patients who were ready to be weaned. No study has yet compared the efficacy of IMV and PSV as a primary means of ventilator support during acute respiratory failure.

3. *Effects on patient effort.* Leung et al[33] carried out a head-to-head comparison of the efficacy of SIMV and PSV in unloading inspiratory effort at various levels of assistance. The rate of change in inspiratory effort with increasing assistance levels, estimated as PTP per minute, did not differ between the two modes. Unloading efficacy, however, differed according to the level of assistance. From 0–60% of maximum, the decrease in PTP per minute was greater with PSV than with SIMV. At higher assistance level, the converse was observed (Fig. 8-9). Frequency decreased linearly with increase in PSV. With SIMV, frequency changed little until a high assistance level was provided (see Fig. 8-9).[122] Thus, when a high assistance level is needed, both SIMV and PSV provide comparable assistance. At low to medium assistance levels, however, a greater decrease in patient effort with PSV makes it more useful clinically than SIMV. Leung et al[33] also

TABLE 8-2 Gas Exchange, Mechanics, and Oxygen Consumption during SIMV and PSV

	SIMV	PSV
$F_{I_{O_2}}$	0.44 ± 0.11	0.44 ± 0.11
pH	7.41 ± 0.02	7.36 ± 0.02[a]
Pa_{CO_2}, mmHg	33.0 ± 2.0	39.0 ± 2.0[a]
Pa_{O_2}, mmHg	102.0 ± 7.0	98.0 ± 8.0
Peak Paw, cmH2O	32.8 ± 1.3	19.4 ± 2.1[a]
Mean Paw, cmH2O	9.6 ± 1.1	8.4 ± 1.0
Ppl, cmH2O	3.8 ± 1.0	3.8 ± 1.1
Ptp, cmH2O	5.8 ± 0.6	4.6 ± 0.5
$\dot{V}_E$, liters/min	9.4 ± 0.6	9.0 ± 0.5
fS, breaths per minute	3.4 ± 1.8	
fM, breaths per minute	8.4 ± 0.4	15.8 ± 0.9[a]
$V_T S$, liters	0.08 ± 0.07	
$V_T M$, liters	1.03 ± 0.03	0.58 ± 0.03[a]
$\dot{V}_{O_2}$, ml/min	269 ± 13	268 ± 14

[a]$p < 0.05$.

NOTE: Values are mean ± SE; $n = 9$.

ABBREVIATIONS: SIMV, synchronous intermittent mandatory ventilation; PSV, pressure-support ventilation; $F_{I_{O_2}}$, inspired oxygen fraction. Paw, airway pressure; Ppl, pleural pressure; Ptp, transpulmonary pressure; $\dot{V}_E$, total minute ventilation; fS, frequency of spontaneous breaths during SIMV; fM, frequency of mandatory breaths or pressure support assisted breaths; $V_T S$, tidal volume of spontaneous breath during SIMV; $V_T M$, tidal volume of mandatory breath or pressure-support assisted breath; $\dot{V}_{O_2}$, oxygen consumption.

SOURCE: Adapted, with permission, from Valentine el al.[121]

assessed the patient's wasted efforts or nontriggered attempts during both SIMV and PSV. The number of nontriggered attempts is proportional to the assistance level and highest at 100% of machine assistance (29% with SIMV and 26% with PSV). The breaths preceding the nontriggered attempts had a shorter total duration and expiratory time, higher V_T, and higher dynamic intrinsic PEEP ($PEEP_I$) than did the breaths preceding triggered breaths. This observation suggests that nontriggered attempts resulted from an inspiratory effort that was insufficient to overcome the elevated recoil pressure associated with dynamic hyperinflation. Thus, increasing the ventilator assistance level de-

FIGURE 8-9 Changes in PTP per minute (*left panel*) and frequency (*right panel*) as intermittent mandatory ventilation (IMV) and pressure-support ventilation (PSV) were increased progressively. PSV of 100% represents the level necessary to achieve a V_T equivalent to that during ACV (10 ml/kg); IMV 100% is the same ventilator rate and V_T as during ACV. (*Adapted, with permission, from Leung et al: Am J Respir Crit Care Med 155:1940–8, 1997; and Tobin et al: Am J Respir Crit Care Med 163:1059–63, 2001.*)

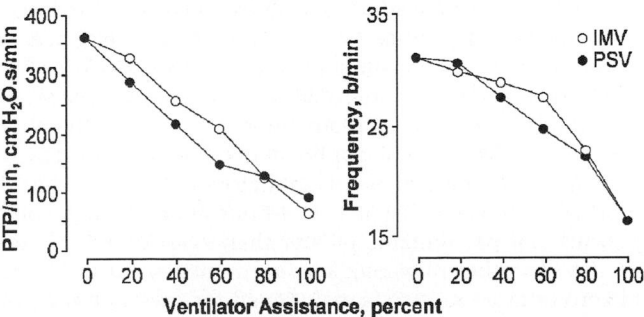

creases inspiratory muscle effort but also increases ineffective triggering. The impact of ineffective triggering on ventilator outcome remains unclear.

IMV AND AIRWAY PRESSURE-RELEASE VENTILATION

Airway pressure-release ventilation (APRV) consists essentially of two CPAP levels with a transient decrease or "release" of airway pressure from a higher CPAP to a lower CPAP for a set release time. Spontaneous breathing is allowed to occur between airway pressure releases.[113,123–125] The pressure gradient between the two CPAP levels and the frequency of releases determine the level of ventilator support (see Chapter 12). The original version of APRV used a short release time, and in the absence of spontaneous breathing, APRV resembled pressure-controlled inverse-ratio ventilation.[123] The modified version, in which the inspiration-to-expiration (I:E) ratio is adjustable, is termed *biphasic intermittent positive airway pressure* (BiPAP).[125] The primary indication for APRV is the provision of ventilation during an oxygenation crisis.[123] Although the indications and operating principles of IMV and APRV differ significantly, both modes allow the patient to breathe spontaneously between machine-cycled breaths.[123,124] Comparison of IMV with APRV will be discussed with regard to its efficacy as a primary means of ventilator support in patients with acute respiratory distress syndrome (ARDS)[126] in relation to gas exchange,[121,126–128] hemodynamics,[126,128,129] breathing comfort,[128,130] intubation duration, and sedative use.[126,131]

Recently, Varpula et al[126] undertook a randomized, controlled comparison of pressure-limited SIMV (with 10 cmH2O of PS added to the unassisted breaths) and APRV in patients with ARDS. The primary endpoint was the number of ventilator-free days from the time of randomization to day 28. The secondary endpoints were the effect on gas exchange, hemodynamics, and sedative use. PEEP was set slightly above the lower inflection point on the pressure-volume curve obtained during paralysis (or if not detected, at 10 cmH2O). The upper inflection point was never exceeded (or if not detected, the inspiratory pressure was set at less than 35 cmH2O). The pressure-release frequency with APRV and the machine assistance rate with SIMV were similar at 12 breaths per minute. The I:E ratio with APRV was set at 4:1; with SIMV, it was set at 1:2 and adjusted to 2:1. Ventilator-free days, gas exchange, hemodynamics, and sedative dosage were comparable with the two modes, although average inspiratory pressure was significantly lower with APRV than with SIMV (25.9 versus 28.6 cmH2O). Moderate hypercapnia developed during the first study day in both groups but returned toward normal after 4 days. Previous studies of patients with lung injury[127,128] or after cardiac surgery[121,129] demonstrated comparable effects of SIMV and APRV on gas exchange and hemodynamics. In contrast to patients with ARDS, application of short-term APRV proved superior to SIMV in patients who underwent coronary artery bypass surgery. Intubation duration was about 4 hours shorter with APRV than with SIMV (mean 10.1 versus 14.7 hours). Analgesic and sedative dosage also was less with APRV than with SIMV. This study, however, was a nonrandomized, open clinical trial.

Breathing comfort during SIMV and APRV were evaluated in inexperienced healthy subjects breathing via a mouthpiece and compared with PSV. SIMV was set at 8 breaths per minute, V_T at 5 ml/kg, and PEEP at 5 cmH_2O. The low and high PEEP levels with APRV were set at 5 and 10 cmH_2O, the release rate was 8 breaths per minute, and the I:E ratio was 1:2. PSV was set at 10 cmH_2O with PEEP of 5 cmH_2O. Breathing comfort was measured with a visual analog scale (0–10 cm). PSV achieved the greatest comfort, SIMV the worst, and APRV fell between PSV and SIMV (2.03, 5.38, and 4.12 cm, respectively). Unfortunately, flow-limited SIMV was employed rather than pressure-limited SIMV (both APRV and PSV are pressure-limited ventilation modes).

IMV AND PROPORTIONAL-ASSIST VENTILATION, ADAPTIVE-SUPPORT VENTILATION, AND PRESSURE-REGULATED VOLUME CONTROL

Proportional-Assist Ventilation

Proportional-assist ventilation (PAV) is a mode in which the ventilator instantaneously generates pressure in proportion to the patient's effort (see Chapter 13).[132] The ventilator amplifies the patient's inspiratory effort without any preselected target volume or pressure. A randomized crossover comparison of continuous-flow IMV versus PAV was conducted in 36 preterm infants.[133] The inspiratory pressure with IMV was set to deliver a V_T of 4 to 6 ml/kg. The IMV rate was not reported. With PAV, the volume-assist gain was adjusted to decrease lung elastance to its normal value, whereas the flow-assist gain was set at −20 $cmH_2O/liter/s$. Each mode was applied for 45 minutes. With PAV, peak and mean airway pressures and transpulmonary pressure were significantly lower, frequency was higher, and V_T was comparable to that with IMV, resulting in a higher $\dot{V}_E$. Pa_{CO_2}, however, remained the same as with IMV, and Pa_{O_2} was higher. There were no significant differences in the number of apneic or hypoxemic episodes. The lower transpulmonary pressure with PAV might help to prevent lung injury during prolonged mechanical ventilation. The results in preterm infants were similar to those in an earlier short-term trial in a few adult patients.[134]

Adaptive-Support Ventilation

Adaptive-support ventilation (ASV) is based on the work by Otis et al[135] and Mead et al,[136] who demonstrated that any given level of alveolar ventilation has an optimal respiratory frequency that is least costly in terms of respiratory work: the frequency at which the respiratory muscles develop the least average force or tension.[136] ASV is a mode that can alternate between pressure control and pressure support, relying on closed-loop regulation of ventilator settings that respond to changes in respiratory system mechanics and spontaneous breathing efforts (see Chapter 16). ASV adjusts inspiratory pressure, I:E ratio, and mandatory rate to maintain the target minute ventilation and respiratory rate within a frame designed to avoid both rapid, shallow breathing and excessive inflation volumes.[137] Tassaux et al[138] com-

pared the short-term effects of ASV versus SIMV plus PS on patient-ventilator interaction in patients ready to be weaned from mechanical ventilation. ASV achieved a $\dot{V}_E$ similar to that of SIMV. Central neural drive, however, estimated as $P_{0.1}$, and sternocleidomastoid electrical activity, measured with surface electrodes, were reduced markedly. Thus ASV provided comparable total $\dot{V}_E$ but with a significantly decreased inspiratory load than did SIMV plus PS.

Pressure-Regulated Volume-Controlled Ventilation

Pressure-regulated volume-controlled ventilation (PRVCV) is a dual-control, breath-to-breath mode. PRVCV has both the benefits of pressure-controlled ventilation, with a constant V_T, and automatic weaning from pressure limit as patient compliance improves and/or patient effort increases (see Chapter 16). Piotrowski et al[139] undertook a randomized, controlled comparison of PRVCV and continuous-flow IMV in neonates with respiratory distress syndrome. Thirty neonates received IMV, and 27 received PRVCV; the average peak inspiratory pressures were 18.6 and 16.2 cmH_2O, respectively. The IMV rate was selected by the clinician. With PRVCV, the V_T was set at 5–6 ml/kg. The primary endpoint was duration of mechanical ventilation and incidence of bronchopulmonary dysplasia. The secondary endpoint was complications from mechanical ventilation, consisting of air leaks, intraventricular hemorrhage, and hemodynamic instability. PRVCV did not decrease duration of mechanical ventilation or incidence of bronchopulmonary dysplasia, although it decreased the incidence of high-grade intraventricular hemorrhage (11% versus 35%). The benefit may have occurred in part because PRVCV delivers a stable volume. In newborn preterm infants, large fluctuations in intrathoracic and arterial pressures cause variations in cerebral blood flow velocity that is a risk factor for intraventricular hemorrhage.[140] In a subgroup of neonates weighing less than 1000 g, duration of mechanical ventilation was reduced and hypotension was less in the PRVCV group than in the IMV group. Unfortunately, the number of neonates in the subgroup was small ($n = 10$). In the preterm infants, PRVCV appears to decrease complications related to mechanical ventilation. A patient-triggered, pressure-controlled ventilation without volume guarantee would have been a better comparison with to assess PRVCV's efficacy.

IMV AS A WEANING METHOD

IMV, PRESSURE SUPPORT, AND T PIECE

IMV was first used in adult patients as a means of discontinuing mechanical ventilation.[5] This method was claimed to be more efficient, safer, and more readily accepted by the patient, and it avoided the necessity of setting up a T-piece circuit. While preceding ventilator support may be with either the ACV or IMV, IMV is applied when the patient is ready to be weaned. The number of mandatory breaths is reduced gradually (1–3 breaths) at 1- to 4-hour intervals, provided that arterial pH remains greater than 7.30[7] or 7.35,[141] regardless of other physiologic measurements. An IMV rate of zero or close to zero is maintained for several hours, or as long as 24 hours, before extubating the patient.

With PSV as a weaning method, the pressure level is set initially at a maximum, defined as the level that produces a V_T of 10–12 ml/kg; then the PS level is reduced according to the patient's respiratory frequency.[142] When the PS level reaches 5 cmH$_2$O, extubation is considered.

With a T piece, once the patient meets predefined weaning criteria, he or she is placed on a T-piece circuit.[143] Progressively longer intervals of spontaneous breathing through a T piece are alternated with ACV. Extubation is considered when the patient can sustain breathing through a T piece for 1–2 hours. The early claim for IMV's superiority over a T piece was not based on a controlled study, and subsequent retrospective[144] and prospective studies[145,146] failed to demonstrate IMV's superiority. Studies comparing IMV and PSV showed either a significantly reduced duration[147] or a tendency for a shorter weaning time[148] with PSV. As PSV grew in popularity, two prospective, randomized, controlled multicenter trials[149,150] simultaneously compared the three weaning modalities: SIMV, PSV, and T piece. These trials laid to rest IMV's claim to superiority over T piece and PSV.

Brochard et al[149] studied 109 patients who met three of the four defined weaning criteria and had failed a 2-hour T-piece trial. Patients were randomized to SIMV ($n = 43$), PSV ($n = 31$), and T piece ($n = 35$). Weaning failure was defined as continued inability to be weaned after 21 days on the same mode, the need for reintubation after 48 hours of extubation, or intercurrent events (e.g., cardiac ischemia or nosocomial pneumonia) within 72 hours in the selected mode. The initial SIMV rate was set at half the total frequency during ACV or CMV, keeping V_T and flow rates constant (mean initial SIMV rate of 9.5 breaths per minute).

Once or twice a day, the SIMV rate was decreased by 2 to 4 breaths per minute if patients did not demonstrate signs of poor tolerance. When a patient demonstrated poor tolerance, the SIMV rate was increased to its preceding level. When a patient tolerated a SIMV rate of 4 breaths per minute or less over 1 day, tracheal extubation was performed. The T-piece method consisted of a gradual lengthening of the periods of disconnection from the ventilator. The initial T-piece trial was set shorter than the initial tolerance duration (mean duration of 38 minutes). The number of T-piece trials depended on the length of disconnection and on nurse availability and varied from three to eight trials per day. The T-piece periods were lengthened incrementally twice a day. Between the T-piece trials, ACV was applied. When the duration of a T-piece trial had reached 2 hours with adequate gas exchange, tracheal extubation was performed. In the patients assigned to PSV, the initial pressure was adjusted until the frequency ranged between 20 and 30 breaths per minute. Twice a day, the pressure was decreased by 2–4 cmH$_2$O if the patient did not show any signs of poor tolerance; if tolerance worsened, pressure was increased to its preceding level. When the patient tolerated a PSV level of 8 cmH$_2$O or less throughout a 24-hour period, tracheal extubation was performed. During the 21-day trial, the probability of being weaned was twice as high with PSV than with SIMV or T piece. Weaning duration did not differ between SIMV and T piece but was significantly shorter with PSV than with the other two modalities (6 versus 9 days, respectively). The number of weaning success patients was significantly larger with PSV (77%) than with SIMV (58%) or T piece (57%) (Table 8-3).

TABLE 8-3 Trials Comparing Three Weaning Methods: Intermittent T Piece, Pressure-Support Ventilation (PSV), and Synchronized Intermittent Mandatory Ventilation (SIMV)

Trial	SUCCESSFUL WEAN [n (%)]		
	T Piece	PSV	SIMV
Brochard et al[149]	20/35 (57)	24/31 (77)	25/43 (58)
Esteban et al[150]	27/33 (82)	23/37 (62)	20/29 (69)

Trial	RISK DIFFERENCE (%)[a]		
	T Piece vs. PSV	T Piece vs. SIMV	PSV vs. SIMV
Brochard et al[149]	−20 (−42, 2)	−1 (−23, 21)	19 (−2, 40)
Esteban et al[150]	14 (−5, 32)	7 (−13, 27)	−7 (−20, 16)

Trial	TIME TO EXTUBATION (DAYS)		
	T Piece	PSV	SIMV
Brochard et al[149]	8.5 ± 8.3	5.7 ± 3.7	9.9 ± 8.2
Esteban et al[150]	3 (2, 6)	4 (2, 12)	5 (3, 11)

[a]Risk differences expressed as the difference in proportions of successfully weaned subjects between respective weaning methods. Negative numbers imply lower success rates and positive numbers higher success rates. The 95% confidence intervals follow risk differences in parentheses. Time to extubation is presented as either mean ± SD[149] or median (first and third quartiles).[150]

SOURCES: Adapted, with permission, from Brochard et al,[149] Esteban et al,[150] and Butler et al[151] for the risk-difference calculations.

In the study by Esteban et al,[150] 130 patients who met two of three weaning criteria and had failed a 2-hour T-piece trial were randomly assigned to one of four methods: SIMV ($n = 29$), PSV ($n = 37$), intermittent T-piece trials (two or more per day) ($n = 37$), and a once-daily T-piece trial ($n = 31$). The initial SIMV rate was set at half the frequency during ACV (average 10 breaths per minute). When the patient tolerated it, SIMV was reduced twice a day by 2 to 4 breaths per minute. Tracheal extubation was performed when the patient tolerated an SIMV rate of 5 breaths per minute for 2 hours without signs of distress. With the PSV, the initial pressure was adjusted to achieve a frequency of 25 breaths per minute or less (average pressure of 18 cmH_2O). According to patient tolerance, pressure was reduced at least twice a day by 2 to 4 cmH_2O. When the patient tolerated a PSV level of 5 cmH_2O for 2 hours, tracheal extubation was performed. With intermittent T-piece trials, the patient breathed through a T-piece circuit or a continuous-flow CPAP of 5 cmH_2O or less at least twice a day. Trial duration was increased gradually, and when the patient tolerated a 2-hour trial, extubation was performed. Between the T-piece trials, ACV was applied. With the once-daily T-piece method, the patient breathed through a T-piece circuit, after which ACV was resumed for 24 hours. Trial duration was increased gradually. When the patient tolerated a 2-hour trial, extubation was performed. Weaning failure was defined as the need for reintubation within 48 hours after extubation or the inability to extubate the patient after 14 days. The median successful weaning duration was 5 days for SIMV, 4 days for PSV, 3 days for intermittent T-piece trials, and 3 days for the once-daily T-piece trials. The rate of successful weaning for the once-daily T-piece method was three times faster than with SIMV (rate ratio 2.83) and two times faster than with PSV (rate ratio 2.05). The rate of success for intermittent or once-daily T-piece trials did not differ significantly. The percentage of patients weaned successfully was 69%, 62%, 82%, and 71% for SIMV, PSV, intermittent T piece, and once-daily T piece, respectively.

These two large randomized studies showed conflicting results. In the study of Brochard et al,[149] PSV was superior to T piece and SIMV. In the study of Esteban et al,[150] T piece was superior to PSV and SIMV. Despite the subtle differences in methodology, both trials demonstrated that weaning time was the longest with SIMV.[151] Thus both T piece and PSV were superior to SIMV (see Table 8-3).[152,153]

In weaning preterm infants, Dimitriou et al[154] compared pressure-limited SIMV with ACV in two separate randomized, controlled trials. With both SIMV and ACV ($n = 20$ each), inspiratory pressure was reduced in decrements of 2 cmH_2O until a defined target pressure tailored to the infant's body weight was reached. With SIMV, in addition to decreasing pressure, the SIMV rate was reduced in decrements of 5 breaths per minute until a target rate of 20 breaths per minute was reached in the first trial. In the second trial, the target was 5 breaths per minute. The frequency of decrements in pressure or SIMV rate was not reported. When the infants tolerated the target pressure (for ACV) or target pressure and rate (for SIMV), ventilation was switched to CPAP for 1 hour before extubation. The end-expiratory

pressure was maintained at 3 cmH_2O throughout the study. Weaning failure was defined as either the failure to achieve a reduction in ventilator support within 48 hours or requirement for reintubation within 48 hours of extubation. Reintubation was indicated when respiratory acidosis developed or frequent apneas or one major apnea occurred. In the first trial, there were no significant differences in the success rate with ACV or SIMV (70% versus 75%) or the duration of successful weaning (median 33 versus 30 hours). In the second trial, differences between the weaning success rates were not significant, but the median weaning duration was significantly shorter with ACV (24 hours) than with SIMV (50 hours) ($P < 0.05$). The results of the second trial are comparable with those of the adult studies,[149,150] demonstrating SIMV's inferiority to T-piece or CPAP weaning methods. A reduction in inspiratory pressure alone is favored in weaning preterm infants from mechanical ventilation.

IMV AND MANDATORY MINUTE VOLUME AND ASV

Mandatory minute ventilation (MMV) allows the patient to breathe spontaneously yet ensures that a preset minute ventilation is maintained should the patient's spontaneous ventilation decline below the set level.[155] MMV was developed to overcome certain ineffective features of IMV.[156] When the set mandatory IMV rate is less than required to achieve adequate ventilation, alveolar hypoventilation will ensue whenever a patient's total minute ventilation falls below a critical level. This drawback of IMV can be circumvented with MMV, which actuates a feedback control so that the ventilator provides pressurized breaths of a fixed volume to achieve a preset total minute ventilation.

Weaning with IMV and MMV was studied prospectively in 40 patients recovering from acute respiratory failure caused by parenchymal lung injury and chronic airflow obstruction.[157] After meeting defined weaning criteria, the patients were randomized to IMV ($n = 18$) or MMV ($n = 22$). In the IMV group, IMV rate was decreased by 2 breaths per minute at 3- to 4-hour intervals during the daytime only until the IMV rate was equal to zero. Weaning was considered complete after 4 hours of breathing on CPAP. In the MMV group, MMV was set at 75% of the total minute volume preceding the weaning trial; this was achieved by decreasing frequency while maintaining a V_T of 12 ml/kg as a reference value. Weaning was considered complete after 4 hours of independent spontaneous breathing. Weaning failure was defined as an inability to complete the trial or the need for ventilator support for the same underlying disease. Successful weaning was comparable: 86% for IMV and 89% for MMV. The weaning trial was longer in the IMV group (33 hours) than in the MMV group (4.75 hours).

SIMV and ASV were compared as weaning modalities in a prospective, randomized study in post–cardiac surgery patients.[158] With both ASV ($n = 18$) and SIMV ($n = 16$), the patients underwent three ventilation phases. With ASV, in phase 1, the initial settings were the ideal body weight (IBW), the desired minute volume at the default value of 100 ml/kg of IBW, and peak airway pressure of less than 25 cmH_2O. Adjustment of minute volume was dictated by a Pa_{CO_2} of less than 38 or greater than 50 mmHg. Phase 1 ended when there were no controlled breaths for 20 minutes. Phase 2 was a continuation of phase 1; it ended when PS was decreased to 10 cmH_2O (±2 cmH_2O) and maintained for 20 minutes. The patient then entered into phase 3, where PS was set manually at 5 cmH_2O for 10 minutes. When the patient showed satisfactory tolerance, tracheal extubation was performed. The initial settings for phase 1 in the SIMV group consisted of a V_T of 8 ml/kg and an SIMV rate adjusted to achieve a Pa_{CO_2} of between 38 and 50 mmHg. The SIMV rate was then set at 12 breaths per minute. When spontaneous breaths exceeded 6 breaths per minute for 20 minute, the patient was switched to PSV of 10 cmH_2O (phase 2). The patient was reassessed 20 minutes later for further reduction of PSV or returned to SIMV. If the patient tolerated it, PSV was reduced to 5 cmH_2O (phase 3), as in the ASV group. There was no difference in duration of tracheal intubation, and all patients except for two (one in each group) were extubated within 6 hours. In the ASV group, patients required fewer manipulations of ventilator settings and endured fewer high inspiratory pressure alarms. This study was performed in postoperative patients who had received mechanical ventilation for less than 24 hours before weaning attempts. Because mechanical ventilation duration before weaning influenced the weaning success rate,[159] the response of critically ill patients to the preceding weaning methods may be different.

Variation in Delivery among Ventilator Brands

To my knowledge, in the SIMV mode, no study has yet evaluated the response of various ventilators to patient flow demand or vice versa. As part of a study evaluating the response of muscle pressure generation to various unloading conditions with assisted ventilation, Mecklenburgh and Mapleson[160] evaluated the response of three ventilators, Hamilton Veolar, Engstrom Elvira, and Puritan Bennett 7200, in the SIMV mode in healthy subjects. V_T was set at 1.5 times the spontaneous V_T and the SIMV rate at 6 breaths per minute. The flow waveform was set to "sine wave." Muscle pressure was calculated using the equation of motion from instantaneous airway pressure, flow, and volume with the respiratory system's known resistance and elastance.[161] Amplitude of muscle pressure generation was similar across the three ventilators. Contraction time for mechanical breaths was shortest with the Engstrom Elvira at 1.03 seconds versus 1.38 seconds for the Hamilton Veolar and 1.37 seconds for the Puritan Bennett. For unassisted breaths, contraction time again was shortest with the Engstrom Elvira (1.33 versus 1.58 seconds for the Hamilton Veolar and 1.70 seconds for the Puritan Bennett). Because V_T was set constant for all three ventilators, the short contraction time led to higher peak airway pressures with the Engstrom Elvira (9.4 versus 3.9 cmH_2O for the Hamilton Veolar and 4.0 cmH_2O for the Puritan Bennett). Despite the set sine wave, the Engstrom

Elvira flow waveform that accounted for the short contraction time was more of a ramp than a sine wave. The investigators concluded that differences in subject responses to different ventilators were related to flow or pressure waveforms and that different subjects may prefer different waveforms.

Adjustment at the Bedside and Troubleshooting

SIMV settings consist of the trigger sensitivity, V_T, flow, and the IMV rate for the flow-limit volume-cycled mandatory breaths. For pressure-limit time-cycled breaths, the ventilator settings include the trigger sensitivity, inspiratory pressure, inspiratory time, pressure attack rate, and IMV rate. V_T is also set if dual hybrid breath-to-breath volume guarantee is applied. With either flow- or pressure-limited mandatory breaths, pressure support, but not volume support, can be added to the spontaneous breaths to overcome circuit and endotracheal tube resistance. Monitoring of the patient and the ventilator output waveforms cannot be overemphasized.[164] For example, palpable abdominal contractions suggest expiratory muscle recruitment and possible encroachment of mechanical inspiratory time into neural expiratory time.[52] Adjustment to reduce mechanical inspiratory time can be made by increasing flow rate (flow-limited breaths) or reducing inspiratory time (pressure-limited breaths). Despite the risk associated with tachypnea when mechanical inspiratory time is reduced, Laghi et al[165] demonstrated an increase in exhalation time and decrease in intrinsic PEEP, changes conducive to improved patient-ventilator interaction.

Important Unknowns

IMV has stood the test of time since its clinical application as a primary means of ventilator support in the early 1970s. To date, advanced technology enables most ventilators to be equipped with closed-loop ventilation that allows full ventilator support with gradual support reduction. Unfortunately, few large randomized, controlled trials have yet compared the efficacy of closed-loop ventilation with SIMV in terms of mechanical ventilation duration, patient-ventilator interaction, sensation of dyspnea, and ventilator-associated complications.

Studies have shown that inspiratory muscle activity is of the same intensity during machine assistance as during the intervening spontaneous breaths[45] and that SIMV prolongs weaning.[149,150] Given that the diaphragm is activated with each breath, it is possible that SIMV protects the respiratory muscles from disuse atrophy, which occurs with CMV.[68–70] Alternatively, the increased workload at low levels of machine assistance actually may cause overload[162,163] and prolong mechanical ventilation duration or weaning time. Which of those two factors plays a role during a low assistance level of SIMV is unknown.

The Future

A ventilator that adapts instantaneously to patient ventilatory demand would be ideal. Because SIMV has simple ventilator settings and the options of combining it with pressure support and of guaranteeing volume with use of pressure-limited mandatory breaths, SIMV will remain an important primary ventilator mode for critically ill patients. If SIMV were to be replaced, clinical trials would be needed that compare SIMV with other modalities, similar to those performed during weaning. If SIMV continues to be used widely, its long-term effects on respiratory muscle function, whether protective or damaging as a result of overload, should be investigated.

Summary and Conclusions

Recent studies have provided a better understanding of patient-ventilator interaction with SIMV. For critically ill patients, SIMV remains one of the most widely used modes of ventilation, as does ACV. To date, no large randomized study has compared SIMV with more technologically advanced modes as primary methods of ventilation. As a weaning technique, SIMV is inferior to T piece and PSV.

Acknowledgment

This work was supported by the Department of Veterans Affairs Medical Research Service.

References

1. Bjork VO, Engstrom CG. The treatment of ventilatory insufficiency after pulmonary resection with tracheostomy and prolonged artificial ventilation. J Thoracic Surg 1955; 30:356–7.
2. Fairley HB. Critique of intermittent mandatory ventilation. Int Anesthesiol Clin 1980; 18:179–89.
3. Kirby RR, Robinson EJ, Shulz J, et al. A new pediatric volume ventilator. Anesth Analg 1971; 50:533–7.
4. Kirby RR, Robinson EJ, Shulz J, et al. Continuous flow as an alternative to assisted or controlled ventilation in infants. Anesth Analg 1972; 51:871–5.
5. Downs JB, Klein EF, Desautels D, et al. Intermittent mandatory ventilation: A new approach to weaning patients from mechanical ventilations. Chest 1973:64:331–5.
6. Downs JB, Block AJ, Vennum KB. Intermittent mandatory ventilation in the treatment of patients with chronic obstructive pulmonary disease. Anesth Analg 1974; 53:437–43.
7. Downs JB, Perkins HM, Modell JH. Intermittent mandatory ventilation: An evaluation. Arch Surg 1974; 109:519–23.
8. Shapiro BA, Harrison RA, Walton JR, et al. Intermittent demand ventilation (IDV): A new technique for support ventilation in critically ill patients. Respir Care 1976; 21:521–5.
9. Harboe S. Weaning from mechanical ventilation by means of intermittent assisted ventilation (IAV). Acta Anaesthesiol Scand 1977; 21:252–6.
10. Esteban A, Anzueto A, Alia I, et al. How is mechanical ventilation employed in the intensive care unit? An international utilization review. Am J Respir Crit Care Med 2000; 161:1450–8.
11. Greenough A, Milner A, Dimitriou G. Synchronized mechanical ventilation for respiratory support in newborn infants. Cochrane Database Syst Rev 2004 Oct 18; 4:CD000456.
12. American Association of Respiratory Care. Consensus statement on the essentials of mechanical ventilators—1992. Respir Care 1992; 37:1000–8.
13. MacIntyre NR, Gropper C, Westfall T. Combining pressure-limiting and volume-cycling features in a patient-interactive mechanical breath. Crit Care Med 1994; 22:353–7.
14. Graybar GB, Smith RA. Apparatus and techniques for intermittent mandatory ventilation. Int Anesthesiol Clin 1980; 18:53–80.
15. Hillman DR, Breakey JN, Lam M, et al. Minimizing the work of breathing with continuous positive airway pressure and intermittent mandatory ventilation: An improved continuous low-flow system. Crit Care Med 1987; 15:665–70.
16. Braschi A, Iotti G, Locatelli A, et al. A continuous flow intermittent mandatory ventilation with continuous positive airway pressure circuit with high-compliance reservoir bag. Crit Care Med 1987; 15:947–50.
17. Weled BJ, Winfrey D, Downs JB. Measuring exhaled volume with continuous positive airway pressure and intermittent mandatory ventilation: Techniques and rationale. Chest 1979; 76:166–9.
18. Petty TL. Intermittent mandatory ventilation—Reconsidered. Crit Care Med 1981; 9:620–1.
19. Petty TL. In defense of IMV. Respir Care 1976; 21:121–2.
20. Page BA, Downs JB. IMV and continuous gas flow: A complication. Anesthesiology 1977; 46:72–3.
21. Heenan TJ, Downs JB, Douglas ME, et al. Intermittent mandatory ventilation: Is synchronization important? Chest 1980; 77:598–602.
22. Bernstein G, Heldt GP, Mannino FL. Increased and more consistent tidal volumes during synchronized intermittent mandatory ventilation in newborn infants. Am J Respir Crit Care Med 1994; 150:1444–8.
23. Cleary JP, Bernstein G, Mannino FL et al. Improved oxygenation during synchronized intermittent mandatory ventilation in neonates with respiratory distress syndrome: A randomized crossover study. J Pediatrics 1995; 126:40–1.
24. Bernstein G, Mannino FL, Heldt GP, et al. Randomized multicenter trial comparing synchronized and conventional intermittent mandatory ventilation in neonates. J Pediatrics 1996; 128:453–63.
25. Stark AR, Bascom R, Frantz ID 3d. Muscle relaxation in mechanically ventilated infants. J Pediatr 1979; 94:439–43.
26. Coggeshall JW, Marini JJ, Newman JH. Improved oxygenation after muscle relaxation in adult respiratory distress syndrome. Arch Intern Med 1985; 145:1718–20.
27. Akashi M, Sakanak K, Noguchi H, et al. Flow-regulated continuous positive airway pressure to minimize imposed work of breathing. Crit Care Med 1990; 18:999–1002.
28. Sassoon CSH. Mechanical ventilator design and function: The trigger variable. Respir Care 1992; 37:1056–69.
29. Sassoon CS, Gruer SE. Characteristics of the ventilator pressure- and flow-trigger variables. Intensive Care Med 1995; 21:159–68.
30. Sassoon CSH, Giron AE, Ely E, et al. Inspiratory work of breathing on flow-by and demand-flow continuous positive airway pressure. Crit Care Med 1989; 17:1108–14.
31. Sassoon CSH, Lodia R, Rheeman CH, et al. Inspiratory muscle work of breathing during flow-by, demand-flow, and continuous-flow systems in patients with chronic obstructive pulmonary disease. Am Rev Respir Dis 1992; 148:1219–22.

32. Marini JJ, Smith TC, Lamb VJ. External work output and force generation during synchronized intermittent mechanical ventilation: Effect of machine assistance on breathing effort. Am Rev Respir Dis 1988; 38:1169–79.

33. Leung P, Jubran A, Tobin MJ. Comparison of assisted ventilator modes on triggering, patient effort, and dyspnea. Am J Respir Crit Care Med 1997; 155:1940–8.

34. Aslanian P, El Atrous S, Isabey D, et al. Effects of flow triggering on breathing effort during partial ventilatory support. Am J Respir Crit Care Med 1998; 157:135–43.

35. Banner MJ, Blanch PB, Kirby RR. Imposed work of breathing and methods of triggering a demand-flow, continuous positive airway pressure system. Crit Care Med 1993; 21:183–90.

36. Messinger G, Banner M. Tracheal pressure triggering a demand-flow continuous positive airway pressure system decreases patient work of breathing. Crit Care Med 1996; 24:1829–34.

37. Bonmarchand G, Chevron V, Chopin C, et al. Increased initial flow rate reduces inspiratory work of breathing during pressure support ventilation in patients with exacerbation of chronic obstructive pulmonary disease. Intensive Care Med 1996; 22:1147–54.

38. Bonmarchand G, Chevron V, Menard JF, et al. Effects of pressure ramp slope values on the work of breathing during pressure support ventilation in restrictive patients. Crit Care Med 1999; 27:715–22.

39. Amato MBP, Barbas CSV, Bonassa J, et al. Volume assisted pressure support ventilation (VAPS): A new approach for reducing muscle workload during acute respiratory failure. Chest 1992; 102:1225–34.

40. Sinha SK, Donn SM. Volume-controlled ventilation: Variations on a theme. Clin Perinatol 2001; 28:547–60.

41. Branson RD, Johannigman JA, Campbell RS, et al. Closed-loop mechanical ventilation. Respir Care 2002; 47:427–53.

42. Herrera CM, Gerhardt T, Claure N, et al. Effects of volume-guaranteed synchronized intermittent mandatory ventilation in preterm infants recovering from respiratory failure. Pediatrics 2002; 110:529–33.

43. Cheema IU, Ahluwalia JS. Feasibility of tidal volume-guided ventilation in newborn infants: A randomized crossover trial using the volume guarantee modality. Pediatrics 2001; 107:1323–8.

44. Weissman IM, Rinaldo JE, Rogers RM, et al. Intermittent mandatory ventilation. Am Rev Respir Dis 1983; 127:641–7.

45. Imsand C, Feihl F, Perret C, et al. Regulation of inspiratory neuromuscular output during synchronized intermittent mechanical ventilation. Anesthesiology 1994; 80:13–22.

46. Uchiyama A, Imanaka H, Taenaka N, et al. Comparative evaluation of diaphragmatic activity during pressure support ventilation and intermittent mandatory ventilation in animal model. Am J Respir Crit Care Med 1994; 150:1564–8.

47. Beck J, Tucci M, Emeriaud G, et al. Prolonged neural expiratory time induced by mechanical ventilation in infants. Pediatr Res 2004; 55:747–54.

48. Shams H, Scheid P. Respiratory response to positive inspiratory pressure in the cat: Effects of CO_2 and vagal integrity. J Appl Physiol 1995; 79:1704–10.

49. Sinderby C, Navalesi P, Beck J, et al. Neural control of mechanical ventilation in respiratory failure. Nature Med 1999; 5:1433–6.

50. Clark FJ, Von Euler C. On the regulation of depth and rate of breathing. J Physiol (Lond) 1972; 222:267–95.

51. Knox CK. Characteristics of inflation and deflation reflexes during expiration in cats. J Neurophysiol 1973; 36:284–95.

52. Parthasarathy S, Jubran A, Tobin MJ. Cycling of inspiratory and expiratory muscle groups with the ventilator in airflow limita-

tion. Am J Respir Crit Care Med 1998; 158:1471–8; erratum in Am J Respir Crit Care Med 1999; 159:1023.

53. Jubran A, Van de Graaff WB, Tobin MJ. Variability of patient-ventilator interaction with pressure support ventilation in patients with chronic obstructive pulmonary disease. Am J Respir Crit Care Med. 1995; 152:129–36.

54. Weiss JW, Rossing TH, Ingram RH. Effect of intermittent mandatory ventilation on respiratory drive and timing. Am Rev Respir Dis 1983; 127:705–8.

55. Imanake H, Nishimura M, Miyano H, et al. Effect of synchronized intermittent mandatory ventilation on respiratory workload in infants after cardiac surgery. Anesthesiology 2001; 95:881–8.

56. Knebel AR, Janson-Bjerklie SL, Malley JD, et al. Comparison of breathing comfort during weaning with two ventilatory modes. Am J Respir Crit Care Med 1994; 149:14–8.

57. Sydow M, Golisch W, Buscher H, et al. Effect of low-level PEEP on inspiratory work of breathing in intubated patients, both with healthy lungs and with COPD. Intensive Care Med 1995; 21:887–95.

58. Petrof BJ, Legare M, Goldberg P, et al. Continuous positive airway pressure reduces work of breathing and dyspnea during weaning from mechanical ventilation in severe chronic obstructive pulmonary disease. Am Rev Respir Dis 1990; 141:281–9.

59. Eldridge FL. Maintenance of respiration by central neural feedback mechanisms. Fed Proc 1977; 36:2400–4.

60. Giuliani R, Mascia L, Recchia F, et al. Patient-ventilator interaction during synchronized intermittent mandatory ventilation: Effects of flow triggering. Am J Respir Crit Care Med 1995; 151:1–9.

61. Sassoon CSH, Del Rosario N, Fei R, et al. Influence of pressure- and flow-triggered synchronous intermittent mandatory ventilation on inspiratory muscle work. Crit Care Med 1994; 22:1933–41.

62. Eldridge FL, Gill-Kumar P. Lack of effect of vagal afferent input on central neural respiratory after discharge. J Appl Physiol 1978; 45:339–44.

63. Hudson LD, Hurlow RS, Craig KC, et al. Does intermittent mandatory ventilation correct respiratory alkalosis in patients receiving assisted mechanical ventilation? Am Rev Respir Dis 1985; 132:1071–4.

64. Kirby RR. Intermittent mandatory ventilation in the neonate. Crit Care Med 1977; 5:18–22.

65. Douglas ME, Downs JB. Cardiopulmonary effects of intermittent mandatory ventilation. Int Anesthesiol Clin 1980; 18:97–121.

66. Downs JB, Douglas ME. Intermittent mandatory ventilation and weaning. Int Anesthesiol Clin 1980; 18:81–95.

67. Downs JB, Stock MC, Tabeling B. Intermittent mandatory ventilation (IMV): A primary ventilatory support mode. Ann Chir Gynaecol 1982; 196(suppl):57–63.

68. Powers SK, Shanely RA, Coombes JS, et al. Mechanical ventilation results in progressive contractile dysfunction in the diaphragm. J Appl Physiol 2002; 92:1851–8.

69. Sassoon CSH, Caiozzo VJ, Manka A, et al. Altered diaphragm contractile properties with controlled mechanical ventilation. J Appl Physiol 2002; 92:2585–95.

70. Sassoon CSH, Zhu E, Caiozzo VJ. Assist-control mechanical ventilation attenuates ventilator-induced diaphragmatic dysfunction. Am J Respir Crit Care Med 2004; 170:626–32.

71. Downs JB, Mitchell LA. Pulmonary effects of ventilatory pattern following cardiopulmonary bypass. Crit Care Med 1976; 4:295–300.

72. Cullen P, Modell JH, Kirby R, et al. Treatment of flail chest: Use of intermittent mandatory ventilation and positive end-expiratory pressure. Arch Surg 1975; 110:1099–103.

73. Douglas ME, Downs JB. Pulmonary function following severe acute respiratory failure and high levels of positive end-expiratory pressure. Chest 1977; 71:18–23.

74. Kirby RR, Downs JB, Civetta JM, et al. High level positive end expiratory pressure (PEEP) in acute respiratory insufficiency. Chest 1975; 67:156–63.

75. Downs JB, Douglas ME, Sanfelippo PM, et al. Ventilatory pattern, intrapleural pressure and cardiac output. Anesth Analg 1977; 56:88–96.

76. Nikki P, Rasanen J, Tahvanainen J, et al. Ventilatory pattern in respiratory failure arising from acute myocardial infarction: Respiratory and hemodynamic effects of IMV_4 versus $IPPV_{12}$ and $PEEP_0$ versus $PEEP_{10}$. Crit Care Med 1982;10:75–8.

77. Marini JJ, Capps JS, Culver BH. The inspiratory work of breathing during assisted mechanical ventilation. Chest 1985; 87:612–8.

78. Marini JJ, Rodriguez RM, Lamb V. The inspiratory work load of patient-initiated mechanical ventilation. Am Rev Respir Dis 1986; 134:902–9.

79. Sassoon CSH, Mahutte CK, Te TT, et al. Work of breathing and airway occlusion pressure during assist-mode mechanical ventilation. Chest 1988; 93:571–76.

80. Luce JM, Pierson DJ, Hudson LD. Intermittent mandatory ventilation. Chest 1981; 79:678–85.

81. Froese AB, Bryan AC. Effects of anesthesia and paralysis on diaphragmatic mechanics in man. Anesthesiology 1974:441: 242–55.

82. Rehder K, Sessler AD, Marsh HM. General anesthesia and the lung. Am Rev Respir Dis 1975; 112:541–63.

83. Downs JB. Ventilatory pattern and modes of ventilation in acute respiratory failure. Respir Care 1983; 28:586–91.

84. Wagner PD, Laravuso RB, Uhl RR, et al. Continuous distribution of ventilation-perfusion ratios in normal subjects breathing air and 100% O_2. J Clin Invest 1974; 54:54–8.

85. Santak B, Radermacher P, Sandmann W, et al. Influence of SIMV plus inspiratory pressure support on $\dot{V}_A/\dot{Q}$ distributions during postoperative weaning. Intensive Care Med 1991; 17:136–40.

86. Brochard L, Pluskwa F, Lemaire F. Improved efficacy of spontaneous breathing with inspiratory pressure support. Am Rev Respir Dis 1987; 36:411–5.

87. Wolff G, Brunner J, Gradel E. Gas exchange during mechanical ventilation and spontaneous breathing: Intermittent mandatory ventilation after open heart surgery. Chest 1986; 90:11–7.

88. Pinsky MR. The effects of mechanical ventilation on the cardiovascular system. Crit Care Clin 1990; 6:663–78.

89. Mathru M, Rao TLK, El-Etr AA, et al. Hemodynamic response to changes in ventilatory patterns in patients with normal and poor left ventricular reserve. Crit Care Med 1982;10:423–6.

90. Mathru M, Rao TLK, Venus B. Ventilator-induced barotrauma in controlled mechanical ventilation versus intermittent mandatory ventilation. Crit Care Med 1983; 11:359–61.

91. Riggs TE, Shafer AW, Guenter CA. Physiologic effects of passive hyperventilation on oxygen delivery and consumption. Proc Soc Exp Biol 1972; 140:1414–7.

92. Laffey JG, Kavanagh BP. Hypocapnia. New Engl J Med 2002; 347:43–53.

93. Andersen JB, Kann T, Rasmussen JP, et al. Intermittent mandatory ventilation assists the diaphragm in weaning patients from mechanical ventilation. Danish Med Bull 1979; 26:363.

94. Anzueto A, Peters JI, Tobin MJ, et al. Effects of prolonged controlled mechanical ventilation on diaphragmatic function in healthy adult baboons. Crit Care Med 1997; 25:1187–90.

95. Shanely RA, Zergeroglu MA, Lennon SL, et al. Mechanical ventilation-induced diaphragmatic atrophy is associated with oxidative injury and increased proteolytic activity. Am J Respir Crit Care Med. 2002; 166:1369–74.

96. Gayan-Ramirez G, de Paepe K, Cadot P, et al. Detrimental effects of short-term mechanical ventilation on diaphragm function and IGF-I mRNA in rats. Intensive Care Med 2003; 29: 825–33.

97. Laghi F, Tobin MJ. Disorders of the respiratory muscles. Am J Respir Crit Care Med. 2003; 168:10–48.

98. Bernard N, Matecki S, Py G, et al. Effects of prolonged mechanical ventilation on respiratory muscle ultrastructure and mitochondrial respiration in rabbit. Intensive Care Med 2003; 29: 111–8.

99. Radell P, Edstrom L, Stibler H, et al. Changes in diaphragm structure following prolonged mechanical ventilation in piglets. Acta Anaesthesiol Scand 2004; 48:430–7.

100. Gibbons WJ, Rotaple MJ, Newman SL. Effect of intermittent mandatory ventilation on inspiratory muscle coordination in prolonged mechanically-ventilated patients (abstract). Am Rev Respir Dis 1986; 122:A123.

101. Steinhoff H, Falke K, Schwarzhoff W. Enhanced renal function associated with intermittent mandatory ventilation acute respiratory failure. Intensive Care Med 1982; 8:69–74.

102. Groeger JS, Levinson MR, Carlon GC. Assist control versus synchronized intermittent mandatory ventilation during acute respiratory failure. Crit Care Med 1989; 17:607–12.

103. Sternberg R, Sahebjami H. Hemodynamic and oxygen transport characteristics of common ventilatory modes. Chest 1994; 105:1798–1803.

104. Shelledy DC, Rau JL, Thomas-Goodfellow L. A comparison of the effects of assist-control, SIMV, and SIMV with pressure support on ventilation, oxygen consumption, and ventilatory equivalent. Heart Lung 1995; 24:67–75.

105. Culpepper JA, Rinaldo JE, Rogers RM. Effect of mechanical ventilator mode on tendency towards respiratory alkalosis. Am Rev Respir Dis 1985; 132:1075–7.

106. Jarreau PH, Moriette G, Mussat P, et al. Patient-triggered ventilation decreases the work of breathing in neonates. Am J Respir Crit Care Med. 1996; 153:1176–81.

107. Kapasi M, Fujino Y, Kirmse M, et al. Effort and work of breathing in neonates during assisted patient-triggered ventilation. Pediatr Crit Care Med. 2001; 2:9–16.

108. Sasse SA, Chen PA, Berry RB, et al. Variability of cardiac output over time in medical intensive care unit patients. Crit Care Med 1994; 22:225–32.

109. Pepe PE, Marini JJ. Occult positive end-expiratory pressure in mechanically ventilated patients with airflow obstruction. Am Rev Respir Dis 1982; 126:166–70.

110. Bhutani VK, Sivieri EM, Abbasi S, et al. Evaluation of neonatal pulmonary mechanics and energetics: a two factor least mean square analysis. Pediatr Pulmonol 1988; 4:150–8.

111. Agostoni E. Volume-pressure relationship of the thorax and lung in the newborn. J Appl Physiol 1959; 14:909–13.

112. MacIntyre NR. Respiratory function during pressure support ventilation. Chest 1986; 89:677–83.

113. Branson RD, Chatburn RL. Technical description and classification of modes of ventilator operation. Respir Care 1992; 37: 1026–44.

114. Younes M. Patient-ventilator interaction with pressure-assisted modalities of ventilatory support. Semin Respir Med 1993; 14:299–322.

115. Rasanen J, Mauricio AL, Cane RD. Adaptation of pressure support ventilation to increasing ventilatory demand during experimental airway obstruction and acute lung injury. Crit Care Med 1993; 21:562–66.

116. Brochard L, Rua F, Lorino H, et al. Inspiratory pressure support compensates for the additional work of breathing caused by the endotracheal tube. Anesthesiology 1991; 75:739–45.

117. Fiastro JF, Habib MP, Quan SF. Pressure support compensation for inspiratory work due to endotracheal tube and demand continuous positive airway pressure. Chest 1983; 83: 499–505.

118. Brochard L, Harf A, Lorino H, et al. Inspiratory pressure support prevents diaphragmatic fatigue during weaning from mechanical ventilation. Am Rev Respir Dis 1989; 139:513–21.

119. Van de Graaff WB, Gordey K, Dornseif SE, et al. Pressure support: Changes in ventilatory pattern and components of the work of breathing. Chest 1991; 100:1082–9.

120. Murphy DF, Dobb GD. Effect of pressure support of spontaneous breathing during intermittent mandatory ventilation. Crit Care Med 1987; 15:612–3.

121. Valentine DD, Hammond MD, Downs JB, et al. Distribution of ventilation and perfusion with different modes of mechanical ventilation. Am Rev Respir Dis 1991; 143:1262–6.

122. Tobin MJ, Jubran A, Laghi F. Patient-ventilator interaction. Am J Respir Crit Care Med 2001; 163:1059–1063.

123. Stock MC, Downs JB, Frolicher DA. Airway pressure release ventilation. Crit Care Med 1987; 15:462–6.

124. Downs JB, Stock MC. Airway pressure release ventilation: A new concept of ventilatory support. Crit Care Med 1987; 15: 459–61.

125. Branson RD, Johannigman JA. What is the evidence base for the newer ventilation modes? Respir Care 2004; 49:742–60.

126. Varpula T, Valta P, Niemi R, et al. Airway pressure release ventilation as a primary ventilatory mode in acute respiratory distress syndrome. Acta Anaesthesiol Scand. 2004; 48:722–31.

127. Rasanen J, Cane RD, Downs JB, et al. Airway pressure release ventilation during acute lung injury: A prospective multicenter trial. Crit Care Med 1991; 19:1234–41.

128. Chiang A, Steinfeld A, Gropper C, et al. Demand-flow airway pressure release ventilation as a partial ventilatory support mode: Comparison with synchronized intermittent mandatory ventilation and pressure support ventilation. Crit Care Med 1994; 22:1431–7.

129. Kazmaier S, Rathgeber J, Buhre W, et al. Comparison of ventilatory and haemodynamic effects of BiPAP and S-IMV/PSV for postoperative short-term ventilation in patients after coronary artery bypass grafting. Eur J Anaesthesiol 2000; 17:601–10.

130. Russell WC, Greer JR. The comfort of breathing: A study with volunteers assessing the influence of various modes of assisted ventilation. Crit Care Med 2000; 28:3645–8.

131. Rathgeber J, Schorn B, Falk V, et al. The influence of controlled mandatory ventilation (CMV), intermittent mandatory ventilation (IMV) and biphasic intermittent positive airway pressure (BiPAP) on duration of intubation and consumption of analgesics and sedatives. A prospective analysis in 596 patients following adult cardiac surgery. Eur J Anaesthesiol 1997; 14:576–82.

132. Younes M. Proportional assist ventilation, a new approach to ventilatory support: Theory. Am Rev Respir Dis 1992; 145: 114–20.

133. Schulze A, Gerhardt T, Musante G, et al. Proportional assist ventilation in low birth weight infants with acute respiratory disease: A comparison to assist/control and conventional mechanical ventilation. J Pediatr 1999; 135:339–44.

134. Younes M, Puddy A, Roberts D, et al. Proportional assist ventilation: Results of an initial clinical trial. Am Rev Respir Dis. 1992; 145:121–9.

135. Otis AB, Fenn WO, Rahn H: Mechanics of breathing in man. J Appl Physiol 1950:2:592–607.

136. Mead J. Control of respiratory frequency. J Appl Physiol 1960; 15:325–6.

137. Brunner JX, Iotti GA. Adaptive support ventilation (ASV). Minerva Anestesiol 2002; 68:365–8.

138. Tassaux D, Dalmas E, Gratadour P, et al. Patient-ventilator interactions during partial ventilatory support: a preliminary study comparing the effects of adaptive support ventilation with synchronized intermittent mandatory ventilation plus inspiratory pressure support. Crit Care Med 2002; 30:801–7.

139. Piotrowski A, Sobala W, Kawezynski P. Patient initiated, pressure regulated, volume controlled ventilation compared with intermittent mandatory ventilation in neonates: A prospective, randomized study. Intensive Cared Med 1997; 23:975–81.

140. Perlman JM, McMenamin JB, Volpe JJ. Fluctuating cerebral blood-flow velocity in respiratory-distress syndrome: Relation to the development of intraventricular hemorrhage. New Engl J Med 1983; 309:204–9.

141. Millbern SM, Downs JB, Jumper LC, et al. Evaluation of criteria for discontinuing mechanical ventilatory support. Arch Surg 1978; 113:1441–3.

142. MacIntyre NR. Weaning from mechanical ventilatory support: Volume-assisting intermittent breaths versus pressure-assisting every breath. Respir Care 1988; 88:121–25.

143. Ely EW, Baker AM, Dunagan DP, et al. Effect on the duration of mechanical ventilation of identifying patients capable of breathing spontaneously. New Engl J Med. 1996; 335:1864–9.

144. Schachter EN, Tucker D, Beck GJ. Does intermittent mandatory ventilation accelerate weaning? JAMA 1981; 246:1210–4.

145. Hastings PR, Bushnell LS, Skillman JJ, et al. Cardiorespiratory dynamics during weaning with IMV versus spontaneous ventilation in good-risk cardiac surgery patients. Anesthesiology 1980; 53:429–31.

146. Tomlinson JR, Miller KS, Lorch DG, et al. A prospective comparison of IMV and T-piece weaning from mechanical ventilation. Chest 1989; 96:348–52.

147. Esen F, Denkel T, Telci L, et al. Comparison of pressure support ventilation (PSV) and intermittent mandatory ventilation (IMV) during weaning in patients with acute respiratory failure. Adv Exp Med Biol 1992; 317:371–6.

148. Jounieaux V, Duran A, Levi-Valensi P. Synchronized intermittent mandatory ventilation with and without pressure support ventilation in weaning patients with COPD from mechanical ventilation. Chest 1994; 105:1204–10; erratum in Chest 1994; 106:984.

149. Brochard L, Rauss A, Benito S, et al. Comparison of three methods of gradual withdrawal from ventilatory support during weaning from mechanical ventilation. Am J Respir Crit Care Med 1994; 150:896–903.

150. Esteban A, Frutos F, Tobin MJ, et al. A comparison of four methods of weaning patients from mechanical ventilation. Spanish Lung Failure Collaborative Group. New Engl J Med 1995; 332:345–350.

151. Butler R, Keenan SP, Inman KJ, et al. Is there a preferred technique for weaning the difficult-to-wean patient? A systematic review of the literature. Crit Care Med 1999; 27:2331–6.

152. Hess D. Ventilator modes used in weaning. Chest 2001; 120(Suppl):474–6S.

153. Meade M, Guyatt G, Sinuff T, et al. Trials comparing alternative weaning modes and discontinuation assessments. Chest 2001; 120(Suppl):425–37S.

154. Dimitriou G, Greenough A, Griffin F, et al. Synchronous intermittent mandatory ventilation modes compared with patient triggered ventilation during weaning. Arch Dis Child Fetal Neonatal Ed 1995; 72:F188–90.

155. Hewlett AM, Platt AS, Terry VG. Mandatory minute volume. Anaesthesia 1977; 32:163–9.

156. Hewlett AM, Platt AS, Terry VG. Intermittent mandatory ventilation: Are IMV, MMV, PEEP, or sighing advantageous? (letter). Anaesthesia 1977; 32:668.

157. Davis S, Potgieter PD, Linton DM. Mandatory minute volume weaning in patients with pulmonary pathology. Anaesth Intensive Care 1989; 17:170–4.

158. Petter AH, Chiolero RL, Cassina T, et al. Automatic "respirator/weaning" with adaptive support ventilation: The effect on duration of endotracheal intubation and patient management. Anesth Analg 2003; 97:1743–50.

159. Vallverdu I, Calaf N, Subirana M, et al. Clinical characteristics, respiratory functional parameters, and outcome of a two-hour T-piece trial in patients weaning from mechanical ventilation. Am J Respir Crit Care Med. 1998; 158:1855–62.

160. Mecklenburgh JS, Mapleson WW. Ventilatory assistance and respiratory muscle activity: 1. Interaction in healthy volunteers. Br J Anaesth 1998; 80:422–33.

161. Mead J, Agostoni E. Dynamics of breathing. In: Fenn WO, Rahn H, editors. Handbook of physiology, Sec 3: Respiration, Vol I. Washington: American Physiological Society 1964;411–27.

162. Orozco-Levi M, Lloreta J, Minguella J, et al. Injury of the human diaphragm associated with exertion and chronic obstructive pulmonary disease. Am J Respir Crit Care Med 2001; 164:1734–9.

163. Reid WD, Huang J, Bryson S, et al. Diaphragm injury and myofibrillar structure induced by resistive loading. J Appl Physiol 1994; 76:176–84.

164. Jubran A. Advances in respiratory monitoring during mechanical ventilation. Chest 1999; 116:1416–25.

165. Laghi F, Segal J, Choe WK, et al. Effect of imposed inflation time on respiratory frequency and hyperinflation in patients with chronic obstructive pulmonary disease. Am J Respir Crit Care Med 2001; 163:1365–70.

Chapter 9

PRESSURE-SUPPORT VENTILATION

LAURENT BROCHARD
FRANÇOIS LELLOUCHE

Pressure-support ventilation (PSV) is a mode of partial ventilator support. Such modes are used widely in intensive-care units (ICUs) for several reasons. First, most ventilated patients (unless deeply sedated and paralyzed) have an intact respiratory drive, and thus it is necessary to synchronize patient activity with that of the ventilator. Second, by allowing the patient to breathe spontaneously, assisted modes may reduce the need for sedation. Third, disuse atrophy of the respiratory muscles can result from controlled ventila-

tion, and maintenance of spontaneous respiratory activity appears to lessen this likelihood.[1,2] Finally, partial support may facilitate the weaning of problematic patients. An ideal mode of partial support should supply both full ventilator support and optimal support during weaning, optimize patient-ventilator synchronization, optimize patient comfort while reducing the need for sedation and the risk of cardiovascular consequences, and if possible, facilitate or reduce the duration of the weaning. PSV may meet these requirements, at least in part, as discussed in this chapter. PSV also has limitations, which are delineated. Improvement in the delivery of PSV continues as a field of research.

Despite more than 20 years of use, PSV remains at times confusing to clinicians. First, although PSV is remarkably effective in reducing patient effort and avoiding respiratory distress, it sometimes delivers support much in excess of patient needs. Problems may relate to excessive delivered volume, duration of inspiration relative to neural inspiratory time (T_I), or both. Much research was undertaken in the late 1990s to understand and analyze the consequences of delivering excessive pressure. Many benefits of PSV, which provides greater freedom to the patient than traditional modes, may have been obscured by improper use.

Second, many clinicians often view PSV primarily as a mode devoted to weaning. Weaning often has been poorly defined and may not be considered until late in a patient's course. Thus possible indications for the early use of PSV have been disregarded by many clinicians. Some clinicians, worrying about the consequences of providing excessive freedom to a patient, have combined PSV with synchronized intermittent mandatory ventilation (SIMV) with little clinical justification. In 1998, an international survey on mechanical ventilation was undertaken in 361 ICUs in 20 countries (published in 2002).[3] On the first day, PSV was used in fewer than 10% of all patients, the combination of SIMV with PSV was used in almost 15%, and assist-control ventilation (ACV) was used in approximately 60%. This result could be interpreted as failure of PSV to gain wide acceptance. The percentage of use was relatively low (and did not vary much over subsequent days), and sole use of PSV was substantially less than use of a combination of SIMV and PSV, for which little physiologic or clinical data exist. Providing a detailed explanation for low PSV use, however, is beyond the scope of this chapter.

Third, in the same survey,[3] a low level of PSV was used to perform a once-daily weaning attempt in 28% of such attempts, a gradual reduction of PSV was used as the sole weaning method in 21% of attempts, and a gradual reduction of SIMV and PSV was used in 22% of attempts. Overall, PSV was used (one way or another) in 45% of weaning attempts, indicating that clinicians consider weaning the main indication for PSV.

Definition and Phases

PSV is a pressure-targeted (or pressure-limited) mode in which each breath is triggered by the patient and supported.[4–9] PSV provides breath-by-breath support by

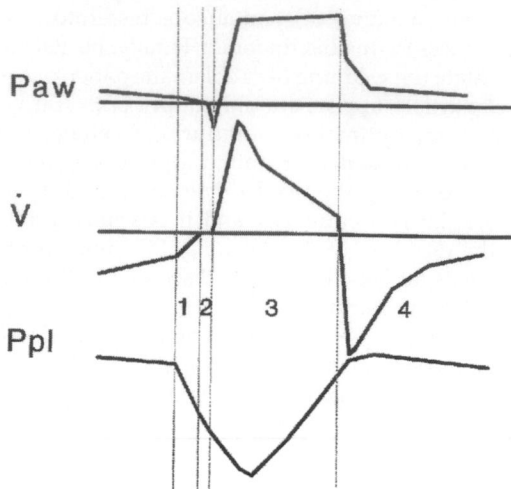

FIGURE 9-1 A pressure-supported breath with tracings of airway pressure (Paw), flow (V̇), and pleural pressure (Ppl). Four phases of patient effort can be discerned. Phase 1 is still expiratory and corresponds to an effort performed against intrinsic positive end-expiratory pressure (PEEP); it occurs before the triggering system of the ventilator can detect any signal that indicates the onset of patient inspiratory effort. Phase 2 is the time required to activate the triggering system of the ventilator (also called the *initiation phase*). Phase 3 is the insufflation phase, during which the ventilator pressurizes the airway at the level set by the clinician. This phase is terminated by the cycling-off criterion. Patient inspiratory effort may terminate before the end of this phase. Phase 4 is the expiratory phase.

means of a positive-pressure boost synchronized with inspiratory effort: patient initiated and flow terminated (Fig. 9-1). During inspiration, airway pressure is raised to a preset level: the pressure-support level. The speed of pressurization initially was fixed and system-specific. Most recent ventilators, however, offer the possibility of adjusting this pressurization rate. Throughout the inspiratory phase, the ventilator works as a pressurized demand-flow system at a predetermined pressure level. PSV is maintained until the machine determines the end of expiration, supposedly reflecting the end of patient demand. This is achieved by means of an expiratory trigger mechanism based on decay of inspiratory flow. When inspiratory flow falls below a threshold value, which may indicate indirectly that the inspiratory muscles have relaxed, the ventilator cycles to the expiratory phase. That is, it releases the PSV and opens its expiratory port. The expiratory phase is free of assistance; a level of positive end-expiratory pressure (PEEP) lower than the inspiratory plateau pressure can be applied. PSV thus can be defined as a patient-initiated (pressure or flow), pressure-targeted, flow-cycled mode of mechanical ventilation.

Three phases of PSV can be distinguished: (1) recognition of the beginning of inspiration, (2) pressurization, and (3) recognition of the end of inspiration. These phases constitute the working principles of PSV and can vary from one ventilator to another (see Fig. 9-1). As discussed below, these variations may induce differences in the effect of PSV for similar levels of pressurization.

INITIATION OF THE CYCLE

Triggering of inspiration is initiated by patient effort and is detected by a pressure or flow sensor. Trigger sensitivity is adjustable. This mechanism requires an active effort by the patient, the intensity of which depends on the characteristics of the valve. The opening time delay varies between 50 and 250 ms depending on the ventilator.[10–15] The most recent data indicate that most ventilators now respond in less than 100 ms.[16–18] Opening of the demand valve can be triggered by a fall in pressure or a difference in the flow signal between inspiratory and expiratory flows (referred to as *flow-by*). For the latter, a constant flow is delivered to the circuit during the expiratory phase; inspiratory effort then is detected as a small difference between inspiratory and expiratory flows. Flow triggering avoids the need for a closed demand valve. Aslanian et al[19] showed that the difference between pressure-triggered and flow-triggered systems has become quite small on modern ventilators. The triggering phase represents less than 10% of a patient's overall effort to breathe. A flow-triggering system makes a statistically significant difference but is of limited clinical importance.

PRESSURIZATION

Once inspiration has been initiated, the ventilator delivers a high inspiratory flow, which decreases rapidly throughout the rest of inspiration. A servo regulatory mechanism ensures that the proper flow reaches the appropriate preset PSV level and keeps this pressure constant until expiration occurs. Flow regulation varies among ventilators, thus determining the pressure waveform. Usually, the servo valve is controlled continuously during the breath such that the delivered pressure closely approximates the target pressure set by the clinician. In general, the aperture of the proportional servo valve is reduced progressively as the monitored pressure gets closer and closer to the target pressure. For this reason, the wave shape often constitutes a pressure ramp rather than a true squarewave. The pressure level can be adjusted between 0 (spontaneous breathing through the ventilator circuit) and a maximum of 30 or 60 cmH₂O (even more with some ventilators). In clinical settings, pressure levels above 30 cmH₂O are rarely reported.

Pressure increases according to a rate that is system-specific; formerly, it was not adjustable. A high speed of pressurization produces a square pressure wave; low achievement of the preset PSV level attenuates this shape.[4] Many ventilators now allow adjustment of the rate of pressurization. The influence of this adjustment on the effectiveness of PSV in reducing the work of breathing is discussed below.

CYCLING OF EXPIRATION

During PSV, cycling to exhalation is triggered primarily by a decrease in inspiratory flow from its peak to a system-specific threshold value. This critical decrease in inspiratory flow is taken as indirect evidence that the inspiratory muscles have begun to relax. Expiration is triggered when either an absolute level of flow (between 2 and 6 liters/min) or a fixed percentage of peak inspiratory flow (12% or 25%) is reached, depending on the ventilator model (Table 9-1). The threshold value for cycling, which can be

TABLE 9-1 Technical Characteristics of Pressure-Support Ventilation and Available Settings on Intensive-Care Ventilators

| Ventilator | Manufacturer | INSPIRATORY TRIGGER | | | Flow Cycle | CYCLING-OFF-CRITERION | |
		Flow (liters/min)	Pressure	Pressurization		Pressure Cycle	Time Cycle
PB 7200	Puritan-Bennet/Tyco	1–15	0.5–20		5 liters/min	+1.5 cmH$_2$O	3 s
PB 740	Puritan-Bennet/Tyco	1–20			10 liters/min or 25% PF	+3 cmH$_2$O	3.5 s
PB 760	Puritan-Bennet/Tyco	1–20		5–100%	Adjust. 1–45% PF	+3 cmH$_2$O	3.5 s
PB 840	Puritan-Bennet/Tyco	1–20		5–100%	Adjust. 1–80% PF	+1.5 cmH$_2$O	3 s
Evita 2	Drager				25% PF	High-pressure limit	
Evita 2dura	Drager	0.3–15		0–2 s	25% PF	High-pressure limit	
Evita 4	Drager	0.3–15		0–2 s	25% PF	High-pressure limit	4 s
Evita XL	Drager	0.3–15		0–2 s	25% PF	High-pressure limit	
Savina	Drager				25% PF	High-pressure limit	
Servo 900C	Maquet	0.6–2	0–20		25% PF	+3 cmH$_2$O	
Servo 300	Maquet	0.6–2	0–20		5% PF	+20 cmH$_2$O	
Servo-i	Maquet	0.6–2	0–20	0–0.4 s	Adjust. 1–80% PF	High-pressure limit	
Servo-s	Maquet	0.6–2	0–20	0–0.4 s	Adjust. 1–80% PF	High-pressure limit	
Veolar	Hamilton				25% PF	High-pressure limit	3 s
Galileo	Hamilton	0.5–15	0.5–10	25–200 ms	Adjust. 10–40% PF	High-pressure limit	3 s
Raphael	Hamilton						
Bird 8400	Viasys Healthcare	1–10	1–20		25% PF	High-pressure limit	3 s
T-Bird	Viasys Healthcare	1–20			5–30% PF (submenu)	High-pressure limit	3 s
Vela	Viasys Healthcare	1–8			Adjust. 5–30% PF	High-pressure limit	0.3–3 s
Avea	Viasys Healthcare	0.1–20	0.1–20	1–9	Adjust. 5–45% PF	High-pressure limit	0.15–5 s
Bear 1000	Viasys Healthcare	Automatic (auto-track)			25% PF		5 s
Bipap Vision	Respironics		0–20	0.05–0.4 s	Automatic (auto-trak)		
Esprit	Respironics	0.5–20		0.1–0.9 s	Adjust. 10–45% PF		
LTV1000	Pulmonetics	1–9			Adjust. 10–40% PF	High-pressure limit	
Elisee	Saime				Adjust. 10–40% PF or automatic		
e500	Newport			1–19	Adjust. 5–50% PF, variable	High-pressure limit	
HT50	Newport		0 to –10		4 liters/min or 10% PF	High-pressure limit	0.1–3 s
Infrasonics star	Infrasonics		–0.5–20				3.5 s
Inspiration	eVent	1–25	–1–20	Fast/medium/low	Adjust. 10–80%		

ABBREVIATION: Adjust., adjustable; PF, peak flow.

223

viewed as the sensitivity of the expiratory trigger, formerly was not adjustable. Adjustment now is offered to clinicians on many ventilators.

Detection of a small degree of pressure (1–3 cmH$_2$O) above the fixed PSV level, consequent to sudden expiratory effort by the patient, also can be used (alone or in combination with the flow criteria) to stop inspiratory assistance. Finally, a time limit for inspiration usually is included. This serves as a safety mechanism if a leak develops in the circuit and the two previous methods of terminating inspiration become inoperative. Complications have been reported in the absence of this time-limit mechanism, whereby constant insufflation (at the PSV level) creates a high level of continuous positive airway pressure (CPAP).[20]

OTHER SETTINGS

Because no mandatory breath is present with PSV, a safety feature often is available in case of apnea. This may be an automatic feature or a minimal frequency or minute ventilation to be set. The time delay for apnea may be adjustable. This safety feature is not available on all ventilators.

PSV can be used in conjunction with SIMV.[21–24] Two approaches have been used: addition of a fixed level of PSV during spontaneous breathing to overcome endotracheal tube (ETT) or circuit resistance[25] or use of a variable level of PSV between the mandatory breaths. The second approach introduces considerable complexity into ventilator management of patients.

Differences Among Mechanical Ventilators

During PSV, specific characteristics of the ventilator may interfere with patient respiratory activity. These differences may be determined by the manufacturer's algorithm to deliver pressure, such as speed of pressurization and/or initial peak-flow setting, ability to maintain a plateau pressure and quality of regulation, and termination criteria used to cycle from inspiration to expiration. Nonspecific features include characteristics of the demand valve and/or triggering mechanism and flow-impeding properties of the expiratory circuits, including PEEP devices. These differences also may vary with the type of ventilator, whether it is designed only for delivery of noninvasive PSV or is a full intensive-care ventilator.[17,18,26,27] The relative weight of each factor is difficult to determine and may vary from one patient to another. This consideration should be kept in mind, however, when interpreting the results of clinical studies of PSV using various ventilators. One study compared three ventilators set at 0 and 15 cmH$_2$O of PSV in seven patients.[28] No significant difference was observed in the work of breathing performed at pressure support (PS) of 0 cmH$_2$O, but major work differences were observed at PS of 15 cmH$_2$O. These data suggest that different characteristics of PSV delivery may have a major influence on its efficacy (Fig. 9-2). Although most recent ventilators have much better systems of regulation, providing more homogeneous delivery of PSV, clinically relevant differences still exist.

As with other assisted modes, the triggering mechanism is a key determinant of the efficacy of PSV. A poorly functioning demand valve has two consequences: It imposes an effort to open the valve, and it prolongs the time before assistance is delivered. Assisted modes, including PSV, are devoted primarily to reducing or optimizing this effort. What happens before delivery of assistance may interfere with efficacy of the mode. Demand valves function with an unalterable delay before delivering gas flow to the patient. For instance, if 200 ms is required between the beginning of an inspiratory effort and opening of the valve, nearly one-third of the duration of inspiratory effort in a tachypneic patient may take place without any gas entering the lungs. If auto (or intrinsic) PEEP is present, another 200 ms may be wasted (while the respiratory muscles work against this positive alveolar pressure) before any inspiratory flow can start. In addition, if the speed of pressurization of PSV is low, another 200 ms is required to reach the plateau pressure. Thus assistance will be delivered to the

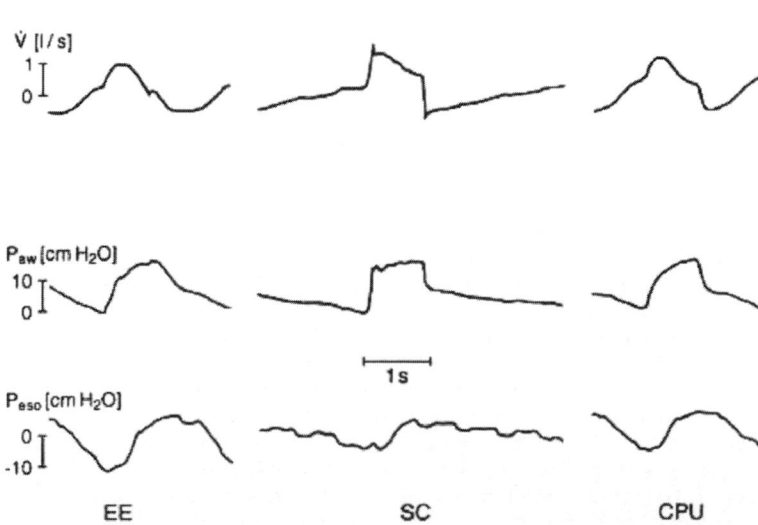

FIGURE 9-2 The influence of a ventilator and its specific algorithm on patient effort. Three ventilators were studied (EE = Erica Engstrom, Bromma, Sweden; SC = Servo 900C, Siemens, Lund, Sweden; and CPU = CPU1, Ohmeda, Maurepas, France) at 15 cmH$_2$O of PSV. Flow, airway pressure (Paw), and esophageal pressure (Pes) are presented. Note the different airway and flow profiles and the impact on esophageal pressure swing. Work of breathing was significantly less with SC (from ref. 28). Although modern ventilators tend to homogenize the delivery of PSV, differences still exist and illustrate the effects of varying the pressure ramp.

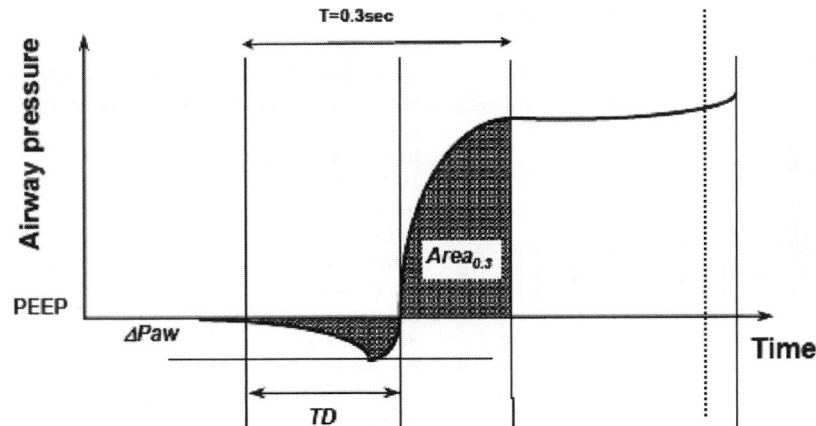

FIGURE 9-3 The method used to calculate the trigger characteristics and pressurization phase during PSV based on the airway pressure-time curve. The total trigger phase is evaluated by the time delay (TD) between the onset of simulated effort and the time at which airway pressure becomes positive after experiencing a pressure fall (ΔPaw). The quality of pressurization is best quantified as the area measured at 0.3 second. (*Modified, with permission, from Richard et al: Intensive Care Med 28:1049–57, 2002.*)

patient 600 ms after the beginning of inspiratory effort, which may correspond to the end of that patient's inspiratory effort.[29]

Comparison of the triggering functions of various ventilators demonstrates that the most recent generation of ventilators, using pressure-sensitive mechanisms, flow-sensitive mechanisms, or both, usually require less effort and open faster than older-generation ventilators. This was studied extensively by Richard et al,[16] who compared different generations of ventilators, including the new turbine ventilators (Figs. 9-3 to 9-6). The ability of different ventilators to pressurize the airway during PSV was investigated. The investigators reasoned that during PSV, unloading efficacy depends on a ventilator's ability to meet inspiratory flow demand. Different levels of simulated inspiratory demand

were used. The net area of the inspiratory airway pressure-time tracing was calculated over the first 0.3, 0.5 and 1 second at three levels of PSV (5, 10, and 15 cmH$_2$O) (see Figs. 9-3 and 9-4). To assess the relative role of PSV delivery and triggering function, triggering sensitivity was assessed independently by measuring the time delay and the pressure fall with different levels of inspiratory drive (see Figs. 9-3, 9-5, and 9-6). All new-generation ventilators (released after 1993) achieved significantly better results than most previous-generation ventilators regarding the pressure-time area at 0.3 second and triggering delay, indicating large improvements in terms of triggering and pressurization. Regarding PSV and trigger performances, new-generation ventilators outperformed most previous-generation ventilators; this also was the case for

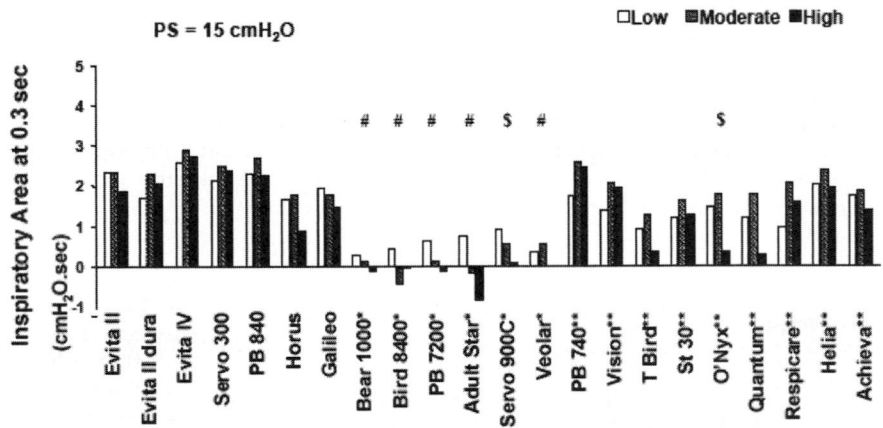

FIGURE 9-4 Inspiratory area, measured as the integral of the airway pressure–time trace over the first 0.3 second of inspiration (see Fig. 9-3), for a PSV level of 15 cmH$_2$O according to the simulated level of inspiratory demand (low, moderate, and high). The number of asterisks indicates ventilator generation (no asterisk, new; one asterisk, previous; two asterisks, piston and turbines), # indicates $p < 0.05$ versus all new-generation ventilators, $ indicates $p < 0.05$ versus at least one of the new-generation ventilators. The following ventilators were tested: *New-generation ventilators:* Evita II, Evita II Dura, and Evita IV (Dräger, Lübeck, Germany); Servo 300 (Siemens-Elema, Solna, Sweden); PB 840 (Puritan-Bennet, Carlsbad, CA); Galileo (Hamilton, Rhäzüns, Switzerland); Horus (Taema, Antony, France). *Previous-generation ventilators:* 8400 ST (Bird, Palm Springs, CA), Servo 900C (Siemens-Elema, Solna, Sweden), PB 7200 (Puritan-Bennet, Carlsbad, CA), Bear 1000 (Bear, Palm Springs, CA), Adult Star 200 (Infrasonics, USA), Veolar (Hamilton, Rhäzüns, Switzerland). *Piston or turbine-based ventilators:* piston: PB 740 (Puritan-Bennett, Carlsbad, CA); turbine: T-Bird (Bird, Palm Springs, CA), BiPAP ST 30 and Vision (Respironics, Murrysville Pittsburgh, PA), Helia (Saime, Savigny-le-Temple, France), O'Nyx (Pierre Medical, Verrières-le-Buisson, France and Puritan-Bennett, Carlsbad, CA), Quantum (Healthdyne Technologies, Marietta, GA), Respicare (Dräger, Lübeck, Germany), Achieva (Puritan-Bennett, Carlsbad, CA). (*Modified, with permission, from Richard et al: Intensive Care Med 28:1049–57, 2002.*)

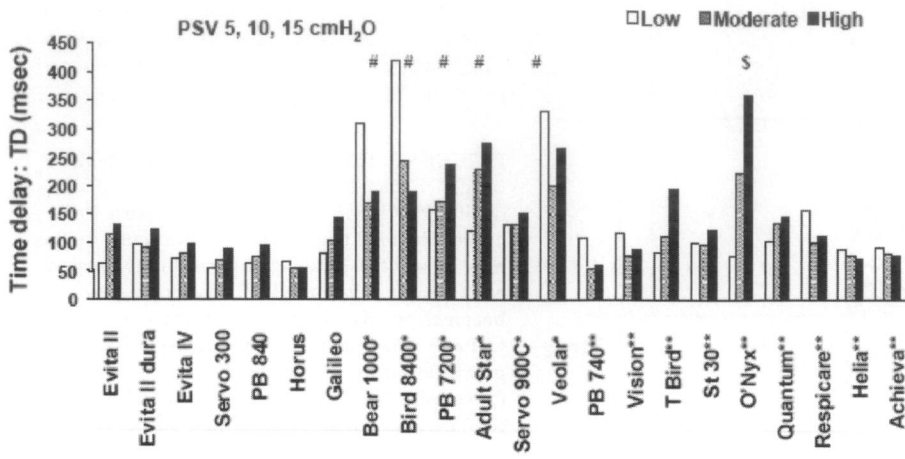

FIGURE 9-5 Total time delay for triggering (TD, expressed in ms; see Fig. 9-3) according to the simulated level of inspiratory demand (low, moderate, and high). Values for measurements obtained at PSV levels of 5, 10 and 15 cmH₂O have been averaged. The number of asterisks indicates ventilator generation (no asterisk, new; one asterisk, previous; two asterisks, piston and turbines), # and $ indicates $p < 0.05$ versus all new-generation ventilators, See legend to Fig. 9-4 for a list of ventilators being tested. (*Modified, with permission, from Richard et al: Intensive Care Med 28:1049–57, 2002.*)

some piston- and turbine-based ventilators, including several of those specially designed for noninvasive ventilation (NIV).

Ventilators delivering PSV and PEEP (termed *bilevel ventilation*) and designed for home ventilation have been evaluated in stable, awake patients with chronic ventilatory failure.[30] Despite some variability in the delivery of pressure, no difference was found in terms of comfort or improvement in inspiratory muscle unloading. These differences, however, might have greater impact in patients with acute respiratory failure.

Main Physiologic Effects

BREATHING PATTERN

During PSV, the patient maintains control over respiratory rate and has partial control of T_I and tidal volume (V_T). As such, PSV seems to allow the patient to breathe in a "physiologic" and natural way. This is only partially true because there is a complex interaction between ventilator support and patient control of breathing. This interaction depends on the pressure level and PSV characteristics. For instance, a change in the criterion for cycling between inspiration and expiration will result in a different T_I and different V_T and may result in more (or less) dynamic hyperinflation.

The addition of PSV modifies the spontaneous breathing pattern.[31–36] Most patients develop an increase in V_T and decrease in respiratory rate with increasing levels of PSV. Numerous authors have shown an inverse relationship between the PSV level and respiratory rate and a positive relationship with V_T.[31–34] This has clinical implications. First, it suggests that breathing pattern adapts rapidly when the respiratory muscles face a new workload.[37] Second, it implies that adjustment of the PSV level can be guided by noting the breathing-pattern response. This information may be obtained very quickly: Changes in breathing pattern in response to loading conditions usually occur within 1–2 minutes.[37,38] Excessive levels of support, however, lead to hyperinflation, respiratory alkalosis, respiratory depression, and periods of apnea.[39] High levels of support-induced hyperinflation may result in inability to trigger the ventilator (so-called ineffective triggering). This will result in a substantial difference in the ventilator's displayed respiratory rate and the patient's true respiratory rate[40] (see below).

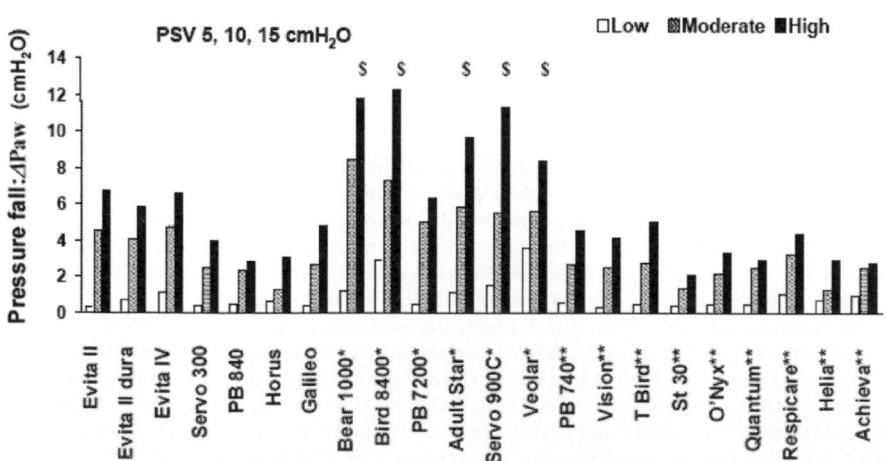

FIGURE 9-6 Pressure fall before PSV delivery (ΔPaw, expressed in cmH₂O; see Fig. 9-1) according to the simulated level of inspiratory demand (low, moderate, and high). Values for measurements obtained at PSV levels of 5, 10 and 15 cmH₂O have been averaged. The number of asterisks indicates ventilator generation (no asterisk, new; one asterisk, previous; two asterisks, piston and turbines), $ indicates $p < 0.05$ versus all new-generation ventilators. (*Modified, with permission, from Richard et al: Intensive Care Med 28:1049–57, 2002.*)

In patients with acute lung injury, factors other than respiratory muscle load influence respiratory drive. Pesenti et al[41] reported that variation in arterial oxygen (O_2) saturation between 85–90% and 100%, obtained by modifying fractional inspired oxygen concentration (F_{IO_2}), had a significant effect on respiratory drive in patients with acute lung injury receiving PSV.

The influence of PSV on the duty cycle (fractional inspiratory time, T_I/T_{TOT}) is variable. It probably depends on differences in working principles of PSV among ventilators. It is, for instance, influenced by the setting of the pressure ramp on the ventilator.[42] A decreasing duty cycle with increasing PSV levels has been observed in several studies.[32–34]

The influence of PSV on minute ventilation is variable, producing an increase or no change.[31–35] An increase in minute ventilation is observed frequently when PSV is compared with unassisted breathing through the ventilator circuit. More frequently, an increase in PSV fails to modify minute ventilation substantially, whereas it modifies alveolar ventilation. Breathing pattern therefore may be modified markedly without significant change in minute ventilation.[31–36] Thus, monitoring minute ventilation is of little help when titrating the level of PSV.

GAS EXCHANGE AND DISTRIBUTION OF VENTILATION AND PERFUSION

The primary goal of PSV is to support patient effort while delivering a satisfactory gas mixture. PSV is not aimed primarily at improving oxygenation. The effects of PSV on gas exchange are explained primarily by increased alveolar ventilation resulting from changes in breathing pattern. Indeed, despite a lack of change in minute ventilation, an increase in V_T produces a decrease in the ratio of dead space to V_T (V_D/V_T). Thus alveolar ventilation often is increased. Other factors may influence arterial blood gases, such as changes in O_2 consumption, modification of total dead space, and altered distribution of ventilation. During the weaning of patients with hypercapnic respiratory failure, addition of PSV produced a correction of Pa_{CO_2} and respiratory acidosis.[31] In normal, nonintubated subjects, PSV of 10 cmH_2O produces significant decreases in Pa_{CO_2}.[39] PSV can induce hyperventilation that is not counteracted by respiratory motor output.[43] Slight hypocapnia was observed in patients following abdominal surgery,[44] whereas normocapnia was observed in other studies. Therefore, although PSV permits correction of hypercapnia resulting from rapid shallow breathing or helps patients with chronic CO_2 retention to choose their own target Pa_{CO_2}, the level of PSV requires fine adjustment to avoid respiratory alkalosis.

Although breathing pattern, and especially respiratory frequency, is controlled in part by the patient, an interaction exists between the level of PSV and alveolar ventilation, Pa_{CO_2}, and pH that is not fully controlled by respiratory center command. MacIntyre and Leatherman[45] showed in a lung model that a biphasic effect can occur with increasing levels of PSV. Above a certain limit, passive (hyper-) inflation will result with high levels of PSV. The fact that excessive assistance with PSV may induce respiratory alkalosis not controlled by the patient's respiratory centers has important consequences. Parthasarathy et al[46] found that during sleep PSV was associated with numerous episodes of apneas, desaturation, and microarousals leading to sleep fragmentation.[46] This could be prevented by adding dead space to the circuit. Although not tested in this study, it is also possible that reductions in the level of PSV might prevent this problem.

The distribution of ventilation and perfusion during PSV has been assessed in several studies.[47–52] Valentine et al[47] compared SIMV, PSV, and airway pressure-release ventilation (APRV) in nine patients a few hours following cardiac surgery. The major characteristics of ventilation-perfusion ($\dot{V}_A/\dot{Q}$) distributions were similar with all modes.[47] Dead space was lower during APRV than during either SIMV or PSV. Gas exchange was assessed with the six-inert-gas technique by Beydon et al[48] in a study comparing controlled mechanical ventilation, unassisted spontaneous breathing, and PSV of 10 cmH_2O. Using isotopic scanning, these authors evaluated regional distribution of $\dot{V}_A/\dot{Q}$ ratios. The study was conducted in eight patients with chronic obstructive pulmonary disease (COPD) who were dependent on mechanical ventilation. Ventilator discontinuation was associated with rapid, shallow breathing and an increase in perfusion to low $\dot{V}_A/\dot{Q}$ regions. Isotopic scans revealed a horizontal craniocaudal difference of $\dot{V}_A/\dot{Q}$ with all modes, and the lowest $\dot{V}_A/\dot{Q}$ ratios were found at the bases. Abnormalities in $\dot{V}_A/\dot{Q}$ distribution observed during spontaneous breathing also were present during 10 cmH_2O of PSV, although to a smaller extent. Whether a higher level of PSV might have been more effective in correcting the maldistribution of $\dot{V}_A/\dot{Q}$ ratios is unknown.

Ferrer et al[50] assessed whether PSV could improve $\dot{V}_A/\dot{Q}$ imbalance during the transition between positive-pressure ventilation and spontaneous breathing in seven intubated patients with COPD during weaning.[50] PSV avoided $\dot{V}_A/\dot{Q}$ worsening during this transition. Hemodynamics, blood gases, and $\dot{V}_A/\dot{Q}$ distributions were equivalent during PSV and ACV when the two modes provided similar levels of assistance. Diaz et al[49] studied the reasons for improvement in P_{O_2} and P_{CO_2} in 10 patients with acute hypercapnic exacerbations of COPD who were switched from spontaneous breathing to PSV during NIV.[49] Improvement in blood gases was mediated primarily by a higher alveolar ventilation and not improvement in $\dot{V}_A/\dot{Q}$ relationships. While O_2 uptake tended to decrease, the respiratory exchange ratio increased, explaining a slight increase in arterial-to-alveolar O_2 difference secondary to increased clearance of body stores of CO_2 during NIV. These results suggested that attaining an efficient breathing pattern rather than high inspiratory pressures should be the primary goal for improving arterial blood gases during NIV with PSV in this type of patient.

The effect of PSV on oxygenation varies and depends on many factors, such as the induced changes in alveolar ventilation, O_2 consumption, dead space, and mean airway pressure.[31–34] Most investigators have not found significant changes in arterial oxygenation when PSV was compared with other modalities (primarily spontaneous breathing or

SIMV) delivered at the same F_{IO_2}. In two studies, an increase in Pa_{O_2} was found when PSV was compared with ACV. Each mode was used for 30 minutes in one study,[33] and two patient groups with identical postoperative characteristics were compared in the other study.[53] Compared with continuous positive-pressure ventilation in surgical ICU patients, Zeravik et al[54] searched for a pulmonary index to predict the effect of PSV on oxygenation in patients with moderate acute respiratory failure. These investigators adjusted PSV and PEEP to achieve a similar V_T and mean airway pressure with both modes. Patients with a low level of extravascular lung water, estimated by bedside thermal dye dilution measurements, had improved oxygenation with PSV, whereas those with an elevated extravascular lung water level deteriorated when shifted from continuous positive-pressure ventilation to PSV. It should be noted that the switch to PSV was accompanied by a reduction in patient sedation, which may have accounted for some of the observed effects.

WORK OF BREATHING AND RESPIRATORY EFFORT

A major goal of PSV is to assist respiratory muscle activity in a way that improves the efficacy of patient effort and decreases workload. Many researchers have focused on this point and have measured work of breathing or indexes of patient effort during PSV.[7,9,31,33,34]

MacIntyre[7] studied the effects of various levels of PSV in patients. The level of PSV was correlated positively with V_T and negatively with respiratory rate. Using a lung model, he suggested that PSV alters the characteristics of work of breathing: The change in the pressure-volume ratio of the work of each breath decreased progressively with increasing levels of PSV.

In eight intubated patients recovering from acute respiratory failure, Brochard et al[9] compared breathing characteristics during 10 cmH$_2$O of PSV, spontaneous unassisted breathing through a Siemens Servo 900C ventilator, and a continuous-flow system without a demand valve. PSV produced significant increases in V_T and Pa_{O_2} and a decreased respiratory rate. Transdiaphragmatic pressure swings (Pdi) and the pressure-time index of the diaphragm were significantly lower during PSV than during the other two modalities. Electromyographic (EMG) activity of the diaphragm decreased markedly in the two patients in whom it was measured.

Subsequently, Brochard et al[31] compared several levels of PSV (0, 10, 15, and 20 cmH$_2$O) in eight patients experiencing weaning difficulties, four of whom had COPD. During unassisted breathing (PS of 0 cmH$_2$O), patients breathed with a small V_T and a high rate, a pattern associated with unsuccessful weaning. This pattern was accompanied by a slight decrease in Pa_{O_2} and a significant increase in Pa_{CO_2} compared with controlled ventilation. All patients exhibited intense activity of their sternocleidomastoid muscles. Work of breathing and O$_2$ cost of breathing were elevated. From the diaphragmatic EMG recordings, the ratio of high-frequency to low-frequency components (H/L), an index of excessive workload that suggests impending high-frequency fatigue, was measured. During PS of 0 cmH$_2$O, seven of eight patients exhibited EMG signs of impending high-frequency diaphragmatic fatigue, a finding consistent with their inability to be weaned from the ventilator. PSV then was delivered at 10, 15, and 20 cmH$_2$O. EMG signs disappeared at 10 cmH$_2$O in four patients and at 20 cmH$_2$O in three others. At this "optimal" PSV level, activity of the sternocleidomastoid muscles was minimized or no longer present. Although work of breathing returned to normal, respiratory rate remained around 30 breaths per minute in some patients. These findings were later confirmed by another study that also included EMG measurements and analysis of centroid frequency as an index of impending high-frequency fatigue.[55]

The respiratory-rate values in the study by Brochard et al emphasize the fact that trying to lower respiratory rate below a point where a patient is no longer in respiratory distress, such as 20 breaths/min or lower arbitrary values, is usually not necessary or useful. This has important clinical implications. In postoperative patients without pre-existing pulmonary disease, PSV 15 cmH$_2$O was shown to take over the major part of work of breathing, quantified as O$_2$ cost of breathing.[56] In patients with COPD, similar findings were demonstrated by Annat et al.[57] In their patients, 15 cmH$_2$O PSV decreased markedly both O$_2$ cost of breathing and diaphragmatic pressure-time index as compared with CPAP.

PSV acts with great efficiency in decreasing work of breathing. This decrease is more or less proportional to the level of PSV and is accompanied by changes in breathing pattern easily measurable at the bedside, together with changes in respiratory muscle recruitment. In the study of Brochard et al,[31] when PSV was absent, large swings in esophageal pressure were associated with a small V_T, whereas with 20 cmH$_2$O of PSV, small excursions in esophageal pressure were associated with a large V_T, suggesting amplification of patient effort. There is an individual limit of pressure, however, above which work of breathing is not decreased and the patient is overassisted.[32] This is associated with dyssynchrony, episodes of apneas and desaturation, and/or occurrence of ineffective efforts (see below).

Different indexes have been used to assess respiratory muscle activity. Beck et al[58] compared crural diaphragmatic electrical activity (EAdi) with Pdi during varying levels of PSV in intubated patients. Changes in PSV did not alter neuromechanical coupling of the diaphragm: EAdi and Pdi decreased proportionally with the addition of PSV. In contrast, Fauroux et al[59] found that diaphragmatic pressure-time product, often used to quantify loading and unloading of the diaphragm, did not exhibit a linear relationship with the diaphragmatic EMG during PSV. These authors suggested that flow measurements are necessary when assessing diaphragmatic unloading during PSV.

COMPENSATION FOR WORK CAUSED BY ETT AND DEMAND VALVE

PSV has been used to predict patient tolerance of unassisted breathing and extubation.[60] The idea is based on selecting a level of PSV just sufficient to overcome the circuit resistance. Thus spontaneous muscular activity should be similar to what a patient would perform in the absence of an ETT or circuit.[61] Measurement of breathing pattern is of major help in assessing work of breathing or ability to tolerate extubation.[62] Therefore, the pressure needed to obtain a "reasonable" breathing pattern can provide insight into a patient's ability to tolerate extubation. This approach raises the question of what is a "reasonable" breathing pattern and of individual values of minimal PSV level, as discussed earlier.

It has long been understood that breathing through an ETT and demand valve increases respiratory muscle work[10,15,63,64] and that PSV can compensate for this increased demand.[61,65,66] This is only partially true. Initially, the level of PSV required to compensate for added inspiratory work (caused by ETT resistance and a demand valve) had been evaluated and calculated using a mechanical model.[65] The resistance offered by the ETT, however, was not compared with the natural resistance opposed by the upper airway.[65] With a lung model, the PSV level needed to compensate for ETT resistance varied from approximately 5–15 cmH_2O for a mean inspiratory flow varying from 0.5–1 liter/s with an ETT size of 8 mm.

Similar reasoning was employed in nine intubated subjects breathing with various levels of PSV who were disconnected from the ventilator and finally extubated.[61] The level of PSV that compensated for the extra work of breathing through the ETT and ventilator circuit was calculated post hoc. It varied among patients. In patients with underlying lung disease, the PSV level that compensated for the additional work ranged from 8–14 cmH_2O, whereas it averaged 5 cmH_2O in patients free of lung disease. The authors concluded that PSV provided the physician with information to predict a patient's tolerance of extubation. For instance, a patient with COPD who exhibits satisfactory clinical and gas-exchange status during PSV of 8 cmH_2O should tolerate extubation, provided there is no major problem with hypoxemia or coughing.

Based on the work of Sassoon et al[67,68] and others, it has been recommended that a PSV level of 5–10 cmH_2O be provided when a patient is breathing through a demand valve. It is important to stress, however, that resistance of the ETT plays little or no role in this pressure requirement. Several subsequent studies compared work of breathing before and immediately after extubation.[66,69,70] These studies demonstrated that the work of breathing was similar or even higher after extubation than before extubation. This indicates that there is no rationale for compensating for the ETT in itself. What needs to be compensated for, however, is the ventilator circuit through which the patient is breathing, including the triggering system.

Despite wide variation among patients in physiologic studies, a simplified approach, based on the same principle, has been applied in several large clinical trials. These studies show that a low level of PSV (7–10 cmH_2O) is as efficient as a T-piece trial in testing whether a patient can be separated from the ventilator and eventually extubated.[71–74] Despite the lack of individual titration of PSV, this approached has performed remarkably well, providing results comparable to a T-piece approach.[71,72,74]

EFFECT OF INSTRUMENTAL DEAD SPACE

Instrumental dead space is usually constituted by the flextube connector, the Y piece, and the humidification system.

Heat and moisture exchangers (HMEs) and heated humidifiers both constitute a resistive load,[75–79] but HMEs also add instrumental dead space because they are positioned between the Y piece and the ETT. The mechanical characteristics of HMEs can modify breathing pattern, effort to breathe, and gas exchange substantially during PSV.[80]

These effects were assessed in six studies during PSV and invasive ventilation[78,81–85] and three studies during NIV.[79,86,87] The studies revealed consistent results. Adding dead space with the HME reproduced the well-known effects of CO_2 on breathing pattern.[88] Acute hypercapnia induced by adding dead space was compared in intubated patients during PSV and proportional-assist ventilation (PAV).[89] Additional dead space produced significantly greater increases of all indexes of effort, respiratory rate, minute ventilation, and Pa_{CO_2} than during PAV. During NIV with PSV, Lellouche et al[79] found that indexes of effort doubled with HMEs compared with heated humidifiers. In intubated patients during PSV, Pelosi et al[82] reported that work of breathing increased from 8.8 ± 9.4 J/min with a heated humidifier to 14.5 ± 10.3 J/min with an HME. They suggested that increasing the level of PSV by 5–10 cmH_2O may be necessary to compensate for the increased work of breathing caused by HME dead space. In a study by Iotti et al,[78] the level of PSV was adjusted automatically by a closed loop to maintain a constant $P_{0.1}$.[78] In comparison with the heated humidifier, PSV was increased by a mean of 3 and 5 cmH_2O when additional dead spaces of HMEs were 37 and 77 ml, respectively.[78] Girault et al[84] observed equivalent work of breathing with an HME and PSV of 15 cmH_2O versus a heated humidifier and PSV of 7 cmH_2O. These studies suggest that use of HMEs should be accompanied by an increase in PSV of 3–10 cmH_2O depending on dead space of the HME. Clinicians should be vigilant about the impact of humidification devices, especially when PSV is used during weaning or with NIV.

During weaning, it may be necessary to avoid HMEs in patients sensitive to dead space, such as patients with severe COPD.[90] Alternatively, the level of PSV should be adjusted according to the humidification device in use.[84] If a weaning trial is performed, the level of PSV should be adjusted according to the humidification device (5–8 cmH_2O with a heated humidifier and 10–12 cmH_2O with an HME). If such adjustments are not made, the outcome of the trial may be misinterpreted.

Patients who present with clinical signs of poor tolerance or persistent hypercapnia during NIV may benefit by a change from an HME to a heated humidifier.

Degree of Patient-Ventilator Synchrony during PSV

The fundamental principle of assisted ventilation is to deliver assistance on a breath-by-breath basis in synchrony with patient effort. As discussed earlier, some patient-ventilator asynchrony often exists with most current assisted modes, which can be aggravated by inappropriate settings, chiefly excessive support. Synchrony has been the subject of several investigations, often not specific to PSV.[24,91–95] Patient-ventilator asynchrony has been described during invasive ventilation[24,94,96–98] and NIV.[99,100]

Synchrony between the patient and ventilator can be defined as the adequacy of matching of patient demand with support provided by the ventilator in terms of synchronization of time, volume, or flow. PSV often is viewed as offering good synchrony with patient activity because it is designed to recognize the beginning and end (more or less) of each spontaneous effort and to adapt mean inspiratory flow rate to patient demand. As discussed earlier, this is far from true in all cases. The incidence of asynchrony has been studied by Chao et al[94] and Thille et al.[95]

During PSV, several forms of asynchrony can be identified by inspecting the airway pressure and flow curves on ventilators. It is often possible to rule out the problem by modifying ventilator settings. Many asynchronies are not specific to PSV.[24,95] Descriptions of these asynchronies may help clinicians to understand their mechanisms and thus undertake remedial steps. A parallel can be made with cardiac arrhythmias, where each type of arrhythmia has a specific

treatment. We describe the asynchronies encountered most frequently during PSV, according to recent publications.[95] Some forms of asynchrony, such as simple delays, are difficult to detect at the bedside and are better recognized by a careful examination of esophageal pressure or diaphragmatic EMG.

AT INITIATION OF THE CYCLE

Triggering delay, ineffective triggering, and auto-triggering are all related to lack of synchrony between onset of patient effort and onset of inspiratory assistance (Figs. 9-7 and 9-8). Short and multiple cycles (Figs. 9-8, 9-9, and 9-10) occur and may be related to problems with inspiratory triggering, setting of the pressurization rate, and cycling criteria.

INSPIRATORY TRIGGER DELAY
Trigger delay can be related to the system (pressure versus flow triggering). Work (or effort) in triggering the ventilator has been evaluated by comparing pressure- and flow-triggering systems.[19,23,101–105] The effort to trigger is significantly reduced with flow-triggering systems compared

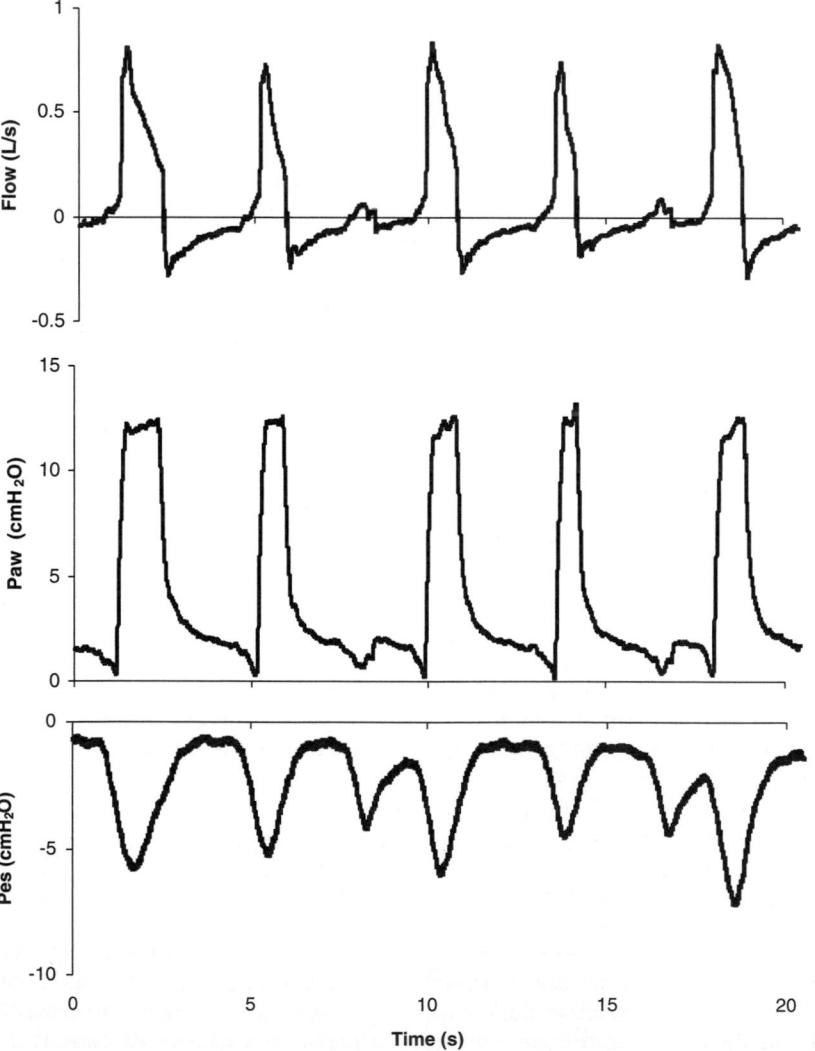

FIGURE 9-7 Ineffective efforts. The third and sixth inspiratory efforts by the patient fail to trigger the ventilator. The efforts by the patient (visible on the esophageal pressure tracing) are not accompanied by ventilator insufflations. A small and transient increase in flow during expiration and a decrease in airway pressure are visible at the time of the failure-to-trigger events.

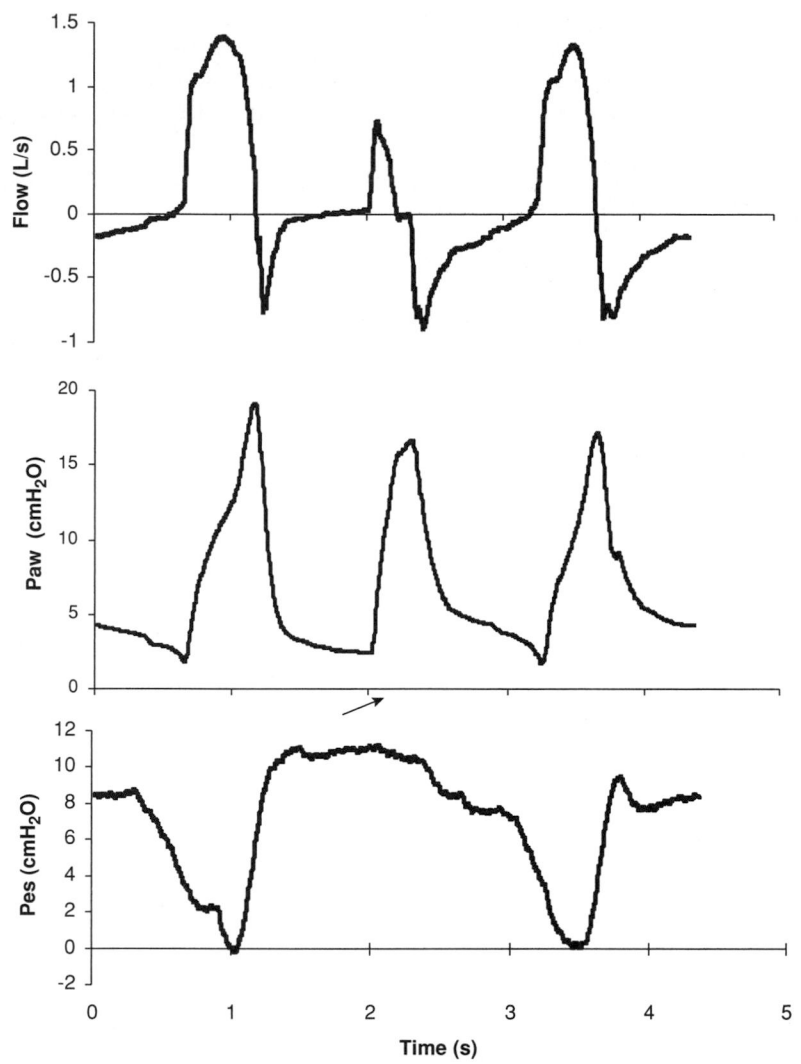

FIGURE 9-8 Auto-triggering. This form of asynchrony can occur when the inspiratory trigger is set too sensitive or in the presence of end-expiratory leaks. As on this tracing, a "short cycle" is a frequent result of an auto-triggered cycle. The "auto-triggered cycle" is accompanied by the absence of an initial airway pressure decay.

with pressure-triggering systems. The specific amount of this effort, however, accounts for 10–30% of total work of breathing, and the clinical impact of this amount is unclear. Ventilator performance is extremely variable. Inspiratory trigger delay varies from 40–200 ms among ventilators[16,19]; it was as long as 400 ms with previous-generation ventilators.[15] In ventilators designed for NIV, Stell et al[18] recently found that inspiratory trigger delay frequently was 120–300 ms; exceptionally, it was up to 500 ms.

Inspiratory effort to overcome intrinsic PEEP is often higher than the effort to trigger the ventilator.[19] The same is true for inspiratory delay. Applied external PEEP may decrease work to trigger the ventilator during invasive ventilation and NIV.[106–109]

INEFFECTIVE TRIGGERING (see Fig. 9-7)
During invasive ventilation with PSV, asynchrony most often results from ineffective triggering, also called *wasted efforts*.[24,91,92,94,96,97,110] The frequency of this asynchrony is influenced directly by the level of PSV and dynamic hyperinflation.[24,40,92,98,111,112] When a patient starts an inspiratory effort, a pressure gradient between the alveoli and

mouth necessitates that the respiratory muscles first counteract this gradient before any inspiratory flow can be generated. This constitutes an inspiratory threshold load that increases breathing effort.[109,113–115] The magnitude of positive pressure generated depends on V_T and therefore set PSV and minute ventilation. Intrinsic PEEP must be overcome first before triggering the ventilator by decreasing airway pressure (in the case of pressure triggering) or generating inspiratory flow (in the case of flow triggering).[23] When patient effort is feeble, it does not reverse expiratory flow or decrease pressure sufficiently to trigger the ventilator. This produces a missed cycle. External PEEP may decrease the frequency of wasted efforts.[92,94,111]

In a study where assistance was varied between 0% and 100%, Leung et al[24] found that there was almost no ineffective efforts below 60% of assistance, but they increased gradually when assistance was 60% to 100%. In a cohort of 62 intubated patients, Thille et al[110] recently found that ineffective triggering represented almost 90% of all asynchronies during PSV. COPD was a risk factor for asynchrony. Patients with ineffective triggering had a higher V_T and higher PSV. This asynchrony has been described with

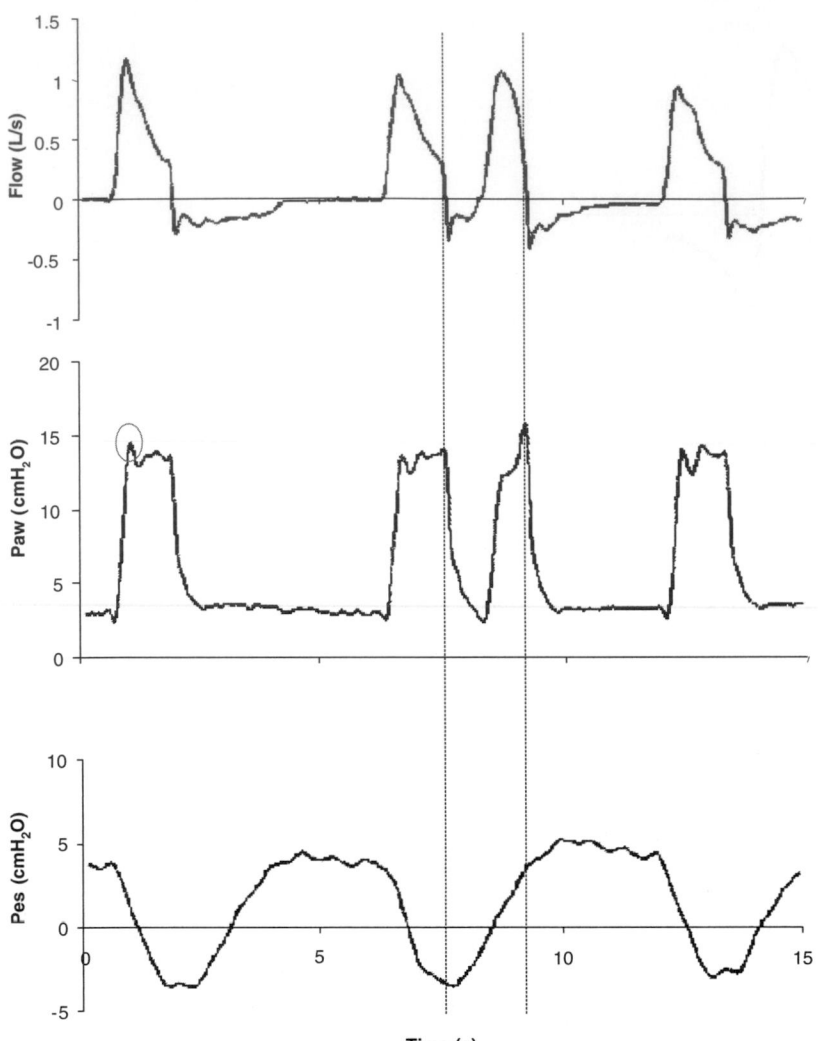

FIGURE 9-9 Double cycles. Two ventilatory cycles occur within a single patient inspiratory effort. Three mechanisms can induce this asynchrony: auto-triggering, high pressurization rate (present here with initial overshoot), and early cycling off (also present in this case).

different diseases but is observed mainly in patients with expiratory flow limitation leading to intrinsic PEEP.[24,94,97] In the study by Leung et al,[24] cycles preceding wasted efforts were characterized by a higher V_T and a lower T_I, which lead to greater levels of hyperinflation. A delay between patient termination and ventilator termination of a cycle can aggravate the problem.[116,117] Indeed, if the ventilator continues the insufflation when the patient has commenced expiration, inspiratory volume will increase and expiratory time will decrease, leading to further hyperinflation. Beck et al[58] found that the greater the level of pressure, the longer was this delay. Therefore, one major reason for ineffective efforts is excessive assistance (PSV), which simultaneously generates dynamic hyperinflation and depresses respiratory drive, both because of high V_T and prolongation of insufflation far beyond the end of patient inspiratory effort.[95]

Ineffective triggering can be detected from irregularities on airway and flow tracings during the expiratory phase[23] (see Fig. 9-7). A respiratory rate lower than 20 breaths per minute or increases in flow and a concomitant decrease in airway pressure on the ventilator screen should rouse suspicion. Giannouli et al[40] found that ineffective triggering could

be detected as accurately on flow and airway tracings as on esophageal pressure tracings. Different approaches can be used to avoid wasted efforts: check trigger sensitivity, increase PEEP,[92,94,111] lower PSV,[23,24] or decrease instrumental dead space.[80–83]

There is no indication that ineffective efforts are more frequent with PSV than with ACV.[95] The clinical consequences are unknown. Thille et al[95] found that a high incidence was associated significantly with prolonged ventilation. Because these asynchronies can be avoided by optimized ventilator settings, their treatment and/or prevention might shorten the time spent on the ventilator.

AUTO-TRIGGERING

Auto-triggered cycles (see Fig. 9-8) represent a default of adequate inspiratory triggering; a cycle is falsely triggered by a signal not coming from a patient's inspiratory effort. These cycles can be caused by expiratory leaks around a mask during NIV, leaks in the ventilator circuit, or motion of liquid in the circuit.[95] An expiratory leak can be misinterpreted by the ventilator as patient effort; an inspiratory cycle then is delivered independently of patient control. Auto-triggered

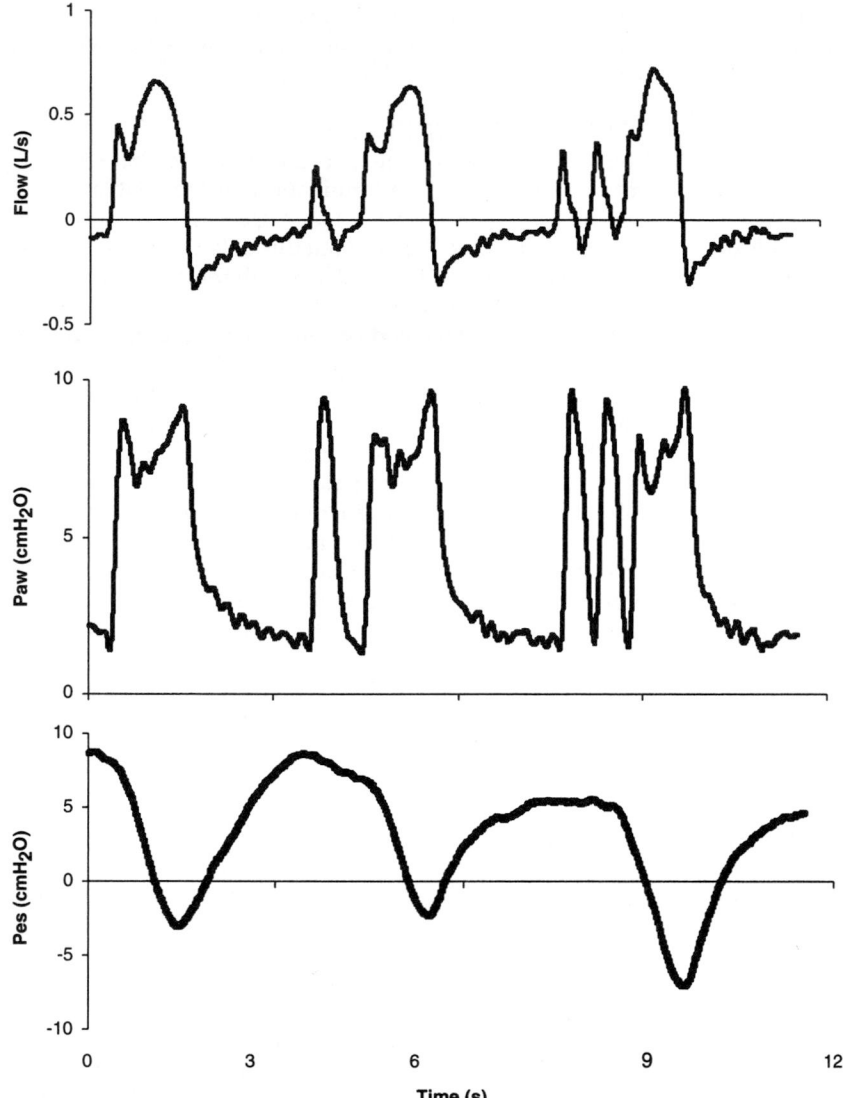

FIGURE 9-10 Multiple cycles. Multiple cycles are frequently associated with auto-triggered cycles and frequent "short cycles." A high pressurization rate can favor this form of asynchrony. In this example, both auto-triggering and high pressurization rate are present.

cycling is also caused by cardiac oscillations[118] and when the setting trigger is excessively sensitive.

Auto-triggering can be difficult to detect on the ventilator tracing. A sudden increase or a persistently high respiratory rate suggests auto-triggering. The absence of airway pressure drop at the beginning of an inspiratory cycle is also suggestive (see Fig. 9-8). In recent-generation ventilators with very sensitive flow-triggering systems, however, this initial decay in airway pressure is very small on triggered cycles and difficult to detect visually.

In cases of auto-triggered cycles, a careful search for a leak must be undertaken. Second, sensitivity of the inspiratory trigger can be reduced both as a diagnostic test and as a remedy. The risk of slightly increasing the work of breathing must be balanced against the advantage of improving synchrony between the patient and ventilator. New automatic inspiratory triggers have been assessed recently. Priniakis et al[119] found that inspiratory triggers based on flow were more sensitive than conventional triggers,

reducing the effort to trigger and ineffective efforts but also increasing the rate of auto-triggering. As with conventional pneumatic inspiratory triggers, a compromise must be found between triggering that is too sensitive (posing a risk of auto-triggering) and triggering that is insensitive (with risk of ineffective efforts or increased effort).

MULTIPLE CYCLES (see Figs. 9-9 and 9-10)
Two or more ventilator insufflations may be delivered within a single patient effort. Auto-triggering can be responsible for multiple cycles (see Fig. 9-10). Ventilator characteristics, such as duration of the refractory period, also may influence this kind of asynchrony. A risk for double-triggering exists with a high inspiratory pressure ramp profile secondary to a reduction in ventilator T_I relative to neural T_I.[120,121] Tokioka et al[122] described double cycles during PSV in intubated patients when the cycling-off criteria were high (35% and 45% of maximal inspiratory flow).

Three mechanisms (auto-triggering, high pressurization rate, and early cycling-off) should be considered when this asynchrony is detected during PSV.

PRESSURIZATION RATE AND INSPIRATORY FLOW

The speed of pressurization determines the initial pressure ramp profile and depends primarily on the initial peak-flow rate. This rate usually is system-specific and is adjustable on several ventilators. Altering this parameter can influence breathing pattern and work of breathing directly.[123–125]

Flow dyssynchrony related to the rise time during PSV, patient respiratory drive, and ventilator performance has been described.[28,42,121,126–128] On new ventilators, rise time can be set to obtain a high rate of pressurization, especially if there is high patient demand.[128] Selecting a low speed of pressurization can cause excessive patient effort, especially when respiratory drive is high and mechanics are poor. Conversely, a very fast rise time may not be optimal[127] and is poorly tolerated by patients.[129] A high speed of pressurization also may make it difficult for the ventilator to regulate the pressure properly throughout inspiration according to its servo-control mechanism, especially in patients with low compliance or high resistance. Differences in pressurization capability among ventilators can be significant.[16,28,39]

MacIntyre and Ho[123] examined the ventilatory-pattern response to seven different levels of delivered initial peak-flow rate. They defined the optimal flow setting as that giving the highest airway pressure-volume product. Settings above and below this optimal flow were associated with tachypnea, smaller V_T, and a tendency for airway pressure not to reach the selected PSV level. Patients with the lowest compliance and highest respiratory drive needed the highest initial flows. Work of breathing was not measured, however, and it is not known if the optimal airway pressure-volume product corresponded to the lowest level of work. By contrast, in two studies, Bonmarchand et al[42,121] showed that the longer the time taken to reach the pressure level set on the ventilator, the greater was the work of breathing in patients with both obstructive and restrictive lung disease. Excessively high pressurization also can lead to an initial overshoot, with possible early termination of the cycle related to high pressure. Chiumello et al[127] found that the highest rate of pressurization did not optimally decrease work of breathing; the relationship between the pressurization rate and dyspnea or work of breathing exhibited a U-shaped pattern. During NIV, Priniakis et al[129] showed that the highest pressurization rate increased the amount of leaks, was poorly tolerated by patients with COPD, and could induce asynchrony such as double-triggering. It could increase respiratory rate, as described previously with ACV.[130,131]

INSPIRATORY CYCLING OFF OR CYCLING TO EXPIRATION

SHORT CYCLES (see Figs. 9-8 and 9-9)

Pertusini et al[100] recently defined a short cycle as one in which T_I (based on flow) was less than half the T_I during spontaneous breathing. These asynchronies can occur during NIV and invasive ventilation. Several mechanisms explain this asynchrony. Auto-triggering is frequently of short cycles.[95] (see Fig. 9-8).

DELAYED EXPIRATION (Fig. 9-11)

This asynchrony is related to the difference between the criterion for inspiration termination on the ventilator and the end of patient neural T_I (see Figs. 9-11, 9-12, and 9-14). Parthasarathy et al[116] quantified this delay in terms of phase angle. When patient T_I ended before the end of ventilator inflation, phase angle was defined as negative. When patient effort ended after the end of ventilator inflation, phase angle was positive. In healthy subjects with simulated airflow obstruction, a negative phase angle was very frequent with early activation of the expiratory muscles during ventilator insufflation.[117] The higher the PSV level, the earlier was activation of the expiratory muscles. Beck et al[58] compared crural diaphragmatic electrical activity with Pdi during varying levels of PSV in 13 intubated patients. With changing PSV, no change in neuromechanical coupling of the diaphragm occurred. From lowest to highest PSV, V_T increased and respiratory rate decreased, but the inspiratory volume calculated during the period when the diaphragmatic EMG increased to its peak did not change. Ventilator assistance continued during the period of diaphragmatic deactivation, a phenomenon that was further exaggerated at higher PSV levels.

In seven intubated patients, Spahija et al[132] recently compared PSV with neurally adjusted ventilatory assist (NAVA), where ventilator support is driven by the diaphragmatic EMG signal. Marked expiratory delays were found with high levels of PSV (1055 ± 1010 ms). These impressive delays may be specific to the ventilator used, the Servo 300 (Maquet, Lund, Sweden), which has a low and nonadjustable cycling-off criterion (5% of peak flow).

The inspiratory-termination criterion frequently is a fixed percentage of peak inspiratory flow rate (12%, 25%, or 30%). This criterion frequently does not correspond accurately with the end of patient inspiratory effort. The effect of this setting is complex and differs between patients with obstructive and restrictive lung diseases. The validity of this criterion has been questioned.[133] Several authors have studied variations of this criterion on breathing pattern.[123,134,135] In 16 patients, MacIntyre and Ho[123] increased the PSV termination criterion from 25–50% of peak flow. T_I was shorter when the criterion was 50% with no change in delivered V_T.

In patients recovering from acute lung injury, Chiumello et al[128] found that a low cycling-off criterion (5% of peak flow) was beneficial in terms of breathing pattern (reduction of respiratory rate and increase in V_T) compared with a threshold at 40%. Tokioka et al[122] found an increase in V_T and a decrease in respiratory rate when the cycling-off criterion was decreased from 45–1%. Work of breathing was less with the low cycling-off criterion. All these observations argue for the use of a low termination criterion in patients with acute lung injury. Conversely, in patients with COPD, the best cycling-off criterion may be above 50%.[136,137] When the cycling-off criterion is set low [5% with the Servo 300 (Maquet, Lund, Sweden) or 5 liters/min with the Puritan-Bennett 7200 (Tyco, Carlsbad, CA)], one can

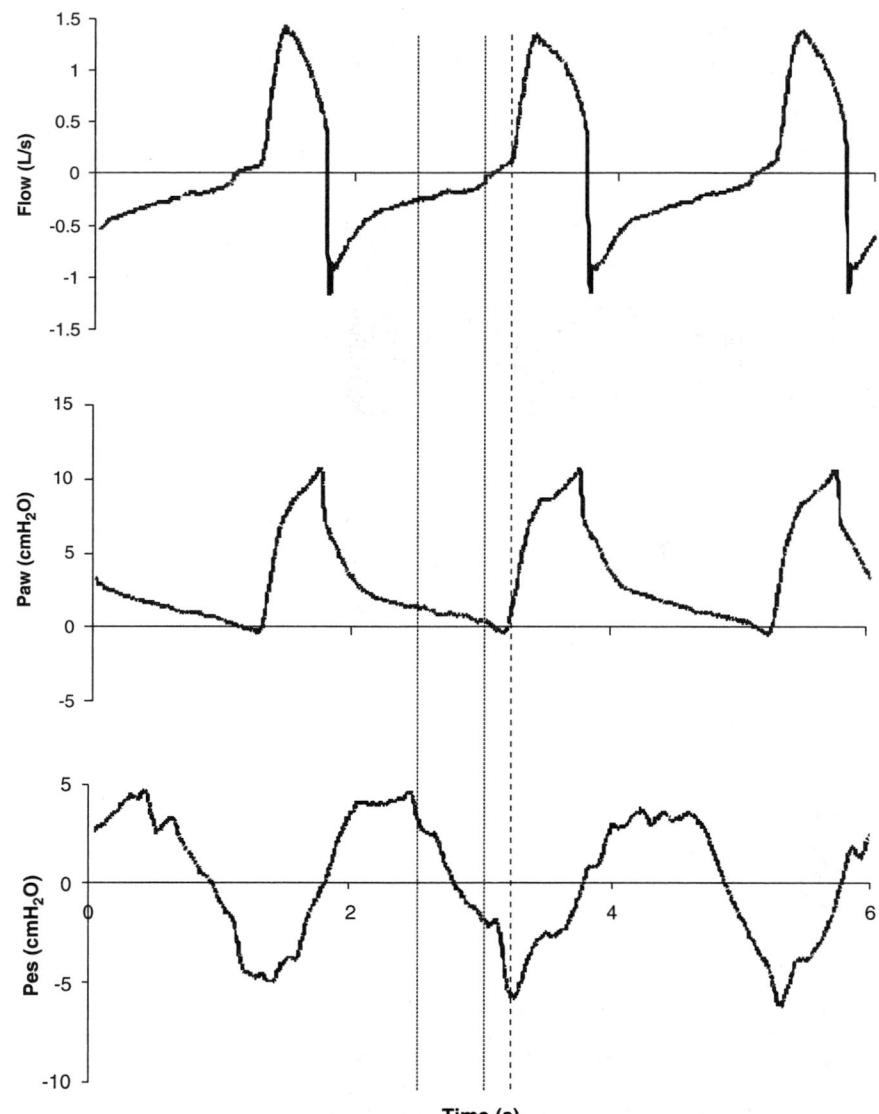

FIGURE 9-11 Inspiratory and expiratory delay. Tracings in an intubated patient with severe COPD receiving PSV. An inspiratory delay secondary to auto-PEEP and triggering delay is evident. The distance between the first and second vertical dotted lines reflects the delay between onset of patient inspiratory effort and positive flow from the ventilator; this delay is caused by auto-PEEP. The delay between the second and third vertical lines is caused by triggering delay (flow triggering). In this patient, mechanical insufflation occurs almost entirely after the patient has terminated inspiratory effort. Consequently, onset of the ventilator's expiratory phase is markedly delayed compared with the patient's neural expiration.

expect the following consequences: Insufflation will continue beyond patient neural T_I, patients will activate their expiratory muscles, and expiratory time will be short; all these factors increase dynamic hyperinflation.[116,138] Conversely, the risk of wasted efforts during subsequent respiratory cycles increases.[117] Some patients exhibit high levels of expiratory muscle activity during PSV[116,138,139] (Fig. 9-13).

PROLONGED INSPIRATION DURING NIV (see Fig. 9-12) Mechanical inflation may be prolonged far beyond the end of patient inspiration, until a limit of maximum T_I has been reached. This limit is sometimes adjustable. This type of asynchrony can occur during invasive ventilation.[20] but is mostly specific to leaks during NIV.[99] It occurs because of the impossibility of reaching the cycling-off criterion. Mechanical inflation usually ends when flow decreases to about 25% of (or below) peak inspiratory flow (see above). In the case of end-inspiratory leaks around a cuff or a mask or in the circuit, the ventilator continues insufflation, and flow does not decrease (because of these leaks). Thus the flow threshold cannot be reached. The breath does not terminate and therefore is prolonged until maximum T_I is reached (which can be several seconds). The patient may "fight" against the ventilator and may even attempt additional inspirations. The inspiration is artificially hung up, and the patient attempts to expire while the expiratory valve remains closed. Ineffective efforts can be observed in this context either within the same ventilator cycle or in following cycles.

Pertusini et al[100] recently found that prolonged inspiration was the most common asynchrony in patients receiving NIV for acute respiratory failure; its frequency correlated with the level of PSV and the amount of leak.

This asynchrony can be detected by inspecting the pressure and flow curves on the ventilator. The first step is to reduce leaks because prolonged inspirations are related directly to end-inspiratory leaks. A decrease in total inspiratory pressure, by decreasing PEEP or PSV, also can

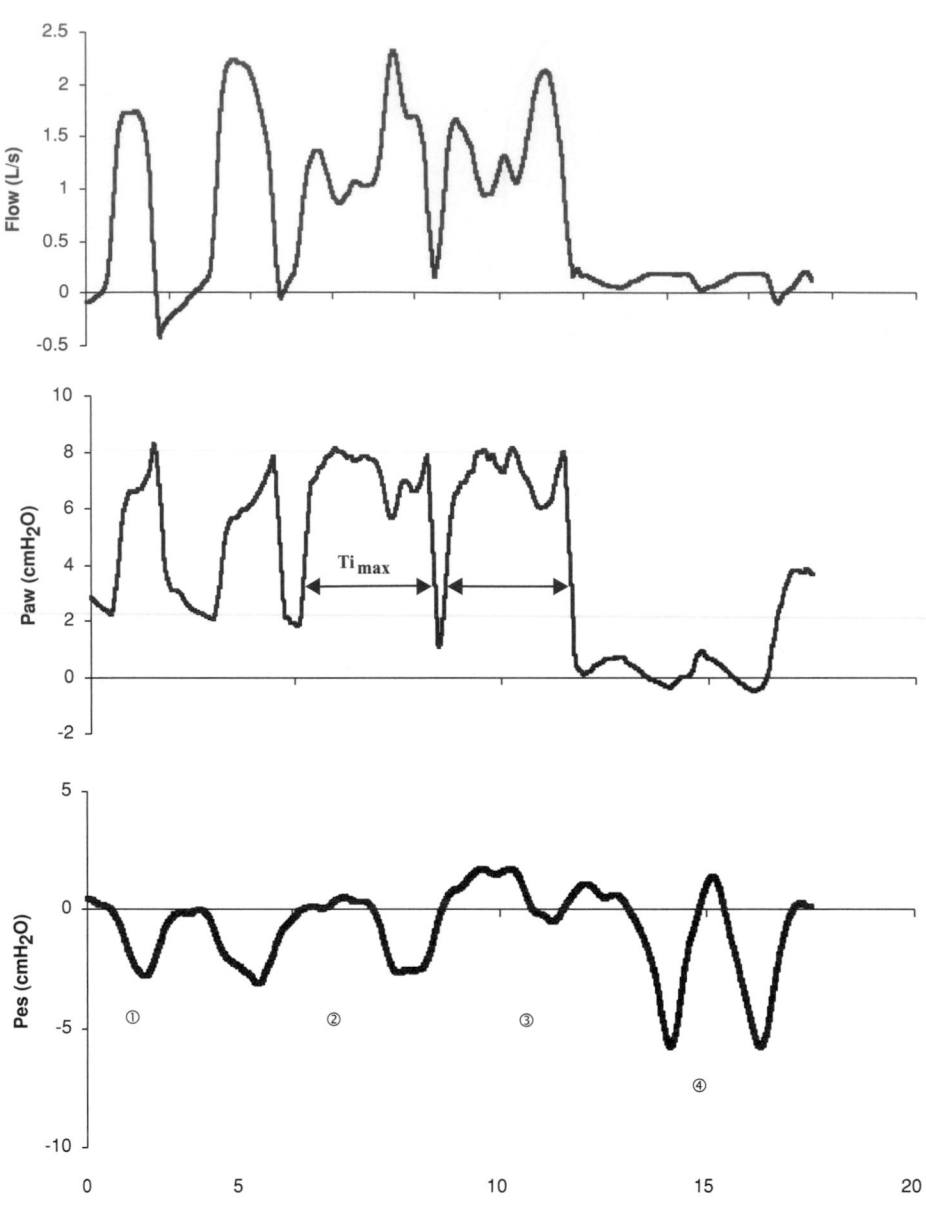

FIGURE 9-12 Prolonged inspiration during noninvasive ventilation. This form of asynchrony during PSV results from a failure to recognize the flow cycling-off criterion. With an end-inspiratory leak, as in this example, the ventilator increases and/or sustains flow to maintain the set airway pressure (here above 2 liters/s). This prevents recognition of the decelerating flow threshold and cycling to expiration. Insufflation is stopped only when maximum inspiratory time (Timax) is reached. Ineffective triggering secondary to hyperinflation may follow the prolonged inspiration, as in this example.

reduce the leaks. This asynchrony can be avoided by adjusting the cycling-off criterion (based on inspiratory-flow decay), which is adjustable in most new ventilators.[99] When leaks are unavoidable, an increase in this threshold to 50% (or more) enables the ventilator to detect the flow threshold. An inappropriately high cycling-off threshold can shorten T_I and decrease V_T.[128,136] A simpler termination criterion is to set a T_I limit, as done with pressure-controlled ventilation. Calderini et al[99] set T_I between 0.8 and 1.2 seconds. This produced better matching between the patient and the ventilator, reducing the work of breathing and improving patient comfort. Assist-controlled pressure ventilation also can be used to deliver pressure with a fixed T_I. Large delays also may result with the use of a helmet for NIV.[140] (Fig. 9-14).

EARLY CYCLING OFF (Fig. 9-15)
If the cycling-off criterion is reached too early, the ventilator stops insufflation and opens the expiratory valve while patient inspiratory effort continues. This produces an initial drop in airway pressure and flow followed by an increase, related to patient inspiration, resulting in a characteristic contour[122] (see Fig. 9-15). This asynchrony is observed during invasive ventilation and NIV. It occurs when the cycling-off criterion is based on either flow decay or time. In patients recovering from acute lung injury,[128] the best cycling-off criterion may be different from the usual default criterion (25% of peak inspiratory flow). Tokioka et al[122] found that the airway pressure shape varied depending on whether the cycling-off criterion was set at 35% or 45%.

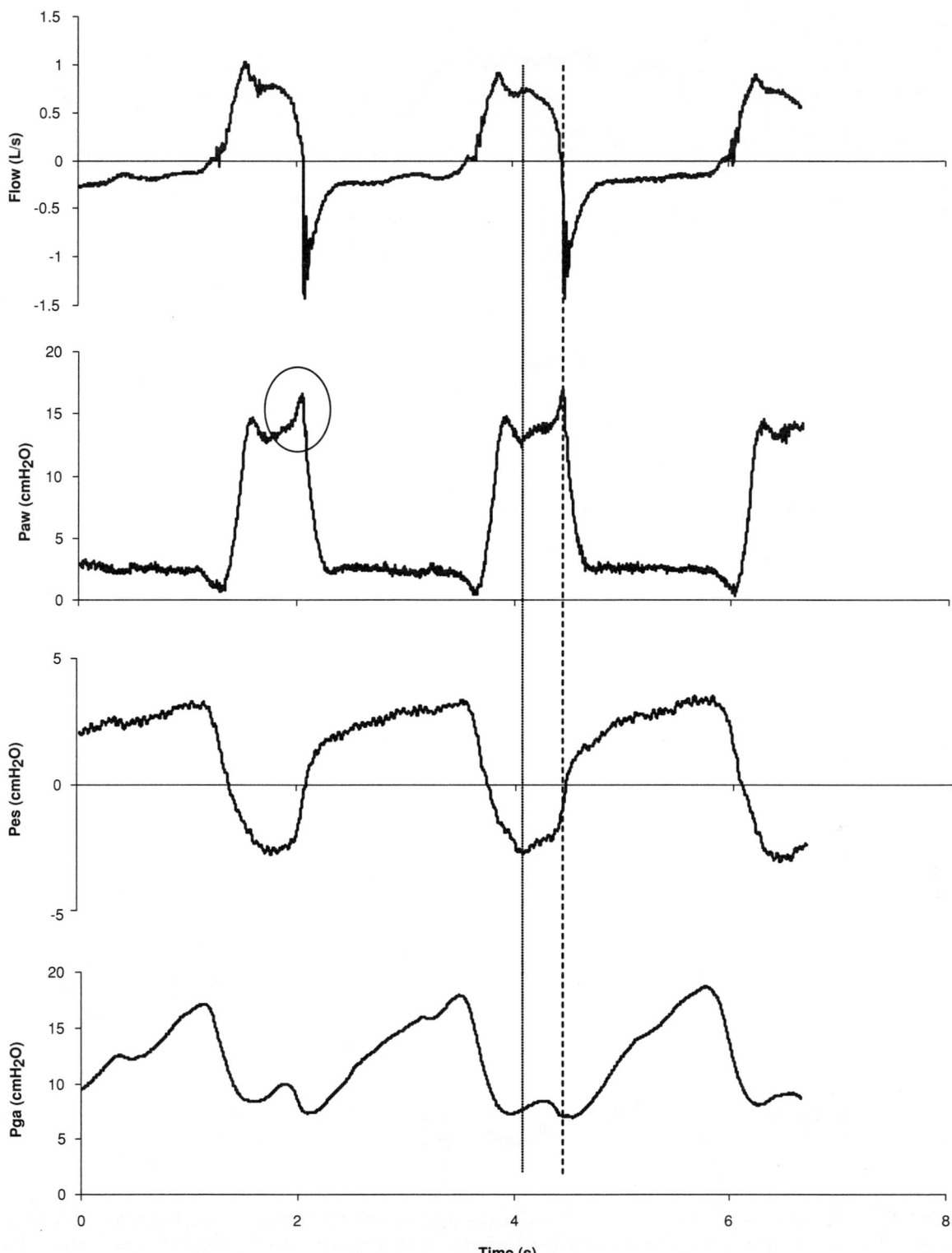

FIGURE 9-13 Expiratory muscle activation. An expiratory increase in gastric pressure (*bottom tracing*) is caused by expiratory muscle activation (at the end of patient inspiration). The apparent "overshoot" on the inspiratory airway pressure tracing (*circle*) indicates, in reality, the abrupt end of patient inspiratory effort. Active expiration is present throughout all of expiration.

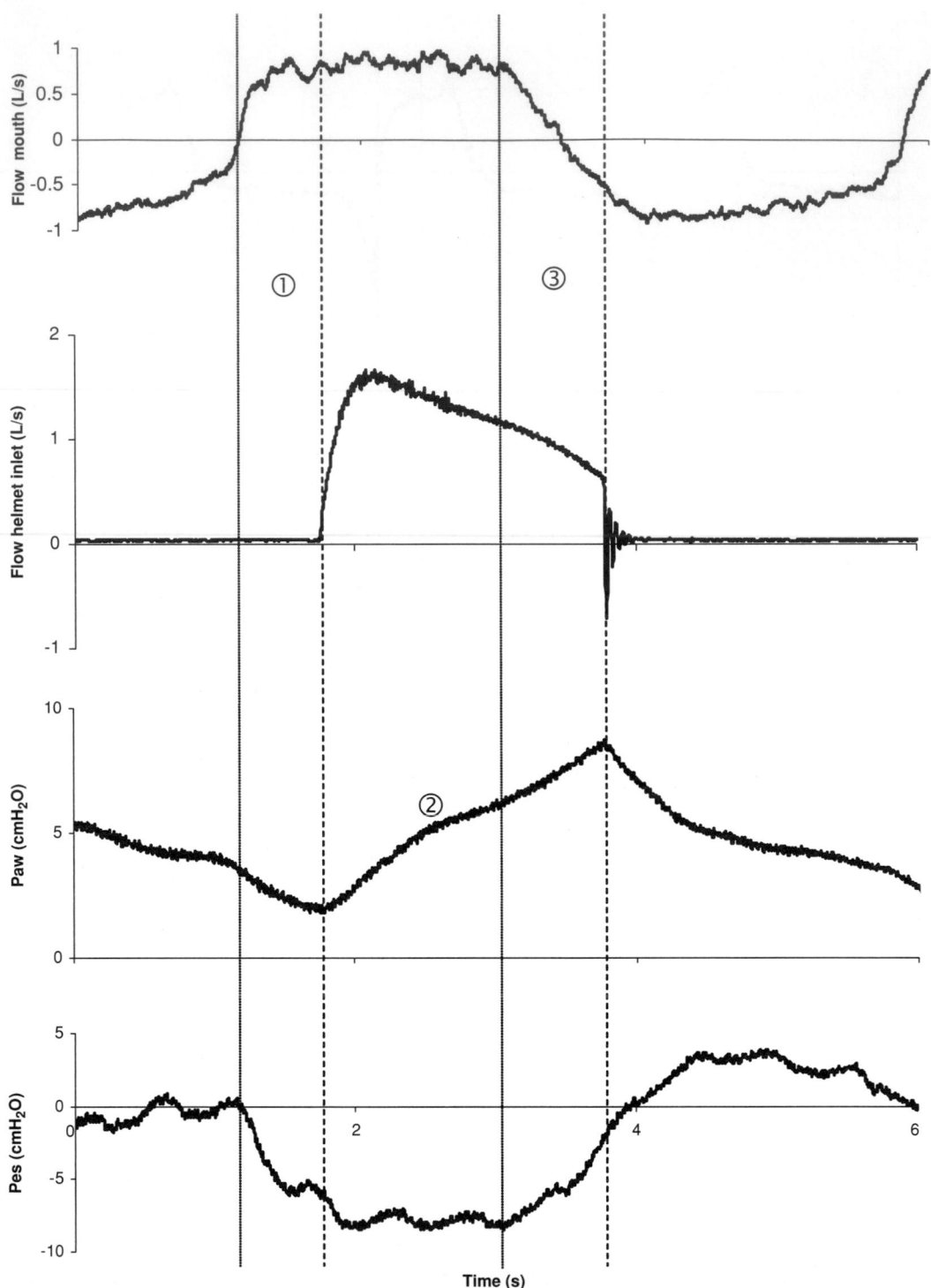

FIGURE 9-14 Inspiratory and expiratory delays and low pressurization during PSV with a helmet system. In this healthy subject, an inspiratory delay is evident between the first vertical dotted line (onset of inspiratory effort) and the second (thicker) vertical line (onset of ventilator assistance) (Interval 1). A low rate of pressurization is evident, typical when PSV is delivered via a helmet system (Interval 2). Expiratory delay corresponds to the time between the third (end of inspiratory effort) and fourth vertical lines (end of insufflation) (Interval 3)

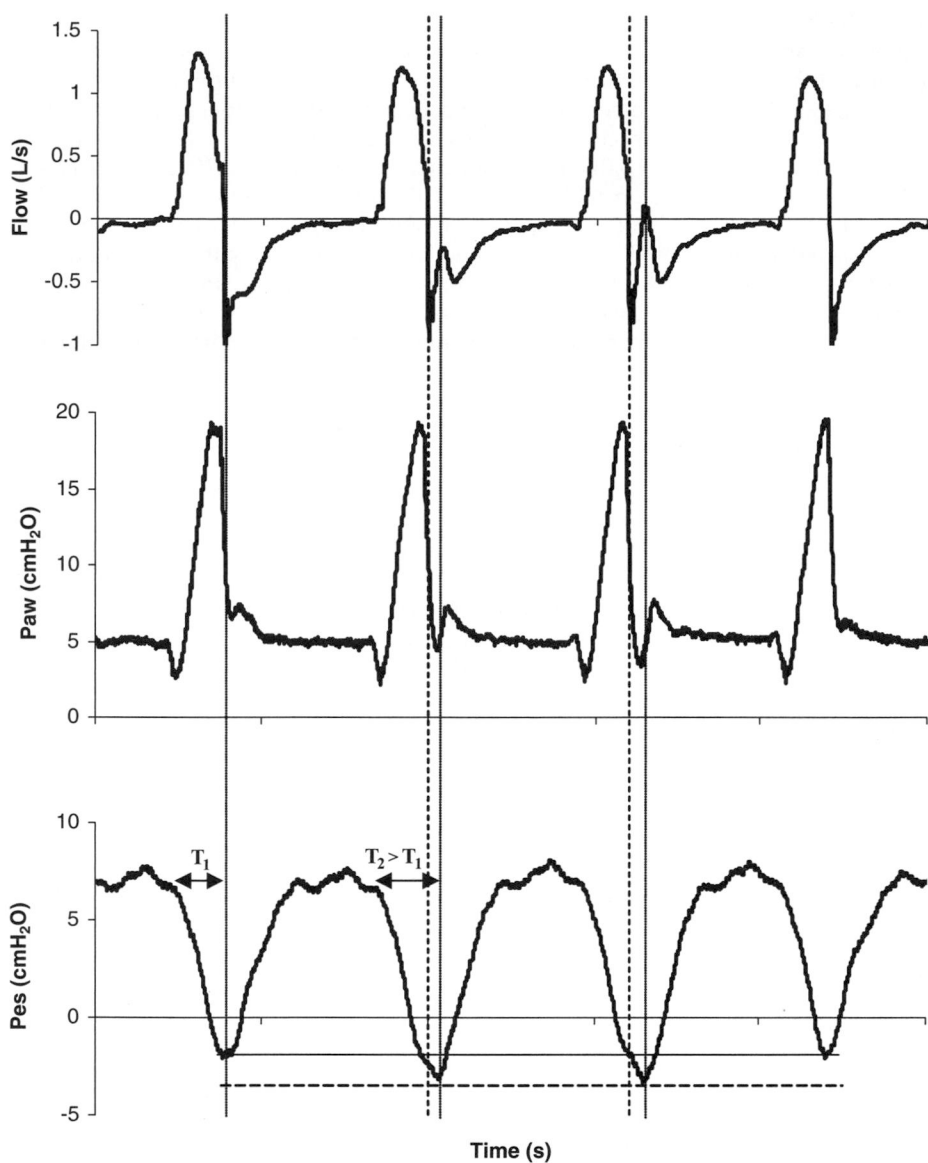

FIGURE 9-15 Early cycling off. The ventilator ends insufflation (*thick vertical dotted line*) before the patient's inspiratory effort ceases (*second vertical line*). The airway pressure tracing then drops transiently below the baseline end-expiratory pressure level because patient effort is still substantial after ventilator insufflation has ceased. The two cycles with this form of asynchrony are associated with increased effort (*dotted horizontal line*) and prolonged neural T_I. The duration of T_I on the second cycle (T_2) is longer than T_I on the first cycle (T_1), as reflected with the greater distance between the arrow heads. A larger T_I favors this form of asynchrony.

The setting of the cycling-off criterion can be difficult. Yamada and Du[137] designed a mathematical model to analyze the mechanisms of expiratory asynchrony during PSV. This model yields several insights.[137] The ratio of flow at the end of patient neural inspiration (neural T_I) to peak inspiratory flow during PSV is determined by the ratio of respiratory time constant (τ) to neural T_I and by the ratio of set PSV to maximal inspiratory muscle pressure. With selected respiratory mechanics, the ratio of flow at the end of neural T_I to peak inspiratory flow ranged from 1–85% and had an excellent linear correlation with τ/neural T_I. A single fixed setting of the flow-termination criterion leads to either synchronized or asynchronized termination depending on patient mechanics. The highest values of the cycling-off criterion corresponded to obstructive patients with high resistances and high compliances (resulting in a high time constant). The lowest values corre-

sponded to patients with acute lung injury, who have low resistances and low compliance (resulting in a short time constant).

Hotchkiss et al[141] used linear and nonlinear mathematical models to investigate the dynamic behavior of PSV. Predicted behavior was confirmed with a test lung. In the setting of airflow obstruction, PSV was accompanied by marked variations in V_T and end-expiratory alveolar pressure, even when patient effort was unvarying. Unstable behavior was observed in the simplest plausible linear mathematical model, and it was an inherent consequence of the underlying dynamics of this mode. Because of its complexity and the frequent changes in ventilatory pattern during PSV,[141] automatic adjustment of triggering based on mathematical models might be helpful.[142] Du et al[143,144] proposed an automatic adjustment of the cycling-off criterion based on the measured time constant in a patient.

Major asynchronies can be detected at the bedside if the ventilator screen displays airway pressure and flow tracings. New ventilators permit clinicians to adjust ventilator settings in order to reduce the frequency of asynchrony. Education, however, is needed to enable clinicians to recognize and treat asynchronies. During invasive PSV, a major goal is recognition of ineffective efforts. During noninvasive PSV, an important issue is recognition of prolonged inspirations caused by leaks. Both problems can be recognized easily. Adjustment of settings (most often a decrease in pressure level) avoids or minimizes the problem. Likely this will improve the efficacy and comfort of PSV.

Differences from Other Modes of Ventilation

Comparison of PSV with other modes helps to define the indications or contraindications of various modes of partial ventilator support and the relative advantages of each.

INTERMITTENT POSITIVE-PRESSURE BREATHING

PSV has some similarities with intermittent positive-pressure breathing (IPPB), an assisted mode used widely in the 1960s for physiotherapy.[145–148] With both IPPB and PSV, cycles are triggered by the patient and limited by pressure, and both can assist patients in acute respiratory failure (with or without endotracheal intubation). They differ in that PSV but not IPPB maintains a constant level of pressure during inspiration. The mechanisms that cycle between inspiration and expiration are also different. The end of inspiration is flow-cycled with PSV and pressure-cycled with IPPB. In normal, nonintubated subjects, work of breathing was lower with PSV than with IPPB.[149] This difference was exaggerated considerably in the presence of CO_2 stimulation, when minute ventilation reached about 25 liters/min. Significant extra work was induced by IPPB devices compared with PSV, as well as compared with unassisted breathing. Expiratory work also was greater and comfort poorer with IPPB devices than with PSV. These differences in operational principles have been made possible by the introduction of reliable flow sensors within the ventilators.

ASSIST-CONTROL VENTILATION

Both PSV and ACV provide full ventilator support; ACV is used far more frequently.[3] The modes differ in ways that explain their relative advantages or disadvantages. During ACV, V_T is guaranteed and independent of respiratory mechanics; thus a minimal frequency and mandatory minute ventilation can be set. During PSV, by contrast, V_T may change with alterations in respiratory compliance or resistance.

For any inspiratory effort, addition of PSV augments the pressure difference between the circuit and the alveoli, leading to a higher inspiratory flow rate and higher V_T than during spontaneous breathing. Whatever the PSV level, it increases inspiratory flow rate in a way that remains partially under patient regulation. During ACV, patient inspiratory effort influences ventilator work, but it does not modify flow or volume. Therefore, the use of volume-assisted ACV is essential when strict control of V_T is considered important, such as in patients with acute respiratory distress syndrome (ARDS) to avoid excessive distension.[150,151] Use of PSV in unstable patients with a high respiratory drive has the major disadvantage of offering no control over V_T. Conversely, PSV may adapt better to variation in patient demand.

Effects of PSV and ACV on breathing pattern, gas exchange, and indices of work or effort have been compared.[44,53] Cinnella et al[152] compared breathing pattern and respiratory muscle effort during ACV and assisted pressure-control ventilation. Although the latter mode differs from PSV in that T_I is preset, this comparison enabled study of the effects of a pressure-targeted mode. Pressure was adjusted to achieve a similar V_T as with ACV; T_I was the same for both. With a high V_T (12 ml/kg), the modes did not differ for respiratory muscle effort. At a moderate V_T (8 ml/kg), work of breathing and pressure-time index were significantly lower with assisted pressure-control ventilation. The decelerating-flow pattern better matched patient demand than did the constant-flow pattern. No difference was found between the modes, however, when T_I was shortened and thus inspiratory peak flow rates increased. Therefore, with adequate settings, both modes could unload the muscles adequately. Leung et al[24] also showed that high levels of assistance were equivalent with PSV, ACV, and SIMV.

Pressure-targeted breaths are more effective than volume-targeted breaths in reducing patient effort during SIMV.[23] In specific circumstances, a switch from ACV to PSV may improve patient-ventilator synchrony. Patients with moderate acute respiratory failure can be ventilated easily with PSV. Some authors report that patients with severe ARDS also benefit from PSV.[5,41]

SIMV

SIMV combines delivery of assisted breaths with spontaneous unassisted breaths.[153,154] SIMV differs from PSV, where every breath is supported to the same extent. Marini et al[155] studied eight patients receiving SIMV delivered at various percentages of total ventilatory requirement. On a breath-to-breath basis, the effort performed by a patient was almost equivalent for assisted and unassisted breathing. Total work performed by a patient depended on the percentage of mechanical assistance delivered. This did not result from a different percentage of unloaded breaths, however, because patient effort remained constant from breath to breath. These findings were confirmed by Imsand et al[156] using diaphragmatic EMGs. Differences in patient effort between assisted and unassisted breaths during SIMV, however, have been found when the mandatory breaths were delivered as pressure-targeted breaths (delivery of a constant pressure during a fixed T_I).[23]

MacIntyre[7] compared SIMV (V_T set at 10–15 ml/kg) and PSV (set at 13–41 cmH_2O) in a crossover study of 15 patients recovering from acute respiratory failure. Sense of comfort was increased, and respiratory rate slower with PSV. There was no change in hemodynamic parameters. In 21 patients ventilated for at least 3 days, Knebel et al[157] compared similar levels of partial support provided by SIMV and PSV in terms of breathing comfort, defined by subjective ratings of dyspnea and anxiety. On a single day, eligible patients experienced, in random order, both SIMV and PSV weaning protocols (sequential 20% reductions in support at timed intervals). Preweaning levels of dyspnea and anxiety did not differ significantly between the modes at any level of support. Surprisingly, comfort was not influenced by the level of support, making it difficult to draw specific conclusions about the comparison of the two modes.

Leung et al[24] compared the effects of PSV and SIMV at varying levels of support in the same patients. They also studied the combination of SIMV and PSV. The level of assistance varied from 0–100%, the latter being equivalent to full support with ACV. Patient effort was similar with SIMV and PSV at high levels of assistance but was higher with SIMV than with PSV at lower levels of assistance (20–40% of maximal support). Although the difference in patients was of smaller magnitude than in animal experiments, the results are consistent with comparisons of IMV and PSV in small animals.[158,159] The studies suggest that when reducing the level of ventilator support, unloading of the respiratory muscles may occur earlier with SIMV than with PSV.[160] Whether this could explain (or partly explain) the different clinical outcomes with the two modes during weaning is unclear (see below).

PAV

PAV was developed several years after PSV.[161,162] Promising initial results and great physiologic interest have characterized this mode. PAV, however, has remained essentially a physiologic tool, and results of the first clinical comparisons with PSV have been disappointing. Most physiologic comparisons of PAV and PSV favor PAV in terms of breathing-pattern variability, patient-ventilator interaction, and comfort. In clinical trials, mainly during NIV, these physiologic effects did not produce any outcome benefit.[163–167]

PAV is designed to deliver assistance in direct proportion to patient effort.[161,162,168] In comparison with PSV, PAV allows more physiologic ventilation, but ventilator settings are more complex.

ADVANTAGES OF PAV COMPARED WITH PSV

During invasive ventilation and NIV, PAV is consistently superior to PSV on physiologic endpoints. In response to variable loads (e.g., dead space and resistive or restrictive loads), PAV adapts the level of assistance to patient demand. With PSV, in contrast, the level of inspiratory pressure remains constant whatever the load. In response to acute hypercapnia (addition of 100 ml of dead space), Ranieri et al[89] showed that PAV adapted more efficiently to ventilatory demand than did PSV. Levels of inspiratory pressure increased during PAV with a relative increase in V_T and no change in respiratory rate, whereas a small increase in V_T and a large increase in rate were observed with PSV. This resulted in lower work of breathing and better comfort with

PAV.[89] In intubated patients, Grasso et al[169] compared the response to a restrictive load (chest and abdominal binding). PAV achieved a higher V_T, lower respiratory rate, and lower pressure-time product of the diaphragm (in response to the load), resulting in better comfort when compared with PSV. Such adaptations to loads with PAV and PSV also were found in healthy subjects[170,171] and with a lung model.[172]

With pneumatic triggering systems, a delay can occur between the onset of patient effort and effective triggering,[173] mainly when auto-PEEP is present.[19,116] Giannouli et al[40] found less ineffective triggering with PAV than with PSV in intubated patients. The authors reasoned that during PSV, in contrast to PAV, ventilator T_I would outlast neural T_I, especially in patients with a long time constant. Thus insufflation continues while the patient has begun to exhale, resulting in hyperinflation and greater risk of ineffective efforts. Other studies also found less ineffective efforts with PAV than with PSV.[174,175] In intubated patients with severe COPD and high intrinsic PEEP (6.8 ± 3.9 cmH_2O), no ineffective triggering occurred with PAV, with or without CPAP[176]; comparison with PSV was not performed.

Many studies reveal a greater variability of V_T with PAV than with PSV[171,177–180] and better patient comfort.[89,163,164,171,178,181–184] PAV also provided better control of P_{CO2} compared with other modes.[185] One study in stable patients with neuromuscular and chest-wall disease noted better unloading and comfort with PSV than with PAV.[186]

DRAWBACKS OF PAV COMPARED WITH PSV

In contrast to any other mode (including PSV), greater knowledge of resistive and elastic characteristics of the respiratory system is necessary when setting PAV. It can be difficult to obtain simple and reliable measurements of these characteristics in awake patients triggering the ventilator. The values also frequently vary. The setting of PAV thus is complex and constitutes an obstacle to its wide acceptance. Porta et al[179] found that the time needed to set PAV was longer than for PSV. Methods to automatically and intermittently determine respiratory resistance and elastance were proposed recently.[187,188] These methods could be incorporated into a closed-loop adjustment of PAV. A major drawback of PAV is the occurrence of a specific asynchrony: *runaway.*[168] Runaway is related mainly to an excess of volume assistance.[40,174,181]

CLINICAL STUDIES

Two prospective, randomized, controlled studies with clinical endpoints have compared PAV and PSV.[163,164] The studies were conducted during NIV. The first study enrolled 44 patients: PAV ($n = 21$) and PSV ($n = 23$). Despite significantly better comfort and less treatment refusal with PAV, intubation and mortality rates were equivalent. Fernandes-Vivas et al[164] used similar methodology in 117 patients. Intubation and mortality rates were equivalent despite better comfort and less intolerance with PAV. Even when used during NIV, in the presence of leaks, few problems related to runaway were reported. These early clinical trials of PAV are disappointing when contrasted with the promising physiologic studies. No clinical study has yet been conducted using the new methods that allow automatic measurement of respiratory mechanics.[187,188]

NAVA

NAVA is a promising but experimental mode of ventilation. It provides assistance in proportion to patient effort. It depends on continuous recording of diaphragmatic electrical activity (EAdi), which is obtained via a nasogastric catheter incorporating a multiple-array esophageal electrode (nine electrodes spaced 10 mm apart). The onset and end of assistance and the level of assistance are driven directly by the EAdi signal.[173] In theory, NAVA should provide better patient-ventilator synchrony than pressure-targeted modes. First results support this expectation. Unlike all other modes (including PAV), NAVA should not be influenced by intrinsic PEEP or by the presence of leaks, as in the case of standard triggering systems. The initial report on NAVA revealed advantages compared with PSV in terms of triggering and cycling off of the ventilator.[173] NAVA and PSV have been compared in a rabbit model of acute lung injury.[189] Diaphragmatic unloading was much more efficient with NAVA than with PSV, with a reduction of indexes of effort and the absence of wasted efforts. In intubated patients, Spahija et al[132] compared the trigger delay and cycling off of inspiration with NAVA and PSV. Both modes were studied at low and high levels of assistance. Inspiratory trigger delay was around 100 ms with NAVA and around 200 ms with PSV. Cycling-off delays were markedly different: 40 ms (whatever the level of assistance) with NAVA and 500–1000 ms with PSV (low and high assistance). Of note, the cycling-off criterion during PSV was set at 5% of peak inspiratory flow (Servo 300), which can cause prolonged expiratory delay, especially in patients with COPD and a long time constant.[137,190] These first physiologic results are encouraging. The same research group recently reported an evaluation of an original closed-loop system using EAdi as a target to select the level of PSV: target-drive ventilation.[191] This system was evaluated in 11 healthy subjects before and during exercise and without ventilator support. Without target-drive ventilation, EAdi increased, as did indexes of effort and end-tidal CO_2 during exercise. With target-drive ventilation, the level of pressure increased during exercise, maintaining the EAdi constant.

Hemodynamic Consequences of PSV

Unique hemodynamic consequences have not been described with PSV.[7,8,33,35,47,60,192,193] Despite a wide range of pressures, most studies have found little or no deleterious effects of PSV on cardiovascular function in patients after cardiac surgery or in patients with respiratory failure. The negativity of pleural pressure during PSV and the control of airway pressure may reduce the risk. One study found that PSV during NIV may lead to a reduction in cardiac output without a change in mixed venous P_{O_2}.[49] Whether this reflects adaptation to a decrease in CO_2 production or a deleterious effect could not be inferred from these data.[194]

Adjustment of Pressure Level at the Bedside

Precise guidelines for the bedside use of PSV are lacking; the pressure level has been adjusted in various ways in many studies.[7,195,196] The maximal PSV level that results in a stable breathing pattern (without bradypnea or apnea) has been proposed.[7] Assessment of accessory muscle activity, especially the sternocleidomastoid, by inspection and palpation was suggested for deciding optimal assistance.[31] In this study, less work also was associated with a decrease in respiratory frequency (below 30–32 breaths per minute). Respiratory frequency can be used as a simple indicator of the adequacy of PSV[31,60]; less than 30 breaths per minute has been recommended.[60,138,197] As indirectly suggested by weaning trials, a target of low frequency (25 breaths per minute or below) may prolong weaning duration. The latter also may be explained by increased occurrence of asynchrony when a low frequency is displayed on the ventilator. In early studies, PSV was adjusted to reach a predetermined V_T (8–12 ml/kg).[8,35,54] A setting of 6–8 ml/kg V_T seems more advisable to avoid patient-ventilator dysynchrony. One study suggested, however, that patients who could be weaned controlled their own V_T and were only mildly influenced by the PSV level.[198]

Closed-Loop Delivery of PSV

The potential for variation in delivered ventilation has led many manufacturers to develop servo-controlled modalities of PSV. In one ventilator, the PSV level was adjusted automatically to achieve a preset breathing frequency.[199] This approach had advantages over fixed PSV when abrupt changes in respiratory demand occurred. More often, servo-controlled modes have been proposed to adjust the PSV level to keep V_T constant. Pressure can be varied from breath to breath using various algorithms. These options have been designed to provide a better ventilator response to changes in respiratory mechanics.[200,201] An increase in resistance or elastance during PSV normally leads to a drop in V_T if no compensation is made by the patient or the ventilator.

These new modes, often called *dual-control modalities*, use closed-loop feedback control systems that enable the ventilator to adapt output based on the difference between measured ventilation and a predefined target. The modes go by different names. To overcome the theoretical limitations of PSV, volume-support ventilation (VSV) was introduced in the 1990s on the Siemens Servo 300 ventilator (Siemens Elema, Solna, Sweden). VSV is a pressure-limited mode that uses a target V_T and minute ventilation for feedback control. The level of PSV is adjusted continuously to deliver a preset V_T. Two anecdotal reports with VSV[202,203] and one randomized, controlled trial[204] have yielded variable results. Other modes working on the same principle—volume-targeted pressure-regulated mode—have been developed extensively by manufacturers without extensive clinical validation. Specifically, physiologic studies have not assessed the efficacy of VSV in terms of adjustment to spontaneous changes in mechanics. The response of such modes to changes in ventilatory demand can be troublesome, such as those occurring with different states of wakefulness, nutrition, episodes of sepsis, pain, and so on. With a fixed level of VSV, but not of PSV, Jaber et al[205] found that an increase in ventilatory demand resulted in a decrease in PSV provided by the ventilator, the opposite of the desired response. Conceivably, VSV may result in respiratory distress in clinical settings.

More complex knowledge-based systems have been developed with the aim of providing an automatically performed, patient-adapted ventilator support that is superimposed on an automated weaning strategy.[73,206–209] Such systems have been implemented in computers that drive a ventilator. These approaches using SIMV plus PSV or PSV alone have been evaluated in patients. Sophisticated modes have been developed through improvements in computer science.[210,211]

When the physiologic and clinical knowledge needed to manage a well-defined clinical situation is acquired, it can be embedded within a computer program that drives the ventilator using artificial intelligence techniques, such as production rules, fuzzy logic, or neural networks.[212] These new techniques allow planning and control. Control is a local task that consists of determining what is the immediate next step. Planning is a strategic task aimed at regulating the time course of the process. For control and planning, numerous techniques have been developed in the fields of control theory and artificial intelligence, respectively. The main difference between these two fields lies in the process models used. Control and planning are two complementary and essential tasks that must be combined to design multilevel controllers for automatically supervising complex systems such as mechanical ventilators. Because the driving process is based on complex physiologic models, it is important to avoid both oversimplification and excessive complexity.[203] Strickland and Hasson[208,209] tried to develop a controller incorporating an active clinical strategy represented by production rules using SIMV and PSV (IF conditions, THEN actions). Their work did not lead to commercial development.[208,209]

The Smart Care® system is an embedded version of the initial NeoGanesh system. The NeoGanesh system drives the ventilator with PSV, keeping a patient within a zone of "respiratory comfort," as defined by respiratory parameters, and superimposing an automated strategy for weaning.[73,207,213] The designers of the knowledge-based NeoGanesh system intended to build a closed-loop system that (1) was efficient for automatically controlling mechanical support and planning of the weaning process, (2) could be evaluated with the goal of gradually improving its reasoning and planning capabilities, and (3) could be subjected at the bedside to performance measurements at each step of its operation. The NeoGanesh system is based on modeling of the medical expertise required to perform mechanical

ventilation in PSV mode. It does not include mathematical equations of a physiologic model. Several types of evaluation have been performed: (1) to determine how well the system adapts the level of assistance to patient needs (evaluation of the control level)[213], (2) to assess the extubation recommendation made by the system (evaluation of the strategic level)[73] and (3) to estimate the impact on clinical outcomes.[214,215] This system has been shown to reduce periods of excessive respiratory efforts and to predict extubation time with good accuracy.[73,213] It has been used safely during prolonged periods of mechanical ventilation and has been shown recently to reduce the time spent on the ventilator.[214,215]

Clinical Applications

WEANING

The usual weaning methods are once-daily trials of spontaneous breathing, most often with a T piece, resulting in abrupt discontinuation of mechanical ventilation, SIMV, and PSV with a gradual reduction in the level of assistance. A low PSV level can be used to mimic spontaneous breathing trials; the latter thus constitutes the final step in the approach of gradual reduction in PSV or as a substitute for a T-piece trial. PSV also can been used in combination with SIMV, although very few data support the use of this combination.[22–24] In a 1998 international survey of the use of mechanical ventilation,[3] PSV was used one way or another in 45% of weaning attempts. These data indicate that PSV is considered an important weaning technique.

Studies comparing T-piece trials, SIMV, and PSV were rare before the mid-1990s. Studies had included a large percentage of postoperative patients who exhibited no persistent weaning problem; no conclusions were drawn regarding the type of ventilator support to use.[216] PSV as a sole mode of ventilation has been tested in two prospective, randomized, controlled trials.[195,196] These trials share common conclusions: (1) Patients who tolerated 2 hours of breathing on a T piece were not enrolled and were considered easy to wean: 60–80% of patients who reached the weaning phase were separated easily from the ventilator on first attempt; (2) weaning outcome in the remaining patients depended heavily on the weaning strategy used; and (3) SIMV was consistently the worst weaning method. The two trials, however, differed regarding efficacy of PSV. PSV was found superior to other methods in the study of Brochard et al[195] but not in the subsequent study of Esteban et al.[196]

Brochard et al[195] compared three methods of gradually withdrawing mechanical ventilation. In one group, PSV was decreased gradually according to patient tolerance. In a second group, SIMV was adjusted to decrease the percentage of total ventilator support gradually. In a third group, T-piece trials of increasing duration were interspersed with ACV. At 21 days, a significantly higher percentage of patients had been separated from the ventilator with PSV than with the other two methods. This was accompanied by a shorter duration of weaning with PSV. Esteban et al[196] did not use the same criteria for adjusting the pressure level in an individual patient. PSV was adjusted to achieve a respiratory rate lower than 25 breaths per minute. PSV was found to be inferior to once-daily T-piece trials and multiple-daily T-piece trials. This PSV approach seemed to lengthen the weaning process compared with once-daily T-piece trials. In the study of Brochard et al,[195] PSV was adjusted to obtain a respiratory rate lower than 35 breaths per minute. In that trial, PSV was superior to all other approaches, including SIMV and intermittent T-piece trials. In the study of Esteban et al,[196] the final test before extubation was a T-piece trial, during which frequency of up to 35 breaths per minute was tolerated. In the same study, the final step with PSV was a level of 5 cmH$_2$O, during which frequency above 25 breaths per minute was considered a sign of poor clinical tolerance. Thus the use of PSV differed markedly in the two studies and likely explains differences in efficacy. No study has compared the PSV approach in the trial of Brochard et al[195] with the once-daily T-piece method in the study of Esteban et al.[196] Another trial, however, found no difference between T-piece trial and PSV in patients with weaning difficulties.[217]

PSV and T piece have been compared as a final step before extubation. Use of a low level of PSV has been found equivalent or slightly superior to a T-piece trial in both adults and infants.[71,72,74] A low level of PSV was slightly superior to T piece in terms of short-term success after extubation.[71,74] At 48 hours, the success rate was not significantly different in the largest trial.[71]

A comparable approach was used in the NeoGanesh closed-loop system that employs automatic adjustment of PSV.[73,213] Although different from standard clinical use of PSV, the results with a computer-driven system constitute a form of validation of PSV weaning in a system that applies it on a 24-hour-a-day basis.

NONINVASIVE VENTILATION

NIV has been used in many patients with acute respiratory failure since the early 1990s.[96,140,218–224] PSV is used preferentially by several groups for NIV. Delivered via a face mask, PSV decreases respiratory muscle activity markedly in patients with COPD in acute distress. During exercise, which also constitutes a high ventilatory workload, noninvasive PSV improves performance in patients with COPD.[225]

Bilevel ventilation, as PSV is often called when combined with PEEP, is by far the most frequent mode of ventilation. In a large multicentric French survey of NIV in ICUs, PSV was used in 67%, ACV in 15%, and CPAP in 18% of patients.[226] PSV frequently is considered better tolerated than ACV during NIV.[227]

Determinants of the success of NIV have been described in several studies. They relate to patient characteristics (e.g., severity scores, etiology of the respiratory failure, and nutritional status)[97,226,228] and immediate outcome variables (e.g., evolution of arterial blood gases over 2 hours, comfort, and level of leaks).[97,226,229–232] These determinants are in part related to technical aspects: ventilator performance, modes,[96,227] settings,[17,27,96,99,111,233] humidification

devices,[86,234] interfaces,[140,235–237] and patient-ventilator asynchrony.[99,100]

USE OF NONINVASIVE VENTILATION WITH PSV FOR WEANING

In patients with acute exacerbations of COPD, prolonged mechanical ventilation is associated with complications. In this setting, Nava et al[223] suggested that deliberate extubation followed by a switch to NIV might improve weaning outcome. Using PSV for such a goal achieved greater weaning success and higher survival rate. A subsequent study did not entirely confirm these results; patients switched to noninvasive PSV experienced a longer time of ventilator support.[238] In patients with stable chronic respiratory disorders who were unable to sustain spontaneous breathing, Vitacca et al[239] found that invasive PSV, delivered while patients were still intubated, and noninvasive PSV were equally effective in reducing respiratory muscle work and improving arterial blood gases. In addition, noninvasive PSV was slightly better tolerated.

Conclusion

PSV is a mode of partial ventilator assistance that has proved very efficient in reducing work of breathing and providing relatively good synchrony with patient effort. PSV provides a good model to increase understanding of patient-ventilator interaction. Its place has been assessed mainly during weaning and NIV. It also can be used early in the course of ventilation, enabling the patient to be ventilated without the need for sedation and in preparation for weaning. In the early phase, its use may be limited by lack of control over the volume delivered. One of its main drawbacks, however, is the possibility of overassisting patients, causing major dyssynchrony between a patient's rhythm and that of the ventilator, inducing hyperventilation, episodes of apneas, and sleep fragmentation, especially in patients with obstructive lung disease.

References

1. Sassoon CS, Zhu E, Caiozzo VJ. Assist-control mechanical ventilation attenuates ventilator-induced diaphragmatic dysfunction. Am J Respir Crit Care Med 2004; 170:626–32.
2. Sassoon CS. Ventilator-associated diaphragmatic dysfunction. Am J Respir Crit Care Med 2002; 166:1017–8.
3. Esteban A, Anzueto A, Frutos F, et al. Characteristics and outcomes in adult patients receiving mechanical ventilation: A 28-day international study. JAMA 2002; 287:345–55.
4. Iotti GA, Brochard L, Lemaire F. Mechanical ventilation and weaning. In: Zapol W, Tinker J, editors. Care of the critically ill, 2nd ed. London: Springer-Verlag, 1991: 457–478.
5. Kacmarek RM. The role of pressure support ventilation in reducing work of breathing. Respir Care 1988; 33:99–120.
6. Whaba R. Pressure support ventilation. J Cardiothorac Anaesth 1990; 4:624–30.

7. MacIntyre NR. Respiratory function during pressure support ventilation. Chest 1986; 89:677–83.

8. Prakash O, Maij S. Cardiopulmonary response to inspiratory pressure support during spontaneous ventilation vs conventional ventilation. Chest 1985; 88:403–8.

9. Brochard L, Pluskwa F, Lemaire F. Improved efficacy of spontaneous breathing with inspiratory pressure support. Am Rev Respir Dis 1987; 136:411–5.

10. Brochard L, Baum T, Bedu C. Les valves à la demande. Réanimation Urgences 1993; 2:97–105.

11. Katz JA, Kraemer RW, Gjerde GE. Inspiratory work and airway pressure with continuous positive airway pressure delivery systems. Chest 1985; 88:519–26.

12. Marini JJ, Capps JS, Culver BH. The inspiratory work of breathing during assisted mechanical ventilation. Chest 1985; 87: 612–8.

13. Beydon L, Chassé M, Harf A, Lemaire F. Inspiratory work of breathing during spontaneous ventilation using demand valves and continuous flow systems. Am Rev Respir Dis 1988; 138: 300–4.

14. Samodelov LF, Falke KJ. Total inspiratory work with modern demand valve devices compared to continuous flow CPAP. Intensive Care Med 1988; 14:632–9.

15. Cox D, Tinloi SF, Farrimond JG. Investigation of the spontaneous modes of breathing of different ventilators. Intensive Care Med 1988; 14:532–7.

16. Richard JC, Carlucci A, Breton L, et al. Bench testing of pressure support ventilation with three different generations of ventilators. Intensive Care Med 2002; 28:1049–57.

17. Lofaso F, Brochard L, Hang T, et al. Home vs intensive-care pressure support devices: Experimental and clinical comparison. Am J Respir Crit Care Med 1996; 153:1591–9.

18. Stell I, Paul G, Lee K, Ponte J, Moxham J. Noninvasive ventilator triggering in chronic obstructive pulmonary disease: A test lung comparison. Am J Respir Crit Car Med 2001; 164:2092–7.

19. Aslanian P, El Atrous S, Isabey D, et al. Effects of flow triggering on breathing effort during partial ventilatory support. Am J Respir Crit Care Med 1998; 157:135–43.

20. Black J, Grover B. A hazard of pressure support ventilation. Chest 1988; 93:333–5.

21. Murphy D, Dobb G. Effect of pressure support support of spontaneous breathing during intermittent mandatory ventilation. Crit Care Med 1987; 15:612–3.

22. Jounieaux V, Duran A, Levi-Valensi P. Synchronized intermittent madatory ventilation with and without pressure support ventilation in weaning patients with COPD from mechanical ventilation. Chest 1994; 105:1204–10.

23. Giuliani R, Mascia L, Recchia F, et al. Patient-ventilator interaction during synchronized intermittent mandatory ventilation: Effects of flow triggering. Am J Respir Crit Care Med 1995; 151:1–9.

24. Leung P, Jubran A, Tobin MJ. Comparison of assisted ventilator modes on triggering, patient effort, and dyspnea. Am J Respir Crit Care Med 1997; 155:1940–8.

25. Marini JJ. Weaning from mechanical ventilation. New Engl J Med 1991; 324:1496–7.

26. Lofaso F, Aslanian P, Richard JC, et al. Expiratory valves used for home devices: Experimental and clinical comparison. Eur Respir J 1998; 11:1382–8.

27. Lofaso F, Brochard L, Hang T, et al. Evaluation of carbon dioxide rebreathing during pressure support with BiPAP devices. Chest 1995; 108:772–8.

28. Mancebo J, Amaro P, Mollo JL, et al. Comparison of the effects of pressure support ventilation delivered by three different ventilators during weaning from mechanical ventilation. Intensive Care Med 1995; 21:913–9.

29. Lessard MR, Brochard L. Assisted ventilation during weaning. Curr Opin Anaesthesiol 1991; 4:266–71.

30. Vitacca M, Barbano L, D'Anna S, et al. Comparison of five bilevel pressure ventilators in patients with chronic ventilatory failure: A physiologic study. Chest 2002; 122:2105–14.

31. Brochard L, Harf A, Lorino H, Lemaire F. Inspiratory pressure support prevents diaphragmatic fatigue during weaning from mechanical ventilation. Am Rev Respir Dis 1989; 139:513–21.

32. Ershowsky P, Krieger B. Changes in breathing pattern during pressure support ventilation. Respir Care 1987; 32:1011–6.

33. Tokioka H, Saito S, Kosaka F. Effect of pressure support ventilation on breathing pattern and respiratory work. Intensive Care Med 1989; 15:491–4.

34. Van de Graaff WB, Gordey K, Dornseif SE, et al. Pressure support: Changes in ventilatory pattern and components of the work of breathing. Chest 1991; 100:1082–9.

35. Hurst J, Branson R, Davis K, Barrette R. Cardiopulmonary effects of pressure support ventilation. Arch Surg 1989; 124:1067–70.

36. MacIntyre N. Pressure support ventilation: Effects on ventilatory reflexes and ventilatory muscle work load. Respir Care 1987; 32:447–57.

37. Tobin MJ, Perez W, Guenther SM, et al. The pattern of breathing during successful and unsuccessful trials of weaning from mechanical ventilation. Am Rev Respir Dis 1986; 134:1111–8.

38. Viale JP, Duperret S, Mahul P, et al. Time course evolution of ventilatory responses to inspiratory unloading in patients. Am J Respir Crit Care Med 1998; 157:428–34.

39. Lofaso F, Isabey D, Lorino H, et al. Respiratory response to positive and negative inspiratory pressure in humans. Respir Physiol 1992; 89:75–88.

40. Giannouli E, Webster K, Roberts D, Younes M. Response of ventilator-dependent patients to different levels of pressure support and proportional assist. Am J Respir Crit Care Med 1999; 159:1716–25.

41. Pesenti A, Rossi N, Calori A, et al. Effects of short-term oxygenation changes on acute lung injury patients undergoing pressure support ventilation. Chest 1993; 103:1185–9.

42. Bonmarchand G, Chevron V, Chopin C, et al. Increased initial flow rate reduces inspiratory work of breathing during pressure support ventilation in patients with exacerbation of chronic obstructive pulmonary disease. Intensive Care Med 1996; 22:1147–54.

43. Lofaso F, Isabey D, Harf A, Scheid P. Airway anesthesia during positive and negative inspiratory pressure breathing in man. Respir Physiol 1992; 89:89–96.

44. Beydon L, Isabey D, Boussignac G, et al. Pressure support ventilation using a new endotracheal gas injection tube. Br J Anaesth 1991; 67:795–800.

45. MacIntyre NR, Leatherman N. Ventilatory muscle load and the frequency–tidal volume pattern during inspiratory pressure-assisted (pressure supported) ventilation. Am Rev Respir Dis 1990; 141:327–31.

46. Parthasarathy S, Tobin MJ. Effect of ventilator mode on sleep quality in critically ill patients. Am J Respir Crit Care Med 2002; 166:1423–9.

47. Valentine DD, Hammond MD, Downs JB, et al. Distribution of ventilation and perfusion with different modes of mechanical ventilation. Am Rev Respir Dis 1991; 143:1262–6.

48. Beydon L, Cinotti L, Rekik N, et al. Changes in the distribution of ventilation and perfusion associated with separation from mechanical ventilation in patients with obstructive pulmonary disease. Anesthesiology 1991; 75:730–8.

49. Diaz O, Iglesia R, Ferrer M, et al. Effects of noninvasive ventilation on pulmonary gas exchange and hemodynamics during acute hypercapnic exacerbations of chronic obstructive pulmonary disease. Am J Respir Crit Care Med 1997; 156:1840–5.

50. Ferrer M, Iglesia R, Roca J, et al. Pulmonary gas exchange response to weaning with pressure-support ventilation in exacerbated chronic obstructive pulmonary disease patients. Intensive Care Med 2002; 28:1595–9.

51. Putensen C, Mutz NJ, Putensen-Himmer G, Zinserling J. Spontaneous breathing during ventilatory support improves ventilation-perfusion distribution in patients with acute respiratory distress syndrome. Am J Respir Crit Car Med 1999; 159:1241–8.

52. Putensen C, Rasanen J, Lopez FA. Interfacing between spontaneous breathing and mechanical ventilation affects ventilation-perfusion distributions in experimental bronchoconstriction. Am J Respir Crit Care Med 1995; 151:993–9.

53. Fargier JJ, Robert D, Boyer F, et al. Positive pressure inspiratory aid vs assisted mechanical ventilation after esophageal surgery. J Crit Care 1987; 2:101–8.

54. Zeravik J, Borg U, Pfeiffer U. Efficacy of pressure support ventilation dependent on extravascular lung water. Chest 1990; 97:1412–9.

55. Hilbert G, Choukroun ML, Benissan GG, et al. Optimal pressure support level for beginning weaning in patients with COPD: Measurement of diaphragmatic activity with step-by-step decreasing pressure support level. J Crit Care 1998; 13:110–8.

56. Viale JP, Annat GJ, Bouffard YM, et al. Oxygen cost of breathing in post-operative patients: Pressure support ventilation vs continuous positive airway pressure. Chest. 1988; 93:506–9.

57. Annat GJ, Viale JP, Derymez CP, et al. Oxygen cost of breathing and diaphragmatic pressure-time index: Measurement in patients with COPD during weaning with pressure support ventilation. Chest 1990; 98:411–4.

58. Beck J, Gottfried SB, Navalesi P, et al. Electrical activity of the diaphragm during pressure support ventilation in acute respiratory failure. Am J Respir Crit Care Med 2001; 164:419–24.

59. Fauroux B, Hart N, Luo YM, et al. Measurement of diaphragm loading during pressure support ventilation. Intensive Care Med 2003; 29:1960–6.

60. Brochard L. Pressure support ventilation. In: Marini JJ, Roussos C, editors. Ventilatory failure. Berlin: Springer-Verlag. 1991: 381–91.

61. Brochard L, Rua F, Lorino H, Lemaire F, Harf A. Inspiratory pressure support compensates for the additional work of breathing caused by the endotracheal tube. Anesthesiology 1991; 75: 739–45.

62. Yang KL, Tobin MJ. A prospective study of indexes predicting the outcome of trials of weaning from mechanical ventilation. New Engl J Med 1991; 324:1445–50.

63. Shapiro M, Wilson RK, Casar G, et al. Work of breathing through different sized endotracheal tubes. Crit Care Med 1986; 14: 1028–31.

64. Moran JL, Homan D, O'Fat Hartaigh M, et al. Inspiratory work imposed by continuous positive airway pressure (CPAP) machines: The effect of CPAP level and endotracheal tube size. Intensive Care Med 1992; 18:148–54.

65. Fiastro JF, Habib MP, Quan SF. Pressure support compensation for inspiratory work due to endotracheal tubes and demand continuous positive airway pressure. Chest 1988; 93:499–505.

66. Nathan SD, Ishaaya AM, Koerner SK, Belman MJ. Prediction of minimal pressure support during weaning from mechanical ventilation. Chest 1993; 103:1215–9.

67. Sassoon CSH, Light RW, Lodia R, et al. Pressure-time product during continuous positive airway pressure, pressure support ventilation and T-piece during weaning from mechanical ventilation. Am Rev Respir Dis 1991; 143:459–75.

68. Sassoon CSH, Lodia R, Rheeman CH, et al. Inspiratory muscle work of breathing during flow-by, demand-flow, and continuous-flow systems in patients with chronic obstructive pulmonary disease. Am Rev Respir 1992; 145:1219–22.

69. Ishaaya AM, Nathan SD, Belman MJ. Work of breathing after extubation. Chest 1995; 107:204–9.

70. Straus C, Louis B, Isabey D, et al. Contribution of the endotracheal tube and the upper airway to breathing workload. Am J Respir Crit Care Med 1998; 157:23–30.

71. Esteban A, Alia I, Gordo F, et al. Extubation outcome after spontaneous breathing trials with T-tube or pressure support ventilation. Am J Respir Crit Care Med 1997; 156:459–65.

72. Farias J-A, Retta A, Alia I, et al. A comparison of two methods to perform a breathing trial before extubation in pediatric intensive care patients. Intensive Care Med 2001; 27:1649–54.

73. Dojat M, Harf A, Touchard D, et al. Evaluation of a knowledge-based system providing ventilatory management and decision for extubation. Am J Respir Crit Car Med 1996; 153:997–1004.

74. Matic I, Majeric-Kogler V. Comparison of pressure support and T-tube weaning from mechanical ventilation: Randomized, prospective study. Croat Med J 2004; 45:162–6.

75. Dennison FH, Taft AA, Mishoe SC, et al. Analysis of resistance to gas flow in nine adult ventilator circuits. Chest 1989; 96: 1374–9.

76. Ploysongsang Y, Branson R, Rashkin MC, Hurst JM. Pressure flow characteristics of commonly used heat-moisture exchangers. Am Rev Respir Dis 1988; 138:675–8.

77. Chiaranda M, Verona L, Pinamonti O, et al. Use of heat and moisture exchanging (HME) filters in mechanically ventilated ICU patients: Influence on airway flow-resistance. Intensive Care Med 1993; 19:462–6.

78. Iotti GA, Olivei MC, Palo A, et al. Unfavorable mechanical effects of heat and moisture exchangers in ventilated patients. Intensive Care Med 1997; 23:399–405.

79. Lellouche F, Maggiore SM, Deye N, et al. Effect of the humidification device on the work of breathing during noninvasive ventilation. Intensive Care Med 2002; 28:1582–9.

80. Iotti GA, Olivei MC, Braschi A. Mechanical effects of heat-moisture exchangers in ventilated patients. Crit Care 1999; 3:R77–82.

81. Le Bourdelles G, Mier L, Fiquet B, et al. Comparison of the effects of heat and moisture exchangers and heated humidifiers on ventilation and gas exchange during weaning trials from mechanical ventilation. Chest 1996; 110:1294–8.

82. Pelosi P, Solca M, Ravagnan I, et al. Effects of heat and moisture exchangers on minute ventilation, ventilatory drive, and work of breathing during pressure-support ventilation in acute respiratory failure. Crit Care Med 1996; 24:1184–8.

83. Campbell RS, Davis K Jr, Johannigman JA, Branson RD. The effects of passive humidifier dead space on respiratory variables in paralyzed and spontaneously breathing patients. Respir Care 2000; 45:306–12.

84. Girault C, Breton L, Richard JC, et al. Mechanical effects of airway humidification devices in difficult to wean patients. Crit Care Med 2003; 31:1306–11.

85. Natalini G, Bardini P, Latronico N, Candiani A. Impact of heat and moisture exchangers on ventilatory pattern and respiratory mechanics in spontaneously breathing patients. Monaldi Arch Chest Dis 1994; 49:561–4.

86. Jaber S, Chanques G, Matecki S, et al. Comparison of the effects of heat and moisture exchangers and heated humidifiers on ventilation and gas exchange during non-invasive ventilation. Intensive Care Med 2002; 28:1590–4.

87. Lellouche F, Pignataro C, Maggiore SM, et al. Influence of the humidification device during non-invasive ventilation. Am J Respir Crit Care Med 2002; 165:A384.

88. Askanazi J, Milic-Emili J, Broell JR, et al. Influence of exercise and CO_2 on breathing pattern of normal man. J Appl Physiol 1979; 47:192–6.

89. Ranieri VM, Giuliani R, Mascia L, et al. Patient-ventilator interaction during acute hypercapnia: Pressure-support vs proportional-assist ventilation. J Appl Physiol 1996; 81:426–36.

90. Hilbert G. Difficult to wean chronic obstructive pulmonary disease patients: Avoid heat and moisture exchangers? Crit Care Med 2003; 31:1580–1.

91. Nava S, Bruschi C, Fracchia C, et al. Patient-ventilator interaction and inspiratory effort during pressure support ventilation in patients with different pathologies. Eur Respir J 1997; 10: 177–83.

92. Nava S, Bruschi C, Rubini F, et al. Respiratory response and inspiratory effort during pressure support ventilation in COPD patients. Intensive Care Med 1995; 21:871–9.

93. Fabry B, Guttmann J, Eberhard L, et al. An analysis of desynchronization between the spontaneously breathing patient and ventilator during inspiratory pressure support. Chest 1995; 107:1387–94.

94. Chao DC, Scheinhorn DJ, Stearn-Hassenpflug M. Patient-ventilator trigger asynchrony in prolonged mechanical ventilation. Chest 1997; 112:1592–9.

95. Thille A, Lellouche F, Brochard L. Patient-ventilator asynchrony during mechanical ventilation: Prevalence and risk factors. Intens Care Med 2004; 30:S71.

96. Nava S, Ambrosino N, Bruschi C, et al. Physiological effects of flow and pressure triggering during non-invasive mechanical ventilation in patients with chronic obstructive pulmonary disease. Thorax 1997; 52:249–54.

97. Ambrosino N, Foglio K, Rubini F, et al. Non-invasive mechanical ventilation in acute respiratory failure due to chronic obstructive pulmonary disease: correlates for success. Thorax 1995; 50: 755–7.

98. Vitacca M, Bianchi L, Zanotti E, et al. Assessment of physiologic variables and subjective comfort under different levels of pressure support ventilation. Chest 2004; 126:851–9.

99. Calderini E, Confalonieri M, Puccio PG, et al. Patient-ventilator asynchrony during noninvasive ventilation: The role of expiratory trigger. Intensive Care Med 1999; 25:662–7.

100. Pertusini E, Lellouche F, Catani F, et al. Patient-ventilator asynchronies during NIV does level of pressure support matter? Intens Care Med 2004; 30:S65.

101. Sassoon CS, Lodia R, Rheeman CH, et al. Inspiratory muscle work of breathing during flow-by, demand-flow, and continuous-flow systems in patients with chronic obstructive pulmonary disease. Am Rev Respir Dis 1992; 145:1219–22.

102. Branson RD, Campbell RS, Davis K Jr, Johnson DJ 2d. Comparison of pressure and flow triggering systems during continuous positive airway pressure. Chest 1994; 106:540–4.

103. Sassoon CS, Gruer SE. Characteristics of the ventilator pressure- and flow-trigger variables. Intensive Care Med 1995; 21:159–68.

104. Ranieri VM, Mascia L, Petruzzelli V, et al. Inspiratory effort and measurement of dynamic intrinsic PEEP in COPD patients: Effects of ventilator triggering systems. Intensive Care Med 1995; 21:896–903.

105. Goulet R, Hess D, Kacmarek RM. Pressure vs flow triggering during pressure support ventilation. Chest 1997; 111:1649–53.

106. MacIntyre NR, Cheng KC, McConnell R. Applied PEEP during pressure support reduces the inspiratory threshold load of intrinsic PEEP. Chest 1997; 111:188–93.

107. Smith TC, Marini JJ. Impact of PEEP on lung mechanics and work of breathing in severe airflow obstruction. J Appl Physiol 1988; 65:1488–99.

108. Rossi A, Gottfried SB, Higgs BD, et al. Respiratory mechanics in mechanically ventilated patients with respiratory failure. J Appl Physiol 1985; 58:1849–58.

109. Brochard L. Intrinsic (or auto-) positive end-expiratory pressure during spontaneous or assisted ventilation. Intensive Care Med 2002; 28:1552–4.

110. Thille A, Lellouche F, Taille S, et al. Incidence des asynchronies patient-ventilateur en ventilation mécanique invasive. Réanimation 2003; 12:243S.

111. Appendini L, Purro A, Patessio A, et al. Partitioning of inspiratory muscle workload and pressure assistance in ventilator-dependent COPD patients. Am J Respir Crit Care Med 1996; 154:1301–9.

112. Vitacca M, Lanini B, Nava S, et al. Inspiratory muscle workload due to dynamic intrinsic PEEP in stable COPD patients: Effects of two different settings of non-invasive pressure-support ventilation. Monaldi Arch Chest Dis 2004; 61:81–5.

113. Fleury B, Murciano D, Talamo C, et al. Work of breathing in patients with chronic obstructive pulmonary disease in acute respiratory failure. Am Rev Respir Dis 1985; 131:822–7.

114. Harf A, Brochard L. Mécanique respiratoire et sevrage. Réanimation Urgences 1992; 1:209–12.

115. Pepe PE, Marini JJ. Occult positive end-expiratory pressure in mechanically ventilated patients with airflow obstruction: The auto-PEEP effect. Am Rev Respir Dis 1982; 216:166–9.

116. Parthasarathy S, Jubran A, Tobin MJ. Cycling of inspiratory and expiratory muscle groups with the ventilator in airflow limitation. Am J Respir Crit Care Med 1998; 158:1471–8.

117. Younes M, Kun J, Webster K, Roberts D. Response of ventilator-dependent patients to delayed opening of exhalation valve. Am J Respir Crit Care Med 2002; 166:21–30.

118. Imanaka H, Nishimura M, Takeuchi M, et al. Autotriggering caused by cardiogenic oscillation during flow-triggered mechanical ventilation. Crit Care Med 2000; 28:402–7.

119. Prinianakis G, Kondili E, Georgopoulos D. Effects of the flow waveform method of triggering and cycling on patient-ventilator interaction during pressure support. Intensive Care Med 2003; 29:1950–9.

120. Jubran A. Inspiratory flow rate: More may not be better. Crit Care Med 1999; 27:670–1.

121. Bonmarchand G, Chevron V, Menard JF, et al. Effects of pressure ramp slope values on the work of breathing during pressure support ventilation in restrictive patients. Crit Care Med 1999; 27:715–22.

122. Tokioka H, Tanaka T, Ishizu T, et al. The effect of breath termination criterion on breathing patterns and the work of breathing during pressure support ventilation. Anesth Analg 2001; 92: 161–5.

123. MacIntyre NR, Ho LI. Effects of initial flow rate and breath termination criteria on pressure support ventilation. Chest 1991; 99:134–8.

124. Messadi AA, Ben Ayed M, Brochard L, et al. Comparison of the efficacy of two waveforms of inspiratory pressure support: Slow versus fast pressure wave (abstract). Am Rev Respir Dis 1990; 141:A519.

125. Braschi A, Iotti G, Rodi G, Salagallini G. Evaluation of the pressure support support function of ventilators (abstract). Intensive Care Med 1988; 14:326.

126. MacIntyre NR, McConnell R, Cheng KC, Sane A. Patient-ventilator flow dyssynchrony: Flow-limited versus pressure-limited breaths. Crit Care Med 1997; 25:1671–7.

127. Chiumello D, Pelosi P, Croci M, et al. The effects of pressurization rate on breathing pattern, work of breathing, gas exchange and patient comfort in pressure support ventilation. Eur Respir J 2001; 18:107–14.

128. Chiumello D, Pelosi P, Taccone P, et al. Effect of different inspiratory rise time and cycling off criteria during pressure support ventilation in patients recovering from acute lung injury. Crit Care Med 2003; 31:2604–10.

129. Prinianakis G, Delmastro M, Carlucci A, et al. Effect of varying the pressurisation rate during noninvasive pressure support ventilation. Eur Respir J 2004; 23:314–20.

130. Corne S, Gillespie D, Roberts D, Younes M. Effect of inspiratory flow rate on respiratory rate in intubated ventilated patients. Am J Respir Crit Care Med 1997; 156:304–8.

131. Laghi F, Segal J, Choe WK, Tobin MJ. Effect of imposed inflation time on respiratory frequency and hyperinflation in patients with chronic obstructive pulmonary disease. Am J Respir Crit Care Med 2001; 163:1365–70.

132. Spahija J, de Marchie M, Bellemare P, et al. Patient-ventilator interaction during pressure support ventilation and neurally adjusted ventilatory assist in acute respiratory failure. Proceedings of the American Thoracic Society, 2005; 2:A847.

133. Younes M. Proportional assist ventilation and pressure support ventilation: Similarities and differences. Intensive Care Emerg Med 1991; 15:361–80.

134. Braschi A, Sala Gallini G, Rodi G, et al. Relationships between sensitivity of the expiratory trigger and breathing pattern during pressure support ventilation (abstract). Am Rev Respir Dis 1989; 139:A361.

135. Imsand C, Feihl F, Perret C, Fitting J. Aide inspiratoire: Le critère utilisé pour détecter la fin de l'inspiration est-il édéquat (abstract)? Réanimation Urgences 1992; 1:995.

136. Tassaux D, Michotte J, Gainnier M, Jolliet P. Effects of adjustable expiratory trigger on delayed cycling during pressure support in obstructive disease. Am J Respir Crit Care Med 2003; 167:A301.

137. Yamada Y, Du HL. Analysis of the mechanisms of expiratory asynchrony in pressure support ventilation: A mathematical approach. J Appl Physiol 2000; 88:2143–50.

138. Jubran A, Van de Graaff WB, Tobin MJ. Variability of patient-ventilator interaction with pressure support ventilation in patients with chronic obstructive pulmonary disease. Am J Respir Crit Care Med 1995; 152:129–36.

139. Lessard MR, Lofaso F, Brochard L. Expiratory muscle activity increases intrinsic positive end-expiratory pressure independently of dynamic hyperinflation in mechanically ventilated patients. Am J Respir Crit Care Med 1995; 151:562–9.

140. Antonelli M, Conti G, Pelosi P, et al. New treatment of acute hypoxemic respiratory failure: Noninvasive pressure support ventilation delivered by helmet—A pilot controlled trial. Crit Care Med 2002; 30:602–8.

141. Hotchkiss JR Jr, Adams AB, Stone MK, et al. Oscillations and noise: Inherent instability of pressure support ventilation? Am J Respir Crit Care Med 2002; 165:47–53.

142. Branson R. Understanding and implementing advances in ventilator capabilities. Curr Opin Crit Care 2004; 10:23–32.

143. Du HL, Amato MB, Yamada Y. Automation of expiratory trigger sensitivity in pressure support ventilation. Respir Care Clin North Am 2001; 7:503–17.

144. Du HL, Ohtsuji M, Shigeta M, et al. Expiratory asynchrony in proportional assist ventilation. Am J Respir Crit Care Med 2002; 165:972–7.

145. Kamat S, Dulfano M, Segal M. The effects of intermittent positive pressure breathing (IPPB/I) with compressed air in patients with severe chronic nonspecific obstructive pulmonary disease. Am Rev Respir Dis 1932; 86:360–80.

146. Ayres S, Kozam R, Lukas D. The effects of intermittent positive pressure breathing on intrathoracic pressure, pulmonary mechanics, and the work of breathing. Am Rev Respir Dis 1963; 87:370–9.

147. Sukumalchantra Y, Park S, Williams MJ. The effects of intermittent positive pressure breathing (IPPB) in acute ventilatory failure. Am Rev Respir Dis 1965; 92:885–93.

148. Jones R, McNamara J, Gaensler E. The effects of intermittent positive pressure breathing on simulated pulmonary obstruction. Am Rev Respir Dis 1960; 92:885–93.

149. Mancebo J, Isabey D, Lorino H, et al. Comparative effects of pressure support ventilation and intermittent positive pressure breathing (IPPB) in non intubated healthy subjects. Eur Respir J 1995; 8:1901–9.

150. Dreyfuss D, Saumon G. Ventilator-induced lung injury: Lessons from experimental studies. Am J Respir Crit Care Med 1998; 157:294–323.

151. Dreyfuss D, Saumon G. From ventilator-induced lung injury to multiple organ dysfunction? Intensive Care Med 1998; 24: 102–4.

152. Cinnella G, Conti G, Lofaso F, et al. Effects of assisted ventilation on the work of breathing: Volume-controlled versus pressure-controlled ventilation. Am J Respir Crit Care Med 1996; 153:1025–33.

153. Weisman IM, Rinaldo JE, Rogers RM, Sanders MH. Intermittent mandatory ventilation. Am Rev Respir Dis 1983; 127:641–7.

154. Schachter EN, Tucker D, Beck CJ. Does intermittent mandatory ventilation accelerate weaning? JAMA 1981; 246:1210–4.

155. Marini JJ, Smith TC, Lamb VT. External work output and force generation during synchronized intermittent mechanical ventilation. Am Rev Respir Dis 1988; 138:1169–79.

156. Imsand C, Feihl F, Perret C, Fitting J. Effect of assisted ventilation in SIMV mode on inspiratory muscle activity (abstract). Am Rev Respir Dis 1991; 143:A603.

157. Knebel AR, Janson-Bjerklie SL, Malley JD, et al. Comparison of breathing comfort during weaning with two ventilatory modes. Am J Respir Crit Care Med 1994; 149:14–8.

158. Uchiyama A, Imanaka H, Taenaka N. Relationship between work of breathing provided by a ventilator and patients' inspiratory drive during pressure support ventilation: Effects of inspiratory rise time. Anaesth Intensive Care 2001; 29:349–58.

159. Uchiyama A, Imanaka H, Taenaka N, et al. Comparative evaluation of diaphragmatic activity during pressure support ventilation and intermittent mandatory ventilation in animal model. Am J Respir Crit Care Med 1994; 150:1564–8.

160. Tobin MJ, Jubran A, Laghi F. Patient-ventilator interaction. Am J Respir Crit Care Med 2001; 163:1059–63.

161. Younes M. Proportional assist ventilation, a new approach to ventilatory support: I. Theory. Am Rev Respir Dis 1992; 145:114–20.

162. Younes M, Puddy A, Roberts D, et al. Proportional assist ventilation: Results of an initial clinical trial. Am Rev Respir Dis 1992; 145:121–9.

163. Gay PC, Hess DR, Hill NS. Noninvasive proportional assist ventilation for acute respiratory insufficiency: Comparison with pressure support ventilation. Am J Respir Crit Care Med 2001; 164:1606–11.

164. Fernandez-Vivas M, Caturla-Such J, Gonzalez de la Rosa J, et al. Noninvasive pressure support versus proportional assist ventilation in acute respiratory failure. Intensive Care Med 2003; 29:1126–33.

165. Ambrosino N, Rossi A. Proportional assist ventilation (PAV): A significant advance or a futile struggle between logic and practice? Thorax 2002; 57:272–6.

166. Vitacca M. New things are not always better: Proportional assist ventilation vs pressure support ventilation. Intensive Care Med 2003; 29:1038–40.

167. Branson RD, Johannigman JA. What is the evidence base for the newer ventilation modes? Respir Care 2004; 49:742–60.

168. Younes M. Proportional assist ventilation. In: Tobin MJ, editor. Principles and practice of mechanical ventilation. New York: McGraw-Hill, 1994: 349–69.

169. Grasso S, Puntillo F, Mascia L, et al. Compensation for increase in respiratory workload during mechanical ventilation: Pressure-support versus proportional-assist ventilation. Am J Respir Crit Care Med 2000; 161:819–26.

170. Wysocki M, Meshaka P, Richard JC, Similowski T. Proportional-assist ventilation compared with pressure-support ventilation during exercise in volunteers with external thoracic restriction. Crit Care Med 2004; 32:409–14.

171. Mols G, von Ungern-Sternberg B, Rohr E, et al. Respiratory comfort and breathing pattern during volume proportional assist ventilation and pressure support ventilation: A study on volunteers with artificially reduced compliance. Crit Care Med 2000; 28:1940–6.

172. Bigatello LM, Nishimura M, Imanaka H, et al. Unloading of the work of breathing by proportional assist ventilation in a lung model. Crit Care Med 1997; 25:267–72.

173. Sinderby C, Navalesi P, Beck J, et al. Neural control of mechanical ventilation in respiratory failure. Nature Med 1999; 5:1433–6.

174. Navalesi P, Hernandez P, Wongsa A, et al. Proportional assist ventilation in acute respiratory failure: Effects on breathing pattern and inspiratory effort. Am J Respir Crit Care Med 1996; 154:1330–8.

175. Passam F, Hoing S, Prinianakis G, et al. Effect of different levels of pressure support and proportional assist ventilation on breathing pattern, work of breathing and gas exchange in mechanically ventilated hypercapnic COPD patients with acute respiratory failure. Respiration 2003; 70:355–61.

176. Purro A, Appendini L, De Gaetano A, et al. Physiologic determinants of ventilator dependence in long-term mechanically ventilated patients. Am J Respir Crit Car Med 2000; 161:1115–23.

177. Wrigge H, Golisch W, Zinserling J, et al. Proportional assist versus pressure support ventilation: Effects on breathing pattern and respiratory work of patients with chronic obstructive pulmonary disease. Intensive Care Med 1999; 25:790–8.

178. Wysocki M, Richard JC, Meshaka P. Noninvasive proportional assist ventilation compared with noninvasive pressure support ventilation in hypercapnic acute respiratory failure. Crit Care Med 2002; 30:323–9.

179. Porta R, Appendini L, Vitacca M, et al. Mask proportional assist vs pressure support ventilation in patients in clinically stable condition with chronic ventilatory failure. Chest 2002; 122:479–88.

180. Delaere S, Roeseler J, D'Hoore W, et al. Respiratory muscle workload in intubated, spontaneously breathing patients without COPD: Pressure support vs proportional assist ventilation. Intensive Care Med 2003; 29:949–54.

181. Ranieri VM, Grasso S, Mascia L, et al. Effects of proportional assist ventilation on inspiratory muscle effort in patients with chronic obstructive pulmonary disease and acute respiratory failure. Anesthesiology 1997; 86:79–91.

182. Ambrosino N, Vitacca M, Polese G, et al. Short-term effects of nasal proportional assist ventilation in patients with chronic hypercapnic respiratory insufficiency. Eur Respir J 1997; 10:2829–34.

183. Bianchi L, Foglio K, Pagani M, et al. Effects of proportional assist ventilation on exercise tolerance in COPD patients with chronic hypercapnia. Eur Respir J 1998; 11:422–7.

184. Hernandez P, Maltais F, Gursahaney A, et al. Proportional assist ventilation may improve exercise performance in severe chronic obstructive pulmonary disease. J Cardiopulm Rehabil 2001; 21:135–42.

185. Mitrouska J, Xirouchaki N, Patakas D, et al. Effects of chemical feedback on respiratory motor and ventilatory output during different modes of assisted mechanical ventilation. Eur Respir J 1999; 13:873–82.

186. Hart N, Hunt A, Polkey MI, et al. Comparison of proportional assist ventilation and pressure support ventilation in chronic respiratory failure due to neuromuscular and chest wall deformity. Thorax 2002; 57:979–81.

187. Younes M, Kun J, Masiowski B, et al. A method for noninvasive determination of inspiratory resistance during proportional assist ventilation. Am J Respir Crit Care Med 2001; 163:829–39.

188. Younes M, Webster K, Kun J, et al. A method for measuring passive elastance during proportional assist ventilation. Am J Respir Crit Care Med 2001; 164:50–60.

189. Beck KC, Offord KP, Scanlon PD. Comparison of four methods for calculating diffusing capacity by the single breath method. Chest 1994; 105:594–600.

190. Tassaux D, Michotte JB, Gainnier M, et al. Expiratory trigger setting in pressure support ventilation: From mathematical model to bedside. Crit Care Med 2004; 32:1844–50.

191. Spahija J, Beck J, de Marchie M, et al. Closed-loop control of respiratory drive using pressure support ventilation:target drive ventilation. Am J Respir Crit Care Med 2005; 171:1009–14.

192. Delafosse B, Bouffard Y, Viale JP, et al. Respiratory changes induced by parenteral nutrition in postoperative patients undergoing inspiratory pressure support ventilation. Anesthesiology 1987; 66:393–6.

193. Fassoulaki A, Eforakopoulorr M. Cardiovascular, respiratory and metabolic changes produced by pressure-supported ventilation in intensive care patients. Crit Care Med 1989; 17:527–9.

194. Wong D, Stemmer E, Gordon I. Acute massive air leak and pressure support ventilation. Crit Care Med 1990; 18:114–5.

195. Brochard L, Rauss A, Benito S, et al. Comparison of three methods of gradual withdrawal from ventilatory support during weaning from mechanical ventilation. Am J Respir Crit Care Med 1994; 150:896–903.

196. Esteban A, Frutos F, Tobin MJ, et al. A comparison of four methods of weaning patients from mechanical ventilation. Spanish Lung Failure Collaborative Group. New Engl J Med 1995; 332:345–50.

197. MacIntyre NR. Weaning from mechanical ventilatory support: Volume-assisting intermittent breaths versus pressure-assisting every breath. Respir Care 1988; 33:121–5.

198. Hörmann C, Baum M, Luz G, et al. Tidal volume, breathing frequency and oxygen consumption at different pressure support levels in the early stage of weaning in patients without chronic obstructive pulmonary disease. Intensive Care Med 1992; 18:226–30.

199. Boyer F, Bruneau B, Gaussorgues P, et al. Aide inspiratoire avec asservissement du niveau de pression: Volume ventilé minute versus fréquence ventilatoire. Rean Soins Intens Med Urgence 1989; 5.

200. Ranieri VM. Optimization of patient-ventilator interactions: Closed-loop technology to turn the century. Intensive Care Med 1997; 23:936–9.

201. Branson R, MacIntyre NR. Dual-control modes of mechanical ventilation. Respir Care 1996; 41:294–305.

202. Keenan H, Martin L. Volume support ventilation in infants and children: Analysis of a case series. Respir Care 1997; 42:281–7.

203. Sottiaux T. Patient-ventilator interactions during volume-support ventilation: Asynchrony and tidal volume instability—A report of three cases. Respir Care 2001; 46:255–62.

204. Randolph AG, Wypij D, Venkataraman ST, et al. Effect of mechanical ventilator weaning protocols on respiratory outcomes

in infants and children: A randomized, controlled trial. JAMA 2002; 288:2561–8.

205. Jaber S, Delay J-M, Matecki S, et al. Volume-guaranteed pressure-support ventilation facing acute changes in ventilatory demand. Intensive Care Med 2005; 31:1181–8.

206. Dojat M, Brochard L, Lemaire F, Harf A. A knowledge based system for assisted ventilation of patients in intensive care units. Int J Clin Monit Comput 1992; 9:239–50.

207. Dojat M, Harf A, Lemaire F, Brochard L. Evaluation of an expert system providing ventilatory management and decision of weaning from mechanical ventilation (abstract). Int J Clin Monit Comput 1992; 18:S64.

208. Strickland JH, Hasson JH. A computer-controlled ventilator weaning system. Chest 1991; 100:1096–9.

209. Strickland JH, Hasson JH. A computer-controlled ventilator weaning system. Chest 1993; 103:1220–6.

210. Brunner JX. Principles and history of closed-loop controlled ventilation. Respir Care Clin North Am 2001; 7:341–62.

211. Dojat M, Brochard L. Knowledge-based systems for automatic ventilatory management. Respir Care Clin North Am 2001; 7:379–96.

212. Nemoto T, Hatzakis GE, Thorpe CW, et al. Automatic control of pressure support mechanical ventilation using fuzzy logic. Am J Respir Crit Care Med 1999; 160:550–6.

213. Dojat M, Harf A, Touchard D, et al. Clinical evaluation of a computer-controlled pressure support mode. Am J Respir Crit Car Med 2000; 161:1161–6.

214. Bouadma L, Lellouche F, Cabello M, et al. A computer driven system to manage weaning during prolonged mechanical ventilation: a pilot study. Intensive Care Med 2005; 31:1446–50.

215. Lellouche F, Mancebo J, Roesler J, et al. Computer-driven ventilation reduces duration of weaning: A multicenter randomized, controlled study. Intensive Care Med 2004; 30:S1–S234.

216. Gluck E, Eubanks DH, Bone RC. Techniques for weaning a patient from mechanical ventilation: When to begin, what method to use, and how to predict outcome. J Crit Illness 1993; 8:121–9.

217. Vitacca M, Vianello A, Colombo D, et al. Comparison of two methods for weaning patients with chronic obstructive pulmonary disease requiring mechanical ventilation for more than 15 days. Am J Respir Crit Care Med 2001; 164:225–30.

218. Leger P, Jennequin J, Gaussorgues P, Robert D. Acute respiratory failure in COPD patient treated with noninvasive intermittent mechanical ventilation (control mode) with nasal mask. Am Rev Respir Dis 1988; 137:A63.

219. Brochard L, Isabey D, Piquet J, et al. Reversal of acute exacerbations of chronic obstructive lung disease by inspiratory assistance with a face mask. New Engl J Med 1990; 323:1523–30.

220. Antonelli M, Conti G, Rocco M, et al. A comparison of noninvasive positive-pressure ventilation and conventional mechanical ventilation in patients with acute respiratory failure. New Engl J Med 1998; 339:429–35.

221. Girou E, Schortgen F, Delclaux C, et al. Association of noninvasive ventilation with nosocomial infections and survival in critically ill patients. JAMA 2000; 284:2361–7.

222. Hilbert G, Gruson D, Vargas F, et al. Noninvasive ventilation in immunosuppressed patients with pulmonary infiltrates, fever, and acute respiratory failure. New Engl J Med 2001; 344:481–7.

223. Nava S, Ambrosino N, Clini E, et al. Noninvasive mechanical ventilation in the weaning of patients with respiratory failure due to chronic obstructive pulmonary disease: A randomized, controlled trial. Ann Intern Med 1998; 128:721–8.

224. Mehta S, Hill NS. Noninvasive ventilation. Am J Respir Crit Care Med 2001; 163:540–77.

225. Maltais F, Reissmann H, Ernst P, Gottfried SB. Pressure support improves exercise performance in severe COPD (abstract). Am Rev Respir Dis 1991; 143:A170.

226. Carlucci A, Richard JC, Wysocki M, et al. Noninvasive versus conventional mechanical ventilation: An epidemiologic survey. Am J Respir Crit Care Med 2001; 163:874–80.

227. Girault C, Richard JC, Chevron V, et al. Comparative physiologic effects of noninvasive assist-control and pressure support ventilation in acute hypercapnic respiratory failure. Chest 1997; 111:1639–48.

228. Brochard L, Mancebo J, Wysocki M, et al. Noninvasive ventilation for acute exacerbations of chronic obstructive pulmonary disease. New Engl J Med 1995; 333:817–22.

229. Hoo GW, Williams AJ. Noninvasive face-mask mechanical ventilation in patients with acute hypercapnic respiratory failure. Chest 1993; 103:1304–5.

230. Anton A, Guell R, Gomez J, et al. Predicting the result of noninvasive ventilation in severe acute exacerbations of patients with chronic airflow limitation. Chest 2000; 117:828–33.

231. Poponick JM, Renston JP, Bennett RP, Emerman CL. Use of a ventilatory support system (BiPAP) for acute respiratory failure in the emergency department. Chest 1999; 116:166–71.

232. Soo Hoo GW, Santiago S, Williams AJ. Nasal mechanical ventilation for hypercapnic respiratory failure in chronic obstructive pulmonary disease: Determinants of success and failure. Crit Care Med 1994; 22:1253–61.

233. L'Her E, Taillé S, Deye N, et al. Physiological response of hypoxemic patients to different modes of non-invasive ventilation. Intensive Care Med 2002; 28:S49.

234. Demoule A, Taillé S, Lellouche F, et al. Non-invasive ventilation. Results from a 2002 new french survey. Am J Respir Crit Care Med 2003; 167:A863.

235. Navalesi P, Fanfulla F, Frigerio P, et al. Physiologic evaluation of noninvasive mechanical ventilation delivered with three types of masks in patients with chronic hypercapnic respiratory failure. Crit Care Med 2000; 28:1785–90.

236. Lellouche F, Fraticelli A, Taillé S, et al. Physiological evaluation of five interfaces during non-invasive ventilation. Am J Respir Crit Care Med 2003; 167:A995.

237. Fraticelli A, Lellouche F, Taillé S, et al. Comparison of different interfaces during NIV in patients with acute respiratory failure. Am J Respir Crit Care Med 2003; 167:A863.

238. Girault C, Daudenthun I, Chevron V, et al. Noninvasive ventilation as a systematic extubation and weaning technique in acute-on-chronic respiratory failure: A prospective, randomized controlled study. Am J Respir Crit Care Med 1999; 160:86–92.

239. Vitacca M, Ambrosino N, Clini E, et al. Physiological response to pressure support ventilation delivered before and after extubation in patients not capable of totally spontaneous autonomous breathing. Am J Respir Crit Care Med 2001; 164:638–41.

Chapter 10 _____

PRESSURE-CONTROLLED AND INVERSE-RATIO VENTILATION

MARCELO B. P. AMATO
JOHN J. MARINI

**TYPES OF CONTROLLED VENTILATION AND
  SELECTION OF THE "CONTROLLED" PARAMETER**
**SPECIFIC CHARACTERISTICS OF
  PRESSURE-CONTROLLED VENTILATION**
  Input Parameters of PCV
  Mean Airway and Alveolar Pressures
  Output Variables of PCV
PHYSIOLOGIC EFFECTS OF PCV
  Advantages of Controlling Airway Pressures
  The controversy on Optimal Distribution of
    Ventilation
  Assisted Versus Controlled (Time-Triggered)
    Ventilation
**VARIANTS OF PCV AND ACTIVATION
  OF EXHALATION VALVE**
  Assisted PCV
  Activation of Exhalation Valve During PCV:
    Airway Pressure-Release Ventilation
  Combined Modes
INVERSE-RATIO VENTILATION
  Implementing Inverse-Ratio Ventilation
  Later Comparative Studies on IRV
  Effects of Total PEEP and ϕ_{aw} on Oxygenation
  Intrinsic PEEP Versus Extrinsic PEEP
  Other Effects of IRV
  Drawbacks
CONCLUSION

The use of pressure-controlled ventilation (PCV) has increased dramatically in the last 10 years. Behind this growing usage, there is an increased awareness of intensivists about the phenomenon of ventilator-induced lung injury and the associated risks of high inspiratory pressures. The recent familiarity with the concept of permissive hypercapnia contributed to this change in attitude, helping physicians to relax about the old and stringent limits for arterial blood gases.[1-3] Tidal volume or minute ventilation requirements were left progressively as secondary goals. Physicians learned that critically ill patients have a surprisingly good tolerance against elevated carbon dioxide (CO_2) levels.[1-3] Recent surveys in intensive-care units (ICUs) around the world have demonstrated that PCV is no longer a pure experimental mode; it is now used in up to 25% of patients receiving prolonged mechanical ventilation, usually

in the most severe cases[4] and including pediatric patients.[5] Many publications address the implications of PCV on the cardiovascular system, work of breathing, regional mechanics, and the risks of ventilator-induced lung injury, which increase physicians' comfort in moving away from volume-controlled ventilation.

In contrast to the growing acceptance of PCV, use of inverse-ratio ventilation (IRV)—that is, the prolongation of inspiratory time to the point of inverting the conventional inspiratory-to-expiratory (I:E) ratio—has declined in the last decade. In 1971, Reynolds[6] reported that ventilation with an extended inspiratory time improved oxygenation in neonates with hyaline membrane disease. A decade later, several investigators embraced this idea, repeatedly showing oxygenation benefits in adults with acute respiratory distress syndrome (ARDS).[7-12] Most studies applied IRV in conjunction with pressure-controlled breaths (PC-IRV) to minimize the risk of overinflation. Initial enthusiasm was followed by a period of skepticism, when investigators suggested that the benefits of IRV could be better ascribed to the generation of intrinsic positive end-expiratory pressure (intrinsic PEEP) or purely to increased alveolar pressures.[13-16] In subsequent comparative studies in patients with ARDS, when equivalent mean airway pressures were applied by different approaches, IRV produced worse oxygenation than did ventilation with conventional I:E ratios plus external positive end-expiratory pressure (external PEEP).[17,18] Over the years, concerns were raised repeatedly about hemodynamic deterioration, elevated mean airway pressures,[14] regional overinflation of lung units,[19,20] and difficulty with clinical implementation of this complex mode in everyday care.[21] The final result was progressive discrediting and a change of focus: Instead of IRV, systematic application of external PEEP and recruiting maneuvers started to receive closer attention.[22,23]

The perspective we present in this chapter is not going to change this scenario. We believe that IRV should be viewed primarily as an experimental mode with few clinical indications. There are safer, more predictable, and more efficient ventilatory solutions to be implemented at the bedside. We also believe that close examination of the rationale and evidence behind the apparently contradictory reports on PC-IRV offers insights on the pathophysiology of injured lungs. Therefore, besides describing our general approach to PCV and its variants, we discuss the history and progressive evidence gathered on IRV.

Types of Controlled Ventilation and Selection of the "Controlled" Parameter

Ventilators currently available regulate either the pressure profile applied in the airways or the pattern of flow delivery. Somewhat imprecisely, flow-controlled ventilation has been designated "volume-controlled" ventilation (VCV). We avoid this convention because the criterion by which the ventilator ceases to pressurize the airway (initiates deflation) may be a specified value of delivered volume, pressure, elapsed time, or flow. The parameter, however, actively controlled by the ventilator during "volume-controlled" breaths is in reality inspiratory flow. Therefore, the modes of ventilation currently used in medical practice should be classified as either *pressure-* or *flow-controlled* and as *time-, volume-, flow-,* or *pressure-cycled.* Pressure-support ventilation (PSV) is an example of a pressure-controlled, *flow-cycled* mode, whereas PCV is an example of pressure-controlled, *time-cycled* mode.

In flow-controlled modes, the waveform theoretically can be of any desired contour; in clinical practice, however, the flow waveforms usually are rectilinear (square), linearly decelerating, and sinusoidal. Setting tidal volume as the "off switch" criterion (*volume-cycled*) means that the pressure applied to the airway opening can rise to any value required by the impedance to inflation that does not exceed the pressure-limit alarm. Very high absolute (if not transmural) alveolar pressures can develop during expulsive efforts or bouts of coughing.

Although once used extensively, *pressure-cycled* ventilation is now considered obsolete for continuous support, and its application in intermittent positive-pressure breathing (IPPB) has been restricted greatly. Currently, pressure cycling serves primarily as a backup cycling-off criterion during flow-controlled, *volume-cycled* ventilation (when airway pressures reach a preset alarm threshold).

In an attempt to improve safety or to decrease the need for repeated adjustments at the bedside, flow- and pressure-controlled algorithms have been combined recently to form new modes (such as "volume-assured pressure support" and "pressure-regulated volume control"), incorporating the desirable characteristics of each category.[24,25]

The equation of motion of the respiratory system confines the clinician to setting independently the inspiratory flow and tidal volume or just the applied pressure profile. Flow and pressure cannot be selected independently at the same time because their relationship is defined by the mechanical properties of the respiratory system. Because modern ventilators can provide online feedback information about output variables (airway pressures during flow-controlled ventilation or flow and tidal volume during pressure-controlled ventilation), either flow-controlled, *volume-cycled* ventilation (VCV) or pressure-controlled, *time-cycled* ventilation (PCV) can be used effectively and interchangeably during specific conditions. For instance, instead of using the original pressure-control algorithms during IRV, some investigators have proposed the equivalent use of IRV through flow-controlled, *volume-cycled* (VCV) breaths,[26] with careful monitoring and frequent readjustments. Depending on particular combinations of compliance and resistance in the respiratory system, the pressure profile generated in the airways can be similar in both modes.

The major differences between *flow-* versus *pressure-*controlled breaths appear during prolonged use, after unpredictable changes in respiratory system characteristics. By using the traditional flow-controlled, *volume-cycled* mode, minute ventilation is guaranteed safely over prolonged periods of time, although airway pressures may rise significantly when respiratory system impedance increases. Conversely, during prolonged use of pressure-controlled, *time-cycled* ventilation, airway pressure limits are guaranteed, although minute ventilation is at risk whenever lung impedance changes.

Independent of selection of the controlled parameter, inspiration can be triggered by elapsed time or by small perturbations in pressure/flow in the airways (usually indicative of patient effort). The former case defines a totally controlled breath, whereas the latter case defines an assisted (i.e., patient-triggered) breath. In recent years, modern ventilators have incorporated algorithms providing pressure-controlled breaths triggered by either elapsed expiratory time, characterizing traditional PCV, or patient effort (*assisted* pressure-controlled ventilation), analogous to the traditional flow-controlled assist-control ventilation (ACV).

Specific Characteristics of Pressure-Controlled Ventilation

Many recently introduced ventilator modes can be considered as variants of pressure-controlled or *pressure-preset* ventilation. This includes traditional PCV,[8,27] pressure-support ventilation,[28,29] biphasic continuous positive airway pressure (BiPAP), and variants of airway pressure-release ventilation.[30,31] In some modes, spontaneous respiratory efforts continue. In others, none occur. These modes vary both in their intended objectives and in their criteria for initiating and terminating the machine's inspiratory cycle. Yet all can be viewed as modes in which the machine applies approximately square waves of pressure to the airway opening. In concept, any pressure profile can be regulated. In current practice, however, most *pressure-controlled* modes build pressure rapidly, toward a preset value, attempting to maintain pressure nearly constant throughout the remainder of the higher-pressure phase. During exhalation, pressure is released abruptly, allowing passive deflation to occur unimpeded or against a set PEEP level. By fixing the level of applied pressure during inspiration, the physician imposes an upper limit to the machine's energy transferred to lung tissue and to the machine component of ventilation that can be achieved.

The specifics of the new pressure-controlled modes are discussed in other chapters. The physical principles governing pressure-controlled, *time-cycled* ventilation—which serves as the prototype for this group—and its major "outcome" variables, such as tidal volume, minute ventilation, and intrinsic PEEP, are addressed here. Some discussion of the concepts of mean airway pressure (ϕ_{aw}) and mean alveolar pressure (ϕ_A) also will be presented because these concepts are essential tools for understanding the physiologic implications of all pressure-controlled modes.

INPUT PARAMETERS OF PCV

Apart from the external PEEP, the clinician sets only three parameters in PCV: the applied inspiratory pressure, backup or mandatory frequency, and fractional inspiratory time (duty cycle, T_I/T_{TOT}). The most salient feature of PCV is that maximal airway and alveolar pressures are restricted by the cap of preset pressure, whereas tidal volume, flow, minute volume, and alveolar ventilation depend on the impedance of the respiratory system in conjunction with the three input variables just described. Once the impedance (i.e., the resistance and compliance characteristics) of the respiratory system is known, the machine's contributions to ventilation and alveolar pressure can be characterized completely from knowledge of just those three input parameters.

Machines vary in the rapidity (*rise time* or *inspiratory slope*) with which airway pressure builds toward the preset maximum value. Faster rates of pressurization are needed in certain situations when flow demands are high (during assisted *pressure-controlled* ventilation) or during low-impedance conditions (in large patients) because of machine limitations. A more gradual pressure buildup is appropriate for quiet breathing and during high-impedance conditions. Some newer machines allow the clinician to adjust rise time to suit the situation at hand, whereas others adjust it automatically.

With most machines today, physicians set the pressure increment above external PEEP to be applied during inspiration. This means that absolute inspiratory pressures increase as external PEEP increases. With a few machines, the physician has to set the absolute inspiratory pressure, which is independent of external PEEP.

MEAN AIRWAY AND ALVEOLAR PRESSURES

When considering a plot of airway-opening pressure (Paw) over time, mean airway pressure is the integral of Paw over time divided by the time span of the breath. Two input parameters that the clinician sets during PCV bear direct relationships to mean airway pressure (ϕ_{aw}): preset inspiratory pressure and T_I/T_{TOT}. Because of the square waveform of pressure during PCV, ϕ_{aw} can be expressed simply as

$$\phi_{aw} = Pset \times T_I/T_{TOT} + PEEP_E \times (1 - T_I/T_{TOT}) \quad (1)$$

where $PEEP_E$ is external PEEP. Therefore, variations in either set pressure (Pset) or T_I/T_{TOT} influence ϕ_{aw} predictably. Frequency variations leave ϕ_{aw} unaffected.[32,33] Under passive conditions, airway pressure represents the total pressure applied across the respiratory system. It can be demonstrated mathematically that this applied pressure, when averaged over both phases of the respiratory cycle, is everywhere the same along the airway once phasic differences are accounted for in nonelastic pressure losses.[32,33] Therefore, mean alveolar pressure (ϕ_A) can be easily estimated from ϕ_{aw} once inspiratory and expiratory resistances are known:

$$\phi_A = \phi_{aw} + \dot{V}_E(R_E - R_I) \quad (2)$$

where R_E and R_I are mean expiratory and mean inspiratory resistances, respectively, and $\dot{V}_E$ is the minute ventilation.

Some practical conclusions can be drawn from this simple formulation. First, changing frequency alters mean alveolar pressure very little if inspiratory and expiratory resis-

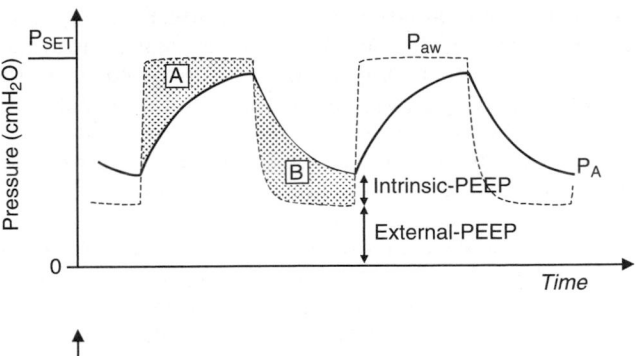

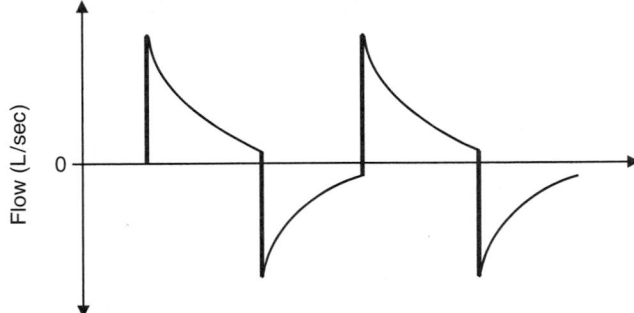

FIGURE 10-1 Airway opening pressure (Paw), alveolar pressure (P$_A$), and flow during pressure-controlled ventilation. Intrinsic PEEP presents a backpressure that opposes the applied pressure (Pset) and reduces the effective ventilating pressure, which is equal to Pset − total PEEP (total PEEP = intrinsic PEEP + extrinsic PEEP). Areas *A* and *B* represent the pressure-time product dissipated during inspiration and exhalation, respectively. These areas are proportional to mean inspiratory and expiratory resistances.

tances are similar. In this particular situation, mean airway pressures will reflect alveolar pressures consistently. Conversely, when expiratory resistance exceeds inspiratory resistance, a frequent condition in chronic obstructive lung disease, mean airway pressures can seriously underestimate mean alveolar pressures, especially when minute ventilation is high. Under such conditions, variations in frequency do influence mean alveolar pressure, and physicians easily could overlook the hemodynamic consequences of a ventilator setting.

Figure 10-1 illustrates some additional features related to alveolar and airway pressures during PCV. Alveolar pressure (P$_A$) can rise no higher than Pset, the pressure to which it equilibrates at end inspiration when sufficient inspiratory time is provided (in Fig. 10-1 there is no equilibrium). Peak P$_A$ falls rather than rises with increasing frequency. One also can grasp from the figure that intrinsic PEEP increases with increasing frequency, reducing the *effective* ventilating pressure (Pset − total PEEP) and consequently reducing tidal volume. As frequency increases further, P$_A$ oscillations decline to the point that ϕ_A sets the upper bounding value for intrinsic PEEP.

Under conditions of passive inflation, mean airway pressure reflects the average distending pressure of the respiratory system. Understandably, therefore, mean airway pressure has been associated with two beneficial physiologic effects (ventilation and oxygenation) and three potentially noxious effects (hemodynamic compromise, fluid retention, and barotrauma). These effects, however, are nonlinear, and there are exceptions. For instance, as discussed later, the relationship between ϕ_{aw} and oxygenation is very dependent on the extent of pressure-volume hysteresis of the lung, which is greatly affected by lung disease. The greater the hysteresis, the greater is the dependency of oxygenation on PEEP and previous lung history (i.e., the maximum alveolar pressure achieved in previous breaths), and the looser is the correlation between the current ϕ_{aw} and oxygenation. In situations of negligible lung hysteresis, for instance, during partial liquid ventilation, the correlation between ϕ_{aw} and oxygenation is straightforward.[34] The complex relationship between ϕ_{aw} and oxygenation will be further elaborated in the discussion of IRV below.

Mean airway pressure is also a measurable correlate of the backpressure for venous return. Raising ϕ_A during passive ventilation increases both lung and chest volumes by similar amounts. Lung expansion tends to increase right-ventricular afterload, which is already high in many patients with acute respiratory failure. More important, the increase in intrapleural pressure raises right-atrial pressure, often impeding venous return. Rising backpressure can have clinical consequences in patients with impaired systemic venous tone and reduced tissue turgor (e.g., consequent to sedation/paralysis). Sodium and water retention also tends to correlate with the magnitude of ϕ_{aw}. Although the place of ϕ_A in the *generation* of barotrauma is not clear, a high level of ϕ_A may *exacerbate* damage or *accentuate* gas leakage through rents in the alveolar tissues, thereby bringing barotrauma to clinical attention.

OUTPUT VARIABLES OF PCV

As discussed earlier, the major "output" variables of PCV are tidal volume, inspiratory flow, minute ventilation, intrinsic PEEP, and ϕ_A.

TIDAL VOLUME

When maximal airway pressure is preset, the tidal volume actually delivered varies with several key variables: the pressure gradient existing between the airway opening and the alveolus at the onset of inflation, the resistance to airflow, the compliance of the respiratory system, and the time available for inspiration. Theoretically, inspiratory time should be longer than the three time constants of the respiratory system to allow near-complete (>95%) lung filling, thus maximizing delivered tidal volume. This scenario would guarantee that alveolar pressures are in equilibrium with airway pressures at the end of inspiration. In adult patients with orotracheal intubation, equilibration usually requires 1.0–1.5 seconds of inspiration. In the presence of severe obstructive lung disease, this value can be as high as 4–5 seconds. In order to improve synchrony during *assisted* PCV, sometimes it is necessary to match the spontaneous inspiratory time of the patient. In this case, inspiratory time rarely should exceed 1.2 seconds, usually resulting in incomplete lung filling but promoting comfort.

Any residual end-expiratory pressure (intrinsic PEEP) detracts from the total pressure difference available to accomplish ventilation (*driving pressure*). Therefore, incomplete lung emptying is also an important factor affecting the delivered tidal volume. To allow near-complete lung emptying, expiratory time should be longer than the three expiratory time constants. The aggravating factor is that expiratory resistance is usually higher than inspiratory resistance, implying that the expiratory time constants are longer. An expiratory time shorter than 1.5 seconds in an adult patient should be considered a potential source of intrinsic PEEP, reducing the potential for tidal volume delivery.

INTRINSIC PEEP

Intrinsic PEEP (auto-PEEP) that results from dynamic hyperinflation is a complex function of the input parameters of PCV in conjunction with the impedance characteristics of the respiratory system.[35] The general principles affecting it can be summarized as follows: (1) higher-frequency, longer T_I/T_{TOT} ratio and higher Pset tend to increase intrinsic PEEP, (2) increments in T_I/T_{TOT} cause a monotonic increase in intrinsic PEEP from external PEEP up to Pset, (3) pure increments in frequency also cause an increase in intrinsic PEEP but with a saturation effect that limits intrinsic PEEP to half (approximately) the range between external PEEP and Pset which arises because as frequency rises, inspiratory time is curtailed, preventing equilibration between applied airway and alveolar pressures, keeping maximum PA well below Pset; (see Fig. 10-2), and (4) the higher the compliance and the higher the expiratory resistance, the higher is the intrinsic PEEP for the same input parameters. Figure 10-2 illustrates some of these relationships.

FIGURE 10-2 Effect of frequency on intrinsic PEEP generation during PCV. Three impedance combinations with moderate airflow obstruction and varying respiratory system compliance (expressed in ml/cmH₂O). A decrease in compliance causes both a reduction in intrinsic PEEP and alteration in the curvature of the intrinsic PEEP/frequency relationship. Note that curves converge to an asymptote at 10 cmH₂O, which corresponds to approximately half Pset. *Simulated conditions:* Pset = 20 cmH₂O above PEEP; T_I/T_{TOT} = 0.4; R_E = 25 cmH₂O/liter/s. (*Adapted, with permission, from Marini et al: Am Rev Respir Dis 147:14–24, 1993.*)

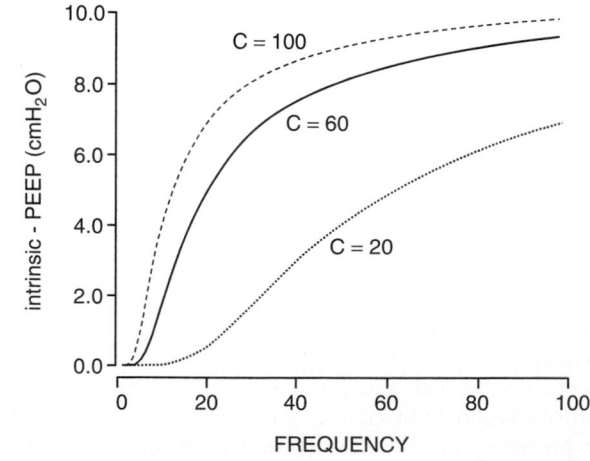

MINUTE VENTILATION

The relationships just described are responsible for important and nonintuitive effects on minute ventilation (Figs. 10-3 and 10-4). When frequency increases at constant values for Pset and T_I/T_{TOT}, the durations of inspiration and expiration both decrease, and intrinsic PEEP rises. As tidal volume falls, minute ventilation exponentially approaches an upper bound mainly determined by resistance.[35] In obstructed adult patients breathing at respiratory rates above

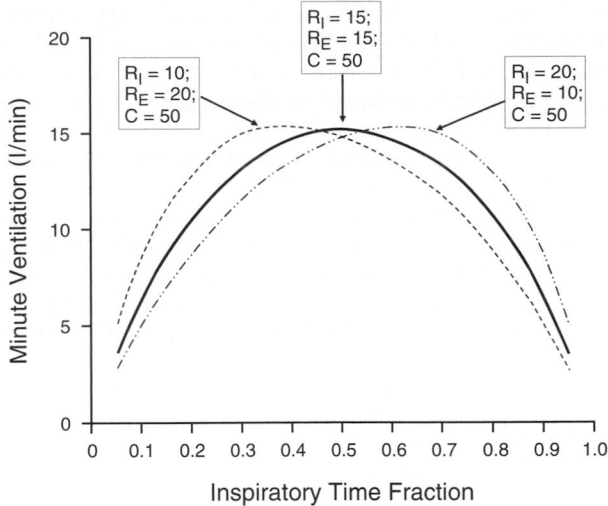

FIGURE 10-4 Effect of inspiratory time fraction (T_I/T_{TOT}) on minute ventilation according to the balance between inspiratory and expiratory resistances (R_I and R_E, respectively). As is true for tidal volume, the apogee of the curve is reached at $T_I/T_{TOT} = 0.5$, provided that $R_I = R_E$. Note that optimal T_I/T_{TOT} is shifted leftward when $R_E > R_I$, exemplifying a common situation in clinical practice. (*Adapted, with permission, from Marini et al: J Appl Physiol 67:1081–92, 1989.*)

40 breaths per minute, changes in compliance have a minor influence on minute ventilation generation. For instance, a decrease in compliance from 100–50 ml/cmH$_2$O will produce a maximum fall in minute ventilation of 10%. Figure 10-3 suggests that in patients with moderate to severe airway obstruction (resistance ≥ 25 cmH$_2$O/liter/s), the benefits of increasing respiratory rate above 12 breaths per minute is negligible (this is an important hint when ventilating patients with asthma). The situation changes considerably, however, under conditions of low compliance (≤ 25 ml/cmH$_2$O), provided that respiratory rates do not exceed 40 breaths per minute: Any increment in frequency becomes an effective mechanism to increase minute ventilation (see Fig. 10-3, *top*).

Important differences between obstructed and restricted patients also can be seen in the relationship between minute ventilation and duty cycle. Minute ventilation becomes very sensitive to changes in duty cycle for obstructed patients but not for restrictive patients. As shown in Fig. 10-4, if one wants to maximize minute ventilation for a given Pset (a common target during intensive care of patients with asthma), T_I/T_{TOT} has to be titrated according to the ratio between inspiratory and expiratory resistances. For patients with fixed obstruction and equivalent values for inspiratory and expiratory resistances, the ideal T_I/T_{TOT} is 0.5.

ALVEOLAR VENTILATION

Over the lower frequency range, increasing frequency tends to improve alveolar as well as total ventilation, decreasing arterial P$_{CO_2}$; however, the same is not necessarily true when high frequencies are used. As frequency rises at a fixed T_I/T_{TOT}, inspiratory time is curtailed, preventing equilibration between applied airway and alveolar pressures.

FIGURE 10-3 (*Upper plot*) Effect of frequency on minute ventilation during PCV. An increase in frequency causes tidal volume to fall so that minute ventilation approaches a mathematically defined plateau value mainly determined by the applied pressure and resistance. The approach is more gradual for a restrictive ventilatory defect with low compliance. (*Bottom plot*) Unlike minute ventilation in the obstructed condition, for which a distinctly optimal T_I/T_{TOT} is evident, minute ventilation in the restricted condition remains essentially unaffected by changes in this parameter. *Simulated conditions:* Pset = 20 cmH$_2$O above PEEP; T_I/T_{TOT} = 0.4; restrictive, C = 20 ml/cmH$_2$O, $R_I = R_E$ = 10 cmH$_2$O/liter/s; obstructed, C = 100 ml/cmH$_2$O, R_I = 15, R_E = 45 cmH$_2$O/liter/s. (*Adapted, with permission, from Marini et al: A general mathematical model for respiratory dynamics relevant to the clinical setting. Am Rev Respir Dis 147:14–24, 1993.*).

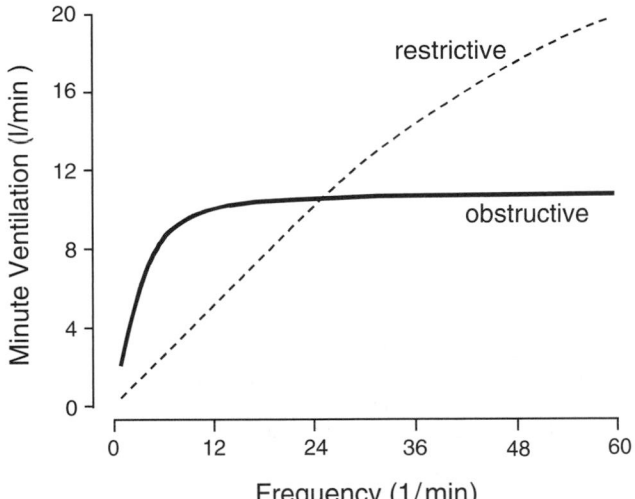

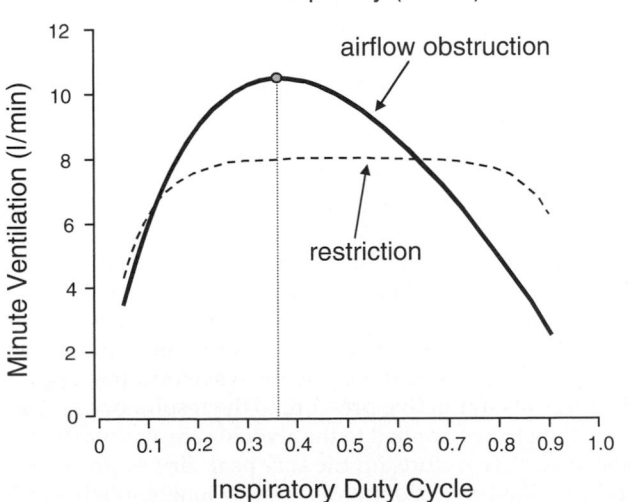

From a practical standpoint, the ventilator itself becomes less able to generate the nominal pressure waveform, especially when flow impedance is low. As tidal volume declines, the wasted fraction of each breath (V_D/V_T) increases owing to the predominance of the series ("anatomic") dead-space component. Under certain conditions, this increase in dead space actually may cause Pa_{CO_2} to rise rather than fall with increasing frequency.[36] In practical terms, there is an important message for the bedside: For a given Pset and T_I/T_{TOT}, increments in frequency may cause a decrease in Pa_{CO_2} up to the point that tidal volume decreases more than approximately 25%. Beyond this limit, even when minute ventilation increases with frequency, it is almost certain that further increments in frequency will be counterproductive because of excessive amounts of dead space.

Because the principles just outlined are rooted in physics and mathematics, hypercapnia can be an unavoidable consequence of a pressure-targeted strategy for managing acute lung injury.

INSPIRATORY FLOW

Decelerating inspiratory flow necessarily is observed during pressure-controlled breaths with rectilinear pressure waveforms—provided that there is no patient effort. Under such conditions, the theoretical maximum of flow associated with a squarewave of pressure (Pset) depends on inspiratory resistance (R_I) and end-expiratory alveolar pressure ($PEEP_{TOT}$) and is achieved at inflation onset:

$$\text{Peak flow} = \frac{P_{set} - PEEP_{TOT}}{R_I} \qquad (3)$$

where $PEEP_{TOT}$ = (intrinsic PEEP + external PEEP). In practice, however, the abruptness of the rise to the nominal peak value is a set characteristic of the particular ventilator, which may be modulated by the *slope* or *inspiratory rise-time* adjustment. Under conditions of quiet breathing, a precipitous buildup to peak flow often is associated with some pressure overshoot, which may be annoying for monitoring purposes because of alarm triggering. Because most of this pressure overshoot represents pressure dissipation as frictional work across the endotracheal tube, it does not cause elevation of peak alveolar pressure and probably is *not* associated with any harm.

Conversely, under high flow demands (especially in large patients), a slow "attack rate" up to peak flow can cause some pressure undershoot or a slow ramp of pressure at the initial phase of the breath, forcing the patient to expend considerable effort or delaying filling of the lung.[37] Because of limitations in the hardware controlling system, the flow performance of most ventilators tends to be poor when Pset is less than 10 cmH$_2$O. Under such conditions, maximizing rise time or slightly increasing Pset can be very helpful.

The decelerating-flow pattern found in PCV usually improves the distribution of ventilation and limits the end-inspiratory gradient of regional pressures among units with heterogeneous time constants. When inspiratory time is long enough, inspiratory flow may decrease down to zero before exhalation, a phenomenon that further favors redis-tribution of air/pressure among heterogeneous units and collateral ventilation. The consequences of such a flow profile are reflected mainly in the CO_2 eliminated per breath (Fig. 10-5). The longer the inspiratory time, the more effective is the clearance of CO_2, although most of the benefit may be seen already when T_I slightly exceeds the point of zero flow (see Fig. 10-5). This topic will be discussed further in the section about distribution of ventilation below.

The effects of resistance and compliance on flow profile are illustrated in Figs. 10-6 and 10-7. Because of the consequent increase in time constant, increments in resistance tend to reduce peak flow, producing a less decelerating (more squared) flow pattern and rendering tidal volume very sensitive to reductions in inspiratory time. In contrast, decrements in compliance tend to accelerate flow decay. It is obvious, therefore, that restrictive patients tolerate a shorter inspiratory time without marked consequences to their tidal volume.

Physiologic Effects of PCV

ADVANTAGES OF CONTROLLING AIRWAY PRESSURES

One of the major features of PCV is that peak alveolar pressure cannot rise any higher than Pset. In critical situations, when one attempts to minimize ventilator-induced lung injury, this aspect of PCV may be very convenient. Specifying the maximum achievable alveolar pressure, however, does not cap the upper limit for *transalveolar* pressure unless the patient's own breathing efforts also have been silenced. As suggested by many studies, transalveolar pressure, rather than alveolar pressure, is the key determinant of ventilator-induced lung injury and barotrauma.[38]

In the absence of patient efforts, keeping peak alveolar pressures within a safe range makes sense. Under these circumstances, controlling airway pressure effectively controls maximal alveolar pressure. Obviously, the same peak alveolar pressure always can be achieved by flow-controlled, volume-cycled ventilation, although more bedside adjustments are necessary. The subtle difference here is that by selecting *pressure* as the controlling parameter, the physician better defines the priority of his or her strategy (i.e., to minimize peak alveolar pressure at the expense of minute ventilation and possible hypercapnia) and probably minimizes violations to the target during ongoing tidal ventilation (see below).

When thinking in peak alveolar pressures as opposed to peak airway pressures, it is important to stress some important aspects of PCV. When inspiratory time is brief, end-inspiratory airway and alveolar pressures fail to equilibrate, so the maximal alveolar pressure is considerably *less* than the set value. This is reflected by persistent end-inspiratory flow. For a given inspiratory time and peak airway pressure, however, PCV is the waveform that applies the greatest cumulative pressure to the respiratory system. Stretching forces applied to the alveolus are also maximally sustained.[39] Therefore, for the *same* peak airway pressure—and provided that inspiratory time is long enough—PCV

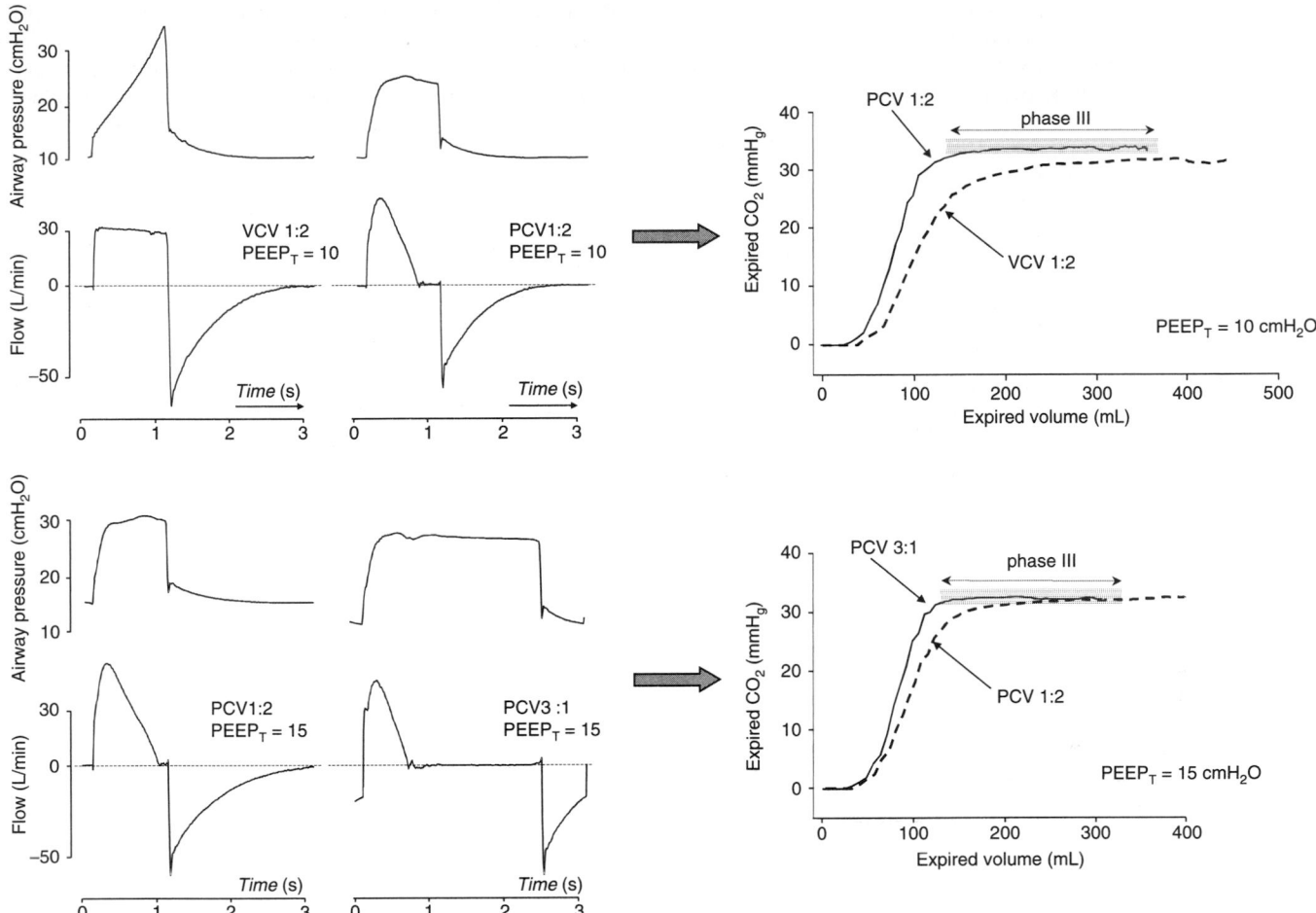

FIGURE 10-5 Effects of inspiratory flow profile on CO_2 elimination per breath (CO_2 single-breath tests obtained in a mainstream capnograph). (*Top*) The change from *flow-controlled, volume-cycled* ventilation (VCV) to PCV, while keeping the same inspiratory time, resulted in more efficient elimination of CO_2 per breath, reflected by the large area under the curve of CO_2 versus exhaled-volume (especially in the first 200 ml—and consequently reflecting a lower dead space). Note that inspiratory flow decayed to zero before exhalation and that phase 3 slope is almost flat during PCV, reflecting less heterogeneity among lung units. Arterial P_{CO_2} was the same (38 mmHg) in both conditions, despite the lower tidal volume during PCV. (*Bottom*) Changing PCV with I:E ratio = 1:2 to PCV 3:1 (when part of external PEEP was replaced by intrinsic PEEP) resulted in a further increase in the area under the curve of CO_2 versus exhaled volume. The benefit, however, was much less evident than in the top panel.

generates a higher peak alveolar pressure than VCV (flow-controlled, volume-cycled breaths delivered with a square-wave profile).

The consequences of PCV on mean airway pressure (ϕ_{aw}) were discussed earlier. It is an important parameter for evaluating the hemodynamic consequences of PCV. Unlike in flow-controlled VCV, ϕ_{aw} relates linearly to Pset and T_I/T_{TOT} (see Eq. 1). As its defining equation indicates, ϕ_{aw} is unaffected by changes of respiratory system impedance and frequency. Provided that changes in inspiratory and expiratory resistance are roughly balanced, mean alveolar pressures follow mean airway pressures very consistently. Consequently, the impact of setting selections on ϕ_{aw} and ϕ_A can be predicted and controlled easily during PCV much more than during VCV.

Such a straightforward relationship between ϕ_{aw} and the input parameters of PCV may be convenient during short-term procedures such as recruiting maneuvers. By adjusting

PEEP, Pset, and T_I/T_{TOT}, one can easily predict the generated ϕ_{aw} (or ϕ_A) and hence the hemodynamic consequences. Recent studies have demonstrated the relative safety of recruitment maneuvers using PCV for 1–2 minutes, which achieved the same efficacy as sustained pressure maneuvers (CPAP) adjusted to equivalent Pset.[40–42] Because the motor of effective recruitment is the surpassing of threshold opening pressures of terminal airspaces,[43] applied long enough to overcome the forces of viscosity and adhesion,[44] repeated cyclic pressurizations with PCV provide an interesting alternative. Theoretically, the only requirement is to adjust Pset above the threshold opening pressures, set PEEP above the closing pressures, and ensure that inspiratory time is long enough to favor slow, sequential stepwise recruitment of clumps of alveolar units.[43] As suggested by Neumann et al,[45] inspiratory times exceeding 0.6 second (ideally closer to 4 seconds)—for instance, obtained during PCV with a frequency of 8–10 breaths per minute and an I:E ratio of

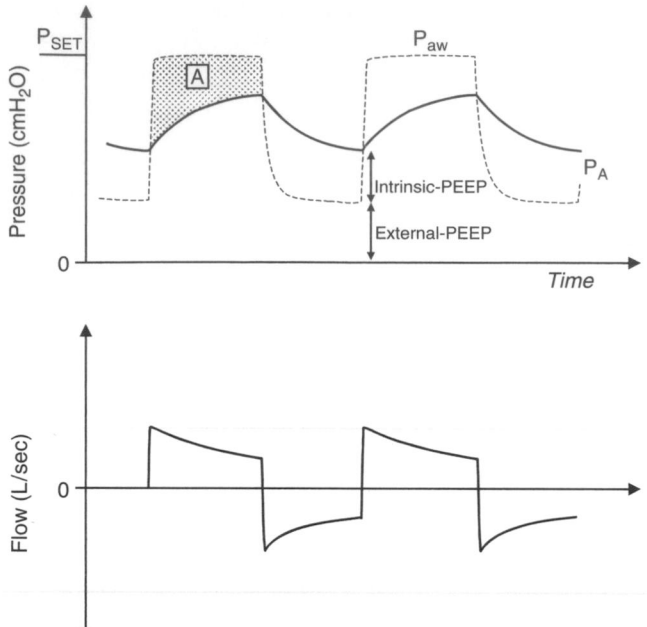

FIGURE 10-6 Typical tracings in an obstructed patient receiving PCV. Note that the flow pattern resembles a square waveform, mimicking flow-controlled, volume-cycled ventilation. Intrinsic PEEP is evident, and end-inspiratory alveolar pressures are much lower than end-inspiratory airway pressures.

FIGURE 10-7 Typical tracings observed in a restricted patient receiving PCV. Note that inspiratory flow decelerates quickly, achieving zero-flow conditions well before the end of inspiration (generating a small area A; compare with Fig. 10-6). There is no intrinsic PEEP, and end-inspiratory alveolar pressures equilibrate with end-inspiratory airway pressures.

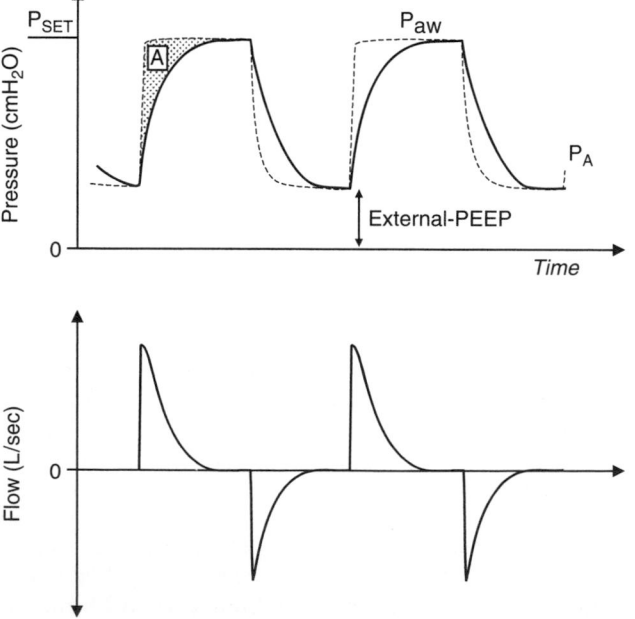

1:1—would be enough to maximize the potential for recruitment at a certain Pset. The great appeal of such PCV maneuvers is their good hemodynamic tolerance: Because ϕ_{aw} generated during a PCV maneuver is usually less than ϕ_{aw} generated during a CPAP maneuver (at equivalent Pset), the hemodynamic consequences are less pronounced.[40,42] Preceding volume expansion with colloids further improves hemodynamic tolerance of the maneuver.[42]

Some investigators, such as Schreiter et al,[46] have applied PCV recruiting maneuvers over much shorter periods (~10 seconds) but reached higher inspiratory pressures (50–80 cmH$_2$O) and reported good success in patients with severe chest trauma. Comparative data of the relative efficacy/safety of such shorter, more intensive application of recruiting pressures versus longer (1–2 minutes) application of less intensive (45–60 cmH$_2$O) recruiting pressures[47–49] do not exist currently.

As with any time-cycled mode of ventilation, PCV invites dyssynchrony when the patient breathes spontaneously. The implications of slow *rising-time* settings was discussed earlier. It is important to think about the other end of the inflation period, however, when the airway continues to be pressurized to the nominal value until the set inspiratory time has elapsed. As with flow-controlled VCV, the patient may attempt to cycle to expiration before the ventilator completes its pressurization cycle. One could imagine, however, that unlike the situation with flow-controlled ventilation, patient effort never could force airway pressure higher than the preset value during PCV. Unfortunately, this is not always true (see immediately below) because of hardware limitations in some ventilators. Notwithstanding these limitations, conflicts between the rhythms of the patient and ventilator are manifested during PCV much more as curtailment of tidal volume rather than as buildup of excessive system pressure.

Another feature related to dyssynchrony is the fact that by fixing T_I, as required with many commercial ventilators, one allows T_I/T_{TOT} to vary with frequency whenever the patient retains control of the cycling rhythm. As frequency increases, T_I/T_{TOT} lengthens, often provoking dynamic overinflation and generation of intrinsic PEEP. Even with ventilators in which the direct input is "duty cycle," most of them calculate the inspiratory time based on the *set* frequency rather than on *measured* frequency. Therefore, the resulting T_I/T_{TOT} can be very different from the originally set T_I/T_{TOT}.

THE CONTROVERSY ON OPTIMAL DISTRIBUTION OF VENTILATION

Several studies have attempted to demonstrate a definitive advantage of PCV over VCV (squared flow pattern) in terms of ventilation distribution, oxygenation, hemodynamics, lung injury, and patient outcome. At first glance, results seem inconclusive. By separating the studies according to key ventilator parameters measured, however, some consistency emerges. First, it is important to distinguish studies that compare PCV-IRV from studies comparing PCV with normal I:E ratio versus other modes. As discussed below, the effects of IRV are complex and depend on intrinsic PEEP generation. Under such conditions, the choice of the controller (*flow* versus *pressure*) is just a minor issue inside a complex picture. Second, it is important to observe whether all the remaining variables (I:E ratio, tidal volume, intrinsic PEEP, total PEEP, frequency, and O_2 fraction) were kept constant during the comparison and whether they were consistent. For example, studies displaying different plateau pressures or tidal volumes during PCV and VCV hardly can be considered to be perfectly matched if one is interested in the effects on oxygenation[50] or lung overdistension.[51]

Keeping such boundaries in mind and first considering only the effects of a pure change in the controller from squared *flow control* to squared *pressure control* (keeping exactly the same I:E ratio, tidal volume, frequency, total PEEP, and plateau pressure), most studies have demonstrated that

- The resulting decelerating flow during PCV decreases peak airway pressures but increases ϕ_{aw}.[15,16,19,27,51–55]
- Pa_{CO_2} and V_D/V_T decrease slightly ($\Delta Pa_{CO_2} \sim 2$–4 mmHg), with modest clinical significance,[15,27,52,53,55] in accordance with the example shown in Fig. 10-5.
- Minor, if any, changes in dynamic (within the breath) or static lung aeration (end-expiratory or end-inspiratory pause) are observed by computed tomography.[19,51,54]
- Minor changes are seen in Pa_{O_2},[15,19,56] slightly favoring PCV.[27,55,57,58]
- No hemodynamic impairment is seen on switching from VCV to PCV, provided that the increments in ϕ_{aw} are moderate (usually the case when using I:E < 1:1).
- No differences are seen in barotrauma or patient outcome.[58] Studies suggesting benefit of PCV had imbalanced randomization,[56] whereas a study suggesting benefit of VCV was poorly controlled (including crossovers and rescue procedures).[59]

Taken together, the evidence suggests a clear physiologic difference between the two modes of flow delivery, although the clinical implications are modest. At the bedside, the most consistent effects are a reduction of peak inspiratory airway pressures, increase in ϕ_{aw}, and small reduction in Pa_{CO_2}. Because of the increment in ϕ_{aw}, Pa_{O_2} tends to increase with PCV, but this depends on PEEP and plateau pressure in the particular case (see Fig. 10-9*b*).

Some concerns are raised repeatedly about the potential generation of greater shear forces at the beginning of inspiration during decelerating-flow patterns. It is suggested that the squared flow waveform might distribute stress more evenly throughout inspiration, theoretically decreasing ventilator-induced lung injury. This hypothesis, however, appears groundless today. The isolated effects of high inspiratory flow rates on ventilator-induced lung injury[62–66] have been investigated. Two studies suggested a deleterious effect,[65,67] whereas other studies suggested a neutral or protective effect.[63,64,66] Because deleterious effects could be demonstrated only under extreme experimental conditions, it is unlikely that the early peak flow achieved during PCV (rarely exceeding 1.5 liters/s because of resistance of the endotracheal tube) causes harm.

Very likely, consistent differences in ventilator-induced lung injury will never be linked to PCV as opposed to VCV. Isolated short-term changes in the controller, from flow to pressure control, probably can induce very mild perturbations in the effective stress applied on the parenchyma. When compared with the potential for iatrogenic damage associated with minor changes in plateau pressures, total PEEP, or pleural pressures commonly found in clinical practice, the controller option may be insignificant.

As discussed earlier, with adequate feedback it is usually possible to obtain the same ventilator output with either a *flow controller* or a *pressure controller* under very specific and restrained conditions. Therefore, a flow-controlled breath with a decelerating-flow waveform can be generated easily by modern ventilators, mimicking some of the physiologic effects of PCV.[55,68] Because it is practically impossible, however, to match the degree of deceleration with the impedance characteristics of different patients (e.g., obstructed patients would require less accentuated deceleration), peak airway pressures frequently are higher during such pressure-control "imitations."[68,69]

Considering the evidence presented, we again suggest that the choice for PCV should be decided in terms of a bedside strategy and not based on subtle physiologic differences. Only in the context of a global strategy do such minor details make a difference. For instance, in a thin patient who requires high PEEP to minimally oxygenate and who also has high dead space and requires plateau pressures greater than 40 cmH_2O to avoid excessive hypercapnia, a strategy prioritizing strict control of transpulmonary pressure makes sense. In this scenario, changing from VCV to PCV might be appropriate because (1) plateau pressures will not exceed the physician-adjusted Pset, (2) considering the entire duration of mechanical ventilation, the number of violations to the Pset target probably will be lower, (3) any decrease in dead space afforded by decelerating flow may allow further reduction in tidal volumes and plateau pressures, (4) an eventual rise in respiratory rate triggered by the patient will not be translated into increased plateau pressures despite the possible generation of intrinsic PEEP, and (5) paralyzing agents and sedation thus may be reduced.

Such advantages, however, may be nullified quickly if spontaneous efforts are excessive. By decreasing pleural pressures, diaphragmatic activity may cause transpulmonary pressures to be excessive despite rigid control of maximum alveolar pressures (capped at Pset). Therefore, after evaluating the spontaneous tidal volume generated by a patient (i.e., observing the extra tidal volume generated during a synchronous effort), one should estimate the extra driving pressure generated by muscle contraction and reduce Pset accordingly. Not observing these principles can make PCV more dangerous than VCV. In fact, during strong patient efforts, a *flow controller* avoids excessive transpulmonary pressure more efficiently than a *pressure controller* simply because airway pressures more closely follow changes in pleural pressure, being transiently reduced during patient effort (i.e., there is no extra "demand" flow to maintain airway pressure).

ASSISTED VERSUS CONTROLLED (TIME-TRIGGERED) VENTILATION

Most reasons to control ventilation can be classified as needs to regulate the ventilatory pattern, reduce agitation and the O_2 cost of breathing, or prevent excursions of the injured chest wall. Perhaps the most common indication is to provide maximal ventilator support to a patient with such marginal cardiorespiratory reserve that breathing efforts compromise comfort, gas exchange, or cardiac function. Reducing O_2 consumption in a patient with critical coronary ischemia, for example, may prove lifesaving, especially in the setting of circulatory shock or acute pulmonary edema. Silencing ventilatory effort also can improve arterial oxygenation and lung volume recruitment in agitated patients with ARDS.[70–72] Controlling minute volume to achieve hyperventilation may be appropriate when reductions in cerebral blood volume and intracranial pressure are urgent priorities, such as after closed-head injury. Controlling ventilation greatly facilitates the monitoring of respiratory mechanics but in itself is seldom sufficient reason to undertake deep sedation or pharmacologic paralysis.

Apart from reducing O_2 consumption and preventing spontaneous efforts from interfering with intended patterns of *conventional* ventilation, establishing ventilatory control facilitates the therapeutic application of "nonphysiologic" breathing patterns. Interventions such as IRV,[7,11] independent lung ventilation,[73] continuous-flow ventilation,[74] and permissive hypercapnia[1–3,75] usually require silencing patient effort.

Sedation is virtually always needed to establish ventilatory control in the conscious patient with moderate to high minute ventilation requirements. Overriding the spontaneous respiratory rate of the patient is always possible but usually results in intrinsic PEEP and wasted ventilation. Use of sedation to improve comfort or inhibit excessive respiratory drive is common practice. Muscle relaxants should be used sparingly, however, because of their injurious potential. These agents must not be used in the conscious or lightly sedated patient.

Better understanding of the sequelae of prolonged paralysis, especially when associated with sepsis and systemic inflammation,[76] high-dose corticosteroids, and hyperglycemia,[77,78] has forced physicians to minimize dosage and duration of paralysis in ventilated patients. Recent work suggests that severe diaphragmatic dysfunction occurs after only 2–3 days of controlled mechanical ventilation,[79,80] independent of the use of paralyzing agents, with loss of more than 40% of power generation. It is likely that paralyzing agents potentialize or trigger such effects[81] by blocking a protective mechanism against atrophy (maintenance of minimal muscle activity). Independent of its precise mechanism, critical illness polyneuropathy, which frequently is associated with diaphragmatic dysfunction, increases the duration of mechanical ventilation and intensive-care stay significantly.[82]

Given such evidence, deep sedation with short-acting sedative drugs is preferable to any form of paralysis. Paralytics should not be used to totally suppress muscle activity but instead to weaken the force of patient effort. Another strategy is to use intermittent dosing, giving only as much as is needed to suppress excessive muscular activity. The periodic withdrawal of paralytics also enables sedation adequacy to be better determined. With either technique, total isolation of the muscle from neural impulses should be avoided. This is also true for sedative agents. Totally controlled ventilation may lead to muscle atrophy with or without paralysis.[80]

Recent evidence suggests that calm assisted ventilation, with efforts just sufficient to trigger the ventilator, can avoid excessive muscle wasting.[80] Because spontaneous efforts also can improve lung aeration during pressure-controlled breaths,[83] probably secondary to increased diaphragmatic tone, it is tempting to conclude that some level of spontaneous effort always should be promoted in patients receiving PCV. An anticipated drawback of such a strategy is an undesirable increase in I:E ratio when the patient respiratory rate is much higher than the set respiratory rate. Another problem is the generation of unpredictably high transpulmonary pressures during strong and synchronous effort by the patient. In both circumstances, however, deeper sedation or partial paralysis could control the situation easily. By keeping the spontaneous respiratory rate close to the set rate, one easily can avoid changes in the I:E ratio. Also, by keeping the exhaled tidal volume close to the tidal volume generated during totally controlled breaths, one may ensure that a patient's spontaneous effort does not cause significant increments in inspiratory transpulmonary pressures.

Variants of PCV and Activation of Exhalation Valve

As discussed earlier, the variants of traditional PCV[8,27] include assisted pressure-controlled ventilation,[84] pressure-support ventilation,[28,29] and variants of airway pressure-release ventilation.[30,31]

ASSISTED PCV

Assisted PCV is similar to pressure-support ventilation (PSV) in that the breaths can be triggered by the patient (physicians set the sensitivity and triggering mechanism). The difference is that cycling off is determined by time instead of flow. Another obvious difference is that assisted PCV possesses the same backup mechanism available with traditional assisted flow-controlled breaths: Breaths can be triggered by patient effort or by elapsed expiratory time, whichever occurs first.

Compared with assisted VCV at equivalent tidal volumes, assisted PCV decreases peak airway pressures. Although irrelevant during invasive ventilation, this characteristic is relevant during noninvasive ventilation, minimizing leaks through the mask[85] or avoiding uncomfortably high pressures in the upper airways.[86] When comparing the level of patient assistance during invasive ventilation, the characteristic decelerating flow (*on demand*) provided by PCV seems to reduce workload more efficiently than most flow-controlled, volume-cycled breaths.[84] The reduction in inspiratory muscle load is especially prominent during moderate tidal volume (8 ml/kg) ventilation or when inspiratory flow rates are set at low levels during VCV (<0.7 liter/s).

The algorithm configured for assisted PCV also may carry some advantages over PSV. First, in patients with unstable respiratory drive, the backup rate works as a safety and stabilizing mechanism, avoiding central apneas and sleep fragmentation, especially in patients with cardiac failure or in those receiving heavy sedation.[87] Second, although PSV is popular during noninvasive ventilation, serious concerns have been raised about potential dyssynchrony at end inspiration. During PSV, transition from inspiration to expiration is triggered by flow (i.e., when inspiratory flow decays below a certain threshold). Hence the presence of mask leaks or severe airway obstruction can render this mechanism inefficient—both conditions falsely create a relatively high inspiratory flow at end inspiration. Leaks simply mislead the inspiratory flow regulator of the ventilator, which cannot detect that inspiratory flow is not being delivered to patient. Conversely, severe obstruction changes the shape of inspiratory flow (see Fig. 10-6), making it less decelerating and pushing end-inspiratory flows closer to peak flow. With both conditions, the default expiratory triggering threshold for PSV (usually 25% of peak inspiratory flow) may never be reached, causing excessive prolongation of inspiratory time and patient overinflation.[88] Under such conditions, pressure-controlled, *time-cycled* ventilation could be convenient: The intensivist needs only to adjust inspiratory time to match the patient's spontaneous inspiratory time, usually 0.6–1.2 seconds.[88] By changing from PSV to PCV, the intensivist necessarily decreases the freedom of ventilation pattern (restraining, for instance, the possibility of a spontaneous sigh and potentially increasing discomfort) but also avoids dangerous prolongation of inspiratory time.[88] This is a difficult balance that has to be judged at the bedside.

During assisted PCV, especially under high flow demands, a fast "attack rate" to peak flow (at the initial phase) of the breath is desirable and decreases the work of breathing.[37] In general, when changing from totally controlled (time-triggered) PCV to assisted PCV, it is common to increase the speed of pressurization (i.e., to decrease the rise time).

ACTIVATION OF EXHALATION VALVE DURING PCV: AIRWAY PRESSURE-RELEASE VENTILATION

OPENING OF THE EXHALATION VALVE
In theory, any pressure-controlled breath should limit airway pressures to Pset independent of patient demand, dyssynchrony, premature expiratory efforts, or cough. In practice, however, hardware and software limitations of most ventilators preclude such ideal configuration. Usually, ventilators can overcome an increase in inspiratory-flow demands efficiently during PCV (caused by leaks or strong inspiratory efforts) by boosting flow through the demand valve. Airway pressures are raised quickly back to Pset. Additionally, during the period in which the demand valve is still open, any sudden increment in alveolar pres-

sure (cough) can be counterbalanced promptly by a sudden decrease in demand flow, attenuating the potential raise in airway pressures. Once the demand valve is already closed, however—because alveolar pressures have equalized airway pressures—the ventilator is no longer able to control airway pressures. Because most ventilators do not actively control the exhalation valve during inspiration (they just close it tightly until the end of inspiratory time), any unexpected increment in airway pressures is counterbalanced only by closure of the demand valve, which is already at its minimum position. The end result is a steep increment in airway pressures, as in *flow-controlled* breaths.

Physicians have to keep this limitation of PCV in mind because it be responsible for undesirable increments in airway pressures above Pset in most ventilators. This situation has been observed during continuous tracheal gas insufflation (TGI),[89] during cough, and during strong efforts in assisted PCV breaths. In the latter circumstance, marked elevations of airway pressures can be found even in the absence of active expiratory efforts. This is so because the patient effort can increase effective driving pressures in early inspiration, increasing tidal volume and, consequently, the elastic recoil pressure at end inspiration (when diaphragmatic contraction already has ceased). An inactive exhalation valve could not release this extra tidal volume before the beginning of next exhalation, thus increasing airway pressures.

To overcome such limitations, some modern ventilators have incorporated improved hardware in their exhalation system that allows the simultaneous control of both valves (the inspiratory demand-flow valve and the exhalation valve) during the inspiratory phase of PCV. The end result is a smoother control of airway pressures during cough or during continuous tracheal gas insufflation.[90] Whenever available, such active control of the exhalation valve enhances ventilator operation.

The opening of the exhalation valve and its active control during inspiration are the technological basis for incorporation of airway pressure-release ventilation (APRV) in microprocessed ventilators.

APRV AND ITS VARIANTS
APRV is a form of partial ventilatory support intended originally to offload a portion of the work required to ventilate during a primary crisis of oxygenation.[30,31] In its original conception, APRV elevated mean airway pressure by maintaining a moderately high level of CPAP, delivered through a specially designed high-flow CPAP system linked to a release valve operated by a time controller. The system was design to work independently of any commercial ventilator. Spontaneous breaths were planned to occur around this pressure baseline. Periodically, the airway was depressurized rapidly during one of the patient's deflation cycles, exhausting waste gas from the expiratory reserve before replacing it with fresh gas as CPAP rebuilt to the baseline level. Total time for both phases of the release cycle generally was brief, ideally occupying only a single breath of the patient's rhythm. The release pattern was repeated at a clinician-selected frequency. As predicated by the mathematics of pressure-preset ventilation,[35] ventilator support (achieved by the machine) was necessarily a function of

the number of release cycles, the magnitude of the pressure drop during release, the duration of the release period, and the impedance to inflation and deflation. Synchronization between the patient's own exhalation and airway depressurization also affects the effectiveness of ventilation. Ineffectual inspiratory efforts during the deflation phase could impair the released volume. Despite such concerns, the original system was not designed to be synchronous.

Subsequently, different names were used for similar systems and arrangements, *biphasic positive airway pressure* and *intermittent mandatory pressure-release ventilation*. (*Bilevel airway pressure*, the commercial *BiPAP*, is different, being simply a combination of pressure-supported ventilation and CPAP; this product is designed for noninvasive use.) The basic difference among these systems was the duration of each phase, although all the systems could be approximated to a periodic alternation between two CPAP levels according to a time controller. A longer period at the lower CPAP level, enough to allow one or more spontaneous breaths, was characteristic of biphasic positive airway pressure ventilation. The specific transition from low to high CPAP levels also was different among these variants, whether it was synchronized or not.

Adjustment of all these features is now possible in modern ventilators, and this does not represent any important conceptual modification. Accordingly, we believe that the confusing profusion of names should be simplified under the acronym, APRV.

Provided that the ventilator works with an active exhalation valve during inspiration, APRV can be perfectly imitated by PCV breaths with a single difference. During APRV, if the expiratory time is set long enough to allow the patient to complete one or more spontaneous breaths during the low-pressure phase, the spontaneous breath will be assisted by an efficient CPAP system (equivalent to PSV set at zero driving pressure). Conversely, during the exhalation phase of PCV, the spontaneous effort cannot be well assisted because the bias flow systems responsible for PEEP maintenance are not designed to support strong efforts. The end result is some drop in PEEP unless sensitivity is adjusted to allow triggered inspirations (i.e., *assisted* PCV).

During the inspiratory phase, both systems perform identically, allowing spontaneous breaths to occur around highly sustained airway pressures. When spontaneous breaths are abolished by paralysis, APRV is not different from PCV.

It is important to remember that spontaneous cycles and ventilator cycles are completely uncoupled in the most frequent usage of APRV. This means that spontaneous breathing can occur at any phase of the ventilator cycle without any synchronization mechanism. Switching between the two CPAP levels obeys a timed-cycled mechanism, and patient inspiratory work is mechanically supported only when it coincides with the restoration of the high CPAP phase.

In view of such inherent dyssynchrony, more sophisticated APRV algorithms have been introduced in recent years, although without a clear rationale or clinical benefit. These include triggered transitions between low and high CPAP levels and use of PSV during one or both phases on top of the corresponding baseline pressures.

Regarding the synchronized transition, it is important to remember that whenever commercial ventilators allow the patient to trigger the CPAP transition, usually during a window that spans the last 25% of the preset low-pressure phase, the actual time intervals at high and low pressures (equivalent to I:E ratio) may vary according to the respiratory drive of the patient.[91] Furthermore, even when some synchronization with CPAP transitions is attempted, most spontaneous breaths during APRV are still nonsynchronous because of the long duration of both phases. Under such conditions, the real advantage of synchronized systems is questionable. From a workload perspective, APRV is an inefficient way of assisting the patient, imposing a higher workload and greater discomfort as compared with equivalent levels of PSV.[92,93] The benefit, if any, of providing some synchronization has to be balanced against the loss of control over T_I/T_{TOT}. Synchronization only makes sense if applied to most spontaneous efforts, meaning that APRV should be set at higher frequencies and shorter inspiratory times, as with assisted PCV.

Whenever APRV is applied in its common configuration, with long time intervals set for both phases, the intermittent mechanical assistance (applied only when the spontaneous effort coincides with transition from low to high pressures) shares some similarities with intermittent mandatory ventilation (IMV). As with synchronized IMV, the presence of alternating levels of assistance probably impairs smooth accommodation of patient drive,[94] potentially causing some distress in patients when sedation is removed. Therefore, it is still an open question as to whether APRV will prove helpful during weaning or for patients with extreme weakness, very high workloads, or conditions in which release cycles are relatively inefficient in achieving ventilation (e.g., severe airflow obstruction).

For the sake of simplicity, whenever the patient gets too distressed during APRV and sedation is contraindicated, it is preferable to change to PSV or assisted PCV, assisting the patient in a more predictable way. The combination of PSV with APRV introduces unnecessary complexity, making little sense in terms of physiologic benefit or as an attempt to minimize driving pressures and ventilator-induced lung injury.

By extending the higher CPAP level further, APRV gets closer to inverse-ratio PCV. The shorter the time at low CPAP levels, the lower is the ventilator contribution to minute ventilation,[91] and the higher is the Pa_{CO_2}. On the other hand, Pa_{O_2} tends to increase because intrinsic PEEP increases. The full consequences of the duty-cycle settings on oxygenation are discussed below.

Comparison of APRV associated *with* spontaneous breaths versus APRV *without* spontaneous efforts (identical to conventional PCV), when both modes are set at equivalent end-expiratory and end-inspiratory airway pressures, showed that the former achieved better oxygenation[95] and increased cardiac output,[95,96] renal blood flow,[97] lung aeration, and functional residual capacity.[83] The hemodynamic benefits may be related to lower intrathoracic pressures generated during spontaneous efforts,[98] and the benefits in lung function may be related to higher transpulmonary pressures.[83]

It is important to stress that equivalent benefits also can be achieved during simple CPAP (matched to the high-pressure phase of APRV), in fact, with better outcomes in terms of oxygenation.[99] These findings demonstrate that most of the benefits attributed to APRV relate to the replacement of mechanically applied driving pressures by patient-generated driving pressures.

When considering the overall implications on hemodynamics, lung injury, and muscle function, APRV still poses a well-defined set of potential problems. Central vascular congestion and exacerbated pulmonary edema are natural consequences of lower intrathoracic pressures and increased cardiac workload. In patients with cardiac failure, APRV should be used with caution. Conversely, to unload inspiratory muscles significantly, the high-pressure CPAP in APRV first must be raised to a considerable degree, obscuring the major advantage of APRV, which is the use of lower airway pressures. Moreover, inspiratory muscles will be disadvantaged by the resulting hyperinflation, promoting a sense of dyspnea that APRV is designed to relieve. In the context of such disadvantages, APRV circuits must be designed carefully to function properly because imperfections in demand flow are not compensated by any mechanically assisted driving pressure, as during PSV. Finally, the intrinsic design of APRV circuits raises an important concern about ventilator-induced lung injury: APRV does not represent any significant advantage in terms of damage related to cyclic lung collapse[100–103] and overdistension.[38,104–107] Therefore, the same principles of conventional mechanical ventilation apply: the need to reduce effective driving pressures, whatever their source of generation, and the need to avoid cyclic collapse and tidal recruitment. The practical implications are that the releasing pressures of APRV should be titrated carefully (as during any PEEP titration), and similarly, driving pressures should be estimated carefully and minimized (as during any attempt to reduce plateau pressures during controlled ventilation).

In conclusion, the important message provided by studies of APRV is that the preservation of spontaneous efforts is an important aspect of mechanical ventilation that should be employed prudently. The simple use of assisted PCV instead of fully controlled PCV can have a positive impact on hemodynamics, lung recruitment, and oxygenation.

COMBINED MODES

In recent years, attempts have been made to combine the desirable features of both flow-controlled, volume-cycled and pressure-controlled, time-cycled ventilation. These modes, which include *pressure-regulated volume-control* and *volume-assured pressure-support* (VAPS)[25] ventilation, guarantee any tidal volume compatible with the physician-set upper pressure limit. The former combination mode accomplishes its dual target over a few breaths, whereas VAPS guarantees its dual-target within the same breath. Despite the very limited research in this field, there is a firm physiologic rationale and a need to apply the benefits of pressure control while avoiding its problems.

A major advantage of such modes is their use in patients in whom some level of spontaneous ventilation is desirable (to promote recruitment or to avoid some problems related to paralysis). Provided that the patient is not extremely agitated, a volume-cycled target promotes a decrease in airway pressure in proportion to the magnitude of patient effort. Such feedback limits transpulmonary pressures and may be a convenient strategy to avoid ventilator-induced lung injury. Also, such feedback usually provides a smooth transition from *ventilator-imposed* driving pressures to *patient-generated* driving pressures.

Inverse-Ratio Ventilation

In 1971, Reynolds suggested that the infant respiratory distress syndrome could be addressed effectively by a ventilator strategy that extended the inspiratory period beyond 50% of total cycle time, that is, inverse-ratio ventilation (IRV).[6] Enthusiastic but largely anecdotal reports or uncontrolled studies followed in the adult literature.[7–10,12,13,108–110] With this mode, T_I/T_{TOT} is prolonged beyond the traditional values of 0.2–0.4, and pressure control has been the modality of choice for its implementation (PC-IRV). Mean inspiratory flow rate (the quotient of tidal volume and inspiratory time) is much lower than conventionally prescribed. IRV has been used with duty cycles ranging from 0.5 (the lower limit consistent with its definition) to 0.8. Extension of T_I/T_{TOT} was supposed to increase ϕ_{aw} and ϕ_A without violating the desired upper limits for airway and alveolar pressures.

IMPLEMENTING INVERSE-RATIO VENTILATION

IRV can be applied either with *pressure-controlled*, time-cycled forms of ventilation (abbreviated in this chapter as PC-IRV) or with *flow-controlled*, volume-cycled ventilation (abbreviated as VC-IRV). During VC-IRV, inspiratory time can be extended by either applying a very low inspiratory flow rate or by prolonging the inspiratory pause. The latter achieves a higher ϕ_{aw} and tends to result in improved CO_2 removal when compared with VC-IRV promoted by low inspiratory flow.[32] When slowing down inspiratory flow, most investigators used *flow-controlled* decelerating waveforms in an attempt to obtain better CO_2 exchange or to better mimic the flow profile of PC-IRV.[111]

Among all forms of IRV, PC-IRV generates the highest possible ϕ_{aw} for any combination of peak pressure, PEEP, and T_I/T_{TOT}. Also, for the same I:E ratio, PC-IRV usually results in the least dead space.[112]

Because most modern ventilators provide PCV, the clinical use of VC-IRV has declined substantially in recent years. When using VC-IRV, any slight variation in expiratory time (frequently found during assisted ventilation or during a physician's attempt to increase CO_2 removal) can cause dramatic variations in airway pressures, imposing a great risk of barotrauma and overinflation. The latter occurs because plateau pressures are not controlled directly during VCV and instead are determined by the end-inspiratory lung volume imposed by the ventilator. Whenever there is further shortening of expiratory time, the additional induced residual volume (intrinsic PEEP) adds to the set or imposed tidal volume, causing large increments in plateau pressures. This is why VC-IRV always has been recommended in association with deep sedation and paralysis.[11] When using PC-IRV at the same settings, one expects some drop in tidal volume and minute ventilation but with safe preservation of end-inspiratory lung volume and plateau pressures. In other words, during PC-IRV, hypercapnia might ensue, but lung structure is better protected.

Minute ventilation is simply a linear function of respiratory rate during VC-IRV, but it is unpredictable during PC-IRV (see Fig. 10-3). Nevertheless, given the adverse effects of deep sedation and paralysis,[78–80,82,113] the risks of high plateau pressures,[38,107] and the tolerance by patients of permissive hypercapnia,[1–3,75] it is hard to justify the use of VC-IRV (instead of PC-IRV) at the present time.

LATER COMPARATIVE STUDIES ON IRV

A decade after the original report on IRV in infants,[6] several investigators demonstrated oxygenation benefits in adult patients with ARDS.[7–10,12] Most of the early clinical studies were not controlled and did not address potential differences in the methods of delivering IRV. No study has specifically addressed the effects of IRV on patient outcome. In most studies, total PEEP and ϕ_{aw} likely increased during PC-IRV application, although the incomplete information provided by the authors precludes a definitive statement.

Over the last 15 years, more rigorous studies attempted to elucidate the mechanism of improved gas exchange during IRV compared with conventional ventilation. Such studies can be divided in two types: (1) studies in which IRV was delivered at equivalent levels of ϕ_{aw} as during conventional ventilation and (2) studies in which IRV was delivered at equivalent levels of total PEEP. In this latter case, most investigators had to apply higher ϕ_{aw} during IRV, associated with lower levels of external PEEP, to compensate for occurrence of intrinsic PEEP.

Whenever IRV was delivered at equivalent levels of ϕ_{aw}, the following pattern of physiologic effects was found consistently: (1) lower peak and plateau pressures for equivalent tidal volumes,[17,114,115] (2) lower external PEEP and total PEEP because of attempts to keep ϕ_{aw} constant,[17,114] (3) a decrease or no change (but never improvement) in arterial P_{O_2} and shunt levels,[17,18,114,115] (4) a slight decreases in dead space and Pa_{CO_2} ($\Delta V_D/V_T \cong -15\%$; $\Delta P_{CO_2} \cong -5$ mm Hg),[17,18,115] and (5) minimal alteration in hemodynamics with no detectable changes in splanchnic perfusion.[18,114]

Conversely, in most studies where IRV was applied at equivalent levels of total PEEP, similar reductions in peak pressures,[14,15,52,112,116–118] dead space, and Pa_{CO_2} levels[14,15,52,112,116,119] were observed, but with three major differences: (1) plateau pressures were kept constant but ϕ_{aw} increased for equivalent tidal volumes (a necessary consequence of study design),[14–16,52,112,116–119] (2) arterial P_{O_2} and shunt sometimes improved,[118,120] and (3) hemodynamics were impaired significantly in most studies.[14–16,112,116,117]

To explain the different responses in P_{O_2} and hemodynamics between the two comparative categories, one could invoke differences in ϕ_{aw}: According to traditional teaching,[32,33] the higher ϕ_{aw} applied during IRV (at equivalent total PEEP) is expected to increase Pa_{O_2} and impair venous return, decreasing cardiac output and arterial pressure. There are many reasons to believe that this is more complex: Many studies in the second category (IRV at equivalent total PEEP) also showed deterioration of Pa_{O_2} and increased shunt levels after IRV application[16,117,119] despite considerable increments in ϕ_{aw}. To reconcile all these findings, a deeper understanding about the process of lung collapse and reopening is necessary.

EFFECTS OF TOTAL PEEP AND ϕ_{aw} ON OXYGENATION

Three potential mechanisms have been invoked traditionally to explain the increase in Pa_{O2} with IRV: (1) higher mean airway pressure, (2) intrinsic PEEP elicited by short expiratory time, and (3) improved intrapulmonary distribution of inspiratory flow. As discussed earlier, the third mechanism is virtually irrelevant in terms of oxygenation, producing just a mild increase in CO_2 elimination.

Regarding the effects of ϕ_{aw} and intrinsic PEEP on oxygenation, we now recognize that neither variable is linearly related to oxygenation, especially in ARDS. Lung *hysteresis* makes the whole system very sensitive to the boundaries of pressures applied during the previous breathing cycles and, therefore, very sensitive to end-expiratory and end-inspiratory alveolar pressures developed previously. The same instantaneous value of intrinsic PEEP or ϕ_{aw} can result in completely different blood gases depending on *lung history* or on the *previous trajectory* of alveolar pressures.

This somewhat complex behavior is linked to the phenomenon of airspace closure and reopening with its inherent hysteresis. A combination of factors, including viscosity of the lining layer inside the alveolar spaces, plastic deformation and folding of alveolar walls, surfactant adsorption, and chaotic sequence of airway reopening (never equivalent to the sequence of closure), always cause some energy to be lost during recruitment/inflation of lung units, and this can never be recovered during the closure/deflation process. This phenomenon prevents the lung from behaving as a perfect elastic system: The same airway pressure results in two different volume states depending on the direction of the previous variation in airway pressures. A given airway pressure always results in lower lung volumes if delivered through an inflation process from lower pressures than if reached from a deflation from higher pressures. Lung inflammation, surfactant deactivation, and massive airspace collapse are frequent conditions favoring the development of such marked lung hysteresis.

An interesting way of interpreting lung hysteresis is provided in Figs. 10-8 and 10-9. One can regard hysteresis as representing an asymmetry of lung status according to the direction of pressure variations in the system. Hysteresis creates a transitional state (defining a corresponding window of pressures) in the system that keeps "memory" of the previous state; if many lungs units were closed in the

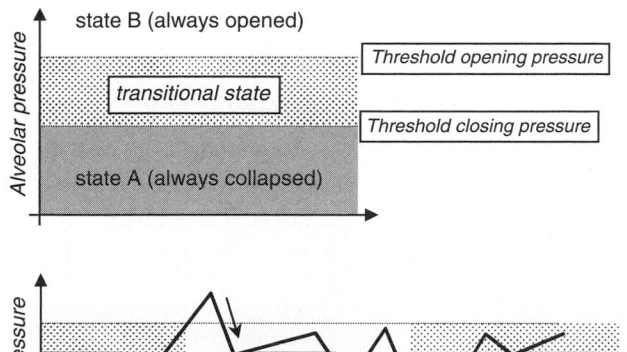

FIGURE 10-8 Representation of lung hysteresis according to the pressures applied on the system. The system changes its status according to the direction of the transition. The transitional state keeps some "memory" of the previous state, behaving as in state *A* when coming from lower pressures or behaving as in state *B* when coming from higher pressures. Once inside the transitional state, the situation can be stable for a long period, provided that pressures do not trespass the boundaries, that is, the threshold opening/closing pressures.

previous state, it is likely that the system will stay partially or totally closed during pressure oscillations up to a certain limit (defined by the transitional window of pressures). And the opposite is also true: A previously opened lung state will favor an open lung state during application of airway pressures brought down to below the opening pressures, provided that they do not trespass closing pressures, that is, that they stay within the transitional window of pressures.

The range of such a transitional window of pressures depends on the distribution of opening and closing pressures of lung units. The higher the mean threshold opening pressures and the lower the mean threshold closing pressures, the larger is this transitional range, and the more the whole system depends on lung history. This transitional window of pressures may exceed 40 cmH$_2$O in severe trauma patients.[46]

Obviously, the actual situation is always complicated by heterogeneities in the distribution of opening/closing pressures among lung units. The basic concept of transitional state, however, is applied easily to complex situations, assuming that there is an *average* behavior of lung units roughly defined by such threshold pressures. For instance, by extending this simple model to clinical examples of pressure tracings (see Fig. 10-9), one can easily grasp the reason for many apparent contradictions in the reports on the physiologic effects of IRV.

Several possible scenarios can be envisioned:

- Two conditions matched for ϕ_{aw} (e.g., A_1 versus B_1 or A_3 versus B_2) could result in completely different Pa$_{O2}$ values, as occurred in some studies.[17,18]
- Two conditions matched for total PEEP (e.g., A_1 versus A_3) could result in equivalent Pa$_{O2}$ values but different

hemodynamics (the higher ϕ_{aw} might impair hemodynamics without further benefit in oxygenation). This situation likely occurred in some studies.[14,112,116]

- Sometimes, when alveolar pressures are confined inside the transitional window (situation B_1), any further lengthening of T_I/T_{TOT} might cause hemodynamic impairment and an eventual drop in Pa$_{O2}$, as occurred in some clinical studies.[16,117,119] The drop in cardiac output should relate to the increased ϕ_{aw}, whereas the drop in Pa$_{O2}$ is easily understood after adding some heterogeneity to the model. During prolonged inspiration, if most damaged units remain closed, the longer compression of capillaries in the preserved units likely would divert perfusion toward the collapsed units, increasing shunt levels.
- Sometimes, when peak alveolar pressures exceed the transitional window but end-expiratory pressures are low enough to allow recollapse (situation B_2), oxygenation improves with prolongation of inspiration, as in some other studies.[118,120] In contrast with the preceding example, now higher inspiratory pressures can transiently recruit damaged lung units,[121] and the prolonged inspiration will favor a longer contact between perfused capillaries and the opened units, decreasing average shunt levels.

Therefore, most reported effects of IRV can be understood according to the preceding rationale. The concept of hysteresis and transitional status also explains why the impact of total PEEP is usually greater than the impact of ϕ_{aw} on oxygenation. The observation of Stewart et al[122] in 1981 remains valid today: In Fig. 10-9, a major difference in oxygenation can be expected when comparing situations in A versus in B simply because of minor changes in total PEEP. In contrast, ϕ_{aw} might be increased largely in situations B_1 or B_2 (either by increasing driving pressures or by prolonging inspiration). As long as total PEEP was not increased, Pa$_{O2}$ could never reach the levels found in situation A. In a recent study using ultrafast P$_{O2}$ sensors, Baumgardner et al[121] have demonstrated that PEEP and respiratory rate (probably via intrinsic PEEP modulation) are the most important factors determining arterial P$_{O2}$ oscillations. Because ϕ_{aw} during PC-IRV does not depend on respiratory rate (see above), frequency could increase considerably without any visible change in ϕ_{aw}. Therefore, oxygenation could increase markedly at fixed levels of ϕ_{aw}. Such relationships explain, once more, the poor correlation between ϕ_{aw} and oxygenation.

In the preceding model, ventilation-perfusion imbalances have not been considered. Because a high F$_{IO2}$ was used in most studies on IRV, however, oxygenation can be assumed to reflect changes in true shunt rather than ventilation-perfusion ratios. Finally, because some minimal alveolar perfusion during inspiration commonly is maintained in most alveolar units, tidal recruitment is an important factor, transiently increasing capillary P$_{O2}$ during inspiration.[121]

INTRINSIC PEEP VERSUS EXTRINSIC PEEP

As discussed earlier, intrinsic PEEP is common during IRV, being responsible for effects on oxygenation. It is possible, however, to extend inspiratory time (use IRV) without

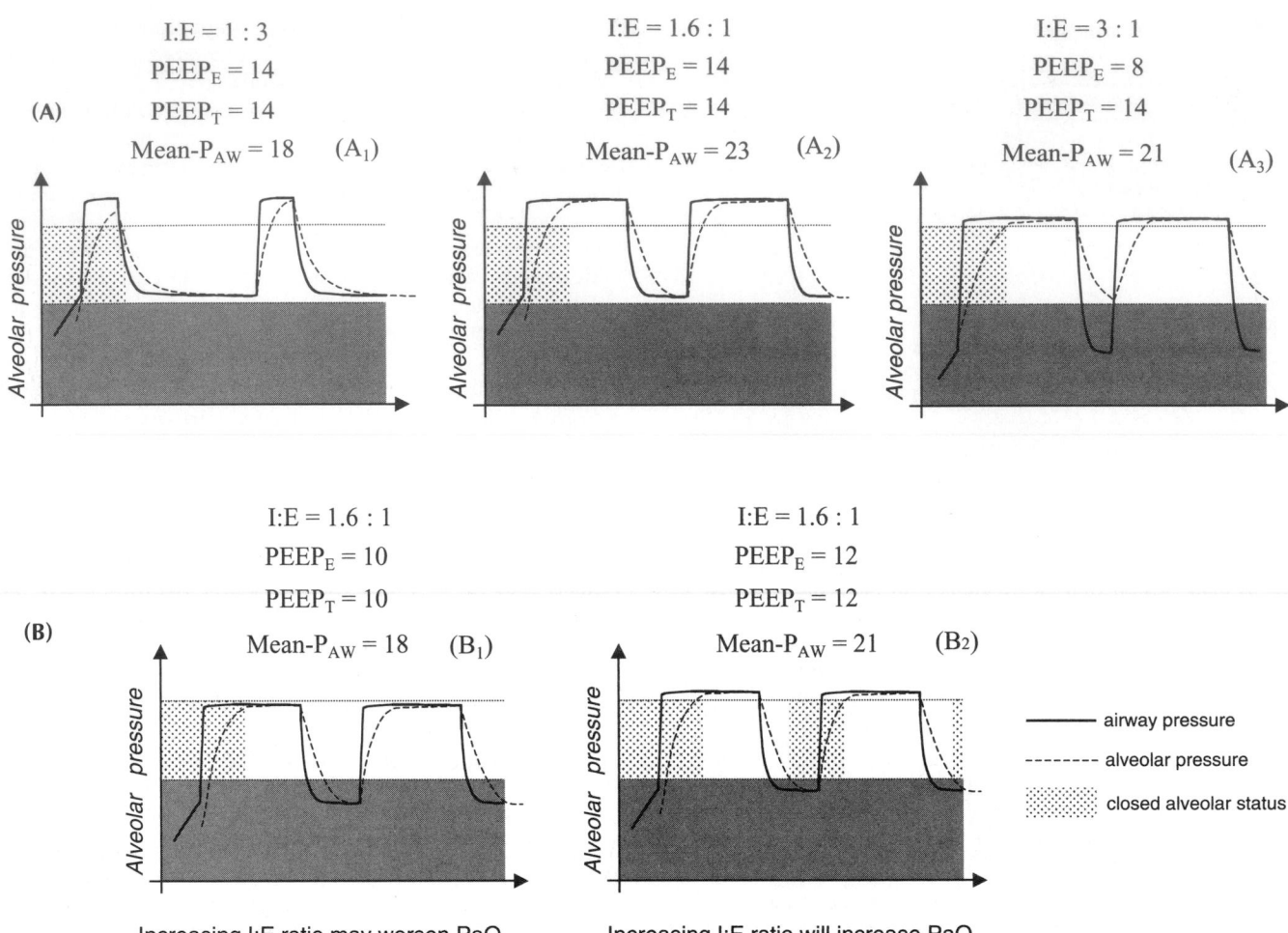

FIGURE 10-9 *A.* **Low-shunt situations: three ventilator settings producing the same effect on Pa$_{O_2}$.** In each, alveolar pressures exceeded the threshold opening pressure after the first breath *and* were kept above the threshold closing pressures for the rest of cycles. Provided that a major part of lung units is adequately represented by the boundaries of threshold pressures indicated, the three settings will result in very low and equivalent shunt levels. Under such conditions, increments in mean airway pressure (produced by increased I:E ratios, as in examples A_2 and A_3) will only put hemodynamics at risk. *B.* **High-shunt situations:** Because *end-expiratory* alveolar pressures are now trespassing on the closing pressures, the situation changes dramatically. The effect of increased mean airway pressure differs according to *end-inspiratory* pressures developed. In B_1, because Pset is below the threshold opening pressures, prolongation of inspiratory time can only impair hemodynamics, but the lung stays closed and producing high shunt levels. Conversely, if Pset and alveolar pressures trespass threshold opening pressures during inspiration (B_2), Pa$_{O_2}$ becomes dependent on mean airway pressure. The longer the inspiratory phase, the longer is the open status, and the higher is the Pa$_{O_2}$.

intrinsic PEEP generation.[119,120] A great controversy has surrounded this subject. Some authors have argued that intrinsic PEEP brings some advantages to the clinical situation. Others argue that intrinsic PEEP is always deleterious.

According to the first perspective, intrinsic PEEP promoted by IRV can be considered a "selective" form of PEEP that preferentially ventilates parts of the lung with short time constants, placing at rest parts with prolonged time constants.[123] In a theoretical exercise, if respiratory rate approaches infinity, alveolar pressures would remain practically constant in the *slow* units, equilibrating at an intermediate value between PEEP and plateau pressures. Because healthier units tend to have slower time constants and to be located in nondependent regions in patients with ARDS, intrinsic PEEP is expected to produce less cyclic overextension

of the nondependent parenchyma, increasing ventilation in dependent and more perfused lung regions. Consequently, selective improvement of ventilation at low $\dot{V}/\dot{Q}$ areas may eliminate CO_2 more efficiently.[124] Another way of formulating such rationale is to propose a strategy in which "the absolute time of the expiratory phase is so short that the stiffest parts of the lung have no time for collapse."[123]

Recent evidence does not support this view but demonstrates the opposite.[20,45,52,119,125–127] Because different time constants in individual lung regions are crucial for a "selective effect" of intrinsic PEEP, intrinsic PEEP may allow the "selective collapse" of regions with short time constants, especially the edematous regions. When comparing intrinsic PEEP with matching levels of external PEEP in patients with ARDS, Zavala et al[52] demonstrated that shunt levels increased by 6% with intrinsic PEEP. There was some increase in the efficiency of CO_2 removal, but this could be ascribed to better inspiratory flow distribution during IRV rather than to intrinsic PEEP. Animal experiments in dogs[119] reproduced the same results. Clinical studies in obstructed patients came to similar conclusions, suggesting that partial or complete substitution of intrinsic PEEP by external PEEP improves gas exchange[126,127] without any impairment in CO_2 removal.

The original perspective of considering absolute time for collapse—instead of end-expiratory pressures—also carries some problems. A recent computed tomographic (CT) investigation has demonstrated that the time window to prevent end-expiratory lung collapse without external PEEP is extremely short (<0.6 second) and might not be feasible during mechanical ventilation of many patients with ARDS.[45,125] To avoid unnecessary confusion, it is also important to prove that time per se, independent of local alveolar pressure, is an important variable affecting lung collapse. To our knowledge, this has never been demonstrated.

After reviewing available evidence, we conclude that there is no rationale supporting the preferential use of intrinsic PEEP. In terms of oxygenation, it seems inferior to external PEEP, slightly increasing the risk of collapse in unstable units.[128] In lung models with different time constants,

it is clear that fast units are at a disadvantage during intrinsic PEEP generation.[20] Figure 10-10 provides further insight: Regional ventilation becomes more heterogeneous with intrinsic PEEP, and ventilation is increased in nondependent regions. A recent CT study revealed more hyperinflation with intrinsic PEEP than with equivalent external PEEP.[19]

In terms of CO_2 removal, it is impossible to draw any conclusion because the concomitant use of IRV in most studies precludes any estimation of the isolated impact of intrinsic PEEP. In clinical practice, one also has to consider that a combination of IRV plus intrinsic PEEP usually results in a higher ϕ_{aw} than conventional I:E ratios plus external PEEP and thus greater hemodynamic compromise.[112] Another major drawback of the intrinsic PEEP approach is its complexity: Much closer monitoring and more frequent adjustments of ventilator settings are required, even with a computerized protocol.[21]

Therefore, external PEEP in association with conventional I:E ratio is preferable. If CO_2 removal is a clinical problem, an increased frequency—even if associated with low tidal volumes—may solve the problem (see Fig. 10-3), especially when using high PEEP levels. By increasing functional residual capacity, external PEEP usually causes a decrease in airway resistance and lung compliance, both factors contributing to a very short time constant. Under such

FIGURE 10-10 Regional ventilation distribution measured by electrical impedance tomography in an animal model (pig) of acute lung injury. The functional images display the standard deviation of each pixel along 1 minute of ventilation. Bright colors represent regions with higher standard deviation and hence higher regional ventilation. Perfusion perturbations were subtracted by temporal filtering. Although total PEEP in both conditions was the same (checked by end-expiratory occlusion), the right image was obtained when 6 cmH_2O intrinsic PEEP was added to 9 cmH_2O external PEEP. The net result was a more heterogeneous ventilation, with preferential ventilation of the right lung and marked hypoventilation of the left lower lung (LL). External PEEP produced a more even pattern of regional ventilation.

PCV 1:2 ; $PEEP_T$ = 15 ; $PEEP_i$ = 0

PCV 3:1 ; $PEEP_T$ = 15 ; $PEEP_i$ = 6

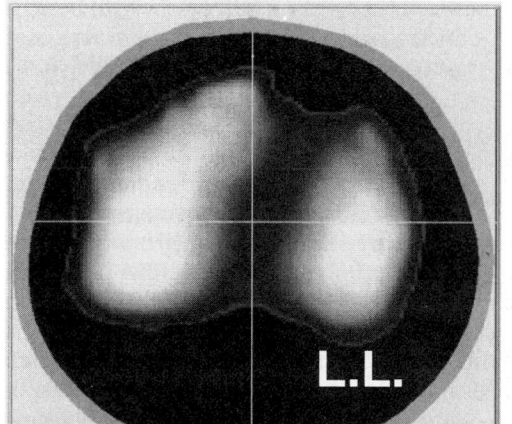
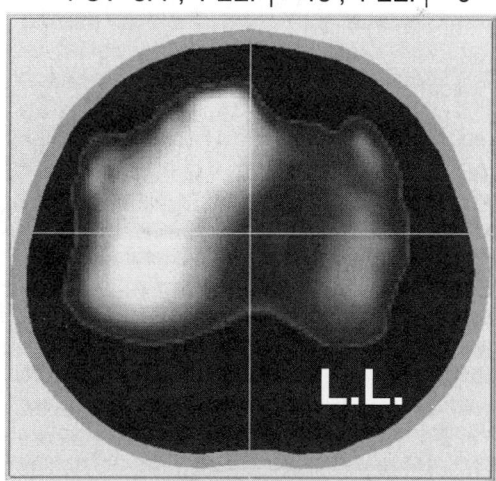
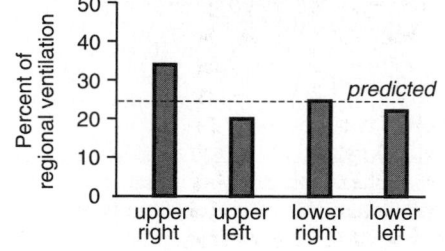
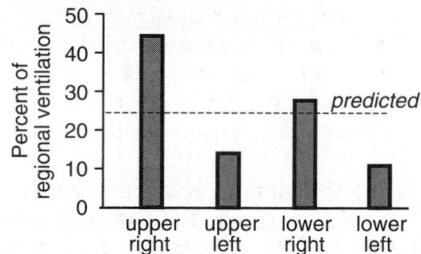

conditions, respiratory rates up to 40–50 cycles per minute could increase minute ventilation considerably, improving CO_2 removal.

OTHER EFFECTS OF IRV

For many years, it was believed that the benefits of IRV were time-dependent and that short-term evaluations would underestimate them.[129] The importance of sustained traction and interdependence to alveolar recruitment was propounded. As discussed earlier, subsequent studies demonstrated no unique effect of IRV that could not be reproduced by conventional I:E ratio plus appropriate PEEP levels.[14,16,120] Slow benefits over time have been observed frequently in many patients with ARDS,[107] especially when recruiting maneuvers are not applied immediately.

DRAWBACKS

With matched levels of total PEEP, IRV always results in higher levels of ϕ_{aw} than conventional I:E ratios. Even when applying equivalent tidal volumes and plateau pressure, traction forces are applied for longer periods of time during IRV. There is some recent evidence suggesting that such prolonged application of pressures may cause some harm to the parenchyma, especially when inspiratory lung volumes approach total lung capacity.[62] The simple prolongation of inspiratory time, despite similar levels of PEEP, end-inspiratory pressures, and tidal volumes, has been associated with gross permeability alterations[117] and ventilator-induced lung injury.[62]

Although there was a high incidence of pneumothorax in initial studies of IRV,[12,118] such studies were performed at a time when high tidal volumes were common. In more recent studies using IRV with careful monitoring and in the hands of physicians experienced to the procedure, IRV has resulted in much better outcomes.[46]

Obviously, the higher levels of ϕ_{aw} imposed by IRV must result in greater hemodynamic compromise. Therefore, for a certain level of total PEEP, IRV is always a worse option for the cardiovascular system[14–16,112,116,117]

Extending T_I/T_{TOT} to the point of inverting the I:E ratio is hazardous and counterproductive in patients with severe airflow obstruction. In this condition, heterogeneities are magnified because ventilation is more dependent on regional time constant than on regional compliance. Dynamic hyperinflation would be accentuated selectively in units with high expiratory resistance. Because these patients often present with serious clinical problems and unnecessary elevations of ϕ_{aw}, it is now common practice to use relatively rapid inspiratory flow rates and short T_I/T_{TOT} to maximize exhalation time.[130] Recent publications suggest that dynamic hyperinflation and localized intrinsic PEEP are also common in patients with ARDS.[131–133]

Conclusion

In contrast with the growing acceptance of PCV, use of IRV has declined. Safer, more predictable, and more efficient ventilator solutions can be implemented at the bedside. At first, physicians were enthusiastic about IRV because internal PEEP and peak pressures were hidden. Later, physicians realized that total PEEP and peak alveolar pressures were not that different, yet IRV necessarily imposed higher levels of ϕ_{aw} and greater hemodynamic consequences for similar clinical benefits. Whereas concepts such as ventilator-induced lung injury and permissive hypercapnia have boosted the use of PCV, the better understanding of the dynamics of alveolar collapse have dampened enthusiasm for and use of IRV.

References

1. Hickling KG. Permissive hypercapnia. Respir Care Clin North Am 2002; 8:155–69.
2. Laffey JG, O'Croinin D, McLoughlin P, Kavanagh BP. Permissive hypercapnia: Role in protective lung ventilatory strategies. Intensive Care Med 2004; 30:347–56.
3. Amato MBP. Permissive hypercapnia. In: Marini JJ, Evans TW, editors. Acute lung injury, Vol 30. Berlin: Springer-Verlag, 1997: 258–75.
4. Esteban A, Anzueto A, Frutos F, et al. Characteristics and outcomes in adult patients receiving mechanical ventilation: A 28-day international study. Jama 2002; 287:345–55.
5. Farias JA, Frutos F, Esteban A, et al. What is the daily practice of mechanical ventilation in pediatric intensive care units? A multicenter study. Intensive Care Med 2004; 30:918–25.
6. Reynolds EO. Effect of alterations in mechanical ventilator settings on pulmonary gas exchange in hyaline membrane disease. Arch Dis Child 1971; 46:152–9.
7. Cole AG, Weller SF, Sykes MK. Inverse ratio ventilation compared with PEEP in adult respiratory failure. Intensive Care Med 1984; 10:227–32.
8. Abraham E, Yoshihara G. Cardiorespiratory effects of pressure controlled inverse ratio ventilation in severe respiratory failure. Chest 1989; 96:1356–9.
9. Gurevitch MJ, Van Dyke J, Young ES, Jackson K. Improved oxygenation and lower peak airway pressure in severe adult respiratory distress syndrome: Treatment with inverse ratio ventilation. Chest 1986; 89:211–3.
10. Lain DC, DiBenedetto R, Morris SL, et al. Pressure control inverse ratio ventilation as a method to reduce peak inspiratory pressure and provide adequate ventilation and oxygenation. Chest 1989; 95:1081–8.
11. Marcy TW, Marini JJ. Inverse ratio ventilation in ARDS: Rationale and implementation. Chest 1991; 100:494–504.
12. Tharratt RS, Allen RP, Albertson TE. Pressure controlled inverse ratio ventilation in severe adult respiratory failure. Chest 1988; 94:755–62.
13. Kacmarek R, Hess D. Pressure-controlled inverse-ratio ventilation: Panacea or auto-PEEP? Respir Care 1990; 35:945–8.
14. Mercat A, Titiriga M, Anguel N, et al. Inverse ratio ventilation (I:E = 2:1) in acute respiratory distress syndrome: A six-hour controlled study. Am J Respir Crit Care Med 1997; 155:1637–42.
15. Mercat A, Graini L, Teboul JL, et al. Cardiorespiratory effects of pressure-controlled ventilation with and without inverse ratio in the adult respiratory distress syndrome. Chest 1993; 104: 871–5.
16. Lessard MR, Guerot E, Lorino H, et al. Effects of pressure-controlled with different I:E ratios versus volume-controlled ventilation on respiratory mechanics, gas exchange, and

hemodynamics in patients with adult respiratory distress syndrome. Anesthesiology 1994; 80:983–91.

17. Neumann P, Berglund JE, Andersson LG, et al. Effects of inverse ratio ventilation and positive end-expiratory pressure in oleic acid-induced lung injury. Am J Respir Crit Care Med 2000; 161:1537–45.

18. Huang CC, Shih MJ, Tsai YH, et al. Effects of inverse ratio ventilation versus positive end-expiratory pressure on gas exchange and gastric intramucosal P_{CO_2} and pH under constant mean airway pressure in acute respiratory distress syndrome. Anesthesiology 2001; 95:1182–8.

19. Edibam C, Rutten AJ, Collins DV, Bersten AD. Effect of inspiratory flow pattern and inspiratory to expiratory ratio on nonlinear elastic behavior in patients with acute lung injury. Am J Respir Crit Care Med 2003; 167:702–7.

20. Kacmarek RM, Kirmse M, Nishimura M, et al. The effects of applied vs auto-PEEP on local lung unit pressure and volume in a four-unit lung model. Chest 1995; 108:1073–9.

21. East TD, Bohm SH, Wallace CJ, et al. A successful computerized protocol for clinical management of pressure control inverse ratio ventilation in ARDS patients. Chest 1992; 101:697–710.

22. Amato MB, Barbas CS, Medeiros DM, et al. Effect of a protective-ventilation strategy on mortality in the acute respiratory distress syndrome. New Engl J Med 1998; 338:347–54.

23. Amato MB, Barbas CS, Medeiros DM, et al. Beneficial effects of the "open lung approach" with low distending pressures in acute respiratory distress syndrome: A prospective, randomized study on mechanical ventilation. Am J Respir Crit Care Med 1995; 152:1835–46.

24. Kocis KC, Dekeon MK, Rosen HK, et al. Pressure-regulated volume control vs volume control ventilation in infants after surgery for congenital heart disease. Pediatr Cardiol 2001;22:233–7.

25. Amato MB, Barbas CS, Bonassa J, et al. Volume-assured pressure support ventilation (VAPSV): A new approach for reducing muscle workload during acute respiratory failure. Chest 1992; 102:1225–34.

26. Marcy TW, Marini JJ. Inverse ratio ventilation in ARDS: Rationale and implementation. Chest 1991; 100:494–504.

27. Abraham E, Yoshihara G. Cardiorespiratory effects of pressure controlled ventilation in severe respiratory failure. Chest 1990; 98:1445–9.

28. MacIntyre NR. Respiratory function during pressure support ventilation. Chest 1986; 89:677–83.

29. Brochard L, Harf A, Lorino H, Lemaire F. Inspiratory pressure support prevents diaphragmatic fatigue during weaning from mechanical ventilation. Am Rev Respir Dis 1989; 139:513–21.

30. Downs JB, Stock MC. Airway pressure release ventilation: A new concept in ventilatory support. Crit Care Med 1987; 15:459–61.

31. Rasanen J, Cane RD, Downs JB, et al. Airway pressure release ventilation during acute lung injury: A prospective multicenter trial. Crit Care Med 1991; 19:1234–41.

32. Marini JJ, Ravenscraft SA. Mean airway pressure: Physiologic determinants and clinical importance: 1. Physiologic determinants and measurements. Crit Care Med 1992; 20:1461–72.

33. Marini JJ, Ravenscraft SA. Mean airway pressure: Physiologic determinants and clinical importance: 2. Clinical implications. Crit Care Med 1992; 20:1604–16.

34. Manaligod JM, Bendel-Stenzel EM, Meyers PA, et al. Variations in end-expiratory pressure during partial liquid ventilation: Impact on gas exchange, lung compliance, and end-expiratory lung volume. Chest 2000; 117:184–90.

35. Marini JJ, Crooke PS 3rd, Truwit JD. Determinants and limits of pressure-preset ventilation: A mathematical model of pressure control. J Appl Physiol 1989; 67:1081–92.

36. Nahum A, Burke WC, Ravenscraft SA, et al. Lung mechanics and gas exchange during pressure-control ventilation in dogs: Augmentation of CO_2 elimination by an intratracheal catheter. Am Rev Respir Dis 1992; 146:965–73.

37. Chiumello D, Pelosi P, Taccone P, et al. Effect of different inspiratory rise time and cycling off criteria during pressure support ventilation in patients recovering from acute lung injury. Crit Care Med 2003; 31:2604–10.

38. Dreyfuss D, Soler P, Basset G, Saumon G. High inflation pressure pulmonary edema: Respective effects of high airway pressure, high tidal volume, and positive end-expiratory pressure. Am Rev Respir Dis 1988; 137:1159–64.

39. Marini JJ, Crooke PS 3rd. A general mathematical model for respiratory dynamics relevant to the clinical setting. Am Rev Respir Dis 1993; 147:14–24.

40. Lim SC, Adams AB, Simonson DA, et al. Transient hemodynamic effects of recruitment maneuvers in three experimental models of acute lung injury. Crit Care Med 2004; 32:2378–84.

41. Lim SC, Adams AB, Simonson DA, et al. Intercomparison of recruitment maneuver efficacy in three models of acute lung injury. Crit Care Med 2004; 32:2371–7.

42. Odenstedt H, Aneman A, Karason S, et al. Acute hemodynamic changes during lung recruitment in lavage and endotoxin-induced ALI. Intensive Care Med 2005; 31:112–20.

43. Suki B, Alencar AM, Tolnai J, et al. Size distribution of recruited alveolar volumes in airway reopening. J Appl Physiol 2000; 89:2030–40.

44. Gaver DP, 3rd, Samsel RW, Solway J. Effects of surface tension and viscosity on airway reopening. J Appl Physiol 1990; 69:74–85.

45. Neumann P, Berglund JE, Mondejar EF, et al. Dynamics of lung collapse and recruitment during prolonged breathing in porcine lung injury. J Appl Physiol 1998; 85:1533–43.

46. Schreiter D, Reske A, Stichert B, et al. Alveolar recruitment in combination with sufficient positive end-expiratory pressure increases oxygenation and lung aeration in patients with severe chest trauma. Crit Care Med 2004; 32:968–75.

47. Medoff BD, Harris RS, Kesselman H, et al. Use of recruitment maneuvers and high-positive end-expiratory pressure in a patient with acute respiratory distress syndrome. Crit Care Med 2000; 28:1210–6.

48. Fujino Y, Goddon S, Dolhnikoff M, et al. Repetitive high-pressure recruitment maneuvers required to maximally recruit lung in a sheep model of acute respiratory distress syndrome. Crit Care Med 2001; 29:1579–86.

49. Villagra A, Ochagavia A, Vatua S, et al. Recruitment maneuvers during lung protective ventilation in acute respiratory distress syndrome. Am J Respir Crit Care Med 2002; 165:165–70.

50. Sharma S, Mullins RJ, Trunkey DD. Ventilatory management of pulmonary contusion patients. Am J Surg 1996; 171:529–32.

51. Roth H, Luecke T, Deventer B, et al. Pulmonary gas distribution during ventilation with different inspiratory flow patterns in experimental lung injury: A computed tomography study. Acta Anaesthesiol Scand 2004; 48:851–61.

52. Zavala E, Ferrer M, Polese G, et al. Effect of inverse I:E ratio ventilation on pulmonary gas exchange in acute respiratory distress syndrome. Anesthesiology 1998; 88:35–42.

53. Dembinski R, Henzler D, Bensberg R, et al. Ventilation-perfusion distribution related to different inspiratory flow patterns in experimental lung injury. Anesth Analg 2004; 98:211–9.

54. Prella M, Feihl F, Domenighetti G. Effects of short-term pressure-controlled ventilation on gas exchange, airway pressures, and gas distribution in patients with acute lung injury/ARDS: Comparison with volume-controlled ventilation. Chest 2002; 122:1382–8.

55. Davis K Jr, Branson RD, Campbell RS, Porembka DT. Comparison of volume control and pressure control ventilation: Is flow waveform the difference? J Trauma 1996; 41:808–14.

56. Yang SC, Yang SP. Effects of inspiratory flow waveforms on lung mechanics, gas exchange, and respiratory metabolism in COPD patients during mechanical ventilation. Chest 2002; 122:2096–104.

57. Al-Saady N, Bennett ED. Decelerating inspiratory flow waveform improves lung mechanics and gas exchange in patients on intermittent positive-pressure ventilation. Intensive Care Med 1985; 11:68–75.

58. Esteban A, Alia I, Gordo F, et al. Prospective, randomized trial comparing pressure-controlled ventilation and volume-controlled ventilation in ARDS. For the Spanish Lung Failure Collaborative Group. Chest 2000; 117:1690–6.

59. Tugrul M, Camci E, Karadeniz H, et al. Comparison of volume controlled with pressure controlled ventilation during one-lung anaesthesia. Br J Anaesth 1997; 79:306–10.

60. Rappaport SH, Shpiner R, Yoshihara G, et al. Randomized, prospective trial of pressure-limited versus volume-controlled ventilation in severe respiratory failure. Crit Care Med 1994; 22:22–32.

61. Sinha SK, Donn SM, Gavey J, McCarty M. Randomised trial of volume controlled versus time cycled, pressure limited ventilation in preterm infants with respiratory distress syndrome. Arch Dis Child Fetal Neonatal Ed 1997; 77:F202–5.

62. Casetti AV, Bartlett RH, Hirschl RB. Increasing inspiratory time exacerbates ventilator-induced lung injury during high-pressure/high-volume mechanical ventilation. Crit Care Med 2002; 30:2295–9.

63. Bilek AM, Dee KC, Gaver DP 3rd. Mechanisms of surface-tension-induced epithelial cell damage in a model of pulmonary airway reopening. J Appl Physiol 2003; 94:770–83.

64. Kay SS, Bilek AM, Dee KC, Gaver DP 3rd. Pressure gradient, not exposure duration, determines the extent of epithelial cell damage in a model of pulmonary airway reopening. J Appl Physiol 2004; 97:269–76.

65. Peevy KJ, Hernandez LA, Moise AA, Parker JC. Barotrauma and microvascular injury in lungs of nonadult rabbits: Effect of ventilation pattern. Crit Care Med 1990; 18:634–7.

66. Medeiros DM, Caramez MPR, Barbas CSV, et al. Flow pattern does not change ventilator induced lung injury (VILI) evolution. Am J Respir Crit Care Med 1998; 157:A45.

67. Rich PB, Reickert CA, Sawada S, et al. Effect of rate and inspiratory flow on ventilator-induced lung injury. J Trauma 2000; 49:903–11.

68. Munoz J, Guerrero JE, Escalante JL, et al. Pressure-controlled ventilation versus controlled mechanical ventilation with decelerating inspiratory flow. Crit Care Med 1993; 21:1143–8.

69. Guerin C, Lemasson S, La Cara MF, Fournier G. Physiological effects of constant versus decelerating inflation flow in patients with chronic obstructive pulmonary disease under controlled mechanical ventilation. Intensive Care Med 2002; 28:164–9.

70. Chandra A, Coggeshall JW, Ravenscraft SA, Marini JJ. Hyperpnea limits the volume recruited by positive end-expiratory pressure. Am J Respir Crit Care Med 1994; 150:911–7.

71. Coggeshall JW, Marini JJ, Newman JH. Improved oxygenation after muscle relaxation in adult respiratory distress syndrome. Arch Intern Med 1985; 145:1718–20.

72. Gainnier M, Roch A, Forel JM, et al. Effect of neuromuscular blocking agents on gas exchange in patients presenting with acute respiratory distress syndrome. Crit Care Med 2004; 32:113–9.

73. Carlon GC, Ray C Jr, Klein R, et al. Criteria for selective positive end-expiratory pressure and independent synchronized ventilation of each lung. Chest 1978; 74:501–7.

74. Lehnert BE, Oberdorster G, Slutsky AS. Constant-flow ventilation of apneic dogs. J Appl Physiol 1982; 53:483–9.

75. Laffey JG, Kavanagh BP. Biological effects of hypercapnia. Intensive Care Med 2000; 26:133–8.

76. de Letter MA, Schmitz PI, Visser LH, et al. Risk factors for the development of polyneuropathy and myopathy in critically ill patients. Crit Care Med 2001; 29:2281–6.

77. Bercker S, Weber-Carstens S, Deja M, et al. Critical illness polyneuropathy and myopathy in patients with acute respiratory distress syndrome. Crit Care Med 2005; 33:711–5.

78. Vassilakopoulos T, Petrof BJ. Ventilator-induced diaphragmatic dysfunction. Am J Respir Crit Care Med 2004; 169:336–41.

79. Sassoon CS, Caiozzo VJ, Manka A, Sieck GC. Altered diaphragm contractile properties with controlled mechanical ventilation. J Appl Physiol 2002; 92:2585–95.

80. Sassoon CS, Zhu E, Caiozzo VJ. Assist-control mechanical ventilation attenuates ventilator-induced diaphragmatic dysfunction. Am J Respir Crit Care Med 2004; 170:626–32.

81. Hund E. Neurological complications of sepsis: Critical illness polyneuropathy and myopathy. J Neurol 2001; 248:929–34.

82. Garnacho-Montero J, Amaya-Villar R, Garcia-Garmendia JL, et al. Effect of critical illness polyneuropathy on the withdrawal from mechanical ventilation and the length of stay in septic patients. Crit Care Med 2005; 33:349–54.

83. Wrigge H, Zinserling J, Neumann P, et al. Spontaneous breathing improves lung aeration in oleic acid-induced lung injury. Anesthesiology 2003; 99:376–84.

84. Cinnella G, Conti G, Lofaso F, et al. Effects of assisted ventilation on the work of breathing: Volume-controlled versus pressure-controlled ventilation. Am J Respir Crit Care Med 1996; 153:1025–33.

85. Schettino GP, Tucci MR, Sousa R, et al. Mask mechanics and leak dynamics during noninvasive pressure support ventilation: A bench study. Intensive Care Med 2001; 27:1887–91.

86. Girault C, Richard JC, Chevron V, et al. Comparative physiologic effects of noninvasive assist-control and pressure support ventilation in acute hypercapnic respiratory failure. Chest 1997; 111:1639–48.

87. Parthasarathy S, Tobin MJ. Effect of ventilator mode on sleep quality in critically ill patients. Am J Respir Crit Care Med 2002; 166:1423–9.

88. Calderini E, Confalonieri M, Puccio PG, et al. Patient-ventilator asynchrony during noninvasive ventilation: The role of expiratory trigger. Intensive Care Med 1999; 25:662–7.

89. Imanaka H, Kacmarek RM, Ritz R, Hess D. Tracheal gas insufflation-pressure control versus volume control ventilation: A lung model study. Am J Respir Crit Care Med 1996; 153:1019–24.

90. Kirmse M, Fujino Y, Hromi J, et al. Pressure-release tracheal gas insufflation reduces airway pressures in lung-injured sheep maintaining eucapnia. Am J Respir Crit Care Med 1999; 160:1462–7.

91. Neumann P, Golisch W, Strohmeyer A, et al. Influence of different release times on spontaneous breathing pattern during airway pressure release ventilation. Intensive Care Med 2002; 28:1742–9.

92. Chiang AA, Steinfeld A, Gropper C, MacIntyre N. Demand-flow airway pressure release ventilation as a partial ventilatory

support mode: comparison with synchronized intermittent mandatory ventilation and pressure support ventilation. Crit Care Med 1994; 22:1431–7.

93. Calzia E, Lindner KH, Witt S, et al. Pressure-time product and work of breathing during biphasic continuous positive airway pressure and assisted spontaneous breathing. Am J Respir Crit Care Med 1994; 150:904–10.

94. Marini JJ, Smith TC, Lamb VJ. External work output and force generation during synchronized intermittent mechanical ventilation: Effect of machine assistance on breathing effort. Am Rev Respir Dis 1988; 138:1169–79.

95. Putensen C, Zech S, Wrigge H, et al. Long-term effects of spontaneous breathing during ventilatory support in patients with acute lung injury. Am J Respir Crit Care Med 2001; 164: 43–9.

96. Kaplan LJ, Bailey H, Formosa V. Airway pressure release ventilation increases cardiac performance in patients with acute lung injury/adult respiratory distress syndrome. Crit Care 2001; 5:221–6.

97. Hering R, Peters D, Zinserling J, et al. Effects of spontaneous breathing during airway pressure release ventilation on renal perfusion and function in patients with acute lung injury. Intensive Care Med 2002; 28:1426–33.

98. Putensen C, Mutz NJ, Putensen-Himmer G, Zinserling J. Spontaneous breathing during ventilatory support improves ventilation-perfusion distributions in patients with acute respiratory distress syndrome. Am J Respir Crit Care Med 1999; 159:1241–8.

99. Neumann P, Hedenstierna G. Ventilatory support by continuous positive airway pressure breathing improves gas exchange as compared with partial ventilatory support with airway pressure release ventilation. Anesth Analg 2001; 92: 950–8.

100. Steinberg JM, Schiller HJ, Halter JM, et al. Alveolar instability causes early ventilator-induced lung injury independent of neutrophils. Am J Respir Crit Care Med 2004; 169:57–63.

101. Taskar V, John J, Evander E, et al. Surfactant dysfunction makes lungs vulnerable to repetitive collapse and reexpansion. Am J Respir Crit Care Med 1997; 155:313–20.

102. Muscedere JG, Mullen JB, Gan K, Slutsky AS. Tidal ventilation at low airway pressures can augment lung injury. Am J Respir Crit Care Med 1994; 149:1327–34.

103. D'Angelo E, Pecchiari M, Baraggia P, et al. Low-volume ventilation causes peripheral airway injury and increased airway resistance in normal rabbits. J Appl Physiol 2002; 92:949–56.

104. Tremblay LN, Slutsky AS. Pathogenesis of ventilator-induced lung injury: Trials and tribulations. Am J Physiol Lung Cell Mol Physiol 2005; 288:L596–8.

105. Ranieri VM, Suter PM, Tortorella C, et al. Effect of mechanical ventilation on inflammatory mediators in patients with acute respiratory distress syndrome: A randomized, controlled trial. Jama 1999; 282:54–61.

106. Tremblay L, Valenza F, Ribeiro SP, et al. Injurious ventilatory strategies increase cytokines and c-fos m-RNA expression in an isolated rat lung model. J Clin Invest 1997; 99:944–52.

107. ARDSNet. Ventilation with lower tidal volumes as compared with traditional tidal volumes for acute lung injury and the acute respiratory distress syndrome. New Engl J Med 2000; 342:1301–8.

108. Duncan SR, Rizk NW, Raffin TA. Inverse ratio ventilation. PEEP in disguise? Chest 1987; 92:390–2.

109. Wang SH, Wei TS. The outcome of early pressure-controlled inverse ratio ventilation on patients with severe acute respiratory distress syndrome in surgical intensive care unit. Am J Surg 2002; 183:151–5.

110. Smith RP, Fletcher R. Pressure-controlled inverse ratio ventilation after cardiac surgery. Eur J Anaesthesiol 2001; 18: 401–6.

111. Ravenscraft SA, Burke WC, Marini JJ. Volume-cycled decelerating flow: An alternative form of mechanical ventilation. Chest 1992; 101:1342–51.

112. Ludwigs U, Klingstedt C, Baehrendtz S, Hedenstierna G. A comparison of pressure- and volume-controlled ventilation at different inspiratory to expiratory ratios. Acta Anaesthesiol Scand 1997; 41:71–7.

113. Kress JP, Pohlman AS, O'Connor MF, Hall JB. Daily interruption of sedative infusions in critically ill patients undergoing mechanical ventilation. New Engl J Med 2000; 342: 1471–7.

114. Mang H, Kacmarek RM, Ritz R, et al. Cardiorespiratory effects of volume- and pressure-controlled ventilation at various I:E ratios in an acute lung injury model. Am J Respir Crit Care Med 1995; 151:731–6.

115. Lichtwarck-Aschoff M, Markstrom AM, Hedlund AJ, et al. Oxygenation remains unaffected by increased inspiration-to-expiration ratio but impairs hemodynamics in surfactant-depleted piglets. Intensive Care Med 1996; 22:329–35.

116. Ludwigs U, Klingstedt C, Baehrendtz S, et al. A functional and morphologic analysis of pressure-controlled inverse ratio ventilation in oleic acid-induced lung injury. Chest 1994; 106: 925–31.

117. Ludwigs U, Philip A. Pulmonary epithelial permeability and gas exchange: A comparison of inverse ratio ventilation and conventional mechanical ventilation in oleic acid–induced lung injury in rabbits. Chest 1998; 113:459–66.

118. Armstrong BW Jr, MacIntyre NR. Pressure-controlled, inverse ratio ventilation that avoids air trapping in the adult respiratory distress syndrome. Crit Care Med 1995; 23:279–85.

119. Yanos J, Watling SM, Verhey J. The physiologic effects of inverse ratio ventilation. Chest 1998; 114:834–8.

120. Mercat A, Diehl JL, Michard F, et al. Extending inspiratory time in acute respiratory distress syndrome. Crit Care Med 2001; 29:40–4.

121. Baumgardner JE, Markstaller K, Pfeiffer B, et al. Effects of respiratory rate, plateau pressure, and positive end-expiratory pressure on Pa_{O_2} oscillations after saline lavage. Am J Respir Crit Care Med 2002; 166:1556–62.

122. Stewart AR, Finer NN, Peters KL. Effects of alterations of inspiratory and expiratory pressures and inspiratory/expiratory ratios on mean airway pressure, blood gases, and intracranial pressure. Pediatrics 1981; 67:474–81.

123. Lachmann B. Open up the lung and keep the lung open. Intensive Care Med 1992; 18:319–21.

124. Vazquez de Anda GF, Hartog A, Verbrugge SJ, et al. The open lung concept: pressure-controlled ventilation is as effective as high-frequency oscillatory ventilation in improving gas exchange and lung mechanics in surfactant-deficient animals. Intensive Care Med 1999; 25:990–6.

125. Neumann P, Berglund JE, Mondejar EF, et al. Effect of different pressure levels on the dynamics of lung collapse and recruitment in oleic-acid-induced lung injury. Am J Respir Crit Care Med 1998; 158:1636–43.

126. Rossi A, Santos C, Roca J, et al. Effects of PEEP on $\dot{V}_A/\dot{Q}$ mismatching in ventilated patients with chronic airflow obstruction. Am J Respir Crit Care Med 1994; 149:1077–84.

127. Brandolese R, Broseghini C, Polese G, et al. Effects of intrinsic PEEP on pulmonary gas exchange in mechanically ventilated patients. Eur Respir J 1993; 6:358–63.

128. Ludwigs U, Klingstedt C, Baehrendtz S, et al. Volume-controlled inverse ratio ventilation in oleic acid induced lung

injury: Effects on gas exchange, hemodynamics, and computed tomographic lung density. Chest 1995; 108:804–9.

129. Sydow M, Burchardi H, Ephraim E, et al. Long-term effects of two different ventilatory modes on oxygenation in acute lung injury: Comparison of airway pressure release ventilation and volume-controlled inverse ratio ventilation. Am J Respir Crit Care Med 1994; 149:1550–6.

130. Leatherman JW. Mechanical ventilation in obstructive lung disease. Clin Chest Med 1996; 17:577–90.

131. Vieillard-Baron A, Jardin F. The issue of dynamic hyperinfla-
tion in acute respiratory distress syndrome patients. Eur Respir J Suppl 2003; 42:43–7s.

132. Vieillard-Baron A, Prin S, Augarde R, et al. Increasing respiratory rate to improve CO_2 clearance during mechanical ventilation is not a panacea in acute respiratory failure. Crit Care Med 2002; 30:1407–12.

133. Vieillard-Baron A, Prin S, Schmitt JM, et al. Pressure-volume curves in acute respiratory distress syndrome: Clinical demonstration of the influence of expiratory flow limitation on the initial slope. Am J Respir Crit Care Med 2002; 165:1107–12.

Chapter 11

POSITIVE END-EXPIRATORY PRESSURE

PAOLO NAVALESI
SALVATORE MAURIZIO MAGGIORE

In the first edition of this book, Rossi and Ranieri began their chapter on positive end-expiratory pressure (PEEP) by stating how difficult it was review the topic because of the enormous number of published studies.[1] Although ancient Romans used to say, "*Excusatio non petita accusatio manifesta* [he who excuses himself accuses himself]," we approach PEEP 12 years later claiming that today it is impossible to cite, not to mention have detailed knowledge of, the entire literature on PEEP.[2] We performed a search through Medline of articles available in English on PEEP published between 1964 and 2004 and found 6788 publications. Publications on PEEP continue to increase (Fig. 11-1). When the search was confined to randomized, controlled trials, the increase is even more pronounced. An identical search for furosemide yielded about the same total number of articles in the last 40 years. Articles on furosemide, however, have declined over the last 10 years (see Fig. 11-1).

PEEP has been defined as "a technique of respiratory therapy, in either spontaneously breathing or mechani-cally ventilated patients, in which airway pressure is main-tained above atmospheric pressure throughout the respi-ratory cycle by pressurization of the ventilatory circuit."[3] This definition makes clear that PEEP is not a ventila-tor mode itself. Rather, it is an adjunctive treatment that can be associated with all forms of mechanical ventila-tion, both controlled and assisted,[4-10] or applied to spon-taneous breathing throughout the entire respiratory cycle, so-called continuous positive airway pressure (CPAP).[11-14] When PEEP is applied to a pressure-preset mode, the pre-set inspiratory pressure is commonly intended as an addi-tion to PEEP. That is, the actual pressure applied during inspiration is the sum of inspiratory and expiratory pre-set pressures. When the terms *expiratory positive airway pres-sure* (EPAP) and *inspiratory positive airway pressure* (IPAP) are encountered—mainly, but not exclusively, with a turbine-driven (so-called bilevel) ventilator—IPAP indicates the to-tal pressure applied during inspiration; thus the actual as-sistance above positive expiratory pressure is the difference between IPAP and EPAP.

Many pathologic conditions benefit from the mainte-nance of a positive expiratory pressure, as shown by the pioneering work of Poulton and Oxon[11] and Barach et al.[15] They demonstrated in the mid-1930s that application of positive pressure to the airway can treat patients with pul-monary edema effectively. Yet the "Medical Subject Head-ing" (MeSH), surprisingly, refers to PEEP as "a method of mechanical ventilation in which pressure is maintained to increase the volume of gas remaining in the lungs at the end of expiration, thus reducing the shunting of blood through the lungs and improving gas exchange." Thus MeSH con-siders only one effect of PEEP, albeit the most widely recog-nized one.

Despite several drawbacks and complications,[16-28] intensive-care unit (ICU) physicians view PEEP as one of the most powerful treatments available for acute respira-tory failure (ARF); in a recent international survey of ICUs on three continents, PEEP was being used in more than 90% patients with acute respiratory distress syndrome (ARDS) and in more than 60% of patients with an exacerbation of chronic obstructive pulmonary disease (COPD).[29]

Overview of Pertinent Pathophysiology

The application of intermittent positive pressure is intended principally to replace, completely or in part, the func-tion of the respiratory muscles and therefore corrects hy-poxemia caused by alveolar hypoventilation. The reversal of hypoxemia caused by intrapulmonary shunt and ve-nous admixture, however, requires interventions that re-cruit more aerated lung units for ventilation. In patients with an acute reduction of the lung volume secondary to lung edema and/or atelectasis, PEEP can improve arterial oxygenation[4,12] by increasing funtional residual capacity (FRC),[30-35] reducing venous admixture,[16,36-39] shifting tidal volume (V_T) to a more compliant portion of the pressure-volume (P-V) curve,[40] preventing the loss of compliance during mechanical ventilation,[8,41] and reducing the work

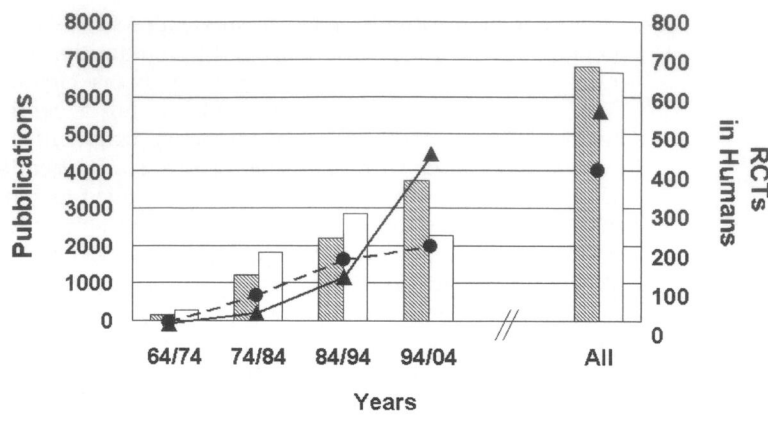

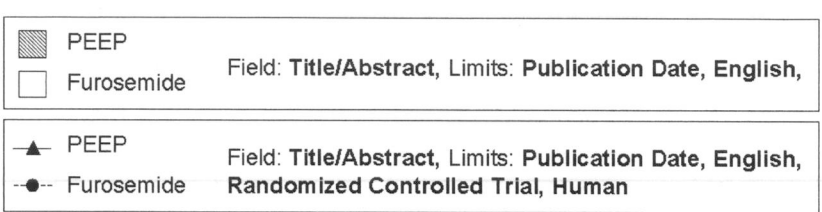

FIGURE 11-1 Publications on PEEP and furosemide from January 1964 to December 2004, obtained from Medline through the National Library of Medicine (*www.ncbi.nlm.nih.gov/ entrez/query.fcgi*). Articles on PEEP and furosemide are indicated by the gray and white bars, respectively (*left axis*). Triangles and circles represent randomized, controlled trials (RCTs) on PEEP and furosemide, respectively (*right axis*). The left side shows articles distributed by decades; the right side presents the sum totals.

of breathing.[42] Figure 11-2A summarizes the rationale for PEEP in patients with ARF secondary to acute lung volume reduction.

Although there is general consensus about the usefulness of PEEP in treating patients with hypoxemic ARF secondary to lung edema and/or atelectasis, several aspects are controversial. For many years it has been recognized that the actions of PEEP on gas exchange and pulmonary mechanics are variable and somewhat unpredictable,[43–47] depending on the cause of ARF, which may be sustained by different pathways[48–50] and pathophysiologic mechanisms.[35,43,48,50] As with any treatment, PEEP is not free of side effects.[24] In patients with acute lung injury (ALI) or ARDS, PEEP recruits nonaerated regions but also distends normally aerated regions,[51,52] contributing to barotrauma through an increase in end-inspiratory plateau pressure.[16,21,26,53,54] High levels of PEEP also have been shown to augment the physiologic dead space[18,39,55] and worsen gas exchange[51] and tissue perfusion.[56–58] Extrapulmonary side effects of PEEP include decreased cardiac output,[17,27,43,59–62] increased intracranial pressure,[19,63] renal dysfunction,[20,64] and decreased splanchnic perfusion[25,65–68] and oxygenation.[56,57]

Benefits and detriments of PEEP have been weighted variously by authors. Both the lowest PEEP resulting in acceptable oxygenation[56,69–71] and a PEEP level exceeding the lower inflection point on the P-V curve (to maximize lung recruitment[9,72] and minimize shear stress caused by repeated opening and collapse of alveolar units during inflation[73]) have been proposed as the best strategy for ALI/ARDS. After many years, debate on optimal PEEP[18] and the best method for detecting it still flourishes.

PEEP is beneficial for reasons other than lung-volume recruitment. In patients with COPD and ARF, hypoxemia is reversed by relatively low concentrations of oxygen (O_2),[74,75] although reversal of the associated respiratory acidosis[76]

FIGURE 11-2 Respiratory effects of PEEP/CPAP in acute respiratory failure secondary to (A) lung volume reduction caused by edema and/or atelectasis and (B) airway obstruction and expiratory flow limitation.

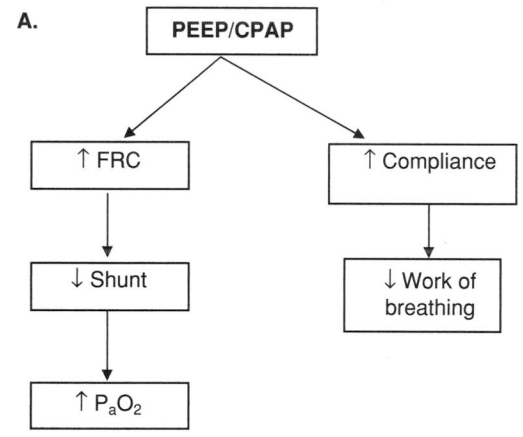

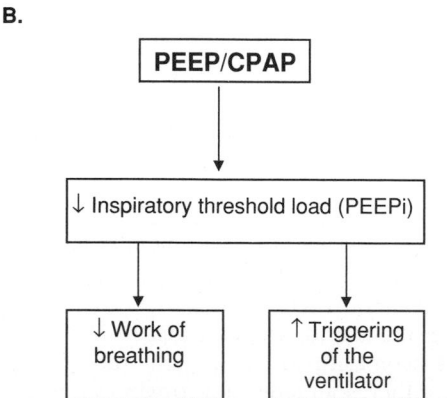

often requires mechanical ventilation.[77,78] In these patients it was thought initially that PEEP produced little or no additional benefit on gas exchange.[79] Following the fundamental work of Pepe and Marini,[80] it was recognized that, particularly in presence of airflow obstruction, the lungs may fail to deflate to FRC at end expiration. Consequently, alveolar pressure remains positive to an extent that depends on the volume of trapped air, a phenomenon referred to as *auto-PEEP* or *intrinsic PEEP* ($PEEP_I$). In this setting, application of external PEEP may be beneficial. Benefit is evident during spontaneous breathing: CPAP has been shown to reduce dyspnea[13,81] and work of breathing.[13,81,82] Benefit is also evident with any patient-triggered mode of ventilation[5,83–85]: PEEP enhances triggering function,[5,83–85] reduces the patient's respiratory drive,[84] reduces inspiratory muscle effort,[5,83–85] and improves patient-ventilator interaction.[85,86] PEEP replaces the amount of pressure that must be generated by the inspiratory muscles to offset $PEEP_I$ (necessary to initiate inspiratory flow or trigger the ventilator).[5,84] The principal effects of PEEP in patients with COPD are summarized in Fig. 11-2B.

If PEEP exceeds $PEEP_I$, it may further hyperinflate the lungs,[87] increase the risk of barotrauma,[88] place the diaphragm at an additional mechanical disadvantage,[28,89] and further impair hemodynamics.[27,87] To achieve the best results, PEEP should be titrated according to a precise evaluation of the level of $PEEP_I$.[90] In passively ventilated patients, this evaluation is straightforward: The expiratory valve of the ventilator is kept occluded at end expiration.[91] Evaluation is not easy when the respiratory muscles are active,[5,92,93] during spontaneous breathing and patient-triggered ventilator assistance, the situation where PEEP is of paramount importance.

PEEP has substantial effects on hemodynamics. When left-ventricular function is normal, an increase in intrathoracic pressure causes a fall in cardiac output largely secondary to a decrease in venous return (i.e., preload).[17,94,95] In patients with poor left-ventricular function, when filling pressure and left-ventricular diastolic volume are elevated, cardiac output is relatively insensitive to a decline in venous return.[96] In this condition the dominant effect of an increase in intrathoracic pressure is to decrease left-ventricular transmural pressure (i.e., afterload), which improves left-ventricular performance.[97–100] These effects (Fig. 11-3C) are also observed with relatively moderate levels of CPAP; the impact on afterload is likely to result primarily from a reduction in the inspiratory negative swings of intrathoracic pressure[101] consequent to improvement in respiratory mechanics.[101] Application of CPAP in patients with severe cardiogenic pulmonary edema may accelerate the physiologic improvement and reduce the need for endotracheal intubation.[14,102–104]

Several investigators have studied the use of CPAP in the treatment of the obstructive sleep apnea syndrome. Sleep apnea is characterized by a reduction or cessation of breathing secondary to periodic narrowing and/or collapse of the upper airway. It can be reversed by CPAP, which keeps the pharynx patent by acting as a "pneumatic splint."[105] In symptomatic patients, CPAP reduces excessive daytime sleepiness,[106] improves cognitive performance[107] and left-ventricular function,[108–110] and decreases daytime blood pressure.[106,108] Detailed discussion of this topic is beyond the scope of this chapter.

Likewise, we do not provide detailed discussion of positive expiratory pressure (PEP), a physiotherapeutic technique aimed at clearance of secretions. PEP is based on the theory that its application might improve collateral ventilation[111] and enhance mucus progression toward the central airways.[112,113] Although using different devices and methods of administration, several studies suggest that PEP might be equally or more effective than other physiotherapeutic techniques for aiding secretion clearance and reducing the risk of atelectasis and superinfection.[114,115] A recent systematic review, however, has weakened enthusiasm for PEP, failing to document any advantage over other physiotherapeutic techniques and raising doubts as to its acceptance by patients.[116]

Physiologic Rationale for PEEP

EFFECT OF PEEP ON GAS EXCHANGE

Ensuring adequate O_2 uptake and carbon dioxide (CO_2) elimination is the chief function of the respiratory system. This function is altered in ARF. Hypoxemia [i.e., an arterial O_2 tension (Pa_{O_2}) lower than 60 mmHg at sea level] is the hallmark of this condition. Mechanical ventilation does not cure the disease that causes ARF. Rather, it buys time and allows the patient to recover. Although correction of gas-exchange abnormalities is not the ultimate goal of the global therapeutic strategy, nevertheless, safe arterial blood-gas values are fundamental for sustaining vital function while waiting for more specific treatment to become effective. The role of PEEP in increasing Pa_{O_2} in patients with pulmonary edema and ARF has long been recognized[117,118] and documented extensively.[18,39,119–122]

The transfer of O_2 from air to mitochondria is termed the O_2 *cascade*.[123] O_2 tension (P_{O_2}) of moist inspired air at sea level is 149 mmHg. P_{O_2} drops to about 100 mmHg in the alveoli, depending on the balance between O_2 supply and removal, which is determined by alveolar ventilation and pulmonary blood flow. Blood equilibrates with the alveolar O_2 while passing through the pulmonary capillaries. Hence, ideally, P_{O_2} in the pulmonary capillaries is the same as in the alveolar gas, whereas Pa_{O_2} is slightly lower (90–95 mmHg) because of some venous admixture from the bronchial and coronary veins. When the arterial blood reaches the peripheral tissues, Pa_{O_2} falls dramatically because of O_2 transfer to the tissues. Any fall in Pa_{O_2} therefore should be reflected by a decrease in tissue P_{O_2}. The aforementioned process moves in the opposite direction for CO_2. Because there is essentially no CO_2 in inspired air, under normal conditions, P_{CO_2} at the arterial and alveolar levels is the same, whereas mixed venous P_{CO_2} is about 45–47 mmHg. Tissue P_{CO_2} is quite variable depending on several factors, such as metabolic rate. Any impairment of lung function that hinders CO_2 removal will increase tissue P_{CO_2}.

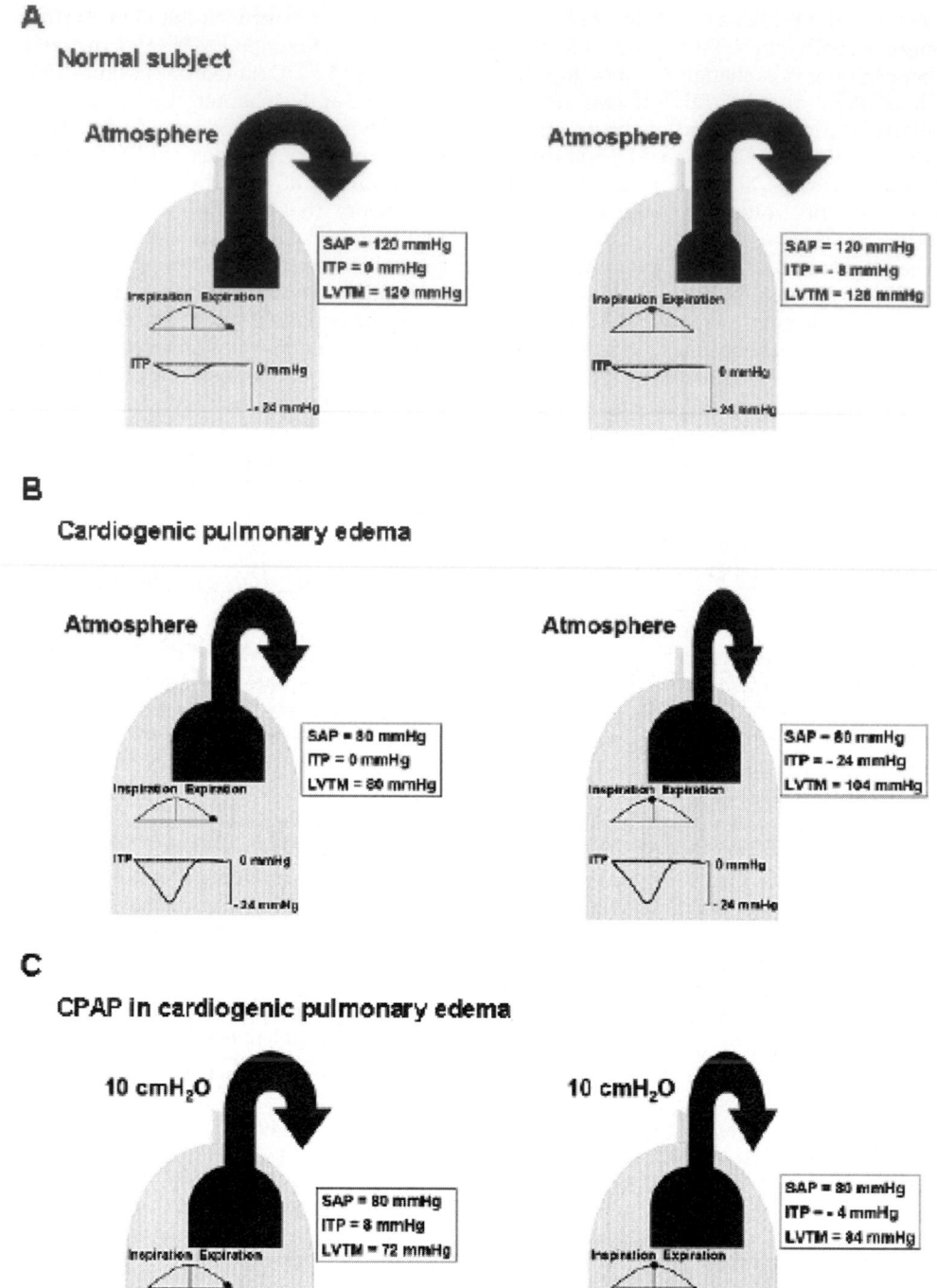

FIGURE 11-3 Heart-lung interactions during spontaneous breathing in a normal subject (*A*) and in a patient with cardiogenic pulmonary edema resulting from low cardiac output in the absence (*B*) and presence (*C*) of CPAP. The effects of variations in intrathoracic pressure (ITP) on left-ventricular systolic function are shown at end expiration (*left panels*) and end inspiration (*right panels*). SAP, systolic arterial (intraventricular) pressure; LVTM, left-ventricular transmural pressure (SAP – ITP). In a normal subject (*A*), tidal excursions in ITP have little effect on left-ventricular systolic function. In a patient with pulmonary edema (*B*), more negative swings in ITP are needed to achieve the same tidal volume. As a result, LVTM (afterload) is increased independently of systemic vascular resistance. The rise in ITP produced by CPAP of 10 cmH₂O (*C*) results in a slight reduction in LVTM during expiration. CPAP remarkably decreases LVTM during inspiration by decreasing negative swings in ITP because of improved lung mechanics.

Physiologic gas exchange requires that (1) air reaches the alveoli, (2) the membrane interposed between alveoli and capillaries is intact, and (3) the flow of blood through the pulmonary capillaries is not altered. Ideally, the greatest efficiency of pulmonary gas exchange occurs when regional ventilation ($\dot{V}_A$) and perfusion ($\dot{Q}$) are completely matched; i.e., $\dot{V}_A/\dot{Q} = 1$. Because of slight heterogeneities in $\dot{V}_A/\dot{Q}$ ratio (secondary to gravity and a small shunt caused by venous blood flow draining from coronary and bronchial veins into systemic circulation), $\dot{V}_A/\dot{Q}$ normally approximates 0.8. Gas exchange is also affected by extrapulmonary factors, such as the inspired O_2 fraction ($F_{I_{O_2}}$), minute ventilation ($\dot{V}_E$), cardiac output, and O_2 consumption ($\dot{V}_{O_2}$) (i.e., metabolic rate). In absence of an intrapulmonary shunt, any increase in $F_{I_{O_2}}$ produces a rise in Pa_{O_2}; the extent depends on the degree of $\dot{V}_A/\dot{Q}$ mismatch.[124–126] $\dot{V}_E$ depends on the activity of the respiratory centers, provided that respiratory mechanics are normal. The effect of change in $\dot{V}_E$ on gas exchange depends on the degree of $\dot{V}_A/\dot{Q}$ inequality.[125–127] The consequences of increase in $\dot{V}_E$ are greater for CO_2 removal than for O_2 uptake because the dissociation curve for CO_2, as opposed to that for O_2, is quite linear.[125] This is true even in case of substantial $\dot{V}_A/\dot{Q}$ mismatch, which explains the high Pa_{CO_2} dependency on $\dot{V}_E$.[128,129] Through effects on mixed venous O_2 tension ($\overline{Pv}_{O_2}$), cardiac output and metabolic rate can influence Pa_{O_2}. $\overline{Pv}_{O_2}$ may decrease as a result of decreased cardiac output, increased O_2 uptake by tissues, or reduced arterial O_2 content. A reduced $\overline{Pv}_{O_2}$, in turn, may decrease Pa_{O_2} to an extent that depends on $\dot{V}_A/\dot{Q}$ mismatch.[124,125,130,131]

EFFECT IN ANESTHETIZED SUBJECTS

Arterial oxygenation often is impaired during anesthesia[132,133] as a result of the intrapulmonary shunt[134–138] caused by atelectasis, predominantly in the dependent zones.[133,139–145] Areas of collapsed parenchyma occur in 90% of all intubated anesthetized subjects during both spontaneous breathing and muscle paralysis.[138,146–148] Other mechanisms, such as regional distribution of ventilation,[149] airway closure,[150–160] and pharmacologic inhibition of hypoxic vasoconstriction[161–164] also may contribute. Application of PEEP during anesthesia can prevent or reverse closing of peripheral airways,[153] decrease atelectasis,[138,148,165] and improve regional $\dot{V}_A/\dot{Q}$ ratios and oxygenation,[166,167] although shunt may be improved only in part.[138] In normal anesthetized dogs, however, Dueck et al[168] found that PEEP of 10 cmH$_2$O or greater produced a reduction in Pa_{O_2} and increases in dead-space ventilation and Pa_{CO_2}. This was caused mainly by a drop in cardiac output associated with an increase in alveolar ventilation of both high $\dot{V}_A/\dot{Q}$ and unperfused lung regions, suggesting overdistension of nondependent lung regions. Similarly, Pelosi et al[169] showed that PEEP values up to 10 cmH$_2$O decreased, although not significantly, Pa_{O_2} during general anesthesia in normal subjects. In contrast, Pa_{O_2} increased in obese patients; this increase was correlated with recruitment of atelectatic lung regions.

Alterations in diaphragmatic position and mechanics during anesthesia also contribute to impaired gas exchange by inducing ventilation abnormalities in the dependent zones.[170,171] This phenomenon has been elegantly studied in anesthetized rabbits by Heneghan et al,[170] who compared PEEP and phrenic nerve stimulation adjusted to produce the same increase in lung volume. Phrenic stimulation caused a greater caudal movement of the diaphragm, particularly in the dependent regions, and produced greater improvement in gas exchange than did PEEP.

Conflicting data on the effect of PEEP have been obtained in postoperative patients who had developed respiratory failure. In two studies, PEEP up to 10 cmH$_2$O did not modify Pa_{O_2} significantly during the early postoperative course of patients who underwent cardiac or vascular surgery.[172,173] Conversely, other investigators found that PEEP, combined with bilevel positive airway pressure ventilation administered via a nasal mask, improved oxygenation in the vast majority of patients who exhibited respiratory distress after various types of surgery.[174–177] A recent randomized clinical trial found that the use of noninvasive positive-pressure ventilation with low PEEP (about 4 cmH$_2$O) increased Pa_{O_2}, reduced the need for intubation, and improved survival of patients who developed ARF after lung resection.[178]

In summary, use of PEEP to improve oxygenation during and after anesthesia in normal subjects has generated contradictory results probably because of the deleterious effects of PEEP on hemodynamics and lung overdistension. PEEP, however, can be effective in improving gas exchange in selected patients.

EFFECT IN HYPOXEMIC RESPIRATORY FAILURE

Most forms of hypoxemic respiratory failure, such as cardiogenic pulmonary edema, ALI/ARDS, and unilateral pneumonia, are characterized by a decrease in lung volume caused by atelectasis, interstitial and alveolar edema, and small airways closure. The pivotal mechanism for hypoxemia in these conditions is intrapulmonary shunt, as demonstrated by the small increase in Pa_{O_2} when pure O_2 is administered[179] and, to a lesser extent, $\dot{V}_A/\dot{Q}$ mismatch.[180,181] Moreover, the high $F_{I_{O_2}}$ frequently used in these patients may decrease lung volume by promoting alveolar denitrogenation and reabsorption atelectasis.[179,182] In ALI/ARDS, the altered blood flow distribution resulting from widespread involvement of the pulmonary vasculature[183] and impaired hypoxic vasoconstriction contributes to gas-exchange worsening.[182]

PEEP has long been recognized as an effective means of increasing lung volume and improving gas exchange.[4] In cardiogenic pulmonary edema, CPAP (alone or in association with an inspiratory assistance) improves gas exchange[14,102,184–195] by increasing aerated lung volume[196] and improving cardiac output[102,184,189] and $\dot{V}_A/\dot{Q}$ distribution.[196,197] A decrease in extravascular lung water is another possible mechanism whereby PEEP reduces intrapulmonary shunt.[198] Yet PEEP does not decrease, and sometimes increases, extravascular lung water when microvascular hydrostatic pressure is high.[199] Malo et al[197] clarified this issue. They showed that PEEP of 13 cmH$_2$O decreased shunt and alveolar flooding without modifying extravascular lung water; indeed, perivascular cuff edema increased.[197] These findings indicate that PEEP redistributes the excess alveolar water into the compliant perivascular space, thus reinflating previously flooded and collapsed airspaces, without decreasing the overall amount of lung edema.[200]

Unilateral pneumonia and ALI/ARDS are characterized by severe impairment of gas exchange because of increased intrapulmonary shunt,[180,182] resulting mainly from flooded and/or collapsed alveoli.[201–204] This observation is corroborated by the correlation between the extent of lung densities found mainly in the dependent regions on a computed tomographic (CT) scan and deterioration in arterial blood gases.[34,121] In fact, the edema increases the total mass of the lung (up to more than twice that of normal lungs); consequently, the dependent zones collapse progressively under the weight of the superimposed lung (compression atelectasis), and aerated lung decreases ("baby lung" concept).[205–207]

Atelectasis in the lower lobes and in dependent lung regions may be caused by other mechanisms, such as external compression by the heart[208,209] and the abdominal compartment.[141,210,211] The severity of intrapulmonary shunt also may be affected by surfactant abnormalities,[212] increased airway resistance,[213–226] hyaline membranes, and inflammatory proteins and cells accumulating within the alveoli. Interstitial edema and the deposition of cells and connective tissue in the interalveolar septa may contribute further to gas-exchange impairment in ALI/ARDS. The amount of nonaerated lung volume also may be increased by the combined effects of reabsorption atelectasis[137,180,182,227] and ventilation occurring at low lung volumes.[228,229] Hypoxic pulmonary vasoconstriction appears greatly impaired in most patients with ALI/ARDS.[182,230] In some patients with diffuse lung injury, however, hypoxic pulmonary vasoconstriction is partially preserved, explaining a lack of hypoxemia despite diffuse loss of aeration. Conversely, hypoxic pulmonary vasoconstriction is constantly impaired in some patients with localized lung injury, explaining severe hypoxemia despite well-preserved lung aeration.[230]

Use of PEEP to correct gas-exchange impairment in ALI/ARDS was proposed initially by Asbaugh et al.[4] It remains the cornerstone of ventilator management of these patients. Extensive literature supports the use of PEEP for improving oxygenation in hypoxemic respiratory failure alone or in combination with various ventilator modes during both invasive[8,18,34,71,119,121,223,231–247] and noninvasive ventilation.[10,178,188,248–260] Several mechanisms may explain the effect of PEEP on gas exchange. PEEP promotes alveolar recruitment and increases aerated lung volume, thereby decreasing intrapulmonary shunt.[31,36,245,261,262] PEEP-induced recruitment of aerated lung volume is strongly correlated with arterial oxygenation[34,71,119,121,236,263–265] (Table 11-1). A redistribution of alveolar edema to the interstitial spaces also may explain the benefit of PEEP on gas exchange.[197] Following the pioneering work of Webb and Tierney,[266] PEEP has been shown to decrease pulmonary edema[267–269] partly because of a concomitant reduction in cardiac output.[268] By recruiting nonaerated alveoli and stabilizing airways, PEEP also affects the regional distribution of tidal ventilation.[210,238,270,271] When the predominant effect of PEEP is recruitment, alveolar ventilation is expected to become more homogeneous, particularly in the dependent zones. Although an increase in lung volume is the main mechanism for PEEP-induced changes in oxygenation, a small decrease in cardiac output also reduces intrapulmonary shunt and improves Pa_{O_2}.[60] Finally, different etiologies and pathophysiologic mechanisms of ALI/ARDS influence the response to PEEP,[50,237] although understanding is far from being conclusive.[272]

Improved efficiency of alveolar ventilation and an expected decrease in alveolar dead space should produce a reduction in Pa_{CO_2}. Several authors, however, have failed to find any significant relationship between Pa_{CO_2} and PEEP. The lack of response probably arises because PEEP both favors lung recruitment, which theoretically reduces Pa_{CO_2}, and promotes pulmonary overdistension, which theoretically increases Pa_{CO_2}.[210,273]

The benefit of PEEP on gas exchange also might be expected in unilateral pneumonia and localized lung injuries. In these conditions, however, high PEEP is more likely to produce overdistension of normally aerated regions because of the coexistence of areas with normal, low, and very low compliance.[210,238] The net effect of PEEP on gas exchange depends on the balance between overdistension of already aerated alveolar units and recruitment of collapsed (nonaerated) alveoli and is also influenced by the level of PEEP.[210,274] In patients with unilateral lung disease, PEEP may be detrimental whenever it hyperinflates the normal lung, thus directing blood flow to the diseased lung and increasing intrapulmonary shunt.[275–279] To limit this risk, unilateral delivery of PEEP to the injured lung has been proposed[280]; the technical complexity of this approach greatly limits its feasibility in the clinical practice.

In summary, PEEP improves gas exchange in hypoxemic ARF mainly through recruitment of previously nonaerated lung areas and the homogenization of regional distribution of tidal ventilation. PEEP remains the cornerstone of ventilator treatment of most forms of hypoxemic ARF. Debate continues about the optimal level of PEEP (see below), not about its usefulness.

EFFECT IN OBSTRUCTIVE LUNG DISEASE

Impaired gas exchange in obstructive lung diseases is caused by complex disturbances of regional $\dot{V}_A/\dot{Q}$ relationships associated with alveolar hypoventilation; diffusion impairment is not a major factor.[281] During an acute exacerbation of COPD, high $\dot{V}_A/\dot{Q}$ areas predominate in patients who mostly have the emphysematous variant with loss of blood flow consequent to alveolar wall destruction.[281–283] Conversely, low $\dot{V}_A/\dot{Q}$ regions are seen mostly in patients with a predominant obstructive component.[281–283] In general, application of PEEP does not affect gas exchange.[5,79,87,284,285] Nevertheless, Rossi et al[286] reported that low PEEP (50% of $PEEP_I$) induced a moderate increase in Pa_{O_2} and a slight decrease in Pa_{CO_2} secondary to improved $\dot{V}_A/\dot{Q}$ distribution without alteration in respiratory mechanics or hemodynamics.[286] Further increases

TABLE 11-1 Studies Assessing the Effect of PEEP on Lung Volumes and Other Physiologic Variables

Reference	Technique	PEEP cmH₂O	FRC ml	ΔEELV ml	Vrec ml	Vrec/ΔEELV %	Voverdist ml	ΔPaO₂ mmHg
Ranieri 1991 (71)	P-V curve	15	—	720	230	0.32	—	50
Ranieri 1994 (239)	P-V curve	15	—	690	248	0.36	—	—
Ranieri 1995 (240)	P-V curve	10	—	1274	756	0.59	—	55
Jonson 1999 (40)	P-V curve	10	—	—	205	—	—	—
Richard 2001 (242)	P-V curve	11	—	—	175	—	—	—
Maggiore 2001 (236)	P-V curve	15	—	764	304	0.40	—	79*
Mergoni 2001 (375)	P-V curve	15	—	—	379	—	—	29
Koutsoukou 2002 (223)	P-V curve	15	—	660	457	0.69	—	57
Richard 2003 (241)	P-V curve	14	—	—	384	—	—	20**
Maggiore 2003 (360)	P-V curve	15	—	650	235	0.36	—	44
Vieillard-Baron 2003 (376)	P-V curve	12	—	358	69	0.19	—	—
Valta 1993 (246)	Static compliance	14	—	500	126	0.25	—	—
Gattinoni 1998 (50)	Static compliance	15	576	721	131	0.18	—	—
Chelucci 2000 (374)	Static compliance	13	—	446	102	0.23	—	—
Vieira 1998 (52)	CT scan	13	—	—	320	—	238	117
Vieira 1999 (274)	CT scan	16	—	—	332	—	13	113
Puybasset 2000 (238)	CT scan	10	1621	659	187	0.28	41	45
Malbouisson 2001 (34)	CT scan	15	1553	820	499	0.61	24	99
Nieszkowska 2004 (371)	CT scan	15	1105	1115	369	0.33	63	80
MEAN		**14**	**1214**	**721**	**290**	**0.37**	**76**	**66**
SD		2	483	249	165	0.16	93	32

ABBREVIATIONS. FRC: functional residual capacity, ΔEELV: change in end-expiratory lung volume, Vrec: recruited volume, Voverdist: volume of lung overdistension, ΔPaO₂: change in arterial oxygen tension compared to PEEP 0 cmH₂O, P-V: pressure-volume, CT: computed tomography, SD: standard deviation.
* compared to PEEP 5 cmH₂O.
** compared to PEEP 10 cmH₂O.

in PEEP (up to 100% of $PEEP_I$) did not produce further improvement in gas exchange.[286] In other small studies, low to moderate PEEP (5–9 cmH$_2$O) produced similar improvements in Pa$_{CO_2}$ and Pa$_{O_2}$.[287–289] Other authors, however, reported little or no change in arterial oxygenation with PEEP[5,81,87,285] unless high levels were applied[87,285]; Pa$_{CO_2}$ did not change with up to 15 cmH$_2$O of PEEP.[5,79,81,87,285]

PEEP may have some benefit on gas exchange. Unless hypoxemia is caused by a large intrapulmonary shunt, the benefit is small and of little clinical importance, and PEEP may have negative hemodynamic effects that worsen oxygen delivery.[79,87,285] The balance between positive and negative effects depends to some extent on the level of PEEP applied; nevertheless, the chief reason for using PEEP in COPD is not to improve gas exchange.

EFFECT OF PEEP ON RESPIRATORY MECHANICS

RESPIRATORY MECHANICS IN HEALTHY SUBJECTS

The static behavior of the respiratory system is described by the P-V curve.[290–292] This curve provides an acceptable description of the elastic properties of the respiratory system.[293] In healthy subjects, the P-V curve, from residual volume (RV) to total lung capacity (TLC), has a sigmoidal shape.[292] Above FRC, however, the curve is linear. Thus the tangential slope of the curve (i.e., the linear or chord compliance, reflecting the elasticity of the respiratory system) is constant over the range of tidal ventilation. FRC is the volume of gas in the lungs at the end of a passive expiration. It corresponds to the point of equilibrium between lung and chest-wall elastic recoil.

The shape of the P-V curve reveals two important features: stiffening of the lungs at high lung volumes and closure of peripheral airways and lung units at low lung volumes.[294] At volumes above 75–80% of TLC, the slope of the P-V curve varies, with a sharp decrease in compliance, indicating that the lungs are close to their maximum stretch limit, whereas the chest wall normally is not stiffer. Further increases in pressure beyond this point, called the *upper inflection point* (UIP), have progressively less effect on lung volume. When lung volume falls below FRC and approaches RV, the smallest airways tend to collapse under the influence of surface tension of alveolar lining fluid.[295–298] During the subsequent inflation, these structures remain closed until a much higher pressure is applied. From this point on, compliance rapidly increases during inflation as the closed lung units progressively pop open. This action produces a knee on the P-V curve termed the *lower inflection point* (LIP). The difference between closing and opening pressure is caused by hysteresis in surface tension, which is greater during inflation than during deflation, and by surface tension and curvature, which are both increased when the airspaces are collapsed.[298]

Static (effective) compliance is the ratio of volume change over pressure change. Graphically, it describes the slope of a line drawn between two points corresponding to end inspiration and end expiration. It is a simplified measure of the elasticity of the respiratory system. In contrast to patients with either ARDS or COPD,[238,294] normal subjects have a linear P-V relationship in the range of V_T at FRC; thus a single value of static compliance may describe the elastic properties of the respiratory system satisfactorily in this range.

The dynamic behavior of the respiratory system depends on its resistive properties. Modeling the airways as a rigid tube, the resistance (R) is described by the equation $R = \Delta P/\dot{V}$, where P is the pressure difference between the extremities of the tube, and $\dot{V}$ is airflow. Poiseuille's law states that R is proportional to fluid viscosity (η) and to the length (l) of the tube and inversely related to tube radius (r) raised to the fourth power ($R = 8\eta l/\pi r^4$). Accordingly, even small variations in airway caliber cause large changes in airway resistance. Because the intrapulmonary airways are tethered to the surrounding parenchyma, they are pulled and widened by lung expansion and narrowed by reduced lung volumes. Therefore, airway (ohmic) resistance decreases with increasing lung volume, and vice versa. A second resistive component exists, defined as tissue or additional resistance, that is consequent to the viscoelastic pressure dissipation (stress relaxation) within the lung and chest-wall tissues.[299–304] Gas redistribution (*pendelluft*) among lung units with different time constants adds to this pressure loss and is included in the calculation of the additional resistance. Additional resistance is proportional to increase in lung volume and inversely related to flow rate[303,304]; it is also characterized by a strong frequency dependency.[305]

During constant-flow controlled ventilation, the elastic and resistive properties of the respiratory system can be assessed using the occlusion technique, which consists of occluding the airway at end inspiration for 3–5 seconds.[299,300,303,304,306–308] As soon as flow is interrupted, there is a rapid drop in airway pressure from the peak (Ppeak) to a lower value (P1), followed by a gradual decay to an apparent plateau (Pplat) (Fig. 11-4). Ohmic (flow-dependent) resistance (Rmax) is calculated as the initial drop in airway pressure (Ppeak − P1) divided by inspiratory flow. The slower pressure change (P1 − Pplat) divided by the inspiratory flow preceding the occlusion yields the additional tissue resistance (ΔR). The sum of airflow and tissue resistances provides the total respiratory resistance [$R_{TOT} = (Ppeak - Pplat)/\dot{V}$]. By occluding the airway at end-expiration, it is possible to determine the total PEEP ($PEEP_{TOT}$), which is the sum of the externally applied PEEP and $PEEP_I$ (Fig. 11-5). The difference between Pplat and $PEEP_{tot}$ is the recoil pressure. It is then possible to compute the static compliance (Cst) of the respiratory system according to the equation $Cst = V_T/(Pplat - PEEP_{TOT})$. The failure to take into account $PEEP_I$ may result in a substantial underestimation of Cst, especially when low or no PEEP is used.[91,309]

The mechanical properties of the respiratory system can be partitioned into lung and chest-wall components by measuring esophageal pressure, a surrogate for intrathoracic (pleural) pressure.[310–312] When the respiratory muscles are not active, esophageal pressure corresponds to intrathoracic (chest-wall) pressure; transpulmonary pressure then can be calculated by subtracting esophageal pressure from airway pressure. It is therefore possible to calculate resistance and compliance of the chest wall and the lung by replacing airway pressure in the aforementioned equations with esophageal and transpulmonary pressure, respectively.

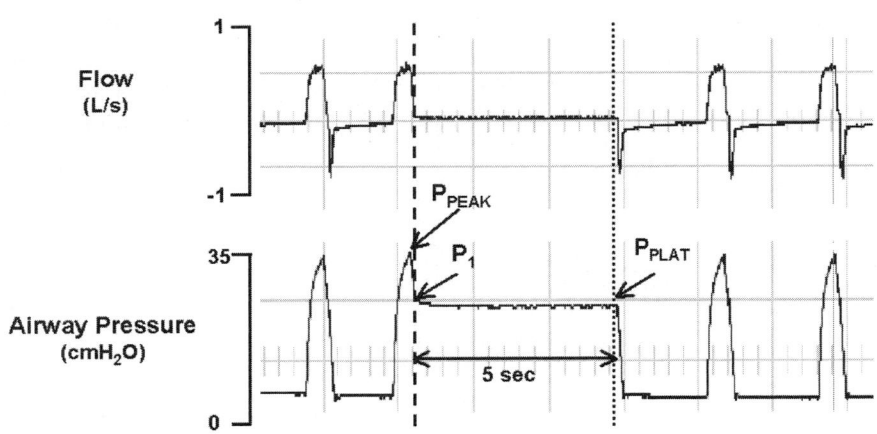

FIGURE 11-4 End-inspiratory occlusion during constant-flow controlled ventilation. As soon as the airway is occluded, flow suddenly falls to zero, and airway pressure drops from a peak (Ppeak) to a lower value (P1) and then declines slowly to an apparent plateau (Pplat).

EFFECTS OF PEEP IN ANESTHETIZED SUBJECTS

Anesthetized healthy subjects may have decreased aerated lung volume consequent to the decline in FRC associated with the supine posture[141,313–318] and the potential for airway closure and atelectasis.[133,138–145,147,148,229,315,319–322] Both anesthesia and paralysis affect the mechanical characteristics of the respiratory system,[133,320–324] which also can be impaired by abdominal and thoracic surgical procedures.[325–329] It is thought that anesthesia primarily alters the elastic properties of the chest wall, causing a fall in FRC, whereas the changes in lung compliance may result from breathing at low lung volumes.[320,330,331] Application of PEEP in anesthetized and paralyzed subjects produces an increase in end-expiratory lung volume (EELV)[169,323,332–336] and upward displacement of respiratory system, lung, and chest-wall P-V relationships[169,322,333,335,336] (Fig. 11-6A). Several authors, however, reported little or no increase in static respiratory compliance with PEEP.[169,322,332,333,335,337,338] In some studies, PEEP increased both chest-wall and lung compliance.[335] In other studies, chest-wall compliance increased and lung compliance decreased,[337] or no effect was observed.[169,332]

The effect of PEEP on the elastic properties of the respiratory system varies with the amount of PEEP applied[336] and preexisting derangement in respiratory mechanics. Compared with zero end-expiratory pressure (ZEEP), D'Angelo et al[336] found that PEEP of 9 cmH$_2$O increased both respiratory system and lung static compliance; the compliance, however, decreased when PEEP was raised above 20 cmH$_2$O, indicating lung overdistension. Dechman et al[321] also observed an increase in lung compliance at PEEP of 10 cmH$_2$O in the patients undergoing closed-chest surgery but not in patients undergoing open-chest surgery, who exhibited a progressive decrease in dynamic lung compliance. The mechanical characteristics of the chest wall may influence the effect of PEEP in subjects with normal lungs during anesthesia.[320] In patients undergoing abdominal surgery, Pelosi et al[169] reported that 10 cmH$_2$O of PEEP did not improve respiratory function in normal subjects, although it increased EELV and lung and chest-wall compliance in morbidly obese patients.

In general, PEEP decreases airway resistance.[169,321,335–337,339] The decrease in airway resistance is related mainly to an increase in lung volume,[335] although other mechanisms, such as a PEEP-induced modification of basal vagal tone,[339] also may play a role.

EFFECT OF PEEP ON LUNG VOLUME IN ALI/ARDS

Since the first description by Asbaugh et al,[4] ARDS has been recognized as a condition characterized by reduction in aerated lung and respiratory system mechanical derangements.[119,122,340–344] In ALI/ARDS, massive lung edema, atelectasis, and tissue consolidation cause a marked decrease in FRC.[119,122] This fall in normally ventilated lung

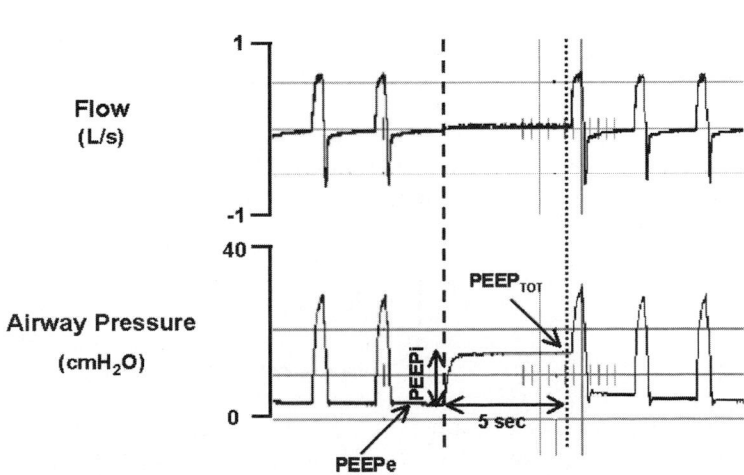

FIGURE 11-5 End-expiratory occlusion. Airway pressure rises following an end-expiratory occlusion and reaches a plateau, which corresponds to total PEEP (PEEP$_{TOT}$). Auto- or intrinsic PEEP (PEEP$_I$) is the difference between PEEP$_{TOT}$ and the externally applied preset PEEP (PEEP$_E$). PEEP$_I$ measured by an end-expiratory occlusion is termed *static PEEP$_I$*.

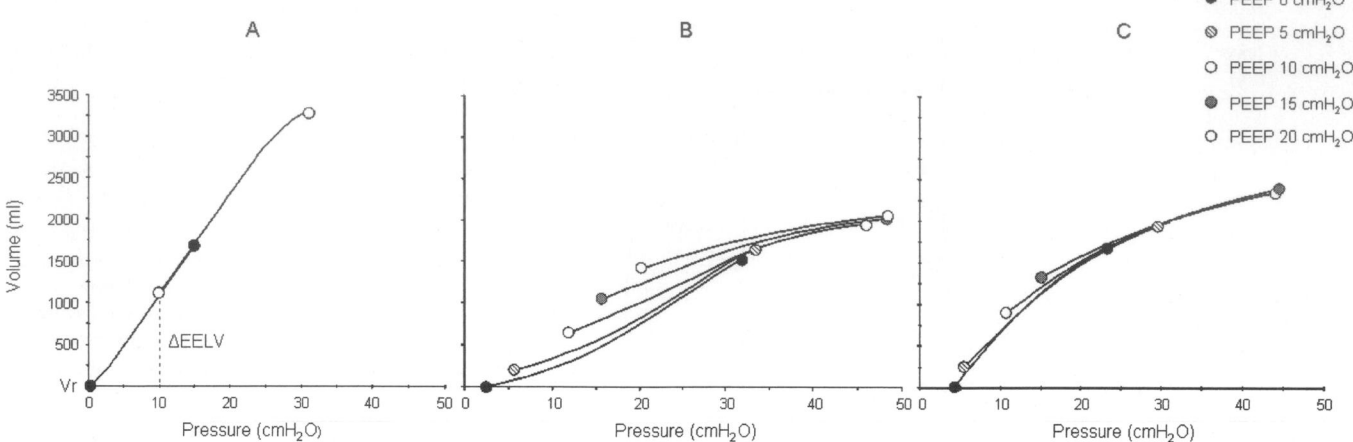

FIGURE 11-6 Pressure-volume (P-V) curves recorded from different PEEP levels in a healthy subject (*A*), a patient with acute respiratory distress syndrome (ARDS) (*B*), and a patient with an acute exacerbation of chronic obstructive lung disease (COPD) (*C*). All curves are related to the relaxation volume of the respiratory system. For each curve, end-expiratory and end-inspiratory points are indicated by circles. In the healthy subject, PEEP of 10 cmH$_2$O generates an increase in end-expiratory lung volume (EELV) and a rightward shift of the P-V curve. The new curve is superimposed on the curve acquired without PEEP, indicating the absence of recruitment. In the patient with ARDS, increasing PEEP produces increases in EELV and a significant lung recruitment, as indicated by the upward shift of the P-V curves. In the patient with COPD, the application of PEEP results in an EELV increase with worsening of hyperinflation, as indicated by the superposition of P-V curves and the progressive decrease in the slope (compliance) of the curves. The reduction in aerated volume in ARDS produces a lower inflection point and flattening of the P-V curve at PEEP of 0 cmH$_2$O. The presence of intrinsic PEEP during ventilation without PEEP in ARDS, and more so in COPD, induces a rightward shift of the initial P-V curve. In the healthy subject (*left panel*), a PEEP-induced increase in EELV is indicated by the dotted line. Vr, relaxation volume of the respiratory system.

volume is the main cause of the impaired respiratory mechanics.[206] Conversely, an increase in aerated lung volume is long recognized as the main cause of the benefit of PEEP on lung function.[18,119] The increase in lung volume may result from two different mechanisms: recruitment of terminal lung units not accessible to ventilation because of collapse or flooding and distension or overdistension of already open lung units.

Several authors have reported an increase in EELV and FRC following the application of PEEP in patients with ARDS[18,30,34,50,52,119,121,122,233,238,246,262,332,340,345–347] (see Fig. 11-6*B*). In absence of PEEP$_I$, the increase in lung volume above FRC at end expiration, or delta end-expiratory lung volume (ΔEELV), depends on the amount of PEEP applied and the compliance of the respiratory system. Different techniques can be used to measure FRC and EELV, such as helium dilution,[348–353] nitrogen[350,353–355] and sulfur hexafluoride,[353,356–359] washout, and CT scan.[52,121,238] These measurements are not obtained routinely in the clinical setting because of technical limitations and/or logistic complexities.

A surrogate approach has been used for assessing PEEP-induced ΔEELV; this involves measuring the volume exhaled between PEEP and the elastic equilibrium volume of the respiratory system[40,71,236,239–242,328,360,361] (Fig. 11-7). While the ventilator is delivering V$_T$, the preset PEEP is brought to zero rapidly. During the following expiration, sufficient time (5–10 seconds) is provided to enable complete exhalation; thus the elastic equilibrium, the relaxation volume, will be reached.[40,71,215,236,240] The difference between

FIGURE 11-7 Measurement of PEEP-induced change in end-expiratory lung volume (ΔEELV). PEEP of 10 cmH$_2$O is abruptly brought to zero. A prolonged expiration ensues, and relaxation volume is achieved. The difference between the volume exhaled during this expiration and the tidal volume delivered by the ventilator equals the increase in EELV induced by PEEP.

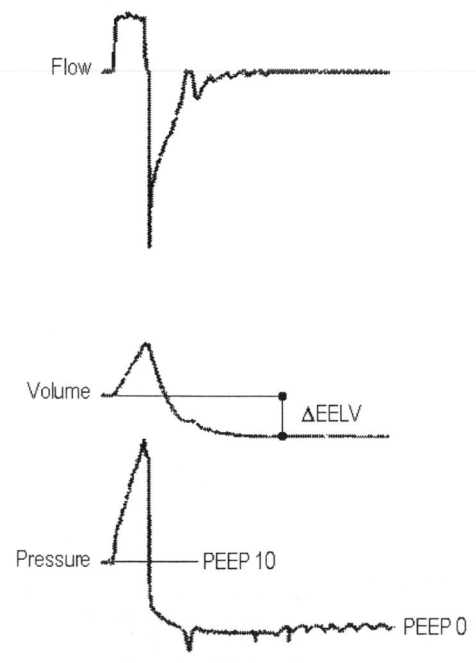

the volume exhaled during this prolonged expiration and the volume insufflated during the preceding inspiration represents the ΔEELV produced by PEEP$_{TOT}$. The excess volume caused by PEEP$_I$ should be assessed separately, and accounted for, to avoid overestimation of PEEP-induced ΔEELV. PEEP-induced variations in EELV also can be measured by inductive[246,360,362–365] or optoelectronic plethysmography.[35,366]

An increase in EELV also may occur when PEEP distends or overdistends already aerated lung regions (see Table 11-1; Fig. 11-8). Hence measurement of ΔEELV without quantification of lung recruitment may be misleading. *Lung recruitment* refers to reaeration of collapsed or fluid-filled terminal airways and alveoli. These areas become accessible to ventilation (anatomic recruitment) and may participate in gas exchange if local perfusion is preserved (functional recruitment). Lung recruitment can be quantified by using P-V curves traced from different levels of PEEP or by CT scan analysis (see Table 11-1).

Measurement of PEEP-induced lung recruitment using P-V curves stems from the pioneering observations of Katz et al[30] on the time course of PEEP-mediated increases in lung volume. After applying PEEP, these authors observed that EELV increased to approximately 66% of its total change within the first breath; it reached 90% in about five breaths and was fully complete only after several minutes, suggesting time dependence for lung recruitment.[30] For a given pressure, lung volume measured during ventilation with 13 cmH$_2$O of PEEP was larger than the volume predicted for that pressure by the static compliance computed at 3 cmH$_2$O of PEEP; this observation suggests that some lung units were not ventilated at the lower PEEP but were recruited by the higher PEEP.[30] Quantification of lung recruit-

ment induced by PEEP was not attempted until Ranieri et al[71,239,240] proposed a simple method using P-V curve analysis. This approach consists of aligning on the same P-V diagram curves obtained at ZEEP and varying PEEP levels. With this technique, which assumes that FRC (i.e., the relaxation volume at ZEEP) remains constant,[30,71,239] the ΔEELV induced by PEEP is added to the volume insufflated during the maneuver for recording the P-V curve at the corresponding PEEP level.[236,294,361] Lung recruitment then is computed as the difference in volume between P-V curves obtained at different PEEP levels at a given value of elastic recoil pressure (generally 20 cmH$_2$O). Anatomic recruitment is reflected by an upward shift of the P-V curve (see Fig. 11-8). If PEEP fails to recruit new regions, no volume gain at a given pressure will be observed; the resulting P-V curve will be shifted rightward and superimposed on the curve acquired at ZEEP.[236,239]

The CT scan is used to measure recruitment.[367,368] PEEP-induced lung recruitment is computed as the decrease in volume of nonaerated lung parenchyma[121,205,264,270,367] or, as proposed recently, as the increase in volume of gas penetrating nonaerated and poorly aerated lung regions.[34,368–371] With this technique, however, recruitment is assessed by comparing scans taken at different pressures (ZEEP and PEEP) and not at the same pressure, as is done with the P-V curve technique. Therefore, no matter how it is computed, recruitment at a given PEEP also will include a certain volume of gas corresponding to lung units that inflate normally from end expiration at ZEEP up to the pressure corresponding to that PEEP. This helps to explain some of the differences in the amounts of recruitment with the CT scan and P-V curve techniques.[372] Conversely, the CT scan offers a unique opportunity to estimate the amount of

FIGURE 11-8 **Pressure-volume (P-V) curves at different levels of PEEP (0, 5, 10, and 15 cmH$_2$O) related to relaxation volume of the respiratory system (Vr) in two patients with acute respiratory distress syndrome (ARDS). In the left panel (A), PEEP induces progressive upward shifts of P-V curves, indicating recruitment. At PEEP of 15 cmH$_2$O, a PEEP-induced increase in end-expiratory lung volume above Vr is indicated by the dotted line between the two open circles. Alveolar recruitment induced by PEEP of 15 cmH$_2$O compared with PEEP of 0 cmH$_2$O and measured at a pressure of 15 cmH$_2$O is shown by the double-arrow solid line. In the right panel (B), P-V curves are particularly flattened, suggesting a marked decrease in aerated lung volume. Increasing PEEP results in minimal recruitment: P-V curves are almost totally superimposed and progressively shifted to right. In both panels, all P-V curves tend to converge at high lung volumes, suggesting that total lung capacity is approached. PEEP-induced recruitment is greater when the slope of the linear segment above the lower inflection point (LIP), that is, linear compliance, of the curve recorded from 0 cmH$_2$O (the lowest curve) is high (A). When the curve at 0 cmH$_2$O has a very low linear compliance, PEEP-induced recruitment is trivial (B). PEEP-induced recruitment also proceeds far above LIP (up to pressures greater than 40 cmH$_2$O), suggesting that lung reopening is a paninspiratory phenomenon (A).**

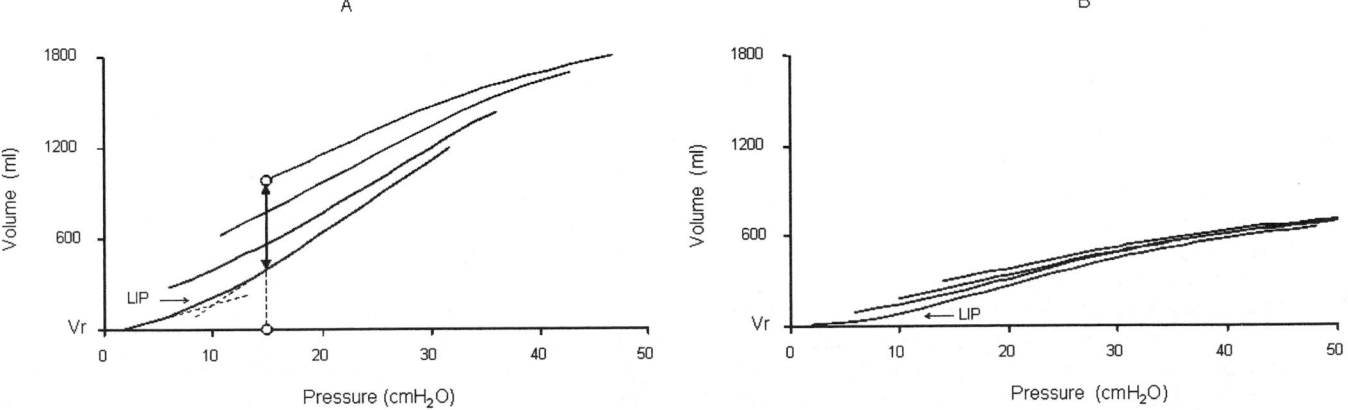

PEEP-induced hyperinflation[34,52,121,238,274,371,373] (see Table 11-1), computed as the increase in gas volume within normally aerated lung regions; hyperinflation, however, does not necessarily mean overstretching.[367]

In patients with ALI/ARDS, PEEP increases EELV and produces varying recruitment[34,40,50,71,119,121,210,236,238–242,246,264, 270,274,332,360,371,373–377] (see Table 11-1). Recent work[236] shows that PEEP achieves progressive recruitment from 84 ml at PEEP of 5 cmH$_2$O (range 41–156 ml) to 304 ml at 15 cmH$_2$O (range 114–545 ml). The large interindividual differences suggest that, in certain patients, PEEP increases lung volume without achieving significant recruitment, likely reflecting overdistension of previously aerated lung regions. Indeed, PEEP-induced overdistension has been shown in several studies.[34,52,71,238,239,240,274,371] In most cases, recruitment and overdistension occur concomitantly rather than sequentially in different regions of the lung following PEEP application.[238,274,368,369,371,373] Vieira et al[52] found that applying PEEP of 10 and 15 cmH$_2$O in patients with ALI who did not have a clear LIP on the P-V curve produced progressive recruitment of nonaerated lung areas and overdistension of aerated lung zones. The interplay between these two phenomena depends on several factors, such as ARDS etiology,[50] lung and chest-wall mechanics,[328,378] stage of disease,[379,380] lung morphology,[238,274,369] and amount of PEEP.[274] The integrated analysis of respiratory mechanics and lung volumes may help in recognizing the effects of PEEP on recruitment and overdistension and hence in selecting optimal PEEP at the bedside.

EFFECT OF PEEP ON RESPIRATORY MECHANICS IN ALI/ARDS

Contrasted with normal subjects, the rate of change per unit of pressure is smaller, and linear compliance of the P-V curve falls to very low values in patients with ARDS (because of the decrease in normally ventilated alveolar units); the whole curve is also flattened and shifted downward, and the inflection knees, normally seen at low (LIP) and high (UIP) lung volumes, may appear in the range of tidal ventilation[294] (see Figs. 11-6B and 11-8). The presence of LIP and UIP in the V$_T$ range suggests considerable susceptibility of the ARDS lung to detrimental shear forces generated by cyclic end-expiratory alveolar opening and collapse[121,206,381] and end-inspiratory overstretching.[239,382] These forces are considered the main mechanism of ventilator-induced lung injury.[383,384] Recent evidence suggests that airspace reopening can occur along the entire P-V curve.[236,264,265,367,385–387] Moreover, the shape and characteristics of the P-V curve can be greatly influenced by several factors, including pathophysiologic mechanisms, stage of disease,[50,381] chest-wall mechanics,[237,328] breathing pattern, and differences in measurement technique.[388]

As already mentioned, one of the typical features of ALI/ARDS is the fall in respiratory system compliance (see Figs. 11-6B and 11-8), described both in experimental[389–392] and clinical settings.[18,119,215,381,393] Decreased compliance was attributed initially to increased lung stiffness.[344] Subsequent studies have demonstrated that the decreased compliance in

ARDS has different pathophysiologic mechanisms.[391,392] In an animal model, Grossman et al[391] showed that the loss of aerated lung units secondary to alveolar flooding accounted for virtually all the decreased static lung compliance. With CT scan analysis, Gattinoni et al[206] found that several parameters of the P-V curve, including linear compliance, were correlated with the amount of aerated areas (mainly distributed in the nondependent, ventral lung regions) but not with nonaerated areas (preferentially distributed in the dependent, dorsal lung regions). Indeed, compliance was in the normal range when normalized to FRC (so-called specific compliance), suggesting that the aerated areas had normal intrinsic elasticity.[206] According to this concept, respiratory system compliance provides an indirect estimate of the amount of aerated lung (see Figs. 11-6B and 11-8).

Through recruitment, PEEP prevents the fall in static compliance[8] and restores the normal P-V pattern by suppressing small airways closure and collapse of unstable lung units.[73,346,394–396] Data suggest that the effects of PEEP on recruitment and overdistension can be predicted by the shape of the P-V curve at ZEEP.[71,236,239,274,385,387,397] Three distinct patterns of P-V curve have been described in patients with ALI/ARDS.[71,239,274] A concave shape with a clear LIP indicates that compliance is increasing progressively above this point, suggesting ongoing recruitment during inflation[71,239,397] (see Fig. 11-8). A convex shape showing a UIP denotes progressive decrease in compliance and likely overstretching[71,239] (see Fig. 11-8). A linear P-V curve with absent or very low LIP may be observed in localized lung injury.[274]

Rouby et al[230,369,370] hypothesized that a linear P-V curve results from two separate regional curves: a concave curve related to normally aerated lung regions and a convex curve related to nonaerated areas. PEEP may have different effects on lung volumes and respiratory mechanics according to these patterns. When a concave shape is observed at ZEEP, PEEP results in lung recruitment, as documented by an upward shift of the P-V curve and disappearance of LIP[71,236,239,274] (see Fig. 11-8). With a convex profile and low linear compliance at ZEEP, PEEP-induced recruitment is minimal or zero: The P-V curve is superimposed on that obtained at ZEEP, with a further decrease in compliance[71,236,239,274] (see Fig. 11-8).

A linear compliance on the P-V curve at ZEEP may be a useful indicator of lung recrutability (see Fig. 11-8). A tight correlation between linear compliance at ZEEP and amount of PEEP-induced recruitment has been suggested recently.[236] Because compliance, as assessed on the P-V curve, is a function of normally aerated lung regions,[206] two different situations can be imagined: (1) The lung is principally characterized by unstable lung regions, which are collapsed at end expiration but pop open progressively during tidal inflation, and (2) the lung is predominantly consolidated with no large areas expanding during inflation (compliance is very low). Application of PEEP results in significant recruitment in the former case; in the latter case, PEEP may overstretch already ventilated areas without producing significant recruitment.[71,239] Independently of its effect on recruitment and overdistension, PEEP constantly and significantly decreases the linear compliance of the P-V curve.[40,236,239,385,387] This contrasts with the classical notion that compliance increases with recruitment and decreases with overdistension.[18] Lung units that pop open at a certain pressure have an infinitely high compliance and contribute to the higher compliance observed at ZEEP, as opposed to that observed when the lung is fully recruited at PEEP. A corollary is that UIP may indicate the end of tidal recruitment and/or the beginning of alveolar overdistension, although both mechanisms may coexist at high pressure[40,385] (see Fig. 11-8). Therefore, a PEEP-related decrease in P-V linear compliance predominantly may reflect recruitment below UIP; a decrease in compliance above this point may reflect overdistension.

LIP has long been considered the pressure at which collapsed lung units open during inflation; it is therefore considered the ideal pressure at which to set PEEP.[381] Recently, however, no relationship between LIP and either opening or closing alveolar pressures was found,[236] indicating that LIP is not useful for optimizing PEEP setting. Other studies confirmed that recruitment and derecruitment are continuous processes unrelated to LIP[40,242,264,265,385,387] (see Fig. 11-8). Nevertheless, the presence of a clear LIP followed by a high inflation compliance on the P-V curve recorded from ZEEP may predict the effect of PEEP on recruitment[206,236,274,387] (see Fig. 11-8). Vieira et al[274] showed that patients with a diffuse loss of aeration had a marked LIP at ZEEP, whereas LIP was absent or blunted in patients with a focal loss of aeration. High PEEP induced progressive recruitment without overdistension in the former group, whereas it caused a significant overdistension of normally aerated regions in the latter group.[274] Some researchers think that LIP is caused by time-constant inequalities within the lung and/or reopening of compressed peripheral airway associated with expiratory flow limitation.[222,223,398,399] Accordingly, the disappearance of LIP following application of low or moderate PEEP might indicate that PEEP can prevent small airways closure and make the distribution of tidal ventilation more homogeneous.[223,399] This also could explain the difference between the reported values of LIP, i.e., 5–15 cmH_2O, and the substantially higher pressures required to reverse atelectasis.[264,291,400]

The mechanical properties of the chest wall may influence the effects of PEEP.[50,237,328] In some patients, Mergoni et al[237] found that the LIP on the P-V curve of the respiratory system at ZEEP reflected the chest wall rather than the lung. Application of PEEP abolished LIP in all instances, but oxygenation significantly improved, suggesting recruitment (only in patients exhibiting a LIP on the lung P-V curve).[237] Gattinoni et al[50] found that increasing levels of PEEP decreased respiratory and lung static compliance without any recruitment in patients with primary pulmonary ARDS; in patients with secondary extrapulmonary ARDS, PEEP induced significant recruitment and increased respiratory, lung, and chest-wall compliance.[50] These findings have not been confirmed by other studies.[40,236,238,274]

The change in static compliance produced by PEEP has been proposed as a guide for optimizing PEEP[18] and as a prognostic factor for predicting mortality in patients with ALI/ARDS.[401] Because of nonlinearity of the P-V relationship in ALI/ARDS, however, and the aforementioned com-plex effect of recruitment on the P-V relationship,[385-387] static compliance (calculated as the P-V differences between two points) may not describe adequately the changes in respiratory mechanics produced by PEEP.[294,361] Indeed, as shown previously[402] and outlined recently,[221,386,403] static compliance may vary for different V_T values. A mathematical model suggests that the highest static compliance computed at a low V_T during a decremental, but not incremental, PEEP trial may help to identify the level of PEEP needed to prevent end-expiratory alveolar collapse.[386] These theoretical findings are supported by data in animals[404] but have not been tested in patients.

Several studies[218,221,224,374,405] reveal that PEEP increases additional resistance through increased viscoelastic dissipation[219] consequent to a PEEP-mediated increase in EELV, as suggested by the correlation between changes in tissue resistance and EELV.[405] Other studies,[332,406] while confirming the rise in tissue resistance, also reported a decrease in airway resistance, especially at high PEEP. When resistances were normalized for lung volume (i.e., specific resistance), these changes disappeared.[332] Partitioning resistance into lung and chest-wall components, Pelosi et al[332] found that the increase in total and tissue respiratory system resistance consequent to PEEP could be ascribed mainly to the lung rather than to the chest wall. Recently, Gattinoni et al[50] found that total respiratory resistance increased with PEEP in pulmonary ARDS mainly because of a marked increase in lung additional resistance.[50] In contrast, patients with extrapulmonary ARDS, characterized by higher chest-wall tissue resistance and lower lung tissue resistance than pulmonary ARDS, did not show any change in total respiratory resistance with PEEP.[50]

EFFECT OF PEEP ON RESPIRATORY MECHANICS IN COPD

In COPD patients, lung and chest-wall static compliance are reported to be similar to those of normal subjects[407] unless expiratory flow limitation and dynamic hyperinflation cause lung overdistension. Depending on the level of PEEP, static compliance may decrease (if overdistension occurs),[87,359,408,409] stay unchanged,[410] or even increase slightly (if recruitment of new lung units occurs)[306] (see Fig. 11-6C).

$PEEP_{TOT}$ may exceed preset PEEP markedly when $PEEP_I$ is present (see Fig. 11-5). Rossi et al[91] demonstrated that failure to take $PEEP_I$ into account caused static compliance to be underestimated by up to 48%. During volume-targeted controlled ventilation, an increase in inspiratory flow resulting in a prolonged expiratory time causes $PEEP_i$ to decrease. Thus the value of static compliance calculated without correcting for $PEEP_I$ will increase falsely (and paradoxically).[91,306] The presence of an LIP on the P-V curve at ZEEP may be partly caused by $PEEP_I$, at least in patients with expiratory flow limitation.[411]

Patients with COPD have a high resistance.[80,87,410,412,413] In patients with expiratory flow limition, PEEP should have little influence on expiratory flow until PEEP exceeds $PEEP_I$.[91] Recent data, however, suggest that PEEP of 5–10 cmH_2O might partly decrease expiratory resistance, particularly at the end expiration, and result in faster and more uniform lung emptying.[359,410,414,415]

EFFECT OF PEEP ON VENTILATOR-INDUCED LUNG INJURY

VENTILATOR-INDUCED LUNG INJURY

Recent decades have brought the recognition that mechanical ventilation per se in ALI/ARDS may damage the lung and/or aggravate preexisting lung injury.[384] This so-called ventilator-induced lung injury (VILI)[384,416,417] is now widely accepted and supported by a large number of animal experimental studies[269,418] and recent data in patients.[9,419,420] Attempts to prevent VILI have modified the ventilator approach to patients with ALI/ARDS.[383] Two main mechanisms for VILI are (1) alveolar[269,418] and bronchial overdistension[421,422] occurring at high volume and transpulmonary pressure and (2) repeated alveolar and small airways collapse and reopening at low end-expiratory volume.[266,421,423] The common pathway for these two mechanisms is mechanical stress on the terminal units (including bronchiolar and alveolar walls).[424,425] Other factors, including elevated F_{IO_2}, high blood flow, high inspiratory flow, and intensity of local inflammation, may play a role in aggravating or inducing lung injury.

EFFECT OF PEEP ON VILI

PEEP may have opposing consequences depending on its effects on the two aforementioned mechanisms of VILI (alveolar overdistension and cyclic alveolar collapse and reopening)[274,373] (Fig. 11-9). In one study, PEEP (13 cmH$_2$O) caused recruitment of nonaerated regions and induced overdistension of already aerated lung areas in three patients.[52]

Since the 1970s, high ventilator pressures have been known to rupture alveoli and cause air leaks.[426] By increasing airway pressure, PEEP may promote alveolar overstretching,[26,239,240,274,371] ultrastructural damage,[422] and worsening of pulmonary edema.[198] Several studies suggest that end-inspiratory lung volume, rather than high intrathoracic pressure, is the major determinant of ventilator-induced lung edema ("volutrauma"), at least in normal lungs.[269,427,428] PEEP, however, also may protect against edema accumulation during ventilation at high end-inspiratory pressure and end-inspiratory lung volume,[266-269] although alteration in microvascular permeability may not be prevented.[268,269] Several factors may explain these apparent contradictions: (1) differences in experimental setup (isolated lung versus intact animals), (2) levels of PEEP and inspiratory airway pressure, and (3) driving pressure (difference between end-inspiratory and end-expiratory alveolar pressures, which, for a given pulmonary elastance, depends on V_T size).[384] In isolated lung with constant perfusion, PEEP augments edema formation probably because of increased filtration across extra-alveolar vessels associated with lung overdistension.[429,430] Conversely, in intact animals, PEEP does not affect edema formation probably because of balancing between the PEEP-induced increase in end-inspiratory lung volume (which increases fluid filtration) and concomitant reduction in cardiac output and blood pressure (which reduce filtration pressure).[431-433]

The role of PEEP-induced changes in hemodynamics on edema accumulation has been suggested by several authors.[268,434] In an animal model, Dreyfuss and Saumon[268]

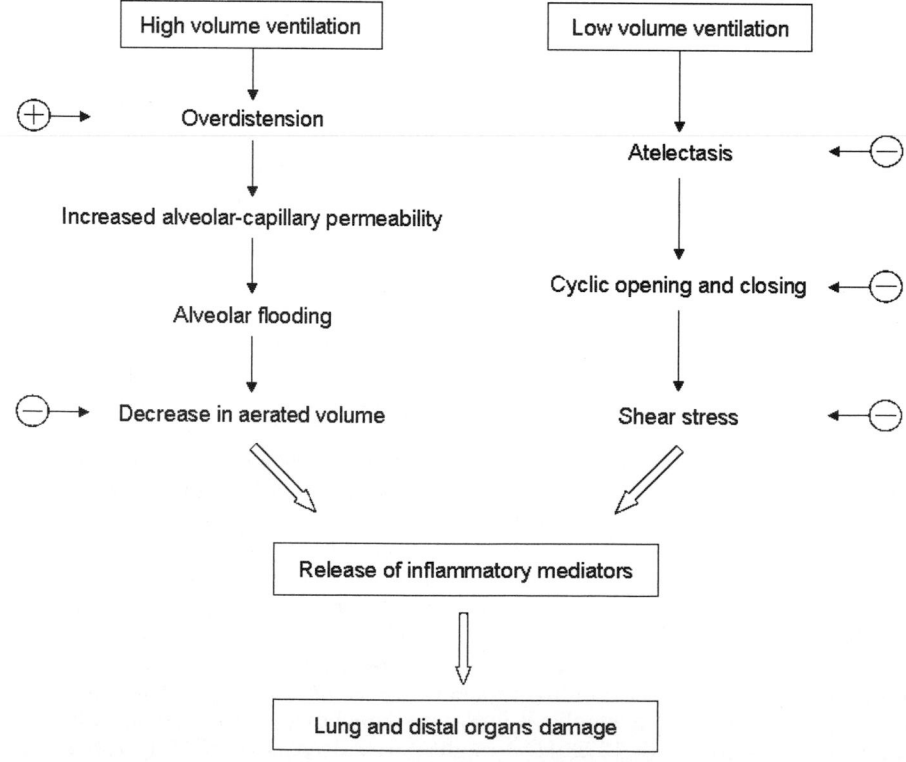

FIGURE 11-9 Postulated mechanisms by which mechanical ventilation may lead to ventilator-associated lung injury and organ injury. Beneficial (minus sign) and detrimental (plus sign) effects of PEEP on these mechanisms are shown.

showed that lung edema was reduced during ventilation with PEEP of 10 cmH$_2$O as opposed to ZEEP despite identical end-inspiratory pressures. When the drop in arterial pressure produced by PEEP was corrected by dopamine infusion, pulmonary edema increased in direct proportion to systemic blood pressure. The increase in permeability edema, however, was less than that observed during ventilation at ZEEP, suggesting that hemodynamic modification is not the only factor explaining the effect of PEEP on edema formation.[268] Indeed, reduction in driving pressure while keeping end-inspiratory lung volume and pressure constant (as obtained by increasing PEEP while reducing V$_T$) may reduce edema and the severity of cellular damage; these findings suggest that a decrease in tissue stress may explain this protective effect of PEEP.[266–269,435] PEEP-associated preservation of surfactant may further explain the benefit of PEEP on high volume–mediated VILI.[266] Thus severity of overinflation is one major determinant of VILI.[436] When ventilator-induced lung edema is produced by high V$_T$, the combination of PEEP and V$_T$ reduction decreases the severity of injury at the same end-inspiratory pressure. When PEEP is not accompanied by V$_T$ reduction, however, excessive inspiratory pressures and additional overstretching occur, further increasing the rate of edema formation and tissue injury.[268]

In a mechanically heterogeneous lung, noninflating, collapsed tissue is surrounded by open airspaces. Mead et al[424] suggested that recruitment of nonaerated lung units induces a local stress to alveoli and bronchioles that is substantially higher than the average transpulmonary or transbronchial pressure, respectively, because of alveolar and small airways interdependence.[421,425] If this process recurs cyclically, high shear forces may damage the alveolar and airway epithelium, overstretch fragile microvessels, deplete surfactant, and initiate or worsen inflammation. By recruiting nonaerated portions and stabilizing airways and lung units prone to repetitive opening and collapse, PEEP plays a key role in protecting the lung from the mechanical shear stress produced by ventilation at low end-expiratory lung volume ("atelectrauma").[423,424,437–439]

A large body of animal data supports the protective effect of PEEP on low volume–mediated VILI.[73,266,267,423,435,437,439–443] By minimizing shear stress associated with cyclic opening and collapse, PEEP may attenuate inequalities in the regional distribution of tidal ventilation, thus avoiding or limiting overdistension in the less injured lung zones.[424,425] By increasing EELV, PEEP also can prevent surfactant loss and preserve surfactant function.[441,444–447] By minimizing mechanical stress, PEEP also may ease the intensity of ventilator-induced lung inflammation[437] and reduce the decompartmentalization of a number of inflammatory mediators[448] and bacteria from the lung into the circulation ("biotrauma").[449,450] These aforementioned mechanisms may play a role in initiating or propagating the systemic inflammatory response that contributes to the multiple organ failure often observed in the terminal stage of ARDS.[451–453] Recent clinical trials have shown that protective ventilator strategies, reduced V$_T$ (to limit the end-inspiratory stretch),[9,419,420] and high PEEP (to avoid cyclic opening and closing)[9,419] were asso-

ciated with decreased pulmonary and systemic cytokine response,[419,420] less organ dysfunction,[454] and reduced mortality in patients with ARDS[9,420] compared with conventional, injurious mechanical ventilation. Although the mechanisms whereby VILI causes organ dysfunction are not completely understood, a recent study suggests that cell apoptosis may be involved.[453] Rabbits ventilated with a low V$_T$ and high PEEP showed less epithelial apoptosis in the kidney and small intestine than did rabbits ventilated with a high V$_T$ and low PEEP.[453] The former rabbits had more apoptotic cells in the lung, whereas the latter rabbits had less lung apoptosis and necrosis of alveolar epithelial type III cells.[453] Analysis of plasma samples from a previous clinical trial[419] revealed higher levels of soluble Fas ligand (a proapoptotic factor) in patients who received conventional ventilation than in patients who received protective ventilation; changes in soluble Fas ligand were correlated with changes in plasma creatinine.[454]

EFFECTS OF PEEP ON CARDIOVASCULAR SYSTEM

The lungs and heart are subject to variations in intrathoracic pressure. How alterations in intrathoracic pressure affect the heart and intrathoracic vessels varies substantially depending on several factors, such as mechanical properties of the lung and chest wall, type of ventilation (spontaneous versus mechanical), blood volume, and left-ventricular function. The complex interplay of these factors and the effects of PEEP on heart-lung interactions have been reviewed extensively.[455–463]

EFFECT ON VENOUS RETURN

Positive airway pressure causes a drop in cardiac output secondary to a decrease in cardiac filling (preload); this was attributed initially to a reduction in the pressure gradient for venous return, determined by the rise in right-atrial pressure consequent to increased intrathoracic pressure.[61,95,464–467] The PEEP-mediated decrease in the gradient for venous return, however, is less than expected because PEEP produces a concomitant rise in mean systemic pressure[468] (the circulatory filling pressure representing the upstream pressure for venous return). In patients without lung disease undergoing implantation of defibrillator devices under general anesthesia, Jellinek et al[469] measured right-atrial pressure and mean systemic pressure at airway pressures of 0 and 15 cmH$_2$O during 15-second periods of apnea when ventricular fibrillation was induced to test the defibrillator. Rising airway pressure produced a drop in left-ventricular stroke volume.[469] Right-atrial and mean systemic pressures, however, increased equally, showing that the reduction in venous return was not determined by a decrease in the pressure gradient.[469] The rise in mean systemic pressure may result from a reduction in vascular capacitance determined by neurovascular reflexes,[470] displacement of blood from the pulmonary to the systemic circulation,[471] and descent of the diaphragm, which increases the upstream pressure for venous return by augmenting intra-abdominal pressure.[472] These homeostatic adaptations, however, may be counteracted by a concomitant increase in venous resistance,[468,473] suggesting that

PEEP may alter venous return by affecting the peripheral venous circulation.

The effects of PEEP on hemodynamics strongly depend on intravascular volume. Cardiac output can be restored by increasing the ventricular filling through volume infusion.[17,474–477] PEEP discontinuation produces a rise in cardiac filling proportional to the pressure withdrawn and the circulating blood volume.[17,478] In hypervolemic and hemodynamically stable patients who underwent cardiac surgery, van der Berg et al[472] recently found that maintaining airway pressure up to 20 cmH$_2$O for 25 seconds produced minimal variations in right-ventricular output despite a concomitant rise in right-atrial pressure.

In summary, PEEP reduces cardiac output through a decrease in venous return that is not a primary consequence of a decrease in its pressure gradient. Regardless of the cause, the drop in cardiac output can be counteracted by blood volume expansion.

EFFECT ON RIGHT-VENTRICULAR AFTERLOAD AND VENTRICULAR INTERDEPENDENCE

PEEP alters both left- and right-ventricular configurations and reduces left-ventricular diastolic compliance by augmenting right-ventricular afterload.[27,479–481] An increase in lung volume causes a rise in pulmonary vascular resistance by directly compressing the alveolar vessels.[482] The interconnections between lung volume and pulmonary blood flow are not straightforward because blood expelled from the alveolar vessels can be retained in the extra-alveolar vessels.[483,484] When airway pressure is augmented, right-ventricular outflow impedence (i.e., afterload) is also increased.[463,485] In patients with ALI/ARDS, high levels of PEEP can cause or worsen tricuspid regurgitation.[486]

The fall in cardiac output with PEEP also has been attributed to the stress exerted by the right ventricle on the interventricular septum,[480] which is displaced leftward and restricts left-ventricular filling.[27] Culver et al[487] altered right-ventricular afterload through a partial occlusion of the main pulmonary arteries and found that this did not produce the same hemodynamic changes induced by increases in lung volume; these findings suggest that ventricular interdependence (caused by an increased right-ventricular afterload) is unlikely to be the main mechanism for the PEEP-mediated fall in cardiac output. Wise et al[488] evaluated the impact of PEEP of 15 cmH$_2$O on left-ventricular compliance in a study where they bypassed the right side of the heart to exclude the effects of interventricular interdependence; they concluded that the elevation in left-ventricular filling pressure was mainly a consequence of pericardial compression. In patients with ARDS, Dhainaut et al[477] did not find any changes in ventricular diastolic compliance and ejection fraction when PEEP was increased up to 20 cmH$_2$O during controlled ventilation; they attributed the reduction in cardiac output mainly to the preload effect.

In summary, PEEP increases pulmonary vascular resistance and right-ventricular afterload and therefore may increase the stress exerted by the right ventricle, which has to maintain an adequate output to guarantee left-ventricular filling. Right-ventricular systolic overload may result in leftward displacement of the interventricular septum; the effect on left-ventricular function seems to be adjunctive rather than a major determinant of the PEEP-mediated reduction in cardiac output.

EFFECT ON CARDIAC CONTRACTILITY

Some researchers think that PEEP causes a humorally mediated impairment in cardiac contractility.[489–491] So far this notion has not been confirmed. Indeed, it has been proven repeatedly to be absent or, at least, irrelevant.[476,488,492–495]

IMPACT OF RESPIRATORY MECHANICS ON THE HEMODYNAMIC EFFECT OF PEEP

Application of positive pressure to the airway (Paw) increases lung volume. When the respiratory muscles are not active, the ventilator generates the entire pressure applied to the respiratory system (Paw = Prs). During inspiration, part of Paw is dissipated in overcoming airflow resistance (Pres), and the remaining part distends the elastic structures of the lung (Pl) and the chest wall (Pcw). Accordingly, Pl + Pcw = Paw − Pres. When the respiratory muscles are not active, as occurs under controlled ventilation, Pcw corresponds to intrathoracic pressure, which affects the heart and intrathoracic vasculature. Because the lung and the chest wall are aligned in series, the pressure is first transmitted to the lung and then to the chest wall. Therefore, Pcw = Paw − Pres − Pl. Pl and Pcw correspond to the product of volume (V) and lung (El) and chest-wall (Ecw) elastance, respectively. Hence V × Ecw = Paw − Pres − (V × El); alternatively, V/Ccw = Paw − Pres − (V/Cl), where C is compliance (the reciprocal of elastance). The lower Cl, the less airway pressure is transmitted to the pleural space (i.e., intrathoracic pressure) and the fewer hemodynamic consequences.

In dogs, a reduction in lung compliance decreased the transmission of airway pressure to the pericardial space.[495] The transmission of PEEP to the pleural space increased when chest-wall compliance was reduced by binding.[496] In another animal model, a decrease in lung compliance decreased transmission of airway pressure to the pleural space; an increase in chest-wall compliance by sternotomy further reduced airway pressure transmission.[497] Venus et al[498] found that the fraction of PEEP transmitted to the pleura was reduced from 62 to 34% and to the pericardium from 54 to 36% in intact and acutely injured lungs, respectively. V$_T$ was kept constant throughout the study, and the reduction in cardiac output produced by PEEP did not differ before and after inducing lung injury because absolute pericardial pressure at end expiration did not differ.[498] When lung compliance diminishes but V$_T$ remains constant, the absolute amount of airway pressure transmitted to the pleural and pericardial spaces at end inspiration remains the same, although it represents a lower fraction of the higher airway pressure.[50,498]

At end expiration, in absence of flow (when Pres = 0), Paw equals PEEP, and then V/Ccw = PEEP − (V/Cl). Accordingly, the fraction of PEEP transmitted to the pleural and pericardial spaces will be determined by the amount of lung recruited at that pressure, which varies substantially with the underlying disorder.[50,499] The reduction in cardiac output with PEEP also depends on overdistension (more likely at high V$_T$).[240]

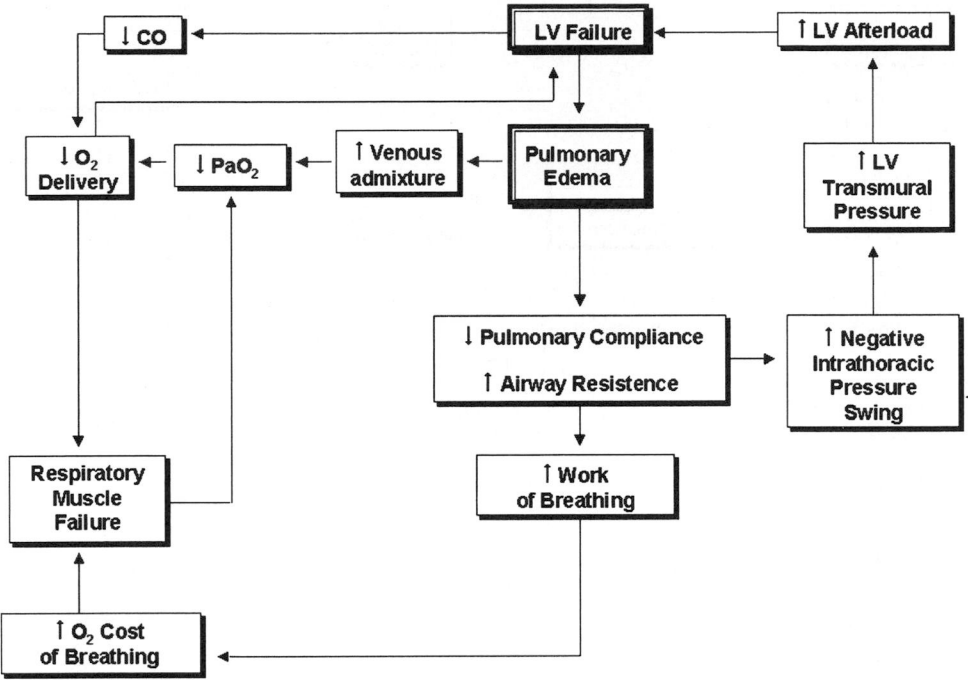

FIGURE 11-10 Pathophysiologic mechanisms and pathways of cardiogenic pulmonary edema. Deterioration in pulmonary mechanics increases negative swings in intrathoracic pressure and left-ventricular afterload. Deterioration in gas exchange decreases oxygen delivery to the heart and the respiratory muscle. See text for further explanation. CO, cardiac output; LV, left ventricle; O_2, oxygen.

EFFECT ON AFTERLOAD

Left-ventricular afterload is the force opposing contraction. It corresponds to the tension developed by the contracting cardiac muscle. It is determined by both the systemic arterial resistance and the transmural pressure exerted on the left-ventricular wall, that is, the difference between the systolic pressure and the pressure surrounding the heart (i.e., intrathoracic pressure). A reduction in left-ventricular afterload is achieved either by decreasing systemic arterial resistance (through vasodilator administration)[500] or by increasing intrathoracic pressure.[99,100,488] In healthy subjects with normal cardiac function, the dominant action of increase in intrathoracic pressure is reduction in venous return; the consequences of the lowered transmural pressure are rather small (see Fig. 11-3*A*). In patients with poor left-ventricular function and congestive heart failure, cardiac output is relatively insensitive to reductions in venous return because left-ventricular filling pressure and diastolic volume are elevated.[96] Thus the net effect of a rise in intrathoracic pressure is a reduction in left-ventricular transmural pressure[97,501,502] (see Fig. 11-3*C*). Conversely, a decrease in intrathoracic pressure raises afterload by augmenting left-ventricular transmural pressure[390,503] (see Fig. 11-3*B*).

When afterload exceeds the capacity of the left ventricle, pulmonary edema ensues, establishing a vicious circle (Fig. 11-10). Because of worsening pulmonary compliance[390,503,504] and resistance,[503,505–507] the inspiratory muscles must exert a stronger effort to achieve adequate alveolar ventilation. Thus inspiratory intrathoracic pressure becomes more negative, and afterload increases. The combination of reduced O_2 delivery[508] and increased metabolic cost of breathing[507–509] may precipitate respiratory muscle failure,[509] which further worsens gas exchange.

The impact on left-ventricular transmural pressure of the increase in intrathoracic pressure produced by CPAP of 10 cmH_2O during expiration is rather small (see Fig. 11-3*C*). Conversely, the improvement in pulmonary mechanics[509] generated by the same CPAP may minimize the swings in intrathoracic pressure[509,510] and hence decrease afterload,[510,511] thereby improving left-ventricular function[101,511] (see Fig. 11-3*C*). CPAP simultaneously may improve gas exchange[101,102,187] by reducing venous admixture[14,187] and avert failure of the respiratory muscles by improving their O_2 balance[14] (Fig. 11-11).

EFFECT ON OXYGEN DELIVERY

O_2 delivery (D_{O_2}) is the product of arterial O_2 concentration (Ca_{O_2}) and cardiac output, where Ca_{O_2} is ($Hb \times 1.39 \times Sa_{O_2}$) + ($Pa_{O_2} \times 0.003$). The effect of PEEP on D_{O_2} depends on its relative effects on cardiac output and Ca_{O_2}, in other words, on the balance between its pulmonary and hemodynamic consequences. Because Ca_{O_2} depends much more on Sa_{O_2} (O_2 bound to hemoglobin) than on Pa_{O_2} (O_2 dissolved in blood), little Ca_{O_2} improvement is observed when an increase in Pa_{O_2} occurs on the upper part of the O_2 dissociation curve. Furthermore, PEEP-induced increase in Pa_{O_2} and Ca_{O_2} may be accompanied by a decrease in D_{O_2} because of concomitant decrease in cardiac output.[59] Several studies indicate that D_{O_2} is more influenced by cardiac output than by Ca_{O_2}.[512–514]

The impact of PEEP on D_{O_2} depends primarily on its hemodynamic effect. PEEP-mediated impairment of cardiac

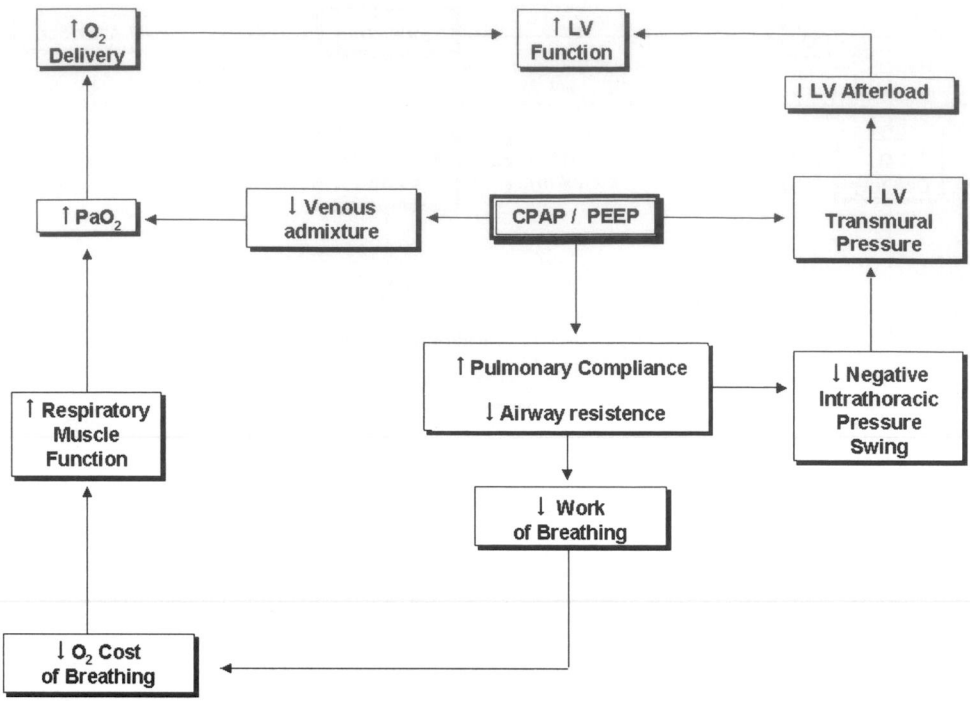

FIGURE 11-11 Cardiopulmonary effects of CPAP in cardiogenic pulmonary edema. By improving pulmonary mechanics, CPAP reduces negative swings in intrathoracic pressure and left-ventricular afterload. By improving gas exchange, CPAP increases oxygen delivery to the heart and the respiratory muscle. See text for further explanation. LV, left ventricle; O_2, oxygen

output is inversely related to pulmonary compliance: The lower lung compliance, the less PEEP is transmitted to the intrathoracic pressure, and the smaller is the decrease in cardiac output. The PEEP-mediated increase in Ca_{O_2} is also greater when producing a large rise in Sa_{O_2} from a low value.[512,515] Therefore, the effect of PEEP on D_{O_2} also depends on ARF severity.[71,239,516–518] In patients with severe ARDS (very low lung compliance and Pa_{O_2}), PEEP increases Ca_{O_2} with a moderate decrease in cardiac output, resulting in a D_{O_2} increase. Conversely, in patients with moderate ARDS (relatively higher lung compliance and Pa_{O_2}), PEEP will decrease cardiac output without causing much change in Ca_{O_2}; the net effect is a more remarkable reduction in D_{O_2}.

Under normal conditions, when the metabolic requirements increase, physiologic homeostatic mechanisms act on central (pulmonary gas exchange, blood flow, hemoglobin concentration, and hemoglobin affinity for O_2)[519] and peripheral (blood flow distribution, capillary-cell distance)[520] determinants of O_2 balance to enhance D_{O_2} and match $\dot{V}_{O_2}$. When $\dot{V}_{O_2}$ is augmented, as during exercise, the first strategy to increase D_{O_2} is to increase cardiac output.[123] If the increase in cardiac output is not sufficient to match the $\dot{V}_{O_2}$ augmentation, tissue O_2 extraction increases; thus $\dot{V}_{O_2}$ is kept constant up to a threshold, above which energy supplies depend on anaerobic metabolism, and lactic acidosis occurs.[521,522] A linear relationship exists between D_{O_2} and $\dot{V}_{O_2}$ (supply dependence) below a critical D_{O_2} threshold; in anesthetized subjects, the threshold is 330 ml/min.[523] In sepsis and ARDS, an altered supply dependence,[43,515,524–536] together with peripheral limitation in O_2 diffusion and increased O_2 hemoglobin affinity,[537] is a major pathophysi-

ologic mechanism for the development of tissue hypoxia and multiple-organ failure.[538] By decreasing cardiac output and consequently D_{O_2}, PEEP may worsen O_2 balance and promote pathologic supply dependence.[43,525,528,533,539]

Recognition of methodologic errors (mathematical coupling of data) subsequently challenged the notion of the pathologic supply dependence.[540–542] Several investigators did not find a correlation between D_{O_2} and $\dot{V}_{O_2}$ when these two parameters were measured independently.[543–548] Two randomized trials failed to demonstrate any clinical benefit of a treatment strategy that achieved supranormal D_{O_2} values.[549,550]

Pathologic $D_{O_2}/\dot{V}_{O_2}$ dependency (assessed from independent measures of the two parameters) was reported recently in brain-dead patients with high plasma lactate levels but not in patients with normal lactate.[551] In the former group, PEEP of 10–15 cmH_2O induced a marked decrease in D_{O_2} and $\dot{V}_{O_2}$; in the latter, the decline in D_{O_2} was associated only with a moderate reducetion in $\dot{V}_{O_2}$.[551]

The effect of protective ventilation (high PEEP and low V_T, permissive hypercapnia) on D_{O_2} was evaluated recently in patients with ARDS.[552–554] In 48 patients with severe ARDS, Carvalho et al[553] found that PEEP of up to 24 cmH_2O (16 cmH_2O on average) produced an increase in cardiac output, heart rate, and D_{O_2} and decreased systemic vascular resistance and plasma lactate. The authors speculated that the good tolerance of high PEEP may have been a consequence of the acute hemodynamic effects of hypercapnia and the observed very low lung compliance.[553] No correlation was found between changes in PEEP and cardiac output. A strong inverse correlation existed between changes in plateau pressure and cardiac output. These findings suggest, in line with other reports,[240,378] that the negative hemodynamic effect classically attributed to PEEP may depend more on the associated high inspiratory pressure (if V_T is not reduced concomitantly).[553]

NON CARDIORESPIRATORY EFFECTS OF PEEP

PEEP may influence regional blood distribution[555] and lead to inequalities in D_{O_2} to the different organs and potentially affect their functions.[22,556] Renal and hepatic failure are independently associated with increased mortality.[29] PEEP-induced alterations in regional blood flows have important implications for the development of multiple-organ failure.[22]

RENAL AND HORMONAL EFFECTS

PEEP decreases urinary output,[17,64,557–582] sodium excretion,[64,557–559,561–563,565–572,575] and creatinine clearance.[557,561,562,565,572] Although there is general consensus about these effects of PEEP, studies investigating the mechanisms are conflicting. Discrepancies are related to differences in experimental design, such as diverse subjects, trial duration, type and severity of underlying disorder, volemic state, use of drugs and anesthetics (which commonly cause sympathetic depression), and level of PEEP. The decrease in urinary output caused by PEEP has been attributed to multiple factors such as fall in cardiac output[558,573,579] and renal blood flow,[558,560,568,573,578] reduced intravascular volume,[579] reflex sympathetic nerve activation,[581] and altered release of hormones, including catecholamines,[557] renin-angiotensin-aldosterone system,[557,569,570,576,582] antidiuretic hormone (ADH),[557,569] and atrial natriuretic factor.[566,567,569,571,572,575]

In dogs receiving a constant fluid infusion, Berry et al[64] observed that the time needed for urinary output to approximate the rate of fluid infusion was 20, 27, and 46 hours during spontaneous breathing, positive-pressure ventilation, and positive-pressure ventilation plus 10 cmH$_2$O of PEEP, respectively. Priebe et al[579] found that renal impairment caused by 10 cmH$_2$O of PEEP in anesthetized dogs resulted primarily from a reduction in intravascular volume. In swine, Venus et al[557] found that the addition of PEEP to positive-pressure ventilation caused a fall in cardiac and urinary output associated with an increase in plasma ADH, renin, epinephrine, and norepinephrine in normovolemic animals but not in animals that received volume expansion through crystalloids. In six neurologic patients with intact cardiopulmonary and renal function receiving positive-pressure ventilation plus 15 cmH$_2$O of PEEP, an increase in lower-body pressure via military antishock trousers improved systemic and renal hemodynamics and decreased plasma norepinephrine, with no change in total blood volume.[576] Urinary output and sodium excretion did not improve. The authors concluded that increased plasma renin and sympathetic activation were the main determinants of renal impairment with PEEP.[576]

Annat et al[558] evaluated the short-term effects of 10 cmH$_2$O of PEEP in normovolemic patients without cardiac and renal abnormalities and little or no respiratory failure who were receiving positive-pressure ventilation. PEEP decreased urinary output by 34%, renal blood flow by 32%, and sodium excretion by 33%; the associated drop in cardiac output was 15%.[558] PEEP also increased urinary ADH and plasma renin and aldosterone levels.[558] In a similar setting, Payen et al[573] found that 15 cmH$_2$O of PEEP reduced urinary output (55%) and fractional sodium excretion (39%); cardiac index fell by 21%. Plasma ADH did not vary, and norepinephrine increased.[573]

PEEP increases sympathetic activity.[583] Nevertheless, the observation by Fewell et al[577] that the effects of PEEP on renal function are mediated by sympathetic activity has not been confirmed.[562,574] PEEP also decreases plasma atrial natriuretic factor.[559,566,567,569,575] This may contribute to the reduction in urinary output and sodium excretion probably as a result of the reduced atrial transmural pressure consequent to the raised intrathoracic pressure.[566]

In summary, PEEP may alter renal function by reducing cardiac output and renal blood flow to an extent that depends on the volemic state and the amount of applied pressure. Other mechanisms, including several hormones, also may play a role.

EFFECTS ON SPLANCHNIC CIRCULATION AND OXYGENATION

PEEP decreases splanchnic blood flow[56,65,67,68,584,585] and causes hepatic congestion.[65] The reduction in splanchnic blood flow is consequent to a fall in cardiac output secondary to impaired central hemodynamic[56,65,67,68,584,585]; it is less pronounced when cardiac output is maintained either by expanding blood volume[67,68] or by inotropic drugs.[585] In hemodynamically stable patients with ALI/ARDS, Kiefer et al[586] found that PEEP of 13 cmH$_2$O (5 cmH$_2$O increment above the preset values) did not decrease cardiac index or splanchnic blood flow and metabolism, suggesting that PEEP does not affect splanchnic blood flow. Other factors, however, such as hepatic outflow resistance may play a role.[68,587] In swine, Brienza et al[587] found that PEEP of 15 cmH$_2$O reduced portal vein flow through an increase in liver venous resistance; the authors postulated a direct compressive effect caused by diaphragmatic descent on the liver.

Sha et al[584] applied increasing PEEP (up to 20 cmH$_2$O) and found proportional decreases in hepatic blood flow. Because the rate of decrease in hepatic D_{O_2} exceeded that of cardiac output and hepatic blood flow, the authors concluded that hepatic D_{O_2} was reduced primarily because of the drop in portal venous O_2 content.[584] More recently, Aneman et al[66] evaluated the impact of PEEP of 10 cmH$_2$O on mesenteric and hepatic blood flow in patients under general anesthesia (during elective surgery for gastric or pancreatic neoplasm). Neither arterial pressure nor arterial, portal, and hepatic venous norepinephrine were significantly affected by PEEP.[66] A decrease in portal blood flow was associated with a rise in mesenteric vascular resistance; conversely, an increase in hepatic arterial flow was associated with a drop in hepatic arterial resistance.[66] Mesenteric D_{O_2} was reduced, and hepatic D_{O_2} remained unchanged.[66] Mesenteric and hepatic $\dot{V}_{O_2}$ did not significantly vary with PEEP.[66] In similar patients, Berendes et al[56] found that hepatic venous lactate did not change with PEEP up to 15 cmH$_2$O and concluded that a critical reduction in splanchnic oxygenation does not occur.

In spontaneously breathing normal subjects, Fournell et al[588] recently reported that CPAP levels of up to 10 cmH$_2$O progressively altered gastric mucosal microvascular O$_2$ saturation, as assessed by reflectance spectrophotometry. Lehtipalo et al[57] found that PEEP of 10 cmH$_2$O had little effect on intestinal perfusion pressure; mesenteric blood flow and oxygenation were maintained until the intestinal perfusion pressure exceeded 33 mmHg. In patients with septic shock, Träger et al[589] increased PEEP up to 15 cmH$_2$O. PEEP decreased cardiac index and hepatic venous O$_2$ saturation.[589] Hepatic metabolic performance, assessed by glucose production, fell at each PEEP level in patients who did not survive, whereas it decreased only at the highest PEEP level among survivors.[589]

In summary, PEEP may reduce hepatic and splanchnic blood flow through a drop in cardiac output, although other mechanisms, such as regional outflow resistance, are likely to be involved.

EFFECTS ON INTRACRANIAL PRESSURE AND CEREBRAL PERFUSION

High intracranial pressure (ICP) and reduced cerebral perfusion pressure (CPP) (the difference between mean arterial pressure and ICP) are common in several acute neurologic and neurosurgical ICU patients, particularly those who have focal or generalized cerebral edema. Hypoxemic respiratory failure secondary to ALI/ARDS is a fearful complication in these patients, leading to use of PEEP.[590]

ICP may be altered by PEEP through a rise in right-atrial pressure, which increases superior vena cava pressure and hence reduces cerebral venous return.[63,591,592] The effects of PEEP on ICP depend on the amount of intracranial compression and are of little importance when cerebral compliance is not altered.[19] In 25 head-injured patients, Apuzzo et al[19] found that PEEP caused an increase in ICP in only 12 patients who had low cerebral compliance and reduced CPP below 60 mmHg in only six of them. In normal, healthy volunteers, Hormann et al[593] found that alterations in ICP and CPP produced by CPAP of 12 cmH$_2$O were slight and not of clinical relevance. Body position also affects the impact of PEEP on ICP. PEEP raises ICP through an increase in the downstream venous pressure; thus, elevating the head above the chest should lessen the transmission of intrathoracic pressure to the venous sinuses and mitigate the effects of PEEP on ICP. In supine anesthetized patients undergoing posterior fossa surgery, Lodrini et al[594] found that PEEP of up to 15 cmH$_2$O caused proportional increases in central venous pressure and ICP; in the sitting position, PEEP also increased central venous pressure, but ICP changed little in most of the patients.

Several studies in neurologic, neurosurgical, or brain-injured patients found that judicious use of PEEP was not detrimental, provided that monitoring was adequate.[595-600]

EFFECTS ON BRONCHIAL CIRCULATION AND THORACIC LYMPH DRAINAGE

By increasing intrathoracic pressure, PEEP alters bronchial blood flow[601-603] and thoracic lymph drainage, which could affect the process of lung repair[604] and edema removal.[605] Blood from the bronchial vessels is drained to the right side of the heart via the azygos and bronchial veins and to the left atrium through anastomoses between the systemic and pulmonary circulation. In ventilated open-chest dogs, Baile et al[601] investigated the effect of increasing PEEP on systemic to pulmonary (anastomotic) flow ($\dot{Q}$ bra) and on bronchial blood flow ($\dot{Q}$ br), which was further partitioned into tracheal, bronchial, and parenchymal fractions. Bronchial and parenchymal but not tracheal fractions of $\dot{Q}$ br decreased with PEEP.[601] $\dot{Q}$ br and $\dot{Q}$ bra did not differ at PEEP of 3 and 10 cmH$_2$O.[601] At PEEP of 15 cmH$_2$O, $\dot{Q}$ br exceeded $\dot{Q}$ bra, indicating a decrease in the anastomotic drainage.[601] In patients undergoing cardiopulmonary bypass, Agostoni et al[603] observed that an increase in alveolar pressure of about 10 cmH$_2$O decreased $\dot{Q}$ bra by 40%.

Local release of mediators, a rise in pulmonary vascular resistance, and reflex bronchial vasoconstriction may explain $\dot{Q}$ bra reduction.[602] To assess the influence of vagal reflexes on PEEP-mediated reductions in $\dot{Q}$ bra, Lakshminarayan et al[606] isolated and perfused the left lower lobe in open-chest dogs and found that increasing PEEP from 5–15 cmH$_2$O halved $\dot{Q}$ bra. At PEEP of 5 cmH$_2$O, bilateral cervical vagal cooling decreased $\dot{Q}$ bra.[606] An increase of PEEP to 15 cmH$_2$O did not further diminish it, suggesting that the effect of PEEP on $\dot{Q}$ bra might be partly vagally mediated.[606]

PEEP may obstruct lymph drainage from the thoracic duct into the jugular vein.[605,607] By altering thoracic lymph return, PEEP might affect edema removal from the lungs.[605]

Intrinsic Positive End-Expiratory Pressure (PEEP$_I$)

During passive exhalation, airflow is driven by the difference between alveolar (Palv) and airway opening (Pao) pressures and opposed by expiratory resistance (Raw,exp). In the absence of expiratory muscle activity and externally applied PEEP, Palv corresponds to the elastic recoil of the respiratory system for a given V$_T$: Palv thus is equal to Ers/V$_T$ or V$_T$/Crs, where Ers and Crs are respiratory system elastance and compliance, respectively. The product of Crs and Raw,exp is the expiratory time constant (τ). During expiration, $V = V_T e^{-(t/\tau)}$, where V is the amount of V$_T$ not yet exhaled (i.e., above FRC), t is the time elapsed from the onset of expiration, and e is the base of natural logarithms (2.7189). When t = τ, V is roughly 37% (1/2.7189) of V$_T$. It takes five τ to almost entirely (99%) exhale V$_T$.

In healthy adult subjects, τ is approximately 0.3 second. Therefore, the time required to exhale V$_T$ is about 1.5 seconds. Assuming a respiratory rate of 12 breaths per minute and an inspiratory duty cycle (T$_I$/T$_{TOT}$) of 40%, expiratory time (T$_E$) is 3 seconds, which considerably exceeds the time necessary for the lungs to deflate to FRC. If either breathing frequency or T$_I$/T$_{TOT}$ increase, T$_E$ diminishes. Any condition causing an increase in expiratory resistance, including an artificial airway,[608] or a loss in elastic recoil prolongs τ and thus the time required for complete V$_T$ exhalation. When shortened T$_E$ and/or prolonged τ impede a complete

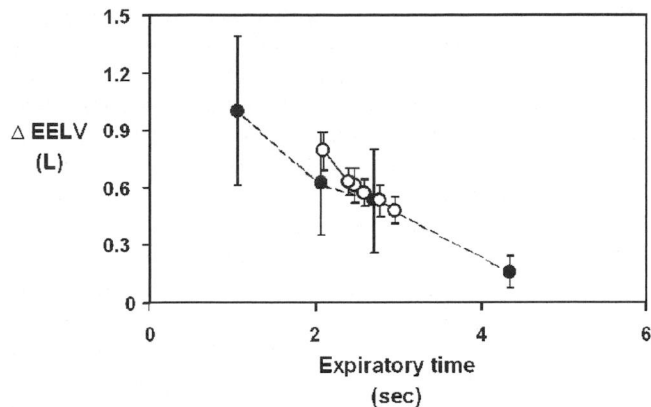

FIGURE 11-12 Effects of varying expiratory time on end-expiratory trapped volume in patients with airway obstruction. ΔEELV indicates end-expiratory lung volume above functional residual capacity. The shorter the expiratory time, the greater is the amount of end-expiratory trapped volume. Data are expressed as mean ± standard deviation (*closed circles*) and mean ± standard error (*open circles*) and taken from refs. 285 and 412, respectively. Tidal volume was always 1 liter in ref. 285 and averaged 0.576 liter (±0.026 liter) in ref. 412. In ref. 412, changes in expiratory time were obtained by manipulating the ventilator preset inspiratory time while leaving respiratory rate (and hence minute ventilation) unmodified. In ref. 285, inspiratory duty cycle remained unchanged, and expiratory time was change by modifying respiratory rate; accordingly, minute ventilation also varied.

exhalation to FRC, dynamic hyperinflation occurs. End-expiratory relaxation volume will exceed FRC to an extent that is proportional to τ and V_T and inversely related to T_E (Fig. 11-12).

Expiratory flow also may be limited in the course of V_T exhalation because the airways collapse at a choke point where intrathoracic pressure equals intrabronchial pressure (so-called equal-pressure point). The airways located downstream of the equal-pressure point are then compressed because intrathoracic pressure exceeds the intrabronchial pressure. Thus Palv − Pao no longer represents the pressure driving expiratory flow. Expiratory flow limitation is very common in patients with an acute exacerbation of COPD.[87,609–612] It also has been reported in patients with asthma,[613,614] obesity,[334,615] and ARDS.[222,223,609,616]

Regardless the underlying mechanism, after a few breaths, a steady state is achieved that depends on the variations in the different components of respiratory mechanics. For a certain trapped volume, the amount of PEEP$_I$ is determined by the corresponding respiratory system compliance.

MEASUREMENT OF PEEP$_I$

PEEP$_I$ can be detected qualitatively by observing the flow-time curve, available on most ventilators. In absence of PEEP$_I$, expiratory flow is zero before the onset of the subsequent inspiration (Fig. 11-13*A*). The persistence of expiratory flow at end expiration indicates the presence of PEEP$_I$ during either mechanical ventilation (see Fig. 11-13*B*) or spontaneous breathing (see Fig. 11-13*C*).

Because the ventilator built-in pressure gauge is open to the atmosphere, PEEP$_I$ cannot be detected simply by in-

specting airway pressure. During controlled ventilation, PEEP$_I$ can be measured by occluding the airway opening at end expiration for a few seconds[80,617] (see Fig. 11-5), the end-expiratory occlusion maneuver. This value is static PEEP$_I$ (PEEP$_{I,stat}$). Unless some alveolar units are not at all communicating with the central airways (because the corresponding peripheral airways are completely occluded),[618] PEEP$_{I,stat}$ represents the average pressure in the different lung regions.[13,87,619–621] A second approach is to measure the difference between preset PEEP and airway pressure at the onset of inspiratory flow[91,620,621]; this value is dynamic PEEP$_I$ (PEEP$_{I,dyn}$). PEEP$_{I,dyn}$ can be considered as the lowest regional end-expiratory alveolar pressure that has to be overcome to begin inspiratory flow.[13,87,619–621] PEEP$_{I,dyn}$ and PEEP$_{I,stat}$ approximate each other in animals[620] and human subjects[621] in the absence of severe airway disorders when PEEP$_I$ is consequent to T_E shortening and/or increasing V_E. In animals receiving high doses of aerosolized methacoline[620] and patients affected by severe airways obstruction,[621] PEEP$_{I,dyn}$ is considerably lower than PEEP$_{I,stat}$. A low ratio of PEEP$_{I,dyn}$ to PEEP$_{I,stat}$ suggests time-constant inequalities within the lung and high lung tissue viscoelastic pressure losses.[222,620–623]

When the inspiratory muscles are contracting, assessing PEEP$_I$ is more complex. When inspiration is active and expiration relaxed, PEEP$_{I,dyn}$ can be measured with a balloon-tipped esophageal catheter.[5,619,624,625] PEEP$_{I,dyn}$ equals the difference in esophageal (pleural) pressure between the onset of negative deflection (indicating the start of the inspiratory effort) and the pressure at the transition between expiratory and inspiratory flow[5,619,625] (Fig. 11-14). When the expiratory muscles are contracting, which is common in flow-limited patients,[93,626–628] especially during partial ventilator support,[5,92,93,629] the pressure developed in the abdomen is transmitted through the relaxed diaphragm and raises intrathoracic pressure. Consequently, assessing PEEP$_I$ via esophageal pressure will overestimate the true end-expiratory elastic recoil pressure.[5,92,93,626–630] With a second balloon-tipped catheter in the stomach, it is possible to measure, and correct for, the amount of intrathoracic pressure rise caused by expiratory muscle contraction[5,92,93]; briefly, the expiratory rise in gastric pressure is subtracted from the esophageal pressure at the onset of the subsequent inspiration[92,93] (Fig. 11-15). Another method is to subtract the rise in gastric pressure during an end-expiratory occlusion from airway pressure.[631] Partitioning the rise in intrathoracic pressure from recording of airway, esophageal, and gastric pressures is complex and is performed infrequently in the clinical setting.

PHYSIOLOGIC EFFECTS OF PEEP$_I$

During volume-targeted controlled ventilation, PEEP$_I$ does not affect V_T, whereas it elevates peak airway pressure, which is a dependent variable (i.e., it varies depending on the impedance of the respiratory system) (Fig. 11-16*A*). Conversely, during pressure-targeted controlled ventilation, the independent variable is the preset positive pressure applied to the airway during inspiration; the presence of PEEP$_I$ decreases the actual lung distending pressure and therefore V_T (see Fig. 11-16*B*).

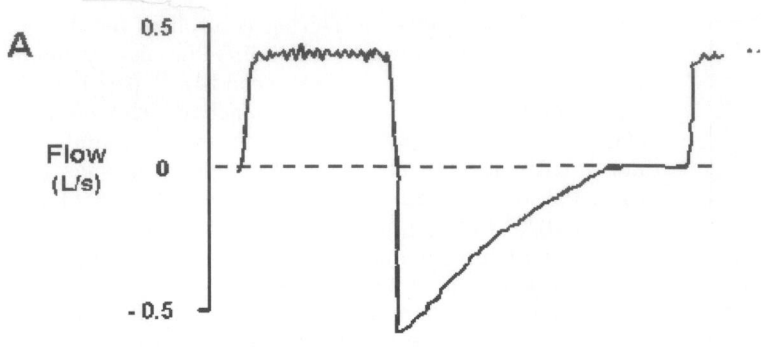

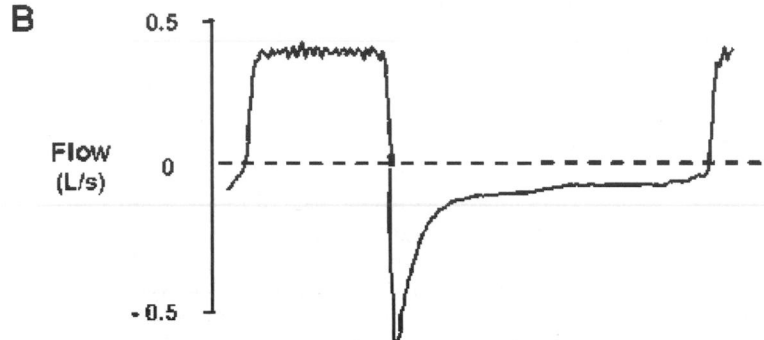

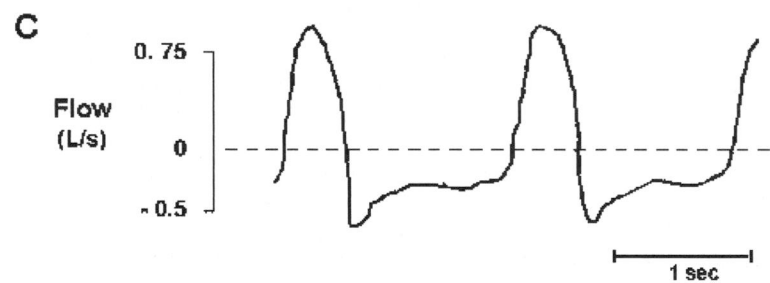

FIGURE 11-13 Flow-time tracings during controlled ventilation in a normal anesthetized subject (*A*) and in a patient with severe COPD during controlled ventilation (*B*) and during spontaneous breathing (*C*). In the normal subject (*A*), expiratory flow reaches zero before expiration ends. In the patient with COPD, expiratory flow remains below zero value before the subsequent inspiration, denoting dynamic hyperinflation, during both controlled ventilation and spontaneous breathing.

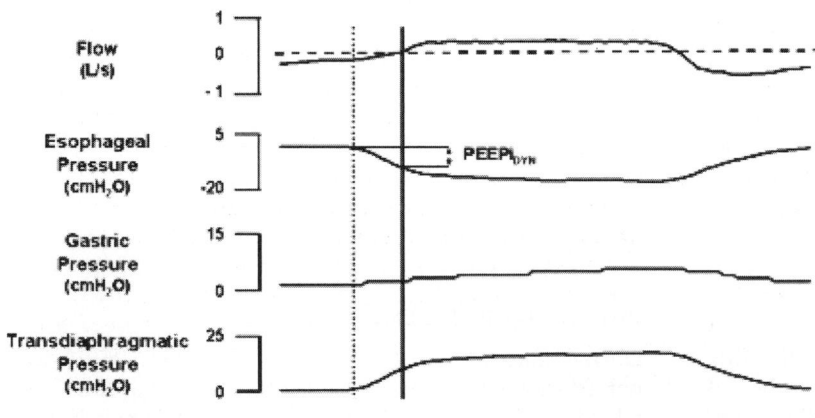

FIGURE 11-14 Measurement of dynamic intrinsic PEEP (PEEP$_{\text{I,dyn}}$) in a spontaneously breathing patient without expiratory muscle activity. The dashed horizontal line indicates zero flow. The dotted vertical line indicates the onset of the inspiratory effort. The solid vertical line indicates the start of inspiratory flow. Gastric pressure rises during inspiration and falls during expiration, indicating that expiratory muscles were not active. PEEP$_{\text{I,dyn}}$ is the difference in esophageal pressure between onset of inspiratory effort and start of inspiratory flow.

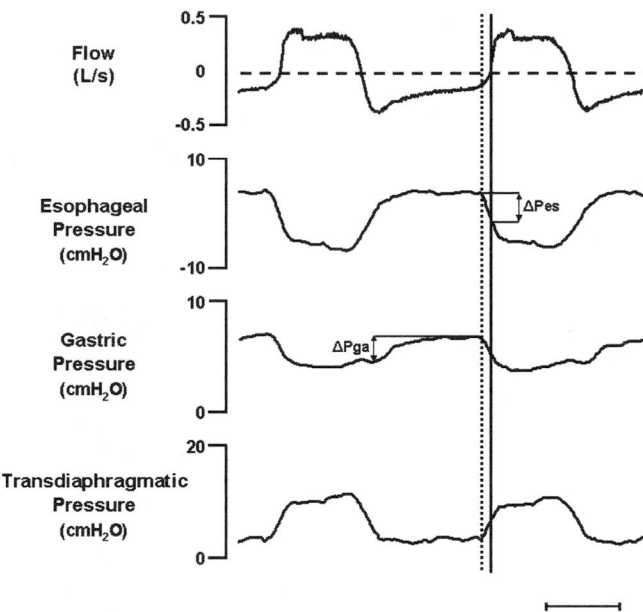

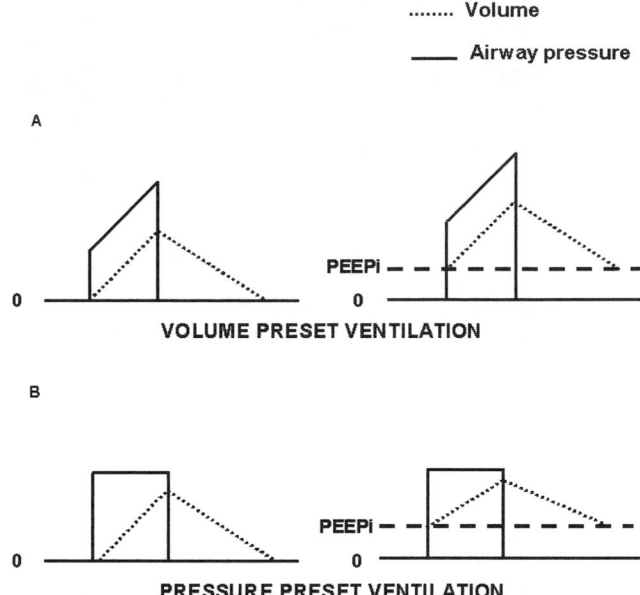

FIGURE 11-15 Measurement of dynamic intrinsic PEEP ($PEEP_{I,dyn}$) in a spontaneously breathing patient with expiratory muscle activity. The dashed horizontal line indicates zero flow. The dotted vertical line indicates onset of inspiratory effort. The solid vertical line indicates the start of inspiratory flow. Unlike in Fig. 11-14, gastric pressure rises during expiration (ΔPga) and descends at the following inspiration, indicating expiratory muscle recruitment. ΔPga must be subtracted from the difference in esophageal pressure between onset of inspiratory effort and start of inspiratory flow to determine $PEEP_{I,dyn}$.

FIGURE 11-16 Simulation of the effects of $PEEP_I$ on volume-targeted (*A*) and pressure-targeted (*B*) controlled ventilation. Volume and airway pressure are indicated by dotted and solid lines, respectively. In the left panels, when $PEEP_I$ is absent, tidal volume is the same for both modes. In the upper-right panel (*A*), during volume-targeted ventilation, $PEEP_I$ causes a rise in airway pressure, whereas preset tidal volume is unchanged. In the lower-right panel (*B*), during pressure-targeted ventilation, preset pressure does not vary, and consequently, tidal volume falls.

$PEEP_I$ resembles in several respects external PEEP. In patients with hypoxemic ARF consequent to ARDS or cardiogenic pulmonary edema, an increase in EELV, produced by T_E shortening, secondary to tachypnea or inverse-ratio ventilation can decrease intrapulmonary shunt as much as can external PEEP.[632] In patients without COPD, Brandolese et al[231] found that external PEEP produced more consistent increases in Pa_{O_2} than did an equivalent level of $PEEP_I$. The authors attributed the less favorable impact of $PEEP_I$ on Pa_{O_2} to less homogeneous gas distribution between different lung units.[231] $PEEP_I$ decreases cardiac output[80,87,231,632] and blood pressure[80,87] to a similar extent to that produced by external PEEP for the same increase in lung volume.[632] Connery et al[633] reported fatal cardiac arrest and life-threatening hypotension during manual ventilation with large V_T and high respiratory frequencies in two patients with severe COPD. By increasing alveolar pressure, $PEEP_I$ also may cause barotrauma.[88]

In spontaneously breathing patients, $PEEP_I$ poses a threshold load that has to be overcome before inspiratory flow can be initiated[13,619,624,634]; this load is perceived as inspiratory difficulty.[635] With any mode of partial ventilator support, this threshold must be overcome before the ventilator can be triggered[5,83,85,625,636–639] (Fig. 11-17). Inspiratory efforts that are not intense enough to overcome $PEEP_I$ fail to trigger the ventilator,[85,86,640–642] a phenomenon referred to as *wasted or ineffective inspiratory efforts* (Fig. 11-18). Wasted efforts occur with all triggered modes[641] and are

more frequent at higher ventilator assistance[85,86,641] because of higher $PEEP_I$ consequent to increased lung volume[85,86,641] and diminished respiratory drive.[641]

Acute hyperinflation impairs the force-generating capacity of the diaphragm by moving the diaphragm to an inefficient part of its force-length relationship[28,643,644] and increasing the O_2 cost of breathing.[645] In healthy volunteers, Beck et al[646] showed that greater diaphragmatic activation to generate a certain amount of pressure increased with increasing lung volume, and pressure generated by maximal diaphragmatic activation decreased with increasing lung volume. In spontaneously breathing dogs, Kawagoe et al[647] found that a threshold load associated with $PEEP_I$ produced pulmonary artery hypertension and decreases in cardiac output and blood flow to the liver, pancreas, and sternomastoid and parasternal muscles with little change in blood flow to the diaphragm.[647] An equivalent resistive load increased diaphragmatic blood flow without changes in cardiac output or regional blood flow.[647] Both loads produced noncompensated respiratory acidosis, but the severity was greater for the threshold load.[647] An acute inspiratory threshold load causes a greater diaphragmatic sarcomere disruption in patients with COPD than in patients without lung disease[648]; hyperinflation explains about 40% of the injury.[648]

The complex interaction of dynamic hyperinflation and $PEEP_I$ on preload has been reviewed by Ranieri et al.[649] During spontaneous breathing or triggered ventilation,

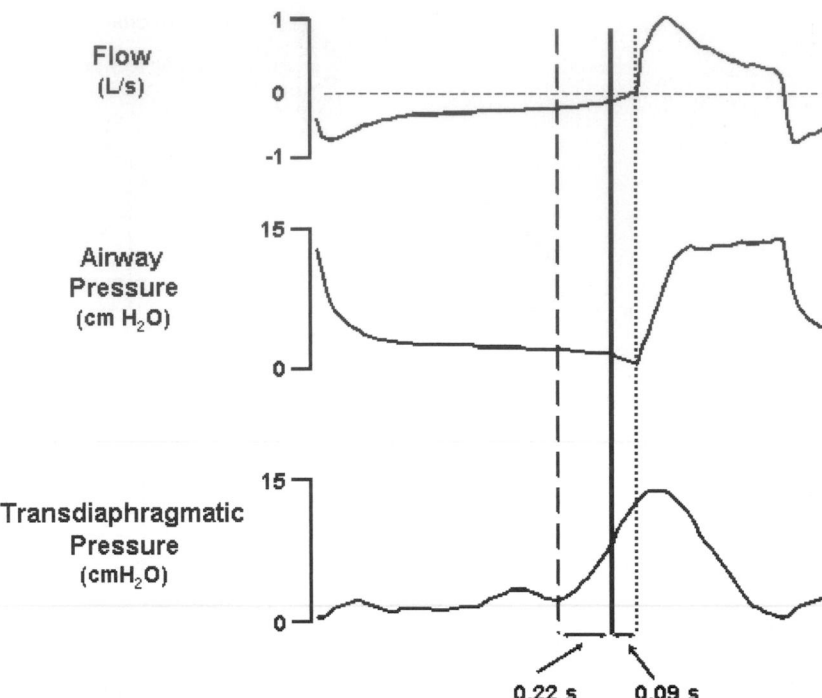

Flow
(L/s)

Airway
Pressure
(cm H₂O)

Transdiaphragmatic
Pressure
(cmH₂O)

0.22 s   0.09 s

FIGURE 11-17 Effect of intrinsic PEEP (PEEP$_I$) on ventilator triggering. The dashed horizontal line indicates zero flow. The dashed vertical line on the left indicates the onset of the inspiratory effort. The dotted vertical line on the right corresponds to the start of inspiratory flow. The solid vertical line indicates the point at which the ventilator is triggered and mechanical assistance is initiated. The amount of effort spent in overcoming PEEP$_I$ corresponds to the difference in transdiaphragmatic pressure between the points crossed by the dashed and solid lines. PEEP$_I$ increases the magnitude of the inspiratory effort and remarkably lengthens the effort-to-assist delay.

FIGURE 11-18 Ineffective or wasted inspiratory efforts. The dashed horizontal line on the flow tracing indicates zero. The dashed vertical line indicates the onset of ventilator assistance. To the left of the dashed line, the patient is breathing spontaneously with the ventilator set in CPAP mode. The breathing pattern is rapid and shallow. Initiation of pressure support increases tidal volume and decreases respiratory rate, as assessed on the flow and airway pressure tracings. The respiratory rate, assessed by swings in esophageal pressure, is higher. The arrows show that half the inspiratory efforts fails to trigger the ventilator. The dotted horizontal lines on the volume tracing indicate that end-expiratory lung volume increased after institution of pressure support (dynamic hyperinflation).

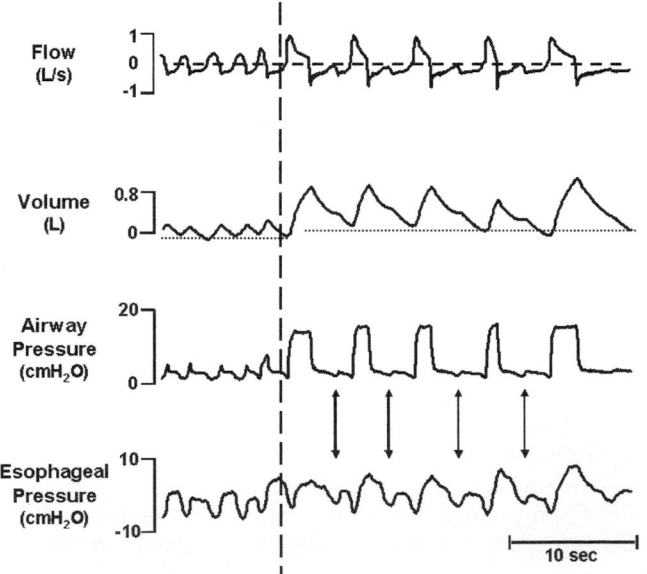

Flow
(L/s)

Volume
(L)

Airway
Pressure
(cmH₂O)

Esophageal
Pressure
(cmH₂O)

10 sec

venous return is decreased by the higher EELV and intrathoracic pressure or increased by the larger negative inspiratory swings in intrathoracic pressure, with the latter dominating.[649] PEEP$_I$ also might affect left-ventricular function by augmenting the afterload, although this possibility has not been studied.

CLINICAL CONSEQUENCES OF PEEP$_I$

The extra load imposed on the respiratory muscles by PEEP$_I$ may be large (Fig. 11-19) and have relevant clinical consequences. In patients with COPD in ARF, Coussa et al[650] found that work of breathing was increased because of increased resistance and PEEP$_I$. PEEP$_I$ accounted for more than 30% of the overall workload (see Fig. 11-19A). In ventilator-dependent patients with COPD, Appendini et al[86] found that the effort to overcome PEEP$_I$ accounted for more than 40% of overall inspiratory effort[86] (see Fig. 11-19B).

Jubran et al[651] studied 31 patients with COPD undergoing a T-tube trial, 17 of whom failed and 14 of whom were extubated successfully (see Fig. 11-19C). At the onset of the trial, PEEP$_I$ was higher in the failure group than in the success group.[651] Between the start and end of the trial, the fraction of inspiratory effort caused by PEEP$_I$ more than doubled in the failure group, whereas it did not change in the success group.[651]

In 30 patients who failed an initial weaning trial but who later succeeded, Vassilakopoulos et al[652] found that dynamic hyperinflation and PEEP$_I$ were higher at the time of weaning failure.

IMPACT OF EXTERNAL PEEP ON DYNAMIC HYPERINFLATION AND PEEP$_I$

Depending on the mechanisms of dynamic hyperinflation and PEEP$_I$, external PEEP can have different effects, as

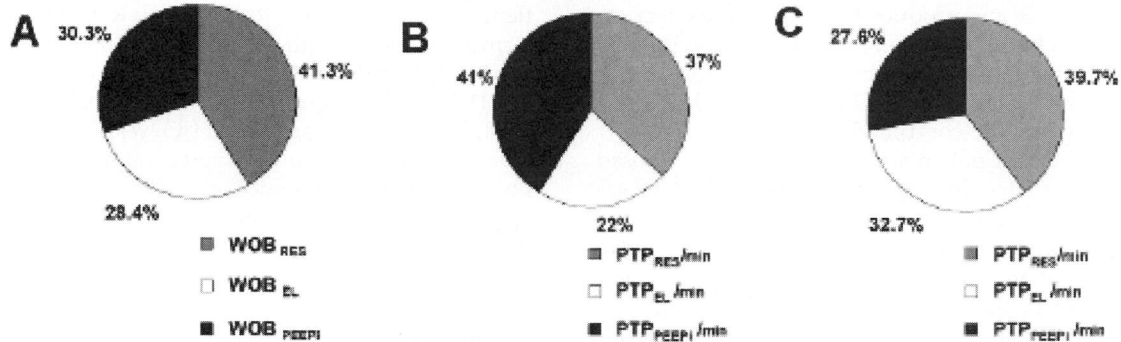

FIGURE 11-19 Fractions of the respiratory load in ventilator-dependent patients with COPD. *A.* Elastic (EL), resistive (RES), and PEEP$_I$ fractions of work of breathing (WOB) in sedated and paralyzed patients with COPD in acute respiratory failure while receiving controlled ventilation. (*From Coussa et al: J Appl Physiol 1993; 75: 1711–9.*) *B.* Elastic (EL), resistive (RES), and PEEP$_I$ components of inspiratory effort, assessed as esophageal pressure-time product (PTP), during a brief period of spontaneous breathing in patients with COPD who could not be weaned (*From Appendini et al: Am J Respir Crit Care Med 1997; 149:1069–76.*). *C.* Same measurement as in *B* in patients with COPD who failed a T-tube trial (*From Jubra et al: Am J Respir Crit Care Med 1997; 155:906.*) Despite the different settings, PEEP$_I$ accounted for a considerable fraction of inspiratory load.

elegantly pointed out by Marini[653] (Fig. 11-20). When PEEP$_I$ is not caused by flow limitation, external PEEP is transmitted entirely to the distal airway, producing a concomitant rise in alveolar pressure (see Fig. 11-20*B*). In six patients with acute asthma or a COPD exacerbation, Tuxen et al[285] increased dynamic hyperinflation and PEEP$_I$ by increasing $\dot{V}_E$ from 10 to 16 and to 22 liters/min. Increasing levels of PEEP up to 15 cmH$_2$O produced increases in EELV and intrathoracic pressure, accompanied by a parallel hemodynamic deterioration.[285] At the lowest $\dot{V}_E$, trapped volume was small, suggesting little, if any, flow limitation.[285]

When flow limitation and dynamic airway compression are present, PEEP is not transmitted to the distal airway and does not increase alveolar pressure as long as it does not exceed the critical pressure corresponding to the choke point[653] (see Fig. 11-20*C*). The waterfall analogy helps in understanding this concept. The equal-pressure point is viewed as the crest of a waterfall, and the airway segment between the choke point and the airway opening is seen as as the downstream water.[654,655] Increasing the level of downstream water (external PEEP) does not alter upstream water flow (airflow) as long as it does not exceed the crest (critical pressure at the choke point).[655] In flow-limited patients with COPD who had PEEP$_I$ of 10 cmH$_2$O and trapped volume of 1 liter, Ranieri et al[87] applied PEEP of 5, 10, and 15 cmH$_2$O. Up to PEEP of 10 cmH$_2$O, changes in peak and plateau airway pressures, EELV, and total PEEP (i.e., PEEP$_I$ + external PEEP) were minimal; hemodynamic impairment was absent. PEEP of 15 cmH$_2$O increased peak and plateau airway pressures, trapped volume, and total PEEP, with worsening of hemodynamics.[87] Changes in EELV and cardiac index started to occur when external PEEP matched about 85% of PEEP$_{I,stat}$.[87] In flow-limited patients with COPD receiving triggered ventilation, Appendini et al[5] found that PEEP slightly lower than PEEP$_{I,dyn}$ did not cause further hyperinflation.

Recent studies show that flow limitation associated with small airways closure and PEEP$_I$ may be present in ventilated patients with ARDS.[222] In patients with ARDS who have flow limitation and PEEP$_I$, Koutsoukou et al[223] found

that PEEP of 10 cmH$_2$O produced a small increase in total PEEP and alveolar recruitment but a significant increase in Pa$_{O_2}$; the latter was attributed to improved regional PEEP$_I$ inhomogeneity. In another group of patients who did not exhibit flow limitation and had little PEEP$_I$, PEEP of 10 cmH$_2$O

FIGURE 11-20 Schematic representation of the effects of PEEP on alveolar pressure in normal conditions (*A*), high airway resistance but no expiratory flow limitation (*B*), and expiratory flow limitation and dynamic airway compression (*C*). The circles represent the alveoli, the rectangles the ventilator, and the tubes the bronchi. PEEP, positive end-expiratory pressure expressed in cmH$_2$O; Rexp, expiratory resistance, expressed in cmH$_2$O/liter/s; ZEEP, zero positive end-expiratory pressure. *A.* At ZEEP (*left panel*), the alveolar pressure falls to zero. Applied PEEP (*right panel*) is transmitted entirely to the alveoli. *B.* At ZEEP (*left panel*), the high expiratory resistance causes alveolar pressure to remain positive at end expiration. Applied PEEP (*right panel*) is transmitted entirely to the alveoli. *C.* At ZEEP (*left panel*), the alveolar pressure is positive. Applied PEEP does not exceed the critical pressure at the choke point and does not affect alveolar pressure.

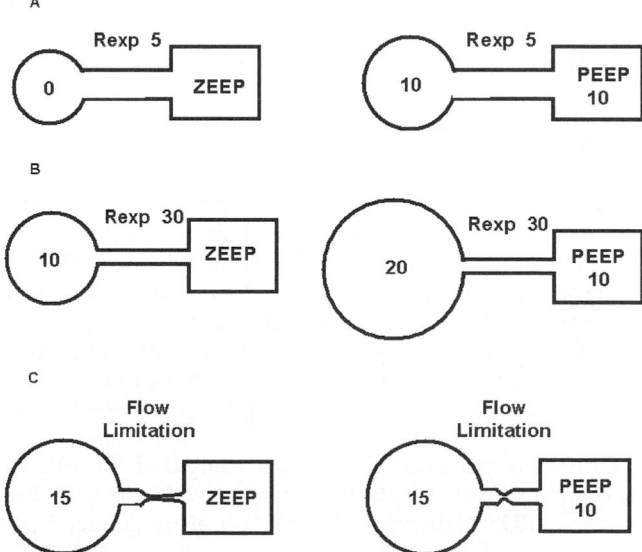

increased total PEEP and produced greater alveolar recruitment, which was the chief reason for an increase in Pa_{O_2}.[223] Analogous results were reported by Vieillard-Baron et al,[399] who found flow limitation and $PEEP_I$ in 73% of patients with ARDS receiving volume-controlled ventilation.

In actively breathing patients, the threshold load imposed by $PEEP_I$ may be offset by applying CPAP[13,81,82,656] or external PEEP.[5,83,85,637] If excessive or improperly applied,[653] external PEEP can worsen hyperinflation,[87,657,658] placing the diaphragm at an additional disadvantage[28,644,646] and causing further hemodynamic impairment.[87,657]

Use of PEEP in the Clinical Setting

ALI/ARDS

The rationale for PEEP in patients with ALI/ARDS is to increase the amount of aerated lung volume,[71,236,270] improve respiratory mechanics,[71,73,236] reduce intrapulmonary shunt[182,659] and ameliorate gas exchange,[4,34,71,119,236] stabilize unsteady lung units,[660] and reduce the risk of VILI.[73,437] From its introduction almost 40 years ago,[4] PEEP remains a cornerstone in management of patients with ALI/ARDS.[661] It is easy to see why no randomized trial evaluated ventilator strategies without PEEP in patients with ALI/ARDS, except in the very early phase.[192,662] Very few studies have assessed the effect of PEEP on clinical outcome of patients with ALI/ARDS[9,70,663,664] (Table 11-2). One early study reported that high PEEP levels did not improve survival and caused more adverse events when compared with patients treated with low PEEP.[70]

In the last decade, research has focused on ventilator strategies that protect the lung from VILI. As stated in a recent editorial,[665] these investigations have shown that ventilator settings per se may affect outcome.[420] Two recent randomized, controlled trials suggest that high levels of PEEP (15–20 cmH_2O), used in the context of a lung-protective strategy, may improve both the physiologic[419] and clinical[9] outcome in patients with ALI/ARDS. Amato et al[9] found that low V_T combined with PEEP set 2 cmH_2O above the LIP (16 cmH_2O, on average) reduced mortality compared with a conventional approach where PEEP was titrated to optimize oxygenation (see Table 11-2). Ranieri et al[419] compared a strategy of high PEEP and low V_T, respectively, based on LIP and UIP against a conventional approach where lower PEEP and higher V_T were targeted to normalize gas exchange (see Table 11-2). The control group exhibited more inflammatory mediators than the lung-protective group.[419] The control group also had a higher rate of organ failure and mortality and fewer ventilator-free days.[419,454] The occurrence of $PEEP_I$, consequent to a high respiratory rate in the low V_T group, may have contributed[666,667] to the positive results in the ARDS Network comparison of low and high V_T in patients with ARDS.[420]

Only one randomized trial has compared the impact of different levels of PEEP on clinical end points.[664] The second ARDS Network (ALVEOLI) trial randomized pa-

tients with ALI/ARDS to high or low PEEP levels to determine whether high PEEP, by enhancing lung recruitment, might reduce VILI and improve outcome[664] (see Table 11-2). In both groups, V_T and plateau pressure were 6 ml/kg and less than 30 cmH_2O, respectively. PEEP was titrated, according to predefined combinations of PEEP and FI_{O_2}, to achieve an identical goal (Pa_{O_2} of 55–88 mmHg or Sp_{O_2} of 88–95%).[664] The study was interrupted after enrollment of 549 patients because no difference was detected in any predefined clinical outcome variable between the two groups.[664] Some methodologic biases cast doubt on the conclusions.[668]

An imbalance occurred in baseline characteristics of the two groups (higher Pa_{O_2}/FI_{O_2} ratio and younger age in favor of the lower PEEP group). The protocol was amended during the study in order to achieve a greater difference in PEEP between the groups, which raises concerns about the validity of the analysis.[669] When analysis is confined to patients enrolled after the protocol was amended and after adjusting for differences in baseline characteristics, the mortality is lower in the high-PEEP than in the low-PEEP group (28% versus 33%), suggesting that the trial was interrupted prematurely.[669] PEEP-induced recruitment was estimated by improvement in oxygenation. It is well known that changes in oxygenation depend not only on recruitment but also on cardiac output.[60,180,182,230] Thus oxygenation may have improved without any lung recruitment.

Grasso et al[378] recently analyzed the physiologic effects of the ALVEOLI protocol. They demonstrated that the protocol has unpredictable effects on lung recruitment. Indeed, the protocol may increase the risk of overdistension when high PEEP is applied in patients with a low potential for recruitment. Moreover, a supplementary analysis of data collected by a large international survey[29] found that the use of low or no PEEP was an independent risk factor for ICU mortality in patients with ARDS.[670]

In ARDS, lung units are unstable and have a strong tendency to collapse. Thus any ventilator circuit disconnection or leakage leading to a complete or partial drop in pressure can cause harmful falls in lung volume and oxygenation.[360]

Several approaches have been proposed for setting PEEP, but none has proved to enhance any clinical outcome[9,16,18,69,70,205,239,369,381,386,664,671–676] (Table 11-3). Optimal PEEP in ALI/ARDS should recruit as much nonaerated lung as possible while avoiding lung overdistension, hemodynamic impairment, and global and regional disturbances of O_2 balance (Fig. 11-21). The choice of optimal PEEP in patients with ALI/ARDS remains an open issue. Two ongoing multicenter trials (in France and Canada) should help to resolve this question.

Despite strong physiologic rationale, no study to date has assessed whether setting PEEP according to respiratory mechanics improves outcome. An approach based on real-time continuous analysis of the dynamic airway pressure-time profile has been proposed for optimizing ventilator settings in ALI/ARDS.[239,397,677] In animal studies, this approach predicts a ventilator strategy that minimizes VILI.[397,677] The implementation of automatic tools that facilitate standardized assessment and continuous monitoring of

TABLE 11-2 Randomized Controlled Trials Evaluating the Effect of PEEP on Clinical and Physiologic Outcomes

Reference	Population	Arm	No. of Patients	Associated Settings	PEEP Setting	Mean PEEP (cmH₂O)	Outcomes
Amato 1995 (72)	Medical	Intervention	15	VT < 6 ml/kg / PIP < 40 cmH$_2$O / CPAP recruiting	2 cmH$_2$O > LIP (minimum 5 cmH$_2$O)	18	Successful weaning: 87% / Mortality: 33% / Barotrauma: 13%
		Control	13	VT = 12 ml/kg / PIP unlimited	Titrated to P/F ratio (minimum 5 cmH$_2$O)	7	Successful weaning: 46% / Mortality: 54% / Barotrauma: 31%
Amato 1998 (9)	Medical	Intervention	29	VT < 6 ml/kg / PIP < 40 cmH$_2$O / CPAP recruiting	2 cmH$_2$O > LIP (minimum 5 cmH$_2$O)	16	Mortality: 45% / Barotrauma: 7%
		Control	24	VT = 12 ml/kg / PIP unlimited	Titrated to P/F ratio (minimum 5 cmH$_2$O)	7	Mortality: 71% / Barotrauma: 42%
Ranieri 1999 (419)	Medical-Surgical	Intervention	18	VT for Pplat < UIP (or VT = 5–8 ml/kg)	2–3 cmH$_2$O > LIP (minimum 15 cmH$_2$O)	15	BAL/systemic levels of inflammatory mediators: → / Ventilator-free days: 12* / Mortality: 38%* / Organ failure score: unchanged
		Control	19	VT for PaCO$_2$ 35–40 mmHg / Pplat < 35 cmH$_2$O	Titrated to SaO$_2$ (minimum 5 cmH$_2$O)	7	BAL/systemic levels of inflammatory mediators: ↑ / Ventilator-free days: 4 * / Mortality: 58%* / Organ failure score: increased (mainly renal)
Brower 2004 (664)	Medical-Surgical	Intervention	270	VT = 6 ml/kg / Pplat < 30 cmH$_2$O	Titrated to oxygenation (minimum 12 cmH$_2$O)	13**	Mortality: 25%*** / Unassisted breathing: 72% / Barotrauma: 11% / Days without organ failure: 16
		Control	273	VT = 6 ml/kg / Pplat < 30 cmH$_2$O	Titrated to oxygenation (minimum 5 cmH$_2$O)	8	Mortality: 28%*** / Unassisted breathing: 73% / Barotrauma: 10% / Days without organ failure: 16

ABBREVIATIONS. VT: tidal volume, PIP: peak inspiratory pressure, CPAP: continuous positive airway pressure, Pplat: plateau pressure, LIP: lower inflection point on the pressure-volume curve, P/F: ratio between arterial oxygen tension and fractional inspired oxygen, SaO$_2$: arterial oxygen saturation, BAL: bronchoalveolar lavage.

* post hoc analysis.

** after protocol amendment.

*** after adjustment for differences in baseline covariates.

TABLE 11-3   Methods for Selecting Optimal PEEP

Reference	Year	PEEP Target	Proposed Method
Suter (18)	1975	Maximal oxygen delivery	Maximal static compliance during stepwise incremental PEEP
Kirby (16)	1975	Intrapulmonary shunt < 15%	Stepwise incremental PEEP to reach the target, while supporting cardiac output with fluids and vasopressors
Hurewitz (674)	1981	Drop of mixed venous oxygen tension	Stepwise incremental PEEP to reach the target
Weisman (675)	1982	Adequate PaO_2 with minimal FiO_2	Stepwise incremental PEEP to reach the target
Murray (676)	1984	Minimal arterial-end-tidal CO_2 gradient	Stepwise incremental PEEP to reach the target
Matamis (381)	1984	Best improvement in gas exchange, intrapulmonary shunt and respiratory mechanics	PEEP set at the lower inflection point on inspiratory P-V curve
Albert (69)	1985	Adequate PaO_2 with FiO_2 < 0.6	Lowest PEEP to reach the target
Hartman (673)	1992	Maximal peripheral tissue perfusion	Maximal subcutaneous oxygen tension during stepwise incremental PEEP
Gattinoni (205)	1993	Prevention of compression atelectasis	Maximal PEEP (equal to superimposed hydrostatic pressure) corresponds to 70% of the dorsal-ventral height of thorax (in cm)
Ranieri (239)	1994	Linear airway pressure-time profile	PEEP variations to reach the target
Amato (9)	1998	Maximal recruitment	PEEP set 2 cmH_2O above the lower inflection point on inspiratory P-V curve
Hickling (386)	2001	Maximal static compliance	Stepwise decremental PEEP trial
Rouby (369)	2002	Best oxygenation with the lowest FiO_2 (> 0.6)	Lung morphology, slope and inflection points of the P-V curve, PEEP trial
Brower (664)	2004	Oxygenation (PaO_2 55–80 mmHg, SpO_2 88–95%)	PEEP-FiO_2 combination table

ABBREVIATIONS. FiO_2: fractional inspired oxygen, CO_2: carbon dioxide, PaO_2: arterial oxygen tension, SpO_2: percutaneous oxygen saturation.

respiratory mechanics might allow this approach to be incorporated into the clinical setting.

POSTOPERATIVE STATE

Postoperative hypoxemia is mainly caused by atelectasis[133,144,678] After various surgical procedures, atelectasis develops in 30–50% of cases[679] and leads to ARF requiring intubation and mechanical ventilation in 8–10% of patients.[679–682] The application of CPAP (5–10 cmH_2O) via a face mask, alone or combined with pressure support, reduces atelectasis and improves oxygenation after both cardiac[176,683] and noncardiac surgery[248,684–687] without increasing surgical complications, such as anastomotic leaks.[688] By reducing atelectasis, CPAP may decrease bacterial growth in the lung, mitigating bacterial translocation into the bloodstream and normalizing alveolocapillary permeability.[689,690]

Onset and duration of CPAP seem to be critical for avoiding or reversing atelectasis. Studies that failed to demonstrate benefit used CPAP several hours after surgery[691] or for a relatively short time.[692–694] Despite well-recognized physiologic benefits, only very recently have randomized trials assessed the effects of CPAP on outcome variables.[695,696] In 70 patients, Fagevik Olsen et al[695] reported that compared with breathing exercises, use of CPAP after thoracoabdominal resection of esophageal cancer resulted in a lower intubation rate. Squadrone et al[696] randomized patients who developed hypoxemia following major abdominal surgery to either O_2 alone (FiO_2 of 50%) or O_2 plus CPAP of 7.5 cmH_2O. The study was interrupted after 209 patients were enrolled because the intubation rate was lower in the CPAP group than in the O_2 group (1% versus 10%).[696] The patients who received CPAP at the end of treatment had higher oxygenation and lower rates of pneumonia, infection, and sepsis than the O_2 group.[696] Although limited to selected patients undergoing elective abdominal surgery, these data show that improvement in physiologic parameters achieved with CPAP can translate into a better clinical outcome. Of note, CPAP was applied almost continuously for a prolonged time (19 ± 22 hours).[696]

In summary, CPAP is a simple, practical, and safe technique for managing postoperative hypoxemia. It may improve outcome in selected patients, provided that it is applied for a sufficient time.

COPD

ARF in patients with COPD is characterized by high airways resistance and $PEEP_I$,[215,619,624,650,697] which increase respiratory muscle load.[5,83,86,624,640] Hyperinflation simultaneously reduces the force-generating capacity of the diaphragm.[28,646] When the force-load balance is altered to a level that severe respiratory acidosis ensues, mechanical ventilation becomes necessary. The ventilator acts as an accessory pump that helps to reverse the unfavorable force-load balance. By reducing O_2 cost of breathing and correcting arterial blood gases, mechanical ventilation can improve respiratory muscle function (force). Inspiratory assistance by the ventilator, however, does not reduce the inspiratory resistive load consequent to airway resistance or the threshold load consequent to $PEEP_I$.

Pharmacotherapy can have favorable effects on both load reduction and force restoration.[698] Agents act on bronchial smooth muscle (β_2 agonists, anticholinergic)[699–702] or inflammatory process (glucocorticoids and

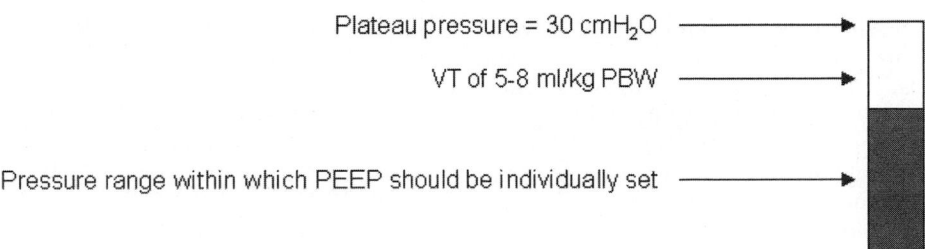

Plateau pressure = 30 cmH$_2$O

VT of 5-8 ml/kg PBW

Pressure range within which PEEP should be individually set

Evaluation of potential for recruitment and overdistension

a. Morphology of lung injury (chest X-ray and/or CT scan)
b. ΔEELV and Vrec with different PEEP (5-10-15-20 cmH$_2$O)
   (P-V curve, equal pressure method)
c. Linear compliance of the P-V curve at ZEEP or low PEEP (i.e. 5 cmH$_2$O)
   (estimated by sequential Cst calculation with incremental VT size)
d. PaO$_2$ and PaCO$_2$ changes with different PEEP (5-10-15-20 cmH$_2$O)

Hemodynamic consequences of PEEP

a. Arterial blood pressure
b. Arterial systolic and pulse pressures variation

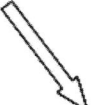
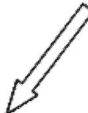

Low potential for recruitment / High risk of overdistension / Hemodynamic impairment: PEEP 7-12 cmH$_2$O

High potential for recruitment / Low risk of overdistension / No hemodynamic impairment : PEEP ≥ 15 cmH$_2$O

FIGURE 11-21 Proposed algorithm for setting PEEP in ALI/ARDS. First, a safe plateau pressure limit of 30 cmH$_2$O is recommended; it should not be exceeded except when chest-wall compliance is very low. Second, V$_T$ is preset, which corresponds to a certain pressure oscillation. Third, PEEP should not exceed the pressure difference between plateau pressure and the tidal pressure oscillation. After hemodynamic stabilization, the potential for recruitment, the risk of overdistension, and the hemodynamic consequences are assessed individually for different levels of PEEP. Potential for recruitment is greater when (1) lung injury is diffuse, (2) alveolar recruitment is large (i.e., >100 ml), (3) the ratio between alveolar recruitment and change in end-expiratory lung volume is high (>15–20%), (4) linear compliance of the pressure-volume curve at 0 cmH$_2$O is high (>40 ml/cmH$_2$O), (5) static compliance measured at low or no PEEP progressively increases with increasing V$_T$, and (6) Pa$_{O_2}$ increases and Pa$_{CO_2}$ decreases concomitantly. By contrast, the risk for overdistension is greater when changes in the preceding parameters go in the opposite direction. PEEP-induced hemodynamic impairment may be considered clinically relevant when arterial systolic pressure falls more than 20 mmHg and/or variations in both arterial systolic pressure or pulse pressure appear or increase. Cst, static compliance; CT, computed tomography; ΔEELV, change in end-expiratory lung volume; PBW, predicted body weight; Vrec, recruited volume; V$_T$, tidal volume.

antibiotics).[699,700,702,703] These agents decrease airways resistance, dynamic hyperinflation, and PEEP$_I$ in ventilated patients.[704–709] Glucocorticoids and antibiotics commonly are administered parenterally. In ventilated patients, bronchodilators are given more effectively and safely via a small-volume nebulizer or a metered-dose inhaler connected to an appropriate spacer.[710]

External PEEP reduces the threshold load imposed on the inspiratory muscles. PEEP, however, does not reduce hyperinflation and its effects on diaphragmatic force-generating capacity. Application of PEEP in patients with COPD may cause a decrease in expiratory resistance and promote a faster and more uniform lung emptying,[410] although the clinical relevance of these findings remains to be determined. CPAP is effective in reducing dyspnea,[13,81,656] decreasing work of breathing,[13,81,82,656] and improving car-

diac function.[649] During triggered ventilation, PEEP reduces inspiratory effort[5,83,85,637] and ventilatory drive[637] and facilitates triggering of the ventilator[5,83,85,637] by reducing both inspiratory effort and the delay between the onset of inspiratory effort and initiation of assistance, improving patient-ventilator interaction and reducing ineffective inspiratory efforts.[85,86]

Despite a large body of physiologic data, no randomized trial has evaluated the effectiveness of PEEP/CPAP in improving outcome in ventilated patients with COPD. Most trials, however, that evaluated the effectiveness of noninvasive ventilation in patients with acute hypercapnia secondary to COPD exacerbation used PEEP of 4–5 cmH$_2$O in addition to pressure support.[711–713]

A new ventilator has been described that uses diaphragmatic electrical activity, measured with an electrode array in the lower esophagus, to trigger the ventilator.[714] The ventilator is triggered, irrespective of $PEEP_I$, as soon as the diaphragm contracts.[714] The "neural trigger" may enhance patient-ventilator coordination markedly by reducing the delay between onset of inspiratory effort and initiation of machine support without the need for external PEEP. Thus this system might eliminate the difficulties in selecting appropriate PEEP and avoid further hyperinflation.[714]

ACUTE SEVERE ASTHMA

Patients with acute severe asthma have high airway resistance, dynamic hyperinflation, and $PEEP_I$, which increase respiratory muscles load and decrease force-generation capacity.[715] These patients generally are less responsive to external PEEP.[285] Although some flow limitation may be present,[613] the main cause of dynamic hyperinflation and $PEEP_I$ is the prolonged time constant secondary to the high expiratory resistance. In the absence of flow limitation, PEEP increases hyperinflation and alveolar pressure.[653,716] Some alveolar units may be entirely occluded by mucus plugs and thus completely disconnected from the central airway.[618]

Low levels of CPAP may decrease breathlessness.[717–719] Lin et al[720] reported that CPAP reduced the bronchial reactivity. In patients with asthma exposed to aerosolized histamine, Martin et al[721] found that CPAP of 12 cmH_2O decreased both esophageal and transdiaphragmatic pressure swings. $\dot{V}_E$ increased, and thus inspiratory work did not fall.[721] Meduri et al,[722] in a series that included 17 patients with acute asthma, reported that CPAP of 3–5 cmH_2O combined with pressure support via a face mask improved gas exchange. Only two patients failed and required endotracheal intubation.[722] In a randomized trial of 30 patients treated in an emergency department for acute asthma, Sorosky et al[723] found that noninvasive ventilation with low CPAP produced greater and faster improvements in lung function and a lower rate of hospitalization than did standard therapy.[723]

In summary, use of PEEP in patients receiving mechanical ventilation for acute severe asthma is often detrimental and thus is not advisable. Very few data suggest that low levels of noninvasive CPAP combined with pressure support in less severe and selected patients might be beneficial, although further evaluation is required.

CARDIOGENIC PULMONARY EDEMA

The benefit of CPAP on the failing left ventricle has been discussed already (see Fig. 11-11). Although most of patients may respond positively to standard medical treatment, some do not and require endotracheal intubation and ventilator assistance.

Over the last two decades, there has been growing interest in the delivery of CPAP via a face mask as a means of avoiding endotracheal intubation and invasive mechanical ventilation. Five randomized, controlled trials have performed head-to-head comparisons of CPAP versus standard therapy in patients with cardiogenic pulmonary edema.[14,102,187,194,724] Two trials[195,725] have compared CPAP versus bilevel positive airway pressure (BiPAP) (i.e., PEEP plus inspiratory pressure support).[195] Two recent trials have compared standard treatment alone versus CPAP and versus BiPAP.[726,727] That is, seven trials have compared CPAP versus standard treatment[14,102,187,194,724,726,727] (Table 11-4) and four trials CPAP versus BiPAP[195,725–727] (Table 11-5).

Only four studies[194,195,725,727] had been powered a priori, according to their primary end points. Three trials were interrupted prematurely after interim analysis. L'Her et al[194] found that mortality after 48 hours was lower in a CPAP group than in the standard therapy group. Park et al[727] suspended their study because the intubation rate was higher in the standard therapy group than in the CPAP and BiPAP groups. Metha et al[195] interrupted their study because myocardial infarction was increased in the BiPAP group. With the exception of the study by Lin et al,[187] the other studies included few patients (risk of type II error).

The seven studies comparing CPAP versus standard treatment[14,102,187,194,724,726,727] included a total of 191 patients receiving CPAP and 197 control patients (see Table 11-4). CPAP was 10 cmH_2O in four studies,[14,102,724,726,727] 7.5 cmH_2O in one study,[194] and varied between 2.5 and 12.5 cmH_2O in one study.[187] CPAP produced a greater and more rapid (10–180 minutes) physiologic improvement in all studies but one.[726] Five studies[14,102,187,194,724] reported a prompter and greater improvement in oxygenation with CPAP, although in only three studies[14,194,724] was $Pa_{O_2}/F_{I_{O_2}}$ assessed. Only Bersten et al,[14] who included patients with the most severe acidemia, observed improvements in pH and Pa_{CO_2} with CPAP. Dyspnea was reduced by CPAP in two studies[194,727] but not in a third study.[726] CPAP produced a lower rate of therapeutic failure and intubation in four studies[14,187,194,727] and decreased hospital mortality in only one study.[726] None of the seven studies revealed differences in the length of hospital stay.

The four studies comparing CPAP with BiPAP[195,725–727] included a total of 82 CPAP and 87 BiPAP patients (see Table 11-5). All studies used CPAP of 10 cmH_2O. The setting of BiPAP varied. Park et al[727] added a small level of IPAP to EPAP of 10 cmH_2O. Mehta et al[195] and Crane et al[726] decreased EPAP from 10 to 5 cmH_2O and raised IPAP to 15 cmH_2O in order to achieve a mean pressure of 10 cmH_2O throughout the entire breath in both groups. Bellone et al[725] also used PEEP of 5 cmH_2O and an initial pressure support of 15 cmH_2O (i.e., IPAP of 20 cmH_2O).

Mehta et al[195] found a more rapid reduction in Pa_{CO_2} and other physiologic variables with BiPAP than with CPAP. The other three studies[725–727] did not find differences in early physiologic variables. Three studies[195,725,727] did not reveal differences in any clinical outcome variable. Crane et al[726] found hospital survival higher in the CPAP than in the BiPAP group. Bellone et al,[725] Park et al,[727] and Crane et al[726] did not find differences in the incidence of myocardial infarction between groups.

In summary, there are sufficient data to support the use of CPAP (10 cmH_2O) for achieving prompt physiologic improvement and a lower rate of endotracheal intubation in patients with cardiogenic pulmonary edema. CPAP should

TABLE 11-4   Randomized Controlled Trials Comparing Medical Therapy Alone versus Medical Therapy Plus CPAP

Source, yr	Sample Size	Intervention SMT	Intervention SMT + CPAP	Early Physiologic Outcomes (10 to 180 minutes)	SMT vs. Baseline	CPAP vs. Baseline	CPAP vs. SMT	Clinical Outcomes	SMT	CPAP
Rasanen, 1985 (ref. 102)	n = 20 SMT n = 19 CPAP		CPAP 10 cmH$_2$O	RR	b	a	ns	Treatment failure no (%)	13 (65)	7 (36)
				HR	a	b	c	Intubation and/or MV no (%)	12 (60)	6 (31)
				SBP	ns	b	ns	Hospital Mortality no (%)	6 (30)	3 (15)
				pH	ns	b	ns	ICU Stay (days) Mean ± SD	NA	NA
				PaCO$_2$	ns	a	ns	Hospital Stay (days) Mean ± SD	NA	NA
				PaO$_2$	ns	a	c			
Bersten, 1991 (ref. 14)	n = 20 SMT n = 19 CPAP		CPAP 10 cmH$_2$O	RR	ns	a	c	Treatment failure no (%)	9 (45)	0 (0) c
				HR	ns	b	d	Intubation and/or MV no (%)	7 (35)	0 (0) c
				SBP	ns	ns	ns	Hospital Mortality no (%)	4 (20)	2 (10)
				PaO$_2$/FiO$_2$	ns	a	c	ICU Stay (days) Mean ± SD	2.7 ± 2.0	1.2 ± 0.4c
				pH	ns	a	c	Hospital Stay (days) Mean ± SD	7.9 ± 4.1	8.7 ± 8.3
				PaCO$_2$	ns	a	c			
Lin, 1995 (ref. 187)	n = 50 SMT n = 50 CPAP		CPAP 2.5 to 12.5 cmH$_2$O	RR	ns	a	c	Treatment failure no (%)	25 (50)	12(24) c
				HR	ns	a	c	Intubation and/or MV no (%)	18 (36)	8 (16) c
				MBP	ns	a	c	Hospital Mortality no (%)	6 (12)	4 (8)
				pH	ns	ns	ns	ICU Stay (days) Mean ± SD	4.5 ± 3.5	4.0 ± 3.0
				PaCO$_2$	ns	ns	ns	Hospital Stay (days) Mean ± SD	9.0 ± 4.5	8.5 ± 4.5
				PaO$_2$	ns	b	c			
Moritz, 2003 (ref. 724)	n = 14 SMT n=14 CPAP		CPAP 9.3 ± 0.3 cmH$_2$O	RR	ns	b	d	Treatment failure no (%)	NA	NA
				HR	ns	b	ns	Intubation and/or MV no (%)	NA	NA
				SBP	ns	ns	ns	Hospital Mortality no (%)	NA	NA
				PaO$_2$/FiO$_2$	ns	b	ns	ICU Stay (days) Mean ± SD	NA	NA
				pH	ns	ns	ns	Hospital Stay (days) Mean ± SD	NA	NA
				PaCO$_2$	ns	ns	ns			
				Dyspnea	NA	NA	NA			
L' Her, 2004 (ref. 194)	n = 46 SMT n = 43 CPAP		CPAP 7.5 cmH$_2$O	RR	NA	NA	c	Treatment failure no (%)	17 (37)	14 (9) c
				HR	NA	NA	c	Intubation and/or MV no (%)	14 (30)	4 (9) c
				MBP	NA	NA	ns	48 h Mortality no (%)	11 (24)	3 (7) c
				PaO$_2$/FiO$_2$	NA	NA	c	Hospital Mortality no (%)	14 (30)	12 (28)
				pH	NA	NA	ns	ICU Stay (days) Mean ± SD	NA	NA
				PaCO$_2$	NA	NA	ns	Hospital Stay (days) Mean ± SD	9.7 ± 7.0	2.0 ± 11
				Dyspnea	NA	NA	c			
Crane, 2004 (ref. 726)	n = 20 SMT n = 19 CPAP		CPAP 10 cmH$_2$O	RR	b	b	ns	Treatment failure no (%)	1 (5)	4 (20)
				HR	NA	NA	ns	Intubation and/or MV no (%)	0 (0)	2 (10)
				SBP	NA	NA	ns	Hospital Mortality no (%)	6 (30)	0(0) d
				pH	NA	NA	ns	ICU Stay (days) Mean ± SD	NA	NA
				PaCO$_2$	NA	NA	ns	Hospital Stay (days) Mean ± SD	NA	NA
				PaO$_2$	NA	NA	ns			
				Dyspnea	NA	NA	ns			
Park, 2004 (ref. 727)	n = 27 SMT n = 27 CPAP		CPAP 10 cmH$_2$O	RR	NA	NA	c	Treatment failure no (%)	11 (42)	2 (7) c
				HR	NA	NA	ns	Intubation and/or MV no (%)	11 (42)	2 (7) c
				MBP	NA	NA	ns	Hospital Mortality no (%)	6 (23)	1 (4)
				PaO$_2$/FiO$_2$	ns	a	c	ICU Stay (days) Mean ± SD	NA	NA
				pH	NA	NA	ns	Hospital Stay (days) Mean ± SD	12.0 ± 8.0	11.0 ± 8.0
				PaCO$_2$	NA	NA	ns			
				Dyspnea	NA	NA	c			

SMT = Standard Medical Treatment, CPAP = Continuous Positive Airway Pressure, RR = Respiratory Rate, HR = Heart Rate, SBP = Systolic Blood Pressure, MBP = Mean Blood Pressure, PaO$_2$/FiO$_2$ = ratio of arterial blood oxygen tension to fractional inspired oxygen concentration, PaO$_2$ = arterial oxygen tension, PaCO$_2$ = arterial carbon dioxide tension, ICU = Intensive Care Unit, SD = Standard Deviation. NA = not available, ns = non significant, a = p ≤ 0.01 within groups, baseline vs. early assessment (10 to 180 minutes), b = p ≤ 0.05 within groups, baseline vs. early assessment (10 to 180 minutes), c = p ≤ 0.01 between CPAP and SMT groups, d = p ≤ 0.05 between CPAP and SMT groups.
See text for further explanation.

TABLE 11-5 Randomized Controlled Trials Comparing CPAP With BiPAP

Source, yr	Sample Size	Intervention CPAP	Intervention BiPAP		Baseline vs. CPAP	Baseline vs. BiPAP	CPAP vs. BiPAP	Clinical Outcomes	CPAP	BiPAP
Metha, 1997 (ref. 195)	n = 13 CPAP n = 14 BiPAP	CPAP 10 cmH$_2$O	IPAP 15 cmH$_2$O EPAP 5 cmH$_2$O	RR	b	b	ns	Hospital Stay (days) Mean ± SD	9 ± 4	10 ± 6
				HR	ns	b	ns	MI no (%)	4 (31)	10 (71)d
				SBP	ns	b	d	Treatment failure no (%)	1 (7)	1 (8)
				pH	ns	b	ns	Hospital Mortality no (%)	1 (7)	2 (15)
				PaCO$_2$	ns	b	ns	Major Complications no (%)	NA	NA
				PaO$_2$	ns	ns	ns			
				Dyspnea	b	b	ns			
Park, 2004 (ref. 727)	n = 27 CPAP n = 29 BiPAP	CPAP 10 cmH$_2$O	IPAP 17 ± 2 cmH$_2$O EPAP 11 ± 2 cmH$_2$O	RR	NA	NA	ns	Hospital Stay (days) Mean ± SD	11 ± 8	10 ± 7
				HR	NA	NA	ns	MI no (%)	0 (0)	0 (0)
				SBP	NA	NA	ns	Treatment failure no (%)	2 (7)	2 (7)
				pH	NA	NA	ns	Hospital Mortality no (%)	1 (4)	2 (7)
				PaCO$_2$	NA	NA	ns	Major Complications no (%)	4 (15)	5 (19)
				PaO$_2$/FiO$_2$	NA	NA	ns			
				Dyspnea	NA	NA	ns			
Crane, 2004 (ref. 726)	n = 20 CPAP n = 20 BiPAP	CPAP 10 cmH$_2$O	IPAP 15 cmH$_2$O EPAP 5 cmH$_2$O	RR	b	a	ns	Hospital Stay (days) Mean ± SD	NA	NA
				HR	ns	ns	ns	MI no (%)	3 (15)	9 (45)
				SBP	ns	ns	ns	Treatment failure no (%)	4 (20)	1 (5)
				pH	ns	ns	ns	Hospital Mortality no (%)	0 (0)	5 (25)d
				PaCO$_2$	ns	ns	ns	Major Complications no (%)	NA	NA
				PaO$_2$	ns	ns	ns			
				Dyspnea	ns	ns	ns			
Bellone, 2004 (ref. 725)	n = 22 CPAP n = 24 BiPAP	CPAP 10 cmH$_2$O	IPAP 20 cmH$_2$O EPAP 5 cmH$_2$O	RR	a	a	ns	Hospital Stay (days) Mean ± SD	NA	NA
				HR	a	a	ns	MI no (%)	3 (14)	2 (8)
				SBP	a	a	ns	Treatment failure no (%)	1 (4)	2 (8)
				pH	a	a	ns	Hospital Mortality no (%)	2 (9)	0 (0)
				PaCO$_2$	a	a	ns	Major Complications no (%)	NA	NA
				PaO$_2$/FiO$_2$	ns	b	ns			
				Dyspnea	NA	NA	NA			

CPAP = Continuous Positive Airway Pressure, IPAP = Inspiratory Positive Airway Pressure, EPAP = Expiratory Positive Airway Pressure, RR = Respiratory Rate, HR = Heart Rate, SBP = Systolic Blood Pressure, MI = Myocardial Infarction, PaO$_2$ = arterial oxygen tension, PaO$_2$/FiO$_2$ = ratio of arterial oxygen tension to fractional inspired oxygen concentration, PaCO$_2$ = arterial carbon dioxide tension, ICU = Intensive Care Unit, SD = Standard Deviation.
NA = not available, ns = non significant, a = p ≤ 0.01 within groups, baseline vs. early assessment (10 to 180 minutes), b = p ≤ 0.05 within groups, baseline vs. early assessment (10 to 180 minutes), d = p ≤ 0.05 between CPAP and BiPAP groups.
See text for further explanation.

be considered first-line ventilator treatment in severe cardiogenic pulmonary edema.

PROPHYLACTIC PEEP

The term *prophylactic PEEP* was used in early studies of PEEP in high-risk patients aimed at reducing the incidence of ARDS.[662,728–733] Both experimental[433,445,734–736] and clinical studies[728–730,737] suggest that PEEP might influence the course of lung injury favorably in patients at risk for ARDS. The hypothesis, however, was refuted by Pepe et al,[662] who randomized 92 ventilated patients at risk for ARDS to receive no PEEP or PEEP of 8 cmH$_2$O. Early use of PEEP improved oxygenation but did not avert the development of ARDS[662] (Table 11-6). Of note, the V$_T$ in the study of Pepe et al[662] was high (12 ml/kg). Such a high V$_T$ might have recruited[240,242] and overdistended the lung, masking any

benefit of prophylactic PEEP. This concern is supported by a barotrauma rate of around 50% in that study.[662]

Use of CPAP in the very early stage of ALI/ARDS was evaluated in spontaneously breathing patients and during fiberoptic bronchoscopy. The investigators tested whether CPAP prevents the severe hypoxemia and respiratory failure requiring intubation.[192,738] CPAP by face mask improved oxygenation but did not improve the need for endotracheal intubation, length of hospital stay, or mortality[192] (see Table 11-6). Early use of noninvasive CPAP, with or without pressure support, may benefit specific high-risk patients, such as immunocompromised patients.[250,254,739,740] In obese patients undergoing gastroplasty, Joris et al[741] found that prophylactic nasal CPAP with pressure support immediately after surgery reduced pulmonary dysfunction and accelerated recovery compared with O$_2$ alone. CPAP is also useful during fiberoptic bronchoscopy,[738] a procedure that can worsen oxygenation and respiratory mechanics.[742–744]

TABLE 11-6 Randomized Controlled Trials Evaluating the Efficacy of Prophylactic PEEP

Reference	Population	Arm	No. of Patients	Associated Settings	PEEP Setting	Mean PEEP (cmH$_2$O)	Outcomes
Pepe 1984 (662)	Medical-Surgical At risk for ARDS	Intervention	44	V$_T$ = 12 ml/kg	Pre-determined	8	Incidence of ARDS: 25% Mortality: 30% Barotrauma: 43%
		Control	48	V$_T$ = 12 ml/kg	—	0	Incidence of ARDS: 27% Mortality: 38% Barotrauma: 50%
Delclaux 2000 (192)	Medical ALI	Intervention	40*	O$_2$ with CPAP for SaO$_2$ > 90%	Clinical response Tolerance	5–10	Endotracheal intubation: 38% ICU length of stay (days): 9 ICU mortality: 23% Hospital mortality: 30%
		Control	41*	O$_2$ alone for SaO$_2$ > 90%	—	0	Endotracheal intubation: 44% ICU length of stay (days): 9 ICU mortality: 22% Hospital mortality: 27%
Maitre 2000 (738)	Medical ALI Undergoing FOB	Intervention	15	O$_2$ with CPAP for SaO$_2$ > 90%	Pre-determined	7.5	Oxygenation: unchanged Ventilatory assistance after FOB: 0%
		Control	15	O$_2$ alone for SaO$_2$ > 90%	—	0	Oxygenation: ↓ Ventilatory assistance after FOB: 33%

ABBREVIATIONS. ALI: acute lung injury, ARDS: acute respiratory distress syndrome, FOB: fiberoptic bronchoscopy, VT: tidal volume, O$_2$: oxygen, CPAP: continuous positive airway pressure, SaO$_2$: arterial oxygen saturation, ICU: intensive care unit.
* subgroup of patients with early ALI.

TABLE 11-7 Complications of PEEP

Pulmonary overdistension
  Barotrauma
  VILI
  Increased dead space
  Impaired CO_2 elimination
Reduced diaphragmatic force-generation capacity
Reduced cardiac output and oxygen delivery
Impaired renal function
Reduced splanchnic blood flow
Hepatic congestion
Decreased lymph drainage

In a double-blind trial, Maitre et al[738] compared mask CPAP with O_2 therapy alone during bronchoscopy in severely hypoxemic spontaneously breathing patients (see Table 11-6). During and immediately after the procedure, oxygenation was well preserved in the CPAP group, whereas it fell in the O_2 group. CPAP prevented subsequent respiratory failure necessitating ventilator support.[738]

PEEP of 5 cmH2O or less is sometimes used in intubated patients to counteract the fall in lung volume secondary to intubation, supine positioning, and/or muscle paralysis. The physiologic foundation is not clear.

PEEP may prevent VILI[745] (see above). Despite robust physiologic rationale, no clinical evidence shows that PEEP protects against VILI. In a retrospective cohort study, Gajic et al[746] reported that approximately 25% of patients ventilated for more than 48 hours developed ALI. V_T size was the only ventilator setting that independently identified risk for ALI.[746] No relationship was found between PEEP and risk for ALI; possibly, scatter was insufficient.[746]

Complications and Contraindications

Table 11-7 summarizes the complications and side effects of PEEP. Complications are directly related to level of PEEP. Table 11-8 lists contraindications to the use of PEEP. In our opinion, there are only two absolute contraindications: severe hypovolemic shock and undrained high-pressure pneumothorax. For all other conditions, there is little risk in using a low level of PEEP (up to 5 cmH2O), but the benefits and drawbacks of higher levels of PEEP need to be weighed carefully in each patient.

TABLE 11-8 Contraindications to PEEP

Absolute contraindications
  Hypovolemic shock
  Undrained high-pressure pneumothorax
Relative contraindications
  Unresolved bronchopleural fistula
  Intracranial hypertension and low cerebral compliance
  Chronic chest-wall restrictive disorders
  Dynamic hyperinflation without expiratory flow limitation

Conclusion

PEEP is used widely in clinical practice.[29] It is an essential component of ventilator management of patients with both hypoxemic ARF, resulting from lung edema caused by increased microvascular permeabilty or hydrostatic pressure, and hypercapnic ARF, secondary to respiratory muscle failure, in obstructive lung diseases.

Seventy years after the pioneering work of Poulton and Oxon[11] and Barach et al,[15] a large body of physiologic data has produced a general consensus on the usefulness of PEEP in the treatment of patients with acute respiratory failure. Doubts remain about the optimal level of PEEP in different clinical situations and the best manner to determine it. In recent years, there has been a growing interest in assessing the effect of varied levels of PEEP on clinical outcome variables, such as survival, complications, length of ICU stay, and costs. Knowledge of pathophysiologic mechanisms and physiologic consequences of PEEP, however, remains an indispensable prerequisite for any decisions made at the bedside. Physiologic principles must serve as the foundation for designing meaningfull randomized, controlled trials.

It is fitting to close with the words of philosopher Charles Pierce (1878)[747]: "It is certainly important how to make our ideas clear, but they may be ever so clear without being true. How to make them so, we have next to study."

Aknowledgments

We are grateful to Pamela Frigerio and Ritana Leo for continuous assistance and help with inserting references and preparing figures and tables. We are also indebted to Massimo Antonelli for invaluable support and to Jennifer Beck for improving the clarity of the manuscript. We thank Mrs. Chiara Vercesi and Mrs. Luciana Capella, from the Scientific Library of Fondazione Salvatore Maugeri-IRCCS (Pavia), who provided hundreds of articles.

References

1. Rossi A, Ranieri MV. Positive end-expiratory pressure. In: Tobin MJ, editor. Principles and practice of mechanical ventilation. New York: McGraw Hill, 1994.
2. Petty TL. The use, abuse, and mystique of positive end-expiratory pressure. Am Rev Respir Dis 1988; 138:475–8.
3. On-Line Medical Dictionary, Dept. of Medical Oncology, University of Newcastle upon Tyne, 1997–2003 (accessed at *www.cancerweb.ncl.ac.uk/omd/index.html*).
4. Ashbaugh DG, Bigelow DB, Petty TL, Levine BE. Acute respiratory distress in adults. Lancet 1967; 2:319–23.
5. Appendini L, Patessio A, Zanaboni S, et al. Physiologic effects of positive end-expiratory pressure and mask pressure support during exacerbations of chronic obstructive pulmonary disease. Am J Respir Crit Care Med 1994; 149:1069–76.
6. Burchardi H. New strategies in mechanical ventilation for acute lung injury. Eur Respir J 1996; 9:1063–72.
7. Navalesi P, Hernandez P, Wongsa A, et al. Proportional assist ventilation in acute respiratory failure: Effects on breathing pattern and inspiratory effort. Am J Respir Crit Care Med 1996; 154:1330–8.

8. Cereda M, Foti G, Musch G, et al. Positive end-expiratory pressure prevents the loss of respiratory compliance during low tidal volume ventilation in acute lung injury patients. Chest 1996; 109:480–5.

9. Amato MB, Barbas CS, Medeiros DM, et al. Effect of a protective-ventilation strategy on mortality in the acute respiratory distress syndrome. New Engl J Med 1998; 338:347–54.

10. Antonelli M, Conti G, Rocco M, et al. A comparison of noninvasive positive-pressure ventilation and conventional mechanical ventilation in patients with acute respiratory failure. New Engl J Med 1998; 339:429–35.

11. Poulton EP, Oxon DM. Left-sided heart failure with pulmonary edema: Its treatment with the "pulmonary plus pressure machine." Lancet 1936; 2:981–3.

12. Gregory GA, Kitterman JA, Phibbs RH, et al. Treatment of the idiopathic respiratory-distress syndrome with continuous positive airway pressure. New Engl J Med 1971; 284:1333–40.

13. Petrof BJ, Legare M, Goldberg P, et al. Continuous positive airway pressure reduces work of breathing and dyspnea during weaning from mechanical ventilation in severe chronic obstructive pulmonary disease. Am Rev Respir Dis 1990; 141:281–9.

14. Bersten AD, Holt AW, Vedig AE, et al. Treatment of severe cardiogenic pulmonary edema with continuous positive airway pressure delivered by face mask. New Engl J Med 1991; 325:1825–30.

15. Barach AL, Martin J, Eckman M. Positive pressure respiration and its application to the treatment of acute pulmonary edema. Ann Intern Med 1938; 12:754–95.

16. Kirby RR, Downs JB, Civetta JM, et al. High level positive end expiratory pressure (PEEP) in acute respiratory insufficiency. Chest 1975; 67:156–63.

17. Qvist J, Pontoppidan H, Wilson RS, et al. Hemodynamic responses to mechanical ventilation with PEEP: The effect of hypervolemia. Anesthesiology 1975; 42:45–55.

18. Suter PM, Fairley B, Isenberg MD. Optimum end-expiratory airway pressure in patients with acute pulmonary failure. New Engl J Med 1975; 292:284–9.

19. Apuzzo JL, Wiess MH, Petersons V, et al. Effect of positive end expiratory pressure ventilation on intracranial pressure in man. J Neurosurg 1977; 46:227–32.

20. Priebe HJ, Heimann JC, Hedley-Whyte J. Mechanisms of renal dysfunction during positive end-expiratory pressure ventilation. J Appl Physiol 1981; 50:643–9.

21. Petersen GW, Baier H. Incidence of pulmonary barotrauma in a medical ICU. Crit Care Med 1983; 11:67–9.

22. Dorinsky PM, Hamlin RL, Gadek JE. Alterations in regional blood flow during positive end-expiratory pressure ventilation. Crit Care Med 1987; 15:106–13.

23. Haider M, Schad H, Mendler N. Thoracic duct lymph and PEEP studies in anaesthetized dogs: I. Lymph formation and the effect of a thoracic duct fistula on lymph flow. Intensive Care Med 1987; 13:183–91.

24. Pingleton SK. Complications of acute respiratory failure. Am Rev Respir Dis 1988; 137:1463–93.

25. Arvidsson D, Almquist P, Haglund U. Effects of positive end-expiratory pressure on splanchnic circulation and function in experimental peritonitis. Arch Surg 1991; 126:631–6.

26. Eisner MD, Thompson BT, Schoenfeld D, et al. Airway pressures and early barotrauma in patients with acute lung injury and acute respiratory distress syndrome. Am J Respir Crit Care Med 2002; 165:978–82.

27. Jardin F, Farcot JC, Boisante L, et al. Influence of positive end-expiratory pressure on left ventricular performance. New Engl J Med 1981; 304:387–92.

28. Macklem PT. Hyperinflation. Am Rev Respir Dis 1984; 129:1–2.

29. Esteban A, Anzueto A, Frutos F, et al. Characteristics and outcomes in adult patients receiving mechanical ventilation: A 28-day international study. JAMA 2002; 287:345–55.

30. Katz JA, Ozanne GM, Zinn SE, Fairley HB. Time course and mechanisms of lung-volume increase with PEEP in acute pulmonary failure. Anesthesiology 1981; 54:9–16.

31. Rose DM, Downs JB, Heenan TJ. Temporal responses of functional residual capacity and oxygen tension to changes in positive end-expiratory pressure. Crit Care Med 1981; 9:79–82.

32. Gattinoni L, Mascheroni D, Torresin A, et al. Morphological response to positive end expiratory pressure in acute respiratory failure: Computerized tomography study. Intensive Care Med 1986; 12:137–42.

33. East TD, in't Veen JC, Pace NL, McJames S. Functional residual capacity as a noninvasive indicator of optimal positive end-expiratory pressure. J Clin Monit 1988; 4:91–8.

34. Malbouisson LM, Muller JC, Constantin JM, et al. Computed tomography assessment of positive end-expiratory pressure-induced alveolar recruitment in patients with acute respiratory distress syndrome. Am J Respir Crit Care Med 2001; 163:1444–50.

35. Dellaca RL, Aliverti A, Pelosi P, et al. Estimation of end-expiratory lung volume variations by optoelectronic plethysmography. Crit Care Med 2001; 29:1807–11.

36. Gilston A. The effects of PEEP on arterial oxygenation: An examination of some possible mechanisms. Intensive Care Med 1977; 3:267–71.

37. McMahon SM, Halprin GM. Modification of intrapulmonary blood shunt by end-expiratory pressure application in patients with acute respiratory failure. Chest 1971; 59:27S +.

38. Pesenti A, Riboni A, Marcolin R, Gattinoni L. Venous admixture (Q̇va/Q̇) and true shunt (Q̇s/Q̇t) in ARF patients: Effects of PEEP at constant FIO2. Intensive Care Med 1983; 9:307–11.

39. Matamis D, Lemaire F, Harf A, et al. Redistribution of pulmonary blood flow induced by positive end-expiratory pressure and dopamine infusion in acute respiratory failure. Am Rev Respir Dis 1984; 129:39–44.

40. Jonson B, Richard JC, Straus C, et al. Pressure-volume curves and compliance in acute lung injury: Evidence of recruitment above the lower inflection point. Am J Respir Crit Care Med 1999; 159:1172–8.

41. Suter PM, Fairley HB, Isenberg MD. Effect of tidal volume and positive end-expiratory pressure on compliance during mechanical ventilation. Chest 1978; 73:158–62.

42. Katz JA, Marks JD. Inspiratory work with and without continuous positive airway pressure in patients with acute respiratory failure. Anesthesiology 1985; 63:598–607.

43. Powers SR Jr, Mannal R, Neclerio M, et al. Physiologic consequences of positive end-expiratory pressure (PEEP) ventilation. Ann Surg 1973; 178:265–72.

44. Horton WG, Cheney FW. Variability of effect of positive end expiratory pressure. Arch Surg 1975; 110:395–8.

45. Wayne KS. Positive end-expiratory pressure (PEEP) ventilation: A review of mechanisms and actions. JAMA 1976; 236:1394–6.

46. Perel A, Olschvang D, Eimerl D, et al. The variable effect of PEEP in acute respiratory failure associated with multiple trauma. J Trauma 1978; 18:218–20.

47. Kuckelt W, Scharfenberg J, Mrochen H, et al. Effect of PEEP on gas exchange, pulmonary mechanics, and hemodynamics in adult respiratory distress syndrome (ARDS). Intensive Care Med 1981; 7:177–85.

48. Lamy M, Fallat RJ, Koeniger E, et al. Pathologic features and mechanisms of hypoxemia in adult respiratory distress syndrome. Am Rev Respir Dis 1976; 114:267–84.

49. Matthay MA. Function of the alveolar epithelial barrier under pathologic conditions. Chest 1994; 105:67–74S.

50. Gattinoni L, Pelosi P, Suter PM, et al. Acute respiratory distress syndrome caused by pulmonary and extrapulmonary disease: Different syndromes? Am J Respir Crit Care Med 1998; 158:3–11.

51. Hasan FM, Beller TA, Sobonya RE, et al. Effect of positive end-expiratory pressure and body position in unilateral lung injury. J Appl Physiol 1982; 52:147–54.

52. Vieira SR, Puybasset L, Richecoeur J, et al. A lung computed tomographic assessment of positive end-expiratory pressure-induced lung overdistension. Am J Respir Crit Care Med 1998; 158:1571–7.

53. Schnapp LM, Chin DP, Szaflarski N, Matthay MA. Frequency and importance of barotrauma in 100 patients with acute lung injury. Crit Care Med 1995; 23:272–8.

54. DiRusso SM, Nelson LD, Safcsak K, Miller RS. Survival in patients with severe adult respiratory distress syndrome treated with high-level positive end-expiratory pressure. Crit Care Med 1995; 23:1485–96.

55. Coffey RL, Albert RK, Robertson HT. Mechanisms of physiological dead space response to PEEP after acute oleic acid lung injury. J Appl Physiol 1983; 55:1550–7.

56. Berendes E, Lippert G, Loick HM, Brussel T. Effects of positive end-expiratory pressure ventilation on splanchnic oxygenation in humans. J Cardiothorac Vasc Anesth 1996; 10:598–602.

57. Lehtipalo S, Biber B, Frojse R, et al. Effects of dopexamine and positive end-expiratory pressure on intestinal blood flow and oxygenation: the perfusion pressure perspective. Chest 2003; 124:688–98.

58. Jedlinska B, Mellstrom A, Jonsson K, Hartmann M. Influence of positive end-expiratory pressure ventilation on peripheral tissue perfusion evaluated by measurements of tissue gases and pH: An experimental study in pigs with oleic acid lung injury. Eur Surg Res 2000; 32:228–35.

59. Lutch JS, Murray JF. Continuous positive-pressure ventilation: Effects on systemic oxygen transport and tissue oxygenation. Ann Intern Med 1972; 76:193–202.

60. Dantzker DR, Lynch JP, Weg JG. Depression of cardiac output is a mechanism of shunt reduction in the therapy of acute respiratory failure. Chest 1980; 77:636–42.

61. Marini JJ, Culver BH, Butler J. Mechanical effect of lung distention with positive pressure on cardiac function. Am Rev Respir Dis 1981; 124:382–6.

62. Dorinsky PM, Whitcomb ME. The effect of PEEP on cardiac output. Chest 1983; 84:210–6.

63. Huseby JS, Pavlin EG, Butler J. Effect of positive end-expiratory pressure on intracranial pressure in dogs. J Appl Physiol 1978; 44:25–7.

64. Berry AJ, Geer RT, Marshall C, et al. The effect of long-term controlled mechanical ventilation with positive end-expiratory pressure on renal function in dogs. Anesthesiology 1984; 61:406–15.

65. Fujita Y. Effects of PEEP on splanchnic hemodynamics and blood volume. Acta Anaesthesiol Scand 1993; 37:427–31.

66. Aneman A, Ponten J, Fandriks L, et al. Hemodynamic, sympathetic and angiotensin II responses to PEEP ventilation before and during administration of isoflurane. Acta Anaesthesiol Scand 1997; 41:41–8.

67. Bredenberg CE, Paskanik AM. Relation of portal hemodynamics to cardiac output during mechanical ventilation with PEEP. Ann Surg 1983; 198:218–22.

68. Matuschak GM, Pinsky MR, Rogers RM. Effects of positive end-expiratory pressure on hepatic blood flow and performance. J Appl Physiol 1987; 62:1377–83.

69. Albert RK. Least PEEP: Primum non nocere. Chest 1985; 87:2–4.

70. Carroll GC, Tuman KJ, Braverman B, et al. Minimal positive end-expiratory pressure (PEEP) may be "best PEEP." Chest 1988; 93:1020–5.

71. Ranieri VM, Eissa NT, Corbeil C, et al. Effects of positive end-expiratory pressure on alveolar recruitment and gas exchange in patients with the adult respiratory distress syndrome. Am Rev Respir Dis 1991; 144:544–51.

72. Amato MB, Barbas CS, Medeiros DM, et al. Beneficial effects of the "open lung approach" with low distending pressures in acute respiratory distress syndrome: A prospective, randomized study on mechanical ventilation. Am J Respir Crit Care Med 1995; 152:1835–46.

73. Muscedere JG, Mullen JB, Gan K, Slutsky AS. Tidal ventilation at low airway pressures can augment lung injury. Am J Respir Crit Care Med 1994; 149:1327–34.

74. Campbell EJ. Respiratory failure: The relation between oxygen concentrations of inspired air and arterial blood. Lancet 1960; 2:10–1.

75. Campbell EJ. The J. Burns Amberson Lecture: The management of acute respiratory failure in chronic bronchitis and emphysema. Am Rev Respir Dis 1967; 96:626–39.

76. Smith JP, Stone RW, Muschenheim C. Acute respiratory failure in chronic lung disease: Observations on controlled oxygen therapy. Am Rev Respir Dis 1968; 97:791–803.

77. Bradley RD, Spencer GT, Semple SJ. Tracheostomy and artificial ventilation in the treatment of acute exacerbations of chronic lung disease: A study in twenty-nine patients. Lancet 1964; 42:854–9.

78. Bone RC, Pierce AK, Johnson RL Jr. Controlled oxygen administration in acute respiratory failure in chronic obstructive pulmonary disease: A reappraisal. Am J Med 1978; 65:896–902.

79. Barat G, Asuero MS. Positive end-expiratory pressure: Effect on arterial oxygenation during respiratory failure in chronic obstructive airway disease. Anaesthesia 1975; 30:183–9.

80. Pepe PE, Marini JJ. Occult positive end-expiratory pressure in mechanically ventilated patients with airflow obstruction: the auto-PEEP effect. Am Rev Respir Dis 1982; 126: 166–70.

81. Goldberg P, Reissmann H, Maltais F, et al. Efficacy of noninvasive CPAP in COPD with acute respiratory failure. Eur Respir J 1995; 8:1894–900.

82. van den Berg B, Aerts JG, Bogaard JM. Effect of continuous positive airway pressure (CPAP) in patients with chronic obstructive pulmonary disease (COPD) depending on intrinsic PEEP levels. Acta Anaesthesiol Scand 1995; 39: 1097–102.

83. Smith TC, Marini JJ. Impact of PEEP on lung mechanics and work of breathing in severe airflow obstruction. J Appl Physiol 1988; 65:1488–99.

84. Appendini L, Purro A, Gudjonsdottir M, et al. Physiologic response of ventilator-dependent patients with chronic obstructive pulmonary disease to proportional assist ventilation and continuous positive airway pressure. Am J Respir Crit Care Med 1999; 159:1510–7.

85. Nava S, Bruschi C, Rubini F, et al. Respiratory response and inspiratory effort during pressure support ventilation in COPD patients. Intensive Care Med 1995; 21:871–9.

86. Appendini L, Purro A, Patessio A, et al. Partitioning of inspiratory muscle workload and pressure assistance in ventilator-dependent COPD patients. Am J Respir Crit Care Med 1996; 154:1301–9.

87. Ranieri VM, Giuliani R, Cinnella G, et al. Physiologic effects of positive end-expiratory pressure in patients with chronic obstructive pulmonary disease during acute ventilatory failure and controlled mechanical ventilation. Am Rev Respir Dis 1993; 147:5–13.

88. Williams TJ, Tuxen DV, Scheinkestel CD, et al. Risk factors for morbidity in mechanically ventilated patients with acute severe asthma. Am Rev Respir Dis 1992; 146:607–15.

89. Similowski T, Yan S, Gauthier AP, et al. Contractile properties of the human diaphragm during chronic hyperinflation. New Engl J Med 1991; 325:917–23.

90. Marini JJ. Should PEEP be used in airflow obstruction? Am Rev Respir Dis 1988; 140:1–3.

91. Rossi A, Gottfried SB, Zocchi L, et al. Measurement of static compliance of the total respiratory system in patients with acute respiratory failure during mechanical ventilation: The effect of intrinsic positive end-expiratory pressure. Am Rev Respir Dis 1985; 131:672–7.

92. Lessard MR, Lofaso F, Brochard L. Expiratory muscle activity increases intrinsic positive end-expiratory pressure independently of dynamic hyperinflation in mechanically ventilated patients. Am J Respir Crit Care Med 1995; 151:562–9.

93. Parthasarathy S, Jubran A, Tobin MJ. Cycling of inspiratory and expiratory muscle groups with the ventilator in airflow limitation. Am J Respir Crit Care Med 1998; 158:1471–8.

94. Cournand A, Motley H, Werko L, Richards D. Physiologic studies of the effects of intermittent positive pressure breathing on cardiac output in man. Am J Physiol 1948; 125:261–73.

95. Braunwald E, Binion JT, Morgan WL Jr, Sarnoff SJ. Alterations in central blood volume and cardiac output induced by positive pressure breathing and counteracted by metaraminol (aramine). Circ Res 1957; 5:670–5.

96. Fessler HE, Brower RG, Wise RA, Permutt S. Effects of systolic and diastolic positive pleural pressure pulses with altered cardiac contractility. J Appl Physiol 1992; 73:498–505.

97. Buda AJ, Pinsky MR, Ingels NB Jr, et al. Effect of intrathoracic pressure on left ventricular performance. New Engl J Med 1979; 301:453–9.

98. Wise RA, Robotham JL, Bromberger-Barnea B, Permutt S. Effect of PEEP on left ventricular function in right-heart-bypassed dogs. J Appl Physiol 1981; 51:541–6.

99. Pinsky MR, Summer WR, Wise RA, et al. Augmentation of cardiac function by elevation of intrathoracic pressure. J Appl Physiol 1983; 54:950–5.

100. Pinsky MR, Matuschak GM, Klain M. Determinants of cardiac augmentation by elevations in intrathoracic pressure. J Appl Physiol 1985; 58:1189–98.

101. Lenique F, Habis M, Lofaso F, et al. Ventilatory and hemodynamic effects of continuous positive airway pressure in left heart failure. Am J Respir Crit Care Med 1997; 155:500–5.

102. Rasanen J, Heikkila J, Downs J, et al. Continuous positive airway pressure by face mask in acute cardiogenic pulmonary edema. Am J Cardiol 1985; 55:296–300.

103. Lin M, Yang YF, Chiang HT, et al. Reappraisal of continuous positive airway pressure therapy in acute cardiogenic pulmonary edema: Short-term results and long-term follow-up. Chest 1995; 107:1379–86.

104. Pang D, Keenan SP, Cook DJ, Sibbald WJ. The effect of positive pressure airway support on mortality and the need for intubation in cardiogenic pulmonary edema: A systematic review. Chest 1998; 114:1185–92.

105. Sullivan CE, Issa FG, Berthon-Jones M, Eves L. Reversal of obstructive sleep apnoea by continuous positive airway pressure applied through the nares. Lancet 1981; 1:862–5.

106. Pepperell JC, Ramdassingh-Dow S, Crosthwaite N, et al. Ambulatory blood pressure after therapeutic and subtherapeutic nasal continuous positive airway pressure for obstructive sleep apnoea: A randomised, parallel trial. Lancet 2002; 359: 204–10.

107. Engleman HM, Martin SE, Deary IJ, Douglas NJ. Effect of continuous positive airway pressure treatment on daytime function in sleep apnoea/hypopnoea syndrome. Lancet 1994; 343:572–5.

108. Tkacova R, Rankin F, Fitzgerald FS, et al. Effects of continuous positive airway pressure on obstructive sleep apnea and left ventricular afterload in patients with heart failure. Circulation 1998; 98:2269–75.

109. Lattimore JD, Celermajer DS, Wilcox I. Obstructive sleep apnea and cardiovascular disease. J Am Coll Cardiol 2003; 41: 1429–37.

110. Mansfield DR, Gollogly NC, Kaye DM, et al. Controlled trial of continuous positive airway pressure in obstructive sleep apnea and heart failure. Am J Respir Crit Care Med 2004; 169:361–6.

111. Morrell NW, Roberts CM, Biggs T, Seed WA. Collateral ventilation and gas exchange during airway occlusion in the normal human lung. Am Rev Respir Dis 1993; 147:535–9.

112. Groth S, Stafanger G, Dirksen H, et al. Positive expiratory pressure (PEP-mask) physiotherapy improves ventilation and reduces volume of trapped gas in cystic fibrosis. Bull Eur Physiopathol Respir 1985; 21:339–43.

113. Fink JB. Positioning versus postural drainage. Respir Care 2002; 47:769–77.

114. McIlwaine PM, Wong LT, Peacock D, Davidson AG. Long-term comparative trial of conventional postural drainage and percussion versus positive expiratory pressure physiotherapy in the treatment of cystic fibrosis. J Pediatr 1997; 131:570–4.

115. van Winden CM, Visser A, Hop W, et al. Effects of flutter and PEP mask physiotherapy on symptoms and lung function in children with cystic fibrosis. Eur Respir J 1998; 12:143–7.

116. Elkins M, Jones A, van der Schans C. Positive expiratory pressure physiotherapy for airway clearance in people with cystic fibrosis. Cochrane Review 2005.

117. Barach AL, Martin J, Eckman M. Positive pressure respiration and its application to the treatment of acute pulmonary edema. Ann Intern Med 1938; 12:754–95.

118. Poulton EP, Oxon DM. Left-sided heart failure with pulmonary edema: Its treatment with the "pulmonary plus pressure machine." Lancet 1936; 2:981–3.

119. Falke KJ, Pontoppidan H, Kumar A, et al. Ventilation with end-expiratory pressure in acute lung disease. J Clin Invest 1972; 51:2315–23.

120. Pontoppidan H. Mechanical aids to lung expansion in non-intubated surgical patients. Am Rev Respir Dis 1980; 122:109–19.

121. Gattinoni L, Pesenti A, Bombino M, et al. Relationships between lung computed tomographic density, gas exchange, and PEEP in acute respiratory failure. Anesthesiology 1988; 69:824–32.

122. Kumar A, Falke KJ, Geffin B, et al. Continuous positive-pressure ventilation in acute respiratory failure. New Engl J Med 1970; 283:1430–6.

123. Cain SM. Gas exchange in hypoxia, apnea and hyperoxia. In: Fishman A, editor. Handbook of physiology, vol 4. Bethesda, MD: American Physiological Society; 1986: 403–20.

124. West JB. Effect of slope and shape of dissociation curve on pulmonary gas exchange. Respir Physiol 1969; 8:66–85.

125. West JB. State of the art: Ventilation-perfusion relationships. Am Rev Respir Dis 1977; 116:919–43.

126. West JB, Wagner PD. Pulmonary gas exchange. In: West JB, editor. Bioengineering aspects of the lung. New York: Marcel Dekker, 1977: 361–457.

127. West JB. Ventilation-perfusion inequality and overall gas exchange in computer models of the lung. Respir Physiol 1969; 7:88–110.

128. West JB. Causes of carbon dioxide retention in lung disease. New Engl J Med 1971; 284:1232–6.

129. Weinberger SE, Schwartzstein RM, Weiss JW. Hypercapnia. New Engl J Med 1989; 321:1223–31.

130. Dantzker D. The influence of cardiovascular function on gas exchange. Clin Chest Med 1983; 4:149–59.

131. Hansen JE, Clausen JL, Levy SE, et al. Proficiency testing materials for pH and blood gases. The California Thoracic Society experience. Chest 1986; 89:214–7.

132. Moller JT, Johannessen NW, Berg H, et al. Hypoxaemia during anaesthesia: An observer study. Br J Anaesth 1991; 66:437–44.

133. Bendixen HH, Hedley-Whyte J, Laver MB. Impaired oxygenation in surgical patients during general anesthesia with controlled ventilation: A concept of atelectasis. New Engl J Med 1963; 269:991–6.

134. Hedenstierna GSJ. Breathing mechanics, dead space and gas exchange in the extremely obese, breathing spontaneously and during anaesthesia with intermittent positive pressure ventilation. Acta Anaesthesiol Scand 1976; 20:248–54.

135. Rehder K, Knopp TJ, Sessler AD, Didier EP. Ventilation-perfusion relationship in young healthy awake and anesthetized-paralyzed man. J Appl Physiol 1979;47:745–53.

136. Gunnarsson L, Tokics L, Lundquist H, et al. Chronic obstructive pulmonary disease and anaesthesia: Formation of atelectasis and gas exchange impairment. Eur Respir J 1991; 4: 1106–16.

137. Rothen HU, Sporre B, Engberg G, et al. Prevention of atelectasis during general anaesthesia. Lancet 1995; 345:1387–91.

138. Tokics L, Hedenstierna G, Strandberg A, et al. Lung collapse and gas exchange during general anesthesia: Effects of spontaneous breathing, muscle paralysis, and positive end-expiratory pressure. Anesthesiology 1987; 66:157–67.

139. Nunn JF, Bergman NA, Coleman AJ. Factors influencing the arterial oxygen tension during anaesthesia with artificial ventilation. Br J Anaesth 1965; 37:898–914.

140. Norlander O, Herzog P, Norden I, et al. Compliance and airway resistance during anaesthesia with controlled ventilation. Acta Anaesthesiol Scand 1968; 12:135–52.

141. Froese AB, Bryan AC. Effects of anesthesia and paralysis on diaphragmatic mechanics in man. Anesthesiology 1974; 41:242–55.

142. Bergman NA. Reduction in resting end-expiratory position of the respiratory system with induction of anesthesia and neuromuscular paralysis. Anesthesiology 1982; 57:14–7.

143. Brismar B, Hedenstierna G, Lundquist H, et al. Pulmonary densities during anesthesia with muscular relaxation: A proposal of atelectasis. Anesthesiology 1985; 62:422–8.

144. Hedenstierna G, Lundquist H, Lundh B, et al. Pulmonary densities during anaesthesia: An experimental study on lung morphology and gas exchange. Eur Respir J 1989; 2:528–35.

145. Sykes MK, Young WE, Robinson BE. Oxygenation during anaesthesia with controlled ventilation. Br J Anaesth 1965; 37: 314–25.

146. Strandberg A, Tokics L, Brismar B, et al. Atelectasis during anaesthesia and in the postoperative period. Acta Anaesthesiol Scand 1986; 30:154–8.

147. Gunnarsson L, Tokics L, Gustavsson H, Hedenstierna G. Influence of age on atelectasis formation and gas exchange impairment during general anaesthesia. Br J Anaesth 1991; 66:423–32.

148. Hedenstierna G, Rothen HU. Atelectasis formation during anesthesia: Causes and measures to prevent it. J Clin Monit Comput 2000; 16:329–35.

149. Heneghan CP, Bergman NA, Jones JG. Changes in lung volume and ($P_{A_{O_2}}–Pa_{O_2}$) during anaesthesia. Br J Anaesth 1984; 56: 437–45.

150. Milic-Emili J, Henderson JA, Dolovich MB, et al. Regional distribution of inspired gas in the lung. J Appl Physiol 1966; 21:749–59.

151. Don H. The mechanical properties of the respiratory system during anesthesia. Int Anesthesiol Clin 1977; 15:113–36.

152. Don HF, Wahba WM, Craig DB. Airway closure, gas trapping, and the functional residual capacity during anesthesia. Anesthesiology 1972; 36:533–9.

153. Hedenstierna G, McCarthy G, Bergstrom M. Airway closure during mechanical ventilation. Anesthesiology 1976; 44:114–23.

154. Gilmour I, Burnham M, Craig DB. Closing capacity measurement during general anesthesia. Anesthesiology 1976; 45:477–82.

155. Juno J, Marsh HM, Knopp TJ, Rehder K. Closing capacity in awake and anesthetized-paralyzed man. J Appl Physiol 1978; 44:238–44.

156. Bergman NA, Tien YK. Contribution of the closure of pulmonary units to impaired oxygenation during anesthesia. Anesthesiology 1983; 59:395–401.

157. Dueck R, Prutow RJ, Davies NJ, et al. The lung volume at which shunting occurs with inhalation anesthesia. Anesthesiology 1988; 69:854–61.

158. Hirshman CA, Bergman NA. Factors influencing intrapulmonary airway calibre during anaesthesia. Br J Anaesth 1990; 65:30–42.

159. Rothen HU, Sporre B, Engberg G, et al. Airway closure, atelectasis and gas exchange during general anaesthesia. Br J Anaesth 1998; 81:681–6.

160. Milic-Emili J, Robatto FM, Bates JH. Respiratory mechanics in anaesthesia. Br J Anaesth 1990; 65:4–12.

161. von Euler U, Liljestrand G. Observations on the pulmonary arterial blood pressure in cat. Acta Physiol Scand 1946; 12: 310–20.

162. Thilenius OG. Effect of anesthesia on response of pulmonary circulation of dogs to acute hypoxia. J Appl Physiol 1966; 21:901–4.

163. Sykes MK, Loh L, Seed RF, et al. The effect of inhalational anaesthetics on hypoxic pulmonary vasoconstriction and pulmonary vascular resistance in the perfused lungs of the dog and cat. Br J Anaesth 1972; 44:776–88.

164. Bjertnaes LJ. Hypoxia-induced vasoconstriction in isolated perfused lungs exposed to injectable or inhalation anesthetics. Acta Anaesthesiol Scand 1977; 21:133–47.

165. Neumann P, Rothen HU, Berglund JE, et al. Positive end-expiratory pressure prevents atelectasis during general anaesthesia even in the presence of a high inspired oxygen concentration. Acta Anaesthesiol Scand 1999; 43:295–301.

166. Tusman G, Bohm SH, Vazquez de Anda GF, et al. "Alveolar recruitment strategy" improves arterial oxygenation during general anaesthesia. Br J Anaesth 1999; 82:8–13.

167. Rusca M, Proietti S, Schnyder P, et al. Prevention of atelectasis formation during induction of general anesthesia. Anesth Analg 2003; 97:1835–9.

168. Dueck R, Wagner PD, West JB. Effects of positive end-expiratory pressure on gas exchange in dogs with normal and edematous lungs. Anesthesiology 1977; 47:359–66.

169. Pelosi P, Ravagnan I, Giurati G, et al. Positive end-expiratory pressure improves respiratory function in obese but not in normal subjects during anesthesia and paralysis. Anesthesiology 1999; 91:1221–31.

170. Heneghan C, Jones J. Pulmonary gas exchange and diaphragmatic position: Effect of tonic phrenic stimulation compared with that of increased airway pressure. Br J Anaesth 1985; 57:1161–6.

171. Kleinman B, Frey K, VanDrunen M, et al. Motion of the diaphragm in patients with chronic obstructive pulmonary disease while spontaneously breathing versus during positive pressure breathing after anesthesia and neuromuscular blockade. Anesthesiology 2002; 97:298–305.

172. Benhamou D, Bourgain JL, Rouby JJ, Viars P. High-frequency jet ventilation vs continuous positive airway pressure for postoperative respiratory support. Chest 1984; 85:733–8.

173. Michalopoulos A, Anthi A, Rellos K, Geroulanos S. Effects of positive end-expiratory pressure (PEEP) in cardiac surgery patients. Respir Med 1998; 92:858–62.

174. Pennock BE, Kaplan PD, Carlin BW, et al. Pressure support ventilation with a simplified ventilatory support system administered with a nasal mask in patients with respiratory failure. Chest 1991; 100:1371–6.

175. Pennock BE, Crawshaw L, Kaplan PD. Noninvasive nasal mask ventilation for acute respiratory failure: Institution of a new therapeutic technology for routine use. Chest 1994; 105:441–4.

176. Matte P, Jacquet L, Van Dyck M, Goenen M. Effects of conventional physiotherapy, continuous positive airway pressure and non-invasive ventilatory support with bilevel positive airway pressure after coronary artery bypass grafting. Acta Anaesthesiol Scand 2000; 44:75–81.

177. Aguilo R, Togores B, Pons S, et al. Noninvasive ventilatory support after lung resectional surgery. Chest 1997; 112:117–21.

178. Auriant I, Jallot A, Herve P, et al. Noninvasive ventilation reduces mortality in acute respiratory failure following lung resection. Am J Respir Crit Care Med 2001; 164:1231–5.

179. Dantzker DR, Wagner PD, West JB. Instability of lung units with low $\dot{V}_A/\dot{Q}$ ratios during O_2 breathing. J Appl Physiol 1975; 38:886–95.

180. Dantzker DR, Brook CJ, Dehart P, et al. Ventilation-perfusion distributions in the adult respiratory distress syndrome. Am Rev Respir Dis 1979; 120:1039–52.

181. Rodriguez-Roisin R. Ventilation-perfusion relationships. In: Pinsky MR, Dhainaut JF, editors. Pathophysiologic foundations of critical care. Baltimore: Williams & Williams; 1993:389–413.

182. Santos C, Ferrer M, Roca J, et al. Pulmonary gas exchange response to oxygen breathing in acute lung injury. Am J Respir Crit Care Med 2000; 161:26–31.

183. Jones R, Zapol WM, Tomashefski JF, et al. Pulmonary vascular pathology: Human and experimental studies. In: Zapol ZM, Falke KJ, editors. Acute respiratory failure. New York: Marcel Dekker, 1985: 23–160.

184. Rasanen J, Vaisanen IT, Heikkila J, Nikki P. Acute myocardial infarction complicated by left ventricular dysfunction and respiratory failure: The effects of continuous positive airway pressure. Chest 1985; 87:158–62.

185. Vaisanen IT, Rasanen J. Continuous positive airway pressure and supplemental oxygen in the treatment of cardiogenic pulmonary edema. Chest 1987; 92:481–5.

186. Lapinsky SE, Mount DB, Mackey D, Grossman RF. Management of acute respiratory failure due to pulmonary edema with nasal positive pressure support. Chest 1994; 105:229–31.

187. Lin M, Yang YF, Chiang HT, et al. Reappraisal of continuous positive airway pressure therapy in acute cardiogenic pulmonary edema: Short-term results and long-term follow-up. Chest 1995; 107:1379–86.

188. Meduri GU, Turner RE, Abou-Shala N, et al. Noninvasive positive pressure ventilation via face mask: First-line intervention in patients with acute hypercapnic and hypoxemic respiratory failure. Chest 1996; 109:179–93.

189. Takeda S, Takano T, Ogawa R. The effect of nasal continuous positive airway pressure on plasma endothelin-1 concentrations in patients with severe cardiogenic pulmonary edema. Anesth Analg 1997; 84:1091–6.

190. Hoffmann B, Welte T. The use of noninvasive pressure support ventilation for severe respiratory insufficiency due to pulmonary oedema. Intensive Care Med 1999; 25:15–20.

191. Rusterholtz T, Kempf J, Berton C, et al. Noninvasive pressure support ventilation (NIPSV) with face mask in patients with acute cardiogenic pulmonary edema (ACPE). Intensive Care Med 1999; 25:21–8.

192. Delclaux C, L'Her E, Alberti C, et al. Treatment of acute hypoxemic nonhypercapnic respiratory insufficiency with continuous positive airway pressure delivered by a face mask: A randomized, controlled trial. JAMA 2000; 284:2352–60.

193. Guntupalli KK. Acute pulmonary edema. Cardiol Clin 1984; 2:183–200.

194. L'Her E, Duquesne F, Girou E, et al. Noninvasive continuous positive airway pressure in elderly cardiogenic pulmonary edema patients. Intensive Care Med 2004; 30:882–8.

195. Mehta S, Jay GD, Woolard RH, et al. Randomized, prospective trial of bilevel versus continuous positive airway pressure in acute pulmonary edema. Crit Care Med 1997; 25:620–8.

196. Bredenberg CE, Kazui T, Webb WR. Experimental pulmonary edema: The effect of positive end-expiratory pressure on lung water. Ann Thorac Surg 1978; 26:62–7.

197. Malo J, Ali J, Wood LD. How does positive end-expiratory pressure reduce intrapulmonary shunt in canine pulmonary edema? J Appl Physiol 1984; 57:1002–10.

198. Rizk NW, Murray JF. PEEP and pulmonary edema. Am J Med 1982; 72:381–3.

199. Demling RH, Staub NC, Edmunds LH Jr. Effect of end-expiratory airway pressure on accumulation of extravascular lung water. J Appl Physiol 1975; 38:907–12.

200. Pare PD, Warriner B, Baile EM, Hogg JC. Redistribution of pulmonary extravascular water with positive end-expiratory pressure in canine pulmonary edema. Am Rev Respir Dis 1983; 127:590–3.

201. Ware LB, Matthay MA. The acute respiratory distress syndrome. New Engl J Med 2000; 342:1334–49.

202. Lewis JF, Jobe AH. Surfactant and the adult respiratory distress syndrome. Am Rev Respir Dis 1993; 147:218–33.

203. Hubmayr RD. Perspective on lung injury and recruitment: A skeptical look at the opening and collapse story. Am J Respir Crit Care Med 2002; 165:1647–53.

204. Wilson TA, Anafi RC, Hubmayr RD. Mechanics of edematous lungs. J Appl Physiol 2001; 90:2088–93.

205. Gattinoni L, D'Andrea L, Pelosi P, et al. Regional effects and mechanism of positive end-expiratory pressure in early adult respiratory distress syndrome. JAMA 1993; 269:2122–7.

206. Gattinoni L, Pesenti A, Avalli L, et al. Pressure-volume curve of total respiratory system in acute respiratory failure: Computed tomographic scan study. Am Rev Respir Dis 1987; 136:730–6.

207. Pelosi P, D'Andrea L, Vitale G, et al. Vertical gradient of regional lung inflation in adult respiratory distress syndrome. Am J Respir Crit Care Med 1994; 149:8–13.

208. Albert RK, Hubmayr RD. The prone position eliminates compression of the lungs by the heart. Am J Respir Crit Care Med 2000; 161:1660–5.

209. Malbouisson LM, Busch CJ, Puybasset L, et al. Role of the heart in the loss of aeration characterizing lower lobes in acute respiratory distress syndrome. CT Scan ARDS Study Group. Am J Respir Crit Care Med 2000; 161:2005–12.

210. Puybasset L, Cluzel P, Chao N, et al. A computed tomography scan assessment of regional lung volume in acute lung injury. The CT Scan ARDS Study Group. Am J Respir Crit Care Med 1998; 158:1644–55.

211. Quintel M, Pelosi P, Caironi P, et al. An increase of abdominal pressure increases pulmonary edema in oleic acid–induced lung injury. Am J Respir Crit Care Med 2004; 169:534–41.

212. Spragg RG, Lewis JF. Pathology of the surfactant system of the mature lung: Second San Diego conference. Am J Respir Crit Care Med 2001; 163:280–2.

213. Bernasconi M, Ploysongsang Y, Gottfried SB, et al. Respiratory compliance and resistance in mechanically ventilated patients with acute respiratory failure. Intensive Care Med 1988; 14:547–53.

214. Broseghini C, Brandolese R, Poggi R, et al. Respiratory resistance and intrinsic positive end-expiratory pressure ($PEEP_I$) in

patients with the adult respiratory distress syndrome (ARDS). Eur Respir J 1988; 1:726–31.

215. Broseghini C, Brandolese R, Poggi R, et al. Respiratory mechanics during the first day of mechanical ventilation in patients with pulmonary edema and chronic airway obstruction. Am Rev Respir Dis 1988; 138:355–61.

216. Chung KF, Keyes SJ, Morgan BM, et al. Mechanisms of airway narrowing in acute pulmonary oedema in dogs: Influence of the vagus and lung volume. Clin Sci (Lond) 1983; 65: 289–96.

217. Delaunois L, Sergysels R, Martin RR. Acute effects on airways mechanics of pulmonary edema induced by intravenous oleic acid in dogs. Bull Eur Physiopathol Respir 1980; 16: 47–55.

218. Eissa NT, Ranieri VM, Corbeil C, et al. Effects of positive end-expiratory pressure, lung volume, and inspiratory flow on interrupter resistance in patients with adult respiratory distress syndrome. Am Rev Respir Dis 1991; 144:538–43.

219. Eissa NT, Ranieri VM, Corbeil C, et al. Analysis of behavior of the respiratory system in ARDS patients: Effects of flow, volume, and time. J Appl Physiol 1991; 70:2719–29.

220. Esbenshade AM, Newman JH, Lams PM, et al. Respiratory failure after endotoxin infusion in sheep: Lung mechanics and lung fluid balance. J Appl Physiol 1982; 53:967–76.

221. Kondili E, Prinianakis G, Athanasakis H, Georgopoulos D. Lung emptying in patients with acute respiratory distress syndrome: Effects of positive end-expiratory pressure. Eur Respir J 2002; 19:811–9.

222. Koutsoukou A, Armaganidis A, Stavrakaki-Kallergi C, et al. Expiratory flow limitation and intrinsic positive end-expiratory pressure at zero positive end-expiratory pressure in patients with adult respiratory distress syndrome. Am J Respir Crit Care Med 2000; 161:1590–6.

223. Koutsoukou A, Bekos B, Sotiropoulou C, et al. Effects of positive end-expiratory pressure on gas exchange and expiratory flow limitation in adult respiratory distress syndrome. Crit Care Med 2002; 30:1941–9.

224. Pesenti A, Pelosi P, Rossi N, et al. The effects of positive end-expiratory pressure on respiratory resistance in patients with the adult respiratory distress syndrome and in normal anesthetized subjects. Am Rev Respir Dis 1991; 144:101–7.

225. Tantucci C, Corbeil C, Chasse M, et al. Flow and volume dependence of respiratory system flow resistance in patients with adult respiratory distress syndrome. Am Rev Respir Dis 1992; 145:355–60.

226. Wright PE, Bernard GR. The role of airflow resistance in patients with the adult respiratory distress syndrome. Am Rev Respir Dis 1989; 139:1169–74.

227. Nunn JF, Payne JP. Hypoxaemia after general anaesthesia. Lancet 1962; 2:631–2.

228. Burger EJ Jr, Macklem P. Airway closure: Demonstration by breathing 100 percent O_2 at low lung volumes and by N_2 washout. J Appl Physiol 1968; 25:139–48.

229. Caro CG, Butler J, Dubois AB. Some effects of restriction of chest cage expansion on pulmonary function in man: An experimental study. J Clin Invest 1960; 39:573–83.

230. Rouby JJ, Puybasset L, Cluzel P, et al. Regional distribution of gas and tissue in acute respiratory distress syndrome: II. Physiological correlations and definition of an ARDS Severity Score. CT Scan ARDS Study Group. Intensive Care Med 2000; 26: 1046–56.

231. Brandolese R, Broseghini C, Polese G, et al. Effects of intrinsic PEEP on pulmonary gas exchange in mechanically-ventilated patients. Eur Respir J 1993; 6:358–63.

232. Burns D, West TA, Hawkins K, O'Keefe GE. Immediate effects of positive end-expiratory pressure and low and high tidal volume ventilation upon gas exchange and compliance in patients with acute lung injury. J Trauma 2001; 51:1177–81.

233. Foti G, Cereda M, Sparacino ME, et al. Effects of periodic lung recruitment maneuvers on gas exchange and respiratory mechanics in mechanically ventilated acute respiratory distress syndrome (ARDS) patients. Intensive Care Med 2000; 26: 501–7.

234. Lim CM, Jung H, Koh Y, et al. Effect of alveolar recruitment maneuver in early acute respiratory distress syndrome according to antiderecruitment strategy, etiological category of diffuse lung injury, and body position of the patient. Crit Care Med 2003; 31:411–8.

235. Luecke T, Roth H, Joachim A, et al. Effects of end-inspiratory and end-expiratory pressures on alveolar recruitment and derecruitment in saline-washout-induced lung injury: A computed tomography study. Acta Anaesthesiol Scand 2004; 48: 82–92.

236. Maggiore SM, Jonson B, Richard JC, et al. Alveolar derecruitment at decremental positive end-expiratory pressure levels in acute lung injury: Comparison with the lower inflection point, oxygenation, and compliance. Am J Respir Crit Care Med 2001; 164:795–801.

237. Mergoni M, Martelli A, Volpi A, et al. Impact of positive end-expiratory pressure on chest wall and lung pressure-volume curve in acute respiratory failure. Am J Respir Crit Care Med 1997; 156:846–54.

238. Puybasset L, Gusman P, Muller JC, et al. Regional distribution of gas and tissue in acute respiratory distress syndrome: III. Consequences for the effects of positive end-expiratory pressure. CT Scan ARDS Study Group. Adult Respiratory Distress Syndrome. Intensive Care Med 2000; 26:1215–27.

239. Ranieri VM, Giuliani R, Fiore T, et al. Volume-pressure curve of the respiratory system predicts effects of PEEP in ARDS: "Occlusion" versus "constant flow" technique. Am J Respir Crit Care Med 1994; 149:19–27.

240. Ranieri VM, Mascia L, Fiore T, et al. Cardiorespiratory effects of positive end-expiratory pressure during progressive tidal volume reduction (permissive hypercapnia) in patients with acute respiratory distress syndrome. Anesthesiology 1995; 83:710–20.

241. Richard JC, Brochard L, Vandelet P, et al. Respective effects of end-expiratory and end-inspiratory pressures on alveolar recruitment in acute lung injury. Crit Care Med 2003; 31:89–92.

242. Richard JC, Maggiore SM, Jonson B, et al. Influence of tidal volume on alveolar recruitment: Respective role of PEEP and a recruitment maneuver. Am J Respir Crit Care Med 2001; 163:1609–13.

243. Rimensberger PC, Cox PN, Frndova H, Bryan AC. The open lung during small tidal volume ventilation: Concepts of recruitment and "optimal" positive end-expiratory pressure. Crit Care Med 1999; 27:1946–52.

244. Schreiter D, Reske A, Stichert B, et al. Alveolar recruitment in combination with sufficient positive end-expiratory pressure increases oxygenation and lung aeration in patients with severe chest trauma. Crit Care Med 2004; 32:968–75.

245. Shah DM, Newell JC, Dutton RE, Powers SR Jr. Continuous positive airway pressure versus positive end-expiratory pressure in respiratory distress syndrome. J Thorac Cardiovasc Surg 1977; 74:557–62.

246. Valta P, Takala J, Eissa NT, Milic-Emili J. Does alveolar recruitment occur with positive end-expiratory pressure in adult respiratory distress syndrome patients? J Crit Care 1993; 8: 34–42.

247. Petty TL, Ashbaugh DG. The adult respiratory distress syndrome: Clinical features, factors influencing prognosis and principles of management. Chest 1971; 60:233–9.

248. Antonelli M, Conti G, Bufi M, et al. Noninvasive ventilation for treatment of acute respiratory failure in patients undergoing solid organ transplantation: A randomized trial. Jama 2000; 283:235–41.

249. Beltrame F, Lucangelo U, Gregori D, Gregoretti C. Noninvasive positive pressure ventilation in trauma patients with acute respiratory failure. Monaldi Arch Chest Dis 1999; 54:109–14.

250. Conti G, Marino P, Cogliati A, et al. Noninvasive ventilation for the treatment of acute respiratory failure in patients with hematologic malignancies: a pilot study. Intensive Care Med 1998; 24:1283–8.

251. Covelli HD, Weled BJ, Beekman JF. Efficacy of continuous positive airway pressure administered by face mask. Chest 1982; 81:147–50.

252. Ferrer M, Esquinas A, Leon M, et al. Noninvasive ventilation in severe hypoxemic respiratory failure: A randomized clinical trial. Am J Respir Crit Care Med 2003; 168:1438–44.

253. Greenbaum DM, Millen JE, Eross B, et al. Continuous positive airway pressure without tracheal intubation in spontaneously breathing patients. Chest 1976; 69:615–20.

254. Hilbert G, Gruson D, Vargas F, et al. Noninvasive ventilation in immunosuppressed patients with pulmonary infiltrates, fever, and acute respiratory failure. New Engl J Med 2001; 344: 481–7.

255. Hurst JM, DeHaven CB, Branson RD. Use of CPAP mask as the sole mode of ventilatory support in trauma patients with mild to moderate respiratory insufficiency. J Trauma 1985; 25: 1065–8.

256. Meduri GU, Conoscenti CC, Menashe P, Nair S. Noninvasive face mask ventilation in patients with acute respiratory failure. Chest 1989; 95:865–70.

257. Rocker GM, Mackenzie MG, Williams B, Logan PM. Noninvasive positive pressure ventilation: Successful outcome in patients with acute lung injury/ARDS. Chest 1999; 115:173–7.

258. Smith RA, Kirby RR, Gooding JM, Civetta JM. Continuous positive airway pressure (CPAP) by face mask. Crit Care Med 1980; 8:483–5.

259. Wood KA, Lewis L, Von Harz B, Kollef MH. The use of noninvasive positive pressure ventilation in the emergency department: Results of a randomized clinical trial. Chest 1998; 113:1339–46.

260. Wysocki M, Tric L, Wolff MA, et al. Noninvasive pressure support ventilation in patients with acute respiratory failure. Chest 1993; 103:907–13.

261. East TD, in't Veen JC, Jonker TA, et al. Computer-controlled positive end-expiratory pressure titration for effective oxygenation without frequent blood gases. Crit Care Med 1988; 16:252–7.

262. Ralph DD, Robertson HT, Weaver LJ, et al. Distribution of ventilation and perfusion during positive end-expiratory pressure in the adult respiratory distress syndrome. Am Rev Respir Dis 1985; 131:54–60.

263. Gattinoni L, Pesenti A, Baglioni S, et al. Inflammatory pulmonary edema and positive end-expiratory pressure: Correlations between imaging and physiologic studies. J Thorac Imaging 1988; 3:59–64.

264. Crotti S, Mascheroni D, Caironi P, et al. Recruitment and derecruitment during acute respiratory failure: A clinical study. Am J Respir Crit Care Med 2001; 164:131–40.

265. Pelosi P, Goldner M, McKibben A, et al. Recruitment and derecruitment during acute respiratory failure: An experimental study. Am J Respir Crit Care Med 2001; 164:122–30.

266. Webb HH, Tierney DF. Experimental pulmonary edema due to intermittent positive pressure ventilation with high inflation pressures: Protection by positive end-expiratory pressure. Am Rev Respir Dis 1974; 110:556–65.

267. Corbridge TC, Wood LD, Crawford GP, et al. Adverse effects of large tidal volume and low PEEP in canine acid aspiration. Am Rev Respir Dis 1990; 142:311–5.

268. Dreyfuss D, Saumon G. Role of tidal volume, FRC, and end-inspiratory volume in the development of pulmonary edema following mechanical ventilation. Am Rev Respir Dis 1993; 148:1194–203.

269. Dreyfuss D, Soler P, Basset G, Saumon G. High inflation pressure pulmonary edema: Respective effects of high airway pressure, high tidal volume, and positive end-expiratory pressure. Am Rev Respir Dis 1988; 137:1159–64.

270. Gattinoni L, Pelosi P, Crotti S, Valenza F. Effects of positive end-expiratory pressure on regional distribution of tidal volume and recruitment in adult respiratory distress syndrome. Am J Respir Crit Care Med 1995; 151:1807–14.

271. Hickling KG, Walsh J, Henderson S, Jackson R. Low mortality rate in adult respiratory distress syndrome using low-volume, pressure-limited ventilation with permissive hypercapnia: A prospective study. Crit Care Med 1994; 22:1568–78.

272. Tugrul S, Akinci O, Ozcan PE, et al. Effects of sustained inflation and postinflation positive end-expiratory pressure in acute respiratory distress syndrome: Focusing on pulmonary and extrapulmonary forms. Crit Care Med 2003; 31: 738–44.

273. Beydon L, Uttman L, Rawal R, Jonson B. Effects of positive end-expiratory pressure on dead space and its partitions in acute lung injury. Intensive Care Med 2002; 28:1239–45.

274. Vieira SR, Puybasset L, Lu Q, et al. A scanographic assessment of pulmonary morphology in acute lung injury: Significance of the lower inflection point detected on the lung pressure-volume curve. Am J Respir Crit Care Med 1999; 159:1612–23.

275. Blanch L, Roussos C, Brotherton S, et al. Effect of tidal volume and PEEP in ethchlorvynol-induced asymmetric lung injury. J Appl Physiol 1992; 73:108–16.

276. Craven KD, Oppenheimer L, Wood LD. Effects of contusion and flail chest on pulmonary perfusion and oxygen exchange. J Appl Physiol 1979; 47:729–37.

277. Kanarek DJ, Shannon DC. Adverse effect of positive end-expiratory pressure on pulmonary perfusion and arterial oxygenation. Am Rev Respir Dis 1975; 112:457–9.

278. Mink SN, Light RB, Cooligan T, Wood LD. Effect of PEEP on gas exchange and pulmonary perfusion in canine lobar pneumonia. J Appl Physiol 1981; 50:517–23.

279. Remolina C, Khan AU, Santiago TV, Edelman NH. Positional hypoxemia in unilateral lung disease. New Engl J Med 1981; 304:523–5.

280. Cinnella G, Dambrosio M, Brienza N, et al. Independent lung ventilation in patients with unilateral pulmonary contusion. Monitoring with compliance and EtCO$_2$. Intensive Care Med 2001; 27:1860–7.

281. Wagner PD, Dantzker DR, Dueck R, et al. Ventilation-perfusion inequality in chronic obstructive pulmonary disease. J Clin Invest 1977; 59:203–16.

282. Barbera JA, Reyes A, Roca J, et al. Effect of intravenously administered aminophylline on ventilation/perfusion inequality during recovery from exacerbations of chronic obstructive pulmonary disease. Am Rev Respir Dis 1992; 145:1328–33.

283. Barbera JA, Roca J, Ramirez J, et al. Gas exchange during exercise in mild chronic obstructive pulmonary disease: Correlation with lung structure. Am Rev Respir Dis 1991; 144:520–5.

284. Esteban A, De Elio FJ, Cerda E, et al. Blood-gas changes with different end-expiratory pressures in patients with chronic bronchitis. Br J Anaesth 1974; 46:159–61.

285. Tuxen DV. Detrimental effects of positive end-expiratory pressure during controlled mechanical ventilation of patients with severe airflow obstruction. Am Rev Respir Dis 1989; 140:5–9.

286. Rossi A, Santos C, Roca J, et al. Effects of PEEP on $\dot{V}_A/\dot{Q}$ mismatching in ventilated patients with chronic airflow obstruction. Am J Respir Crit Care Med 1994; 149:1077–84.

287. Miro AM, Shivaram U, Hertig I. Continuous positive airway pressure in COPD patients in acute hypercapnic respiratory failure. Chest 1993; 103:266–8.

288. de Lucas P, Tarancon C, Puente L, et al. Nasal continuous positive airway pressure in patients with COPD in acute

respiratory failure: A study of the immediate effects. Chest 1993; 104: 1694–7.

289. Shivaram U, Cash ME, Beal A. Nasal continuous positive airway pressure in decompensated hypercapnic respiratory failure as a complication of sleep apnea. Chest 1993; 104:770–4.

290. Fenn WO. Mechanics of respiration. Am J Med 1951; 10:77–91.

291. Radford EP Jr. Static mechanical properties of mammalian lungs. In: Fenn WO, Rahn H, editors. Handbook of physiology, vol 1. Washington: American Physiological Society, 1964: 429–49.

292. Rahn H, Fenn WO, Otis AB. The pressure-volume diagram of the thorax and the lung. Am J Physiol 1946; 146:161–78.

293. Agostoni E, Mead J. Statics of the respiratory system. In: Fenn WO, Rahn H, editors. Handbook of physiology, vol 1. Washington: American Physiological Society, 1964: 387– 409.

294. Maggiore SM, Brochard L. Pressure-volume curve in the critically ill. Curr Opin Crit Care 2000; 6:1–10.

295. Anthonisen NR. Changes in shunt flow, compliance, and volume of lungs during apneic oxygenation. Am J Physiol 1964; 207:235–8.

296. Clements JA, Hustead RF, Johnson RP, Gribetz I. Pulmonary surface tension and alveolar stability. J Appl Physiol 1961; 16: 444–50.

297. Mead J, Collier C. Relation of volume history of lungs to respiratory mechanics in anesthetized dogs. J Appl Physiol 1959; 14:669–78.

298. Williams JV, Tierney DF, Parker HR. Surface forces in the lung, atelectasis, and transpulmonary pressure. J Appl Physiol 1966; 21:819–27.

299. Bates JH, Baconnier P, Milic-Emili J. A theoretical analysis of interrupter technique for measuring respiratory mechanics. J Appl Physiol 1988; 64:2204–14.

300. Bates JH, Rossi A, Milic-Emili J. Analysis of the behavior of the respiratory system with constant inspiratory flow. J Appl Physiol 1985; 58:1840–8.

301. Hildebrandt J. Pressure-volume data of cat lung interpreted by a plastoelastic, linear viscoelastic model. J Appl Physiol 1970; 28:365–72.

302. Hughes R, May AJ, Widdicombe JG. Stress relaxation in rabbits' lungs. J Physiol 1959; 146:85–97.

303. Kochi T, Okubo S, Zin WA, Milic-Emili J. Chest wall and respiratory system mechanics in cats: Effects of flow and volume. J Appl Physiol 1988; 64:2636–46.

304. Kochi T, Okubo S, Zin WA, Milic-Emili J. Flow and volume dependence of pulmonary mechanics in anesthetized cats. J Appl Physiol 1988; 64:441–50.

305. Sharp JT, Johnson FN, Goldberg NB, Van Lith P. Hysteresis and stress adaptation in the human respiratory system. J Appl Physiol 1967; 23:487–97.

306. Rossi A, Gottfried SB, Higgs BD, et al. Respiratory mechanics in mechanically ventilated patients with respiratory failure. J Appl Physiol 1985; 58:1849–58.

307. D'Angelo E, Calderini E, Torri G, et al. Respiratory mechanics in anesthetized paralyzed humans: effects of flow, volume, and time. J Appl Physiol 1989; 67(6):2556–64.

308. D'Angelo E, Robatto FM, Calderini E, et al. Pulmonary and chest wall mechanics in anesthetized paralyzed humans. J Appl Physiol 1991; 70:2602–10.

309. Jonson B, Nordstrom L, Olsson SG, Akerback D. Monitoring of ventilation and lung mechanics during automatic ventilation: A new device. Bull Physiopathol Respir (Nancy) 1975; 11:729–43.

310. Mead J, Mc IM, Selverstone NJ, Kriete BC. Measurement of intraesophageal pressure. J Appl Physiol 1955; 7:491–5.

311. Milic-Emili J, Mead J, Turner JM. Topography of esophageal pressure as a function of posture in man. J Appl Physiol 1964; 19:212–6.

312. Milic-Emili J, Mead J, Turner JM, Glauser EM. Improved technique for estimating pleural pressure from esophageal balloons. J Appl Physiol 1964; 19:207–11.

313. Whitfield AG, Waterhouse JA, Arnott WM. The total lung volume and its subdivisions; A study in physiological norms; the effect of posture. Br J Soc Med 1950; 4:86–97.

314. Leblanc P, Ruff F, Milic-Emili J. Effects of age and body position on "airway closure" in man. J Appl Physiol 1970; 28:448–51.

315. Don HF, Wahba M, Cuadrado L, Kelkar K. The effects of anesthesia and 100 percent oxygen on the functional residual capacity of the lungs. Anesthesiology 1970; 32:521–9.

316. Craig DB, Wahba WM, Don HF, et al. "Closing volume" and its relationship to gas exchange in seated and supine positions. J Appl Physiol 1971; 31:717–21.

317. Ibanez J, Raurich JM. Normal values of functional residual capacity in the sitting and supine positions. Intensive Care Med 1982; 8:173–7.

318. Behrakis PK, Baydur A, Jaeger MJ, Milic-Emili J. Lung mechanics in sitting and horizontal body positions. Chest 1983; 83:643–6.

319. Rehder K, Hatch DJ, Sessler AD, et al. Effects of general anesthesia, muscle paralysis, and mechanical ventilation on pulmonary nitrogen clearance. Anesthesiology 1971; 35:591–601.

320. Westbrook PR, Stubbs SE, Sessler AD, et al. Effects of anesthesia and muscle paralysis on respiratory mechanics in normal man. J Appl Physiol 1973; 34:81–6.

321. Dechman GS, Chartrand DA, Ruiz-Neto PP, Bates JH. The effect of changing end-expiratory pressure on respiratory system mechanics in open- and closed-chest anesthetized, paralyzed patients. Anesth Analg 1995; 81:279–86.

322. Sigurdsson S, Svantesson C, Larsson A, Jonson B. Elastic pressure-volume curves indicate derecruitment after a single deep expiration in anaesthetised and muscle-relaxed healthy man. Acta Anaesthesiol Scand 2000; 44:980–4.

323. Valta P, Takala J, Eissa NT, Milic-Emili J. Effects of PEEP on respiratory mechanics after open heart surgery. Chest 1992; 102: 227–33.

324. Svantesson C, Sigurdsson S, Larsson A, Jonson B. Effects of recruitment of collapsed lung units on the elastic pressure-volume relationship in anaesthetised healthy adults. Acta Anaesthesiol Scand 1998; 42:1149–56.

325. Zin WA, Caldeira MP, Cardoso WV, et al. Expiratory mechanics before and after uncomplicated heart surgery. Chest 1989; 95: 21–8.

326. Berrizbeitia LD, Tessler S, Jacobowitz IJ, et al. Effect of sternotomy and coronary bypass surgery on postoperative pulmonary mechanics: Comparison of internal mammary and saphenous vein bypass grafts. Chest 1989; 96:873–6.

327. Locke TJ, Griffiths TL, Mould H, Gibson GJ. Rib cage mechanics after median sternotomy. Thorax 1990; 45:465–8.

328. Ranieri VM, Brienza N, Santostasi S, et al. Impairment of lung and chest wall mechanics in patients with acute respiratory distress syndrome: Role of abdominal distension. Am J Respir Crit Care Med 1997; 156:1082–91.

329. Ranieri VM, Vitale N, Grasso S, et al. Time-course of impairment of respiratory mechanics after cardiac surgery and cardiopulmonary bypass. Crit Care Med 1999; 27:1454–60.

330. Rehder K, Sittipong R, Sessler AD. The effects of thiopental-meperidine anesthesia with succinylcholine paralysis on functional residual capacity and dynamic lung compliance in normal sitting man. Anesthesiology 1972; 37:395–8.

331. Rehder K, Mallow JE, Fibuch EE, et al. Effects of isoflurane anesthesia and muscle paralysis on respiratory mechanics in normal man. Anesthesiology 1974; 41:477–85.

332. Pelosi P, Cereda M, Foti G, et al. Alterations of lung and chest wall mechanics in patients with acute lung injury: Effects of

positive end-expiratory pressure. Am J Respir Crit Care Med 1995; 152:531–7.

333. Dyhr T, Laursen N, Larsson A. Effects of lung recruitment maneuver and positive end-expiratory pressure on lung volume, respiratory mechanics and alveolar gas mixing in patients ventilated after cardiac surgery. Acta Anaesthesiol Scand 2002; 46:717–25.

334. Koutsoukou A, Koulouris N, Bekos B, et al. Expiratory flow limitation in morbidly obese postoperative mechanically ventilated patients. Acta Anaesthesiol Scand 2004; 48:1080–8.

335. D'Angelo E, Calderini E, Tavola M, et al. Effect of PEEP on respiratory mechanics in anesthetized paralyzed humans. J Appl Physiol 1992; 73:1736–42.

336. D'Angelo E, Tavola M, Milic-Emili J. Volume and time dependence of respiratory system mechanics in normal anaesthetized paralysed humans. Eur Respir J 2000; 16:665–72.

337. Musch G, Foti G, Cereda M, et al. Lung and chest wall mechanics in normal anaesthetized subjects and in patients with COPD at different PEEP levels. Eur Respir J 1997; 10:2545–52.

338. Fahy BG, Barnas GM, Flowers JL, et al. Effects of PEEP on respiratory mechanics are tidal volume and frequency dependent. Respir Physiol 1997; 109:53–64.

339. Cohendy R, Ripart J, Eledjam JJ. The effect of positive end-expiratory pressure on respiratory resistive properties in anaesthetized paralysed humans. Eur Respir J 1994; 7:286–91.

340. Ramachandran PR, Fairley HB. Changes in functional residual capacity during respiratory failure. Can Anaesth Soc J 1970; 17:359–69.

341. Pontoppidan H, Geffin B, Lowenstein E. Acute respiratory failure in the adult, part 3. New Engl J Med 1972; 287:799–806.

342. Pontoppidan H, Geffin B, Lowenstein E. Acute respiratory failure in the adult, part 2. New Engl J Med 1972; 287:743–52.

343. Pontoppidan H, Geffin B, Lowenstein E. Acute respiratory failure in the adult, part 1. New Engl J Med 1972; 287:690–8.

344. Petty TL, Silvers GW, Paul GW, Stanford RE. Abnormalities in lung elastic properties and surfactant function in adult respiratory distress syndrome. Chest 1979; 75:571–4.

345. Ibanez J, Raurich JM, Moris SG. A simple method for measuring the effect of PEEP on functional residual capacity during mechanical ventilation. Crit Care Med 1982; 10:332–4.

346. Dall'ava-Santucci J, Armaganidis A, Brunet F, et al. Mechanical effects of PEEP in patients with adult respiratory distress syndrome. J Appl Physiol 1990; 68:843–8.

347. Benito S, Lemaire F. Pulmonary pressure-volume relationship in acute respiratory distress syndrome in adults: Role of positive end expiratory pressure. J Crit Care 1990; 5:27–34.

348. Heldt GP, Peters RM. A simplified method to determine functional residual capacity during mechanical ventilation. Chest 1978; 74:492–6.

349. Weaver LJ, Pierson DJ, Kellie R, et al. A practical procedure for measuring functional residual capacity during mechanical ventilation with or without PEEP. Crit Care Med 1981; 9:873–7.

350. Ibanez J, Raurich JM, Moris SG. Measurement of functional residual capacity during mechanical ventilation: Comparison of a computerized open nitrogen washout method with a closed helium dilution method. Intensive Care Med 1983; 9:91–3.

351. Macnaughton PD, Morgan CJ, Denison DM, Evans TW. Measurement of carbon monoxide transfer and lung volume in ventilated subjects. Eur Respir J 1993; 6:231–6.

352. Macnaughton PD, Evans TW. Measurement of lung volume and DL_{CO} in acute respiratory failure. Am J Respir Crit Care Med 1994; 150:770–5.

353. Kendrick AH. Comparison of methods of measuring static lung volumes. Monaldi Arch Chest Dis 1996; 51:431–9.

354. Fretschner R, Deusch H, Weitnauer A, Brunner JX. A simple method to estimate functional residual capacity in mechanically ventilated patients. Intensive Care Med 1993; 19:372–6.

355. Wrigge H, Sydow M, Zinserling J, et al. Determination of functional residual capacity (FRC) by multibreath nitrogen washout in a lung model and in mechanically ventilated patients: Accuracy depends on continuous dynamic compensation for changes of gas sampling delay time. Intensive Care Med 1998; 24:487–93.

356. Jonmarker C, Castor R, Drefeldt B, Werner O. An analyzer for in-line measurement of expiratory sulfur hexafluoride concentration. Anesthesiology 1985; 63:84–8.

357. Jonmarker C, Jansson L, Jonson B, et al. Measurement of functional residual capacity by sulfur hexafluoride washout. Anesthesiology 1985; 63:89–95.

358. East TD, Wortelboer PJ, van Ark E, et al. Automated sulfur hexafluoride washout functional residual capacity measurement system for any mode of mechanical ventilation as well as spontaneous respiration. Crit Care Med 1990; 18:84–91.

359. Beydon L, Svantesson C, Brauer K, et al. Respiratory mechanics in patients ventilated for critical lung disease. Eur Respir J 1996; 9:262–73.

360. Maggiore SM, Lellouche F, Pigeot J, et al. Prevention of endotracheal suctioning-induced alveolar derecruitment in acute lung injury. Am J Respir Crit Care Med 2003; 167:1215–24.

361. Maggiore SM, Richard JC, Brochard L. What has been learnt from P/V curves in patients with acute lung injury/acute respiratory distress syndrome. Eur Respir J Suppl 2003; 42:22–6S.

362. Tobin MJ, Jenouri G, Birch S, et al. Effect of positive end-expiratory pressure on breathing patterns of normal subjects and intubated patients with respiratory failure. Crit Care Med 1983; 11:859–67.

363. Hoffman RA, Ershowsky P, Krieger BP. Determination of auto-PEEP during spontaneous and controlled ventilation by monitoring changes in end-expiratory thoracic gas volume. Chest 1989; 96:613–6.

364. Cereda M, Villa F, Colombo E, et al. Closed system endotracheal suctioning maintains lung volume during volume-controlled mechanical ventilation. Intensive Care Med 2001; 27:648–54.

365. Nunes S, Uusaro A, Takala J. Pressure-volume relationships in acute lung injury: Methodological and clinical implications. Acta Anaesthesiol Scand 2004; 48:278–86.

366. Aliverti A, Dellaca R, Pelosi P, et al. Optoelectronic plethysmography in intensive care patients. Am J Respir Crit Care Med 2000; 161:1546–52.

367. Gattinoni L, Caironi P, Pelosi P, Goodman LR. What has computed tomography taught us about the acute respiratory distress syndrome? Am J Respir Crit Care Med 2001; 164:1701–11.

368. Rouby JJ, Puybasset L, Nieszkowska A, Lu Q. Acute respiratory distress syndrome: Lessons from computed tomography of the whole lung. Crit Care Med 2003; 31:S285–95.

369. Rouby JJ, Lu Q, Goldstein I. Selecting the right level of positive end-expiratory pressure in patients with acute respiratory distress syndrome. Am J Respir Crit Care Med 2002; 165:1182–6.

370. Rouby JJ, Lu Q, Vieira S. Pressure/volume curves and lung computed tomography in acute respiratory distress syndrome. Eur Respir J Suppl 2003; 42:27–36S.

371. Nieszkowska A, Lu Q, Vieira S, et al. Incidence and regional distribution of lung overinflation during mechanical ventilation with positive end-expiratory pressure. Crit Care Med 2004; 32:1496–503.

372. Lu Q, Constantin JM, Malbouisson L, et al. Comparison of two methods for assessing alveolar recruitment in ARDS:

Pressure-volume curve vs CT scan analysis (abstract). Am J Respir Crit Care Med 2000; 161:A487.

373. Dambrosio M, Roupie E, Mollet JJ, et al. Effects of positive end-expiratory pressure and different tidal volumes on alveolar recruitment and hyperinflation. Anesthesiology 1997; 87: 495–503.

374. Chelucci GL, Dall'Ava-Santucci J, Dhainaut JF, et al. Association of PEEP with two different inflation volumes in ARDS patients: Effects on passive lung deflation and alveolar recruitment. Intensive Care Med 2000; 26:870–7.

375. Mergoni M, Volpi A, Bricchi C, Rossi A. Lower inflection point and recruitment with PEEP in ventilated patients with acute respiratory failure. J Appl Physiol 2001; 91:441–50.

376. Vieillard-Baron A, Prin S, Chergui K, et al. Early patterns of static pressure-volume loops in ARDS and their relations with PEEP-induced recruitment. Intensive Care Med 2003; 29: 1929–35.

377. Albaiceta GM, Taboada F, Parra D, et al. Tomographic study of the inflection points of the pressure-volume curve in acute lung injury. Am J Respir Crit Care Med 2004; 170:1066–72.

378. Grasso S, Fanelli V, Cafarelli A, et al. Effects of high versus low positive end-expiratory pressure in acute respiratory distress syndrome. Am J Respir Crit Care Med 2005;171:1002–8.

379. Gattinoni L, Bombino M, Pelosi P, et al. Lung structure and function in different stages of severe adult respiratory distress syndrome. JAMA 1994; 271:1772–9.

380. Grasso S, Mascia L, Del Turco M, et al. Effects of recruiting maneuvers in patients with acute respiratory distress syndrome ventilated with protective ventilatory strategy. Anesthesiology 2002; 96:795–802.

381. Matamis D, Lemaire F, Harf A, et al. Total respiratory pressure-volume curves in the adult respiratory distress syndrome. Chest 1984; 86:58–66.

382. Roupie E, Dambrosio M, Servillo G, et al. Titration of tidal volume and induced hypercapnia in acute respiratory distress syndrome. Am J Respir Crit Care Med 1995; 152:121–8.

383. International consensus conferences in intensive care medicine. Ventilator-associated lung injury in ARDS. Am J Respir Crit Care Med 1999; 160:2118–24.

384. Dreyfuss D, Saumon G. Ventilator-induced lung injury: Lessons from experimental studies. Am J Respir Crit Care Med 1998; 157:294–323.

385. Hickling KG. The pressure-volume curve is greatly modified by recruitment: A mathematical model of ARDS lungs. Am J Respir Crit Care Med 1998; 158:194–202.

386. Hickling KG. Best compliance during a decremental, but not incremental, positive end-expiratory pressure trial is related to open-lung positive end-expiratory pressure: A mathematical model of acute respiratory distress syndrome lungs. Am J Respir Crit Care Med 2001; 163:69–78.

387. Jonson B, Svantesson C. Elastic pressure-volume curves: What information do they convey? Thorax 1999; 54:82–7.

388. Servillo G, Svantesson C, Beydon L, et al. Pressure-volume curves in acute respiratory failure: Automated low flow inflation versus occlusion. Am J Respir Crit Care Med 1997; 155: 1629–36.

389. Cheney FW Jr, Martin WE. Effects of continuous positive-pressure ventilation on gas exchange in acute pulmonary edema. J Appl Physiol 1971; 30:378–81.

390. Cook CD, Mead J, Schreiner GL, et al. Pulmonary mechanics during induced pulmonary edema in anesthetized dogs. J Appl Physiol 1959; 14:177–86.

391. Grossman RF, Jones JG, Murray JF. Effects of oleic acid-induced pulmonary edema on lung mechanics. J Appl Physiol 1980; 48:1045–51.

392. Slutsky AS, Scharf SM, Brown R, Ingram RH Jr. The effect of oleic acid–induced pulmonary edema on pulmonary and chest wall mechanics in dogs. Am Rev Respir Dis 1980; 121: 91–6.

393. Lemaire F, Harf A, Simonneau G, et al. Echanges gazeux, courbe statique pression-volume et ventilation en pression positive de fin d'expiration: Etude dans seize cas d'insuffisance respiratoire aigue de l'adulte. Ann Anesthesiol Fr 1981; 22:435–41.

394. Benito S, Lemaire F. Pulmonary pressure-volume relationship in acute respiratory distress syndrome in adults: Role of positive end expiratory pressure. J Crit Care 1990; 5:27–34.

395. Dall'ava-Santucci J, Armaganidis A, Brunet F, et al. Causes of error of respiratory pressure-volume curves in paralyzed subjects. J Appl Physiol 1988; 64:42–9.

396. Hartog A, Vazquez de Anda GF, Gommers D, et al. At surfactant deficiency, application of "the open lung concept" prevents protein leakage and attenuates changes in lung mechanics. Crit Care Med 2000; 28:1450–4.

397. Grasso S, Terragni P, Mascia L, et al. Airway pressure-time curve profile (stress index) detects tidal recruitment/hyperinflation in experimental acute lung injury. Crit Care Med 2004; 32: 1018–27.

398. Glaister DH, Schroter RC, Sudlow MF, Milic-Emili J. Bulk elastic properties of excised lungs and the effect of a transpulmonary pressure gradient. Respir Physiol 1973; 17:347–64.

399. Vieillard-Baron A, Prin S, Schmitt JM, et al. Pressure-volume curves in acute respiratory distress syndrome: Clinical demonstration of the influence of expiratory flow limitation on the initial slope. Am J Respir Crit Care Med 2002; 165:1107–12.

400. Glaister DH, Schroter RC, Sudlow MF, Milic-Emili J. Transpulmonary pressure gradient and ventilation distribution in excised lungs. Respir Physiol 1973; 17:365–85.

401. Mancebo J, Benito S, Martin M, Net A. Value of static pulmonary compliance in predicting mortality in patients with acute respiratory failure. Intensive Care Med 1988; 14:110–4.

402. Suter PM, Fairley HB, Isenberg MD. Effect of tidal volume and positive end-expiratory pressure on compliance during mechanical ventilation. Chest 1978; 73:158–62.

403. Thille A, Richard J, Maggiore S, Brochard L. Pulmonary versus extrapulmonary ARDS: Recruitment measured using PV curve or effective compliance? (abstract). Intensive Care Med 2004; 30:S71.

404. Downie JM, Nam AJ, Simon BA. Pressure-volume curve does not predict steady-state lung volume in canine lavage lung injury. Am J Respir Crit Care Med 2004; 169:957–62.

405. Eissa NT, Ranieri VM, Corbeil C, et al. Effect of PEEP on the mechanics of the respiratory system in ARDS patients. J Appl Physiol 1992; 73:1728–35.

406. Pesenti A, Pelosi P, Rossi N, et al. Respiratory mechanics and bronchodilator responsiveness in patients with the adult respiratory distress syndrome. Crit Care Med 1993; 21: 78–83.

407. Guerin C, Coussa ML, Eissa NT, et al. Lung and chest wall mechanics in mechanically ventilated COPD patients. J Appl Physiol 1993; 74:1570–80.

408. Jolliet P, Watremez C, Roeseler J, et al. Comparative effects of helium-oxygen and external positive end-expiratory pressure on respiratory mechanics, gas exchange, and ventilation-perfusion relationships in mechanically ventilated patients with chronic obstructive pulmonary disease. Intensive Care Med 2003; 29:1442–50.

409. Guerin C, LeMasson S, de Varax R, et al. Small airway closure and positive end-expiratory pressure in mechanically ventilated patients with chronic obstructive pulmonary disease. Am J Respir Crit Care Med 1997; 155:1949–56.

410. Kondili E, Alexopoulou C, Prinianakis G, et al. Pattern of lung emptying and expiratory resistance in mechanically ventilated patients with chronic obstructive pulmonary disease. Intensive Care Med 2004; 30:1311–8.

411. Fernandez R, Mancebo J, Blanch L, et al. Intrinsic PEEP on static pressure-volume curves. Intensive Care Med 1990; 16:233–6.

412. Georgopoulos D, Giannouli E, Patakas D. Effects of extrinsic positive end-expiratory pressure on mechanically ventilated patients with chronic obstructive pulmonary disease and dynamic hyperinflation. Intensive Care Med 1993; 19:197–203.

413. Lourens MS, Berg BV, Hoogsteden HC, Bogaard JM. Detection of flow limitation in mechanically ventilated patients. Intensive Care Med 2001; 27:1312–20.

414. Aerts JG, van den Berg B, Bogaard JM. Controlled expiration in mechanically-ventilated patients with chronic obstructive pulmonary disease (COPD). Eur Respir J 1997; 10:550–6.

415. Kaczka DW, Ingenito EP, Body SC, et al. Inspiratory lung impedance in COPD: Effects of PEEP and immediate impact of lung volume reduction surgery. J Appl Physiol 2001; 90:1833–41.

416. Parker JC, Hernandez LA, Peevy KJ. Mechanisms of ventilator-induced lung injury. Crit Care Med 1993; 21:131–43.

417. Dos Santos CC, Slutsky AS. Invited review: Mechanisms of ventilator-induced lung injury: a perspective. J Appl Physiol 2000; 89:1645–55.

418. Dreyfuss D, Basset G, Soler P, Saumon G. Intermittent positive-pressure hyperventilation with high inflation pressures produces pulmonary microvascular injury in rats. Am Rev Respir Dis 1985; 132:880–4.

419. Ranieri VM, Suter PM, Tortorella C, et al. Effect of mechanical ventilation on inflammatory mediators in patients with acute respiratory distress syndrome: A randomized, controlled trial. JAMA 1999; 282:54–61.

420. The Acute Respiratory Distress Syndrome Network. Ventilation with lower tidal volumes as compared with traditional tidal volumes for acute lung injury and the acute respiratory distress syndrome. New Engl J Med 2000; 342:1301–8.

421. Goldstein I, Bughalo MT, Marquette CH, et al. Mechanical ventilation-induced air-space enlargement during experimental pneumonia in piglets. Am J Respir Crit Care Med 2001; 163:958–64.

422. Rouby JJ, Lherm T, Martin de Lassale E, et al. Histologic aspects of pulmonary barotrauma in critically ill patients with acute respiratory failure. Intensive Care Med 1993; 19:383–9.

423. Argiras EP, Blakeley CR, Dunnill MS, et al. High PEEP decreases hyaline membrane formation in surfactant deficient lungs. Br J Anaesth 1987; 59:1278–85.

424. Mead J, Takishima T, Leith D. Stress distribution in lungs: A model of pulmonary elasticity. J Appl Physiol 1970; 28:596–608.

425. Marini JJ. Ventilator-induced airway dysfunction? Am J Respir Crit Care Med 2001; 163:806–7.

426. Pierson DJ. Barotrauma and bronchopleural fistula. In: Tobin MJ, editor. Principles and practice of mechanical ventilation. New York: McGraw-Hill, 1994: 813–36.

427. Carlton DP, Cummings JJ, Scheerer RG, et al. Lung overexpansion increases pulmonary microvascular protein permeability in young lambs. J Appl Physiol 1990; 69:577–83.

428. Hernandez LA, Peevy KJ, Moise AA, Parker JC. Chest wall restriction limits high airway pressure-induced lung injury in young rabbits. J Appl Physiol 1989; 66:2364–8.

429. Caldini P, Leith JD, Brennan MJ. Effect of continuous postive-pressure ventilation (CPPV) on edema formation in dog lung. J Appl Physiol 1975; 39:672–9.

430. Toung T, Saharia P, Permutt S, et al. Aspiration pneumonia: beneficial and harmful effects of positive end-expiratory pressure. Surgery 1977; 82:279–83.

431. Hopewell PC. Failure of positive end-expiratory pressure to decrease lung water content in alloxan-induced pulmonary edema. Am Rev Respir Dis 1979; 120:813–9.

432. Hopewell PC, Murray JF. Effects of continuous positive-pressure ventilation in experimental pulmonary edema. J Appl Physiol 1976; 40:568–74.

433. Luce JM, Huang TW, Robertson HT, et al. The effects of prophylactic expiratory positive airway pressure on the resolution of oleic acid-induced lung injury in dogs. Ann Surg 1983; 197:327–36.

434. Luce JM. The cardiovascular effects of mechanical ventilation and positive end-expiratory pressure. JAMA 1984; 252:807–11.

435. Colmenero-Ruiz M, Fernandez-Mondejar E, Fernandez-Sacristan MA, et al. PEEP and low tidal volume ventilation reduce lung water in porcine pulmonary edema. Am J Respir Crit Care Med 1997; 155:964–70.

436. Dreyfuss D, Saumon G. Barotrauma is volutrauma, but which volume is the one responsible? Intensive Care Med 1992; 18:139–41.

437. Tremblay L, Valenza F, Ribeiro SP, et al. Injurious ventilatory strategies increase cytokines and c-fos m-RNA expression in an isolated rat lung model. J Clin Invest 1997; 99:944–52.

438. Tobin MJ. Advances in mechanical ventilation. New Engl J Med 2001; 344:1986–96.

439. McCann UG 2d, Schiller HJ, Carney DE, et al. Visual validation of the mechanical stabilizing effects of positive end-expiratory pressure at the alveolar level. J Surg Res 2001; 99:335–42.

440. Sandhar BK, Niblett DJ, Argiras EP, et al. Effects of positive end-expiratory pressure on hyaline membrane formation in a rabbit model of the neonatal respiratory distress syndrome. Intensive Care Med 1988; 14:538–46.

441. Taskar V, John J, Evander E, Robertson B, Jonson B. Surfactant dysfunction makes lungs vulnerable to repetitive collapse and reexpansion. Am J Respir Crit Care Med 1997; 155:313–20.

442. Woo SW, Hedley-Whyte J. Macrophage accumulation and pulmonary edema due to thoracotomy and lung over inflation. J Appl Physiol 1972; 33:14–21.

443. Lachmann B. Open up the lung and keep the lung open. Intensive Care Med 1992; 18:319–21.

444. Faridy EE. Effect of ventilation on movement of surfactant in airways. Respir Physiol 1976; 27:323–34.

445. Wyszogrodski I, Kyei-Aboagye K, Taeusch HW Jr, Avery ME. Surfactant inactivation by hyperventilation: Conservation by end-expiratory pressure. J Appl Physiol 1975; 38:461–6.

446. Faridy EE, Permutt S, Riley RL. Effect of ventilation on surface forces in excised dogs' lungs. J Appl Physiol 1966; 21:1453–62.

447. Verbrugge SJ, Bohm SH, Gommers D, et al. Surfactant impairment after mechanical ventilation with large alveolar surface area changes and effects of positive end-expiratory pressure. Br J Anaesth 1998; 80:360–4.

448. Sugiura M, McCulloch PR, Wren S, et al. Ventilator pattern influences neutrophil influx and activation in atelectasis-prone rabbit lung. J Appl Physiol 1994; 77:1355–65.

449. Nahum A, Hoyt J, Schmitz L, et al. Effect of mechanical ventilation strategy on dissemination of intratracheally instilled Escherichia coli in dogs. Crit Care Med 1997; 25:1733–43.

450. Verbrugge SJ, Sorm V, van 't Veen A, et al. Lung overinflation without positive end-expiratory pressure promotes bacteremia after experimental *Klebsiella pneumoniae* inoculation. Intensive Care Med 1998; 24:172–7.

451. Slutsky AS, Tremblay LN. Multiple system organ failure: Is mechanical ventilation a contributing factor? Am J Respir Crit Care Med 1998; 157:1721–5.

452. Chiumello D, Pristine G, Slutsky AS. Mechanical ventilation affects local and systemic cytokines in an animal model of acute

respiratory distress syndrome. Am J Respir Crit Care Med 1999; 160:109–16.

453. Imai Y, Parodo J, Kajikawa O, et al. Injurious mechanical ventilation and end-organ epithelial cell apoptosis and organ dysfunction in an experimental model of acute respiratory distress syndrome. JAMA 2003; 289:2104–12.

454. Ranieri VM, Giunta F, Suter PM, Slutsky AS. Mechanical ventilation as a mediator of multisystem organ failure in acute respiratory distress syndrome. JAMA 2000; 284:43–4.

455. Cassidy SS, Schwiep F. Cardiovascular effects of positive end-expiratory pressure. In: Scharf SM, Cassidy SS, editors. Heart-lung interactions in health and disease. New York: Marcel Dekker, 1989: 463–506.

456. Dhainaut JF, Aouate P, Brunet FP. Circulatory effects of positive end-expiratory pressure in patients with acute lung injury. In: Scharf SM, Cassidy SS, editors. Heart-lung interactions in health and disease. New York: Marcel Dekker, 1989: 809–38.

457. Cassidy SS. Heart-lung interactions in health and disease. Am J Med Sci 1987; 294:451–61.

458. Fessler HE, Permutt S. Interactions between the circulatory and ventilatory pumps: The thorax. In: Roussos C, Macklem PT, editors. Lung biology in health and disease, 2d ed. New York: Marcel Dekker, 1995: 1621–39.

459. Fessler HE. Heart-lung interactions: Applications in the critically ill. Eur Respir J 1997; 10:226–37.

460. Michard F, Teboul JL. Using heart-lung interactions to assess fluid responsiveness during mechanical ventilation. Crit Care 2000; 4:282–9.

461. Pinsky MR. Recent advances in the clinical application of heart-lung interactions. Curr Opin Crit Care 2002; 8:26–31.

462. Vieillard-Baron A, Prin S, Chergui K, et al. Echo-Doppler demonstration of acute cor pulmonale at the bedside in the medical intensive care unit. Am J Respir Crit Care Med 2002; 166:1310–9.

463. Jardin F, Vieillard-Baron A. Right ventricular function and positive pressure ventilation in clinical practice: From hemodynamic subsets to respirator settings. Intensive Care Med 2003; 29: 1426-34.

464. Cournand A, Motley H, Werko L, Richards D. Physiologic studies of the effects of intermittent positive pressure breathing on cardiac output in man. Am J Physiol 1948; 125: 261–73.

465. Powers SR Jr, Mannal R. Neclerio M, et al. Physiologic consequences of positive end-expiratory pressure (PEEP) ventilation. Ann Surg 1973; 178:265–72.

466. Liebman PR, Patten MT, Manny J, et al. The mechanism of depressed cardiac output on positive end-expiratory pressure (PEEP). Surgery 1978; 83:594–8.

467. Guyton AC, Lindsey AW, Abernathy B, Richardson T. Venous return at various right atrial pressures and the normal venous return curve. Am J Physiol 1957; 189:609–15.

468. Scharf SM, Caldini P, Ingram RH Jr. Cardiovascular effects of increasing airway pressure in the dog. Am J Physiol 1977; 232:H35–43.

469. Jellinek H, Krenn H, Oczenski W, et al. Influence of positive airway pressure on the pressure gradient for venous return in humans. J Appl Physiol 2000; 88:926–32.

470. Fessler HE, Brower RG, Wise RA, Permutt S. Effects of positive end-expiratory pressure on the gradient for venous return. Am Rev Respir Dis 1991; 143:19–24.

471. Peters J, Hecker B, Neuser D, Schaden W. Regional blood volume distribution during positive and negative airway pressure breathing in supine humans. J Appl Physiol 1993; 75: 1740–7.

472. van den Berg PC, Jansen JR, Pinsky MR. Effect of positive pressure on venous return in volume-loaded cardiac surgical patients. J Appl Physiol 2002; 92:1223–31.

473. Nanas S, Magder S. Adaptations of the peripheral circulation to PEEP. Am Rev Respir Dis 1992; 146:688–93.

474. Sykes MK, Adams AP, Finlay WE, et al. The effects of variations in end-expiratory inflation pressure on cardiorespiratory function in normo-, hypo-and hypervolaemic dogs. Br J Anaesth 1970; 42:669–77.

475. Schreuder JJ, Jansen JR, Versprille A. Hemodynamic effects of PEEP applied as a ramp in normo-, hyper-, and hypovolemia. J Appl Physiol 1985; 59:1178–84.

476. Haynes JB, Carson SD, Whitney WP, et al. Positive end-expiratory pressure shifts in left ventricular diastolic pressure-area curves. J Appl Physiol 1980; 48:670–6.

477. Dhainaut JF, Devaux JY, Monsallier JF, et al. Mechanisms of decreased left ventricular preload during continuous positive pressure ventilation in ARDS. Chest 1986; 90:74–80.

478. Lemaire F, Teboul JL, Cinotti L, et al. Acute left ventricular dysfunction during unsuccessful weaning from mechanical ventilation. Anesthesiology 1988; 69:171–9.

479. Taylor RR, Covell JW, Sonnenblick EH, Ross J Jr. Dependence of ventricular distensibility on filling of the opposite ventricle. Am J Physiol 1967; 213:711–8.

480. Scharf SM, Brown R. Influence of the right ventricle on canine left ventricular function with PEEP. J Appl Physiol 1982; 52: 254–9.

481. Cassidy SS, Mitchell JH, Johnson RL Jr. Dimensional analysis of right and left ventricles during positive-pressure ventilation in dogs. Am J Physiol 1982; 242:H549–56.

482. Whittenberger JL, Mc Gregor M, Berglund E, Borst HG. Influence of state of inflation of the lung on pulmonary vascular resistance. J Appl Physiol 1960; 15:878–82.

483. Permutt S, Howell JB, Proctor DF, Riley RL. Effect of lung inflation on static pressure-volume characteristics of pulmonary vessels. J Appl Physiol 1961; 16:64–70.

484. Brower R, Wise RA, Hassapoyannes C, et al. Effect of lung inflation on lung blood volume and pulmonary venous flow. J Appl Physiol 1985; 58:954–63.

485. Vieillard-Baron A, Loubieres Y, Schmitt JM, et al. Cyclic changes in right ventricular output impedance during mechanical ventilation. J Appl Physiol 1999; 87:1644–50.

486. Artucio H, Hurtado J, Zimet L, et al. PEEP-induced tricuspid regurgitation. Intensive Care Med 1997; 23:836–40.

487. Culver BH, Marini JJ, Butler J. Lung volume and pleural pressure effects on ventricular function. J Appl Physiol 1981; 50:630–5.

488. Wise RAR, Bromberger-Barnea B, Permutt S. Effect of PEEP on left ventricular function in right-heart-bypassed dogs. J Appl Physiol 1981; 51:541–6.

489. Powers SR Jr, Dutton RE. Correlation of positive end-expiratory pressure with cardiovascular performance. Crit Care Med 1975; 3:64–8.

490. Patten MT, Liebman PR, Manny J, et al. Humorally mediated alterations in cardiac performance as a consequence of positive end-expiratory pressure. Surgery 1978; 84:201–5.

491. Manny J, Patten MT, Liebman PR, Hechtman HB. The association of lung distention, PEEP and biventricular failure. Ann Surg 1978; 187:151–7.

492. Calvin JE, Driedger AA, Sibbald WJ. Positive end-expiratory pressure (PEEP) does not depress left ventricular function in patients with pulmonary edema. Am Rev Respir Dis 1981; 124: 121–8.

493. Marini JJ, Culver BH, Butler J. Effect of positive end-expiratory pressure on canine ventricular function curves. J Appl Physiol 1981; 51:1367–74.

494. Fewell JE, Abendschein DR, Carlson CJ, et al. Continuous positive-pressure ventilation does not alter ventricular pressure-volume relationship. Am J Physiol 1981; 240: H821–6.

495. Cabrera MR, Nakamura GE, Montague DA, Cole RP. Effect of airway pressure on pericardial pressure. Am Rev Respir Dis 1989; 140:659–67.

496. O'Quin RJ, Marini JJ, Culver BH, Butler J. Transmission of airway pressure to pleural space during lung edema and chest wall restriction. J Appl Physiol 1985; 59:1171–7.

497. Chapin JC, Downs JB, Douglas ME, et al. Lung expansion, airway pressure transmission, and positive end-expiratory pressure. Arch Surg 1979; 114:1193–7.

498. Venus B, Cohen LE, Smith RA. Hemodynamics and intrathoracic pressure transmission during controlled mechanical ventilation and positive end-expiratory pressure in normal and low compliant lungs. Crit Care Med 1988; 16: 686–90.

499. Ranieri VM, Brienza N, Santostasi S, et al. Impairment of lung and chest wall mechanics in patients with acute respiratory distress syndrome: Role of abdominal distension. Am J Respir Crit Care Med 1997; 156:1082–91.

500. Miller RR, Vismara LA, Zelis R, et al. Clinical use of sodium nitroprusside in chronic ischemic heart disease: Effects on peripheral vascular resistance and venous tone and on ventricular volume, pump and mechanical performance. Circulation 1975; 51:328–36.

501. Summer WR, Permutt S, Sagawa K, et al. Effects of spontaneous respiration on canine left ventricular function. Circ Res 1979; 45:719–28.

502. Hall MJ, Ando S, Floras JS, Bradley TD. Magnitude and time course of hemodynamic responses to Mueller maneuvers in patients with congestive heart failure. J Appl Physiol 1998; 85: 1476–84.

503. Noble WH, Kay JC, Obdrzalek J. Lung mechanics in hypervolemic pulmonary edema. J Appl Physiol 1975; 38:681–7.

504. Bernard GR, Pou NA, Coggeshall JW, et al. Comparison of the pulmonary dysfunction caused by cardiogenic and noncardiogenic pulmonary edema. Chest 1995; 108:798–803.

505. Hogg JC, Agarawal JB, Gardiner AJ, et al. Distribution of airway resistance with developing pulmonary edema in dogs. J Appl Physiol 1972; 32:20–4.

506. Tang GJ, Freed AN. The role of submucosal oedema in increased peripheral airway resistance by intravenous volume loading in dogs. Eur Respir J 1994; 7:311–7.

507. Pellegrino R, Dellaca R, Macklem PT, et al. Effects of rapid saline infusion on lung mechanics and airway responsiveness in humans. J Appl Physiol 2003; 95:728–34.

508. Aubier M, Trippenbach T, Roussos C. Respiratory muscle fatigue during cardiogenic shock. J Appl Physiol 1981; 51:499–508.

509. Rutledge FS, Hussain SN, Roussos C, Magder S. Diaphragmatic energetics and blood flow during pulmonary edema and hypotension. J Appl Physiol 1988; 64:1908–15.

510. Lockhat D, Roussos C, Ianuzzo CD. Metabolite changes in the loaded hypoperfused and failing diaphragm. J Appl Physiol 1988; 65:1563–71.

511. Supinski GS. Respiratory muscle blood flow. Clin Chest Med 1988; 9:211–23.

512. Spec-Marn A, Tos L, Kremzar B, et al. Oxygen delivery-consumption relationship in adult respiratory distress syndrome patients: The effects of sepsis. J Crit Care 1993; 8:43–50.

513. Russell JA, Ronco JJ, Lockhat D, et al. Oxygen delivery and consumption and ventricular preload are greater in survivors than in nonsurvivors of the adult respiratory distress syndrome. Am Rev Respir Dis 1990; 141:659–65.

514. Steltzer H, Krafft P, Fridrich P, et al. Right ventricular function and oxygen transport patterns in patients with acute respiratory distress syndrome. Anaesthesia 1994; 49:1039–45.

515. Ranieri VM, Giuliani R, Eissa NT, et al. Oxygen delivery-consumption relationship in septic adult respiratory distress syndrome patients: The effects of positive end-expiratory pressure. J Crit Care 1992; 7:150–7.

516. Brienza A, Dambrosio M, Bruno F, et al. Right ventricular ejection fraction measurement in moderate acute respiratory failure (ARF): Effects of PEEP. Intensive Care Med 1988; 14:478–82.

517. Pinsky M, Vincent JL, De Smet JM. Estimating left ventricular filling pressure during positive end-expiratory pressure in humans. Am Rev Respir Dis 1991; 143:25–31.

518. Lloyd TC Jr. Effect of oleic acid injury on lung-heart interaction during ventricular filling. J Appl Physiol 1982; 52:1519–23.

519. Finch CA, Lenfant C. Oxygen transport in man. New Engl J Med 1972; 286:407–15.

520. Bruns FJ, Fraley DS, Haigh J, et al. Control of organ blood flow. In: Snyder JV, Pinsky MR, editors. Oxygen transport in the critically ill. Chicago: Year Book Medical Publishers, 1987: 87–124.

521. Astrand PO, Cuddy TE, Saltin B, Stenberg J. Cardiac output during submaximal and maximal work. J Appl Physiol 1964; 19:268–74.

522. Rowell LB. Human cardiovascular adjustments to exercise and thermal stress. Physiol Rev 1974; 54:75–159.

523. Shibutani K, Komatsu T, Kubal K, et al. Critical level of oxygen delivery in anesthetized man. Crit Care Med 1983; 11:640–3.

524. D'Orio V, Wahlen C, Naldi M, et al. Contribution of peripheral blood pooling to central hemodynamic disturbances during endotoxin insult in intact dogs. Crit Care Med 1989; 17: 1314–9.

525. Schumacker PT, Cain SM. The concept of a critical oxygen delivery. Intensive Care Med 1987; 13:223–9.

526. Nelson DP, Beyer C, Samsel RW, et al. Pathological supply dependence of O_2 uptake during bacteremia in dogs. J Appl Physiol 1987; 63:1487–92.

527. Nelson DP, Samsel RW, Wood LD, Schumacker PT. Pathological supply dependence of systemic and intestinal O_2 uptake during endotoxemia. J Appl Physiol 1988; 64:2410–9.

528. Danek SJ, Lynch JP, Weg JG, Dantzker DR. The dependence of oxygen uptake on oxygen delivery in the adult respiratory distress syndrome. Am Rev Respir Dis 1980; 122:387–95.

529. Vincent JL, Roman A, De Backer D, Kahn RJ. Oxygen uptake/supply dependency: Effects of short-term dobutamine infusion. Am Rev Respir Dis 1990; 142:2–7.

530. Clarke C, Edwards JD, Nightingale P, et al. Persistence of supply dependency of oxygen uptake at high levels of delivery in adult respiratory distress syndrome. Crit Care Med 1991; 19:497–502.

531. Kruse JA, Haupt MT, Puri VK, Carlson RW. Lactate levels as predictors of the relationship between oxygen delivery and consumption in ARDS. Chest 1990; 98:959–62.

532. Krachman SL, Lodato RF, Morice R, et al. Effects of dobutamine on oxygen transport and consumption in the adult respiratory distress syndrome. Intensive Care Med 1994; 20:130–7.

533. Mohsenifar Z, Goldbach P, Tashkin DP, Campisi DJ. Relationship between O_2 delivery and O_2 consumption in the adult respiratory distress syndrome. Chest 1983; 84:267–71.

534. Ronco JJ, Montaner JS, Fenwick JC, et al. Pathologic dependence of oxygen consumption on oxygen delivery in acute respiratory failure secondary to AIDS-related *Pneumocystis carinii* pneumonia. Chest 1990; 98:1463–6.

535. Weg JG. Oxygen transport in adult respiratory distress syndrome and other acute circulatory problems: Relationship of oxygen delivery and oxygen consumption. Crit Care Med 1991; 19:650–7.

536. Cain SM, Curtis SE. Experimental models of pathologic oxygen supply dependency. Crit Care Med 1991; 19:603–12.

537. Gutierrez G, Andry JM. Increased hemoglobin O_2 affinity does not improve O_2 consumption in hypoxemia. J Appl Physiol 1989; 66:837–43.

538. Schumacker PT, Samsel RW. Oxygen supply and consumption in the adult respiratory distress syndrome. Clin Chest Med 1990; 11:715–22.

539. Gilston A. PEEP and oxygen balance: Where are the emperor's clothes? Intensive Crit Care Dig 1990; 9:7–13.

540. Moreno LF, Stratton HH, Newell JC, Feustel PJ. Mathematical coupling of data: Correction of a common error for linear calculations. J Appl Physiol 1986; 60:335–43.

541. Stratton HH, Feustel PJ, Newell JC. Regression of calculated variables in the presence of shared measurement error. J Appl Physiol 1987; 62:2083–93.

542. Archie JP Jr. Mathematic coupling of data: A common source of error. Ann Surg 1981; 193:296–303.

543. Marik PE, Sibbald WJ. Effect of stored-blood transfusion on oxygen delivery in patients with sepsis. JAMA 1993; 269: 3024–9.

544. Annat G, Viale JP, Percival C, et al. Oxygen delivery and uptake in the adult respiratory distress syndrome: Lack of relationship when measured independently in patients with normal blood lactate concentrations. Am Rev Respir Dis 1986; 133:999–1001.

545. Ronco JJ, Phang PT, Walley KR, et al. Oxygen consumption is independent of changes in oxygen delivery in severe adult respiratory distress syndrome. Am Rev Respir Dis 1991; 143: 1267–73.

546. Hanique G, Dugernier T, Laterre PF, et al. Significance of pathologic oxygen supply dependency in critically ill patients: Comparison between measured and calculated methods. Intensive Care Med 1994; 20:12–8.

547. Ronco JJ, Fenwick JC, Wiggs BR, et al. Oxygen consumption is independent of increases in oxygen delivery by dobutamine in septic patients who have normal or increased plasma lactate. Am Rev Respir Dis 1993; 147:25–31.

548. Wysocki M, Besbes M, Roupie E, Brun-Buisson C. Modification of oxygen extraction ratio by change in oxygen transport in septic shock. Chest 1992; 102:221–6.

549. Hayes MA, Timmins AC, Yau EH, et al. Elevation of systemic oxygen delivery in the treatment of critically ill patients. New Engl J Med 1994; 330:1717–22.

550. Gattinoni L, Brazzi L, Pelosi P, et al. A trial of goal-oriented hemodynamic therapy in critically ill patients. $\overline{S}v_{O_2}$ Collaborative Group. New Engl J Med 1995; 333:1025–32.

551. Langeron O, Couture P, Mateo J, et al. Oxygen consumption and delivery relationship in brain-dead organ donors. Br J Anaesth 1996; 76:783–9.

552. Thorens JB, Jolliet P, Ritz M, Chevrolet JC. Effects of rapid permissive hypercapnia on hemodynamics, gas exchange, and oxygen transport and consumption during mechanical ventilation for the acute respiratory distress syndrome. Intensive Care Med 1996; 22:182–91.

553. Carvalho CR, Barbas CS, Medeiros DM, et al. Temporal hemodynamic effects of permissive hypercapnia associated with ideal PEEP in ARDS. Am J Respir Crit Care Med 1997; 156:1458–66.

554. Puybasset L, Stewart T, Rouby JJ, et al. Inhaled nitric oxide reverses the increase in pulmonary vascular resistance induced by permissive hypercapnia in patients with acute respiratory distress syndrome. Anesthesiology 1994; 80:1254–67.

555. Bersten AD, Gnidec AA, Rutledge FS, Sibbald WJ. Hyperdynamic sepsis modifies a PEEP-mediated redistribution in organ blood flows. Am Rev Respir Dis 1990; 141:1198–208.

556. Beyer J, Beckenlechner P, Messmer K. The influence of PEEP ventilation on organ blood flow and peripheral oxygen delivery. Intensive Care Med 1982; 8:75–80.

557. Venus B, Mathru M, Smith RA, et al. Renal function during application of positive end-expiratory pressure in swine: Effects of hydration. Anesthesiology 1985; 62:765–9.

558. Annat G, Viale JP, Bui Xuan B, et al. Effect of PEEP ventilation on renal function, plasma renin, aldosterone, neurophysins and urinary ADH, and prostaglandins. Anesthesiology 1983; 58: 136–41.

559. Andrivet PAS, Sanker SP. Chabrier E, et al. Hormonal interactions and renal function during mechanical ventilation and ANF infusion in humans. J Appl Physiol 1991; 70:287–92.

560. Gammanpila S, Bevan DR, Bhudu R. Effect of positive and negative expiratory pressure on renal function. Br J Anaesth 1977; 49:199–205.

561. Hemmer M, Suter PM. Treatment of cardiac and renal effects of PEEP with dopamine in patients with acute respiratory failure. Anesthesiology 1979; 50:399–403.

562. Jacob LP, Chazalet JJ, Payen DM, et al. Renal hemodynamic and functional effect of PEEP ventilation in human renal transplantations. Am J Respir Crit Care Med 1995; 152:103–7.

563. Jarnberg PO, de Villota ED, Eklund J, Granberg PO. Effects of positive end-expiratory pressure on renal function. Acta Anaesthesiol Scand 1978; 22:508–14.

564. Kaczmarczyk G, Vogel S, Krebs M, et al. Vasopressin and renin-angiotensin maintain arterial pressure during PEEP in nonexpanded, conscious dogs. Am J Physiol Regul Integr Comp Physiol 1996; 271:R1396–402.

565. Kaukinen S, Eerola R. Positive end expiratory pressure ventilation, renal function and renin. Ann Clin Res 1979; 11:58–62.

566. Kharasch ED, Yeo KT, Kenny MA, Buffington CW. Atrial natriuretic factor may mediate the renal effects of PEEP ventilation. Anesthesiology 1988; 69:862–9.

567. Andrivet PAS, Brun-Buisson C, Chabrier PE, et al. Involvement of ANF in the acute antidiuresis during PEEP ventilation. J Appl Physiol 1988; 65:1967–74.

568. Payen DM, Brun-Buisson CJ, Carli PA, et al. Hemodynamic, gas exchange, and hormonal consequences of LBPP during PEEP ventilation. J Appl Physiol 1987; 62:61–70.

569. Shirakami G, Magaribuchi T, Shingu K, et al. Positive end-expiratory pressure ventilation decreases plasma atrial and brain natriuretic peptide levels in humans. Anesth Analg 1993; 77:1116–21.

570. Rossaint RKM, Forther J, Unger V, et al. Inferior vena caval pressure increase contributes to sodium and water retention during PEEP in awake dogs. J Appl Physiol 1993; 75:2484–92.

571. Ramamoorthy C, Rooney MW, Dries DJ, Mathru M. Aggressive hydration during continuous positive-pressure ventilation restores atrial transmural pressure, plasma atrial natriuretic peptide concentrations, and renal function. Crit Care Med 1992; 20:1014–9.

572. Leithner C, Frass M, Pacher R, et al. Mechanical ventilation with positive end-expiratory pressure decreases release of alpha-atrial natriuretic peptide. Crit Care Med 1987; 15:484–8.

573. Payen DM, Farge D, Beloucif S, et al. No involvement of antidiuretic hormone in acute antidiuresis during PEEP ventilation in humans. Anesthesiology 1987; 66:17–23.

574. Boemke W, Krebs MO, Djalali K, et al. Renal nerves are not involved in sodium and water retention during mechanical ventilation in awake dogs. Anesthesiology 1998; 89: 942–53.

575. Christensen G, Bugge JF, Ostensen J, Kiil F. Atrial natriuretic factor and renal sodium excretion during ventilation with PEEP in hypervolemic dogs. J Appl Physiol 1992; 72:993–7.

576. Farge D, Beloucif S, Fratacci MD, Payen DM. Interactions between hemodynamic and hormonal modifications during PEEP-induced antidiuresis and antinatriuresis. Chest 1995; 107:1095–100.

577. Fewell JE, Bond GC. Renal denervation eliminates the renal response to continuous positive-pressure ventilation. Proc Soc Exp Biol Med 1979; 161:574–8.

578. Mullins RJ, Dawe EJ, Lucas CE, et al. Mechanisms of impaired renal function with PEEP. J Surg Res 1984; 37:189–96.

579. Priebe HJ, Hedley-Whyte J. Mechanisms of renal dysfunction during positive end-expiratory pressure ventilation. J Appl Physiol 1981; 50:643–9.

580. Rossaint R, Jorres D, Nienhaus M, et al. Positive end-expiratory pressure reduces renal excretion without hormonal activation after volume expansion in dogs. Anesthesiology 1992; 77: 700–8.

581. Aibiki M, Koyama S, Ogli K, Shirakawa Y. Reflex mechanisms for changes in renal nerve activity during positive end-expiratory pressure. J Appl Physiol 1988; 65:109–15.

582. Kaczmarczyk G, Rossaint R, Altmann C, et al. ACE inhibition facilitates sodium and water excretion during PEEP in conscious volume-expanded dogs. J Appl Physiol 1992; 73: 962–7.

583. Chernow B, Soldano S, Cook D, et al. Positive end-expiratory pressure increases plasma catecholamine levels in non-volume-loaded dogs. Anaesth Intensive Care 1986; 14:421–5.

584. Sha M, Saito Y, Yokoyama K, et al. Effects of continuous positive-pressure ventilation on hepatic blood flow and intrahepatic oxygen delivery in dogs. Crit Care Med 1987; 15:1040–3.

585. Steinberg S, Azar G, Love R, et al. Dopexamine prevents depression of mesenteric blood flow caused by positive end-expiratory pressure in rats. Surgery 1996; 120:597–601.

586. Kiefer P, Nunes S, Kosonen P, Takala J. Effect of positive end-expiratory pressure on splanchnic perfusion in acute lung injury. Intensive Care Med 2000; 26:376–83.

587. Brienza N, Revelly JP, Ayuse T, Robotham JL. Effects of PEEP on liver arterial and venous blood flows. Am J Respir Crit Care Med 1995; 152:504–10.

588. Fournell A, Schwarte LA, Kindgen-Milles D, et al. Assessment of microvascular oxygen saturation in gastric mucosa in volunteers breathing continuous positive airway pressure. Crit Care Med 2003; 31:1705–10.

589. Trager K, Radermacher P, Georgieff M. PEEP and hepatic metabolic performance in septic shock. Intensive Care Med 1996; 22:1274–5.

590. Cooper KR, Boswell PA. Reduced functional residual capacity and abnormal oxygenation in patients with severe head injury. Chest 1983; 84:29–35.

591. Holt J. The effect of positive and negative intrathoracic pressure on peripheral venous pressure in man. Am J Physiol 1943; 139:209–11.

592. Luce JM, Huseby JS, Kirk W, Butler J. Mechanism by which positive end-expiratory pressure increases cerebrospinal fluid pressure in dogs. J Appl Physiol 1982; 52:231–5.

593. Hormann C, Mohsenipour I, Gottardis M, Benzer A. Response of cerebrospinal fluid pressure to continuous positive airway pressure in volunteers. Anesth Analg 1994; 78:54–7.

594. Lodrini S, Montolivo M, Pluchino F, Borroni V. Positive end-expiratory pressure in supine and sitting positions: Its effects on intrathoracic and intracranial pressures. Neurosurgery 1989; 24:873–7.

595. Cooper KR, Boswell PA, Choi SC. Safe use of PEEP in patients with severe head injury. J Neurosurg 1985; 63:552–5.

596. McGuire G, Crossley D, Richards J, Wong D. Effects of varying levels of positive end-expiratory pressure on intracranial pressure and cerebral perfusion pressure. Crit Care Med 1997; 25:1059–62.

597. Videtta W, Villarejo F, Cohen M, et al. Effects of positive end-expiratory pressure on intracranial pressure and cerebral perfusion pressure. Acta Neurochir Suppl 2002; 81: 93–7.

598. Huynh T, Messer M, Sing RF, et al. Positive end-expiratory pressure alters intracranial and cerebral perfusion pressure in severe traumatic brain injury. J Trauma 2002; 53:488–92.

599. Georgiadis D, Schwarz S, Baumgartner RW, et al. Influence of positive end-expiratory pressure on intracranial pressure and cerebral perfusion pressure in patients with acute stroke. Stroke 2001; 32:2088–92.

600. Frost EA. Effects of positive end-expiratory pressure on intracranial pressure and compliance in brain-injured patients. J Neurosurg 1977; 47:195–200.

601. Baile EM, Albert RK, Kirk W, et al. Positive end-expiratory pressure decreases bronchial blood flow in the dog. J Appl Physiol 1984; 56:1289–93.

602. Cassidy SS, Haynes MS. The effects of ventilation with positive end-expiratory pressure on the bronchial circulation. Respir Physiol 1986; 66:269–78.

603. Agostoni P, Arena V, Biglioli P, et al. Increase of alveolar pressure reduces systemic-to-pulmonary bronchial blood flow in humans. Chest 1989; 96:1081–5.

604. Rossi A, Ranieri, MV. Positive end-expiratory pressure. In: Tobin M, editor. Principles and practice of mechanical ventilation. New York: McGraw-Hill, 1994.

605. Haider M, Schad H, Mendler N. Thoracic duct lymph and PEEP studies in anaesthetized dogs: II. Effect of a thoracic duct fistula on the development of a hyponcotic-hydrostatic pulmonary edema. Intensive Care Med 1987; 13:278–83.

606. Lakshminarayan S, Agostoni PG, Kirk W. Vagal cooling and positive end-expiratory pressure reduce systemic to pulmonary bronchial blood flow in dogs. Respiration 1990; 57:85–9.

607. van der Zee H, Cooper JA, Hakim TS, Malik AB. Alterations in pulmonary fluid balance induced by positive end-expiratory pressure. Respir Physiol 1986; 64:125–33.

608. Navalesi P, Hernandez P, Laporta D, et al. Influence of site of tracheal pressure measurement on in situ estimation of endotracheal tube resistance. J Appl Physiol 1994; 77:2899–906.

609. Valta P, Corbeil C, Lavoie A, et al. Detection of expiratory flow limitation during mechanical ventilation. Am J Respir Crit Care Med 1994; 150:1311–7.

610. Gay PC, Rodarte JR, Hubmayr RD. The effects of positive expiratory pressure on isovolume flow and dynamic hyperinflation in patients receiving mechanical ventilation. Am Rev Respir Dis 1989; 139:621–6.

611. Alvisi V, Romanello A, Badet M, et al. Time course of expiratory flow limitation in COPD patients during acute respiratory failure requiring mechanical ventilation. Chest 2003; 123:1625–32.

612. Ninane V, Leduc D, Kafi SA, et al. Detection of expiratory flow limitation by manual compression of the abdominal wall. Am J Respir Crit Care Med 2001; 163:1326–30.

613. Maltais F, Sovilj M, Goldberg P, Gottfried SB. Respiratory mechanics in status asthmaticus: Effects of inhalational anesthesia. Chest 1994; 106:1401–6.

614. Pellegrino R, Violante B, Nava S, et al. Expiratory airflow limitation and hyperinflation during methacholine-induced bronchoconstriction. J Appl Physiol 1993; 75:1720–7.

615. Ferretti A, Giampiccolo P, Cavalli A, et al. Expiratory flow limitation and orthopnea in massively obese subjects. Chest 2001; 119:1401–8.

616. Marini JJ. Auto-positive end-expiratory pressure and flow limitation in adult respiratory distress syndrome: Intrinsically different? Crit Care Med 2002; 30:2140–1.

617. Gottfried SB, Reissman H, Ranieri VM. A simple method for the measurement of intrinsic positive end-expiratory pressure during controlled and assisted modes of mechanical ventilation. Crit Care Med 1992; 20:621–9.

618. Leatherman JW, Ravenscraft SA. Low measured auto-positive end-expiratory pressure during mechanical ventilation of patients with severe asthma: hidden auto-positive end-expiratory pressure. Crit Care Med 1996; 24:541–6.

619. Haluszka J, Chartrand DA, Grassino AE, Milic-Emili J. Intrinsic PEEP and arterial P_{CO_2} in stable patients with chronic obstructive pulmonary disease. Am Rev Respir Dis 1990; 141: 1194–7.

620. Hernandez P, Navalesi P, Maltais F, et al. Comparison of static and dynamic measurements of intrinsic PEEP in anesthetized cats. J Appl Physiol 1994; 76:2437–42.

621. Maltais F, Reissmann H, Navalesi P, et al. Comparison of static and dynamic measurements of intrinsic PEEP in mechanically ventilated patients. Am J Respir Crit Care Med 1994; 150: 1318–24.

622. Jubran A, Laghi F, Mazur M, et al. Partitioning of lung and chest-wall mechanics before and after lung-volume-reduction surgery. Am J Respir Crit Care Med 1998; 158:306–10.

623. Yan S, Kayser B, Tobiasz M, Sliwinski P. Comparison of static and dynamic intrinsic positive end-expiratory pressure using the Campbell diagram. Am J Respir Crit Care Med 1996; 154: 938–44.

624. Fleury B, Murciano D, Talamo C, et al. Work of breathing in patients with chronic obstructive pulmonary disease in acute respiratory failure. Am Rev Respir Dis 1985; 131:822–7.

625. MacIntyre NR, Cheng KC, McConnell R. Applied PEEP during pressure support reduces the inspiratory threshold load of intrinsic PEEP. Chest 1997; 111:188–93.

626. Ninane V, Rypens F, Yernault JC, De Troyer A. Abdominal muscle use during breathing in patients with chronic airflow obstruction. Am Rev Respir Dis 1992; 146:16–21.

627. Ninane V, Yernault JC, de Troyer A. Intrinsic PEEP in patients with chronic obstructive pulmonary disease: Role of expiratory muscles. Am Rev Respir Dis 1993; 148:1037–42.

628. Gorini M, Misuri G, Duranti R, et al. Abdominal muscle recruitment and $PEEP_I$ during bronchoconstriction in chronic obstructive pulmonary disease. Thorax 1997; 52:355–61.

629. Zakynthinos SG, Vassilakopoulos T, Zakynthinos E, Roussos C. Accurate measurement of intrinsic positive end-expiratory pressure: how to detect and correct for expiratory muscle activity. Eur Respir J 1997; 10:522–9.

630. Zakynthinos SG, Vassilakopoulos T, Zakynthinos E, et al. Contribution of expiratory muscle pressure to dynamic intrinsic positive end-expiratory pressure: Validation using the Campbell diagram. Am J Respir Crit Care Med 2000; 162:1633–40.

631. Zakynthinos SG, Vassilakopoulos T, Zakynthinos E, et al. Correcting static intrinsic positive end-expiratory pressure for expiratory muscle contraction: Validation of a new method. Am J Respir Crit Care Med 1999; 160:785–90.

632. Cole AG, Weller SF, Sykes MK. Inverse ratio ventilation compared with PEEP in adult respiratory failure. Intensive Care Med 1984; 10:227–32.

633. Connery LE, Deignan MJ, Gujer MW, Richardson MG. Cardiovascular collapse associated with extreme iatrogenic $PEEP_I$ in patients with obstructive airways disease. Br J Anaesth 1999; 83:493–5.

634. Dal Vecchio L, Polese G, Poggi R, Rossi A. "Intrinsic" positive end-expiratory pressure in stable patients with chronic obstructive pulmonary disease. Eur Respir J 1990; 3:74–80.

635. Chen RC, Yan S. Perceived inspiratory difficulty during inspiratory threshold and hyperinflationary loadings. Am J Respir Crit Care Med 1999; 159:720–7.

636. Appendini L. About the relevance of dynamic intrinsic PEEP ($PEEP_{I,dyn}$) measurement. Intensive Care Med 1999; 25: 252–4.

637. Appendini L, Purro A, Gudjonsdottir M, et al. Physiologic response of ventilator-dependent patients with chronic obstructive pulmonary disease to proportional assist ventilation and continuous positive airway pressure. Am J Respir Crit Care Med 1999; 159:1510–7.

638. Brochard L. Intrinsic (or auto-) positive end-expiratory pressure during spontaneous or assisted ventilation. Intensive Care Med 2002; 28:1552–4.

639. Sydow M, Golisch W, Buscher H, et al. Effect of low-level PEEP on inspiratory work of breathing in intubated patients, both with healthy lungs and with COPD. Intensive Care Med 1995; 21:887–95.

640. Fernandez R, Benito S, Blanch L, Net A. Intrinsic PEEP: A cause of inspiratory muscle ineffectivity. Intensive Care Med 1988; 15:51–2.

641. Leung P, Jubran A, Tobin MJ. Comparison of assisted ventilator modes on triggering, patient effort, and dyspnea. Am J Respir Crit Care Med 1997; 155:1940–8.

642. Nava S, Ambrosino N, Bruschi C, et al. Physiological effects of flow and pressure triggering during non-invasive mechanical ventilation in patients with chronic obstructive pulmonary disease. Thorax 1997; 52:249–54.

643. Kim H, Bach JR. Central alveolar hypoventilation in neurosarcoidosis. Arch Phys Med Rehabil 1998; 79:1467–8.

644. Smith J, Bellemare F. Effect of lung volume on in vivo contraction characteristics of human diaphragm. J Appl Physiol 1987; 62:1893–900.

645. Collett PW, Engel LA. Influence of lung volume on oxygen cost of resistive breathing. J Appl Physiol 1986; 61:16–24.

646. Beck J, Sinderby C, Lindstrom L, Grassino A. Effects of lung volume on diaphragm EMG signal strength during voluntary contractions. J Appl Physiol 1998; 85:1123–34.

647. Kawagoe Y, Permutt S, Fessler HE. Hyperinflation with intrinsic PEEP and respiratory muscle blood flow. J Appl Physiol 1994; 77:2440–8.

648. Orozco-Levi M, Lloreta J, Minguella J, et al. Injury of the human diaphragm associated with exertion and chronic obstructive pulmonary disease. Am J Respir Crit Care Med 2001; 164:1734–9.

649. Ranieri VM, Dambrosio M, Brienza N. Intrinsic PEEP and cardiopulmonary interaction in patients with COPD and acute ventilatory failure. Eur Respir J 1996; 9:1283–92.

650. Coussa ML, Guerin C, Eissa NT, et al. Partitioning of work of breathing in mechanically ventilated COPD patients. J Appl Physiol 1993; 75:1711–9.

651. Jubran A, Tobin MJ. Pathophysiologic basis of acute respiratory distress in patients who fail a trial of weaning from mechanical ventilation. Am J Respir Crit Care Med 1997; 155:906–15.

652. Vassilakopoulos T, Zakynthinos S, Roussos C. The tension-time index and the frequency/tidal volume ratio are the major pathophysiologic determinants of weaning failure and success. Am J Respir Crit Care Med 1998; 158:378–85.

653. Marini JJ. Should PEEP be used in airflow obstruction? Am Rev Respir Dis 1989; 140:1–3.

654. Pride NB, Permutt S, Riley RL, Bromberger-Barnea B. Determinants of maximal expiratory flow from the lungs. J Appl Physiol 1967; 23:646–62.

655. Tobin MJ, Lodato RF. PEEP, auto-PEEP, and waterfalls. Chest 1989; 96:449–51.

656. Reissmann HK, Ranieri VM, Goldberg P, Gottfried SB. Continuous positive airway pressure facilitates spontaneous breathing in weaning chronic obstructive pulmonary disease patients by improving breathing pattern and gas exchange. Intensive Care Med 2000; 26:1764–72.

657. Baigorri F, de Monte A, Blanch L, et al. Hemodynamic responses to external counterbalancing of auto-positive end-expiratory pressure in mechanically ventilated patients with chronic obstructive pulmonary disease. Crit Care Med 1994; 22:1782–91.

658. Tan IK, Bhatt SB, Tam YH, Oh TE. Effects of PEEP on dynamic hyperinflation in patients with airflow limitation. Br J Anaesth 1993; 70:267–72.

659. Mancini M, Zavala E, Mancebo J, et al. Mechanisms of pulmonary gas exchange improvement during a protective ventilatory strategy in acute respiratory distress syndrome. Am J Respir Crit Care Med 2001; 164:1448–53.

660. Halter JM, Steinberg JM, Schiller HJ, et al. Positive end-expiratory pressure after a recruitment maneuver prevents both alveolar collapse and recruitment/derecruitment. Am J Respir Crit Care Med 2003; 167:1620–6.

661. Artigas A, Bernard GR, Carlet J, et al. The American-European Consensus Conference on ARDS: 2. Ventilatory, pharmacologic, supportive therapy, study design strategies, and issues related to recovery and remodeling—Acute respiratory distress syndrome. Am J Respir Crit Care Med 1998; 157:1332–47.

662. Pepe PE, Hudson LD, Carrico CJ. Early application of positive end-expiratory pressure in patients at risk for the adult respiratory-distress syndrome. New Engl J Med 1984; 311:281–6.

663. Springer RR, Stevens PM. The influence of PEEP on survival of patients in respiratory failure: A retrospective analysis. Am J Med 1979; 66:196–200.

664. Brower RG, Lanken PN, MacIntyre N, et al. Higher versus lower positive end-expiratory pressures in patients with the acute respiratory distress syndrome. New Engl J Med 2004; 351:327–36.

665. Tobin MJ. Culmination of an era in research on the acute respiratory distress syndrome. New Engl J Med 2000; 342:1360–1.

666. de Durante G, del Turco M, Rustichini L, et al. ARDSNet lower tidal volume ventilatory strategy may generate intrinsic positive end-expiratory pressure in patients with acute respiratory distress syndrome. Am J Respir Crit Care Med 2002; 165: 1271–4.

667. Richard JC, Brochard L, Breton L, et al. Influence of respiratory rate on gas trapping during low volume ventilation of patients with acute lung injury. Intensive Care Med 2002; 28:1078–83.

668. Gattinoni L, Caironi P, Carlesso E. How to ventilate patients with acute lung injury and acute respiratory distress syndrome. Curr Opin Crit Care 2005; 11:69–76.

669. Levy MM. PEEP in ARDS—How much is enough? New Engl J Med 2004; 351:389–91.

670. Ferguson ND, Frutos-Vivar F, Esteban A, et al. Airway pressures, tidal volumes, and mortality in patients with acute respiratory distress syndrome. Crit Care Med 2005; 33:21–30.

671. Downs JB, Klein EF Jr, Modell JH. The effect of incremental PEEP on Pa_{O_2} in patients with respiratory failure. Anesth Analg 1973; 52:210–5.

672. Gallagher TJ, Civetta JM, Kirby RR. Terminology update: Optimal PEEP. Crit Care Med 1978; 6:323–6.

673. Hartmann M, Rosberg B, Jonsson K. The influence of different levels of PEEP on peripheral tissue perfusion measured by subcutaneous and transcutaneous oxygen tension. Intensive Care Med 1992; 18:474–8.

674. Hurewitz A, Bergofsky EH. Adult respiratory distress syndrome: Physiologic basis of treatment. Med Clin North Am 1981; 65:33–51.

675. Weisman IM, Rinaldo JE, Rogers RM. Current concepts: Positive end-expiratory pressure in adult respiratory failure. New Engl J Med 1982; 307:1381–4.

676. Murray IP, Modell JH, Gallagher TJ, Banner MJ. Titration of PEEP by the arterial minus end-tidal carbon dioxide gradient. Chest 1984; 85:100–4.

677. Ranieri VM, Zhang H, Mascia L, et al. Pressure-time curve predicts minimally injurious ventilatory strategy in an isolated rat lung model. Anesthesiology 2000; 93:1320–8.

678. Lindberg P, Gunnarsson L, Tokics L, et al. Atelectasis and lung function in the postoperative period. Acta Anaesthesiol Scand 1992; 36:546–53.

679. Arozullah AM, Daley J, Henderson WG, Khuri SF. Multifactorial risk index for predicting postoperative respiratory failure in men after major noncardiac surgery. The National Veterans Administration Surgical Quality Improvement Program. Ann Surg 2000; 232:242–53.

680. O'Donohue WJ Jr. National survey of the usage of lung expansion modalities for the prevention and treatment of postoperative atelectasis following abdominal and thoracic surgery. Chest 1985; 87:76–80.

681. Thompson JS, Baxter BT, Allison JG, et al. Temporal patterns of postoperative complications. Arch Surg 2003; 138:596–602.

682. Lang M, Niskanen M, Miettinen P, et al. Outcome and resource utilization in gastroenterological surgery. Br J Surg 2001; 88:1006–14.

683. Pasquina P, Merlani P, Granier JM, Ricou B. Continuous positive airway pressure versus noninvasive pressure support ventilation to treat atelectasis after cardiac surgery. Anesth Analg 2004; 99:1001–8.

684. Stock MC, Downs JB, Gauer PK, et al. Prevention of postoperative pulmonary complications with CPAP, incentive spirometry, and conservative therapy. Chest 1985; 87:151–7.

685. Dehaven CB Jr, Hurst JM, Branson RD. Postextubation hypoxemia treated with a continuous positive airway pressure mask. Crit Care Med 1985; 13:46–8.

686. Lindner KH, Lotz P, Ahnefeld FW. Continuous positive airway pressure effect on functional residual capacity, vital capacity and its subdivisions. Chest 1987; 92:66–70.

687. Ricksten SE, Bengtsson A, Soderberg C, et al. Effects of periodic positive airway pressure by mask on postoperative pulmonary function. Chest 1986; 89:774–81.

688. Huerta S, DeShields S, Shpiner R, et al. Safety and efficacy of postoperative continuous positive airway pressure to prevent pulmonary complications after roux-en-Y gastric bypass. J Gastrointest Surg 2002; 6:354–8.

689. van Kaam AH, Lachmann RA, Herting E, et al. Reducing atelectasis attenuates bacterial growth and translocation in experimental pneumonia. Am J Respir Crit Care Med 2004; 169:1046–53.

690. Duggan M, McCaul CL, McNamara PJ, et al. Atelectasis causes vascular leak and lethal right ventricular failure in uninjured rat lungs. Am J Respir Crit Care Med 2003; 167:1633–40.

691. Drummond GB, Stedul K, Kingshott R, et al. Automatic CPAP compared with conventional treatment for episodic hypoxemia and sleep disturbance after major abdominal surgery. Anesthesiology 2002; 96:817–26.

692. Carlsson C, Sonden B, Thylen U. Can postoperative continuous positive airway pressure (CPAP) prevent pulmonary complications after abdominal surgery? Intensive Care Med 1981; 7:225–9.

693. Pinilla JC, Oleniuk FH, Tan L, et al. Use of a nasal continuous positive airway pressure mask in the treatment of postoperative atelectasis in aortocoronary bypass surgery. Crit Care Med 1990; 18:836–40.

694. Jousela I, Rasanen J, Verkkala K, et al. Continuous positive airway pressure by mask in patients after coronary surgery. Acta Anaesthesiol Scand 1994; 38:311–6.

695. Fagevik Olsen M, Wennberg E, Johnsson E, et al. Randomized clinical study of the prevention of pulmonary complications

after thoracoabdominal resection by two different breathing techniques. Br J Surg 2002; 89:1228–34.

696. Squadrone V, Coha M, Cerutti E, et al. Continuous positive airway pressure for treatment of postoperative hypoxemia: A randomized, controlled trial. JAMA 2005; 293:589–95.

697. Similowski T, Milic-Emili J, Derenne JP. Respiratory mechanics during acute respiratory failure of chronic obstructive pulmonary disease. In: Derenne JP, Whitelaw WA, Similowski T, editors. Acute respiratory failure in chronic obstructive pulmonary disease. New York: Marcel Dekker, 1996: 23–46.

698. Nava S, Navalesi P. Bronchodilators and mechanical ventilation in COPD patients. Emptying, pumping or both? Intensive Care Med 1999; 25:1206–8.

699. Soto FJ, Varkey B. Evidence-based approach to acute exacerbations of COPD. Curr Opin Pulm Med 2003; 9:117–24.

700. Sherk PA, Grossman RF. The chronic obstructive pulmonary disease exacerbation. Clin Chest Med 2000; 21:705–21.

701. Lu CC. Bronchodilator therapy for chronic obstructive pulmonary disease. Respirology 1997; 2:317–22.

702. Bach PB, Brown C, Gelfand SE, McCrory DC. Management of acute exacerbations of chronic obstructive pulmonary disease: A summary and appraisal of published evidence. Ann Intern Med 2001; 134:600–20.

703. Niewoehner DE, Erbland ML, Deupree RH, et al. Effect of systemic glucocorticoids on exacerbations of chronic obstructive pulmonary disease. Department of Veterans Affairs Cooperative Study Group. New Engl J Med 1999; 340:1941–7.

704. Dhand R, Duarte AG, Jubran A, et al. Dose-response to bronchodilator delivered by metered-dose inhaler in ventilator-supported patients. Am J Respir Crit Care Med 1996; 154:388–93.

705. Mouloudi E, Katsanoulas K, Anastasaki M, et al. Bronchodilator delivery by metered-dose inhaler in mechanically ventilated COPD patients: Influence of tidal volume. Intensive Care Med 1999; 25:1215–21.

706. Mouloudi E, Maliotakis C, Kondili E, et al. Duration of salbutamol-induced bronchodilation delivered by metered-dose inhaler in mechanically ventilated COPD patients. Monaldi Arch Chest Dis 2001; 56:189–94.

707. Mouloudi E, Prinianakis G, Kondili E, Georgopoulos D. Effect of inspiratory flow rate on β_2-agonist-induced bronchodilation in mechanically ventilated COPD patients. Intensive Care Med 2001; 27:42–6.

708. Rubini F, Rampulla C, Nava S. Acute effect of corticosteroids on respiratory mechanics in mechanically ventilated patients with chronic airflow obstruction and acute respiratory failure. Am J Respir Crit Care Med 1994; 149:306–10.

709. Guerin C, Chevre A, Dessirier P, et al. Inhaled fenoterol-ipratropium bromide in mechanically ventilated patients with chronic obstructive pulmonary disease. Am J Respir Crit Care Med 1999; 159:1036–42.

710. Fink JB, Dhand R, Duarte AG, et al. Aerosol delivery from a metered-dose inhaler during mechanical ventilation: An in vitro model. Am J Respir Crit Care Med 1996; 154:382–7.

711. Celikel T, Sungur M, Ceyhan B, Karakurt S. Comparison of non-invasive positive pressure ventilation with standard medical therapy in hypercapnic acute respiratory failure. Chest 1998; 114:1636–42.

712. Plant PK, Owen JL, Elliott MW. Early use of non-invasive ventilation for acute exacerbations of chronic obstructive pulmonary disease on general respiratory wards: A multicentre randomised controlled trial. Lancet 2000; 355:1931–5.

713. Conti G, Antonelli M, Navalesi P, et al. Noninvasive vs conventional mechanical ventilation in patients with chronic obstructive pulmonary disease after failure of medical treatment in the ward: A randomized trial. Intensive Care Med 2002; 28:1701–7.

714. Sinderby C, Navalesi P, Beck J, et al. Neural control of mechanical ventilation in respiratory failure. Nature Med 1999; 5:1433–6.

715. Hill AR. Respiratory muscle function in asthma. J Assoc Acad Minor Phys 1991; 2:100–8.

716. Peigang Y, Marini JJ. Ventilation of patients with asthma and chronic obstructive pulmonary disease. Curr Opin Crit Care 2002; 8:70–6.

717. Shivaram U, Donath J, Khan FA, Juliano J. Effects of continuous positive airway pressure in acute asthma. Respiration 1987; 52:157–62.

718. Shivaram U, Miro AM, Cash ME, et al. Cardiopulmonary responses to continuous positive airway pressure in acute asthma. J Crit Care 1993; 8:87–92.

719. Lougheed DM, Webb KA, O'Donnell DE. Breathlessness during induced lung hyperinflation in asthma: The role of the inspiratory threshold load. Am J Respir Crit Care Med 1995; 152:911–20.

720. Lin HC, Wang CH, Yang CT, et al. Effect of nasal continuous positive airway pressure on methacholine-induced bronchoconstriction. Respir Med 1995; 89:121–8.

721. Martin JG, Shore S, Engel LA. Effect of continuous positive airway pressure on respiratory mechanics and pattern of breathing in induced asthma. Am Rev Respir Dis 1982; 126:812–7.

722. Meduri GU, Cook TR, Turner RE, et al. Noninvasive positive pressure ventilation in status asthmaticus. Chest 1996; 110:767–74.

723. Soroksky A, Stav D, Shpirer I. A pilot prospective, randomized, placebo-controlled trial of bilevel positive airway pressure in acute asthmatic attack. Chest 2003; 123:1018–25.

724. Moritz F, Benichou J, Vanheste M, et al. Boussignac continuous positive airway pressure device in the emergency care of acute cardiogenic pulmonary oedema: A randomized pilot study. Eur J Emerg Med 2003; 10:204–8.

725. Bellone A, Monari A, Cortellaro F, et al. Myocardial infarction rate in acute pulmonary edema: Noninvasive pressure support ventilation versus continuous positive airway pressure. Crit Care Med 2004; 32:1860–5.

726. Crane SD, Elliott MW, Gilligan P, et al. Randomised, controlled comparison of continuous positive airways pressure, bilevel non-invasive ventilation, and standard treatment in emergency department patients with acute cardiogenic pulmonary oedema. Emerg Med J 2004; 21:155–61.

727. Park M, Sangean MC, Volpe Mde S, et al. Randomized, prospective trial of oxygen, continuous positive airway pressure, and bilevel positive airway pressure by face mask in acute cardiogenic pulmonary edema. Crit Care Med 2004; 32:2407–15.

728. Schmidt GB, O'Neill WW, Kotb K, et al. Continuous positive airway pressure in the prophylaxis of the adult respiratory distress syndrome. Surg Gynecol Obstet 1976; 143:613–8.

729. Shah DM, Powers SR Jr. Prevention of pulmonary complications in high risk patients. Surg Clin North Am 1980; 60:1359–72.

730. Weigelt JA, Mitchell RA, Snyder WH 3d. Early positive end-expiratory pressure in the adult respiratory distress syndrome. Arch Surg 1979; 114:497–501.

731. McAslan TC, Cowley RA. The preventive use of PEEP in major trauma. Am Surg 1979; 45:159–67.

732. Demling RH. Improved survival after massive burns. J Trauma 1983; 23:179–84.

733. Goris RJ, Gimbrere JS, van Niekerk JL, et al. Early osteosynthesis and prophylactic mechanical ventilation in the multitrauma patient. J Trauma 1982; 22:895–903.

734. Askanazi J, Wax SD, Neville JF Jr, et al. Prevention of pulmonary insufficiency through prophylactic use of PEEP and rapid respiratory rates. J Thorac Cardiovasc Surg 1978; 75:267–72.

735. Barash PG, Bunke MC, Tilson MD, et al. The salutary effects of positive end expiratory pressure (PEEP) in experimentally

induced pseudomonas pneumonia. Anesth Analg 1979; 58: 208–15.

736. Luce JM, Robertson HT, Huang T, et al. The effects of expiratory positive airway pressure on the resolution of oleic acid-induced lung injury in dogs. Am Rev Respir Dis 1982; 125:716–22.

737. Valdes ME, Powers SR Jr, Shah DM, et al. Continuous positive airway pressure in prophylaxis of adult respiratory distress syndrome in trauma patients. Surg Forum 1978; 29: 187–9.

738. Maitre B, Jaber S, Maggiore SM, et al. Continuous positive airway pressure during fiberoptic bronchoscopy in hypoxemic patients: A randomized double-blind study using a new device. Am J Respir Crit Care Med 2000; 162:1063–7.

739. Gachot B, Clair B, Wolff M, et al. Continuous positive airway pressure by face mask or mechanical ventilation in patients with human immunodeficiency virus infection and severe *Pneumocystis carinii* pneumonia. Intensive Care Med 1992; 18: 155–9.

740. Hilbert G, Gruson D, Vargas F, et al. Noninvasive continuous positive airway pressure in neutropenic patients with acute respiratory failure requiring intensive care unit admission. Crit Care Med 2000; 28:3185–90.

741. Joris JL, Sottiaux TM, Chiche JD, et al. Effect of bi-level positive airway pressure (BiPAP) nasal ventilation on the postoperative pulmonary restrictive syndrome in obese patients undergoing gastroplasty. Chest 1997; 111:665–70.

742. Lindholm CE, Ollman B, Snyder JV, et al. Cardiorespiratory effects of flexible fiberoptic bronchoscopy in critically ill patients. Chest 1978; 74:362–8.

743. Matsushima Y, Jones RL, King EG, et al. Alterations in pulmonary mechanics and gas exchange during routine fiberoptic bronchoscopy. Chest 1984; 86:184–8.

744. Verra F, Hmouda H, Rauss A, et al. Bronchoalveolar lavage in immunocompromised patients: Clinical and functional consequences. Chest 1992; 101:1215–20.

745. Valenza F, Guglielmi M, Irace M, et al. Positive end-expiratory pressure delays the progression of lung injury during ventilator strategies involving high airway pressure and lung overdistention. Crit Care Med 2003; 31:1993–8.

746. Gajic O, Dara SI, Mendez JL, et al. Ventilator-associated lung injury in patients without acute lung injury at the onset of mechanical ventilation. Crit Care Med 2004; 32: 1817–24.

747. Pierce C. How to make our ideas clear. Popular Science Monthly 1878 January.

PART V
ALTERNATIVE METHODS OF VENTILATOR SUPPORT

Chapter 12
AIRWAY PRESSURE-RELEASE VENTILATION

CHRISTIAN PUTENSEN
HERMANN WRIGGE

Controlled mechanical ventilation (CMV) traditionally is provided via an artificial airway to completely unload a patient's work of breathing and ensure adequate gas exchange during the acute phase of respiratory insufficiency until the underlying respiratory function has resolved.[1] The criteria used to determine when to terminate mechanical ventilation essentially are based on the clinical and often subjective assessment by the intensive-care physician or by standardized weaning methods.[2,3] The actual process of weaning the patient from CMV is carried out by allowing spontaneous breathing attempts with a T piece or continuous positive airway pressure (CPAP) or by gradually reducing mechanical assistance.[4,5] Not surprisingly, gradual reduction of partial ventilator support has been shown to benefit only patients who have difficulty in sustaining unassisted breathing.[4] Although introduced as weaning techniques, partial support modes have become standard methods of providing primary mechanical ventilatory support in critically ill patients.

Basic Principles of Airway Pressure-Release Ventilation

Airway pressure-release ventilation (APRV)[6] ventilates by time-cycled switching between two pressure levels in a high-flow (or demand-valve) CPAP circuit, and therefore, unrestricted spontaneous breathing is permitted in any phase of the mechanical ventilator cycle (Fig. 12-1). The degree of ventilator support with APRV is determined by the duration of the two CPAP levels and the mechanically delivered tidal volume (V_T).[6,7] V_T depends mainly on respiratory compliance and the difference between the CPAP levels. By design, changes in ventilatory demand do not alter the level of mechanical support during APRV. When spontaneous breathing is absent, APRV is not different from conventional pressure-controlled, time-cycled mechanical ventilation.[7,8]

Synonyms used for APRV are *biphasic positive airway pressure* (BiPAP)[7] and bilevel airway pressure (bilevel). BiPAP is identical to APRV except that no restriction is imposed on the duration of the low CPAP level (release pressure).[8] Based on the initial description, APRV keeps the duration of the low CPAP level (release time) at 1.5 seconds or less.

Physiologic Effects

VENTILATION DISTRIBUTIONS

Radiologic studies demonstrate that ventilation is distributed differently during pure spontaneous breathing and CMV.[9] During spontaneous breathing, the posterior muscular sections of the diaphragm move more than the anterior tendon plate.[9] Consequently, when patients are supine, the dependent lung regions tend to be better ventilated during spontaneous breathing (Fig. 12-2). If the diaphragm is relaxed, it will be moved by the weight of the abdominal cavity and intra-abdominal pressure toward the cranium; mechanical V_T will be distributed more to the anterior, nondependent, and less perfused lung regions.[10] When compared with spontaneous breathing, the latter leads to lung areas in the dorsal lung regions close to the diaphragm being less ventilated (or atelectatic) in both patients with healthy

CPAP_{high}

$\Delta FRC = V_T$

CPAP_{low}

T_{low} T_{high}

Determinants of V_T
- ΔP_{aw}
- Compliance
- Resistance

FIGURE 12-1 Airway pressure-release ventilation ventilates by time-cycled switching between a high and low level of continuous positive airway pressure (CPAP) in the circuit. Thus unrestricted spontaneous breathing is permitted in any phase of the mechanical ventilator cycle. Change between the two CPAP levels results in a change in functional residual capacity (ΔFRC) that equals the mechanical delivered tidal volume (V_T). V_T depends mainly on respiratory compliance and resistance and the airway pressure difference (ΔPaw) between the CPAP levels. Setting the time for the low (T_{low}) and high (T_{high}) CPAP produces adjustment of the ventilator rate.

lungs and patients undergoing mechanical ventilation. Recent results demonstrate that the posterior muscular sections of the diaphragm move more than the anterior tendon plate when large breaths or sighs are present during spontaneous breathing.[11]

Computed tomography (CT) of patients with acute respiratory distress syndrome (ARDS) reveals radiographic densities corresponding to alveolar collapse localized primarily in the dependent lung regions, which correlates with intrapulmonary shunting and accounts entirely for the observed arterial hypoxemia.[12,13] Formation of radiographic densities is attributed to alveolar collapse caused by superimposed pressure on the lung and a cephalad shift of the diaphragm, most evident in dependent lung areas during CMV.[14] The cephalad shift of the diaphragm may be even more pronounced in patients with extrapulmonary induced ARDS, in whom an increase in intra-abdominal pressure is invariably observed. Persisting spontaneous breathing is considered to improve the distribution of ventilation to dependent lung areas and thereby improve ventilation-perfusion ($\dot{V}_A/\dot{Q}$) matching, presumably by diaphragmatic contraction that opposes alveolar compression.[9,15] This concept

is supported by CT observations in anesthetized patients demonstrating that contractions of the diaphragm induced by phrenic nerve stimulation favor distribution of ventilation to dependent, well-perfused lung areas, decreasing atelectasis formation.[16]

Spontaneous breathing with APRV in experimental induced lung injury is associated with less atelectasis formation on end-expiratory spiral CT of the whole lungs and on CT scans above the diaphragm[17] (Fig. 12-3). Although other inspiratory muscles may contribute to improvement in aeration during spontaneous breathing, the craniocaudal gradient in aeration, aeration differences, and the marked differences in aeration in regions close to the diaphragm between APRV with and without spontaneous breathing suggest that diaphragmatic contractions play a dominant role in the observed aeration differences.[17] Spontaneous breathing results in significant improvement of end-expiratory lung volume in experimental lung injury.[17] Experimental data suggest that recruitment of dependent lung areas may be caused essentially by an increase in transpulmonary pressure secondary to the decrease in pleural pressure with spontaneous breathing during APRV.[18]

PULMONARY GAS EXCHANGE

In patients with ARDS, APRV with spontaneous breathing of 10–30% of the total minute ventilation ($\dot{V}_E$) accounts for an improvement in $\dot{V}_A/\dot{Q}$ matching, intrapulmonary shunting, and arterial oxygenation.[15] These results confirm earlier investigations in animals with induced lung injury[19–21] that demonstrated improvement in intrapulmonary shunt and arterial oxygenation during spontaneous breathing with APRV. An increase in arterial oxygenation in conjunction with greater pulmonary compliance indicates recruitment of previously nonventilated lung areas. Clinical studies in patients with ARDS show that spontaneous breathing during APRV does not necessarily lead to instant improvement in gas exchange. Instead, improvement in oxygenation continues over the 24 hours after the start of spontaneous breathing.[22]

In patients at risk of developing ARDS, maintaining spontaneous breathing with APRV resulted in lower venous admixture and better arterial oxygenation over a period of more than 10 days as compared with CMV with subsequent weaning.[23] These results show that even in patients requiring ventilator support, maintaining spontaneous breathing

FIGURE 12-2 During spontaneous breathing, the posterior muscular sections of the diaphragm move more than does the anterior tendon plate. Consequently, in the supine position, spontaneous ventilation preferably is directed to well-perfused, dependent lung regions. Conversely, a mechanically delivered tidal volume is directed primarily to nondependent lung areas, away from regions with maximal blood flow. Thus spontaneous breathing contributes to better ventilation-perfusion ($\dot{V}_A/\dot{Q}$) matching.

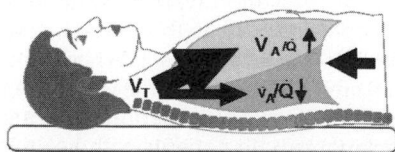

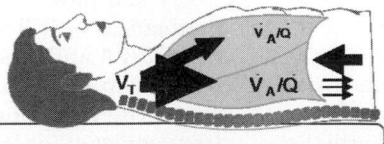

APRV *with* spontaneous breathing   **APRV *without* spontaneous breathing**

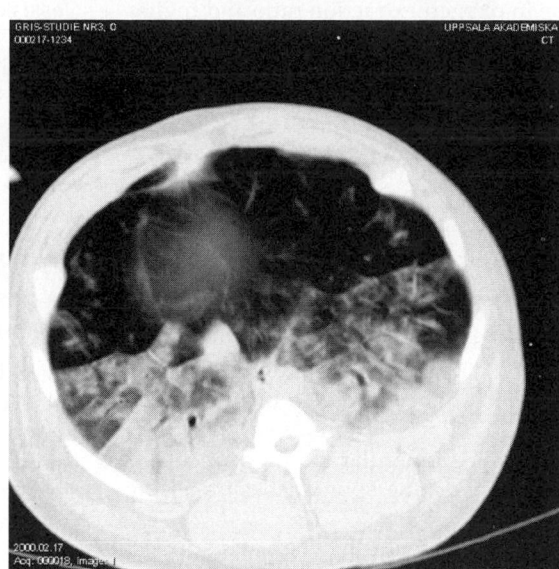

FIGURE 12-3 Computed tomography of a lung region above the diaphragm at end expiration in oleic acid–induced lung injury with and without spontaneous breathing during APRV. Atelectasis formation is reduced with spontaneous breathing.

can counteract progressive deterioration in pulmonary gas exchange.

Automatic tube compensation (ATC) compensates for endotracheal tube resistance. The ventilator increases airway pressure during inspiration, reduces it during expiration, and aims to keep the tracheal pressure constant and independent of tube resistance. In patients with acute lung injury (ALI), ATC during APRV achieved considerable inspiratory muscle unloading and increased alveolar ventilation without decreasing functional residual capacity or worsening pulmonary gas exchange.[24] Apparently, the transient lowering of airway pressures during expiration with ATC does not promote alveolar collapse or worsen gas exchange when superimposed on APRV.

CARDIOVASCULAR EFFECTS

Application of a ventilator breath generates an increase in airway pressure and therefore in intrathoracic pressure, which, in turn, reduces venous return to the heart. In normo- and hypovolemic patients, this action produces a reduction in right- and left-ventricular filling and results in decreased stroke volume, cardiac output, and oxygen delivery (D_{O_2}).[25] To normalize systemic blood flow during mechanical ventilation, intravascular volume often needs to be increased and/or the cardiovascular system needs pharmacologic support. Reducing mechanical ventilation to a level that provides adequate support for existing spontaneous breathing should help to reduce the cardiovascular side effects of ventilator support.[26]

Periodic reduction of intrathoracic pressure, achieved by maintaining spontaneous breathing during ventilator support, promotes venous return to the heart and right- and left-ventricular filling, thereby increasing cardiac output and D_{O_2}.[27] Experimental[21,28,29] and clinical[15,22] studies show

that when spontaneous breathing during APRV achieves 10–40% of total $\dot{V}_E$, with no change in $\dot{V}_E$ or airway pressure limits, cardiac index increases. A simultaneous rise in right-ventricular end-diastolic volume during spontaneous breathing with APRV indicates improved venous return to the heart.[15] In addition, outflow from the right ventricle, which depends mainly on lung volume (the major determinant of pulmonary vascular resistance), may benefit from decrease in intrathoracic pressure during APRV.[15]

Patients with left-ventricular dysfunction may not benefit from the augmentation of venous return to the heart and increase in left-ventricular afterload that occurs with lowering of intrathoracic pressure. Thus, switching abruptly from CMV to pressure support (PS) with a simultaneous reduction in airway pressure can cause further decompensation in patients with existing cardiac insufficiency.[30] Räsänen et al[31,32] showed a need for adequate ventilator support and CPAP levels in patients with respiratory and cardiogenic failure. Provided that spontaneous breathing receives adequate support and that satisfactory CPAP levels are applied, maintaining spontaneous breathing during APRV should not be a disadvantage and is not contraindicated per se in patients with ventricular dysfunction.[31–33]

OXYGEN SUPPLY AND DEMAND

An increase in cardiac index and arterial oxygen tension (Pa_{O_2}) during APRV improves the relationship between tissue oxygen supply and demand because oxygen consumption remains unchanged despite the work of spontaneous breathing. In accordance with previous experimental[20] and clinical[15] findings, total oxygen consumption is not measurably altered by adequately supported spontaneous breathing in patients with low lung compliance. An increase in D_{O_2} with unchanged oxygen consumption indicates an improved tissue oxygen supply and demand balance, as reflected by a decrease in oxygen extraction ratio and higher mixed venous P_{O_2}.

ORGAN PERFUSION

By reducing cardiac index and venous return to the heart, CMV can have a negative effect on the perfusion and functioning of extrathoracic organ systems. An increase in venous return and cardiac index secondary to the periodic fall in intrathoracic pressure during spontaneous inspiration should improve organ perfusion and function significantly during partial ventilator support. In patients with ARDS, spontaneous breathing with intermittent mandatory ventilation (IMV) leads to an increase in glomerular filtration rate and sodium excretion.[34] Compatible with these results, renal perfusion and glomerular filtration rate of patients with ARDS improve during spontaneous breathing with APRV.[35]

Preliminary data in patients requiring ventilator support for ALI suggest that maintained spontaneous breathing may be beneficial for liver function. These clinical data are supported by experimental observations using colored microspheres in pigs with oleic acid–induced lung injury that demonstrated improved perfusion of the splanchnic area.[36]

Rationale, Advantages, and Limitations

Based on physiologic observations, APRV is advantageous for recruiting atelectasis adjacent to the diaphragm, thereby improveing pulmonary gas exchange in patients with ALI, ARDS, and atelectasis after major surgery. Because the increase in transalveolar pressure is localized to areas near the diaphragm and is caused by a decrease in intrapleural pressure, the concomitant decrease in intrathoracic pressure contributes to improved cardiovascular function. Areas of atelectasis not adjacent to the diaphragm may not be recruited successfully by spontaneous breathing during APRV.

To enable spontaneous breathing, lower levels of sedation (Ramsay score of 2 or 3) are required. Less sedation helps in reduceing the doses of vasopressor and inotropic agents while maintaining cardiovascular function stable and reduces the duration of ventilator support. The use of APRV, however, has to be limited to patients who do not require deep sedation for management of their underlying disease (e.g., cerebral edema with increased intracranial pressure).

Two periods during the APRV cycle are particularly vulnerable to patient-ventilator asynchrony. When airway pressure release occurs during spontaneous inspiration and when restoration of CPAP occurs during spontaneous expiration, ventilation may be impaired because spontaneous and ventilator efforts oppose each other. Rarely, a reduction in ventilatory efficiency, indicated by a decrease in alveolar ventilation and an increase in the work of breathing, may result from temporary asynchrony. Synchronized APRV and optimizing ventilator settings and sedation may be required in this rare event.[29]

As a concept, APRV does not provide breath-to-breath assistance of spontaneous inspiration. Previous investigations have demonstrated that separation from mechanical ventilation in difficult-to-wean patients may be prolonged with the use of IMV and may be expedited with breath-to-breath assistance of inspiratory efforts during pressure-support ventilation (PSV).[4] Thus APRV is not expected to be an advantage in difficult-to-wean patients.

Indications and Contraindications

INDICATIONS

Based on the clinical[15,22,23,37] and experimental[20,21] data, APRV is indicated in patients with acute lung injury, ARDS, and atelectasis after major surgery. APRV recruits atelectasis adjacent to the diaphragm, thereby restoring pulmonary gas exchange, and improves cardiovascular and extrathoracic organ function in patients with acute lung injury, ARDS, and atelectasis after major surgery.

CONTRAINDICATIONS

Because lower levels of sedation (Ramsay score of 2 or 3) are used to allow spontaneous breathing, APRV should not be used in patients who require deep sedation for management of their underlying disease (e.g., cerebral edema with increased intracranial pressure).

To date, no data are available on use of APRV in patients with obstructive lung disease. Theoretically, use of a short release time should not be beneficial in patients with obstructive lung disease who have prolonged expiratory time constants. Currently, use of APRV is not supported by clinical research.

Likewise, use of APRV has not been investigated in patients with neuromuscular disease and is not supported by any evidence.

Comparison with Other Modes

APRV VERSUS PSV

APRV and PSV were compared in 24 patients with ALI/ARDS using equal $\dot{V}_E$ or airway pressure limits. Because insufflation during PSV is flow-cycled, alveolar end-inspiratory pressure may not reach the preset level. Thus, in patients with reduced lung compliance, equal airway pressure limits achieve a lower V_T during PSV as compared with APRV. Consequently, a compensatory increase in respiratory rate is required during PSV to maintain alveolar ventilation. To deliver APRV and PSV with comparable V_T at an acceptable respiratory rate, the pressure level has to be increased during PSV.[15]

In contrast to spontaneous breathing with APRV, assisted inspiration with PSV did not produce significant improvement in intrapulmonary shunt, gas exchange, and cardiac output when compared with CMV.[15] Apparently, the spontaneous contribution to a mechanically assisted breath was not sufficient to counteract the $\dot{V}_A/\dot{Q}$ maldistribution and cardiovascular depression caused by positive-pressure ventilation. A possible explanation might be that inspiration is terminated by the decrease in inspiratory gas flow during PSV, which may reduce ventilation in areas of the lung that have a slow time constant.

APRV VERSUS IMV

In a randomized multicenter trial in 52 patients with ALI, APRV with lower peak airway pressures resulted in better alveolar ventilation and equal arterial oxygenation as compared with IMV.[38] A similar trial in 58 patients with ALI supports these findings but did not show a difference in mortality.[39] In eight patients recovering from open-heart surgery, APRV provided adequate ventilation with lower airway pressures and less dead-space ventilation than did IMV or PSV.[40] Arterial oxygenation was not different between the modalities.

Variation in Delivery among Ventilator Brands

SYNCHRONIZED APRV

Asynchronous interferences between spontaneous and mechanical ventilation may increase the work of breathing and reduce the effective support during APRV.[41] Synchronization of the switching between the two CPAP levels to spontaneous inspiration or expiration has been incorporated in all commercially available demand-valve APRV circuits to avoid asynchronous interferences between spontaneous and mechanical breaths. A trigger window of 0.25 second usually is used to enable synchronization of the switching between the two CPAP levels and spontaneous breathing efforts. Bench-model data indicate that the synchronization of spontaneous inspiration with the switch to the high CPAP level, but not the synchronization of spontaneous expiration with pressure release, may be beneficial. Patient data on the advantage of synchronized APRV are lacking currently.[41] Because patient-triggered mechanical cycles during IMV are not advantageous for patients, there is no reason why this should be different for APRV.[41] Synchronization during APRV may produce inconstant times for the high and low CPAP levels. Synchronization of APRV is switched off in the APRV mode of the Dräger EVITA IV and XL ventilators. In the Puritan-Bennett 840 and the Viasys Vela and Avea, APRV is synchronized with spontaneous ventilation.

MODIFICATIONS OF APRV

Most commercially available ventilators offer hybrid modes of ventilation such as APRV + PSV and APRV + ATC (Table 12-1). Very few of these combinations have been shown to benefit patients.[24] It is doubtful that simply combining different modalities will achieve an addition of their positive effects.[42,43] Indeed, it is possibile that proven physiologic benefits of one modality may be minimized or even neutralized when it is by combined with another mode.

TABLE 12-1   Modifications of APRV

Synchronized airway pressure-release ventilation (APRV)
Change between CPAP levels is synchronized with spontaneous breathing.
Advantage of synchronization is not proven.[29]
Intermittent mandatory pressure-release ventilation (IMPRV)
Spontaneous breathing on the high CPAP level is assisted with PSV.
Advantage is not supported by data.[42,43]
APRV + pressure-support ventilation (PSV)
Spontaneous breathing on the low CPAP level is assisted with PSV.
Advantage is not supported by data.
APRV + automatic tube compensation (ATC)
Spontaneous breathing on both CPAP levels is assisted with ATC.
May reduce work of breathing in selected patients without deteriorating gas exchange.[24]

ABBREVIATIONS: CPAP, continuous positive airway pressure.

Adjustments at the Bedside

SETTING VENTILATION PRESSURES AND TIDAL VOLUMES DURING APRV

Mechanical ventilation with positive end-expiratory airway pressure titrated above the lower inflection pressure of a static pressure-volume curve and a low V_T is thought to prevent tidal alveolar collapse at end expiration and overdistension of lung units at end inspiration in patients with ARDS.[44] This lung-protective strategy causes improvement in lung compliance, venous admixture, and Pa_{O_2} without causing cardiovascular impairment in ARDS.[44] Mechanical ventilation using a V_T of 6 ml/kg (ideal body weight) has been shown to result in a better outcome when compared with a V_T of 12 ml/kg in patients with ARDS.[44,45] Based on these results, CPAP levels during APRV should be titrated to prevent end-expiratory alveolar collapse and tidal alveolar overdistension.[44,45] When CPAP levels during APRV were adjusted in patients with ARDS according to a lung-protective strategy, occurrence of spontaneous breathing led to improved cardiorespiratory function without affecting total oxygen consumption secondary to the work of breathing.[15] Moreover, pulmonary compliance should be greatest in this range of airway pressures, and thus a small change in transpulmonary pressure achieves normal tidal breathing with minimal elastic work of breathing[46] (Fig. 12-4). Because APRV does not provide assistance on every inspiratory effort, the CPAP levels need to be adjusted carefully to achieve efficient spontaneous ventilation with minimal work of breathing.

SETTING TIMES DURING APRV

The duration of the high CPAP level needs to allow at least complete inflation of the lungs, as indicated by an end-inspiratory phase of no flow when spontaneous breathing is absent. Spontaneous breathing occurs normally on the high CPAP level. Thus duration of the high CPAP level should be adjusted so that it is long enough to allow spontaneous

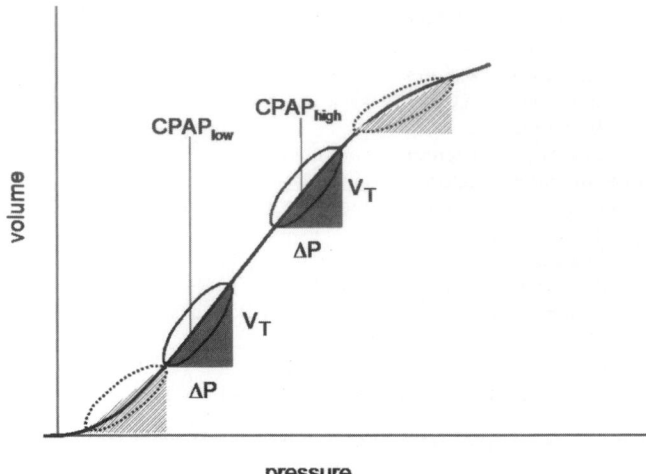

FIGURE 12-4 During airway pressure-release ventilation, both CPAP levels should be titrated to achieve the greatest compliance. Thus a small change in transpulmonary pressure achieves normal tidal breathing, whereas elastic work of breathing (*shaded area*) is minimal. If the CPAP levels are too high or too low (*dashed line*), elastic work of breathing will be increased unnecessarily (*shaded area*).

breathing. If the release time is shorter than four times the time constant of the lungs (τ = compliance × resistance), alveolar pressure will not equilibrate at the low CPAP level, and intrinsic PEEP ($PEEP_I$) will result.[47,48] Incomplete expiration and the likelihood of $PEEP_I$ are indicated by gas flow at end expiration (Fig. 12-5). In the presence of $PEEP_I$, alveolar pressure amplitude will be reduced; consequently, alveolar ventilation decreases, and Pa_{CO_2} increases. To date, data do not indicate that $PEEP_I$ is superior to external PEEP in preventing derecruitment of the lungs. Thus duration of the low CPAP level should be adjusted to allow complete expiration to the resting lung volume.

OTHER CONCEPTS OF SETTING APRV

Earlier approaches used high CPAP levels, which were released briefly to near-ambient pressure during APRV. Depending on the time constant of the lungs, brief release times may cause $PEEP_I$.[47] Clinical studies, however, demonstrate that external PEEP is superior to $PEEP_I$ in restoring gas exchange in patients with acute lung injury. Not surprisingly, in patients with ARDS, Cane et al[49] observed an increase in atelectasis on briefly releasing high CPAP levels to near-ambient pressure during APRV. Based on available scientific and clinical data, this approach of adjusting ventilator settings during APRV cannot be recommended.

Troubleshooting

ANALGESIA AND SEDATION DURING APRV

Analgesia and sedation are used not only to ensure satisfactory pain relief and anxiolysis but also to help the patient adapt to mechanical ventilation.[50,51] The level of analgesia

FIGURE 12-5 Computer simulation of airway pressure (Paw), volume (V), and gas flow ($\dot{V}$) for the respiratory system and both a fast and slow lung compartment with a short release time. Expiration in the slow compartment is not completed at end expiration; consequently, gas flow is still present at end expiration, associated with intrinsic PEEP.

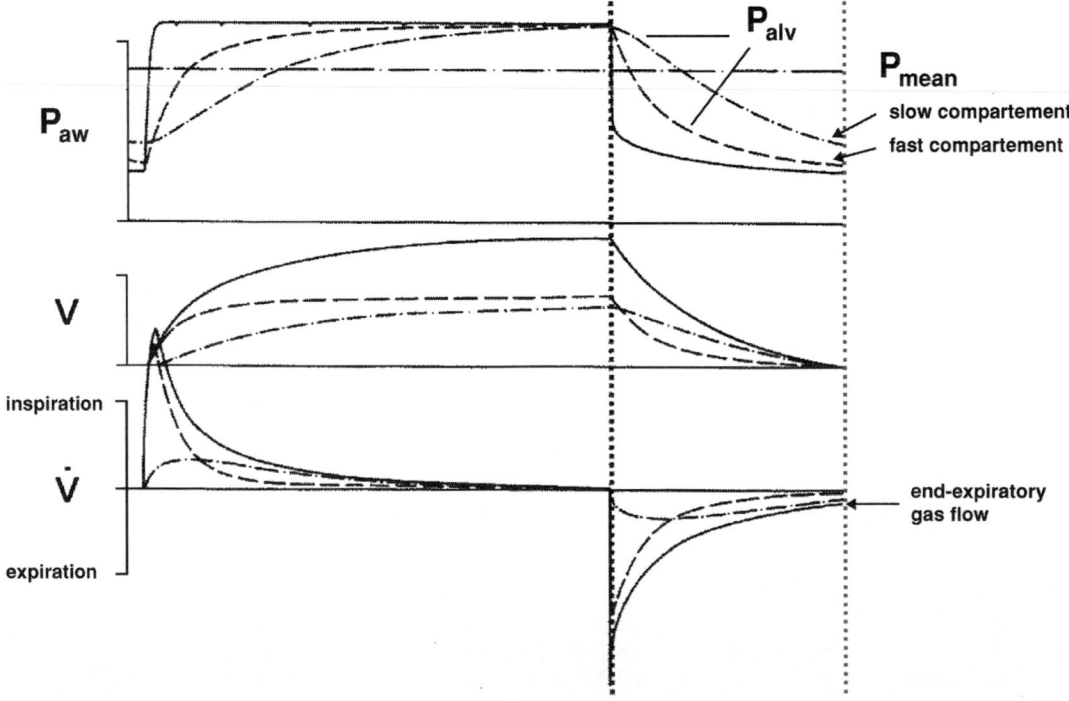

and sedation required during CMV is equivalent to a Ramsay score of between 4 and 5, that is, a deeply sedated patient who is unable to respond when spoken to and who has no sensation of pain. During APRV, a Ramsay score of between 2 and 3 can be targeted, that is, an awake patient who is responsive and cooperative. In nearly 600 post–cardiac surgery patients[37] and in patients with multiple injuries,[23] maintaining spontaneous breathing during APRV led to less consumption of analgesics and sedatives as compared with initial use of CMV followed by weaning with partial ventilator support. Higher doses of analgesics and sedatives used in patients managed with CMV are associated with the use of higher doses of vasopressors and inotropic agents to maintain stable cardiovascular function.[23]

Important Unknowns

Compared with an initial period of CMV followed by weaning, maintaining spontaneous breathing with APRV is associated with significantly fewer days of ventilator support, earlier extubation, and a shorter stay in the intensive-care unit (ICU).[23] These findings may be explained by a lower level of sedation required during APRV.

The Future

Small randomized, controlled studies have demonstrated that early spontaneous breathing with APRV in patients with ALI/ARDS and in patients with pulmonary dysfunction after major surgery leads to improved arterial oxygenation and cardiovascular function. Also, sedation is less, and duration of ventilator support and ICU stay is shorter. In the future, large-scaled randomized multicenter studies are needed to test the validity of these results in critically ill patients.

Summary and Conclusion

Based on available data, it is suggested that spontaneous breathing during ventilator support should not be suppressed, even in patients with severe pulmonary dysfunction, if there are no contraindications (e.g., increased intracranial pressure). Improvement in pulmonary gas exchange, systemic blood flow, and oxygen supply to the tissue, which have been observed when spontaneous breathing is allowed during ventilator support, are reflected in improvement in the patient's condition. Maintaining spontaneous breathing with APRV may help to decrease days of ventilator support and stay in the ICU. CMV followed by weaning with partial ventilator support is the standard in ventilation therapy, but the place of spontaneous breathing with APRV should be reconsidered in view of available data. Today's standard practice should be to maintain spon-

taneous breathing from the onset of ventilator support and to adapt the level of support continuously according to the individual needs of the patient.

References

1. Marini JJ. New options for the ventilatory management of acute lung injury. New Horizons 1993; 1:489–503.
2. Ely EW, Baker AM, Dunagan DP, et al. Effect on the duration of mechanical ventilation of identifying patients capable of breathing spontaneously. New Engl J Med 1996; 335:1864–9.
3. Kollef MH, Shapiro SD, Silver P, et al. A randomized, controlled trial of protocol-directed versus physician-directed weaning from mechanical ventilation. Crit Care Med 1997; 25: 567–74.
4. Brochard L, Rauss A, Benito S, et al. Comparison of three methods of gradual withdrawal from ventilatory support during weaning from mechanical ventilation. Am J Respir Crit Care Med 1994; 150:896–903.
5. Esteban A, Frutos F, Tobin MJ, et al. A comparison of four methods of weaning patients from mechanical ventilation. Spanish Lung Failure Collaborative Group. New Engl J Med 1995; 332:345–50.
6. Stock MC, Downs JB. Airway pressure release ventilation. Crit Care Med 1987; 15:462–6.
7. Baum M, Benzer H, Putensen C, Koller W. Biphasic positive airway pressure (BiPAP): A new form of augmented ventilation. Anaesthesist 1989; 38:452–8.
8. Stock MC, Downs JB. Airway pressure release ventilation. Crit Care Med 1987; 15:462–6.
9. Froese AB, Bryan AC. Effects of anesthesia and paralysis on diaphragmatic mechanics in man. Anesthesiology 1974; 41:242–55.
10. Reber A, Nylund U, Hedenstierna G. Position and shape of the diaphragm: Implications for atelectasis formation. Anaesthesia 1998; 53:1054–61.
11. Kleinman BS, Frey K, VanDrunen M, et al. Motion of the diaphragm in patients with chronic obstructive pulmonary disease while spontaneously breathing versus during positive pressure breathing after anesthesia and neuromuscular blockade. Anesthesiology 2002; 97:298–305.
12. Bernard GR, Artigas A, Brigham KL, et al. Report of the American-European consensus conference on ARDS: Definitions, mechanisms, relevant outcomes and clinical trial coordination. Intensive Care Med 1994; 20:225–32.
13. Gattinoni L, Presenti A, Torresin A, et al. Adult respiratory distress syndrome profiles by computed tomography. J Thorac Imaging 1986; 1:25–30.
14. Puybasset L, Cluzel P, Chao N, et al. A computed tomography scan assessment of regional lung volume in acute lung injury. The CT Scan ARDS Study Group. Am J Respir Crit Care Med 1998; 158:1644–55.
15. Putensen C, Mutz NJ, Putensen-Himmer G, Zinserling J. Spontaneous breathing during ventilatory support improves ventilation-perfusion distributions in patients with acute respiratory distress syndrome. Am J Respir Crit Care Med 1999; 159:1241–8.
16. Hedenstierna G, Tokics L, Lundquist H, et al. Phrenic nerve stimulation during halothane anesthesia: Effects of atelectasis. Anesthesiology 1994; 80:751–60.
17. Wrigge H, Zinserling J, Neumann P, et al. Spontaneous breathing improves lung aeration in oleic acid–induced lung injury. Anesthesiology 2003; 99:376–84.
18. Henzler D, Dembinski R, Bensberg R, et al. Ventilation with biphasic positive airway pressure in experimental lung injury:

Influence of transpulmonary pressure on gas exchange and haemodynamics. Intensive Care Med 2004; 30:935–43.

19. Putensen C, Räsänen J, Lopez FA. Interfacing between spontaneous breathing and mechanical ventilation affects ventilation-perfusion distributions in experimental bronchoconstriction. Am J Respir Crit Care Med 1995; 151:993–9.

20. Putensen C, Räsänen J, Lopez FA. Effect of interfacing between spontaneous breathing and mechanical cycles on the ventilation-perfusion distribution in canine lung injury. Anesthesiology 1994; 81:921–30.

21. Putensen C, Räsänen J, Lopez FA. Ventilation-perfusion distributions during mechanical ventilation with superimposed spontaneous breathing in canine lung injury. Am J Respir Crit Care Med 1994; 150:101–8.

22. Sydow M, Burchardi H, Ephraim E, Zielmann S. Long-term effects of two different ventilatory modes on oxygenation in acute lung injury: Comparison of airway pressure release ventilation and volume-controlled inverse ratio ventilation. Am J Respir Crit Care Med 1994; 149:1550–6.

23. Putensen C, Zech S, Wrigge H, et al. Long-term effects of spontaneous breathing during ventilatory support in patients with acute lung injury. Am J Respir Crit Care Med 2001; 164:43–9.

24. Wrigge H, Zinserling J, Hering R, et al. Cardiorespiratory effects of automatic tube compensation during airway pressure release ventilation in patients with acute lung injury. Anesthesiology 2001; 95:382–9.

25. Pinsky MR. Determinants of pulmonary arterial flow variation during respiration. J Appl Physiol 1984; 56:1237–45.

26. Kirby RR, Perry JC, Calderwood HW, Ruiz BC. Cardiorespiratory effects of high positive end-expiratory pressure. Anesthesiology 1975; 43:533–9.

27. Downs JB, Douglas ME, Sanfelippo PM, Stanford W. Ventilatory pattern, intrapleural pressure, and cardiac output. Anesth Analg 1977; 56:88–96.

28. Falkenhain SK, Reilley TE, Gregory JS. Improvement in cardiac output during airway pressure release ventilation. Crit Care Med 1992; 20:1358–60.

29. Putensen C, Leon MA, Putensen-Himmer G. Timing of pressure release affects power of breathing and minute ventilation during airway pressure release ventilation. Crit Care Med 1994; 22:872–8.

30. Lemaire F, Teboul JL, Cinotti L, et al. Acute left ventricular dysfunction during unsuccessful weaning from mechanical ventilation. Anesthesiology 1988; 69:171–9.

31. Räsänen J, Heikkila J, Downs J, et al. Continuous positive airway pressure by face mask in acute cardiogenic pulmonary edema. Am J Cardiol 1985; 55:296–300.

32. Räsänen J, Nikki P. Respiratory failure arising from acute myocardial infarction. Ann Chir Gynaecol Suppl 1982; 196:43–7.

33. Nikki P, Tahvanainen J, Räsänen J, Makelainen A. Ventilatory pattern in respiratory failure arising from acute myocardial infarction: II. Ptc_{O_2} and Ptc_{CO_2} compared to Pa_{O_2} and Pa_{CO_2} during IMV4 vs IPPV12 and PEEP0 vs PEEP10. Crit Care Med 1982; 10:79–81.

34. Steinhoff H, Falke K, Schwarzhoff W. Enhanced renal function associated with intermittent mandatory ventilation in acute respiratory failure. Intensive Care Med 1982; 8:69–74.

35. Hering R, Peters D, Zinserling J, et al. Effects of spontaneous breathing during airway pressure release ventilation on renal perfusion and function in patients with acute lung injury. Intensive Care Med 2002; 28:1426–33.

36. Hering R, Viehofer A, Zinserling J, et al. Effects of spontaneous breathing during airway pressure release ventilation on intestinal blood flow in experimental lung injury. Anesthesiology 2003; 99:1137–44.

37. Rathgeber J, Schorn B, Falk V, et al. The influence of controlled mandatory ventilation (CMV), intermittent mandatory ventilation (IMV) and biphasic intermittent positive airway pressure (BiPAP) on duration of intubation and consumption of analgesics and sedatives: A prospective analysis in 596 patients following adult cardiac surgery. Eur J Anaesthesiol 1997; 14:576–82.

38. Räsänen J, Cane RD, Downs JB, et al. Airway pressure release ventilation during acute lung injury: A prospective multicenter trial. Crit Care Med 1991; 19:1234–41.

39. Varpula T, Valta P, Niemi R, et al. Airway pressure release ventilation as a primary ventilatory mode in acute respiratory distress syndrome. Acta Anaesthesiol Scand 2004; 48:722–31.

40. Valentine DD, Hammond MD, Downs JB, Sears NJ. Distribution of ventilation and perfusion with different modes of mechanical ventilation. Am Rev Respir Dis 1991; 143:1262–6.

41. Putensen C, Leon MA, Putensen-Himmer G. Timing of pressure release affects power of breathing and minute ventilation during airway pressure release ventilation. Crit Care Med 1994; 22:872–8.

42. Räsänen J. IMPRV: Synchronized APRV, or more? Intensive Care Med 1992; 18:65–6.

43. Rouby JJ, Ben Ameur M, Jawish D, et al. Continuous positive airway pressure (CPAP) vs intermittent mandatory pressure release ventilation (IMPRV) in patients with acute respiratory failure. Intensive Care Med 1992; 18:69–75.

44. Amato MB, Barbas CS, Medeiros DM, et al. Effect of a protective-ventilation strategy on mortality in the acute respiratory distress syndrome. New Engl J Med 1998; 338:347–54.

45. ARDS network. Ventilation with lower tidal volumes as compared with traditional tidal volumes for acute lung injury and the acute respiratory distress syndrome. The Acute Respiratory Distress Syndrome Network. New Engl J Med 2000;342:1301–8.

46. Katz JA, Marks JD. Inspiratory work with and without continuous positive airway pressure in patients with acute respiratory failure. Anesthesiology 1985; 63:598–607.

47. Martin LD, Wetzel RC. Airway pressure release ventilation in a neonatal lamb model of acute lung injury. Crit Care Med 1991; 19:373–8.

48. Neumann P, Golisch W, Strohmeyer A, et al. Influence of different release times on spontaneous breathing pattern during airway pressure release ventilation. Intensive Care Med 2002; 28:1742–9.

49. Cane RD, Peruzzi WT. Airway pressure release ventilation in severe acute respiratory failure. Chest 1991;100:460–3.

50. Wheeler AP. Sedation, analgesia, and paralysis in the intensive care unit. Chest 1993; 104:566–77.

51. Burchardi H, Rathgeber J, Sydow M. The concept of analgosedation depends on the concept of mechanical ventilation. In: Vincent JL, editor. Yearbook of intensive care and emergency medicine. New York: Springer-Verlag, 1995: 155–64.

Chapter 13

PROPORTIONAL-ASSIST VENTILATION

MAGDY YOUNES

Proportional-assist ventilation (PAV) is a form of synchronized ventilator support in which the ventilator generates pressure in proportion to *instantaneous* patient effort[1] (Fig. 13-1). The ventilator simply amplifies inspiratory efforts. Unlike other modes of partial support, there is no target flow, tidal volume, or ventilation or airway pressure. Rather, PAV's objective is to allow the patient to comfortably attain whatever ventilation and breathing pattern his or her control system desires.[1] The main operational advantages of PAV are automatic synchrony with inspiratory efforts and adaptability of the assist to changes in ventilatory demand (see Fig. 13-1).

How Can a Ventilator Deliver Pressure in Proportion to Patient Effort without Directly Measuring Effort?

A simple PAV delivery system illustrates how this happens[2] (Fig. 13-2). Alveoli and chest wall are represented as an elastic compartment that opposes expansion. Elastic recoil pressure (Pel; *hatched arrow*) is a function of how much lung volume deviates from passive functional residual capacity (FRC) and the stiffness of the system (elastance E): Pel = V × E. In a passive system, Pel increases alveolar pressure as the lung is artificially inflated. During assisted ventilation, inspiratory muscles are active. These muscles decrease alveolar pressure by an amount corresponding to their pressure output (Pmusc) (see Fig. 13-2). At any instant, alveolar pressure (Palv) is the difference between Pel (V × E), which tends to increase it, and Pmusc, which tends to decrease it:

$$Palv = (V \times E) - Pmusc \qquad (1)$$

The elastic compartment is connected to the external tubing via airways and the endotracheal tube. The ventilator controls pressure at the external airway (Paw). Air flows into the lungs when Paw exceeds Palv. Flow is a function of the difference between Paw and Palv (resistive pressure Pres) and the resistance of the intervening tubing (R). Thus

$$Flow = (Paw - Palv)/R \qquad (2)$$

Substituting Eq. (1) for Palv in Eq. (2) and rearranging, we get

$$Flow \times R = Paw - (V \times E) + Pmusc$$

or

$$Pmusc + Paw = flow \times R + V \times E \qquad (3)$$

This equation simply states that the distending force is the sum of patient-generated (Pmusc) and ventilator-generated (Paw) pressures and that this distending force is opposed by the sum of resistive pressure drop (Pres, or flow × R) and elastic recoil pressure (Pel, or V × E).

The gas-delivery system in Fig. 13-2 is a freely moving piston pressurized by a fast-responding linear motor. This arrangement emphasizes that PAV gas-delivery systems must allow rapid and free flow of gas in response to changes in downstream (i.e., alveolar) pressure. Flow and volume leaving the ventilator are measured. The gains of the flow and volume signals are adjustable by separate amplifiers: flow assist (FA) and volume assist (VA). The summed output of the two amplifiers is the input to the motor. Thus the ventilator's pressure output is a function of instantaneous flow and volume that left the ventilator since triggering.

With this arrangement (see Fig. 13-2), a greater effort (more reduction in alveolar pressure) will draw more gas from the ventilator. This, in turn, results in more assist. This

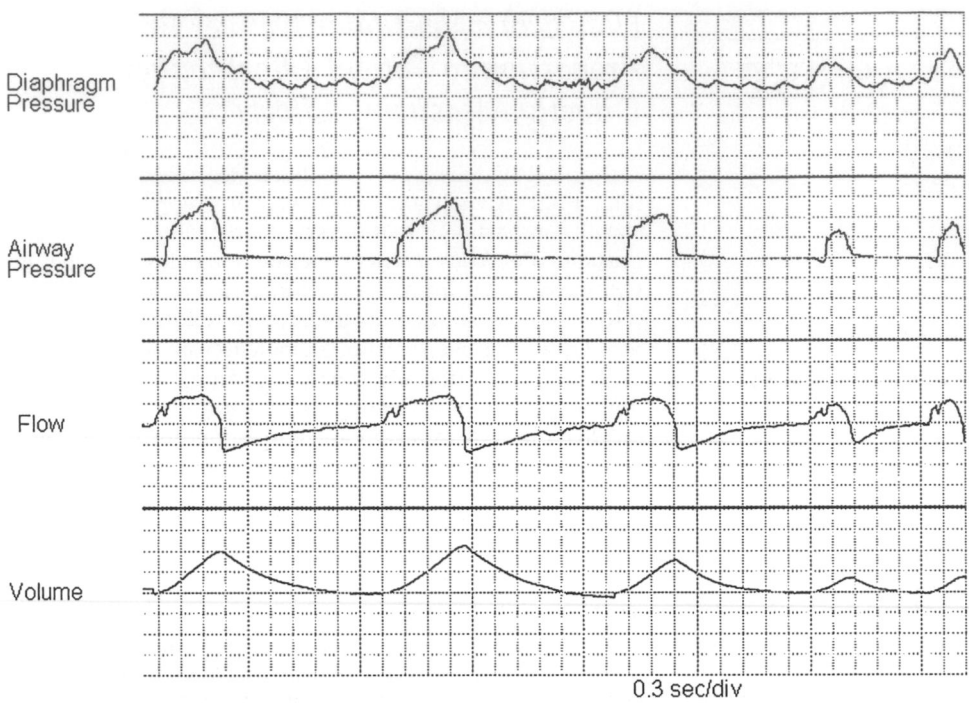

Diaphragm
Pressure

Airway
Pressure

Flow

Volume

0.3 sec/div

FIGURE 13-1 Relation between assist provided (airway pressure) and independently measured diaphragmatic pressure in proportional-assist ventilation. Note that amplitude and duration of assist correspond to amplitude and duration of inspiratory efforts.

provides a positive relation between effort and assist but does not per se cause the assist to be proportional to instantaneous effort. Proportionality is achieved through customized adjustment of the flow- (FA) and volume-assist (VA) gains. The basis for these adjustments is as follows:

FA is the assist pressure per unit flow (in cmH$_2$O/liter/s). These are resistance units. If FA is 50% of R, the ventilator provides 50% of the resistive pressure (i.e., 50% of flow × R, Eq. 3). At 80% R, the ventilator assumes 80% of resistive work, and so on. Likewise, setting VA gain to 50% of E causes the ventilator to assume 50% of elastic pressure (i.e., 50% of V × E, Eq. 3), and so on. The total assist (Paw) is the sum of the flow and volume assists:

$$Paw = \%flow \times R + \%V \times E \qquad (4)$$

During the inspiratory phase, volume rises progressively, peaking at end inspiration. By contrast, flow peaks in early

to middle inspiration and falls later. Thus the relative contributions of resistive and elastic pressures vary considerably during the inspiratory phase. If the same percent is used for both components, total assist (Paw) represents the same percent of total pressure regardless of the relative contribution of each. Percent assist then is constant throughout. If different percent values are used for FA and VA, however, total assist (Paw) will represent a different percent of total applied pressure at different times. When percent assist (ventilator's contribution) is constant throughout inspiration, patient's percent contribution (i.e., 100 − %assist) is also constant throughout and the relation between Paw and Pmusc (i.e., proportionality becomes constant) as given by

$$Proportionality = \%assist/(100 - \%assist)$$

Thus at 50% assist, proportionality is 1.0; Paw equals Pmusc throughout. At 80% assist, proportionality is 4, and

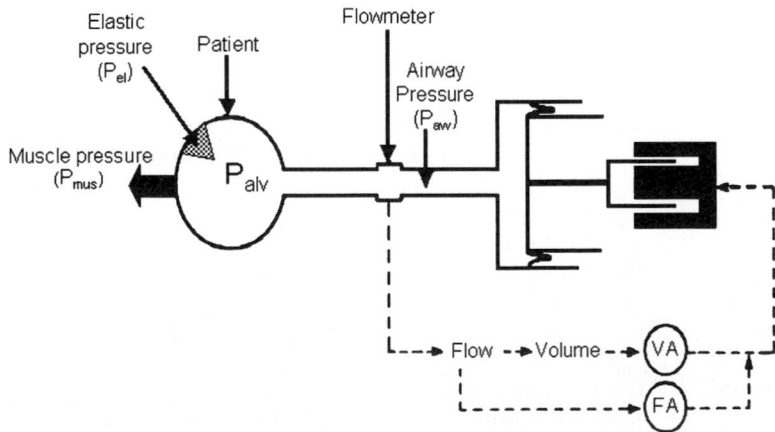

Elastic
pressure
(P$_{el}$)

Patient

Flowmeter

Airway
Pressure
(P$_{aw}$)

Muscle pressure
(P$_{mus}$)

P$_{alv}$

Flow → Volume → VA

FA

FIGURE 13-2 Diagram illustrating how a PAV delivery system generates pressure in proportion to effort. The gas-delivery system consists of a freely moving piston pressurized by a fast-acting motor. Force exerted by motor is a function of flow and volume leaving the ventilator. A stronger effort results in greater reduction in alveolar pressure (Palv), drawing more gas from the piston and resulting in more assist. If the volume-assist (VA) and flow-assist (FA) components are set to the same fraction of elastance and resistance, respectively, the pressure generated becomes proportional to effort (Pmusc). See text.

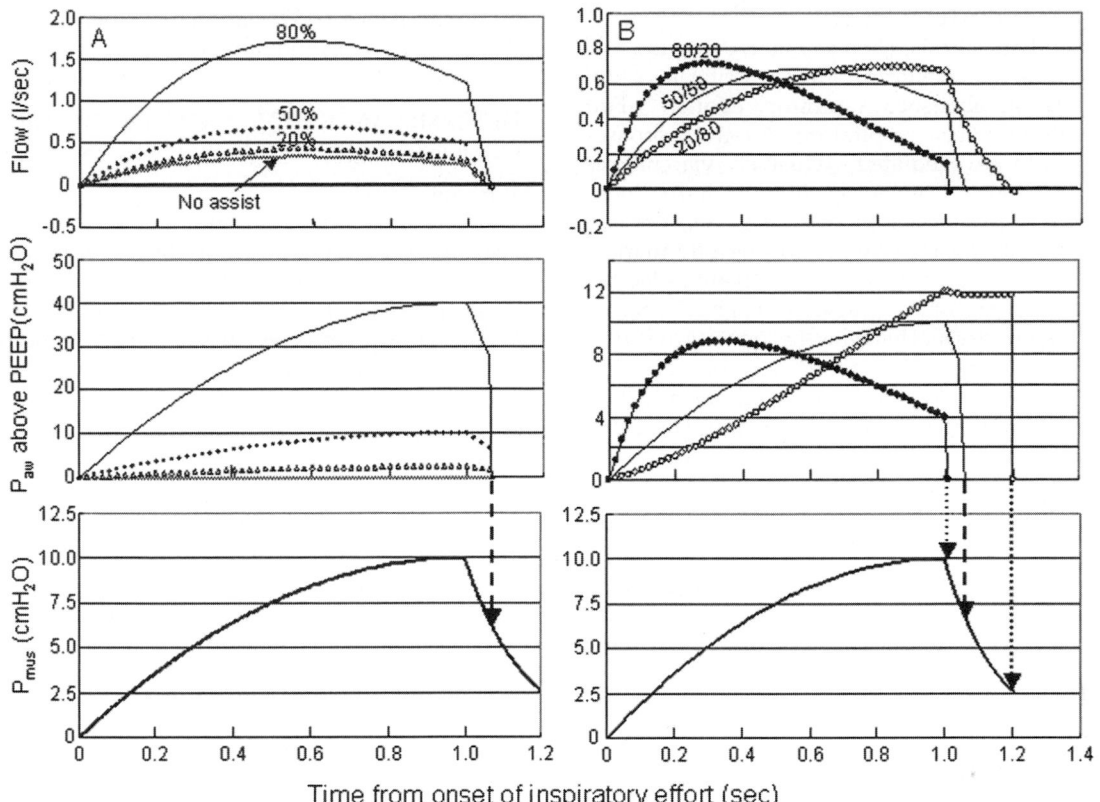

FIGURE 13-3 Model simulation showing the impact of using equal (*A*) versus unequal (*B*) percent assist for the flow and volume components. *A.* Three assist levels are shown: 20%, 50%, and 80%. When the same percent assist is applied to both components, the shape of the assist [airway pressure (Paw)] is identical to that of muscle pressure (Pmusc), but the proportionality is different (Paw/Pmusc = 0.25, 1.0, and 4.0, respectively). Note also that flow reaches zero (end of mechanical inspiration) at the same time during the declining phase of Pmusc at all assist levels, including the no-assist situation (*top panel*). *B.* Flow assist is 80% of resistance, and volume assist is 20% of elastance (*solid dots*). Note that the assist (Paw) is more aggressive early in inspiration and terminates sooner relative to the balanced assist (50/50 line). A relatively greater volume assist (*open circles*) offers less assist early while cycling off is delayed.

so on. Under these conditions, the shapes of the Pmusc and Paw waveforms are identical, and the decline in Pmusc at end inspiration will be associated with a decline in Paw, ensuring synchrony (Fig. 13-3*A*). By contrast, if percent assist varies through inspiration (such as by using different percent values for FA and VA), proportionality between Paw and Pmusc is no longer constant, and the shapes of the two waveforms differ (see Fig. 13-3*B*).

Another reason why FA and VA need to be customized to patient's R and E is to avoid the occurrence of *runaway*.[1] Runaway occurs if FA exceeds the patient's R and/or V̇A exceeds the patient's E.[1] So long as FA is less than R and V̇A is less than E, the pressure assist (Paw, Eq. 4) is only a fraction of the total pressure required to offset the prevailing resistive and elastic pressures, and the patient must contribute the difference. Under these conditions, if the patient withdraws his or her contribution, the pressure provided by the ventilator can no longer offset the prevailing resistive and elastic pressures, and the cycle must end. If, however, FA is greater than R and/or V̇A is greater than E, Paw single-handedly may exceed the total opposing forces (right side of Eq. 3). A patient's contribution is no longer necessary to continue the inflation. The excess pressure provided by the

ventilator generates more flow (and volume), causing more pressure to be generated, and so on. Inflation continues until terminated by a ventilator or physiologic limiting mechanism. Under runaway conditions, technically, the patient is no longer in the PAV mode because assist no longer tracks effort. The various runaway patterns and their mechanisms are discussed under "Limitations," below.

Physiologic Effects

RELEVANT PHYSIOLOGIC PRINCIPLES
(see ref. 3 for more details)

These principles will be discussed first because they not only help to explain PAV's reported effects but also make it possible to gain useful insights from a patient's responses to this mode. Responses to PAV may be mediated by changes in blood-gas tensions (chemical factors) or through modification of nonchemical sources of respiratory drive. Chemical responses are highly predictable, whereas the others are not. What happens, therefore, depends on what sources of respiratory drive are operative at the time of application.

SOURCES OF RESPIRATORY DRIVE

During sleep and anesthesia, chemical factors are the sole source of respiratory drive; artificially reducing P_{CO_2} under these conditions abolishes respiratory efforts.[4–6] Furthermore, in these states, respiratory muscle responses to changes in load are mediated exclusively via changes in blood-gas tensions.[7] Conversely, in alert individuals, other sources of respiratory drive exist; it is very difficult to produce apnea by assisted ventilation despite marked hypocapnia.[8–11] These drive inputs, collectively called the *consciousness factor*,[4] presumably arise from behavioral centers and from respiratory mechanisms that operate only during consciousness (e.g., nonchemical load-compensatory mechanisms[7]). Patients who require mechanical ventilation cover a wide spectrum of levels of consciousness. Therefore, it is difficult to make general conclusions about their drive inputs. The next few sections describe what should happen in response to PAV if respiratory output were driven solely by chemical factors. Deviation from this expected behavior then might be attributed to nonchemical factors.

DETERMINANTS OF V_E AND Pa_{CO_2} IN THE ABSENCE OF NONCHEMICAL DRIVE SOURCES

Without Assist

A steady state in P_{CO_2} and minute ventilation ($\dot{V}_E$) can occur only if pulmonary carbon dioxide (CO_2) removal [the product of alveolar ventilation ($\dot{V}_A$) and alveolar CO_2 concentration (FA_{CO_2})] equals the CO_2 produced by the tissues ($\dot{V}_{CO_2}$). At a given $\dot{V}_{CO_2}$, if ventilation is increased artificially, FA_{CO_2}, and hence Pa_{CO_2}, must decrease before a steady state is reached. Accordingly, at a given $\dot{V}_{CO_2}$, there is an inverse relation between $\dot{V}_E$ and Pa_{CO_2} in the steady state: the metabolic hyperbola.[12] The actual equation is $Pa_{CO_2} = 0.86 [\dot{V}_{CO_2}/\dot{V}_E(1 - V_D/V_T)]$,[12] where V_D/V_T is the dead-space ratio. Figure 13-4A illustrates this relation.

FIGURE 13-4 Effect of proportional assist on steady-state ventilation ($\dot{V}_E$) and Pa_{CO_2}. A metabolic hyperbola is shown for a subject with CO_2 production ($\dot{V}_{CO_2}$) of 200 ml/min and dead-space ratio (V_D/V_T) of 0.4. *A.* Unassisted breathing. The ventilatory responses to CO_2 in four subjects are shown: (*a*) normal, (*b*) acute hypercapnic failure, (*c*) chronic hypercapnic failure, and (*d*) acute non-hypercapnic failure with metabolic acidosis. In each case, the *x* intercept of the ventilatory response is the apneic threshold (AT). AT is shifted up in subject *c* and down in subject *d*. The intersection of ventilatory response line and the hyperbola gives steady-state values of $\dot{V}_E$ and Pa_{CO_2}. Vertical dotted lines represent additional nonchemical inputs that cause ventilation to be higher and Pa_{CO_2} to be lower than in their absence. *B, C.* Effect of 50% and 80% assist in the four subjects. In each case the ventilatory-response slope doubles with 50% assist and increases fivefold at 80%. Open circles off the hyperbola are immediate responses not consistent with steady state. Open circles on the hyperbola are the steady-state values with assist. Note that the magnitude of change in $\dot{V}_E$ and Pa_{CO_2} is a function of the difference between unassisted Pa_{CO_2} (*solid circle*) and the AT. *D.* Response to proportional assist in the presence of nonchemical input (*vertical solid line*). Note that the response is highly unpredictable (see text).

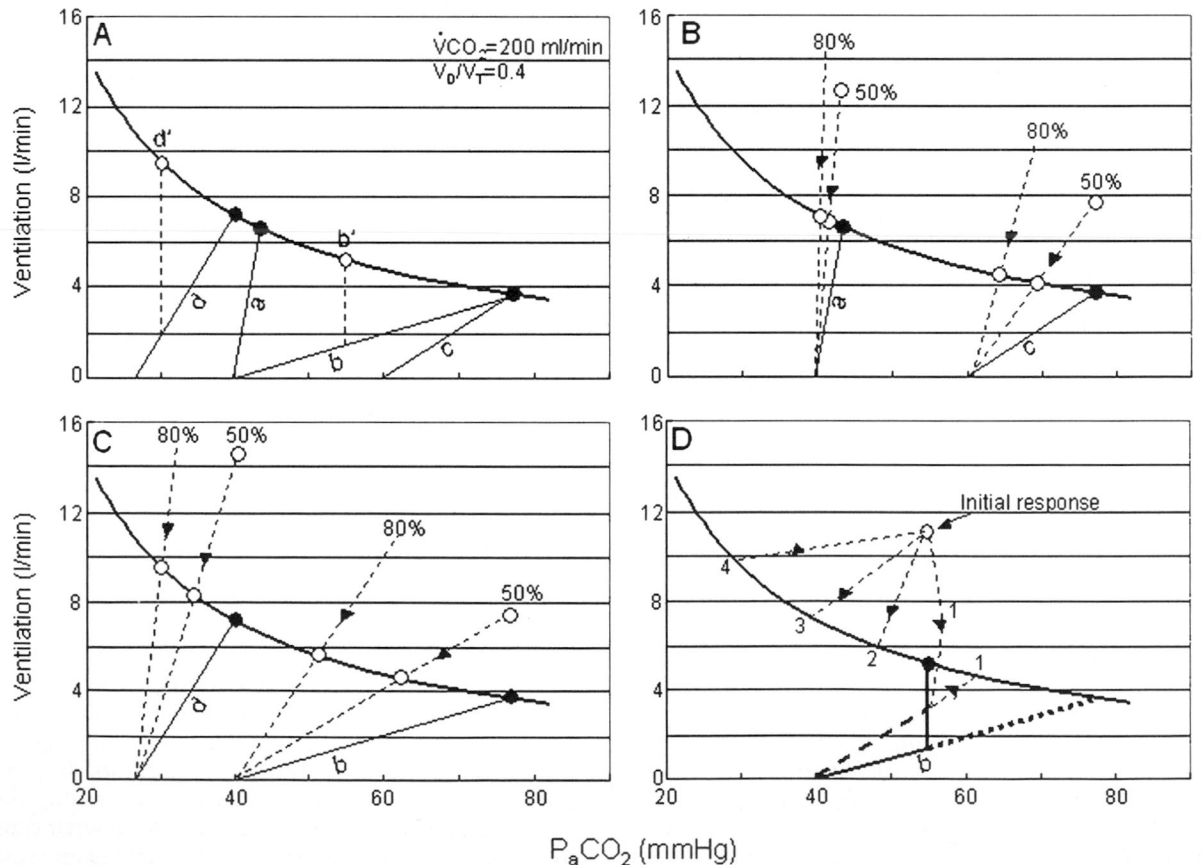

Ventilation increases progressively as a function of P_{CO_2}.[13] The slope of the response depends on the sensitivity of chemoreceptors (the sensory arm) and the effectiveness of the motor arm in generating ventilation. Thus, for a given chemoreceptor response, ventilatory response is less if respiratory muscles are weaker or mechanics are abnormal. Without nonchemical drive sources, there is a Pa_{CO_2} below which apnea develops,[4-6] the apneic threshold (AT; see Fig. 13-4).

Four subjects with different disorders are illustrated in Fig. 13-4*A*. For each subject, there is only one possible steady state, namely, the point of intersection of the CO_2 response line and the hyperbola.[13] At this point, pulmonary CO_2 elimination equals tissue CO_2 production.

Line *a* represents a normal subject. Ventilatory response is normal (2.2 liters/min/mmHg), and AT is 40 mmHg. The intersection point is at a Pa_{CO_2} of 43 mmHg and a $\dot{V}_E$ of 6.6 liters/min. The difference between unassisted (no assist, NA) steady-state P_{CO_2} and AT (i.e., $\Delta P_{CO_2, NA-AT}$) is very small (3 mmHg). Line *b* represents a patient with severe acute hypercanic respiratory failure. AT is the same, but the ventilatory response to CO_2 is much depressed because of abnormal mechanics. The intersection point is 76 mmHg at a $\dot{V}_E$ of 3.8 liters/min. $\Delta P_{CO_2, NA-AT}$ is very large (36 mmHg). Line *c* describes a patient with chronic respiratory failure. Ventilatory response to CO_2 is depressed because of abnormal mechanics and/or weak respiratory muscles. In this case, however, AT is higher. $\Delta P_{CO_2, NA-AT}$ is larger than normal (16 mmHg), but for the same steady-state Pa_{CO_2}, it is lower than in the patient represented by line *b*. Line *d* represents a patient with a reduced ventilatory response to CO_2 (0.6 liter/min/mmHg) because of abnormal mechanics or weak muscles but in whom the apneic threshold is low, for example, because of concomitant metabolic acidosis.[14] Steady-state P_{CO_2} and $\dot{V}_E$ are near normal, but $\Delta P_{CO_2, NA-AT}$ is large.

Expected Response to PAV Application

With PAV, respiratory motor output is amplified by an amount that is related to percent assist (see Fig. 13-3*A*). Within the linear range of the pressure-volume and pressure-flow relations, the amplification of pressure results in a corresponding amplification of ventilation (see Fig. 13-3*A*). Thus the net effect of PAV is to increase the slope of the ventilatory response to CO_2 (as well as to P_{O_2} and pH). For simplicity, we will assume that P_{CO_2} is the only stimulus and that resistance and elastance are constant in the tidal volume range. Under these conditions, at 50% assist, delivered assist equals Pmusc, and the combined pressure (patient + ventilator) is twice Pmusc. Accordingly, the slope of the CO_2 response is doubled. At 80% assist, Paw is four times Pmusc (see Fig. 13-3*A*), and pressure output is amplified by a factor of 5. The ventilatory response should increase nearly fivefold, and so on.

In the normal subject (line *a*), 50% assist doubles the CO_2 response (see Fig. 13-4*B*). $\dot{V}_E$ immediately doubles (*upper open circle*). Pulmonary CO_2 output now exceeds $\dot{V}_{CO_2}$. Pa_{CO_2} falls. Respiratory efforts decrease, and $\dot{V}_E$ follows along the new CO_2 response line until the metabolic hyperbola. A steady state is now possible. The same would happen at

higher percent assist. Because steady-state values must be above the apneic threshold, and $\Delta P_{CO_2, NA-AT}$ is very small, $\dot{V}_E$ and Pa_{CO_2} cannot change much. Furthermore, since $\dot{V}_E$ hardly changes, virtually all the assist (Paw) is used to reduce respiratory motor output, and percent reduction in Pmusc is similar to percent assist.

A similar analysis for the patient with chronic respiratory failure (line *c* in Fig. 13-4*B*) shows that at 50% assist, Pa_{CO_2} decreases by 7 mmHg and $\dot{V}_E$ increases by 10%, whereas at 80% assist, Pa_{CO_2} decreases by 13 mmHg and $\dot{V}_E$ increases by 20%. Because $\dot{V}_E$ increased significantly, the decrease in respiratory muscle output (Pmusc) is less than percent assist. For example, at 50% assist, Pmusc is contributing 50% to a higher $\dot{V}_E$ (110%). The decrease in Pmusc is 45% instead of 50%. Because the difference between Pa_{CO_2} at 80% assist and AT is now very small, increasing assist beyond 80% would have little further effect, even though Pa_{CO_2} is still high. Thus, when AT is high, it is not possible to acutely normalize Pa_{CO_2} using PAV (or any other strictly assist mode).

In the patient with severe acute hypercapnic failure (line *b* in Fig. 13-4*C*), the changes are even greater. At 50% and 80%, assist, Pa_{CO_2} decreases by 14 and 25 mmHg, respectively, and $\dot{V}_E$ increases by 23% and 50%. Even at 80% assist, the difference between Pa_{CO_2} and AT is still large, and further reduction in Pa_{CO_2} is possible. Because $\dot{V}_E$ increases substantially, the decrease in Pmusc is much less than percent assist (39% and 70%, for the 50% and 80% assist, respectively).

Finally, in the patient represented by line *d* in Fig. 13-4*C*, increasing PAV assist results in progressive hypocapnia. By normalizing mechanics, the effect of the concomitant metabolic acidosis is now exposed.

In summary, *in the absence of nonchemical drive sources*, whether and by how much ventilation and Pa_{CO_2} change following institution of a given percent assist are determined by the unassisted ventilatory response to CO_2, the apneic threshold, and the position of the metabolic hyperbola. These determine the difference between unassisted Pa_{CO_2} and AT. Because the more $\dot{V}_E$ increases, the less Pmusc decreases, the same three factors determine the extent to which the assist is used to increase ventilation versus decrease muscle output.

EFFECT OF NONCHEMICAL DRIVES ON RESPONSE TO PAV

The action of nonchemical drive inputs can be viewed as additive with chemical drive. They cause ventilation to be higher at a given Pa_{CO_2} than if chemical drive were the sole source (points *b'* and *d'* in Fig. 13-4*A*). Total drive is made up of a CO_2-sensitive component and a component that reflects consciousness-related reflexes and unpredictable behavioral influences.

Figure 13-4*D* illustrates how these inputs may modify the response to PAV. Without nonchemical influences, Pa_{CO_2} would be 76 mmHg. Because of the nonchemical input (*solid vertical line*), however, steady-state $\dot{V}_E$ is 5.5 liters/min at a Pa_{CO_2} of 55 mmHg. A 50% assist results in an immediate increase in $\dot{V}_E$ to 11 liters/min (both components are amplified). Pa_{CO_2} must fall. What happens then depends on the response of the nonchemical component. At one extreme, it may disappear (e.g., the patient may fall asleep when assisted). $\dot{V}_E$ would fall to the new CO_2 response line (*diagonal dashed line*). Should $\dot{V}_E$ at this point be below the hyperbola, Pa_{CO_2} and $\dot{V}_E$ will rise along the CO_2 response line, reaching the hyperbola at point 1. Here, the assist is followed by an increase in Pa_{CO_2}, but the patient is working much less. If the nonchemical stimulus remains the same, Pa_{CO_2} and $\dot{V}_E$ will decrease along a path parallel to the CO_2 response line, meeting the hyperbola at point 3. Here, there is no longer a CO_2 stimulus, and ventilation is sustained by the twice-amplified nonchemical influence. An intermediate value (point 2) may result if the nonchemical influence partially decreases. Finally, at the other extreme, the patient may become agitated with the assist, increasing the nonchemical stimulus, and this, when amplified, may reduce Pa_{CO_2} to very low levels (point 4). It is clear that with nonchemical stimuli (alert individuals), the ventilatory response to PAV is theoretically unpredictable.

REPORTED PHYSIOLOGIC RESPONSES

RESPIRATORY MUSCLE OUTPUT

PAV resulted in significant reduction in muscle output in all studies where this was tested.[15–26] Typically, Pmusc decreased by 30–45% at 50% assist and by 55–70% at 80% assist. The less than expected reduction is caused by (1) differences between assumed and actual E and R (see "Accuracy and Stability of Respiratory Mechanics Values," below), (2) imperfect delivery by the ventilator (see "Ventilator Response Time," below), (3) dynamic hyperinflation [see "Dynamic Hyperinflation (DH)," below] or nonlinearity in the pressure-volume relation [see "Nonlinearity in the Pressure-Volume (P-V) Relation within the Tidal Volume Range," below], and (4) an associated increase in $\dot{V}_E$ (see "Ventilation and P_{CO_2}," below). As indicated earlier, when some of the assist is used to increase $\dot{V}_E$, less is used to reduce muscle output.

VENTILATION AND P_{CO_2}

Application of PAV to normal sleeping subjects results in an immediate increase in V_T and $\dot{V}_E$, which decrease over several breaths to near-baseline levels.[17] Steady-state responses are minimal,[6,17] and the decrease in Pet_{CO_2} is very modest (~3 mmHg[6,17]). These results are consistent with a small difference between unassisted Pa_{CO_2} and AT secondary to a normal ventilatory response to CO_2 (subject represented by line *a* in Fig. 13-4*B*).

By contrast, in experienced, awake normal subjects, PAV results in an important increase in $\dot{V}_E$ and a more pronounced reduction in Pa_{CO_2}, and the decrease in respiratory muscle output is only modest.[18] Pa_{CO_2} generally decreases below the apneic threshold (e.g., 30 ± 5 mmHg[18]), reflecting the presence of nonchemical drive inputs that fail to be eliminated. PAV applied to inexperienced, awake subjects is followed by unpredictable responses extending to severe hyperventilation (personal observations), reflecting erratic behavioral responses.

There are numerous reports on the changes in $\dot{V}_E$ and Pa_{CO_2} with PAV in patients with respiratory failure.[15,16,19–33] Responses ranged from virtually no change or even a decrease in $\dot{V}_E$ as assist increased[27–30] to large increases in $\dot{V}_E$ and decreases in Pa_{CO_2}.[16,19,25,31] These differences can be explained readily if one considers the experimental circumstances of the various studies or patients:

1. *Intubated ventilator-dependent patients with normocapnia.* It is clearly not possible to establish steady-state values of $\dot{V}_E$ and Pa_{CO_2} during unassisted breathing in these patients; they rapidly develop distress. The effect of PAV is, accordingly, determined over a range of assist above a minimum value (e.g., 80% versus 40%). Furthermore, in such patients, Pa_{CO_2} at the minimum tolerable assist is normal. All such studies demonstrated very little change or even a small decrease in $\dot{V}_E$ as assist increased.[27–30] Pa_{CO_2} decreased, but the change was small (2–4 mmHg). These patients, therefore, behave like the subject represented by line *a* in Fig. 13-4, who has no nonchemical inputs and a small $\Delta P_{CO_2, NA-AT}$. This state, however, is reached only at some finite assist. It therefore would appear that these patients become comfortable only when their Pa_{CO_2} is a few millimeters of mercury above AT. Under these conditions, $\dot{V}_E$ cannot increase further; the extra assist is used simply to decrease muscle output. The decrease in $\dot{V}_E$ observed in some cases[28,30] is caused by a reduction in V_D/V_T and/or $\dot{V}_{CO_2}$ (secondary to decreased respiratory muscle work) because in all such cases Pa_{CO_2} was lower even though $\dot{V}_E$ was lower.[28,30]

The preceding observations lead to an interesting conclusion: Ventilator-dependent patients who show little change in $\dot{V}_E$ and Pa_{CO_2} over a relatively wide PAV assist do not tolerate a Pa_{CO_2} that is much above AT. This indicates a high degree of chemosensitivity that likely contributes to their ventilator dependence. *Chemosensitivity*, as used here, does not refer to ventilatory responses (which are affected by mechanics and muscle strength) but to central effects of Pa_{CO_2} on respiratory sensation and muscle activation.

2. *Chronic hypercapnia with and without acute exacerbation.* In virtually all reported studies, $\dot{V}_E$ and Pa_{CO_2} on PAV were compared with values obtained during a period of unassisted breathing.[16,19–21,23,25,26,34] Unlike the preceding group, there always was a significant increase in $\dot{V}_E$ and a decrease in Pa_{CO_2}. The changes were modest, however (~25% increase in $\dot{V}_E$ and 3–6 mmHg decrease in Pa_{CO_2}). Such a response is consistent with a somewhat larger difference between AT and unassisted P_{CO_2} (subject represented by line *c* in Fig. 13-4*B*). Pa_{CO_2} remained abnormally high in all cases, consistent with a high AT. The changes in $\dot{V}_E$ and Pa_{CO_2} likely would have been greater if the hypoxic stimulus did not change. In all but one study,[19] Pa_{O_2} was quite low during unassisted breathing and improved with PAV. Because a higher Pa_{O_2} decreases the ventilatory response to CO_2,[13] an increase in Pa_{O_2} mitigates the increase in CO_2 response produced by PAV, resulting in a smaller increase in ventilatory response. The assist provided in this case is used preferentially to decrease muscle output as opposed to increasing $\dot{V}_E$. In one study,[19] the hypoxic drive was negligible at baseline ($Pa_{O_2} = 99.5$ mmHg). Here, the increase in $\dot{V}_E$ was much greater (38%[19]). Although the changes in Pa_{CO_2} and Pa_{O_2} undoubtedly contributed to the reduction in respiratory muscle output, most of these patients were alert, so a reduction in nonchemical inputs may have been partly responsible.

3. *Acute hypercapnic failure.* Gay et al[32] reported an average 8 mmHg decrease in Pa_{CO_2} (60–52 mmHg) within a half hour of instituting noninvasive PAV. Considering that only 60% of patients were hypercapnic and that the nonhypercaneic patients likely did not contribute to the average decrease (see 4, below), the decrease in Pa_{CO_2} in the hypercapnic group must have been greater. In another study,[31] there were four patients with acute hypercapnic failure not associated with central depression. In them, Pa_{CO_2} declined 17 mmHg on average (66–49 mmHg) within a half hour of instituting PAV. Although these observations are not rigorous, they suggest that patients with acute hypercapnia secondary to severe acute mechanical abnormalities do sustain large increases in $\dot{V}_E$ and reductions in Pa_{CO_2} on institution of PAV. Interestingly, Pa_{CO_2} remained above normal (~50 mmHg) for a few hours.[31] It is possible that the apneic threshold increased somewhat during the preceding period of severe hypercapnia.

4. *Acute hypoxemic failure.* Information about this group is scant. Although many were included in three previous reports,[31–33] only in one study were the results of the normocapnic group (four patients) separated from those of hypercapnic patients.[31] In these four patients, Pa_{CO_2} did not change despite distress decreasing dramatically. The likely explanation for failure of Pa_{CO_2} to decrease is that respiratory muscle output to a large extent was related to nonchemical inputs, which decreased substantially on unloading (pathway 1 in Fig. 13-4D).

RESPIRATORY RATE AND BREATHING PATTERN

With one exception,[16] when there was no clinical distress at the lowest level of assist, application of PAV or further increases in percent assist did not result in appreciable changes in respiratory rate (i.e., >2–3 breaths per minute). This applied to normal sleeping subjects,[6,17] intensive-care unit (ICU) patients in whom percent assist was changed over a wide range above a comfortable level,[27–30] and ambulatory patients with chronic respiratory failure in whom the lowest level was spontaneous breathing.[19,20,24–26,34] In the only exception,[16] respiratory rate (RR) deceased substantially when PAV was applied, but in this case there were clear signs of runaway (i.e., patient was no longer in the PAV mode).

In patients with acute exacerbation of chronic obstructive pulmonary disease (COPD), RR on PAV was lower than during spontaneous breathing (3–5 breaths per minute[21,23]). The pH, however, was low at baseline, and some degree of distress may have been present then. When PAV is applied to patients with clear respiratory distress, RR decreases dramatically along with relief of distress.[31–33]

From these observations it is clear that PAV does not per se change RR. RR changes only when PAV relieves respiratory distress. In physiologic studies in which respiratory drive is deliberately increased, RR does not increase until moderate levels of stimulation.[18,35] This applies whether stimulation is produced by hypercapnia, hypoxemia, academia, or an increase in metabolic rate.[36] Thus a change in RR with assist level indicates that respiratory drive is in a range where RR

is sensitive to drive and hence probably excessive, whereas failure of RR to change over a range of PAV assist indicates that respiratory drive is only modest over this range. There are important clinical implications to these observations on PAV:

1. Failure of RR to change over a range of PAV assist indicates that respiratory drive is only modest over this range and that the RR observed in this range is the undistressed value preferred by the patient's control system. Importantly, undistressed RR, so defined, ranges from 12–46 breaths per minute.[27,28] That undistressed RR varies widely among patients is consistent with the wide range in normal subjects (8–25 breaths per minute).[37] The main difference between ICU patients and normal subjects is that the average undistressed rate is 10 breaths per minute higher.[27] A number of factors may contribute to this, including body temperature, irritation of tracheal receptors by the endotracheal tube, disease-related effects on pulmonary and other receptors, neuropathology, drug effects, and so on.[27]

2. Because the undistressed RR can be quite low, a change in RR as assist level is changed is more important than absolute RR at the low assist. For example, an increase from 20–25 breaths per minute may indicate distress, although 25 breaths per minute is not usually considered a sign of distress. By contrast, RR in excess of the usual cutoff of 35 breaths per minute need not reflect distress.

Tidal volume responses mirror the $\dot{V}_E$ responses and obviously share the same mechanisms (see "Ventilation and P_{CO_2}," above). It is important to note that in normocapnic patients, once a distress-free assist level is reached, further increases have little effect on V_T.[27,28] Accordingly, every patient has a preferred or target V_T that cannot be exceeded with more PAV assist. As with normal subjects,[37] the preferred V_T varies widely among patients (4–15 ml/kg[27,28]).

PAV has made it possible to determine the undistressed breathing pattern in ICU patients. This proved quite variable. Figure 13-5 shows two extremes. With this wide range, a one-size-fits-all strategy of mechanical ventilation (e.g., setting a target V_T) is clearly not ideal (see "Physiologic Consequences of Operational Differences," below).

Large breath-by-breath variability in V_T is characteristic of normal breathing, particularly in wakefulness.[38,39] Variability decreases in patients with abnormal mechanics.[40,41] Probably because PAV improves neuroventilatory coupling, breath-by-breath variability tends to be large in this mode (see, for example, Fig. 13-1). Coefficients of variation of 25% or more are not unusual,[23,25,29–31] and spontaneous sighs may be frequent. As with normal subjects,[42] breathing variability on PAV is less in sleeping and obtunded patients (personal observations).

VENTILATORY INSTABILITY

The tendency for the respiratory system to become unstable is described by the so-called loop gain.[43–45] A value of 1.0 indicates that recurrent cycling will occur spontaneously [e.g., Cheyne-Stokes breathing (CSB)]. The

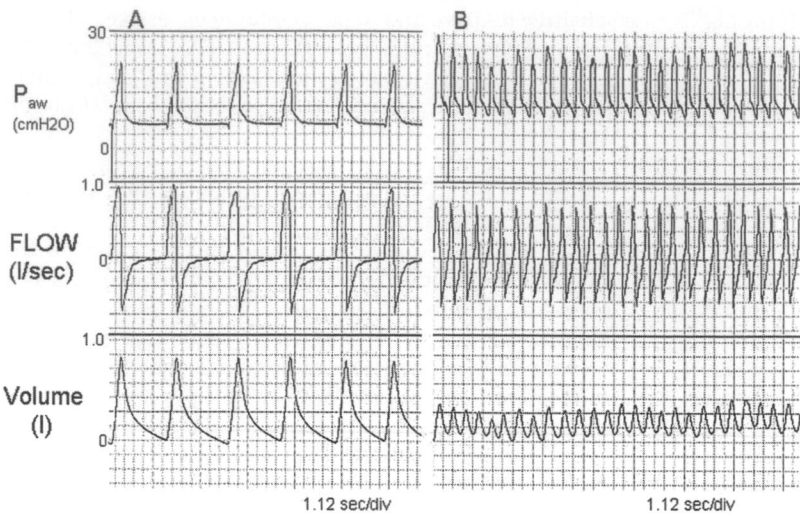

FIGURE 13-5 Tracings from two patients on high PAV assist showing extremes of undistressed breathing pattern. Paw, airway pressure.

lower the value, the more stable is the system. Ventilatory response to chemical stimuli is an important determinant of loop gain.[43-45] Because PAV increases ventilatory responses, we were concerned initially that it might precipitate periodic breathing.[1] This, however, did not materialize. Although PAV may aggravate preexisting CSB,[46] there are no reports of PAV-induced CSB in the usual ICU patient, and we have observed only a few in whom breathing became periodic on high PAV support.

The resistance to CSB has been explained recently. Normal subjects require three- to fourfold amplification of ventilatory responses to develop periodic breathing.[6,17,47] Thus, when respiratory muscles and mechanics are normal, native loop gain is less than 0.3. In the average ICU patient, respiratory muscle strength is 50% of normal,[48] resistance is four times normal (14 versus 3–4 cmH_2O/liter/s[49]), and elastance is two to three times normal (28 versus 10–14 cmH_2O/liter[50]). Collectively, these abnormalities should decrease ventilatory responses to 20% of the normal value. For PAV to induce periodic breathing in the average patient, it first must normalize ventilatory responses (i.e., a fivefold increase in the average patient) and then three to four times more, a greater than 10-fold amplification. This is impossible because of technical and physiologic limitations (see "Limitations," below).

Accordingly, if periodic breathing develops on PAV, it suggests that (1) respiratory muscles and mechanics are near normal, and the patient likely does not need ventilator support, and/or (2) the chemical control system is inherently unstable, and one should suspect disorders that result in CSB, chiefly heart failure. A third condition that may precipitate periodic breathing is runaway. Here, large tidal volumes may result, precipitating hypocapnia and recurrent central apneas. The pattern is unlike the crescendo-decrescendo CSB variety, however, and more like that produced by pressure support (several large breaths alternating with apnea[6,51]).

The ability of PAV to increase loop gain by measurable quantities is currently being used to study mechanisms of instability during sleep.[45,52]

RESPONSES DURING EXERCISE

Application of PAV during submaximal exercise in patients with severe COPD increased endurance time and reduced the rate of progression of dyspnea.[53-55] Patients with very severe COPD who received PAV during exercise in a rehabilitation program demonstrated greater improvement in unassisted exercise tolerance relative to a control group.[56] A beneficial effect of assist was not evident in mild COPD.[57] Apart from its potential therapeutic role, PAV also has been used to examine the role of respiratory muscles in limiting exercise in normal subjects.[58-60]

Comparison with Other Modes

OPERATIONAL DIFFERENCES BETWEEN PAV AND OTHER MODES

With PAV, the assist (i.e., Paw) varies directly with the intensity of patient effort (see Fig. 13-1). By contrast, with pressure-support ventilation (PSV), the assist is the same breath after breath regardless of intensity of effort. With volume-cycled ventilation (VCV), assist varies inversely with effort (Fig. 13-6). This is so because flow and volume are preset. If the patient's contribution increases, the ventilator must deliver less assist (Paw), and vice versa. Otherwise, delivered flow and volume will deviate from set values. These different relations have been well documented.[18,22,61]

With PAV, the end of the ventilator cycle is synchronized automatically with the end of patient effort (see Fig. 13-1), whereas with other modes it is not. Although ventilator response delays tend to delay cycling off somewhat,[62] the effect is fairly trivial compared with the situation in other modes (see "Ventilator Response Time," below). In VCV, there is no relation whatsoever; the patient determines the end of his effort, whereas the caregiver determines the end of the ventilator's cycle. Any synchrony is happenstance. The ventilator may continue inflation well after the end of effort, when patient wants to exhale (e.g., breath 1 in Fig. 13-6), or may cycle off, withdrawing support before

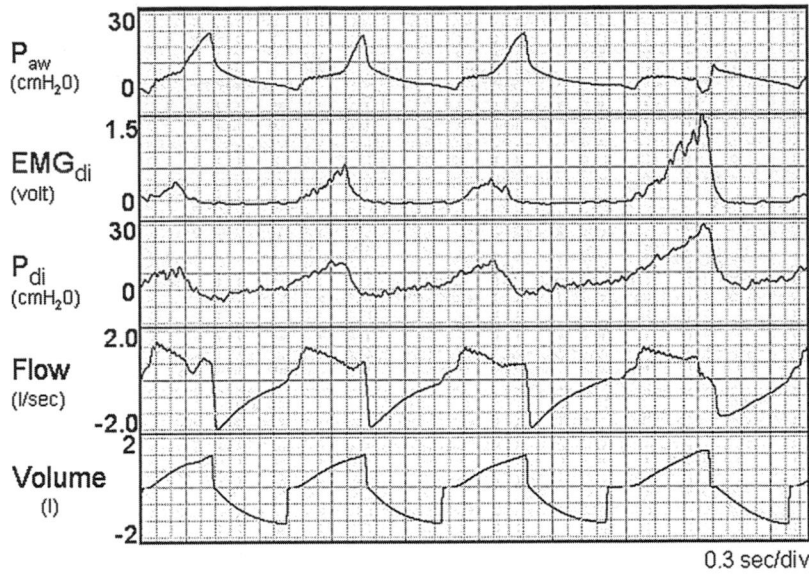

FIGURE 13-6 Tracings from a patient on volume-cycled ventilation. EMGdi, diaphragmatic activity; Paw, airway pressure; Pdi: diaphragmatic pressure. Note that ventilator cycles extend beyond inspiratory effort in the first three breaths while terminating during the effort in the last breath. Note also that patient received little or no assist when his effort was greatest (last breath).

the end of effort while patient is still trying to inhale (e.g., breath 4 in Fig. 13-6).

With PSV, synchrony between the ends of the ventilator's and the patient's inspiratory phases may or may not occur depending on the patient's respiratory mechanics and the relation between PSV level and Pmusc.[63,64] Ventilator cycles often extend well beyond inspiratory effort[28,65] or may be almost completely out of phase with them[65] (Fig. 13-7A). At times, inflation extends over two or more efforts[28] (Fig. 13-8A).

PHYSIOLOGIC CONSEQUENCES OF OPERATIONAL DIFFERENCES

RESPONSE TO DIFFERENT LEVELS OF ASSIST

Figure 13-9 illustrates what, theoretically, should happen when assist level is varied in different modes (see refs. 3 and 66 for more details). The response of RR to changes in Pa_{CO_2} near the AT is key to understanding these plots. As indicated earlier, RR is fairly constant over a range of Pa_{CO_2} above the AT. For example, average difference between spontaneous RR and RR just before apnea is less than 1.0 breath per minute.[6] At AT, breathing simply stops. There is no gradual reduction in RR.

The effect of different levels of PAV (see Fig. 13-9A) was discussed earlier (see Fig. 13-4). A steady state is possible at all assist levels, except in rare cases where chemical control is highly unstable (see "Ventilatory Instability," above). Once the AT is approached, it is not possible to increase $\dot{V}_E$ further.

The relation between P_{CO_2} and ventilation during PSV is extremely complex.[3,28,63,66] For simplicity, it is shown as a parallel shift in the ventilatory response, reflecting the fact that the assist is independent of P_{CO_2}. Exactly what happens, however, to the slope of the ventilatory response is not terribly important here. What is important is that with PSV a finite (i.e., minimum) V_T is delivered once the ventilator is triggered. This minimum V_T is a function of PSV level and respiratory mechanics.[6,63] For example, in a pa-

tient with an elastance of 25 cmH_2O/liter and a resistance of 12 cmH_2O/liter/s, the minimum V_T at PSV of 7, 14, and 20 cmH_2O will be approximately 0.22, 0.43, and 0.64 liter, respectively.[6,63] If the patient's RR near the AT is a conservative 16 breaths per minute, and every effort triggers the ventilator, minimum $\dot{V}_E$ near the AT will be 3.5, 6.9, and 10.2 liters/minute for the three levels, respectively (see Fig. 13-9). A higher minimum RR (range 12–46 breaths per minute; see "Respiratory Rate and Breathing Pattern," above) would increase minimum $\dot{V}_E$ correspondingly.

For the patient in Fig. 13-9, applying PSV at level 1 will boost ventilation initially above the metabolic hyperbola. Pa_{CO_2} falls along the response line of that level. Because minimum $\dot{V}_E$ is below the hyperbola (*left end of line 1*), a steady state can be reached (*solid dot on line 1*). For level 2, a steady state still can be reached, but Pa_{CO_2} will be just above the AT, and efforts will be very feeble. At level 3, a steady state is not possible because minimum $\dot{V}_E$ is above the metabolic hyperbola. When Pa_{CO_2} is above the AT, $\dot{V}_E$ is above the hyperbola, and P_{CO_2} must fall. When it falls below the AT, $\dot{V}_E$ becomes zero. The only steady-state $\dot{V}_E$ is the open circle. This is not possible, however, if all efforts trigger the ventilator. For average $\dot{V}_E$ to equal $\dot{V}_E$ at the open circle, ventilator rate must decrease below the patient's minimum RR. This occurs in one of two ways depending on the time constant of the respiratory system (resistance/elastance (R/E)). If R/E is very short (e.g., severe restrictive disease), ventilator cycles will not encroach on neural expiration,[63,64] allowing lung volume to return to FRC before the next effort. Here, it is possible to continue triggering until the AT, and recurrent central apneas develop. When R/E is long, the ventilator cycle is also long[63,64] and extends into neural expiration. As efforts weaken, more and more efforts fail to trigger the ventilator. Here, ineffective efforts are scattered between triggered breaths. Depending on R/E, ineffective efforts may appear well before the AT. Because R/E is more commonly long than short, intermittent ineffective efforts are more common than recurrent central apneas.[28,67]

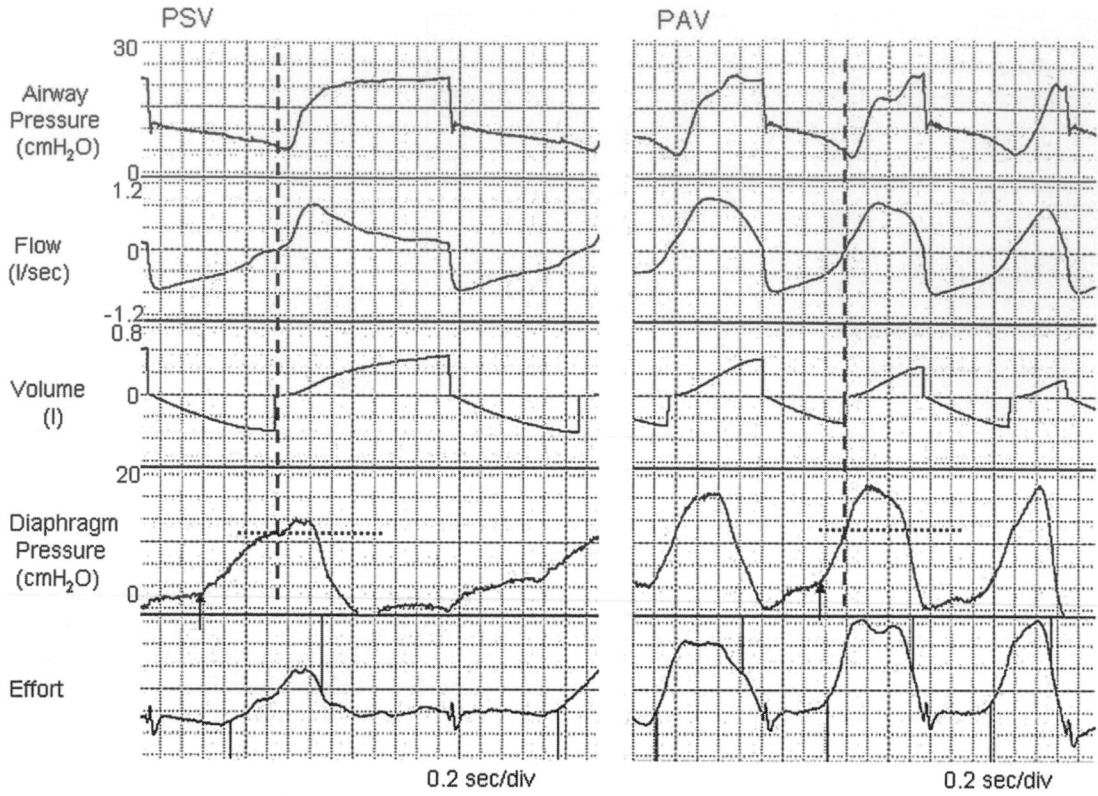

FIGURE 13-7 Comparison of pressure-support (PSV) and proportional-assist ventilation (PAV) in a patient with severe dynamic hyperinflation. With both modes, inspiratory muscles had to generate 10 cmH$_2$O before inspiratory flow could be generated and the ventilator triggered (*vertical dashed lines*). Note that in PSV, ventilator cycle extends well into neural expiration. There also were many ineffective efforts (not shown). This is not the case in PAV. Note also that diaphragmatic output is considerably higher in PAV. As a result, delay between onset of effort (*arrows*) and triggering is much less. In addition, respiratory rate is higher with PAV. With severe dynamic hyperinflation, it is difficult to maintain respiratory muscle output at a low level in PAV. See Fig. 13-13 for transition from PSV to PAV in this patient. (*Bottom tracing*) A semiquantitative effort signal generated without knowledge of respiratory mechanics[92] that can be used to identify onset and end of efforts noninvasively in real time (*event marks*). Note that the onset of effort (*downgoing marks*) can be identified well before inspiratory flow crossing. If used for triggering, this essentially can eliminate the extra work associated with dynamic hyperinflation.

In summary, with neither PAV nor PSV is it possible to decrease average Pa$_{CO_2}$ below the AT. What is different is that with PAV, V$_T$ is independent of assist level near the AT, and ventilator cycles cannot extend substantially into neural expiration. Thus a steady state can be reached at all levels without nonsynchrony.[28] With PSV, by contrast, V$_T$ increases monotonically with assist. At some level the product V$_T$ × minimum RR exceeds the V̇$_E$ required for steady state, and nonsynchrony must occur. These differences have been demonstrated experimentally.[28]

With VCV, V̇$_E$ is constant over the range where RR is independent of drive and is given by patient RR × set V$_T$. As set V$_T$ increases, V̇$_E$ increases and remains at that level as efforts decline (*horizontal lines, right panel*, Fig. 13-9). If steady-state Pa$_{CO_2}$ associated with this fixed V̇$_E$ is above the AT, a steady state with maintained synchrony can result (e.g., line 1). If not (lines 2 and 3), and there is no or minimal backup rate, ineffective efforts or recurrent central apneas must result (as with PSV), and nonsynchrony will increase as set V$_T$ increases.[67] With a backup rate, once the AT is reached, V̇$_E$ will decrease to set V$_T$ × backup rate. If this V̇$_E$ is below the hyperbola at the AT, periods in which the ventilator is triggered by the patient will alternate with periods

in which it is self-triggered as Pa$_{CO_2}$ oscillates about the AT. If backup V̇$_E$ is above the hyperbola (line *BU* in Fig. 13-9), Pa$_{CO_2}$ must fall further. Depending on ventilator settings, marked hypocapnia may develop.

In summary, with PSV and VCV there is a limited range of assist that is consistent with synchrony. Above this range, ineffective efforts or recurrent central apneas must develop. It is evident that the "appropriate" assist range depends on the metabolic hyperbola (a function of metabolic rate and V$_D$/V$_T$) and minimum patient RR near the AT (see Fig. 13-9). Because these may change with time, a suitable level may become unsuitable at another time. Several studies have confirmed that nonsynchrony is quite common with PSV and VCV[24,28,65,67] while being virtually nonexistent at all levels of PAV.[19,24,28] Ineffective efforts do occur at times during PAV, but they are very infrequent[28] and usually occur when a large breath (spontaneous sigh or runaway breath) is followed by a weak effort.

RESPONSE TO CHANGES IN VENTILATORY DEMAND
Figure 13-10 is a representative example of spontaneous changes in V̇$_E$ over a 2-hour period. The changes are not trivial; the highest level was almost twice the lowest. This

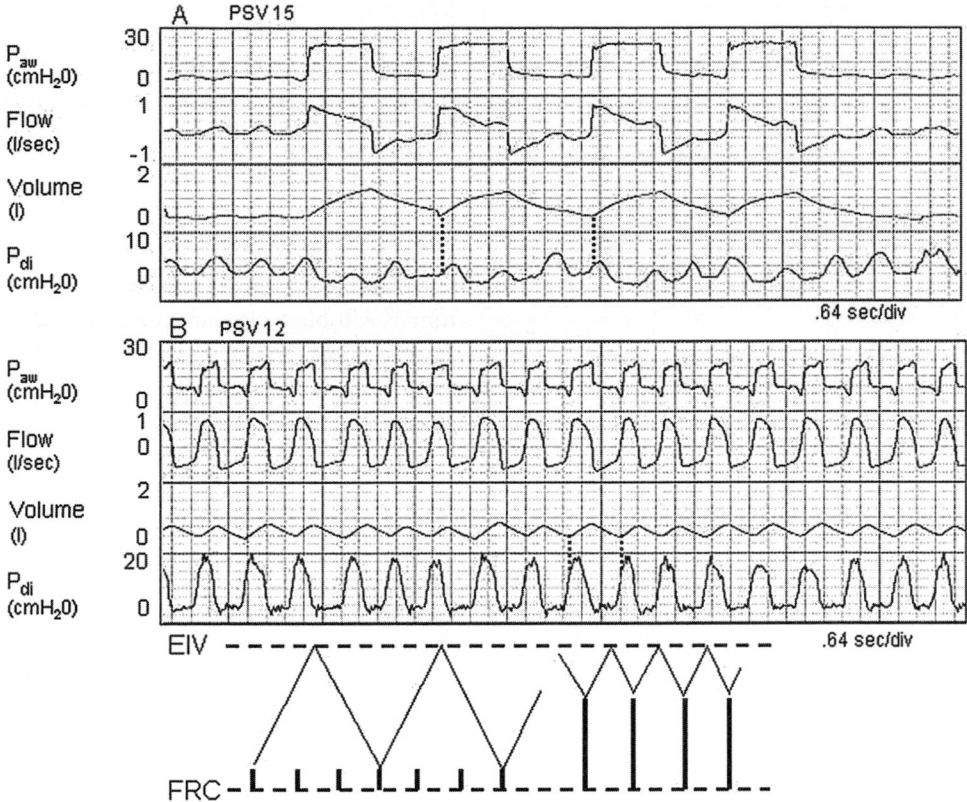

FIGURE 13-8 A dramatic example of a marked shift from slow, deep breathing to very rapid, shallow breathing following a small reduction in pressure support (PSV). Paw, airway pressure; Pdi, diaphragmatic pressure. The increase in respiratory rate was artifactual and related to improved synchrony (note that the rate of diaphragmatic efforts was unchanged). The small tidal volumes are related to dynamic hyperinflation (note that Pdi increases substantially before flow becomes inspiratory) (*vertical dotted lines*). Inset shows schematically the mechanism of shallow breathing. Height of solid lines represents effort amplitude. EIV, end-inspiratory volume; FRC, functional residual capacity. See text for additional details.

is not surprising because many influences that affect ventilatory demand can change in these patients, for example, pain, anxiety, sleep-wake cycles, metabolic rate, pH, drugs, and so on. It is therefore useful to examine what happens with the three modes in response to such changes.

Figure 13-11 illustrates two metabolic hyperbolas. Initial settings resulted in identical $\dot{V}_E$ (6 liters/min) and Pa_{CO_2} (48 mmHg). Ventilatory demand increases by 50%. Efforts increase, but RR initially does not. With PAV, assist increases, and $\dot{V}_E$ increases along a relatively steep response

FIGURE 13-9 Responses to different levels of assist with proportional-assist (PAV), pressure-support (PSV), and volume-cycled ventilation (VCV). The ventilatory response to CO_2 is shown for three assist levels in each case. The format is as in Fig. 13-4. Note that in PAV the ventilatory-response line intersects the metabolic hyperbola at all levels of assist. A steady state thus is possible at all levels. In PSV and VCV, the response lines intersect the hyperbola over a limited range of assist. At higher levels, a steady state is not possible, and nonsynchrony must result (see text). In this simulation, respiratory rate is shown to increase when Pa_{CO_2} exceeds 53 mmHg. This accounts for the increase in ventilation above this Pa_{CO_2} in VCV. BU, backup rate.

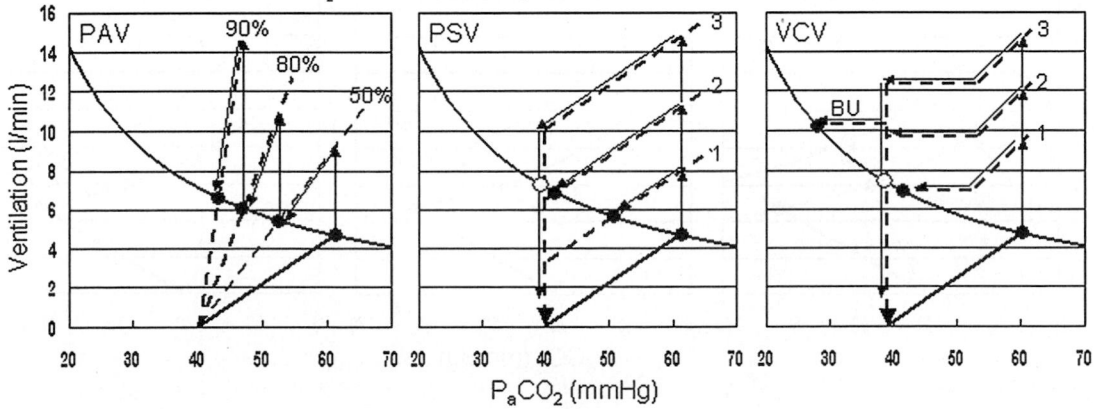

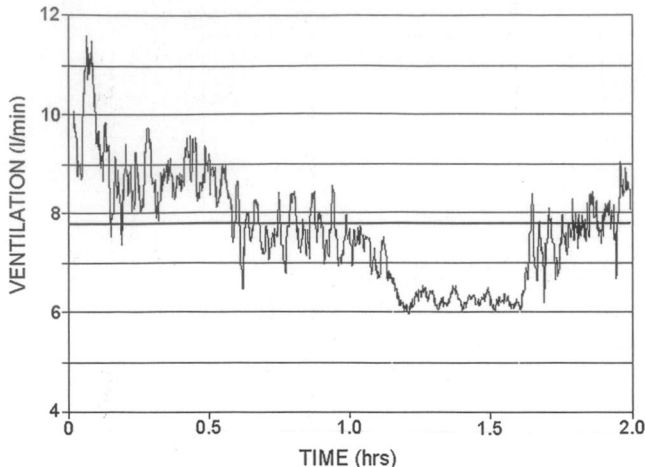

FIGURE 13-10 One-minute moving average of ventilation over a 2-hour period on PAV. Note large spontaneous changes in ventilatory demand.

line, reaching the higher hyperbola at a Pa_{CO_2} of 51 mmHg. With PSV, assist is constant. As a result, the ventilatory response is no better than the unassisted slope. The higher hyperbola is reached at 57 mmHg. With VCV, ventilation cannot increase until RR increases. Without tachypnea, the metabolic hyperbola is reached at a Pa_{CO_2} of 70 mmHg.

It is clear that the likelihood of respiratory distress and tachypnea developing is higher with VCV and PSV. With VCV, there is the added problem that ventilator inspiratory time (T_I) does not change as patient respiratory cycle time (T_{TOT}) decreases. Less time remains for exhalation, promoting nonsynchrony.[67] Nonsynchrony occurring at a time of high respiratory drive may trigger anxiety. Of course, both PSV and VCV can be readjusted to provide adequate support at the higher demand. This level, however, will be excessive when ventilatory demand returns to the lower level.

The different responses to CO_2 challenge under the three modes were well illustrated in normal subjects.[18] In ventilator-dependent patients, Ranieri et al[61] showed that

following addition of dead space during PAV, V_T increased with no change in RR (20.1–19.8 breaths per minute). When added during PSV in the same patients, there was little change in V_T, and RR increased dramatically (16.4–33.2 breaths per minute).

RESPONSE TO CHANGES IN RESPIRATORY MECHANICS

Substantial changes in resistance (R) may occur from time to time.[49] Although similar information about elastance (E) is not available, there is every expectation that it also changes from time to time (e.g., secondary to changes in lung water, abdominal pressure, or atelectasis). Accordingly, it is important to consider the response to changes in mechanics.

Figure 13-12 illustrates the effect of a combined 50% increase in R and E. At a given Pmusc, ventilation is inversely related to mechanical properties. Thus a 50% increase in E and R reduces the unassisted ventilatory response to CO_2 to 67% of baseline.

An increase in R and E will reduce the slope of the ventilatory response under PAV for two reasons. First, percent assist is now lower. For example, if $\dot{V}_A$ were 70% E, and E increased by 50%, $\dot{V}_A$ would become 47% (70/150). This reduces the amplification factor [from 3.3 to 1.88 in this case; amplification factor = 100/(100 − %assist)]. Second, the slope of the ventilatory response that is being amplified also has decreased to 67% of the initial value. As a result, ventilatory response on PAV is now 38% of its initial value. $\dot{V}_E$ must fall, Pa_{CO_2} must rise, and distress may develop.

The situation is comparable with PSV. The already low ventilatory slope becomes even lower because the unassisted slope is now lower. Furthermore, the same pressure assist will be less effective in boosting V_T because of worse mechanics. As a result, the ventilatory response is displaced downward as well (e.g., Figure 4 in ref. 22). A new steady state is reached at a lower $\dot{V}_E$ and higher Pa_{CO_2}. The changes in $\dot{V}_E$ and Pa_{CO_2} are comparable in the two modes.

FIGURE 13-11 Responses to a 50% increase in ventilatory demand with proportional-assist (PAV), pressure-support (PSV), and volume-cycled ventilation (VCV). The unassisted ventilatory response to CO_2 is given by the solid diagonal line in each panel. The three modes were set during the low-demand period to produce the same ventilation and Pa_{CO_2} (*solid circles/dashed lines*). Because of the higher ventilatory-response slope on PAV, the new ventilation could be reached with a much smaller increase in Pa_{CO_2} (*open circles*). See text for more details.

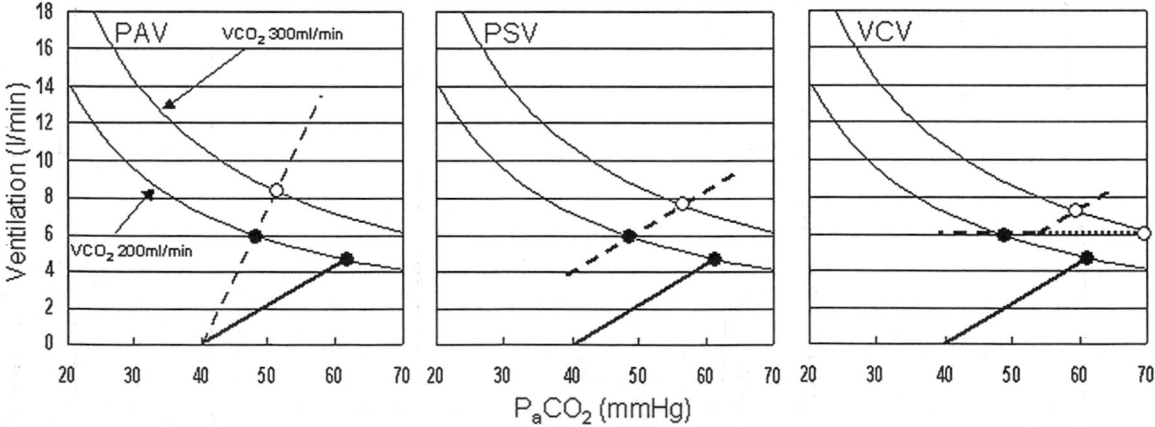

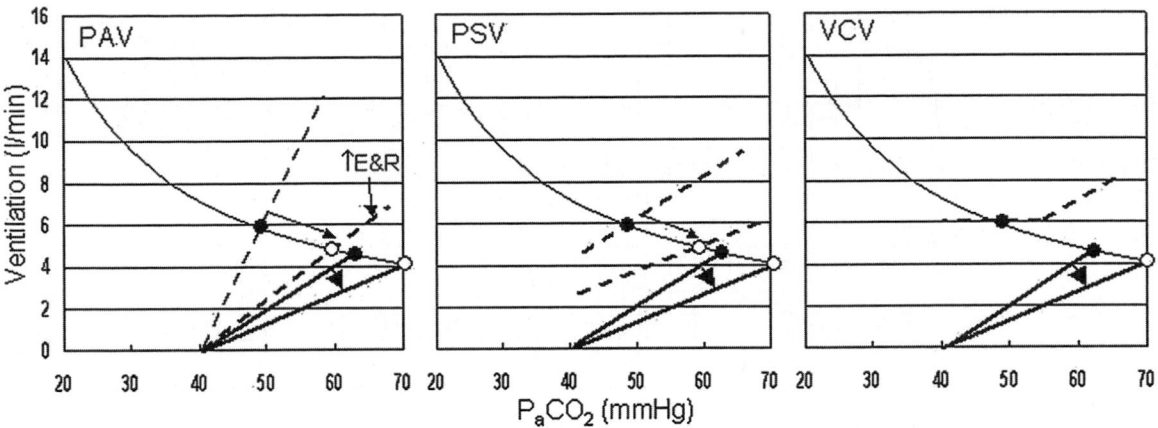

FIGURE 13-12 Responses to a 50% increase in elastance and resistance with proportional-assist (PAV), pressure-support (PSV), and volume-cycled ventilation (VCV). (*Solid diagonal lines*) Unassisted ventilatory responses before and after the change in mechanics. (*Dashed lines*) Ventilatory responses on assisted ventilation. All modes were set before the change to produce the same ventilation and Pa_{CO_2} (*solid circles/dashed lines*). As mechanics worsen, Pa_{CO_2} increases and ventilation decreases with PAV and PSV (*open circles*) but not with VCV.

By contrast, with VCV, a change in E and R will have no effect on ventilation. The ventilator will deliver the same V_T. Because there is no change in Pa_{CO_2}, there is no increase in effort. In this respect, therefore, VCV is superior to both PAV and PSV.

Grasso et al[22] compared responses to an increase in elastance with PAV and PSV. Surprisingly, they found that with PAV, V_T decreased less, RR increased less, and the increase in dyspnea was less. It is not clear why this was so. Regardless, the better results in this study were not expected and should not be viewed as intrinsic to PAV.

An improvement in mechanics also can create problems with PAV and PSV but not with VCV. If percent assist is high before the change, a reduction in R or E may cause the percent assist to exceed 100% of the new R or E, resulting in runaway. With PSV, improvement in mechanics at the same assist level will increase $\dot{V}_E$ and decrease Pa_{CO_2}. Asynchrony may appear.

In summary, on PAV, changes in mechanics may be followed by distress or excessive ventilator alarming (runaways). This problem for PAV is mitigated by the possibility of monitoring passive R and E continuously and adjusting assist accordingly (see "Noninvasive Monitoring of Respiratory Mechanics, Pmusc, and Work of Breatheing," below).

RESPIRATORY RATE IN DIFFERENT MODES

With all modes, patient RR will increase if assist is inadequate. Patient RR, however, is also sensitive to reflexes, independent of chemical drive. Continued inflation during neural expiration prolongs neural expiration and, by extension, reduces RR.[68–70] This reflex is less pronounced in ICU patients[70] than in alert patients[68,69] but is still quite evident. Its gain varies widely among patients.[70] Figure 13-8 shows a very weak response. Note that patient RR was the same whether efforts occurred during inflation or deflation. By contrast, Figure 13-13 illustrates a strong response. Here, on PSV, ventilator cycle extended well into neural T_E. When PSV was discontinued, there was a marked increase in patient RR (20–33 breaths per minute). This cannot represent distress because it occurred immediately, and diaphragmatic swings were still very low (~5 cmH$_2$O). Thus, with PSV, nonsynchrony may reduce patient RR for reasons that have little to do with relieving distress. As a corollary, reduction in asynchrony, as would occur if PSV levels were reduced,[28,63] may result in acceleration of RR that is unrelated to distress. This is not a problem with PAV because the ends of patient and ventilator inspiratory phases are synchronized. Therefore, changes in RR on PAV reflect level of distress more reliably.

TIDAL VOLUME IN DIFFERENT MODES

As indicated earlier (under "Respiratory Rate and Breathing Pattern"), with PAV, V_T is determined by the patient, and the preferred V_T ranges from 4–15 ml/kg, with an average of 7 ml/kg.[27,28] With VCV, V_T is set without knowledge of the patient's preferred V_T. PSV is also usually adjusted to yield a given V_T. In either case, the set V_T almost always will be larger than necessary. For example, if V_T is set to 10 ml/kg, it will be greater than preferred V_T in most patients. In the others, it will be inadequate. If one individualizes the assist to comfort level, V_T still will be higher than with PAV for two reasons: First, when V_T is titrated to the lowest level consistent with comfort, the chosen V_T is greater than the average V_T during spontaneous breathing.[8,71] Second, if V_T or PSV level is set to comfort level at a given point, a change in ventilatory demand (see, for example, Figs. 13-10 and 13-11) will cause it to become either excessive or too little later. If it becomes excessive, it will not be adjusted down. If it becomes inadequate (increase in demand), however, it will be increased and remain at the high level after, when demand decreases again. On average, V_T will be larger than if it were allowed to vary with demand (i.e., PAV).

Another peculiarity unique to PSV is that dynamic hyperinflation may cause tidal volume to be inversely related to inspiratory effort (see, for example, Fig. 13-8). This is so because at a given PSV, the end-inspiratory volume, relative

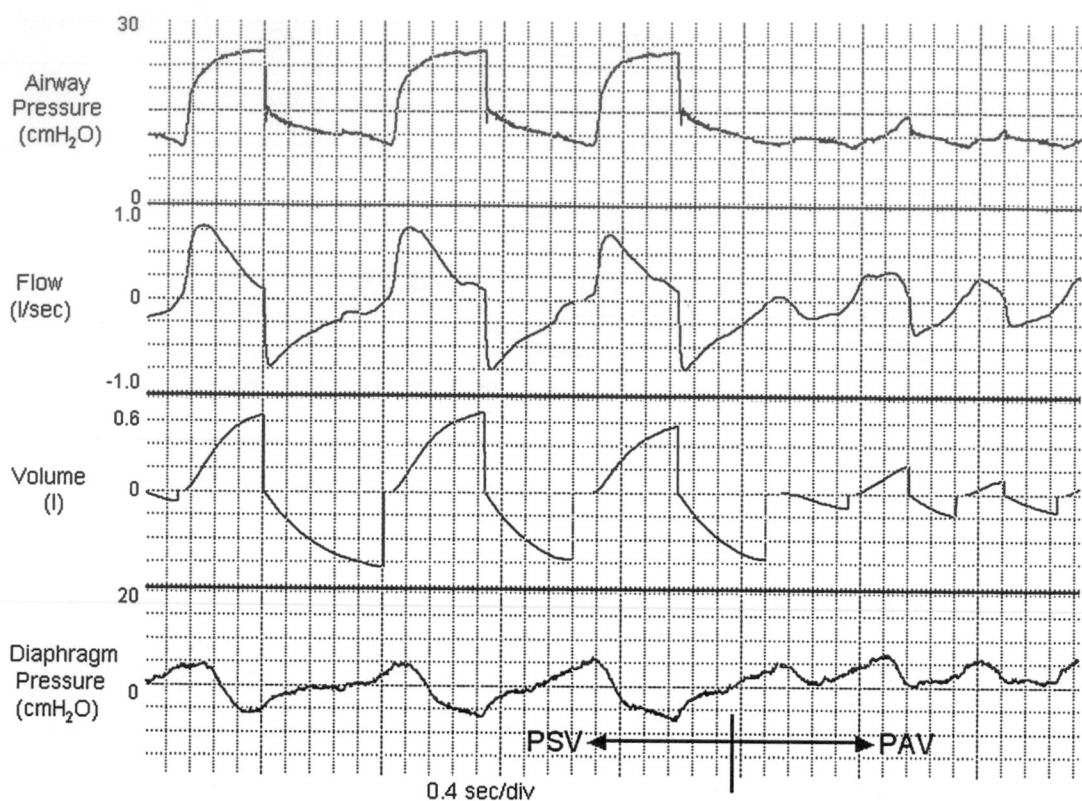

FIGURE 13-13 Transition from pressure-support ventilation (PSV) to PAV in the same patient as in Fig. 13-7 with marked dynamic hyperinflation. Efforts were quite weak on PSV and barely succeeded in triggering the ventilator. On switching to PAV, the patient receives very little assist because, unlike PSV, assist cannot outlast inspiratory effort. Effort must increase in order to advance triggering and obtain adequate ventilation (see Fig. 13-7*B*). Note that respiratory rate increased suddenly on the switch. Because efforts were still quite weak and the response was immediate, the increase in rate was not caused by a high respiratory drive (i.e., distress) and almost certainly was reflexic in origin secondary to removal of inflation during neural expiration (see text).

to passive FRC, at which the ventilator cycles off, in the absence of effort (Vth), is fixed.[63] A stronger effort will trigger the ventilator at a higher volume relative to FRC, leaving less difference between the onset of the breath and Vth (see inset of Fig. 13-8). With high PSV, it is possible to reduce chemical drive to very near the AT, resulting in very weak efforts (see, for example, Fig. 13-8*A*). Triggering then can occur only when volume is very close to FRC. When a breath is triggered, volume must increase by a large amount before the ventilator cycles off. Large protracted V_TS result (see Fig. 13-8*A*). If efforts increase, either spontaneously or after reducing PSV level, breaths can be triggered at a higher volume and hence closer to Vth. A small V_T will cause Vth to be reached. Once effort ceases, flow decreases to the cycling-off threshold, and the ventilator cycle ends. Synchrony is reestablished, but breathing becomes faster and shallower (see Fig. 13-8). Thus, paradoxically, under these conditions V_T is largest when effort is weakest, and changes in V_T no longer reflect effort.

This scenario can never happen with PAV in part because in the presence of dynamic hyperinflation it is not possible to reduce efforts to the very low levels that can be reached with high-level PSV [see "Dynamic Hyperinflation (DH)," below] and in part because the inflation cycle ends when pa-

tient effort ceases regardless of the end-inspiratory volume reached.

COMFORT

Comfort, of course, cannot be compared in obtunded patients. Whenever PSV and PAV were compared in alert patients with respiratory distress, however, PAV was preferred.[23,32,33]

HEMODYNAMIC EFFECTS

Mechanical ventilation has complex effects on the circulation (see Chapter 38). Data comparing hemodynamics on PAV with other modes are very limited. Patrick et al[72] found that cardiac output was 22% higher during PAV than during VCV in eight patients with septic shock (see Fig. 15-9 in ref. 73). Blood pressure also was higher. These results likely were secondary to lower airway pressure, and hence mean intrathoracic pressure, during PAV promoting higher venous return. There is no information on the effect of PAV versus other modes in left-ventricular dysfunction. Such information is needed because, in theory, a lower intrathoracic pressure may not be helpful in these patients (higher afterload).

CLINICAL CONSEQUENCES OF THE PHYSIOLOGIC DIFFERENCES

PATIENT MANAGEMENT ISSUES

Noninvasive Monitoring of Respiratory Mechanics, Pmusc, and Work of Breathing

PAV has unique features that allow estimation of passive mechanics noninvasively.[49,50] In PAV, end of ventilator cycle occurs during the declining phase of inspiratory Pmusc (see Figs. 13-1 and 13-14A). A brief end-inspiratory occlusion coincides with the terminal part of the declining phase. This phase ends shortly after the onset of occlusion, and its end is readily recognizable[50] (Fig. 13-14A). Paw at the end of this phase provides the passive recoil pressure associated with occluded volume. This is not the case with VCV or PSV because the end of the ventilator cycle may occur during an active inspiratory or expiratory phase. This approach has been validated,[50] and an automated version was included in new 840 PAV + software (Tyco). A multicenter study confirmed its reliability ($r^2 = 0.92$ compared with elastance measured by esophageal catheter[74]).

Because V_T is usually variable on PAV, random end-inspiratory occlusions frequently produce a wide range of V_Ts and plateau pressures from which confident estimates of the slope and pressure intercept can be obtained (Fig. 13-15). A positive intercept indicates either dynamic hyperinflation or a respiratory system that is stiffer in the lower part of tidal ventilation [see "Nonlinearity in the Pressure-Volume (P-V) Relation within the Tidal Volume Range," below]. Because both abnormalities respond to increasing PEEP, changes in intercept can be used to set the PEEP level associated with best elastance.

Because Paw at the end of brief occlusions reflects passive recoil at end inspiration, it is possible to estimate passive *expiratory* resistance[75] (see Fig. 13-14A). This approach was incorporated in the newly released 840 PAV+ option (Tyco). Its main limitation is that expiratory resistance may overestimate inspiratory resistance when flow limitation exists.[76] When used to adjust flow assist in these patients, flow runaway may occur. To circumvent this possibility, the manufacturer limited the maximum R to be used for PAV adjustment, a reasonable but not ideal solution. An alternate method that estimates inspiratory resistance from brief pulses has been described and validated.[49] It was incorporated in a new Japanese PAV system (see "Commercially Available PAV Delivery Systems," below).

FIGURE 13-14 Tracings from a patient on the 840 PAV+ option (Tyco) illustrating the random brief end-inspiratory occlusions. *A.* 40% assist. *B.* 80% assist. Note the minimal change in breathing and lower amplitude of diaphragmatic pressure swings. Airway pressure rises early during the occlusion in panel *A*, reflecting the fact the inspiratory phase ended during the declining phase of inspiratory pressure *(vertical dashed line)*. During occlusion, airway pressure is inversely related to muscle pressure. By the end of occlusion, airway pressure had plateaued, corresponding to inspiratory pressure reaching its baseline level. In panel *B*, there is no rising phase during the occlusion because inspiratory pressure had returned to baseline already; at high assist, the inspiratory phase tends to end at a later point on the declining phase.[62] Note that airway pressure is approximately the same at end occlusion in both cases. Elastance is determined from [(end-occlusion pressure – PEEP)/V_T]. Expiratory resistance is determined from flow early in expiration and ΔP (the difference between airway pressure and elastic recoil at the same point). Elastic recoil is obtained from end-occlusion pressure minus an amount corresponding to the volume expired and elastance *(dotted line)*.

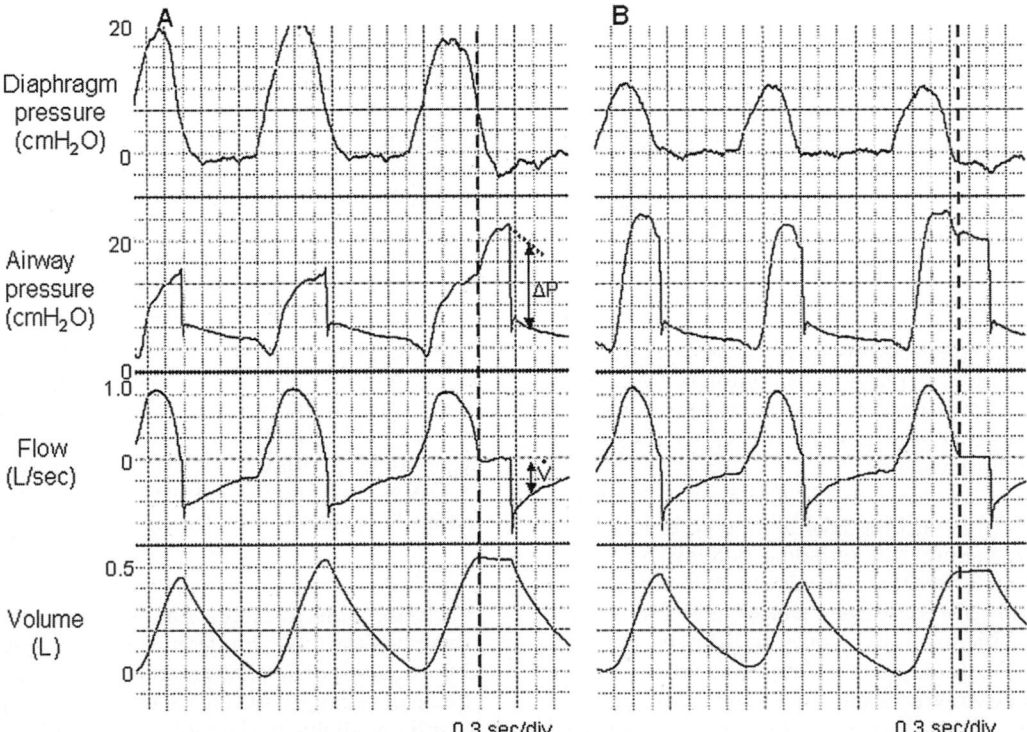

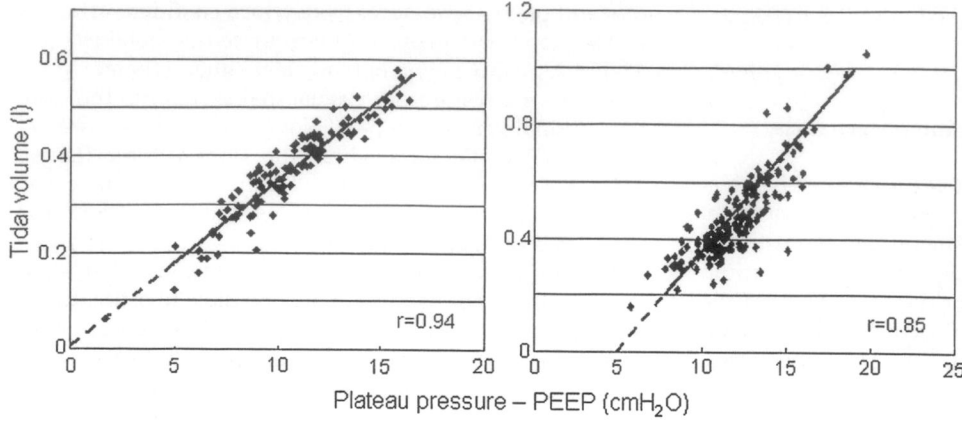

FIGURE 13-15 Relation between occlusion pressure and tidal volume. Data collected over approximately an hour of recording with randomly applied occlusions. The range of volumes was the result of spontaneous tidal volume variability. In both cases, a highly significant correlation was obtained. *A.* Pressure intercept not different from PEEP, indicating no dynamic hyperinflation. *B.* Patient with dynamic hyperinflation. Note the positive intercept.

Apart from overcoming the major practical limitation to implementing PAV, namely, knowing passive mechanics, continuous monitoring of passive R and E should help in monitoring disease progression and in the timely identification of complications (e.g., changes in lung water, accumulation of secretions, bronchospasm, and so on). If a patient's condition deteriorates, it should be possible to sort out what happened to mechanics by observing recent trends in R and E. Furthermore, when R and E are known, it is possible to calculate patient-generated pressure (Pmusc) and work of breathing in real time.

Improved Reliability of Ventilator Rate as a Measure of Distress and Weaning Failure

As indicated earlier (under "Physiologic Consequences of Operational Differences"), an increase in ventilator rate is not specific to distress in PSV and VCV. In either mode, a simple increase in effort, occurring spontaneously or as result of reduction in assist, may decrease ineffective efforts and result in an artifactual, sometimes dramatic increase in ventilator rate (see Fig. 13-8). Although this artifact can be identified from flow and Paw tracings,[28] considerable expertise is required. Furthermore, even if true RR is counted and found to have increased, the increase may be reflexic and not secondary to true distress (see "Respiratory Rate in Different Modes," above). With PAV, ineffective efforts are very rare, and inflation extends minimally into neural expiration. Accordingly, ventilator rate faithfully reflects patient rate.[20,28] When it increases, distress can be inferred more reliably. Because a substantial increase in ventilator rate following a reduction in assist is used commonly to infer continued ventilator dependence, this feature of PAV should reduce false weaning failure verdicts.

The occurrence of an absolute RR of more than 35 breaths per minute during a weaning trial is used commonly as a sign of weaning failure.[77,78] Yet some patients breathe at rates greater than 35 breaths per minute even when assist is very high and efforts are very weak[28] (see Fig. 13-8*A*). Thus, in some patients, a high absolute RR need not indicate distress. PAV can be used to determine whether absolute tachypnea observed during a weaning trial is distress-related. Failure of RR to decrease as PAV assist is increased to high levels would indicate that tachypnea is not distress-

related (see "Respiratory Rate and Breathing Pattern," above). Such a test would not be feasible with other modes because in such patients (high intrinsic RR), ventilator or even patient rate invariably will decrease as assist increases because of nonsynchrony. It remains to be determined, however, whether tachypnea that is not relieved by ventilator support is a reason to continue mechanical ventilation.

Choice of Ventilator Settings

With VCV and PSV, one does not know what is appropriate for each patient. Given what we know now about variability in undistressed (preferred) breathing pattern and time-to-time changes in demand, no general guidelines will be suitable for all patients; in most cases, the assist delivered will exceed what is necessary (see "Tidal Volume in Different Modes," above). With PAV, there is no uncertainty about what the patient wants or needs or how to set the level of assist. There is only one variable to consider (percent assist), and when percent assist is increased to a point where V_T and RR no longer respond to further increases, the values observed are what the patient needs.

This apparent simplicity of setting PAV has been mitigated by a number of practical limitations, however, that proved problematic when simple PAV delivery systems were used (see "Limitations," below). In some patients these can cause frequent ventilator alarming and/or the presence of distress in the face of supposedly high assist levels. To compound matters, troubleshooting these problems requires considerable expertise. At present, there is a consensus that PAV delivery systems must be able to monitor respiratory mechanics continuously and automatically[16,79] and that their alarm systems must be adapted to take into account the spontaneous variability of breathing in patients on PAV. Such systems have just become available (see "Commercially Available PAV Delivery Systems," below).

CLINICAL OUTCOME

It is reasonable to enquire as to whether the physiologic advantages of PAV translate into better clinical outcome. Unfortunately, information about outcomes is either inadequate or nonexistent. This is so chiefly because, until very recently, available ICU ventilators [Winnipeg ventilator and Evita (Drager)] were not equipped with means to provide smooth, nuisance-free PAV delivery over the extended periods required for outcome studies. It is hoped that with newly available systems such studies will be carried out. In the meantime, one is limited to speculation about how physiologic advantages may improve outcome.

Noninvasive Ventilation

Two studies compared outcomes with PSV and PAV in acute respiratory failure.[32,33] Both found greater comfort and acceptance rate and a lower incidence of facial ulcers and conjunctivitis with PAV. One study found faster improvement in respiratory rate and Pa_{CO_2} with PAV.[32] Neither study found a difference in intubation rate. Both studies, however, were seriously underpowered in this respect. When faced with a choice between severe distress and a somewhat uncomfortable way to relieve it, most people will opt for relief of dyspnea. Thus nonacceptance rate with PSV is low (15% versus 3% in PAV[33]). Furthermore, intubation rate in such patients is also low (~20–30%[32,33]). It is estimated that more than 1000 patients are required to determine whether a new intervention reduces rate of intubation.[33]

Clinical Outcome in the ICU Setting

PAV may improve clinical outcome in a number of ways:

1. *Sedative use.* Most ICU patients are heavily sedated if they are not spontaneously unconscious. Sedatives may affect clinical outcome adversely.[80,81] It is not clear to what extent patient-ventilator interactions contribute to need for sedation. To the extent that they may, PAV may result in less sedative use and reduction in sedation-related complications.
2. *Impact on sleep.* Poor patient-ventilator interaction may affect sleep adversely in the ICU.[51,82] Sleep deprivation

may increase blood pressure, depress immune function, and promote a negative nitrogen balance, actions that can affect morbidity adversely (for review, see ref. 82). By improving patient-ventilator interaction, PAV may help to reduce these complications.

3. *Barotrauma and ventilator-induced lung injury.* Excessive lung distension may result in further lung injury (see Chapter 46) and possibly multisystem organ failure[83] (see Chapter 44). There are a number of reasons why V_T will, on average, be smaller in PAV (see "Tidal Volume in Different Modes," above). Furthermore, neural reflexes terminate inspiratory muscle activity if lung distension exceeds a certain threshold that is well below physiologic total lung capacity (TLC) (e.g., Hering-Breuer reflex). For example, when tidal expansion approaches TLC during exercise, further increases in ventilation are achieved automatically via increases in RR.[84] Because the assist terminates automatically with PAV when respiratory muscles are inhibited, overdistension beyond physiologic TLC (transpulmonary pressure $\approx$ 40 cmH_2O) is virtually impossible. Figure 13-16 shows average plateau pressure on PAV in 48 patients with a wide range of elastance. Plateau pressure was less than 30 cmH_2O above positive end-expiratory pressure (PEEP) in all and less than 20 cmH_2O above PEEP in all but four. Considering that plateau pressure also includes chest-wall recoil, lung distension was even less. It is reasonable to expect that this behavior will reduce barotrauma. It also may make it possible to achieve the objectives of permissive hypercapnia (small V_T) without the need for sedation or even hypercapnia (because RR increases automatically as end-inspiratory volume approaches TLC).

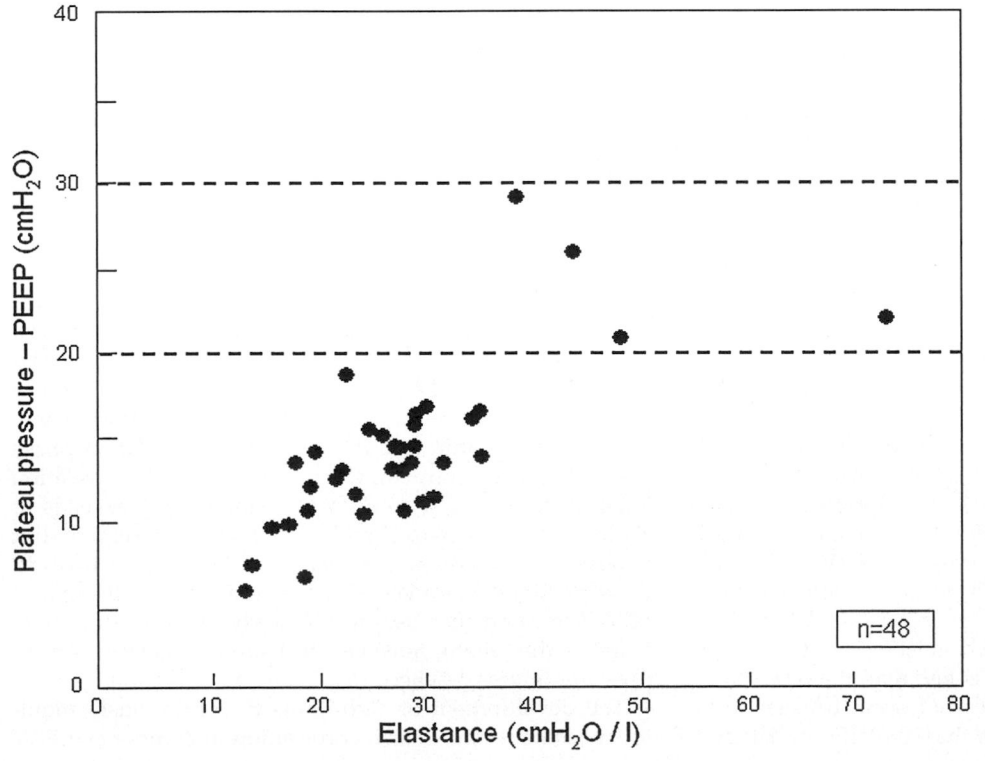

FIGURE 13-16 Average plateau pressure (minus PEEP) in 48 patients with a wide range of elastance.

4. *Weaning.* The greater reliability of ventilator rate as a measure of distress (see "Improved Reliability of Ventilator Rate as a Measure of Distress and Weaning Failure," above) should decrease instances of false ventilator dependence. Tachypnea as the sole reason for a declaration of weaning failure accounted for 37% of all weaning failures in two large trials[77,78] (A. Esteban, personal communication). It is tempting to speculate that some of these patients were not ventilator-dependent, so their identification under PAV will reduce ventilator time.

With PSV and VCV, Pa_{CO_2} may decrease to very near the AT, resulting in extremely weak efforts, particularly during periods of reduced demand (see "Physiologic Consequences of Operational Differences," above). With VCV in the assist-control mode, it is also possible to produce protracted apnea. With PAV, a modest to moderate level of activation is present at all times, including during sleep. The likelihood of disuse atrophy of respiratory muscles (see Chapter 45) may be less, and this may facilitate weaning.

Most ineffective efforts occur during mechanical expiration. Accordingly, the inspiratory muscles are being lengthened during their activation. This type of contraction has been associated with muscle injury.[85,86] Because ineffective efforts are very common with PSV and VCV[67] but not with PAV, this type of injury may be mitigated.

5. Continuous noninvasive monitoring of passive mechanics, made possible by PAV, may lead to better PEEP management and early detection and management of complications.

Limitations

The following mechanisms often result in excessive sounding of alarms and occasional instances in which patients are in distress despite a high percent assist. Fortunately, the underlying reasons for these difficulties are well understood, and auxiliary algorithms have become available that should mitigate most, if not all, of these problems.

RUNAWAY PHENOMENON

Runaway is a limitation because (1) it often results in triggering of alarms, which can be annoying and may promote anxiety in alert patients, (2) excessive delivered pressure, flow, or volume may disturb the patient, and (3) the patient is no longer in the PAV mode.

The runaway pattern depends on whether the resistive or elastic component is overassisted. With elastic overassist, the elastic pressure provided (V × VA) exceeds actual elastic pressure (V × E) by an amount that increases as a function of volume [excess elastic pressure = V(VA − E)]. If flow is not overassisted (FA < R), the resistive pressure provided is less than actual resistive pressure by an amount that is related to flow [deficit in resistive assist = flow(R − FA)]. So long as excess elastic pressure is less than the deficit in resistive pressure, a runaway does not occur because total applied pressure (Paw) is less than the sum of actual resistive and elastic pressures. Runaway occurs when excess elastic pressure cannot be absorbed by the deficit (or reserve) in resistive pressure.

With elastic overassist, excess elastic pressure increases progressively during inspiration because volume rises throughout. By contrast, reflecting flow pattern, deficit/reserve in resistive pressure is highest in early and middle inspiration and decreases later. The point at which elastic overassist will exceed the reserve in resistive pressure (i.e., runaway) necessarily will occur late in inspiration. When VA is just greater than E, the runaway will occur at the very end of the inspiratory phase when flow is near zero (Fig. 13-17A). This fact has been put to use to measure actual patient E in sleeping or obtunded patients.[6,17,73] VA is dialed up in small steps until the characteristic runaway pattern appears (see Fig. 13-17B). At this point, VA is just greater than E. The more the elastic overassist, the sooner, in the inspiratory phase, runaway will develop (see Fig. 13-17). Likewise, runaway occurs earlier if the difference between R and FA is small because the deficit in resistive pressure will be less and more readily overcome by excess elastic pressure.

By analogy, with resistive overassist, runaway will occur when the excess resistive pressure provided by the ventilator [flow(FA − R)] exceeds the deficit/reserve in applied elastic pressure [V(E − VA)]. This point invariably will occur at the very beginning of inspiration, where volume, and hence elastic assist, is near zero, and there is no possibility for the elastic deficit/reserve to absorb the excess resistive pressure.

Notwithstanding the danger implied by the term, there is in fact no danger for two reasons:

1. Modern ventilators limit the pressure and/or volume that can be delivered. During normal PAV operation (i.e., no runaway), the high-pressure limit rarely needs to be greater than 40 cmH_2O.
2. The naturally nonlinear pressure-volume relation of the respiratory system[87] and the nonlinear pressure-flow relation in intubated patients[88] effectively preclude dangerous overdistension. Figure 13-18 illustrates this.

The pattern of flow runaway depends on whether the pressure-flow relation is linear (Fig. 13-19). A linear pressure-flow relation occurs when breathing via the mouth, thereby excluding the nonlinear nasal pressure-flow relation, or when the nonlinear relation of the endotracheal tube is offset independently by automatic tube compensation (ATC). Here, as FA just exceeds resistance, there is a very rapid increase in flow and pressure that can be aborted only by a ventilator limit (see Fig. 13-19A). The inflation phase is very brief. By contrast, when the pressure-flow relation is nonlinear, there is no discrete change as FA exceeds R. Rather, change is gradual and consists of a progressive shift in peak flow to earlier points in inspiration (see Fig. 13-19B). Flow pattern at high levels of overassist resembles that of PSV. The rapid increase in flow early in inspiration may truncate the breath, however, and sound an alarm if peak pressure limit is reached.

The development of algorithms to continuously monitor mechanics and their incorporation in commercial PAV

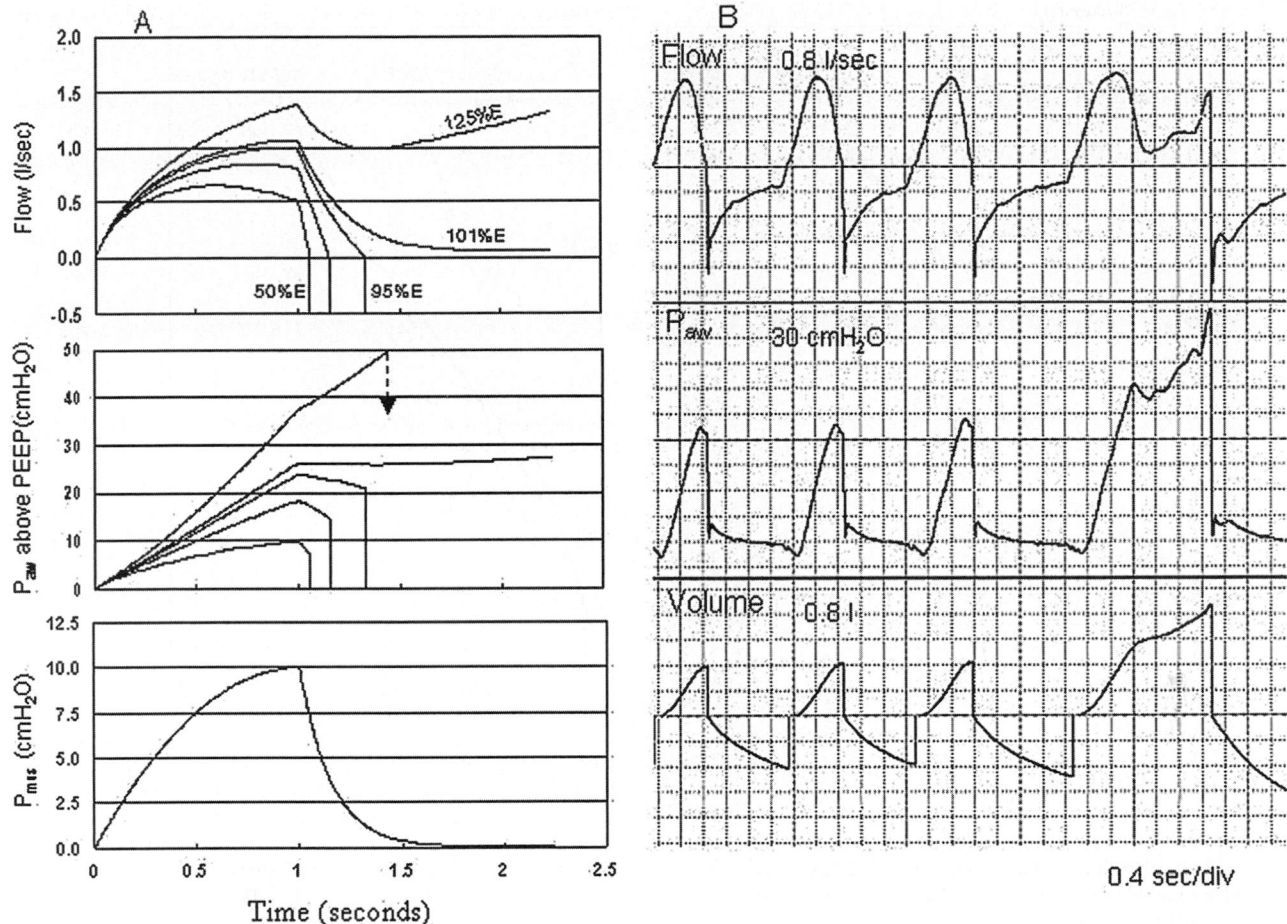

FIGURE 13-17 Runaway. *A.* Model simulation of effect of increasing percent of elastance used for volume assist (VA). Note that as soon as VA exceeds elastance (101% E), flow fails to return to zero at the end of inspiratory phase. At higher levels, the runaway begins earlier, and flow and pressure increase progressively until the cycle is terminated by a physiological or ventilator limit. *B.* Patient with COPD and moderate dynamic hyperinflation, 90% assist. Note the spontaneous occurrence of a runaway breath (last breath). The pattern is intermediate between the 101% and 125% in the left panel. Note that in the breath preceding the runaway, exhaled volume exceeded inhaled volume, suggesting less dynamic hyperinflation at the beginning of the runaway breath. See text for more details. The runaway breath was terminated by the ventilator's high-pressure limit.

delivery systems (see "Noninvasive Monitoring of Respiratory Mechanics, Pmusc, and Work of Breathing," above) should greatly reduce this problem.

Runaways need not occur on every breath (see, for example, Fig. 13-17). Because elastance (E) may vary breath by breath [see "Dynamic Hyperinflation (DH)" and "Nonlinearity in the Pressure-Volume (P-V) Relation within the Tidal Volume Range," above], volume assist may exceed E in some breaths even though it is less than 100% of average E. Assume that average E, determined from a number of end-inspiratory occlusions, is 30 cmH$_2$O/liter, with a range of 24–36 cmH$_2$O/liter. At 90% assist (i.e., 27 cmH$_2$O/liter), some breaths may develop runaway. The closer VA is to average E, the more frequent are the runaways.

ACCURACY AND STABILITY OF RESPIRATORY MECHANICS VALUES

Knowledge of R and E is not necessary in noninvasive applications. Feedback from the alert patient ensures that VA and FA are appropriate. In the usually obtunded ICU patient, subjective feedback is not possible, and setting PAV properly requires knowledge of passive mechanics. This has created problems for two reasons: First, measuring passive mechanics in the usual way (under sedation, hyperventilation, and/or paralysis) is cumbersome, requires expertise, cannot be done frequently, and the results may not reflect the E and R values on PAV (because of differences in V$_T$, flow rate, dynamic hyperinflation, and so on). Second, passive mechanics frequently change (see "Response to Changes in Respiratory Mechanics," above). Values that are accurate at one point may become inaccurate later.

When differences between actual and assumed R and E values are small (e.g., <25%) and percent assist is not high, the impact is operationally insignificant. For example, with a 20% error at 50% assist, actual assist will be 42% or 60%. Either value is consistent with proper functioning, and if the assist is insufficient, there is room to increase it. By contrast, with a 50% error at 80% assist, actual assist will be 40%

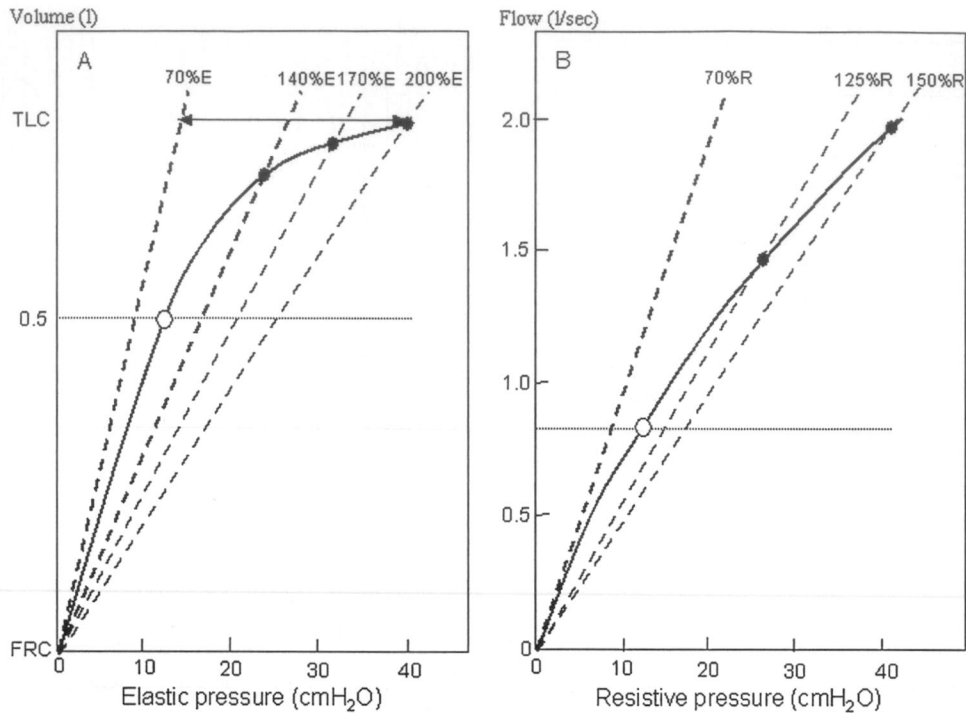

FIGURE 13-18 Physiologic limits to runaway. *A.* Typical pressure-volume curve in an average ventilated patient. Elastance (E) at a tidal volume (V$_T$) of 0.5 liter (the average V$_T$ on PAV in this case) is 25 cmH$_2$O/liter (*open circle*). FRC, functional residual capacity; TLC, total lung capacity. (*Left diagonal line*) Volume assist = 70% E. The elastic pressure delivered by the ventilator is less than elastic recoil at all volumes (no runaway). The next three diagonal lines represent progressively increasing overassist. An excess elastic pressure is delivered in the spontaneous tidal volume range (horizontal distance between diagonal lines and pressure-volume line), forcing a volume runaway. Because of the stiffening of the system near TLC, however, excess pressure decreases as volume increases. Runaway ends when the diagonal line meets the pressure-volume line because there is no longer an excess pressure. Note that even with a marked overassist (200% E), runaway stops at an elastic pressure of 40 cmH$_2$O, corresponding to a physiologic TLC value. *B.* Typical pressure-flow relation in an average patient (airway resistance is 10 cmH$_2$O/liter/s with a no. 8 endotracheal tube). Total resistance at a flow of 0.8 liter/s is 15 cmH$_2$O/liter/s. A flow assist in excess of this value will cause a flow runaway (*right two diagonal lines*). Because the pressure-flow relation is not linear, excess resistive pressure decreases as flow increases. Flow runaway stops when the diagonal line meets the pressure-flow line. Excessive overdistension of the lung is also mitigated in this case by nonlinearity of the pressure-volume curve. Note that if VA is less than than E (*left diagonal line*, panel *A*), the deficit in elastic pressure increases dramatically near TLC (*horizontal arrow*, panel *A*). This helps offset the excess resistive pressure and aborts the flow runaway below physiologic TLC.

or 120%. In the former case, assist may be insufficient, resulting in distress when the patient is "supposedly" receiving high assist, and there is little room for further increases. In the latter case, runaway will develop, with frequent sounding of the alarms, even though it should not happen (percent assist <100). In our opinion, the discrepancy between assumed and actual R and E is the most important source of implementation difficulties. Fortunately, this has now been largely resolved (see "Noninvasive Monitoring of Respiratory Mechanics, Pmusc, and Work of Breathing," above).

LEAKS

Leaks affect PAV delivery in much the same way overestimation of E and R does. For example, if half the gas leaving the ventilator leaks out, assist will be twice that intended, or analogous to 100% overestimation of E and R. Thus the magnitude of overestimation is related directly to the magnitude of the leak. As in the case of overestimation of E and

R (see preceding section), a small leak will not have much impact if percent assist is low or moderate and will cause runaway if assist is high. Large leaks would result in runaway at all but the lowest assist levels.

In noninvasive applications, leaks can be huge. For this reason, noninvasive PAV delivery systems must be equipped with leak-compensation algorithms. In the ICU setting, leaks are usually very small, except in bronchocutaneous fistulas. Nonetheless, checking for leaks should be undertaken if alarms begin sounding excessively when they did not before.

Inclusion of automatic mechanics in PAV delivery systems essentially should eliminate leak-related problems. Thus, when a leak exists, the end-inspiratory occlusion technique (see Fig. 13-14) will underestimate E by an amount corresponding to the leak (provided inspired volume is used to compute E). This should offset the error at the ventilator level. Likewise, the pulse technique (resistance) will underestimate inspiratory resistance in the presence of leaks, thereby offsetting the pressure-delivery error at the ventilator level.

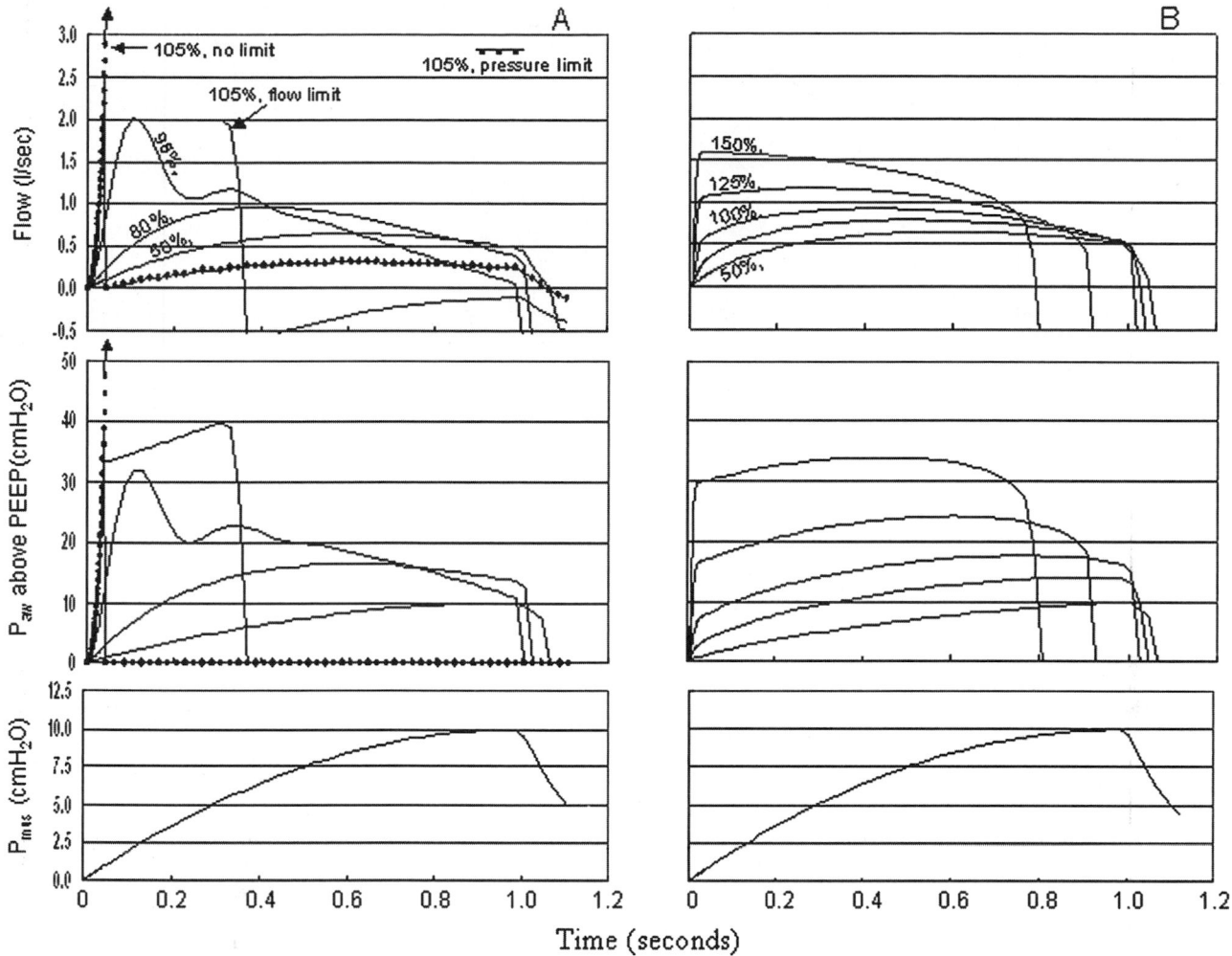

FIGURE 13-19 Patterns of flow runaway. Paw, airway pressure; Pmusc; respiratory muscle pressure. Percent denotes ratio of flow assist to resistance at a reference flow (0.5 liter/s in panel *B*). *A.* Linear pressure-flow relation. FA is increased in steps beginning with 50% R. As the assist approaches 100% R, some oscillations become apparent. At just above 100% R, there is a sudden change in response. Without any ventilator limits, flow and pressure increase very rapidly to extremely high levels at the beginning of inspiration. Termination of runaway depends on ventilator limits. With activation of peak-pressure limit, the cycle is aborted rapidly. If the maximum flow capability of the ventilator (e.g., 2 liters/s) is reached before the peak-pressure limit, the cycle continues a while more at the maximum flow and then self-terminates rapidly. With a constant resistance, therefore, transition of assist to above 100% is abrupt. *B.* Nonlinear pressure-flow relation (e.g., in the presence of an endotracheal tube). Runaway is blunted by the increasing resistance at higher flow (see Fig. 13-18*B*). There is no clear change in response at 100% assist. Rather, change is gradual and consists of a progressive shift in peak flow to earlier points in inspiration.

DYNAMIC HYPERINFLATION (DH)

DH presents occasional implementation difficulties, particularly when severe and associated with marked respiratory muscle weakness. Thus

1. By definition, DH means that elastic recoil pressure is greater than zero at inspiratory onset. Inspiratory muscles must generate enough pressure to offset this elastic recoil before the ventilator is triggered (see, for example, Figs. 13-7 and 13-8). Therefore, by the time the ventilator is triggered, a finite fraction of the patient's inspiratory phase will have elapsed. This delay is a function of magnitude of DH and the rate of rise of Pmusc (see Fig. 13-7). When DH is large (e.g., 10 cmH$_2$O in Fig. 13-7*A*) and the

rate of rise of Pmusc is low, triggering may not occur until near the end of inspiratory effort (see, for example, Fig. 13-7*A*). In PSV and VCV, once triggering occurs, a substantial breath will be delivered. Although volume delivery will be almost entirely during the patient's expiratory phase, adequate ventilation nonetheless will be delivered, making it possible for chemical drive to remain low. In PAV, the ventilator will provide support only for the remaining duration of inspiratory effort. When triggering is much delayed, the duration of support may be very brief, resulting in inadequate ventilation (see, for example, Fig. 13-13). The only way the patient can receive reasonable ventilation is to increase the rate of rise of inspiratory effort in order to advance triggering (see, for example, Fig. 13-7*B*). This will occur naturally at the

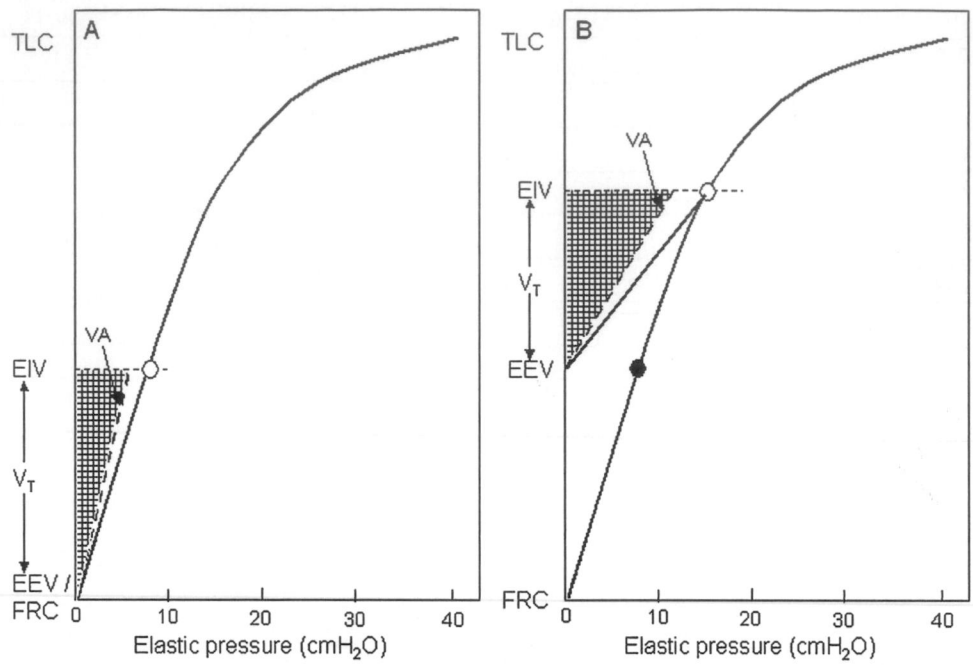

FIGURE 13-20 Impact of dynamic hyperinflation (DH) on PAV delivery. EEV, end-expiratory volume; FRC, functional residual capacity; TLC, total lung capacity; V_T, tidal volume; VA, volume assist. *A.* No DH (FRC and end-expiratory volume are the same). If 80% assist is dialed, the elastic work done by the ventilator (*shaded triangle*) is 80% of the total elastic work (*sum of shaded and open triangles*). DH: Elastic recoil pressure at end-expiratory volume is 8 cmH_2O (*solid circle*). Measured elastance (E = plateau pressure/V_T) overestimates actual elastance because V_T, the denominator, underestimates the difference between end-inspiratory volume and FRC (compare the solid diagonal line with the slope of the main pressure-volume curve in the V_T range). At 80% of this inflated elastance (*VA line*), the ventilator is providing only 50% of elastic work (compare the shaded triangle with the pressure-volume area in the V_T range). There is little room to increase the assist. Forcing VA to exceed measured elastance will result in runaway. In such cases, therefore, the maximum assist that can be delivered is limited.

expense of a higher chemical drive. When respiratory muscle reserve is high, the required increase in respiratory muscle output may be tolerated. When DH is very high and muscle reserve is quite low, distress may develop.

2. As illustrated in Fig. 13-20, the effective assist received is less than the percent assist dialed in. This is so because the ventilator is unaware of the Pmusc generated before triggering; the assist is applied only to that part of Pmusc in excess of that required for triggering. Thus not only does the patient have to generate more pressure to advance triggering, but the maximum percent assist that can be delivered effectively also is less. Distress may occur even at the highest possible assist.

3. Even if an assist level is found with which the patient is comfortable, runaway still may develop in occasional breaths, causing confusion (since VA is technically less that 100% E). The duration of expiration of spontaneous efforts can be quite variable. A breath preceded by a long expiratory time begins at a lower absolute volume (less DH). The same VA that was not associated with runaway when end-expiratory volume (EEV) was higher may now cause runaway (see Fig. 13-17*B*). This can be appreciated by moving the VA line downwards in Fig. 13-20*B*. It will be noted that at some point the VA line will cross to the right of the pressure-volume line.

The preceding account should not suggest that patients with severe COPD or other causes of DH are difficult to support. As judged by numerous reports[19–21,24–26,30,33,34] and our own experience, the vast majority can be supported very comfortably. Even in patients with severe COPD, elastic recoil at end expiration is usually approximately 3–5 cmH_2O,[89–91] a level that is accommodated easily by most patients. Nonetheless, a very high expiratory resistance combined with a high ventilatory demand and weak muscles may make it difficult to achieve adequate support.

The adverse impact of severe DH on PAV's performance can be mitigated in some patients by increasing PEEP. This is effective only when the high expiratory resistance is related to expiratory flow limitation in the lung, however. Where the high resistance is in the tubing, raising PEEP simply increases lung volume without relieving DH. The impact of DH can be eliminated completely if the ventilator is made to trigger at the onset of inspiratory effort instead of being triggered by inspiratory flow or airway pressure. A method for noninvasive identification of the onset of effort in real time has been developed recently[92] (see "effort channel" in Fig. 13-7). With such a system, PAV assist continues to be a function of flow and volume, but the reference flow is the expiratory flow at onset of effort (as opposed to zero flow, as is currently practiced). In this fashion, assist would apply throughout inspiratory effort.

NONLINEARITY IN THE PRESSURE-VOLUME (P-V) RELATION WITHIN THE TIDAL VOLUME RANGE

The relation between volume and elastic recoil is sigmoid.[87] Most patients breathe in the linear midrange, and E is nearly constant within the V_T range. In others, the P-V relation is not linear within V_T. This creates some difficulties because there is no fixed E to use for the sake of setting the volume assist. The difficulties depend on whether V_T falls within the stiff upper range (high-end nonlinearity) or the stiff lower range (low-end nonlinearity).

1. *High-end nonlinearity* (Fig. 13-21 A). This occurs when end-inspiratory volume approaches total lung capacity (TLC), such as when external PEEP is excessive or in very severe restrictive disease (e.g., severe ARDS). Here, the maximum elastic assist that can be provided without runaway is limited, and the highest V_T, with or without runaway, is constrained by physiologic TLC (see Fig. 13-21 A). Should this V_T be inadequate for the patient's ventilatory demand, distress will develop and cannot be relieved by increasing percent assist. Unless heavily sedated, such patients (high demand plus very stiff respiratory system) require supraphysiologic distending pressures for adequate ventilation, and PAV is not suitable.
2. *Low-end nonlinearity* (see Fig. 13-21 B). Here, the system is stiffest in the low range of tidal volume, for example,

when end-expiratory volume is close to residual volume (abdominal distension and obesity[93–95]) or when derecruitment of airways or alveoli occurs within the tidal volume range. The impact of this abnormality on PAV delivery is similar to that of dynamic hyperinflation [see "Dynamic Hyperinflation (DH)," above]; the assist received by patient is less than intended (see Fig. 13-21 B). When assist requirement is low, this behavior presents no difficulty. When assist level must be high (e.g., 80%), however, the patient may be comfortable, but because of the usually large breath-by-breath variability in V_T, runaways may occur during large breaths, triggering alarms (see Fig. 13-21 B). Therefore, in some patients it may be difficult to reach an assist level that is both adequate and free of frequent alarming. This problem can be eliminated by increasing PEEP, thereby placing V_T in the linear P-V range.

VENTILATOR RESPONSE TIME

Response delays are unavoidable in electromechanical systems. In the original Winnipeg ventilator, the delay was approximately 40 ms. We had assumed that the delay simply would result in a parallel shift relative to the target Paw waveform[73] and felt that this would be acceptable. However, Du et al[62] recently demonstrated that ventilator response delay becomes compounded during the inspiratory

FIGURE 13-21 **Impact of nonlinearity in the pressure-volume (P-V) relation within tidal volume. EEV, end-expiratory volume; FRC; functional residual capacity; TLC, total lung capacity; VA, volume assist; V_T; tidal volume. A. High-end nonlinearity. The P-V relation becomes quite flat within 0.5 liter of FRC. Elastance at a volume of 0.5 liter is 75 cmH$_2$O/liter (pressure and volume values at the open circle). The maximum VA that can be given without runaway is 50%. At higher assist, runaway develops until the flat region is reached. In either case, the maximum V_T that can be obtained with PAV is limited by physiologic TLC. B. Low-end non-linearity. Elastance is determined at an average V_T given by the open circle. At a VA of 80% E, the elastic assist received is only 55% (compare the hatched area with the total area inside the P-V line). Furthermore, if the patient makes a larger effort and obtains a larger V_T, elastic assist may exceed elastic recoil, and runaway may occur (*arrow*). At 50% assist, runaways would not occur, but the patient receives only 35% assist (not shown).**

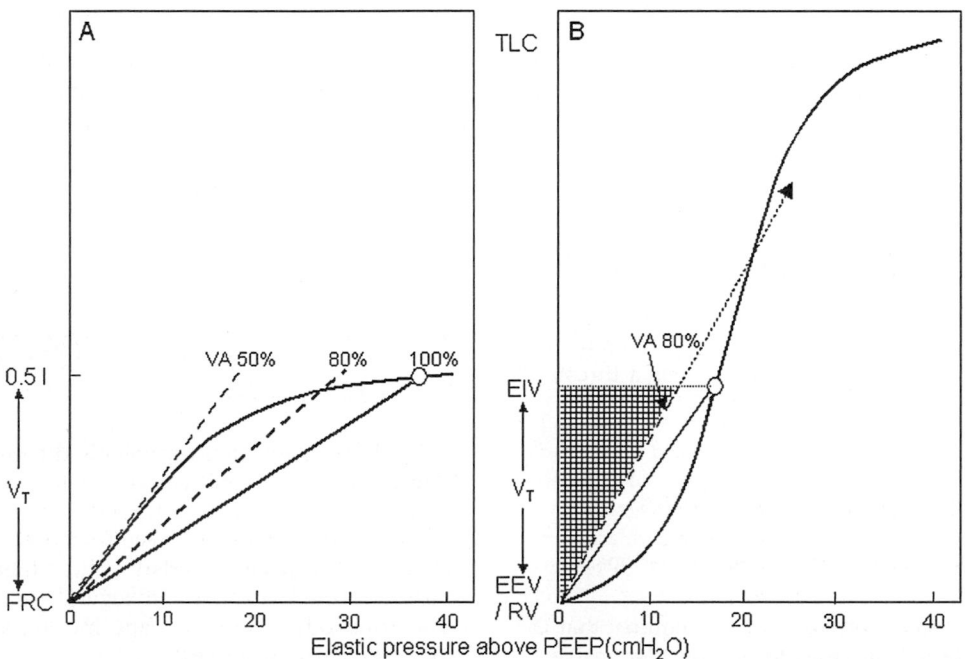

phase, resulting in cycling-off delays that are longer than the nominal ventilator delay. In their study, cycling-off delay was calculated as the difference between inspiratory flow reaching zero and the end of neural inspiration, defined as peak Pmusc. This presentation ignores the fact that even without a ventilator, transition from inspiration to expiration does not occur at peak Pmusc but during the declining phase of inspiratory activity.[42,96,97] The authors did not subtract this physiologic delay. If one does that, the cycling-off delay attributable to the ventilator is 0.2 second under the worst conditions (80% assist, highest R/E). [The authors[62] also reported data in normal volunteers. These are meaningless because the time constant of the system was increased to unrealistic values (2–3 seconds) by addition of a high resistance, and the rate of decline in Pmusc was not reported. In normal, awake subjects, Pmusc declines very slowly.[98]]

That response delays become compounded during PAV delivery[62] emphasizes the need for fast-responding gas-delivery systems in this mode. In practice, however, the reported cycling-off delays when the nominal delay is 40 ms (0.2 second under worst case) would be of little consequence,[20] particularly when one considers the performance of PSV under comparable circumstances (i.e., high assist in a patient with a high R/E ratio). Here, inflation may extend for greater than 1.0 second into neural expiration (e.g., compare PSV and PAV panels in Fig. 13-7) or even into the next inspiratory effort (see, for example, Fig. 13-8A).

EXCESSIVE ALARMING

Standard ventilator alarms that sound off every time a limit is reached proved to be a considerable nuisance in the PAV mode. Because of the spontaneous variability in breathing pattern, one or more limits may be reached frequently. Furthermore, without automatic mechanics, runaway breaths were frequent. With incorporation of automatic mechanics (see "Noninvasive Monitoring of Respiratory Mechanics, Pmusc, and Work of Breathing," above), occurrence of runaway will be greatly reduced, but some may still occur [see "Dynamic Hyperinflation (DH)" and "Nonlinearity in the Pressure-Volume (P-V) Relation within the Tidal Volume Range," above], and spontaneous variability will remain as a possible source for activating alarms. Accordingly, alarms in the PAV mode should take into account the breath-by-breath variability in breathing pattern and mechanics. A reasonable approach (e.g., 840 PAV+ option) is to use special filters whereby ventilator limits still function as such for safety reasons, but alarms sound off only when the frequency of reaching a ventilator limit exceeds a threshold value.

Indications and Contraindications

PAV is appropriate to use in all but a few situations:

1. *Respiratory depression.* Safe use of PAV requires that the patient's respiratory muscle output be responsive to

changes in Pa_{CO_2}, Pa_{O_2}, and pH. Absolute contraindications therefore are patients with central apnea or very weak efforts and *no respiratory distress despite an abnormally low pH.* Patients who are intubated for respiratory depression (e.g., overdose or neuropathology) or who had to be heavily sedated for intubation should not be placed on PAV initially. The situation is different in patients already being ventilated with another mode. Here, weak efforts and even no efforts (e.g., on assist-control ventilation or having recurrent central apneas on PSV[51]) are almost invariably secondary to overventilation. The assist with the other mode should be reduced first to establish that efforts resume at a reasonably normal pH before switching to PAV.

Care should be exercised when initiating PAV in a patient with known or suspected chronic CO_2 retention whose Pa_{CO_2} and pH were normalized by another ventilation mode. Such patients often respond poorly to CO_2 until Pa_{CO_2} reaches a level commensurate with their preintubation value. This may result in acute hypercapnia and acidemia following a switch to PAV. Chronic CO_2 retention per se is clearly not a contraindication, and many such patients were treated adequately with PAV. Patients who develop shallow, relatively slow breathing *with no distress* on PAV should have their blood gases checked, and if they are acidemic, they should be switched to another mode. These patients likely had undocumented prior chronic CO_2 retention.

2. *Bronchocutaneous fistulas.* Patients with bronchocutaneous fistulas should have their leak measured before switching to PAV. If the leak is high on another mode (e.g., exhaled volume less than 75% of inhaled volume), it is better not to use PAV unless the ventilator is equipped with automatic mechanics or leak-compensation algorithms.

USE OF SEDATIVES IN PATIENTS ON PAV

Sedatives are not contraindicated when PAV is used. When the response of a patient to sedatives is not known, the dose should be titrated initially until the amount required to attain the desired effect without severe depression is learned. Because backup systems always must be available on PAV delivery systems, the inadvertent use of an excessive amount of sedatives should not be hazardous.

Commercially Available PAV Delivery Systems

The BiPAP Vision (Respironics) is the only ventilator currently suitable for noninvasive use. ICU ventilators have no leak-compensation capability. The Vision is equipped with well-validated leak-compensation algorithms. It also has excellent response characteristics and trigger sensitivity and has performed very well in several clinical trials.[21,23,32,33] The Vision offers pathology-specific default startup settings as well as custom settings.

Until very recently, the Evita ventilator (Drager) was the only commercial ICU ventilator capable of delivering PAV. It is a basic system with no capability to monitor passive mechanics in real time and with standard alarms. As indicated earlier, such basic systems (including the Winnipeg ventilator) have proven difficult to use except by experts and for short periods.

Tyco recently released (outside the United States) a PAV+ option for the 840 ventilator. The ventilator monitors mechanics continuously by applying random brief end-inspiratory occlusions (see Fig. 13-14). The results have been validated.[74] In addition, the alarms were modified to allow for pressure and volume limits to be reached occasionally without the alarms sounding off. With this option, the maximum possible airway pressure, including PEEP, is 35 cmH$_2$O. This may be a limitation in a few patients on high PEEP whose resistance is also high. Another limitation is that the resistance measured is expiratory, so in patients with severe expiratory-flow limitation, inspiratory resistance may be overestimated.

A new ventilator capable of PAV delivery is about to be released in Japan (SSV, Kawasaki Safety Services). It is also equipped with the automatic mechanics function, but the resistance is measured with an inspiratory-pulse technique.[49]

Adjustment at the Bedside

NONINVASIVE APPLICATION

General instructions regarding noninvasive ventilation are similar to those for other modes and will not be discussed here (see Chapter 19). The following procedure pertains to BiPAP Vision (Respironics).

STARTUP

It is neither necessary nor recommended to attempt to measure respiratory mechanics. Patients are alert, and settings are best accomplished using patient feedback. Before attaching the ventilator to the mask, the limits should be set initially to a maximum pressure of 20 cmH$_2$O, a maximum volume of 1.5 liters, and a maximum inspiratory duration of 3 seconds. EPAP should be set to the minimum value (4 cmH$_2$O). Many patients prefer a lower EPAP, but 4 cmH$_2$O is the lowest setting on the BiPAP Vision. Set the ventilator in the "custom" mode to permit manual adjustment. Percent assist should be set to 99%. In this fashion, the E and R inserted in the ventilator are the actual VA and FA delivered to the patient. Set E and R initially to 2 and 1, respectively.

After attaching the ventilator to the patient and waiting a few breaths for the patient to adapt, inform him or her that the assist will be increased in steps and that he or she should signal approval/disapproval by some agreed-on system. Increase E in steps of one, waiting a few breaths between steps, until the patient signals that the assist is too high. Go back one or two steps. Repeat using the R input. Increase EPAP by 1 cmH$_2$O. If the patient signals approval, keep increasing EPAP. Most will not want more. Finally, perform final adjustment of E. Some patients will prefer a somewhat lower E setting once the other variables are optimized.

Observe the screen display for the range of airway pressure and V$_T$. Set the high limits a reasonable amount above the observed ranges. For example, if peak Paw ranges up to 15 cmH$_2$O and V$_T$ ranges up to 0.7 liter, set the pressure limit to 20 cmH$_2$O and the volume limit to 1.0 liter.

SUBSEQUENT MANAGEMENT

This is guided by clinical course. If distress progresses or reappears, the values of E and R should be retitrated. Nasal congestion should be avoided. Ask the patient if his or her nose is congested. If so, use decongestant, or switch to full face mask. If distress persists, then other methods of therapy should be considered. With clinical improvement, percent assist is reduced in steps guided by patient feedback. Because improvement may occur rapidly, it is a good idea to ask the patient at intervals whether the assist is too much and to see whether a lower percent assist is tolerated.

TROUBLESHOOTING

Although the ventilator corrects for leaks, it takes it three to five breaths to adjust to a leak change. A sudden change (e.g., mouth opening or loosening of mask) may result in a transient increase in applied pressure (up to the set limit). Patients should be instructed to keep their mouth closed. For talking or feeding, percent assist can be reduced to zero (or the ventilator disconnected) temporarily. When the problem occurs without mouth opening, the straps need to be tightened.

Frequent activation of alarms may be secondary to the alarm levels being set too low relative to the prevailing ventilatory demand (V$_E$ and V$_T$ demands may have increased) or to improvement of mechanics since the last titration, with the assist now becoming excessive. Note the range of V$_T$ on the display, in particular the highest volumes. Reduce percent assist by 20% or so. If the large V$_T$s are eliminated and alarming stops, the problem was an improvement in mechanics, and the large breaths were runaways. Retitrate E and R. Conversely, if the large volumes continue to occur, then the problem is large ventilatory demand or marked breath-by-breath variability. In such cases, the limits should be adjusted upward.

INTUBATED PATIENTS

The following pertains to the PAV+option on the 840 ventilator because it is currently the only ventilator available with automatic mechanics and "smart" alarms. The procedure for setting basic PAV systems has been described elsewhere.[99] As indicated earlier, such systems are difficult to manage for extended periods. If other systems are used, *full* (i.e., 100%) automatic tube compensation (ATC) should be avoided. With complete compensation for the nonlinear component of resistance, very small errors in estimated R may cause aggressive flow runaway with rapid loss of the assist secondary to ventilator limits (see "Runaway Phenomenon," above).

STARTUP
1. Enter ideal body weight (IBW). *This is an important step.* IBW does not have to be precise but should be a

reasonable approximation of reality. It takes the ventilator four breaths to determine actual E and R. In the interim, it uses default values based on normal E and R values for a patient of the specified size. Should the specified IBW value be for a much smaller patient, the first few breaths may be overassisted.

2. Enter endotracheal or tracheostomy tube size. This input is also quite important because part of the delivered assist is based on stated tube size.

3. Set expiratory sensitivity (Esense) to 3 (default value).

4. Set triggering to flow modality at 3 liters/min.

5. Enter humidifier volume if applicable.

6. Set high tidal volume limit (V_{TI} limit) to a value corresponding to 15 ml/kg IBW.

7. Set high peak pressure (HIP) limit to 40 cmH$_2$O (default). The ventilator caps the assist at the HIP limit less 5 cmH$_2$O or 35 cmH$_2$O, whichever is less (i.e., breath is not terminated, but pressure cannot increase beyond this level). Setting HIP to a higher value has no effect in this option. Setting it to a lower value may restrict the assist given unnecessarily.

8. Set percent assist to 60%. It is better to start on the low side and increase if necessary. Most patients do very well at 60%. The use of higher values at the outset, before enough mechanics values have accumulated, may result in overassist.

9. Set PEEP to 5 cmH$_2$O unless a higher value is deemed necessary for oxygenation.

10. Activate the PAV mode.

SUBSEQUENT MANAGEMENT AND TROUBLESHOOTING

1. *Patient appears comfortable at initial settings.* This is the typical response. Subsequent management is similar to that for other modes and consists of gradual reduction in assist (percent assist in this case) as warranted by clinical condition. In clinically stable patients, percent assist is reduced in 10–20% decrements. If respiratory rate does not increase and other manifestations of distress do not appear over a few hours, it may be reduced further. If sustained tachypnea (relative to the previous level) or other distress manifestations appear, percent assist should be increased again, preferably to 20% higher than the level that resulted in tachypnea to maintain some reserve. The following are some additional recommendations that pertain specifically to PAV:
   - Patients with suspected prior chronic hypercapnia should have arterial blood gases checked a half hour after initiation of PAV to exclude significant acidemia (see "Indications and contraindications").
   - If breathing pattern is rapid and shallow (e.g., RR > 30 breaths per minute and/or V_T < 5 ml/kg) but the patient is comfortable, increase percent assist to 85%. If the pattern remains the same, then it is not distress-related. Return to 60%. Whether to maintain the patient on PAV in this case is debatable. There is currently no information to indicate that such a pattern is harmful, but some practitioners may prefer to be on the safe side

and switch to another mode until this issue is addressed scientifically (see "Important Unknowns," below).
   - Breathing may be highly variable in some patients. This is normal.

2. *Patient shows signs (other than tachypnea) of inadequate support.* No one, including the writer, has yet much direct experience with the new 840 PAV+ option. The following are tentative recommendations based on previously documented mechanisms of distress on PAV and our understanding of the functioning of the 840 PAV+ option. These apply whether distress develops soon after initiation of PAV or develops later:
   - Increase percent assist to 85%. Further increases add very little actual assist and increase the likelihood of runaway and instability. If the patient still appears to be in distress or uncomfortable:
   - Ensure that the HIP limit is 40 cmH$_2$O. Inspect the Paw waveform display for several breaths. If Paw does not reach 35 cmH$_2$O or reaches it only in the occasional breath, proceed to the next step. If it reaches 35 cmH$_2$O in the latter part of inspiration in most breaths, the patient needs more assist than can be provided by the PAV+ option. This scenario should be very rare and indicates high-end nonlinearity [see "Nonlinearity in the Pressure-Volume (P-V) Relation within the Tidal Volume Range," above] plus high ventilatory demand. The patient needs to be sedated. If heavy sedation must be used, consider switching to another mode (e.g., assist control). If Paw reaches 35 cmH$_2$O *immediately* after triggering and stays there until the cycle ends (i.e., squarewave pattern), flow runaway exists because of overestimation of inspiratory resistance (the 840 PAV+ option uses expiratory resistance to infer inspiratory resistance). Unfortunately, there is no direct way to address this problem in the current version of the PAV+ option. The patient is not in the PAV mode but is essentially receiving pressure-support ventilation (PSV) of 30 cmH$_2$O plus 5 cmH$_2$O of PEEP. The problem is more likely discomfort with excessive pressure rather than inadequate assist. Either switch to a different mode or reduce the HIP limit. This reduces the pressure cap. For example, if HIP is reduced to 30 cmH$_2$O, the cap is 25 cmH$_2$O, and this is equivalent to PSV of 20 cmH$_2$O + PEEP of 5 cmH$_2$O.
   - If Paw is not capped at 35 cmH$_2$O or reaches this level only occasionally, the problem is either severe dynamic hyperinflation or low-end nonlinearity (see "Limitations," above). PEEP needs to be titrated to an optimal level. Note the displayed average E. Increase PEEP by 3 cmH$_2$O, and follow the change in E over a few minutes. If it decreases, increase PEEP another 2 cmH$_2$O. Repeat until E no longer decreases. Go back to the immediately preceding PEEP. If this procedure does not relieve the distress, the problem is almost certainly severe dynamic hyperinflation not responsive to PEEP [i.e., high resistance is in the tubing (including the endotracheal tube)]. Until triggering is linked to onset of effort [see "Dynamic Hyperinflation (DH)," above and Fig. 13-7], such patients cannot be supported adequately with PAV.

Important Unknowns

Whereas the physiologic advantages of PAV have been proven, it is not clear whether these necessarily translate into clinical benefits. There are reasons to believe that clinical outcome will improve (see "Clinical Outcome," above). This needs to be confirmed, however. Questions may be of a general nature (e.g., "Are mortality, length of intubation, and length of ICU stay less with PAV?") or may be directed at specific aspects that we know affect outcome (e.g., by comparison with optimal protocols with other modes):

- If sedation is used on an "as needed" basis, will patients need less sedation on PAV?
- Will tidal volume over the course of illness be smaller on average?
- Is weaning faster?

We believe that two other questions need to be addressed. These relate to management of tachypnea that is unrelated to distress, a phenomenon that is evident only when PAV is used:

- If a patient decides to breathe in a rapid, shallow manner while on high PAV support (see, for example, Fig. 13-5*B*), should he or she be left on PAV or switched to another mode?
- If tachypnea (e.g., >35 breaths per minute) with no other signs of distress is present during a weaning trial and does not decrease on high PAV, does the patient need to stay on a ventilator?

The Future

With the inclusion of automatic mechanics and "smart" alarms, PAV should become the easiest mode to set and use. There is only one variable to adjust: percent assist. The mode adapts automatically to changes in ventilatory demand and respiratory mechanics. A problem will remain, however, in the management of patients with severe DH secondary to very high expiratory resistance and high ventilatory demand. Future PAV delivery systems should include algorithms to begin the assist at the onset of inspiratory effort.

It is also possible that adjustment of percent assist can be automated. PAV offers two features that would facilitate the complete automation of ventilator adjustment. First, ventilator rate, something ventilators can keep track of easily, is an accurate reflection of the patient's respiratory rate. Thus ventilator rate may be used as one feedback element for automatic adjustment of percent assist. Second, because PAV makes it possible to obtain passive mechanics on an ongoing basis, it is also possible to monitor respiratory muscle output and the work of breathing continuously. These can be used as additional feedback signals to automatically adjust percent assist.

Summary and Conclusion

When we wrote this chapter in the first edition of this book,[73] PAV was only an idea with very limited clinical data. The chapter was mostly theory and speculation. In the intervening 12 years, many studies have confirmed PAV's feasibility and its operational features and physiologic superiority over other modes. These studies, however, also have identified a number of practical limitations that precluded it use as a routine method of support or even for extended use in research studies. These limitations have made it difficult to ask the most important question: Does better physiology lead to better clinical outcome? Now that the practical limitations have been resolved, it will be possible to carry out such studies. Although there are good reasons to believe that clinical outcome will be better, critical illness is very complex, and it may be that poor patient-ventilator interaction is an insignificant contributor to overall outcome. Only time will tell.

Acknowledgment

This work was supported by the Canadian Institutes of Health Research.

References

1. Younes M. Proportional assist ventilation, a new approach to ventilatory support: Theory. Am Rev Respir Dis 1992; 145:114–20.
2. Younes M, Puddy A, Roberts D, et al. Proportional assist ventilation: Results of an initial clinical trial. Am Rev Respir Dis 1992; 145:121–9.
3. Younes M, Georgopoulos D. Control of breathing relevant to mechanical ventilation. In: Marini J, Slutsky A, editors. Physiological basis of ventilatory support, lung biology in health and disease. New York: Marcel Dekker, 1998: 1–74.
4. Fink BR. Influence of cerebral activity in wakefulness on regulation of breathing. J Appl Physiol 1961; 16:15–20.
5. Skatrud JB, Dempsey JA. Interaction of sleep state and chemical stimuli in sustaining rhythmic ventilation. J Appl Physiol 1983; 55:813–22.
6. Meza S, Mendez M, Ostrowski M, Younes M. Susceptibility to periodic breathing with assisted ventilation during sleep in normal subjects. J Appl Physiol 1998; 85:1929–40.
7. Younes M. Mechanisms of respiratory load compensation. In: Dempsey JA, Pack AI, editors. Regulation of breathing, lung biology in health and disease. New York: Marcel Dekker, 1995: 867–922.
8. Puddy A, Patrick W, Webster K, Younes M. Respiratory control during volume-cycled ventilation in normal humans. J Appl Physiol 1996; 80:1749–58.
9. Lofaso F, Isabey D, Lorino H, et al. Respiratory response to positive and negative inspiratory pressure in humans. Respir Physiol 1992; 89:75–88.
10. Morrell MJ, Shea SA, Adams L, Guz A. Effects of inspiratory support upon breathing in humans during wakefulness and sleep. Respir Physiol 1993; 93:57–70.
11. Scheid P, Lofaso F, Isabey D, Harf A. Respiratory response to inhaled CO_2 during positive inspiratory pressure in humans. J Appl Physiol 1994; 77:876–82.

12. Otis AB. Quantitative relationships in steady state gas exchange. In: Fenn WO, Rahn H, editors. Handbook of physiology: Respiration, vol 1. Bethesda, MD: American Physiological Society, 1964: 681–98.

13. Cunningham DJC, Robbins PA, Wolff CB. Integration of respiratory responses to changes in alveolar partial pressures of CO_2 and O_2 and in arterial pH. In: Cherniack NS, Widdicombe JG, editors. Handbook of physiology: Respiration, vol 2. Bethesda, MD: American Physiological Society, 1986: 475–528.

14. Nakayama H, Smith CA, Rodman JR, et al. Effect of ventilatory drive on carbon dioxide sensitivity below eupnea during sleep. Am J Respir Crit Care Med 2002; 165:1251–60.

15. Navalesi P, Hernandez P, Wongsa A, et al. Proportional assist ventilation in acute respiratory failure: Effects on breathing pattern and inspiratory effort. Am J Respir Crit Care Med 1996; 154:1330–8.

16. Ranieri VM, Grasso S, Mascia L, et al. Effects of proportional assist ventilation on inspiratory muscle effort in patients with chronic obstructive pulmonary disease and acute respiratory failure. Anesthesiology 1997; 86:79–91.

17. Meza S, Giannouli E, Younes M. Control of breathing during sleep assessed by proportional assist ventilation. J Appl Physiol 1998; 84:3–12.

18. Mitrouska J, Xirouchaki N, Patakas D, et al. Effects of chemical feedback on respiratory motor and ventilatory output during different modes of assisted mechanical ventilation. Eur Respir J 1999; 13:873–82.

19. Appendini L, Purro A, Gudjonsdottir M, et al. Physiologic response of ventilator-dependent patients with chronic obstructive pulmonary disease to proportional assist ventilation and continuous positive airway pressure. Am J Respir Crit Care Med 1999; 159:1510–7.

20. Polese G, Vitacca M, Bianchi L, et al. Nasal proportional assist ventilation unloads the inspiratory muscles of stable patients with hypercapnia due to COPD. Eur Respir J 2000; 16:491–8.

21. Vitacca M, Clini E, Pagani M, et al. Physiologic effects of early administered mask proportional assist ventilation in patients with chronic obstructive pulmonary disease and acute respiratory failure. Crit Care Med 2000; 28:1791–7.

22. Grasso S, Puntillo F, Mascia L, et al. Compensation for increase in respiratory workload during mechanical ventilation: Pressure-support versus proportional-assist ventilation. Am J Respir Crit Care Med 2000; 161:819–26.

23. Wysocki M, Richard JC, Meshaka P. Noninvasive proportional assist ventilation compared with noninvasive pressure support ventilation in hypercapnic acute respiratory failure. Crit Care Med 2002; 30:323–9.

24. Passam F, Hoing S, Prinianakis G, et al. Effect of different levels of pressure support and proportional assist ventilation on breathing pattern, work of breathing and gas exchange in mechanically ventilated hypercapnic COPD patients with acute respiratory failure. Respiration 2003; 70:355–61.

25. Porta R, Appendini L, Vitacca M, et al. Mask proportional assist vs pressure support ventilation in patients in clinically stable condition with chronic ventilatory failure. Chest 2002; 122: 479–88.

26. Serra A, Polese G, Braggion C, Rossi A. Non-invasive proportional assist and pressure support ventilation in patients with cystic fibrosis and chronic respiratory failure. Thorax 2002; 57: 50–4.

27. Marantz S, Patrick W, Webster K, et al. Response of ventilator-dependent patients to different levels of proportional assist. J Appl Physiol 1996; 80:397–403.

28. Giannouli E, Webster K, Roberts D, Younes M. Response of ventilator-dependent patients to different levels of pressure support and proportional assist. Am J Respir Crit Care Med 1999; 159:1716–25.

29. Delaere S, Roeseler J, D'hoore W, et al. Respiratory muscle workload in intubated, spontaneously breathing patients without COPD: Pressure support vs proportional assist ventilation. Intensive Care Med 2003; 29:949–54.

30. Wrigge H, Golisch W, Zinserling J, et al. Proportional assist versus pressure support ventilation: Effects on breathing pattern and respiratory work of patients with chronic obstructive pulmonary disease. Intensive Care Med 1999; 25:790–8.

31. Patrick W, Webster K, Ludwig L, et al. Noninvasive positive-pressure ventilation in acute respiratory distress without prior chronic respiratory failure. Am J Respir Crit Care Med 1996; 153:1005–11.

32. Gay PC, Hess DR, Hill NS. Noninvasive proportional assist ventilation for acute respiratory insufficiency: Comparison with pressure support ventilation. Am J Respir Crit Care Med 2001; 164:1606–11.

33. Fernandez-Vivas M, Caturla-Such J, Gonzalez de la Rosa J, et al. Noninvasive pressure support versus proportional assist ventilation in acute respiratory failure. Intensive Care Med 2003; 29:1126–33.

34. Ambrosino N, Vitacca M, Polese G, et al. Short-term effects of nasal proportional assist ventilation in patients with chronic hypercapnic respiratory insufficiency. Eur Respir J 1997; 10:2829–34.

35. Patrick W, Webster K, Puddy A, et al. Respiratory response to CO_2 in the hypocapnic range in awake humans. J Appl Physiol 1995; 79:2058–68.

36. Hey EN, Lloyd BB, Cunningham DJC, et al. Effects of various respiratory stimuli on the depth and frequency of breathing in man. Respir Physiol 1966; 1:193–205.

37. Jammes Y, Auran Y, Gouvermet J, et al. The ventilatory pattern of conscious man according to age and morphology. Bull Eur Physiopathol Respir 1979; 15:527–40.

38. Davis JN, Stagg D. Interrelationships of the volume and time components of individual breaths in resting man. J Physiol 1975; 245:481–98.

39. Tobin MJ, Mador MJ, Guenther SM, et al. Variability of resting respiratory drive and timing in healthy subjects. J Appl Physiol 1988; 65:309–17.

40. Brack T, Jubran A, Tobin MJ. Dyspnea and decreased variability of breathing in patients with restrictive lung disease. Am J Respir Crit Care Med 2002; 165:1260–4.

41. Loveridge B, West P, Anthonisen NR, Kryger MH. Breathing patterns in patients with chronic obstructive pulmonary disease. Am Rev Respir Dis 1984; 130:730–3.

42. Read DJ, Freedman S, Kafer ER. Pressures developed by loaded inspiratory muscles in conscious and anesthetized man. J Appl Physiol 1974; 37:207–18.

43. Khoo MC, Kronauer RE, Strohl KP, Slutsky AS. Factors inducing periodic breathing in humans: A general model. J Appl Physiol 1982; 53:644–59.

44. Younes, M: The physiologic basis of central apnea and periodic breathing. Curr Pulmonol 1989; 10:265–326.

45. Younes M, Ostrowski M, Thompson W, et al. Chemical control stability in patients with obstructive sleep apnea. Am J Respir Crit Care Med 2001; 163:1181–90.

46. Haberthur C, Fabry B, Zappe D, Guttmann J. Effects of mechanical unloading/loading on respiratory loop gain and periodic breathing in man. Respir Physiol 1998; 112:23–36.

47. Wellman A, Malhotra A, Fogel RB, et al. Respiratory system loop gain in normal men and women measured with proportional-assist ventilation. J Appl Physiol 2003; 94:205–12.

48. Purro A, Appendini L, De Gaetano A, et al. Physiologic determinants of ventilator dependence in long-term mechanically

ventilated patients. Am J Respir Crit Care Med 2000; 161: 1115–23.

49. Younes M, Kun J, Masiowski B, et al. A method for noninvasive determination of inspiratory resistance during proportional assist ventilation. Am J Respir Crit Care Med 2001; 163:829–39.

50. Younes M, Webster K, Kun J, et al. A method for measuring passive elastance during proportional assist ventilation. Am J Respir Crit Care Med 2001; 164:50–60.

51. Parthasarathy S, Tobin MJ. Effect of ventilator mode on sleep quality in critically ill patients. Am J Respir Crit Care Med 2002; 166:1423–9.

52. Wellman A, Jordan AS, Malhotra A, et al. Ventilatory control and airway anatomy in obstructive sleep apnea. Am J Respir Crit Care Med 2004; 170:1225–32.

53. Dolmage TE, Goldstein RS. Proportional assist ventilation and exercise tolerance in subjects with COPD. Chest 1997; 111:948–54.

54. Bianchi L, Foglio K, Pagani M, et al. Effects of proportional assist ventilation on exercise tolerance in COPD patients with chronic hypercapnia. Eur Respir J 1998; 11:422–7.

55. Hernandez P, Maltais F, Gursahaney A, et al. Proportional assist ventilation may improve exercise performance in severe chronic obstructive pulmonary disease. J Cardiopulm Rehabil 2001; 21:135–42.

56. Hawkins P, Johnson LC, Nikoletou D, et al. Proportional assist ventilation as an aid to exercise training in severe chronic obstructive pulmonary disease. Thorax 2002; 57:853–9.

57. Bianchi L, Foglio K, Porta R, et al. Lack of additional effect of adjunct of assisted ventilation to pulmonary rehabilitation in mild COPD patients. Respir Med 2002; 96:359–67.

58. Harms CA, Babcock MA, McClaran SR, et al. Respiratory muscle work compromises leg blood flow during maximal exercise. J Appl Physiol 1997; 82:1573–83.

59. Wetter TJ, Harms CA, Nelson WB, et al. Influence of respiratory muscle work on V_{O_2} and leg blood flow during submaximal exercise. J Appl Physiol 1999; 87:643–51.

60. Babcock MA, Pegelow DF, Harms CA, Dempsey JA. Effects of respiratory muscle unloading on exercise-induced diaphragm fatigue. J Appl Physiol 2002; 93:201–6.

61. Ranieri VM, Giuliani R, Mascia L, et al. Patient-ventilator interaction during acute hypercapnia: Pressure-support vs proportional-assist ventilation. J Appl Physiol 1996; 81:426–36.

62. Du HL, Ohtsuji M, Shigeta M, et al. Expiratory asynchrony in proportional assist ventilation. Am J Respir Crit Care Med 2002; 165:972–7.

63. Younes M. Patient-ventilator interaction with pressure-assisted modalities of ventilatory support. Semin Respir Med 1993; 14:299–322.

64. Yamada Y, Du HL. Analysis of the mechanisms of expiratory asynchrony in pressure support ventilation: A mathematical approach. J Appl Physiol 2000; 88:2143–50.

65. Jubran A, Van de Graaff WB, Tobin MJ. Variability of patient-ventilator interaction with pressure support ventilation in patients with chronic obstructive pulmonary disease. Am J Respir Crit Care Med 1995; 152:129–36.

66. Younes M. Interactions between patients and ventilators. In: Roussos C, editor. The Thorax: Lung Biology in Health and Disease, vol. 85. New York: Marcel Dekker, 1995: 2367–2420.

67. Leung P, Jubran A, Tobin MJ. Comparison of assisted ventilator modes on triggering, patient effort, and dyspnea. Am J Respir Crit Care Med 1997; 155:1940–8.

68. Laghi F, Karamchandani K, Tobin MJ. Influence of ventilator settings in determining respiratory frequency during mechanical ventilation. Am J Respir Crit Care Med 1999; 160:1766–70.

69. Laghi F, Segal J, Choe WK, Tobin MJ. Effect of imposed inflation time on respiratory frequency and hyperinflation in patients with chronic obstructive pulmonary disease. Am J Respir Crit Care Med 2001; 163:1365–70.

70. Younes M, Kun J, Webster K, Roberts D. Response of ventilator-dependent patients to delayed opening of exhalation valve. Am J Respir Crit Care Med 2002; 166:21–30.

71. Fernandez R, Mendez M, Younes M. Effect of ventilator flow rate on respiratory timing in normal humans. Am J Respir Crit Care Med 1999; 159:710–9.

72. Patrick W, Webster K, Wiebe P, et al. Effect of proportional assist ventilation on the hemodynamics of patients in septic shock. Am Rev Respir Dis 1993; 147:A611.

73. Younes M. Proportional assist ventilation. In: Tobin M, editor. Principles and practice of mechanical ventilation. New York: McGraw-Hill, 1994: 349–70.

74. Grasso S, Ranieri VM, Brochard L, et al. Closed loop proportional assist ventilation (PAV): Results of a phase II multicenter trial. Am J Respir Crit Care Med 2001; 163:A303.

75. Younes M, Riddle W, Polacheck J. A model for the relation between respiratory neural and mechanical outputs: III. Validation. J Appl Physiol 1981; 51:990–1001.

76. Gottfried SB, Rossi A, Higgs BD, et al. Noninvasive determination of respiratory system mechanics during mechanical ventilation for acute respiratory failure. Am Rev Respir Dis 1985; 131:414–20.

77. Esteban A, Alia I, Gordo F, et al. Extubation outcome after spontaneous breathing trials with T-tube or pressure support ventilation. The Spanish Lung Failure Collaborative Group. Am J Respir Crit Care Med 1997; 156:459–65.

78. Esteban A, Alia I, Tobin MJ, et al. Effect of spontaneous breathing trial duration on outcome of attempts to discontinue mechanical ventilation. Spanish Lung Failure Collaborative Group. Am J Respir Crit Care Med 1999; 159:512–8.

79. Grasso S, Ranieri VM. Proportional assist ventilation. Respir Care Clin North Am 2001; 7:465–73.

80. Kollef MH, Levy NT, Ahrens TS, et al. The use of continuous IV sedation is associated with prolongation of mechanical ventilation. Chest 1998; 114:541–8.

81. Kress JP, Pohlman AS, O'Connor MF, Hall JB. Daily interruption of sedative infusions in critically ill patients undergoing mechanical ventilation. New Engl J Med 2000; 342:1471–7.

82. Parthasarathy S, Tobin MJ. Sleep in the intensive care unit. Intensive Care Med 2004; 30:197–206.

83. Imai Y, Slutsky AS. Systemic effects of mechanical ventilation. In: Slutsky AS, Brochard L, editors. Update in intensive care and emergency medicine, vol 40. New York: Springer, 2004: 259–71.

84. Younes M. Determinants of thoracic excursion during exercise. In: Whipp BJ, Wasserman K, editors. Pulmonary physiology and pathophysiology of exercise (lung biology in health and disease), vol 52. New York: Marcel Dekker, 1991: 1–67.

85. Van Der Meulen JH, McArdle A, Jackson MJ, Faulkner JA. Contraction-induced injury to the extensor digitorum longus muscles of rats: The role of vitamin E. J Appl Physiol 1997; 83:817–23.

86. Devor ST, Faulkner JA. Regeneration of new fibers in muscles of old rats reduces contraction-induced injury. J Appl Physiol 1999; 87:750–6.

87. Agostoni E, Mead J. Statics of the respiratory system. In: Fenn WO, Rahn H, editors. Handbook of physiology: Respiration. Bethesda, MD: American Physiological Society, 1964: 387–409.

88. Wright PE, Marini JJ, Bernard GR. In vitro versus in vivo comparison of endotracheal tube airflow resistance. Am Rev Respir Dis 1989; 140:10–16.

89. Appendini L, Patessio A, Zanaboni S, et al. Physiologic effects of positive end-expiratory pressure and mask pressure support during exacerbations of chronic obstructive pulmonary disease. Am J Respir Crit Care Med 1994; 149:1069–76.

90. Lessard MR, Lofaso F, Brochard L. Expiratory muscle activity increases intrinsic positive end-expiratory pressure independently of dynamic hyperinflation in mechanically ventilated patients. Am J Respir Crit Care Med 1995; 151:562–9.

91. Zakynthinos SG, Vassilakopoulos T, Zakynthinos E, et al. Contribution of expiratory muscle pressure to dynamic intrinsic positive end-expiratory pressure: Validation using the Campbell diagram. Am J Respir Crit Care Med 2000; 162:1633–40.

92. Younes M. Method and device for monitoring and improving patient-ventilator interaction. PCT application no PCT/CA 2003/000976.

93. Bates DV, Macklem PT, Christie RV. Respiratory function in disease. Philadelphia: Saunders, 1971.

94. Gattinoni L, Pelosi P, Suter PM, et al. Acute respiratory distress syndrome caused by pulmonary and extrapulmonary disease: Different syndromes? Am J Respir Crit Care Med 1998; 158: 3–11.

95. Pelosi P, Croci M, Ravagnan I, et al. Respiratory system mechanics in sedated, paralyzed, morbidly obese patients. J Appl Physiol 1997; 82:811–8.

96. Mead J, Agostoni E. Dynamics of breathing. In: Fenn WO, Rahn H, editors. Handbook of physiology: Respiration. Bethesda, MD: American Physiological Society, 1964: 411–27.

97. Polacheck J, Strong R, Arens J, et al. Phasic vagal influence on inspiratory motor output in anesthetized human subjects. J Appl Physiol 1980; 49:609–19.

98. Im Hof V, West P, Younes M. Steady-state response of normal subjects to inspiratory resistive load. J Appl Physiol 1986; 60:1471–81.

99. Younes M. Proportional assist ventilation. Update in intensive care and emergencies medicine. 2002; vol 36: p 39–73.

Chapter 14

CLOSED-LOOP VENTILATION

JASON H. T. BATES

CONTROL OF SPONTANEOUS RESPIRATION
CLOSED-LOOP CONTROL ALGORITHMS
　　Control by Explicit Formulas
　　PID Control
　　Fuzzy Logic Control
VENTILATION CONTROL STRATEGIES
THE FUTURE
SUMMARY AND CONCLUSIONS

We breathe according to our needs. Thus breathing frequency (f) and tidal volume (V_T) are chosen to produce an alveolar minute ventilation ($\dot{V}_A$) appropriate to the prevailing metabolic demands. In simple terms, we can say that

$$\dot{V}_A = f(V_T - V_D) \qquad (1)$$

where V_D is the volume of the dead space in the lungs. Through independent choice of f and V_T, the normal, healthy individual can adjust $\dot{V}_A$ manyfold from rest to severe exercise. Failure to choose an appropriate level of $\dot{V}_A$ has significant negative consequences, so tight control of ventilation is essential. When the respiratory control system fails to function properly, respiratory failure itself may ensue.

Patients in respiratory failure can be managed for extended periods with mechanical ventilation. This practice has reached high levels of sophistication and effectiveness, with closed-loop control being a key component of the current state of the art. Mechanical ventilation, however, is still far from being a perfect substitute for the real thing and is associated with significant morbidity and mortality. Indeed, weaning patients from the ventilator as quickly as possible is always a key management goal. Thus the development of improved methods of mechanical ventilation remains an active area of research. It is likely that closed-loop control will play an increasingly important role in this effort.

Control of Spontaneous Respiration

The control of spontaneous respiration is undertaken, for the most part, by the central pattern generator in the brain stem. Periodic commands from this controller are sent via the respiratory motoneurons to the respiratory muscles, which act as effectors in bringing about the alternating processes of inspiration and expiration (Fig. 14-1). The central pattern generator and respiratory muscles on their own, however, can operate only in an open loop in which there is a unidirectional flow of information from controller to effector. Responding appropriately to the changing ventilatory demands of life requires a third crucial element, the sensors, which continually provide the controller with an assessment of how well the effectors are doing their job. This feedback of information closes the control loop, allowing actions to be modified continuously in light of their consequences.

There are a number of respiratory sensors, the most important for every day life being the central chemoreceptors that track carbon dioxide (CO_2) levels in the blood via their effect on the pH of cerebrospinal fluid.[1] When these levels move above or below the narrow normal range, the controller commands the effectors to either increase or decrease their pumping action, as the case may be, to return the arterial partial pressure of CO_2 (Pa_{CO_2}) to normal. Of course, the control of ventilation depends on other factors such as the arterial partial pressure of oxygen (Pa_{O_2}) and the degree of lung inflation[1] and can be overridden temporarily by conscious decision making. Also, there are an infinite number of combinations of f and V_T in Eq. (1) that will produce a given value of $\dot{V}_A$, yet f and V_T vary remarkably little within and between individuals, possibly because of additional constraints related to minimization of muscular work.[2] Nevertheless, the controller-effector-sensor paradigm in Fig. 14-1 embodies the essential elements involved in the closed-loop control of natural ventilation.

Mechanical ventilation replaces, either partially or completely, the respiratory muscles in their role as effectors. It also does away with the natural controller and sensors, replacing both with the attending health care professional; medical opinion becomes the controller, whereas the role of sensor is assumed by clinical acumen aided by such technical devices as the blood-gas analyzer and saturation monitor. These artificial controllers and sensors, however, fall far short of their natural counterparts for a variety of reasons, not the least of which concerns their availability. It is typical for patients in the intensive-care unit (ICU) to be seen by the attending physician once or twice per day and to be evaluated by other health care staff only somewhat more often unless there is a crisis. Resource limitations make this inevitable, of course, but the result is a poor substitute for the moment-to-moment control of the ventilatory pattern (f, V_T, etc.) that occurs naturally in the healthy individual.

Thus, although the control loop in Fig. 14-1 can be considered closed with respect to conventional mechanical ventilation in one sense, a complete circuit of the loop for a typical patient often takes so long that the control is effectively open loop for much of the time. It seems logical to suppose that this state of affairs would be improved markedly if sensing could rely entirely on medical devices, and the physician could be replaced by a computer algorithm (see Fig. 14-1). This is much easier said than done, however, and the complete implementation and acceptance of automatic closed-loop ventilation are likely some distance in the future. Nevertheless, many currently employed modes of ventilation use closed-loop control in some way or other. Understanding the principles of closed-loop control is thus

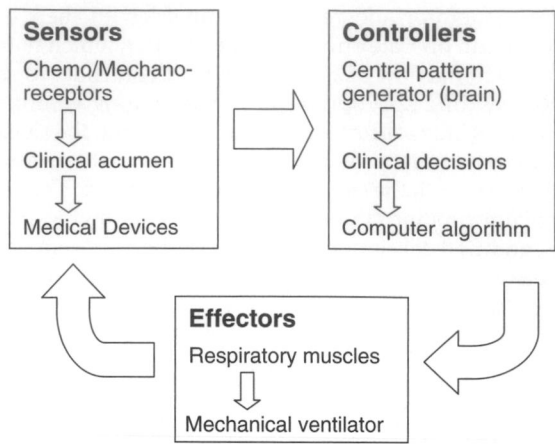

FIGURE 14-1 The controller-effector-sensor paradigm of ventilatory control. (*Adapted, with permission, from Bates et al: Respir Care Clin North Am 7:363–77, 2001.*)

important for appreciating the limitations and promise of current and future approaches to mechanical ventilation.

Closed-Loop Control Algorithms

The essence of closed-loop control is feedback, which allows the pursuit of a target to be adjusted continuously according to the movement of the target itself. Good control is achieved when the pursuer is able to respond rapidly to changes in target position and depends to a large extent on the capabilities of the effectors that are being controlled. Thus, for example, good control of airway pressure during mechanical ventilation requires a pump that is able to generate any desired pressure within a small fraction of the breath cycle. Even when all the physical engineering requirements are met, however, effective closed-loop control will not be realized without a suitable servo-control algorithm that determines how the pump is going to be driven.

CONTROL BY EXPLICIT FORMULAS

In some situations, there may be an explicit formula that tells the controller how to track the target precisely. An example is the choice of f during adaptive-support ventilation,[3–5] which is determined by the following formula based on the notion of minimization of the work of breathing[2]:

$$f = \frac{\sqrt{1 + 2aRC(\dot{V}_A/V_D)} - 1}{aRC} \qquad (2)$$

where RC is the respiratory time constant (the product of resistance R and compliance C), and a is a constant that depends on the flow waveform. In order to implement this formula, the values of R, C, $\dot{V}_A$, and V_D must be known. Although not a trivial undertaking, it is possible to measure all these quantities in an individual patient. If such measurements could be made for each breath, then, in principle, one could feed these values back into the preceding formula to

calculate how f should be set for the subsequent breath. Ideally, this information should be available before mechanical ventilation is initiated so that the initial ventilatory parameters are suitable for the situation at hand.[6]

Another example of control by explicit formula is that involved in proportional-assist ventilation,[7–9] also known as *negative-impedance ventilation*.[10] Tracheal flow ($\dot{V}$) and volume (V) above functional residual capacity are monitored continuously so that a ventilator can be directed to generate an airway pressure (P) according to

$$P(t) = \alpha Rrs\dot{V}(t) + \beta ErsV(t) \qquad (3)$$

where Rrs and Ers are respiratory system resistance and elastance, respectively, and α and β are constants between 0 and 1. The ventilator thus takes care of a fraction α of the resistive load of breathing and a fraction β of the elastic load, leaving the patient's respiratory muscles to deal with the remainder. The values of α and β are chosen by the physician on the basis of how much ventilator assistance the patient needs. The great advantage of proportional-assist ventilation is that although the patient remains in charge of how much flow and volume are going to enter his or her lungs, he or she does not have to do all the work required.

The principal difficulty with implementation of proportional-assist ventilation, however, is that the algorithm becomes unstable if either α or β in Eq. (3) is greater than unity.[11] Ensuring that this does not happen requires that Rrs and Ers be known. Both these quantities may change during the course of ventilator support, causing the work required of the patient's respiratory muscles to change accordingly. Proportional-assist ventilation thus would be enhanced by feedback on the values of Rrs and Ers so that the values of α and β could be adjusted appropriately. Unfortunately, evaluating Rrs and Ers during proportional-assist ventilation is problematic, which has made it difficult to realize the full potential of this mode.[11] A promising approach to dealing with this problem is to use the patient's own neural drive as an index of how much ventilator assistance is required,[12] although this demands instrumentation of the esophagus with electrodes to measure the diaphragmatic electromyogram.

PID CONTROL

In most pursuit situations, the pursuer cannot reach the target immediately but rather can only move in the direction of the current target position. Consequently, when the target position is finally reached, the target has already moved on to a new position. The pursuer therefore must be content with being constantly on the target's tail but never actually catching it. The classic way this is achieved is through a proportional-integral-differential (PID) servo-control algorithm,[13] some subset of which is used widely in the control of mechanical ventilators.[14]

To see how PID servo control works, suppose that a piston pump is to be used to generate a specified-volume waveform. In fact, precisely this approach has been taken to apply proportional-assist ventilation in humans[15] and to measure

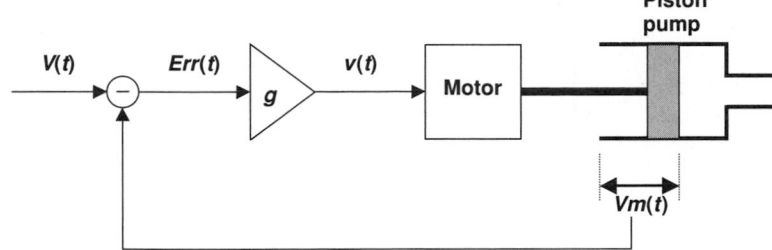

FIGURE 14-2 Proportional feedback control of a mechanical volume ventilator. The volume output Vm(t) is compared with a desired volume signal V(t). The difference between these two signals, Err(t), is then amplified (gain factor g) to produce a voltage signal v(t) that controls a motor that, in turn, drives the ventilator piston.

respiratory input impedance in small laboratory animals.[16] The effector in this case is a motor that drives the piston back and forth (Fig. 14-2). The volume change generated by the piston can be measured by a variety of sensors, but it is perhaps easiest to imagine that a displacement transducer is used to register the position of the piston face. The product of the face area and the change of piston position then provides volume as a function of time. This measured volume signal (Vm) provides feedback to a controller that must direct the motor to move the piston in a prescribed manner. The question is, How should the controller use Vm to direct the motor?

A simple algorithm suitable for this situation is proportional control (i.e., the *P* in PID). Here, the controller tries to make the difference between Vm and the desired volume signal (V) as small as possible by always directing the motor to move in the direction that reduces V − Vm. The voltage signal v(t) sent to the motor is thus

$$v(t) = g[V(t) - Vm(t)]$$

$$= gErr(t) \qquad (4)$$

where Err(t) is the error signal, and g is a gain factor that determines how vigorously the motor is going to make the piston pursue V(t). This strategy is called *P control* because it acts in direct proportion to the distance between the target and the current position of the object being controlled.

A limitation of P control is that the force driving the piston tends toward zero as the target is approached. If there is a force and velocity below which the piston suddenly sticks, such as often occurs owing to static friction, then there will be a limit to how close P control can get the piston to the target position. What is required when the piston sticks is a control signal that increases until the piston starts to move again. Such a signal is provided by adding a second term to v(t) that is proportional to the time integral of Err(t) (the *I* in PID). When the piston initially becomes stuck, this term may be very small, but it will build up linearly with time until the piston is finally able to break free from the bonds of static friction and proceed on toward the target.

Control of the piston in Fig. 14-2 also depends on its mass. If the piston has significant inertia, it will take time to accelerate, which will increase the time it takes to reach the target. Increasing the value of g can help to a certain degree. If the acceleration is too great, however, then the piston will have difficulty decelerating as the target volume is approached, causing it to overshoot. Thus, instead of a smooth, asymptotic approach to the target volume, the piston executes a series of damped oscillations known as *ringing* (Fig. 14-3). Indeed, if g is large enough, the oscillations may not even be damped but may increase in size indefinitely as the system becomes unstable. Instability also can be caused by a delay between the time the controller issues a command to the motor and when it responds. The result is often a sequence of exaggerated oscillations known as *hunting* as the controller attempts to chase a target that is always several steps ahead of it. An equivalent situation is seen in the spontaneous control of respiration; periodic Cheyne-Stokes breathing may be caused either by oversensitivity of the central chemoreceptor (equivalent to an increase in g) or by a delay in the circulation time from the lung to the central chemoreceptor.[1]

Further improvement in control of the piston thus may be achieved by considering not only how far it is from the target at any given instant but also how fast it is moving. Clearly, for a given distance from the target, a smaller push from the controller is required if the piston is already approaching the target rapidly than if it is stationary. Thus the v(t) sent to the motor should be supplemented by an additional term proportional to the time derivative of Err(t) (the *D* in PID).

The complete algorithm for PID control thus is

$$v(t) = g_1 Err(t) + g_2 \int_0^t Err(t)\, dt + g_3 \frac{dErr(t)}{dt} \qquad (5)$$

FIGURE 14-3 If the ventilator in Fig. 14-2 begins with its piston at Vm(t) = 0 and is given a command at time = 0 to produce Vm(t) = 1, it may response sluggishly if the value of g is small (*dotted line*), briskly if g is increased (*solid line*), and with an oscillating overshoot if g is too large (*dashed line*).

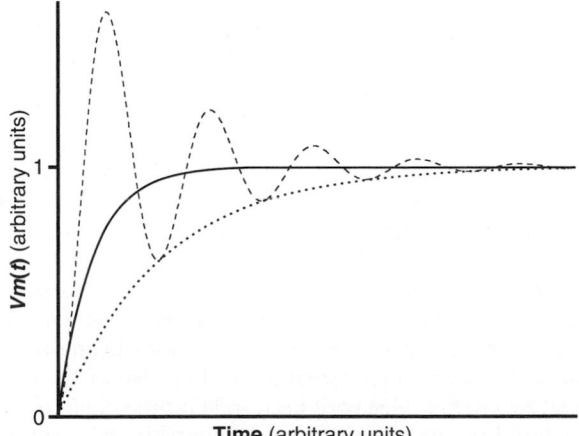

where g_1, g_2, and g_3 are separate gain factors that have optimal values depending on the physics of the particular control situation at hand. This combined strategy of PID control may result in significantly better target tracking than P control alone when the piston is affected by friction and has significant mass. Note also that we have used Err(t) here to represent the difference between target and actual piston positions, but this error signal could be based on other targets, such as flow measured at the airway opening.

PID-type controllers obviously are well suited to the control of ventilators for the purposes of producing prescribed flow or volume waveforms and have been used in various guises for these purposes.[15–17] They also have been used in the pursuit of physiologic goals, such as the control of arterial oxygen saturation and end-tidal CO_2,[18,19] as well as positive end-expiratory pressure (PEEP).[20,21]

FUZZY LOGIC CONTROL

Although PID controllers are the mainstay of servo-control algorithms, they have some limitations. First, they are linear, which means that they drive the effectors in direct proportion to Err(t) and its integral and derivative. This is not always appropriate. Second, evaluation of optimal values for the gain coefficients g_1, g_2, and g_3 in Eq. (5) may be difficult when the control variables are not readily quantifiable. A useful heuristic alternative to PID control is provided by fuzzy logic,[22,23] the principles of which are best explained through a simple example.[22]

Suppose that we wish to control the minute ventilation ($\dot{V}_E$) that a patient receives and that the only information available about the patient's status is an hourly measurement of arterial P_{CO_2}. Each hour an adjustment must be made to $\dot{V}_E$ based on the current reading of P_{CO_2} and how it has changed since the last reading (ΔP_{CO_2}). In some cases the appropriate course of action will be obvious, whereas for others there may be no clear guidelines, so the physician will have to rely on intuition and experience to make a decision.

Fuzzy logic deals with this situation by dividing the range of possible values for P_{CO_2} and ΔP_{CO_2} into overlapping fuzzy sets that are represented in terms of level of membership. For example, a value of P_{CO_2} will have a membership level of 1.0 in the *normal* set for a range of values that are definitely normal, whereas either side of this range the membership level decreases gradually to zero in a manner that reflects increasing levels of doubt about normality. Sets corresponding to *high* and *low* values of P_{CO_2} can be constructed similarly. Figure 14-4*A* shows an example of such a fuzzification, whereas Fig. 14-4*B* shows a corresponding construction for ΔP_{CO_2}.

Because the fuzzy sets depicted in Fig. 14-4 overlap, some values of P_{CO_2} and ΔP_{CO_2} have membership in two sets simultaneously, with the respective levels of membership reflecting the probability of belonging to either set. Each pair of P_{CO_2} and ΔP_{CO_2} measurements thus leads to one or more pairs of fuzzy set memberships. In the case of the example shown in Fig. 14-4 with P_{CO_2} = 38 mmHg and ΔP_{CO_2} = −0.5 mmHg/min, there is finite membership in the set com-

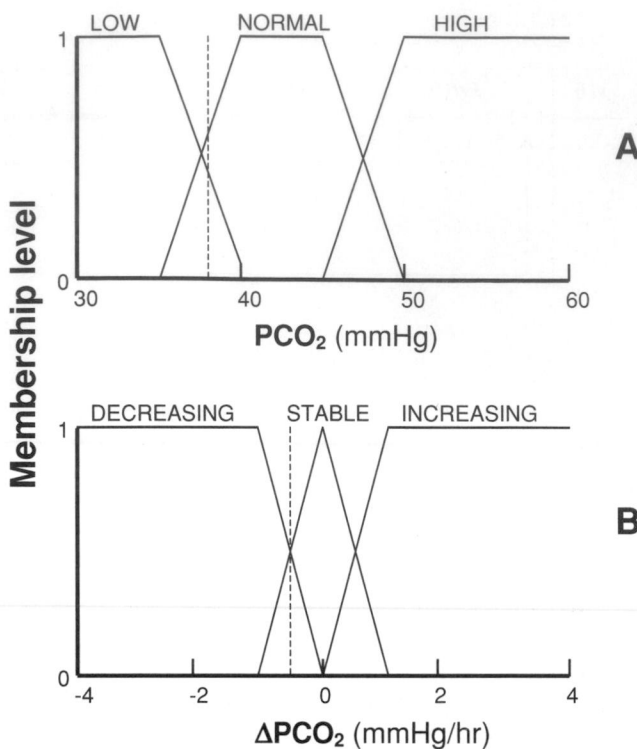

FIGURE 14-4 Example fuzzifications of (A) P_{CO_2} and (B) ΔP_{CO_2}. Representative measurements of each variable are indicated by the vertical dashed lines, which give membership levels of about 0.45 in *low* and 0.55 in *normal* for P_{CO_2} and 0.5 in both *decreasing* and *stable* for ΔP_{CO_2}. (Adapted, with permission, from Bates et al: *Respir Care Clin North Am* 7:363–77, 2001.)

binations *low* and *decreasing, low* and *stable, normal* and *decreasing,* and *normal* and *stable.*

The next step is to decide what action should be taken for each pair of set memberships. For example, if P_{CO_2} is *normal* and ΔP_{CO_2} is *stable,* then $\dot{V}_E$ probably should be maintained unchanged, whereas if P_{CO_2} is *high* and ΔP_{CO_2} is *increasing,* then $\dot{V}_E$ should be increased a lot, and so on. We thus can specify rules for every possible pair of fuzzy set memberships for P_{CO_2} and ΔP_{CO_2}, as show in Table 14-1.

For the rules in Table 14-1 to be implemented, such terms as *increase a lot* must be translated into precise changes in $\dot{V}_E$ in terms of liters per minute. This is achieved again using fuzzy sets. For the purposes of this illustration, we will divide the range of $\Delta \dot{V}_E$ into five fuzzy sets labeled *increase a lot, increase a little, maintain, decrease a little,* and *decrease a*

TABLE 14-1 Rule Table for All Pairs of Fuzzy Set Memberships in Fig. 14-4

| | P_{CO_2} | | |
ΔP_{CO_2}	Low	Normal	High
Decreasing	Decrease a lot	Decrease a little	Maintain
Stable	Decrease a little	Maintain	Increase a little
Increasing	Maintain	Increase a little	Increase a lot

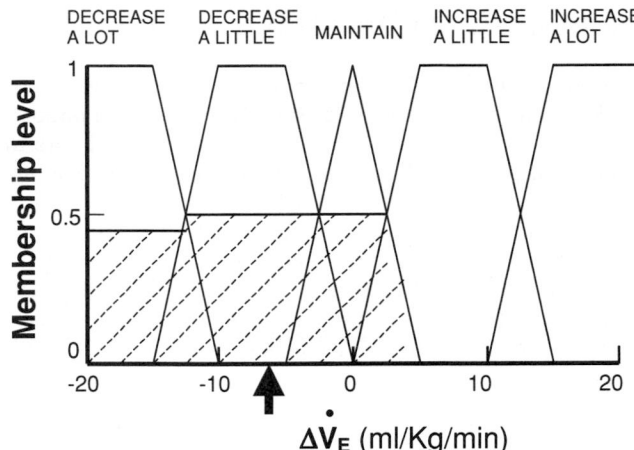

FIGURE 14-5 Example fuzzification of $\dot{V}_E$ into five fuzzy sets. The hatched area indicates the weighting of the sets that contribute to the final action to be taken. The precise value of the final action for the example measurements of P_{CO_2} and ΔP_{CO_2} (indicated by the dashed lines in Fig. 14-4) is equal to the area's centroid located at the position of the arrow. (*Adapted, with permission, from Bates et al: Respir Care Clin North Am 7:363–77, 2001.*)

lot. Considering the example shown in Fig. 14-5, this leads to fuzzy set memberships of

P_{CO_2}: 0.45 in *low*
0.55 in *normal*
ΔP_{CO_2}: 0.50 in *decreasing*
0.50 in *stable*

Invoking every pair combination of these sets in the rule table (see Table 14-1) gives the following actions:

Low and *decreasing* = *decrease a lot*
Low and *stable* = *decrease a little*
Normal and *decreasing* = *decrease a little*
Normal and *stable* = *maintain*

The final action clearly is going to be some weighted sum of these four actions. The weighting factor for each action is taken as the smallest of the two set memberships in P_{CO_2} and ΔP_{CO_2} that produced it. Thus, for example, the action *decrease a lot* came from a membership of 0.45 in *low* for P_{CO_2} and 0.50 in *decreasing* for ΔP_{CO_2}. Therefore, *decrease a lot* receives a weighting of 0.45.

These weightings finally are converted into "crisp" values of $\Delta \dot{V}_E$ as indicated in Fig. 14-5, where each of the fuzzy action sets is highlighted to a level equal to its weighting factor. If an action set is invoked more than once, as occurs in this example with *decrease a little*, then the largest of the weighting factors is used. This defines a polygonal shape whose centroid gives the precise value of $\Delta \dot{V}_E$ to be applied to the patient, which in this example is close to -7 ml/kg/min (see Fig. 14-5).

Although fuzzy logic control can be used with systems amenable to the classic PID algorithm, it really comes into its own when the nature of the control problem is similar to that of a human engaging in subjective judgment. As such, fuzzy logic is especially suited to certain aspects of medical decision making[24] and has been used in a variety of medical applications.[25–30] Fuzzy logic also appears to have promise as a means of automatically controlling mechanical ventilation. For example, Nemoto et al[31] developed a fuzzy logic algorithm for controlling pressure-support ventilation based on ongoing assessments of V_T, f, heart rate, and arterial O_2 saturation, together with their respective rates of change. Similarly, Schaublin et al[32] used fuzzy logic to control V_T and f during anesthesia to try to maintain end-tidal CO_2 at a predetermined level.

Ventilation Control Strategies

The preceding discussion has focused on the engineering problem of getting a mechanical ventilator to achieve a specified goal, for which the well-developed techniques of PID control and fuzzy logic are at our disposal. A more significant challenge for the future of closed-loop ventilation, however, is the medical problem of deciding what the ventilation goal, or goals, should be. A dog chasing a rabbit represents a complex closed-loop control problem for the dog, but the overall strategy is obvious—catch the rabbit. In mechanical ventilation, the goal frequently is less clear and depends on the clinical situation. During elective surgery, for example, the goal of mechanical ventilation simply may be to maintain normal blood gases. Indeed, the earliest applications of closed-loop ventilatory control aspired to precisely this[11] and date back as much as 50 years.[11,33–35] Some of these early efforts were rather impressive, such as that of Frumin et al,[34] who were able to maintain end-tidal CO_2 within 3 mmHg of the desired value by controlling airway pressure. More recently, Anderson and East[21] used a closed-loop PID controller to adjust PEEP and inspired O_2 fraction automatically in order to control Pa_{O_2} and were able to maintain control in 84% of a small group of patients with acute respiratory distress syndrome.

During surgery for major trauma, on the other hand, ventilating the lung in a manner that minimizes the risk for ventilator-induced lung injury is likely to be an additional consideration. For example, Jandre et al[20] recently developed a control scheme based on the simultaneous control of end-tidal P_{CO_2} and PEEP, together with minimization of the ratio of peak alveolar pressure to peak inspiratory resistive pressure. The latter condition was postulated to minimize the risk of ventilator-induced lung injury. They tested their controller in piglets and found that it compared favorably with manual titration of ventilation, being able to respond to step changes in inspired CO_2 with a rapidity similar to that of the normal physiologic response. Along the same lines, Tehrani et al[18] developed a scheme that chooses values for V_T and f based on ventilatory needs while simultaneously attempting to minimize the work of breathing. They also achieved encouraging results in pigs, finding that under steady-state conditions, arterial O_2 saturation and end-tidal P_{CO_2} exhibited standard deviations of 1.76% and 1.78%, respectively. Another example of control of multiple targets is that developed by Iotti et al,[36–38] who developed an algorithm for incrementally adjusting the applied pressure level during pressure-support ventilation. Their goal was to achieve satisfactory levels of both $\dot{V}_E$ and patient effort simultaneously, the latter being assessed in terms of $P_{0.1}$ (the airway occlusion pressure measured 0.1 second after the start of inspiratory effort). They were able to maintain $P_{0.1}$ at between 1.5 and 4.5 cmH_2O while preventing hypoventilation.[38]

Closed-loop ventilation thus can involve the simultaneous pursuit of multiple situation-specific goals. A basic premise behind any form of closed-loop ventilation, however, is that the information necessary to implement the ultimate control strategy is contained within the quantities providing feedback to the controller. A case in point is automatic weaning of patients from mechanical ventilation. It is compelling to think that automating either the gradual withdrawal of ventilator support or the decision to extubate would be advantageous in terms of both reducing time on the ventilator and relieving the workload on medical personnel. Indeed, much work toward this end has been done already,[39,40] and even the knowledge-based systems currently being implemented by medical personnel at the bedside are, for the most part, readily adapted to a computer algorithm.[41–45] Nevertheless, many practitioners feel that the optimal control of mechanical ventilation always will rest to some extent on the evaluation of quantities that are not readily measured by machines, such as patient comfort and general air of well-being. How essential these factors are for control of mechanical ventilation is still debated (see discussion at the end of ref. 11).

The Future

The ultimate goal of closed-loop ventilation is to replace the physician in his or her role as controller with a computer algorithm (see Fig. 14-1). One thus can imagine a future in which the mechanical ventilation of a patient is monitored by a computer that integrates incoming information about patient status, makes a decision about the actions required to improve that status, and directs a mechanical ventilator to deliver ventilation accordingly, all without human intervention. Of course, this also requires electronic sensors capable of detecting appropriate physiologic variables with the necessary accuracy and rapidity, as well as a ventilator that can be controlled by an external signal. Even if all the difficult technical problems are resolved, however, there remain some key cultural issues concerning of the role of physician as caregiver. These issues can lead to widespread misgivings about a future in which the course of mechanical ventilation is dictated entirely by a machine. It is difficult therefore to say whether human decision making ever will be excluded completely from the mechanical ventilation control loop. Nevertheless, closed-loop methods are already demonstrating that they can control many of the ventilator-related functions that traditionally have relied on human intervention, guaranteeing that significant efforts will continue to be applied to their development.

Summary and Conclusions

Closed-loop mechanical ventilation involves the use of feedback to control how a ventilator delivers flow to a patient. PID-type control is used widely in modern ventilators to produce a prescribed flow or volume waveform. The actual control strategy (i.e., which flow or volume waveform should be applied), however, is still largely up to the attending health care professionals. Using a computer algorithm to decide on the control strategy (i.e., replacing the physician as controller) remains in the experimental stage, although a number of promising approaches are being developed. Among these are knowledge-based systems for weaning, fuzzy logic for control of ventilator assist, neural control of proportional-assist ventilation, and the use of PID control to pursue the control of blood gases and the minimization of lung injury simultaneously.

References

1. West JB. Respiratory physiology: The essentials, 6th ed. Baltimore: Williams & Wilkins, 1995.
2. Otis AB, Fenn WO, Rahn H. Mechanics of breathing in man. J Appl Physiol 1950; 2:592–607.
3. Laubscher TP, Frutiger A, Fanconi S, et al. Automatic selection of tidal volume, respiratory frequency and minute ventilation in intubated ICU patients as start up procedure for closed-loop controlled ventilation. Int J Clin Monit Comput 1994; 11:19–30.
4. Laubscher TP, Heinrichs W, Weiler N, et al. An adaptive lung ventilation controller. IEEE Trans Biomed Eng 1994; 41:51–9.
5. Campbell RS, Branson RD, Johannigman JA. Adaptive support ventilation. Respir Care Clin North Am 2001; 7:425–40, ix.
6. Laubscher TP, Frutiger A, Fanconi S, Brunner JX. The automatic selection of ventilation parameters during the initial phase of mechanical ventilation. Intensive Care Med 1996; 22:199–207.
7. Marantz S, Patrick W, Webster K, et al. Response of ventilator-dependent patients to different levels of proportional assist. J Appl Physiol 1996; 80:397–403.
8. Younes M. Proportional assist ventilation, a new approach to ventilatory support: Theory. Am Rev Respir Dis 1992; 145:114–20.
9. Younes M, Puddy A, Roberts D, et al. Proportional assist ventilation: Results of an initial clinical trial. Am Rev Respir Dis 1992; 145:121–9.
10. Poon CS, Lebowitz HH, Sidney DA, Li SX. Negative-impedance ventilation and pressure support ventilation: A comparative study. Respir Physiol 1997; 108:117–27.
11. Branson RD, Johannigman JA, Campbell RS, Davis K Jr. Closed-loop mechanical ventilation. Respir Care 2002; 47:427–51; discussion 51–3.
12. Sinderby C, Navalesi P, Beck J, et al. Neural control of mechanical ventilation in respiratory failure. Nature Med 1999; 5:1433–6.
13. Shaw J. The PID control algorithm: How it works, how to tune it, and how to use it, 2d ed. Rochester, NY: Process Control Solutions 2005; available and updated on the Web at *www.jashaw.com/pidbook/2005*.
14. Brunner JX. Principles and history of closed-loop controlled ventilation. Respir Care Clin North Am 2001; 7:341–62, vii.
15. Younes M, Bilan D, Jung D, Kroker H. An apparatus for altering the mechanical load of the respiratory system. J Appl Physiol 1987; 62:2491–9.

16. Schuessler TF, Bates JH. A computer-controlled research ventilator for small animals: Design and evaluation. IEEE Trans Biomed Eng 1995; 42:860–6.

17. Kaczka DW, Lutchen KR. Servo-controlled pneumatic pressure oscillator for respiratory impedance measurements and high-frequency ventilation. Ann Biomed Eng 2004; 32:596–608.

18. Tehrani F, Rogers M, Lo T, et al. A dual closed-loop control system for mechanical ventilation. J Clin Monit Comput 2004; 18:111–29.

19. Tehrani F, Rogers M, Lo T, et al. Closed-loop control if the inspired fraction of oxygen in mechanical ventilation. J Clin Monit Comput 2002; 17:367–76.

20. Jandre FC, Pino AV, Lacorte I, et al. A closed-loop mechanical ventilation controller with explicit objective functions. IEEE Trans Biomed Eng 2004; 51:823–31.

21. Anderson JR, East TD. A closed-loop controller for mechanical ventilation of patients with ARDS. Biomed Sci Instrum 2002; 38:289–94.

22. Bates JH, Hatzakis GE, Olivenstein R. Fuzzy logic and mechanical ventilation. Respir Care Clin North Am 2001; 7(3):363–77, vii.

23. Bates JH, Young MP. Applying fuzzy logic to medical decision making in the intensive care unit. Am J Respir Crit Care Med 2003; 167:948–52.

24. Steinmann F. On the use and usefulness of fuzzy sets in medical AI. Artif Intell Med 2001; 21:131–7.

25. Mason DG, Ross JJ, Edwards ND, et al. Self-learning fuzzy control with temporal knowledge for atracurium-induced neuromuscular block during surgery. Comput Biomed Res 1999;32: 187–97.

26. Chan W, Naghdy F. Prognosis of body fluid level by fuzzy logic technique. Methods Inf Med 2001; 40:52–8.

27. Martin JF. Fuzzy control in anesthesia. J Clin Monit 1994; 10:77–80.

28. Tsutsui T, Arita S. Fuzzy-logic control of blood pressure through enflurane anesthesia. J Clin Monit 1994; 10:110–7.

29. Ohayon MM. Improving decisionmaking processes with the fuzzy logic approach in the epidemiology of sleep disorders. J Psychosom Res 1999; 47:297–311.

30. Velasevic DM, Saletic DZ, Saletic SZ. A fuzzy sets theory application in determining the severity of respiratory failure. Int J Med Inform 2001; 63:101–7.

31. Nemoto T, Hatzakis GE, Thorpe CW, et al. Automatic control of pressure support mechanical ventilation using fuzzy logic. Am J Respir Crit Care Med 1999; 160:550–6.

32. Schaublin J, Derighetti M, Feigenwinter P, et al. Fuzzy logic control of mechanical ventilation during anaesthesia. Br J Anaesth 1996; 77:636–41.

33. Saxton G, Myers G. An electromechanical substitute for the human respiratory center. Clin Res Proc 1953; 1:116–7.

34. Frumin MJ, Bergman NA, Holaday DA. Carbon dioxide and oxygen blood levels with a carbon dioxide controlled artificial respirator. Anesthesiology 1959; 20:313–20.

35. Noshiro M. Design of a control system for maintaining a normal arterial pCO_2 by artificial respiration. Med Biol Eng Comput 1984; 22:418–25.

36. Iotti G, Braschia A, Galbusera C. $P_{0.1}$, breathing pattern and pressure support ventilation. Intensive Care Med 1996;22:1131–2.

37. Iotti GA, Braschi A. Closed-loop support of ventilatory workload: The $P_{0.1}$ controller. Respir Care Clin North Am 2001; 7:441–64, ix.

38. Iotti GA, Brunner JX, Braschi A, et al. Closed-loop control of airway occlusion pressure at 0.1 second ($P_{0.1}$) applied to pressure-support ventilation: Algorithm and application in intubated patients. Crit Care Med 1996; 24:771–9.

39. Linton DM. Adaptive lung ventilation. Respir Care Clin North Am 2001; 7:409–24, viii.

40. Linton DM, Potgieter PD, Davis S, et al. Automatic weaning from mechanical ventilation using an adaptive lung ventilation controller. Chest 1994; 106:1843–50.

41. Dojat M, Brochard L. Knowledge-based systems for automatic ventilatory management. Respir Care Clin North Am 2001; 7: 379–96, viii.

42. Dojat M, Brochard L, Lemaire F, Harf A. A knowledge-based system for assisted ventilation of patients in intensive care units. Int J Clin Monit Comput 1992; 9:239–50.

43. Dojat M, Harf A, Touchard D, et al. Evaluation of a knowledge-based system providing ventilatory management and decision for extubation. Am J Respir Crit Care Med 1996; 153:997–1004.

44. Dojat M, Harf A, Touchard D, et al. Clinical evaluation of a computer-controlled pressure support mode. Am J Respir Crit Care Med 2000; 161:1161–6.

45. Krishnan JA, Moore D, Robeson C, et al. A prospective, controlled trial of a protocol-based strategy to discontinue mechanical ventilation. Am J Respir Crit Care Med 2004; 169:eak 673–8.

Chapter 15

PERMISSIVE HYPERCAPNIA

JOHN G. LAFFEY
BRIAN P. KAVANAGH

Carbon dioxide (CO_2) is the "waste product" of aerobic respiration. In health, arterial carbon dioxide tension (Pa_{CO_2})
is tightly regulated, with minute ventilation potently enhanced in response to small elevations in CO_2 tension. Although usually well tolerated, hypercapnia traditionally has been considered to be adverse. In fact, the extent and severity of acidosis are predictive of adverse outcome in diverse clinical contexts, including cardiac arrest,[1,2] sepsis,[3–5] and in the neonate.[6] Traditional approaches to CO_2 management in the operating room and for patients with acute respiratory failure have focused on the deleterious effects of hypercapnia, therefore targeting normocapnia or even hypocapnia.

This approach, however, has been questioned increasingly. The potential for high tidal volumes to injure the lung directly, a phenomenon termed *ventilator-induced lung injury,* is clear from experimental[7,8] and clinical[9–13] studies. Strategies with lower tidal volumes (V_T) generally necessitate hypoventilation and tolerance of hypercapnia. This "permissive hypercapnia" has been accepted progressively in critical care for adult, pediatric, and neonatal patients requiring mechanical ventilation.

Rationale

The potential for mechanical ventilation to contribute to lung and systemic organ injury and to worsen outcome in patients with the acute respiratory distress syndrome (ARDS) is clear. The use of high V_T may cause injury via several mechanisms.[7,8] Increased mechanical stress may activate the cellular and humoral immune response directly in the lung,[7,14–16] although the exact role of this mechanism in the pathogenesis of lung and systemic organ injury has been disputed.[17,18] Intrapulmonary mediators and pathogens, such as prostaglandins,[19] cytokines,[20] endotoxin,[21] and bacteria,[22] have been demonstrated to access the systemic circulation following high-stretch mechanical ventilation. The demonstration that high-stretch mechanical ventilation causes systemic organ dysfunction in animal models may explain in part the high rate of multiorgan failure in ARDS. Currently, hypercapnia is tolerated as the lesser of two evils in order to realize the benefits of low lung stretch.

Basic Principles

PERMISSIVE HYPERCAPNIA

Conventionally, the protective effect of ventilator strategies incorporating permissive hypercapnia is solely secondary to reductions in lung stretch, with hypercapnia permitted in order to achieve this goal. Protective ventilator strategies, however, that involve hypoventilation cause both limitation of lung stretch and elevation of systemic P_{CO_2}. Lung stretch is distinct from elevated P_{CO_2} and, by manipulation of respiratory variables (frequency, V_T, dead space, and inspired CO_2) can be controlled separately, at least to some extent.

THERAPEUTIC HYPERCAPNIA

If hypercapnia were proven to have independent benefit, then deliberately elevating Pa_{CO_2}, termed *therapeutic hypercapnia*, might provide an additional advantage over reducing lung stretch alone. Conversely, in patients managed with conventional permissive hypercapnia, adverse effects of elevated Pa_{CO_2} may be concealed by the benefits of lessened lung stretch. These issues are further underlined by the fact that hypercapnia potentially has severe adverse effects in some clinical settings, such as critically elevated intracranial pressure or pulmonary vascular resistance. Because patient outcome from critical illness may be related to systemic injury rather than to lung injury alone, the clinician also must consider the effects on the brain and cardiovascular systems.

These issues have led several investigators to study the direct effects of induced hypercapnia per se in models of lung and systemic organ injury. These studies raise the potential that hypercapnia may exert active roles—beneficial and adverse—in the pathogenesis of inflammation and tissue injury. Thus therapeutic hypercapnia may constitute a testable clinical approach to critically ill patients.[23]

ACCIDENTAL HYPERCAPNIA

This is reported most commonly in the context of errors in mechanical ventilation, such as circuit disconnects or malconnects, that permit rebreathing of exhaled gases.[24] A second cause is hypoventilation secondary to drug-induced respiratory depression,[25] severe respiratory failure (e.g., status asthmaticus),[26] or massive aspiration (e.g., grain inhalation).[27]

DETERMINANTS OF HYPERCAPNIA

The determinants of hypercapnia can de described as the balance of CO_2 production versus elimination.

$$Pa_{CO_2} \propto \frac{CO_2 \text{ production}}{CO_2 \text{ elimination}} + \text{inspired } [CO_2]$$

Inspired CO_2 (FI_{CO_2}) usually is negligible. Increased CO_2 production is a potential contributor to hypercapnia, particularly in hypermetabolic disease states such as hyperpyrexia. Therefore, for practical purposes, Pa_{CO_2} reflects the rate of elimination of CO_2; there are no common "physiologic" causes of hypercapnia. Hypercapnia is seen most commonly in the context of acute or chronic respiratory failure associated with reduced minute ventilation or increased dead space.

EFFECTS ON ALVEOLAR GAS EXCHANGE

The effects of hypercapnia on systemic oxygenation are discussed below. It is often forgotten that decreasing V_T can reduce oxygenation of pulmonary venous blood. This has two contributing elements: the composition of the alveolar gas and the increase in intrapulmonary shunt. Decreased V_T increases propensity to atelectasis, which increases intrapulmonary shunt.[28] In addition, when V_T is decreased, there is a proportionate decrease in alveolar ventilation ($\dot{V}_A$), resulting in an elevated alveolar CO_2 tension (PA_{CO_2}). As pointed out by Bidani et al,[29] the alveolar gas equation

$$PA_{O_2} = FI_{O_2}(P_B - 47) - (Pa_{CO_2}/R)$$

where PA_{O_2} is the alveolar oxygen tension, P_B is the barometric pressure, and R is the respiratory quotient, can be combined with the following relationship:

$$PA_{CO_2} = (\dot{V}_{CO_2}/\dot{V}_A) \times P_B$$

where $\dot{V}_{CO_2}$ is CO_2 production, to express alveolar O_2 as a function of FI_{O_2} and $\dot{V}_A$:

$$PA_{O_2} = FI_{O_2}(P_B - 47) - (\dot{V}_{CO_2}/\dot{V}_A) \times (P_B/R)$$

Thus, with the exception of very low levels of minute ventilation, increases in $\dot{V}_A$ have minor impact on alveolar—and consequently pulmonary venous—oxygenation. In contrast, modest increases in FI_{O_2} can have a far more significant impact on oxygenation and can compensate easily for reduced $\dot{V}_A$[29] (Fig. 15-1).

Physiologic Effects

The physiologic effects of hypercapnia are complex and not completely understood, with direct effects often counterbalanced by indirect effects. If, however, hypercapnia—whether permissive or therapeutic—is to be used rationally and safely in critically ill patients, the effects of pH and Pa_{CO_2} need to be considered.

FIGURE 15-1 Relationship of alveolar oxygen tension (PA_{O_2}) and alveolar ventilation ($\dot{V}_A$) at FI_{O_2} (0.21 and 0.30), calculated assuming a constant carbon dioxide production ($\dot{V}_{CO_2}$ of 200 mL/min). At either FI_{O_2}, decreasing $\dot{V}_A$ to low values significantly reduces PA_{O_2}, especially with very low levels of $\dot{V}_A$. A small increase in FI_{O_2} (21–30%) easily compensates for the fall in PA_{O_2} resulting from hypoventilation. *Symbols*: solid line, relationship between PA_{O_2} and $\dot{V}_A$; dotted line, relationship between Pa_{CO_2} and $\dot{V}_A$. (*Reproduced, with permission, from Bidani et al: JAMA 272:957–62, 1994.*)

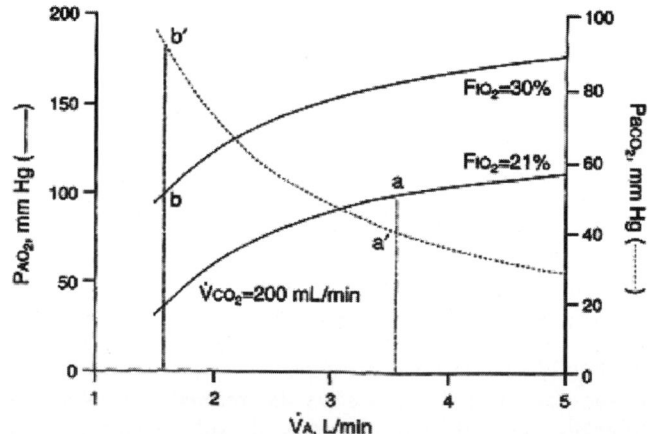

CO₂ VERSUS HYDROGEN ION

Hypercapnia generally results in acidosis (greater H^+ concentration) via its spontaneous and carbonic anhydrase–catalyzed combination with water to form carbonic acid. The protons thus generated can react with titratable groups in certain amino acids, resulting in structural changes in many proteins and enzymes in cell membranes and cellular aqueous environments.[30] Because acidosis suppresses most cellular functions, the body uses a number of strategies to defend its intracellular and extracellular pH within remarkably narrow limits.[23] The intracellular acidosis produced by hypercapnia may be corrected within a few hours, as opposed to 1–2 days for renal compensation.[31] This buffering occurs via active cell-membrane ion transporters that extrude protons and exchange them for extracellular sodium.

During hypercapnia, CO_2 per se may react directly with some free amine groups in proteins to form carbamate residues.[32–34] This binding of CO_2 also modifies protein structure and function and may explain some of the differences in the observed effects of CO_2 and H^+ when both lead to equal changes in pH. A good example is the Bohr effect, where increased Pa_{CO_2} results in a rightward shift of the $Hb-O_2$ dissociation curve, reflecting a lowered affinity of hemoglobin for O_2.

PULMONARY EFFECTS

HYPERCAPNIA AND THE NORMAL LUNG

Pulmonary Vascular Effects

In contrast to the systemic circulation, hypercapnic acidosis produces vasoconstriction and increased resistance in the pulmonary circulation[35]; such effects are exacerbated in the setting of preexisting pulmonary hypertension.[35] Hypercapnic vasoconstriction generally is weaker than hypoxic pulmonary vasoconstriction; its more important effect may be in augmenting hypoxic vasoconstriction.[30] Little is understood about how CO_2 acts on pulmonary vascular smooth muscle.

Pulmonary Gas Exchange

Acute respiratory acidosis can alter shunt via autonomic or direct effects on pulmonary vasculature and on the airways. Acidosis enhances hypoxic pulmonary vasoconstriction and therefore usually reduces shunt and increases Pa_{O_2}, whereas alkalosis has the opposite effect.[36] CO_2 administration improves matching of ventilation and perfusion and increases arterial oxygenation by this mechanism in both health[37–39] and disease.[40] A dose-response relationship exists wherein increased $F_{I_{CO_2}}$ results in progressive augmentation of Pa_{O_2}.[39,41] In fact, administration of $F_{I_{CO_2}}$ during late inspiration—limiting its exposure to the conducting airways—results in most of the beneficial pulmonary effects (i.e., $\dot{V}_A/\dot{Q}$ matching and oxygenation) and less systemic acidosis[42] (Fig. 15-2). Permissive hypercapnia in patients with ARDS appears to increase shunt secondary to a reduction in V_T and airway closure rather than from hypercapnia.[43]

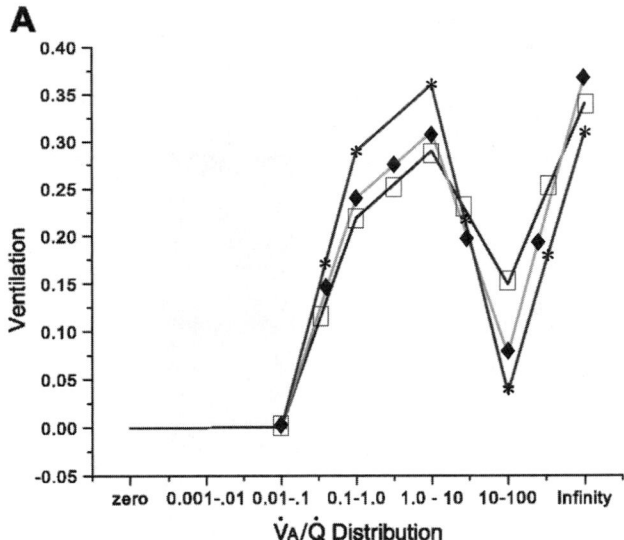

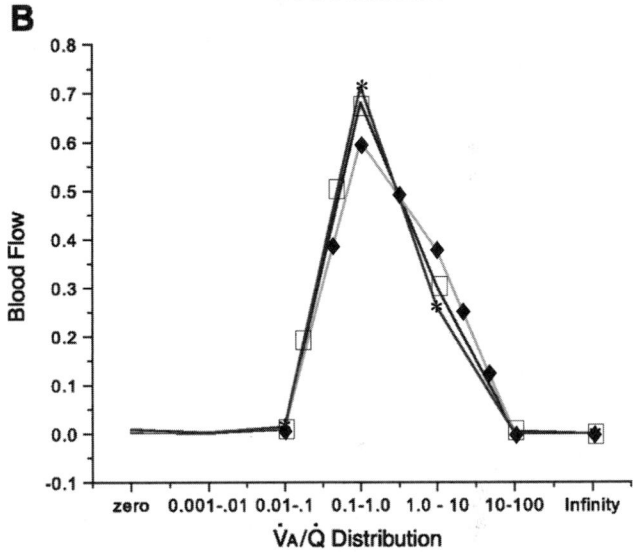

FIGURE 15-2 Effects of room air and inspired CO_2 on the distribution of ventilation (*A*) and of perfusion (*B*). The lowest values of $\dot{V}_A/\dot{Q}$ correspond to regions of intrapulmonary shunt and the highest to regions of alveolar dead space. Addition of CO_2 to inspired gas (throughout the respiratory cycle, *; restricted to late inspiration, □) resulted in more homogeneous ventilation and perfusion compared to no added CO_2 (room air ◆). $\dot{V}_A/\dot{Q}$, ratio of ventilation to perfusion. (*Reproduced, with permission, from Brogan et al: J Appl Physiol 96:1894–8, 2004.*)

Airway Tone

Hypercapnia has been reported to either increase[44] or decrease[45] airway resistance. These effects may be explained the direct dilation of small airways and the indirect (i.e., vagally mediated) large airway constriction.[30] These opposing but balanced actions may produce little net alteration in airway resistance.[46]

Lung Compliance

Parenchymal lung compliance increases in response to hypercapnic acidosis. This may be secondary to increased surfactant secretion or more effective surface tension–lowering properties under acidic conditions.[47]

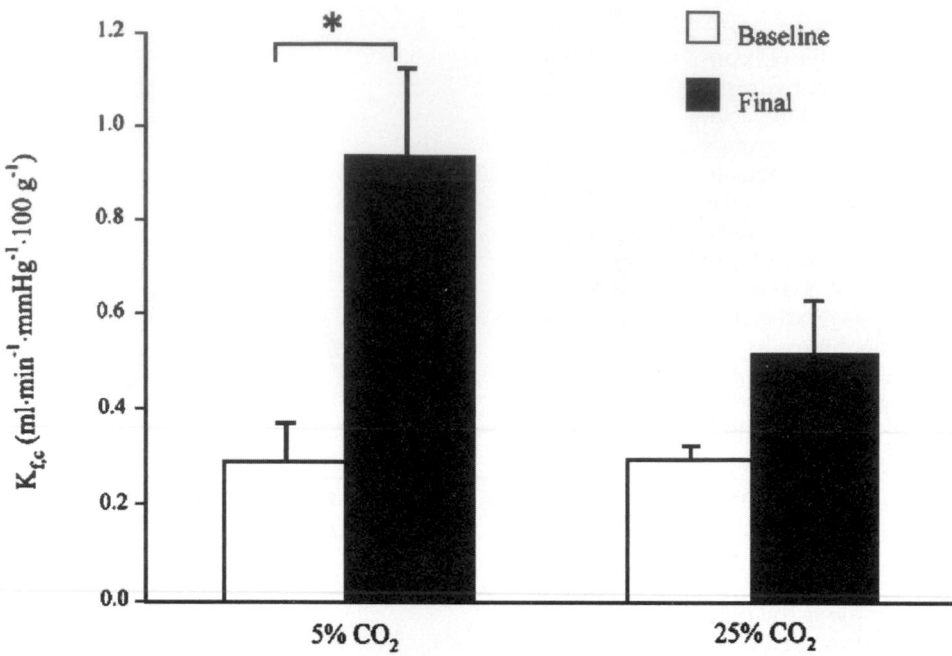

FIGURE 15-3 Effects of CO_2 on ischemia-reperfusion in the isolated perfused lung. Pulmonary microvascular permeability is significantly less following reperfusion in the presence of hypercapnia (25% CO_2) compared with normocapnia (5% CO_2). $K_{f,c}$, pulmonary microvascular filtration coefficient. (*Reproduced, with permission, from Shibata et al: Am J Respir Crit Care Med 158:1578–84, 1998.*)

Physiologic Role of Hypercapnia in the Lung

In health, CO_2 alters lung compliance as well as pulmonary vascular and airway tone.[30] The combined effect of small airways constriction and decreased compliance explains the phenomenon of hypocapnic bronchoconstriction and pneumoconstriction that occurs following acute regional pulmonary artery occlusions.[48,49] These effects either may alter regional ventilation to keep pace with a primary change in perfusion or may alter regional perfusion to match a primary change in ventilation.[30]

HYPERCAPNIA AND THE INJURED LUNG: LABORATORY DATA

Hypercapnic acidosis attenuates the increased lung permeability consequent to free radical–mediated lung injury[50] (Fig. 15-3). Although hypercapnic acidosis attenuates xanthine oxidase activity,[50] this does not account for all its protective effects.[51]

Subsequent in vivo studies confirmed and further characterized the protective effects of hypercapnic acidosis in ischemia-reperfusion–induced lung injury. Hypercapnic acidosis preserved lung mechanics, attenuated protein leakage, reduced pulmonary edema, and improved oxygenation in comparison with control conditions following in vivo pulmonary ischemia-reperfusion,[52] as well as in secondary lung injury.[41] Such protective effects of hypercapnic acidosis are not mediated via a decrease in pulmonary artery resistance; on the contrary, protection occurred despite elevated pulmonary artery pressures.[41]

The direct effects of hypercapnic acidosis in the setting ventilator-associated lung injury have been examined in both ex vivo and in vivo models. In two key studies, the addition of inspired CO_2 resulted in lessened ventilator-induced lung injury in the isolated rabbit lung[53] and in the in vivo rabbit[54] (Fig. 15-4). All the data are not positive. Supplemental CO_2 exhibits more modest protective effects in the setting of more clinically relevant tidal stretch. Strand et al[55] demonstrated that significant hypercapnic acidosis (mean Pa_{CO_2} of 95 mmHg) was well tolerated in preterm lambs and also appeared to reduce lung injury. In the context of a clinically relevant high V_T strategy [V_T of 12 ml/kg, positive end-expiratory pressure (PEEP) of 0 cm H_2O, respiration rate (RR) of 42 breaths per minute] in an adult model, Laffey et al[41] reported that hypocapnia was potentially deleterious and hypercapnic acidosis somewhat protective. Furthermore, inspired CO_2 did not significantly attenuate lung injury induced by an atelectasis-prone model of lung injury that mimics the neonatal respiratory distress syndrome.[56] Taken together, these findings suggest that while hypercapnic acidosis substantially attenuates injury secondary to excessive stretch, its effects in the context of more clinically relevant lung stretch or extensive atelectasis may be more modest.

In lung injury induced by oleic acid, metabolic alkalosis increased shunt fraction and decreased Pa_{O_2}.[57] Whereas metabolic acidosis decreased shunt and increased Sa_{O_2} and Pv_{O_2}, hypercapnic acidosis did not affect $\dot{Q}_S/\dot{Q}_T$, Sa_{O_2}, or Sv_{O_2}. Both Pa_{O_2} and Pv_{O_2}, however, increased with hypercapnic acidosis possibly in part because of a rightward shift of the Hb-O_2 dissociation curve and increased cardiac output. When the hypercapnia was buffered with bicarbonate to maintain constant pH, gas exchange deteriorated during hypercapnia, shunt increased, and Sa_{O_2} fell.[57] The authors suggested that the direct vasodilator effect of hypercapnia in hypoxic lung regions is opposed by acidosis and results in little overall effect on shunt from respiratory acidosis. When the acidosis was buffered, the vasodilator effect of

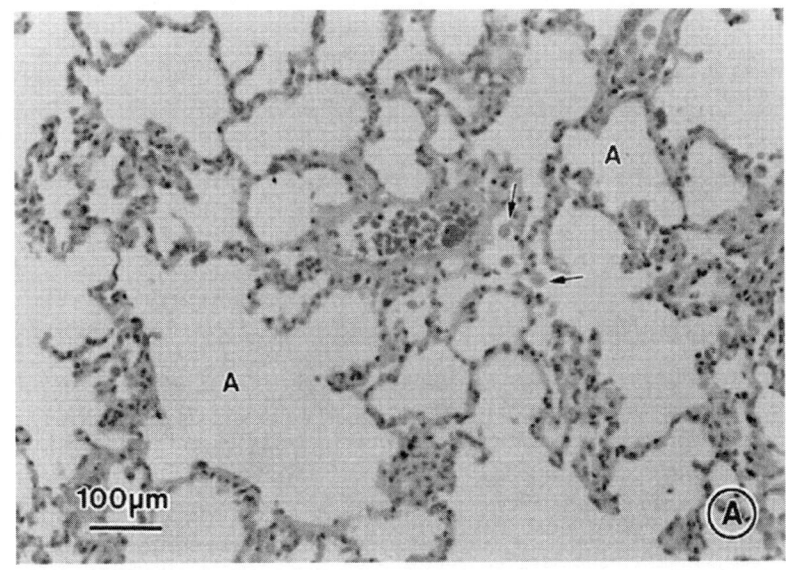

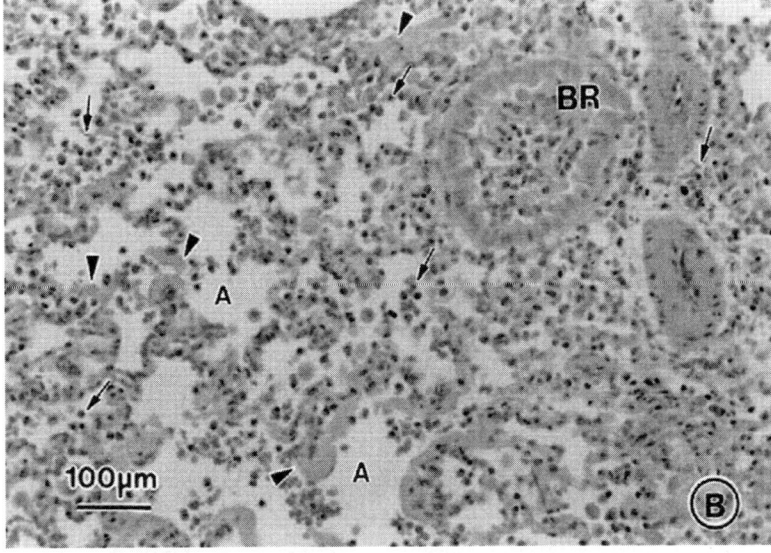

FIGURE 15-4 Lung histology following high tidal volume ventilation in the in vivo rabbit. The extent of histologic injury is far less with addition of inspired CO$_2$ (Pa$_{CO_2}$ of 80–100 mmHg) (*A*) than with a Pa$_{CO_2}$ of 40 mmHg (*B*). *Symbols*: Arrow, macrophage; arrowhead, hyaline membrane formation; BR, bronchiole. (*Reproduced, with permission, from Sinclair et al: Am J Respir Crit Care Med 166:403–8, 2002.*)

CO$_2$ was unopposed, hypoxic pulmonary vasoconstriction was inhibited, and shunt increased.[57]

ARDS commonly develops in the context of severe sepsis, where the potential for deleterious effects has been raised.[58] The mechanisms of lung injury in sepsis-induced ARDS are quite distinct from those in many experimental models. Lipopolysaccharide, a key endotoxin of gram-negative bacteria, initiates lung injury by activating a specific receptor called *toll-like receptor-4.*[59] Hypercapnia appears to exert different effects in lung injury caused by pulmonary versus systemic administration of endotoxin. Hypercapnic acidosis, induced by the administration of CO$_2$, protects directly against acute lung injury induced by intratracheal endotoxin instillation.[60] Conversely, hypercapnia induced by reduced V$_T$ and respiratory rate appears to worsen lung damage induced by systemic endotoxin administration.[61] Inspired CO$_2$ is distributed uniformly through all ventilated

regions, whereas hypercapnia caused by reducing alveolar ventilation may not be.[58] These issues underline the need to consider the means of achieving hypercapnia, as well as the diversity of experimental models.[62]

HYPERCAPNIA AND THE INJURED LUNG: CLINICAL DATA

Reduction of V$_T$ results in permissive hypercapnia. The lung alterations, however, involve the reduced V$_T$, the ensuing hypercapnic acidosis, and the potential influence of altered respiratory frequency. No clinical studies to date have dissected out these changes; it is difficult to conceive of how this would be done. Nonetheless, conventional application of permissive hypercapnia involves reduction of V$_T$, some increase in respiratory frequency, and tolerance of hypercapnic acidosis.

Pulmonary Vascular Effects

Pulmonary hypertension is almost invariable in ARDS. While protective ventilation may augment pulmonary vascular flow, the net effect of hypercapnic acidosis is usually to increase pulmonary vascular resistance. Inhaled nitric oxide usually can overcome such hypercapnia-induced pulmonary hypertension and may increase cardiac output.[63] Pulmonary hypertension may result in high capillary wall stress; therefore, worsening of such stress by hypercapnia theoretically could exacerbate stretch-induced lung injury.[31,64]

Pulmonary Gas Exchange in ARDS

In ARDS, hypercapnia usually results in a slight increase in Pa_{O_2} and a somewhat larger increase in venous and tissue P_{O_2}.[65] The increase in Pa_{O_2} occurs partly because of an increase in cardiac output and partly because of a rightward shift of the Hb-O_2 dissociation curve, which facilitates oxygen unloading to the tissues.[23,66] The overall effect, therefore, is likely to enhance tissue oxygen uptake. In patients with ARDS, the reduction in mean airway pressure after initiation of pressure-limited ventilation (without high PEEP) may result in lung derecruitment and increased shunt.[67] Three clinical studies shed light on these mechanisms.

Feihl et al[43] provided a detailed assessment of pulmonary physiology associated with a large reduction in V_T (mean of 10–6 ml/kg). Induction of permissive hypercapnia markedly increased intrapulmonary shunt, although there was no effect on dispersion of $\dot{V}_A/\dot{Q}$[43] (Fig. 15-5). Permissive hypercapnia increased cardiac output and decreased Pa_{O_2} from 109–92 mmHg apparently owing to a combined effect of reduced V_T, increased shunt fraction, and decreased alveolar ventilation.[43] Thorens et al[65] studied the rapid induction of hypercapnia in 11 patients with ARDS. V_T was reduced such that Pa_{CO_2} rose from 40.3–59.3 mmHg, and pH decreased from 7.4 to 7.26.[65] There were significant increases in venous mixture, cardiac index, and mean pulmonary artery pressure, prompting the authors to caution against rapid induction of permissive hypercapnia. Pfeiffer et al[68] studied the effect of permissive hypercapnia consequent to V_T reduction in 22 patients with ARDS categorized into septic (i.e., hyperdynamic) or nonseptic groups. Multiple inert-gas uptake measurements revealed an increase in intrapulmonary shunt but maintained—or increased—Pa_{O_2}.[68] Overall, these data support two opposing effects on oxygenation: Reduced V_T worsens atelectasis and increases intrapulmonary shunt, countered by elevated cardiac output (and perhaps reduced O_2 consumption), which increases mixed venous O_2 content.[68] These concepts have been supported by mathematical models of oxygen kinetics in ARDS.[66]

CENTRAL NERVOUS SYSTEM EFFECTS

HYPERCAPNIA AND THE NORMAL BRAIN

Neurovascular Regulation

Hypercapnic acidosis causes cerebral vasodilation. The increase in cerebral blood flow and blood volume must be considered carefully in any patient as a risk for raised in-

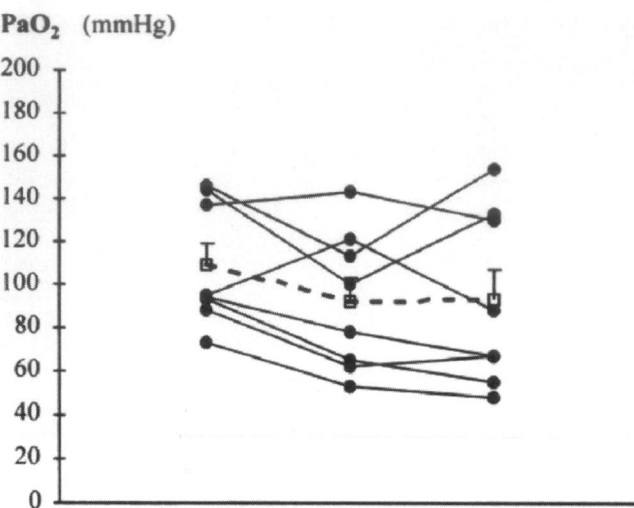

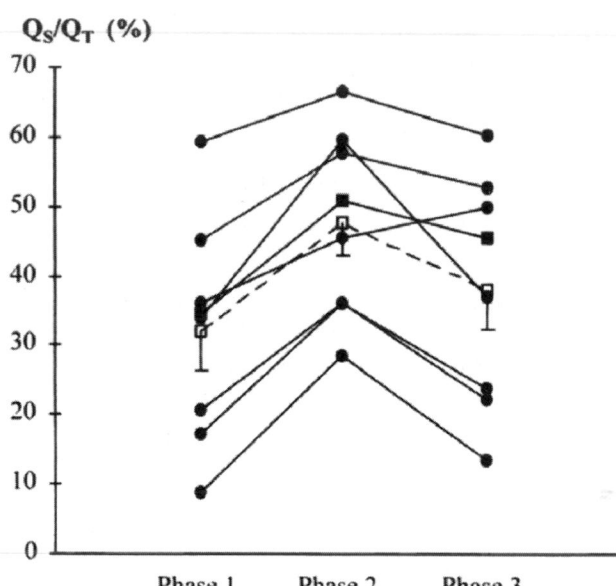

FIGURE 15-5 The effects of permissive hypercapnia and dobutamine on arterial oxygen tension (Pa_{O_2}) and venous admixture $\dot{Q}_S/\dot{Q}_T$. Phase 1 (high V_T, 10.3 ml/kg) represents baseline conditions. Phase 2 (low V_T, 6.5 ml/kg) represents a change to permissive hypercapnia, which was associated with a slight decrease in mean Pa_{O_2} and a large increase in $\dot{Q}_S/\dot{Q}_T$. Phase 3 represents resumption of baseline high V_T (10.3 ml/kg) plus infusion of dobutamine; it resulted in stabilization of Pa_{O_2} despite residual elevation of $\dot{Q}_S/\dot{Q}_T$. $\dot{Q}_S/\dot{Q}_T$, intrapulmonary shunt. (*Reproduced, with permission, from Feihl et al: Am J Respir Crit Care Med 162:209–15, 2000.*)

tracranial pressure.[23] The mechanism of cerebral vasodilation depends on the arterial bed and type of artery. Nakahata et al[69] demonstrated that hypercapnic acidosis induced cerebral precapillary arteriolar vasodilation, which depended on acidosis rather than CO_2. They demonstrated that the ATP-sensitive potassium channel plays a major role. Others have suggested roles for both ATP-sensitive and calcium-activated potassium channels[70] and the neuronal isoform of nitric oxide synthase.[71]

Regulation of Ventilation

Hypercapnia is a potent regulator of ventilation. Mild hypercapnia (increase in end-tidal P_{CO_2} of 8 mmHg) in healthy volunteers resulted in a compensatory metabolic alkalosis over 24–48 hours that was maintained over the course of exposure.[72] While there was a modest increase in ventilatory chemosensitivity to acute hypoxia, no change occurred in response to acute elevations in CO_2.

Cerebral Tissue Oxygenation

Hare et al[39] demonstrated that hypercapnic acidosis increases cerebral tissue P_{O_2} through augmentation of Pa_{O_2} and increased cerebral blood flow (Fig. 15-6).

NEUROMUSCULAR EFFECTS OF HYPERCAPNIA

Recent studies highlight the potential for hypercapnia to exert potentially deleterious neuromuscular effects. Diaphragm of rats exposed to prolonged hypercapnia (7.5% CO_2 for 6 weeks) undergoes significant changes.[73] Hypercapnia depressed diaphragmatic tension and time to contraction and relaxation; it altered diaphragmatic composition, increasing slow-twitch and decreasing fast-twitch fibers. In fact, even short-term exposure (7% inspired CO_2) may impair neuromuscular function transiently through effects on afferent transmission or synaptic integrity in healthy volunteers.[74]

HYPERCAPNIA AND THE INJURED BRAIN: LABORATORY DATA

Several studies have demonstrated protective effects of hypercapnia in brain injury. Hypercapnic acidosis attenuates

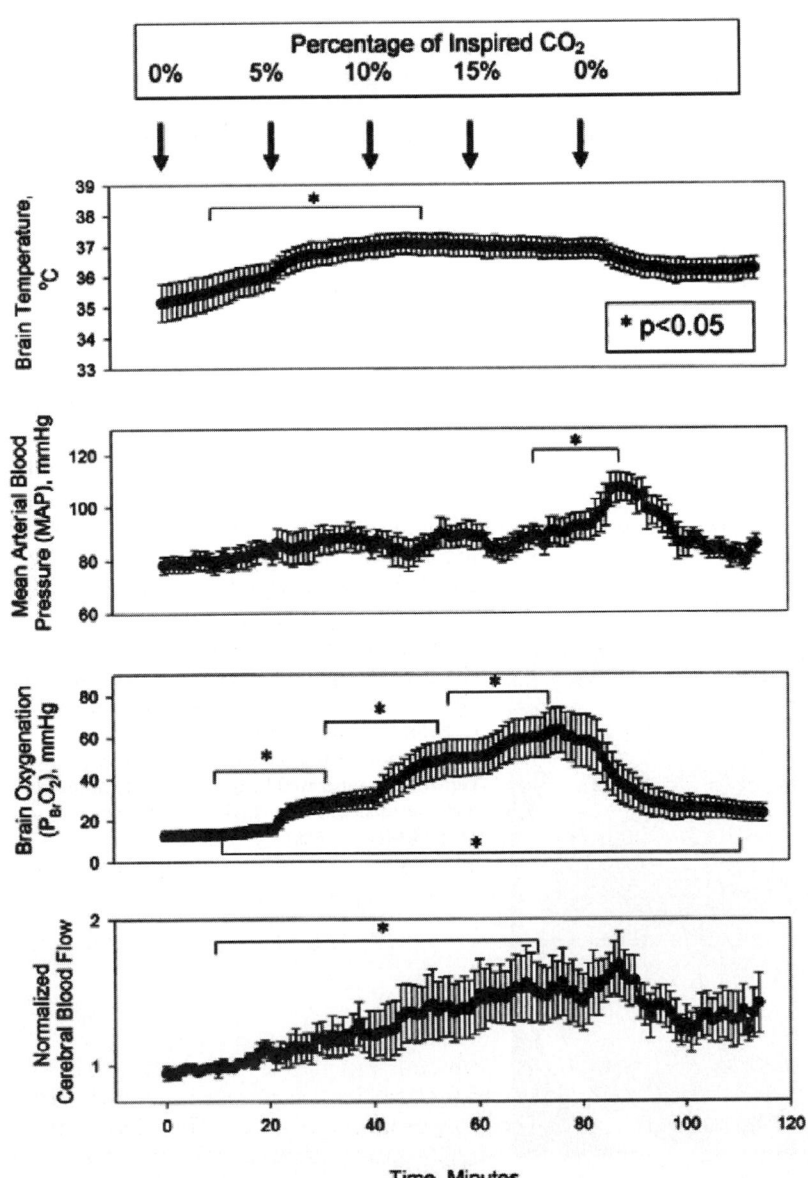

FIGURE 15-6 Increases in inspired CO_2 concentration produce progressive increases in brain tissue O_2 tension and cerebral perfusion. (*Reproduced, with permission, from Hare et al: Can J Anaesth 50:1061–8, 2003.*)

hypoxic-ischemic brain injury in the immature rat. Vannucci et al[75,76] developed a model of hypoxic-ischemic injury in the immature rat consisting of unilateral common carotid artery ligation, exposure to hypoxia (F_{IO_2} of 0.8%), and thereafter exposure to varying concentrations of inspired CO_2 (0%, 3%, 6%, or 9%) for 2 hours.[75,76] Neuropathologic assessment at 30 days of age demonstrated that hypocapnia was deleterious and that elevated CO_2 was protective.[76] The experimental model caused hyperventilation. Without supplemental CO_2, the animals were frankly hypocapnic, which was harmful. Therefore, exposure to supplemental CO_2 may have provided protection by preventing hypocapnia rather than by producing hypercapnia per se. The investigators subsequently demonstrated that cerebral flood flow was better preserved during hypercapnia; the greater oxygen delivery promoted cerebral glucose utilization and oxidative metabolism for optimal maintenance of tissue high-energy phosphate reserves.[75] Cerebrospinal fluid glutamate levels were lowest with hypercapnia. It is possible that inhibition of excitatory amino acid neurotransmitter secretion may contribute to neural protection.[75] Additional mechanisms of neural protection may involve inhibition of free radicals[77] or attenuation of neuronal apoptosis.[78]

HYPERCAPNIA AND THE INJURED BRAIN: CLINICAL DATA

Hypercapnia greatly increases cerebral blood flow and, if critical, may raise intracranial pressure, resulting in papilloedema and headache. In the clinical setting, cerebral effects of hypercapnia often overlap with the effects of hypoxemia.[79] The resulting abnormalities include restlessness, tremor, slurred speech, and fluctuations of mood. High levels of Pa_{CO_2} cause narcosis.[79] Raised intracranial pressure, however, is not an absolute contraindication to permissive hypercapnia; in fact, it has been used successfully for management of acute lung injury in a patient with acute meningoencephalitis and cerebral edema[80] (Fig. 15-7).

CARDIOVASCULAR EFFECTS

NORMAL CARDIOVASCULAR PHYSIOLOGY

Hemodynamic Effects

Hypercapnic acidosis directly reduces the contractility of cardiac and vascular smooth muscle.[30] This is counterbalanced by the hypercapnic-mediated sympathoadrenal effects, causing increased preload, increased heart rate, and decreased afterload, which lead to a net increase in cardiac output.[30] In intact animals and human subjects, myocardial contractility and cardiac output increase during hypercapnia because of increased sympathetic activity.[81]

Effects on Tissue Oxygenation

Hypercapnia results in a complex interaction of altered cardiac output, hypoxic pulmonary vasoconstriction, and intrapulmonary shunt, with a net increase in Pa_{O_2}. Because hypercapnia generally elevates cardiac output, global O_2 delivery is increased.[82] Regional (including mesenteric) blood flow also is increased,[83] thereby increasing organ oxygen delivery. Because hypercapnia and acidosis shift the Hb-O_2 dissociation curve rightward and may cause an elevation in hematocrit,[84] tissue oxygen delivery is further facilitated. Acidosis may reduce cellular respiration and oxygen consumption,[85] which further benefit a supply-demand imbalance, in addition to enhanced O_2 delivery. Acidosis may protect against ongoing tissue production of *further* organic acids by a negative-feedback loop, providing a mechanism of cellular metabolic shutdown at times of nutrient shortage (e.g., ischemia).[86] In addition, hypercapnic acidosis increases P_{O_2} in both subcutaneous tissues and the intestinal wall.[87]

CARDIOVASCULAR EFFECTS: LABORATORY DATA

Hypercapnic acidosis protects the heart against ischemia-reperfusion injury. This has been demonstrated in isolated perfused neonatal lamb hearts, where greater degrees of hypercapnic acidosis were associated with progressively greater protection.[88] Exposure to comparable metabolic

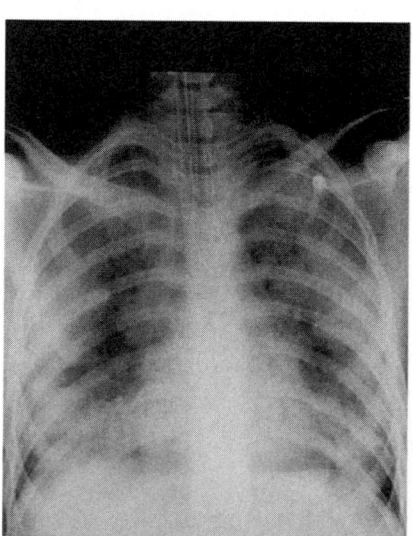
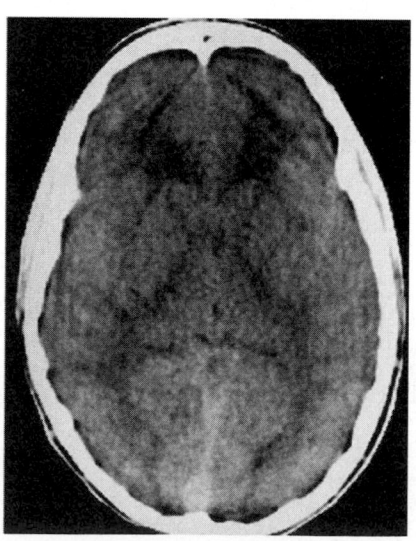

FIGURE 15-7 A chest radiograph and brain computed tomographic (CT) scan of a child with both ARDS and cerebral edema illustrating the tradeoff that occurs when permissive hypercapnia is instituted to protect against ventilator-associated lung injury. (*Reproduced, with permission, from Tasker et al: Intensive Care Med 24:616–9, 1998.*)

acidemia (pH 6.8), however, followed by buffering to normal pH with bicarbonate and tris-hydroxymethyl aminomethane (THAM), is not protective.[88] In contrast, metabolic acidosis (pH 6.6) without buffering prevented myocardial stunning following global ischemia in the isolated perfused ferret heart.[89] The latter investigators have since demonstrated that both hypercapnic and metabolic acidosis were equally effective in reducing infarct size in an in vivo canine model of coronary artery ischemia-reperfusion.[90] Possible mechanisms for the protective effects of acidosis include reduction of calcium loading to the myocardium through H^+ inhibition of calcium uptake and, in the case of hypercapnic acidosis, induction of coronary vasodilation. Nomura et al[88] found that the greatest coronary artery flow occurred with maximal hypercapnia. In contrast, increases in regional coronary artery flow do not contribute to the protective effects of normocapnic acidosis.[91]

CARDIOVASCULAR EFFECTS: CLINICAL DATA

Critical Illness

The potential for hypercapnia to exert detrimental effects on cardiac output[92] and the peripheral circulation[93] may be overstated, particularly when hypercapnia develops gradually. As discussed earlier, the net hemodynamic effect is probably beneficial.[43,82] Nevertheless, hypercapnic acidosis may exert adverse hemodynamic effects in critically ill patients, particularly where myocardial function is already depressed. In addition, acute hypercapnia may cause hypotension where endogenous catecholamine production has been maximized or where β-blocking drugs reduce the potential for sympathetic activation to overcome the direct depressive effects of hypercapnia. Even in critically ill patients requiring inotropic drug infusions, however, cardiac output increases almost invariably after an acute rise in Pa_{CO_2}, although the mean arterial pressure may fall because of direct hypercapnia-induced systemic vasodilation.[63]

In patients with ARDS, the rapid induction of hypercapnia to a target Pa_{CO_2} of 80 mmHg for 2 hours resulted in decreased systemic vascular resistance and increased cardiac output.[94] In addition, myocardial contractility was decreased, and mean pulmonary artery pressure was increased.[94] In stable patients with ARDS, reduction of V_T (10–7.7 ml/kg) associated with an increase in Pa_{CO_2} (37.9–56.7 mmHg) was not associated with changes in hemodynamics or measures of oxygen delivery or consumption.[95]

RENAL, HEPATIC, AND SPLANCHNIC EFFECTS

In isolated hepatocytes exposed to anoxia[96] and chemical hypoxia,[97] acidosis delays the onset of cell death markedly. Correction of pH accelerated cell death. This phenomenon may represent a protective adaptation against hypoxic and ischemic stress. Isolated renal cortical tubules exposed to anoxia have improved ATP levels on reoxygenation at a pH of 6.9 when compared with tubules incubated at pH 7.5.[96]

The marked sympathetic activation of hypercapnic acidosis, particularly when combined with arterial hypoxemia, can lead to intense renal vasoconstriction (unlike elsewhere in the circulation) and avid tubular sodium reabsorption, causing depressed glomerular filtration and increased fluid retention.[98] Patients with ARDS exposed to permissive hypercapnia demonstrated no important alterations in splanchnic circulation, although CO_2 was increased by the addition of dead space and not by reduction of V_T.[99]

CELLULAR AND MOLECULAR EFFECTS OF HYPERCAPNIA

A clear understanding of cellular and biochemical mechanisms underlying the effects of hypercapnia is essential. It is a prerequisite for successful translation of laboratory findings to the bedside. It enables prediction of potential side effects, so identifying patients in whom hypercapnia should be avoided.

ACIDOSIS VERSUS HYPERCAPNIA

The protective effects of hypercapnic acidosis in experimental lung and systemic organ injury is primarily a function of the acidosis generated.[51,100] In the isolated lung, the protective effect of hypercapnic acidosis in ischemia-reperfusion was greatly attenuated if the pH was buffered toward normal.[51] No significant protective effect was detected with buffered hypercapnia. Metabolic acidosis, however, attenuates ischaemia-reperfusion injury, although less effectively than hypercapnic acidosis.[51] The myocardial protective effects of hypercapnic acidosis are also seen with metabolic acidosis both in ex vivo[89] and in vivo[90,91] models. Metabolic acidosis exerts protective effects in other models of organ injury. Metabolic acidosis delays the onset of cell death in isolated hepatocytes exposed to anoxia[96] or chemical hypoxia.[97] Isolated renal cortical tubules exposed to anoxia have improved ATP levels on reoxygenation at acidotic (compared with alkalotic) pH.[96] In contrast to the lung, the type of acidosis (i.e., hypercapnic versus metabolic) appears to be of importance in the renal tubule.

ANTI-INFLAMMATORY EFFECTS

Several key components of the inflammatory response are attenuated by hypercapnic acidosis. Hypercapnic acidosis inhibits the release of tumor necrosis factor α (TNF-α) and interleukin-1 (IL-1) from stimulated macrophages in vitro,[101] as well levels of TNF-α in the bronchoalveolar fluid following in vivo pulmonary ischaemia-reperfusion.[52]

Cellular and molecular mechanisms underlying the inhibitory effects of hypercapnic acidosis in the neutrophil are increasingly well understood. Both hypercapnia and acidosis impair neutrophil intracellular pH regulation. Intracellular pH decreases when neutrophils are activated by immune stimuli.[102] If pH is normal, there tends to be a recovery in neutrophil intracellular pH back toward normal. Hypercapnia decreases extracellular and intracellular pH in the local milieu, resulting in a rapid fall in neutrophil cytosolic pH,[103] potentially overwhelming the capacity of neutrophils—especially when activated[104]—to regulate cytosolic pH. This failure impairs important neutrophil

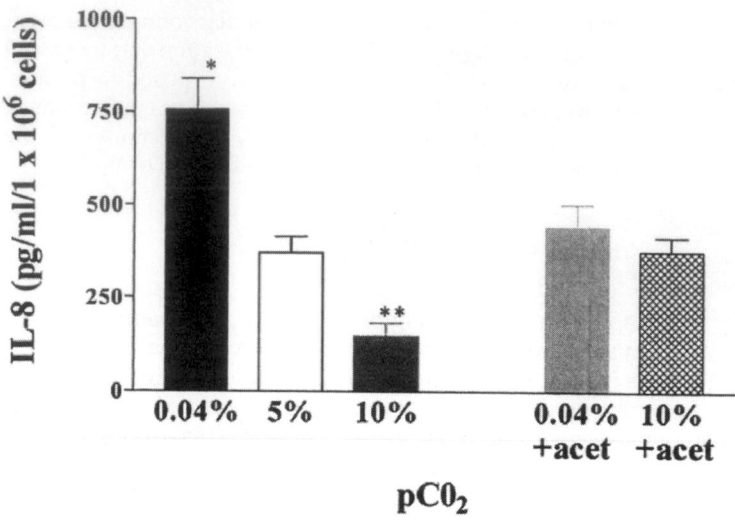

FIGURE 15-8 Hypercapnia (10% CO_2) inhibits, whereas hypocapnia (0.04% CO_2) potentiates, the release of interleukin-8 from endotoxin-stimulated neutrophils. Incubation with acetazolamide, which impairs the effect of extracellular CO_2 on intracellular pH, abolished the influence of extracellular CO_2. IL-8, interleukin 8. (*Reproduced, with permission, from Coakley et al: J Leuk Biol 71:603–10, 2002.*)

functions, such as chemotaxis[105] and release of IL-8 following endotoxin stimulation[102] (Fig. 15-8). Such effects also occur in vivo because lung neutrophil recruitment is inhibited during ventilator-induced[54] and endotoxin-induced[60] lung injury.

FREE-RADICAL GENERATION AND ACTIVITY

In common with most biologic enzymes, the enzymes that produce oxidizing free radicals function optimally at physiologic pH. Oxidant generation by both basal and stimulated neutrophils appears to be regulated by ambient CO_2 levels, with oxidant generation reduced by hypercapnia and increased by hypocapnia.[102] Production of superoxide by stimulated neutrophils in vitro is decreased at acidic pH.[106] In the brain, hypercapnic acidosis attenuates glutathione depletion and lipid peroxidation,[77] which reflect free-radical activity and tissue damage, respectively. In the lung, hypercapnic acidosis reduces free-radical tissue injury following ischemia-reperfusion[52] and attenuates the production of the higher oxides of nitric oxide, such as nitrate and nitrite, following both ventilator-induced[53] and endotoxin-induced[60] injury. Hypercapnic acidosis inhibits injury mediated by xanthine oxidase and directly inhibits the enzyme.[50]

Peroxynitrite-Mediated Tissue Nitration

Concerns exist regarding the potential for hypercapnia to potentiate tissue nitration by peroxynitrite, a potent free radical. Peroxynitrite is produced in vivo largely by the reaction of nitric oxide with superoxide radical and causes tissue damage by oxidizing a variety of biomolecules and by nitrating phenolic amino acid residues in proteins.[107] The potential for buffered hypercapnia to promote the formation of nitration products from peroxynitrite has been clearly demonstrated in vitro.[100,108] The potential, however, for hypercapnic acidosis to promote nitration of lung tissue in vivo depends on the injury. Hypercapnic acidosis decreased tissue nitration following pulmonary ischemia-reperfusion[52] but increased nitration following endotoxin exposure[60,61,100] (Fig. 15-9).

REGULATION OF GENE EXPRESSION

The effects of hypercapnia may be mediated by regulation of gene expression. Several unidentified proteins are upregulated by hypercapnia in the normal lung.[109] Hypercapnia may regulate this process at the level of gene transcription via alterations in the half-life of messenger RNA (mRNA) or by modulating protein synthesis. Molecular mechanisms underlying hypercapnic acidosis–mediated control of gene transcription include membrane acid–sensing ion channels and acid-responsive gene promoter regions.[110–112] Furthermore, the coding for certain proteins for mRNA has pH-sensitive regions.[110]

Hypercapnic acidosis has been demonstrated to regulate the expression of genes central to the inflammatory response in models of cell injury. Nuclear factor-$\kappa\beta$ (NF-$\kappa\beta$) is a key regulator of the expression of multiple genes involved in inflammatory response, and its activation represents a pivotal early step in activation of the inflammatory response.[113] NF-$\kappa\beta$ is found in the cytoplasm in an inactive form bound to inhibitory proteins called *inhibitory protein $\kappa\beta$* (I$\kappa\beta$). The important isoforms are I$\kappa\beta$-α and I$\kappa\beta$-β. I$\kappa\beta$ proteins are phosphorylated by the I$\kappa\beta$ kinase complex and subsequently degraded, thus allowing NF-$\kappa\beta$ to translocate into the nucleus, bind to specific promoter sites, and activate target genes.[113] Hypercapnic acidosis inhibits endotoxin-induced NF-$\kappa\beta$ activation and DNA binding in pulmonary endothelial cells by decreasing I$\kappa\beta$-α degradation[114] (Fig. 15-10). Hypercapnic acidosis also suppressed endothelial production of intercellular adhesion molecule 1 (ICAM-1) and IL-8, which are critically regulated by the NF-$\kappa\beta$ pathway.[114]

Use in Specific Clinical Settings

ACUTE SEVERE ASTHMA

Although much current work on ventilator strategies involving permissive hypercapnia concentrates on lung injury, its use was first described in status asthmaticus by Darioli and Pettet.[115] Permissive hypercapnia decreases

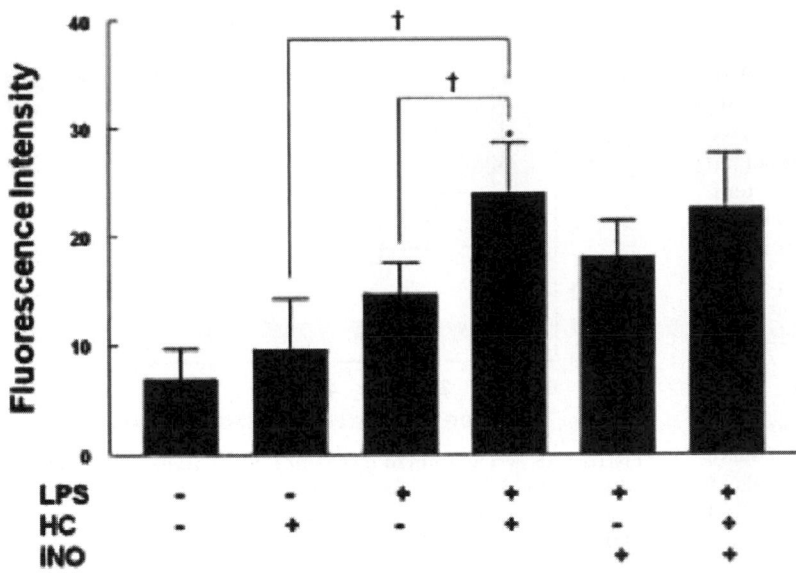

FIGURE 15-9 Hypercapnia and inhaled nitric oxide significantly increased the formation of 3-nitrotyrosine following LPS pretreatment. HC, hypercapnia; iNO, inhaled nitric oxide; LPS, lipopolysaccharide. (*Reproduced, with permission, from Lang et al: Am J Respir Crit Care Med 171:147–57, 2005.*)

dynamic hyperinflation in ventilated patients with acute severe asthma by increasing expiratory time and decreasing V_T. This reduces end-inspiratory lung volume and auto-PEEP. Other investigators have confirmed that morbidity and mortality are reduced with the use of permissive hypercapnia in ventilated patients with acute severe asthma.[116] Modest levels of permissive hypercapnia (~60 mmHg) are employed widely in ventilated patients with acute severe asthma.[117]

ACUTE RESPIRATORY DISTRESS SYNDROME

The potential for protective lung ventilation strategies with varying degrees of permissive hypercapnia to improve survival in patients with acute lung injury and ARDS was sug-

gested initially by Hickling et al.[11,12] Two studies by this group, one retrospective[11] and one prospective,[12] strongly indicated that use of low V_T was beneficial. In the retrospective study, 50 patients with severe ARDS (lung injury score ≥ 2.5, mean $Pa_{O_2}/F_{I_{O_2}} = 94$) were managed with limitation of peak airway pressure to less than 30 cmH$_2$O. The mean maximum Pa_{CO_2} was 62 mmHg, and the hospital mortality (16%) was less than predicted by APACHE II score (39.6%). Importantly, the authors reported no differences between survivors and nonsurvivors in terms of lung injury score, ventilator score, $Pa_{O_2}/F_{I_{O_2}}$, or maximum Pa_{CO_2}.[11] The prospective study[12] investigated comparable patients and also limited peak airway pressures to less than 30 cmH$_2$O, did not buffer hypercapnic acidosis, and commenced with a V_T of 7 ml/kg (as opposed to 12 ml/kg in the retrospective

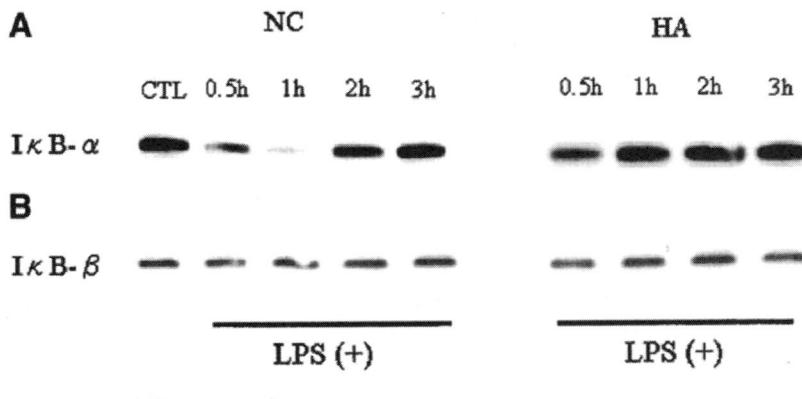

FIGURE 15-10 Hypercapnia suppresses the degradation of I$\kappa\beta$-α (*A*) but not I$\kappa\beta$-β (*B*) following exposure to lipopolysaccharide, thereby inhibiting the nuclear translocation of NF-$\kappa\beta$ and downstream cytokine production. The effects of isocapnic acidosis and buffered hypercapnia (*C*) on I$\kappa\beta$-α degradation were intermediate between normocapnic control and hypercapnic acidosis conditions. BH, buffered hypercapnia; HA, hypercapnic acidosis; IA, isocapnic acidosis; LPS, lipopolysaccharide; NC, normocapnia; NF-$\kappa\beta$, nuclear factor $\kappa\beta$. (*Reproduced, with permission, from Takeshita et al: Am J Respir Cell Mol Biol 29:124–32, 2003.*)

study). Again, hospital mortality rates were lower than predicted by APACHE II score (26.4% versus 53.3%).[12]

The five prospective, randomized, controlled trials[9,10,118–120] that measured survival in ARDS are discussed in detail elsewhere (see Chapter 73). Two were positive (the ventilator strategy had an impact on mortality),[9,10] and three were not.[118–120] To some extent, permissive hypercapnia developed in all the trials, although there was much variability. Among the four major trials, the postrandomization Pa_{CO_2} values (mean ± SD) in the control (higher V_T) trial groups were $35.8 ± 8.0$,[9] $36.0 ± 1.5$,[10] $41.0 ± 7.5$,[119] and $46.0 ± 10$[118] mmHg. The postrandomization Pa_{CO_2} values in the protective (lower V_T) trial groups were $40.0 ± 10$,[9] $58.0 ± 3.0$,[10] $59.5 ± 15$,[119] and $54.5 ± 19$[118] mmHg. It is clear that ventilation strategy can have an impact on mortality (in the positive trials), yet there was no discernible relationship between levels of hypercapnia and survival. Also, there was no controlled approach to the administration of buffers. Finally, one of the reports suggested (without convincing evidence) that the permissive hypercapnia might have increased the incidence of renal failure.[118]

The database of the largest of these studies[9] has been analyzed subsequently to determine whether, in addition to the effect of V_T, there might be an independent effect of hypercapnic acidosis.[121] Mortality was examined as a function of permissive hypercapnia on the day of enrollment using multivariate analysis and controlling for other comorbidities and severity of lung injury. It was found that permissive hypercapnia reduced mortality in patients randomized to the higher V_T but not in those receiving lower V_T.[121] If these data are confirmed, there may be a good case for using hypercapnic acidosis to attenuate ventilator-associated lung injury.

NEONATAL AND PEDIATRIC PRACTICE

Use of permissive hypercapnia in neonatology has been recognized since the study by Wung et al.[13] They described lower than previous mortality and lower incidence of chronic lung disease in neonates suffering from persistent fetal circulation who were treated with low V_T entailing a high Pa_{CO_2}.[13]

NEONATAL RESPIRATORY DISTRESS SYNDROME

Infants with neonatal respiratory distress syndrome have been studied in a randomized, controlled trial.[122] Although not powered to detect differences in survival, duration of mechanical ventilation was shorter in the permissive hypercapnia group, and no obvious adverse effects were seen (Fig. 15-11). Although encouraging, such a small study would not detect a subtle increase in adverse effect. More recently, a prospective multicenter study of extremely premature neonates in Denmark (1994–1995) reported that a ventilator strategy incorporating permissive hypercapnia and early use of nasal continuous positive airway pressure and surfactant reduced the incidence of chronic lung disease significantly.[123]

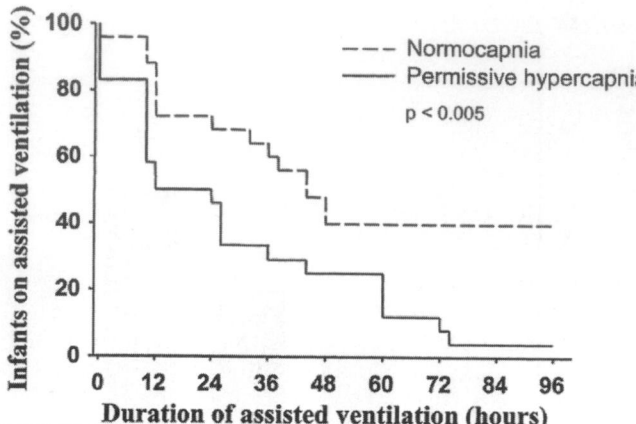

FIGURE 15-11 Duration of mechanical ventilation in neonates with respiratory failure randomized to conventional therapy or permissive hypercapnia. (*Reproduced, with permission, from Mariani et al: Pediatrics 104:1082–8, 1999.*)

CONGENITAL DIAPHRAGMATIC HERNIA

Permissive hypercapnia plays an increasing role in the ventilator management of infants with congenital diaphragmatic hernia.[124] This contrasts sharply with traditional management, which involved aggressive hyperventilation with the aim of producing systemic alkalinization. High levels of barotrauma, poor long-term respiratory outcomes, and poor survival rates, however, have prompted the recognition that the hypoplastic lung is the major pathophysiologic defect. Accordingly, avoidance of barotrauma has assumed increasing importance, and ventilator strategies involving permissive hypercapnia are used increasingly. A retrospective analysis of three treatment protocols in high-risk infants with congenital diaphragmatic hernia reported that permissive hypercapnia was associated with a substantial increase in survival, decreased barotrauma, and decreased morbidity at 6 months. In contrast, the earlier introduction of high-frequency oscillatory ventilation (which readily controls Pa_{CO_2}) had minimal impact. Despite limitations, the increased survival associated with the use of permissive hypercapnia is persuasive.[125]

CONGENITAL HEART DISEASE

Four studies of patients with congenital heart disease are relevant.[126–129] In the context of single-ventricle physiology, pulmonary vascular resistance can be controlled by inducing alveolar hypoxia or alveolar hypercapnia. Two studies documented that the addition of inspired CO_2 increased cerebral oxygenation and mean arterial pressure compared with reducing FI_{O_2} in hypoplastic left-heart syndrome[128] and following cavopulmonary connection.[126] Hypoventilation also improves systemic oxygenation after bidirectional superior cavopulmonary connection, potentially via a hypercarbia-induced decrease in cerebral vascular resistance, thus increasing cerebral, superior vena caval, and pulmonary blood flow.[127] Finally, a detailed recent study demonstrated that without altering V_T or mean airway pressure, the addition of CO_2 to inspired gas resulted in improved cerebral blood flow and systemic oxygenation following cavopulmonary connection.[129]

Complications

The complications of hypercapnia relate primarily to those caused by hypercapnic acidosis per se and those caused by the use of low V_T.

COMPLICATIONS ASSOCIATED WITH HYPERCAPNIC ACIDOSIS

Although many physiologic effects are associated with hypercapnic acidosis, there are few complications. The most notable complications include intracranial and pulmonary hypertension. Complications are of most concern in patients with specific risk factors, especially where acidosis is acute, severe, or not buffered.

COMPLICATIONS ASSOCIATED WITH LOW TIDAL VOLUMES

Reduced V_T may lead to increased intrapulmonary shunt, reducing Pa_{O_2}.[43] This is generally not a difficult problem and can be countered by a recruitment maneuver, elevation of PEEP or mean airway pressure, prone positioning, or other strategies. A more serious issue is whether small V_T values increase mortality. This has been the source of significant controversy. It was a major issue in the meta-analysis by Eichacker et al.[130] They suggested that not only were very high V_T values dangerous, but so too were very small V_T values. This was the basis of the U-shaped curve that depicts a relationship between V_T and mortality. The investigators suggested that the ARDS Network 6 ml/kg V_T protocol was potentially dangerous, should not be used, and should not be considered the standard of care.[130] Considerable controversy ensued. Another group published an abbreviated meta-analysis pooling the results of important clinical trials.[131] They countered the analysis of Eichacker et al and concluded that there was no statistical basis for the assertion that low V_T values are harmful.

Limitations and Contraindications

LIMITATIONS

A substantial body of literature emphasizes the potential for full recovery following exposure to extreme levels of hypercapnia, termed *supercarbia*, in both adults and children. Several children exposed to extremes of Pa_{CO_2} (155–269 mmHg)[132] and one patient with asthma with a Pa_{CO_2} of 293 mmHg (pH 6.77)[26] have been described, with excellent recovery and no long-term sequelae. In adults, in the early 1950s, the accidental development of severe respiratory acidosis was not uncommon in patients undergoing certain surgical procedures; Pa_{CO_2} as high as 200 mmHg was reported during thoracotomy without apparent adverse effects.[133] More recently, reports exist of survival without sequelae following exposure to Pa_{CO_2} values of up to 375 mmHg (pH 6.6).[134,135] Indeed, a case report indicates complete recovery following a pH of 6.46 secondary to ethylene glycol poisoning.[136] These numbers, impressive though

they are, do not suggest that all patients—certainly not those who are already critically ill—would survive such exposure without incident or even survive at all. Nonetheless, they do indicate that severe hypercapnic acidosis per se is not invariably harmful.

CONTRAINDICATIONS

As with almost any situation, there are few absolute contraindications and many relative contraindications. Some authorities suggest that intracranial hypertension is an absolute contraindication,[137] although this is disputed.[80] In any case, the risks and benefits of hypercapnia in the setting of intracranial hypertension must be weighed and monitored carefully. Additional contraindications include pulmonary hypertension, significant hypovolaemia, or uncontrolled severe metabolic acidosis.[137]

Adjunctive Therapies

BUFFERING HYPERCAPNIC ACIDOSIS

Buffering of the acidosis induced by hypercapnia in patients with ARDS remains a common, albeit controversial, clinical practice.[138,139] The effects of buffering hypercapnic acidosis need to be considered because both hypercapnia and acidosis per se may exert distinct biologic effects. As discussed earlier, there is evidence that the protective effects of hypercapnic acidosis in ARDS are a function of the acidosis rather than the elevated CO_2 per se.[51,100]

SODIUM BICARBONATE

Buffering with sodium bicarbonate was permitted in the ARDS Network study.[9] Concerns with the use of bicarbonate, however, have caused its removal from routine use in cardiac arrest algorithms.[140,141] Effectiveness of bicarbonate as a buffer depends on the ability to excrete CO_2, rendering it less effective in buffering hypercapnic acidosis. In fact, bicarbonate may further raise Pa_{CO_2} where alveolar ventilation is limited, as in ARDS.[142] Bicarbonate may correct arterial pH but worsen intracellular acidosis[143] because the CO_2 produced when bicarbonate reacts with metabolic acids diffuses readily across cell membranes, whereas bicarbonate cannot.[144]

In metabolic acidosis, the situation is also complex. Bicarbonate infusion can augment the production of lactic acid.[145–151] In ketoacidosis it can slow the clearance of ketoacids.[152] Of greater concern, bicarbonate administration is associated with a fourfold increase in risk of cerebral edema in children with diabetic ketoacidosis.[153] When compared with an equimolar dose of sodium chloride, bicarbonate administration does not improve the hemodynamic status of critically ill patients who have lactic acidosis.[154]

TROMETHAMINE

There may be a role for the amino alcohol tromethamine [tris-hydroxymethyl aminomethane (THAM)] in hypercapnic acidosis. THAM penetrates cells easily and can buffer pH changes and simultaneously reduce P_{CO_2}.[155] Unlike

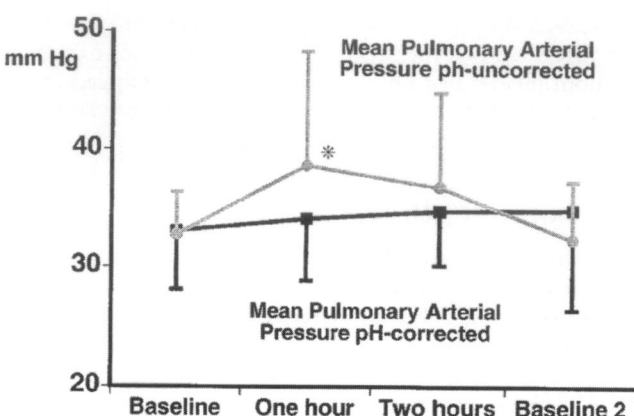

FIGURE 15-12 Pulmonary artery pressure is elevated by rapid institution (over 2 hours) of permissive hypercapnia (*gray line*) in patients with ARDS. Institution of a comparable degree of permissive hypercapnia buffered with tromethamine (THAM, *black line*) attenuated the effects. (*Reproduced, with permission, from Weber et al: Am J Respir Crit Care Med 162:1361–5, 2000.*)

bicarbonate, which requires an open system for CO_2 elimination in order to exert its buffering effect, THAM is effective in a closed or semiclosed system.[155] THAM rapidly restores pH and acid-base regulation in acidemia caused by CO_2 retention.[155] In a small but carefully performed clinical study of 12 patients with ARDS, rapid induction of a hypercapnic acidosis resulted in decreased systemic vascular resistance, increased cardiac output, decreased myocardial contractility, decreased mean arterial pressure, and increased mean pulmonary arterial pressure.[94] Buffering of the hypercapnic acidosis with THAM rapidly attenuated but did not fully reverse these changes[94] (Fig. 15-12). Thus it could be argued that although permissive hypercapnia generally is well tolerated in patients with ARDS, buffering with THAM[94] might be a useful cotherapy where hemodynamic instability supervenes.

CARBICARB

Carbicarb is an equimolar mixture of sodium carbonate and sodium bicarbonate (Na_2CO_3 0.33 M, $NaHCO_3$ 0.33 M) and may have advantages over the latter. Carbicarb has been studied in mixed respiratory and metabolic acidosis and has proved effective in raising arterial pH and preventing lactate elevation.[142] Carbicarb corrects the systemic and intracellular acidosis seen with hypercapnia[156] without elevating Pa_{CO_2}. This contrasts with sodium bicarbonate.[143] Carbicarb, however, did not appear to possess any advantages in terms of restoration of hemodynamic stability over iso-osmolar amounts of hypertonic saline or sodium bicarbonate in a canine shock model.[147] The similar responses may relate to their identical sodium content, with no additional benefit attributable to correction of pH.[147]

In summary, although common clinical practice, no outcome data (e.g., survival or duration of hospital stay) support buffering of a hypercapnic acidosis. In the absence of correcting the primary problem, buffering a hypercapnic acidosis with bicarbonate is not likely to be of benefit. If the clinician elects to buffer a hypercapnic acidosis, the ratio-

nale should be clear (e.g., to ameliorate potentially deleterious hemodynamic consequences) and the responses measured. THAM and Carbicarb may have a role in these clinical situations.

AUGMENTING CO_2 CLEARANCE

DEAD-SPACE GAS REPLACEMENT

At the end of expiration, the ventilator circuit distal to the Y piece and the anatomic dead space both contain alveolar gas. This CO_2-rich gas then constitutes the first part of the next breath delivered to the distal lung. The contribution of this dead-space gas to ventilation increases with decreased V_T, given that dead space is relatively fixed. Techniques that aim to replace dead-space gas with fresh gas have been advocated as an adjunct to protective ventilator strategies. These techniques may increase effective alveolar ventilation and facilitate further reductions in V_T, minimizing transpulmonary pressures.

Tracheal gas insufflation (TGI) delivers fresh gas into the central airways either continuously or in a phasic fashion during expiration (see Chapter 24). Experimental studies in animal models of ARDS and in lung models highlight the potential role of TGI in clinical practice.[157] In a recent experimental study, Zhu et al[108] reported that TGI, either alone or in combination with partial liquid ventilation, attenuated the development of lung injury resulting from mechanical ventilation of surfactant-depleted lungs. Despite extensive investigation, however, concerns persist with regard to the safety and monitoring of TGI that have impeded its introduction into clinical practice.[158]

Aspiration of dead-space gas (ASPIDS) during expiration and controlled replacement with fresh gas are a related technique designed to minimize dead space. A feasibility study of eight patients with COPD who were managed with permissive hypercapnia demonstrated that ASPIDS resulted in a similar decrease in Pa_{CO_2} but with less intrinsic PEEP compared to TGI.[159]

Coaxial double-lumen endotracheal tubes, which eliminate the contribution to dead space from the ventilator circuit distal to the Y piece, may improve the efficiency of ventilation. No adverse hemodynamic effects or auto-PEEP has been detected with use of the coaxial tube.[160] Reduction in Pa_{CO_2} is inversely proportional to V_T. Initial safety and efficacy evaluations of this promising adjunct in patients with ARDS are required.

ADDITIONAL TECHNIQUES

High-frequency oscillatory ventilation and extracorporeal CO_2 removal ($ECCO_2R$) are discussed in Chapters 20 and 22, respectively.

Adjustments at the Bedside

Adjustments at the bedside are specific to the patient and the clinical context. The following principles may guide therapy, although in the end the physician must individualize the risks and benefits for each patient.

First, in a patient who is being mechanically ventilated, confirm correct placement of the endotracheal tube and the ventilation of both lungs. Consider and, where possible, correct reversible conditions that might have an impact on oxygenation or CO_2 removal (e.g., pleural effusion, atelectasis, and/or pneumothorax). Next, decide whether the patient is comfortable and whether there is patient-ventilator dyssynchrony. Then note the ventilator settings (i.e., plateau pressure, V_T, and rate) and the arterial blood-gas values, and consider whether these are appropriate. Concurrent with these considerations, evaluate the patient for causes of high Pa_{CO_2}, and reduce or eliminate any that are present. Such conditions include increased production of CO_2 (e.g., fever, sepsis, shivering, or more rarely, thyroid storm, malignant hyperthermia, or neuroleptic malignant syndrome) or decreased CO_2 elimination (e.g., increased V_D/V_T).

The next step involves arbitrary decisions made by the clinician at the bedside on the target tidal distension (V_T, or plateau pressure). It is important to recognize that optimal values are unknown, which is not to say that the values are unimportant. They are definitely important. Across populations, adverse effects are associated with very high V_T.[9,10] We do not advise on the ideal V_T or plateau pressure, recognizing that these issues are both difficult and controversial. After clinicians select an appropriate V_T for a given patient, they next decide on the "maximal" allowable Pa_{CO_2} and the degree of acidosis that they believe the patient can tolerate. This is empirical. Although some authors suggest arbitrary limits, in the end the decision is based on patient comfort, presence of contraindications, and clinician "comfort." When considering ventilator settings, consider the relative values of V_T, plateau pressure, and rate, and estimate the relative contributions of changes in each. For example, if the rate is inappropriately low, then increasing it will allow further reduction in V_T with less elevation in Pa_{CO_2}. Conversely, increasing the rate may induce a degree of hyperinflation (auto-PEEP),[161] which, although potentially protective, can complicate ventilator management and could induce elevation of the Pa_{CO_2}.

Finally, having decided on the desired ventilator settings and the permissible limits of toleration, decide on the trade-offs involved and the time scale. One trades the benefits of the approach—reduction of ventilator-associated lung injury—against the cost—conditions caused or exacerbated by permissive hypercapnia. Such tradeoffs are inherent in the practice of medicine[162] but are addressed seldom by clinical trials. Finally, the clinician decides on the rate of introducing permissive hypercapnia. In some situations, there is little choice. For example, in acute severe asthma, permissive hypercapnia is initiated immediately; otherwise, the patient is subjected to incredibly high airway pressures. Having decided on the target V_T or plateau pressure, increase the rate and decrease the V_T slowly. There is no formula. Extremes of V_T or plateau pressure should be reduced immediately, and less extreme elevations should be reduced more gradually. For example, in ARDS, a V_T of 15 ml/kg could be reduced immediately to 10 ml/kg and further reduced over several hours with a concomitant increase in rate.

Troubleshooting

To address problems that develop, it is key to understand the pathophysiology. This amounts to management of dyspnea, intracranial hypertension, pulmonary hypertension, and sometimes, hypoxemia. Troubleshooting follows logically the principles used in initiating permissive hypercapnia. In reality, it represents a work in progress, wherein the clinician considers risks versus benefits (real and potential) for each patient at the bedside.

TIDAL VOLUME AND RESPIRATORY RATE

The first issue is to determine whether the V_T (or perhaps plateau pressure) is actually in the range desired by the clinician. If V_T is far lower than desired, increasing it will alleviate "unnecessary" hypercapnic acidosis. If the respiratory rate is too low, increasing it also will lower the Pa_{CO_2}.

RATE OF CHANGE

Was the permissive hypercapnia introduced too quickly? Overly rapid introduction of hypercapnia results in a greater degree of acidosis because the physiologic buffering systems are unable to cope. All unfavorable effects of hypercapnic acidosis (e.g., dyspnea and intracranial hypertension) are far more pronounced where acidosis is greater. More gradual introduction of permissive hypercapnia may prevent these problems.

ADJUVANT THERAPIES: CONTROL OF METABOLIC ACIDOSIS

Buffering sometimes can be appropriate for modifying the adverse effects of significant acidosis. The clinician needs to identify conditions other than ventilator settings and Pa_{CO_2} per se that have an impact on acid-base status. Hyperchloremic acidosis may have developed consequent to high volumes of intravenous saline, total parental nutrition, or renal tubular acidosis and can be buffered easily or possibly prevented. Renal impairment, which slows the generation of endogenous bicarbonate or excretion of hydrogen ion—or generates endogenous organic acids—can be alleviated by renal replacement therapy.

ADJUVANT THERAPIES: ALTERNATIVE ELIMINATION OF CO_2

Adjuvant therapies can be directed at the elevated Pa_{CO_2}. Examples include high-frequency oscillation, transtracheal gas insufflation, and extracorporeal techniques.

SPECIFIC EVALUATION OF THE COMPLICATION

In some circumstances, clinicians suspect a problem, such as pulmonary or intracranial hypertension, that leads them to completely avoid permissive hypercapnia. Such an approach may not be appropriate in the absence of clear proof of the feared condition because the patient may be at a far greater risk of ventilator-associated lung injury than of the feared condition or potential complication. In such a setting, the clinician should consider appropriate monitoring. For example, insertion of an intracranial pressure monitor or jugular oximetry catheter may provide evidence that allows the clinician to gradually introduce, titrate, or clearly avoid hypercapnia in a patient with head injury. Such an approach has been described when managing children suffering from meningococcal septicemia complicated by elevated intracranial pressure and severe acute lung injury[80] (see Fig. 15-7). Concerns about pulmonary hypertension can be addressed by measuring, and monitoring the degree of pulmonary hypertension or its sequelae (e.g., right-ventricular failure, tricuspid regurgitation, or right-to-left shunting). In this case, transthoracic echocardiography or pulmonary artery catheterization may be indicated.

SPECIFIC TREATMENT OF THE COMPLICATION

Direct testing for a feared complication may enable early detection. It also permits the direct "independent" treatment if permissive hypercapnia is still deemed necessary. Specific treatment might include inhaled nitric oxide for pulmonary hypertension[63] or sedation, osmotherapy, or hypothermia for intracranial hypertension. Of course, the most common complaint, dyspnea, can be treated directly with sedatives and opioids[163]; neuromuscular blockade, while paralyzing respiratory muscle contraction, of course, does not alter the perception of dyspnea.

Important Unknowns

While much is known about hypercapnia, much remains unknown. The principles underlying the approach to permissive hypercapnia have been established.[23,29,31,137,164–166] Such principles are inherently limited by the state of our knowledge. The unknowns relating to permissive hypercapnia can be grouped as follows.

HYPERCAPNIA VERSUS ACIDOSIS

Most of the acute physiologic effects of hypercapnic acidosis can be attributed to the effects of pH. CO_2 itself, however, has significant biochemical effects, especially on tissue nitration. In the context of endogenous or exogenous buffering, the effects of elevated CO_2 are not understood.

THERAPEUTIC HYPERCAPNIA

The role of the deliberate elevation of CO_2, as opposed to passive elevation of CO_2 resulting from reduced V_T, is experimentally exciting but essentially conjectural.[23] The state of knowledge is insufficient to justify a clinical study with mortality as an outcome.[62]

MECHANISMS OF BENEFIT (OR HARM)

Although evolving studies are providing better understanding of the mechanisms of benefit and harm associated with hypercapnia and acidosis, clinical definitions of lung injury do not take into account the biologic processes that cause the injury. While some mechanisms are understood, it is not possible for the clinician to extrapolate from mechanisms discovered in the laboratory to the care of a patient with lung injury.

MONITORING DURING HYPERCAPNIA

There are no specific monitors for patients being ventilated with permissive hypercapnia. Regular arterial blood-gas analysis is a requirement, and clinicians will monitor parameters that lead them to detect or prevent complications such as intracranial hypertension.

The Future

Future advances in the early diagnosis of acute respiratory failure and the development of specific therapies may reduce the need for ventilator strategies involving permissive hypercapnia. In the interim, ventilator strategies involving hypercapnia appear likely to play a central role in the management of these disease states. This highlights the need to improve our understanding of the biology of hypercapnia, which should lead us to a better understanding of the advantages, disadvantages, and contraindications pertaining to its use in the clinical context. If the requirement for ventilator strategies that are adverse lessens, the requirement for permissive hypercapnia will lessen, and concerns related to its use will become less relevant. Nonetheless, a fuller profile of biochemical and physiologic responses to elevated CO_2 is needed for the clinician to decide whether hypercapnia is particularly dangerous—or likely beneficial—in the management of a specific patient.

Summary and Conclusions

Permissive hypercapnia simply means reducing V_T in order to lessen the likelihood of ventilator-associated lung injury; in so doing, the clinician accepts the inevitable development of higher Pa_{CO_2}. Elevated P_{CO_2} is associated with a long list of physiologic alterations. Some of these effects are harmful, others may be neutral, and some may turn out to be beneficial. In any case, there is ample evidence that high tidal volumes harm patients. In avoiding such high tidal volumes, the clinician must decide for each patient what is the appropriate tradeoff between the benefits of avoiding high V_Ts and the cost (and benefits) of the associated hypercapnia.

References

1. Jorgensen EO, Holm S. The course of circulatory and cerebral recovery after circulatory arrest: Influence of pre-arrest, arrest and post-arrest factors. Resuscitation 1999; 42:173–82.
2. Suljaga-Pechtel K, Goldberg E, Strickon P, et al. Cardiopulmonary resuscitation in a hospitalized population: Prospective study of factors associated with outcome. Resuscitation 1984; 12:77–95.
3. Balakrishnan I, Crook P, Morris R, et al. Early predictors of mortality in pneumococcal bacteraemia. J Infect 2000; 40:256–61.

4. Mathur NB, Singh A, Sharma VK, et al. Evaluation of risk factors for fatal neonatal sepsis. Indian Pediatr 1996; 33:817–22.

5. Friedman G, Berlot G, Kahn RJ, et al. Combined measurements of blood lactate concentrations and gastric intramucosal pH in patients with severe sepsis. Crit Care Med 1995; 23:1184–93.

6. Anyaegbunam A, Fleischer A, Whitty J, et al. Association between umbilical artery cord pH, five-minute Apgar scores and neonatal outcome. Gynecol Obstet Invest 1991; 32:220–3.

7. Dreyfuss D, Saumon G. Ventilator-induced lung injury: Lessons from experimental studies. Am J Respir Crit Care Med 1998; 157:294–323.

8. Pinhu L, Whitehead T, Evans T, et al. Ventilator-associated lung injury. Lancet 2003; 361:332–40.

9. The Acute Respiratory Distress Syndrome Network. Ventilation with lower tidal volumes as compared with traditional tidal volumes for acute lung injury and the acute respiratory distress syndrome. New Engl J Med 2000; 342:1301–8.

10. Amato MB, Barbas CS, Medeiros DM, et al. Effect of a protective-ventilation strategy on mortality in the acute respiratory distress syndrome. New Engl J Med 1998; 338:347–54.

11. Hickling KG, Henderson SJ, Jackson R. Low mortality associated with low volume pressure limited ventilation with permissive hypercapnia in severe adult respiratory distress syndrome. Intensive Care Med 1990; 16:372–7.

12. Hickling KG, Walsh J, Henderson S, et al. Low mortality rate in adult respiratory distress syndrome using low-volume, pressure-limited ventilation with permissive hypercapnia: A prospective study. Crit Care Med 1994; 22:1568–78.

13. Wung JT, James LS, Kilchevsky E, et al. Management of infants with severe respiratory failure and persistence of the fetal circulation, without hyperventilation. Pediatrics 1985; 76:488–94.

14. Ricard JD, Dreyfuss D, Saumon G. Ventilator-induced lung injury. Curr Opin Crit Care 2002; 8:12–20.

15. Slutsky AS, Tremblay LN. Multiple system organ failure: Is mechanical ventilation a contributing factor? Am J Respir Crit Care Med 1998; 157:1721–5.

16. Tremblay LN, Slutsky AS. Ventilator-induced injury: From barotrauma to biotrauma. Proc Assoc Am Phys 1998; 110:482–8.

17. Dreyfuss D, Ricard JD, Saumon G. On the physiologic and clinical relevance of lung-borne cytokines during ventilator-induced lung injury. Am J Respir Crit Care Med 2003; 167:1467–71.

18. Ricard JD, Dreyfuss D. Cytokines during ventilator-induced lung injury: A word of caution. Anesth Analg 2001; 93:251–2.

19. Edmonds JF, Berry E, Wyllie JH. Release of prostaglandins caused by distension of the lungs. Br J Surg 1969; 56:622–3.

20. Tremblay L, Valenza F, Ribeiro SP, et al. Injurious ventilatory strategies increase cytokines and c-fos mRNA expression in an isolated rat lung model. J Clin Invest 1997; 99:944–52.

21. Murphy D, Cregg N, Tremblay L, et al. Adverse ventilator strategy causes pulmonary to systemic translocation of endotoxin. Am J Respir Crit Care Med 2000; 162:27–33.

22. Nahum A, Hoyt J, Schmitz L, et al. Effect of mechanical ventilation strategy on dissemination of intratracheally instilled *Escherichia coli* in dogs. Crit Care Med 1997; 25:1733–43.

23. Laffey JG, Kavanagh BP. Carbon dioxide and the critically ill: Too little of a good thing? (hypothesis paper). Lancet 1999; 354: 1283–6.

24. Han SR, Ho CS, Jin CH, et al. Unexpected intraoperative hypercapnia due to undetected expiratory valve dysfunction: A case report. Acta Anaesthesiol Scand 2003; 41:215–8.

25. McCrimmon DR, Alheid GF. On the opiate trail of respiratory depression. Am J Physiol Regul Integr Comp Physiol 2003; 285:R1274–5.

26. Mazzeo AT, Spada A, Pratico C, et al. Hypercapnia: What is the limit in paediatric patients? A case of near-fatal asthma successfully treated by multipharmacological approach. Paediatr Anaesth 2004; 14:596–603.

27. Slinger P, Blundell PE, Metcalf IR. Management of massive grain aspiration. Anesthesiology 1997; 87:993–5.

28. Duggan M, Kavanagh BP. Atelectasis: A pathogenic perioperative entity. Anesthesiology 2005; 102:838–54.

29. Bidani A, Tzouanakis AE, Cardenas VJ Jr, et al. Permissive hypercapnia in acute respiratory failure. JAMA 1994; 272:957–62.

30. Kregenow DA, Swenson ER. The lung and carbon dioxide: Implications for permissive and therapeutic hypercapnia. Eur Respir J 2002; 20:6–11.

31. Hickling KG. Permissive hypercapnia. Respir Care Clin North Am 2002; 8:155–69, v.

32. Gros G, Forster RE, Lin L. The carbamate reaction of glycylglycine, plasma, and tissue extracts evaluated by a pH stopped flow apparatus. J Biol Chem 1976; 251:4398–407.

33. Clark RW, Volpi M, Berlin RD. Carbamate formation on tubulin: CO_2/bicarbonate buffers protect tubulin from inactivation by reductive methylation and carbamoylation and promote microtubule assembly at alkaline pH. Biochemistry 1988; 27:1025–33.

34. Max B. This and that: the neurotoxicity of carbon dioxide. Trends Pharmacol Sci 1991; 12:408–11.

35. Lee KJ, Hernandez G, Gordon JB. Hypercapnic acidosis and compensated hypercapnia in control and pulmonary hypertensive piglets. Pediatr Pulmonol 2003; 36:94–101.

36. Prys-Roberts C, Kelman GR, Greenbaum R, et al. Hemodynamics and alveolar-arterial P_{O_2} differences at varying Pa_{CO_2} in anesthetized man. J Appl Physiol 1968; 25:80–7.

37. Domino KB, Swenson ER, Polissar NL, et al. Effect of inspired CO_2 on ventilation and perfusion heterogeneity in hyperventilated dogs. J Appl Physiol 1993; 75:1306–14.

38. Swenson ER, Robertson HT, Hlastala MP. Effects of inspired carbon dioxide on ventilation-perfusion matching in normoxia, hypoxia, and hyperoxia. Am J Respir Crit Care Med 1994; 149: 1563–9.

39. Hare GM, Kavanagh BP, Mazer CD, et al. Hypercapnia increases cerebral tissue oxygen tension in anesthetized rats. Can J Anaesth 2003; 50:1061–8.

40. Keenan RJ, Todd TR, Demajo W, et al. Effects of hypercarbia on arterial and alveolar oxygen tensions in a model of gram-negative pneumonia. J Appl Physiol 1990; 68:1820–5.

41. Laffey JG, Jankov RP, Engelberts D, et al. Effects of therapeutic hypercapnia on mesenteric ischemia-reperfusion injury. Am J Respir Crit Care Med 2003; 168:1383–90.

42. Brogan TV, Robertson HT, Lamm WJ, et al. Carbon dioxide added late in inspiration reduces ventilation-perfusion heterogeneity without causing respiratory acidosis. J Appl Physiol 2004; 96:1894–8.

43. Feihl F, Eckert P, Brimioulle S, et al. Permissive hypercapnia impairs pulmonary gas exchange in the acute respiratory distress syndrome. Am J Respir Crit Care Med 2000; 162:209–15.

44. Rodarte JR, Hyatt RE. Effect of acute exposure to CO_2 on lung mechanics in normal man. Respir Physiol 1973; 17:135–45.

45. van den Elshout FJ, van Herwaarden CL, Folgering HT. Effects of hypercapnia and hypocapnia on respiratory resistance in normal and asthmatic subjects. Thorax 1991; 46:28–32.

46. Butler J, Caro CG, Alcala R, et al. Physiological factors affecting airway resistance in normal subjects and in patients with obstructive respiratory disease. J Clin Invest 1960; 39:584–91.

47. Wildeboer-Venema F. The influences of temperature and humidity upon the isolated surfactant film of the dog. Respir Physiol 1980; 39:63–71.

48. Swenson EW, Finley TN, Guzman SV. Unilateral hypoventilation in man during temporary occlusion of one pulmonary artery. J Clin Invest 1961; 40:828–35.

49. Swenson ER, Graham MM, Hlastala MP. Acetazolamide slows $\dot{V}_A/Q$ matching after changes in regional blood flow. J Appl Physiol 1995; 78:1312–8.

50. Shibata K, Cregg N, Engelberts D, et al. Hypercapnic acidosis may attenuate acute lung injury by inhibition of endogenous xanthine oxidase. Am J Resp Crit Care Med 1998; 158:1578–84.

51. Laffey JG, Engelberts D, Kavanagh BP. Buffering hypercapnic acidosis worsens acute lung injury. Am J Resp Crit Care Med 2000; 161:141–6.

52. Laffey JG, Tanaka M, Engelberts D, et al. Therapeutic hypercapnia reduces pulmonary and systemic injury following in vivo lung reperfusion. Am J Resp Crit Care Med 2000; 162:2287–94.

53. Broccard AF, Hotchkiss JR, Vannay C, et al. Protective effects of hypercapnic acidosis on ventilator-induced lung injury. Am J Respir Crit Care Med 2001; 164:802–6.

54. Sinclair SE, Kregenow DA, Lamm WJ, et al. Hypercapnic acidosis is protective in an in vivo model of ventilator-induced lung injury. Am J Respir Crit Care Med 2002; 166:403–8.

55. Strand M, Ikegami M, Jobe AH. Effects of high P_{CO_2} on ventilated preterm lamb lungs. Pediatr Res 2003; 53:468–72.

56. Rai S, Laffey JG, Engelberts D, et al. Therapeutic hypercapnia is not protective in the in vivo surfactant-depleted rabbit lung. Pediatr Res 2003; 55:42–9.

57. Brimioulle S, Vachiery JL, Lejeune P, et al. Acid-base status affects gas exchange in canine oleic acid pulmonary edema. Am J Physiol 1991; 260:H1080–6.

58. Swenson ER. Therapeutic hypercapnic acidosis: Pushing the envelope. Am J Respir Crit Care Med 2004; 169:8–9.

59. Beutler B. Innate immune responses to microbial poisons: Discovery and function of the Toll-like receptors. Annu Rev Pharmacol Toxicol 2003; 43:609–28.

60. Laffey JG, Honan D, Hopkins N, et al. Hypercapnic acidosis attenuates endotoxin-induced acute lung injury. Am J Respir Crit Care Med 2004; 169:46–56.

61. Lang JD, Figueroa M, Sanders KD, et al. Hypercapnia via reduced rate and tidal volume contributes to lipopolysaccharide-induced lung injury. Am J Respir Crit Care Med 2005; 171: 147–57.

62. Kavanagh BP. Therapeutic hypercapnia: Careful science, better trials. Am J Respir Crit Care Med 2005; 171:96–7.

63. Puybasset L, Stewart T, Rouby JJ, et al. Inhaled nitric oxide reverses the increase in pulmonary vascular resistance induced by permissive hypercapnia in patients with acute respiratory distress syndrome. Anesthesiology 1994; 80:1254–67.

64. Hotchkiss JR Jr, Blanch L, Murias G, et al. Effects of decreased respiratory frequency on ventilator-induced lung injury. Am J Respir Crit Care Med 2000; 161:463–8.

65. Thorens JB, Jolliet P, Ritz M, et al. Effects of rapid permissive hypercapnia on hemodynamics, gas exchange, and oxygen transport and consumption during mechanical ventilation for the acute respiratory distress syndrome. Intensive Care Med 1996; 22:182–91.

66. Joyce CJ, Hickling KG. Permissive hypercapnia and gas exchange in lungs with high $\dot{Q}_S/\dot{Q}_T$: A mathematical model. Br J Anaesth 1996; 77:678–83.

67. Marcy TW, Marini JJ. Inverse ratio ventilation in ARDS: Rationale and implementation. Chest 1991; 100:494–504.

68. Pfeiffer B, Hachenberg T, Wendt M, et al. Mechanical ventilation with permissive hypercapnia increases intrapulmonary shunt in septic and nonseptic patients with acute respiratory distress syndrome. Crit Care Med 2002; 30:285–9.

69. Nakahata K, Kinoshita H, Hirano Y, et al. Mild hypercapnia induces vasodilation via adenosine triphosphate-sensitive K^+ channels in parenchymal microvessels of the rat cerebral cortex. Anesthesiology 2003; 99:1333–9.

70. Lindauer U, Vogt J, Schuh-Hofer S, et al. Cerebrovascular vasodilation to extraluminal acidosis occurs via combined activation of ATP-sensitive and Ca^{2+}-activated potassium channels. J Cereb Blood Flow Metab 2003; 23:1227–38.

71. Sato E, Sakamoto T, Nagaoka T, et al. Role of nitric oxide in regulation of retinal blood flow during hypercapnia in cats. Invest Ophthalmol Vis Sci 2003; 44:4947–53.

72. Crosby A, Talbot NP, Balanos GM, et al. Respiratory effects in humans of a 5-day elevation of end-tidal P_{CO_2} by 8 torr. J Appl Physiol 2003; 95:1947–54.

73. Shiota S, Okada T, Naitoh H, et al. Hypoxia and hypercapnia affect contractile and histological properties of rat diaphragm and hind limb muscles. Pathophysiology 2004; 11: 23–30.

74. Beekley MD, Cullom DL, Brechue WF. Hypercapnic impairment of neuromuscular function is related to afferent depression. Eur J Appl Physiol 2004; 91:105–10.

75. Vannucci RC, Brucklacher RM, Vannucci SJ. Effect of carbon dioxide on cerebral metabolism during hypoxia-ischemia in the immature rat. Pediatr Res 1997; 42:24–9.

76. Vannucci RC, Towfighi J, Heitjan DF, et al. Carbon dioxide protects the perinatal brain from hypoxic-ischemic damage: An experimental study in the immature rat. Pediatrics 1995; 95:868–74.

77. Barth A, Bauer R, Gedrange T, et al. Influence of hypoxia and hypoxia/hypercapnia upon brain and blood peroxidative and glutathione status in normal weight and growth-restricted newborn piglets. Exp Toxicol Pathol 1998; 50:402–10.

78. Xu L, Glassford AJ, Giaccia AJ, et al. Acidosis reduces neuronal apoptosis. Neuroreport 1998; 9:875–9.

79. West JB. Respiratory failure. In: Respiratory pathophysiology: The Essentials. Baltimore: Williams & Wilkins 2003: 145–58.

80. Tasker RC, Peters MJ. Combined lung injury, meningitis and cerebral edema: How permissive can hypercapnia be? Intensive Care Med 1998; 24:616–9.

81. Cullen DJ, Eger EI 2d. Cardiovascular effects of carbon dioxide in man. Anesthesiology 1974; 41:345–9.

82. Hickling KG, Joyce C. Permissive hypercapnia in ARDS and its effects on tissue oxygenation (review). Acta Anaesthesiol Scand 1995; 107:201–8.

83. Cardenas VJ, Zwischenberger JB, Tao W, et al. Correction of blood pH attenuates changes in hemodynamics and organ blood flow during permissive hypercapnia. Crit Care Med 1996; 24:827–34.

84. Tobarti D, Mangino MJ, Garcia E, et al. Acute hypercapnia increases the oxygen-carrying capacity of the blood in ventilated dogs. Crit Care Med 1998; 26:1863–7.

85. Hillered L, Ernster L, Siesjo BK. Influence of in vitro lactic acidosis and hypercapnia on respiratory activity of isolated rat brain mitochondria. J Cereb Blood Flow Metab 1984; 4:430–7.

86. Hood VL, Tannen RL. Protection of acid-base balance by pH regulation of acid production (review). New Engl J Med 1998; 339:819–26.

87. Ratnaraj J, Kabon B, Talcott MR, et al. Supplemental oxygen and carbon dioxide each increase subcutaneous and intestinal intramural oxygenation. Anesth Analg 2004; 99:207–11.

88. Nomura F, Aoki M, Forbess JM, et al. Effects of hypercarbic acidotic reperfusion on recovery of myocardial function after cardioplegic ischemia in neonatal lambs. Circulation 1994; 90: 321–7.

89. Kitakaze M, Weisfeldt ML, Marban E. Acidosis during early reperfusion prevents myocardial stunning in perfused ferret hearts. J Clin Invest 1988; 82:920–7.

90. Kitakaze M, Takashima S, Funaya H, et al. Temporary acidosis during reperfusion limits myocardial infarct size in dogs. Am J Physiol 1997; 272:H2071–8.

91. Preckel B, Schlack W, Obal D, et al. Effect of acidotic blood reperfusion on reperfusion injury after coronary artery occlusion in the dog heart. J Cardiovasc Pharmacol 1998; 31:179–86.

92. Prys-Roberts C, Kelman GR, Greenbaum R, et al. Circulatory influences of artificial ventilation during nitrous oxide anaesthesia in man: II. Results: The relative influence of mean intrathoracic pressure and arterial carbon dioxide tension. Br J Anaesth 1967; 39:533–48.

93. Ebata T, Watanabe Y, Amaha K, et al. Haemodynamic changes during the apnoea test for diagnosis of brain death. Can J Anaesth 1991; 38:436–40.

94. Weber T, Tschernich H, Sitzwohl C, et al. Tromethamine buffer modifies the depressant effect of permissive hypercapnia on myocardial contractility in patients with acute respiratory distress syndrome. Am J Respir Crit Care Med 2000; 162:1361–5.

95. McIntyre RC Jr, Haenel JB, Moore FA, et al. Cardiopulmonary effects of permissive hypercapnia in the management of adult respiratory distress syndrome. J Trauma 1994; 37:433–8.

96. Bonventre JV, Cheung JY. Effects of metabolic acidosis on viability of cells exposed to anoxia. Am J Physiol 1985; 249:C149–59.

97. Gores GJ, Nieminen AL, Wray BE, et al. Intracellular pH during "chemical hypoxia" in cultured rat hepatocytes: protection by intracellular acidosis against the onset of early cell death. J Clin Invest 1989; 83:386–96.

98. DiBona GF, Kopp UC. Neural control of renal function. Physiol Rev 1997; 77:75–197.

99. Kiefer P, Nunes S, Kosonen P, et al. Effect of an acute increase in P_{CO_2} on splanchnic perfusion and metabolism. Intensive Care Med 2001; 27:775–8.

100. Lang JD Jr, Chumley P, Eiserich JP, et al. Hypercapnia induces injury to alveolar epithelial cells via a nitric oxide–dependent pathway. Am J Physiol Lung Cell Mol Physiol 2000; 279:L994–1002.

101. West MA, Baker J, Bellingham J. Kinetics of decreased LPS-stimulated cytokine release by macrophages exposed to CO_2. J Surg Res 1996; 63:269–74.

102. Coakley RJ, Taggart C, Greene C, et al. Ambient pCO_2 modulates intracellular pH, intracellular oxidant generation, and interleukin-8 secretion in human neutrophils. J Leuk Biol 2002; 71:603–10.

103. Trevani AS, Andonegui G, Giordano M, et al. Extracellular acidification induces human neutrophil activation. J Immunol 1999; 162:4849–57.

104. Hackam DJ, Grinstein S, Nathens A, et al. Exudative neutrophils show impaired pH regulation compared with circulating neutrophils. Arch Surg 1996; 131:1296–301.

105. Demaurex N, Downey GP, Waddell TK, et al. Intracellular pH regulation during spreading of human neutrophils. J Cell Biol 1996; 133:1391–402.

106. Leblebicioglu B, Lim JS, Cario AC, et al. pH changes observed in the inflamed gingival crevice modulate human polymorphonuclear leukocyte activation in vitro. J Periodontol 1996; 67:472–7.

107. Squadrito GL, Pryor WA. Oxidative chemistry of nitric oxide: The roles of superoxide, peroxynitrite, and carbon dioxide. Free Rad Biol Med 1998; 25:392–403.

108. Zhu G, Shaffer TH, Wolfson MR. Continuous tracheal gas insufflation during partial liquid ventilation in juvenile rabbits with acute lung injury. J Appl Physiol 2004; 96:1415–24.

109. Rounds S, Piggott D, Dawicki DD, et al. Effect of hypercarbia on surface proteins of cultured bovine endothelial cells. Am J Physiol 1997; 273:L1141–6.

110. Curthoys NP, Gstraunthaler G. Mechanism of increased renal gene expression during metabolic acidosis. Am J Physiol Renal Physiol 2001; 281:F381–90.

111. Bassler EL, Ngo-Anh TJ, Geisler HS, et al. Molecular and functional characterization of acid-sensing ion channel (ASIC) 1b. J Biol Chem 2001; 276:33782–7.

112. Yiangou Y, Facer P, Smith JA, et al. Increased acid-sensing ion channel ASIC-3 in inflamed human intestine. Eur J Gastroenterol Hepatol 2001; 13:891–6.

113. Tak PP, Gerlag DM, Aupperle KR, et al. Inhibitor of nuclear factor $\kappa\beta$ kinase β is a key regulator of synovial inflammation. Arthritis Rheum 2001; 44:1897–907.

114. Takeshita K, Suzuki Y, Nishio K, et al. Hypercapnic acidosis attenuates endotoxin-induced nuclear factor-$\kappa\beta$ activation. Am J Respir Cell Mol Biol 2003; 29:124–32.

115. Darioli R, Perret C. Mechanical controlled hypoventilation in status asthmaticus. Am Rev Respir Dis 1984; 129:385–7.

116. Tuxen DV, Williams TJ, Scheinkestel CD, et al. Use of a measurement of pulmonary hyperinflation to control the level of mechanical ventilation in patients with acute severe asthma. Am Rev Respir Dis 1992; 146:1136–42.

117. Gupta D, Keogh B, Chung KF, et al. Characteristics and outcome for admissions to adult, general critical care units with acute severe asthma: a secondary analysis of the ICNARC Case Mix Programme Database. Crit Care 2004; 8:R112–21.

118. Stewart TE, Meade MO, Cook DJ, et al. Evaluation of a ventilation strategy to prevent barotrauma in patients at high risk for acute respiratory distress syndrome: Pressure- and volume-limited ventilatory strategy. New Engl J Med 1998; 338:355–61.

119. Brochard L, Roudot-Thoraval F, Roupie E, et al. Tidal volume reduction for prevention of ventilator-induced lung injury in acute respiratory distress syndrome. The Multicenter Trail Group on Tidal Volume reduction in ARDS. Am J Respir Crit Care Med 1998; 158:1831–8.

120. Brower RG, Shanholtz CB, Fessler HE, et al. Prospective, randomized, controlled clinical trial comparing traditional versus reduced tidal volume ventilation in acute respiratory distress syndrome patients. Crit Care Med 1999; 27:1492–8.

121. Kregenow DA, Rubenfeld GD, Hudson LD, Swenson ER. Hypercapnic acidosis and mortality in acute lung injury. Crit Care Med. 2006; 34:1–7.

122. Mariani G, Cifuentes J, Carlo WA. Randomized trial of permissive hypercapnia in preterm infants. Pediatrics 1999; 104:1082–8.

123. Kamper J, Feilberg Jorgensen N, Jonsbo F, et al. The Danish national study in infants with extremely low gestational age and birthweight (the ETFOL study): Respiratory morbidity and outcome. Acta Paediatr 2004; 93:225–32.

124. Bohn D. Congenital diaphragmatic hernia. Am J Respir Crit Care Med 2002; 166:911–5.

125. Bagolan P, Casaccia G, Crescenzi F, et al. Impact of a current treatment protocol on outcome of high-risk congenital diaphragmatic hernia. J Pediatr Surg 2004; 39:313–8; discussion 313–8.

126. Ramamoorthy C, Tabbutt S, Kurth CD, et al. Effects of inspired hypoxic and hypercapnic gas mixtures on cerebral oxygen saturation in neonates with univentricular heart defects. Anesthesiology 2002; 96:283–8.

127. Bradley SM, Simsic JM, Mulvihill DM. Hypoventilation improves oxygenation after bidirectional superior cavopulmonary connection. J Thorac Cardiovasc Surg 2003; 126:1033–9.

128. Tabbutt S, Ramamoorthy C, Montenegro LM, et al. Impact of inspired gas mixtures on preoperative infants with hypoplastic left heart syndrome during controlled ventilation. Circulation 2001; 104:I159–64.

129. Hoskote A, Li J, Hickey C, et al. The effects of carbon dioxide on oxygenation and systemic, cerebral, and pulmonary vascular hemodynamics after the bidirectional superior cavopulmonary anastomosis. J Am Coll Cardiol 2004; 44:1501–9.

130. Eichacker PQ, Gerstenberger EP, Banks SM, et al. Meta-analysis of acute lung injury and acute respiratory distress syndrome trials testing low tidal volumes. Am J Respir Crit Care Med 2002; 166:1510–4.

131. Amato M, Brochard L, Stewart T, et al. Meta-analysis of tidal volume in ARDS. Am J Respir Crit Care Med 2003; 168:612; author reply 612–3.

132. Goldstein B, Shannon DC, Todres ID. Supercarbia in children: Clinical course and outcome. Crit Care Med 1990; 18:166–8.

133. Ellison RG, Ellison LT, Hamilton WF. Analysis of respiratory acidosis during anesthesia. Ann Surg 1955; 141:375–82.

134. Potkin RT, Swenson ER. Resuscitation from severe acute hypercapnia: Determinants of tolerance and survival. Chest 1992; 102:1742–5.

135. Urwin L, Murphy R, Robertson C, et al. A case of extreme hypercapnia: Implications for the prehospital and accident and emergency department management of acutely dyspnoeic patients. Emerg Med J 2004; 21:119–20.

136. Blakeley KR, Rinner SE, Knochel JP. Survival of ethylene glycol poisoning with profound acidemia. New Engl J Med 1993; 328:515–6.

137. Feihl F, Perret C. Permissive hypercapnia: How permissive should we be? Am J Respir Crit Care Med 1994; 150:1722–37.

138. Kollef MH, Schuster DP. The acute respiratory distress syndrome (review). New Engl J Med 1995; 332:27–37.

139. Tobin MJ. Mechanical ventilation (review). New Engl J Med 1994; 330:1056–61.

140. Levy MM. An evidence-based evaluation of the use of sodium bicarbonate during cardiopulmonary resuscitation. Crit Care Clin 1998; 14:457–83.

141. Grillo JA, Gonzalez ER. Changes in the pharmacotherapy of CPR. Heart Lung 1993; 22:548–53.

142. Sun JH, Filley GF, Hord K, et al. Carbicarb: An effective substitute for $NaHCO_3$ for the treatment of acidosis. Surgery 1987; 102:835–9.

143. Shapiro JI, Whalen M, Kucera R, et al. Brain pH responses to sodium bicarbonate and Carbicarb during systemic acidosis. Am J Physiol 1989; 256:H1316–21.

144. Goldsmith DJ, Forni LG, Hilton PJ. Bicarbonate therapy and intracellular acidosis. Clin Sci 1997; 93:593–8.

145. Abu Romeh S, Tannen RL. Amelioration of hypoxia-induced lactic acidosis by superimposed hypercapnea or hydrochloride acid infusion. Am J Physiol 1986; 250:F702–9.

146. Arieff AI, Leach W, Park R, et al. Systemic effects of $NaHCO_3$ in experimental lactic acidosis in dogs. Am J Physiol 1982; 242:F586–91.

147. Benjamin E, Oropello JM, Abalos AM, et al. Effects of acid-base correction on hemodynamics, oxygen dynamics, and resuscitability in severe canine hemorrhagic shock. Crit Care Med 1994; 22:1616–23.

148. Graf H, Leach W, Arieff AI. Evidence for a detrimental effect of bicarbonate therapy in hypoxic lactic acidosis. Science 1985; 227:754–6.

149. Graf H, Leach W, Arieff AI. Metabolic effects of sodium bicarbonate in hypoxic lactic acidosis in dogs. Am J Physiol 1985; 249:F630–5.

150. Fraley DS, Adler S, Bruns FJ, et al. Stimulation of lactate production by administration of bicarbonate in a patient with a solid neoplasm and lactic acidosis. New Engl J Med 1980; 303: 1100–2.

151. Rhee KH, Toro LO, McDonald GG, et al. Carbicarb, sodium bicarbonate, and sodium chloride in hypoxic lactic acidosis: Effect on arterial blood gases, lactate concentrations, hemodynamic variables, and myocardial intracellular pH. Chest 1993; 104: 913–8.

152. Okuda Y, Adrogue HJ, Field JB, et al. Counterproductive effects of sodium bicarbonate in diabetic ketoacidosis. J Clin Endocrinol Metab 1996; 81:314–20.

153. Glaser N, Barnett P, McCaslin I, et al. Risk factors for cerebral edema in children with diabetic ketoacidosis. The Pediatric Emergency Medicine Collaborative Research Committee of the American Academy of Pediatrics. New Engl J Med 2001; 344:264–9.

154. Cooper DJ, Walley KR, Wiggs BR, et al. Bicarbonate does not improve hemodynamics in critically ill patients who have lactic acidosis: A prospective, controlled clinical study. Ann Intern Med 1990; 112:492–8.

155. Nahas GG, Sutin KM, Fermon C, et al. Guidelines for the treatment of acidaemia with THAM. Drugs 1998; 55:191–224.

156. Shapiro JI. Functional and metabolic responses of isolated hearts to acidosis: Effects of sodium bicarbonate and Carbicarb. Am J Physiol 1990; 258:H1835–9.

157. Nahum A. Tracheal gas insufflation as an adjunct to mechanical ventilation. Respir Care Clin North Am 2002; 8:171–85, v–vi.

158. Dyer IR, Esmail M, Findlay G, et al. Effect of catheter design on tracheal pressures during tracheal gas insufflation. Eur J Anaesthesiol 2003; 20:740–4.

159. Liu YN, Zhao WG, Xie LX, et al. Aspiration of dead space in the management of chronic obstructive pulmonary disease patients with respiratory failure. Respir Care 2004; 49:257–62.

160. Lethvall S, Lindgren S, Lundin S, et al. Tracheal double-lumen ventilation attenuates hypercapnia and respiratory acidosis in lung injured pigs. Intensive Care Med 2004; 30:686–92.

161. de Durante G, del Turco M, Rustichini L, et al. ARDSNet lower tidal volume ventilatory strategy may generate intrinsic positive end-expiratory pressure in patients with acute respiratory distress syndrome. Am J Respir Crit Care Med 2002;165: 1271–4.

162. Kavanagh BP. Goals and concerns for oxygenation in acute respiratory distress syndrome. Curr Opinion Crit Care 1998;4: 16–20.

163. Kress JP, Pohlman AS, O'Connor MF, et al. Daily interruption of sedative infusions in critically ill patients undergoing mechanical ventilation. New Engl J Med 2000; 342:1471–7.

164. Chonghaile MN, Higgins B, Laffey JG. Permissive hypercapnia: role in protective lung ventilatory strategies. Curr Opin Crit Care 2005;11:56–62.

165. Laffey JG, Kavanagh BP. Biological effects of hypercapnia (review). Intensive Care Med 2000; 26:133–8.

166. Laffey JG, O'Croinin D, McLoughlin P, et al. Permissive hypercapnia: Role in protective lung ventilatory strategies. Intensive Care Med 2004; 30:347–56.

FEEDBACK ENHANCEMENTS ON VENTILATOR BREATHS

NEIL MACINTYRE
RICHARD D. BRANSON

Conventional Positive-Pressure Breath-Delivery Strategies/Modes

Positive-pressure breaths delivered by mechanical ventilators can be classified by the behavior of three variables: (1) the trigger variable (what initiates the breath), (2) the target or limit variable (what controls gas delivery during the breath), and (3) the cycle variable (what terminates the breath).[1–3] Trigger variables are either patient effort (detected by the ventilator as a pressure or flow change) or a set machine timer. Target or limit variables generally are either a set flow or a set inspiratory pressure. Cycle variables generally are a set volume, a set inspiratory time, or a set flow rate. Pressure is often a backup safety-cycle variable. Figure 16-1 uses this classification scheme to describe the five most common breath types available on the current generation of mechanical ventilators.

Conceptually, flow and pressure strategies incorporate a simple feedback system. With flow targeting (breaths 1 and 2 in Fig. 16-1), the clinician sets an inspiratory flow and generally a cycling volume. Under these conditions, airway pressure becomes the dependent variable that the machine adjusts according to respiratory system mechanics and patient effort to maintain the set target flow and cycling volume. With pressure targeting (breaths 3–5

in Fig. 16-1), the clinician sets an inspiratory pressure target (with either time or flow as the cycling criteria). Under these conditions, flow and volume become dependent variables that the machine adjusts according to respiratory system mechanics and patient effort to maintain the set pressure target.

The putative advantage of a flow-targeted, volume-cycled breath is that a guaranteed volume is delivered (even though applied airway pressures may change). The putative advantages of a pressure-targeted breath (either time- or flow-cycled) are that an airway pressure limit is guaranteed (even though volumes may change), that the rapid initial flow may enhance gas mixing, and that the variable flow pattern may enhance patient-ventilator synchrony.[3] It must be emphasized, however, that clinical outcome studies showing benefit of one breath-targeting strategy over the other do not exist.

The availability and delivery logic of different breath types define the "mode" of mechanical ventilator support.[1–3] The mode controller is an electronic, pneumatic, or microprocessor-based system that is designed to provide the proper combination of breaths according to both set and various feedback algorithms. Newer ventilators now can provide very sophisticated feedback and automatic controllers of both the breath-delivery pattern and the mode behavior. These range from complex breath-rate adjusters to various algorithms designed to better match positive-pressure breath delivery with patient effort and respiratory system mechanics. It is important to note that the engineering data supporting all these developments far exceed the clinical data to support widespread application of any of them. Nevertheless, there is at least some rationale for many of these newer feedback features, and the remainder of this chapter reviews their design and the available data supporting their clinical utility.

Feedback Control of Respiratory Rate

Several generations of positive-pressure ventilators have had simple feedback systems for control of the mandatory breath rate in assist-control ventilation (ACV) or synchronized intermittent mandatory ventilation (SIMV).[4–6] These feedback systems use a single input variable, spontaneous patient effort, to set the controlled breath rate. In ACV, every patient efforts triggers an assisted breath, and the machine provides a backup control rate. In SIMV, patient efforts trigger assisted breaths up to the backup control rate. Patient efforts above this backup control rate trigger either unassisted breaths (pure SIMV) or pressure-support (PS) breaths (SIMV + PS).

Mandatory minute ventilation (MMV) is an extension of these feedback controllers of rate. With MMV, however, the feedback input variable is now total minute ventilation (frequency and tidal volume), and a clinician-set target minute ventilation is required.[7–10] With most MMV systems, the ventilator monitors minute ventilation over a 30-second moving time window. If the set minimum minute

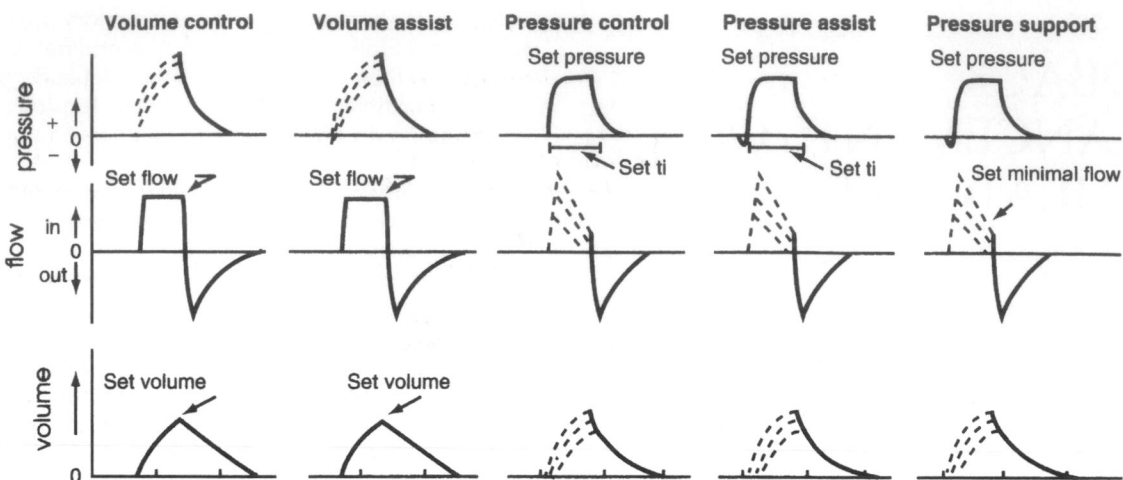

FIGURE 16-1 Airway pressure (*upper panel*), flow (*middle panel*), and volume (*lower panel*) profiles over time of the five "basic breaths" available on most modern mechanical ventilators. Note that patient-initiated breaths have a small deflection in airway pressure preceding the ventilator flow delivery, whereas machine-initiated breaths do not. The solid lines and arrows represent clinician-set parameters; the dashed lines represent the variable ventilator adjustments to respiratory system mechanics and patient effort. (*Reproduced, with permission, from MacIntyre.*[3])

ventilation is being met by either spontaneous or pressure-supported breaths, no further ventilator control breaths are given. If the set target minute ventilation is not being met, clinician-set volume- or pressure-controlled breaths are delivered to provide it. MMV is available as MMV (Drager), augmented minute volume (AMV; Bear/Viasys), and extended mandatory minute ventilation (EMMV). A point of confusion is that *mandatory minimum ventilation* (MMV) is also the term used by one manufacturer to describe its dual-control breath-to-breath algorithm (see below).

Conceptually, the MMV feedback control of rate offers the appeal of a positive-pressure breath-delivery strategy that supplies control breaths only when needed and allows either unassisted breathing or PS to be the predominant form of support. Uncomfortable or excessively large control breaths thus can be minimized. The breath-delivery pattern with this form of MMV, however, depends heavily on how the clinician sets the PS level and the desired minute ventilation, and this can lead to undesired effects. For example, insufficient PS leading to respiratory muscle fatigue may lead to tachypnea but a minute ventilation that remains above the set minimum.[11] Needed additional support thus may not be given. Alternatively, setting the minute ventilation excessively high (i.e., above that desired by the patient's oxygen and carbon dioxide needs) may lead to unnecessary pressure application, intrinsic positive end-expiratory pressure (PEEP), or a reduction in spontaneous drive and virtually complete takeover by the control rate.[11]

A number of observational studies have demonstrated that the MMV feedback control of rate works as designed and can be set to provide an appropriate backup feature to PS.[7–10] Studies showing improvements in clinical outcome from this approach, however, are lacking. Because of this, and because of the concerns noted earlier regarding proper setup, the popularity of MMV has been waning, especially since the introduction of more sophisticated feedback approaches (described below).

Feedback Control of Combination Pressure- and Flow-Targeted Breaths

As noted earlier, the downside to pressure targeting (and either time or flow cycling) is the lack of any control of volume; the downside to flow targeting and volume cycling is the lack of any control of pressure. Over the last two decades, a number of engineering innovations have attempted to produce feedback algorithms that allow some control of volume with pressure targeting and some control of pressure with flow targeting. Collectively, these are often referred to as *hybrid breaths* or *dual-control breaths*.[11–15] On the current generation of mechanical ventilators, there are two basic approaches to providing these types of breaths: dual control within a breath (DCWB; intrabreath control) and dual control from breath to breath (DCBB; interbreath control). The former uses a measured flow input to switch from pressure targeting to flow targeting in the middle of the breath. The latter uses a measured volume input to manipulate the pressure level of subsequent pressure-targeted breaths.

DUAL CONTROL WITHIN A BREATH (DCWB)

The currently available DCWB breath begins with either patient or machine triggering and is followed by a pressure-targeted flow-delivery algorithm. There is thus a high initial flow to rapidly pressurize the airway and then subsequent flow adjustments according to respiratory system mechanics and patient effort to maintain the target pressure. As the lungs fill, flow decelerates until a flow-cycling mechanism terminates the breath. In these respects, this breath type is similar to the PS breath. Unlike PS, however, the clinician also must set a minimum tidal volume, flow, and backup rate with the DCWB breath. These backup settings take over control of the breath should the pressure-targeted flow

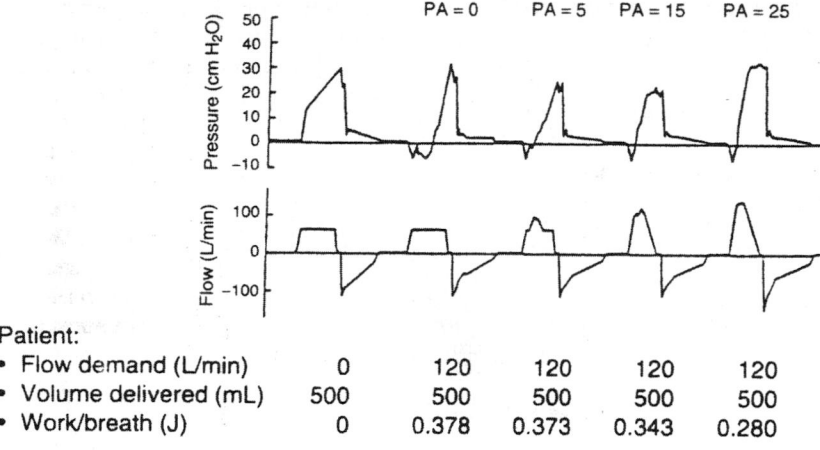

FIGURE 16-2   Airway pressure (*upper panel*) and flow (*lower panel*) profiles over time of the DCWB feature compared to volume assist-control ventilation (VACV). Data are from a lung model with a set guaranteed tidal volume of 500 ml and a set flow of 50 liters/min under all conditions. The simulated flow demand is zero in the first breath and 120 liters/min in the next four breaths. The pressure target is inactive in the first two breaths (i.e., stand-alone volume-cycled ACV). Note that during the simulated patient breath with stand-alone volume-cycled ACV (breath 2), the simulated effort outstrips the delivered flow, and the airway pressure graphic is "sucked down." This is reflected in a simulated patient work of 0.378 J/breath. In breaths 3 through 5, a DCWB pressure target (PA) is set (5, 15, and 25 cmH$_2$O, respectively) that increasingly pressurizes the airway early in the breath and reduces simulated patient work. If the flow associated with the pressure target is inadequate for the set 500-ml tidal volume, the minimum flow activates and guarantees this tidal volume (breaths 3 and 4). If the flow associated with the pressure target is adequate for the 500-ml tidal volume, the breath will terminate on flow like a PS breath (breath 5). (*Reproduced, with permission, from MacIntyre et al: Crit Care Med 22:353–7, 1994.*)

drop below the minimum required to deliver the set tidal volume in the allotted inspiratory time. The breath thus begins like PS and can either flow cycle like PS (if the volume exceeds the set minimum) or volume cycle like a flow-targeted breath (if necessary to deliver the set volume).[11–13] This breath type is depicted in Fig. 16-2 and is available as *volume-assured pressure support* (VAPS; Bird/Viasys), *pressure augmentation* (PA; Bear/Viasys), and *machine volume* (Viasys).

The original description of DCWB used two flow sources in parallel.[23] The first source provided a constant flow set by the clinician (10–120 liters/min) to provide the minimal volume. The second source of flow (up to 200 liters/min) was set to reach a pressure target. When the patient initiated a breath, both flow sources were activated. If the pressure-targeted flow was sufficient to deliver a tidal volume (V$_T$) greater than or equal to the set minimum V$_T$ before the flow-cycling criterion was met, then the breath flow cycled and was essentially only a pressure-supported breath. In contrast, if the pressure-targeted flow was insufficient for the set V$_T$, then the constant flow from the other source continued until the desired V$_T$ was delivered.

The reasoning behind DCWB breaths is that the high initial flow would provide better gas mixing and also reduce flow dyssynchrony during assisted breaths, whereas the volume guarantee ensures a constant V$_T$.[17–22] DCWB breaths thus can be considered to be "more comfortable" flow-targeted, volume-cycled breaths. Alternatively, they could be considered PS with a V$_T$ "safety net."

Both bench studies and small clinical trials have evaluated DCWB breaths. In a lung model study with varying simulated patient effort,[23] DCWB breaths allowed for more effective matching of ventilator output to simulated patient demand than did flow-targeted, volume-cycled

breaths regardless of set flow pattern. In the original clinical trial of DCWB breaths, Amato et al[16] found that DCWB breaths reduced patient work markedly during assisted breaths as compared with flow-targeted, volume-cycled assist-control ventilation (ACV). This was attributed to both better patient-ventilator flow synchrony, as well as to higher inspiratory flows, resulting in a shorter inspiratory time and reduced auto-PEEP with the DCWB breaths. It must be pointed out, however, that the set flows during ACV in this study may have been inappropriately slow.

A subsequent larger study of 17 patients compared DCWB breaths with flow-targeted, volume-cycled ACV, with the set flows adjusted to match patient demand.[24] A significant reduction in the patient's pressure-time product (PTP), a measure of effort, was observed with the DCWB breaths, along with a trend toward lower auto-PEEP. Of note, V$_T$ with DCWB varied considerably above the set minimum. This may be important in that as patient demands vary, the ability to increase V$_T$ may play an important role in controlling the sensation of breathlessness.[25]

Both these clinical studies suggested that the initial set pressure target should be less than peak pressure (and closer to plateau pressure) during flow-targeted, volume-cycled ACV. An inspiratory flow of at least 40 liters/min seems reasonable in order to have the constant flow activate at a reasonable point in the inspiratory cycle.

As noted earlier, DCWB breath algorithms exist on several ventilators, but their clinical role remains unclear, and use is driven primarily by a clinician's belief in the underlying concept. More important, however, the dual-control breath-to-breath (DCBB) approach described below appears to be a simpler approach to dual control and has appeared on more devices in recent years than the DCWB approach.

DUAL CONTROL BREATH TO BREATH (DCBB)

DCBB breaths are standard pressure-targeted breaths (either PS or pressure-targeted ACV), but the ventilator has the ability to adjust the pressure target according to a clinician-set V_T and the delivered V_T of previous breaths.[12,13,26–32]

With this approach, instead of setting a target pressure, the clinician selects a V_T. The ventilator then delivers one or more "test breaths" with a small amount of inspiratory pressure. The delivered V_T is measured, and total system compliance is calculated. Thereafter, each subsequent breath

FIGURE 16-3 Behavior of DCBB breaths in a lung model simulation of changing lung compliance. In both the top and bottom panels, pressure (Paw), flow, and volume (Vol) are plotted over time. The target tidal volume in both panels is 600 ml. In the top panel, lung compliance decreases after the fourth breath. Initially, there is a drop in tidal volume, but then the DCBB algorithm gradually increases the target inspiratory pressure to restore the volume. In the bottom panel, lung compliance increases after the fourth breath. Initially, there is an increase in tidal volume, but then the DCBB algorithm gradually reduces the inspiratory pressure target to restore the volume. (*Reproduced, with permission, from Branson et al: Respir Care 50:187–201, 2005.*)

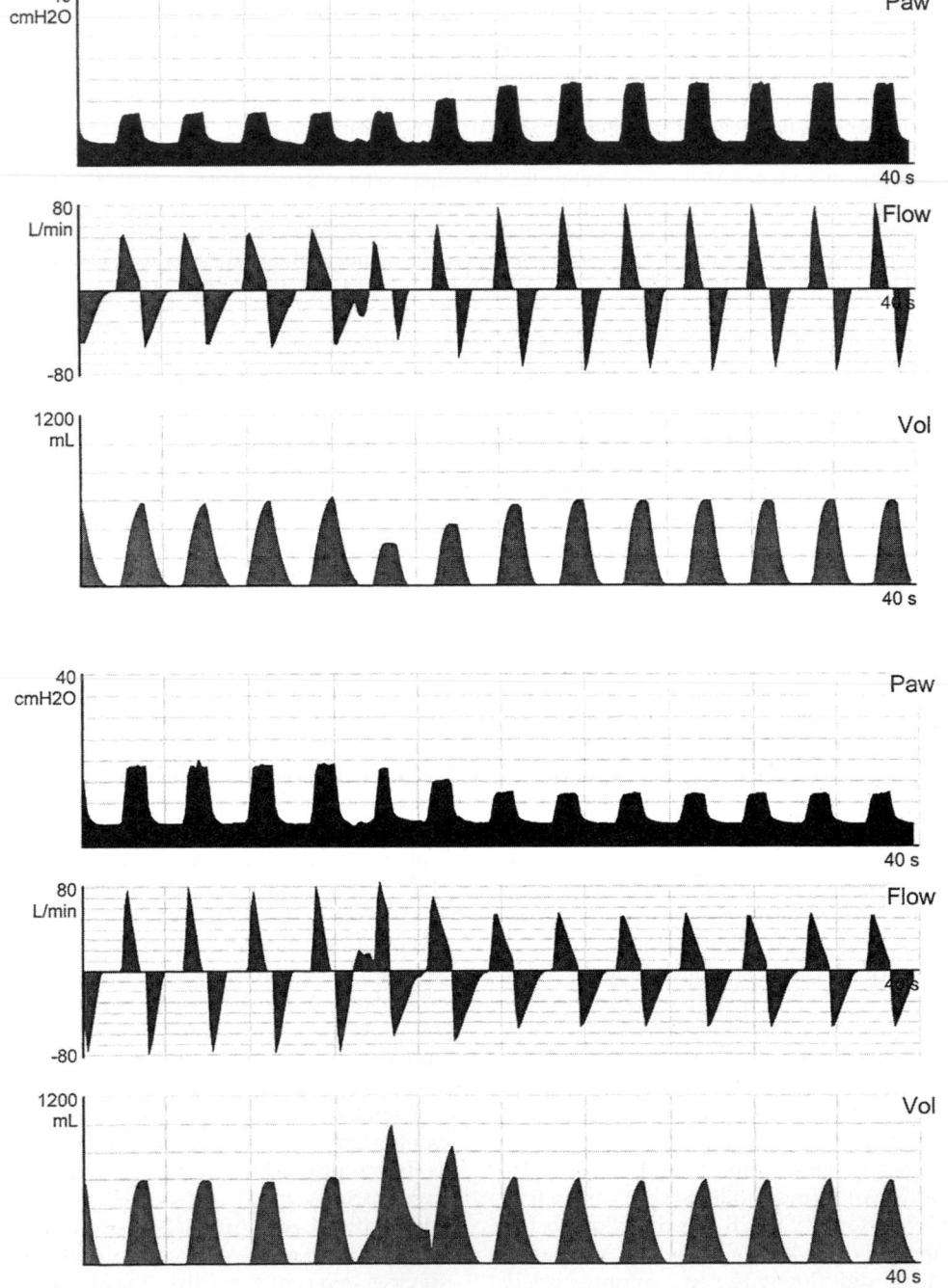

uses the previous calculation of system compliance to manipulate the ensuing pressure target to achieve the desired V_T (Fig. 16-3). The maximum pressure change from breath to breath on most systems generally is limited to a few centimeters of water to prevent large swings in pressure and volume. The volume signal used for DCBB feedback control is not exhaled V_T but V_T exiting the ventilator. This prevents a runaway effect, which could occur if a leak in the circuit prevented accurate measurement of exhaled V_T.

If the DCBB breath is flow-cycled, the flow-cycling criterion is manufacturer-specific (e.g., 25–35% of peak flow), or it can be clinician-adjusted on many newer machines. A secondary cycling mechanism may be present on some devices if inspiratory time exceeds a certain fraction (e.g., 80%) of a set total cycle time. Also, as with other pressure-targeted breaths, a rate-of-rise adjustment usually is available on DCBB breaths.

DCBB breaths are available in a variety of modes that can supply patient-triggered, flow-cycled DCBB breaths and patient- or machine-triggered, time-cycled DCBB breaths either as stand-alone breaths or combined with each other, with PS breaths, or with assist-control breaths (Table 16-1). Although a clinician-set V_T is always required to control the DCBB breath pressure level, these modes also may require a minimum rate setting by the clinician to either control the type of breath that will be given or, on some systems, to enable automatic adjustments in the target V_T.

When time-cycled (ACV-like) DCBB breaths are interspersed with either spontaneous unsupported or pressure-supported breaths, or when flow-cycled (PS-like) DCBB breaths are interspersed with conventional ACV breaths, algorithms similar to SIMV or MMV are often used to determine which breath type will be delivered. Airway occlusion pressure ($P_{0.1}$),[33] oxygen saturation (Sp_{O_2}),[34-36]

TABLE 16-1   Proprietary Names and Characteristics of Newer Dual-Control Breath-to-Breath (DCBB) Modes

DCBB Breath Type	Examples of Proprietary Names
Patient- or machine-triggered, time-cycled[a]	Pressure-regulated volume control (Macquet/Siemens, Viasys)
	Adaptive pressure ventilation (Hamilton)
	Volume control plus (Puritan-Bennett)
	Autoflow (Drager)
Patient-triggered, flow-cycled[b]	Volume support (Macquet/Siemens, Puritan-Bennett)
	Flow-cycled, pressure-regulated volume control (Viasys)
	Minimum mandatory ventilation (Hamilton)
Combined patient/ machine-triggered, time-cycled and patient-triggered, flow-cycled	Automode (Macquet/Siemens)

[a]Some manufacturers allow pressure-support breaths to be provided in addition to the DCBB breaths.

[b]Some manufacturers allow synchronized intermittent mandatory breaths to be provided in addition to the DCBB breaths.

and end-tidal CO_2 concentrations[37,38] also may be incorporated into the mode-control algorithm to adjust either the target V_T or the breath-delivery pattern. If time-cycled (ACV-like) and flow-cycled (PS-like) DCBB breaths are interspersed in a single mode, the machine is designed to switch between the two breath types depending on the presence or absence of patient effort (flow-cycled breaths being delivered in response to patient effort, and time-cycled breaths being delivered in response to a machine-initiated breath).[39,40]

As with the DCWB breath, the putative advantage of DCBB breath modes is to provide the mixing and synchrony features of pressure targeting with the volume guarantee of flow-targeted volume cycling. More specifically, proponents of DCBB modes argue that applied pressure can be minimized "automatically" as mechanics improve or effort increases.[12,13,39] This, in turn, should keep the ventilator-applied stretch of the lung to the minimum necessary for the desired V_T and also may facilitate weaning.

Both animal and human studies have shown that DCBB breaths function as designed using both flow-cycled and time-cycled approaches.[26-32,34-40] These studies emphasize that the DCBB breath is similar to other pressure-targeted breaths with enhanced gas mixing and better patient-ventilator flow synchrony as compared with flow-targeted, volume-cycled breaths and confirm that DCBB breaths do provide a volume guarantee without untoward side effects. Not surprisingly, several of these studies showed lower peak pressures with DCBB breaths than with volume assist-control breaths.[26,28] This, however, is a finding consistent with the decelerating flow patterns of all pressure-targeted breaths (e.g., PS or PACV).

Flow-cycled DCBB breaths, either alone or in combination with time-cycled DCBB breaths or various SIMV/PS modes, have been used in several weaning studies; in general, they have performed as well as (or sometimes better than) stand-alone SIMV or PS protocols.[30,32,34-39] A common finding in these weaning studies is that the DCBB breath modes required fewer ventilator manipulations. One must be cautious, however, in interpreting these weaning studies. The SIMV or SIMV + PS control strategies have been shown in a number of clinical trials to delay weaning inappropriately compared with spontaneous breathing trials or stand-alone PS strategies.[41-43] A more appropriate evaluation of DCBB breath weaning strategies would be a comparison with spontaneous breathing trials delivered according to a protocol.[42,44,45] Further studies on the effect of both stand-alone and automated-switching algorithms for DCBB breaths on important clinical outcomes are clearly needed before widespread use is recommended.

Importantly, the DCBB breath may have unintentional outcomes under certain circumstances.[11] For instance, if the set V_T in a patient-triggered DCBB breath is higher than patient demand, a recovering patient may never attempt to take over the work of breathing for that sized V_T, and thus ventilator-support reduction and weaning may not progress. In addition, if the pressure level increases in an attempt to maintain an inappropriately high V_T in a patient with airflow obstruction, intrinsic PEEP may result. This may be further complicated by the intrinsic PEEP reducing

TABLE 16-2 Boundary Conditions for Adaptive Lung/Support Ventilation

Parameter	Minimum	Maximum
Inspiratory pressure (cmH$_2$O)	5 above baseline airway pressure (PEEP/CPAP)	10 below P$_{max}$ alarm setting
Tidal volume (ml)	4.4 • IBW	15.4 • IBW or $\dot{V}_E$/5, whichever is lower (may be limited by Pmax alarm)
Target respiratory rate (bpm)	5 bpm	22 bpm • % min vol/100 (If IBW > 15 kg) 45 bpm • % min vol/100 (if IBW < 15 kg)
Mandatory breath rate (bpm)	5 bpm	60 bpm
Inspiratory time (s)	0.5 seconds or 1 • RCe, whichever is longer	2.0 s
Expiratory time (s)	2 • RCe (possibly 3 • RCe)	12 s
I:E ratio range	1:4	1:1

NOTE: These parameters set the limits on the various parameters used during ASV. Pmax, clinician-set maximal inspiratory pressure; IBW, ideal body weight; $\dot{V}_E$, exhaled minute volume; bpm, allowable breaths per minute; % min vol, clinician-set proportion of predicted minute volume needed by the patient that will be supplied by the ventilator; the percent minute volume is based on predicted body weight, e.g., for a 80-kg patient, 100% of minute volume is a minute ventilation of 8 liters/min; I:E, inspiratory to expiratory time ratio.

the V$_T$, which causes yet further increases in airway pressure and intrinsic PEEP.[31] Conversely, if the set V$_T$ is below patient demand, a patient may receive inadequate support. Under these conditions, a patient will perform excessive work to maintain a certain V$_T$ even as the inspiratory pressure is being reduced because the delivered V$_T$ exceeds that set by the clinician.

Despite these concerns and the fact that no outcome studies have been performed using DCBB breaths, there are specific clinical situations where they may have some utility (e.g., fluctuating patient demand and rapidly recovering patient). Clinicians, however, need to be aware of the behavior of DCBB breaths under a variety of circumstances to use these modes properly.

Feedback Control of DCBB Breaths Based on Respiratory System Mechanics and Effort

A novel approach to automated feedback control of ventilator support combines the switching algorithm between DCBB patient-triggered, flow-cycled and machine-triggered, time-cycled breaths described earlier with an automated V$_T$/frequency/inspiratory-to-expiratory (I:E) ratio setup based on respiratory system mechanics. Known as *adaptive lung ventilation*[46] or *adaptive support ventilation* (ASV),[11,47] the breath-control algorithm attempts to partition the frequency, tidal volume, and I:E ratio in order to minimize the potential for the combination of ventilator-patient inspiratory work and intrinsic PEEP. ASV does this by calculating respiratory system mechanics using several "test breaths." It then uses a "mimimal work" calculation[47] to set the frequency–tidal volume pattern that minimizes the combined resistance and compliance components of work. The ASV algorithm then uses a measurement of the expira-

tory time constants (RCe = resistance × compliance) to ensure an inspiratory time of at least one RCe and an expiratory time of at least three RCes.[48] Boundary rules exist to prevent excessive (runaway) settings (Table 16-2). Clinicians must set the desired minute ventilation and the proportion of that minute ventilation that the machine is to supply. Ideal body weight also can be used to calculate the desired minute ventilation based on metabolic demands and predicted dead space. Clinicians also must set the PEEP and F$_{IO_2}$.

Conceptually, ASV has been proposed as a way to minimize ventilator-delivered inspiratory pressure for a given minute ventilation through the use of the "minimal work" frequency–tidal volume pattern and the minimization of intrinsic PEEP.[11,46,47] It thus may reduce overdistension and associated ventilator-induced lung injury. ASV also might be considered an automatic weaning mode because the algorithm responds with lower pressures and fewer mandatory breaths as patient effort increases.

ASV has been evaluated in a number of ways. Initial lung model testing[49] demonstrated that the ASV algorithm responded properly to abrupt changes in lung mechanics. Several clinical studies have compared initial ASV settings with traditional clinician-selected settings and have found that ASV tends to select a lower tidal volume and faster rate (and thus lower inspiratory pressures) than do clinicians.[49–52] Two other studies suggest that ASV also appropriately adapts to changes in patient position and double- to single-lung anesthesia.[52–54] One other study suggested that the I:E algorithm of ASV produced less air trapping in patients with chronic obstructive pulmonary disesae (COPD).[55]

Longer-duration clinical studies with ASV have shown that the algorithm provided appropriate ventilator support in anesthetized patients,[49,52] as well as in patients with respiratory failure.[56] One study noted decreased patient loading with ASV.[57] A number of studies have evaluated ASV in patients being weaned from mechanical ventilation.[46,56–61] In general, these studies showed that ASV safely provided adequate ventilator support and had similar (or faster) weaning times as compared with various SIMV and SIMV + PS protocols. These studies also generally showed fewer ventilator manipulations with ASV. As noted earlier for other DCBB approaches, a more appropriate evaluation of ASV weaning strategies would be a comparison with use of spontaneous breathing trials delivered by protocol,[42,44,45] not with SIMV or SIMV + PS. Larger trials in patients with lung injury clearly are needed to establish the appropriateness of the ASV algorithms in various disease states and the effects of ASV on outcome.

Automatic Adjustments in Pressure and Flow Based on Artificial Airway Geometry

The endotracheal tube (ETT) imposes a significant inspiratory resistance on a spontaneously breathing patient[62,63] (Fig. 16-4, *left panel*). This imposed load can have an impact on flow synchrony during interactive assisted/supported breaths and can make it difficult to assess potential for ventilator withdrawal during periods of unassisted/unsupported breathing.

Low level (e.g., 5–8 cmH$_2$O) PS has been proposed as a way of eliminating the ETT resistive load.[64–66] Unfortunately, the PS algorithm supplies a constant inspiratory pressure, which, because of the high fixed resistance of the ETT, tends to undercompensate the load at the beginning of the breath and overcompensate the load at the end of the breath (see Fig. 16-4, *middle panel*). Patient muscle unloading thus is uneven and may be suboptimal.

One way to address this is to use a pressure sensor at the distal end of the ETT to target the PS applied pressure. This approach would provide a more even pressure bias to the contracting inspiratory muscles. Unfortunately, this approach is unreliable because intra-airway sensors are subject to errors from positioning and mucus occlusion. An alternative is to have the ventilator calculate the ETT resistance properties and use those calculations to manipulate applied pressure in such a way as to compensate for the ETT effects[67,68] (see Fig. 16-4, *right panel*). To accomplish this, the clinician must input the tube geometry (length and diameter) and the percentage of compensation desired (10–100%). The ventilator then uses these data to calculate ETT resistance and incorporates this with measurements of instantaneous flow to apply pressure proportional to resistance throughout the total respiratory cycle.

The ETT-compensation concept was first introduced in 1993 by Guttmann et al[67] and was applied during both inspiration and expiration. It was believed that the expiratory effect (i.e., circuit pressure actually going below set baseline pressure to "assist" expiratory flow) might further improve patient-ventilator interactions by reducing expiratory work and hyperinflation. In a series of ventilated patients, this approach was shown to improve subjective patient comfort substantially.[69]

FIGURE 16-4 Effects of the endotracheal tube (ETT) resistance on the application of continuous positive airway pressure (CPAP), pressure support (PS), and CPAP with ETT compensation (CPAP-ATC) in a spontaneously breathing patient. Depicted are airway pressure profiles over time in the ventilator circuit (*upper panels*) and the distal trachea (*lower panels*). In the left breath, the CPAP tracing in the ventilator circuit is appropriately constant, whereas the tracheal pressure downswing reflects the patient work required to effect flow trough the ETT. In the middle breath, PS is applied in the ventilator circuit. This reduces some of the patient work, but because the "squarewave" PS breath does not adequately pressurize the trachea rapidly enough, there still can be significant work required by the patient early in the breath. In the right breath, a similar mean inspiratory pressure to the PS breath is applied, but the pressure profile is altered to provide a higher pressure early and a lower pressure later (CPAP-ATC). This profile is machine-determined, and knowledge of ETT geometry accounts more appropriately for the effects of ETT resistance. It thus creates a truer CPAP pattern in the trachea. Note that this ETT-compensation feature also can be combined with PS on some ventilators. (*Reproduced, with permission, from MacIntyre: Respir Care 50:275–86, 2005.*)

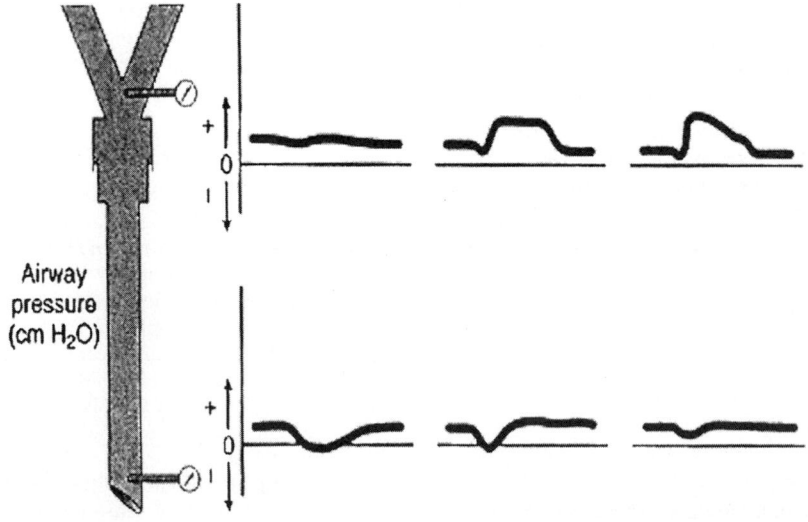

Airway pressure (cm H$_2$O)

Variations on this computational approach to manipulating applied pressure are now available as automatic tube compensation (ATC; Drager, Puritan-Bennett, Maquet/Siemens) and automatic airway compensation (AAC; Viasys). Bench and clinical studies have verified that the ETT-compensation algorithms on these commercial systems generally perform as designed during both continuous positive airway pressure (CPAP) and PS.[70–72] Not all systems, however, have the expiratory feature, and the response characteristics of commercial systems may not be as robust as the Guttman design.[67]

It also must be recognized that the ETT-compensation strategy is based on the input geometry of the artificial airway and cannot account for changes in tube characteristics induced by kinks or partial occlusions or the relationship of the tube opening against the tracheal wall. Thus this strategy should not be considered a perfect surrogate for a tracheal pressure sensor, especially as the duration of intubation increases. Nevertheless, despite these limitations, and despite the fact that ETT compensation has not been subjected to outcome studies, the simplicity of the concept and safety of the design would seem to warrant its application during PS and CPAP and even during trials of weaning.

An interesting extension of the ETT-compensation concept is to use a pleural pressure to target the positive-pressure breath.[73] This approach requires an esophageal balloon to measure esophageal pressure, a surrogate for pleural pressure. Conceptually, a pleural pressure target could be used to control the breath directly in such a way as to account for all the components of patient work, not just that caused by the ETT. At the present time, this approach has been explored only with prototype systems in experimental animals.

Conclusion

A positive-pressure breath ideally should provide a V_T that is adequate for gas exchange and appropriate muscle unloading while minimizing any risk for injury or discomfort. The latest generation of ventilators is now using sophisticated feedback systems to "sculpt" positive-pressure breaths according to patient effort and respiratory system mechanics. At the present time, these new control strategies are not totally "closed-loop" systems because the automatic input variables are still limited, some clinician settings are still required, and the specific features of the "perfect" breath design still are not entirely clear. Despite these limitations, there is at least some rationale for many of these newer feedback features, even though all of them await outcome studies to justify their widespread use.

References

1. Chatburn RL. A new system for understanding mechanical ventilators. Respir Care 1991; 36:1123–55.
2. Branson RD, Chatburn RL. Technical description and classification of modes of ventilator operation. Respir Care 1992; 37:1026–44.
3. MacIntyre NR. Principles of mechanical ventilation. In: Murray J, Nadel J, editors. Textbook of respiratory medicine, 4th ed. New York: Elsevier, 2005.
4. Luce JM, Pierson DJ, Hudson LD. Intermittent mandatory ventilation. Chest 1981; 79:678–85.
5. Weisman IM, Rinaldo JE, Rogers RM, et al. Intermittent mandatory ventilation. Am Rev Respir Dis 1983; 127:641–7.
6. Heenan TJ, Downs JB, Douglas ME, et al. Intermittent mandatory ventilation: Is synchronization important? Chest 1980; 77:598–602.
7. Hewlett AM, Platt AS, Terry VG. Mandatory minute volume: A new concept in weaning from mechanical ventilation. Anaesthesia. 1977; 32:163–9.
8. Ravenscroft PS. Simple mandatory minute volume. Anesthesia 1978; 33:246–9.
9. Sassoon CSH. Positive pressure ventilation: alternate modes. Chest 1991; 100:1421–9.
10. Sassoon CSH, Mahutte CK, Light RW. Ventilator modes, old and new. Crit Care Clin 1990; 6:605–34.
11. Branson RD, Johannigman JA. Role of ventilator graphics when setting dual control modes. Respir Care 2005; 50:187–201.
12. Branson RD, MacIntyre NR. Dual control modes of mechanical ventilation. Respir Care 1996; 41:294–305.
13. Branson RD, Davis K. Dual control modes: Combining volume and pressure breaths. Respir Care Clin North Am. 2001; 7:397–401.
14. Raneri VM. Optimization of patient ventilator interactions: Closed loop technology. Intensive Care Med 1997; 23:936–9.
15. Iotti GA, editor. Closed-loop control mechanical ventilation. Respir Care Clin North Am 2001; 7:341–519.
16. Amato MBP, Barbos CSV, Bonassa J, et al. Volume assisted pressure support ventilation (VAPSV): A new approach for reducing muscle workload during acute respiratory failure. Chest 1992; 102:1225–34.
17. Marini JJ, Rodriguez RM, Lamb V. The inspiratory workload of patient-initiated mechanical ventilation. Am Rev Respir Dis 1986; 134:902–9.
18. Marini JJ, Capps JS, Culver BH. The inspiratory work of breathing during assisted mechanical ventilation. Chest 1985; 87:612–8.
19. Knebel AR, Janson-Bjerklie SL, Malley JD, et al. Comparison of breathing comfort during weaning with two ventilatory modes. Am J Respir Crit Care Med 1994; 149:14–8.
20. Cinnella G, Conti G, Lofaso F, et al. Effects of assisted ventilation on the work of breathing: Volume-controlled versus pressure-controlled ventilation. Am J Respir Crit Care Med 1996; 153:1025–33.
21. Kallet RH, Campbell AR, Alonso JA, et al. The effects of pressure control versus volume control assisted ventilation on patient work of breathing in acute lung injury and acute respiratory distress syndrome. Respir Care 2000; 45:1085–96.
22. MacIntyre NR, McConnell R, Cheng KC, et al. Patient-ventilator flow dyssynchrony: Flow-limited versus pressure-limited breaths. Crit Care Med 1997; 25:1671–7.
23. MacIntyre NR, Gropper C, Westfall T. Combining pressure limiting and volume cycling features in a patient-interactive mechanical ventilation. Crit Care Med 1994; 22:353–7.
24. Haas CF, Branson RD, Folk LM, et al. Patient determined inspiratory flow during assisted mechanical ventilation. Respir Care 1995; 40:716–21.
25. Manning HL, Molinary EJ, Leiter JC. Effects of inspiratory flow rate on respiratory sensation and pattern of breathing. Am J Respir Crit Care Med 1995; 151:751–7.

26. Piotrowski A, Sobala W, Kawczynski P. Patient initiated, pressure regulated, volume controlled ventilation compared with intermittent mandatory ventilation in neonates: A prospective, randomized study. Intensive Care Med 1997; 23:975–81.

27. East TD, Elkhuizan PHM, Pace CL. Pressure support in mandatory minute ventilation supplied by the Ohmeda CPU-1 prevents alveolar hypoventilation due to respiratory depression in a canine model. Respir Care 1989; 34:795–800.

28. Kocis KC, Dekeon MK, Rosen HK, et al. Pressure-regulated volume control vs volume control ventilation in infants after surgery for congenital heart disease. Pediatr Cardiol 2001; 22:233–7.

29. Guldager H, Nelso SL, Carl P, et al. A comparison of volume controlled ventilation and pressure regulated volume control in acute respiratory failure. Crit Care 1997; 1:75–7.

30. Randolph AG, Wypij D, Venkataraman ST, et al. Effect of mechanical ventilator weaning protocols on respiratory outcomes in infants and children: A randomized, controlled trial. JAMA. 2002; 288:2561–8.

31. Sottiaux TM. Patient-ventilator interactions during volume-support ventilation: Asynchrony and tidal volume instability—A report of three cases. Respir Care 2001; 46:232–3.

32. Abubakar KM, Keszler M. Patient-ventilator interactions in new modes of patient-triggered ventilation. Pediatr Pulmonol 2001; 32:71–5.

33. Iotti GA, Braschi A. Closed loop support of ventilatory workload: The $P_{0.1}$ controller. Respir Care Clin North Am 2001; 7:441–51.

34. Strickland JH, Hasson JH. A computer-controlled ventilator weaning system. Chest. 1991; 100:1096–9.

35. Tong DA. Weaning patients from mechanical ventilation: A knowledge-based system approach. Comput Methods Prog Biomed 1991; 35:267–78.

36. Strickland JH, Hasson JH. A computer-controlled ventilator weaning system: A clinical trial. Chest 1993; 103:1220–6.

37. Dojat M, Harf A, Touchard D, et al. Evaluation of a knowledge-based system providing ventilatory management and decision for extubation. Am J Respir Crit Care Med 1996; 153:997–1004.

38. Dojat M, Harf A, Touchard D, et al. Clinical evaluation of a computer-controlled pressure support mode. Am J Respir Crit Care Med. 2000; 161:1161–6.

39. Holt SJ, Sanders RC, Thurman TL, Heulitt MJ. An evaluation of automode, a computer-controlled ventilator mode, with the Siemens Servo 300A ventilator, using a porcine model. Respir Care 2001; 46:26–36.

40. Roth H, Luecke T, Lansche G, et al. Effects of patient-triggered automatic switching between mandatory and supported ventilation in the postoperative weaning period. Intensive Care Med 2001; 27:47–51.

41. Esteban A, Frutos F, Tobin MJ, et al. A comparison of four methods of weaning patients from mechanical ventilation. New Engl J Med 1995; 332:345–50.

42. ACCP/SCCM/AARC Task Force. Evidence based guidelines for weaning and discontinuing mechanical ventilation. Chest 2001; 120:375–95S.

43. Brochard L, Rauss A, Benito S, et al. Comparison of three methods of gradual withdrawal from ventilatory support during weaning from mechanical ventilation. Am J Respir Crit Care Med 1994; 150:896–903.

44. Ely EW, Baker AM, Dunagan DP, et al. Effect on the duration of mechanical ventilation of identifying patients capable of breathing spontaneously. New Engl J Med 1996; 335:1864–9.

45. Kollef MH, Shapiro SD, Silver P, et al. A randomized, controlled trial of protocol-directed versus physician-directed weaning from mechanical ventilation. Crit Care Med 1997; 25:567–74.

46. Linton DM. Adaptive lung ventilation. Respir Care Clin North Am 2001; 7:409–20.

47. Campbell RS, Branson RD, Johannigman JA. Adaptive support ventilation. Respir Care Clin North Am 2001; 7:425–40.

48. Brunner JX, Laubscher TP, Banner MJ, et al. A simple method to measure total expiratory time constant based on the passive expiratory flow-volume curve. Crit Care Med 1995; 23:1117–22.

49. Laubscher TP, Heinrichs W, Weiler N, et al. An adaptive lung ventilation controller. IEEE Trans Biomed Eng 1995; 41:51–9.

50. Laubscher TP, Frutiger A, Fanconi S, et al. Automatic selection of tidal volume, respiratory frequency and minute volume in intubated ICU patients as startup procedure for closed-loop controlled ventilation. Int J Clin Monit Comput 1994; 11:19–30.

51. Laubscher TP, Frutiger A, Fanconi S, Brunner JX. The automatic selection of ventilation parameters during the initial phase of mechanical ventilation. Intensive Care Med 1996; 22:199–207.

52. Weiler N, Eberle B, Latorre F, et al. Adaptive lung ventilation. Anaesthetist 1996; 45:950–6.

53. Weiler N, Eberle B, Heinrichs W. Adaptive lung ventilation (ALV) during anesthesia for pulmonary surgery: Automatic response to transitions to and from one-lung ventilation. Int J Clin Monit Comput 1998; 14:245–52.

54. Weiler N, Henrichs W, Kebler W. The ALV mode: A safe closed loop algorithm for ventilation during total intravenous anesthesia. Int J Clin Monit Comput 1994; 11:85–8.

55. Belliato M, Maggio G, Neri S, et al. Evaluation of the adaptive support ventilation (ASV) mode in paralyzed patients. Intensive Care Med 2000; 26:S327.

56. Linton DM, Brunner JX, Laubscher TP. Continuous use of an adaptive lung ventilation controller in critically ill patients in a multi-disciplinary intensive care unit. S Afr Med J 1995; 85:430–3.

57. Tassaux D, Dalmas E, Gratadour P, Jolliet P. Patient-ventilator interactions during partial ventilatory support: A preliminary study comparing the effects of adaptive support ventilation with synchronized intermittent mandatory ventilation plus inspiratory pressure support. Crit Care Med 2002; 30:801–7.

58. Linton DM, Potgieter PD, Davis S, et al. Automatic weaning from mechanical ventilation using an adaptive lung controller. Chest 1994; 106:1843–50.

59. Sulzer CF, Chiolero R, Cassot PG, et al. Adaptive support ventilation for fast tracheal extubation after cardiac surgery: A randomized, controlled study. Anesthesiology 2001; 95:1339–45.

60. Cassina T, Chiolero R, Mauri R, Revelly JP. Clinical experience with adaptive support ventilation for fast-track cardiac surgery. J Cardiother Vasc Anesth 2003; 17:571–5.

61. Petter AH, Chiolero RL, Cassina T, et al. Automatic "respirator/weaning" with adaptive support ventilation: The effect on duration of endotracheal intubation and patient management. Anesth Analg 2003; 97:1743–50.

62. Bersten AD, Rutten AJ, Vedig AE, Skowronski GA. Additional work of breathing imposed by endotracheal tubes, breathing circuits, and intensive care ventilators. Crit Care Med 1989; 17:671–80.

63. Shapiro M, Wilson RK, Casar G, et al. Work of breathing through different sized endotracheal tubes. Crit Care Med 1986; 14:1028–31.

64. Bersten AD, Rutten AJ, Vedig AE. Efficacy of pressure support in compensating for apparatus work. Anaesth Intensive Care 1993; 21:67–71.

65. Brochard L, Rua F, Lorini H, et al. Inspiratory pressure support compensates for the additional work of breathing caused by the endotracheal tube. Anesthesiology 1991; 75:739–45.

66. Fiastro JF, Habib MP, Quan SF. Pressure support compensation for inspiratory work due to endotracheal tubes and demand continuous positive airway pressure. Chest 1988; 93:499–505.

67. Guttmann, Ebehard L, Fabry B, et al. Continuous calculation of intratracheal pressure in tracheally intubated patients. Anesthesiology 1993; 79:503–13.

68. Guttmann J, Haberthur C, Mols G. Automatic tube compensation. Respir Care Clin North Am 2001; 7:475–83.

69. Guttmann J, Bernhard H, Mols G, et al. Respiratory comfort of automatic tube compensation and inspiratory pressure support in conscious humans. Intensive Care Med 1997; 23:1119–23.

70. Fabry B, Guttmann J, Eberhard L, Wolff G. Automatic compensation of endotracheal tube resistance in spontaneously breathing patients. Technol Health Care 1994; 1:281–5.

71. Fabry B, Haberthur G, Zappe D, et al. Breathing pattern and additional work of breathing in spontaneously breathing patients with different ventilatory demands during inspiratory pressure support and automatic tube compensation. Intensive Care Med. 1997; 23:545–50.

72. Stocker R, Fabry B, Eberhard L, Haberthur C. Support of spontaneous breathing in the intubated patient: Automatic tube compensation (ATC) and proportional assist ventilation (PAV). Acta Anaesthesiol Scand Suppl 1997; 111:123–9.

73. Takahashi T, Takezawa J, Kimura T, et al. Comparison of inspiratory work of breathing in T-piece breathing, PSV, and pleural pressure support ventilation (PPSV). Chest 1991; 100:1030–4.

74. MacIntyre NR. Respiratory mechanics in the patient who is weaning from the ventilator. Respir Care 2005; 50:275–86.

PART VI
NONINVASIVE METHODS OF VENTILATOR SUPPORT

Chapter 17
NEGATIVE-PRESSURE VENTILATION

ANTONIO CORRADO, MASSIMO GORINI

Conventional mechanical ventilation via endotracheal intubation or tracheostomy in the treatment of acute respiratory failure (ARF) is a lifesaving procedure. Yet it exposes patients to severe complications, including upper airway trauma and nosocomial pneumonia, and may prolong the length of stay in the intensive-care unit (ICU) and hospital because additional time may be necessary for weaning.[1–4]

Noninvasive ventilator techniques have been used recently to treat ARF, and while their benefits, as compared with intubation, have not been firmly established, their use is attractive. Advantages include the possibility of avoiding sedative agents, facilitating communication between patients and care providers, and preserving such functions as swallowing and coughing. Noninvasive mechanical ventilation consists of both negative- and positive-pressure ventilators. We discuss the basic principles, the physiologic effects, and the more recent clinical application of negative-pressure ventilation (NPV).

Basic Principles

NPV works by exposing the surface of the thorax to subatmospheric pressure during inspiration. This pressure causes thoracic expansion and a decrease in pleural and alveolar pressures, creating a pressure gradient for air to move from the airway opening into the alveoli. When the pressure surrounding the thorax increases and becomes atmospheric or greater, expiration occurs passively owing to the elastic recoil of the respiratory system. The inspiratory changes with NPV, in pleural and alveolar pressures, replicate those during spontaneous breathing. On the contrary, positive-pressure ventilation (PPV) causes an increase in intrathoracic pressures during inspiration (Fig. 17-1).

All negative-pressure ventilators have two major components: an airtight, rigid chamber that encloses the rib cage and abdomen and a pump that generates pressure changes in the chamber.[5,6]

NEGATIVE-PRESSURE VENTILATORS

TANK VENTILATOR
Tank ventilators enclose the body up to the neck. The advantage is that chest-wall expansion is not limited by contact with the sides of the chamber, and only one airtight seal is required around the neck. Most modern tank ventilators are constructed of aluminium and plastic and are lighter than previously. The patient's body rests on a thin mattress, and the head protrudes through a porthole at one end of the ventilator. A head and neck rest is provided in most designs to ensure comfort and to prevent upper airway collapse. Most tank ventilators have windows allowing patient observation and portholes for catheters and monitor leads and where procedures can be performed[7] (Fig. 17-2).

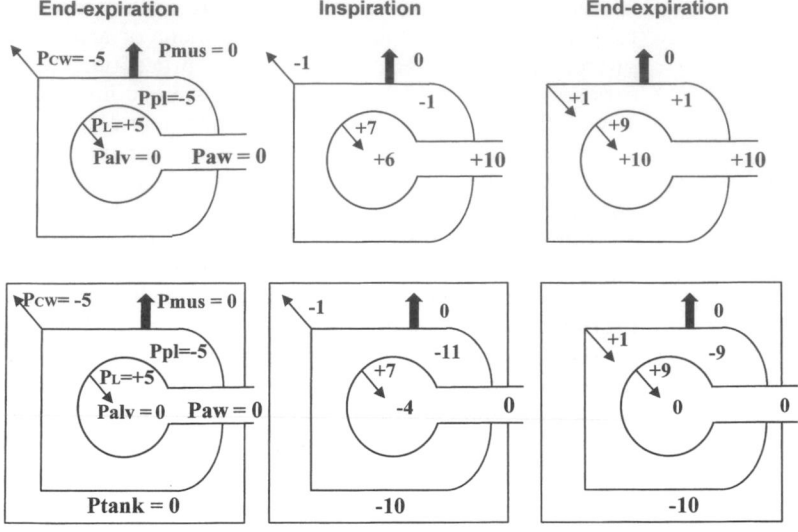

FIGURE 17-1 Airway and intrathoracic pressures during positive-pressure ventilation (*upper panel*) and during negative-pressure ventilation (*bottom panel*). Palv, alveolar pressure; PL, elastic recoil pressure of the lung; PCW, elastic recoil pressure of the chest wall; Ppl, pleural pressure; Pmusc, muscle pressure; Paw, airway pressure; Ptank, tank ventilator pressure.

JACKET VENTILATOR (PULMO-WRAP, PONCHO-WRAP)

This ventilator is a windproof, water-permeable nylon parka suspended over a rigid grid that includes the rib cage and abdomen. It allows the application of negative pressure over the anterior portion of the chest wall.[8] Airtight seals around the neck, arms, and hips are required to prevent air leakage. The jackets do not restrain expansion of the rib cage and abdomen but are awkward for many patients to put on and often cold to wear because of air leaks. They are preferable to tank ventilators for home use but less efficient for treating patients with ARF. The tidal volume they develop at any given level of negative pressure is less than that of a tank ventilator, and the peak pressure that patients can tolerate also usually is slightly less.[6]

CUIRASS

This consists of a rigid shell fitting firmly over the anterior portion of the chest. It applies negative pressure over a smaller surface area than either the iron lung or jacket and is the least efficient negative-pressure ventilator.[8] Its efficiency improves if the anterior abdominal wall is enclosed in the device and movement of the lateral aspect of the upper rib cage is not restrained. Proper fitting can be difficult, and tailor-made fiberglass shells often are necessary, particularly in patients with kyphoscoliosis.

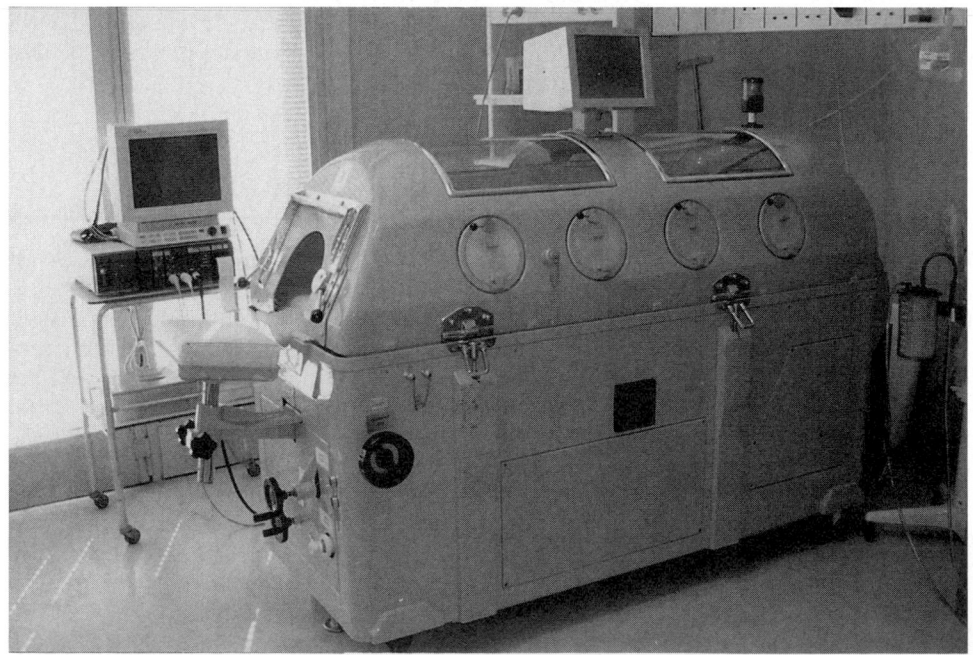

FIGURE 17-2
Microprocessor-based iron lung (Coppa CA 1001, Coppa, Biella, Italy).

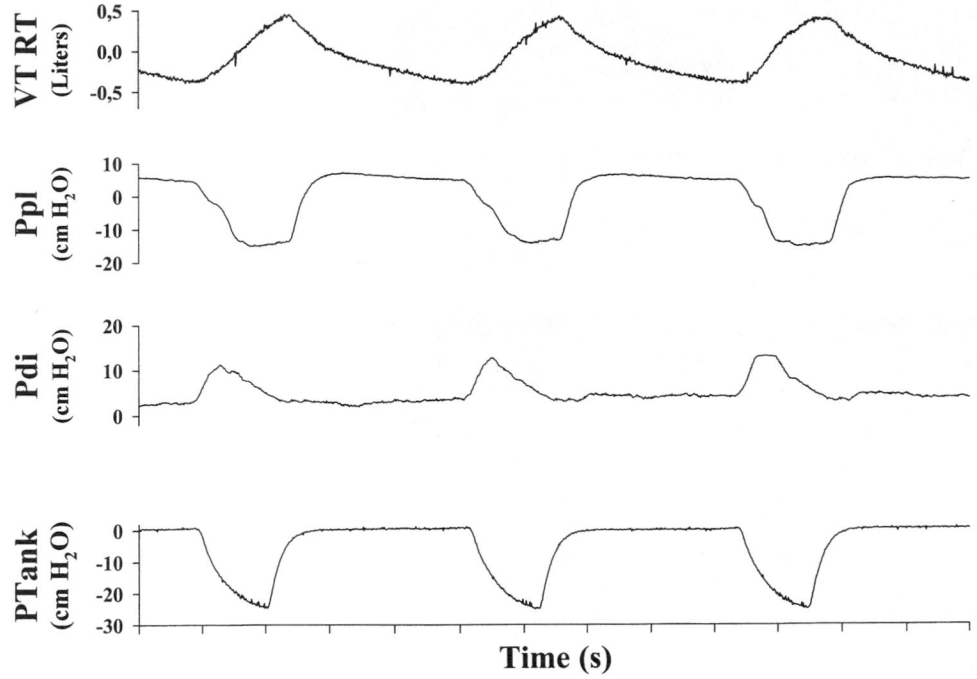

FIGURE 17-3 Recordings of tidal volume by Respitrace (V_T RT), pleural pressure (Ppl), transdiaphragmatic pressure (Pdi), and tank pressure (Ptank) in a patient with an acute exacerbation of COPD during assist negative-pressure ventilation provided by iron lung.

NEGATIVE-PRESSURE VENTILATOR PUMPS

Negative pressure is generated by bellows or rotary pumps that are separate or incorporated into the structure of the ventilator. Modern rotary pumps perform pressure-preset ventilation.[9] After a breath is initiated, these pumps apply and maintain a targeted amount of subatmospheric pressure around the chest wall to meet a specified time-cycling criterion (Fig. 17-3). This mode is equivalent to pressure-controlled ventilation available with the latest positive-pressure ventilators. As with positive-pressure-preset ventilation, tidal volume during NPV is a complex function of applied pressure and its rate of approach to target pressure, available inspiratory time, and the impedance to breathing [compliance of the respiratory system, airway resistance, dynamic hyperinflation with intrinsic positive end-expiratory pressure (PEEP)].

MODES FOR DELIVERING NEGATIVE-PRESSURE VENTILATION

Traditionally, NPV is controlled mechanical ventilation, and the device provides a fixed number of breaths per minute. If mechanical and spontaneous respiratory cycles do not match, the patient "fights" the ventilator, resulting in discomfort. For this reason, airway pressure or flow generally is used in positive-pressure ventilators to detect inspiratory efforts and to trigger the mechanical breath (assist and assist-control ventilation).[1] Unlike PPV, during NPV, the airway opening is free; consequently, it is not possible to monitor airway pressure or flow continuously and to use these signals to trigger a mechanical breath. This patient-triggering inability may contribute to poor patient synchrony and induction of upper airway collapse sec-

ondary to the lack of coordinated activity between the upper airway and the inspiratory muscles.[10] To overcome this limitation, some negative-pressure ventilators have incorporated patient-triggered modes using pressure change sensed via nasal prongs. There are data indicating that this technology is slow and relatively insensitive to patient inspiratory efforts.[11] Recently, the performance of a prototype microprocessor-based iron lung capable of thermistor triggering was evaluated.[12] The device used to trigger the iron lung was thermally sensitive and similar to that used in sleep studies, and it was activated by temperature changes caused by the onset of inspiratory airflow (Fig. 17-4). In normal subjects and patients with chronic obstructive pulmonary disease (COPD) recovering from ARF, we measured (1) the time delay between airflow onset and start of an assisted breath, (2) pressure-time product for the diaphragm per minute (PTPdi) during triggered breaths, and (3) nontriggering inspiratory efforts (Fig. 17-5). At maximum trigger sensitivity, the time delay was about 0.21 second in both groups. PTPdi was reduced markedly. Nontriggering inspiratory efforts were 1.1% and 2.3% of total breaths, respectively. Although the time delay of the thermistor trigger is longer than most recent flow- and pressure-triggering systems of positive-pressure ventilators,[13] the study suggests that this system permits the use of assisted NPV with an acceptable patient-ventilator interaction.

Presently, NPV can be delivered by five modes: (1) intermittent negative pressure, (2) negative/positive pressure, (3) continuous negative pressure (CNEP), (4) negative pressure/negative end-expiratory pressure (Fig. 17-6), and (5) external high-frequency oscillation.

INTERMITTENT NEGATIVE PRESSURE

The ventilator generates targeted subatmospheric pressure for the selected inspiratory time. Pressure around the chest

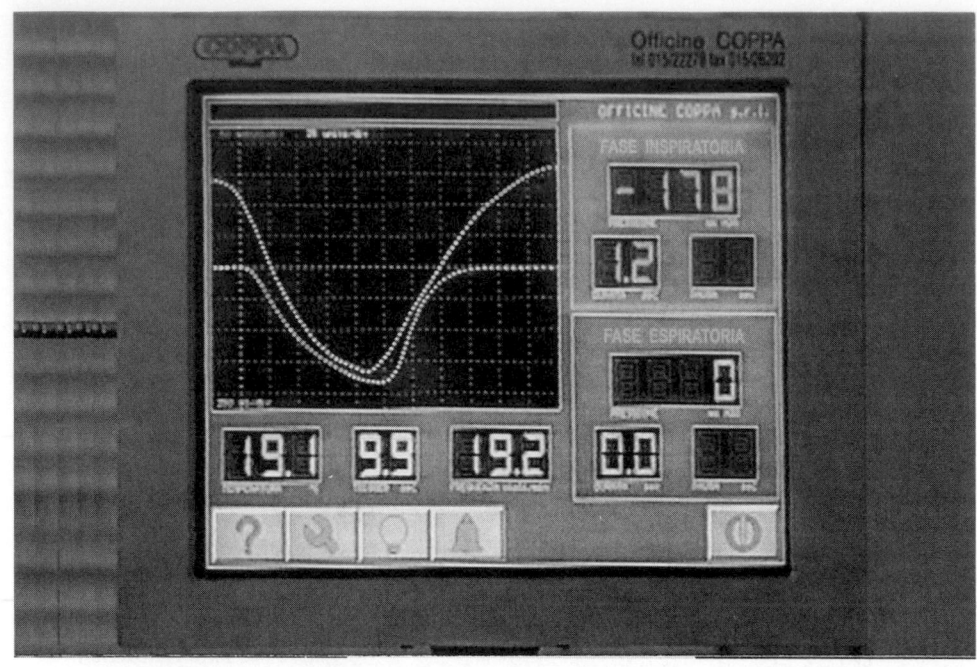

FIGURE 17-4 Control panel of a microprocessor-based iron lung (Coppa CA 1001, Coppa, Biella, Italy) capable of thermistor triggering. The upper trace is the thermistor signal, and the lower trace is the tank pressure.

wall becomes atmospheric during expiration, which occurs passively owing to the elastic recoil of the respiratory system.

NEGATIVE/POSITIVE PRESSURE

The ventilator generates the preset extrathoracic subathmospheric pressure during inspiration and preset extrathoracic positive pressure during expiration. In patients with chest-wall disorders, this combination has been found to increase tidal volume more than intermittent negative pressure alone by reducing the end-expiratory volume of the respiratory system.[14] On a theoretical basis, it is unlikely that positive extrathoracic pressure during expiration can increase expiratory flow in patients with severe COPD and tidal expiratory-flow limitation. A useful application of this option is to assist cough and promote clearance of

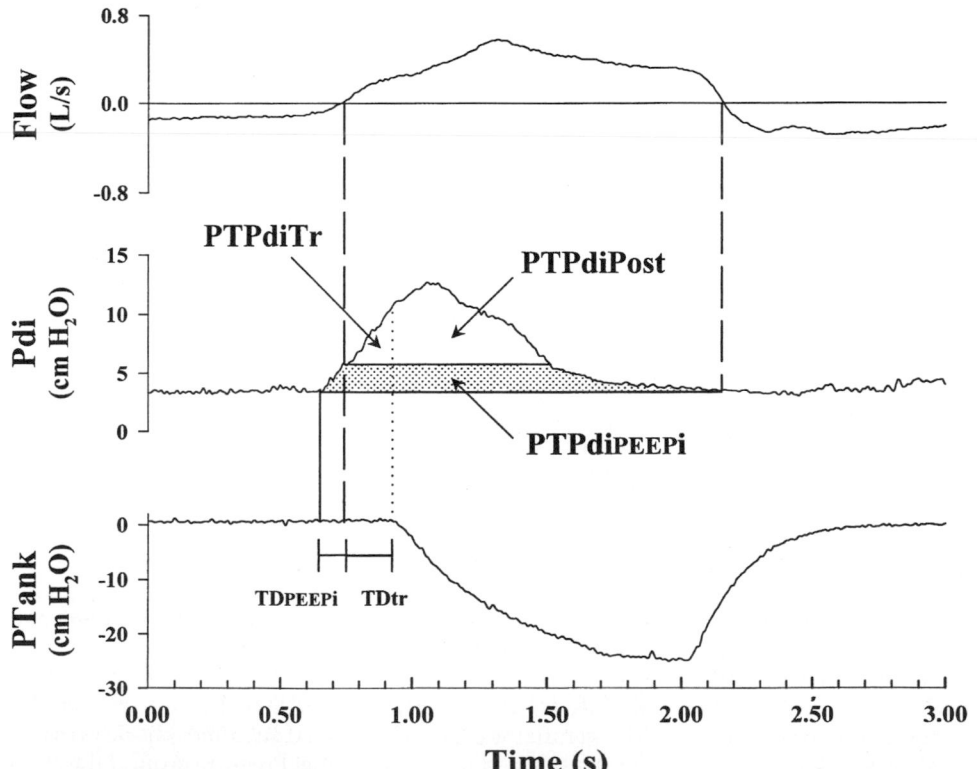

FIGURE 17-5 Recordings of flow, transdiaphragmatic pressure (Pdi), and tank pressure (Ptank) in a patient with COPD receiving assist NPV. The continuous vertical line indicates the onset of inspiratory effort, the dashed vertical line indicates the start of inspiratory flow, and the dotted vertical line indicates the start of an assisted breath. The partitioning of the pressure-time product of the diaphragm is shown: effort required to overcome $PEEP_I$ ($PTPdiPEEP_I$), effort required to trigger the assisted breath (PTPdiTr), and effort exerted in the post–trigger phase (PTPdiPost). $TDPEEP_I$ and TDtr indicate the time delay between the onset of inspiratory effort and the start of inspiratory flow and the time delay between the onset of inspiratory flow and the start of assisted breath, respectively. (*Used, with permission, from Gorini et al: Thorax 57:258–62, 2002.*)

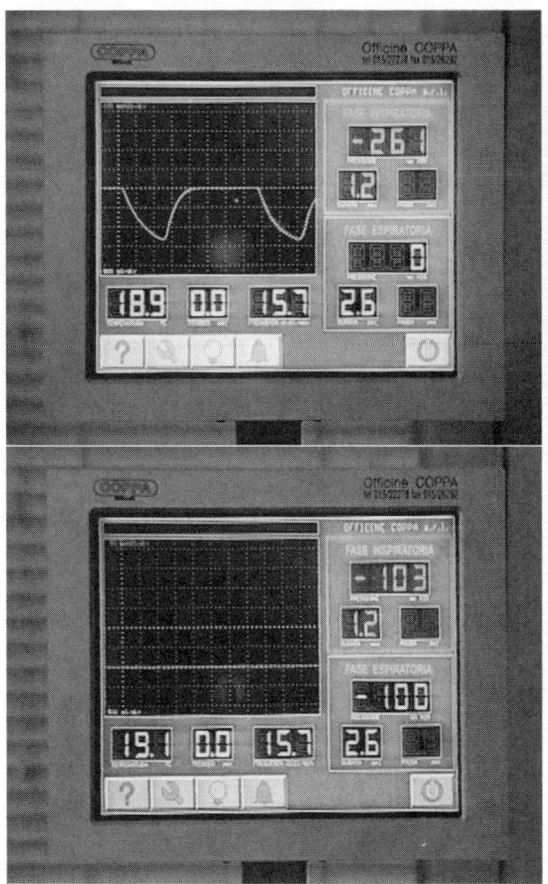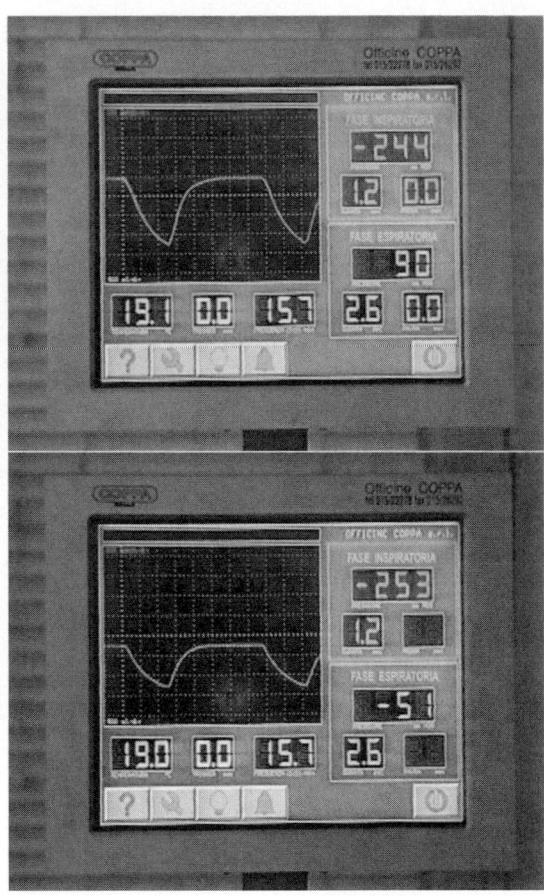

FIGURE 17-6 Control panel of a microprocessor-based iron lung (Coppa CA 1001, Coppa, Biella, Italy) during intermittent negative-pressure (*upper-left panel*), negative/positive-pressure (*upper-right panel*), continuous negative extrathoracic pressure (*lower-left panel*), and negative-pressure/negative extrathoracic end-expiratory pressure (*lower-right panel*) ventilation.

sputum in patients with copious secretions (i.e., cystic fibrosis, bronchiectasis).[8]

CONTINUOUS NEGATIVE EXTRATHORACIC PRESSURE (CNEP)

The ventilator provides a constant subatmospheric pressure throughout the respiratory cycle, and the patient breathes spontaneously.

NEGATIVE PRESSURE/NEGATIVE EXTRATHORACIC END-EXPIRATORY PRESSURE

The ventilator generates the preset subatmospheric pressure during inspiration and maintains a preset level of negative pressure throughout the expiration.

EXTERNAL HIGH-FREQUENCY OSCILLATION

High-frequency ventilation using a jet system can be applied via a tracheal tube or a tracheotomy. Alternatively, a cuirass can be used to apply high-frequency oscillation externally.[15] The Hayek oscillator includes a cuirass, power unit, and control unit. The power unit has (1) a diaphragmatic pump, which can operate over a wide range of frequencies to generate an oscillating pressure wave, and (2) a vacuum pump, which enables the oscillation to be superimposed on a negative-pressure baseline. Peak inspiratory (up

to $-70 \, cmH_2O$) and peak expiratory (up to $70 \, cmH_2O$) pressures, frequency (8–999 cycles per minute), and inspiratory-expiratory (I:E) ratio (1:6–6:1) can be set on the control unit.

Two studies suggest that external high-frequency oscillation can provide effective ventilation in healthy subjects[15] and improve end-tidal carbon dioxide (CO_2) and oxygen (O_2) saturation (Sa_{O_2}) in patients with severe stable COPD.[16] In five patients with ARF, short-term application of external high-frequency oscillation improved oxygenation by 16% and reduced Pa_{CO_2} by 6% compared with conventional PPV.[15] In a randomized, controlled study, a 4-hour period of external high-frequency oscillation improved cardiac index and tissue perfusion in adult patients after coronary artery bypass grafting compared with conventional PPV.[17]

Physiologic Effects

GAS EXCHANGE

Pioneering studies showed NPV, particularly that provided by tank ventilators, to be a highly effective form of mechanical ventilation, capable of maintaining normal arterial blood-gas tensions in patients with little or no spontaneous respiratory activity.[18–20] In stable COPD patients with chronic respiratory failure, poncho-wrap NVP is able to

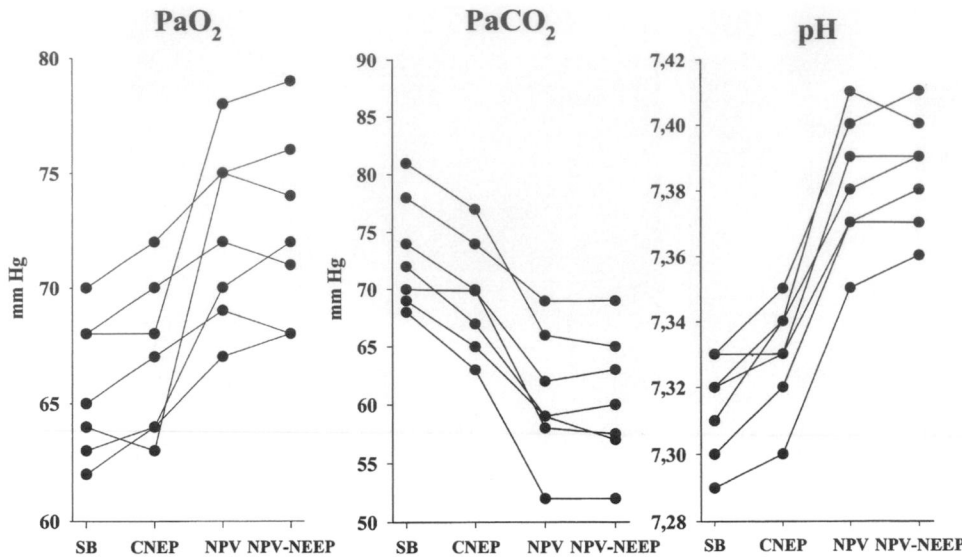

FIGURE 17-7   Values for Pa_{O_2}, Pa_{CO_2}, and pH in seven patients with acute exacerbation of chronic obstructive pulmonary disease during spontaneous breathing (SB), continuous negative extrathoracic pressure (CNEP), negative-pressure ventilation (NPV), and negative extrathoracic end-expiratory pressure added to NPV (NPV-NEEP). (*Used, with permission, from Gorini et al: Am J Respir Crit Care Med 163:1614–8, 2001.*)

improve the pattern of breathing, minute ventilation, and arterial blood-gas tensions.[21,22] Recently, the physiologic effects of CNEP, NPV, and NPV plus negative extrathoracic end-expiratory pressure (NEEP) provided by a microprocessor-based iron lung in seven patients with COPD recovering from ARF were studied.[23] The different types of NPV were able to improve ventilatory pattern, arterial blood gases, and pH significantly (Fig. 17-7).

RESPIRATORY MUSCLES

Two studies reported that NPV, carried out continuously for 6 hours by iron lung[24] or intermittently for 7 days by poncho-wrap,[25] was effective in improving respiratory muscle strength and in decreasing Pa_{CO_2}. In patients with chronic respiratory failure secondary to COPD and restrictive diseases, NPV reduced electrical and mechanical activity of the inspiratory muscles.[26–30] Rodenstein et al[31] showed that controlled NPV provided by an old iron lung requires a short period of adaptation to obtain inspiratory muscle rest. Other studies have shown that when inspiratory and expiratory times were adjusted carefully to approximate the subject's spontaneous timing components, NPV results in a substantial suppression of electromyographic activity of inspiratory muscles.[27,28] Assist-control NPV provided by a cuirass is effective in relief of dyspnea induced experimentally in normal subjects by a combination of inspiratory resistive loading and hypercapnia, probably reducing inspiratory muscle workload.[32]

The effects of NPV provided by a microprocessor-based iron lung capable of providing CNEP and assist-control NPV on respiratory mechanics and inspiratory muscle effort in patients with COPD with ARF were evaluated by measuring the pressure-time product of the diaphragm and the electromyographic activity of parasternal muscles.[23] Compared with spontaneous breathing, CNEP (-5 cmH$_2$O) resulted in a significant decrease in dynamic intrinsic PEEP and pressure-time product of the diaphragm, whereas assist-control NPV caused a significant improvement in

the pattern of breathing associated with a marked reduction in both pressure-time product of the diaphragm and electromyographic activity of the parasternal muscles. The application of -5 cmH$_2$O of negative extrathoracic end-expiratory pressure during NPV further decreased the pressure-time product of the diaphragm slightly and improved patient-ventilator interaction by reducing dynamic intrinsic PEEP and nontriggering inspiratory effort (Fig. 17-8). Reduction in diaphragmatic effort obtained during assist-control NPV[23] is similar to that measured in patients with an acute exacerbation of COPD with pressure-support ventilation.[33,34]

UPPER AIRWAY

The application of NPV during sleep in normal subjects[35] and in patients with chronic respiratory failure secondary to COPD[10] and neuromuscular disorders[36,37] may result in the development of recurrent episodes of apnea and hypopnea, as well as altered sleep quality. Most obstructive events during NPV were associated with mild oxygen desaturation (<3%), and only one subject had marked desaturation.[10,36] Moreover, a recent controlled study in patients with neuromuscular disorders showed that NPV resulted in a general improvement in sleep quality and oxygen saturation.[38] It has been reported that in normal subjects during voluntary respiratory muscle relaxation, NPV caused a decrease in the caliber of the upper airway at the glottic or supraglottic level.[39] In normal, awake subjects, the glottis width did not decrease with the increase in negative pressure applied to the chest wall.[40] Consequently, the increasing level of NPV resulted in progressive increases in tidal volume and minute ventilation. On the contrary, control positive-pressure ventilation provided by mask caused inspiratory adduction of the vocal cords, which reduced the tidal volume effectively reaching the lungs.[41,42]

The mechanisms of upper airway obstruction observed with NPV at supraglottic level have not been elucidated fully. During spontaneous breathing, activation of the

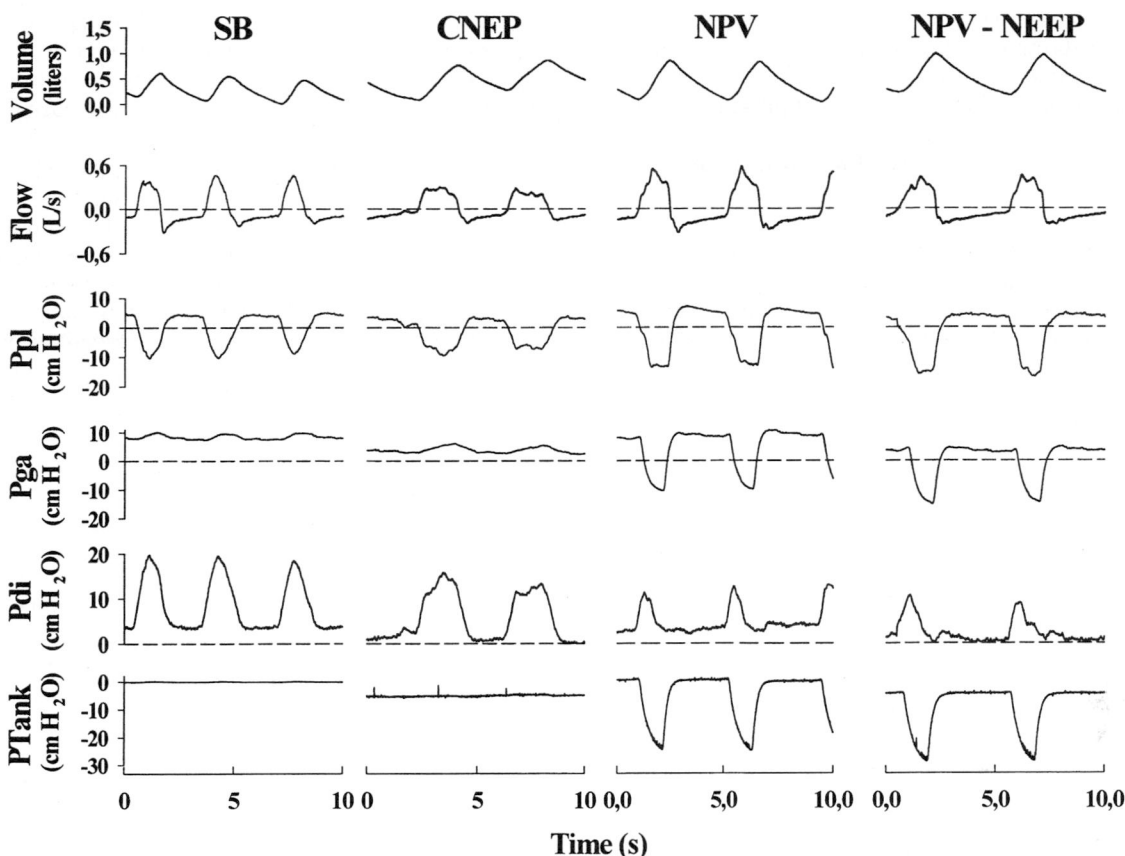

FIGURE 17-8 Recordings of volume, flow, pleural pressure (Ppl), gastric pressure (Pga), transdiaphragmatic pressure (Pdi), and tank pressure (Ptank) in a patient with an acute exacerbation of COPD during spontaneous breathing (SB), continuous negative extrathoracic pressure (CNEP), negative-pressure ventilation (NPV), and negative extrathoracic end-expiratory pressure added to NPV (NPV-NEEP). The dashed lines indicate the level of zero in flow, Ppl, Pga, and Pdi recordings. (*Used, with permission, from Gorini et al: Am J Respir Crit Care Med 163:1614–8, 2001.*)

pharyngeal and laryngeal muscles precedes activation of the inspiratory muscles, resulting in stiffening of the upper airway walls. When NPV is applied during sleep or in completely relaxed subjects, this coordinated respiratory muscle activity may be abolished. Consequently, the subatmospheric pressure developed in the upper airway during inspiration may result in their collapse.[5,10,36,39] Upper airway obstruction has been reported in 2 of 10 patients with acute-on-chronic respiratory failure during treatment with NPV[43] and was the reason for NPV failure in 16% of patients in a large prospective cohort study.[44]

LOWER ESOPHAGEAL SPHINCTER

NPV may induce a lower esophageal sphincter dysfunction in healthy subjects[45] and patients with COPD.[46] This dysfunction may cause regurgitation of stomach contents and expose patients to the risk of aspiration. It can be prevented completely with metoclopramide.[46]

CARDIOVASCULAR

The hemodynamic effects of mechanical ventilation are complex and are the result of changes in intrathoracic pressure and lung volume, which independently can affect the determinants of cardiovascular performance.[47–49] The increase in intrathoracic pressure caused by PPV decreases both venous return to the right ventricle and left-ventricular afterload. The net effect of this reduction depends on the cardiac function. When left-ventricular function is impaired, cardiac output increases in response to the rise in intrathoracic pressure because the decrease in left-ventricular afterload secondary to the reduction in transmural pressure has a greater effect than the decrease in venous return.[50] When left-ventricular function is normal, the increase in intrathoracic pressure reduces cardiac output because the decrease in venous return has more effect than the decrease in left-ventricular afterload.[51] In clinical situations such as hypovolemia, septic shock, and gas trapping associated with airflow obstruction, the reduction in cardiac output is more relevant.[52]

Although the hemodynamic effects of NPV have not been studied extensively,[53] the effects are assumed to be the opposite of those of PPV, that is, more physiologic and more likely to maintain a normal cardiac output. The exposure of the entire body (except for the airway opening) to NPV by tank ventilators, however, results in the same hemodynamic effects as occurs with PPV.[54] These effects occur because intrathoracic pressure actually is raised relative to body surface pressure, reducing the gradient for venous return. This consequence is not seen when NPV is confined to the thorax and upper abdomen using a cuirass or poncho-wrap.[55,56] Unlike tank ventilators, these machines selectively decrease intrathoracic pressure so that right-atrial pressure becomes more negative relative to the rest of body, potentially enhancing the gradient for venous return. In an animal model of acute lung injury, NPV plus NEEP, provided by poncho-wrap, resulted in a similar improvement in gas exchange and in higher cardiac output compared with PPV plus PEEP.[55] In anaesthetized dogs, PPV plus PEEP and NPV plus NEEP applied by iron lung had a similar effect on cardiac output, whereas the latter was higher with NPV plus NEEP applied by poncho-wrap compared with the other two modes.[56]

NPV provided by cuirass does not induce adverse hemodynamic effects in stable patients with COPD,[57] whereas a significant reduction in cardiac output has been reported with mask ventilation with PEEP in patients with COPD both when stable[58] and during acute exacerbations.[59] Short-term studies have compared the effects of CNEP provided by cuirass[60] or poncho-wrap[61,62] with those of PEEP in intubated patients with acute lung injury receiving volume-controlled ventilation. CNEP was adjusted to obtain the same change in transpulmonary pressure[62] or functional residual capacity[60] as with PEEP. The combination of volume-controlled ventilation with CNEP, compared with volume-controlled ventilation with PEEP, resulted in significant increases in oxygen delivery and cardiac index, whereas arterial oxygen content and Pa_{O_2}/F_{IO_2} ratio did not differ between the two modes of ventilation.[60-62] Further studies are required to define the feasibility of long-term clinical treatment with CNEP during controlled ventilation via endotracheal intubation and its effects on clinical outcomes. Children with congenital heart diseases, submitted to right-sided heart surgery with Fontan-type procedures, have unique cardiopulmonary physiology. In the absence of a right ventricle, pulmonary blood flow, the major determinant of cardiac output, is exquisitely sensitive to changes in intrathoracic pressure. In these patients, NPV, provided by cuirass, markedly increased pulmonary blood flow and cardiac output compared with volume-controlled PPV.[63,64]

Rationale, Advantages, and Limitations

RATIONALE

NPV can be used to widen the field of application of noninvasive ventilator techniques. It is well known that compared with standard medical treatment, mask ventilation reduces the need for endotracheal intubation[65-67] and reduces hospital mortality[65-68] in selected patients with an acute exacerbation of COPD. A recent randomized study comparing mask with conventional mechanical ventilation in patients with exacerbations of COPD who failed medical treatment has shown that mask ventilation avoided endotracheal intubation in 48% of patients.[69] Mask ventilation, however, is not without its problems, and failure rates of 7–50% have been reported.[70] Severe respiratory acidosis[71-73] and illness at presentation,[71,74] excessive airway secretions,[74] and in-

ability to minimize the amount of air leakage[74] are major factors associated with failure of this technique. In clinical studies, NPV has been used successfully in patients with severe respiratory acidosis or impaired level of consciousness.[75-77] During NPV, the airway opening is free, unlike in PPV, and consequently, performing bronchial aspiration or fiberoptic bronchoscopy to remove excessive airway secretions is easy. Finally, NPV can be used in patients who cannot tolerate a mask because of facial deformity or as a rescue therapy to avoid endotracheal intubation in those in whom mask ventilation fails. Routine implementation of noninvasive PPV in critically ill patients with acute exacerbations of COPD or severe cardiogenic pulmonary edema was associated with improved survival and reduction of nosocomial infection.[78] For these reasons, mask ventilation is recommended as the standard method of ventilator support for exacerbations of COPD; invasive mechanical ventilation is regarded as second-line rescue therapy when mask ventilation fails.[79] To verify the hypothesis that using both noninvasive mask and iron-lung ventilation should further reduce the need for endotracheal intubation in patients with acute on chronic respiratory failure, a prospective cohort study was carried out in 258 consecutive patients[44]: 77% of patients were treated exclusively with noninvasive ventilation (40% with NPV, 23% with mask, and 14% with the sequential use of both) and 14% with invasive ventilation. In patients in whom NPV or mask ventilation failed, sequential use of the alternative technique allowed a significant reduction in the failure of noninvasive mechanica ventilation (from 23.4% to 8.8%, $p = .002$, and from 25.3% to 5%, $p = .0001$, respectively). Overall hospital mortality (21%) was lower than that estimated by APACHE II score (28%). This study shows that use of NPV and mask ventilation made it possible to avoid endotracheal intubation in the vast majority of unselected patients with acute-on-chronic respiratory disorders needing ventilator support.[44] Another recent study reported that using both modalities of noninvasive ventilation in patients with acute-on-chronic respiratory failure, the total rate of success in avoiding endotracheal intubation was 81.6%.[80]

ADVANTAGES

As with other modalities of noninvasive ventilation, the major advantage of NPV is the avoidance of endotracheal intubation and its related complications[1-4] while preserving physiologic functions such as speech, cough, swallowing, and feeding. Moreover, because the airway opening is free, airway suction and therapeutic and diagnostic maneuvers by fiberoptic bronchoscopy are performed more easily during NPV[43] than during mask ventilation.

LIMITATIONS

The following limitations should be considered when treating patients with NPV. First, the lack of upper airway protection, as with all modalities of noninvasive ventilation, may result in aspiration, especially in unconscious patients. Second, upper airway obstruction may occur or be enhanced in unconscious patients, patients with neurologic disorders that cause bulbar dysfunction, and patients with obstructive

TABLE 17-1 Side Effects and Complications during Negative-Pressure Ventilation in 153 Patients Treated with Iron Lung for Acute-on-Chronic Respiratory Failure

	Number of Patients (%)
Patients with complications	38 (25%)
Upper airway obstruction	24 (16%)
Large air leaks	0 (0%)
Back pain	8 (5%)
Claustrophobia	17 (11.4%)
Gastric insufflation	2 (1.3%)
Major complications	
Patients with complications	3 (2%)
Pneumonia	1 (0.6%)
Pneumothorax	0 (0%)
Gastrointestinal bleeding	3 (2%)

SOURCE: Used, with permission, from Gorini et al.[44]

sleep apnea syndrome.[10,35–37] This effect compromises the effectiveness of ventilation with negative-pressure ventilators and requires shifting to PPV. In unconscious patients with normal bulbar function, the positioning of an oropharyngeal airway can minimize the risk of airway collapse. Third, tank and wrap ventilators restrict patients to the supine position, which may induce muscular back and shoulder pain. Fourth, severe obesity and kyphoscoliosis often compromise the possibility to put the patients in an iron lung or other negative-pressure ventilators.

Most reports of side effects of NPV come from stable, chronically ventilated patients. In these studies, the most common side effects were poor compliance secondary to claustrophobia, upper airway obstruction, and musculoskeletal pain. NPV has been associated with rib fractures and pneumothorax.[21] In an acute setting, 2 of 26 patients

with ARF had uneasiness and back pain, and a further 2 suffered from vomiting during NPV.[76] The incidence of complications and side effects of NPV delivered by iron lung has been evaluated recently in 153 patients with acute-on-chronic respiratory failure[44] (Table 17-1). While NPV outcomes, such as complications and mortality rate, are within the ranges reported for noninvasive PPV,[81] it must be stressed that there are some difficulties in introducing this modality in the vast majority of ICUs, where mask ventilation is preferred as a noninvasive means of ventilation.[82,83] The main reasons are that the iron lung is cumbersome and needs a large amount of space, and most caregivers presently have little or no experience with NPV, rather than problems associated with NPV per se.

Indications and Contraindications

ACUTE RESPIRATORY FAILURE

CHRONIC OBSTRUCTIVE PULMONARY DISEASE
Sauret et al[84] studied 17 patients with severe COPD in hypercapnic ARF. All patients underwent NPV, delivered by poncho-wrap for 6 hours, with significant improvement in arterial blood gases and pH, suggesting that this technique may prevent the need for more aggressive ventilation.

Large studies with different experimental designs have confirmed the effectiveness of NPV in the treatment of patients with acute-on-chronic respiratory failure caused mainly by COPD[44,76,80,85–90] (Table 17-2). In a pioneer study in 560 patients, 475 of whom had exacerbations of COPD, NPV, provided by iron lung, was applied successfully, resulting in improved gas exchange with an overall mortality rate of 10.5%.[85] This rate was comparable with that reported in a more recent study that analyzed retrospectively

TABLE 17-2 Clinical Studies on the Effects of NPV in Patients with Acute-on-Chronic Respiratory Failure

Authors	Experimental Design	Number of Patients	COPD (%)	Setting	Ventilator	Success[a] (%)
Gunella et al: Ann Med Physique, 1980	RS	560	84	Respiratory ICU	Iron lung	90
Corrado et al: Monaldi Arch Chest Dis, 1994	RS	2564	78	Respiratory ICU	Iron lung	90
Corrado et al: Chest, 1992	RS	105	100	Respiratory ICU	Iron lung	89
Corrado et al: Thorax, 1996	RS	150	79	Respiratory ICU	Iron lung	70
Todisco et al: Chest, 2004	PCS	152	72	Respiratory ICU	Iron lung	84
Gorini et al: Intensive Care Med, 2004	PCS	258	70	Respiratory ICU	Iron lung	77
Corrado et al: Eur Respir J, 1998	CCS (NPV vs invasive MV)	66	100	Respiratory ICU	Iron lung	77 vs 73
Corrado et al: Chest, 2002	CCS (NPV vs mask ventilation)	106	100	Respiratory ICU	Iron lung	79 vs 75
Corrado et al: Eur Respir J, 1998	RCS (NPV vs invasive MV)	44	100	Respiratory ICU	Iron lung	82 vs 73

[a] Avoiding endotracheal intubation or death; RS, retrospective study; PCS, prospective cohort study; CCS, case-control study; RCS, prospective, randomized, controlled study.

16 years of activity in a respiratory ICU.[86] Between 1975 and 1991, 2564 patients with ARF (2011 with COPD and 553 with restrictive thoracic disorders) were treated with NPV, provided by iron lung, and hospital mortality rate was 9.9%.[86] NPV used as first-line treatment in patients with severe COPD in ARF is also associated with a good long-term prognosis.[87] In 105 patients with COPD treated with an iron lung for ARF, the survival rates after 1 and 5 years were 82% and 37%, respectively.[87] Although comparisons with previous studies can be subjected to biases, this long-term survival is better than that reported previously in patients with COPD treated with conventional ventilation.[91]

The effectiveness of NPV provided by iron lung in patients with hypercapnic encephalopathy was evaluated retrospectively in 150 consecutive patients (79% with COPD).[75] On admission, severe hypoxemia ($Pa_{O_2} = 56 \pm 22$ mmHg) and hypercapnia ($Pa_{CO_2} = 112 \pm 21$ mmHg) with respiratory acidosis (pH 7.13 ± 0.13) were present, Glasgow coma score ranged from 3 to 8, and the mean APACHE II score was 31.6 ± 5.3. The failure rate of NPV (death or need for endotracheal intubation) was 45 of 150 (30%); the observed mortality rate was 24% versus 67.5% predicted mortality based on APACHE II. Nine patients (6%) required intubation because of a lack of control of the airway. In recent years, the effectiveness of NPV for the treatment of acute-on-chronic respiratory failure in patients with COPD has been confirmed in two case-control studies and in one randomized, prospective control study[76,89,90] (see Table 17-2).

NEUROMUSCULAR DISORDERS

Few uncontrolled studies have investigated the effect of NPV in the treatment of neuromuscular patients with ARF. NPV, provided by iron lung[92–94] or pneumowrap,[95] was successful in avoiding endotracheal intubation and in facilitating weaning from invasive ventilation in small groups of patients. We have reported in a retrospective study the effects of NPV provided by iron lung in the treatment of 15 neuromuscular patients with ARF.[96] On admission, all patients exhibited severe hypoxemia ($Pa_{O_2} = 37.6 \pm 12.4$ mmHg) and hypercapnia ($Pa_{CO_2} = 88.2 \pm 20.4$ mmHg) with uncompensated respiratory acidosis (pH 7.25 ± 0.08). The treatment was successful in 12 of 15 patients (80%). A recent retrospective study, published in abstract form, analyzed the outcome of 65 neuromuscular patients with ARF treated with NPV or mask ventilation.[97] There was no significant difference in mortality rate and need for endotracheal intubation between the groups despite more severe clinical condition on admission in the NPV than in the mask ventilation group. Although these reports suggest that NPV can be effective in the treatment of ARF in patients with neuromuscular diseases, prospective, controlled studies are needed to clarify the impact of noninvasive ventilation on clinical outcome in these patients.

PEDIATRIC DISEASES

During the 1970s, several uncontrolled[98–100] and controlled[101,102] studies showed that NPV was effective in the management of the neonatal respiratory distress syndrome. In 1989, Samuels and Southall[103] reported, in an uncontrolled clinical trial, the effects of NPV in patients with respira-

tory failure secondary to bronchopulmonary dysplasia and neonatal distress syndrome. Of 40 patients intubated at the start of treatment, 28 were extubated successfully with the aid of NPV and 24 survived. More recently, Samuels et al[104] performed a prospective, randomized, controlled trial over a period of 4 years in 244 neonates comparing CNEP (−4 to −6 cmH$_2$O) with standard therapy that included CPAP of 4 cmH$_2$O. They found that need for intubation was slightly less with CNEP than with standard therapy (86% versus 91%).

Infants with ARF who fail to respond to conventional ventilation are considered elective candidates for extracorporeal membrane oxygenation. Although this technique can be lifesaving, it is associated with significant complications[105] and a high mortality rate.[106] In 1989, an uncontrolled study reported that the use of CNEP administered by a tank ventilator in conjunction with invasive ventilation was successful in five neonates suffering from respiratory failure and persistent pulmonary hypertension, thus avoiding the use of extracorporeal membrane oxygenation.[107] The benefit of combining invasive ventilation and CNEP in these patients has been confirmed by the same group in a crossover prospective, randomized study.[108] Patients treated with CNEP showed a greater increase in Pa_{O_2} than those treated with PEEP without any increase in morbidity.

CHRONIC RESPIRATORY FAILURE

CHRONIC OBSTRUCTIVE PULMONARY DISEASE

Based on the hypothesis that chronic hypercapnia in patients with severe COPD may be caused by an excessive load on the inspiratory muscles, several studies have evaluated the effects of NPV provided by poncho-wrap in terms of improvement in arterial blood gases, muscle function, and exercise performance.[21,28,109–111] These studies, carried out in small number of patients, produced conflicting results. In 1992, Shapiro et al[112] published the results of the largest trial on the effects of NPV in 184 patients with COPD (92 patients and 92 controls, with mean Pa_{CO_2} of 44 ± 7 mmHg). The distance walked in 6 minutes was the primary outcome variable, with severity of dyspnea, quality of life, arterial blood gases, and respiratory muscle strength as secondary outcomes. There was no evidence of significant difference in any outcome measurements between the two groups. Compliance of the patients was poor, and the mean duration of the ventilator use was 2.4 and 3.0 hours in the active and control groups, respectively. In summary, there is no evidence that long-term NPV treatment can improve respiratory muscle function, exercise endurance, quality of life, and survival in patients with severe COPD. Also NPV, provided in control mode by cuirass or pneumowrap, is poorly tolerated by stable patients with COPD in a typical outpatient setting. It is important to stress that until now, no other ventilator techniques has been shown to be effective in the long-term treatment of stable patients with COPD.

RESTRICTIVE DISORDERS

Many studies, although uncontrolled, have shown that NPV can be used successfully for long-term home ventilation in patients with restrictive ventilatory impairment secondary to neuromuscular and chest-wall diseases.[113–118] NPV devices, however, are more cumbersome and difficult to use than recent home positive-pressure ventilators. Although direct comparisons between the efficiency of NPV and mask ventilation are rare, in patients with muscular dystrophy and bulbar weakness, NPV tends to predispose patients to obstructive apneas during sleep.[119] For these reasons, NPV largely has been supplanted by mask ventilation in the last decade. In experienced hands, NPV remains a second choice in patients who, for technical or other reasons, cannot be offered mask ventilation. Brief discontinuation of mask ventilation secondary to intolerable nasal irritation or upper airway congestion may result in significant worsening of the arterial blood gases in some patients with chronic respiratory failure.[120] In these patients and in those with other clinical conditions, such as facial deformity or lack of teeth, NPV should be used as an alternative to mask ventilation.

OTHER APPLICATIONS

NPV DURING RIGID BRONCHOSCOPY

Some studies have evaluated the effectiveness of NPV provided by poncho-wrap[121–123] or cuirass[123] compared with spontaneous assisted ventilation (manual assisted ventilation with an anesthesia bag if Sa_{O_2} fell below 90%) in patients submitted to interventional rigid bronchoscopy under general anesthesia. In nonparalyzed patients, NPV was able to prevent apnea and significant intraoperative derangement of acid-base balance.[121] A subsequent study has shown that NPV reduced administration of opioids, shortened recovery time, and prevented respiratory acidosis in anesthetized and paralyzed patients who underwent rigid bronchoscopy.[122] Both intermittent NPV and external high-frequency oscillation ensure effective ventilation and a comfortable operating condition in most patients during rigid broncoschopy.[123]

Comparison with Other Modes

NPV VERSUS IMV

Two studies have compared the effects of NPV and conventional mechanical ventilation in patients with COPD and severe ARF.[76,90] A retrospective case-control study was carried out in 66 patients who underwent NPV or invasive mechanical ventilation (IMV).[76] The primary end points were in-hospital death for both groups and the need for endotracheal intubation in patients treated with NPV. Mortality rate was 23.1% in the NPV group and 26.9% in the group treated with IMV. The duration of ventilation in survivors was significantly lower with NPV than with IMV, with a median of 22.5 hours (range 2–114 hours) versus 96 hours (range 12–336 hours). Length of hospital stay was similar in both groups. These findings have been confirmed recently in a prospective, randomized, controlled study.[90] Forty-four patients with an exacerbation of COPD and severe respiratory acidosis (mean pH 7.20 ± 0.04) were assigned either to iron-lung ventilation (22 patients) or IMV (22 patients). Primary end points were improvement in gas exchange and compli-

cations related to mechanical ventilation. Compared with baseline, NPV and IMV induced a similar and significant improvement in Pa_{O_2}/Fi_{O_2}, Pa_{CO_2}, and pH after 1 hour and at discontinuation of treatments. Among patients treated with NPV, four (18.2%) needed endotracheal intubation. Major complications tended to be more frequent in patients treated with IMV than in those treated with NPV (27.3% versus 4.5%), whereas mortality rate was similar (27.3% versus 18.2%). Ventilator-free days and length of hospital stay were significantly lower in the iron-lung group than in the IMV group. This study suggests that iron-lung ventilation is as effective as IMV in improving gas exchange in patients with COPD and ARF and is associated with a tendency toward a lower rate of major complications.

NPV VERSUS NONINVASIVE PPV

A direct comparison between the two noninvasive ventilator techniques in the treatment of patients with COPD in ARF has been recently reported in a retrospective case-control study involving 53 pairs of patients treated with iron-lung and mask ventilation.[89] The two groups were matched according to age, sex, causes of ARF, APACHE II score, pH (7.26 ± 0.05 versus 7.27 ± 0.04), and Pa_{CO_2} (88.1 ± 11.5 versus 85.1 ± 13.5 mmHg) on admission. Treatment failure (death and/or need for endotracheal intubation) was 20.7% in the NPV group and 24.5% in the mask ventilation group. Duration of mechanical ventilation (29.6 ± 28.6 versus 62.3 ± 35.7 hours) and length of hospital stay (10.4 ± 4.3 versus 15 ± 5.2 days) were significantly lower in patients treated with NPV than in those treated with mask ventilation. These findings suggest that both ventilator techniques are equally effective in avoiding endotracheal intubation and death in patients with COPD in ARF. This finding has been confirmed recently by preliminary results of a multicenter prospective, randomized, controlled study[124] carried out in 73 patients (39 assigned to NPV and 34 to mask ventilation). The rate of success was similar for the two techniques. Among the failures of the first ventilator treatment, endotracheal intubation was avoided in 64.3% of patients when one of the two techniques was used as rescue of the other. Hospital mortality rate and hospital stay were similar for patients treated with NPV and mask ventilation. These data show that NPV is as effective as mask ventilation for the treatment of patients with COPD in ARF; when the two techniques are combined, endotracheal intubation can be avoided in a high percentage of patients.

Variations in Delivery among Ventilator Brands

The characteristics of modern negative-pressure pumps are reported in Table 17-3. A study by Smith et al[9] on five negative-pressure ventilator pumps, using a lung model, showed that tidal volume during NPV is related both to target pressure and the pressure waveform generated by the pump. For the same target negative pressure, pumps able to generate a square wave produce a tidal volume up to

TABLE 17-3 Characteristics of Some Negative-Pressure Ventilator Pumps

Model	Inspiratory Pressure, cmH_2O	Expiratory Pressure, cmH_2O	CNEP, cmH_2O	T_I, s	T_E, s	Ventilation Modes	Inspiratory Trigger	Pump	Alarms
Iron Lung Coppa CA 1001	0 to −80	−30 to +80	0 to −30	0.4–9.9	0.4–9.9	C, A/C, CNEP	Thermistor	Inside the model	Pmax, MF
Porta Lung Emerson 33=CR	0 to −90	—	Yes	Up to 5	[a]	C, A/C, A, CNEP	Pressure	Outside	No
Porta Lung Life Care NEV-100, Respironics	−5 to −100	−30 to +30	−5 to −30	0.5–5	[b]	C, A/C, C+S, A/C+S	Pressure	Outside	Pmin, MF
New Negavent Respirator Mod DA-3, Dima	−5 to −99	−25 to +99	−5 to −99	[c]	[c]	C, A/C, CNEP	Pressure	Outside	Pmax, Pmin

[a] Rate 0–49 cycles/min; I/E ratio: 1/3 to inverse ratio.
[b] Rate 4–60 cycles/min; I/E ratio: 1/0.5 to 1/29.
[c] Rate 5–50 cycles/min; I/E ratio 1/99 to 5/1.
ABBREVIATIONS: CNEP, continuous negative extrathoracic pressure; T_I, inspiratory time; T_E, expiratory time; I/E, inspiratory expiratory ratio; C, control; A/C, assist control; A, assist; S, sigh; Pmax, maximum pressure; Pmin, minimum pressure; MF, machine failure.

30% greater than pumps that generate a half sine wave.[9] Most modern negative-pressure ventilator pumps respond rapidly to changing leaks to maintain the preset pressure[9] and allow independent setting of the pressure to be delivered during inspiration and expiration, as well as inspiratory and expiratory duration.

Adjustments at the Bedside

Guidelines concerning the bedside management of patients ventilated with NPV are scarce.[6,8] The effectiveness of NPV depends on strict supervision by well-trained nurses and physiotherapists with considerable expertise in this technique. Proper fit of the airtight seal around the neck and correct position of the head and neck rest are very important in optimizing comfort and preventing kinking and upper airway obstruction.[6] Values ranging from −30 to −40 cmH_2O have been recommended for the setting of negative pressure during inspiration.[6] In our experience, the setting of pressures and timing depends on the clinical condition and chest-wall impedance of patients. In patients with severe respiratory acidosis and hypercapnic encephalopathy, we used control NPV with a frequency of 12–15 cycles per minute and an I:E ratio of 1:3–1:4, whereas assist-control NPV is used preferentially in patients with tachypnea and respiratory distress to facilitate patient-ventilator synchrony. Inspiratory negative pressure is set initially at values ranging from −30 to −40 cmH_2O and then adjusted in each patient to obtain a tidal volume of about 6 ml/kg.[89] Positive expiratory pressures of 10–15 cmH_2O are set to assist cough in patients with excessive secretions[8] or to increase tidal volume in restrictive disorders[14]; negative extrathoracic expiratory pressure is set to counterbalance intrinsic PEEP in patients with COPD (usually ranging from −4 to −6 cmH_2O)[12] or to improve oxygenation in patients with severe hypoxemia (ranging from −5 to −10 cmH_2O). Arterial blood gases are checked approximately 30 minutes after mechanical ventilation starts and after any setting

changes. During NPV, oxygen is supplemented by nasal cannula, venturi mask, or mask with reservoir. The flow is adjusted to keep O_2 saturation usually between 92% and 94%. Bronchodilators also can be administered by metered-dose inhaler or by aerosol.

Troubleshooting

Many problems must be considered when treating acute patients with negative-pressure ventilators.

SETTING IN CONTROL MODE

The old iron-lung models have only this mode of ventilation, which may cause patients to "fight the ventilator," resulting in discomfort and ineffective ventilation. In order to "capture" the patient to the superimposed frequency of the machine, we can operate mainly on the timing. Table 17-4 reports some examples of iron-lung settings in the control mode to overcome this concern.

TABLE 17-4 Typical Setting of Iron Lung Used in Control Mode for the Treatment of Patients with Acute-on-Chronic Respiratory Failure

- Negative inspiratory pressure: Usually from −30 to −40 cmH_2O at first and then adjusted in order to obtain a tidal volume of about 6 ml/kg
- Expiratory positive pressure: From +10 to +15 cmH_2O in patients with excessive secretions to assist cough or to improve patient-ventilator synchrony
- The timing must be adjusted some breaths below patient's spontaneous rate
- Typical setting for a ventilatory rate of 15 cycles/min: $T_I = 1.2$ s; $T_E = 2.8$ s; ($T_I/T_{TOT} = 30\%$)
- Typical setting for a ventilatory rate of 27 cycles/min: $T_I = 0.8$ s; $T_E = 1.4$ s; ($T_I/T_{TOT} = 36\%$); when patient is "captured," respiratory rate is reduced progressively

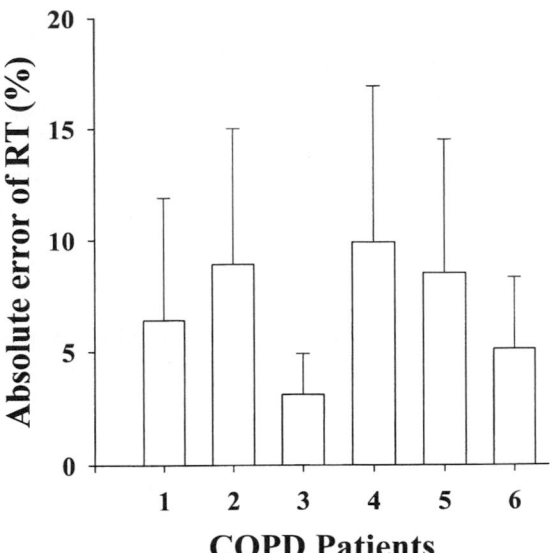

FIGURE 17-9 Error of inductance plethysmography (Respitrace, RT) in estimating tidal volume during NPV in patients with an acute exacerbation of COPD. The error of the Respitrace was assessed as $(V_{T,Respitrace} - V_{T,pneumotachograph})/V_{T,pneumotachograph} \times 100$. Individual values are shown.

MONITORING OF TIDAL VOLUME

During NPV, the patient airway opening is free, which is a disadvantage for continuous monitoring of tidal volume. Currently, tidal volume is monitored intermittently using a Wright spirometer connected to a face mask. Continuous monitoring can be achieved with the use of inductance plethysmography (Respitrace), which permits an indirect evaluation of tidal volume. Recently, we have compared tidal volume measured by a pneumotachograph and by Respitrace in patients with COPD in acute exacerbation treated by iron lung. The error of the Respitrace, assessed as $(V_{T,Respitrace} - V_{T,pneumotachograph})/V_{T,pneumotacograph} \times 100$, ranged from 3% to 10% (Fig. 17-9). These observations suggest that inductance plethysmography may be a useful tool, allowing continuous estimate of tidal volume during NPV.

NURSING CARE

The major problems related to the assistance of patients with NPV by iron lung are transfer from the bed to inside the chamber of the tank ventilator and access to patients for nursing procedures during ventilation. Well-trained nurses, however, can manage both transfer, by using aids (e.g., a roll mattress and a mechanical elevator), and nursing procedures (e.g., insertion of a urinary catheter and venous lines, placement of electrocardiograph electrodes and Sa_{O_2} probe for monitoring the level of oxygenation) easily using the portholes in the tank ventilator. We have measured the time spent by nurses in the second day after admission in patients with COPD in ARF treated with the iron lung.[77] The following procedures were considered: transfer of patients from the bed to inside the tank ventilator, measurement of tidal volume and minute ventilation by a Wright spirometer, tracheobronchial suction, arterial blood-gas sampling,

drug administration, and other procedures. The total time spent by nurses for these procedures was 250 minutes. Even though there are no studies comparing nursing workload in patients submitted to NPV and IMV, Nava et al[125] have reported that nursing workload in patients treated with IMV was 527.5 ± 51.1 minutes in the first 48 hours after admission.

Important Unknowns

It is completely unknown if NPV may play a role in the treatment of patients with acute lung injury. Physiologic studies[60–62] have shown the advantageous hemodynamic effects of NPV applied to the chest wall in patients with acute lung injury, although studies on clinical outcomes are completely lacking. The absence of this information is particularly relevant because some physiologic studies suggest that NPV may result in reduced lung biotrauma compared with PPV.[126–129] Physiologic studies[54,56] show that NPV by iron lung has the same hemodynamic effects as PPV. Future studies should determine whether iron-lung ventilation may be applied successfully to patients with cardiogenic pulmonary edema.

The Future

INSPIRATORY TRIGGER SYSTEM

Sinderby et al[130] used diaphragmatic electrical activity, recorded by electrodes attached to a nasogastric tube, to trigger ventilatory support. This signal is directly related to phrenic nerve activity and probably to the output of the respiratory center; unlike airway pressure or flow, it is not affected by mechanical dysfunction (dynamic hyperinflation and intrinsic PEEP). By overcoming the problem associated with the current technology for triggering, this "neural trigger" has the potential to improve patient-ventilator interaction during both positive- and negative-pressure mechanical ventilation.

DESIGN OF TANK VENTILATOR

Most iron lungs, although improved in design, remain cumbersome and need a large amount of space. A lighter and completely transparent chamber incorporated into the ICU bed would enable the posture of patients to be changed from supine to semirecumbent. This step should permit a major implementation of NPV in the ICU.

POTENTIAL CLINICAL APPLICATION

The clinical relevance of intra-abdominal pressure, which may cause organ dysfunction, is being recognized increasingly in the ICU settings.[131,132] Decompressive laparatomy is recommended when intra-abdominal pressure exceeds 25 mmHg,[133] although there are no definite techniques of intervention for pressures between 12 and 25 mmHg. It has been suggested that NPV applied around the abdomen by a cuirass might be a potential tool to treat intra-abdominal hypertension.[134] This hypothesis has been investigated recently in a physiologic study of 30 patients admitted to an ICU.[135] Continuous NPV decreased intra-abdominal pressure from 8.7 ± 4.3 to 6 ± 4.2 mmHg ($p < .001$). There was a further decrease in intra-abdominal pressure when more negative pressure was applied. These data suggest that in a population of critically ill patients, NPV may be used to decrease intra-abdominal pressure. Future studies with clinical outcome will be necessary to assess the effectiveness of this technique for the treatment of increased abdominal pressure.

Summary and Conclusions

Evidence now exists that (1) NPV unloads respiratory muscles and improves gas exchange in patients with COPD and ARF, (2) volume-controlled ventilation with CNEP, compared with volume-controlled ventilation with PEEP, increases oxygen delivery and cardiac index in patients with acute lung injury and children submitted to right-sided heart surgery, (3) iron-lung ventilation, in expert hands, is as effective as mask ventilation and invasive ventilation in the treatment of acute-on-chronic respiratory failure, and (4) NPV can been used successfully for home mechanical ventilation in patients with chronic respiratory failure who are unable to tolerate mask ventilation. Furthermore, the use of both NPV and mask ventilation may avoid endotracheal intubation and its complications in most of these patients, widening the field of application of noninvasive ventilator techniques.

References

1. Tobin MJ. Mechanical ventilation. New Engl J Med 1994; 330:1056–61.
2. Mehta S, Hill NS. Noninvasive ventilation. Am J Respir Crit Care Med 2001; 163:540–77.
3. Pingleton SK. Complications of acute respiratory failure. Am Rev Respir Dis 1988; 137:1463–93.
4. Fagon JY, Chastre J, Hance AJ, et al. Nosocomial pneumonia in ventilated patients: A cohort study evaluating attributable mortality and hospital stay. Am J Med 1993; 94:281–8.
5. Levine S, Henson D. Negative pressure ventilation. In: Tobin MJ, editor. Principles and practice of mechanical ventilation, 1st ed. New York: McGraw–Hill, 1994: 393.
6. Shneerson JM. Non-invasive and domiciliary ventilation: Negative pressure techniques. Thorax 1991; 46:131–5.
7. Corrado A, Gorini M, Villella G, et al. Negative pressure ventilation in the treatment of acute respiratory failure: An old noninvasive technique reconsidered. Eur Respir J 1996; 9:1531–44.
8. Hill NS. Clinical applications of body ventilators. Chest 1986; 90:897–905.
9. Smith IE, King MA, Shneerson JM. Choosing a negative pressure ventilation pump: Are there any important differences? Eur Respir J 1995; 8:1792–5.
10. Levy RD, Cosio MG, Gibbons L, et al. Induction of sleep apnea with negative pressure ventilation in patients with chronic obstructive lung disease. Thorax 1992; 47:612–5.
11. Aaron J, McCool FD, Benditt J, Hill NS. Evaluation of trigger sensitivity of patient-triggered negative pressure ventilators. Am J Respir Crit Care Med 1995; 151:A237.
12. Gorini M, Villella G, Ginanni R, et al. Effects of assist negative pressure ventilation by microprocessor-based iron lung on breathing effort. Thorax 2002; 57:258–62.
13. Aslanian P, Atrous S, Isabey D, et al. Effects of flow triggering on breathing effort during partial ventilatory support. Am J Respir Crit Care Med 1998; 157:135–43.
14. Kinnear W, Petch M, Taylor G, Shneerson J. Assisted ventilation using cuirass respirators. Eur Respir J 1988; 1:198–203.
15. Al-Saady NM, Fernando SSD, Petros AJ, et al. External high frequency oscillation in normal subjects and in patients with acute respiratory failure. Anaesthesia 1995; 50:1031–5.
16. Spitzer SA, Fink G, Mittelman M. External high-frequency ventilation in severe chronic obstructive pulmonary disease. Chest 1993; 104:1698–1701.
17. Sideno B, Vaage J. Ventilation by external high-frequency oscillations improves cardiac function after coronary artery bypass grafting. Eur J Cardiothorac Surg 1997; 11:248–57.
18. Lassen HCA. A preliminary report on the 1952 epidemic of poliomyelitis in Copenhagen with special reference to the treatment of acute respiratory insufficiency. Lancet 1953; 1:37–41.
19. Lovejoy FW, Yu PNG, Nye RE, et al. Pulmonary hypertension: III. Physiological studies in three cases of carbon dioxide narcosis treated by artificial respiration. Am J Med 1954; 16:4–11.
20. Marks A, Bocles J, Morganti L. A new ventilatory assister for patients with respiratory acidosis. New Engl J Med 1963; 268: 61–7.
21. Zibrack JD, Hill NS, Federman EC, et al. Evaluation of intermittent long-term negative pressure ventilation in patients with severe chronic obstructive pulmonary disease. Am Rev Respir Dis 1988; 138:1515–8.
22. Cooper CB, Harris ND, Howard P. Acute effects of external negative pressure ventilation in chronic obstructive pulmonary disease compared with normal subjects. Eur Respir J 1991; 4:63–8.
23. Gorini M, Corrado A, Villella G, et al. Physiologic effects of negative pressure ventilation in acute exacerbation of COPD. Am J Respir Crit Care Med 2001; 163:1614–8.
24. Corrado A, Bruscoli G, De Paola E, et al. Respiratory muscle insufficiency in acute respiratory failure of subjects with severe COPD: Treatment with intermittent negative pressure ventilation. Eur Respir J 1990; 3:644–8.
25. Montserrat JM, Martos JA, Alarcon A, et al. Effect of negative pressure ventilation on arterial blood gas pressure and inspiratory muscle strength during an exacerbation of chronic obstructive lung disease. Thorax 1991; 46:6–8.
26. Nava S, Ambrosino N, Zocchi L, et al. Diaphragmatic rest during negative pressure ventilation by pneumowrap: Assessment in normal and COPD patients. Chest 1990; 98:850–6.
27. Gigliotti F, Duranti R, Fabiani A, et al. Suppression of ventilatory muscle activity in healthy subjects and COPD patients with negative pressure ventilation. Chest 1991; 99:1186–92.
28. Gigliotti F, Spinelli A, Duranti R, et al. Four-week negative pressure ventilation improves respiratory function in severe hypercapnic COPD patients. Chest 1994; 105:87–94.
29. Belman MJ, Soo Hoo GW, Kuei JH, et al. Efficacy of positive vs negative pressure evaluation in unloading respiratory muscles. Chest 1990; 98:850–6.
30. Rochester DF, Braun NMT, Laine S. Diaphragmatic energy expenditure in chronic respiratory failure: The effect of assisted ventilation with body respirators. Am J Med 1977; 63: 223–32.
31. Rodenstein DO, Stanescu DC, Cuttita G, et al. Ventilatory and diaphragmatic EMG responses to negative pressure ventilation in airflow obstruction. J Appl Physiol 1988; 65:1621–6.

32. Nishino T, Isono S, Ide T. Effects of negative pressure assisted ventilation on dyspnoeic sensation and breathing pattern. Eur Respir J 1998; 12:1278–83.

33. Appendini L, Patessio A, Zanaboni S, et al. Physiologic effects of positive end-expiratory pressure and mask pressure support during exacerbations of chronic obstructive pulmonary disease. Am J Respir Crit Care Med 1994; 149:1069–76.

34. Leung P, Jubran A, Tobin MJ. Comparison of assisted ventilator modes on triggering, patient effort, and dyspnea. Am J Respir Crit Care Med 1997; 155:1940–8.

35. Levy RD, Bradley TD, Newman SL, et al. Negative pressure ventilation: Effects on ventilation during sleep in normal subjects. Chest 1989; 95:95–9.

36. Hill NS, Redline S, Carskadon MA, et al. Sleep-disordered breathing in patients with Duchenne muscular dystrophy using negative pressure ventilators. Chest 1992; 102:1656–62.

37. Bach JR, Penek J. Obstructive sleep apnea complicating negative pressure ventilatory support in patients with chronic paralytic/restrictive ventilatory dysfunction. Chest 1991; 99:1386–93.

38. Schiavina M, Fabbri A. Intermittent negative pressure ventilation in patients with respiratory failure. Monaldi Arch Chest Dis 1993; 48:169–75.

39. Sanna A, Veriter C, Stanescu D. Upper airway obstruction induced by negative-pressure ventilation in awake healthy subjects. J Appl Physiol 1993; 75:546–52.

40. Glerant JC, Jounieaux V, Parreira VF, et al. Effects of intermittent negative pressure ventilation on effective ventilation in normal awake subjects. Chest 2002; 122:99–107.

41. Jounieaux V, Aubert G, Dury M, et al. Effects of nasal positive-pressure hyperventilation on the glottis in normal awake subjects. J Appl Physiol 1995; 79:176–85.

42. Parreira VF, Jounieaux V, Aubert G, et al. Nasal two-level positive-pressure ventilation in normal subjects. Am J Respir Crit Care Med 1996; 153:1616–23.

43. Todisco T, Eslami A, Scarcella L, et al. Flexible bronchoscopy during iron lung mechanical ventilation in nonintubated patients. J Bronchol 1995; 2:200–5.

44. Gorini M, Ginanni R, Villella G, et al. Non-invasive negative and positive pressure ventilation in the treatment of acute on chronic respiratory failure. Intensive Care Med 2004; 30:875–81.

45. Marino WD, Jain NK, Pitchumoni CS. Induction of lower esophageal sphincter (LES) dysfunction during use of the negative pressure body ventilator. Am J Gastroenterol 1988; 83:1376–80.

46. Marino WD, Pitchumoni CS. Reversal of negative pressure ventilation induced lower esophageal sphincter dysfunction with metoclopramide. Am J Gastroenterol 1992; 87:190–4.

47. Pinsky MR. The effects of mechanical ventilation on the cardiovascular system. Crit Care Med 1990; 6:663–78.

48. Pinsky MR. The hemodynamic consequences of mechanical ventilation an evolving story. Intensive Care Med 1997; 23:493–503.

49. Takata M, Robotham JL. Effects of inspiratory diaphragmatic descent on inferior vena caval venous return. J Appl Physiol 1992; 72:597–607.

50. Pinsky MR, Summer WR. Cardiac augmentation by phasic high intrathoracic support in man. Chest 1983; 84.370–5.

51. Cassidy SA, Wead WB, Seibert GB, et al. Geometric left ventricular responses to interaction between the lung and left ventricle: Positive pressure breathing. Ann Biomed Eng 1987; 15:373–83.

52. Jardin F, Farcot JC, Boisante L, et al. Influence of positive end-expiratory pressure on left ventricular performance. New Engl J Med 1981; 304.387–92.

53. Krumpe PE, Zidulka A, Urbanetti J, et al. Comparison of the effects of continuous negative external chest pressure and positive end-expiratory pressure on cardiac index in dogs. Am Rev Respir Dis 1977; 115:39–45.

54. Maloney JV, Whittenberger JL. Clinical implication of pressures used in the body respirator. Am J Med Sci 1951; 221:425–30.

55. Skabursis M, Helal R, Zidulka A. Hemodynamic effects of external continuous negative pressure ventilation compared with those of continuous positive pressure ventilation in dogs with acute lung injury. Am Rev Respir Dis 1987; 136:886–91.

56. Lockhat D, Langleben D, Zidulka A. Hemodynamic differences between continuous positive and two types of negative pressure ventilation. Am Rev Respir Dis 1992; 146:677–80.

57. Ambrosino N, Cobelli F, Torbicki A, et al. Hemodynamic effects of negative-pressure ventilation in patients with COPD. Chest 1990; 97:850–6.

58. Ambrosino N, Nava S, Torbicki A, et al. Haemodynamic effects of pressure support and PEEP ventilation by nasal route in patients with stable chronic obstructive pulmonary disease. Thorax 1993; 48:523–8.

59. Diaz O, Iglesia R, Ferrer M, et al. Effects of noninvasive ventilation on pulmonary gas exchange and hemodynamics during acute hypercapnic exacerbations of chronic obstructive pulmonary disease. Am J Respir Crit Care Med 1997; 156:1840–5.

60. Scholz SE, Knothe C, Thiel A, Hempelmann G. Improved oxygen delivery by positive pressure ventilation with continuous negative external chest pressure. Lancet 1997; 349:1295–6.

61. Torelli L, Zoccali G, Casarin M, et al. Comparative evaluation of the haemodynamic effects of continuous negative external pressure (CNEP) and positive end-expiratory pressure (PEEP) in mechanically ventilated trauma patients. Intensive Care Med 1995; 21:67–70.

62. Borelli M, Benini A, Denkevitz T, et al. Effects of continuous negative extrathoracic pressure versus positive end-expiratory pressure in acute lung injury patients. Crit Care Med 1998; 26:1025–31.

63. Shekerdemian LS, Shore DF, Lincoln C, et al. Negative pressure ventilation improves cardiac output after right hearth surgery. Circulation 1996; 94:49–55.

64. Shekerdemian LS, Bush A, Shore DF, et al. Cardiopulmonary interaction after Fontan operations: Augmentation of cardiac output using negative pressure ventilation. Circulation 1997; 96:3934–42.

65. Brochard L, Mancebo J, Wysochi M, et al. Noninvasive ventilation for acute exacerbations of chronic obstructive pulmonary disease. New Engl J Med 1995; 333:817–22.

66. Kramer N, Meyer TJ, Meharg J, et al. Randomized, prospective trial of noninvasive positive pressure ventilation in acute respiratory failure. Am J Respir Crit Care Med 1995; 151:1799–806.

67. Plant PK, Owen JL, Elliott MW. Early use of non-invasive ventilation for acute exacerbations of chronic obstructive pulmonary disease on general respiratory wards: A multicentre randomised, controlled trial. Lancet 2000; 355:1931–5.

68. Bott J, Carroll MP, Conway JH, et al. Randomised, controlled trial of nasal ventilation in acute ventilatory failure due to chronic obstructive airways disease. Lancet 1993; 341:1555–7.

69. Conti G, Antonelli M, Navalesi P, et al. Noninvasive vs conventional mechanical ventilation in patients with chronic obstructive pulmonary disease after failure of medical treatment in the ward: A randomized trial. Intensive Care Med 2002; 28:1701–7.

70. Lightowler JVJ, Elliott MW. Predicting the outcome of NIV for acute exacerbations of COPD. Thorax 2000, 55:815–6.

71. Ambrosino N, Foglio K, Rubini F, et al. Non-invasive mechanical ventilation in acute respiratory failure due to chronic obstructive pulmonary disease: Correlates for success. Thorax 1995; 50:755–7.

72. Plant PK, Owen JL, Elliott MW. Non-invasive ventilation in acute exacerbations of chronic obstructive pulmonary disease:

Long-term survival and predictors of in-hospital outcome. Thorax 2001; 56:708–12.

73. Carlucci A, Richard JC, Wysocki M, et al. Noninvasive versus conventional mechanical ventilation: An epidemiologic survey. Am J Respir Crit Care Med 2001; 163:874–80.

74. Soo Hoo GW, Santiago S, Williams A. Nasal mechanical ventilation for hypercapnic respiratory failure in chronic obstructive pulmonary disease: Determinants of success and failure. Crit Care Med 1994; 22:1253–61.

75. Corrado A, De Paola E, Gorini M, et al. Intermittent negative pressure ventilation in the treatment of hypoxic hypercapnic coma in chronic respiratory insufficiency. Thorax 1996; 5: 1077–82.

76. Corrado A, Gorini M, Ginanni R, et al. Negative pressure ventilation versus conventional mechanical ventilation in the treatment of acute respiratory failure in COPD patients. Eur Respir J 1998; 12:519–25.

77. Corrado A, Gorini M. Negative pressure ventilation: Is there still a role? Eur Respir J 2002; 20:187–97.

78. Girou E, Brun Buisson C, Taille S, et al. Secular trends in nosocomial infections and mortality associated with noninvasive ventilation in patients with exacerbation of COPD and pulmonary edema. JAMA 2003; 290:2985–91.

79. Elliott MW. Non-invasive ventilation in acute exacerbations of chronic obstructive pulmonary disease: A new gold standard? Intensive Care Med 2002; 28:1691–3.

80. Todisco T, Baglioni S, Eslami A, et al. Treatment of acute exacerbations of chronic respiratory failure. Chest 2004; 125: 2217–23.

81. Mehta S, Hill NS. Noninvasive ventilation. Am J Respir Crit Care Med 2001; 163:540–77.

82. Nava S, Confalonieri M, Rampulla C. Intermediate respiratory intensive care units in Europe: A European perspective. Thorax 1998; 53:798–802.

83. European Respiratory Task Force. Respiratory intermediate care units: A European survey. Eur Respir J 2002; 20:1343–50.

84. Sauret JM, Guitart AC, Frojan GR, et al. Intermittent short-term negative pressure ventilation and increased oxygenation in COPD patients with severe hypercapnic respiratory failure. Chest 1991; 100:455–9.

85. Gunella G. Traitement de l'insuffisancé respiratoire aiguë des pulmonaires chroniques avec le poumon d'acier: Résultat dans une série de 560 cas. Ann Med Phys 1980; 2:317–27.

86. Corrado A, Gorini M, De Paola E, et al. Iron lung treatment of acute on chronic respiratory failure: 16 years of experience. Monaldi Arch Chest Dis 1994; 49:552–5

87. Corrado A, Bruscoli G, Messori A, et al. Iron lung treatment of subjects with COPD in acute respiratory failure: Evaluation of short and long-term prognosis. Chest 1992; 101:692–6

88. Corrado A, De Paola E, Messori A, et al. The effect of intermittent negative pressure ventilation and long-term oxygen therapy for patients with COPD: A 4-year study. Chest 1994; 105: 95–9.

89. Corrado A, Confalonieri M, Marchese S, et al. Iron lung versus mask ventilation in the treatment of acute on chronic respiratory failure in COPD patients: A multicenter study. Chest 2002; 121:189–95.

90. Corrado A, Ginanni R, Villella G, et al. Iron lung versus conventional mechanical ventilation in acute exacerbation of COPD. Eur Respir J 2004; 23:419–24.

91. Menzies R, Gibbons W, Goldberg P. Determinants of weaning and survival among patients with COPD who require mechanical ventilation for acute respiratory failure. Chest 1989; 95: 398–405.

92. Del Bufalo C, Fasano L, Quarta CC, et al. Use of extrathoracic negative pressure ventilation in weaning COPD and kyphosco-liotic patients from mechanical ventilation. Respir Care 1994; 39:21–9.

93. Garay SM, Turino GM, Goldring RM. Sustained reversal of chronic hypercapnia in patients with alveolar hypoventilation syndromes: Long-term maintenance with noninvasive nocturnal mechanical ventilation. Am J Med 1981; 70:269–74.

94. Libby BM, Briscoe WA, Boyce B, et al. Acute respiratory failure in scoliosis or kyphosis. Am J Med 1982; 73:532–8.

95. Braun SR, Sufit RL, Giovannoni R, et al. Intermittent negative pressure ventilation in the treatment of respiratory failure in progressive neuromuscular disease. Neurology 1987; 37:1874–5.

96. Corrado A, Gorini M, De Paola E. Alternative techniques for managing acute neuromuscular respiratory failure. Semin Neurol 1995; 15:84–9.

97. Corrado A, Vianello A, Arcaro G, et al. Noninvasive mechanical ventilation for the treatment of acute respiratory failure in neuromuscular diseases. Eur Respir J 2000; 16:542s.

98. Brancalari E, Gerhardt T, Monkus E. Simple device for producing continuous negative pressure in infants with IRDS. Pediatrics 1973; 52:128–30.

99. Alexander G, Gerhardt T, Brancalari E. Hyaline membrane disease: Comparison of continuous negative pressure and nasal positive airway pressure in its treatment. Am J Dis Chest 1979; 133:1156–9.

100. Outerbridge EW, Roloff DW, Stern L. Continuous negative pressure in the management of severe respiratory distress syndrome. J Pediatr 1972; 81:384–91.

101. Fanaroff AA, Cha CC, Sosa R, et al. Controlled trial of continuous negative external pressure in the treatment of severe respiratory distress syndrome. J Pediatr 1973; 82:921–8.

102. Silverman WA, Sinclair JC, Gandy GM, et al. A controlled trial of management of respiratory distress syndrome in a body-enclosing respirator: I. Evaluation of safety. Pediatrics 1967; 39:740–8.

103. Samuels MP, Southall DP. Negative extrathoracic pressure in the treatment of respiratory failure in infants and young children. Br Med J 1989; 299:1253–7.

104. Samuels MP, Raine J, Wright T. Continuous negative extrathoracic pressure in neonatal respiratory failure. Pediatrics 1996; 98:1154–60.

105. Sell LL, Cullen ML, Whittlessey GC, et al. Hemorrhagic complications during extracorporeal membrane oxygenation: Prevention and treatment. J Pediatr Surg 1986; 21:1087–91.

106. Nading JH. Historical controls for extracorporeal membrane oxygenation in neonates. Crit Care Med 1989; 17:423–5.

107. Sillis JH, Cvetnic WG, Pietz J. Continuous negative pressure in the treatment of infants with pulmonary hypertension and respiratory failure. J Perinatol 1989; 9:43–8.

108. Cvetnic WG, Shouptaugh M, Sills JH. Intermittent mandatory ventilation with continuous negative pressure compared with positive end-expiratory pressure for neonatal hypoxemia. J Perinatol 1992; 12:316–24.

109. Cropp AJ, Dimarco AF. Effect of intermittent negative pressure ventilation on respiratory muscle function in patients with severe COPD. Am Rev Respir Dis 1987; 135:1056–61.

110. Gutierrez M, Beroiza T, Contreras G. Weekly cuirass ventilation improves blood gases and inspiratory muscle strength in patients with chronic airflow limitation and hypercarbia. Am Rev Respir Dis 1988; 138:617–23.

111. Celli B, Lee H, Criner G, et al. Controlled trial of external negative pressure ventilation in patients with severe chronic airflow obstruction. Am Rev Respir Dis 1989; 140:1251–6.

112. Shapiro SH, Ernst P, Gray-Donald K, et al. Effect of negative pressure ventilation in severe chronic obstructive pulmonary disease. Lancet 1992; 340:1425–9.

113. Garay SM, Turino GM, RM. Sustained reversal of chronic hypercapnia in patients with alveolar hypoventilation syndromes: Long-term maintenance with noninvasive nocturnal mechanical ventilation. Am J Med 1981; 70:269–74.

114. Curran FJ, Colbert AP. Ventilatory management in Duchenne muscular dystrophy: Twelve years' experience. Arch Phys Med Rehabil 1989; 70:180–5.

115. Jackson M, Kinnear W, King M, et al. The effects of five years of nocturnal cuirass-assisted ventilation in chest wall disease. Eur Respir J 1993; 6:630–5.

116. Splaingard ML, Frates RC, Jefferson LS, et al. Home negative pressure ventilation: Report of 20 years' experience in patients with neuromuscular disease. Arch Phys Med Rehabil 1985; 66:239–42.

117. Schiavina M, Fabiani A. Intermittent negative pressure ventilation in patients with restrictive respiratory failure. Monaldi Arch Chest Dis 1993; 48:169–75.

118. Baydur A, Layne E, Aral H, et al. Long term non-invasive ventilation in the community for patients with musculoskeletal disorders: 46-year experience and review. Thorax 2000; 55:4–11.

119. Ellis ER, Bye PTP, Bruderer JW, et al. Treatment of respiratory failure during sleep in patients with neuromuscular disease: Positive pressure ventilation through a nose mask. Am Rev Respir Dis 1987; 135:148–52.

120. Karakurt S, Fanfulla F, Nava S. Is it safe for patients with chronic hypercapnic respiratory failure undergoing home noninvasive ventilation to discontinue ventilation briefly? Chest 2001; 119:1379–86.

121. Vitacca M, Natalini G, Cavaliere S, et al. Breathing pattern and arterial blood gases during Nd-YAG laser photoresection of endobronchial lesions under general anaesthesia: Use of negative pressure ventilation—A preliminary study. Chest 1997; 112:1466–73.

122. Natalini G, Cavaliere S, Vitacca M, et al. Negative pressure ventilation vs spontaneous assisted ventilation during rigid bronchoscopy. Acta Anaesthesiol Scand 1998; 42:1063–9.

123. Natalini G, Cavaliere S, Seramondi V, et al. Negative pressure ventilation vs external high-frequency oscillation during rigid bronchoscopy: A controlled, randomized trial. Chest 2000; 118:18–23.

124. Corrado A, Consigli GF, Todisco T, et al. Negative pressure ventilation (NPV) by iron lung versus noninvasive positive-pressure ventilation (NPPV) in the treatment of acute respiratory failure (ARF) in COPD patients: A prospective, randomised multicentre study. Eur Respir J 2001; 18:185S.

125. Nava S, Evangelisti I, Rampulla C, et al. Human and financial costs of noninvasive mechanical ventilation in patients affected by COPD and acute respiratory failure. Chest 1997; 111: 1631–8.

126. Uhlig S. Ventilation-induced lung injury and mechanotransduction: Stretching it too far? Am J Physiol Lung Cell Mol Physiol 2002; 282: L893–L896.

127. Culver BH, Butler J. Mechanical influence on the pulmonary microcirculation. Ann Rev Physiol 1980; 42:187–98.

128. Koyama S, Hildebrandt J. Air interface and elastic recoil affect vascular resistance in three zone of rabbit lung. J Appl Physiol 1991; 70:2422–31.

129. Von Bethmann AN, Brasch F, Nusing R, et al. Hyperventilation reduces release of cytokines from perfused mouse lung. Am J Respir Crit Care Med 1998; 157:263–72.

130. Sinderby C, Navalesi P, Beck J, et al. Neural control of mechanical ventilation in respiratory failure. Nature Med 1999; 5: 1433–6.

131. Malbrain ML. Abdominal pressure in the critically ill: Measurement and clinical relevance. Intensive Care Med 1999; 25:1453–8.

132. Bailey J, Shapiro MJ. Abdominal compartment syndrome. Critical Care 2000; 4:23–9.

133. Meldrum DR, Moore FA, Moore EE, et al. Prospective characterization and selective management of the abdominal compartment syndrome. Am J Surg 1997; 174:667–72.

134. Bloomfield G, Saggi B, Blocher C, et al. Physiologic effects of externally applied continuous negative abdominal pressure for intra-abdominal hypertension. J Trauma 1999; 46:1009–14.

135. Valenza F, Bottino N, Canavesi K, et al. Intra-abdominal pressure may be decreased non-invasively by continuous negative extra-abdominal pressure (NEXAP). Intensive Care Med 2003; 29:2063–7.

Chapter 18

NONINVASIVE RESPIRATORY AIDS: ROCKING BED, PNEUMOBELT, AND GLOSSOPHARYNGEAL BREATHING

NICHOLAS S. HILL

ROCKING BED AND PNEUMOBELT
    Historical Development
    Mechanism of Action
    Application
    Indications
GLOSSOPHARYNGEAL BREATHING

Rocking Bed and Pneumobelt

The rocking bed and pneumobelt are noninvasive ventilators that were developed and saw their greatest use during the latter years of the polio epidemics but are used rarely today. They both rely on the effect of gravity to assist diaphragmatic motion and are particularly well suited to patients with severe diaphragmatic weakness or paralysis. Neither one should be used in the management of acute respiratory failure, and both have limited present-day applicability. Despite the similarities, there are also important differences, such as portability and suitability for nocturnal versus daytime use. This chapter reviews the historical development, mechanisms of action, and present-day uses of the rocking bed and pneumobelt. Glossopharyngeal breathing, another noninvasive approach to ventilator assistance, will be discussed briefly at the end of the chapter.

HISTORICAL DEVELOPMENT

The conceptual groundwork for development of the rocking bed was laid during the early 1930s by Eve,[1] who described the use of manual rocking to assist ventilation in two patients with acute respiratory paralysis. The technique consisted of placing the patient supine on a stretcher that was pivoted on a fulcrum placed at waist level. The patient then was rocked up and down approximately 45° in either direction. Eve noted that the "weight of the viscera pushed the flaccid diaphragm alternatively up and down," achieving artificial respiration.[1] The technique was adopted subse-

quently by the British Navy as the recommended means of resuscitation for drowning victims.[2] Later studies demonstrated that this tilting method compared quite favorably with other resuscitation methods of the day, and it remained an acceptable means of resuscitation until mouth-to-mouth resuscitation gained acceptance during the 1960s.[3,4]

Automatic rocking beds were first introduced as ventilatory aids during the late 1940s. Wright[5] was the first to describe the management of respiratory insufficiency using an oscillating bed that had been designed originally to assist circulation. This experience led to the development of the McKesson Respiraid rocking bed, which was accepted by the Council on Physical Medicine and Rehabilitation in 1950.[6] Intended mainly as an aid to weaning patients with poliomyelitis from dependence on the tank respirator,[7] it facilitated nursing care and enhanced patient freedom but was quite noisy, bulky, and heavy (455 kg).[6,7] The Emerson rocking bed (J. H. Emerson Co., Cambridge, MA), also introduced during the late 1940s, was quieter and lighter than the McKesson bed and became the dominant model during the 1950s. Hundreds of rocking beds were manufactured between 1950 and 1960 (Emerson JH, personal communication), but after introduction of the Salk and Sabin vaccines and control of the polio epidemics, demand fell drastically. Many survivors of the polio epidemics continued to use rocking beds for ventilator support, sometimes for decades,[8] but most have since died or switched to other ventilators, and present-day use is rare.

The intermittent abdominal pressure respirator or insufflator (pneumobelt) was introduced at the end of the polio epidemics in an attempt to address the limitations of existing ventilators.[9] The pneumobelt was designed to allow complete freedom of the upper extremities and mouth during use in the sitting position and was intended mainly as a daytime ventilatory aid during meals or wheelchair use. Several modifications of the pneumobelt have been reported since the original description, but these have never gained wide acceptance. These include a piston-like device that compresses the abdomen while the patient sits in a wheelchair[10] and a combination of the pneumobelt and intermittent positive-pressure breathing.[11] Like the rocking bed, the pneumobelt has seen only limited use since control of the polio epidemics.

MECHANISM OF ACTION

Eve compared the rocking-induced motion of the abdominal viscera within the thorax with that of a piston within a cylinder.[1] As the head moves down, the viscera and diaphragm slide cephalad, assisting exhalation (Fig. 18-1). In the foot-down position, the abdominal contents and diaphragm slide caudad, assisting inhalation (Fig. 18-2).

A number of early studies on the efficacy of rocking compared it as a method of resuscitation with others then used commonly.[3,4] These studies used fresh corpses or live subjects with pharmacologically induced paralysis or voluntarily suspended respirations to show that rocking produced tidal volumes ranging from a few hundred milliliters to a liter, and success in the resuscitation of near-drowning victims was reported.[2] Later, Plum and

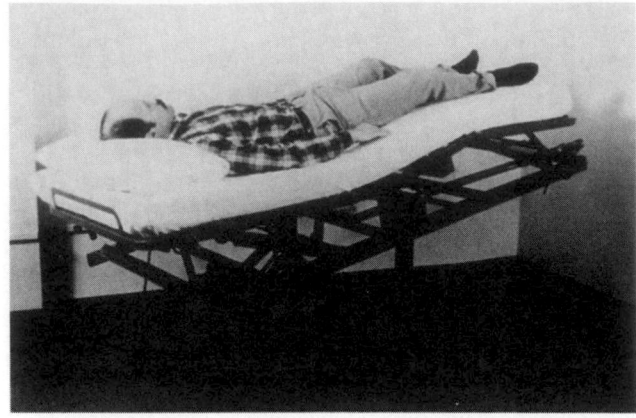

FIGURE 18-1 Rocking bed in 10° head-down position. Sliding of the viscera and diaphragm cephalad assists exhalation.

Whedon[12] found that the automatic rocking bed was not as effective as the tank respirator but produced adequate alveolar ventilation in 11 convalescent patients with respiratory paralysis secondary to poliomyelitis. The bed, however, was unable to sustain adequate ventilation in 5 patients during the acute stages of respiratory paralysis. Plum and Whedon recommended that use of the rocking bed be reserved for stable patients who are capable of at least some spontaneous breathing, a recommendation that holds true today.

Colville et al[13] subsequently examined the physiologic effects of rocking on respiratory mechanics and identified factors responsible for the wide individual variations in tidal volumes generated during rocking. They found that the greatest displacement of the diaphragm occurred during rocking from horizontal to the 40° foot-down position (Fig. 18-3). Beyond this angle, relatively little further displacement of the diaphragm occurred. Likewise, relatively little displacement of the diaphragm occurred during rocking from the horizontal to the head-down position. This indicated that in the horizontal position, the resting diaphragm was fairly close to its uppermost position, so

FIGURE 18-2 Rocking bed in 27° foot-down position. Sliding of the abdominal viscera and diaphragm caudad assists inhalation. (*Used, with permission, from Hill: Chest 90:897–905, 1986.*)

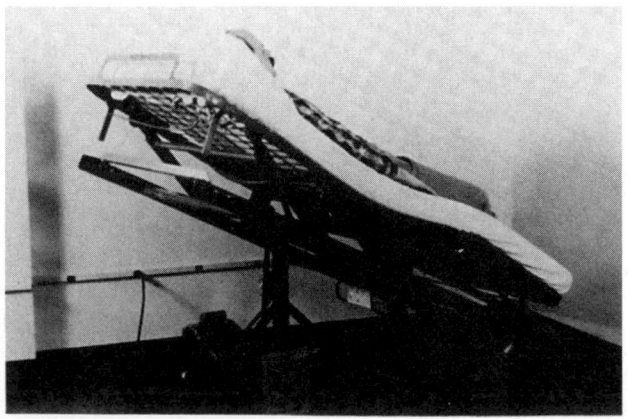

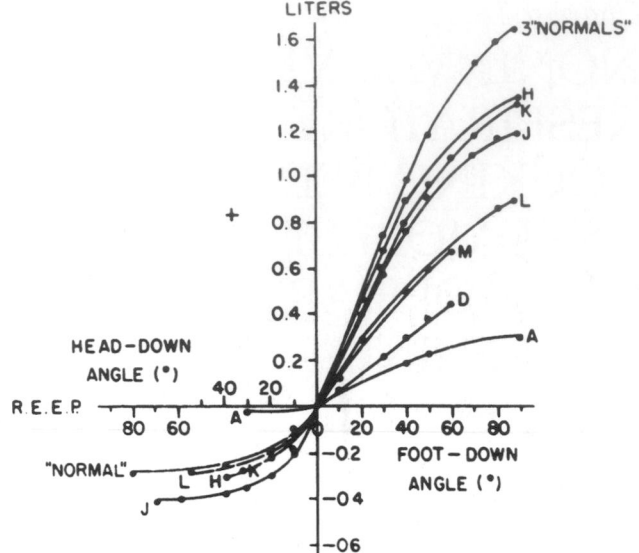

FIGURE 18-3 Relationship between angle of rocking bed and static lung volume in three normal individuals and in patients with poliomyelitis, as indicated by letters. Note that the greatest volume shift occurs between 0° and the 40° foot-down angle. Note also the marked variability between individuals. REEP, resting end-expiratory position. (*Used, with permission, from Colville et al: J Appl Physiol 9:19–24, 1956.*)

the greatest passive motion could be achieved by applying gravitational force in the caudad direction.

Along these lines, Joos et al[14] found that tidal volumes were greater in some patients when rocking was achieved entirely in the head-up position (5–42° above the horizontal plane) rather than between the head-down and head-up positions (10° below to 27° above the horizontal plane). In addition, others found that relatively little increase in minute volume could be achieved by increasing the rate of rocking beyond 15–16 per minute.[3] At higher rocking frequencies, the tidal volume tended to diminish, negating the effects of the increased rocking rate.

With regard to the large individual variation (see Fig. 18-3), Colville et al[13] found that as the compliance of the abdominal wall increased, the greater was the tidal volume during rocking. Thus rocking was relatively ineffective in patients with severe kyphoscoliosis, who have low abdominal and diaphragmatic compliance and short abdominal lengths. Taken together, these findings indicate that the efficacy of the rocking bed is highly dependent on patient body characteristics and that function is likely to be optimal when rocking is between the near-horizontal and the 40° foot-down positions at rates between 12 and 16 per minute. Wider manipulations of rocking rate and arc, however, may be useful in optimizing alveolar ventilation in some patients.

The pneumobelt[9] operates by a mechanism similar to that of the rocking bed in that it assists diaphragmatic motion by causing piston-like motions of the abdominal viscera within the thoracic "cylinder." The major difference is that the pneumobelt assists exhalation by applying positive pressure to the abdominal surface rather than using

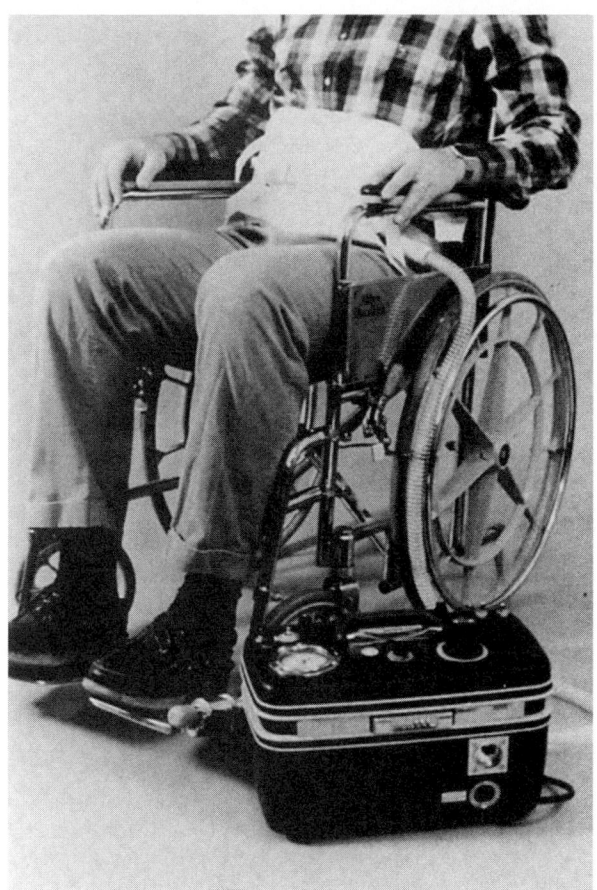

FIGURE 18-4 Pneumobelt is shown attached via a connecting hose to a Bantam positive-pressure ventilator (Puritan-Bennett Corp, Lenexa, KS). (*Used, with permission, from Rondinelli et al. In: Delisa JA, editor. Rehabilitation medicine: Principles and practice. Philadelphia: Lippincott, 1988.*)

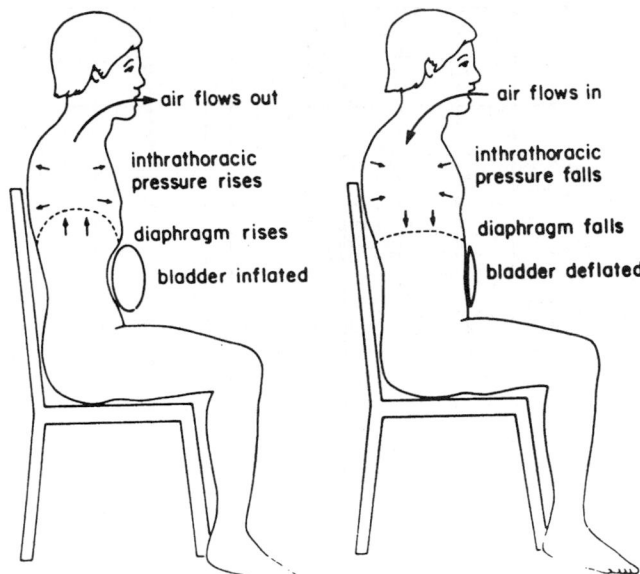

FIGURE 18-5 The pneumobelt functions by exerting positive pressure on the abdominal viscera, forcing the diaphragm up and assisting exhalation (*left*). When the bladder deflates, gravity returns the diaphragm to its original position, assisting inhalation (*right*). (*Used, with permission, from Hill: Chest 90:897–905, 1986.*)

gravitational force. It consists of an inflatable rubber bladder held firmly over the abdomen by an adjustable corset (Fig. 18-4s). Inflation of the bladder squeezes the viscera, forcing the diaphragm cephalad and actively assisting exhalation. On deflation of the bladder, gravity pulls the viscera and diaphragm back to their original positions, assisting inhalation (Fig. 18-5). Because of this dependence on gravitational force, the pneumobelt must be used in a sitting position, optimally at angles of 45° or greater. Below 30°, the ability to assist ventilation is diminished markedly (Fig. 18-6B). Thus nocturnal use of the pneumobelt is limited to patients who can sleep in a sitting position.[15]

Despite this limitation, the pneumobelt can be a very useful device in appropriately selected patients. As shown in Fig. 18-7A, the ability of the pneumobelt to augment tidal volume is linearly related to the inflation pressure of the bladder between pressures of approximately 15 and 50 cmH$_2$O. Pressures exceeding 50 cmH$_2$O are rarely tolerated because of abdominal discomfort. As with the rocking bed, the ability of the device to augment tidal volume varies considerably among individuals (see Fig. 18-6A). Important factors that contribute to the variability among individuals include abdominal and chest-wall compliances.

High abdominal compliance favors efficient functioning of the device, but high chest-wall compliance may allow expansion of the chest wall during bladder inflation, reducing efficiency.[9] Thus, like the rocking bed, body habitus is also an important determinant of ventilator efficiency for the pneumobelt. Although thin patients can be ventilated effectively,[16] both devices work less efficiently in extremely thin or obese patients and in those with severe kyphoscoliosis. The sitting position in patients with severe kyphoscoliosis often brings the lower rib cage in contact with the thighs, rendering proper positioning of the pneumobelt impossible.

APPLICATION

Rocking beds are no longer available commercially. The former manufacturer, J. H. Emerson Company, can no longer makes them (Emerson G, personal communication). Pneumobelts (small, medium, or large) can be obtained via home medical equipment vendors from Respironics, Inc. (Murrysville, PA). Respironics supplies the NEV-100 ventilator to power the pneumobelt, but other positive-pressure ventilators with sufficient pressure- and volume-generating capabilities can be used. Most portable "bilevel" positive-pressure devices, however, are insufficient.

Consisting of a bed frame that is suspended on an axis 100 cm above the ground, rocking beds are bulky (193 cm long by 84 cm wide) and heavy (approximately 136 kg). Although the axis of rotation can be adjusted, they usually are set to rotate 10° in the head-down direction and 27° foot-down. As noted previously, maintaining the rocking arc in the head-up range may improve efficacy in some patients.[14] Adjustable cranks allow raising of the head and knees to

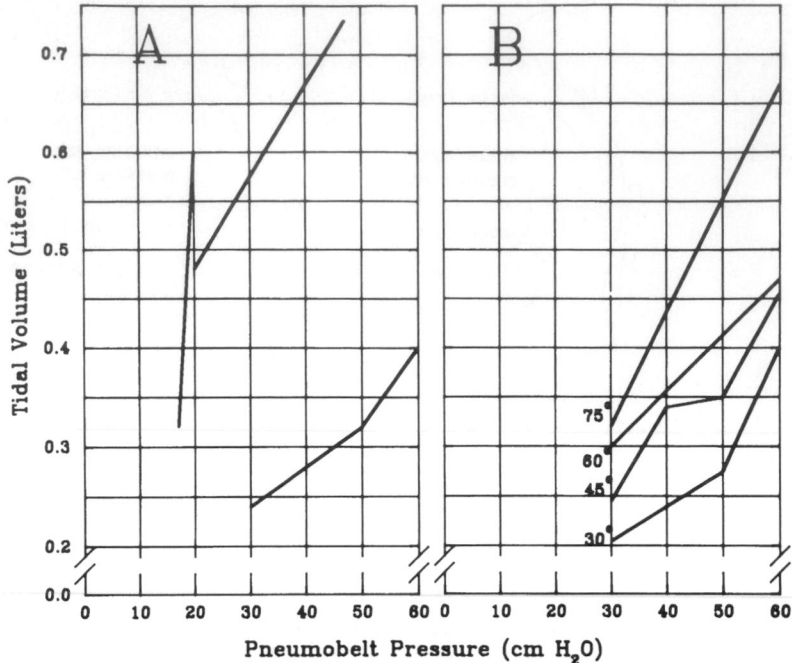

FIGURE 18-6 *A.* Pressure-volume curves for individual patients show that augmentation of tidal volume is linearly related to the increase in pneumobelt pressure within certain pressure ranges, but variations between individuals are wide. *B.* Pressure-volume curves obtained at different trunk angles in an individual patient. Efficiency of the pneumobelt falls with trunk angle. (*Redrawn, with permission, from Adamson et al: JAMA 169:1613–7, 1959.*)

minimize slippage. Excessive flexion of the hips, however, may impair functioning.[14] A foot rest also may be attached to prevent downward sliding, but with proper positioning of the head and knees, this is usually unnecessary.

The most attractive feature of the rocking bed is its ease of application. With use of a foot stool, most patients can position themselves on it with minimal assistance. Paralyzed patients require help from one or two attendants depending on body weight. The patient lies supine with the head and knees raised slightly to maximize comfort. A baseline minute volume is measured using a portable spirometer. Rocking then is commenced at rates between 12 and 16 per minute, again adjusted to optimize patient comfort. The patient is coached to exhale during head-down rocking and

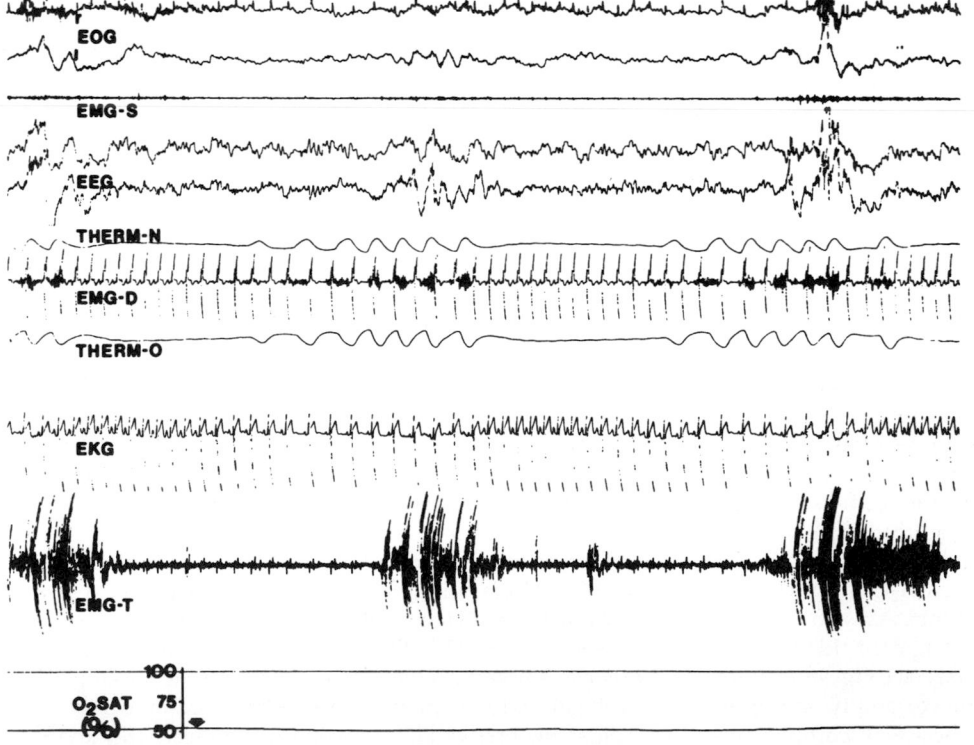

FIGURE 18-7 Nocturnal polysomnogram in patient 1 obtained in August of 1991 during spontaneous room-air breathing shows periodic breathing with sustained severe oxygen desaturation. EOG, electro-oculogram; r, right; l, left; EMG-S, submental electromyogram; EEG, electronencephalogram; THERM-N, nasal thermistor; EMG-D, diaphragmatic EMG; THERM-O, oral thermistor; EKG, electrocardiogram; EMG-T, temporal EMG; O_2SAT, oxygen saturation.

to inhale while the head moves up. When synchronization has been achieved, further adjustments in rocking rate may be made to optimize minute volume. An arterial blood-gas determination may be helpful after an hour or two during the initial trial to assess adequacy of alveolar ventilation.

Patients then are encouraged to initiate rocking at bedtime and to extend the hours of use gradually until they are able to sleep through the night. Most patients find the rocking bed quite comfortable and encounter little difficulty in learning to sleep while rocking. Motion sickness is unusual presumably because the bed rocks in one plane only, but it may disturb some patients. The bed limits daytime mobility, so most patients use it only nocturnally. If daytime ventilatory assistance is necessary, another technique, such as noninvasive positive-pressure ventilation or the pneumobelt, is recommended for daytime supplementation.

Application of the pneumobelt is slightly more difficult than that of the rocking bed, usually requiring at least one attendant unless the patient has full upper extremity strength. The corset is positioned while the patient is sitting comfortably. The rubber bladder is positioned over the abdomen with the curved lower border of the corset over the pubis and the horizontal upper border over the xiphoid. Some coverage of the lower rib cage may serve to minimize paradoxical motion of the ribs during assisted exhalation, although some authors have found more efficient functioning if the corset is placed below the xiphoid.[16] If the corset extends too far below or above the lower rib margin, another of the three available sizes should be tried. The corset then is tightened using the three straps that surround the abdomen until the rubber bladder is held firmly but not uncomfortably against the abdomen. After baseline spontaneous respiratory rate and tidal volume are measured, the rubber bladder is attached to a positive-pressure ventilator using a connecting hose. Volume-limited positive-pressure ventilators that generate adequate pressures and volumes will operate the pneumobelt successfully, but portable "bilevel-type" pressure-limited devices that are popular to provide noninvasive positive-pressure ventilation are not adequate because their pressure-generating capabilities are too limited.

The ventilator is set at a rate that approximates spontaneous respiratory frequency and an inspiratory-expiratory (I:E) ratio of approximately 1:1.5. Some authors have found that function is optimal at rates of 12 to 14 breaths per minute,[16] but this may depend on the underlying respiratory disorder. Some patients prefer rates as high as the low 20s per minute (see Case 2). Ventilator assistance is initiated by intermittently inflating the rubber bladder with peak inflation pressures of 20–25 cmH$_2$O. Inflation pressure then is raised gradually until the patient's assisted tidal volume increases to the desired range, usually 30–50% over spontaneous breathing or the patient reaches the limit of tolerance. Peak pressures of 30–50 cmH$_2$O are usually sufficient, but pressures up to 60 cmH$_2$O may be necessary in some patients.[16] Pressures exceeding 60 cmH$_2$O rarely are tolerated because of discomfort. Considerable coaching usually is necessary during initial adaptation to encourage synchronization of patient breathing with ventilator cycling. Patients who will be successful usually learn to synchronize their breathing with the ventilator after a few sessions.

In addition to measurement of minute volume, efficacy is assessed using arterial blood-gas determinations that are done as soon as the patient is comfortable and synchronizing well. The desired amount of ventilator assistance will vary depending on the patient, but a decrease in arterial carbon dioxide tension (Pa$_{CO_2}$) of approximately 5–10 mmHg below spontaneous breathing levels is acceptable during the initial sessions. Subsequent use of the device also will depend on the patient. Most often, because the pneumobelt must be used in the sitting position, it is used as a daytime ventilator aid to supplement another device used nocturnally. As illustrated by Case 2 (see below) and another case report,[15] however, occasional patients may adapt to nocturnal use. The monthly rental for the belt itself is less than $100, but ventilator costs and associated respiratory therapy services raise monthly charges to the $500–$1000 range.

Long-term follow-up of patients using either the rocking bed or pneumobelt should include assessment for symptoms or signs of chronic hypoventilation such as morning headache, hypersomnolence, and ankle swelling. Daytime spontaneous arterial blood gas determinations are particularly useful for assessing the adequacy of ventilatory assistance,[17,18] and attempts should be made to increase assisted minute volume if Pa$_{CO_2}$ remains substantially above 50 mmHg. Nocturnal oximetry or polysomnography are useful not only to assess adequacy of nocturnal oxygenation but also to detect obstructive apneas that may be induced by negative-pressure ventilators[19] and also may occur during use of the rocking bed or pneumobelt.

Complications of rocking bed or pneumobelt use are relatively few. Some patients using the pneumobelt for many consecutive hours develop skin abrasions, and others have trouble coordinating their breathing with either of the ventilators so that efficacy may be inadequate. If appropriate patients are selected, the risk of worsened respiratory failure or arrest during use is low because such patients should be capable of some spontaneous breathing. As deterioration occurs with progressive neuromuscular syndromes or acute respiratory infections, however, patients may have to switch to other, more effective ventilators.

INDICATIONS

Considering that the rocking bed and pneumobelt share similar mechanisms of action, it is not surprising that they also share indications for use (Table 18-1). Because both assist ventilation essentially by augmenting diaphragmatic motion, they are particularly useful in patients with bilateral diaphragmatic weakness or paralysis. Abd et al[20] have demonstrated the utility of this application in patients with bilateral diaphragmatic paralysis following open-heart surgery. In this study, 10 patients were weaned from conventional positive-pressure ventilation to the rocking bed and continued to use it nocturnally until phrenic nerve function recovered after 4–27 months.

The rocking bed and pneumobelt also may be used in the management of chronic respiratory failure caused by a variety of slowly progressive neuromuscular syndromes that weaken the diaphragm and leave upper airway function intact. Chalmers et al[21] described their experience with

TABLE 18-1 Indications and Contraindications for the Rocking Bed and Pneumobelt

Indications
 Chronic respiratory failure[a] caused by
  Bilateral diaphragmatic paralysis
  Muscular dystrophies
   Duchenne
   Limb-Girdle
   Myotonic
  Postpolio syndrome
  Amyotrophic lateral sclerosis
  Multiple sclerosis
 Traumatic quadriplegia[b]
Contraindications
 Acute respiratory failure or rapidly progressive neuromuscular
  disease
 Excessive secretions
 Upper airway dysfunction
 Excessive obesity or thinness
 Severe kyphoscoliosis

[a] With intact upper airway and appropriate body habitus.
[b] Pneumobelt only.

53 neuromuscular patients, 30 with postpolio syndrome, 12 with various muscular dystrophies, 4 with adult-onset acid maltase deficiency, and 4 with motoneuron disease [amyotrophic lateral sclerosis (ALS)]. Forty-three of the patients used the rocking bed for an average of 16 years with good control of symptoms and stabilization of gas exchange in most patients. Seventeen patients discontinued use: 9 because of discomfort and 8 because progression of respiratory insufficiency necessitated more efficacious therapy. The pneumobelt has been used in patients with high spinal cord lesions, mainly as a daytime supplement, often in combination with positive-pressure ventilation administered noninvasively or via a tracheostomy.[16] In this setting, the pneumobelt frees the face of encumbrances and improves speech and mobility. It also may be used for total ventilator support.[22] Surprisingly, those with the least ability to sustain spontaneous breathing adapt best to pneumobelt use.[22]

Because both ventilators have limitations that are influenced heavily by the patient's body habitus, however, a number of caveats should be borne in mind (see Table 18-1). Neither device is suitable for use in acute respiratory failure mainly because a period of adaptation is necessary for optimal efficiency and also because excessive secretions interfere with function.[12] In addition, care should be exercised to select patients who have an appropriate body habitus, adequate upper airway function, and a condition that is sufficiently stable or slowly progressive so that the anticipated duration of use will justify the effort and time required for adaptation.

Because the rocking bed is suited for nocturnal use and the pneumobelt for daytime use, the two may be used in complementary fashion. A patient might use the rocking bed during sleep and the pneumobelt for daytime desk work or wheelchair use.

Many choices are available currently for noninvasive ventilation of patients with chronic respiratory failure

secondary to idiopathic diaphragmatic paralysis or slowly progressive neuromuscular conditions. Noninvasive positive-pressure ventilation administered via a nasal mask is unquestionably the mode of first choice because of its convenience, ease of application, portability, and avoidance of the intermittent upper airway obstructions and oxygen desaturations associated with the use of negative-pressure ventilators.[19,23] Nevertheless, other noninvasive ventilators still should be considered in patients with chronic respiratory failure who are unable to use noninvasive positive-pressure ventilation, as illustrated in a recent report of a woman with scapuloperoneal muscular dystrophy who used a rocking bed successfully when loss of upper extremity strength rendered her incapable of applying her nasal ventilator.[24]

Efficacy comparisons between the rocking bed and pneumobelt and other noninvasive ventilators are limited because few relevant studies are available. In acutely anesthetized intubated subjects, Bryce-Smith and Davis[25] showed that the rocking bed produced barely adequate tidal volumes when rocking through an arc of 40° and was much less effective than negative-pressure ventilators, including the tank ventilator and chest cuirass. Goldstein et al[26] demonstrated that cuirass-type negative-pressure ventilators augment tidal volumes and suppress diaphragmatic electromyographic activity more effectively than did the rocking bed in patients with neuromuscular disease. Both types of ventilators, however, were deemed effective, and considering that this was an acute daytime study, the rocking bed may have been more effective at reducing diaphragmatic electrical activity had patients been monitored overnight after a suitable adaptation period. Even so, the conclusion that the rocking bed is less effective than negative-pressure ventilators seems justified. In one case, the rocking bed was combined with noninvasive positive-pressure ventilation via a nasal mask to enhance efficacy and achieve "necessary ventilatory support."[27]

In summary, both the pneumobelt and rocking bed currently have limited indications (see Table 18-1). They are unsuitable for use in acute respiratory failure, must be used in patients with a relatively "normal" body habitus, and have marginal efficacy even under optimal circumstances. Noninvasive positive-pressure ventilation has convenience and efficacy advantages over these devices. Nonetheless, there are occasional patients who are unable to tolerate a nasal mask or negative-pressure ventilator who may prefer the relatively greater comfort of the rocking bed or the daytime freedom that the pneumobelt affords. The following cases illustrate such applications.

CASE 1: USE OF THE ROCKING BED
J.F., a 47-year-old man with myotonic dystrophy, first presented with symptoms of chronic hypoventilation, including morning headache and daytime hypersomnolence. He was found to have global muscular weakness, although he was still able to walk with a cane. Pulmonary function studies demonstrated a severe restrictive defect with a forced vital capacity (FVC) of 1.5 liters (31% of predicted) and a forced expiratory volume in 1 second (FEV_1) of 1.3 liters. Room-air

arterial blood-gas determinations revealed a pH of 7.36, a Pa_{CO_2} of 53 mmHg, and a Pa_{O_2} of 69 mmHg. Nocturnal polysomnography showed mild obstructive sleep apnea and sustained mild oxygen desaturations consistent with hypoventilation. A trial of noninvasive positive-pressure ventilation via a nasal mask was initiated. Despite much coaching and trials with different masks, the patient declined further use after 2 months because of intolerable mask discomfort. Megestrol, 40 mg PO tid, then was begun, followed within a month by normalization of blood gases and resolution of symptoms.

Two years later, the patient again developed symptoms of morning headache and daytime hypersomnolence. A daytime arterial blood-gas determination showed a pH of 7.36, a Pa_{CO_2} of 65 mmHg, and a Pa_{O_2} of 42 mmHg. Nocturnal polysomnography was repeated (Fig. 18-7), showing periodic breathing and sustained severe oxygen desaturations. Oxygen supplementation was begun, but the Pa_{CO_2} rose to 76 mmHg. Nasal ventilation was tried once more and was rejected rapidly by the patient. Initiation of negative-pressure ventilation

using a pneumowrap brought about a rapid improvement in symptoms and daytime gas exchange, with a room-air arterial blood-gas determination showing a pH of 7.42, a Pa_{CO_2} of 55 mmHg, and a Pa_{O_2} of 65 mmHg. The patient's wife, however, refused to consider use of the pneumowrap at home because placing the patient in it each night seemed too difficult.

Nocturnal ventilation using the rocking bed then was begun at a rocking rate of 16 per minute. Tidal volume during the initial rocking trial ranged from 300–350 ml. The patient's wife found the rocking bed more acceptable because of simpler application. After a several-day adaptation period, the patient was able to sleep for 4 to 5 hours using the device, and he was discharged home. Nocturnal polysomnography obtained after several months of use showed good synchronization of chest-wall motion with the rocking bed, but some obstructive hyponeas and apneas continued to occur (Fig. 18-8). The oxygen desaturations associated with the obstructive events were ameliorated by 2 liters/min of nasal oxygen used

FIGURE 18-8 Continuous nocturnal recording of case 1 during rocking bed use without oxygen supplementation. Tracing shows consistent regular chest-wall motions at a rate of 16 breaths per minute, indicating good synchronization with the rocking bed. However, periodic obstructive hypopneas are signified by decreases in airflow followed by oxygen desaturations and arousals, as evidenced by disruption of chest-wall synchrony. Channel 1 is chest-wall impedance, channel 2 is combined nasal and oral thermistor, and channel 3 is finger pulse oximetry. Vertical lines indicate 30-s intervals. Monitoring performed using Edentec monitor (Edentec, Inc., Eden Prairie, MN).

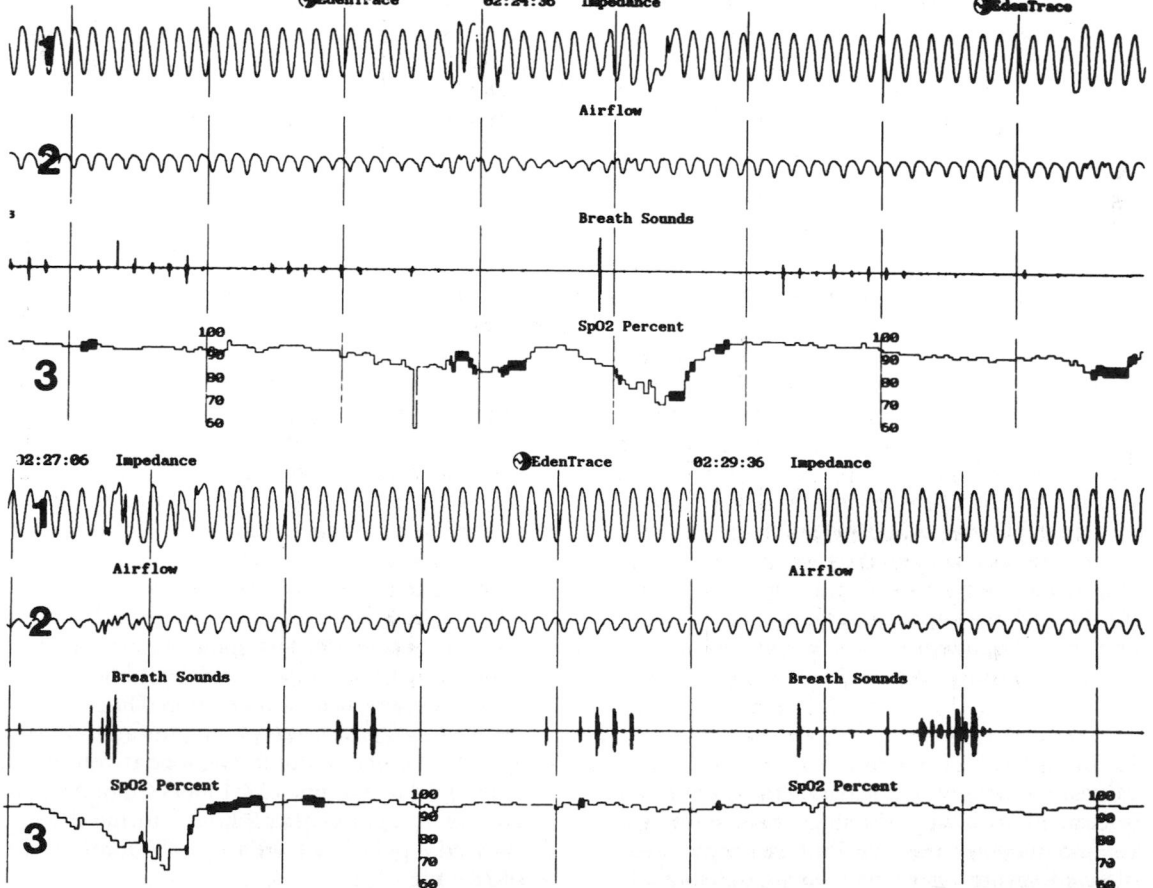

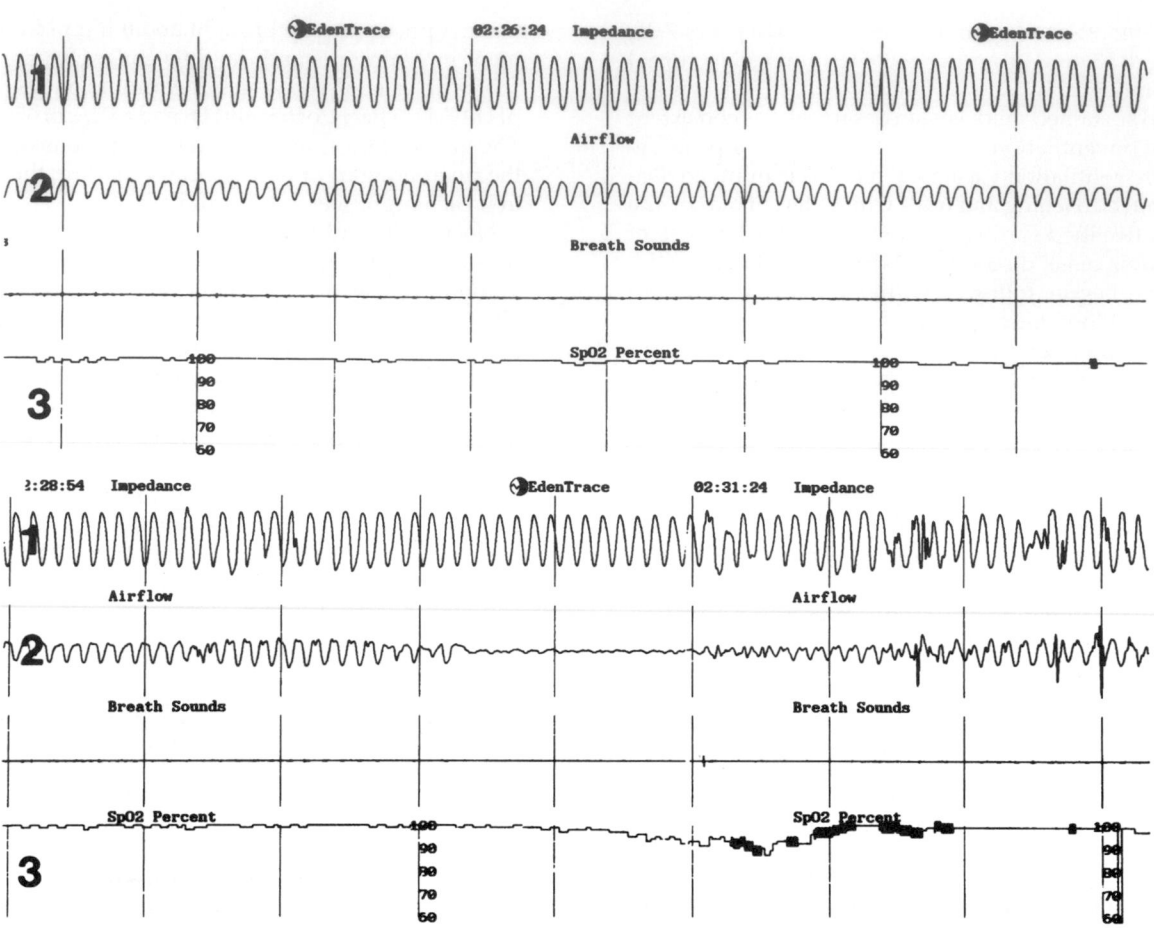

FIGURE 18-9 Nocturnal recording of case 1 using rocking bed and 2 liters/min O$_2$ via nasal cannula. Tracing again shows excellent synchrony of chest-wall motion with rocking. A 50-s obstructive apnea ia apparent in the lower tracing but is associated with only a mild oxygen desaturation to 90%. Channels are the same as in Fig. 18-8.

nocturnally (Fig. 18-9). The patient slept 7 to 8 hours nightly using the rocking bed with supplemental oxygen, and a daytime unassisted room-air arterial blood-gas determination after 15 months showed a pH of 7.42, a Pa$_{CO_2}$ of 52 mmHg, and a Pa$_{O_2}$ of 78 mmHg. After 3 years of clinical stability with nocturnal rocking bed use, the patient was hospitalized with pneumonia and progressive respiratory failure; he declined intubation and died. This case illustrates that trials of a variety of noninvasive ventilators may be necessary before an acceptable one is identified. It also shows that many considerations, including pragmatic limitations in the home, help to determine the final selection. Here the rocking bed was selected not because of greater efficacy or patient preference but because of greater ease of application as perceived by the patient's wife.

CASE 2: USE OF THE PNEUMOBELT

M.C., a 24-year-old man with Duchenne muscular dystrophy, presented with a weakening voice, morning headaches, and hypersomnolence. Pulmonary function studies showed severe restriction with reductions of

both FVC and FEV$_1$ to 0.5 liter (14% of predicted). Arterial blood-gas determinations on room air showed a pH of 7.36, a Pa$_{CO_2}$ of 68 mmHg, and a Pa$_{O_2}$ of 55 mmHg. The patient was admitted to the hospital for a trial of noninvasive ventilation.

Noninvasive positive-pressure ventilation was tried initially, but the patient could not tolerate a face mask or lip seal. (Comfortable nasal masks were not available commercially at that time.) Negative-pressure ventilators were tried, but the patient found the iron lung too bulky and the pneumowrap too restricting and uncomfortable. Standard chest shells fit poorly because of his mild scoliosis. Only the pneumobelt, which was quite effective in augmenting his minute volume, was acceptable to the patient. His spontaneous respiratory rate was 28 breaths per minute, tidal volume was 90 ml, and minute volume was 2.5 liters/min. The pneumobelt was set at a rate of 22 breaths per minute and a positive pressure of 35 cmH$_2$O, producing a tidal volume of 200 ml and a minute volume of 4.4 liters/min. Arterial blood-gas determination after 2 hours during the initial trial showed a pH of 7.41, a Pa$_{CO_2}$ of 59 mmHg, and a Pa$_{O_2}$ of 78 mmHg.

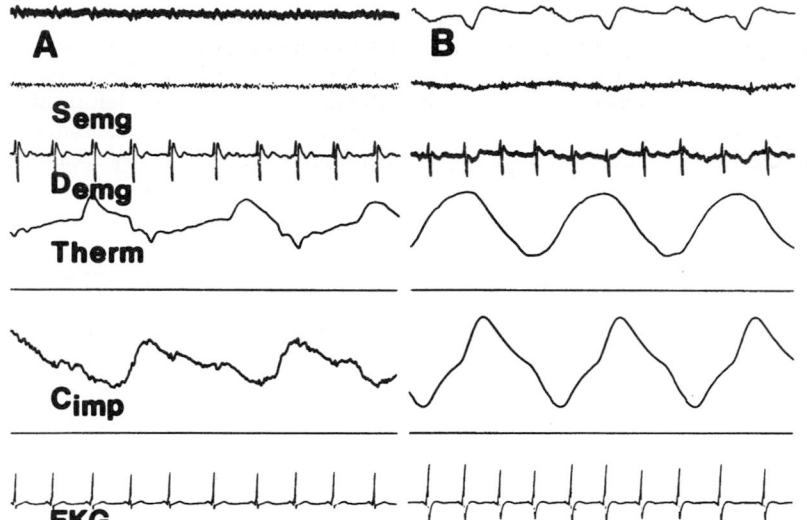

FIGURE 18-10 Nocturnal recording of case 2. *A.* Spontaneous breathing at a rate of 20 breaths per minute. As expected, airflow increases, whereas chest-wall dimensions decrease. *B.* During use of pneumobelt at a rate of 22 breaths per minute, chest wall and ventilator are synchronized. However, chest-wall motion is paradoxical, expanding during expiration. Diaphragmatic electromyogram (D_{emg}) failed to detect electrical muscular discharge during either spontaneous breathing or ventilator use. S_{emg}, submental EMG; D_{emg}, diaphragmatic EMG; THERM, nasal thermistor; C_{imp}, chest-wall impedance; EKG, electrocardiogram.

The patient was discharged with instructions to use the pneumobelt at night and as needed during the daytime. Arrangements were made to attach a ventilator platform to his wheelchair to facilitate daytime use. The patient rapidly adapted to nocturnal use and encountered little difficulty in sleeping while sitting upright. In addition to nocturnal use, he used the ventilator for 2–3 hours during the daytime. A daytime room-air arterial blood-gas determination during spontaneous breathing after full adaptation 7 months after initiation showed a pH of 7.37, a Pa_{CO_2} of 49 mmHg, and a Pa_{O_2} of 84 mmHg. A nocturnal polysomnogram showed excellent synchrony of chest-wall movement with the ventilator and no evidence of obstructive apneas (Fig. 18-10). Oxygen saturations remained between 95% and 98% throughout the night while the patient was breathing room air.

The patient continued to use the pneumobelt both nocturnally and during the daytime for the next 2 years and found it particularly useful for reducing dyspnea associated with eating. During this time, his pulmonary function deteriorated gradually, necessitating more and more daytime use of the pneumobelt. Eventually, he had very little free time from the ventilator, amounting to 1–2 hours/day. Shortly, in September of 1985, the patient developed pneumonia and required endotracheal intubation because of airway secretions that were unmanageable with either the pneumobelt or an iron lung despite manual cough assistance (mechanical assistance was not tried). He was unable to resume pneumobelt use, and a tracheostomy was performed. He lived at home for an additional 3 years following tracheostomy placement but died unexpectedly when his ventilator inadvertently became detached from his tracheostomy tube.

This case shows that the pneumobelt may be used as the main mode of ventilator support in exceptional patients who prefer it to other forms of noninvasive ventilation. This patient was able to adapt quickly to noctur-

nal use while sleeping in the sitting position. The pneumobelt was an appropriate choice for him not only because he preferred it but also because he had a favorable body habitus and slowly progressive respiratory failure that allowed a several-week adaptation period. The pneumobelt proved to be temporizing in this patient, although it provided adequate ventilator assistance even when he was almost entirely dependent on ventilator support. It was inadequate, however, when he developed a pulmonary infection, illustrating the limitations of the device in the face of acute respiratory failure.

Glossopharyngeal Breathing

Glossopharyngeal, or "frog," breathing was first described by Dail et al[28] after they observed a polio patient who had begun using it spontaneously. The technique consists of repetitive gulping motions in which the tongue thrusts small boluses of air into the lungs (Fig. 18-11). The 40- to 80-ml boluses take roughly 0.5 second and are repeated 8 to 12 times in succession to achieve a tidal volume of 500–600 ml, followed by passive exhalation. Roughly 10 of these tidal volume maneuvers are performed each minute so that a minute volume of 4–8 liters/min can be attained (Fig. 18-12). In this way, persons with severely weakened respiratory muscles can use the technique to sustain ventilation and free themselves from the need for continuous ventilator assistance. Patients who become adept at the technique typically use it for periods ranging from a few minutes to several hours, but some ventilator-dependent patients can use it for up to 14 consecutive hours without other aids to ventilation (Sternburg L, personal communication).

Glossopharyngeal breathing also may be used to aid spontaneous breathing in patients with marginal pulmonary reserve by supplementing each tidal breath with one to two boluses of air or to assist coughing. Coughing is assisted by repeating boluses until tidal volumes of

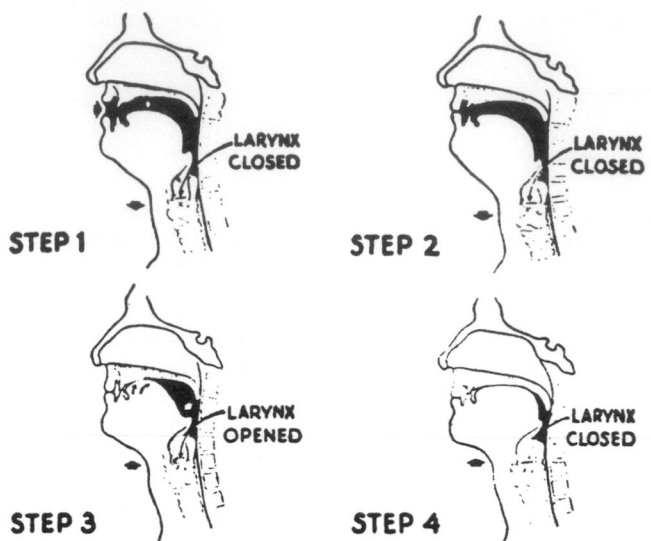

FIGURE 18-11 Steps taken during one "stroke" of glossopharyngeal breathing. In step 1, lips are open, and air fills the mouth and oropharynx as the tongue and jaw are maximally depressed. In step 2, lips are closed, and soft palate is raised to trap air. In step 3, the tongue is raised against roof of the mouth as the larynx is opened, forcing air into lungs. In step 4, the larynx is closed, trapping air in lungs, and the cycle is then repeated. (*Used, with permission, from Dail et al: JAMA 158:445–9, 1953.*)

2–2.5 liters/min are achieved, allowing greater expiratory flows.[28,29] Complications are infrequent, with occasional patients complaining of aerophagia or chest tightness when fully inflating their lungs to assist cough.

Glossopharyngeal breathing requires intact function of upper airway structures, including the glottis, and therefore

FIGURE 18-12 Spirogram tracing obtained during glossopharyngeal breathing in a paralyzed patient. Each small increment during the inspiratory cycle represents a single "stroke" during glossopharyngeal breathing. As can be seen from the tracing, expiratory tidal volumes ranging from 500 to 800 ml are achieved by this patient. (*Used, with permission, from Dail et al: JAMA 158:445–9, 1953.*)

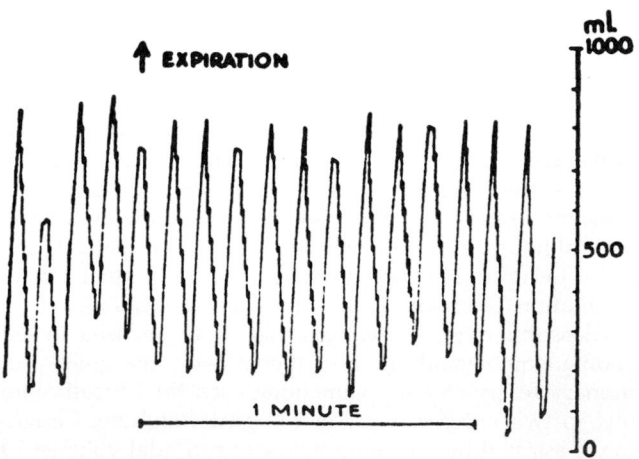

is of little value in patients with severe global weakness or bulbar dysfunction. Efficiency is also impaired by reduced chest-wall or lung compliance or increased airway resistance, limiting use in patients with chest-wall deformities or chronic obstructive pulmonary disease. In addition, because the upper airway contractions are voluntary, it cannot be used during sleep. Use of the technique complements any of the noninvasive aids to ventilation to extend "free time" from the ventilator.[30]

Glossopharyngeal breathing was used widely during the 1950s when it was taught to many patients with respiratory paralysis secondary to poliomyelitis. It is used less commonly today, however, partly because skilled teachers are few and also because most conditions leading to chronic respiratory insufficiency are associated with global muscle weakness or alterations in respiratory system compliance or airway resistance. Nonetheless, occasional glossopharyngeal breathers are found among survivors of the polio epidemics,[29] and some patients with muscular dystrophy or cervical spinal cord lesions learn to use the technique, sometimes spontaneously. Illustrative is a recent case study of a 6-year-old boy with a high cervical lesion secondary to tumor resection who learned glossopharyngeal breathing on his own and was able to use it for ventilator-free breathing for up to 12 hours a day during a 16-year period. Despite having a tracheostomy, he was able to achieve a vital capacity of 3.3 liters to augment cough. [30]

References

1. Eve FC. Actuation of the inert diaphragm. Lancet 1932; 2:995–7.
2. Eve FC. Resuscitation methods for rescue boats. Br Med J 1945; 1:21–2.
3. Gordon AS, Fainer DC, Ivy AC. Artificial respiration: A new method and a comparative study of different methods in adults. JAMA 1950; 144:1455–65.
4. Gordon AS, Raymon F, Savode M, Ivy AC. Manual of artificial respiration: Comparison of effectiveness of various methods on apneic normal adults. JAMA 1950; 144:1447–52.
5. Wright J. The respiraid rocking bed in poliomyelitis. Am J Nurs 1947; 47:454–5.
6. Carter HA. McKesson respiraid rocking bed accepted. JAMA 1950; 144:1181.
7. Lewis L, Hirschberg GG, Adamson JP. Respiratory rehabilitation in poliomyelities. Arch Phys Med Rehabil 1957; 38:243–9.
8. Sternburg L, Sternburg D. View from the seesaw. New York: Dodd, Mead, 1986.
9. Adamson JP, Lewis L, Stein JD. Application of abdominal pressure for artificial respiration. JAMA 1959; 169:1613–7.
10. Janelli HV, Krouskop TA, Canzoneri J, Jameson J. Positive pressure respiratory assist for wheelchair-mobile persons. Arch Phys Med Rehabil 1980; 61:143–4.
11. Gray FD, Field AS. The use of mechanical assistance in treating cardiopulmonary disease. Am J Med Sci 1959; 288:146–52.
12. Plum F, Whedon GD. The rapid-rocking bed: Its effect on the ventilation of poliomyelitis patients with respiratory paralysis. New Engl J Med 1951; 245;235–41.
13. Coville P, Shugg C, Ferris BG. Effects of body tilting on respiratory mechanics. J Appl Physiol 1956; 9:19–24.
14. Joos TH, Dickinson DG, Talner NS, Wilson JL. The rocking bed and head position. New Engl J Med 1956; 255:1089–90.

15. Yang G-FW, Alba A, Lee M, Khan A. Pneumobelt for sleep in the ventilatory user: Clinical experience. Arch Phys Med Rehabil 1989; 70:707–11.

16. Miller HJ, Thomas E, Wilmot CB. Pneumobelt use among high quadriplegic population. Arch Phys Med Rehabil 1988; 69: 369–72.

17. Hill NS. Clinical application of body ventilators. Chest 1986; 90:897–905.

18. Mohr CH, Hill NS. Long-term follow-up of nocturnal ventilatory assistance in patients with respiratory failure due to Duchenne-type muscular dystrophy. Chest 1990; 97:91–6.

19. Hill NS, Redline S, Carskadon MA, et al. Sleep-disordered breathing in patients with Duchenne muscular dystrophy using negative pressure ventilators. Chest 1992; 102:1656–62.

20. Abd AG, Braun NMT, Baskin MI, et al. Diaphragmatic dysfunction after open heart surgery: Treatment with a rocking bed. Ann Intern Med 1989; 111:881–6.

21. Chalmers RM, Howard RS, Wiles CM, Spencer GT. Use of the rocking bed in the treatment of neurogenic respiratory insufficiency. Q J Med 1994; 87:423–9.

22. Bach JR, Alba AS. Total ventilatory support by the intermittent abdominal pressure ventilator. Chest 1991; 99:630–6.

23. Ellis ER, Bye PT, Bruderer JW, Sullivan CE. Treatment of respiratory failure during sleep in patients with neuromuscular disease: Positive-pressure ventilation through a nose mask. Am Rev Respir Dis 1987; 135:148–52.

24. Cormican LJ, Higgins S, Davidson AC, et al. Rocking bed and prolonged independence from nocturnal non-invasive ventilation in neurogenic respiratory failure associated with limb weakness. Postgrad Med J 2004; 80:360–2.

25. Bryce-Smith R, Davis HS. Tidal exchange in respirators. Curr Res Anaesth Analg 1954; 33:73–85.

26. Goldstein RS, Molotiu N, Skrastins R, et al. Assisting ventilation in respiratory failure by negative pressure ventilation and by rocking bed. Chest 1987; 92:470–4.

27. Goldberg AI, Cane RD, Childress D, et al. Combined nasal intermittent positive-pressure ventilation and rocking bed in chronic respiratory insufficiency: Nocturnal ventilatory support of a disabled person at home. Chest 1991; 99:627–9.

28. Dail CW, Affeldt JE, Collier CR. Clinical aspects of glossopharyngeal breathing: Report of use by one hundred postpoliomyelitis patients. JAMA 1953; 158:445–9.

29. Bach JR, Alba AS, Bodofsky E, et al. Glosopharyngeal breathing and noninvasive aids in the management of post-polio respiratory insufficiency. Birth Defects 1987; 23:99–113.

30. Bianchi C, Grandi M, Felisari G. Efficacy of glossopharyngeal breathing for a ventilator-dependent, high-level tetraplegic patient after cervical cord tumor resection and tracheotomy. Am J Phys Med Rehabil 2004; 83:216–9.

Chapter 19

NONINVASIVE POSITIVE-PRESSURE VENTILATION

NICHOLAS S. HILL

Noninvasive ventilation (NIV) refers to the provision of mechanical ventilation without the need for an invasive artificial airway. Many different approaches to assisting ventilation noninvasively have been used in the past, including negative-pressure ventilators, pneumobelts, and rocking beds[1] (see Chapters 17 and 18). By virtue of its effectiveness and convenience compared with other noninvasive approaches, however, noninvasive positive-pressure ventilation (NPPV) using a mask (or *interface*) that conducts gas from a positive-pressure ventilator into the nose or mouth has become the predominant means of administering NIV throughout the world. NPPV has long been used to treat chronic respiratory failure caused by chest-wall deformities, slowly progressive neuromuscular disorders, or central hypoventilation.[2] In more recent years, NPPV has been increasingly used to treat patients with various forms of acute respiratory failure.[3] For the purposes of this discussion, *noninvasive positive-pressure ventilation* (NPPV) refers to active ventilator assistance achieved by the noninvasive provision of a mechanical positive-pressure breath during inhalation, and *continuous positive airway pressure* (CPAP) refers to the provision of a nonfluctuating positive pressure. This chapter discusses the rationale for use, evidence for efficacy of noninvasive positive-pressure techniques in both acute and chronic settings, selection of appropriate patients, techniques for administration, and pitfalls and complications.

Why Use Noninvasive Ventilation and How It Works?

RATIONALE

NIV has become an integral component of ventilator support in both acute and chronic settings because it avoids the complications of invasive ventilation. Invasive mechanical ventilation is highly effective and reliable in supporting alveolar ventilation, but endotracheal intubation carries well-known risks of complications that have been described elsewhere in detail[4] (see Chapter 39). These complications have been lumped into three main categories: complications related to insertion of the tube and mechanical ventilation, those caused by loss of airway defense mechanisms, and those that occur after removal of the endotracheal tube.[4]

In the first category, aspiration of gastric contents; trauma to the teeth, hypopharynx, esophagus, larynx, and trachea; arrhythmias; hypotension; and barotrauma may occur during placement of a translaryngeal tube.[5–7] Tracheostomy tube placement incurs risks of hemorrhage, stomal infection, intubation of a false lumen, mediastinitis, and acute injury to the trachea and surrounding structures, including the esophagus and blood vessels.[7] In the second category, endotracheal tubes serve as a source of continual irritation, interfere with airway ciliary function, and require frequent suctioning that contributes to airway injury, patient discomfort, and mucus hypersecretion. They also provide a direct channel to the lower airways for microorganisms and other foreign materials, leading to biofilm formation, chronic bacterial colonization, and ongoing inflammation. As a consequence, health care–acquired pneumonias are seen in up to 20% of mechanically ventilated intensive-care unit (ICU) patients[8] (see Chapter 46), and sinusitis is seen in 5–25% of nasally intubated patients, related to blockade of the sinus ostia and accumulation of infected secretions in the paranasal sinuses[9] (see Chapter 47). In the third category, hoarseness, sore throat, cough, sputum production, hemoptysis, upper airway obstruction secondary to vocal cord dysfunction or laryngeal swelling, and tracheal stenosis all may follow extubation.[10]

In addition, from the point of view of the patient, translaryngeal intubation is uncomfortable and compromises the ability to eat and communicate, contributing to feelings of powerlessness, isolation, and anxiety.[11] This increases the need for sedation, delaying weaning, prolonging the duration of invasive mechanical ventilation, and potentiating the risks of further complications. If tracheostomy placement becomes necessary, sophisticated equipment including suctioning paraphernalia and a high level of technical expertise among caregivers are required. Tracheostomies promote upper airway colonization with gram-negative bacteria, increasing the risk of pneumonias.[8] Further, long-term tracheostomies are complicated by tracheomalacia, granulation tissue formation, and tracheal stenoses that sometimes obstruct the airway, chronic pain, and tracheoesophageal or even tracheoarterial fistulas.[10] These considerations and potential complications may limit the options for chronic-care placement, add substantially to the costs of care,[12] and even preclude home discharge in patients with limited caregiver and financial resources.

NIV can avoid many of these complications if candidates are selected properly using guidelines that will be discussed in detail later. NIV leaves the upper airway intact, preserves airway defense mechanisms, and allows patients to eat, drink, verbalize, and expectorate secretions. NPPV reduces the infectious complications of mechanical ventilation, including nosocomial pneumonia and sinusitis[13,14] (Fig. 19-1).

FIGURE 19-1 Percent of initiations of mechanical ventilation that were noninvasive (*top panel*), mortality (*middle panel*), and occurrence of health care–acquired pneumonias (*bottom panel*) in patients with COPD and cardiogenic pulmonary edema over an 8-year period in the ICU of Henri Mondor Hospital in Paris. (*Used, with permission, from Girou et al: JAMA 290:2985–91, 2003.*)

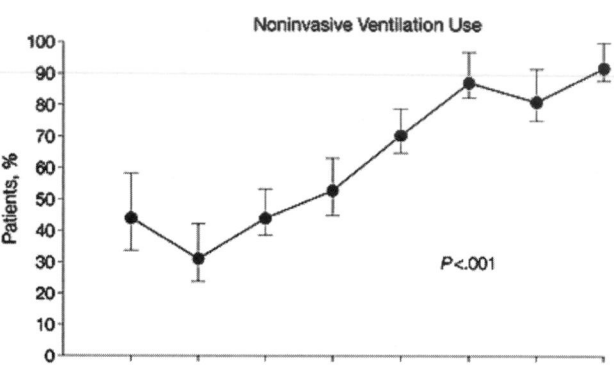

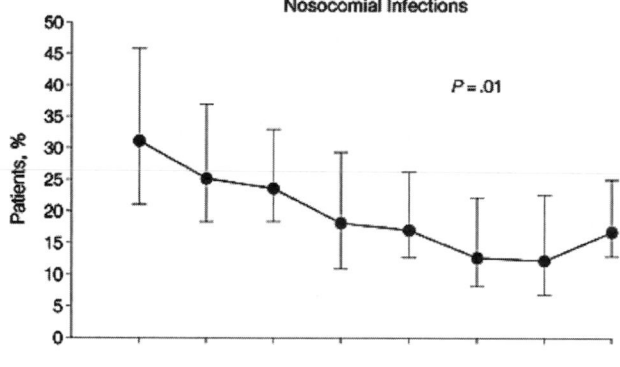

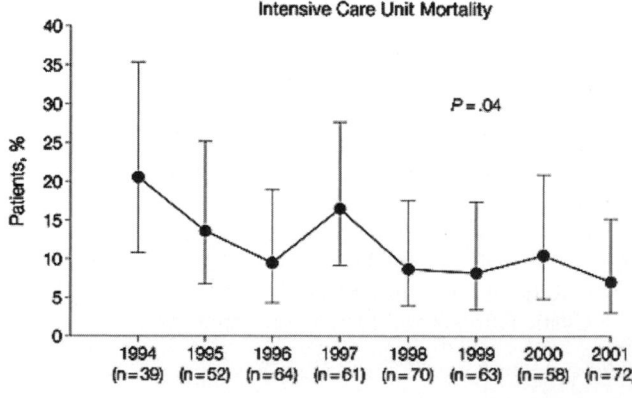

It also enhances patient comfort, convenience, and mobility at no greater[15] or even less[12] cost than endotracheal intubation. NIV can be administered outside the ICU setting as long as adequate nursing and respiratory therapy support can be provided, allowing for more rational use of acute-care beds, and it greatly simplifies care for patients with chronic respiratory failure in the home.

MECHANISMS OF NPPV ACTION

ACUTE RESPIRATORY FAILURE

NPPV improves the respiratory status of failing patients via a number of mechanisms. Most important, NPPV reduces the work of breathing by the same mechanism as invasive positive-pressure ventilation (PPV): By applying supra-atmospheric pressure intermittently to the airways, it increases transpulmonary pressure, inflates the lungs, augments tidal volume, and unloads the inspiratory muscles. Exhalation is achieved by passive lung recoil. Studies in patients with severe stable chronic obstructive pulmonary disease (COPD) or restrictive thoracic disorders show that NPPV reduces or, if inflation pressure is sufficient, even eliminates diaphragmatic work.[16,17] In patients with severe COPD exacerbations, the addition of positive end-expiratory pressure (PEEP) to inspiratory pressure support further reduces the work of breathing by counteracting the effects of auto-PEEP. This combination (pressure support plus PEEP) lowers diaphragmatic pressure swings even more than with either pressure support or PEEP alone.[18] These actions lead to a prompt reduction in respiratory rate, sternocleidomastoid muscle activity, dyspnea, and carbon dioxide (CO_2) retention.

Other beneficial actions include an increase in functional residual capacity (FRC) that opens collapsed alveoli, reducing shunt and enhancing ventilation-perfusion ratios in certain forms of respiratory failure, such as acute cardiogenic pulmonary edema. These effects improve oxygenation and may further reduce the work of breathing because the respiratory system is shifted to a more compliant position on its pressure-volume curve. In addition, CPAP alone (and with NPPV) may improve left-ventricular function by virtue of an afterload-reducing effect of increased intrathoracic pressure.[19] This effect occurs mainly in patients with dilated, hypocontractile left ventricles whose heart function is more dependent on afterload than on preload. The increased intrathoracic pressure reduces both preload and afterload, but the latter effect predominates, lowering transmyocardial pressure and enhancing cardiac output.[20]

A major effect of NPPV that appears to be responsible for benefits reported in many studies, including reduced complication rates, mortality, and hospital lengths of stay, is a reduction in health care–acquired infections. Two prospective surveys[13,14] observed roughly a fourfold reduction in the risk of health care–acquired pneumonia compared with physiologically matched endotracheally intubated patients, even after controlling for severity of illness. Patients treated with NPPV also tend to receive fewer other invasive interventions, such as urinary bladder catheters or central intravenous lines,[14] and this also likely contributes to a lower rate of health care–acquired infections and episodes of sepsis.

Despite the advantages of NPPV related to the avoidance of airway invasion, the lack of a direct connection to the lower airway also poses a number of challenges. The patient must be able to protect his or her airway and clear secretions adequately, or failure is inevitable. The patient's upper airway must permit airflow into the lungs, so NPPV cannot be used in patients with high-grade fixed upper-airway obstructions. In addition, air leaks around the interface seal or via other routes are nearly ubiquitous with NPPV and may interfere with the efficacy of ventilation. Further, the patient must be able to cooperate and synchronize breathing with the ventilator, or no reduction in the work of breathing can be achieved, but the patient cannot be heavily sedated or paralyzed in order to achieve synchrony. Thus patients to receive NPPV must be selected carefully and managed with an eye to these limitations in ways that differ from the approach used for invasive mechanical ventilation.

CHRONIC RESPIRATORY FAILURE

Long-term NPPV is used mainly nocturnally during sleep, when intermittent air leaking through the mouth or under the mask seal is universal, but sufficient air usually enters the lungs to assist ventilation.[21] The adaptations that permit air entry into the lungs while NPPV is administered during sleep are poorly understood, but resistance to airflow in the upper airway is undoubtedly an important factor. In one study, large amounts of air leaking through the mouth during nasal CPAP increased nasal resistance,[22] an effect that was countered by provision of heated, humidified air, consistent with the idea that nasal mucosal cooling was responsible. Increases in nasal resistance secondary to this mechanism, upper airway infection, or allergy is likely to reduce delivered tidal volumes during nasal NPPV. Passive positioning of the soft palate is also important in maintaining patency of the upper airway,[23] as underlined by the observation that patients treated with nasal CPAP experience increased air leaking through the mouth after uvulopharyngoplasty.[24]

Glottic aperture is also important in determining the flow of gas into the lower airways during NPPV. Compared with the awake state, the glottic aperture narrows and delivered tidal volume falls when NPPV is administered during stage 1 or 2 sleep.[25,26] In deeper sleep (stages 3 or 4), the glottic aperture widens, permitting more ventilation; if minute volume is increased excessively, however, the glottic aperture narrows once again, partly related to the reduction in Pa_{CO_2}. These findings indicate that both sleep stage and the amount of ventilator assistance influence glottic aperture, which is a potentially important determinant of the efficacy of NIV. They also apply mainly to controlled modes of ventilation[27]; glottic aperture is not as important when NPPV is administered via a pressure-limited "bilevel" ventilator in the spontaneous mode.[28]

Three theories have been proposed to explain the mechanism by which stabilization of daytime gas exchange is achieved in patients with chronic respiratory failure who are receiving ventilator assistance for as little as 4–6 hours nightly. One postulates that NIV rests chronically fatigued respiratory muscles, thereby improving daytime respiratory muscle function.[29,30] Supporting this theory are studies demonstrating that respiratory muscles do indeed rest during NIV[31–33]; also, indices of respiratory muscle strength and endurance may improve in patients with chronic respiratory failure after varying periods of noninvasive ventilatory assistance.[31–33] Conversely, chronic respiratory muscle fatigue has never been defined adequately or demonstrated convincingly; other studies have failed to demonstrate improvement in respiratory muscle function after initiation of NIV,[35] and some studies have demonstrated that patients with neuromuscular disease have stable Pa_{CO_2} values for years despite a progressive decline in pulmonary function.[36]

A second theory proposes that NIV improves respiratory system compliance by reversing microatelectasis of the lung, thereby diminishing daytime work of breathing.[37] This theory derives from studies showing improvements in forced vital capacity (FVC) without changes in indices of respiratory muscle strength after periods of PPV. Once again, however, data are conflicting, with a number of studies showing no changes in vital capacity after periods of NIV.[34,35] In addition, computed tomographic (CT) scanning of the chest indicates that microatelectasis is not an important contributor to chest-wall restriction in patients with respiratory muscle weakness.

A third theory proposes that NIV lowers the respiratory center "set point" for CO_2 by reversing chronic hypoventilation.[29,38] During deeper stages of sleep, particularly rapid-eye-movement (REM) sleep, upper airway muscle tone and the activity of nondiaphragmatic inspiratory muscles diminish.[39] This response may be exaggerated in patients with ventilatory impairment, leading to progressive nocturnal hypoventilation. Repeated episodes of nocturnal hypoventilation are thought to lead to a gradual accumulation of bicarbonate, desensitization of the respiratory center to CO_2, and worsening of daytime hypoventilation.[38] Nocturnal ventilator assistance reverses nocturnal hypoventilation and allows excretion of bicarbonate and a gradual downward resetting of the respiratory center set point for CO_2, thereby reducing daytime hypercarbia. In addition, NPPV may improve the quantity and quality of sleep by preventing hypoventilation-related arousals that lead to sleep fragmentation,[40] reducing fatigue and improving daytime function. Evidence for this theory derives from studies showing that when ventilator assistance is discontinued for a night in patients with chronic respiratory failure who have been using nightly NIV, the degree of nocturnal hypoventilation is less than before initiation, suggesting a resetting of respiratory center sensitivity for CO_2.[41] Also, nocturnal ventilation, oxygen (O_2) saturation, sleep quality, and daytime symptoms deteriorate without reductions in respiratory muscle strength or vital capacity when nocturnal NPPV is discontinued temporarily in patients with restrictive thoracic disease and improve promptly when NPPV is resumed.[34,40] Moreover, in 16 patients with chronic respiratory failure secondary to restrictive thoracic disorders followed prospectively for 3 years after starting NPPV, Pa_{CO_2} improved in association with an increase in the slope of the ventilatory response

curve, whereas the maximal inspiratory pressure remained unchanged.[42] These studies suggest that amelioration of nocturnal hypoventilation with resetting of respiratory center CO_2 sensitivity and improved sleep quality may be the most important mechanisms contributing to the efficacy of long-term NPPV. The three theories, however, are not mutually exclusive, and all could contribute more or less, depending on the patient.

Clearly, much remains to be learned regarding specific mechanisms of action of NIV. Understanding of these mechanisms is complicated by the application of NIV in both acute and chronic settings using many different techniques for patients with varying etiologies of respiratory failure. The ability to unload respiratory muscles appears to be key, particularly in the acute setting. Mechanisms controlling upper airway responses and respiratory center adaptations are less well understood but appear to be critical to success in the long-term setting.

Noninvasive Positive-Pressure Ventilation in the Acute-Care Setting

EVIDENCE FOR EFFICACY

Numerous acute applications of NPPV have been described, but only a few are supported by strong evidence (Table 19-1). The following will discuss important applications according to the type of respiratory failure.

OBSTRUCTIVE DISEASES

CHRONIC OBSTRUCTIVE PULMONARY DISEASE
Patients with exacerbations of chronic obstructive pulmonary disease (COPD) usually are good candidates for NPPV because they respond to partial ventilator support, hypoxemia is usually mild to moderate, and the condition is most often reversible within a few days. Thus numerous earlier uncontrolled studies have reported that NPPV avoids intubation in patients with COPD, with success rates ranging from 58–93%. Some studies have reported the use of CPAP alone to treat acute exacerbations of COPD,[43,44] based on the rationale that by counterbalancing auto-PEEP, it will reduce the work of breathing.[45] In these studies, relatively low levels of nasal CPAP (5–9.3 cmH_2O) were associated with improvements in Pa_{CO_2} and arterial oxygen tension (Pa_{O2}), and few patients required intubation. The lack of controls, however, renders these studies inconclusive.

The first controlled study on NPPV for acute exacerbations of COPD reported that patients treated with facemask NPPV were endotracheally intubated less often (1 of 13 versus 11 of 13), weaned from the ventilator faster, and spent less time in the ICU than historically matched controls.[46] Historical controls, however, may bias results in favor of the treatment group.[47] Subsequently, these findings have been buttressed by randomized, controlled trials that lend support to the earlier observations. In a study by Bott et al,[48] patients with acute exacerbations of COPD randomized to receive nasal NPPV had improvements in Pa_{CO_2} (65–55 mmHg in the first hour) and dyspnea scores,

TABLE 19-1 Types of Acute Respiratory Failure Treated with Noninvasive Ventilation Graded

	References
A. Strong Evidence—Recommended	
Exacerbation of COPD	46,48–62
Acute cardiogenic pulmonary edema	90–105
Immunocompromised (hematologic malignancy, bone marrow or solid-organ transplant, AIDS)	109–114
Facilitation of weaning/extubation patients with COPD	130–136
B. Intermediate Evidence—Guideline	
Asthma	66–70
Community-acquired pneumonia in patients with COPD	105
Extubation failure in patients with COPD	141[a]
Hypoxemic respiratory failure	81–88
Do-not-intubate patients (COPD and CHF)	117–122
Postoperative respiratory failure (lung resection, bariatric, CABG)	123–129
C. Weaker Evidence—Optional	
Acute-respiratory distress syndrome (ARDS) with single-organ involvement	115
Community-acquired pneumonia (non-COPD)	105–109
Cystic fibrosis	72–74
Facilitation of weaning/extubation failure (non-COPD)	137–140,142
Neuromuscular disease/chest-wall deformity	77–79
Obstructive sleep apnea/obesity hypoventilation	75,76
Trauma	116
Upper airway obstruction	
D. Not Recommended	
Acute deterioration in end-stage interstitial pulmonary fibrosis	80
Severe ARDS with multiple organ dysfunction	
Postoperative upper airway or esophageal surgery	
Upper airway obstruction with high risk for occlusion	

Level of evidence: A = multiple randomized, controlled trials and meta-analyses; B = single controlled trial and cohort series or multiple randomized studies with conflicting findings; C = anecdotal reports and case series; D = not recommended based on contrary evidence or expert opinion.
ABBREVIATIONS: AIDS, acquired immune deficiency syndrome; COPD, chronic obstructive pulmonary disease; CHF, congestive heart failure; CABG, coronary artery bypass graft.

whereas no significant changes occurred among controls. In addition, mortality rate was lower among NPPV-treated patients than in controls (10% versus 30%), although this reduction became statistically significant only after exclusion of four NPPV patients who never actually received the therapy. Kramer et al[49] randomized 31 patients with various etiologies for respiratory failure, 21 of whom had COPD, to receive NPPV or conventional therapy. Among COPD patients who received NPPV in their study, respiratory rate and Pa_{CO_2} fell more rapidly during the first hour of therapy than among controls, and intubation rates were reduced to 9% compared with 67% in controls. In a multicenter European trial[16] of 85 patients with COPD randomized to receive face-mask pressure-support ventilation (PSV) or conventional therapy, respiratory rate but not Pa_{CO_2} fell significantly in the NPPV

group during the first hour; intubation (26% versus 74%), complication (16% versus 48%), and mortality (9% versus 29%) rates and hospital lengths of stay (35 versus 23 days) all were significantly lower in the NPPV versus control group.

Additional controlled trials have compared the effects of NPPV with those of doxapram over 4 hours in patients with acute exacerbations of COPD; although doxapram transiently improved Pa_{O_2}, it had no effect on Pa_{CO_2}.[50] Also, three deaths occurred in the doxapram group. NPPV was deemed more effective than doxapram because it brought about sustained improvements in both Pa_{CO_2} and Pa_{O_2}. Another randomized, controlled trial compared the efficacy of standard medical therapy with NPPV in 30 patients with acute hypercapnic respiratory failure caused by exacerbations, pneumonia, or congestive heart failure.[51] Those randomized to NPPV had greater improvements in pH and respiratory rate within 6 hours, higher success rate (93%), and shorter hospital lengths of stay (11.7 versus 14.6 days, $p < .05$) than controls. The largest study to date on NPPV for exacerbations of COPD randomized 236 patients to receive NPPV or standard therapy at 14 British centers.[52] NPPV was administered in general respiratory wards by nurses who had a few hours of in-servicing training with the technique. Patients treated with NPPV had lower intubation (15% versus 27%) and mortality (10% versus 20%) rates than controls, but the benefit was seen only in patients with pH values of 7.30 or greater. The authors concluded that although NPPV proved to be effective in their study, these sicker patients probably should have been treated in an ICU.

In addition to the favorable findings regarding the use of NPPV for acute exacerbations of COPD, some studies have found that 1-year survival rates are better and the need for rehospitalization and consumption of ICU beds over the next year are less for patients treated with NPPV as opposed to conventional therapy.[53,54] Although these latter studies were not randomized, so the results could have reflected a selection bias favoring less ill patients in the NPPV group, it is also possible that NPPV avoids late complications of invasive ventilation, such as sustained muscle weakness or swallowing dysfunction.[9]

Among the many controlled and uncontrolled studies examining the efficacy of NPPV in exacerbations of COPD, only two have obtained unfavorable results. In one,[55] 25 of 49 consecutive COPD patients with acute exacerbations were treated with nasal NPPV, and 24 were intolerant and served as the "control" group. Blood gases in both groups improved at similar rates, and no differences in outcome were apparent between the two groups. In the second, Barbe et al[56] randomized 24 patients with acute exacerbations of COPD to receive nasal NPPV or standard therapy. Four of 14 patients randomized to NPPV were intolerant; among the remaining patients, blood-gas improvements and hospital lengths of stay were similar, and no differences in intubation or mortality rates were apparent, leading the authors to conclude that NPPV is ineffective in COPD. Both studies, however, enrolled consecutive patients who, on average, had less severe blood-gas abnormalities than patients enrolled in favorable studies; none of the patients in the study of Barbe et al[56] required intubation, as did almost three-quarters of the controls in the studies of Kramer et al[49] and

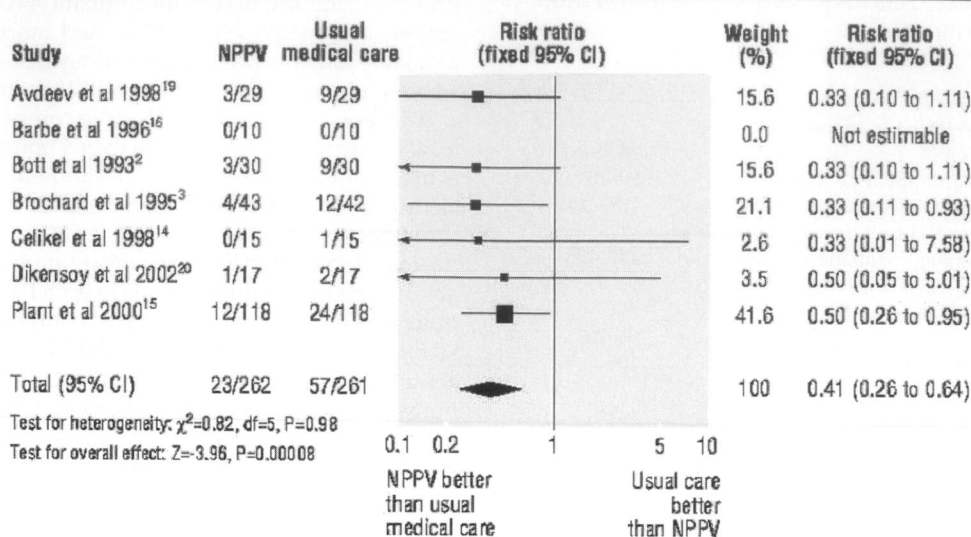

Study	NPPV	Usual medical care	Risk ratio (fixed 95% CI)	Weight (%)	Risk ratio (fixed 95% CI)
Avdeev et al 1998[19]	3/29	9/29		15.6	0.33 (0.10 to 1.11)
Barbe et al 1996[16]	0/10	0/10		0.0	Not estimable
Bott et al 1993[2]	3/30	9/30		15.6	0.33 (0.10 to 1.11)
Brochard et al 1995[3]	4/43	12/42		21.1	0.33 (0.11 to 0.93)
Celikel et al 1998[14]	0/15	1/15		2.6	0.33 (0.01 to 7.58)
Dikensoy et al 2002[20]	1/17	2/17		3.5	0.50 (0.05 to 5.01)
Plant et al 2000[15]	12/118	24/118		41.6	0.50 (0.26 to 0.95)
Total (95% CI)	23/262	57/261		100	0.41 (0.26 to 0.64)

Test for heterogeneity: χ^2=0.82, df=5, P=0.98
Test for overall effect: Z=-3.96, P=0.00008

NPPV better than usual medical care — Usual care better than NPPV

FIGURE 19-2 Forest plot of eight randomized, controlled studies on NPPV in patients with acute respiratory failure secondary to COPD. The reduction in mortality rate was consistent among studies. (*Used, with permission, from Lightowler: Br Med J 185–9, 2003.*)

Brochard et al.[16] These observations support the contention that the patients in the two unfavorable studies were less ill than those in the favorable studies and argue that NPPV should be reserved for sicker patients with COPD who are at risk of requiring intubation.

Multiple randomized, controlled trials lend themselves to meta-analysis. An earlier meta-analysis by Keenan et al[57] concluded that NPPV significantly reduces mortality and reduces the cost of hospitalization by an average of $3244 Canadian dollars compared with conventional therapy. Peter et al[58] examined both COPD and non-COPD causes of acute respiratory failure in their meta-analysis, concluding that NPPV significantly reduces the need for intubation as well as mortality. More recent meta-analyses by Keenan et al[59] and Lightowler et al[60] (Cochrane analysis) observed absolute and relative risk reductions of 28% and 0.42 for intubation, 10% and 0.41 for mortality, and 4.57 and 3.21 hospital days, respectively (all $p < .05$) (Fig. 19-2). The analysis of Keenan et al also concluded that there is little evidence to support NPPV use in milder COPD, although they analyzed only two studies of mild patients. The analysis of Lightowler et al also found that Pa_{CO_2}, heart rate, and dyspnea scores improved more rapidly than in conventionally treated patients. These studies lend strong support to the use of NPPV for patients with COPD in the acute-care setting, leading consensus groups to recommend that the modality "be considered" in selected patients.[61,62] The need for careful patient selection cannot be overemphasized (see "Selection Guidelines," below). NPPV is best used to avoid intubation, not to replace it. Although NPPV should be viewed as the ventilator therapy of first choice for appropriate COPD patients, those with contraindications to NPPV should be intubated and ventilated without delay.

In view of the idea that NPPV is best used to avoid intubation, Squadrone et al[63] asked whether it can serve as an alternative to intubation in patients with COPD and advanced acute hypercapnic respiratory failure (pH ≤ 7.25, Pa_{CO_2} ≥ 70 mmHg, respiratory rate ≥ 35 breaths per minute). Sixty-four such patients had similar mortality rates and hospital lengths of stay but fewer serious complications (mainly infectious) and a trend toward a higher weaning rate at 30 days compared with a historically matched control group of invasively ventilated patients. The authors concluded that NPPV can be used as an alternative to invasive mechanical ventilation in severely ill patients with COPD, but considering that the failure rate approached two-thirds in the NPPV group, this approach should be applied with great caution. As pointed out previously, the use of historical controls is a serious design limitation that may favor the treatment group.

Few data provide guidance on selecting patients who might benefit from continued use of NPPV after hospital discharge. In an uncontrolled retrospective study, Tuggey et al[64] found that patients treated with NIV during their acute admissions and sent home with it had many fewer hospital days per year (25 versus 78 days; $p = .004$) and incurred much lower costs per year ($7407 versus $23,065) after starting domiciliary NIV than before. Despite the small number of patients and uncontrolled design, these results support the idea that domiciliary NIV should be considered in "revolving-door patients" who require repeated hospital admissions and highlight the need for more definitive studies addressing this question.

ASTHMA

Although acute asthma would be anticipated to respond favorably to NPPV because it shares pathophysiologic features with COPD, much less evidence supports this application. One earlier study of 158 patients with acute respiratory failure of diverse etiologies treated with face-mask NPPV included 5 patients with acute asthma (average initial Pa_{CO_2} of 67 mmHg).[65] Only one of these required intubation, and there were no mortalities. The same group later described 17 patients with asthma who had an average initial pH of

7.25 and a Pa_{CO_2} of 65 mmHg and were treated with face-mask PSV.[66] Only two required intubation (for increasing Pa_{CO2}), average duration of ventilation was 16 hours, and no complications occurred.

More recently, Fernandez et al[67] reported on 58 patients with status asthmaticus, 33 of whom were retrospectively deemed candidates for NPPV because of persisting CO_2 retention ($Pa_{CO_2} > 50$ mmHg) and because they met other clinical criteria.[67] Of these, 11 were intubated according to clinician preference, and 22 were managed noninvasively. The noninvasively and invasively treated groups had similar initial Pa_{CO_2} values, which improved less rapidly in the noninvasive group. Only 14% of the NPPV-treated patients eventually required intubation, and they had shorter ICU and hospital lengths of stay than the intubated group. Thus far two randomized, controlled trials have been reported. Holley et al[68] were able to enroll only one-tenth of the roughly 350 patients their power analysis had projected. Not surprisingly, their major outcome variable, intubation rate, was not reduced significantly in their NPPV group (1 of 19 versus 2 of 16 in controls), and they observed no deaths. Their major finding was that physicians who a priori believed that NPPV was effective were less likely to enroll patients in the trial because of concern that the patients might require intubation if randomized to the control group. Soroksky et al[69] randomized 33 patients with severe acute asthma [average initial forced expiratory volume in 1 second (FEV_1) roughly 33%] to receive NPPV or sham therapy via a face mask. The NPPV group had a significantly greater increase in FEV_1 within the first hour (53.5% versus 28.5%) and fewer hospitalizations (3 of 17 versus 10 of 16) compared with the sham group. Both groups received aerosolized bronchodilators via a nebulizer, not the ventilator. The authors speculated that the greater improvement in airflow in the NPPV group might be related to a bronchodilator effect of positive pressure.

These studies suggest that NPPV may be effective in improving airflow, correcting gas-exchange abnormalities, avoiding intubation, and reducing the need for hospitalization in patients with acute severe asthma. Published studies, however, are either uncontrolled or underpowered or the findings have not been replicated. A recent Cochrane analysis concluded that evidence for use of NPPV for acute asthma was "very promising" but "controversial" and tat more controlled studies are needed.[70] Furthermore, medical therapy alone may be quite effective.[71] Lacking more evidence, no firm conclusions can be drawn regarding the relative effectiveness of NPPV versus conventional therapy in exacerbations of asthma. The British Thoracic Society Standards of Care Committee opined that NPPV should not be used routinely for acute asthma.[62] Nonetheless, a trial of NPPV might be considered in patients not responding promptly to standard medical therapy if selected according to commonly used criteria (see "Selection Guidelines," below).

CYSTIC FIBROSIS

NPPV has been used to treat acutely deteriorating patients with end-stage cystic fibrosis (CF). In one study, six patients with FEV_1 ranging from 350–800 ml and severe acute-on-chronic CO_2 retention (initial Pa_{CO_2} ranging from 63–112 mmHg) were treated with NPPV for periods of 3–36 days; four survived until a heart-lung transplant could be performed.[72] The same investigators reported more recently on 113 patients with CF treated with NPPV for acute deteriorations.[73] Ninety of these patients (median FEV_1/FVC ratio of 0.5) were listed for lung transplantation, 28 survived to transplant, 10 remained on the list at the time of reporting, and the remainder expired. NPPV improved hypoxia but not hypercapnia. These case series suggest that NPPV may serve as a rescue therapy to provide a "bridge to transplantation" for patients with acutely deteriorating CF, but mortality still will be substantial if the wait is prolonged.

UPPER AIRWAY OBSTRUCTION

NPPV has been deemed contraindicated for patients with upper airway obstruction in the past,[65] and the inappropriate use of NPPV in patients with tight, fixed upper airway obstruction should be avoided so as not to delay the institution of definitive therapy. In the author's experience, however, NPPV can be used to treat patients with reversible upper airway obstruction, such as that caused by glottic edema following extubation, sometimes in combination with aerosolized medication and/or heliox. Although no controlled trials demonstrate the efficacy of this approach in adults, a controlled trial in 10 infants with respiratory failure showed that NPPV[74] and CPAP were equally efficacious in lowering respiratory rate, but NPPV contributed to patient-ventilator asynchrony. If used, NPPV should be administered cautiously and monitored closely because these patients are at risk for precipitous deteriorations.

DECOMPENSATED OBSTRUCTIVE SLEEP APNEA OR OBESITY HYPOVENTILATION SYNDROME

Patients with acute-on-chronic respiratory failure caused by sleep apnea syndrome, often in combination with obesity hypoventilation, have been treated successfully with NPPV and transitioned to CPAP once stabilized.[75] but no controlled trials have evaluated this application. Sturani et al[76] described the successful use of nasal NPPV administered with the BiPAP device (18 cmH_2O inspiratory and 6 cmH_2O expiratory pressures) in five morbidly obese patients [mean body mass index (BMI) of 50 mg/m^2] with severe sleep apnea. Anecdotally, high inflation pressures, sometimes necessitating use of volume-limited ventilators that have greater pressure-generating capabilities than portable pressure-limited ventilators, may be needed because of high respiratory system impedance.

RESTRICTIVE DISEASES

Although NPPV to treat patients with chronic respiratory failure secondary to restrictive thoracic diseases is well accepted (see "Chronic Respiratory Failure," above), it is used for only a small portion of patients admitted to acute-care hospitals with respiratory failure. Accordingly, few studies on the management of acute respiratory failure in these patients have been reported. In the large trial that treated all eligible patients admitted to an ICU over a 2-year period, only 5 of 158 patients had restrictive lung disease.[65] Small uncontrolled series have reported success using NPPV to alleviate gas-exchange abnormalities and to avoid intubation in patients with acute respiratory failure secondary to neuromuscular disease[77] and kyphoscoliosis.[78] Despite the lack of evidence, the British Thoracic Society Standards of Care Committee considers that NPPV "is indicated" in patients with acute or acute-on-chronic respiratory failure secondary to restrictive thoracic diseases.[62]

A regimen for managing acute deteriorations in patients with chronic respiratory failure secondary to neuromuscular disease, reported by Bach et al,[79] requires that patients receive NIV at home 24 hours a day during the exacerbation. When O_2 saturation falls below 90% as determined by continuous pulse oximetry, airway secretions are removed aggressively using manually assisted coughing and mechanical aids such as the cough insufflator-exsufflator until O_2 saturation returns to the 90% range. In this small series of patients, the need for hospitalization was reduced dramatically after institution of the regimen.[79]

Limited information is available on NPPV therapy for patients with acutely deteriorating restrictive lung diseases such as interstitial fibrosis. Such patients fare poorly with mechanical ventilation.[80] It is discouraged unless an acutely reversible superimposed condition is thought to be responsible for the deterioration, or the patient or family desires temporizing therapy, perhaps to finalize affairs.

HYPOXEMIC RESPIRATORY FAILURE

Hypoxemic respiratory failure is defined as a $Pa_{O_2}/F_{I_{O_2}}$ ratio of less than 200 and a respiratory rate greater than 35 breaths per minute, and diagnoses include acute pneumonia, acute pulmonary edema, acute respiratory distress syndrome (ARDS), and trauma.[81] It is an extremely broad category of acute respiratory failure. Hence, perhaps not surprisingly, studies of NPPV to treat it have yielded conflicting results. Meduri et al[82] were the first to report the successful application of NPPV in such patients. Subsequently, Wysocki et al[83] found that hypercapnia was a strong predictor of NPPV success in patients with hypoxemic respiratory failure: seven of nine patients with an initial Pa_{CO_2} of greater than 45 mmHg having been treated successfully and seven of eight patients with a Pa_{CO_2} of less than 45 mmHg having failed. In a later randomized trial,[84] the same authors found no benefit of NPPV over conventional therapy among all entered patients. Once again, initial hypercapnia predicted a favorable outcome: Patients with an initial Pa_{CO_2} of greater than 45 mmHg had significantly lower intubation and ICU mortality rates and shorter ICU lengths of stay than normocapnic patients. The authors concluded that hypoxemic respiratory failure without CO_2 retention responds poorly to NPPV.

Conversely, Antonelli et al[81] randomized 64 patients with hypoxemic respiratory failure to NPPV or immediate intubation. Improvements in oxygenation were similar in the two groups, and only 31% of the NPPV-treated patients required intubation. NPPV-treated patients had significantly fewer septic complications such as pneumonia or sinusitis (3% versus 31%), and there were trends toward decreased mortality and ICU length of stay (27% versus 45% and

9 versus 15 days, respectively) compared with intubated controls. Another randomized, controlled trial of 61 patients with various forms of acute respiratory failure found a significantly reduced intubation rate when patients with acute hypoxemic respiratory failure were treated with NPPV as opposed to conventional therapy (7.5 versus 22.6 intubations per 100 ICU days); mortality rates, however, were not significantly different.[85]

More recently, Ferrer et al[86] randomized patients with severe hypoxemia (defined as a Pa_{O_2} of less than 60 mmHg or an Sa_{O_2} of less than 90% on 50% $F_{I_{O_2}}$ for at least 6–8 hours) to receive NPPV or conventional therapy. Intubation rate was decreased from 52–25%, the incidence of septic shock was reduced, and both ICU (39% versus 18%) and 90-day mortality were lower in the NPPV group compared with controls. In contrast to some previous studies, substantial benefit was observed in patients with severe pneumonia, whereas patients with cardiogenic pulmonary edema had no reduction in intubation rate.

The favorable results of these latter studies might be interpreted to show broad support for the use of NPPV in patients with hypoxemic respiratory failure. A systematic review, however, noted that although intubations in patients with acute hypoxemic respiratory failure seem to be reduced by NPPV, the heterogeneity between studies precluded any firm conclusions and recommended against the routine use of NPPV in these patients.[87] Also, when overall results are favorable in a heterogeneous group of patients, it cannot be assumed that each subgroup benefits equally. It is possible that harm to a particular subgroup could be obscured by benefit in other subgroups. The following subsections examine evidence regarding the use of NPPV in specific subgroups of patients with acute hypoxemic respiratory failure that may be more appropriate to apply to individual patients.

Acute Cardiogenic Pulmonary Edema

Continuous positive airway pressure (CPAP), although not a form of mechanical ventilatory assistance per se, was described as a treatment for acute pulmonary edema dating back to the 1930s.[88] Over the past 15 years, a number of studies have demonstrated that CPAP (10–12.5 cmH$_2$O) is effective in treating acute pulmonary edema. Rasanen et al[89] randomized 40 patients with cardiogenic pulmonary edema to either face-mask CPAP or standard medical therapy and demonstrated that CPAP more rapidly improves oxygenation and respiratory rate. In a study on 55 patients with pulmonary edema, Lin and Chang[90] found that those randomized to face-mask CPAP (adjusted to maintain a Pa_{O_2} of 80 mmHg or greater) had a lower intubation rate (17.5% versus. 42.5%, $p < .05$) than conventionally treated controls. Bersten et al[91] and Lin et al[92] subsequently performed randomized studies on 39 and 100 patients, respectively, demonstrating more rapid improvements in respiratory rates and oxygenation and a reduced need for intubation in patients treated with CPAP. The study of Bersten et al[91] also showed a significant reduction in the length of ICU stay among CPAP-treated patients, and the study of Lin et al[94] showed a trend for a lower hospital mortality rate. The average reduction in intubation rate among these studies was 28% (from 47% in controls to 19% for CPAP). These studies provide strong evidence to support the use of CPAP to treat acute cardiogenic edema.

As discussed earlier, the combination of increased inspiratory pressure and positive expiratory pressure (i.e., pressure support plus PEEP or NPPV) might be expected to reduce work of breathing more effectively than CPAP alone, bringing about more rapid relief of dyspnea and improvement in gas exchange. Thus more recent studies have focused on the use of NPPV to treat acute cardiogenic pulmonary edema. One prospective, uncontrolled study found that face-mask PSV improved pulse oximetry, pH, and Pa_{CO_2} within 30 minutes in 29 patients with acute pulmonary edema, only one of whom required intubation.[93] A second prospective, uncontrolled study[94] reported similar effects on gas exchange, but 5 of 26 patients required intubation, and successfully treated patients had higher Pa_{CO_2} (54 versus 32 mmHg) and lower creatine phosphokinase levels (176 versus 1282 IU) (both $p < .05$) than failure. Further, four patients died in the first study and five in the second, three and four with myocardial infarctions, respectively. The authors concluded that NPPV is a "highly effective technique." The accompanying editorialist, however, cautioned about applying NPPV to patients with acute myocardial infarctions.[95]

Several randomized, controlled trials have been performed subsequently comparing NPPV with conventional O_2 therapy to treat patients with acute cardiogenic pulmonary edema. Masip et al[96] found that inspiratory and expiratory pressures of 15 and 5 cmH$_2$O, respectively, lowered the intubation rate from 33% in 18 controls to 5% among 22 patients randomized to NPPV ($p = .037$). NPPV also improved oxygenation more rapidly, but hospital lengths of stay and mortality rates were similar in the two groups. Sharon et al[97] randomized 40 patients to receive NPPV plus low- or high-dose nitroglycerin. The NPPV group had higher rates of intubation (80% versus 20%), myocardial infarction (55% versus 10%), and death (10% versus none) compared with the nitroglycerin controls (all $p < .05$), leading the authors to conclude that NPPV was less effective and potentially harmful compared with high-dose nitroglycerin. This inference, however, is suspect because the treatments were not comparable, and the inordinately high intubation rate in the NPPV group (80%) is difficult to explain. In the largest study to date, Nava et al[98] randomized 130 patients with acute pulmonary edema to receive NPPV (average 14.5 cmH$_2$O of pressure support and 6.1 cm H$_2$O of PEEP) or O_2 therapy; hypercapnic and normocapnic patients were prospectively distributed equally between groups. As in the earlier studies, NPPV improved oxygenation, respiratory rate, and dyspnea more rapidly than conventional therapy, but mortality and hospital lengths of stay did not differ between the groups. Overall, the rates of intubation were not significantly different (25% in controls versus 20% for NPPV); in the hypercapnic subgroup, however, the intubation rate was lower in the NPPV group than in controls (6% versus 29%, $p = .015$). These studies suggest that NPPV is effective therapy for acute pulmonary edema, but whether this is true only for hypercapnic patients awaits further evaluation.

The question of whether NPPV (the combination of pressure support and PEEP) is superior to CPAP alone is important because CPAP can be delivered more simply and less expensively. An earlier randomized trial comparing the two to treat acute pulmonary edema showed significantly more rapid reductions in respiratory rate, dyspnea scores, and hypercapnia in the NPPV group compared with the CPAP-treated group.[99] The study was stopped prematurely after enrollment of 27 patients, however, because of a greater myocardial infarction rate in the NPPV group (71% versus 31% in controls). This difference may have been attributable to unequal randomization because more patients in the NPPV group presented with chest pain. The results nonetheless raise concerns about the safety of ventilator techniques used to treat acute pulmonary edema.

More recent randomized, controlled trials comparing NPPV with CPAP have not detected similar differences in the myocardial infarction rate. Crane et al[100] randomized 60 patients with cardiogenic pulmonary edema to three different therapies: conventional, CPAP (10 cmH$_2$O), or bilevel ventilation (15 cmH$_2$O inspiratory and 5 cmH$_2$O expiratory pressures). Treatment success was 15% in the control group, 35% in the CPAP group, and 45% in the bilevel group ($p = .116$). Although myocardial infarction rate did not differ among the groups, hospital mortality was 30% in the control group, 0% in the CPAP group, and 25% in the bilevel group ($p = .029$). The difference in mortality was not statistically significant until after the first week of hospitalization, after patients had stopped using the devices. Two additional studies that randomized 46 patients with acute cardiogenic pulmonary edema to CPAP or noninvasive PSV plus PEEP found similar myocardial infarction rates.[101,102] Physiologic variables improved equally in both groups, intubation and mortality rates were similar, and troponin I levels and the speed of clinical resolution were nearly identical. In addition to finding no increase in the myocardial infarction rate in NIV-treated patients, these latter studies also found no clear advantage of NIV over CPAP alone. These findings must be interpreted with caution, however, because patients with myocardial infarction or acute ischemia were excluded.

Deciding which patients with acute cardiogenic pulmonary edema should receive NPPV can be challenging because they may respond rapidly to conventional therapy. Using their single-center registry, Masip et al[103] obtained data on 80 conventionally treated patients with cardiogenic pulmonary edema to identify those at risk for intubation. Patients with a pH of less than 7.25 or hypercapnia and a systolic blood pressure of less than 180 mmHg were found to be at high risk. The authors recommended that such patients should be "promptly considered" for NIV. Because studies have not shown definitively that NIV is more effective than CPAP, however, the most sensible current recommendation is to use CPAP (10 cmH$_2$O) initially and consider switching to NPPV if the patient has unrelenting dyspnea or persisting tachypnea or hypercapnia. Furthermore, either CPAP or NPPV should be used with great caution, if at all, in patients with acute myocardial infarction or active ischemia. These recommendations are in line with the conclusion of a meta-analysis by Pang et al,[104] as well as the consensus of the British Thoracic Society Standards of Care

Committee, which recommended that NPPV be reserved for CPAP failures.[62]

Pneumonia

An earlier retrospective study found that acute severe pneumonia is a predictor of NIV failure, perhaps because NPPV does little to facilitate the clearance of secretions.[105] Confalonieri et al[106] randomized 56 patients with severe community-acquired pneumonia to receive NPPV or standard O_2 therapy. The NPPV group had fewer intubations (21% versus 50%) and shorter ICU lengths of stay (1.8 versus 6 days) than controls (both $p < .05$). In addition, NPPV-treated patients with COPD had significantly better survival at 2 months, thought to be related to fewer late complications of intubation. The most important observation, though, was that all the benefit was attributable to the subgroup with COPD, and no clear benefit of NPPV was seen in patients without COPD patients. More recently, a prospective study on NPPV to treat patients with severe community-acquired pneumonia but without COPD found that oxygenation and respiratory rates improved initially in 22 of 24 patients after starting NPPV, but 66% eventually required intubation.[107] Based on the preceding evidence, initiation of NPPV is justifiable in appropriate patients with pneumonia and COPD. The benefit of NPPV in patients with pneumonia but without COPD has not been established. As such, NPPV should be used selectively and with caution in such patients.

The severe acute respiratory syndrome (SARS) epidemic was characterized by a high rate of respiratory failure among afflicted individuals, many of whom were otherwise healthy health care workers. Initially, use of NPPV was discouraged because of concerns about aerosolization and transmission of the highly contagious coronavirus to other health care workers. Two retrospective studies, however, one from Beijing on 28 patients treated with NPPV[108] and the other from Hong Kong on 20 patients,[109] suggest that NPPV is effective in avoiding intubation in some patients. Intubation was required in only 33% and 30% of NPPV-treated patients in the two studies, respectively. Stringent infection-control measures, including the use of a face mask, an in-line viral/bacterial filter in the bilevel ventilator tubing, and a high-efficiency particulate accumulator mask by all health care workers having contact with the patients, prevented transmission of SARS to any caregivers. Both studies reported high rates of barotraumas, 22% and 20%, respectively; it was unclear that this was related to NPPV. Given the lack of controls, these studies cannot be used to assess the efficacy of NPPV in SARS, although the lack of transmission to health care workers should allay fears about NPPV spreading the virus so long as stringent isolation and prevention measures are employed.

Immunocompromised Patients

The use of NPPV to avoid endotracheal intubation in immunocompromised patients is appealing because, by assisting ventilation without having to invade the airway, it reduces infectious and hemorrhagic complications. Encouraging results derived from an uncontrolled series that reported NPPV success rates as high as 67% (in 48 patients with AIDS and *Pneumocystis carinii* pneumonia).[110] Conti et al[111] avoided intubation in 15 of 16 patients treated with NPPV with acute respiratory failure complicating hematologic malignancies, although patients were excluded if they had more than two organ-system failures or were responding poorly to antineoplastic therapy. More recently, Antonelli et al[112] randomized 40 patients with acute respiratory failure of various etiologies following solid-organ transplantation to receive NPPV or standard therapy. NPPV reduced the need for intubation and lowered ICU mortality rate (both 20% versus 50% in controls, $p < .05$), but total hospital mortality was similar. Trends for fewer health care–associated pneumonias and episodes of severe sepsis also were apparent among NPPV-treated patients. In a subsequent study of 52 immunocompromised patients with respiratory failure, 58% with hematologic malignancies, randomized to receive NPPV for at least 2 hours three times daily or standard O_2 therapy, those treated with NPPV had fewer intubations (46% versus 77%) and mortalities (50% versus 81%, both $p < .05$).[113]

The sizable reductions in mortality among these high-risk patients strongly supports the use of NIV as the ventilatory modality of first choice in selected imunocompromised patients with acute respiratory failure. Patients developing respiratory insufficiency should be started on NPPV relatively early,[105] before progression to severe respiratory failure, watched closely, and intubated without delay if needed.

Acute Respiratory Distress Syndrome (ARDS)

No controlled trials have been reported on the efficacy of NPPV to treat ARDS. One cohort series reported that NPPV maintained adequate oxygenation and averted intubation in 6 of 12 episodes of ARDS in 10 patients.[114] Thus, although NPPV can be tried in patients with early, relatively mild ARDS in an attempt to avoid intubation, routine use is not advised. NPPV should be avoided in patients with multiple organ-system failure and very severe oxygenation defects who are likely to require prolonged ventilatory support using sophisticated ventilator modes. If a trial of NPPV is initiated, patients should be monitored closely and intubated without undue delay if they deteriorate or even fail to improve sufficiently.

Trauma

Traumatic chest-wall injuries such as flail chest or mild acute lung injury might respond favorably to NPPV, but other etiologies might not. In a retrospective survey on 46 trauma patients with respiratory insufficiency treated with NPPV, Beltrame et al[115] found rapid improvements in gas exchange and a 72% success rate, but burn patients responded poorly. Despite these promising initial results, the lack of controlled studies limits the ability to draw conclusions or make recommendations on the use of NPPV in trauma patients.

Noninvasive Positive-Pressure Ventilation for Categories of Patients with Acute Respiratory Failure

DO-NOT-INTUBATE PATIENTS

One could argue that there is little to lose by using NPPV in almost any terminal patient. NPPV could be used to lessen dyspnea, preserve patient autonomy, and permit verbal communication with loved ones during a terminal patient's final hours.[116] Some patients might be salvaged in the near term who otherwise would die without ventilatory assistance. This application is controversial, however, with some arguing that it merely could prolong the dying process, diminish patients' comfort in their waning hours, and promote excessive resource utilization.[117]

Among reports on NPPV to treat patients who have declined or are reluctant to undergo intubation, Benhamou et al[118] retrospectively studied 30 such patients, mostly elderly men (mean age 76 years) with COPD. Despite severe respiratory failure (mean Pa_{O_2} of 43 mmHg and Pa_{CO_2} of 75 mmHg), NPPV was successful initially in 60% of patients. The authors considered NPPV to be preferable to endotracheal intubation because short-term prognosis was better, and the modality appeared to be more comfortable with fewer complications. In another uncontrolled series, Meduri et al[119] observed a similar response to NPPV among 26 patients with acute hypercapnic and hypoxemic respiratory failure who refused intubation. In their randomized, controlled trial in patients with acute exacerbations of COPD, Bott et al[48] used invasive mechanical ventilation in only one of the nine control patients who died. Thus the survival advantage they observed among NPPV-treated patients was, in effect, in comparison with do-not-intubate patients.

In a prospective survey of 113 do-not-intubate patients treated with NIV,[120] amounting to 10% of all patients treated with NPPV, survival to hospital discharge was 72% and 52% for patients with acute pulmonary edema and COPD, respectively, whereas it was less than 25% for patients with pneumonia or cancer. In addition, the absence of an effective cough and the inability to be awakened were significantly associated with hospital mortality. Thus the use of NIV may be justifiable in do-not-intubate patients who have a high likelihood of surviving the hospitalization. Longer-term survival of these hospital survivors, however, is poor; Chu et al[121] found a 30% 1-year survival for do-not-intubate patients with COPD as compared with 65% for patients desiring intubation. Also, no studies have yet assessed effects on patient comfort or family satisfaction. Nonetheless, NPPV may offer significant benefits such as the ability to finalize affairs or alleviation of dyspnea even in patients who do not survive the hospitalization. If NIV is to be used for such patients, patients and/or their families should be informed that it is being used as a form of life support that may be uncomfortable and can be removed at any time.

POSTOPERATIVE PATIENTS

Several early case series on the use of NPPV to treat respiratory insufficiency in postoperative patients with Pa_{CO_2} values of greater than 50 mmHg, Pa_{O_2} values of less than 60 mmHg, or evidence of respiratory muscle fatigue reported prompt reductions in respiratory rate and dyspnea scores, improvement in gas exchange, and high success rates (roughly 75%) in avoiding the need for reintubation.[122-124] Subsequent studies found that NPPV was more effective than CPAP or chest physiotherapy in improving lung mechanics and oxygenation after coronary artery bypass

surgery[125] and better than O_2 therapy alone in improving oxygenation after lung-resection surgery.[126] NPPV also ameliorated postgastroplasty pulmonary dysfunction in morbidly obese patients.[127] More recently, a randomized trial of NPPV in 48 post-lung-resection patients with acute respiratory insufficiency, most with COPD, showed significant improvements in oxygenation and reductions in the need for intubation (21% versus 50%) and mortality rate (13% versus 38%) compared with conventionally treated controls (both $p < .05$).[128] Thus, accumulating evidence now supports the use of NPPV in selected postoperative patients to maintain improved gas exchange and avoid reintubation and its attendant complications.

FACILITATION OF WEANING AND EXTUBATION

FACILITATION OF WEANING

Udwadia et al[129] first reported the use of NPPV to facilitate weaning from mechanical ventilation in tracheostomized difficult-to-wean patients. Restrick et al[130] found that NPPV was successful in weaning 13 of 14 difficult-to-wean patients, expanding this experience to patients with translaryngeal tubes. Munshi et al[131] found that 451 hypoxemic postextubation trauma patients could be treated with NPPV rather than O_2, saving an estimated $50,000, although the cost calculation did not allow for therapist, nurse, or physician time attributable to the administration of NPPV.

These reports suggested that NPPV could be used to shorten the duration of invasive ventilation, thus reducing the occurrence of associated complications. Nava et al[132] tested this hypothesis in a randomized, controlled trial of 50 patients intubated for acute respiratory failure secondary to COPD. If they failed a T-piece weaning trial performed 48 hours after intubation, patients were randomized to extubation followed by face-mask PSV or continued intubation and routine weaning. The NPPV patients had higher overall weaning rates (88% versus 68%), shorter durations of mechanical ventilation (10.2 versus 16.6 days), briefer stays in the ICU (15.1 versus 24 days), and improved 60-day survival rates (92% versus 72%) (NPPV-treated versus controls, all $p < 0.05$). In addition, no NPPV-treated patients had nosocomial pneumonia compared with 7 pneumonias among the controls. In a similar trial, Girault et al[133] randomized 33 patients with acute-on-chronic respiratory failure to remain intubated or to be extubated to NPPV after failure of a 2-hour T-piece trial. The NPPV group had a shorter duration of endotracheal intubation (4.6 versus 7.7 days, $p = .004$), but the total duration of mechanical ventilation was longer in the NPPV group, and weaning and mortality rates and ICU and hospital lengths of stay were similar between the groups.

More recently, Ferrer et al[134] randomized 43 patients with "persistent" weaning failure (three consecutive failed T-piece trials) to be extubated to NIV or to remain intubated and be weaned using conventional methods. Patients randomized to NIV had shorter periods of intubation (9.5 versus 20.1 days), shorter ICU (14 versus 25 days) and hospital stays (14.6 versus 40.8 days), a lower rate of nosocomial pneumonia (24% versus 59%), and improved ICU and 90-day survivals (roughly 80% versus 50%, all $p < .05$). This study lends strong support to the use of NIV to facilitate extubation, but it is worth noting that two-thirds of the patients had COPD or congestive heart failure. In a preliminary study examining the use of NPPV as a routine measure to facilitate weaning in selected patients failing T-piece trials, the extubation failure rate was significantly greater than in the conventionally weaned group (41% versus none).[135] Thus, overall, the evidence is strong to support the use of NPPV to facilitate weaning and extubation in difficult-to-wean patients with COPD. The following caveats, however, should be borne in mind: (1) This approach should be reserved mainly for COPD patients, (2) patients should be selected carefully, ascertaining that they are good candidates for NPPV (see "Selection Guidelines," below), (3) patients should not have been difficult intubations, and (4) patients should be comfortable on levels of PSV that can used via mask after extubation.

NONINVASIVE POSITIVE-PRESSURE VENTILATION TO TREAT EXTUBATION FAILURE

Another potential application of NPPV in the weaning process is to avoid reintubation in patients who fail extubation. Epstein et al[136] reported that extubation failure is associated with much higher morbidity and mortality rates (43%) than successful extubations (approximately 10%). Some investigators have used NPPV prophylactically to see if extubation failure can be avoided. Jiang at al[137] randomized consecutive extubated patients to receive NPPV or conventional therapy and found a trend for a higher reintubation rate in the NPPV group (28% versus 15%), suggesting that indiscriminate use of NPPV is not effective for preventing extubation failure. Other investigators have attempted to prevent extubation failure by initiating NPPV when patients develop risk factors for extubation failure. Esteban et al[138] tried this approach in a multicenter, multinational randomized trial of 221 patients developing risk factors for respiratory failure within 48 hours after they were extubated, including hypercapnia, tachypnea, or hypoxemia. Reintubation rates (48%) and ICU lengths of stay (18 days) were identical in both groups, and the study was terminated prematurely because of a significantly increased ICU mortality in the NIV group (25% versus 15%, $p = .048$). The mortality difference was attributable to a higher mortality in the reintubated NIV patients, reintubation occurring almost 10 hours later than in the standard-therapy group. The authors concluded that NIV is not effective in unselected patients at risk for extubation failure and speculated that the greater delay in reintubation was responsible for the higher mortality rate. It is worth noting, however, that 28 patients in the control group crossed over to NPPV when they met failure criteria. Thus the controls likely would have had a substantially higher reintubation rate if not crossed over to NPPV. The overall results are not really relevant to patients with COPD, which comprised only 10% of the enrollees and had a trend toward lower reintubation rates than in controls. In a preliminary report, Nava et al[139] used NPPV prophylactically in patients deemed to be at "high risk" for respiratory failure by virtue of their having failed at least one weaning trial after more than 72 hours of intubation. These authors demonstrated significant reductions in reintubation rate, ICU mortality, and hospital length of stay. The conflicting results render any firm conclusions difficult, but

evidence to support the routine use of NPPV to avoid extubation failure is lacking. Conversely, this approach still holds promise in patients with COPD and in those at high risk of extubation failure, although further studies examining these subgroups are needed.

Another approach to treating extubation failure is to await the development of overt respiratory failure before initiating NPPV. Hilbert et al[140] found that NPPV used in this fashion lowered reintubation rate (20% versus 67%) and shortened ICU lengths of stay in 30 patients with COPD and postextubation hypercapnic respiratory insufficiency compared with 30 historically matched controls. Keenan et al[141] randomized 81 patients to receive NPPV or conventional therapy if they developed respiratory failure within 48 hours of extubation. The reintubation rate in this trial was roughly 70% in both the NPPV group and controls, and no significant differences were found in hospital length of stay or survival. Patients with COPD, however, were excluded after the first year for ethical reasons, and only 12% of the patients had COPD. Furthermore, the pressures used (10 cmH_2O inspiratory and 5 cmH_2O expiratory) may have been insufficient to provide adequate ventilatory assistance. Thus, once again, firm evidence is lacking to guide the use of NPPV in patients with overt extubation failure, but patients with COPD appear to be helped, and a trial seems reasonable in patients with other diagnoses that are likely to be reversible, such as congestive heart failure or glottic edema.

PEDIATRIC APPLICATIONS

Fewer reports of pediatric than adult applications of NPPV for acute respiratory failure have appeared. A 1993 case series of acute pediatric applications of NPPV by Akingbola et al[142] reported the successful use of nasal ventilation in two 12-year-old boys with atelectasis and pulmonary edema. In a retrospective series of 28 pediatric patients with hypoxemic respiratory failure ranging in age from 4 months to 16 years, Fortenberry et al[143] found that respiratory rate, Pa_{CO_2}, and oxygenation improved promptly after initiation of nasal bilevel NPPV, and only 3 patients required intubation. Padman et al[144] subsequently reported similar results in a prospective series of 34 pediatric patients with both hypoxemic and hypoventilatory respiratory insufficiency, again with only 3 patients requiring intubation.

Favorable responses to NPPV in older children are not surprising, particularly when they are suffering from conditions reported to be treated successfully by NPPV in adults. Concerns have been raised, however, about treating very young children and infants with NPPV because of increased nasal resistance[145] and inability to cooperate.[146] In a series reported by Fortenberry et al[143] of 28 patients, NPPV was successful in avoiding intubation in the 10 children younger than 5 years of age. More recently, a retrospective trial observed successful application of NPPV in infants following liver transplantation.[147] In a randomized, prospective trial on infants (median age 9.5 months) with various causes of upper airway obstruction, CPAP and BiPAP proved to be equally efficacious in reducing respiratory rate and breathing effort; both were well tolerated, although BiPAP was associated with more asynchrony.[148] The lack of controlled trials makes it difficult to formulate selection guidelines for

NPPV in children, although reported success rates appear to be comparable with those in adults, and tentative guidelines have been proposed[149] that are based on those used for adults.

Patients Undergoing Bronchoscopy

NPPV administered via T connector attached to a face mask can be used to assist ventilation and enhance oxygenation during fiberoptic bronchoscopy in high-risk patients. First reported to improve oxygenation and be well tolerated in a small series of immunocompromised hypoxemic patients, NPPV was shown subsequently to improve and sustain oxygenation better than conventional O_2 supplementation in a randomized, prospective trial in 26 patients with Pa_{O_2}/Fi_{O_2} ratios of 200 or less and suspected nosocomial pneumonia.[150] More recently, NPPV to assist ventilation during fiberoptic bronchoscopy was administered successfully using a "helmet" device (see techniques section below).[151] NPPV also has been used to assist ventilation during upper endoscopy for gastric tube placement in patients with neuromuscular disease.[152]

Selection of Patients for Noninvasive Positive-Pressure Ventilation in the Acute Setting

DETERMINANTS OF SUCCESS

Retrospective[105,153] and prospective[154–156] studies have identified predictors of NPPV success (Table 19-2). Patients with baseline hypercapnia fare better than those with hypoxemia alone, but successful patients have lower baseline Pa_{CO_2} values (79 versus 98 mmHg) and higher pH values (7.28 versus 7.22) than failure patients.[105] Pneumonia predisposes to failure whether alone or in combination with COPD (odds ratio 5.63 for COPD).[154,156] The strongest predictor of success, though, is prompt improvement in gas exchange and heart and respiratory rates within an hour or

TABLE 19-2   Predictors of Success during Acute Applications of NPPV

Younger age
Lower activity of illness (APACHE score)
Able to cooperate, better neurologic score
Able to coordinate breathing with ventilator
Less air leaking, intact dentition
Tachypnea, but not excessively rapid (>24 but <35 breaths per minute)
Hypercarbia, but not too severe (Pa_{CO_2} > 45 but < 92 mmHg)
Acidemia, but not too severe (pH < 7.35 but > 7.10)
Improvements in gas exchange, heart and respiratory rates within first 2 hours[a]

[a] Most powerful predictor
SOURCE: Adapted, with permission, from refs. 106, 154, and 156.

two of NPPV initiation.[105,153–156] Confalonieri et al[155] have incorporated some of these predictors (APACHE II score ≥ 29, pH < 7.25, Glasgow coma score ≤ 11, and respiratory rate ≥ 35 breaths per minute) into two risk charts for NPPV failure, one to be used at baseline and the other at 2 hours (Fig. 19-3). If these abnormalities were all present at baseline, the likelihood of failure was 82% and rose to 99% if they persisted at 2 hours.

Timing of initiation is another determinant of success. Ambrosino et al[105] advised that NPPV "should be instituted early in every patient before a severe acidosis ensues." Initiation of NPPV should be viewed as taking advantage of a "window of opportunity." The window opens when acute respiratory distress occurs and shuts when the patient deteriorates to the point of necessitating immediate intubation. In this context, it should be emphasized that NPPV is used as a way of preventing intubation, not replacing it.

SELECTION GUIDELINES

The preceding predictors of success and failure and the entry criteria used for enrollment of patients into the many studies have served as a basis for consensus guidelines on the selection of patients to receive NPPV for acute respiratory failure.[157] These guidelines use a simple two-step approach outlined in Table 19-3. The first step identifies patients at risk of needing intubation. Patients with mild respiratory distress are excluded from consideration because they should do well without ventilator assistance. Those needing ventilator assistance are identified using clinical indicators of acute respiratory distress and gas-exchange derangement, as listed in Table 19-3. These criteria are most applicable to patients with COPD but can be used to screen those with other forms of expiratory failure, although some modifications are advisable. For example, studies on NPPV in acute pulmonary edema and acute hypoxemic respiratory failure have used higher respiratory rates as enrollment criteria (>30–35 instead of >24 breaths per minute) and a Pa_{O_2}/Fi_{O2} ratio of less than 200.[96–99]

The second step is to screen out patients in whom use of NPPV is contraindicated (see Table 19-3). Most are relative contraindications, and judgment should be exercised in implementing them. Also, some conditions that have been listed as contraindications in the past no longer preclude the use of NPPV. For example, patients with coma, if related to hypercapnia, may be managed successfully with NPPV. Diaz et al[158] demonstrated that patients (mainly with COPD) with hypercapnic coma (Glasgow coma scores ≤ 8) had outcomes just as good as those with higher Glasgow coma scores. In another report,[118] nearly half the patients were obtunded or somnolent initially, yet most were managed successfully with NPPV.

The underlying etiology and potential reversibility of acute respiratory failure are also important considerations in patient selection. As discussed previously, the strongest evidence supports the use of NPPV for COPD and either NPPV or CPAP for acute cardiogenic pulmonary edema. As illustrated in Fig. 19-4, a reversible etiology permits the use of NPPV as a "crutch" that assists the patient through a critical interval, allowing time for other therapies such as bronchodilators, steroids, or diuretics to reverse the

Admission

	RR	pH admission <7.25		pH admission 7.25–7.29		pH admission >7.30	
		APACHE ≥29	APACHE <29	APACHE ≥29	APACHE <29	APACHE ≥29	APACHE <29
GCS 15	<30	29	11	18	6	17	6
	30–34	42	18	29	11	27	10
	≥35	52	24	37	15	35	14
GCS 12–14	<30	48	22	33	13	32	12
	30–34	63	34	48	22	46	21
	≥35	71	42	57	29	55	27
GCS ≤11	<30	64	35	49	23	47	21
	30–34	76	49	64	35	62	33
	≥35	82	59	72	44	70	42

1 Hour

	RR	pH after 2 h <7.25		pH after 2 h 7.25–7.29		pH after 2 h ≥7.30	
		APACHE ≥29	APACHE <29	APACHE ≥29	APACHE <29	APACHE ≥29	APACHE <29
GCS 15	<30	72	35	27	7	11	3
	30–34	88	59	49	17	25	7
	≥35	93	73	64	27	38	11
GCS 12–14	<30	84	51	41	13	19	5
	30–34	93	74	65	28	39	12
	≥35	96	84	78	42	54	20
GCS ≤11	<30	93	74	65	28	39	12
	30–34	97	88	83	51	63	26
	≥35	99	93	90	66	76	40

FIGURE 19-3 Charts showing percentage likelihood of NPPV failure in patients with COPD based on pH and APACHE score and Glasgow Coma Score (GCS). Chart on top refers to values at the time of admission, and bottom chart is at 2 hours. Numbers in boxes are percentages for likelihood of failure. At 2 hours, the combination of an APACHE score of less than 11, APACHE score of 29 or greater, and a Glasgow Coma Score of less than 11 predicts failure with a likelihood of 99%. Based on 1,033 patients with COPD treated with NPPV in 13 different experienced units. (*Used, with permission, from Antonelli et al: Intensive Care Med 27:1718–28, 2001.*)

underlying condition. More severe, less easily reversed forms of respiratory failure that will require prolonged periods of ventilatory support, such as status asthmaticus requiring controlled hypoventilation, complicated pneumonias, or ARDS, are best managed using invasive ventilation.

TABLE 19-3 Selection Guidelines: Noninvasive Ventilation for Patients with Acute Respiratory Failure (ARF)

Step 1. Identify patients with reversible causes for ARF in need of ventilator assistance.
  a. Reversible cause for ARF such as COPD or acute cardiogenic pulmonary edema
  b. Symptoms and signs of acute respiratory distress:
    i. Moderate to severe dyspnea, increased over usual
    ii. Rate > 24 for COPD, rate > 30 for hypoxemic ARF
    iii. Accessory muscle use, paradoxical breathing
  c. Gas-exchange abnormalities:
    i. $Pa_{CO_2} > 45$ mmHg, pH < 7.35
    ii. $Pa_{O_2}/F_{IO_2} < 200$
Step 2. Exclude those at increased risk with noninvasive ventilation:
  a. Respiratory arrest
  b. Medically unstable (hypotensive shock, uncontrolled cardiac ischemia or arrhythmias)
  c. Unable to protect airway (impaired cough or swallowing mechanism)
  d. Excessive secretions
  e. Agitated or uncooperative
  f. Facial trauma or burns or anatomic abnormalities interfering with mask fit

SOURCE: Adapted, with permission, from Mehta and Hill.[1]

Marginal patients might be considered for a trial of NPPV but should be watched closely for further deterioration so that needed intubation is not delayed unduly.

Noninvasive Positive-Pressure Ventilation for Chronic Respiratory Failure

EVIDENCE FOR EFFICACY

RESTRICTIVE THORACIC DISEASES

Restrictive thoracic disorders limit expansion of the thoracic cage either because of increased elastance (as with chest-

FIGURE 19-4 Schema to illustrate importance of reversibility in success of NPPV for acute respiratory failure. (*Left*) Relentless downhill clinical course of underlying process (severe ARDS). NPPV initiated when window of opportunity opens still fails because it is not sufficient to support the patient when the underlying process has progressed too far. (*Right*) NPPV succeeds when medical therapy reverses the underlying process (COPD exacerbation).

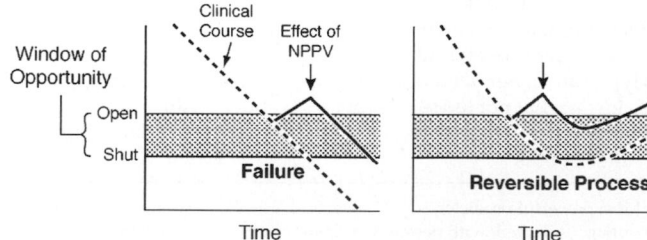

wall deformity), muscle weakness (as with neuromuscular diseases), or both. Experience gained during the polio epidemics of the 1930s through 1950s and subsequently with other neuromuscular disorders demonstrated that "body ventilators," even when used intermittently, were effective at stabilizing or even reversing chronic respiratory failure secondary to restrictive thoracic disorders.[159,160] Although NPPV had been available for the therapy of restrictive thoracic diseases for decades,[161] its use beyond a few centers with special expertise was quite limited until the late 1980s. Mouthpieces or full-face masks designed mainly for administration of anesthesia were the only interfaces available, posing challenges for patient adaptation. Despite this, one center reported remarkable success with mouthpiece ventilation in a cohort of 257 patients with neuromuscular disease and chronic respiratory failure that was treated for an average of 9.6 years.[162] Bulbar function was intact, including speech and swallowing, but the patients were otherwise severely compromised. One-hundred and forty-four of these patients required 20–24 hours of ventilator support daily and had vital capacities of only 10.5% of predicted. Nonetheless, 67 were switched successfully from tracheostomies to NPPV, and only 38 died during the follow-up interval of up to 37 years. Although the study was uncontrolled, the authors concluded that mouthpiece NPPV prolonged survival and enhanced convenience and communication in these severely compromised patients.

Despite this favorable experience, however, wider use of NPPV awaited further developments during the early 1980s. One was the development of nasal CPAP for therapy of obstructive sleep apnea that encouraged the creation of more comfortable commercially available nasal masks.[163] Another was the suggestion by French investigators that nasal ventilation could be used in patients with muscular dystrophy to halt progression of the disease.[22] In 1987, several small series and case reports appeared describing successful management with nocturnal nasal ventilation of patients with chronic respiratory failure secondary to a variety of restrictive thoracic disorders.[164–166] Subsequently, additional small series have confirmed the earlier findings, but no prospective, randomized series have been performed, mainly for ethical reasons. Despite this, NPPV has gained wide acceptance as the modality of first choice to treat patients with chronic respiratory failure.[157] Because most series have combined patients with different etiologies, the following will discuss evidence for benefits attributed to NPPV for restrictive thoracic diseases in general, making reference to individual diagnoses as appropriate. Table 19-4 lists individual diagnoses of neuromuscular diseases reported to benefit from NPPV.

EFFECTS ON SYMPTOMS AND DAYTIME GAS EXCHANGE

Numerous studies on the efficacy of NPPV in a wide variety of neuromuscular and chest-wall disorders have shown that intermittent NPPV consistently improves symptoms of fatigue, daytime hypersomnolence, and morning headache.[32,167–169] Daytime gas exchange also improves, Pa_{CO_2} dropping on average from 63 mmHg to 48 mmHg and Pa_{O_2} increasing from 54–71 mmHg among multiple studies.[1] The improvement in gas exchange is gradual, usu-

TABLE 19-4 Restrictive Thoracic Diseases Treated with Noninvasive Ventilation

Recommended for the following diagnoses:
Chest wall deformity
   Kyphoscoliosis
   Post thoracoplasty for tuberculosis
Slowly progressive neuromuscular disorders
   Postpolio syndrome
   High spinal cord injury
   Spinal muscular atrophy
   Slowly progressive muscular dystrophies
      Duchenne muscular dystrophy
      Limb-girdle muscular dystrophy
      Myotonic dystrophy
   Multiple sclerosis
   Bilateral diaphragmatic paralysis
More rapidly progressive neuromuscular disorders[a]
   Amyotrophic lateral sclerosis
Not recommended for[b]:
Rapidly progressive neuromuscular disorders
   Guillain-Barré syndrome
   Myasthenia gravis

[a] Tracheostomy ventilation should be considered in far-advanced cases.
[b] Unless upper airway protective mechanisms intact

ally occurring over a period of weeks, as patients increase their hours of use, mainly at night. In addition, nasal NPPV has been shown to ameliorate chronic hypoventilation in patients with severe kyphoscoliosis who fail to improve with nasal CPAP alone.[171]

EFFECTS ON NOCTURNAL GAS EXCHANGE AND SLEEP

Neuromuscular and chest-wall disorders cause protean sleep-related breathing disturbances depending on the specific syndrome and the involvement of respiratory muscles.[172] Abnormalities include obstructive and central sleep apneas, intermittent desaturations, particularly during REM sleep in patients with diaphragmatic weakness, and sustained hypoventilation as global weakness and/or chest-wall restriction advances. These abnormalities often lead to sleep disruption, characterized by diminished sleep duration, fragmentation related to arousals, and poor sleep quality secondary to diminished slow-wave and REM sleep.

NPPV ameliorates nocturnal hypoventilation and has been shown to eliminate the intermittent obstructive apneas and severe O_2 desaturations that occur during negative-pressure ventilation, particularly during REM sleep.[172] Although no randomized, prospective trials have been performed, investigators have evaluated efficacy using temporary withdrawal of nocturnal nasal NPPV from long-term users with restrictive thoracic diseases whose gas exchange had been improved by prior NPPV use.[34,173] Temporary withdrawal of NPPV caused a deterioration of nocturnal oxygenation and ventilation[34] (Fig. 19-5) and increased frequency of arousals.[173] All changes were reversed promptly on resumption of NPPV. These findings indicate that NPPV is important in preventing deterioration of nocturnal gas exchange that is thought to predispose to chronic hypoventilation and contribute to frequent arousals and

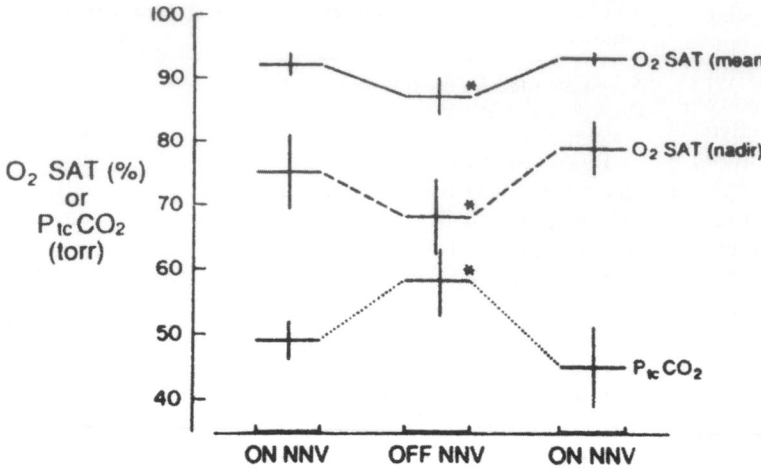

FIGURE 19-5 Effect of withdrawal of nocturnal nasal ventilation (NNV) on mean and nadir O_2 saturations and mean transcutaneous P_{CO_2} levels obtained during nocturnal monitoring. Values on the left labeled "on NNV" were obtained during NNV use on the night before NNV withdrawal, values in the middle were obtained on the last night of the NNV withdrawal period, and values on the right labeled "on NNV" were obtained a week after NNV was resumed. Data are mean ± SE. Asterisk indicates $p < .05$ compared with "on NNV" values ($n = 6$). (*Used, with permission, from Hiel et al: Am Rev Respis Dis 145:365–71, 1992.*)

fragmented sleep. Stabilization of nocturnal gas exchange and improved sleep quality are thought to be major reasons for the improvement in symptoms associated with NPPV use. Although sleep quality is improved compared to no ventilator assistance, air leaking during NPPV, however, can contribute to sleep fragmentation.[174]

EFFECTS ON QUALITY OF LIFE

NPPV improves health-related quality of life in patients with restrictive thoracic disorders.[175,176] The nature and duration of improvement, however, depend on the natural history of the underlying disorder. Among patients with amyotrophic lateral sclerosis (ALS), the mental-component summary score[177] and the vitality score[178] on the SF-(short form-36) questionnaire register sustained improvements. These improvements are seen even when the functional rating declines (Fig. 19-6), but attrition rates are high over time related to the high mortality of the underlying condition.[179] More sustained benefits would be expected, of course, in conditions with lower rates of progression. Likewise, musculoskeletal functional gains would not be expected unless the underlying condition offers the potential for improvement (i.e., no quadriplegia).

Some studies have compared quality of life during use of NPPV with that during use of tracheostomy PPV among patients with restrictive thoracic diseases.[180–182] Both groups have high levels of satisfaction, but NPPV was rated as preferable to ventilation via a tracheostomy with regard to comfort, convenience, portability, and overall acceptability.[180] Although tracheostomy ventilation received higher scores for quality of sleep and providing a sense of security, the vast majority of patients preferred NPPV. Another survey of 35 ventilator users, with 29 NPPV users and 6 with tracheostomy ventilation, found satisfactory levels of psychosocial functioning and mental well-being, as determined by standard questionnaires.[181] The ratings compared favorably with those of a general population, and NPPV and tracheostomy ventilation received similar scores. In another survey of home mechanical ventilation users, patients with scoliosis receiving tracheostomy ventilation had higher health-index ratings than those receiving

FIGURE 19-6 Serial data for the Short Form-36 Mental Component Summary (SF-36 MCS), Sleep Apnea Quality of Life Index (SAQLI) symptoms domain, and ALS Functional Rating Scale (ALSFRS) immediately before starting noninvasive ventilation (NIV) and after 1, 3, 5, and 7 months of NIV. The slight improvement in the ALSFRS score at 7 months is secondary to a survivor effect. (*Used, with permission, from Lyall et al: Neurology 57:153–6, 2001.*)

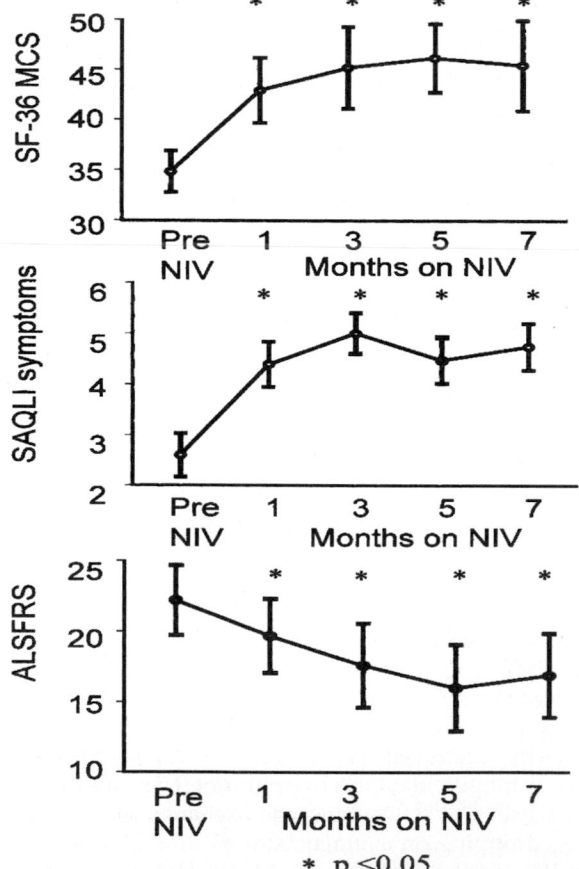

NPPV.[182] Thus NPPV offers many advantages over invasive mechanical ventilation, including comfort, portability, cost, and convenience, but some ratings, including overall health and sense of security, may favor invasive mechanical ventilation.

EFFECT ON HOSPITAL UTILIZATION

In their long-term follow-up study of patients with kyphoscoliosis, sequelae of tuberculosis, and Duchenne muscular dystrophy, Leger et al[183] observed significant reductions in hospital days per patient per year from 34, 31, and 18 days for the year before starting NPPV to 6, 10, and 7 days for the year after, respectively. These findings suggest that NPPV may cut health care resource utilization in these patients, with the potential for substantial cost savings. More recently, Janssens et al[184] observed a similar reduction in hospital days per patient per year (median of 17 for the year before and 6 for the year after NPPV) for patients with restrictive thoracic disorders in a long-term retrospective study from Switzerland. Although these uncontrolled studies do not preclude the possibility that changes in hospitalization practices over time could have been responsible for the reductions, it appears highly likely that NPPV reduces the need for hospitalization among these patients.

EFFECT ON SURVIVAL

Despite the lack of randomized, controlled trials, long-term follow-up series provide strong evidence that NPPV prolongs survival in comparison with unventilated patients. The ability to prolong survival is obvious in patients using NPPV continuously who would die if ventilator assistance stops for more than a few minutes.[162] Studies from France[183] and England[185] have reported on several hundred patients with chronic respiratory failure of various etiologies treated with intermittent nasal NPPV for periods of up to 5 years (Fig. 19-7). Rather than survival rates, these studies used the rate for continuation of NPPV, thought to

correspond closely with survival for most diagnoses. The studies found very favorable continuation rates for postpolio and kyphoscoliosis patients (approximately 100% and 80%, respectively, after 5 years). Patients with sequelae of old tuberculosis had higher continuation rates in the British compared with the French study (94% versus 60%, respectively), perhaps reflecting the greater morbidity of the French patients at the time of enrollment. Also, patients with Duchenne muscular dystrophy (DMD) in the French study had lower continuation rates (47%) than those with other neuromuscular diseases, with 28% undergoing tracheostomy and the remaining 25% dying. A more recent follow-up on the English cohort observed much better survival rates for patients with DMD treated with NPPV than those previously reported by the French group: 85% for 1 year and 73% for 5 years.[186] This disparity may reflect differences in the severity of illness between patients when begun on NPPV, how cough was assisted, or practices on switching to tracheostomy. Overall, the continuation rates from these long-term follow-up studies are similar to those observed for patients treated with invasive ventilation reported earlier by the French group.[187]

Survival would be anticipated to be shorter in patients with ALS than in those with more slowly progressive neuromuscular diseases. In a prospective, nonrandomized trial on 20 consecutive patients, Pinto et al[188] treated the first 10 with medical therapy alone and the next 10 with NPPV. After 2 years, 50% of the NPPV patients were alive, whereas all the medical therapy patients had died. Aboussouan et al[189] compared the survival of 31 patients with ALS who continued NPPV with that of 21 patients who were intolerant of NPPV. The intolerant patients had a significantly greater risk of dying over the 3-year study period than those who remained on NPPV (relative risk 3.1). As might be anticipated, patients with bulbar involvement were unlikely to be tolerant of NPPV (only 6 of 20); if they could tolerate the therapy, however, it imparted an apparent survival

FIGURE 19-7 *A. Survival after tracheostomy in 222 patients with chronic respiratory failure of various etiologies followed for as long as 10 years. (Redrawn, with permission, from Robert et al: Rev Fr Mal Respir 11:923–36, 1993) B. Likelihood of continuing noninvasive positive pressure ventilation (NPPV) in 276 patients with chronic respiratory failure followed for as long as 3 years. (Redrawn, with permission, from Leger et al: Chest 105:100–5, 1994.)* BRO, bronchiectasis; COPD, chronic obstructive pulmonary disease; DMD, Duchenne muscular dystrophy; KS, kyphoscoliosis; MYO, myopathy; PP, postpolio syndrome; TB, history of tuberculosis.

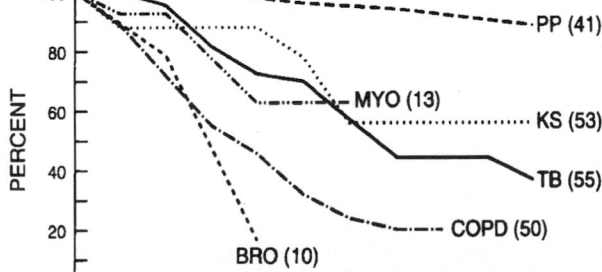

A SURVIVAL AFTER TRACHEOSTOMY

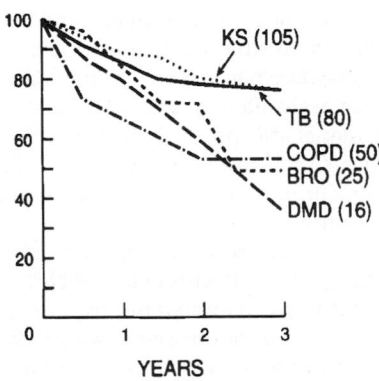

B CONTINUATION OF NPPV

advantage. Bach[190] has reported that NPPV prolongs survival and postpones the need for tracheostomy in ALS. Based on these observations, NPPV is now used in approximately 15% of patients with ALS compared with only 2% using invasive mechanical ventilation, according to one recent cross-sectional U.S. survey.[191] On the other hand, Bach[190] also found that after 5 years of follow-up, only 8 of 25 (32%) patients with ALS using NPPV were alive compared with 27 of 50 (54%) patients receiving tracheostomy ventilation. This suggests that NPPV is less effective at prolonging survival than tracheostomy ventilation, as might be anticipated among patients with neuromuscular diseases such as ALS that impair bulbar function.

SELECTION OF PATIENTS WITH RESTRICTIVE THORACIC DISEASE TO RECEIVE NONINVASIVE POSITIVE-PRESSURE VENTILATION

Guidelines for the selection of patients with restrictive thoracic disorders to receive NIV based on American College of Chest Physicians (ACCP) consensus and Medicare guidelines in the United States are listed in Table 19-5.[192] Patients should have symptoms attributable to chronic hypoventilation and poor sleep quality, such as morning headache, daytime hypersomnolence, and low energy in combination with daytime or sustained nocturnal hypoventilation. The duration of nocturnal O_2 desaturation used as an indicator of nocturnal hypoventilation (<88% for more than 5 consecutive minutes) was suggested by consensus[192] but has never been validated. Even if symptoms are minimal or lacking, patients with severe CO_2 retention (>50 mmHg) and those recovering from bouts of acute respiratory failure are considered for long-term NIV, particularly if there is persistent CO_2 retention or a history of repeated hospitalizations. The consensus group also recommended NPPV for patients with severe pulmonary dysfunction (FVC < 50% of predicted or maximal inspiratory pressure < 60 cmH_2O), even in the absence of CO_2 retention, despite the lack of evidence from clinical studies to support the initiation of NIV on the basis of pulmonary function alone.

Relative contraindications to the use of NPPV for chronic respiratory failure (Table 19-5) include inability to protect the upper airway because of impaired cough or swallowing or excessive secretions. Aggressive treatment with techniques or devices to assist cough[193] may permit the use of NPPV in such patients who otherwise would not be candidates, but if the condition is too severe, tracheostomy is indicated if the patient desires maximal prolongation of life. Tracheostomy ventilation has been recommended when the need for ventilator assistance exceeds 16 hours daily,[194] although many patients still prefer NPPV.[180] Other relative contraindications to NPPV are listed in Table 19-5. The clinician must render a judgment as to whether these are sufficient to preclude a trial of NIV.

The natural history of the restrictive thoracic disorder also should be considered when deciding about NPPV. Patients with chest-wall deformities and stable or slowly progressive neuromuscular disorders respond well to NPPV and remain stable for long periods of time.[183,185] Patients with more rapidly progressive neuromuscular disorders such as

TABLE 19-5 Selection Guidelines: Long-Term Noninvasive Ventilation for Restrictive Thoracic Disorders or Obesity Hypoventilation

Indications
1. Symptoms: fatigue, morning headache, hypersomnolence, nightmares, enuresis, dyspnea, and so on
2. Signs: cor pulmonale
3. Gas-exchange criteria:
   Daytime $Pa_{CO_2} \geq 45$ mmHg
   Nocturnal oxygen desaturation ($Sa_{O_2} \leq 88\%$ for more than 5 minutes sustained or >10% of total monitoring time)
4. Sleep evaluation:
   Unnecessary in restrictive thoracic disorders if other criteria met
   Should be obtained for obesity hypoventilation to assess OSA[a]
5. Other possible indications
   Recovering from acute respiratory failure with persistent CO_2 retention
   Repeated hospitalizations for acute respiratory failure

Contraindications
Inability to protect airway
  Impaired cough
  Impaired swallowing with chronic aspiration
Copious secretions
Need for continuous or nearly continuous ventilatory assistance
Anatomic abnormalities that interfere with mask fitting
Poorly motivated patient or family
Inability to cooperate or comprehend therapy
Inadequate financial or caregiver resources

[a] If OSA (obstructive sleep apnea) is present, trial of CPAP may be warranted see (Table 6).
SOURCE: Adapted, with permission, from Mehta and Hill.[1]

ALS may respond well temporarily, but as debility progresses and bulbar function deteriorates, NPPV loses its efficacy. Those who wish to optimize their chances for survival may prefer invasive ventilation, and others may desire hospice care. Patients with rapidly progressive neuromuscular conditions such as Guillain-Barré syndrome or myasthenia gravis in crisis usually are poor candidates for NIV because swallowing frequently is impaired when ventilatory dysfunction becomes severe.

WHEN TO START LONG-TERM NONINVASIVE POSITIVE-PRESSURE VENTILATION FOR RESTRICTIVE THORACIC DISORDERS

NPPV to treat chronic respiratory failure secondary to restrictive thoracic diseases has gained wide acceptance, but the optimal time for initiation has been debated. Prophylactic initiation in progressive neuromuscular diseases, before the onset of symptoms or daytime hypoventilation, has been proposed to retard the progression of respiratory dysfunction. Raphael et al[195] tested this hypothesis in 76 patients with DMD who had not yet developed symptoms or daytime hypoventilation, randomizing them to receive nasal NPPV or standard therapy. Not only did NPPV fail to slow disease progression, but it also was associated with greater mortality, leading to premature termination of the trial. The authors surmised that mortality was increased because NPPV gave patients a false sense of security that caused them to delay seeking medical attention when they developed respiratory infections. The study had numerous shortcomings, including failure to document patient adherence or to consistently use techniques to assist cough, but it has stemmed any enthusiasm about using prophylactic NPPV in patients with DMD.

Early initiation of NPPV also has been proposed to treat patients with ALS.[196] Current guidelines based on expert consensus recommend starting NPPV if FVC drops below 50% of predicted[197] or maximal inspiratory pressure drops below 60 cmH$_2$O. In a preliminary study,[196] 20 patients with ALS and FVC values ranging between 70% and 100% of predicted were randomized to receive NPPV if they had an Sa$_{O2}$ of less than 90% for more than 1 minute during nocturnal oximetry ("early intervention") or to await a drop in FVC to less than 50% of predicted ("standard of care"). The early-intervention group had a significant increase in the vitality subscale on the SF-36, suggesting that earlier intervention might be beneficial in patients with ALS, but more research is necessary.

Presently, awaiting the onset of symptoms of nocturnal hypoventilation before initiation of NPPV is the most pragmatic approach because adherence to therapy is often poor unless patients are motivated by the desire for symptom relief. Symptomatic patients who have only nocturnal but no daytime hypoventilation, as demonstrated by frequent, sustained nocturnal O$_2$ desaturations, are good candidates for initiation. Masa et al[198] showed improvements in dyspnea scores, morning headache, and confusion after 2 weeks of nocturnal NPPV in 21 such patients, whose proportion of sleep time with an Sa$_{O2}$ of less than 90% averaged 40–50% on room air before initiation of NPPV and fell to 6% afterwards. The timing of initiation requires a judgment based on the anticipated progression of the disease (sooner for more rapid progression), the patient's symptoms, pulmonary function, and daytime and nocturnal gas exchange. The aim is to begin when there are symptoms with significant pulmonary function and/or gas-exchange abnormalities when the patient still has time to adapt but well before the occurrence of a respiratory crisis.

Central Hypoventilation, Obstructive Sleep Apnea, and Obesity Hypoventilation

CENTRAL HYPOVENTILATION/OBSTRUCTIVE SLEEP APNEA

The first case reports describing the use of nasal ventilation for chronic respiratory failure were in young children with central hypoventilation, who had resolution of gas-exchange abnormalities and symptoms after initiation of therapy.[199,200] No controlled studies have examined this application, but enough anecdotal evidence has accrued that consensus groups consider therapy of central hypoventilation as an appropriate indication for NPPV.[157,192]

Nasal CPAP is considered the therapy of first choice for obstructive sleep apnea. NPPV, however, may be successful in improving daytime gas exchange and symptoms in hypoventilating patients with obstructive sleep apnea who have persistent CO$_2$ retention after use of nasal CPAP alone. Among 13 patients with severe obstructive sleep apnea whose hypercapnia (average Pa$_{CO2}$ of 62 mmHg) was unresponsive to CPAP, NPPV using volume-limited ventilators lowered the Pa$_{CO2}$ to 46 mmHg, and 9 of the patients eventually stabilized on CPAP alone.[201]

Independently adjusted inspiratory and expiratory pressure or "bilevel" positive-pressure ventilation was first developed as a way of controlling obstructive sleep apnea while using lower expiratory pressures than with CPAP alone, thus potentially enhancing comfort and adherence with therapy.[202] Reeves-Hoche et al[203] were unable to demonstrate improved adherence rates in patients with obstructive sleep apnea treated with bilevel ventilation compared with CPAP alone. Even so, bilevel devices are still used commonly to treat patients intolerant of CPAP alone, but a stronger rationale supports the use of bilevel NPPV for obstructive apnea if patients have persisting hypoventilation despite adequate CPAP therapy.

OBESITY-HYPOVENTILATION SYNDROME

Respiratory impairment is common among obese patients, including those with restricted lung volumes secondary to increased chest-wall and lung elastance, abnormal blood gases, and breathing disturbances during sleep. When obese patients hypoventilate, the term *obesity-hypoventilation syndrome* is applied, a condition that is multifactorial in etiology. The altered chest-wall mechanics are accompanied by reductions in respiratory drive (either acquired or congenital), as well as obstructive sleep apnea (in 80–90% of patients), giving rise to the hypoventilation.[204] This is a morbid condition associated with cor pulmonale and a high mortality rate over time, but it responds favorably to NIV.

Morbidly obese subjects have significantly increased work of breathing at baseline, and NPPV (inspiratory pressure of 9–12 cmH$_2$O, expiratory pressure of 4 cmH$_2$O) lowers that work.[205] NPPV also raises tidal volumes and lowers end-tidal P$_{CO2}$ more in patients with obesity hypoventilation than in obese patients without sleep-disordered breathing or in nonhypoventilating subjects with obstructive sleep apnea.[205] NPPV lowers Pa$_{CO2}$ and improves symptoms as effectively in patients with obesity hypoventilation as in those with severe kyphoscoliosis,[206] associated with an increase in respiratory drive.[207] CPAP alone, however, may be as effective as NPPV in some patients.[204] Some investigators also have started with NPPV and converted to CPAP once hypoventilation has been controlled.[201] These studies support the use of NPPV for obesity hypoventilation to improve symptoms and gas exchange.

As obesity has become an increasingly prevalent problem, obesity-hypoventilation sundrome has become an increasingly common indication for using long-term NPPV. A Swiss survey found that during the 1990s it became the most common diagnosis among patients using long-term NPPV at home in the Geneva region[184] (Fig. 19-8). Adherence was excellent with the therapy, exceeding 70%, average Pa$_{CO2}$ normalized, and hospital days fell significantly following NPPV initiation.

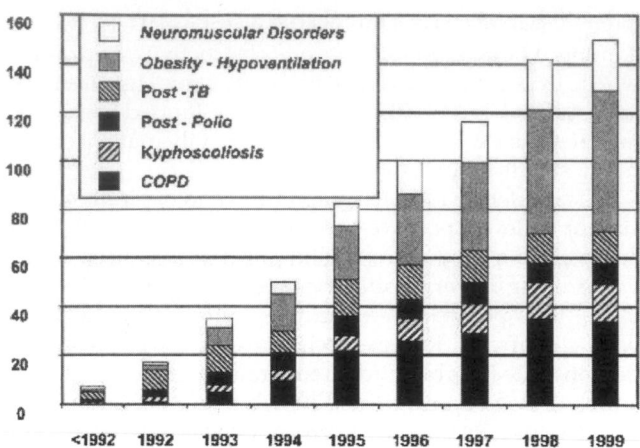

FIGURE 19-8 Yearly count of the cumulative population of patients treated by NPPV during the study period (1992–2000) according to diagnostic category. (*Used, with permission, from Janseens et al: Chest 128:67–79, 2003.*)

SELECTION OF PATIENTS WITH CENTRAL SLEEP APNEA/OBESITY-HYPOVENTILATION SYNDROME FOR NONINVASIVE POSITIVE-PRESSURE VENTILATION

Firm indications and selection guidelines for central hypoventilation/central sleep apnea/obesity-hypoventilation syndrome have not been established. The contentious issue is that patients with obstructive apneas might respond to CPAP alone. Patients who are symptomatic with frank hypoventilation or who have prolonged central apneas clearly are good candidates for NPPV. The more severe the hypoventilation, the more important it would be to start with a mode that augments minute volume, and using a backup rate would be important for those with prolonged central apneas. Medicare guidelines in the United States (Table 19-6) require a polysomnogram to document the central apneas, prolonged O_2 desaturations ($\leq$ 88% for more than 5 minutes) as evidence of nocturnal hypoventilation and, if the patient has obstructive sleep apnea, evidence of CPAP failure with improvement on NPPV, as determined by oximetry or a repeat polysomnogram.

Obstructive Lung Diseases

CHRONIC OBSTRUCTIVE PULMONARY DISEASE

During the 1960s, McClement et al[208] speculated that improved ventilation-perfusion relationships, reduced O_2

TABLE 19-6 Guidelines for Noninvasive Positive-Pressure Ventilation in Obstructive Sleep Apnea/Central Sleep Apnea[a]

1. Polysomnogram demonstrating OSA, CSA, or mixed apneas
2. If OSA, patient failed to improve or tolerate CPAP alone
3. Sustained oxygen desaturation nocturnally ($\leq$ 88% for >5 min)
4. Significant improvement in nocturnal gas exchange during NPPV use, as documented by oximetry or polysomnography

[a] Based on Center for Medicare and Medicaid Services Guidelines.
ABBREVIATIONS: OSA, obstructive sleep apnea; CSA, central sleep apnea.

consumption, and mobilization of secretions would benefit patients with COPD treated with negative-pressure ventilators. During the early 1980s, Braun and Marino[209] tested the theory that respiratory muscles are chronically fatigued and will benefit from intermittent rest. They treated 16 patients with severe COPD using wrap negative-pressure ventilators for 5 hours daily over 5 months and observed improvements in vital capacity, maximal inspiratory and expiratory pressure, and daytime Pa_{CO_2} during spontaneous breathing. Although these results were interpreted as supporting the "muscle rest" hypothesis, controls were lacking, and other aspects of rehabilitation or passage of time alone could have been responsible for the improvements.

Subsequently, several controlled studies showed improvement in respiratory muscle strength after short-term (days to a week) use of negative-pressure ventilation.[210–212] These studies documented respiratory muscle rest by showing significant reductions in the diaphragmatic electromyographic (EMG) signal. Subsequent controlled trials, however, of longer duration (up to several months) showed no benefit.[213–215] Notably, baseline Pa_{CO_2} among the latter unfavorable trials was approximately 47 mmHg, substantially lower than that in the favorable studies (57 mmHg). This raises the possibility that respiratory muscles in patients with severe CO_2 retention are more likely to benefit from intermittent negative-pressure ventilation than patients with little or no CO_2 retention, perhaps because of relief of the unfavorable effect of hypercapnia on respiratory muscle function.[216]

Negative-pressure ventilation was tolerated poorly in the preceding trials, so subsequent trials tested NPPV to see if better tolerance might achieve more consistent benefits. In addition, patients with severe COPD are known to have more frequent nocturnal desaturations related to hypoventilation than normal subjects. These desaturations are associated with arousals that shorten the duration and diminish the quality of sleep, an effect that can be ameliorated by O_2 supplementation, at least in "blue and bloated" patients.[217] Furthermore, patients with COPD have a 32% drop in inspiratory flow rate during REM sleep associated with a reduced tidal volume.[218] By assisting ventilation, NPPV offers the potential of restoring inspiratory flow, eliminating episodes of hypoventilation, and improving nocturnal gas exchange, as well as the duration and quality of sleep.

Studies using NPPV in patients with severe obstructive lung diseases have yielded conflicting results. Initial small uncontrolled cohort series on the use of nasal NPPV in patients with severe stable COPD lent support to the idea that NPPV would improve sleep efficiency and daytime and nocturnal gas exchange.[219,220] A 3-month crossover trial by Strumpf et al,[35] however, found improvement only in neuropsychological function but not in nocturnal or daytime gas exchange, sleep quality, pulmonary functions, exercise tolerance, or symptoms. This study also encountered a high dropout rate, with 7 patients withdrawing because of mask intolerance and only 7 of 19 entered patients actually completed the trial. In contrast, in a study of nearly identical design, Meecham-Jones et al[221] enrolled 18 patients with severe COPD, 14 of whom completed the study. Nocturnal and daytime gas exchange, total sleep time, and symptoms improved during NPPV use. These salutary effects of NPPV on sleep duration and efficiency in patients with severe stable COPD also were observed in a 2-night crossover trial in 6 patients with an initial Pa_{CO_2} of 58 mmHg.[222] Some of the disparity between these studies may be explained by the observation that patients in the study of Strumpf et al had more severe airway obstruction (FEV_1 of 0.54 versus 0.81 liter) despite having less CO_2 retention (Pa_{CO_2} of 47 versus 57 mmHg) than did patients in the study of Meecham-Jones et al. This suggests that different subsets of patients with COPD were entered into the studies and that those with greater CO_2 retention ("blue bloaters") may be more likely to benefit from NPPV.

Two other randomized, controlled trials failed to substantiate the hypothesis that greater CO_2 retention predicts NPPV success in patients with severe COPD, despite attempts to enroll hypercapnic subjects. Gay et al[223] screened 32 hypercapnic patients, but only 13 remained after exclusion for obstructive sleep apnea or other terminal illness. Only 4 of the 7 patients randomized to NPPV completed the trial, and not surprisingly, no significant differences emerged. Lin et al[224] performed an 8-week crossover trial consisting of consecutive, randomized 2-week periods of no therapy, O_2 alone, NPPV alone, and NPPV combined with O_2. Among 12 patients with a mean initial Pa_{CO_2} of 50.5 mmHg, NPPV not only conferred no added benefit over O_2 alone with regard to oxygenation, ventricular function, or sleep quality, but it also reduced sleep efficiency and total sleep time. The authors, however, used inspiratory pressures of only 12 cmH_2O, which may have provided insufficient ventilator assistance, and 2 weeks may have been too brief to permit adequate adaptation to NPPV.

Several longer-term controlled trials have been performed subsequently. Casanova et al[225] performed a randomized year-long trial in 44 patients with severe COPD, finding no improvements in gas exchange, survival, or hospitalization rate, although one test of neuropsychological function improved. This study, however, also used relatively low inspiratory pressures and did not assess sleep quality or health status. In an Italian multicenter trial, Clini et al[226] screened 120 patients with severe COPD and chronic CO_2 retention (Pa_{CO_2} of 50 mmHg or more). Ninety patients were enrolled. After dropouts and deaths, 47 were left, divided between the NPPV plus O_2 and O_2 alone groups. Patients treated with NPPV had less of an increase in Pa_{CO_2} over the 2-year period than controls (55–56 versus 55–60 mmHg, respectively, $p < .05$), less deterioration in the MRF-28 functional score (although the St. George's Respiratory Questionnaire was no different), and a trend toward fewer hospital days per patient per year (20 days before and 14 days after intiation of NPPV). No differences were detected in the 6-minute walk distance, dyspnea score, sleep symptoms, or mortality rate. One other multicenter European trial reported thus far only in preliminary form observed no significant difference overall, but a post-hoc analysis revealed a reduction in mortality in the subgroup of patients older than 65 years of age.[227]

These studies have lacked statistical power, and even in those with favorable results, benefit has been shown only for physiologic variables such as respiratory muscle strength and Pa_{CO_2} or total sleep time and symptoms but not for functional status, resource utilization, morbidity, or

mortality. In addition, the two large follow-up studies on NIV[183,185] found that patients with COPD had substantially lower continuation rates than patients with neuromuscular or chest-wall disorders (see Fig. 19-7). This suggests that patients with COPD are less tolerant of or benefit less from NPPV than most neuromuscular patients. Criner at al[228] initiated NPPV in 20 patients with neuromuscular disease and 20 with COPD during a several-week stay in a specialized ventilator unit. Despite these optimal conditions, only 50% of patients with COPD as compared with 80% of those with neuromuscular disease were still using NPPV after 6 months.

Overall, the results of these long-term trials testing the efficacy of NPPV in severe stable COPD have been disappointing, and this application remains controversial.[229] A meta-analysis of these trials concluded that the studies were too small to discern a "clear clinical direction."[230] It should be acknowledged, however, that two randomized trials[221,226] have yielded favorable findings, and several small uncontrolled series show promise among the patients with marked CO_2 retention.[231,232] The conflicting results highlight the need for more studies with greater statistical power to test outcomes such as reductions in hospital days per year and event-free survival rather than just physiologic or sleep-related outcome variables.

NONINVASIVE POSITIVE-PRESSURE VENTILATION TO ENHANCE REHABILITATION IN COPD

NPPV may serve as an adjunct to exercise training in rehabilitation for patients with severe stable COPD. Two different approaches have been used: One employs NPPV to unload the inspiratory muscles during exercise and to permit a greater exercise intensity to magnify the training effect; the other rests muscles between sessions (mainly at night) to enhance daytime function during the sessions. Investigations show that CPAP and PSV singly and in combination increase exercise capacity in patients with severe COPD.[233,234] Bianchi et al[235] showed that compared with CPAP or PSV, proportional-assist ventilation (PAV) brought about the greatest improvement in cycling endurance and reduction in dyspnea in 15 stable hypercapnic patients with COPD. This enhanced exercise capacity during ventilator use, however, has not yet been shown to translate into a greater training effect or functional improvement during spontaneous breathing.[236] Garrod et al[237] tested the second approach among 45 patients with severe COPD ($FEV_1 < 50\%$ of predicted), showing that nocturnal NPPV between rehabilitation sessions increased the shuttle-walk distance and improved quality of life compared with standard therapy. These studies indicate that NPPV, used either during or between exercise sessions, has the potential to enhance benefits accruing from pulmonary rehabilitation, but confirmatory studies are needed.

CYSTIC FIBROSIS AND DIFFUSE BRONCHIECTASIS

Small case series[238,239] have reported stabilization and sometimes even improvement of gas-exchange abnormalities for periods ranging up to 15 months in severely hypercapnic ($Pa_{CO_2} > 54$ mmHg) patients with end-stage cystic fibrosis (CF) awaiting lung transplantation. Gozal et al[240] observed markedly improved gas exchange in all sleep stages in 6 patients with CF treated with NPPV plus O_2 therapy in comparison with patients treated with O_2 therapy alone, although sleep duration and architecture were similar in the two conditions. CF is now a common reason among children for the use of NPPV at home, constituting 17% of such children in a recent French survey.[241]

The mechanism by which NPPV assists CF patients is not entirely clear. NPPV reduces the work of breathing significantly,[242] but a study in 13 hypercapnic patients with CF (average Pa_{CO_2} of 51 mmHg) found no improvements in sleep quality, daytime arterial blood gases, pulmonary function tests, respiratory muscle strength, or exercise tolerance after 2 months of NPPV, even though 8 of the patients felt improved symptomatically.[243] Madden et al[244] found improved hypoxemia but again no improvement in hypercapnia among 113 patients treated long term with NPPV; these authors still considered NPPV useful as a bridge to lung transplantation. NPPV also can be useful for administration of aerosol to CF patients. Fauroux et al[245] found that it was superior to a standard nebulizer in a small group of CF patients. Thus NPPV appears to have a role in supporting deteriorating patients with CF and serving as a bridge to transplantation, even though improvements in gas exchange and sleep parameters are not seen consistently.

In diffuse bronchiectasis patients, Benhamou et al[246] found that the use of NPPV was associated with improved Karnovsky function scores and a reduction in days of hospitalization from 46 for the year before to 21 for the year after starting NPPV. Compared with a historical control group, however, rates of deterioration in oxygenation were similar, and no survival benefit was apparent. In fact, in the long-term English follow-up study,[185] patients with end-stage bronchiectasis had poorer survivals than other patient subgroups, most dying within 2 years. Dupont et al[247] retrospectively reviewed the outcomes of 48 patients with diffuse bronchiectasis following their first ICU admission over a 10-year period; 27% were treated with NPPV, and 54% required intubation. One-year mortality was 40%. Age greater than 65 years, a higher simplified acute physiology score (SAPS) II score (>32), and the need for intubation were identified as predictors of mortality. These studies suggest a role for NPPV in treating patients with CF and diffuse bronchiectasis who have developed severe CO_2 retention, as well as in serving as a bridge to transplantation, but the capacity to prolong life may be limited. Lacking controlled trials, definitive recommendations on how to select patients with CF or diffuse bronchiectasis for NPPV or when to start are unavailable; most clinicians use guidelines similar to those used for severe COPD (see below), paying particular attention to the inclusion of techniques to aid in secretion clearance.

SELECTION OF PATIENTS WITH CHRONIC RESPIRATORY FAILURE AND OBSTRUCTIVE LUNG DISEASES TO RECEIVE NONINVASIVE VENTILATION

An earlier consensus statement noted the discordant results of the available trials and concluded that more study is needed before NPPV can be recommended in severe stable COPD.[157] A subsequent consensus conference agreed that the data are scanty and conflicting but opined that the available evidence suggests that certain subgroups of patients with COPD may benefit.[192] Most trials that have observed benefit from either negative- or positive-pressure NIV in severe stable COPD have enrolled patients with more CO_2 retention at baseline than trials with negative results. Thus the consensus opinion was that a trial of NPPV in severe stable COPD patients is justified if CO_2 retention is severe (i.e., $Pa_{CO_2} > 55$ mmHg).

Considering that one of the two controlled trials reporting beneficial effects of NPPV in severe stable COPD patients[221] enrolled patients with frequent hypopneas (10 per hour) and O_2 desaturations during sleep, another indication suggested by the consensus group was sustained, severe nocturnal O_2 desaturation (<88% for more than 5 consecutive minutes). O_2 therapy alone, however, has been shown to improve sleep quality, reduce drowsiness, and improve neuropsychological function in such patients.[217,218] Therefore, the recommendation was made that sleep monitoring be performed during O_2 supplementation and that NPPV not be initiated unless symptoms failed to respond to a trial of long-term O_2 therapy. This includes patients who retain more CO_2 during O_2 therapy, a group that responded favorably to NPPV in an uncontrolled trial.[232] If patients have a Pa_{CO_2} of between 50 and 54 mmHg, the consensus group opined that NPPV should be used if such patients have evidence of nocturnal hypoventilation, as indicated by nocturnal oximetry, or if there is a history of repeated hospitalizations.

In the absence of more controlled trials with favorable findings, however, these guidelines are tentative. Also, even for patients who meet the criteria, patient tolerance of NPPV may be poor.[228] In order to maximize patient compliance, only motivated symptomatic patients, such as those with fatigue or daytime hypersomnolence, who can cooperate and comprehend the purpose of the therapy should be selected. As outlined in Table 19-7, NIV should not be initiated unless other therapies have been optimized, including O_2 supplementation and CPAP (if indicated). These guidelines have led to reduced use of NPPV for severe stable COPD

TABLE 19-7 Recommended Guidelines for Selection of Patients with Obstructive Lung Diseases to Receive Long-Term NPPV[a]

1. Symptoms: fatigue, hypersomnolence, dyspnea, and so on
2. Failure to respond to optimal medical therapy:
   Maximal bronchodilator therapy and/or steroids
   O_2 supplementation if indicated
3. Gas-exchange abnormalities:
   $Pa_{CO_2} \geq 52$ mmHg
   $Sa_{O_2} < 88\%$ for more than 5 consecutive minutes nocturnally despite O_2 supplementation
4. Obstructive sleep apnea excluded on clinical grounds or failure to respond to CPAP therapy if moderate to severe obstructive sleep apnea detected on sleep study
5. Reassess after 2 months' therapy; continue if adequate compliance (>4 hours a day) and favorable therapeutic response

[a] Based on Center for Medicaid and Medicare Services reimbursement guidelines.

in the United States since the late 1990s, when certain home respiratory companies were encouraging widespread use. Use is currently more prevalent in certain European countries, such as Switzerland, where a recent survey found that COPD was the second most common reason for use of NPPV in the home.[184] A recent pan-European survey on home mechanical ventilation showed enormous variability between countries in the proportion of patients receiving ventilation for neuromuscular versus lung diseases and between those receiving noninvasive versus tracheostomy ventilation.[248]

CONGESTIVE HEART FAILURE

As discussed earlier, evidence supports the use of NIV (either CPAP alone or NPPV) in the therapy of acute heart failure, and it also may have a role in chronic congestive heart failure (CHF). Increases in intrathoracic pressure have long been known to have salutary hemodynamic effects in some patients with congestive heart failure. Naughton et al[20] found that CPAP (10 cmH$_2$O) reduced both ventilatory work (by minimizing negative intrathoracic pressure swings) and cardiac load (by reducing transmural pressure) in 15 patients with congestive heart failure. A subsequent study found that longer-term nocturnal CPAP (9 cmH$_2$O) improved inspiratory muscle strength (maximal inspiratory pressure increased from 79.3–90.7 cmH$_2$O) in a group of 8 patients with CHF.[249] One month of nocturnal CPAP also increased left-ventricular ejection fraction (33.8% versus 25%) and lowered systolic systemic pressure (116 versus 126 mmHg) in patients with CHF and obstructive sleep apnea compared with healthy subjects.[250]

Whether NPPV is better than CPAP alone in these patients has been controversial. Willson et al[251] found dramatic improvements in sleep parameters (apnea-hypopnea index 49–6, arousal index 42–17) in patients with CHF and Cheynes-Stokes respiration after treatment with a portable bilevel device. Conversely, Kohnlein et al[252] performed a crossover trial consisting of randomized 2-week periods of NPPV and CPAP in 35 patients with Cheynes-Stokes respiration. Both modalities improved apnea-hypopnea and arousal indexes dramatically, but there was no difference between the two. Teschler et al[253] randomized 14 patients with CHF and Cheynes-Stokes respiration to control, O$_2$ alone, CPAP alone, bilevel NPPV, and adaptive pressure-support servo ventilation (ASV) on five separate randomly ordered nights. They observed equal reductions in apnea-hypopnea and arousal indexes with O$_2$ alone and CPAP alone, a greater reduction with bilevel ventilation, and the greatest improvement with ASV. This study supports the idea that customized modes designed to respond to the apneas of Cheynes-Stokes respiration (such as ASV) may be especially effective, but no adequately powered trials addressing important clinical outcomes have yet been performed. The Canadian CPAP (CanPAP) trial is a large randomized trial examining the effects of long-term CPAP in patients with CHF; it has provided disappointing preliminary findings, with only a trend for improved left-ventricular function and no improvement in functional status.[254] Thus the role of NPPV in CHF patients is currently unclear. Most clinicians currently use CPAP alone for patients with CHF and obstructive sleep apnea and optimal medical therapy, in-

cluding O$_2$ supplementation, for those with Cheynes-Stokes breathing. Despite the promising findings with ASV modes, further studies are needed before they can be recommended.

PEDIATRIC USES OF NONINVASIVE POSITIVE-PRESSURE VENTILATION FOR CHRONIC RESPIRATORY FAILURE

Since the first case reports on the successful use of nasal NPPV in children with central hypoventilation,[199,200] relatively few reports of NPPV have appeared in the pediatric literature. Nonetheless, some of the experience in adults can be applied to children because such conditions as DMD or CF may impair respiratory function in older children, and these have been included in a number of the published reports.[183,185] In their experience with 15 children having neuromuscular disease or CF treated with nasal NPPV and followed for periods ranging from 1–21 months, Padman et al[144] found that average Pa$_{CO_2}$ and hospital utilization fell; only one child required an artificial airway. Fauroux et al[255] undertook a French survey on the use of NPPV by children at home. Of 102 children followed at 15 centers, 7% were younger than 3 years of age, 35% were 4–11 years of age, and 58% were 12 years of age, and 34% had neuromuscular disease, 30% had obstructive sleep apnea or craniofacial abnormalities, 17% had CF, 9% had central hypoventilation, and 8% had scoliosis. In a subsequent report, Fauroux et al[256] described flattening of the face in 48% of patients. Nevertheless, pediatric patients appear to respond as well to NPPV as most adults with chronic respiratory failure. In a long-term follow-up study of 30 pediatric patients (average age 12.3 years) with mainly non-Duchenne's neuromuscular syndromes, Mellies et al[257] observed clinical stability exceeding an average of 2 years in duration. Nocturnal and diurnal gas exchange, quality of sleep, and symptoms were improved, and these deteriorated promptly on temporary withdrawal of NPPV. The authors concluded that NPPV is effective and should be used in children with symptomatic sleep-disordered breathing associated with neuromuscular syndromes.

Practical Application of Noninvasive Positive-Pressure Ventilation

Despite the accumulating evidence on NPPV indications that helps in selecting appropriate patients, the delivery of NPPV remains very much an art. After the decision is made to treat a patient with NPPV, the clinician must decide on a mask (or interface), ventilator, settings, and adjuncts. NPPV must be delivered in a safe and adequately monitored location. Implementation of each step requires knowledge and experience. More than with invasive ventilation, the interaction between patient and clinician is central to success. The following will provide an overview of the steps in this process.

INITIATION

Although little scientific evidence is available to guide the decisions surrounding initiation, they should be made

TABLE 19-8   Goals of Noninvasive Ventilation

Acute applications
Relieve dyspnea
Optimize patient comfort
Reduce work of breathing
Improve or stabilize gas exchange
Minimize complications
Avoid intubation
Avoid delay of needed intubation
Long-term applications
Ameliorate symptoms
Improve or stabilize gas exchange
Improve sleep duration and quality
Maximize quality of life
Enhance functional status
Prolong survival

SOURCE: Adapted, with permission, from Mehta and Hill.[1]

carefully because success or failure depends on them. Focusing on the major goals of NIV may help (Table 19-8). NIV shares with invasive ventilation the goals of improving gas exchange, either nocturnal, daytime, or both, and minimizing complications. Even more than with invasive ventilation, though, NIV seeks to alleviate symptoms and optimize comfort. Because of the open-circuit design of noninvasive positive-pressure ventilators, success depends largely on patient cooperation and acceptance. Patient tolerance is an important goal because the other goals are not achievable unless the patient accepts the therapy. The goals of acute and long-term applications are overlapping, but alleviation of increased work of breathing is an important goal in acute applications, whereas improvement in sleep duration and quality is more important during long-term applications. The following gives recommendations for initiation, citing evidence when available, pointing out controversy where it exists, and offering opinion where necessary. Most sections offer comments on both acute and long-term applications.

LOCATION

ACUTE

NIV can be initiated wherever the patient presents with acute respiratory distress—in the emergency department,[49,258] ICU,[16,51] intermediate- or respiratory-care unit, or hospital ward.[52] A survey of acute-care hospitals in Massachusetts and Rhode Island found that a third of NPPV initiations were in the emergency department, and half were in the ICU.[259] Following initiation, transfer to a location that offers continuous monitoring is recommended until the patient stabilizes. The patient's acuity of illness and risk of deterioration if an accidental disconnection occurs should dictate the intensity of monitoring. During transfers, ventilator assistance and monitoring should be continued because rapid deteriorations can occur. Recent preliminary evidence suggests that less acutely ill patients with COPD can be managed on a general medical ward, but if pH is less than 7.30, admission to a more intensively monitored setting is advised.[52]

LONG TERM

Stable patients with chronic respiratory failure may start NPPV during an inpatient admission, in a sleep laboratory during the daytime or an overnight stay, in a physician's outpatient office (with therapists from the home respiratory vendor present), or at home. Although there are strong proponents for one location or another, no evidence is available to dictate the choice. Routine hospitalization is unnecessary unless warranted by the patient's medical condition, although some clinicians believe that this increases subsequent adherence rates and prefer the closer initial monitoring and opportunity for early adjustment that it affords. Use of a sleep laboratory offers the advantage of precise titration of initial pressure or volume settings during sleep monitoring but adds to costs and may delay implementation because of scheduling problems. Also, no titration protocol has been validated, and selecting pressures to eliminate apneas and hypopneas, as is done with sleep apnea, may not be adequate to reverse hypoventilation in patients with chronic respiratory failure. Until outcome studies demonstrate the superiority of one location over another, the choice of location will be based on practitioner preference. Perhaps more important than the specific location is the availability of skilled, attentive practitioners to help during the initiation and adaptation processes.

MASKS (INTERFACES)

A daunting array of interfaces has become available to deliver NPPV, and detailed descriptions can be found elsewhere.[260] In brief, the most commonly used interfaces in both acute and long-term settings are nasal and oronasal (or full-face) masks. Nasal masks usually are triangular clear plastic domes that have soft silicone sealing surfaces. Oronasal (or full-face) masks are similar in appearance but are larger and fit over the nose and mouth. Nasal interfaces offer many modifications, however, including nasal pillows with soft rubber cones that insert directly into the nares, so-called minimasks that fit over the tip of the nose, and gel-filled seals designed to enhance comfort. Various oronasal masks are available, including those with foam- or air-filled seals and a chin support. A larger version of the full-face mask is available that seals around the perimeter of the face, potentially enhancing comfort and eliminating the development of nasal bridge ulcers.[261] Oral interfaces also are used occasionally, mainly in the long-term setting in patients with neuromuscular disease.[162]

More recently, a number of studies have evaluated the "helmet," a novel interface for NIV that consists of a clear plastic cylinder that fits over the head and seals on the shoulders. The Food and Drug Administration has not yet approved this application in the United States. It avoids contact with the nose and mouth, eliminating nasal ulceration and potentially enhancing comfort.[262] CPAP delivered via the helmet to patients with acute respiratory failure is better tolerated than the full-face mask in historically matched controls.[263] Compared with the full-face mask used to deliver PSV in patients with COPD in acute respiratory failure[264] the helmet similarly improved vital signs, achieved similar intubation and mortality rates, and reduced complications. Pa_{CO_2} tended to be higher, however, in patients treated with the helmet, raising concerns about rebreathing. High flow rates must be used to avoid this problem,[265] but this contributes to noise levels exceeding 100 dB.[266]

Oral interfaces have been used successfully for many years in patients with slowly progressive neuromuscular diseases.[162] Long-term nasal ventilation appears to offer improved tolerance compared with mouthpiece ventilation in some patients,[168] although no studies have directly compared nasal and mouthpiece NPPV. Either may be effective, even in patients with minimal pulmonary reserve, and both may be used in the same patient, nasal ventilation during sleep at night, for example, with mouthpiece ventilation used as needed during the daytime.[168]

SELECTION OF INTERFACES

ACUTE

Ideally, interfaces for the acute setting should be inexpensive and disposable or reusable without sacrificing comfort. A recent randomized, controlled trial in 70 patients with acute respiratory failure showed that full-face and nasal masks similarly improve dyspnea, vital signs, and gas exchange, but the nasal mask had a higher initial intolerance rate (34% versus 12%), attributed to air leaking through the mouth.[267] Thus the full-face mask usually is the mask of first choice in the acute setting, although claustrophobic patients or those with a need to expectorate frequently may fare better with nasal masks. The larger full-face mask that seals around the perimeter of the face was rated by patients as more comfortable than the standard full-face mask in a preliminary report.[268] Concerns have been raised about the dead space attributable to the large volumes of these face masks, but "streaming" of airflow directly from the inlet to the patient's nose and mouth appears to minimize this problem.[269,270] The oral interface is used sometimes in the acute setting to facilitate initial patient adaptation.[271] Clinicians should have a variety of interfaces readily available; a "mask bag" can be suspended from the ventilator so that individual patient needs can be accommodated. Whichever interface is chosen, optimal fit and comfort are critical to the eventual success of NPPV.

CHRONIC

Comfort and tolerance are even more important in the long-term setting because interfaces must be used for months, mainly during sleep, before being replaced. Many different interfaces are available partly because of the demand driven by the large population of patients with obstructive sleep apnea using similar technology. Standard nasal masks are the most commonly used interfaces in the chronic setting, and a short-term controlled trial on naive patients with restrictive and obstructive forms of chronic respiratory failure found that patients rated these nasal masks as more comfortable than nasal prongs or full-face masks.[272] A polysomnographic comparison of the two masks in patients with chronic respiratory failure[273] found that nasal and full-face masks were equivalent with regard to apnea-hypopnea index, gas exchange, and sleep quality, but the nasal mask required chin straps to control mouth leaks, and sleep efficiency was less with the full-face mask.

Once again, clinicians must be prepared to try a number of different interfaces to optimize comfort. Fitting gauges should be used when available to facilitate proper sizing, and strap tension should be the minimum that controls leaks. Headstrap materials, tightness, and attachments to the head and mask are also important for comfort. Many different types of headstraps are available, although they usually are designed for a particular mask.

SELECTION OF A VENTILATOR

ACUTE

A steadily expanding number of ventilators are available for NPPV in the acute setting. Bilevel devices are portable PSV ventilators, first developed for home applications, that cycle between higher inspiratory and lower expiratory pressures.[202] These ventilators have been used widely in acute settings because of their ease of administration and low cost, but they have been limited by a lack of alarms, monitoring capabilities, and O_2 blenders. Newer bilevel devices have been designed specifically for acute applications of NPPV. They have features aimed at enhancing leak compensation and patient comfort, such as adjustable triggering and cycling mechanisms and rise times (the time to reach the preset inspiratory pressure).

"Critical care" ventilators are those designed for invasive ventilation and, by virtue of microprocessor technology, offer a wide variety of modes, extensive alarm and monitoring capabilities, and O_2 blenders. In the past, these devices have been limited by triggering of nuisance alarms and limited leak-compensating abilities when used for NPPV.[274] Many, however, now offer "NIV modes" that use a PSV mode, silence alarms, and add leak compensation and algorithms that facilitate triggering and cycling, even in the face of leaks. A laboratory study that compared a number of bilevel ventilators with a critical-care ventilator found that triggering, cycling, and leak-compensatory mechanisms were superior in several of the bilevel ventilators.[275]

Because they use a single tube for both inspiration and expiration, bilevel ventilators contribute to CO_2 rebreathing unless used with a nonrebreathing exhalation valve that may increase expiratory resistance and expiratory work of breathing.[276,277] This rebreathing can be minimized by using an expiratory pressure greater than 4 cmH_2O[276] and masks with an in-mask exhalation valve situated over the bridge of the nose.[269,270] Comparisons of bilevel and critical-care ventilators in intubated patients have demonstrated that gas exchange is equivalent, but work of breathing is increased during bilevel ventilation if minimal expiratory pressure levels (2–3 cmH_2O) are used.[278] When expiratory pressures of 5 cmH_2O are used, however, the two types perform equally well in supporting gas exchange and reducing work of breathing, presumably because of counterbalancing of auto-PEEP. For delivery of NIV, clinical outcome studies using bilevel ventilators report success rates that compare favorably with those for critical-care ventilators,[49,52] although no randomized, controlled trials have compared the two directly. Thus the selection of either system can be justified, and the choice is often based on availability and financial considerations. Further, recent developments have blurred the distinctions between the ventilators, with bilevel ventilators adding monitoring and alarm capabilities as well as O_2 blenders.

CHRONIC

Blower- or turbine-based portable pressure-limited bilevel ventilators are used most often in the long-term setting to deliver NPPV. In a 9-year Swiss survey,[184] volume-limited devices predominated initially, but pressure-limited devices accounted for over 90% of ventilator applications during the latter years. This shift has been driven by the low cost, ease of use, and portability of the pressure-limited devices. In addition, manufacturers have steadily been adding features that enhance monitoring. Some now offer wireless Internet connections that permit home monitoring of respiratory rate, oximetry, airway pressures, tidal volumes, and air leaks. Portable volume-limited positive-pressure ventilators are still preferred by some clinicians for specific applications. Because they offer sophisticated monitoring, they are used in patients requiring nearly continuous ventilator support. Because of their high pressure-generating capabilities, they may be preferred in patients with high respiratory system impedances, such those with morbid obesity or chest-wall deformity, or they may be used to "stack" breaths to attain a higher inspired lung volume to increase cough flows.[193] Also, because volume-limited ventilators usually are driven by intermittent piston action rather than continuously operating blowers, backup battery life can be considerably longer. Studies in the long-term setting have shown no consistent benefit of one type of ventilator over the other,[279,280] however, and the choice usually becomes one of clinician and/or patient preference.

SELECTION OF A VENTILATOR MODE

ACUTE

Although no studies have demonstrated superior efficacy of one ventilator mode over another in the acute setting, some practitioners have found enhanced patient comfort or compliance with PSV.[281,282] Thus, although either volume- and pressure-limited modes can be used with the expectation of similar rates of success, pressure-limited modes appear to be accepted more readily by patients. Some newer hybrid ventilators designed specifically for NIV are able to deliver both volume- or pressure-limited modes, with the capability of adjusting triggering and cycling sensitivity, rise time, and inspiratory duration to optimize patient comfort.[283] PAV, a unique mode that tracks instantaneous patient airflow, is capable of closely matching patient breathing pattern and hence potentially enhancing synchrony and comfort[284] (see Chapter 13). The flow signal is fed back to the ventilator as a raw signal (flow assist) or integrated over time (volume assist). Gains are imposed on both these signals and on a composite signal (proportional assist) that can be adjusted to assist a "proportion" of the patient's breathing effort. Theoretically, flow and volume assist are adjusted to match resistive and elastic work, respectively, which must

be measured. These specific adjustments, however, are unnecessary when PAV is used to deliver NPPV clinically. PAV has been shown to be as effective and a more comfortable means of administering NPPV than PSV delivered via a critical-care ventilator[285] or a bilevel device.[286] Ventilators offering PAV are currently available in Europe and Canada but have not yet been approved by the Food and Drug Administration in the United States.

CHRONIC

In the long-term setting, pressure-support and volume-limited ventilators achieve similar levels of overnight oxygenation.[280] Thirty consecutive patients, mainly with restrictive forms of chronic respiratory failure, received nasal volume-limited ventilation for 1 month followed by pressure-limited ventilation.[279] Only 2 patients failed to improve with volume-limited ventilation, whereas 10 had increased Pa_{CO_2} or symptomatic deterioration when switched to pressure-limited ventilation. Conversely, 10 patients in another study had improved daytime blood gases when switched from volume- to pressure-limited ventilation.[287] Although these were not prospective, randomized trials, they show no clear advantage of one ventilator mode over the other. Thus the choice between the two hinges on clinician preference and consideration of specific ventilator properties such as portability, pressure-generating capabilities, backup-battery life, ability to stack breaths, and other factors. In general, though, volume-limited ventilators have greater pressure-generating and alarm capabilities.

VENTILATOR SETTINGS

ACUTE

Two strategies have been described: the *high-low approach*, which starts with a higher inspiratory pressure (20–25 cm H_2O) and lowers it if patients are intolerant,[16] and the *low-high approach*, which starts with a low inspiratory pressure (8–10 cmH$_2$O) and raises it gradually as tolerated by the patient.[49] The former approach prioritizes rapid alleviation of respiratory distress; the latter aims to optimize patient comfort in an effort to maximize patient tolerance. Reported success rates for the two approaches are similar, although no studies have compared them directly. Paramount with both approaches is the realization that subsequent adjustments are necessary depending on patient response. Higher initial pressure often must be adjusted downward, and it is very important that low initial pressure be raised (usually to 12–20 cmH$_2$O) within the first hour, if possible, to provide adequate ventilator assistance.

Expiratory pressure (or PEEP) is used routinely with bilevel ventilators and is optional with volume-limited ventilators. Bilevel ventilators require a bias flow during expiration to flush CO_2 from the single ventilator tube and avoid rebreathing.[276] Minimal expiratory pressure with these ventilators is in the 3–4 cmH$_2$O range. Higher expiratory pressures (typically 4–8 cmH$_2$O) are used to counterbalance intrinsic PEEP during treatment of exacerbations of COPD or to enhance oxygenation. It is important to recall that the difference between inspiratory and expiratory pressure is the level of PSV, so inspiratory pressure must be increased in tandem with expiratory pressure if the same level of ventilatory assistance is to be maintained. Adjusting the rate of pressurization (or rise time) may be useful to enhance comfort; patients with COPD prefer slightly more rapid rise times than restrictive patients. Very rapid pressurization rates minimize the work of breathing in patients with COPD but may be sensed as less comfortable by patients than slightly lower pressurization rates.[288]

CHRONIC

No consensus has been reached on how to select ventilator settings for patients in the long-term setting. In the sleep laboratory, one approach is to increase expiratory pressure until apneas are eliminated and inspiratory pressure until hypopneas are eliminated without inducing excessive arousals. This approach, however, does not ensure that the pressures selected will alleviate hypoventilation, nor does it facilitate initial adaptation if the patient finds the recommended initial pressures are intolerable. Thus the author prefers a gradual uptitration of pressures over weeks or even months as tolerated by the patient. Initial inspiratory pressure is 6–10 cmH$_2$O, with increases weekly by 1–2 cmH$_2$O as tolerated. Expiratory pressure is set at 3–4 cmH$_2$O and rarely is increased above 6 cmH$_2$O unless sleep apnea is deemed an important contributor. For volume-limited ventilation, an initial tidal volume of 10–15 ml/kg has been recommended, in excess of the standard recommendations for invasive ventilation, because of the need to compensate for air leaks.[289] Parreira et al[290] found that a tidal volume of 13 ml/kg optimized assisted minute volume in a group of patients with restrictive thoracic disorders.

A backup rate sufficiently high to control breathing nocturnally has been recommended for patients with neuromuscular disease to maximize respiratory muscle rest and prevent apneas. In patients with severe stable COPD, on the other hand, the need for a backup rate is not clear, considering that one controlled trial of NPPV found significant benefit using a spontaneous ventilator mode without a backup rate.[221] Compared with a spontaneous mode, these authors found that use of a backup rate had no effect on nocturnal gas exchange in patients with COPD and chronic respiratory failure. On the other hand, Parreira et al[290] found that minute volume was optimized when patients with restrictive thoracic disorders used a relatively high backup rate of 23 breaths per minute.

ADJUNCTS TO NONINVASIVE VENTILATION

With bilevel ventilators, supplemental O$_2$ can be provided directly through tubing connected to a nipple in the mask or to a T connector in the ventilator tubing, with liter flow adjusted to keep Sa$_{O2}$ above 90–92%. Maximal F$_{IO2}$ using this setup is only 45–50%. F$_{IO2}$ delivered via bilevel ventilators depends on a number of factors, including O$_2$ flow rate, breathing pattern, ventilator settings, and location of the O$_2$ connection (connection to the mask gives a higher F$_{IO2}$).[291] With critical-care ventilators and some bilevel devices designed for acute applications, standard O$_2$ blenders are used to accurately provide the desired F$_{IO2}$. Thus these latter ventilators are preferred for patients with hypoxemic respiratory failure. Humidification may enhance comfort during NPPV and is advised if NPPV is to be used for more than a few hours. A heated humidifier is preferred over a heat and moisture exchanger because the latter adds to work of breathing[292] and may interfere with triggering and cycling. Also, with excessive air leaking, a heated humidifier lowers nasal resistance.[22] In the long-term setting, humidification usually is provided, particularly during the winter months in colder climates. Nasogastric tubes are not recommended routinely as adjuncts to NIV, even when oronasal masks are used.

NONINVASIVE TECHNIQUES TO ASSIST COUGH

Because it provides no direct access to the lower airways, as does invasive ventilation, NPPV depends on the integrity of airway protective reflexes for its success. In the acute setting, patients with excessive secretions or severe cough impairment are intubated rather than managed noninvasively. In the long-term setting, however, a number of techniques have been developed to enhance secretion removal in patients with compromised secretion-clearance capabilities. These techniques are of greatest value in patients with neuromuscular disease and weakened expiratory muscles. Severe bulbar involvement such as occurs with ALS is treated most effectively with invasive ventilation. Secretion retention related to abnormal mucus, such as occurs with CF, is beyond the scope of this chapter.

An effective cough depends on the ability to generate adequate expiratory airflow, estimated at more than 160 liters/min.[293] Expiratory airflow is determined by lung and chest-wall elasticity, airway conductance, and at least at higher lung volumes, expiratory muscle force. By generating an adequate vital capacity (>2.5 liters) to take advantage of respiratory system elasticity, inspiratory muscle function also contributes to cough adequacy. In addition, an effective cough requires the ability to close the glottis so that explosive release of intrathoracic pressure can generate high peak expiratory cough flows.[294] When patients with severe neuromuscular disease are too weak to take advantage of these mechanisms and have insufficient cough flows, techniques to assist cough should be applied.

The simplest maneuver to augment cough flow is manually assisted or "quad" coughing. This consists of firm, quick thrusts applied to the abdomen using the palms of the hands, timed to coincide with the patient's cough effort.[193] The technique should be taught to caregivers of patients with severe respiratory muscle weakness with instructions to use it whenever the patient has difficulty expectorating secretions. With practice, the technique can be applied effectively and frequently with minimal discomfort to the patient. Peak expiratory flows can be increased severalfold when manually assisted coughing is applied successfully.[295] To minimize the risk of regurgitation and aspiration of gastric contents, the patient should be semiupright when manually assisted coughing is applied, and the technique should be used cautiously after meals. The technique can be used, though, in patients with gastric feeding tubes.

Although manually assisted coughing may enhance expiratory force, it does not augment inspired volume. Thus patients with severely restricted volumes may not achieve sufficient cough flows even when assisted by skilled caregivers. To overcome this problem, the inhaled volume should be augmented. One approach is to "stack" breaths using glossopharyngeal breathing[296] or volume-limited ventilation and then to augment the cough using manual assistance. Another is to use a mechanical insufflator-exsufflator, a device that was developed during the polio epidemics to aid in airway secretion removal.[295] This device delivers a positive inspiratory pressure of 30–40 cmH$_2$O via a face mask and then rapidly switches to an equal negative pressure. The positive pressure ensures delivery of an adequate tidal volume, and the negative pressure has the effect of simulating the rapid expiratory flows generated by a cough. Use of the insufflator-exsufflator has been combined with manually assisted coughing in an effort to further augment cough flows.[295]

The mechanical insufflator-exsufflator increases cough flows in patients with neuromuscular weakness but is less effective in patients with kyphoscoliosis and in one study actually decreased cough flows of patients with COPD.[297] In another study, however, mechanical insufflation-exsufflation decreased dyspnea and improved oxygenation not only in neuromuscular patients but also in patients with airflow obstruction.[298] Although no controlled trials have evaluated the efficacy of the cough insufflator-exsufflator, anecdotal evidence suggests that it enhances removal of secretions in patients with impaired cough. It has been reported to reduce failures (need for intubation) in neuromuscular patients in critical-care settings,[299] reduce the occurrence of atelectasis and pneumonias in children with neuromuscular disease,[300] and improve cough flows in patients with ALS unless there is bulbar dysfunction, which may predispose to upper airway collapse.[301] It has been particularly useful in patient homes to treat episodes of acute bronchitis, permitting avoidance of hospitalization.[302] Other devices that aid expectoration, such as the percussive ventilator, Hayek oscillator, and vibratory vest, have some theoretical advantages over other techniques for assisting secretion removal.[193] Their use of high-frequency vibrations (up to 10–15 Hz) may facilitate mobilization of airway secretions. Unfortunately, even anecdotal evidence to support their use is lacking.

Clinicians caring for patients with severely impaired cough should be familiar with the various techniques available to assist expectoration. These are particularly important with NIV because there is no direct access to the airway, and secretion retention is a frequent complication and common cause for failure. Although controlled data are lacking, these techniques appear to help in maintaining airway patency in patients with cough impairment during use of NIV in both acute and chronic settings.

ROLE OF THE CLINICIAN: TIME DEMANDS, IMPORTANCE OF EXPERIENCE, AND GUIDELINES

An experienced clinician conveying an air of assuredness to patients is thought to be crucial to the success of NPPV. The clinician should motivate the patient, explaining the purpose of each piece of equipment and preparing the patient for each step in the initiation process. Patients should be reassured, encouraged to communicate any discomfort or fears, and coached in ways to coordinate their breathing with the ventilator. When using nasal masks, patients are instructed to keep their mouths shut.

Time demands on medical personnel have been a concern for the delivery of NPPV. Chevrolet et al[303] were the first to draw attention to this potential problem, reporting large time demands on nurses during administration of NPPV. Bott et al[48] subsequently found that nurses rated NPPV as no more demanding to administer than conventional therapy. Conversely, Kramer et al[49] found that compared with controls, NPPV patients tended to require more time from respiratory therapists during the first 8 hours, an amount that fell significantly during the second 8 hours. Nava et al[304] also found that respiratory therapists spent more time during the first 48 hours caring for NPPV patients than invasively ventilated patients. These findings indicate that NPPV initially requires more time to administer than conventional therapy, for interface fitting and initial ventilator adjustment, although these demands diminish rapidly after the first few hours. Nurses, respiratory therapists, physicians, or some combination of these must spend the additional time, depending on institutional practices.

As might be anticipated, the experience of personnel also appears to be important for the success of NPPV. Girou et al[14] reviewed the experience of a 26-bed French ICU between January 1994 and December 2001 on 479 patients with either COPD or cardiogenic pulmonary edema requiring ventilator assistance, invasively or noninvasively. Use of NIV increased from approximately 20–90% (of the patients) during the course of the study, associated with a decrease in the rate of nosocomial pneumonias from 20–8% and in ICU mortality from 21–7% (all $p < .05$). The authors speculated that a "learning effect" over the course of the study was responsible for the improved outcomes. Over an 8-year period in their ICU, Carlucci et al[305] found that NPPV success rates increased in patients with COPD despite a worsening of the severity of illness as staff gained experience with the technique. Whether or not guidelines for NPPV implementation can improve patient outcomes remains to be established. Sinuff et al[306] found that clinician behavior changed after implementation of a guideline at their single academic institution, but overall patient outcomes were not altered.

Monitoring

Patients receiving NIV are monitored to determine whether the goals are being achieved (see Table 19-8).

SUBJECTIVE RESPONSES

The key aims of NPPV are alleviation of respiratory distress in the acute setting and of fatigue, hypersomnolence, and other symptoms of impaired sleep in the chronic setting while achieving patient tolerance. Agitation and mask discomfort are challenges during NPPV. These aspects can be assessed easily using bedside observation and patient queries. Some patients minimize or deny discomfort and still may have great difficulty adapting successfully to NIV, so clinicians not should only query patients but also should observe for nonverbal signs of distress or discomfort.

PHYSIOLOGIC RESPONSES

Evidence of physiologic improvement within the first hour or two, including decreases in respiratory and heart rates, diminished sternocleidomastoid muscle activity, and elimination of abdominal paradox, portends a favorable NPPV outcome.[105,153] Patients should be breathing in synchrony with the ventilator, and air leaking should be minimal. Some clinicians also monitor tidal volumes, aiming for delivered volumes in excess of 7 ml/kg.[307] Relying on ventilator monitoring to follow tidal volumes may be misleading, however, particularly during use of bilevel ventilators, because these integrate the inspired flow signal and may be very inaccurate in the face of air leaks.

GAS EXCHANGE

Improvement in gas exchange as determined by continuous oximetry and occasional blood gases is a key aim in acute application of NPPV, although improvement in ventilation may occur gradually over hours.[16] In chronic stable patients, the improvement in daytime gas exchange occurs even more slowly, over a period of weeks, depending on the duration of daily ventilator use. Some patients adapt slowly and require up to several months before they sleep through the night using the ventilator. Arterial blood-gas measurement should be delayed until the patient is consistently using the ventilator for a period of time likely to improve gas exchange: usually at least 4–6 hours a day. No consensus on an ideal level for daytime Pa_{CO_2} has been reached; most investigators target levels in the middle 40s. In the author's experience, a daytime Pa_{CO_2} of up to 60 mmHg or higher may be tolerated without hypersomnolence or evidence of cor pulmonale as long as oxygenation is adequate. Noninvasive CO_2 monitoring may be useful for trending purposes in patients with normal lung parenchyma such as those with neuromuscular disease. Transcutaneous Pa_{CO_2} is probably the most useful because variable air leaks and breathing patterns and dilution secondary to bias flow with some ventilators render end-tidal CO_2 recordings inaccurate, particularly if the patient has parenchymal lung disease.[308]

SLEEP

Little is known about sleep during NPPV in the acute setting, and the role of sleep monitoring in the long-term setting is controversial. As noted earlier, some clinicians prefer to use the sleep laboratory to decide on initial settings for NPPV. Others begin most patients, particularly those with neuromuscular disease, without a polysomnographic evaluation. If both approaches prove to be equal in achieving the goals of NIV, it would be difficult to argue that routine sleep studies are necessary. The relative utilities of polysomnograhy, multichannel portable recordings, and

nocturnal oximetry are also unclear in follow-up of longterm NPPV, but one pragmatic approach is to screen patients using home oximetry and to perform more sophisticated studies when the oximetry results indicate the need for further evaluation.

Adaptation

ACUTE

It is critically important to ascertain that the delivered pressures are sufficient to alleviate respiratory distress; a common mistake is to fail to increase pressures quickly enough, and the patient fails because of inadequate ventilator support. The patient also should use the ventilator for more time initially, with increasing periods of time off the ventilator as the underlying condition improves. Some clinicians encourage use most of the time initially, as dictated by the degree of respiratory distress during ventilator-free intervals.[49] Others employ sequential use,[309] wherein periods of use alternate with lengthy ventilator-free periods; total daily use averages only 6 hours, although this would be suitable only for mildly ill patients. When no respiratory distress recurs during ventilator-free intervals, ventilator assistance is discontinued. Total duration of ventilator assistance depends on the speed of resolution of the respiratory failure. Patients with acute pulmonary edema require an average of 6–7 hours of ventilator use,[99] whereas patients with COPD average 2 or more days.[49] Some patients may continue nocturnal ventilation after discharge from the hospital, following guidelines for long-term use of NPPV.

LONG TERM

Patients start more gradually and increase periods of use as tolerated. Anxious patients may begin with only an hour or two of daytime use followed by gradually increasing periods of nocturnal use over several weeks or even months. Compared with the acute setting, urgency in the chronic setting is less, and because the intent is to use the ventilator during sleep, great care must be exercised in optimizing patient comfort. During this period, visits from a home respiratory therapist are helpful to assess comfort and address any problems that arise. Criner et al[228] found that 36% of patients required further adjustments in mask or ventilator settings, even after discharge from a several-week stay in an inpatient ventilator unit.

Adverse Effects and Complications

In properly selected patients, NPPV is safe and well tolerated, and most of the adverse effects are related to the interface or ventilator (Table 19-9). Approximately 10–15% of patients fail to tolerate interfaces despite adjustments in strap tension, repositioning, and trials of different sizes and types of interfaces. These patients may have claustrophobia or high levels of anxiety and fail even after multiple attempts at mask readjustment and judicious use of sedation. Other mask-related adverse effects include erythema, pain, or

TABLE 19-9 Frequency of Adverse Side Effects and Complications of NPPV with Possible Remedies

Complication	Occurrence (%)[a]	Possible Remedy
Mask-related		
Discomfort	30–50%	Check fit, adjust strap, new mask type
Facial skin erythema	20–34%	Loosen straps, apply artifical skin
Claustrophobia	5–10%	Smaller mask, sedation
Nasal bridge ulceration	5–10%	Loosen straps, artificial skin, change mask type
Acneiform rash	5–10%	Topical steroids or antibiotics
Air pressure– or flow-related		
Nasal congestion	20–50%	Nasal steroids, decongestant/antihistamines
Sinus/ear pain	10–30%	Reduce pressure if intolerable
Nasal/oral dryness	10–20%	Nasal saline/emollients, add humidifier, decrease leak
Eye irritation	10–20%	Check mask fit, readjust straps
Gastric insufflation	5–10%	Reassure, simethacone, reduce pressure if intolerable
Air leaks	80–100%	Encourage mouth closure, try chin straps, oronasal mask
		If using nasal mask, reduce pressures slightly
Major complications		
Aspiration pneumonia	<5%	Careful patient selection
Hypotension	<5%	Reduce pressure
Pneumothorax	<5%	Stop ventilation if possible, reduce pressure if not
		Thoracostomy tube if indicated

[a] Occurrences estimated from literature and author's experience
SOURCE: Adapted, with permission, from Mehta and Hill.[1]

ulceration on the bridge of the nose. Minimizing strap tension and advances in mask technology, with softer silicon seals and routine use of artificial skin on the bridge of the nose, have been associated with less frequent nasal bridge ulceration, which had been as high as 40% in earlier studies.[310]

Air pressure– and flow-related adverse effects include oronasal dryness or congestion that may respond to humidification or decongestants, sinus and ear pain, eye irritation from air leakage under the mask seal on the sides of the nose, and gastric insufflation. Readjusting the mask seal to reduce air leaking or reducing inspiratory pressure, if possible, may help.

Air leaking is ubiquitous during NIV, either under the seal or through the mouth with nasal ventilation. Air leaking adds to discomfort and may interfere with ventilator triggering and cycling, as well as efficacy of ventilation. The leaks usually are tolerated as long as the ventilator compensates adequately, as most bilevel ventilators do. As discussed earlier, bilevel ventilators cannot function properly without a small intentional leak in the tubing, which is necessary for removal of CO_2 to prevent rebreathing. Most volume-limited modes compensate poorly for leaks, but large air leaks may compromise the effectiveness of any form of NPPV. Attempts to control air leaks should start with a reassessment of mask fit and readjustment of the head straps. To reduce air leaking through the mouth during nasal ventilation, edentulous patients should not be treated with nasal masks, others are coached to keep their mouths shut, chin straps may be used, or an oronasal mask may be tried.

Major complications such as pneumothoraces are unusual probably because inflation pressures are low compared with those used with invasive ventilation. Lack of patient cooperation interferes with efficacy and may be ameliorated by judicious use of sedation, such as low doses of benzodiazapines. Unremitting agitation should be considered an indication for intubation. Aspiration is a reported complication[311] but should be unusual if patients with swallowing dysfunction and problems clearing secretions are excluded. Routine insertion of nasogastric tubes has been recommended at some centers to lower the risk of aspiration during use of face masks,[307] but there are no data available to support this practice, and it is no longer recommended. Progressive hypoventilation occurs in a small minority of patients, usually necessitating intubation. Uncooperativeness, lack of synchronization with the ventilator, inability to tolerate adequate inflation pressures, and excessive air leaking are common causes for this predicament, and measures aimed at correcting these may be helpful. Rarely, nasal obstruction contributes and may respond to decongestant sprays.

In the acute setting, NPPV fails in roughly a third to a quarter of patients depending on many factors, including skill and experience of the team, occurrence of adverse effects and complications as discussed earlier, and underlying severity of the patient's illness. Progression of the underlying process, such as worsening hypoxemia, also may be responsible for failure. Close monitoring with proactive efforts to address and minimize adverse effects should minimize failure rates.

Summary and Conclusions

In the acute setting, evidence now supports NPPV in the treatment of respiratory failure secondary to acute exacerbations of COPD, acute cardiogenic pulmonary edema (which can be managed with CPAP as well), and immunocompromised states and to facilitate weaning in patients with COPD. Weaker evidence supports NPPV in the treatment of other forms of respiratory failure, including respiratory insufficiency in patients with asthma, post-lung resection, or those who decline intubation. NPPV should not be used routinely in ARDS or severe pneumonia. Regardless of the underlying cause of the respiratory failure, patients to receive NPPV must be selected carefully. Those with mild deteriorations likely will succeed without ventilator assistance, and prompt intubation usually is preferred in severely ill patients. Patients with unstable medical conditions, inability to protect the airway or clear secretions, or uncooperativeness are excluded from consideration. Patients selected according to these guidelines and monitored closely can be managed with NPPV with the expectation that intubation and its inherent complications will be avoided.

In the chronic setting, NPPV has long been considered the modality of first choice for patients with respiratory failure secondary to neuromuscular disease or chest-wall deformity. Randomized, controlled trials have not been done because of ethical concerns, but the ability of NPPV to improve symptoms, gas exchange, quality of life, and survival in these patients is widely accepted. NPPV for patients with severe stable COPD has been more controversial because of conflicting data, but it may prevent deterioration of gas exchange, improve quality of life, and reduce the need for hospitalization in patients with severe CO_2 retention and nocturnal hypoventilation who adhere to therapy (which is often not the case). In some countries, the obesity-hypoventilation syndrome has become the largest diagnostic category for NPPV at home, perhaps because of increasing recognition and the obesity epidemic.

In both the acute and chronic settings, experience and skill with the implementation of NPPV are important. Proper fit and application of the mask are keys to success. Although the type of ventilator is not as important, ventilator mode and settings affect comfort and effectiveness. In carefully selected patients initiated according to current recommendations and monitored in an appropriate setting, NPPV can be delivered safely with no or minor adverse effects. The failure rate remains substantial at roughly a quarter to a third but hopefully will decline as clinicians gain experience, selection criteria are refined, and technology improves. NPPV has assumed an important role in acute- and chronic-care settings and should be considered a lung-protective strategy for certain forms of respiratory failure, and clinicians caring for patients with respiratory failure should have skill and experience with NPPV applications.

References

1. Mehta S, Hill NS. Noninvasive ventilation: State of the art. Am J Respir Crit Care Med 2001; 163:540–77.
2. Shneerson JM, Simonds AK. Noninvasive ventilation for chest wall and neuromuscular disorders. Eur Respir J 2002; 20:480–7.
3. Liesching T, Kwok H, Hill NS. Acute applications of noninvasive positive pressure ventilation. Chest 2003; 124:699–713.
4. Pingleton SK. Complications of acute respiratory failure. Am Rev Respir Dis 1988; 137:1463–93.
5. Zwillich CW, Pierson DJ, Creagh CE, et al. Complications of assisted ventilation. Am J Med 1974; 57:161–70.
6. Colice GL, Stukel TA, Dain B. Laryngeal complications of prolonged intubation. Chest 1989; 96:877–84.
7. Heffner JE, Miller KS, Sahn SA. Tracheostomy in the intensive care unit: 2. Complications. Chest 1986; 90:430–6.
8. Patel PJ, Leeper Jr KV, McGowan JE Jr. Epidemiology and microbiology of hospital-acquired pneumonia. Semin Respir Crit Care Med 2002; 23:415–26.
9. Colice GL, Stukel TA, Dain B. Laryngeal complications of prolonged intubation. Chest 1989; 96:877–84.
10. Stauffer JL, Silvestri RC. Complications of endotracheal intubation, tracheostomy, and artificial airways. Respir Care 1982; 27:417–34.
11. Criner GJ, Tzouanakis A, Kreimer DT. Overview of improving tolerance of long-term mechanical ventilation. Crit Care Clin 1994; 10:845–66.
12. Bach JR, Intintola P, Alba AS, Holland I. The ventilator-assisted individual cost analysis of institutionalization versus rehabilitation and in-home management. Chest 1992; 101: 26–30.
13. Nourdine K, Combes P, Carton MJ, et al. Does noninvasive ventilation reduce the ICU nosocomial infection risk? A prospective clinical survey. Intensive Care Med 1999; 25:567–77.
14. Girou E, Brun-Buisson C, Taille S, et al. Secular trends in nosocomial infections and mortality associated with noninvasive ventilation in patients with exacerbation of COPD and pulmonary edema. JAMA 2003; 290:2985–91.
15. Nava S, Evangesliti I, Rampulla C, et al. Human and financial costs of noninvasive mechanical ventilation in patients affected by COPD and acute respiratory failure. Chest 1997; 111: 1631–8.
16. Brochard L, Mancebo J, Wysocki M, et al: Noninvasive ventilation for acute exacerbations of chronic obstructive pulmonary disease. New Engl J Med 1995; 333:817–22.
17. Carrey Z, Gottfried SB, Levy RD. Ventilatory muscle support in respiratory failure with nasal positive pressure ventilation. Chest 1990; 97:150–8.
18. Appendini L, Palessio A, Zanaboni S, et al: Physiologic effects of positive end-expiratory pressure and mask pressure support during exacerbations of chronic obstructive pulmonary disease. Am J Respir Crit Care Med 1994; 149:1069–76.
19. Bradley TD. Sleep: Hemodynamic and sympathoinhibitory effects of nasal CPAP in congestive heart failure. 1996; 19:S232–5.
20. Naughton MT, Rahman MA, Hara K, et al. Effect of continuous positive airway pressure on intrathoracic and left ventricular transmural pressures in patients with congestive heart failure Circulation 1995; 91:1725–31.
21. Meyer TJ, Pressman MR, Benditt J, et al. Air leaking through the mouth during nocturnal nasal ventilation: Effect on sleep quality. Sleep 1997; 20:561–9.
22. Richards GN, Cistulli PA, Ungar G, et al. Mouth leak with nasal continuous positive airway pressure increases nasal airway resistance. Am J Respir Crit Care Med 1996; 154:182–6.
23. Rodenstein DO, Stanescu DC, Delguste P, et al: Adaptation to intermittent positive pressure ventilation applied through the nose during day and night. Eur Respir J 1989; 2:473–8.
24. Mortimore IL, Bradley PA, Murray JAM, Douglas NH. Uvulopalatopharyngoplasty may compromise nasal CPAP therapy in sleep apnea syndrome. Am J Respir Crit Care Med 1996; 154:1759–62.
25. Jounieaux V, Aubert G, Dury M, et al. Effects of nasal positive-pressure hyperventilation on the glottis in normal awake subjects. J Appl Physiol 1995; 79:176–85.

26. Jounieaux V, Aubert G, Dury M, et al. Effects of nasal positive-pressure hyperventilation on the glottis in normal sleeping subjects. J Appl Physiol 1995; 79:186–3.
27. Parreira VF, Delguste P, Jounieaux V, et al. Effectiveness of controlled and spontaneous modes in nasal two-level positive pressure ventilation in awake and asleep normal subjects. Chest 1997; 112:1267–77.
28. Parriera VF, Delguste P, Jounieaux V, et al. Glottic aperature and effective minute ventilation during nasal two-level positive pressure ventilation in spontaneous mode. Am J Respir Crit Care Med 1996; 154:1857–63.
29. Roussos C. Function and fatigue of respiratory muscles. Chest 1985; 88:124–32S.
30. Rochester DF. Does respiratory muscle rest relieve fatigue or incipient fatigue? Am Rev Respir Dis 1988; 138:516–7.
31. Hoeppner VH, Cockcroft DW, Dosman JA, et al. Nighttime ventilation improves respiratory failure in secondary kyphoscoliosis. Am Rev Respir Dis 1984; 129:240–3.
32. Heckmatt JZ, Loh L, Dubowitz V. Nighttime nasal ventilation in neuromuscular disease. Lancet 1990; 335:579–81.
33. Goldstein RS, DeRosie JA, Avendano MA, Dolmage TE. Influence of noninvasive positive pressure ventilation on inspiratory muscles. Chest 1991; 99:408–15.
34. Hill NS, Eveloff SE, Carlisle CC, et al. Efficacy of nocturnal nasal ventilation in patients with restrictive thoracic disease. Am Rev Respir Dis 1992; 101:516–21.
35. Strumpf DA, Millman RP, Carlisle CC, et al. Nocturnal positive-pressure ventilation via nasal mask in patients with severe chronic obstructive pulmonary disease. Am Rev Respir Dis 1991; 144:1234–9.
36. Mohr CH, Hill NS. Long-term follow-up of nocturnal ventilatory assistance in patients with respiratory failure due to Duchenne-type muscular dystrophy. Chest 1990; 97:91–6.
37. Bergofsky EH. Respiratory failure in disorders of the thoracic cage. Am Rev Respir Dis 1979; 119:643–69.
38. NHLBI Workshop Summary. Respiratory muscle fatigue: Report of the Respiratory Muscle Fatigue Workshop Group. Am Rev Respir Dis 1990; 142:474–80.
39. McNicholas WT. Impact of sleep in respiratory failure. Eur Respir J 1997; 10:920–33.
40. Jimenez JFM, de Cos Escuin JS, Vicente CD, et al. Nasal intermittent positive pressure ventilation: Analysis of its withdrawal. Chest 1995; 107:382–8.
41. Goldstein RS, Molotiu N, Skrastins R, et al. Reversal of sleep-induced hypoventilation and chronic respiratory failure by nocturnal negative pressure ventilation in patients with restrictive ventilatory impairment. Am Rev Respir Dis 1987; 135:1049–55.
42. Annane D, Quera-Salva MA, Lofaso F, et al. Mechanisms underlying effects of nocturnal ventilation on daytime blood gases in neuromuscular diseases. Eur Respir J 1999; 13:157–62.
43. Miro AM, Shivarum U, Hertig I. Continuous positive airway pressure in COPD patients in acute hypercapnic respiratory failure. Chest 1993; 103:266–8.
44. DeLucas P, Tarancon C, Puente L, et al. Nasal continuous positive airway pressure in patients with COPD in acute respiratory failure. Chest 1993; 104:1694–7.
45. Petrof BJ, Legare M, Goldberg P, et al. Continuous positive airway pressure reduces work of breathing and dyspnea during weaning from mechanical ventilation in severe chronic obstructive pulmonary disease. Am Rev Respir Dis 1990; 141:281–9.
46. Brochard L, Isabey D, Piquet J, et al. Reversal of acute exacerbations of chronic obstructive lung disease by inspiratory assistance with a face mask. New Engl J Med 1990; 95:865–70.
47. Sacks H, Chalmers TC, Smith H Jr. Randomized versus historical controls for clinical trials. Am J Med 1982; 72:233–40.
48. Bott J, Carroll MP, Conway JH, et al. Randomized, controlled trial of nasal ventilation in acute ventilatory failure due to chronic obstructive airways disease. Lancet 1993; 341:1555–7.
49. Kramer N, Meyer TJ, Meharg J, et al. Randomized, prospective trial of noninvasive positive pressure ventilation in acute respiratory failure. Am J Respir Crit Care Med 1995; 151:1799–806.
50. Angus RM, Ahmed AA, Fenwick LJ, Peacock AJ. Comparison of the acute effects on gas exchange of nasal ventilation and doxapram in exacerbations of chronic obstructive pulmonary disease. Thorax 1996; 51:1048–50.
51. Celikel T, Sungur M, Ceyhan B, Karakurt S. Comparison of noninvasive positive pressure ventilation with standard medical therapy in hypercapnic acute respiratory failure. Chest 1998; 114:1636–42.
52. Plant PK, Owen JL, Elliott MW. Early use of noninvasive ventilation for acute exacerbations of chronic obstructive pulmonary disease on general respiratory wards: A multicenter randomized, controlled trial. Lancet 2000; 355:1931–5.
53. Vitacca M, Rubini F, Foglio K, et al. Noninvasive modalities of positive pressure ventilation improved the outcome of acute exacerbations in COPD patients. Intensive Care Med 1993; 19:450–5.
54. Vitacca M, Clini E, Rubini F, et al. Non-invasive mechanical ventilation in severe chronic obstructive lung disease and acute respiratory failure: Short- and long-term prognosis. Intensive Care Med 1996; 22:94–100.
55. Foglio C, Vitacca M, Quadri A, et al. Acute exacerbations in severe COPD patients: Treatment using positive pressure ventilation by nasal mask. Chest 1992; 101:1533–8.
56. Barbe F, Togores B, Rubi M, et al. Noninvasive ventilatory support does not facilitate recovery from acute respiratory failure in chronic obstructive pulmonary disease. Eur Respir 1996; 9:1240–5.
57. Keenan SP, Kernerman PD, Cook DJ, et al. The effect of noninvasive positive pressure ventilation on mortality in patients admitted with acute respiratory failure: A meta-analysis. Crit Care Med 1997; 25:1685–92.
58. Peter JV, Moran JL, Phillips-Hughes J, Warn D. Noninvasive ventilation in acute respiratory failure: A meta-analysis update. Crit Care Med. 2002; 30:555–62.
59. Keenan SP, Sinuff T, Cook DJ, Hill N. Which patients with acute exacerbation of chronic obstructive pulmonary disease benefit from noninvasive positive pressure ventilation? A systematic review of the literature. Ann Intern Med 2003; 138:861–70.
60. Lightowler J, Wedzicha TA, Elliott MW, Ram FS. Noninvasive positive pressure ventilation for the treatment of respiratory failure due to exacerbations of chronic obstructive pulmonary disease (Cochrane review). Br Med J 2003; 326:185–9.
61. International Consensus Conferences in Intensive Care Medicine. Noninvasive positive pressure ventilation in acute respiratory failure. Am J Respir Crit Care Med 2001; 163:283–91.
62. British Thoracic Society Standards of Care Committee. BTS guideline: Non-invasive ventilation in acute respiratory failure. Thorax 2002; 57:192–211.
63. Squadrone E, Frigerio P, Fogliati C, et al. Noninvasive versus invasive ventilation in COPD patients with severe acute respiratory failure deemed to require ventilatory assistance. Intensive Care Med 2004; 30:1303–10.
64. Tuggey JM, Plant PK, Elliot MW. Domiciliary non-invasive ventilation for recurrent acidotic exacerbations of COPD: An economic analysis. Thorax 2003; 58:867–71.
65. Meduri GU, Turner RE, Abou-Shala N, et al. Noninvasive positive pressure ventilation via face mask. Chest 1996; 109:179–93.

66. Meduri GU, Cook TR, Turner RE, et al. Noninvasive positive pressure ventilation in status asthmaticus. Chest 1996; 110: 767–74.

67. Fernandez MM, Villagra A, Blanch L, et al. Non-invasive mechanical ventilation in status asthmaticus. Intensive Care Med 2001; 27:486–92.

68. Holley MT, Morrissey TK, Seaberg DC, et al. Ethical dilemmas in a randomized trial of asthma treatment: Can Bayesian statistical analysis explain the results? Acad Emerg Med 2001; 8: 1128–35.

69. Soroksky A, Stav D, Shpirer I. A pilot prospective, randomized, placebo-controlled trial of bilevel positive airway pressure in acute asthmatic attack. Chest 2003; 123:1018–25.

70. Ram FS, Wellington S, Rowe BH, Wedzicha JA. Non-invasive positive pressure ventilation for treatment of respiratory failure due to severe acute exacerbations of asthma. Cochrane Database Syst Rev 2005; 1:CD004360.

71. Wenzel S. Severe asthma in adults. Am J Respir Crit Care Med 2005; 172:149–60.

72. Hodson ME, Madden BP, Steven MH, et al. Non-invasive mechanical ventilation for cystic fibrosis patients: A potential bridge to transplantation. Eur Respir J 1991; 4:524–7.

73. Madden BP, Kariyawasam H, Siddiqi AJ, et al. Noninvasive ventilation in cystic fibrosis patients with acute or chronic respiratory failure. Eur Respir J 2002; 19:310–3.

74. Essouri S, Nicot F, Clement A, et al. Noninvasive positive pressure ventilation in infants with upper airway obstruction: Comparison of continuous and bilevel positive pressure. Intensive Care Med 2005; 31:574–80.

75. Piper AJ, Sullivan CE. Effects of short-term NIPPV in the treatment of patients with severe obstructive sleep apnea and hypercapnia. Chest 1994, 105:434–44.

76. Sturani C, Galavotti V, Scarduelli C, et al. Acute respiratory failure, due to severe obstructive sleep apnoea syndrome, managed with nasal positive pressure ventilation. Monaldi Arch Chest Dis 1994; 49:558–60.

77. Mazia CG, De Vito EL, Varela M. BiPAP in acute respiratory failure due to myasthenic crisis may prevent intubation. Neurology 2003; 8:61–144.

78. Finlay G, Conconnon D, McDonell TJ. Treatment of respiratory failure due to kyphoscoliosis with nasal intermittent positive pressure ventilation (NIPPV). Irish J Med Sci 1995; 164:28–30.

79. Bach JR, Ishikawa Y, Kim H. Prevention of pulmonary morbidity for patients with Duchenne muscular dystrophy. Chest 1997; 112:1024–8.

80. Al-Hameed FM, Sharma S. Outcome of patients admitted to the intensive care unit for acute exacerbation of idiopathic pulmonary fibrosis. Can Respir J 2004; 11:117–22.

81. Antonelli M, Conti G, Rocco M, et al. A comparison of noninvasive positive-pressure ventilation and conventional mechanical ventilation in patients with acute respiratory failure. New Engl J Med 1998; 339:429–35.

82. Meduri GU, Conoscenti CC, Menashe P, Nair S. Noninvasive face mask ventilation in patients with acute respiratory failure. Chest. 1989; 95:865–70.

83. Wysocki M, Tric L, Wolff MA, et al. Noninvasive pressure support ventilation in patients with acute respiratory failure. Chest 1993; 103: 907–13.

84. Wysocki M, Laurent T, Wolff MA, et al. Noninvasive pressure support ventilation in patients with acute respiratory failure: A randomized comparison with conventional therapy. Chest 1995; 107:761–8.

85. Martin TJ, Hovis JD, Constantino JP, et al. A randomized, prospective evaluation of noninvasive ventilation for acute respiratory failure. Am J Respir Crit Care Med 2000; 161:807–13.

86. Ferrer M, Esquinas A, Leon M, et al. Noninvasive ventilation in severe hypoxemic respiratory failure: A randomized clinical trial. Am J Respir Crit Care Med 2003; 168:1438–44.

87. Keenan SP, Sinuff T, Cook DJ, Hill NS. Does noninvasive positive pressure ventilation improve outcome in acute hypoxemic respiratory failure? A systematic review. Crit Care Med 2004; 32:2516–23.

88. Barach AL, Martin J, Eckman M. Positive pressure respiration and its application to the treatment of acute pulmonary edema. Ann Intern Med 1938; 12:754–95.

89. Rasanen J, Heikkila J, Downs J, et al. Continuous positive airway pressure by face mask in acute cardiogenic pulmonary edema. Am J Cardiol 1985; 55:296–300.

90. Lin M, Chiang HT. The efficacy of early continuous positive airway pressure therapy in patients with acute cardiogenic pulmonary edema. J Formos Med Assoc 1991; 90:736–43.

91. Bersten AD, Holt AW, Vedig AE, et al. Treatment of severe cardiogenicpulmonary edema with continuous positive airway pressure delivered by face mask. New Engl J Med 1991; 325:1825–30.

92. Lin M, Yang YF, Chiang HT, et al. Reappraisal of continuous positive airway pressure therapy in acute cardiogenic pulmonary edema: Short-term results and long-term follow-up. Chest 1995; 107:1379–86.

93. Hoffmann B, Welte T. The use of noninvasive pressure support ventilation for severe respiratory insufficiency due to pulmonary edema. Intensive Care Med 1999; 25:15–20.

94. Rusterholtz T, Kempf J, Berton C, et al. Noninvasive pressure support ventilation (NIPSV) with face mask in patients with acute cardiogenic pulmonary edema (ACPE). Intensive Care Med 1999; 25:21–8.

95. Wysocki M. Noninvasive ventilation in acute cardiogenic pulmonary edema: Better than continuous positive airway pressure? Intensive Care Med 1999; 25:1–2.

96. Masip J, Betbese AJ, Paez J, et al. Non-invasive pressure support ventilation versus conventional oxygen therapy in acute cardiogenic pulmonary oedema: A randomised trial. Lancet 2000; 356:2126–32.

97. Sharon A, Shpirer I, Kaluski E, et al. High-dose intravenous isosorbide-dinitrate is safer and better than BiPAP ventilation combined with conventional treatment for severe pulmonary edema. J Am Coll Cardiol 2000; 36:832–7.

98. Nava S, Carbone G, DiBattista N, et al. Noninvasive ventilation in cardiogenic pulmonary edema: A multicenter randomized trial. Am J Respir Crit Care Med 2003; 168:1432–7.

99. Mehta S, Jay GD, Woolard RH, et al. Randomized, prospective trial of bilevel versus continuous positive airway pressure in acute pulmonary edema. Crit Care Med 1997; 25: 620–8.

100. Crane SD, Elliott MW, Gilligan P, et al. Randomised, controlled comparison of continuous positive airways pressure, bilevel noninvasive ventilation, and standard treatment in emergency department patients with acute cardiogenic pulmonary edema. Emerg Med J 2004; 21:155–61.

101. Bellone A, Monari A, Cortellaro F, et al. Myocardial infarction rate in actue pulmonary edema: Noninvasive pressure support ventilation versus continuous positive airway pressure. Crit Care Med 2004; 32:1860–5.

102. Bellone A, Vettorello M, Monari A, et al. Noninvasive pressure support ventilation vs continuous positive airway pressure in acute hypercapnic pulmonary edema. Intensive Care Med 2005; 31:807–11.

103. Masip J, Paez J, Merino M, et al. Risk factors for intubation as a guide for noninvasive ventilation in patients with severe acute cardiogenic pulmonary disease. Intensive Care Med 2003; 29:1921–8.

104. Pang D, Keenan SP, Cook DJ, et al. The effect of positive pressure airway support on mortality and the need for intubation in cardiogenic pulmonary edema: A systematic review. Chest 1998; 114:1185–92.

105. Ambrosino N, Foglio K, Rubini F, et al. Non-invasive mechanical ventilation in acute respiratory failure due to chronic obstructive pulmonary disease: Correlates for success. Thorax 1995; 50: 755–7.

106. Confalonieri M, Potena A, Carbone G, et al. Acute respiratory failure in patients with severe community-acquired pneumonia: A prospective, randomized evaluation of noninvasive ventilation. Am J Respir Crit Care Med 1999; 160:1585–91.

107. Jolliet P, Abajo B, Pasquina P, et al. Non-invasive pressure support ventilation in severe community-acquired pneumonia. Intensive Care Med 2001; 27:812–21.

108. Han F, Jiang HF, Zheng JH, et al. Noninvasive positive pressure ventilation treatment for acute respiratory failure in SARS. Sleep Breath 2004; 8:97–106.

109. Cheung TM, Yam LY, So LK, et al. Effectiveness of noninvasive positive pressure ventilation in the treatment of acute respiratory failure in severe acute respiratory syndrome. Chest 2004; 126:845–50.

110. Confalonieri M, Calderini E, Terraciano S, et al. Noninvasive ventilation for treating acute respiratory failure in AIDS patients with *Pneumocystis carinii* pneumonia. Intensive Care Med 2002; 28:1233–8.

111. Conti G, Marino P, Cogliati A, et al. Noninvasive ventilation for the treatment of acute respiratory failure in patients with hematologic malignancies: A pilot study. Intensive Care Med 1998; 24:1283–8.

112. Antonelli M, Conti G, Bufi M, et al. Noninvasive ventilation for treatment of acute respiratory failure in patients undergoing solid organ transplantation: A randomized trial. JAMA 2000; 283:235–41.

113. Hilbert G, Gruson D, Vargas F, et al. Noninvasive ventilation in immunosuppressed patients with pulmonary infiltrates, fever, and acute respiratory failure. New Engl J Med 2001; 344: 481–7

114. Rocker GM, Mackenzie MG, Williams B, et al. Noninvasive positive pressure ventilation: Successful outcome in patients with acute lung injury/ARDS. Chest 1999; 115:173–7.

115. Beltrame F, Lucangelo U, Gregori D, et al. Noninvasive positive pressure ventilation in trauma patients with acute respiratory failure. Monaldi Arch Chest Dis 1999; 54:1109–48.

116. Freichels TA. Pallative ventilatory support use of noninvasive positive pressure ventilation in terminal respiratory insufficiency. Am J Crit Care 1984; 3:6–10.

117. Clarke DE, Vaughan L, Raffin TA. Noninvasive positive pressure ventilation for patients with terminal respiratory failure: The ethical and economic costs of delaying the inevitable are too great. Am J Crit Care 1994; 3:4–5.

118. Benhamou D, Girault C, Faure C, et al. Nasal mask ventilation in acute respiratory failure: Experience in elderly patients. Chest 1992; 102:912–7.

119. Meduri GU, Fox RC, Abou-Shala N, et al. Noninvasive mechanical ventilation via face mask in patients with acute respiratory failure who refused endotracheal intubation. Crit Care Med 1994; 22:1584–90.

120. Levy M, Tanios MA, Nelson D, et al. Outcomes of patients with do-not-intubate orders treated with noninvasive ventilation. Crit Care Med 2004; 32:2002–7.

121. Chu CM, Chan VL, Wong IW, et al. Noninvasive ventilation in patients with acute hypercapnic exacerbation of chronic obstructive pulmonary disease who refused endotracheal intubation. Crit Care Med 2004; 32:372–7.

122. Pennock BE, Kaplan PD, Carlin BW, et al. Pressure support ventilation with a simplified ventilatory support system administered with a nasal mask in patients with respiratory failure. Chest 1991; 100:1371–6.

123. Pennock BE, Crawshaw L, Kaplan PD. Noninvasive nasal mask ventilation for acute respiratory failure: Institution of a new therapeutic technology for routine use. Chest 1994; 105: 441–4.

124. Gust R, Gottschalk A, Schmidt H, et al. Effects of continuous (CPAP) and bilevel positive airway pressure (BiPAP) on extravascular lung water after extubation of the trachea in patients following coronary artery bypass grafting. Intensive Care Med 1996; 22:1345–50.

125. Matte P, Jacquet L, Van Dyck M, et al. Effects of conventional physiotherapy, continuous positive airway pressure and noninvasive ventilatory support with bilevel positive airway pressure after coronary artery bypass grafting. Acta Anaesthesiol Scand 2000; 44:75–81.

126. Aguilo R, Togores B, Pons S, et al. Noninvasive ventilatory support after lung resectional surgery. Chest 1997; 112:117–21.

127. Joris JL, Sottiaux TM, Chiche JD, et al. Effect of bilevel positive airway pressure (BiPAP) nasal ventilation on the postoperative pulmonary restrictive syndrome in obese patients undergoing gastroplasty. Chest 1997; 111:665–70.

128. Auriant I, Jallot A, Herve P, et al. Noninvasive ventilation reduces mortality in acute respiratory failure following lung resection. Am J Respir Crit Care Med 2001; 164:1231–5.

129. Udwadia ZF, Santis GK, Stevan MH, et al: Nasal ventilation to facilitate weaning in patients with chronic respiratory insufficiency. Thorax 1992; 47:715–8.

130. Restrick LJ, Scott AD, Ward EM, et al. Nasal intermittent positive-pressure ventilation in weaning intubated patients with chronic respiratory disease from assisted intermittent positive-pressure ventilation. Respir Med 1993; 87:199–204.

131. Munshi IA, DeHaven B, Kirton O, et al. Reengineering respiratory support following extubation avoidance of critical care unit costs. Chest 1999; 116:1025–8.

132. Nava S, Ambrosino N, Clini E, et al. Noninvasive mechanical ventilation in the weaning of patients with respiratory failure due to chronic obstructive pulmonary disease: A randomized, controlled trial. Ann Intern Med 1998; 128:721–8.

133. Girault C, Daudenthun I, Chevron V, et al. Noninvasive ventilation as a systematic extubation and weaning technique in acute-on-chronic respiratory failure: A prospective, randomized, controlled study. Am J Respir Crit Care Med 1999; 160: 86–92.

134. Ferrer M, Esquinas A, Arancibia F, et al. Noninvasive ventilation during persistent weaning failure: A randomized, controlled trial. Am J Respir Crit Care Med 2003; 168:70–6.

135. Hill N, Lin D, Levy M, et al. Noninvasive positive pressure ventilation (NPPV) to facilitate extubation after acute respiratory failure: a feasibility study. Am J Respir Crit Care Med 2000; 161:A263.

136. Epstein SK, Ciubotaru RL, Wong JB. Effect of failed extubation on the outcome of mechanical ventilation. Chest 1997; 112:186–92.

137. Jiang JS, Kao SJ, Wang SN. Effect of early application of biphasic positive airway pressure on the outcome of extubation in ventilator weaning. Respirology 1999; 4:161–5.

138. Esteban A, Frutos-Vivar F, Ferguson ND, et al. Noninvasive positive-pressure ventilation for respiratory failure after extubation. New Engl J Med 2004; 350:2452–60.

139. Nava S, Gregoretti C, Fanfulla F, et al. Noninvasive ventilation to prevent respiratory failure after extubation in high risk patients. Crit Care Med 2005; 33:2465–70.

140. Hilbert G, Gruson D, Gbikpi-Benissan G, et al. Sequential use of noninvasive pressure support ventilation for acute exacerbations of COPD. Intensive Care Med 1997; 23:955–61.

141. Keenan SP, Powers C, McCormack DG, Block G. Noninvasive positive-pressure ventilation for postextubation respiratory distress: A randomized, controlled trial. JAMA. 2002; 287:3238–44.

142. Akingbola OA, Sevant GM, Custer JR, Palmisano JM. Noninvasive bilevel positive pressure ventilation: Management of two pediatric patients. Respir Care 1993; 38:1092–8.

143. Fortenberry JD, Del Toro J, Jefferson LS, et al. Management of pediatric acute hypoxemic respiratory insufficiency with bilevel positive pressure (BiPAP) nasal mask ventilation. Chest 1995; 108:1059–64.

144. Padman R, Lawless ST, Kettrick RG. Noninvasive ventilation via bilevel positive airway pressure support in pediatric practice. Crit Care Med 1998; 26:169–73.

145. Stocks J, Godfrey S. Nasal resistance during infancy. Respir Physiol 1978; 34:233–46.

146. Teague GW. Pediatric application of noninvasive ventilation. Respir Care 1997; 42:414–23.

147. Chin K, Uemoto S, Takahashi K, et al. Noninvasive ventilation for pediatric patients including those under 1-year-old undergoing liver transplantation. Liver Transplant 2005; 11:188–95.

148. Essouri S, Nicot F, Clement A, et al. Noninvasive positive pressure ventilation in infants with upper airway obstruction: Comparison of continuous and bilevel positive pressure. Intensive Care Med 2005; 31:574–80.

149. Teague WG. Noninvasive ventilation in the pediatric intensive care unit for children with acute respiratory failure. Pediatr Pulmonol 2003; 35:418–26.

150. Antonelli M, Conti G, Rocco M, et al. Noninvasive positive-pressure ventilation vs conventional oxygen supplementation in hypoxemic patients undergoing diagnostic bronchoscopy. Chest 2002; 121:1149–54.

151. Antonelli M, Pennisi MA, Conti G, et al. Fiberoptic bronchoscopy during noninvasive positive pressure ventilation delivered by helmet. Intensive Care Med 2003; 29:126–9.

152. Gregory S, Siderowf A, Golaszewski AL, McCluskey L. Gastrostomy insertion in ALS patients with low vital capacity: Respiratory support and survival. Neurology 2002; 58:485–7.

153. Soo Hoo GW, Santiago S, Williams AJ. Nasal mechanical ventilation for hypercapnic respiratory failure in chronic obstructive pulmonary disease: determinants of success and failure. Crit Care Med 1994; 22:1253–61.

154. Phua J, Kong K, Lee KH, et al. Noninvasive ventilation in hypercapnic acute respiratory failure due to chronic obstructive pulmonary disease vs other conditions: Effectiveness and predictors of failure. Intensive Care Med 2005; 31:533–9.

155. Confalonieri M, Garuti G, Cattaruzza MS, et al. Italian noninvasive positive pressure ventilation (NPPV) study group. A chart of failure risk for noninvasive ventilation in patients with COPD exacerbation. Eur Respir J 2005; 25:348–55.

156. Antonelli M, Conti G, Moro ML, et al. Predictors of failure of noninvasive positive pressure ventilation in patients with acute hypoxemic respiratory failure: A multi-center study. Intensive Care Med 2001; 27:1718–28.

157. American Respiratory Care Foundation. Consensus conference: Non-invasive positive pressure ventilation. Respir Care 1997; 42: 364–9.

158. Diaz GG, Alcaraz AC, Talavera JC, et al. Noninvasive positive-pressure ventilation to treat hypercapnic coma secondary to respiratory failure. Chest 2005; 127:952–60.

159. Splaingard ML, Frates RC Jr, Harrison GM, et al. Home-positive-pressure ventilation: Twenty years' experience. Chest 1983; 84: 376–84.

160. Curran FJ, Colbert AP. Ventilator management in Duchenne muscular dystrophy and post-poliomyelitis syndrome: Twelve years' experience. Arch Phys Med Rehabil 1989; 70:180–5.

161. Alba A, Khan A, Lee M. Mouth IPPV for sleep. Rehabil Gaz 1984; 24:47–9.

162. Bach JR, Alba AS, Saporito LR: Intermittent positive pressure ventilation via the mouth as an alternative to tracheostomy for 257 ventilator users. Chest 1993; 103:174–82.

163. Sullivan CE, Issa FG, Berthon-Jones M, et al: Reversal of obstructive sleep apnea by continuous positive airway pressure applied through the nares. Lancet 1981; 1:862–5.

164. Bach JR, Alba AS. Management of chronic alveolar hypoventilation by nasal ventilation. Chest 1990; 97:52–7.

165. Kerby GR, Mayer LS, Pingleton SK. Nocturnal positive pressure ventilation via nasal mask. Am Rev Respir Dis 1987; 135:738–40.

166. Ellis ER, Bye PT, Bruderer JW, et al: Treatment of respiratory failure during sleep in patients with neuromuscular disease: Positive-pressure ventilation through a nose mask. Am Rev Respir Dis 1987; 135:148–52.

167. Leger P, Jennequin J, Gerard M, Robert D. Home positive pressure ventilation via nasal masks in patients with neuromuscular weakness and restrictive lung or chest wall disease. Respir Care 1989; 34:73–9.

168. Bach JR, Alba AS. Noninvasive options for ventilatory support of the traumatic high level quadriplegic. Chest 1990; 98:613–9.

169. Gay PC, Patel AM, Viggiano RW, Hubmayr RD. Nocturnal nasal ventilation for treatment of patients with hypercapnic respiratory failure. Mayo Clin Proc 1991; 144:1234–9.

170. Finlay G, Concannon D, McDonell TJ. Treatment of respiratory failure due to kyphoscoliosis with nasal intermittent positive pressure ventilation (NIPPV). Irish J Med Sci 1995; 164:28–30.

171. Perrin C, D'Ambrosio C, White A, Hill NS. Sleep in restrictive and neuromuscular respiratory disorders. Semin Respir Crit Care Med 2005; 26 117–30.

172. Hill NS, Redline S, Carskadon MA, et al. Sleep-disordered breathing in patients with Duchenne muscular dystrophy using negative pressure ventilators Chest 1992; 102:1656–62.

173. Masa Jimenez JF, de Cos Escuin JS, Vicente CD, et al. Nasal intermittent positive pressure ventilation: Analysis of its withdrawal. Chest 1995; 107:382–8.

174. Meyer TJ, Pressman MR, Benditt J, et al. Air leaking through the mouth during nocturnal nasal ventilation: Effect on sleep quality. Sleep 1997; 20:561–9.

175. Pehrsson K, Olofson J, Larsson, Sullivan M. Quality of life of patients treated by home mechanical ventilation due to restrictive ventilatory disorders. Respir Med 1994; 88:21–6.

176. Nauffal D, Domenech R, Martinez Garcia MA, et al. Noninvasive positive pressure home ventilation in restrictive disorders: Outcome and impact on health-related quality of life. Respir Med. 2002; 96:777–83.

177. Bourke SC, Bullock RE, Williams TL, et al. Noninvasive ventilation in ALS: Indications and effect on quality of life. Neurology 2003; 61:171–7.

178. Lyall RA, Donaldson N, Fleming T, et al. A prospective study of quality of life in ALS patients treated with noninvasive ventilation. Neurology 2001; 57:153–6.

179. Butz M, Wollinsky KH, Wiedemuth-Catrinescu U, et al. Longitudinal effects of noninvasive positive-pressure ventilation in patients with amyotrophic lateral sclerosis. Am J Phys Med Rehabil 2003; 82:597–604.

180. Bach JR. A comparison of long-term ventilatory support alternatives from the perspective of the patient and care giver. Chest 1993; 104:1702–6.

181. Cazzoli PA, Oppenheimer EA. Home mechanical ventilation for amyotrophic lateral sclerosis: Nasal compared to

tracheostomy-intermittent positive pressure ventilation. J Neurol Sci 1996; 139:123–8.

182. Markstrom A, Sundell K, Lysdahl M, et al. Quality-of-life evaluation of patients with neuromuscular and skeletal diseases treated with noninvasive and invasive home mechanical ventilation. Chest 2002; 122:1695–700.

183. Leger P, Bedicam JM, Cornette A, et al. Nasal intermittent positive pressure: Long-term follow-up in patients with severe chronic respiratory insufficiency. Chest 1994; 105:100–5.

184. Janssens JP, Derivaz S, Breitenstein E, et al. Changing patterns in long.-term noninvasive ventilation: A 7-year prospective study in the Geneva Lake area. Chest 2003; 123:67–79.

185. Simonds AK, Elliott MW. Outcome of domiciliary nasal intermittent positive pressure ventilation in restrictive and obstructive disorders. Thorax 1995; 50:604–9.

186. Simonds AK, Muntoni F, Heather S, Fielding S. Impact of nasal ventilation on survival in hypercapnic Duchenne muscular dystrophy. Thorax 1998; 53:949–52.

187. Robert D, Gerard M, Leger P, et al. La Ventilation mechanique a domicile definitive par tracheostomie de l'insuffisant respiratoir chronique. Rev Fr Mal Respir 1983; 11:923–36.

188. Pinto AC, Evangelista T, Carvalho M, et al. Respiratory assistance with a noninvasive ventilator (BiPAP) in MND/ALS patients: Survival rates in controlled trial. J Neurol Sci 1995; 129: 19–26.

189. Aboussouan LS, Khan SU, Meeker DP, et al. Effect of noninvasive positive pressure ventilation on survival in amyotrophic lateral sclerosis. Ann Intern Med 1997; 127:450–3.

190. Bach JR. Amyotrophic lateral sclerosis: Prolongation of life by noninvasive respiratory AIDS. Chest 2002; 122:92–8.

191. Lechtzin N, Wiener CM, Clawson L, et al. ALS CARE Study Group. Use of noninvasive ventilation in patients with amyotrophic lateral sclerosis. Amyotroph Lateral Scler Other Motor Neuron Disord 2004; 5:9–15.

192. American College of Chest Physicians. Clinical indications for noninvasive positive pressure ventilation in chronic respiratory failure due to restrictive lung disease, COPD, and nocturnal hypoventilation—A consensus conference report Chest 1999; 116:521–34.

193. Bach JR. Update and perspective on noninvasive respiratory muscle aids: 2. The expiratory aids. Chest 1994; 105:1538–44.

194. Branthwaite MA. Noninvasive and domiciliary ventilation: Positive pressure techniques. Thorax 1991; 46:208–12.

195. Raphael JC, Chevret S, Chastang CI, Bouvet F. Home mechanical ventilation in Duchenne's muscular dystrophy: In search of a therapeutic strategy. Eur Respir Rev 1993; 12:270–4.

196. Jackson CE, Rosenfeld J, Moore DH, et al. A preliminary evaluation of a prospective study of pulmonary function studies and symptoms of hypoventilation in ALS/MND patients. J Neurol Sci 2001; 191:75–8.

197. Miller RG, Rosenberg JA, Gelinas DF, et al. Practice parameter: The care of the patient with amyotrophic lateral sclerosis (an evidence-based review): Report of the Quality Standards Subcommittee of the American Academy of Neurology: ALS Practice Parameters Task Force. Neurology 1999; 52:1311–23.

198. Masa JF, Celli BR, Riesco JA, et al. Noninvasive positive pressure ventilation and not oxygen may prevent overt ventilatory failure in patients with chest wall diseases. Chest 1997; 112: 207–13.

199. Ellis ER, McCauley VB, Mellis C, Sullivan CE. Treatment of alveolar hypoventilation in a six-year-old girl with intermittent positive pressure ventilation through a nose mask. Am Rev Respir Dis 1987; 136:188–91.

200. DiMarco AF, Connors AF, Alrose MD. Management of chronic alveolar hypoventilation with nasal positive pressure breathing. Chest 1987; 92:952–4.

201. Piper AJ, Sullivan CE. Effects of short-term NIPPV in the treatment of patients with severe obstructive sleep apnea and hypercapnia. Chest 1994; 105:434–40.

202. Sanders MH, Kern NB. Obstructive sleep apnea treated by independently adjusted inspiratory and expiratory positive airway pressure via nasal mask. Chest 1990; 98:317–24.

203. Reeves-Hoche MK, Hudgel DW, Meck R, et al. Continuous versus bilevel positive airway pressure for obstructive sleep apnea. Am J Respir Crit Care Med 1995; 151:443–9.

204. Berger KI, Ayappa I, Chatr-amontri B, et al. Obesity hypoventilation syndrome as a spectrum of respiratory disturbances during sleep. Chest 2001; 120:1231–8.

205. Pankow W, Hijjeh N, Schuttler F, et al. Influence of noninvasive positive pressure ventilation on inspiratory muscle activity in obese subjects. Eur Respir J 1997; 10:2847–52.

206. Masa JF, Celli BR, Riesco JA, et al. The obesity hypoventilation syndrome can be treated with noninvasive mechanical ventilation. Chest 2001; 119:1102–7.

207. de Lucas-Ramos P, de Miguel-Diez J, Santacruz-Siminiani A, et al. Benefits at 1 year of nocturnal intermittent positive pressure ventilation in patients with obesity-hypoventilation syndrome. Respir Med 2004; 98:961–7.

208. McClement JH, Christianson LC, Hubaytar RT, Simpson DG. The body-type respirator in the treatment of chronic obstructive pulmonary disease. Ann NY Acad Sci 1965; 121: 746–50.

209. Braun NM, Marino WD. Effect of daily intermittent rest of respiratory muscles in patients with severe chronic airflow limitation (CAL). Chest 1984; 85:59–60S.

210. Cropp A, Dimarco AF. Effects of intermittent negative pressure ventilation on respiratory muscle function in patients with severe chronic obstructive pulmonary disease. Am Rev Respir Dis 1987; 135:1056–61.

211. Ambrosino N, Montagna T, Nava S, et al. Short term effect of intermittent negative pressure ventilation in COPD patients with respiratory failure. Eur Respir J 1990; 3:502–8.

212. Sauret JM, Guitart AC, Rodriguez-Frojan G, et al. Intermittent short-term negative pressure ventilation and increased oxygenation in COPD patients with severe hypercapnic respiratory failure. Chest 1991; 100:455–9.

213. Celli B, Lee H, Criner G, et al. Controlled trial of external negative pressure ventilation in patients with severe airflow obstruction. Am Rev Respir Dis 1989; 140:1251–6.

214. Zibrak JD, Hill NS, Federman ED, et al. Evaluation of intermittent long-term negative pressure ventilation in patients with severe chronic obstructive pulmonary disease. Am Rev Respir Dis 1988; 138:1515–8.

215. Shapiro SH, Ernst P, Gray-Donald K, et al. Effect of negative pressure ventilation in severe chronic obstructive pulmonary disease. Lancet 1992; 340:1425–9.

216. Juan G, Calverley P, Talamo C, et al. Effect of carbon dioxide on diaphragmatic function in human beings. New Engl J Med 1984; 310:874–9.

217. Calverley PMA, Brezinova V, Douglas NJ, et al. The effect of oxygenation on sleep quality in chronic bronchitis and emphysema. Am Rev Respir Dis 1982; 126:204–10.

218. Hudgel DW, Martin RJ, Capehart M, et al. Contribution of hypoventilation to sleep oxygen desaturation in chronic obstructive pulmonary disease. J Appl Physiol 1983; 83:669–77.

219. Elliott MW, Mulvey DA, Moxham J, et al. Domiciliary nocturnal nasal intermittent positive pressure ventilation in COPD: Mechanisms underlying changes in arterial blood gas tensions. Eur Respir J 1991; 4:1044–52.

220. Elliott MW, Simonds AK, Carroll MP, et al. Domiciliary nocturnal nasal intermittent positive pressure ventilation in

hypercapnic respiratory failure due to chronic obstructive lung disease: Effects on sleep and quality of life. Thorax 1992; 47:342–8.

221. Meecham Jones DJ, Paul EA, Jones PW. Nasal pressure support ventilation plus oxygen compared with oxygen therapy along in hypercapnic COPD. Am J Respir Crit Care Med 1995; 152: 538–44.

222. Krachman SL, Quaranta AJ, Berger TJ, Criner GJ. Effects of non-invasive positive pressure ventilation on gas exchange and sleep in COPD patients. Chest 1997; 112:623–8.

223. Gay PC, Patel AM, Viggiano RW, et al. Nocturnal nasal ventilation for treatment of patients with hypercapnic respiratory failure. Mayo Clinic Proc 1991; 66: 695–703.

224. Lin CC. Comparison between nocturnal nasal positive pressure ventilation combined with oxygen therapy and oxygen monotherapy in patients with severe COPD. Am J Respir Crit Care Med 1996; 154:353–8.

225. Casanova C, Celli BR, Tost L, et al. Long-term controlled trial of nocturnal nasal positive pressure ventilation with severe COPD. Chest 2000; 118:1582–90.

226. Clini E, Sturani C, Rossi A, et al. Rehabilitation and Chronic Care Study Group, Italian Association of Hospital Pulmonologists (AIPO). The Italian multicentre study on noninvasive ventilation in chronic obstructive pulmonary disease patients. Eur Respir J 2002; 20:529–38.

227. Muir JF, Cuvelier A, Tengang B, et al. Long-term home nasal intermittent positive pressure ventilation (NPPV) + oxygen therapy (L$_{TOT}$) versus L$_{TOT}$ alone in severe hypercapnic COPD: Preliminary results of a European multicenter trial. Respir Crit Care Med 1997; 155:A408.

228. Criner GJ, Brennan K, Travaline JM, Kreimer D. Efficacy and compliance with noninvasive positive pressure ventilation in patients with chronic respiratory failure. Chest 1999; 116:667–5.

229. Rossi A, Hill NS. Noninvasive ventilation has been shown to be ineffective in stable COPD: Pro-con debate. Am J Respir Crit Care Med 2000; 161:689–91.

230. Wijkstra PJ, Lacasse Y, Guyatt GH, et al. A meta-analysis of nocturnal noninvasive positive pressure ventilation in patients with stable COPD. Chest 2003; 124:337–43.

231. Jones SE, Packham S, Hebden M, Smith AP. Domiciliary nocturnal intermittent positive pressure ventilation in patients with respiratory failure due to severe COPD: Long term follow-up and effect on survival. Thorax 1998; 53:495–8.

232. Sivasothy P, Smith IE, Shneerson JM. Mask intermittent positive pressure ventilation in chronic hypercapnic respiratory failure due to chronic obstructive pulmonary disease. Eur Respir J 1998; 11:34–40.

233. Ambrosino N. Exercise and noninvasive ventilatory support. Monaldi Arch Chest Dis 2000; 55:242–6.

234. Maltais F, Reissmann H, Gottfried SB. Pressure support reduces inspiratory effort and dyspnea during exercise in chronic airflow obstruction. Respir Med 2002; 96:359–67.

235. Bianchi L, Foglio K, Pagani M, et al. Effects of proportional assist ventilation on exercise tolerance in COPD patients with chronic hypercapnia. Eur Respir J 1998; 11:422–7.

236. Bianchi L, Foglio K, Porta R, et al. Lack of additional effect of adjunct of assisted ventilation to pulmonary rehabilitation in mild COPD patients. Respir Med 2002; 96:359–67.

237. Garrod R, Mikelsons C, Paul EA, Wedzicha JA. Randomized, controlled trial of domiciliary noninvasive positive pressure ventilation and physical training in severe COPD. Am J Respir Crit Care Med 2000; 162:1335–41.

238. Piper AJ, Parker S, Torzillo PJ, et al. Nocturnal nasal IPPV stabilizes patients with cystic fibrosis and hypercapnic respiratory failure. Chest 1992; 102:846–50.

239. Padman R, Nadkarni VM, Von Nessen S, Goodill J. Noninvasive positive pressure ventilation in end-stage cystic fibrosis: A report of seven cases. Respir Care 1994; 39:736–9.

240. Gozal D. Nocturnal ventilatory support in patients with cystic fibrosis: Comparison with supplemental oxygen. Eur Respir J 1997; 10:1999–2003.

241. Fauroux B, Boffa C, Desguerre I, et al. Long-term noninvasive mechanical ventilation for children at home: A national survey. Pediatr Pulmonol 2003; 35:119–25.

242. Granton JT, Kesten S. The acute effects of nasal positive pressure ventilation in patients with advanced cystic fibrosis. Chest 1998; 113:1013–8.

243. Granton JT, Shapiro C, Kesten S. Noninvasive nocturnal ventilatory support in advanced lung disease from cystic fibrosis. Respir Care 2002; 47:675–81.

244. Madden BP, Kariyawasam H, Siddiqi AJ, et al. Noninvasive ventilation in cystic fibrosis patients with acute or chronic respiratory failure. Eur Respir J 2002; 19:310–3.

245. Fauroux B, Itti E, Pigeot J, et al. Optimization of aerosol deposition by pressure support in children with cystic fibrosis: An experimental and clinical study. Am J Respir Crit Care Med 2000; 162:2265–71.

246. Benhamou D, Muri JF, Raspaud C, et al. Long-term efficiency of home nasal mask ventilation in patients with diffuse bronchiectasis and severe chronic respiratory failure. Chest 1997; 112:1259–66.

247. Dupont M, Gacouin A, Lena H, et al. Survival of patients with bronchiectasis after the first ICU stay for respiratory failure. Chest 2004; 125:1815–20.

248. Lloyd-Owen SJ, Donaldson GC, Ambrosino N, et al. Patterns of home mechanical ventilation use in Europe: Results from the Eurovent survey. Eur Respir J 2005; 25:1025–31.

249. Granton JT, Naughton MT, Benard DC, et al. CPAP improves inspiratory muscle strength in patients with heart failure and central sleep apnea. Am J Respir Crit Care Med 1996; 153:277–82.

250. Kaneko Y, Floras JS, Usui K, et al. Cardiovascular effects of continuous positive airway pressure in patients with heart failure and obstructive sleep apnea. New Engl J Med 2003; 348:1233–41.

251. Willson GN, Wilcox I, Piper AJ, et al. Noninvasive pressure preset ventilation for the treatment of Cheyne-Stokes respiration during sleep. Eur Respir J 2001; 17:1250–7.

252. Kohnlein T, Welte T, Tan LB, Elliott MW. Assisted ventilation for heart failure patients with Cheyne-Stokes respiration. Eur Respir J 2002; 20:934–41.

253. Teschler H, Dohring J, Wang YM, Berthon-Jones M. Adaptive pressure support servo-ventilation: A novel treatment for Cheyne-Stokes respiration in heart failure. Am J Respir Crit Care Med 2001; 164:614–9.

254. Cleland JG, Coletta AP, Freemantle N, et al. Clinical trials update from the American College of Cardiology meeting: CARE-HF and the Remission of Heart Failure, Women's Health Study, TNT, COMPASS-HF, VERITAS, CANPAP, PEECH and PREMIER. Eur J Heart Failure 2005; 7:931–6.

255. Fauroux B, Boffa C, Desguerre I, et al. Long-term noninvasive mechanical ventilation for children at home: A national survey. Pediatr Pulmonol 2003; 35:119–25.

256. Fauroux B, Lavis JF, Nicot F, et al. Facial side effects during noninvasive positive pressure ventilation in children. Intensive Care Med 2005; 31:965–9.

257. Mellies U, Ragette R, Dohna Schwake C, et al. Long-term noninvasive ventilation in children and adolescents with neuromuscular disorders. Eur Respir J 2003; 22:631–6.

258. Wood KA, Lewis L, Von Harz B, Kollef MH. The use of noninvasive positive pressure ventilation in the emergency department. Chest 1998; 113:1339–46.

259. Maheshwari V, Piaoli D, Hill NS. Survey of the use of noninvasive ventilation in acute care hospitals of Massachusetts and Rhode Island. Chest (in press).

260. Schonhofer B, Sortor-Leger S. Equipment needs for noninvasive mechanical ventilation. Eur Respir J 2002; 20:1029–36.

261. Criner GJ, Travaline JM, Brennan KJ, Kreimer DT. Efficacy of a new full face mask for noninvasive positive pressure ventilation. Chest. 1994; 106:1109–15.

262. Tonnelier JM, Prat G, Nowak E, et al. Noninvasive continuous positive airway pressure ventilation using a new helmet interface: A case prospective pilot study. Intensive Care Med 2003; 29:2077–80.

263. Principi T, Pantanetti S, Catani F, et al. Noninvasive continuous positive airway pressure delivered by helmet in hematological malignancy patients with hypoxemic acute respiratory failure. Intensive Care Med 2004; 30:147–50.

264. Antonelli M, Pennisi MA, Pelosi P, et al. Noninvasive positive pressure ventilation using a helmet in patients with acute exacerbation of chronic obstructive pulmonary disease. Anesthesiology 2004; 100:16–24.

265. Taccone P, Hess D, Caironi P, Bigatello LM. Continuous positive airway pressure delivered with a "helmet": Effects on carbon dioxide rebreathing. Crit Care Med 2004; 32:2090–6.

266. Cavaliere F, Conti G, Costa R, et al. Noise exposure during noninvasive ventilation with a helmet, a nasal mask, and a facial mask. Intensive Care Med 2004; 30:1755–60.

267. Kwok H, McCormack J, Cece R, et al. Controlled trial of oronasal versus nasal mask ventilation in the treatment of acute respiratory failure. Crit Care Med 2003; 31:468–73.

268. Liesching TN, Cromier K, Nelson D, et al. Total face mask TM vs standard full face mask for noninvasive therapy of acute respiratory failure. Am J Respir Crit Care Med 2003; 167:A996.

269. Schettino GPP, Chatmongkolchart S, Hess D, Kacmarek RM. Position of exhalation port and mask design affect CO_2 rebreathing during noninvasive positive pressure ventilation. Crit Care Med 2003; 31:2178–82.

270. Saatci E, Miller DM, Sztell IM, et al. Dynamic dead space in face masks used with noninvasive ventilators: A lung model study. Eur Respir J 2004; 23:129–35.

271. Patrick W, Webster K, Ludwig L, et al. Noninvasive positive-pressure ventilation in acute respiratory distress without prior chronic respiratory failure. Am J Respir Crit Care Med 1996; 153:1005–11.

272. Navalesi P, Fanfulla F, Frigerio P, et al. Physiologic evaluation of noninvasive mechanical ventilation delivered by three types of masks in patients with chronic hypercapnic respiratory failure. Crit Care Med 2000, 28:1785–90.

273. Willson GN, Piper AJ, Norman M, et al. Nasal versus full face mask for noninvasive ventilation in chronic respiratory failure. Eur Respir J 2004; 23:605–9.

274. Mehta S, McCool FD, Hill NS. Leak compensation in positive pressure ventilators: A lung model study. Eur Respir J 2001;17:259–67.

275. Bunburaphong T, Imanaka H, Nishimura M, et al. Performance characteristics of bilevel pressure ventilators: A lung model study. Chest 1997;111:1050–60.

276. Ferguson GT, Gilmartin M: CO_2 rebreathing during BiPAP ventilatory assistance. Am J Respir Crit Care Med 1995; 151:1126–35.

277. Lofaso F, Brochard L, Touchard D, et al. Evaluation of carbon dioxide rebreathing during pressure support ventilation with BiPAP devices. Chest 1995; 108:772–8.

278. Patel RG, Petrini MF. Respiratory muscle performance, pulmonary mechanics, and gas exchange between the BiPAP S/T-D system and Servo Ventilator 900C with bilevel positive airway pressure ventilation following gradual pressure support weaning. Chest 1998; 114:1390–6.

279. Schoenhofer B, Sonneborn M, Haide P, et al. Comparison of two different modes for noninvasive mechanical ventilation in chronic respiratory failure: Volume versus pressure controlled device. Eur Respir J 1997; 10:184–91.

280. Restrick LJ, Fox NC, Braid G, et al. Comparison of nasal pressure support ventilation with nasal intermittent positive pressure ventilation in patients with nocturnal hypoventilation. Eur Respir J 1993; 6:365–70.

281. Vitacca M, Rubini F, Foglio K, et al. Noninvasive modalities of positive pressure ventilation improved the outcome of acute exacerbations in COLD patients. Intensive Care Med 1993; 19:450–5.

282. Girault C, Richard J-C, Chevron V, et al. Comparative physiologic effects of noninvasive assist-control and pressure support ventilation in acute hypercapnic respiratory failure. Chest 1997; 111:1639–48.

283. Kacmarek R, Hill NS. Ventilators for noninvasive positive pressure ventilation: Technical aspects. In: Muir JR, Simonds A, Ambrosino N, editors. Noninvasive mechanical ventilation. European Respiratory Monograph Series. Sheffield, UK: European Respiratory Society, 2001.

284. Younes M. Proportional assist ventilation, a new approach to ventilatory support. Am Rev Respir Dis 1992; 145:114–20.

285. Gay P, Hess D, Hollets S, et al. A randomized, prospective trial of noninvasive proportional assist ventilation (PAV) to treat acute respiratory insufficiency (ARI). Am J Respir Crit Care Med 1999; A14:159.

286. Fernandez-Vivas M, Caturia-Such J, de la Rosa JG, et al. Noninvasive pressure support versus proportional assist ventilation in acute respiratory failure. Intensive Care Med 2003; 29:1126–33.

287. Smith IE, Shneerson JM. Secondary failure of nasal intermittent positive pressure ventilation using the Monnal D: Effects of changing ventilator. Thorax 1997; 52:89–91.

288. Prinianakis G, Delmastro M, Carlucci A, et al. Effect of varying the pressurization rate during noninvasive pressure support ventilation. Eur Respir J 2004; 23:314–20.

289. Leger P, Jennequin J, Gerard M, et al: Home positive pressure ventilation via nasal mask for patients with neuromuscular weakness or restrictive lung or chest wall deformities. Respir Care 1989; 34:73–7.

290. Parreira VF, Jounieaux V, Delguste P, et al. Determinants of effective ventilation during nasal intermittent positive pressure ventilation. Eur Respir J 1997; 10:1975–82.

291. Schwartz AR, Kacmarek RM, Hess DR. Factors affecting oxygen delivery with bilevel positive airway pressure. Respir Care 2004; 49:270–5.

292. Lellouche F, Maggiore SM, Deye N, et al. Effect of the humidification device on the work of breathing during noninvasive ventilation. Intensive Care Med 2002; 28:1582–9.

293. Barach AL, Beck GJ. Exsufflation with negative pressure: Physiologic and clinical studies in poliomyelitis bronchial asthma, pulmonary emphysema and bronchiectasis. Arch Intern Med 1954; 93:825–41.

294. Leith DE. Cough. In: Brain JD, Proctor D, Reid L, editors. Lung biology in health and disease: Respiratory defense mechanisms, Part 2. New York: Marcel Dekker, 1977: 545–92.

295. Bach JR. Mechanical insufflation-exsufflation: Comparison of peak expiratory flows with manually assisted and unassisted coughing techniques. Chest 1993; 104:1553–64.

296. Bach JR, Alba AS, Bodofsky E, et al. Glossopharyngeal breathing and noninvasive aids in the management of post-polio respiratory insufficiency. Birth Defects 1987; 23:99–113.

297. Sivasothy P, Brown L, Smith IE, Shneerson JM. Effect of manually assisted cough and mechanical insufflation on cough flow of normal subjects, patients with chronic obstructive pulmonary disease (COPD), and patients with respiratory muscle weakness. Thorax 2001; 56:438–44.

298. Winck JC, Goncalves MR, Lourenco C, et al. Effects of mechanical insufflation-exsufflation on respiratory parameters for patients with chronic airway secretion encumbrance. Chest 2004; 126:774–80.

299. Vianello A, Corrado A, Arcaro G, et al. Mechanical insufflation-exsufflation improves outcomes for neuromuscular disease patients with respiratory tract infections. Am J Phys Med Rehabil 2005; 84:83–8

300. Miske LJ, Hickey EM, Kolb SM, et al. Use of the mechanical in-exsufflator in pediatric patients with neuromuscular disease and impaired cough. Chest 2004; 125:1406–12.

301. Sancho J, Servera E, Diaz J, Marin J. Efficacy of mechanical insufflation-exsufflation in medically stable patients with amyotrophic lateral sclerosis. Chest 2004; 125:1400–5.

302. Bach JR, Ishikawa Y, Kim H. Prevention of pulmonary morbidity for patients with Duchenne muscular dystrophy. Chest 1997; 112:1024–8.

303. Chevrolet JC, Jolliet P, Abajo B, et al. Nasal positive pressure ventilation in patients with acute respiratory failure: Difficult and time-consuming procedure for nurses. Chest 1991; 100: 445–54.

304. Nava S, Evangelisti I, Rampulla C, et al. Human and financial costs of noninvasive mechanical ventilation in patients affected by COPD and acute respiratory failure. Chest 1997; 111: 1631–8.

305. Carlucci A, Delmastro M, Rubini F, et al. Changes in the practice of non-invasive ventilation in treating COPD patients over 8 years. Intensive Care Med 2003; 29:419–25.

306. Sinuff T, Cook DJ, Randall J, Allen CJ. Evaluation of a practice guideline for noninvasive positive pressure ventilation for acute respiratory failure. Chest 2003; 123:2062–73.

307. Meduri GU, Abou-Shala N, Fox RC, et al: Noninvasive face mask mechanical ventilation in patients with acute hypercapnic respiratory failure. Chest 1991; 100:445–54.

308. Prause G, Hetz H, Lauda P, et al. A comparison of the end-tidal CO_2 documented by capnometry and the arterial pCO_2 in emergency patients. Resuscitation 1997; 35:145–8.

309. Hilbert G, Gruson D, Gbikpi-Benissan G, Cardinaud JP. Sequential use of noninvasive pressure support ventilation for acute exacerbations of COPD. Intensive Care Med 1997; 23: 955–61.

310. Gregoretti C, Confalonieri M, Navalesi P, et al. Evaluation of patient skin breakdown and comfort with a new face mask for non-invasive ventilation: A multi-center study. Intensive Care Med 2002; 28:278–84.

311. Hill NS. Complications of noninvasive positive pressure ventilation. Respir Care 1997; 42:432–42.

PART VII
UNCONVENTIONAL METHODS OF VENTILATOR SUPPORT

Chapter 20

HIGH-FREQUENCY VENTILATION

ALISON B FROESE

High-frequency ventilation (HFV) has been an unconventional option for over 30 years. Several varieties of high-frequency ventilators have come and gone over that period. Currently, interest in HFV in adult critical care is part of a larger search for ventilator patterns that can support gas exchange in the severely hypoxemic patient without contributing additional ventilator-induced lung injury (VILI).

Over the past 25 years, high-frequency ventilators provided an experimental tool that identified many of the mechanisms that contribute to VILI. It became clear that VILI is minimized by ventilator patterns that achieve homogeneous aeration of as much of the lung as possible, avoiding both injury from overdistension (volutrauma) and that arising from the repetitive opening and closing of lung units in regions of ongoing atelectasis (atelectrauma)[1] (Fig. 20-1). Failure to operate in the "safe zone" initiates biotrauma.[2,3]

The concept of a "safe zone" within which to ventilate the atelectasis-prone lung has been reflected in numerous clinical trials of lung-protective ventilation over the last 10 years. Conventional ventilator protocols have found survival benefit from shrinking the tidal volume and minimizing peak or plateau distending pressures.[4] Studies such as that of Roupie et al[5] suggest that very small tidal volumes may be needed in some patients to avoid overdistension. Very high positive end-expiratory pressure (PEEP) levels would be needed in some patients to avoid derecruitment.[6] Concurrently, HFV—both in oscillatory and jet forms—has become an established lung-protective modality in neonatal and pediatric intensive care[7–11] (see Chapter 25). The question now arises: In severe acute respiratory distress syndrome (ARDS) in adult patients, will use of a high-frequency device result in clinically important outcome differences compared with lung-protective conventional ventilation?

Historical Overview

Several existing reviews detail the history of HFV.[12,13] Early developments often were driven by issues peripheral to pulmonary critical care. Sjöstrand et al[14] wanted to eliminate respiration-related variations in vascular pressures so that they could investigate carotid sinus reflexes and developed high-frequency positive-pressure ventilation (HFPPV). Lunkenheimer et al[15] wanted to use the lungs as a route to deliver oscillatory pressure pulses to the myocardium. They needed apnea for this and were amazed to find gas exchange occurring while they applied their high-frequency flow oscillations. Emerson[16] thought that high-frequency flow oscillations might provide internal physiotherapy and help to mobilize secretions. In Toronto, Bryan[17] initially was curious to see whether an external "shaker" could enhance the gas mixing produced by cardiogenic oscillations. Klain and Smith[18] explored jet ventilation at increasing frequencies to solve the problem of achieving alveolar ventilation in respiratory systems with a big leak, such as a bronchopleural fistula.

These devices often became intriguing phenomena in search of a reason for being. Devices such as HFPPV and high-frequency jet ventilation (HFJV) were particularly useful for surgical procedures when both anesthesiologist and surgeon needed access to the airway. The notion, however, that high rates and small tidal volumes might be of broader therapeutic value needed a pathophysiologic rationale. An emerging concept in the 1970s was that many of the pulmonary perturbations that put patients into intensive-care units (ICUs) were problems of low lung volume. Low lung

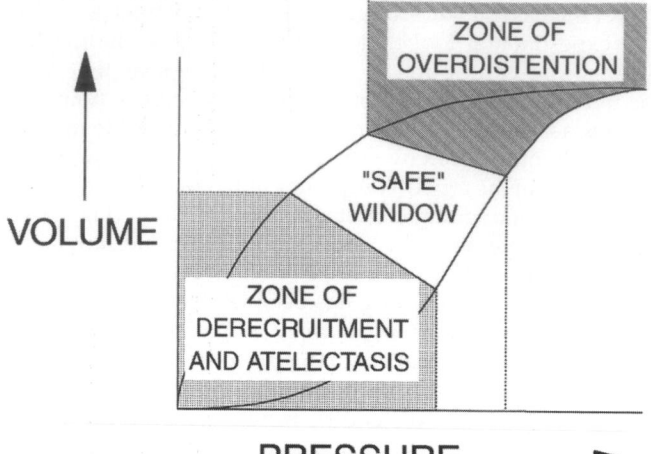

FIGURE 20-1 Pressure-volume curve of a moderately diseased lung, as in a patient with acute lung injury. Ventilator-induced lung injury (VILI) occurs at both extremes of lung volume. In the *zone of overdistension,* damage arises from edema fluid accumulation, surfactant degradation, and mechanical disruption. In the *zone of derecruitment and atelectasis,* lung injury arises from the direct trauma of repeated closure and re-expansion of small airways and alveoli, through accumulation and activation of inflammatory cells with release of cytokines (biotrauma), through interactions with local hypoxemia, by inhibition of surfactant, and through compensatory overexpansion of the rest of the lung as the lung "shrinks." High end-expiratory pressures plus small tidal volume cycles are needed to stay in the *safe window.* (*Reproduced, with permission, from Froese: Crit Care Med 25:906–8, 1997.*)

volumes were associated with poor lung compliance, increasing airway and vascular resistances, increased work of breathing, airway closure, low ventilation-perfusion ($\dot{V}_A/\dot{Q}$) ratios, atelectasis, hypoxemia, and high oxygen (O_2) exposure. Neonatal outcome was improving simply from the introduction of continuous positive airway pressure

(CPAP) to improve alveolar aeration.[19] A crucial insight occurred early in our experience with high-frequency oscillatory ventilation (HFOV) when we explored a variety of mean airway pressure settings while ventilating an infant with neonatal respiratory distress syndrome[20] (Fig. 20-2). The infant was stable in terms of both hemodynamics and carbon dioxide (CO_2) elimination over the whole range of mean pressures tested, but oxygenation varied markedly. One could either ventilate with a low mean airway pressure and high fractional inspired oxygen concentration (F_{IO_2}) or a higher mean pressure and low F_{IO_2}. A choice had to be made. We gave priority to the reversal of low lung volumes. We argued that the small-volume cycles of HFOV should allow one to optimize alveolar aeration by using higher mean pressures than were considered safe during conventional mechanical ventilation (CMV) while still keeping peak pressures less than those needed to eliminate CO_2 at conventional rates. This pathophysiologic rationale continues to guide high-frequency applications to this day.

Many devices invented along the way, such as HFPPV, have since disappeared from use. HFJV was explored in many adult ICUs in the 1980s for difficult cases of bronchopleural fistula or tracheal disruption.[21] It gradually became clear that any oxygenation benefits occurring during HFJV resulted from increases in mean lung volume, not from some unusual properties of gas distribution.[22] With an HFJV device, the end-expiratory lung volume is a complex product of jet diameter and placement, driving pressure, jet frequency, and the time available for expiration.[23,24] Safe use requires accurate intrapulmonary pressure monitoring, which was rarely provided with early devices. Inadvertent hyperinflation could cause problems with both circulatory depression and/or barotrauma. No North American commercial adult-sized jet ventilator was ever marketed with a safe, effective humidification system such as that available in Europe. The largest early comparative trial of HFJV versus CMV in hypoxemic lung disease was performed before the importance of atelectasis reversal was established.

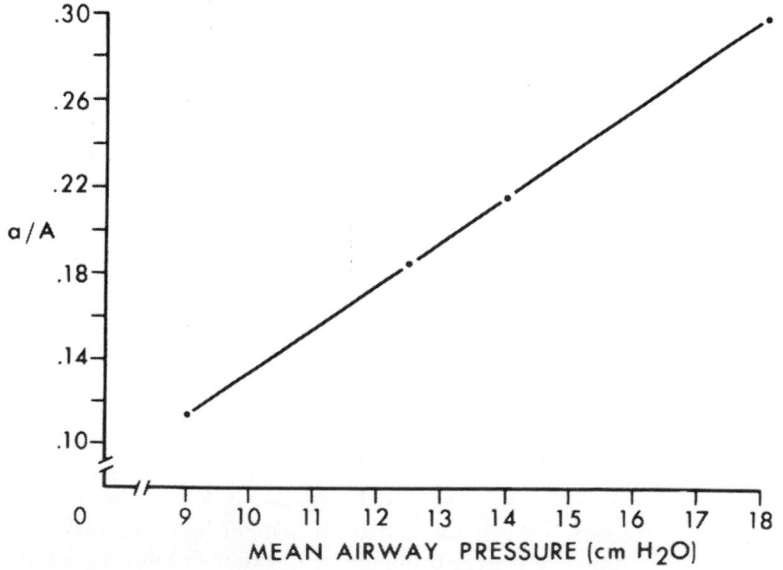

FIGURE 20-2 Relationship of oxygenation, as reflected in the arterial-alveolar P_{O_2} (a–A) ratio, to the mean airway pressure applied during HFOV, at constant tidal volume and frequency, in an infant with respiratory distress syndrome. No circulatory instability occurred over the entire range of mean pressures. CO_2 elimination could be achieved equally well using a high F_{IO_2} and a low mPaw or a low F_{IO_2} and a higher mPaw. A choice of operating conditions had to be made. (*Reproduced, with permission, from Marchak et al: J Pediatr 99:287–92, 1981.*)

It therefore was carried out with the goal of supporting gas exchange with the lowest possible peak and mean pressures and proved of no benefit.[25] For all these reasons, HFJV in adults has become a rare event. Jet ventilation at high or low frequencies continues to be a useful approach to situations in which airway access must be shared during surgical procedures[26] or alveolar ventilation needs to be maintained in the presence of severe bronchopleural fistulas.[23]

HFJV has persisted in neonatal and pediatric critical care largely because of the continuous design refinements of the Bunnell Life Pulse device.[27] Early problems with poor humidification causing desiccation of tracheal mucosa were corrected, appropriate pressure-monitoring systems were devised, and expert training and technical support were provided.

A hybrid device combining HFV and conventional pressure-cycled ventilation [e.g., the high-frequency percussive ventilation/volume diffusive respirator (HFPV/VDR; Percussionaire 4, Bird Technologies, Sandpoint ID)] is used in many burn units. It has been reviewed recently.[28] Currently, the main high-frequency ventilatory options in the critical care of adults or larger children are HFOV or the HFPV/VDR Percussionaire. In neonatology and small infants, high-frequency oscillatory ventilators, high-frequency jet ventilators, and the high-frequency percussive ventilator remain available. In view of its increasing role in adult intensive care, this chapter will focus on HFOV.

Basic Principles of HFOV

HFOV achieves gas transport with stroke volumes approximating anatomic dead space. Quasi-sinusoidal flow oscillations applied at the airway opening induce rapid gas mixing within the lungs. A number of physical transport mechanisms contribute to this mixing process. They have been reviewed in detail elsewhere.[29] In practical terms, HFOV can be viewed as a mixing device that rapidly blends high-O_2/low-CO_2 gas from the top of the endotracheal tube with gas in the alveoli (Fig. 20-3). Net transport occurs along the partial-pressure gradients for O_2 and CO_2, with CO_2 moving out of the lung along its partial-pressure gradient and O_2 moving inward to the alveolar-capillary interface. These flow oscillations cause symmetric oscillations of intrapulmonary pressure around a mean distending airway pressure (mPaw) (Fig. 20-4). Although subambient pressures can occur in the circuit, intrapulmonary air trapping or "choke points" are unlikely with appropriate mPaw settings.[30,31] One can view HFOV as a means of delivering "CPAP" with built-in CO_2 elimination. In contrast to current conventional approaches to supplying CPAP with assisted CO_2 elimination, the mean distending pressure during HFOV is midway between the minimal and maximum values, introducing less risk of derecuitment during the expiratory phase for any given peak distending volume/pressure.[32] One attraction of HFOV in neonatal and pediatric use has been the way in which it uncouples the regulation of oxygenation and CO_2 elimination into two

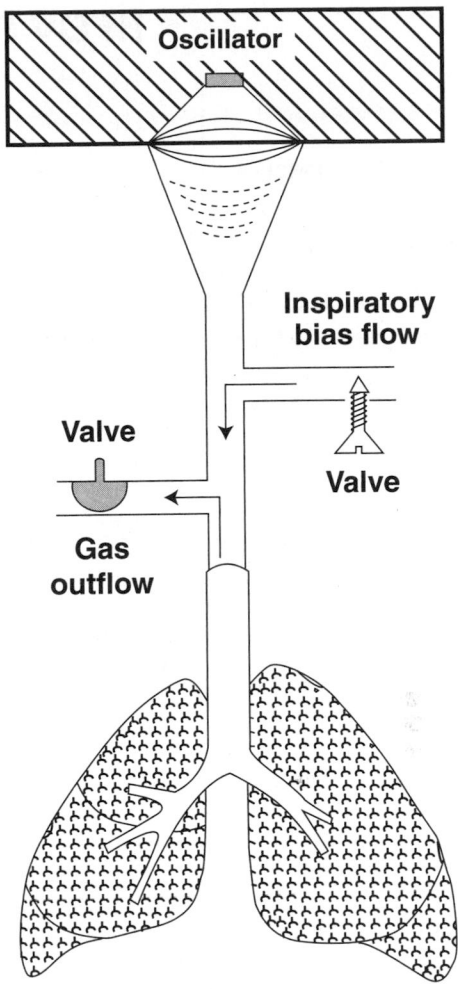

FIGURE 20-3   Schematic of a circuit for delivery of HFOV. Quasi-sinusoidal flow oscillations are generated by a diaphragm or piston pump and directed to the endotracheal tube. A bias flow of humidified gas flushes the CO_2 that is transported out of the lungs out of the circuit. Mean airway pressure is regulated by adjustments of the bias flow and the resistance of the expiratory limb. (*Reproduced, with permission, from Krishnan et al: Chest 118:795–807, 2000.*)

separate control systems, unlike the situation with conventional ventilators, where it is often difficult to adjust one (i.e., the CO_2 level) without also affecting the other. Oxygenation is regulated by reversing atelectasis and then finding the mean distending pressure that maintains alveolar expansion. The F_{IO_2} then is set at a level that maintains appropriate arterial oxygenation goals. CO_2 elimination is relatively independent of mean airway pressure,[33] being regulated by frequency and stroke volume (i.e., power or ΔP) adjustments.[34,35]

OXYGENATION

ACHIEVING ALVEOLAR AERATION
Although lung-volume optimization has become an accepted goal of HFOV, the "best way" to achieve this optimization remains controversial (Fig. 20-5).

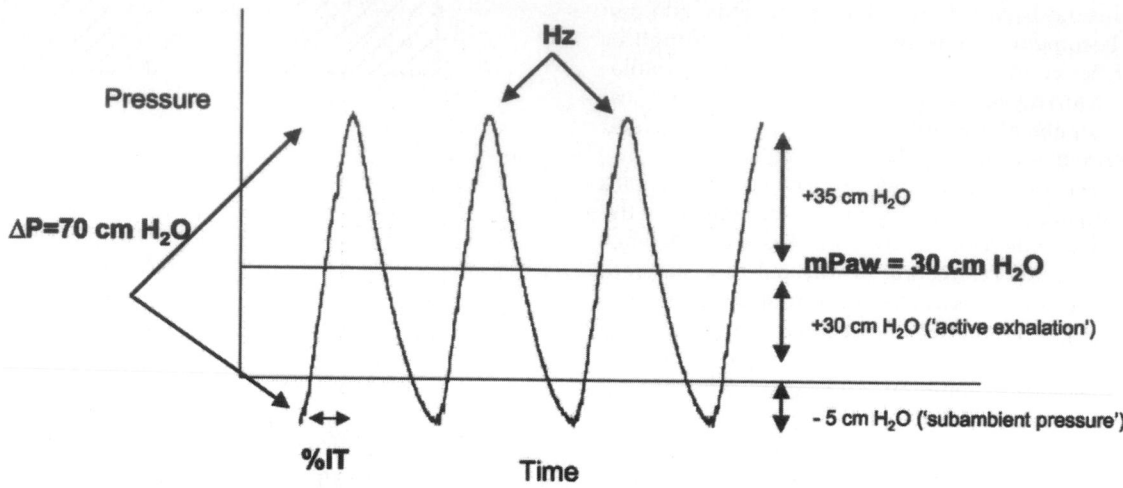

HFOV Pressure Waveform

FIGURE 20-4 Waveform of high-frequency pressure oscillations in the circuit above the endotracheal tube. Both inspiratory and expiratory flows are actively driven by the oscillator diaphragm. Pressure cycles equally above and below the mean level. When the oscillatory pressure amplitude (ΔP) is more than twice the mean airway pressure (mPaw), subambient pressures may occur in the circuit without inducing air trapping or choke points in the lung.[30] The endotracheal tube filters the pressure swings, decreasing ΔP in the trachea and alveoli. Filtering is greater with smaller endotracheal tubes[63,79] and higher frequencies (D Hager, personal communication). (*Reproduced, with permission, from Derdak: Crit Care Med 31:S317–23, 2003*).

Ventilating on the "Deflation Limb"

All initial animal studies and one early human trial used a brief recruitment maneuver to near-total lung capacity, followed by reduction of mPaw to a maintenance level that prevented derecruitment.[36–40] This is termed getting the lung *onto the deflation limb* of its pressure-volume (P-V) relationship.[41] Recent investigations in both animal models and humans reinforce the value of ventilating on the deflation limb.[42–49] After a recruitment maneuver, oxygenation goals are achieved at substantially lower maintenance mPaw values (near the point of maximum curvature),[43,46,47] alveolar expansion becomes more homogeneous (which

FIGURE 20-5 Schematic representation of two approaches to alveolar re-expansion during HFOV. The horizontal dashed line indicates the desired maintenance mean lung volume. The solid line is the pressure-volume (P-V) relationship of a moderately diseased lung that still exhibits hysteresis. The dashed line indicates the P-V relationship after some recovery has occurred. A. A brief sustained increase in mean airway pressure (mPaw) from *a* to *b* inflates the lung to near total lung capacity (TLC), putting it on the deflation limb of its P-V curve. After this discrete recruitment maneuver, the target volume *c* is maintained at an mPaw of 11 cmH$_2$O. If the P-V relationship happens to change (as with position, diuresis, etc), the operational lung volume remains constant. This is the approach used in the recent TOOLS Trial.[49] *B*. A gradual march up the inflation limb of the P-V relationship. Progressive increases in mPaw are used to achieve the target lung volume. An mPaw of 19 cmH$_2$O is now needed to maintain lung volume at *c*. Also, if the P-V relationship of the respiratory system changes, overdistension of the lung could occur (i.e., movement from point 5 to point 6). This is the approach used in the majority of neonatal and adult trials of HFOV to date. When actual lung volumes are measured, settings felt to have optimized lung volume clinically by these stepwise increases in mPaw often prove to be inadequate.[55] (*Reproduced, by permission of Routledge/Taylor & Francis Group, LLC*).

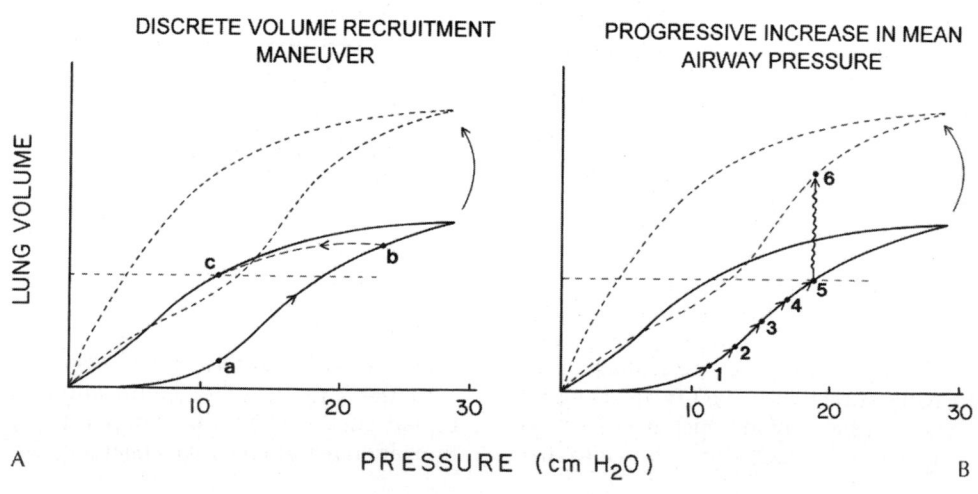

should reduce shear forces during ventilation),[45,50] and the percentage transmission of HFOV pressure cycles into the lung is decreased relative to settings producing equal shunt reduction on the inflation limb.[44]

Ventilating on the "Inflation Limb"

Following the HIFI Trial of the late 1980s,[51] fear of intraventricular hemorrhage in the fragile brain of the premature patient led most neonatologists to pursue stepwise increases in mPaw until either x-ray and blood-gas evidence of lung reexpansion was achieved or the mPaw level reached whatever level was deemed the "maximum allowable" level for a given institution.[52] Physiologically, this can be described as "marching up the inflation limb" of the P-V curve, as in Fig. 20-5B. Most post-HIFI Trial neonatal/pediatric trials (including the largest recent randomized, controlled trials in 2002[53,54]) used stepwise increases in mPaw to "optimize" lung volume to oxygenation and chest x-ray targets. Unfortunately, when the actual lung volumes achieved by such clinical protocols are measured, many lungs prove to be suboptimally expanded.[55] All early adult trials of HFOV started at mPaw levels of 3–5 cmH$_2$O above the mPaw on conventional ventilation and then increased mPaw incrementally—again marching up the inflation limb.[56–60]

A few human trials have used protocols that rapidly place the lung "on the deflation limb" of its P-V relationship.[48,49] Although large comparative trials of the relative safety of these different recruitment protocols are not available, no evidence of risk from either barotrauma or IVH has emerged using any of the neonatal/pediatric approaches since optimization of lung volume became an accepted goal of HFOV.[7,8] What we do know is that lung-volume optimization is essential for HFOV to be protective of the lung. The small volume cycles of HFOV simply are not powerful enough to reopen atelectatic alveoli without some type of recruitment measure.

Atelectrauma: The Costs of Inadequate Recruitment

Ongoing atelectasis strongly affects the phasic pressures exerted on intrapulmonary structures.[61–63] Sakai et al[64] measured "swing pressures" (i.e., peak-to-trough ΔP) at intratracheal, bronchial, and pleural sites in rabbits with normal and lavaged lungs. ΔP values at intratracheal and bronchial sites were much higher in lavaged lung than in normal lung at low levels of mPaw. These pressure swings reduced rapidly to normal values following lung recruitment. The authors postulated that failure to reverse atelectasis during HFOV would expose airways and alveoli unnecessarily to potentially damaging shear forces. Similar messages come from the data of van Genderingen et al,[44] who analyzed intrapulmonary pressure transmission in terms of the ratio of intratracheal and proximal airway ΔP values, termed the *oscillatory pressure ratio*. Pressure transmission into the lung increased sharply at low lung volume. In vivo, adequate alveolar re-expansion optimized oxygenation while also minimizing intrapulmonary pressure swings. For a given level of shunt reduction, both the oscillatory pressure ratio and the mPaw were substantially lower after a recruitment maneuver (Fig. 20-6).

Inadequate alveolar recruitment also may trigger inappropriate increases in ΔP or decreases in frequency because of hypercapnia, when what was really needed was alveolar re-expansion. All high-frequency oscillators currently available are load-dependent and deliver less tidal volume at any given setting when the lung is stiffer, as with ongoing atelectasis.[65,66] If one's goal is to explore HFOV for the potential lung-protective effects of maintaining O$_2$ and CO$_2$ transport at the smallest possible intrapulmonary pressure and volume swings, then lung-volume optimization is essential.

Volutrauma: The Cost of Excessive Recruitment

It costs less to pursue lung recruitment vigorously than to accept ongoing atelectasis.[67] All clinical trials done to date—from neonate to adult—that have mandated lung-volume optimization have reported similar or decreased incidences of barotrauma, a transient need for inotropic support, and a decreased need for nitric oxide to reduce pulmonary vascular resistance despite using mean pressures in the thirties or forties when necessary to achieve oxygenation.[10,56,57,68–70] Recent computed tomographic (CT) studies during HFOV in eight adult patients with ARDS documented substantial (~800 ml) increases in normally aerated volume with only a minor increase in hyperinflated lung (<50 ml).[71] Overdistension certainly can occur, particularly as the lung normalizes during treatment. Avoidance of this requires awareness and periodic reassessment of lung expansion. Some algorithms warn against using mean distending pressures on HFOV higher than the plateau pressure limit of 30 cmH$_2$O currently advocated for conventional ventilation. This warning may produce inadequate volume optimization. It fails to take into account that the risk of a given "maximum pressure" will vary with the size of the lung and the size and rate of delivery of the tidal volume engendering that plateau pressure. If 60% or 70% of the lung is not participating in gas exchange, then a tidal volume of even 6 ml/kg may induce dangerous overdistension of the ventilated alveolar units, as well as exerting shear forces on any alveolar units re-expanded during the course of the breath. If, instead, 70% or 80% of the lung is kept expanded throughout the ventilatory cycle, then a mean distending pressure of 30 cmH$_2$O or more is safe, as proven in numerous clinical trials of HFOV,[56–58,68] presumably because that distending pressure is now accommodated within many more participating lung units, fewer units are sheared open during the course of a cycle,[32] and volume swings of only 1.5–2 ml/kg at high rates minimize peak distension. Conversely, if one fails to open the lung during HFOV and then keep it open, one will expose the lung to unwanted shear forces many more times per minute, particularly if forced to use lower rates and larger volume cycles because of inadequate recruitment.

MAINTENANCE MEAN AIRWAY PRESSURE (mPaw)

Numerous studies have tried to predict an optimal maintenance mPaw from some feature of the static P-V curve of the respiratory system, such as the inflection point on the inflation limb.[46] These studies demonstrate a general

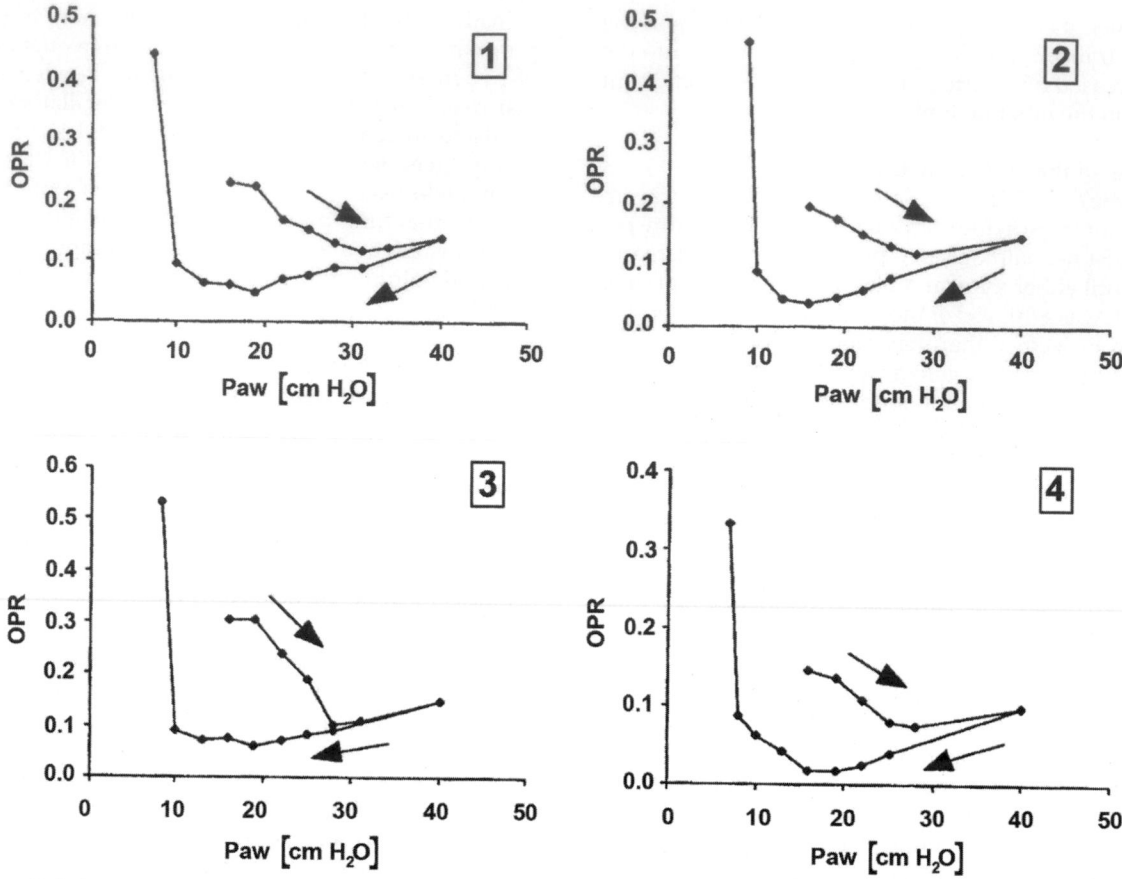

FIGURE 20-6 Relationship of the oscillatory pressure ratio (OPR) to the mean airway pressure (Paw) during HFOV in pigs with lung injury induced by saline lavage. Data are shown for four animals. Arrows show the order of Paw application starting from the baseline mean Paw value. The OPR is the ratio of ΔP in the trachea to the ΔP (i.e., the pressure amplitude) at the top of the endotracheal tube. Intrapulmonary oscillatory pressure swings are strongly influenced by the degree of alveolar re-expansion and are substantially smaller when the lung is operating on its deflation limb. (*Reprinted with permission of Wiley–Liss, Inc., a subsidiary of John Wiley & Sons, Inc.*)

property of the respiratory system, namely, that the mPaw needed to maintain a given level of oxygenation is substantially less after the lung has been inflated briefly to a pressure of 30–40 cmH₂O so that it is "operating on the deflation limb."[44] Because recruitment/derecruitment pressures vary markedly between lung regions[45,72] and between lung-injury models, however, generalizations to human ventilator management must be made cautiously. In clinical practice, a gradual deterioration in oxygenation over time that corrects with a recruitment maneuver indicates that the mPaw needs to be increased 2–3 cmH₂O to keep alveoli/airways above their closing pressures. Bedside regional lung-volume monitoring techniques have the potential to clarify mPaw adjustments.[43,73,74]

CO₂ ELIMINATION

The basic transport studies of the 1980s were executed with accurate measurements of delivered stroke volumes over a wide range of frequencies using sinusoidal flow oscillations.[35,75,76] They established that the volume of CO_2 eliminated per minute ($\dot{V}_{CO_2}$) was proportional to the product of oscillatory frequency and the approximate square of the stroke volume ($\dot{V}_{CO_2} = V_T{}^{\sim 2} \cdot f$). The endotracheal tube contributes a substantial impedance to gas transport during HFOV.[77] If one uses an uncuffed endotracheal tube such that the fresh-gas front moves to the bottom of the tube and CO_2 exits around rather than through the tube, the stroke volume needed to achieve normocapnia decreases by up to 50% (Fig. 20-7). The bias gas-flow rate also influences transport efficiency through its effect on gas tensions at the fresh-gas front.[78] Uncuffed tubes are used routinely in neonates and infants. Cuff leaks substantially assist CO_2 elimination in adults as well[34,59] and reduce intrapulmonary pressure swings.[79]

FREQUENCY SELECTION

Early HFOV trials used a frequency of 15 Hz and an inspiration-expiration (I:E) ratio of 1:1. Demonstration of small inter-regional mean pressure gradients at 15 Hz and 50% inspiratory period (T_I)[80] subsequently induced a shift to a lower operating frequency of 10 Hz and a 33% T_I in many centers. It is worth noting that although pressure gradients definitely occur in the lung during HFOV, their magnitude is small (i.e., on the order of 1–3 cmH₂O from apex to base).[81] With a 33% inspiratory period, the mPaw displayed on the

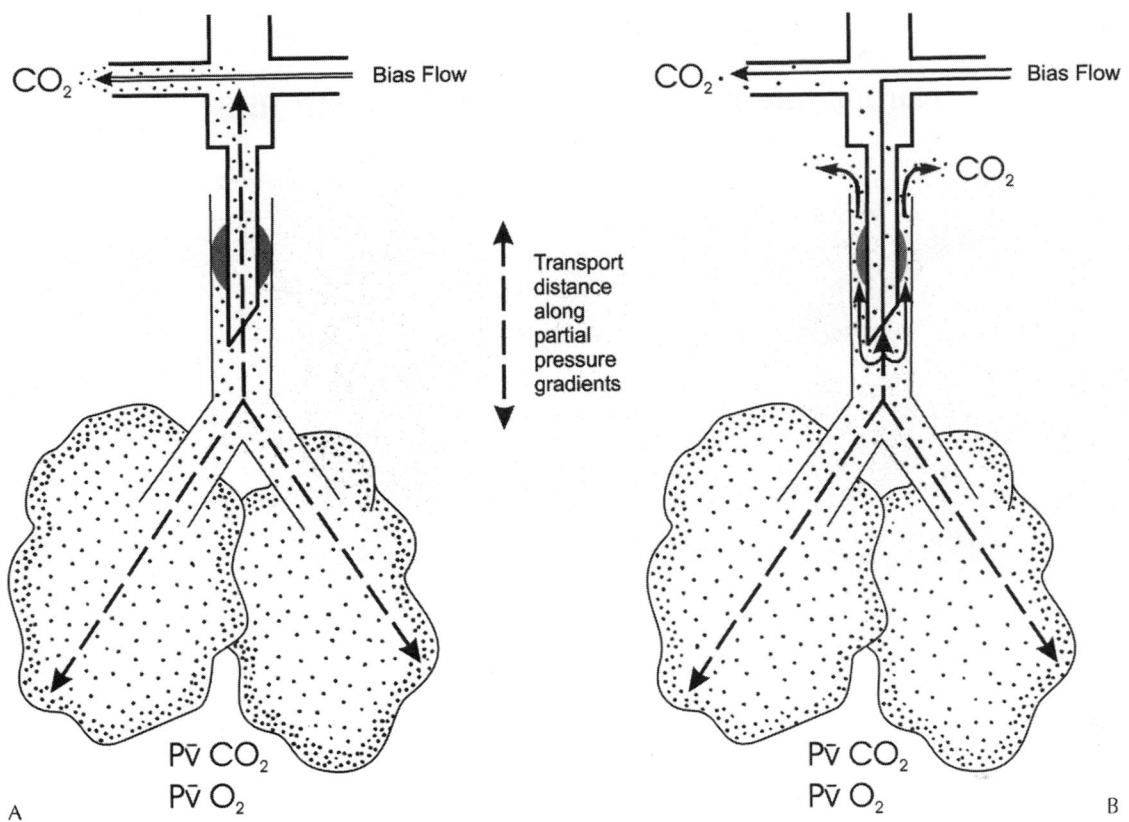

FIGURE 20-7 Schematic of the gas transport pathways during HFOV before and after establishment of a cuff leak. Transport distances are shown for CO_2. On the left, with the endotracheal tube (ETT) cuff occluding the trachea, the fresh-gas front for both CO_2 and O_2 is at the top of the ETT. Gas-transport mechanisms must bring CO_2 from the alveoli to the top of the ETT before CO_2 is flushed away by the bias flow. On the right, with partial ETT cuff deflation, some of the bias flow passes down the ETT and flushes CO_2 molecules out beside the ETT, in effect reducing the transport distance substantially. The ETT represents 50% of the transport impedance during HFOV.[63,77] Introduction of a cuff leak reduces the tidal volume needed to support CO_2 elimination and decreases the intrapulmonary ΔP imposed on lung tissue.[79] A cuff leak also may increase tracheal contamination by oral secretions. The risk-benefit ratio of a cuff leak is not yet established.

ventilator exceeds the mPaw within the lung by an amount that increases with tidal volume, frequency, and smaller endotracheal tube diameters.[82]

Frequency selection directly affects the pressure cycles applied to the lung. A smaller percentage of the circuit ΔP is transmitted down an endotracheal tube at higher frequencies (D Hager, personal communication).

The most useful theoretical approach to conceptualizing the optimal frequency for HFOV has been that of Venegas and Fredberg.[83] They approached the optimization question as a problem of providing adequate alveolar ventilation at a minimal pressure cost. Their approach addressed the whole lung, not just flow in a tube, and incorporated elements such as alveolar recruitment and derecruitment into the "cost functions," as well as the effects of lung inflation and frequency on dead-space volume and the dependence of lung compliance on lung volume. The lung characteristics used were those of infants with a variety of clinical scenarios. Results were expressed as a series of three-dimensional plots of safe combinations of frequency and PEEP, with *safe* being defined as settings that resulted in a *peak* alveolar distension of less than 90% of total lung capacity (Fig. 20-8). The importance of this approach is that it provides graphic depictions

of the shifting boundary conditions for safe ventilator settings with varying lung pathology. These plots demonstrate the familiar reality that the normal lung can be ventilated over a wide range of frequencies and PEEP levels without inducing dangerous overdistension. The lung with poor compliance but relatively normal airways, however, such as the infant or child with respiratory distress syndrome (RDS), has a very limited zone of safe frequency/PEEP combinations. With this pathophysiology, the selection of PEEP becomes critical, particularly at lower frequencies, with penalties in terms of pressure cost and overdistension with either too low or too high a level of PEEP. As seen in Fig. 20-8, at high frequencies, the zone of safe PEEP widens, making it easier to maintain more of the lung homogeneously aerated. In lungs with increased airways resistance, the optimal frequency moves to a lower rate. This complex modeling supports practices that had evolved clinically in neonatology, where frequencies of 10–15 Hz are standard practice in the management of diffuse alveolar disease. Currently, this analysis has been done only for the infant lung. One would predict that similar plots would shift to a somewhat lower frequency in adults. These plots concur with the perception of many neonatologists that it is simply easier to

$$D_{alv} = \left(V_{EE} + V_T\right)/TLC$$

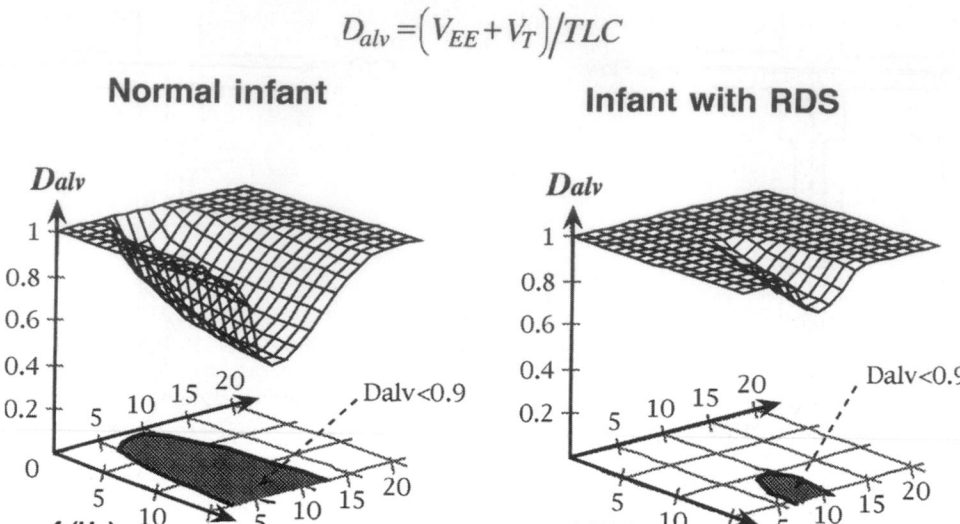

FIGURE 20-8 Three-dimensional plots providing a conceptual basis for the selection of frequency (f) and positive end-expiratory pressure (PEEP) settings during mechanical ventilation. Normalized peak alveolar distension (Dalv) is plotted against f and PEEP for a normal infant (*left*) and one with respiratory distress syndrome (RDS) (*right*). Normalized peak alveolar distension (Dalv) is defined as lung volume at end expiration (V_{EE}) plus the tidal volume (V_T) normalized by TLC. The safe zone for peak alveolar distension was set at 90% of TLC. For clarity, combinations of f and PEEP producing alveolar distension that exceeds this safe level are arbitrarily assigned a value of 1. The combinations of f and PEEP that produce peak volumes within this limit are given by the shaded zones projected onto the *xz* plane. In the normal infant, the range of safe f-PEEP choices is very large (i.e., the shaded zone projected on the *xz* plane). Because of the tendency to atelectasis in the infant with RDS (*right*), lung peak distension encroaches on TLC for all but a small range of f-PEEP combinations. The width of the safe zone becomes greater as frequency increases. This formulation graphically depicts the twin dangers of both too little and too much PEEP. Both lead to potentially damaging alveolar overdistension. (*Reproduced, with permission, from Venegas et al: Crit Care Med 22:S49–57, 1994.*)

keep an atelectasis-prone lung in the safe zone using the higher frequencies of HFOV than to attempt to track the "right" frequency–PEEP–tidal volume combination at conventional rates.[9]

TIDAL VOLUME

Tidal volume delivery during HFOV is influenced by many factors[20,84] (Table 20-1). Recent publications have challenged the notion that HFOV supports CO_2 elimination with small tidal volumes.[85] At a ΔP of 60 cmH$_2$O and 4 Hz, the SensorMedics 3100B oscillator delivered tidal volumes of 4.4 ml/kg to 29-kg sheep. No Pa_{CO_2} data were provided at those settings. Such settings equate to a tidal volume approximating 1.7 ml/kg in an 80-kg adult. Any ventilator has to be adjusted to appropriate Pa_{CO_2} targets. Old data with piston oscillators of known volume delivery,[86,87] plus a recent case report from Japan,[88] demonstrate that adequate CO_2 elimination is achieved in adults with ALI/ARDS using tidal volumes of 1.5–2 ml/kg during HFOV. For optimal

lung protection, one should use the smallest tidal volume and highest frequency that achieves Pa_{CO_2} elimination targets. Introduction of a cuff leak should be considered before decreasing frequency below 6 Hz. Even higher frequencies and small tidal volumes may be preferable, but the relative risk/benefit of early cuff leak versus lower frequencies requires further investigation.[89,90] Resonant amplification of the delivered volume has been demonstrated[91,92] at a median of 19 Hz in babies. Heliox can increase the tidal volume delivered at a given power setting by decreasing circuit/lung impedance.[93]

Although inability to eliminate CO_2 occurred in 1 of 17 patients in the original report of Fort et al,[56] the incidence of ventilation failure (i.e., pH $\leq$ 7.15 with bicarbonate $\geq$ 19 meq/liter) was the same in both HFOV and conventional ventilation groups in the subsequent larger MOAT trial[57] and is rare if one follows current recommendations (see "Troubleshooting," below).

Physiologic Effects of HFOV

CARDIOPULMONARY INTERACTIONS

HFOV is a sensitive detector of hypovolemia. Patients need intravascular volume repletion before one initiates HFOV and optimizes lung volume. Fortunately, clinical experience and animal studies demonstrate that despite this need for

TABLE 20-1 Factors Decreasing Delivered Tidal Volume

↓ Endotracheal tube diameter (includes secretions, edema fluid)
↑ Endotracheal tube length
↑ Frequency (most HFOV devices)
↓ Power or amplitude
↓ Percent inspired time
↓ Respiratory system compliance

an adequate volume status, treatment with HFOV does not induce "wet lungs."[94] Alveolar expansion has a powerful impact on pulmonary vascular resistance. Pulmonary vascular resistance goes up both in areas of atelectasis and overdistension. Therefore, the impact of HFOV on pulmonary artery pressure will be influenced strongly by the extent to which homogeneous alveolar expansion can be achieved. This will vary with lung pathophysiology, decisions made about mPaw and recruitment techniques, and body position. In clinical experience, pulmonary hypertension secondary to the use of higher mPaw during HFOV has not been a problem. Rather, HFOV often has enhanced the responsiveness to inhaled nitric oxide in both infants and adults.[59,95–97] As with conventional lung-protective ventilator patterns, patients with pre-existing right-ventricular failure need to be watched closely for the possible adverse effects of measures to optimize lung volume on right-ventricular output.

Cardiac output decreases as mPaw increases with any ventilator modality.[98] In early HFOV trials in the premature baboon, cardiac output was less during HFOV[39] unless mPaw was weaned as lung aeration improved.[99] Similar interactions of cardiac output and mPaw occur in infants.[100] Lesser hemodynamic impact can be expected when ventilating "on the deflation limb," where alveolar expansion can be maintained at a lower mPaw cost.[47] In adult clinical trials, such as MOAT[57] and the recent TOOLS trial,[49] there were no significant deleterious effects on mean arterial pressure, central venous pressure, pulmonary artery occlusion pressure, or cardiac output compared with conventional ventilation. Small (1–2 mmHg), often transient increases in central venous pressure and pulmonary artery occlusion pressure were observed after transition to HFOV.[60] Transesophageal echocardiography has proven useful to assess preload adequacy when clarification is needed.

INTERACTION WITH SPONTANEOUS BREATHING

Spontaneous breaths contribute useful re-expanding forces.[101,102] Spontaneous breaths [as with airway pressure-release ventilation (APRV)] help to maintain end-expiratory alveolar expansion in dependent lung regions[103] and improve $\dot{V}_A/\dot{Q}$ distributions.[104] A significant decrease in ventilator days occurred when spontaneous efforts were maintained in patients with ALI/ARDS.[102] Unfortunately, with current HFOV circuit designs, vigorous respiratory efforts in large patients may cause pressure swings that activate alarms, interrupt oscillations, and produce significant desaturations. Initial oscillator trials in adults recommended muscle paralysis for this reason. Current protocols attempt to maintain these valuable spontaneous breaths.[34,90] Such an approach also minimizes potential problems from the myopathy of prolonged neuromuscular blockade.

Rationale, Advantages, and Limitations

If we accept that both overdistension and ongoing atelectasis damage lung tissue, then HFOV offers the ability to cycle the largest possible percentage of the total lung within

TABLE 20-2   Pulmonary Therapies Decreasing Mortality in Neonatal RDS since 1970

Early use of CPAP
Exogenous surfactant replacement therapy
HFOV/HFJV with "optimized lung volume"
Conventional ventilation with "optimized lung volume" strategy

NOTE: All these produced more homogeneous lung aeration.

that "safe" range of volume excursion. The key is to decipher exactly when small pressure and volume excursions will make a difference. All therapeutic advances in neonatal and pediatric critical care over the past 30 years that have had a significant impacted on survival exhibit one unifying feature: all have produced more homogeneous lung expansion (Table 20-2).

ADVANTAGES OF HFOV

It is much easier in theory than in practice to ventilate the lung within the safe zone of pressure and volumes in *all* lung regions.[105] Although much has been written about using the static P-V curve of the respiratory system to guide ventilator settings, any single curve is only a crude composite of the family of P-V curves occurring in different parts of the lungs. A safe peak or plateau pressure will be lower in nondependent and more normal lung regions; closing pressures will be higher in dependent, inflamed, or edematous regions than suggested by a single overall curve.[6,42,45,50,71] Studies in adults with ALI/ARDS demonstrate that derecruitment often begins at PEEP levels substantially above the values recommended as protective of the lung.[6,106] As one raises PEEP levels, even acceptable degrees of permissive hypercapnia may be unattainable without exceeding safe peak/plateau pressures at conventional ventilator rates. In such patients, HFOV has the potential to keep that lung in the safe zone with a much larger margin of safety simply because of its ability to sustain gas transport with small volume cycles[32] (Fig. 20-9). This is particularly so at higher frequencies because of the impact of time-constant variability on alveolar filling.

A very old but elegant study demonstrated some fundamental features of lung re-expansion risk.[107] In essence, unless one exceeds airway/alveolar opening pressures, re-expansion will not occur. If one exceeds opening pressure with a long inspiratory period, atelectatic areas open, but normal areas become overdistended. Even very high pressures, however, will not overdistend normal lung if applied very briefly (<0.15 second in this study) because the time constant of highly compliant alveoli is long. Therefore, pressures high enough to exceed opening pressures are safer if applied as brief pulses, as with HFOV. As one turns down the frequency, this safety feature diminishes.

Lung-volume optimization and outcomes equivalent to HFOV have been achieved using recruitment maneuvers followed by rapid conventional ventilation with careful PEEP titration in saline-lavaged animal models.[108–110] Whether this equivalency extends to more established disease with greater inhomogeneity of opening and closing pressures has not been tested.

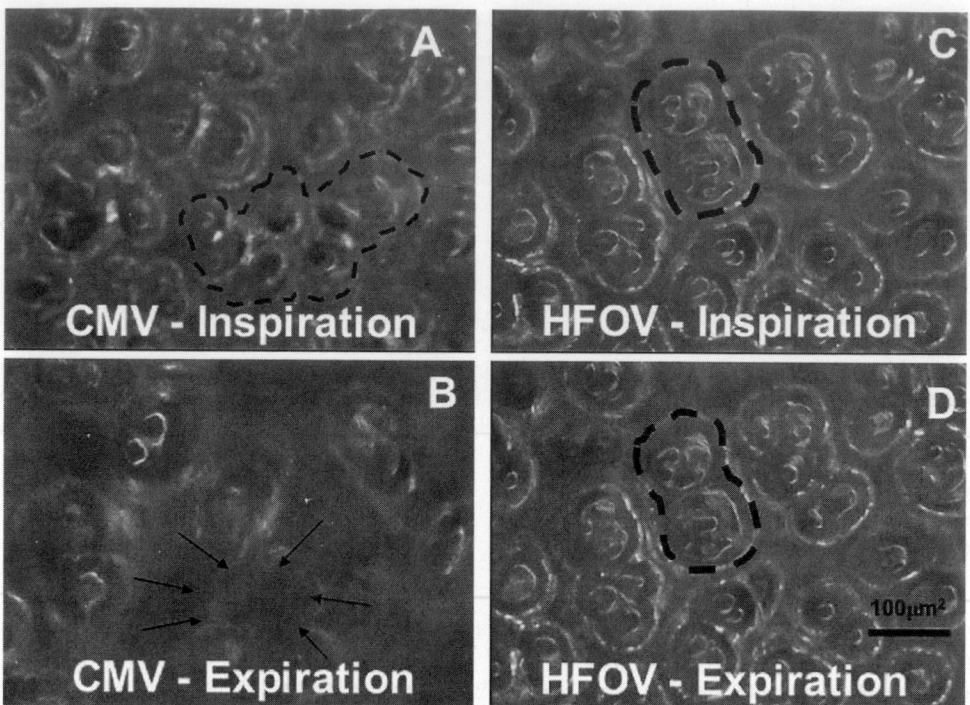

FIGURE 20-9 In vivo photomicrographs of subpleural alveoli of a rat after inducing lung injury by saline lavage. Animals were ventilated to equal oxygenation and Pa_{CO_2} targets using either conventional mechanical ventilation (CMV) or high-frequency oscillatory ventilation (HFOV). Alveoli in (*A*) were inflated at end inspiration during CMV to a peak pressure of 34 cmH$_2$O but collapsed during expiration (*B*) with a PEEP of 9 cmH$_2$O (*arrows*). Alveoli were very stable during HFOV at a mean airway pressure of 19 cmH$_2$O. The same alveolus is seen at inspiration and expiration in panels (*C*) and (*D*) (*dots*). (*Reproduced, with permission, from Carney et al: Crit Care Med 33:S122–8, 2005.*)

LIMITATIONS

Most of the perceived limitations of HFOV currently are really limitations of the machines available rather than the technique per se. Even minor modifications trigger expensive Food and Drug Administration (FDA) approval processes. Therefore, oscillator design in North America has been frozen for years.

INCREASED USE OF MUSCLE PARALYSIS

A significant limitation of the adult-sized oscillator currently available in North America is its inability to facilitate spontaneous ventilation. Infants and children are rarely paralyzed during HFOV. Paralysis of adults on HFOV can be minimized by titrating sedative agents, using higher bias flows to minimize air hunger, and reserving paralytic agents for as-needed bolus use rather than constant infusions.[34,90,111] Shallow breathing is tolerated in some adults without significant desaturation, particularly during the recovery phase of their disease. The lack of demand flow to augment spontaneous breaths requires adults to be transitioned to conventional ventilation or APRV for final weaning and extubation.[90]

INFECTION CONTROL

The lack of an expiratory filter initially limited the use of HFOV in patients with infections such as Severe Acute Respiratory Syndrome (SARS). A suitable filter is now available (SensorMedics, Yorba Linda, CA).

AEROSOL DELIVERY

Metered-dose inhalers are ineffective during HFOV. The Aeroneb nebulizer (Aeroneb Pro, Aerogen, Sunnyvale, CA) delivered the highest percentage of drug in test lung studies.[112]

TRANSPORT DURING HFOV

It is simplest to execute anticipated transports such as for CT scan before starting HFOV. There is no transport version of HFOV. Cartotto et al[59] describe an effective protocol for transport during HFOV, such as to the operating room. It involves clamping the endotracheal tube while on HFOV, transition to a self-inflating bag with a 20 cmH$_2$O PEEP valve, unclamping of the endotracheal tube with vigorous manual ventilation during transport, and reversal of these procedures once an oscillator has been set up at the destination. Recruitment maneuvers then are used as needed to reestablish oxygenation at the pretransport HFOV settings.

MONITORING

High-frequency oscillatory ventilators have few ventilator alarms to alert one to a mainstem intubation, tension pneumothorax, or endotracheal tube obstruction. Patterns of possible changes in ventilator readouts with such events have been modeled.[90] Also, ventilator noise necessitates brief piston interruption to auscultate heart or breath sounds.

UNFAMILIARITY OF PERSONNEL

A major limitation to the use of HFOV is the level of discomfort of personnel (i.e., physicians, respiratory therapists, and nurses) who encounter it rarely and usually as a measure of last resort.[113] If one does not understand that a mean pressure of 35 cmH$_2$O that is stenting 70–80% of a stiff lung open while supporting CO$_2$ elimination with small volume cycles may well induce less lung injury than a PEEP of 15 cmH$_2$O, plateau pressure of 30 cmH$_2$O, and larger tidal volumes being distributed to 30–40% of that lung, then HFOV "feels" dangerous. Only experience gained in less dire circumstances can produce a comfortable level of understanding of the interaction of ventilator decisions and lung pathophysiology. Then and only then can one really test the applicability of any high-frequency modality.[89]

PROTOCOL/ALGORITHM LIMITATIONS

When protocols are generalized to patients outside the population on which the protocol was devised, HFOV may be used inappropriately. Several HFOV protocols specify maximum mean airway pressure limits that were derived in patients with primary pulmonary diffuse airspace disease. If these limits are applied to patients with major extrapulmonary factors, such as abdominal distension or chest-wall burn eschar, adequate atelectasis reversal is unlikely because 30–70% of the applied mPaw will be lost to inflate the chest wall.[71]

Indications and Contraindications

INDICATIONS

Is HFOV still needed in the current era of "gentler" conventional ventilation? When HFOV first came into clinical use, large tidal volumes were considered safe during conventional ventilation as long as high peak pressures were avoided.[10] In this milieu, randomized, controlled trials in neonates demonstrated substantial outcome advantages from HFOV.[114] Conventional ventilator protocols then were modified to pursue the same lung protection. In two recent randomized, prospective studies, significant differences between lung volume–optimizing HFOV and conventional ventilation protocols were seen only in the study in which just 40% of the infants meeting very low birth weight criteria were randomized. These neonates required an F$_{IO_2}$ of approximately 0.6 on an mPaw of 8 cmH$_2$O. In this trial, more neonates managed with HFOV (until extubation) survived without chronic lung disease and were extubated successfully 1 week earlier than neonates receiving lung-protective ventilation at conventional frequencies.[54] When all very low birth weight babies were randomized regardless of O$_2$ requirements, outcome with both ventilators was the same.[53] This neonatal experience reflects the predictions of the Venegas-Fredberg analysis.[83] If the lung is fairly normal, a wide range of tidal volumes, PEEP levels, and frequencies can be used without inducing atelectasis or overdistension. Ventilator choice becomes a matter of user preference. As the lung becomes more prone to atelectasis, the range of safe PEEP values shrinks, and injurious extremes of alveolar volume

are avoided more reliably at higher frequencies. These are the lungs in which HFOV improves outcome.

NEONATAL/PEDIATRIC PATIENTS

Current criteria for using HFOV vary among institutions. A switch from conventional ventilation to HFOV generally occurs at some combination of F$_{IO_2}$ and airway pressures needed to achieve goals for oxygenation and CO$_2$ elimination. Experience in animal models, infants, and children has demonstrated the importance of instituting HFOV early in the lung at risk.[52,69,70,115] In infants, an mPaw of 10–12 cmH$_2$O or greater with an F$_{IO_2}$ of more than 0.6 and/or a falling aerated lung volume trigger a switch to HFOV in some units. Duval et al[113] switched to HFOV at an oxygenation index of greater than 13 or a pH of less than 7.25 despite a bicarbonate level of 20 mmol/liter or greater and peak pressures of more than 30 cmH$_2$O. In older children, Doctor and Arnold[116] recommend institution of HFOV if an "open-lung strategy" using conventional ventilation generates a peak pressure of greater than 35 cmH$_2$O despite permissive hypercapnia or mPaw values approach 15–18 cmH$_2$O and the F$_{IO_2}$ still exceeds 0.6. Some pediatric units convert to HFOV at oxygen requirements of more than 0.4 with peak pressures of 30–35 cmH$_2$O, PEEP levels of 12–15 cmH$_2$O, and a pH approaching 7.30 in pediatric patients with acute respiratory failure. The same group considers a switch to HFOV earlier in neonates, in particular in premature infants presenting with iRDS. In this patient population there frequently is echocardiographic evidence of pulmonary hypertension. Such pulmonary hypertension can generally be reversed using HFOV to achive better CO$_2$ elimination and normalize pH values. (Rimensberger, personal communication). Randomized, prospective studies indicate that when inhaled nitric oxide is needed, therapeutic response is improved with concurrent institution of HFOV in both neonates and children.[95,117,118] All these guidelines represent an attempt to define the characteristics of a lung for which HFOV might be more protective than a conventional lung-protective strategy.

ADULT PATIENTS

Indications for HFOV are evolving in adult lung disease. A consistent theme in studies to date is that survival is better with early (<3 days) rather than late (>7 days) institution of HFOV.[56,58] Currently, a trial of HFOV is recommended if F$_{IO_2}$ requirements remain greater than 0.6, the plateau pressure is approaching 30 cmH$_2$O, PEEP is greater than 15 cmH$_2$O, or the high pressure is greater than 30 cmH$_2$O on APRV.[89,90] The current challenge is to define the pulmonary characteristics that indicate that the lung is at risk of VILI using conventional frequencies and then to test whether HFOV is of benefit in that population. Indicators such as PEEP responsiveness,[119] dead-space measurements,[120] and biomarkers[121] are being explored. Indicators ideally would include an accurate bedside method to determine the extent of inhomogeneity of alveolar expansion across lung regions both at end inspiration and at end expiration.[42,71,74]

CONTRAINDICATIONS

Early literature advised against the use of HFOV in obstructive airway diseases such as asthma because of the theoretical risk of inadvertant gas trapping and hyperinflation. Recent reports demonstrate that HFOV can be used in such patients, even in patients demonstrating gas trapping on conventional settings. Case reports of patients with severe asthma and a series of infants with respiratory syncytial virus infection with severe bronchiolitis describe what is being termed the *open-airway strategy* for the management of such patients.[30,122] The goal in these patients is to find the narrow window of mean airway pressure that stents the diseased airways open enough to support high-frequency gas transport without inducing excessive lung distension with hemodynamic impairment. Extensive experience with HFOV is recommended before one pursues this application.[30]

Before development of an expiratory gas filter, SARS and other highly contagious airborne pathogens were a relative contraindication to HFOV.[123]

Comparison with Other Modes

Limited comparisons are available among various high-frequency modalities. When HFJV was introduced into adult and neonatal use, the primary goal was to support gas exchange at the lowest possible peak and mean airway pressures to facilitate resolution of barotrauma. When HFOV was introduced in an early neonatal clinical trial, the primary goal was to optimize the volume of aerated lung. Both devices, in fact, can be used with either a low-pressure or open-lung strategy.[52] The strategy must be matched to the patient's pathophysiology. Only one study systematically compared three high-frequency options in an animal model of the atelectasis-prone lung.[124] Optimal outcome occurred with the mode (HFO) in which the end-expiratory pressure was closest to the mean pressure level and the least time was spent at the end-expiratory level.

Variations in Delivery

The performance of several commercially available devices for delivery of HFOV to neonates has been evaluated both in bench studies and in animal models. Substantial differences in performance have been demonstrated.[65,66,125] Any ventilator introduced into an ICU should be thoroughly understood before clinical use. For example, all neonatal ventilators tested by Hatcher et al[65] and Pillow et al[66] showed a decrease in delivered volume with a decrease in lung compliance, but one ventilator (no longer available) exhibited the reverse phenomenon.[125] That outlier characteristic may explain puzzling episodes of hypercapnia during the weaning of infants with that ventilator.[125] One ventilator failed to increase delivered volume at settings between 50% and 100% of its amplitude dial. It also was the only ventilator that markedly increased tidal volume as mean pressure increased.[65,125] Ventilators varied in the relationship of displayed mPaw and intrapulmonary mean pressure measured during endotracheal tube occlusion.[65] Threefold

differences were documented in maximum tidal volume among ventilators tested at 15 Hz,[65,66] and frequency dependence of tidal volume varied substantially. It is amazing that HFOV has been used as safely and effectively as it has considering these major discrepancies in ventilator performance among the devices used.

Adjustments at the Bedside

PREPARATION FOR INITIATION OF HFOV (TABLE 20-3)

Documentation of a patent endotracheal or tracheostomy tube is essential.[34] Partial obstructions impede gas transport much more during HFOV than with conventional modes. Tubes that allow passage of a suction catheter still may have a narrow lumen. A preemptive bronchoscopy will verify tube patency as well as provide opportunity for removal of any mucus plugs if the patient has been intubated for more than 2–3 days. Hypovolemic patients will not tolerate the high mean mPaw used with HFOV; adequate volume status should be ensured before initiating HFOV.

Sedative and analgesic drugs should be titrated while the patient is still receiving conventional ventilation. Although muscle paralysis was used in most adult published trials, subsequent experience has found continuous paralytic infusions unnecessary in many cases when appropriate levels of sedation are established.[34] Small as-needed doses of muscle relaxants may facilitate the initial period of adjustment to HFOV and may be needed intermittently during periods of agitation to facilitate retitration of sedative and analgesic agents.[90,111] Preservation of some spontaneous respiratory effort is valuable as with any type of prolonged ventilation, provided those efforts do not produce marked fluctuations in mPaw (>5 cmH$_2$O) or O$_2$ saturation (>3–5%). Careful observation for spontaneous breathing following transition to HFOV allows proper adjustment of high- and low-pressure alarms. Patient comfort may be enhanced when bias flows of 40–60 liters/min are used to achieve the target mPaw in adults.

OXYGENATION

Two conceptually different approaches are described for initiation of HFOV in adult patients with respect to oxygenation adjustments. The approach used in most published algorithms and trials to date uses an F$_{IO_2}$ of 1.0 during transition to HFOV with the mPaw set approximately 5 cmH$_2$O higher than the mean pressure during conventional ventilation.[89] F$_{IO_2}$ levels are reduced as much a possible, keeping Sa$_{O_2}$ at 88–90%. Inability to reduce the F$_{IO_2}$ below 0.6 is managed primarily with stepwise increases in mPaw, in essence, gradually moving the respiratory system up the inflation limb of the P-V relationship as the first intervention. Derdak et al[90] currently recommend initiating HFOV at an mPaw of 30 cmH$_2$O. When hypoxemia is severe at the time of initiating HFOV, intermittent lung-recruitment maneuvers are used along with rapid upward titration of mPaw. Recruitment maneuvers are performed by resetting the high-pressure alarm to a higher value (i.e., 50 cmH$_2$O), eliminating a cuff leak if present, turning off

TABLE 20-3 Algorithm(s) for High-Frequency Oscillatory Ventilation in Adult Patients

Initial Steps	Oxygenation	Ventilation	Weaning
Adequate analgesia and sedation Ensure adequate volume status	Set initial mPaw 5 cmH_2O higher than on CV[89] Set initial mPaw at 30 cmH_2O after setting cuff leak[90] % IT = 33	Goal is highest frequency with lowest ΔP for lung protection	Goal is F_{IO_2} of 40%, Sp_{O_2} of >88%, mPaw of 20–24 cmH_2O before CV transition
Neuromuscular blocker as required (if desaturation with movement or spontaneous breathing)	F_{IO_2} at 100% during transition period	Set initial ET cuff leak (5–8 cmH_2O)[90] Use cuff leak before reducing f below 5 Hz[89]	If required mPaw of > 35 cmH_2O, give equal priority to reducing mPaw and F_{IO_2} Reduce mPaw earlier with circulatory failure
Establish transcutaneous CO_2 monitoring to guide ΔP and f adjustments during transition	Recruiting maneuvers (40–50 cmH_2O for 40–60 s with piston off)—if severe hypoxemia, desaturation with suction, postbronchoscopy, or circuit disconnection[89,90] or on initiation of HFOV[49]	Set initial ΔP at 20 cmH_2O + Pa_{CO_2} or to "chest vibration" (usual range, 60–90 cmH_2O)	Reduce mPaw 2–3 cmH_2O every 4–6 h
Bronchoscopy to evaluate ET tube patency (especially if prolonged time on CV)	If Sp_{O_2} < 88%, increase mPaw 3 cmH_2O every 30–60 min (maximum, 45 cmH_2O) and consider additional recruiting maneuvers	Use f-ΔP algorithm in ref. 90 Set initial frequency at 5 Hz Adjust f and ΔP as in ref. 89	When mPaw approaches 20 cmH_2O, transition to CV (e.g., TV, 6 ml/kg; PEEP, 10 cmH_2O; Pplat, <30 cmH_2O; I:E, 1:1; rate, 15–25 breaths/min) or to APRV (e.g., Phi, 20 cmH_2O; Plow 0 cmH_2O; Thi, 4 s, Tlo, 0.8 s)
Bag-mask with attached PEEP valve at head of bed	Prone position if F_{IO_2} remains >0.6 or mPaw of >35 cmH_2O[90] Prone patient if F_{IO_2} > 0.9[89]	ABG 15 min after initiating HFOV: adjust ΔP (5–10 cmH_2O steps) and frequency (1–2 Hz steps) based on Pa_{CO_2} trends and pH (goal, pH > 7.2) Bronchoscopy if refractory hypercapnea	Conventional weaning progressin g to spontaneous breathing trials

ABBREVIATIONS: mPaw, mean airway pressure; CV, conventional ventilation; ΔP, oscillatory pressure amplitude; ET, endotracheal; PEEP, positive end-expiratory pressure; TV, tidal volume; I:E, inspiratory-expiratory ratio; Pplat, inspiratory pressure plateau; Sp_{O_2}, oxygen saturation; Phi, high pressure; Plow, low pressure; Thi, high pressure time; Tlo, low pressure time; ABG, arterial blood gas; APRV, airway pressure-release ventilation; HFOV, high-frequency oscillatory ventilation; %IT, percent inspiratory time.

NOTE: This table outlines an overall approach while indicating areas in which different "experts" use somewhat different decision algorithms.

the piston, raising the mPaw to 40–45 cmH_2O (maximum 50 cmH_2O) for 40–60 seconds, returning the mPaw to the original setting (or 3 cmH_2O higher), and then restarting the piston and restoring cuff leak and alarms to the original levels. Recruitment maneuvers should be considered if desaturation occurs after suctioning, bronchoscopy, circuit disconnects, or patient repositioning.

An alternative approach in the recently published TOOLS trial used one to three recruitment maneuvers immediately on initiating HFOV.[49] The initial maintenance mPaw was set at 30 cmH_2O regardless of mean pressures on conventional ventilation. The conceptual framework here is to use initial recruitment maneuver(s) to re-expand atelectatic regions and then titrate the maintenance mPaw "down the deflation limb" of the P-V relationship in a timely fashion according to the patient's oxygenation response. This methodology matches protocols used in many animal studies of lung protection using HFOV. With this protocol, an F_{IO_2} of less than 0.6 was achieved in 68% of patients by the end of the initial recruitment cycle, which delivered 2.4 recruitment maneuvers over a mean of 1.5 hours (Fig. 20-10).

With both approaches, the accepted target has been projection of the diaphragm onto the eighth or ninth rib posteriorly on an anteroposterior film. An alternative reference in adults is visualization of the fifth rib above the diaphragm anteriorly or an apical-diaphragm distance not greater than 25 cm.[126] Emerging techniques for the evaluation of regional expansion hopefully will soon replace these crude measures.[74] Information on the relative timing, efficacy in terms of achieving the most homogeneous lung-expansion pattern, and complication rate of these two approaches is needed before it will be possible to define an "optimal" approach. The potential hazard of the first approach is too little recruitment too slowly. The potential hazard of the second approach is excessive lung distension at a rote value of 30 cmH_2O mPaw if that value is not reduced expeditiously enough in a lung that is very responsive to recruitment. What is becoming clear is the importance of ventilating "on the deflation limb," whether with conventional ventilation or with HFOV.[47,127]

It remains speculative whether the target F_{IO_2} for optimal lung protection should be 0.4 or 0.6. A substantial amount of

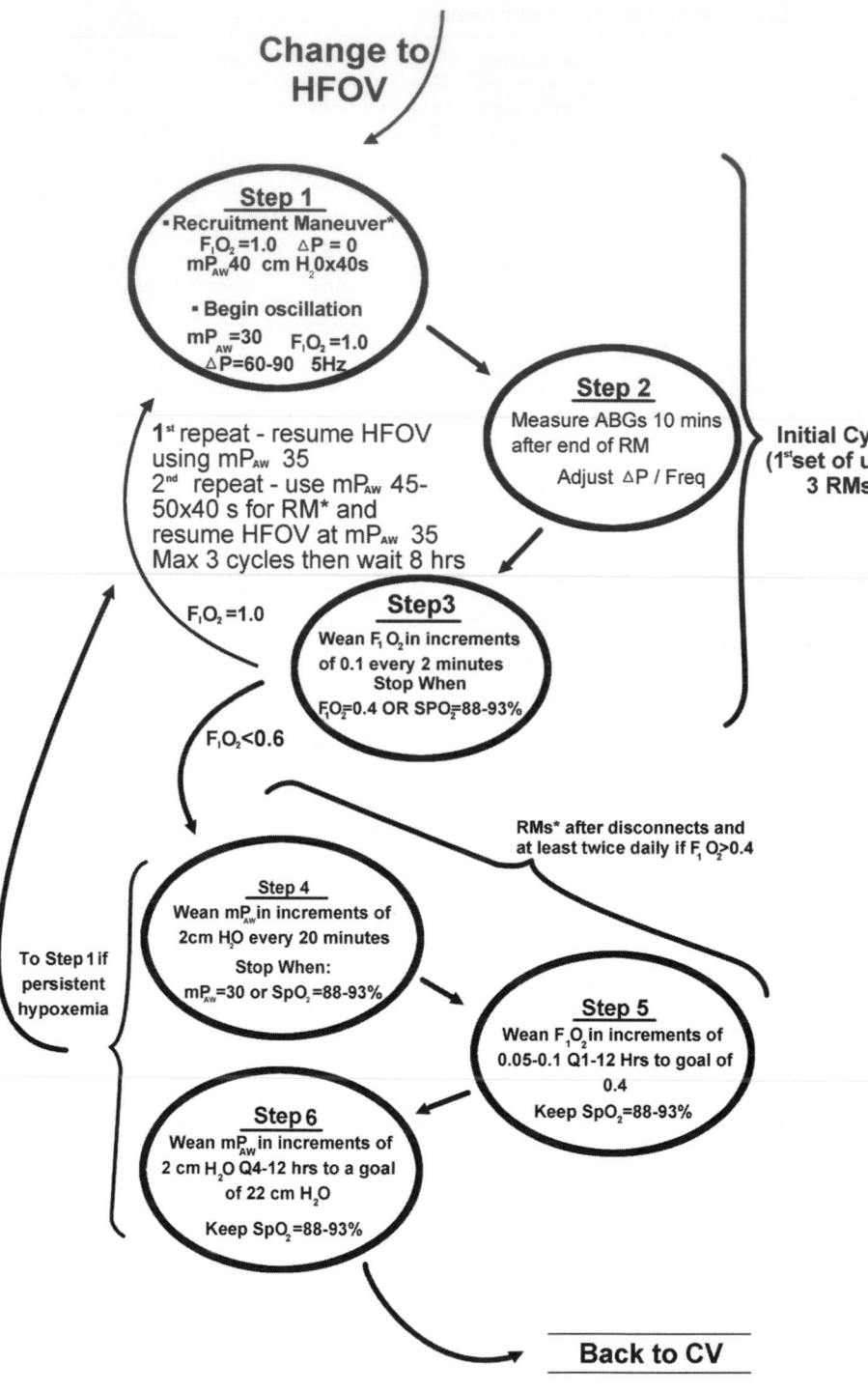

Change to HFOV

Step 1
- Recruitment Maneuver*
  F_1O_2=1.0 ΔP = 0
  mP_{AW} 40 cm H_2Ox40s

- Begin oscillation
  mP_{AW}=30 F_1O_2=1.0
  ΔP=60-90   5Hz

1st repeat - resume HFOV using mP_{AW} 35
2nd repeat - use mP_{AW} 45-50x40 s for RM* and resume HFOV at mP_{AW} 35
Max 3 cycles then wait 8 hrs

Step 2
Measure ABGs 10 mins after end of RM
Adjust ΔP / Freq

Initial Cycle (1st set of up to 3 RMs)

F_1O_2=1.0

Step3
Wean F_1O_2 in increments of 0.1 every 2 minutes
Stop When
F_1O_2=0.4 OR SPO_2=88-93%

F_1O_2<0.6

RMs* after disconnects and at least twice daily if F_1O_2>0.4

To Step 1 if persistent hypoxemia

Step 4
Wean mP_{AW} in increments of 2cm H_2O every 20 minutes
Stop When:
mP_{AW}=30 or SpO_2=88-93%

Step 5
Wean F_1O_2 in increments of 0.05-0.1 Q1-12 Hrs to goal of 0.4
Keep SpO_2=88-93%

Step 6
Wean mP_{AW} in increments of 2 cm H_2O Q4-12 hrs to a goal of 22 cm H_2O
Keep SpO_2=88-93%

Back to CV

* Recruitment Maneuvers
- Pre-oxygenated with F_1O_2 = 1.0 x 5 mins
- Aborted immediately if hemodynamic compromise
- Not performed if an active airleak present

FIGURE 20-10 Protocol outlining the sequence of recruitment maneuvers and HFOV settings used in the TOOLS Trial to re-expand atelectatic alveoli at the time of initiation of HFOV to get the lung onto its deflation limb.[49] Patients underwent an initial cycle of up to three sustained inflation recruitment maneuvers (RM) (steps 1 to 3). Ten minutes after the first RM, F_{IO_2} was decreased in decrements of 0.10 every 2 minutes, stopping when either the F_{IO_2} was 0.40 or the arterial oxygen saturation (Sp_{O_2}) was 88–93% (step 3). If the F_{IO_2} requirement remained greater than 0.60 after a third RM to 45–50 cmH$_2$O, the recruitment procedure was repeated every 8 hours. Once the F_{IO_2} was less than 0.60, maintenance mean airway pressure (mPaw) was reduced in 2 cmH$_2$O steps to 30 cmH$_2$O, keeping Sp_{O_2} at 88–93% (step 4). F_{IO_2} was then weaned to 0.40 before further reductions in mPaw (steps 5 and 6). MPaw, mean airway pressure; RM, recruitment maneuver; ΔP, pressure amplitude in cmH$_2$O; Freq, frequency (Hz); CV, conventional ventilation; ABG, arterial blood gas. (*Reproduced, with permission, from Ferguson et al: Crit Care Med 33:479–86, 2005.*)

ongoing atelectasis remains at an F_{IO_2} of 0.6. As one moves toward an earlier transition to HFOV—as in current neonatal and pediatric experience in many centers—lower F_{IO_2} targets become achievable at "reasonable" mean pressures. At high F_{IO_2} requirements, mPaw levels are reduced only when doing so does not increase F_{IO_2} requirement. When the F_{IO_2} is stable at 0.6, some protocols recommend reduction of mPaw before further F_{IO_2} decreases if the mPaw is greater than 35 cmH$_2$O. Whether this compromise between ongoing atelectasis and the risk of higher pressures is necessary likely will be best resolved when bedside methods of assessing areas of overdistension become available. One protocol that recommends this mPaw/F_{IO_2} compromise also recommends placing the patient in a prone position if the F_{IO_2} requirement remains 0.6 or more (in order to potentiate alveolar recruitment in dorsal lung regions).[34]

CO$_2$ ELIMINATION

The optimal approach to CO$_2$ elimination is currently controversial. When should the transport advantages of an endotracheal tube cuff leak be introduced? Inasmuch as the lung-protective potential of HFOV lies in its small volume cycles, it would seem logical to introduce it at the time of initiating HFOV in a large patient. With a cuff leak of 5–8 cmH$_2$O, one can eliminate CO$_2$ at a higher frequency, deliver the smallest possible tidal volumes, and produce the lowest possible ratio of intratracheal to airway opening pressure swings.[79] With this approach, even very heavy patients generally can be ventilated at frequencies of 6 Hz or more. If reductions in frequency are required at any stage, the first response to a decrease in Pa$_{CO_2}$ with recovery should be an increase in frequency. Whether the frequency target in adults should be 8 Hz or higher is presently unknown.[89] Detailed protocols differing in their relative weighting of amplitude (ΔP) and frequency are available.[89,90]

An alternative approach is progressive reduction of frequency to 3 Hz as needed to achieve target CO$_2$ levels, with a cuff leak being added only when these much larger stroke volumes prove inadequate.

The advantage of instituting a cuff leak when initiating HFOV is the ability to use higher frequencies and smaller volume cycles. The disadvantages are a need for more nursing care to ensure removal of oral secretions and respiratory therapy involvement to remove and then reset the cuff leak whenever a recruitment maneuver is performed. Endotracheal tubes with infraglottic suction ports may prove useful in this context. In cases of severe upper airway swelling, a pharyngeal airway positioned just above the larynx can be used to provide an exit pathway for a cuff leak, as described by Cartotto et al[59] in a burn patient. Failure of mPaw to drop when instituting a cuff leak indicates swelling around the cuff or upper airway.

Protocols also differ in their approach to setting power or ΔP. Some advocate starting at maximal power so that one can use the highest frequency possible[89]; other algorithms manipulate both ΔP and frequency settings.[34,90] Transcutaneous P$_{CO_2}$ sensors can provide useful trend information (not absolute values) to guide power/frequency adjustments during the initiation phase. Lower Pa$_{CO_2}$ targets are needed in patients with elevated intracranial pressure or head injury, as well as in neonates, in whom the risk of retinopathy of prematurity may increase at high Pa$_{CO_2}$.[7]

PATIENT POSITIONING

Patients should be placed at 30° head up unless hemodynamically unstable. The prone position also can be used during HFOV to optimize expansion of dorsal lung regions, with appropriate protocols for caring for the prone patient.[128] If the prone position is not feasible but hypoxemia remains severe, switching the patient from side to side in true lateral positions (i.e., 90° to the mattress) may improve lung recruitability.

Troubleshooting

Pa$_{CO_2}$ PROBLEMS

It is particularly important to troubleshoot Pa$_{CO_2}$ problems appropriately (Table 20-4).

TABLE 20-4 Pa$_{CO_2}$ Problems

Pa$_{CO_2}$ Too Low	Pa$_{CO_2}$ Too High	Acute Increase in Pa$_{CO_2}$
↑ f in increments of 1–2 Hz to 8[90] or 12 Hz[89]	↑ ΔP if not already at 90 cmH$_2$O in increments of 5 cmH$_2$O	Verify ETT is patent: • Pass suction catheter • Quick bronchoscopy
↓ ΔP in 5 cmH$_2$O increments	Institute a cuffleak if not present	• Can one ventilate adequately with manual bag/mask?
	Try RM(s) to reverse atelectasis Is a higher maintenance mPaw needed? (CXR or other measure of lung volume)	Is there a pneumothorax? • Decreased vibrations unilaterally? • CXR
	↓ f to a minimum of 3 Hz in 1–2 Hz decrements	Progressive Increase Pa$_{CO_2}$ Is chest wall compliance decreasing? • Abdominal compartment syndrome • Burn eschar

DECREASED Pa_{CO_2}

As Pa_{CO_2} levels decrease during the course of lung recovery, the first response should be to increase frequency back up to the 7–8 Hz range (1- to 2-Hz increments) and then to decrease power (5–10 cmH$_2$O ΔP decrements) in order to minimize volume and pressure swings in the lung. A decrease in ΔP at a constant power setting may be an indicator that lung volume is increasing.

INCREASED Pa_{CO_2}

An abrupt substantial increase in Pa_{CO_2} in a previously stable patient may reflect plugging of the endotracheal tube, development of a pneumothorax, or atelectasis. One should ensure passage of a suction catheter, check one's ability to manually bag/mask ventilate, and perform a quick bronchoscopy while waiting for a chest x-ray to clarify the etiology. Before decreasing frequency or increasing power in response to a gradual increase in Pa_{CO_2}, one must ensure that the lung is expanded adequately. An abdominal compartment syndrome should be considered. Available oscillators all decrease delivered stroke volume when faced with a greater load.[65,66] Appropriate recruitment procedures often can resolve Pa_{CO_2} problems while at the same time decreasing the phasic pressure swings within the airways and alveoli. A cuff leak should be considered before lowering frequency.

OXYGENATION PROBLEMS

As discussed earlier, oxygenation depends on achieving and then maintaining end-expiratory lung volume. A gradual downward drift of O$_2$ saturation after a recruitment maneuver is indicative of too low a maintenance mPaw. Recruitment should be repeated with a return to an mPaw 2–3 cmH$_2$O higher than the previous level. If the F_{IO_2} requirement remains greater than 0.60 despite recruitment maneuvers, prone positioning should be considered. Inhaled nitric oxide can be added, although whether this improves outcome as well as oxygenation remains unknown.[97]

AIR LEAKS

Barotrauma occurs during HFOV but may be more subtle in its manifestations. Displayed mPaw will remain stable even with a tension pneumothorax. The gradual development of hypotension and desaturation, with or without a unilateral decrease in chest-wall motion, should trigger a portable chest x-ray. In an experimental model of pneumothorax during HFOV, air leak was minimized by the use of higher frequency, lower ΔP, lower mPaw, and shorter inspiratory period.[129] Excessive decreases in mPaw will promote atelectasis with a resulting increase in intrapulmonary pressure cost, delaying resolution of the air leak. In general, recruitment maneuvers are not advised in the presence of air leak. This is not an absolute contraindication. In the presence of severe hypoxemia and unilateral air leak, recruitment maneuvers performed with the patient in a full lateral position with the leak side down may achieve significant benefit by re-expansion of the nondependent lung.

HEMODYNAMIC COMPROMISE

Inability to tolerate the institution of HFOV or application of recruitment maneuvers may reflect an inadequate intravascular volume. Duval et al[122] reported a need for a transient increase in fluids and inotropic agents in some infants during transition to HFOV. Interpretation of filling pressures (central venous pressure, pulmonary artery occlusion pressure) may be difficult in the setting of high mPaw. A fluid challenge or transesophageal echo study may be needed in ambiguous situations.[34]

Important Unknowns

HFOV protocols are under constant revision through animal experiments and clinical trials that evaluate both the gas-exchange and VILI impact of ventilator setting decisions. We need criteria that indicate when any given ventilator pattern needs to be replaced by one with a greater potential for lung protection. This is a complex question considering that we do not even know when permissive hypercarbia becomes deleterious for patients.

The optimal frequency or frequencies for minimizing the intrapulmonary pressure and distension "cost" of HFOV in the adult lung with varying pathophysiologies remain unknown. Such information would clarify the risk-benefit ratio of early use of a cuff leak. Existing algorithms differ substantially in their management of f.[89,90]

Optimal methods of aerosol delivery during HFOV need further evaluation. Better bedside knowledge of which techniques [e.g., recruitment maneuvers, ventilator settings, position changes (prone/supine), and so on] produce the most homogeneous lung expansion across all lung regions would greatly aid decision making. Emerging technologies such as electrical impedance tomography show promise.

Neonates often are maintained on HFOV until extubation. Premature transition to conventional ventilation can negate the benefit of HFOV. Because spontaneous breaths are not augmented during HFOV, this approach is not feasible in large patients. The "optimal" timing of transition to conventional ventilation may be difficult to determine until this device limitation is resolved. It is well recognized that gross deterioration of oxygenation after transition to conventional ventilation should trigger an immediate re-evaluation of the patient and possible return to HFOV. Whether keeping the lung splinted open with low F_{IO_2} and small volume/pressure cycles in a spontaneously breathing patient for an extra few days (as with APRV)[90] would facilitate lung recovery biochemically and/or structurally during the resolution of ARDS remains to be tested.

Future Directions

Hopefully, further pilot studies will clarify some of the issues outlined herein before large-scale comparative trials of HFOV and other lung-protective options are performed. To date, no large randomized, controlled trial of HFOV has been performed with lung-volume optimization "on the deflation limb" of the P-V relationship. Validation of various mPaw, recruitment maneuver, ΔP, and frequency algorithms for their effect on VILI in large animal models is needed. Prospective, randomized trials can only be done in centers comfortable with HFOV. Currently, many centers use HFOV rarely and only for severe, refractory oxygenation failure or air-leak syndromes associated with end-stage lung disease. This is not the way to develop a cadre of physicians, nurses, and respiratory therapists who can skillfully troubleshoot interactions between the machinery and the patient's pathophysiology.

REDESIGNED MACHINES

Currently, high-frequency oscillators are still classified as class 3 devices by the FDA. This means that any redesign triggers expensive review costs, much in excess of that required for bringing a new conventional ventilator to market. Revision of this classification would greatly facilitate improvements in device design.

CLINICAL LUNG-VOLUME MONITORING

Developments in this area should take a lot of guesswork out of lung-volume optimization during both conventional and high-frequency ventilation. Hopefully, future guidelines for the initiation of HFOV will be able to include some measure of interregional inhomogeneity of alveolar expansion as one of the criteria, not just a plateau pressure, Fi_{O_2}, or pH value.

References

1. Froese AB. High-frequency oscillatory ventilation for adult respiratory distress syndrome: Let's get it right this time! Crit Care Med 1997; 25:906–8.
2. Ranieri VM, Suter PM, Tortorella C, et al. Effect of mechanical ventilation on inflammatory mediators in patients with acute respiratory distress syndrome: A randomized, controlled trial. JAMA 1999; 282:54–61.
3. Imai Y, Slutsky AS. High-frequency oscillatory ventilation and ventilator-induced lung injury. Crit Care Med 2005; 33:S129–34.
4. Ventilation with lower tidal volumes as compared with traditional tidal volumes for acute lung injury and the acute respiratory distress syndrome. The Acute Respiratory Distress Syndrome Network. New Engl J Med 2000; 342:1301–8.
5. Roupie E, Dambrosio M, Servillo G, et al. Titration of tidal volume and induced hypercapnia in acute respiratory distress syndrome. Am J Respir Crit Care Med 1995; 152:121–8.
6. Crotti S, Mascheroni D, Caironi P, et al. Recruitment and derecruitment during acute respiratory failure: A clinical study. Am J Respir Crit Care Med 2001; 164:131–40.
7. Clark RH, Gerstmann DR, Jobe AH, et al. Lung injury in neonates: Causes, strategies for prevention, and long-term consequences. J Pediatr 2001; 139:478–86.
8. Ventre KM, Arnold JH. High frequency oscillatory ventilation in acute respiratory failure. Paediatr Respir Rev 2004; 5:323–32.
9. Rimensberger PC. ICU cornerstone: High frequency ventilation is here to stay. Crit Care (Lond) 2003; 7:342–4.
10. Froese AB, Kinsella JP. High-frequency oscillatory ventilation: Lessons from the neonatal/pediatric experience. Crit Care Med 2005; 33:S115–21.
11. Clark RH, Slutsky AS, Gerstmann DR. Lung protective strategies of ventilation in the neonate: What are they? Pediatrics 2000; 105:112–4.
12. Froese AB, Bryan AC. High frequency ventilation. Am Rev Respir Dis 1987; 135:1363–74.
13. Slutsky AS. Nonconventional methods of ventilation. Am Rev Respir Dis 1988; 138:175–83.
14. Sjöstrand U. Review of the physiological rationale for and development of high-frequency positive-pressure ventilation— HFPPV. Acta Anaesthesiol Scand Suppl 1977; 64:7–27.
15. Lunkenheimer PP, Rafflenbeul W, Keller H, et al. Application of transtracheal pressure oscillations as a modification of "diffusing respiration." Br J Anaesth 1972; 44:627.
16. Emerson J. Apparatus for vibrating portions of a patients' airway. U.S. patent no 2,918,917, January 1959.
17. Bryan AC. The oscillations of HFO. Am J Respir Crit Care Med 2001; 163:816–7.
18. Klain M, Smith RB. High frequency percutaneous transtracheal jet ventilation. Crit Care Med 1977; 5:280–7.
19. Gregory GA, Kitterman JA, Phibbs RH, et al. Treatment of the idiopathic respiratory-distress syndrome with continuous positive airway pressure. New Engl J Med 1971; 284:1333–40.
20. Marchak BE, Thompson WK, Duffty P, et al. Treatment of RDS by high-frequency oscillatory ventilation: A preliminary report. J Pediatr 1981; 99:287–92.
21. Carlon GC, Kahn RC, Howland WS, et al. Clinical experience with high frequency jet ventilation. Crit Care Med 1981; 9:1–6.
22. Rouby JJ, Simonneau G, Benhamou D, et al. Factors influencing pulmonary volumes and CO_2 elimination during high-frequency jet ventilation. Anesthesiology 1985; 63:473–82.
23. Rouby JJ, Viars P. Clinical use of high frequency ventilation. Acta Anaesthesiol Scand Suppl 1989; 90:134–9.
24. Krishnan JA, Brower RG. High-frequency ventilation for acute lung injury and ARDS. Chest 2000; 118:795–807.
25. Carlon GC, Howland WS, Ray C, et al. High-frequency jet ventilation: A prospective, randomized evaluation. Chest 1983; 84:551–9.
26. Flatau E, Lewinsohn G, Konichezky S, et al. Mechanical ventilation in fiberoptic-bronchoscopy: Comparison between high frequency positive pressure ventilation and normal frequency positive pressure ventilation. Crit Care Med 1982; 10:733–5.
27. Keszler M, Durand DJ. Neonatal high-frequency ventilation: Past, present, and future (review). Clin Perinatol 2001; 28:579–607.
28. Salim A, Martin M. High-frequency percussive ventilation. Crit Care Med 2005; 33:S241–5.
29. Chang HK. Mechanisms of gas transport during ventilation by high-frequency oscillation. J Appl Physiol 1984; 56:553–63.
30. Duval EL, van Vught AJ. Status asthmaticus treated by high-frequency oscillatory ventilation. Pediatr Pulmonol 2000; 30:350–3.
31. Bryan AC, Slutsky AS. Long volume during high frequency oscillation. Am Rev Respir Dis 1986; 133:928–30.
32. Carney D, DiRocco J, Nieman G. Dynamic alveolar mechanics and ventilator-induced lung injury. Crit Care Med 2005; 33:S122–8.
33. Boynton BR, Villanueva D, Hammond MD, et al. Effect of mean airway pressure on gas exchange during high-frequency oscillatory ventilation. J Appl Physiol 1991; 70:701–7.
34. Derdak S. High-frequency oscillatory ventilation for acute respiratory distress syndrome in adult patients. Crit Care Med 2003; 31:S317–23.
35. Boynton BR, Hammond MD, Fredberg JJ, et al. Gas exchange in healthy rabbits during high-frequency oscillatory ventilation. J Appl Physiol 1989; 66:1343–51.
36. Kolton M, Cattran CB, Kent G, et al. Oxygenation during

high-frequency ventilation compared with conventional mechanical ventilation in two models of lung injury. Anesth Analg 1982; 61:323–32.

37. Hamilton PP, Onayemi A, Smyth JA, et al. Comparison of conventional and high-frequency ventilation: Oxygenation and lung pathology. J Appl Physiol 1983; 55:131–8.

38. McCulloch PR, Forkert PG, Froese AB. Lung volume maintenance prevents lung injury during high frequency oscillatory ventilation in surfactant-deficient rabbits. Am Rev Respir Dis 1988; 137:1185–92.

39. Meredith KS, deLemos RA, Coalson JJ, et al. Role of lung injury in the pathogenesis of hyaline membrane disease in premature baboons. J Appl Physiol 1989; 66:2150–8.

40. Froese AB, Butler PO, Fletcher WA, Byford LJ. High-frequency oscillatory ventilation in premature infants with respiratory failure: A preliminary report. Anesth Analg 1987; 66:814–24.

41. Froese AB. Neonatal and pediatric ventilation: Physiological and clinical perspectives. In: Marini JJ, Slutsky AS, editors. Physiological Basis of Ventilatory Support. New York: Marcel Dekker, 1998: 1315–57.

42. Albaiceta GM, Taboada F, Parra D, et al. Tomographic study of the inflection points of the pressure-volume curve in acute lung injury. Am J Respir Crit Care Med 2004; 170:1066–72.

43. Gothberg S, Parker TA, Griebel J, et al. Lung volume recruitment in lambs during high-frequency oscillatory ventilation using respiratory inductive plethysmography. Pediatr Res 2001; 49:38–44.

44. van Genderingen HR, van Vught AJ, Duval EL, et al. Attenuation of pressure swings along the endotracheal tube is indicative of optimal distending pressure during high-frequency oscillatory ventilation in a model of acute lung injury. Pediatr Pulmonol 2002; 33:429–36.

45. van Genderingen HR, van Vught AJ, Jansen JR. Regional lung volume during high-frequency oscillatory ventilation by electrical impedance tomography. Crit Care Med 2004; 32:787–94.

46. Goddon S, Fujino Y, Hromi JM, Kacmarek RM. Optimal mean airway pressure during high-frequency oscillation: Predicted by the pressure-volume curve. Anesthesiology 2001; 94:862–9.

47. van Genderingen HR, van Vught JA, Jansen JR, et al. Oxygenation index, an indicator of optimal distending pressure during high-frequency oscillatory ventilation? Intensive Care Med 2002; 28:1151–6.

48. Rimensberger PC, Beghetti M, Hanquinet S, Berner M. First intention high-frequency oscillation with early lung volume optimization improves pulmonary outcome in very low birth weight infants with respiratory distress syndrome. Pediatrics 2000; 105:1202–8.

49. Ferguson ND, Chiche JD, Kacmarek RM, et al. Combining high-frequency oscillatory ventilation and recruitment maneuvers in adults with early acute respiratory distress syndrome: The Treatment with Oscillation and an Open Lung Strategy (TOOLS) Trial pilot study. Crit Care Med 2005; 33:479–86.

50. Lim CM, Soon LS, Seoung LJ, et al. Morphometric effects of the recruitment maneuver on saline-lavaged canine lungs: A computed tomographic analysis. Anesthesiology 2003; 99: 71–80.

51. High-frequency oscillatory ventilation compared with conventional mechanical ventilation in the treatment of respiratory failure in preterm infants. The HIFI Study Group. New Engl J Med 1989; 320:88–93.

52. Gerstmann DR, deLemos RA, Clark RH. High-frequency ventilation: Issues of strategy. Clin Perinatol 1991; 18:563–80.

53. Johnson AH, Peacock JL, Greenough A, et al. High-frequency oscillatory ventilation for the prevention of chronic lung disease of prematurity. New Engl J Med 2002; 347:633–42.

54. Courtney SE, Durand DJ, Asselin JM, et al. High-frequency oscillatory ventilation versus conventional mechanical ventilation for very-low-birth-weight infants. New Engl J Med 2002; 347:643–52.

55. Thome U, Topfer A, Schaller P, Pohlandt F. Effects of mean airway pressure on lung volume during high-frequency oscillatory ventilation of preterm infants. Am J Respir Crit Care Med 1998; 157:1213–8.

56. Fort P, Farmer C, Westerman J, et al. High-frequency oscillatory ventilation for adult respiratory distress syndrome: A pilot study. Crit Care Med 1997; 25:937–47.

57. Derdak S, Mehta S, Stewart TE, et al. High-frequency oscillatory ventilation for acute respiratory distress syndrome in adults: A randomized, controlled trial. Am J Respir Crit Care Med 2002; 166:801–8.

58. Mehta S, Lapinsky SE, Hallett DC, et al. Prospective trial of high-frequency oscillation in adults with acute respiratory distress syndrome. Crit Care Med 2001; 29:1360–9.

59. Cartotto R, Cooper AB, Esmond JR, et al. Early clinical experience with high-frequency oscillatory ventilation for ARDS in adult burn patients. J Burn Care Rehabil 2001; 22:325–33.

60. Chan KP, Stewart TE. Clinical use of high-frequency oscillatory ventilation in adult patients with acute respiratory distress syndrome. Crit Care Med 2005; 33:S170–4.

61. Pillow JJ, Sly PD, Hantos Z. Monitoring of lung volume recruitment and derecruitment using oscillatory mechanics during high-frequency oscillatory ventilation in the preterm lamb. Pediatr Crit Care Med 2004; 5:172–80.

62. Pillow JJ, Sly PD, Hantos Z, Bates JH. Dependence of intrapulmonary pressure amplitudes on respiratory mechanics during high-frequency oscillatory ventilation in preterm lambs. Pediatr Res 2002; 52:538–44.

63. Pillow JJ. High-frequency oscillatory ventilation: Mechanisms of gas exchange and lung mechanics. Crit Care Med 2005; 33: S135–41.

64. Sakai T, Kakizawa H, Aiba S, et al. Effects of mean and swing pressures on piston-type high-frequency oscillatory ventilation in rabbits with and without acute lung injury. Pediatr Pulmonol 1999; 27:328–35.

65. Hatcher D, Watanabe H, Ashbury T, et al. Mechanical performance of clinically available, neonatal, high-frequency, oscillatory-type ventilators. Crit Care Med 1998; 26:1081–8.

66. Pillow JJ, Wilkinson MH, Neil HL, Ramsden CA. In vitro performance characteristics of high-frequency oscillatory ventilators. Am J Respir Crit Care Med 2001; 164:1019–24.

67. Bond DM, Froese AB. Volume recruitment maneuvers are less deleterious than persistent low lung volumes in the atelectasis-prone rabbit lung during high-frequency oscillation. Crit Care Med 1993; 21:402–12.

68. Mehta S, Granton J, MacDonald RJ, et al. High-frequency oscillatory ventilation in adults: The Toronto experience. Chest 2004; 126:518–27.

69. Arnold JH, Hanson JH, Toro-Figuero LO, et al. Prospective, randomized comparison of high-frequency oscillatory ventilation and conventional mechanical ventilation in pediatric respiratory failure. Crit Care Med 1994; 22:1530–9.

70. Arnold JH, Anas NG, Luckett P, et al. High-frequency oscillatory ventilation in pediatric respiratory failure: A multicenter experience. Crit Care Med 2000; 28:3913–9.

71. Luecke T, Herrmann P, Kraincuk P, Pelosi P. Computed tomography scan assessment of lung volume and recruitment during high-frequency oscillatory ventilation. Crit Care Med 2005; 33:S155–62.

72. Maggiore SM, Richard JC, Brochard L. What has been learnt from P/V curves in patients with acute lung injury/acute respiratory distress syndrome. Eur Respir J Suppl 2003; 42: 22s–26s.

73. Frerichs I, Dargaville PA, Dudykevych T, Rimensberger PC. Electrical impedance tomography: A method for monitoring regional lung aeration and tidal volume distribution? Intensive Care Med 2003; 29:2312–6.

74. Wolf GK, Arnold JH. Noninvasive assessment of lung volume: Respiratory inductance plethysmography and electrical impedance tomography. Crit Care Med 2005; 33:S163–9.

75. Kolton M, McGhee I, Bryan AC. Tidal volumes required to maintain isocapnia at frequencies from 3 to 30 Hz in the dog. Anesth Analg 1987; 66:523–8.

76. Slutsky AS, Kamm RD, Rossing TH, et al. Effects of frequency, tidal volume, and lung volume on CO_2 elimination in dogs by high frequency (2–30 Hz), low tidal volume ventilation. J Clin Invest 1981; 68:1475–84.

77. Rossing TH, Solway J, Saari AF, et al. Influence of the endotracheal tube on CO_2 transport during high-frequency ventilation. Am Rev Respir Dis 1984; 129:54–7.

78. Solway J, Gavriely N, Slutsky AS, et al. Effect of bias flow rate on gas transport during high-frequency oscillatory ventilation. Respir Physiol 1985; 60:267–76.

79. Van de Kieft M, Dorsey D, Morison D, et al. High-frequency oscillatory ventilation: Lessons learned from mechanical test lung models. Crit Care Med 2005; 33:S142–7.

80. Gerstmann DR, Fouke JM, Winter DC, et al. Proximal, tracheal, and alveolar pressures during high-frequency oscillatory ventilation in a normal rabbit model. Pediatr Res 1990; 28:367–73.

81. Allen JL, Frantz ID, III, Fredberg JJ. Heterogeneity of mean alveolar pressure during high-frequency oscillations. J Appl Physiol 1987; 62:223–8.

82. Pillow JJ, Neil H, Wilkinson MH, Ramsden CA. Effect of I/E ratio on mean alveolar pressure during high-frequency oscillatory ventilation. J Appl Physiol 1999; 87:407–14.

83. Venegas JG, Fredberg JJ. Understanding the pressure cost of ventilation: Why does high-frequency ventilation work? Crit Care Med 1994; 22:S49–57.

84. Gavriely N, Solway J, Loring SH, et al. Pressure-flow relationships of endotracheal tubes during high-frequency ventilation. J Appl Physiol 1985; 59:3–11.

85. Sedeek KA, Takeuchi M, Suchodolski K, Kacmarek RM. Determinants of tidal volume during high-frequency oscillation. Crit Care Med 2003; 31:227–31.

86. Butler WJ, Bohn DJ, Bryan AC, Froese AB. Ventilation by high-frequency oscillation in humans. Anesth Analg 1980; 59:577–84.

87. Rehder K, Didier EP. Gas transport and pulmonary perfusion during high-frequency ventilation in humans. J Appl Physiol Exerc Physiol 1984; 57:1231–7.

88. Nagano O, Fujii F, Morimatsu H, et al. An adult with ARDS managed with high-frequency oscillatory ventilation and prone position. J Anesth 2002; 16:75–8.

89. Fessler HE, Brower RG. Protocols for lung protective ventilation. Crit Care Med 2005; 33:S223–7.

90. Higgins J, Estetter B, Holland D, et al. High-frequency oscillatory ventilation in adults: Respiratory therapy issues. Crit Care Med 2005; 33:S196–203.

91. Lee S, Alexander J, Blowes R, et al. Determination of resonance frequency of the respiratory system in respiratory distress syndrome. Arch Dis Child Fetal Neonatal Ed 1999; 80:F198–202.

92. Brusasco V, Beck KC, Crawford M, Rehder K. Resonant amplification of delivered volume during high-frequency ventilation. J Appl Physiol 1986; 60:885–92.

93. Katz AL, Gentile MA, Craig DM, et al. Heliox does not affect gas exchange during high-frequency oscillatory ventilation if tidal volume is held constant. Crit Care Med 2003; 31:2006–9.

94. Bauer K, Buschkamp S, Marcinkowski M, et al. Postnatal changes of extracellular volume, atrial natriuretic factor, and diuresis in a randomized, controlled trial of high-frequency oscillatory ventilation versus intermittent positive-pressure ventilation in premature infants <30 weeks gestation. Crit Care Med 2000; 28:2064–8.

95. Dobyns EL, Anas NG, Fortenberry JD, et al. Interactive effects of high-frequency oscillatory ventilation and inhaled nitric oxide in acute hypoxemic respiratory failure in pediatrics. Crit Care Med 2002; 30:2425–9.

96. Kinsella JP, Abman SH. High-frequency oscillatory ventilation augments the response to inhaled nitric oxide in persistent pulmonary hypertension of the newborn: Nitric Oxide Study Group. Chest 1998; 114:100S.

97. Fan E, Mehta S. High-frequency oscillatory ventilation and adjunctive therapies: Inhaled nitric oxide and prone positioning. Crit Care Med 2005; 33:S182–7.

98. Arnold JH, Truog RD, Thompson JE, Fackler JC. High-frequency oscillatory ventilation in pediatric respiratory failure. Crit Care Med 1993; 21:272–8.

99. Kinsella JP, Gerstmann DR, Clark RH, et al. High-frequency oscillatory ventilation versus intermittent mandatory ventilation: Early hemodynamic effects in the premature baboon with hyaline membrane disease. Pediatr Res 1991; 29:160–6.

100. Simma B, Fritz M, Fink C, Hammerer I. Conventional ventilation versus high-frequency oscillation: Hemodynamic effects in newborn babies. Crit Care Med 2000; 28:227–31.

101. Putensen C, Hering R, Wrigge H. Controlled versus assisted mechanical ventilation (review). Curr Opin Crit Care 2002; 8:51–7.

102. Putensen C, Zech S, Wrigge H, et al. Long-term effects of spontaneous breathing during ventilatory support in patients with acute lung injury. Am J Respir Crit Care Med 2001; 164:43–9.

103. Wrigge H, Zinserling J, Neumann P, et al. Spontaneous breathing improves lung aeration in oleic acid-induced lung injury. Anesthesiology 2003; 99:376–84.

104. Putensen C, Mutz NJ, Putensen-Himmer G, Zinserling J. Spontaneous breathing during ventilatory support improves ventilation-perfusion distributions in patients with acute respiratory distress syndrome. Am J Respir Crit Care Med 1999; 159:1241–8.

105. Nieszkowska A, Lu Q, Vieira S, et al. Incidence and regional distribution of lung overinflation during mechanical ventilation with positive end-expiratory pressure. Crit Care Med 2004; 32:1496–503.

106. Tugrul S, Akinci O, Ozcan PE, et al. Effects of sustained inflation and postinflation positive end-expiratory pressure in acute respiratory distress syndrome: focusing on pulmonary and extrapulmonary forms. Crit Care Med 2003; 31:738–44.

107. Day R, Goodfellow AM, Apgar V, Beck GJ. Pressure-time relations in the safe correction of atelectasis in animal lungs. Pediatrics 1952; 10:593–602.

108. van Kaam AH, de Jaegere A, Haitsma JJ, et al. Positive pressure ventilation with the open lung concept optimizes gas exchange and reduces ventilator-induced lung injury in newborn piglets. Pediatr Res 2003; 53:245–53.

109. Sedeek KA, Takeuchi M, Suchodolski K, et al. Open-lung protective ventilation with pressure control ventilation, high-frequency oscillation, and intratracheal pulmonary ventilation results in similar gas exchange, hemodynamics, and lung mechanics. Anesthesiology 2003; 99:1102–11.

110. Rimensberger PC, Pristine G, Mullen BM, et al. Lung recruitment during small tidal volume ventilation allows minimal positive end-expiratory pressure without augmenting lung injury. Crit Care Med 1999; 27:1940–5.

111. Sessler CN. Sedation, analgesia, and neuromuscular blockade for high-frequency oscillatory ventilation. Crit Care Med 2005; 33:S209–16.

112. Lowson SM. Inhaled alternatives to nitric oxide. Crit Care Med 2005; 33:S188–95.

113. Duval EL, Markhorst DG, Gemke RJ, van Vught AJ. High-frequency oscillatory ventilation in pediatric patients. Netherlands J Med 2000; 56:177–85.

114. Gerstmann DR, Minton SD, Stoddard RA, et al. The Provo multicenter early high-frequency oscillatory ventilation trial: Improved pulmonary and clinical outcome in respiratory distress syndrome. Pediatrics 1996; 98:1044–57.

115. deLemos RA, Coalson JJ, deLemos JA, et al. Rescue ventilation with high frequency oscillation in premature baboons with hyaline membrane disease. Pediatr Pulmonol 1992; 12:29–36.

116. Doctor A, Arnold J. Mechanical support of acute lung injury: Options for strategic ventilation. New Horizons 1999; 7:359–73.

117. Kinsella JP, Abman SH. Recent developments in the pathophysiology and treatment of persistent pulmonary hypertension of the newborn. J Pediatr 1995; 126:853–64.

118. Kinsella JP, Walsh WF, Bose CL, et al. Inhaled nitric oxide in premature neonates with severe hypoxaemic respiratory failure: A randomised, controlled trial. Lancet 1999; 354:1061–5.

119. Ferguson ND, Kacmarek RM, Chiche JD, et al. Screening of ARDS patients using standardized ventilator settings: Influence on enrollment in a clinical trial. Intensive Care Med 2004; 30:1111–6.

120. Kallet RH, Alonso JA, Pittet JF, Matthay MA. Prognostic value of the pulmonary dead-space fraction during the first 6 days of acute respiratory distress syndrome. Respir Care 2004; 49:1008–14.

121. Ware LB. Prognostic determinants of acute respiratory distress syndrome in adults: Impact on clinical trial design. Crit Care Med 2005; 33:S217–22.

122. Duval EL, Leroy PL, Gemke RJ, van Vught AJ. High-frequency oscillatory ventilation in RSV bronchiolitis patients. Respir Med 1999; 93:435–40.

123. Sweeney AM, Lyle J, Ferguson ND. Nursing and infection-control issues during high-frequency oscillatory ventilation. Crit Care Med 2005; 33:S204–8.

124. Simma B, Luz G, Trawoger R, et al. Comparison of different modes of high-frequency ventilation in surfactant-deficient rabbits. Pediatr Pulmonol 1996; 22:263–70.

125. Jouvet P, Hubert P, Isabey D, et al. Assessment of high-frequency neonatal ventilator performances. Intensive Care Med 1997; 23:208–13.

126. Johnson MM, Ely EW, Chiles C, et al. Radiographic assessment of hyperinflation: Correlation with objective chest radiographic measurements and mechanical ventilator parameters. Chest 1998; 113:1698–704.

127. Rouby JJ. Optimizing lung aeration in positive end-expiratory pressure. Am J Respir Crit Care Med 2004; 170:1039–40.

128. Messerole E, Peine P, Wittkopp S, et al. The pragmatics of prone positioning. Am J Respir Crit Care Med 2002; 165:1359–63.

129. Ellsbury DL, Klein JM, Segar JL. Optimization of high-frequency oscillatory ventilation for the treatment of experimental pneumothorax. Crit Care Med 2002; 30:1131–5.

Chapter 21

EXTRACORPOREAL MEMBRANE OXYGENATION AND EXTRACORPOREAL LIFE SUPPORT

ROBERT BARTLETT
THEODOR KOLOBOW

The earliest development of the artificial lung (Fig. 21-1) was directed to its use in the repair of congenital heart defects in the surgical operating room using filming or "bubble" oxygenators.[1-3] Such early blood oxygenators served their purpose well because most cardiac surgical repairs could be completed in a few hours. Limitations in the use of both bubble and the subsequently introduced filming oxygenators for more that a few hours produced deterioration in organ function, with coagulopathy, hemolysis, thrombocytopenia, and fluid retention being the more conspicuous findings. There was a general consensus that direct exposure of blood to oxygen largely was responsible for those complications.[4,5]

The earliest prototype membrane artificial lung was based on a relatively low-permeability polyethylene membrane.[6] Such membranes were replaced subsequently by far more gas-permeable silicone rubber membranes.[7,8] More recently, the latter membranes have been complemented by microporous polymeric capillary tubes (the capillary membrane lung) of various designs,[9] the use of which now assumes a commanding lead in cardiovascular surgery. Not only did membrane-based artificial-lung technology allow for longer and safer cardiotho-

racic surgical procedures, but it also raised the possibility that patients with severe acute respiratory failure not responding to mechanical ventilation also might benefit from extracorporeal blood oxygenation and carbon dioxide removal.

The first successful clinical application of long-term extracorporeal membrane lung gas exchange for severe acute respiratory failure was reported by Hill et al[10] in 1970 in a young man following a motorcycle accident, with use of the Bramson membrane lung. Subsequently, membrane lung bypass was applied successfully in the treatment of acute respiratory distress syndrome (ARDS) of various causes.[11,12]

The many sporadic attempts at extracorporeal membrane lung assist led to a concerted effort by the National Institutes of Health (NIH) to launch a randomized, controlled multicenter study[13] in patients with severe ARDS (1975–1977). One group of patients was managed with conventional methods; the other group, with extracorporeal membrane oxygenation (ECMO). Of the total of 90 patients divided between the study and control groups, 4 patients in each group survived. It was concluded that patients entered into this trial were far too advanced in their illness to benefit from any form of therapy.

To address fears that the study groups represented patients who were unlikely to benefit from any extracorporeal gas exchange, a follow-up study (as part of the same study) was performed on 702 patients who had required only intubation for 24 hours or more and a fractional inspired oxygen concentration (F_{IO_2}) of 0.5 or greater. Overall, that study showed a mortality rate of 61%, much higher than anticipated.

Over the years, a hard core of ECMO centers has continued to apply lessons learned through experience, as well as lessons learned from animal research, to the use of ECMO in patients with ARDS or acute respiratory failure who were believed to be salvageable. Results have been encouraging. ECMO, when applied in a timely manner by experienced clinicians and investigators, remains an important adjunct in the care of the patients with severe ARDS. A registry of cases in all age groups is compiled through the Extracorporeal Life Support Organization (ELSO).[14]

Current Status of Extracorporeal Life Support

Extracorporeal life support (ECLS)/ECMO is now used routinely in every major childrens hospital, and use is growing in adult intensive-care units (ICUs). The indication for ECLS is acute severe cardiac or pulmonary failure when reversibility and recovery (or organ replacement) can be expected within a few weeks. The measurements of severity of illness and the likelihood of recovery (or replacement) are different for patients with respiratory or cardiac failure and also are different among patients of different ages groups. Hence evaluation of the use of ECLS requires information on a variety of patient groups. Through the ELSO, which

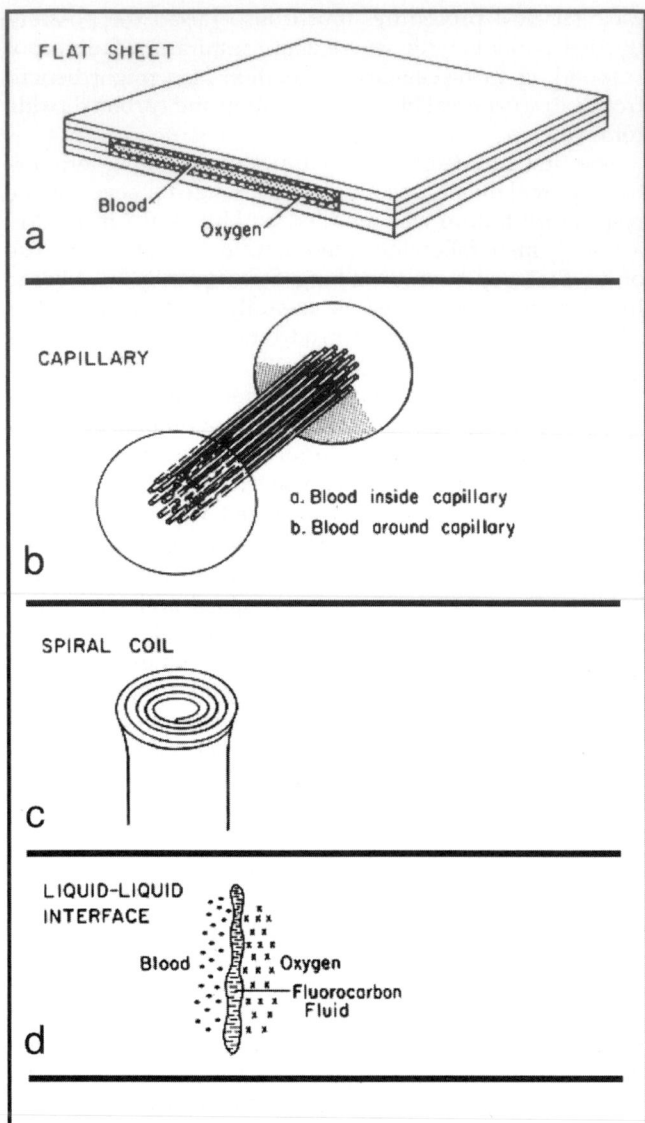

FIGURE 21-1 The four basic membrane lung design concepts.
A. **The flat-sheet membrane lung. Venous blood flows between two sheets of gas-permeable membrane with oxygen-enriched gas on the outside. For increased surface area, such units are stacked one on top of the other with a screen spacer providing space for gas (air, oxygen) flow.** *B.* **Capillary membrane lung. Venous blood flows either through the inside of gas-permeable plastic capillary fibers or outside with oxygen-enriched gas on the other side.**
C. **Spiral coiled membrane lung. A long ribbon of plastic screen is covered on both sides with a fabric-reinforced silicone rubber membrane that is rolled into a spiral coil. Oxygen flows within the coiled screen, with blood flow perpendicular to oxygen flow on the outside.** *D.* **Liquid-liquid interface membrane lung. Blood is exposed to microdroplets of well-oxygenated and CO_2-depleted fluorocarbon fluid to pick up O_2 and wash out CO_2.**

maintains a registry of ECLS patients, this information is readily available.

The technology and personnel involved with ECLS are evolving continuously. The concept of replacing cardiac and/or lung function by extracorporeal circulation is basic to all applications, but the methods of vascular access, monitoring variables, control of blood flow, goals of management, and personnel are custom made for each application.

VENOARTERIAL ACCESS

Venoarterial access (VA) is required for cardiac support or in patients with respiratory failure who are in profound shock. In babies, VA is achieved by cannulation of the right atrium through the right internal jugular vein and the aortic arch via the right common carotid artery. These vessels are exposed directly, ligated distally, and cannulated.[15] There is abundant collateral circulation around the common carotid artery, and the incidence of right cerebral ischemia is less than 1%. Brain blood flow does not depend on an intact circle of Willis because forward flow is established in the internal carotid artery distal to the ligated common carotid artery. In adults and children older than 3 or 4 years, the femoral artery is large enough for arterial access, although perfusion to the distal leg poses a significant risk. The best method for VA access is to cannulate the right atrium through the right internal jugular vein and to cannulate the femoral artery at the groin. Access to both vein and artery are achieved by the percutaneous Seldinger technique, although direct exposure may be necessary in very small children. Draining blood from the right atrium via the jugular vein avoids the problem of differential circulation, which can occur when the inferior vena cava is cannulated via the femoral vein. When the femoral artery is used for cannulation, distal perfusion can be established by direct cutdown and placement of a catheter in the superficial femoral artery. An alternative technique is to cannulate the posterior tibial artery by direct cutdown after the patient is on extracorporeal support. If the pressure in the posterior tibial artery is greater than 50 mmHg, distal perfusion is usually not necessary. If the pressure is less than 50 mmHg, then the leg can be perfused via the catheter in the posterior tibial artery, employing a tubing extension off the arterial perfusion line.

During VA bypass, extracorporeal flow is managed by measuring venous blood saturation; saturation should be between 70% and 80%. Patients usually exhibit some cardiac function, and blood flow is regulated to maintain an arterial pulse contour. This is usually equivalent to about 20–30% of the venous return going through the native circulation rather than through the extracorporeal circuit.

During VA access through the femoral artery, blood is perfused retrogradely up the aorta. Unless the patient is on total bypass, however, blood in the aortic root perfuses the coronary vessels and carotid vessels. This blood has a gas content of blood passing through the lungs and out through the left ventricle. If the patient is on ECLS for cardiac failure and the lungs are working adequately, the blood is well oxygenated. If the patient is in combined cardiopulmonary failure, however, some method must be undertaken to ensure adequate oxygenation of the blood in the root of the aorta. This can be accomplished by arterial perfusion via the carotid artery or by perfusing oxygenated blood off the arterial line into the venous circulation, a technique we refer to as *VAV access.*

Often during the use of ECLS for cardiac failure, the heart stops working altogether. If this occurs, the left atrium and left ventricle will overdistend gradually with blood returning from bronchial and thebesian veins. The pulmonary vascular pressure can reach very high levels, creating pulmonary edema and lung dysfunction. This is avoided by draining blood from the left side of the heart, generally by doing a blade atrial septostomy in the cardiac catheterization laboratory. The creation of an atrial-septal defect decompresses the left atrium into the right atrium. This atrial-septal defect can be repaired at a later date when the heart recovers, although most patients who require this extensive step ultimately undergo cardiac transplantation.

When an infant has recovered and it is time to decannulate the VA bypass, this is done under direct exposure. The catheters are removed, and the vessels are ligated proximally. Although it is possible to repair both the vein and artery, our practice is to leave the vessels ligated because of the potential risks of distal embolization in a repaired vessel. If VA access has been achieved via the percutaneous route in a large child or adult, it is usually possible to remove the catheters and apply local pressure. Even with a large catheter in the femoral artery, hemostasis usually is achieved without need for direct repair.

VENOVENOUS ACCESS

Venovenous (VV) acces is the preferred method for patients in respiratory failure who have adequate cardiac function. Even patients who require high doses of pressors and inotropes to maintain the circulation before ECLS are managed successfully by VV access. The inotropes and pressors can be discontinued as soon as the ventilator is returned to resting settings. A major advantage of VV access is that all the blood flow passes through the pulmonary circulation and left side of the heart, minimizing the risks of intrapulmonary and left-sided cardiac thrombosis and embolism. In addition, sustaining the pulmonary circulation may produce some beneficial effect on the healing of acute lung injury. In infants and small children, VV access is best achieved by cannulation of the right atrium through the right internal jugular vein using a double-lumen catheter.[16] The larger lumen is for venous drainage, and the smaller lumen for blood return. Blood return is aimed toward the tricuspid valve to minimize recirculation. Total gas-exchange support can be achieved easily in this fashion, although there is some mixing with the rest of venous blood.

In the future, VV access in larger children and adults will be achieved through large-bore double-lumen catheters. At present, however, these catheters do no exist, so VV access is achieved by cannulating the inferior vena cava via the femoral vein; the vena cava blood is drained, with reinfusion into the right atrium via the right internal jugular vein.[17] During VV support, cardiac function is normal; indeed, the patients are dependent on their own cardiac function for systemic perfusion. Pulse contour therefore is normal. VV flow is regulated to maintain the desired gas exchange: Arterial saturation remains in the 85% range for hypoxemic respiratory failure and normocapnia in hypercapnic respiratory failure. Membrane oxygenators are very efficient at removing carbon dioxide. Thus patients with hypercapnic respiratory failure (secondary to asthma, for example) can be managed with relatively low blood flow. Percutaneously placed VV catheters can be removed when the patient has recovered. Hemostasis is achieved by local pressure.

The Perfusion Circuit

The extracorporeal perfusion circuit includes a membrane oxygenator, a blood pump, and conduit tubing. The circuit usually includes a heat exchanger to maintain normal body temperature. Monitors include pre- and postoxygenator pressure sensors, which are useful for detecting signs of oxygenator thrombosis or failure. Blood-gas or saturation sensors can be inserted directly into the venous drainage tubing. The extracorporeal circuit requires systemic anticoagulation. A device to measure whole-blood activated clotting time (ACT) is an important part of the bedside apparatus. A continuous infusion of heparin is titrated to maintain the ACT at approximately 50% above normal. With the usual ACT system, for example, the upper level of normal is 120 seconds, and ACT during ECLS is maintained at 180 seconds. It is essential to use whole-blood ACT rather than partial thromboplastin time or some other measure of plasma anticoagulation.

The Team

The team caring for the patient on ECLS varies from standard ICU staff with extra training in ECLS to a independent team of ECLS specialists. In most programs, the latter approach is favored because the patient is totally dependent on the circuit, and someone needs to be on hand to respond to circuit emergencies within seconds. Improvements in technology to simplify the bedside system will make it possible for any ICU team to manage patients on extracorporeal support.

Clinical Results

The most recent data from the ELSO registry and the University of Michigan are shown in Table 21-1. Participation in the ELSO is voluntary, and yet, almost all patients treated with ECLS in established centers are included in the registry. There are now over 30,000 patients who have been managed with ECLS. Extensive data are available on gas exchange, perfusion, coagulation, and so on, but the only important outcome is survival at hospital discharge because this technique is applied only to patients who are not expected to survive otherwise. The indication for ECLS is a high risk (80–100%) of dying with continued conventional treatment. The mortality risk is quantified differently in different age groups.

TABLE 21-1 ECLS: Overall Survival results in ELSO Registry and University of Michigan, January 2005

Patients	ELSO REGISTRY		UNIVERSITY OF MICHIGAN	
	Number	Survival Percentage	Number	Survival Percentage
Neonatal				
Respiratory	19,463	77	701	84
Cardiac	2,518	39	136	46
Pediatric				
Respiratory	2,883	56	192	75
Cardiac	3,381	42	148	41
Adult				
Respiratory	1,025	53	266	54
Cardiac	638	33	147	39
Overall	29,908	66	1,590	72

Neonatal Respiratory Failure

The largest group of patients treated with ECLS are newborn infants in respiratory failure. There are only a few causes of severe respiratory failure in newborn infants. Survival for these diagnoses is 64–94% and 52% for congenital diaphragmatic hernia (Fig. 21-2). The reason for the excellent results is that respiratory failure in neonates does not destroy lung tissue. The primary pathophysiology in neonates is pulmonary hypertension with right-to-left shunting through the ductus arterious (persistent fetal circulation). During ECLS, the pulmonary vasculature relaxes, the ductus closes, and lung recovery occurs promptly. The problem in congenital diaphragmatic hernia is mechanical because the hernia compresses the lungs and causes lung hypoplasia in utero, in addition to pulmonary vasospasm. Hypoplastic lungs may be too small to support the infant.

The early neonatal ECMO patients are now adults with children of their own. There is abundant information on long-term follow-up. About 10% of survivors have some

FIGURE 21-2 Survival with use of extracorporeal life support in neonatal respiratory failure according to diagnosis. MAS, meconium aspiration syndrome; CDH, congenital diaphragmatic hernia; PPHN, persistent pulmonary hypertension in the neonate; RDS, respiratory distress syndrome.

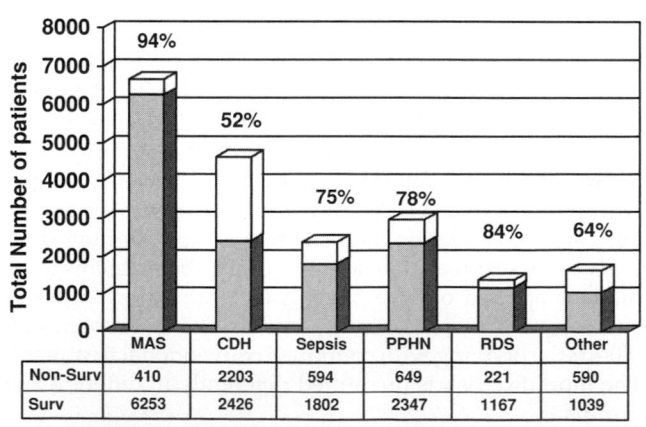

	MAS	CDH	Sepsis	PPHN	RDS	Other
Non-Surv	410	2203	594	649	221	590
Surv	6253	2426	1802	2347	1167	1039

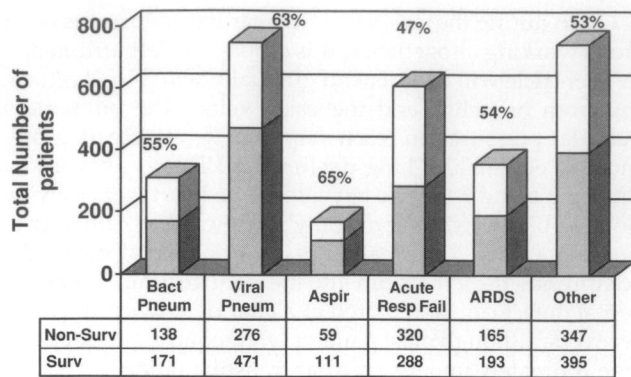

FIGURE 21-3 Survival with use of extracorporeal life support in pediatric patients with respiratory failure according to diagnosis.

	Bact Pneum	Viral Pneum	Aspir	Acute Resp Fail	ARDS	Other
Non-Surv	138	276	59	320	165	347
Surv	171	471	111	288	193	395

neurologic disability; the most common is some hearing loss. This is lower than the incidence of complications in critically ill infants not treated with ECLS, indicating that the complications are those of profound illness in the newborn.[18] The use of ECLS in neonatal respiratory failure has decreased after the introduction of nitric oxide inhalation for treating pulmonary hypertension.[19] At present, approximately 1000 patients per year are entered into the ELSO registry.

Pediatric Respiratory Failure

Severe respiratory failure in older children is relatively rare compared with the incidence in newborn infants and adults. The most common cause is viral or bacterial pneumonia. Status asthmaticus is another life-threatening problem in children. ECLS is used when a patient is not responding to other methods of management. The survival rate is approximately 55%, varying to some extent with the primary condition (Fig. 21-3). Most children with respiratory failure can be managed successfully with VV access. In children who do not survive, the most common cause of death is progressive lung destruction from the primary infection or brain damage from hypoxia and ischemia that preceded ECLS. These children are essentially all normal at follow-up. Specifically, once the lungs recover pulmonary function, exercise tolerance returns to normal.

Adult Respiratory Failure

ARDS is a primary pulmonary disorder in about half the patients (e.g., pneumonia and so on) and secondary to extrapulmonary causes in the rest (e.g., shock trauma, pancreatitis, and so on). Overall mortality for ARDS is 30–40% even with excellent management. ECLS is indicated for patients at high risk of mortality within the first 5 days of intubation. These patients are relatively easy to identify. They have an alveolar-arterial oxygen gradient of greater than 600 on the second to fourth day following initial intubation. The mortality risk is approximately 80%, and the recovery rate with ECLS in these patients is approximately 70%.[20–22] Patients

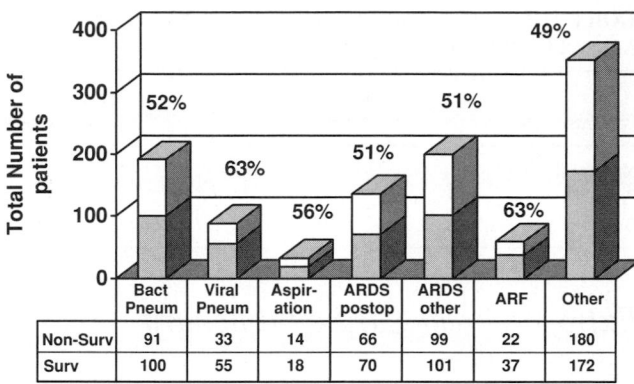

FIGURE 21-4 Survival with use of extracorporeal life support in patients with adult respiratory failure according to diagnosis.

TABLE 21-2 Extracorporeal Life Support for Cardiac Failure: Infant ELSO Registry, January 2005

Patients	Number	Survival Percentage
Posttransplantation	80	50
Other postoperative		
Not bridged	1263	40
Bridged	29	38
Not postoperative		
Not bridged	271	48
Bridged	27	44

on the ventilator for more than 5 days before ECLS have a lower chance of recovery. Hence the overall survival rate for ECLS treatment of ARDS is approximately 55%[23,24] (Fig. 21-4). The University of Michigan has reported the largest experience with ECLS for ARDS. In their series, overall survival was 52%.[23] A prospective, randomized trial of ECLS for ARDS is currently underway in the United Kingdom.[25]

Another important application for ECLS in children and adults is status asthmaticus. These patients are unresponsive to bronchodilators, intubation, ventilation, sedation, heliox, general anesthesia, and the other extreme measures. Pneumothorax occurs often and usually is fatal. Approximately 4000 patients die of acute asthma in the United States every year. This condition ideally is treated with ECLS. Simple VV cannulation and relatively low blood flow are all that are required to achieve normal CO_2 clearance and restore normal blood gases. Once this occurs, bronchospasm invariably clears within a day or two.[26] Because the risk of pneumothorax and death are significant, and because the risk of ECLS is low, ECLS should be considered in any patient who has a severe asthma attack with a Pa_{CO_2} of greater than 80 mmHg despite mechanical ventilation and other optimal treatment. When ECLS is used for status asthmaticus, the gas flow to the membrane lung is increased slowly over hours to avoid sudden changes in Pa_{CO_2} and pH.

Cardiac Failure: Children

VA ECLS is the only mechanical support system available for children in the United States. The experience with cardiac failure in children is listed in Tables 21-2 and 21-3. Most children treated with ECLS have cardiac failure following cardiac operation, usually for congenital heart disease. ECLS patients have myocardial injury from their primary disease or during cardiopulmonary bypass. These patients cannot be weaned off cardiopulmonary bypass in the operating room, or if they are weaned, they remain in profound cardiac failure despite full inotropic support. Patients who cannot be weaned from cardiopulmonary bypass are attached to the ECLS machine using the same catheters used for bypass, typically in the right atrium and aorta. If

the patient has been weaned off bypass and the chest is closed, vascular access is achieved by cannulation of the right internal jugular vein and right common carotid artery, as in newborn respiratory failure. This vascular access is also used for children with myocarditis or myocardiopathy. Because ECLS commonly is used directly after cardiopulmonary bypass, bleeding is a more common occurrence in cardiac patients than in respiratory patients. This is best managed by maintaining the chest open with a sterile plastic sheet over the open wound and with blood drainage tubes placed in the chest. In this manner, bleeding can be observed directly; it is easy to reexplore the chest, which frequently is required every 8–12 hours during the first day on ECLS. Bleeding is managed by maintaining the heparinization at very low levels (1.25 times the upper limit of normal ACT), maintaining platelet count above 100,000, and adding aprotinin to enhance platelet function and amicar to minimize fibrinolysis. A combination of amicar, aprotinin, and low-level heparinization can lead to thrombus formation in the extracorporeal circuit. It is important to keep a primed extracorporeal circuit available so that the perfusion circuit can be changed should clotting occur.

Generalized fluid overload is a common problem associated with cardiac failure in children. Diuresis is begun immediately with ECLS. If satisfactory negative fluid balance cannot be achieved with continuous infusion of diuretics, continuous hemofiltration is instituted.

When ECLS is used for cardiac support, pulmonary and left-ventricular blood flow decreases in proportion to the extracorporeal flow. As described earlier, this can lead to two problems. First, if the heart stops altogether, the left atrium and the left ventricle gradually distends, and bronchial venous blood produces high pulmonary venous pressures and

TABLE 21-3 Extracorporeal Life Support for Cardiac Failure in Children Aged 1–16 years ELSO Registry, January 2005

Patients	Number	Survival Percentage
Posttransplantation	160	51
Other postoperative		
Not bridged	786	40
Bridged	47	40
Not postoperative		
Not bridged	326	48
Bridged	115	55

pulmonary edema. This condition is diagnosed by the lack of pulsatility in the systemic arterial system. If the arterial pressure is nonpulsatile, VA flow is decreased gradually until pulsatility is established. If left-ventricular function is inadequate to maintain emptying of the left side of the heart, some system must be used to vent the left side of the heart, either direct catheterization of the left atrium or creation of an atrial-septal defect. Another problem with VA bypass in the totally failing heart is thrombosis in the left atrium or left ventricle. This can occur even during systemic heparinization. Thrombosis is diagnosed by echocardiography. If a patient has a left-atrial or left-ventricular thrombus, it is important to avoid spontaneous left-ventricular function because the thrombus can embolize and enter the systemic circulation. Usually these patients are candidates for left-ventricular assist devices or cardiac replacement, and the clot is removed before embolism occurs.

Cardiac Failure: Adults

The experience with ECLS for cardiac failure in adults is listed in Table 21-4. The most common indication is acute cardiac failure following myocardial infarction or cardiac surgery. Vascular access usually is achieved by cannulation of the right atrium via the right internal jugular vein, and arterial return is retrograde via the femoral artery. If function is severely impaired, it may be necessary to use the system of VAV access described earlier.

Intra-aortic balloon pumping is possible in adults and will support approximately 40% of cardiac output. Most patients treated with ECLS have already failed balloon pumping and full inotropic support. If a balloon pump is in place through a femoral artery, it is best to keep it in place because of the risk of bleeding after pump removal. The contralateral femoral artery is used for arterial access.

Adult patients in acute cardiac failure are candidates for a left-ventricular assist device as a bridge to recovery or to transplantation. In acute cardiac failure, however, it is best to institute ECLS first to stabilize the circulation and gas exchange and to determine if other organs are functioning, especially the brain. If severe brain injury has occurred during the period of acute cardiac failure, ECLS is discontinued, thus avoiding futile thoracotomy and the expense of the left-ventricular assist device. Survival for ECLS in adult cardiac failure is 40–50%.[27–29]

TABLE 21-4   Extracorporeal Life Support for Cardiac Failure in Adults, ELSO Registry, January 2005

Patients	Number	Survival Percentage
Posttransplant	79	32
Other postoperative		
Not bridged	278	31
Bridged	22	50
Not postoperative		
Not bridged	167	32
Bridged	25	36

TABLE 21-5   Extracorporeal Life Support as Resuscitation Adjunct (ECPR), ELSO Registry, 2005

Patients	Number	Survival Percentage
Neonatal	174	41
Pediatric	322	39
Adult	139	37

Extracorporeal Cardiopulmonary Resuscitation

ECLS can be used in association with resuscitation to support cardiac and pulmonary function in cases of cardiac arrest or profound shock. For this application, the ECLS circuit must be primed and available within minutes. Hence extracorporeal cardiopulmonary resuscitation (ECPR) is used primarily in established ECLS centers that have the equipment and a team to institute ECLS at a moment's notice. The limiting factor in establishing ECLS is vascular access. It is difficult to achieve rapid arterial and venous access in a patient in cardiac arrest. Successful ECPR has occurred mostly in patients who arrested and were resuscitated briefly, in whom simple vascular access had been gained following initial resuscitation. The ECLS catheters can be placed through smaller catheters if and when the patient arrests again or proceeds to cardiogenic shock or intractable arrhythmias. At the University of Michigan Hospitals, we consider ECPR for patients who have been in cardiac arrest for less than 5 minutes. A few patients who arrested and received full resuscitation for over an hour have been treated successfully. If the arrest is prolonged and profound metabolic acidosis exists, establishing ECLS is often futile. Overall healthy survival after ECPR is approximately 40%, much better than the 5% success rate of external massage[30,31] (Table 21-5).

Other Applications of ECLS

The ability to totally control perfusion and gas exchange with an extracorporeal system offers unique opportunities. Profound hypothermia can be treated. This is particularly important because hypothermic patients may develop ventricular fibrillation during external warming. Hypothermia associated with exsanguinating hemorrhage in the operating room can be treated successfully with ECLS.[32] Perfusion is maintained until bleeding is controlled, and hypothermia can be maintained to protect organ function. Blood then is returned to the patient to avoid the coagulopathy caused by low temperature. With a heat exchanger, hyperthermic perfusion also can be established either for total-body warming or for regional warming as an adjunct to cancer chemotherapy.

Septic shock was once considered a contraindication to ECLS. Sepsis often clears during ECLS, however, and this has become a standard indication in our institution. It is common for patients in septic shock to regain normal vascular tone and to come off all vasopressors within a day or two of instituting ECLS.[33] This is partly related to establishing normal perfusion and gas exchange and partly related to adsorption of inflammatory mediators by the plastic in the circuit.

ECLS also has been applied in potential organ donors, in particular following cardiac arrest subsequent to elective withdrawal of ventilator support.[34]

Conclusions

ECLS can sustain cardiac and pulmonary function by mechanical means in patients with profound cardiac or respiratory failure. This technology centers on extracorporeal vascular access, perfusion devices, and management of anticoagulation. ECLS does not treat cardiac or pulmonary failure but offers hours or days to establish a diagnosis and allow time for organ recovery or replacement. Overall success is measured in survival because ECLS is used only in patients at high risk of dying from acute heart or lung failure. Survival ranges between 95% in some patients with newborn respiratory failure to 40% with use of ECLS as an adjunct to cardiac resuscitation.

It is tempting to blame the failure of any new treatment, as occurred in the adult ECMO study, on device/concept failure. Performance of newborn ECMO has been precisely evaluated in terms of O_2 delivery and CO_2 removal and has achieved uniformly outstanding results. In the adult ECMO study, however, recovery of respiratory status and survival did not significantly differ from patients treated by traditional means.[13] Indeed, peak airway pressure in the ECMO group did not differ much from that in the control group. The findings of this study remained highly disturbing; ECMO did not buy the time for lungs to heal.

It has been shown in rats[35] and sheep[36,37] that healthy lungs can be severely injured by mechanical ventilation with high peak airway pressures as low as 30 cmH$_2$O. Recently, lung injury was induced at peak airway pressures as low as 25 cmH$_2$O.[38] The uniform increase in total static lung compliance over the first 12 hours of mechanical ventilation in sheep is deceptive. The increase in compliance was a harbinger of overdistension, which led to progressive decrease in functional residual capacity over the ensuing hours and days and impaired gas exchange. Ventilator-induced lung injury in patients also may be masked by early improvement in gas exchange.

It is disappointing to note how little survival from severe ARDS with or without ECMO has improved over the years.[39,40] One possible cause is the need for prolonged tracheal intubation. It is probable that new knowledge emerging from the research laboratory will improve our understanding of how to manage patients with acute respiratory failure and also will lead to improvement of extracorporeal membrane lung gas exchange with enhanced survival.

References

1. Gibbon JH Jr. Artificial maintenance of circulation during experimental occlusion of pulmonary artery. Arch Surg 1937; 34:1105–31.
2. Gibbon JH. Application of a mechanical heart and lung apparatus to cardiac surgery. Minn Med 1954; 37:171–80.
3. Dennis C. A heart lung machine for open-heart operation: How it came about. ASAIO Trans 1989: 35:767–77.
4. Lee WH Jr, Krumhar D, Fonkalsrud EW, et al. Denaturation of plasma proteins as a cause of morbidity and death after intracardiac operations. Surgery 1961; 50:29–39.
5. Dobell ARC, Mitri M, Galva R, et al. Biological evaluation of blood after prolonged recirculation through film and membrane oxygenators. Ann Surg 1965; 161:617–22.
6. Clowes GHA, Hopkins AL, Kolobow T. Oxygen diffusion through plastic films. Trans Am Soc Artif Intern Organs 1955; 1:23–4.
7. Kammermeyer K. Silicone rubber as a selective barrier: Gas and vapor transfer. Ind Eng Chem 1957; 49:1685–6.
8. Kolobow T, Bowman RL. Construction and evaluation of an alveolar membrane artificial heart-lung. ASAIO Trans 1963; 238–43.
9. Gille JP, Trudell L, Snider MT, et al. Capability of the micropourous, membrane-lined, capillary oxygenator in hypercapnic dogs. Trans Am Soc Artif Intern Organs 1970; 16:365–71.
10. Hill JD, O'Brien TG, Murray JJ, et al. Extracorporeal oxygenation for acute post traumatic respiratory failure (shock-lung syndrome): Use of the Bramson membrane lung. New Engl J Med 1972; 286:629–34.
11. Schulte HD. Membrane oxygenators in prolonged assisted extracorporeal circulation. Dtsch Med Wochenschr 1973; 98:508–13.
12. Kolobow T, Stool E, Sacks K, Vurek GG. Acute respiratory failure: Survival following ten days support with membrane lung. J Thorac Cardiovasc Surg 1975; 69:947–53.
13. National Heart Lung and Blood Institute, National Institutes of Health. Extracorporeal support for respiratory insufficiency. Bethesda, MD: Department of Health, Education and Welfare, 1980.
14. Extracorporeal Life Support Organization. Ann Arbor, Michigan.
15. German JD, Worcester C, Gazzaniga AB, et al. Technical aspects in the management of the meconium aspiration syndrome with extracorporeal circulation. J Pediatr Surg 1980; 15:378–83.
16. Anderson HL, Otsu T, Chapman RA, Bartlett RH. Venovenous extracorporeal life support in neonates using a double lumen catheter. Trans ASAIO 1989; 35:650–3.
17. Rich PB, Awad SS, Crotti S, et al. A prospective comparison of atrial-femoral and femora-atrial flow in adult venovenous extracorporeal life support. J Thorac Cardiovasc Surg 1998; 116:628–32.
18. Rais-Bahrami K, Wagner AE, Coffman C, et al. Neurodevelopmental outcome in ECMO vs near-miss ECMO patients at 5 years of age. Clin Pediatr 2000; 39:145–52.
19. Inhaled nitric oxide in term and near-term infants: Neurodevelopmental follow-up of the neonatal inhaled nitric oxide study group (NINOS). J Pediatr 2000; 136:611–7.
20. Peek GJ, Moore HM, Sosnowski AW, et al. Extracorporeal membrane oxygenation for adult respiratory failure. Chest 1997; 112:759–64.
21. Ullrich R, Lorber C, Roder G, et al. Controlled airway pressure therapy, nitric oxide inhalation, prone position, and extracorporeal membrane oxygenation (ECMO) as components of an integrated approach to ARDS. Anesthesiology 1999; 91:1577–86.
22. Linden V, Palmer K, Reinhard J, et al. High survival in adult patients with acute respiratory distress syndrome treated by extracorporeal membrane oxygenation, minimal sedation, and pressure supported ventilation. Intensive Care Med 2000; 26:1630–7.

23. Hemmila MR, Rowe SA, Boules TN, et al. Extracorporeal life support for severe acute respiratory syndrome in adults. Ann Surg 2004; 240:595–605.

24. Lewandowski K, Rossaint R, Pappert D, et al. High survival rate in 122 ARDS patients managed according to a clinical algorithm including extracorporeal membrane oxygenation. Intensive Care Med 1997; 23:819–35.

25. Conventional ventilation or ECMO for severe adult respiratory failure. Available at *www.cesar-trial.org/*; accessed April 12, 2004.

26. Shapiro MB, Kleaveland AC, Bartlett RH. Extracorporeal life support for status asthmaticus. Chest 1993; 103:1651–4.

27. Pagani FD, Aaronson KD, Dyke DB, et al. Assessment of an extracorporeal life support LVAD bridge to heart transplant strategy. Ann Thorac Surg 2000; 70:1977–984; discussion 1984–5.

28. Muehreke DD, McCarthy PM, Stewart RW, et al. Extracorporeal membrane oxygenation for postcardiotomy cardiogenic shock. Ann Thorac Surg 1996; 61:684–91.

29. Magovern GJ, Simpson KA. Extracorporeal membrane oxygenation for adult cardiac support: The Allegheny experience. Ann Thorac Surg 1999; 68:655–61.

30. Younger JG, Schreiner RJ, Swaniker F, et al. Extracorporeal resuscitation of cardiac arrest. Acad Emerg Med 1999; 6:700–7.

31. Massetti M, Tasle M, LePage O, et al. Back from irreversibility: Extracorporeal life support for prolonged cardiac arrest. Ann Thorac Surg 2005; 79:178–83.

32. Hines M, Pranikoff T. Personal communication, 2004.

33. Rich PB, Younger J, Soldes OS, et al. The use of extracorporeal life support for adult patients with respiratory failure and sepsis. ASAIO J 1998; 44:263–6.

34. Magliocca JF, Magee JC, Rowe SA, et al. Extracorporeal support for organ donation after cardiac death safely expands the donor pool. J Trauma (in press).

35. Dreyfuss D, Basset G, Soler P, Saumon G. High inflation pressure pulmonary edema: Respective effects of high airway pressure, high tidal volume, and positive end-expiratory pressure. Am Rev Respir Dis 1988; 137:1159–64.

36. Kolobow T, Moretti MP, Fumagalli D, et al. Severe impairment in lung function induced by peak airway pressure during mechanical ventilation. Am Rev Respir Dis 1987; 135:312–5.

37. Tsuno K, Prato P, Kolobow T. Acute lung injury from mechanical ventilation at moderately high airway pressure. J Appl Physiol 1990; 69:956–61.

38. Berra L, De Marchi L, Curto F, et al. Adverse changes in lungs of sheep ventilated for 72 hours at a moderately high peak inspiratory pressure and prolonged inspiratory time. Am J Respir Crit Care Med 2004; 7:A785.

39. Lee WL, Slutsky AS. Ventilator induced lung injury and recommendations for mechanical ventilation of patients with ARDS. Semin Respir Crit Care Med 2001; 22;269–80.

40. Brower RG, Matthay MA, Morris A, et al. Ventilation with lower tidal volumes for acute lung injury and the acute respiratory distress syndrome. The Acute Respiratory Distress Syndrome Network. New Engl J Med 2000; 342;1301–308.

Chapter 22

EXTRACORPOREAL CARBON DIOXIDE REMOVAL

ANTONIO PESENTI
LUCIANO GATTINONI
MICHELA BOMBINO

Artificial Organs for Respiratory Failure

Extracorporeal carbon dioxide removal (ECCO$_2$R) refers to a technique of extracorporeal life support focused on the removal of CO$_2$ from blood rather than improving blood oxygenation.[1] In this chapter we introduce the concept of ECCO$_2$R and discuss some of the experience and future perspectives on this exciting topic. ECCO$_2$R has been developed mainly with a view to applying it in patients with the most severe form of acute respiratory distress (ARDS).[2] The possible role of ECCO$_2$R in the prevention of hyaline membrane disease[3] or in the treatment of severe asthma[4–8] or multiple bronchopleural fistulas[9] remains experimental or anecdotal.

The mainstay of supportive treatment in ARDS is mechanical ventilation, a lifesaving procedure introduced in the management of patients with bulbar polio in the great epidemic that struck Copenhagen in 1952. These patients, paralyzed by polio, required long-term artificial ventilation[10]; they became the first critical-care patients. The use of mechanical ventilators later was extended to all pa-

tients with severe acute respiratory failure, whose main problem often was altered gas exchange and not respiratory muscle weakness or paralysis. The critical-care profession witnessed both the pros and cons of optimizing gas exchange through use of the ventilator: The focus shifted from high to low tidal volumes, from high to low airway pressures, and from high to lower inspired oxygen fractions (F$_{I_{O_2}}$). It is provocative to consider how we support the failing lung. In ARDS, we use an artificial organ (the ventilator), which is designed to substitute for the respiratory muscles rather than to act as a gas exchanger. Technology has been the limiting factor for a widespread application of artificial gas exchange,[11] but research and development continues at a promising pace.

MEMBRANE OXYGENATORS, MEMBRANE GAS EXCHANGE, AND MEMBRANE LUNGS

Extracorporeal oxygenation was first provided as a heart-lung machine to render major cardiovascular surgery feasible and safe.[12] The first oxygenators were based on bubbling of oxygen through the blood or filming of blood in an oxygen atmosphere. To avoid the problems caused by the direct contact between blood and gas,[13,14] Kolff designed a membrane oxygenator,[15] which Clowes[16] and Kolobow[17] developed further into clinically applicable membrane gas exchangers.[18–20] Attention was focused on extracorporeal oxygenation, and the term *extracorporeal membrane oxygenation* (ECMO) was coined. Very little attention was paid to concurrent CO$_2$ removal: Hypocapnia was recognized as a common annoyance to be prevented by adding CO$_2$ to the gas ventilating the oxygenator.

PIONEERS

In 1967, Ashbaugh et al[21] described ARDS. Soon this became a very common diagnosis in critical care, and mechanical ventilation moved to center stage as the main supportive therapy.[22] To optimize oxygenation, tidal volumes of 10–15 ml/kg were recommended. The high minute volumes often required the addition of dead space to avoid hypocapnia. Recommended levels of positive end-expiratory pressure (PEEP) ranged from 5–60 cmH$_2$O.[23,24] With these ventilator settings, patients with ARDS experienced high inspiratory pressures and gross disruption of lung parenchyma. Barotrauma was common.[25–27] In 1972, Hill et al[28] published the first successful ECMO application in a patient with ARDS. Over the next few years, 217 patients with acute respiratory failure were supported with ECMO.[29] In 1973, a group of pioneers initiated a National Institutes of Health (NIH)–sponsored randomized trial of ECMO in severe ARDS. The entry criteria (Table 22-1) were intended to enroll a population with a 70% mortality rate. In fact, final mortality was 90% in both the control and ECMO groups.[30] The NIH-ECMO study proved that long-term extracorporeal life support was feasible, but it did not show any benefit on survival. Consequently, adult ECMO almost stopped,[31] with the exception of a few centers, such as the one where Bartlett (see Chapter 21), conducted innovative studies on extracorporeal life support in infants and adults.

TABLE 22-1   ECMO Entry Criteria: $Pa_{O_2} \leq 50$ mmHg (Repeated Three Times)

Study Entry Speed	Entry Testing Period, h	$F_{I_{O_2}}$	PEEP, cmH_2O	$^aQs/Qt$	Pa_{CO_2} mmHg	ICU Care Duration Before Entry Testing, h
Rapid	2	1.0	≥5	—	30–45	—
Slow	12	≥0.6	≥5	≥0.3	30–45	≥48

ECMO EXCLUSIONS

Contraindication to anticoagulation (e.g., gastrointestinal
   bleeding, recent cerebrovascular accident, chronic bleeding
   disorder
Pulmonary artery wedge pressure >25 mmHg
Mechanical ventilation >21 days
Severe chronic systemic disease or another clinical condition that
   in itself greatly limits survival, for example,
     Irreversible central nervous system disease
     Severe chronic pulmonary disease ($^bFEV_1$
       <1 liter, $FEV_1/^cFVC$ <30% of predicted, chronic Pa_{CO_2}
       >45 mmHg, chest x-ray evidence of overinflation or
       interstitial infiltration, previous hospitalization for
       chronic respiratory insufficiency)
     Total body surface burns >40%
     Rapidly fatal malignancy
     Chronic left-ventricular failure
     Chronic renal failure
     Chronic liver failure

$^aQs/Qt$ = right-to-left shunt fraction.
$^bFEV_1$ = forced expiratory volume in 1 s.
^cFVC = forced vital capacity.
SOURCE: From Zapol et al.[30] and NHLBI.[83]

Meanwhile, astute observers pondered the question: Why did the NIH-ECMO study fail?[32]

WHY DID THE NIH-ECMO STUDY FAIL?

ECMO was aimed at buying time for the lung to rest and heal.[33] This could not be achieved under the persisting damage caused by high tidal volumes and pressures, however. Lung management in the ECMO group was not much different from that in the control group; this fact could explain the similarities in survival.[32] The choice of a venoarterial bypass, aimed in part at lowering pulmonary blood flow and pulmonary artery pressure, might have contributed to severe maldistribution of pulmonary blood flow. In turn, this might have deprived the lungs of enough blood flow to defend against the damage of high-tidal-volume, high-pressure ventilation.[34]

The Concept of $ECCO_2R$

In 1976, Kolobow et al[1] noted that membrane oxygenators more appropriately constituted membrane lungs than just oxygenators. They observed that a membrane lung can exchange CO_2 much more easily than it can oxygenate blood. They explored the potential of $ECCO_2R$ in a series of innovative experiments.

Dissociating Respiratory Functions

Blood oxygenation and CO_2 removal take place through different mechanisms.[35] When normal venous blood reaches the lungs, its mixed venous oxygen tension (Pv_{O_2}) is typically 47 mmHg, and Pv_{CO_2} is 43 mmHg (Fig. 22-1). Let's assume that oxygen consumption and CO_2 production

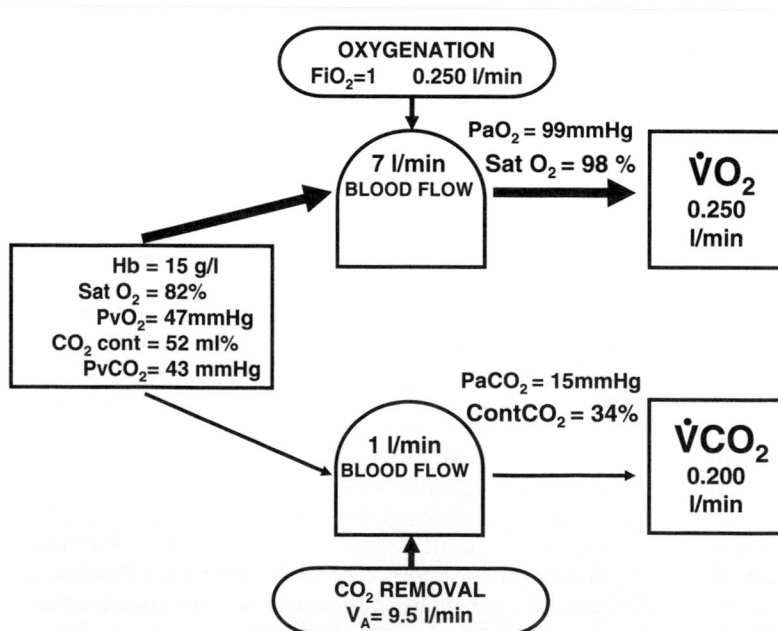

FIGURE 22-1 Dissociation of oxygenation and CO_2 removal. For normal mixed venous blood (v), oxygenation requires normal pulmonary blood flow and a continuous O_2 supply equal to O_2 consumption (250 ml/min in this example) without any ventilation. Removal of CO_2 can be accomplished by a reduced pulmonary blood flow if this is matched by a sufficiently high alveolar ventilation. (*Reproduced, with permission, from Gattinoni et al: Int Anesthesiol Clin 21:97–117, 1983.*)

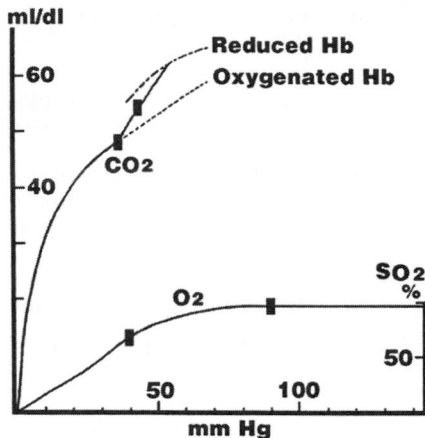

FIGURE 22-2 Gas dissociation curves for O_2 and CO_2 in blood. The solid rectangles represent arterial and mixed venous blood points. The line connecting the CO_2 dissociation curves for reduced and oxygenated hemoglobin (Hb) represents the nominal in vivo CO_2 dissociation curve as mixed venous blood becomes oxygenated in the lung (Haldane effect).

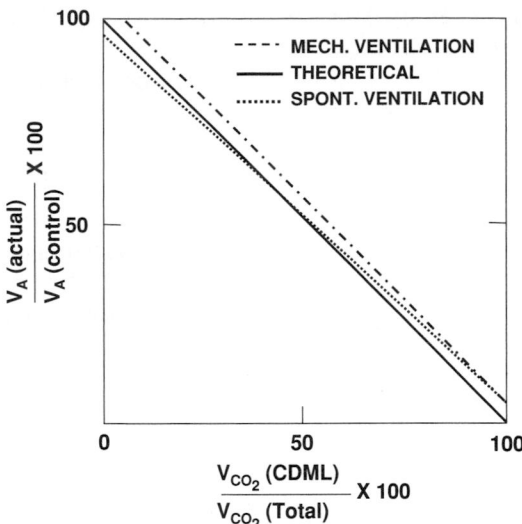

FIGURE 22-3 Alveolar ventilation (percent of control values) as a function of extracorporeal CO_2 removal [percent of total CO_2 production, i.e., V_{CO_2} of carbon dioxide membrane lung (CDML) plus natural lung]. The theoretical values are computed assuming that Pa_{CO_2} and total V_{CO_2} are constant throughout the procedure. (*Reproduced, with permission, from Gattinoni et al: Int Anesthesiol Clin 21:97–117, 1983.*)

amount to 250 and 200 ml/min, respectively. The hemoglobin carried in venous blood (150 g/liter) is normally 70–85% saturated; the lungs therefore can add just 40–60 ml of oxygen per liter of venous blood. Thus, to fulfill the requirements for oxygenation, we need a blood flow of at least 4–7 liters/min. Note that ventilation is not required to oxygenate blood, whereas what is strictly needed is enough oxygen to compensate for its consumption and maintain a constant alveolar concentration. In summary, oxygenation requires a high blood flow (4–7 liters/min) and a small supply of oxygen (250 ml/min). The opposite applies to CO_2 removal. Mixed venous CO_2 content is at least double the maximum O_2 content (Fig. 22-2). The normal CO_2 production per minute therefore can be removed easily from less than 1 liter of blood, provided that ventilation is high enough.

In conclusion, oxygenation requires a high blood flow, whereas CO_2 removal can be achieved at low blood flows. Kolobow et al[36] exploited the concept that if CO_2 is removed by a membrane lung through a low-flow, high-ventilation venovenous bypass, then oxygenation can be maintained by the natural lung without any ventilatory constraint. Physicians now had an opportunity to adjust the ventilator settings free of the constraints of tidal ventilation.

ECCO₂R and the Control of Spontaneous Breathing

When CO_2 was removed by the membrane lung, unsedated lambs decreased their spontaneous ventilation, reducing both respiratory frequency and tidal volume.[37] Changes in alveolar ventilation were highly predictable, targeted toward a constant pH and Pa_{CO_2}. The greater the removal of CO_2 by the membrane lung, the greater was the decrease in alveolar ventilation (Fig. 22-3). The amount of CO_2 excreted by the natural lung decreased to maintain the total CO_2 re-

moval (sum of membrane lung plus natural lung) constant and equal to the rate of CO_2 production by the body.

APNEIC OXYGENATION

When CO_2 production is entirely removed by a membrane lung, then ventilation is no longer needed. The lung can be kept motionless, provided the alveolar oxygen concentration is kept constant by continuously supplying oxygen to match the body's O_2 consumption.[36] This process, known as *apneic oxygenation*,[38] is otherwise normally limited by the CO_2 rise. In this case, an increase in CO_2 is avoided by the membrane lung. Apneic oxygenation therefore can be maintained at will by ECCO₂R: The lung can be kept completely motionless, the ultimate goal being lung rest and recovery.

LOW-FREQUENCY POSITIVE-PRESSURE VENTILATION

A decrease in respiratory compliance and functional residual capacity (FRC) was noticed during apneic oxygenation. This led to the introduction of low-frequency positive-pressure ventilation (LFPPV). LFPPV with ECCO₂R[39] is simply apneic oxygenation to which a few (deep) breaths per minute are added. The intent is to provide the physiologic role of sighs rather than remove CO_2. With LFPPV-ECCO₂R, respiratory compliance and FRC can be maintained at baseline for days or weeks.

ALVEOLAR P_{O_2} CONTROL DURING ECCO₂R

During ECCO₂R, the respiratory quotient (R), that is, the ratio of CO_2 removal from the natural lung to oxygen uptake, changes according to the amount of CO_2 removed by the

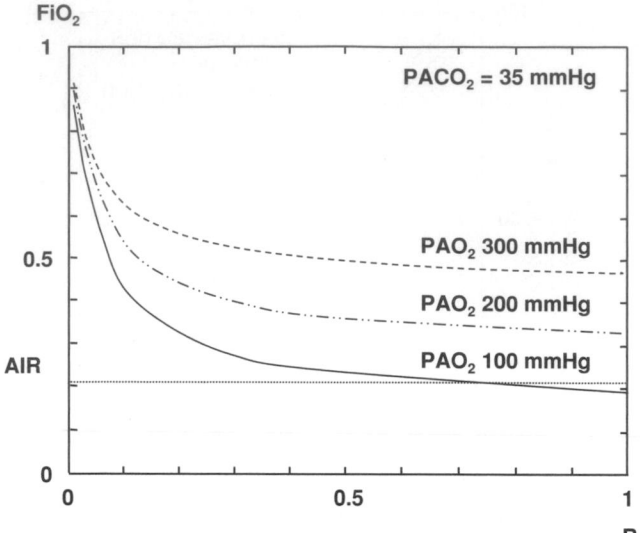

FIGURE 22-4 F_{IO_2} required to maintain a P_{AO_2} of 100, 200, and 300 mmHg at constant P_{ACO_2} as function of pulmonary respiratory quotient (R) according to Riley's alveolar air equation. (*Reproduced, with permission, from Gattinoni et al: Int Anesthesiol Clin 21:97–117, 1983.*)

TABLE 22-2   Natural (Patient) Lung Treatment and Goals: ECMO versus LFPPV-ECCO$_2$R

	ECMO[30]	LFPPV-ECCO$_2$R
	GOALS	
Ventilation	Minimize F_{IO_2}, TRADITIONAL VT	Minimize F_{IO_2}, LUNG REST
Extracorporeal circulation	Arterial Oxygenation	CO$_2$ removal (to rest he lung)
	TREATMENT	
Lung ventilation	VT = 0.6 liters Ppeak = 50 cmH$_2$O PEEP = 10 cmH$_2$O VR = 15/min	VT low Ppeak = 35–40 cmH$_2$O PEEP = 17 cmH$_2$O VR = 2–4/min
Lung perfusion	Low (0.1 Qt)	High (all Qt)

VT = tidal volume; VR = ventilator rate; Q$_t$ = cardiac output.

membrane lung. If baseline R equals 1, when we remove 50% of the body's CO$_2$ production by ECCO$_2$R, the new R of the natural lung will be 0.5. This affects alveolar oxygen tension (P_{AO_2}), which follows Riley's alveolar gas equation: At any given F_{IO_2}, when R decreases, P_{AO_2} decreases. Figure 22-4 shows the changes in F_{IO_2} required to maintain a constant P_{AO_2} at varying R values. Note that P_{aCO_2} is held constant through the effect of ECCO$_2$R.[35]

When ECCO$_2$R equals 100% of the CO$_2$ produced by the body, then alveolar ventilation is nil, and F_{IO_2} must be raised to 1 to compensate for oxygen consumption. This does not at all mean that the alveolar oxygen concentration must be 100%. At this extreme of physiology, the gas mixture ventilating the membrane lung is of the utmost importance. At a steady state and during apneic oxygenation, the only gas exchange taking place in the lung is oxygen consumption. No nitrogen, CO$_2$, or water exits or enters the alveolar gas. If the gas ventilating the membrane lung is 100% humidified oxygen, then alveolar gas will be 100% oxygen minus CO$_2$ and water. If nitrogen (N$_2$) is added to the gas ventilating the membrane lung, then mixed venous blood P_{N_2} will equilibrate with P_{N_2} of the gas in the membrane lung, causing a corresponding change in P_{AO_2}.[36] During apneic oxygenation, despite the need to keep F_{IO_2} at 1, P_{AO_2} will be determined by the P_{N_2} of gas in the membrane lung. The role of membrane lung P_{N_2} in preventing reabsorption atelectasis during ECCO$_2$R is entirely speculative but based on accepted physiology.[40]

Because of the Haldane effect, P_{aCO_2} (and P_{ACO_2}) will be higher than P_{vO_2} secondary to changes in the CO$_2$ dissociation curve related to the oxygenation of hemoglobin. During LFPPV-ECCO$_2$R, P_{AO_2} is mostly regulated by F_{IO_2}. If a continuous oxygen flow is added to compensate for oxygen consumption taking place between breaths, then many fac-

tors come into play. Experimental data exemplify the complexity of these mechanisms.[41]

Rationale for ECCO$_2$R Use

The goals of ECCO$_2$R are different from those of the 1974–1977 ECMO trial (Table 22-2). The reasons for these differences are rooted in ARDS pathophysiology. As already outlined, mechanical ventilation was developed by many workers[42–49] who pointed out how positive pressure and tidal volume interact in optimizing oxygenation. At the same time, however, the dangers and drawbacks of mechanical ventilation became apparent.[25] This was no surprise. Teplitz, a U.S. Army pathologist during the Vietnam war, described ARDS as "an end-stage pathologic picture which ... is not a new disease process ... but a result of iatrogenic modification of the pathology of noncardiogenic pulmonary edema." This view underlined the interaction between the original insult and the evolution and damages caused by treatment.[50]

Pontoppidan[47] suggested a tidal volume of 12–15 ml/kg as ideal for patients with ARDS. He also issued warnings[26,27] about the side effects of continuous positive-pressure ventilation and the appearance of lung damage related to high F_{IO_2}, high pressure, and high volumes.

In the late 1970s and early 1980s, the deleterious effects of mechanical ventilation were elucidated, and the concept of barotrauma evolved to that of volutrauma.[51,52] A third mechanism of damage was proposed later: the release of inflammatory mediators from the ventilated lung, leading eventually to multiple-organ failure and possibly death.[53–57] The term *ventilator-induced lung injury* (VILI) became popular. In the meantime, a revolutionary idea was gathering momentum: Why strive to maintain a normal P_{aCO_2} in patients with ARDS? Trying to achieve this goal can damage the lung severely, whereas accepting a higher than normal P_{aCO_2} may induce only minor side effects. In 1990, Hickling et al[58] reported that a better outcome could be achieved by lowering tidal ventilation and tolerating high P_{aCO_2} levels. They proposed the term *permissive hypercapnia,* indicating the price to be paid for limiting barotrauma. The targets of gas exchange in ARDS changed quickly.[59] A similar approach had been suggested previously for severe asthma.[60]

Several studies were performed to investigate the effects of lung-protective (low-pressure, low-tidal-volume) ventilation.[61–66] Only two studies[61,63] demonstrated benefit, but their effect has been striking. For the first time, the mode of ventilation was shown to affect outcome. One limitation with lung-protective ventilation, however, is hypercapnia. In selected patients, low-flow $ECCO_2R$ offers a very powerful tool for overcoming these limitations while offering total lung rest.

Hypoxemia, however, is the main characteristic of ARDS. Supportive therapy in ARDS is directed to its relief because hypoxemia is a major determinant of organ dysfunction and even may be the direct cause of death. Mechanical ventilation can be tailored to correct hypoxemia primarily by increasing F_{IO_2} and airway pressures.[67] Use of high airway pressure, however, is limited by several factors mainly related to hemodynamics and barotrauma. When PEEP is increased, then peak and plateau pressures also increase to maintain ventilation. The solution is often to decrease tidal volume and increase frequency; this solution culminates in the use of high-frequency ventilation or oscillation. With high-frequency oscillation, the mean airway pressure is in principle much higher than during positive-pressure ventilation. High-frequency ventilation has proven safe and effective in the treatment of adult patients with ARDS.[68,69] Use of high airway pressures, however, combined with inspiratory pressure limitation may lead to insufficient carbon dioxide removal.

In summary, the major aims of $ECCO_2R$ are to prevent barotrauma by avoiding the maldistribution of ventilation in a nonhomogeneous lung, to put the lung to rest, and to foster healing while maintaining a selected Pa_{CO_2}. In addition, $ECCO_2R$ enables the application of a constant mean airway pressure targeted to optimal oxygenation and free of the constraints dictated by tidal ventilation.

Clinical Applications: Venovenous Bypass

The main indication for $ECCO_2R$ is severe ARDS secondary to a potentially reversible cause. The main criteria are based on the original ECMO entry criteria, to which additional restrictions have been added over the years.[70,71] Generally accepted contraindications to extracorporeal life support and $ECCO_2R$ include the presence of significant bleeding, surgery in the preceding 72 hours, severe brain damage, uncontrolled severe sepsis, unresolved malignancies, severe chronic systemic disease, and ARDS of a known irreversible origin. The length of the preceding mechanical ventilation generally is not considered a contraindication to $ECCO_2R$.

BYPASS TECHNIQUE

In 1979, Gattinoni et al[2] reported the use of LFPPV-$ECCO_2R$ in an adult patient with ARDS. The technique involved venovenous bypass: The common femoral and jugular veins were cannulated both distally and centrally through surgical cutdowns. Blood was drained from the two femoral cannulas and from the distal jugular cannula, and it was returned centrally to the jugular vein. The wounds and the multiple cannulation involved continuous oozing of blood and limitations in nursing care and patient mobility.[72] Subsequently, we developed a double-lumen cannulation of the femoral vein that allowed a single cutdown.[73] With saphenosaphenous bypass,[74] surgery became very superficial, distal drainage was unnecessary, and access to the inferior vena cava was excellent. The number of cannulas therefore was reduced to two. The most significant improvement in cannulation, however, came with the spring-wire-reinforced percutaneous cannulas,[9,75,76] which were placed by a modified Seldinger technique.

The main advantages of percutaneous cannulation are a shorter procedure time, practically no bleeding, a reduced risk of cannulation-site infection, and very simple decannulation. When a roller pump is used, a small (100–250 ml) reservoir is placed in the drainage line; when it collapses, a servo control stops the pump. Blood is pumped through the membrane lung(s) and then returned to the patient; flow is normally kept at 15–30% of the patient's cardiac output. The system must have a capability of running at 50–60 ml/kg per minute should we need to substitute for the natural lung oxygenation (Fig. 22-5).

We have experience in using both roller pumps and Biomedicus centrifugal pumps, as well as Sci Med Kolobow spiral membrane lungs and Carmeda surface-heparinized[77,78] hollow-fiber membrane lungs. Our current standard includes the use of two spring-wire-reinforced percutaneous femoral cannulas (20–28F; Biomedicus), a Jostra centrifugal pump, and a plasma tight hollow-fiber polymethylpentene Quadrox D Jostra oxygenator. The entire circuit is surface heparinized (Bioline coating) to minimize the need for systemic anticoagulation.[79]

ANTICOAGULATION

Anticoagulation is achieved by 100 IU/kg intravenous heparin bolus at the time of cannulation. A heparin infusion is then started, aiming at the selected activated clotting time (ACT) (150–200 seconds in the case of Jostra Bioline surfaces). Surface-heparinized circuits can be run without any systemic anticoagulation[80] for at least 12–48 hours as needed to stop or prevent incidental bleeding. Because heparinized surfaces need a normal antithrombin III plasma level, we routinely infuse antithrombin III at a rate of 500–1000 U/day. Platelets are transfused when lower than $50,000/\mu l$. When heparinized surfaces are not in use, ACT and/or partial thromboplastin times (PTTs) of 1.5–2 times normal must be maintained at all times. In all instances, ACT is measured at least four times per day. A laboratory screen is ordered twice a day, including prothrombin time (PT), PTT, fibrinogen, platelet count, fibrinogen degradation product or equivalent, and antithrombin III. A continuous prostaglandin I_2 (PGI_2) infusion may be effective in both decreasing a high pulmonary artery pressure and preventing platelet aggregation.[81]

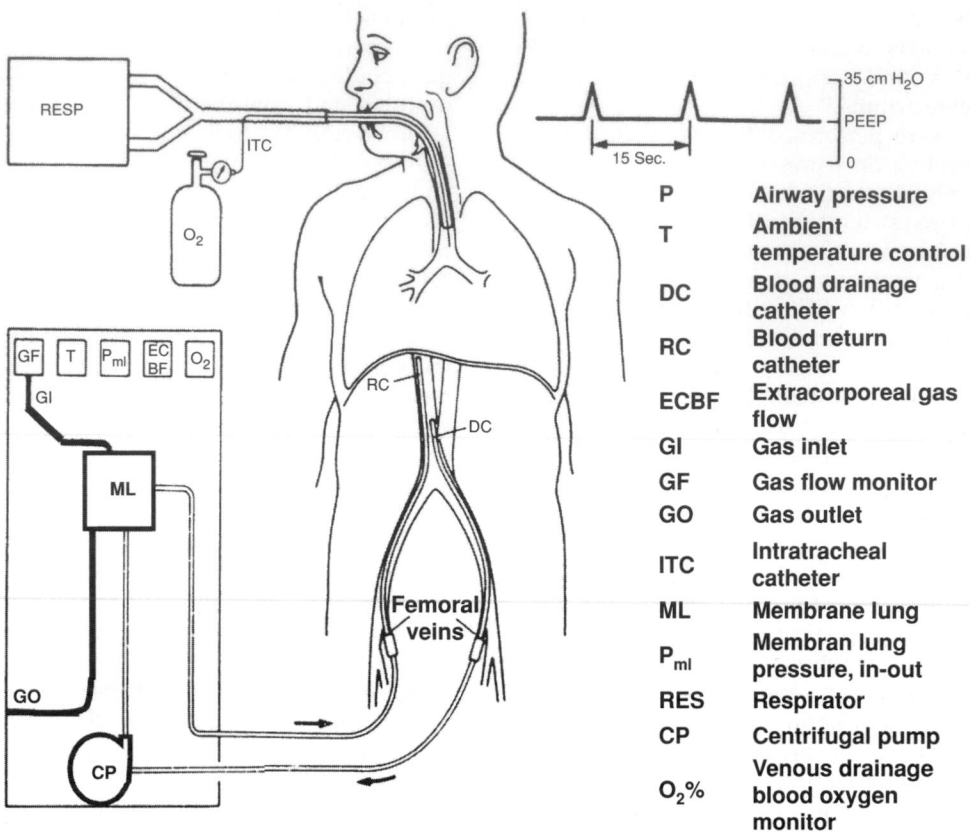

FIGURE 22-5 LFPPV-ECCO$_2$R circuit. (*Reproduced, with permission, from Gattinoni et al: JAMA 256:881–6, 1986.*)

CLINICAL MANAGEMENT

ECCO$_2$R normally is started in a sedated, paralyzed patient. After the initial adjustments (which normally take 1–2 hours), the ventilator is set to provide a low-frequency sigh over a baseline constant PEEP [e.g., using intermittent mandatory ventilation (IMV) or biphasic positive airway pressure (i.e., BiPAP)]. PEEP is adjusted to maintain mean airway pressure at the prebypass level and to prevent acute worsening of lung edema. A catheter inserted into the inspiratory line provides a constant O$_2$ supply and constant PEEP during the long expiratory pause. As soon as possible, attempts are made to reestablish spontaneous respiratory activity, most often in the form of pressure supported breathing with an intermittent sigh (e.g., BiPAP plus assisted breathing or IMV plus pressure support).

Hemodynamics are not affected by the venovenous bypass, and cardiac output can be measured by regular thermodilution. Changes in lung function can be followed with venous admixture measurements. Very high values of mixed venous saturation and arterial O$_2$ saturation suggest decreased cardiac output with an increased proportion of extracorporeal blood flow/total cardiac output. When lung function improves, weaning is attempted by decreasing FI$_{O_2}$ and PEEP and by decreasing the CO$_2$ removal from the membrane lung.[82] When necessary, the extracorporeal circuit setup allows low-flow venovenous ECCO$_2$R to be converted into high-flow venovenous ECMO, and management then is focused on achieving a viable oxygenation despite an extremely reduced or even absent natural-lung oxygen transfer.

COMPLICATIONS OF VENOVENOUS ECCO$_2$R

We have never stopped ECCO$_2$R because of a technical accident. From day to day, however, various changes of circuit elements may be required, mainly involving the membrane lung and/or the centrifugal pump(s).

Bleeding always has been the major complication with extracorporeal life-support techniques. The NIH-ECMO study reported an average blood-product transfusion of 3575 ml/day.[83] Half the 38 patients were managed in three of the nine participating centers; their average blood transfusion requirement was only 1896 ml/day, indicating that experience had a lot to do with blood loss. In 1986, we reported[84] an average blood-product requirement of 1.8 liters/day in our first 43 patients. The use of percutaneous cannulation coupled with heparinized surfaces decreased the packed-red-cell requirement to 200–300 ml/day.[71] Bleeding from the chest drainage tubes is a major complication that often demands a surgical approach.[85] We performed 17 thoracotomies or redo thoracotomies to control bleeding in 10 patients, of whom 4 survived.

The major threat posed by extracorporeal support remains intracranial hemorrhage. In our experience, this complication accounted for 26% of deaths. We reported that a prebypass Pa_{CO_2} of greater than 75 mmHg, disseminated intravascular coagulation, or a positive brain computed tomographic (CT) scan before bypass increase the risk of fatal intracranial hemorrhage during bypass.[71]

CLINICAL RESULTS

It is difficult to isolate from the literature the experience with venovenous $ECCO_2R$ because of undefined boundaries between venovenous $ECCO_2R$, venovenous ECMO, and partial extracorporeal CO_2 removal ($PECO_2R$).[82] $ECCO_2R$ refers more to a way of managing the diseased lung rather than to technical details, and the flexible handling of the circuitry is one of the advantages of $ECCO_2R$. We have suggested a minimum of three classification criteria[71]: type of bypass (venovenous versus venoarterial or arteriovenous), proportion of cardiac output pumped, and the ventilator regimen for the natural lung. The technique can shuttle back and forth between venovenous $ECCO_2R$, venovenous ECMO, and $PECO_2R$ in the same patient.

Table 22-3 is an attempt to collect the available experience on $ECCO_2R$, defined as such by authors, including our own data (see also Table 22-4). Survival ranges between 33% and 76%. Variation probably is explained by differences in selection criteria and in management of the patients supported by extracorporeal means. Selection criteria, although derived from the original ECMO entry criteria (see Table 22-1), have been modified over the years and among centers.[70] Our present, very restrictive criteria are based on the original ECMO criteria; in addition, we require a total static respiratory compliance of less than 30 ml/cmH$_2$O plus lack of improvement with PEEP, permissive hypercapnia, extravascular lung-water reduction, prone positioning, recruitment maneuvers, and nitric oxide inhalation.

Newer therapies and better understanding of ARDS pathophysiology not only have changed the criteria for $ECCO_2R$ but also have restricted it more and more to a last-ditch salvage role. Whether this is wise or not, we have our doubts. Patients are starting on $ECCO_2R$ later and later in their illness, and the time spent on bypass gets longer and longer (50 days for our longest survival run), probably indicating increases in unmeasured elements of disease severity at the time of connection. Despite these considerations, many patients with ARDS suffer from complications related to VILI and are doomed to an unfavorable outcome. ARDS carries a substantial mortality, 31–39.8% in the ARDS Network studies.[63]

TABLE 22-4 Outcome with $ECCO_2R$ in Milan-Monza

	Survivors	Non Survivors	p
No. Patients	46 (39%)	72 (61%)	
Age	31.9 ± 14.7	29.1 ± 15.2	NS
Days from intubation	12.5 ± 13.8	10.9 ± 7.5	NS
Qs/Qt[a]	0.46 ± 0.12	0.51 ± 0.11	0.0284
PaCO$_2$ mmHG	53.6 ± 16.2	63.2 ± 21.4	0.0117
PEEP cmH$_2$O	11.3 ± 5.1	13.5 ± 4.0	0.0104
Cardiac Index l/min	5.27 ± 1.62	5.04 ± 1.35	NS
Heart Rate bpm	134 ± 18	131 ± 20	NS
BP[b] mmHg	84.2 ± 14.9	79.4 ± 14.2	NS
CVP[c] cmH$_2$O	10.9 ± 5.4	11.4 ± 5.1	NS
PAP[d] mmHg	32.8 ± 8.2	35.3 ± 8.3	NS
WP[e] mmHg	12.6 ± 6.1	13.8 ± 5.0	NS
No receiving Vasopressor	2 (4%)	20 (28%)	0.0012
Days of $ECCO_2R$	13.8 ± 13.0	13.8 ± 13.3	NS

[a]Qs/Qt = intrapulmonary shunt.
[b]BP = arterial blood pressure, mean.
[c]CVP = central venous pressure.
[d]PAP = pulmonary artery pressure, mean.
[e]WP = pulmonary artery wedge pressure.

Only one controlled, randomized trial has been conducted on the effect of LFPPV-$ECCO_2R$ in patients with severe ARDS.[86] The investigators enrolled 40 patients meeting the original NIH-ECMO entry criteria. Nineteen patients were randomized to LFPPV-$ECCO_2R$ and 21 to control mechanical ventilation. Survival was equivalent in the two groups: 7 survivors in the $ECCO_2R$ and 8 in the control group. The investigators and accompanying editorialists[87] concluded that extracorporeal support is not recommended in ARDS.

A more balanced interpretation of this study, however, must take into account several considerations.[88–90] The incidence of uncontrollable bleeding, leading to premature interruption of the treatment in 7 of 19 patients, was extremely high. More surprisingly, of 7 $ECCO_2R$ survivors, 5 had been disconnected as an emergency because of severe bleeding. Average transfused blood products (packed red cells plus fresh-frozen plasma) was 3.39 liters/day (4.79 liters/day in the survivors). A problem in the management of blood clotting or the surgical procedure to control bleeding appears obvious when related to contemporary published experience. This study suggests that despite a high rate of catastrophic bleeding in the $ECCO_2R$ group, the net outcome was not worse in the $ECCO_2R$ group. As such,

TABLE 22-3 Veno-Venous ECCO2R for ARDS: International Experience

Author	Year	Center	No.[a]	Survivors	%Survival
Wagner (85)	1990	Marburg (Germany)	76	38	50%
Bindslev (78)	1991	Stockolm (Sweden)	14	6	43%
Brunet (103)	1993	Paris (France)	23	12	52%
Morris (86)	1994	Salt Lake City (USA)	21	7	33%
Guinard (104)	1997	Paris (France)	10	4	40%
Gattinoni, Pesenti	2004	Milan, Monza (Italy)	118	46	39%
Total			262	113	43%

[a]No = Number of patients.

$ECCO_2R$ may prove beneficial, provided that the associated bleeding problems are handled effectively.

Recent Clinical Developments: Arteriovenous Bypass

Venovenous $ECCO_2R$ still remains a complex procedure, reserved for centers with experience and capabilities to run it safely in very diseased patients. In an effort to simplify extracorporeal respiratory assist, Barthelemy et al[91] reported that an animal could be supported for up to 24 hours by a pumpless artery-to-vein extracorporeal system in combination with apneic oxygenation. Subsequently, Awad et al[92] demonstrated the feasibility of arteriovenous CO_2 removal ($AVCO_2R$) for up to 7 days in sheep. Young et al[93] evaluated $AVCO_2R$ in a femorofemoral arteriovenous (AV) model, both with and without a blood pump. A step forward in pumpless $AVCO_2R$ came with the design of very low-resistance membrane lungs.[94] A pumpless system is expected to minimize the foreign-surface interactions and blood-element shear stress.

$AVCO_2R$ [also termed *interventional lung assist* or *pumpless extracorporeal lung assist* (ECLA)] was studied in normal animals and in experimental lung-injury models.[95–98] Short-term feasibility and safety phase I trials were performed successfully in patients,[99] showing that an AV shunt coupled with a low-resistance membrane lung can achieve an $ECCO_2R$ between 70% and 100% of the total CO_2 production. Reng et al[100] published a collection of 10 patients treated by what they named "pumpless ECLA." In a second paper,[101] they reported a 60% survival rate in 20 patients with severe ARDS who fulfilled modified NIH-ECMO entry criteria. The technique included the use of 17–21F arterial cannulas and 19–21F venous cannulas. The membrane oxygenator was a modified Quadrox Jostra, and the entire circuit was surface heparinized. A third paper[102] from the same institution reports on 30 patients, with 50% mortality, and stresses the low costs and reduced personnel requirements of the pumpless technique.

AV bypass can be established quickly, it is simple, and it provides sufficient CO_2 removal to achieve complete apnea at normal or near-normal Pa_{CO_2} levels. The clinical application is limited to patients whose cardiovascular system can tolerate the increased cardiac output and whose arterial blood pressure can drive enough blood to achieve a sufficiently high CO_2 removal (shunt flows are 1–2.5 liters/min). While vasopressors can be added to increase shunt blood flow, no direct intervention is possible to otherwise regulate it. Lastly, $AVCO_2R$ consists of pure CO_2 removal: With the exception of extremely severe hypoxemia, the amount of oxygen that can be transferred to arterial blood can influence the systemic oxygenation only marginally. In contrast to venovenous $ECCO_2R$, no simple conversion to ECMO is possible. The technique is fascinating and promising in its extreme simplicity, however. Very low-resistance, surface-heparinized membrane lungs are now available for clinical use.[94]

Conclusions

$ECCO_2R$ is a fascinating approach to the management of respiratory failure and is a powerful tool for overcoming any ventilatory problem. In contrast with venoarterial ECMO, $ECCO_2R$ can be performed at comparatively low blood flows and with a relatively simple technique. In its purest conceptual application, $ECCO_2R$ is achieved by an arteriovenous pumpless shunt. For patients with the most severe form of ARDS, a venovenous circuit with the possibility of shifting to modern full venovenous ECMO (if needed) may be a better solution. Venovenous $ECCO_2R$ should be limited to centers where appropriate technical skills, motivations, personnel, and experience are available. The arteriovenous approach appears very promising, but experience is still limited; the simpler approach and the essential technology involved increase the feasibility of a formal prospective trial.

References

1. Kolobow T, Gattinoni L, Tomlinson T, et al. The carbon dioxide membrane lung (CDML): A new concept. Trans Am Soc Artif Intern Organs 1977; 23:17–21.
2. Gattinoni L, Kolobow T, Agostoni A, et al. Clinical application of low frequency positive pressure ventilation with extracorporeal CO_2 removal (LFPPV-$ECCO_2R$) in treatment of adult respiratory distress syndrome (ARDS). Int J Artif Organs 1979; 2:282–3.
3. Pesenti A, Kolobow T, Buckhold DK, et al. Prevention of hyaline membrane disease in premature lambs by apneic oxygenation and extracorporeal carbon dioxide removal. Intensive Care Med 1982; 8:11–7.
4. Sakai M, Ohteki H, Doi K, Narita Y. Clinical use of extracorporeal lung assist for a patient in status asthmaticus. Ann Thorac Surg 1996; 62:885–7.
5. Tajimi K, Kasai T, Nakatani T, Kobayashi K. Extracorgreal lung assist for patient with hypercapnia due to status asthmaticus. Intensive Care Med 1988; 14:588–9.
6. Kukita I, Okamoto K, Sato T, et al. Emergency extracorporeal life support for patients with near-fatal status asthmaticus. Am J Emerg Med 1997; 15:566–9.
7. Lukomskii GI, Alekseeva ME, Vaisberg LA, et al. [Extracorporeal elimination of CO_2 as a component of the intensive therapy of status asthmaticus]. Anestesiol Reanimatol 1990; 4:6–8.
8. Knoch M, Konder H, Holtermann W, et al. [Successful treatment of a most severe therapy-refractory status asthmaticus by extracorporeal CO_2 elimination]. Prax Klin Pneumol 1987; 41:187–90.
9. Pesenti A, Rossi GP, Pelosi P, et al. Percutaneous extracorporeal CO_2 removal in a patient with bullous emphysema with recurrent bilateral pneumothoraces and respiratory failure. Anesthesiology 1990; 72:571–3.
10. Trubuhovich RV. August 26, 1952 at Copenhagen: "Bjorn Ibsen's Day": A significant event for anaesthesia. Acta Anaesthesiol Scand 2004; 48:272–7.
11. Kolobow T. The artificial lung: The past. A personal retrospective. ASAIO J 2004; 50:xliii–viii.
12. Haworth WS. The development of the modern oxygenator. Ann Thorac Surg 2003; 76:S2216–9.
13. Dobell AR, Galva R, Sarkozy E, Murphy DR. Biologic evaluation of blood after prolonged recirculation through film and membrane oxygenators. Ann Surg 1965; 161:617–22.

14. Lee WH Jr, Krumhaar D, Fonkalsrud EW, et al. Denaturation of plasma proteins as a cause of morbidity and death after intracardiac operations. Surgery 1961; 50:29–39.

15. Effler DB, Groves LK, Kolff WJ, Sones FM Jr. Disposable membrane oxygenator (heart-lung machine) and its use in experimental surgery. J Thorac Surg 1956; 32:620–9.

16. Clowes GH Jr, Hopkins AL, Neville WE. An artificial lung dependent upon diffusion of oxygen and carbon dioxide through plastic membranes. J Thorac Surg 1956; 32:630–7.

17. Kolobow T, Bowman RL. Construction and evaluation of an alveolar membrane artificial heart-lung. Trans Am Soc Artif Intern Organs 1963; 9:238–43.

18. Lande AJ, Dos SJ, Carlson RG, et al. A new membrane oxygenator-dialyzer. Surg Clin North Am 1967; 47:1461–70.

19. Bramson ML, Osborn JJ, Main FB, et al. A new disposable membrane oxygenator with integral heat exchange. J Thorac Cardiovasc Surg 1965; 50:391–400.

20. Peirce EC. A modification of the Clowes membrane lung. J Thorac Cardiovasc Surg 1960; 39:438–48.

21. Ashbaugh DG, Bigelow DB, Petty TL, Levine BE. Acute respiratory distress in adults. Lancet 1967, 2:319–23.

22. Ashbaugh DG, Petty TL, Bigelow DB, Harris TM. Continuous positive-pressure breathing (CPPB) in adult respiratory distress syndrome. J Thorac Cardiovasc Surg 1969; 57:31–41.

23. Kirby RR, Downs JB, Civetta JM, et al. High level positive end expiratory pressure (PEEP) in acute respiratory insufficiency. Chest 1975; 67:156–63.

24. Gallagher TJ, Civetta JM. Goal-directed therapy of acute respiratory failure. Anesth Analg 1980; 59:831–4.

25. Kumar A, Pontoppidan H, Falke KJ, et al. Pulmonary barotrauma during mechanical ventilation. Crit Care Med 1973; 1:181–6.

26. Nash G, Blennerhassett JB, Pontoppidan H. Pulmonary lesions associated with oxygen therapy and artifical ventilation. New Engl J Med 1967; 276:368–74.

27. Sladen A, Laver MB, Pontoppidan H. Pulmonary complications and water retention in prolonged mechanical ventilation. New Engl J Med 1968; 279:448–53.

28. Hill JD, O'Brien TG, Murray JJ, et al. Prolonged extracorporeal oxygenation for acute post-traumatic respiratory failure (shocklung syndrome): Use of the Bramson membrane lung. New Engl J Med 1972; 286:629–34.

29. Gille JP. World census of long term perfusion for respiratory support. In: Zapol WM, Qvist J, editors. Artificial lungs for acute respiratory failure. New York: Academic Press, 1976: 513–24.

30. Zapol WM, Snider MT, Hill JD, et al. Extracorporeal membrane oxygenation in severe acute respiratory failure: A randomized, prospective study. JAMA 1979; 242:2193–6.

31. Zapol WM, Snider MT. Membrane lungs for acute respiratory failure: Current status. Am Rev Respir Dis 1980; 121:907–9.

32. Kolobow T, Solca M, Gattinoni L, Pesenti A. Adult respiratory distress syndrome (ARDS): Why did ECMO fail? Int J Artif Organs 1981; 4:58–9.

33. Zapol WM, Kitz RJ. Buying time with artificial lungs. New Engl J Med 1972; 286:657–8.

34. Kolobow T, Spragg RG, Pierce JE. Massive pulmonary infarction during total cardiopulmonary bypass in unanesthetized spontaneously breathing lambs. Int J Artif Organs 1981; 4:76–81.

35. Gattinoni L, Pesenti A, Kolobow T, Damia G. A new look at therapy of the adult respiratory distress syndrome: Motionless lungs. Int Anesthesiol Clin 1983; 21:97–117.

36. Kolobow T, Gattinoni L, Tomlinson T, Pierce JE. An alternative to breathing. J Thorac Cardiovasc Surg 1978; 75:261–6.

37. Kolobow T, Gattinoni L, Tomlinson TA, Pierce JE. Control of breathing using an extracorporeal membrane lung. Anesthesiology 1977; 46:138–41.

38. Frumin MJ, Epstein RM, Cohen G. Apneic oxygenation in man. Anesthesiology 1959; 20:789–98.

39. Gattinoni L, Kolobow T, Tomlinson T, et al. Low-frequency positive pressure ventilation with extracorporeal carbon dioxide removal (LFPPV-ECCO$_2$R): An experimental study. Anesth Analg 1978; 57:470–7.

40. West JB. State of the art: Ventilation-perfusion relationships. Am Rev Respir Dis 1977; 116:919–43.

41. Peters J, Radermacher P, Pesenti A, et al. Tracheal and alveolar gas composition during low-frequency positive pressure ventilation with extracorporeal CO$_2$ removal (LFPPV-ECCO$_2$R). Intensive Care Med 1985; 11:213–7.

42. Falke KJ, Pontoppidan H, Kumar A, et al. Ventilation with end-expiratory pressure in acute lung disease. J Clin Invest 1972; 51:2315–23.

43. Kumar A, Falke KJ, Geffin B, et al. Continuous positive-pressure ventilation in acute respiratory failure. New Engl J Med 1970; 283:1430–6.

44. Kumar A, Falke KJ, Geffin B, et al. Hemodynamics and lung function during continuous positive pressure ventilation (CPPV) in acute respiratory failure. Nord Med 1970; 84:1637.

45. Suter PM, Fairley B, Isenberg MD. Optimum end-expiratory airway pressure in patients with acute pulmonary failure. New Engl J Med 1975; 292:284–9.

46. Suter PM, Fairley HB, Isenberg MD. Effect of tidal volume and positive end-expiratory pressure on compliance during mechanical ventilation. Chest 1978; 73:158–62.

47. Pontoppidan H, Geffin B, Lowenstein E. Acute respiratory failure in the adult, part 3. New Engl J Med 1972; 287:799–806.

48. Pontoppidan H, Geffin B, Lowenstein E. Acute respiratory failure in the adult, part 2. New Engl J Med 1972; 287:743–52.

49. Pontoppidan H, Geffin B, Lowenstein E. Acute respiratory failure in the adult, part 1. New Engl J Med 1972; 287:690–8.

50. Teplitz C. The core pathobiology and integrated medical science of adult acute respiratory insufficiency. Surg Clin North Am 1976; 56:1091–133.

51. Kolobow T, Moretti MP, Fumagalli R, et al. Severe impairment in lung function induced by high peak airway pressure during mechanical ventilation: An experimental study. Am Rev Respir Dis 1987; 135:312–5.

52. Dreyfuss D, Saumon G. Ventilator-induced lung injury: Lessons from experimental studies. Am J Respir Crit Care Med 1998; 157:294–323.

53. Ranieri VM, Giunta F, Suter PM, Slutsky AS. Mechanical ventilation as a mediator of multisystem organ failure in acute respiratory distress syndrome. JAMA 2000; 284:43–4.

54. Ranieri VM, Suter PM, Tortorella C, et al. Effect of mechanical ventilation on inflammatory mediators in patients with acute respiratory distress syndrome: A randomized, controlled trial. JAMA 1999; 282:54–61.

55. Plotz FB, Slutsky AS, van Vught AJ, Heijnen CJ. Ventilator-induced lung injury and multiple system organ failure: A critical review of facts and hypotheses. Intensive Care Med 2004; 30:1865–72.

56. Dos Santos CC, Slutsky AS. Invited review. Mechanisms of ventilator-induced lung injury: A perspective. J Appl Physiol 2000; 89:1645–55.

57. Tremblay LN, Slutsky AS. Ventilator-induced injury: From barotrauma to biotrauma. Proc Assoc Am Phys 1998; 110:482–8.

58. Hickling KG, Henderson SJ, Jackson R. Low mortality associated with low volume pressure limited ventilation with permissive hypercapnia in severe adult respiratory distress syndrome. Intensive Care Med 1990; 16:372–7.

59. Pesenti A. Target blood gases during ARDS ventilatory management. Intensive Care Med 1990; 16:349–51.

60. Darioli R, Perret C. Mechanical controlled hypoventilation in status asthmaticus. Am Rev Respir Dis 1984; 129:385–7.

61. Amato MB, Barbas CS, Medeiros DM, et al. Effect of a protective-ventilation strategy on mortality in the acute respiratory distress syndrome. New Engl J Med 1998; 338:347–54.

62. Stewart TE, Meade MO, Cook DJ, et al. Evaluation of a ventilation strategy to prevent barotrauma in patients at high risk for acute respiratory distress syndrome. Pressure- and Volume-Limited Ventilation Strategy Group. New Engl J Med 1998; 338:355–61.

63. Ventilation with lower tidal volumes as compared with traditional tidal volumes for acute lung injury and the acute respiratory distress syndrome. The Acute Respiratory Distress Syndrome Network. New Engl J Med 2000; 342:1301–8.

64. Brower RG, Lanken PN, MacIntyre N, et al. Higher versus lower positive end-expiratory pressures in patients with the acute respiratory distress syndrome. New Engl J Med 2004; 351:327–36.

65. Brochard L, Roudot-Thoraval F, Roupie E, et al. Tidal volume reduction for prevention of ventilator-induced lung injury in acute respiratory distress syndrome. The Multicenter Trail Group on Tidal Volume reduction in ARDS. Am J Respir Crit Care Med 1998; 158:1831–8.

66. Petrucci N, Iacovelli W. Ventilation with lower tidal volumes versus traditional tidal volumes in adults for acute lung injury and acute respiratory distress syndrome. Cochrane Database Syst Rev 2003; 3:CD003844.

67. Pesenti A, Marcolin R, Prato P, et al. Mean airway pressure vs positive end-expiratory pressure during mechanical ventilation. Crit Care Med 1985; 13:34–7.

68. Derdak S, Mehta S, Stewart TE, et al. High-frequency oscillatory ventilation for acute respiratory distress syndrome in adults: A randomized, controlled trial. Am J Respir Crit Care Med 2002; 166:801–8.

69. David M, Weiler N, Heinrichs W, et al. High-frequency oscillatory ventilation in adult acute respiratory distress syndrome. Intensive Care Med 2003; 29:1656–65.

70. Lewandowski K. Extracorporeal membrane oxygenation for severe acute respiratory failure. Crit Care 2000; 4:156–68.

71. Pesenti A, Bombino M, Gattinoni L. Extracorporeal support of gas exchange. In: Marini JJ, Slutsky AS, editors. Physiological basis of ventilatory support. New York: Marcel Dekker, 1998: 997–1020.

72. Gattinoni L, Pesenti A, Bombino M, et al. Role of extracorporeal circulation in adult respiratory distress syndrome management. New Horizons 1993; 1:603–12.

73. Pesenti A, Kolobow T, Riboni A. Single vein cannulation for extracorporeal respiratory support. ESAO Proceedings, Bruxelles, Belgium 1982: 65–7.

74. Pesenti A, Romagnoli G, Fox U. Sapheno-saphenous cannulation for LFPPV-ECCO2R. Paper presented at 10th Congress of the European Society of Artificial Organs, Bologna, Italy, 1983.

75. Bombino M, Marcolin R, Pesenti A. Percutaneous cannulation for long term bypass. Paper presented at the 2nd European Congress on Extracorporeal Lung Support, Marburg, Germany, 1992.

76. Pranikoff T, Hirschl R, Remenapp R, et al. Venovenous extracorporeal life support via percutaneous cannulation in 94 patients. Chest 1999; 115:818–22.

77. Rossaint R, Slama K, Lewandowski K, et al. Extracorporeal lung assist with heparin-coated systems. Int J Artif Organs 1992; 15:29–34.

78. Bindslev L, Bohm C, Jolin A, et al. Extracorporeal carbon dioxide removal performed with surface-heparinized equipment in patients with ARDS. Acta Anaesthesiol Scand Suppl 1991; 95:125–30; discussion 130–1.

79. Palatianos GM, Foroulis CN, Vassili MI, et al. A prospective, double-blind study on the efficacy of the bioline surface-heparinized extracorporeal perfusion circuit. Ann Thorac Surg 2003; 76:129–35.

80. Marcolin R, Cugno M, Pesenti A, et al. Extracorporeal circulation in sheep with normal bleeding time using a surface heparinized circuit. ASAIO Trans 1991; 37:584–7.

81. Uziel L, Agostoni A, Pirovano E, et al. Effect of PGI2 infusion during long term extracorporeal circulation with membrane lung in sheep. Int J Artif Organs 1981; 4:142–5.

82. Marcolin R, Mascheroni D, Pesenti A, et al. Ventilatory impact of partial extracorporeal CO2 removal (PECOR) in ARF patients. ASAIO Trans 1986; 32:508–10.

83. ECMO Technology, 1977: The state of the art and future directions. In: Extracorporeal support for respiratory insufficiency: A collaborative study in response to RFP-NHLI-73-20. NHLBI, Bethesda, MD: Division of Lung Diseases, 1979: 185–94.

84. Gattinoni L, Pesenti A, Mascheroni D, et al. Low-frequency positive-pressure ventilation with extracorporeal CO2 removal in severe acute respiratory failure. JAMA 1986; 256:881–6.

85. Wagner PK, Knoch M, Sangmeister C, et al. Extracorporeal gas exchange in adult respiratory distress syndrome: Associated morbidity and its surgical treatment. Br J Surg 1990; 77:1395–8.

86. Morris AH, Wallace CJ, Menlove RL, et al. Randomized clinical trial of pressure-controlled inverse ratio ventilation and extracorporeal CO2 removal for adult respiratory distress syndrome. Am J Respir Crit Care Med 1994; 149:295–305.

87. Donahoe M, Rogers RM. An anecdote is an anecdote is an anecdote . . . but a clinical trial is data. Am J Respir Crit Care Med 1994; 149:293–4.

88. Brunet F, Mira JP, Dhainaut JF, Dall'ava-Santucci J. Efficacy of low-frequency positive-pressure ventilation-extracorporeal CO2 removal. Am J Respir Crit Care Med 1995; 151:1269–70.

89. Habashi NM, Reynolds HN, Borg U, Cowley RA. Randomized clinical trial of pressure-controlled inverse ration ventilation and extracorporeal CO2 removal for ARDS. Am J Respir Crit Care Med 1995; 151:255–6.

90. Falke KJ. Randomized clinical trial of pressure-controlled inverse ratio ventilation and extracorporeal CO2 removal for adult respiratory distress syndrome. Am J Respir Crit Care Med 1997; 156:1016–7.

91. Barthelemy R, Galletti PM, Trudell LA, et al. Total extracorporeal CO2 removal in a pumpless artery-to-vein shunt. Trans Am Soc Artif Intern Organs 1982; 28:354–8.

92. Awad JA, Deslauriers J, Major D, et al. Prolonged pumpless arteriovenous perfusion for carbon dioxide extraction. Ann Thorac Surg 1991; 51:534–40.

93. Young JD, Dorrington KL, Blake GJ, Ryder WA. Femoral arteriovenous extracorporeal carbon dioxide elimination using low blood flow. Crit Care Med 1992; 20:805–9.

94. Matheis G. New technologies for respiratory assist. Perfusion 2003; 18:245–51.

95. Zwischenberger JB, Conrad SA, Alpard SK, et al. Percutaneous extracorporeal arteriovenous CO2 removal for severe respiratory failure. Ann Thorac Surg 1999; 68:181–7.

96. Conrad SA, Brown EG, Grier LR, et al. Arteriovenous extracorporeal carbon dioxide removal: A mathematical model and experimental evaluation. ASAIO J 1998; 44:267–77.

97. Alpard SK, Bidani A, Conrad SA, Zwischenberger JB. Arteriovenous carbon dioxide removal. ASAIO J 1998; 44:223–4.

98. Brunston RL Jr, Zwischenberger JB, Tao W, et al. Total arteriovenous CO2 removal: Simplifying extracorporeal support for respiratory failure. Ann Thorac Surg 1997; 64:1599–1604.

99. Conrad SA, Zwischenberger JB, Grier LR, et al. Total extracorporeal arteriovenous carbon dioxide removal in acute respiratory failure: A phase I clinical study. Intensive Care Med 2001; 27:1340–51.

100. Reng M, Philipp A, Kaiser M, et al. Pumpless extracorporeal lung assist and adult respiratory distress syndrome. Lancet 2000; 356:219–20.

101. Liebold A, Reng CM, Philipp A, et al. Pumpless extracorporeal lung assist: Experience with the first 20 cases. Eur J Cardiothorac Surg 2000; 17:608–13.

102. Bein T, Prasser C, Philipp A, et al. [Pumpless extracorporeal lung assist using arterio-venous shunt in severe ARDS. Experience with 30 cases]. Anaesthetist 2004; 53:813–9.

103. Brunet F, Belghith M, Mira JP, et al. Extracorporeal carbon dioxide removal and low-frequency positive-pressure ventilation: Improvement in arterial oxygenation with reduction of risk of pulmonary barotrauma in patients with adult respiratory distress syndrome. Chest 1993; 104:889–98.

104. Guinard N, Beloucif S, Gatecel C, et al. Interest of a therapeutic optimization strategy in severe ARDS. Chest 1997; 111:1000–7.

Chapter 23

LIQUID VENTILATION

RUPA SEETHARAMAIAH
STEFANO TREDICI
RONALD B. HIRSCHL

HISTORY OF LIQUID VENTILATION
PHYSIOLOGY OF PERFLUOROCARBON
   VENTILATION
PARTIAL LIQUID VENTILATION
   Laboratory Studies
   Clinical Studies
TOTAL LIQUID VENTILATION
   Laboratory Studies
   Clinical Studies
CONCLUSION

Acute respiratory distress syndrome (ARDS) is a complex life-threatening illness with many different etiologies associated with the diffuse alveolar damage leading to hypoxemic respiratory failure. It affects an estimated 43,000–107,000 patients per year.[1] Despite advancement in supportive therapy, including positive end-expiratory pressure (PEEP), inverse-ratio ventilation (IRV), permissive hypercapnia, and extracorporeal life support (ECLS), ARDS remains a highly lethal condition in the nonneonatal population, with a mortality rate of approximately 30–50%.[2,3]

Liquid ventilation using fluorinated organic liquids (perfluorocarbons) is an alternative technique for the management of respiratory failure. Because of the high solubility of respiratory gases and low surface tension,[4] perfluorocarbons are an attractive choice for gas exchange in liquid ventilation. Liquid ventilation has been performed by two methods. The first is *total liquid ventilation* (TLV), in which the lungs are filled with perfluorocarbon to a volume equivalent to functional residual capacity (FRC) on which a specialized mechanical liquid ventilator delivers perfluorocarbon tidal volumes to the lungs.[5] The second technique, in which conventional mechanical ventilators supply gas tidal volumes to lungs filled with perfluorocarbons, usually to a volume equivalent to FRC, is known as *partial liquid ventilation* (PLV).[6,7] There is growing evidence in laboratory and clinical studies to suggest that liquid ventilation may be effective as a supportive and therapeutic technique for patients with severe respiratory failure. In this chapter, the history and methods of liquid ventilation, as well as a summary of laboratory and early clinical evidence to support its development as a new therapy for severe respiratory failure, are discussed.

History of Liquid Ventilation

The concept of liquid ventilation has been investigated for almost 40 years. Although intrapulmonary saline was used in the early twentieth century for both lung-lavage therapy and physiologic studies,[8–12] the use of liquid as an alternative medium was not investigated until 1962. Kylstra[13] demonstrated the ability to sustain gas exchange in dogs spontaneously breathing hyperbarically oxygenated saline. These animals did not survive beyond the experimental period because of hypercarbia and acidosis, which was attributed to the low solubility of carbon dioxide (CO_2) in saline and to drainage limitations. Repeating the experiment with a mechanical-assist device yielded similar results.[14]

Subsequently, effort was directed toward finding a liquid for supporting gas exchange. Silicone and vegetable oils were found to be too toxic for in vivo use.[15] Interest then turned toward perfluorocarbons, which were first produced as a by-product of reactions used during the Manhattan Project (World War II). These liquids were noted to be clear, colorless, odorless, and biologically inert with remarkably low surface tension (15–19 dyn/cm at 25°C) and high solubility for both oxygen (45–55 ml O_2/dl at 25°C) and CO_2 (140–200 ml CO_2/dl at 25°C).[16–18] Clark and Gollan[19] in 1966 demonstrated that spontaneously breathing mice could survive when submerged in perfluorocarbon under normobaric conditions. This established an acceptable medium for gas exchange during liquid ventilation.

Although effective in oxygenating an animal, the relative high densities and low CO_2 content of perfluorocarbons imposed limitations in CO_2 clearance and acidosis in a spontaneously breathing model.[19] In an effort to improve expiratory flow and limit work of breathing, demand-regulated ventilators were developed in the early 1970s by Moscowitz and Shaffer.[20–23] Variations of the original device were developed subsequently to allow the study of TLV in a number of animal models ranging from preterm lambs to adult sheep.[24–30] The use of inhaled perfluorocarbons for preventing decompression sickness during deep-water diving also has been explored.[31,32] The ability of TLV to improve gas exchange and pulmonary compliance, as well as homogeneous alveolar inflation of the lungs, in premature animal models with neonatal respiratory distress syndrome (RDS) has been demonstrated.[24,25,33,34] Studies also have been performed in adult animal models with ARDS with encouraging results.[26–28] Extensive investigation of the toxicology, uptake, and elimination of perfluorocarbons has shown no significant adverse pulmonary or systemic effects.[35–39] The first demonstration of the ability to sustain gas exchange during liquid ventilation in humans was demonstrated in 1989 by Greenspan et al. Even though the severity of pulmonary injury precluded a successful outcome, this trial of TLV in three moribund, preterm newborns demonstrated the ability to support gas exchange and exhibited a trend toward improved pulmonary compliance.[40,41]

In contrast to TLV, PLV avoids the use of relatively large and complex ventilators with associated large perfluorocarbon priming volumes. Even though the concept

513

TABLE 23-1 Properties of Perfluorocarbon Liquids

Property	FC-77	RM-101	FC-75	PFdecalin	Perflubron
Boiling point (°C)	97	101	102	142	143
Density at 25°C (g/ml)	1.78	1.77	1.78	1.95	1.93
Kinematic viscosity (centistokes at 25°C)	0.80	0.82	0.82	2.90	1.10
Vapor pressure (torr at 37°C)	85	64	63	14	11
Surface tension (dynes/cm at 25°C)	15	15	15	15	18
O_2 solubility at 25°C (ml gas/100 ml liq.)	50	52	52	49	53
CO_2 solubility at 37°C (ml gas/100 ml liq.)	198	160	160	140	210

ABBREVIATIONS: PFC, perfluorochemical, including FC77 and FC75 from 3M Corp., USA, RM101 from Miteni, Italy; PFdecalin, perfluorodecalin from Green Gross Corp., Japan, and Air Products and Chemicals Inc., Allentown, PA; Perflubron, generic name for perfluoroctylbromide, developed for medical applications by Alliance Pharmaceutical Corp., USA.
SOURCE: Used with permission, from Shaffer TH, et al: Pediatr Pulmonol 14:102–9, 1992.

of transition from TLV to gas ventilation via PLV had been explored by Shaffer, the technique was first reported in 1991 by Fuhrman et al.[42] Numerous laboratory studies of PLV in animal models of both neonatal and adult lung injury induced by intravenous oleic acid administration, gastric aspiration, and saline lavage have demonstrated enhanced lung compliance and gas exchange during PLV compared with gas ventilation.[43–49] Human trials were conducted in neonatal, pediatric, and adult patients maintained with ECLS for severe respiratory failure.[50–53] Further trials followed with mixed results, as outlined later in this chapter.[54–59]

Physiology of Perfluorocarbon Ventilation

Perfluorocarbons are produced by fluorination of common organic hydrocarbons. This is accomplished through a highly exothermic vapor-phase method using fluorine gas or through a less exothermic, more stable cobalt trifluoride technique.[61] More recently, these compounds have been produced by electrochemical fluorination, as first described by Simmons in 1950.[62] This results in a more homogeneous product with less carbon-carbon bond cleavage. A large number of perfluorocarbon compounds have been produced using this technique for liquid-ventilation research. The carbon chain may vary in length, and any additional moiety that attaches gives each perfluorocarbon its unique properties.

Perfluorocarbons are clear, odorless, inert liquids with unique physical properties.[61] These compounds have a density approximately twice that of water and a kinematic viscosity (ratio of viscosity to density) similar to that of water.[63,64] These fluids have remarkably low surface tension (15–19 dyn/cm) secondary to weak intermolecular forces created by peripheral fluorine atoms and are relatively volatile, with vapor pressures ranging from 11–85 torr at 37°C. The vapor pressure of an individual perfluorocarbon determines the rapidity with which it evaporates after intratracheal administration. In addition, the peripheral fluorine atoms make them both thermally stable and chemically nonreactive. Perfluorocarbons are immiscible in aqueous- and alcohol-based solutions but have varying degrees of solubility for hydrocarbons. Solubilities of respiratory gases in perfluorocarbons are greater when compared

with water or a nonpolar solvent. They have excellent O_2 (45–55 ml O_2/dl) and CO_2 (160–210 ml CO_2/dl) carrying capacity.[61] The oxygen content of perfluocarbons at 1 atm of oxygen is approximately 20 times that of water, twice that of blood, and one-half that of an equal volume of oxygen gas. Some of the important physical properties of perfluorocarbons used in liquid-ventilation research are shown in Table 23-1. An ideal perfluorocarbon for respiratory application should have the properties of high gas solubility and moderate vapor pressure and viscosity. These properties, however, may not be found in a single pure perfluorocarbon. Thus recent studies are focusing on the development of new perfluorocarbons with physical properties that are tailored to better suit a particular application.

The potential toxicity of perfluorocarbons has been studied extensively in animals and in patients. They are absorbed in small quantities during TLV, reaching a steady state after 15–30 minutes of liquid breathing.[38,39] These compounds deposit preferentially in tissues with high lipid content[109] (Table 23-2 and Fig. 23-1) and do not appear to undergo biotransformation.[38] Perfluorocarbons are eliminated primarily by evaporation from the lungs and are scavenged by macrophages in both lungs and other tissues. Perfluorocarbons evaporate from the lungs of humans in approximately 3 weeks after discontinuing liquid ventilation.[74–76]

TABLE 23-2 Perfluorocarbon Tissue Levels as a Function of Time

Tissue	24h ($n = 6$)	72h ($n = 3$)	p Value
Blood	6 ± 0.24		
Heart	109 ± 18	117 ± 26	NS
Liver	63 ± 15	44 ± 15	NS
Intestine	67 ± 18	112 ± 6	NS
Kidney	79 ± 15	73 ± 5	NS
Spleen	61 ± 16	67 ± 6	NS
Thymus	110 ± 36	175 ± 63	NS
Brain	119 ± 13	245 ± 19	<0.01
Skeletal muscle	29 ± 3	56 ± 12	NS
Mean[a]	81 ± 7	108 ± 15	<0.01

NOTE: Perflubron levels expressed in microgram per gram of tissue. All data are presented as mean ± SEM.
[a]Mean across tissues.
SOURCE: Used with permission, from Cox C, et al: Biol Neonate 84:232–242, 2003.

PFC Levels as a Function of Lipids

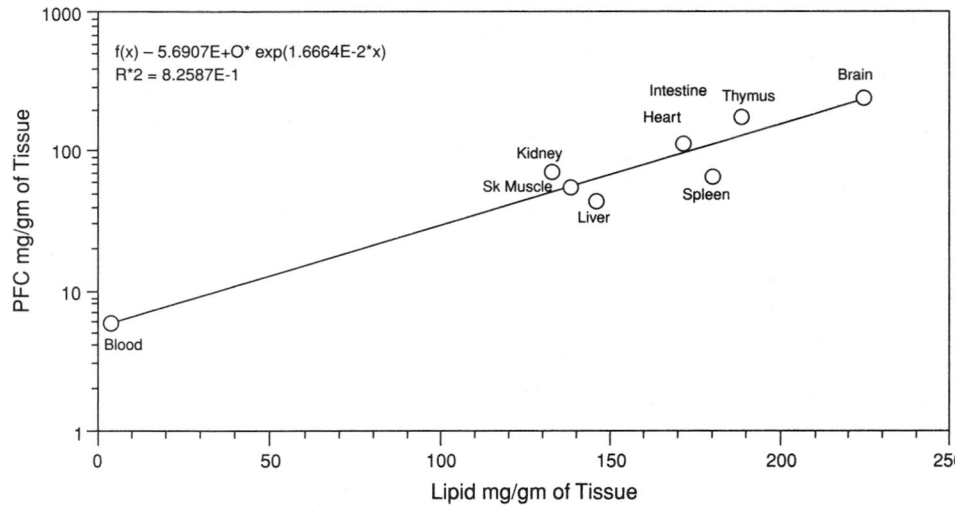

$f(x) - 5.6907E+O^* \exp(1.6664E\text{-}2^*x)$

$R^*2 = 8.2587E\text{-}1$

FIGURE 23-1 **Perflubron concentrations as a function of tissue lipid content. Perfluorocarbon concentration varied significantly among different tissues ($p < .001$), and these differences were related to tissue lipid content ($r = 0.93$, $p < .01$).** (*Used, with permission, from Cox et al: Biol Neonat 84:232–42, 2003.*)

Perfluorocarbons have the potential to support gas exchange under normobaric conditions because of the high solubility of respiratory gases.[22] High densities of perfluorocarbons facilitate their distribution to the dependent region of the lung, which leads to the recruitment of alveoli that otherwise tend to be collapsed or filled with inflammatory exudate in the setting of severe pulmonary injury.[3,27] Perfluorocarbons-filled lungs redistribute pulmonary blood flow to the better inflated, nondependent lung segments.[65–67] Albumin leak and water content are reduced during liquid ventilation in the setting of acute lung injury.[67,68] These effects lead to improvement in ventilation-perfusion matching and oxygenation in the setting of severe respiratory failure.

Since fluid-filled lungs exhibit a reduction in the gas-liquid interface, surface tension and surface-active forces favoring alveolar collapse are reduced.[9,10] Perfluorocarbons increase alveolar stability by acting as an artificial surfactant, and they do not appear to reduce endogenous surfactant production or activity.[62,69] This results in enhanced alveolar recruitment at lower inflation pressures.

A pulmonary-protective effect, by reducing lung injury, is another potential benefit of using perfluorocarbons. This is related to improved alveolar inflation and to enhanced displacement and lavage of inflammatory mediators and exudates from the affected lung. Perfluorocarbons facilitate exudate clearance secondary to their relative densities, through lavage during TLV, or through simple displacement of dependent exudates during PLV. They also have been shown to have in vitro anti-inflammatory activity, such as reductions in neutrophil chemotaxis, nitric oxide production, and endotoxin-stimulated macrophage production of cytokines.[70,71] In vivo evaluation has shown a reduction in release of tumor necrosis factor α, interleukin-1, and interleukin-6 in human alveolar macrophages in perfluorocarbon-exposed lungs.[72,73]

Besides their use in liquid ventilation, perfluorocarbons have been used in the cosmetic industry for their water-retention properties and also as cooling agents and insula-

tors. They also have been explored in patients as possible blood substitutes, as ultrasound and oral contrast media, as vitreal replacement in vitreoretinal surgery, to enhance oxygenation via peritoneal lavage, for organ preservation, and to distend and grow lungs in patients with congenital diaphragmatic hernia.[77–81]

Partial Liquid Ventilation

PLV refers to a hybrid method of gas exchange achieved through gas ventilation of perfluorocarbon-filled lungs. Shaffer et al[82] observed that there was a smooth transition from TLV to gas ventilation during animal experiments, even though a significant amount of perflorocarbon was still present in the respiratory tree. In 1991, Fuhrman et al[42] reported the first experience with PLV, achieving equivalent gas exchange and pulmonary compliance compared with gas ventilation in healthy piglets. With this technique, the lungs are filled with perfluorocarbon, in general to a volume equivalent to FRC (5–30 ml/kg) depending on the disease process, age, and weight, and then gas ventilated with a standard ventilator. During early clinical trials, perfluocarbon dosing consisted of 5–10 ml/kg aliquots, with repeat dosing every 30 minutes to 3 hours as tolerated hemodynamically or until the weight-adjusted estimated FRC was reached or by visually identifying a perfluorocarbon meniscus in the endotracheal tube at end expiration with zero PEEP.[52,54–56] Daily redosing was based on overall clinical status, degree of dependent-lung filling on lateral chest radiography, and the presence of a perfluorocarbon meniscus in the endotracheal tube.

The advantage of PLV over TLV consists of relative simplicity because the need for use of a new, complex device or an understanding of physiology of fluid mechanics in airways or the endotracheal tube is eliminated. A number of studies have demonstrated the efficacy of PLV in respiratory failure by improving gas exchange and pulmonary

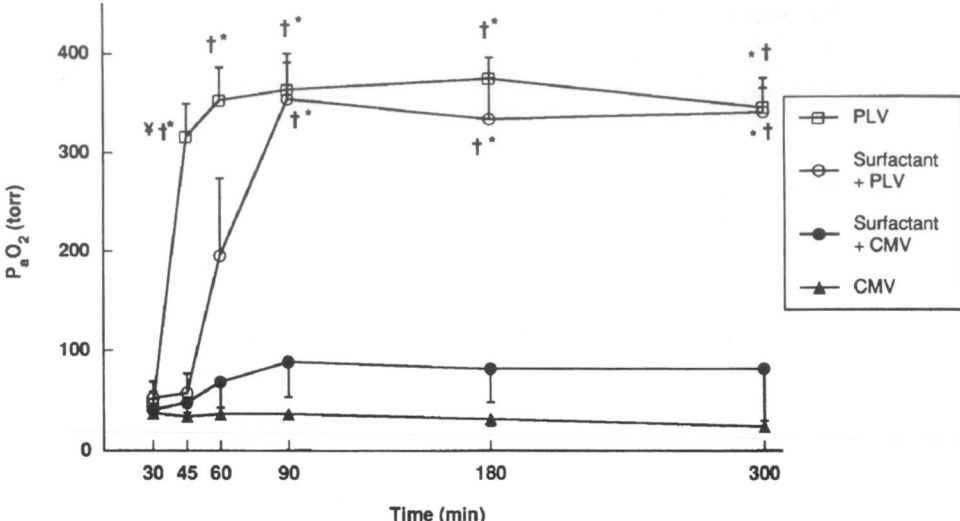

FIGURE 23-2 PaO_2 in four groups of premature lambs. Surfactant was administered at 30 minutes. PLV was initiated at 30 minutes in the PLV group and at 45 minutes (15 minutes after surfactant) in the surfactant plus PLV group. $*p < .05$ compared with baseline value within group; $\dagger p < .008$ compared with the CMV group at the same time point; $p < .008$ compared with the surfactant plus CMV group at the same time point. (*Used, with permission, from Leach et al: J Pediatr 126:412–20, 1995.*)

compliance by recruiting atelectatic lung regions, redistributing pulmonary blood flow, and lowering surface tension.

LABORATORY STUDIES

PLV has been studied in preterm and full-term neonatal, pediatric, and adult lung-injury models. Leach et al[44] reported significant improvement in gas exchange and pulmonary compliance during PLV in premature newborn lambs with RDS above those associated with pulmonary administration of surfactant (Fig. 23-2). PLV in piglets after lung injury by gastric acid aspiration demonstrated a significant increase in arterial oxygenation when compared with gas-ventilated controls over a 6-hour period as the injury matured.[47] Comparison of standard mechanical ventilation and high-frequency ventilation during PLV in a neonatal model of RDS showed improvements in gas exchange and pulmonary mechanics, even though high-frequency ventilation did not offer an advantage over conventional ventilation.[48,49]

Evaluation of PLV in an oleic acid–injured canine model of ARDS by Curtis et al[83] reported a dose-dependent increase in arterial oxygenation, with the highest P_{O_2} in the canines receiving the largest dose of perfluorocarbon (60 ml/kg). Maximum improvement in pulmonary compliance was seen after the 40 ml/kg dose of perfluorocarbon; further dosing resulted in a decrease in compliance. Hirschl et al[50] studied PLV for 2.5 hours in oleic acid–injured young-adult sheep on venovenous ECLS using a smaller FRC (35 ml/kg). They demonstrated an improvement in gas exchange and pulmonary function, manifested by decreased pulmonary shunt ($\dot{Q}ps/\dot{Q}t$) and slightly improved compliance.[50] In a separate study from the same institution in similarly injured sheep receiving PLV, the investigators identified a dose-related increase in O_2 delivery and mixed venous O_2 saturation that peaked at a perfluorocarbon lung volume of 40 ml/kg[84] (Fig. 23-3). These studies demonstrated that arterial oxygenation and CO_2 clearance

were facilitated during PLV in various neonatal and adult models of respiratory failure.

Gas exchange and pulmonary function appear to be improved during PLV by various mechanisms. Perfluorocarbons are effectively distributed into collapsed lung regions during PLV with associated alveolar recruitment.[3,85] Gauger et al[86] demonstrated an increase in total lung volume during PLV in an oleic acid model of lung injury. Administration of perfluorocarbon tends to redistribute pulmonary blood flow from the collapsed dependent to the better recruited nondependent lung regions.[87] These data suggest that administration of perfluorocarbon during PLV results in recruitment of atelectatic, consolidated lung tissue and redistributes pulmonary blood flow, resulting in improvement in ventilation-perfusion matching and gas exchange.

Pulmonary compliance is increased during PLV in smaller-animal models of respiratory failure, such as the newborn model of congenital diaphragmatic hernia[88,89] and preterm RDS.[43] In midsized and large animal models of oleic acid lung injury, however, only a small increase or even a decrease in pulmonary compliance has been observed during PLV.[26,50] This may be related to inhomogeneous distribution of perfluorocarbon in the lungs, most of which pools in the dependent portion of the lungs, whether the patient is supine or upright.[52] The effect of this dependent/nondependent distribution of gas and perfluorocarbon is less in patients with a smaller anteroposterior diameter, which may contribute to the observed increase in pulmonary compliance in newborns and infants.

Of interest is the recent demonstration of enhanced gas exchange with aerosolized perfluorocarbon in saline-lavaged, surfactant-depleted piglets. Arterial O_2 content was higher and CO_2 lower during both PLV and administration of aerosolized perfluorocarbon when compared with animals receiving standard mechanical ventilation.[90] This response was sustained after discontinuation of aerosolization but not standard PLV.

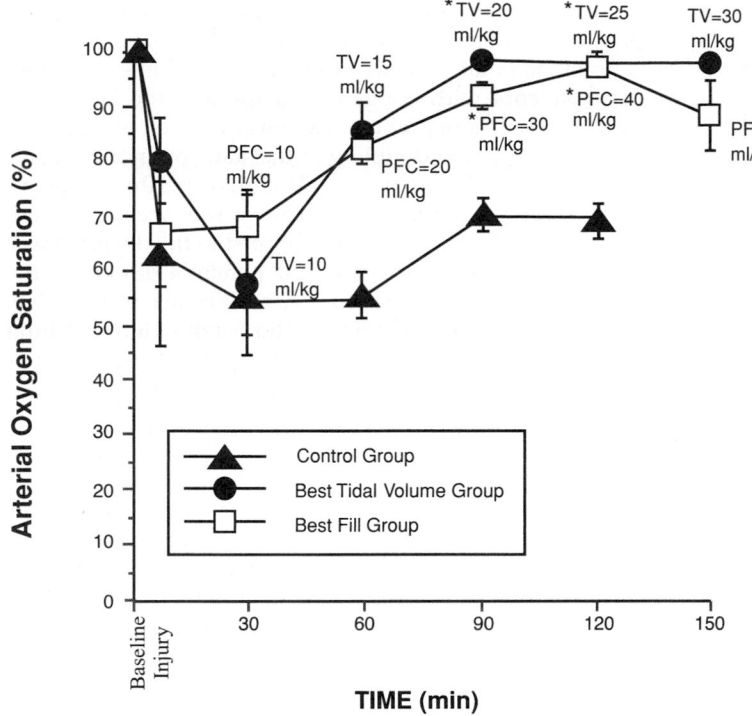

FIGURE 23-3 Arterial oxygen saturation at baseline, after lung injury, and for 150 minutes during conventional gas ventilation (control group), PLV with 10 ml/kg incremental increases in perflubron dose from 10–50 ml/kg (best fill, BF group), or PLV with 35 ml/kg Perflubron dose followed by 5 ml/kg incremental increase in gas tidal volume from 10–30 ml/kg (best tidal volume, BTV group). Values are mean ± SEM. (BF: $p = .01$ by repeated-measures ANOVA; $p = .020$ and $.020$ at 90 and 120 minutes when BF and control data were compared post hoc; BTV: $p = .001$ by repeated-measures ANOVA; $p = .025$ and $.022$ at 90 and 120 minutes when BTV and control data were compared post hoc). $*p < .025$. (*Used, with permission, from Parent et al: Surgery 121:320–7, 1997.*)

CLINICAL STUDIES

PEDIATRIC AND ADULT TRIALS

In 1995, the first clinical study of PLV for respiratory failure was reported.[51] PLV was used as an adjunctive therapy to ECLS in 19 patients (10 adults, 4 children, and 5 neonates) with severe respiratory failure. Patients receiving PLV demonstrated a significant decrease in the alveolar-arterial oxygen gradient [(A–a)D$_{O_2}$] and an increase in pulmonary compliance when ECLS was discontinued for short periods. Associated complications were limited to pneumofluorothoraces. Overall survival was 58%.

Safety and efficacy of PLV have been evaluated by a number of phase I and II clinical trials in adults and children with respiratory insufficiency.[7,51] Initial studies in adult and pediatric patients demonstrated a decrease in (A–a)D$_{O_2}$ within the first 48 hours after initiation of PLV.[54,55] Prospective, controlled, randomized studies to evaluate the safety and efficacy of PLV in adult and pediatric patients have been performed. A total of 200 pediatric patients were randomized to receive either PLV or conventional mechanical ventilation. A low mortality, 20% in the conventional group compared with 26% in the PLV group, made successful completion of the study impossible. The pediatric trial therefore was discontinued, which led to simultaneous pausing of all other clinical PLV studies. In a randomized trial in adult patients, no difference in pulmonary mechanics, gas exchange, or survival was noted between the PLV ($n = 65$) and conventional ($n = 25$) groups.[60] A multicenter prospective, randomized trial involving 311 patients with ARDS showed no significant difference in mortality or 28-day ventilator-free days between PLV and conventional ventilation groups.[91] Migliori et al[92] recently demonstrated an improvement in

gas exchange with reduction in O$_2$ indices with use of high-frequency PLV in two infants with chronic lung disease and severe respiratory failure.

PREMATURE NEWBORN TRIALS

In a multicenter noncontrolled trial, Leach et al[57] reported significant improvement in gas exchange, a decrease in mean oxygen index (OI = mean airway pressure × F$_{I_{O_2}}$ × 100/Pa$_{O_2}$), and a twofold increase in pulmonary compliance during PLV in 13 premature infants (24–34 weeks of gestation) with surfactant-refractory RDS (Fig. 23-4). Significant complications occurring during the trial attributed to PLV included mucus plugging in 5 patients and pneumothorax in 1 patient. The overall survival of the infants was 80%. A prospective, randomized trial involving 24 premature newborns (gestational age 24–34 weeks and birth weight 600–2000 g) who had failed surfactant administration showed a 62% survival with PLV when compared with a 100% survival in the control group. This study was placed on hold secondary to discontinuation of the pediatric trials, as noted earlier.

FULL-TERM NEWBORN TRIALS

In a phase I–II noncontrolled study in full-term newborns (two patients with congenital diaphragmatic hernia and four with ARDS) receiving ECLS but failing to improve, PLV was evaluated for 96 hours. All patients demonstrated improved lung compliance[59] (Fig. 23-5). Four infants were weaned from ECLS, and two were long-term survivors. In a prospective, randomized trial in 24 full-term newborn patients, 100% survival was noted in the control patients as opposed to 86% in the PLV patients. Fewer patients

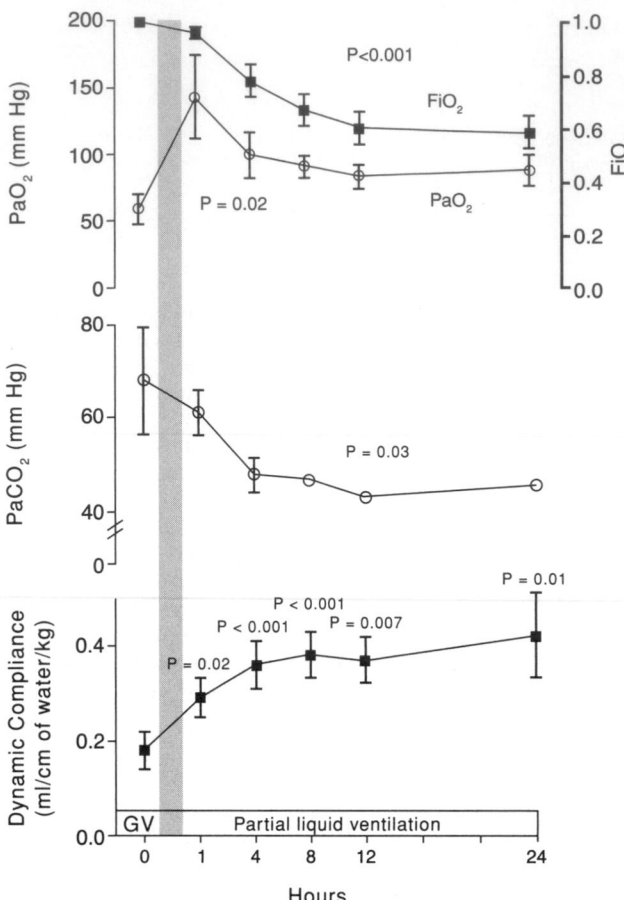

FIGURE 23-4 Mean (± SE) values for arterial oxygen tension (Pa$_{O_2}$), arterial carbon dioxide tension (Pa$_{CO_2}$), fractional inspired oxygen concentration (F$_{I_{O_2}}$), and dynamic compliance during gas ventilation (GV) in the initial 24 hours of partial liquid ventilation in 10 infants. P values present comparisons between partial liquid ventilation and gas ventilation. The gray bar denotes the period during which the liquid functional residual capacity was established. (*Used, with permission, from Leach et al: New Engl J Med 335:761–7, 1996.*)

growth factor also has been reported in animals undergoing perfluorocarbon-induced lung growth.[98]

Pranikoff et al[93] evaluated the use of PLV in seven newborn patients with congenital diaphragmatic hernia on ECLS for respiratory failure. Patients exhibited a significant increase in P$_{O_2}$ and doubling of the static pulmonary compliance during 5–6 days of PLV and/or perfluorocarbon-induced lung growth. This therapy was well tolerated. Significant complications were limited to the development of pulmonary hemorrhage in one patient 4 days after the final dose of perfluorocarbon. A multicenter prospective, randomized trial evaluating perfluorocarbon-induced lung growth in 13 newborns with congenital diaphragmatic hernia was performed. Patients were randomized for treatment with standard conventional gas ventilation on ECLS ($n = 5$) or perfluorocarbon-induced lung growth on ECLS ($n = 8$). Survival was 75% in the experimental group as opposed to 40% in the control group. The duration of ECLS was 9.8 ± 2.3 days in experimental group and 14.5 ± 3.5 days in the control patients. This trial was placed on hold when the definitive pediatric trial closed, and the study numbers were not adequate to demonstrate a significant difference in any parameter between the two groups.

Total Liquid Ventilation

TLV refers to the process of instilling and removing perfluorocarbon liquid tidal volumes from lungs for the purpose of gas exchange. During liquid ventilation, a volume equal to the estimated FRC of preoxygenated, prewarmed perfluorocarbon is instilled into the lung while residual gas bubbles are removed by gentle manipulation of the chest and gravitational positioning. The liquid ventilation then is initiated with the inspiratory phase in order to prevent massive pulmonary hemorrhage secondary to excessive negative pressure.[99] Unlike gas ventilation, in which minute ventilation and oxygenation can be achieved using a wide variety of ventilator settings, the mechanics of the fluid-filled lung dictate the use of long inspiratory and expiratory times, low flow rates secondary to the relatively high resistance to the flow of the liquid medium in the airways, and large tidal volumes owing to the diffusional limitations of perfluorocarbons. The elimination of the gas-liquid interface at the alveolar level minimizes the inflation pressure despite the high tidal volume (i.e., 15–20 ml/kg) necessary to maintain adequate minute ventilation. Thus pulmonary compliance and alveolar recruitment are enhanced markedly. Maintenance of lung distension also is facilitated. In addition, the distribution of the perfluorocarbon is relatively homogeneous throughout the liquid-filled lung. Finally, TLV has the ability to lavage very effectively the exudate and potential intra-alveolar inflammatory mediators from the lungs. Together these advantages make TLV a potentially effective tool in the treatment of lung injury and ARDS.

The need of a fresh-liquid tidal volume requires the use of a specialized device. Although simple gravitational drainage can be effective, a more complex device is essential to better control the tidal volume and the flow profile over

receiving PLV (43%) required ECLS compared with the control patients (70%). This study also was closed before completion because of discontinuation of the pediatric ARDS trial.

CONGENITAL DIAPHRAGMATIC HERNIA

In utero tracheal ligation has been used to correct structural and physiologic effects of pulmonary hypoplasia.[94,95] Fauza et al[96] evaluated the ability to induce lung growth via distension of the isolated upper lobe in newborn sheep with perfluorocarbon to a pressure of 7–10 mmHg. This study also demonstrated an increase in the size and number of alveoli in the right upper lobe while maintaining the airspace fraction, the protein-DNA ratio, and the (A–a)D$_{O_2}$ ratio compared with nondistended control animals.[96,97] Patients exposed to perfluorocarbon-induced lung growth (PILG) demonstrated radiologic evidence of ipsilateral lung growth[96] (Fig. 23-6). An increased expression of insulin-like

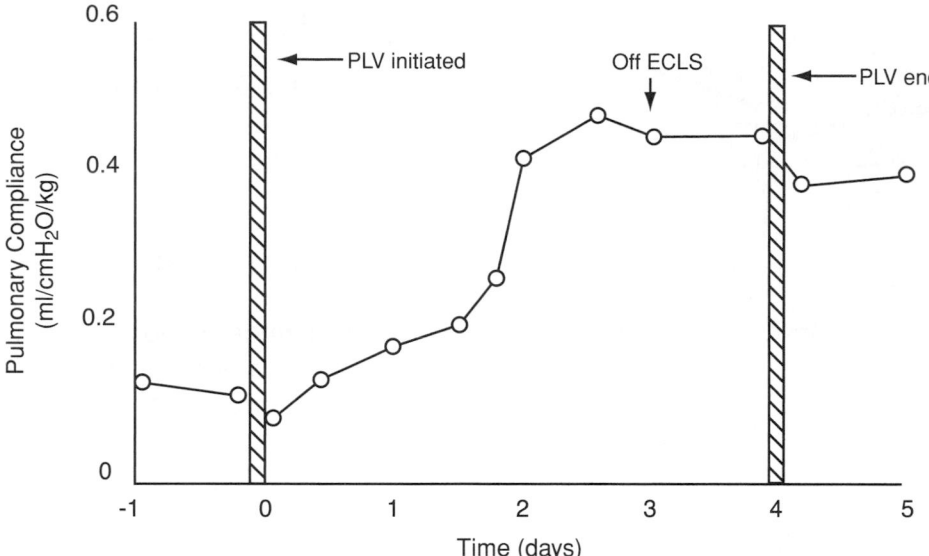

FIGURE 23-5 Change in pulmonary compliance with partial liquid ventilation (PLV) in an infant with the acute respiratory distress syndrome (ARDS). There is no change while receiving extracorporeal life support before PLV. With PLV, there is a slow increase in compliance during the first 48 hours. The infant was weaned off extracorporeal life support after 72 hours of PLV, and PLV was stopped after 96 hours. Recovery continued, and the infant survived. (*Used, with permission, from Greenspan et al: Pediatrics 99:E2, 1997.*)

FIGURE 23-6 Progression of the distended lungs ipsilateral to a hernia over time (the perfluorocarbon is radiopaque) in the three patients who received 7 days of pulmonary distention. Notice the increase in lung size, which was not observed in the contralateral lung. (*Used, with permission, from Fauza et al: J Pediatr Surg 36:1237–40, 2001.*)

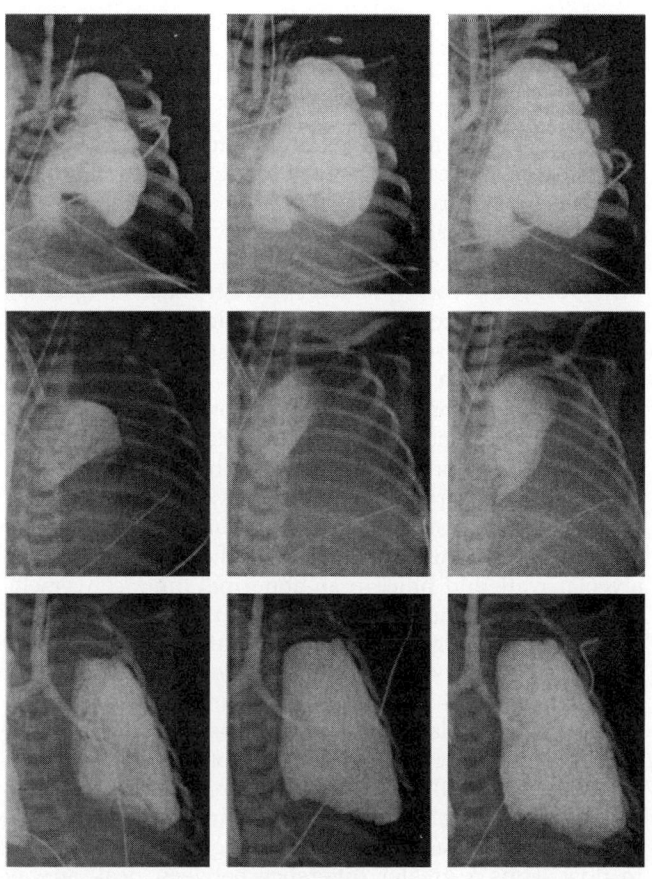

DAY 1   DAY 3   DAY 7

time. The development of liquid ventilators for the study of TLV is progressing continuously. Efforts have centered on improving CO_2 clearance, limiting the work of liquid breathing, and simplifying the design. The first true mechanical ventilator for liquid breathing was developed by Moskowitz in 1970.[20] This demand-regulated ventilator was modified by Shaffer et al and was used extensively in premature animal models of RDS.[21–23] The second-generation devices using a modified ECLS circuit described by Curtis et al in 1990 was simplified by Hirschl et al in the last decade. Meinhardt et al[99,100] were among the first to explore the use of piston-driven liquid ventilation and found enhanced expiratory flow when compared with a roller-pump technique. A double-piston pump ventilator, combined with the development of more sophisticated computer programming, then was used for the study of TLV in adult animal models of acute respiratory distress. Recently, a multicenter study was undertaken to evaluate the effectiveness of the double-piston device in an oleic acid lung-injury model. Liquid ventilation improved P_{CO_2}, O_2 delivery, Sa_{O_2}, Sv_{O_2}, and cardiac output with no change in pH and CO_2 clearance when compared with control ventilation. In addition, histologic evidence of decreased lung injury was noted. Lately, the advent of solid-silicone membrane technology has led to a simplified liquid ventilator with a single-piston design[30] (Fig. 23-7).

During liquid ventilation, not only is a simple design essential, but also CO_2 clearance and low resistance to flow are critical aspects. Thus research design is currently focusing on optimizing the gas exchanger used in the TLV system. Several investigators are using commercial blood-circuit membrane oxygenators, but excessive evaporative loss, leakage though the porous membrane, and material compatibility are problems. As an alternative, spray-bubbler column gas exchangers have been constructed, although gas-exchange efficiency is reduced and perfluorocarbon loss is increased when compared with membrane gas-exchange devices.[101] Thus, in the most recent devices, a silicone hollow-fiber gas-exchange device[30] has provided low resistance to flow and excellent gas-exchange efficiency.

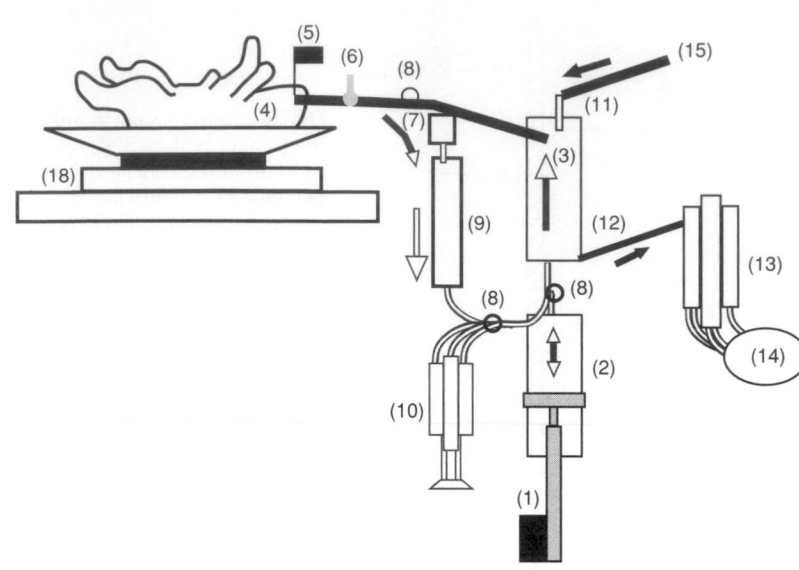

(1) Actuator
(2) Piston
(3) Membrane Oxygenator
(4) ETT
(5) Pressure transducer
(6) Flowmeter
(7) Bubble trap
(8) One-way Valves
(9) Heater
(10) PFC syringe pump
(11) Oxygen sweep Gas Inlet
(12) Oxygen sweep Gas Outlet
(13) PFC vapor Condenser
(14) Recovery bag
(15) Oxygen Tubing
(16) PFC tubing
(17) Oxygen Tubing
(18) Weighing Table

FIGURE 23-7 Schematic diagram of the single-piston liquid ventilator. PFC is pumped by the actuator (1) from the piston (2) through the oxygenator (3) and then directly to the animal via the endotracheal tube (4). During the expiratory phase, PFC is actively drained from the animal back to the piston, passing through a bubble trap (7) and heat exchanger (9). One-way valves (8) are used to control the direction of flow (PFC flow direction is indicated by the unfilled arrows). Additional PFC volume is added to the system by a syringe-pump system (10) connected to the expiratory limb. PFC vapor exhaled from the oxygenator is condensed by a cooler coil (13) and collected in a recovery bag (14). Countercurrent sweep gas flow (indicated by filled arrows), 5 liters/min of 100% of oxygen from a tank (15), is passed through the oxygenator from the gas inlet (11) sited on the top of the oxygenator to the gas outlet (12) at the bottom. PFC tidal volume and end-expiratory and end-inspiratory volumes are recorded by a scale (18). (*Used, with permission, from Tredici et al: Crit Care Med 32:2104–9, 2004.*)

The low resistance to flow, combined with simple design and ability to precisely control tidal volume and flow, provides a ventilator that allows maintenance of dynamic airway pressures in an appropriate range. One factor that limits the respiratory rate during TLV is flow limitation during expiration. This is also known as *choked flow* and leads to upstream expiratory airway collapse. According to the wave-speed theory of Dawson and Elliot,[102,103] maximal expiratory flow is limited by the wave speed of the liquid. Airway collapse is induced if the drainage flow exceeds the maximum flow determined by the wave speed. When choked flow occurs, tracheal pressure decreases (becoming very negative) and results in the closure of airways, located more in the large airways than at the alveolar level. Liquid is trapped in the lungs, increasing the end-expiratory lung volume, which, in turn, increases the risk of barotrauma and compromises hemodynamics, similar to that seen with auto-PEEP. Choked flow is avoided by allowing an adequate expiratory time, although the initial lung volume, tidal volume, perfluorocarbon, and expiratory waveforms all affect the development of expiratory flow limitation.[105,106]

LABORATORY STUDIES

The use of TLV in healthy animals or in models of respiratory distress (e.g., surfactant deficiency, meconium aspira-

tion, or oleic acid injury) has demonstrated improvement in gas exchange, cardiovascular stability, and pulmonary recruitment; effective lavage of pulmonary debris (i.e., exudate, meconium, or mucus); and preservation of pulmonary architecture when compared with gas ventilation and/or PLV. During TLV, as explained by Kylstra et al[14] (Fig. 23-8), the O_2 gradient between the inspired liquid and the alveolar surface is large secondary to a lower diffusion coefficient when compared with gas ventilation. As a consequence, during TLV in a normal lung, Pa_{O_2} is lower (approximately 300–400 mmHg) than during gas ventilation with 100% O_2 (~600 mmHg). Considering the alveolus as a sphere, with gas exchange occurring at the periphery, the initial and final O_2 concentrations depend on the radius of the sphere, the diffusion coefficient of O_2 in the fluid, the flux of O_2 into the alveolar wall, and time. In an abnormal lung, conversely, the more homogeneous distribution of the perfluorocarbon as compared with gas overcomes the diffusional limitation, resulting in more efficient gas exchange during TLV.

Despite the use of a large tidal volume during TLV, the airway and alveolar pressures are less than those generated during gas ventilation. Because of the high viscosity and density of perfluorocarbons, the proximal airway pressures generally are high during liquid breathing when compared with the alveolar pressures, reflecting high resistance to flow. Thus a greater difference between peak airway

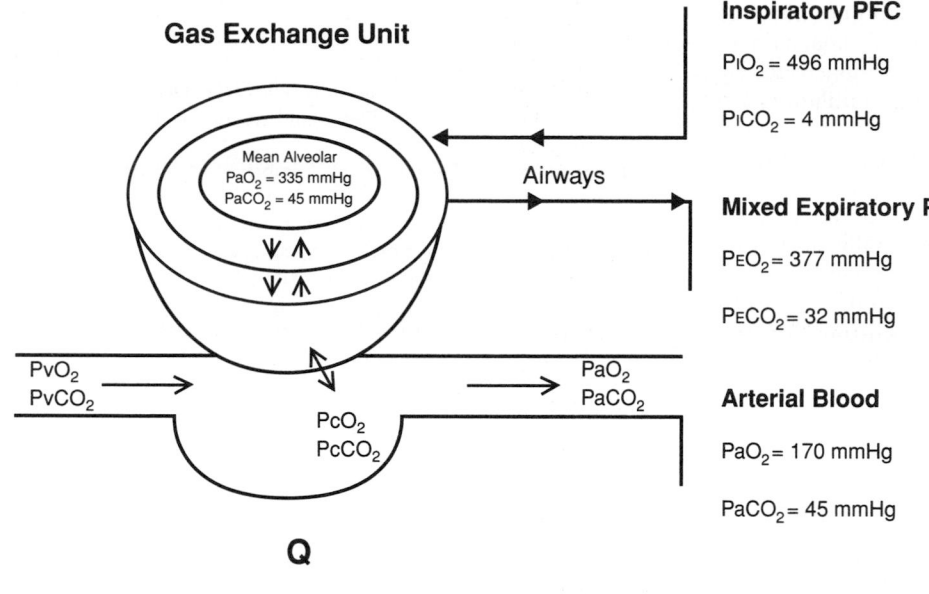

Gas Exchange Unit

Mean Alveolar
PaO_2 = 335 mmHg
$PaCO_2$ = 45 mmHg

PvO_2
$PvCO_2$

PcO_2
$PcCO_2$

PaO_2
$PaCO_2$

Q

Airways

Inspiratory PFC

PIO_2 = 496 mmHg

$PICO_2$ = 4 mmHg

Mixed Expiratory PFC

PEO_2 = 377 mmHg

$PECO_2$ = 32 mmHg

Arterial Blood

PaO_2 = 170 mmHg

$PaCO_2$ = 45 mmHg

FIGURE 23-8 The theoretical model of Kylstra et al[14,109] of an alveolus in which a sphere, or alveolus, is gas or liquid filled at a uniform oxygen concentration. A gradient from the center of the sphere to the periphery is created as gas exchange occurs. This gradient depends on the radius of the sphere, the diffusion coefficient of oxygen in the fluid, the flux of oxygen into the alveolar wall, and time. (*Used, with permission, from Cox et al: Biol Neonat 84:232–42, 2003.*).

pressure and alveolar pressure generally is observed during TLV. It is important to obtain an optimal balance between gas exchange and hemodynamic effects during TLV. Respiratory rate, tidal volume, and inspiratory-expiratory (I:E) ratio can be adjusted to alter the effect of TLV on hemodynamics.

Use of large tidal volumes induces cyclic changes in lung volume and intrathoracic pressure, producing a respiratory-related fluctuation in arterial blood pressure (Traube-Hering waves)[104] (Fig. 23-9). These effects are exacerbated during liquid ventilation secondary to the relatively high density of perfluorocarbons. The weight of the lung at end expiration is increased, and this may lead to compression of central structures such as the heart, great veins, and aorta. This may affect both ventricular filling and cardiac ejection.

It has been suggested that during the delivery of a liquid tidal volume that the venous return is impaired and transmural right-atrial pressure is increased, leading to a reduction in the right-ventricular preload and right-ventricular stroke volume. While the lungs inflate, the left-ventricular preload initially increases secondary to the shift of the pulmonary blood content. Consequently, the initial stroke volume is increased. After this initial increase in left-ventricular stroke volume, the preload of the left side is impaired by the low right-side stroke volume, resulting in a decrease in left-ventricular stroke volume.

The use of a high respiratory rate with consequent reduction in expiratory time and development of auto-PEEP also can impair hemodynamics. Such impairments, however, can be corrected by providing an adequate circulating

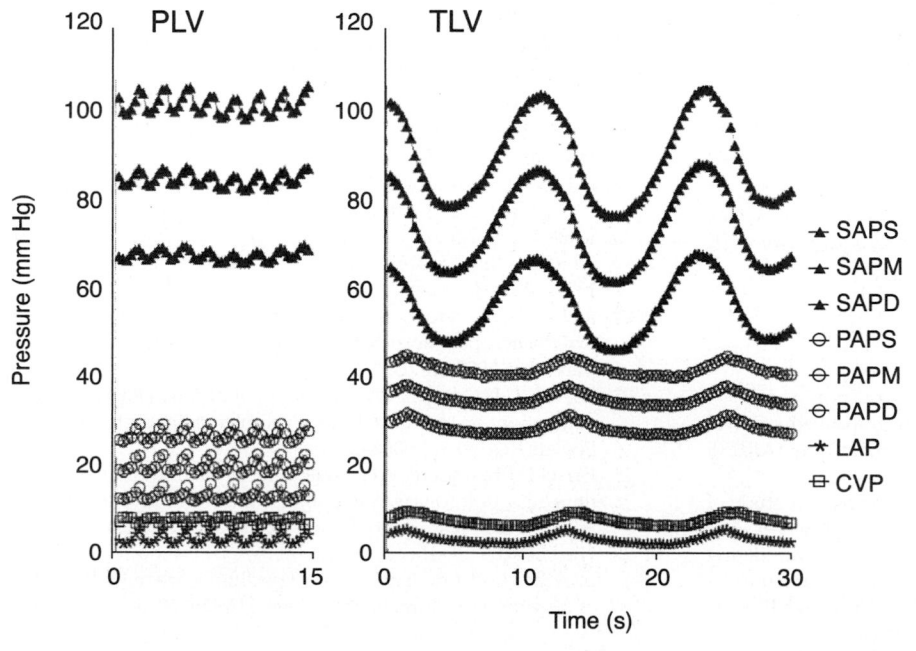

FIGURE 23-9 Typical tracing of beat-to-beat trend data of hemodynamic variables: systolic, mean, and diastolic systemic arterial pressures (SAPS, SAPM, and SAPD), pulmonary arterial pressures (PAPS, PAPM, and PAPD), and mean values for central venous pressure (CVP) and left atrial pressure (LAP). The time scale is constant for both PLV (*left*) and TLV (*right*). (*Used, with permission, from Degraeuwe et al: Pediatr Pulmonol 30:114–21, 2000.*)

blood volume. The ability of liquid ventilation to improve pulmonary mechanics with homogeneous expansion of the lungs during early development was demonstrated by Wolfson et al.[107] When compared with gas ventilation, liquid ventilation was able to sustain oxygenation and maintain CO_2 clearance and acid-base status without altering the cardiovascular status independent of the gestational age. Achievement of a balance between optimal gas exchange and hemodynamic effects is especially important with the use of TLV in premature newborns, where the oscillation of blood pressure can result in intraventricular hemorrhage. Another study showed that O_2 consumption and CO_2 production do not change during TLV.[108]

CLINICAL STUDIES

Unfortunately, clinical application of TLV is limited to one study performed in 1990 by Greenspan et al[41] on three moribund premature infants. TLV using a gravity-assisted device was performed for two separate 3- to 5-minute intervals in these three infants with severe RDS that was refractory to both high-frequency jet ventilation and surfactant therapy. All three infants exhibited increased pulmonary compliance during liquid-breathing trials, and two showed improved oxygenation. Although positive, this study, because of its short duration and small sample size, cannot be considered conclusive. The fact that the infants tolerated the trial, however, is encouraging and indicates the potential for further application of this technique in the clinical setting.

Conclusion

Liquid ventilation is in the early stages of its evolution. Although PLV in early clinical trials in pediatric and adult patients with respiratory failure has not yielded encouraging results, further evaluation of its efficacy in neonates needs to occur. Newer treatment modality of enhancing lung growth in newborns with congenital diaphragmatic hernia appears promising and, hopefully, will be evaluated in clinical trials. With TLV, there is much to be learned about the technical aspects of device design and overall technique. Once these technical aspects are refined, TLV has the potential to enter the clinical arena. Preliminary preclinical experience with TLV suggests that this novel intervention carries a promise of enhancing our ability to manage patients with respiratory failure effectively and efficiently.

References

1. Milberg JA, Davis DR, Steinberg KP, et al. Improved survival of patients with acute respiratory distress syndrome (ARDS): 1983–1993. JAMA 1995; 273:306–9.
2. Bartlett RH, Morris AH, Fairly HB, et al. A prospective study of acute hypoxemic respiratory failure. Chest 1986; 89:684–9.
3. The Acute Respiratory Distress Syndrome Network. Ventilating with lower tidal volumes for acute lung injury and the acute respiratory distress syndrome. New Engl J Med 2000; 342:1301–8.
4. Wolfson MR, Shaffer TH. Liquid ventilation during early development: Theory, physiologic processes and application. J Appl Physiol 1990; 13:1–12.
5. Hirschl RB, Merz SI, Montoya JP, et al. Development and application of a simplified liquid ventilator. Crit Care Med 1995; 23:157–63.
6. Fuhrman BP, Paczan PR, DeFrancisis M. Perfluorocarbon associated gas exchange. Crit Care Med 1991; 19:712–22.
7. Gauger PG, Pranikoff T, Schreiner RJ, et al. Initial experience with partial liquid ventilation in pediatric patients with the acute respiratory distress syndrome. Crit Care Med 1996; 24:16–22.
8. Winternitz MC, Smith GH. Preliminary studies in intratracheal therapy. In: Winternitz MC, editor. Pathology of war gas poisoning. New Haven: Yale University Press, 1920: 144–60.
9. Clements JA. Surface tension in lung extracts. Proc Soc Exp Biol Med 1957; 10:170–2.
10. Avery ME, Mead J. Surface properties in relation to atelectasis and hyaline membrane disease. Am J Dis Child 1959; 97:517–32.
11. Clements JA, Tierney DF. Alveolar stability associated with altered surface tension. In: Clements JA, editor. Handbook of physiology: Respiration. Bethesda, MD: American Physiological Society, 1964: 1565–83.
12. Mead J, Whittenberger JL, Radford EP. Surface tension as factor in pulmonary volume-pressure hysteresis. J Appl Physiol 1957; 10:191–6.
13. Kylstra JA, Tissing MO. Fluid breathing. In: Boerema I, Brummelkamp WH, Meyne NG, editors. Clinical applications of hyperbaric oxygen. Amsterdam, Elsevier, 1964:371–9.
14. Kylstra JA, Pagenelli CV, Lanphier EH. Pulmonary gas exchange in dogs ventilated with hyperbarically oxygenated liquid. J Appl Physiol 1966; 21:177–84.
15. Clark LC. Introduction to federation proceedings. Fed Proc 1970; 29:698.
16. Kylstra JA, Schoenfish WH. Alveolar surface tension in perfluorocarbon-filled lung. J Appl Physiol 1972; 33:32–5.
17. Zander R. O_2-Loslichkeit in fluorocarbonen. Res Exp Med (Berl) 1974; 164:97–109.
18. Tham MK, Walker RD, Modell JH. Physical properties of and gas solubilities in selected fluorinated ethers. J Chem Eng Data 1973; 18:385–6.
19. Clark LC, Gollan F. Survival of mammals breathing organic liquid equilibrated with oxygen at atmospheric pressures. Science 1966; 152:1755–6.
20. Moskowitz GD. A mechanical respirator for control of liquid breathing. Fed Proc 1970; 29:1751–2.
21. Moskowitz GD, Shaffer TH, Dublin SE. Liquid breathing trials and animal studies with a demand-regulated breathing system. Med Instrum 1973; 9:28–33.
22. Shaffer TH, Moskowitz GD. Demand-controlled liquid ventilation of the lungs. J Appl Physiol 1974; 36:208–13.
23. Shaffer TH, Moskowitz GD. An electromechanical demand-regulated liquid breathing system. IEEE Trans Biomed Eng 1975; 22:24–8.
24. Richman PS, Wolfson MR, Shaffer TH. Lung lavage with oxygenated perfluorochemical liquid in acute lung injury. Crit Care Med 1993; 21:768–76.
25. Shaffer TH, Douglas PR, Lowe CA, et al. The effects of liquid ventilation on cardiopulmonary function in preterm lambs. Pediatr Res 1983; 17:303–6.
26. Hirschl RB, Parent AP, Tooley R, et al. Liquid ventilation improves pulmonary function, gas exchange and lung injury in a model of respiratory failure. Ann Surg 1995; 221:79–88.
27. Hirschl RB, Overbeck M, Parent A, et al. Liquid ventilation provides uniform distribution of perfluorocarbon in the setting of respiratory failure. Surgery 1994; 116:159–68.

28. Hirschl RB, Tooley R, Parent A, et al. Evaluation of gas exchange, pulmonary compliance and lung injury during total followed by partial liquid ventilation in acute respiratory distress syndrome. Crit Care Med 1996; 24:1001–8.

29. Hirschl RB, Mey SI, Montoya JP, et al. Development and application of simplified liquid ventilator. Crit Care Med 1995; 23:157–63.

30. Tredici S, Komori E, Funakubo A, et al. A prototype of a liquid ventilator using a novel hollow fiber oxygenator in a rabbit model. Crit Care Med 2004; 32:2104–9.

31. Gollan F, Clark LC. Prevention of bends by breathing an organic liquid. Trans Assoc Am Phys 1967; 29:102–9.

32. Harris DJ, Coggin RR, Roby J, et al. Liquid ventilation in dogs: An apparatus for normobaric and hyperbaric studies. J Appl Physiol 1983; 54:1141–8.

33. Wolfson MR, Tran N, Bhutani VK, et al. A new experimental approach for the study of cardiopulmonary physiology during early development. J Appl Physiol 1988; 65:1436–43.

34. Wolfson MR, Shaffer TH. Liquid ventilation during early development on theory, physiologic process and application. J Dev Physiol 1990; 13:1–12.

35. Modell JH, Newby EJ, Ruiz BC. Long term survival of dogs after breathing oxygenated fluorocarbon liquid. Fed Proc 1970; 29:1731–6.

36. Modell JH, Hood CI, Kuck EJ, et al. Oxygenation by ventilation with fluorocarbon liquid (FX-80). Anesthesiology 1971; 34: 312–20.

37. Calderwood HW, Ruiz BC, Tham MK, et al. Residual levels and biochemical changes after ventilation with a perfluorinated liquid. J Appl Physiol 1975; 39:603–7.

38. Holaday DA, Fiserova-Bergerova V, Modell JH. Uptake, distribution and excretion of fluorocarbon FX-80 (perfluorobutyl perfluorotetrahydrofuran) during liquid breathing in dog. Anesthesiology 1972; 13:387–94.

39. Shaffer TH, Wolfson MR, Greenspan JS, et al. Liquid ventilation: Uptake, biodistribution and elimination of perfluorocarbon liquid (PFC). Pediatr Res 1992; 31:223A.

40. Greenspan JS, Wolfson MR, Rubenstein SD, et al. Liquid ventilation of preterm baby. Lancet 1989; 2:1095.

41. Greenspan JS, Wolfson MR, Rubenstein SD, et al. Liquid ventilation of human preterm neonates. J Pediatr 1990; 117:106–11.

42. Fuhrman BP, Paczan PR, De Francisis M. Perfluorocarbon-associated gas exchange. Crit Care Med 1991; 19:712–22.

43. Leach CL, Fuhrman BP, Morin FC III. Perfluorocarbon-associated gas exchange (partial liquid ventilation) in respiratory syndrome: A prospective, randomized, controlled study. Crit Care Med 1993; 21:1270–8.

44. Leach CL, et al. Partial liquid ventilation in premature lambs with respiratory distress syndrome: Efficacy and compatibility with exogenous surfactant. J Pediatr 1995; 126:412–20.

45. Tutuncu AS, Faithfull NS, Lachman B. Comparison of ventilatory support with intratracheal perfluorocarbon administration and conventional mechanical ventilation in animals with acute respiratory failure. Am Rev Respir Dis 1993; 148:785–92.

46. Tutuncu AS, Faithfull NS, Lachman B. Intratracheal perfluorocarbon combined with mechanical ventilation in experimental respiratory distress syndrome: Dose dependent improvement of gas exchange. Crit Care Med 1993; 21:962–9.

47. Nesti FD, Fuhrman BP, Steinhorn DM, et al. Perfluorocarbon-associated gas exchange in gastric acid aspiration. Crit Care Med 1994; 22:1445–52.

48. Smith K, et al. Prolonged partial liquid ventilation using conventional and high-frequency ventilatory techniques: Gas exchange and lung pathology in an animal model of respiratory distress syndrome. Crit Care Med 1997; 25:1888–97.

49. Smith K, et al. Partial liquid ventilation: A comparison using conventional and high-frequency techniques in an animal model of acute respiratory failure. Crit Care Med 1997; 25:1179–86.

50. Hirschl RB, Tooley R, Parent AC, et al. Improvement in gas exchange, pulmonary function and lung injury with partial liquid ventilation. Chest 1995; 108:500–8.

51. Hirschl RB, Pranikoff T, Gauger P, et al. Liquid ventilation in adults, children and neonates. Lancet 1995; 346:1201–2.

52. Hirschl RB, Pranikoff T, Wise C, et al. Initial experience with partial liquid ventilation in adult patients with the acute respiratory distress syndrome. JAMA 1996; 275:383–9.

53. Gauger PG, Pranikoff T, Schreiner RJ, et al. Initial experience with partial liquid ventilation in pediatric patients with the acute respiratory distress syndrome. Crit Care Med 1996; 24: 16–22.

54. Hirschl RB, Conrad S, Kaiser R, et al. Partial liquid ventilation in adult patients with ARDS: A multicenter phase I/II trial. Ann Surg 1998; 228:692–700.

55. Toro-Figueroa LO, Melinoes JN, Curtis SE, et al. Perflubron partial liquid ventilation (PLV) in children with ARDS: A safety and efficacy pilot study. Crit Care Med 1996; 24:150A.

56. Bartlett R, Croce M, Hirschl R, et al. A phase II randomized, controlled trial of partial liquid ventilation (PLV) in patients with acute hypoxemic respiratory failure (AHRF). Crit Care Med 1997; 25:A35.

57. Leach CL, Greenspan JS, Rubenstein SD, et al. Partial liquid ventilation with Perflubron in infants with severe respiratory distress syndrome. New Eng J Med 1996; 335:761–7.

58. Gross GW, Greenspan JS, Fox WW, et al. Use of liquid ventilation with perflubron during extracorporeal membrane oxygenation: Chest radiographic appearances. Radiology 1995; 194: 717–20.

59. Greenspan JS, Fox WW, Rubenstein SD, et al. Partial liquid ventilation in critically ill infants receiving extracorporeal life support. Pediatrics 1997; 99:E2.

60. Hirschl RB, Croce M, Gore D, et al, for the Adult PLV Study Group. Prospective, randomized, controlled pilot study evaluating the safety and efficacy of partial liquid ventilation with the acute respiratory distress syndrome (ARDS). Am J Respir Crit Care Med 2002; 165:781–7.

61. Sargent JW, Seffl RJ. Properties of perfluorinated liquids. Fed Proc 1970; 29:1699–1703.

62. Simmons JH, editor. Fluorine chemistry, vols I, II, and V. New York: Academic Press, 1950.

63. Shaffer TH, Wolfson MR, Clark LC. State of art review: Liquid ventilation. Pediatr Pulmonol 1992; 14:102–9.

64. Wolfson MR, Shaffer TH. Liquid ventilation: An adjunct to respiratory management. J Pediatr Anesth 2004; 14:15–23.

65. West JB, Dolley CT, Matthew CME, et al. Distribution of blood flow and ventilation in the saline filled lung. J Appl Physiol 1965; 20:1107–17.

66. Lowe CA, Shaffer TH. Redistribution of pulmonary blood flow in the fluorocarbon-filled lung. Fed Proc 1981; 40:587A.

67. Gauger PG, Overbeck MC, Koeppe RA, et al. Distribution of pulmonary blood flow and total lung water during partial liquid ventilation in acute lung injury. Surgery 1997; 122: 313–23.

68. Colton DM, Till GO, Johnson KJ, et al. Partial liquid ventilation decreases albumin leak in the setting of acute lung injury. J Crit Care 1998; 13:136–9.

69. Leach CL, Holm B, Morin FC. Partial liquid ventilation in premature neonates with respiratory distress syndrome: Efficacy and compatibility with exogenous surfactant. J Pediatr 1995; 126:412–20.

70. Rossman JE, Caty MG, Rich GA, et al. Neutrophil activation and chemotaxis in in vitro treatment with perfluorocarbon. J Pediatr Surg 1996; 31:1147–51.

71. Smith TM, Steinhorn DM, Thusu K, et al. A liquid perfluorochemical decreases the in vitro production of reactive oxygen species by alveolar macrophages. Crit Care Med 1995; 23:1533–9.

72. Thomassen MJ, Buhrow LT, Weidemann HP. Perflubron decreases inflammatory cytokine production by human alveolar macrophages. Crit Care Med 1997; 25:2045–7.

73. Kawamae K, Pristine G, Chiumello D, et al. Partial liquid ventilation decreases serum tumor necrosis factor-α concentrations in a rat acid aspiration lung injury model. Crit Care Med 2000; 28:479–83.

74. Hood CI, Modell JH. A morphologic study of long-term retention of fluorocarbon after liquid ventilation. Chest 2000; 118:1436–40.

75. Reickert C, Pranikoff T, Overbeck M, et al. The pulmonary and systemic distribution and elimination of perflubron from adult patients treated with partial liquid ventilation. Chest 2001; 119:515–22.

76. Stavis RL, Wolfson MR, Cox C, et al. Physiology, biochemical and histologic correlates associated with tidal liquid ventilation. Pediatr Res 1998; 43:132–8.

77. Winslow RM. Blood substitutes. Curr Opin Hematol 2002; 9:146–51.

78. Brazitikos PD, Androudi S, D'Amico DJ, et al. Perfluorocarbon liquid utilization in primary vitrectomy repair of retinal detachment with multiple breaks. Retina 2003; 23:615–21.

79. Hirschl RB, Philip WF, Glick L, et al. A prospective, randomized pilot trial of perfluorocarbon-induced lung growth in newborns with congenital diaphragmatic hernia. J Pediatr Surg 2003; 38:283–9.

80. Soman N, Banerjee R. Artificial vitreous replacements. Biomed Mater Eng 2003; 13:59–74.

81. Anderson CM, Brown JJ, Balfe DM, et al. MR imaging of Crohn disease: Use of Perflubron as gastrointestinal contrast agent. J Magn Reson Imaging 1994; 4:491–6.

82. Curtis SE, Fuhrman BP, Howland DF, et al. Cardiac output during liquid (perfluorocarbon) breathing in newborn piglets. Crit Care Med 1991; 19:225–30.

83. Curtis SE, Peek JT, Kelly DR. Partial liquid breathing with Perflubron improves arterial oxygenation in acute canine lung injury. Am J Physiol 1993; 75:2696–702.

84. Parent AC, Overbeck MC, Hirschl RB. Oxygen dynamics during partial liquid ventilation in a sheep model of severe respiratory failure. Surgery 1997; 121:320–7.

85. Quintel M. Hirschl RB, Roth H, et al. Computed tomographic assessment of Perflubron and gas distribution during partial liquid ventilation for acute respiratory failure. Am J Respir Crit Care Med 1998; 158:249–55.

86. Gauger PG, et al. Perfluorocarbon partial liquid ventilation improves gas exchange while augmenting decreased functional residual capacity in an animal model of acute lung injury. Surg Forum 1995; 46:669–71.

87. Doctor A, Ibla JC, Grenier BM, et al. Pulmonary blood flow distribution during partial liquid ventilation. J Appl Physiol 1998; 184:1540–50.

88. Wilcox DT, Glick PL, Karamanoukian HL, et al. Partial liquid ventilation and nitric oxide in congenital diaphragmatic hernia. J Pediatr Surg 1997; 32:1211–5.

89. Wilcox DT, Glick PL, Karamanoukian HL, et al. Perfluorocarbon-associated gas exchange improves pulmonary mechanics, oxygenation, ventilation and allow nitric oxide delivery in hypoplastic lung congenital diaphragmatic hernia lamb model. Crit Care Med 1995; 23:1858–63.

90. Kandler MA, von der Hardt K, Schoof E, et al. Persistent improvement of gas exchange and lung mechanics by aerosolized perfluorocarbon. Am J Respir Crit Care Med 2001; 164:31–5.

91. Wiedemann, Alliance Pharmaceutical Corp. Announced preliminary results of LiquiVent phase 2–3 clinical study. San Diego, CA, 2001.

92. Migliori C, Bottino R, Angeli A, et al. High frequency liquid ventilation in two infants. J Perinatol 2004; 24:118–20.

93. Pranikoff T, Gauger P, Hirschl RB. Partial liquid ventilation in newborn patients with congenital diaphragmatic hernia. J Pediatr Surg 1996; 31:613–8.

94. DiFiore JW, et al. Experimental fetal tracheal ligation reverses the structural and physiological effect of pulmonary hypoplasia in congenital diaphragmatic hernia. J Pediatr Surg 1994; 29:248–56; discussion 256–7.

95. Hedrick MH, et al. Plug the lung until it grows (PLUG): A new method to treat congenital diaphragmatic hernia in utero. J Pediatr Surg 1994; 29:612–7.

96. Fauza D, Hirschl RB, Wilson J. Continuous intrapulmonary distension with perfluorocarbon accelerates lung growth in infants with congenital diaphragmatic hernia. J Pediatr Surg 2001; 36:1237–40.

97. Nobuhara KK, Fauza DO, DiFiore JW, et al. Continuous intrapulmonary distension with perfluorocarbon accelerates neonatal (but not adult) lung growth. J Pediatr Surg 1998; 33: 292–8.

98. Nobuhara KK, DiFiore JW, Ibla JC, et al. Insulin-like growth factor-I gene expression in three models of accelerated lung growth. J Pediatr Surg 1998; 33:1057–60.

99. Meinhardt JP, Quintel M, Hirschl RB. Development and application of a double-piston configured, total liquid ventilatory support device. Crit Care Med 2000; 28:1483–8.

100. Meinhardt JP, Sawada S, Quintel M, Hirschl RB. Comparison of static airway pressures during total liquid ventilation while applying different expiratory modes and time patterns. ASAIO J 2004; 50: 68–75.

101. Wolfson MR, Miller TF, Peck G, et al. Multifactorial analysis of exchanger efficiency and liquid conservation during perflorochemical liquid-assisted ventilation. Biomed Instrum Tech 1999; 33:260–267.

102. Dawson SV, Elliot EA. Wave-speed limitation on expiratory flow: A unifying concept. J Appl Physiol 1977; 43:498–515.

103. Dawson SV, Elliot EA. Use of the choke point in the prediction of flow limitation in elastic tube. Fed Proc 1980; 39:2765–70.

104. Degraeuwe PL, Vos GD, Geskens GG, et al. Effect of perfluorochemical liquid ventilation on cardiac output and blood pressure variability in neonatal piglet with respiratory insufficiency. Pediatr Pulmonol 2000; 30:114–24.

105. Baba Y, Brant D, Brah SS, et al. Assessment of development of choked flow during total liquid ventilation. Crit Care Med 2004; 32:201–8.

106. Foley DS, Brah R, Bull JL, et al. Total liquid ventilation: Dynamic airway pressure and development of expiratory flow limitation. ASAIO J 2004; 50:485–90.

107. Wolfson MR, Greenspan JS, Deoras KS, et al. Comparison of gas and liquid ventilation: Clinical, physiological and histological correlates. J Appl Physiol 1992; 72:1024–31.

108. Hirschl RB, Grover B, McCracken M, et al. Oxygen consumption and carbon dioxide production during liquid ventilation. J Pediatr Surg 1993; 28:513–9.

109. Cox C, Stavis RL, Wolfson MR, et al. Long-term tidal liquid ventilation in premature lambs: Physiology, biochemical and histological correlates. Biol Neonat 2003; 84:232–42.

Chapter 24 _____

TRANSTRACHEAL GAS INSUFFLATION

LLUIS BLANCH
AVI NAHUM

Strategies for lung-protective mechanical ventilation use small tidal volumes (V_T) to avoid high alveolar pressures at end inspiration and alveolar overdistension, together with moderate or high levels of positive end-expiratory pressure (PEEP) to keep alveoli open at end expiration and thereby maintain alveolar recruitment.[1,2] These strategies have resulted in improved outcomes in patients with acute lung injury (ALI) and in patients with acute respiratory distress syndrome (ARDS).[3–6] Unfortunately, they also can decrease alveolar ventilation, leading to carbon dioxide (CO_2) retention and eventually severe respiratory acidosis. Patients with unstable hemodynamics or associated cerebrovascular diseases might not tolerate moderate elevations in Pa_{CO_2}.

In this context, tracheal gas insufflation (TGI) has a role as an adjunct to mechanical ventilation. This technique consists of the continuous or phasic injection of fresh gas into the central airways for the purpose of improving the efficiency of alveolar ventilation and/or minimizing the ventilator pressure requirements.[7]

Variants of TGI have been investigated for several decades. In nonhospitalized, stable patients with chronic lung diseases, administration of fresh gas into the trachea reduced inspired minute ventilation, improved dyspnea and exercise tolerance, and lessened the work of breathing.[8–10] Continuous apneic ventilation delivers oxygen and maintains adequate blood oxygenation at a stable level of hypercapnia.[11–13] This chapter discusses TGI as an adjunct to mechanical ventilation; other forms of transtracheal gas (air/oxygen) administration are considered briefly.

Basic Principles

MECHANISM OF ACTION

TGI attempts to minimize dead space by delivering fresh gas through an intratracheal catheter to flush the anatomic dead space free of CO_2. During TGI, low to moderate flows of fresh gas introduced near the carina, either continuously or in phases, dilute the CO_2 residing in the anatomic dead space proximal to the catheter tip. Because CO_2 is washed out during expiration, less CO_2 is recycled back into the alveoli during the subsequent inspiration (Fig. 24-1). Any catheter flow during inspiration contributes to the inspired V_T but bypasses the anatomic dead space proximal (mouthward) of the catheter tip. At higher catheter flow rates, turbulence generated at the tip of the catheter by the jet stream can enhance gas mixing in regions distal to the catheter tip, thereby contributing to CO_2 removal.[14,15] The fresh-gas stream exiting the catheter tip rapidly establishes an expiratory front beyond the catheter tip between CO_2-rich alveolar gas and CO_2-free fresh catheter gas.[15] This front is practically abolished by inverting the catheter tip and directing the catheter jet mouthward, thus eliminating the distal effect of TGI.[14] Consequently, the straight catheter consistently outperforms the inverted catheter. Under experimental conditions, the observed difference in Pa_{CO_2} between the straight and inverted catheters during continuous TGI amounted to 25% of the total decrease in Pa_{CO_2} with a catheter flow rate of 10 liters/min.[14] End-expiratory CO_2 values at the tip of the endotracheal tube (ETT) during continuous TGI in dogs were comparatively higher using the straight catheter than the inverted catheter, indicating that projecting the TGI jet distally improved CO_2 removal at end expiration.[16] Furthermore, a study on the penetration and mixing behavior of TGI gas in a simulated trachea has shown that mixing of expiratory and TGI gases occurred close to the TGI orifice; the oxygenated domain extended several centimeters beyond the ETT, even at high expiratory flows, but had a definite distal limit. Moreover, more distally from the site of gas injection, the TGI gas tended to propagate along the tracheal wall rather than projecting centrally.[17] These observations indicate that the primary mechanism of CO_2 elimination during TGI is expiratory washout, and the forward-directed TGI penetrates a

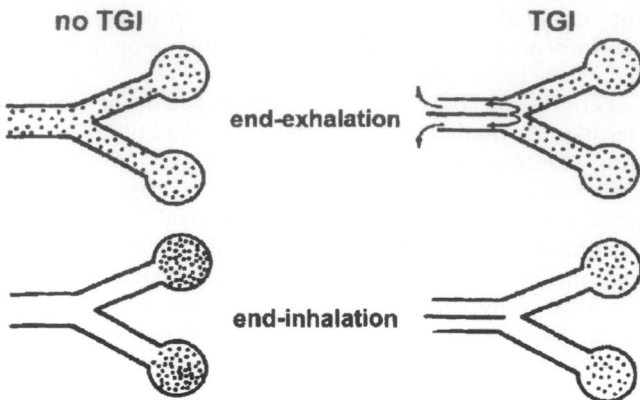

FIGURE 24-1 (*Left*) With no tracheal gas insufflation (no TGI), the central airways contain CO_2 at end-expiration; this CO_2 is delivered to alveoli during subsequent inspirations. (*Right*) with TGI, the CO_2 from the central airways is flushed during the expiratory phase, which reduces the CO_2 delivered to alveoli during the subsequent inspiration. (*Used, with permission, from Ravenscraft: Respir Care 41:105–11, 1996.*)

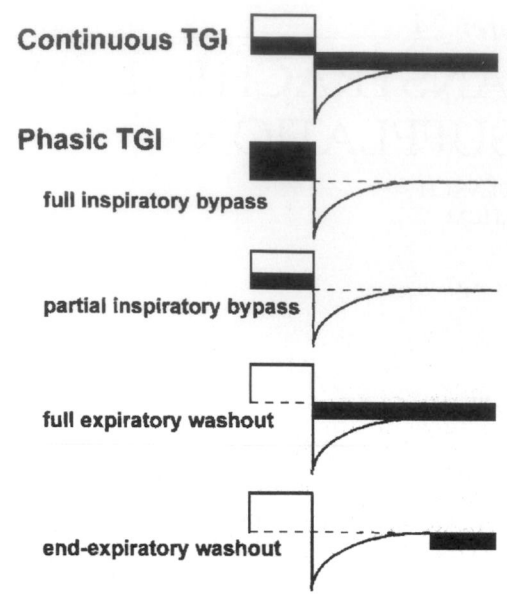

FIGURE 24-2 Tracheal gas insufflation (TGI) can be provided as a continuous flow of gas into the airway or specific to the phase of the respiratory cycle. Different approaches can be used to provide phasic TGI. (*Used, with permission, from Ravenscraft: Respir Care 41:105–11, 1996.*)

substantial distance into the central airways, extending the compartment susceptible to CO_2 washout with a smaller contribution of turbulence beyond the straight catheter tip. Consequently, Pa_{CO_2} during TGI falls as a nonlinear function of catheter flow rate. Initially, modest flow rates achieve large decrements in Pa_{CO_2}, but once the anatomic dead space is flushed free of CO_2, the effect on Pa_{CO_2} diminishes as catheter flow rate is increased.[7,18]

MODES OF OPERATION

During TGI, fresh gas can be delivered continuously, or delivery can be timed to occur in phases during a specific portion of the respiratory cycle by gating a solenoid valve that either directs the flow to the catheter or diverts it to the atmosphere.[19,20] During continuous TGI, closure of the expiratory valve during inspiration causes catheter flow to deliver a variable portion of the inspired V_T.[21,22] The analog output of the ventilator or flow signal from a pneumotachograph can be used to operate a metering device that controls the solenoid (Fig. 24-2).

Phasic inspiratory TGI can be used as the only source of fresh gas, thereby bypassing the anatomic dead space proximal to the catheter tip.[20] It also can be combined with a conventional ventilator to augment alveolar ventilation. During continuous or phasic inspiratory TGI, the catheter-delivered portion of the inspired V_T is a function of catheter flow rate and inspiratory time. During phasic expiratory TGI, catheter flow is timed to occur during all or part of expiration and does not contribute appreciably to the inspired V_T. As an alternative to using a catheter, the apparatus dead space and part of the tracheal dead space can be eliminated by using a double-lumen ETT to separate the inspiratory and expiratory limbs of the ventilator circuit.[22]

The effect of insufflating fresh gas during specific phases of the respiratory cycle has been examined using three catheter-flow conditions: (1) continuous TGI, (2) flow only during inspiration (see Fig. 24-2), and (3) flow during the final third of expiration[20,23] (Fig. 24-3). When catheter flow

occurred only during inspiration (inspiratory bypass), the "anatomic" dead space proximal to the catheter tip (extending from the ventilator's Y piece) was effectively avoided. When insufflation occurred during late expiration (expiratory washout), fresh gas washed the proximal dead space free of CO_2. Limiting TGI to the final 60% of expiration achieved effective Pa_{CO_2} reduction (not significantly different from panexpiratory TGI) while limiting exposure of the trachea to TGI gas and reducing the potential for TGI-induced hyperinflation.[23] Differences between these phasic methods tended to narrow at higher catheter flow rates. Early expiratory injection (i.e., where catheter flow was timed to occur early in expiration and terminated before end expiration) was less effective, however, than late expiratory injection.[16] Even though CO_2-containing gas is washed out of the airways during early expiratory injection by TGI, CO_2-laden alveolar gas refills the proximal anatomic dead space later in the expiratory period. This CO_2-rich expired gas is then "rebreathed" during the subsequent inspiration. Consequently, fresh gas delivered too early in expiration cannot participate fully in dead-space reduction.[24] Lung-model studies have shown that the marked increases in system pressures and volumes caused by continuous TGI could be avoided with expiratory-phase TGI and volume-adjusted TGI.[25]

Continuous TGI produced an effect superior to both inspiratory bypass and late-expiratory washout in augmenting alveolar ventilation.[20] When catheter flow is set to occur selectively throughout expiration (panexpiratory TGI), however, the increase in alveolar ventilation is very similar to that achieved by continuous TGI.[20] Because TGI does not contribute appreciably to inspired V_T during panexpiratory TGI, it allows the use of high catheter flows without increasing peak alveolar pressure. Studies are needed to define the

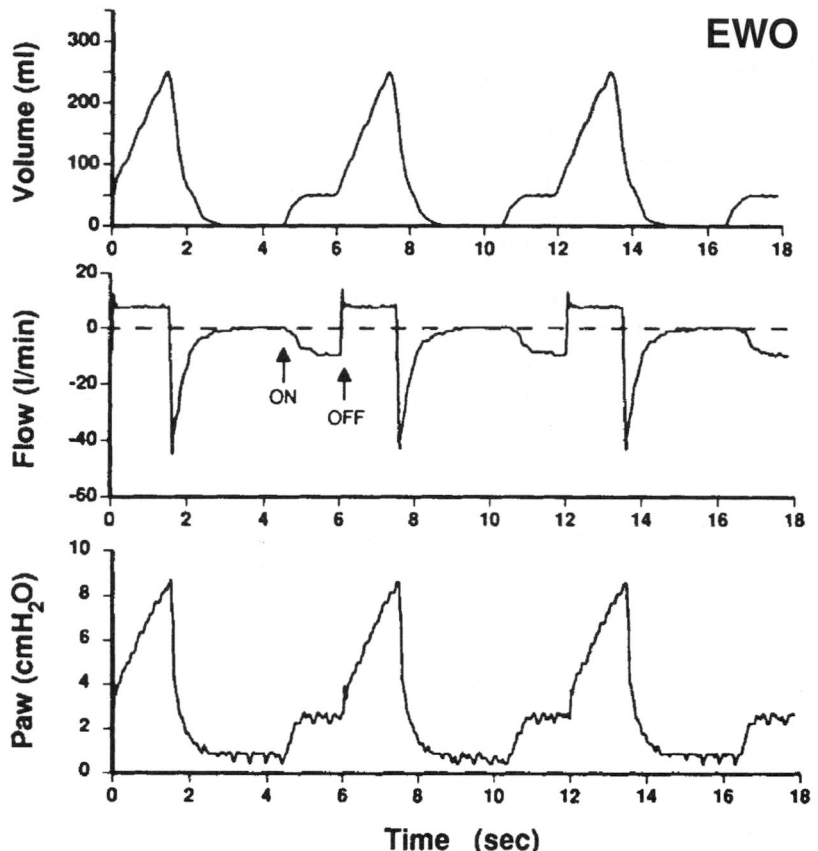

FIGURE 24-3 Simultaneous tracings during expiratory washout (EWO) at 10 liters/min catheter flow. (*Above*) Plethysmographic lung volume relative to the end-expiratory lung volume measured without catheter flow. (*Center*) Flow tracing measured in the inspiratory and expiratory limbs of the external circuit. (*Below*) Proximal airway pressure. Note that lung volume and proximal airway pressure tracings show preinspiratory step changes. These deflections indicate that gas flows both antegrade (volume tracing) and retrograde (flow tracing) from the catheter tip during this period. (*Used, with permission, Burke et al: Am Rev Respir Dis 148:561–8, 1993.*)

optimal coordination of catheter injection with respect to the cycling pattern of the ventilator.

Physiologic Effects

The physiologic dead space consists of conducting airways (instrumental and anatomic dead space) and well-ventilated alveoli that receive minimal blood flow. In the second, or intrapulmonary, shunt compartment, little or no gas exchange takes place because alveoli are perfused but not ventilated. Because the anatomic dead space remains relatively constant as V_T is reduced, low V_Ts are associated with a high dead-space-to-tidal-volume ratio.[18] TGI applied together with conventional mechanical ventilation effectively reduces the size of the dead-space compartment and improves overall CO_2 elimination by replacing the CO_2 that normally occupies the anatomic dead space with fresh gas during expiration. Consequently, less CO_2 is recycled to the alveoli during the next inspiration, and the ventilatory efficiency of each tidal respiration is improved. Therefore, TGI reduces anatomic dead space and increases alveolar ventilation for a given frequency and V_T combination. The main effect of TGI is to flush the dead space from the carina to the Y of the ventilator circuit to enhance CO_2 removal.

The presence of the catheter and the TGI jet effect, however, oppose expiratory flow and favor air trapping at end expiration and auto-PEEP.[7,18,25–30]

Rationale, Advantages, and Limitations

TGI reduces Pa_{CO_2} during hypoventilation.[20,31–34] This effect occurs whether hypoventilation is caused by a decrease in minute ventilation or an increase in respiratory rate at constant minute ventilation. The efficacy of TGI in lowering Pa_{CO_2}, however, diminishes when an increased alveolar component dominates the total physiologic dead space.[22,34,35]

The volume of gas injected per breath during expiration and the volume of gas flushed out of the dead space during the expiratory period determine the effectiveness of TGI, provided that inspired minute ventilation remains unchanged and end expiration is included in the catheter flush period.[36] Increasing catheter flow in clinical situations where only a brief expiratory time is available may maintain TGI efficiency. In fact, an inverse correlation between respiratory rate and Pa_{CO_2} has been observed,[37] indicating that lower breathing frequencies (or longer expiratory times) favor TGI efficiency (defined as reductions in Pa_{CO_2} and physiologic dead space).

A significant increase in airway pressure and in lung volumes is a well-known side effect of TGI and correlates with the flow used.[14,33] When TGI is limited to the expiratory phase, V_T remains virtually unchanged during volume-control ventilation (VCV), but airway pressures still can increase through expiratory flow limitation and auto-PEEP. Therefore, successful application of TGI is limited by the potential for overpressurization of the airways and production of dynamic hyperinflation.[33] An increase in total PEEP either may increase alveolar dead space, which counteracts the TGI clearance of CO_2, or may recruit collapsed alveoli and improve CO_2 clearance.

Increase in lung volume is a serious limitation of TGI and should be avoided. Solutions to minimize expiratory TGI-induced auto-PEEP include using lower TGI flows, delivering TGI during pressure-controlled ventilation (PCV), and optimizing mechanical ventilation during TGI. During PCV, a TGI-induced increase in airway pressure automatically results in a decrease in V_T, and the lack of expiratory TGI-induced auto-PEEP is associated with a reduction in the efficiency of CO_2 elimination. Likewise, if TGI flow is reduced, the ability to clear CO_2 also will be diminished.[28,38–40]

Indications and Contraindications

END-STAGE PULMONARY DISEASE

Continuous insufflation of fresh gas (oxygen/air) through an intratracheal catheter has been used in patients with end-stage pulmonary disease and chronic CO_2 retention to provide continuous oxygen therapy and to decrease oxygen flow requirements.[8–10,41] In patients with end-stage lung disease, TGI provides a method for oxygen delivery and confers the additional benefits of decreasing dyspnea and increasing exercise tolerance.[42] A continuous low flow (4–5 liters/min) delivered to the tracheostomy tube produces a reduction in dead space, V_T, and minute ventilation without affecting Pa_{CO_2} in the acute state, whereas it maintains or reduces Pa_{CO_2} in the chronic state presumably secondary to reductions in dead space. In patients with the most severe forms of chronic obstructive pulmonary disease (COPD), TGI brought about a reduction in oxygen consumption and CO_2 production, as well as a less demanding respiratory pattern.[10] These findings help to explain the improvements in exercise tolerance and decreased dyspnea and support the use of transtracheal gas therapy for indications other than oxygenation. Interestingly, when TGI was combined with periodic tracheal occlusions in spontaneously breathing tracheostomized animals,[43] a progressive increase in minute ventilation and reductions in Pa_{CO_2} that ultimately led to the cessation of spontaneous breathing efforts were observed. Further studies are necessary to determine the efficacy of TGI in supporting patients with chronic hypercapnic respiratory insufficiency during sleep and wakefulness.

ACUTE LUNG INJURY AND ACUTE RESPIRATORY DISTRESS SYNDROME

Studies of TGI in patients with ARDS have focused on demonstrating a reduction in V_T and subsequently on airway pressure while Pa_{CO_2} is maintained constant or a reduction in Pa_{CO_2} during permissive hypercapnia[36,39,44,45] (Fig. 24-4). Despite the fact that TGI was first tested in humans

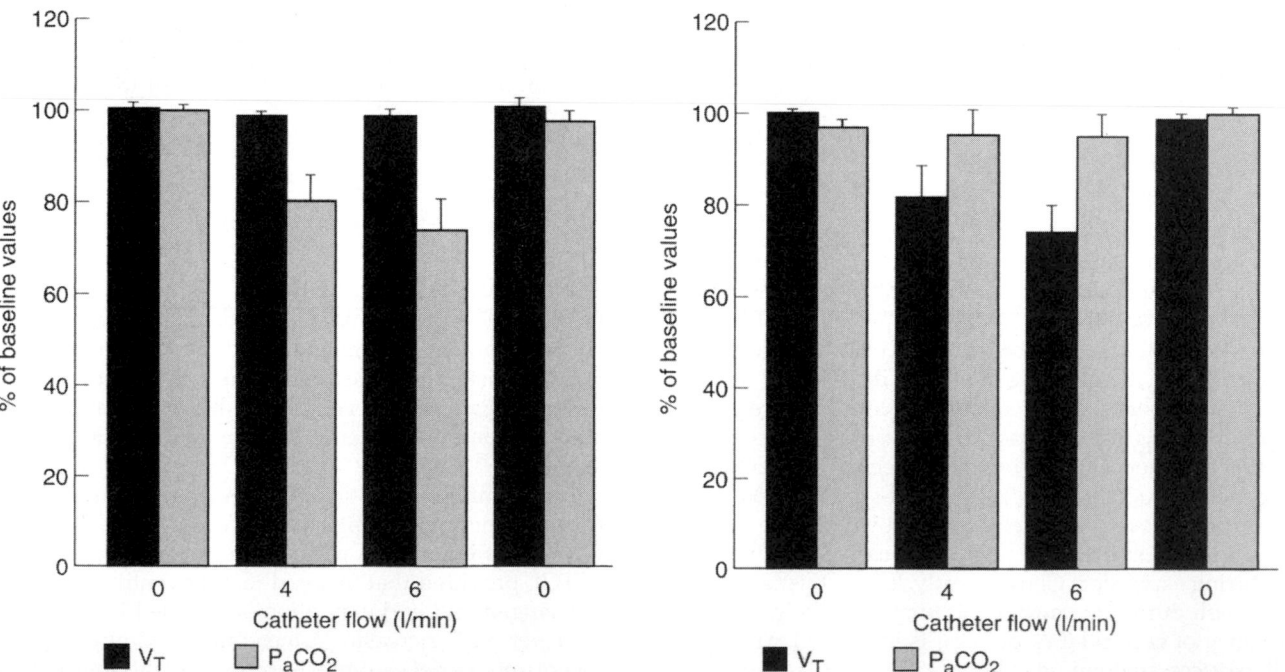

FIGURE 24-4 The effect of different TGI catheter flows in patients with acute respiratory failure. (*Left*) percent reductions in Pa_{CO_2} while tidal volume (V_T) was maintained constant. (*Right*) Percent reductions in V_T while Pa_{CO_2} was maintained constant. (*Used, with permission, from Nakos et al: Intensive Care Med 20:407–13, 1994.*)

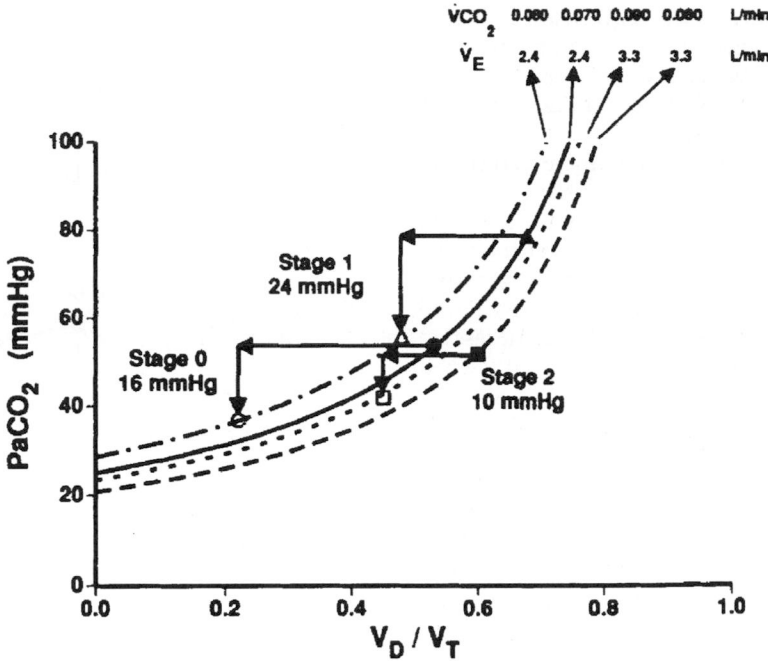

FIGURE 24-5 The effect of TGI on Pa_{CO_2} as a function of the total physiologic dead-space fraction (V_D/V_T). The lines were constructed using the equation $Pa_{CO_2} = 863 V_{CO_2}[\dot{V}_E(1 - V_D/V_T)]$. The CO_2 production rate (V_{CO_2}) and the minute ventilation ($\dot{V}_E$) used for each line are specified.   Symbols respectively represent before (stage 0, *circles*) and after (stage 1, *triangles*) oleic acid injury in experimental animals and after oleic acid injury with increased tidal volume (stage 2, *squares*). Solid and open symbols correspond to baseline and TGI conditions, respectively. Despite a smaller decrease in V_D/V_T during TGI after oleic acid injury (stage 1), the decrement in Pa_{CO_2} was larger because the respiratory system operated on the most curvilinear portion of the curve. During stage 2, the increase in $\dot{V}_E$ shifted the curve to the right, causing the system to operate on the flatter portion of the curve. Consequently, the decrement in Pa_{CO_2} resulting from TGI was much smaller than it would have been if $\dot{V}_E$ had remained constant. During all TGI stages, the increase in V_{CO2} shifted the curve to the left and attenuated the observed decrement in Pa_{CO_2} for a given decrease in V_D/V_T caused by TGI. (*Used, with permission, from Nahum et al: Am J Respir Crit Care Med 152:489–95, 1995.*)

receiving mechanical ventilation in 1969,[46] randomized clinical trials are still lacking.

In patients with ARDS, part of the dead space resides in the alveoli (alveolar dead space). The alveolar gas originating from those ventilated but hypoperfused lung regions is poor in CO_2, diminishing the impact of washing proximal airways. Adopting a permissive hypercapnia strategy increases the amount of CO_2 that can be removed from the proximal anatomic dead space and counterbalances the decreased efficacy of TGI for CO_2 removal caused by increased alveolar dead space[7,47] (Fig. 24-5). Several studies[39,44,48] have shown that one of the most important features of TGI

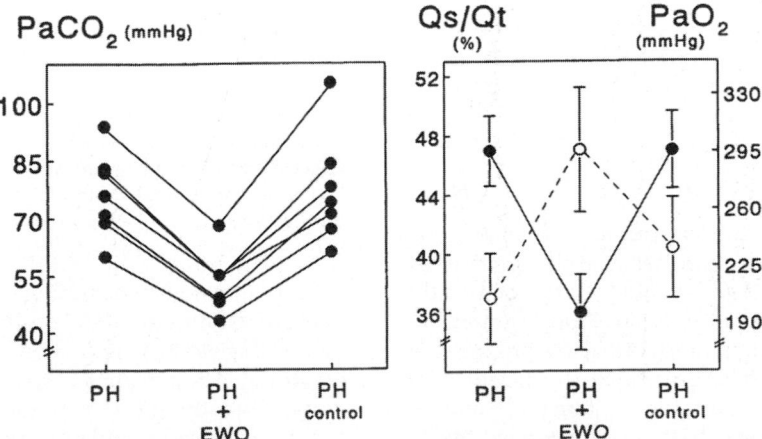

FIGURE 24-6 Individual changes in Pa_{CO_2}, true pulmonary shunt ($\dot{Q}s/\dot{Q}t$), and Pa_{O_2} during permissive hypercapnia (PH) and PH plus expiratory washout at 15 liters/min (EWO) in patients with acute respiratory distress syndrome. PH plus EWO reduced Pa_{CO_2} and pulmonary shunt and improved oxygenation. These effects were associated with a parallel increase in plateau and mean airway pressures, suggesting the development of auto-PEEP and air trapping during EWO. (*Used, with permission, from Kalfon et al: Anesthesiology 87:6–17, 1997.*)

is that it can maintain normocapnia or a given level of Pa_{CO_2} while V_T is decreased, allowing a reduction in minute ventilation. Therefore, TGI can be used to decrease the forces acting on the lung and thereby minimize ventilator-induced lung injury in patients with ARDS.

In patients with ARDS ventilated with a permissive hypercapnia strategy,[30] high expiratory washout flows (15 liters/min) are very useful in reducing Pa_{CO_2}, although there may be a considerable risk of favoring air trapping, auto-PEEP, and a subsequent increase in plateau pressure (Fig. 24-6). The combination of increasing respiratory rate to the limit of originating auto-PEEP, eliminating unnecessary instrumental dead space, and reducing external PEEP when TGI-induced auto-PEEP rises (to maintain the total PEEP constant) seems to be a suitable approach to delivering a pressure-limited ventilator strategy in combination with TGI in hypercapnic patients with severe ARDS[39,49] (Fig. 24-7).

Severe unilateral lung pathology, such as lung contusion, unilateral pneumonia, or refractory atelectasis, is common in the intensive-care setting and often requires mechanical ventilation with a high fraction of inspired oxygen (F_{IO_2}). In this context, the application of PEEP usually does not improve oxygenation because it may cause overdistension of compliant lung regions and redistribute blood flow to collapsed or fluid-filled alveoli.[50] In experimental studies on unilateral lung injury,[51,52] selective TGI application improved oxygenation and decreased P_{CO_2} and airway pressures, and functional residual capacity (FRC) remained constant, whereas V_T could be further decreased. Although selective TGI improved pulmonary function without any side effects, it is hazardous to extrapolate experimental data to the clinical setting because it is not known whether high TGI flows could be maintained for a long period.

TGI-associated reduction in Pa_{CO_2} may be a potentially important maneuver in patients with cerebrovascular injury with intracranial hypertension and concomitant ALI/ARDS. These patients need aggressive treatment to maintain intracranial pressure as low as possible, together with protective lung ventilation. Both anecdotal case reports[53,54] and case series[55] have shown that TGI in patients with ALI/ARDS and severe head trauma allowed a more protective ventilator strategy while Pa_{CO_2} was reduced or remained constant; more important, no short-term deleterious effects on hemodynamics or cerebral parameters were seen (Fig. 24-8).

LIBERATION FROM MECHANICAL VENTILATION

Failure of the respiratory muscle pump is probably the most common cause of failure to wean from mechanical ventilation. Indeed, patients with COPD who subsequently fail a weaning trial exhibit not only an almost immediate rapid and shallow breathing pattern but also a progressive worsening of pulmonary mechanics with inefficient CO_2 clearance. Deterioration in respiratory system mechanics in patients who fail the weaning trial is characterized by increases in auto-PEEP and in inspiratory resistance, together with a decrease in dynamic lung compliance.[56] Therefore, TGI could facilitate liberation from ventilator support by enhancing CO_2 clearance.

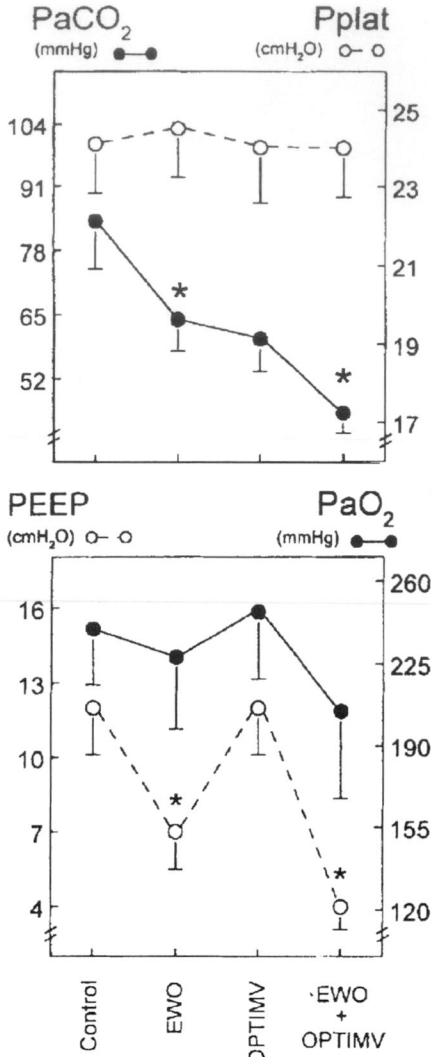

FIGURE 24-7 Changes in Pa_{CO_2}, inspiratory plateau airway pressure (Pplat), PEEP, and Pa_{O_2} induced by optimized mechanical ventilation (OPTIMV), expiratory washout (EWO), and the combination of OPTIMV and EWO in six patients with severe acute respiratory distress syndrome. Extrinsic PEEP had to be reduced by 5.3 ± 2.1 cmH$_2$O during EWO and by 7.3 ± 1.3 cmH$_2$O during the combination of OPTIMV and EWO, whereas it remained unchanged during OPTIMV alone. Plateau pressure did not change significantly, suggesting that lung hyperinflation was not produced. In patients with severe ARDS, the combination of OPTIMV and EWO has additive effects and resulted in Pa_{CO_2} levels close to normal values. (*Used, with permission, from Richecoeur et al: Am J Respir Crit Care Med 160:77–85, 1999.*)

In spontaneously breathing sheep with ALI,[57] the combination of continuous-flow positive airway pressure (CPAP) and TGI yielded a reduction in the inspiratory work of breathing. The beneficial effect of TGI with CPAP on the work of breathing was attributed to a favorable balance between decreased ventilatory requirements and low workload superimposed by the apparatus and TGI. In fact, when CPAP is delivered in combination with TGI, additional inspiratory effort is required to overcome the insufflation flow and trigger the ventilator valves. TGI may increase the work

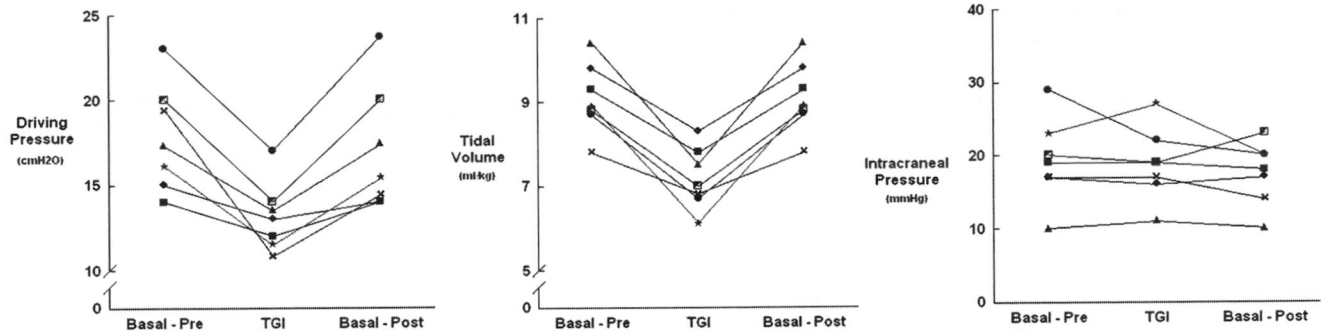

FIGURE 24-8 Individual values of driving airway pressure (difference between plateau pressure and PEEP) (*left*), tidal volume (*center*), and intracranial pressure before (basal-pre), during (TGI), and after (basal-post) application of expiratory TGI in patients with severe head trauma and acute lung injury. Expiratory TGI allowed the targeted Pa_{CO_2} level to be maintained, together with substantial reductions in tidal volume and driving pressure, without deleterious effects on cerebral parameters. (*Used, with permission, from Martinez et al: Intensive Care Med 30:2021–7, 2004.*)

needed to open the demand valve and trigger the ventilator; this problem may be surmounted by a system that stops TGI flow before the end of expiration[58] (Fig. 24-9).

Case series[37,59] on the effects of TGI on lung function in patients undergoing weaning from mechanical ventilation have reported that V_T, minute ventilation, Pa_{CO_2}, and physiologic dead space were reduced in a flow-dependent manner when gas was delivered through an orotracheal tube. Moreover, distal positioning of the TGI catheter was more effective than proximal positioning, and the effects were less pronounced in patients with tracheostomy. Interestingly, the improvement in ventilatory efficiency resulting from the reduction of dead space yielded a decrease in Pa_{CO_2} at the same respiratory rate and at lower V_T.

Operational Characteristics of TGI

CATHETER POSITION

In TGI, a single catheter usually is placed above the main carina, making this technique simple to use. Nonetheless, more distal catheter placement may improve the efficiency of TGI in two ways[33] (Fig. 24-10). First, with more distal placement, a greater volume lies proximal to the catheter tip, permitting additional expiratory flushing of CO_2-laden dead space. Moving the catheter toward the carina also advances the jet-generated turbulence zone closer to the lung periphery, thereby improving TGI efficacy. In support of this hypothesis, advancing the catheter tip from 0.5 cm proximal

FIGURE 24-9 Flow and inductive plethysmographic lung-volume tracing in a mechanically ventilated patient (pressure support of 4 cmH$_2$O) during panexpiratory TGI of 8 liters/min. In 6 of 11 breaths, TGI flow meets the patient's inspiratory flow demand and provides the total inspiratory volume for the breath, and the ventilator is not triggered. (*Used, with permission, from Hoyt et al: Chest 110:775–83, 1996.*)

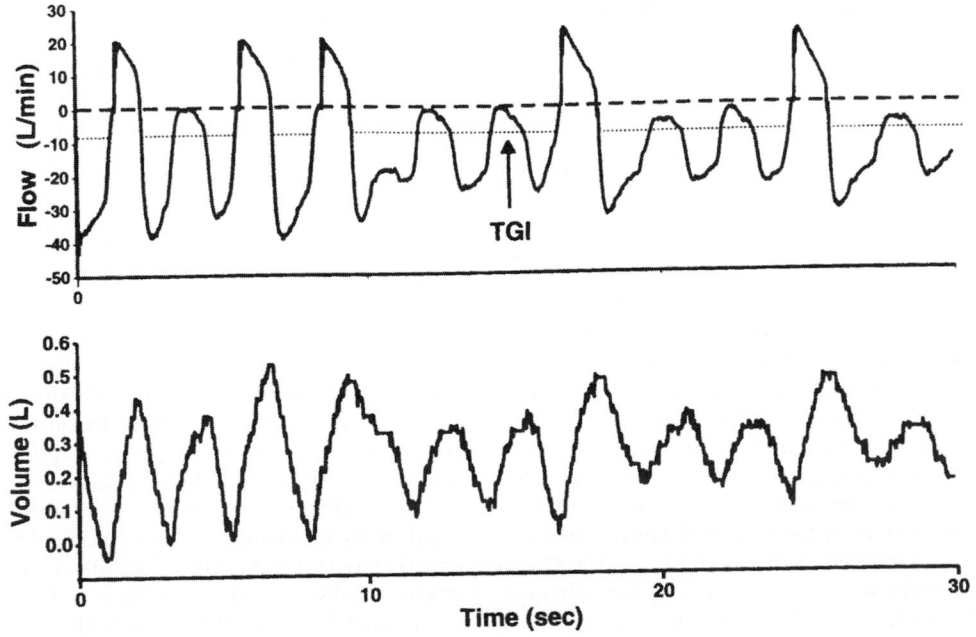

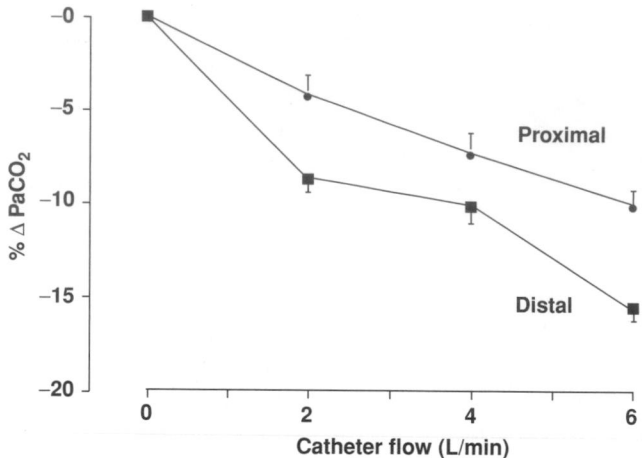

FIGURE 24-10 Percent reduction in Pa_{CO_2} from the baseline value as a function of catheter flow. Distal and proximal catheter positions were 1 and 10 cm above the carina, respectively. Increasing catheter flow caused a reduction in the percent change of Pa_{CO_2} from baseline at both catheter positions. At studied catheter flows, the distal position provided a larger percentage reduction in Pa_{CO_2}. (*Used, with permission, from Ravenscraft et al: Am Rev Respir Dis 148:345–51, 1993.*)

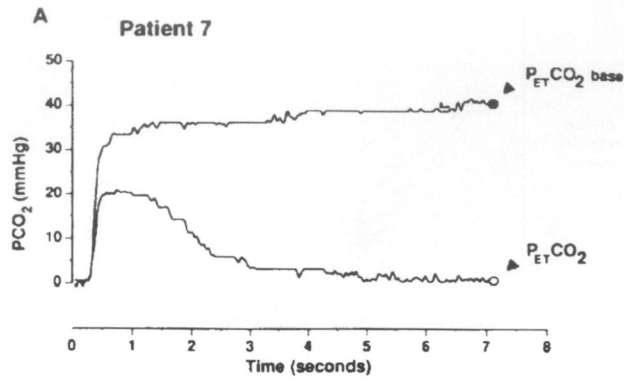

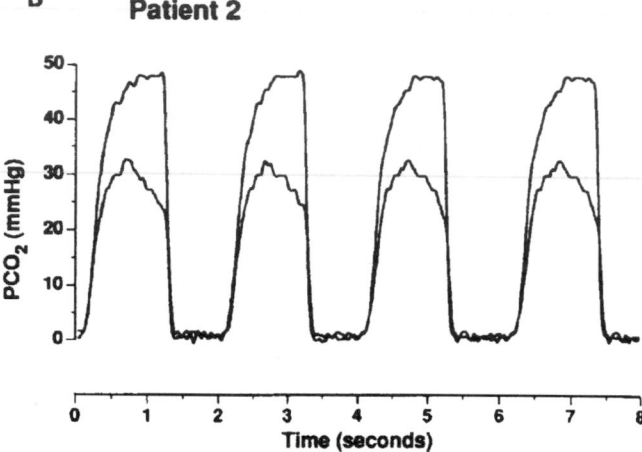

FIGURE 24-11 Representative exhaled capnograms in two patients without TGI and with TGI at 6 liters/min insufflation flow. A greater reduction in end-tidal CO_2 (Pet_{CO_2}) from the Pet_{CO_2} base value corresponded with a larger reduction in Pa_{CO_2}. At a given insufflation flow, efficiency to clear CO_2 is a function of the time available to flush proximal dead space. (*Used, with permission, from Ravenscraft et al: Am Rev Respir Dis 148:345–51, 1993.*)

to 4.0 cm distal to the main carina in normal dogs moved the peak resistance to gas transport from second- to fourth-generation airways.[15] The clinical benefit of introducing TGI catheters deeper than the main carina is doubtful, however. In a series of animal studies, the effect of TGI on Pa_{CO_2} was strongly dependent on catheter flow rate, but catheter tip position was not crucial as long as it was within a few centimeters below or above the main carina.[15,27,33] Similar findings have been reported in critically ill patients.[36] In summary, these results indicate that during TGI, bronchoscopic guidance may not be necessary for TGI catheter placement; this helps to keep its clinical application simple because the position of the catheter can be verified on a recent chest radiograph by estimating the distance from the tip of the ETT to the main carina.

CATHETER FLOW RATE

TGI usually employs modest catheter flow rates. Most animal and human studies of TGI have used a flow rates of 4–10 liters/min. Carbon dioxide elimination during TGI depends primarily on catheter flow rate,[33,36,44,60] with turbulence generated at higher flows enhancing distal gas mixing and CO_2 elimination.[14] Once fresh gas sweeps the proximal anatomic dead-space compartment free of CO_2, further increases in flow rate are unlikely to wash more CO_2 out of the proximal anatomic dead space. Because expiratory washout of the proximal anatomic dead space is the primary mechanism of action of TGI, both curtailing expiratory time and prolonging lung deflation may diminish the efficacy of TGI unless catheter flow rate is very high. Decreasing expiratory time would decrease the volume of fresh gas delivered to the central airways per respiratory cycle (Fig. 24-11). The presence of expiratory flow at end expiration would deliver additional CO_2 into the proximal anatomic dead space and thus decrease the efficacy of TGI. The effect of ongoing lung

deflation on TGI efficacy has been studied in normal dogs using short and extended duty cycles at a fixed respiratory frequency.[16] The expiratory flush volume of fresh gas, however, rather than its delivery pattern or flow rate determined the observed decline in Pa_{CO_2} with TGI. These observations suggest that as expiratory time is shortened, higher flow rates are required to preserve TGI efficacy. At high catheter flow rates, bronchotrauma is possible because of the high impact pressure and shear of the inflow jet on the bronchial mucosa.[61,62]

The optimal flow rate in terms of the decrement in Pa_{CO_2} afforded by TGI is a complex function of the volume of anatomic dead space proximal to catheter tip, volume of fresh gas delivered per expiration, pattern of CO_2 exhalation from the lungs, and the CO_2 exchange characteristics of the respiratory system before initiation of TGI. Once dead space proximal to the catheter tip has been almost completely flushed by the fresh gas during expiration, any catheter-flow dependence of Pa_{CO_2} is likely to be secondary to enhanced turbulent mixing in the airways distal to the catheter tip. Consequently, Pa_{CO_2} continues to decrease with

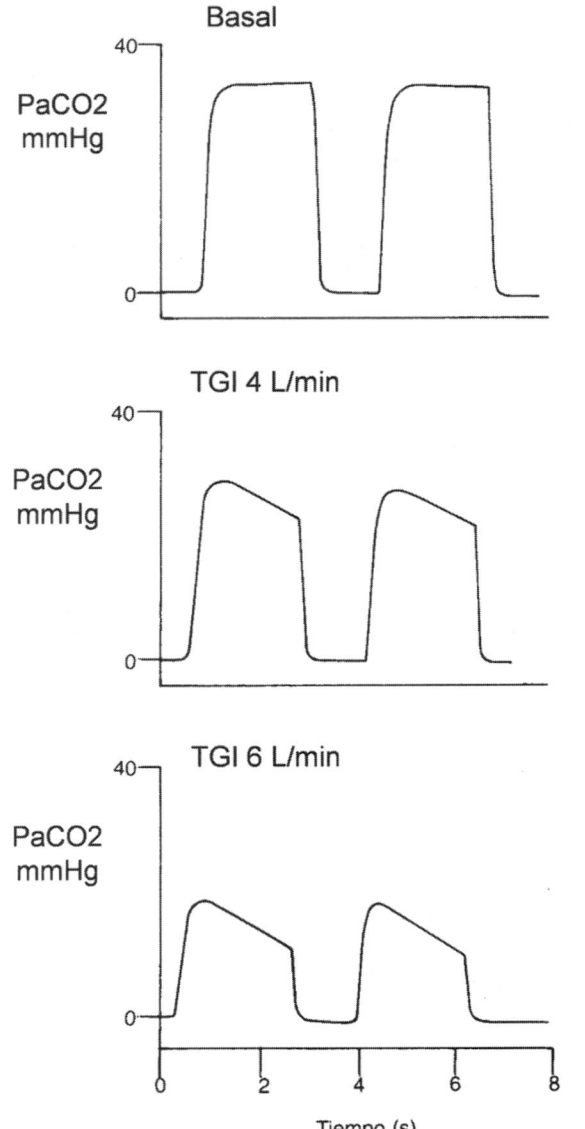

Basal

PaCO2 mmHg

TGI 4 L/min

PaCO2 mmHg

TGI 6 L/min

PaCO2 mmHg

Tiempo (s)

FIGURE 24-12 Effect of continuous TGI on exhaled capnogram in patients with acute respiratory failure. Increasing catheter flows produced greater clearance of exhaled CO_2. (*Used, with permission, from Saura et al: Med Intensiva 20:246–51, 1996.*)

increasing flow rate as catheter flow rate rises but at a slower pace[14,33] (Fig. 24-12). In most TGI systems, the effect of increasing flow rate diminishes considerably when flow rate exceeds 10 liters/min. If TGI-induced turbulent mixing contributes sufficiently to CO_2 removal during expiration, it is possible to calculate a negative physiologic dead space using the Enghoff modification of the Bohr equation corrected for the catheter's dilutional effect on mixed expired CO_2.[49]

CATHETER SHAPE

In order to benefit from the distal turbulence produced by TGI, the catheter needs to direct the jet stream toward the periphery of the lung.[14] Inverting the catheter mouthward eliminates the distal effects and decreases CO_2 removal. Inverting the catheter within the ETT, however, avoids direct-

ing the jet stream onto the bronchial mucosa, which may cause bronchial injury.[61-63] Alternatively, the catheter tip can be positioned within the ETT so that the jet hits the ETT wall. The orientation of the ETT holes with respect to the catheter (end or side) appears to have little impact on catheter efficiency.[33] Nevertheless, catheter shape directly influences the extent (or lack of) dynamic hyperinflation caused by TGI.[13,64]

HUMIDIFICATION

The fresh gas delivered by TGI should be heated and humidified to prevent mucous plug formation and to prevent TGI gas from causing bronchial injury via cooling and dehydration of the bronchial mucosa. Few studies have examined the occurrence of bronchial mucosal injury systematically during TGI. Similarly, not many studies have examined the effect of conditioning TGI gas on the extent of injury to bronchial mucosa. TGI can cool tracheal gas significantly. The extent of cooling was greatest at high catheter flow rates with continuous TGI and could be compensated only partially by conditioning the ventilator-delivered inspired gas during panexpiratory TGI.[65,66] Case series have reported either no damage or no encrustation,[63] whereas other investigators found intratracheal catheter obstruction after 2 days of continuous use.[48]

The drying and cooling effect of TGI can be eliminated if the gas can be heated and humidified. Most humidifiers, however, cannot withstand the pressures needed to drive gas at 5–10 liters/min through small-bore catheters. Most commercially available humidifiers leak or burst when the pressure within their chamber exceeds 140 cmH_2O. This pressure limit restricts the rate of catheter flow that can be used. For example, approximately 140 cmH_2O of driving pressure is required to deliver air through 40-cm-long 6.5F and 8.0F catheters at flow rates of 3.6 and 6.4 liters/min, respectively. Therefore, the pressure tolerance limits of currently available humidifiers cannot withstand the flow rates of 5–10 liters/min necessary for most TGI systems.

ENDOTRACHEAL TUBE DESIGN

There is no standard method of introducing the TGI catheter into the trachea. In most human studies, a small-caliber catheter is introduced through an angled sidearm adapter attached to the ETT and positioned just above the main carina.[36,44,45,48] Catheter placement usually is performed under bronchoscopic guidance or estimated from a chest radiograph. This type of system is simple to construct and can be duplicated in most intensive-care units but suffers from some drawbacks. Placement of a catheter through the ETT interferes with suctioning of patients and can increase airway resistance by partially occluding the airway. Moreover, the catheter is not fixed in space and may cause injury to bronchial mucosae if it whips within the trachea at high flows. Alternatively, the catheter can be placed outside the ETT along the trachea. This technique requires visualization of the vocal cords and deflation of the ETT cuff and risks puncturing the cuff.

New designs that incorporate channels within the ETT wall would solve these problems and simplify TGI

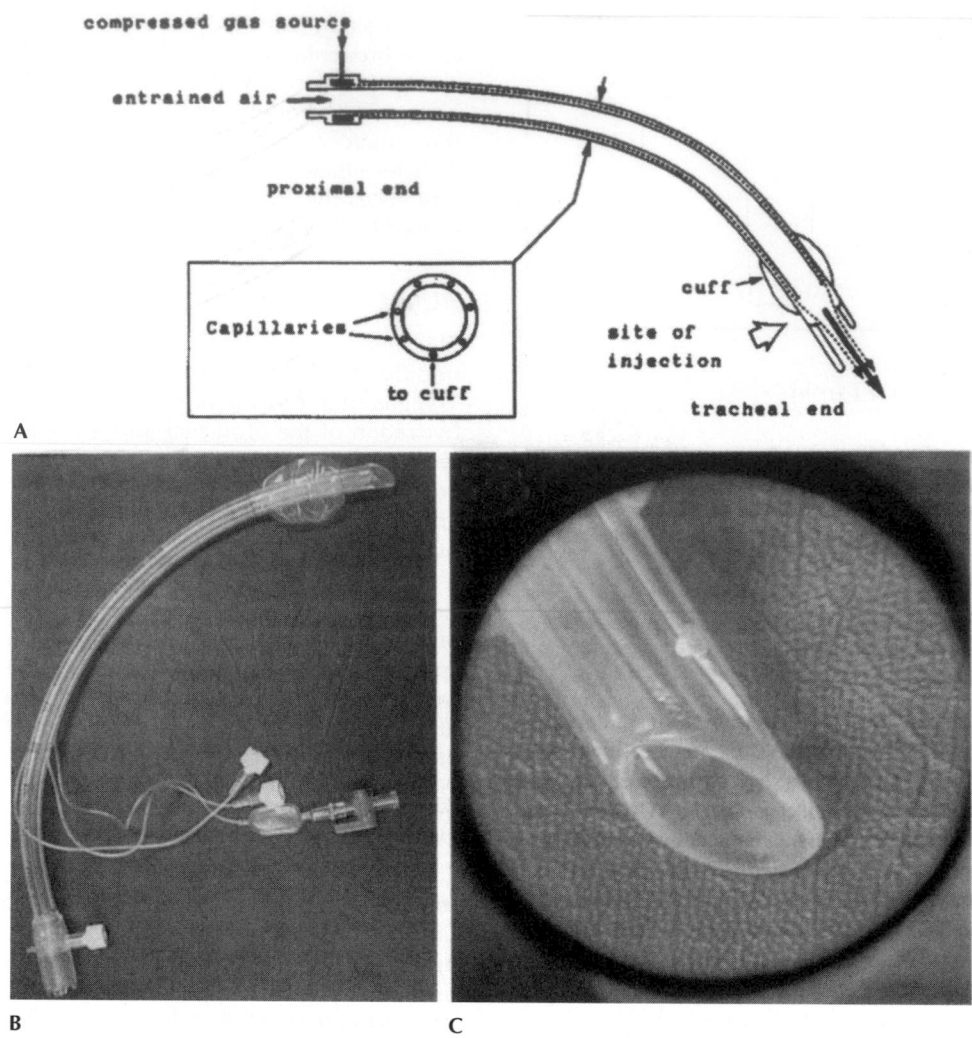

FIGURE 24-13 The LaBrune-Boussignac endotracheal tube. *A.* Schematic of the entire tube with a midtube cross section. *B.* Photograph of the tube. *C.* Photograph of the tube tip. (*Used, with permission, from Adams: Respir Care 46:177–84, 2001.*)

application. Boussignac et al[67,68] embedded small capillaries in the walls of an ETT for TGI (Fig. 24-13). The same group also has used this modified ETT to deliver high-velocity jets of O_2 at the carinal orifice in order to prevent arterial O_2 desaturation during suctioning.[69] Although lung volumes did not change during suctioning when O_2 was delivered in this fashion, the rate of increase in Pa_{CO_2} was similar to that observed during apnea. The modified ETT can be used to reduce the aggressive nature of mechanical ventilation in different clinical scenarios.[70,71] Most likely, future clinical applications of TGI will use a modified ETT that incorporates the catheter in its wall attached to a standardized circuit for gas delivery. In any case, application of TGI should never require reintubation of the patient.[72]

Kolobow et al[63] developed a reverse-thrust catheter that directs gas flow from the distal to the proximal part of the ETT, creating a venturi effect (Fig. 24-14). Inverted flow is less effective at expiratory flushing compared with straight flow but has the advantage that it avoids hyperinflation.[64,73] Finally, ETTs for single-lung anesthesia have been used suc-

cessfully to provide selective TGI in experimental models of ALI.[51,52]

The combination of aspiration of anatomic and instrumental dead space in the late part of expiration and replacement of the aspired volume with fresh gas through the inspiratory line of the ventilator improves CO_2 clearance.[74] This aspiration system has allowed reductions in airway pressure and V_T while keeping Pa_{CO_2} constant in healthy humans,[75] as well as in patients with ARDS[76] and COPD.[77] The aforementioned aspiration system has the potential for avoiding the problems associated with jet streams of gas or with gas humidification without developing auto-PEEP (Fig. 24-15).

Adjustments at the Bedside

INSPIRED OXYGEN FRACTION

The actual $F_{I_{O_2}}$ during TGI depends on two factors: contribution of TGI to total inspired V_T and the $F_{I_{O_2}}$ of the catheter

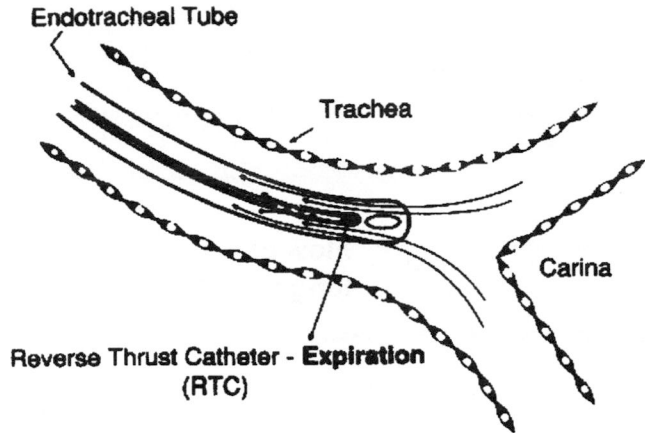

FIGURE 24-14 The reverse-thrust catheter used for intratracheal pulmonary ventilation. Reverse-thrust catheter design allows gas exiting the distal end of the catheter to be directed cephalad. (*Used, with permission, from Hess et al: Respir Care 46:119–29, 2001.*)

gas. However, if the F_{IO_2} of the catheter gas is matched to that of the ventilator, the actual inspired F_{IO_2} always will be identical to that delivered by the ventilator. On the other hand, if 100% O_2 is used as the insufflated gas, the actual inspired F_{IO_2} will be increased by an amount determined by the contribution of TGI to total inspired V_T. This effect will be most prominent during continuous TGI and will be minimized during expiratory TGI.

AIRWAY OPENING PRESSURE

During TGI, the jet stream increases flow through the ventilator circuit during expiration and creates a region where bidirectional flows exist. Both effects change the resistance characteristics of the respiratory system and modify the relationship between airway opening (Pao) and alveolar (Palv) pressures observed at baseline at a catheter flow rate of 0 liter/min. Because expiratory resistance increases during TGI, Pao tends to underestimate Palv (and FRC) when the system is switched from baseline to TGI conditions. In an experimental study, monitoring tracheal pressure 2 cm beyond the tip of the catheter seemed to predict

lung-volume changes at end expiration accurately, suggesting that tracheal pressures should be monitored beyond the jet stream during TGI.[14] During panexpiratory TGI, catheter flow ceases during inspiration, and inspiratory Pao provides as much useful information regarding Palv as during conventional mechanical ventilation. In contrast, during continuous TGI, inspiratory Pao (measured at the tip of the ETT) differs from the tracheal pressure (Fig. 24-16). The magnitude of this difference depends on the flow through the circuit spanning the two pressure-measurement points and is usually less than 3 cmH₂O. During expiration under both continuous and expiratory TGI conditions, however, catheter flow pressurizes the respiratory system, and as a result, Pao underestimates tracheal pressure.[61] During expiration, the extent Pao underestimates tracheal pressure increases with catheter flow rate and depends on the geometry of the system and the orientation of the catheter with respect to the trachea.

EFFECT OF TGI ON LUNG VOLUME

In both animal and human experiments, TGI increased FRC in a flow-dependent fashion.[14,36] TGI can increase FRC in three ways. First, part of the momentum of the discharging jet stream is transferred to the alveoli.[78] Second, the catheter decreases the cross-sectional area of the trachea, increases expiratory resistance, and delays emptying. Third, catheter flow through the ETT, expiratory circuit, and expiratory valve can build up a backpressure that impedes deflation and is the major determinant of dynamic hyperinflation.[79] Continuous TGI increased FRC more than expiratory TGI, especially when the inspiratory time fraction was prolonged.[79]

Dynamic hyperinflation caused by TGI may present either a problem or a therapeutic option[39] and can be manipulated by using an inverted-jet insufflator to achieve a venturi effect.[14,63] Monitoring dynamic hyperinflation during TGI requires a means of external lung-volume measurement such as impedance plethysmography. Guided by the plethysmograph signal, ventilator-set PEEP can be adjusted to maintain FRC constant as flow rate is varied.[27,34] Alternatively, if the TGI system allows an end-expiratory hold maneuver to be performed, the ventilator-set PEEP can be

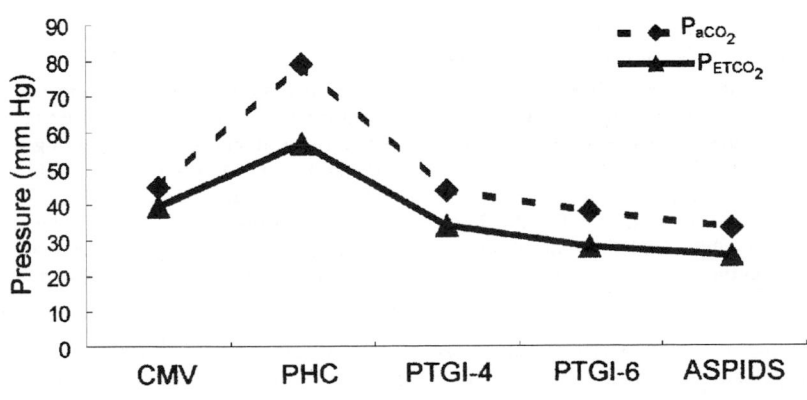

FIGURE 24-15 Comparison between aspiration of dead space (ASPIDS) and phasic tracheal gas insufflation (PTGI) during conventional mechanical ventilation (CMV) and permissive hypercapnia (PHC) that was induced by decreasing tidal volume by 30% in patients with severe COPD. The mean Pa_{CO_2} reductions with PTGI flows of 4.0 and 6.0 liters/min and during ASPIDS (at 4.0 liters/min) were 32.7%, 51.8%, and 53.5%, respectively. Auto-PEEP increased with PTGI but not with ASPIDS. (*Used, with permission, from Liu et al: Respir Care 49:257–62, 2004.*)

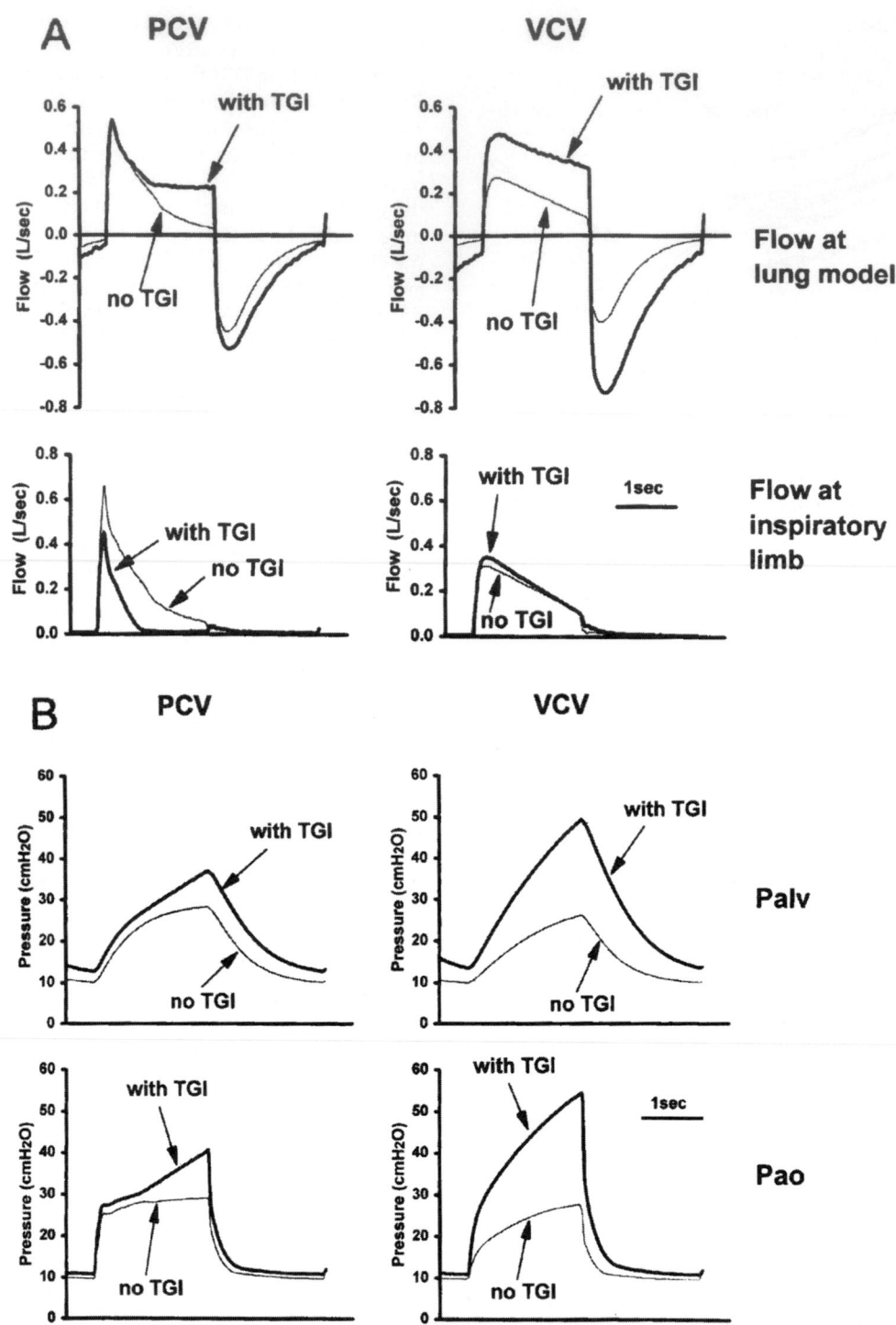

FIGURE 24-16 *A.* Flow-versus-time tracings of delivered gas flow measured both at airway opening and distal to the entrance of tracheal gas insufflation (TGI) during both pressure-controlled ventilation (PCV) and volume-controlled ventilation (VCV) with and without the addition of 12 liters/min TGI in a lung model. *B.* Pressure-versus-time tracings of system pressure measured both at the airway opening (Pao) and distal to the entrance of the TGI flow (Palv) during both PCV and VCV with and without the addition of 12 liters/min of TGI flow in a lung model. Regardless of whether VCV or PCV was used, continuous TGI increases Pao and peak carinal pressure (*B*). In association with these changes there is an increase in tidal volume. During VCV (*A*), the flow from TGI is additive to the flow from the ventilator. During PCV, the addition of the TGI flow caused the flow from the ventilator to decelerate more rapidly; once ventilator flow reached zero, a squarewave flow pattern derived entirely from the TGI system persisted. (*Used, with permission, from Kacmarek: Respir Care 46:167–76, 2001.*)

adjusted to maintain total PEEP constant.[40,80] Alternatively, during PCV, a flow-relief valve automatically compensates for the extra gas that is introduced into the system by TGI and eliminates the need to make ventilator adjustments to control total PEEP.[81]

TIDAL VOLUME

Catheter flow delivered during inspiration contributes to total inspired V_T. This contribution is eliminated if TGI is timed to occur only during expiration.[20] Even in this case, however, decompression of the TGI circuit within the ventilator circuit during the inspiratory phase of solenoid closure contributes to total inspired V_T.[27] In most TGI circuits, however, this volume is rather small (about 10–20 ml at a catheter flow rate of 10 liters/min). These problems are obviated if an independent measure of V_T such as inductive plethysmography is used. The effect of TGI on total inspired V_T depends on the ventilator operation mode.

FLOW-CONTROLLED, VOLUME-CYCLED VENTILATION

During continuous TGI, total inspired V_T is the sum of two components: that delivered by the ventilator and that delivered by the catheter (V_{TC}). The contribution of continuous TGI to total inspired V_T can be estimated from the volume of gas that is insufflated by the catheter during inspiration. Consequently, during flow-controlled, volume-cycled ventilation, total inspired V_T can be maintained relatively constant during continuous TGI by decreasing the ventilator-set V_T by that amount.[27,44]

PRESSURE-CONTROLLED VENTILATION

During pressure-controlled ventilation (PCV), TGI application does not change the total inspired V_T, provided that TGI does not pressurize the respiratory system beyond the set pressure. As catheter flow rate is increased, the ventilator-delivered V_T declines, but the total inspired V_T remains the same.[27,60] The respiratory system behaves in this manner as long as catheter-delivered V_T is less than the V_T generated by the set pressure under PCV conditions without TGI. If V_{TC} exceeds the V_T generated by PCV in the absence of TGI, then TGI will overpressurize the circuit, and peak Pao will be greater than that produced by the ventilator-set pressure. Almost all ventilators allow pressures higher than that generated by the set pressure as long as Pao remains below the high-pressure limit of the ventilator. Consequently, excessive pressures can be produced within the respiratory system if V_{TC} is too large. When this happens, the Pao-time profile becomes a hybrid of PCV and constant-flow volume-cycled ventilation, resembling that generated during volume-assured pressure-support ventilation. This problem can be circumvented by introducing a pressure-release valve into the ventilator circuit that dumps circuit pressure above a set threshold.[82]

TGI-VENTILATOR INTERACTIONS

The interactions between TGI and ventilator mode, V_T, and Pao that result in development of auto-PEEP deserve mention. During volume-controlled ventilation, when ventilator PEEP is left constant, V_T remains constant, but there is an increase in end-expiratory pressure and Pao because of TGI-induced auto-PEEP. During PCV, when ventilator PEEP and peak airway pressure are kept the same as baseline, V_T excursions (and hence minute ventilation) are reduced because of TGI-induced auto-PEEP. When ventilator PEEP is reduced by an amount equivalent to TGI-induced auto-PEEP, V_T, peak airway pressure, and total PEEP remain the same as baseline during PCV[40,65] (Fig. 24-17).

During CPAP delivered by a mechanical ventilator in combination with TGI, additional inspiratory effort is required to overcome the insufflation flow and trigger the ventilator valves. Bench studies have found that TGI might interfere with ventilator triggering at low peak inspiratory flow rates, and this suggests that weak patients may fail to open the demand valve at high catheter flow rates[83] (Fig. 24-18).

Monitoring and Troubleshooting

TGI is a simple and apparently safe method of reducing both minute ventilation and Pa_{CO_2}. Regardless of the approach used, TGI has the potential to alter volumes as well as airway and alveolar pressures; careful monitoring of delivered volumes and pressures therefore is necessary to ensure safe clinical application and to evaluate the effect on lung function. Moreover, the position of the TGI catheter within the ETT should be controlled carefully. The presence of a catheter inside the ETT may increase both inspiratory and expiratory resistances, particularly when small endotracheal or tracheostomy tubes are used.[7,18,32,84,85]

Because TGI introduces an external flow source independent of the ventilator, it can adversely effect the ventilator's ability to monitor pressures and volumes and may cause the ventilator alarm to go off incessantly. The presence of catheter flow during expiration disables the monitoring role of the ventilator's expiratory pneumotachograph, triggering some ventilator alarms when the difference between the measured inspired and exhaled volumes exceeds a certain value. More important, the presence of an external flow that can pressurize the ventilator circuit interferes with the ventilator's ability to detect a leak. Using the end-expiratory occlusion technique to measure auto-PEEP may increase lung volume dramatically if TGI flow is not interrupted simultaneously. The same effect will occur with continuous TGI during end-inspiratory occlusions.[7,32]

Tracheal gas can be delivered throughout the respiratory cycle, throughout expiration, or only during a specific portion of the expiratory period. Continuous-flow TGI is the easiest method to implement but has the greatest potential to cause complications. Continuous-flow TGI could increase delivered V_T, airway and alveolar pressures, and total PEEP with both PCV and with VCV. Moreover, in PCV, when ventilator flow reaches zero, continuous flow from

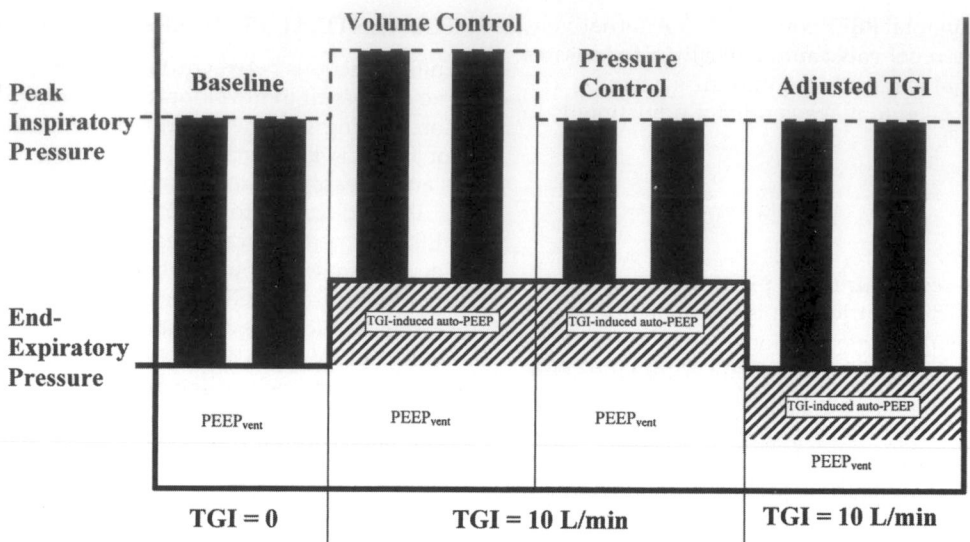

FIGURE 24-17 Theoretical framework that illustrates interactions between tracheal gas insufflation (TGI), ventilator mode, minute ventilation (tidal volume), and auto-PEEP. During volume-controlled ventilation, when ventilator PEEP is left constant, tidal volume (*black bars*) remains constant, but there is an increase in end-expiratory pressure and, consequently, in peak inspiratory pressure. During pressure-controlled ventilation, when set PEEP and peak airway pressure are kept the same as baseline, tidal volume excursions are reduced because of TGI-induced auto-PEEP. When set PEEP is reduced by an amount equivalent to TGI-induced auto-PEEP, tidal volume, peak airway pressure, and total PEEP remain the same as baseline during pressure-controlled ventilation. (*Used, with permission, from Delgado et al: Respir Care 46:185–92, 2001.*)

the continuous TGI increases V_T and airway pressures. A similar phenomenon occurs during end-inspiratory pauses in VCV. These increases occur because the exhalation valve of the ventilator is not active during the inspiratory phase.[25] Overpressurization can be identified by examining the airway pressure tracing[18] and can be remedied by placing a pressure-relief valve in the ventilator circuit to dissipate insufflated flow that produces excess pressure.[57,86] A complete obstruction of the outflow can cause overinflation of the lungs in seconds, with the potential for pneumothorax or hemodynamic compromise.

TGI also may interfere with the clinician's ability to measure lung mechanics. Respiratory system compliance and auto-PEEP measurements require a pause at end inspiration and/or at end expiration. If catheter flow persists during these measurements, the pressure within the respiratory system builds up with time. Consequently, a plateau pressure cannot be reached, and alveolar pressure can increase to hazardous levels if unnoticed. During panexpiratory TGI, depending on the timing and nature of the signal that gates the solenoid to divert catheter flow to the atmosphere, these measurements still can be made safely. Nevertheless, it is advisable to test the TGI-ventilator system using a mechanical lung model under controlled conditions before measuring lung mechanics at the bedside.

The efficacy of TGI can be monitored by capnography (see Figs. 24-11 and 24-12). Expiratory capnograms provide an indicator of the effect of TGI on the CO_2 concentration of the gas remaining in the proximal anatomic dead-space compartment at the onset of inspiration.[36,45,48] Although Pet_{CO_2} is a poor estimate of Pa_{CO_2}[87,88] in patients with respiratory failure, changes in Pet_{CO_2} induced by TGI correlate significantly with changes in Pa_{CO_2} and justify routine measurement of Pet_{CO_2} during TGI as a marker of its effectiveness[35,36,45,48] (Fig. 24-19).

Important Unknowns

The effect of different gas mixtures (helium and oxygen) during TGI has been studied in patients with respiratory failure.[89] Helium is an inert gas that has a much lower density than oxygen or air. When given at the same flow rate as a nitrogen-oxygen mixture, a helium-oxygen mixture produces a much lower Reynolds number and laminar flow.[90] TGI with helium seems to be more effective than TGI with oxygen in treating hypercarbia because the use of helium leads to a smaller increase in airway pressure accompanying the decrease in Pa_{CO_2}.[89] Because the combination helium and oxygen for TGI has the potential to decrease Pa_{O2}, precautions in the use of helium should be taken, particularly in patients who require high F_{IO2} values to provide adequate oxygenation.

The delivery of catheter gas at higher flows needs to be examined with regard to the need for humidification and the potential for tracheal damage with long-term use. Only limited data are available on the clinical safety of TGI. Application of TGI using a large-caliber reverse-thrust catheter resulted in no damage to tracheobronchial mucosa when minute ventilation was adjusted to achieve a similar level of gas exchange during intratracheal pulmonary ventilation to that achieved with conventional mechanical ventilation.[64,91] A similar experiment, however, performed in different species and lasting several hours was associated with a significantly greater difference in tracheobronchial damage at the carina and main bronchus.[62] Turbulent

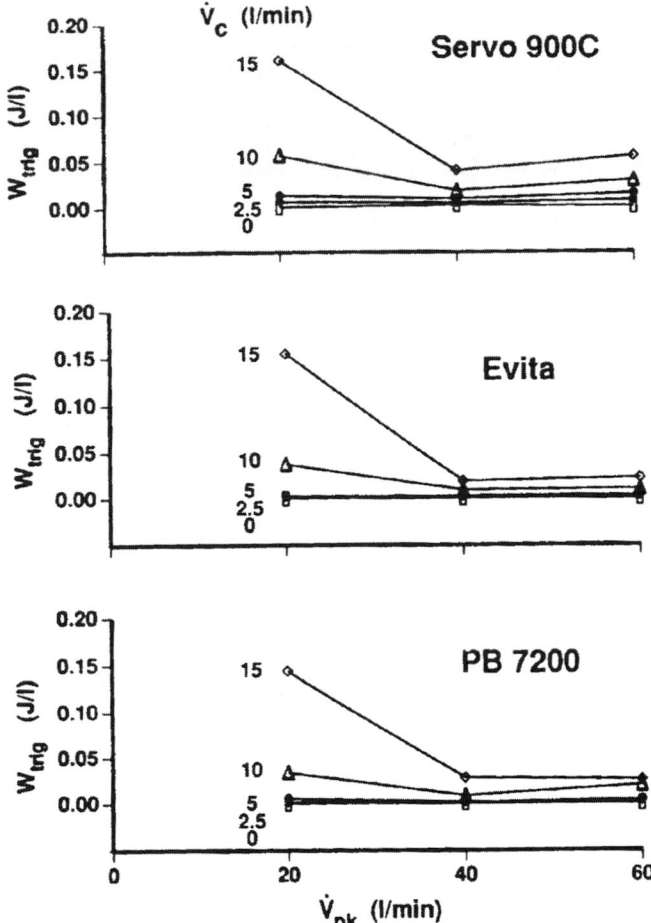

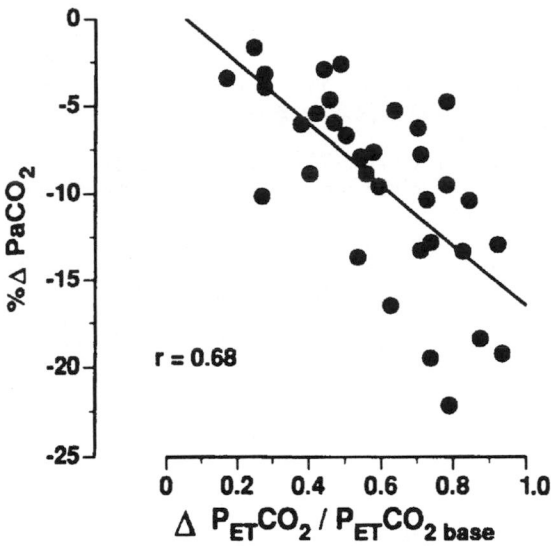

FIGURE 24-19 Percentage reduction in arterial P_{CO_2} (Pa_{CO_2}) from baseline as a function of the reduction in partial pressure of end-tidal P_{CO_2} (Pet_{CO_2}) from the baseline value ($Pet_{CO_2,base}$). As the difference between Pet_{CO_2} and $Pet_{CO_2,base}$ widened, larger reductions in arterial P_{CO_2} were observed. (*Used, with permission from Ravenscraft et al: Am Rev Respir Dis 148:345–51, 1993.*)

FIGURE 24-18 Work of triggering (W-trig) measured from the respiratory muscle compartment (bench) connected to a ventilator (RM-ventilator) for three demand-flow continuous positive airway pressure systems at catheter flow rates ($\dot{V}c$) of 0, 2.5, 5, 10, and 15 liters/min expressed as a function of peak flow rate ($\dot{V}pk$) of the RM-ventilator. None of the ventilators were triggered using a $\dot{V}pk$ and a $\dot{V}c$ of 20 and 15 liters/min, respectively. (*Used, with permission, from Hoyt et al: Chest 110:775–83, 1996.*)

conditions promote shear stress, increased gas impact on the walls of the airway, and the transfer of a higher kinetic energy to the tracheal mucosa.[78,92] The end-hole TGI catheter mode could, in theory, cause more airway damage than large-caliber reverse-thrust catheters because the flow exiting the end-hole catheter is closer to the carina and points directly at it. Further studies in patients are needed to assess clinical safety.[93] Until this information is available, all TGI techniques should be considered investigational.

The Future

TGI should be weighed against therapeutically proven, currently available invasive and noninvasive modes of ventilation. Evidence demonstrating better patient-ventilator interaction with TGI and the absence of significant TGI-related adverse effects needs to be accumulated before TGI can be considered suitable for standard intensive-care practice.

Future TGI systems for clinical applications ideally should include a number of features.[32,61,94] First, intimate coordination with the ventilator is mandatory. This could be accomplished by either a built-in or external device for triggering and breath delivery. Moreover, safety and monitoring capabilities must include an automatic TGI flow shut-off to prevent overpressurization of the ventilator circuit and airways,[82,86] as well as to display precise volume and pressure measurements. Finally, ideal TGI catheters should form part of the artificial airway and be made available commercially.

Summary and Conclusion

TGI is a promising complementary technique to mechanical ventilation. TGI is very effective during permissive hypercapnia in patients with ARDS, diminishing the complications associated with both mechanical ventilation and respiratory acidosis. Furthermore, some studies suggest that TGI-aided weaning may allow a reduction in the patient's respiratory demands. Further studies, however, including randomized trials in patients receiving mechanical ventilation or with weaning difficulties, are necessary to improve technical problems and to demonstrate the clinical benefits and absence of adverse effects of TGI before this technique can be employed routinely in intensive-care units.

Acknowledgment

This work was supported by Fondo de Investigación Sanitaria (FIS) G03/063 Red-Gira.

References

1. Dreyfuss D, Saumon G. Ventilator-induced lung injury: Lessons from experimental studies. Am J Respir Crit Care Med 1998; 157:294–323.

2. International Consensus Conferences in Intensive Care Medicine. Ventilator-associated lung injury in ARDS. Am J Respir Crit Care Med 1999; 160:2118–24.

3. Amato MBP, Barbas CS, Medeiros DM, et al. Effect of a protective-ventilation strategy on mortality in the acute respiratory distress syndrome. New Engl J Med 1998; 338:347–54.

4. Acute Respiratory Distress Syndrome Network. Ventilation with lower tidal volume as compared with traditional tidal volumes for acute lung injury and the acute respiratory distress syndrome. New Engl J Med 2000; 342:1301–8.

5. Ranieri VM, Suter P, Tortorella C, et al. Effect of mechanical ventilation on inflammatory mediators in patients with acute respiratory distress syndrome: A randomized, controlled trial. JAMA 1999; 282:54–61.

6. Brower RG, Lanken PN, MacIntyre N, et al. Higher versus lower positive end-expiratory pressures in patients with the acute respiratory distress syndrome. New Engl J Med 2004; 351:327–36.

7. Nahum A, Marini JJ, Slutsky AS. Tracheal gas insufflation. In: Marini JJ, Slutsky AS, editors. Physiological basis of ventilatory support. New York, Marcel Dekker, 1998; 1021.

8. Bergofsky EH, Hurewitz AN. Airway insufflation: Physiologic effects on acute and chronic gas exchange in humans. Am Rev Respir Dis 1989; 140:885–90.

9. Hurewitz AN, Bergofsky EH, Vomero E. Airway insufflation: Increasing flow rates progressively reduce dead space in respiratory failure. Am Rev Respir Dis 1991; 144:1229–32.

10. Benditt J, Pollock M, Roa J, et al. Transtracheal delivery of gas decreases the oxygen cost of breathing. Am Rev Respir Dis 1993; 147:1207–10.

11. Slutsky AS. Nonconventional methods of ventilation. Am Rev Respir Dis 1988; 138:175–83.

12. Hess DR, Gillette MA. Tracheal gas insufflation and related techniques to introduce gas flow into the trachea. Respir Care 2001; 46:119–29.

13. Velarde CA, Short BL, Rivera O, et al. A comparison of intra-tracheal pulmonary ventilation to conventional ventilation in a surfactant deficient animal model. Crit Care Med 2000; 28:1455–8.

14. Nahum A, Ravenscraft SA, Nakos G, et al. Effect of catheter flow direction on CO_2 removal during tracheal gas insufflation in dogs. J Appl Physiol 1993; 75:1238–46.

15. Eckmann DM, Gavriely N. Intra-airway CO_2 distribution during airway insufflation in respiratory failure. J Appl Physiol 1995; 78:546–54.

16. Ravenscraft SA, Shapiro R, Nahum A, et al. Tracheal gas insufflation: Catheter effectiveness is determined by expiratory flush volume. Am J Respir Crit Care Med 1996; 153:1817–24.

17. Carter CS, Hotchkiss JR, Adams AB, et al. Distal projection of insufflated gas during tracheal gas insufflation. J Appl Physiol 2002; 92:1843–50.

18. Ravenscraft SA. Tracheal gas insufflation: Adjunct to conventional mechanical ventilation. Respir Care 1996; 41:105–11.

19. Stresemann E. Washout of anatomical dead space: Design of a method and experimental study using an external dead space. Respiration 1968; 25:281–91.

20. Burke WC, Nahum A. Ravenscraft SA, et al. Modes of tracheal gas insufflation: Comparison of continuous and phase-specific gas injection in normal dogs. Am Rev Respir Dis 1993; 148:562–8.

21. Sznajder JI, Becker CJ, Crawford GP, et al. Combination of constant flow and continuous positive pressure ventilation in canine pulmonary edema. J Appl. Physiol 1989; 67:817–23.

22. Lethvall S, Sondergaad S, Karason S, et al. Dead-space reduction and tracheal pressure measurements using coaxial inner tube in an endotracheal tube. Intensive Care Med 2002; 28:1042–8.

23. Carter CS, Adams AB, Stone M, et al. Tracheal gas insufflation during late exhalation efficiently reduces Pa_{CO_2} in experimental acute lung injury. Intensive Care Med 2002; 28:504–8.

24. Nahum A. Animal and lung model studies of tracheal gas insufflation. Respir Care 2001; 46:149–57.

25. Imanaka H, Kacmarek RM, Riggi V, et al. Expiratory phase and volume adjusted tracheal gas insufflation: A lung model study. Crit Care Med 1998; 26:939–46.

26. Kirmse M, Fujino Y, Hromi J, et al. Pressure-release tracheal gas insufflation reduces airway pressures in lung injured sheep maintaining eucapnia. Am J Respir Crit Care Med 1999; 160:1462–7.

27. Nahum A, Ravenscraft SA, Adams AB, et al. Inspiratory tidal volume sparing effects of tracheal gas insufflation in dogs with oleic acid–induced lung injury. J Crit Care 1995; 10:115–21.

28. Imanaka HM, Kirmse M, Mang D, et al. Expiratory phase tracheal gas insufflation and pressure control ventilation in lung lavage sheep with permissive hypercapnia: Effects of TGI flow direction and inspiratory time. Am J Respir Crit Care Med 1999; 159:49–54.

29. Slutsky A, Menon A. Catheter position and blood gases during constant-flow ventilation. J Appl Physiol 1987; 62:513–9.

30. Kalfon P, Umamaheswara GS, Gallart L, et al. Permissive hypercapnia with and without expiratory washout in patients with severe acute respiratory distress syndrome. Anesthesiology 1997; 87:6–17.

31. Stresemann E, Sattler FP. Effect of washout of anatomic dead space on ventilation, pH and blood gas composition in anesthesized dogs. Respiration 1969; 26:116–21.

32. Dorne R, Liron L, Pommier C. Insufflation tracheale de gaz associee a la ventilation mecanique pour l'epuration du CO_2. Ann Fr Anesth Reanim 2000; 19:115–27.

33. Nahum A, Ravenscraft SA, Nakos G, et al. Tracheal gas insufflation during pressure-control ventilation: Effect of catheter position, diameter, and flow rate. Am Rev Respir Dis 1992; 146:1411–8.

34. Nahum A, Chandra A, Niknam J, et al. Effect of tracheal gas insufflation on gas exchange in canine oleic acid–induced lung injury. Crit Care Med 1995; 23:348–56.

35. Nahum A, Shapiro RS, Ravenscraft SA, et al. Efficacy of expiratory tracheal gas insufflation in a canine model of lung injury. Am J Respir Crit Care Med 1995; 152:489–95.

36. Ravenscraft SA, Burke WC, Nahum A, et al. Tracheal gas insufflation augments CO_2 clearance during mechanical ventilation. Am Rev Respir Dis 1993; 148:345–51.

37. Nakos G, Lachana A, Prekates A, et al. Respiratory effects of tracheal gas insufflation in spontaneously breathing COPD patients. Intensive Care Med 1995; 21:904–12.

38. Findlay GP, Dingley J, Smithies MN, et al. Expiratory washout in patients with severe acute respiratory distress syndrome. Anesthesiology 1998; 88:835–6.

39. Richecoeur J, Lu Q, Vieira SRR, et al. Expiratory washout versus optimization of mechanical ventilation during permissive hypercapnia in patients with severe acute respiratory distress syndrome. Am J Respir Crit Care Med 1999; 160:77–85.

40. Miro AM, Hoffman LA, Tasota FJ, et al. Auto-positive end-expiratory pressure during tracheal gas insufflation: Testing a hypothetical model. Crit Care Med 2000; 28:3474–9.

41. Hoffman LA, Johnson JT, Wesmiller SW, et al. Transtracheal delivery of oxygen: Efficacy and safety for long-term continuous theraphy. Ann Otol Rhinol Laryngol 1991; 100:108–15.

42. Wesmiller SW, Hoffman LA, Sciurba FC, et al. Exercise tolerance during nasal cannula and transtracheal oxygen delivery. Am Rev Respir Dis 1990; 141:789–91.

43. Tagaito Y, Schneider H, O'Donnell CP, et al. Ventilating with tracheal gas insufflation and periodic tracheal occlusion during sleep and wakefulness. Chest 2002; 122:1742–50.

44. Nakos G, Zakinthinos S, Kotanidou A, et al. Tracheal gas insufflation reduces the tidal volume while Pa_{CO_2} is maintained constant. Intensive Care Med 1994; 20:407–13.

45. Saura P, Lucangelo, Blanch L, et al. Factores determinantes de la reducción de la Pa_{CO_2} con la insuflación de gas traqueal en pacientes con lesión pulmonar aguda. Med Intensiva 1996; 20: 246–51.

46. Stresemann E, Votteri BA, Sattler FP. Washout of anatomical dead space for alveolar hypoventilation. Respiration 1969; 26:425–34.

47. Blanch L. Clinical studies of tracheal gas insufflation. Respir Care 2001; 46:158–66.

48. Kuo PH, Wu HD, Yu CJ, et al. Efficacy of tracheal gas insufflation in acute respiratory distress syndrome with permissive hypercapnia. Am J Respir Crit Care Med 1996; 154:612–6.

49. Gavriely N, Eckmann D, Grotberg JB. Gas exchange by intratracheal insufflation in a ventilatory failure dog model. J Clin Invest 1992; 90:2376–83.

50. Blanch L, Aguilar JL, Villagra A. Unilateral lung injury. Curr Opin Crit Care 2003; 9:33–8.

51. Blanch L, Van der Kloot TE, Youngblood M, et al. Application of tracheal gas insufflation to acute unilateral lung injury in an experimental model. Am J Respir Crit Care Med 2001; 164: 642–7.

52. Blanch L, Van der Kloot TE, Youngblood M, et al. Selective tracheal gas insufflation during partial liquid ventilation improves lung function in an animal model of unilateral acute lung injury. Crit Care Med 2001; 29:2251–7.

53. Levy B, Bollaert P-E, Nace L, et al. Intracranial hypertension and adult respiratory distress syndrome: Usefulness of tracheal gas insufflation. J Trauma 1995; 39:799–801.

54. Chomel A, Combes JC, Yeguiayan JM, et al. L'insufflation trachéale de gas permet d'éviter l'hypercapnie chez le traumatisé crânien grave avec syndrome de détresse respiratoire aiguë. Can J Anesth 2001; 48:1040–4.

55. Martinez M, Bernabe F, Peña R, et al. Effects of expiratory tracheal gas insufflation in patients with severe head trauma and acute lung injury. Intensive Care Med 2004; 30:2021–7.

56. Jubran A, Tobin MJ: Discontinuation of ventilatory support. In: Marini JJ, Slutsky AS, editors. Physiological basis of ventilatory support. New York, Marcel Dekker, 1998: 1283.

57. Cereda MF, Sparacino M, Frank A, et al. Efficacy of tracheal gas insufflation in spontaneously breathing sheep with lung injury. Am J Respir Crit Care Med 1999; 159:845–50.

58. Epstein SK. TGIF: Tracheal gas insufflation. For whom? Chest 2002; 122:1515–7.

59. Hoffman LA, Tasota FJ, Delgado E, et al. Effect of tracheal gas insufflation during weaning from prolonged mechanical ventilation: A preliminary study. Am J Crit Care 2003; 12:31–9.

60. Nahum A, Burke W, Ravenscraft SA, et al. Lung mechanics and gas exchange during pressure-controlled ventilation in dogs: Augmentation of CO_2 elimination by an intratracheal catheter. Am Rev Respir Dis 1992; 146:965–73.

61. Kacmarek RM. Complications of tracheal gas insufflation. Respir Care 2001; 46:167–76.

62. Olarte JL, Gelvez J, Fakioglu H, et al. Tracheobronchial injury during intratracheal pulmonary ventilation in rabbits. Crit Care Med 2003; 31:916–23.

63. Kolobow T, Powers T, Mandava S, et al. Intratracheal pulmonary ventilation (ITPV): Control of positive end-expiratory pressure at the level of the carina through the use of a novel ITPV catheter design. Anesth Analg 1994; 78:455–61.

64. Rossi N, Musch G, Sangalli F, et al. Reverse-thrust ventilation in hypercapnic patients with acute respiratory distress syndrome:

Acute physiological effects. Am J Respir Crit Care Med 2000; 162:363–8.

65. Delgado E, Hoffman LA, Tasota FJ, et al. Monitoring and humidification during tracheal gas insufflation. Respir Care 2001; 46:185–92.

66. Blanch L, Murias G, Romero P, et al. Application of tracheal gas insufflation for critical care patients. In: Mancebo J, Net A, Brochard L, editors. Mechanical ventilation and weaning. Berlin : Springer-Verlag, 2002: 87.

67. Boussignac G, Bertrand C, Huguenard P. Etude preliminaire d'une nouvelle sonde d'intubation endotracheale. Conv Med 1988; 7:111–3.

68. Isabey D, Boussignac G, Harf A. Effect of air entrainment on airway pressure during endotracheal gas injection. J Appl Physiol 1989; 67:771–9.

69. Brochard L, Mion G, Isabey D, et al. Constant-flow insufflation prevents arterial oxygen desaturation during endotracheal suctioning. Am Rev Respir Dis 1991; 144:395–400.

70. Dassieu G, Brochard L, Agudze E, et al. Continuous tracheal gas insufflation enables a volume reduction strategy in hyaline membrane disease: Technical aspects and clinical results. Intensive Care Med 1998; 24:1076–82.

71. Dassieu G, Brochard L, Benani M, et al. Continuous tracheal gas insufflation in preterm infants with hyaline membrane disease: A prospective, randomized trial. Am J Respir Crit Care Med 2000; 162:826–31.

72. Adams AB. Catheters for tracheal gas insufflation. Respir Care 2001; 46:177–84.

73. Slutsky AS. Techniques of ventilation using constant flow, In: Marini JJ, Roussos C, editors. Ventilatory failure. Berlin: Springer-Verlag 1991: 293.

74. De Robertis E, Sigurdur E, Sigurdsson E, et al. Aspiration of airway dead space: A new method to enhance CO_2 elimination. Am J Respir Crit Care Med 1999; 159:728–32.

75. De Robertis E, Servillo G, Jonson B, et al. Aspiration of dead space allows normocapnic ventilation at low tidal volumes in man. Intensive Care Med 1999; 25:674–9.

76. De Robertis E, Servillo G, Tufano R, et al. Aspiration of dead space allows isocapnic low tidal volume ventilation in acute lung injury: Relationships to gas exchange and mechanics. Intensive Care Med 2001; 27:1496–1503.

77. Liu YN, Zhao WG, Xie LX, et al. Aspiration of dead space in the management of chronic obstructive pulmonary disease patients with respiratory failure. Respir Care 2004; 49:257–62.

78. Nahum A, Sznajder JI, Solway J, et al. Pressure, flow, and density relationships in airway models during constant-flow ventilation. J Appl Physiol 1988; 64:2066–73.

79. Fujino Y, Nishimura M, Hirao O, et al. Functional residual capacity measurement during tracheal gas insufflation. J Clin Monit 1998; 14:225–32.

80. Bunegin L, Gelineau J, Stone E, et al. The effect of endotracheal catheter position on Pa_{CO_2} and Pa_{O_2} during continuous flow apneic ventilation. Crit Care Med 1986; 14:372–6.

81. Delgado E, Hete B, Hoffman LA, et al. Effects of continuous, expiratory, reverse, and bidirectional tracheal gas insufflation in conjunction with a flow relief valve on delivered tidal volume total positive end-expiratory pressure, and carbon dioxide elimination: A bench study. Respir Care 2001; 46:577–85.

82. Gowski DT, Delgado E, Miro MA, et al. Tracheal gas insufflation during pressure-controlled ventilation: Effect of using a pressure relief valve. Crit Care Med 1997; 25:145–52.

83. Hoyt JD, Marini JJ, Nahum A. Effect of tracheal gas insufflation on demand valve triggering and total work during continuous positive airway pressure ventilation. Chest 1996; 110: 775–83.

84. Adams AB. Tracheal gas insufflation. Respir Care 1996; 41:285–92.

85. Lucangelo U, Blanch L, Artigas A, et al. Resistencia al flujo aereo sobreañadida por los diferentes materiales del circuito ventilatorio de pacientes en ventilacion mecanica. Med Intensiva 1995; 19:125–9.

86. Delgado E, Miro AM, Hoffman LA, et al. Continuous and expiratory tracheal gas insufflation produce equal levels of total PEEP. Respir Care 1999; 44:428–33.

87. Blanch L, Fernandez R, Saura P, et al. Relationship between expired capnogram and respiratory system resistance in critically ill patients during total ventilatory support. Chest 1994; 105: 219–23.

88. Hess D. Capnometry and capnography: Technical aspects, physiologic aspects, and clinical applications. Respir Care 1990; 35: 557–76.

89. Pizov R, Oppenheim A, Eidelman LA, et al. Helium versus oxygen for tracheal gas insufflation during mechanical ventilation. Crit Care Med 1998; 26:290–5.

90. Jaber S, Fodil R, Carlucci A, et al. Noninvasive ventilation with helium-oxygen in acute exacerbations of chronic obstructive pulmonary disease. Am J Respir Crit Care Med 2000; 161:1191–1200.

91. Trawoger R, Kolobow T, Cereda M, et al. Clearance of mucus from endotracheal tubes during intratracheal pulmonary ventilation. Anesthesiology 1997; 86:1367–74.

92. Sznajder JI, Nahum A, Crawford G, et al. Alveolar pressure inhomogeneity and gas exchange during constant-flow ventilation in dogs. J Appl Physiol 1989; 67:1489–94.

93. Nahum A. Tracheal gas insufflation as an adjunct to mechanical ventilation. Respir Care Clin 2002; 8:171–85.

94. Hess DR, MacIntyre NR. Tracheal gas insufflation: Overcoming obstacles to clinical implementation. Respir Care 2001; 46:198–9.

PART VIII

VENTILATOR SUPPORT IN SPECIFIC SETTINGS

Chapter 25

MECHANICAL VENTILATION IN THE NEONATAL AND PEDIATRIC SETTING

PETER C. RIMENSBERGER
JUERG HAMMER

Respiratory disease in its various forms remains the most common cause of pediatric and neonatal morbidity and mortality. One of the most common reasons for admission to an intensive-care unit (ICU) is the need for mechanical ventilation for acute or impending respiratory failure. Respiratory failure, characterized by inadequacy of oxygenation and/or ventilation, can occur as a result of airway and lung disease, cardiac dysfunction, multiorgan failure, neurologic and neuromuscular disorders, or the effects of surgery and/or cardiopulmonary bypass. Pediatric respiratory failure is divided in two major pathophysiologic entities: lung failure and pump failure. Primary *lung failure* can result from multiple causes, including pneumonia, inhalational injury, near-drowning, hemorrhage, aspiration, and chest trauma. *Pump failure* can result from upper airway obstruction, cardiovascular dysfunction, or systemic septic disease characterized by increased work of breathing that may lead, especially in the newborn and small child, to respiratory fatigue; it also can result from neurologic injury or neuromuscular disease. Such patients may require mechanical ventilation not only for hypoventilation but also for airway protection.

The three major indications for mechanical ventilation in the pediatric and neonatal field are to improve gas exchange, reduce work of breathing, and secure the upper airways. Common objectives of ventilation are

1. To support or manipulate gas exchange by improving alveolar ventilation in order to achieve acceptable oxygenation
2. To restore or maintain adequate functional residual capacity (FRC) in order to prevent or reopen atelectasis and improve oxygenation and lung compliance
3. To reduce work of breathing in the presence of high airway resistance and/or reduced compliance, which causes ineffective spontaneous breathing

The aim of mechanical ventilation is not only to support impaired vital function and maintain adequate gas exchange. It is also to provide time for resolution of the underlying disorder without adding further injury by the ventilator. The respiratory strategy takes into account the type and severity of the underlying pathology, the clinical condition (e.g., neuromuscular weakness), and the age [i.e., for age-specific pathologies and conditions such as neonatal respiratory distress syndrome (RDS) or bronchiolitis in infants and toddlers].

Despite worldwide daily use of mechanical ventilation in pediatric and neonatal ICUs, many questions are unresolved, and answers often are extrapolated from adult studies. The latter may seem sensible for older children but not for infants and toddlers, in whom age-specific

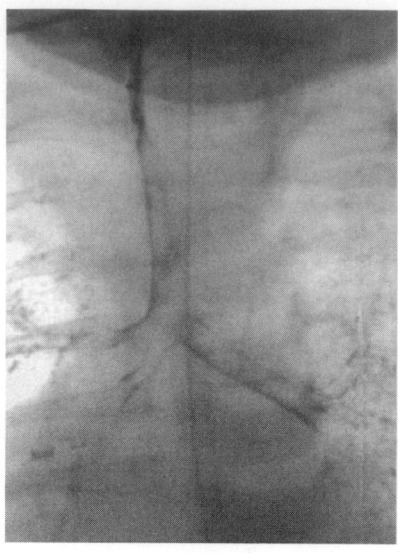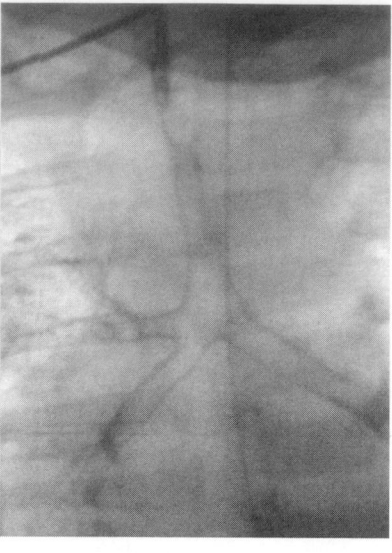

FIGURE 25-1 Bronchography in patient with tracheobronchomalacia without application of positive airway pressure (*left*) and with 10 cmH$_2$O of positive airway pressure (*right*). Application of positive airway pressure produces stenting of the trachea and bronchial tree. (*Courtesy of Queen Mok, Great Ormond Street Hospital for Children, United Kingdom.*)

considerations of function and physiology in the developing respiratory system have to be taken into account.

Unique Pathophysiology

Physiology of the respiratory system differs among babies, children, and adults in a number of important respects. First, infants and small children have less respiratory reserve than adults and are prone to respiratory failure during any critical illness of pulmonary or nonpulmonary origin. Second, some differences in the anatomic structure of the airways and respiratory mechanics of the respiratory system among infants, children, and adults must be stressed.

UPPER LARGE AIRWAYS: ANATOMIC AND FUNCTIONAL CONSIDERATIONS

Infants are thought to be mainly nose breathers because the large omega-shaped, soft epiglottis, positioned high in the larynx (at the level of C4 in the infant versus C6 in the adult), tends to obscure the laryngeal inlet. Partial or complete occlusion of the nasopharyngeal airway (congenital or acquired) may increase work of breathing and contribute to respiratory failure.

The narrowest part of the infant airway is not the laryngeal inlet (vocal cords) but the cone-shaped cricoid cartilage in the subglottic region. Any decrease in airway diameter—acquired or congenital—results in a dramatic increase in airway resistance in infants because resistance is inversely related to the fourth power of the radius.

The cross-sectional area between the vocal cords is widened during inspiration and narrowed during expiration. This narrowing allows infants to brake flow during expiration. By this action, infants can generate intrinsic positive end-expiratory pressure (PEEP) (grunting) to stabilize their cartilaginous, relatively elastic and flaccid chest, which has a tendency to collapse.

SMALL AND PERIPHERAL AIRWAYS: ANATOMIC AND FUNCTIONAL CONSIDERATIONS

In the presence of intrathoracic airway obstruction (e.g., tracheobronchomalacia or asthma), the pressure within the airways above the site of obstruction (during expiration) becomes lower than pleural pressure. This predisposes the compliant airways of children to collapse. Such expiratory flow limitation produces wheezing, prolonged expiratory times, and air trapping with dynamic hyperinflation. PEEP may help to stent collapsing airways during expiration in some patients[1] (e.g., those with tracheobronchomalcia; Fig. 25-1); in other patients who have dynamic hyperinflation without expiratory flow limitation, PEEP may lead to further air trapping.[2]

In infants and children up to about 6 years of age, the small airways account for up to 50% (compared with about 20% in adults) of total airway resistance.[3] Therefore, diseases affecting predominantly the small airways, such as viral bronchiolitis, can cause a significant increase in total airway resistance and work of breathing and may lead to severe respiratory failure in children.

STATIC PROPERTIES OF LUNG AND CHEST WALL

The ribs in infants are aligned horizontally, allowing for less anteroposterior movement during respiration and rendering the intercostal muscles less efficient than in adults. Breathing is primarily diaphragmatic. The combination of a soft and compliant chest wall and predominant diaphragmatic breathing can cause two specific pathologic conditions: (1) rapid and sometimes serious impairment of breathing efficiency (in the case of abdominal distension) and (2) inward distortion of the rib cage and waste of energy through sucking in of the ribs rather than of air, as manifested by paradoxical thoracoabdominal movements. The latter is a typical sign of upper airway obstruction. This renders breathing less efficient because chest-wall distortion represents a pressure-induced change in volume,

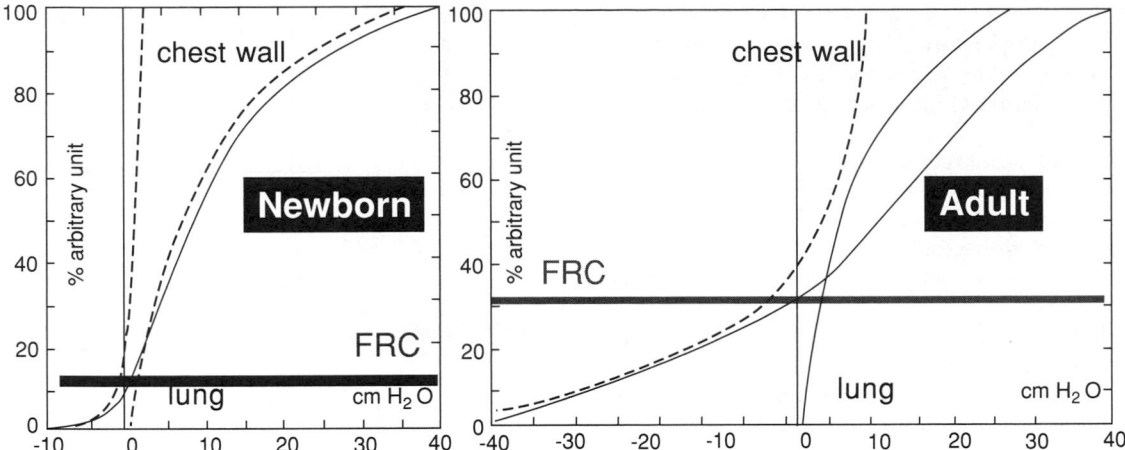

FIGURE 25-2 Characterisitcs of lung and chest-wall mechanics in newborns compared with adults. The compliant chest wall in the newborn leads to lower functional residual capacity in the newborn. (*Adapted, with permission, from Agostini: J Appl Physiol 14:909–13, 1959.*)

constituting a form of work with an energy cost; this is thought to be one reason for poor weight gain and development of fatigue in infants recovering from respiratory distress syndrome (RDS).[4]

Static and elastic properties of the respiratory system change with maturation and the state of health (Fig. 25-2). In infants, the chest wall generates little outward recoil compared with adults, whereas inward recoil of the lungs varies little with respect to size and age. Therefore, the relaxation volume of the thorax is smaller than in the adult, resulting in a lower FRC in the infant (around 15% of vital capacity compared with 35% in the adult). This imposes a clear disadvantage in terms of alveolar stability, making the infant more vulnerable to changes in muscle coordination and tone during rapid-eye-movement (REM) sleep, anesthesia, sedation, or central nervous system depression.

Whereas the volume-pressure relationship of the lungs is similar in infants and adults, the volume-pressure relationship of the chest wall is much steeper in the infant. Relatively large changes in intrathoracic pressure therefore are accompanied by only small variations in chest-wall pressure. Consequently, large changes in ventilator pressures have only a limited effect on pleural pressure. This explains the generally high cardiovascular tolerance of infants to the application of high airway pressures.

The tidal volume (V_T) necessary to achieve a given increase in airway pressure is less in a small person than in a large person. Thus noncorrected compliance values of the respiratory system cannot be compared between infants and adults. Correction is commonly made to body weight. It is better to correct to a unit of lung volume, however, such as FRC. Thus specific static compliance (Cst/FRC) is comparable between adults and children independent of age and disease stage.

PERTINENT PULMONARY MECHANICS FOR PEDIATRIC VENTILATION

A basic understanding of pulmonary mechanics is necessary when ventilating an infant or child. The most impor-

tant elements are elastic recoil, compliance, resistance, and time constant.

ELASTIC RECOIL

The newborn has a low elastic recoil of the chest wall because it is nonossified and has low total muscle mass, with a low percentage of slow-muscle fibers in both the diaphragm and intercostal muscles. Very little airway pressure therefore is needed to expand the chest wall during inspiration; this explains why muscle relaxation is rarely needed in the young infant during (nonassisted) controlled ventilation.

The major force contributing to elastic recoil in the newborn is surface tension at the air-liquid interface in distal bronchioli and alveoli. As described by LaPlace's law (P = 2T/r), the pressure (P) needed to counteract the tendency of bronchioli to collapse is directly proportional to the surface tension (T) and inversely related to its radius (r). A decrease in surface tension in surfactant deficiency states (infant RDS) or after inactivation of surfactant [acute respiratory distress syndrome (ARDS)] results in decreased stability of the small terminal airways and alveoli, producing a tendency to collapse.

COMPLIANCE

Lung compliance is very low (3.5 ml/cmH$_2$O) at birth and increases rapidly during the first week to about 5–6 ml/cmH$_2$O (corresponding to about 1.5–2 ml/cmH$_2$O per kilogram of body weight) in the full-term infant. Reduced lung compliance is seen in neonates with congenital pathologies characterized by small lung volumes (e.g., congenital pulmonary hypoplasia and diaphragmatic hernia), with primary or secondary surfactant deficiency (e.g., RDS and congenital pneumonia), with restrictive lung disease (including ARDS and viral or bacterial pneumonia), with bronchopulmonary dysplasia (BPD; often a combination of restrictive and obstructive lung disease), or after correction of congenital diaphragmatic hernia. Reduced compliance also can be seen in obstructive lung disease combined with high lung volumes, such as asthma and bronchiolitis.

RESISTANCE

Airway resistance in spontaneously breathing infants is normally 20–30 cmH$_2$O/liter per second; values in intubated infants are 50–150 cmH$_2$O/liter per second, consequent to a narrow endotracheal tube (ETT).[5] For many years it was thought that small infants could not breathe spontaneously through a small ETT (because of high resistance imposed by the small lumen), but this view is no longer maintained. Under normal tidal-flow conditions, resistance imposed by a small tube is not substantially higher than that with larger tube.

Clinically, an increase in airway resistance is manifested by retractions of the soft tissue, contractions of accessory muscles, and active participation of the abdominal muscles during expiration.

TIME CONSTANT

An understanding of time constant, the product of lung compliance and airway resistance, is important when ventilating infants and children, especially at high respiratory frequencies. If lung compliance is decreased (RDS or ARDS) and resistance is normal or only slightly altered, the time constant, and the corresponding time for pressure equilibrium between proximal airways and the alveolar space, will be shorter than for healthy lungs. Therefore, high respiratory frequencies leading to short inspiratory times (T$_I$) may be appropriate when RDS or ARDS is at peak severity. During recovery from RDS or ARDS (increasing compliance), however, high ventilator rates can lead to two major problems. First, insufficient T$_I$ may limit delivery of an adequate volume.[6,7] Second, excessively short expiratory times (T$_E$) will not allow complete emptying of peripheral airspaces at end expiration (as indicated by the absence of expiratory flow termination before the next inspiration), with the risk of generating intrinsic PEEP (Fig. 25-3).

Long time constants (slower filling and emptying) can be seen in diseases characterized by increased airway resistance (e.g., BPD, bronchiolitis, or asthma), and low respiratory rates should be selected. In some pathologies (e.g., meconium aspiration) that can exhibit both obstructive and restrictive features, careful adaptation of frequency and inspiratory-expiratory (I:E) ratio will be necessary in some patients. An intervention that improves compliance (e.g., surfactant treatment or lung-recruitment maneuvers) produces a longer time constant by improving compliance.[8–10] Therefore, respiratory rates, especially expiratory times, may need rapid adjustment, in addition to adjusting airway pressure. This must be taken in account when ventilating infants and small children at any stage of an evolving or resolving lung disease. Thus use of fixed high rates (leading to relatively short T$_I$ and T$_E$ values), which has become commonplace since the advent of small V$_T$ ventilation, is not always appropriate.

Considerations Peculiar to Neonates

The neonate is not a small adult. Specific characteristics include (1) small and soft upper and lower airways, (2) compliant chest wall and a low FRC, making the neonate susceptible to airway collapse and atelectasis, and (3) poor

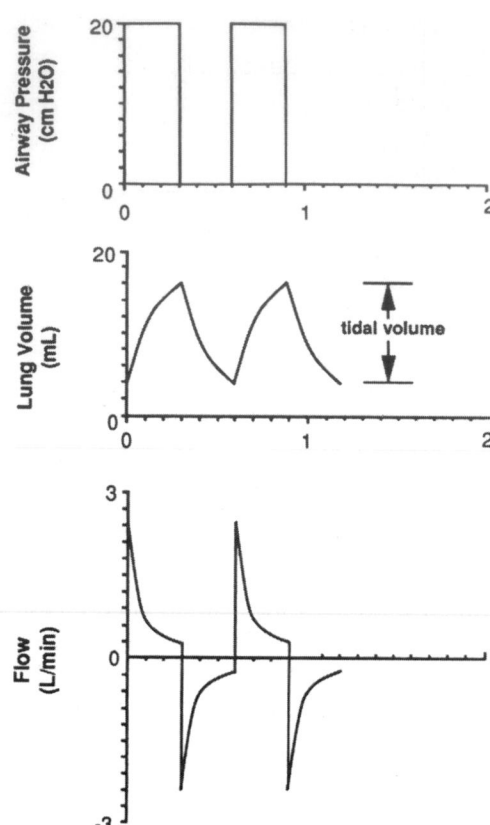

FIGURE 25-3 Pressure, volume, and flow curves illustrating the phenomenon of alveolar gas trapping. Note that both inspiratory and expiratory times are so short that flow does not decay to zero. As a result, the tidal volume is less than it would be if complete inspiration and expiration were permitted. (*Reprinted, with permission, from Chatburn: Respir Care 36:580, 1991.*)

effectiveness of the respiratory pump. Other characteristics include circulatory changes after birth, special features of fetal hemoglobin (HbF) when considering oxygen (O$_2$) transport, and control of breathing.

CIRCULATORY CHANGES PERTINENT TO VENTILATION

Aeration of the lung must be matched to perfusion for satisfactory gas exchange. Before birth, only about 10% of blood flow passes through the lungs as a result of high pulmonary vascular resistance, patent ductus arteriosus, open foramen ovale, and the low-resistance placental component to the systemic circulation. After birth, clamping of the umbilical cord removes the low systemic resistance, and aeration of the lungs leads to opening of the pulmonary capillary bed with consecutive reduction in pulmonary vascular resistance. The increase in left-atrial pressure (by increased pulmonary venous return) and the reduction in right-atrial pressure (by reduced systemic venous return) lead to closure of the foramen ovale. Blood oxygenation lowers pulmonary vascular resistance and initiates ductus closure. Although pulmonary vascular resistance falls rapidly in the first minutes of life, it is still elevated and falls only gradually to normal levels over days to weeks. During the first days

TABLE 25-1 Main Determinants of Pulmonary Vascular Resistance

Increase in Pulmonary Vascular Resistance	Decrease in Pulmonary Vascular Resistance
High interstitial pressure	Low interstitial pressure
High lung volumes (alveolar overdistension)	Normal lung volumes
Low lung volumes (atelectasis)	
Low Pa_{O_2} –alveolar P_{O_2}	High P_{O_2} –alveolar P_{O_2}
Low arterial pH	High arterial pH

and weeks, the pulmonary circulation is therefore unstable. Under certain circumstances (e.g., birth asphyxia, chronic hypoxia, or neonatal septicemia with or without metabolic acidosis), pulmonary vascular resistance increases or remains high, leading to right-to-left shunting through the ductus arteriosus and sometimes even through the foramen ovale. This persistent pulmonary hypertension of the newborn (PPHN) leads to poor systemic oxygenation, as revealed by low postductal transcutaneous saturation levels (e.g., lower limbs and left upper limb) or desaturation of all four extremities when the right-to-left shunt at the level of the foramen ovale is important. In this situation (poor oxygenation because of an extrapulmonary shunt), a low arterial O_2 tension (Pa_{O_2}) cannot be overcome by administration of high O_2 concentrations, although supplemental O_2 may be useful in lowering pulmonary vascular resistance. High inflation pressures to recruit lung volume and improve oxygenation should be used with caution because of the risk of increased pulmonary vascular resistance by overdistension and compromised cardiac output. First-line treatment is directing toward known determinants of pulmonary vascular resistance (Table 25-1) such as acidosis or high interstitial pressures. Second-line therapy includes specific pulmonary vasodilators, such as nitric oxide (NO),[11–13] after excluding congenital heart disease with duct-dependent systemic circulation, which may deteriorate when pulmonary vascular resistance is lowered (e.g., total anomalous pulmonary venous return or hypoplastic left heart syndrome).[14]

OXYGEN TRANSPORT

Fetal hemoglobin (HbF) is the predominant type of Hb at birth. It decreases steadily over the first 6 months, with adult hemoglobin (HbA) predominating after about 3 months. 2,3-diphosphglycerate (2,3-DPG) has a lower affinity to HbF and shifts the dissociation curve to the left, resulting in higher O_2 affinity and a lower P_{50} (P_{O_2} at which Hb is 50% saturated). This left shift facilitates loading and unloading of O_2, ensuring, together with the high O_2-carrying capacity of HbF, adequate tissue oxygenation despite low P_{O_2} values in utero (15–30 mmHg). The predominance of HbF makes it possible, if necessary, to tolerate lower P_{O_2} values (but not really Sa_{O_2}) more in early postnatal life than is possible later in life.

CONTROL OF BREATHING

Control of breathing depends on the interaction of brainstem centers, the reticular activating system that can be activated by various nonspecific factors (e.g., REM sleep, arousal, temperature, and pain), chemoreceptors, and mechanoreceptors of the lung and chest wall. Function of these components may be impaired when maturation is not complete.

Brain-stem neurons undergo rapid maturation between 30 weeks of gestation and term.[15] Accordingly, preterm infants are subject to "physiologic apnea." When this is associated with recurrent severe bradycardia and hypoxemia, continuous positive airway pressure (CPAP) or intubation and mechanical ventilation may be necessary.

Carbon dioxide (CO_2), through its effect on brain-tissue pH, is the major metabolic respiratory stimulant in neonates and adults. In pretem infants, a decreased response to hypercapnia, which improves with postconceptional age, is observed often.[16] This fact may account for hypercapnia during quiet breathing in the absence of underlying lung disease or sedatives.

In contrast to hyperventilation in infants, children, and adults[17] (Fig. 25-4), hypoxemia induces respiratory depression in the newborn that may lead to apnea. This phenomenon is best explained by the presence of brain-stem inhibitory reflexes in the fetus that prevent breathing in utero.[18] As a result, the brain-stem response to carotid afferent stimulation is still altered after birth.

Feedback from vagal stretch reflexes, rib-cage muscles, and the changing mechanical state of the respiratory system during each breath influence respiratory activity. If inflation is small, there is less inhibitory vagal feedback. Inspiratory activity of the next breath increases to overcome the increased respiratory load. If inflation is excessive, inspiration is inhibited. This inspiratory-inhibitory reflex, the *Hering-Breuer inflation reflex*, is potent in the newborn and infant during the first weeks of life[19] and may persist for longer in preterm babies.[20] This inflation reflex facilitates passive measurement of respiratory mechanics (e.g., airway occlusion technique) without a paralytic agent.

Conversely, the increased ability of infants to adjust to increased inspiratory load during support with CPAP suggests a diminished Hering-Breuer reflex.[21] This reflex

FIGURE 25-4 Age-related response to the breathing of hypoxic gases for 5 minutes. (*Adapted, with permission, from Henderson-Smart: Regulation of breathing in the perinatal period. In: Saunders NA, Sullivan CE, editors. Sleep and breathing: Lung biology in health and disease, Vol 20. New York: Marcel Dekker, 1983: 605–647.*)

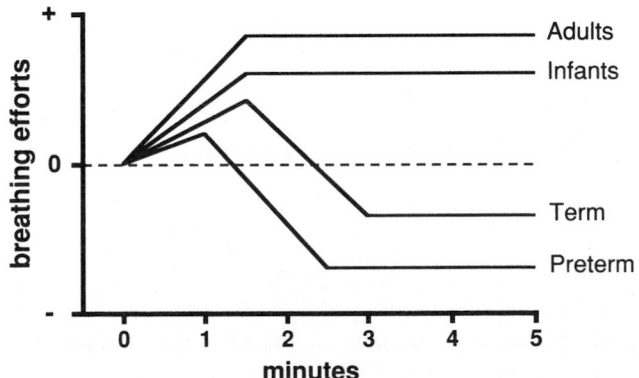

activity also may interfere with successful ventilator triggering because an infant may become apneic secondary to inhibitory activity (after an inflation),[22] especially if the clinician selects an excessively long T_I, despite a nonalkalotic pH.

Do Ventilator Goals Differ between Infants and Children?

The basic objectives of ventilator support remain the same from early life to adulthood.[23,24] The physiologic objectives are to (1) support gas exchange in terms of alveolar ventilation and arterial oxygenation, (2) achieve sufficient end-inspiratory lung expansion to prevent or treat atelectasis, (3) maintain sufficient end-expiratory lung volumes to restore reduced FRC, (4) reduce work of breathing by unloading the respiratory muscles in the setting of increased airway resistance or reduced compliance and to reduce work of breathing and thus O_2 consumption in patients with heart failure or sepsis, and (5) to prevent small or large airway collapse in certain situations (laryngotracheobronchomalacia; see Fig. 25-1).

Historically, the main objective has been to restore normal physiology by normalizing oxygenation and alveolar ventilation. With recognition that the ventilator has side effects, this target of normalizing blood gases has become relative. There is, however, still debate about how permissive one should be in terms of accepting hypoxemia or hypercapnia. Other objectives include to (1) relieve signs of distress (e.g., indrawing, use of accessory muscles, or tachypnea), (2) reverse or avoid respiratory muscle fatigue, (3) reduce systemic O_2 consumption, and (4) permit sedation, analgesia, and neuromuscular blockade (intra- or postoperatively).

The same guidelines can be used in infants and children as in adults. The oxygenation goal is an Sa_{O_2} of more than 90% (equivalent to a Pa_{O_2} of 60 mmHg, assuming a normal "adult" O_2 dissociation curve). The ventilation goals are a V_T below 8 ml/kg (8–10 ml/kg being about physiologic) and plateau pressures of 35 cmH_2O or less; permissive hypercapnia entails accepting respiratory acidosis (pH $\geq$ 7.25). A rapid rise in Pa_{CO_2} should be avoided. Contraindications to increased Pa_{CO_2} (and/or low pH) include increased intracranial pressure and increased risk for pulmonary hypertension. Conversely, any rapid reduction in Pa_{CO_2}, which may occur with surfactant therapy or change in ventilator mode, may lead to cerebral vasoconstriction, increasing the risk of cerebral hemorrhage and/or leukomalacia in premature babies.

Common Clinical Conditions

NEONATES

RESPIRATORY DISTRESS SYNDROME
(HYALINE MEMBRANE DISEASE)
RDS is characterized by pulmonary surfactant deficiency and transudation of plasma proteins into the alveolar spaces. It typically occurs in preterm infants. The result is a stiff lung and a tendency to atelectasis in the early stages. The main goals of therapy are to recruit collapsed alveoli, restore FRC, and achieve adequate alveolar ventilation. Technical and pharmacologic advances, with improved understanding of pathophysiology and causes of lung injury, have altered the strategy for ventilating preterm infants with RDS dramatically. Therapy is titrated to disease severity and includes noninvasive and invasive ventilator support.

CPAP is the primary respiratory support for RDS, although a conclusive controlled trial has not been undertaken. Several uncontrolled studies indicate that nasal CPAP reduces respiratory failure and the duration and invasiveness of respiratory support without impairing neonatal outcome.[25-28] Nasal CPAP improves respiration in preterm infants by increasing FRC and chest-wall stability, as well as decreasing upper-airway collapsibility and upper-airway resistance.[29]

When positive-pressure ventilation (PPV) was first introduced in newborn infants with RDS, high peak inspiratory pressures (PIPs) were used to oxygenate the stiff lungs. This was associated with high mortality rates, air leaks, and the development of BPD.[30] In the 1970s, uncontrolled studies in a small number of infants demonstrated a reduction in the incidence of pneumothoraces through use of long T_I values and slow rates.[31] This strategy was widely adopted until PEEP was shown to have greatest effect on mean airway pressure.[32] The availability of exogenous surfactant and ventilator capability of synchronizing ventilator breaths with spontaneous breaths has further altered ventilator management of RDS. It is now widely accepted that RDS, characterized by poorly compliant lungs and very short time constants (0.26–0.34 second), is best managed with short T_I values, rapid rates, and PEEP.[33,34] The availability of flow sensors in neonatal ventilators enables continuous measurement of V_T, eliminating much of the guesswork in setting the ventilator.

The underlying pathophysiology, decreased lung compliance, high chest-wall compliance, and dynamically maintained FRC above closing volume make RDS a perfect candidate for an open-lung strategy and use of high-frequency oscillatory ventilation (HFOV). Nevertheless, most studies to date have not demonstrated a significant difference in outcome measures with the use of HFOV versus conventional ventilation and a lung-protective strategy.[35-38] HFOV seems to have a small benefit on pulmonary outcome in very low-birth-weight infants without increasing the complications of premature birth.[36,39]

Exogenous surfactant therapy has been part of routine care of preterm neonates with RDS since the early 1990s. Animal-derived exogenous surfactants are the present treatment of choice, with few adverse effects largely related to changes in oxygenation and heart rate during surfactant administration.[40] The optimal dose is usually 100 mg/kg. Both prophylaxis and treatment are successful in infants with established RDS, but prophylaxis appears to produce greater clinical benefit.[41]

Persistent fetal circulation is a complication of RDS in preterm infants. At present, there is no clear-cut evidence in favor of using inhaled nitric oxide (iNO) for preterm infants requiring mechanical ventilation.[42] Clinicians will continue to make case-by-case decisions for the treatment of preterm infants with hypoxia unresponsive to other therapies.[43]

PERSISTENT PULMONARY HYPERTENSION OF THE NEWBORN (PPHN)

PPHN is the result of elevated pulmonary vascular resistance to the point that venous blood is shunted to some degree through fetal channels (e.g., ductus arteriosus and foramen ovale) into the systemic circulation. By bypassing the lungs, it causes systemic arterial hypoxemia. It is associated with (1) pulmonary parenchymal disease such as RDS or meconium aspiration and (2) hypoplasia of the lungs, most often in the form of diaphragmatic hernia, and (3) it also can occur without evident underlying disease.

Traditionally, these infants have been hyperventilated to achieve mild hypocapnic alkalosis in an attempt to attenuate hypoxic pulmonary vasoconstriction. iNO is an approved adjunct to improve oxygenation in term infants with severe hypoxemic respiratory failure secondary to PPHN and has been shown to reduce the need for extracorporeal membrane oxygenation (ECMO).[44] Alveolar recruitment should be optimized before iNO because it improves responsiveness.[14] An open-lung approach generally is recommended, and HFOV has become the favorite method.

MECONIUM ASPIRATION SYNDROME

Meconium aspiration syndrome affects mature infants and is characterized by a mixture of inflammatory pulmonary disease, secondary surfactant deficiency, obstruction of small airways, and pulmonary hypertension. The result is a very inhomogeneous lung with areas of atelectasis and hyperinflation. Setting the ventilator in disease with different time constants is challenging; the aim is provide sufficient alveolar ventilation without development of intrinsic PEEP. Studies have not conclusively demonstrated any form of ventilation to be superior to others, but strategies that recruit alveoli are recommended. Surfactant replacement or lavage may be beneficial.[45,46] When hypoxic respiratory failure is progressive, iNO may improve oxygenation and avoid ECMO.

CONGENITAL DIAPHRAGMATIC HERNIA (CDH)

CDH is characterized by lung hypoplasia, surfactant deficiency, and an extremely reactive hypoplastic pulmonary vascular system. The hypoplastic lungs are very vulnerable to injury from aggressive ventilation with high inspiratory pressures. Treatment is no longer focused on immediate surgery but rather on delaying repair until all reversible problems are resolved.[47] These include pulmonary hypertension and parenchymal injury from inappropriately high inflation pressures.[48] The new strategy has increased survival of infants with early respiratory failure from below 50% to as high as 80%.[47,49] Increased survival appears equivalent to that with ECMO, HFOV, and pressure-support ventilation (PSV) with permissive hypercapnia.[49–52] Although high airway pressures may be required with secondary parenchymal injury to ensure adequate oxygenation, special care is necessary to avoid alveolar distension in the set-

ting of pulmonary hypoplasia. Inappropriately high airway pressures also increase pulmonary vascular resistance and aggravate hemodynamic instability and lung injury.[53] iNO is less effective in avoiding the need for ECMO than in patients with meconium aspiration syndrome.[54]

PEDIATRIC PATIENTS

VIRUS-INDUCED HYPOXEMIC FAILURE

Two distinct patterns of disease occur in infants with virus-induced respiratory failure.[55,56] The primary causative agent is respiratory syncytial virus (RSV). The most frequent pattern is acute bronchiolitis characterized by an obstruction of small airways with air trapping and a moderate degree of parenchymal disease from atelectasis. This leads to increased respiratory resistance, a prolonged time constant, intrinsic PEEP, and decreased respiratory compliance.[57] Radiographic findings include hyperinflation, perihilar infiltrates, and atelectasis. The second pattern, which affects about 25–30% of infants with RSV-induced respiratory failure, consists of severe restrictive parenchymal disease (usually termed *RSV-pneumonia*). Typically, respiratory compliance and lung volumes are decreased markedly without significant airway obstruction or air trapping. Alveolar consolidation is the main radiographic feature. This subgroup also usually fulfills the criteria of ARDS. Patients require prolonged ventilation compared with a brief duration (4–8 days) for the bronchiolitic pattern.[55,56]

No consensus exists on optimal ventilator strategy. Nasal CPAP appears useful in the early stages of severe bronchiolitis. It decreases work of breathing needed to overcome intrinsic PEEP but may increase dead space. In patients with restrictive disease, nasal CPAP improves hypoxemia by recruiting lung volume and increasing FRC above closing volume. Reports do not provide definite conclusions on the benefit of CPAP in avoiding intubation and mechanical ventilation in children with hypoxemic respiratory failure.[58–62]

Pressure-controlled ventilation (PCV) is the mode used most commonly in virus-induced respiratory failure because the decelerating flow pattern achieves a lower mean airway pressure than does volume-controlled ventilation (VCV). Most patients need PIPs of 25–35 cmH$_2$O to achieve adequate ventilation. Infants with obstructive disease have long time constants. They are best ventilated with slow rates and inspiratory-expiratory (I:E) ratios of at least 1:3 to prevent breath "stacking" and further hyperinflation. Conversely, patients with restrictive disease may require faster rates and shorter I:E ratios. Cautious application of PEEP may decrease work of breathing (if intrinsic PEEP) in triggering of PSV and improving oxygenation in restrictive disease. Permissive hypercapnia, to avoid high PIPs and barotrauma, can be used with both pathophysiologic patterns. Obstructive patients usually do poorly with HFOV. Patients with more restrictive disease might benefit from HFOV. iNO has no role in obstructive disease. Although it can improve hypoxemia in ARDS, it does not improve outcome in restrictive disease.[14,63,64] Other adjuvant strategies awaiting proof of benefit include glucocorticoids, surfactant (both under trial), and heliox.

PEDIATRIC ARDS

The causes of ARDS in pediatric patients are the same as in adults, although viral or bacterial respiratory infections are more common in children.[65] Ventilator strategies are almost the same as in adult patients and include PEEP to recruit and keep open collapsed lung tissue and limiting peak inflation pressure to below 30–35 cmH$_2$O to avoid overinflation. Although no single ventilation mode has proven superior, the most common modes are PCV and HFOV[66] despite the absence of solid data on the use of HFOV in pediatric patients beyond the neonatal period. HFOV, using a high-volume strategy, can be used safely.[67] Despite higher mean airway pressures during HFOV than during conventional mechanical ventilation (CMV), barotrauma is less frequent.[68] Whether HFOV alters morbidity or mortality awaits prospective studies.

Prone positioning is used commonly, but without proven benefit.[69,70] iNO cannot be recommended for routine use, although it is used as rescue therapy (for a short time) in the very early stages of life-threatening hypoxemia and severe pulmonary hypertension.

STATUS ASTHMATICUS

Most complications in patients with asthma receiving ventilation occur during or immediately after intubation. They result largely from gas trapping causing hypotension, O$_2$ desaturation, pneumothorax, and cardiac arrest. Institution of positive-pressure ventilation in patients with asthma alters cardiocirculatory and respiratory dynamics dramatically, leading to diminished venous return and hypotension.

The optimal ventilator mode for status asthmaticus is not established. Randomized, controlled trials comparing different modes in pediatric asthma patients are virtually impossible.[71] Most clinicians prefer pressure-limited ventilation, keeping PIP below 35–40 cmH$_2$O and accepting hypercapnia.[72] Because of their decelerating flow pattern, PCV and pressure-regulated VCV allow for lower PIPs but result in higher mean airway pressures than VCV with identical V$_T$. Ventilator rates are set well below normal and require an extremely long expiratory time. A T$_I$ of 0.75–1.5 seconds allows ample time for inflation. Externally applied PEEP should be just below auto-PEEP to decrease trigger work but not increase hyperinflation. Duration of mechanical ventilation for status asthmaticus is usually of 1–4 days. Children with rapid-onset near-fatal asthma may have a shorter duration of ventilation than children with asthma that progresses slowly to respiratory failure.[73]

HFOV, PSV, and noninvasive ventilation have been tried in status asthmaticus. HFOV is believed to be contraindicated in children with severe airflow obstruction, although recent experience challenges this belief.[74] PSV enables active exhalation, which may decrease hyperinflation. PSV allows patients to determine their own respiratory pattern (rate, T$_I$, and V$_T$) and may decrease patient-ventilator dyssynchrony. PSV decreases work of breathing by partially unloading the respiratory muscles. Careful selection of PEEP decreases the work of triggering during PSV. PSV of 22–37 cmH$_2$O has been used successfully in children with asthma requiring full or near-full support, resulting in rapid improvement in gas exchange.[75] Noninvasive PSV is often poorly tolerated without sedation, and its role in avoiding intubation in children with status asthmaticus remains unclear.[76]

CHRONIC RESPIRATORY INSUFFICIENCY: LONG-TERM VENTILATION

Chronic respiratory insufficiency can be defined as a life-affecting or growth-affecting situation caused by a long-term problem with oxygenation and/or ventilation. Different ventilation techniques such as positive-pressures ventilation via tracheostomy, noninvasive positive-pressure mask ventilation (NIPPV), negative-pressure ventilation, and diaphragmatic pacing are available for long-term or home ventilator support in children. Selecting a technique depends on the underlying disease, age, expected duration of assistance, patient acceptability, local experience, availability of equipment, and cost. The simplest technology capable of supporting the patient's lifestyle needs should dictate choice.

Diseases that cause chronic respiratory insufficiency in infancy, such as BPD, may improve with age and allow withdrawal from mechanical ventilation. The respiratory system of infants is immature and prone to respiratory failure but has great potential for recovery as a result of growth of small airway size and increase in alveolar number during the first decade of life.[77] Long-term ventilation enables children to grow, preserves physiologic function, and prevents further damage from respiratory deterioration. In older children with chronic lung disease, such as cystic fibrosis, home ventilation can improve sleep-related hypoxemia and hypercapnia and serve as a short-term bridge to transplantation.[78–80]

Similar expectations for growth and development can be made for the infant's chest wall, which becomes stiffer and more stable with increasing age. The most common reasons for home ventilation in children are neuromuscular disorders and congenital central hypoventilation syndrome (CCHS). In children with neuromuscular disorders, nocturnal NIPPV may prevent respiratory deterioration secondary to atelectasis or respiratory infections and decrease hospitalization rates. Ethical concerns regarding the institution of long-term invasive ventilation through a tracheotomy in infants and small children with progressive neuromuscular disorders relate to the fear of prolonging suffering from a miserable and unfavorable disease. Intermittent NIPPV offers an alternative and serves as a comfort measure to relieve anxiety from hypoventilation and hypoxemia and probably has little impact on long-term survival. Death usually results from ineffective cough and clearing of secretions in patients with progressive respiratory muscle weakness rather than from insufficient ventilation.

CCHS is a rare disorder characterized by inadequate autonomic control of respiration. It is a common indication for pediatric home ventilation. Most infants need ventilator support from birth and demonstrate adequate ventilation during wakefulness but not during sleeping. Nevertheless,

CCHS varies in severity, ranging from complete apnea during sleep and severe hypoventilation during wakefulness to mild hypoventilation during quiet sleep. Some infants require 24-hour ventilator support from birth. Some develop awake hypoventilation at age 2–4 years as a result of increased physical activity. Therapy includes diaphragmatic pacing, negative-pressure ventilation, and various methods of noninvasive and invasive ventilation. Long-term prognosis of CCHS is reasonable, and the necessary therapeutical options should be offered.[81]

Common Ventilator Modes

The following invasive and noninvasive techniques are used in infants and children:

1. CPAP during spontaneous breathing
2. PSV or volume-support ventilation to assist spontaneous breathing
3. Intermittent mandatory ventilation (IMV) and synchronized intermittent mandatory ventilation (SIMV) using pressure or volume control
4. High-frequency ventilation (HFV) with or without spontaneous breathing

Clinical experience with these modes in neonates and infants, although less in children, is distinctly different from that in adults. There is a long-standing neonatal experience of nasal CPAP and HFV. Conversely, assist modes only recently became available in the neonatal field because of difficulties in providing sufficiently sensitive trigger systems, especially for end-expiratory flow termination during PSV.

CPAP IN NEONATES

In 1971, CPAP was first used to support breathing in preterm neonates presenting with RDS.[82] In infants, CPAP is commonly applied via the nasal route with a short binasal cannula (nasal prongs) or a soft nasal mask. Three systems are used:

1. An infant flow-driver system that generates CPAP in the nasal interface. This needs relatively high constant or variable flow rates (often above 8 liters/min) to ensure sufficient flow during inspiration and avoid excessive work of breathing.
2. An underwater bubble CPAP device, with an underwater blow-off system, positioned at a specific level on the expiratory side to create PEEP. Flow has to be suffcient to create continuous bubbling.
3. A conventional neonatal ventilator that offers a continuous flow to create CPAP.

Randomized trials of appropriate design that compare various CPAP systems (e.g., bubble versus infant flow) have not been conducted, and no clear evidence favors one or the other system of nasal interfaces[83] or design-related flow patterns.[84] Nasal CPAP is now used as first-line support in the neonatal field, mainly for premature infants presenting with various forms of respiratory distress (classically, infant RDS). Many unanswered questions remain, such as the optimal pressure and/or flow to be used,[85] whether early CPAP for RDS reduces mortality and morbidity (chronic lung disease remaining a significant problem in neonatal intensive care) as compared with intubation and mechanical ventilation,[26,28,86,87] and the lack of clear criteria to indicate when an infant is unresponsive to nasal CPAP. Empirical criteria of failure in infants with RDS are presented as the rule of 60s ($Pa_{CO_2} > 60$ mmHg or $F_{IO_2} > 60$ mmHg to maintain acceptable O_2 saturation). Persistence of serious apneic episodes is also a clear indication.[88]

After the neonatal period, observational reports of successful nasal CPAP in infants with viral bronchiolitis[58,62] have started to appear, opening a wider field for nasal CPAP use.

CONVENTIONAL VENTILATION IN NEONATES AND INFANTS

TIME-CYCLED, PRESSURE-LIMITED VENTILATION
Pressure-control techniques have been used in neonates for many years. Such neonatal *pressure controllers* deliver a continuous, constant flow during inspiration and expiration, and the inspiratory and expiratory pressure levels cycle at regular intervals [time-cycled, pressure-limited (TCPL) ventilation]. In that inspiratory flow characteristics of TCPL ventilation differ from classic PCV, which modulates inspiratory flow in a decelerating pattern (Fig. 25-5), a classic neonatal ventilator that offers TCPL ventilation is nothing more than a simple and easy-to-operate *flow driver*. To achieve an inspiratory plateau pressure, relatively high flow rates are required (6–10 liters/min), especially when short T_I values (0.3–0.4 second) are used to keep mean airway pressures low. On several occasions, pressure-limited ventilators have failed to provide adequate alveolar ventilation in newborn babies; this can be a problem when T_I is too short or with insufficient inspiratory flows. A second and perhaps more important problem with TCPL ventilation is that delivered V_T varies from breath to breath, coupled with the fact that many flow drivers do not offer measurements or display of delivered V_T. The same problems, however, hold true for any pressure-control mode. A third problem with TCPL ventilation is the slow buildup of pressure and cycle to pause as the pressure target is achieved. There is argument as to whether this leads to slow intratidal recruitment of the airways during the insufflation phase, the quantity of which depends on the pressure delivered. This may create less shear force in the airways than does classic PCV with a decelerating flow pattern. Conversely, a potential disadvantage of TCPL ventilation is that as soon as the inspiratory pause time commences, unstable airways are prone to collapse as gas is redistributed to areas with longer time constants. Consequently, a situation arises whereby collapse is already commencing during the inspiratory phase. Conversely, if a fast regulation system is used (variable flow delivery in a pressure-controlled mode) that promptly delivers flow, tightly regulated by pressure, previously collapsed airways will continue to expand; others with a longer

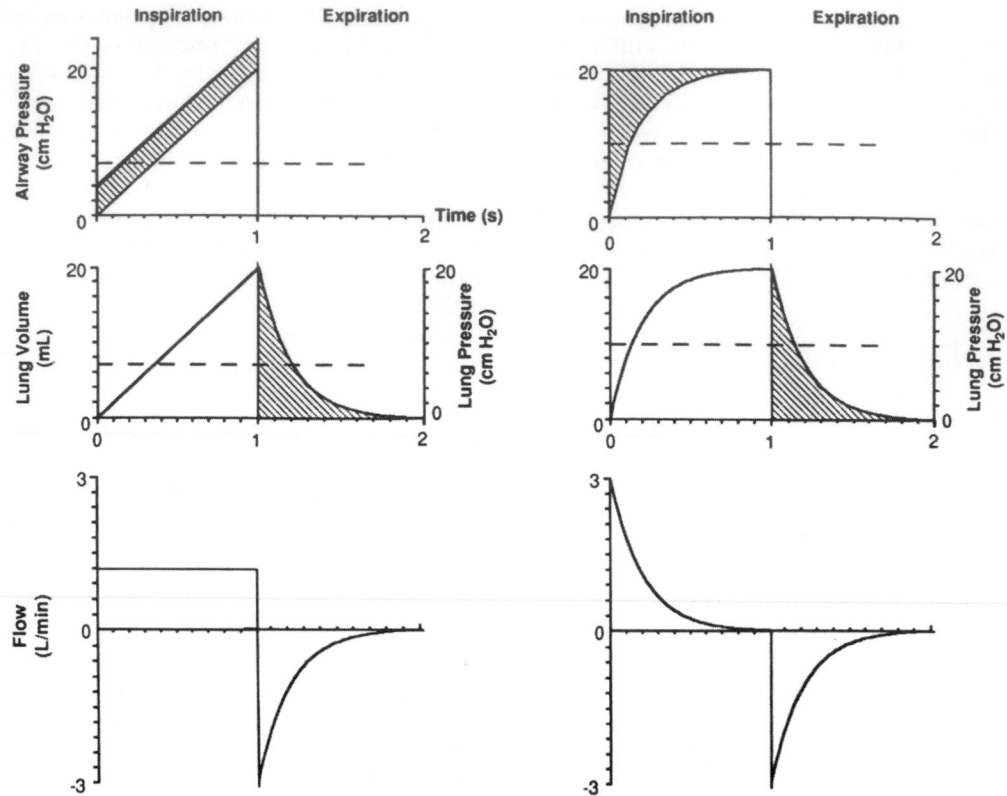

FIGURE 25-5 Graphic respresentation of the equation of motion for a constant inspiratory flow pattern (*left*) and a constant inspiratory pressure pattern (*right*). The dotted lines indicate mean airway and lung pressures. The shaded sections represent equal geometric areas proportional to the pressure required to overcome flow resistance. The unshaded sections represent equal geometric areas proportional to the pressure required to overcome elastic recoil. Note that for the same tidal volume and mean inspiratory flow rate (i.e., tidal volume/inspiratory time, V_T/T_I), the constant-flow pattern produces a higher peak airway pressure and lower mean airway pressure but the same peak lung pressure. (*Reprinted, with permission, from Chatburn: Respir Care 36:577, 1991.*)

time constant experience a chance of opening throughout inspiration. This implies that there is no pause during the inspiratory period and that the regulation system is active even during the "no flow" phase. Flow during this "no flow" phase is seen only on high resolution but adds to the efficacy of recruitment by providing extra time for lung inflation; this behavior is best explained by the power law of avalanches.[89]

PRESSURE-CONTROLLED VENTILATION
Classic PCV has been introduced in neonatal ventilation only recently. It differs from TCPL ventilation in that inspiratory flow is variable (decelerating flow pattern). PIP can be reached early during inspiration. This leads to fast increases in circuit and airway pressures, which may help to overcome high airway resistance. For years, this was considered harmful, but no evidence supports this concern.

VOLUME-CONTROLLED VENTILATION
VCV in neonatology was abandoned in the early 1980s mainly because of difficulties in measuring very small V_T values under low-flow conditions. A second argument was the slow rise to peak pressures (with constant inspiratory flow), eventually causing unequal lung volume distribution within the lung. A third argument was the frequent occur-

rence of an ETT leak (not using cuffed tubes), which can alter effective delivery of volume substantially. All these concerns are mere assumptions and not supported by clear scientific evidence. Because of technological advances and discussion of small V_T values for lung protection, there is growing interest in this mode again. A recent single-center randomized, controlled trial has compared pressure-limited ventilation versus VCV, with identical V_T values in both arms, in newborns presenting with RDS.[90] There was a small benefit, in terms of ventilator duration and significantly less intraventricular hemorrhages and abnormal periventricular echodensities on ultrasound scans, in favor of VCV. The lower rate of cerebral complications with VCV may reflect better P_{CO_2} stability.

VOLUME-TARGETED VENTILATION
Recognition that volume rather than pressure causes ventilator-induced lung injury has led to the development of various techniques that combine features of pressure- and volume-limited ventilation in a mode, usually referred to as *volume-targeted ventilation* (i.e., volume guarantee, pressure-regulated volume control, or volume-assured pressure support). With this, delivery of a set V_T is guaranteed by adjusting inspiratory pressure according to changes in compliance, resistance, or respiratory drive. This usually

requires a learning period over a number of breaths, during which dynamic compliance and respiratory system resistance are assessed by the ventilator. A few randomized studies in limited numbers of patients showed that these modes can be used safely[91-93] and may decrease ventilator-associated complications. Despite small studies showing only small breath-to-breath variability in V_T,[94,95] there is concern about overshooting volume delivery over several breaths (learning-period effect) if compliance or resistance change rapidly. The safety of these devices may need to be rethought.

PATIENT-TRIGGERED VENTILATION

Babies often breathe asynchronously with the ventilator or against the ventilator.[96] Such asynchrony may cause poor gas exchange and air trapping, leading to pneumothorax, hemodynamic instability, changes in cerebral blood flow, and intracranial hemorrhage in newborns.[97] Synchronization of spontaneous inspiration with the ventilator has been attempted, such as with SIMV, which conducts a search for a spontaneous effort within a predefined time frame (Fig. 25-6). Although SIMV was thought to be superior to IMV, no evidence supports this suspicion.[98]

Assist-control ventilation (ACV) was developed to assist all spontaneous breaths that exceed a trigger threshold; in the case of apnea, a mechanical breath is provided by the machine. Asynchrony occurs when the machine's T_I exceeds the infant's T_I. It is possible to terminate a machine breath based on a decline in inspiratory flow to below a certain percentage of peak inspiratory flow. Algorithms such as this help to synchronize patient effort with ventilator assistance.[96]

PSV increases inspiratory pressure to a preset level and is intended to overcome the work imposed by the ventilator and tubing system. Flow delivery is variable and proportional to patient effort. Initially, PSV was viewed mainly as a weaning mode, but subsequently, it was used more widely.[99] Since the development of sensitive flow triggers and variable inspiratory flow termination, PSV can be used even in neonates.[100]

SIMV, ACV, and PSV can be grouped under the generic term of *patient-triggered ventilation* (PTV). In neonates and especially in preterm infants, the trigger needs to sense any weak spontaneous breathing effort. It also must minimize artifacts that may result from other sources: heartbeat-induced variations in intrathoracic pressure or variations in pressure oscillations induced by rain-out in the ventilator tubing. Various trigger signals have been used: flow or pressure triggers, abdominal or thoracic impedance methods, and detection of abdominal motion. Flow triggering is more sensitive than pressure triggering for neonatal ventilation.[101] Two major sources of patient-ventilator dyssynchrony are (1) inappropriate long delays in inspiratory triggering (preterm infants with a short T_I may have completed much of the inspiratory phase before ventilator assistance commences) and (2) inappropriately selected inspiratory flow termination ("cycling off" setting that is given as a percentage of maximum inspiratory flow; if set too low, inflation times will be too long). With this, the flow at which

FIGURE 25-6 Volume (*above*) and flow (*below*) waveforms in a patient receiving synchronized intermittent mandatory ventilation. The SIMV breaths occur at somewhat irregular intervals because of the timing windows, during which the machine waits to detect a spontaneous effort by the patient. V_T, tidal volume; $\dot{V}$, flow; Paw, airway pressure. (*Used, with permission, from Respir Care 48:426–39, 2003.*)

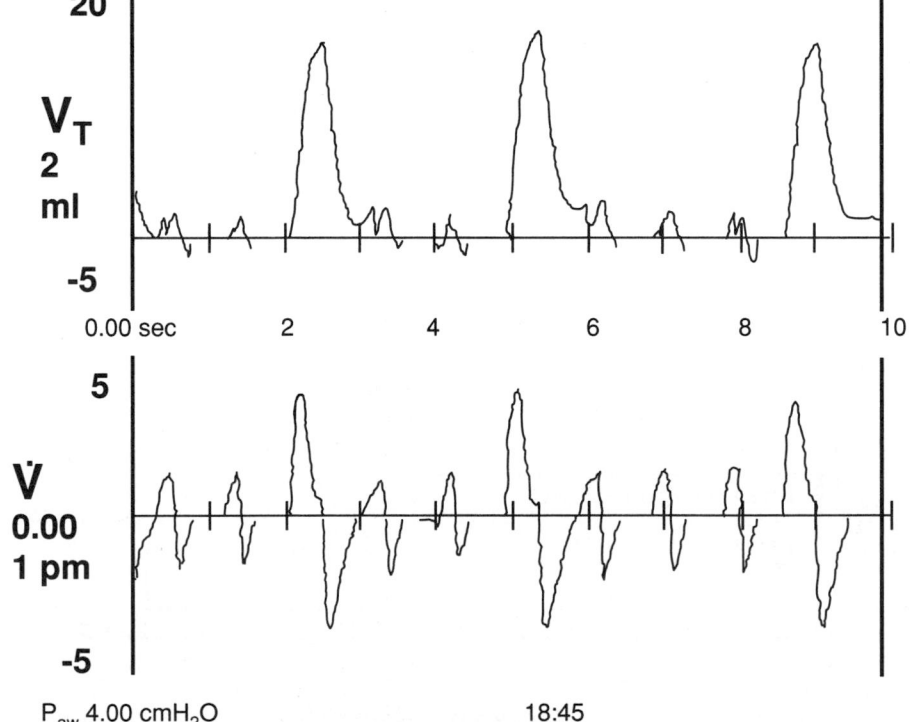

the ventilator cycles to exhalation does not coincide with the end of patient T_I.

NONCONVENTIONAL MODES: HIGH-FREQUENCY VENTILATION

HFV is defined by a frequency that greatly exceeds the normal respiratory rate and a V_T that approximates anatomic dead space (see Chapter 20). There are three major types of HFV:

1. High-frequency positive-pressure ventilation (HPPV; rate 60–150/minute)
2. High-frequency jet ventilation (HFJV; rate 100–600/minute)
3. High-frequency oscillatory ventilation (HFOV; rate 180–1500/minute or 3–25 Hz)

HFOV is the most commonly used method in pediatric and neonatal ICUs. HPPV and HFJV promote gas exchange in a conventional way with V_T greater than dead-space volume. Expiration is passive. In contrast, HFOV uses V_T values that are less than dead space, and expiration is active (Fig. 25-7).

HFJV is used mainly during (adult) laryngeal surgery; few randomized, controlled trials exist in neonates, with conflicting results.[102,103] Concerns have been raised about prolonged HFJV not only in neonates but also in adults regarding airway damage, ranging from focal necrosis to complete airway obstruction with mucus and severe necrotizing tracheobronchitis.[104,105] Increased risk of adverse cerebral outcome[106] has been reported. Studies have not used consistent criteria for assessment, however, and HFJV systems have varied widely.

HFOV has become the most widely used mode of HFV, and considerable experience with HFOV in acute neonatal respiratory failure now exists. The success of HFOV depends on its ability to recruit lung volume, which is not always easy late in disease when substantial ventilator-induced damage is superimposed on preexisting injury. The first randomized study of HFOV, the HiFi trial,[107] failed to stress early intervention, volume-recruitment maneuvers, and maintaining high mean airway pressures, as was clearly suggested from experimental data.[108–111] Recent trials, designed to ensure "opening the lung and keeping it open," showed that HFOV is efficient and safe.[35,36,68,112–117] Recent neonatal data suggest improved pulmonary outcome[36] compared with nonprotective, conventional ventilation.[115] It is still unclear, however, whether HFOV achieves better overall outcome in infants with RDS than does careful conventional ventilation.[38,118] Use of HFOV in pediatric patients with diffuse alveolar disease or ARDS is safe and improves physiologic endpoints but has not been shown to improve clinical outcome.[68]

All these methods are highly effective in eliminating CO_2, but the effect on oxygenation is less uniform. This is one reason that these modes (especially HFOV) have failed to sustain their initial attraction. Within the context of ventilator-induced lung injury and lung-protective strategies, HFV could be viewed as the optimal protective mode. By providing very small V_T values, it is possible to ventilate the lung within a safe zone with the pressure-volume curve of the respiratory system[119] (see Chapter 20). Side effects such as from respiratory acidosis (permissive hypercapnia) are not associated with HFOV and spontaneous ventilation can

FIGURE 25-7 Range of respiratory rate and tidal volume for various methods of mechanical ventilation. HFO, high-frequency oscillation; HFJV, high-frequency jet ventilation; HFPPV, high-frequency positive-pressure ventilation; V_D, dead space. (*Adapted, with permission, from Slutsky: Am Rev Respir Dis 138:175–83, 1988.*)

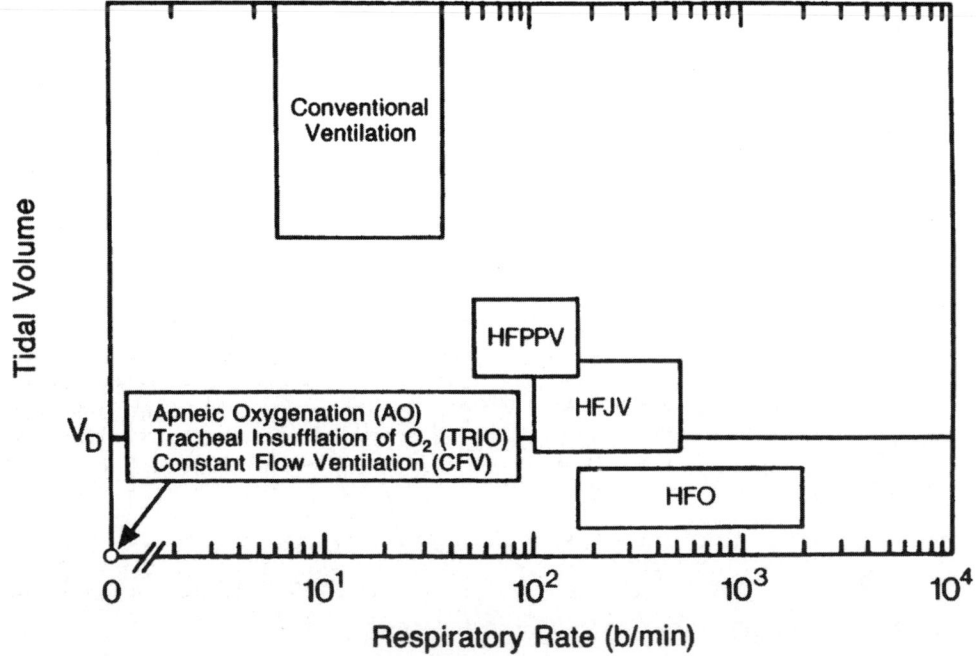

TABLE 25-2   Inital Settings of Frequency during Transition from CMV to HFO According to Age Group

	Frequency
Preterm infant	12–5 Hz
Neonate at term and small children	10–12 Hz
Children	8–10 Hz
Adolescents	5–8 Hz

be often maintained, at least in neonates and small children. Thus use of sedation is decreased, and muscle relaxants are avoided. In larger patients, inspiratory flow demands are higher; thus spontaneous breathing is not managed as easily, and heavy sedation and/or paralysis may be required.

INDICATIONS AND TIMING FOR HFOV

HFOV is still used mainly as rescue therapy despite clear indicators from experimental and clinical experience that it is most beneficial when initiated before major lung injury has developed[68,115,120,121] because no ventilator strategy can repair pre-existing lung injury.[118,122] Classic indications for HFOV in neonatal patients include

1. *RDS* characterized by surfactant deficiency, high chest-wall compliance, and low FRC. This is the constellation for easy and efficient lung recruitment, at least with early disease.[115,118]
2. *CDH,* usually associated with alveolar and pulmonary vascular hypoplasia,[123] resulting in increased risk of ventilator-induced lung injury[48] and presenting with PPHN requiring aggressive P_{CO_2} control. Lung recruitment should be applied with great caution because of the difficulty in estimating the degree of lung hypoplasia.
3. *Air-leak syndrome,* such as pneumothorax or interstitial emphysema. HFOV can achieve early improvement and resolution of air leak in patients with interstitial emphysema, enabling better gas exchange and lower airway pressures than with CMV.[124]
4. *PPHN.* Although iNO is the classic treatment for PPHN, HFOV can enhance delivery of iNO by achieving adequate lung recruitment[125] and enable easier CO_2 control and correction of respiratory acidosis.

The classic indication for HFOV in pediatric patients is *diffuse alveolar disease (primary or secondary ARDS)*[68,126] as rescue therapy to improve oxygenation. The only pediatric randomized, controlled trial[68] did not show any difference in survival or ventilator duration, although duration of supplemental O_2 was shorter with HFOV than with CMV. Recommended strategies for use of HFOV (Fig. 25-8 and Table 25-2) are empirical and derive mainly from the neonatal field and experience with HFOV in adult patients.[116]

Weaning from Mechanical Ventilation

Weaning is largely determined by institutional practices or individual preferences. There is a traditional belief that support should be withdrawn gradually, certainly after prolonged respiratory failure, to enable children to regain respiratory muscle strength. Technological advances, however, in patient-ventilator synchronization and improved management of sedative and narcotic drugs carry considerable potential for shortening weaning and reducing extubation failure.[127]

CORRECT TIMING OF EXTUBATION

Avoidance of unnecessary weaning delays is important for reducing the risk of nosocomial infection, ETT damage to the airway, development of chronic lung disease in neonates, and prolonged dependency on narcotic drugs.[128,129] Aggressiveness with early weaning, however, must be balanced against the risk of extubation failure that occurs in 6–15% of children and up to 40% of neonates[130–132] and is associated with increased mortality.

Extubation failure may be caused by (1) reduced respiratory drive (e.g., sedation, central nervous system infection or trauma, and hypocapnia), (2) increased respiratory muscle load (e.g., unresolved lung disease, upper airway obstruction including postextubation stridor, thick secretions, and pulmonary edema including left-to-right shunt), abdominal distension, sepsis, and metabolic acidosis, and (3) impaired respiratory muscle function (e.g., neuromuscular disorders, diaphragmatic paralysis, cervical spinal injury, malnutrition and severe electrolyte abnormalities).

Extubation failure is more frequent with chronic respiratory disorders, neuromuscular and chronic neurologic disorders, and upper airway problems.[131] The most common cause of extubation failure in preterm infants is apnea/bradycardia.[132]

Objective weaning criteria have not been established for infants and children. A trial of spontaneous breathing with a T piece and use of 10 cmH2O of PSV for up to 2 hours have been successful in allowing assessment of extubation readiness and in predicting extubation failure.[133] Baumeister et al[134] modified the rapid shallow breathing index (RSBI) and the compliance, rate, oxygenation and, pressure (CROP) index for weaning prediction in children. RSBI is also known as the *frequency-to-V_T ratio*; the threshold that best discriminated between successful and failed extubation was less than 11 breaths per minute per milliliter per kilogram. CROP is calculated as $[C_{dyn} \times P_{I,max} \times (Pa_{O_2}/Pa_{O_2})]/RR$, where C_{dyn} is dynamic compliance (corrected for body weight), $P_{I,max}$ is maximum negative inspiratory pressure, Pa_{O_2}/Pa_{O_2} is the ratio of arterial to alveolar O_2 tension, and RR is the patient's respiratory rate. All children with a modified CROP index of 0.1 ml × mmHg per breath per minute per kilogram or greater were extubated successfully. As part of a study not designed for weaning prediction, the PALISI investigators changed Fi_{O_2} to 0.5 and decreased PEEP to 5 cmH2O. Children who maintained an S_{O_2} of 95% or greater were placed on minimal PSV for 2 hours. They were extubated if they maintained an S_{O_2} of 95% or greater, an exhaled V_T of 5 ml/kg or greater, and a respiratory rate within the acceptable range for age.[127]

Developing reliable thresholds for indices for weaning extremely low-birth-weight infants has proven more difficult.[135] The percentage of time spent below a target value of spontaneous expiratory minute ventilation

High Frequency Oscillatory Ventilation

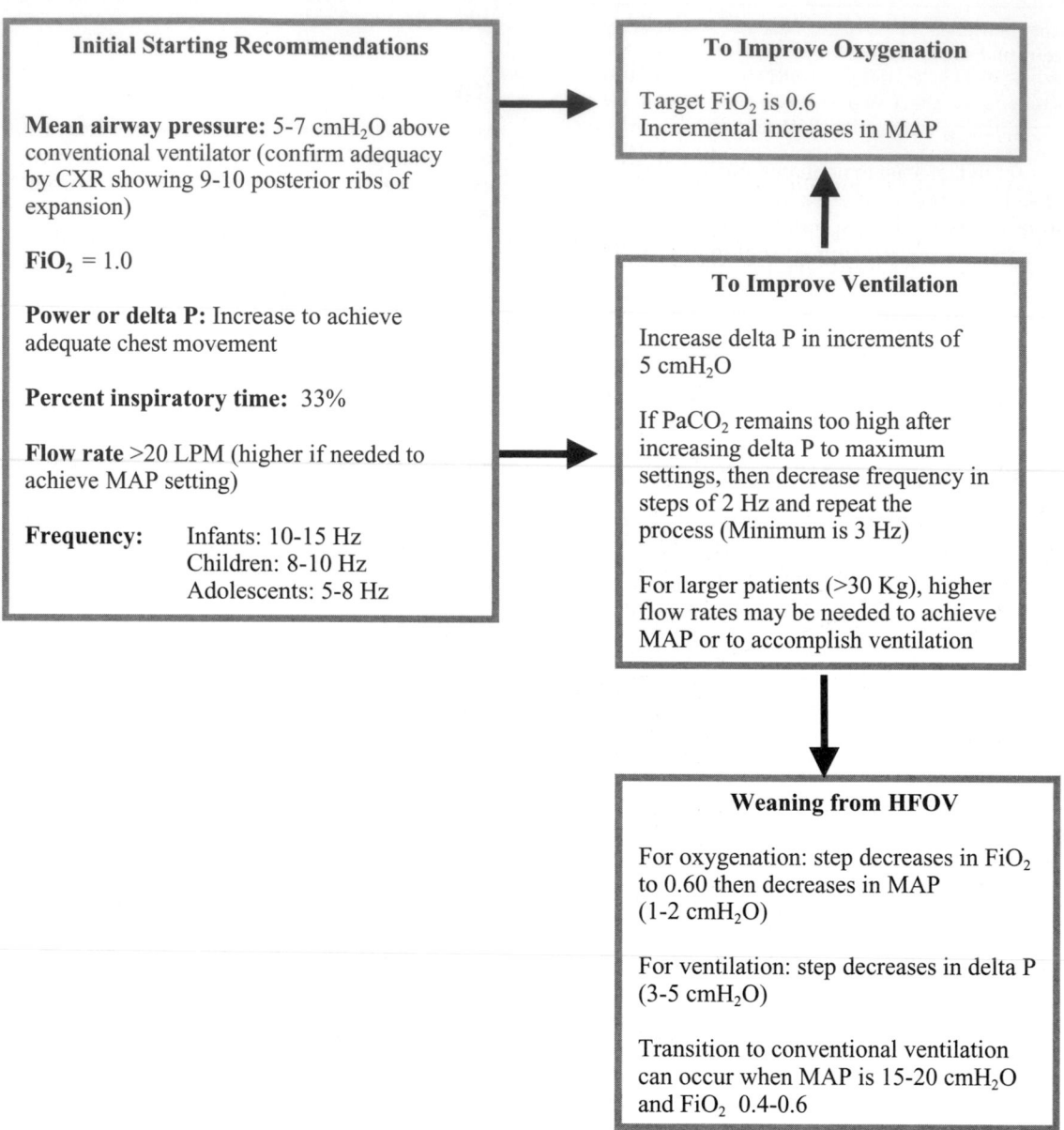

FIGURE 25-8 Guidelines for instituting high-frequency oscillatory ventilation and the transition to conventional ventilation. (*Courtesy of Martha Curley, Children's Hospital Boston, Harvard Medical School; see ref. 70.***)**

(<125 ml/min/kg) during a 2-hour CPAP trial appears promising but requires further testing.[136,137]

WEANING MODES AND ADJUNCTS TO WEANING

Weaning methods include PSV and volume-support ventilation (VSV). Both methods involve patient-triggered pressure support. With PSV, the level of PSV is adjusted gradually by the physician to a minimal level that achieves acceptable respiratory parameters. With VSV, the level of PSV is adjusted continually by the ventilator to achieve a minimum minute ventilation. Today, many ventilator modes have been developed to facilitate weaning by reducing work imposed by respiratory apparatus, but their use has not been investigated in children.[138,139] Some studies in adult patients suggest that protocol-directed weaning implemented by nurses and respiratory therapists might achieve extubation more rapidly than physician-directed weaning.[140,141] One pediatric study (using as study endpoint the time at which minimal settings were achieved but not the time of extubation)[142] reached a similar conclusion. The largest pediatric weaning study, however, showed that weaning protocols were no better than physician-directed weaning and suggested that gradual weaning is not indicated in most infants and children.[127] Studies have not included children who are difficult to wean, especially those with disorders of the respiratory muscles. NIPPV may prove helpful in weaning such children. Diaphragmatic plication can be of benefit in children with diaphragmatic paralysis and may facilitate weaning.[143]

The classic approach to weaning neonates from CMV is to extubate them from a rate of about 15 breaths per minute to supplemental O_2 or nasal CPAP. Weaning strategies involve decreasing rate (except for patient-trigger ventilation) and positive inspiratory pressure to maintain the V_T at 4 ml/kg or greater. PSV may be combined with SIMV. Newer options include volume-assured pressure support and proportional-assist ventilation.[144,145] In neonates, direct extubation from a low ventilator rate showed a trend toward greater successful extubation than did extubation after a period of endotracheal CPAP.[146] Weaning from HFOV is performed by switching to CMV or by direct extubation directly after gradual reduction of mean airway pressure and amplitude to very low values.

In preterm infants, methylxanthines, nasal CPAP, and nasal NIPPV have been used to facilitate weaning and extubation, although only the latter two are recommended for routine use.[147] There is no role for glucocorticoids.[148,149] Methylxanthines (especially caffeine because of its wide therapeutic margin[150]) increase the chance of successful extubation of preterm infants within 1 week, but there is insufficient information on side effects or long-term effects on child development. Nasal CPAP stabilizes the upper airway, improves lung function, and reduces apnea.[151] It can prevent extubation failure in preterm infants, but the optimal levels and best methods of administration remain to be determined.[152] Synchronized NIPPV can augment the beneficial effects of nasal CPAP in preterm infants after extubation.[153]

In conclusion, neonates and children can be weaned much quicker than adults, and weaning protocols have proven to be of little or limited value in pediatric patients.

Unique Neonatal and Pediatric Machines and Interfaces

Conventional pediatric and/or neonatal ventilators can be divided in three groups: (1) neonatal ventilators, (2) pediatric ventilators (which generally are identical to adult ventilators), and (3) all-age-group ventilators (from neonates to adults). Traditionally, a neonatal ventilator was used for neonates or toddlers up to a body weight of 10 kg. Neonatal ventilators were mainly constant-flow generators, which build up pressure and cycle to pause as the pressure target is achieved (TCPL ventilators). Today, some neonatal ventilators, mainly all-age-group ventilators, also offer classic pressure- and volume-control modes.

The following are the characteristics of a good neonatal ventilator: (1) small apparatus dead space, (2) stiff but flexible circuit tubing, (3) reliable tidal-volume measurement device (hot-wire or pressure-differential flowmeter or fixed- or variable-orifice device) placed between the Y piece and ETT, (4) highly sensitive trigger device (flow triggering preferred to pressure triggering at least in premature infants,[154] which provides adjustable inspiratory and expiratory trigger criteria, ranging from 5–25% or more of peak inspiratory flow), (5) built-in leak compensation, which can be turned off if there is a large leak around the ETT (this is important with PSV to enable inspiratory flow termination so as to avoid excessive T_I in relation to patient need), and (6) airway humidification with cascade humidifiers and heated-wire ventilator circuitry.[155]

The new-generation all-patient units offer all these neonatal requirements and perform as well as those designed specifically for neonatal/pediatric patients.[156] Detailed specifications on "only neonatal" and "all-patient" ventilators are listed in Tables 25-3 and 25-4. Ventilator companies have provided these data in response to the authors' request.

HIGH-FREQUENCY VENTILATORS

Important differences in performance characteristics of devices for HFV have been shown repeatedly.[157–160] Thus it is not possible to compare settings from one form to another. Three major systems are used: HFOV, HFJV, and HFV with a flow-interrupter device (HFFI).

HFOV
HFOV is characterized by use of mean airway pressure (continuous distending pressure), on top of which squarewave or sinusoidal pressure swings are added by means of a piston, diaphragm, or bidirectional high-velocity flow in the expiratory limb. This leads to a more or less active aspiration during the "expiratory" phase of the oscillatory cycle. The best studied and most widely applied HFOV system is the Sensormedics 3100 high-frequency oscillator (VIASYS Healthcare, Palm Springs, CA). This exists in two versions: the 3100A for neonatal use and the 3100B for pediatric and adult use. The Humming V (Metran Medical Instruments, Saitama, Japan) exhibits similar performance to the Sensormedics 3100A in in vitro and bench studies and also can be switched to CMV. A new neonatal ventilator offers a slightly different technique of HFOV: The SLE 5000 (Specialized Laboratory Equipment Limited, South-Croydon, Surrey, UK) uses a bidirectional high-velocity flow in the expiratory limb to generate sinusoidal ventilation with active expiration. This ventilator also allows combined use of CMV and HFOV. No clinical or experimental data exist for this new ventilator, nor have safety issues been addressed.

HFJV
HFJV is characterized by the delivery of small, high-velocity breaths at fast rates coupled with passive exhalation. HFJV allows the application of relatively low airway pressure to maintain reasonable oxygenation. Pulses of gas are delivered at high velocity through an orifice at frequencies of 10–100 Hz. The orifice may be in a T piece connected to a conventional ETT or a narrow tube incorporated in the wall of a special ETT or at end of a fine-bore catheter placed in the trachea. Available HFJVs for neonatal and pediatric use include the Acutronic Monsoon Deluxe Jet Ventilator,

TABLE 25-3 Conventional Ventilators: Limited to Neonatal (and Partially Pediatric) Use

Ventilator	Babylog 8000 plus	Bear Cub 750psv	Christina	Fabian	Sechrist Millenium	SLE 5000	Stephanie
	Dräger Medical, Lübeck, Germany	VIASYS Healthcare, PalmSprings, CA	Stephan GmbH, Medizintechnik, Gackenbach, Germany	Acutronic Medical Systems, Hirzel, Switzerland	Sechrist, Anaheim CA	Specialised Laboratory Equipment Limited, South-Croydon, Surrey, UK	Stephan Biomedical Incorporation, Gackenbach, Germany
Control principle	Continuous flow, time/flow cycled, pressure-limited	Continuous flow	Continuous flow	Continuous flow, time/flow-cycled, pressure-limited	Continuous flow	Continuous flow	Auto-/continuous flow
Modes	IPPV/IMV SIPPV/ SIMV PSV, CPAP Volume guarantee (VG)	IPPV/IMV SIPPV/ SIMV PSV, CPAP Volume limit	IPPV/IMV, SIPPV/ SIMV, assist-control, CPAP with backup ventilations,	IPPV/IMV SIPPV/ SIMV PSV, CPAP, CPAP with backup frequency Volume limit	SIMV/IMV, assist control, CPAP and CPAP with backup ventilation	IPPV/IMV SIPPV/ SIMV PSV, CPAP target tidal volume ventilation	IPPV/IMV, SIPPV/ SIMV, assist-control, PSV Volume target in P-CMV, leak-adapted volume-control in V-CMV, CPAP with minute volume target, and PAV with several backup ventilations
Trigger type (type/response sensibility/time)	Leak-adapted flow/volume trigger. (heated wire/0.2 l/min + 0.02–3 ml/ 40–60 ms)	Flow trigger (heated wire/0.02–5 liters/min)	Flow trigger (0.1– 2.0 ml)/pressure trigger optional (0.1–2.0 mbar) Pneumotachograph (PNT)	Leak-adapted flow trigger (heated wire/5–30% of the tidal volume/ 10 ms)	Pressure trigger (pressure differential/0.1 cmH$_2$O/5–40 ms)	Leak-adapted flow trigger (heated wire/0.2– 20 liters/min)	Flow trigger (0.1– 2.9 ml)/pressure cycling optional (0.1–2.9 mbar) Pneumotachograph
Inspiratory flow	1–30 liters/min	1–30 liters/min	0–20 liters/min	Neonatal: 1–20 liters/min Pediatric: 4–40 liters/min	2–32 liters/min	8–60 liters/min	0–20 liters/min
Expiratory flow (base flow), independently adjustable	1–30 liters/min	1–30 liters/min		2–20 liters/min	Continuous flow (equals inspiratory flow)	Continuous flow (equals inspiratory flow)	3–5 liters/min cross-flow to wash out the Y piece

End-expiratory pressure control device	Servo-controlled nonoccluding expiratory valve		Electrically controlled expiratory valve	Servo-controlled nonoccluding expiratory valve	0–20 cmH$_2$O (non occluding expiratory valve)	Valveless expiratory valve	Servo-controlled combined Inspiratory and expiratory propotional valve
Mechanical dead space of flow/pressure-sensing device	0.9 ml (with ISO 15 flow sensor) 1.5 ml (with integrated Y-piece sensor)	1.0 ml	0.56 ml (PNT B) 1.1 ml (PNT C)	0.9 ml	1.5 ml	1.0 ml	0.56 ml (PNT B) 1.1 ml (PNT C)
Incorporated graph monitoring	Flow and pressure, integrated waveforms (only one curve displayed without optional screen) optional screen provides three simultaneous waveforms and loops	Pressure, flow, and volume waveform; pressure and flow volume loops	Pressure, flow, and volume waveforms over time; volume/pressure, flow/volume, and flow/pressure loops	Pressure, flow, and volume waveforms; flow/volume, flow/pressure, and volume/flow loops (max. 2 curves displayed simultaneously)	n/a	Pressure, flow, and volume waveforms; flow/volume, flow/pressure, and volume/flow loops	Pressure, flow, and volume waveforms over time; volume/pressure, flow/volume, and flow/pressure loops
Lung function parameters	Compliance C20/C Resistance time constant Correlation coefficient	n/a	Compliance, resistance	Compliance C20/C, resistance	n/a	Compliance C20/C, resistance	Compliance, resistance, intrapulmonary pressure, inadvertant PEEP (insp. or exp. occlusion maneuver)
Additional features	HFV (HFFI) — optional (not available in the US)	Graphics display	HFOV—optional	Battery pack Transport option	—	HFOV—optional	HFOV Variable ventilatory resistance and elastance (negative ventilator impedance, PAV)
Upper body weight limitation	20 kg 10 kg (in the US)	30 kg	16 kg	30 kg	50 kg		42 kg

TABLE 25-4 Conventional Ventilators: All Patient Ventilators

Ventilator	AVEA	EvitaXL	Galileo Gold	Newport e500	Puritan Benett 840	Servo i
	VIASYS Healthcare, PalmSprings, CA	Dräger Medical, Lübeck, Germany	Hamilton Medical, Rhäzüns, Switzerland	Newport Medical Instruments, Costa Mesa, CA	Puritan-Benett, Pleasanton, CA	Maquet Critical Care, Solna, Sweden
Control principle	Variable-flow (adult/pediatric) Continuous-flow time-cycled (neonate)	Time-cycled, volume-constant, pressure-controlled NeoFlow: baseflow combined with demand system	Variable-flow	Servo-controlled, mandatory and spontaneous variable-flow, time-cycled, pressure- or volume- (flow) controlled Bias flow with Automatic Leak Compensation to provide a stable 3 L/min between breaths	Time-cycled controlled flow or algorithmically controlled flow	Variable-flow
Modes	A/C, PCV, VCV, SIMV, TCPL (only neonate) SPONT, CPAP assist (pressure or volume) PRVC (= volume-targeted ventilation, only adult/pediatric) APRV Noninvasive ventilation (NIV) Apnea backup	CMV, SIMV, A/C, PCV+ (BIPAP), PCV+ assist (BIPAP assist), MMV, CPAP, ASB (PS) Automode (= volume-targeted ventilation) BIPAP/ BIPAP-ASB APRV Proportional pressure support (PPS) (optional, not available in the US) Noninvasive ventilation (NIV) Apnea backup Independent lung ventilation (ILV)	CMV, SIMV, PCV, SPONT, CPAP Assist (pressure or volume) APV (= volume-targeted ventilation) ASV DuoPAP/APRV Noninvasive ventilation (NIV) Apnea backup	Volume control: A/CMV SIMV (± Psupport) SPONT (± psupport) Pressure control: A/CMV SIMV (± psupport) SPONT (± psupport) Volume target pressure controll and volume target pressure support Noninvasive ventilation (NIV) Apnea backup	A/C, PCV, VCV, SIMV, SPONT, CPAP assist (pressure or volume) Optional: bilevel, APRV Volume-ventilation plus (= volume-targeted ventilation) as volume cotroll plus or voulme support Apnea backup ventilation	A/C VCV, PCV, SIMV SPONT, CPAP PS and VS assist (pressure or volume) PRVC (= volume- targeted ventilation) SIMV(PRVC) + PS Bi-vent (optional) Auto-mode (= automatic switch from control to spontaneous and spontanoues to control according patient's respiratory activity, optional) Noninvasive ventilation (NIV) PC and PS Nasal CPAP (optional for infant only) Apnea backup ventilation

Trigger type	Pressure or flow trigger (neonate: flow trigger only) Optional: Proximal variable orifice (all patients) or proximal hot-wire sensor (for neonate only) Variable inspiratory backup trigger (flow or pressure, respectively)	Leak-adapted flow trigger, Proximal heated-wire flow sensor (for neonatal and optionally pediatric patients)	Flow trigger and pressure trigger, leak-adapted Proximal variable orifice flow sensor	Leak-adapted, pressure or flow trigger	Pressure or flow trigger (neonate: flow trigger only) No special neonatal flow sensor, only Neo-Mode Software Fixed inspiratory backup trigger (pressure)	Flow or pressure trigger (leak-adapted flow trigger) Proximal fixed orifice flow and pressure sensor (for neonate, pediatric and adult) Expiratory Ultrasound flow sensor
Trigger sensitivity	0.1–20 liters/min flow 0.1–20.0 cmH$_2$O pressure below PEEP	0.3–15 liters/min flow	0.5–15 liters/min flow 0.5–10 mbar pressure below PEEP	0.1–2.0 liters/min (pediatric/infant) 0–5 cmH$_2$O pressure below PEEP Response time 10 msec	1–20 liters/min (adult and pediatric) 0.1–10 liters/min (neonatal) 0.1–20 cmH$_2$O pressure below PEEP	Flow trigger sensitivity level (fraction of bias flow 0–100% of 33 ml/s (2 liters/min) adult 8 ml/s (0.5 liters/min) infant Pressure trigger 0–20 (cmH$_2$O) below PEEP
Inspiratory flow	3–150 liters/min (adult) 1–75 liters/min (pediatric) 0.4–30.0 liters/min (neonate)	6–120 liters/min (adult) 6–30 liters/min (pediatric)	1–180 liters/min (peak flow for adult and pediatric applications)	1–100 liters/min (pediatric/infant)	3–150 liters/min (adult) 3–60 liters/min (pediatric) 1–30 liters/min (neonate) (Continuous flow rate is automatically ajusted to 1.5 liters/min above flow trigger sensitivity)	0–3.3 liters/s (0–200 liters/min) (adult/pediatric) 0–0.55 liters/s (0–33 liters/min) (neonate)
Expiratory trigger (flow termination)	Variable (0–45% of peak flow)	Fixed at 25% of peak flow	Variable (5–70% of peak flow)	No proximal flow/pressure device available	Variable (1–80%)	Variable (1–70% of peak flow)
Mechanical dead-space of flow/pressure sensing device	VarFlex: 0.7 ml (neonate), 9.6 ml (adult) Hot wire: 0.8 ml (neonate)	9 ml (including optional mainstream capnograph) Neoflow: 0.9 ml flow sensor (neonate)	9–11 ml (adult and pediatric) 1.93 ml (neonate)		None (flow/pressure sensing is integral to the pneumatic system)	N/A Proximal fixed orifice sensor <0.75 ml infant <6.9 ml adult

(Continued)

TABLE 25-4 (Continued)

Ventilator	AVEA	EvitaXL	Galileo Gold	Newport e500	Puritan Benett 840	Servo i
Incorporated graph monitoring	Pressure-, flow-, and volume-time waveforms Flow/volume, airway; esophageal, tracheal, and/or transpulmonary pressure/volume loops	Pressure-, flow-, and volume-time waveforms Pressure/volume, volume/flow, tracheal pressure/volume, flow/pressure, volume/CO_2 (optional) or flow/tracheal pressure loops Long and short trends	Pressure-, flow-, and volume-time waveforms Any pair of three basic parameters for loops: airway pressure, flow and volume presented	Pressure-, flow-, and volume-time waveforms with auto or manual scaling (multiloops: up to 5 displayed simultaneously Pressure/volume, flow/volume loops with trace function and store function for two sets of loops, all with auto or manual scaling	Pressure, flow, and volume, waveforms (two waveforms simultaneoulsy displayed) Pressure-volume loop (with calculation of inspiratory area)	Pressure, flow, volume, and CO_2 waveforms Flow/volume, pressure/volume loops
Lung function parameters/ weaning parameters	Lung function package (inclusive in comprehensive model) with compliance, resistance, rapid-shallow breathing index, negative inspiratory force, auto-PEEP, chest-wall compliance, lung compliance, imposed resistance, lung resistance, peak inspiratory flow, peak expiratory flow, delta airway pressure, delta auto-PEEP, esoPhageal auto-PEEP, transpulmonary plateau pressure, Occlusion pressure ($P_{0.1}$), ventilator work of breathing, patient work of breathing, imposed work of breathing, transpulmonary auto-PEEP, C20/C	Compliance Resistance Intrinsic $PEEP—PEEP_I$ Vtrap (volume trapped due to $PEEP_I$); Rapid-shallow breathing index (RSBI); Negative inspiratory force (NIF); Occlusion pressure $P_{0.1}$	Compliance (Cstat) Inspiratory resistance (Rinsp) Expiratory resistance (Rexp) Auto-PEEP Inspiratory time constant (RCinsp) Expiratory time constant (RCexp) Occlusion pressure ($P_{0.1}$); Rapid shallow breathing index (RSBI); Imposed work of breathing (WOBimp) PV tool (with inflation and deflation limb of quasi-static pressure-volume curve)	Compliance (Cstat, Cdyn effective); Inspiratory resistance (Rinsp) Expiratory resistance (Rexp); $PEEP_{TOT,stat}$; Imposed work of breathing (WOBim); Peak inspiratoy flow, peak expiratory flow; Delta airway pressure Minimum expiratory time (time constant *3); f/VT (rapid shallow breathing index); Peak negative pressure WW version (optional) : manual slow inflation creates static PV curve	Compliance Resistance Rapid shallow breathing index (f/Vt)	Dynamic characteristics T_I/T_{TOT} WOB patient WOB ventilator Rapid shallow breathing index Total PEEP Static Compliance Inspiratory Resistance Expiratory Resistance I:E ratio Elastance Time constant O_2 concentration EtCO_2 concentration VCO_2 minute elimination CO_2 elimination Mv$_e$sp/Mv$_e$ Spontaneous exp. minute volume Leakage fraction in NIV $P_{0.1}$ Dynamic Compliance

Additional features	Heliox modul (inclusive in comprehensive model)	Automatic tube compensation CO_2 incorporated (optional) SmartCare/PS knowledge-based weaning system (optional, down to 15-kg patients, not available in the US) Lung-protection package (optional)	Tube resistance compensation Sigh feature Built in jetnebulizer flow driver (cycled)	Separately adjusted expiratory bias flow with automatic leak compensation (up to 8 liters/min) to provide stable 3 liters/min between breaths Sigh feature (1.5 × tidal volume setting every 100 breaths) Dual control breath management (VTPC/VTPS) Event History WW version (optional): FlexCycle (automatic exp threshold adjustment) Automatic Slope/Rise adjustment, noninvasive ventilation, open exhalation valve (for biphasic pressure release ventilation)	Tube compensation (assisting proportioanl to patients inspiratory flow) Proportional-assist ventilation (PAV+) with automatic calculation of elastance and resistance (optional)	Automatic tube and leak compensation Open lung tool (optional) CO_2 incorporated (optional) Ultrasound nebulizer (optional) and/or aeroneb (nebulization with vibration technology) Ventilation record card recording data and waveforms Time constant controlled exhalation valve Consumable or nonconsumable sensor for O_2 measurement Event log
Infant/neonate ventilation	Standard	Optional	Standard	Standard	Optional	Standard

the Acutronic Medical Systems (Hirzel, Switzerland), and the Life Pulse High Frequency Ventilator (Bunnell, Salt Lake City, UT).

HFFI

HFFI offers CMV as the basic mode. Expiration is mainly passive, but negative pressure generated by a venturi effect may enhance lung emptying. Examples include the Draeger Babylog 8000 (Drägerwerk, Lubeck, Germany), the Stephanie (Stephan Biomedical Incorporation, Gackenbach, Germany), and the Infrasonics Infant Star 950 (Nellcor Puritan-Bennett, Inc., Pleasanton, PA). HFFIs are available only for neonatal ventilation, and little data exist on their clinical use.[161,162]

AIRWAY HUMIDIFICATION SYSTEMS

The objective of humidification in infants and children is to achieve a physiologic situation: 100% water saturation of the inspired gas at 37°C, corresponding to 44 mg H_2O/liter. $\geq$ 30 mg H_2O/liter are considered to be acceptable.[163,164] This can be achieved with heated- moisture-exchange (HME) filters that allow retention of the temperature and humidity of a patient's expired gas.[164] HME filters, however, add considerable dead space and resistance to the circuit,[165] which is problematic in neonates and small children. Cascade humidifiers interposed in the inspiratory limb, therefore adding no resistance or dead space, are more efficient for airway humidification[166] and should be preferred. To avoid rain-out during transport of humidified and heated gas, gas temperature needs to be maintained by a heated wire in the inspiratory limb. Most recent circuits also allow for heating of the expiratory limb.

Monitoring of Mechanical Ventilation

Several specific pediatric and neonatal issues about respiratory monitoring must be noted. First, ventilator-circuit dead space should kept as small as possible when monitoring devices are added. Second, flow measurements must be made as close as possible to the airway opening to get true delivered V_T.[167–169] Third, CO_2 production is lower in neonates ($\sim$15 ml/min) and toddlers than in adults ($\sim$200 ml/min). Accurate measurements of exhaled CO_2 in pediatric patients is more challenging because of limitations in size of the analyzer chamber, the amount of flow that must be suctioned by sidestream devices, and the need for fast response times because of rapid respiratory rates. Therefore, mainstream sensors, which have a faster response time (than side-stream devices) and do not need suction flow, are preferred.[170]

Complications of Mechanical Ventilation

In addition to barotrauma (e.g., pneumothorax and interstitial emphysema), three other complications include pos-

textubation stridor, development of chronic lung disease or BPD (classic in the preterm infant), and ventilator-associated pneumonia.

POSTEXTUBATION STRIDOR

Acquired subglottic stenosis became a well-recognized problem with use of long-term endotracheal intubation. Serious tube trauma and postextubation stridor have decreased markedly with improvements in material and tube design, greater care in choosing appropriately sized tubes, and meticulous care of the intubated patient. The old dictum, "Cuffed ETTs should not be used in children under the age of 8 years," is incorrect given the development of high-volume, low-pressure cuffs.[171,172] Tube complications usually arise from incorrect size, traumatic or multiple intubations, up-and-down movements of the tube, and inadequate analgesia and sedation, causing intubated infants to struggle. Poor design can result in a cuff being positioned too high within the larynx (Fig. 25-9), causing severe trauma.[173] Other risk factors of postextubation stridor include duration of intubation, gastroesophageal reflux, and tracheobronchial infection. Checking for a cuff leak is of little help in predicting postextubation problems in young children.[174]

Most injuries causing postextubation stridor are superficial and include nonspecific changes such as laryngeal edema, granulation tissue, and ulcerations. Stridor usually resolves with medical therapy. Inhaled epinephrine is successful in treating subglottic edema. If reintubation is required, a smaller ETT should be used to prevent additional trauma. The nasal route is preferred to optimize tube stabilization and to minimize the tube shifting with head movement. The child should be weaned rapidly from the ventilator to humidified O_2 delivered via a light T tube. These measures prevent infants from pushing out the tube with their tongue and allow for better head movements, thereby

FIGURE 25-9 Positioning of the cuff on various endotacheal tubes: (1) uncuffed tracheal tube, ID 4.5 mm, (2) Rueschelit Super Safety Clear, ID 4.0 mm, (3) Mallinkrodt Hi-Contour P, ID 4.0, (4) Microcuff PET, ID 4.0 mm, and (5) Sheridan CF, ID 4.0 mm. Note that only tube 4 has a cuff off appropriate size and positioning. (*Courtesy of Markus Weiss, Pediatric Anesthesia, Children's Hospital of Zurich, Switzerland.*)

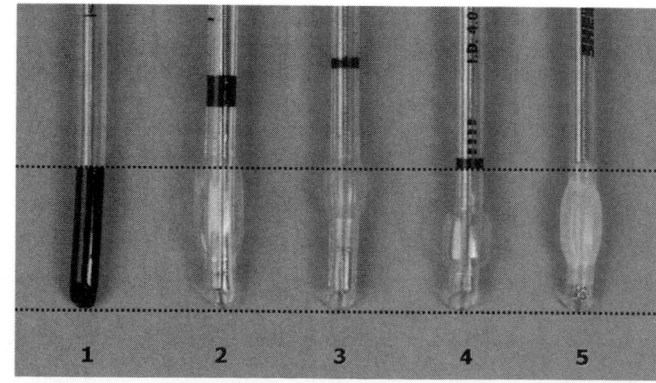

minimizing risk of further trauma. Alternatively, the child can be heavily sedated and eventually receive neuromuscular blockade. In most cases of simple subglottic edema, extubation is successful after a rest period of about 2–3 days with or without a short course of dexamethasone (1–2 mg/kg per day in divided doses). It is reasonable to administer dexamethasone to patients at risk of stridor for 24 hours before and 24 hours after extubation. Such prophylactic steroids may reduce postextubation stridor and the rate of reintubation.[175]

Endoscopy is recommended after failed attempts at extubation. Soft granulation tissue secondary to early intubation injury often can be treated with a CO_2 laser. Severe and lasting trauma from prolonged intubation, such as perichondritis, subglottic stenosis, necrotizing tracheobronchitis, subglottic cysts, tracheal perforation, and tracheal stenosis, is rare. Surgical options for subglottic stenosis include anterior cricoid split, laryngotracheal reconstruction, tracheal resection, and cricotracheal resection.

BRONCHOPULMONARY DYSPLASIA IN THE PRETERM BABY

The etiology of BPD is multifactorial. The principal risk factors are lung immaturity, barotrauma, volutrauma, O_2 toxicity, prenatal and nosocomial infections, and increased pulmonary blood flow secondary to a patent ductus arteriosus.[176,177] The complex interaction between inflammatory mediators and fibrosis has not been defined. Neither has the interference of inflammation with postnatal lung development, especially alveolarization.

Changes in neonatal care of very low-birth-weight infants, including antenatal corticosteroids, postnatal surfactant, and modified respiratory support, have improved survival. BPD is still frequent in very premature infants, although the more severe forms are less frequent. The incidence of BPD varies from 0–56%.[35,36,62,178–180] This wide range reflects the heterogeneity of study populations, management practices, and disease definitions. The initial description of BPD by Northway et al[30] and subsequently by Bancalari et al[181] was based on O_2 requirements at 28 days of age. As newborns of lower gestational age survived, Shennan[182] later proposed the term *chronic lung disease*, defined as O_2 dependency at 36 weeks' postconceptional age. This definition seemed to better predict pulmonary outcome. Jobe and Bancalari[183] introduced grading of BPD severity.

Management of BPD includes minimizing ventilator duration and avoiding high O_2 concentrations. Fluid restriction, diuretics, and bronchodilators are helpful but do not alter disease course. Pulmonary vasodilators are not beneficial for BPD-associated pulmonary hypertension.[184] Dexamethasone can accelerate ventilator weaning and shorten the period of O_2 supplementation but is associated with worse neurologic outcome (increased leukomalacia, impaired brain growth) and more frequent severe gastrointestinal complications.[185–189] Dexamethasone therapy, if given at all, should be brief and early.[190] Adequate nutrition helps lung injury protection and recovery.[181]

VENTILATOR-ASSOCIATED PNEUMONIA

Although ventilator-associated pneumonia is the second most common nosocomial infection in the pediatric ICU,[191–193] it has been little studied. *Pseudomonas aeruginosa*, enteric gram-negative bacilli, and *Staphylococcus aureus* are isolated most commonly from endotracheal aspirates in ventilator-associated pneumonia, particularly when of late onset.[191] Mortality and cost in pediatric patients are unknown. Blind protected bronchoalveolar lavage[194] has been proposed as the most reliable diagnostic method. Diagnostic bronchoscopy usually is not required[195] because protected bronchoalveolar lavage is reasonably reproducible and provides acceptable sensitivity (72%) and specificity (88%).[196] Treatment can be adapted from ATS guidelines for adults. (American Thoracic Society, Infectious Diseases Society of America. Guidelines for the management of adults with hospital-acquired, ventilator associated, and health-associated pneumonia. Am J Respir Crit Care Med 2005; 171: 388–416.)

Important Unknowns

Mechanical ventilation has increased survival of acutely ill neonates and children. A better understanding of pathophysiology has led to newer ventilator strategies. Many of these strategies, however, have not been tested in the pediatric setting but simply adapted from adult experience. Recent research suggests that comparable ventilator settings are more injurious in the adult than in the infant lung.[197]

Approaches to optimizing ventilation are based on bedside assessment of respiratory mechanics and blood-gas response. Unfortunately, no characteristic of the pressure-volume curve can predict end-expiratory atelectasis, overstretching, or optimal airway pressure.[198,199] Despite improved understanding of pediatric diseases and mechanical ventilation, we still do not know the best settings for an individual child. To date, evidence is confined to bad ventilator settings.

Noninvasive ventilation has proven safe and feasible in pediatric settings and can help to avoid intubation.[200,201] Ventilator discontinuation is believed to decrease several complications, but proof is limited.

The Future

Respiratory monitoring has been used to decrease complications and improve patient-ventilator interactions. We need to develop approaches whereby this knowledge can be used to improve patient outcome. Tools that provide continuous recordings of pulmonary function have yet to be incorporated into ventilator equipment. For example, the continuous monitoring of FRC might improve ventilator strategies and enhance assessment of lung recruitment. Newer imaging techniques, such as electrical impedance tomography[202–204] and bedside ultrasound, may help to monitor regional ventilation. In the end, such techniques will need to prove cost-effective and/or improve outcome. Furthermore, we need a better description of what constitutes "standard" care.

Summary and Conclusion

Mechanical ventilation of infants or small children requires fundamental knowledge of the anatomic and functional characteristics of the respiratory system in a growing child. Clinicians also require good knowledge of specific pediatric pathologies, which sometimes results in a different approach to ventilation than in an adult patient. Nevertheless, adult experience has influenced many strategies applied in pediatric and even neonatal settings because it remains difficult to do well-controlled trials of mechanical ventilation in the pediatric ICU.

References

1. Mok Q, Negus S, McLaren CA, et al. Computed tomography versus bronchography in the diagnosis and management of tracheobronchomalacia in ventilator dependent inflants. Arch Dis Child Fetal Neonatal Ed. 2005; 90:I290–3.
2. Marini J. Should PEEP be used in airflow obstruction? Am Rev Respir Dis 1989; 140:1–3.
3. Hogg J, Williams J, Richardson J, et al. Age as a factor in the distribution of lower-airway conductance and in the pathologic anatomy of obstructive lung disease. New Engl J Med 1970; 282:1283–7.
4. Heldt G, McIlroy M. Distortion of chest wall and work of diaphragm in preterm infants. J Appl Physiol 1987; 62:164–9.
5. Manczur T, Greenough A, Nicholson G, et al. Resistance of pediatric and neonatal endotracheal tubes: Influence of flow rate, size, and shape. Crit Care Med 2000; 28:1595–8.
6. Boros S, Bing D, Mammel M, et al. Using conventional infant ventilators at unconventional rates. Pediatrics 1984; 74:487–92.
7. Field D, Milner A, Hopkin I. Inspiratory time and tidal volume during intermittent positive pressure ventilation. Arch Dis Child 1985; 60:259–61.
8. Couser R, Ferrara T, Ebert J, et al. Effects of exogenous surfactant therapy on dynamic compliance during mechanical breathing in preterm infants with hyaline membrane disease. J Paediatr 1990; 116:119–24.
9. Szymankiewicz M, Gadzinowski J, Kowalska K. Pulmonary function after surfactant lung lavage followed by surfactant administration in infants with severe meconium aspiration syndrome. J Matern Fetal Neonatal Med 2004; 16: 125–30.
10. Rimensberger PC, Cox PN, Frndova H, et al. The open lung during small tidal volume ventilation: Concepts of recruitment and "optimal" PEEP. Crit Care Med 1999; 27:1946–52.
11. Wessel D, Adatia I, Marter LV, et al. Improved oxygenation in a randomized trial of inhaled nitric oxide for persistent pulmonary hypertension of the newborn. Pediatrics 1997:E7.
12. Davidson D, Barefield E, Kattwinkel J, et al. Inhaled nitric oxide for the early treatment of persistent pulmonary hypertension of the term newborn: A randomized, double-masked, placebo-controlled, dose-response, multicenter study. The I-NO/PPHN Study Group. Pediatrics 1998; 101:325–34.
13. Kinsella J, Abman S. Inhaled nitric oxide: Current and future uses in neonates. Semin Perinatol 2000; 24:387–95.
14. Macrae D, Field D, Mercier J, et al. Inhaled nitric oxide therapy in neonates and children: Reaching a European consensus. Intensive Care Med 2004; 30:372–80.
15. Henderson-Smart D, Pettigrew A, Campbell D. Clinical apnea and brain-stem neural function in preterm infants. New Engl J Med 1983; 17:353–7.
16. Frantz Ir, Adler S, Thach B, et al. Maturational effects on respiratory responses to carbon dioxide in premature infants. J Appl Physiol 1976; 41:41–5.
17. Henderson-Smart D. Regulation of breathing in the prenatal period. In: Saunders N, Sullivan C, editors. Sleep and breathing, Vol 20. New York: Marcel Dekker, 1983: 605–47.
18. Dawes G. The central control of fetal breathing and skeletal muscle movements. J Physiol 1984; 346:1–18.
19. Trippenbach T. Pulmonary reflexes and control of breathing during development. Biol Neonate 1994; 65:205–10.
20. Stocks J, Dezateux C, Hoo A, et al. Delayed maturation of Hering-Breuer inflation reflex activity in preterm infants. Am J Respir Crit Care Med 1996; 154:1411–7.
21. Martin R, Nearman H, Katona P, et al. The effect of a low continuous positive airway pressure on the reflex control of respiration in the preterm infant. J Pediatr 1977; 90:976–81.
22. Chan V, Greenough A, Muramatsu K. Influence of lung function and reflex activity on the success of patient-triggered ventilation. Early Hum Dev 1994; 37:9–14.
23. Slutsky A. Consensus conference on mechanical ventilation— January 28–30, 1993 at Northbrook, Illinois, USA, Part I: European Society of Intensive Care Medicine, the ACCP and the SCCM. Intensive Care Med 1994; 20:64–79.
24. Slutsky A. Consensus conference on mechanical ventilation— January 28–30, 1993 at Northbrook, Illinois, USA, Part 2. Intensive Care Med 1994; 20:150–62.
25. Gittermann MK, Fusch C, Gittermann AR, et al. Early nasal continuous positive airway pressure treatment reduces the need for intubation in very low birth weight infants. Eur J Pediatr 1997; 156:384–8.
26. Ho J, Subramaniam P, Henderson-Smart D, et al. Continuous distending pressure for respiratory distress syndrome in preterm infants. Cochrane Database Syst Rev 2002; 2:CD002271.
27. De Klerk AM, De Klerk RK. Nasal continuous positive airway pressure and outcomes of preterm infants. J Paediatr Child Health 2001; 37:161–7.
28. Subramaniam P, Henderson-Smart D, Davis P. Prophylactic nasal continuous positive airways pressure for preventing morbidity and mortality in very preterm infants. Cochrane Database Syst Rev 2000; 2:CD001243.
29. Hammer J. Nasal CPAP in preterm infants: Does it work and how? Intensive Care Med 2001; 27:1689–91.
30. Northway WHJ, Rosan RC, Porter DY. Pulmonary disease following respirator therapy of hyaline-membrane disease: Bronchopulmonary dysplasia. New Engl J Med. 1967; 276: 357–68.
31. Reynolds E. Effect of alterations in mechanical ventilator settings on pulmonary gas exchange in hyaline membrane disease. Arch Dis Child 1971; 46:152–9.
32. Stewart A, Finer N, Peters K. Effects of alterations of inspiratory and expiratory pressures and inspiratory/expiratory ratios on mean airway pressure, blood gases, and intracranial pressure. Pediatrics 1981; 67:474–81.
33. Ahluwalia J, Morley C, Mockridge J. Computerised determination of spontaneous inspiratory and expiratory times in premature neonates during intermittent positive pressure ventilation: II. Results from 20 babies. Arch Dis Child Fetal Neonat Ed 1994; 71:F161–4.

34. Kamlin C, Davis P. Long versus short inspiratory times in neonates receiving mechanical ventilation. Cochrane Database Syst Rev 2004; 4: CD004503.

35. Johnson AH, Peacock JL, Greenough A, et al. High-frequency oscillatory ventilation for the prevention of chronic lung disease of prematurity. New Engl J Med 2002; 347:633–42.

36. Courtney SE, Durand DJ, Asselin JM, et al. High-frequency oscillatory ventilation versus conventional mechanical ventilation for very low-birth-weight infants. New Engl J Med 2002; 347:643–52.

37. Henderson-Smart D, Bhuta T, Cools F, et al. Elective high frequency oscillatory ventilation versus conventional ventilation for acute pulmonary dysfunction in preterm infants. Cochrane Database Syst Rev 2003; (4):CD00104.

38. Bollen C, Uiterwaal C, Vught AV. Cumulative meta-analysis of high-frequency versus conventional ventilation in premature neonates. Am J Respir Crit Care Med 2003; 168:1105–6.

39. Moriette G, Paris-Llado J, Walti H, et al. Prospective, randomized multicenter comparison of high-frequency oscillatory ventilation and conventional ventilation in preterm infants of less than 30 weeks with respiratory distress syndrome. Pediatrics 2001; 107:363–72.

40. Soll RF, Blanco F. Natural surfactant extract versus synthetic surfactant for neonatal respiratory distress syndrome (Cochrane review). Cochrane Database Syst Rev 2001; 2.

41. Gortner L, Wauer R, Hammer H, et al. Early versus late surfactant treatment in preterm infants of 27 to 32 weeks' gestational age: A multicenter controlled clinical trial. Pediatrics 1998; 102:1153–60.

42. Hascoet J, Fresson J, Claris O, et al. The safety and efficacy of nitric oxide therapy in premature infants. J Pediatr 2005; 146:318–23.

43. Finer N. Inhaled nitric oxide for preterm infants: A therapy in search of an indication? The search continues. J Pediatr 2005; 146:301–3.

44. Finer N, Barrington K. Nitric oxide for respiratory failure in infants born at or near term. Cochrane Database Syst Rev 2000; CD000399.

45. Rais-Bahrami K, Rivera O, Seale W, et al. Effect of nitric oxide in meconium aspiration syndrome after treatment with surfactant. Crit Care Med 1997; 25:1744–7.

46. Lejeune T, Pfister R. Surfactant lavage for extracorporeal membrane oxygenation—requiring meconium aspiration syndrome —a cheap alternative. Eur J Pediatr 2005; 164:331–3.

47. Reyes C, Chang L, Waffarn F, et al. Delayed repair of congenital diaphragmatic hernia with early high-frequency oscillatory ventilation during preoperative stabilization. J Pediatr Surg 1998; 33:1010–4.

48. Sakurai Y, Azarow K, Cutz E, et al. Pulmonary barotrauma in congenital diaphragmatic hernia: A clinicopathological correlation. J Pediatr Surg 1999; 34:1813–7.

49. Wilson J, Lund D, Lillehei C, et al. Congenital diaphragmatic hernia—a tale of two cities: The Boston experience. J Pediatr Surg 1997; 32:401–5.

50. Azarow K, Messineo A, Pearl R, et al. Congenital diaphragmatic hernia—a tale of two cities: The Toronto experience. J Pediatr Surg 1997; 32:395–400.

51. Cacciari A, Ruggeri G, Mordenti M, et al. High-frequency oscillatory ventilation versus conventional mechanical ventilation in congenital diaphragmatic hernia. Eur J Pediatr Surg 2001; 11:3–7.

52. Desfrere L, Jarreau P, Dommergues M, et al. Impact of delayed repair and elective high-frequency oscillatory ventilation on survival of antenatally diagnosed congenital diaphragmatic hernia: First application of these strategies in the more "severe" subgroup of antenatally diagnosed newborns. Intensive Care Med 2000; 26:934–41.

53. Ventre K, Arnold J. High frequency oscillatory ventilation in acute respiratory failure. Paediatr Respir Rev 2004; 5:323–32.

54. Inhaled nitric oxide and hypoxic respiratory failure in infants with congenital diaphragmatic hernia. The Neonatal Inhaled Nitric Oxide Study Group (NINOS). Pediatrics 1997; 99:838–45.

55. Hammer J, Numa A, Newth C. Acute respiratory distress syndrome induced by respiratory syncytial virus. Pediatr Pulmonol 1997; 23:176–83.

56. Tasker R, Gordon I, Kiff K. Time course of severe respiratory syncytial virus infection in mechanically ventilated infants. Acta Paediatr 2000; 89:938–41.

57. Hammer J, Numa A, Newth C. Albuterol responsiveness in infants with respiratory failure due to RSV infection. J Pediatr 1995; 127:485–90.

58. Beasley J, Jones S. Continuous positive airway pressure in bronchiolitis. Br Med J (Clin Res Ed) 1981; 283:1506–8.

59. Outwater K, Crone R. Management of respiratory failure in infants with acute viral bronchiolitis. Am J Dis Child 1984; 138:1071–5.

60. Soong W, Hwang B, Tang R. Continuous positive airway pressure by nasal prongs in bronchiolitis. Pediatr Pulmonol 1993; 16:163–6.

61. Kristensen K, Dahm T, Frederiksen P, et al. Epidemiology of respiratory syncytial virus infection requiring hospitalization in East Denmark. Pediatr Infect Dis J 1998; 17:996–1000.

62. Rimensberger P. Noninvasive pressure support ventilation for acute respiratory failure in children. Schweiz Med Wochenschr 2000; 130:1880–6.

63. Patel N, Hammer J, Nichani S, et al. Effect of inhaled nitric oxide on respiratory mechanics in ventilated infants with RSV bronchiolitis. Intensive Care Med 1999; 25:81–7.

64. Abman S, Griebel J, Parker D, et al. Acute effects of inhaled nitric oxide in children with severe hypoxemic respiratory failure. J Pediatr 1994; 124:881–8.

65. Hammer J. Acute lung injury: Pathophysiology, assessment and current therapy. Paediatric Respir Rev 2001; 2:10–21.

66. Harel Y, Niranjan V, Evans B. The current practice patterns of mechanical ventilation for respiratory failure in pediatric patients. Heart Lung 1998; 27:238–44.

67. Arnold J, Truog R, Thompson J, et al. High-frequency oscillatory ventilation in pediatric respiratory failure. Crit Care Med 1993; 21:272–8.

68. Arnold JH, Hanson JH, Toro-Figuero LO, et al. Prospective, randomized comparison of high-frequency oscillatory ventilation and conventional mechanical ventilation in pediatric respiratory failure. Crit Care Med 1994; 22:1530–9.

69. Numa A, Hammer J, Newth C. Effect of prone and supine positions on functional residual capacity, oxygenation and respiratory mechanics in ventilated infants and children. Am J Respir Crit Care Med 1997; 156:1185–9.

70. Curley M, Hibberd P, Fineman L, et al. Effect of prone positioning on clinical outcomes in children with acute lung injury: A randomized, controlled trial. JAMA 2005; 294:229–37.

71. Ackerman A. Mechanical ventilation of the intubated asthmatic: How much do we really know? Pediatr Crit Care Med 2004; 5:501.

72. Sarnaik A, Daphtary K, Meert K, et al. Pressure-controlled ventilation in children with severe status asthmaticus. Pediatr Crit Care Med 2004; 5:133–8.

73. Maffei F, Jagt Evd, Powers K, et al. Duration of mechanical ventilation in life-threatening pediatric asthma: Description of an acute asphyxial subgroup. Pediatrics 2004; 114:762–7.

74. Duval E, Vught Av. Status asthmaticus treated by high-frequency oscillatory ventilation. Pediatr Pulmonol 2000; 30: 350–3.

75. Wetzel R. Pressure-support ventilation in children with severe asthma. Crit Care Med 1996; 24:1603–5.

76. Teague W. Noninvasive ventilation in the pediatric intensive care unit for children with acute respiratory failure. Pediatr Pulmonol 2003; 35:418–26.

77. Hammer J, Eber E. The pecularities of infant respiratory physiology. In: Hammer J, Eber E, editors. Paediatric pulmonary function testing. Prog Respir Res 2005; 33:2–7.

78. Gozal D. Nocturnal ventilatory support in patients with cystic fibrosis: comparison with supplemental oxygen. Eur Respir J 1997; 10:1999–2003.

79. Hodson M, Madden B, Steven M, et al. Non-invasive mechanical ventilation for cystic fibrosis patients: A potential bridge to transplantation. Eur Respir J 1991; 4:524–7.

80. Hill A, Edenborough F, Cayton R, et al. Long-term nasal intermittent positive pressure ventilation in patients with cystic fibrosis and hypercapnic respiratory failure (1991–1996). Respir Med 1998; 92:523–6.

81. Gozal D. Congenital central hypoventilation syndtrome: An update. Pediatr Pulmonol 1998; 26:273–82.

82. Gregory GA, Kitterman JA, Phibbs RH, et al. Treatment of idiopathic respiratory distress syndrome with continuous positive airway pressure. New Engl J Med 1971; 284:1333–40.

83. De Paoli AG, Davis P, Faber B, et al. Devices and pressure sources for administration of nasal continuous positive airway pressure (NCPAP) in preterm neonates. Cochrane Database Syst Rev 2002; 4:CD002977.

84. Courtney S, Aghai Z, Saslow J, et al. Changes in lung volume and work of breathing: A comparison of two variable-flow nasal continuous positive airway pressure devices in very low birth weight infants. Pediatr Pulmonol 2003; 36:248–52.

85. Elgellab A, Riou Y, Abbazine A, et al. Effects of nasal continuous positive airway pressure (NCPAP) on breathing pattern in spontaneously breathing premature newborn infants. Intensive Care Med 2001; 27:1782–7.

86. Thomson M. Continuous positive airway pressure and surfactant: Combined data from animal experiments and clinical trials. Biol Neonate 2002; 81:16–9.

87. Dani C, Bertini G, Pezzati M, et al. Early extubation and nasal continuous positive airway pressure after surfactant treatment for respiratory distress syndrome among preterm infants <30 weeks' gestation. Pediatrics 2004; 113:E560–3.

88. De Paoli AG, Morley C, Davis P. Nasal CPAP for neonates: What do we know in 2003? Arch Dis Child Fetal Neonatal Ed 2003; 88:F168–72.

89. Suki B, Barabasi AL, Hantos Z, et al. Avalanches and power-law behaviour in lung inflation. Nature 1994; 368:615–8.

90. Sinha S, Donn S, Gavey J, et al. Randomised trial of volume controlled versus time cycled, pressure limited ventilation in preterm infants with respiratory distress syndrome. Arch Dis Child Fetal Neonatal Ed 1997; 77:F202–5.

91. Cheema I, Ahluwalia J. Feasibility of tidal volume-guided ventilation in newborn infants: A randomized, crossover trial using the volume guarantee modality. Pediatrics 2001; 107:1323–8.

92. Herrera C, Gerhardt T, Claure N, et al. Effects of volume-guaranteed synchronized intermittent mandatory ventilation in preterm infants recovering from respiratory failure. Pediatrics 2002; 110:529–33.

93. Riley C, Pilcher J. Volume-guaranteed ventilation. Neonatal Netw 2003; 22:17–22.

94. Abubakar K, Keszler M. Patient-ventilator interactions in new modes of patient-triggered ventilation. Pediatr Pulmonol 2001; 32:71–5.

95. Keszler M, Abubakar K. Volume guarantee: Stability of tidal volume and incidence of hypocarbia. Pediatr Pulmonol 2004; 38:240–5.

96. Donn S, Nicks J, Becker M. Flow-synchronized ventilation of preterm infants with respiratory distress syndrome. J Perinatol 1994; 14:90–4.

97. Lipscomb A, Thorburn R, Reynolds E, et al. Pneumothorax and cerebral haemorrhage in preterm infants. Lancet 1981; 21:414–6.

98. Greenough A, Milner A, Dimitriou G. Synchronized mechanical ventilation for respiratory support in newborn infants. Cochrane Database Syst Rev 2004; 18:CD000456.

99. Putensen C, Hering R, Muders T, et al. Assisted breathing is better in acute respiratory failure. Curr Opin Crit Care 2005; 11:63–8.

100. Migliori C, Cavazza A, Motta M, et al. Effect on respiratory function of pressure support ventilation versus synchronised intermittent mandatory ventilation in preterm infants. Pediatr Pulmonol 2003; 35:364–7.

101. Dimitriou G, Greenough A, Laubscher B, et al. Comparison of airway pressure-triggered and airflow-triggered ventilation in very immature infants. Acta Paediatr 1998; 82:1256–60.

102. Carlo W, Siner B, Chatburn R, et al. Early randomized intervention with high-frequency jet ventilation in respiratory distress syndrome. J Pediatr 1990; 117:765–70.

103. Keszler M, Modanlou H, Brudno D, et al. Multicenter controlled clinical trial of high-frequency jet ventilation in preterm infants with uncomplicated respiratory distress syndrome. Pediatrics 1997; 100:593–9.

104. Kercsmar C, Martin R, Chatburn R, et al. Bronchoscopic findings in infants treated with high-frequency jet ventilation versus conventional ventilation. Pediatrics 1988; 82:884–7.

105. Delafosse C, Chevrolet J, Suter P, et al. Necrotizing tracheobronchitis: A complication of high frequency jet ventilation. Virchows Arch [A] 1988; 413:257–64.

106. Wiswell T, Graziani L, Kornhauser M, et al. High-frequency jet ventilation in the early management of respiratory distress syndrome is associated with a greater risk for adverse outcomes. Pediatrics 1996; 98:1035–43.

107. Hifi SG. High-frequency oscillatory ventilation compared with conventional ventilation in the treatment of respiratory failure in preterm infants. New Engl J Med 1989; 320: 88–93.

108. Hamilton PP, Onayemi A, Smyth JA, et al. Comparison of conventional and high-frequency ventilation: Oxygenation and lung pathology. J Appl Physiol 1983; 55:131–8.

109. Kolton M, Cattran CB, Kent G, et al. Oxygenation during high-frequency ventilation compared with conventional mechanical ventilation in two models of lung injury. Anesth Analg 1982; 61:323–32.

110. McCulloch PR, Forkert PG, Froese AB. Lung volume maintenance prevents lung injury during high frequency oscillatory ventilation in surfactant-deficient rabbits. Am Rev Respir Dis 1988; 137:1185–92.

111. Meredith KS, deLemos RA, Coalson J, et al. Role of lung injury in the pathogenesis of hyaline membrane disease in premature baboons. J Appl Physiol 1989; 66:2150–8.

112. Clark RH, Gerstmann DR, Null DMJ, et al. Prospective, randomized comparison of high-frequency oscillatory ventilation in infants with severe respiratory distress syndrome. Pediatrics 1992; 89:5–12.

113. Gerstmann DR, Minton SD, Stoddard RA, et al. The Provo multicenter early high-frequency oscillatory ventilation trial: Improved pulmonary and clinical outcome in respiratory distress syndrome. Pediatrics 1996; 98:1044–57.

114. Plavka R, Kopecky P, Sebron V, et al. A prospective, randomized comparison of conventional mechanical ventilation and very early high frequency oscillatory ventilation in extremely premature newborns with respiratory distress syndrome. Intensive Care Med 1999; 25:68–75.

115. Rimensberger PC, Beghetti M, Hanquinet S, et al. First intention high-frequency oscillation with early lung volume optimization improves pulmonary outcome in very low birth weight infants with respiratory distress syndrome. Pediatrics 2000; 105: 1202–8.

116. Derdak S, Mehta S, Stewart TE, et al. The Multicenter Oscillatory Ventilation for Acute Respiratory Distress Syndrome Trial (MOAT) Study Investigators. High-frequency oscillatory ventilation for acute respiratory distress syndrome in adults: A randomized, controlled trial. Am J Respir Crit Care Med 2002; 166:801–8.

117. Ferguson D, Chiche J, Kacmarek R, et al. Combining high-frequency oscillatory ventilation and recruitment maneuvers in adults with early acute respiratory distress syndrome: The Treatment with Oscillation and an Open Lung Strategy (TOOLS) Trial pilot study. Crit Care Med 2005; 33:479–86.

118. Rimensberger P. Neonatal respiratory failure. Curr Opin Pediatr 2002; 14:315–21.

119. Froese A. High-frequency oscillatory ventilation for adult respiratory distress syndrome: Let's get it right this time! Crit Care Med 1997; 25:906–8.

120. Fedora M, Klimovic M, Seda M, et al. Effect of early intervention of high-frequency oscillatory ventilation on the outcome in pediatric acute respiratory distress syndrome. Bratisl Lek Listy 2000; 101:8–13.

121. Mehta S, Lapinsky SE, Hallett DC, et al. Prospective trial of high-frequency oscillation in adults with acute respiratory distress syndrome. Crit Care Med 2001; 29:1360–9.

122. Rimensberger P. ICU cornerstone: High frequency ventilation is here to stay. Crit Care Clin 2003; 7:342–4.

123. Nobuhara K, Wilson J. Pathophysiology of congenital diaphragmatic hernia. Semin Pediatr Surg 1996; 5:234–42.

124. Clark R, Gerstmann D, Null D, et al. Pulmonary interstitial emphysema treated by high-frequency oscillatory ventilation. Crit Care Med 1986; 14:926–30.

125. Kinsella J, Truog W, Walsh W, et al. Randomized multicenter trial of inhaled nitric oxide and high-frequency oscillatory ventilation in severe, persistent pulmonary hypertension of the newborn. J Pediatr 1997; 131:55–62.

126. Rosenberg R, Broner C, Peters K, et al. High-frequency ventilation for acute pediatric respiratory failure. Chest 1993; 104: 1216–21.

127. Randolph A, Wypij D, Venkataraman S, et al. Pediatric Acute Lung Injury and Sepsis Investigators (PALISI) Network. Effect of mechanical ventilator weaning protocols on respiratory outcomes in infants and children: A randomized, controlled trial. JAMA 2002; 288:2561–8.

128. Rivera R, Tibballs J. Complications of endotracheal intubation and mechanical ventilation in infants and children. Crit Care Med 1992; 20:193–9.

129. Tobias J, Deshpande J, Gregory D. Outpatient therapy of iatrogenic drug dependency following prolonged sedation in the pediatric intensive care unit. Intensive Care Med 1994; 20:504–7.

130. Fontela P, Piva J, Garcia P, et al. Risk factors for extubation failure in mechanically ventilated pediatric patients. Pediatr Crit Care Med 2005; 6:166–70.

131. Kurachek S, Newth C, Quasney M, et al. Extubation failure in pediatric intensive care: A multiple-center study of risk factors and outcomes. Crit Care Med 2003; 31:2657–64.

132. Stefanescu B, Murphy W, Hansell B, et al. A randomized, controlled trial comparing two different continuous positive airway pressure systems for the successful extubation of extremely low birth weight infants. Pediatrics 2003; 112:1031–8.

133. Farias J, Retta A, Alia I, et al. A comparison of two methods to perform a breathing trial before extubation in pediatric intensive care patients. Intensive Care Med 2001; 27:1649–54.

134. Baumeister B, el-Khatib M, PG PS, et al. Evaluation of predictors of weaning from mechanical ventilation in pediatric patients. Pediatr Pulmonol 1997; 24:344–52.

135. Sinha S, Donn S. Weaning newborns from mechanical ventilation. Semin Neonatol 2002; 7:421–8.

136. Vento G, Tortorolo L, Zecca E, et al. Spontaneous minute ventilation is a predictor of extubation failure in extremely-low-birth-weight infants. J Matern Fetal Neonatal Med 2004; 15:147–54.

137. Gillespie L, White S, Sinha S, et al. Usefulness of the minute ventilation test in predicting successful extubation in newborn infants: a randomized controlled trial. J Perinatol 2003; 23:205–7.

138. Elsasser S, Guttmann J, Stocker R, et al. Accuracy of automatic tube compensation in new-generation mechanical ventilators. Crit Care Med 2003; 31:2619–26.

139. Jarreau P, Moriette G, Mussat P, et al. Patient-triggered ventilation decreases the work of breathing in neonates. Am J Respir Crit Care Med 1996; 153:1176–81.

140. Kollef M, Shapiro S, Silver P, et al. A randomized, controlled trial of protocol-directed versus physician-directed weaning from mechanical ventilation. Crit Care Med 1997; 25:567–74.

141. MacIntyre N, Cook D, Ely EW, et al. Evidence-based guidelines for weaning and discontinuing ventilatory support: A collective task force facilitated by the American College of Chest Physicians, the American Association for Respiratory Care, and the American College of Critical Care Medicine. Chest 2001; 120:375–95S.

142. Schultz T, Lin R, Watzman H, et al. Weaning children from mechanical ventilation: A prospective randomized trial of protocol-directed versus physician-directed weaning. Respir Care 2001; 46:772–82.

143. Simansky D, Paley M, Refaely V, et al. Diaphragm plication following phrenic nerve injury: A comparison of paediatric and adult patients. Thorax 2002; 57:613–6.

144. Schulze A, Gerhardt T, Musante G, et al. Proportional assist ventilation in low birth weight infants with acute respiratory disease: A comparison to assist/control and conventional mechanical ventilation. J Pediatr 1999; 135:339–44.

145. Schulze A, E EB. Proportional assist ventilation in infants. Clin Perinatol 2001; 28:561–78.

146. Davis P, Henderson-Smart D. Extubation from low-rate intermittent positive airways pressure versus extubation after a trial of endotracheal continuous positive airways pressure in intubated preterm infants. Cochrane Database Syst Rev 2001; 4:CD001078.

147. Halliday H. What interventions facilitate weaning from the ventilator? A review of the evidence from systematic reviews. Paediatr Respir Rev 2004; 5:S347–52.

148. Davis P, Henderson-Smart D. Intravenous dexamethasone for extubation of newborn infants. Cochrane Database Syst Rev 2001; 4:CD000308.

149. Tellez D, Galvis A, Storgion S, et al. Dexamethasone in the prevention of postextubation stridor in children. J Pediatr 1991; 118:289–94.

150. Henderson-Smart D, Davis P. Prophylactic methylxanthines for extubation in preterm infants. Cochrane Database Syst Rev 2003; 1:CD000139.

151. Hammer J. Nasal CPAP in preterm infants: Does it work and how? Intensive Care Med 2001; 27:1689–91.

152. Davis P, Henderson-Smart DJ. Nasal continuous positive airways pressure immediately after extubation for preventing morbidity in preterm infants. Cochrane Database Syst Rev 2003; 2:CD000143.

153. De Paoli AG, Davis P, Lemyre B. Nasal continuous positive airway pressure versus nasal intermittent positive pressure ventilation for preterm neonates: A systematic review and meta-analysis. Acta Paediatr 2003; 92:70–5.

154. Dimitriou G, Greenough A, Cherian S. Comparison of airway pressure and airflow triggering systems using a single type of neonatal ventilator. Acta Paediatr 2001; 90:445–7.

155. Schulze A. Respiratory gas conditioning in infants with an artificial airway. Semin Neonatol 2002; 7:369–77.

156. Neonatal/pediatric intensive care ventilators. Health Devices 2002; 31:237–55.

157. Fredberg J, Glass G, Boynton B, et al. Factors influencing mechanical performance of neonatal high-frequency ventilators. J Appl Physiol 1987; 62:2485–90.

158. Jouvet P, Hubert P, Isabey D, et al. Assessment of high-frequency neonatal ventilator performances. Intensive Care Med 1997; 23:208–13.

159. Hatcher D, Watanabe H, Ashbury T, et al. Mechanical performance of clinically available, neonatal, high-frequency, oscillatory-type ventilators. Crit Care Med 1998; 26:1081–8.

160. Pillow J, Wilkinson M, Heather L, et al. In vitro performance characteristics of high-frequency oscillatory ventilators. Am J Respir Crit Care Med 2001; 164:1019–24.

161. Thome U, Kossel H, Lipowsky G, et al. Randomized comparison of high-frequency ventilation with high-rate intermittent positive pressure ventilation in preterm infants with respiratory failure. J Pediatr 1999; 135:39–46.

162. Craft A, Bhandari V, Finer NN. The Sy-Fi study: A randomized, prospective trial of synchronized intermittent mandatory ventilation versus a high-frequency flow interrupter in infants less than 1000 g. J Perinatol 2003; 23:14–9.

163. Beydon L, Tong D, Jackson N, et al. Correlation between simple clinical parameters and the in vitro humidification characteristics of filter heat and moisture exchangers. Groupe de Travail sur les Respirateurs. Chest 1997; 112:739–44.

164. Schiffmann H, Rathgeber J, Singer D, et al. Airway humidification in mechanically ventilated neonates and infants: A comparative study of a heat and moisture exchanger vs a heated humidifier using a new fast-response capacitive humidity sensor. Crit Care Med 1997; 25:1755–60.

165. Le Bourdelles G, Mier L, Fiquet B, et al. Comparison of the effects of heat and moisture exchangers and heated humidifiers on ventilation and gas exchange during weaning trials from mechanical ventilation. Chest 1996; 110:1294–8.

166. Ricard J, Markowicz P, Djedaini K, et al. Bedside evaluation of efficient airway humidification during mechanical ventilation of the critically ill. Chest 1999; 115:1646–52.

167. Cannon M, Cornell J, Tripp-Hamel D, et al. Tidal volumes for ventilated infants should be determined with a pneumotachometer placed at the endotracheal tube. Am J Respir Crit Care Med 2000; 162:2109–12.

168. Castle R, Dunne C, Mok Q, et al. Accuracy of displayed values of tidal volume in the pediatric intensive care unit. Crit Care Med 2002; 30:2566–74.

169. Neve V, Leclerc F, Noizet O, et al. Influence of respiratory system impedance on volume and pressure delivered at the Y piece in ventilated infants. Pediatr Crit Care Med 2003; 4:418–25.

170. Pascucci R, Schena J, Thompson J. Comparison of sidestream and mainstream capnometer in infants. Crit Care Med 1989; 17:560–2.

171. Deakers T, Reynolds G, Stretton M, et al. Cuffed endotracheal tubes in pediatric intensive care. J Pediatr 1994; 125:57–62.

172. Dullenkopf A, Gerber A, Weiss M. Fit and seal characteristics of a new paediatric tracheal tube with high volume-low pressure polyurethane cuff. Acta Anaesthesiol Scand 2005; 49:232–7.

173. Dillier C, Trachsel D, Baulig W, et al. Laryngeal damage due to an unexpectedly large and inappropriately designed cuffed pediatric tracheal tube in a 13-month-old child. Can J Anaesth 2004; 51:72–5.

174. Mhanna M, Zamel Y, Tichy C, et al. The "air leak" test around the endotracheal tube, as a predictor of postextubation stridor, is age dependent in children. Crit Care Med 2002; 30:2639–43.

175. Markovitz B, Randolph A. Corticosteroids for the prevention of reintubation and postextubation stridor in pediatric patients: A meta-analysis. Pediatr Crit Care Med 2002; 3:223–6.

176. Bancalari. E. Corticosteroids and neonatal chronic lung disease. Eur J Pediatr 1998; 157:S31–7.

177. Lyon A. Chronic lung disease of prematurity: The role of intrauterine infection. Eur J Pediatr 2005; 159:798–802.

178. Lee S, McMillan D, Ohlsson A, et al. Variations in practice and outcomes in the Canadian NICU network: 1996–1997. Pediatrics 2000; 106:1070–9.

179. Lemons J, Bauer C, Oh W, et al. Very low birth weight outcomes of the National Institute of Child Health and Human Development Neonatal Research Network, January 1995 through December 1996. NICHD Neonatal Research Network. Pediatrics 2001; 107:E1.

180. Berger T, Bachmann I, Adams M, et al. Impact of improved survival of very low-birth-weight infants on incidence and severity of bronchopulmonary dysplasia. Biol Neonate 2004; 86:124–30.

181. Bancalari E, Abdenour G, Feller R. Bronchopulmonary dysplasia: Clinical presentation. J Pediatr 1979; 95:819–23.

182. Shennan A, Dunn M, Ohlsson A, et al. Abnormal pulmonary outcomes in premature infants: Prediction from oxygen requirement in the neonatal period. Pediatrics 1988; 82:527–32.

183. Jobe A, Bancalari E. Bronchopulmonary dysplasia. Am J Respir Crit Care Med 2001; 163:1723–9.

184. Athavale K, Claure N, D'Ugard C, et al. Acute effects of inhaled nitric oxide on pulmonary and cardiac function in preterm infants with evolving bronchopulmonary dysplasia. J Perinatol 2004; 24:769–74.

185. Stark A, Carlo W, JE Tyson, et al for the National Institute of Child Health Human Development Neonatal Research Network. Adverse effects of early dexamethasone treatment in extremely-low-birth-weight infants. New Engl J Med 2001; 344:95–101.

186. Murphy B, Inder T, Huppi P. Impaired cerebral cortical gray matter growth after treatment with dexamethasone for neonatal chronic lung disease. Pediatrics 2001; 107:217–21.

187. Watterberg K, Gerdes J, Cole C, et al. Prophylaxis of early adrenal insufficiency to prevent bronchopulmonary dysplasia: A multicenter trial. Pediatrics 2004; 114:1649–57.

188. Roberts R. Early closure of the Watterberg trial. Pediatrics 2004; 114:1670–1.

189. Grier D, Halliday H. Management of bronchopulmonary dysplasia in infants: Guidelines for corticosteroid use. Drugs 2005; 65:15–29.

190. Anttila E, Peltoniemi O, Haumont D, et al. Early neonatal dexamethasone treatment for prevention of bronchopulmonary dysplasia: Randomised trial and meta-analysis evaluating the duration of dexamethasone therapy. Eur J Pediatr 2005; 164:472–81.

191. Richards M, Edwards J, Culver D, et al. Nosocomial infections in pediatric intensive care units in the United States. Pediatrics 1999; 103:E39.

192. Almuneef M, Memish Z, Balkhy H, et al. Ventilator-associated pneumonia in a pediatric intensive care unit in Saudi Arabia: A 30-month prospective surveillance. Infect Control Hosp Epidemiol 2004; 25:753–8.

193. Abramczyk M, Carvalho W, Carvalho E, et al. Nosocomial infection in a pediatric intensive care unit in a developing country. Braz J Infect Dis 2003; 7:375–80.

194. Gauvin F, Dassa C, Chaibou M, et al. Ventilator-associated pneumonia in intubated children: Comparison of different diagnostic methods. Pediatr Crit Care Med 2003; 4:437–43.

195. Gauvin F, Lacroix J, Guertin M, et al. Reproducibility of blind protected bronchoalveolar lavage in mechanically ventilated children. Am J Respir Crit Care Med 2002; 165:1618–23.

196. Labenne M, Poyart C, Rambaud C, et al. Blind protected specimen brush and bronchoalveolar lavage in ventilated children. Crit Care Med 1999; 27:2537–43.

197. Kornecki A, Tsuchida S, Ondiveeran H, et al. Lung development and susceptibility to ventilator-induced lung injury. Am J Respir Crit Care Med 2005; 17:743–52.

198. Rimensberger PC, Bryan AC. Measurement of functional residual capacity in the critically ill: Relevance for the assessment of respiratory mechanics during mechanical ventilation. Intensive Care Med 1999; 25:540–2.

199. Markhorst D, Genderingen HV, Vught AV. Static pressure volume curve characteristics are moderate estimators of optimal airway pressures in a mathematical model of (primary/pulmonary) acute respiratory distress syndrome. Intensive Care Med 2004; 30:2086–93.

200. Fortenberry J, Toro JD, Jefferson L, et al. Management of pediatric acute hypoxemic respiratory insufficiency with bilevel positive pressure (BiPAP) nasal mask ventilation. Chest 1995; 108:1059–64.

201. Padman R, Lawless S, Kettrick R. Noninvasive ventilation via bilevel positive airway pressure support in pediatric practice. Crit Care Med 1998; 26:169–73.

202. Frerichs I, Hahn G, Schroder T, et al. Electrical impedance tomography in monitoring experimental lung injury. Intensive Care Med 1998; 24:829–36.

203. Frerichs I, Schiffmann H, Hahn G, et al. Non-invasive radiation-free monitoring of regional lung ventilation in critically ill infants. Intensive Care Med 2001; 27:1385–94.

204. Frerichs I, Dargaville P, Dudykevych T, et al. Electrical impedance tomography: A method for monitoring regional lung aeration and tidal volume distribution? Intensive Care Med 2003; 29:2312–6.

INDEPENDENT LUNG VENTILATION

DAVID V. TUXEN

BASIC PRINCIPLES OF ILV
APPLICATIONS OF ILV
    Thoracic Surgery
    Selective Airway Protection
    Bronchopleural Fistula
    Asymmetric Lung Disease
    Bilateral Symmetric Lung Disease
TECHNIQUES AND PROBLEMS WITH ILV
    Lung Separation
    Techniques for ILV
    Problems with ILV
CONCLUSION

Independent lung ventilation (ILV) was first reported for thoracic surgery by Gale and Waters in 1931. They passed a single-lumen endobronchial tube into the main bronchus of the nonoperative lung. They ventilated that lung in the dependent position while preventing drainage of purulent secretion (if present) from the operative lung. In 1936, Magill[1] reported endobronchial placement of a suction catheter with a balloon to occlude the operative bronchus and tracheal placement of an endotracheal tube to ventilate the nonoperative lung. In 1947, Moody[2] encased the endobronchial balloon with metal studs to reduce the risk of balloon dislodgment.

A series of double-lumen tubes (DLTs) enabling ILV of both lungs was reported next. The first, reported by Carlens[3] in 1949, was a DLT similar to current left DLTs but with a rubber "hook" to engage the carina for accurate placement. This was a major advance, but it was unsuitable for left pneumonectomy. Moreover, the carinal hook caused trauma and difficulties with surgical dissection. It was not until 1960 that White[4] reported a right DLT that did not occlude the right upper-lobe bronchus. In 1962, Robertshaw[5] reported right and left DLTs, which served as the prototype of today's DLTs. Current DLTs have replaced red rubber with polyvinyl chloride (PVC) to reduce mucosal injury and improve malleability and airflow (Fig. 26-1).

For many years, DLTs and ILV were used entirely for thoracic surgery.[2,6,7] In 1976, Glass and Trew[8,9] and their coworkers reported ILV for nonsurgical purposes: respiratory insufficiency from unilateral lung disease. Since then, application of ILV has broadened to a wide range of conditions (Table 26-1) employing a variety of techniques. It was used in about 0.5% of all ventilated patients[10] in an institution familiar with ILV. In most intensive-care units (ICUs), ILV is used in less than 0.5% of all ventilated patients.

Basic Principles of ILV

All indications for ILV (see Table 26-1) are based on one or two fundamental requirements:

1. *The need to protect one lung from harmful effects of fluid in the other lung* (blood, purulent or malignant secretions, lavage fluid). Placing a fluid-filled lung in the dependent position (lateral decubitus) minimizes the risk of unwanted fluid entering the other lung but also maximizes hypoxia[11] by maximizing blood diversion to the less functional lung. Placing the fluid-filled lung in the nondependent position improves oxygen saturation (Sa_{O_2}), but the risk from fluid spillage in this position is unacceptably high.[11] The supine position is usually the best compromise, except during thoracic surgery, where the operative lung must be in the uppermost position.

2. *Potential benefit from different ventilator patterns to each lung.* This could range from one-lung ventilation (OLV; e.g., thoracic surgery, whole-lung lavage) to ventilation to each lung differing in only a single variable [e.g., positive end-expiratory pressure (PEEP)] or ventilation requirements differing in every variable [e.g., single-lung transplant for chronic airflow obstruction (CAO)].

If OLV is required, a bronchial blocker and endobronchial tube or DLT (see "Lung Separation," below) may be used. If ILV is required, a DLT usually is used [some bronchial blockers can allow limited ventilation such as continuous positive airway pressure (CPAP) or jet ventilation].

Irrespective of technique, tube or blocker position usually is checked using fiberoptic bronchoscopy immediately after instigation, and lung isolation is leak tested (see "Lung Separation," below). This is important for all indications for ILV but is most critical when protection from secretions is required.

Applications of ILV

Applications of ILV (see Table 26-1) fall into five categories.

THORACIC SURGERY

A number of thoracic surgical procedures require OLV, usually in the lateral position. The common thoracic surgical indications for OLV are listed in Table 26-1.[12,13] Although OLV is required during surgery, ILV may be required before and sometimes after the surgical procedure.[14]

OLV may be undertaken with a DLT, bronchial blocker, or endobronchial tube. A DLT has the advantage of enabling ILV, which may be important in alleviating hypoxia; it has the disadvantage of high-resistance airways with more difficult suctioning. An endotracheal tube (ETT) with a bronchial blocker (see "Lung Separation," below) has the advantage of a wide-bore, low-resistance endotracheal lumen with better bronchoscopic and suction access, through which either OLV (bronchial blocker inflated) or double-lung ventilation (bronchial blocker deflated)[15] can be

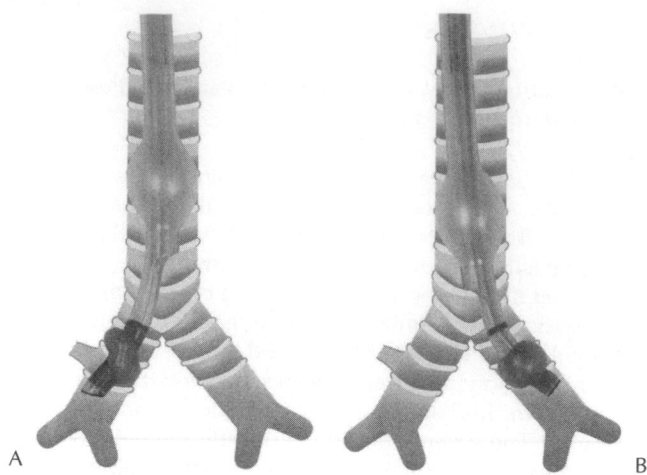

FIGURE 26-1 (*A*) Right and (*B*) left polyvinyl chloride (PVC) (Mallinckrodt) double-lumen tubes (DLT) shown against a schematic of the trachea and major airways.

delivered. The narrow lumen in some bronchial blockers can enable lung inflation, deflation, CPAP, or high-frequency jet ventilation (HFJV) but does not allow conventional ILV. OLV may be delivered to either lung, but repositioning of the bronchial blocker is required.[15] When the blocker is an integral part of the ETT (Univent tube),[15–17] it is easier to insert and maintains a more stable position compared

TABLE 26-1 Indications for Independent Lung Ventilation

Thoracic Surgery
  Pneumonectomy
  Some lobectomies
  Thoracic aortic surgery
  Thoracoscopy
  Some esophageal surgery
Selective airway protection
  Secretions (tuberculosis, bronchiectasis, abscess)
  Whole lung lavage
  Massive hemoptysis
  Bronchial repair protection
Bronchopleural fistula
Asymmetrical lung disease
  Unilateral parenchymal injury
    Aspiration
    Pulmonary contusion
    Pneumonia
    Massive pulmonary embolism
    Reperfusion edema
    Asymmetrical ARDS
    Asymmetrical pulmonary edema
  Atelectasis
  Unilateral airflow obstruction
    Single lung transplant for chronic airway obstruction
    Unilateral bronchospasm
Severe bilateral lung disease
  ARDS
  Aspiration
  Pneumonia

with intra- or extraluminal blockers that are more subject to movement and dislodgment, especially during suctioning, bronchoscopy, or patient movement.[15] Bronchoscopy is easier and required less.[12,15] A disadvantage is that the inflated blocking balloon near the site of intended bronchial surgery (e.g., pneumonectomy, single-lung transplant) may hamper that procedure, and a DLT placed in the opposite lung may be technically easier.

PHYSIOLOGIC EFFECTS OF THE LATERAL DECUBITUS POSITION

When a patient is in the erect or supine position, gravitational differences in ventilation and perfusion occur vertically within each lung. In the lateral decubitus position, these gravitational differences occur between the two lungs.[18,19] Up to two-thirds of perfusion shifts to the dependent lung.[18,20,21] During *spontaneous ventilation*, a smaller increase in ventilation also occurs in the dependent lung in the lateral position, thereby reducing ventilation-perfusion mismatch.[18,19] When the patient is anesthetized and *mechanically ventilated* in the lateral decubitus position, however, reduced diaphragmatic activity allows the weight of abdominal contents to retard expansion of the dependent lung,[18,19] and most ventilation is diverted to the nondependent lung. In this situation, the nondependent lung may receive up to two-thirds of ventilation.[20,22,23] Opening the nondependent thorax further reduces ventilation to the dependent lung by facilitating expansion of the nondependent lung.[21,24] The net effect of these changes is overperfusion relative to ventilation (or shunting) in the dependent lung and overventilation relative to perfusion (or dead-space ventilation) in the nondependent lung with adverse effects on gas exchange.

Other factors affect the degree of hypoxia during OLV in the lateral decubitus position. Left thoracotomy achieves a higher Pa_{O_2} during OLV than does right thoracotomy because the left lung normally receives 10% less cardiac output than the right lung.[25] The presence of CAO is associated with better Pa_{O_2} during OLV possibly because of dynamic hyperinflation in the dependent lung.[25] Pa_{O_2} during double-lung ventilation is also predictive of Pa_{O_2} during OLV.

Some forms of ILV cannot be applied when the nondependent lung is immobile, deflated, or removed, yet ILV has been shown to improve many of these abnormalities. Application of PEEP to both lungs improves dependent-lung ventilation and oxygenation.[20] Synchronized ILV (SILV; see "Techniques for ILV," below) with delivery of equal tidal volumes (V_T) to both lungs[26] or PEEP to the dependent lung[23,27–30] or both[29] improves oxygenation when compared with double-lung ventilation or generalized PEEP.

When OLV is undertaken and the nondependent lung is excluded from ventilation, the reduction in ventilation to the dependent lung is eliminated, but all perfusion through the nondependent lung constitutes a shunt. In this situation, the amount of perfusion of the nondependent lung is a major determinant of hypoxia. Hypoxic vasoconstriction (not opposed by anesthetic agents), lung collapse, and surgical occlusion of blood flow (pneumonectomy) to the nondependent lung all have the potential to reduce shunt and improve Pa_{O_2} in OLV.

PEEP in the dependent lung may be beneficial by increasing functional residual capacity (FRC) and improving distribution of ventilation or be detrimental by increasing alveolar pressure and diverting blood flow to the nonventilated lung.[19,31-36] Consequently, PEEP to the dependent lung during OLV may improve Pa_{O_2},[31,36] decrease Pa_{O_2},[31,32,36] or cause no change.[34-36] During OLV, Cohen et al[27] compared PEEP (10 cmH$_2$O) to the dependent lung, CPAP (10 cmH$_2$O) to the nondependent lung, and both. All three maneuvers increased Pa_{O_2} compared with OLV alone. PEEP caused the smallest (nonsignificant) increase in Pa_{O_2}. CPAP and PEEP + CPAP caused larger (significant) increases in Pa_{O_2}, whereas PEEP + CPAP reduced cardiac output and oxygen (O$_2$) delivery significantly, which CPAP alone did not. Cohen et al[27] concluded that CPAP alone (to the nondependent lung) had the most beneficial effect by diverting blood flow to the dependent lung without reducing cardiac output. More recently, PEEP has been shown to benefit oxygenation during OLV to the dependent lung during thoracotomy.[37]

Because of these variable effects, it has been recommended that CPAP (5-10 cmH$_2$O) be applied to the nondependent lung, combined with no, low, or high PEEP (5-15 cmH$_2$O) to the dependent lung, depending on patient response.

Although function of the two lungs commonly differs after thoracotomy, conventional mechanical ventilation or spontaneous ventilation usually are resumed after surgery. ILV is required occasionally in the postoperative period for marked asymmetry of lung function with hypoxia,[8,9,38] bronchopleural fistula,[39-43] or following esophagectomy.[14]

SELECTIVE AIRWAY PROTECTION

WHOLE-LUNG LAVAGE

Pulmonary alveolar proteinosis is the most common indication for whole-lung lavage. This condition was first described in 1958,[44] and soon after, bronchopulmonary lavage became established as the main treatment.[45-53]

Pulmonary alveolar proteinosis is most often acquired (90%) but may be congenital or secondary to conditions such as acute silicosis and other inhalational syndromes, immunodeficiency disorders, malignancies, hematopoietic disorders, and lysinuric protein intolerance.[54] Recent studies suggest that acquired pulmonary alveolar proteinosis may be caused by deficiency of granulocyte-macrophage colony-stimulating factor,[54,55] and administration of this factor is of value in about 50% of patients. Despite these advances, lavage remains the most effective therapy.[54,55]

The clinical course is variable: increasing dyspnea progressing to respiratory insufficiency, static disease with minimal symptoms, asymptomatic disease, and spontaneous resolution in some patients.[54,56] Because the course is variable, the decision to undertake bronchopulmonary lavage is based on disease progression and symptoms.

Whole-lung lavage has been used for asthma,[57,58] chronic bronchitis, and cystic fibrosis[11,51,57-63] but with doubtful benefit, and it is no longer recommended. Radioactive dust inhalation is another indication.[64]

Procedure for Whole-Lung Lavage

To minimize hypoxia during the procedure, the worst lung should be lavaged first. The worst lung can be identified by chest x-ray, ventilation-perfusion scan, or oxygenation[3,65,66] during OLV to each lung before the procedure.

The procedure usually is performed with anesthesia, neuromuscular paralysis,[11,57,67] and a left DLT in the supine position. The supine position is chosen to balance the risk between hypoxia and fluid spillage[11] (see "Basic Principles of ILV," above).

Complete lung isolation to prevent spillage from the lavaged lung into the ventilated lung is essential (see "Lung Separation," below). Correct DLT position should be established using both auscultation and bronchoscopy, and leak testing should be verified by ventilating one lung at a plateau pressure of 40-50 cmH$_2$O[11,12] and connecting the airway of the contralateral lung to an underwater seal to ensure the absence of bubbling. Both lungs should be preoxygenated with 100% O$_2$ to maximize gas exchange and eliminates nitrogen, which may prevent full access of lavage fluid to the lung to be lavaged.

Isotonic saline, warmed to body temperature, then should be infused through wide-bore tubing into the lung to be lavaged from a gravitational height 30 cm above the midaxillary line[11] in volumes compatible with the infusion pressure (30 cmH$_2$O) and compliance of the lung (usually 500-1000 ml). Efflux of fluid may be commenced as soon as fluid influx is complete; the drainage tube is placed below the patient, assisted by head-down posturing and percussion and vibration of the hemithorax.[11,67] Fluid flow may be achieved using separate clamped inlet and outlet lines or a single line that is elevated for fluid influx and lowered for fluid efflux. Total fluid exchange may range from 10-50 liters and should be continued until efflux fluid is relatively clear.

When fluid influx into the lavaged lung is complete, the alveolar pressure usually exceeds the pulmonary capillary pressure, minimizing shunt through this lung and maximizing arterial oxygenation at this stage of the procedure.[57,67-70] When the lavaged lung is emptied of fluid, blood flow returns, and significant hypoxemia can occur.[11,57,67-69]

On conclusion of the lavage, double-lung ventilation should be recommenced with the DLT in situ using a single ventilator and a bifurcated circuit. If oxygenation is satisfactory, the patient may be weaned and extubated or reintubated with a regular ETT and later weaned. If oxygenation is unsatisfactory, ILV may need to be recommenced. Up to 1000 ml of saline may be retained in the lavaged lung[67]; although this is absorbed rapidly, lung function may not improve for hours or days. The procedure is repeated on the second lung after an interval of 1-3 days.

Leakage of fluid into the ventilated lung may be recognized by desaturation, crepitations, and rhonchi in the ventilated lung; fluid in the tubing to the ventilated lung; or air bubbles in the fluid from the lavaged lung.[11] If this occurs, lavage should be ceased, and the patient should be placed in the lateral decubitus position with the lavaged lung dependent and the head down to facilitate drainage from both lungs. Active suctioning of both lungs should be undertaken. If the leak is only minor and adequate oxygenation is restored, the correct DLT position may be re-established, lung isolation rechecked, and the procedure continued. With a major leak and failure to restore adequate oxygenation once fluid removal is complete, double-lung ventilation with PEEP should be resumed and further lavage delayed until hypoxia has improved.

Hypoxemia during the procedure is common. Some patients with severe lung disease are too hypoxemic before the procedure to tolerate OLV. Several options exist for such patients. Extracorporeal membrane oxygenation (ECMO) may be instituted before lavaging the first lung.[11,71-75] ECMO may or may not be required for lavage of the second lung depending on the effect of the first lung lavage on subsequent oxygenation. Cohen et al[73] reported successful lavage of both lungs with ECMO during a single session, avoiding the need for a second procedure. Because of the complexity and limited availability of ECMO, an alternative is to perform limited bronchoalveolar lavage using a fiberoptic bronchoscope,[76,77] with or without an inflatable cuff on the bronchoscope, under local anesthesia. This may be undertaken in a spontaneously breathing patient or during conventional mechanical ventilation (CMV) through a single-lumen ETT. Limiting lavage to a lobe or several subsegments necessitates multiple procedures but minimizes hypoxemia. Nadeau et al[78] reported that the combination of inhaled nitric oxide and inflation of a balloon in the right pulmonary artery during right whole-lung lavage improved oxygenation sufficiently to avoid ECMO.

Randomized studies of whole-lung lavage for pulmonary alveolar proteinosis have not been undertaken. Seymour and Presneill[54] analyzed survival of 231 patients in multiple reports; 5-year actuarial survival from diagnosis was $94\% \pm 2\%$ in patients who underwent whole-lung lavage ($n = 146$) compared with $85\% \pm 5\%$ for patients who did not ($n = 85$). In 55 patients in whom duration of benefit was reported,[54] median duration of benefit from lavage was 15 months; fewer than 20% of patients followed beyond 3 years remained symptom-free. In a series of 21 patients followed prospectively after whole-lung lavage, Beccaria et al[79] found that more than 70% remained free from recurrent pulmonary alveolar proteinosis at 7 years. Although whole-lung lavage is labor-intensive, these data suggest that it is worthwhile.

MASSIVE HEMOPTYSIS

Massive hemoptysis carries a high mortality[80-82] and requires prompt intervention. Common causes include tuberculosis, bronchiectasis, lung abscess, mycetoma, pulmonary carcinoma, cystic fibrosis, arteriovenous malformations, and trauma.[56,80,83] The source of bleeding is the bronchial arterial system in 90% of patients.[84] Iatrogenic causes are uncommon but include pulmonary artery rupture by a pulmonary artery catheter[80,85,86] and transbronchial lung biopsy. Death results from acute asphyxia and is related to the rate and volume of blood loss and the underlying condition.[80,81,87-89] Factors increasing mortality include pre-existing pulmonary insufficiency, obtundation from any cause, poor cough, and coagulopathy.[81,88,90,91]

Management consists of general measures, diagnosing the site of bleeding, isolating the bleeding lung, and controlling the bleeding. The patient should be given 100% O_2,

placed in the head-down lateral-decubitus position, bleeding side down, clotting studies performed, blood typed, wide-bore intravenous access established, and cough suppressed with an opiate, and resuscitation and suction equipment should be in close proximity.

A number of alternatives exist for localization, isolation, and control of the bleeding. Their choice depends on the rate of bleeding, ready availability, and skill of the personnel involved.

1. Fiberoptic bronchoscopy and placement of an endobronchial blocker (Fogarty catheter or Arndt endobronchial blocker) in the bleeding lung or segment should be done.[92-96] This can be performed in a patient who is not intubated but is easier in one who is. Fiberoptic bronchoscopy is limited by the narrow suction channel and rapid visual loss secondary to occlusion of the lens by clot.[91] Bronchoscopy allows accurate localization of bleeding,[56,80,91,97,98] catheter placement in a bronchial segment,[80,92,99] and lavage with iced isotonic saline or epinephrine.[80,99]

2. Rigid bronchoscopy has advantages over fiberoptic bronchoscopy when blood loss is massive because of better suction, visual access, and airway control.[88,90,91,97,100,101] It allows easier placement of endobronchial blockers, iced saline, or epinephrine lavage and also allows diathermy, laser and cryotherapy[82] and placement of endobronchial tampons soaked in vasoconstrictor drugs.[88] As use of embolization increases, rigid bronchoscopy is required less, although it still has a place.[97,100]

3. Endotracheal intubation may be required where bleeding is sufficient to compromise oxygenation, particularly if mentation is depressed or cough inadequate. If bleeding is so rapid that acute asphyxic arrest is imminent despite intubation,[80] the ETT can be advanced beyond the carina (usually into the right main bronchus) and OLV commenced.[80,102] If blood does not flow out of the ETT (implying blood loss from the contralateral side), the cuff is inflated and the ETT left in situ. If bleeding continues through the ETT, a Fogarty or Foley catheter is passed, the main bronchus is occluded, and the ETT is withdrawn to the trachea to ventilate the contralateral side.

4. Selective intubation is performed with a small (6–7 mm) ETT, with or without fiberoptic bronchoscope guidance, or with a selective left or right endobronchial tube.[80,88] Selective intubation must be preceded by accurate bronchoscopic localization of bleeding because it excludes one lung from ventilation. Selective intubation has the advantage of reliable protection of the nonbleeding lung[88,91] but the disadvantage of permitting OLV only and excluding the bleeding lung from endobronchial procedures and suctioning. Bleeding then must be controlled by tamponade, bronchial angiography, and embolization or surgery.

5. DLT insertion is an alternative that isolates the lungs but preserves access to both. In the past, DLTs were not recommended as an early alternative[80,88] to control bleeding. Problems included difficulties with insertion under adverse circumstances, requirement for an experienced operator, difficulties with suction and bronchoscopy access, and easy blockage of DLT lumen with clot. More

recently, use of PVC DLTs has been successful.[83,87,103] A DLT enables lateralizing of the bleeding, protects the non-bleeding lung, allows ILV, and allows therapeutic procedures to address the bleeding lung without compromising the healthy lung.[87,103] A left DLT is the tube of choice.[83,87,88,103] Most commonly, a single ventilator with a Y connection to the DLT lumens is used[87] with distribution of ventilation according to the relative impedance of the two lungs (see "Lung Separation," below). If there is risk of blood overflowing to the nonbleeding lung, or if differential ventilation is required, a second ventilator with asynchronous ILV (AILV) should be used. OLV must be present during bronchial blockade or endobronchial intubation and may be required during iced-saline lavage or massive blood loss.

6. Embolization. Since 90% of major hemoptyses arise from bronchial arteries,[84] once bleeding has been localized, bronchial artery embolization has a high success rate.[56,84,98,104–106]

7. Emergency surgery. Urgent resection is undertaken if bleeding overwhelms airway control or fails to respond to other measures. Resection is associated with a low mortality in many series.[56,81,91,97,105,107] It should not be unduly delayed if bleeding is not readily controlled.

Localization of bleeding usually is achieved by history, fiberoptic bronchoscopy, or radiology [chest x-ray, computed tomographis (CT) scan, or angiography]. Bleeding is controlled by conservative measures, embolization, or surgery.[56,98,105] The relative requirement for these three treatments varies widely[56,98,105] depending on cause, amount of bleeding, and local expertise. Supportive care, correction of coagulopathy, and time as the only measure ranged from 13–87% of patients with major hemoptysis. Embolization was used in 7–51% with success rates of over 80%. Surgery was required in 6–50%.

LUNG PROTECTION FROM SECRETIONS

Spread of purulent secretions from a lung abscess, empyema, bronchiectasis, cavitating tuberculosis, or cavitating malignant disease to the dependent normal lung during chest surgery is associated with considerable risk.[1,2,6,7,108] A DLT not only allows thoracic surgery but also protects the dependent normal lung[1,42,108] and allows perioperative ILV if required.[1,42,108] Although these conditions have become less common, the requirement for ILV for lung protection, during or outside thoracic surgery, occurs occasionally.[109] Essential during thoracic surgery, it is problematic outside that setting because viscous or tenacious secretions drain poorly through the narrower lumen of a DLT. Appropriate antibiotic therapy, postural drainage, and a standard ETT may be preferable.

BRONCHIAL REPAIR PROTECTION

Main-stem bronchi and lower trachea (near the carina) can be ruptured by severe blunt chest trauma, resulting in tension pneumothoraces, massive air leak, and the need for urgent surgical repair. Selective airway intubation usually is required for the repair, and ILV has been used postoperatively to protect the anastomoses.[110–113] Pizov et al[113] used one-lung high-frequency ventilation in the management of a traumatic tear of the bronchus in a child. After a right main-stem bronchial rupture, Moerer et al[110] used a left DTL with bilevel ventilation to the left lung and CPAP alone to the right lung for 48 hours before switching to CMV. In three patients with lower tracheal rupture (near the carina), Wichert et al[111] reported that standard DLTs position the cuff too close to the site of carinal injury and used bronchoscopy-guided selective endobronchial intubation with two tubes to undertake the repairs. After repair, the tubes were reintroduced via tracheostomy, and ILV was performed for 9–14 days to allow recovery from respiratory and other complications.

BRONCHOPLEURAL FISTULA

Bronchopleural fistulas (BPFs) can result from trauma, necrotizing pneumonia, lung abscess, tuberculosis, acute respiratory distress syndrome (ARDS), thoracic surgery, overinflation from mechanical ventilation, central venous catheter insertion, and intercostal catheters. Persisting BPF often leads to infection of the pleural space.[114] If massive air leak from a BPF occurs during mechanical ventilation, the consequences include respiratory insufficiency and sometimes tension pneumothorax. Persisting failure of lung expansion can occur despite intercostal catheters if the rate of air leak exceeds the rate of drainage through the catheters. BPFs are estimated to occur in 2% of ventilated patients.[115] Mortality depends on the size of the leak[115] and the cause and is reported to be 18–67%.[114,115]

Management includes antibiotics, pleural sclerosing agents, surgical control of air leaks at thoracotomy, intercostal catheter insertion, underwater seal drainage with suction, conventional ventilation strategies to reduce air leak, patient positioning[114] positive pleural pressure during inspiration,[114,116] HFJV, a variety of bronchoscopic occlusion techniques, and ILV. ILV generally is employed when massive air leak persists despite conservative measures and results in respiratory insufficiency. Before instigating ILV, conservative measures should be optimized.

Inadequate drainage can occur despite actively bubbling intercostal catheters and can lead to failure of lung expansion and respiratory insufficiency. Intercostal catheters must be adequate in number and diameter; their patency must be visualized and demonstrated by active bubbling. Underwater-seal drainage systems and wall-suction units must have an adequate maximum flow capacity. Air-filter patency must be checked. High resistances and low maximum flow rates in either the drainage system or wall-suction unit actually can retard thoracic drainage and increase pneumothorax size. Ideally, maximum flow capacity should approximate or exceed the percentage of V_T lost to the BPF multiplied by the inspiratory flow rate. Drainage devices vary widely in maximum flow capacity but rarely exceed a capacity of 35 liters/min. Increased bubbling or radiologic improvement after suction disconnection suggests retardation by the device. Persisting negative pressure on a wall-suction unit after disconnection suggests an occluded air filter. With massive air leaks, more than one underwater-seal drainage system may be required.

The conventional ventilator strategy for a BPF has three goals: reduce air-leak rate (to facilitate healing), reduce pneumothorax size, and maintain adequate gas exchange. These goals often have conflicting needs. The usual strategy is directed toward lowering alveolar and airway pressure to reduce air leak. V_T and PEEP should be minimized and the rate reduced, especially if dynamic hyperinflation is present, although these steps may impair gas exchange. Inspiratory flow is controversial. Increasing flow may decrease air leak by decreasing inspiratory time or increase proximal air leak by increasing peak airway pressure. The impact of any change on all three goals must be assessed.

HFJV without ILV appears to benefit patients with a proximal BPF and otherwise relatively normal lungs.[114] Reported success of HFJV in patients with parenchymal lung disease, whose BPFs usually are peripheral, is variable.[114] ILV has been used in many patients with a BPF.[39–43,115,117–130] Conditions in which ILV has been used for BPF include pneumonia with and without CAO,[41,122,126] ARDS,[119] trauma,[41,115,117,120,124] pulmonary contusion,[128] emphysema, asthma,[118] staphylococcal pneumatoceles,[121] and thoracic surgery.[39–43] Most patients had air leaks exceeding 50% of V_T, lung collapse despite multiple intercostal catheter insertions, and hypercapnic acidosis and hypoxia despite attempts at optimizing mechanical ventilation.

The most common form of ILV for BPF is asynchronous ILV (AILV) using two ventilators[40,42,123–125] with low V_T, low rates, and low or no PEEP for the lung with the BPF. The BPF lung also has been ventilated with synchronous ILV (SILV) with low V_T, PEEP, and inspiratory flow[43,126,129]; HFJV[41,127]; and high-frequency oscillation[119] or excluded from ventilation by a Fogarty catheter passed through a DLT after failing to respond to both CPAP and jet ventilation.[122] Successful use of a DLT with a single ventilator and a variable-resistance valve in the inspiratory circuit to the BPF lung has been reported in an animal model[131] and in one patient[39] with a large BPF.

Almost all authors report reduction in air leak with improvement in gas exchange. ILV was continued from 2 hours[42] up to 10 days[40] in some patients before CMV could be resumed. Improvement was reported in most patients with ILV. Overall survival was about 50%, although a large BPF is as a poor prognostic factor.[114] Outcome mainly was related to the prognosis of the underlying condition.

ASYMMETRIC LUNG DISEASE

ILV has been used for a variety of unilateral or asymmetric lung diseases (see Table 26-1). Three main indications are unilateral pulmonary parenchymal injury, unilateral atelectasis, and unilateral airflow obstruction.

UNILATERAL PARENCHYMAL INJURY
Patients who receive ILV for asymmetric pulmonary injury have poor compliance on the affected side, hypoxemia refractory to high O_2 concentrations, and high levels of PEEP. Under these circumstances, PEEP may cause hyperinflation of the unaffected lung, collapse of the affected lung,[132,133] barotrauma,[132–135] and worsening of hypoxemia[132] consequent to increased pulmonary vascu-

lar resistance in the unaffected lung (diverting blood flow to the injured lung). This hyperinflation also can elevate intrathoracic pressure, reduce arterial pressure and cardiac output,[129,130,132,133] and combined with arterial desaturation reduce O_2 delivery.[19,129,130,136–141]

The prime objective of ILV under these circumstances is differential PEEP, although different ventilator patterns have been applied to achieve a similar effect and optimize gas exchange and minimize barotrauma. ILV allows lung recruitment maneuvers and high PEEP to the affected lung, permitting maximum benefit to that lung without adverse effects on the contralateral lung, intrathoracic pressure, cardiac output, and the distribution of ventilation between the two lungs. PEEP applied to the diseased lung can improve oxygenation by alveolar recruitment and diverting blood flow to the more normal lung. Low or no PEEP in the more normal lung avoids hyperinflation and the adverse effects of high intrathoracic pressure.

ILV has been used in various unilateral or asymmetric lung diseases (see Table 26-1). The most common indication has been *pulmonary contusion*. Of 45 patients who received ILV for asymmetric lung injury,[10,41,117,132–135,142–144] three received SILV,[132,133] but most received AILV.[10,117,134,135,142] Two patients received no mechanical ventilation and breathed spontaneously through a DLT with different levels of CPAP applied to the expired limb of each circuit.[144] All methods improved gas exchange, and overall mortality was only 10%. In 12 trauma patients with unilateral contusion requiring ILV, Cinnella et al[142] monitored end-tidal CO_2 and static compliance in each lung and reverted to conventional ventilation when these became similar in the two lungs.

ILV has been reported in patients with *aspiration*[38,123,129,130] and *pneumonia* or *consolidation*.[10,126,129,130,145–150] As with contusion, a mixture of AILV and SILV has been used. In one patient, high-frequency oscillatory ventilation (HFOV) was used with a higher mean airway pressure to the affected lung.[147] SILV has been used in patients with unilateral consolidation on a background of congenital heart disease with asymmetric lung blood supply.[145,146] Mortality was 48%.

SILV has been reported in patients with asymmetric ARDS secondary to trauma and sepsis (56% mortality[151]), asymmetric acute pulmonary edema,[130,145,152] and massive pulmonary embolism.[153] In a patient with a single-lung transplant it enabled weaning from ECMO.[152]

All patients received differential PEEP: 0–10 cmH_2O on the unaffected side and 7–25 cmH_2O on the affected side. In all cases, higher PEEP was used on the affected side. V_T values to the two lungs were equal in some studies, smaller to the affected lung in some, and larger in one study.[133] In two studies, PEEP administered to each affected lung was carefully adjusted to the compliance response of that lung. Carlon et al[130] increased PEEP in the affected lung until its compliance was similar to that of the unaffected lung. Siegal et al[151] found that increasing PEEP in the affected lung initially improved compliance, but then it decreased secondary to overinflation. They set PEEP at the level that achieved maximum compliance. Both methods improved oxygenation, shunt fraction, and cardiac output. The duration of ILV ranged from 1 hour[133] to 12 days.[135]

From these reports, several factors emerge as requirements for ILV:

1. *Differential PEEP* with a higher level applied to the affected lung is a key factor. PEEP may be applied to the affected lung until gas exchange improves, to an inflection point[151] on a compliance curve, until lung compliance is equal on the two sides,[130] or based on CO_2 excretion. PEEP most commonly is 10–20 cmH_2O. A recruitment maneuver and PEEP level that maximizes arterial oxygenation can be recommended.[154] PEEP may or may not be required in the contralateral lung.
2. *Equal V_T* to both lungs was used most commonly and was most likely to maximize gas exchange[22,23,26] compared smaller or larger V_T values to the affected lung. Maintenance of plateau pressure below 30 cmH_2O is an important goal.[155,156]
3. *AILV or SILV* is equally acceptable because there is no requirement for a different respiratory rate. AILV holds no disadvantages when compared with SILV[38,157] and is simpler and more flexible.

The primary goal of ILV and differential PEEP or CPAP is improvement in gas exchange and hemodynamics and physical expansion of collapsed lung regions.

UNILATERAL ATELECTASIS

Unilateral atelectasis that has failed to respond to standard ventilator support, bronchoscopy, or both[9,38,103,129,130,133,136,149,158–161] is another indication for ILV. High PEEP has been applied to the atelectatic lung, primarily for the purpose of reinflation without the risk of overinflating the contralateral lung and generalized elevation of intrathoracic pressure.

In some studies,[129,130,136,149,159,162] high PEEP was applied to the atelectatic lung during AILV or SILV with mechanical ventilation of both lungs. The collapsed lung received 10–30 cmH_2O of PEEP, whereas the unaffected side received 0–10 cmH_2O of PEEP. In other studies, the collapsed lung received transient CPAP alone[9,103,159–161] (20–80 cmH_2O) without mechanical or spontaneous ventilation. Miranda et al[160] applied 30 cmH_2O of CPAP via a DLT to reinflate a collapsed lung and subsequently used HFJV with 25 cmH_2O of PEEP (to the same lung after expansion) to improve gas exchange. Millen et al[161] transiently applied 60–70 cmH_2O of CPAP to individual lungs in two nonintubated, spontaneously breathing patients via a cuffed fiberoptic bronchoscope with good results. Narr et al[159] required 80 cmH_2O of CPAP to reinflate an asthmatic lung that collapsed during pleurodesis and then subsequently used AILV with a very low rate to the same lung to reduce its hyperinflation. Plotz et al[158] used HFOV (mean airway pressure of 28 cmH_2O) to the atelectatic lung of a child, with CMV to the unaffected lung. There was no report of lung injury despite transient application of very high inflation pressures, and there were only 2 deaths in this group of 14 patients with atelectasis.[9,38,103,130,136,149,158–160,162]

These reports demonstrate success with a range of recruitment maneuvers. Application of CPAP up to 50–60 cmH_2O to both lungs for a few minutes has no prolonged consequences of raised intrathoracic pressure and is recommended for lung collapse.[154] In unilateral atelectasis, recruitment maneuvers should be undertaken routinely during double-lung ventilation (unless contraindicated by a problem in the nonatelectatic lung) before attempting ILV and may prevent the need for ILV in many patients.

UNILATERAL AIRFLOW OBSTRUCTION

Unilateral airflow obstruction occurs most commonly following single-lung transplantation (SLT) but may occur with a mechanical or chemical insult to one lung in a patient with asthma or partial occlusion of a major bronchus. Under these circumstances, standard ventilation can cause dynamic hyperinflation and high intrinsic PEEP in the obstructed lung. This can elevate intrathoracic pressure, reduce cardiac output, and compress the contralateral lung.

To achieve hypoventilation of the obstructed lung, SILV can be used with a much lower V_T to the obstructed lung. It is better achieved with AILV using reduced rate and V_T (or CPAP alone) to the obstructed lung.[159,163]

Single-Lung Transplantation

Early reports suggested that SLT was contraindicated in chronic obstructive pulmonary disease (COPD) because of the risk of dynamic hyperinflation in the native lung with mediastinal shift.[74,164] Initial experience supported these concerns.[165–168] Subsequent series[164,169–178] combined with 210 SLTs at our institution result in a total of 733 patients. Overall early mortality is 18% and only 13% when the primary diagnosis is CAO (emphysema, α_1-antitryspin deficiency, leiomyoangiomyomatosis) (Table 26-2). Thirty-day mortality varies widely (0%[172] to 50%[169]). Small series reveal that early mortality[164,169,176,177] ranges from being slightly lower with SLT than with bilateral lung transplant (BLT)[164,176,177] to higher with SLT.[169] Larger series suggest lower mortality with BLT,[179–182] although selection criteria such as age may have contribute.[179]

Despite this uncertainty, SLT is now a popular alternative to BLT, especially in patients over 50 years of age. SLT is technically easier than BLT and benefits more recipients when donor availability is a limiting factor. The most common indication for SLT is some form of CAO, which accounts for 77% of SLTs.[164,169–178] Although lung function is better after BLT, SLT substantially improves quality of life[164,176] and achieves equivalent maximum work capacity and maximum O_2 consumption.[183]

Over 30 reports[152,159,163–178,184–196] plus experience from our institution provide information on 768 patients receiving SLTs, 601 for CAO. ILV was required almost exclusively in patients who received SLT for CAO.[163,169,171–173,177,178,184,186–189,191,193] There are few reports of patients requiring ILV after BLT for any reason, nor after SLT for restrictive lung disease. In one patient,[193] ILV was required for a large, unresolving BPF arising in the native lung after SLT that eventually necessitated pneumonectomy of the native lung. In another patient,[152] ILV was required for reperfusion edema after SLT for primary pulmonary hypertension. Use of ILV in SLT series for CAO (see Table 26-2) varies widely: 0%[164,170,174–176] to 43%,[169] with an overall frequency of 9%.[164,169–178]

TABLE 26-2 Incidence of acute native lung hyperinflation (ANLH) and incidence and mortality with independent lung ventilation (ILV) in patients undergoing single lung transplantation (SLT) for airflow obstruction.

Authors	SLT FOR AIRFLOW OBSTRUCTION			RADIOLOGICAL ANHL		SYMPTOMATIC ANHL		ILV		ILV MORTALITY	
	No. Pts	No. Died	Mortality	No.	%	No.	%	No.	%	No.	%
Kaiser et al	11	0	0%	—		—		1	9%	0	0%
Patterson et al	7	1	14%	1		1		0			
Egan et al	4	0	0%	—		—		1	25%	0	0%
Marinelli et al	7	1	14%	—		—		0			
Low et al	16	2	13%	—		—		0			
Montoya et al	39	1	3%	—		—		0			
Yonan et al	27	5	19%	12	44%	12	44%	8	30%	2	25%
Weill et al	51	0	0%	16	31%	8	16%	1	2%	0	0%
Mitchell et al	132	34	26%	—		—		13	10%	6	46%
Hansen et al	90	1	1%	—		—		0			
Angles et al	14	7	50%	9	64%	9	64%	6	43%		
Author's institution	170	21	12%	78/95	82%	20	12%	20	12%	7	35%
Totals	**568**	**73**	**13%**	**116**	**60%**	**50**	**19%**	**50**	**9%**	**15**	**30%**

From Kaiser et al [178], Patterson et al [164], Egan et al [177], Marinelli et al [175], Low et al [176], Montoya et al [174], Yonan et al [173], Weill et al [179], Mitchell et al [171], Hansen et al [170], Angles et al [169] and the author's institution (unpublished).

The phenomenon leading to use of ILV has been termed *acute native lung hyperinflation* (ANHL), which is defined as radiologic mediastinal shift with flattening of the ipsilateral hemidiaphragm (Fig. 26-2 A) associated with signs of hemodynamic instability or respiratory dysfunction.[169,172,173] Evolution of this phenomenon can be divided into three stages:

1. *Asymptomatic ANLH.* Dynamic hyperinflation of the native lung with mediastinal shift is seen commonly in the postoperative period without transplant-lung collapse, hypoxia, or hypotension and without the need for ILV.[164,195] This phenomenon arises because of asymmetry of lung disease following transplantation. The native lung with severe airflow obstruction undergoes dynamic hyperinflation during CMV, just as both lungs would do during CMV before transplantation.[197] A healthy transplanted lung with normal compliance and airflow resistance will receive most of the blood flow and ventilation, thereby reducing the degree of dynamic hyperinflation that would have occurred if both lungs received the same ventilation. Nevertheless, the transplanted lung does

FIGURE 26-2 Chest x-rays of a patient with a right single-lung transplant before (*A*) and (*B*) after insertion of a right double-lumen tube and independent lung ventilation, as suggested in Table 26-4.

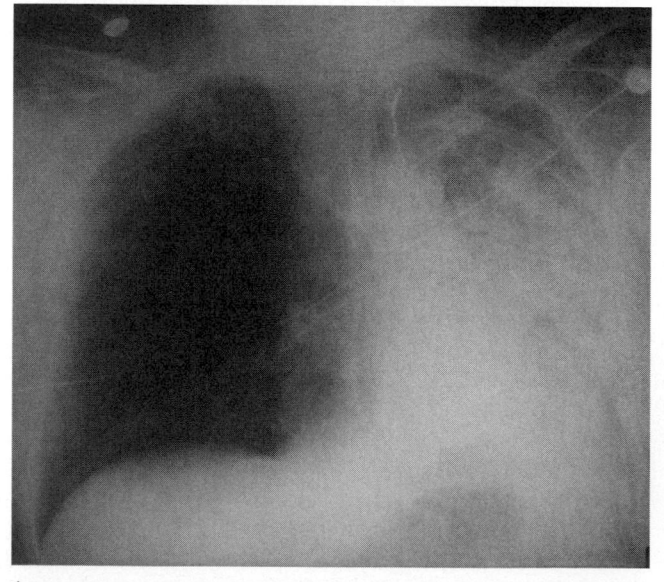

A

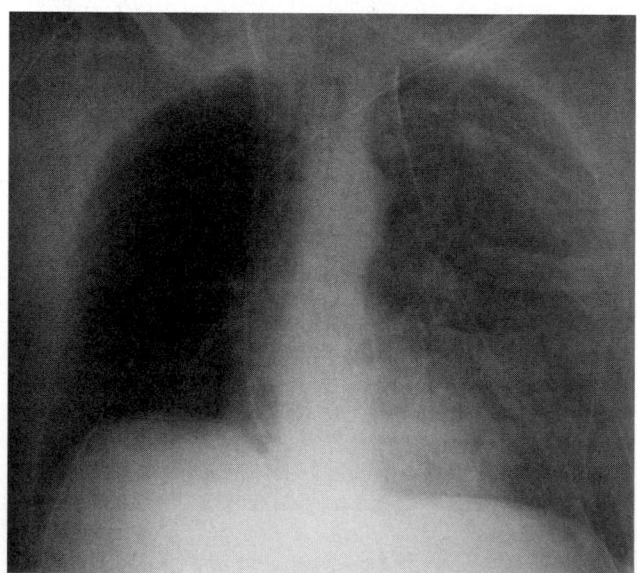

B

TABLE 26-3   Incidence of radiological and symptomatic acute native lung hyperinflation (ANLH) in left and right single lung transplantation (SLT) for airflow obstruction.

| | RADIOLOGICAL ANHL | | | | | | |
| | LEFT | | | RIGHT | | | |
	No.	Total	%	No.	Total	%	P value
Weill et al	10	27	37	6	24	25	NS
Author's instituition	45	54	83	33	41	80	NS
TOTAL	**55**	**81**	**68**	**39**	**65**	**60**	**NS**

| | SYMPTOMATIC ANHL | | | | | | |
| | LEFT | | | RIGHT | | | |
	No.	Total	%	No.	Total	%	P value
Weill et al	4	27	15	4	24	17	NS
Angles et al	5	6	83	4	8	50	NS
Author's institution	14	82	17	7	88	8	NS
TOTAL	23	115	20	15	120	13	<0.05

From Weill et al [179], Angles et al[169] and the author's institution (unpublished)

not have a "balancing" degree of dynamic hyperinflation, and mediastinal shift occurs commonly. The occurrence of asymptomatic ANHL is reported infrequently (Table 26-3). Weill et al[172] reported asymptomatic ANHL in 16 of 51 patients (31%), although smaller series have reported symptomatic ANHL in 44%[173] and 64%[169] of SLTs for CAO. In our institution, mediastinal shift (shift of right heart border relative to the spine by 1 cm or greater toward the transplanted lung) occurred in 78 of 95 consecutively evaluated SLTs (82%) for CAO (see Table 26-3). The asymmetry usually improves or resolves over time, but it persists indefinitely in some patients. In some patients it can arise weeks or months after transplant.[169]

2. *Transplanted lung dysfunction.* Any dysfunction in the transplanted lung, whether parenchymal (e.g., reperfusion edema, contusion, rejection, pneumonia, or collapse) or airway (e.g., anastomosis narrowing or sputum obstruction), impedes ventilation in the transplanted lung and redistributes ventilation to the native lung, especially during volume-controlled ventilation. This necessarily increases dynamic hyperinflation in the native lung and increases mediastinal shift and collapse and further impairs gas exchange in the transplanted lung. A vicious cycle results, redistributing more ventilation to the native lung with greater dynamic hyperinflation and mediastinal shift. Progressive compromise of the transplanted lung can lead to refractory hypoxia and hypercapnia, whereas dynamic hyperinflation, mediastinal shift, and pulmonary vessel compression can lead to circulatory compromise with hypotension (see Fig. 26-2A). Primary dysfunction of the transplanted lung,[189] severe postimplantation syndrome,[188] and ARDS have been identified as major contributors to native-lung hyperinflation and mediastinal shift.[177,178,186,188,189,191] It usually results in hypotension, collapse of the transplanted lung with hypoxia, or both. This has been termed *symptomatic ANLH*[172,173] (see Table 26-3). Almost all such problems have occurred only during mechanical ventilation in the immediate or early postoperative period.

3. *Mechanical ventilation response.* The typical response to a lung collapse with worsening hypoxemia and hypercapnia includes increasing PEEP, increasing rate, and/or increasing V_T. Each response increases dynamic hyperinflation in the native lung,[197,198] which can worsen gas exchange, precipitate circulatory collapse, and necessitate ILV. Although the requirement for ILV usually is attributed to step 2 (above), the precipitant often is the failure to improve (or deterioration) with mechanical ventilation. Risk factors for this problem, in addition to injury to the transplanted lung (above), include severity of airflow obstruction in the native lung, size of the transplanted lung, and side of the transplant. Severity of airflow obstruction directly affects the degree of dynamic hyperinflation.[197,198] Yonan et al[173] found that patients who developed ANHL had higher pulmonary artery pressures, higher residual volumes, and lower forced expiratory volumes (FEV_1) than did patients who did not develop symptomatic ANHL. Weill et al[172] suspected more symptomatic ANHL in patients with bullous emphysema, but lung function and pulmonary artery pressure were equivalent among patients with and without symptomatic ANHL. Angles et al[169] found no preoperative predictors of ANLH. The size of the donor lung[164,178,188] is an important factor. A donor's predicted vital capacity (VC) that approximates[178] or is smaller than[188] the recipient's predicted VC is associated with the need for ILV. Donor-to-recipient predicted VC ratio of 1.4[178] or a donor-lung predicted VC exceeding recipient-lung predicted VC by 2 liters[164] is associated with the absence of mediastinal shift following SLT. Others have found no difference in donor size.[172]

Several reports have suggested a higher incidence of ANLH with left SLTs (see Table 26-3). Weill et al[172] found radiographic ANLH in 37% of left SLTs and 25% of right SLTs and no difference in symptomatic ANLH (Table 26-4). Angles et al[169] did not report radiographic ANLH but found symptomatic ANLH in 83% of left SLTs and 50% of

TABLE 26-4   Ventilator settings for independent ventilation after single lung transplantation for airflow obstruction.

	Native Lung	Transplanted Lung
Ventilator rate (b/min)	2–4	14–20
Tidal volume (ml/kg)	2–3	3–4
Plateau pressure (cm H_2O)	<25	<30
Inspiratory flow rate (L/min)	80	40–50
PEEP (cm H_2O)	0	10–17
Recruitment maneuver (cm H_2O)	No	±35-50*

* Stability of the anastomosis and the presence of air leak need to be considered before undertaking a recruitment maneuver. Lower than normal recruitment pressures may be initially chosen.

right SLTs. At our institution, mediastinal shift did not differ between left and right SLTs for CAO, but ILV was required twice as often with left SLTs (see Table 26-4).

Severe symptomatic ANLH commonly requires urgent intervention. Options include

1. *Permissive hypercapnia.*[170] Permissive hypercapnia reduces dynamic hyperinflation in the native lung and may improve mild symptomatic ANLH but is unlikely to be adequate for severe ANLH. Although ILV was not used in this study, four patients required ECMO.
2. *ILV.*[163,167,169,171–173,177,178,184,186–189,191,193] Although technically complex, ILV commonly results in immediate resolution or improvement in gas exchange and circulatory problems and provides the most rapidly available and chosen solution (see Fig. 26-2).
3. *ECMO.*[170] ECMO is a complex and invasive solution but provides an alternative to ILV.
4. *Contralateral lung-reduction surgery.*[171–173] This has been reported recently. It has been undertaken concurrently with SLT, during the post-operative period, and late after SLT. It may offer the best long-term solution to ANLH but is less readily applicable in urgent or life-threatening situations.
5. *Contralateral lung transplantation.*[171,173] After primary SLT, this offers a solution but depends on availability of a donor lung and subjects the recipient to two major surgical procedures and two sets of foreign antigens.
6. *Retransplantation of the SLT.*[173] This has been used for early graft dysfunction associated with ANLH.

The choice of DLT for ILV is different following SLT. A left DLT normally is easier to position correctly. With a left SLT, however, this can compromise the anastomosis and airway distal to the anastomosis, which has a tenuous blood supply in the immediate postoperative period. Thus a DLT opposite to the side of the SLT normally is chosen in the early postoperative period. If ILV is required more than 2–3 weeks after left SLT when the anastomosis is stable, a left DLT may be used, although a smaller size is chosen in case the anastomosis is narrower than the adjacent airway.

ILV after SLT usually consists of CMV to the transplanted lung and AILV,[177,178,188,189] SILV,[191] bronchial

blockade,[178,186] CPAP,[193] or spontaneous ventilation (SV)[188] to the native lung. All methods are viable options. The ventilatory requirements of each lung differ so much, however, that AILV is the method of choice primarily because of different rate requirements of the two lungs (see Table 26-4). AILV was the method of choice in 27 patients in three recent series[169,171,173] and in the 20 patients at our institution who received ILV. The donor lung commonly requires PEEP at a sufficient level to expand collapsed regions and improve oxygenation, a V_T sufficiently low to avoid pressure injury to the lung, and a rate high enough for adequate CO_2 elimination without causing flow limitation. A recruitment maneuver may maximize the benefit from PEEP, provided that it is safe to undertake.[154] The native lung should be ventilated with a pattern that maximizes its contribution to gas exchange without excessive dynamic hyperinflation. This necessitates low V_T, high inspiratory flow rate, and a very low rate[198] (see Table 26-4). The goals of native-lung ventilation are to maintain a low plateau pressure, restore the mediastinum to the midline (see Fig. 26-2B), and allow restoration of circulatory instability (that caused by dynamic hyperinflation). If this is not achieved, rate should be reduced further (even to 0). The goals of SLT ventilation are a safe plateau pressure (see Table 26-4) and restoration of adequate Sa_{O_2} and Pa_{CO_2}. If this is not achieved, further recruitment maneuvers and higher PEEP should be explored. The introduction and stabilization of these different ventilator strategies to each lung generally necessitate sedation and paralysis during the early stages of ILV. If Sa_{O_2} or circulation is not satisfactory, ECMO may be needed.

Withdrawal of ILV can be initiated when function of the transplanted lung improves and its ventilatory requirements decrease. This can be assessed with a DLT in situ by ventilating both lungs with a single ventilator and a bifurcated ventilator circuit. Since spontaneous ventilation is difficult with a DLT, patients usually require reintubation with a single-lumen ETT for weaning before extubation. Others experience recurrent dynamic hyperinflation with double-lung ventilation and must wean with the DLT in situ. ILV has been required for as little as 1 day.[178] In most instances, prolonged ILV has been required; periods exceeding 1 month[188,189,191,193] have been reported with eventual resolution and good functional outcome. Patients who require prolonged ILV should undergo a tracheostomy and receive a double-lumen tracheostomy tube.[188,191,199] (Fig. 26-3).

Outcome of ANLH

Three series[169,172,173,188,191,199] reported a longer duration of mechanical ventilation and ICU stay in patients with symptomatic ANLH. One series reported a higher mortality in ANLH patients.[173] In a second series,[169] mortality was not significantly higher because of small numbers. In a third series, no difference was noted.[172] Combining all three series plus data from our institution reveals differences in mortality: 7% mortality in 213 SLT patients without symptomatic ANLH and 37% mortality in 49 SLT patients with symptomatic ANLH ($P < .05$). Yonan et al[173] reported lower FEV_1 values and higher residual volumes after transplantation in

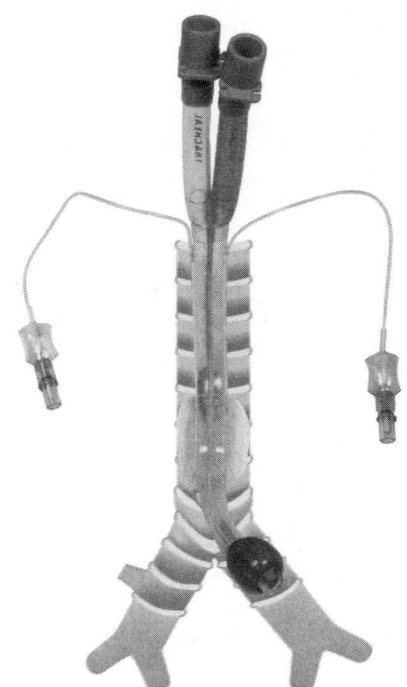

FIGURE 26-3 A double-lumen tracheostomy tube.

ANLH patients, whereas Weill et al,[172] in a larger series, found no differences in long-term lung function.

Outcome of ILV

Fifteen papers[163,167,169,171–173,177,178,184,186–189,191,193] plus data from our institution report 63 patients with ILV following an SLT for CAO. Overall mortality was 30%. Including only recent case series in which all SLT patients and ILV survival were reported,[171–173] plus our data, ILV patients had higher mortality (15 of 42 patients, or 36% mortality) than non-ILV patients (45 of 338 patients, or 13% mortality). This difference is not surprising because ILV patients are sicker and show a higher incidence of graft dysfunction.

In summary, SLT for airflow obstruction poses a risk of ANLH with mediastinal shift. When this is sufficient to compromise gas exchange and/or circulation, AILV is the initial method of choice and may reduce the need for ECMO.

UNILATERAL BRONCHOSPASM

In patients with asthma, airways respond locally to local stimuli; irritants applied to one lung may create a different degree of bronchospasm in the two lungs.[200] During mechanical ventilation, this can lead to different levels of dynamic hyperinflation and mediastinal shift, and during thoracic surgery, this can lead to difficulty with thoracotomy closure and the need for ILV. Narr et al[159] reported unilateral bronchospasm during unilateral pleurodesis. The pleurodesed lung initially collapsed; following DLT insertion and ILV with 80 cmH$_2$O of CPAP applied to the collapsed lung, that lung inflated and would not deflate. Low-level CPAP to the affected lung, CMV to the unaffected lung, and aggressive bronchodilator therapy allowed deflation of the

affected lung, maintenance of gas exchange, and thoracotomy closure.[159]

PATIENT SELECTION FOR ILV IN UNILATERAL LUNG DISEASE

Asymmetric lung disease usually is easy to recognize, but criteria for ILV are not so clear. Not all patients with asymmetric lung disease require ILV. Commonly used criteria are unilateral or clearly asymmetric lung disease, which is evident on chest x-ray or known from the patient's condition (e.g., SLT), plus one of the following:

1. Severe hypoxemia despite 100% O$_2$ and different levels of PEEP
2. Circulatory failure/hypotension secondary to dynamic hyperinflation

Factors that suggest that a patient is likely to benefit from ILV include

1. Worsening hypoxemia and/or circulatory status by increasing PEEP, rate, or V$_T$
2. Improvement in gas exchange but marked deterioration in circulatory status with increasing PEEP and the opposite when PEEP is reduced

BILATERAL SYMMETRIC LUNG DISEASE

Acute bilateral lung injury may appear diffuse, uniform, and symmetric on chest x-ray but contain significant inhomogeneity on CT scan.[201,202] Many of these changes result from a uniformly injured lung collapsing in dependent zones as a result of increased lung weight. Because patients commonly are nursed on their back, collapse occurs in posterior zones and is not apparent on anteroposterior chest x-rays. In this case, no PEEP is required to open alveoli in the least dependent regions, and high PEEP may be required in the most dependent regions. Generalized PEEP may fail to inflate the most dependent regions and may overinflate nondependent regions. There is now increasing evidence that the injury can result from prolonged collapse[203] and repetitive collapse/re-expansion and overexpansion[204,205] and that lung injury may contribute to multiple-organ failure and death.[155,206] Considerable effort has been devoted to ventilator strategies that reduce prolonged collapse, collapse/re-expansion, and overexpansion.[155,156,207] While some strategies have been successful, all have the same problem of conflicting pressure requirements within different regions of the same lung.

The application of ILV under these circumstances is based on two principles:

1. Differences in compliance, ventilation-perfusion ratios, and gas exchange between the two lungs may be present and not be suspected from plain x-rays.[23,26,130,151]
2. Placing the patient in the lateral decubitus position will redistribute much of the collapsed (high-PEEP-requiring) lung regions to the dependent lung and the open (low-PEEP-requiring) regions to the nondependent lung.[23,26,208,209]

When a patient with normal lungs is ventilated in the lateral decubitus position, up to two-thirds of perfusion goes to the dependent lung, and up to two-thirds of ventilation goes to the nondependent lung,[18,22] creating significant ventilation-perfusion mismatch and shunt. Application of global PEEP improves distribution of ventilation,[210] but perfusion inequality may be increased and cardiac output reduced[22] with little net benefit.

ILV with equal V_T to each lung and selective PEEP to the dependent lung proved additive in improving shunt fraction, arterial oxygenation, cardiac output, and O_2 delivery compared with CMV in both the supine and lateral positions.[28,29] These maneuvers have been applied on a long-term basis in bilateral lung injury with some early success.[209] Wickerts et al[208] and Diaz-Reganon Valverde et al[211] prospectively studied 11 and 45 patients, respectively, with severe bilateral ARDS who received ILV. These patients were assessed in the supine position on global PEEP and then reintubated with a DLT and placed in the lateral decubitus position. PEEP was applied to the dependent lung and no PEEP to the nondependent lung. Both groups reported improved oxygenation, and Diaz-Reganon Valverde et al [211] reported a good response in 83% of patients.

ILV is difficult and labor-intensive to apply.[208] Accordingly, it has not gained widespread acceptance for symmetric bilateral lung injury.

Techniques and Problems with ILV

LUNG SEPARATION

Use of ILV must be preceded by the introduction of a DLT or alternative device. These must be introduced, correctly positioned, and then tested to demonstrate they have achieved their intended purpose: isolation of lung ventilation.

The preferred DLT is the PVC type (e.g., Mallinckrodt, Sheridan, Rusch, Concord, Portex, and Marraro; see Fig. 26-1). These DLTs are more flexible, have better internal-external diameter ratios, better gas-flow characteristics, and easier suction and bronchoscopy access,[87] allow airway seal with lower cuff pressures,[212] are less irritating to respiratory mucosa, have a lower risk of trauma, and are easier and quicker to position[213] compared with their red-rubber counterparts.[3–5] Despite this airway injury from PVC DLTs still may occur.[214,215]

For most indications, a left DLT (see Fig. 26-1B) should be used because placement is easier and less critical than with a right DLT, which has a high risk of right upper-lobe occlusion.[216] A right DLT (see Fig. 26-1A) is required for thoracic surgical procedures that include the left main bronchus (left pneumonectomy, left main bronchial lesions, stenosis, or rupture), thoracic aortic aneurysm repair, or anatomic abnormalities that prevent satisfactory access to the left main bronchus[12,13,217] A right DLT is also required for ILV with a recent left SLT to avoid injury to the anastomosis and distal airway. To minimize airflow resistance and maximize endobronchial access, the largest DLT that will not cause laryngeal or airway injury should be chosen (see Table 26-3).

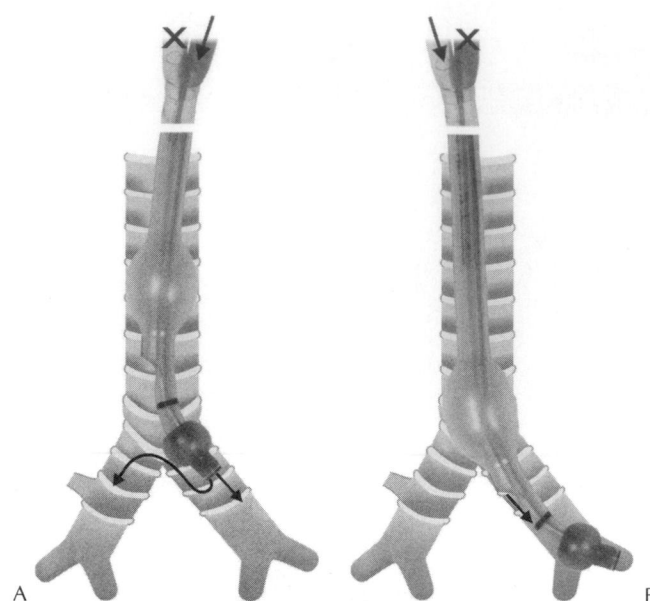

FIGURE 26-4 Flow patterns that may occur during auscultatory verification of a left DLT position (*A*) when DLT is insufficiently inserted and the left lumen is ventilated (right lumen clamped) and (*B*) when DLT is inserted too far and the right lumen is ventilated (left lumen clamped).

PVC DLTs usually are introduced with the endobronchial curvature angled anteriorly and a rigid stylet in situ to facilitate passage of the tip through the vocal cords. Once through the cords, the stylet is removed and the DLT is rotated through 90° so that the endobronchial curvature is directed toward the appropriate side. The tube then is advanced until an increase in resistance is detected.

DLT tube position and function then must be confirmed by one or more of three techniques:

1. *Auscultation.* Following cuff inflation, the tracheal port should be clamped and the bronchial port ventilated.[12] Bilateral or contralateral breath sounds indicate incorrect placement and the need to reposition the tubes (Fig. 26-4A), whereas breath sounds heard only on the correct side indicate correct placement (see Fig. 26-1). Difficulty with ventilation should be resolved by deflating the bronchial cuff: Bilateral breath sounds indicate that placement is too proximal (see Fig 26-4A), whereas breath sounds heard only on the side of the endobronchial tube indicate that placement is too distal (see Fig. 26-4B). Lung auscultation always should include both upper and lower lobes to ensure correct placement of the endobronchial port within the bronchus, especially with a right DLT, with which the right upper lobe is occluded easily.

2. *Bronchoscopy.* Following DLT insertion, a small fiberoptic bronchoscope may be passed through the tracheal lumen to confirm position of the tracheal port and that the endobronchial tube is in the correct position.[12,218] The endobronchial cuff should be visible just distal to the carina. Subsequent insertion of the bronchoscope down the endobronchial lumen may be used to confirm that

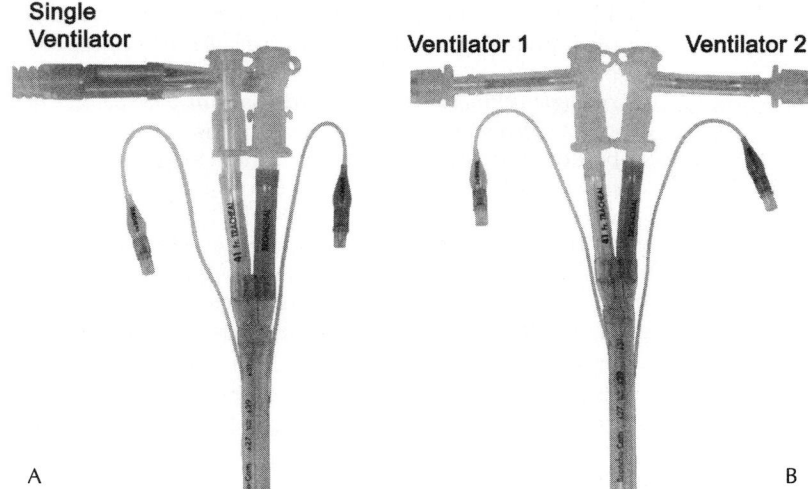

**Single
Ventilator**

Ventilator 1   **Ventilator 2**

A   B

FIGURE 26-5 (A) Both lumens of a double-lumen tube connected to a single ventilator airway. (B) Each lumen of a double-lumen tube connected to separate ventilators.

endobronchial placement is not too distal and that, with right DLTs, the right upper-lobe bronchus is over the corresponding fenestration. Although not essential for DLT placement, bronchoscopy reliably confirms accurate placement and should be used routinely. It has an advantage with anatomic variations and in detecting partial airway occlusions.[216]

3. *Leak test.* While ventilating one lung, a connection to the second airway can be placed under water. Any bubbling indicates air leak from the ventilated lung to the opposite side. Such leaks may not be detected by auscultation or bronchoscopy and may be important, particularly when one of the goals is to protect one lung against fluid (whole-lung lavage, blood, or purulent secretions) from the other lung. Bubbling may indicate the need for tube repositioning or higher bronchial-cuff inflation.

Chest x-ray may be used to visualize DLT position but is insufficient to verify critical tube placement or functional isolation.

DLTs may be connected to a single ventilator (e.g., for hemoptysis or at the beginning and end of whole-lung lavage; Fig. 26-5*A*) or connected to two separate ventilators (see Fig. 26-5*B*).

Bronchial blocking techniques and selective endobronchial intubation are alternatives to a DLT. The right or left main bronchus may be blocked by placement of a balloon-tipped catheter into that bronchus. This allows OLV and is suitable for thoracic surgery, bleeding, or fistula control. The catheter (Arndt endobronchial blocker, Magill blocker, Cohen Flexitip Endobronchial Blocker, Fogarty or Foley catheter)[93,94,186,219,220] may be placed outside or within a standard cuffed ETT lumen or passed down a specially designed second small lumen in the ETT (Univent tube).[15–17] A Univent tube (Fig. 26-6) has a coudé-tipped bronchial blocker that allows blind guidance of the blocker into the desired bronchus with auscultatory confirmation of correct positioning. Bronchoscopic confirmation of best position within the airway, however, is still recommended. In addition, the Univent's axial-blocker shaft has a

lumen that allows irrigation, suction, O_2 insufflation, CPAP, and high-frequency ventilation.[16] The Arndt endobronchial blocker[93,94,219] (Fig. 26-7) requires bronchoscopic guidance for placement. The kit comes with an ETT adaptor that allows access for mechanical ventilation, the blocker, and the bronchoscope through separate ports (see Fig. 26-7). The bronchoscope is passed into the airway that requires blocking, and the blocker is then guided into that airway via a snare over the bronchoscope (see Fig. 26-7*A*). The bronchoscope then is withdrawn, the balloon is inflated, and its position is confirmed by bronchoscopy before withdrawal (see Fig. 26-7*B*). This has the advantage of being performed via the ETT in situ, thereby avoiding reintubation, provided that the ETT is sufficiently large to admit both the blocker

FIGURE 26-6 The Univent tube with the balloon inflated in the left main bronchus.

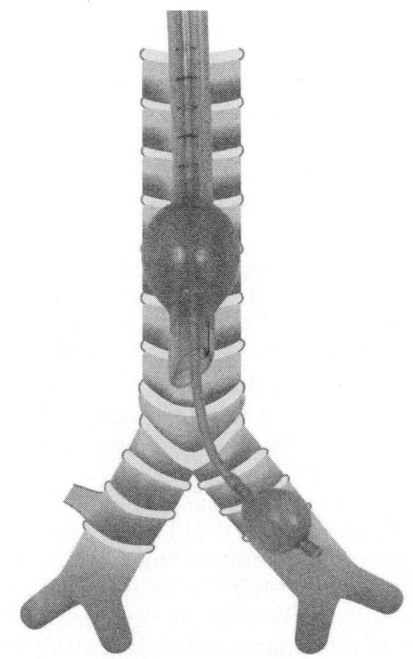

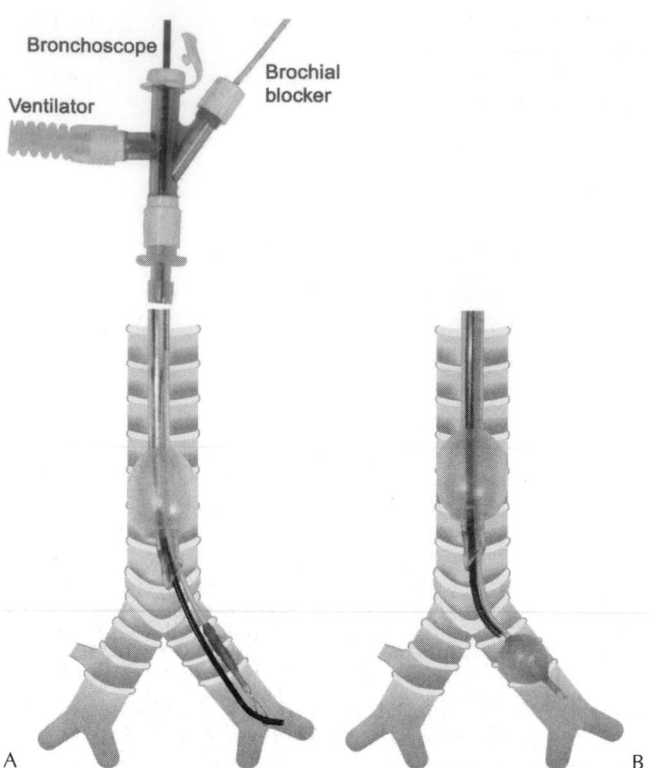

Bronchoscope

Brochial blocker

Ventilator

A   B

FIGURE 26-7 The Arndt endobronchial blocker shown (*A*) during bronchoscope guidance into the left main bronchus and (*B*) after partial bronchoscope withdrawal and balloon inflation, with the bronchoscope remaining to check balloon position.

and the available bronchoscope. The Cohen Flexitip Endobronchial Blocker[220] has a flexible tip that can be guided under bronchoscopy but independently of the bronchoscope.

TECHNIQUES FOR ILV

Several techniques have been reported.

SYNCHRONIZED ILV (SILV)

SILV consists of synchronous initiation of inspiration into each lung. Each lung necessarily must have the same respiratory rate but can have different V_T, PEEP, and inspiratory flow. SILV may be achieved by a variety of techniques.

1. *Two ventilators of the same type linked to cycle synchronously.* This may be achieved by electronically "slaving" the rate control of a second ventilator to a primary ("master") ventilator.[22,23,26,28,29,126,145,151,211,216] Alternatively, synchronization may be achieved by the rate of two ventilators being electronically controlled by an external device[132,162] or by manually resetting the respiratory cycle on paired ventilators and relying on accurate internal timing devices to maintain synchronization.[148,221] This method allows different V_T, PEEP, inspiratory flow, and hence inspiratory/expiratory time (T_I/T_E) combinations.
   Another form of SILV is one in which the lungs are ventilated alternately with the two ventilators synchronized 180° out of phase with each other.[222,223] Although

successful in animals, this technique holds no advantages over other forms of ILV, and its use has not been reported in humans.

2. *A single ventilator linked to a twin circuit with devices that create different flows into each circuit.* This may be achieved by flow dividing: Variable resistances are placed in each inspiratory line, which divide inspiratory flow from the ventilator in a variable manner.[39,131,224] Since the flow (and hence volume) that each lung receives will be determined both by the resistance in the circuit and by impedance in the lung, V_T must be measured independently in each circuit and resistance adjusted accordingly. Gallagher et al[133,136] described an alternative to this technique by placing flow controllers in both inspiratory lines. V_T delivered to each lung was simply the product of set flow in each circuit and inspiratory time. Separate PEEP in each circuit was achieved by expiratory flow controllers. This method allows different V_T and PEEP to each lung but necessarily must have the same T_I/T_E.

3. *A single ventilator linked to two circuits, each with a separate PEEP valve or other PEEP-generating device.*[150,225] This arrangement allows different PEEP to each lung. The division of V_T between the lungs is not controlled independently, being determined by both the relative inherent impedance of each lung and the effect of PEEP on that impedance.

4. *A single ventilator linked to two circuits with no attempt to influence the distribution of ventilation..*[87] This method generally is used during selective airway protection. The division of V_T between the two lungs is determined solely by their relative impedance.

While many indications for ILV are suited to having the same ventilator rate to each lung, there is usually no particular benefit for exact coordination of two ventilators. The only exception may be the uncommon circumstance where patient-triggered ventilation is attempted.

ASYNCHRONOUS ILV (AILV)

AILV consists of completely independent ventilator techniques applied to each lung. It requires two separate ventilation devices. Options include

1. *Controlled or intermittent mechanical ventilation to both lungs (CMV, IMV)*[10,38,40,123–125,128,149,157,163]
2. *CMV or IMV to one lung and HFJV to the other*[41,42,124,127,160]
3. *CMV or IMV to one lung and CPAP to the other*[9,40,124,159]
4. *High-frequency oscillatory ventilation to both lungs*[147]

AILV permits different rate, V_T, inspiratory flow, and PEEP to each lung. Lack of synchronization between the two lungs offers the greatest flexibility and appears to hold no disadvantage and a number of advantages compared with SILV.[38,157]

ONE-LUNG VENTILATION (OLV)

With OLV, one lung is ventilated mechanically while the other is either occluded or open to atmosphere with an option of spontaneous ventilation. OLV is used mainly in thoracic surgery to keep the lung collapsed and immobile. It also may be used in BPF to prevent air leak or for selective airway protection if secretions from the affected lung prevent any useful ventilation (e.g., massive haemoptysis). Options include

1. *Intubation with DLT, and CMV applied to only one lumen.*[11,13,19,25,217,226]
2. *Endotracheal intubation with a bronchial blocker inserted into one of the major bronchi.* The occlusive balloon excludes that lung from mechanical ventilation, and the blocker lumen allows deflation (and inflation) of that lung.[1,13,15,93,94,219]
3. *Endobronchial intubation with a single-lumen tube* (e.g., Mackintosh-Leatherdale left endobronchial tube and Gordon Green right endobronchial tube).[13]

SPONTANEOUS VENTILATION

Spontaneous ventilation with a DLT and differential CPAP applied to each lung was first reported by Venus et al.[227] It has been used in spontaneously breathing patients with unilateral pulmonary contusion and atelectasis with good results.[144,227] It is not recommended because of increased work of breathing through a long, narrow tube.

PROBLEMS WITH ILV

Many of the problems with ILV are related to the DLT. The technique of DLT placement and verifying its correct position is complex, time-consuming, and requires experienced personnel.[12,13,213,218] These considerations can limit the use of DLTs and ILV when required urgently or under adverse circumstances, such as massive hemoptysis.[88,91]

Trauma of the larynx and upper airways was a common problem with red-rubber tubes[12,58] but is uncommon with PVC tubes.[213,228,229] Rare complications have included cardiovascular collapse after a DLT displaced a mediastinal tumor into the mediastinal vessels[230] and exsanguination following inclusion of the DLT in sutures during pneumonectomy with subsequent vessel laceration when the DLT was removed.[231,232]

Placement of right DLTs is critical with respect to right upper-lobe ventilation. Benumof et al[233] estimated a right upper-lobe occlusion rate of 11% with PVC tubes. McKenna et al[216] assessed occlusion of the right upper lobe by bronchoscopy: Occlusion was 89% with Mallinckrodt PVC DLTs and only 10% with right Robertshaw red-rubber DLTs. This has become an uncommon problem now that most DLT insertions are assessed routinely by bronchoscopy. Left upper-lobe occlusion also has been reported[234,235] with left PVC DLTs from overinsertion, wedging the tip of the DLT in the left lower-lobe bronchus. Saito et al[236] found 27 ± 6 mm movement of the tip of a left DLT, proximally with neck extension and distally with flexion, with a total potential range of movement of up to 4.5–7 cm. This range of movement is sufficient to either occlude the left upper-lobe bronchus or lose lung isolation. Similar problems are more likely with a right DLT, with which tube position is more critical.

High cuff pressures are a significant problem with DLTs. In routinely placed tubes with cuffs inflated to avoid air leak, bronchial cuff pressures were 56 ± 21 mmHg in left

TABLE 26-5 Polyvinyl chloride double-lumen tubes: choice of size

Tube Size (French)	Circumference (mm)	Lumen Diameter (mm)	Use
28	—	—	Children <40 kg
35	38	50	Children >40 kg
37	40	55	Small adult
39	44	60	Medium adults, usual female size
41	45	65	Large adult, usual male size

SOURCE: Adapted from Burton NA[229].

PVC DLTs and 130 ± 41 mmHg in Carlens tubes.[212,237] This study suggests a considerably lower risk to the airway from PVC tubes, although the pressures required to prevent leaks still were well above safe limits.

Bronchial rupture was reported regularly[229,238–243] and there is one report of bronchial stenosis[143] with red-rubber tubes. Bronchial rupture is uncommon with PVC DLTs, although they are not free of this complication[229,231,244] (Table 26-5).

Although lumen diameter has improved considerably with PVC tubes, difficult suction access, retained secretions,[43,125,132,148] and lumen blockage remain a problem and can lead to difficult ventilation, the need for regular bronchoscopic toilet, and the need to change the DLT.[87]

When ILV is continued for some time, several difficulties related to patient care arise. Head movement, patient movement, and routine patient turning all threaten DLT position and can lead to loss of lung isolation and lobe occlusion.[43,125,148,236] Frequent bronchoscopy may be required to maintain DLT position.[148,229] Running two ventilators requires additional space, O$_2$, air and, suction outlets, and standard patient charts usually are inadequate.[125] There are significant increases in nursing time requirement and workload,[125,245,246] and the patient may find the DLT more uncomfortable and restrictive than normal intubation.[43]

Conclusion

ILV has been used in a wide range of conditions (see Table 26-1). Although ILV is required infrequently, AILV can be undertaken with any ventilator and used for all indications. ILV has an established and occasional lifesaving role for many conditions. Users of mechanical ventilation must be familiar with the complexities of ILV so that it can be instigated promptly and appropriately when the need arises.

References

1. Magill I. Anaesthesia in thoracic surgery, with special reference to lobectomy. Proc R Soc Med 1936; 19:643–53.
2. Moody J, Trent J, Newton G. An endobronchial balloon for the control of bronchial secretions during lobectomy and pneumonectomy. J Thoracic Surg 1947; 16:258.

3. Carlens E. A new flexible double-lumen tube for bronchospirometry. J Thorac Surg 1949; 18:742–6.

4. White G. A new double-lumen endobronchial tube. Br J Anaesth 1960; 32:232.

5. Robertshaw F. Low resistance double lumen endobronchial tubes. Br J Anaesth 1962; 34:576.

6. Moody J. Endobronchial occlusion during pulmonary resection. J Thoracic Surg 1949; 18:82.

7. Moody J. A method of bronchial occlusion for the prevention of transbronchial spread during lobectomy and pneumonectomy: Clinical application. J Thoracic Surg 1948; 17:681.

8. Trew F, Warren B, Potter W. Differential ventilation in the lungs of man. Crit Care Med 1976; 4:112.

9. Glass D, Tonnesen A, Gabel J, Arens J. Therapy of unilateral pulmonary insufficiency with a double lumen endotracheal tube. Crit Care Med 1976; 4:323–6.

10. Hartenauer U, Wendt M, Lawin P, Reinhold P. Treatment of unilateral pulmonary insufficiency with differential ventilation via a double lumen tube (abstract). Crit Care Med 1982; 9:189.

11. Alfery D, Benumof J, Spragg R. Anesthesia for bronchopulmonary lavage. In: Kaplan J, editor. Thoracic anaesthesia. New York: Churchill-Livingstone, 1983: 403–19.

12. Strange C. Double-lumen endotracheal tubes. Clin Chest Med 1991; 12:497–506.

13. Wilson R. Endobronchial Intubation. In: Kaplan J, editor. Thoracic anesthesia. New York: Churchill-Livingstone, 1983: 371–88.

14. Neidhardt A. Prevention of early respiratory complications in esophageal surgery by ventilation of the independent lung. Can Anaesthesiol 1984; 32:613–6.

15. Scheller M, Kriett J, Smith C, Jamieson S. Airway management during anesthesia for double-lung transplantation using a single-lumen endotracheal tube with an enclosed bronchial blocker. J Cardiothorac Vasc Anaesth 1992; 6:204–7.

16. Gayes J. Pro: One-lung ventilation is best accomplished with the Univent endotracheal tube. J Cardiothorac Vasc Anaesth 1993; 7:103–7.

17. Inoue H, Shotsu A, Ogawa J, et al. New device for one-lung anesthesia: Endotracheal tube with movable blocker. J Thorac Cardiovasc Surg 1982; 83:940–1.

18. Benumof J. Physiology of the lateral decubitous position, the open chest, and one lung ventilation. In: Kaplan J, editor. Thoracic anesthesia. New York: Churchill-Livingstone, 1983: 193–221.

19. Benumof J. One lung ventilation: Which lung should be PEEPed? Anesthesiology 1982; 56:161–3.

20. Rehder K, Wenthe F, Sessler A. Function of each lung during mechanical ventilation with ZEEP and with PEEP in a man anesthetized with thiopental-meperidine. Anesthesiology 1973; 39:597–606.

21. Wulff K, Aulin I. The regional lung function in the lateral decubitus position during anesthesia and operation. Acta Anaesthesiol Scand 1972; 16:195–205.

22. Hedenstierna G, Baehrendtz S, Klingstedt C, et al. Ventilation and perfusion of each lung during differential ventilation with selective PEEP. Anesthesiology 1984; 61:369–76.

23. Baehrendtz S, Bindslev L, Hedenstierna G, Santesson J. Selective PEEP in acute bilateral lung disease: Effect on patients in the lateral posture. Acta Anaesthesiol Scand 1983; 27:311–7.

24. Nunn J. The distribution of inspired gas during thoracic surgery. Ann R Coll Surg Engl 1961; 28:223–37.

25. Slinger P, Suissa S, Adam J, Triolet W. Predicting arterial oxygenation during one-lung ventilation with continuous positive airway pressure to the nonventilated lung. J Cardiothorac Anesth 1990; 4:436–40.

26. Baehrendtz S, Santesson J, Bindslev L, et al. Differential ventilation in acute bilateral lung disease: Influence on gas exchange and central haemodynamics. Acta Anaesthesiol Scand 1983; 27:270–4.

27. Cohen E, Eisenkraft J, Thys D, et al. Oxygenation and hemodynamic changes during one-lung ventilation: Effects of CPAP 10, PEEP 10, and CPAP 10/PEEP 10. J Cardiovasc Anesth 1988; 2:34–40.

28. Baehrendtz S, Klingstedt C. Differential ventilation and selective PEEP during anaesthesia in the lateral decubital posture. Acta Anaesthesiol Scand 1984; 28:252–9.

29. Baehrendtz S, Hedenstierna G. Differential ventilation and selective positive end-expiratory pressure: Effects on patients with acute bilateral lung disease. Anesthesiology 1984; 61:511–7.

30. Brown D, Kafer E, Roberson V, et al. Improved oxygenation during thoracotomy with selective PEEP to the dependent lung. Anesth Analg 1977; 56:26–31.

31. Katz J, Laverne R, Fairley H, Thomas A. Pulmonary oxygen exchange during endobronchial anesthesia: Effects of tidal volume and PEEP. Anesthesiology 1982; 56:164–71.

32. Capan L, Turdorf H, Chandrakant P, et al. Optimization of arterial oxygenation during one lung anesthesia. Anesth Analg (1980; 59:847–51.

33. Benumof J, Rogers S, Moyce P, et al. Hypoxic pulmonary vasoconstriction and regional and whole lung PEEP in the dog. Anesthesiology 1979; 51:503–7.

34. Aalto-Setala M, Heinonen J, Salorinne Y. Cardiorespiratory function during thoracic anaesthesia: A comparison of two lung ventilation and one lung ventilation with and without PEEP. Acta Anaesthesiol Scand 1975; 19:287–95.

35. Khanam T, Branthwaite M. Arterial oxygenation during one lung anaesthesia, part 2. Anaesthesia 1973; 28:280–90.

36. Tarhan S, Lundborg R. Effects of increased expiratory pressure on blood gas tensions and pulmonary shunting during thoracotomy with use of the Carlens catheter. Can Anaesth Soc J 1970; 17:4–11.

37. Valenza F, Ronzoni G, Perrone L, et al. Positive end-expiratory pressure applied to the dependent lung during one-lung ventilation improves oxygenation and respiratory mechanics in patients with high FEV_1. Eur J Anaesthesiol 2004; 21:938–43.

38. Hillman K, Barber J. Asynchronous independent lung ventilation (AILV). Crit Care Med 1990; 8:390–5.

39. Carvalho P, Thompson W, Riggs R, et al. Management of bronchopleural fistula with a variable-resistance valve and a single ventilator. Chest 1997; 111:1452–4.

40. Feeley T, Keating D, Nishimura T. Independent lung ventilation using high-frequency ventilation in the management of bronchopleural fistula. Anesthesiology 1988; 69:420–2.

41. Crimi G, Candiani A, Conti G, et al. Clinical applications of independent lung ventilation with unilateral high-frequency jet ventilation (ILV-UHFJV). Intensive Care Med 1986; 12:90–4.

42. Benjaminsson E, Klain M. Intraoperative dual-mode independent lung ventilation of a patient with bronchopleural fistula. Anesth Analg 1981; 60:118–9.

43. Rafferty T, Palma J, Motoyama E, et al. Management of a bronchopleural fistula with differential lung ventilation and PEEP. Respir Care 1980; 25:654–7.

44. Rosen S, Castleman B, Liebow A. Pulmonary alveolar proteinosis. New Engl J Med 1958; 258:1123–42.

45. Smith L, Ankin M, Katzenstein A, et al. Management of pulmonary alveolar proteinosis. Chest 1980; 78:765–70.

46. Kao D, Wasserman K, Costley D, et al. Advances in the treatment of pulmonary alveolar proteinosis. Am Rev Respir Dis 1975; 111:361–3.

47. Farca A, Maher G, Miller A. Pulmonary alveolar proteinosis. JAMA 1973; 224:1283–5.

48. Ramirez R. Alveolar proteinosis: Importance of pulmonary lavage. Am Rev Respir Dis 1971; 103:666–78.

49. Ramirez R, Obenour W. Bronchopulmonary lavage in asthma and chronic bronchitis: Clinical and physiologic observations. Chest 1971; 59:146–52.

50. Wasserman K, Blank N, Fletcher G. Lung lavage (alveolar washing) in alveolar proteinosis. Am J Med 1968; 44:611–4.

51. Ramirez R. Pulmonary alveolar proteinosis: Treatment by massive bronchopulmonary lavage. Arch Intern Med 1967; 119:147–55.

52. Ramirez R, Kieffer R, Ball W. Bronchopulmonary lavage in man. Ann intern Med 1965; 63:819–28.

53. Ramirez R. Pulmonary alveolar proteinosis: A roentgenologic analysis. AJR 1964; 92:571–7.

54. Seymour J, Presneill J. Pulmonary alveolar proteinosis: Progress in the first 44 years. Am J Respir Crit Care Med 2002; 166: 215–35.

55. Trapnell B, Whitsett J, Nakata K. Pulmonary alveolar proteinosis. New Engl J Med 2003; 349:2527–39.

56. Reechaipichitkul W, Latong S. Etiology and treatment outcomes of massive hemoptysis. Southeast Asian J Trop Med Public Health 2005; 36:474–80.

57. Rogers R, Szidon J, Shelburne J, et al. Hemodynamic response of the pulmonary circulation to bronchopulmonary lavage in man. New Engl J Med 1972; 286:1230–3.

58. Thompson H, Pryor W, Hill J. Bronchial lavage in the treatment of obstructive lung disease. Thorax 1966; 21:557.

59. Millman M, Goodman A, Goldstein I, et al. Status asthmaticus: Use of acetylcysteine during bronchoscopy and lavage to remove mucous plugs. Ann Allergy 1983; 50:85–93.

60. Nariman S, Bell H. Bronchopulmonary lavage in the treatment of chronic asthma. Br J Hosp Med 1975:170–2.

61. Williams N. Bronchial lavage in asthma. Postgrad Med J 1971; 47:188–9.

62. Rogers R, Tatum K. Bronchopulmonary lavage: A "new" approach to old problems. Med Clin North Am 1970; 54:755–71.

63. Rausch D, Spick A, Kylstra J. Lung lavage in cystic fibrosis. Am Rev Respir Dis 1970; 101:1006.

64. Muggenberg B, McWhinney J, Slavson D. The removal of 239 Pu from beagle dogs by bronchopulmonary lavage and chelation therapy. Health Phys 1976; 31:315–21.

65. Kylstra J, Rausch D, Hall K. Volume controlled lung lavage in the treatment of asthma, bronchiectasis, mucoviscidosis. Am Rev Respir Dis 1971; 103:651–65.

66. Rogers R, Kuhl D, Hyde R, Mayock R. Measurement of the vital capacity and perfusion of each lung by fluoroscopy and microaggregated albumin scanning: An alternative to bronchospirometry for evaluating individual lung function. Ann Intern Med 1967; 67:947–56.

67. Claypool W, Rogers R, Matuschak G. Update on the clinical diagnosis, management, and pathogenesis of pulmonary alveolar proteinosis (phospholipidosis). Chest 1984; 85:550–8.

68. Alfrey D, Zamost B, Benumof J. Unilateral lung lavage: Blood flow manipulation by ipsilateral pulmonary artery balloon inflation. Anesthesiology 1981; 55:376–81.

69. Seidman J, Sasahara A. Bronchopulmonary lavage. J Med 1972; 236:23.

70. Smith J, Miller J, Safer P. Intrathoracic pressure, pulmonary vascular pressures and gas exchange during pulmonary lavage. Anesthesiology 1970; 33:401–5.

71. Kim K, Kim J, Kim Y. Use of extracorporeal membrane oxygenation (ECMO) during whole lung lavage in pulmonary alveolar proteinosis associated with lung cancer. Eur J Cardiothorac Surg 2004; 26:1050–1.

72. Cai H-R, Cui S-Y, Jin L, et al. Pulmonary alveolar proteinosis treated with whole-lung lavage utilizing extracorporeal membrane oxygenation: A case report and review of literatures. Chin Med J 2004; 117:1746–9.

73. Cohen E, Elpern E, Silver M. Pulmonary alveolar proteinosis causing severe hypoxemic respiratory failure treated with sequential whole-lung lavage utilizing venovenous extracorporeal membrane oxygenation: A case report and review. Chest 2001; 120:1024–6.

74. Cooper J, Duffin J, Glynn M. Combination of membrane oxygenator support and pulmonary lavage for acute respiratory failure. J Thorac Cardiovasc Surg 1976; 71:304–8.

75. Altose M, Hicks R, Edwards M. Extracorporeal membrane oxygenation during bronchopulmonary lavage. Arch Surg 1976; 111:1148–53.

76. Vast C, Demonet B, Mouveroux J. Value of selective pulmonary lavage under fiberoptic control in alveolar proteinosis. Poumon Coeur 1978; 34:305–7.

77. Brach B, Harrell J, Moser K. Alveolar proteinosis: Lobar lavage by fiberoptic bronchoscopic technique. Chest 1976; 69: 224–7.

78. Nadeau M, Cote D, Bussieres J. The combination of inhaled nitric oxide and pulmonary artery balloon inflation improves oxygenation during whole-lung lavage. Anesth Analg 2004; 99: 676–9.

79. Beccaria M, Luisetti M, Rodi G, et al. Long-term durable benefit after whole lung lavage in pulmonary alveolar proteinosis. Eur Respir J 2004; 23:526–31.

80. Strollo P. Hemoptysis. In: Civetta J, Taylor R, Kirby R, editors. Critical care. Philadelphia: Lippincott, 1988 :1127–32.

81. Crocco J, Rooney J, Fankhusen D, et al. Massive hemoptysis. Arch Intern Med 1968; 121:495–98.

82. Hassine E, Marniche K, Bousnina S, et al. Management of massive hemoptysis: Current role of interventional endoscopy. Tunis Med 2003; 81:94–100.

83. Laplace C, Martin L, Sachet M, et al. Lung separation after reintubation with airway exchange catheter in multiple trauma patient with massive haemoptysis. Ann Fr Anaesth Reanim 2004; 23:920–4.

84. Yoon W, Kim J, Kim Y, et al. Bronchial and nonbronchial systemic artery embolization for life-threatening hemoptysis: A comprehensive review. Radiographics 2002; 22:1395–409.

85. Abreu A, Campos M, Krieger B. Pulmonary artery rupture induced by a pulmonary artery catheter: A case report and review of the literature. J Intensive Care Med 2004; 19:291–6.

86. Hannan A, Brown M, Bigman O, et al. Pulmonary artery catheter-induced hemorrhage. Chest 1984; 85:128.

87. Shivaram U, Finch P, Nowak P. Plastic endobronchial tubes in the management of life-threatening hemoptysis. Chest 1987; 92:1108–9.

88. Conlan A. Massive hemoptysis: Diagnosis and therapeutic implications. Surg Ann 1985; 17:337–54.

89. Wolfe J, Simmons D. Hemoptysis: Diagnosis and management. West J Med 1977; 127:383.

90. Conlan A, Hurwitz S, Krige L, et al. Massive hemoptysis: Review of 123 cases. J. Thorac Cardiovasc Surg 1983; 85:120.

91. Garzon A, Cennuti N, Golding M. Exsanguinating hemoptysis. J Thorac Cardiovasc Surg 1982; 84:829–33.

92. Lee S, Kim H, Ahn Y. Parallel technique of endobronchial balloon catheter tamponade for transient alleviation of massive hemoptysis. J Korean Med Sci 2002; 17:823–5.

93. Arndt G, Kranner P, Rusy D, Love R. Single-lung ventilation in a critically ill patient using a fiberoptically directed wire-guided endobronchial blocker. Anesthesiology 1999; 90:1484–6.

94. Arndt G, DeLessio S, Kranner P, et al. One-lung ventilation when intubation is difficult: Presentation of a new endobronchial blocker. Acta Anaesthesiol Scand 1999; 43:356–8.

95. Bobrowitz I, Ramakrishna S, Shim Y, et al. Comparison of mecical vs surgical treatment of major hemoptysis. Arch Intern Med 1983; 143:1343.

96. Kato R, Sawafuji M, Kawamura M, et al. Massive hemoptysis successfully treated by modified bronchoscopic balloon tamponade technique. Chest 1996; 109:842–3.

97. Ayed A. Pulmonary resection for massive hemoptysis of benign etiology. Eur J Cardiothorac Surg 2003; 24:689–93.

98. Ong T, Eng P. Massive hemoptysis requiring intensive care. Intensive Care Med 2003; 29:317–20.

99. Imgrund S, Goldberg S, Walkenstein M, et al. Clinical diagnosis of massive hemoptysis using the fiberoptic bronchoscope. Crit Care Med 1985; 13:438.

100. Karmy-Jones R, Cuschieri J, Vallieres E. Role of bronchoscopy in massive hemoptysis. Chest Surg Clin North Am 2001; 11:873–906.

101. Conlan A, Hurwitz S. Management of massive haemoptysis with the rigid bronchoscope and cold saline lavage. Thorax 1980; 35:901.

102. Brenner B. Comprehensive management of respiratory emergencies. Rockville MD: Aspen Systems Corp, 1985.

103. Miller R, Nelson L, Rutherford E, Morris JJ. Synchronized independent lung ventilation in the management of a unilateral pulmonary contusion with massive hemoptysis. J Tenn Med Assoc 1992; 374–5.

104. Mossi F, Maroldi R, Battaglia G, et al. Indicators predictive of success of embolisation: Analysis of 88 patients with haemoptysis. Radiol Med (Torino) 2003; 105:48–55.

105. Lee T, Wan S, Choy D, et al. Management of massive hemoptysis: A single-institution experience. Ann Thorac Cardiovasc Surg 2000; 6:232–5.

106. Uflacker R, Kaemmerer A, Picon P, et al. Bronchial artery embolization in the management of hemoptysis: Technical aspects and long term results. Radiology 1985; 157:637.

107. Endo S, Otani S, Saito N, et al. Management of massive hemoptysis in a thoracic surgical unit. Eur J Cardiothorac Surg 2003; 23:467–72.

108. Bjork V, Carlens E. The prevention of spread during pulmonary resection by the use of a double-lumen catheter. J Thorac Surg 1950; 20:151–7.

109. Pfitzner J, Peacock M, Tsirgiotis E, Walkley I. Lobectomy for cavitating lung abscess with haemoptysis: Strategy for protecting the contralateral lung and also the non-involved lobe of the ipsilateral lung. Br J Anaesth 2000; 85:791–4.

110. Moerer O, Heuer J, Benken I, et al. Blunt chest trauma with total rupture of the right main stem bronchus: A case report. Anaesthesiol Reanim 2004; 29:12–5.

111. Wichert A, Bittersohl J, Lukasewitz P, et al. Intra- and postoperative airway management of tracheal carina ruptures from bilateral endobronchial intubation. Anasthesiol Intensivmed Notfallmed Schmerzther 1999; 34:678–83.

112. Wulf H, Elfeldt R, Huckstadt A. Diagnosis and therapy of tracheal rupture after blunt thoracic trauma. Anasthesiol Intensivmed Notfallmed Schmerzther 1997; 32:258–62.

113. Pizov R, Shir Y, Eimerl D, et al. One-lung high-frequency ventilation in the management of traumatic tear of bronchus in a child. Crit Care Med 1987; 15:1160–1.

114. Baumann M, Sahn S. Medical management and therapy of bronchopleural fistulas in the mechanically ventilated patient. Chest 1990; 97:721–8.

115. Pierson D, Horton C, Bates P. Persistent bronchopleural air leak during mechanical ventilation. Chest 1986; 90:321–3.

116. Phillips Y, Lonigan R, Joyner L. A simple technique for managing a bronchopleural fistula while maintaining positive pressure ventilation. Crit Care Med 1979; 7:351–3.

117. Katsaragakis S, Stamou K, Androulakis G. Independent lung ventilation for asymmetrical chest trauma: Effect on ventilatory and haemodynamic parameters. Injury 2005; 36:501–4.

118. Dedrick D, Brown L, Mapel D. A 47-year-old woman with wheezing and respiratory failure unresponsive to conventional ventilatory modalities. Chest 2002; 121:1688-91.

119. Wippermann C, Schranz D, Baum V, Huth R. Independent right lung high frequency and left lung conventional ventilation in the management of severe air leak during ARDS. Paediatr Anaesth 1995; 5:189–92.

120. Pierson D. Management of bronchopleural fistula in the adult respiratory distress syndrome. New Horizons 1993; 1:512–21.

121. Lohse A, Klien W, Hermann E, et al. Pneumatoceles and pneumothoraces complicating staphylococcal pneumonia: Treatment by synchronous independent lung ventilation. Thorax 1993; 48:578–80.

122. Otruba Z, Oxorn D. Lobar bronchial blockade in bronchopleural fistula. Can J Anaesth 1992; 39:176–8.

123. Bonnet R, Wilms D. Langzeitanwendung der asynchronen seitendifferenten Beatmung: Auswirkungen auf Gasaustausch und Hamodynamik. Pneumologie 1990; 44:665–7.

124. Wendt M, Hachenberg T, Winde G, Lawin P. Differential ventilation with low-flow CPAP and CPPV in the treatment of unilateral chest trauma. Intensive Care Med 1989; 15:209–11.

125. de Bruyn G, Prins N, Lipman J. Nursing problems encountered with asynchronous independent lung ventilation. Nurs RSA Verpleg 1987; 2:16–7.

126. Parish J, Gracey D, Southorn P, et al. Differential mechanical ventilation in respiratory failure due to severe lung disease. Mayo Clin Proc 1984; 59:822–8.

127. Mortimer A, Laurie P, Garrett H, Kerr J. Unilateral high frequency jet ventilation. Intensive Care Med 1984; 10:39–41.

128. Dodds C, Hillman K. Management of massive air leak with asynchronous independent lung ventilation. Intensive Care Med 1982; 8:287–90.

129. Carlon G, Ray C, Klein R, et al. Acute life-threatening ventilation-perfusion inequality: An indication for independent lung ventilation. Crit Care Med 1978; 6:380–3.

130. Carlon G, Kahn R, Howland W, et al. Criteria for selecting positive end-expiratory pressure and independent synchronized ventilation of each lung. Chest 1978; 74:501–7.

131. Charan N, Carvalho C, Hawk P, et al. Independent lung ventilation with a single ventilator using a variable resistance valve. Chest 1995; 107:256–60.

132. Frame S, Marshall W, Clifford T. Synchronized independent lung ventilation in the management of pediatric unilateral pulmonary contusion: Case report. J Trauma 1989; 29:395–5.

133. Branson R, Hurst J, DeHaven C. Synchronous independent lung ventilation in the treatment of unilateral pulmonary contusion: A report of two cases. Respir Care 1984; 29:361–7.

134. Zandstra D, Stoutenbeek C. Reflection of differential pulmonary perfusion in polytrauma patients on differential lung ventilation (DLV). Intensive Care Med 1989; 15:151–4.

135. Zandstra D, Stoutenbeek C, van Saene H, Bams J. Selective decontamination of the digestive tract improves survival in patients receiving differential lung ventilation. Intensive Care Med 1988; 15:15–8.

136. Gallagher T, Banner M, Smith R. A simplified method of independent lung ventilation. Crit Care Med 1980; 8:396–9.

137. Powers S, Dutton R. Correlation of PEEP with cardiovascular performance. Crit Care Med 1975; 3:64.

138. Kanarek D, Shannon D. Adverse effect of positive end-expiratory pressure on pulmonary perfusion and arterial oxygenation. Am Rev Respir Dis 1975; 112:457–9.

139. Baeza O, Wagner R, Lowery B, et al. Pulmonary hyperinflation: A form of barotrauma during mechanical ventilation. J Thorac Cardiovasc Surg 1975; 70:790.

140. Powers S, Mannal R, Neclerio M, et al. Physiologic consequences of positive end-expiratory pressure (PEEP) ventilation. Ann Surg 1973; 178:265.

141. Falke K, Pontoppidan H, Kumar A, et al. Ventilation with end-expiratory pressure in acute lung disease. J Clin Invest 1972; 51:2315.

142. Cinnella G, Dambrosio M, Brienza N, et al. Independent lung ventilation in patients with unilateral pulmonary contusion. Monitoring with compliance and $EtCO_2$. Intensive Care Med 2001; 27:1860–7.

143. Evrard C, Pelouze G, Quesnel J. Stenoses iatrogenes tracheale et bronchique gauche: Complication exceptionelle d'une sonde Carlens. Ann Chir Chir Thorac Cardiovasc 1990; 44:149–56.

144. Crimi G, Conti G, Candiani A, et al. Clinical use of differential continuous positive airway pressure in the treatment of unilateral acute lung injury. Intensive Care Med 1987; 15:90–4.

145. Levine D, Carmichael T, Laussen P. Independent lung ventilation in a patient with complex congenital heart disease. Respir Care 2002; 47:688–92.

146. Almodovar M, Laussen P, Roth S. Synchronized independent lung ventilation in palliated congenital heart disease with variable sources of pulmonary blood flow. Pediatr Crit Care Med 2000; 1:79–83.

147. Graciano A, Barton P, Luckett P, et al. Feasibility of asynchronous independent lung high-frequency oscillatory ventilation in the management of acute hypoxemic respiratory failure: A case report. Crit Care Med 2000; 28:3075–7.

148. Nielsen M, Acklin L, Kelly P. Synchronized independent lung ventilation (SILV). Crit Care 1992; 4:6–8.

149. Lev A, Barzilay E, Geber D, et al. Differential lung ventilation: A review and 2 case reports. Resuscitation 1987; 15:77–86.

150. Powner D. Differential lung ventilation with PEEP in the treatment of unilateral pneumonia. Crit Care Med 1977; 4:170–2.

151. Siegel J, Stokkosa J, Borg U, et al. Quantification of asymmetric lung pathophysiology as a guide to the use of simultaneous independent lung ventilation in post-traumatic and septic ARDS. Am Surg 1985; 202:425–39.

152. Badesch D, Zamora M, Jones S, et al. Independent ventilation and ECMO for severe unilateral pulmonary edema after SLT for primary pulmonary hypertension. Chest 1995; 107:1766–70.

153. Zandstra D, Stoutenbeek C. Treatment of massive unilateral pulmonary embolism by differential lung ventilation. Intensive Care Med 1987; 13:422–4.

154. Barbas C, de Matos, GF, Pincelli M, et al. Mechanical ventilation in acute respiratory failure: Recruitment and high positive end-expiratory pressure are necessary. Curr Opin Crit Care 2005; 11:18–28.

155. Ventilation with lower tidal volumes as compared with traditional tidal volumes for acute lung injury and the acute respiratory distress syndrome. The Acute Respiratory Distress Syndrome Network. New Engl J Med 2000; 342:1301–8.

156. Amato M, Barbas C, Medeiros D, et al. Effect of a protective-ventilation strategy on mortality in the acute respiratory distress syndrome. New Engl J Med 1998; 338:347–54.

157. East T, Pace N, Westenskow D. Synchronous versus asynchronous differential lung ventilation with PEEP after unilateral acid aspiration in the dog. Crit Care Med 1983; 11:441–4.

158. Plötz F, Hassing M, Sibarani-Ponsen R, Markhorst D. Differentiated HFO and CMV for independent lung ventilation in a pediatric patient. Intensive Care Med 2003; 29:1855.

159. Narr B, Fromme G, Peters S. Unilateral bronchospasm during pleurodesis in an asthmatic patient. Chest 1990; 98:767–8.

160. Miranda D, Stoutenbeek C, Kingma L. Differential lung ventilation with HFPPV. Intensive Care Med 1981; 7:139–41.

161. Millen J, Vandree J, Glauser F. Fibreoptic bronchoscopic balloon occlusion and reexpansion of refractory unilateral atelectasis. Crit Care Med 1978; 6:50–5.

162. Bochenek K, Brown M, Skupin A. Use of a double-lumen endotracheal tube with independent lung ventilation for treatment of refractory atelectasis. Anesth Analg 1987; 66:1014–7.

163. Smiley R, Navedo A, Kirby T, Schulman L. Postoperative independent lung ventilation in a single-lung transplant recipient. Anesthesiology 1991; 74:1144–8.

164. Patterson G, Maurer J, Williams T, et al. Comparison of outcomes of double and single lung transplantation for obstructive lung disease. J Thorac Cardiovasc Surg 1991; 101:623–32.

165. Veith J, Koerner S, Siegleman S, et al. Single lung transplantation in experimental and human emphysema. Ann Surg 1971; 178:463–76.

166. Vanderhoeft R, Rocmans P, Nemry C, et al. Left lung transplantation in a patient with emphysema. Arch Surg 1971; 103:505–9.

167. Wilevuur R, Benfield J. A review of 23 human lung transplantations by 20 surgeons. Ann Thorac Surg 1970; 9:489–515.

168. Stevens P, Johnson P, Bell R, et al. Regional ventilation and perfusion after lung transplantation in patients with emphysema. New Engl J Med 1970; 282:245–9.

169. Angles R, Tenorio L, Roman A, et al. Lung transplantation for emphysema. Lung hyperinflation: Incidence and outcome. Transplant Int 2005; 17(12):810–814.

170. Hansen L, Ravn J, Yndgaard S. Early extubation after single-lung transplantation: Analysis of the first 106 cases. J Cardiothorac Vasc Anesth 2003; 17:36–9.

171. Mitchell J, Shaw A, Donald S, Farrimond J. Differential lung ventilation after single-lung transplantation for emphysema. J Cardiothorac Vasc Anesth 2002; 16:459–62.

172. Weill D, Torres F, Hodges T, et al. Acute native lung hyperinflation is not associated with poor outcomes after single lung transplant for emphysema. J Heart Lung Transplant 1999; 18:1080–7.

173. Yonan N, el-Gamel A, Egan J, et al. Single lung transplantation for emphysema: Predictors for native lung hyperinflation. J Heart Lung Transplant 1998; 17:192–201.

174. Montoya A, Mawulawde K, Houck J, et al. Survival and functional outcome after single and bilateral lung transplantation. Surgery 1994; 116:712–8.

175. Marinelli W, Hertz M, Shumway S, et al. Single lung transplantation for severe emphysema. J Heart Lung Transplant 1992; 11:577–83.

176. Low D, Trulock E, Kaiser L, et al. Morbidity, mortality, and early results of single versus bilateral lung transplantation for emphysema. J Thorac Cardiovasc Surg 1992; 103:1119–26.

177. Egan T, Westerman J, Lambert C, et al. Isolated lung transplantation for end-stage lung disease: A viable therapy. Ann Thorac Surg 1992; 53:590–6.

178. Kaiser L, Cooper J, Trulock E, et al. The evolution of single lung transplantation for emphysema. J Thorac Cardiovasc Surg 1991; 102:333–41.

179. Weill D, Keshavjee S. Lung transplantation for emphysema: Two lungs or one. J Heart Lung Transplant 2001; 20:739–42.

180. Hosenpud J, Bennett L, Keck B, et al. The Registry of the International Society for Heart and Lung Transplantation: Eighteenth Official Report—2001. J Heart Lung Transplant 2001; 20:805–15.

181. Sundaresan R, Shiraishi Y, Trulock E, et al. Cardiac and pulmonary replacement: Single or bilateral lung transplantation for emphysema? J Thorac Cardiovasc Surg 1996; 112:1485–95.

182. Bando K, Paradis I, Keenan R, et al. Comparison of outcomes after single and bilateral lung transplantation for obstructive lung disease. J Heart Lung Transplant 1995; 14:692–8.

183. Williams T, Patterson G, McClean P, et al. Maximal exercise testing in single and double lung transplant recipients. Am Rev Respir Dis 1992; 145:101–5.

184. Officer T, Wheeler D, Frost A, Rodarte J. Respiratory control during independent lung ventilation. Chest 2001; 120:678–81.

185. Estenne M, Cassart M, Poncelet P, Gevenois P. Volume of graft and native lung after single-lung transplantation for emphysema. Am J Respir Crit Care Med 1999; 159:641–5.

186. Boujoukos A, Keenan R. Use of a bronchial blocker to improve gas exchange in respiratory failure and differential lung disease. Chest 1996; 110:1110–1.

187. Popple C, Higgins T, McCarthy P, et al. Unilateral auto-PEEP in the recipient of a single lung transplant. Chest 1993; 103:297–9.

188. Gavazzeni V, Iapichino G, Mascheroni D, et al. Prolonged independent lung respiratory treatment after single lung transplantation in pulmonary emphysema. Chest 1993; 103:96–100.

189. Zannini P, Baisi A, Melloni G, et al. Single lung transplantation for emphysema lessons learned on the field. Int Surg 1992; 77:28–36.

190. Raffin L, Michel-Cherqui M, Sperandio M, et al. Anesthesia for bilateral lung transplantation without cardiopulmonary bypass: Initial experience and review of intraoperative problems. J Cardiothorac Vasc Anaesth 1992; 6:409–17.

191. Harwood R, Graham T, Kendall S, et al. Use of double-lumen tracheostomy tube after single lung transplantation. J Thorac Cardiovasc Surg 1992; 103:1224–33.

192. Thomas B, Siegel L. Anesthetic and postoperative management of single-lung transplantation. J Cardiothorac Vasc Anesth 1991; 5:266–7.

193. Novick R, Menkis A, Sandler D, et al. Contralateral pneumonectomy after single-lung transplantation for emphysema. Ann Thorac Surg 1991; 52:1317–9.

194. Egan T, Cooper J. Surgical aspects of single lung transplantation. Clin Chest Med 1990; 11:195–205.

195. Trulock E, Egan T, Kouchoukos N, et al. Single lung transplantation for severe chronic obstructive pumonary disease. Chest 1989; 96:738–42.

196. Mal H, Andreassin M, Fabrice P, et al. Unilateral lung transplantation in end-stage pulmonary emphysema. Am Rev Respir Dis 1989; 140:797–802.

197. Tuxen D. Detrimental effects of positive end-expiratory pressure during controlled mechanical ventilation of patients with severe airflow obstruction. Am Rev Respir Dis 1989; 140:5–9.

198. Tuxen D, Lane S. The effects of ventilatory pattern on hyperinflation, airway pressures, and circulation in mechanical ventilation of patients with severe airflow obstruction. Am Rev Respir Dis 1987; 136:872–9.

199. Coe V, Brodsky J, Mark J. Double-lumen endobronchial tubes for patients with tracheostomies. Anesth Analg 1984; 63:882–3.

200. Samanek M, Aviado D, Peskin G. Bronchopulmonary effects of tobacco and related substances. Arch Environ Health 1965; 11:160–6.

201. Gattinoni L, Pesenti A, Torresin A, et al. Adult respiratory distress syndrome profiles by computed tomography. J Thorac Imag 1986; 3:25–30.

202. Gattinoni L, Mascheroni D, Torresin A, et al. Morphological response to positive end-expiratory pressure in acute respiratory failure: Computerized tomography study. Intensive Care Med 1986; 12:137–42.

203. Gattinoni L, Bombino M, Pelosi P, et al. Lung structure and function in different stages of severe adult respiratory distress syndrome. JAMA 1994; 271:1772–9.

204. Dreyfuss D, Saumon G. Ventilator-induced lung injury: Lessons from experimental studies. Am J Respir Crit Care Med 1998; 157:294–323.

205. Webb H, Tierney D. Experimental pulmonary edema due to intermittent positive pressure ventilation with high inflation pressures: Protection by positive end-expiratory pressure. Am Rev Respir Dis 1974; 110:556–65.

206. Ranieri V, Suter P, Tortorella C, et al. Effect of mechanical ventilation on inflammatory mediators in patients with acute respiratory distress syndrome: A randomized, controlled trial. JAMA 1999; 282:54–61.

207. Barbas C, de Matos G, Okamoto V, et al. Lung recruitment maneuvers in acute respiratory distress syndrome. Respir Care Clin North Am 2003; 9:401–18.

208. Wickerts C, Blomqvist H, Baehrendtz S, et al. Clinical application of differential ventilation with selective positive end-expiratory pressure in adult respiratory distress syndrome. Acta Anaesthesiol Scand 1995; 39:307–11.

209. Hedenstierna G, Baehrendtz S, Frostell C, Mebius C. Differential ventilation in acute respiratory failure: Indications and outcome. Bull Eur Physiopathol Respir 1985; 21:281–5.

210. Bindsley L, Santesson J, Hedenstierna G. Distribution of inspired gas to each lung in anesthetized human subjects. Acta Anaesthesiol Scand 1981; 25:297–302.

211. Diaz-Reganon Valverde G, Fernandez-Rico R, Iribarren-Sarrias J, et al. Ventilacion pulmonar independiente sincronizada en el tratamientom del sindrome respiratorio del adulto [Synchronized independent pulmonary ventilation in the treatment of adult respiratory distress syndrome]. Rev Espanol Anestesiol Reanim 1997; 44:392–5.

212. Neto P. Bronchial cuff pressure: Comparison of Carlens and polyvinylchloride (PVC) double lumen tubes. Anesthesiology 1987; 66:255–6.

213. Clapham M, Vaughan R. Bronchial intubation: A comparison between polyvinyl chloride and red rubber double lumen tubes. Anaesthesia 1985; 40:1111–4.

214. Probert D, Hardman J. Failed extubation of a double-lumen tube requiring a cricoid split. Anaesth Intensive Care 2003; 31:584–7.

215. Yuceyar L, Kaynak K, Canturk E, Aykac B. Bronchial rupture with a left-sided polyvinylchloride double-lumen tube. Acta Anaesthesiol Scand 2003; 47:622–5.

216. McKenna M, Wilson R, Botelho R. Right upper lobe obstruction with right-sided double-lumen endobronchial tubes: A comparison of two tube types. J Cardiovasc Anesth 1988; 2:734–40.

217. Benumof J. One lung ventilation and hypoxic pulmonary vasoconstriction. Anesth Analg 1985; 64:821–33.

218. Slinger P. Fiberoptic bronchoscopic positioning of double-lumen tubes. J Cardiothorac Anesth 1989; 3:486–96.

219. Arndt G, Kranner P, Valdes-Mura H. Reversal of hypoxemia using insufflation of oxygen during one-lung ventilation with a wire-guided endobronchial blocker. J Cardiothorac Vasc Anesth 2001; 15:144.

220. Cohen E. Methods of lung separation. Minerva Anestesiol 2004; 70:313.

221. Henk J. SILV comes to the 7200. Progr Notes 1991; 3:15.

222. Reinhold P. Alternierende seitengetrennte Lungenbeatmung. Berlin: Thieme Copytek, 1986.

223. Muneyki M, Konishi K, Horiguchi R, et al. Effects of alternating lung ventilation on cardiopulmonary function in dogs. Anaesthesiology 1983; 58:353–6.

224. Darowski M, Hedenstierna G, Baehrendtz S. Development and evaluation of a flow-dividing unit for differential ventilation and selective PEEP. Acta Anaesthesiol Scand 1985; 29:61–6.

225. Cavanilles J, Garrigosa F, Prieto C, Oncins J. A selective ventilation distribution circuit (SVDC). Intensive Care Med 1979; 5:95.

226. Pawar D, Marraro G. One lung ventilation in infants and children: Experience with Marraro double lumen tube. Paediatr Anaesth 2005; 15:204–8.

227. Venus B, Pratap K, Op'Tholt T. Treatment of unilateral pulmonary insufficiency by selective administration of CPAP through a double-lumen tube. Anaesthesiology 1980; 52: 74–7.

228. Wagner D, Gammage G, Wong M. Tracheal rupture following insertion of a disposable double-lumen endotracheal tube. Anesthesiology 1985; 63:698–700.

229. Burton N, Watson DC, Brodsky J, et al. Advantages of a new polyvinyl chloride double-lumen tube in thoracic surgery. Ann Thorac Surg 1983; 36:78.

230. Wells D, Zelcer J, Podolakin W, et al. Cardiac arrest from pulmonary outflow tract obstruction due to a double-lumen tube. Anesthesiology 1987; 66:422.

231. Scherer R, Reinhold P, Buchholz B. Einseitiges Lungenödem nach Thoraxtrauma: Eine Indikation zur seitendifferenten Beatmung. Anästh Intensivther Notfallmed 1983; 18:65–7.

232. Dryden G. Circulatory collapse after pneumonectomy (an unusual complication from the use of a Carlens catheter): Case report. Anesth Analg 1977; 56:451.

233. Benumof J, Partridge B, Salvatierra C, et al. Margin of safety in positioning modern double-lumen endotracheal tubes. Anesthesiology 1987; 67:729–38.

234. Greene E, Gutierrez F. Tip of polyvinyl chloride double lumen endotracheal tube inadvertently wedged in left lower lobe bronchus. Anaesthesiology 1986; 64:406.

235. Brodsky J, Shulman M, Mark J. Malposition of left-sided double-lumen endobronchial tubes. Anaesthesiology 1985; 62:223.

236. Saito S, Dohi S, Naito H. Alteration in double-lumen endobronchial tube position by flexion and extension of the neck. Anaesthesiology 1985; 62:696–7.

237. Brodsky J, Adkins M, Gaba D. Bronchial cuff pressures of double-lumen tubes. Anesth Analg 1989; 69:608–10.

238. Jooss D, Zeiler D, Muhrer K, Hempelmann G. Die Bronchialruptur. Diagnose und Therapie einer seltenen Komplikation bei der Anwendung von Doppellumentuben. Anaesthetist 1991; 40:291–3.

239. Hannallah M, Gomes M. Bronchial rupture associated with the use of a double-lumen tube in a small adult. Anesthesiology 1989; 71:457–9.

240. MacGillivray R, Rocke D, Mohomedy A. Endobronchial tube placement in repair of ruptured bronchus. Anaesth Intensive Care 1987; 15:459-62.

241. Foster J, Lau O, Alimo E. Rupture of bronchus following endobronchial intubation. Br J Anaesth 1983; 55:687–8.

242. Heiser M, Steinberg J, McVaugh H, Klineberg P. Bronchial rupture, a complication of the use of the Robertshaw double-lumen tube. Anesthesiology 1979; 51:88.

243. Guernelli N, Bragaglia R, Briccoli A, et al. Tracheobronchial ruptures due to cuffed Carlens tube. Ann Thorac Surg 1979; 28:66–8.

244. Rommelscheim K. A new double-lumen tracheostomy tube for long-term use. Anaesth Intensiv Notfallmed 1985; 20:342–4.

245. Twomey C. Preventing complications in double-lumen endotracheal tubes with independent lung ventilation. Dimens Crit Care Nur 1994; 13:309–14.

246. Mays L, Eckert S. Synchronous independent lung ventilation. Dimens Crit Care Nurs 1994; 13:249–55.

Chapter 27 _____

MECHANICAL VENTILATION DURING RESUSCITATION

ACHIM VON GOEDECKE
VOLKER WENZEL

SPECTRUM OF EMERGENCY-CARE SKILLS
DISTINCTION BETWEEN AIRWAY PROTECTION
    AND ASSISTED VENTILATION
      Cricoid Pressure/Sellick Maneuver
ROLE IN DIFFERENT SETTINGS
      Prehospital Care
      Cardiopulmonary Resuscitation (CPR)
      Trauma
      Cervical Spine Injury
      Open Penetrating Chest Wounds and
        Tension Pneumothorax
      Traumatic Brain Injury
      Burns
      Drowning
ADJUNCTS FOR OYXGENATION, VENTILATION,
    AND AIRWAY CONTROL
      Oxygenation Devices
      Ventilation Devices
      Airway Control Devices
CONCLUSION

Before the arrival of an emergency medical service unit, ventilation given by bystanders must employ techniques that do not require special equipment. Safar, Elam, and Ruben first showed that obstruction of the upper airway by the tongue and soft palate occurs commonly in victims who lose consciousness or muscle tone and that ventilation with manual techniques is markedly reduced or prevented by such obstruction.[1–3] Subsequently, Safar et al[4,5] developed techniques that prevent obstruction by extending the neck and jaw and applied these in conjunction with mouth-to-mouth ventilation. The "gold standard" today for airway maintenance during resuscitation is intubation of the trachea, which provides a route for ventilation with oxygen, allows suctioning of the upper airway, protects the airway from aspiration of gastric contents, and prevents inflation of the stomach.

Spectrum of Emergency-Care Skills

Airway management should be mastered by all properly trained prehospital personnel. This involves both airway assessment and airway control. Compromise of the airway may occur suddenly or slowly and progress over time;

therefore, continuous assessment of the airway is vitally important. Pulse oximetry is helpful in identifying hypoxia, although hypoxia may be a relatively late sign of airway compromise. It is therefore important to evaluate breathing pattern, level of consciousness, and shortness of breath continuously.

When endotracheal intubation of children was added to paramedic practice, 15 of 177 (~8%) children either were intubated esophageally or dislodgment of the endotracheal tube went unrecognized; 14 of these 15 children died subsequently.[6] Accordingly, invasive pediatric airway equipment was removed from emergency medical service units in Los Angeles County; instead, bag-valve-mask ventilation was recommended. A similarly alarming experience was seen in Orlando, Florida, when the esophagus was intubated in 18 of 108 (~16%) patients being managed by the emergency medical services.[7] This suggests that the skills and experience of a rescuer performing basic and advanced airway management may determine if these maneuvers achieve effective oxygenation and carbon dioxide elimination or result in extremely serious complications, such as severe neurologic impairment, or even death.[8]

Endotracheal intubation is the "gold standard" for providing emergency ventilation. Thus every advanced emergency medical service provider must acquire and, especially, maintain intubation skills. Such a goal may be difficult to guarantee because of the large numbers of individuals who require training and/or the infrequent performance of intubations. This experience is similar to observations of the emergency medical services in Houston, Texas, where airway device–related complications were associated more with training with the devices than with the devices themselves.[9] This confirms that the success rate of airway management interventions depends on several factors: (1) initial training, (2) continuous quality assurance, and (3) actual frequency of performing the specific intervention. For example, when the actual frequency of performing endotracheal intubation is relatively low, as in the case of the Los Angeles County emergency medical services (e.g., 2584 trained individuals performing 420 actual endotracheal intubations over 33 months), it is not surprising that endotracheal intubation performed by paramedics (who were allowed to perform bag-valve-mask ventilation) did not improve survival or neurologic outcome; instead, it caused some catastrophes.[6] This actually may tip the scales toward bag-valve-mask ventilation for emergency ventilation of patients with a respiratory or even cardiac arrest performed by emergency medical services personnel without excellent intubation skills. Thus, teaching emergency medical services personnel a limited number or even a single airway procedure may follow the axiom "The simpler, the better" and ensure adequate oxygenation and avoid airway-related catastrophes.

Distinction between Airway Protection and Assisted Ventilation

Discussion of whether health care professionals or lay bystanders should or should not perform mouth-to-mouth

TABLE 27-1 Rescuer and Patient Variables Affecting Respiratory Mechanics during Mouth-to-Mouth Ventilation and Bag-Value-Mask Ventilation

Rescuer	Patient	Conscious	Anesthetized	Cardiac Arrest
Chin support	LESP (cmH$_2$O)	~20–25	~20	5?
Tidal volume	Crs (ml/cmH$_2$O)	~100–150	~50	~20–50
Inflation time	Raw (cmH$_2$O/liter/s)	~2–4	~15	?
Ventilator setting				
Bag-valve-mask size				

ABBREVIATIONS: LESP, lower esophageal sphincter pressure; Crs, compliance of the respiratory system; Raw, airway resistance.

ventilation has emotional connotations. The question of whether satisfactory lung ventilation in an unintubated cardiac arrest patient can be achieved, however, is clearly a scientific issue. If it is possible to identify ventilation strategies that are beneficial to patients and not harmful, then resuscitation outcomes may be improved.

The distribution of ventilation volume between lungs and stomach in a patient with an unprotected airway depends on factors such as lower esophageal sphincter pressure, airway resistance, and respiratory system compliance.[10] Of equal importance are specifics of techniques used for basic or advanced airway support, such as head position, tidal volume, inflation flow rate, and duration, all of which determine upper airway pressure.[11,12] The combination of these variables determines gas distribution between the lungs and the esophagus and, subsequently, the stomach.[13] Several fundamental differences exist between respiratory mechanics in a healthy, awake adult, an anesthetized supine patient, and a victim of a cardiac arrest (Table 27-1).

Lower esophageal sphincter pressure is the pressure that prevents regurgitation of stomach contents into the pharynx and insufflation of air into the gastrointestinal tract during ventilation. Sphincter pressure in a healthy adult is approximately 20–25 cmH$_2$O but may be lower in patients with chronic esophageal reflux disease, during induction of anesthesia, and after insertion of a laryngeal mask airway.[14] It is unclear, however, whether these changes in sphincter pressure result from induction of anesthesia. Animal investigations showed that the lower esophageal sphincter pressure deteriorated rapidly from a baseline level of 20 to 5 cmH$_2$O within 5 minutes of untreated cardiac arrest.[15,16] This decrease in lower esophageal sphincter pressure also was measured in human subjects following cardiac arrest.[17] In a healthy adult, air flows freely from the lips to the alveoli, and therefore, minimal inspiratory pressure is required to move gas during spontaneous ventilation. In a patient with chronic obstructive lung disease, airflow through the respiratory system may be impaired by mucus or airway spasm.[18] Data from clinical studies showed an airway resistance of 2–4 cmH$_2$O/liter per second in healthy volunteers, 8–15 cmH$_2$O/liter per second in patients with varying degrees of lung disease, and 17 cmH$_2$O/liter per second with positive-pressure bag-valve-mask ventilation in a patient during induction of anesthesia.[19] In a healthy awake adult, 1 cmH$_2$O of inspiratory pressure moves approximately 100 ml of air into the lungs; compliance decreases to 50 ml in an anesthetized supine adult and may decrease to approximately 20–50 ml in a cardiac arrest patient.[20]

Many factors can change lung compliance. Pulmonary vascular congestion during cardiac arrest increases the volume of the parenchymal interstitium and reduces compliance. Chest compressions and pulmonary edema secondary to left-ventricular failure also contribute to a reduction in compliance.[21]

Chin support and backward tilt of the head are the two most important maneuvers during rescue ventilation of paralyzed and nonparalyzed patients with an unprotected airway. Moreover, a slight lateral tilt of the head may reduce upper airway obstruction arising from backward relaxation of the tongue and soft tissues.[22] The settings of an automatic ventilator or the technique of bag-valve-mask ventilation governs inflation flow rate, inflation time, and tidal volume, all of which affect peak inflation pressure, assuming that there is no significant upper airway obstruction.[23] The relationship between peak inflation pressure and lower esophageal sphincter pressure determines gas distribution between the stomach and lungs.[24] For example, when peak inflation pressure exceeds sphincter pressure, some air will flow into the stomach; if sphincter pressure is higher than peak inflation pressure, inspiratory air will flow completely into the lungs. The preceding scenario, however, depends on the assumption that the lower esophageal sphincter pressure acts like a mechanical valve, which may not be the case. For example, Safar[25] stated that stomach inflation in healthy volunteers was self-limiting, but lower esophageal sphincter pressure was not reported. This observation implies that the physiology of respiratory mechanics in human subjects may be more complex than has been considered previously. Until a better understanding of these mechanisms is obtained, the goal of ventilation with an unprotected airway is to keep it permanently patent and to keep peak inflation pressure to a minimum at all times to prevent stomach inflation.

Stomach inflation is a complex problem that may cause regurgitation,[26] aspiration,[27] pneumonia,[28] and possibly death.[29] Stomach inflation will increase intragastric pressure,[30] elevate the diaphragm, restrict lung movements, and so reduce respiratory system compliance.[31] A reduced respiratory compliance may direct even more ventilation volume into the stomach when the airway is unprotected,[10] thereby inducing a *vicious cycle with each breath*[32] (Fig. 27-1). The life-threatening complication of stomach inflation, regurgitation, and subsequent aspiration pneumonia (induced by gastric acid) causes a loss of alveolocapillary integrity and pulmonary surfactant. As a result, fluid and proteins pass into the interstitial spaces, alveoli, and

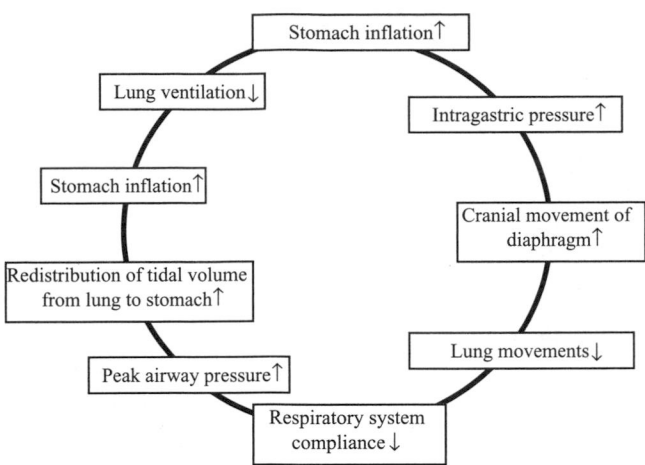

FIGURE 27-1 Vicious circle of increasing stomach inflation and decreasing lung ventilation during ventilation of an unintubated cardiac arrest patient. (*Reprinted from Wenzel et al: Resuscitation 38:113–8, 1998, with permission from Elsevier Science, Ireland.*)

bronchi, causing pulmonary edema, decreased pulmonary compliance, increased lung weight, and significant intrapulmonary shunting or ventilation-perfusion mismatching. Consequently, alveolar gas exchange is impaired markedly. Data from an animal model showed that aspiration of more than 0.8 ml/kg of body weight resulted in 50% mortality. Extrapolation of these results to humans suggest a critical aspiration volume of 50 ml at a pH of 1.0.[33] The results from recent studies of anesthetic practice, however, suggest that the true morbidity from acid aspiration has been exaggerated greatly.[34]

CRICOID PRESSURE/SELLICK MANEUVER

A maneuver for preventing stomach inflation during ventilation with an unprotected airway is to apply cricoid pressure; this is a simple, effective maneuver to prevent stomach inflation[35] that was first described 200 years ago.[36] In a model of human cadavers, an intraesophageal pressure of 75 cmH$_2$O was required to overcome cricoid pressure, indicating that the Sellick maneuver may be able to prevent gastric distension even when ventilating with a high peak inflation pressure[37] (Fig. 27-2). One study investigating the efficacy and minimum inflation pressure at which gas entered the stomach in pediatric patients found that appropriately applied cricoid pressure was invariably effective in preventing gas insufflation into the stomach in all children with and without paralysis. The minimum inflation pressure at which gas entered the stomach decreased significantly from 31 cmH$_2$O in nonparalyzed patients to 24 cmH$_2$O in paralyzed patients; thus neuromuscular blockade and *functional paralysis*, such as cardiac arrest, may increase the risk of stomach inflation.[38,39] The value of cricoid pressure has been questioned[40] because of the risk of esophageal rupture when vomiting occurs.[41] Stomach inflation, asphyxia, and aspiration after ventilation with an unprotected airway are relatively common; however, esophageal rupture after applying cricoid pressure is ex-

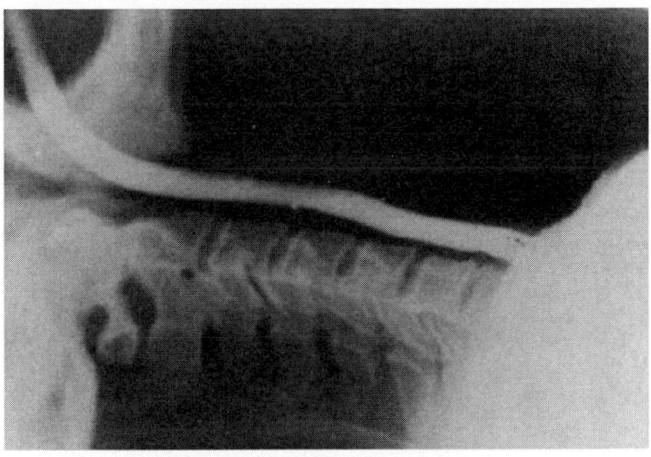

A

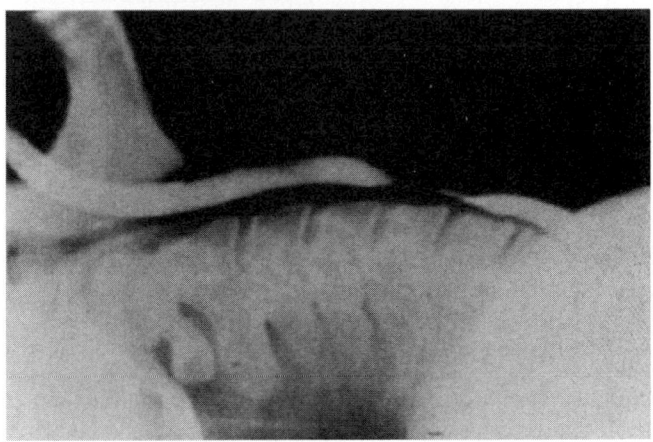

B

FIGURE 27-2 *A.* Latex tube inflated to 100 cmH$_2$O, filled with a contrast agent, and inserted into the esophagus. *B.* Manual obstruction of the latex tube in the esophagus with cricoid pressure. Only approximately 3–5 kg of pressure on the cricoid cartilage, but not on the thyroid cartilage (Adam's apple), is needed to obstruct the esophagus. (*Reprinted, with permission, from Sellick: Lancet 2:404–6, 1961.*)

tremely rare. It also should be remembered that active vomiting does not occur in patients during cardiac arrest. This may tip the balance of risks during ventilation with an unprotected airway in favor of cricoid pressure,[42] a maneuver proven to prevent stomach inflation,[43,44] which outweighs the risk of esophageal rupture.

One possible complication of cricoid pressure is airway obstruction. In 52 anesthetized patients, airway obstruction did not occur without cricoid pressure, occurred in 1 patient (2%) with cricoid pressure of 30 N (3 kg or ~7 lb), in 29 patients (56%) with cricoid pressure of 30 N (3 kg or ~7 lb) applied in an upward and backward direction, and in 18 (35%) patients with cricoid pressure of 44 N (4.4 kg or ~10 lb).[45] This indicates that cricoid pressure needs to be applied carefully and accurately. Finally, administration of both cricoid pressure and bag-mask ventilation by a single rescuer is nearly impossible and requires a second person to assist.

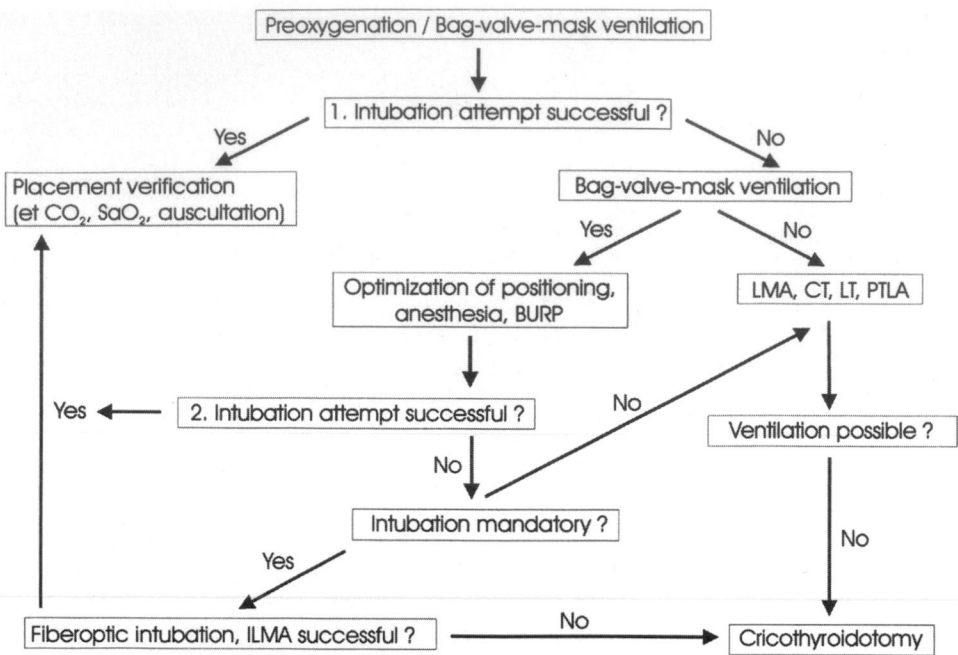

FIGURE 27-3 Algorithm for airway management. ILMA, intubating laryngeal mask airway; CT, combitube; LMA, laryngeal mask airway; LT, laryngeal tube; PTLA, pharyngotracheal lumen airway; BURP, backward, upward, rightward pressure maneuver; Pet_{CO_2}, end-tidal carbon dioxide; S_{O_2}, oxygen saturation.

Role in Different Settings

PREHOSPITAL CARE

Securing the airway by tracheal intubation in the prehospital setting may be very difficult. If airway management is difficult in a prehospital patient, maintenance of oxygenation can be in doubt despite use of a bag-valve-mask. Definite securing of the airway can be done later in the emergency department with more experienced personnel and equipment. In acute life-threatening situations, however, a standardized procedure, such as an algorithm, may be fast and reliable (Fig. 27-3).

CARDIOPULMONARY RESUSCITATION (CPR)

Outcome after CPR in adults with chest compression alone was similar to that after chest compressions combined with mouth-to-mouth ventilation; the authors concluded that chest compressions alone may be the preferred approach for bystanders inexperienced in CPR.[46] It has been suggested that more lives could be saved if only rapid chest compressions are performed (producing immediate reperfusion of vital organs but with decreased oxygen content) in contrast to the "gold" solution of rapid chest compressions combined with ventilation, which may produce less perfusion but with higher oxygen content. Most likely, the value of ventilation increases over time because ischemia and hypoxic hypercarbia increase.[47] Until a prospective trial proves when and how ventilation should be done, assisted ventilation should be provided whenever possible.[48]

The reluctance to perform mouth-to-mouth-ventilation does not represent a problem in most cases because most arrests of cardiac etiology occur at home. Unreliable recommendations for mouth-to-mouth-ventilation, lack of train-ing, poor retention of skills and knowledge,[49] and limited motivation are the main causes of the disappointingly low rates of bystander CPR worldwide. This situation cannot necessarily be rectified simply by eliminating ventilation.[50]

One argument that ventilation during CPR could be abandoned is that gasping provides sufficient gas exchange. The value of gasping in human subjects has to be interpreted with caution because fundamental differences in human and animal upper airway anatomy make it difficult to extrapolate results from laboratory studies, where gasping was beneficial. The human upper airway is kinked and is subject to rapid occlusion by the tongue and/or head position in the supine position, whereas the upper airway in swine, dogs, and rats is straight and may not be occluded by the tongue or head position in the supine position.[51] In addition, animal studies were performed in fasting animals that are therefore extremely unlikely to aspirate gastric contents. Furthermore, it is unknown if humans gasp as frequently or as deeply as animals during cardiac arrest. Whether gasping in humans results in effective gas exchange has not been studied, and for ethical reasons, such a study would be extremely difficult to perform. If a patient is gasping and the rescuer is unwilling or unable to perform mouth-to-mouth ventilation during basic life-support CPR, one strategy is to keep the airway open and perform chest compressions alone until emergency medical services arrive in order to provide a minimum of ventilation.[52] In the absence of a dedicated airway, extending the head by placing a pillow under the shoulder or gently tilting it laterally could reduce the acute pharyngeal obstruction from the tongue falling backward over the palate.

Ventilation consumes time during CPR that could be devoted to chest compressions.[53] Because only rapid chest compressions are effective, some argue that time spent for ventilation should be decreased and the time for chest compressions increased. Because cardiac output during CPR is at best approximately 25% of normal, some argue that the low cardiac output does not need to be accompanied with a normal minute ventilation. This argument has yet to be proven in a clinical study. Until evidence is available, assisted ventilation should be performed during CPR whenever possible, although the rate of chest compressions should not be decreased critically by ventilation attempts.

TRAUMA

The underlying principle for care of trauma patients is the ABCs (*a*irway, *b*reathing, *c*irculation) of resuscitation. Initial priorities after trauma are the same for the field and the hospital, but field providers usually have only limited equipment and limited assistance. They also provide care in the least controlled circumstances, such as the roadside. Airway management is the highest priority and should occur as early as possible; in severe cases, it may be necessary in the field. Physical examination may reveal subcutaneous emphysema, absent breath sounds, and unilateral hyperresonance, identifying a tension pneumothorax, which can be decompressed. Progressive clouding of consciousness indicates nearly always a loss of airway protection, risking aspiration; endotracheal intubation is required. Oral intubation is the most common method because adequately sized tubes can be placed under direct vision. Nasal intubation requires significant expertise, especially when performed blind, and may exacerbate agitation; it is contraindicated in patients with midface fractures. Laryngoscopy in an awake patient nearly always worsens agitation; in these instances, rapid-sequence intubation (RSI) is advised. RSI involves administration of a sedative followed by a short-acting muscle relaxant, typically succinylcholine. If endotracheal intubation fails, however, the patient must be ventilated with a bag-valve-mask device until short-term paralysis resolves. A retrospective analysis of trauma patients revealed that RSI in the field and in hospital were equally successful (97.9% versus 98.5%) and safe.[54] Other studies reported success rates of 84–90.5% for field intubations, suggesting that training and experience are the major determinants of success.[55–57] Failed intubation was associated mainly with inadequate relaxation and difficult anatomy (i.e., morbid obesity or inability to visualize the vocal cords). Although the length of hospital stay and mortality were comparable, pneumonia occurred more frequent with RSI in the field than in hospital (28% versus 6%).[54,58] In a prospective study of severely injured trauma patients who were intubated in the field via RSI or immediately intubated on admission to the hospital, total out-of-hospital times were twice as high for the field group versus the hospital group (26 versus 13 minutes).[59] Patients intubated in the field versus in the hospital had more ventilator, hospital, and intensive-care-unit (ICU) days, higher mortality (23% versus 12.4%), and a 1.5-fold increased risk of nosocomial pneumonia.[60] These data argue against spending extra time in the field with severely or even moderately injured patients (injury severity score 15–25).[61] Of more than 6000 intubations in emergency departments, the success rate was 98.7%, with a 1% cricothyroidotomy rate.[62]

Proper ventilation and perfect intubation skills in the field are of utmost importance, although not possible in all cases. Rescue personnel must recognize the importance of skill retention. Before intubation attempts, a risk-benefit assessment is needed to prevent harm with multiple failed attempts. For example, if conditions are difficult (morbid obesity or midface fractures), it may be prudent to use a bag-valve-mask device and subsequently intubate immediately after arrival in the emergency department. Health care personnel, however, must understand that bag-valve-mask ventilation needs to be performed carefully. In laboratory shock models, excessive ventilation with a bag-valve-mask caused increasing positive intrathoracic pressure, inhibition of venous return, decreased coronary perfusion, and thereby decreased survival.[63,64]

CERVICAL SPINE INJURY

Cervical spine injuries occur in 2–5% of blunt trauma patients,[65] and 7–14% of these are unstable.[66,67] The most common fracture was C2, accounting for 24% of fractures. Dislocations are most common at C5–6 and C6–7.[68] Missed cervical spine injury can have disastrous consequences. The incidence of missed or delayed diagnosis is 1–5%, and up to 30% of these patients develop secondary neurologic damage.[69] The primary objective when managing the airway of such a patient is to minimize neck movement while the airway is secured rapidly and efficiently. Flight paramedics had only a 52% success rate with blind nasal intubation in spontaneously breathing patients in an out-of-hospital setting but were successful with this procedure in 14 of 15 patients in the hospital.[70] Traumatologists working in a prehospital environment used RSI with a success rate of 97–99%.[71] When emergency physicians were compared with anesthesiologists using RSI in an out-of-hospital environment, the nonanesthesiologists were twice as likely to fail to intubate and needed to undertake a surgical airway.[72]

During normal direct laryngoscopy and oral intubation, significant extension occurs between the occiput and C1 and between C1 and C2.[73] In an emergency department, the most common approach to intubating the multiple-injury patient with a potential cervical spine injury is RSI while maintaining cricoid pressure and manual inline neck stabilization. Manual inline neck stabilization is provided by an assistant who holds the patient's mastoid processes firmly down, opposing the upward forces generated during laryngoscopy.[74] In anesthetized patients, this maneuver reduced head extension by 50% and should increase the safety of direct laryngoscopy.[75] Axial traction must be avoided because excessive distraction may injure the spinal cord. The view at laryngoscopy is better with manual inline neck stabilization than with rigid-collar immobilization[76]; if a cervical collar is left on during laryngoscopy, the view often will be grade 3 or 4.[77] Once manual inline neck stabilization has been applied, the rigid collar should be removed and then reapplied when successful placement of the tracheal tube has been confirmed. Direct laryngoscopy and oral intubation are the quickest method for securing the airway in a patient with potential cervical spine injury. Cricoid pressure is applied during RSI; in a recent cadaver study using lateral cervical spine x-rays, cricoid pressure caused negligible cervical spine movement.[78] By accepting a view of only the arytenoids and using a gum-elastic bougie for intubation, the laryngoscopist uses less force and minimizes cervical spine movement.[75,79]

Many clinicians advocate awake intubation as the safest approach in a patient with a cervical spine injury. It is thought that preservation of muscle tone provides protection, and spinal integrity can be monitored during airway manipulation.[80] Prolonged hypotension or malposition after intubation is at least as likely to cause neurologic injury as the intubation itself.[81] Awake techniques are particularly favored when the need for intubation is not urgent. Awake intubation is slower than RSI. In the acute trauma patient it may increase the risk of aspiration and can increase intracranial pressure. Awake techniques, such as blind nasal, blind oral, and fiberoptic intubation, require considerable training and the patient has to be cooperative. Of the awake techniques, fiberoptic intubation is best in the patient with a cervical spine injury. The laryngeal mask airway (LMA), intubating LMA, and ProSeal LMA are useful alternatives if tracheal intubation is not possible. The LMA can be inserted easily in the neutral position and is an option in patients with cervical spine instability.[82] The standard LMA and intubating LMA cause temporary pressures of greater than 250 cmH$_2$O against the posterior pharyngeal wall during insertion in cadavers. This pressure is sufficient to induce up to 2 mm of displacement of C3.[83] During insertion, the intubating LMA causes some movement of the upper cervical spine, but it is less than that produced during direct laryngoscopy.[84] Neck-stabilization methods make insertion of the LMA and intubating LMA more difficult, although the effect on the intubating LMA is less.[85]

OPEN PENETRATING CHEST WOUNDS AND TENSION PNEUMOTHORAX

An open penetrating chest wound is a challenging injury that is potentially associated with life-threatening airway compromise requiring complicated emergency airway management.[86] Intubation is challenging because preoxygenation may be less effective than usual; further, if mask ventilation is attempted, air may be forced into the subcutaneous tissue, further distorting the anatomy.[87] In one study of thoracic trauma, approximately 20% of the patients suffered a pneumothorax and/or hemothorax, injuries were penetrating in approximately 10%, and only approximately 3% required a thoracotomy.[88] Dyspnea, hemoptysis, subcutaneous emphysema, pneumomediastinum, and pneumothorax are found commonly in patients with open penetrating chest wounds (secondary to blunt trauma). Such a difficult airway needs to be secured; alternative airway techniques have been recommended as first-line approach, in particular fiberoptic laryngoscopy. Fiberoptic intubation is the "gold standard" whenever the airway is expected to be difficult; direct airway injury can be diagnosed definitively, and an endotracheal tube can be placed into one of the bronchi if there is a major injury of the opposite side.[89] The patient should breathe spontaneously for as long as possible and ideally undergo a gas induction of anesthesia

followed by bronchoscopy; a rigid scope may be useful if there is blood or copious secretions in the pharynx.

TRAUMATIC BRAIN INJURY

Outcome of traumatic brain injury depends heavily on initial and admission Glasgow Coma Scale (GCS) score and age.[90] Direct trauma-related destruction of brain structures (primary lesion) cannot be saved therapeutically. Secondary brain injury, however, defined as the damage to neurons owing to a systemic physiologic response to the initial injury, can be influenced. Hypotension and hypoxia are major causes of secondary brain injury.[91] One of the first tasks of trauma resuscitation is airway management. Approximately 50% of traumatic brain injury patients are reported to be hypoxic in the field, a finding associated with increased mortality.[92] Indications for intubation include an inability to maintain and to protect the airway but also may include inadequate ventilation, need to hyperventilate, hemodynamic instability, and need for radiographic imaging and subsequent surgery. The common coexistence of cervical spine injury requires vigilance. Early orotracheal intubation is recommended if GCS score 8 or less, although retrospective studies revealed increased mortality with field intubation.[93,94] Intubation usually can be accomplished without sedation and pharmacologic paralysis. Sedation and neuromuscular blockade can be useful in optimizing transport of the head-injured patient, but they interfere with neurologic examination and influence initial evaluation and management.[95] Hemodynamic stability similarly is ranked as a priority before and after intubation. These priorities should not be compromised in an attempt to prevent an increase in intracranial pressure.

Intracranial hypertension itself is not harmful unless it causes cerebral perfusion pressure to fall below a critical value. Cerebral ischemia leads to neuronal injury and cerebral edema, which further increases intracranial pressure, progressing to irreversible neurologic damage. Proper maintenance of gas exchange is more important than pharmacotherapy aimed at intracranial pressure control. Hyperventilation reduces intracranial pressure by causing cerebral vasoconstriction with a subsequent reduction in cerebral blood flow. Long-term hyperventilation is no longer recommended because outcome is worse than with normocapnia[96,97]; initial target Pa$_{CO_2}$ should be 35–40 mmHg.[98] Short-term hyperventilation, however, may have a role in reducing intracranial pressure in patients who are deteriorating rapidly before other measures can be instituted.[99] The lowest level of positive end-expiratory pressure that maintains adequate oxygenation and prevents end-expiratory alveolar collapse should be used.[92] Hemodynamic stability has particular importance in serious traumatic brain injury patients because outcome is worse with systolic pressures of less than 90 mmHg[100] and cerebral perfusion pressures of less than 70 mmHg.[101] Thus perfusion pressures should be kept higher by employing either intravascular volume replacement or vasopressors. Evidence of elevated intracranial pressure includes progressive coma and pupillary dilatation. Maneuvers that decrease intracranial pressure include raising the head to 30°, ensuring unobstructed venous drainage, and infusion of mannitol, which may reduce cerebral blood flow in patients at high risk of secondary ischemic brain injury.[102,103]

BURNS

In a burn patient, airway and respiratory complications remain a common cause of morbidity and mortality. Multiple variables have an impact on resuscitation, including delay in its initiation, inhalation injury, and the depth and vapor-transmission characteristics of the wound itself. Inaccurate volume administration causes substantial airway, respiratory, and other morbidity; thus burn resuscitations must be guided by hourly evaluation of resuscitation endpoints.[104] Constricting circumferential or near-circumferential torso wounds can reduce chest-wall compliance as soft tissues swell beneath the inelastic eschar. Improvement in ventilation is common after escharotomy of the chest and abdomen. In the initial evaluation and resuscitation phase, the key point of airway management is assessment of airway patency and inhalation injury. The latter results from aspiration of superheated gases, steam, or noxious products of incomplete combustion. Inhalation injury adversely affects gas exchange and hemodynamics. It also profoundly influences mortality from that predicted by age and burn size.[105] Physical signs of particular importance are singed nasal hair, facial burns, and soot in the mouth and between the teeth. Stridor mandates rapid intubation. In questionable cases, direct laryngoscopy and fiberoptic bronchoscopy can be very helpful; the bronchoscope can serve as a stylet for intubation. Patients at risk for progressive edema should be observed closely and intubated early. After securing the airway, the following require close attention: bronchospasm, small airway obstruction, carbon monoxide poisoning, and respiratory failure. If massive edema is associated with burn resuscitation, reintubation after unplanned extubation can be especially difficult; prevention by endotracheal tube security is the best approach, such as securing the endotracheal tube with an umbilical tie harness. Adjunctive techniques in case of difficult intubation, such as laryngeal mask airway or a needle or open cricothyroidotomy, can be lifesaving.

DROWNING

Worldwide, 3.5 deaths per 100,000 population are caused by drowning accidents. Death by submersion is the second most common cause of accidental death in children.[106] Victims of drowning accidents usually show an initial phase of panic and swimming movements. Apnea and breath holding often are followed by swallowing of large amounts of fluid with subsequent vomiting, gasping, and fluid aspiration. Ultimately, severe hypoxia leads to unconsciousness, loss of airway reflexes, and further movement of water into the lungs. Aspirated hypotonic or hypertonic fluids result in bronchospasm, leading to an increase in relative shunt and alveolar edema.[107] These events cause hypoxemia, decreased lung compliance, and increased work of breathing. Up to 70% of drowning victims aspirate foreign material such as mud, algae, and vomitus. Patients usually develop

acute lung injury followed by acute respiratory distress syndrome within a very short time. Because hypoxia is the major cause of death, the primary goal is to restore oxygen delivery. Immediate rescue out of the water is critical. After initial resuscitation, continuing heat loss must be prevented by adequate insulation against the environment.[108] Patients presenting awake or somnolent but with clinical signs of respiratory distress should receive oxygen at a high concentration using a tight-fitting mask and a reservoir bag. In the case of progressive deterioration of respiratory or neurologic function, RSI under cricoid pressure has to be performed and ventilation with positive end-expiratory pressure and 100% oxygen initiated without delay. A nasogastric tube will decompress a full stomach and aid ventilation in these patients. Asystole and ventricular fibrillation warrant aggressive CPR because the prognosis is dismal; unfortunately, CPR is underused in drowning victims.[109] In a recent investigation of unwitnessed out-of-hospital cardiac arrest, near-drowning was an independent predictor of survival.[110]

The level of consciousness on hospital admission is a rough predictor of outcome. Patients awake or with blunted consciousness on admission usually survive without neurologic pathology. In hemodynamically stable but hypothermic patients, reheating should be performed using warmed humidified inspiratory gases, warmed intravenous fluids, heating blankets, or forced-air surface rewarming. With these methods, body temperature may increase by approximately 1–2°C per hour.[111] In the presence of hemodynamic instability, more aggressive reheating strategies, including bladder irrigation, gastric or pleural lavage, peritoneal dialysis, and extracorporal rewarming using hemofiltration, are mandatory.[108] In severely hypothermic patients with cardiocirculatory arrest, rewarming employing cardiopulmonary bypass is the method of choice.[112]

Adjuncts for Oyxgenation, Ventilation, and Airway Control

OXYGENATION DEVICES

During resuscitation, 100% inspired oxygen ($F_{IO_2} = 1.0$) should be used as soon as possible. Exhaled air contains approximately 17% oxygen and approximately 4% carbon dioxide.[113,114] Small tidal volumes (500 ml) of 17% oxygen and 4% carbon dioxide in animals[115] and healthy, conscious volunteers resulted in insufficient oxygenation and ventilation.[116] Short-term therapy with pure oxygen is beneficial and not toxic. Oxygen toxicity occurs only during prolonged therapy with a high F_{IO_2}. During bag-valve-mask ventilation using room air (21% oxygen) and a normal cardiac output, tidal volumes of 700–1000 ml (~8.5 ml/kg) were required to maintain adequate oxygenation.[117,118]

VENTILATION DEVICES

BAG-VALVE-MASK VENTILATION
A simple, portable bag-valve-mask device usually is available in hospital wards and in every emergency medical

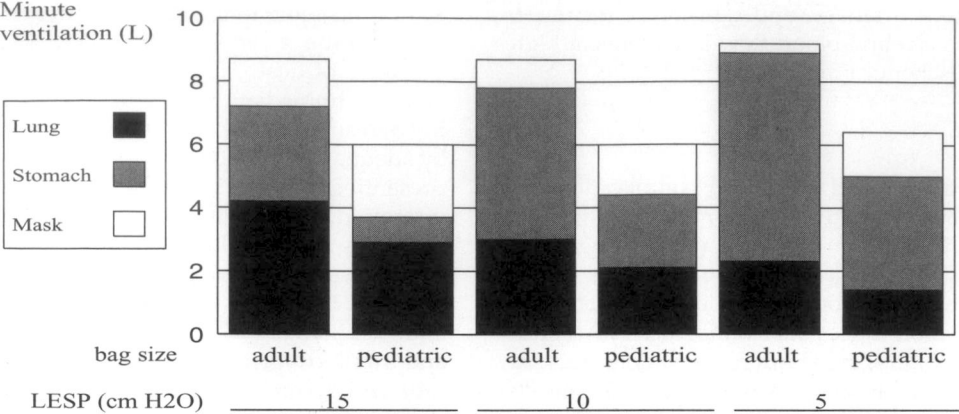

FIGURE 27-4 Mask, lung, and stomach tidal volume applied with an adult and pediatric self-inflatable bag at lower esophageal sphincter pressure (LESP) levels of 15, 10, and 5 cmH$_2$O. Bars representing lung (*black columns*) and stomach tidal volumes (*gray columns*) for a given bag size, and LESP levels are superimposed; mask tidal volumes (*white columns*) start from 0. Data are shown only as means. (*Reprinted, with permission, from Lippincott Williams & Wilkins and Wenzel et al: Crit Care Med 26:364–8, 1998.*)

service. Proper bag-valve-mask ventilation is a fundamental skill of resuscitation and should receive a high priority in training. Unfortunately, these skills are poorly performed even after retraining, and inadvertent hyperventilation is detrimental to morbidity and mortality. With an unprotected airway, the risk of stomach inflation and aspiration is high using standard bag-valve-mask resuscitators. Short inspiratory times, high flow rates, and high airway pressures, caused by squeezing the bag too hard and too fast, are the main causes of stomach inflation. Reduced expiratory times produced by inadvertent hyperventilation stacks air in the lungs, creating decreasesd cardiac refill and decreased coronary perfusion pressure. A small self-inflatable bag was advantageous over a large one when paramedics undertook bag-valve-mask ventilation with a pediatric versus an adult-sized self-inflatable bag using an in vitro model of ventilation with an unprotected airway. Pulmonary ventilation was similar with both bags, but stomach inflation was much less with the pediatric bag[119,120] (Fig. 27-4).

Depending on lung compliance, different tidal volumes caused stomach inflation in patients, but most often at a peak inflation pressure of greater than 20 cmH$_2$O. Data from an in vitro model of an unprotected airway confirmed that longer inflation times produced increased lung ventilation and reduced stomach inflation, especially when intrapulmonary airway resistance was high. While the bag-valve mask is the simplest and most-cost effective ventilation device available, its efficacy is diminished by lack of skill of the user, the "incident stress" associated with treating a patient in cardiac arrest, and the subsequent inadvertent hyperventilation that these issues cause. A relatively new bag-valve-mask technology exists that assists rescuers in ventilating correctly by responding to squeeze and release of the bag and controlling the flow of gas from the bag, reducing airway pressure, increasing inspiratory times, and nearly completely eliminating the risk of stomach insufflation.[121]

AUTOMATIC TRANSPORT VENTILATORS

In prehospital care, mechanically powered devices are as effective as other devices for ventilating intubated patients. In unintubated patients, it depends on the mode of power; that is, in pressure-cycled devices, because these device must achieve a relatively high airway pressure (usually greater than the reported lower esophageal sphincter pressure) to turn off the flow and cycle to an exhalation, they create large amounts of stomach inflation, especially as the airway resistance increases or lung compliance decreases. The guidelines for resuscitation recommend avoiding these devices. On the other hand, tidal volume should be restricted in volume- and time-cycled ventilators. In an in vitro model of an unprotected airway, significantly less stomach inflation was found when applying a tidal volume of approximately 500 ml versus approximately 1000 ml.[122] Controlling inflation time, flow rate, and flow waveform with a mechanical ventilator may be the best solution to control and limit peak inflation pressure for a given tidal volume, but these variables are not controlled easily during manual ventilation.

AIRWAY CONTROL DEVICES

OROPHARYNGEAL AND NASOPHARYNGEAL AIRWAYS

These airway adjuncts can be used in unintubated patients requiring ventilation. The oropharyngeal airway should be inserted only in unconscious patients; otherwise, gagging and vomiting can be evoked. The nasopharyngeal airway is better tolerated in somnolent patients. The devices should be inserted carefully by trained personnel; lubricants ease insertion.

ENDOTRACHEAL TUBE

As early as possible during resuscitation, trained personnel should intubate the trachea. Before commencing intubation, the patient should be preoxygenated either by spontaneously breathing pure oxygen or by controlled bag-valve-mask ventilation with a high inspired concentration of oxygen. Preoxygenation increases the alveolar pressure of oxygen; elimination of nitrogen increases the reservoir of oxygen fivefold and generates a grace period of several minutes before a patient becomes hypoxic (Fig. 27-5). The

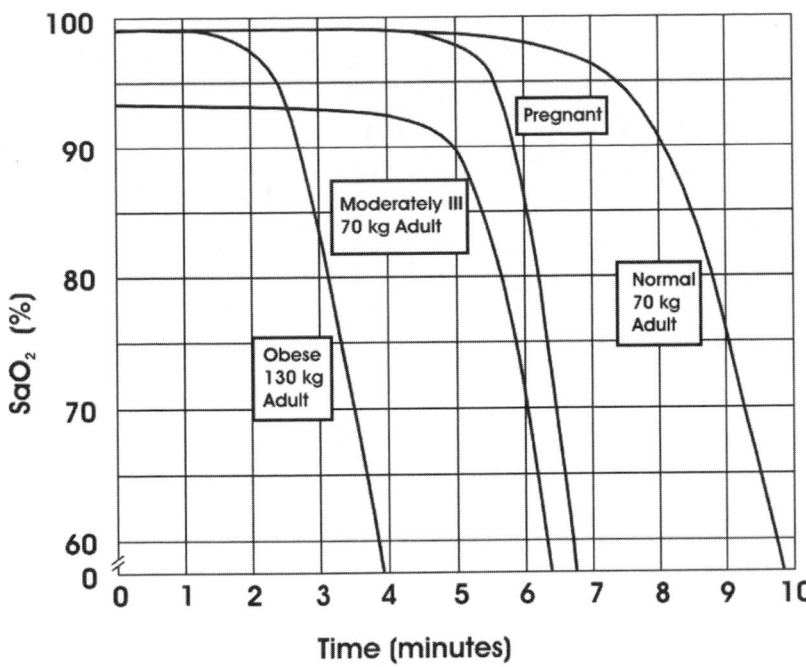

FIGURE 27-5 Desaturation after preoxygenation. Time in minutes until oxygen saturation (Sa_{O_2}) drops during apnea.

grace period depends on the alveolar volume, shunts, oxygen consumption, and oxygen-carrying capacity. The interruption of ventilation should be as brief as possible, and adequate ventilation and oxygenation must be provided if more than one intubation attempt is necessary. To facilitate intubation, the sniffing position and hyperextension of the head at the atlanto-occipital joint is beneficial. A stylet, which should not extend over the distal end, can be used to provide some stiffness to the tube and makes control during insertion easier. A second rescuer applies cricoid pressure during bag-valve-mask ventilation and intubation to prevent regurgitation and subsequent aspiration. When the cuff of the tracheal tube is inflated and the airway thus secured, cricoid pressure can be removed. Tube placement is confirmed by chest excursion and auscultation; over the epigastrium, no stomach gurgling should be heard during inspiration. These clinical signs are not always reliable[123]; unrecognized misplacement of the endotracheal tube occured in up to 6–25% of intubated patients in the field.[6,7] Verification by direct visualization of the tube passing through the vocal cords and use of end-tidal carbon dioxide monitoring also are recommended.[124,125] Clinical assessment and esophageal detector devices may be used but are not reliable in all patients.

LARYNGEAL MASK AIRWAY

The laryngeal mask airway (LMA) now is used widely for managing failed intubations or difficult airways.[126,127] It should be considered first among the alternative airway devices. Placement and use of an LMA are simpler than tracheal intubation because laryngoscopy and visualization of the vocal cords are unnecessary. The LMA is introduced into the hypopharynx, and the cuff seals the larynx after inflation. While the arrow is positioned at the upper esophageal sphincter without sealing it, the distal open-

ing of the tube is just above the glottis, providing ventilation and oxygenation. The main limitation of the LMA is a lack of protection against aspiration,[128] although regurgitation is less likely than with bag-valve-mask ventilation.[129] A recently developed ProSeal LMA has an additional lumen to introduce a nasogastric tube to drain the stomach or regurgitated fluids[130] away from the respiratory tract.[131] The bowl of the mask is deeper than that of a standard LMA, with an additional cuff on the dorsal side. Because of these modifications, the airway sealing pressures achievable with the ProSeal LMA are at least 10 cmH_2O higher than with the standard LMA. As with the standard LMA, the ProSeal LMA can be inserted in the neutral position, making it attractive in potential cervical spine injury. Another limitation of the LMA is the relatively low leak pressure 19–22 cmH_2O,[132,133] which may decrease tidal volume and increase stomach inflation.[134] The intubating LMA is a modified conventional LMA; once inserted, it allows passage of a tracheal tube, either blindly or by fiberoptic bronchoscopy. Standard insertion requires a neutral position; manipulation of the head and neck is not needed.

COMBITUBE

The Combitube is essentially a double-lumen tube that is inserted blindly through the mouth and is more likely to pass into the esophagus (~95%) than into the trachea (~5%). The esophageal lumen is closed distally and perforated at the hypopharyngeal level with several small openings; the tracheal lumen is open distally. First, the proximal large pharyngeal balloon is inflated, thereby filling the space between the base of the tongue and the soft palate. Second, the distal cuff is inflated. These cuffs provide a good seal of the hypopharynx from the oropharynx and stability in the trachea or esophagus, respectively. The most common reason for failure to ventilate is placing the Combitube too deeply;

the entire perforated pharyngeal section enters the esophagus. Pulling the Combitube back 3–4 cm usually resolves the problem. The success of insertion and ventilation with the Combitube is comparable with that of other upper airway devices[135] and is 100% in an urban environment where trauma patients receive care.[136] The Combitube, however, is not well tolerated by patients with a persistent strong gag reflex. It should be exchanged to an alternative airway as early as possible. Advantageously, the Combitube can be a routine device in emergency medicine[137] and in "cannot ventilate, cannot intubate" situations.[138] The Combitube has the same limitations as the LMA. Thus it may be unsuitable in patients with hypopharyngeal pathology or preexisting esophageal pathology, such as a malignancy or esophageal varices.[139]

LARYNGEAL TUBE

The recently introduced single-lumen laryngeal tube can be inserted orally without additional equipment and is effective for ventilating and oxygenating patients who experience a respiratory arrest during induction of anesthesia.[140] Thus the laryngeal tube may be used as an alternative airway device during routine or emergency airway management. Handling of the laryngeal tube has been simplified by blocking two cuffs with one instead of two catheters; the first secures inflation of the oropharyngeal cuff, and the second secures inflation of the esophageal cuff because of different resistance characteristics of the connected tubing. Given its design, the laryngeal tube may not be the best device for spontaneously breathing patients.[141] The blind ending in the esophageal inlet also may cause esophageal rupture in the case of vomiting.[142] Accordingly, the laryngeal tube has been fitted with a second lumen for suctioning and free stomach drainage (laryngeal tube S) but not for ventilation, as with the Combitube. In contrast to the Combitube, the laryngeal tube S has only one adapter, which may be connected with a ventilation device, whereas the remaining connector can only be connected to a suction adapter. This may achieve additional patient safety; it prevents an inexperienced user from inadvertently attaching a ventilator or bag-valve-mask device to the esophageal tubing, which could result in stomach inflation and subsequent ventilation-related complications.

PHARYNGOTRACHEAL LUMEN AIRWAY

The pharyngotracheal lumen airway is an improvement on the design of the esophageal obturator airway and the esophageal gastric tube airway. Both devices are double-lumen airways that are inserted blindly, preferably into the esophagus. The pharyngotracheal lumen airway has an oral balloon that provides a seal for the airway. An inflatable distal cuff prevents aspiration of stomach contents. Just like the Combitube, the rescuer should evaluate carefully if the device is in the esophagus or in the trachea, and based on this evaluation, ventilate through the appropriate lumen. Once popular, the pharyngotracheal lumen airway is now used rarely.

TRACHEOSTOMY AND CRICOTHYROIDOTOMY

When the airway is compromised by trauma, or when massive oropharyngeal or hypopharyngeal pathology is present, emergency access may be possible only through an emergency tracheostomy or cricothyroidotomy. Emergency tracheostomy usually is performed via a vertical incision from the cricoid cartilage down in the direction of the sternal notch. A skilled operator can insert a small, cuffed endotracheal tube rapidly. Emergency cricothyroidotomy is a valid alternative for a less skilled operator. The cricothyroid membrane, palpable directly under the skin, is incised in its inferior third to minimize the possibility of bleeding. The cricothyroid membrane is not always easy to appreciate (in obese patients or those with short necks). Cricothyroidotomy is performed infrequently; in inexperienced hands, success is only 60–70%.[143] The main advantage of this technique is the blunt dissection of the subcutaneous tissues all the way to the cricoid membrane. An airway catheter is then introduced over a dilator threaded over the guidewire.[144] This technique allows the ultimate insertion of an airway that is considerably larger than the initial needle or catheter. Its internal diameter often is sufficient to allow ventilation with conventional ventilation devices, suctioning, and spontaneous ventilation. Needle cricothyroidotomy is another alternative, regardless of whether it is surgical or percutaneous. Needle cricothyroidotomy always requires the use of a jet device to provide ventilation. It is associated with a high incidence of complications, such as massive subcutaneous emphysema, barotrauma with pneumothorax or tension pneumothorax, and air trapping with severe hemodynamic instability.

Conclusion

The goal of ventilation strategy during resuscitation is to optimize oxygenation and carbon dioxide elimination. This can be achieved in an unprotected airway with techniques such as mouth-to-mouth ventilation but preferably with bag-valve-mask ventilation. Because ventilation of an unprotected airway may result in stomach inflation and subsequent severe complications, securing the airway with an endotracheal tube is the "gold standard"; however, other airway devices are acceptable if rescuers are trained properly. Of importance, airway device complications are more related to training than to the devices themselves. Excellent success in emergency ventilation depends on initial training, retraining, and actual frequency of performing a given procedure on the job.

References

1. Safar P. Failure of manual respiration. J Appl Physiol 1959; 14: 84–8.
2. Safar P, Brown TC, Holtey WJ, Wilder RJ. Ventilation and circulation with closed-chest cardiac massage in man. JAMA 1961; 176:574–6.
3. Safar P, Escarraga LA, Chang F. Upper airway obstruction in the unconscious patient. J Appl Physiol 1959; 14:760–4.

4. Safar P, Escarraga LA, Elam JO. A comparison of the mouth-to-mouth and mouth-to-airway methods of artificial respiration with the chest-pressure arm-lift methods. New Engl J Med 1958; 258:671–7.

5. Safar P, Brown TC, Holtey WJ. Failure of closed chest cardiac massage to produce pulmonary ventilation. Dis Chest 1962; 41:1–8.

6. Gausche M, Lewis RJ, Stratton SJ, et al. Effect of out-of-hospital pediatric endotracheal intubation on survival and neurological outcome: a controlled clinical trial. JAMA 2000; 283:783–90.

7. Katz SH, Falk JL. Misplaced endotracheal tubes by paramedics in an urban emergency medical services system. Ann Emerg Med 2001; 37:32–7.

8. Cummins RO, Hazinski MF. Guidelines based on the principle "first, do no harm": New guidelines on tracheal tube confirmation and prevention of dislodgment. Circulation 2000; 102: I380–4.

9. Pepe PE, Zachariah BS, Chandra NC. Invasive airway techniques in resuscitation. Ann Emerg Med 1993; 22:393–403.

10. Wenzel V, Idris AH, Banner MJ, et al. Respiratory system compliance decreases after cardiopulmonary resuscitation and stomach inflation: Impact of large and small tidal volumes on calculated peak airway pressure. Resuscitation 1998; 38:113–8.

11. von Goedecke A, Voelckel WG, Wenzel V, et al. Mechanical versus manual ventilation via a face mask during the induction of anesthesia: A prospective, randomized, crossover study. Anesth Analg 2004; 98:260–3.

12. von Goedecke A, Wagner-Berger HG, Stadlbauer KH, et al. Effects of decreasing peak flow rate on stomach inflation during bag-valve-mask ventilation. Resuscitation 2004; 63:131–6.

13. Wenzel V, Idris AH, Lindner KH. Ventilation with an unprotected airway during cardiac arrest. In: Vincent J-L, editor. Yearbook of intensive care and emergency medicine. Berlin: Springer-Verlag, 1997: 483–92.

14. Rabey PG, Murphy PJ, Langton JA, et al. Effect of the laryngeal mask airway on lower oesophageal sphincter pressure in patients during general anaesthesia. Br J Anaesth 1992; 69: 346–8.

15. Bowman FP, Menegazzi JJ, Check BD, Duckett TM. Lower esophageal sphincter pressure during prolonged cardiac arrest and resuscitation. Ann Emerg Med 1995; 26:216–9.

16. Melker RJ. Alternative methods of ventilation during respiratory and cardiac arrest. Circulation 1986; 74:IV63–5.

17. Gabrielli A, Wenzel V, Layon AJ, et al. Lower esophageal sphincter pressure measurement during cardiac arrest in humans: Potential implications for ventilation of the unprotected airway Anesthesiology 2005;103:897–9.

18. von Goedecke A, Bowden K, Keller C, et al. Decreased inspiratory time during ventilation of an unprotected airway: Effect on stomach inflation and lung ventilation in a bench model. Anaesthesist 2005; 54:117–22.

19. Weiler N, Heinrichs W, Dick W. Assessment of pulmonary mechanics and gastric inflation pressure during mask ventilation. Prehosp Disaster Med 1995; 10:101–5.

20. Ornato JP, Bryson BL, Donovan PJ, et al. Measurement of ventilation during cardiopulmonary resuscitation. Crit Care Med 1983; 11:79–82.

21. Davis K Jr, Johannigman JA, Johnson RC Jr, Branson RD. Lung compliance following cardiac arrest. Acad Emerg Med 1995; 2:874–8.

22. Idris AH, Florete OG, Melker RJ, Chandra NC. Physiology of ventilation, oxygenation, and carbon dioxide elimination during cardiac arrest. In: Paradis NA, Halperin HR, Nowak RM, editors. Cardiac arrest: The science and practice of resuscitation medicine. Baltimore: Williams & Wilkins, 1996: 382–419.

23. von Goedecke A, Keller C, Wagner-Berger HG, et al. Developing a strategy to improve ventilation in an unprotected airway with a modified mouth-to-bag resuscitator in apneic patients. Anesth Analg 2004; 99:1516–20.

24. von Goedecke A, Bowden K, Wenzel V, et al. Effects of decreasing inspiratory times during simulated bag-valve-mask ventilation. Resuscitation 2005; 64:321–5.

25. Safar P. Ventilatory efficacy of mouth-to-mouth artificial respiration: Airway obstruction during manual and mouth-to-mouth artificial respiration. JAMA 1958; 167:335–41.

26. Morton HJ, Wylie WD. Anaesthetic deaths due to regurgitation or vomiting. Anaesthesia 1951; 6:190–201.

27. Lawes EG, Baskett PJ. Pulmonary aspiration during unsuccessful cardiopulmonary resuscitation. Intensive Care Med 1987; 13:379–82.

28. Bjork RJ, Snyder BD, Campion BC, Loewenson RB. Medical complications of cardiopulmonary arrest. Arch Intern Med 1982; 142:500–3.

29. Krischer JP, Fine EG, Davis JH, Nagel EL. Complications of cardiac resuscitation. Chest 1987; 92:287–91.

30. Spence AA, Moir DD, Finlay WE. Observations on intragastric pressure. Anaesthesia 1967; 22:249–56.

31. Ruben H, Knudsen EJ, Carugati G. Gastric inflation in relation to airway pressure. Acta Anaesthesiol Scand 1961; 5:107–14.

32. Johannigman JA, Branson RD, Davis K Jr, Hurst JM. Techniques of emergency ventilation: A model to evaluate tidal volume, airway pressure, and gastric insufflation. J Trauma 1991; 31: 93–8.

33. Raidoo DM, Rocke DA, Brock-Utne JG, et al. Critical volume for pulmonary acid aspiration: Reappraisal in a primate model. Br J Anaesth 1990; 65:248–50.

34. Engelhardt T, Webster NR. Pulmonary aspiration of gastric contents in anaesthesia. Br J Anaesth 1999; 83:453–60.

35. Sellick BA. Cricoid pressure to control regurgitation of stomach contents during induction of anaesthesia. Lancet 1961; 2:404–6.

36. Salem MR, Sellick BA, Elam JO. The historical background of cricoid pressure in anesthesia and resuscitation. Anesth Analg 1974; 53:230–2.

37. Fanning GL. The efficacy of cricoid pressure in preventing regurgitation of gastric contents. Anesthesiology 1970; 32:553–5.

38. Moynihan RJ, Brock-Utne JG, Archer JH, et al. The effect of cricoid pressure on preventing gastric insufflation in infants and children. Anesthesiology 1993; 78:652–6.

39. Schwartz DE, Matthay MA, Cohen NH. Death and other complications of emergency airway management in critically ill adults: A prospective investigation of 297 tracheal intubations. Anesthesiology 1995; 82:367–76.

40. Roewer N. Can pulmonary aspiration of gastric contents be prevented by balloon occlusion of the cardia? A study with a new nasogastric tube. Anesth Analg 1995; 80:378–83.

41. Ralph SJ, Wareham CA. Rupture of the oesophagus during cricoid pressure. Anaesthesia 1991; 46:40–1.

42. Notcutt W. Oesophageal rupture and cricoid pressure. Anaesthesia 1991; 46:424–5.

43. Lawes EG, Campbell I, Mercer D. Inflation pressure, gastric insufflation and rapid sequence induction. Br J Anaesth 1987; 59:315–8.

44. Salem MR, Wong AY, Mani M, Sellick BA. Efficacy of cricoid pressure in preventing gastric inflation during bag-mask ventilation in pediatric patients. Anesthesiology 1974; 40:96–8.

45. Hartsilver EL, Vanner RG. Airway obstruction with cricoid pressure. Anaesthesia 2000; 55:208–11.

46. Hallstrom A, Cobb L, Johnson E, Copass M. Cardiopulmonary resuscitation by chest compression alone or with mouth-to-mouth ventilation. New Engl J Med 2000; 342:1546–53.

47. von Goedecke A, Wenzel V. ["Above too please"! Artificial respiration during cardiopulmonary resuscitation]. Anaesthesist 2004; 53:925–6.

48. Safar P, Bircher N, Pretto E Jr, et al. Reappraisal of mouth-to-mouth ventilation during bystander-initiated CPR. Circulation 1998; 98:608–10.

49. Wenzel V, Lehmkuhl P, Kubilis PS, et al. Poor correlation of mouth-to-mouth ventilation skills after basic life support training and 6 months later. Resuscitation 1997; 35:129–34.

50. Dick WF, Brambrink AM, Kern T. ["Topless" cardiopulmonary resuscitation? Should heart-lung resuscitation be preformed without artificial resuscitation?]. Anaesthesist 1999; 48:290–300.

51. Safar P. Resuscitation medicine research: Quo vadis. Ann Emerg Med 1996; 27:542–52.

52. Assar D, Chamberlain D, Colquhoun M, et al. A rationale for staged teaching of basic life support. Resuscitation 1998; 39: 137–43.

53. van Alem AP, Sanou BT, Koster RW. Interruption of cardiopulmonary resuscitation with the use of the automated external defibrillator in out-of-hospital cardiac arrest. Ann Emerg Med 2003; 42:449–57.

54. Sloane C, Vilke GM, Chan TC, et al. Rapid sequence intubation in the field versus hospital in trauma patients. J Emerg Med 2000; 19:259–64.

55. Burton JH, Baumann MR, Maoz T, et al. Endotracheal intubation in a rural EMS state: Procedure utilization and impact of skills maintenance guidelines. Prehosp Emerg Care 2003; 7:352–6.

56. Wang HE, Sweeney TA, O'Connor RE, Rubinstein H. Failed prehospital intubations: An analysis of emergency department courses and outcomes. Prehosp Emerg Care 2001; 5:134–41.

57. Wang HE, Kupas DF, Paris PM, et al. Multivariate predictors of failed prehospital endotracheal intubation. Acad Emerg Med 2003; 10:717–24.

58. Karch SB, Lewis T, Young S, et al. Field intubation of trauma patients: Complications, indications, and outcomes. Am J Emerg Med 1996; 14:617–9.

59. Ochs M, Davis D, Hoyt D, et al. Paramedic-performed rapid sequence intubation of patients with severe head injuries. Ann Emerg Med 2002; 40:159–67.

60. Bochicchio GV, Ilahi O, Joshi M, et al. Endotracheal intubation in the field does not improve outcome in trauma patients who present without an acutely lethal traumatic brain injury. J Trauma 2003; 54:307–11.

61. Demetriades D, Chan L, Cornwell E, et al. Paramedic vs private transportation of trauma patients: Effect on outcome. Arch Surg 1996; 131:133–8.

62. Walls RM, Gurr DE, Kulkarni RG, et al. 6,294 Emergency department intubations: Second report of the Ongoing National Emergency Airway Registry (NEAR) II Study. Ann Emerg Med 2000; 36(suppl):S51.

63. Aufderheide TP, Sigurdsson G, Pirrallo RG, et al. Hyperventilation-induced hypotension during cardiopulmonary resuscitation. Circulation 2004; 109:1960–5.

64. Pepe PE, Raedler C, Lurie KG, Wigginton JG. Emergency ventilatory management in hemorrhagic states: Elemental or detrimental? J Trauma 2003; 54:1048–55.

65. Lowery DW, Wald MM, Browne BJ, et al. Epidemiology of cervical spine injury victims. Ann Emerg Med 2001; 38:12–6.

66. Ajani AE, Cooper DJ, Scheinkestel CD, et al. Optimal assessment of cervical spine trauma in critically ill patients: A prospective evaluation. Anaesth Intensive Care 1998; 26:487–91.

67. Berne JD, Velmahos GC, El-Tawil Q, et al. Value of complete cervical helical computed tomographic scanning in identifying cervical spine injury in the unevaluable blunt trauma patient with multiple injuries: A prospective study. J Trauma 1999; 47:896–902.

68. Goldberg W, Mueller C, Panacek E, et al. Distribution and patterns of blunt traumatic cervical spine injury. Ann Emerg Med 2001; 38:17–21.

69. Davis JW, Phreaner DL, Hoyt DB, Mackersie RC. The etiology of missed cervical spine injuries. J Trauma 1993; 34:342–6.

70. Brown J, Thomas F. What happens with failed blind nasal tracheal intubations? Air Med J 2001; 20:13–6.

71. Gerich TG, Schmidt U, Hubrich V, et al. Prehospital airway management in the acutely injured patient: The role of surgical cricothyrotomy revisited. J Trauma 1998; 45:312–4.

72. Mackay CA, Terris J, Coats TJ. Prehospital rapid sequence induction by emergency physicians: is it safe? Emerg Med J 2001; 18:20–4.

73. Lennarson PJ, Smith D, Todd MM, et al. Segmental cervical spine motion during orotracheal intubation of the intact and injured spine with and without external stabilization. J Neurosurg Spine 2000; 92:201–6.

74. Criswell JC, Parr MJ, Nolan JP. Emergency airway management in patients with cervical spine injuries. Anaesthesia 1994; 49: 900–3.

75. Hastings RH, Wood PR. Head extension and laryngeal view during laryngoscopy with cervical spine stabilization maneuvers. Anesthesiology 1994; 80:825–31.

76. Gerling MC, Davis DP, Hamilton RS, et al. Effects of cervical spine immobilization technique and laryngoscope blade selection on an unstable cervical spine in a cadaver model of intubation. Ann Emerg Med 2000; 36:293–300.

77. Heath KJ. The effect of laryngoscopy of different cervical spine immobilisation techniques. Anaesthesia 1994; 49:843–5.

78. Helliwell V, Gabbott DA. The effect of single-handed cricoid pressure on cervical spine movement after applying manual in-line stabilisation: A cadaver study. Resuscitation 2001; 49:53–7.

79. Nolan JP, Wilson ME. Orotracheal intubation in patients with potential cervical spine injuries: An indication for the gum elastic bougie. Anaesthesia 1993; 48:630–3.

80. Meschino A, Devitt JH, Koch JP, et al. The safety of awake tracheal intubation in cervical spine injury. Can J Anaesth 1992; 39:114–7.

81. McLeod AD, Calder I. Spinal cord injury and direct laryngoscopy: The legend lives on. Br J Anaesth 2000; 84:705–9.

82. Brimacombe J, Berry A. Laryngeal mask airway insertion: A comparison of the standard versus neutral position in normal patients with a view to its use in cervical spine instability. Anaesthesia 1993; 48:670–1.

83. Keller C, Brimacombe J, Keller K. Pressures exerted against the cervical vertebrae by the standard and intubating laryngeal mask airways: A randomized, controlled, cross-over study in fresh cadavers. Anesth Analg 1999; 89:1296–300.

84. Kihara S, Watanabe S, Brimacombe J, et al. Segmental cervical spine movement with the intubating laryngeal mask during manual in-line stabilization in patients with cervical pathology undergoing cervical spine surgery. Anesth Analg 2000; 91: 195–200.

85. Asai T, Wagle AU, Stacey M. Placement of the intubating laryngeal mask is easier than the laryngeal mask during manual in-line neck stabilization. Br J Anaesth 1999; 82:712–4.

86. Tayal VS, Riggs RW, Marx JA, et al. Rapid-sequence intubation at an emergency medicine residency: Success rate and adverse events during a two-year period. Acad Emerg Med 1999; 6:31–7.

87. Demetriades D, Velmahos GG, Asensio JA. Cervical pharyngoesophageal and laryngotracheal injuries. World J Surg 2001; 25:1044–8.

88. Kulshrestha P, Munshi I, Wait R. Profile of chest trauma in a level I trauma center. J Trauma 2004; 57:576–81.

89. Ovassapian A. The flexible bronchoscope: A tool for anesthesiologists. Clin Chest Med 2001; 22:281–99.

90. Baker A. Ischemic preconditioning in the brain. Can J Anaesth 2004; 51:201–5.

91. Chesnut RM, Marshall LF, Klauber MR, et al. The role of secondary brain injury in determining outcome from severe head injury. J Trauma 1993; 34:216–22.

92. Marik PE, Varon J, Trask T. Management of head trauma. Chest 2002; 122:699–711.

93. Davis DP, Hoyt DB, Ochs M, et al. The effect of paramedic rapid sequence intubation on outcome in patients with severe traumatic brain injury. J Trauma 2003; 54:444–53.

94. Murray JA, Demetriades D, Berne TV, et al. Prehospital intubation in patients with severe head injury. J Trauma 2000; 49:1065–70.

95. Marion DW, Carlier PM. Problems with initial Glasgow Coma Scale assessment caused by prehospital treatment of patients with head injuries: Results of a national survey. J Trauma 1994; 36:89–95.

96. Muizelaar JP, Marmarou A, Ward JD, et al. Adverse effects of prolonged hyperventilation in patients with severe head injury: A randomized clinical trial. J Neurosurg 1991; 75:731–9.

97. Davis DP, Dunford JV, Poste JC, et al. The impact of hypoxia and hyperventilation on outcome after paramedic rapid sequence intubation of severely head-injured patients. J Trauma 2004; 57:1–8.

98. The Brain Trauma Foundation. The American Association of Neurological Surgeons. The Joint Section on Neurotrauma and Critical Care. Hyperventilation. J Neurotrauma 2000; 17:513–20.

99. Qureshi AI, Geocadin RG, Suarez JI, Ulatowski JA. Long-term outcome after medical reversal of transtentorial herniation in patients with supratentorial mass lesions. Crit Care Med 2000; 28:1556–64.

100. Pietropaoli JA, Rogers FB, Shackford SR, et al. The deleterious effects of intraoperative hypotension on outcome in patients with severe head injuries. J Trauma 1992; 33:403–7.

101. Rosner MJ, Rosner SD, Johnson AH. Cerebral perfusion pressure: Management protocol and clinical results. J Neurosurg 1995; 83:949–62.

102. Ng I, Lim J, Wong HB. Effects of head posture on cerebral hemodynamics: Its influences on intracranial pressure, cerebral perfusion pressure, and cerebral oxygenation. Neurosurgery 2004; 54:593–7.

103. Skippen P, Seear M, Poskitt K, et al. Effect of hyperventilation on regional cerebral blood flow in head-injured children. Crit Care Med 1997; 25:1402–9.

104. Sheridan RL. Airway management and respiratory care of the burn patient. Int Anesthesiol Clin 2000; 38:129–45.

105. Shirani KZ, Pruitt BA Jr, Mason AD Jr. The influence of inhalation injury and pneumonia on burn mortality. Ann Surg 1987; 205:82–7.

106. Sibert JR, Lyons RA, Smith BA, et al. Preventing deaths by drowning in children in the United Kingdom: Have we made progress in 10 years? Population based incidence study. Br Med J 2002; 324:1070–1.

107. Hasibeder W, Friesenecker B, Mayr A. [Near drowning: Epidemiology—pathophysiology—therapy]. Anasthesiol Intensivmed Notfallmed Schmerzther 2003; 38:333–40.

108. Giesbrecht GG. Cold stress, near drowning and accidental hypothermia: A review. Aviat Space Environ Med 2000; 71:733–52.

109. Wyatt JP, Tomlinson GS, Busuttil A. Resuscitation of drowning victims in southeast Scotland. Resuscitation 1999; 41:101–4.

110. Kuisma M, Jaara K. Unwitnessed out-of-hospital cardiac arrest: Is resuscitation worthwhile? Ann Emerg Med 1997; 30:69–75.

111. Kornberger E, Schwarz B, Lindner KH, Mair P. Forced air surface rewarming in patients with severe accidental hypothermia. Resuscitation 1999; 41:105–11.

112. Vretenar DF, Urschel JD, Parrott JC, Unruh HW. Cardiopulmonary bypass resuscitation for accidental hypothermia. Ann Thorac Surg 1994; 58:895–8.

113. Wenzel V, Idris AH, Banner MJ, et al. The composition of gas given by mouth-to-mouth ventilation during CPR. Chest 1994; 106:1806–10.

114. Htin KJ, Birenbaum DS, Idris AH, et al. Rescuer breathing pattern significantly affects O_2 and CO_2 received by the patient during mouth-to-mouth ventilation (abstract). Crit Care Med 1998; 26:A56–60.

115. Idris AH, Gabrielli A, Caruso L. Smaller tidal volume is safe and effective for bag-valve-mask ventilation, but not for mouth-to-mouth ventilation: An animal model of basic life support (abstract). Circulation 1999:I-664.

116. Stallinger A, Wenzel V, Oroszy S, et al. The effects of different mouth-to-mouth ventilation tidal volumes on gas exchange during simulated rescue breathing. Anesth Analg 2001; 93:1265–9.

117. Dorges V, Ocker H, Hagelberg S, et al. Optimisation of tidal volumes given with self-inflatable bags without additional oxygen. Resuscitation 2000; 43:195–9.

118. Dorges V, Ocker H, Hagelberg S, et al. Smaller tidal volumes with room-air are not sufficient to ensure adequate oxygenation during bag-valve-mask ventilation. Resuscitation 2000; 44:37–41.

119. Wenzel V, Idris AH, Banner MJ, et al. Influence of tidal volume on the distribution of gas between the lungs and stomach in the nonintubated patient receiving positive-pressure ventilation. Crit Care Med 1998; 26:364–8.

120. Dorges V, Ocker H, Wenzel V, et al. Emergency airway management by non-anaesthesia house officers: A comparison of three strategies. Emerg Med J 2001; 18:90–4.

121. Wagner-Berger HG, Wenzel V, Voelckel WG, et al. A pilot study to evaluate the SMART BAG: A new pressure-responsive, gas-flow limiting bag-valve-mask device. Anesth Analg 2003; 97:1686–9.

122. Idris AH, Wenzel V, Banner MJ, Melker RJ. Smaller tidal volumes minimize gastric inflation during CPR with an unprotected airway (abstract). Circulation 1995; 92:I-759.

123. Takeda T, Tanigawa K, Tanaka H, et al. The assessment of three methods to verify tracheal tube placement in the emergency setting. Resuscitation 2003; 56:153–7.

124. ECC committee, subcommittees and task forces of the American Heart Association. 2005 American Heart Association guidelines for cardiopulmonary resuscitation and emergency cardiovascular care. Circulation 2005; 112(suppl):VI-203.

125. Nolan JP, Deakin CD, Soar J, Bottiger BW, Smith G. European resuscitation council. European resuscitation council guidelines for resuscitation 2005. Section 4. Adult advanced life suppport. Resuscitation 2005;67(suppl):S39–86.

126. Parmet JL, Colonna-Romano P, Horrow JC, et al. The laryngeal mask airway reliably provides rescue ventilation in cases of unanticipated difficult tracheal intubation along with difficult mask ventilation. Anesth Analg 1998; 87:661–5.

127. Martin SE, Ochsner MG, Jarman RH, et al. Use of the laryngeal mask airway in air transport when intubation fails. J Trauma 1999; 47:352–7.

128. Keller C, Brimacombe J, Bittersohl J, et al. Aspiration and the laryngeal mask airway: Three cases and a review of the literature. Br J Anaesth 2004; 93:579–82.

129. Stone BJ, Chantler PJ, Baskett PJ. The incidence of regurgitation during cardiopulmonary resuscitation: A comparison between the bag valve mask and laryngeal mask airway. Resuscitation 1998; 38:3–6.

130. Brimacombe J, Keller C. The ProSeal laryngeal mask airway: A randomized, crossover study with the standard laryngeal

mask airway in paralyzed, anesthetized patients. Anesthesiology 2000; 93:104–9.

131. Keller C, Brimacombe J, Kleinsasser A, Loeckinger A. Does the ProSeal laryngeal mask airway prevent aspiration of regurgitated fluid? Anesth Analg 2000; 91:1017–20.

132. Ocker H, Wenzel V, Schmucker P, et al. A comparison of the laryngeal tube with the laryngeal mask airway during routine surgical procedures. Anesth Analg 2002; 95:1094–7.

133. Asai T, Kawashima A, Hidaka I, Kawachi S. The laryngeal tube compared with the laryngeal mask: insertion, gas leak pressure and gastric insufflation. Br J Anaesth 2002; 89:729–32.

134. Devitt JH, Wenstone R, Noel AG, O'Donnell MP. The laryngeal mask airway and positive-pressure ventilation. Anesthesiology 1994; 80:550–5.

135. Rumball CJ, MacDonald D. The PTL, Combitube, laryngeal mask, and oral airway: A randomized prehospital comparative study of ventilatory device effectiveness and cost-effectiveness in 470 cases of cardiorespiratory arrest. Prehosp Emerg Care 1997; 1:1–10.

136. Blostein PA, Koestner AJ, Hoak S. Failed rapid sequence intubation in trauma patients: Esophageal tracheal Combitube is a useful adjunct. J Trauma 1998; 44:534–7.

137. Rabitsch W, Schellongowski P, Staudinger T, et al. Comparison of a conventional tracheal airway with the Combitube in an urban emergency medical services system run by physicians. Resuscitation 2003; 57:27–32.

138. Della Puppa A, Pittoni G, Frass M. Tracheal esophageal Combitube: A useful airway for morbidly obese patients who cannot intubate or ventilate. Acta Anaesthesiol Scand 2002; 46:911–3.

139. Vezina D, Lessard MR, Bussieres J, et al. Complications associated with the use of the esophageal-tracheal Combitube. Can J Anaesth 1998; 45:76–80.

140. Asai T, Murao K, Shingu K. Efficacy of the laryngeal tube during intermittent positive-pressure ventilation. Anaesthesia 2000; 55:1099–102.

141. Miller DM, Youkhana I, Pearce AC. The laryngeal mask and VBM laryngeal tube compared during spontaneous ventilation: A pilot study. Eur J Anaesthesiol 2001; 18:593–8.

142. Dorges V, Ocker H, Wenzel V, Schmucker P. The laryngeal tube: A new simple airway device. Anesth Analg 2000; 90:1220–2.

143. Eisenburger P, Laczika K, List M, et al. Comparison of conventional surgical versus Seldinger technique emergency cricothyrotomy performed by inexperienced clinicians. Anesthesiology 2000; 92:687–90.

144. Chan TC, Vilke GM, Bramwell KJ, et al. Comparison of wire-guided cricothyrotomy versus standard surgical cricothyrotomy technique. J Emerg Med 1999; 17:957–62.

Chapter 28

TRANSPORT OF THE VENTILATOR-SUPPORTED PATIENT

RICHARD D BRANSON
JAY A JOHANNIGMAN

Mechanical ventilation of the critically ill patient is best practiced in the safe confines of the intensive-care unit (ICU). Transport of ventilated patients, however, remains a frequent challenge.[1-3] Successful transport requires effective communication, appropriate planning, key personnel, and compact, rugged equipment. Clinicians should be aware of the physiologic effects of transport, frequency of adverse events, and methods to prevent complications.

Intrahospital Transport

Intrahospital transport of the ventilated patient includes movement between the operating room and recovery room or ICU, a routine procedure accomplished in minutes.[4] Transport of critically ill patients from the ICU for diagnostic techniques represents a greater challenge.[2,3] Intrahospital transport from the ICU is accomplished most commonly for computed tomography (CT) with a mean duration of 90 minutes.[5-7] CT is ordered most frequently for evaluation of head injury, identification of bleeding, and location and drainage of fluid collections.[4-14] Table 28-1 lists investigations of intrahospital transports, indicating the type and number of patients along with most frequent destinations.

Magnetic resonance imaging (MRI) is an increasingly common destination for the critically ill ventilated patient. The prohibition of ferrous materials in the MRI scanner represents a significant challenge in providing mechanical ventilation.

Interhospital Transport

Interfacility transport has increased in recent years owing to the regionalization of specialty care and the growth of hospital systems. Neonatal intensive-care and extracorporeal membrane oxygenation centers are the classic examples of this model. More recently, specialty care in respiratory failure, trauma, transplant, and cardiac disorders at tertiary-care medical facilities has increased interhospital transports.[15,16] The growth of hospital systems with acute- and chronic-care facilities represents another reason for interhospital transport as patients travel back and forth based on acuity.

Interhospital transport can be accomplished using ground or air transport. Each method possesses unique advantages and new challenges. Choice of transport vehicle should include an assessment of urgency, weather, traffic, geography, and cost. Ground transport using a specially equipped ambulance and personnel can provide "mobile intensive care" and is the most common mode of transport. Ground transport is the most readily available and cost-effective while also the least influenced by weather.[3]

Air transport should be considered when distances exceed 50 miles or ground transport requires greater than 2 hours. Rotor-wing or helicopter transport is preferred in areas where access is limited or distances are between 50 and 150 miles. Helicopter transport reduces transport time, but the environment is cramped and noisy compared with ground transport. Additionally, rotor-wing aircraft are expensive to purchase, operate, and maintain and have a poorer safety record.[3] Fixed-wing transport is considered when distances exceed 150 miles. While some hospitals maintain a fixed-wing aircraft as a consequence of geography, air ambulances frequently are private corporations

TABLE 28-1 Comparison of Studies Evaluating Intrahospital Transport of Critically Ill Patients

Year, Author (Reference)	Number of Patients	Patient Population	Number of Transports	Transport Destination	Duration of Transport Mean (Range)
1986, Insel (4)	47	Adult, postoperative	47	Radiology 30%, OR 70%	NR
1987, Braman (8)	36	Adult, ICU	36	Radiology 100%	NR
1988, Indeck (6)	56	Adult, trauma	103	Radiology 100%	81 min
1989, Weg (9)	20	Adult, ICU	20	Radiology 100%	50 min (15–80 min)
1990, Andrews (10)	27	Adult, closed head injury	35	OR 51%, radiology 49%	NR
1990, Smith (7)	127	Adult, ICU	127	OR 25%, radiology 75%	95 min
1992, Hurst (5)	83	Adult, surgical/trauma	100	Radiology 100%	74 min (20–225 min)
1995, Szem (11)	175	Adult, surgical	203	OR 39%, radiology 61%	NR
1995, Evans (12)	36	Adult, ICU	36	Radiology 100%	62 min (26–166 min)
1995, Wallen (13)	139	Pediatric	180	OR 49%, radiology 30%	NR
1998, Stearly (14)	237	Adult, ICU	237	Radiology 100%	NR

available for hire. When using a fixed-wing aircraft, the distance for ground transport from the airport to the hospital must be considered.

Preparation and Planning

The key to a successful, safe transport is preparation and planning. Before movement, goals of transport should be established and appropriate personnel and equipment assembled. Communication with the receiving institution or department is critical to reduce unnecessary delays.[1,17] During intrahospital transport to radiology, goals include obtaining a quality examination while maintaining stability, continuing care, and avoiding mishaps. Elective transports should be delayed until patient stability is achieved.[16] In emergent situations, current care and resuscitation should be continued and plans to treat further deterioration agreed on. Uneventful transport often is attributed to planning and communication.[18]

Guidelines

The American College of Critical Care Medicine (ACCM) guidelines state that "each hospital should have a formalized plan for intra- and interhospital transport."[19] This includes pretransport coordination and communication and guidelines for defining the appropriate personnel, equipment, and monitoring. ACCM further suggests that these plans should be developed by multidisciplinary teams and subjected to continuous quality improvement.

The ACCM guidelines are based on research suggesting that protocols reduce mishaps and facilitate transport.[7,21] Transport protocols should match patient acuity with the personnel and equipment necessary to achieve appropriate monitoring and safety. A survey of 152 ICUs, showed that 95% expressed being quite concerned or very concerned (51%) about the dangers of transporting critically ill patients. In the same survey, only 45% had policies defining personnel requirements.[21]

Transport policies should describe the type and level of training for personnel involved.[1,16,19,20] The American Association for Respiratory Care (AARC) clinical practice guide-

line recommends that at least one member of the transport team be certified in advanced cardiac life support (ACLS) or pediatric advanced life support (PALS).[20] The AARC also recommends that one member be proficient in endotracheal intubation. Several groups have suggested that a registered nurse and a respiratory therapist accompany all ventilated patients.[1,5,19–21] Requiring a physician to attend transports may increase patient safety and decrease the number of unnecessary transports but is impractical outside of academic centers.[5,21]

Risk-Benefit of Transport

Considerable effort has been expended to catalog the risks of transport.[1,4–14] These are considered in detail below. Benefits of transport include discovery of pathology or verifying diagnoses that guide treatment. Several investigations have noted that in two-thirds of transports to radiology, the patient's treatment course is unaltered.[5,6,11] Head CT is least likely to result in a change in therapy, whereas abdominal CT is most likely to result in new findings and guide intervention. Negative findings, however, rule out sources of clinical deterioration and lead the physician to search for other etiologies.

Cost-benefit ratio is difficult to measure and includes not only the cost for the procedure but also the costs of transport equipment, transport personnel, and personnel to cover the workload of caregivers attending the patient outside the ICU. This additional burden to remaining ICU staff frequently is associated with reduced staffing levels and end-of-shift overtime.[5,6]

Physiologic Effects and Complications of Transport

Transport of the ventilated patient requires exchange of existing monitoring and support equipment to portable equipment, as well as the physical movement of the patient. These interruptions in care and change in patient position can alter the patient's condition. Patients typically are transported in the supine position, which changes respiratory mechanics

TABLE 28-2 Commonly Reported Complications during Transport of the Mechanically Ventilated Patient

Cardiovascular
  Arrythmia
  Hypotension
  Hypertension
  Tachycardia
  Bradycardia
  Myocardial ischemia
  Worsening heart failure
  Cardiac arrest

Respiratory
  Hypoventilation
  Hyperventialion
  Hypoxemia
  Barotrauma

Neurologic
  Elevated intracranial pressure
  Increased anxiety

Other
  Increased risk of ventilator associated pneumonia
  Bleeding or hemorrhage
  Hypothermia
  Effects of altitude on physiology[a]

Equipment failure/mishaps
  Airway obstruction
  Extubation
  Intubation of right main-stem bronchus
  Gastric aspiration around endotracheal tube cuff
  Loss of battery power to monitoring equipment or ventilator
  Damage to equipment due to mishandling or falls
  Loss of oxygen supply
  Failure to reproduce ICU ventilation parameters with a portable
    ventilator or manual ventilator (loss of PEEP, failure to trigger,
    inappropriate tidal volume or frequency)
  Effects of altitude on equipment performance[a]
  Loss of venous access/indwelling vascular catheters
  Interruption of medications—continuous and intermittent
  Inadequate chest tube drainage

[a]Unique to air transport.

and may alter hemodynamics. Many departments where procedures are done are distant from the ICU, located in facilities never designed to house the critically ill patient. Both remote location and poor physical plant may contribute to untoward outcomes following a complication. Complications of transport are frequently recalled as "the catastrophe in radiology." The spectrum of complications ranges from minor changes in heart rate to cardiac arrest. A list of common complications is given in Table 28-2.

CARDIOVASCULAR COMPLICATIONS

Cardiovascular events are the most frequent complication of transport and are reported in up to 50% of cases.[6,8,9,11] An increase in heart rate is seen frequently as a result of anxiety, pain, and activity. Arrhythmias are common during the transport of high-risk cardiac patients, a finding complicated by the fact that routine lead II monitoring may be unable to detect early changes.[23,24] Acute respiratory alkalosis resulting from hyperventilation alters myocardial ir-

ritability, leading to dysrhythmias.[8,25–28] This finding commonly is associated with unmonitored manual ventilation but can occur with a ventilator when minute ventilation is unreliable.[28]

Hypotension during transport may result from loss of intravenous access, interruption of vasoactive agents, pneumothorax, or bleeding. Alkalemia associated with hyperventilation likewise can cause hypotension.[8,28,29] Hypertension can result from stress and anxiety, as well as from patient movement that encounters "bumps" in the transport path and jostling of patients that causes pain.[5,6,10,22] Cardiac arrest has been reported during transport, but patient movement per se has not been directly implicated.

RESPIRATORY COMPLICATIONS

Hypoxemia may occur during transport as a consequence of loss of positive end-expiratory pressure (PEEP), changes in patient position, impaired secretion removal, and failure to reproduce ventilator settings adequately.[2,5,6,8,29–31] During transport of adult patients, high inspired oxygen concentrations (F_{IO_2}) are used commonly as a matter of convenience.[1,32] Elevated F_{IO_2} may lead to masking of deterioration in lung function and contribute to absorption atelectasis. Patients requiring PEEP of more than 10 cmH_2O have demonstrated a deterioration in oxygenation during transport that lasted for up to 24 hours.[10]

Hyperventilation is a frequent complication associated with manual ventilation[8,28,31,33] and with poor control of minute ventilation by portable ventilators.[31] Sudden respiratory alkalosis can result in changes in cardiovascular function. During resuscitation, hyperventilation has been shown to impair hemodynamics and contribute to the development of electromechancial disassociation and poor outcome.[34] Hyperventilation increases intrathoracic pressure, produces air trapping, reduces cardiac output, shifts the oxyhemoglobin dissociation curve to the left hindering oxygen unloading, and causes cerebral and myocardial vasoconstriction. These combined effects may affect patient outcome adversely.[34]

Hypoventilation is reported less frequently and generally is better tolerated.[4–14] Too small a tidal volume may contribute to atelectasis and respiratory acidosis. In acute acidosis, cardiac function may be compromised. Hypoventilation may result from the increased use of sedation and neuromuscular blocking agents to achieve patient comfort and facilitate quality examinations.

Loss of the artificial airway is an infrequent but catastrophic complication of transport. Inability to establish an adequate airway is associated with hypoxemia and poor outcome in head-injured patients.[17,35] Unintubated patients with marginal airway control may benefit from intubation before transport. Radiologic procedures requiring the patient to remain supine may compromise the tenuous airway.

NEUROLOGIC COMPLICATIONS

Increases in intracranial pressure have been reported during transport and are associated with supine positioning, changes in ventilation, airway compromise, and hypoxemia.[10,17,35] Anxiety may contribute to hemodynamic alterations as well as increased intracranial pressure (ICP). Anxiety results from patient movement and uncertainty, as well as adjustment from ICU to transport equipment.

OTHER COMPLICATIONS

Hypothermia during transport occurs because hallways and examination areas have less precise environmental controls.[13] Exposure of skin surfaces for adequate radiologic examinations and use of skin preparations for procedures further contribute to temperature loss. Blood loss has been reported during movement of patients with unstable fractures.[13] A late complication of transport is ventilator-associated pneumonia. Transport from the ICU is an independent predictor for the development of pneumonia.[36] Possible causes include supine positioning, aspiration around artificial airways, contaminated manual resuscitators, manipulation of the ventilator circuit, and inadequate infection control policies.[37-39] It is also possible that the need for transport implies a greater severity of illness and prolonged ventilaton, increasing the risk of pneumonia.

Air transport introduces the unique issues of physiologic alterations at altitude. Fixed-wing aircraft employ pressurized cabins equivalent to an altitude of 8000 ft (barometric pressure of 565 mmHg).[40] Rotor-wing aircraft may operate at higher altitudes during movement over rugged terrain.

The hypobaric environment can cause hypoxic hypoxemia and expansion of gases in closed spaces. A change in altitude from sea level to 8000 ft is associated with hypoxemia in patients with normal and abnormal pulmonary function.[41,42] At similar altitude changes, gas trapped in closed spaces can expand in volume by 30%. Gas trapped in the body, such as a small pneumothorax, can become significant at altitude. Gas in equipment is also affected, including the volume and pressure inside airway cuffs and urinary catheters, which may result in pain, discomfort, or rupture. Ventilator performance can be adversely affected by changes in barometric pressure. In particular, pneumatically operated devices will have alterations in tidal volume, frequency, and inspiratory time as altitude increases. Newer ventilators include a barometric pressure sensor that automatically compensates for hypobaric effects on gas density.[43]

Contraindications to Transport

There are few absolute contraindications to transport. Appropriate planning, equipment, personnel, and monitoring allow safe transport. Transport of the ventilated patient is best considered as transferring the ICU with the patient, not transferring the patient from the ICU. Patients occasionally are deemed too sick to transport. The specific contraindications to transport are (1) inability to maintain acceptable hemodynamic status, (2) inability to establish an adequate airway, (3) inadequate personnel, (4) inability to maintain adequate gas exchange, and (5) inability to monitor patient status effectively.

Equipment Malfunction/Mishaps

Mishaps range from the benign to the catastrophic. The frequency of mishaps varies widely with the definition. *Mishap* has been defined as "the occurrence of any unplanned event that potentially could have a detrimental effect on patient care stability."[7,9] Using a broad definition of mishap, early studies found that half of patients suffered a mishap during transport. Most of these, however, were minor (e.g., electrocradiograph electrode disconnection), and only 24% of mishaps resulted in any change in patient physiology.[7] Other common mishaps include loss of vascular access, disconnection from oxygen supply, disconnection from the ventilator, and improper care of chest tubes.[6-9,22]

Equipment failure remains a common mishap during transport, frequently attributed to poor planning and carlessness.[9,22] Reported failures include depletion of battery power of ventilator or monitoring equipment, exhaustion of portable oxygen supplies, and damage to devices resulting from falls to the floor.[4-9] Exhaustion of a compressed oxygen supply during use of a pneumatically powered ventilator terminates ventilation and can be a life-threatening mishap. Table 28-3 provides a comparison of studies evaluating complications and mishaps in intrahospital transport of critically ill patients.

Equipment and Monitoring During Transport

Approriate equipment and monitoring are important to maintaining homeostasis and ensuring safety. Monitoring during transport should emulate the ICU. Minimum requirements include electrocardiographic (ECG) monitoring (lead II) of heart rhythm and rate, invasive or noninvasive blood pressure monitoring, and pulse oximetry. Monitoring should adapt to the needs of the patient and include additional pressure monitoring if ICP or central venous pressure catheters are present. Battery-powered intravenous pumps for medication delivery also are required.

Equipment for transport should be rugged, lightweight, reliable, and operate from battery power for at least 1 hour. Required equipment includes the physiologic monitor, pulse oximeter, and ventilator. Additional equipment includes a manual resuscitator with a PEEP valve, oxygen supplies, stethoscope, and emergency airway-management equipment. A spirometer to monitor tidal volume during manual resuscitation also should be available.

A drug box with the patient's current medications and agents for resuscitation should accompany the patient. Agents for sedation or paralysis and intravenous fluids for resuscitation and ongoing management also should be available.

A dedicated transport cart or trolley may simplify transport but is an inefficient use of resources.[6,23,33,43,44] The advantage of the cart is immediate availability of required devices. The disadvantages are cumbersome size and cost. A dedicated trolley for transport perhaps is best suited for interhospital transport.[45] Table 28-4 lists the monitoring and

TABLE 28-3 Comparison of Studies Evaluating Complications and Mishaps in Intrahospital Transport of Critically Ill Patients

Year, Author (Reference)	Complication Rate	COMPLICATIONS				Type of Ventilation	Attendants
		Cardiovascular	Respiratory	Equipment	Other		
1975, Waddell (22)	7.2%	7.2% hypotension, hypertension, tachycardia	0%	0%	Bleeding 1.6%	NR	RN, MD
1986, Insel (4)	24%	24% hypotension, arrhythmia	0%	0%	0%	Manual	RN, MD
1987, Braman (8)	66%	25% hypotension, arrythmia	56% hypocarbia, hypercarbia	5.5% ventilator battery failure, disconnected oxygen supply	0%	Manual, $n = 20$ Ventilator, $n = 16$	RN, MD, RRT
1988, Indeck (6)	68%	61% tachycardia, hypotension, hypertension	37% hypoxemia, tachypnea	0%	0%	Ventilator	RN, MD RRT
1989, Weg (9)	15%	0%	10% hypoxemia hypocarbia	5% disconnected oxygen supply	0%	Manual	RN, RRT
1990, Andrews (10)	51%	9% hypotension, 23% rise in ICP, 14% hypertension	9% hypoxemia	NR	0%	Ventilator	NR
1990, Smith (7)	34%	NR	NR	34% ECG lead disconnected, monitor battery failure, ventilator disconnection	NR	NR	RN, MD, RRT
1992, Hurst (5)	66%	27% tachycardia, 36% hypotension, hypertension	20% tachypnea 2% hypoxemia	5% pulse oximeter failure, monitor battery failure	0%	Ventilator	RN, MD, RRT
1995, Szem (11)	5.9%	1% hypotension, 1.5% cardiac arrest	4% hypoxemia	NR	NR	Manual or ventilator	MD, RRT
1995, Evans (12)	53%	5.5% arrhythmia, 25% tachycardia, 39% hypotension	17% hypoxemia	11%	0%	Ventilator	NR
1995, Wallen (13)	76%	47% tachycardia, 21% hypotension	29% tachypnea 6% hypoxemia	10% monitoring battery failure, ventilator disconnection	10% hypothermia	Manual	RN, MD
1998, Stearly (14)	15.5%	NR	NR	NR	NR	NR	RN

ABBREVIATIONS: ECG, electrocardiograph; ICP, intracranial pressure; MD, physician; NR, not reported; RN, registered nurse; RRT, registered respiratory therapist.

TABLE 28-4 Monitoring and Life-Support Equipment for Transport of the Ventilator-Dependent Patient

Monitoring
- ECG monitoring (rate and rhythm)
- Arterial blood pressure monitoring (invasive or noninvasive)
- Pulse oximetry
- Additional pressure monitoring (e.g., pulmonary artery, intracranial)
- Stethoscope
- End-tidal CO_2 monitor (optional)
- Portable spirometer

Support equipment
- Portable ventilator capable of providing required mode, F_{IO_2}, tidal volume, and PEEP
- Airway maintenance (should include a difficult airway kit)
- Manual resuscitator and mask
- Oxygen supplies (one or two cylinders)
- Drug box (emergency drugs, patient specific drugs, sedatives, IV fluids)
- Infusion pumps (battery operated)
- Defibrillator (optional)
- Portable suction (optional)

life-support equipment necessary for transport of the ventilated patient.

Rationale for Use of a Portable Ventilator

Manual ventilation historically has been used during transport. It is inexpensive, simple, and requires only human power. During manual ventilation, however, the volume, frequency, and pressure applied are unknown. Several investigators have noted hyperventilation and acute respiratory alkalosis during manual ventilation resulting in cardiovascular complications.[2,23,28,29,31,33–35] Aggressive manual ventilation can result in excessive airway pressures, causing barotrauma or volutrauma and worsening air trapping.[46]

Manual ventilation can be successful in the hands of a skilled clinician with additional volume- and pressure-monitoring capabilities.[9,13] Monitoring end-tidal CO_2 also may prove helpful in preventing hyperventilation. Simple reasoning, however, dictates that manual ventilation cannot replicate the tidal volume, frequency, F_{IO_2}, PEEP, and mode of ventilation with the consistency and precision of a ventilator. Maintaining constant PEEP with a manual resuscitator is difficult and can lead to hypoxemia.[1,2,30] Finally, manual resuscitators were not meant to allow spontaneous breathing, causing excessive work of breathing.[47,48]

Comparisons of manual ventilation with a transport ventilator uniformly support the use of a ventilator to preserve normal gas exchange.[8,28,31] A mechanical ventilator also allows monitoring and alarms. Recently introduced portable ventilators provide volume- and pressure-control ventilation along with flow triggering and pressure-support ventilation.[32] A portable ventilator also can provide a constant F_{IO_2} and maintain PEEP.

Portable ventilators are more expensive than manual resuscitators, and many require a high-pressure (50 psig) gas supply. While manual ventilation of the postoperative pa-

tient with normal lungs during transport to the recovery room is safe, ventilation of the patient requiring PEEP, elevated F_{IO_2}, and constant volume is best accomplished by a ventilator.

Transport Ventilators

Technically, any ventilator that operates from a battery and either an internal gas source or a compressed gas cylinder could be considered a transport ventilator. Because of the demands of patient transport, however, these simple criteria are inadequate. Using performance to discriminate transport ventilators yields three categories: automatic resuscitators, pneumatically powered transport ventilators, and sophisticated transport ventilators.

AUTOMATIC RESUSCITATOR

An automatic resuscitator is a device that provides ventilation at a set pressure. A few automatic resuscitators do not have the ability to set or control frequency. These devices are flow-limited and pressure-cycled. Frequency varies with lung impedance: When impedance is high, tidal volume is small and frequency rapid; when impedance is low, tidal volume is high and frequency slow. These devices are powered pneumatically (requiring no electricity), have only a mechanical, audible high-pressure alarm, and have only disposable pressure manometers.

INTENDED USE
These devices are designed for use in a prehospital setting by personnel with limited expertise in mechanical ventilation.

EXAMPLES OF AUTOMATIC RESUSCITATORS
Examples include the Vortran and Oxylator EM-100 (Fig. 28-1). Both these devices are flow-limited and pressure-cycled. As such, rate cannot be set, and tidal volume varies with changes in patient resistance and compliance. The Vortran has proven unreliable when the ventilator's orientation is changed, failing to cycle.[49,50] Both devices are inexpensive (Vortran $45 and Oxylator $600). In the presence of a leak, if the set peak pressure cannot be reached, both devices will remain stuck in inspiration. Successful use of the Vortran in intubated, closely monitored subjects has been reported.[51]

The Ambu Matic is a pneumatically powered automatic resuscitator delivering controlled mandatory ventilation (Fig. 28-2). It consists of a patient valve and a control module with a single-slide control for frequency and tidal volume settings and a control for manually triggering a breath. An F_{IO_2} of 0.6 (prolonging the duration of oxygen supply) or 1.0 is available. There is a fixed pressure-limiting valve, set at 60 cmH_2O. Performance in the laboratory suggests that this device can provide set tidal volumes up to a peak pressure of 50 cmH_2O.[52] A comparison of the physical and operational characteristics of automatice resuscitators is given in Tables 28-5 and 28-6.

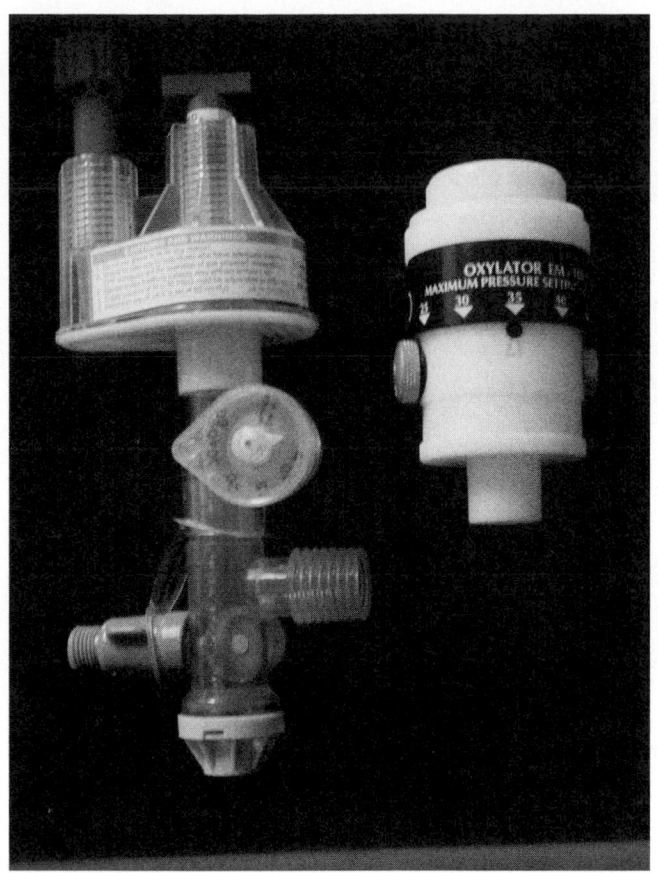

FIGURE 28-1 Examples of automatic resuscitators, the Vortran (*left*) and the Oxylator (*right*).

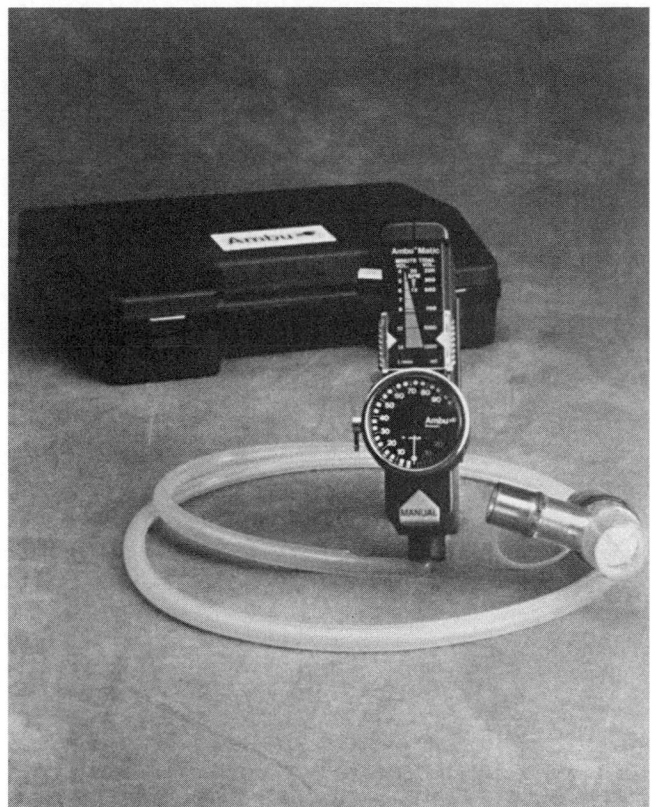

FIGURE 28-2 The AmbuMatic automatic resuscitator.

SIMPLE TRANSPORT VENTILATOR

The simplest transport ventilator is a device that supplies mechanical ventilation at a specified rate and volume and includes a pressure-relief valve with an audible mechanical alarm. Most simple transport ventilators are powered and controlled pneumatically. In some instances, a battery allows for simple low- and high-pressure alarms, as well as monitoring and display of airway pressure.

INTENDED USE

These devices also are used primarily in prehospital settings by personnel with some training in mechanical ventilation.

More complex than automatic resuscitators, these devices offer a range of breath rate and tidal volume adjustment and also can be used with spontaneously breathing patients. A comparison of the physical and operational characteristics of automatic resuscitators is given in Tables 28-7 and 8.

EXAMPLES OF SIMPLE TRANSPORT VENTILATORS

The Auto Vent 2000 (Fig. 28-3) and 3000 are pneumatically powered transport ventilators operating in the intermittent mandatory ventilation (IMV) mode. Mandatory breaths are time-triggered, flow- or pressure-limited, and time-cycled at an F_{IO_2} of 1.0. A demand valve at the airway opens at -2 cmH$_2$O. Spontaneous breaths are pressure-triggered, pressure-limited, and pressure-cycled. During spontaneous breaths, the patient breathes from the demand valve at

TABLE 28-5   Physical Characteristics of Automatic Resuscitators

	Dimensions (cm)	Weight (kg)	Supply Pressure (psig)	Operating Temperature (°C)	Gas Consumption	Minimum Patient Weight (kg)
Ambu Matic	16 × 9 × 4	1.2	39–94	−18–50	0.8 liters/cycle	15
VAR Model RT	16.8 × 8.4 × 6.4	0.074	50	−18–50 (storage −40–60)	NS	40
VAR Model RC	6.6 × 3.3× 2.5	0.074	50	−18–50 (storage −40–60)	NS	40
Oxylator EM-100	5.7 × 10.8	0.5	45–80	−30–60 (storage −40–70)	NS	10
Oxylator FR-300	4.8 × 10.0 (round)	0.18	45–80	−30–60 (storage −40–70)	NS	10
paraPAC Responder	4 × 6 × 18	1.9 (Patient valve 0.08)	37–87	−10–65	Max of 2 liters/min in excess of minute volume	23

NS, not specified.

TABLE 28-6 Operational Characteristics of Automatic Resuscitators

	Cycling Variables	Modes	Rate (breaths/min)	Tidal Volume (ml)	Inspiratory Time (s)	Peak Flow (liters/min)
Ambu Matic	Pressure	CMV	4 or 20	200–1200	NS	40
VAR Model RT	Pressure	CMV, AMV	Varies with impedance	170–2000	0.5–3	40
VAR Model RC	Pressure	CMV, AMV	Varies with impedance	170–2000	0.5–3	40
Oxylator EM-100	Pressure (20–50 cmH$_2$O)	CMV	Varies with impedance	Depends on respiratory system compliance	I:E 1:1 or 1:2	40
Oxylator FR 300	Pressure (20 cmH$_2$O)	CMV	Varies with impedance	Depends on respiratory system compliance	1:1.5	30
paraPAC Responder	Time	CMV	11–21	340–1450	0.5–2.2	40

	F$_{IO_2}$	PEEP/CPAP (cmH$_2$O)	Alarms	Monitoring	Demand-Flow Valve	Manual Breath
Ambu Matic	0.6 or 1.0	External PEEP/CPAP valve	Audible high pressure Accessory module available	Accessory module available	No (does allow entrainment of ambient air)	Yes
VAR Model RT	1	1/10 of PIP, 2–5 cmH$_2$O	Audible high pressure	Optional airway pressure manometer	Yes	No
VAR Model RC	0.5 or 1.0	1/10 of PIP, 2–5 cmH$_2$O	Audible high pressure	Optional airway pressure manometer	Yes	No
Oxylator EM-100	1	2–4	Audible high pressure	None	No (does allow entrainment of ambient air)	Yes
Oxylator FR 300	1	2–4	Audible high pressure	None	No (does allow entrainment of ambient air)	Yes
paraPAC Responder	1	No	Audible high pressure	None	No	No

ABBREVIATIONS: CMV, continuous mandatory ventilation; AMV, assisted mandatory ventilation; NS, not specified.

48 liters/min. If patient demand exceeds 48 liters/min, ambient air is drawn into the valve, diluting the F$_{IO_2}$. A mechanical visual indicator on the patient valve turns green during the inspiratory phase. If the 50 cmH$_2$O pressure relief is violated, an audible alarm caused by gas escaping can be heard. There is no monitoring.

The AutoVent 2000 is designed for adults with a control for breath rate and one for tidal volume. The AutoVent 3000 is designed for adults and children and has three controls: breath rate, tidal volume, and inspiratory time. Both consist of a control module, patient valve, and connecting hoses.

The AutoVent ventilators consume approximately 0.5 liter/min of gas to operate the logic. The higher the frequency setting, the higher is the gas consumption. The inspiratory flow is fixed at 48 liters/min. If patient inspiratory

TABLE 28-7 Physical Characteristics of Simple Transport Ventilators

	Dimensions (cm)	Weight (kg)	Supply Pressure (psig)	Operating Temperature (°C)	Gas Consumption (liters/min)	Minimum Patient Weight (kg)
AutoVent 2000	15 × 9 × 4.5	0.68	40–90	36°C	0.5 liter/min depending on breath rate	Child
AutoVent 3000	15 × 9 × 4.5	0.68	40–90	−34–36°C	0.5 liter/min depending on breath rate	Child
paraPAC Medic	9.2 × 22.0 × 16.2	2.8	39–87	−10–65°C	Delivered volume plus 10 ml/cycle	4.5
Uni-Vent 706	20 × 13 × 5.5	1.45	50–100	−60–65°C	0	Infant

TABLE 28-8   Operational Characteristics of Simple Transport Ventilators

	Cycling Variables	Modes	Rate (breaths/min)	Tidal Volume (ml)	Inspiratory Time (s)	Peak Flow (liters/min)
AuttoVent 2000	Time	CMV, IMV	8, 9, 10, 12, 14, 16, 20	400, 600, 800, 1000, 1200	1.5	48
AutoVent 3000	Time	CMV, IMV	Child 9, 11, 14, 17, 20, 23, 27 Adult 8, 9, 10, 12, 14, 16, 20	Child 200, 300, 400, 500, 600 Adult 400, 600, 800, 1000, 1200	Child 0.75 Adult 1.5	48
ParaPAC Medic	Time	Synchronized minimum mandatory ventilation	8–40	70–1300	0.6 to 1.6	60
Uni-Vent 706	Time	CMV	Child/infant 14, 20, 30 Adult 12, 18	10–1250	Child 0.75 to 2.7; Adult 1.5 to 3.5	90

	$F_{I_{O_2}}$	PEEP/CPAP (cmH$_2$O)	Alarms	Monitoring	Demand-Flow Valve	Manual Breath
AutoVent 2000	1	No	Audible high pressure	Green light indicating inspiratory phase	Yes	No
AutoVent 3000	1	No	Audible high pressure	Green light indicating inspiratory phase	Yes	No
ParaPAC Medic	0.5 or 1.0	Add on PEEP valve to 20 cm H$_2$O	Audible high airway pressure	Airway pressure	Yes	No
Uni-Vent 706	1	No	Audible high airway pressure, low battery[a]	None	No	Yes

ABBREVIATIONS: CMV, continuous mandatory ventilation; IMV, intermittent mandatory ventilation.
[a]Battery duration 10 hours.

flow exceeds 48 liters/min, the patient entrains ambient air, increasing the imposed work of breathing. The limited number of rate–tidal volume combinations that can be set is a limitation.

The Uni-Vent 706 (Fig. 28-4) is a pneumatically powered, electronically controlled ventilator delivering an $F_{I_{O_2}}$ of 1.0. Controls set inspiratory flow and a series of rate, inspira-

FIGURE 28-3 The AutoVent 2000 simple transport ventilator.

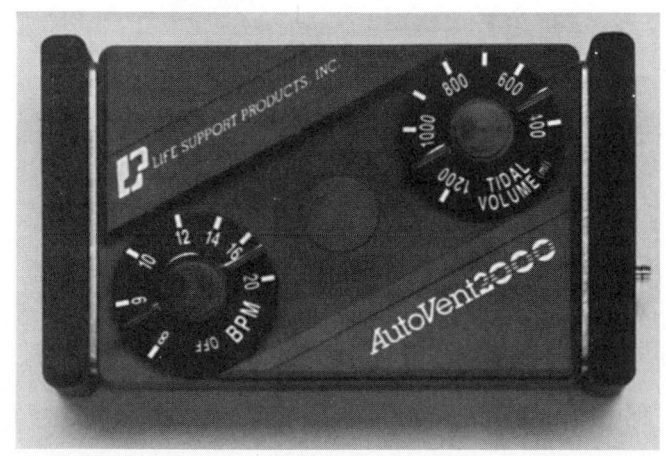

tory time, and inspiratory-expiratory (I:E) ratio combinations corresponding to those predicted to be appropriate for adult and pediatric ventilation. Inspiratory flow is limited from 0–90 liters/min, and a high-pressure limit can be set (60 or 80 cmH$_2$O) at the patient valve, which activates an audible alarm when exceeded. Indicator lamps illuminate signaling inhalation and exhalation. There is a low-battery alarm. Prehospital use of the Uni-Vent 706 by paramedics during cardiopulmonary resuscitation of intubated victims has proven successful.[53]

SOPHISTICATED TRANSPORT VENTILATOR

A sophisticated transport ventilator is capable of performance comparable with that of an ICU ventilator. These devices may have built-in compressors or turbines to generate positive pressure without compressed gas and contain an air-oxygen blender.

INTENDED USE

Sophisticated transport ventilators are intended for inter- or intrahospital transport of critically ill patients. These devices should be capable of ventilating the sickest patients.

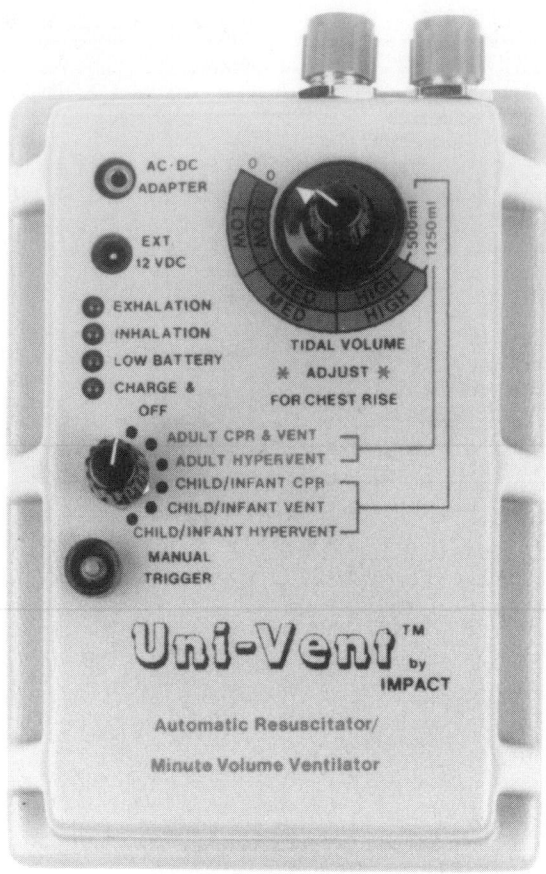

FIGURE 28-4 The Uni-Vent 706 simple transport ventilator.

EXAMPLES OF SOPHISTICATED TRANSPORT VENTILATORS

The IC-2A is a flow controller that can be triggered by pressure or time or manually; it is also pressure- or flow-limited and time-cycled (Fig. 28-5). It requires a compressed-gas source for delivery to the patient, as well as for the fluidic logic circuit. The IC-2A delivers an F_{IO_2} of 1.0. Controls include the mode of ventilation, inspiratory and expiratory time, inspiratory flow, sensitivity, and PEEP/continuous positive airway pressure (CPAP) level. A single control on the rear panel adjusts the mechanical pressure limit. Mode is selected by toggle switches and inspiratory flow; inspiratory and expiratory times are adjusted with calibrated dials. Controls for sensitivity, PEEP/CPAP, and pressure limit are uncalibrated. Airway pressure is displayed on an aneroid pressure gauge. Pressure-activated indicators alert the operator to the type of breath delivered (mandatory or spontaneous).

The IC-2A is used most often for ventilation in the MRI scanner because it has no ferrous components. The excessive gas consumption should be considered when gas supplies are limited. The system for delivering gas during spontaneous breaths is not a demand valve. If the patient's inspiratory effort exceeds the sensitivity setting, the IC-2A will deliver gas at the set inspiratory flow and inspiratory time on the ventilator. Mandatory and spontaneous breaths differ

only in that the latter are pressure-triggered, and the fluidic logic prevents pressurization of the exhalation valve.

The LTV 1000 is a flow-triggered, flow- or pressure-limited, flow- or time-cycled microprocessor-controlled device that has an integral turbine (Fig. 28-6). Oxygen can be supplied from a low-flow or compressed-gas source. The ventilator provides SIMV, controlled mechanical ventilation (CMV), pressure-support, and CPAP modes. Pressure- and volume-controlled breaths are possible. Operator controls include primarily a keypad and rotating knob. Controls include ventilation mode, F_{IO_2}, rate, tidal volume, inspiratory time, peak flow, PEEP, sensitivity, pressure support, and peak pressure. Parameters monitored and displayed include airway pressure, total breath rate, exhaled tidal volume, total minute volume, I:E ratio, calculated peak flow, and patient effort. There are indicators for electrical power status. A full set of alarms is available. An optional color display is available that displays measured values in a graphic or numerical format. The LTV 1000 offers the performance of a critical-care ventilator at a size and weight appropriate for a transport ventilator.

The Uni-Vent 754 is an electrically powered flow or pressure controller that is triggered by pressure or time or manually; it is also time- or pressure-cycled and has an internal compressor and oxygen-air blender (Fig. 28-7). Modes of ventilation include CMV, SIMV, and CPAP. Calibrated dials and pushbuttons select mode of ventilation, breath rate, inspiratory time, tidal volume, sensitivity, PEEP, sigh, F_{IO_2}, and peak inspiratory-pressure limit. Airway pressure is displayed, as well as the airway pressure waveform, ventilator breath rate, inspiratory time, I:E ratio, tidal volume, F_{IO_2}, external air on/off, set plateau pressure, high- and low-pressure alarm setting, mean airway pressure, and baseline airway pressure. A full set of alarms is present.

The Uni-Vent 754 has a proven track record in transporting ventilated military casualties by U.S. Air Force critical-care air-transport teams. A comparison of the physical and operational characteristics of sophisticated transport ventilators is given in Tables 28-9 and 28-10.

Attributes Common to All Transport Ventilators

WEIGHT

These devices must be person-portable and able to be mounted on a variety of platforms. A maximum weight of 8 kg facilitates these requirements.

DURABILITY

These devices should be compact, simple to operate, durable, and unaffected by extremes of heat and cold or vibration. Proper shielding is required to limit emission of unacceptable levels of electromagnetic energy. Automatic resuscitators in particular should function properly after prolonged storage with minimal maintenance.

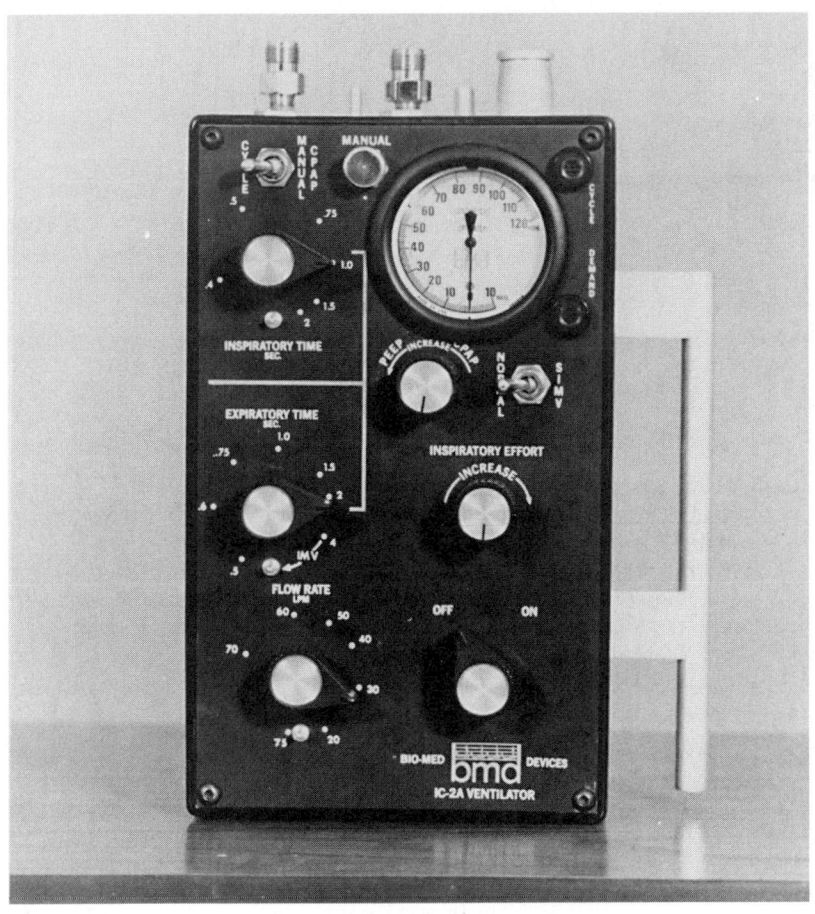

FIGURE 28-5 The IC-2A ventilator used for transport of patients to magnetic resonance imaging (MRI).

POWER REQUIREMENTS

Automatic resuscitators are pneumatically powered, negating the need for batteries. Simple and sophisticated transport ventilators often are powered electrically and pneumatically. Battery life should be sufficient for the duration of the expected transport. Battery life of ventilators with a built-in air source is shortened by increased lung impedance, use of pressure-control ventilation, and increased PEEP.[53]

Transport ventilators use a variety of battery supplies. Sealed lead-acid (SLA) batteries have a low energy density but are durable and inexpensive. SLA batteries hold a charge even when stored for long periods of time. Nickel-cadmium (NiCad) batteries have a higher energy density but are more expensive. Nickel–metal hydride (NiMH) batteries have even a higher energy density than NiCad batteries and are more expensive. Lithium-ion (Li-ion) batteries have the highest energy density and are the most expensive. NiCad and to a lesser extent NiMH batteries (but not SLA or Li-ion batteries) can suffer from voltage memory and should be stored in the discharged state. Both Li-ion and NiCad batteries will self-discharge during storage.

Oxygen consumption should be less than 5 liters/min, keeping in mind that oxygen consumption varies with ventilation mode and the use of PEEP. The device should have the capability of generating flow without a compressed-gas source and offer a means of enriching the inspired-gas mix-

ture with oxygen from a low-pressure source such as a concentrator.

CONTROLS

Controls should be large and not easily adjusted accidentally. Any display should be viewable from an angle and in variable ambient light.

SAFETY

Automatic resuscitators and simple transport ventilators have basic safety features, whereas sophisticated transport ventilators possess safety features comparable with those of critical-care ventilators. A pressure-relief valve that vents gas to the atmosphere at a preselected peak inspiratory pressure is essential. Violation of the high-pressure limit should be signaled by a visual or audible alarm. An antiasphyxia valve that allows the patient to breathe from ambient air in the event of power-source failure is desirable.[55] Battery-powered ventilators should be equipped with a "low battery" alarm as the battery nears depletion. If the compressed-gas source falls below operating pressure of the ventilator or is empty/disconnected, an audible or visual alarm should sound. Visual alarms are critical when

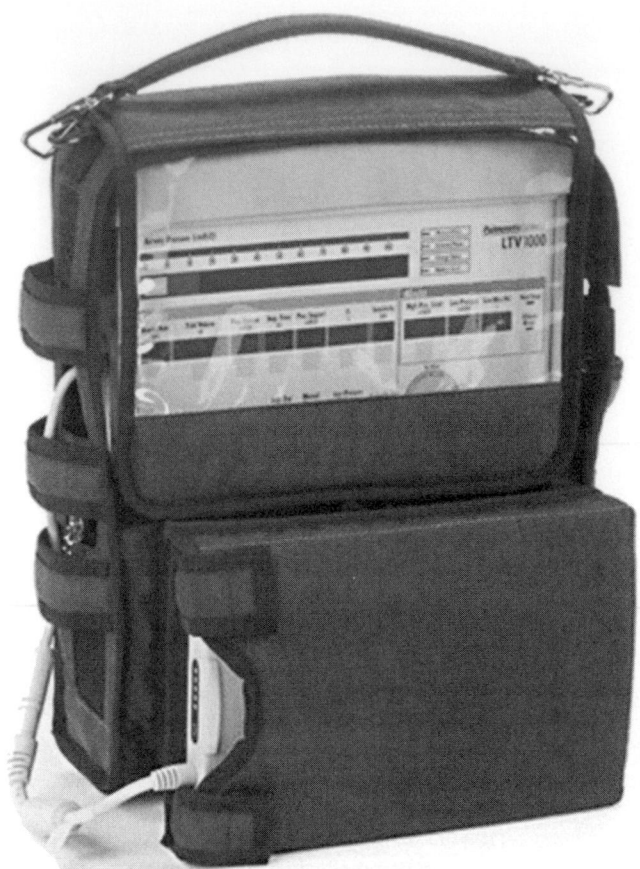

FIGURE 28-6 The LTV-1000 sophisticated transport ventilator.

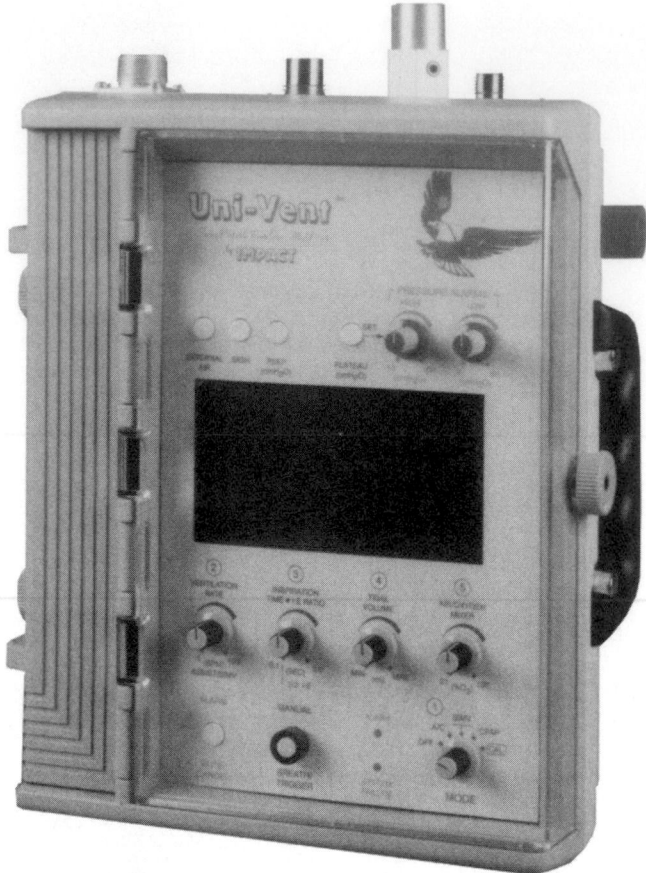

FIGURE 28-7 The Impact 754 sophisticated transport ventilator.

ventilators are used in environments with high levels of ambient noise such as aircraft.

ASSEMBLY AND DISASSEMBLY

These devices should be designed so that incorrect circuit installation is impossible. Typically, there is a single-limb circuit with an external expiratory valve. Patient valves located at the endotracheal tube should be cleared of secretions easily.

Performance Issues Relevant to All Types of Transport Ventilators

DELIVERED TIDAL VOLUME

Several investigators have demonstrated unreliable tidal volume delivery with transport ventilators, encouraging monitoring with a portable spirometer.[21,56-58] This includes low tidal volumes in the face of low lung compliance and excessive tidal volume under normal loads.

IMPOSED WORK OF BREATHING

Transport and home-care ventilators often used for transport have been shown to have an unacceptable imposed

work of breathing.[59] In recent studies of new devices there remains a wide range of capabilities among transport ventilators.[60-62] Transport ventilators with flow triggering and PEEP compensation consistently offer the least imposed work of breathing.

Ancillary Equipment for Transport

OXYGEN SUPPLY

All ventilators require an oxygen supply source. Both compressed-gas cylinders and liquid systems can fulfill this need. Intrahospital transport usually is accomplished with an E cylinder or two E cylinders yoked together. These provide 630 and 1260 liters of gas, respectively. An H cylinder contains 6900 liters and may be required for longer transports. The H cylinder is 152 cm in height, weighs 68 kg, and requires its own attendant.

Liquid-oxygen systems can provide 860 ft^3 of gaseous oxygen for every liquid cubic foot. Most liquid systems, however, cannot operate at 50 psig.

HUMIDIFICATION

A passive humidification device, or "artificial nose," is ideal for transport. Use of an artificial nose may result in a

TABLE 28-9   Physical Characteristics of Sophisticated Transport Ventilators

	Dimensions (cm)	Weight (kg)	Supply Pressure (psig)	Operating Temperature (°C)	Gas Consumption (liters/min)	Battery Duration Using Nominal Ventilator Settings (h)	Minimum Patient Weight (kg)
Avian	25.4 × 30.5 × 12.7	5	40–60	−20–40	3.8–6.6	11	NS
Crossvent 4	22.5 × 16.25 × 10.6	3.6	44–66	−10–50	NS	15	Infant to adult
IC-2A	8.6 × 15.5 × 26	4.1	45–55	NS	12	No battery	Pediatric to adult
IVent$_{201}$	35 × 24 × 29	11	40–60 (also uses low-pressure O$_2$ source) Internal compressor	18–50	0	1–2	10
LTV 1000	7.62 × 25.4 × 30.48	5.72	40–70 (also uses low-pressure O$_2$ source) Internal compressor	5–40	0	1.6	10
MVP-10	20 × 23 × 7.4	2.3	45–55	NS	3, changes with breath per minute	No battery	Neonatal to pediatric
Oxylog 2000	21.5 × 12 × 20.5	4.3	40–87	−18–50	0	4	7.5
paraPAC Transport	9.2 × 22.0 × 16.2	2.8	40–90	−10–65	Delivered volume plus 10 ml/cycle	No battery	4.5
Uni-Vent 750	23.9 × 11.5 × 4.5	4.4	50–90	−60–60	0	12	NS
Uni-Vent 754	23 × 29 × 11	5.8	50 Internal compressor	−60–60	0	3 (Compressor on) 12 (Compressor off)	Infant to adults

NS, not specified.

621

TABLE 28-10 Operational Characteristics of Sophisticated Transport Ventilators

	Cycling Variables	Modes	Rate (breaths/min)	Tidal Volume (ml)	Inspiratory Time (s)	Peak Flow (liters/min)
Avian	Time	CMV, AMV, SIMV, CPAP	0–150	50–2000	0.1–3	100
Crossvent 4	Time, pressure	CMV, SIMV/CPAP, PSV, PCV	5–150 CMV 0.6–30 SIMV	5–2500	0.1–3	120
IC-2A	Time, pressure	SIMV, CMV/CPAP	1–666	130–2500	0.4–2	75
IVent$_{201}$	Time, pressure, flow	VCV, PCV, AMV, SIMV, CPAP, PSV	1–50	100–2000	0.3–3	180
LTV 1000	Time, pressure, flow	VCV, PCV, AMV, CMV, SIMV, CPAP, NPPV	0–80	50–2000	0.3–9.9	140
MVP-10 (pediatric/neonatal)	Time	IMV, CMV	0–120	0–666	0.2–2	25
Oxylog 2000	Time, pressure	CMV, SIMV, CPAP	5–40	100–1500	0.5–2	60
paraPacTransport	Time	Synchronized minimum mandatory ventilation	7–60	50–3000	0.5–3	>120
Uni-Vent 750	Time, pressure	CMV, SIMV, AMV	1–150	10–3000	0.1–3	100
Uni-Vent 754	Time	CMV, AMV, SIMV, CPAP	1–150	70–1300	0.1–3	60

Operational Characteristics of Sophisticated Transport Ventilators (Continued)

	F$_{I_{O_2}}$	PEEP/CPAP (cmH$_2$O)	Demand-Flow Valve	Manual Breath
Avian	1.0	0–20	Yes	Yes
Crossvent 4[a]	1.0 (0.5 optional)	0–35	Yes	Yes
IC-2A	1	Yes	Yes	Yes
IVent$_{201}$	0.21 to 1.0	0–20	Yes	Yes
LTV 1000[b]	0.21 to 1.0	0–20	Yes	Yes
MVP-10 (Pediatric/neonatal)	0.21 to 1	0–25	No (continuous flow)	No
Oxylog 2000	0.6 and 1.0	0–15	Yes	Yes
paraPacTransport	0.5 or 1.0	Add on, 0–20	Yes	No
Uni-Vent 750	1	Add on	Yes	Yes
Uni-Vent 754	0.21 to 1.0	0 to 20	Yes	Yes

ABBREVIATIONS: VCV, volume controlled ventilation; PCV, Pressure controlled ventilation; AMV, assisted mandatory ventilation; CMV, controlled mandatory ventilation; SIMV, synchronized intermittent mandatory ventilation; CPAP, continuous positive airway pressure; NPPV, noninvasive positive pressure ventilation.
[a]CV 3, Pediatric and adult; CV 2, Neonate, pediatric
[b]LTV 900, CMV, AMV, SIMV, CPAP (VCV, PCV, PSV); no O$_2$ blender, low flow O$_2$ only; LTV 950 CMV, AMV, SIMV, CPAP (VCV, PSV) no O$_2$ blender, low flow O$_2$ only

progressive increase in breathing circuit resistance, and the patient should be monitored for signs of expiratory-flow restriction. Dead space should be accounted for during low-volume ventilation. Premoistening an artificial nose is inadvisable, does not improve efficiency, and only serves to further increase flow resistance.

Summary

Safe transport of the mechanically ventilated patient requires effective communication, appropriate planning, the presence of key personnel, and compact, rugged equipment. Equipment should meet the demands of patient acuity, and personnel should have the requisite skills and training for the task at hand. Clinicians should be aware of the most frequent complications of transport along with methods of prevention and treatment. The nuances of individual ventilators from battery life and oxygen consumption to imposed work of breathing must be appreciated.

References

1. Branson RD. Intrahospital transport of critically ill, mechanically ventilated patients. Respir Care 1992; 37:775–90.
2. Waydhas C. Intrahospital transport of critically ill patients. Crit Care 1999; 3:R83–9.
3. Wallace PGM, Ridley SA. ABC of intensive care: Transport of critically ill patients. Br Med J 1999; 319:368–71.
4. Insel J, Weissman C, Kemper M, et al. Cardiovascular changes during transport of critically ill and postoperative patients. Crit Care Med 1986; 14:539–42.
5. Hurst JM, Davis K, Johnson DJ, et al. Cost and complications during in-hospital transport of critically ill patients: A prospective cohort study. J Trauma 1992; 33:582–5.

6. Indeck M, Peterson S, Smith J, et al. Risk, cost, and benefit of transporting ICU patients for special studies. J Trauma 1988; 28: 1020–4.

7. Smith S, Fleming S, Cernaianu A. Mishaps during transport from the intensive care unit. Crit Care Med 1990; 18:278–81.

8. Braman SS, Dunn SM, Amico C, Millman RP. Complications of inter-hospital transport in critically ill patients. Ann Intern Med 1987; 107:469–73.

9. Weg JG, Haas CF. Safe Intra-hospital transport of critically ill ventilator dependent patients. Chest 1989; 96:631–5.

10. Andrews PJD, Piper IR, Dearden NM, et al. Secondary insults during intrahospital transport of head-injured patients. Lancet 1990; 335:327–30.

11. Szem JW, Hydo LJ, Fischer E, et al. High-risk intrahospital transport of critically ill patients: Safety and outcomes of the necessary "road trip." Crit Care Med 1995; 23:1660–6.

12. Evans A, Winslow EH. Oxygen saturation and hemodynamic response in critically ill, mechanically ventilated adults during intrahospital transport. Am J Crit Care 1995; 4:106–11.

13. Wallen E, Venkataraman ST, Grosso MJ, et al. Intrahospital transport of critically ill pediatric patients. Crit Care Med 1995; 23:1588–95.

14. Stearley HE. Patients' outcomes: Intrahospital transportation and monitoring of critically ill patients by a specially trained ICU nursing staff. Am J Crit Care 1998; 7:282–7.

15. Pearl RG, Mihm FG, Rosenthal MH. Care of the adult patient during transport. Int Anaesthesiol Clin 1987; 44:822–77.

16. Fromm RE Jr, Dellinger RP. Transport of critically ill patients. J Intensive Care Med 1992; 7:223–33.

17. Venkataraman ST, Orr RA. Intrahospital transport of critically ill patients. Crit Care Clin 1992; 8:525–32.

18. Bion JF, Edlin SA, Ramsay G, et al. Validation of a prognostic score in critically ill patients undergoing transport. Br Med J 1985; 291:432–6.

19. Guidelines Committee of the American College of Critical Care Medicine, Society of Critical Care Medicine and American Association of Critical Care Nurses Transfer Guidelines Task Force. Guidelines for the transfer of critically ill patients. Crit Care Med 1993; 21:931–7.

20. AARC Clinical Practice Guideline. Transport of the mechanically ventilated patient. Respir Care 1993; 38:1169–75.

21. Smith IU, Fleming S, Bekes CE. Written policy and patient transport from the intensive care unit (letter). Crit Care Med 1987; 15:1162.

22. Waddell G. Movement of critically ill patients within hospital. Br Med J 1975; 2:417–9.

23. Taylor JO, Landers CF, Chulay JD, et al. Monitoring high-risk cardiac patients during transportation in hospital. Lancet 1970; 2:1205–7.

24. Carson KL, Drew BJ. Electrocardiographic changes in critically ill adults during intrahospital transport. Prog Cardiovasc Nurs 1994; 9:4–12.

25. Freeman LJ, Nixon PGF. Are coronary artery spasm and progressive damage to the heart associated with the hyperventilation syndrome? Br Med J 1985; 291:851–5.

26. Hisano K, Matsuguchi T, Ootsbo H, et al. Hyperventilation-induced variant angina with ventricular tachycardia. Am Heart J 1984; 108:423–9.

27. Samuelson RG, Nagy G. Effects of respiratory alkalosis and acidosis on myocardial excitation. Acta Physiol Scand 1976; 97:158–65.

28. Gervais HW, Eberle B, Konietzke D, et al. Comparison of blood gases of ventilated patients during transport. Crit Care Med 1987; 15:761–5.

29. Palmon SC, Liu M, Moore LE, et al. Capnography facilitates tight control of ventilation during transport. Crit Care Med 1996; 24:608–12.

30. Waydhas C, Schneck G, Duswald KH. Deterioration of respiratory function after intra-hospital transport of critically ill surgical patient. Intensive Care Med 1995; 21:784–9.

31. Hurst JM, Davis K, Branson RD. Comparison of blood gases during transport using two methods of ventilatory support. J Trauma 1989; 29:1637–40.

32. Austin PA, Campbll RS, Johannigman JA, Branson RD. Transport ventilators. Respir Care Clin North Am 2002; 8:119–50.

33. Dockery WK, Futterman C, Keller SR, et al. A comparison of manual and mechanical ventilation during pediatric transport. Crit Care Med 1999; 27:802–5.

34. Aufderheide TP, Sigurdsson G, Pirrallo RG, et al. Hyperventilation-induced hypotension during cardiopulmonary resuscitation. Circulation 2004; 109:1960–5.

35. Davis DP, Dunford JV, Poste JC, et al. The impact of hypoxia and hyperventilation on outcome after paramedic rapid sequence intubation of severly head injured patients. J Trauma 2004; 57: 1–8.

36. Kollef MH, Von Harz B, Prentice D, et al. Patient transport from intensive care increases the risk of developing ventilator-associated pneumonia. Chest 1997; 112:765–73.

37. Branson RD. The ventilator circuit and ventilator associated pneumonia. Respir Care 2005; 50:323–31.

38. Weber DJ, Wilson MB, Rutala WA, Thomann CA. Manual ventilation bags as a source for bacterial colonization of intubated patients. Am Rev Respir Dis 1990; 142:892–4.

39. Woo AH, Yu VL, Goetz A. Potential in-hospital modes of transmission of *Legionella pneumophila:* Demonstration experiments for dissemination by showers, humidifiers, and rinsing of ventilation bag apparatus. Am J Med 1986; 80:567–73.

40. Kirby RR, DiGiovanni AJ, Bancroft RW, et al. Function of the Bird respirator at high altitude. Aerospace Med 1969; 40: 463–9.

41. Saltzman AR, Grant BJB, Aquilina AT, et al. Ventilatory criteria for aeromedical evacuation. Aviat Space Environ Med 1987; 58: 958–63.

42. Thomas G, Brimacombe J. Function of the Drager Oxylog Ventilator at high altitude. Anesth Intensive Care 1994; 22:276–80.

43. Link J, Krause H, Wagner W, et al. Intrahospital transport of critically ill patients. Crit Care Med 1990; 18:1427–30.

44. Hanning CD, Gilmour DG, Hothersall AP, et al. Movement of the critically ill within hospital. Intens Care Med 1978; 4:137–42.

45. Uusaro A, Parviainedn I, Takala J, Ruokonen E. Safe long distance interhospital ground transfer of critically ill patients with acute severe unstable respiratory and circulatory failure. Intensive Care Med 2002; 28:1122–5.

46. Turki M, Young MP, Wagers SS, Bates JH. Peak pressures during manual ventilation. Respir Care 2005; 50:340–4.

47. Hess D, Hirsch C, Marquis-D'Amico C, Kacmarek RM. Imposed work and oxygen delivery during spontaneous breathing with adult disposable manual ventilators. Anesthesiology 1994; 81:1256–63.

48. Mills PJ, Baptiste J, Preston J, Barnas GM. Manual resuscitators and spontaneous ventilation: An evaluation. Crit Care Med 1991; 19:1425–31.

49. Mellor S, Holland D, Boynton J. Effects of positioning on the reliability and effectiveness of the Vortran Automatic Resuscitator (abstract). Respir Care 2001; 45:A1021.

50. Blackson T, Speakman B, Iverson J, et al. Effect of positional changes on the performance of the Vortran Automatic Resuscitator (abstract). Respir Care 2004; 49:A1231.

51. Romano M, Raabe OG, Walby W, et al. The stability of arterial blood gases during transport of patients during the RespirTech PRO. Am J Emerg Med 2000; 18:273–7.

52. Nolan JP, Baskett PJF. Gas powered and portable ventilators: An evaluation of six models. Prehosp Disaster Med 1992; 7:25–34.

53. Johannigman JA, Branson RD, Johnson DJ, et al. Out-of-hospital ventilation: Bag valve devices vs transport ventilators. Acad Emerg Med 1995; 2:719–24.

54. Campbell RS, Austin PA, Matacia GM, et al. Battery life of eight portable ventilators: Effect of control variable, PEEP, and F_{IO_2}. Respir Care 2002; 47:1173–83.

55. Austin PA, Campbell RS, Johannigman JA, Branson RD. Work of breathing during ventilator failure in portable and ICU ventilators. Respir Care 2002; 47:667–74.

56. McGough EK, Banner MJ, Melker RJ. Variations in tidal volume with portable transport ventilators. Respir Care 1992; 37:233–9.

57. Heinrichs W, Mertzluft F, Dick W. Accuracy of delivered versus preset minute ventilation of portable emergency. Crit Care Med 1989; 29:1637–40.

58. Attebo L, Bengtsson M, Johnson A. Comparison of portable emergency ventilators using a lung model. Br J Anaesth. 1993; 70: 372–7.

59. Branson RD, Davis K. Work of breathing imposed by five ventilators used for long term support: The effects of PEEP and patient demand. Respir Care 1995; 40:1270–8.

60. Austin PA, Campbell RS, Johannigman JA, Branson RD. Work of breathing during ventilator failure in portable and ICU ventilators. Respir Care 2002; 47:667–74.

61. Nakamura T, Fujino Y, Uchiyama A, et al. Intrahospital transport of critically ill patients using ventilator with patient-triggering function. Chest 2003; 123:159–64.

62. Miyoshi E, Fujino Y, Mashimo T, Nishimura M. Performance of transport ventilator with patient-triggered ventilation. Chest 2000; 118:1109–15.

MECHANICAL VENTILATION IN THE ACUTE RESPIRATORY DISTRESS SYNDROME

JOHN J. MARINI

Few areas of critical-care medicine have been the subject of as much investigative attention or clinical concern as the set of problems grouped under the label *acute respiratory distress syndrome* (ARDS). This syndrome, first formally described in 1967,[1] continues to be recognized clinically as a rapidly developing impairment of pulmonary oxygen (O_2) exchange accompanied by diffuse infiltrates and altered respiratory system mechanics that cannot be attributed solely to hydrostatic forces. Fueled by better characterization of innate pathophysiology and of iatrogenic factors, considerable progress has been made in recent years toward reducing the adverse consequences of this condition. Yet, after almost four decades, active debate continues regarding key elements of the ventilatory prescription and appropriate therapeutic targets.

From the outset, mechanical ventilation with positive pressure has been essential in addressing the life-threatening gas-exchange abnormalities and otherwise unsustainable workloads associated with acute lung injury (ALI). Only in the relatively recent past, however, has there been clear documentation that the tidal pressures with which mechanical ventilation is conducted can have an impact on morbidity and survival.[2,3] This awareness gradually has resulted in a conceptual shift away from attempting to maintain or restore normal blood-gas values at high pressure and O_2 costs and toward adopting the avoidance of preventable iatrogenicity ("lung protection") as the first priority.

Many aspects of the debate concerning appropriate ventilator management of this group of conditions can be traced to the heterogeneity of the patient population, to our still imperfect comprehension of the mechanisms of ventilator-associated lung injury, and to the relative imprecision of the criteria on which the ARDS/ALI label is assigned.[4] Despite an incomplete and still evolving understanding, a rich experimental and clinical database—much of it collected over the past decade—allows for the development of a rational set of principles on which to formulate an effective ventilation strategy.[5,6] Definitive answers for many important clinical questions related to this topic are not available; what is presented here reflects a pathophysiology-guided approach to accomplish essential clinical objectives while avoiding ventilator-induced lung injury (VILI) (Table 29-1).

General Objectives for Ventilator Support

In the clinical setting, mechanical ventilation ensures adequate oxygenation of arterial blood, provides sufficient O_2 transport to vital organs and tissues, assists in eliminating carbon dioxide (CO_2), relieves excessive burdens placed on the respiratory muscles, helps to maintain alveolar stability, and facilitates therapeutic measures where ventilatory control is required. It has become clear, however, that despite its undeniable value, mechanical ventilation also has the potential to inflict adverse clinical outcomes. The task of accomplishing ventilation safely in patients with injured lungs is made far more difficult by the mechanical heterogeneity of the respiratory system and the diversity of pathophysiology encountered among different patients who satisfy extisting operational criteria for this condition.

TABLE 29-1   Conceptual Principles in ARDS Ventilation

ARDS is a heterogeneous problem
  Between patients
  Over time
  Between lung regions
Risk for VILI is proportional to *transalveolar* pressure
Lung recruitment is essential to avoid VILI
  The chest wall influences regional lung volumes, tolerated
    pressures, and recruitability

ABBREVIATION: VILI, ventilator-induced lung injury.

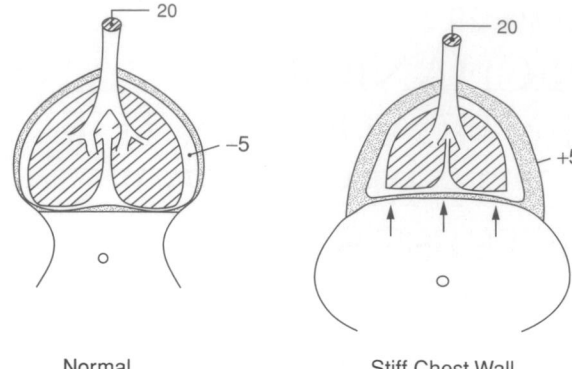

Normal   Stiff Chest Wall

FIGURE 29-1 Influence of chest-wall compliance on transpulmonary pressure and lung volume. Any specified airway pressure is associated with less transpulmonary pressure in the presence of chest wall stiffness or expiratory effort.

Defining the Problem

The terms *ALI* and *ARDS*, diagnoses based on physiologic and radiographic criteria, comprise a category of patients with varied pathoanatomy and mechanical characteristics. According to the widely used American-European consensus guideline,[4] the primary criteria on which this diagnosis is based relate to pulmonary O_2 exchange, the appearance of the plain chest radiograph, and a clinical assessment of left-ventricular function. Although such broadly inclusive criteria may be useful for some purposes, they prove problematic for others. In formal definitions, for example, no provision is made for the level of positive end-expiratory pressure (PEEP) at which the arterial sample is obtained or the chest radiograph is exposed. No stipulation requires that the defining criteria be met under standardized conditions and remain reproducible over time. Chest-wall properties and body weight are left unaccounted for. Yet pulmonary O_2 exchange is influenced not only by the properties of the lung but also by end-expiratory lung volume, body position, mixed venous O_2 content, pulmonary blood flow, and the integrity and intensity of hypoxic pulmonary constriction. The chest radiograph is interpreted subjectively, and experts often differ with respect to their assessments.[7] Moreover, it is clear that the lungs of different patients with ARDS vary with regard to radiographic appearance, inherent recruitability, and histopathology. Even within the same individual, assessed at the same moment, the pathoanatomy and mechanical environment vary from site to site within the injured lung. Such regional differences are explained in part by the properties of the surrounding chest wall, which profoundly influence the inflation characteristics of the integrated respiratory system as well as their regional distribution.[8,9]

Similar clinical presentations can mask radical differences in lung pathology, mechanical properties, and response to ventilator settings and maneuvers. Lungs of patients with ARDS resulting from pneumonic consolidation, for example, are less likely to inflate easily than are lungs made edematous by the circulating mediators of extrapulmonary sepsis.[10] Computed tomographic (CT) patterns may reflect these differences.[11] Moreover, inflexibility of the chest wall may increase dramatically the pressures required to inflate the respiratory system[12] (Fig. 29-1). From these considerations, it is clear that inflexible guidelines for selecting PEEP and tidal volume that advise specific numerical values of these settings will be variably effective in accomplishing the

goal of minimizing tissue stresses, depending on the type and severity of lung injury, the compliance of the chest wall, and the ranges for opening pressures and closing tendencies among the multiplicity of the lung units that comprise the injured lung.

Pathophysiologic Features Relevant to Ventilator Support

One of the major conceptual advances of the past 20 years is the recognition that the lungs of patients with ARDS are mechanically heterogeneous and vary enormously in their patterns of infiltration, their inflation and collapse properties, and their regional expressions of pathology. CT scanning has revealed densities that may be localized or diffuse—with implications for response to ventilator interventions such as PEEP.[11] Variation in the underlying conditions that give rise to the clinical problem described as ARDS precludes categorical histologic descriptions that apply across the full range of clinical experience. A few salient characteristics, however, are shared by most. In its earliest phase, noncardiogenic (high-permeability) edema gives rise to a lung whose parenchymal airspace is partially occupied by proteinaceous edema and cellular infiltrate. A relatively large proportion of the lung—often exceeding 50%—is airless at end expiration, with the exact percentage depending jointly on severity, disease stage, and etiology. Destruction of surfactant-producing type 2 alveolar cells leads to its diminished production, whereas exuded proteins and inflammatory products compromise the viability of the surfactant that remains.[13] Surfactant plays several important biologic and physiologic roles. From a purely mechanical standpoint, the loss of functional surfactant increases surface tension, thereby contributing to alveolar flooding, increased tissue elastance, small-airway closure, and atelectasis—particularly at low lung volumes.

The relative proportions of airless and aerated tissue also vary with disease type and stage. Although some controversy persists, CT scan estimates of gas and tissue volumes suggest that potentially "recruitable" tissue comprises only a minority of radiographic density at functional residual capacity (FRC) in most patients.[14] Flooded and consolidated lung units comprise the remainder. Although clearly a minority viewpoint, a plausible argument has been advanced that "reopening" of lung units by alveolar pressure may occur primarily by redistributing alveolar liquid and shifting fluid volume from the alveolar to the interstitial compartments of the lung—not by atelectasis reversal ("recruitment").[15] The rapidity with which CT scan tissue density develops and resolves, however, as changes in alveolar pressure are imposed, as well as direct observations by intravital microscopy of alveoli at the lung's surface,[16] cast doubt on the primacy of the "fluid-shift hypothesis."

MECHANICAL PROPERTIES OF THE INJURED LUNG

Replacement of airspaces by inflammatory debris, cells, and fluid results in a lung whose aeratable capacity and compliance (measured in terms of volume accepted per unit of pressure) is severely reduced. The compliance of the respiratory system (lungs and chest wall) falls during ARDS for two reasons: First, infiltrated and surfactant-depleted tissue is inherently more elastic than healthy tissue. Second—and more important—many functional lung units operate near their elastic limit because many fewer are available to accept the tidal volume. Under normal conditions, surfactant-modified surface forces allow the lung to inflate and deflate at similar pressures. In contrast, the injured lung is characterized by a right-shifted pressure-volume loop, made so by its reduced aeratable capacity and by surfactant depletion.[12,17,18] For the same tidal volume, therefore, the mechanical work of breathing is increased dramatically.

Although clinicians characterize the mechanics of the injured lung by airway pressure and flow measurements made at the airway opening—the common entry and exit points for gas exchange with the environment—the mechanical properties of the lung's individual subunits are hardly uniform, even in health. In part, this heterogeneity relates to regional variations of pleural (and therefore transpulmonary) pressure that arise from interactions of the chest wall with the injured lung and from the need for dependent tissues to support the weight of the mediastinal contents and the edematous lung (Fig. 29-2). This underlying mechanical heterogeneity is implied by quantitative CT imaging techniques that characterize the topographic anatomy in response to changing patterns of airway pressure or more directly in real time by imaging of ventilation with radiotracer gases or electrical impedance tomography.[19,20]

For any specified airway pressure, there exist lung units that are closed and those that are open. Among the population of open units, there exists a range of states of lung-unit expansion depending on the local transpulmonary pressures that distend them. Even at airway pressures that generally are considered modest, some of the open lung units verge on overdistension, whereas others are on the compliant portion of their pressure-volume relationship (Fig. 29-3). While alveolar distension that approaches the elastic limit stimulates surfactant production, the repetitive appli-

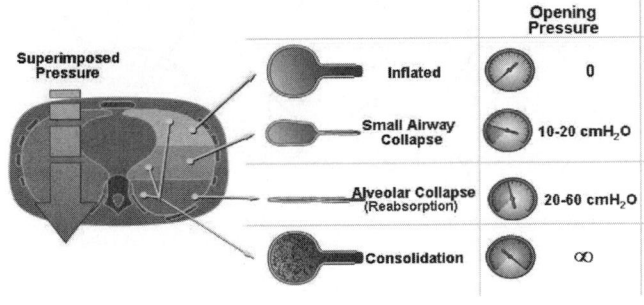

(*modified from Gattinoni*)

FIGURE 29-2 Spectrum of opening pressures associated with lung units within the injured lung. Lung units located in dependent areas are compressed by the weight of the overlying lung and mediastinum. Local transpulmonary pressures vary considerably; some lung units remain fully inflated throughout the tidal cycle, whereas others cannot be aerated. Less pressure is required to open small airways when the alveoli remain aerated than when all alveolar gas has been absorbed. (*Image courtesy of Luciano Gattinoni.*)

cation of nonphysiologic stretching forces, as during high tidal volume/high-pressure tidal ventilation, is currently believed to initiate molecular signaling of a local inflammatory response.[21,22] Mechanical interdependence among the lung units of a heterogeneously affected lung amplifies the stresses of high pressure at the junctions of closed and

FIGURE 29-3 Mechanical characteristics of lung units in dependent (*below*) and nondependent (*above*) lung regions. As the lung is inflated by constant flow of gas, electrical impedance increases in proportion to aerated volume. Although the relationship between volume and impedance for the total lung appears roughly linear (*center tracing*), upper lung regions are relatively overdistended (*upper tracing*), whereas lower lung regions are relatively underrecruited until total lung capacity is achieved (*lower tracing*). (*Image courtesy of Marcelo Amato.*)

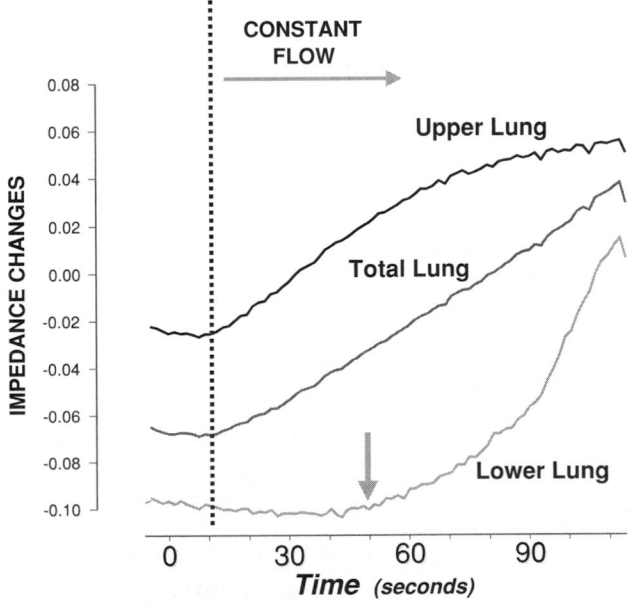

$$P_{eff} = P_{appl} \, (V/V_o)^{2/3}$$

FIGURE 29-4 Amplification of tension at the boundaries of open and collapsing lung tissue. Normally distended (*left*), collapsing (*center*), and overdistended (*right*) states of inflation. Because of interdependence, the tensions applied to a collapsing alveolus are amplified. A simple mathematical model predicts that the tensions resulting from an alveolar pressure (Pappl) produce a tension comparable with an effective pressure (Peff) described by the equation. At 30 cmH$_2$O applied pressure, the volume of an aerated alveolus (V) is approximately 10 times that of a collapsed alveolus (V$_0$). Thus the estimated pressure necessary to mimic the tensions at the interface is approximately 4.5 times as great as that applied (140 cmH$_2$O). (*Used, with permission, from J. Mead et al JAP 1970 Am J Respir Crit Care Med 163:1609–13, 2001.*)

open lung units in a nonlinear fashion[23] (Fig. 29-4). Such recurring forces not only strain the lung's structural meshwork to signal inflammation but also assist in reopening potentially recruitable (atelectatic) lung units.[24] When atelectatic tissues are subjected to high pressures, amplified shearing forces within these zones at high risk for damage may be of sufficient magnitude to tear the delicate terminal airways or alveoli themselves, creating microwounds that produce tissue hemorrhage and incite inflammation as a secondary phenomenon. Stress amplification at the margins of dissimilar tissues is at least partially a function of their relative volumes. (A flooded, gasless alveolus of volume similar to its air-filled neighbors may experience forces that are no more intense.) Whether injury results from the process of repetitive popping open of lung units under high pressure or simply is the cumulative result of high-

tension stretching at the interface remains to be resolved. It appears, therefore, that there are at least two critical elements that place the injured lung at risk for ventilation-associated lung damage: high inflating pressures and the prevalence of collapsed lung units that interface with open ones.

ATELECTASIS

At the microscopic level, lung-unit collapse may be thought of in two broad categories: "Loose" atelectasis arises primarily from compressive forces of the heavy lung acting to close small airways and responds to relatively low levels of transpulmonary pressure, conversely, adhesive or "sticky" atelectasis results from gas absorption and requires very high pressures to reverse.[25] High concentrations of inspired O$_2$ encourage the latter in poorly ventilated regions, as well as interfere with surfactant kinetics. These hard-to-recruit units may be among the first to close as high airway pressure is withdrawn. Loose and sticky types of atelectasis often coexist, perhaps accounting for the fact that lung units open throughout the entire range of total lung capacity (TLC)[26,27] (Fig. 29-5). In the setting of severe ARDS, pressures that exceed 60 cmH$_2$O may be needed to complete the recruiting process. Although opening of lung units is primarily a function of transalveolar pressure, the duration with which pressure is applied also contributes; that is, a lower pressure may be sufficient if applied for an adequate period. Moreover, atelectatic lung units tend to "yield" (open) in a stuttering, discontinuous fashion, with high sustained pressure causing a serial snapping open of small blocks of units.[28] Discontinuous lung opening during the tidal cycle may give rise to audible crackles, usually best heard in dependent regions.

PULMONARY EDEMA

The increased microvascular permeability of ALI/ARDS renders it vulnerable to edema formation and impedes its relative rate of edema clearance. The weight of the normal lung does not begin to rise significantly until pulmonary venous pressure exceeds 20 mmHg. Unlike the healthy lung,

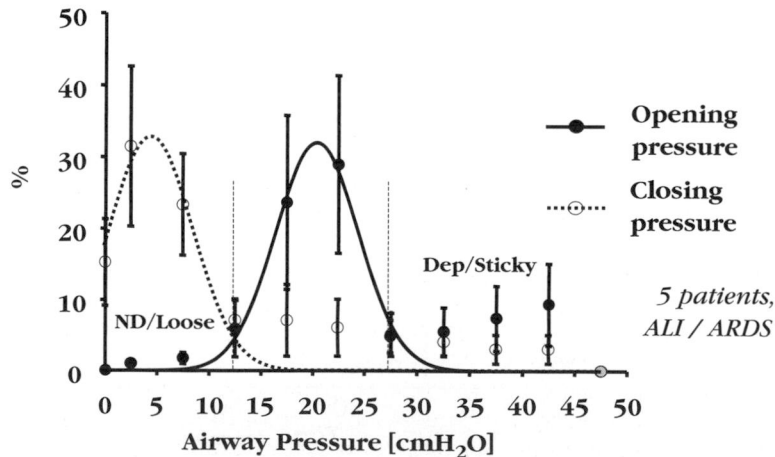

FIGURE 29-5 Histograms relating percentage of potentially recruitable lung units to inflation (opening) and deflation (closing) airway pressures. Unstable airways open at relatively modest pressures, whereas alveoli that have undergone absorption collapse require much higher pressures to open. The spectrum of closing pressures is shifted to the left. Note that some lung units begin to collapse at relatively high airway pressures (*Adapted, with permission, from Crotti et al: Am J Respir Crit Care Med 164:131–40, 2001.*)

however, extravascular water in the injured lung bears a strong quasi-linear dependence on hydrostatic microvascular pressure, a relationship that begins from capillary pressures that are considered low by most clinical standards.[29] The term *noncardiogenic pulmonary edema*, therefore, does not imply that gas exchange cannot be improved by lowering the hydrostatic pressure gradient across the injured lung. Because extra-alveolar microvessels as well as capillaries can leak,[30] numerous factors influence the vascular pressures relevant to edema formation. These include left-ventricular filling pressure, cardiac output (which increases the pressure needed to drive blood flow through the lung with limited capillary recruiting reserve), plasma oncotic pressure, interstitial fluid pressure, and the integrity of the alveolar and lymphatic lung-water clearance mechanisms. Clearance mechanisms are influenced by the degree of lung stretch. Translocation of blood from infradiaphragmatic vascular capacitance beds to the central vessels of the thorax can occur as intra-abdominal pressure rises.[31]

Mechanisms and Consequences of Ventilator-Induced Lung Injury

For more than three decades, experimental studies have shown that *excessive mechanical stresses* developed during mechanical ventilation can inflict injury on both normal and acutely injured lungs and, once the lungs are injured, retard their healing.[32,33] Injury may result from overstretching of tissues that are already open, from shear forces at the junctions of expandable and unyielding tissue, and from repeated percussion of closed terminal airways (Fig. 29-6). Repeated application of transalveolar pressures exceeding those corresponding to the inflation capacity of a healthy lung may disrupt the alveolar epithelial barrier, especially in the absence of sufficient end-expiratory pressure to reduce stress focusing by holding open mechanically unstable lung units.[32,34] From a theoretical standpoint, sustained recruitment reduces the potential for damaging forces to concentrate at the boundaries of inflating lung and unyield-

FIGURE 29-6 Forms of tissue stress that occur near the junctions of open and closed lung units.

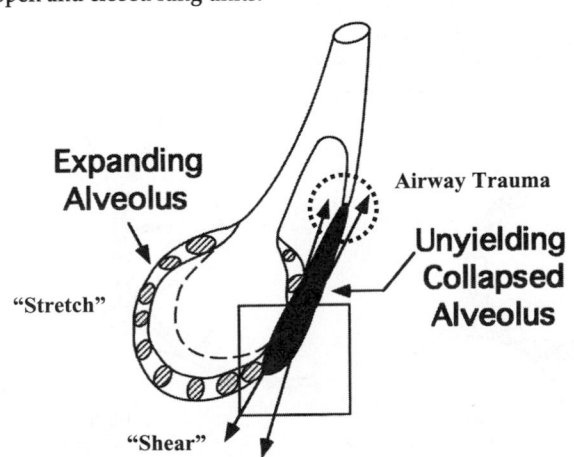

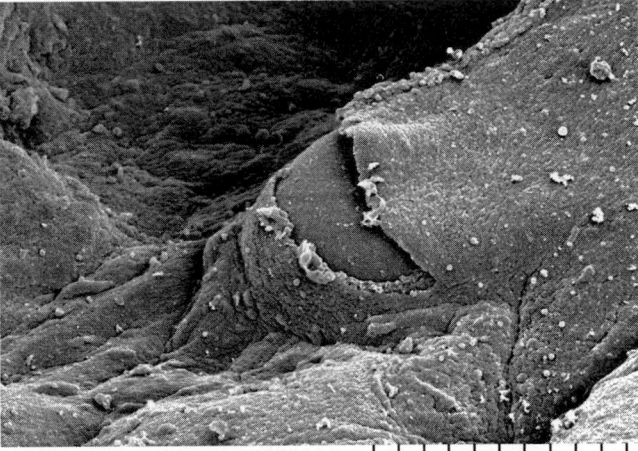

S4700-38 2.0kV 10.6mm x 10.0k SE(M) 12/18/00   5.00um

FIGURE 29-7 Stress fracture of the alveolar-capillary membrane resulting from ventilator-induced lung injury in a previously normal rat lung. Similar tears also have been demonstrated to occur in human patients with ARDS.

ing or collapsed structures. Indeed, an overwhelming body of experimental work indicates the lung-protective effect of sustained "recruitment" when high tidal inflation pressures are used.[32,35] Mechanosignaling at moderately high airway pressures may induce the formation and release of inflammatory mediators,[21,22] initiate programmed cell death (apoptosis), or produce necrosis.[36] Excessive strain may exceed cytoskeletal tolerances, causing physical tears and stress fractures of endothelium, epithelium, and intercellular matrix[37,38] (Fig. 29-7). Experiments conducted in animals and in patients indicate that translocation of inflammatory mediators and bacteria into the bloodstream is influenced by the ventilatory pattern.[39,40-42] Although brisk controversy continues, such observations suggest possible links between adverse patterns of ventilation and dysfunction in remote vital organs.

PATHOPHYSIOLOGY AND PREVENTION OF VILI

From available data, VILI appears to be a complex process initiated by the repetitive application of excessive stress/strain to the lung's fibroskeleton, microvasculature, terminal airways, and delicate juxta-alveolar tissues. Defining the linkage between stress, strain, and diffuse alveolar damage is currently a subject of intense investigation.[36,43,44] On the strength of excellent laboratory evidence, however, it seems undeniable that high levels of mechanical stress may disrupt the normal functioning of cells that populate the pulmonary microenvironment and that sufficient dimensional strain triggers the release of inflammatory mediators and destructive enzymes[43-45] (Fig. 29-8). Under moderate degrees of strain, such mechanosignaling may be the primary pathway to injury. When the applied mechanical stress is very high, fibroelastic structural integrity may be breached directly, with the inflammatory process a consequence rather than initiator of the observed histopathology (Fig. 29-9). These high tissue-rupturing forces are especially likely to be generated in dependent lung regions, where

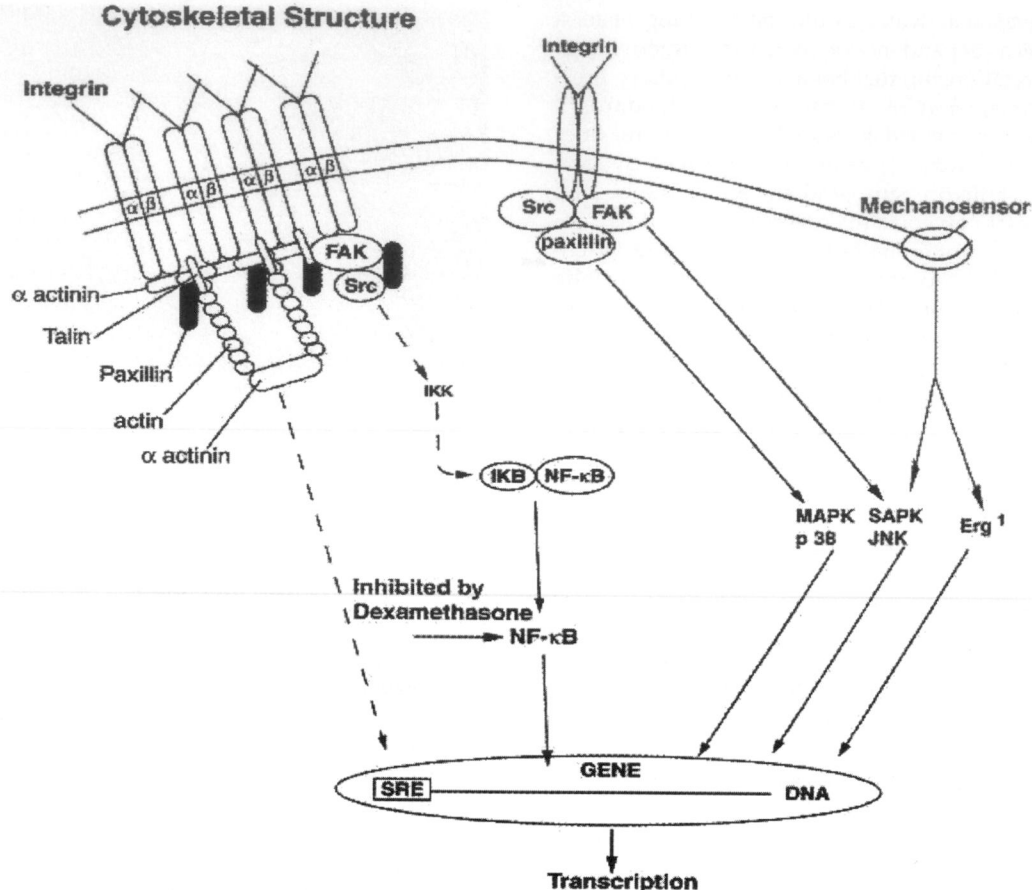

FIGURE 29-8 Mechanosignaling pathways of inflammation under conditions of excessive tissue strain. (*Used, with permission, from Dos Santos et al: J Appl Physiol 89:1645–55, 2000.*)

unstable alveoli are most prevalent (Fig. 29-10). Another important mechanism in the causation of lung-tissue damage may occur at the level of the terminal airways as they open and reclose with each tidal cycle.[34] Damaging shear forces (those that run tangential to the plane of the structure) appear to rip the epithelium from its attachments.

From an engineering perspective, mechanical *stress* is a function of transstructural tension; *strain* is the dimension-altering consequence of high transstructural pressure, conditioned by the elastance of the element in question. Although by no means the only determinant of tissue forces, the measurable analogue of the stress across the entire lung

FIGURE 29-9 Excised heart-lung block from a previously normal animal subjected to high inflation pressure and low levels of PEEP. Specimen is shown inflated at 20 cmH$_2$O airway pressure in the supine (*left panel*) and prone (*right panel*) conditions. Note the sharp demarcation of hemorrhagic edema from relatively normal appearing lung. Damage may progress sequentially from dependent to nondependent regions, as indicated by the sequence of arrows.

FIGURE 29-10 Mechanical behavior of capillaries embedded in the wall of inflatable alveoli and of microvessels within the interstitial spaces. Capillaries embedded in the alveolar walls are compressed, whereas extra-alveolar microvessels (and perhaps corner vessels) are dilated by lung expansion.

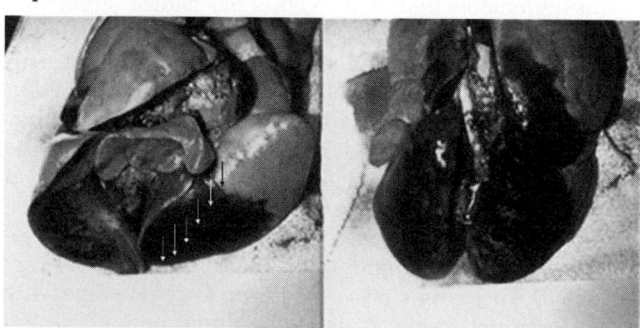

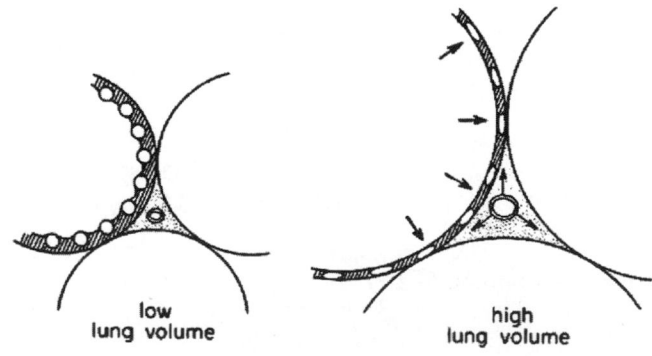

is transpulmonary pressure—crudely estimated as the difference between static airway pressure (the "plateau" pressure) and the average pleural pressure (often estimated by use of an esophageal balloon). Regional transpulmonary pressures vary considerably secondary to the influence of gravity, chest-wall irregularities, intra-abdominal pressure, mediastinal weight, and vascular-filling pressure[46] (see Fig. 29-2). Available laboratory data illustrate that pleural pressure, however measured, does not accurately reflect interstitial pressure when the lung is edematous and inflamed.[47] Even directional changes of pleural and interstitial pressures may not track together in a nonuniform environment. Although not directly measurable, strain correlates with aerated volume as a fraction of aeratable capacity.

HOW DOES TIDAL VOLUME RELATE TO TISSUE STRESS?

Once this latter concept is understood, it becomes clear that tissue stress is not a predictable function of tidal volume but rather is influenced strongly by tidal volume in relation to the size (and compliance) of the compartment forced to accept it. Even this, however, is not the full story— stress amplification and shearing forces at the boundaries of tissues with differing capacities to expand must be considered. Peak tidal transalveolar pressure interacts with end-expiratory transalveolar pressure to determine *local* stress, which varies markedly from site to site across the damaged lung. The alveolar pressures resulting from tidal volume and PEEP, therefore, are both interactive elements in the injury process, but even when considered together, they cannot estimate tissue stresses precisely because interstitial pressure is an unmeasured variable that differs throughout.

Moreover, the damaging *strain* that results from a given stress depends on tissue fragility. In the setting of ARDS, tissue integrity is likely to be at least normally delicate or even compromised, especially in its earliest phase. The low compliance typically associated with ALI results primarily from the reduced number of aeratable lung units—not from increased stiffness of the individual lung units themselves.[48] The tidal volumes pulled during exercise by a healthy athlete may exceed 25–30 ml/kg of lean body weight, whereas much smaller breaths eventually would cause damage or lung rupture in the setting of ALI. In the same individual, increasing tidal volume invariably will cause tissue stresses to rise in some lung units; a raised tidal volume, however, actually may cause the stresses in other units to *fall*. This apparent paradox results from the recruiting effect of the higher pressures and perhaps improved ventilation of marginally ventilated units predisposed to absorption collapse. At any clinically selected tidal volume, tissue stresses may be reduced or accentuated by the application of PEEP, depending on whether PEEP effectively recruits vulnerable tissue or simply raises plateau pressure. Quests for a universally applicable predetermined tidal volume or PEEP value applicable to all patients would seem destined to be a fruitless exercise.

Modifying the characteristics of the chest wall (e.g., by prone positioning[49,50]) is a potent mechanism for altering regional differences in transpulmonary pressure. Even within the same small region, inflationary stresses can vary markedly in magnitude and even in direction between structures situated within microns of one another. Shearing forces, one of the varied forms of mechanical stress resulting from lung inflation, intensify at the junctions of tissues with different compliance values and anchoring attachments.[23] Minimizing or eliminating these irregularities reduces the potential for adverse "stress focusing" and tissue strain. In such a microenvironment, limiting end-tidal alveolar pressure assumes major importance for two primary reasons: (1) A high plateau pressure may overstretch open alveoli, and (2) perhaps more important, because junctional tension rises in nonlinear proportion to airway pressure,[23] the plateau pressure acts as a potent lever arm at stress focus points.

By reducing the number of junctional interfaces and by preventing the repetitive opening of terminal lung units at high pressure, recruitment of lung tissue—defined as the sustained reversal of atelectasis on whatever scale it occurs—may be lung protective. When nearly all potentially recruitable tissue is aerated, the lung is said to be "open."[51] A given transpulmonary pressure applied to a fully open lung should be associated with less stress than the same pressure applied to a lung with closed units juxtaposed to open ones. Some authors argue that the injured lung should be fully "opened" in order to reduce the potential for repetitive opening and reclosure.[51] Presently, however, it is not clear that this always should be given highest priority; to what extent repetitive opening and closing of small airways produces injury and whether the prevention of such behavior is the key to lung protection remain debatable, especially when peak tidal pressures are restrained; modest airway pressures may not inflict shearing injury when opening occurs at low pressure. In addition, because the difference between opening and closing pressures is often quite narrow in units that do open at higher pressure, some degree of tidal recruitment may be unavoidable. Therefore, how much of the lung should be "opened" and what pressure cost is acceptable are key unresolved questions.

PATHOGENETIC COFACTORS OF VILI

Experimentally, a number of cofactors apart from end-inspiratory and end-expiratory tidal transpulmonary pressures are important in the generation or prevention of VILI (Table 29-2). Prone positioning confers a protective advantage in both normal and preinjured animals.[52,53] The potential role of high inspired O_2 as a contributor to iatrogenic injury has been intimated for many years but never

TABLE 29-2 Clinically Modifiable Cofactors Influence the Expression of VILI

Vascular pressure
   High inflow or low outflow pressures
Ventilation frequency and/or minute ventilation
   Hypercapnia may be protective
Position
Body temperature
Inspired oxygen percentage
Pharmacological interventions

ABBREVIATION: VILI, ventilator-induced lung injury.

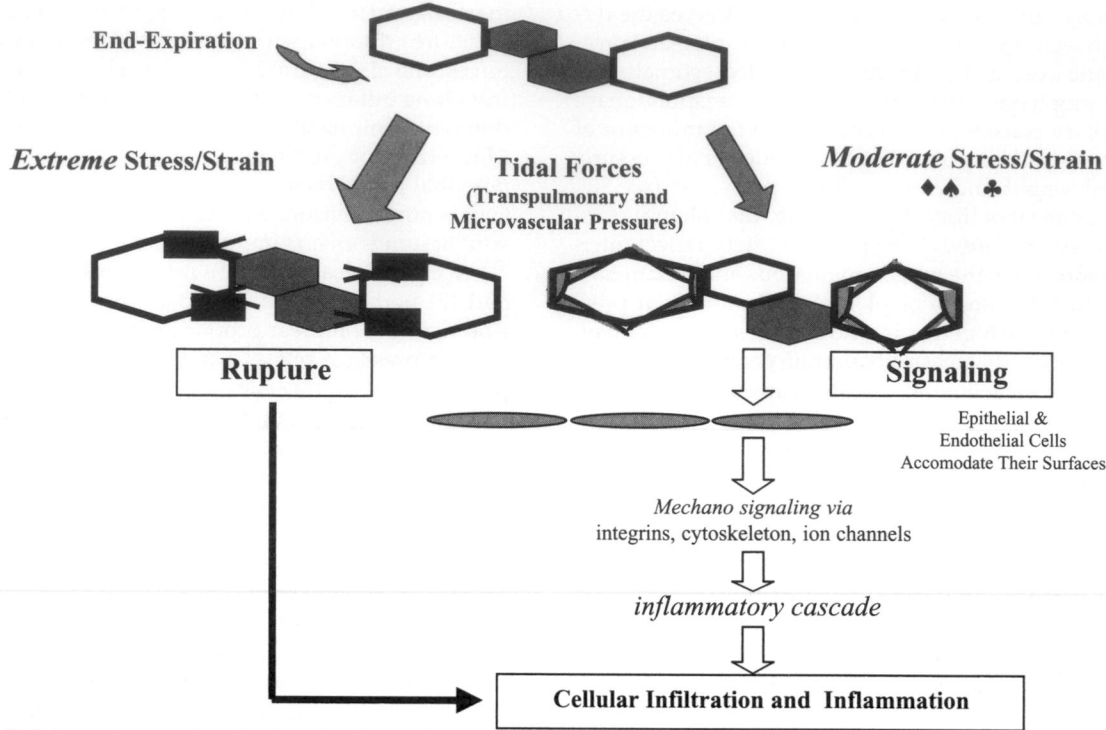

FIGURE 29-11 Hypothetical relationship between tissue damage and the severity of mechanical stress/strain during the tidal cycle. Moderate forces applied repeatedly to junctional tissues may result in mechanosignaling of inflammation. Extreme stress/strain causes microwounds to develop, with inflammation occurring as an epiphenomenon. (*Used, with permission, from Marini et al: Crit Care Med 32:250–5, 2004.*)

documented convincingly in the clinical setting.[1,35] As other examples, higher precapillary[54] and lower postcapillary[55] vascular pressures intensify the injury inflicted by a fixed ventilatory pattern. As the lung expands, alveolar and extra-alveolar microvessels are compressed and dilated, respectively (Fig. 29-11). At some intermediate point on the luminal pathway that links them, the pushes and pulls are oppositely directed, giving rise to forces that stress the microvascular endothelium. Energy dissipation across the waterfall created by intermittent zone 2 conditions, vascular interdependence, and opening and closing of the microvascular endothelium potentially could explain the damaging influence of reduced postalveolar vascular pressure. For identical tidal inflation and end-expiratory pressures, reducing respiratory frequency attenuates or delays damage, provided that the tidal ventilatory stresses are sufficiently high.[56] This observation seems logical, in that some large tidal breaths and sighs occur infrequently as part of an inherent pattern of normal breathing. Sighs, for example, are inherent to the natural breathing pattern and are not injurious.[57] Multiple high-tension tidal cycles are required to signal inflammation. Experimental evidence also demonstrates that effective repair of minor defects of the cell membrane may occur within seconds of reducing stress,[58,59] and reducing respiratory frequency may allow these repair processes sufficient time to run to completion. Alternatively, less *cumulative* damage to the lung may occur per unit time

as injurious forces unzip structural elements of the lung's fibroskeleton.

What level of transpulmonary pressure is likely to be damaging, therefore, depends on variables other than the tidal "plateau" pressure. Moreover, when the lung is comprised of large numbers of recruitable units, PEEP attenuates the tendency for high plateau pressures or tidal volumes to cause injury.[60–62] It is therefore difficult to specify an exact level of transpulmonary pressure that serves as an appropriate threshold criterion for safety. From a theoretical standpoint, a *transpulmonary* pressure of 20 cmH$_2$O (corresponding in a patient with a normal chest wall to a plateau pressure that may be in the range of 25–35 cmH$_2$O) gives cause for concern because some higher-compliance regions of the injured lung may approach their elastic limits at this pressure. It is worth noting that a *transpulmonary* pressure of only 15 cmH$_2$O subjects the *normal* lung to about two-thirds of its total capacity and is associated with a tidal volume exceeding 2500 ml.[12]

In addition to these pathogenetic cofactors, intriguing experimental data suggest that lung tissues can be injured by mechanical stretching forces more easily in the setting of other noxious influences. In other words, it takes a higher stretching force to cause injury in a previously healthy lung than in one that has been exposed previously or concurrently to another inflammatory stimulus, such as endotoxin, hyperoxia, or cytotoxic drug.[63,64] Such data have given rise

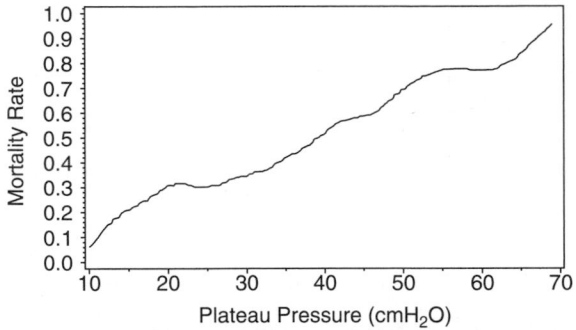

FIGURE 29-12 Relationship between mortality rate and plateau pressure generated during the NIH-sponsored ARDS Network multicenter trial of high versus low tidal volumes. Note the quasi-linear relationship of mortality rate to plateau pressure. (*Used, with permission, from Brower et al: Am J Respir Crit Care Med 166:1515–7, 2002.*)

to the "two-hit hypothesis" for VILI and underscore the potential vulnerability of the preinjured lung to imprudent ventilatory prescriptions. At the same time, such vulnerability can be viewed as an opportunity to modulate the severity of VILI by altering nonventilatory as well as ventilatory factors.

A *post hoc* analysis of the ARDS Network tidal volume trial (ARMA) indicates that observed mortality paralleled plateau pressure to very low values—considerably lower than 20 cmH_2O[65] (Fig. 29-12). This correlation, which is difficult to explain entirely by indices of disease severity, suggests the possibility that for the injured lung there is no obvious safety threshold below which ventilator-associated lung damage does not occur. Other data have shown a similar relationship but argue that plateau pressures of less than 30 cmH_2O have little impact on mortality once PEEP and disease severity are accounted for.[66] [Tidal volume must correlate with plateau pressure in any given individual; prestudy tidal volume and plateau pressure data from the ARMA trial, however, showed remarkably poor correlation because compliance is the missing parameter (Fig. 29-13).]

FIGURE 29-13 Scatter plot of tidal volume versus plateau pressure before randomization to the limbs of the (NIH-ARDS Network) ARMA trial. (*Used, with permission, from Brower et al: Am J Respir Crit Care Med 166:1515–7, 2002.*)

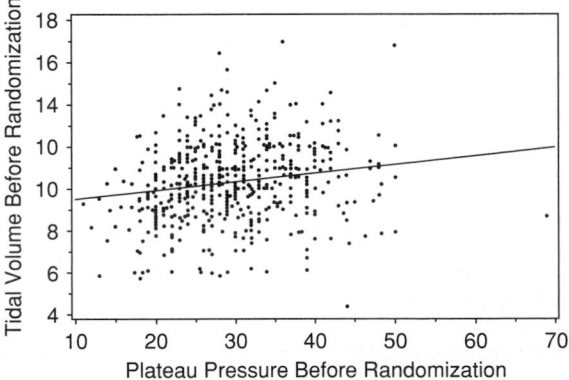

ACTIONS OF PEEP

Elevating the pressure baseline from which breaths are taken or delivered raises mean and end-expiratory lung volumes. Doing so nearly always improves oxygenation to some extent—primarily a function of keeping the lung open. When the breaths are drawn spontaneously or with pressure support, it is customary to call the end-expiratory pressure *continuous positive airway pressure* (CPAP); during breaths of predetermined length, the term is *PEEP*. Both are instrumental in the supportive care of patients with ARDS.

Gas Exchange

The potential clinical utility of PEEP in improving oxygenation was mentioned in the paper that first brought ARDS to widespread clinical attention.[1] Subsequent work demonstrated its potential to increase ventilation dead space and impair cardiac output by several mechanisms, the most important of which are impeded venous return and increased right-ventricular afterload.[67] In patients in whom PEEP stabilizes lung units that are susceptible to collapse, the response to increasing PEEP is generally to improve pulmonary O_2 exchange efficiency. Many patients show limited or negligible response, however, presumably because the recruitable population of lung units under baseline conditions is small. Infrequently, increasing PEEP actually can cause Pa_{O_2} to fall presumably by redirecting pulmonary blood flow, by causing pulmonary arterial pressure to rise high enough to shunt venous blood through a patent foramen ovale, or by causing sufficient reduction in O_2 delivery to force an increase in systemic O_2 extraction and desaturate venous blood (see Chapter 37).

The benefit of PEEP on oxygenation depends on improving FRC. When patients labor to breathe, as during hyperpnea, expiratory efforts made against PEEP may force lung volume to fall below its equilibrium value, effectively storing elastic energy to aid inspiration but interfering with improvement in O_2 exchange. Under these circumstances, eliminating forceful expiratory muscle action (such as by sedation) tends to improve O_2 exchange efficiency.[68]

Alteration of Tissue Stress

Because PEEP has the potential to maintain recruitment of unstable lung units (thereby reducing "stress amplification"), there has been intense interest in its role as a core element of a lung-protective ventilating strategy. When plateau pressure is held constant, raising PEEP not only reduces the number of closed lung units but also shortens the lever arm applied to the unstable lung units at risk to open forcefully (Fig. 29-14). Yet, when tidal driving pressure is preserved, PEEP raises both mean and peak tidal pressures, distends lung units that are already open, redirects blood flow, and alters cardiac loading conditions. Moreover, those lung units that continue to undergo repeated tidal recruitment despite an increase of PEEP are subjected to any PEEP-related elevation of end-inspiratory pressure, increasing the tendency for damage to those specific units. Thus PEEP has the clear potential for benefit or harm depending on the balance among its multiple effects. Prone positioning tends to even the distribution of ventilation and reduce the gradient of transpulmonary pressure across the lung that exists

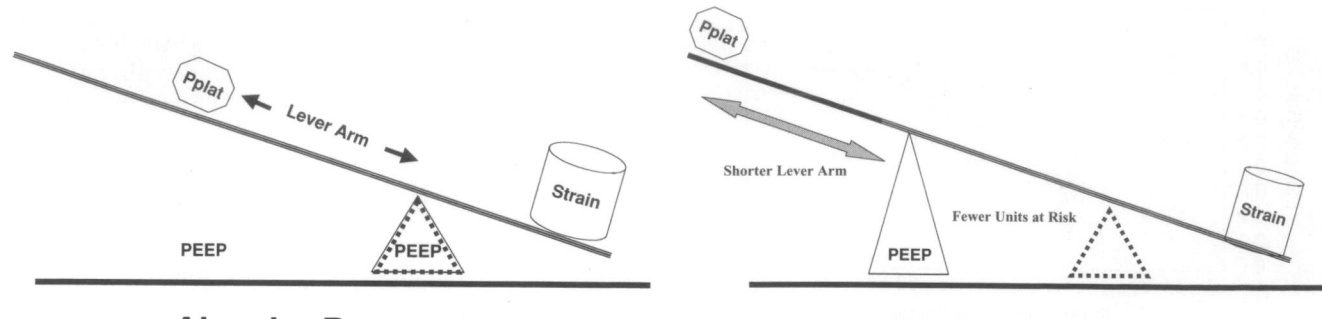

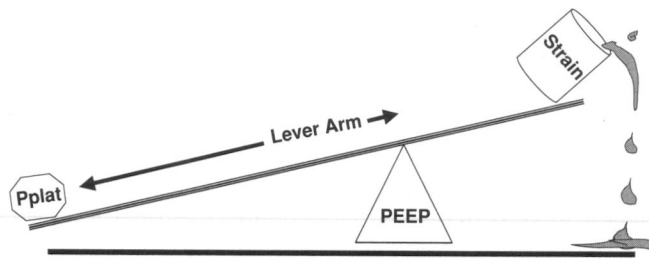

FIGURE 29-14 Conceptual relationship between plateau pressure, PEEP, and tissue strain. In the generation of tissue strain, the driving pressure for tidal volume (the difference between plateau pressure and PEEP) acts as a force lever arm, whereas PEEP acts as the fulcrum. (*Upper-left*) Levels of plateau pressure and PEEP produce strain within acceptable limits. (*Bottom-center*) Increasing plateau pressure while keeping PEEP at a level insufficient to hold open unstable units lengthens the lever arm and produces excessive tissue strain. (*Upper-right*) When PEEP is increased, the same high plateau pressure that caused damage previously is better tolerated in that fewer lung units are placed at risk after recruitment, and the lever arm of driving pressure is shortened.

in the supine position.[50,69] Airway and lymphatic drainage also tend to improve (Fig. 29-15). This improved uniformity facilitates the selection of a single combination of PEEP and tidal volume that achieves a protective strategy for the *entire* organ.

FIGURE 29-15 CT slices obtained in supine and prone positions in two patients without ARDS. In both patients, the heart and mediastinal contents are supported by dependent lung tissue in the supine position. In the prone position, the sternum bears the compressive weight, allowing the lung to expand. Lymphatic drainage also may be improved in the prone position in that the heart resides below rather that above the midplane that divides the lung tissue into superior and inferior portions. (*Modified, with permission, from Albert et al: Am J Respir Crit Care Med 161:1660–5, 2000.*)

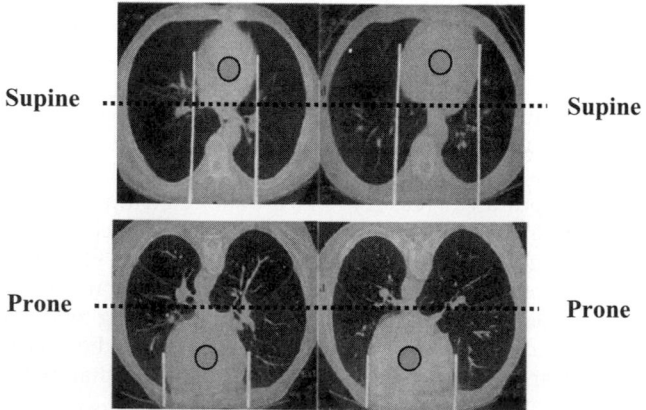

RECRUITING MANEUVERS

A major clinical challenge is to apply sufficient pressure to keep the lung fully recruited without either increasing the stress applied to tissue that remains closed or overdistending alveoli that remain patent. Certain steps can be taken to minimize the number of unstable units by reversing those conditions that predispose to compressive and absorptive atelectasis (Table 29-3). PEEP cannot keep lung units open that were not open at an earlier point in the respiratory cycle, and the recruiting process is not completed until pressures are reached that considerably exceed the total capacity of the healthy lung (Fig. 29-16). Although most lung units open at pressures less than 25 cmH$_2$O, some refractory units of the acutely injured lung may require much higher pressures to establish patency. To reach the "yield" (opening) pressures of refractory lung units requires the initial application of pressures that would be hazardous during tidal ventilation.[14,27,70] Once opened, the lung units tend to close at lower pressures, allowing ventilation with the same tidal volume and PEEP to occur in the context of a more open

TABLE 29-3 How Is the Injured Lung Best Recruited?

Prone position
Adequate PEEP
Adequate tidal volume (and/or sighs?)
Recruiting maneuvers
Minimize edema (?)
Lowest acceptable Fi$_{O_2}$ (?)
Spontaneous efforts (?)

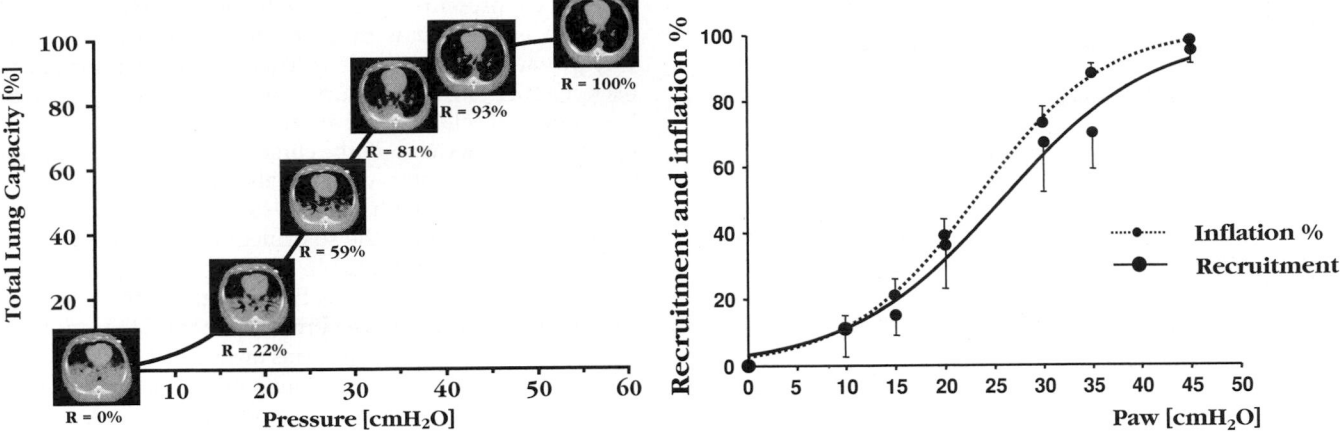

FIGURE 29-16 (*Left*) CT slices obtained after oleic acid injury of the lung superimposed on the pressure-volume relationship of the respiratory system. Consolidation and radiographic density are greatest in the dependent lung regions, and high pressures must be applied even in this "highly recruitable" lung model to fully reverse the radiographic evidence of collapse. Percentages denote aerated recruitable tissue. (*Right*) Recruitment and inflation percentages as functions of static airway pressure. The pressure-recruitment curve parallels the pressure-inflation curve when both are expressed as percentages of their maximum ranges. (*Used, with permission, from Pelosi et al: Am J Respir Crit Care Med 164:122–30, 2001; and Crotti et al: Am J Respir Crit Care Med 164:131–40, 2001.*)

lung with fewer lung units at risk for opening and closure (Fig. 29-17).

Because of viscoelastance and other time-dependent force-distributing phenomena, the tendency of a previously collapsed airway to open (or "yield") is a jointly hyperbolic function of transmural pressure and time. A number of techniques known as *recruiting maneuvers* are designed to "open" the lung so that safe and effective combinations of PEEP and tidal volume can be used. Each recognizes that recruitment depends not only on the magnitude of transpulmonary pressure but also on the duration of its application (Fig. 29-18). To consolidate benefit after a successful "recruiting maneuver," end-expiratory pressure must remain high enough to hold open these newly recruited units once safe tidal plateau pressures are resumed. With few ex-

ceptions, this "stabilizing" value of PEEP is higher than the initial one before recruitment.[71,72] The effect of a recruiting maneuver is extremely short lived if PEEP returns to its original value.

While most unstable lung units can be kept open with end-expiratory alveolar pressures (total PEEP) of approximately 10 cmH$_2$O (assuming a normally compliant chest wall), some units close at pressures considerably higher than those that are safe to apply with each tidal breath[27]

FIGURE 29-17 Effect on the tidal pressure-volume relationship (*small loops*) before and after a sustained-inflation (SI) recruiting maneuver during controlled mechanical ventilation (CMV). Hypothetically, first opening the lung by increasing pressure to high values (by means of a sustained-inflation recruiting maneuver) allows tidal ventilation to occur at similar or lower pressures with more lung units open at an expiration.

FIGURE 29-18 Time course of changes in functional residual capacity (FRC) in respiratory failure following a step increase of PEEP from 3–13 cmH$_2$O. Multiple tidal cycles are required to fully achieve the ultimate increase in an expiratory lung volume. Although tidal volume would affect the time needed to equilibrate, in this instance, approximately 40 seconds was required. (*Used, with permission, from Katz et al: Anesthesiology 54:9–16, 1981.*)

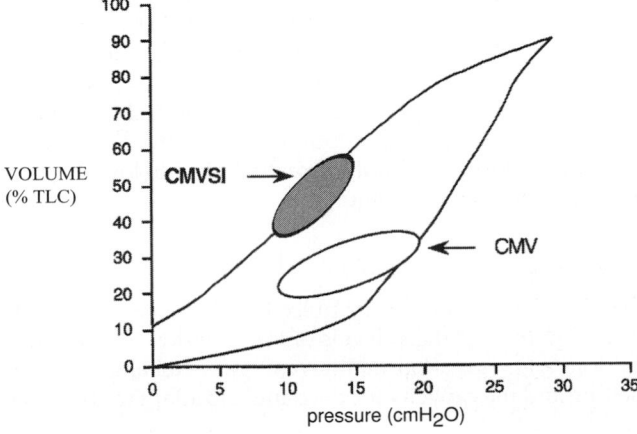

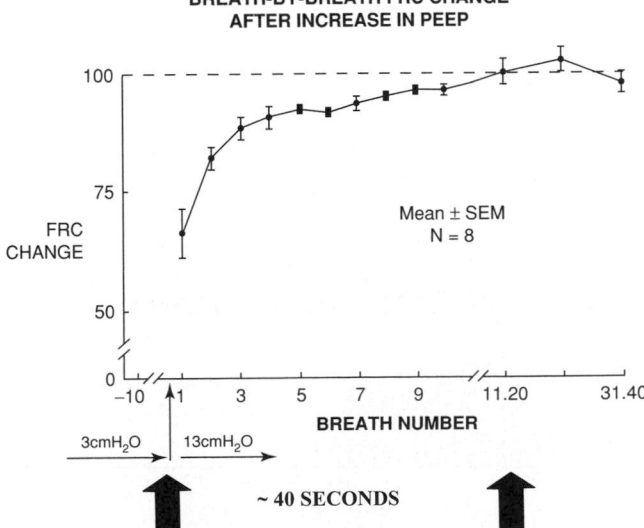

TABLE 29-4   Determinants of Recruitment Maneuver Effectiveness

ARDS category
  Inherent *potential* for response
ARDS stage
  Responsiveness diminishes over time
Starting PEEP and tidal volume
  Was the lung well recruited to start with?
  How much higher than the tidal plateau is the recruiting pressure?
  How many more units can be opened?
Postrecruitment PEEP
  Duration of response
Aggressiveness and type of recruiting method
  Often limited by tolerance

(see Fig. 29-5). It is a fallacy to consider all injured tissue as potentially recruitable. Unlike most experimental models of ALI,[27,73] only a small fraction of the lungs of pneumonia-caused ("primary") ARDS, for example, can be "opened."[74,75]

Although a number of recruitment maneuvers have been described, their efficacy depends on numerous factors (Table 29-4). Moreover, even when indicated, the best technique with which to perform a recruitment maneuver is currently unknown and may well vary with specific circumstances, and repeated maneuvers may be required for maximum benefit. The two most commonly used are the sustained-inflation and the incremental-PEEP/fixed-driving-pressure methods[76] (Fig. 29-19). The latter is often

FIGURE 29-19 Three types of recruiting maneuvers that combine high pressures with extended application time. Recruitment that employs tidal ventilation with pressure-control ventilation (PCV) achieves the same peak pressure for the same cumulative time as sustained inflation but at considerably lower mean airway pressure. PCV also provides multiple recruiting cycles and ventilates during the maneuver. (*Used, with permission, from Lim et al: Crit Care Med 32:2371–7, 2004.*)

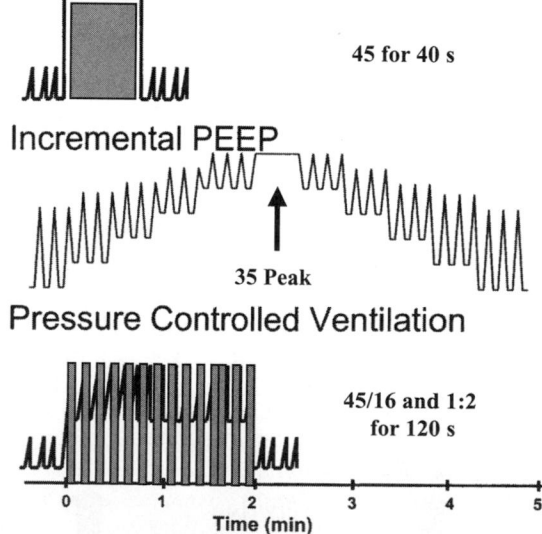

applied by pressure-control ventilation. When sustained pressure is applied without relief, mean and peak airway pressures are equivalent. This imposes extraordinary backpressure to venous return and poses a high afterload to the right ventricle for the period of its application. Both in experimental models and the clinical setting, ARDS caused by pneumonia (a primary form of alveolar damage) appears to be the condition with greatest risk for hypotension and least responsiveness to the sustained-inflation recruitment maneuver.[77]

Sustaining high pressure is believed to be an important component of the recruiting process, whereas the length of time required for its effect remains unsettled. Moreover, it is possible that for the same maximum pressure, briefer applications more frequently may be as effective as fewer cycles with a longer inspiratory time. Mean airway pressure can be reduced considerably while maintaining the same peak airway pressure value—the actual recruiting pressure—using a limited period of tidal ventilation with a constant driving pressure [e.g., 1–2 minutes of pressure control with a driving pressure of 30 cmH$_2$O and high PEEP (e.g., 25 cmH$_2$O)]. Thus the pressure-control recruitment maneuver may hold an advantage if pressures beyond those tolerated during the sustained high-pressure method are needed to complete lung opening.[75,77]

SPONTANEOUS VENTILATORY EFFORTS

Preservation of spontaneous breathing efforts during assisted ventilation may help to improve ventilation-perfusion matching by preferentially ventilating the peridiaphragmatic regions that receive disproportionate blood flow.[78,79] Whether this redistribution of ventilation aids *sustained* recruitment and thus whether it reduces or augments the tendency for VILI currently remain unknown. The answer may well vary with the intensity of the breathing efforts and the vigor of expiratory muscle activity.

Ventilating Objectives and Decisions in ARDS

The foregoing discussion suggests that a rational lung-protective ventilator strategy should include the following elements: (1) avoidance of high tidal end-inspiratory alveolar pressures, (2) provision of adequate end-expiratory pressure to avoid extensive end-expiratory tidal collapse, (3) reduction of regional nonuniformity of mechanical properties, and (4) to the extent possible, avoidance of cofactors that abet the development of VILI, such as high inspired concentrations of O$_2$ and increased metabolic demands for ventilation and cardiac output. Choice of the appropriate therapeutic targets is fundamentally linked to lowering the risk for iatrogenic lung injury.

THERAPEUTIC TARGETS

There is little evolutionary precedent for surviving ARDS that requires advanced levels of life support. Yet the limits of tolerance to abnormalities of gas exchange in this setting and the capacity for the patient to adapt to abnormal blood gases have not been explored extensively and remain largely unknown. Tradeoffs must be made when intervening to sustain life because the supports applied to maintain oxygenation and ventilation—inspired O_2 and positive pressure—are both potentially injurious to the lung.[64,80] The discipline of intensive care evolved as an extension of postoperative care. Therefore, it was natural to employ ventilator parameters that serve well in that setting, where the general aim is to hold arterial blood gases reasonably close to their preoperative values, and large tidal volumes are needed to forestall atelectasis and avert dyspnea. Three decades ago, awareness of O_2 toxicity was well entrenched, and the acutely injured lung was viewed on the basis of plain frontal chest radiographs as mechanically uniform—diffusely stiff and therefore tolerant of the high ventilating pressures needed to maintain normal blood gases.

Over the ensuing decades these assumptions eventually were challenged. Premature infants ventilated for infantile respiratory distress syndrome (IRDS) clearly were vulnerable to the application of high ventilating pressure. In adults, the high mortality rate of diseases with intrinsically high survivability, such as asthma,[81] the high incidence of radiographically evident barotrauma,[82] and newfound awareness of dynamic hyperinflation[83,84] brought the wisdom of traditional practices and therapeutic targets into question. The concept of reducing ventilatory requirements by allowing Pa_{CO_2} to rise was first implemented successfully in the care of patients with status asthmaticus.[85] Five years later, the same strategy was reported to have been implemented successfully in patients with ARDS.[86] Subsequent research has emphasized that acute hypercapnic acidosis occurring in this setting is a complex phenomenon with diverse physiologic effects that include those with potential benefit (e.g., inhibiting inflammation) as well as those with potentially undesirable consequences (e.g., stimulation of ventilatory drive and cerebral vasodilation)[87] (see Chapters 41, 44, 46, and 47). Although guidelines for selecting the most appropriate values for pH and Pa_{CO_2} are elusive and undoubtedly should vary with the individual in question, it is clear from accumulated experience that mild to moderate deviations from the normal ranges of both parameters are generally well tolerated. At present, the dangers of VILI are perceived to outweigh those attributable to either inspired O_2 or hypercapnia.

IMPLEMENTING VENTILATOR SUPPORT

Important principles gathered from laboratory experiments, shared clinical experience, observational studies, and randomized clinical trials have emerged regarding the application of ventilator support to lung-injured patients (see Table 29-1). Noninvasive ventilation has been reported to be successful in patients with mild to moderate severity of injury,[88–90] and when feasible to employ, benefit is likely to accrue from the need for less sedation and the lower incidence of infection associated with this approach.[90] Although the interface between ventilator and patient continues to improve, only limited pressure can be tolerated for longer than brief periods, many patients cannot protect the upper airway, and the lung must be kept well recruited to avoid hypoxemia, precluding intermittent removal. For these reasons, airway intubation is virtually always required in severe cases of lung injury.

Patterns of lung expansion differ for passive and actively assisted breathing. Preservation of muscular effort conceptually holds an advantage regarding the matching of ventilation to perfusion—at least in the healthy lung. The same advantage also may hold for the acutely injured lung, provided that breathing remains comfortable and unlabored. Vigorous efforts, however, are undesirable for several reasons: increased ventilatory workload, O_2 consumption, and CO_2 production; increased cardiac output and pulmonary blood flow (which may accelerate edema formation and possibly VILI); and expiratory muscle contraction that counters the effects of PEEP.[91] Whether gentle or vigorous, it has yet to be shown convincingly that patients who expend effort in breathing benefit from doing so.

MODES OF VENTILATION FOR ARDS

An extensive array of ventilator options is available for treating patients with ARDS. Each method is described in detail elsewhere in this textbook. As a general statement, it is accurate to state that the choice of ventilating mode is of much less importance than how the selected mode is implemented. When guided by the principles of attaining efficient gas exchange, targeting appropriate therapeutic objectives, and protecting the lung against iatrogenic damage, many different selections can be justified. What is presented here is a brief outline of some of the more important characteristics applicable to ALI.

For the past two decades, four modes have served to ventilate patients with ARDS at conventional frequencies: (1) flow-controlled, time- or volume-cycled ventilation (*volume control*), (2) pressure-targeted, time-cycled ventilation (*pressure control*), (3) pressure-targeted, flow-cycled ventilation (*pressure support*), and (4) combination modes in which a specified number of stereotyped time-limited machine cycles (pressure- or volume-controlled) that are specified by the clinician and synchronized to be triggered by patient effort are delivered intermittently at evenly spaced intervals among additional breaths of variable size and depth taken by the patient [*synchronized intermittent mechanical ventilation* (SIMV)]. As described in detail elsewhere in this book, flow and pressure cannot be controlled simultaneously because the energetics of ventilation require one or the other to become a dependent variable in order to satisfy the equation of motion for ventilating the respiratory system.[92]

Flow control ensures that the desired tidal volume will be delivered reliably but obligates the patient to that specified contour, independent of flow demand. Therefore, alveolar pressure, a function of delivered volume and compliance during passive ventilation, has the potential to ascend to dangerous levels. The flow profile delivered may be unchanging ("square") or decelerating. Pressure control offers the flexibility to satisfy flow demand and *under passive conditions* ensures that alveolar pressure rises no higher than a known peak airway pressure. [During active breathing (assisted cycles), the maximum transpulmonary pressure is not regulated by pressure control.] Flow is inherently decelerating, which may improve distribution of ventilation moderately among heterogeneous lung units compared with constant flow. The potentially adverse tradeoff with using pressure control is that the delivered volume is a function of the impedance to breathing and any backpressure opposing inspiratory flow, so tidal volume may change abruptly with muscular activity, airway resistance, lung and chest-wall compliance, or auto-PEEP.

In recent years, the imperative to maintain consistent ventilation and nearly normal levels of Pa_{CO_2} has declined in relative importance. Awareness of the potential for high ventilating pressures to inflict iatrogenic lung injury, coupled with a growing clinical experience that suggests the safety of higher than normal Pa_{CO_2} values (permissive hypercapnia), has caused many clinicians to adopt pressure control as the default mode. In the absence of effort and provided that both tidal volume and end-inspiratory pause pressure are monitored, the choice of pressure or volume control makes little practical difference to physiology or outcome.

Inverse-ratio ventilation (IRV), a mode that extends inspiratory time with the intent of raising mean airway pressure and capping applied airway pressure while maintaining adequate ventilation typically is applied with pressure control.[93,94] To prevent airway closure at end expiration, however, may require generation of auto-PEEP that narrows the inspiratory pressure difference and limits tidal volume (Fig. 29-20). Although there may be rare exceptions, IRV appears not to offer any notable advantage over conventional-ratio ventilation that is applied with adequate PEEP.

During vigorous breathing, as during the first days of severe ARDS, it may be difficult to avoid patient-ventilator dyssynchrony with either assist volume control or pressure control because both require preset inspiratory times. Pressure limitation and failure to deliver full tidal volumes then may occur. In these instances, high-level pressure-support ventilation (PSV), a flow-cycled mode, offers response flexibility. When used alone or in combination with intermittent time-limited mandatory machine cycles (SIMV), PSV may minimize the timing collisions that otherwise occur between the cycling phases of patient and machine. In any form of pressure-targeted or flow-regulated breathing, the ventilator's alarms should be set carefully so as to avoid overapplication of pressure or underventilation.

FIGURE 29-20 Concept of inverse-ratio ventilation using pressure-control ventilation. As airway pressure is applied and released, alveolar pressure rises and falls exponentially (*heavy line*). Extending the inspiratory time fraction increases mean airway pressure and levels of auto-PEEP without changing peak alveolar pressure.

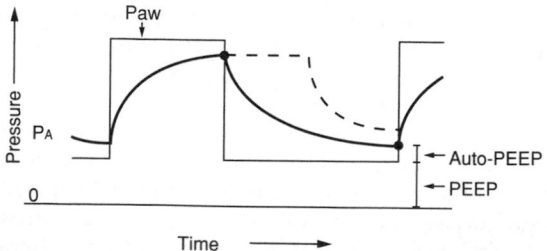

NEWER MODES OF VENTILATION

For patients capable of sustained ventilatory effort, it is an option to elevate the airway pressure baseline, allowing the patient to draw breaths from that higher volume level. When airway pressure is maintained relatively constant throughout both phases of the breathing cycle, the condition is termed *CPAP*.[95] If the baseline shifts periodically, with the patient able to draw breaths unimpeded through a valveless system at each level, ventilator assistance is given to an extent governed by the difference between pressure baselines and the frequency with which these baseline shifts occur. This mode is known as *biphasic airway pressure* (BiPAP).[96] When a high CPAP baseline is released only for a very brief period and then restored quickly to its original level, BiPAP contracts into airway pressure-release ventilation (APRV).[97,98] The putative advantage of each of these modes for the care of patients with ARDS is that they encourage maintenance of an open lung with their high-pressure baselines and ensure that the spontaneous breathing pattern is preserved. As with so many mode options, however, no definitive evidence exists to confirm their relative advantage over a well-adjusted traditional approach (see Chapters 10 and 12).

High-frequency Ventilation

Awareness of the tissue-damaging potential of applying high end-inspiratory plateau pressures with insufficient end-expiratory pressure to keep unstable alveoli open ignited interest in using methods that apply very small tidal volumes so rapidly that alveolar collapse has no time to occur. Over the past three decades, various techniques for providing high-frequency ventilation have been explored with enthusiasm, tried tentatively in the clinical setting, and then set aside reluctantly.[99–103] These have included positive-pressure ventilation with valved-circuit closure to separate the phases of the ventilatory cycle (as traditionally done) but applied at nonconventional frequencies and tidal volumes. The technical demands of such high-frequency valving have limited its operating frequency range, efficiency, and safety. Another form of high-frequency ventilation, jet ventilation, uses a lung-directed injector of conditioned gas pulsating at rapid frequencies into an open circuit. Problems with gas trapping, drying of airway secretions, and limited efficacy have dampened enthusiasm for its use in critically ill patients. At present, a third form, high-frequency oscillation, is in most widespread clinical use for patients with ARDS.[101,102] This "open-circuit" technique uses a rapidly reciprocating piston-like action to vibrate the air column at high amplitude, building and releasing small alveolar pressure excursions in the process. A fresh-gas source allows effective gas exchange via mechanisms that complement the bulk flow that accounts for ventilation at lower frequencies[103] (see Chapter 20). Although the experimental and clinical data available amply document the feasibility of high-frequency oscillation for the setting of ALI in adults,[101–103] the prevailing opinion is that this unfamiliar and seemingly exotic technique seems to offer little advantage over ventilation performed conventionally with equivalent attention to the principles of lung protection.

TABLE 29-5   Therapeutic Adjuncts to Mechanical Ventilation of ARDS

Minimize O_2 demands
Optimize O_2 delivery
Recruiting maneuvers
Prone positioning
Inhaled nitric oxide/inhaled prostacyclin
Tracheal gas insufflation
Corticosteroids and (?) other drugs

ADJUNCTS TO MECHANICAL VENTILATION

Attention to limiting tissue strain mandates that the pressure driving each tidal cycle (the difference between end-inspiratory and end-expiratory pressures), as well as the number of high-pressure cycles applied per unit time, be kept within acceptable bounds. These requirements limit tidal volume and minute ventilation and stimulate interest in methods that reduce the requirements for ventilation and oxygenation, reduce local tissue stresses, and improve the efficiency of pulmonary gas exchange, all without the need for additional ventilating pressures or higher ventilating frequency (Table 29-5). The majority of these "adjunctive" techniques are discussed in detail elsewhere in this book. Here it should be emphasized that perhaps the most effective and universally applicable means for avoiding the need for high ventilatory pressures is to reduce the *demand* for them by the patient or to readjust the clinician's therapeutic targets for ventilator support. Thus avoidance of high fever, pain, agitation, and metabolic acidosis reduces O_2 and ventilation demands, as well as the need for cardiac output—an important potential cofactor for VILI in the experimental setting. Optimizing O_2 delivery by improving cardiac performance and providing adequate hemoglobin concentration also minimize the ventilatory requirements.

Using the prone position evens the distribution of transpulmonary pressure, reducing local tissue strains and effectively recruiting well-perfused dorsal parenchyma, thereby improving oxygenation in most patients.[50] Methods for improving gas-exchange efficiency include those directed at oxygenation (inhaled nitric oxide[104–106] or inhaled prostacyclin[107]), and those that lessen wasted ventilation (tracheal gas insufflation[108–110] or reduction of apparatus deadspace[110]). Although often considered to be a ventilatory adjunct of limited value, recruiting maneuvers are incorporated by many practitioners, including this author, as an entrenched part of clinical practice.[111] In difficult situations, the recruiting maneuver affords a logical means of reopening the atelectatic lung so that the appropriate values of PEEP and tidal volume may be selected (see below).

Setting the Ventilator: Recommendations for Practice

Given the joint potential for the ventilator to offer life support or to extend the severity and duration of the illness, the machine settings for the ventilatory cycle are of unquestioned importance. How best to achieve the appropri-ate tradeoff, however, remains a topic of active debate. The available clinical database, albeit difficult to reconcile, appears broadly to agree with the highly consistent scientific body of information that addresses ventilator use in the setting of ALI.

INSIGHTS FROM CLINICAL TRIALS OF LUNG PROTECTION

With the rise of "evidence-based practice," physicians have sought guidance from clinical trials that have addressed the relative merits of different ventilation strategies.[2,3,112–115] Studies in which the highest tidal volumes and pressures were applied in the "control arm" have shown benefit from low-tidal-volume ventilation.[2,3] Results have been particularly impressive when higher PEEP was used in conjunction with small tidal volumes in a setting where emphasis was placed on establishing stable recruitment, avoiding high ventilating pressures, and managing clinical cointerventions consistently.[2,115]

Only one of the several studies that randomized *selectively* on tidal volume—by far the largest yet published—successfully demonstrated mortality benefit for a smaller-tidal-volume approach.[3] In retrospect, this hardly should come as a surprise because the physiologic impact of tidal volume depends on compliance (see Fig. 29-13). Furthermore, provocative examinations of the data collected in the ARDS Network ARMA study and a meta-analysis of all published trials addressing the selection of tidal volume have suggested that "lower is not necessarily better," especially when compliance is less severely impaired and periodic sighs or recruiting maneuvers are not employed.[116,117] Knowing that tidal volume is only indirectly linked to tissue strain, inflammation, and rupture (consider the noninjurious effects of high tidal volumes during exercise), it is interesting to speculate that the recruiting effects of higher tidal volumes actually might have a salutary effect on inflammatory signaling if peak transpulmonary pressure were kept below the "overstretch" signaling threshold and an appropriate level of PEEP were used. Whatever the validity of this controversial argument, the collective results of these clinical studies have focused attention on transalveolar stresses rather than on tidal volume per se. They also have demonstrated that the levels and effects of hypercapnia experienced during low-tidal-volume ventilation, although complex,[87,118–120] generally are modest and well tolerated.

The National Institutes of Health (NIH)–sponsored trial of high versus moderate PEEP failed to demonstrate a significant survival advantage for patients allocated to the high-PEEP group.[121] Important considerations, however, were (1) neither group was exposed to plateau pressures that were clearly in a dangerous range, (2) recruitment potential was not stratified, so patients who were not likely to benefit were assigned to both groups, and (3) no recruiting maneuver preceded PEEP application, nor was PEEP regulated as in conventional clinical practice. Unfortunately, there also was a failure of the randomization process so that a disproportionate number of older patients were assigned to the high-PEEP limb. The importance of PEEP is likely to depend on the plateau pressure achieved. A recently

TABLE 29-6 Common Effects of Prone Positioning in Early ARDS

More homogeneous transpulmonary pressure
Increased and sustained traction on dorsal lung units
 Better $\dot{V}/\dot{Q}$ matching
 Tendency for *recruitment*
Improved airway drainage
Improved lymphatic drainage
Modestly increased functional residual capacity (FRC)
Reduced tidal tissue strain [V_T/FRC (and VILI?)]

ABBREVIATIONS: $\dot{V}/\dot{Q}$, ventilation-perfusion ratio; V_T, tidal volume; VILI, ventilator-induced lung injury.

completed Spanish multicenter trial appears to confirm that PEEP is an integral part of a lung-protective approach,[115] an implication supported by an analysis of "real world" ventilatory practice and outcomes.[66]

Recruitment maneuvers also have been examined in a clinical trials format as a substudy of the high-PEEP NIH investigation.[122] The recruiting maneuvers were applied only in the high-PEEP limb, and the peak pressure achieved was limited to 35 cmH$_2$O. The small separation between plateau pressure and PEEP, the underlying disease characteristics of the study population, the relatively high level of PEEP at baseline, and the failure to augment PEEP after the recruiting maneuver undoubtedly biased the result against showing a significant benefit.[123]

Finally, notwithstanding considerable theoretical appeal (Table 29-6), oxygenation benefit,[124] and suggestive experimental evidence,[52,53,125] three relatively large randomized trials[126–128] have failed to demonstrate a statistically significant mortality benefit for prone positioning in broad samples of patients with ARDS. A French study reported a lower incidence of ventilator-associated pneumonia in the prone cohort,[127] but this did not translate into a survival advantage for that trial limb. An Italian trial used prone positioning for less than one-third of each day, and a prematurely truncated Spanish trial,[128] in which prone positioning was maintained for three-quarters of the day, showed an impressive separation (25% relative risk of death) between the supine and prone treatment arms. Unfortunately, nei-

ther study entered its targeted number of patients. Moreover, because post hoc analyses of the large Italian trial strongly suggested that the most seriously affected patients, those exposed to higher ventilating pressures, and those who demonstrate improved ventilation efficiency are most likely to benefit[126,129] (Fig. 29-21), a follow-up trial focused on this subset has now been initiated. This important question remains unsettled. Therefore, despite the lack of trial evidence, there is a strong rationale to use prone positioning to improve oxygenation, to allow reductions in F$_{IO_2}$ and ventilating pressure, and for its as yet unproven potential to protect the lung.

Disappointingly, clinical trials of various other adjuncts to ventilation also have not demonstrated major outcome advantages.[130–134] From a physiologic perspective, this is hardly surprising. Precise numerical guidelines for selecting PEEP, tidal volume, and ventilatory position that are applicable to any given individual patient should not be expected from the results of studies conducted in a diverse sample population whose inclusion criteria are broadly inclusive and for whom management details are unconstrained. In the end, the best that can be hoped for is a proof of principle—not a prescription for care. However internally valid such trials may be, they do not correspond to the "real world" environment wherein comorbidities impinge and management of potentially influential variables (such as PEEP, Pa$_{CO_2}$, and fluid management) is not protocolized. What follows is an approach to care of the individual patient with ARDS based on an understanding of the physiologic principles that must be brought to bear in the complex clinical environment.

GENERAL GUIDELINES FOR VENTILATOR MANAGEMENT

Key guiding principles include the following: First, adjust ventilator parameters empirically rather than by formula-driven rules; prioritize patient comfort and safety. Second, assign the prevention of mechanical trauma precedence over maintenance of normocapnia and avoidance of O$_2$ toxicity. Although no exact upper limits for acceptable plateau pressure or F$_{IO_2}$ can be specified, very high settings of F$_{IO_2}$

FIGURE 29-21 Effect of prone positioning on mortality as functions of illness severity (*left*) and tidal volume (*right*). In patients who were most critically ill (highest SAPS quartile) or receiving tidal volumes that risk ventilator-induced lung injury (highest tidal volume quartile), prone positioning may offer a survival advantage. (*Data from Italian multicenter clinical trial of prone versus supine positioning in ARDS.*[126])

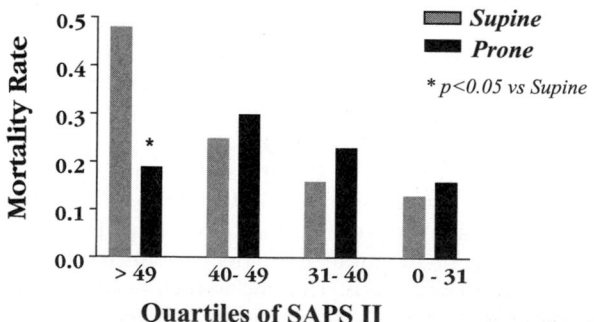
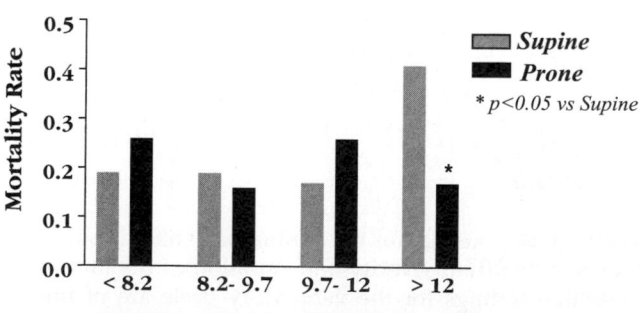

pose a risk for absorption atelectasis as well as O_2 toxicity. Therefore, F_{IO_2} should be held to less than 0.70 whenever possible. Third, consider the impact of chest-wall stiffness (including abdominal contents) on transpulmonary pressure and gas-exchange efficiency. In questionable situations, determine abdominal (bladder) and/or esophageal pressures to help estimate the transalveolar pressure.[43] Fourth, monitor hemodynamics as well as mechanics and gas exchange when regulating ventilatory therapy. Wide respiratory variation in the arterial pulse pressure suggests the need for additional volume.[135] A surrogate for measuring hemodynamics directly may be to monitor the central venous O_2 saturation. A value greater than 70% and a difference of 25% or less between arterial and mixed-venous saturations almost invariably is associated with an adequate cardiac index (>2.5 liters/m^2/min).[136] Fifth, in severe cases, attempt to minimize ventilatory demands and thereby reduce airway pressures, high rates of gas flow, and cardiac output requirements. Sixth, incorporate the "challenge" principle in making therapeutic decisions regarding both the intensification and the withdrawal of therapeutic measures. Examples of such challenges include recruiting maneuvers to assess lung-unit instability and closely monitored challenges of fluid administration or removal. Seventh, unless otherwise contraindicated, use prone positioning when high values for ventilatory pressure, PEEP and F_{IO_2} are needed to maintain adequate supine arterial O_2 tension. Eighth, assess pulmonary interventions in the volume-control mode of ventilation so as to better track thoracic mechanics and the lung's gas-exchanging efficiency for CO_2. At other times, employ pressure-limited forms of ventilation (e.g., pressure control, pressure support, or BiPAP/APRV) for ongoing management.

As a general rule, the desired goal is to use the least PEEP and tidal volume needed to achieve acceptable gas exchange while avoiding tidal collapse and reopening of unstable lung units. Knowing that moderate hypercapnia generally is well tolerated, therapeutic targeting priorities are directed toward lung protection and maintenance of appropriate hemodynamics and O_2 delivery. Recruiting maneuvers help to characterize PEEP responsiveness, to determine the relative status of intravascular filling and response to altered cardiac loading conditions, and to set the PEEP–tidal-volume combination. Prone positioning is strongly considered in all but the mildest cases and patients who rapidly improve. On rare occasions, noninvasive mechanical ventilation using a comfortable full face mask (or a helmet, if available) may overcome short-lived deficits of O_2 exchange without the need for intubation. In practice, however, the needs to control the airway, to reduce ventilatory requirements, to apply high levels of end-expiratory pressure, and to sustain support for extended periods usually preclude the use of noninvasive ventilation.

In the first phase of ventilatory support, patient comfort must be ensured and ventilatory effort kept to a minimum. Modes such as APRV, BIPAP, and high-frequency oscillation have persuasive advocates and considerable theoretical appeal.[96,98,137,138] The existing database and shared personal experience, however, have not provided convincing evidence that they offer a great deal beyond that which can be

accomplished with carefully adjusted pressure-controlled ventilation in a well-sedated patient.

All patients should be assessed for severity of disease and for recruitment potential. After deficits in intravascular volume have been addressed and hemodynamics have been optimized, recruitment potential is gauged by applying high-level pressure-control ventilation: PEEP of 15–20 cmH$_2$O, driving pressure of 30 cmH$_2$O, and plateau pressure of 50–60 cmH$_2$O for 1–2 minutes, as tolerated. Even higher pressures may be appropriate for some severely affected patients and for patients with very stiff chest walls—for example, burn victims with chest-wall edema or eschar. Although sustained inflation with high pressure has been used traditionally, employed widely, and selected for most reported research,[139] it is no more effective and tends to be less well tolerated hemodynamically than a recruiting method based on pressure-controlled ventilation that achieves lower average pressure but similar peak pressure during its inspiratory phase.[77] If oxygenation and lung mechanics do not improve substantially with high-level pressure-controlled ventilation as a recruiting technique, the patient is considered to have low recruiting potential *in that position and at that specific time*. Management goals in the "recruitable" group emphasize the maintenance of high-level end-expiratory pressure, whereas in poorly recruitable patients, PEEP is maintained as low as feasible—generally in the range of 5–10 cmH$_2$O. In both groups, end-inspiratory plateau pressure is kept less than 30 cmH$_2$O, except when chest-wall compliance is very low. Periodic sighs may be advisable when very low tidal volumes are in use.[140,141]

ADJUSTING PEEP (TABLE 29-7)
Patients with an extensive "recruitable" population of lung units should respond to increased PEEP and recruiting maneuvers by demonstrating improved alveolar mechanics and improved gas exchange, reflected both by increased Pa$_{O_2}$ and a reduction of the ratio of minute ventilation to Pa$_{CO_2}$. These salutary changes are accompanied by only marginal effects on hemodynamics, as judged by systemic blood pressure and central venous O_2 saturation.[126] Assuming an unchanged rate of CO_2 production, the latter index—like a dead-space calculation—reflects the efficiency of CO_2 elimination, which is expected to improve with recruitment and deteriorate with overdistention. Inspiratory crackles

TABLE 29-7 How Should PEEP be Adjusted? A Practical Compromise

Ensure adequate preload.
Use small to moderate V_T or driving pressure.
Recruit by increasing PEEP/PCV to plateau of $\sim$ 50–60 cmH$_2$O for $\sim$ 1–2 minutes.
Reduce driving pressure to 15–20 cmH$_2$O.
Reduce PEEP until arterial O_2 or compliance falls significantly.
Rerecruit and select next higher PEEP if hemodynamics are acceptable.
   Ensure that plateau pressure remains below acceptable maximum (e.g., <30 cmH$_2$O)

ABBREVIATIONS: V_T, tidal volume; PCV, pressure-controlled ventilation.

(rales) audible over the dependent zones of the chest suggest that recruitment and derecruitment are occurring with each breath and indicate that recruitment maneuvers and higher levels of end-expiratory pressure may be indicated to silence them.[140] Crackles occurring late in inspiration are of particular concern because they may originate in units opening under relatively high pressures. In gauging response to PEEP, it is important to consider CO_2 exchange as well as oxygenation response. With rare exception (e.g., when PEEP-impaired cardiac output causes mixed-venous O_2 content to fall), Pa_{O_2} tends to increase when PEEP is applied. This oxygenation improvement, however, may be accounted for either by recruitment of lung units or by reduced or redirected blood flow within the injured lung. In the latter circumstance, Pa_{CO_2} also may rise. When recruitment is the explanation for O_2 improvement, however, CO_2 exchange is not compromised and even may improve, reflecting increased alveolar ventilation. Similar principles apply during prone positioning.

The prone position should be considered in patients with severe gas-exchange impairment regardless of their "recruiting test" result in the supine position. Patients requiring more than 10 cmH_2O of PEEP at an $F_{I_{O_2}}$ of 0.6 to maintain O_2 saturation at 90% or greater should be considered for prone positioning unless there is a clear contraindication or the patient is improving rapidly. The prone position should be considered independently of supine recruiting potential because prone positioning will help lymphatic drainage and secretion removal and release the lower lobes of the lungs from the need to support the weight of the heart. Although provocative experimental data have challenged the concept recently,[143] the preferred angle for head elevation in supine

patients is 30° to horizontal (Fowler) with frequent (at least every 2–4 hours) lateral turning. Similar rules apply in the prone position; reverse Trendelenberg at 15–30° is preferred to flat (0°) horizontal. Tidal volume is adjusted to the same value used in the supine position. An increase in plateau pressure strongly suggests that chest-wall compliance has been altered by proning. In these instances, a proportional increase in PEEP also may be justified. (For example, if plateau pressure rises by 10%, PEEP would be increased by 10%.)

SUGGESTED SEQUENCE OF MANAGEMENT DECISIONS (FIG. 29-22)

INITIAL PHASE OF STABILIZATION AND SUPPORT

1. Determine whether the patient with oxygenation impairment has ALI, and if so, determine whether it is complicated by such reversible comobidities as volume overload, pleural effusion, abdominal distension, or pneumothorax.
2. Initiate ventilation with face mask or intubate as severity warrants.
3. Decide on controlled versus spontaneous ventilation. Use controlled or nearly controlled ventilation to subdue respiratory efforts for the most severely involved patients during the early stage of support.
4. Initial ventilatory settings: $F_{I_{O_2}}$ 0.80, PEEP 5–8 cmH_2O (depending on concern regarding hemodynamic tolerance), and tidal volume 6–10 ml/kg (depending on inspiratory plateau pressure).
5. Estimate volemic status initially from arterial blood pressure, respiratory variations of pulmonary and

FIGURE 29-22 A suggested decision sequence for ventilation decisions in ARDS. (*Used, with permission, from Marini et al: Crit Care Med 32:250–5, 2004.*)

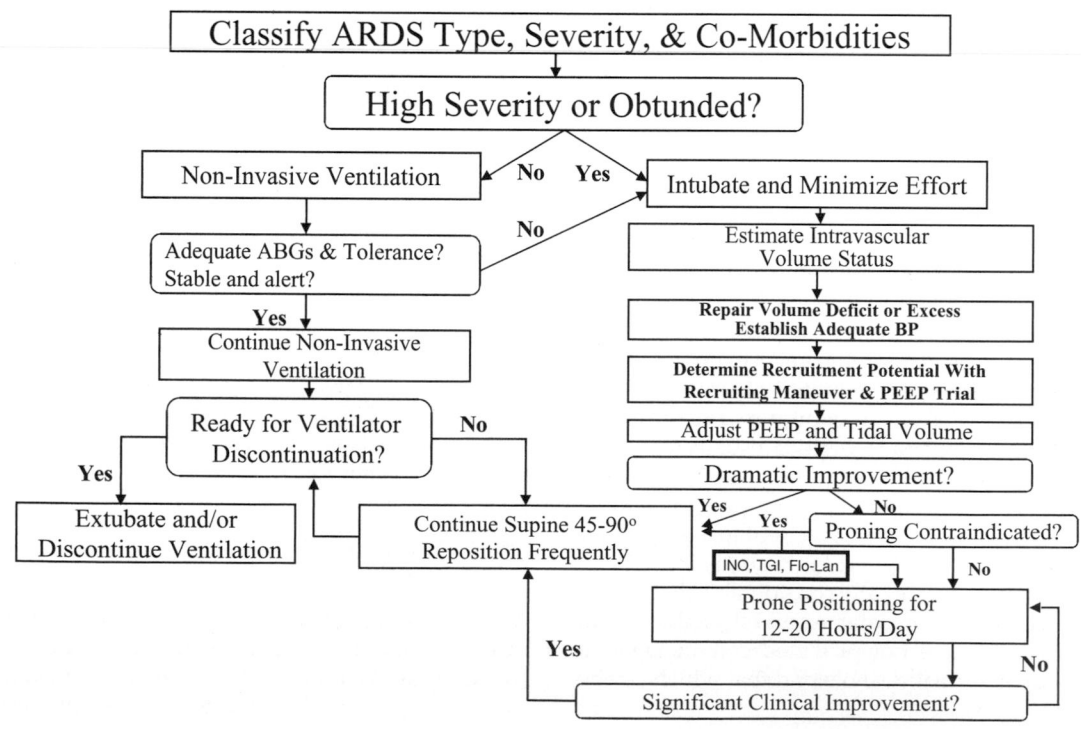

systemic arterial pulse pressures, central venous pressure, urinary output, and urinary electrolytes.

6. Confirm adequacy of intravascular volume using echocardiography, results from a volume challenge, and central venous and pulmonary artery catheter data (cardiac index, mixed-venous O_2 saturation, and occlusion pressure), if available.

7. Replete any volume deficits, and support the circulation with vasopressors and inotropes to the extent necessary to perform the ventilator manipulations safely.

8. Determine the recruitment potential of the patient by using a recruiting maneuver/PEEP trial.

9. Selected tidal volume should be inversely proportional to individual thoracic compliance and may range from 5–8 ml/kg of ideal body weight. During the PEEP trial, consider together the oxygenation change, the Pa_{CO_2} change, the alterations in mechanics, and the hemodynamic response. Adjust the PEEP and tidal volume combination to the lowest tolerated values that sustain the recruitment benefit.

10. Proning is advisable in patients with no contraindications and moderate to severe disease regardless of recruiting test unless they are already improving rapidly. If the patient does not respond to the prone position, another recruiting maneuver is attempted while the patient is prone. The PEEP and tidal volume combination is readjusted, as before.

11. When proning is used, scheduled reversion to the supine position is conducted at least once a day for cleanup, dressing changes, edema clearance, diagnostic procedures, transport to imaging, and so on. Many patients require almost continuous proning to maintain adequate gas exchange during the first several days of illness. Proning can be discontinued when it no longer makes an impressive difference to oxygenation, and plateau pressure can be kept in a "safe" range when the patient is supine.

SUBSEQUENT CARE

Recovery onset is recognized by improving Pa_{O_2}/FI_{O_2} and minute-ventilation-to-Pa_{CO_2} ratios, clearing radiographic opacity, and rising compliance of the total respiratory system. Appropriate adjustments then are made to sedation and ventilating pressures, and spontaneous breathing is encouraged by conversion to PSV or to pressure-controlled ventilation with lower driving pressures as tolerated. Proning is discontinued when the alterations in Pa_{O_2} observed during position changes are less than 10%, status is clearly improved, or no obvious benefit has been achieved after a lengthy trial (>48 hours). Reductions in FI_{O_2} to an acceptable range are undertaken before cutbacks in PEEP.

Weaning of PEEP is initiated when FI_{O_2} is 40% or less and Pa_{O_2} is 80 mmHg or greater.

Future Directions and Research

Numerous questions related to the practical application of mechanical ventilation remain incompletely answered. These include the following.

PATHOGENESIS AND DETECTION OF VILI

Experimental data suggest that numerous intersecting variables can influence the severity of VILI. For a given combination of PEEP and tidal volume, vascular pressure, breathing frequency, and body temperature appear to be important covariables in the expression of VILI. Although both mechanical and inflammatory disruptions of the air-blood interface are likely to be in some part responsible, how mechanical forces cause structural alterations and signal inflammation is not well elucidated. Markers for damaging patterns of ventilation are badly needed.

LONG-TERM DAMAGE TO AIRWAYS AND PARENCHYMA

The determinants of alveolar and small airway damage occurring in patients ventilated for ARDS are not clear—peak pressure, end-expiratory pressure, or both. Future outcome studies should target the incidence of obstructive, restrictive, and disordered gas exchange following recovery from ARDS.

RELATIONSHIP OF VILI TO MULTISYSTEM ORGAN DYSFUNCTION

Although laboratory studies have shown the release into the systemic circulation of gas, bacteria, and inflammatory mediators from injured lungs ventilated at high pressures with insufficient PEEP, the causative role of VILI in multiple-organ failure must be investigated further for the clinical setting.

VENTILATOR-ASSOCIATED PNEUMONIA

The incidence of ventilator-associated pneumonia is high in intubated patients, especially among those with ALI. Whether and how ventilator-related injury predisposes to pneumonia needs to be clarified and the measures necessary to reduce its incidence identified.

ENVIRONMENTAL MODIFICATIONS

Multiple factors have been shown in the laboratory to be important in the expression of VILI, including elevations in precapillary pressure, reduced left-atrial pressure, and elevated body temperature. Whether such factors play a role in the clinical setting is not clear. Do such cofactors as edema, FI_{O_2}, vasoactive and anti-inflammatory drugs, and plasma protein concentrations determine the severity of expression of VILI? Are there additive or synergistic interactions among these variables?

APPROPRIATE LEVELS OF PEEP AND TIDAL VOLUME

How to select the most lung-protective combination of PEEP and tidal volume remains an area of active controversy. Although considerable progress has been made, the debate needs to be settled regarding the relative importance of limiting peak inflation pressure, optimizing PEEP, reducing driving pressure, or limiting tidal volume. Should arterial oxygenation, thoracic mechanics, or bedside imaging (such as by electrical impedance tomography or acoustic mapping) be used to guide these selections?

RECRUITMENT MANEUVERS

Sustained inflation with high airway pressure is an effective means of opening collapsed tissue and may be integral to selecting PEEP. The value of repeated recruiting maneuvers and the best means of doing so, however, have not been studied carefully. The effectiveness of recruitment maneuvers may well vary with the type or stage of ALI. Moreover, the incidence of lung rupture, hemodynamic compromise, and other complications requires documentation. How should such maneuvers be performed? In which patients? How often, and at what F_{IO_2}? Whether sighs help to maintain recruitment in patients with low tidal volumes and unstable airways should be clarified.

PRONE POSITIONING

The duration of proning (e.g., how long each day and when to cease proning in each patient) remains unsettled. Most investigators favor proning for most of each day, at least until there are clear improvements in mechanics and gas exchange, allowing adequate arterial oxygenation with an F_{IO_2} of less than 0.50–0.60 at tolerated levels of PEEP in the supine position. Whether proning confers an advantage on key outcomes other than oxygenation and in which categories of patient are other questions that merit investigation.

NONINVASIVE VENTILATION

Noninvasive ventilation has been applied successfully to problems of acute respiratory failure, including some patients with ALI and ARDS.[88–90] Although vastly better than before, interfaces must be improved to ensure reliability and patient comfort. More information is needed to guide clinicians regarding optimal selection of patients, timing, equipment, and monitoring.

THERAPEUTIC VALUE OF HYPERCAPNIA AND TOLERANCE OF HYPOXEMIA

Laboratory data suggest that hypercapnic intracellular acidosis protects against some forms of oxidant injury.[130,131] Its therapeutic value for the clinical setting requires further investigation. Adaptation to hypoxemia occurs gradually in healthy individuals exposed to altitude and in many patients with chronically impaired O_2 exchange. Can patients who are acutely ill adapt to gradual imposition of hypoxemia? If so, how fast do they do so?

HIGH-FREQUENCY VENTILATION

The physiologic rationale for high-frequency ventilation in ARDS is strong. It is not yet clear, however, that it confers benefits beyond those achieved with conventional ventilator-based lung-protective strategies. Definitive comparisons of high-frequency ventilation versus lung-protective strategies using a conventional ventilator are needed to identify possible benefits and hazards, as well as to learn the best approach to using this technology in the clinical setting.

VALUE OF ADJUNCTIVE AND PHARMACOLOGIC MEASURES

Tested as isolated interventions, nitric oxide, partial-liquid ventilation, aerosolized surfactant, corticosteroids, almitrine, and prone positioning have not been demonstrated to influence mortality in multicentric trials.[130] The physiologic rationale for these measures, however, is strong for certain types of patients and for certain clinical conditions. Moreover, few of these adjuncts have been tested in combination. (Prone positioning, for example, adds to the oxygenation benefit of inhaled nitric oxide.) The utility of such measures—used alone and in combination—requires further study in populations most likely to benefit.

Summary and Conclusion

Injury to the alveolar-capillary membrane originates from diverse causes that initially may disrupt either the epithelial or endothelial surfaces. Managing the spectrum of conditions grouped together under the all-encompassing label of ARDS is a challenging assignment that must take into account the severity of illness as well as the interactions among the ventilatory and nonventilatory variables that influence the progress of this condition. Prevention of excessive tissue strain during the tidal cycle entails the avoidance of intolerable peak transalveolar pressures and repetitive opening and closing of unstable lung units, as well as attention to pathogenetic cofactors that may exacerbate injury or retard healing. Because of the diversity of mechanical problems presented by different patients, as well as the heterogeneity of mechanical properties among the lung units within the same individual, a logical approach requires mastery of key physiologic principles, awareness of the guidelines provided by well-conducted clinical trials, and integrated clinical judgment at the patient's bedside.

References

1. Ashbaugh DB, Bigelow DB, Petty TL. Acute respiratory distress in adults. Lancet 1967; 2:319–23.
2. Amato MBP, Barbas CSV, Medeiros DM, et al. Effect of a protective-ventilation strategy on mortality in the acute respiratory distress syndrome. New Engl J Med 1998; 338:347–54.
3. The ARDS network. Ventilation with lower tidal volumes as compared with traditional tidal volumes for acute lung injury and the acute respiratory distress syndrome. New Engl J Med 2000; 342:1301–8.
4. Artigas A, Bernard GR, Carlet J, et al and the Consensus Committee. The American-European Consensus Conference on ARDS, Part 2. Am J Respir Crit Care Med 1998; 157:1332–47.

5. Marini JJ, Gattinoni L. Ventilatory management of ARDS: A consensus of two. Crit Care Med 2004; 32:250–5.

6. Rouby JJ, Constantin JM, Roberto De A, et al. Mechanical ventilation in patients with acute respiratory distress syndrome. Anesthesiology 2004; 101:228–34.

7. Rubenfeld GD, Caldwell E, Granton J, et al. Interobserver variability in applying a radiographic definition for ARDS. Chest 1999; 116:1347–53.

8. Kallet RH. Katz JA. Respiratory system mechanics in acute respiratory distress syndrome. Respir Care Clin North Am 2003; 9:297–319.

9. Ranieri M, Brienza N, Santostasi S, et al. Impairment of lung and chest wall mechanics in patients with acute respiratory distress syndrome: Role of abdominal distension. Am J Respir Crit Care Med 1997; 156:1082–91

10. Gattinoni L, Pelosi P, Suter PM, et al. Acute respiratory distress syndrome caused by pulmonary and extrapulmonary disease different syndromes? Am J Respir Crit Care Med 1998; 158:3–11.

11. Rouby JJ, Puybasset L, Nieszkowska A, Lu Q. Acute respiratory distress syndrome: Lessons from computed tomography of the whole lung. Crit Care Med 2003; 31:S285–95.

12. Rahn H, Otis AB, Chadwick LE, Fenn WO. The pressure-volume diagram of the thorax and lung. Am J Physiol 1946; 146:161–78.

13. Griese M. Pulmonary surfactant in health and human lung diseases: State of the art. Eur Respir J 1999; 13:1455–76.

14. Crotti S, Mascheroni D, Caironi P, et al. Recruitment and derecruitment during acute respiratory failure: A clinical study. Am J Respir Crit Care Med 2001; 164131–40.

15. Hubmayr RD. Perspective on lung injury and recruitment: A skeptical look at the opening and collapse story. Am J Respir Crit Care Med 2002; 165:1647–53.

16. Halter JM, Steinberg JM, Schiller HJ, et al. Positive end-expiratory pressure after a recruitment maneuver prevents both alveolar collapse and recruitment/derecruitment. Am J Respir Crit Care Med 2003; 167:1620–6.

17. Lewis JF, Brackenbury A. Role of exogenous surfactant in acute lung injury. Crit Care Med 2003; 31:S324–8.

18. Matamis D, Lemaire F, Harf A, et al. Total respiratory pressure-volume curves in the adult respiratory distress syndrome. Chest 1984; 86:58–66.

19. Wolf GK, Arnold JH. Noninvasive assessment of lung volume: Respiratory inductance plethysmography and electrical impedance tomography. Crit Care Med 2005; 33:S163–9.

20. Victorino JA, Borges JB, Okamoto VN, et al. Imbalances in regional lung ventilation: A validation study on electrical impedance tomography. Am J Respir Crit Care Med 2004; 169:791–800.

21. Uhlig S. Ventilation-induced lung injury: Stretching it too far? Am J Physiol Lung Cell Mol Physiol 2002; 282:L892–6.

22. Pugin J. Molecular mechanisms of lung cell activation induced by cyclic stretch. Crit Care Med 2003; 31:S200–6.

23. Mead J, Takishima T, Leith D. Stress distribution in the lungs: A model of pulmonary elasticity J Appl Physiol 1970; 28: 596–608.

24. Richard JC, Maggiore SM, Johnson B, et al. Influence of tidal volume on alveolar recruitment: Respective role of PEEP and a recruitment maneuver. Am J Respir Crit Care Med 2001; 163:1609–13.

25. Duggan M, Kavanagh BP. Pulmonary atelectasis: A pathogenic perioperative entity. Anesthesiology 2005; 102:838–54.

26. Hickling KG. Recruitment greatly alters the pressure volume curve: A mathematical model of ARDS lungs. Am J Respir Crit Care Med 1998; 158:194–202.

27. Pelosi P, Goldner M, McKibben A, et al. Recruitment and derecruitment during acute respiratory failure: An experimental study. Am J Respir Crit Care Med 2001; 164:122–30.

28. Mutch WA, Harms S, Lefevre GR, et al. Biologically variable ventilation increases oxygenation over that seen with positive end-expiratory pressure alone in a porcine model of acute respiratory distress syndrome. Crit Care Med 2000; 28:2457–64.

29. Brigham KL, Staub NC. Pulmonary edema and acute lung injury research. Am J Respir Crit Care Med 1998; 157:S109–13.

30. Lamm WJ, Luchtel D, Albert RK. Sites of leakage in three models of acute lung injury. J Appl Physiol 1988; 64:1079–83.

31. Valenza F, Guglielmi M, Maffioletti M, et al. Prone position delays the progression of ventilator-induced lung injury in rats: Does lung strain distribution play a role? Crit Care Med 2005; 33:361–7.

32. Webb HH, Tierney DF. Experimental pulmonary edema due to intermittent positive pressure ventilation with high pressures. Am Rev Respir Dis 1974; 110:556.

33. Kolobow T, Moretti MP, Fumagalli R, et al. Severe impairment in lung function induced by high peak airway pressuring during mechanical ventilation: An experimental study. Am Rev Respir Dis 1987; 135:312–5.

34. McCulloch PR, Forkert PG, Froese AB. Lung volume maintenance prevents lung injury during high frequency oscillatory ventilation in surfactant-deficient rabbits. Am Rev Respir Dis 1988; 137:1185–92.

35. Dreyfuss D, Saumon G. Ventilator-induced lung injury: Lessons from experimental studies Am J Respir Crit Care Med 1998; 157:294–323.

36. Dos Santos CC, Slutsky AS. Invited review: Mechanisms of ventilator-induced lung injury: A perspective. J Appl Physiol 2000; 89:1645–55.

37. Vlahakis NE, Hubmayr RD. Invited review: Plasma membrane stress failure in alveolar epithelial cells. J Appl Physiol 2000; 89:2490–6.

38. Hotchkiss JR, Simonson DA, Marek DJ, et al. Pulmonary microvascular fracture in a patient with acute respiratory distress syndrome. Crit Care Med 2002; 30:2368–70.

39. Imai Y, Kawano T, Miyasaka K, et al. Inflammatory chemical mediators during conventional ventilation and during high frequency oscillatory ventilation. Am J Respir Crit Care Med 1994; 150: 1550–4.

40. Tremblay L, Valenza F, Ribeiro SP, et al. Injurious ventilatory strategies increase cytokines and c-fos m-RNA expression in an isolated rat lung model. J Clin Invest 1997; 99:944–52.

41. Ranieri VM, Suter P, Tortorella C, et al. Effect of mechanical ventilation on inflammatory mediators in patients with acute respiratory distress syndrome. JAMA 1999; 282:54–61.

42. Nahum A, Hoyt J, Schmitz L, et al. Effect of mechanical ventilation strategy on dissemination of intratracheally instilled *Escherichia coli* in dogs. Crit Care Med 1997; 25:1733–43.

43. Matthay MA, Bhattacharya S, Gaver D, et al. Ventilator-induced lung injury: In vivo and in vitro mechanisms. Am J Physiol Lung Cell Mol Physiol 2002; 283:L678–82.

44. Vlahakis NE, Hubmayr RD. Response of alveolar cells to mechanical stress. Curr Opin Crit Care 2003; 9:2–8.

45. Whitehead T, Slutsky AS. The pulmonary physician in critical care: 7. Ventilator-induced lung injury. Thorax 2002; 57:635–42.

46. Gattinoni L, Pelosi P, Crotti S, Valenza F. Effects of positive end-expiratory pressure on regional distribution of tidal volume and recruitment in adult respiratory distress syndrome. Am J Respir Crit Care Med 1995; 151:1807–14.

47. Lai-Fook SJ, Rodarte JR. Pleural pressure distribution and its relationship to lung volume and interstitial pressure. J Appl Physiol 1991; 70:967–78.

48. Gattinoni L, Pesenti A, Avalli L, et al. Pressure-volume curve of total respiratory system in acute respiratory failure: Computed tomographic scan study. Am Rev Respir Dis 1987; 136: 730–6.

49. Albert RK, Hubmayr RD. The prone position eliminates compression of the lungs by the heart. Am J Respir Crit Care Med 2000; 161:1660–5.

50. Lamm WJ, Graham MM, Albert RK. Mechanism by which the prone position improves oxygenation in acute lung injury. Am J Respir Crit Care Med 1994; 150:184–93.

51. Lachmann B. Open up the lung and keep the lung open. Intensive Care Med 1992; 18:319–21.

52. Broccard AF, Shapiro RS, Schmitz LL, et al. Influence of prone position on the extent and distribution of lung injury in a high tidal volume oleic acid injury model of acute respiratory distress syndrome. Crit Care Med 1997; 25:16–27.

53. Broccard AF, Shapiro RS, Schmitz LL, et al. Prone positioning attenuates and redistributes ventilator-induced lung injury in dogs. Crit Care Med 2000; 28:295–303.

54. Hotchkiss JR, Blanch LL, Naviera A, et al. Relative roles of vascular and airspace pressures in ventilator induced lung injury. Crit Care Med 2001; 29:1593–8.

55. Broccard A, Vannay C, Feihl F, Schaller MD. Impact of low pulmonary vascular pressure on ventilator-induced lung injury. Crit Care Med 2002; 30:2183–90.

56. Hotchkiss JR, Blanch LL, Murias G, et al. Effects of decreased respiratory frequency on ventilator induced lung injury Am J Respir Crit Care Med 2000; 161:463–8.

57. Foti G, Cereda M, Sparacino ME, et al. Effects of periodic lung recruitment maneuvers on gas exchange and respiratory mechanics in mechanically ventilated acute respiratory distress syndrome (ARDS) patients. Intensive Care Med 2000; 26:501–7.

58. Dreyfuss D, Soler P, Saumon G. Spontaneous resolution of pulmonary edema caused by short periods of cyclic overinflation. J Appl Physiol 1992; 72:2081–9.

59. Gajic O, Lee J, Doerr CH, et al. Ventilator-induced cell wounding and repair in the intact lung. Am J Respir Crit Care Med 2003; 167:1057–63.

60. Dreyfuss D, Soler P, Basset G, Saumon G. High inflation pressure pulmonary edema: Respective effects of high airway pressure, high tidal volume, and positive end-expiratory pressure. Am Rev Respir Dis 1988; 137:1159–64.

61. Muscedere JG, Mullen JB, Gan K, Slutsky AS. Tidal ventilation at low airway pressures can augment lung injury. Am J Respir Crit Care Med 1994; 149:1327–34.

62. Simonson DA, Adams AB, Wright LA, et al. Effects of ventilatory pattern on experimental lung injury caused by high airway pressure. Crit Care Med 2004; 32:781–6.

63. Sinclair SE, Altemeier WA, Matute-Bello G, Chi EY. Augmented lung injury due to interaction between hyperoxia and mechanical ventilation. Crit Care Med 2004; 32:2496–501.

64. Dreyfuss D, Soler P, Saumon G. Mechanical ventilation–induced pulmonary edema: Interaction with previous lung alterations. Am J Respir Crit Care Med 1995; 151:1568–75.

65. Brower RG, Matthay M, Schoenfeld D. Meta-analysis of acute lung injury and acute respiratory distress syndrome trials. Am J Respir Crit Care Med 2002; 166:1515–7.

66. Ferguson ND, Frutos-Vivar F, Esteban A, et al. Mechanical Ventilation International Study Group. Airway pressures, tidal volumes, and mortality in patients with acute respiratory distress syndrome. Crit Care Med 2005; 33:21–30.

67. Pinsky MR. The effects of mechanical ventilation on the cardiovascular system. Crit Care Clin 1990; 6:663–78.

68. Coggeshall JW, Marini JJ, Newman JH. Improved oxygenation after muscle relaxation in the adult respiratory distress syndrome. Arch Intern Med 1985; 145:1718–20.

69. Pelosi P, Tubiolo D, Mascheroni D, et al. Effects of the prone position on respiratory mechanics and gas-exchange during acute lung injury. Am J Respir Crit Care Med 1998; 157:387–93.

70. Gaver DP, Samsel RW, Solway J. Effects of surface tension and viscosity on airway reopening. J Appl Physiol 1990; 69: 74–85.

71. Takeuchi M, Goddon S, Dolhnikoff M, et al. Set positive end-expiratory pressure during protective ventilation affects lung injury. Anesthesiology 2002; 97:682–92.

72. Fujino Y, Goddon S, Dolhnikoff M, et al. Repetitive high-pressure recruitment maneuvers required to maximally recruit lung in a sheep model of acute respiratory distress syndrome. Crit Care Med 2001; 29:1579–86.

73. Rimensberger PC, Pristine G, Brendan J, et al. Lung recruitment during small tidal volume ventilation allows minimal positive end-expiratory pressure without augmenting lung injury. Crit Care Med 1999; 27:1940–5.

74. Van der Kloot TE, Blanch L, Youngblood AM, et al. Recruitment maneuvers in three experimental models of acute lung injury. Am J Respir Crit Care Med 2000; 161:1485–94.

75. Lim S-C, Adams AB, Simonson DA, et al. Intercomparison of recruitment maneuvers in three models of acute lung injury. Crit Care Med 2004; 32:2371–7.

76. Lim CM, Jung H, Koh Y, et al. Effect of alveolar recruitment maneuver in early acute respiratory distress syndrome according to antiderecruitment strategy, etiological category of diffuse lung injury, and body position of the patient. Crit Care Med 2003; 31:411–8.

77. Lim S-C, Alexander B, Simonson DA, et al. Transient hemodynamic effects of recruitment maneuvers in three experimental models of acute lung injury. Crit Care Med 2004; 32: 2378–84.

78. Puybasset L, Gusman P, Muller JC, et al. Regional distribution of gas and tissue in acute respiratory distress syndrome: III. Consequences for the effects of positive end-expiratory pressure. Intensive Care Med 2000; 26:1215–27.

79. Putensen C, Mutz N, Putensen-Himmer G, Zinserling J. Spontaneous breathing during ventilatory support improves ventilation-perfusion distributions in patients with acute respiratory distress syndrome. Am J Respir Crit Care Med 1999; 159:1241–8.

80. Barber RE, Lee J, Hamilton WK. Oxygen toxicity in man. New Engl J Med 1970; 283:1478–84.

81. Scoggin CH, Sahn SA, Petty TL. Status asthmaticus: A nine-year experience. JAMA 1977; 238:1158–62.

82. Johnson TH, Altman AR, McCaffree RD. Radiologic considerations in the adult respiratory distress syndrome treated with positive end expiratory pressure (PEEP). Clin Chest Med 1982; 3:89–100.

83. Pepe PE, Marini JJ. Occult positive end-expiratory pressure in mechanically ventilated patients with airflow obstruction (the auto-PEEP effect). Am Rev Respir Dis 1982; 126:166–70.

84. Kimball WR, Leith DE, Robins AG. Dynamic hyperinflation and ventilator dependence in chronic obstructive pulmonary disease. Am Rev Respir Dis 1982; 126:991–5.

85. Darioli R, Perret C. Mechanical controlled hypoventilation in status asthmaticus. Am Rev Respir Dis 1984; 129:385–7.

86. Hickling KG, Henderson SJ, Jackson R. Low mortality associated with low volume pressure limited ventilation with permissive hypercapnia in severe adult respiratory distress syndrome. Intensive Care Med 1990; 16:372–7.

87. Laffey JG, Engelberts D, Kavanagh BP. Buffering hypercapnic acidosis worsens acute lung injury. Am J Respir Crit Care Med 2000; 161:141–6.

88. Antonelli M, Conti G, Rocco M, et al. A comparison of noninvasive positive-pressure ventilation and conventional mechanical ventilation in patients with acute respiratory failure. New Engl J Med 1998; 339:429–35.

89. Hilbert G, Gruson D, Vargas F, et al. Noninvasive ventilation in immunosuppressed patients with pulmonary infiltrates, fever, and acute respiratory failure. New Engl J Med 2001; 344:481–7.

90. Girou E, Schortgen F, Delclaux C, et al. Association of noninvasive ventilation with nosocomial infections and survival in critically ill patients. JAMA 2000; 284:2361–7.

91. Chandra A, Coggeshall JW, Ravenscraft SA, Marini JJ. Hyperpnea limits the volume recruited by positive end-expiratory pressure. Am Rev Respir Dis 1994; 150:911–7.

92. Otis AB. The work of breathing. Physiol Rev 1954; 34:449–61.

93. Marini JJ. Inverse ratio ventilation: Simply an alternative or something more? Crit Care Med 1995; 23:224–8.

94. Marcy TW, Marini JJ. Inverse ratio ventilation in ARDS: Rationale and implementation. Chest 1991; 100:494–504.

95. Downes JJ. CPAP and PEEP: A perspective. Anesthesiology 1976; 44:1–5.

96. Hormann C, Baum M, Putensen C, et al. Biphasic positive airway pressure (BIPAP): A new mode of ventilatory support. Eur J Anaesthesiol 1994; 11:37–42.

97. Stock MC, Downs JB, Frolicher DA. Airway pressure release ventilation. Crit Care Med 1987; 15:462–6.

98. Habashi NM. Other approaches to open-lung ventilation: Airway pressure release ventilation. Crit Care Med 2005; 33:S228–40.

99. Salim A, Martin M. High-frequency percussive ventilation. Crit Care Med 2005; 33:S241–5.

100. Froese AB, Kinsella JP. High-frequency oscillatory ventilation: Lessons from the neonatal/pediatric experience. Crit Care Med 2005; 33:S115–21.

101. Fort P, Farmer C, Westerman J, et al. High-frequency oscillatory ventilation for adult respiratory distress syndrome: A pilot study. Crit Care Med 1997; 25:937–94.

102. Derdak S, Mehta S, Stewart TE, et al and the Multicenter Oscillatory Ventilation for Acute Respiratory Distress Syndrome Trial (MOAT) study investigators. High frequency oscillatory ventilation for acute respiratory distress syndrome in adults: A randomized clinical trial. Am J Respir Crit Care Med 2002; 166:801–8.

103. Chan KP, Stewart TE. Clinical use of high-frequency oscillatory ventilation in adult patients with acute respiratory distress syndrome. Crit Care Med 2005; 33:S170–4.

104. Ichinose F, Roberts JD Jr, Zapol WM. Inhaled nitric oxide: A selective pulmonary vasodilator. Current uses and therapeutic potential. Circulation 2004; 109:3106–11.

105. Koh Y, Hurford WE. Inhaled nitric oxide in acute respiratory distress syndrome: From bench to bedside. Int Anesthesiol Clin 2003; 41:91–102.

106. Gallart L, Lu Q, Puybasset L, et al. Intravenous almitrine combined with inhaled nitric oxide for acute respiratory distress syndrome. Am J Respir Crit Care Med 1998; 158:1770–7.

107. Zwissler B, Kemming G, Habler O, et al. Inhaled prostacyclin (PGI2) versus inhaled nitric oxide in adult respiratory distress syndrome. Am J Respir Crit Care Med 1996; 154:1671–7.

108. Kalfon P, Rao GS, Gallart L, et al. Permissive hypercapnia with and without expiratory washout in patients with severe acute respiratory distress syndrome. Anesthesiology 1997; 87:6–17.

109. Marini JJ. Tracheal gas insufflation: A useful adjunct to ventilation? (editorial). Thorax 1994; 49:735–7.

110. Richecoeur J, Lu Q, Vieira SR, et al. Expiratory washout versus optimization of mechanical ventilation during permissive hypercapnia in patients with severe acute respiratory distress syndrome. Am J Respir Crit Care Med 1999; 160:77–85.

111. Marini JJ. Are recruiting maneuvers needed when ventilating acute respiratory distress syndrome? (editorial). Crit Care Med 2003; 31:2701–2.

112. Brochard L, Roudot-Thoraval F, Roupie E, et al. Tidal volume reduction for prevention of ventilator-induced lung injury in acute respiratory distress syndrome: The multicenter trial group on tidal volume reduction in ARDS. Am J Respir Crit Care Med 1998; 158:1831–8.

113. Stewart TE, Meade MO, Cook DJ, et al. Evaluation of a ventilation strategy to prevent barotrauma in patients at high risk for acute respiratory distress syndrome. New Engl J Med 1998; 338:355–61.

114. Brower RG, Shanholtz CB, Fessler HE, et al. Prospective, randomized, controlled clinical trial comparing traditional versus reduced tidal volume ventilation in acute respiratory distress syndrome. Crit Care Med 1999; 27:1492–8.

115. Villar J, Kacmarek RM, Perez-Mendez L, Aguirre-Jaime and the ARIES Network. A high PEEP-low tidal volume ventilatory strategy improves outcome in persistent ARDS. Crit Care Med 2006 (in press)

116. Eichacker PQ, Gerstenberger, Banks SM, et al. Meta-analysis of acute lung injury and acute respiratory distress syndrome trials with low tidal volumes. Am J Respir Crit Care Med 2002; 166:1510–4.

117. Deans KJ, Minneci PC, Cui X, et al. Mechanical ventilation in ARDS: One size does not fit all. Crit Care Med 2005; 33:1141–3.

118. Broccard AF, Hotchkiss JR, Vannay C, et al. Protective effects of hypercapnic acidosis on ventilator-induced lung injury. Am J Resp Crit Care Med 2001; 164:802–6.

119. Feihl F, Perret C. Permissive hypercapnia: How permissive should we be? Am J Respir Critical Care Med 1994; 150:1722–37.

120. Sinclair SE, Kregenow DA, Lamm WJ, et al. Hypercapnic acidosis is protective in an in vivo model of ventilator-induced lung injury. Am J Respir Crit Care Med 2002; 166:403–8.

121. Brower RG, Lanken PN, MacIntyre N, et al. National Heart, Lung, and Blood Institute ARDS Clinical Trials Network. Higher versus lower positive end-expiratory pressures in patients with the acute respiratory distress syndrome. New Engl J Med 2004; 351:327–36.

122. Brower RG, Morris A, MacIntyre N, et al. ARDS Clinical Trials Network, National Heart, Lung, and Blood Institute, National Institutes of Health. Effects of recruitment maneuvers in patients with acute lung injury and acute respiratory distress syndrome ventilated with high positive end-expiratory pressure. Crit Care Med 2003; 31:2592–7.

123. Chatte G, Sab JM, Dubois JM, et al. Prone position in mechanically ventilated patients with severe acute respiratory failure. Am J R Crit Care Med 1997; 155:473–8.

124. Gainnier M, Michelet P, Thirion X, et al. Prone position and positive end-expiratory pressure in acute respiratory distress syndrome. Crit Care Med 2003; 31:2719–26.

125. Valenza F, Guglielmi M, Maffioletti M, et al. Prone position delays the progression of ventilator-induced lung injury in rats: Does lung strain distribution play a role? Crit Care Med 2005; 33:361–7.

126. Gattinoni L, Tognoni G, Pesenti A, et al. Effect of prone positioning on the survival of patients with acute respiratory failure. New Engl J Med 2001; 345:568–73.

127. Guerin C, Gaillard S, Lemasson S, et al. Effects of systematic prone positioning in hypoxemic acute respiratory failure: A randomized, controlled trial. JAMA. 2004; 292:2379–87.

128. Mancebo J, Rialp G, Fernández R, et al. Prone vs supine position in ARDS patients: Results of a randomized multicenter trial (abstract). Am J Respir Crit Care Med 2003; 168:167.

129. Gattinoni L, Vagginelli F, Carlesso E, et al. Prone-Supine Study Group. Decrease in Paco₂ with prone position is predictive of improved outcome in acute respiratory distress syndrome. Crit Care Med 2003; 31:2727–33.

130. McIntyre RC Jr, Pulido EJ, Bensard DD, et al. Thirty years of clinical trials in acute respiratory distress syndrome. Crit Care Med 2000; 28:3314–31.

131. Taylor RW, Zimmerman JL, Dellinger RP, et al. Inhaled nitric oxide in ARDS Study Group: Low-dose inhaled nitric oxide in patients with acute lung injury: A randomized, controlled trial. JAMA 2004; 291:1603–9.

132. Dellinger RP, Zimmerman JL, Taylor RW, et al. Effects of inhaled nitric oxide in patients with acute respiratory distress syndrome: Results of a randomized phase II trial. Inhaled Nitric Oxide in ARDS Study Group. Crit Care Med 1998; 26:15–23.

133. Anzueto A, Baughman RP, Guntupalli KK, et al. Aerosolized surfactant in adults with sepsis-induced acute respiratory distress syndrome. Exosurf Acute Respiratory Distress Syndrome Sepsis Study Group. New Engl J Med 1996; 334:1417–21.

134. Bernard GR. Luce JM, Sprung CL, et al. High-dose corticosteroids in patients with the adult respiratory distress syndrome. New Engl J Med 1987; 317:1565–70.

135. Michard F, Chemla D, Richard C, et al. Clinical use of respiratory changes in arterial pulse pressure to monitor the hemodynamic effects of PEEP. Am J Respir Crit Care Med 1999; 159:935–9.

136. Rivers EP, Ander DS, Powell D. Central venous oxygen saturation monitoring in the critically ill patient. Curr Opin Crit Care 2001; 7:204–11.

137. Froese AB, Kinsella JP. High-frequency oscillatory ventilation: Lessons from the neonatal/pediatric experience. Crit Care Med 2005; 33:S115–21.

138. Putensen C, Hering R, Wrigge H. Controlled versus assisted mechanical ventilation. Curr Opin Crit Care 2002; 8:51–7.

139. Grasso S, Mascia L, Del Turco M, et al. Effects of recruiting maneuvers in patients with acute respiratory distress syndrome ventilated with protective ventilatory strategy. Anesthesiology 2002; 96:795–802.

140. Pelosi P, Cadringher P, Bottino N, et al. Sigh in acute respiratory distress syndrome. Am J Respir Crit Care Med 1999; 159: 872–80.

141. Patroniti N, Foti G, Cortinovis B, et al. Sigh improves gas exchange and lung volume in patients with acute respiratory distress syndrome undergoing pressure support ventilation. Anesthesiology 2002; 96:788–94.

142. Lichtenstein D, Goldstein I, Mourgeon E, et al. Comparative diagnostic performances of auscultation, chest radiography, and lung ultrasonography in acute respiratory distress syndrome. Anesthesiology 2004; 100:9–15.

143. Panigada M, Berra L, Greco G, et al. Bacterial colonization of the respiratory tract following tracheal intubation: Effect of gravity. An experimental study. Crit Care Med 2003; 31: 729–37.

Chapter 30 _____

MECHANICAL VENTILATION FOR SEVERE ASTHMA

JAMES W. LEATHERMAN

LIFE-THREATENING ASTHMA
VENTILATOR MANAGEMENT
    Pulmonary Hyperinflation: Mechanism and
       Assessment
    Ventilator Settings
    Gas Exchange: hypercapnia
NONVENTILATOR MANAGEMENT
    Standard Therapy
    Alternative Therapies
DEATH AND COMPLICATIONS
    Mortality
    Complications
POSTHOSPITALIZATION PROGNOSIS

It is estimated that 6000–10,000 patients require mechanical ventilation for acute asthma in the United States each year.[1] Although often lifesaving, mechanical ventilation for severe asthma is associated with many complications and a fatal outcome in some patients. An understanding of salient principles regarding ventilator support of patients with severe asthma may reduce the risk of an adverse outcome.[2]

Life-Threatening Asthma

Asthma attacks that lead to mechanical ventilation may have a gradual onset over one or more days or occur suddenly over minutes to hours (Table 30-1). Onset is gradual in 80% of patients, with viral infections being the most common identifiable trigger.[3] Slow-onset status asthmaticus is characterized by extensive mucus plugging with eosinophilic infiltration and edema, a limited immediate response to bronchodilators, and slow resolution over days.[4] The remaining 20% of patients have rapid-onset attacks that often are triggered by aeroallergens, nonsteroidal antiinflammatory agents, or airway irritants.[3,5] These "sudden asphyxial" attacks are caused by profound bronchospasm with minimal mucus plugging, explaining the often rapid resolution.[4]

Regardless of the mode of onset, life-threatening asthma is associated with a markedly increased airway resistance, pulmonary hyperinflation, and high physiologic dead space, which together lead to hypercapnia and risk of respiratory arrest.[6] Hypercapnia per se, however, is not an indication for intubation because most episodes respond to bronchodilator therapy.[7] In addition, some hypercapnic patients may avoid intubation through use of noninvasive ventilation[8–10] (Fig. 30-1). Inhalation of a helium-oxygen gas mixture (heliox) also may reduce work of breathing and decrease the likelihood of intubation.[11,12]

The decision to intubate a patient with status asthmaticus is made primarily on clinical grounds. Indications for intubation include respiratory arrest, a depressed level of consciousness, marked agitation and inability to cooperate with therapy, and progressive fatigue and exhaustion. Endotracheal intubation may be performed by either the oral or nasal route. One advantage of oral intubation is that it allows insertion of a larger endotracheal tube that facilitates suctioning and offers less airways resistance.[2,13] A rapid-sequence technique is advocated by some experts, and fiberoptic guidance also has been used.[13] Regardless of the technique used, intubation should be performed by the most skilled operator present. Repeated airway manipulation and failed intubation in patients with fulminant asthma may prove catastrophic.

Various drugs have been used to facilitate intubation of patients with severe asthma. One approach uses ketamine, an anesthetic that does not cause respiratory depression or hypotension, in conjunction with a benzodiapine to prevent emergence hallucinations.[13] Ketamine, however, may increase laryngeal reflexes and predispose to laryngospasm with excessive upper airway manipulation.[14] Propofol, a potent and fast-acting sedative, decreases airways resistance after intubation as compared with etomidate or thiopental.[15] Propofol, however, may cause hypotension, and etomidate may be a better alternative in hemodynamically unstable patients.[14] Although succinylcholine can cause histamine release, this is likely of little clinical significance, and this depolarizing paralytic agent is appropriate for rapid-sequence intubation of patients with severe asthma.[14] Many of the sedative drugs used to facilitate intubation reduce vascular tone and, in conjunction with decreased venous return secondary to marked pulmonary hyperinflation, may contribute to hemodynamic instability at the time of intubation.[16] Postintubation hypotension should be anticipated and managed by rapid fluid administration and manual ventilation via an Ambu bag at a slow rate to limit the severity of hyperinflation.[17]

Ventilator Management

Traditional goals of mechanical ventilation for patients with acute respiratory failure are to provide adequate oxygenation with nontoxic levels of inspired oxygen and sufficient minute ventilation to achieve a normal arterial carbon dioxide tension (Pa_{CO_2}) and arterial pH. In status asthmaticus, however, attempts to correct respiratory acidosis by increasing minute ventilation may lead to extreme pulmonary hyperinflation, with the attendant risks of tension pneumothorax and hemodynamic collapse.[18] For this reason, controlled hypoventilation with permissive hypercapnia was first proposed 20 years ago and subsequently gained widespread acceptance.[19]

TABLE 30-1 Patterns of Near-Fatal Asthma

	Slow-Onset	Rapid-Onset
Time course (onset)	One or more days	Minutes to hours
Triggers	Virus, unknown	Aeroallergen, NSAID, airway irritant, emotional stress, unknown
Frequency	∼ 80%	∼ 20%
Mechanisms of airflow obstruction	Mucous plugging and airway edema > bronchospam	Bronchospasm ("dry airways")
Airway inflammation	Eosinophils	Neutrophils
Response to treatment	Slow: minimal response to initial bronchodilators	Rapid: good response to initial bronchodilators
Prevention	Steroids early in exacerbation	Avoid triggers
Duration intubation	Often several days	Often < 24 hours

ABBREVIATION: NSAID, nonsteroid anti-inflammatory drug.

In brief, the rationale for this approach is that hypercapnia poses less risk than does markedly increased lung volume.[20,21] Although there have been no prospective, randomized studies of controlled hypoventilation in asthma, a retrospective analysis suggested that it is associated with better outcomes than a conventional ventilator strategy.[20] To apply controlled hypoventilation rationally, it is essential to understand methods for monitoring the severity of pulmonary hyperinflation and how the latter is influenced by the choice of ventilator settings.[22–24] Although anecdotal experience with pressure-control or pressure-support ventilation has been reported, there may be some theoretical advantages to use of a volume-cycled mode (assist-control or synchronized intermittent mandatory ventilation),[2] and the great preponderance of clinical experience has been with the latter approach.[2,9,22–29] Subsequent discussion of ventilator techniques and monitoring will be limited to use of volume-cycled ventilation.

PULMONARY HYPERINFLATION: MECHANISM AND ASSESSMENT

Spontaneously breathing patients with severe asthma undergo tidal ventilation near their total lung capacity; with mechanical ventilation, lung volumes may increase further[2] (Fig. 30-2). During mechanical ventilation, dynamic hyperinflation is initiated when there is insufficient time during expiration for complete exhalation of delivered tidal volume, resulting in an increase in end-expiratory lung volume and positive end-expiratory alveolar pressure (auto-PEEP). With subsequent breaths, a progressive increase in lung volume leads to an improvement in expiratory gas flow because of higher elastic recoil pressure and an increase in airways diameter, permitting the entire tidal volume to be exhaled (Fig. 30-3). Therefore, dynamic hyperinflation may be viewed as an adaptive process that enhances expiratory flow in the setting of airways obstruction but one that also exposes the patient to increased risk of complications related to alveolar overdistension.

The severity of hyperinflation in severe asthma varies among patients and within individual patients over time. Serial monitoring of dynamic hyperinflation is important to identify those patients with marked hyperinflation who may be at increased risk of complications and to assess the response to treatment and the evolution of airflow obstruction.

Two principal methods of monitoring the severity of airflow obstruction in status asthmaticus have been used: measurement of total exhaled volume during a prolonged apnea beginning at end inspiration and assessment of airway

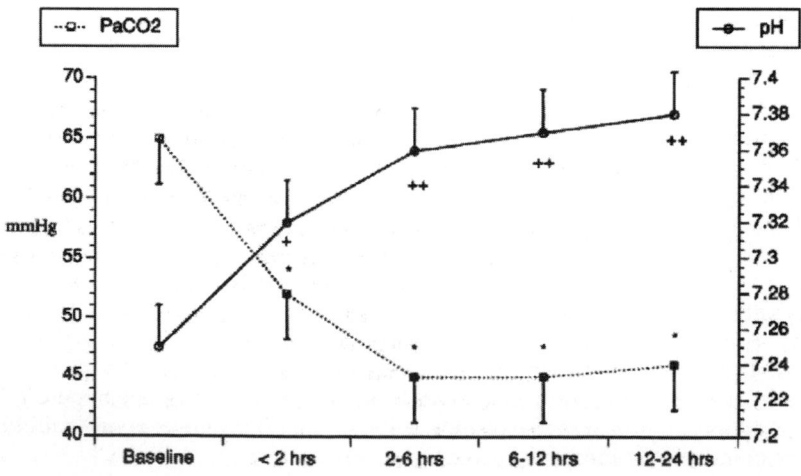

FIGURE 30-1 Change in Pa$_{CO_2}$ and pH associated with the use of noninvasive positive-pressure ventilation by face mask in patients with severe asthma. (*Used, with permission, from Meduri et al: Chest 110:767–74, 1996.*)

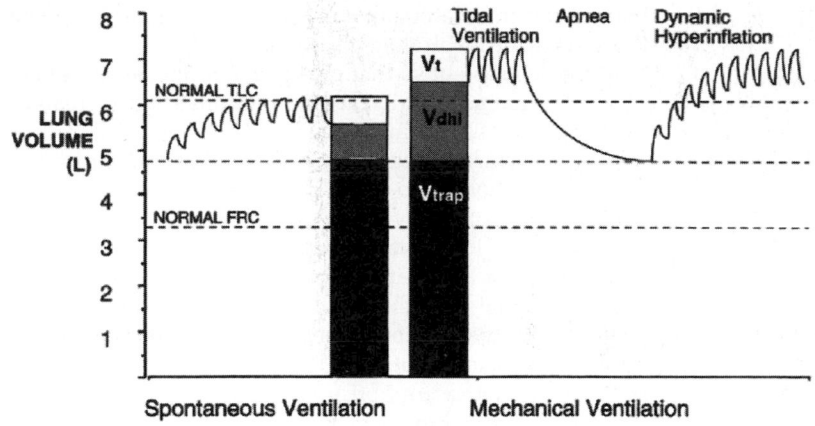

FIGURE 30-2 Lung volumes in severe asthma during spontaneous ventilation and with mechanical ventilation. Tidal breathing occurs near total lung capacity (TLC) during spontaneous ventilation and above TLC during mechanical ventilation. After delivery of tidal volume (V_T) during mechanical ventilation, a prolonged apnea permits exhalation of volume produced by dynamic hyperinflation (V_{DHI}); lung volume at the end of apnea, however, remains well above normal functional residual capacity (FRC) because of gas trapped behind occluded airways (Vtrap) (*Adapted, with permission, from Tuxen et al.*[2])

pressures during volume-cycled ventilation. Tuxen et al[18,22,23] have used a prolonged apnea to assess dynamic hyperinflation in patients with severe asthma. With this method, the total amount of gas exhaled during an apnea represents the volume (above functional residual capacity) at end inspiration (V_{EI}). The volume at end expiration (V_{EE}) is calculated by subtracting tidal volume from the V_{EI} and represents the increase in lung volume caused by dynamic hyperinflation (Figs. 30-3 and 30-4). In one study, V_{EI} predicted the development of hypotension and barotrauma better than did airway pressures.[18] Measurement of V_{EI} and V_{EE}, however, has not gained widespread clinical acceptance for serial monitoring of dynamic hyperinflation in part because of the need for paralysis.[2]

A more common method of monitoring patients with severe asthma is assessment of airway pressures (Fig. 30-5). As described initially,[19] controlled hypoventilation in status asthmaticus limited peak airway pressure to less than 50 cmH$_2$O, a target used by others subsequently.[25] Such a strategy, however, may be problematic in patients with asthma because peak pressure is highly dependent on inspiratory flow-resistive properties and therefore does not reliably reflect the degree of hyperinflation.[2] Indeed, the combination of markedly increased airways resistance and

use of a high inspiratory flow rate commonly results in a peak pressure above 50 cmH$_2$O but without increased risk of barotrauma.[26] In addition, a recent study found that peak pressure may not reflect the reduction in dynamic hyperinflation that follows prolongation of expiratory time, presumably because of an increase in airways resistance as lung volume decreases[24] (Fig. 30-6).

Unlike peak pressure, plateau airway pressure (Pplat) is not affected by inspiratory flow-resistive properties and may be a better parameter for monitoring lung hyperinflation in status asthmaticus.[2,26–30] Because patients with severe airflow obstruction typically have near-normal respiratory system compliance, an increase in Pplat is usually a result of dynamic hyperinflation. At constant tidal volume, changes in the degree of dynamic hyperinflation in response to bronchodilators or manipulation of expiratory time can be inferred from changes in Pplat.[24] Because Pplat represents end-inspiratory elastic recoil pressure and provides an estimate of average peak alveolar pressure, it also might (in theory) help to predict risk of alveolar rupture. Although the threshold Pplat that predicts increased risk of barotrauma is not well defined in status asthmaticus, an acceptable upper limit of 25–30 cmH$_2$O has been suggested most often[2,26,27,29,30] (Table 30-2).

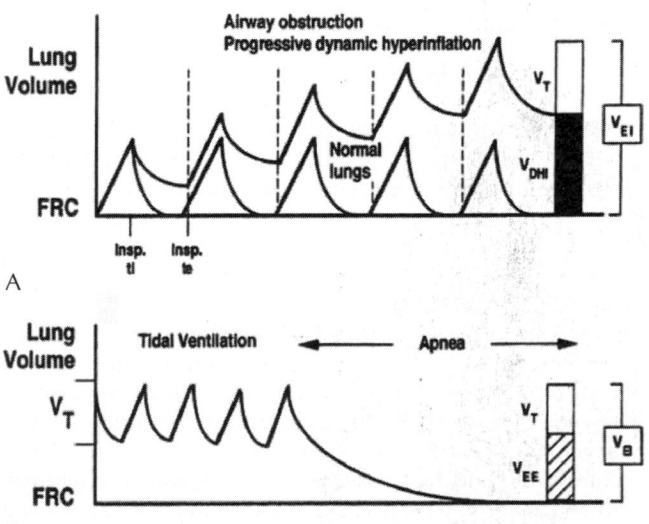

FIGURE 30-3 *A.* Dynamic hyperinflation. FRC, functional residual capacity; V_T, tidal volume; V_{EI}, volume (above FRC) at end inspiration; V_{DHI}, volume (above FRC) caused by dynamic hyperinflation. (*Used, with permission, from Tuxen: Am J Respir Crit Care Med 150:1722–37, 1994.*) *B.* Measurement of V_{EI} and V_{EE} (volume above FRC at end expiration) by use of a prolonged apnea. V_{EE} and V_{DHI} are equivalent. (*Used, with permission, from Tuxen et al: Am Rev Respir Dis 136:872–9, 1987.*)

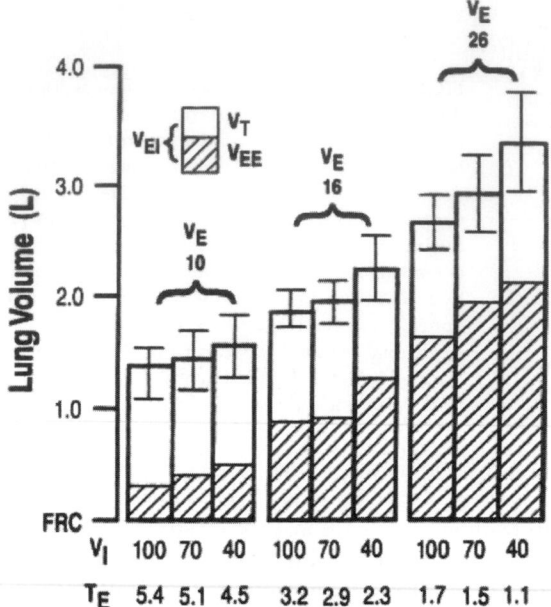

FIGURE 30-4 Effect of minute ventilation ($\dot{V}_E$) and inspiratory flow rate (V_I) on dynamic hyperinflation during mechanical ventilation for severe asthma. V_{EI}, volume at end inspiration; V_{EE}, volume at end expiration. V_T, tidal volume. (*Used, with permission, from Tuxen et al: Am Rev Respir Dis 136:872–9, 1987.*)

The end-inspiratory airway occlusion used to measure Pplat results in an initially rapid fall in airway pressure, followed by a slower decline until a final, stable pressure is reached (see Fig. 30-5). The initial drop in pressure is a function of inspiratory flow and inspiratory airway resistance, whereas intrapulmonary gas redistribution (pendeluft) and stress relaxation are responsible for the subsequent fall in pressure. The marked time-constant heterogeneity of status athmaticus requires several seconds for a stable pressure to be reached. A shorter (0.4–0.5 second) inspiratory pause often has been used to measure Pplat.[2] Although the latter overestimates *average* end-inspiratory alveolar pressure, it may reflect more closely those lung units with the

highest end-inspiratory alveolar pressure. Regardless of the duration of the inspiratory pause that is selected, it is important to be consistent so that changes in Pplat caused solely by varying pause duration are not misconstrued as changes in the degree of hyperinflation.

When measured by the "static" method of end-expiratory airway occlusion, auto-PEEP provides an estimate of the average end-expiratory alveolar pressure. Although there is relatively little published data regarding levels of auto-PEEP in status asthmaticus, one study found an average value of 15 cmH$_2$O on the first day of mechanical ventilation when minute ventilation approximated 10 liters/min.[24] In general, changes in auto-PEEP track closely with changes in Pplat, and either (or both) may be helpful for following the degree of dynamic hyperinflation. There are, however, certain caveats regarding the measurement of auto-PEEP that must be considered.

First, the duration of the end-expiratory pause influences the auto-PEEP value; a pause of at least 2–3 seconds should be used to avoid its underestimation. (Unlike Pplat, a higher value for auto-PEEP will be obtained with the longer pause.) Ventilators whose auto-PEEP function is automated may terminate the pause prematurely, and this may lead to gross underestimation of end-expiratory alveolar pressure. Second, the measured value is influenced by the circuit compression factor; use of a highly compliant ventilator circuit may lead to underestimation of auto-PEEP.[31] Third, patients with status asthmaticus who have radiographic evidence of hyperinflation and elevated Pplat on occasion may have unexpectedly low values of measured auto-PEEP when ventilated at very low respiratory rates. This phenomenon arises presumably because very long expiratory times may encourage airway closure that prevents accurate assessment of end-expiratory alveolar pressure.[32] Fourth, and perhaps most important, expiratory muscle activity may influence measured auto-PEEP markedly and cause gross overestimation of the severity of dynamic hyperinflation, potentially leading to unnecessary restriction of minute ventilation.[33] It is therefore imperative that the patient's expiratory muscles be relaxed during the measurement.

VENTILATOR SETTINGS

In severe asthma, three key factors determine the degree to which V_{EE} increases during mechanical ventilation: resistance to airflow during expiration, tidal volume that must be exhaled, and time for expiration. The key ventilator settings that influence the severity of hyperinflation are tidal volume, respiratory rate, and inspiratory flow rate.

MINUTE VENTILATION: TIDAL VOLUME AND RESPIRATORY RATE

Tuxen and Lane[22] examined various ventilator settings in severe asthma and found that minute ventilation was the most important determinant of dynamic hyperinflation (see Fig. 30-4). For a given minute ventilation, V_{EE} was similar regardless of the specific combination of respiratory rate and tidal volume.[22] V_{EI}, however, obviously will be greater when a given minute ventilation is achieved

FIGURE 30-5 Proximal airway pressure during an end-inspiratory and end-expiratory airway occlusion. End-inspiratory occlusion is followed by an initial rapid fall in airway pressure, secondary to intrinsic airways resistance and then a more gradual fall in pressure secondary to gas redistribution and tissue resistance. Ppk, peak airway pressure; Pplat, plateau airway pressure; auto-PEEP, auto-positive end-expiratory

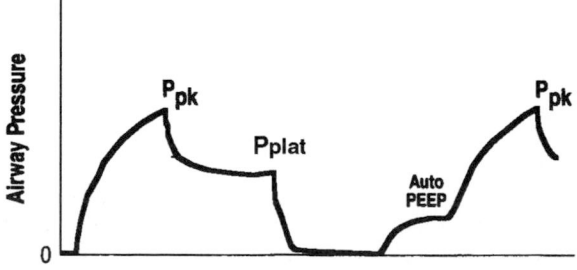

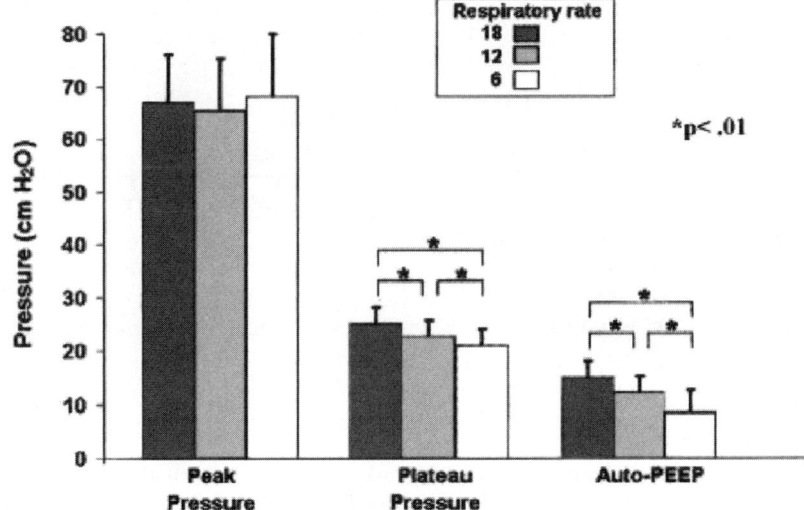

FIGURE 30-6 Peak airway pressure, plateau pressure, and auto-PEEP at respiratory rates of 18, 12, and 6 breaths per minute during mechanical ventilation for severe asthma (*n* = 12). (*Used, with permission, from Leatherman et al: Crit Care Med 32:1542–5, 2004.*)

through use of a higher tidal volume and lower rate. In this study, the degree of hyperinflation became quite marked when minute ventilation was increased from 10 to 16 and 26 liters/min; at the highest minute ventilation, both hypotension and barotrauma were noted[22] (see Fig. 30-4). This clearly demonstrates the potential risk of progressively increasing minute ventilation in an attempt to correct hypercapnia.

While very high levels of minute ventilation clearly pose a risk in the ventilated patient, the benefit of extreme limitation of minute ventilation, as advocated by some authors,[34]

TABLE 30-2   **Mechanical Ventilation for Severe Asthma: One Approach**

Ventilator settings (initial)

Mode	Assist-control
V_T	8–9 ml/kg
Rate	12–14 breaths/min
$\dot{V}_E$	0.1–0.13 liter/kg/min
V_I	60–70 liters/min
Waveform	Decelerating or square
PEEP	$\leq$5 cmH$_2$O
FI$_{O_2}$	Sa$_{O_2}$ > 90%

Sedation/paralysis

Propofol	2–5 mg/kg/h infusion
Fentanyl	50–200 μg/h infusion
Vecuronium	0.1 mg/kg bolus prn

Therapy of airflow obstruction

Albuterol-ipratroprium MDI	6 puffs qh $\times$ 4, then q1–2h
Methylprednisolone	1–2 mg/kg/day

Ventilator adjustments
Goals: Pplat < 30 cmH$_2$O ($\leq$ 25 ideal) and pH $\geq$ 7.2
- Pplat > 30 cmH$_2$O $\rightarrow$ decrease $\dot{V}_E$ (rate)
- pH < 7.2 and Pplat < 25 $\rightarrow$ increase $\dot{V}_E$(rate)
- pH < 7.2 and Pplat 25–30 $\rightarrow$ no change
  (consider buffer if adverse effects of acidosis suspected clinically)

ABBREVIATIONS: V_T, tidal volume; $\dot{V}_E$, minute ventilation; V_I, inspiratory flow rate; MDI, metered-dose inhaler; and Pplat, plateau airway pressure.

is less certain. A recent study examined the effect of prolongation of expiratory time on dynamic hyperinflation—as assessed by Pplat and auto-PEEP—when the baseline minute ventilation approximated 10 liters/min.[24] As expected, Pplat and auto-PEEP decreased when expiratory time was prolonged, but the magnitude of this reduction was not profound (see Fig. 30-6). For example, when respiratory rate was reduced from 12 to 6 breaths per minute (adding 5 seconds to expiratory time), Pplat and auto-PEEP fell by only 2–3 cmH$_2$O.[24] The relatively modest effect on dynamic hyperinflation is understandable given the low expiratory flow rates after a few seconds of expiration (Fig. 30-7). Also, because expiratory flow decreases progressively throughout expiration, the reduction in hyperinflation resulting from a given prolongation of expiratory time depends on the baseline respiratory rate (i.e., less benefit at a lower respiratory rate) (see Fig. 30-7).

Another factor that limits the extent to which prolongation of expiratory time can reduce lung hyperinflation is the presence of gas trapped behind occluded airways. Total pulmonary hyperinflation has two components: a dynamic component that is amenable to ventilator manipulation and a second component caused by trapped gas behind occluded airways, which is therefore not influenced by prolongation of expiratory time (see Fig. 30-2). One study used a prolonged apnea to measure the dynamic component and a postapnea radiographic estimate of lung volume to estimate the fixed component.[23] The results of this study suggested that trapped gas contributed a greater percentage of total pulmonary hyperinflation than did dynamic hyperinflation.[23]

In essence, available data suggest that while very high respiratory rates (and very short expiratory times) should be avoided, there is often little to be gained by reducing the respiratory rate below 12–14 breaths per minute when a tidal volume of 8–9 ml/kg is used (see Table 30-2). An exception might be when hyperinflation is marked (e.g., Pplat > 30 cmH$_2$O) or has resulted in complications because then even a small reduction in hyperinflation could have a meaningful clinical impact. Truly dramatic reductions in

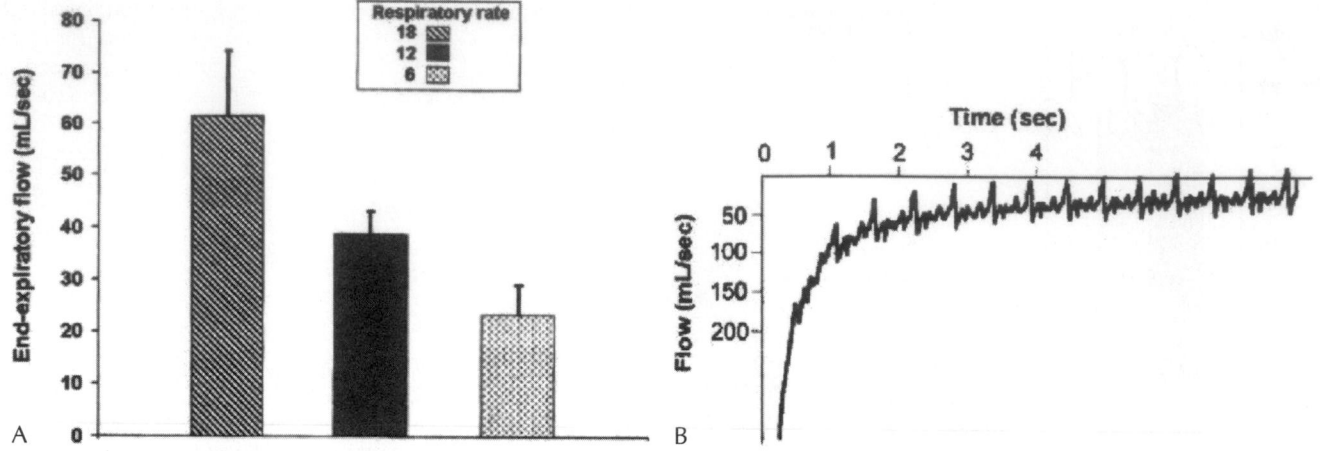

FIGURE 30-7 *A.* End-expiratory flow rates at respiratory rates of 18, 12, and 6 breaths per minute during mechanical ventilation for severe asthma (*n* = 7). *B.* Expiratory flow tracing from an individual patient. (*Used, with permission, from Leatherman et al: Crit Care Med 32:1542–5, 2004.*)

hyperinflation, however, may not be easily achieved by ventilator manipulation alone and usually must await improvement in airflow obstruction.

INSPIRATORY FLOW RATE

At any given respiratory rate, shortening of inspiratory time through the use of a high inspiratory flow rate of necessity will lengthen expiratory time. Similarly, inspiratory time will be shorter when the inspiratory waveform is square rather than decelerating. Accordingly, it has been advocated that a flow rate of approximately 100 liters/min and a square waveform be used in patients with status asthmaticus.[2,26,27] Although this strategy will produce a more favorable inspiratory-expiratory (I:E) ratio, the effect on dynamic hyperinflation in patients whose minute ventilation already has been restricted will be modest.[24] With a tidal volume of 600 ml, for example, a change from a flow rate of 60 liters/min with a decelerating wave to a flow rate of 120 liters/min with a square wave will add less than 1 second to expiratory time. Because end-expiratory flow rates typically are 60 ml/s or less at a respiratory rate of 12–14 breaths per minute (Fig. 30-7), this degree of prolongation will result in a negligible reduction in lung volume (Table 30-3). In brief, a high inspiratory flow rate and square waveform offer no significant advantage over a decelerating waveform and more conventional flow rate (~60 liters/min) in patients with asthma whose minute ventilation already has been limited.

APPLIED PEEP

External positive end-expiratory pressure (PEEP) is used often during mechanical ventilation of patients with chronic obstructive pulmonary disease (COPD) to decrease the effort required to trigger the ventilator and does not increase lung volume as long as applied PEEP is less than auto-PEEP.[35,36] There is no clear-cut rationale for the use of external PEEP, however, when a patient is receiving controlled mechanical ventilation under the influence of deep sedation or paralysis. Furthermore, the impact of applied PEEP on lung volume may be different in asthma and COPD[35,37,38] (Fig. 30-8). One study of found that external PEEP of 10–15 cmH$_2$0 increased the lung volumes of ventilated patients with severe asthma, suggesting that minimal PEEP (≤5 cmH$_2$O) levels should be used in this setting[38] (see Table 30-2).

GAS EXCHANGE: HYPERCAPNIA

Hypercapnia is common during mechanical ventilation of patients with severe asthma. Two studies found average values for Pa$_{CO_2}$ and pH of 61 mmHg and 7.2 (mean minute ventilation 11.4 liters/min) and 68 mmHg and 7.18 (mean minute ventilation 9 liters/min).[18,24] There is considerable variation in the degree of respiratory acidosis, and Pa$_{CO_2}$ values may range from normal to over 100 mmHg. Hypercapnia despite normal or increased minute ventilation can only result from an increase in carbon dioxide (CO$_2$)

TABLE 30-3 Effect of Inspiratory Flow Rate in Severe Asthma

V$_I$ and Waveform	T$_I$(s)	T$_E$(s)	I:E Ratio	ΔDHI (ml)	Δauto-PEEP (cmH$_2$O)
60 liters/min, decelerating	1.1	3.2	1:3	—	—
120 liters/min, square	0.3	4.0	1:13	~ −50	~ −1

NOTE: Assume V$_T$ 600 ml, respiratory rate 14 breaths/min, respiratory compliance 60 ml/cmH$_2$O, and end-expiratory flow rate ~ 60 ml/s.

ABBREVIATIONS: V$_I$, inspiratory flow rate; T$_I$, inspiratory time; T$_E$, expiratory time; I:E ratio, inspiratory-to-expiratory ratio; and DHI, dynamic hyperinflation.

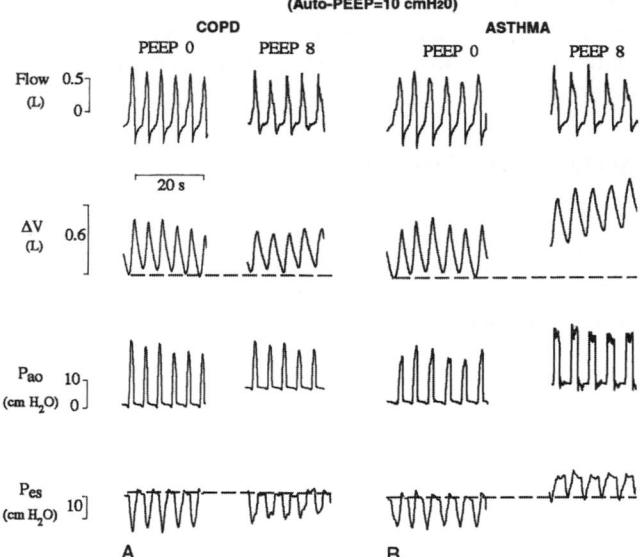

FIGURE 30-8 Response to 8 cmH₂O of PEEP in COPD and asthma during proportional-assist ventilation. Esophageal pressure (Pes) indicates a similar reduction in inspiratory effort in both patients. External PEEP did not affect lung volume (V) or airway pressure (Pao) in COPD, but both were increased by PEEP in asthma. (*Adapted, with permission, from Ranieri, et al: Clin Chest Med 17(3):381, 1996.*)

production or an increase in physiologic dead space. It is presumed that hypercapnia during mechanical ventilation of patients with status asthmaticus is caused by marked increases in dead space that result from alveolar overdistension. Normally, an increase in minute ventilation will lower Pa_{CO_2} (doubling the rate should decrease Pa_{CO_2} by 50%). This may not by the case in patients with status asthmaticus, however, because when minute ventilation is increased, the resulting increase in dynamic hyperinflation may further increase dead space. Although the precise effect of minute ventilation on Pa_{CO_2} in status asthmaticus has not been well documented, anecdotal experience has shown that efforts to reduce an elevated Pa_{CO_2} by increasing minute ventilation may be relatively ineffective. In truth, the hypercapnia of severe asthma may not be "permissive" because one may not be able to normalize the Pa_{CO_2} through ventilator manipulation.

Because the ability to correct hypercapnia may be limited and fraught with potential hazards, a reasonable approach may be simply to choose ventilator settings that usually provide a safe level of dynamic hyperinflation (tidal volume of 8–9 ml/kg, respiratory rate of 12–14 breaths per minute) and accept the resulting Pa_{CO_2} (see Table 30-2) . Fortunately, hypercapnia in status asthmaticus seems to be generally well tolerated, with truly serious adverse consequences being quite uncommon.[20] Perhaps the most serious risk of hypercapnia is an increase in cerebral blood flow and intracranial pressure in patients with acute neurologic pathology. Although unlikely to occur in the setting of status asthamticus, there are rare reports of cerebral edema or subarachnoid hemorrhage attributed to hypercapnia.[39–41] Profound hypercapnia is of greatest concern if the patient has experienced profound cerebral anoxia secondary to res-

piratory arrest before intubation. In this situation, it is best to avoid hypercapnia, if at all possible. As mentioned earlier, this may not be easy to accomplish without extracorporeal CO_2 removal unless the patient has rapidly reversible bronchospasm.

Hypercapnia in status asthmaticus is acute in onset and therefore is not compensated for by increased bicarbonate. One approach to acute hypercapnia in status asthmaticus is to ignore the elevated Pa_{CO_2} and administer buffering agents to correct acidosis. Unlike metabolic acidosis, however, buffering acute respiratory acidosis with bicarbonate is relatively inefficient. Discounting the loss of administered bicarbonate in the urine and generation of CO_2 through buffering of protons, even partial correction of severe respiratory acidosis will require a minimum of several hundred milliequivalents of sodium bicarbonate in an adult.[20] One animal study did find that administration of sufficient sodium bicarbonate (14 mEq/kg) to preserve a normal pH during induction of acute hypercapnia (Pa_{CO_2} = 80 mmHg) prevented an increase in cerebral blood flow and intracranial pressure.[42] The effect on intracranial pressure was less certain, however, if a lesser amount of bicarbonate was given slowly to only partially correct pH to 7.15–7.20, as is usually recommended.[20,42] Another problem with the use of large amounts of bicarbonate is that with resolution of airflow obstruction and hypercapnia, the patient is left with a therapeutically induced metabolic alkalosis.

As a general rule, unless there is some compelling reason to correct underlying respiratory acidosis (e.g., arrhythmia, hyperkalemia, or otherwise unexplained hemodynamic instability), it is probably reasonable to forego attempts to correct serum pH and wait for the Pa_{CO_2} to decrease as airflow obstruction improves. Fortunately, many patients experience substantial improvement in their hypercapnia during the first 12 hours of intubation.[43] If bicarbonate therapy is given, ideally it should be administered by slow infusion rather than by rapid bolus administration because the latter may lead to an acute increase in CO_2 production and a transient fall in intracellular pH as a consequence of rapid diffusion of CO_2 into cells. An alternative to sodium bicarbonate is tromethamine (THAM), a buffer that does not generate CO_2 during the buffering process.[20] Even though THAM may offer some theoretical advantages over sodium bicarbonate for buffering respiratory acidosis, its use may lead to the same problem of a posthypercapnic metabolic alkalosis.

Nonventilator Management

All ventilated patients with severe asthma require bronchodilators, corticosteroids, and sedation. In rare instances, other nonconventional approaches may be considered.

STANDARD THERAPY

BRONCHODILATORS AND GLUCOCORTICOIDS
There have been no studies specifically examining the use of inhaled bronchodilators during mechanical ventilation of

patients with severe asthma. Studies in patients with COPD suggest that either metered-dose inhaler or nebulization is beneficial and that the optimal dose of albuterol given by metered-dose inhaler is likely to be 4–6 puffs.[44–46] Because the dose-response characteristics in ventilated patients with asthma is unknown, assessment of lung mechanics during incremental dosing of inhaled β_2 agonists may be useful in determining the optimal number of puffs and dosing interval for individual patients using an "$n = 1$" trial. A similar approach might be used when assessing other agents with bronchodilator properties, such as ipratroprium or intravenous magnesium sulfate.

Glucocorticoids are an essential component of the treatment of severe asthma, with an effect being evident within 12 hours of administration.[47] Based on data from nonintubated patients, an initial dose of 1–2 mg/kg per day of methylprednisolone or equivalent seems appropriate.[48]

SEDATION AND PARALYSIS

No studies have specifically examined various sedation regimens in status asthmaticus. As with other causes of respiratory failure, minimal goals in status asthmaticus would include provision of amnesia, anxiolysis, and analgesia and prevention of patient-ventilator dyssynchrony. Patients with status asthmaticus present an additional challenge because of the need to enforce controlled hypoventilation despite acute respiratory acidosis that increases respiratory drive.[9] A combination of propofol or a benzodiazepine (midazolam or lorazepam) with a narcotic (fentanyl or morphine) often proves optimal, and very large doses may be required[9] (see Table 30-2). Because most patients improve significantly within 24–48 hours,[26,43] prolonged residual sedation that delays extubation is undesirable. One advantage of propofol over benzodiazepines in severe asthma is that this agent often allows deep sedation that reverses promptly on its discontinuation. A maximal propofol dose of approximately 5 mg/kg per hour is recommended because prolonged infusion of very high doses of propofol can lead to life-threatening complications.[49]

Large doses of sedatives and narcotics in combination with marked lung hyperinflation may lead to hypotension secondary to decreased venous return. When additional muscle relaxation is needed in the face of hemodynamic instability, it may be safer to administer a nondepolarizing neuromuscular blocking agent (NMBA) than increase the dose of sedatives and narcotics. Even when hypotension is not present, intermittent administration of one or more boluses of an NMBA may help to provide a period of temporary muscle relaxation, during which time sedative doses can be escalated gradually to achieve target levels. Prolonged use of an NMBA may increase the likelihood of myopathy in status asthmaticus (see below), but short-term use does not carry significant risk.[50,51] The specific NMBA selected is likely not important, although vecuronium perhaps should be avoided in patients with renal failure.[52] Intermittent bolusing is preferred to a continuous infusion because this permits ongoing assessment of the adequacy of sedation and lessens the likelihood that the patient will undergo unnecessarily prolonged neuromuscular paralysis. When sedatives and narcotics are used liberally, supplemented by short-term intermittent boluses of an NMBA if needed, very few patients with status asthmaticus will require prolonged, continuous neuromuscular paralysis.

ALTERNATIVE THERAPIES

The great majority of ventilated patients with severe asthma respond to standard treatment with inhaled bronchodilators and corticosteroids. Occasionally, however, patients with very fulminant asthma may be considered for one of several nontraditional approaches in order to reduce extreme hyperinflation and lessen marked hypercapnia. Strategies that have been reported ancecdotally to be beneficial in severe fulminant asthma include the use of a helium-oxygen mixture (heliox), inhalational anesthetics or ketamine, nitric oxide, mucolytic agents, bronchoscopy, and extracorporeal support.

HELIOX

The lower gas density of heliox reduces frictional resistance where gas flow is turbulent and, by lowering the Reynolds number, also encourages laminar flow.[12,53] One study reported that heliox produced a rapid fall in peak airway pressure and Pa_{CO_2} of ventilated patients with asthma.[54] The effects on Pplat and auto-PEEP, however, were not reported, and it is unclear whether changes in Pa_{CO_2} were at constant minute ventilation.[54] A second study of heliox in severe asthma found little change in Pa_{CO_2} when tidal volume and respiratory rate were held constant.[55] Two prospective studies found that a 70:30 mixture of heliox significantly reduced auto-PEEP during mechanical ventilation of patients with COPD[56,57] (Fig. 30-9). This suggests that heliox may have a measurable benefit in some patients and might be considered for use when conventional

FIGURE 30-9 Change in trapped volume and intrinsic PEEP in response to heliox in mechanically ventilated patients with COPD (*n = 25*). (*Used, with permission, from Lee et al: Crit Care Med 33:968–73, 2005.*)

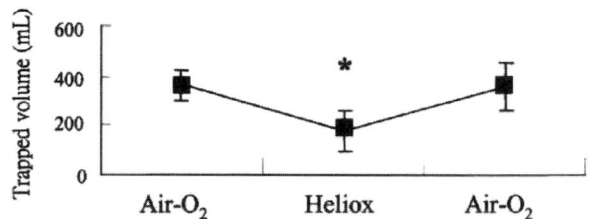

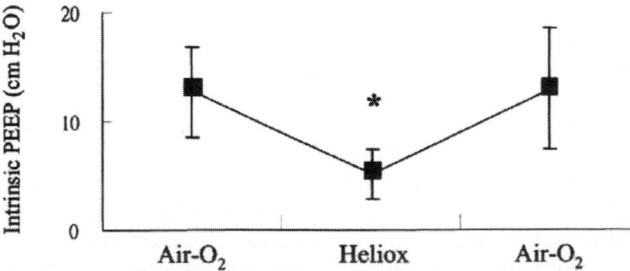

management results in an unacceptable degree of dynamic hyperinflation in patients with status asthmaticus.[2]

Before using heliox, it is crucial to fully understand how performance of the ventilator will be affected.[58] Some ventilators become inoperable with heliox, and others require adjustments in tidal volume or inspiratory flow rates. Because the ventilator's pneumotachographs may not interpret exhaled tidal volume accurately when heliox is used, use of a density-independent spirometer in the expiratory limb of the ventilator circuit is advisable to ensure accurate setting of tidal volume.[12,57]

GENERAL ANESTHETICS

Inhalational anesthetics have potent bronchodilating properties, and several anecdotal reports have described their use in status asthmaticus.[59,60] In the only study to carefully assess lung mechanics, isoflurane resulted in a decrease in airways resistance and auto-PEEP in three patients with asthma, although only one had a marked response[61] (Fig. 30-10). It is possible that unsuccessful trials of inhalational anesthetics have not been reported, and the overall likelihood of benefit is unknown. Nonetheless, there are unquestionably individual patients with fulminant asthma who may derive benefit from general anesthetics.

Isoflurane and sevoflurane are less arrythmogenic than halothane and have equal or greater bronchodilator properties. All these agents may cause hypotension secondary to their peripheral vascular effects, and an increase in venous capacitance may be particularly detrimental when marked dynamic hyperinflation already has compromised venous return. The adverse hemodynamic effects generally can be mitigated through liberal administration of fluid and with vasoactive support if necessary. It is mandatory, of course, that personnel highly skilled in the use of anesthetic agents be responsible for their administration. Some intensive-care unit (ICU) ventilators (e.g., Servo 300 and 900) have a port to which the anesthesia vaporizer can be attached, and with appropriate scavenging of anesthetic gases, the general anesthetic can be administered in the ICU.

Ketamine, an intravenous dissociative anesthetic, also has been advocated for use in severe asthma. This drug, however, can lead to significant increases in blood pressure, heart rate, and intracranial pressure. There seems little justification for the use of ketamine in ventilated patients with status asthmaticus.

MUCOLYTICS

The potential benefit of *N*-acetycysteine as a mucolytic is unknown; in an anecdotal report, it seemed to enhance bronchoscopic extraction of mucus plugs.[62] Benefit from rh-DNAse also has been reported.[63]

NITRIC OXIDE

Although nitric oxide is a relatively weak bronchodilator, it was reported to be of significant benefit in one small series of patients with very severe asthma.[64]

BRONCHOSCOPY

Patients with fatal asthma often have extensive mucoid impaction.[65] Removal of impacted mucus by bronchoscopy has been reported to lower airway pressures and improve gas exchange in ventilated patients with severe asthma.[62] Although probably safe in most instances, there is a potential for worsening bronchospasm, and several large series have reported good outcomes without use of bronchoscopy.[18,26,43] Patients who fail to improve after several days of mechanical ventilation might be considered for diagnostic bronchoscopy to inspect the airways for mucus plugs that might be extracted, the goal being to reduce the duration of ventilator support.

EXTRACORPOREAL MEMBRANE OXYGENATION

Extracorporeal membrane oxygenation (ECMO) has been used in severe asthma.[66] Because severe asthma is fully reversible, this approach clearly would be justified if there were an imminently lethal impairment in gas exchange. Refractory hypoxemia, however, is unusual in asthma, and hypercapnia generally is well tolerated (see above). One scenario in which ECMO might be considered would be combined severe impairment in gas exchange together with extreme hyperinflation resulting in bartorauma or hemodynamic instability. In this situation, ECMO conceivably could provide a period of stability during which bronchoscopy could be performed to extract as much inspissated mucus as possible.

Death and Complications

MORTALITY

Published mortality rates for patients undergoing mechanical ventilation for severe asthma have varied greatly, ranging from 0–38%. A literature review of over 1220 patients reported an average mortality of 12.4%.[2] Although the outcome seems to have improved over the last two decades, perhaps because of more widespread use of controlled hypoventilation,[2,20] mortality rates as high as 15–20% have been reported in series published during the last 5 years.[67,68]

FIGURE 30-10 The effect of isoflurane on auto-PEEP and change in lung volume (ΔV) in three patients with severe asthma. (*Adapted, with permission, from Maltais et al: Chest 105:1401–6, 1994.*)

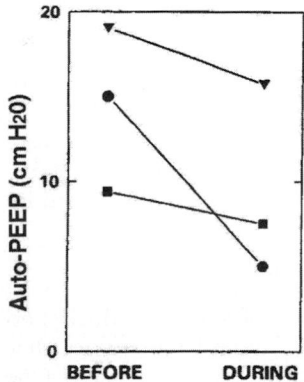
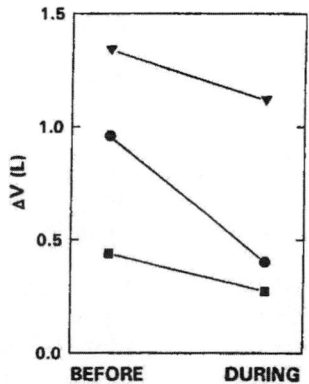

Most fatalities result from cerebral anoxia secondary to cardiorespiratory arrest before intubation. Indeed, in a recent analysis of 1223 patients who underwent mechanical ventilation for severe asthma, 80% of in-hospital deaths were preceded by cardiorespiratory arrest before admission to the ICU.[68] This is not to minimize the importance of controlled hypoventilation. Instead, it merely emphasizes that ICU management ultimately may be less important than steps taken in the outpatient setting to prevent asthma deterioration and avoidance of patient delay in activating the emergency transport system in response to an acute asthma attack.

COMPLICATIONS

Patients with severe asthma are at risk for many of the same complications affecting other ventilated patients, including nosocomial pneumonia, sinusitis, pulmonary embolism, and gastrointestinal bleeding. Additional complications that result from severe asthma itself or from medications used to treat airflow obstruction and provide muscle relaxation include ventilator-associated hypotension, barotrauma, myocardial injury, rhabdomyolysis, lactic acidosis, neurologic injury, and acute myopathy (Table 30-4).

HYPOTENSION

Hypotension during mechanical ventilation for status asthmaticus most often results from excessive pulmonary hyperinflation that impedes venous return. In one series, mild to moderate hypotension was documented at some point during the course of mechanical ventilation in 35% of patients, with risk being greatest in patients whose V_{EI} exceeded approximately 20 ml/kg[18] (Fig. 30-11). Although unusual,

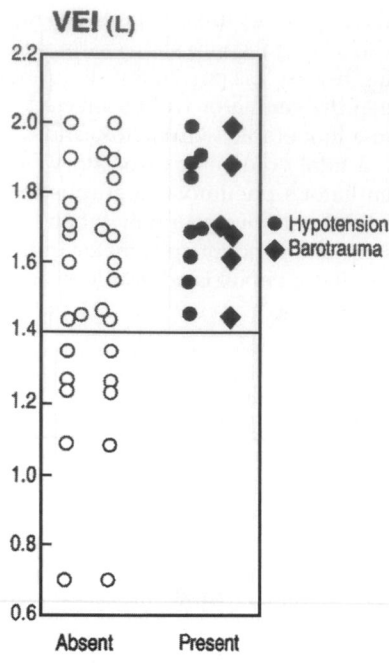

Complications

FIGURE 30-11 Relationship between hypotension, barotrauma, and lung volume at end inspiration (V_{EI}). (*Used, with permission, from Williams et al: Am Rev Respir Dis 146:607–15, 1992.*)

extreme hyperinflation can lead to cardiac arrest with pulseless electrical activity.[17] When a ventilated patient with severe asthma develops significant hypotension, a 1-minute apnea trial is recommended.[2] If the apnea trial and a rapid infusion of fluid do not restore blood pressure, then less common causes of hypotension (e.g., pneumothorax, myocardial depression) must be considered.

BAROTRAUMA

Pneumothorax also occurs most often in patients with the highest end-inspiratory lung volume[18] (Fig. 30-11). The incidence of pneumothorax was as high as 30% in some early series[69] but is relatively infrequent (<10%) when a strategy of controlled hypoventilation is used.[9,20,25,26,43] In a recent analysis of barotrauma in various types of respiratory failure, pneumothorax was documented in only 6% of patient with status asthmaticus.[70] Nonetheless, a pneumothorax may be particularly dangerous in patients with severe asthma because the hyperinflated lungs resist collapse and allow even a small pneumothorax to be under tension, resulting in rapid deterioration and sometimes death.[2,67] For this reason, clinical (and radiographic) diagnosis of tension pneumothorax may be particularly challenging in severe asthma.[2] Chest tubes always should be placed by blunt dissection rather than by the blind trocar method to avoid injuring the hyperinflated lungs.[2]

CARDIAC COMPLICATIONS

Despite the common occurrence of severe acidosis and the use of high-dose inhaled β_2-agonist therapy, cardiac arrhythmias in status asthmaticus are uncommon. One

TABLE 30-4 Complications of Mechanical Ventilation for Severe Asthma

Complications	Likely Mechanism
Hypotension	Primary: Excessive hyperinflation, sedatives
	Secondary: Pneumothorax, myocardial depression
Barotrauma	Excessive hyperinflation
Myocardial dysfunction	Primary: "Stunned myocardium" secondary to massive catecholamine release
	Secondary: Severe myocardial hypoxia/acidosis
Rhabdomyolysis	Primary: Extreme muscle exertion with or without hypoxia
	Secondary: High dose propofol
Lactic acidosis	Primary: Excessive β_2 agonists
	Secondary: Extreme muscle exertion/hypoxia
CNS injury	Primary: Cerebral anoxia secondary to respiratory arrest
	Secondary: Hypercapnia-related cerebral edema, subarachnoid hemorrhage
Acute myopathy	Glucocorticoids plus prolonged paralysis or deep sedation

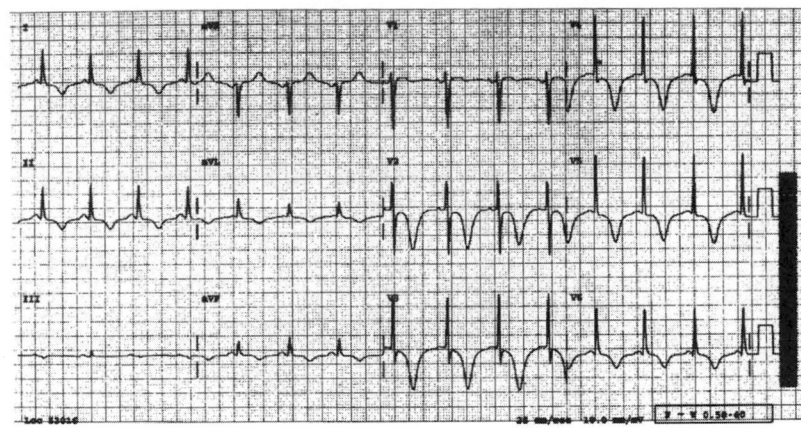

FIGURE 30-12 Electrocardiogram of a patient with acute reversible left-ventricular dysfunction caused by status asthmaticus. Deep inverted T waves in anterior precordial leads are seen commonly in this condition. (*Used, with permission, from Levine et al: Chest 107:1469–73, 1995.*)

reported cardiac complication of status asthmaticus is decreased myocardial contractility with reversible segmental myocardial wall-motion abnormalities and deep T-wave inversions in the electrocardiogram, simulating myocardial ischemia[71,72] (Fig. 30-12). The "stunned myocardium" of status asthmaticus is similar to that seen after subarachnoid hemorrhage, severe psychological stress, and other conditions associated with massive endogenous sympathetic activation and typically has a benign course and no long-term cardiac sequelae.[72]

RHABDOMYOLYSIS

Rhabdomyolysis has been reported in patients with status asthmaticus, presumably as a result of extreme muscular exertion coupled with hypoxia.[73] Rhabdomyolysis also has been noted in patients who had received prolonged infusions of propofol in very high doses.[49]

LACTIC ACIDOSIS

Mild lactic acidosis is relatively common in status asthmaticus.[74] Lactic acidosis has been attributed to lactate production by respiratory muscles[75,76] but also can occur as a result of excessive use of β_2 agonists. Although more common when the latter are given intravenously, lactic acidosis also can follow high-dose inhalational therapy with albuterol.[77] Even a moderate degree of lactic acidosis may be problematic in patients with significant hypercapnia.

CENTRAL NERVOUS SYSTEM INJURY

As noted earlier, cerebral anoxia is the most common cause of death in patients with status asthmaticus.[68] Hypercapnia-induced increases in intracranial pressure potentially could worsen brain injury following a cardiorespiratory arrest; overall, however, hypercapnia appears to pose little risk of long-term neurologic sequelae.[20] Nonetheless, rare instances of cerebral edema or subarachnoid hemorrhage in status asthmaticus that occurred in the absence of prior cerebral anoxia have been attributed to hypercapnia[39-41] (Fig. 30-13).

MYOPATHY

Acute myopathy probably is the most common cause of morbidity affecting patients with asthma who undergo mechanical ventilation. The pathogenesis of myopathy is incompletely understood, but it usually has been attributed to the combined effects of glucocorticoids and prolonged neuromuscular paralysis[50,51] (Fig. 30-14). Myopathy, however, also can occur in glucocorticoid-treated patients with asthma who have undergone prolonged (>5–7 days) mechanical ventilation under deep sedation without paralysis.[78,79] It is possible that prolonged near-total muscle inactivity, whether induced by neuromuscular paralysis or by deep sedation, may increase the sensitivity of muscles to the myotoxic effects of corticosteroids.[79]

FIGURE 30-13 Subarachnoid hemorrhage in an 11-year-old boy with status asthmaticus who was managed with controlled hypoventilation and permissive hypercapnia (Pa_{CO_2} = 75–35 mmHg). (Use of ketamine may have contributed to increased intracranial pressure.) (*Used, with permission, from Edmunds et al: Pediatr Crit Care Med 4:100–3, 2003.*)

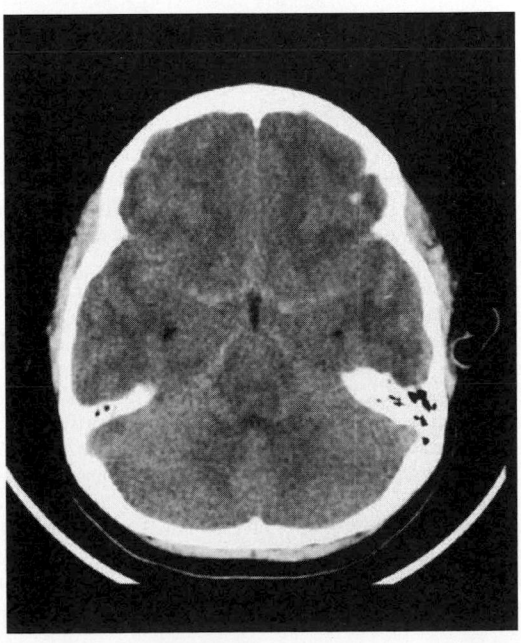

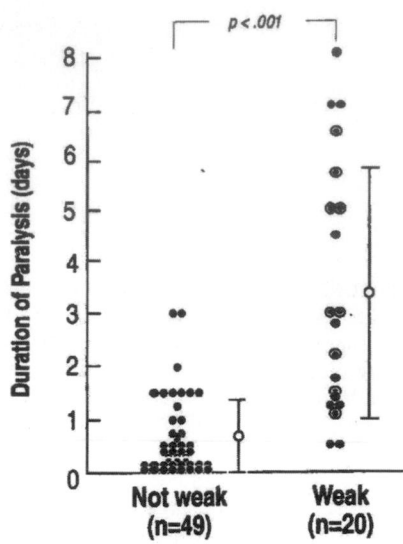

FIGURE 30-14 Duration of paralysis in patients with and without weakness (defined clinically) after undergoing mechanical ventilation for severe asthma. (*Used, with permission, from Leatherman et al: Am J Respir Crit Care Med 153:1686–90, 1996.*)

Posthospitalization Prognosis

Although in-hospital mortality of patients who receive mechanical ventilation for severe asthma is relatively low, various studies have estimated the mortality from recurrent attacks to be between 10% and 25% over the subsequent decade.[80] Indeed, prior intubation has been identified as the strongest risk factor for death from asthma.[1] These data emphasize the crucial importance of outpatient management—including regular use of inhaled glucocorticoids, avoidance of smoking and other factors known to increase airway responsiveness, close supervision, and intensive education—following hospital discharge of patients with asthma who undergo mechanical ventilation.

References

1. Pendergraft TB, Stanford RH, Beasley R, et al. Rates and characteristics of intensive care unit admissions and intubations among asthma-related hospitalizations. Ann Allergy Asthma Immunol 2004; 93:29–35.
2. Tuxen DV, Andersen MB, Scheinkestel CD Mechanical ventilation for severe asthma. In: Hall JB, Corbridge TC, Rodrigo C, Rodrigo GV, editors. Acute asthma: Assessment and management. New York: McGraw-Hill, 2000.
3. Plaza V, Serrano J, Picado C, Sanchis J. High Risk Asthma Research Group. Frequency and clinical characteristics of rapid-onset fatal and near-fatal asthma. Eur Respir J 2002; 19:846–52.
4. Sur S, Crotty TB, Kephart GM, et al. Sudden-onset fatal asthma: A distinct entity with few eosinophils and relatively more neutrophils in the airway submucosa? Am Rev Respir Dis 1993; 148:713–9.
5. O'Hollaren MT, Yunginger JW, Offord KP, et al. Exposure to an aeroallergen as a possilble precipitating factor in respiratory arrest in young patients with asthma. New Engl J Med 1991; 324:359–63.
6. Molfino NA, Nannini LJ, Martelli AN, Slutsky AS. Respiratory arrest in near-fatal asthma. New Engl J Med 1991; 324:285–8.
7. Mountain RD, Sahn SA. Clinical features and outcome in patients with acute asthma presenting with hypercapnia. Am Rev Respir Dis 1988; 138:535–9.
8. Meduri GU, Cook TR, Turner RE, et al. Noninvasive positive pressure ventilation by face mask: First-line intervention in patients with acute hypercapnic and hypoxemic respiratory failure. Chest 1996; 110:767–74.
9. Gehlbach B, Kress JP, Kahn J, et al. Correlates of prolonged hospitalization in inner-city ICU patients receiving noninvasive and invasive positive pressure ventilation for status asthmaticus. Chest 2002; 122:1709–14.
10. Fernandez MM, Villagra A, Blanch L, Fernandez R. Non-invasive mechanical ventilation in status asthmaticus. Intensive Care Med 2001; 27:486–92.
11. Kass JE, Castriotta RJ. Heliox therapy in acute severe asthma. Chest 1995; 107:757–60.
12. Hess D, Chatmongkolchart S. Techniques to avoid intubation: Noninvasive positive pressure ventilation and heliox therapy. Int Anesthesiol Clin 2000; 38:161–87.
13. Jagoda A, Shepherd SM, Spevitz A, Joseph MM. Refractory asthma: 2. Airway interventions and management. Ann Emerg Med 1997; 29:275–81.
14. Marik PE, Varon J, Fromm R Jr. The management of acute severe asthma. J Emerg Med 2002; 23:257–68.
15. Eames WO, Rooke GA, Wu RS, Bishop MJ. Comparison of the effects of etomidate, propofol, and thiopental on respiratory resistance after tracheal intubation. Anesthesiology 1996; 84:1307–11.
16. Franklin C, Samuel J, Hu T. Life-threatening hypotension associated with emergency intubation and the initiation of mechanical ventilation. Am J Emerg Med 1994; 12:425–8.
17. Rosengarten PL, Tuxen DV, Dzulkas L, et al. Circulatory arrest induced by intermittent positive-pressure ventilation in a patient with severe asthma. Anaesth Intensive Care 1991; 19:118–21.
18. Williams TJ, Tuxen DV, Scheinkestel CD. Risk factors for morbidity in mechanically ventilated patients with acute severe asthma. Am Rev Respir Dis 1992; 146:607–15.
19. Darioli R, Perret C. Mechanical controlled hypoventilation in status asthmaticus. Am Rev Respir Dis 1984; 129:385–7.
20. Feihl F, Perret C. Permissive hypercapnia: How permissive should we be? Am J Respir Crit Care Med 1994; 150:1722–37.
21. Tuxen DV. Permissive hypercapnic ventilation. Am J Respir Crit Care Med 1994; 150:870–1.
22. Tuxen DV, Lane S. The effects of ventilatory pattern on hyperinflation, airway pressures, and circulation in mechanical ventilation of patients with severe airflow obstruction. Am Rev Respir Dis 1987; 136:872–9.
23. Tuxen DV, Williams TJ, Scheinkestel CD. Use of a measurement of pulmonary hyperinflation to control the level of mechanical ventilation in patients with acute severe asthma. Am Rev Respir Dis 1992; 146:1136–42.
24. Leatherman JW, McArthur C, Shapiro RS. Effect of prolongation of expiratory time on dynamic hyperinflation in mechanically ventilated patients with severe asthma. Crit Care Med 2004; 32:1542–5.
25. Braman SS, Kaemmerlen JT. Intensive care of status asthmaticus: A 10-year experience. JAMA 1990; 264:366–8.
26. Leatherman JW. Life-threatening asthma. Clin Chest Med 1994; 15:453–79.

27. Corbridge TC, Hall JB. The assessment and management of adults with status asthmaticus. Am J Respir Crit Care Med 1995; 151:1296–1316.

28. Slutsky AS. Mechanical ventialtion. ACCP consensus conference. Chest 1993; 104:1833–57

29. Manthous CA. Management of severe exacerbations of asthma. Am J Med 1995; 99:298–308.

30. Oddo M, Feihl F, Schaller M-D, Perret C. Management of mechanical ventilation in severe asthma: Practical aspects. Intensive Care Med 2006; 27:1–10.

31. Grootensdorst AF, Lugtigheid G, van der Weygert EJ. Error in ventilator measurement of intrinsic PEEP: Cause and remedy. Respir Care 1993; 38:348–50.

32. Leatherman, JW, Ravenscraft SA. Low measured auto-positive end-expiratory pressure during mechanical ventilation of patients with severe asthma: Hidden auto-positive end-expiratory pressure? Crit Care Med 1996; 24:541–6.

33. Lessard MR, Lofaso F, Brochard L. Expiratory muscle activity increases intrinsic positive end-expiratory pressure independently of dynamic hyperinflation in mechanically ventilated patients. Am J Respir Crit Care Med 1995; 151:562–9.

34. Phipps P, Garrard CS. The pulmonary physician in critical care: 12. Acute severe asthma in the intensive care unit. Thorax 2003; 58:81–8.

35. Ranieri VM, Graasso S, Fiore T, Giuliani R. Auto-positive end-expiratory pressure and dynamic hyperinflation. Clin Chest Med 1996; 17: 379–94.

36. Ranieri VM, Giuliani R, Cinnella G, et al. Physiologic effects of positive end-expiratory pressure in patients with chronic obstructive pulmonary disease during acute ventilatory failure and controlled mechanical ventilation. Am Rev Respir Dis 1993; 147:5–13.

37. Marini JJ. Should PEEP be used in airflow obstruction? Am Rev Respir Dis. 1989; 140:1–3.

38. Tuxen DV. Detrimental effects of positive end-expiratory pressure during controlled mechanical ventilation of patients with severe airflow obstruction. Am Rev Respir Dis 1989; 140:5–9.

39. Edmunds SM, Harrison R. Subarachnoid hemorrhage in a child with status asthmaticus: Significance of permissive hypercapnia. Pediatr Crit Care Med 2003; 4:100–3.

40. Rodrigo C, Rodrigo G. Subarachnoid hemorrhage following permissive hypercapnia in a patient with severe acute asthma. Am J Emerg Med. 1999; 17:697–9.

41. Gaussorgues P, Piperno D, Fouqu P, et al. Hypertension intracranienne au cours de l',tat asthmatique. Ann Fr Anesth Reanim 1987; 6:38–41

42. Cardenas VJ Jr, Zwischenberger JB, Tao W, et al. Correction of blood pH attenuates changes in hemodynamics and organ blood flow during permissive hypercapnia. Crit Care Med 1996; 24:827–34.

43. Bellomo R, McLaughlin P, Tai E, et al. Asthma requiring mechanical ventilation: A low-morbidity approach. Chest 1994; 105:891–6.

44. Manthous CA, Chatila W, Schmidt G, et al. Treatment of bronchospasm by metered-dose inhaler albuterol in mechanically ventilated patients. Chest 1995; 107:210–3.

45. Dhand R, Duarte AG, Jubran A, et al. Dose-response to bronchodilator delivered by metered-dose inhaler in ventilator-supported patients. Am J Respir Crit Care Med 1996; 154:388–93.

46. Dhand R, Tobin MJ. Inhaled bronchodilator therapy in mechanically ventilated patients. Am J Respir Crit Care Med 1997; 156:3–10.

47. Fanta CH, Rossing TH, McFadden ER Jr. Glucocorticoids in acute asthma: A critical controlled trial. Am J Med 1983; 74:845–51.

48. Barnes NC. Effects of corticosteroids in acute severe asthma. Thorax 1992; 47582–3.

49. Stelow EB, Johari VP, Smith SA, et al. Propofol-associated rhabdomyolysis with cardiac involvement in adults: Chemical and anatomic findings. Clin Chem 2000; 46:577–81.

50. Douglas JA, Tuxen DV, Horne M. Myopathy in severe asthma. Am Rev Respir Dis 1992; 146:517–9.

51. Leatherman JW, Fleugel WW, David WD, et al. Muscle weakness in ashmatic patients who undergo mechanical ventilation. Am J Respir Crit Care Med 1966; 153:1686–90.

52. Segredo V, Caldwell JE, Matthay MA, et al. Persistent paralysis in critically ill patients after long-term administration of vecuronium. New Engl J Med. 1992; 327:524–8.

53. Reuben AD, Harris AR. Heliox for asthma in the emergency department: A review of the literature Emerg Med J 2004; 21:131–5.

54. Gluck EH, Onorato DJ, Castriotta R. Helium-oxygen mixtures in intubated patients with status asthmaticus and respiratory acidosis. Chest 1990; 98:693–8.

55. Schaeffer EM, Pohlman A, Morgan S, Hall JB. Oxygenation in status asthmaticus improves during ventilation with helium-oxygen. Crit Care Med 1999; 27:2666–70.

56. Tassaux D, Jolliet P, Roeseler J, Chevrolet JC. Effects of helium-oxygen on intrinsic positive end-expiratory pressure in intubated and mechanically ventilated patients with severe chronic obstructive pulmonary disease. Crit Care Med 2000; 28:2721–8.

57. Lee DL, Lee H, Chang HW, et al. Heliox improves hemodynamics in mechanically ventilated patients with chronic obstructive pulmonary disease with systolic pressure variations. Crit Care Med 2005; 33:968–73.

58. Tassaux D, Jolliet P, Thouret JM, et al. Calibration of seven ICU ventilators for mechanical ventilation with helium-oxygen mixtures. Am J Respir Crit Care Med. 1999; 160:22–32.

59. Saulnier FF, Durocher AV, Deturck RA, et al. Respiratory and hemodynamic effects of halothane in status asthmaticus. Intensive Care Med 1990; 16:104–7.

60. Parnass SM, Feld JM, Chamberlin WH, Segil LJ. Status asthmaticus treated with isoflurane and enflurane. Anesth Analg 1987; 66:1193–5.

61. Maltais F, Sovilj M, Goldberg P, et al. Respiratory mechanics in status asthmaticus: Effects of inhalational anesthesia. Chest 1994; 105:1401–6.

62. Henke CA, Hertz M, Gustafson P. Combined bronchoscopy and mucolytic therapy for patients with severe refractory status asthmaticus on mechnical ventilation: A case report and review of the literature. Crit Care Med 1994; 22:1880–3.

63. Durward A, Forte V, Shemie SD. Resolution of mucus plugging and atelectasis after intratracheal rhDNase therapy in a mechanically ventilated child with refractory status asthmaticus. Crit Care Med 2000; 28:560–2.

64. Nakagawa TA, Johnston SJ, Falkos SA, et al. Life-threatening status asthmaticus treated with inhaled nitric oxide. J Pediatr 2000; 137:119–22.

65. Kuyper LM, Pare PD, Hogg JC, et al. Characterization of airway plugging in fatal asthma. Am J Med 2003; 115:6–11.

66. Shapiro MB, Kleaveland AC, Bartlett RH. Extracorporeal life support for status asthmaticus. Chest 1993; 103:1651–4.

67. Afessa B, Morales I, Cury JD. Clinical course and outcome of patients admitted to an ICU for status asthmaticus. Chest 2001; 120:1616–21.

68. Gupta D, Keogh B, Chung KF, et al. Characteristics and outcome for admissions to adult, general critical care units with acute severe asthma: A secondary analysis of the ICNARC Case Mix Programme Database. Crit Care 2004; 8:R112–21.

69. Scoggin CH, Sahn SA, Petty TL. Status asthmaticus: A nine-year experience. JAMA 1977; 238:1158–62.

70. Anzueto A, Frutos-Vivar F, Esteban A, et al. Incidence, risk factors and outcome of barotrauma in mechanically ventilated patients. Intensive Care Med 2004; 30:612–9.

71. Levine GN, Powell C, Bernard SA, et al. Acute, reversible left ventricular dysfunction in status asthmaticus. Chest 1995; 107:1469–73.

72. Sharkey SW, Shear W, Hodges M, Herzog CA. Reversible myocardial contraction abnormalities in patients with an acute noncardiac illness. Chest 1998; 114:98–105.

73. Barrett SA, Mourani S, Villareal CA, et al. Rhabdomyolysis associated with status asthmaticus. Crit Care Med 1993; 21:151–3.

74. Rabbat A, Laaban JP, Boussairi A, Rochemaure J. Hyperlactatemia during acute severe asthma. Intensive Care Med 1998; 24:304–12.

75. Mountain RD, Heffner JE, Brackett NC Jr, Sahn SA. Acid-base disturbances in acute asthma. Chest 1990; 98:651–5.

76. Appel D, Rubenstein R, Schrager K, Williams MH Jr. Lactic acidosis in severe asthma. Am J Med. 1983; 75:580–4.

77. Stratakos G, Kalomenidis J, Routsi C, et al. Transient lactic acidosis as a side effect of inhaled salbutamol. Chest 2002; 122:385–6.

78. Hanson P, Dive A, Brucher JM, et al. Acute corticosteroid myopathy in intensive care patients. Muscle Nerve 1997; 20:1371–80.

79. Marinelli WA, Leatherman JW. Neuromuscular disorders in the intensive care unit. Crit Care Clin 2002; 18:915–29.

80. Marquette CH, Saulnier F, Leroy O, et al. Long-term prognosis of near-fatal asthma: A 6-year follow-up study of 145 asthmatic patients who underwent mechanical ventilation for a near-fatal attack of asthma. Am Rev Respir Dis 1992; 146: 76–81.

Chapter 31

MECHANICAL VENTILATION IN CHRONIC OBSTRUCTIVE PULMONARY DISEASE

SONIA KHIRANI
GUIDO POLESE
LORENZO APPENDINI
ANDREA ROSSI

PATHOPHYSIOLOGY
  Hypoxemia
  Hypercapnia
  Respiratory Acidosis
VENTILATOR ASSISTANCE
  Noninvasive Positive-Pressure Ventilation
  Pressure-Support Ventilation
  Proportional-Assist Ventilation
  Other Modes of Ventilation
  Role of PEEP
  Controlled Mechanical Ventilation and Monitoring
  Home Mechanical Ventilation
  Failure and Success of Mechanical Ventilation
  Weaning
  Bronchodilators
  Mortality
CONCLUSION

Acute exacerbation of chronic obstructive pulmonary disease (COPD) is a common cause of respiratory failure. Many such patients need admission to the intensive-care unit (ICU). The institution of mechanical ventilation should be considered when hypercapnia and respiratory acidosis, often associated with breathlessness and tachypnea, persist or worsen despite aggressive and optimal medical therapy.[1–5] In some patients, ventilator assistance is instituted primarily to alleviate distressing breathlessness. On occasion, respiratory frequency can be abnormally low because of extreme hyperinflation.[6] Therefore, an arterial blood-gas (ABG) sample should be obtained in all patients considered for mechanical ventilation to confirm that dyspnea is related to respiratory acidosis and not to other causes that would not benefit from mechanical ventilation.

In the last 20 years, use of mechanical ventilation in patients with exacerbations of COPD and hypercapnic respiratory acidosis has undergone profound changes. The principal change has been the reevaluation of noninvasive mechanical ventilation (NIMV),[6,7] its rapid rise in popularity,[8] and its extensive application.[9,10] International guidelines for management of COPD,[11–13] as well as for NIMV,[14,15] recommend the early institution of NIMV as first-line treatment of exacerbations of COPD associated with respiratory failure and acidosis.

The decision-making process about the mode and setting of ventilator support requires knowledge of the pathophysiology of decompensated COPD, which has some peculiarities compared with acute respiratory failure from other causes.[14]

Pathophysiology

Inefficient gas exchange is a cardinal feature of patients with an exacerbation of COPD needing mechanical ventilation. The associated respiratory failure is characterized by hypoxemia (ratio of arterial oxygen tension to fractional inspired oxygen concentration, Pa_{O_2}/FI_{O_2}, less than 300 mmHg), often associated with hypercapnia (arterial carbon dioxide tension, Pa_{CO_2}, greater than 45 mmHg) and respiratory acidosis (arterial pH < 7.36).[1,16]

HYPOXEMIA

In general terms, hypoxemia results from the combination of *pulmonary* ventilation-perfusion ($\dot{V}_A/\dot{Q}$) mismatching, shunt, and reduced alveolar-capillary diffusion capacity and *extrapulmonary* [FI_{O_2}, minute ventilation, cardiac output, mixed venous $P_{O_2}(Pv_{O_2})$] determinants of Pa_{O_2}.[17] During exacerbations of COPD, both intrapulmonary and extrapulmonary factors contribute to the hypoxemia.

Stable COPD is characterized by an abnormal distribution of $\dot{V}_A/\dot{Q}$ ratios.[18] The abnormal distribution of pulmonary capillary blood flow and alveolar ventilation is the result of parenchymal destruction and small airways disease, respectively.[19–21] Figure 31-1 presents the four possible patterns of $\dot{V}_A/\dot{Q}$ mismatching. When an exacerbation occurs, $\dot{V}_A/\dot{Q}$ mismatching worsens, further impairing gas exchange (lung failure). Using the multiple inert-gas elimination technique (MIGET), hypoxemia during an exacerbation was found to be caused by the combination of $\dot{V}_A/\dot{Q}$ mismatching (46%), low Pv_{O_2} (26%), and increased peripheral oxygen (O_2) uptake (because of increased effort by the inspiratory muscles to bear the increased mechanical load[14]) (28%).[16] The true shunt fraction is consistently negligible. Thus administration of O_2-enriched air generally is effective in keeping oxyhemoglobin saturation (Sa_{O_2}) greater than 90%.

Pulse oximetry, although noninvasive and useful for monitoring oxygen saturation,[22] cannot replace periodic sampling of the arterial blood in patients with an exacerbation of COPD receiving ventilator assistance.[23–25] Indeed, oxygenation is only part of the problem. Hypercapnia and respiratory acidosis are also major concerns.

HYPERCAPNIA

Without supplemental O_2 (while breathing room air), patients with an exacerbation of COPD can develop hypercapnia, which is the result of the ineffective ventilatory pattern characterized by a rapid (high respiratory frequency) and

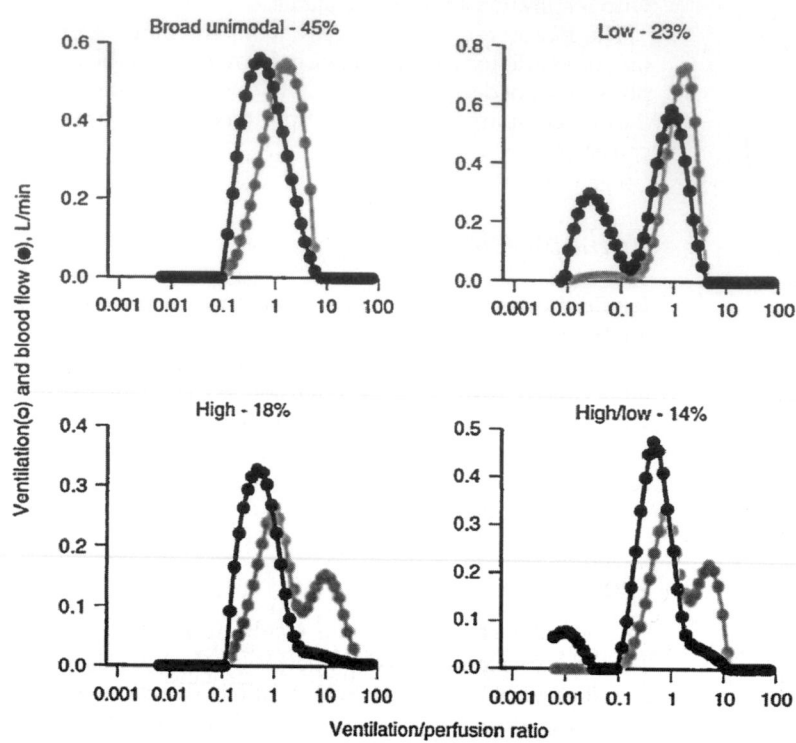

Patterns of Ventilation-Perfusion Distribution in COPD

FIGURE 31-1 Characteristic patterns of ventilation-perfusion mismatching in patients with COPD. Ventilation ($\dot{V}_A$; *gray circles*) and perfusion ($\dot{Q}$ *black circles*) distributions plotted against $\dot{V}_A/\dot{Q}$ ratios expressed on a logarithmic scale. (*Upper left panel*) Approximately 45% of patients show abnormally broad unimodal $\dot{V}_A$ and $\dot{Q}$ distributions centered on lung units with $\dot{V}_A/\dot{Q}$ ratios close to 1. (*Upper right panel*) In 23% of patients, a bimodal perfusion distribution with blood flow diverted to lung units with low $\dot{V}_A/\dot{Q}$ ratios (<0.1) is seen. (*Lower left panel*) A broad unimodal $\dot{Q}$ distribution together with a bimodal ventilation distribution with alveolar ventilation diverted to lung units with high $\dot{V}_A/\dot{Q}$ ratios is observed in 18% of patients. (*Lower right panel*) Approximately 14% of patients show both bimodal ventilation and perfusion distributions. Perfusion to nonventilated areas (shunt) is absent in these patients and negligible in general. (*Used, with permission, from Rossi et al: Respir Care Clin North Am 8:379–404, 2002.*)

shallow (low tidal volume, V_T) breathing (Fig. 31-2) leading to reduced alveolar ventilation.

An exacerbation of COPD almost invariably is associated with increased inflammation and altered mucus transport, particularly in the small airways. Hence airway resistance increases, leading to an augmented inspiratory effort to ven-

tilate the lungs[14,26] and a retarded rate of lung emptying. Thus the time between two inspiratory efforts is not sufficient to decompress the lungs to the relaxation volume,[27] generating dynamic pulmonary hyperinflation.[28–30] Consequently, positive end-expiratory alveolar pressure [conventionally named *intrinsic positive end-expiratory pressure* (PEEP$_I$)] is present. This pressure must be counterbalanced by the contracting inspiratory muscles in order to produce inspiratory flow[31] (Fig. 31-3).

A few cmH$_2$O of PEEP$_I$ usually are present in stable moderate to severe COPD.[32–34] During acute exacerbations, PEEP$_I$ increases significantly. Consequently, the inspiratory threshold load produces increased work of breathing and challenges the ability of the respiratory muscles to clear carbon dioxide (CO$_2$)[33] (see Fig. 31-2). The degree of PEEP$_I$ is related to the severity of resting hypercapnia.[28] Compensatory mechanisms exist[35,36] but are inadequate. The combination of increased mechanical load and reduced respiratory muscle force may lead to respiratory muscle fatigue and eventual exhaustion of the ventilatory pump.[37] Assisted ventilation needs to be instituted promptly as a lifesaving procedure.[14]

Purro et al[38] showed that the main characteristics of ventilator-dependent patients with extreme COPD are shallow breathing pattern; high (P$_{0.1}$), airway occlusion pressure, an index of overall neuromuscular drive[39]; high effective inspiratory impedance (P$_{0.1}$/V$_T$/T$_I$ ratio, where V$_T$ is tidal volume, T$_I$ is inspiratory duration, and V$_T$/T$_I$ is mean inspiratory flow)[40]; and high P/Pmax for both transdiaphragmatic (Pdi) and total pleural (Ppl) pressure.[41] A P$_{0.1}$/V$_T$/T$_I$ ratio greater than 10 cmH$_2$O/liter/s and a

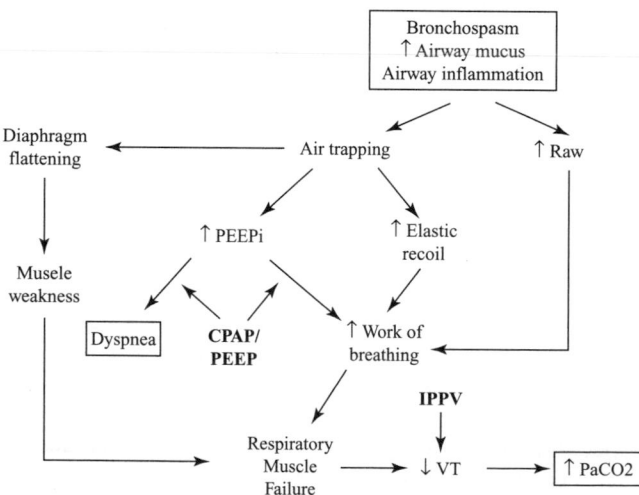

FIGURE 31-2 General mechanism leading to an increase in Pa$_{CO_2}$ in patients with COPD and ventilatory failure. Raw, airway resistance; PEEP$_I$, intrinsic positive end-expiratory pressure; CPAP, continuous positive airway pressure; IPPV, intermittent positive-pressure ventilation; V$_T$, tidal volume. (*Used, with permission, from International Consensus Conferences in Intensive Care Medicine: Am J Respir Crit Care Med 163:283–91, 2001.*)

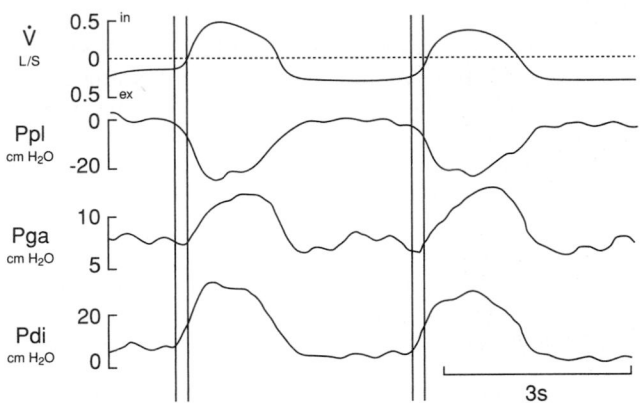

FIGURE 31-3 Method to determine dynamic intrinsic PEEP ($PEEP_{I,dyn}$) during spontaneous unoccluded breathing in a patient with COPD. (*From top to bottom*) Records of flow, pleural pressure (Ppl), gastric pressure (Pga), and transdiaphragmatic pressure (Pdi). The first vertical line indicates the point corresponding to the onset of the inspiratory effort (Pdi swing). The second vertical line indicates the point corresponding to the start of the inspiratory flow. The dotted horizontal line represents zero flow. In, inspiratory flow; ex, expiratory flow. Note that expiratory flow ends abruptly before inspiration, whereas the Pdi and Ppl swings have already begun, and Pga remains constant during the interval. $PEEP_{I,dyn}$ is measured as the negative deflection in Ppl between the onset of the Pdi swing and the point of zero flow. (*Used, with permission, from Saetta et al: Am Rev Respir Dis 132:894–900, 1985.*)

Pdi/Pdi,max of greater than 40% were associated with inability to sustain spontaneous breathing for more than a few minutes.[38] The ineffective compensatory mechanism with the low V_T caused chronic CO_2 retention. The data of Purro et al[38] were collected in a special long-term weaning unit. Nevertheless, the results are in line with many other studies showing that patients with COPD develop a high respiratory drive in trying to cope with an excessive mechanical load.

RESPIRATORY ACIDOSIS

When the lungs cannot remove all the CO_2 produced by the body, or when alveolar ventilation is decreased, respiratory acidosis occurs. Respiratory acidosis represents a Pa_{CO_2} that is higher than normal (>45 mmHg), leading to an arterial blood pH of less than 7.36. If a patient with respiratory acidosis breathes ambient air, life-threatening hypoxemia ensues. One reason for hypercapnia is inappropriately increased supplemental oxygen.[42] Supercabia (Pa_{CO_2} > 150 mmHg) can occur.

Correction of respiratory acidosis should be performed carefully.[1] The goal is to return pH toward normal limits, not to return P_{CO_2} to normal.[3,43,44] Vigorous increases in minute ventilation should be avoided because of the risk of dynamic hyperinflation. When dynamic hyperinflation is a concern, and provided that intracranial hypertension and overt hemodynamic instability do not exist, acceptance of acidemia (pH > 7.2) may be reasonable.[45]

Ventilator Assistance

Ventilator assistance can be delivered to patients with an exacerbation of COPD in different ways[1]: traditional or conventional invasive mechanical ventilation (via an endotracheal tube) or noninvasive mechanical ventilation (NIMV) by means of either negative (intermittent) pressure ventilation (iron lung) or noninvasive positive-pressure ventilation (NPPV). The latter is by far the most common mode of assistance in patients with exacerbations of COPD. Negative-pressure ventilation is effective clinically[46] and physiologically[47] in the hands of a well-trained team but has not gained wide popularity.

NONINVASIVE POSITIVE-PRESSURE VENTILATION

Although available for many years, only in the late 1980s and early 1990s was NIMV reintroduced successfully in the treatment of hypercapnic respiratory failure.[6,48] It soon became clear that patients with exacerbations of COPD derive most benefit from NIMV.[7–10,49–51] NIMV can produce significant decreases in in-hospital and 1-year mortality, need of endotracheal intubation, rate of ventilator-related complications, rate of ICU admission, and length of ICU and hospital stay.[51,52] These significant achievements were the result of a synergic effort: major advances in the knowledge of the pathophysiology of respiratory failure caused by exacerbation of COPD, improvement in the technology of noninvasive ventilators, improvement in the interfaces for the patient-ventilator connection, and the organization of prospective randomized clinical trials.

The best candidates for NIMV are patients with dyspnea, increased breathing frequency, hypercapnia, and respiratory acidosis who are able to cooperate with their caregivers and interact with the ventilator. The patient shares the act of breathing with the ventilator and must trigger each mechanical breath. According to international guidelines on COPD[11–13] and NPPV,[15] NPPV is a first-line intervention, together with optimal medical therapy and O_2 supplementation, for the management of patients with hypercapnic respiratory failure secondary to exacerbations of COPD. In the first few hours, NPPV requires the same level of assistance as conventional ventilation.[53,54] In appropriate settings, NPPV can be as effective as conventional ventilation in reversing acute respiratory failure secondary to decompensation of COPD.[55]

Despite the widespread use of NPPV, many patients with exacerbations of COPD and respiratory acidosis still need endotracheal intubation and conventional ventilation,[56] which may be more appropriate.[8] It always must be promptly available in any environment administering NIMV. Controlled ventilation can be delivered only in intubated patients, whereas assisted ventilation can be applied either through an endotracheal tube or noninvasively.

In patients receiving NPPV, intubation should be considered when NPPV seems to fail,[57–59] as shown by worsening of ABGs over 1–2 hours or lack of improvement in ABGs after 4 hours.

In many instances, the choice of the ventilator mode depends more on local organizational considerations than on scientific guidelines (e.g., physician preference and experience, available types of ventilators, team training, and so on). Recent approaches tend to give to the patient greater control of the ventilator either mechanically or through respiratory center drive.[60]

NPPV can be considered successful when ABGs and pH improve, dyspnea is relieved, the exacerbation resolves without intubation, mechanical ventilation can be discontinued, and the patient is discharged from the hospital.

PRESSURE-SUPPORT VENTILATION

The most popular mode of delivering NPPV is pressure-support ventilation (PSV).[61] It was introduced by Brochard et al[62] as a mode of conventional ventilation. In patients with COPD, optimal PSV decreases O_2 cost of breathing, diaphragmatic pressure-time index,[62–67] and work of breathing.[4,62,64,68,69] PSV does not worsen dynamic hyperinflation and $PEEP_I$ in some patients with COPD.[70–72]

PSV was used preferentially by several groups for NPPV in patients with acute exacerbations of COPD admitted to an ICU.[4,7,73–77] PSV by face mask decreases respiratory muscle activity and workload.[61,77–79] The most effective mode of NPPV is the combination of PSV (10–15 cmH_2O) and continuous positive airway pressure (CPAP) (4–8 cmH_2O).[80] The only study addressing the effect of noninvasive PSV on gas exchange with the MIGET technique showed that NPPV does not improve $\dot{V}_A/\dot{Q}$ mismatching significantly, but it increases alveolar ventilation by correcting breathing pattern, which achieves more efficient clearance of arterial CO_2.[81]

In patients with COPD ventilated through a tracheotomy, Appendini et al[82] showed that 5 cmH_2O of CPAP plus 10 cmH_2O of PSV were more effective in unloading the inspiratory muscles than 15 cmH_2O of PSV. In other words, the same global level of pressure assistance achieved a better physiologic result if partitioned between CPAP and PSV rather than when delivered as PSV alone. This confirms the important role of the inspiratory threshold load in COPD patents.

Brochard et al[78] reported differences between various devices for noninvasive PSV. These differences have an impact on patient effort.[83]

PROPORTIONAL-ASSIST VENTILATION

Proportional-assist ventilation (PAV) was proposed as a means of bringing one oscillatory pump (the ventilator) under the control of another (the patient's controller).[84,85] With PAV, responsibility for guiding the ventilatory pattern is shifted completely from the caregiver to the patient, with the aim of improving patient-ventilator interaction (Fig. 31-4). NPPV was considered as an application in which PAV should display advantages over conventional modes.[86–89] Nevertheless, the few clinical studies performed during invasive ventilation[90–93] and NPPV in patients with acute or chronic respiratory failure[94–97] did not find PAV to be significantly superior to PSV. Invasive PAV, however, enabled greater V_T variability than invasive PSV in the face of increased ventilatory demand.[90–93] Both invasive and noninvasive PAV improved ABGs and alveolar ventilation and unloaded the respiratory muscles in both acute[86,87,98] and chronic patients.[88,89] Wysocki et al[99] found that NPPV-PAV

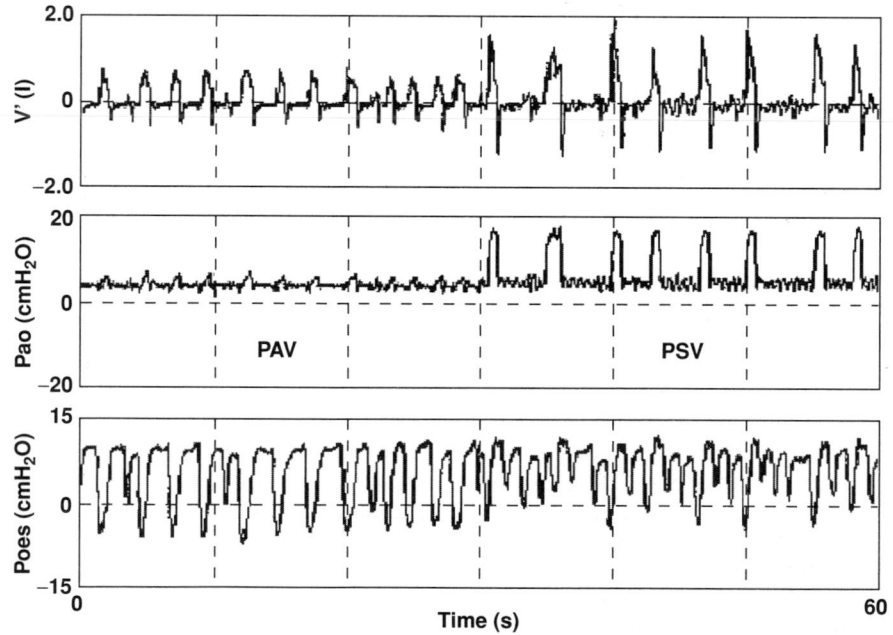

FIGURE 31-4 Representative tracing in a patient with COPD and chronic ventilatory failure during proportional-assist ventilation (PAV) (*left*) and pressure-support ventilation (PSV) (*right*) showing pressure at the airway opening (Pao) and esophageal pressure (Poes). With greater assistance during PSV, the occurrence of ineffective efforts increases compared with PAV. (*Used, with permission, from Ambrosino et al: Thorax 57:272–6, 2002.*)

and NPPV-PSV achieved similar improvements in work of breathing and ABGs. Patient comfort, however, was better with PAV.[100]

In conclusion, the most common ventilator setting of NPPV for patients with COPD in acute respiratory failure remains a few cmH$_2$O of CPAP, to counterbalance intrinsic PEEP, and PSV on top of CPAP to support the inspiratory effort and increase V$_T$.[14,80] The role for PAV requires further exploration.

OTHER MODES OF VENTILATION

ASSIST-VOLUME CONTROL

With assist-volume control (AVC) ventilation, V$_T$, inspiratory flow rate, flow waveform, and trigger sensitivity are set. In patients with COPD and high levels of PEEP$_I$, AVC ventilation with high inspiratory flow rates is recommended (provided that plateau pressure is not increased excessively) because it shortens inspiratory time and increases expiratory time, potentially reducing PEEP$_I$.[101] A V$_T$ of about 7–9 ml/kg is prudent in COPD. AVC ventilation was used in some studies of NPPV in decompensated COPD,[77,102] although PSV is now used much more commonly.[51]

PRESSURE CONTROL

With pressure-control ventilation (PCV), the maximal pressure generated by the ventilator, the frequency, and the inspiratory time are set. V$_T$ is the primary output and depends on patient impedance, PEEP$_I$, and ventilator settings. Maximal airway and alveolar pressures are controlled. With rapid variations in patient impedance, as in acute COPD, PCV will not deliver a consistent V$_T$.[103] This mode basically is restricted to conventional ventilation.

INTERMITTENT MANDATORY VENTILATION

With intermittent mandatory ventilation (IMV), unsynchronized breaths were feared to predispose patients to hyperinflation and barotrauma.[4] Synchronized intermittent mandatory ventilation (SIMV), an evolution of IMV, was designed to avoid dyssynchrony. It was believed that SIMV would facilitate weaning by allowing patients to assume graded increases in the work of breathing. Aslanian and Brochard[64] considered this mode to represent "an interesting example of the discrepancy which can be found between the objectives of a modality of partial ventilatory support and its real physiological effects." Two studies showed that SIMV was the least effective weaning method,[104,105] although another study found SIMV to be useful in weaning of patients with COPD.[106] In the latter study, addition of PSV tended to produce a slight but not significantly shorter weaning time.

ROLE OF PEEP

PEEP is one of the most successful clinical applications of respiratory physiology. It was introduced 40 years ago in the management of patients with acute respiratory failure.[107] The effect of PEEP in COPD depends on the mechanism of PEEP$_I$ and its magnitude.[108–110] Several studies documented that PEEP$_I$ is common in ventilator-dependent patients with COPD.[32,38,111–114] In some instances, the level

TABLE 31-1 Factors Determining Dynamic Pulmonary Hyperinflation and Intrinsic PEEP

Patient respiratory mechanics
  Pulmonary flow resistance
  Expiratory flow limitation
  Total respiratory system compliance
Added flow resistance
  Endotracheal tube
  Ventilator tubings and circuits
Patient breathing pattern and ventilator setting
  Tidal volume
  Frequency
  T$_I$/T$_{TOT}$
  End-inspiratory pause

ABBREVIATIONS: PEEP, positive end-expiratory pressure; T$_I$/T$_{TOT}$, fractional inspiratory time.
SOURCE: Used, with permission, from ref. 209.

of PEEP$_I$ is so high that without the addition of PEEP, the patient cannot trigger the ventilator. The resulting ineffective efforts unduly increase the respiratory workload. PEEP$_I$ is caused by both intrapulmonary and extrapulmonary factors[32] (Table 31-1) in patients with acute respiratory failure, including those with acute respiratory distress syndrome[115,116] and acute severe asthma.[116]

In the presence of expiratory flow limitation, stepwise application of PEEP does not increase end-expiratory lung volume (EELV) until a level close to PEEP$_I$ is reached.[108,111,117] When PEEP exceeds initial PEEP$_I$, EELV may increase, worsening pulmonary hyperinflation. In ventilator-dependent patients with COPD, several studies showed that low levels of PEEP induced a reduction of the inspiratory threshold load without affecting EELV.[111–113,118–120] Although there is still debate on "optimal PEEP" in ventilated patients with COPD, a reasonable approach is to set a few cmH$_2$O of PEEP and ensure that the patient is comfortable and able to trigger all ventilator breaths. Alternatively, PEEP$_I$ can be measured.[121–124] The more accurate method requires an esophageal balloon and sometimes an additional gastric balloon to assess changes in abdominal and transdiaphragmatic pressures.[125–127] Measurement of changes in abdominal pressure allows correction of PEEP$_I$ for expiratory muscle activity[125,126,128] and a more exact computation of PEEP$_I$.[24,33,129]

During controlled mechanical ventilation (CMV), the respiratory muscles are inactive and cannot be unloaded. Nevertheless, Rossi et al[130] showed that replacement of PEEP$_I$ with PEEP (of 50–100% of the measured static PEEP$_I$) may improve, slightly but significantly, $\dot{V}_A/\dot{Q}$ mismatching and oxygenation without any effect on cardiac output.

In conclusion, low levels of CPAP/PEEP are recommended in patients with COPD needing mechanical ventilation, either conventionally or by NPPV.

CONTROLLED MECHANICAL VENTILATION AND MONITORING

CMV is used less commonly in the ICU than in the past because of wider use of NIMV and improved pharmacologic

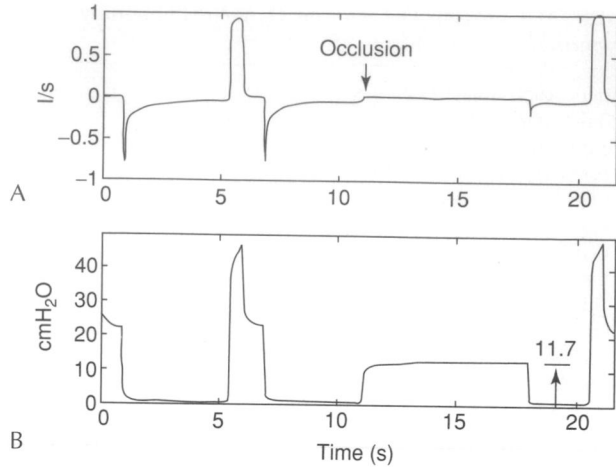

FIGURE 31-5 Measurement of static intrinsic positive end-expiratory pressure (PEEP$_{I,st}$) by the end-expiratory occlusion maneuver in a patient with COPD. The arrow in *B* indicates the value of PEEP$_{I,st}$. (*Used, with permission, from Nucci et al: J Appl Physiol 89:985–95, 2000.*)

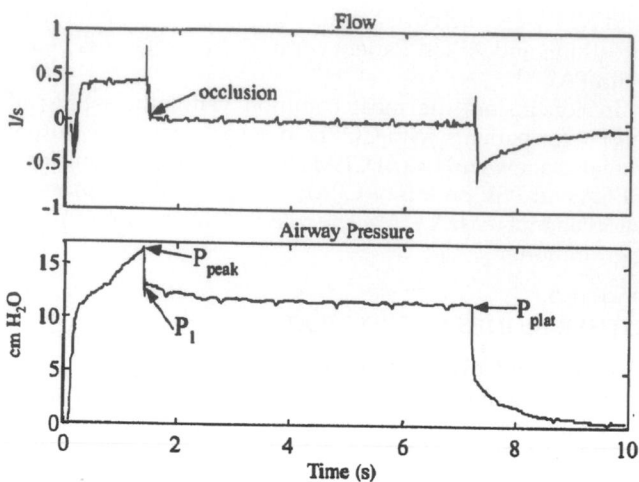

FIGURE 31-6 Tracings of flow and pressure at the airway opening in a ventilated patient with COPD in whom an end-inspiratory occlusion during constant-flow inflation has been performed. After end-inspiratory occlusion, there was an immediate drop in pressure from the maximum value (Ppeak) to a lower value (P$_1$) and then by a slow decay to an apparent plateau (Pplat), which is achieved after 2 seconds. (*Used, with permission, from Rossi et al.[133]*)

treatment of COPD.[80] CMV, however, provides a unique opportunity to measure passive respiratory mechanics.[24,129] Measurements can be performed using offline (i.e., ventilator facilities, physiologic equipment, or interfering maneuvers) or online (i.e., acquisition equipment, mathematical models, and continuous breath-by-breath analysis) techniques. Several studies have shown that respiratory mechanics are severely abnormal in ventilated patients with COPD, particularly in the early days of ventilation[131] and at the end stage of the disease.[38]

The rapid airway-occlusion technique is a simple method for assessing respiratory mechanics based on airway opening pressure and flow measurements.[132,133] When applied at the end of expiration [end-expiratory occlusion (EEO); Fig. 31-5], this technique provides a measure of the static PEEP$_I$, also known as *auto-PEEP*.[132] If applied just before the end of inspiration [end-inspiratory occlusion (EIO); Fig. 31-6], it enables measurement of most variables of respiratory mechanics [static elastance (Est), interrupter resistance (Rint), and total flow resistance (Rtot)].[24,129]

Rint represents airway resistance. Rtot represents total respiratory system resistance after subtracting flow resistance of the endotracheal tube.[134–140] In ventilated patients with COPD, ΔR (the difference between Rtot and Rint, caused by tissue-stress adaptation and time-constant inhomogeneity within the lungs) amounts to almost 50% of Rtot; this indicates that the periphery of the lungs contributes significantly to total flow resistance.[133]

During CMV, dynamic PEEP$_I$ (PEEP$_{I,dyn}$) represents the lowest regional PEEP$_I$ that has to be counterbalanced by the positive pressure of the ventilator to start inspiratory flow (Fig. 31-7). This can be assessed by superimposing flow–airway pressure loops and looking at the point where pressure tracings cross the zero flow[33] (Fig. 31-8). With severe airflow limitation, considerable regional variations in mechanical time constants exist. Thus the value of PEEP$_I$ may vary between different measurements and be underestimated.[5]

During relaxed expiration, dynamic pulmonary hyperinflation, if present, can be computed from the difference in volume between the end-expiratory volume of relaxed expiration and the end-expiratory volume of the preceding breath. Expiratory flow limitation also can be disclosed by the lack of change in flow with alteration in pressure at the airway opening (PEEP, NEP: negative expiratory pressure)[28,141] or flow resistance.[121,141]

The measurements just mentioned are not suitable for continuous monitoring.[142,143] Accordingly, new interest has focused on online monitoring of respiratory mechanics in ventilated patients[33,122,144] because it enables early detection of changes in a patient's status, thus enabling rapid therapeutic intervention. The monitoring systems currently used, however, are based on the assumption of a first-order linear model of respiratory mechanics, whereas resistance and elastance are known to be dependent on volume and airflow.

One algorithm to track respiratory parameters in real time is the recursive least-squares (RLS) algorithm.[145] Nucci et al[33,144] have adopted a modified RLS algorithm based on nonlinear behavior of respiratory mechanics,[146] combined with a classic first-order model and continuous measurement of airflow and airway pressure, to estimate respiratory mechanics in ventilated patients, including those with COPD. The mean estimated values weighted on inspiration are updated on a cycle-by-cycle basis. Nucci et al[33] compares different methods of measuring PEEP$_I$ (Fig. 31-9). The varying numbers reflect different physiologic connotations of the data obtained with the different techniques.

Recently, Volta et al[147] applied a different method based on least-squares fitting with a first-order model, keeping resistance and compliance constant over the whole breathing cycle. They concluded that data weighted on inspiration

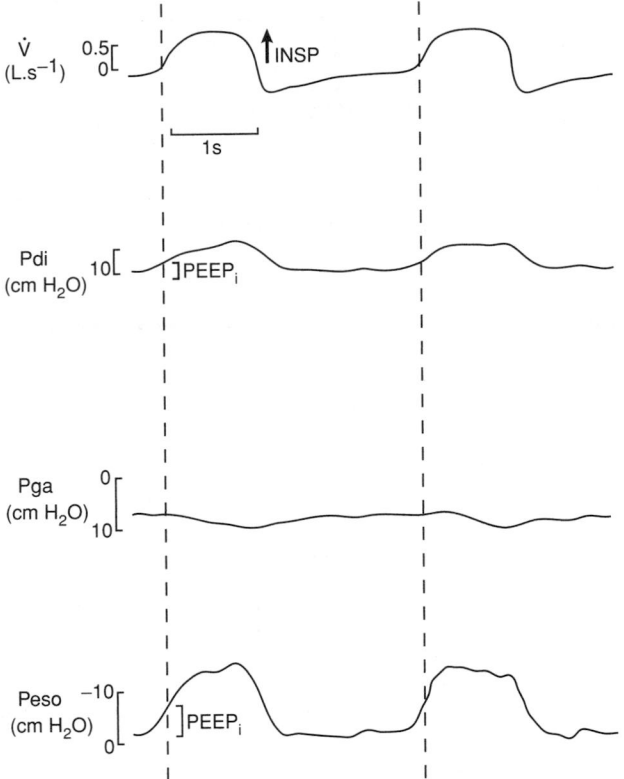

FIGURE 31-7 Tracings of flow, transdiaphragmatic (Pdi), gastric (Pga), and esophageal (Pes) pressures in a representative patient with COPD during tidal breathing. Tidal volume was 0.75 liter. The vertical dashed lines correspond to the start of inspiratory flow. Note that expiratory flow ends abruptly at the end of expiration ("truncated" appearance), whereas the Pdi and Pes swings (inspiratory effort) already have begun, and Pga remains constant in the interval. The difference between the onset of swings in Pdi and Pes and the point of zero flow on the Pes tracing represents the intrinsic PEEP (dynamic), which has to be counterbalanced by the inspiratory muscles in order to start inspiration. (*Used, with permission, from Rossi et al.[218]*)

were acceptable in patients with and without expiratory flow limitation.

Khirani et al[148] proposed a new method based on a mathematical model for noninvasive detection of expiratory airflow limitation. The model parameters were identified via a nonlinear curve-fitting method (Levenberg-Marquardt). Expiratory airflow limitation was correlated with a sharp increase in a parameter of the model, which represents resistance of the compressible airway. Agreement was found between flow-volume curve indications and model simulations for severe expiratory airflow limitation.

Future studies should focus on online monitoring when respiratory activity is present because most modes involve assisted ventilation.

HOME MECHANICAL VENTILATION

Most patients treated with NIMV can be weaned within a few days. If NIMV is needed for more than 1 week, this suggests that long-term NIMV may be necessary, and the patient may need to be referred to a center providing home NIMV. Long-term domiciliary NIMV should be considered in patients with COPD who have had three or more episodes of acute hypercapnic respiratory failure in the preceding year. The role of long-term nocturnal NIMV in COPD is not yet clearly established.[15] Chronic NPPV should not be prescribed systematically in patients with COPD and chronic ventilatory failure, although it may produce benefit in selected yet-to-be defined patients.[149] Some patients with end-stage COPD undergo tracheotomy and become chronically ventilator-dependent.[6]

Because home ventilation is applied long term and deteriorations can occur quickly and out of sight, it is important to include a monitoring strategy.[150] Peak flow, oximetry, and leaks can be monitored by patients themselves. Spirometry and muscular pressure measurements can be monitored frequently by staff visiting the home.

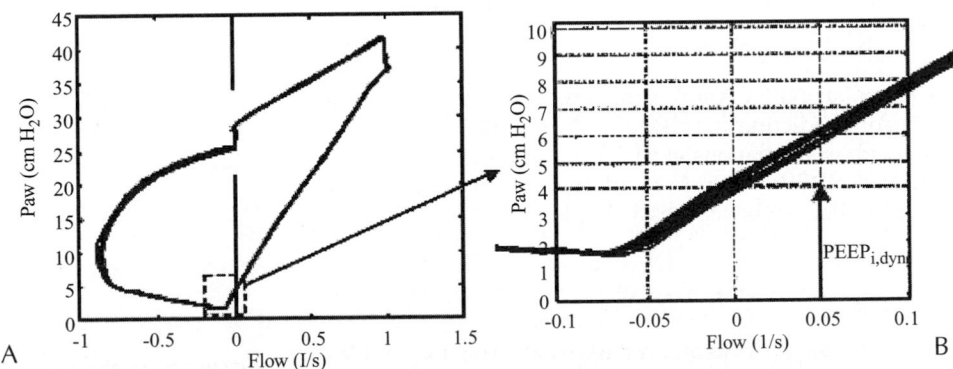

FIGURE 31-8 Determination of dynamic PEEP$_I$ (PEEP$_{I,dyn}$). *A.* Airway pressure (Paw) versus flow diagram. Twenty-two consecutive ventilatory cycles are superimposed. Inspiration is rightward. Note that the start of inspiration precedes the zero flow (*dotted line*). The dashed box in panel *A* is magnified in *B.* Dynamic PEEP$_I$ (PEEP$_{I,dyn}$) is measured as the difference between the value of Paw at zero flow and end-expiratory pressure. The small end-expiratory pressure reflects the resistive pressure consequent to end-expiratory flow and is included in the value of PEEP$_{I,dyn}$. (*Used, with permission, from Nucci et al: J Appl Physiol 89:985–95, 2000.*)

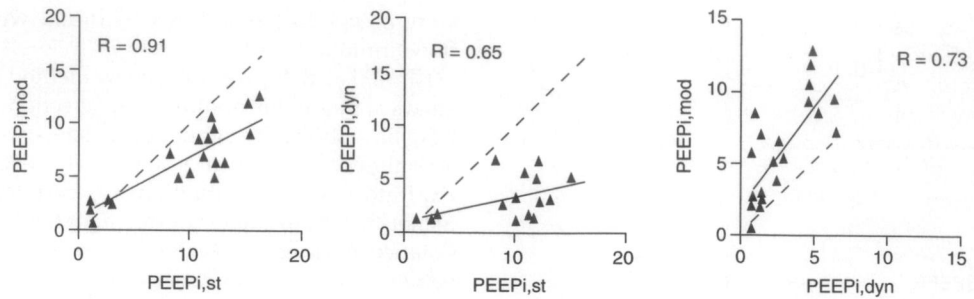

FIGURE 31-9 Identity plots comparing values of static (st), dynamic (dyn), and model (mod) PEEP$_I$ at zero end-expiratory pressure (ZEEP). Model PEEP$_I$ was computed according to the RLS as suggested by Nucci et al.[33] The values obtained by the three methods are significantly correlated. Dashed line is the identity line, and solid line is computed according to regression analysis. R, coefficient of correlation. For further explanations see text. (*Used, with permission, from Nucci et al: J Appl Physiol 89:985–95, 2000.*)

FAILURE AND SUCCESS OF MECHANICAL VENTILATION

Complications during mechanical ventilation in patients with COPD are similar to those in other groups of patients.[1,2,5] Dynamic hyperinflation is a major factor responsible for ventilator dependency and weaning failure.[162] In the presence of dynamic hyperinflation, high alveolar pressures ensue and may cause pneumothorax, ventilator-induced lung injury, or hypotension. The latter occurs most often immediately after intubation.[1]

NPPV decreases mortality from acute respiratory failure, need for endotracheal intubation (in more than 50% of patients when used as initial treatment[151]), treatment failure, and complications of intubation and ventilation.[152] A face mask achieves more rapid correction of hypercapnia than a nasal mask during NPPV[7,74,153,154] and can be more effective.[76] Use of helium-oxygen (HeO$_2$) during NPPV markedly enhances the ability of NPPV to reduce patient effort and improve gas exchange.[155]

Factors associated with success of NPPV include younger age, ability to cooperate, lower acuity of illness, an experienced team of caregivers, and availability of resources (monitoring). NPPV fails when the patient either needs intubation or dies because intubation is not performed (i.e., for ethical reasons or because it is not available). Adjustments of the mask and ventilator settings are essential during the first 30–60 minutes of NPPV; patients who show improvement in gas exchange within the first hour are more likely to avoid intubation.[8]

The Italian NPPV study group recently proposed two charts for predicting the risk of failure with NIMV in patients with exacerbations of COPD (at admission and after 2 hours of NPPV).[57] Figure 31-10 presents an example of a flowchart that can be used as a simple tool.

WEANING

Most ventilated patients are weaned easily from the ventilator, although some require considerable time.[156,157] Difficult-to-wean patients have a high hospital mortality and poor long-term prognosis.[158,159] Reintubation should be avoided because it carries a 6 to 12-fold increased risk of mortality. Continuation of unnecessary ventilator support also car-

ries risks.[160] Weaning failure is associated with increased work of breathing and a high tension-time index.[161] Dynamic hyperinflation is a major determinants of weaning failure.[116,145,162] Decreasing the breathing load and increasing respiratory muscle capacity are the major strategies for achieving successful weaning. Purro et al[38] suggested that measurement of P$_{0.1}$ and breathing pattern may help to discover why some patients are ventilator-dependent.

Three randomized trials suggest a place for NPPV in weaning selected patients with COPD.[163–165] NPPV weaning was associated with a shorter duration of invasive ventilation. Two other studies failed to show a benefit of NPPV.[166,167] Further studies are needed to assess the role of NPPV.[168]

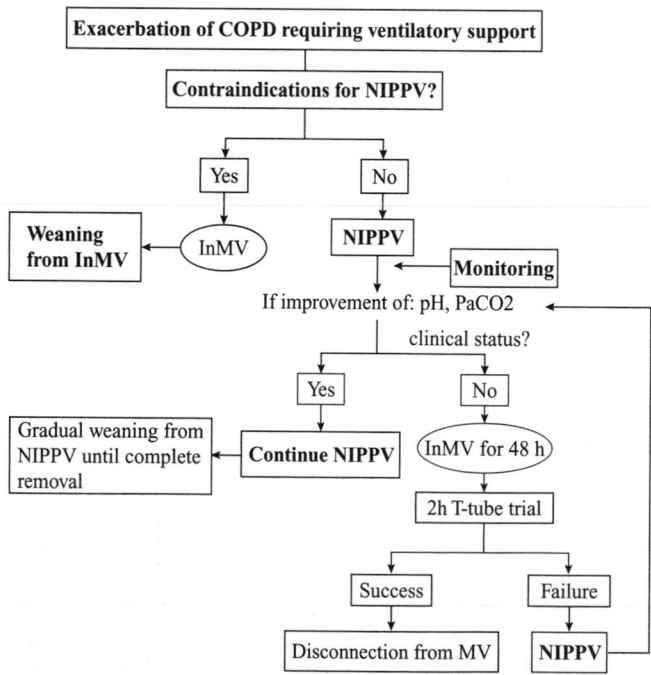

FIGURE 31-10 Flowchart for the use of noninvasive positive-pressure ventilation (NIPPV) during exacerbation of COPD with acute respiratory failure. MV, mechanical ventilation; InMV, invasive MV; Pa$_{CO_2}$, arterial carbon dioxide tension. (*Modified, with permission, from Celli et al: Eur Respir J 23:932–46, 2004.*)

Ceriana et al[169] assessed the value of a decision flowchart in deciding whether to wean tracheotomized patients receiving long-term ventilation. They removed the tracheotomy cannula in about 80% of patients without major complication. It is important to note that "protocols (and the weaning parameters therein) are meant to help guide and expedite, and they never should substitute for common sense."[170]

BRONCHODILATORS

Guidelines[80,171] recommend inhaled bronchodilators as first-line therapy in the management of COPD and discourage the use of systemic corticosteroids in stable patients. Short-acting bronchodilators (β-agonists, anticholinergics, or the combination) are the key component.[172] Bach et al[173] found no significant difference between β-agonists and anticholinergics. No substantial data demonstrate the superiority of combination therapy over either agent alone.[174] Turner et al[175] showed no difference between administration via a nebulizer versus metered-dose inhaler with spacer.

Administering bronchodilators to intubated patients is challenging.[172,176] To improve drug delivery to the airways, a spacer device is helpful during conventional ventilation or NPPV.[177,178] Several studies document that the inhaled route is at least as effective and safe as parenteral administration in ventilated patients.[177–181]

MORTALITY

COPD is a leading cause of death worldwide and the only major cause of death still rising.[80,171] The rate of hospitalization for acute exacerbations of COPD is high, although knowledge about critical determinants is incomplete.

Connors et al[182] studied the outcome of patients hospitalized for acute exacerbations of severe COPD in five hospitals. They found that 11% of the patients died within 6 months of the in-hospital period and 43% after 1 year. Seneff et al[183] observed a mortality of 24% after 1 year among patients hospitalized for an acute exacerbation of COPD; in patients 65 years of age or older, mortality doubled at 1 year. The need for mechanical ventilation on admission did not influence short- or long-term outcomes.

Only one study has compared the outcomes between NPPV and conventional ventilation in an ICU environment; no difference in mortality or complications was observed.[55] Table 31-2 shows 1-year survival in patients with COPD receiving conventional therapy or NIMV in four studies.[52,184–186] Survival was better in the NIMV group. Some studies showed a 1-year survival rate of 44–66% after invasive ventilation in patients with COPD and respiratory failure.[186–188] Plant and Elliott[189] found that survival after invasive ventilation was worse than after NIMV.

NPPV reduces mortality in patients with COPD in hypercapnic acute respiratory failure.[10,14,152,190–192] Several studies support the early use of NPPV in this setting.[107–116] The benefit of early application of NPPV appears to be greater than in the case with invasive ventilation.[193] Keenan et al[194]

TABLE 31-2   Controlled Clinical Trials of Conventional Therapy versus Noninvasive Mechanical Ventilation: 1-Year Survival

Author (Ref.)	n	Conventional Therapy	NIMV
Plant (184)	118/118	54%	62%
Bardi (52)	15/15	53%	87%
Confalonieri (185)	24/24	50%	71%
Vitacca (186)	27/30	37%[a]	70%

ABBREVIATIONS: *n*, number of patients in each group, NIMV, noninvasive mechanical ventilation.
[a] All patients were intubated in the conventional therapy group.
SOURCE: Used, with permission, from ref. 189.

and Plant et al[51,184] showed that addition of NPPV to standard therapy in patients with acute respiratory failure improved in-hospital survival only in the subgroup with an exacerbation of COPD.[195] Antón et al[196] found the evolution of ABGs, particularly pH, after 1 hour of NIMV to be the best predictor of outcome. Although NIMV reduces in-hospital mortality, its effectiveness needs to be monitored.[51,55,184]

Girou et al[152] and Carlucci et al[197] recently reported a learning effect with the use of NIMV over an 8-year period. The efficacy of NIMV technique also depends on the skill and motivation of the care team.[78]

Table 31-3 presents the risk differences for hospital mortality rates between NPPV and control groups in several studies and clearly shows the benefit of NPPV. Those studies concluded that NPPV was indicated in patients with a severe acute exacerbation of COPD but not in patients with mild exacerbations of COPD. Esteban et al[198] reported that survival of ventilated patients is related to factors at baseline (start of mechanical ventilation) and to the development of complications and patient management in the ICU.

NIMV is now well established in the management of COPD, and more patients should survive an acute exacerbation.[199] Because patients who receive NIMV for an acute exacerbation of COPD are at high risk for hospital

TABLE 31-3   Hospital Mortality Rates, Expressed as Risk Difference, for Severe and Nonsevere Exacerbations of COPD

Study (Ref.)	Risk Difference
Severe exacerbations	
Bott et al (210)	25
Servillo et al (211)	0
Brochard et al (190)	22
Angus et al (212)	45
Avdeev et al (213)	20
Celikel et al (214)	10
Plant et al (51)	12
Confalonieri et al (58)	12
Dikensoy et al (215)	8
Nonsevere exacerbations	
Barbé et al (216)	0
Keenan et al (217)	2

NOTE: Risk differences, with the exception of 0%, indicate an outcome in favor of NPPV.
SOURCE: : Modified, with permission, from Keenan et al.[8]

readmission and death,[199,200] Elliott suggested that home NIMV might improve their long-term outcome.[199] Ram et al,[201] however, found equivalent readmission rates and mortality at 2–3 months between home management and in-hospital care of such patients. Tarnow-Mordi et al[202] demonstrated a negative effect of excessive workload of hospital staff on hospital mortality.

Conclusion

Two major changes have occurred in the mechanical ventilation of patients with COPD in ventilatory failure and respiratory acidosis in recent years. First, PEEP and CPAP, formerly banned, are now used commonly to counterbalance $PEEP_I$. Second, NIMV, particularly as NPPV, is successful when optimal medical therapy and oxygenation fail to reverse respiratory failure. All international guidelines recommend the use of NPPV in such patients. The results of NPPV should be monitored carefully to assess success or failure.[203,204] Local organization and expertise of the caregiver team are the major determinants of how, when, and where to ventilate decompensated patients with COPD.

Randomized clinical trials form the backbone of modern therapy. They were based on innovative observation of a few original investigators who dared to propose unorthodox thinking and found open-minded journal editors. Examples include the pioneering work by Darioli and Perret,[205] who first proposed permissive hypercapnia in status asthmaticus, and Meduri et al,[73] who used mask ventilation in critically ill patients refusing intubation. The data of Darioli and Perret[205] were so convincing, though uncontrolled, that no randomized trial in acute severe asthma followed that study. The concept of controlled hypoventilation and permissive hypercapnia also has met with success in acute respiratory distress syndrome (ARDS).[206]

Progress in the field of mechanical ventilation (NPPV, low V_T, PEEP/CPAP in COPD) contributes to the contemporary debate between physiology[207] and cell biology[208] and supports the view that physiologic studies play a substantial role to advancement in clinical medicine.[207] Specifically, more physiologic studies are needed to better understand changes in lung mechanics and gas exchange in exacerbations of COPD so as to better identify which individual patients are likely to benefit from knowledge generated by randomized clinical trials.

References

1. Georgopoulos D, Rossi A. Invasive mechanical ventilation in acute exacerbation of chronic obstructive pulmonary disease. In: Anthonisen NR, Siafakas N, editors. Acute exacerbations of COPD: Lung biology in heath and disease. Basel, Switzerland: Marcel Dekker AG, 2003.
2. Aldrich TK, Prezant DJ. Indications for mechanical ventilation. In: Tobin MJ, editor. Principles and practice of mechanical ventilation. New York: McGraw-Hill, 1994: 155.
3. Georgopoulos D, Rossi A, Moxham J. Ventilatory support in COPD. European Respiratory Monograph 1998; 7:189–208.
4. Ambrosino N, Simonds AK. Mechanical ventilation. In: Muir J-F, Ambrosino N, Simonds AK, editors. The European Respiratory Monograph, vol 13. Sheffield, UK: European Respiratory Society Journals, Ltd., 2000: 155.
5. Leatherman JW. Mechanical ventilation in obstructive lung disease. In: Nahum A, Marini JJ, editors. Clinics in chest medicine: Recent advances in mechanical ventilation, vol 17. Philadelphia: Saunders, 1996: 577.
6. Meduri GU. Noninvasive positive-pressure ventilation in patients with acute respiratory failure. In: Marini JJ, Slutsky AS, editors. Lung biology in health and disease, Vol 118: Physiological basis of ventilatory support. New York: Marcel Dekker, 1998: 921.
7. Brochard L, Isabey D, Piquet J, et al. Reversal of acute exacerbations of chronic obstructive pulmonary disease by inspiratory assistance with a face mask. New Engl J Med 1990; 323:1523–30.
8. Keenan SP, Sinuff T, Cook DJ, et al. Which patients with acute exacerbation of chronic obstructive pulmonary disease benefit from noninvasive positive-pressure ventilation? Ann Intern Med 2003; 138:861–70.
9. Peters JV, Moran JL. Noninvasive ventilation in exacerbations of chronic obstructive pulmonary disease: Implications of different meta-analytic strategies. Ann Intern Med 2004; 141:W-78–79.
10. Lightowler JV, Wedzicha JA, Elliott MW, et al. Noninvasive positive pressure ventilation to treat respiratory failure resulting from exacerbations of chronic obstructive pulmonary disease: Cochrane systematic review and metaanalysis. Br Med J 2003; 326:185–90.
11. Celli BR, MacNee W. ATS/ERS Task Force: Standards for the diagnosis and treatment of patients with COPD: A summary of the ATS/ERS position paper. Eur Respir J 2004; 23:932–46.
12. Global Initiative for Chronic Obstructive Lung Disease (GOLD). Global strategy for the diagnosis, management, and prevention of chronic obstructive pulmonary disease. NHLBI/WHO Workshop report, NIH Publication update 2004.
13. NICE (National Institute for Clinical Excellence) guideline on COPD. National clinical guideline on management of chronic obstructive pulmonary disease in adults in primary and secondary care. Thorax 2004; 59:1–232.
14. International Consensus Conferences in Intensive Care Medicine. Noninvasive positive pressure ventilation in acute respiratory failure. Organized jointly by the American Thoracic Society, the European Respiratory Society, the European Society of Intensive Care Medicine, and the Société de Réanimation de Langue Française and approved by the ATS Board of Directors, December 2000. Am J Respir Crit Care Med 2001; 163: 283–91.
15. British Thoracic Society Standards of Care Committee. Noninvasive ventilation in acute respiratory failure. Thorax 2002; 57:192–211.
16. Rossi A, Poggi R, Roca J. Physiologic factors predisposing to chronic respiratory failure. Respir Care Clin North Am 2002; 8:379–404.
17. Rodriguez-Roisin R, Ballester E, Roca J, et al. Mechanisms of hypoxemia in patients with status asthmaticus requiring mechanical ventilation. Am Rev Respir Dis 1989; 139:732–9.
18. Roca J. Gas-exchange in mechanically ventilated patients. In: Milic-Emili J, Lucangelo U, Pesenti A, Zin WA, editors. Basics of respiratory mechanics and artificial ventilation: Topics in Anaesthesia and Critical Care. Milan: Springer-Verlag Italia, 1999: 207.
19. Barbera JA, Roca J, Ferrer A, et al. Mechanisms of worsening gas exchange during acute exacerbations of chronic obstructive pulmonary disease. Eur Respir J 1997; 10:1285–91.
20. Saetta M, Ghezzo H, Kim WD, et al. Loss of alveolar attachments in smokers: A morphometric correlate of lung function impairment. Am Rev Respir Dis 1985; 132:894–900.

21. Hogg JC. Pathophysiology of airflow limitation in chronic obstructive pulmonary disease. Lancet 2004; 364:709–21.

22. Tobin MJ. Respiratory monitoring in the intensive care unit. Am Rev Respir Dis 1988; 138:1625–42.

23. Jubran A, Tobin MJ. Reliability of pulse oximetry in titrating supplemental oxygen in ventilator-dependent patients. Chest 1990; 97:1420–5.

24. Shapiro RS, Kacmarek RM. Monitoring of the mechanically ventilated patient. In: Marini JJ, Slutsky AS, editors. Physiological basis of ventilatory support: Lung biology in health and disease, Vol 118. New York: Marcel Dekker, 1998: 709.

25. Jubran A. Pulse oximetry. In: Tobin MJ, editor. Principles and practice of intensive care monitoring. New York: McGraw-Hill, 1998: 261.

26. Agostoni E, Hyatt RE. Static behaviour of the respiratory system. In: Macklem PT, Mead J, editors. Handbook of physiology, Sec 3: The Respiratory System: Mechanics of breathing, Part 1, vol. III. Bethesda, MD: American Physiological Society, 1986: 295.

27. Appendini L, Patessio A, Zanaboni S, et al. Physiologic effects of positive end-expiratory pressure and mask pressure support during exacerbations of chronic obstructive pulmonary disease. Am J Respir Crit Care Med 1994; 149:1069–76.

28. Calverley PM, Koulouris NG. Flow limitation and dynamic hyperinflation: Key concepts in modern respiratory physiology. Eur Respir J 2005; 25:186–99.

29. Kimball WR, Leith DE, Robins AG. Dynamic hyperinflation and ventilator dependence in chronic obstructive pulmonary disease. Am Rev Respir Dis 1982; 126:991–5.

30. Agostoni E, Mead J. Statics of the respiratory system. In: Macklem PT, Mead J, editors. Handbook of physiology, Sec 3, Vol I: The respiratory system: Mechanics of breathing. Bethesda, MD: American Physiology Society, 1964: 387.

31. Dal Vecchio L, Polese G, Poggi R, et al. "Intrinsic" positive end-expiratory pressure in stable patients with chronic obstructive pulmonary disease. Eur Respir J 1990; 3:74–80.

32. Rossi A, Polese G, Brandi G, et al. Intrinsic positive end-expiratory pressure (PEEP$_i$). Intensive Care Med 1995; 21:522–36.

33. Nucci G, Mergoni M, Bricchi C, et al. Online monitoring of intrinsic PEEP in ventilator-dependent patients. J Appl Physiol 2000; 89:985–95.

34. Tobin MJ, Brochard L, Rossi A. Assessment of respiratory muscle function in the intensive care unit. In: ATS/ERS statement on respiratory muscle testing. Am J Respir Crit Care Med 2002; 166:518–624.

35. Farkas GA, Roussos C. Adaptability of the hamster diaphragm to exercise and/or emphysema. J Appl Physiol 1982; 53:1263–72.

36. Similowski T, Yan S, Gauthier AP, et al. Contractile properties of the human diaphragm during chronic hyperinflation. New Engl J Med 1991; 325:917–23.

37. Rochester DF. The diaphragm in COPD: Better than expected, but not good enough. New Engl J Med 1991; 325:961–2.

38. Purro A, Appendini L, De Gaetano A, et al. Physiologic determinants of ventilator dependence in long-term mechanically ventilated patients. Am J Respir Crit Care Med 2000; 161:1115–23.

39. Whitelaw WA, Derenne JP, Milic-Emili J. Occlusion pressure as a measure of respiratory center output in conscious man. Respir Physiol 1975; 23:181–99.

40. Milic-Emili J. Recent advances in clinical assessment of control of breathing. Lung 1982; 160:1–17.

41. Roussos CS, Macklem PT. Diaphragmatic fatigue in man. J Appl Physiol 1977; 43:189–97.

42. Calverley PM. Respiratory failure in chronic obstructive pulmonary disease. Eur Respir J Suppl 2003; 47:26S–30.

43. Slutsky AS. Mechanical ventilation: ACCP consensus conference. *Chest* 1993; 104:1833–59.

44. Georgopoulos D, Brochard L. Ventilator strategies in acute exacerbations of COPD. Eur Resp Monogr 1998; 8:12–44.

45. Feihl F, Perret C. Permissive hypercapnia: How permissive should we be? Am J Respir Crit Care Med 1994; 150:1722–37.

46. Gorini M, Ginanni R, Villella G, et al. Non-invasive negative and positive pressure ventilation in the treatment of acute or chronic respiratory failure. Intensive Care Med 2004; 30:875–81.

47. Corrado A, Ginanni R, Villella G, et al. Iron lung versus conventional mechanical ventilation in acute exacerbation of COPD. Eur Respir J 2004; 23:419–24.

48. Elliott MW. Non-invasive ventilation in acute exacerbations of chronic obstructive pulmonary disease: A new gold standard? Intensive Care Med 2002; 28:1691–4.

49. Peter JV, Moran JL, Philips-Hughes J, et al. Noninvasive ventilation in acute respiratory failure: A meta-analysis update. Crit Care Med 2002; 30:555–2.

50. Martin TJ, Hovis JD, Constantino JP, et al. A randomized, prospective evaluation of noninvasive ventilation for acute respiratory failure. Am J Respir Crit Care Med 2000; 161:807–13.

51. Plant PK, Owen JL, Elliott MW. Early use of non-invasive ventilation for acute exacerbations of chronic obstructive pulmonary disease on general respiratory wards: A multicenter randomized, controlled trial. Lancet 2000; 355:1931–5.

52. Bardi G, Pierotello R, Desideri M, et al. Nasal ventilation in COPD exacerbations: Early and late results of a prospective, controlled study. Eur Respir J 2000; 15:98–104.

53. Nava S, Ceriana P. Causes of failure of noninvasive mechanical ventilation. Respir Care 2004; 49:295–303.

54. Jolliet P, Abajo B, Pasquina P, et al. Non-invasive pressure-support ventilation in severe community-acquired pneumonia. Intensive Care Med 2001; 27:812–21.

55. Conti G, Antonelli M, Navalesi P, et al. Noninvasive vs conventional mechanical ventilation in patients with chronic obstructive pulmonary disease after failure of medical treatment in the ward: A randomized trial. Intensive Care Med 2002; 28:1701–7.

56. Squadrone E, Frigerio P, Fogliati C, et al. Noninvasive vs invasive ventilation in COPD patients with severe acute respiratory failure deemed to require ventilatory assistance. Intensive Care Med 2004; 30:1303–10.

57. Confalonieri M, Garuti G, Cattaruzza MS, et al on behalf of the Italian Noninvasive Positive Pressure Ventilation (NPPV) Study Group. A chart of failure risk for noninvasive ventilation in patients with COPD exacerbation. Eur Respir J 2005; 25:348–55.

58. Confalonieri M, Potena A, Carbone G, et al. Acute respiratory failure in patients with severe community-acquired pneumonia: A prospective, randomized evaluation of noninvasive ventilation. Am J Respir Crit Care Med 1999; 160:1585–91.

59. Ambrosino N, Foglio K, Rubini F, et al. Non-invasive mechanical ventilation in acute respiratory failure due to chronic obstructive pulmonary disease: Correlates for success. Thorax 1995; 50:755–7.

60. Heyer L, Baconnier PF, Eberhard A, et al. Non-invasive detection of respiratory muscles activity during assisted ventilation. C R Biol 2002; 325:383–91.

61. Brochard L. Pressure support ventilation. In: Tobin MJ, editor. Principles and practice of mechanical ventilation. New York: McGraw-Hill, 1994: 239.

62. Brochard L, Harf A, Lorino H, et al. Inspiratory pressure support prevents diaphragmatic fatigue during weaning from mechanical ventilation. Am Rev Respir Dis 1989; 139:513–21.

63. Vitacca M, Bianchi L, Zanotti E, et al. Assessment of physiologic variables and subjective comfort under different levels of pressure support ventilation. Chest 2004; 126:851–9.

64. Aslanian P, Brochard L. Partial ventilatory support. In: Marini JJ, Slutsky AS, editors. Lung biology in health and disease,

Vol 118: Physiological basis of ventilatory support. New York: Marcel Dekker, 1998: 817.

65. Jubran A, Van de Graaf W, Tobin MJ. Variability of patient-ventilator interaction with pressure support ventilation in patients with chronic obstructive pulmonary disease. Am J Respir Crit Care Med 1995; 152:129–36.

66. Kimura T, Takezawa J, Nishiwaki K, et al. Determination of the optimal pressure support level evaluated by measuring transdiaphragmatic pressure. Chest 1991; 100:112–7.

67. Annat GJ, Viale JP, Derymez CP, et al. Oxygen cost of breathing and diaphragmatic pressure-time index: Measurement in patients with COPD during weaning with pressure support ventilation. Chest 1990; 98:411–4.

68. Mancebo J, Isabey D, Lorino H, et al. Comparative effects of pressure support ventilation and intermittent positive pressure breathing (IPPB) in nonintubated healthy subjects. Eur Respir J 1995; 8:1901–9.

69. Brochard L, Rua F, Lorino H, et al. Inspiratory pressure support compensates for the additional work of breathing caused by the endotracheal tube. Anesthesiology 1991; 75:739–45.

70. Sassoon CS, Lodia R, Rheeman H, et al. Inspiratory muscle work of breathing during flow-by, demand-flow, and continuous-flow systems in patients with chronic obstructive pulmonary disease. Am Rev Respir Dis 1992; 145:1219–22.

71. Poggi R, Polese G, Brandolese R, et al. Comparison between continuous positive airway pressure and inspiratory pressure support in patients with chronic obstructive pulmonary disease during weaning (abstract). Am Rev Respir Dis 1991; 143: A690.

72. Tokioka H, Saito S, Kosaka F. Effect of pressure support ventilation on breathing pattern and respiratory work. Intensive Care Med 1989; 15:491–4.

73. Meduri GU, Conoscenti CC, Menashe P, et al. Noninvasive face mask ventilation in patients with acute respiratory failure. Chest 1989; 95:865–70.

74. Meduri GU, Abou-Shala N, Fox RC, et al. Noninvasive face mask mechanical ventilation in patients with acute hypercapnic respiratory failure. Chest 1991; 100:445–54.

75. Fernandez R, Blanch LL, Valles J, et al. Pressure support ventilation via facial mask in acute respiratory failure in hypercapnic COPD patients. Intensive Care Med 1993; 19:456–61.

76. Vitacca M, Rubini F, Foglio K, et al. Non-invasive modalities of positive pressure ventilation improve the outcome of acute exacerbation of COLD patients. Intensive Care Med 1993; 19: 450–5.

77. Girault C, Richard JC, Chevron V, et al. Comparative physiologic effects of noninvasive assist-control and pressure support ventilation in acute hypercapnic respiratory failure. Chest 1997; 111:1639–48.

78. Brochard L. Noninvasive pressure support ventilation: Physiological and clinical results in patients with COPD and acute respiratory failure. Monaldi Arch Chest Dis 1997; 52:64–7.

79. Vitacca M, Lanini B, Nava S, et al. Inspiratory muscle workload due to dynamic intrinsic PEEP in stable COPD patients: Effects of two different settings of non-invasive pressure support ventilation. Monaldi Arch Chest Dis 2004; 61:81–5.

80. American Thoracic Society, European Thoracic Society Task Force. Standards for the diagnosis and management of patients with COPD [internet]. Version 1.2. New York: American Thoracic Society; 2004 [updated 2005 September 8]. Available from: http://www-test.thoracic.org/copd/.

81. Diaz O, Iglesia R, Ferrer M, et al. Effects of noninvasive ventilation on pulmonary gas exchange and hemodynamics during acute hypercapnic exacerbations of chronic obstructive pulmonary disease. Am J Respir Crit Care Med 1997; 156:1840–5.

82. Appendini L, Purro A, Patessio A, et al. Partitioning of inspiratory muscle workload and pressure assistance in ventilator-dependent COPD patients. Am J Respir Crit Care Med 1996; 154:1301–9.

83. Brochard L. Non-invasive ventilation for acute exacerbations of COPD: A new standard of care. Thorax 2000; 55:817–8.

84. Younes M. Proportional assist ventilation, a new approach to ventilatory support: I. Theory. Am Rev Respir Dis 1992; 145:114–20.

85. Younes M. Proportional assist ventilation. In: Tobin MJ, editor. Principles and practice of mechanical ventilation. New York: McGraw-Hill, 1994: 349.

86. Vitacca M, Clini E, Pagani M, et al. Physiologic effects of early administered mask proportional assist ventilation in patients with chronic obstructive pulmonary disease and acute respiratory failure. Crit Care Med 2000; 28:1791–7.

87. Patrick W, Webster K, Ludwig L, et al. Noninvasive positive-pressure ventilation in acute respiratory distress without prior chronic respiratory failure. Am J Respir Crit Care Med 1996; 153:1005–11.

88. Ambrosino N, Vitacca M, Polese G, et al. Short-term effects of nasal proportional assist ventilation in patients with chronic hypercapnic respiratory insufficiency. Eur Respir J 1997; 10:2829–34.

89. Polese G, Vitacca M, Bianchi L, et al. Nasal proportional assist ventilation unloads the inspiratory muscles of stable patients with hypercapnia due to COPD. Eur Respir J 2000; 16:491–8.

90. Ranieri V, Giuliani R, Mascia L, et al. Patient-ventilator interaction during acute hypercapnia: Pressure support vs proportional assist ventilation. J Appl Physiol 1996; 81:426–36.

91. Wrigge H, Golisch W, Zinserling J, et al. Proportional assist versus pressure support ventilation: Effects on breathing pattern and respiratory work of patients with chronic obstructive pulmonary disease. Intensive Care Med 1999; 25:790–8.

92. Giannouli E, Webster K, Roberts D, et al. Response of ventilator-dependent patients to different levels of pressure support and proportional assist. Am J Respir Crit Care Med 1999; 159:1716–25.

93. Grasso S, Puntillo F, Mascia L, et al. Compensation for increase in respiratory workload during mechanical ventilation: Pressure-support versus proportional-assist ventilation. Am J Respir Crit Care Med 2000; 161:819–26.

94. Porta R, Appendini L, Vitacca M, et al. Mask proportional assist vs pressure support ventilation in patients in clinically stable condition with chronic ventilatory failure. Chest 2002; 122:479–88.

95. Serra A, Polese G, Braggion C, et al. Non-invasive proportional assist and pressure support ventilation in patients with cystic fibrosis and chronic respiratory failure. Thorax 2002; 57:50–4.

96. Winck JC, Vitacca M, Morais A, et al. Tolerance and physiologic effects of nocturnal mask pressure support vs proportional assist ventilation in chronic ventilatory failure. Chest 2004; 126:382–8.

97. Passam F, Hoing S, Prinianakis G, et al. Effect of different levels of pressure support and proportional assist ventilation on breathing pattern, work of breathing and gas exchange in mechanically ventilated hypercapnic COPD patients with acute respiratory failure. Respiration 2003; 70: 355–61.

98. Navalesi P, Hernandez P, Wongsa A, et al. Proportional assist ventilation in acute respiratory failure: effects on breathing pattern and inspiratory effort. Am J Respir Crit Care Med 1996; 154:1330–8.

99. Wysocki M, Richard JC, Meshaka P. Noninvasive proportional assist ventilation compared with noninvasive pressure support ventilation in hypercapnic acute respiratory failure. Crit Care Med 2002; 30:323–9.

100. Ambrosino N, Rossi A. Proportional assist ventilation (PAV): A significant advance or a futile struggle between logic and practice? Thorax 2002; 57:272–6.

101. Mador MJ. Assist-control ventilation. In: Tobin MJ, editor. Principles and practice of mechanical ventilation. New York: McGraw-Hill, 1994: 207.

102. Girault C, Chevron V, Richard JC, et al. Physiologic effects and optimisation of nasal assist-control ventilation for patients with chronic obstructive pulmonary disease in respiratory failure. Thorax 1997; 52:690–6.

103. McKibben AW, Ravenscraft SA. Pressure-controlled and volume-cycled mechanical ventilation. In: Nahum A, Marini JJ, editors. Clinics in chest medicine: Recent advances in mechanical ventilation, vol 17. Philadelphia: Saunders, 1996: 395.

104. Esteban A, Frutos F, Tobin MJ, et al. A comparison of four methods of weaning patients from mechanical ventilation. New Engl J Med 1995; 332:346–89.

105. Brochard L, Rauss A, Benito S, et al. Comparison of three methods of gradual withdrawal from ventilatory support during weaning from mechanical ventilation. Am J Respir Crit Care Med 1994; 150:896–903.

106. Jounieaux V, Duran A, Levi-Valensi V. Synchronized intermittent mandatory ventilation with and without pressure support ventilation in weaning patients with COPD from mechanical ventilation. Chest 1994; 105:1204–10.

107. Rossi A, Ranieri MV. Positive end-expiratory pressure. In: Tobin MJ, editor. Principles and practice of mechanical ventilation. New York: McGraw-Hill, 1994: 259.

108. Marini JJ. Should PEEP be used in airflow obstruction? Am Rev Respir Dis 1989; 140:1–3.

109. Wrigge H, Putensen C. What is the "best PEEP" in chronic obstructive pulmonary disease? Intensive Care Med 2000; 26:1167–9.

110. Smith TC, Marini JJ. Impact of PEEP on lung mechanics and work of breathing in severe airflow obstruction. J Appl Physiol 1988; 65:1488–99.

111. Georgopoulos D, Giannouli E, Patakas D. Effects of extrinsic positive end-expiratory pressure on mechanically ventilated patients with chronic obstructive pulmonary disease and dynamic hyperinflation. Intensive Care Med 1993; 19:197–203.

112. Muñoz J, Guerrero JE, De La Calle B, et al. Interaction between intrinsic positive end-expiratory pressure and externally applied positive end-expiratory pressure during controlled mechanical ventilation. Crit Care Med 1993; 21:348–56.

113. Ranieri VM, Giuliani R, Cinnella G, et al. Physiologic effects of positive end-expiratory pressure in patients with chronic obstructive pulmonary disease during acute ventilatory failure and controlled mechanical ventilation. Am Rev Respir Dis 1993; 147:5–13.

114. Guerin C, LeMasson S, de Varax R, et al. Small airway closure and positive end-expiratory pressure in mechanically ventilated patients with chronic obstructive pulmonary disease. Am J Respir Crit Care Med 1997; 155:1949–56.

115. Koutsoukou A, Armaganidis A, Stavrakaki-Kallergi C, et al. Expiratory flow limitation and intrinsic positive end-expiratory pressure at zero positive end-expiratory pressure in patients with adult respiratory distress syndrome. Am J Respir Crit Care Med 2000; 161:1590–6.

116. Rossi A, Ganassini, Polese G, et al. Pulmonary hyperinflation and ventilator-dependent patients. Eur Respir J 1997; 10:1663–74.

117. Hyatt RE. Forced expiration. In: Macklem PT, Mead J, editors. Handbook of physiology, Sec 3: The respiratory system: Mechanics of breathing, Part 1, Vol III. Bethesda, MD: American Physiological Society, 1986: 295.

118. MacIntyre NR, Cheng KC, McConnell R. Applied PEEP during pressure support reduces the inspiratory threshold load of intrinsic PEEP. Chest 1997; 111:188–93.

119. Guerin C, Milic-Emili J, Fournier G. Effect of PEEP on work of breathing in mechanically ventilated COPD patients. Intensive Care Med 2000; 26:1207–14.

120. Tan IK, Bhatt SB, Tam YH, et al. Effects of PEEP on dynamic hyperinflation in patients with airflow limitation. Br J Anaesth 1993; 70:267–72.

121. Gottfried SB, Rossi A, Higgs BD, et al. Noninvasive determination of respiratory system mechanics during mechanical ventilation for acute respiratory failure. Am Rev Respir Dis 1985; 131:414–20.

122. Appendini L, Confalonieri M, Rossi A. Clinical relevance of monitoring respiratory mechanics in the ventilator-supported patient: an update (1995–2000). Curr Opin Crit Care 2001; 7:41–8.

123. Purro A, Appendini L, Patessio A, et al. Static intrinsic PEEP in COPD patients during spontaneous breathing. Am J Respir Crit Care Med 1998; 157:1044–50.

124. Hoffman RA, Ershowsky P, Krieger BP. Determination of auto-PEEP during spontaneous and controlled ventilation by monitoring changes in end-expiratory thoracic gas volume. Chest 1989; 96:613–6.

125. Zakynthinos SG, Vassilakopoulos T, Zakynthinos E, et al. Correcting static intrinsic positive end-expiratory pressure for expiratory muscle contraction: Validation of a new method. Am J Respir Crit Care Med 1999; 160:785–90.

126. Zakynthinos SG, Vassilakopoulos T, Zakynthinos E, et al. Contribution of expiratory muscle pressure to dynamic intrinsic positive end-expiratory pressure: Validation using the Campbell diagram. Am J Respir Crit Care Med 2000; 162:1633–40.

127. Ninane V, Leduc D, Kafi SA, et al. Detection of expiratory flow limitation by manual compression of the abdominal wall. Am J Respir Crit Care Med 2001; 163:1326–30.

128. Lessard MR, Lofaso F, Brochard L. Expiratory muscle activity increases intrinsic positive end-expiratory pressure independently of dynamic hyperinflation in mechanically ventilated patients. Am J Respir Crit Care Med 1995; 151:562–9.

129. Tobin MJ, Van de Graaff WB. Monitoring of lung mechanics and work of breathing. In: Tobin MJ, editor. Principles and practice of mechanical ventilation. New York: McGraw-Hill, 1994: 967.

130. Rossi A, Santos C, Roca J, et al. Effects of PEEP on $\dot{V}_A/\dot{Q}$ mismatching in ventilated patients with chronic airflow obstruction. Am J Respir Crit Care Med 1994; 149:1077–84.

131. Broseghini C, Brandolese R, Poggi R, et al. Respiratory mechanics during the first day of mechanical ventilation in patients with pulmonary edema and chronic airway obstruction. Am Rev Respir Dis 1988; 138:355–61.

132. Pepe PE, Marini JJ. Occult positive end-expiratory pressure in mechanically ventilated patients with airflow obstruction. Am Rev Respir Dis 1982; 126:166–70.

133. Rossi A, Polese G, Milic-Emili J. Mechanical ventilation in the passive patient: Theory and clinical investigation. In: Derenne JP, Whitelaw WA, Similowski T, editors. Acute respiratory failure in chronic obstructive pulmonary disease: Lung biology in health and disease, Vol 92. New York: Marcel Dekker, 1996: 709.

134. Bates JHT, Baconnier P, Milic-Emili J. A theoretical analysis of interrupter technique for measuring respiratory mechanics. J Appl Physiol 1988; 64:2204–14.

135. Bates JHT, Milic-Emili J. The flow interruption technique for measuring respiratory resistance. J Crit Care 1991; 6:227–38.

136. Milic-Emili J, Robatto FM, Bates JHT. Respiratory mechanics in anaesthesia. Br J Anesth 1990; 65:4–12.

137. Milic-Emili J. Pulmonary flow resistance. Lung 1989; 167:141–8.

138. D'Angelo E, Calderini E, Torri G, et al. Respiratory mechanics in anesthetized paralyzed humans: effects of flow, volume and time. J Appl Physiol 1989; 67:2556–64.

139. D'Angelo E, Robatto FM, Calderini E, et al. Pulmonary and chest wall mechanics in anesthetized paralyzed humans. J Appl Physiol 1991; 70:2602–10.

140. D'Angelo E, Calderini E, Tavola M, et al. Effect of PEEP on respiratory mechanics in anesthetized paralyzed humans. J Appl Physiol 1992; 73:1736–42.

141. Valta P, Corbeil C, Lavoie A, et al. Detection of expiratory flow limitation during mechanical ventilation. Am J Respir Crit Care Med 1994; 150:1311–7.

142. Tobin MJ: Respiratory monitoring during mechanical ventilation. Crit Care Clin 1990; 6:679–709.

143. Marini JJ. Lung mechanics determinations at the bedside: Instrumentation and clinical application. Respir Care 1990; 35:669–93.

144. Nucci G, Mergoni M, Polese G, et al. Online monitoring of respiratory mechanics. In: Aliverti A, Brusasco V, Macklem PT, Pedotti A, editors. Mechanics of breathing: Pathophysiology, diagnosis and treatment. Milan: Springer-Verlag Italia, 2002: 326.

145. Kaczka DW, Barnas GM, Suki B, et al. Assessment of time-domain analyses for estimation of low-frequency respiratory mechanical properties and impedance spectra. Ann Biomed Eng 1995; 23:135–51.

146. Avanzolini G, Barbini P, Cappello A, et al. A new approach for tracking respiratory mechanical parameters in real time. Ann Biomed Eng 1997; 25:154–63.

147. Volta CA, Marangoni E, Alvisi V, et al. Respiratory mechanics by least squares fitting in mechanically ventilated patients: Application on flow-limited COPD patients. Intensive Care Med 2002; 28:48–52.

148. Khirani S, Biot L, Lavagne P, et al. Identification of a non-linear model as a new method to detect expiratory airflow limitation in mechanically ventilated patients. Acta Biotheor 2004; 52:241–54.

149. Jones SE, Packham S, Hebden M, et al. Domiciliary nocturnal intermittent positive pressure ventilation in patients with respiratory failure due to severe COPD: Long-term follow-up and effect on survival. Thorax 1998; 53:495–8.

150. Teschler H. Monitoring of the home mechanical ventilated patient. In: Muir J-F, Ambrosino N, Simonds AK, editors. Noninvasive mechanical ventilation. European Respiratory Monograph, Vol. 6. Sheffield, UK: European Respiratory Society, 2001: 274.

151. Cuvelier A, Muir J-F. Non invasive ventilation and chronic respiratory failure: Indications and obstructive lung diseases. Eur Respir Monit 2001; 16:187–203.

152. Girou E, Brun-Buisson C, Taillé S, et al. Secular trends in nosocomial infections and mortality associated with noninvasive ventilation in patients with exacerbation of COPD and pulmonary edema. JAMA 2003; 290:2985–91.

153. Kramer N, Meyer TJ, Meharg J, et al. Randomized, prospective trial of noninvasive positive pressure ventilation in acute respiratory failure. Am J Respir Crit Care Med 1995; 151:1799–1806.

154. Benhamou D, Girault C, Faure C, et al. Nasal mask ventilation in acute respiratory failure: Experience in elderly patients. Chest 1992; 102:912–7.

155. Jaber S, Fodil R, Carlucci A, et al. Noninvasive ventilation with helium-oxygen in acute exacerbations of chronic obstructive pulmonary disease. Am J Respir Crit Care Med 2000; 161:1191–1200.

156. Nevins ML, Epstein SK. Predictors of outcome for patients with COPD requiring invasive mechanical ventilation. Chest 2001; 119:1840–9.

157. Esteban A, Alia I, Ibanez J, et al. Modes of mechanical ventilation and weaning: A national survey of Spanish hospitals. The Spanish Lung Failure Collaborative Group. Chest 1994; 106:1188–93.

158. Hill NS. Following protocol: Weaning difficult-to wean patients with chronic obstructive pulmonary disease. Am J Respir Crit Care Med 2001; 164:186–7.

159. Schonhofer B, Euteneuer S, Nava S, et al. Survival of mechanically ventilated patients admitted to a specialized weaning center. Intensive Care Med 2002; 28:908–16.

160. A Collective Task Force Facilitated by the American College of Chest Physicians, the American Association for Respiratory Care, and the American College of Critical Care Medicine. Section I: Guidelines: Evidence-based guidelines for weaning and discontinuing ventilatory support. Chest 2001; 120:375S–95.

161. Vassilakopoulos T, Zakynthinos S, Roussos C. The tension-time index and the frequency/tidal volume ratio are the major pathophysiologic determinants of weaning failure and success. Am J Respir Crit Care Med 1998; 158:378–85.

162. Gay PC, Rodarte R, Hubmayr RD. The effects of positive expiratory pressure on isovolume flow and dynamic hyperinflation in patients receiving mechanical ventilation. Am Rev Respir Dis. 1989; 139:621–6.

163. Nava S, Ambrosino N, Clini E, et al. Noninvasive mechanical ventilation in the weaning of patients with respiratory failure due to chronic obstructive pulmonary disease: A randomized, controlled trial. Ann Intern Med 1998; 128:721–8.

164. Girault C, Daudenthun I, Chevron V, et al. Noninvasive ventilation as a systematic extubation and weaning technique in acute-on-chronic respiratory failure: A prospective, randomized, controlled study. Am J Respir Crit Care Med 1999; 160:86–92.

165. Ferrer M, Esquinas A, Arancibia F, et al. Noninvasive ventilation during persistent weaning failure: A randomized, controlled trial. Am J Respir Crit Care Med 2003; 168:70–6.

166. Keenan SP, Powers C, McCormack DG, et al. Noninvasive positive-pressure ventilation for postextubation respiratory distress: A randomized, controlled trial. JAMA 2002; 287:3238–44.

167. Esteban A, Frutos-Vivar F, Ferguson ND, et al. Non-invasive positive-pressure ventilation for respiratory failure after extubation. New Engl J Med 2004; 350:2452–60.

168. Burns KE, Adhikari NK, Meade MO. Noninvasive positive pressure ventilation as a weaning strategy for intubated adults with respiratory failure. Cochrane Database Syst Rev 2003; (4):CD004127.

169. Ceriana P, Carlucci A, Navalesi P, et al. Weaning from tracheotomy in long-term mechanically ventilated patients: Feasibility of a decisional flowchart and clinical outcome. Intensive Care Med 2003; 29:845–8.

170. Manthous CA. The anarchy of weaning techniques (editorials). Chest 2002; 121:1738–40.

171. Ferguson GT. Recommendations for the management of COPD. Chest 2000; 117:23S–28.

172. Schumaker GL, Epstein SK. Managing acute respiratory failure during exacerbation of chronic obstructive pulmonary disease. Respir Care 2004; 49:766–82.

173. Bach PB, Brown C, Gelfand SE, McCrory DC, American College of Physicians-American Society of Internal Medicine, and American College of Chest Physicians. Management of acute exacerbations of chronic obstructive pulmonary disease: A summary and appraisal of published evidence. Ann Intern Med 2001; 134:600–20.

174. McCrory DC, Brown CD. Anti-cholinergic bronchodilators versus β_2-sympathomimetic agents for acute exacerbations of chronic obstructive pulmonary disease. Cochrane Database Syst Rev 2002; (4):CD003900.

175. Turner MO, Patel A, Ginsburg S, et al. Bronchodilator delivery in acute airflow obstruction: A meta-analysis. Arch Intern Med 1997; 157:1736–44.

176. Hamill RJ, Houston ED, Georghiou PR, et al. An outbreak of *Burkholderia* (formerly *Pseudomonas*) *cepacia* respiratory tract

colonization and infection associated with nebulized albuterol therapy. Ann Intern Med 1995; 122:762–6.

177. Dhand R, Duarte AG, Jubran A, et al. Dose-response to bronchodilator delivered by metered-dose inhaler in ventilator-supported patients. Am J Respir Crit Care Med 1996; 154:388–93.

178. Nava S, Karakurt S, Rampulla C, et al. Salbutamol delivery during non-invasive mechanical ventilation in patients with chronic obstructive pulmonary disease: A randomized, controlled study. Intensive Care Med 2001; 27:1627–35.

179. Barnes PJ. New treatments for COPD. Thorax 2003; 58:803–8.

180. Dhand R, Jubran A, Tobin MJ. Bronchodilator delivery by metered-dose inhaler in ventilator-supported patients. Am J Respir Crit Care Med 1995; 151:1827–33.

181. Dhand R, Tobin MJ. Bronchodilator delivery with metered-dose inhalers in mechanically ventilated patients. Eur Respir J 1996; 9:585–95.

182. Connors AF, Dawson NV, Thomas C, et al for the SUPPORT Investigators. Outcome following acute exacerbation of severe chronic obstructive lung disease. Am J Respir Crit Care Med 1996; 154:956–67.

183. Seneff MG, Wagner DP, Wagner RP, et al. Hospital and 1-year survival of patients admitted to intensive care units with acute exacerbation of chronic obstructive pulmonary disease. JAMA 1995; 274:1852–7.

184. Plant PK, Owen JL, Elliott MW. Non-invasive ventilation in acute exacerbations of chronic obstructive pulmonary disease: Long term survival and predictors of in-hospital outcome. Thorax 2001; 56:708–12.

185. Confalonieri M, Parigi P, Scartabellati A, et al. Noninvasive mechanical ventilation improves the immediate and long-term outcome of COPD patients with acute respiratory failure. Eur Respir J 1996; 9:422–30.

186. Vitacca M, Clini E, Rubini F, et al. Non-invasive mechanical ventilation in severe chronic obstructive lung disease and acute respiratory failure: Short- and long-term prognosis. Intensive Care Med 1996; 22:94–100.

187. Stauffer JL, Fayter NA, Graves B, et al. Survival following mechanical ventilation for acute respiratory failure in adult men. Chest 1993; 104:1222–9.

188. Nava S. Noninvasive techniques of weaning from mechanical ventilation. Monaldi Arch Chest Dis 1998; 53:355–7.

189. Plant PK, Elliott MW. Chronic obstructive pulmonary disease: 9. Management of ventilatory failure in COPD. Thorax 2003; 58:537–42.

190. Brochard L, Mancebo J, Wysocki M, et al. Noninvasive ventilation for acute exacerbations of chronic obstructive pulmonary disease. New Engl J Med 1995; 333:817–22.

191. Antonelli M, Conti G, Rocco M, et al. A comparison of noninvasive positive-pressure ventilation and conventional mechanical ventilation in patients with acute respiratory failure. New Engl J Med 1998; 339:429–35.

192. Hill NS. Noninvasive ventilation for chronic obstructive pulmonary disease. Respir Care 2004; 49:72–87.

193. Brochard L, Mancebo J, Elliott MW. Noninvasive ventilation for acute respiratory failure. Eur Respir J 2002; 19:712–21.

194. Keenan SP, Kernerman PD, Cook DJ, et al. Effect of noninvasive positive pressure ventilation on mortality in patients admitted with acute respiratory failure: A meta-analysis. Crit Care Med 1997; 25:1685–92.

195. Afessa B, Morales JJ, Scanlon PD, et al. Prognostic factors, clinical course, and hospital outcome of patients with chronic obstructive pulmonary disease admitted to an intensive care unit for acute respiratory failure. Crit Care Med 2002; 30:1610–5.

196. Anton A, Guell R, Gomez J, et al. Predicting the result of noninvasive ventilation in severe acute exacerbations of patients with chronic airflow limitation. Chest 2000; 117:828–33.

197. Carlucci A, Delmastro M, Rubini F, et al. Changes in the practice of non-invasive ventilation in treating COPD patients over 8 years. Intensive Care Med 2003; 29:419–25.

198. Esteban A, Anzueto A, Frutos F, et al for the Mechanical Ventilation International Study Group. Characteristics and outcomes in adult patients receiving mechanical ventilation: A 28-day international study. JAMA 2002; 287:345–55.

199. Elliott MW. Non-invasive ventilation in acute exacerbations of COPD: What happens after hospital discharge? Thorax 2004; 59:1006–8.

200. Chu CM, Chan VL, Lin AWN, et al. Readmission rates and life threatening events in COPD survivors treated with non-invasive ventilation for acute hypercapnic respiratory failure. Thorax 2004; 59:1020–5.

201. Ram FSF, Wedzicha JA, Wright J, et al. Hospital at home for patients with acute exacerbations of chronic obstructive pulmonary disease: Systematic review of evidence. Br Med J 2004; 329:315–20.

202. Tarnow-Mordi WO, Hau C, Warden A, et al. Hospital mortality in relation to staff workload: A 4-year study in adult intensive-care unit. Lancet 2000; 356:185–9.

203. Groenewegen KH, Schols AMWJ, Wouters EFM. Mortality and mortality-related factors after hospitalization for acute exacerbation of COPD. Chest 2003; 124:459–67.

204. Nash EF. Non-invasive ventilation. Thorax 2002; 57:919–20.

205. Darioli R, Perret C. Mechanical controlled hypoventilation in status asthmaticus. Am Rev Respir Dis 1984; 129:385–7.

206. The Acute Respiratory Distress Syndrome Network. Ventilation with lower tidal volumes as compared with traditional tidal volumes for acute lung injury and the acute respiratory distress syndrome. New Engl J Med 2000; 342:1301–8.

207. Macklem PT. Cell and molecular biology is not the only way to a better understanding of pathogenesis of lung disease. Am J Respir Crit Care Med 2004; 170:ii–iii; author reply iv.

208. Snider GL. Only cell and molecular biology can lead to an understanding of pathogenesis of lung disease. Am J Respir Crit Care Med 2004; 170:i–ii.

209. Rossi A, Appendini L, Ranieri MV. PEEP and CPAP in severe airflow obstruction. In: Marini JJ, Slutsky AS, editors. Lung biology in health and disease, Vol 118: Physiological basis of ventilatory support. New York: Marcel Dekker, 1998: 847.

210. Bott J, Carroll MP, Conway JH, et al. Randomised, controlled trial of nasal ventilation in acute ventilatory failure due to chronic obstructive airways disease. Lancet 1993; 341:1555–7.

211. Servillo G, Ughi L, Rossano F, et al. Noninvasive mask pressure support ventilation in COPD patients. Intensive Care Med 1994; 50:S54.

212. Angus RM, Ahmed AA, Fenwick LJ, et al. Comparison of the acute effects on gas exchange of nasal ventilation and doxapram in exacerbations of chronic obstructive pulmonary disease. Thorax 1996; 51:1048–50.

213. Avdeev SN, Tret'iakov AV, Grigor'iants RA, et al. Study of the use of noninvasive ventilation of the lungs in acute respiratory insufficiency due exacerbation of chronic obstructive pulmonary disease. Anesteziol Reanimatol 1998; 3:45–51.

214. Celikel T, Sungur M, Ceyhan B, et al. Comparison of noninvasive positive pressure ventilation with standard medical therapy in hypercapnic acute respiratory failure. Chest 1998; 114:1636–42.

215. Dikensoy O, Ikidag B, Filiz A, et al. Comparison of non-invasive ventilation and standard medical therapy in acute

hypercapnic respiratory failure: A randomised, controlled study at a tertiary health centre in SE Turkey. Int J Clin Pract 2002; 56: 85–8.

216. Barbé F, Togores B, Rubì M, et al. Noninvasive ventilatory support does not facilitate recovery from acute respiratory failure in chronic obstructive pulmonary disease. Eur Respir J 1996; 9:1240–5.

217. Keenan SP, Powers C, McCormack DG. Noninvasive ventilation in milder COPD exacerbations: An RCT (abstract). Am J Respir Crit Care. 2001; 163:A250.

218. Rossi A, Polese G, Brandi G. Dynamic hyperinflation. In: Marini JJ, and Roussos C, editors. Ventilatory failure: Update in intensive care and emergency medicine, Vol 15. Berlin: Springer-Verlag, 1991: 199.

Chapter 32

MECHANICAL VENTILATION IN NEUROMUSCULAR DISEASE

AHMET BAYDUR

OVERVIEW OF PERTINENT PATHOPHYSIOLOGY
VENTILATOR TARGETS IN
   NEUROMUSCULAR DISEASE
EXPERIENCE WITH TRADITIONAL
   MODES OF VENTILATION
ROLE FOR NEWER MODES OF VENTILATION
ROLE FOR PEEP
SELECTING VENTILATOR SETTINGS
VULNERABILITY TO VENTILATOR
   COMPLICATIONS
ADJUNCTIVE THERAPY
     Glossopharyngeal Breathing (GPB)
     Assisted Coughing
     Mechanical Insufflation-Exsufflation Devices
TIMING OF TRANSFER FROM ICU
   TO THE COMMUNITY
LONG-TERM SURVIVAL AND QUALITY OF LIFE
IMPORTANT UNKNOWNS AND THE FUTURE
SUMMARY AND CONCLUSION

The earliest application of assisted ventilation in patients with neuromuscular disease was with the iron lung during the poliomyelitis epidemic in the 1940s and 1950s. While cumbersome and associated with problems related to nursing and bronchial hygiene, this device saved many lives, permitting most patients with severe respiratory insufficiency to recover, become ventilator-free, and go on to lead productive lives.[1] In most cases, the device was used for durations of a few weeks to up to 2 years, with eventual recovery of ventilatory function. Many polio patients with disability continue to reside in iron lungs in the community after several decades.[2] Others have converted to tracheostomy-assisted positive-pressure ventilation, achieving mobility and the ability to clear the airway of secretions. With appropriate weaning techniques, some have switched to noninvasive positive-pressure ventilation (NIPPV),[3] particularly those experiencing the late effects of poliomyelitis (postpolio syndrome). NIPPV is now the preferred means to support most patients with chronic neuromuscular disorders and is used increasingly to support patients with acute ventilatory insufficiency, such as with Guillain-Barré syndrome and myasthenia gravis. Table 32-1 lists neuromuscular conditions associated with respiratory impairment and failure.

Overview of Pertinent Pathophysiology

The primary muscle of inspiration is the diaphragm, which is innervated by the third through fifth cervical nerves. In addition, the external intercostal muscles provide stability to the rib cage and prevent its inward collapse during diaphragmatic contraction. With ascending paralysis, such as with Guillain-Barré syndrome or traumatic quadriplegia above the T10 level,[4] there are reductions in vital capacity and other volume subdivisions, as well as rib-cage distortion with inspiratory effort. These changes result in regional ventilation-perfusion mismatching, particularly in the dependent portions of the lungs. An early increase in the alveolar-arterial oxygen (O_2) gradient can be found in some patients with neuromuscular impairment long before hypercapnia develops.[5,6] Gas exchange worsens during sleep secondary to alveolar hypoventilation, inhibited intercostal and accessory muscle activity, and dead-space ventilation induced by rapid shallow breathing[6–8] (Fig. 32-1). Despite muscle weakness, central drive in patients with neuromuscular and chest-wall disorders often is increased.[9]

With reduction in lung volume, respiratory compliance decreases, adding to the elastic load of already weakened inspiratory muscles.[10] Thoracic scoliosis, often associated with disorders such as poliomyelitis and muscular dystrophy (Fig. 32-2), further reduces respiratory compliance, resulting in an increase in inspiratory drive and altered force-length and force-velocity relationships.[11,12] The diaphragm has to carry most of this respiratory load and eventually may fatigue. The fatigue threshold of the diaphragm in quadriplegic individuals is lower than in normal subjects (0.10–0.12 versus 0.15, respectively).[13]

Respiratory impairment in patients with neuromuscular disease generally is proportional to the number of respiratory muscles involved. Measurement of maximal static mouth pressures (Pmax) provides a guide to the degree of respiratory muscle weakness (although not necessarily of general muscle weakness) and is an adjunct to assessing the need for assisted ventilation. In chronic stable neuromuscular disease, maximal expiratory mouth pressures are lower in myopathy than in polyneuropathy and in proximal than in distal muscle weakness.[14] In healthy people, expiratory Pmax increases hyperbolically with lung volume. In patients with neuromuscular disease, however, the lung volume is reduced by 10–20% for the corresponding predicted Pmax, a finding thought to be related to intercostal muscle weakness.[10]

Weakened abdominal muscles reduce the ability to cough, as reflected by decreased peak expiratory flow rates. Bach et al[15] showed that patients with peak expiratory flows of less than 160 liters/min need cough assistance to prevent accumulation of airway secretions. Cough impairment is worsened by inspiratory muscle weakness and glottic dysfunction. Bulbar muscle involvement impairs swallowing and speech and increases risk of aspiration and upper

TABLE 32-1 Neuromuscular Diseases Associated with Respiratory Impairment or Failure

1. Muscle diseases
   a. Dystrophies (Ducehenne, fascioscapulohumeral, limb girdle)
   b. Myotonias
   c. Autoimmune/inflammatory myopathies (dermatomyositis, polymyositis)
   d. Metabolic myopathies (hypophosphatemia, glycogen-storage disorders, disturbed lipid metabolism)
   e. Endocrine myopathies (hypothyroidism, hyperthyroididsm)
   f. Periodic paralysis
   g. Toxic myopathies (alcohol)
2. Peripheral neuropathies
   a. Autoimmune/inflammatory (Guillan-Barré)
   b. Toxic (heavy metal, organophosphates, nitrofurantoin, hexocarbons)
   c. Acute intermittent porphyria
   d. Tick paralysis
   e. Shellfish poisoning
   f. Hereditary (Charcot-Marie-Tooth)
   g. Endocrine (hypothyroidism, hyperthyroidism)
3. Neuromuscular junction (myasthenia gravis, botulism)
4. Motor neuron disease
   a. Poliomyelitis
   b. Amyotrophic lateral sclerosis
   c. Spinal muscle atrophies
5. ICU-related weakness
   a. Critical illness polyneuropathy (sepsis, multisystem organ failure)
   b. Neuromuscular blocking agent–related neuropathy
   c. Status asthmaticus–associated neuromyopathy (high-dose steroids, aminoglycosides, paralytic agents)
6. Spinal cord injury

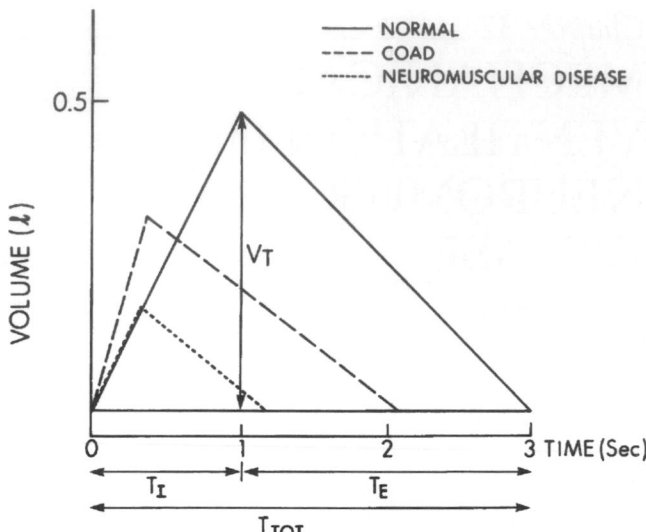

FIGURE 32-1 The respiratory cycle (spirogram) in a normal individual, a patient with chronic obstructive airway disease (COAD), and a patient with neuromuscular disease. The normal spirogram is divided into its components. V_T, tidal volume; T_I, duration of inspiration; T_E, duration of expiration; T_{TOT}, duration of total respiratory cycle. Note the decreased V_T, increased V_T/T_I, and decreased T_I/T_{TOT} of the patient with COAD and the decreased V_T but normal V_T/T_I and T_I/T_{TOT} of the patient with neuromuscular disease. (*Reproduced, with permission, from Baydur: Semin Respir Med 9:223–238, 1988.*)

airway collapse. These conditions can be exacerbated by the use of negative-pressure ventilators.

Dysregulation of breathing in muscular dystrophy and myotonic dystrophy has been attributed to abnormal feedback from respiratory muscle receptors and abnormal central ventilatory control, respectively.[16,17] Sleep-disordered breathing can be related to many factors, including respiratory muscle weakness, chest-wall deformities, obesity, craniofacial abnormalities, bulbar dysfunction, and abnormalities in control of ventilation.[18,19] Loss of rib-cage and bulbar muscle tone, particularly during rapid-eye motion (REM) sleep, results in hypoventilation, decreased inspiratory flow, fragmented sleep, and daytime symptoms, well described in myotonic dystrophy, diaphragmatic paralysis, and amyotrophic lateral sclerosis.[20–22] Obstructive events during sleep can occur in Duchenne muscular dystrophy and amyotrophic lateral sclerosis.[23,24]

Ventilator Targets in Neuromuscular Disease

Initiating ventilation in a patient with progressive respiratory impairment depends on recognition of clinical find-

ings and key physiologic variables. The patient developing progressive respiratory failure will experience dyspnea, increased use of accessory neck muscles, paradoxical breathing, tachycardia, sweating, and inability to say more than a few words in a row. These findings, however, are nonspecific. Altered mental status is a sign of severe hypercapnia and acidosis and/or hypoxemia. Individuals with slowly progressive respiratory impairment can tolerate severe weakness without overt signs but may complain of headaches or sleep disturbances or exhibit cognitive impairment associated with daytime hypercapnia with partial

FIGURE 32-2 Patient with Duchenne muscular dystrophy and severe scoliosis.

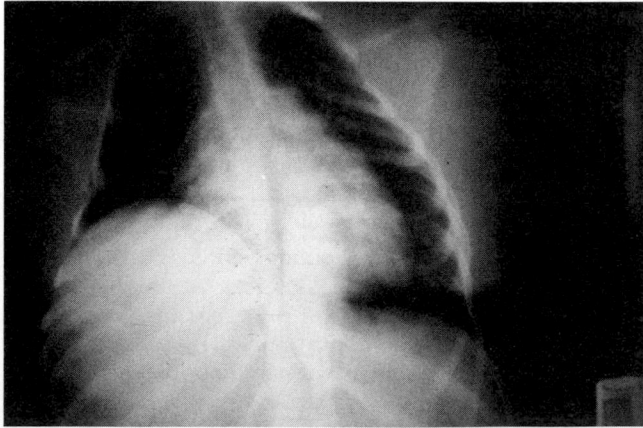

compensation. Those with generalized muscle weakness often experience orthopnea because of a combination of diaphragmatic fatigue, an unstable chest wall, and cephalad pressure exerted by abdominal contents on the diaphragm. By contrast, patients with quadriplegia often prefer the supine position because the diaphragm assumes a greater appositional area with respect to the abdominal wall, increasing its resting length and force generation. Another explanation has been a reduction in the residual volume occuring in the recumbent position.[25]

Measurements of vital capacity (VC) and total lung capacity (TLC) provide a guide to the progression of respiratory muscle weakness, although as much as a 50% reduction of respiratory muscle strength occurs before these values are reduced.[26] In general, patients with less than 10% of predicted VC have little tolerance off assisted ventilation.[2,3] Measurements of inspiratory and expiratory Pmax are noninvasive and have established normal values for adults and children. They are, however, influenced by posture, lung volume, and effort. Poor effort or air leaks around the mouthpiece give rise to submaximal measurements. The maximal sniff test is easier to perform and better reflects global inspiratory muscle strength.[27] Tests of respiratory muscle strength that correlate best with the degree of hypercapnia include the measurement of maximal sniff esophageal (Pes) and transdiaphragmatic pressures (Pdi) and Pdi after bilateral cervical magnetic stimulation of the phrenic nerves.[28] Measurements of Pdi during transcutaneous phrenic nerve stimulation are more reliable and require no patient effort but have the disadvantage of being dependent on chest-wall impedance.[29] Measurements of Pes and Pdi, however, are invasive. For clinical purposes, in patients with amyotrophic lateral sclerosis without significant bulbar involvement, the noninvasive nasal pressure measured during a sniff has been found to have greater predictive power than percent predicted VC and maximal mouth pressures in identifying the risk of ventilatory failure.[28] Table 32-2 lists physical and functional findings used in the evaluation of patients with impending respiratory failure secondary to neuromuscular disease. A useful guide to diaphragmatic weakness is the comparison of the VC measured in the seated and supine positions. Reductions in VC of 12–65% have been recorded in patients with neuromuscular disease[3,4,30–32] (except in those with traumatic quadriplegia[4,25]) on assuming the supine position.

Electromyography and nerve conduction studies provide diagnostic assistance with respect to a neuropathic or myopathic cause of muscle weakness, particularly in acute illnesses (e.g., Guillain-Barré syndrome, myasthenia gravis, and critical-illness polyneuropathy or myopathy). They are also of prognostic value in patients with acute and chronic denervation, as in amyotrophic lateral sclerosis and critical-illness neuropathies and myopathies.

Experience with Traditional Modes of Ventilation

With increasing use of positive-pressure ventilators during the 1960s, many patients with poliomyelitis supported with negative-pressure devices such as iron lungs (Fig. 32-3) and cuirasses (Fig. 32-4) and, subsequently, individuals with

FIGURE 32-3 An iron lung (negative-pressure) ventilator.

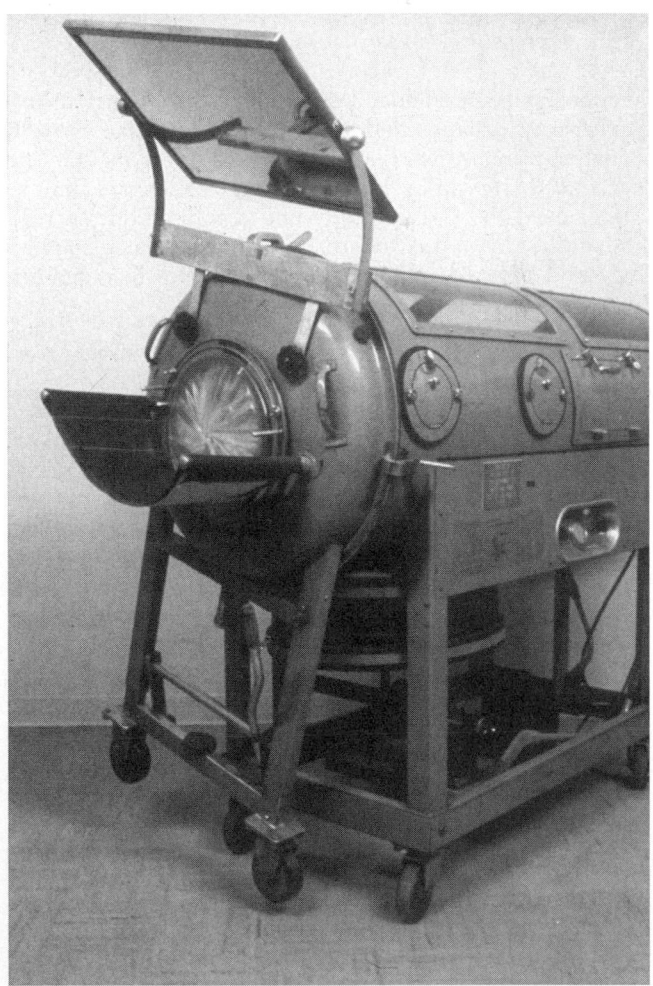

TABLE 32-2   Indications for Initiating Mechanical Ventilation in Neuromuscular Diseases

Relative subjective symptoms [orthopnea, frequent arousals from sleep, morning headaches, daytime somnolence/napping, impaired cognitive function (memory, concentration), fatigue]
Cor pulmonale
Vital capacity < 25% of predicted
Maximal inspiratory mouth pressure < 25 cmH$_2$O
Nasal "sniff" pressure < 25 cmH$_2$O
Changes in gas exchange indicating progressive respiratory failure:
   Daytime Pa$_{CO_2}$ > 45 mmHg
   Sustained nocturnal hemoglobin desaturation (> 5 minutes or >10% of total study time)
Recurrent acute respiratory failure episodes requiring intervention
Failure to respond to continuous positive pressure alone in patients with documented sleep apnea syndrome before neuromuscular weakness is detected

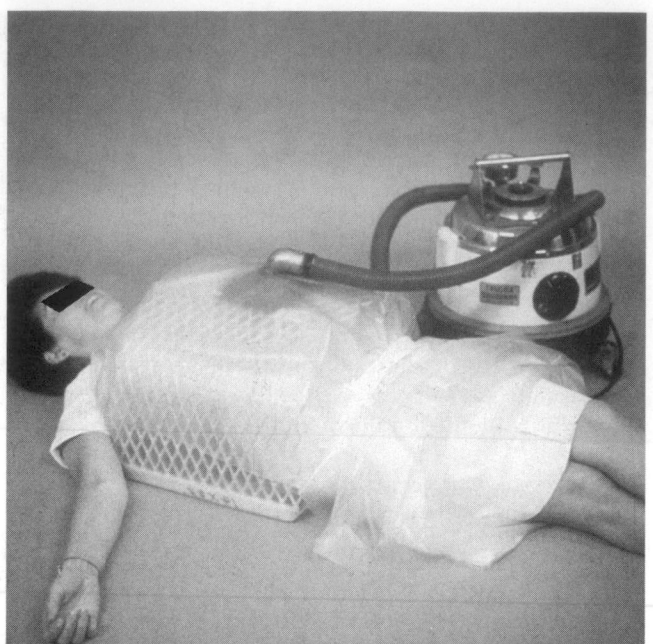

FIGURE 32-4 A cuirass (negative-pressure) ventilator.

other neuromuscular disorders received tracheostomies for positive-pressure support (Fig. 32-5). Until the 1980s, most positive-pressure ventilators were of the volume-cycled variety. Advantages of tracheostomies include the ability to suction tracheobronchial secretions and avoidance of upper airway collapse and hypercapnia encountered with negative-pressure ventilation. Disadvantages include the necessity of teaching the patient and caregivers how to maintain of the tracheostomy and complications such as stomal infections, airway erosions (from repeated suctioning), and difficulty with speech and swallowing (that can

be overcome with proper speech and bulbar training and use of a one-way speaking valve). Airway vascular fistulas (with fatal hemorrhage) and tracheobronchomalacia are infrequent but potentially devastating complications that can occur even with uncuffed tracheostomies.[33]

Not all patients with poliomyelitis, however, elected to undergo tracheostomy for ventilation. Many learned to use oral, lip, nasal, or full-face interfaces with positive-pressure ventilators. Some adopted this technique to maintain ventilatory support when removed from negative-pressure ventilation, whereas others used these devices solely for part- or full-time ventilation (Fig. 32-6). Some individuals use a lip seal during sleep. The use of such interfaces in other neuromuscular disorders has been successful in avoiding tracheostomies. They also have been used to wean patients off tracheostomy-assisted ventilation.[3] An open mouthpiece circuit can be used in respiratory-dependent neuromuscular patients with a portable volume ventilator. It has the disadvantage, however, of alarming when the circuit pressure drops during a system disconnection. Only volume-cycled ventilators with negative-pressure triggering should be used because flow-triggered volume ventilators autocycle when used with an open-circuit mouth-positive system. Most ventilators can support mouth-positive ventilation in the assist-control mode.[3]

Soon after the advent of continuous positive airway pressure (CPAP) for the management of sleep apnea, bilevel positive airway pressure (BiPAP) was introduced to ventilate patients with neuromuscular disorders. In contrast with volume-cycled ventilators, these pressure-limited machines exhibit tidal volume variability secondary to changes in respiratory compliance or the presence of airway secretions or collapse. Patients with severe scoliosis or other causes of increased respiratory elastance are likely to benefit more from a volume-cycled ventilator than from a BiPAP machine. The latter device may generate an insufficient pressure "span"

FIGURE 32-5 A patient with Duchenne muscular dystrophy receiving tracheostomy positive ventilation.

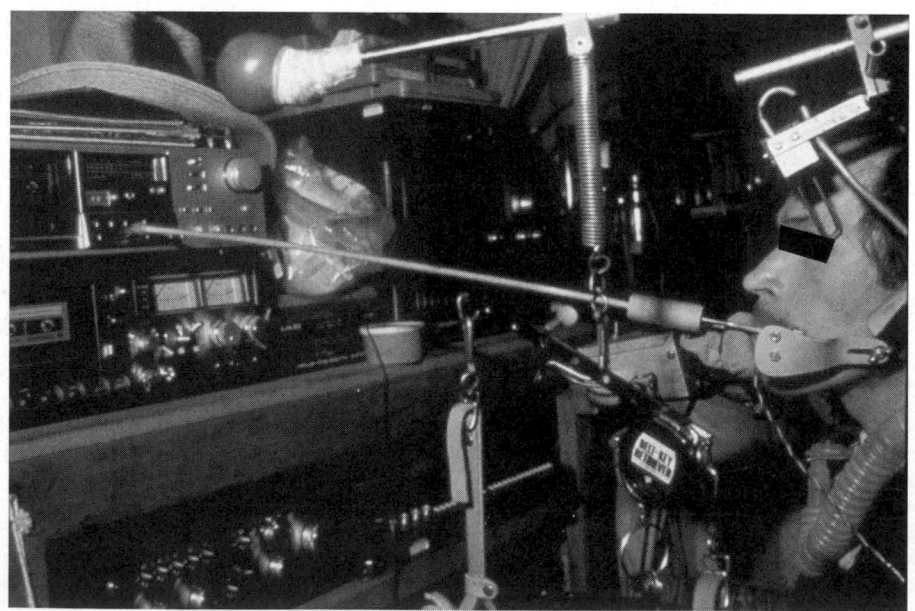

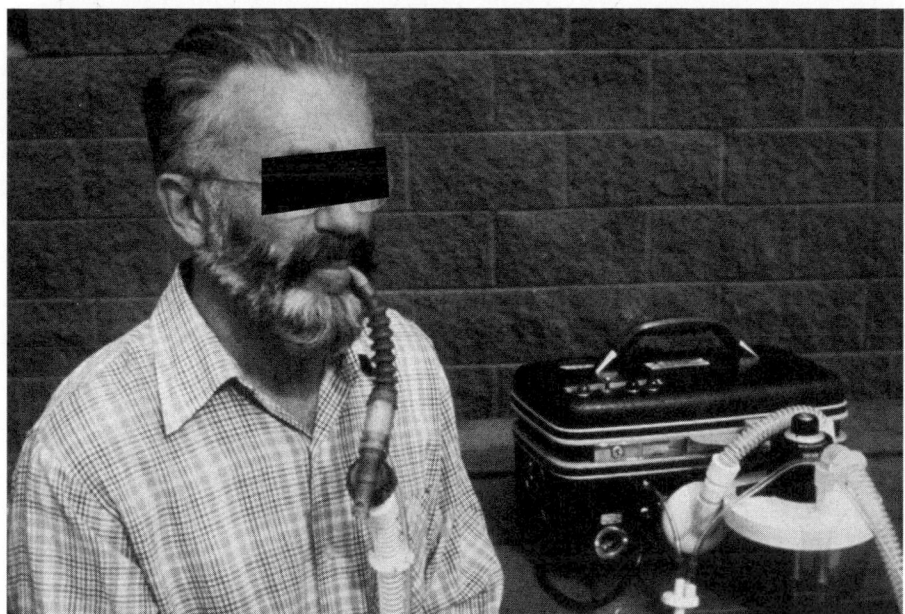

FIGURE 32-6 An individual with late effects of poliomyelitis receiving mouth positive ventilation through a mouthpiece.

(i.e., the difference between the end-inspiratory and end-expiratory pressures) to ventilate the lungs.[3] Volume-cycled ventilators have the advantage of delivering higher volumes and can provide air "stacking" to maximum insufflations via an oral interface.[3] In general, they operate more quietly than pressure-cycled devices, use less electricity, and have alarm systems that are useful for nighttime ventilation. There is a subgroup of patients with more severe chronic respiratory failure for whom pressure-controlled ventilation is also inadequate.[34] A period of 1 month is enough for judging the efficacy of a specific type of noninvasive ventilation, such as pressure-cycled ventilation, a more comfortable and less expensive mode. Ventilators can be used with a variety of nasal, oral, and full-face interfaces (Figs. 32-7 and 8).

FIGURE 32-7 A full-face mask used in noninvasive ventilation. (*Used, with permission, from Hans Rudolph, Inc.*)

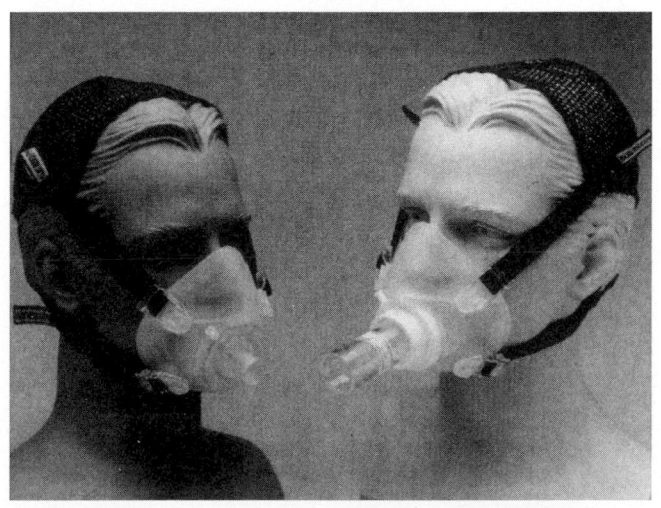

Patients who tolerate NIPPV have a significant survival advantage compared with patients who do not tolerate it. With a close working relationship between the patient and caregivers, machine tolerance can be achieved in virtually all patients with neuromuscular diseases, including those with hypercapnic amyotrophic lateral sclerosis.[35] The prognosis in the latter group is particularly poor if they do not tolerate or accept mask ventilation (death usually within less than a year). One study found a survival disadvantage in patients treated early with NIPPV for Duchenne muscular dystrophy,[36] but this finding may have resulted from the exclusion of hypercapnic patients.

Current evidence concerning the benefits of NIPPV is weak but consistent, suggesting relief of symptoms of hypoventilation in the short term and, for the most part, improvement in survival in a few small studies.[37] Development of a home protocol in which oxygen desaturations are prevented or reversed using NIPPV and manual and mechanically assisted coughing techniques results in fewer and shorter hospitalizations than if such a protocol were not used.[3]

Role for Newer Modes of Ventilation

Although pressure-cycled ventilation is the most common mode of providing ventilatory assistance in the long-term setting, patient-ventilation asynchrony sometimes occurs.[38] Proportional-assist ventilatory mode improves patient-ventilatory synchrony by providing inspiratory flow and pressure in proportion to the patient's effort.[39] In patients with stable chronic respiratory failure (most with chronic obstructive pulmonary disease), application of daytime nasal proportional-assist ventilation results in improvements in gas exchange and respiratory muscle

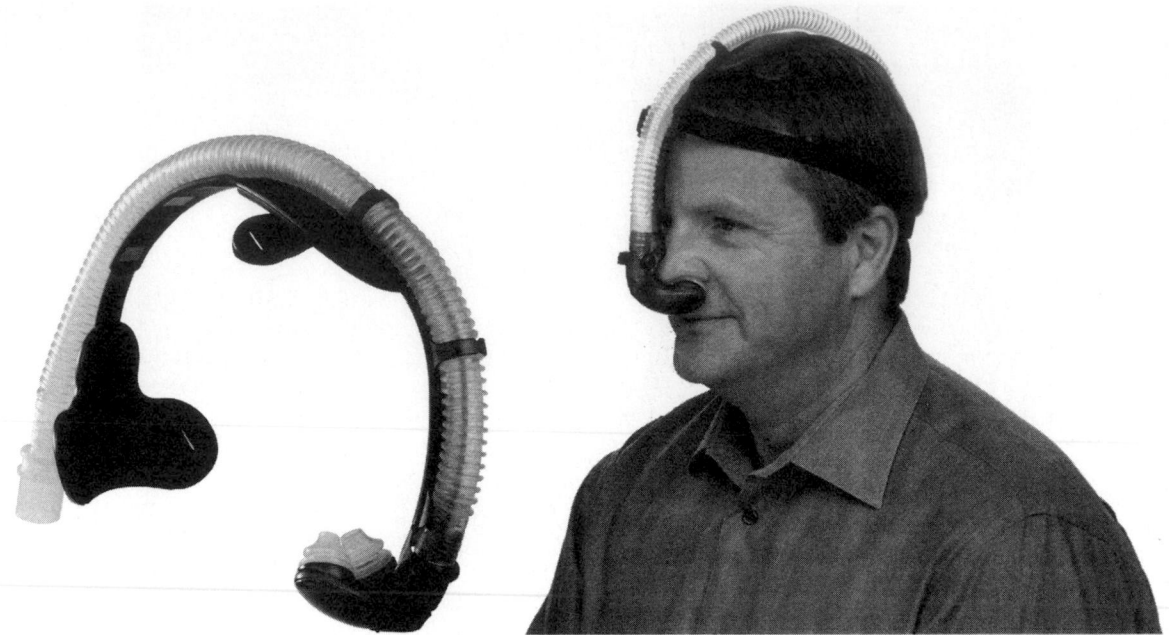

FIGURE 32-8 Nasal adaptor ("pillows") used with noninvasive ventilation. (*Used, with permission, from Puritan-Bennett Corporation.*)

function.[40–42] A lower level of mean airway pressure is counteracted by more time needed to set the ventilator.[42] In a recent crossover study of 14 patients with chronic ventilatory insufficiency (10 with restrictive thoracic disorders) comparing 5 consecutive nights of pressure-cycled with proportional-assist ventilation, both modes were shown to result in similar tolerance and were equally effective in reducing daytime hypercapnia and improving nocturnal saturation and symptoms.[43]

Role for PEEP

Positive end-expiratory pressure (PEEP) is used primarily to improve oxygenation in patients with severe and refractory hypoxemia. Given that patients with acute respiratory distress syndrome have decreased functional residual capacities, application of PEEP maintains alveolar patency during expiration and reverses the ventilation-perfusion mismatch that results in hypoxemia. Similarly, PEEP should have a beneficial effect on reversing dependent alveolar collapse in neuromuscular weakness because most patients have reduced functional residual capacities and dependent alveolar units that fail to open during inspiration.

The most practical application of PEEP is in the form of the expiratory positive airway pressure (EPAP) delivered by BiPAP. To the extent that EPAP is applied during noninvasive ventilation, there must be a parallel increase in the inspiratory airway pressure (IPAP) to provide adequate ventilation. While pressure-cycled ventilators can compensate partially for mask leaks, excessive leaks can prolong the inspiratory phase and worsen intrinsic PEEP and patient-ventilator asynchrony. The latter problem can be corrected with the use of time-cycled expiratory trig-

gers better than with flow-cycled expiratory triggers.[44] As in any patient with impaired left-ventricular function receiving high levels of PEEP, excess EPAP (and the concomitantly increased IPAP) can lead to a decrease in cardiac output. This could be a problem in muscular dystrophy–associated cardiomyopathy.

Selecting Ventilator Settings

For most patients who present with findings of respiratory impairment as shown in Table 32-2, ventilator assistance usually is begun nocturnally. The choice of volume-cycled versus pressure-cycled mode seems to be arbitrary, and there are no controlled, randomized trials demonstrating the advantage of one over the other. Bach,[3] however, recommends that most patients be started on a volume-cycled ventilator to achieve air "stacking" for maximum insufflations (see below) and for eventual daytime use. Occasional patients will benefit more from a pressure-cycled ventilator if they have glottic incompetence and cannot stack breaths. If they do use a pressure-cycled device, the pressure spans must be high enough to generate adequate volumes. The EPAP should be set as low as possible (e.g., 2 cmH_2O) unless the patient has underlying lung disease or documented sleep apnea. The spontaneous-timed mode is recommended. Mask leaks must be prevented to ensure consistent volume delivery. Patients with oral leaks can be switched to a full-face mask or, if this turns out to be uncomfortable, to mouth or lip seals. Because the use of such interfaces results in an open system, and patients can take in as much volume as they want, the set volume should be able to compensate for leaks (starting at 600–1000 ml, with eventual increases to 800–1500 ml).[3]

Ideally, the effects of NIPPV should be followed up by nocturnal monitoring with pulse oximetry and, if available, end-tidal capnography. This enables optimization of ventilator settings. For patients who tolerate being off the ventilator during the day, a daytime arterial blood-gas analysis will determine the longer-term effects of NIPPV. With progressive reductions in lung volume and compliance, the patient may need to be switched to a volume-cycled ventilator to ensure consistent ventilation.

Noninvasive ventilation may be initiated in the hospital, a sleep laboratory, the outpatient office, or the patient's home depending on the resources available. Ideally, the procedure should be initiated with the patient alert, under the guidance and supervision of experienced personnel. The goals should be to familiarize and encourage the patient with the technique and to establish initial ventilator settings (determined by optimizing both by physiology and patient comfort). Inspiratory pressures are increased gradually over days or weeks, usually during daytime hours. Once gas-exchange and patient-comfort goals have been reached, transition to nocturnal use is initiated. Evaluations should be conducted under monitored conditions, ideally using nocturnal oximetry and daytime arterial gases. Polysomnography (and where available continuous CO_2 monitoring) are recommended in patients in whom sleep hypoventilation is suspected.[45,46]

Vulnerability to Ventilator Complications

Hyperventilation is a frequent complication in neuromuscular patients receiving tracheostomy-assisted ventilation. Chronic ventilation at fixed tidal volumes, whether hypocapnic or isocapnic in nature, results in loss of respiratory compliance and an increase in airway resistance,[47] thought to result from insufficient lung expansion to predicted inspiratory capacities. The progressive weight loss in patients with many chronic neuromuscular disorders also may result in a decrease in tidal volume requirements. In such patients, the delivered tidal volume is better based on the actual rather than the ideal weight. Reducing the ventilation of patients who have been chronically hyperventilated results in immediate dyspnea and demands to restore the previous ventilator settings.[48–50] Dyspnea probably occurs as a result of the loss of inhibition of inspiratory cell discharge through the Hering-Breuer reflex.[51] In contrast to tracheostomy-assisted ventilation, NIPPV provides an open system of ventilation with maintenance of more optimal levels of P_{CO_2}, allowing restoration of the ventilatory drive.[3] The correction should be done with small (e.g., 50 ml) decrements in tidal volume and/or respiratory rate over a period of weeks to restore serum bicarbonate concentrations to sufficient buffering capacity. Sometimes mild sedation is required to tolerate this maneuver. Periodic assessments of blood gases or end-tidal or rebreathe P_{CO_2} values[52] should be done to optimize ventilation. Ventilator volumes higher than those used in tracheostomy-assisted ventilation and the use of pressure-limited ventilation can compensate for leakage around the interface.[53]

Adverse effects of the interface, while not life-threatening, can lead to serious discomfort and the possibility of discontinuation. They include skin and eye irritation, drying of mucus membranes, aerophagia, leaks around the nasal and full-face interfaces, and abdominal distension with colic.[54] Leaks can be prevented with the use of chin straps or oral/lip seals.[3]

Volume-cycled ventilation in control mode may result in a decrease in effective ventilation secondary to glottic closure.[55,56] Mechanical dysfunction and power outages occur occasionally, leaving the ventilator-dependent patient vulnerable to acute or progressive respiratory failure. In patients with little or no tolerance off the ventilator, a backup device is recommended. The physician may have to exert influence as the patient's advocate to persuade third-party payors to provide reimbursement for the spare ventilator.

Other respiratory aids such as rocking beds, pneumobelts, diaphragmatic pacing, and negative-pressure ventilators are covered in other chapters of this book. In general, they are not as effective as NIPPV, particularly in patients with severe scoliosis and bulbar dysfunction. Negative-pressure ventilators and diaphragmatic pacers can promote obstructive apneas, whereas the disadvantages of diaphragmatic pacers also include their high cost, lack of alarms, and potential to fail.

Adjunctive Therapy

GLOSSOPHARYNGEAL BREATHING (GPB)

Originally taught to persons with poliomyelitis, GPB may be useful in other neuromuscular diseases in maintaining ventilation. In individuals with weak inspiratory muscles and no tolerance off the ventilator, GPB is a nonmechanical form of breathing that can be handy in the case of sudden ventilator failure or to augment spontaneous breathing.[57] With each closure of the glottis (a "gulp"; 40–200 ml) can be inhaled and then exhaled to augment breathing. GPB can be used to stack breaths (up to 1.6 liters) and promote cough.[3]

ASSISTED COUGHING

As noted earlier, respiratory complications are the principal causes of morbidity and mortality in advanced neuromuscular diseases, in particular, inability to eliminate airway secretions because of ineffective coughing. Effectiveness of secretion clearance depends on the peak expiratory flow rate. A peak flow of less than 160 liters/min has been recommended as an indication to provide manually or mechanically applied cough assistance.[58] Baseline peak flows of less than 270 liters/min are also associated with poor secretion elimination during chest infections. These values should be used as guidelines and not as absolute cutoffs because some patients may develop difficulty eliminating secretions despite higher peak flows.

Assisted coughing can augment peak flows during coughing and increase airway clearance ability. Manually assisted coughing requires cooperation on the part of the patient and caregiver coordination. The patient achieves a maximal inspiratory capacity, preferably with use of a positive-pressure device and breath "stacking," closes his or her glottis, and then "lets go" with the help of an externally applied upward and inward abdominal thrust.[59] A mouth pressure of 60 cmH$_2$O or more during relaxation at peak insufflation against a closed shutter usually indicates a recoil pressure adequate to generate a good cough flow.[59] Clearance of secretions with assisted coughing can prevent respiratory failure and delay or avoid the need for a tracheostomy.

MECHANICAL INSUFFLATION-EXSUFFLATION DEVICES

A mechanical insufflation-exsufflation (MI-E) device is a positive-pressure generator that produces a deep inspiration followed by a powerful sucking action that achieves a high expiratory flow rate. Minimum pressures of 35–40 cmH$_2$O are required to expel secretions but should be increased gradually over time according to the patient's comfort level.[60] Such pressures would be required to overcome small lungs and stiff chest walls, as in scoliosis. Flows that exceed 160 liters/min decrease the risk for respiratory complications and the need for intubation and bronchoscopy.[15] The MI-E device can be used with tracheostomies (Fig. 32-9) and full-face masks, avoiding the mucosal trauma that results from suctioning. Frequency of use can range from once a day to every 4 hours depending on the amount of secretions produced. Many patients note that they can breathe more easily after using the MI-E device. These devices are useful in patients with most neuromuscular conditions,[61] including amyotrophic lateral sclerosis with bulbar dysfunction.[62] For optimal results, use of the MI-E device can be augmented with application of manual cough technique and proper positioning of the patient to promote drainage of airway secretions.

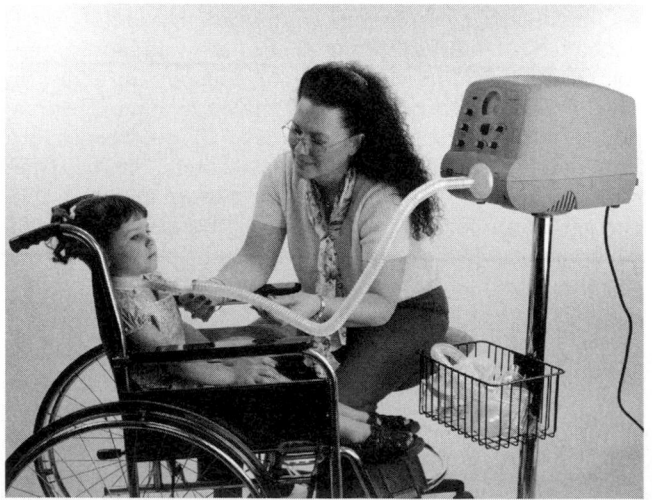

FIGURE 32-9 A mechanical insufflation-exsufflation device shown in use through a tracheostomy. (*Used, with permission, from J. H. Emerson Co.*)

Complications with MI-E devices are rare and include nausea, bradycardia, tachycardia, and abdominal distension. The most common reason for intolerance of the MI-E device is inadequate caregiver training regarding its application. As with any respiratory device used for life support, education of the patient and caregivers is important to ensure best results.

Bronchoscopy is useful only in selected cases of atelectasis caused by mucus plugging and should be tried after other methods of secretion removal have failed.

Patients with quadriplegia can contract the clavicular portion of the pectoralis major to compress the rib cage during forced expiration and cough.[63] They have decreased ability to increase intrathoracic pressure, however, because of paralysis of expiratory rib-cage and abdominal muscles. Electrical or magnetic stimulation can increase intrathoracic pressure inversely proportional to the degree of abdominal muscle atrophy and may be used to augment dynamic airway compression and clearance of airway secretions.[64]

Timing of Transfer from ICU to the Community

Patients may be hospitalized for a number of acute consequences of respiratory muscle weakness, including pneumonia, atelectasis, hypoventilation, and sleep apnea. After the complication has resolved, the patient must be prepared for discharge into the community using a multidisciplinary approach incorporating potential caregivers in the planning. This goal is best achieved in special care units that may be part of the medical facility to which the patient was admitted or a separate facility designed for this purpose. During this period, there should be clarification of the patient's advance directives, particularly with regard to interventions for long-term survival. If the patient is supported with NIPPV, attention must be given to maintenance of appropriate ventilator settings, the oral/nasal interface, seating, mobility, and nutrition (including gastrostomy or jejunostomy feeding). Caregivers must be trained in techniques of manual and mechanical cough assistance. Only if such measures are unsuccessful in clearing secretions (as in severe bulbar involvement with amyotrophic lateral sclerosis or postpolio syndrome) should tracheostomies be resorted to. If the patient has been on long-term tracheostomy-assisted or negative-pressure ventilation, attempts to transition to NIPPV may be appropriate.[3] Many patients have expressed a preference to NIPPV, even after many years of having lived with tracheostomies.

Long-Term Survival and Quality of Life

While home NIPPV probably improves survival in amyotrophic lateral sclerosis[35,65,66] and Duchenne muscular dystrophy,[67–69] its impact on quality of life in such patients is not clear. Because assisted ventilation does not prevent the progression of disease, it is difficult to distinguish dissatisfaction related to disease progression and family stress related to the implementation of mechanical ventilation itself and the various methods needed to maintain the patient's airways clear of secretions. Another problem is that there is marked variability in clinical practice among physicians[70–72] most likely because of a perception that mechanical ventilation may prolong suffering in a progressive disease such as Duchenne muscular dystrophy, spinal muscular atrophy, and amyotrophic lateral sclerosis. In general, health care workers tend to underestimate quality-of-life scores of life satisfaction.[73]

Patients usually appreciate having meaningful discussions about assisted ventilation throughout the course of their illness. Discussions concerning mechanical ventilation should occur before the onset of respiratory impairment. Care of the patient with progressive neuromuscular disease should be implemented and continued in a multidisciplinary setting involving neurologists, pulmonologists, psychologists, social workers, physical and occupational therapists, speech pathologists, nutritionists, and respiratory therapists.[74–77] In some respects, working closely with the family and other caregivers is even more vital than working with the patient, not only for educational purposes but also for providing support during a stressful period.

Important Unknowns and the Future

While it is agreed that NIPPV is the preferred means of managing ventilatory impairment and failure in neuromuscular disease, many patients have difficulty in tolerating mask ventilation. Inability or unwillingness to use the ventilator detracts from quality of life as well as survival. Glottic closure, patient-ventilator asynchrony leading to increased work of breathing in those patients with remaining respiratory muscle function, a sensation of suffocation, and facial pressure points and abrasions contribute to this lack of success. Increased use of spontaneous-timed ventilator mode ventilation and of oral/lip seals may circumvent some of these problems. Controlled and comparative studies of ventilators and interfaces would help to increase the acceptability of NIPPV at an earlier stage of respiratory impairment, enabling the patient to increase its use with disease progression. Such studies also would increase physician acceptance of the use of NIPPV as a routine means of improving quality of life and possibly survival. A change in physician attitudes will lead to greater acceptance among patients who, unfortunately, still face indifferent and even negative attitudes concerning life support.

Summary and Conclusion

Noninvasive ventilation is now the accepted form of respiratory support for people with neuromuscular and chest-wall disorders. Improvements in ventilator modes, interfaces, and adjunctive secretion-removal techniques have facilitated care and increased the quality of life in such individuals. An interdisciplinary approach aimed at not only the patient but also the family and other caregivers is essential for coping with the rigors of providing care under potentially stressful conditions. Close involvement by third-party payors and private community-based and governmental agencies is also crucial to ease the cost of home care.

References

1. Affeldt JE, Bower AG, Dail CW. Prognosis for respiratory recovery in severe poliomyelitis. Arch Phys Med Rehabil 1957; 38:290–5.
2. Baydur A, Layne E, Aral H, et al. Long term non-invasive ventilation in the community for patients with musculoskeletal disorders: 46 year experience and review. Thorax 2000; 55:4–11.
3. Bach J. Management of patients with neuromuscular disease. Philadelphia: Hanley and Belfus, 2004: Chap 10,11, pp. 211–308.
4. Baydur A, Adkins RH, Milic-Emili J. Lung mechanics in individuals with spinal cord injury: Effects of injury level and posture. J Appl Physiol 2001; 90:405–11.
5. Gibson GJ, Pride NB, Newsom Davis J, et al. Pulmonary mechanics in patients with respiratory muscle weakness. Am Rev Respir Dis 1977; 115:389–95.
6. Loh L, Hughes JMB, Newsom Davis J. Gas exchange problems in bilateral diaphragm paralysis. Bull Eur Physiopathol Respir 1979; 15:137–41.
7. Bye PTP, Ellis ER, Issa FG, et al. Respiratory failure and sleep in neuromuscular disease. Thorax 1990; 45:241–7.
8. Smith PEM, Edwards RHT, Calverley PMA. Ventilation and breathing pattern during sleep in Duchenne muscular dystrophy. Chest 1989; 96:1346–51.
9. Baydur A. Respiratory muscle strength and control of ventilation in patients with neuromuscular disease. Chest 1991; 99:330–8.
10. De Troyer A, Borenstein S, Cordier R. Analysis of lung volume restriction in patients with respiratory muscle weakness. Thorax 1980; 35:603–10.
11. Baydur A, Swank, Stiles CM, Sassoon CSH. Respiratory elastic load compensation in anesthetized patients with kyphoscoliosis. J Appl Physiol 1989; 67:1024–31.
12. Baydur A, Carlson M. Immediate response to inspiratory resistive loading in anesthetized patients with kyphoscoliosis: Spirometric and neural effects. Lung 1996; 174:99–118.
13. Nava S, Rubini F, Zanotti, et al. The tension-time index of the diaphragm revisited in quadriplegic patients with diaphragm pacing. Am J Respir Crit Care Med 1996; 153:1322–7.
14. Vincken W, Elleker MG, Cosio MG. Determinants of respiratory muscle weakness in stable chronic neuromuscular disorders. Am J Med 1987; 82:53–8.
15. Bach JR, Saporito LR. Criteria for extubation and tracheostomy tube removal for patients with ventilatory failure: A different approach to weaning. Chest 1996; 110:1566–71.
16. Begin P, Mathieu J, Almirall J, et al. Relationship between chronic hypercapnia and inspiratory muscle weakness in myotonic dystrophy. Am J Respir Crit Care Med 1997; 156:133–9.
17. Veale D, Cooper BG, Gilmartin JJ, et al. Breathing pattern awake and asleep in patients with myotonic dystrophy. Eur Respir J 1995; 8:815–8.
18. Bourke SC, Gibson GJ. Sleep and breathing in neuromuscular disease. Eur Respir J 2002; 19:1194–201.
19. Piper A. Sleep abnormalities associated with neuromuscular disease: Pathophysiology and evaluation. Semin Respir Crit Care Med 2002; 23:211–9.
20. Fergusson KA, Strong MJ, Ahmad D, et al. Sleep-disordered breathing in amyotrophic lateral sclerosis. Chest 1996; 110:664–9.

21. Finnimore AJ, Jackson RV, Morton A, Lynch E. Sleep hypoxia in myotonic dystrophy and its correlation with awake respiratory function. Thorax 1994; 49:66–70.

22. White JES, Drinnan MJ, Smithson AJ, et al. Respiratory muscle activity and oxygenation during sleep in patients with muscle weakness. Eur Respir J 1995; 8:807–14.

23. Gay PC, Westbrook PR, Daube JR, et al. Effects of alterations in pulmonary function and sleep variables on survival in patients with amyotrophic lateral sclerosis. Mayo Clin Proc 1991; 66:686–94.

24. Khan Y, Heckmatt JZ. Obstructive apneas in Duchenne muscular dystrophy. Thorax 1994; 49:157–61.

25. Estenne M, De Troyer A. Mechanism of the postural dependence of vital capacity in tetraplegic subjects. Am Rev Respir Dis 1987; 135:367–71.

26. Braun NMT, Arora NS, Rochester DF. Respiratory muscle and pulmonary function in polymyositis and other proximal myopathies. Thorax 1983; 38:616–23.

27. Stefanutti D, Benoist MR, Scheinmann P, et al. Usefulness of sniff nasal pressure in patients with neuromuscular or skeletal disorders. Am J Respir Crit Care Med 2000; 162:1507–11.

28. Lyall RA, Donaldson N, Polkey MI, et al. Respiratory muscle strength and ventilatory failure in amyotrophic lateral sclerosis. Brain 2001; 124:2000–13.

29. DePalo VA, McCool FD. Respiratory muscle evaluation of the patient with neuromuscular disease. Semin Respir Crit Care 2002; 23:201–9.

30. Newsom-Davis J, Goldman M, Loh L, et al. Diaphragm function and alveolar hypoventilation. Q J Med 1976; 45:87–100.

31. Lechtzin N, Wiener CM, Shade DM, et al. Spirometry in the supine position improves the detection of diaphragmatic weakness in patients with amyotrophic lateral sclerosis. Chest 2002; 121:436–42.

32. Maeda CJ, Baydur A, Waters RL, et al. The effect of the halovest and body position on pulmonary function in quadriplegia. J Spinal Disord 1990; 3:47–51.

33. Baydur A, Kanel G. Tracheobronchomalacia and tracheal hemorrhage in patients with Duchenne muscular dystrophy receiving long-term ventilation with uncuffed tracheostomies. Chest 2003; 123:1307–11.

34. Schönhofer B, Geibel M, Sonneborn M, et al. Daytime mechanical ventilation in chronic respiratory insufficiency. Eur Respir J 1997; 10:2840–6.

35. Aboussouan LS, Khan SU, Meeker DP, et al. Effect of noninvasive positive-pressure ventilation on survival in amyotrophic lateral sclerosis. Ann Intern Med 1997; 127:450–3.

36. Raphael JC, Chevret S, Chastang C, et al. Randomized trial of preventive nasal ventilation in Duchenne muscular dystrophy. French Multicentre Cooperative Group on Home Mechanical Ventilation Assistance in Duchenne de Boulogne Muscular Dystrophy. Lancet 1994; 343:1600–4.

37. Annane D, Chevrolet JC, Chevret S, et al. Nocturnal mechanical ventilation for chronic hypoventilation in patients with neuromuscular and chest wall disorders. The Cochrane Library, Issue 1, 2006.

38. Jubran A, Van de Graaff WB, Tobin MJ. Variablity of patient-ventilator interaction with pressure support ventilation in patients with chronic obstructive pulmonary disease. Am J Respir Cri Care Med 1995; 152:129–36.

39. Younes M. Proportional assist ventilation, a new approach to ventilatory support: Theory. Am Rev Respir Dis 1992; 145:114–20.

40. Ambrosino N, Vitacca M, Polese G, et al. Short-term effects of nasal proportional assist ventilation in patients with chronic hypercapnic respiratory insufficiency. Eur Respir J 1997; 10:2829–34.

41. Polese G, Vitacca M, Bianchi L, et al. Nasal proportional assist ventilation unloads the inspiratory muscles of stable patients with hypercapnia due to COPD. Eur Respir J 2000; 16:491–8.

42. Porta R, Appendini L, Vitacca M, et al. Mask proportional assist vs pressure support ventilation in patients in clinically stable condition with chronic ventilatory failure. Chest 2002; 122:479–88.

43. Winck JC, Vitacca M, Morais A, et al. Tolerance and physiologic effects of nocturnal mask pressure support vs proportional assist ventilation in chronic ventilatory failure. Chest 2004; 126:382–8.

44. Calderini E, Confalonieri M, Puccio PG, et al. Patient-ventilator asynchrony during noninvasive ventilation: The role of the expiratory trigger. Intensive Care Med 1999; 25:662–7.

45. American Thoracic Society Statement. Respiratory care of the patient with Duchenne muscular dystrophy. Am J Respir Crit Care Med 2004; 170:456–65.

46. Perrin C, Unterborn JN, Ambrosio CD, et al. Pulmonary complications of chronic neuromuscular diseases and their management. Muscle Nerve 2004; 29:5–27.

47. Sinha R, Bergofsky EH. Prolonged alteration of lung mechanics in kyphoscoliosis by positive pressure hyperinflation. Am Rev Respir Dis 1972; 106:47–57.

48. Bach JR, Haber II, Wang TG, et al. Alveolar ventilation as a function of ventilatory support method. Eur J Phys Med Rehabil 1995; 5:80–4.

49. Bach JR, Kang SW. Disorders of ventilation: Weakness, stiffness, and mobilization. Chest 2000; 117:301–3.

50. Manning HL, Shea SA, Schwartzstein RM, et al. Reduced tidal volume increases air hunger at fixed pCO_2 in ventilated quadriplegics. Respir Physiol 1992; 90:9–30.

51. Patterson JL, Mullinax PF, Bain T, et al. Carbon dioxide–induced dyspnea in a patient with respiratory muscle paralysis. Am J Med 1962; 32:811–6.

52. Hackney JD, Seares CH, Collier CR. Estimation of arterial CO_2 tension by rebreathing technique. J Appl Physiol 1958; 12:425–30.

53. Tzeng AC, Bach JR. Prevention of pulmonary morbidity for patients with neuromuscular disease. Chest 2000; 118:1390–6.

54. Leger P, Langevin B, Guez A, et al. What to do when nasal ventilation fails for neuromuscular patients? Eur Respir Rev 1993; 3:279–83.

55. Jounieaux V, Aubert G, Dury M, et al. Effects of nasal positive-pressure hyperventilation on the glottis in normal awake subjects. J Appl Physiol 1995; 79:176–85.

56. Parreira VF, Jounieaux V, Aubert G, et al. Nasal two-level positive-pressure ventilation in normal subjects. Am J Respir Crit Care Med 1996; 153:1616–23.

57. Dail C, Rodgers M, Guess V, et al. Glossopharyngeal breathing. Downey, CA: Rancho Los Amigos Department of Physical Therapy, 1979.

58. Bach JR, Smith WH, Michaels J, et al. Airway secretion clearance by mechanical exsufflation for post-poliomyelitis ventilator-assisted individuals. Arch Phys Med Rehabil 1993; 74:170–77.

59. Kang SW, Bach JR. Maximum insufflation capacity. Chest 2000; 118:213–9.

60. Miske L, Hickey EM, Kolb SM, et al. Use of the mechanical inexsufflator in pediatric patients with neuromuscular disease and impaired cough. Chest 2004; 125:1406–12.

61. Bach JR, Ishikima Y, Kim H. Prevention of pulmonary morbidity for patients with Duchenne muscular dystrophy. Chest 1997; 112:1024–8.

62. Sancho J, Servera E, Diaz J, et al. Efficacy of mechanical insufflation-exsufflation in medically stable patients with amyotrophic lateral sclerosis. Chest 2004; 125:1400–5.

63. De Troyer A, Estenne M, Heilporn A. Mechanism of active expiration in tetraplegic subjects. New Engl J Med 1986; 314:740–4.

64. Estenne M, Pinet C, De Troyer A. Abdominal muscle strength in patients with tetraplegia. Am J Respir Crit Care Med 2000; 161:707–12.

65. Kleopa KA, Sherman M, Neal B, et al. Bipap improves survival and rate of pulmonary function decline in patients with ALS. J Neurol Sci 1999; 164:82–8.

66. Pinto AC, Evangelista T, Carvalho MA, et al. Respiratory assistance with a noninvasive ventilator (BiPAP) in MND/ALS patients: Survival rates in a controlled trial. J Neurol Sci 1995; 129:19–26.

67. Simonds AK, Muntoni F, Heather S, et al. Impact of nasal ventilation on survival in hypercapnic Duchenne muscular dystrophy. Thorax 1998; 53:949–52.

68. Jeppesen J, Green A, Steffensen BF, Rahbek J. The Duchenne muscular dystrophy population in Denmark, 1997–2001: Prevalence, incidence and survival in relation to the introduction of ventilator use. Neuromusc Disord 2003; 13:804–12.

69. Eagle M, Baudoin SV, Chandler C, et al. Survival in Duchenne muscular dystrophy: Improvements in life expectancy since 1967 and the impact of home nocturnal ventilation. Neuromusc Disord 2003; 13:804–12.

70. Bourke SC, Shaw PJ, Williams TL, et al. Non-invasive ventilation in motor neurone disease: Current UK practice. Amyotrophic Lateral Scler Other Motor Neuron Disord 2002; 3:145–9.

71. Cedarbaum JM, Stambler N. Disease status and use of ventilatory support by ALS patients. Amyotroph Lateral Scler Other Motor Neuron Disord 2001; 2:19–22.

72. Hardart MKM, Burns, J, Truog RD. Respiratory support in spinal muscular atrophy type I: A survey of physician practices and attitudes. Pediatrics 2002; 110:e24–30.

73. Bach JR, Campagnolo DI, Hoeman S. Life satisfaction of individuals with Duchenne muscular dystrophy using long-term mechanical ventilatory support. Am J Phys Med Rehabil 1991; 70: 129–35.

74. Traynor BJ, Alexander M, Corr B, et al. Effect of a multidisciplinary amyotrophic lateral sclerosis (ALS) clinic on ALS survival: A population study, 1996–2000. J Neurol Neurosurg Psychiatry 2003; 74:1258–61.

75. Gilgoff I, Prentice W, Baydur A. Patient and family participation in the management of respiratory failure in Duchenne's muscular dystrophy. Chest 1989; 95:519–24.

76. Baydur A, Gilgoff I, Prentice W, et al. Decline in respiratory function and experience with long-term assisted ventilation in advanced Duchenne's muscular dystrophy. Chest 1990; 97:884–9.

77. Bradley MD, Orrell RW, Clarke J, et al. Outcome of ventilatory support for acute respiratory failure in motor neurone disease. J Neurol Neurosurg Psychiatr 2002; 72:752–6.

78. Baydur A. Respiratory muscle function in systemic disorders. Semin Respir Med 1988; 9:223–38.

Chapter 33

CHRONIC VENTILATOR FACILITIES

STEFANO NAVA
MICHELE VITACCA

Chronic ventilator facilities (CVFs) are meant to be "protected" environments for the treatment of patients requiring prolonged mechanical ventilation. Rarely in medicine has there been so great a confusion in terminology and wording to define a relatively simple concept of patient care. On this particular subject, researchers in different countries or even in different areas within the same country are essentially speaking in different medical tongues.

Numerous names are included under the umbrella of CVFs: long-term acute-care facilities, respiratory special care units, chronic ventilator-dependent units, regional weaning centers, ventilator-dependent rehabilitation hospitals, prolonged respiratory-care units, noninvasive respiratory-care units, high-dependency units, and respiratory intensive-care units. And this is without even considering nursing homes and hospice care.

Because "Language is the source of misunderstandings" (Le Petit Prince, Antoine de Saint-Exupery, 1900–1944),[1] the aim of this chapter is to review the available scientific evidence about the role of CVFs and to try to dissipate as much confusion as possible in this field so that we do not get "lost in translation."[2]

A 16-year study showed that the number of acute-care hospital beds in the United States has decreased over time, but the number of critical-care beds has increased progressively in both absolute and proportional terms. Indeed, the total number of non-critical-care beds decreased by 31%, whereas critical-care beds increased by 26%[3]; nevertheless, admissions to an intensive-care unit (ICU) are very strongly influenced by bed shortages. Most beds in an ICU are occupied by patients requiring mechanical ventilation.

Several reports indicate that ICU patients, especially those needing mechanical ventilation for acute respiratory failure, have a relatively poor outcome.[4-8] There is a subset of patients who require prolonged mechanical ventilation (i.e., >14 days) because of complex cardiopulmonary disease or multisystem problems. These patients represent less than 10% of ICU admissions but consume a large amount of financial resources. For example Cohen and Booth[9] demonstrated that this small group consumed about 50% of ICU patient-days and resources. The extent to which this relatively small population cuts into hospital costs has attracted the attention of experts in the field. Wagner has openly stated that "there is some level of costs of acute care that is beyond our society's economic capacity."[10]

More important, when these "chronically ill" patients are discharged from the ICU because the precipitating cause of their acute episode of respiratory failure has been reversed, they still have the need of mechanical ventilation. Thus they either require transfer to a long-term care or rehabilitation facility[11] or need frequent ICU or hospital readmissions over the subsequent weeks.[12]

Given the dramatically higher number of inpatient critical-care days in 2000 than in 1985,[3] the absolute number of patients receiving mechanical ventilation has increased. It is also likely to continue to increase in the near future. For example, it was demonstrated recently that the incidence of tracheostomy for prolonged mechanical ventilation increased by nearly 200% over the past decade in North Carolina.[13] One reason for the sudden rise in tracheotomy is an attempt by physicians to relieve congestion in busy ICUs through the transfer of ventilator-dependent patients to CVFs.

Rationale

ICUs are not specifically focused on the care of chronically ill patients for several reasons. First, the "closed" environment does not allow optimal comprehensive care for these patients. Weaning from mechanical ventilation is a prolonged, time-consuming process that involves not only selecting the best ventilation method for a particular patient[14,15] but also attention to aggressive physiotherapy,[16] nursing care, counseling, a return to normal eating habits,[17] and open visiting hours for family members and/or caregivers. Second, patient comfort is enhanced by a return to a more physiologic circadian rhythm. The latter may be facilitated through lower noise and activity levels, especially during night hours, than found in an ICU (Table 33-1). Third, the disproportionate number of days of care required by chronically ventilated patients contributes to overcrowding and the limited availability of ICU beds.[23] Last, but not least, the system of reimbursement by third-party carriers, even through the diagnostic-related group (DRG) system, clearly results in significant monetary loss.[24]

Recently, there has been an increase of facilities in both the United States and Europe that specialize in the care of chronically ventilated patients. Being DRG-exempt, these facilities are reimbursed using a cost-based system. Although the

TABLE 33-1 Sound Intensity in Different Environments

Authors (Ref)	Environment	Mean Day Noise Level (dBA)	Mean Night Noise Level (dBA)	Mean Peak Noise Level (dBA)
Gabor et al (ref. 18)	ICU	56 ± 2	54 ± 2	67 ± 3
Freedman et al (ref. 19)	ICU	60 ± 6	57 ± 5	84 ± 5
Aaron et al (ref. 20)	Intermediate ICU			many episodes ≥ 80
Balogh et al (ref. 21)	ICU	60–65	60–65	~96
Ceriana and Frigerio (unpublished data)	CVF (Weaning Center)	47 ± 5	44 ± 2	57 ± 6
Environmental Protection Agency (ref. 22)		<45	<35	

NOTE: Reference 22 is the recommended noise level in a hospital environment according to the Environmental Protection Agency. ICU, intensive-care unit; CVF, chronic ventilator facility.

quality of care in these facilities has never been explored in detail or demonstrated scientifically, these facilities appear to be very effective. Chronically ill patients in these facilities are treated at lower costs than in ICUs but achieve similar outcomes.[25]

Organization of Chronic Ventilator Facilities

The term *CVF* is not necessarily synonymous with the so-called intermediate-care unit or high-dependency unit, which are meant for patients who do not require full ICU care but are thought to need more care than usually can be offered in a general ward.[26–30] Not all patients in the latter units may be ventilator-dependent, but they may require either noninvasive monitoring or noninvasive mechanical ventilation. There is no agreement about the classification of facilities for patients needing prolonged mechanical ventilation because of geographic differences, lack of consensus regarding the appropriate timing of transfer from the ICU, and different criteria of admission. For example, the American College of Critical Care Medicine States in its guidelines for admission to and discharge from adult intermediate-care units that "medically stable ventilator patients for weaning and chronic care" are the ideal candidates for these environments.[31] Unfortunately, these units were described only generically as "progressive-care units or single-organ subspecialty floors or chronic ventilator respiratory-care units." Details were not provided on how these units should be organized or financially reimbursed.

Timing of discharge from the ICU is also critical. Long-term ventilator patients are often old and have various underlying chronic comorbidities that may complicate or exacerbate their respiratory condition at any time after discharge from the ICU.[32,33] The 6-month rate of readmission to an acute-care hospital is close to 40%, and readmission is often within the first 2 months after discharge from the ICU.[12] Surprisingly, this rate was not influenced by the initial discharge disposition. That is, it did not differ for patients discharged to a nursing home, a CVF, or their own home. These findings indirectly suggest that not all CVFs are presently prepared to cope with the burden of a new "acute exacerbation" in such patients. For example, Nasraway et al[34]

found that despite a 31-fold increase in the number of all adults transferred from ICUs to extended-care facilities in the Boston area between 1990 and 1996, the level of care of these facilities varied greatly depending mainly on the availability of skilled nurses.

There is still disagreement about the definition of a ventilator-dependent patient. The ninth revision of the *International Classification of Diseases*[35] defines long-term ventilation patients as those who have received 5 or more days of ventilation. Various authors, however, have used limits as short as 48–72 hours and as long as 40 days.[36–38] Realistically, about 20% of patients in an ICU require mechanical ventilation for more than 1 week, and about half of them are weaned successfully over the following few days.[39] Therefore, a limit of 2 weeks has been chosen by most authors to define the threshold for ventilator dependency. The Health Care Financing Administration[40] has expanded this limit to 21 days of mechanical ventilation for at least 6 hours a day. A definition based only on time, however, does not consider that for a particular patient to be regarded as ventilator dependent (and therefore eligible for transfer to a chronic-care facility), the precipitating cause of the respiratory failure must have been reversed.

CVFs have been described in the literature only in North America,[25] Europe,[41] and Asia.[42] Substantial differences exist in their organization, location, and criteria of admission. A recent editorial entitled, "The Challenge of Prolonged Mechanical Ventilation: A Shared Global Experience,"[43] stressed the need for common international consensus. Yet international evidence-based guidelines and/or "position papers" are lacking.

Given the confusion of terminology, we submit that the most logical classification of CVFs is one based on the location of the different facilities, specifically whether the facility is inside or outside a so-called acute-care hospital. Figure 33-1 illustrates the possible sites of care for patients who are chronically ventilator dependent. It should be borne in mind that access to these different environments may differ internationally or even regionally within the same country.

FACILITIES WITHIN ACUTE-CARE HOSPITALS

Mechanical ventilation is initiated outside the hospital in a relatively small proportion of patients; ventilation is mostly started and stabilized in an ICU.[44] The timing of discharge of

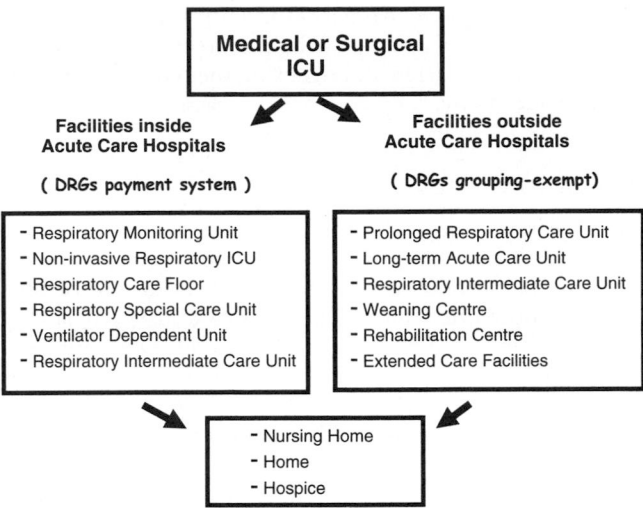

FIGURE 33-1 Potential sites of care for ventilator-dependent patients when discharged from an intensive-care unit (ICU). DRG, Diagnostic-Related Grouping

ventilator-dependent patients from the ICU is linked strictly to the criteria of admission of each single CVF, which are described in Chapter 34.

In the late 1980s, CVFs started to emerge in acute-care hospitals as an attempt to provide an alternative therapeutic environment for ICU patients requiring prolonged mechanical ventilation. Krieger et al[45,46] probably were the first to establish a CVF within an acute-care hospital (Central Respiratory Monitoring Unit at the Miami Mount Sinai Medical Center). They were followed shortly after by Elpern et al[47,48]) (Noninvasive Respiratory Care Unit of St. Luke's Medical Center in Chicago). These units were devoted mainly to patients requiring prolonged mechanical ventilation. In 1990, the Mayo Clinic opened a ventilator-dependent unit (VDU) inside Saint Mary's Hospital.[49–52] Their mission was to create an environment conducive to the rehabilitation of patients with respiratory failure and also to lower the costs of ventilator-dependent patients.[53] Shortly thereafter, new CVFs were opened. These went under different names at Saint Vincent's Hospital and Medical Center in New York[54] (Non-Monitored Respiratory Care Floor) and at Cleveland Clinic Foundation[55] (Respiratory Special Care Unit). As discussed later (in outcome and effectiveness), the overall rate of weaning success was high (>50%), with a mortality rate below 40%.

In Europe, the first report on this subject was published in 1995 by Smith and Shneerson[56] from England. Rather than opening a special unit for patients requiring prolonged ventilation, they described the institution of a progressive-care multidisciplinary program carried out within the ICU by a dedicated team of respiratory physicians and nurses. As soon as patients were judged ready for discharge from the ICU, they were transferred to a respiratory unit, where they continued the multidisciplinary program. The program was very successful with regard to discharge to home (80% of the patients) and 1-year survival (76%). The recent survey[41] of the European Respiratory Society on respiratory intermediate-care units (RICUs) showed that during 1999, the majority (58%) of the 11,890 patients admitted to 55 RICUs received invasive mechanical ventilation. These units almost always (>90%) were inside an acute-care hospital. Unfortunately, no data were available on how many of these patients actually were ventilator dependent. Nevertheless, an Italian survey published in 2001[57] reported that 61% of patients receiving invasive mechanical ventilation in Italian RICUs were tracheotomized and therefore were considered ventilator dependent. The percentages may be similar in other European countries.

Irrespective of location on either side of the Atlantic, the organization and staffing of CVFs inside acute-care hospitals appear to be homogeneous and more similar to that of an ICU than to that of a CVF located outside an acute-care hospital.[58,59] The majority of these CVFs provide noninvasive monitoring, the nurse-patient ratio is usually 1:2 to 1:4,[41,47,50,54,55] and a lead respiratory therapist is assigned permanently and present in the unit. General medical care is provided around the clock by medical house staff under the direction of a an attending physician in either critical care or pulmonology. The nursing staff usually is specially trained through orientation and in-service programs to address the needs of this particular population of patients. The approach to the patients is multidisciplinary, involving dieticians, psychologists, physical therapists, speech therapists, social workers, and clergy as needed. Because these CVFs are located within an acute-care hospital, all the diagnostic (e.g., computed tomographic scans, nuclear magnetic resonance imaging) and therapeutic (e.g., major surgery) options are readily available. In Europe, the nurse-patient ratio varies slightly according to the three levels of care of RICUs.[27,41] Because of the different education and responsibilities of respiratory therapists (rarely present around the clock), an attending physician is always present in the units.[60,61]

FACILITIES OUTSIDE ACUTE-CARE HOSPITALS

This classification consists of several CVFs going under names such as regional weaning centers, prolonged respiratory-care units, long-term acute-care units, and respiratory intensive-care units inside rehabilitation hospitals. The need for these special facilities outside the acute-care health system was recognized a long time ago in North America but only recently in Europe. For example, the Comprehensive Critical Care of the British Department of Health[62] recently stated that "the effectiveness of specialist weaning and progressive care programs for long-term ventilation of patients has been demonstrated by research, and NHS Trusts should review the need for provision of such services."

The first experience of a CVF dedicated to the problem of ventilator-dependent patients was reported by Indihar,[63–65] who described 10 years of activity, starting in 1979, of a unit located in Bethesda Lutheran Medical Center. In the late 1980s there was substantial growth of regional weaning centers in the United States. Examples include the Barlow Respiratory Hospital in Los Angeles,[66,67] the Medical Center of Central Massachusetts,[68] and the Hospital for Special Care, New Britain, Connecticut.[69,70] Later, there was an impressive burgeoning of new long-term acute-care units. By 1997, these had a capacity of about 15,000 patients per year.[71] These units were established either as free-standing hospitals, as in the case of most regional weaning centers, or within an acute-care hospital but operating with total independence. As such, their governance is independent of the host hospital, and reimbursement is not based on a DRG system.

CVFs within a rehabilitation hospital are also popular in the United States and Europe, especially in Germany and Italy, where about 15% of RICUs are located inside rehabilitation centers.[41,72–74]

Unlike CVFs located within acute-care hospitals, CVFs located outside appear to have a rather heterogeneous organization and staffing. This heterogeneity occurs despite these facilities espousing a program based on the common ideal of providing comprehensive medical, nursing, and respiratory care to ventilator-dependent patients. For example, New England[34] has several "extended-care facilities" outside acute hospitals; the skills and level of care vary dramatically among different centers. Despite the personnel being fully licensed health care practitioners, they may not all be completely familiar with the complexities of ventilator-dependent patients. Patient outcome is likely to depend on the different levels of care provided.

In most North American centers, the nurse-patient ratio is about 1:4 during the day and 1:8 at night and on weekends. A full-time respiratory therapist[66,75] usually is present. The primary physicians are either internists or specialists in pulmonary and/or critical-care medicine, whereas nighttime coverage commonly is provided by junior doctors. The comprehensive-care team includes physical therapists, occupational therapists, speech and swallowing therapists, and clinical psychologists. Screening for admission is performed either by an attending physician or by a nurse in consultation with an attending physician.[75] Weaning protocols and the selection of ventilator settings during this process are implemented by respiratory therapists.[76] Discharges are planned by nurses or social-work care managers. With the exception of a few facilities, which may have operating rooms for minor surgery, most CVFs located outside acute-care hospitals cannot offer surgery or sophisticated diagnostic procedures.

In Europe, CVFs outside acute-care hospitals are run mainly by full-time attending physicians who are specialists in respiratory and/or critical-care medicine.[27,41,57] These physicians are in charge of the admission and discharge of patients and the weaning protocols. They are on duty 24 hours a day. The doctor-patient ratio is at least 1:8. The nurse-patient ratio is usually similar to that of North American centers. Because of their different educational training, respiratory therapists in Europe tend to be involved mainly in rehabilitation programs, for about 8 hours a day (excluding Sundays and holidays), rather than in the weaning process.[77] In common with North American facilities, most European CVFs do not offer major surgery.

Irrespective of their geographic location, CVFs located outside acute-care hospitals are intended to provide privacy, rest, and longer visiting hours for relatives and friends.

Above all, they provide physical and pulmonary rehabilitation, which has been shown to help in freeing patients from mechanical ventilation and restoring them to an acceptable level of autonomy.[78]

NURSING HOMES

A small percentage of ventilator-dependent patients are discharged from an ICU[12] directly to a nursing home. Nursing homes, however, are more likely to receive such patients once they have left a CVF. In 1991, a survey by the American Association for Respiratory Therapists[79] found that nearly 30% of ventilator-dependent patients remained in CVFs for nonmedical reasons, such as reimbursement obstacles to discharge or lack of postdischarge placement options. Indeed, about 20% of patients cared for in a ventilator-dependent unit are transferred to nursing home simply because they are not ready to go home.[12]

Nursing homes have been established all over the United States[80] either as independent units inside larger facilities or as stand-alone facilities. To the best of our knowledge, very few exist in Europe.[81] Apparently, there is no standardization of admission criteria, staffing, or organization of these units apart from the person needing "24-hour nursing care for a cognitive or a physical impairment."[82] Nurses working in this specialized area should be trained by respiratory therapists to perform specific procedures such as suctioning, tracheotomy care, and monitoring of ventilator parameters. In some cases, for example, Lakeside Hospital in Wisconsin,[80] weekly care rounds have been introduced; these are led by a pulmonary physician with the participation of the care team, including not only the certified nurses but also respiratory therapists, dieticians, social workers, and when possible, family members. In the very few observational studies performed in this kind of facility, weaning outcomes are very promising.[83] Further studies are needed to define the characteristics of ventilator-dependent patients who are most likely to benefit from admission to this environment.

Criteria for Admission

Table 33-2 presents criteria for defining the "ideal" candidate for a CVF. The concept of ventilator dependency is the primary criterion for selecting admissions to a CVF. Accordingly, most centers accept only tracheotomized patients because tracheotomy per se is assumed as evidence of ventilator dependency. Indeed, the dramatic increase in tracheotomies performed over the last 10 years[13] suggests that ICU physicians tend to perform an early tracheotomy before trying a complete weaning protocol. This change may reflect attempts to decongest busy ICUs more rapidly by allowing transfer of ventilator-dependent patients to extended-care facilities. To avoid this problem, some units request proof that a patient has failed at least two weaning trials before being admitted.[51]

TABLE 33-2   Criteria for Defining the Ideal Candidate to a Chronic Ventilator Facility

Patients ventilated for more than 14 days, necessitating prolonged weaning
Presence of a tracheostomy
Potential weaning possibility
Defined diagnosis
Single-organ failure
Hemodynamically stable (no pressor infusion)
No sepsis or active infections
Absence of surgical problems
No need of continuous sedation
Absence of chronic renal failure necessitating hemodialysis
$Pa_{O_2}/F_{IO_2} > 200$ and need for external PEEP < 10 cmH$_2$O
Need for aggressive rehabilitation program
Potential to benefit from a rehabilitation program

TABLE 33-3   Classification of Patients Admitted to a Chronic Ventilator Facility

Acute lung injury
    Acute respiratory distress syndrome
    Pneumonia
    Aspiration injury
    Burns
Chronic lung disease
    Chronic obstructive pulmonary disease
    Asthma
    Pulmonary fibrosis
    Fibrothorax
Postoperative
    Lobectomy or pneumectomy
    Cardiac surgery
    Major abdominal surgery
Neuromuscular diseases
    Amyotrophic lateral sclerosis
    Multiple sclerosis
    Postpolio syndrome
    Spinal cord injuries
    Kyphoscoliosis
    Critically Ill polyneuropathy
    Guillain-Barre' syndrome
Cardiovascular disorders
    Chronic congestive heart failure
    Ischemic cardiomyopathy

SOURCE: Adapted, with permission, from ref. 89.

Other criteria used for selecting patients for admission to CVFs are clinical stability and potential to benefit from a rehabilitation program.[49,55] Clinical stability is defined as reversal of the precipitating cause of respiratory failure, hemodynamic stability (not needing invasive measurements of blood pressure or pulmonary artery pressure, not requiring vasoactive drug infusion before transfer), and absence an arrhythmia requiring telemetry. Patients with multiple-organ failure often are not admitted. Patients receiving hemodialytic support usually are accepted, particularly if the unit is inside an acute-care hospital.

The idea of the ability to benefit from a rehabilitation or other comprehensive program is subjective and depends strongly on the judgement of the proposing or accepting physician. In some facilities, the proposing physician must make a written statement that he or she believes that the patient is either capable of being weaned from the ventilator or is likely to return to the community despite receiving ventilator assistance.[50] Other facilities specifically ask that patients are returned to their referring hospital once they have been weaned successfully or when it becomes clear that weaning will not be possible. To ensure that all parties understand this policy, a letter of confirmation may be required from the referring physician, countersigned by the patient or his or her surrogate.[84] A more liberal attitude is shown by other facilities, for example, the Worcester County Ventilator Unit,[68] where "specifically no admission decision is based on prognosis, weaning potential or rehabilitation potential." Also, at the Long-Term Acute Care Unit of the University of Chicago,[75] "patients are accepted regardless of the severity of their illness, provided they are stable for transfer." The latter institution theoretically accepts patients requiring positive end-expiratory pressure of more than 10 cmH$_2$O or an F$_{IO_2}$ of greater than 60%. Finally, methods have been proposed for identifying patients suitable for admission to CVFs based on severity-of-illness scores or activity of treatments.[85–88]

With small local differences, the classification of ventilator-dependent patients admitted to CVFs follows that proposed by Gillespie et al[89] in Table 33-3.

Outcomes and Effectiveness

COMPARISONS WITH ICUs

Commenting on the rationale for opening an intermediate-care unit, Vincent and Buchardi[90] stated they "would recommend that instead of fragmenting ICU facilities by separating 'intensive' from 'intermediate,' with the potential risk of reduced staff morale and less adequate patient care, intensive and intermediate care beds should be combined in one unit." As stated earlier, intermediate-care units are not necessarily equivalent to CVFs. Despite the lack of strong scientific evidence, specific facilities for ventilator-dependent patients do have some clinical and financial advantages over ICU care (they are not, however, "in competition").[91–95] The main differences between ICUs and CVFs located inside or outside acute-care hospitals are listed in Table 33-4.

A recent retrospective review[95] of 429 ICU patients tracheotomized for respiratory failure and needing prolonged mechanical ventilation showed that only 57% of survivors had been freed from mechanical ventilation by the time of discharge from the ICU. Patients who were finally weaned and had their tracheostomy tubes removed had better survival than patients who did not. Improved survival, however, came at higher hospital cost and longer ICU stay. This study illustrated the need to compare the clinical outcomes and financial burdens of these "difficult to wean" patients when treated exclusively in a traditional ICU or transferred during hospitalization to a CVF. The study also demonstrated that the emotional status of these patients at ICU

TABLE 33-4 Differences in Services Provided by Intensive-Care Unit and Chronic Ventilator Facilities

	ICU	CVFs Inside an Acute-Care Hospital	CVFs Outside an Acute-Care Hospital
Medical-centred care	+ + + +	+ +	+
Dedicated multidisciplinary team	+	+ + +	+ + + +
Nurse-patient ratio	+ + + +	+ +	+ +
Invasive monitoring	+ + + +	+ +	+
Diagnostic availability	+ + + +	+ + +	+ +
Privacy	+	+ +	+ + +
Family contact	+/−	+ +	+ + + +
Noise and artificial light	+ + + +	+ +	+ +
Surgical availability	+ + + +	+ + +	+
Hemodialysis	+ + + +	+ + +	+
Physiotherapy and rehabilitation	+	+ + +	+ + + +
Costs	+ + + +	+ +	+ +

discharge was generally good, whereas physical function was quite limited.[95]

The only randomized, controlled study directly comparing the outcomes of chronically ill patients, most of them ventilator dependent, managed entirely in the ICU or transferred when clinically stable to a special care unit (SCU), managed mainly by specialized nurses, was performed by Rudy et al.[96] The SCU had a case-management approach for clinical problems, a full rehabilitation program, weaning protocols, and control of resource use. A total of 220 patients were assigned randomly to the SCU or to the ICU. Overall mortality rates were similar in the two groups, but the rate of readmission was lower and hospital stay shorter in the SCU group. The average cost of delivering care was US$5000 less per patient in the SCU than in the ICU, and the cost to produce a survivor was US$19,000 less. It makes sense that specialized care may achieve better outcomes. It is difficult to draw up standardized recommendations, however, based on a relatively small single-center study where the two groups were not fully comparable in either number or baseline conditions.

Using a retrospective chart review and questionnaires, Seneff et al[24] analyzed 6-month mortality and hospital costs in 54 acute-care referral hospitals and 26 long-term acute-care institutions. Hospital costs included the amount of uncompensated care incurred by the ICU under the Medicare prospective payment DRG system. They compared 432 patients ventilated for an average of 3 weeks who where referred but not transferred to CVFs (Vencor) with 1702 patients who where referred and transferred to CVFs. Six-month mortality was not adversely affected by transfer to a CVF. Because patients had long hospital stays and consumed much resources, overall cost of care was very high. Acute-care hospitals, however, theoretically can reduce the amount of uncompensated care for these patients by timely referral to an appropriate CVF. Only about 10% of the two groups were discharged directly home; most patients were transferred to a nursing home or another CVF.

This study[24] leaves three major issues unresolved. First, the "appropriate" timing of transfer has not been clearly defined because some CVFs accept sicker patients with "overt" nonpulmonary dysfunction, whereas others only accept patients with the "single organ failure." Second, although the authors showed that transfer to CVFs is associated with a reduction of ICU uncompensated costs of care, the issue of best reimbursement system for CVFs was not assessed. Third, even after patients were transferred to a CVF, the rate of discharge home was disappointingly low; there is an urgent need to identify the best location of care for these patients once they are discharged from a CVF.

OBSERVATIONAL STUDIES

Table 33-5 provides a summary of outcome indices for patients admitted to an acute-care setting for weaning. Although comparisons between studies is difficult, the rate of weaning success ranged from 25–92%. Variability of hospital mortality was equally great, ranging from 10–50%. In a controlled study, Gracey et al[51] found that mortality decreased dramatically after the opening of a dedicated ventilator unit within an acute-care hospital. The percentage of patients discharged home is also extremely variable, and about about 40% usually are discharged to long-term facilities with skilled nursing care.

Of patients discharged home, Dasgupta et al[55] found that only 10% were still ventilated; more than 40% of patients discharged to a skilled nursing facility or nursing home were partially or totally ventilator dependent. Latriano et al[54] reported an alternative location to ease pressures on the ICU: use of a nonmonitored general medical floor to treat hemodynamically stable mechanically ventilated patients. The strategy was associated with financial savings. To our knowledge, this model has not been repeated elsewhere.

Table 33-6 provides a summary of outcome indices for patients admitted to nonacute settings for weaning. There is overall agreement that a rehabilitation-based weaning unit can assist with weaning and maximal functional independence and prepare the family for discharge of the ventilated patient to home.[68]

Clinical outcome of patients requiring prolonged ventilation depends on the underlying disease. Weaning success is highest in postoperative patients (58%) and patients with acute lung injury (57%) and lowest in patients with chronic obstructive pulmonary disease (COPD) or neuromuscular disease (22%).[68] Chronically ventilated patients with respiratory failure caused by COPD have a worse prognosis than patients with respiratory failure from other causes.[69] This observation is consistent with the findings of Schonofer et al[72] that long-term survival rate was worse in patients with severe COPD than in other patients. In a homogeneous group of 42 patients with COPD, Nava et al[73] observed a successful weaning rate of 55% when a rehabilitation program was continued for a long period outside the ICU.

The possibility that patient outcomes is influenced by a staff learning is suggested indirectly by several studies. De Vivo et al[98] demonstrated that mortality decreased dramatically over years secondary to the development

TABLE 33-5 Outcomes for Ventilator-Dependent Patients Admitted to a Chronic Ventilatory Facility within an Acute-Care Hospital

Author (Ref)	Year	Patients (n)	Age(yrs)	Patients	Patients Weaned (%)	Patients Died in Hospital (%)	Patients Died within 1 Year (%)	Duration of Mechanical Ventilation (days)	Post Discharge Location (%)
Elpern (47)	1989	95	71.6	Mixed	31%	67%	?	8.1	?
Rudy (96)	1995	145	64 ± 12	Mixed	?	44%	?	?	?
Latriano (54)	1996	224	66 ± 17	Mixed	51% (all pts) 92% (survived)	50%	?	50 ± 66	H = 31%; CVFo = 64%; other = 5%
Douglas (5)	1997	57	61 ± 20	Mixed	?	44%	50%	28	H = 33%; CVFo = 42%; NH = 18%; other = 7%
Gracey (51)	1997	206	65 ± 14	Mixed	74%	8%	31%	?	?
Dasgupta (55)	1999	212	68	Mixed	60%	18%	?	17	H = 34%; other = 66%
Robson (91)	2003	161	69	Mixed	89%	14%	?	8	?
Engoren (95)	2004	429	68	Mixed	57%	22%	36%	29	?

ABBREVIATIONS: H, home; NH, nursing home hospital; CVFo, chronic ventilator facility outside an acute-care hospital.

TABLE 33-6 Outcomes for Ventilator-Dependent Patients Admitted to a Chronic Ventilatory Facility outside an Acute-Care Hospital

Author (Ref)	Year	Patients (n)	Age (yrs)	Patients	Patients Weaned (%)	Patients Died in Hospital (%)	Patients Died within 1 Year (%)	Duration of Mechanical Ventilation (days)	Discharge Location (%)
Indihar (65)	1991	171	60	Mixed	34%	60%	?	55	?
Freichels (97)	1993	442	?	Mixed	?	31.7%	?	48	H = 20%; CVFo = 35%; other = 45%
Nava (73)	1994	42	67 ± 9	COPD	55%	29%	35%	44	?
Scheinorn (66)	1994	421	68 ± 0.9	Mixed	74%	28%	72%	?	H = 50%; other = 50%
De Vivo (98)	1995	435	40	SCI	?	?	25%	?	?
Bagley (68)	1997	278	67	Mixed	38%	31%	?	(11–75)	H = 29%; CVFo = 71%;
Scheinorn (67)	1997	1123	69 ± 13	Mixed	56%	29%	62%	29 (1–226)	?
Escarrabil (99)	1998	10	59 ± 8	ALS	0%	10%	70%	90 (15–150)	H = 100%
Votto (69)	1998	293	(45–70)	Mixed	?	?	29–60%	?	?
Carson (75)	1999	133	71	Mixed	70% (discharged); 38% (total)	50%	77%	?	H = 18%; CVFo = 63%; other = 19%
Modowal (100)	2002	145	66 ± 16	Mixed	50%	34%	?	94 ± 82	?
Schonofer (72)	2002	403	66	Mixed	68%	24%	51%	41	H = 28%; CVFo = 16%; other = 56%
Stoller (101)	2003	162	65 ± 14	Mixed	?	17%	57%	?	H = 28%; CVFo = 63%; CVFi = 9%
Ceriana (102)	2003	40	67 ± 12	Mixed	67%	15%	?	38	?
Lindsay (83)	2004	102	?	Mixed	67%	20%	?	46	H = 36%; NH = 20%; other = 44%

ABBREVIATIONS: H, home; NH, nursing home; CVFi, chronic ventilator facility inside an acute care hospital; CVFo, chronic ventilator facility outside an acute-care hospital; COPD, chronic obstructive pulmonary disease; ALS, amyotrophic lateral sclerosis; SCI, spinal cord injuries.

of improved methods of prevention and management of respiratory complications, particularly pneumonia. Sheinhorn et al[67] reported that a overall survival after discharge improves over time probably because of the improved expertise and care of personnel.

Not all the authors have described the postdischarge destination of their surviving patients. In most cases, when stated, it was home; alternatives include extended-care facilities or a nursing home. Ceriana et al[77] highlighted the possibility of removing the tracheotomy cannula from almost 80% of patients breathing autonomously among a group of 72 patients recovering from weaning. It is often possible to use and adapt a tracheotomy speaking valve that facilitates verbal communication by ventilator-dependent subjects. This step facilitates care and greatly enhances the mental outlook of patients.[103]

Physical function is limited and reduced in most patients[56,104,105] but is sometimes good or improved after discharge.[56,75,100,105] Quality of life is defined as good, quite good, reasonable, or normal, although severe impairment is reported in a minority of studies[56,75,100,105]; often it is improved 1 year after discharge.[106] Ambrosino et al[105] conducted a prospective, controlled cohort study in a respiratory intermediate intensive-care unit in 63 patients with COPD requiring mechanical ventilation. Perceived health status and cognitive function were worse in patients recovering from acute-on-chronic respiratory failure (requiring mechanical ventilation) than in stable patients receiving long-term oxygen therapy who never required ICU admission. After discharge, cognition and mobility improved to levels found in stable COPD patients on oxygen therapy.

Chronic ventilator units provide settings in which an interdisciplinary team develops and implements tools that assist the patient and caregivers. A planned discharge gives the patient and caregivers confidence and skills before discharge[107] and helps with the emotional burden caused by the heavy responsibility of home caregivers. The time spent in these units helps to prepare patients and their families, educates them about various aspects of care after discharge, and helps them with decisions about future placement.[108,109]

Problems Unique to Chronic Facilities

FINANCES

A major issue facing medicine today is containing costs, particularly with regard to critical-care beds. In this respect, CVFs have a peculiar system of reimbursement that deserves special attention.[110] As shown in Table 33-7, most observational studies estimate that the daily cost of care for ventilator-dependent patients is lower in a CVF than in an ICU. Dasgupta et al[55] reported that for 11 patients transferred from an ICU to a respiratory special care unit, the difference in the mean daily costs for the first 3 days in the special unit and for the last 3 days of ICU care was US$469. Gracey et al[52] showed that over a 6-year period, more than US$4 million were saved in patient-care costs by transferring care for 964 patients from ICUs to their chronic

ventilator-dependent unit (CVDU). They also observed that all ICU daily costs (medical, neurosurgical, coronary care, and cardiovascular surgery ICUs) rose dramatically between 1993 and 1998; the only exception was the CVDU. This lower cost of the CVDU was related mainly to the lower salaries, decreased room charges, lower overheads, simpler, usually noninvasive monitoring, and changes in the pattern of diagnostics and therapeutics. Given these findings, it has been suggested that CVFs may be a cost-effective alternative to ICUs. Unfortunately, we still lack randomized comparisons of the real costs of care in the two environments.

The DRG-based system is used for payment in most ICUs round the world. The Medicare prospective payment system is designed to compensate hospitals for overall cost of care for patients who share a common diagnosis. DRG 483, "tracheotomy except for mouth, larynx, or pharynx disorder," is the group usually applied to ventilator-dependent patients.[112] Because of large variation in time spent in an ICU, whether a hospital renders uncompensated care in a given year depends on the case mix, average duration of hospital stay, and availability of alternative locations for patient care. Seneff et al[24] reported that Medicare uncompensated care in an ICU was an average of US$16,000 per ventilator-dependent patient.

To address the problem of under-reimbursement, some CVFs are now licensed as DRG-grouping-exempt[52] and are required by the Health Care Financial Administration to maintain a mean length of stay more than 25 days and usually fewer than 90 days. In the United States, long-term acute-care facilities are reimbursed under regulations of the Tax Equity and Fiscal Responsibility Act (TEFRA)[113] for care provided to Medicare patients. Charges are reimbursed up to the annual maximum cap for the facility, calculated during a 12-month period designated as the base year. Hospitals incur penalties when charges for Medicare exceed the discharge target amount and receive incentives if charges are reduced in subsequent years. This policy, unfortunately, has led, as it did for rehabilitation hospitals, to substantial extra costs, including increases in payments to hospitals and doctors and numbers of hospital days for the average patient.[113] In most European countries, the health care system is funded primarily by government. Therefore, the vast majority of public hospitals and some private hospitals receive most of their funds through a national health service. Most beds are devoted to the treatment of acutely ill patients, independent of the baseline disease (i.e., medical or surgical), and are reimbursed through a DRG-based system. A minor share is devoted to the care of chronically ill patients. The latter beds are located inside rehabilitation wards of acute-care hospitals or within independently structured rehabilitation hospitals. For acute care, the DRG-based reimbursement per case is applied. For chronic care, reimbursement is on a per diem basis, allowing for some increase according to DRG classification. This per diem fee applies for only a limited number of days (40–60), after which the fee is curtailed drastically.

Mean duration of stay in CVFs differs considerably, with an impressively high standard deviation. Nasraway et al[34] reported the duration of hospital stay to range from 1–2125 days. Because the time spent in CVFs differs so greatly,

TABLE 33-7 Costs per Day for a Ventilator-Dependent Patient Admitted to an Intensive-Care Unit (ICU) or to a Chronic Ventilator Facility

Authors	Year of Publication	Year of Analysis	Type of Unit	Daily Costs(US$)
Sheinhorn et al (ref. 66)	1994	?	WC (outside acute-care H)	980
Latriano et al (ref. 54)	1996	?	Non-monitored care floor (inside acute-care H)	453
Bagley et al (ref. 68)	1997	1995	WC (outside acute-care H)	630
Nava et al (ref. 111)	1997	1995	RICU (outside acute-care H)	865
Gracey et al (ref. 52)	2000	1998	CVDU (inside acute-care H)	1084
Engoren et al (ref. 104)	2000	?	Cardiac stepdown unit (inside acute-care H)	439
Seneff et al (ref. 24)	2000	?	ICU	4174
Linsday et al (ref. 83)	2004	?	Nursing home	303
Halpern et al (ref. 3)	2004	2000	Daily cost per patient admitted to a critical-care bed	2647

NOTE: Reference 3 is the actual daily cost of a critical-care bed in year 2000 in the United States. WC, weaning center; RICU, respiratory intensive-care unit; CVDU, chronic ventilator-dependent unit.

it is clear that exemption from the DRG-based payment system is granted to avoid massive losses. The per diem reimbursement up to relatively small ceiling of days, however, may not achieve reasonable reimbursement.

STAFFING

CVFs, especially those outside acute-care hospitals, are still characterized by heterogeneous staffing. Most of the centers share common views about the equipment to be used (i.e., ventilators and monitoring systems) and the overall multidisciplinary organization, aimed at improving the autonomy of patients, privacy, and environment. There is, however, considerable discrepancy concerning the training of personnel, especially of nurses. Table 33-8 shows the availability of skilled nurses in extended-care facilities in the

TABLE 33-8 Range of Skilled Nursing Care in the Extended-Care Facilities

Skilled Nursing Care	Nursing Hours/Patient/Day
Subactute care Patients technologically complex; stable patients with prolonged mechanical ventilation; potential for rehabilitation	4.0–5.0
Acute rehabilitation Intensive rehabilitation; hospital level of care; presence of attending physician	6.0–7.0
Long-term acute care Hospital level of care with ICU and the possibility of minor surgical procedures; stable patients with prolonged mechanical ventilation	7.5–8.3
Intensive care Tertiary Care; artificial life support; major surgery; full ancillary services	14–18

Based on a random survey in several extended care facilities in each category in the New England Region.
SOURCE: Adapted, with permission, from ref. 34.

Boston area, as determined by an informal survey.[34] Marked differences exist in the care that each center provides to long-term ventilated patients. The authors[34] state that "some facilities may accept ventilator-dependent patients but may not be able to provide for all their needs, especially when serious infections or other setbacks ensue." Nurses working in a CVF should be specifically trained not only in acute lifesavings procedures, such as resuscitation, but also in specific "chronic" procedures, such as bronchial toilet, prevention of sores at the tracheotomy site, and positioning of the tracheal cannula.

Vitacca et al[114] studied the allocation of nursing time in a respiratory unit located in a rehabilitation center. In the first two days after admission, time devoted to care of a ventilator-dependent patient consumed about 45% of a nursing shift.

Respiratory therapists should be skilled in weaning protocols that have been shown to shorten the duration of mechanical ventilation. The hospital team should be trained in clinical tests (i.e., bronchoscopy, fluoroscopy, assessment of expiratory muscle function) that may help the clinicians to decide whether or not a patient can have the tracheotomy removed.[77] Special attention should be paid to the diagnosis of ICU-acquired neuromuscular abnormalities, which have been shown to increase the time to weaning. Diagnosis may require electrophysiologic studies and needle electromyography of the limb and respiratory muscles.[115,116]

SIZE OF THE PROBLEM

The number of "actual" ventilator-dependent patients" and "post-ICU patients" who might benefit from an admission to a CVF is unknown because most published data are anecdotal and not derived from structured surveys or rigorous epidemiology data. Figure 33-2 reports the estimated number of ventilator-dependent patients in the United States and the theoretical need for CVF beds per head of population, calculated on the available data. It is believed that the ideal number of CVF beds per head of population for European countries would be equivalent to that in the United States. This estimate is based on the observation that in the subset of patients (~15%)

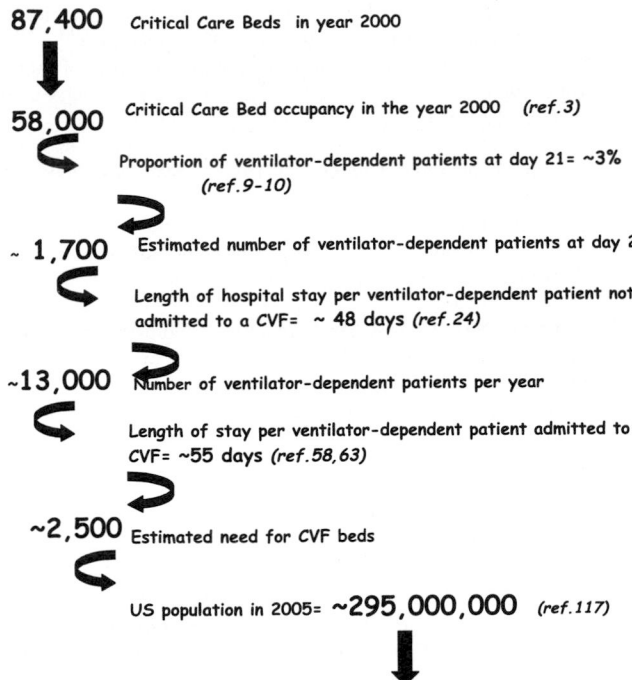

87,400   Critical Care Beds in year 2000

58,000   Critical Care Bed occupancy in the year 2000   *(ref.3)*

Proportion of ventilator-dependent patients at day 21= ~3%
(ref.9-10)

~ 1,700   Estimated number of ventilator-dependent patients at day 21

Length of hospital stay per ventilator-dependent patient not
admitted to a CVF= ~ 48 days *(ref.24)*

~13,000   Number of ventilator-dependent patients per year

Length of stay per ventilator-dependent patient admitted to a
CVF= ~55 days *(ref.58,63)*

~2,500   Estimated need for CVF beds

US population in 2005= **~295,000,000**   *(ref.117)*

1/150,000-1/200,000   Estimated number of CVF beds

**FIGURE 33-2 Estimated need for chronic ventilator facility (CVF)
beds in the United States. The number of ventilator-dependent
patients on day 21 after intubation was estimated as 3%[9,10] of the
ICU bed occupancy in the year 2000 in the United States.[3] In that
average hospital stay for a ventilator-dependent patient not
transferred to a CVF is about 48 days,[24] the estimated number of
ventilator-dependent patients per year is approximately 13,000.
Mean length of hospital stay for patients transferred from the
ICU to a CVF is approximately 55 days,[58,63,102] and CVF beds
needed are about 2-500. Given the estimated U.S. population in
January 2005,[116] the estimated number of CVF beds per head of
population is 1 per 150,000-200,000.**

requiring prolonged mechanical ventilation, 60–70% of the
time spent in an ICU is related to the post–acute phase of
the illness.[118] A precise calculation of available CVF beds,
both in North America and in Europe, is impossible. Based
on a recent European survey, we estimate that the ratio is
roughly 1:1 million, with very large discrepancies among
countries.

Two steps are urgent. First, we must quantify precisely
how many patients are potential candidates for CVF admission. Seconfd, we must determine how many beds are
presently available in these facilities.[119,120] Once obtained,
these data can be used to convince administrators and health
care system politicians of the need for this neglected form
of care. Knowing that patients with COPD constitute the
largest proportion of ventilator-dependent patients and that
COPD is the fifth cause of death in the Western world,[121] the
problem of ventilator dependency should be introduced to
the media so that the subject can be disseminated to the
public. Beforehand, we need to design randomized, controlled studies to assess the clinical and financial benefits of
CVFs.

Conclusion

Over the last 10 years, the availability of ICU beds, new technology, and improved levels of care have increased a new
population of patients termed *survivors of catastrophic illness.*
These patients commonly require prolonged weaning.

The rate of achieving complete ventilator independence in specific, dedicated weaning units is generally
high. It has been demonstrated that these units are cost-
saving alternatives to an ICU for carefully selected patients. Survivors have an acceptable long-term quality of
life. Weaning success, however, does not in itself solve
other severe problems such as the heavy financial and
human burdens that the high level of dependency impose on families, caregivers, and health service organizations once these patients are discharged from a protected
environment.

In conclusion, the main benefits of chronic ventilator facilities are (1) the possibility of relieving congestion of ICU
beds, (2) maintaining a high level of nursing assistance,
(3) responding to sudden changes in a patient's clinical
condition, (4) allowing enough time for a multidisciplinary
rehabilitation approach, and (5) acting as a bridge to home-
care programs or other forms of continuous chronic assistance (e.g., telemedicine or dedicated long-term units).

References

1. De Saint-Exupery A. The little prince (Le petit prince). New
   York: Harvest Books, 2000.
2. Coppola S. Lost in translation. Los Angeles: Universal Studios
   Movies, 2003.
3. Halpern NA, Pastores SM, Greenstein RJ. Critical care medicine
   in the United States 1985–2000: An analysis of bed numbers, use,
   and costs. Crit Care Med 2004; 32:1254–9.
4. Stauffer JL, Fayter NA, Graves B, et al Survival following mechanical ventilation for acute respiratory failure in adult man.
   Chest 1993; 104:1222–9.
5. Douglas SL, Daly BJ, Brennan PF, et al. Outcomes of long-term
   ventilator patients: A descriptive study. Am J Crit Care 1997;
   6:99–105.
6. Angus DC, Musthafa AA, Clermont G, et al. Quality adjusted
   survival in the first year after the acute respiratory distress syndrome. Am J Respir Crit Care Med 2001; 163:1389–94.
7. Esteban A, Anzueto A, Alia I, et al. How is mechanical ventilation employed in the intensive care unit? An international
   utilization review. Am J Respir Crit Care Med 2000; 161:
   1450–8.
8. Lipsett PA, Swoboda SM, Dickerson J, et al. Survival and functional outcome after prolonged intensive care unit stay. Ann
   Surg 2000; 231:262–8.
9. Cohen IL, Booth FV. Cost containment and mechanical ventilation in the United States. New Horizons 1994; 2:283–90.
10. Wagner DP. Economics of prolonged mechanical ventilation.
    Am Rev Respir Dis 1989; 140:514–8.
11. Epstein SK, Ciubataru RL, Wong JB. Effect of failed extuba-
    tion on the outcome of mechanical ventilation. Chest 1997; 112:
    186–92.
12. Douglas SL, Daly BJ, Brennan PF, et al. Hospital readmission
    among long-term ventilator patients. Chest 2001; 120:1278–86.

13. Cox CE, Carson SS, Holmes GM, et al. Increase in tracheostomy for prolonged mechanical ventilation in North Carolina, 1993–2002. Crit Care Med 2004; 32:2219–26.

14. Brochard L, Rauss A, Benito S, et al. Comparison of three methods of gradual withdrawal from ventilatory support during weaning from mechanical ventilation. Am J Respir Crit Care Med 1994; 150:896–903.

15. Esteban A, Frutos F, Tobin MJ, et al. A comparison of four methods of weaning from mechanical ventilation. Spanish Lung Failure Collaborative Group. New Engl J Med 1995; 332: 345–50.

16. Lee Bishop K. Pulmonary rehabilitation in the intensive care unit. In: Fishman AP, editor. Pulmonary rehabilitation, 1st ed. New York: Marcel Dekker, 1996: 725.

17. Vitacca M, Callegari G, Sarva M, et al. Physiological effects of meals in difficult-to-wean tracheostomised patients with chronic obstructive pulmonary disease. Intensive Care Med 2005; 31:236–42.

18. Gabor JY, Cooper AB, Crombach SA, et al. Contribution of the intensive care unit environment to sleep disruption in mechanically ventilated patients and healthy subjects. Am J Respir Crit Care Med 2003; 167:708–15.

19. Freedman NS, Gazendam J, Levan L, et al. Abnormal sleep/wake cycles and the effect of environmental noise on sleep disruption in the intensive care unit. Am J Respir Crit Care Med 2001; 163:451–7.

20. Aaron JN, Carlisle CC, Carskadon MA, et al. Environmental noise as a cause of sleep disruption in an intermediate respiratory care unit. Sleep 1996; 19:707–10.

21. Balogh D, Kittinger E, Benzer A, et al. Noise in the ICU. Intensive Care Med 1993; 19:343–6.

22. Environmental Protection Agency. Information on environmental noise requisite to protect public health and welfare with an adequate margin of safety. No 550/9-74-004. Washington: US Government Printing Office, 1974.

23. Vincent JL. Forgoing life support in western European intensive care units: The results of an ethical questionnaire. Crit Care Med 1999; 27:1626–33.

24. Seneff MG, Wagner D, Thompson D, et al. The impact of long-term acute care facilities on the outcome and cost of care for patients undergoing prolonged mechanical ventilation. Crit Care Med 2000; 28:342–50.

25. Scheinhorn D, Chao DC, Stearn-Hassenpflug M, Gracey DR. Post-ICU weaning from mechanical ventilation: The role of long term facilities. Chest 2001; 120:4828–48.

26. Bone RC, Balk RA. Noninvasive respiratory care unit: A cost-effective solution for the future. Chest 1988; 93:390–4.

27. Nava S, Rampulla C, Confalonieri M. Intermediate respiratory intensive care units in Europe: A European perspective. Thorax 1998; 53:798–802.

28. Byrick RJ, Power JD, Ycas JO, et al. Impact of an intermediate care area on ICU utilization after cardiac surgery. Crit Care Med 1986; 14:869–72.

29. Byrick RJ, Mazer CD, Caskennette GM. Closure of an intermediate care unit: Impact on critical care utilization. Chest 1993; 104:876–81.

30. Fox AJ, Owen-Smith O, Spiers P. The immediate impact of opening an adult high dependency unit on intensive care unit occupancy. Anaesthesia 1999; 54:266–96.

31. Nasraway SA, Cohen IL, Dennis RC, et al. Guidelines on admission and discharge for adult intermediate care units. Crit Care Med 1998; 26:607–10.

32. Rady MY, Johnson DJ. Hospital discharge to care facility: A patient-centered outcome for the evaluation of intensive care for octogenarians. Chest 2004; 126:1583–91.

33. Klenhenz ME, Younger Lewis C. Chronic ventilator dependence in elderly patients. Clin Geriatr Med 2000; 16:735–55.

34. Nasraway SA, Button GJ, Rand WM, et al. Survivors of catastrophic illness: Outcome after direct transfer from intensive care to extended care facilities. Crit Care Med 2000; 28:19–25.

35. Classifications of diseases and functioning and disability. ICD-9-CM National Center for Health Statistics, 2004; at *www.cdc.gov/nchs/icd9.htm.*

36. Quality of life after mechanical ventilation in the aged study investigators: 2-month mortality and functional status of critically ill adult patients receiving prolonged mechanical ventilation. Chest 2002; 121:549–58.

37. Sapijaszko MJA, Brant R, Sandham D, et al. Nonrespiratory predictor of mechanical ventilation dependency in intensive care unit patients. Crit Care Med 1996; 24:601–7.

38. Douglas SL, Daly B, Gordon N, et al. Survival and quality of life: Short-term versus long-term ventilator patients. Crit Care Med 2002; 30:2655–62.

39. Ely WE, Baker AM, Dunagan DP, et al. Effect on the duration of mechanical ventilation of identifying patients capable of breathing spontaneously. New Engl J Med 1996; 335:1864–69.

40. Scheinhorn DJ, Stearn-Hassenpffug M. Provision of long-term mechanical ventilation. Crit Care Clin 1998; 14:819–33.

41. European Respiratory Task Force on Epidemiology of Respiratory Intermediate Care in Europe. Respiratory intermediate care units: A European survey. Eur Respir J 2002; 20: 1343–50.

42. Wu CP, Yang SH, Chen CH, et al. The outcome of patients with long-term mechanical ventilation admitted to a respiratory care center in medical center: 3-year experience Am J Respir Crit Care Med 2002; 165:A385.

43. Chao DC, Stearn-Hassenpflug M, Scheinhorn DJ. The challenge of prolonged mechanical ventilation: A shared global experience. Respir Care 2003; 48:668–9.

44. Carlucci A, Richard JC, Wysocki M, et al. SRLF Collaborative Group on Mechanical Ventilation. Noninvasive versus conventional mechanical ventilation: An epidemiologic survey. Am J Respir Crit Care Med 2001; 163:874–80.

45. Krieger BP, Ershowsky P, Spivack D, et al. Initial experience with a central respiratory monitoring unit as a cost-saving alternative to the intensive care unit for Medicare patients who require long-term ventilator support. Chest 1988; 93:395–7.

46. Krieger BP, Ershowsky P, Spivack D. One year's experience with a noninvasively monitored intermediate care unit for pulmonary patients. JAMA 1990; 264:1143–6.

47. Elpern EH, Larson R, Douglass P, et al. Long-term outcomes for elderly survivors of prolonged ventilator assistance. Chest 1989; 96:1120–4.

48. Elpern EH, Silver MR, Rosen RL, et al. The non-invasive respiratory care unit: Patterns of use and financial implications. Chest 1991; 99:205–8.

49. Gracey DR, Viggiano RW, Naessens JM, et al. Outcomes of patients admitted to a chronic ventilator dependent unit in an acute care hospital. Mayo Clin Proc 1992; 67:131–6.

50. Gracey DR, Naessens JM, Viggiano RW, et al. Outcome of patients cared for in a ventilator-dependent unit in a general hospital. Chest 1995; 107:494–9.

51. Gracey DR, Hardy D, Naessens JM, et al. The Mayo ventilator-dependent rehabilitation unit: A 5-year experience. Mayo Clin Proc 1997; 72:13–9.

52. Gracey DR, Hardy DC, Koenig GE. The chronic ventilator-dependent unit: A lower-cost alternative to intensive care. Mayo Clin Proc 2000; 75:445–9.

53. Gracey DR. The problem with diagnosis related group 475. Chest 2002; 122:299–301.

54. Latriano B, McCauley P, Astiz ME, et al. Non ICU care in hemodynamically stable mechanically ventilated patients. Chest 1996; 109:1591–6.

55. Dasgupta A, Rice R, Mascha E, et al. Four-year experience with a unit for long-term ventilation (respiratory special care unit) at the Cleveland Clinic Foundation. Chest 1999; 116: 447–55.

56. Smith IE, Shneerson JM. A progressive care programme for prolonged ventilatory failure: analysis of outcome. Br J Anaesth 1995;75:399–404.

57. Confalonieri M, Gorini M, Mollica C, et al for the Scientific group on Respiratory Intensive Care of the Italian Association of Hospital Pneumologists (AIPO). Respiratory intensive care unit in Italy: A national census and prospective cohort study. Thorax 2001; 56:373–8.

58. Iapichino G, Radrizzani D, Ferla L, et al. Description of trends in the course of illness of critically ill patients: Markers of intensive care organization and performance. Intensive Care Med 2002; 28:985–9.

59. Carson SS, Stocking C, Podsadecki T, et al. Effects of organizational change in the medical intensive care unit of a teaching hospital: A comparison of "open" and "closed" formats. JAMA 1996; 276:322–8.

60. Norrenberg M, Vincent JL. A profile of European intensive care unit physiotherapists. European Society of Intensive Care Medicine. Intensive Care Med 2000; 26:988–94.

61. Nava S, Ambrosino N. Rehabilitation in the ICU: The European phoenix. Intensive Care Med 2000; 26:841–4.

62. Department of Health. Comprehensive critical care: A review of adult critical care services. London: Department of Health, 2000: 45.

63. Indihar FJ, Forsberg DP. Experience with a prolonged respiratory care unit. Chest 1982; 81:189–92.

64. Indihar FJ, Walker NE. Experience with a respiratory care unit revisited. Chest 1984; 86:616–20.

65. Indihar FJ. A 10-year report of patients in a prolonged respiratory care unit. Minn Med 1991; 74:23–7.

66. Scheinhorn DJ, Artinian BM, Catlin JL. Weaning from prolonged mechanical ventilation: The experience at a regional weaning center. Chest 1994; 105:534–9.

67. Scheinhorn, D, Chao DC, Stearn-Hassenpflug M. Post-ICU mechanical ventilation: Treatment of 1123 patients at a regional weaning center. Chest 1997; 111:1654–9.

68. Bagley PH, Cooney E. A community-based regional ventilator weaning unit: Development and outcomes. Chest 1997; 111:1024–9.

69. Votto J, Brancifort JM, Scalise PJ, et al. COPD and other diseases in chronically ventilated patients in a prolonged respiratory care unit: A retrospective 20-year survival study. Chest 1998; 113:86–90.

70. Scalise PJ, Gerardi DA, Wollschlager CM, et al. A regional weaning center for patients requiring mechanical ventilation: An 18 month experience. Conn Med 1997; 61:387–9.

71. Campbell S. HCFA clamping down on long-term acute care "hospitals within hospitals." Health Care Strateg Manage 1997; 15:12–23.

72. Schonofer B, Euteneur S, Nava S, et al. Survival of mechanically ventilated patients admitted to a specialized weaning centre. Intensive Care Med 2002; 28:908–16.

73. Nava S, Rubini F, Zanotti E, et al. Survival and prediction of successful ventilator weaning in COPD patients requiring mechanical ventilation for more than 21 days. Eur Respir J 1994; 7:1645–52.

74. Vitacca M, Clini E, Scalvini S, et al. Cardiopulmonary intermediate intensive unit: Time course of two years activity. Monaldi Arch Chest Dis 1993; 48:296–300.

75. Carson SS, Bach PB, Brzozowski L, et al. Outcomes after long-term acute care: An analysis of 133 mechanically ventilated patients. Am J Respir Crit Care Med 1999; 159:1568–73.

76. Scheinhorn DJ, Chao DC, Stearn-Hassenpflug M, et al. Outcomes in post-ICU mechanical ventilation: A therapist-implemented weaning protocol. Chest 2001; 119:236–42.

77. Ceriana P, Carlucci A, Navalesi P, et al. Weaning from tracheostomy in long-term ventilated patients: Feasibility of decisional flowchart and clinical outcome. Intensive Care Med 2003; 29:845–8.

78. Nava S. Rehabilitation of patients admitted to a respiratory intensive care unit. Arch Phys Med Rehabil 1998; 79:849–54.

79. Milligan S. AARC and Gallup numbers and costs of caring for chronic ventilator patients. AARC Times 1991; 15: 32–36.

80. Sevik MA, Sereika S, Matthews Talbot J, et al. Home-based ventilator dependent patients: Measurement of the emotional aspects of home caregivers. Heart Lung 1994; 23:269–78.

81. Schmidt-Ohlemann M. Ventilation in nursing home: Management of ventilator-dependent patients in inpatients facilities for handicapped—a report of experiences. Med Klin 1996; 91:56–8.

82. Baldwin D. Long-term ventilator-dependent care in nursing homes. Geriatr Nurs 1996; 17:20–1.

83. Linsday ME, Bijwadia JS, Schauer WW, et al. Shifting care of chronic ventilator-dependent patients from the intensive care unit to nursing home. Joint Commis J Qual Saf 2004; 30:257–65.

84. Weaning program for mechanically ventilated patients, Montreal Chest Institute, MUHC; at *www.meakins.mcgill.ca/respdiv/;* updated June 7, 2000.

85. LeGall JR, Lomeshow S, Saulnier F. A new simplified acute physiology score (SAPS II) based on a European/North American multicenter study. JAMA 1993; 270:2957–63.

86. Knaus WA, Wagner DP, Draper EA, et al. The APACHE III prognostic system: Risk prediction of hospital mortality for critically ill hospitalized adults. Chest 1991; 100:1619–36.

87. Cullen DJ, Nemeskal AR, Zaslavsky AM. Intermediate TISS: A new therapeutic intervention scoring system for non-ICU patients. Crit Care Med 1994; 22:1406–11.

88. Zimmerman JE, Wagner DP, Knaus WA, et al. The use of risk predictions to identify candidates for intermediate care units: Implications for intensive care utilization and costs. Chest 1995; 108:490–9.

89. Gillepsie DJ, Marsh HM, Divertie MB, et al. Clinical outcome of respiratory failure in patients requiring prolonged (>24 hours) mechanical ventilation. Chest 1986; 90:364–9.

90. Vincent JL, Burchardi H. Do we need intermediate care units? Intensive Care Med 1999; 25:1345–9.

91. Robson V, Poynter J, Lawler PG, et al. The need for a regional weaning centre, a one-year survey of intensive care weaning delay in northern region of England. Anaesthesia 2003; 58:161–82.

92. Franklin CM, Rackow EC, Mamdani B, et al. Decreases in mortality in a large urban medical service by facilitating access to critical care: An alternative to rationing. Arch Intern Med 1988; 148:1403–5.

93. Fox AJ, Owen-Smith O, Spiers P. The immediate impact of opening an adult high dependency unit on intensive care unit occupancy. Anaesthesia 1999; 54:L280–3.

94. Heyland DK, Konopad E, Noseworthy TW, et al. Is it "worthwhile" to continue treating patients with a prolonged stay (>14 days) in the ICU? An economic evaluation. Chest 1998; 114:192–8.

95. Engoren M, Arslanan-Engoren C, Fenn-Buderer N. Hospital and long-term outcome after tracheostomy for respiratory failure. Chest 2004; 125:220–7.

96. Rudy E, Daly B, Douglas S, et al. Patient outcomes for chronically ill: Special care unit versus intensive care unit. Nurs Res 1995; 44:324–31.

97. Freichels T. Financial implications and recommendations for care of ventilator dependent patients. JONA 1993; 23:16–20.

98. De Vivo MJ, Ivie CS. Life expectancy of ventilator dependent persons with spinal cord injuries. Chest 1995; 108:226–32.

99. Escarrabill J, Estopà R, Farrero E, et al. Long term mechanical ventilation in amyotrophic lateral sclerosis. Respir Med 1998; 92:438–41.

100. Modawal A, Candadai NP, Mandell KM, et al. Weaning success among ventilator-dependent patients in a rehabilitation facility. Arch Phys Med Rehabil 2002; 83:154–7.

101. Stoller JK, Meng Xu, Mascha E, et al. Long-term outcomes for patients discharged from a long term hospital based weaning unit. Chest 2003; 124:1892–9.

102. Ceriana P, Delmastro M, Rampulla C, et al. Demographics and clinical outcomes of patients admitted to a respiratory intensive care unit located in a rehabilitation center. Respir Care 2003; 48:670–6.

103. Passy V, Baydur A, Prentice W, et al. Muir tracheostomy speaking valve on ventilator dependent patients. Laryngoscope 1993; 103:653–8.

104. Engoren M. Marginal cost of liberating ventilator dependent patients after cardiac surgery in a stepdown unit. Ann Thorac Surg 2000; 70:182–5.

105. Ambrosino N, Bruletti G, Scala V, et al. Cognitive and perceived health status in patients recovering from an acute exacerbation of COPD: A controlled study. Intensive Care Med 2002; 28: 170–7.

106. Chatila W, Kreimer DT, Criner GJ. Quality of life in survivors of prolonged mechanical ventilatory support. Crit Care Med 2001; 29:737–42.

107. Warren ML, Jarrett C, Senegal R, et al. An interdisciplinary approach to transitioning ventilator dependent patients to home. J Nurs Care Qual 2003; 19:67–73.

108. Douglas S, Daly BJ, Flatley Brennan P, et al. Outcomes of long-term ventilator patients: A descriptive study. Am J Crit Care 1997; 6:99–105.

109. Douglas S, Daly BJ. Caregivers of long-term ventilator patients: Physical and psychological outcomes. Chest 2003; 123: 1073–81.

110. Understanding costs and cost-effectiveness in critical care. Report from the second American Thoracic Society workshop on outcomes research. Am J Respir Crit Care Med 2002; 165:540–50.

111. Nava S, Evangelisti I, Rampulla C, et al. Human and financial costs of noninvasive mechanical ventilation in patients affected by COPD and acute respiratory failure. Chest 1997; 111: 1631–8.

112. Baskin JZ, Panagopoulos G, Parks C, et al. Clinical outcomes for the elderly patient receiving a tracheotomy. Head Neck 2004; 26:71–6.

113. Chan L, Koepsell DT, Deyo R, et al. The effect of Medicare's payment system for rehabilitation hospitals on length of stay, charges and total payments. New Engl J Med 1997; 337:978–85.

114. Vitacca M, Clini E, Porta R, et al. Preliminary results on nursing workload in a dedicated weaning center. Intensive Care Med 2000; 26:796–9.

115. Maher J, Rutledge F, Remtulla H, et al. Neuromuscular disorders associated with failure to wean from the ventilator. Intensive Care Med 1995; 21:737–43.

116. De Jonghe B, Bastuji-Garin S, Sharshar T, et al. Does ICU-acquired paresis lengthen weaning from mechanical ventilation. Intensive Care Med 2004; 30:1117–21.

117. US Census Bureau. US POPClock Projection; available at *www.census.gov/cgi-bin/popclock*.

118. Iapichino G, Apolone G, Melotti R, et al. Intermediate intensive care units: Definition, legislation and need in Italy. Monaldi Arch Chest Dis 1994; 49:493–5.

119. Lindquist R, Banasik J, Barnsteiner J, et al. Determining research priority for the 90s. Am J Crit Care 1993; 2:110–7.

120. Parrillo JE. Research in critical care medicine: Present status of critical care investigation. Crit Care Med 1991; 19:569–77.

121. Pauwels R, Buist SA, Calverley PM, et al. Global strategy for the diagnosis, management, and prevention of chronic obstructive pulmonary disease. NHLBI/WHO Global Initiative for Chronic Obstructive Lung Disease (GOLD) workshop summary. Am J Respir Crit Care Med 2001; 163:1256–76.

Chapter 34

NONINVASIVE VENTILATION ON A GENERAL WARD

MARK ELLIOTT

EVIDENCE AND RATIONALE FOR NONINVASIVE
VENTILATION ON A GENERAL WARD
Acute Noninvasive Ventilation
Elective Ventilation For Chronic Ventilatory Failure
WHERE SHOULD NONINVASIVE VENTILATION
BE PERFORMED?
Acute NIV: ICU or General Ward?
Elective NIV: General Ward or Chronic-Care Facility?
The Advantage of The General Ward
SELECTION OF PATIENTS FOR NIV
IN A GENERAL WARD
Acute Respiratory Failure
Chronic Respiratory Failure: Elective Institution of
NIV
IMPLICATIONS FOR STAFFING AND TRAINING
ECONOMIC CONSIDERATIONS
CONCLUSION

In any discussion about location of a noninvasive ventilation (NIV) service, it is important to note that the model of hospital care differs between countries and that there may be significant differences even between hospitals within the same country. There will be variations in staffing levels; the skills of doctors, nurses, and paramedical staff; and the sophistication of monitoring. The terms *intensive-care unit* (ICU), *high-dependency unit* (HDU), and *general ward* have a different meaning to different people. Care therefore must be taken when extrapolating experience and results obtained in one environment to other hospitals and countries. The United Kingdom's King's Fund panel[1] defines intensive care as "a service for patients with potentially recoverable diseases who can benefit from more detailed observation and treatment than is generally available in the standard wards and departments." The definition of HDU is less clear, with some HDUs allowing invasive monitoring, whereas in others only noninvasive monitoring is performed. In some countries, specific respiratory ICUs and intermediate ICUs have been developed.[2,3] Specifically, within the King's Fund definition is the consideration of intensive care as a service rather than a place; critical care is provided within a continuum of primary, secondary, and tertiary care, and patients are categorized on the basis of their needs[4] (Table 34-1). Movement through the different levels usually means transfer from one location to another. Critical-care outreach teams can advise on care as patients cross organizational boundaries and also facilitate transfer when this is needed.[5,6] Although most acute NIV services are situated in a specific clinical area, a peripatetic model has been described and has some advantages.[7,8]

For the purposes of this chapter, the following definitions are used:

- *Intensive care.* High ratio of staff to patients, facility for invasive ventilation and sophisticated monitoring.
- *Intermediate respiratory ICU or HDU.* Continuous monitoring of vital signs, with a staffing ratio intermediate between an ICU and a general ward, in a specified clinical area. Intubated patients (unless with tracheostomy) usually are not cared for in this environment.
- *General ward.* Takes unselected emergency admission, and although most wards will have a particular speciality interest, it is likely that because of the unpredictability of demand, patients with a variety of conditions and degrees of severity will be cared for in the same clinical area. Nurse staffing levels vary, but the intensity of nursing input available in HDU and ICUs is not possible. Only basic monitoring is available.

Another important issue when considering NIV in different locations is the severity and acuteness of the insult leading to ventilatory failure. Ventilatory failure can be considered *acute* when it occurs on a background of normal function, *acute-on-chronic* when there is a sudden deterioration on a background of impaired function, or *chronic* when there is ventilatory failure but with no precipitating acute event. Assisted ventilation can be considered *necessary* when without it death will ensue over a few hours or *desirable* when the primary aim is to improve quality of life and also to improve survival over the longer term.

Evidence and Rationale for Noninvasive Ventilation on a General Ward

ACUTE NONINVASIVE VENTILATION

CHRONIC OBSTRUCTIVE PULMONARY
DISEASE (COPD)
The respiratory muscle pump in patients with severe COPD often is functioning close to the point at which it can no longer maintain effective ventilation. There is an excessive elastic and resistive load on it because of hyperinflation and airways obstruction, respectively, and reduced capacity because of the adverse effect of hyperinflation on the configuration of the respiratory muscles, causing them to operate at a mechanical disadvantage.[9,10] In addition, the presence of intrinsic positive end-expiratory pressure (intrinsic PEEP) causes an inspiratory threshold load.[11] In an acute exacerbation, when the load on the respiratory muscles becomes excessive, effective ventilation can no longer be maintained, worsening hypoxia, and hypercapnia and, most important, acidosis ensue. Acidosis in particular is deleterious to muscle function,[12] and the capacity of the

TABLE 34-1   Classification of Individual Patient Dependency

Level 0:   Patients whose needs can be met through normal ward care in an acute hospital

Level 1:   Patients at risk of their condition deteriorating or patients recently relocated from higher levels of care whose needs can be met in an acute ward with additional advice and support from the critical-care team

Level 2:   Patients requiring more detailed observation or intervention, including support for a single failing organ system or postoperative care, and those stepping down from higher levels of care

Level 3:   Patients requiring advanced respiratory support alone or basic respiratory support, together with the support of at least two organ systems. This level includes all complex patients requiring support for multiorgan failure

---

respiratory muscle pump is reduced further. Respiratory muscle function also may be compromised by the development of muscle fatigue because of the increased load. A vicious cycle develops, worsening acidosis causing further impairment of respiratory muscle function, which, in turn, has an adverse effect on pH and arterial blood-gas tensions. Early randomized, controlled trials (RCTs) comparing NIV with conventional therapy in the ICU showed that successful NIV is possible. Most striking was a reduction in the need for intubation,[13,14] which in the largest study translated into improved survival and reduced length of both ICU and hospital stays.[13] Complications, particularly pneumonia and other infectious complications, were reduced markedly.[13,15–17] It is striking that NIV was administered for only a relatively small proportion (mean 6 hours) of each day[13] or at modest levels for a longer period.[14] With NIV, paralysis and sedation are not needed, and ventilation outside the ICU is an option. Given the considerable pressure on ICU beds in some countries, the high costs, and that for some patients admission to ICU is a distressing experience.[18] this is an attractive option.

There have been seven prospective, randomized, controlled studies of NIV outside the ICU.[19–25] Bott et al[19] randomized 60 patients with COPD to either conventional treatment or NIV. NIV initiation, by research staff, took 90 minutes, on average (range 15 minutes to 4 hours). NIV led to a more rapid correction of pH and Pa_{CO_2}. On an intention-to-treat analysis, there was no significant benefit from NIV. When patients unable to tolerate NIV were excluded, a significant survival benefit was seen (9 of 30 versus 1 of 26). Generalizabilty from this study, although performed on general wards, to routine practice is difficult because staff additional to the normal ward complement set up NIV. The high mortality (30%) in the control group was surprising considering that the mean pH was only 7.34. In addition, the low intubation rate, while probably reflecting British practice, has been criticized.

Barbe et al[20] initiated NIV in the emergency department in patients presenting with an acute exacerbation of COPD and continued it in a general ward. To ease some of the problems of workload and compliance, NIV was administered for 3 hours twice a day. In this small study ($n = 24$), there were no intubations nor deaths in either group. Arterial blood-gas tensions improved equally in both the NIV group and the control group. The mean pH at entry, however, in each group was 7.33; at this level of acidosis, significant mortality is not expected; in other words, it was unlikely that such a small study would show an improved outcome because recovery was to be expected anyway.[26]

Wood et al[21] randomized 27 patients with acute respiratory distress secondary to various conditions to conventional treatment or NIV in the emergency department. Intubation rates were similar (7 of 16 versus 5 of 11), but there was a nonsignificant trend toward increased mortality in those given NIV (4 of 16 versus 0 of 11; $p = .123$). The authors attributed the excess mortality to delay in intubation because conventional patients requiring invasive ventilation were intubated after a mean of 4.8 hours compared with 26 hours in those on NIV ($p = .055$). It is difficult to draw many conclusions from this study given its small size, that the numbers of patients in each group were different, and that patients were not matched for etiology of respiratory failure. It does highlight the danger of prolonging NIV inappropriately.

Another possible reason why the two studies in which NIV was initiated in the emergency room[20,21] failed to show any advantage for NIV over conventional therapy is the fact that patients usually are admitted to an ICU when other therapies have failed, whereas most of those presenting to the emergency room have not received any treatment. A proportion is going to improve with medical therapy. In a 1-year-period prevalence study[27] of patients with acute exacerbations of COPD, of 954 patients admitted through the emergency department (Leeds, England), 20% were acidotic on arrival in the department; of these, 25% had completely corrected their pH by the time of arrival on the ward. There was a weak relationship between Pa_{O_2} on arrival at hospital and the presence of acidosis, suggesting that, in at least some patients, respiratory acidosis had been precipitated by high-flow oxygen therapy administered in the ambulance on the way to hospital.

Angus et al[22] compared NIV and doxapram in patients with COPD and type II (hypercapnic) respiratory failure in a small randomized trial in a general ward. NIV caused significant improvement in Pa_{O_2} and Pa_{CO_2} at 4 hours. In contrast, no fall in Pa_{CO_2} occurred in patients treated with doxapram, and initial improvement in Pa_{O_2} was not sustained at 4 hours. At both 1 and 4 hours, pH was significantly better in the NIV group compared with the doxapram group. All the patients in the NIV group were discharged home, although one required doxapram in addition to NIV during the acute illness. Of eight patients treated with doxapram, three died, and another two received NIV. Currently, respiratory stimulants are not recommended routinely, although they may have a role if there is no access to NIV.[28]

Bardi et al[23] found no significant differences in hospital outcome between NIV and conventional therapy in a study of 30 patients with COPD; most patients in both groups recovered without the need for invasive ventilation. Given that mean pH in the two groups was 7.36 and 7.39 and that no patient in either group had a pH of less than 7.30, these results are not surprising (as with the study of Barbe et al[20]).

In a study performed in an intermediate-care unit, Avdeev et al[25] randomly assigned 29 patients to NIV and 29 to conventional therapy alone. The patients were well matched, and pH indicated a severe exacerbation (7.28 versus 7.26). The mean duration of NIV was 29 ± 25 hours. Three patients refused NIV, of whom two required intubation and one died. In patients receiving NIV, there was a significant rise in pH and fall in Pa_{CO_2} after 1 hour compared with no change or a worsening in the conventional group. Fewer patients in the NIV group required intubation (12% versus 28%; $p = .18$) or died (8% versus 31%), and hospital stay was shorter (26 ± 7 versus 34 ± 10 days).

Plant et al[24] undertook the largest study to date ($n = 236$) on general respiratory wards in 13 centers. NIV was applied, by the usual ward staff, using a bilevel device in spontaneous mode according to a simple protocol. "Treatment failure," a surrogate for the need for intubation, defined by a priori criteria, was reduced from 27–15% by NIV. In-hospital mortality was reduced from 20–10%. This study suggests that with adequate staff training, NIV can be applied with benefit outside the ICU by the usual ward staff and that early introduction of NIV in a general ward results in better outcomes than providing no ventilator support for acidotic patients outside the ICU.

CONDITIONS OTHER THAN COPD

There are no RCTs of NIV outside the ICU in hypoxemic respiratory failure. The study of Antonelli et al[16] showed that NIV was as effective as conventional ventilation in improving gas exchange in patients with acute hypoxic respiratory failure. Patients receiving NIV had significantly lower rates of serious complications, and those treated successfully with NIV had shorter ICU stays. Post hoc analysis of patients grouped according to the simplified acute physiologic scores (SAPS) showed that NIV was superior to conventional mechanical ventilation in patients with SAPS < 16. In patients with a SAPS ≥ 16, outcome was similar, irrespective of the type of ventilation. As with acute exacerbations of COPD, it appears that it is possible to manage patients successfully with NIV. Further data are needed. Yet it is reasonable for selected patients to have a trial of NIV in an experienced noninvasive unit outside the ICU; rapid access to intubation and mechanical ventilation must be available.

Cardiogenic pulmonary edema (CPE) represents a special case because the onset and recovery usually are both rapid. Most patients present to the emergency room, but some develop CPE in the ward while an inpatient. The first focus is delivery of standard medical therapy, particularly nitrates.[29,30] Continuous positive airway pressure (CPAP) probably is the noninvasive mode of choice, although NIV may have a role in patients with significant hypercapnia.[31] Patients usually should receive ventilator support where they are because by the time arrangements have been made and transfer effected, most patients will have either improved or deteriorated to the point at which intubation is needed. Sufficient patients will attend the emergency room

with CPE or develop CPE in the coronary-care unit to make staff training in NIV in these areas worthwhile and to ensure enough throughput to maintain skills. When patients develop CPE outside these areas (e.g., in a surgical ward), it is likely to be sufficiently infrequent that it is not worth training the staff, or if trained, staff will not have had sufficient opportunity to use and develop their skills. This is a situation in which the peripatetic NIV team or critical-care outreach service may have a role. It is important that personnel are able to recognize and treat arrythmias and myocardial ischemia.[32]

ELECTIVE VENTILATION FOR CHRONIC VENTILATORY FAILURE

There have been a number of small and two large[33,34] series reporting the use of NIV in the successful treatment of diurnal ventilatory failure by the adequate control of nocturnal hypoventilation in patients with chest-wall deformity, neuromuscular disorders, and morbid obesity. Although there are no prospective RCTs, NIV is an accepted treatment for chronic hypercapnic ventilatory failure. It is unlikely that such trials will ever be performed, with most researchers considering such a study to be unethical. Comparative studies of patients with amyotrophic lateral sclerosis (ALS) who are treated with NIV shows a clear survival advantage when compared with patients who do not opt for assisted ventilation.[35,36] A prospective RCT of NIV in ALS has been reported in abstract form and shows clear advantages in terms of both survival and quality of life with NIV.[37] There have been a number of small prospective RCTs of NIV in patients with hypercapnia secondary to COPD.[38–41] Only one showed any benefit from the combination of NIV and long-term oxygen therapy,[40] with the others failing to show any advantage to NIV. All can be criticized primarily because of small numbers and because, in most, the adequacy of effective ventilator support overnight was not confirmed.[42] There have been two longer-term studies.[43,44] Neither showed benefit from NIV, although, again, both can be criticized[42] for similar reasons to those outlined earlier. There may be a role for NIV in patients who suffer recurrent exacerbations of sufficient severity to warrant hospitalization and acute NIV because these patients are at high risk for future hospitalization and death.[45] In the study of Clini et al,[44] there was a trend toward a lesser time in hospital in the NIV group compared with an increase in the oxygen-therapy group when compared with the period before the study. ICU stay was reduced in both groups but more in the NIV group than in the oxygen-therapy group. In an uncontrolled study, the provision of NIV reduced the need for hospitalization in the year after compared with the year before home NIV was instituted and reduced costs.[46] Further studies are needed, but at present, NIV should not be considered for most patients with COPD.

In summary there is no prospective RCT evidence to support the chronic use of NIV in any patient group. Most practitioners, however, would consider it unethical not to offer NIV to patients with chest-wall deformity and neuromuscular disease, and it is unlikely that there will ever be any RCTs of NIV in these conditions. Chronic NIV is not appropriate for most patients with COPD.

Where Should Noninvasive Ventilation Be Performed?

ACUTE NIV: ICU OR GENERAL WARD?

There have been no direct comparisons of outcome with NIV delivered in the ICU, intermediate units, and in a general ward. It is unlikely that there ever will be such a trial. It should be appreciated that while there is some overlap, the skills needed for NIV are different from those required for invasive ventilation. Familiarity with and confidence in NIV by all members of the multidisciplinary team is the most important factor. Nurses, physiotherapists, or respiratory therapists may be the primary caregiver; this will depend on local availability, enthusiasm, and expertise. The outcome from NIV is likely to be better on a general ward where the staff has a lot of experience of NIV than in an ICU with high nurse-, therapist-, and doctor-patient ratios and a high level of monitoring, but little experience of NIV. The patient's perspective is also important; many find their experience of ICU to be unpleasant,[18] and the less intensive atmosphere of a noninvasive unit may not be as distressing for patients and their relatives. NIV may be quite time-consuming in the early stages, and patients may benefit from the extra attention from caregivers, which is possible in an ICU compared with less well staffed clinical areas.

Assuming that the skills to deliver NIV are equal in the various possible locations, there are a number of other factors to be considered. These include whether or not intubation is considered appropriate should NIV fail, the presence of other system failure, comorbidity, severity of the respiratory failure, and likelihood of success with NIV (Fig. 34-1). Patients who cannot sustain ventilation for more than a few minutes when acutely unwell require continuous observation. This level of support is more likely to be available in the ICU than in other ward environments.

Although there are no published data, anecdotally there may be a tendency to abandon NIV more readily in an ICU because intubation is easily available, and in some ways it is easier for staff to manage a paralyzed, sedated patient than one who is struggling with NIV. When intubation is not immediately an option, there is a need to keep going a little longer, and a number of patients who at first sight appear to be failing can be managed successfully with a bit of persistence. It certainly has been the experience of the author that problems have been solved between the time that the ICU staff has been contacted and its arrival in the ward to intubate and/or transfer the patient (10–15 minutes).

Another important difference between the ICU and the general ward is the complexity of monitoring and the types of ventilators available. Monitoring serves two roles: (1) safety, to warn of impending catastrophe, and (2) optimization of ventilator settings. Vitacca et al[47] have shown that setting a ventilator on the basis of physiologically derived information resulted in more complete respiratory muscle unloading than when the ventilator was set by experienced operators using clinical judgement alone. ICU ventilators differ from the portable devices designed primarily for home use but frequently used in general wards. The principal limitation to the use of home ventilators during acute respiratory failure is the lack of direct online monitoring of pressure, volume, and flow provided by these devices. The evaluation of patient-ventilator asynchrony is easier with visualization of flow and pressure waveforms.[48] This may be important, particularly during the initiation of ventilation, when it is important to assess patient-ventilator

FIGURE 34-1 The spectrum of provision for an acute NIV service.

Intensive Care ←——————————————————————————————————→ General Ward

Intensive Care	General Ward
Lower pH	Higher pH
Comorbidities	No comorbidities
Acute	
Chronic	
Need for intensive monitoring	
NIV technically difficult	NIV technically easier
Invasive ventilation deemed appropriate if NIV fails	Invasive ventilation not deemed appropriate
	NIV the ceiling of intervention
Advantages	**Advantages**
Higher nurse / patient ratio	Cost saving compared with ICU
More monitoring	Specific interest / expertise lung disease
Ready access to invasive ventilation	Absence of immediate easy intubation encourages greater persistence and problem solving
	More "pleasant" environment
Disadvantages	**Disadvantages**
Cost	Low nurse to patient ratio
Less pleasant environment	Care needs of other patients may be neglected
Easier to abandon NIV and intubate	Lack of ready access to invasive ventilation

TABLE 34-2   Monitoring During NIV

Essential
- Regular clinical observation
- Continuous pulse oximetry
- Arterial blood gases after 1 to 4 hours of NIV and after 1 hour of any change in ventilator settings or F_{IO_2}.
- Respiratory rate—continuous or intermittent

Desirable
- ECG
- More detailed physiologic information such as leak, expired tidal volume, and measure of ventilator-patient asynchrony

---

interaction, respiratory mechanics, and the expired tidal volume.[49] Further work is needed to establish which variables should be monitored to optimize NIV. It should be appreciated that high-technology monitoring is never a substitute for good clinical observation.[50] For safety, it is recommended that all patients receiving NIV for acute ventilatory failure should have continuous monitoring of oxygen saturation (S_{O_2}) by pulse oximetry, regular assessments of arterial blood-gas tensions (because there is no accurate and reliable noninvasive measure of P_{CO_2} or, more important, pH), and respiratory rate.[51] The S_{O_2} should be maintained at around 92%[52] to avoid the twin dangers of dangerous hypoxia and the risk of worsening hypercapnia secondary to altering the dead-space-to-tidal-volume ratio.[53] There is no reason why this level of monitoring cannot be provided in a general ward (Table 34-2).

If NIV is only to be provided in the ICU, the number of patients needing ICU care will increase, and this may not be necessary or appropriate. The study of Plant et al[24] has shown that NIV is an option outside the ICU, but the outcome for patients with a pH of less than 7.30 was not as good as that seen for comparable patients in the studies performed in a higher-dependency setting. Also, for reasons of training, throughput, quality of service, and skill retention, NIV is best performed in a single location.[27] An intermediate unit with ready access to an ICU may provide the best compromise, but such units are not widely available.[54] They can be effective, and data from the United States suggest that they are cost-effective.[55] A study[3] of 756 consecutive patients admitted to 26 respiratory intermediate-care units in Italy with a nurse-patient ratio ranging from 1:2.5 to 1:4 per shift, availability of adequate continuous noninvasive monitoring, expertise in NIV and for intubation in case of NIV failure, and physician availability 24 hours a day showed a better outcome than that expected on the basis of APACHE II scores. The median APACHE II score was 18 (range 1–43). The predicted inpatient mortality was 22.1%, whereas the actual mortality was 16%. All but 48 patients had chronic respiratory disease, mainly COPD ($n = 451$). These units are different from other similar units in being able to care for intubated patients; this has major implications for training of medical and nursing staff and may not be possible in many health care systems.

ELECTIVE NIV: GENERAL WARD OR CHRONIC-CARE FACILITY?

The onset of established chronic ventilatory failure usually is insidious. Patients at risk are best seen and regularly reviewed in specialist centers so that the onset of significant nocturnal hypoventilation and the development of diurnal ventilatory failure can be anticipated. As a result, NIV usually should be instituted before the patient becomes critically ill requiring HDU or ICU admission. It is advisable to acclimatize patients to NIV at an early stage once the development of significant ventilatory failure becomes likely. Decompensation may occur with an intercurrent event, most commonly respiratory tract infection. NIV is much easier in the acute situation if the patient has experienced it previously when reasonably well. In such patients, if they are clinically stable, there is no need for assisted ventilation to "work" immediately; indeed, it does not matter if the patient is hardly able to use the ventilator at all initially. More detailed description of the use of NIV in chronic respiratory failure can be found in Chapters 19 and 32.

There is little reason to admit these patients to the ICU, and it is questionable whether, with appropriate teams in place, the patient even needs admission to hospital. Some patients, particularly those with severe neuromuscular disease, have complex nursing needs, and their home environment may be better adapted to their needs than a hospital bed. It is more pleasant for relatives and caregivers to stay in their own home. Particular issues for that patient concerning positioning of equipment, ensuring adequate access to electrical power, and so on can be addressed.[56] If the patient is to be admitted to hospital, the choice may be between a chronic-care facility and a general ward. As for acute NIV, local staff expertise is the most important factor determining the best location (Table 34-3). Staffing and expertise being equal, advantages of the general ward include access to the ICU if things go wrong and more ready access to other specialist teams because some of these patients have other complex needs that the need to start NIV brings into focus. Adequate control of nocturnal hypoventilation needs to be confirmed. For some patients, overnight oximetry may suffice; for others, particularly those receiving supplemental oxygen, monitoring of P_{CO_2} is necessary. Patients also will need intermittent arterial blood-gas analyses. These advantages, however, are generalizations; depending on the nature of the chronic-care facility, it may be better suited than a general ward for providing the care and support for the other needs of patients.

TABLE 34-3   Elective Ventilation for Chronic Ventilatory Failure

---

There is likely to be great local variation. Factors that determine the best location:
- Enthusiastic and trained staff
- Possibility of colocating with acute NIV unit
- Access to expertise in the management of nonrespiratory aspects of care
- Diagnostics, e.g., sleep laboratory
- Access to ICU

THE ADVANTAGE OF THE GENERAL WARD

An acute and a chronic NIV service depends critically on local factors, particularly the skill levels of doctors, nurses, and therapists. The major advantage of the general ward is that it sits in the middle of the spectrum of locations for NIV provision and is likely to treat the greatest number of patients. Use of skills is a key factor in developing and retaining them. The skills learned looking after patients needing NIV acutely are equally relevant for patients being started electively on NIV. Familiarity with the nonrespiratory needs of patients with complex neuromuscular or musculoskeletal disorders, learned when patients are admitted electively to start NIV, are transferable to the care of such patients needing NIV acutely or for weaning. Continuity of care is also important. Some patients start home ventilation after an acute event, and the option of dealing with both aspects in the same place and with the same care team probably is advantageous to the patient and caregivers.

Selection of Patients for NIV in a General Ward

ACUTE RESPIRATORY FAILURE

COPD

The place of NIV in the management of COPD is now well established.[57,58] The pH at the time NIV is initiated is the best single predictor of severity and the likelihood of success with the noninvasive approach.[59] Moreover, changes in pH and respiratory rate are easily measurable and useful in predicting the likelihood of a successful outcome from NIV. Arterial blood gases should be checked at baseline and after 1–4 hours because a number of studies have shown that the change in arterial blood-gas values, particularly pH, after a short period of NIV predicts a successful outcome.[13,19,60–64] Patients who have been intubated and are likely to fail a weaning attempt adopt a pattern of rapid shallow breathing when disconnected from the ventilator,[65] suggesting that they are breathing against an unsustainable load. A reduction in respiratory rate with NIV has been variably observed in a number of studies; larger falls generally are associated with a successful outcome from NIV,[13,61,62] although this is not always seen.[66] Data from the largest study[67] showed that hydrogen ion concentration at enrollment (odds ratio 1.22 per nmol/liter) and Pa_{CO_2} (odds ratio 1.14 per kPa) were associated with treatment failure. After 4 hours of therapy, improvement in acidosis (odds ratio 0.89 per nmol/liter) and/or fall in respiratory rate (odds ratio 0.92 per breath per minute) were associated with success. If at least one of these two variables was improving, successful NIV was likely. pH therefore is useful in determining, first, who should receive NIV, second, in what location, and finally, when the patient can or should move to a more or less intensive location. Generally speaking, the lower the pH, the greater is the risk to the patient of needing invasive ventilation if NIV is not offered or, if it is attempted, of failure. The more acidotic the patient, the greater is the need for that patient to be managed in an ICU because the risk of failure of NIV and the potential need for endotracheal intubation is higher.[68] If it has been decided that NIV is the ceiling of treatment, this is not necessary; indeed, if NIV is failing, the patient may be allowed to die in a slightly less high-tech environment than that afforded by most ICUs.

HYPOXEMIC RESPIRATORY FAILURE

These patients are best managed in an ICU because the risks of failure are higher and because the major problem is a failure of oxygenation. Patients are more likely to need prompt invasive ventilation if they are deteriorating or have other organ failure; moreover, ventilators usually used on general wards are those designed primarily for home use, and a high F_{IO_2} cannot be delivered. One further consideration was highlighted by Delclaux et al[69] in a study on the use of noninvasive CPAP in patients with hypoxemic respiratory failure; there was a trend toward more cardiorespiratory arrests in the CPAP group. The increase was attributed to the improvement in oxygenation and other physiologic parameters while the patients were using CPAP, which led to a false sense of security; when patients take the mask off, even for a short period, S_{O_2} may fall rapidly, putting them at high risk. Any patient who desaturates within seconds of removing a mask should be monitored very carefully, usually in an ICU, and probably this should be considered an indication for intubation. From a study performed by Hilbert et al[70] in immunocompromised patients, it is clear that the institution of intermittent NIV earlier than would be the case for invasive ventilation conferred a clear survival benefit in patients who are known to have a very poor prognosis,[71] and this could be performed safely outside the ICU.

CHRONIC RESPIRATORY FAILURE: ELECTIVE INSTITUTION OF NIV

The choice of location is usually between an institution (general ward or chronic-care facility, depending on local factors) and the home. Patients will need admission to an institution if NIV is likely to be problematic, requires 24-hour nursing support, there is a risk of significant decompensation, there are other care needs best addressed in an institution, or there is no infrastructure in place to support the patient at home. Some patients also will require more detailed investigation, such as polysomnography, before NIV is started.

Implications for Staffing and Training (Table 34-4)

NIV has been reported to be a time-consuming procedure[72]; as with any new technique, there is a learning curve, and the same authors subsequently published more encouraging results.[73] A number of ICU studies have shown that a significant amount of time is required to establish the patient on NIV, but this drops off substantially in subsequent days.[14,74,75] It is possible, therefore, that NIV may have a

TABLE 34-4   Key Training Requirements

Understanding the rationale for assisted ventilation
Mask and headgear selection and fitting
Ventilator circuit assembly
Theory of operation and adjusting ventilation to achieve desired outcome
Principles and practice of humidification
Inhaled therapy for the patient receiving NIV
Cleaning and general maintenance
Understanding how to monitor progress
Ethical issues relevant to the care of patients with incurable disease
Problem solving—the ability to recognize serious situations and act accordingly

---

much greater impact on nursing workload outside the ICU, where nurses have responsibility for a larger number of patients. In the study of Bott et al,[19] there was no difference in nursing workload, assessed by asking the senior nurse to rate, on a visual analogue scale, the amount of care needed in the conventional and NIV groups. This, however, is an insensitive way of measuring nursing needs; in addition, some of the potential extra work associated with NIV was performed by supernumerary research staff. In the study of Plant et al,[24] NIV resulted in a modest increase in nursing workload, assessed using an end-of-bed log, in the first 8 hours of the admission, equivalent to 26 minutes, but no difference was identified thereafter. No data exist, however, on the effect NIV on the care of other patients on the ward, nor whether outcome would have been better had nurses spent more time with patients receiving NIV. Most of the centers that participated in the study had little or no previous experience of NIV and therefore required training in mask fitting and application of NIV. Formal training in the first 3 months of opening a ward by a research doctor and nurse was 7.6 hours (SD 3.6). Thereafter, each center received 0.9 hour per month (SD 0.82) to maintain skills. It should be appreciated that there was no need to make subtle adjustments to ventilator settings, which all was done according to protocol. Much more training would be needed if sophisticated ventilators are used. This underlines the fact, however, that NIV, in whatever location, is not just a question of purchasing the necessary equipment but also of staff training.

Although considerable input is likely when a unit commences to provide an NIV service, thereafter, as long as a critical mass of nurses and therapists remains, new staff will gain the necessary skills from their colleagues. Given that NIV in the more severely ill patient may require as much input as an invasively ventilated patient,[74] there usually should be one nurse responsible for no more than three or four patients, although this will depend on the other care needs of the patients. In the less severely affected patient, NIV can be successful with a lower level of staffing.[24]

Economic Considerations

Economic analysis is complex. As a result, many diagnostic and therapeutic technologies have been adopted into practice without any consideration of the economic implications. Even techniques with a clear clinical advantage may not be endorsed in the current health care climate without a favorable cost-effectiveness analysis. The first step in an economic analysis is to calculate the cost of an intervention. Relevant costs for ventilation include equipment, supplies, capital, and overhead. More complex is the calculation of the costs of the care for patients, including medical and paramedic time and the level of assistance, laboratory and pharmacy costs, nutrition costs, and ventilation costs. The daily cost of NIV is similar to that of standard medical therapy[14] or invasive ventilation (calculated only on the first day of treatment).[74] According to the different studies and countries, the mean daily cost of NIV varies from about $850[74] to $1500[14,76]; the difference results mainly from salaries of the personnel, which are much higher in the United States than in Europe. The second step is to evaluate the outcome for patients. Outcomes may be calculated in terms of economic resources saved or created, efficacy of treatment in improving survival or, in the case of NIV, rate of intubation, or as impact of a technique on quality of life.

Although the findings are not consistent, some of the larger studies have shown that NIV can shorten length of ICU and/or hospital stay compared, for example, with medical therapy or invasive ventilation.[13,14,16,17,70,77] In no study has NIV been shown to lengthen hospital stay. Although not the primary aim of the studies, the finding of reduced hospital, and particularly ICU, length of stay creates or saves resources and thereby indicates a cost benefit from NIV.

There have been two detailed cost-effectiveness studies of NIV: one in North America in the ICU the other in the United Kingdom, where NIV was delivered on general wards. In the former, base care was modeled for a tertiary-care teaching hospital.[78] The two alternatives considered were NIV and standard medical therapy, whereas the main outcomes were modeled, and calculated were costs, mortality, and intubation rates. To determine clinical effectiveness, the authors used a meta-analysis of randomized trials. Then a decision tree was constructed, and probabilities were applied at each chance node using research evidence and a comprehensive regional database. The authors concluded that NIV was more effective than standard treatment in reducing hospital mortality and also less expensive, with a cost saving of about $2500 per patient admission.

Intensive care is also expensive care. Intermediate units may provide an alternative to the classic ICU at reduced cost.[54] The daily costs of a ventilated patient may be reduced by two-thirds when NIV is performed in a specialized respiratory unit rather than in an ICU.[55] These costs can be reduced still further when NIV is performed on a general ward,[79] although effectiveness may not be as good as in higher-dependency settings. Outcome in patients with a pH of less than 7.30 in the study of Plant et al[24] was not as good as the results obtained in the ICU in patients with a similar severity of ventilatory failure, at least as evidenced by the pH.[13,14,77] Carlucci et al[80] showed that over time, as practitioners develop the necessary skills and grow in confidence with NIV, practice changes. They found that after a few years, patients with more severe acidosis were ventilated successfully with NIV; more patients, usually those with a higher pH, received NIV on general wards, with significant cost savings, compared with when they first started providing an acute NIV service.

Conclusion

Staff training and experience are more important than location. Adequate numbers of staff, skilled in NIV, must be available throughout 24 hours. Because of the demands of looking after acutely ill patients, and to aid training and skill retention, acute NIV usually is best carried out in one single-sex location with one nurse responsible for three to four patients. Basic monitoring, at least pulse oximetry and facilities for arterial blood-gas analysis, should be available. Because the skills, both for NIV and for the other care needs of the patient population likely to need NIV, are transferable, there are significant advantages to locating both the acute and elective NIV service in the same place. This is probably best sited in a general ward with close geographic and organizational links with the ICU. The best location for both an acute and chronic NIV service will vary from institution to institution, and local expertise, enthusiasm, and hospital geography will be the major determinants of where the service should be located and how it is delivered.

References

1. Anonymous. Intensive care in the United Kingdom: Report from the King's Fund panel. Anaesthesia 1989; 44:428–31.
2. Corrado A, Roussos C, Ambrosino N, et al. Respiratory intermediate care units: A European survey. Eur Respir J 2002; 20:1343–50.
3. Confalonieri M, Gorini M, Ambrosino N, et al. Respiratory intensive care units in Italy: A national census and prospective cohort study. Thorax 2001; 56:373–8.
4. Department of Health, London. Comprehensive critical care: A review of adult critical care services. 2000.
5. Ball C, Kirkby M, Williams S. Effect of the critical care outreach team on patient survival to discharge from hospital and readmission to critical care: Non-randomised population based study. Br Med J 2003; 327:1014.
6. Pittard AJ. Out of our reach? Assessing the impact of introducing a critical care outreach service. Anaesthesia 2003; 58:882–5.
7. Shee CD, Green M. NIV guidelines. Thorax 2002; 57:1002.
8. Elliott MW. Improving the care for patients with acute severe respiratory disease. Thorax 2003; 58:285–8.
9. Tobin MJ, Perez W, Guenther SM, et al. The pattern of breathing during successful and unsuccessful trials of weaning from mechanical ventilation. Am Rev Respir Dis 1986; 134:1111–8.
10. Macklem PT. Hyperinflation. Am Rev Respir Dis 1984; 129:1–2.
11. Smith TC, Marini JJ. Impact of PEEP on lung mechanics and work of breathing in severe airflow obstruction. J Appl Physiol 1988; 65:1488–99.
12. Juan G, Calverley P, Talamo C, et al. Effect of carbon dioxide on diaphragmatic function in human beings. New Engl J Med 1984; 310:874–9.
13. Brochard L, Mancebo J, Wysocki M, et al. Noninvasive ventilation for acute exacerbations of chronic obstructive pulmonary disease. New Engl J Med 1995; 333:817–22.
14. Kramer N, Meyer TJ, Meharg J, et al. Randomized, prospective trial of noninvasive positive pressure ventilation in acute respiratory failure. Am J Respir Crit Care Med 1995; 151:1799–806.
15. Nava S, Ambrosino N, Clini E, et al. Noninvasive mechanical ventilation in the weaning of patients with respiratory failure due to chronic obstructive pulmonary disease: A randomized, controlled trial. Ann Intern Med 1998; 128:721–8.
16. Antonelli M, Conti G, Rocco M, et al. A comparison of noninvasive positive-pressure ventilation and conventional mechanical ventilation in patients with acute respiratory failure. New Engl J Med 1998; 339:429–35.
17. Antonelli M, Conti G, Bufi M, et al. Noninvasive ventilation for treatment of acute respiratory failure in patients undergoing solid organ transplantation: A randomized trial. JAMA 2000; 283:235–41.
18. Easton C, MacKenzie F. Sensory-perceptual alterations: Delirium in the intensive care unit. Heart Lung 1988; 17:229–37.
19. Bott J, Carroll MP, Conway JH, et al. Randomised, controlled trial of nasal ventilation in acute ventilatory failure due to chronic obstructive airways disease. Lancet 1993; 341:1555–7.
20. Barbe F, Togores B, Rubi M, et al. Noninvasive ventilatory support does not facilitate recovery from acute respiratory failure in chronic obstructive pulmonary disease. Eur Respir J 1996; 9:1240–5.
21. Wood KA, Lewis L, Von Harz B, Kollef MH. The use of noninvasive positive pressure ventilation in the emergency department. Chest 1998; 113:1339–46.
22. Angus RM, Ahmed AA, Fenwick LJ, Peacock AJ. Comparison of the acute effects on gas exchange of nasal ventilation and doxapram in exacerbations of chronic obstructive pulmonary disease. Thorax 1996; 51:1048–50.
23. Bardi G, Pierotello R, Desideri M, et al. Nasal ventilation in COPD exacerbations: Early and late results of a prospective, controlled study. Eur Respir J 2000; 15:98–104.
24. Plant PK, Owen JL, Elliott MW. Early use of non-invasive ventilation for acute exacerbations of chronic obstructive pulmonary disease on general respiratory wards: A multicentre randomised, controlled trial. Lancet 2000; 355:1931–5.
25. Avdeev SN, Tret'iakov AV, Grigor'iants RA, et al. [Study of the use of noninvasive ventilation of the lungs in acute respiratory insufficiency due exacerbation of chronic obstructive pulmonary disease]. Anesteziol Reanimatol 1998; 3:45–51.
26. Jeffrey AA, Warren PM, Flenley DC. Acute hypercapnic respiratory failure in patients with chronic obstructive lung disease: Risk factors and use of guidelines for management. Thorax 1992; 47:34–40.
27. Plant PK, Owen J, Elliott MW. One year period prevalance study of respiratory acidosis in acute exacerbation of COPD: Implications for the provision of non-invasive ventilation and oxygen administration. Thorax 2000; 55:550–4.
28. Greenstone M, Lasserson TJ. Doxapram for ventilatory failure due to exacerbations of chronic obstructive pulmonary disease. Cochrane Database of Systematic Reviews 2003; CD000223.
29. Sharon A, Shpirer I, Kaluski E, et al. High-dose intravenous isosorbide-dinitrate is safer and better than Bi-PAP ventilation combined with conventional treatment for severe pulmonary edema. J Am Coll Cardiol 2000; 36:832–7.
30. Crane SD, Elliott MW, Gilligan P, et al. Randomised, controlled comparison of continuous positive airways pressure, bilevel non invasive ventilation, and standard treatment in emergency department patients with acute cardiogenic pulmonary oedema. Emerg Med J 2004; 21:155–61.

31. Nava S, Carbone G, DiBattista N, et al. Noninvasive ventilation in cardiogenic pulmonary edema: A multicenter randomized trial. Am J Respir Crit Care Med 2003; 168:1432–7.

32. Bersten AD. Noninvasive ventilation for cardiogenic pulmonary edema: Froth and bubbles? Am J Respir Crit Care Med 2003; 168:1406–8.

33. Leger P, Bedicam JM, Cornette A, et al. Nasal intermittent positive pressure ventilation: Long-term follow-up in patients with severe chronic respiratory insufficiency. Chest 1994; 105: 100–5.

34. Simonds AK, Elliott MW. Outcome of domiciliary nasal intermittent positive pressure ventilation in restrictive and obstructive disorders. Thorax 1995; 50:604–9.

35. Pinto AC, Evangelista T, Carvalho M, et al. Respiratory assistance with a non-invasive ventilator (BiPAP) in MND/ALS patients: Survival rates in a controlled trial. J Neurol Sci 1995; 129: 19–26.

36. Kleopa KA, Sherman M, Neal B, et al. Bipap improves survival and rate of pulmonary function decline in patients with ALS. J Neurol Sci 1999; 164:82–8.

37. Bourke SC, Tomlinson M, Williams TL, et al. Randomised, controlled trial of noninvasive ventilation in motor neurone disease. Thorax 2004; 59:ii–30.

38. Strumpf DA, Millman RP, Carlisle CC, et al. Nocturnal positive-pressure ventilation via nasal mask in patients with severe chronic obstructive pulmonary disease. Am Rev Respir Dis 1991; 144:1234–9.

39. Lin CC. Comparison between nocturnal nasal positive pressure ventilation combined with oxygen therapy and oxygen monotherapy in patients with severe COPD. Am J Respir Crit Care Med 1996; 154:353–8.

40. Meecham Jones DJ, Paul EA, Jones PW, Wedzicha JA. Nasal pressure support ventilation plus oxygen compared with oxygen therapy alone in hypercapnic COPD. Am J Respir Crit Care Med 1995; 152:538–44.

41. Gay PC, Hubmayr RD, Stroetz RW. Efficacy of nocturnal nasal ventilation in stable, severe chronic obstructive pulmonary disease during a 3-month controlled trial. Mayo Clin Proc 1996; 71:533–42.

42. Elliott MW. Noninvasive ventilation in chronic ventilatory failure due to chronic obstructive pulmonary disease. Eur Respir J 2002; 20:511–4.

43. Casanova C, Celli BR, Tost L, et al. Long-term controlled trial of nocturnal nasal positive pressure ventilation in patients with severe COPD. Chest 2000; 118:1582–90.

44. Clini E, Sturani C, Rossi A, et al. The Italian multicentre study on noninvasive ventilation in chronic obstructive pulmonary disease patients. Eur Respir J 2002; 20:529–38.

45. Chu CM, Chan VL, Lin AWN, et al. Readmission rates and life threatening events in COPD survivors treated with non-invasive ventilation for acute hypercapnic respiratory failure. Thorax 2004; 59:1020–5.

46. Tuggey JM, Plant PK, Elliott MW. Domiciliary non-invasive ventilation for recurrent acidotic exacerbations of COPD: An economic analysis. Thorax 2003; 58:867–71.

47. Vitacca M, Nava S, Confalonieri M, et al. The appropriate setting of noninvasive pressure support ventilation in stable COPD patients. Chest 2000; 118:1286–93.

48. Kacmarek RM. NIPPV: Patient-ventilator synchrony, the difference between success and failure? Intensive Care Med 1999; 25:645–7.

49. Calderini E, Confalonieri M, Puccio PG, et al. Patient-ventilator asynchrony during noninvasive ventilation: The role of expiratory trigger. Intensive Care Med 1999; 25:662–7.

50. Tobin MJ. Respiratory monitoring. JAMA 1990; 264:244–51.

51. British Thoracic Society Standards of Care Committee. Non-invasive ventilation in acute respiratory failure. Thorax 2002; 57:192–211.

52. Jubran A, Tobin MJ. Reliability of pulse oximetry in titrating supplemental oxygen therapy in ventilator-dependent patients. Chest 1990; 97:1420–5.

53. Stradling JR. Hypercapnia during oxygen therapy in airways obstruction: A reappraisal. Thorax 1986; 41:897–902.

54. Nava S, Confalonieri M, Rampulla C. Intermediate respiratory intensive care units in Europe: A European perspective. Thorax 1998; 53:798–802.

55. Elpern EH, Silver MR, Rosen RL, Bone RC. The noninvasive respiratory care unit: Patterns of use and financial implications. Chest 1991; 99:205–8.

56. Elliott MW, Latham M. Assisted ventilation for patients with motor neurone disease. CME Bull Palliative Care Med 1999; 1: 78–81.

57. Brochard L. Non-invasive ventilation for acute exacerbations of COPD: A new standard of care. Thorax 2000; 55:817–8.

58. Elliott MW. Non-invasive ventilation in acute exacerbations of chronic obstructive pulmonary disease: A new gold standard? Intensive Care Med 2002; 28:1691–4.

59. Lightowler JV, Elliott MW. Predicting the outcome from NIV for acute exacerbations of COPD. Thorax 2000; 55:815–6.

60. Ambrosino N, Foglio K, Rubini F, et al. Non-invasive mechanical ventilation in acute respiratory failure due to chronic obstructive airways disease: Correlates for success. Thorax 1995; 50:755–7.

61. Meduri GU, Abou-Shala N, Fox RC, et al. Noninvasive face mask mechanical ventilation in patients with acute hypercapneic respiratory failure. Chest 1991; 100:445–54.

62. Soo Hoo GW, Santiago S, Williams AJ. Nasal mechanical ventilation for hypercapnic respiratory failure in chronic obstructive pulmonary disease: Determinants of success and failure. Crit Care Med 1994; 22:1253–61.

63. Meduri GU, Turner RE, Abou-Shala N, et al. Noninvasive positive pressure ventilation via face mask: First line intervention in patients with acute hypercapnic and hypoxemic respiratory failure. Chest 1996; 109:179–93.

64. Poponick JM, Renston JP, Bennett RP, Emerman CL. Use of a ventilatory support system (BiPAP) for acute respiratory failure in the emergency department. Chest 1999; 116:166–71.

65. Yang KL, Tobin MJ. A prospective study of indexes predicting the outcome of trials of weaning from mechanical ventilation. New Engl J Med 1991; 324:1445–50.

66. Anton A, Guell R, Gomez J, et al. Predicting the result of noninvasive ventilation in severe acute exacerbations of patients with chronic airflow limitation. Chest 2000; 117:828–33.

67. Plant PK, Owen JL, Elliott MW. Non-invasive ventilation in acute exacerbations of chronic obstructive pulmonary disease: Long term survival and predictors of in-hospital outcome. Thorax 2001; 56:708–12.

68. Conti G, Antonelli M, Navalesi P, et al. Noninvasive vs. conventional mechanical ventilation in patients with chronic obstructive pulmonary disease after failure of medical treatment in the ward: A randomized trial. Intensive Care Med 2002; 28:1701–7.

69. Delclaux C, L'Her E, Alberti C, et al. Treatment of acute hypoxemic nonhypercapnic respiratory insufficiency with continuous positive airway pressure delivered by a face mask: A randomized, controlled trial. JAMA 2000; 284:2352–60.

70. Hilbert G, Gruson D, Vargas F, et al. Noninvasive ventilation in immunosuppressed patients with pulmonary infiltrates, fever, and acute respiratory failure. New Engl J Med 2001; 344: 481–7.

71. Hill NS. Noninvasive ventilation for immunocompromised patients. New Engl J Med 2001; 344:522–4.

72. Chevrolet JC, Jolliet P, Abajo B, et al. Nasal positive pressure ventilation in patients with acute respiratory failure. Chest 1991; 100:775–82.

73. Chevrolet JC, Jolliet P. Workload on non-invasive ventilation. In: Vincent JL, editor. Year book of intensive and emergency medicine. Berlin: Springer, 1997: 505–13.

74. Nava S, Evangelisti I, Rampulla C, et al. Human and financial costs of noninvasive mechanical ventilation in patients affected by COPD and acute respiratory failure. Chest 1997; 111:1631–8.

75. Hilbert G, Gruson D, Vargas F, et al. Noninvasive ventilation for acute respiratory failure: Quite low time consumption for nurses. Eur Respir J 2000; 16:710–6.

76. Criner GJ, Kreimer DT, Tomaselli M, et al. Financial implications of noninvasive positive pressure ventilation (NPPV). Chest 1995; 108:475–81.

77. Celikel T, Sungur M, Ceyhan B, Karakurt S. Comparison of noninvasive positive pressure ventilation with standard medical therapy in hypercapnic acute respiratory failure. Chest 1998; 114:1636–42.

78. Keenan SP, Gregor J, Sibbald WJ, et al. Noninvasive positive pressure ventilation in the setting of severe, acute exacerbations of chronic obstructive pulmonary disease: More effective and less expensive. Crit Care Med 2000; 28:2094–2102.

79. Plant PK, Owen JL, Parrott S, Elliott MW. Cost-effectiveness of ward based non-invasive ventilation for acute exacerbations of chronic obstructive pulmonary disease: Economic analysis of randomised, controlled trial. Br Med J 2003; 326:956–61.

80. Carlucci A, Delmastro M, Rubini F, et al. Changes in the practice of non-invasive ventilation in treating COPD patients over 8 years. Intensive Care Med 2003; 29:419–25.

PART IX
PHYSIOLOGIC EFFECTS OF MECHANICAL VENTILATION

Chapter 35

EFFECTS OF MECHANICAL VENTILATION ON CONTROL OF BREATHING

DIMITRIS GEORGOPOULOS

The main reasons for instituting mechanical ventilation are to decrease the work of breathing, support gas exchange, and buy time for other interventions to reverse the cause of respiratory failure.[1] Mechanical ventilation can be applied in patients who are making or not making respiratory efforts, whereby assisted or controlled modes of support are used, respectively.[1] In patients without respiratory efforts, the respiratory system represents a passive structure, and thus the ventilator is the only system that controls breathing. During assisted modes of ventilator support, the patient's system of control of breathing is under the influence of the ventilator pump.[2–4] In the latter instance, ventilatory output is the final expression of the interaction between the venti-lator and the patient's system of control of breathing. Thus physicians who deal with ventilated patients should know the effects of mechanical ventilation on control of breathing, as well as their interaction. Ignorance of these issues may prevent the ventilator from achieving its goals and also lead to significant patient harm.

Physiology

The respiratory control system consists of a motor arm, which executes the act of breathing, a control center located in the medulla, and a number of mechanisms that convey information to the control center.[5,6] Based on information, the control center activates spinal motor neurons that subserve the respiratory muscles (inspiratory and expiratory); the intensity and rate of activity vary substantially between breaths and between individuals. The activity of spinal motor neurons is conveyed, via peripheral nerves, to respiratory muscles, which contract and generate pressure (Pmus). According to equation of motion, Pmus at time t during a breath is dissipated in overcoming the resistance (Rrs) and elastance (Ers) of the respiratory system (inertia is assumed to be negligible) as follows:

$$\text{Pmus(t)} = \text{Rrs} \times \dot{V}(t) + \text{Ers} \times \Delta V(t) \qquad (1)$$

where $\Delta V(t)$ is instantaneous volume relative to passive functional residual capacity (FRC) and $\dot{V}(t)$ is instantaneous flow. Equation (1) determines the volume-time profile and, depending on the frequency of respiratory muscle activation, ventilation. Volume-time profile affects Pmus via neuromechanical feedback; inputs generated from other sources (cortical inputs) may modify the function of control center. Ventilation, gas-exchange properties of the lung, and cardiac function determine arterial blood gases, termed *arterial oxygen tension* (Pa_{O_2}) and *arterial carbon dioxide tension* (Pa_{CO_2}), which, in turn, affect the activity of control center via peripheral and central chemoreceptors (chemical feedback). This system can be influenced at any level by diseases or therapeutic interventions.

During mechanical ventilation, the pressure provided by the ventilator (Paw) is incorporated into the system.[3] Thus the total pressure applied to respiratory system at time t [$\text{P}_{\text{TOT}}(t)$] is the sum of Pmus(t) and Paw(t). As a result, the equation of motion is modified as follows:

$$\text{P}_{\text{TOT}}(t) = \text{Pmus(t)} + \text{Paw(t)} = \dot{V}(t) \times \text{Rrs} + \Delta V(t) \times \text{Ers} \quad (2)$$

The relationships of Eq. (2) determine the volume-time profile during mechanical ventilation, which via neuromechanical, chemical and behavioral feedback systems affects the Pmus waveform (Fig. 35-1). The ventilator pressure, by changing flow and volume, may influence these feedback systems and thus alter either the patient's control of breathing itself or its expression. In addition, Pmus, depending on several factors, alters the Paw

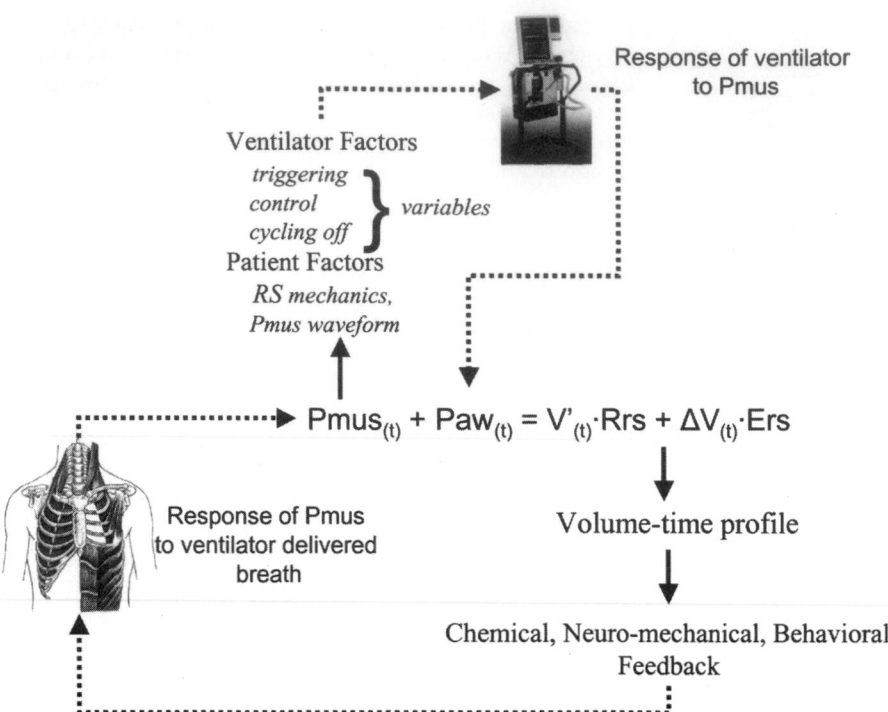

FIGURE 35-1 Schematic representation of variables that determine the volume-time profile during mechanical ventilation. Pmus(t), instantaneous respiratory muscle pressure; Paw(t), airway (ventilator) pressure; V̇(t), instantaneous flow; ΔV(t), instantaneous volume relative to passive functional residual capacity of respiratory system; Rrs, resistance of the respiratory system; Ers, elastance of the respiratory system; RS, respiratory system. Neuromechanical, chemical, and behavioral feedback systems are the main determinants of Pmus. The functional operation of the ventilator mode (triggering, control, and cycling-off variables) and patient-related factors (namely, respiratory system mechanics and the Pmus waveform) determine the response of the ventilator to Pmus.

waveform (see Fig. 35-1). Thus, during assisted mechanical ventilation (i.e., Pmus ≠ 0), ventilatory output is not under the exclusive influence of patient's control of breathing; instead, it represents the final expression of an interaction between ventilator-delivered pressure and patient respiratory effort.

Effects of Mechanical Ventilation on Feedback Systems

CHEMICAL FEEDBACK

Chemical feedback refers to the response of Pmus to Pa_{O_2}, Pa_{CO_2} and pH.[5-7] In spontaneously breathing and mechanically ventilated patients, this system is an important determinant of respiratory motor output both during wakefulness and sleep.[8-13]

Mechanical ventilation can influence chemical feedback simply by altering the three variables Pa_{O_2}, Pa_{CO_2}, and pH. Hypoxemia, hypercapnia, or acidemia may be corrected by mechanical ventilation and thus modify activity of the medulary respiratory controller via peripheral and central chemoreceptors.[7] The effects of mechanical ventilation on gas-exchange properties of the lung are beyond the scope of this chapter and are discussed in Chapter 37. In this chapter, the fundamental elements of the response of respiratory motor output to chemical stimuli, their relationship to unstable breathing, and the operation of chemical feedback during mechanical ventilation are reviewed.

RESPONSE OF RESPIRATORY MOTOR OUTPUT TO CHEMICAL STIMULI

CO₂ STIMULUS
Carbon dioxide (CO_2) is a powerful stimulus of breathing.[7] This stimulus, expressed by Pa_{CO_2}, largely depends on the product of tidal volume (V_T) and breathing frequency (f) (i.e., minute ventilation) according to the Eq.(3):

$$Pa_{CO_2} = 0.863\, \dot{V}_{CO_2}/[V_T \times f(1 - V_D/V_T)] \qquad (3)$$

where $\dot{V}_{CO_2}$ is CO_2 production, and V_D/V_T is dead space to V_T ratio. Because minute ventilation is an adjustable variable in ventilated patients, understanding the relationship between respiratory motor output and CO_2 stimuli is of fundamental importance.

Several studies have examined the respiratory motor output to CO_2 in ventilated conscious healthy subjects.[8,15-18] Major findings include

1. Manipulation of Pa_{CO_2} over a wide range has no appreciable effect on respiratory rate. Despite hypocapnia, subjects continue to trigger the ventilator with a rate similar to that of eucapnia. Respiratory rate increases slightly when Pa_{CO_2} approaches values well above eucapnia (Fig. 35-2).

2. The intensity of respiratory effort (respiratory drive) increases progressively as a function of P_{CO_2}. This response is evident even in hypocapnic range. Over the range of CO_2 stimuli examined, it was not possible to identify a threshold below which the response of respiratory motor output did not exist. The response slope increases progressively with increasing CO_2 stimuli,

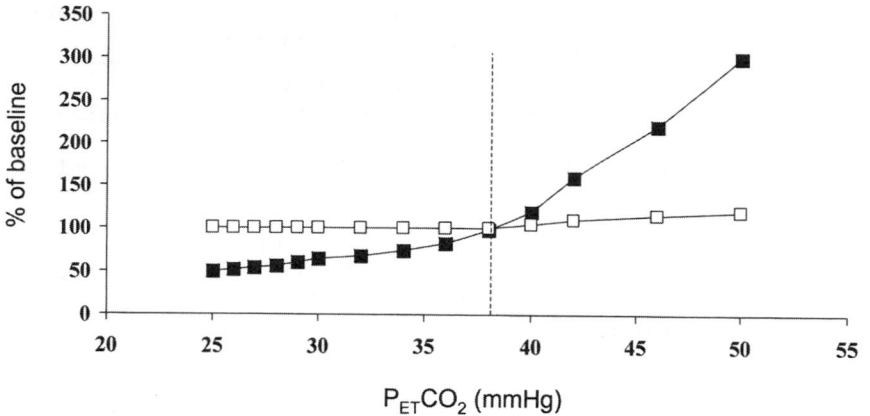

FIGURE 35-2 Schematic representation of the response of respiratory frequency (*open squares*) and pressure-time product of the inspiratory muscles per breath (an index of the intensity of patient effort, *closed squares*), both expressed as a percentage of values during spontaneous eupnea (baseline), to CO_2 challenge in conscious healthy subjects ventilated with a high level of ventilator assistance. $P_{ET}CO_2$ is end-tidal P_{CO_2}, and the dotted vertical line is $P_{ET}CO_2$ during spontaneous breathing (eupnea). Contrast the vigorous response of intensity of inspiratory effort to CO_2, even in the hypocapnic range, with the response of respiratory frequency, which remains at eucapnic level over a broad range of CO_2 stimuli. The response is based on data from refs. 8 and 15–18.

reaching its maximum in the vicinity of eucapnic values (see Fig. 35-2).

3. There is no fundamental difference in the response to CO_2 between various ventilator modes.

4. Above eupnea, the slope of the response does not differ significantly with that observed during spontaneous breathing, suggesting that mechanical ventilation per se does not considerably modify the sensitivity of respiratory system to CO_2.

During sleep (or sedation), the response of respiratory motor output to CO_2 differs substantially from that during wakefulness, secondary to loss of the suprapontine neural input to the medullary respiratory controller (loss of the wakefulness drive to breathe).[11,19] In ventilated sleeping subjects, a decrease in Pa_{CO_2} by a few millimeters of mercury causes apnea.[11] Sleep unmasks a highly Pa_{CO_2}-sensitive apneic threshold, whereby apnea is induced by small transient reductions in Pa_{CO_2} below eupnea.[11,19] Respiratory rhythm is not restored until Pa_{CO_2} has increased significantly above eupneic levels. The difference between eupneic Pa_{CO_2} and Pa_{CO_2} at apneic threshold, referred to as *CO_2 reserve*,[20] depends on several factors (see below). This reserve determines the propensity of an individual to develop breathing instability during sleep; propensity increases as CO_2 reserve decreases. Similar to wakefulness, the response of respiratory motor output to CO_2 is mediated mainly by the intensity of respiratory effort, whereas respiratory rate decreases abruptly to zero (apnea) when the CO_2 apneic threshold is reached.[21]

OTHER CHEMICAL STIMULI

The effects of mechanical ventilation on the response of respiratory motor output to stimuli other than CO_2 have not been studied adequately. In a steady state during wakefulness, the effects of oxygen (O_2) and pH on breathing pattern are similar qualitatively to that observed with CO_2: Changes in O_2 and pH mainly alter the intensity of pa-

tient effort, whereas respiratory rate is affected considerably less.[7] There is no reason to expect a different response pattern during mechanical ventilation. Indeed, this is the case regarding the hypoxic response in normal conscious subjects ventilated in assist-control mode during eucapnia.[22] Indirect data also revealed that during eucapnia, the sensitivity of respiratory motor output to hypoxia was not modified by mechanical ventilation.[22] During mild hypocapnia, however, the response was attenuated, whereas at moderate hypocapnia (end-tidal $P_{CO_2} \sim$ 31 mmHg) the response was negligible. The latter observations may be relevant clinicaly because ventilated patients do not always keep Pa_{CO_2} at eucapnic levels and can become hypocapnic.[18]

CHEMICAL STIMULI AND UNSTABLE BREATHING

The response pattern of respiratory motor output to CO_2 during sleep is relevant to the occurrence of periodic breathing in mechanically ventilated patients. Unstable breathing in critically ill patients did not receive much attention in the past. Recent evidence, however, indicates that this breathing pattern might increase the morbidity and mortality of critically ill patients because it can cause sleep fragmentation and patient-ventilator dyssynchrony.[23,24] Sleep deprivation may cause serious cardiorespiratory,[25,26] neurologic,[27,28] immunologic, and metabolic consequences.[29–32]

The following is a brief review of the factors that can lead to unstable breathing. In a closed system governed mainly by chemical control (such as occurs during sleep or sedation), a transient change in ventilation at a given metabolic rate ($\Delta \dot{V}_{initial}$) will result in a transient change in alveolar gas tensions. This change is sensed by peripheral and central chemoreceptors, which, after a variable delay, exert a corrective ventilatory response ($\Delta \dot{V}_{corrective}$) that is in the opposite direction to the initial perturbation[33–35] (Fig. 35-3). The ratio of $\Delta \dot{V}_{corrective}$ to $\Delta \dot{V}_{initial}$ defines the loop gain of the system, an engineering concept introduced by Khoo et al.[33] Loop gain is a dimensionless index that is the mathematical

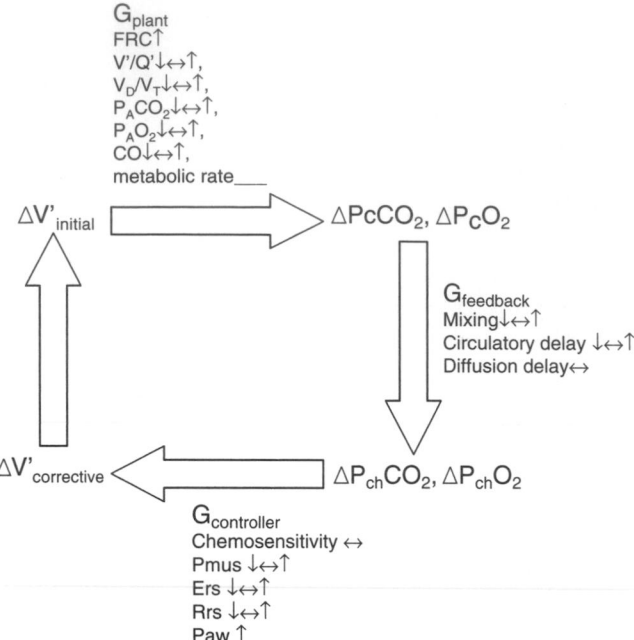

FIGURE 35-3 Schematic representation of the variables that determine the propensity of an individual to develop periodic breathing in a closed system dominated by chemical feedback. Loop gain is the product of three gains: plant, feedback, and controller. Instability occurs when $\Delta V_{corrective}$ (the final response) is 180° out of phase with $\Delta V_{initial}$ (the transient initial perturbation) and $\Delta V_{corrective}/\Delta V_{initial} > 1$. Mechanical ventilation, by affecting almost all variables of the system (↑ Increase, ↔ no change, ↓ decrease), may change both the magnitude and the dynamic component of loop gain and thus the propensity of an individual to develop periodic breathing. LG, G_{plant}, $G_{feedback}$, and $G_{controller}$, loop, plant, feedback, and controller gains, respectively; ΔPc_{CO_2} and ΔPc_{O_2}, the difference in partial pressures of CO_2 and O_2 in mixed pulmonary capillary blood, respectively; ΔPch_{CO_2} and ΔPch_{O_2}, the difference in partial pressure of CO_2 and O_2 at chemoreceptors (peripheral and central), respectively; FRC, functional residual capacity; $\dot{V}/\dot{Q}$, ventilation-perfusion ratio; CO, cardiac output; V_D/V_T, dead-space fraction, Pa_{CO_2} and Pa_{O_2}, alveolar partial pressure of CO_2 and O_2, respectively; Pmus, pressure developed by respiratory muscles; Paw, airway (ventilator) pressure; and Ers and Rrs, elastance and resistance of respiratory system, respectively.

TABLE 35-1   Effects of Mechanical Ventilation on Gain Factors and Gain Changes

Gain Factors (Influence)	Ventilator Effect[a]	Gain Change
Lung volume (stabilizing)	↑	↓G_{plant}
Cardiac output (destabilizing)	↓	↑G_{plant}, ↑$G_{feedback}$
Thoracic blood volume (destabilizing)	↓	↑$G_{feedback}$
Paw response to Pmus (destabilizing)	↑	↑$G_{controller}$
Alveolar PCO_2 (stabilizing)	↓	↓G_{plant}
Alveolar PO_2 (stabilizing)	↑	↓G_{plant}, ↓$G_{controller}$
Respiratory elastance (destabilizing)	↓	↑$G_{controller}$

ABBREVIATIONS: Paw, airway pressure; Pmus, respiratory muscle pressure; ↓, decrease; ↑, increase.
[a] Mechanical ventilation may also exert opposite effects on the various gain factors.

Positive-pressure breathing exerts multiple effects on loop gain by influencing almost all the factors that determine plant, feedback, and controller gains. The effects are complex and at times opposing and variable (Table 35-1; see also Fig. 35-3). Nevertheless, the effect of mechanical ventilation on controller gain exerts the most powerful influence on the propensity to develop breathing instability.[12,21,24] The magnitude and direction of the change in controller gain depends on the ventilator mode, the level of assistance, the mechanics of the respiratory system, and the Pmus waveform (see below).[12,18,21,24] The disease states also may interfere with the effects of mechanical ventilation on loop gain. For example, positive-pressure ventilation may increase or decrease cardiac output, causing corresponding changes in circulatory delay depending on cardiac function and intravascular volume[36–39] (see Chapter 36). It has been shown that nocturnal mechanical ventilation in patients with congestive heart failure decreases the frequency of Cheyne-Stokes breathing, presumably by causing an increase in cardiac output secondary to afterload reduction.[40–42]

In addition to CO_2, O_2 and pH can play a key role in producing unstable breathing in ventilated patients during sleep (or sedation). It is well known that hypoxia, acting via peripheral chemoreceptor stimulation, decreases Pa_{CO_2}. The result reduces the plant gain (stabilizing influence); for a given change in alveolar ventilation, Pa_{CO_2} will change less when baseline Pa_{CO_2} is low than when it is high.[20] Hypoxia, however, increases the controller gain to a much greater extent[43] because the slope of ventilatory response to CO_2 below eupnea increases,[7] a highly destabilizing influence.[33–35] Similar principles apply if pH is considered as a chemical stimulus; acidemia decreases the plant gain (lowers Pa_{CO_2}) and increases, to a much lesser extent, the controller gain.[20,43] During mechanical ventilation, the propensity to unstable breathing in the face of changing O_2 and pH stimuli depends on a complex interaction

product of three types of gains: plant gain (the relationship between the change in gas tensions in mixed pulmonary capillary blood and $\Delta\dot{V}_{initial}$), feedback gain (the relationship between gas tensions at the chemoreceptor level and those at the mixed pulmonary capillary level), and controller gain (the relationship between $\Delta\dot{V}_{corrective}$ and the change in gas tensions at the chemoreceptor level) (see Fig. 35-3). Loop gain has both a magnitude and a dynamic component.[33–35] In this system, instability occurs when the corrective response is 180° out of phase with initial disturbance (dynamic component) and loop gain is greater than 1 (magnitude component). This instability leads to fluctuation in chemical stimuli, namely, P_{CO_2}. If P_{CO_2} reaches the apneic threshold, apnea occurs.

between the effects of these stimuli and mechanical ventilation on plant, feedback, and controller gains (Fig. 35-4; see also Table 35-1).

OPERATION OF CHEMICAL FEEDBACK

The ventilator mode is a major determinant of driving pressure for flow and thus arterial blood gases. Before discussing the operation of chemical feedback, it is useful to review briefly the functional features of three modes of assisted ventilation, namely, assist-control ventilation (ACV), pressure-support ventilation (PSV), and proportional-assist ventilation (PAV) (for detailed descriptions, see Chapters 7, 9, and 13). Figure 35-5 shows the response of the ventilator to respiratory effort in a representative subject ventilated with each mode in the presence and absence of CO_2 challenge.[18] With CO_2 challenge, Paw decreases with ACV, it remains constant with PSV, and it increases with PAV. Pressure-time product of inspiratory muscle pressure (PTP-$Pmus_I$) is an accurate index of the intensity of inspiratory effort.[44] With ACV, the ratio of V_T to PTP-$Pmus_I$ per breath decreases with increasing Pmus (see Chapter 7); the ratio is largely independent of inspiratory effort with PAV (see Chapter 13). With PSV, V_T/PTP-$Pmus_I$ per breath may change in either direction with increasing Pmus, depending on factors such as the level of pressure assist and cycling-off criterion, change in Pmus, and mechanics of the respiratory system (see Chapter 9). With PSV, in the absence of active termination of pressure delivery (with expiratory muscle contraction), the ventilator delivers a minimum V_T, which may be quite high, depending on the pressure level, mechanics of the respiratory system, and cycling-off criterion.[21]

Assume that in a ventilated patient Pa_{CO_2} drops because of an increase in the set level of assistance or decrease in metabolic rate and/or V_D/V_T ratio.[14] During wakefulness, patients will react to this drop by decreasing the intensity of their inspiratory effort, whereas the breathing frequency will remain relatively constant (see "Response of Respiratory Motor Output to Chemical Stimuli," above). The extent to which a patient is able to prevent respiratory alkalosis via operation of chemical feedback depends almost exclusively on the relationship between the intensity of patient inspiratory effort and the volume delivered by the ventilator (i.e., V_T/PTP-$Pmus_I$). Similarly, if Pa_{CO_2} increases (decrease in assistance level, increase in metabolic rate and/or V_D/V_T ratio), the patient will increase the intensity of inspiratory effort and, to much lesser extent, respiratory frequency. Thus V_T/PTP-$Pmus_I$ per breath is critical for the effectiveness of chemical feedback to compensate for changes in chemical stimuli (Pa_{CO_2}). For given respiratory system mechanics, V_T/PTP-$Pmus_I$ is heavily dependent on the mode of support. Thus the effectiveness of chemical feedback in compensating for changes in chemical stimuli should be mode-dependent. Modes of support that permit the intensity of patient inspiratory effort to be expressed on ventilator-delivered volume improve the effectiveness of chemical feedback in regulating Pa_{CO_2} and particularly in preventing respiratory alkalosis. In normal

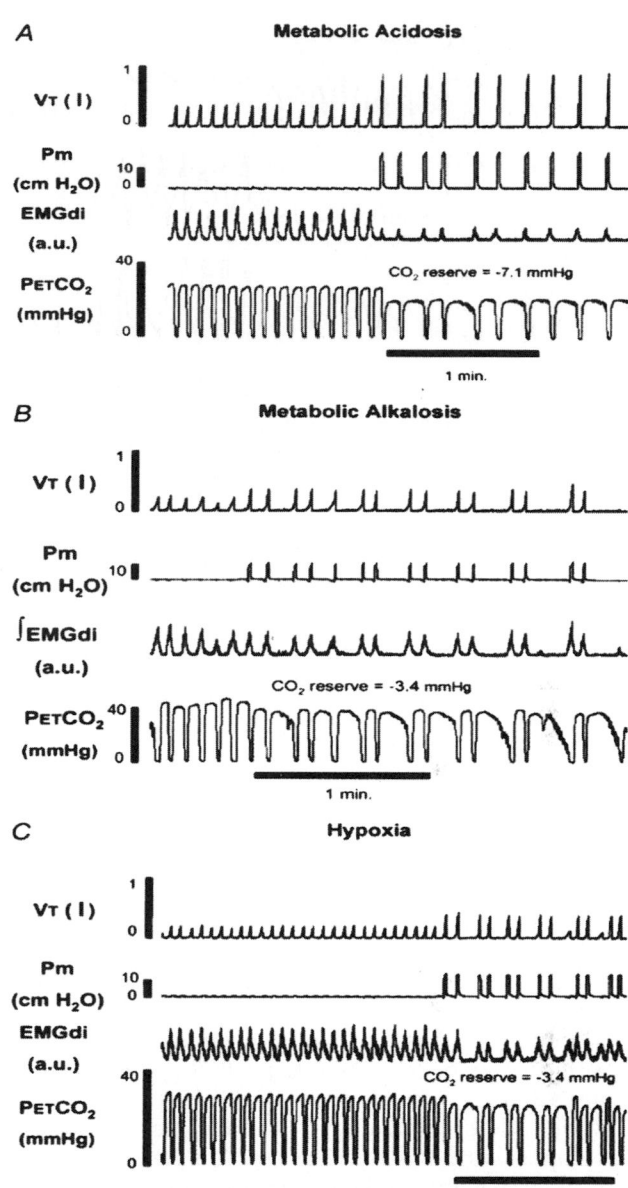

FIGURE 35-4 Tidal volume (V_T), airway pressure (Pm), diaphragmatic EMG (EMGdi, arbitrary units), and partial pressure of end-tidal CO_2 ($P_{ET_{CO_2}}$) in a tracheostomized dog during non-REM sleep without and with pressure-support ventilation at a pressure level that caused periodic breathing. *A.* At a background of 5 hours of metabolic acidosis (pH 7.34, HCO_3^- 16 mEq/liter, Pa_{CO_2} 30 mmHg). *B.* At a background of 1 hour of metabolic alkalosis (pH 7.51, HCO_3^- 35 mEq/liter, Pa_{CO_2} 44 mmHg). *C.* During hypoxia (Pa_{O_2} 47 mmHg, Pa_{CO_2} 31 mmHg). At a background of metabolic acidosis, CO_2 reserve was quite high; consequently, the pressure level that caused periodic breathing (20 cmH$_2$O) was significantly higher than the corresponding values (~10 cmH$_2$O) during metabolic alkalosis or hypoxia. Hyperventilation during spontaneous breathing was similar during metabolic acidosis and hypoxia (similar stabilization influence via a decrease in plant gain secondary to low Pa_{CO_2}), indicating that the destabilizing influence of hypoxia was caused by an increase in controller gain (hypoxic increase in the slope of CO_2 below eupnoea). (*Used, with permission, from Dempsey et al: J Physiol 560:1–11, 2004, based on data from ref. 43.*)

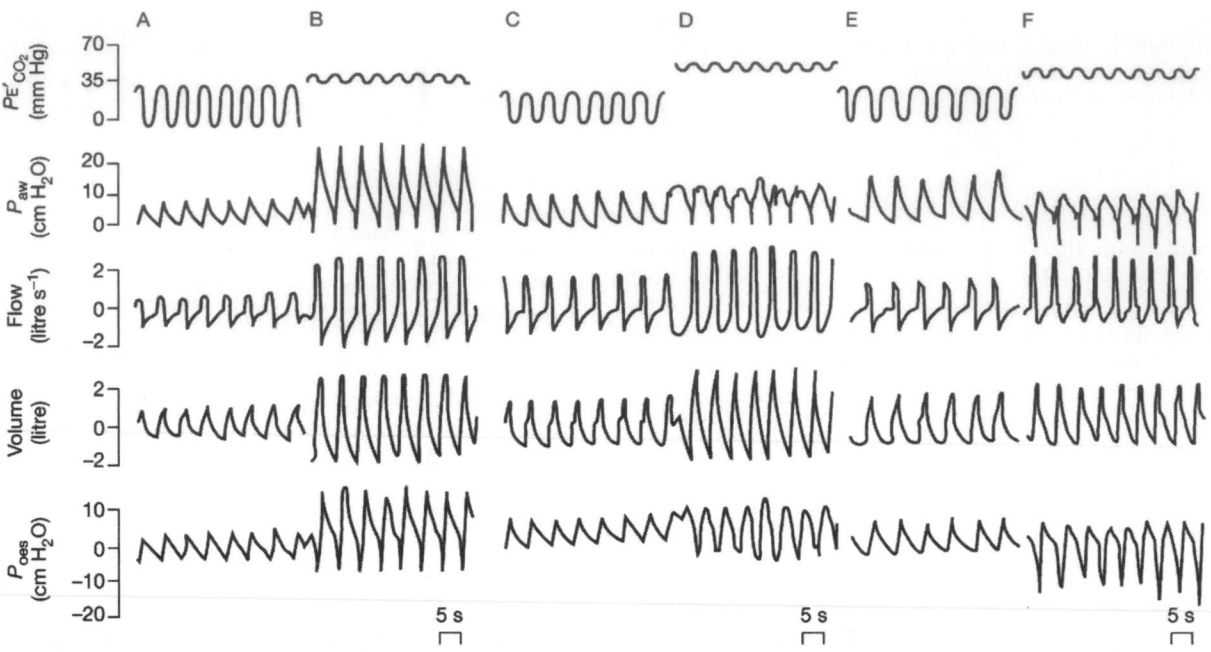

FIGURE 35-5 End-tidal carbon dioxide tension (PET_{CO_2}), airway pressure (Paw), flow (inspiration up), volume (inspiration up), and esophageal (Pes) pressure in a representative subject during proportional-assist ventilation (*A, B*), pressure-support ventilation (*C, D*), and volume-control ventilation (*E, F*) in the absence (*A, C, E*) and presence (*B, D, F*) of CO_2 challenge. With CO_2 challenge, Paw decreases with assist-control ventilation (the ventilator antagonizes patient's effort); it remains constant with pressure-support ventilation (no relationship between patient effort and level of assist); and it increases with proportional-assist ventilation (positive relationship between effort and pressure assist). (*Used, with permission from Mitrouska et al: Eur Respir J 13:873–82, 1999.*)

conscious subjects receiving maximum assistance on the three main ventilator modes,[18] the ability of the subject to regulate Pa_{CO_2} depends on the operational principles of each mode, specifically in terms of V_T/PTP-Pmus$_I$ (Fig. 35-6). At all levels of CO_2 stimulation, preservation of neuroventilatory coupling increased progressively from ACV to PSV to PAV; the ability of subjects to regulate Pa_{CO_2} followed the same pattern.[18]

During sleep or sedation, the tendency to develop hypocapnia with ACV and PSV (see Chapter 57 for the effects of mechanical ventilation on sleep) may have serious consequences because a drop of a few millimeters of mercury in Pa_{CO_2} leads to apnea and periodic breathing.[12,21] Thus excessive assistance with ACV and PSV promotes unstable breathing secondary to impaired neuroventilatory coupling; controller gain remains high in the face of low inspiratory effort (Fig. 35-7). Unstable breathing, however, during sleep secondary to mechanical ventilation may be prevented or attenuated with PAV that does not guarantee a minimum V_T.[12,21] Modes that decrease the volume delivered by a ventilator in response to any reduction in the intensity of patient effort enhance breathing stability. Nevertheless, if the assist setting during PAV is such that controller gain increases considerably, and the inherent loop gain of the patient is relatively high, the patient will be at risk of developing unstable breathing.[35,45,46]

These principles may be altered by disease states and therapeutic interventions. Although little is known about the interaction between disease states and mechanical ventilation on control of breathing, two examples help in illustrating the point. First, in conscious patients with sleep apnea syndrome, a drop in Pa_{CO_2} because of brief (40 second) hypoxic hyperventilation resulted, contrary to healthy subjects, in significant hypoventilation and triggering of periodic breathing in some patients.[47] This hypoventilation was interpreted as evidence of a defect (or reduced effectiveness) of short-term poststimulus potentiation, a brain-stem mechanism that promotes ventilatory stability.[48] In this situation, a level of assistance that causes a significant decrease in Pa_{CO_2} may promote unstable breathing in awake patients with sleep apnea syndrome, a situation closely resembling that observed during sleep. Second, studies in ventilated critically ill patients have shown that when awake patients are unable to increase V_T appropriately as a result of the mode used (i.e., PSV), they increase respiratory rate in response to a chemical challenge. Behavioral feedback, however, may underlie this response pattern. In sedated patients with acute respiratory distress syndrome (in whom behavioral feedback is not an issue) receiving PSV, considerable variation in Pa_{CO_2} elicited a steady-state response limited to the intensity of breathing effort, a response pattern similar to that observed in normal subjects.[10]

NEUROMECHANICAL FEEDBACK

INTRINSIC PROPERTIES OF RESPIRATORY MUSCLES

For a given neural output, Pmus decreases with increasing lung volume and flow, as dictated by the force-length and force-velocity relationships of inspiratory muscles, respectively.[49] Therefore, for a given level of muscle

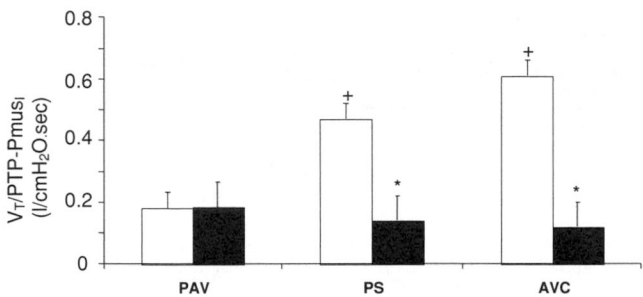

FIGURE 35-6 Ratio (mean $\pm$ SD) of tidal volume to pressure-time product of inspiratory muscles (V_T/PTP-Pmus$_I$) in normal conscious subjects ventilated with three modes of assisted ventilation in the absence and presence of CO_2 challenge (inspired CO_2 concentration increased in small steps until intolerance developed). Open and closed bars represent zero and final (highest) concentration of inspired CO_2, respectively. PAV, proportional-assist ventilation; PS, pressure-support ventilation; and AVC, assist volume control. Asterisk indicates significant difference from the value without CO_2 challenge. Plus sign indicates significant difference from the corresponding value with PAV. With each mode, subjects were ventilated at the highest comfortable level of assistance (corresponding to 80% reduction of patient resistance and elastance with PAV, 10 cmH$_2$O of pressure support, and 1.2-liter tidal volume with AVC). With CO_2 challenge, V_T/PTP-Pmus$_I$ decreased significantly when the subjects were ventilated with PS and AVC, but it remained relatively constant with PAV. Without CO_2 challenge, V_T/PTP-Pmus$_I$ was significantly higher with PS and AVC than with PAV. This response pattern caused severe respiratory alkalosis with PS and AVC (PET_{CO_2} decreased to $\sim$ 22 mmHg with both modes) but not with PAV (PET_{CO_2} $\sim$ 30 mmHg). Unlike with PS and PAV, subjects ventilated with AVC could not tolerate high values of PET_{CO_2} (final PET_{CO_2} was $\sim$7, 11, and 13 mmHg higher than baseline eupnea, respectively with AVC, PS, and PAV). Based on data from ref. 18.

activation, Pmus should be smaller during mechanical ventilation than during spontaneous breathing if pressure provided by the ventilator results in greater flow and volume. It has been shown in healthy subjects ventilated with PSV that compared with spontaneous breathing, the relationship between electrical activity (EMGdi) and pressure-time product of diaphragm (PTPdi) is shifted to the left; thus, at any given level of EMGdi, PTPdi is reduced.[50]

The influence and consequences of mechanical feedback during mechanical ventilation have not been studied satisfactorily. It is possible that this type of feedback is of clinical significance in patients with dynamic hyperinflation (high end-expiratory lung volume), high ventilatory requirements (requirements for high flow and volume), and/or impaired neuromuscular capacity.

The intrinsic properties of respiratory muscles must be considered when pressure measurements are used to infer changes in respiratory muscle activation; otherwise, errors in estimation of respiratory muscle activity may occur. These errors may be significant when ventilation is elevated secondary to high volume and flow. During hypercapnic hyperventilation, intrinsic properties of inspiratory muscles may decrease peak Pmus by about 20%.[8] Fauroux et al[50] reported correction factors for higher flows and volumes that

facilitate proper interpretation of respiratory motor output during mechanical ventilation. These authors showed that the left shift of the EMGdi-PTPdi relationship was decreased significantly by the addition of inspiratory flow to pressure analysis.[50]

REFLEX FEEDBACK

The characteristics of each breath are influenced by various reflexes that are related to lung volume or flow and mediated, after a latency of a few milliseconds, by receptors located in the respiratory tract, lung, and chest wall.[5,6] Mechanical ventilation may stimulate these receptors by changing flow and volume. In addition, changes in ventilator settings, inevitably associated with changes in volume and flow, also may elicit acute Pmus responses mediated by reflex feedback. In sedated patients with acute respiratory distress syndrome, manipulation of ventilator settings altered immediately (within one breath) the neural respiratory timing, whereas respiratory drive remained constant.[10,51] Specifically, decreases in V_T and pressure support and increases in inspiratory flow caused an increase in respiratory frequency. Depending on the type of alteration, changes in respiratory frequency were mediated via alteration in neural inspiratory and expiratory time; increases in inspiratory flow caused increases in respiratory frequency mainly by decreasing neural inspiratory time; decreases in V_T and pressure support caused increases in respiratory frequency by decreasing neural expiratory time. This reflex response was similar, at least qualitatively, to that observed in healthy subjects during wakefulness and sleep.[52–56] There was a strong dependency of neural expiratory time on the time that mechanical inflation extended into neural expiration; neural expiratory time increased proportionally to the increase in the delay between the ventilator cycling off and the end of neural inspiratory time[10,51] (Fig. 35-8). This finding indicates that expiratory asynchrony may elicit a reflex timing response. A subsequent study in a general ICU population confirmed the dependency of neural expiratory time on expiratory asynchrony.[57] The most likely explanation for the timing response is the Herring-Breuer reflex.

The final response may be unpredictable depending on the magnitude and type of lung volume change, the level of consciousness, and the relative strength of the reflexes involved. Nevertheless, reflex feedback should be taken into account when ventilator strategies are planned. A few examples may help in illustrating the importance of reflex feedback in patient-ventilator interaction. Assume that the patient is receiving pressure support that is being decreased during weaning. This results in lower V_T, which through reflex feedback decreases neural expiratory time, causing an increase in respiratory frequency.[10,51] This increase should not be interpreted as patient intolerance to the decrease in pressure support. Consider another patient with obstructive lung disease receiving ACV. V_T is decreased at a constant inspiratory flow in order to reduce the magnitude of dynamic hyperinflation (less volume is exhaled over a longer period). The lower V_T usually results in less delay in breath termination as compared with the end of neural inspiration, which through vagal feedback will decrease neural

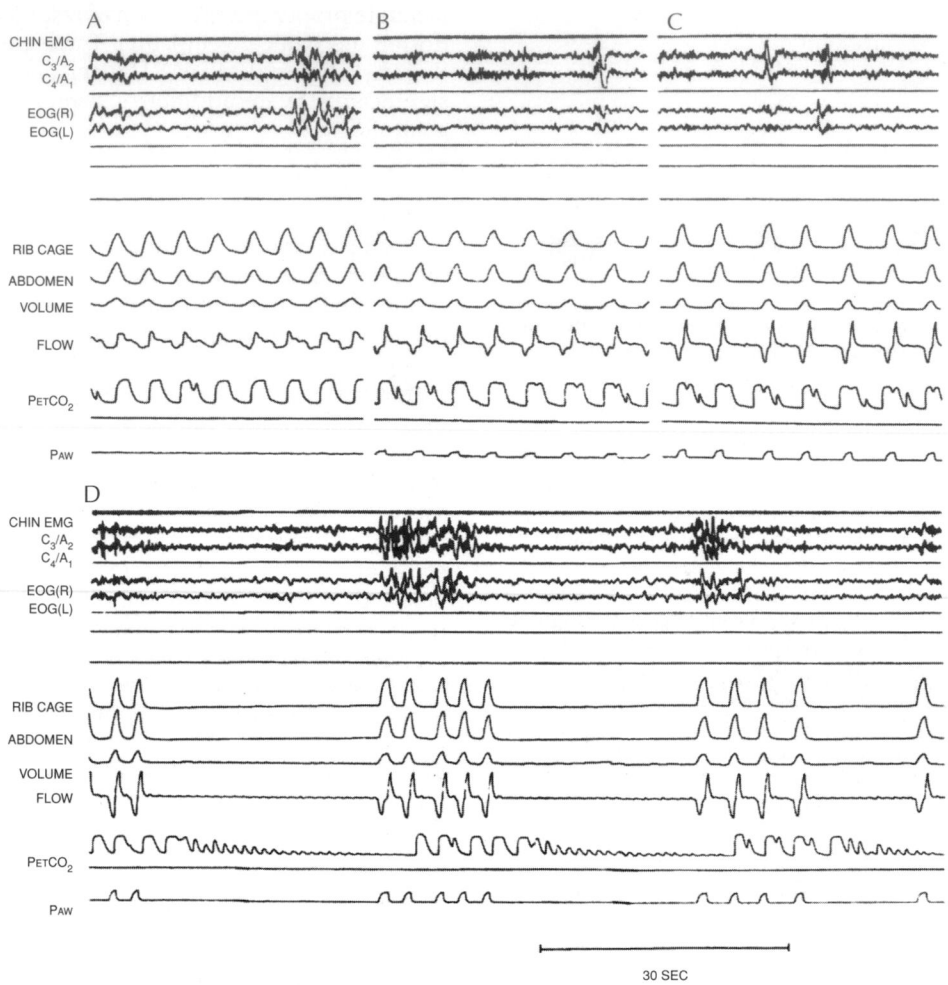

FIGURE 35-7 Polygraph tracings in a healthy subject during non-REM sleep with and without pressure-support ventilation. *A.* Spontaneous breathing with CPAP. B–D. Pressure support of 3, 6, and 8 cmH2O, respectively. Periodic breathing with central apneas developed with pressure support of 8 cmH2O. C3/A2 and C4/A1, electroencephalogram channels; EOG; electroocculogram [right (R) and left (L)]; Paw, airway pressure; EMG, electromyogram; P_{ETCO_2}, end-tidal P_{CO_2}. (*Used, with permission, from Meza et al: J Appl Physiol 167:1193–9, 2003.*)

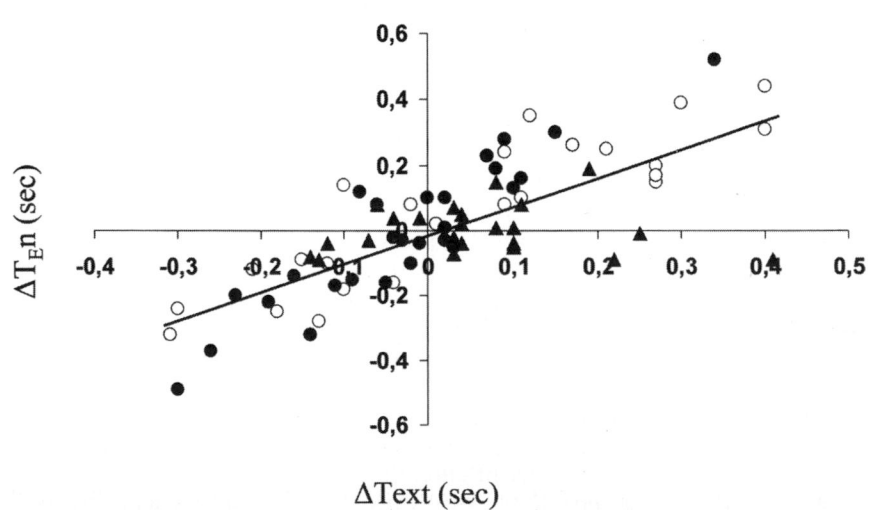

FIGURE 35-8 Relationship between the changes in the time that mechanical inspiration extended into neural expiration (ΔText, expiratory asynchrony) and neural expiratory time (ΔTen) in mechanically ventilated patients with ARDS. Closed circles, open circles, and open triangles represent ΔText induced by changes in volume (at constant flow), flow (at constant volume), and pressure support, respectively. Solid line, regression line. Based on data from ref. 51.

y=-0.004+0.897x, P<0.001

expiratory time, limiting the effectiveness of this strategy for reducing dynamic hyperinflation.[51] Assume in another patient receiving ACV that inspiratory flow is increased at a constant V_T, with the intent of reducing inflation time and providing more time for expiration so as to reduce dynamic hyperinflation. This step causes a reflex decrease in neural inspiratory time and an increase in respiratory frequency. Mechanical expiratory time may change in either direction depending mainly on the relation between neural and mechanical inspiratory time. In patients receiving ACV, expiratory time showed a variable response to changes in flow rate; some patients actually demonstrate a reduced expiratory time with a higher flow,[58] which cancels the desired reduction in dynamic hyperinflation.

NEUROMECHANICAL INHIBITION

Mechanical ventilation at relatively high tidal volume and ventilator frequency results in a non–chemically mediated decrease in respiratory motor output.[59–61] This decrease, referred to as *neuromechanical inhibition,* is manifested both in respiratory frequency and in amplitude of respiratory motor output. Neuromechanical inhibition lasts for several breaths after termination of mechanical ventilation, thus constituting a type of control-system inertia and resetting of the spontaneous respiratory rhythm.[62] Neuromechanical inhibition has been observed both with controlled and assisted modes of ventilation—at V_T considerably greater than that during spontaneous breathing and at a ventilator frequency of just 1 breath per minute higher than baseline breathing.[62] In sleeping subjects, controlled ventilation is able to totally suppress respiratory motor output, and it leads to apnea after cessation of support[62] (Fig. 35-9*A*). With assisted ventilation, neuromechanical inhibition is expressed mainly in terms of the intensity of breathing effort[62] (see Fig. 35-9*B*). Although the mechanism underlying neuromechanical inhibition is not entirely clear, the Hering-Breuer reflex is the most plausible explanation. It also has been shown that repeated augmented ventilatorcycles delivered at a frequency higher than eupnea exert a cumulative, time-dependent inhibition of respiratory motor output.[63]

Mechanical ventilation has been shown to influence the excitability of the motor cortex supplying the diaphragm. In healthy subjects, Sharshar et al[64] assessed cortical control of the diaphragm by measuring its electrical response, the motor evoked potential, to transcranial magnetic stimulation during spontaneous breathing and isocapnic ACV. Mechanical ventilation was associated with a decrease in motor evoked potential amplitude and hyperexcitability of intracortical facilitatory neurons. The findings indicate that unloading of the respiratory muscles reduces the excitability of cortical motor areas representing these muscles.[64] It is possible that mechanoreceptor feedback accounts for the depression of the motor evoked potential of the diaphragm via vagal and other proprioceptive afferents to the respiratory center. This effect of mechanical ventilation represents neuromechanical inhibition at the level of the motor cortex, and it may contribute to a non–chemically mediated decrease in respiratory motor output in awake subjects.

The clinical relevance of neuromechanical inhibition is currently unknown. Available evidence suggests that its contribution to respiratory motor output in ventilated critically ill patients is rather minimal.[10,13,51] That neuromechanical inhibition is observed at relatively high tidal volumes and when ventilator frequency exceeds spontaneous respiratory rate[62] raises questions of its clinical relevance, particularly with assisted modes of ventilation. In critically ill patients ventilated with PSV or ACV at relatively low tidal volumes, neuromechanical inhibition was not evident.[10,51]

ENTRAINMENT OF RESPIRATORY RHYTHM TO VENTILATOR RATE

Entrainment of respiratory rhythm to the ventilator rate implies a fixed, repetitive, temporal relationship between the onset of respiratory muscle contraction and the onset of a mechanical breath.[65–67] Human subjects exhibit one-to-one entrainment over a considerable range above and below the spontaneous breathing frequency.[68,69] This entrainment response is affected by state (sleep or wakefulness) and is independent of mild increases in respiratory drive induced by CO_2 stimulation.[68] Cortical influences (learning or adaptation response) and the Hering-Breuer reflex are postulated as the predominant mechanisms of entrainment. Theoretically, one-to-one entrainment should facilitate patient-ventilator synchrony, but studies of the entrainment response in critically ill patients are lacking.

BEHAVIORAL FEEDBACK

The effects of behavioral feedback on control of breathing in ventilated patients are unpredictable, depending on several factors related to the individual patient and surroundings. Alteration in ventilator settings, planned to achieve a particular goal, might be ineffective in awake patients because of behavioral feedback.[70,71] Inappropriate ventilator settings may cause breathing discomfort in awake patients. Consequent panic reactions further aggravate the unpleasant breathing sensation and create a vicious cycle. Behavioral feedback also may be altered considerably from time to time secondary to changes in the level of sedation, sleep/awake state, patient status, and environmental stimuli. The many factors involved in behavioral feedback complicate its study and the interpretation of its effects on the system that controls breathing in mechanically ventilated patients.

Interactive Effects of Patient-Related Factors and Ventilator on Control of Breathing

MECHANICS OF RESPIRATORY SYSTEM

The mechanical properties of the respiratory system may influence the pressure delivered by the ventilator independent of patient effort and thus may modify the effects of

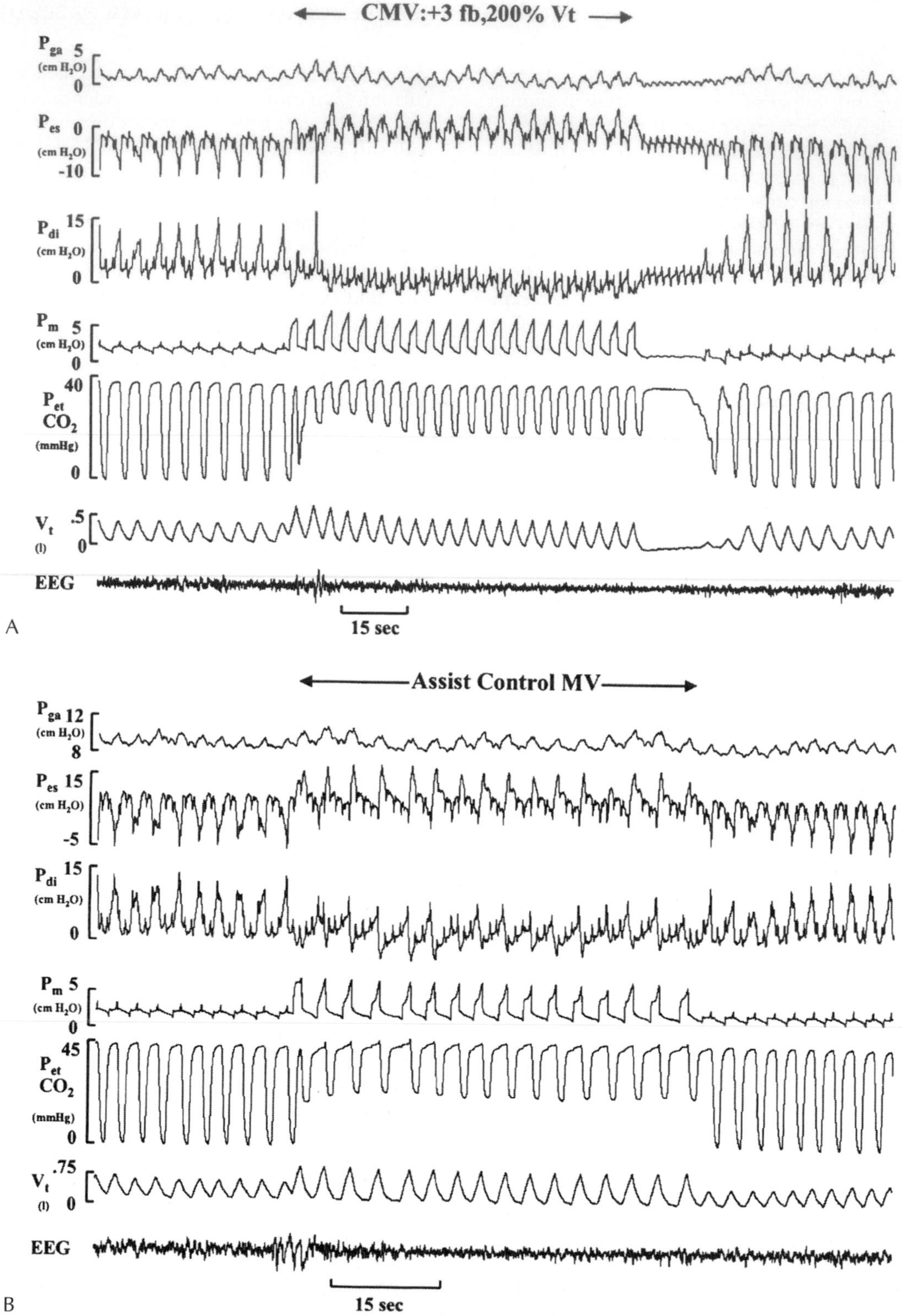

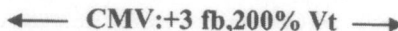

FIGURE 35-9 Gastric pressure (Pga), esophageal pressure (Pes), transdiaphragmatic pressure (Pdi), mouth pressure (Pm), partial pressure of end-tidal CO_2 ($P_{ET_{CO_2}}$), tidal volume (V_T), and electroencephalogram (EEG) in a subject during non-REM sleep. *A.* Spontaneous breathing with continuous positive airway pressure (CPAP) followed by controlled mechanical ventilation (CMV) at a respiratory frequency that is three breaths per minute above spontaneous eupnea and a V_T that is 200% of spontaneous eupnea. Note the immediate reduction in Pdi at CMV onset and the apnea that followed the cessation of CMV. Inspired CO_2 was added to prevent the $P_{ET_{CO_2}}$ from falling when V_T was raised with CMV. *B.* Spontaneous breathing with CPAP followed by assist volume-control ventilation (ACV) at a V_T that was 195% of spontaneous eupnea. Note the sudden decrease in Pdi and increase in Pes at the onset of ACV; these values were maintained throughout ACV and gradually returned to normal during spontaneous breathing after the cessation of ACV. $P_{ET_{CO_2}}$ was maintained at or slightly above than eupneic levels through the addition of inspired CO_2. (*Used, with permission, from Rice et al: Am J Respir Crit Care Med 168:92–101, 2003.*)

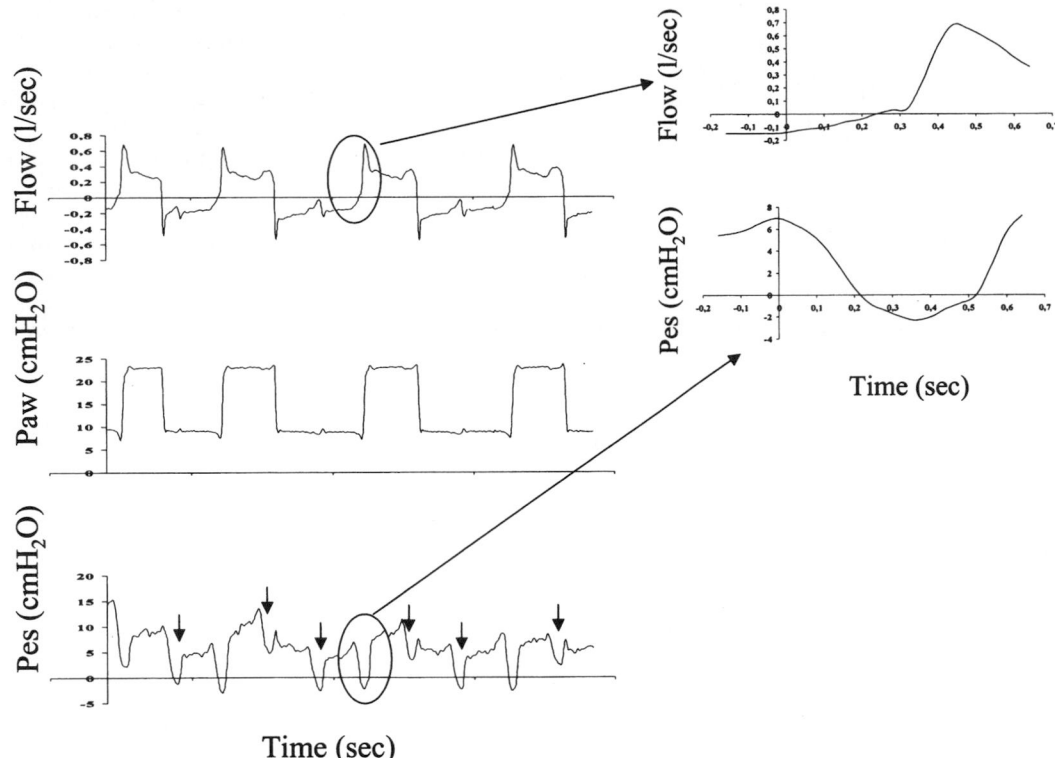

FIGURE 35-10 Airflow (inspiration up), airway pressure (Paw), and esophageal pressure (Pes) in a patient with obstructive lung disease ventilated with pressure support. Note the triggering delay with every mechanical breath (see the magnified tracing of flow and Pes) and the ineffective efforts (*arrows*). The ventilator rate was 12 breaths per minute, whereas the patient's respiratory frequency was 35 breaths per minute. Extrapolation from ventilator rate to the patient's system of control of breathing is misleading.

mechanical ventilation on the various feedback loops. Excessive triggering delay and ineffective triggering are common in patients with obstructive lung disease and dynamic hyperinflation (Fig. 35-10). In the setting of airflow obstruction, mathematical models predict that PSV can be accompanied by marked variation in V_T and intrinsic PEEP even when patient effort is constant.[72] This dynamic instability increases as the time constant of the respiratory system increases and produces patient-ventilator asynchrony of variable magnitude and type. The demonstration of increased arousals during PSV, but not during volume-cycled ventilation, may be caused in part by dynamic patient-ventilator asynchrony.[24]

Ineffective triggering has been observed with all modes of assisted ventilation. It is particularly common with tachypnea and when the level of assistance is relatively high and mechanical inflation extends well into neural expiration.[13,73] With PAV, the likelihood of ineffective efforts is reduced significantly because mechanical inflation time is terminated close to the end of neural inspiration, and tidal volume in most cases remains relatively small.[73]

The phenomenon of ineffective efforts considerably influences the interpretation of ventilatory output in relation to the control of breathing during mechanical ventilation.[3,74] In the presence of ineffective efforts, ventilator frequency does not reflect the patient's spontaneous respiratory rate (see Fig. 35-10). Moreover, with ineffective efforts, signifi-

cant alteration in a patient's respiratory effort occurs secondary to changes in feedback loop.

CHARACTERISTICS OF THE MUSCLE PRESSURE WAVEFORM

The characteristics of the Pmus waveform influence the ventilator-delivered volume in a complex manner, depending on several patient and ventilator factors. Extensive review of these factors is beyond the scope of this chapter, but some examples are provided.

The initial rate of increase in Pmus interacts with triggering of the ventilator.[13] A low rate of initial increase in Pmus occurs with a concave upward shape of Pmus or a low respiratory drive (such as with low Pa_{CO_2}, sedation, sleep, or a high level of assistance); this increases the time delay between the onset of patient inspiratory effort and ventilator triggering and promotes asynchrony. In the presence of dynamic hyperinflation, a prolonged triggering time, particularly when associated with a relatively short neural inspiratory time and low peak Pmus, may result in ineffective efforts. Alternatively, an increase in the intensity of inspiratory effort, such as occurs with an increase in metabolic rate, high Pa_{CO_2}, or decrease in the level of sedation or assistance, is manifested both in the rate of rise and in the peak of Pmus. The change may cause a decrease in the time delay, thus promoting patient-ventilator synchrony.[13] If, however, patient inspiratory effort is vigorous and longer than

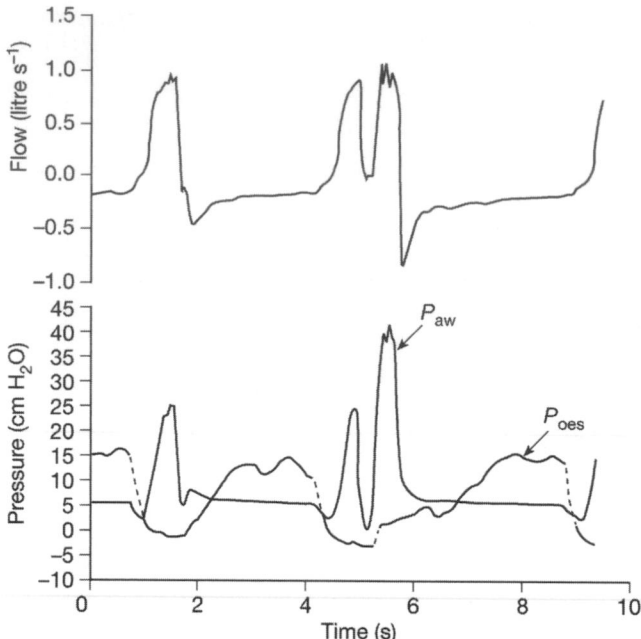

FIGURE 35-11 Flow, airway pressure (Paw), and esophageal pressure (Pes) in a patient recovering from acute lung injury and ventilated on assist volume control at constant inspiratory flow. In the second breath, tidal volume (volume was not shown) was decreased at constant inspiratory flow. As a result, there was premature termination of mechanical inspiration. Because the inspiratory muscles continued to contract, they developed sufficient pressure to overcome elastic recoil at end inspiration. As a result, Paw decreased below the triggering threshold, and the ventilator delivered a new mechanical breath. The ventilator was triggered three times by the two inspiratory efforts. Note the high Paw of the third mechanical breath secondary to high lung volume (the volume of the third breath was added to that of the second). Total breath duration of the second respiratory effort was considerably longer than that of the first effort owing to activation of Hering-Breuer reflex by the high volume. (*Used, with permission, from Kondili et al: Br J Anaesth 91:106–19, 2003.*)

mechanical inflation time, the ventilator may be triggered more than once during the same inspiratory effort (Fig. 35-11). It follows that changes in the characteristics of the Pmus waveform may influence the ventilator rate and ventilatory output despite no change in a patient's breathing frequency. Alterations in ventilatory output may secondarily modify patient effort through changes in feedback loops (see Fig. 35-1).

The Future

Over the last decade, many studies have been performed in animals and human subjects with an aim of improving a patient's ability to control the ventilator. Various ventilator modes target either an improvement in the response of the ventilator to patient effort or tight coupling between the ventilator-delivered pressure and patient instantaneous ventilatory demands. Studies of these modes have yielded

promising results. New methods of triggering, through use of the flow waveform or mechanical activity (Pdi-driven servoventilation) or electrical activity (neurally adjusted ventilatory assistance) of the diaphragm as triggering signals, have been shown to improve the response of the ventilator to patient effort.[75–77] Algorithms that automatically adjust the criterion for cycling off have been designed with a goal of reducing expiratory asynchrony.[78] Mechanical[77] and electrical[75,79] activity of the diaphragm has been used experimentally to control the level and duration of inspiratory assistance. This approach is challenging and further emphasizes the advantages of PAV. With PAV, methods for noninvasive automatic estimation of elastance and resistance of the respiratory system have been introduced that enable controller gain to be maintained constant in the face of changes in the mechanical load of respiratory system.[80,81] By achieving tight coupling between neural output and ventilator-delivered pressure, the ventilator is able to serve as a respiratory muscle with high capabilities and operate in harmony with the system that controls breathing.

Negative-feedback methods, such as adaptive pressure-support servoventilation, have been designed recently with a goal of reducing periodic breathing through appropriate changes in the level of assistance and maintaining a target minute ventilation in the face of waxing and waning respiratory efforts.[82] Incorporation of this approach in assisted modes may decrease the propensity of high-risk individuals to develop periodic breathing. It is not known whether this mode could decrease morbidity in critically ill patients, although it should enhance sleep efficiency.[23]

Conclusion

Incorporating an auxiliary pressure into the system that controls breathing changes the volume-time profile of a breath. It also alters, via chemical, neuromechanical, and behavioral feedback, the pressure developed by the respiratory muscles. The latter, depending on ventilator and patient factors, may or may not modify the auxiliary pressure. The response of patient effort to a ventilator-delivered breath and the response of a ventilator to patient effort are the two essential components of control of breathing during mechanical ventilation. The physician dealing with a ventilated patient should be aware that both the basic features of control of breathing and its expression can be altered considerably by the process of mechanical ventilation.

References

1. Tobin MJ. Advances in mechanical ventilation. New Engl J Med 2001; 344:1986–96.
2. Tobin MJ, Jubran A, Laghi F. Patient-ventilator interaction. Am J Respir Crit Care Med 2001; 163:1059–63.
3. Kondili E, Prinianakis G, Georgopoulos D. Patient-ventilator interaction. Br J Anaesth 2003; 91:106–19.
4. Georgopoulos D, Roussos C. Control of breathing in mechanically ventilated patients. Eur Respir J 1996; 9:2151–60.

5. Berger A. Control of breathing. In: Murray JF, Nadel JA, editors. Respiratory medicine. Philadelphia: Saunders, 1988: 49–166.

6. Younes M, Remmers J. Control of tidal volume and respiratory frequency. In: Hornbein TF, editor. Regulation of breathing. New York: Marcel Dekker, 1981: 621–71.

7. Cunningham DJC, Robbins PA, Wolff CB. Intergration of respiratory responses to changes in alveola partial pressures of CO_2 and O_2 and in the arterial pH. Bethesda, MD: American Physiologica Society, 1986.

8. Georgopoulos D, Mitrouska I, Webster K, et al. Effects of inspiratory muscle unloading on the response of respiratory motor output to CO_2. Am J Respir Crit Care Med 1997; 155:2000–9.

9. Milic-Emili J, Tyler JM. Relation betwen work out-put of respiratory muscles and end-tidal CO_2 tension. J Appl Physiol 1963; 18:497–504.

10. Xirouhaki N, Kondili E, Mitrouska I, et al. Response of respiratory motor output to varying pressure in mechanically ventilated patients. Eur Respir J 1999; 14:508–16.

11. Skatrud JB, Berssenbrugge AD. Effect of sleep state and chemical stimuli on breathing. Prog Clin Biol Res 1983; 136:87–95.

12. Meza S, Giannouli E, Younes M. Control of breathing during sleep assessed by proportional assist ventilation. J Appl Physiol 1998; 84:3–12.

13. Leung P, Jubran A, Tobin MJ. Comparison of assisted ventilator modes on triggering, patient effort, and dyspnea. Am J Respir Crit Care Med 1997; 155:1940–8.

14. Otis A. Quantitative relationships in steady state gas exchange. In Fenn WO, Rahn H, editors. Handbook of physiology: Respiration, Vol. I. Washington: American Physiological Society, 1964: 681–98.

15. Georgopoulos D, Mitrouska I, Bshouty Z, et al. Respiratory response to CO_2 during pressure-support ventilation in conscious normal humans. Am J Respir Crit Care Med 1997; 156:146–54.

16. Puddy A, Patrick W, Webster K, Younes M. Respiratory control during volume-cycled ventilation in normal humans. J Appl Physiol 1996; 80:1749–58.

17. Patrick W, Webster K, Puddy A, Sanii R, Younes M. Respiratory response to CO_2 in the hypocapnic range in awake humans. J Appl Physiol 1995; 79:2058–68.

18. Mitrouska J, Xirouchaki N, Patakas D, et al. Effects of chemical feedback on respiratory motor and ventilatory output during different modes of assisted mechanical ventilation. Eur Respir J 1999; 13:873–82.

19. Dempsey JA, Skatrud JB. A sleep-induced apneic threshold and its consequences. Am Rev Respir Dis 1986; 133:1163–70.

20. Dempsey JA, Smith CA, Przybylowski T, et al. The ventilatory responsiveness to CO_2 below eupnoea as a determinant of ventilatory stability in sleep. J Physiol 2004; 560:1–11.

21. Meza S, Mendez M, Ostrowski M, Younes M. Susceptibility to periodic breathing with assisted ventilation during sleep in normal subjects. J Appl Physiol 1998; 85:1929–40.

22. Corne S, Webster K, Younes M. Hypoxic respiratory response during acute stable hypocapnia. Am J Respir Crit Care Med 2003; 167:1193–9.

23. Parthasarathy S, Tobin MJ. Sleep in the intensive care unit. Intensive Care Med 2004; 30:197–206.

24. Parthasarathy S, Tobin MJ. Effect of ventilator mode on sleep quality in critically ill patients. Am J Respir Crit Care Med 2002; 166:1423–9.

25. Sin DD, Logan AG, Fitzgerald FS, et al. Effects of continuous positive airway pressure on cardiovascular outcomes in heart failure patients with and without Cheyne-Stokes respiration. Circulation 2000; 102:61–6.

26. Leung RS, Bradley TD. Sleep apnea and cardiovascular disease. Am J Respir Crit Care Med 2001; 164:2147–65.

27. McGuire BE, Basten CJ, Ryan CJ, Gallagher J. Intensive care unit syndrome: A dangerous misnomer. Arch Intern Med 2000; 160:906–9.

28. Helton MC, Gordon SH, Nunnery SL. The correlation between sleep deprivation and the intensive care unit syndrome. Heart Lung 1980; 9:464–8.

29. Irwin M, McClintick J, Costlow C, et al. Partial night sleep deprivation reduces natural killer and cellular immune responses in humans. FASEB J 1996; 10:643–53.

30. Irwin M, Rinetti G, Redwine L, et al. Nocturnal proinflammatory cytokine-associated sleep disturbances in abstinent African-American alcoholics. Brain Behav Immun 2004; 18:349–60.

31. Redwine L, Hauger RL, Gillin JC, Irwin M. Effects of sleep and sleep deprivation on interleukin-6, growth hormone, cortisol, and melatonin levels in humans. J Clin Endocrinol Metab 2000; 85:3597–603.

32. Scrimshaw NS, Habicht JP, Pellet P, et al. Effects of sleep deprivation and reversal of diurnal activity on protein metabolism of young men. Am J Clin Nutr 1966; 19:313–9.

33. Khoo MC, Kronauer RE, Strohl KP, Slutsky AS. Factors inducing periodic breathing in humans: A general model. J Appl Physiol 1982; 53:644–59.

34. Younes M. The physiologic basis of central apnea. Curr Pulmonol 1989; 10:265–326.

35. Younes M, Ostrowski M, Thompson W, et al. Chemical control stability in patients with obstructive sleep apnea. Am J Respir Crit Care Med 2001; 163:1181–90.

36. Grace MP, Greenbaum DM. Cardiac performance in response to PEEP in patients with cardiac dysfunction. Crit Care Med 1982; 10:358–60.

37. Lenique F, Habis M, Lofaso F, et al. Ventilatory and hemodynamic effects of continuous positive airway pressure in left heart failure. Am J Respir Crit Care Med 1997; 155:500–5.

38. Pinsky MR. The effects of mechanical ventilation on the cardiovascular system. Crit Care Clin 1990; 6:663–78.

39. Pinsky MR. Instantaneous venous return curves in an intact canine preparation. J Appl Physiol 1984; 56:765–71.

40. Mansfield D, Naughton MT. Effects of continuous positive airway pressure on lung function in patients with chronic obstructive pulmonary disease and sleep disordered breathing. Respirology 1999; 4:365–70.

41. Javaheri S. Effects of continuous positive airway pressure on sleep apnea and ventricular irritability in patients with heart failure. Circulation 2000; 101:392–7.

42. Kohnlein T, Welte T, Tan LB, Elliott MW. Assisted ventilation for heart failure patients with Cheyne-Stokes respiration. Eur Respir J 2002; 20:934–41.

43. Nakayama H, Smith CA, Rodman JR, et al. Effect of ventilatory drive on carbon dioxide sensitivity below eupnea during sleep. Am J Respir Crit Care Med 2002; 165:1251–60.

44. ATS/ERS statement on respiratory muscle testing. Am J Respir Crit Care Med 2002; 166:518–624.

45. Wellman A, Jordan AS, Malhotra A, et al. Ventilatory control and airway anatomy in obstructive sleep apnea. Am J Respir Crit Care Med 2004; 170:1225–32.

46. Wellman A, Malhotra A, Fogel RB, et al. Respiratory system loop gain in normal men and women measured with proportional-assist ventilation. J Appl Physiol 2003; 94:205–12.

47. Georgopoulos D, Giannouli E, Tsara V, et al. Respiratory short-term poststimulus potentiation (after-discharge) in patients with obstructive sleep apnea. Am Rev Respir Dis 1992; 146: 1250–5.

48. Georgopoulos D, Bshouty Z, Younes M, Anthonisen NR. Hypoxic exposure and activation of the afterdischarge mechanism in conscious humans. J Appl Physiol 1990; 69:1159–64.

49. Younes M, Riddle W. Relation between respiratory neural output and tidal volume. J Appl Physiol 1984; 56:1110–9.

50. Fauroux B, Hart N, Luo YM, et al. Measurement of diaphragm loading during pressure support ventilation. Intensive Care Med 2003; 29:1960–6.

51. Kondili E, Prinianakis G, Anastasaki M, Georgopoulos D. Acute effects of ventilator settings on respiratory motor output in patients with acute lung injury. Intensive Care Med 2001; 27:1147–57.

52. Georgopoulos D, Mitrouska I, Bshouty Z, et al. Effects of non-REM sleep on the response of respiratory output to varying inspiratory flow. Am J Respir Crit Care Med 1996; 153:1624–30.

53. Georgopoulos D, Mitrouska I, Bshouty Z, et al. Effects of breathing route, temperature and volume of inspired gas, and airway anesthesia on the response of respiratory output to varying inspiratory flow. Am J Respir Crit Care Med 1996; 153:168–75.

54. Fernandez R, Mendez M, Younes M. Effect of ventilator flow rate on respiratory timing in normal humans. Am J Respir Crit Care Med 1999; 159:710–9.

55. Corne S, Webster K, Younes M. Effects of inspiratory flow on diaphragmatic motor output in normal subjects. J Appl Physiol 2000; 89:481–92.

56. Tobert DG, Simon PM, Stroetz RW, Hubmayr RD. The determinants of respiratory rate during mechanical ventilation. Am J Respir Crit Care Med 1997; 155:485–92.

57. Younes M, Kun J, Webster K, Roberts D. Response of ventilator-dependent patients to delayed opening of exhalation valve. Am J Respir Crit Care Med 2002; 166:21–30.

58. Corne S, Gillespie D, Roberts D, Younes M. Effect of inspiratory flow rate on respiratory rate in intubated ventilated patients. Am J Respir Crit Care Med 1997; 156:304–8.

59. Wilson CR, Satoh M, Skatrud JB, Dempsey JA. Non-chemical inhibition of respiratory motor output during mechanical ventilation in sleeping humans. J Physiol 1999; 518:605–18.

60. Leevers AM, Simon PM, Dempsey JA. Apnea after normocapnic mechanical ventilation during NREM sleep. J Appl Physiol 1994; 77:2079–85.

61. Manchanda S, Leevers AM, Wilson CR, et al. Frequency and volume thresholds for inhibition of inspiratory motor output during mechanical ventilation. Respir Physiol 1996; 105:1–16.

62. Rice AJ, Nakayama HC, Haverkamp HC, et al. Controlled versus assisted mechanical ventilation effects on respiratory motor output in sleeping humans. Am J Respir Crit Care Med 2003; 168:92–101.

63. Satoh M, Eastwood PR, Smith CA, Dempsey JA. Nonchemical elimination of inspiratory motor output via mechanical ventilation in sleep. Am J Respir Crit Care Med 2001; 163:1356–64.

64. Sharshar T, Ross ET, Hopkinson NS, et al. Depression of diaphragm motor cortex excitability during mechanical ventilation. J Appl Physiol 2004; 97:3–10.

65. Petrillo GA, Glass L. A theory for phase locking of respiration in cats to a mechanical ventilator. Am J Physiol 1984; 246:R311–20.

66. Muzzin S, Trippenbach T, Baconnier P, Benchetrit G. Entrainment of the respiratory rhythm by periodic lung inflation during vagal cooling. Respir Physiol 1989; 75:157–72.

67. Muzzin S, Baconnier P, Benchetrit G. Entrainment of respiratory rhythm by periodic lung inflation: Effect of airflow rate and duration. Am J Physiol 1992; 263:R292–300.

68. Simon PM, Zurob AS, Wies WM, et a. Entrainment of respiration in humans by periodic lung inflations: Effect of state and CO_2. Am J Respir Crit Care Med 1999; 160:950–60.

69. Simon PM, Habel AM, Daubenspeck JA, Leiter JC. Vagal feedback in the entrainment of respiration to mechanical ventilation in sleeping humans. J Appl Physiol 2000; 89:760–9.

70. Manning HL, Molinary EJ, Leiter JC. Effect of inspiratory flow rate on respiratory sensation and pattern of breathing. Am J Respir Crit Care Med 1995; 151:751–7.

71. Jubran A, Van de Graaff WB, Tobin MJ. Variability of patient-ventilator interaction with pressure support ventilation in patients with chronic obstructive pulmonary disease. Am J Respir Crit Care Med 1995; 152:129–36.

72. Hotchkiss JR Jr, Adams AB, Stone MK, et al. Oscillations and noise: Inherent instability of pressure support ventilation? Am J Respir Crit Care Med 2002; 165:47–53.

73. Giannouli E, Webster K, Roberts D, Younes M. Response of ventilator-dependent patients to different levels of pressure support and proportional assist. Am J Respir Crit Care Med 1999; 159:1716–25.

74. Georgopoulos DB, Anastasaki M, Katsanoulas K. Effects of mechanical ventilation on control of breathing. Monaldi Arch Chest Dis 1997; 52:253–62.

75. Sinderby C, Navalesi P, Beck J, et al. Neural control of mechanical ventilation in respiratory failure. Nature Med 1999; 5:1433–6.

76. Prinianakis G, Kondili E, Georgopoulos D. Effects of the flow waveform method of triggering and cycling on patient-ventilator interaction during pressure support. Intensive Care Med 2003; 29:1950–9.

77. Sharshar T, Desmarais G, Louis B, et al. Transdiaphragmatic pressure control of airway pressure support in healthy subjects. Am J Respir Crit Care Med 2003; 168:760–9.

78. Du HL, Amato MB, Yamada Y. Automation of expiratory trigger sensitivity in pressure support ventilation. Respir Care Clin North Am 2001; 7:503–17, x.

79. Spahija JBJ, de Marchie M, Comtois A, Sinderby C. Closed loop control of respiratory drive using pressure support ventilation: Target drive ventilation. Am J Respir Crit Care Med 2005 (in press).

80. Younes M, Webster K, Kun J, et al. A method for measuring passive elastance during proportional assist ventilation. Am J Respir Crit Care Med 2001; 164:50–60.

81. Younes M, Kun J, Masiowski B, et al. A method for noninvasive determination of inspiratory resistance during proportional assist ventilation. Am J Respir Crit Care Med 2001; 163:829–39.

82. Pepperell JC, Maskell NA, Jones DR, et al. A randomized, controlled trial of adaptive ventilation for Cheyne-Stokes breathing in heart failure. Am J Respir Crit Care Med 2003; 168:1109–14.

EFFECT OF MECHANICAL VENTILATION ON HEART-LUNG INTERACTIONS

MICHAEL R. PINSKY

The heart and lungs are intimately coupled by their anatomic proximity within the thorax, and more importantly, by their responsibility to deliver the oxygen (O_2) requirements of individual cells and organs. During critical illness, if these two organ systems fail either alone or in combination, the end result is an inadequate O_2 delivery to the body with inevitable tissue ischemia, progressive organ

dysfunction, and if untreated, death. Thus, restoration and maintenance of normalized cardiopulmonary function is an essential and primary goal in the management of critically ill patients. Heart failure can impair gas exchange by inducing pulmonary edema and limiting blood flow to the respiratory muscles. Ventilation can alter cardiovascular function by altering lung volume and intrathoracic pressure (ITP), and by increasing metabolic demands. These processes will be discussed from the perspective of the impact that ventilation has on the cardiovascular system.

Relevance

The ventilatory apparatus and the cardiovascular system have profound effects on each other.[1,2] Acute hypoxia impairs cardiac contractility and vascular smooth muscle tone, promoting cardiovascular collapse. Hyperinflation increases pulmonary vascular resistance which impedes right ventricular (RV) ejection, and also compresses the heart inside the cardiac fossa in a fashion analogous to tamponade. Lung collapse also increases pulmonary vascular resistance, impeding RV ejection.[3] Acute RV failure, or *cor pulmonale*, is not only difficult to treat, but it can induce immediate cardiovascular collapse and death.

Mechanical ventilation technologies and numerous vasoactive drugs have been developed as means to improve oxygenation of arterial blood. These advances are the subjects of other chapters in this book. The complex interactions, however, between the heart, circulation, and lungs often lead to a paradoxical worsening of one organ system function while the function of the other system is either maintained or even improved by the use of these technologies and drugs. To minimize these deleterious events, and in the hope of more efficiently and effectively treating critically ill patients with cardiorespiratory failure, a better knowledge and understanding of the integrated behavior of the cardiopulmonary system, during both health and critical illness, is essential. Based on this perspective, the health care provider can more appropriately manage this complex and challenging group of patients.

Respiratory function alters cardiovascular function and cardiovascular function alters respiratory function. A useful way to consider the cardiovascular effects of ventilation is to group them by their impact on the determinants of cardiac performance. The determinants of cardiac function can be grouped into four interrelated processes: *heart rate, preload, contractility,* and *afterload*. Phasic changes in lung volume and ITP can simultaneously change all four of these hemodynamic determinants for both ventricles. Our current understanding of cardiovascular function also emphasizes both the independence and interdependence of RV and left ventricular (LV) performance on each other and to external stresses. Complicating these matters further, the direction of interdependence, from right to left or left to right, can be similar or opposite in direction, depending on the baseline cardiovascular state. It is clear, therefore, that a comprehensive understanding of the specific cardiopulmonary interactions and their relative importance in defining a specific cardiovascular state is a nearly impossible goal to achieve in most patients. By understanding the components of this process, however, one can come to a better realization of its determinants, and, to a greater or lesser degree for any individual patient, predict the limits of these interactions, and how the patient may respond to stresses imposed by either adding or removing artificial ventilator support.

Physiology of Heart-Lung Interactions

Both spontaneous and positive-pressure ventilation increase lung volume above an end-expiratory baseline. Many of the hemodynamic effects of all forms of ventilation are similar despite differences in the mode of ventilation. ITP, however, decreases during spontaneous inspiration, while it increases during positive-pressure ventilation. Thus, the primary reasons for different hemodynamic responses seen during spontaneous and positive-pressure breathing are related to the changes in ITP and the energy necessary to produce those changes.

EFFECT OF LUNG VOLUME

Changing lung volume phasically alters autonomic tone and pulmonary vascular resistance. At very high lung volumes, the expanding lungs compress the heart in the cardiac fossa, limiting absolute cardiac volumes. This action is analogous to cardiac tamponade, except that with hyperinflation both pericardial pressure and ITP increase by a similar amount.

AUTONOMIC TONE

Although neurohumoral processes define a few immediate effects of ventilation on the heart, these processes probably play a primary function in all of the long-term effects of ventilation on the cardiovascular system. Most of the immediate effects of ventilation of the heart are due to changes in autonomic tone. The lungs are richly innervated with somatic and autonomic fibers, which originate, traverse through, and end in the thorax. These networks mediate multiple homeostatic processes through the autonomic nervous system, altering instantaneous cardiovascular function. The most commonly known of these are the vagally-mediated heart rate changes during ventilation.[4,5] Inflation of the lung to a normal tidal volume (<10 ml/kg) induces vagal-tone withdrawal, accelerating heart rate. This phenomenon is known as *respiratory sinus arrhythmia*.[6] It can be used to document normal autonomic control,[7] especially in patients with diabetes who are at risk of peripheral neuropathy.[8] Inflation to larger tidal volumes (>15 ml/kg), however, decreases heart rate by a combination of both increased vagal tone[10] and sympathetic withdrawal. Sympathetic withdrawal also creates arterial vasodilation.[4,9,11,12,14] This inflation-vasodilation response can reduce LV contractility in healthy volunteers,[15] and in ventilator-dependent patients with the initiation of high-frequency ventilation[4] or hyperinflation.[12] This inflation-vasodilation response is presumed to be the cause of the initial hypotension seen when infants are placed on mechanical ventilation. It appears to be mediated at least partially by afferent vagal

fibers, because it is abolished by selective vagotomy. Hexamethonium, guanethidine, and bretylium, however, also block this reflex.[16,17] These data suggest that lung inflation mediates its reflex cardiovascular effects by modulating central autonomic tone. Interestingly, the almost total lack of measurable hemodynamic effects of unilateral hyperinflation in subjects with normal lungs receiving split-lung ventilation[18] suggests that these autonomic cardiovascular effects require a generalized increase in lung volume to be realized. This is not a minor point because selective hyperinflation within lung units commonly occurs in subjects with acute lung injury (ALI) and chronic obstructive pulmonary disease (COPD). If localized hyperinflation were able to induce cardiovascular impairment, these subjects would be profoundly compromised.

Humoral factors, including compounds blocked by cyclooxygenase inhibition,[19] released from pulmonary endothelial cells during lung inflation, may also induce this depressor response,[20-22] within a short (15-second) time frame. These interactions, however, do not appear to grossly alter cardiovascular status.[23] Ventilation also alters the more chronic control of intravascular fluid balance via hormonal release. The right atrium functions as the body's effective circulating blood volume sensor. Circulating levels of a family of natriuretic peptides decrease in heart failure states, secondary to right atrial stretch. These hormones promote sodium and water diuresis. The levels of these hormones vary inversely with the degree of heart failure. Both positive-pressure ventilation and sustained hyperinflation decrease right atrial stretch, mimicking hypovolemia. Plasma norepinephrine, plasma activity,[24,25] and plasma atrial natriuretic peptide[26] increase during positive-pressure ventilation. This humoral response is the primary reason why ventilator-dependent patients gain weight early in the course of respiratory failure, despite protein catabolism being common. Interestingly, when subjects with congestive heart failure are given nasal continuous positive airway pressure (CPAP), plasma atrial natriuretic peptide activity decreases in parallel with improvements in blood flow.[27,28] This finding suggests that some of the observed benefit of CPAP therapy in heart failure is mediated in part through humoral mechanisms, owing to the mechanical effects of CPAP on cardiac function.

PULMONARY VASCULAR RESISTANCE

Changing lung volume alters pulmonary vascular resistance.[3] Marked increases in pulmonary vascular resistance, as may occur with hyperinflation, can induce acute cor pulmonale and cardiovascular collapse. The reasons for these changes are multifactorial. They can reflect conflicting cardiovascular processes, and almost always reflect both humoral and mechanical interactions.

Lung volume can only increase if its distending pressure increases. Lung-distending pressure, called the *transpulmonary pressure*, equals the pressure difference between alveolar pressure (Palv) and ITP. If lung volume does not change, then transpulmonary pressure does not change. Thus, occluded inspiratory efforts (Mueller maneuver) and expiratory efforts (Valsalva maneuver) cause ITP to vary by an amount equal to Palv, but do not change pulmonary vascular resistance. Although obstructive inspiratory efforts, as occur during obstructive sleep apnea, are usually associated with increased RV afterload, the increased afterload is caused primarily by either increased vasomotor tone (hypoxic pulmonary vasoconstriction) or backward LV failure.[29,30]

RV afterload is maximal RV systolic wall stress.[31,32] By Laplace's law, wall stress equals the product of the radius of curvature of a structure and its transmural pressure. Systolic RV pressure equals transmural pulmonary artery pressure. Increases in transmural pulmonary artery pressure increases RV afterload, impeding RV ejection,[33] decreasing RV stroke volume,[34] inducing RV dilation, and passively causing venous return to decrease.[34] If such acute increases in transmural pulmonary artery pressure are not reduced, or if RV contractility is not increased by artificial means, then acute cor pulmonale rapidly develops.[35] If RV dilation and RV pressure overload persist, RV free-wall ischemia and infarction can develop.[36] These concepts are of profound clinical relevance because rapid fluid challenges in the setting of acute cor pulmonale can precipitate profound cardiovascular collapse secondary to excessive RV dilation, RV ischemia, and compromised LV filling. Ventilation can alter pulmonary vascular resistance by either altering pulmonary vasomotor tone, via a process known as *hypoxic pulmonary vasoconstriction*, or mechanically altering vessel cross-sectional area, by changing transpulmonary pressure.

Hypoxic Pulmonary Vasoconstriction

Unlike systemic vessels that dilate under hypoxic conditions, the pulmonary vasculature constricts. Once alveolar P_{O_2} ($P_{A_{O_2}}$) decreases below 60 mmHg, or acidemia develops, pulmonary vasomotor tone increases.[37] Hypoxic pulmonary vasoconstriction is mediated, in part, by variations in the synthesis and release of nitric oxide, by endothelial nitric oxide synthase localized on pulmonary vascular endothelial cells, and in part by changes in intracellular calcium fluxes in the pulmonary vascular smooth muscle cells. The pulmonary endothelium normally synthesizes a low basal amount of nitric oxide, keeping the pulmonary vasculature actively vasodilated. Loss of nitric oxide allows the smooth muscle to return to its normal resting vasomotor tone. Nitric oxide synthesis is dependent on adequate amounts of O_2 and is inhibited by both hypoxia and acidosis. Presumably hypoxic pulmonary vasoconstriction developed to minimize ventilation-perfusion mismatches caused by local alveolar hypoventilation. Generalized alveolar hypoxia, however, increases global pulmonary vasomotor tone, impeding RV ejection.[33] At low lung volumes terminal bronchioles collapse, trapping gas in the terminal alveoli. With continued blood flow, these alveoli lose their O_2 and also may collapse. Patients with acute hypoxemic respiratory failure have small lung volumes and are prone to both alveolar hypoxia and spontaneous alveolar collapse.[38,39] This is one of the main reasons why pulmonary vascular resistance is increased in patients with acute hypoxemic respiratory failure.

Based on the above considerations mechanical ventilation may reduce pulmonary vasomotor tone by a variety of mechanisms. First, hypoxic pulmonary vasoconstriction can be inhibited if the patient is ventilated with gas enriched with O_2, increasing $P_{A_{O_2}}$.[40–43] Second, mechanical breaths and positive end-expiratory pressure (PEEP) can refresh hypoventilated lung units and recruit collapsed alveolar units, causing local increase in $P_{A_{O_2}}$,[3,44–46] especially if small lung volumes are returned to resting functional residual capacity.[47] Third, mechanical ventilation often reverses respiratory acidosis by increasing alveolar ventilation.[43] Fourth, decreasing central sympathetic output, by sedation or decreased stress of breathing against high-input impedance during mechanical ventilation, will also reduce vasomotor tone.[48,49] Importantly, these effects do not require endotracheal intubation to occur; they may occur with mere re-expansion of collapsed alveoli.[50,51] Thus, PEEP, CPAP, recruitment maneuvers, and noninvasive ventilation may all reverse hypoxic pulmonary vasoconstriction and may all improve cardiovascular function.

Volume-Dependent Changes in Pulmonary Vascular Resistance

Changes in lung volume directly alter pulmonary vasomotor tone by compressing the alveolar vessels.[38,45,46] The actual mechanisms by which this occurs have not been completely resolved, but appear to reflect vascular compression induced by a differential extraluminal pressure gradient. The pulmonary circulation lives in two environments, separated from each other by the pressure that surrounds them.[45] The small pulmonary arterioles, venules, and alveolar capillaries sense Palv as their surrounding pressure, and are called *alveolar vessels*. The large pulmonary arteries and veins, as well as the heart and intrathoracic great vessels of the systemic circulation, sense interstitial pressure or ITP as their surrounding pressure, and are called *extra-alveolar vessels*. Because the pressure difference between Palv and ITP is transpulmonary pressure, increasing lung volume increases this extraluminal pressure gradient. Increases in lung volume progressively increase alveolar vessel resistance by increasing this pressure difference once lung volumes increase much above functional residual capacity (FRC)[41,52] (Fig. 36-1). Similarly, increasing lung volume, by stretching and distending the alveolar septa, may also compress alveolar capillaries, although this mechanism is less well substantiated. Hyperinflation can create significant pulmonary hypertension, and may precipitate acute RV failure (acute cor pulmonale)[53] and RV ischemia.[36] Thus, PEEP may increase pulmonary vascular resistance if it induces overdistention of the lung above its normal FRC.[54]

Extra-alveolar vessels are also influenced by changes in transpulmonary pressure. Normally, radial interstitial forces of the lung, which keep the airways patent, only make the large vessel more distended as lung volume increases,[44,55,56] just as increasing lung volume increases airway diameter. These radial forces also act upon the extra-alveolar vessels, causing them to remain dilated, increasing their capacitance.[57] This tethering is reversed with lung deflation, thereby increasing extra-alveolar vascular resistance.[41,44] Thus, at small lung volumes, pulmonary vascular resistance is increased owing to the combined effect of hypoxic pulmonary vasoconstriction and extra-alveolar vessel collapse, and at high lung volumes by alveolar compression.

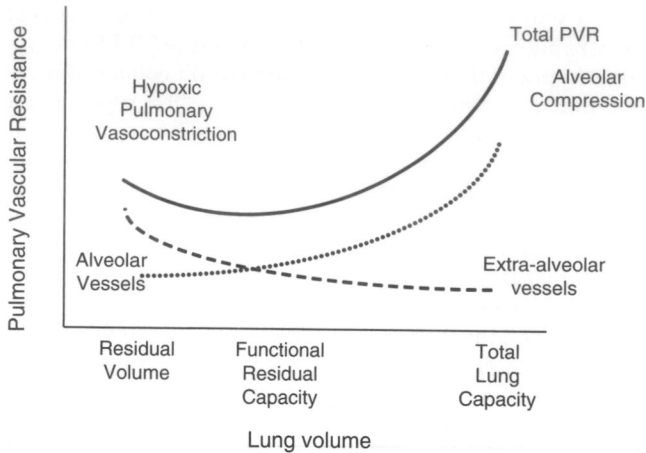

FIGURE 36-1 Schematic diagram of the relation between changes in lung volume and pulmonary vascular resistance, where the extra-alveolar and alveolar vascular components are separated. Pulmonary vascular resistance is minimal at resting lung volume or functional residual capacity. As lung volume increases toward total lung capacity or decreases toward residual volume, pulmonary vascular resistance also increases. The increase in resistance with hyperinflation is caused by increased alveolar vascular resistance, whereas the increase in resistance with lung collapse is caused by increased extra-alveolar vessel tone.

VENTRICULAR INTERDEPENDENCE

Because RV output is linked to LV output serially, if RV output decreases, LV output must eventually decrease. The two ventricles, however, are also linked in parallel through their common septum and pericardium, which limits total cardiac volume. The most common manifestation of ventricular interdependence is *pulsus paradoxus*. Changes in RV end-diastolic volume inversely alter LV diastolic compliance.[58] Because venous return can and often does vary by as much as 200% between inspiration and expiration, owing to associated changes in the pressure gradient for venous return (infra vide), RV filling also changes in parallel. Increasing RV end-diastolic volume, as occurs during spontaneous inspiration and spontaneous inspiratory efforts, will reduce LV diastolic compliance, immediately decreasing LV end-diastolic volume. Positive-pressure ventilation may decrease venous return, causing RV volumes to also decrease, increasing LV diastolic compliance. Except in volume overloaded LV failure states, however, the impact of positive-pressure ventilation on LV end-diastolic volume is minimal. Ventricular interdependence functions through two separate processes. First, increasing RV end-diastolic volume will induce an intraventricular septal shift into the LV, thereby decreasing LV diastolic compliance[59] (Fig. 36-2). Second, if pericardial restraint or absolute cardiac fossal volume restraint limits absolute biventricular filling, then RV dilation will increase pericardial pressure (Ppc) without a septal shift.[60,61] Because spontaneous inspiration increases venous return, causing RV dilation, LV end-diastolic compliance decreases during spontaneous inspiration. Because RV volumes usually do not increase during positive-pressure inspiration, ventricular interdependence is usually less.

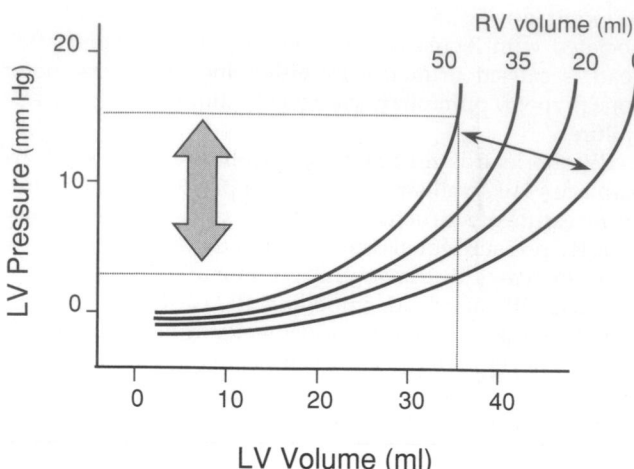

FIGURE 36-2 Schematic diagram of the effect of increasing right ventricular (RV) volumes on the relationship between left ventricular (LV) diastolic pressure and volume (filling). Increases in RV volumes decrease LV diastolic compliance, such that a higher filling pressure is required to generate a constant end-diastolic volume. (*Adapted, with permission, from Taylor et al.*[58])

MECHANICAL HEART-LUNG INTERACTIONS SECONDARY TO LUNG VOLUME

With inspiration, the expanding lungs compress the heart in the cardiac fossa,[62] increasing juxtacardiac ITP. Because the chest wall and diaphragm can move away from the expanding lungs, whereas the heart is trapped within this cardiac fossa, juxtacardiac ITP usually increases more than these peripheral ITPs.[63,64] This effect is caused by increasing lung volume. It is not affected by the means whereby lung volume is increased. Both spontaneous[65] and positive-pressure–induced hyperinflation[65,66] induce similar compressive effects on cardiac filling. If one measured only intraluminal LV pressure then it would appear as if LV diastolic compliance was reduced, because the associated increase in pericardial pressure and ITP would not be seen.[66–68] When LV function, however, is assessed as the relation between end-diastolic volume and output, no evidence for impaired LV contractile function is seen,[69,66] despite the continued application of PEEP.[70] These compressive effects can be considered analogous to cardiac tamponade.[71–73]

EFFECT OF INTRATHORACIC PRESSURE

The heart lives within the thorax, a pressure chamber inside a pressure chamber. Thus, changes in ITP will affect the pressure gradients for both systemic venous return to the right ventricle and systemic outflow from the left ventricle, independent of the heart itself (Fig. 36-3). Increases in ITP, by increasing right atrial pressure (Pra) and decreasing transmural LV systolic pressure, will reduce the pressure gradients for venous return and LV ejection, decreasing intrathoracic blood volume. Using the same argument, decreases in ITP will augment venous return and impede LV ejection, increasing intrathoracic blood volume. The increases in ITP during positive-pressure ventilation show marked

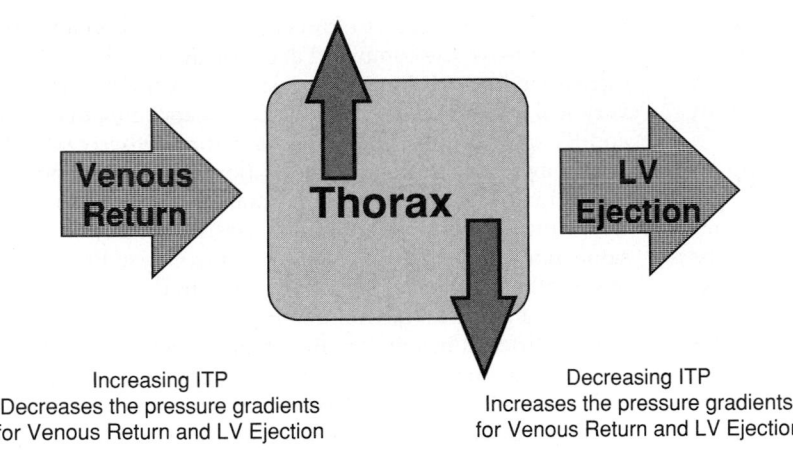

Increasing ITP
Decreases the pressure gradients
for Venous Return and LV Ejection

Decreasing ITP
Increases the pressure gradients
for Venous Return and LV Ejection

FIGURE 36-3 Schematic diagram of the effect of increasing or decreasing intrathoracic pressure on left ventricular (LV) filling (venous return) and ejection pressure.

regional differences: juxtacardiac ITP increases more than lateral chest-wall ITP as inspiratory flow rate and tidal volume increase.[63] Interestingly, lung compliance plays a minimal role in defining the positive-pressure–induced increase in ITP. For the same increase in tidal volume, ITP usually increases similarly if tidal volume is kept constant.[74,75] If, however, chest wall compliance decreases, then ITP will increase for a fixed tidal volume.[76,77]

SYSTEMIC VENOUS RETURN

Guyton et al described the determinants of venous return almost 50 years ago.[79] Blood flows back from the systemic venous reservoirs into the right atrium through low-pressure, low-resistance venous conduits.[79] Pra is the backpressure, or downstream pressure, for venous return. Pressure in the upstream venous reservoirs is called *mean systemic pressure*, which, itself, is a function of blood volume, peripheral vasomotor tone, and the distribution of blood within the vasculature.[80] Ventilation alters both Pra and the pressure in the venous reservoirs. Many of the observed ventilation-induced changes in cardiac performance can be explained by these changes. Mean systemic pressure does not change rapidly during positive-pressure ventilation, whereas Pra does, owing to parallel changes in ITP[81,82] (Fig. 36-4). Positive-pressure inspiration increases both ITP and Pra, decreasing venous-blood flow,[34] RV filling, and consequently, RV stroke volume.[34,81,83–91] During normal spontaneous inspiration, the opposite effects occur. Spontaneous inspiration decreases ITP and Pra, accelerating venous blood flow, and increasing RV filling and RV stroke volume.[34,35,60,85,88,92–94]

If changes in Pra were the only process that altered venous return, then positive-pressure ventilation would induce profound hemodynamic insufficiency in most patients. The decrease in venous return during positive-pressure ventilation, however, is often lower than one might expect based on the increase in Pra.

The reasons for this preload-sparing effect seen during positive-pressure ventilation are twofold. First, when cardiac output does decrease, increased sympathetic tone decreases venous capacitance, increasing mean systemic pressure, which tends to restore the pressure gradient for venous return, even in the face of an elevated Pra. Increases

in sympathetic tone, however, would increase steady-state cardiac output, and would not alter the phasic changes in venous return seen during positive-pressure ventilation. The decreased phasic reductions in venous return are caused by associated increases in mean systemic pressure during inspiration. Diaphragmatic descent and abdominal muscle contraction increase intra-abdominal pressure, decreasing intra-abdominal vascular capacitance.[95,96] Because a large proportion of venous blood is in the abdomen, the net effect of both inspiration and PEEP is to increase mean systemic pressure and Pra in a parallel but unequal fashion. Accordingly, the pressure gradient for venous return may not be reduced as much as predicted from a pure increase

FIGURE 36-4 A venous return curve, describing the relationship between the determinants of right ventricular preload. Right atrial pressure inversely changes the magnitude of venous return, and is influenced by changes in intrathoracic pressure (ITP). Positive-pressure ventilation shifts the ventricular function curve to the right (A), increasing right-atrial pressure but decreasing blood flow. Spontaneous inspiration decreases ITP and shifts the ventricular function curve to the left (B), decreasing right atrial pressure but increasing blood flow. As right atrial pressure becomes negative, as may occur during forced inspiratory efforts against resistance or impedance, a maximal blood flow is reached; further decreases in right atrial pressure no longer augment venous return.

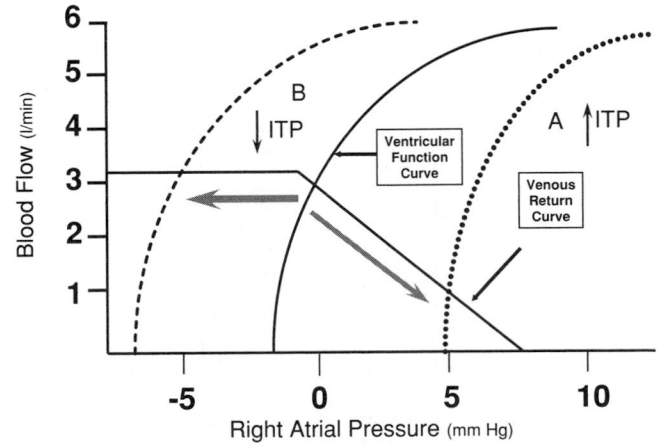

in Pra. This preload-sparing effect is especially well demonstrated in patients with hypervolemia. In fact, abdominal pressurization by diaphragmatic descent may be the major mechanism by which the decrease in venous return is minimized during positive-pressure ventilation.[97–101] In fact, Van den Berg et al[102] documented that up to 20 cmH$_2$O CPAP did not significantly decrease cardiac output, as measured 30 seconds into an inspiratory-hold maneuver, in fluid-resuscitated, postoperative cardiac surgery patients. Although CPAP induced an increase in Pra, intra-abdominal pressure also increased, preventing a significant change in RV volumes (Fig. 36-5). Interest in inverse-ratio ventilation has raised questions as to its hemodynamic effect, because its use constitutes a large component of hyperinflation. Mang et al,[103] however, demonstrated in an animal model of ALI that if total PEEP (intrinsic PEEP plus additional extrinsic PEEP) was similar, no hemodynamic difference between conventional ventilation and inverse-ratio ventilation was seen.

Relevance of Intrathoracic Pressure on Venous Return

It is axiomatic that the heart can only pump out that amount of blood that it receives and no more. Thus, venous return is the primary determinant of cardiac output.[80] Because Pra is the backpressure to venous return, venous return is maintained near maximal levels at rest,[12,79] because RV filling occurs with minimal changes in filling pressure.[73] Venous blood flow is maximal if Pra is kept near zero or less.[79,86]

Spontaneous inspiratory efforts usually increase venous return because of the combined decrease in Pra[60,104,86–88] and increase in intra-abdominal pressure.[95,96] For Pra to remain very low, however, RV diastolic compliance must be high and RV output must equal venous return. Otherwise, sustained increases in venous blood flow would distend the RV and increase Pra. During normal spontaneous inspiration, although venous return increases, ITP decreases at the same time, minimizing any potential increase in Pra, which might otherwise occur if ITP were not to decrease.[81] Aiding in this process of minimizing RV workload, the pulmonary arterial inflow circuit is highly compliant and can accept large increases in RV stroke volume without changing pressure.[34,105] Thus, increases in venous return proportionally increase pulmonary arterial inflow without significant changes in RV filling or ejection pressures. Accordingly, this compensatory system fails if RV diastolic compliance decreases or if Pra increases independent of changes in RV end-diastolic volume. These differential effects of negative (spontaneous inspiration) and positive (positive-pressure inspiration) swings in ITP on dynamic RV and LV performance are illustrated in Fig. 36-6.

Note further in Fig. 36-6 that not only does RV stroke volume increase with spontaneous inspiration and decrease with positive-pressure inspiration, but also that LV stroke volume decreases only during spontaneous inspiration (ventricular interdependence); during positive-pressure inspiration, however, any change in LV stroke volume occurs late, as the decrease in RV output finally reaches the left

FIGURE 36-5 Effect of increasing levels of continuous positive airway pressure (CPAP) on the relations between increasing airway pressure (Paw) and right atrial pressure (Pra) (*left graph*), Paw and intra-abdominal pressure (Pabd) (*center graph*), and Paw and changes in right ventricular end-diastolic volume (RVEDV) (*right graph*) in 43 postoperative fluid-resuscitated cardiac surgery patients. (*Data derived, with permission, from Van den Berg et al.[102]*)

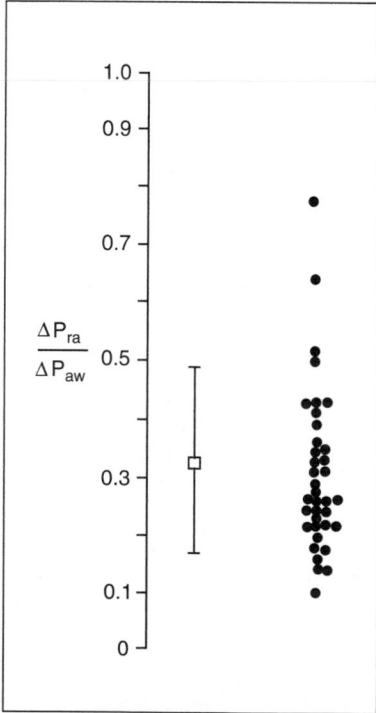
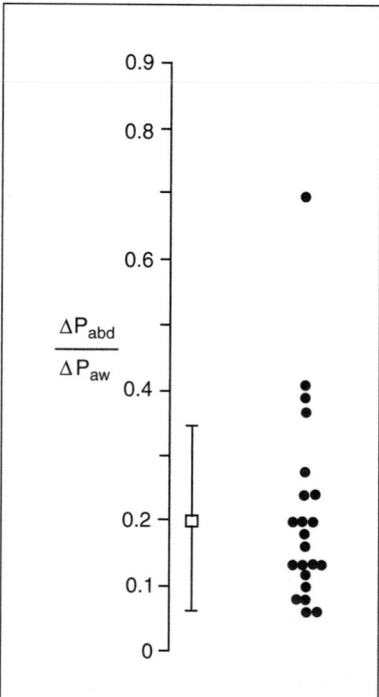
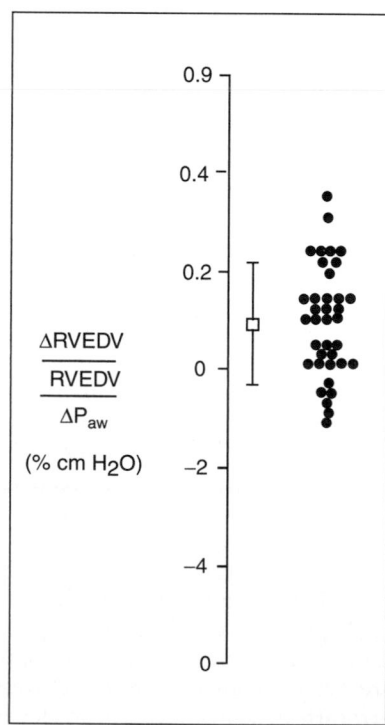

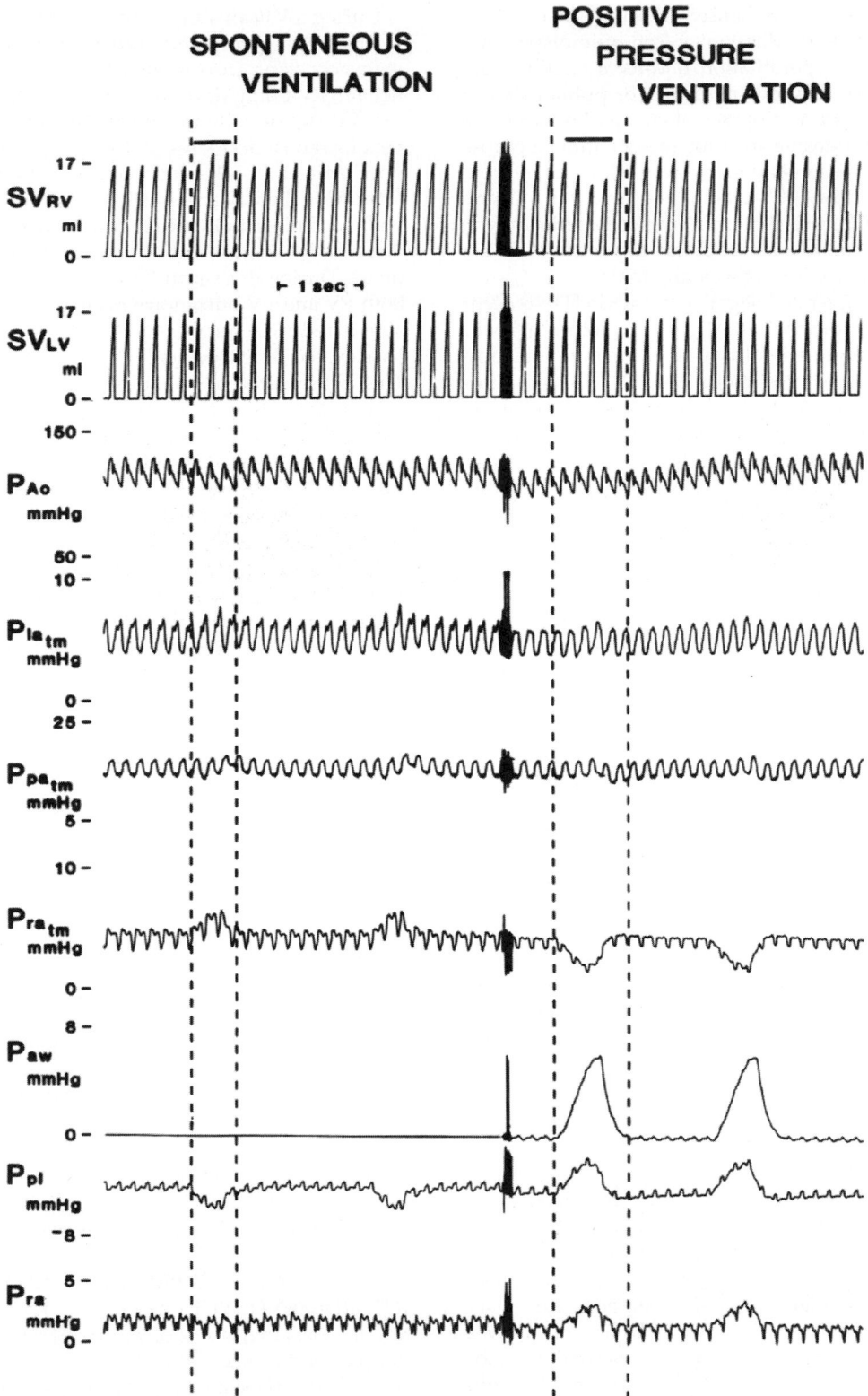

FIGURE 36-6 Strip chart recording of right and left ventricular stroke volumes (SVrv and SVlv, respectively), aortic pressure (P_{Ao}), left atrial, pulmonary arterial, and right atrial transmural pressures (Pla_{tm}, Ppa_{tm}, and Pra_{tm}, respectively), airway pressure (Paw), pleural pressure (Ppl), and right atrial pressure (Pra) during spontaneous ventilation (*left*) and similar tidal volume positive-pressure ventilation (*right*) in an anesthetized, intact canine model. (*Reproduced, with permission, from Pinsky et al.*[123])

ventricle. RV diastolic compliance can acutely decrease in the setting of acute RV dilation or cor pulmonale (pulmonary embolism, hyperinflation, and RV infarction). Importantly, acute RV dilation and acute cor pulmonale can not only induce rapid cardiovascular collapse, but they are singularly not responsive to fluid resuscitation. Because spontaneous inspiration and inspiratory efforts cause both ITP and Pra to decrease, RV dilation may occur in subjects with occult heart failure. Accordingly, some patients who were previously stable and ventilator dependent can develop acute RV failure during weaning trials.

Finally, with exaggerated negative swings in ITP, as occur with obstructed inspiratory efforts, venous return behaves as if abdominal pressure is additive to mean systemic pressure in augmenting venous blood flow.[106–109] These findings have led some investigators to suggest that obstructive breathing may be a therapeutic strategy in sustaining cardiac output in patients in hemorrhagic shock.[110] Interestingly, negative-pressure ventilation, by augmenting venous return, increases cardiac output by 39% in children following repair of tetralogy of Fallot.[111] It this condition, impaired RV filling secondary to RV hypertrophy and reduced RV chamber size are the primary factors limiting cardiac output. This augmentation of venous return, however, is limited,[107,108] because as ITP decreases below atmospheric pressure, venous return becomes flow-limited because the large systemic veins collapse as they enter the thorax.[79] This vascular flow limitation is a safety valve for the heart, because ITP can decrease greatly with obstructive inspiratory efforts,[13] and if not flow-limited, the RV could become overdistended and fail.[13,112] Finally, having subjects breathe through an airway that selectively impedes inspiration will result in exaggerated negative swings in both ITP and Pra, and associated greater increases in intra-abdominal pressure secondary to recruitment of accessory muscles of respiration (to sustain a normal tidal volume).[110]

Positive-pressure ventilation tends to create the opposite effects: increase in ITP increases Pra, thus decreasing venous return, RV volumes, and ultimately, LV output. The detrimental effect of positive-pressure ventilation on cardiac output can be minimized by either fluid resuscitation, to increase mean systemic pressure,[92,83,102,106] or by keeping both mean ITP and swings in lung volume as low as possible. Accordingly, prolonging expiratory time, decreasing tidal volume, and avoiding PEEP all minimize this decrease in systemic venous return to the right ventricle.[1,81,85–89,113,114] Increases in lung volume during positive-pressure ventilation primarily compress the two ventricles into each other, decreasing bi-ventricular volumes.[115] The decrease in cardiac output commonly seen during PEEP is caused by a decrease in LV end-diastolic volume, because both LV end-diastolic volume and cardiac output are restored by fluid resuscitation[116,117] without any measurable change in LV diastolic compliance.[66]

A common respiratory maneuver, called the Valsalva maneuver, which is forced expiration against an occluded airway (such as while straining at stool), displays most of the hemodynamic effects commonly seen in various disease states and with different types of positive-pressure ventilation.

During a Valsalva maneuver, airway pressure (Paw) and ITP increase equally, and pulmonary vascular resistance remains constant. During the first phase of the Valsalva maneuver, RV filling decreases first with no change in LV filling, LV stroke volume, or arterial pulse pressure because venous return decreases. Although LV stroke volume does not change, LV peak ejection pressure increases equal to the amount of the increase in ITP.[118] As the strain is sustained, both LV filling and cardiac output decrease owing to the decrease in venous return,[62,119] which results in the second phase. During this second phase of the Valsalva maneuver, both RV and LV output are decreased; arterial pulse pressure is reduced, but peak systolic pressure is sustained at an elevated level owing to the sustained increase in ITP. This phase delay in LV output decrease compared to RV output decrease is also seen during positive-pressure ventilation; it is exaggerated if tidal volumes increase or if the pressure gradient for venous return was already low, as is the case in hypovolemia.[1,66–68,90,113,120–126] With release of the strain in phase three of the Valsalva maneuver, arterial pressure abruptly declines because the low LV stroke volume cannot sustain an adequate ejection pressure on its own. Furthermore, with the release of the increased ITP, venous return increases, increasing RV volume, and, through the process of ventricular interdependence, decreases LV diastolic compliance, making LV end-diastolic volume even less. Conceptually, then ventricular interdependence usually becomes apparent with sudden increases in RV volume from apneic baseline, as would occur during spontaneous inspiration, but less so when RV volumes decrease below these volumes. As described above, because RV volumes are usually decreased during positive-pressure ventilation, ventricular interdependence is not a prominent feature of this form of breathing[58,124–127] (see Fig. 36-6). Although PEEP results in some degree of right-to-left intraventricular septal shift, echocardiographic studies demonstrate that the shift is small.[69,120] It follows that positive-pressure ventilation decreases intrathoracic blood volume[86] and PEEP decreases it even more[129] without altering LV diastolic or contractile function.[128,130] During spontaneous inspiration, however, RV volumes increase transiently shifting the intraventricular septum into the LV,[59] decreasing LV diastolic compliance and LV end-diastolic volume.[47,131,127] This transient RV dilation-induced septal shift is the primary cause of inspiration-associated decreases in arterial pulse pressure, which, if greater than 10 mmHg or 10% of the mean pulse pressure, is referred to as *pulsus paradoxus*[60,78] (see Fig. 36-6).

LEFT VENTRICULAR PRELOAD AND VENTRICULAR INTERDEPENDENCE

Strictly speaking, issues of ventricular interdependence are not part of the effects of ITP on venous return and LV ejection. But the associated rapid changes in RV filling induced by phasic changes in ITP cause marked changes in LV output, which are a hallmark of ventilation-induced hemodynamic changes. The fundamental interactions defining ventricular interdependence were described above.

LEFT VENTRICULAR AFTERLOAD

LV afterload is defined as the maximal LV systolic wall tension, which equals the maximal product of LV volume and transmural LV pressure. Under normal conditions, maximal LV wall tension occurs at the end of isometric contraction, with the opening of the aortic valve. During LV ejection, as LV volumes rapidly decrease, LV afterload also decreases despite an associated increase in ejection pressure. Importantly, when LV dilation exists, as in CHF, maximal LV wall stress occurs during LV ejection because the maximal product of pressure and volume occurs at that time. LV ejection pressure is the transmural LV systolic pressure. This is the main reason why patients with dilated cardiomyopathies are very sensitive to changes in ejection pressure, whereas patients with primarily diastolic dysfunction are not. Normal baroreceptor mechanisms, located in the extrathoracic carotid body, function to maintain arterial pressure constant with respect to atmosphere. Accordingly, if arterial pressure were to remain constant as ITP increased, then transmural LV pressure would decrease. Similarly, if transmural arterial pressure were to remain constant as ITP increased, then LV wall tension would decrease.[132] Thus, increases in ITP decrease LV afterload, and decreases in ITP increase LV afterload.[118,133] These two opposing effects of changes in ITP on LV afterload have important clinical implications.

The concept that increases in ITP decrease both LV preload and LV afterload can be clearly illustrated with the use of high-frequency jet ventilation (HFJV), which can increase ITP but does not result in large swings in lung volume.[123] When HFJV is delivered in synchrony with the cardiac cycle, such that heart rate and ventilatory frequency are identical, one can dissect out the effects of ITP on preload and afterload. Under hypovolemic and normovolemic conditions with intact cardiovascular reserve, positive-pressure ventilation usually decreases steady-state cardiac output by decreasing the pressure gradient for venous return. When one compares the hemodynamic effects of HFJV synchronized to occur during diastole when ventricular filling occurs, cardiac output decreases to levels seen during end-inspiration for normal large-tidal-volume (10 ml/kg) ventilation. In the same subject, however, if the increases in ITP occur during systole, the detrimental effects of the same mean Paw, mean ITP, and tidal volume do not impede venous return[134,135] (Fig. 36-7). Furthermore, in heart failure states, positive-pressure ventilation does not impede cardiac output because the same decreases in venous return do not alter LV preload. If these increases in ITP, however, reduce LV afterload, then cardiac output will also increase. These points are illustrated in Fig. 36-8, wherein synchronous HFJV is delivered either during pre-ejection systole (presystolic) or ejection (systolic). The only difference between the two ventilatory states is that arterial pulse pressure does not change despite increases in LV stroke volume with presystolic increases in Paw, consistent with a decreased LV afterload, whereas with systolic increases in Paw, arterial pulse pressure increases, and peak arterial pressure increases by an amount equal to the increase in ITP, consistent with mechanically augmented LV ejection.

Relevance of Intrathoracic Pressure on Myocardial Oxygen Cosumption

Decreases in ITP increase both LV afterload and myocardial O_2 consumption (MVO$_2$). Accordingly, spontaneous ventilation increases not only global O_2 demand by its exercise

component,[136,113,72] but also increases MVO$_2$. Profound decreases in ITP commonly occur during spontaneous inspiratory efforts with bronchospasm, obstructive breathing, and acute hypoxemic respiratory failure. Under these disease conditions, the cardiovascular burden can be great and may induce acute heart failure and pulmonary edema.[13,29] Because weaning from positive-pressure ventilation to spontaneous ventilation may induce dramatic changes in ITP swings, from positive to negative, independent of the energy requirements of the respiratory muscles, weaning is a selective LV stress test.[132,137,138] Similarly, improved LV systolic function is observed in patients with severe LV failure placed on mechanical ventilation.[138] Very negative swings in ITP, as seen with vigorous inspiratory efforts in the setting of airway obstruction (asthma, upper airway obstruction, or vocal cord paralysis) or stiff lungs (interstitial lung disease, pulmonary edema, or ALI), selectively increase LV afterload, and may be the cause of LV failure and pulmonary edema,[13,29,30,139] especially if LV systolic function is already compromised.[140,141]

Pulsus paradoxus seen during spontaneous inspiration under conditions of marked pericardial restraint reflects primarily ventricular interdependence.[142–146] The negative swings in ITP, however, also increase LV ejection pressure, increasing LV end-systolic volume.[118] Other systemic factors may influence LV systolic function during loaded inspiratory efforts. These associated factors also contribute to a greater or lesser degree to the inhibition of normal LV systolic function, including increase in aortic input impedance,[147] altered synchrony of contraction of the global LV myocardium,[148] and hypoxemia-induced decreased global myocardial contractility.[149] Hypoxia also directly reduces LV diastolic compliance.[150] Experimental repetitive periodic airway obstructions induce pulmonary edema in normal animals.[29,30] Furthermore, removing the negative swings in ITP by applying nasal CPAP results in improved global LV performance in patients with combined obstructive sleep apnea and CHF.[150]

Effects of Intrathoracic Pressure on Left Ventricular Afterload

If arterial pressure remains constant, then increases in ITP decrease transmural LV ejection pressure, decreasing LV afterload. These points are easily demonstrated in a subject with an indwelling arterial pressure catheter during cough or Valsalva maneuvers. During a cough, ITP increases rapidly without changes in intrathoracic blood volume. Arterial pressure also increases by a similar amount, as described above for phase 1 of the Valsalva maneuver. Thus, transmural LV pressure (LV pressure relative to ITP)[118,151,152] and aortic blood flow[62] would remain constant. Sustained increases in ITP, however, must eventually decrease aortic blood flow and arterial pressure secondary to the associated decrease in venous return.[118] If ITP increased arterial pressure without changing transmural arterial pressure, then baroreceptor-mediated vasodilation would induce arterial vasodilation to keep extrathoracic arterial pressure-flow relations constant.[122] Because coronary perfusion pressure reflects the ITP gradient for blood flow, and is not increased by ITP-induced increases in arterial pressure, such sustained increases in ITP can cause

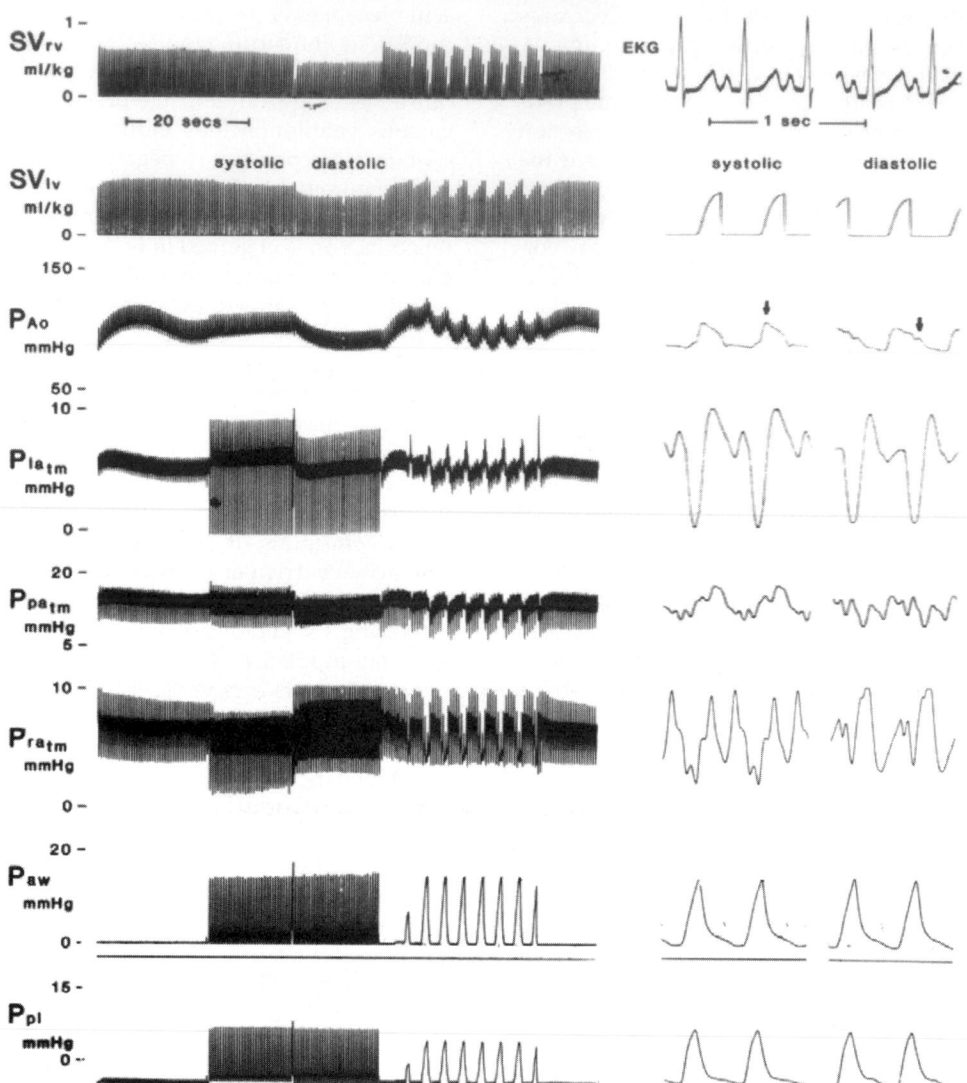

FIGURE 36-7 Strip chart recording of right and left ventricular stroke volumes (SVrv and SVlv, respectively), aortic pressure (P_{Ao}), left atrial, pulmonary arterial, and right atrial transmural pressures (Pla_{tm}, Ppa_{tm}, and Pra_{tm}, respectively), airway pressure (Paw), and pleural pressure (Ppl) during apnea (*left*), and both systolic (*systole*) and diastolic (*diastole*) high-frequency jet ventilation (HFV) (*middle*), and intermittent positive-pressure ventilation (IPPV) with similar mean Paw (*right*) in an anesthetized, intact canine model with normal cardiovascular function. Note that the cardiac cycle–specific increases in Paw created by systole HFV minimally impede cardiac output, whereas diastole HFV markedly decreases venous return (SVrv decreases first, then SVlv decreases). The rapid strip chart speed shown on the left is to illustrate the exact timing of synchronous HFV. (*Reproduced, with permission, from Pinsky et al.*[134])

decreased coronary perfusion pressure and induce myocardial ischemia.[153–155]

Spontaneous Breathing versus Mechanical Ventilation

Both spontaneous and mechanical ventilation increase lung volume above resting end-expiratory lung volume (FRC). During both spontaneous and positive-pressure ventilation,

end-expiratory lung volume can be artificially increased by the addition of end-expiratory airway pressure. Thus, the primary hemodynamic differences between spontaneous ventilation and positive-pressure ventilation are caused by the changes in ITP and the muscular contraction needed to create these changes. Importantly, even if a patient is receiving mechanical ventilation support, spontaneous respiratory efforts can persist and may result in marked increases in metabolic load, and contribute to sustained respiratory muscle fatigue.[156] Still, one of the primary reasons for instituting mechanical ventilation is to remove the work of

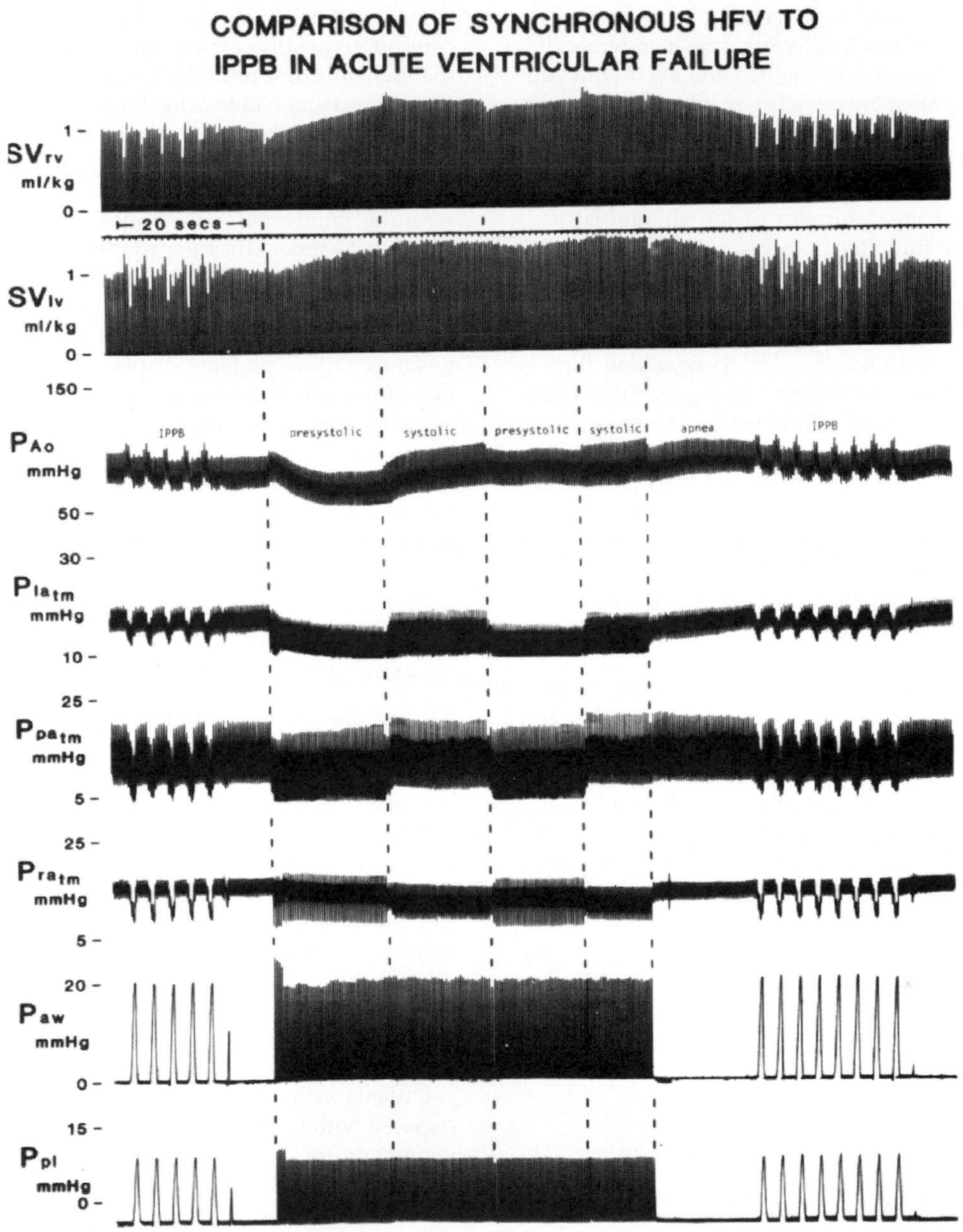

COMPARISON OF SYNCHRONOUS HFV TO IPPB IN ACUTE VENTRICULAR FAILURE

FIGURE 36-8 Continuous strip chart recording of right and left ventricular stroke volumes (SVrv and SVlv, respectively), aortic pressure (P_{Ao}), left atrial, pulmonary arterial, and right atrial transmural pressures (Pla_{tm}, Ppa_{tm}, and Pra_{tm}, respectively), airway pressure (Paw), pleural pressure (Ppl), and right atrial pressure (Pra) during intermittent positive-pressure ventilation (V_T 10 ml/kg) (IPPV), apnea (*left*), and then both pre-ejection systole (presystolic) and LV ejection (systolic) synchronous high-frequency jet ventilation (HFV) (*middle*), and then IPPV again (*right*) in an anesthetized, intact canine model with fluid-resuscitated acute ventricular failure. Note that the cardiac cycle–specific increases in Paw created by both presystolic and systolic HFV increase steady-state SVrv and SVlv (i.e., cardiac output), but affect P_{Ao} differently. Presystolic HFV does not change P_{Ao} pulse pressure despite an increase in SVlv (reduced afterload), whereas systolic HFV increases P_{Ao} pulse pressure for a similar increase in SVlv. (*Reproduced, with permission, from Pinsky et al.[134]*)

breathing. Normal spontaneous ventilation augments venous return and vigorous inspiratory efforts account for most of the increased blood flow seen in exercise. Conversely, positive-pressure ventilation may impair ventricular filling and induce hypovolemic cardiac dysfunction in normal or hypovolemic subjects while augmenting LV function in patients with heart failure.[92] Finally, heart failure, whether primary or induced by ventilation, may induce

acute respiratory muscle fatigue, causing acute respiratory failure or failure to wean from mechanical ventilation, and overtax the ability of the circulation to deliver O_2 to the rest of the body.

Fundamental to this concept is the realization that spontaneous ventilation is exercise. Spontaneous ventilatory efforts are induced by contraction of the respiratory muscles, of which the diaphragm and intercostal muscles comprise the bulk.[136] Although ventilation normally requires less than 5% of total O_2 delivery to meet its demand[136] (and is difficult to measure at the bedside even with calibrated metabolic measuring devices), in lung disease states in which the work of breathing is increased (such as pulmonary edema or bronchospasm), the metabolic demand for O_2 can increase to 30% of total O_2 delivery.[72,113,136,157] With marked hyperpnea, muscles of the abdominal wall and shoulder girdle function as accessory respiratory muscles. Blood flow to these muscles is derived from several arterial circuits, whose absolute flow exceeds the highest metabolic demand of maximally exercising skeletal muscle under normal conditions.[158,159,136] Thus, blood flow is usually not the limiting factor determining maximal ventilatory effort. In severe heart failure states, however, blood flow constraints may limit ventilation because blood flow to other organs and to the respiratory muscles may be compromised, inducing both tissue hypoperfusion and lactic acidosis.[158,159] Aubier et al demonstrated that if cardiac output is severely limited by the artificial induction of tamponade in a canine model that respiratory muscle failure develops despite high central neuronal drive.[159] The animals die a respiratory death before cardiovascular standstill.[159] The institution of mechanical ventilation for ventilatory and hypoxemic respiratory failure may reduce metabolic demand on the stressed cardiovascular system, increasing mixed venous oxygen saturation (Sv_{O_2}) for a constant cardiac output and arterial oxygen content (Ca_{O_2}).[160] Intubation and mechanical ventilation, when adjusted to the metabolic demands of the patient, may dramatically decrease the work of breathing, resulting in increased O_2 delivery to other vital organs and decreased serum lactic acid levels. Under conditions in which fixed right-to-left shunts exist, the obligatory increase in Sv_{O_2} will result in an increase in the Pa_{O_2}, despite no change in the ratio of shunt blood flow to cardiac output.

Detection and Monitoring

WEANING FAILURE

Ventilator-dependent patients who fail to wean often have impaired baseline cardiovascular performance that is readily apparent,[141] but commonly patients develop overt signs of heart failure during weaning, such as pulmonary edema,[141,161] myocardial ischemia,[162–165] tachycardia, and gut ischemia.[166] Pulmonary artery occlusion pressure may rise rapidly to nonphysiologic levels within 5 minutes of instituting weaning.[141] Although all patients increase their cardiac output in response to a weaning trial, those that subsequently fail to wean demonstrate a reduction in mixed venous O_2 saturation, consistent with a failing cardiovascular response to an increased metabolic demand.[167] Weaning from mechanical ventilation can be considered a cardiovascular stress test. Again, investigators have documented weaning-associated ECG and thallium cardiac blood flow scan–related signs of ischemia in both patients with known coronary artery disease[162] and in otherwise normal patients.[164,165] Using this same logic, placing patients with severe heart failure and/or ischemia on ventilator support, by either intubation and ventilation[168] or noninvasive continuous positive airway pressure,[169] can reverse myocardial ischemia. Importantly, the increased work of breathing may come from endotracheal tube flow resistance.[170] Thus, some subjects who fail a spontaneous breathing trial may actually be able to breathe on their own if extubated.

It follows, that if spontaneous ventilation is exercise, then weaning failure patients should display signs of circulatory insufficiency during a trial of spontaneous breathing. Patients with chronic obstructive pulmonary disease who fail to wean often develop gut hypoperfusion, as assessed by gastric tonometry, during weaning trials.[166] Similarly, weaning failure patients display an increase in arteriovenous O_2 content difference, a commonly used method of assessing cardiovascular stress.[167] Much of the increased work of breathing can be caused by the endotracheal tube.[170] Thus, some patients who fail spontaneous breathing trials can be extubated successfully, but there is no known method of identifying this subgroup.

USING VENTILATION TO DEFINE CARDIOVASCULAR PERFORMANCE

Because the cardiovascular response to positive-pressure breathing is determined by the baseline cardiovascular state, these responses can be used to define such cardiovascular states. Sustained increases in airway pressure will reduce venous return, allowing one to assess LV ejection over a range of end-diastolic volumes. If echocardiographic measures of LV volumes are simultaneously made, then one can use an inspiratory-hold maneuver to measure cardiac contractility, as defined by the end-systolic pressure-volume relationship (ESPVR),[171] which is similar to that created by transient inferior vena caval occlusion.[172,173] Furthermore, these measures can be made during the respiratory cycle to define dynamic interactions.[173]

Patients with relative hypervolemia, a condition often associated with CHF, are at less risk of developing impaired venous return during initiation of mechanical ventilation, whereas hypovolemic patients are at increased risk. If positive airway pressure augments LV ejection in heart failure states by reducing LV afterload, then systolic arterial pressure should not decrease, but actually increase, during inspiration, so-called reverse pulsus paradoxus. This was what Abel et al[174] saw in 10 post–cardiac surgery patients. Perel et al[175,176,177] suggested that the relation between respiratory efforts and systolic arterial pressure may be used to identify which patients may benefit from cardiac-assist maneuvers. Patients who increase their systolic arterial pressure during ventilation, relative to an apneic baseline, tend to have a greater degree of volume overload[176] and heart failure,[177] whereas patients who decrease systolic arterial pressure tend to be volume responsive. Perhaps more relevant to usual clinical practice is the identification of subjects whose cardiac output will increase if given a volume challenge. Identification of preload-responsiveness is important because only half of the hemodynamically unstable patients studied in several clinical series were actually preload responsive.[178] Thus, nonspecific fluid loading will not only be ineffective at restoring cardiovascular stability in half the subjects, it will also both delay definitive therapy and may promote cor pulmonale or pulmonary edema. Finally, Michard et al[179] found, in a series of ventilator-dependent septic patients, that the greater the degree of arterial pulse-pressure variation during positive-pressure ventilation, the greater the subsequent increase in cardiac output in response to volume-expansion therapy. The recent literature has documented that both arterial pulse pressure[180] and LV stroke volume variations[181,182] induced by positive-pressure ventilation are sensitive and specific markers of preload responsiveness. The greater the degree of flow or pressure variation over the course of the respiratory cycle for a fixed tidal volume, the more likely a subject is to increase cardiac output in response to a volume challenge, and the greater that increase. The overarching principles of this clinical tool have not been previously described. There are several important caveats and limitations to this approach, which need to be considered before the clinician proceeds to monitoring arterial pulse pressure or stroke volume variation during ventilation as a routine means for predicting preload responsiveness.

First, and perhaps most importantly, being preload responsive does not mean that the subject should be given volume. Otherwise normal subjects under general anesthesia without evidence of cardiovascular insufficiency are also preload responsive, but do not need a volume challenge. The presence of positive-pressure–induced changes in aortic flow or arterial pulse pressure does not itself define therapy. Independent documentation of cardiovascular insufficiency needs to be sought before the clinician attempts fluid resuscitation based on these measures. Second, these indices, which quantify the variation in aortic flow, stroke volume, and arterial systolic and pulse pressures, have routinely been demonstrated to outperform more traditional measures of LV preload, such as pulmonary occlusion pressure, Pra, total thoracic blood volume, RV end-diastolic volume, and LV end-diastolic area.[180,181] There appears to be little relation between ventricular preload and preload responsiveness. Ventricular filling pressures poorly reflect ventricular volumes,[183] and measures of absolute ventricular volumes do not define diastolic compliance.[184] Patients with small LV volumes that are also stiff, as may occur with acute cor pulmonale, tamponade, LV hypertrophy, and myocardial fibrosis, will show poor volume responsiveness. Conversely, patients with large LV volumes, as often occurs with CHF and afterload reduction, may be quite volume responsive. Thus, preload does not equal preload responsiveness. Third, all the reported studies used positive-pressure ventilation to vary venous return. For such changes in venous return, however, to induce LV output changes, the changes in venous return must be of sufficient magnitude to cause measurable changes in preload.[185] If the increase in lung volume with each tidal breath is either not great enough to induce changes in pulmonary venous flow,[186] or if the positive-pressure breath is associated with spontaneous inspiratory efforts that minimize the changes in venous return,[81] then the cyclic perturbations to cardiac filling may not be sufficient to induce the cyclic variations in LV filling needed to identify preload responsiveness. Further-

more, the degree of pressure or flow variation will be proportional to tidal volume, with greater tidal volumes inducing greater changes for the same cardiovascular state.[188,183] Thus, the means by which cyclic changes in lung volume and ITP are induced will affect the magnitude of arterial pressure and flow variations. Fourth, although the primary determinant of arterial pulse pressure variation over a single breath is LV stroke volume variation, because changes in aortic impedance and arterial tone cannot change that rapidly[190] over time, this limitation no longer applies. As arterial tone decreases, for example, then for the same aortic flow and stroke volume both mean arterial pressure and pulse pressure will be less. Accordingly, flow variation becomes more sensitive than pulse pressure variation as hemorrhage progresses.[182]

Clinical Scenarios

INITIATING MECHANICAL VENTILATION

NORMO- AND HYPOVOLEMIC PATIENTS

The process of initiating mechanical ventilation is a complex physiologic process for a variety of reasons. First, pharmacologic factors needed to allow for endotracheal intubation also blunt sympathetic responses, exaggerating the hemodynamic effects induced by increasing airway pressure and defining tidal volume and respiratory frequency. This point is clearly demonstrated by comparing the relatively benign impact of re-instituting ventilator support in a patient with a pre-existent tracheotomy, with the impact of the initial intubation and ventilation of the same patient a few days or weeks earlier. As noted above, positive-pressure ventilation increases ITP, which must alter venous return. If a patient has reduced vasomotor tone, as commonly exists during induction of anesthesia, the associated increase in Pra will induce a proportional decrease in venous return, pulmonary blood flow, and subsequently cardiac output.[34,81,191] If the associated tidal volumes are excessive for the duration of expiratory time available for passive deflation, then dynamic hyperinflation will occur, increasing pulmonary vascular resistance and compressing the heart in the cardiac fossa, further decreasing bi-ventricular volumes.[115] If one were to examine the dynamic effects of ventilation on the LV pressure-volume relation over the course of a single breath, one would see a more complex effect, characterized by alterations in LV diastolic compliance, end-diastolic volume, stroke volume, and LV afterload (as exemplified by the leftward shift of the end-systolic pressure-volume relations) (Fig. 36-9). Importantly, the impact of ventilation on LV performance, as described in the first part of this chapter, is overly simplified by this assumption that breathing alters only LV preload. Clearly, other factors also function simultaneously. The preload-reducing effects of tidal volume, however, are best described during hypovolemic states, as illustrated in the right hand panel of Fig. 36-10. Note that increasing tidal volumes limit ventricular filling, decreasing LV stroke volume under both normovolemic (left) and hypovolemic (right) conditions (see Fig. 36-10), but this effect is markedly exaggerated by hypovolemia.

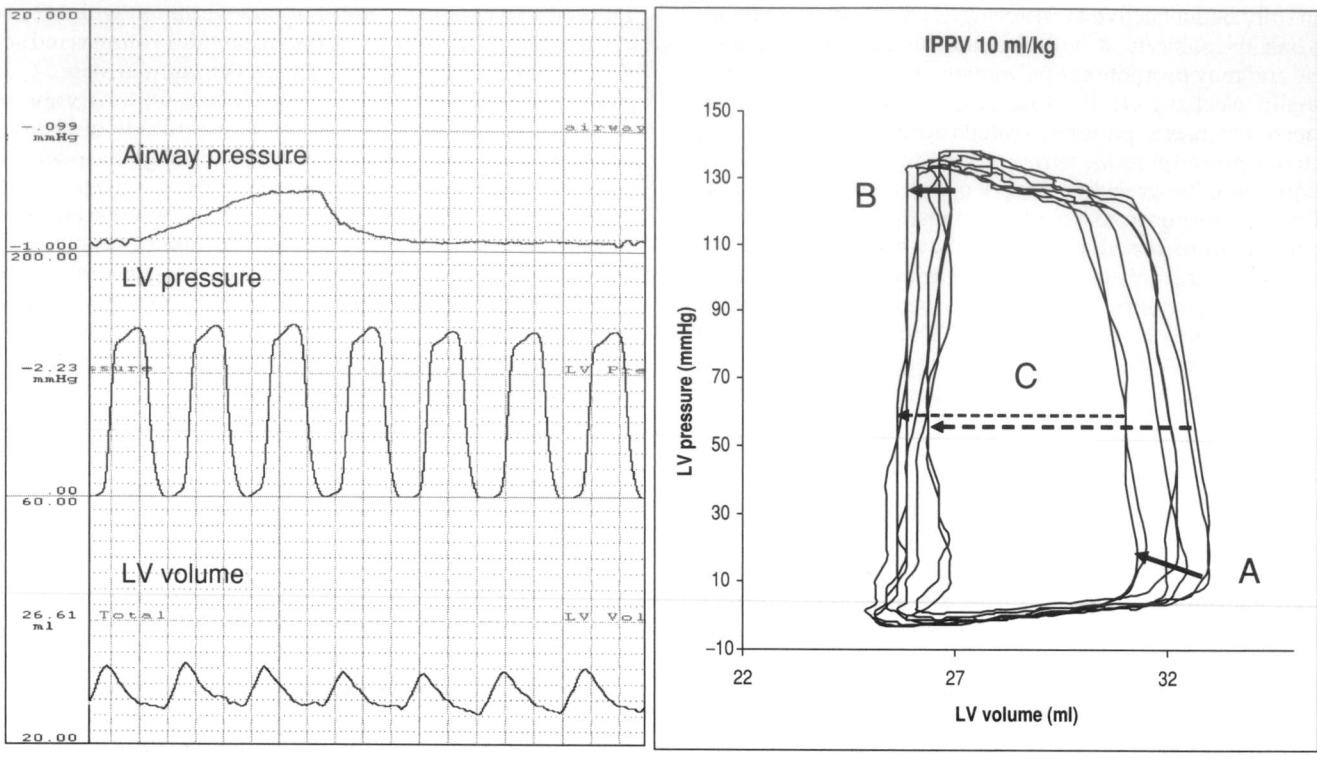

FIGURE 36-9 Dynamic effect of positive-pressure ventilation on the LV pressure-volume relation from end-expiration through a ventilatory cycle. Note that during the breath, as airway pressure rises and then falls (*left panel*) LV diastolic compliance (*right panel*) decreases minimally (the slope of the LV pressure-volume relation as LV volume increases during filling; *lower horizontal line*), while LV preload markedly decreases (*arrow A*), and LV end-systolic pressure-volume domains do not decrease but shift to the left (*arrow B*), associated with a decrease in LV stroke volume (*arrow C*). Thus, all four processes occur during a single positive-pressure breath. Refer to Fig. 36-10 to see how changes in tidal volume and intravascular volume alter these changes differently.

FIGURE 36-10 Effect of increasing tidal volume on the LV pressure-volume relation during normovolemic (*left*) and hypovolemic (*right*) conditions in an intact anesthetized canine model. Under normovolemic conditions, the preload-reducing effects of positive-pressure inspiration become more pronounced at end-inspiration as tidal volume increases. Under hypovolemic conditions, similar increases in tidal volume also tend to decrease the overall size and performance of the heart along lines consistent with pure reductions in LV preload (end-diastolic volume); that is, steady-state LV end-diastolic and end-systolic volumes decrease, end-systolic pressure decreases, and stroke volume decreases with increasing tidal volumes and airway pressures.

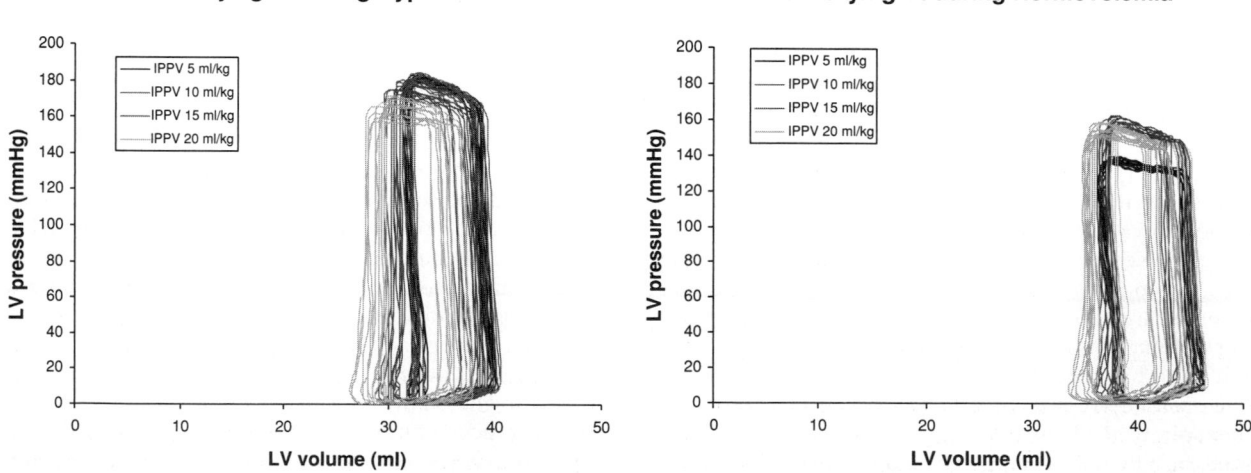

HYPERVOLEMIC AND HEART FAILURE PATIENTS

Initiating mechanical ventilation in hypervolemic patients has far less effect on cardiac output than that seen during normovolemic or hypovolemic conditions, because the impact of ventilation on venous return is much less (right hand panel of Fig. 36-6). Moreover, if such patients also have a component of acute RV volume overload, one may actually see LV diastolic compliance increase and LV output markedly improve. It is not clear, however, if these often-seen improvements in LV performance and cardiac output in hypervolemic conditions represents improved LV filling, reduced metabolic demands, or improved LV contraction. Regrettably, no clinical trials have examined the mechanisms by which such improvement occurs.

COMPARING DIFFERENT MODES OF MECHANICAL VENTILATION

Any hemodynamic differences between different modes of mechanical ventilation at a constant airway pressure and PEEP are caused by differential effects on lung volume and ITP.[134] When two different modes of total or partial ventilatory support have similar changes in ITP and respiratory effort, their hemodynamic effects are also similar despite markedly different airway waveforms. Partial ventilator support, with intermittent mandatory ventilation or pressure-support ventilation, give similar hemodynamic responses when matched for similar tidal volumes.[194] Similar tissue oxygenation occurred in ventilator-dependent patients when switched between assist-control, intermittent mandatory ventilation and pressure-support ventilation, with matched tidal volumes.[195] Numerous studies have documented cardiovascular equivalence when different ventilator modes were matched for tidal volume and level of PEEP.[196,197] Different ventilator modes will affect cardiac output to a similar extent for similar increases in lung volume.[198,199] When pressure-control with a smaller tidal volume, however, was compared to volume-control, pressure-control was associated with a higher cardiac output.[199,200] Davis et al[238] compared effects of volume-control versus pressure-control ventilation in 25 patients with ALI. When matched for the same mean Paw, both methods gave the same cardiac output. When Paw, however, was increased during volume-control ventilation from a sine-wave to a square-wave flow pattern, cardiac output fell. Furthermore, Kiehl et al[244] found that cardiac output was better during biphasic positive airway pressure than volume-control ventilation, leading to an increased Sv_{O_2} and indirectly increasing Pa_{O_2}. In 18 ventilator-dependent but hemodynamically stable patients, Singer et al[240] showed that the degree of hyperinflation, not the Paw, determined the decrease in cardiac output.

UPPER AIRWAY OBSTRUCTION

The cardiovascular effects of upper airway obstruction were recently reviewed.[201] To understand the effects, it is useful to examine the effect of spontaneous inspiratory efforts against an occluded airway, referred to as a Mueller maneuver. This maneuver is easy to create in a graded fashion in the laboratory by having the subject inspire against an occluded airway while connected to a manometer; the negative swings in Paw can be controlled by the subject. Based on the above physiologic discussion, it is clear that a Mueller maneuver will result in an increase in both venous return and LV afterload. The hemodynamic effects, however, of positive and negative swings in ITP may not be mirror opposites of each other; the interactions are nonlinear. As ITP becomes more negative, venous return becomes flow limited as the veins collapse because their transmural pressure becomes negative. LV afterload, however, increases progressively and linearly.[118] These nonlinear effects are illustrated in Fig. 36-4. Changes in ITP will appear to shift the LV Frank-Starling curve to the left or right, with Pra on the x axis, equal to the change in ITP, because the heart is in the chest and acted upon by ITP, whereas venous return is from the body, which is outside of this pressure chamber. Accordingly, large negative swings in ITP will selectively increase LV ejection pressure without greatly increasing RV preload or LV diastolic compliance. This concept is important. Removing large negative swings in ITP, without inducing positive swings in ITP, as would occur by endotracheal intubation or tracheotomy to bypass any upper airway obstruction, should selectively reduce LV ejection pressure (LV afterload) and not reduce venous return (LV preload).

Large negative swings in ITP commonly occur in critically ill patients. Upper airway obstruction is a medical emergency. The most common cause of upper airway obstruction is pharyngeal obstruction due to loss of muscle tone, which is manifest as snoring and/or obstructive sleep apnea. Laryngeal edema or vocal cord paralysis following extubation commonly present as acute upper airway obstruction immediately following extubation. Other causes of upper airway obstruction include epiglottitis, retropharyngeal hematomas, tumors of the neck and vocal cords, and foreign body aspiration. Because the site of obstruction is in the extrathoracic airway, increasing inspiratory efforts only cause the obstruction to become more pronounced. By markedly increasing LV afterload, inspiration against an occluded airway rapidly leads to acute pulmonary edema.[118,202–209] During an acute asthma attack in a child, peak negative ITP can be –40 cmH$_2$O and mean tidal ITP maintained between –24 and –7 cmH$_2$O,[13] increasing LV afterload[118] and promoting pulmonary edema.[202]

CHRONIC OBSTRUCTIVE PULMONARY DISEASE

The hemodynamic consequences of COPD reflect complex issues related to hyperinflation, a propensity to further dynamic hyperinflation and increased airway resistance. Hyperinflation, within the context of pre-existing reduced pulmonary vascular cross-sectional area and increased pulmonary vasomotor tone, are the primary reasons for ventilation-induced pulmonary hypertension and RV failure. RV afterload is often increased owing to loss of pulmonary parenchyma and hyperinflation. Ventilation-perfusion mismatch can promote further increases in pulmonary vasomotor tone through hypoxic pulmonary vasoconstriction. The ultimate effects of this process are to impede RV ejection and induce RV dilation, and, if pulmonary hypertension persists, induce RV hypertrophy. An immediate increase in lung volume may decrease RV end-diastolic volume because of cardiac compression and an associated increase in Pra. Neurohumoral reflex mechanisms, however, acting through right atrial stretch receptors cause salt and water retention, causing blood volume and Pra to increase. The goal of this exercise is to restore venous return to its baseline level. Accordingly, the elevated Pra commonly seen in patients with COPD reflects a survival strategy analogous to LV dilation in heart failure.

During exacerbations of COPD, hypoxemia, respiratory acidosis, increased intrinsic sympathetic tone, and increased, but inefficient, respiratory efforts combine to increase the work of breathing. The net result is often unpredictable, but certain scenarios often present themselves, which suggests the dominance of one process over the others. These differences are relevant because they identify specific, and often opposite, therapeutic strategies that are used to reverse the associated cardiovascular insufficiency. On a global level, however, any treatments that can reduce airways obstruction and bronchospasm will reduce the work of breathing, minimize hyperinflation, and reverse respiratory acidosis and hypoxemia, decreasing RV afterload. Accordingly, the aggressive use of supplemental O_2, bronchodilating agents, and antibiotics to reduce airway infections and the volume and viscosity of secretions will improve cardiovascular function. If mechanical ventilation can reverse hyperinflation and alveolar hypoxia, one will see reductions in Pra, increases in cardiac output, and less radical arterial pressure swings during ventilation. If, however, hyperinflation persists or is exaggerated by mechanical ventilation, then acute RV failure may occur.

ACUTE COR PULMONALE

Hyperinflation, in the setting of pre-existing pulmonary hypertension or decreased pulmonary vessel cross-sectional area, can induce profound increases in pulmonary arterial pressure, promoting acute cor pulmonale. With the initiation of mechanical ventilation, it is easy to set tidal volume too large and inspiratory times too long, promoting dynamic hyperinflation.[210] Every effort should be made to minimize this life-threatening complication. Cardiovascular management is to reduce RV wall strain and maintain or improve RV coronary perfusion. These topics require extensive review, but certain aspects are briefly summarized here. First, one almost always sees acute elevations of Pra, often accompanied by acute tricuspid regurgitation at end-inspiration. If a pulmonary artery catheter is present, Pra will equal or exceed pulmonary artery occlusion pressure. Furthermore, if the catheter has the ability to measure RV ejection fraction, it almost always reduced (<40%). Importantly, acute volume infusions will only compromise the dilated right ventricle further, such that both stroke volume and RV ejection fraction are decreased. These are clear signs of impending or existing cardiovascular collapse secondary to acute cor pulmonale. Because most RV myocardial blood flow occurs in systole, maintaining aortic pressure higher than pulmonary artery pressure to sustain RV myocardial perfusion is an essential aspect of the initial cardiovascular management.

LEFT-VENTRICULAR FAILURE

Although COPD is usually characterized by right-sided dysfunction owing to the alterations in pulmonary vascular biology, these patients tend to be smokers, elderly, and male, three demographic qualities placing them at high risk of coronary artery disease. With the exception of intubation-induced hypotension and reactive tachycardia, the risk of LV ischemia during intubation and sustained mechanical ventilation is relatively low in these patients. Because they are usually volume overloaded with reduced cardiac reserve before intubation, these patients usually benefit from a combined marked reduction in metabolic demands and a reduced ventricular interdependence owing to the smaller RV volumes when being supported on mechanical ventilation. Similarly, upon weaning, the risk of exposing occult LV failure can also occur. Patients with COPD may fail weaning attempts because their work of breathing exceeds their cardiovascular reserve.[211,212] Just as these patients cannot climb two flights of stairs, they may not be able to wean because of impaired cardiovascular reserve. Weaning-trial–associated hypoxemia or transient pulmonary edema are due to the increased cardiovascular demand on the heart caused by spontaneous ventilation, coupled with the augmented venous-return–associated increased intrathoracic blood volume induced by the negative swings in ITP and positive swings in intra-abdominal pressure. Beach et al demonstrated many years ago that heart failure patients who are ventilator dependent may be weaned after pharmacologic support of the heart.[140]

AUTO-PEEP

The hemodynamic effects of positive-pressure ventilation are caused by changes in ITP, not airway pressure. This concept greatly influences our analysis of heart-lung interactions in patients with lung disease. As discussed early in this chapter, the primary determinants of the hemodynamic responses to ventilation are changes in ITP and lung volume,[3] not Paw. The relation between Paw, ITP, pericardial pressure, and lung volume varies with spontaneous ventilatory effort, lung compliance, and chest-wall compliance. Lung parenchymal compliance and thoracic compliance determine the relation between end-expiratory Paw and lung volume in the sedated and paralyzed patient. If a ventilated patient, however, actively resists lung inflation or sustains expiratory muscle activity at end-inspiration, then end-inspiratory Paw will exceed resting Paw for that lung volume. Similarly, if the patient activity prevents full exhalation by expiratory braking, then for the same end-expiratory Paw, lung volume may be much higher than that predicted from end-expiratory Paw values alone. Finally, even if inspiration is passive and no increased airway resistance is present, Paw may rapidly increase over minutes as chest wall compliance decreases. During inspiration, positive-pressure Paw increases as a function of both total thoracic compliance and airway resistance. Patients with marked bronchospasm will display a peak Paw greater than end-inspiratory (plateau) Paw. The difference between measured Paw and alveolar pressure is called *auto-PEEP*. Changes in transpulmonary pressure and total thoracic compliance alter functional residual capacity (FRC), and FRC is the primary volume about which all hemodynamic interactions revolve.

FRC is a nefarious value. When one reclines from a standing position, FRC may decrease by as much as 500 ml in a 70-kg healthy man. PEEP and CPAP increase FRC by offsetting Palv. If a subject does not have sufficient time to exhale completely to FRC, however, then the next breath will stack upon the extra lung volume already present. Bergman described this concept of dynamic hyperinflation many years ago.[210] Pepe et al[210] coined the term "occult PEEP" to illustrate the similarities between dynamic hyperinflation (also called occult PEEP) and extrinsically applied PEEP. Auto-PEEP is not measured by the ventilator, as part of the usual variables, and may go unappreciated. Yet, it functions identically to extrinsic PEEP in altering pulmonary vascular resistance and recruiting alveoli. The hemodynamic effect of this hyperinflation is to increase ITP and pulmonary vascular resistance and compress the heart within the cardiac fossa. Thus, one may see Pra and pulmonary artery occlusion pressure progressively increase as arterial pulse pressure and urine output decrease. One may then make the erroneous diagnosis of acute heart failure, when in fact all that is occurring is hyperinflation and the unaccounted increase in ITP. If one adds extrinsic PEEP to the ventilator circuit of subjects with auto-PEEP, no measurable hemodynamic effects are seen until extrinsic PEEP exceeds auto-PEEP levels.[213] These data suggest that auto-PEEP and extrinsic PEEP have identical hemodynamic effects during controlled ventilation.

During assisted ventilator support or spontaneous breathing, however, auto-PEEP adds an additional elastic workload on the respiratory muscles. This increased workload is often the cause of failure to wean from mechanical ventilation because spontaneous breathing trials are often associated with tachypnea, which prevents adequate time for complete exhalation. Clinical signs and symptoms suggestive of hemodynamically significant auto-PEEP include increased anxiety and agitation during spontaneous breathing associated with a marked increase in respiratory efforts and paradoxical chest wall motion. Because changes in ITP are occurring even though no air movement initially takes place, an arterial pressure recording will show immediate decreases in diastolic pressure without changes in pulse pressure until the inspiratory air flow finally occurs. Finally, by adding progressive increases in extrinsic PEEP to the ventilator circuit during a spontaneous breathing trial, changes in arterial diastolic pressure and pulse pressure will start to occur in unison as ventilatory efforts re-couple with the ability to cause airflow.

ACUTE RESPIRATORY DISTRESS SYNDROME AND ACUTE LUNG INJURY

Patients with ALI have decreased aerated lung volumes owing at alveolar collapse and flooding secondary to the lung injury. Because lung expansion during positive-pressure inspiration pushes on the surrounding structures, distorting them, this expansion causes thoracic surface pressures to increase. The degree of lateral chest wall, diaphragmatic, or juxtacardiac ITP increase, relative to each other as lung volume increases, will be a function of the compliance and inertness of their opposing structures.[63] Changes in pleural

pressure (Ppl) induced by positive-pressure inflation are different among differing lung regions (Fig. 36-11). Pleural pressure close to the diaphragm increases least during inspiration, and juxtacardiac Ppl increases most, presumably because the diaphragm is very compliant whereas the mediastinal contents are not. If abdominal distention develops, however, then the diaphragm will become relatively noncompliant and ITP will increase similarly across the entire thorax. Increasing Paw to overcome chest wall stiffness (abdominal distention) in secondary ARDS should produce a greater increase in ITP, with greater hemodynamic consequences, but it should not improve gas exchange, because the alveoli are not damaged. Conversely, if lung compliance is reduced, as in primary ARDS, then for a similar increase in Paw, ITP will increase less, creating fewer hemodynamic effects, but also recruiting more collapsed and injured alveolar units, improving gas exchange. If lung injury induces alveolar flooding or increased pulmonary parenchymal stiffness, then greater increases in Paw will be required to distend the lungs to a constant end-inspiratory volume. Romand et al[74] demonstrated that although Paw increased more during ALI than under control conditions for a constant tidal volume, the increases in lateral chest wall Ppl and pericardial pressure (Ppc) were equivalent for the two conditions if tidal volume was held constant (Fig. 36-12). The primary determinant of the increase in Ppl and Ppc during positive-pressure ventilation is lung volume change, not Paw change.[76]

The distribution of alveolar collapse and lung compliance in ALI is nonhomogeneous. Accordingly, lung distention during positive-pressure ventilation must reflect overdistention of some regions at the expense of poorly compliant regions because aerated lung units display a normal specific compliance.[77] Accordingly, Paw will reflect distention of lung units that were aerated before inspiration, but may not reflect the degree of lung inflation of non-aerated lung units. Pressure-limited ventilation assumes that this is the case and aims to limit Paw in ALI states so as to prevent overdistention of aerated lung units, with the understanding that tidal volume, and thus minute ventilation, must decrease. Thus, pressure-limited ventilation will hypoventilate the lungs, leading to "permissive" hypercapnia. In an animal model of ALI, when tidal volume was either kept constant at preinjury levels or reduced to match preinjury plateau pressure (pressure-limited ventilation), both Ppl and Ppc increased less as compared with either the pre–lung injury state or the ALI state, but with tidal volume set at the preinjury level.[74] These points underlie the fundamental hemodynamic differences seen when different ventilator modes are compared to each other.

ALI is often nonhomogeneous, with aerated areas of the lung displaying normal specific compliance. Accordingly, vascular structures that are distended will have a greater increase in their surrounding pressure than collapsible structures that do not distend.[215] Romand et al[74] and Scharf et al,[75] however, demonstrated that, despite this nonhomogeneous alveolar distention, if tidal volume is kept constant, then Ppl increases equally, independently of the mechanical properties of the lung. Thus, under constant tidal volume conditions, changes in peak and mean Paw will reflect changes in the mechanical properties of the lungs and

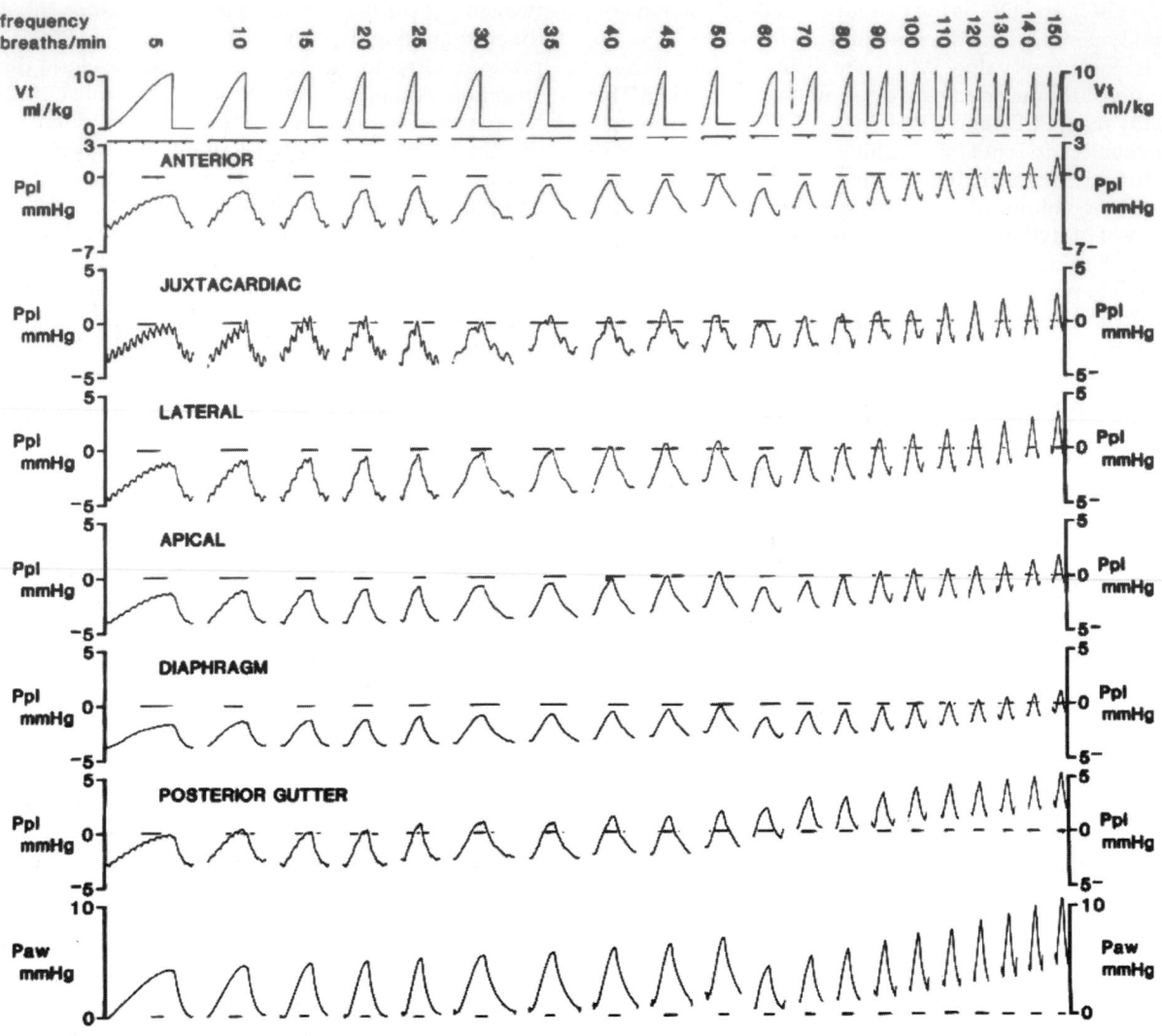

FIGURE 36-11 Effect of increasing ventilatory frequency on regional pleural pressure (Ppl) changes in the lung of an intact dog. Ppl (mean ± SE) for 6 pleural regions of the right hemothorax of an intact supine canine model. (*Reproduced, with permission, from Novak et al.[63]*)

patient coordination, but may not reflect changes in ITP. Similarly, these changes in Paw may not alter global cardiovascular dynamics.

Positive-pressure ventilation can also have beneficial effects on hemodynamics in patients with ALI. Intentional hyperinflation in patients with ALI, induced by the use of PEEP to treat hypoxemia, may reduce pulmonary vascular resistance, if lung recruitment and aeration of hypoxic alveolar units reduce hypoxic pulmonary vasoconstriction; eventually, however, pulmonary vascular resistance must increase as all lung units are expanded above their normal resting lung volumes.[216] Applying the least amount of PEEP necessary to achieve an adequate Pa_{O_2} and $F_{I_{O_2}}$ combination should be associated with the least detrimental hemodynamic effects.

CONGESTIVE HEART FAILURE

CHF patients are difficult to wean from the ventilator because the increases in work of breathing, venous return,

and intrathoracic blood volume during the transition between assisted to spontaneous breathing may cause acute pulmonary edema. Rasanen et al documented that decreasing levels of ventilator support in patients with myocardial ischemia and acute LV failure worsened ischemia and promoted the development of pulmonary edema.[168,217] These acute LV failure effects of spontaneous ventilation could be minimized by preventing spontaneous inspiratory effort–induced negative swings in ITP by the use of CPAP while still allowing the subject to continue to breathe spontaneously.[170] Thus, in these patients, it is not the work of breathing that is inducing heart failure, but the negative swings in ITP. Presumably, the ability of CPAP to decrease ventricular afterload explains the beneficial effects of CPAP during weaning trials.

If increases in ITP during positive-pressure ventilation decrease LV afterload, why then does positive-pressure ventilation not induce an increase in cardiac output in patients with CHF? The answer is that it does. Increases in cardiac output with increases in Paw suggest the presence of

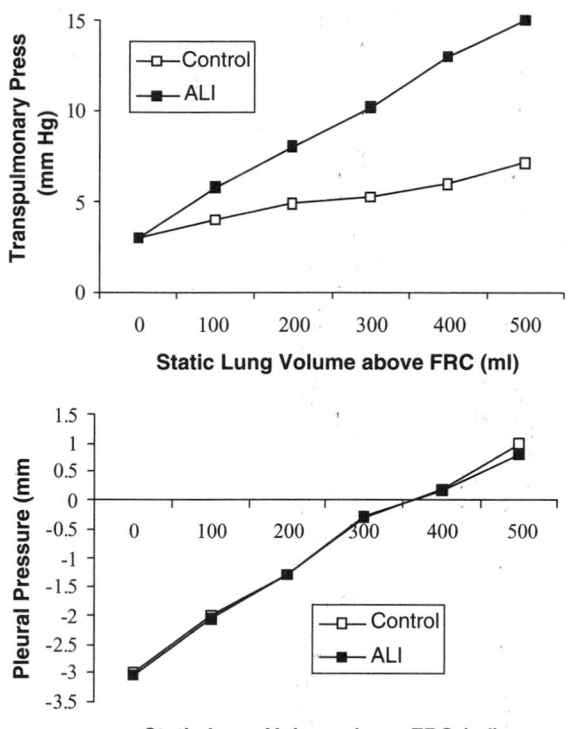

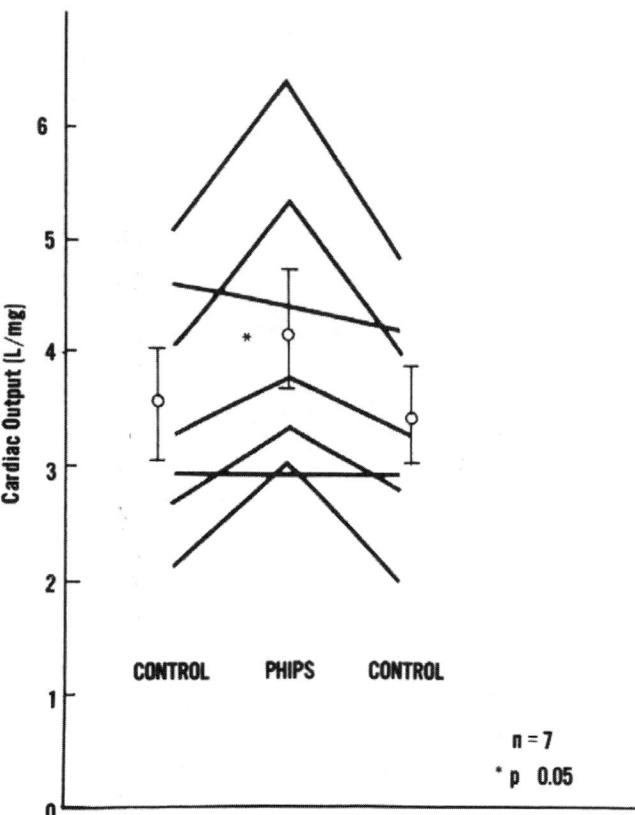

FIGURE 36-12 Relation between transpulmonary pressure (*top*) and pleural pressure (*bottom*) and lung volume as lung volume is progressively increased above functional residual capacity (FRC) in control and oleic acid–induced acute lung injury (ALI) conditions in a canine model. Note that despite greater increases in transpulmonary pressure for the same increase in lung volume during ALI as compared to control conditions, pleural pressure increases similarly during both control and ALI conditions for the same increase in lung volume. (*Reproduced, with permission, from Romand et al.*[74])

FIGURE 36-13 Effect of phasic high intrathoracic pressure support (PHIPS) on cardiac output in ventilator-dependent patients. (*Reprinted, with permission, from Pinsky et al.*[221])

CHF.[169,174] Grace et al[218] noted that adding PEEP to patients with CHF did not decrease cardiac output; cardiac output actually increased if pulmonary artery occlusion pressure exceeded 18 mmHg. Similarly, Calvin et al[219] noted that patients with cardiogenic pulmonary edema had no decrease in cardiac output when given PEEP.[220] Finally, Pinsky et al demonstrated that ventilator-induced increases in ITP, using ventilatory frequencies of 12–20/minute (phasic high intrathoracic pressure support; PHIPS) (Fig. 36-13), and increases in ITP synchronized to occur with each cardiac systole (cardiac cycle–specific, where ventilatory frequency equals heart rate) greatly increased cardiac output in patients with cardiomyopathy[221,222] (Fig. 36-14). Note the similarities of the increase in mean cardiac output seen with systolic synchronized ventilation (see Fig. 36-11) with the cardiovascular responses to similar systolic synchronized ventilation shown in Fig. 36-8, which was derived from an acute animal model, wherein many more hemodynamic measurements were made.

These beneficial effects do not require endotracheal intubation. They are realized with the use of mask CPAP. In fact, CPAP levels as low as 5 cmH$_2$O can increase cardiac output in patients with CHF. Cardiac output, how-

ever, decreases with similar levels of CPAP in both normal subjects and patients with heart failure who are not volume overloaded. Nasal CPAP can also accomplish the same results in patients with obstructive sleep apnea and heart failure,[223] although the benefits do not appear to be related to changes in obstructive breathing pattern.[224] Prolonged nighttime nasal CPAP can selectively improve respiratory muscle strength and LV contractile function in patients who have pre-existent heart failure.[225,226] These benefits are associated with reductions of serum catecholamine levels.[227] There is no special effect of non-intubated CPAP on cardiac performance. In patients with hypovolemic CHF, as manifest by a pulmonary artery occlusion pressure $\leq$12 mmHg, CPAP and biphasic positive airway pressure (BiPAP), at the same mean airway pressure, decrease cardiac output equally.[228]

If noninvasive ventilation improves LV performance in patients with both obstructive sleep apnea and CHF, can noninvasive ventilation then be useful to treat acute cardiogenic pulmonary edema? Several workers have asked this question. Rasanen et al[169] used mask CPAP to treat patients with acute coronary insufficiency and cardiogenic pulmonary edema. They demonstrated that myocardial ischemia was reversed by CPAP, but only after the level of CPAP was adjusted to prevent negative swings in ITP. CPAP levels below this threshold did not improve LV performance. The amount of CPAP needed to abolish negative

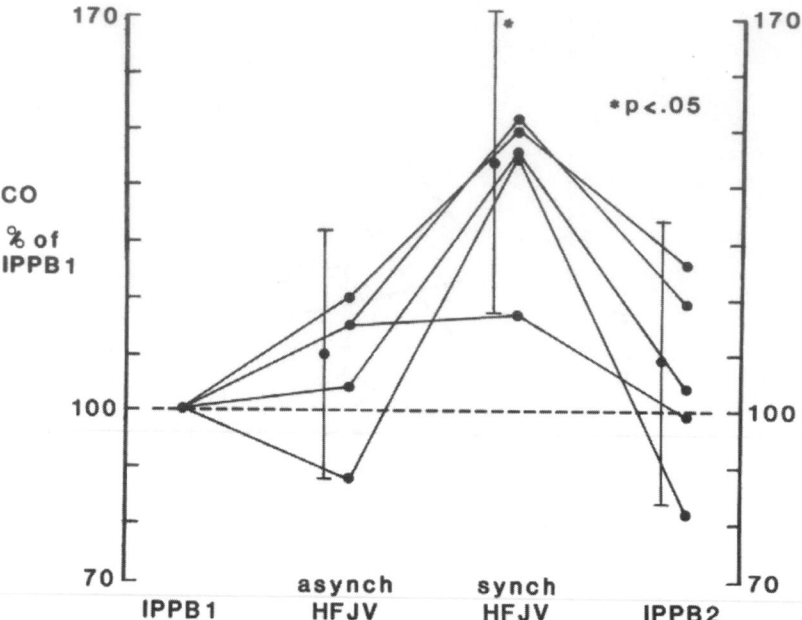

FIGURE 36-14 Effect of cardiac cycle–specific increases in airway pressure, delivered by a synchronized high-frequency jet ventilator in intraoperative patients with congestive heart failure. Note that for the same mean airway pressure, tidal volume, and ventilatory frequency, the placement of the inspiratory pulse within the cardiac cycle has profoundly different effects. (*Reproduced, with permission, from Pinsky et al.[222]*)

swings in ITP, however, varied among patients. This is important, because subsequent clinical trials of CPAP to treat cardiogenic pulmonary edema used only fixed levels of CPAP, not CPAP levels titrated to abolish negative swings in ITP. Several early studies demonstrated that mask CPAP improved gas exchange and reduced the need for endotracheal intubation.[229,230] Mortality and hospital length of stay, however, were usually similar among patients on CPAP and conventional O_2,[231–233] suggesting that prevention of intubation is not a determinant of outcome from cardiogenic pulmonary edema. Consistent with an afterload-sparing effect of blocking negative swings in ITP, both static CPAP and BiPAP, which decrease equally the negative swings in ITP, demonstrated similar improvement in oxygenation without changing long-term outcome.[234] The lack of long-term benefit from CPAP therapy in acute cardiogenic pulmonary edema underscores the importance of separating outcome from acute processes determined by clinical symptoms (cardiogenic pulmonary edema) from the underlying pathology (congestive heart failure). In fact, it would be surprising if mask CPAP would have improved outcome as long as endotracheal intubation remained the default option for CHF. Still, abolishing negative swings in ITP acutely improves cardiac function in heart failure patients.

However, one cannot readily apply increasing ITP to augment LV performance because the effect rapidly becomes self-limited as venous return declines. This is analogous to phase 3 of the Valsalva maneuver. The effect of removing large negative levels of ITP, however, does not have the same effect on venous return as does increasing ITP. Because venous return is flow-limited below an ITP of zero, removing large negative swings in ITP will not alter venous return. The effect, however, of removing negative ITP swings on LV afterload will be identical millimeter of mercury for millimeter of mercury to adding positive ITP. Thus, any relative increase in ITP from very negative values to zero, relative to atmosphere, will minimally alter venous return, but markedly reduce LV afterload. Removing large negative swings in ITP, by either bypassing upper airway obstruction (endotracheal intubation) or instituting mechanical ventilation or PEEP-induced loss of spontaneous inspiratory efforts, should selectively reduce LV afterload, without significantly decreasing either venous return or cardiac output.[92,79,105,119,154,169,235] The cardiovascular benefits of positive airway pressure on nonintubated patients can be seen by withdrawing negative swings in ITP, as created by using increasing levels of CPAP.[236,237]

INTRAOPERATIVE STATE

Most elective surgical patients are kept relatively hypovolemic before surgery because of the risk of aspiration pneumonia during induction. They are not allowed food for 8–12 hours nor anything by mouth for 6 hours before surgery, and they rarely are given intravenous fluids before coming into the operating room. Moreover, with the induction of general anesthesia, basal sympathetic tone is markedly reduced. Thus, it is amazing how little cardiovascular compromise occurs in this setting. Two factors may explain the lack of significant cardiovascular compromise. First, almost all patients are supine, and do not perform work; thus venous return is maximized, and metabolic demand reduced. Second, almost all anesthesiologists insert an intravenous catheter to infuse anesthetic agents; usually they use this port to rapidly infuse large volumes of saline as part of the induction. Nevertheless, to the extent that vasomotor tone is compromised, venous return will decrease, causing cardiac output to become a limiting cardiovascular variable.

Independent of these initial blood volume and vasomotor tone effects, other common events can profoundly alter cardiovascular status. Both laparotomies and thoracotomies cause cardiac output to decrease by altering heart-lung interactions. Recall that the primary determinant of venous return is the pressure gradient between the venous reservoirs and Pra (see Fig. 36-2). Because a little over half of the venous blood resides in the abdomen, intra-abdominal pressure represents a significant determinant of mean systemic pressure.[102] This point was illustrated earlier, when it was shown that diaphragmatic descent during positive-pressure inspiration pressurized the intra-abdominal compartment, minimizing the decrease in venous return predicted by the associated increase in Pra (see Fig. 36-5). During abdominal surgery, however, the act of opening the abdomen and keeping it open abolishes the effect of diaphragmatic descent on intra-abdominal pressure. Accordingly, an open laparotomy induces a fall in cardiac output by making the pressure gradient for venous return dependent only on changes in Pra. From the opposite side of the venous return curve, changes in Pra are dependent on changes in ITP. Thus, an open thoracotomy, by abolishing the end-expiratory negative ITP, induces an immediate increase in Pra, causing cardiac output to decrease.

During general anesthesia, most intubated patients have their ventilation completely controlled by the ventilator. Under these conditions, assuming that tidal volume and PEEP remain constant, the hemodynamic effects of ventilation remain remarkably constant. Thus, one can use this phasic-forcing function to assess preload responsiveness, as discussed above. Specifically, positive-pressure ventilation induces a cyclic change in LV end-diastolic volume, owing to complex and often different processes. But these ventilation phase–specific changes in LV end-diastolic pressure occur anyway. Thus, in subjects whose global cardiovascular system is preload responsive, they will also manifest ventilation-induced changes in LV stroke volume and arterial pulse pressure. When quantified as positive-pressure–induced stroke volume variation or pulse-pressure variation, numerous studies have shown that these measures reflect both robust and profoundly simple means to assess preload responsiveness.[180–182,188,238,239]

Steps to Limit or Overcome Detrimental Heart-Lung Interactions

Two major approaches can be used to minimize deleterious cardiovascular interactions while augmenting the beneficial ones: those focusing on ventilation, and those focusing on cardiovascular status. All these approaches, however, are relative.

MINIMIZE WORK OF BREATHING

The most obvious technique for minimizing the work of breathing during spontaneous ventilation is to decrease airway resistance and recruit collapsed alveolar units. Because ventilation is exercise, minimizing the metabolic load on the respiratory muscles allows blood flow to be diverted to other organ systems in need of O_2. Bronchodilator therapy and recruitment maneuvers accomplish these effects.

MINIMIZE NEGATIVE SWINGS IN INTRATHORACIC PRESSURE

It is important to minimize the negative swings in ITP that reflect increased work of breathing during spontaneous breathing, because these swings account for the increased intrathoracic blood volume and increased LV afterload, and can induce acute LV failure and pulmonary edema. Still, allowing normal negative swings in ITP at end-expiration promotes normal venous return and maintains cardiac output higher than during positive-pressure ventilation in patients with hemorrhagic shock. Although promoting inspiratory strain to augment cardiac output is the logical extension of this concept,[240] this logic is self-limiting because the associated increase in metabolic demand exceeds the associated increase in blood flow. Numerous studies, cited above, document the improvements in myocardial O_2 demand, ischemia, and cardiovascular reserve achieved by this strategy. All these effects can be achieved in nonintubated patients using noninvasive mask CPAP and BiPAP.

PREVENT HYPERINFLATION

By preventing overdistension of the lungs, pulmonary vascular resistance will not increase, cardiac filling will not be impeded, and venous return will remain at or near maximal levels. Several important clinical caveats, however, need to be listed. First, hyperinflation is not PEEP. Recruitment of collapsed alveoli and stabilization of injured alveoli in an aerated state often requires the use of PEEP, which itself may reduce pulmonary vascular resistance. Overdistension of aerated alveoli to further improve gas exchange, however, will increase pulmonary vascular resistance. Thus, one should use the lowest level of PEEP required to create adequate oxygenation. Second, in CHF, lung inflation improves LV ejection effectiveness[241] and may itself reflect a type of ventricular support.

FLUID RESUSCITATION DURING INITIATION OF POSITIVE-PRESSURE VENTILATION

The act of endotracheal intubation is often accompanied by complex manipulations, including the use of anesthetic and analgesic agents, and institution of positive-pressure ventilation. The consequent reduction in sympathetic tone and increase in Pra act synergistically to reduce venous return. These combined effects can be life-saving in patients with cardiogenic pulmonary edema. In otherwise healthy subjects or in patients with hypovolemia (e.g., trauma), however, these additive effects can induce hypovolemic cardiovascular collapse. The clinician should be prepared to rapidly infuse intravascular volume to potentially hypovolemic patients during the act of endotracheal intubation.

PREVENT VOLUME OVERLOAD DURING WEANING

The transition from positive-pressure to spontaneous ventilation must reduce ITP and increase volume of oxygen utilization. Thus, patients are at risk of developing or worsening pulmonary edema, myocardial ischemia, and acute LV failure during weaning trials. Before initiating a spontaneous breathing trial, it is important to ensure that a patient is not volume overloaded. Steps to minimize volume overload include limiting fluids before weaning trials, forced diuresis in the setting of overt volume overload and pleural effusion, and gradual reduction in the level of positive-pressure through the use of partial support modes, so as to allow fluid shifts to be excreted in the urine. Furthermore, in patients with markedly increased total body water, common in critically ill patients after aggressive fluid resuscitation during the early phases of an illness or in the immediate postoperative state, fluid resorption often accelerates as Pra decreases. Thus, attention to subsequent fluid overload during the days following extubation, and the use of limited intravascular fluids or forced diuresis is often needed to prevent reintubation. A clinician cannot presume that a patient with clear evidence of increased extravascular water has been successfully extubated when an endotracheal tube is removed or even several hours later. Although detailed studies of the pathophysiology of extubation failure have not been conducted, and while failure may be multifactorial, cardiovascular compromise secondary to subsequent volume overload from either fluid resorption or intravascular volume loading (often manifest by increased secretions, wheezing, and hypoxemia) is likely to be one important cause.

AUGMENT CARDIAC CONTRACTILITY

Because breathing is exercise, a spontaneous breathing trial may precipitate acute coronary insufficiency, even in patients who are successfully weaned from the ventilator. Over 30 years ago, Beach et al[140] demonstrated that many ventilator-dependent patients can be successfully weaned if they are simultaneously given a positive inotropic agent, such as dobutamine. Although only case reports and no prospective clinical trials have ever been done to address this issue, many physicians support such patients with dobutamine infusions for 12–24 hours before a spontaneous breathing trial. If one were to use this approach, then the inotropic agent may still be needed following extubation and weaned thereafter, because the work of breathing may remain high even if the endotracheal tube is not contributing to the increase in airway resistance.

Important Unknowns

Perhaps the most important unknown in assessing the hemodynamic effect of ventilation is the assessment of cardiovascular reserve and the effects of breathing on hyperinflation and the swings in ITP. To date no set of physiologic variables derived from measures of respiratory performance or ventilatory reserve have proved reliable in predicting weaning outcome in the setting of acute ventricular failure. In large part, I believe, this failure reflects an underappreciation of the role that cardiovascular responsiveness plays in weaning and inadequate methods for assessing cardiovascular reserve. In essence, physicians have chosen an oversimplistic approach to weaning, and now institute blind daily spontaneous breathing trials to define whether

a patient is capable of weaning. Although this approach is commendable in its simplicity, it still places patients who would obviously fail such trials at risk of coronary ischemia, ongoing respiratory muscle fatigue, and impaired gas exchange secondary to LV failure and hydrostatic pulmonary edema. Moreover, pre-existing fatigue or ischemia-induced heart failure can also be causes of failure to wean as well as the consequences of such an approach. Because the breathing pattern can change in just one breath, and physiologically significant hyperinflation can occur in a single breath, it is probably impossible to predict with accuracy whether a patient can be weaned or not using static measures.

The Future

The future of heart-lung interactions is wedded to both new and evolving methods of mechanical ventilation and our increasing reliance on clinical trials, like the spontaneous breathing trial, to predict weaning success and the need for supplemental cardiovascular support. To the extent that new assisted techniques of ventilator support follow the principles of proportional assist ventilation they will limit the detrimental effects of positive-pressure ventilation and patient-ventilator synchrony, minimizing the work of breathing. Mask CPAP will need to be titrated to minimize negative swings in ITP. To the extent that mask CPAP abolishes negative swings in ITP, it promotes LV ejection efficiency and minimizes LV failure. The use of pressure-limited ventilation in patients with ALI has resulted in marked decreases in delivered tidal volume. Because increases in ITP are linked to changes in lung volume, these newer ventilator strategies must result in less cardiovascular dysfunction than were seen with use of higher tidal volumes and peak airway pressures, that were commonly used in the past.

Acute care medicine is evolving from a static treatment and monitoring center into a proactive diagnostic and treatment center. We now use pulse pressure and stroke volume variation during positive-pressure ventilation to identify those hemodynamically unstable patients who are likely to respond to a volume challenge with an increase in cardiac output, and by how much. In the future, patients would be better served if clinicians were to examine the immediate hemodynamic effects of spontaneous breathing trials before patients progressed to ventilatory and cardiovascular deterioration. Invasive and noninvasive measures of tissue oxygenation, using data derived from pulmonary artery catheters, central venous catheters, pulse oximetry, and newer evolving noninvasive technologies provide dynamic assessment of impending respiratory failure and its causes. The future is upon us, and will be led by firms that are developing newer noninvasive technologies, which address these specific issues.[241]

Summary and Conclusion

Our understanding of clinically relevant cardiopulmonary interactions has advanced far over the last 30 years. What was once cloaked with much mystery, now seems obvious. Still, complacency in the application of these principles at the bedside should be avoided. Just as we thought we knew all there was to know about COPD 15 years ago, the entire management scheme was altered with a better understanding of dynamic hyperinflation and auto-PEEP.[242] Similarly, the exact nature by which heart-lung interactions define myocardial ejection efficiency and myocardial O_2 requirements in both ALI states and severe airflow obstruction remain to be defined.

The hemodynamic effects of ventilation are multiple and complex, but can be grouped into four clinically relevant concepts. First, spontaneous ventilation is exercise. In patients with increased work of breathing, initiation of mechanical ventilation improves O_2 delivery to the remainder of the body by decreasing O_2 consumption. To the extent that mixed venous P_{O_2} increases, arterial P_{O_2} will also increase without any improvement in pulmonary gas exchange. Similarly, weaning from mechanical ventilation is a cardiovascular stress test. Patients who fail to wean exhibit cardiovascular insufficiency during the failed weaning attempts. Improving cardiovascular reserve or supplementing support with inotropic therapy may enable patients to wean.

Second, changes in lung volume alter autonomic tone and pulmonary vascular resistance, and high lung volumes compress the heart in the cardiac fossa, similarly to cardiac tamponade. As lung volume increases, so does the pressure difference between airway and pleural pressure. When this pressure difference exceeds pulmonary artery pressure, pulmonary vessels collapse as they pass from the pulmonary arteries into the alveolar space, increasing pulmonary vascular resistance. Thus, hyperinflation increases pulmonary vascular resistance and pulmonary artery pressure, which impede RV ejection. Decreases in lung volume below FRC, as occurs in ALI and alveolar collapse, also increases pulmonary vasomotor tone by the process of hypoxic pulmonary vasoconstriction. Recruitment maneuvers, PEEP, and CPAP may reverse hypoxic pulmonary vasoconstriction and reduce pulmonary artery pressure.

Third, spontaneous inspiration and spontaneous inspiratory efforts decrease intrathoracic pressure. Because diaphragmatic descent increases intra-abdominal pressure, these combined effects cause right atrial pressure inside the thorax to decrease, but venous pressure in the abdomen to increase, which markedly increases the pressure gradient for systemic venous return. Furthermore, the greater the decrease in intrathoracic pressure, the greater the increase in LV afterload for a constant arterial pressure. Mechanical ventilation, by abolishing the negative swings in intrathoracic pressure, selectively decreases LV afterload, as long as the increases in lung volume and intrathoracic pressure are small.

Finally, positive-pressure ventilation increases intrathoracic pressure. Because diaphragmatic descent increases intra-abdominal pressure, the decrease in the pressure gradient for venous return is less than would otherwise occur if the only change were an increase in right atrial pressure.[3] In hypovolemic states, however, positive-pressure ventilation can induce profound decreases in venous return. Increases in intrathoracic pressure decrease LV afterload and augment LV ejection. In patients with hypervolemic heart failure, this afterload-reducing effect can result in improved LV ejection, increased cardiac output, and reduced myocardial O_2 demand.

Acknowledgments

This work was supported by grants HL67181-02 and HL07820-06

References

1. Cournand A, Motley HL, Werko L, et al. Physiologic studies of the effect of intermittent positive pressure breathing on cardiac output in man. Am J Physiol 1948; 152:162–74.
2. Tyberg JV, Grant DA, Kingma I, et al. Effects of positive intrathoracic pressure on pulmonary and systemic hemodynamics. Respir Physiol 2000; 119:171–9.
3. Whittenberger JL, McGregor M, Berglund E, et al. Influence of state of inflation of the lung on pulmonary vascular resistance. J Appl Physiol 1960; 15:878–82.
4. Glick G, Wechsler AS, Epstein DE. Reflex cardiovascular depression produced by stimulation of pulmonary stretch receptors in the dog. J Clin Invest 1969; 48:467–72.
5. Paintal AS. Vagal sensory receptors and their reflex effects. Physiol Rev 1973; 53:59–88.
6. Anrep GV, Pascual W, Rossler R. Respiratory variations in the heart rate. In: The reflex mechanism of the respiratory arrhythmia. Proc R Soc Lond B Biol Sci 1936; 119:191–217.
7. Taha BH, Simon PM, Dempsey JA, Skatrud JB, Iber C. Respiratory sinus arrhythmia in humans: an obligatory role for vagal feedback from the lungs. J Appl Physiol 1995; 78:638–45.
8. Bernardi L, Calciati A, Gratarola A, et al. Heart rate-respiration relationship: computerized method for early detection of cardiac autonomic damage in diabetic patients. Acta Cardiol 1986; 41:197–206.
9. Persson MG, Lonnqvist PA, Gustafsson LE. Positive end-expiratory pressure ventilation elicits increases in endogenously formed nitric oxide as detected in air exhaled by rabbits. Anesthesiology 1995; 82:969–74.
10. Cassidy SS, Eschenbacher WI, Johnson Jr RL. Reflex cardiovascular depression during unilateral lung hyperinflation in the dog. J Clin Invest 1979; 64:620–26.
11. Daly MB, Hazzledine JL, Ungar A. The reflex effects of alterations in lung volume on systemic vascular resistance in the dog. J Physiol (London) 1967; 188:331–51.
12. Shepherd JT. The lungs as receptor sites for cardiovascular regulation. Circulation 1981; 63:1–10.
13. Stalcup SA, Mellins RB. Mechanical forces producing pulmonary edema in acute asthma. N Engl J Med 1977; 297:592–96.
14. Vatner SF, Rutherford JD. Control of the myocardial contractile state by carotid chemo- and baroreceptor and pulmonary inflation reflexes in conscious dogs. J Clin Invest 1978; 63:1593–601.
15. Karlocai K, Jokkel G, Kollai M. Changes in left ventricular contractility with the phase of respiration. J Auton Nerv Syst 1998; 73:86–92.
16. Rankin JS, Olsen CO, Arentzen CE, et al. The effects of airway pressure on cardiac function in intact dogs and man. Circulation 1982; 66:108–20.
17. Ashton JH, Cassidy SS. Reflex depression of cardiovascular function during lung inflation. J Appl Physiol 1985; 58:137–45.

18. Fuhrman BP, Everitt J, Lock JE. Cardiopulmonary effects of unilateral airway pressure changes in intact infant lambs. J Appl Physiol 1984; 56:1439–48.

19. Said SI, Kitamura S, Vreim C. Prostaglandins: Release from the lung during mechanical ventilation at large tidal ventilation. J Clin Invest 1972; 51:83a.

20. Bedetti C, Del Basso P, Argiolas C, Carpi A. Arachidonic acid and pulmonary function in a heart-lung preparation of guinea-pig. Modulation by PCO2. Arch Int Pharmacodyn Ther 1987; 285:98–116.

21. Berend N, Christopher KL, Voelkel NF. Effect of positive end-expiratory pressure on functional residual capacity: Role of prostaglandin production. Am Rev Respir Dis 1982; 126:641–47.

22. Pattern MY, Liebman PR, Hetchman HG. Humorally-mediated decreases in cardiac output associated with positive end-expiratory pressure. Microvasc Res 1977; 13:137–44.

23. Berglund JE, Halden E, Jakobson S, Svensson J. PEEP ventilation does not cause humorally mediated cardiac output depression in pigs. Intensive Care Med 1994; 20:360–64.

24. Payen DM, Brun-Buisson CJL, Carli PA, et al. Hemodynamic, gas exchange, and hormonal consequences of LBPP during PEEP ventilation. J Appl Physiol 1987; 62:61–70.

25. Frage D, de la Coussaye JE, Beloucif S, Fratacci MD, Payen DM. Interactions between hormonal modifications during peep-induced antidiuresis and antinatriuresis. Chest 1995; 107: 1095–100.

26. Frass M, Watschinger B, Traindl O, et al. Atrial natriuretic peptide release in response to different positive end-expiratory pressure levels. Crit Care Med 1993; 21:343–47.

27. Wilkins MA, Su XL, Palayew MD, Yamashiro Y, et al. The effects of posture change and continuous positive airway pressure on cardiac natriuretic peptides in congestive heart failure. Chest 1995; 107:909–15.

28. Shirakami G, Magaribuchi T, Shingu K, et al. Positive end-expiratory pressure ventilation decreases plasma atrial and brain natriuretic peptide levels in humans. Anesth Analg 1993; 77:1116–121.

29. Fletcher EC, Proctor M, Yu J, et al. Pulmonary edema develops after recurrent obstructive apneas. Am J Respir Crit Care Med 1999; 160:1688–96.

30. Chen L, Shi Q, Scharf SM. Hemodynamic effects of periodic obstructive apneas in sedated pigs with congestive heart failure. J Appl Physiol 2000; 88:1051–60.

31. Maughan WL, Shoukas AA, Sagawa K, Weisfeldt ML. Instantaneous pressure-volume relationships of the canine right ventricle. Circ Res 1979; 44:309–15.

32. Sibbald WJ, Driedger AA. Right ventricular function in disease states: Pathophysiologic considerations. Crit Care Med 1983; 11:339.

33. Piene H, Sund T. Does pulmonary impedance constitute the optimal load for the right ventricle? Am J Physiol 1982; 242: H154–60.

34. Pinsky MR. Determinants of pulmonary arterial flow variation during respiration. J Appl Physiol 1984; 56:1237–45.

35. Theres H, Binkau J, Laule M, et al. Phase-related changes in right ventricular cardiac output under volume-controlled mechanical ventilation with positive end-expiratory pressure. Crit Care Med 1999; 27: 953–8.

36. Johnston WE, Vinten-Johansen J, Shugart HE, Santamore WP. Positive end-expiratory pressure potentates the severity of canine right ventricular ischemia-reperfusion injury. Am J Physiol 1992; 262:H168–76.

37. Madden JA, Dawson CA, Harder DR. Hypoxia-induced activation in small isolated pulmonary arteries from the cat. J Appl Physiol 1985; 59:113–18.

38. Hakim TS, Michel RP, Chang HK. Effect of lung inflation on pulmonary vascular resistance by arterial and venous occlusion. J Appl Physiol 1982; 53:1110–15.

39. Quebbeman EJ, Dawson CA. Influence of inflation and atelectasis on the hypoxic pressure response in isolated dog lung lobes. Cardiovas Res 1976; 10:672–77.

40. Brower RG, Gottlieb J, Wise RA, Permutt W, Sylvester JT. Locus of hypoxic vasoconstriction in isolated ferret lungs. J Appl Physiol 1987; 63:58–65.

41. Hakim TS, Michel RP, Minami H, Chang K. Site of pulmonary hypoxic vasoconstriction studied with arterial and venous occlusion. J Appl Physiol 1983; 54:1298–302.

42. Marshall BE, Marshall C. A model for hypoxic constriction of the pulmonary circulation. J Appl Physiol 1988; 64:68–77.

43. Marshall BE, Marshall C. Continuity of response to hypoxic pulmonary vasoconstriction. J Appl Physiol 1980; 49:189–96.

44. Dawson CA, Grimm DJ, Linehan JH. Lung inflation and longitudinal distribution of pulmonary vascular resistance during hypoxia. J Appl Physiol 1979; 47:532–36.

45. Howell JBL, Permutt S, Proctor DF, et al. Effect of inflation of the lung on different parts of the pulmonary vascular bed. J Appl Physiol 1961; 16:71–76.

46. West JB, Dollery CT, Naimark A. Distribution of blood flow in isolated lung; relation to vascular and alveolar pressures. J Appl Physiol 1964; 19:713–24.

47. Canada E, Benumnof JL, Tousdale FR. Pulmonary vascular resistance correlated in intact normal and abnormal canine lungs. Crit Care Med 1982; 10:719–23.

48. Fuhrman BP, Everitt J, Lock JE. Cardiopulmonary effects of unilateral airway pressure changes in intact infant lambs. J Appl Physiol 1984; 56:1439–48.

49. Fuhrman BP, Smith-Wright DL, Kulik TJ, Lock JE. Effects of static and fluctuating airway pressure on the intact, immature pulmonary circulation. J Appl Physiol 1986; 60:114–22.

50. Thorvalson J, Ilebekk A, Kiil F. Determinants of pulmonary blood volume. Effects of acute changes in airway pressure. Acta Physiol Scand 1985; 125:471–79.

51. Hoffmann B, Jepsen M, Hachenberg T, Huth C, Welte T. Cardiopulmonary effects of non-invasive positive pressure ventilation (NPPV)—a controlled, prospective study. Thorac Cardiovasc Surg 2003; 51:142–46.

52. Lopez-Muniz R, Stephens NL, Bromberger-Barnea B, Permutt S, Riley RL. Critical closure of pulmonary vessels analyzed in terms of Starling resistor model. J Appl Physiol 1968; 24:625–35.

53. Block AJ, Boyson PG, Wynne JW. The origins of cor pulmonale, a hypothesis. Chest 1979; 75:109–14.

54. Vieillard-Baron A, Loubieres Y, Schmitt JM, et al. Cyclic changes in right ventricular output impedance during mechanical ventilation. J Appl Physiol 1999; 87:1644–50.

55. Hoffman EA, Ritman EL. Heart-lung interaction: effect on regional lung air content and total heart volume. Ann Biomed Eng 1987; 15:241–57.

56. Olson LE, Hoffman EA. Heart-lung interactions determined by electron beam x-ray CT in laterally recumbent rabbits. J Appl Physiol 1995; 78:417–27.

57. Grant BJB, Lieber BB. Compliance of the main pulmonary artery during the ventilatory cycle. J Appl Physiol 1992; 72:535–42.

58. Taylor RR, Corell JW, Sonnenblick EH, Ross Jr J. Dependence of ventricular distensibility on filling the opposite ventricle. Am J Physiol 1967; 213:711–18.

59. Brinker JA, Weiss I, Lappe DL, et al. Leftward septal displacement during right ventricular loading in man. Circulation 1980; 61:626–33.

60. Wise RA, Robotham JL, Summer WR. Effects of spontaneous ventilation on the circulation. Lung 1981; 159:175–92.

61. Takata M, Harasawa Y, Beloucif S, Robotham JL. Coupled vs. uncoupled pericardial restraint: effects on cardiac chamber interactions. J Appl Physiol 1997; 83:1799–813.

62. Butler J. The heart is in good hands. Circulation 1983; 67: 1163–68.

63. Novak RA, Matuschak GM, Pinsky MR. Effect of ventilatory frequency on regional pleural pressure. J Appl Physiol 1988; 65:1314–23.

64. Tsitlik JE, Halperin HR, Guerci AD, et al. Augmentation of pressure in a vessel indenting the surface of the lung. Ann Biomed Eng 1987; 15:259–84.

65. Cassidy SS, Wead WB, Seibert GB, Ramanathan M. Changes in left ventricular geometry during spontaneous breathing. J Appl Physiol 1987; 63:803–11.

66. Marini JJ, Culver BN, Butler J. Mechanical effect of lung distention with positive pressure on cardiac function. Am Rev Respir Dis 1980; 124:382–86.

67. Cassidy SS, Robertson CH, Pierce AK, et al. Cardiovascular effects of positive end-expiratory pressure in dogs. J Appl Physiol 1978; 4:743–49.

68. Conway CM. Hemodynamic effects of pulmonary ventilation. Br J Anaesth 1975; 47:761–66.

69. Jardin F, Farcot JC, Boisante L. Influence of positive end-expiratory pressure on left ventricular performance. N Engl J Med 1981; 304:387–92.

70. Berglund JE, Halden E, Jakobson S, Landelius J. Echocardiographic analysis of cardiac function during high PEEP ventilation. Intensive Care Med 1994; 20:174–80.

71. Pinsky MR, Vincent JL, DeSmet JM. Estimating left ventricular filling pressure during positive end-expiratory pressure in humans. Am Rev Respir Dis 1991; 143:25–31.

72. Shuey CB, Pierce AK, Johnson RL. An evaluation of exercise tests in chronic obstructive lung disease. J Appl Physiol 1969; 27:256–61.

73. Jayaweera AR, Ehrlich W. Changes of phasic pleural pressure in awake dogs during exercise: potential effects on cardiac output. Ann Biomed Eng 1987; 15:311–18.

74. Romand JA, Shi W, Pinsky MR. Cardiopulmonary effects of positive pressure ventilation during acute lung injury. Chest 1995; 108:1041–48.

75. Scharf SM, Ingram RH Jr. Effects of decreasing lung compliance with oleic acid on the cardiovascular response to PEEP. Am J Physiol 1977; 233:H635–41.

76. O'Quinn RJ, Marini JJ, Culver BH, et al. Transmission of airway pressure to pleural pressure during lung edema and chest wall restriction. J Appl Physiol 1985; 59:1171–77.

77. Gattinoni L, Mascheroni D, Torresin A, et al. Morphological response to positive end-expiratory pressure in acute respiratory failure. Intensive Care Med 1986; 12:137–42.

78. Rebuck AS, Read J. Assessment and management of severe asthma. Am J Med 1971; 51:788–98.

79. Guyton AC, Lindsey AW, Abernathy B, et al. Venous return at various right atrial pressures and the normal venous return curve. Am J Physiol 1957; 189:609–15.

80. Goldberg HS, Rabson J. Control of cardiac output by systemic vessels: Circulatory adjustments of acute and chronic respiratory failure and the effects of therapeutic interventions. Am J Cardiol 1981; 47:696.

81. Pinsky MR. Instantaneous venous return curves in an intact canine preparation. J Appl Physiol 1984; 56:765–71.

82. Kilburn KH. Cardiorespiratory effects of large pneumothorax in conscious and anesthetized dogs. J Appl Physiol 1963; 18: 279–83.

83. Chevalier PA, Weber KC, Engle JC, et al. Direct measurement of right and left heart outputs in Valsalva-like maneuver in dogs. Proc Soc Exper Biol Med 1972; 139:1429–37.

84. Guntheroth WC, Gould R, Butler J, et al. Pulsatile flow in pulmonary artery, capillary and vein in the dog. Cardiovascular Res 1974; 8:330–37.

85. Guntheroth WG, Morgan BC, Mullins GL. Effect of respiration on venous return and stroke volume in cardiac tamponade. Mechanism of pulsus paradoxus. Circ Res 1967; 20:381–90.

86. Guyton AC. Effect of cardiac output by respiration, opening the chest, and cardiac tamponade. In: Circulatory physiology: cardiac output and its regulation. Philadelphia: Saunders, 1963: 378–86.

87. Holt JP. The effect of positive and negative intrathoracic pressure on cardiac output and venous return in the dog. Am J Physiol 1944; 142:594–603.

88. Morgan BC, Abel FL, Mullins GL, et al. Flow patterns in cavae, pulmonary artery, pulmonary vein and aorta in intact dogs. Am J Physiol 1966; 210:903–9.

89. Morgan BC, Martin WE, Hornbein TF, et al. Hemodynamic effects of intermittent positive pressure respiration. Anesthesiology 1960; 27:584–90.

90. Scharf SM, Brown R, Saunders N, Green LH. Hemodynamic effects of positive pressure inflation. J Appl Physiol 1980; 49:124–31.

91. Jardin F, Vieillard-Baron A. Right ventricular function and positive-pressure ventilation in clinical practice: from hemodynamic subsets to respirator settings. Intensive Care Med 2003; 29:1426–34.

92. Braunwald E, Binion JT, Morgan WL, Sarnoff SJ. Alterations in central blood volume and cardiac output induced by positive pressure breathing and counteracted by metraminol (Aramine). Circ Res 1957; 5:670–75.

93. Scharf SM, Brown R, Saunders N, et al. Effects of normal and loaded spontaneous inspiration on cardiovascular function. J Appl Physiol 1979; 47:582–90.

94. Groeneveld AB, Berendsen RR, Schneider AJ, et al. Effect of the mechanical ventilatory cycle on thermodilution right ventricular volumes and cardiac output. J Appl Physiol 2000; 89:89–96.

95. Fessler HE, Brower RG, Wise RA, Permutt S. Effects of positive end-expiratory pressure on the canine venous return curve. Am Rev Respir Dis 1992; 146:4–10.

96. Takata M, Robotham JL. Effects of inspiratory diaphragmatic descent on inferior vena caval venous return. J Appl Physiol 1992; 72:597–607.

97. Matuschak GM, Pinsky MR, Rogers RM. Effects of positive end-expiratory pressure on hepatic blood flow and hepatic performance. J Appl Physiol 1987; 62:1377–83.

98. Chihara E, Hasimoto S, Kinoshita T, et al. Elevated mean systemic filling pressure due to intermittent positive-pressure ventilation. Am J Physiol 1992; 262:H1116–21.

99. Takata M, Wise RA, Robotham JL. Effects of abdominal pressure on venous return: abdominal vascular zone conditions. J Appl Physiol 1990; 69:1961–72.

100. Barnes GE, Laine GA, Giam PY, Smith EE, Granger HJ. Cardiovascular responses to elevation of intra-abdominal hydrostatic pressure. Am J Physiol 1985; 248:R208–13.

101. Lichtwarck-Aschoff M, Zeravik J, Pfeiffer UJ. Intrathoracic blood volume accurately reflects circulatory volume status in critically ill patients with mechanical ventilation. Intensive Care Med 1992; 18:142–45.

102. Van den Berg P, Jansen JRC, Pinsky MR. The effect of positive-pressure inspiration on venous return in volume loaded post-operative cardiac surgical patients. J Appl Physiol 2002; 92:1223–31.

103. Mang H, Kacmarek RM, Ritz R, Wilson RS, Kimball WP. Cardiorespiratory effects of volume- and pressure-controlled ventilation at various I/E ratios in an acute lung injury model. Am J Respir Crit Care Med 1995; 151:731–36.

104. Brecher GA, Hubay CA. Pulmonary blood flow and venous return during spontaneous respiration. Circ Res 1955; 3:40–214.

105. Sibbald WH, Calvin J, Driedger AA. Right and left ventricular preload, and diastolic ventricular compliance: Implications of therapy in critically ill patients. Critical Care State of the Art. Fullerton, Calif. Society of Critical Care, 1982, Vol. 3.

106. Magder S, Georgiadis G, Cheong T. Respiratory variation in right atrial pressure predict the response to fluid challenge. J Crit Care 1992; 7:76–85.

107. Terada N, Takeuchi T. Postural changes in venous pressure gradients in anesthetized monkeys. Am J Physiol 1993; 264:H21–H25.

108. Scharf S, Tow DE, Miller MJ, et al. Influence of posture and abdominal pressure on the hemodynamic effects of Mueller's maneuver. J Crit Care 1989; 4:26–34.

109. Tarasiuk A, Scharf SM. Effects of periodic obstructive apneas on venous return in closed-chest dogs. Am Rev Respir Dis 1993; 148:323–29.

110. Convertino VA, Ratliff DA, Ryan KL, et al. Hemodynamics associated with breathing through an inspiratory impedance threshold device in human volunteers. Crit Care Med. 2004; 32(9 Suppl):S381–6.

111. Shekerdemian LS, Bush A, Shore DF, Lincoln C, Redington AN. Cardiorespiratory responses to negative pressure ventilation after tetralogy of Fallot repair: a hemodynamic tool for patients with low-output state. J Am Coll Cardiol 1999; 33:549–55.

112. Lores ME, Keagy BA, Vassiliades T, et al. Cardiovascular effects of positive end-expiratory pressure (PEEP) after pneumonectomy in dogs. Ann Thorac Surg 1985; 40:464–73.

113. Grenvik A. Respiratory, circulatory and metabolic effects of respiratory treatment. Acta Anaesth Scand (Suppl) 1966.

114. Harken AH, Brennan MF, Smith N, Barsamian EM. The hemodynamic response to positive end-expiratory ventilation in hypovolemic patients. Surgery 1974; 76:786–93.

115. Bell RC, Robotham JL, Badke FR, Little WC, Kindred MK. Left ventricular geometry during intermittent positive pressure ventilation in dogs. J Crit Care 1987; 2:230–44.

116. Qvist J, Pontoppidan H, Wilson RS, Lowenstein E, Laver MB. Hemodynamic responses to mechanical ventilation with PEEP: the effects of hypovolemia. Anesthesiology 1975; 42:45–53.

117. Denault AY, J Gorcsan III, Deneault LG, Pinsky MR. Effect of positive pressure ventilation on left ventricular pressure-volume relationship. Anesthesiology 1993; 79:A315.

118. Buda AJ, Pinsky MR, Ingels NB, et al. Effect of intrathoracic pressure on left ventricular performance. N Engl J Med 1979; 301:453–59.

119. Sharpey-Schaffer EP. Effects of Valsalva maneuver on the normal and failing circulation. Br Med J 1955; 1:693–99.

120. Jardin FF, Farcot JC, Gueret P, et al. Echocardiographic evaluation of ventricles during continuous positive pressure breathing. J Appl Physiol 1984; 56:619–27.

121. Prec KJ, Cassels DE. Oximeter studies in newborn infants during crying. Pediatrics 1952; 9:756–61.

122. Peters J, Kindred MK, Robotham JL. Transient analysis of cardiopulmonary interactions II. Systolic events. J Appl Physiol 1988; 64:1518–26.

123. Pinsky MR, Matuschak GM, Klain M. Determinants of cardiac augmentation by increases in intrathoracic pressure. J Appl Physiol 1985; 58:1189–98.

124. Rankin JS, Olsen CO, Arentzen CE, et al. The effects of airway pressure on cardiac function in intact dogs and man. Circulation 1982; 66:108–20.

125. Robotham JL, Rabson J, Permutt S, Bromberger-Barnea B. Left ventricular hemodynamics during respiration. J Appl Physiol 1979; 47:1295–303.

126. Ruskin J, Bache RJ, Rembert JC, Greenfield JC Jr. Pressure-flow studies in man: Effect of respiration on left ventricular stroke volume. Circulation 1973; 48:79–85.

127. Olsen CO, Tyson GS, Maier GW, et al. Dynamic ventricular interaction in the conscious dog. Circ Res 1983; 52:85–104.

128. Tyberg JV, Taichman GC, Smith ER, et al. The relationship between pericardial pressure and right atrial pressure: An intraoperative study. Circulation 1986; 73:428–32.

129. Pinsky MR, Vincent JL, DeSmet JM. Effect of positive end-expiratory pressure on right ventricular function in man. Am Rev Respir Dis 1992; 146:681–87.

130. Dhainaut JF, Devaux JY, Monsallier JF, et al. Mechanisms of decreased left ventricular preload during continuous positive pressure ventilation in ARDS. Chest 1986; 90:74–80.

131. Janicki JS, Weber KT. The pericardium and ventricular interaction, distensibility and function. Am J Physiol 1980; 238:H494–H503.

132. Beyar R, Goldstein Y. Model studies of the effects of the thoracic pressure on the circulation. Ann Biomed Eng 1987; 15:373–83.

133. Pinsky MR, Summer WR, Wise RA, Permutt S, Bromberger-Barnea B. Augmentation of cardiac function by elevation of intrathoracic pressure. J Appl Physiol 1983; 54:950–55.

134. Pinsky MR, Matuschak GM, Bernardi L, Klain M. Hemodynamic effects of cardiac cycle-specific increases in intrathoracic pressure. J Appl Physiol 1986; 60:604–12.

135. Matuschak GM, Pinsky MR, Klain M. Hemodynamic effects of synchronous high-frequency jet ventilation during acute hypovolemia. J Appl Physiol 1986; 61:44–53.

136. Roussos C, Macklem PT. The respiratory muscles. N Engl J Med 1982; 307:786–97.

137. Cassidy SA, Wead WB, Seibert GB, Ramanathan M. Geometric left-ventricular responses to interactions between the lung and left ventricle: positive pressure breathing. Ann Biomed Eng 1987; 15:285–95.

138. Scharf SM, Brown R, Warner KG, Khuri S. Intrathoracic pressure and left ventricular configuration with respiratory maneuvers. J Appl Physiol 1989; 66:481–91.

139. Bromberger-Barnea B. Mechanical effects of inspiration on heart functions: A review. Fed Proc 1981; 40:2172–77.

140. Beach T, Millen E, Grenvik A. Hemodynamic response to discontinuance of mechanical ventilation. Crit Care Med 1973; 1:85–90.

141. Lemaire F, Teboul JL, Cinoti L, et al. Acute left ventricular dysfunction during unsuccessful weaning from mechanical ventilation. Anesthesiology 1988; 69:171–79.

142. Pinsky MR, Matuschak GM, Itzkoff JM. Respiratory augmentation of left ventricular function during spontaneous ventilation in severe left ventricular failure by grunting: An auto-EPAP effect. Chest 1984; 86:267–69.

143. Blaustein AS, Risser TA, Weiss JW, et al. Mechanisms of pulsus paradoxus during resistive respiratory loading and asthma. J Am Coll Cardiol 1986; 8:529–36.

144. Strohl KP, Scharf SM, Brown R, Ingram RH Jr. Cardiovascular performance during bronchospasm in dogs. Respiration 1987; 51:39–48.

145. Scharf SM, Graver LM, Balaban K. Cardiovascular effects of periodic occlusions of the upper airways in dogs. Am Rev Respir Dis 1992; 146:321–29.

146. Viola AR, Puy RJM, Goldman E. Mechanisms of pulsus paradoxus in airway obstruction. J Appl Physiol 1990; 68:1927–31.

147. Scharf SM, Graver LM, Khilnani S, Balaban K. Respiratory phasic effects of inspiratory loading on left ventricular hemodynamics in vagotomized dogs. J Appl Physiol 1992; 73:995–1003.

148. Latham RD, Sipkema P, Westerhof N, Rubal BJ. Aortic input impedance during Mueller maneuver: an evaluation of "effective strength." J Appl Physiol 1988; 65:1604–10.

149. Virolainen J, Ventila M, Turto H, Kupari M. Effect of negative intrathoracic pressure on left ventricular pressure dynamics and relaxation. J Appl Physiol 1995; 79:455–60.

150. Gomez A, Mink S. Interaction between effects of hypoxia and hypercapnia on altering left ventricular relaxation and chamber stiffness in dogs. Am Rev Respir Dis 1992; 146:313–20.

151. Kingma I, Smiseth OA, Frais MA, Smith ER, Tyberg JV. Left ventricular external constraint: relationship between pericardial, pleural and esophageal pressures during positive end-expiratory pressure and volume loading in dogs. Ann Biomed Eng 1987; 15:331–46.

152. Denault AY, Gorcsan J 3rd, Pinsky MR. Dynamic effects of positive-pressure ventilation on canine left ventricular pressure-volume relations. J Appl Physiol 2001; 91:298–308.

153. Abel FL, Mihailescu LS, Lader AS, Starr RG. Effects of pericardial pressure on systemic and coronary hemodynamics in dogs. Am J Physiol 1995; 268:H1593–605.

154. Khilnani S, Graver LM, Balaban K, Scharf SM. Effects of inspiratory loading on left ventricular myocardial blood flow and metabolism. J Appl Physiol 1992; 72:1488–92.

155. Satoh S, Watanabe J, Keitoku M, et al. Influences of pressure surrounding the heart and intracardiac pressure on the diastolic coronary pressure-flow relation in excised canine heart. Circ Res 1988; 63:788–97.

156. Marini JJ, Rodriguez RM, Lamb V. The inspiratory workload of patient-initiated mechanical ventilation. Am Rev Respir Dis 1986; 134:902–9.

157. Stock MC, David DW, Manning JW, Ryan ML. Lung mechanics and oxygen consumption during spontaneous ventilation and severe heart failure. Chest 1992; 102:279–83.

158. Kawagoe Y, Permutt S, Fessler HE. Hyperinflation with intrinsic PEEP and respiratory muscle blood flow. J Appl Physiol 1994; 77:2440–48.

159. Aubier M, Vires N, Sillye G, Mozes R, Roussos C. Respiratory muscle contribution to lactic acidosis in low cardiac output. Am Rev Respir Dis 1982; 126:648–52.

160. Vires N, Sillye G, Rassidakis A, et al. Effect of mechanical ventilation on respiratory muscle blood flow during shock. Physiologist 1980; 23:1–8.

161. Richard C, Teboul JL, Archambaud F, et al. Left ventricular dysfunction during weaning in patients with chronic obstructive pulmonary disease. Intensive Care Med 1994; 20:171–2.

162. Hurford WE, Lynch KE, Strauss HW, Lowenstein E, Zapol WM. Myocardial perfusion as assessed by thallium-201 scintigraphy during the discontinuation of mechanical ventilation in ventilator-dependent patients. Anesthesiology 1991; 74:1007–16.

163. Abalos A. Leibowitz AB, Distefano D, Halpern N, Iberti TJ. Myocardial ischemia during the weaning period. Am J Crit Care 1992; 1:32–6.

164. Chatila W, Ani S, Guaglianone D, et al. Cardiac ischemia during weaning from mechanical ventilation. Chest 1996; 109:1421–2.

165. Srivastava S, Chatila W, Amoateng-Adjepong Y, et al. Myocardial ischemia and weaning failure in patients with coronary disease: an update. Crit Care Med 1999; 27:2109–12.

166. Mohsenifar Z, Hay A, Hay J, Lewis MI, Koerner SK. Gastric intramural pH as a predictor of success or failure in weaning patients from mechanical ventilation. Ann Intern Med 1993; 119:794–98.

167. Jubran A, Mathru M, Dries D, Tobin MJ. Continuous recordings of mixed venous oxygen saturation during weaning from mechanical ventilation and the ramifications thereof. Am J Respir Crit Care Med 1998; 158:1763–9.

168. Rasanen J, Nikki P, Heikkila J. Acute myocardial infarction complicated by respiratory failure. The effects of mechanical ventilation. Chest 1984; 85:21–28.

169. Rasanen J, Vaisanen IT, Heikkila J, et al. Acute myocardial infarction complicated by left ventricular dysfunction and respiratory failure. The effects of continuous positive airway pressure. Chest 1985; 87:156–62.

170. Straus C, Lewis B, Isebey D, et al. Contribution of the endotracheal tube and the upper airway to breathing workload. Am J Respir Crit Care Med 1998; 157:23–30.

171. Suga H, Sagawa K. Instantaneous pressure-volume relationships and their ratio in the excised supported canine left ventricle. Circ Res 1974; 35:117–34.

172. Haney MF, Johansson G, Haggmark S, Biber B. Heart-lung interactions during positive-pressure ventilation: left ventricular pressure-volume momentary response to airway pressure elevation. Acta Anaesthesiol Scand 2001; 45:702–9.

173. Haney MF, Johansson G, Haggmark S, Biber B. Method of preload reduction during LVESPVR analysis of systolic function: airway pressure elevations and vena caval occlusion. Anesthesiology 2002; 97:436–46.

174. Abel JG, Salerno TA, Panos A, et al. Cardiovascular effects of positive pressure ventilation in humans. Ann Thorac Surg 1987; 43:36–43.

175. Baeaussier M, Coriat P, Perel A, et al. Determinants of systolic pressure variation in patients ventilated after vascular surgery. J Cardiothorac Vasc Anesth 1995; 9:547–51.

176. Coriat P, Vrillon M, Perel A, et al. A comparison of systolic blood pressure variations and echocardiographic estimates of end-diastolic left ventricular size in patients after aortic surgery. Anesth Analg 1994; 78:46–53.

177. Szold A, Pizov R, Segal E, Perel A. The effect of tidal volume and intravascular volume state on systolic pressure variation in ventilated dogs. Intensive Care Med 1989; 15:368–71.

178. Michard F, Teboul JL. Predicting fluid responsiveness in ICU patients: a critical analysis of the evidence. Chest 2002; 121:2000–8.

179. Michard F, Boussat S, Chemla D, et al. Relation between respiratory changes in arterial pulse pressure and fluid responsiveness in septic patients with acute circulatory failure. Am J Respir Crit Care Med 2000; 162:134–8.

180. Michard F, Boussat S, Chemla D, et al. Relation between respiratory changes in arterial pulse pressure and fluid responsiveness in septic patients with acute circulatory failure. Am J Respir Crit Care Med 2000; 162:134–38.

181. Reuter DA, Felbinger TW, Schmidt C, et al. Stroke volume variation for assessment of cardiac responsiveness to volume loading in mechanically ventilated patients after cardiac surgery. Intensive Care Med 2002; 28:392–98.

182. Slama M, Masson H, Teboul JL, et al. Monitoring of respiratory variations of aortic flow velocity using oesophageal Doppler. Intensive Care Med 2004; 30:1182–87.

183. Hansen RM, Viquerat CE, Matthay MA, et al. Poor correlation between pulmonary arterial wedge pressure and left ventricular end-diastolic volume after coronary artery bypass graft surgery. Anesthesiology 1986; 64:764–70.

184. Pinsky MR. Clinical significance of pulmonary artery occlusion pressure. Intensive Care Med 2003; 29:175–78.

185. Pinsky MR. Determinants of pulmonary artery flow variation during respiration. J Appl Physiol 1984; 56:1237–45.

186. Romand JA, Shi W, Pinsky MR. Cardiopulmonary effects of positive pressure ventilation during acute lung injury. Chest 1995; 108:1041–48.

188. Rooke GA, Schwid HA, Shapira Y. The effect of graded hemorrhage and intravascular volume replacement on systolic pressure variation in humans during mechanical and spontaneous ventilation. Anesth Analg 1995; 80:925–32.

190. Sylvester JT, Gilbert RD, Traystman RJ, Permutt S. Effects of hypoxia on the closing pressure of the canine systemic arterial circulation. Circ Res 1981; 49:980–87.

191. Pinsky MR, Guimond JG. The effects of positive end-expiratory pressure on heart-lung interactions. J Crit Care 1991; 6:1–11.

194. Dries DJ, Kumar P, Mathru M, et al. Hemodynamic effects of pressure support ventilation in cardiac surgery patients. Am Surg 1991; 57:122–25.

195. Sternberg R, Sahebjami H. Hemodynamic and oxygen transport characteristics of common ventilatory modes. Chest 1994; 105:1798–803.

196. Lessard MR, Guerot E, Lorini H, Lemaire F, Brochard L. Effects of pressure-controlled with different I:E ratios versus volume-controlled ventilation on respiratory mechanics, gas exchange and hemodynamics in patients with adult respiratory distress syndrome. Anesthesiology 1994; 80:983–91.

197. Chan K, Abraham E. Effects of inverse ratio ventilation on cardio-respiratory parameters in severe respiratory failure. Chest 1992; 102:1556–61.

198. Hartmann M, Rosberg B, Jonsson K. The influence of different levels of PEEP on peripheral tissue perfusion measured by subcutaneous and transcutaneous oxygen tension. Intensive Care Med 1992; 18:474–78.

199. Abraham E, Yoshihara G. Cardiorespiratory effects of pressure controlled ventilation in severe respiratory failure. Chest 1990; 98:1445–49.

200. Poelaert JI, Visser CA, Everaert JA, Koolen JJ, Colardyn FA. Acute hemodynamic changes of pressure-controlled inverse ratio ventilation in the adult respiratory distress syndrome. A transesophageal echocardiographic and Doppler study. Chest 1993; 104:214–19.

201. Blum RH, McGowan FX Jr. Chronic upper airway obstruction and cardiac dysfunction: anatomy, pathophysiology and anesthetic implications. Paediatr Anaesth 2004; 14:75–83.

202. Conzanitis DA, Leijala M, Pesoner E, Saki HA. Acute pulmonary edema due to laryngeal spasm. Anesthesia 1982; 37:1198–99.

203. Jackson FN, Rowland V, Corssen G. Laryngospasm-induced pulmonary edema. Chest 1980; 78:819–24.

204. Leatherman JW, Schwartz S. Pulmonary edema due to upper airway obstruction. South Med J 1983; 76:1058–60.

205. Lee KWT, Downes JJ. Pulmonary edema secondary to laryngospasm in children. Anesthesiology 1983; 59:347–49.

206. Oswalt CE, Gates GA, Holstrom FMG. Pulmonary edema as a complication of acute upper airway obstruction. JAMA 1977; 238:1833–35.

207. Poulton TJ. Laryngospasm-induced pulmonary edema. Chest 1981; 80:762–63.

208. Stradling J, Bolton P. Upper airways obstruction as cause of pulmonary edema. Lancet 1982; 1:1353–54.

209. Sofer S, Bar-Ziv J, Scharf SM. Pulmonary edema following relief of upper airway obstruction. Chest 1984; 86:401–3.

210. Bergman NA. Intrapulmonary gas trapping during mechanical ventilation at rapid frequencies. Anesthesiology 1969; 37:626–33.

211. Frazier SK, Stone KS, Schertel ER, Moser DK, Pratt JW. A comparison of hemodynamic changes during the transition from mechanical ventilation to T-piece, pressure support, and continuous positive airway pressure in canines. Biol Res Nurs 2000; 1:253–64.

212. Magder S, Erian R, Roussos C. Respiratory muscle blood flow in oleic acid-induced pulmonary edema. J Appl Physiol 1986; 60:1849–56.

213. Baigorri F, De Monte A, Blanch L, et al. Hemodynamic responses to external counterbalancing of auto-positive end-expiratory pressure in mechanically ventilated patients with chronic obstructive pulmonary disease. Crit Care Med 1994; 22:1782–91.

215. Globits S, Burghuber OC, Koller J, et al. Effect of lung transplantation on right and left ventricular volumes and function measured by magnetic resonance imaging. Am J Respir Crit Care Med 1994; 149:1000–4.

216. Calvin JE, Driedger AA, Sibbald WJ. Positive end-expiratory pressure (PEEP) does not depress left ventricular function in patients with pulmonary edema. Am Rev Respir Dis 1981; 124:121–28.

217. Rasanen J. Respiratory failure in acute myocardial infarction. Appl Cardiopulm Pathophysiol 1988; 2:271–79.

218. Grace MP, Greenbaum DM. Cardiac performance in response to PEEP in patients with cardiac dysfunction. Crit Care Med 1982; 20:358–60.

219. Calvin JE, Driedger AA, Sibbald WJ. Positive end-expiratory pressure (PEEP) does not depress left ventricular function in patients with pulmonary edema. Am Rev Respir Dis 1981; 124:121–28.

220. Loick HM, Wendt M, Rotker J, Theissen JL. Ventilation with positive end-expiratory airway pressure causes leukocyte retention in human lung. J Appl Physiol 1993; 75:301–6.

221. Pinsky MR, Summer WR. Cardiac augmentation by phasic high intrathoracic support (PHIPS) in man. Chest 1983; 84:370–75.

222. Pinsky MR, Marquez J, Martin D, Klain M. Ventricular assist by cardiac cycle-specific increases in intrathoracic pressure. Chest 1987; 91:709–15.

223. Lin M, Yang Y-F, Chiang H-T, et al. Reappraisal of continuous positive airway pressure therapy in acute cardiogenic pulmonary edema. Chest 1995; 107:1379–86.

224. Buckle P, Millar T, Kryger M. The effect of short-term nasal CPAP on Cheyne-Stokes respiration in congestive heart failure. Chest 1992; 102:31–35.

225. Granton JT, Naughton MT, Benard DC, et al. CPAP improves inspiratory muscle strength in patients with heart failure and central sleep apnea. Am J Respir Crit Care Med 1996; 153:277–82.

226. Kaneko Y, Floras JS, Usui K, et al. Cardiovascular effects of continuous positive airway pressure in patients with heart failure and obstructive sleep apnea. N Engl J Med 2003; 348:1233–41.

227. Naughton MT, Benard DC, Liu PP, et al. Effects of nasal CPAP on sympathetic activity in patients with heart failure and central sleep apnea. Am J Respir Crit Care Med 1995; 152:473–79.

228. Joet-Philip FF, Paganelli FF, Dutau HL, Saadjian AY. Hemodynamic effects of bi-level nasal positive airway pressure ventilation in patients with heart failure. Respiration 1999; 66:136–43.

229. Bersten AD, Holt AW, Vedig AE, Skowronski GA, Baggoley CJ. Treatment of severe cardiogenic pulmonary edema with continuous positive airway pressure delivered by facemask. N Engl J Med 1991; 325:1825–30.

230. Lin M, Yang YF, Chiang HT, et al. Reappraisal of continuous positive airway pressure therapy in acute cardiogenic pulmonary edema: short-term results and long term follow-up. Chest 1995; 107:1379–86.

231. Masip J, Betbese AJ, Paez J, et al. Non-invasive pressure support versus conventional oxygen therapy in acute cardiogenic pulmonary oedema: a randomized trial. Lancet 2000; 356:2126–32.

232. Giacomini M, Iapichino G, Cigada M, et al. Short-term noninvasive pressure support prevents ICU admittance in patients with acute cardiogenic pulmonary edema. Chest 2003; 123:2057–61.

233. Nava S, Carbone G, DiBattista N, et al. Noninvasive ventilation in cardiogenic pulmonary edema: A multicenter randomized trial. Am J Respir Crit Care Med 2003; 168:1432–7.

234. Park M, Sangean MC, de Volpe M, et al. Randomized, prospective trial of oxygen, continuous positive airway pressure,

and bilevel positive airway pressure by face mask in acute cardiogenic pulmonary edema. Crit Care Med 2004; 32: 2407–15.

235. Garpestad E, Parker JA, Katayama H, et al. Decrease in ventricular stroke volume at apnea termination is independent of oxygen desaturation. J Appl Physiol 1994; 77:1602–8.

236. DeHoyos A, Liu PP, Benard DC, Bradley TD. Haemodynamic effects of continuous positive airway pressure in humans with normal and impaired left ventricular function. Clin Sci Colch 1995; 88:173–78.

237. Naughton MT, Rahman MA, Hara K, Flora JS, Bradley TD. Effect of continuous positive airway pressure on intrathoracic and left ventricular transmural pressures in patients with congestive heart failure. Circulation 1995; 91:1725–31.

238. Pinsky MR. Functional hemodynamic monitoring: asking the right question. Intensive Care Med 2002; 28:386–88.

239. Pinsky MR. Probing the limits of arterial pulse contour analysis to predict preload-responsiveness. Anesth Analg 2003; 96:1245–47.

240. Convertino VA, Ratliff DA, Ryan KL, et al. Hemodynamics associated with breathing through an inspiratory impedance threshold device in human volunteers. Crit Care Med 2004; 32: S381–86.

241. Pinsky MR. The hemodynamic consequences of mechanical ventilation: An evolving story. Intensive Care Med 1997; 23:493–503.

242. Pinsky MR. Though the past darkly: Ventilatory management of patients with chronic obstructive pulmonary disease. Crit Care Med 1994; 22:1714–17.

243. Davis K Sr, Branson RD, Campbell RS, Porembka DT. Comparision of volume control and pressure control ventilation is flow wave from the difference? J Trauma 1996, 41:808–814.

244. Kichl M, Schiele C, Stenzinger W, Klenast J. Volume-controlled versus biphase positive airway pressure ventilation in leukopenic patients with severe respiratory failure. NVC Crit Care Med 1996; 24:780–4.

245. Singer M, Vermaat J, Hall G, Latter G, Patel M, Hemodynamic effects of manual hyperinflation in critically ill Mechanically Ventilated Patients Chest 1994; 106:1182–7.

246. Pepe PE, Marini JJ. Occult positive end-expiratory pressure in mechanically ventilated patients with airflow obstruction. Am Rev Respir Dis 1982; 126:166–170.

EFFECT OF MECHANICAL VENTILATION ON GAS EXCHANGE

ROBERT RODRÍGUEZ-ROISIN
ANTONI FERRER

PHYSIOLOGIC CONCEPTS
    Ventilation-Perfusion Relationships
    Inspired Oxygen
    Reabsorption Atelectasis
    Mixed Venous Oxygen
    Oxygen Consumption
    Cardiac Output
MULTIPLE INERT GAS ELIMINATION TECHNIQUE
NATURE OF GAS EXCHANGE IN DISEASE STATES
    Acute Respiratory Failure ("Wet Lung")
    Chronic Airflow Limitation ("Dry Lung")
    Acute Severe Asthma
EFFECT OF SPECIAL MODES OF VENTILATION
    High Frequency Ventilation
    Continuous-Flow Ventilation
CONCLUSION

The major function of the lung is to exchange physiologic (respiratory) gases, namely oxygen (O_2) and carbon dioxide (CO_2). Once the lungs fail as a gas exchanger, arterial hypoxemia, hypercapnia, or both appear and respiratory failure ensues. Arterial P_{O_2} (Pa_{O_2}) and P_{CO_2} (Pa_{CO_2}) are the measurable end-point variables used routinely by clinicians to manage patients with acute respiratory failure. When the latter is severe, mechanical ventilation is then considered the final strategy for treating patients.

Physiologic Concepts

Classically, the mechanisms of hypoxemia are alveolar hypoventilation, limitation of alveolar to end-capillary O_2 diffusion, intrapulmonary shunt, and ventilation-perfusion ($\dot{V}_A/\dot{Q}$) imbalance; the major causes of hypercapnia are alveolar hypoventilation and $\dot{V}_A/\dot{Q}$ mismatching.[1] Ideally, it would be of great interest to solely manage respiratory blood gas measurements, such as alveolar-arterial P_{O_2} dif-

R Rodríguez-Roisin MD, FRCPE is supported by the Red Respira-ISCIII–RTIC-03/11, the Comissionat per a Universitats i Recerca de la Generalitat de Catalunya (2001 SGR00386), and holds a career scientist award from the Generalitat de Catalunya.

ference [$P(\text{A-a})_{O_2}$], venous admixture ratio ($\dot{Q}_S/\dot{Q}_T$), and physiologic dead space (V_D/V_T), as a general marker of the overall function of the lung. Thus, impaired or improved results of these variables, whose principal merits are their simplicity and relative ease of measurement, could reflect impaired or improved pulmonary gas exchange. Unfortunately, all these variables reflect not only the state of the lung, but also the conditions under which the lung is operating. These conditions, which uniquely determine the P_{O_2} and P_{CO_2} in any single gas-exchange unit of the lung, are the $\dot{V}_A/\dot{Q}$ ratio, the composition of inspired gas, and the composition of mixed venous blood.[2] It is important to appreciate the key role played by these three factors governing the respiratory gases in any single gas-exchange unit.

VENTILATION-PERFUSION RELATIONSHIPS

Figure 37-1 illustrates the behavior of the end-capillary P_{O_2} and P_{CO_2} in a single functional unit of the lung as the $\dot{V}_A/\dot{Q}$ ratio is increased. As the $\dot{V}_A/\dot{Q}$ ratio rises above 0.1, P_{O_2} increases sharply, but there is little change in P_{CO_2} until a $\dot{V}_A/\dot{Q}$ ratio of 1.0 is approached. Notice that if the overall $\dot{V}_A/\dot{Q}$ ratio increases (right-shift) because minute ventilation increases and/or cardiac output decreases (common when ventilator support is applied), this will tend to increase P_{O_2} and decrease P_{CO_2}, other things being equal. Conversely, if minute ventilation decreases (or is inefficient) and/or cardiac output increases (discontinuing ventilator support or administering vasodilators) (left-shift), then gas exchange worsens and respiratory gases become abnormal or further deteriorate.

Increases in overall ventilation have a powerful effect on gas exchange when $\dot{V}_A/\dot{Q}$ distributions are normal, with increases in Pa_{O_2} and decreases in Pa_{CO_2} (Fig. 37-2).[3] Abnormal $\dot{V}_A/\dot{Q}$ distributions, however, are usually accompanied by an increase in Pa_{CO_2}, and other factors being equal, this is rapidly brought down to normal values by increases in ventilation. Arterial P_{O_2} also increases with further increases in ventilation. When $\dot{V}_A/\dot{Q}$ distributions are altered, however, normal values of Pa_{O_2} cannot be regained easily, and further increases in ventilation have little effect on Pa_{O_2}. Because increasing $\dot{V}_A/\dot{Q}$ mismatch reduces the transfer of O_2 and CO_2, it might be expected that such mismatch will lead always to both hypoxemia and hypercapnia. Small increases in Pa_{CO_2}, however, may activate the chemoreceptors, thus increasing minute ventilation as long as the ventilatory system works adequately and the patient is able to respond. The distribution of this increase in ventilation to well-ventilated areas will increase the $\dot{V}_A/\dot{Q}$ ratios, causing an increase in end-capillary P_{O_2} and a fall in Pa_{CO_2}. When the ability to increase ventilation is exceeded by the degree of $\dot{V}_A/\dot{Q}$ mismatch, Pa_{CO_2} will increase. Maintaining increased minute ventilation effectively prevents simultaneous increases in the level of Pa_{CO_2}, provided that there is no parallel increase in the work of breathing. In patients who cannot maintain a high level of ventilation, because of increased work of breathing, and in patients whose respiratory drive increases slightly when Pa_{CO_2} is high, hypercapnia can ensue.

759

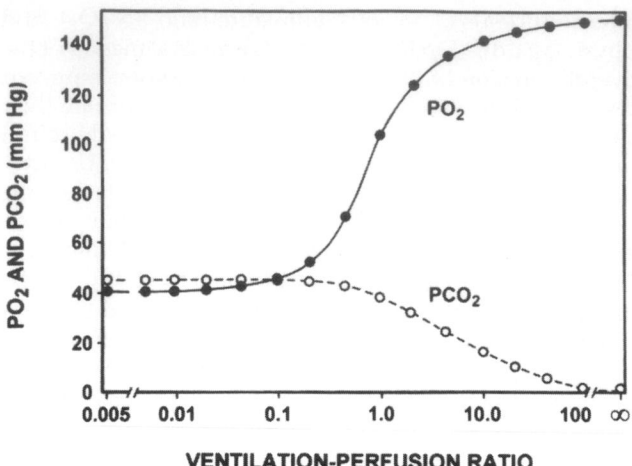

FIGURE 37-1 Variations in end-capillary P_{O_2} and P_{CO_2} in a single gas-exchange lung unit as a function of $\dot{V}_A/\dot{Q}$ ratio. For further explanation, see text. (*Reproduced, with permission, from West.*[2])

The effects of increasing total blood flow on $\dot{V}_A/\dot{Q}$ relationships are less marked on arterial blood gases than the effects of increases in ventilation.[3] Mixed venous P_{O_2} is an exception, however, because it can increase threefold when cardiac output is doubled. Otherwise, changes in Pa_{O_2} and Pa_{CO_2} are much smaller than those observed for increasing overall ventilation. When $\dot{V}_A/\dot{Q}$ inequalities are absent, increases in overall blood flow do not induce changes in arterial gases; if $\dot{V}_A/\dot{Q}$ mismatch is present, there is a mild positive effect on Pa_{O_2} together with a fall in Pa_{CO_2}.

INSPIRED OXYGEN

The influence of inspired O_2 on Pa_{O_2} depends on the degree of underlying $\dot{V}_A/\dot{Q}$ mismatch. End-capillary oxygen content rises as the fractional inspired O_2 concentration ($F_{I_{O_2}}$) is increased for conditions wherein $\dot{V}_A/\dot{Q}$ inequality is mild to moderate (up to 0.1). In contrast, as $\dot{V}_A/\dot{Q}$ mismatch

becomes more severe (below 0.1), the increase in the end-capillary O_2 content is much slower; accordingly, to reach similar levels to those obtained during less critical conditions, $F_{I_{O_2}}$ needs to be much higher.

Figure 37-2 illustrates the relationship between $F_{I_{O_2}}$ and Pa_{O_2} in the presence of different levels of intrapulmonary shunt.[4] As $F_{I_{O_2}}$ is increased, Pa_{O_2} increases as long as the amount of shunt is limited (below 20% of cardiac output). In contrast, increases in $F_{I_{O_2}}$ produce little change in Pa_{O_2} at greater levels of shunt. Even small increases in Pa_{O_2} in the presence of a large shunt, however, will markedly increase the arterial O_2 content, hence optimizing the O_2 delivery to peripheral tissues. Because of the shape of the oxyhemoglobin dissociation curve, O_2 delivery will improve as much for an increase in $F_{I_{O_2}}$ in clinical conditions with large shunts as in conditions with modest shunts.[4]

When assessing the influence of $F_{I_{O_2}}$ on $\dot{V}_A/\dot{Q}$ distributions, bear in mind that this can be determined through three different mechanisms: hypoxic pulmonary vasoconstriction,[5,6] reabsorption atelectasis secondary to instability of alveolar units with very low $\dot{V}_A/\dot{Q}$ ratios,[7] and airway-wall tone.[8–11]

One of the main adjustments for $\dot{V}_A/\dot{Q}$ mismatch in the normal lung is the ability of the pulmonary vasculature to reduce perfusion and to shift blood flow away from nonventilated areas (atelectasis) or alveolar units with very low $\dot{V}_A/\dot{Q}$ ratios, where P_{O_2} values are modest. This phenomenon minimizes the amount of $\dot{V}_A/\dot{Q}$ inequality in a diseased lung and limits the fall of Pa_{O_2}, other things being equal. Hypoxic pulmonary vasoconstriction represents a response of the pulmonary blood vessels that, although variable, is present in all mammalian species. Its mechanism, however, remains obscure. The site of the vasoconstriction is still not well defined, although there is a large body of evidence to suggest that the major site is the small pulmonary arteries at the precapillary level.[12,13] There are, however, considerable species differences in the stimulus-response curves.

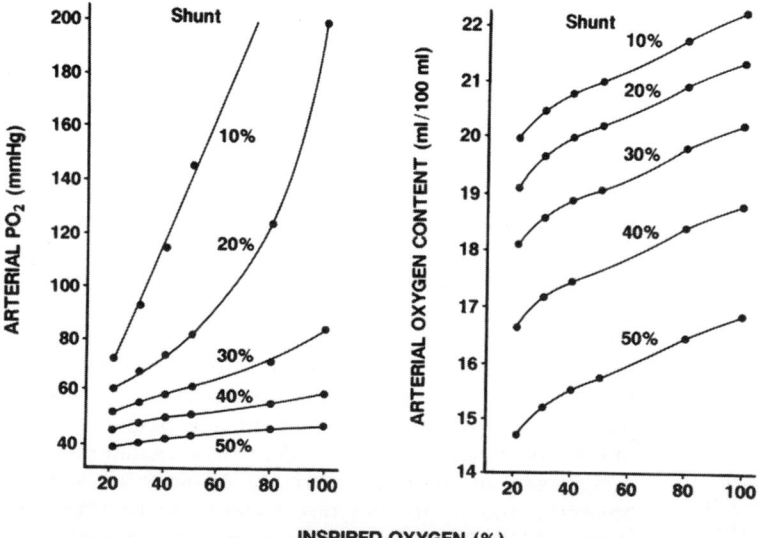

FIGURE 37-2 Influence of inspired oxygen on Pa_{O_2} (*left panel*) and oxygen content (*right panel*) as a function of the severity of shunt expressed as percentage of cardiac output. For further explanation, see text. (*Reproduced, with permission, from Dantzker et al.*[7])

REABSORPTION ATELECTASIS

A theoretical analysis of the gas-exchange factors involved in the development of shunt while breathing 100% oxygen showed that low inspired $\dot{V}A/\dot{Q}$ ratios (designated critical) could produce an absence of expired ventilation and alveolar denitrogenation, hence inducing reabsorption atelectasis in the alveoli.[7] By increasing FI_{O_2}, such a critical unit will no longer eliminate gas but may continue gas uptake. Moreover, this unit becomes unstable and may ultimately collapse, thereby causing reabsorption atelectasis.[14] These critical $\dot{V}A/\dot{Q}$ units are quite dependent on the FI_{O_2}, and they increase considerably as the latter approaches 100%. Alternatively, these critical units may remain open and not collapse because of increases in inspired ventilation to these units from other units. The time to collapse of an alveolar unit for a given inspired volume becomes progressively shorter as the FI_{O_2} is increased.

An additional mechanism that might enhance the rate of collapse is the instability of these small alveolar units at very small lung volumes as a result of surface tension, which may cause the units to collapse even before zero volume is reached.[15] Gas uptake would be reduced in these open critical units because some of their inspired gas will have come from units in which gas exchange has already taken place.

MIXED VENOUS OXYGEN

The pivotal role played by the mixed venous P_{O_2} on Pa_{O_2} is a well-known concept, yet too often ignored in the clinical setting.[16] From the Fick principle,

$$\dot{Q}_T = \frac{\dot{V}_{O_2}}{Ca_{O_2} - C\bar{v}_{O_2}} \tag{1}$$

and,

$$C\bar{v}_{O_2} = Ca_{O_2} - \frac{\dot{V}_{O_2}}{\dot{Q}_T} \tag{2}$$

where $\dot{V}_{O_2}$ denotes oxygen consumption, and $\dot{Q}_T$ cardiac output. It follows from equation 2 that mixed venous hypoxemia ($C\bar{v}_{O_2}$) may result from decreased Ca_{O_2}, increased $\dot{V}_{O_2}$, or decreased $\dot{Q}_T$. Moreover, Ca_{O_2} may be conditioned by changes in the factors that modulate the oxyhemoglobin dissociation curve, such as hemoglobin concentration, temperature, P_{50}, or pH, although these factors are considered less influential.

OXYGEN CONSUMPTION

In a lung model of pure shunt,[17] Pa_{O_2} is fairly sensitive to changes in O_2 consumption; an increase in O_2 consumption from 300 to 600 ml/min, acting alone, decreases Pa_{O_2} by 10 mmHg. In contrast, in a model characterized by pure $\dot{V}A/\dot{Q}$ mismatch, a 10% change in O_2 consumption can change the Pa_{O_2} by 10 mmHg in either direction. The different results in each model (less sensitivity of Pa_{O_2} in the model of shunt) may be related to the different levels of Pa_{O_2} in each condition and its unique relationship with arterial O_2 saturation. When Pa_{O_2} is located at the lower, steeper, linear part of the oxyhemoglobin dissociation curve in the shunt model, variations in O_2 consumption induce less change in Pa_{O_2}. Increased O_2 consumption is a common finding in patients with acute respiratory failure when discontinuing ventilator support.[18]

CARDIAC OUTPUT

There are three potential ways by which cardiac output modulates pulmonary gas exchange.[19] The most influential way is by means of the effect on O_2 content of the mixed venous blood, discussed above. This may occur directly through changes in cardiac output and its effect on arterial-venous oxygen content difference, or as a result of failure of the cardiovascular system (cardiac output) to respond to changes in O_2 delivery or changes in O_2 extraction by the tissues.

A second way in which cardiac output influences pulmonary gas exchange is by modifying the transit time of the red blood cell spent in the pulmonary capillary. If cardiac output increases, the transit time decreases. Thus, abnormal gas exchange secondary to incomplete O_2 diffusion may, at least in theory, occur. This mechanism, however, is only possible when there is a combined limitation for O_2 diffusion, as in interstitial pulmonary disorders, both at rest and during exercise,[20] or in normal humans during extreme exercise conditions.[21]

A third possibility, common in critically ill patients, is redistribution of pulmonary blood flow within the lungs. Alterations in blood flow may be achieved in different ways. One is through the well-known, although poorly understood, strong positive association between shunt and cardiac output. If shunt fraction increases, then cardiac output increases, and vice versa.[22,23] Another way may be through modification of the pulmonary vascular tone, basically resulting from alterations of alveolar P_{O_2}. Mixed venous P_{O_2}, however, may also influence, at least partly, pulmonary hypoxic vasoconstrictor tone through an undetermined pathway.[24] Finally, increases and decreases in intracardiac and pulmonary artery pressures may lead to redistribution of pulmonary blood flow.[19]

Another relationship of paramount interest, with marked influence on Pa_{O_2}, is the interaction between the arterial-venous O_2 content difference (the inverse of cardiac output if O_2 consumption remains unchanged) and shunt. Figure 37-3 depicts the interaction of these three variables while breathing 100% O_2.[25] It is clear that Pa_{O_2} may reach considerable levels (approaching 500 mmHg or above) with an inordinately high cardiac output (or very low arterial-mixed venous O_2 content difference), even in the presence of moderate to severe gas-exchange abnormalities (shunt above 20% of cardiac output). In an animal model of abnormal gas exchange induced by methacholine,[26] the dependence of combined shunt and $\dot{V}A/\dot{Q}$ mismatch on cardiac output was studied at varying levels of FI_{O_2}. For a 1-L/min increase in blood flow the increase in shunt was much greater while breathing 100% O_2 than during hypoxic conditions. This dependency of the "shunt-cardiac output" relationship on FI_{O_2} suggests that the increase in shunt following increase in cardiac output is more dependent on pulmonary vascular tone of intact lung areas than on tone of injured regions.

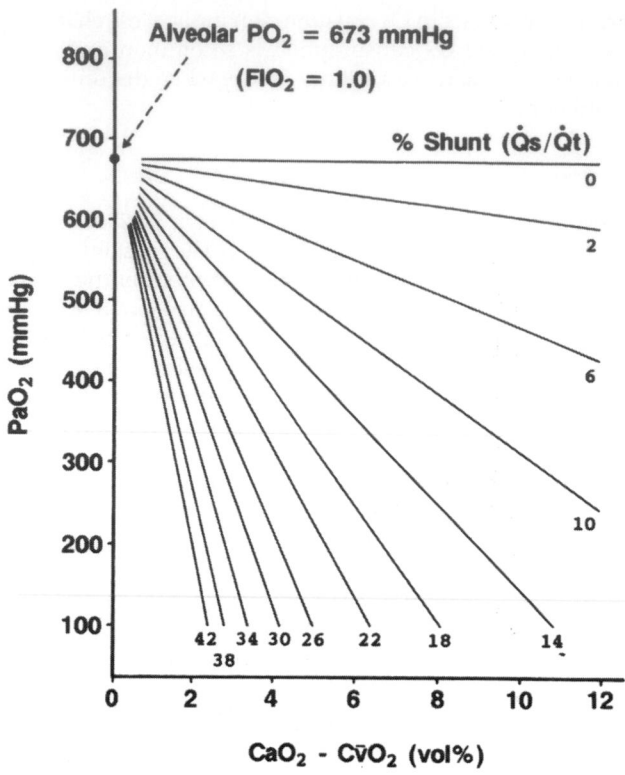

FIGURE 37-3 Relationships between Pa_{O_2} and arterial-venous oxygen content difference as a function of the severity of shunt, expressed as percentage of cardiac output. For further explanation, see text. (*Reproduced, with permission, from Laver et al.*[25])

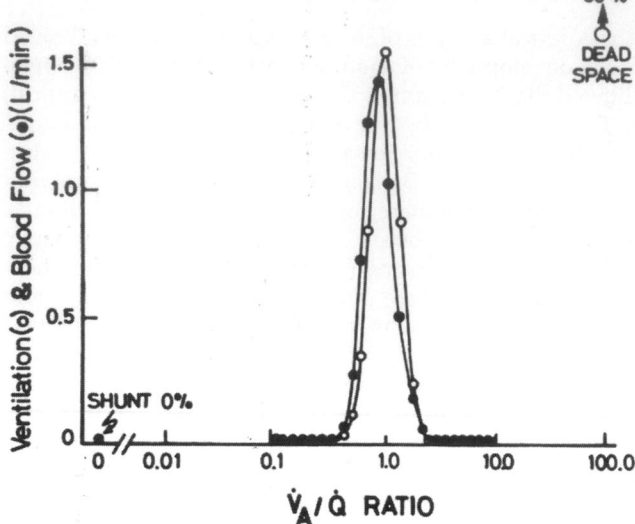

FIGURE 37-4 Distributions of alveolar ventilation and pulmonary blood flow plotted versus $\dot{V}A/\dot{Q}$ ratio. For further explanation, see text.

Multiple Inert Gas Elimination Technique

This chapter reviews the effect of ventilator support on pulmonary gas exchange using all the aforementioned concepts instead of those based exclusively on the classical four causes of hypoxemia and hypercapnia ($\dot{V}A/\dot{Q}$ mismatch, intrapulmonary shunt, alveolar hypoventilation, and O_2 diffusion limitation). Assessment of the intrapulmonary factors of abnormal gas exchange with the multiple inert gas elimination technique (MIGET) represents a major conceptual breakthrough in our understanding of pulmonary medicine pathophysiology in disease states.[27–30]

MIGET has three major advantages. First, it estimates the pattern of pulmonary blood flow and alveolar ventilation and calculates the mismatch of $\dot{V}A/\dot{Q}$ relationships. Second, it partitions the alveolar-arterial P_{O_2} difference into components of intrapulmonary shunt, $\dot{V}A/\dot{Q}$ inequality and diffusion limitation to O_2. And third, it apportions and unravels arterial oxygenation into intrapulmonary and extrapulmonary components. Of paramount importance is the ability to perform measurements at any $F_{I_{O_2}}$ without perturbing the vascular and bronchomotor tones.

Figure 37-4 illustrates the $\dot{V}A/\dot{Q}$ distribution obtained with MIGET in a healthy, young individual at rest breathing room air. Each data point represents a particular amount of blood flow or alveolar ventilation. Both overall pulmonary perfusion and total ventilation correspond to the sum of the respective data points (the lines have been drawn for clarity only). These quantities (distributions) are plotted against a broad range (50) of $\dot{V}A/\dot{Q}$ ratios, from zero (shunt) to infinity (dead space), on a log scale. The unimodal profile of each distribution has three main characteristics: symmetry, location around a $\dot{V}A/\dot{Q}$ ratio of 1.0, and narrowness (very little dispersion). Note that there is no inert-gas shunt (contrasted with the concept of venous admixture ratio), because the tracer nature of inert gases utilized for MIGET is insensitive to the presence of postpulmonary shunt (i.e., the bronchial and thebesian circulations). Inert-gas physiologic dead space is also slightly lower than Bohr dead space because it does not include the alveolar units which have an alveolar P_{CO_2} that is lower than the arterial P_{CO_2}.

Nature of Gas Exchange in Disease States

From a clinical standpoint, the three principal mechanisms of altered arterial respiratory gases during spontaneous breathing in any pulmonary disease state are $\dot{V}A/\dot{Q}$ mismatching, increased intrapulmonary shunt, and alveolar hypoventilation. The role of diffusion limitation to O_2 is modest and plays a role in patients with pulmonary fibrosis[20] and in healthy individuals under very extreme conditions.[21] During mechanical ventilation, however, alveolar hypoventilation is controlled in such a way that Pa_{CO_2} does not represent a problem. $\dot{V}A/\dot{Q}$ inequality plays a pivotal role in disorders characterized by chronic lung disease ("dry lung"), namely exacerbations of chronic obstructive pulmonary disease (COPD) and bronchial asthma, which have in common expiratory airflow limitation and large pulmonary volumes. Increased intrapulmonary shunt is a key determinant of hypoxemia in conditions characterized by acute lung injury ("wet lung"), such as acute lung injury (ALI), acute respiratory distress syndrome (ARDS), and

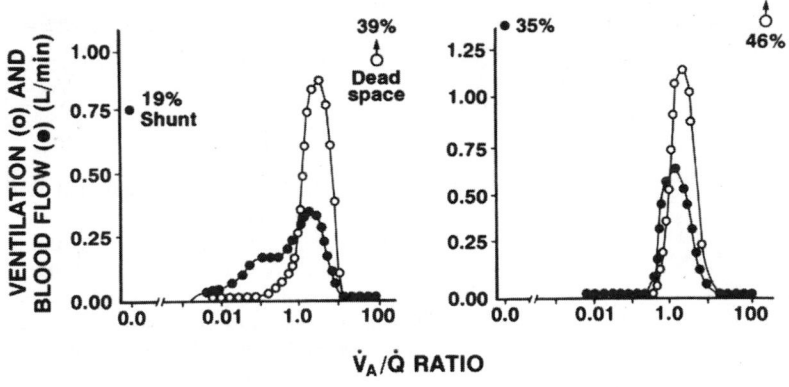

FIGURE 37-5 Two patterns of $\dot{V}_A/\dot{Q}$ distributions in patients with ARDS (with PEEP). Note that intrapulmonary shunt and dead space were considerably increased in both individuals. Notice also the presence of some amount of blood flow distributed to units with low $\dot{V}_A/\dot{Q}$ (*left panel*). (*Reproduced, with permission, from Reyes et al.*[33])

life-threatening pneumonia, all of which have small lung volumes.[24]

This section will extensively review the main mechanisms of pulmonary gas exchange during mechanical ventilation in ALI/ARDS, pneumonia, COPD, and asthma–the most common conditions in the critical-care setting. The characteristic gas-exchange abnormalities at maintenance F_{IO_2} and while breathing 100% O_2 will be reviewed. Likewise, the effects of external positive end-expiratory pressure (PEEP) and intrinsic PEEP ($PEEP_i$) on gas exchange, and the effects of several ventilator settings will be reviewed.

ACUTE RESPIRATORY FAILURE ("WET LUNG")

This section will review the two most frequent disorders seen in the intensive-care unit, ARDS and severe life-threatening pneumonia, together with a short review of gas exchange in patients with head trauma and following cardiac surgery. It can be difficult to differentiate ALI/ARDS from the other disorders–after all, ALI/ARDS is a constellation of many entities, among which pneumonia and the other conditions of acute respiratory failure are common causes. From a gas-exchange viewpoint, however, ALI/ARDS and pneumonia show different functional findings. Furthermore, the response to high F_{IO_2} differs substantially.

ACUTE LUNG INJURY/ACUTE RESPIRATORY DISTRESS SYNDROME
Severe acute respiratory failure in previously healthy subjects may result from a primary infectious lung process or a more widespread, noninfectious process, namely either ALI or ARDS. The latter entity is characterized by severe hypoxemia refractory to high F_{IO_2}, and differences are related to the severity of gas-exchange abnormalities.[31]

MECHANISMS OF HYPOXEMIA
The main cause of hypoxemia in patients with ALI/ARDS is a considerable intrapulmonary shunt, averaging 20% or more of cardiac output. In approximately half the patients, however, there are considerable additional areas with low $\dot{V}_A/\dot{Q}$ ratios: a moderate percentage of total pulmonary blood flow is distributed to areas of the lung with reduced ventilation.[32]

Figure 37-5 illustrates the profiles of two representative $\dot{V}_A/\dot{Q}$ distributions of patients with ARDS during mechanical ventilation with PEEP (at F_{IO_2}, 0.5).[33] While both patterns show marked amounts of shunt and dead space, the main body of the dispersion of blood flow is different. In one patient, the dispersion is narrowly unimodal (right panel). In the other, the pattern of perfusion is broadly unimodal, i.e., blood flow is distributed to areas with low $\dot{V}_A/\dot{Q}$ ratios (usually less than 10% of cardiac output) (left panel). The former profile reflects an "all-or-none" phenomenon; pulmonary perfusion is essentially diverted to two lung areas, those with ventilation that is normal and proportional to blood flow, and those that are completely unventilated.[34] The presence of areas with low $\dot{V}_A/\dot{Q}$ ratios suggests the coexistence of areas with partially filled alveolar spaces or alveolar units in which ventilation is reduced compared to blood flow (because of increased airways resistance) or both. A few patients showed an increase of alveolar ventilation distributed to high $\dot{V}_A/\dot{Q}$ ratios, including a bimodal pattern of the dispersion of ventilation; in contrast, dead space was increased in most patients. These two findings may reflect areas with reduced pulmonary blood flow secondary to the effects of external PEEP, although an additional influence of pulmonary vascular derangement cannot be ruled out.[32]

There was no limitation to the diffusion of O_2, as reflected by the close agreement between predicted Pa_{O_2} (according to MIGET, this reflects the underlying amount of intrapulmonary shunt and $\dot{V}_A/\dot{Q}$ mismatch only) and measured Pa_{O_2} (Fig. 37-6).[34,35] When measured Pa_{O_2} is not significantly different from the predicted Pa_{O_2}, this suggests that other potential causes of hypoxemia, namely diffusion limitation for O_2, increased postpulmonary shunt, and/or augmented intrapulmonary O_2 consumption,[36] are not occurring.

BREATHING 100% OXYGEN
The concept of an increase in intrapulmonary shunt while breathing 100% oxygen in patients with acute respiratory failure is old.[14,37] Earlier data using MIGET, however, did not support this view.[32] It was considered that areas with critical inspiratory $\dot{V}_A/\dot{Q}$ ratios may remain partly open and facilitate O_2 transfer; potential mechanisms include the efficiency of collateral ventilation, interdependence of surrounding lung parenchyma, or the interaction of mechanical

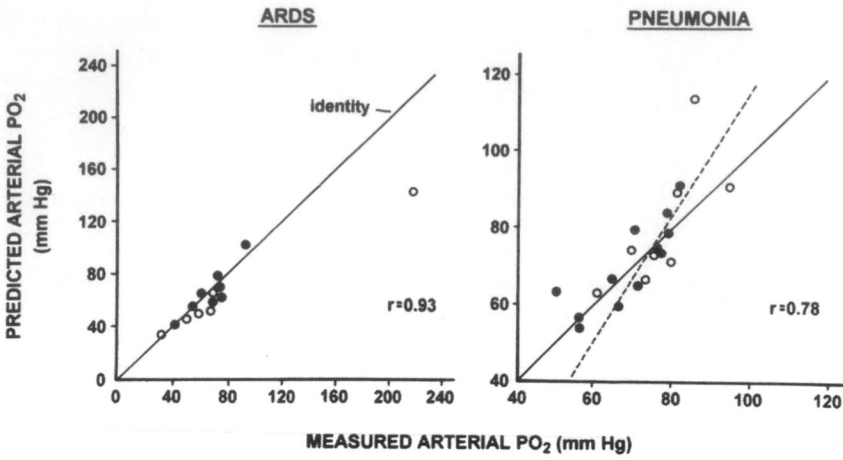

FIGURE 37-6 Plots of predicted (estimated by MIGET) Pa_{O_2} versus measured Pa_{O_2} in patients with ARDS (*left panel; open symbols* = without PEEP; *closed symbols* = with PEEP) and with severe pneumonia (*right panel; open symbols* = with mechanical ventilation ; *closed symbols* = without mechanical support). Note the good agreement between both variables in each clinical condition (*dashed line* = regression line). (*Reproduced, with permission, from Dantzker et al.[34] and Gea et al.[35]*)

forces exerted during artificial ventilation.[7] No studies, however, properly addressed this question.

Our group has shown that Pa_{O_2} increases modestly (~300 mmHg) and intrapulmonary shunt increases considerably (about 35%) during hyperoxic breathing over 1 hour, suggesting the development of reabsorption atelectasis (Fig. 37-7).[7,38] The increase in shunt was noticed within less than half an hour, confirming the theoretical analysis on the minimum time required for collapse of alveolar units with various fixed inspired $\dot{V}_A/\dot{Q}$ ratios according to the different levels of $F_{I_{O_2}}$.[7] The limited increase in Pa_{O_2} while breathing 100% O_2 indicates that increased intrapulmonary shunt is the key determinant of hypoxemia in ALI/ARDS. Further, the increments in shunt persisted for 1 hour after resuming maintenance $F_{I_{O_2}}$, indicating the persistence of atelectasis. Of note, this worsening of shunt was also accompanied by a small but significant increase in Pa_{CO_2}, possibly explained by the Haldane effect (Fig. 37-8). The Haldane effect is the increase in Pa_{CO_2} at a given arterial CO_2 content that occurs in response to an increase in arterial O_2 saturation. The dispersions of blood flow and alveolar ventilation remained unchanged.

The increase in shunt not accompanied with release of hypoxic pulmonary vasoconstriction in patients with ALI/ARDS is compatible with the concept that, at any level of $F_{I_{O_2}}$, units with low $\dot{V}_A/\dot{Q}$ cannot redistribute blood flow from areas of shunt or very low $\dot{V}_A/\dot{Q}$ ratios, because their vascular resistance remains unchanged.[7]

EFFECTS OF PEEP

The gas-exchange response to external PEEP illustrates one of the best examples of the complex interplay between intrapulmonary and extrapulmonary determinants of respiratory gases.[16,32] Several studies have assessed this action in patients with ALI/ARDS.

In a seminal study,[34] which measured $\dot{V}_A/\dot{Q}$ distributions at increasing levels of PEEP, two distinct patterns were shown (Fig. 37-9). In some patients, the $\dot{V}_A/\dot{Q}$ pattern remained unchanged despite progressive increases of PEEP. In others, there was a broadening of the dispersion of ventilation because areas with high $\dot{V}_A/\dot{Q}$ ratios increased and ventilation was redistributed to infinity $\dot{V}_A/\dot{Q}$ ratios. In each patient, however, PEEP led ultimately to a marked decrement in cardiac output distributed to unventilated (shunt) areas or poorly ventilated $\dot{V}_A/\dot{Q}$ units and to a considerable increase in dead space. The final result was a substantial optimization of Pa_{O_2}.

Subsequently, the $\dot{V}_A/\dot{Q}$ response to external PEEP was investigated while cardiac output was kept constant at control values with dopamine.[39] During PEEP, Pa_{O_2}, mixed venous P_{O_2}, and oxygen delivery increased significantly,

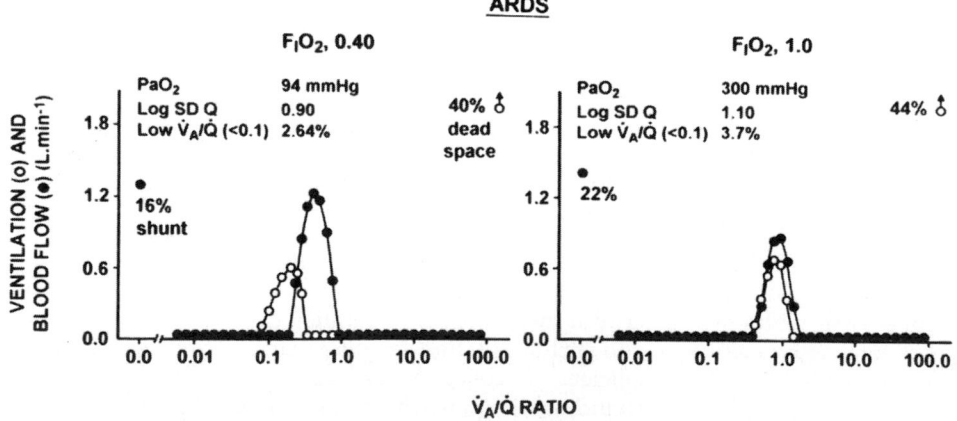

FIGURE 37-7 Effect of breathing 100% oxygen (*right panel*) in a representative patient with ARDS (with PEEP). Compared with low $F_{I_{O_2}}$ (*left panel*), Pa_{O_2} increased modestly (~300 mmHg), but intrapulmonary shunting increased moderately; in contrast, both the dispersion of blood flow (*Log SD Q*) and the amount of blood flow distributed to areas with low $\dot{V}_A/\dot{Q}$ ratios remained unchanged. This suggests the development of reabsorption atelectasis without release of hypoxic vasoconstriction. Dead space tended to increase.

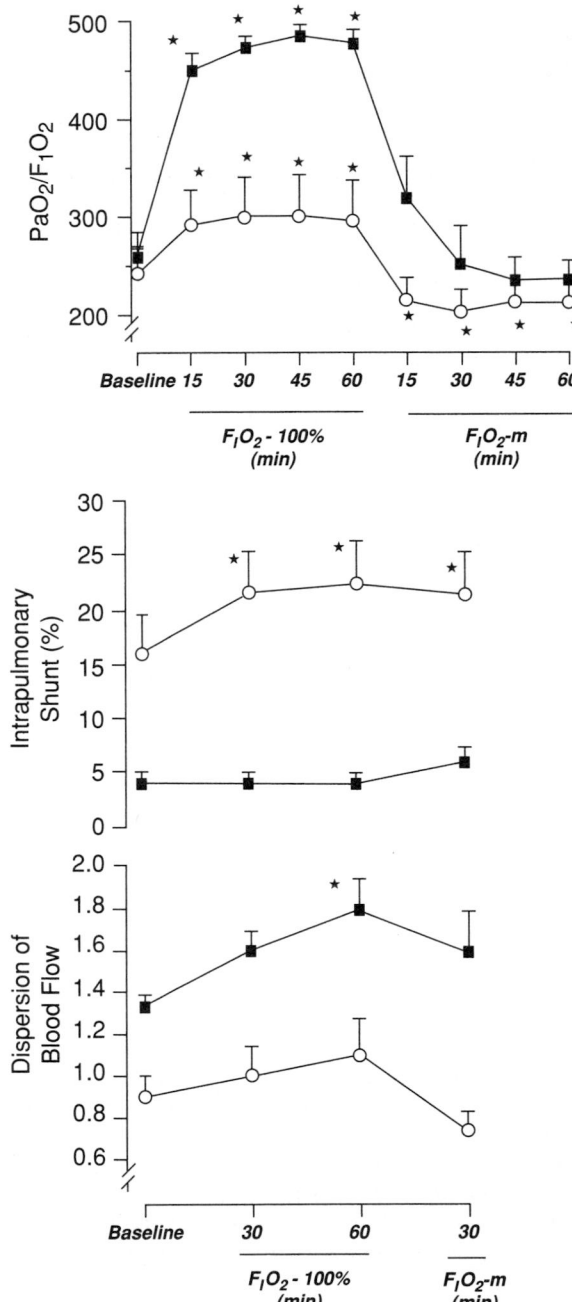

FIGURE 37-8 Sequence of Pa_{O_2}/F_{IO_2} (in millimeters of mercury), shunt (in percentage of cardiac output) and Log SD Q (dimensionless). In patients with ALI (*open circles*) arterial oxygenation and Log SD Q remained almost unchanged, whereas shunt increased significantly, suggesting reabsorption atelectasis. In contrast, in patients with COPD (*solid squares*), Log SD Q and arterial oxygenation substantially increased whereas shunt remained low and unvaried, indicating release of hypoxic vasoconstriction. For further explanation, see text. (*Reproduced, with permission, from Santos et al.*[38])

whereas the venous admixture ratio decreased markedly. Similarly, shunt decreased substantially, and pulmonary blood flow was redistributed from nonventilated units with zero $\dot{V}_A/\dot{Q}$ ratios to areas with normal $\dot{V}_A/\dot{Q}$ ratios. Dead space increased slightly, but the dispersion of the alveolar ventilation did not vary. Because PEEP causes redistribution of extravascular lung water from alveoli to peribronchial and perivascular spaces,[40] these data suggest that the improvement in pulmonary gas exchange with external levels of PEEP results from the reopening of collapsed airways and alveoli. The key message from this study is that the avoidance of the reduction of cardiac output during PEEP application enhances a more optimal gas exchange.

In another study,[41] the gas-exchange response to increments in PEEP was studied. In most patients, Pa_{O_2} improved substantially because of a decrease in intrapulmonary shunt or in the zone of low $\dot{V}_A/\dot{Q}$ ratio, or a derecruitment of blood flow from areas with shunt to those with low or normal $\dot{V}_A/\dot{Q}$ ratio; blood flow reductions to low $\dot{V}_A/\dot{Q}$ areas were less predictable. When Pa_{O_2} did not vary in response to PEEP, there were no variations in the $\dot{V}_A/\dot{Q}$ relationships. An increase either in poorly perfused $\dot{V}_A/\dot{Q}$ units or in dead space was shown in only a few individuals. The beneficial effect of PEEP on Pa_{O_2} could not be predicted by the etiology of ARDS or the severity of abnormal gas exchange. As expected, cardiac output and mixed venous P_{O_2} decreased progressively as PEEP was increased. The mean change in cardiac output was essentially similar between PEEP trials irrespective of the improvement in Pa_{O_2}.

Experimentally, low levels of PEEP (5–10 cmH₂O) decrease physiologic dead space by reducing both shunt and $\dot{V}_A/\dot{Q}$ mismatch.[42] At higher levels of PEEP, however, physiologic dead space increases because both ventilation to high $\dot{V}_A/\dot{Q}$ regions and anatomic dead space increase while the efficiency of CO_2 elimination by the lungs is diminished.

All in all, these studies are of interest for two reasons. First, these findings indicate that the beneficial effects of PEEP in ALI/ARDS essentially result from a redistribution of blood flow from severely injured (shunt) areas to poorly or normally ventilated alveolar units. This seems to be related to the reopening of collapsed alveoli and airways rather than to a decrease of cardiac output by itself. Alternatively, the depression of cardiac output may reduce shunt or blood flow distributed to units with poorly ventilated $\dot{V}_A/\dot{Q}$ ratios.[19] It has been shown both clinically and experimentally, using pharmacologic or mechanical techniques, that changes in cardiac output lead to directionally similar changes in shunt. Likewise, in many instances, the shunt fraction also changes in a similar direction to changes in the mixed venous P_{O_2} and negatively with pulmonary vascular resistance.[43]

Second, in two of the studies in which the values of mixed venous P_{O_2} were reported, this variable either increased[39] or remained stable.[41] when cardiac output was reduced. Arterial P_{O_2} increased during PEEP because the beneficial effects on gas exchange, essentially secondary to the reduction in shunt (intrapulmonary factor), were not offset by the simultaneous deleterious effect on Pa_{O_2} secondary to decreased cardiac output (extrapulmonary factor), which had allowed mixed venous P_{O_2} to decrease, other factors

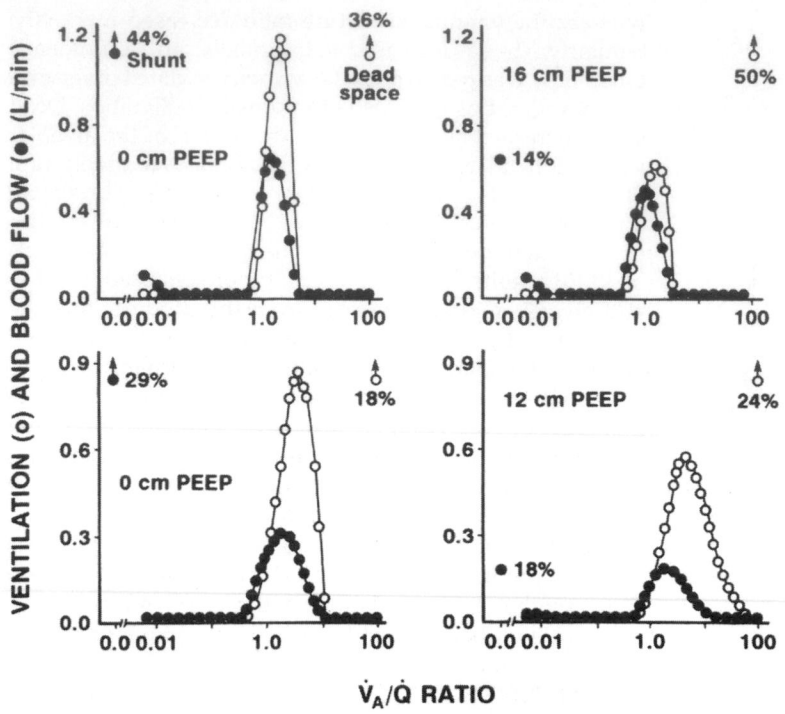

FIGURE 37-9 The application of 16 cmH$_2$O of PEEP in a patient with ARDS induced a reduction of shunt and an increase of dead space, whereas V̇$_A$/Q̇ distributions remain essentially unaltered (*top, from left to right*). In another patient, 12 cmH$_2$O of PEEP caused similar effects on shunt and dead space, but V̇$_A$/Q̇ distributions are broadened (*bottom, from left to right*). For further explanation, see text. (*Reproduced, with permission, from Dantzker et al.[34]*)

being equal. If the reduction in cardiac output had been more severe, Pa$_{O_2}$ would have remained unaltered or even decreased despite the reduction in shunt.[32] Alternatively, the observation that mixed venous P$_{O_2}$ values did not always vary in the same direction as cardiac output raises the question of the pathologic supply dependence between O$_2$ delivery and the O$_2$ consumption.[44] Such patients may respond to the depression of cardiac output during PEEP by reducing O$_2$ consumption.

The development of high V̇$_A$/Q̇ peaks, and the moderate-to-severe increments of dead space during PEEP, are consistent with experimental data indicating that the reduction of cardiac output and the depression of perfusion in the uppermost regions of the lung determine changes in the pattern of ventilation with PEEP.[45]

VENTILATOR MODALITIES

Over the last 10 years, increasing emphasis has been placed on avoiding ventilator-associated lung injury (VALI) and the use of a protective ventilator strategy, accepting an increase in Pa$_{CO_2}$ if necessary (permissive hypercapnia), in patients with ALI/ARDS. VALI[46] is defined as lung damage with characteristic features of ARDS that can occur in patients receiving mechanical ventilation. The two most important mechanical factors responsible for VALI are thought to be: (1) the association of alveolar overdistension and high transpulmonary pressure; and (2) repeated alveolar collapse and reopening owing to ventilation at inappropriate tidal ranges of transpulmonary pressure. The prevention of alveolar overdistension by reducing tidal volume has been investigated in combination with relatively low levels of PEEP and high levels of PEEP. We will describe them separately.

Permissive Hypercapnia with Low Tidal Volume and Low PEEP

Four recent controlled studies[47–50] have compared the outcome with use of low (6–7 ml/kg) versus high (10–12 ml/kg) tidal volumes with standard levels of PEEP (8–11 cmH$_2$O). Only one study[50] showed a significant (20%) decrease in mortality, likely because of a superior statistical power and a larger difference between the low- and high-tidal-volume branches. Use of low tidal volume, however, can worsen pulmonary gas exchange, necessitating higher F$_{IO_2}$ requirements, secondary to reduction in alveolar ventilation and increased shunt caused by both alveolar collapse and increased cardiac output, which may further worsen intrapulmonary shunt in patients with ARDS.[34]

The induction of permissive hypercapnia by reducing tidal volume and maintaining constant standard levels of PEEP was shown to increase cardiac output, decrease Pa$_{O_2}$, and increase shunt, but had no effect on the dispersion of blood flow (Log SD Q).[51] When baseline tidal volume was reinstated and cardiac output was maintained with use of dobutamine, both shunt and Pa$_{O_2}$ remained unchanged. Thus, low tidal volume with standard PEEP increased intrapulmonary shunt and the deterioration in gas exchange was caused by the combined effects of increased cardiac output and decreased alveolar ventilation. In another study,[52] the effects of permissive hypercapnia were compared in two groups of patients with ARDS, with and without hyperdynamic sepsis. Permissive hypercapnia was induced by decreasing tidal volume and increasing PEEP to prevent alveolar recruitment. In both groups of patients, permissive hypercapnia increased shunt but did not worsen Pa$_{O_2}$ because of an increase in mixed venous P$_{O_2}$ secondary to an increased cardiac output. In septic patients, Pa$_{O_2}$ remained unchanged, and in nonseptic patients, it increased. Dead

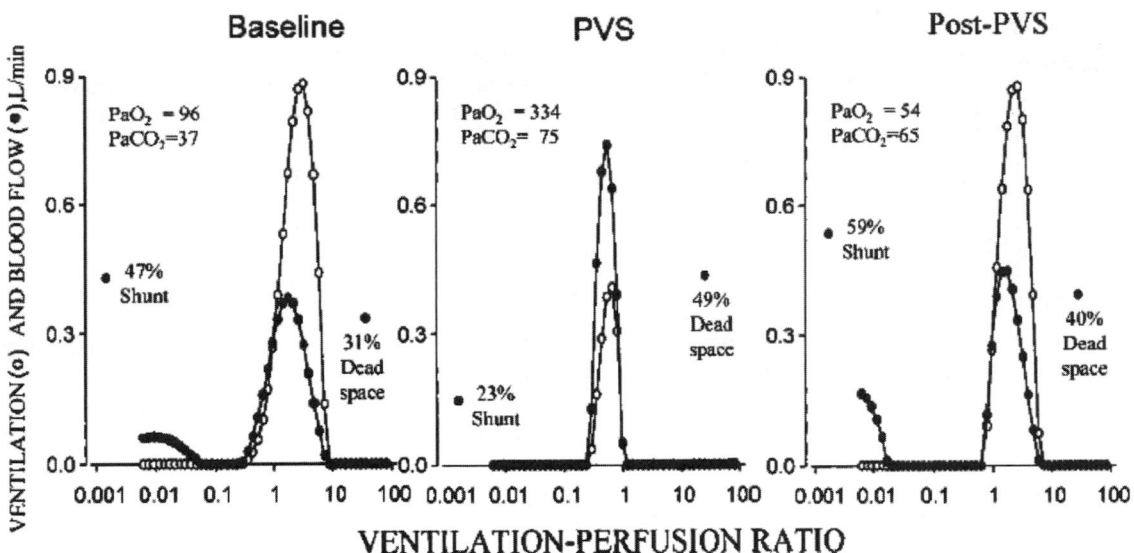

FIGURE 37-10 Representative patient with ARDS at baseline (*left*), during protective ventilator support (PVS) (*center*), and after PVS (*right*). During PVS, shunt decreased and arterial oxygenation improved; dead space increased as a result of low tidal volume and high PEEP. (*Reproduced, with permission, from Mancini et al.[55]*)

space and the descriptors of $\dot{V}A/\dot{Q}$ imbalance remained unchanged in both subsets of patients.

Permissive Hypercapnia With Low Tidal Volume and High PEEP

The combination of low tidal volume, to avoid alveolar overdistension, and high PEEP, to prevent sequential collapse and reopening of alveolar units throughout the ventilatory cycle has been advocated as an alternative strategy to decrease VALI. In patients with ARDS,[53] this approach achieved a significant reduction in mortality at 4 weeks but hospital mortality was not decreased. The protective ventilation group had a higher rate of weaning from mechanical ventilation and a lower rate of barotrauma. This type of permissive hypercapnia produced an acute hyperdynamic state,[54] with transient systemic vasodilatation and increased cardiac output. The acute hemodynamic effects were in part related to acute respiratory acidosis, and progressively attenuated during the first 36 hours of ventilation despite persisting hypercapnia. The gas-exchange response to this ventilator strategy[55] revealed superior efficacy in early ARDS (Fig. 37-10), mainly through recruitment of previously collapsed alveoli and redistribution of pulmonary blood flow from unventilated alveolar units to normal units. Arterial P_{O_2} improved and intrapulmonary shunt decreased. Recruitment of previously collapsed alveolar units was the key factor underlying the decreased intrapulmonary shunt. The beneficial effects of this approach on gas exchange fully overcame the deleterious effect of permissive hypercapnia on arterial oxygenation (i.e., reduced alveolar P_{O_2}). Moreover, the increase in cardiac output secondary to systemic vasodilatation[54] did not result in a proportional increase in intrapulmonary shunt, as one might expect in patients with ARDS,[34] likely because pulmonary blood flow was appropriately redistributed to normal alveolar units secondary to the concomitant efficiency of alveolar recruitment (Fig.

37-11). The substantial improvement in $\dot{V}A/\dot{Q}$ imbalance, indicated by decreased blood flow dispersion (Log SD Q), may have been caused by the reduction of the overall $\dot{V}A/\dot{Q}$ ratio secondary to the concomitant effects of both decreased alveolar ventilation and increased cardiac output (induced by this ventilator modality). Under these circumstances, a more efficient distribution of pulmonary blood flow toward areas with normal $\dot{V}A/\dot{Q}$ ratios cannot be ruled out. Likewise, the marked increase in dead space observed with the protective strategy can be explained by the combination of a decrease in alveolar ventilation and an increase in functional residual capacity induced by high levels of PEEP. This study showed a strong relationship between improvement of alveolar gas exchange and the amount of PEEP-induced alveolar recruitment. Overall, these findings strongly support the combination of low tidal volumes and high PEEP levels as the most appropriate approach, at least in early ARDS, although further studies are warranted. The growing knowledge that therapeutic hypercapnia per se may prevent pulmonary and systemic damage in patients with ARDS[56,57] adds further complexities.

Inverse Inspiratory:Expiratory Ratio Ventilation

Before the advantages of protective ventilation with permissive hypercapnia were known, inverse inspiratory:expiratory (I:E) ratio ventilation was used in ARDS to improve oxygenation at lower-than-conventional peak airway pressures. Because of discrepant results in several studies, the gas-exchange response was investigated.[58] Compared to conventional volume-controlled ventilation with PEEP, the application of equivalent levels of PEEP during inverse-ratio ventilation did not result in a superior Pa_{O_2}. Pressure-controlled ventilation with inverse I:E ratio did not affect Pa_{O_2} either, although it decreased Pa_{CO_2} because of a concomitant decrease in dead space with a shift to the right of $\dot{V}A/\dot{Q}$ distributions.

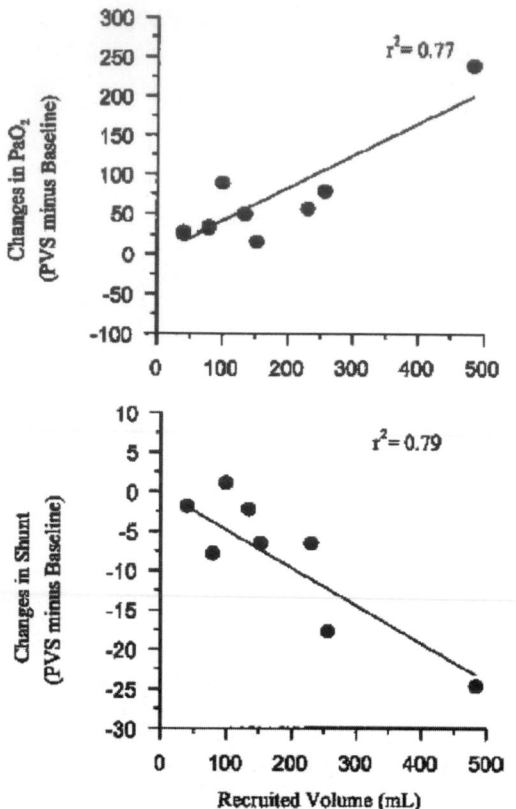

FIGURE 37-11 Correlations between increased Pa_{O_2} (*top*) and decreased shunt (*bottom*) and recruited lung volume during protective ventilator support (PVS) in patients with ARDS (*dots: individual patients; lines: regression lines*). (*Reproduced, with permission, from Mancini et al.[55]*)

Postural Changes

The $\dot{V}A/\dot{Q}$ distributions during pressure-controlled ventilation in the prone position[59] revealed an improvement in Pa_{O_2} of more than 10 mmHg after 30 minutes in two-thirds of patients (responders), whereas the remaining patients showed no change in Pa_{O_2} (nonresponders). In the responders, the prone position caused a substantial decrease in shunt regions with a concomitant increase of areas with normal $\dot{V}A/\dot{Q}$ ratios in the dorsal zones, which were now less gravitationally dependent. Returning the patient to the supine position reversed the improvement in gas exchange. These changes suggest that the redistribution of blood flow away from shunt areas is most likely caused by efficient recruitment of previously atelectatic, but nondiseased, zones induced by altered gravitational forces. Continuous axial rotation might be another method for acutely reducing $\dot{V}A/\dot{Q}$ imbalance in patients with ALI/ARD[60]; continuous axial rotation on a kinetic-treatment table reduced intrapulmonary shunt and improved Pa_{O_2}. The positive response to continuous rotation was only demonstrated in patients with mild-to-moderate ALI; in patients with progressive ARDS, the acute response was limited.

Partial Ventilator Support

A study comparing the effects of airway pressure release ventilation (APRV), with and without spontaneous breathing, and pressure support ventilation, in which both modal-

ities were delivered with equal airway pressure limits or minute ventilation, on pulmonary gas exchange in patients with ARDS[61] showed that spontaneous breathing with APRV improved $\dot{V}A/\dot{Q}$ mismatching, as revealed by decreases in intrapulmonary shunt, dead space, and the dispersions of blood flow and ventilation. Pressure support did not improve $\dot{V}A/\dot{Q}$ imbalance when compared with APRV without spontaneous breathing. These findings indicated that uncoupling of spontaneous and mechanical ventilation during APRV improves $\dot{V}A/\dot{Q}$ inequalities in ARDS, presumably by recruiting nonventilated lung units. As compared with controlled ventilation, inspiratory assistance during pressure support is not sufficient to counteract the $\dot{V}A/\dot{Q}$ imbalance caused by alveolar collapse in patients with ARDS, and does not provide any complementary advantage in cardiopulmonary function or pulmonary gas exchange.

PNEUMONIA

Mechanisms of Hypoxemia

In pneumonia, arterial hypoxemia is basically determined by the presence of a considerable shunt (average, 20% of cardiac output) together with moderate to severe amounts (range 10–20% of cardiac output) of blood flow distributed to units with low $\dot{V}A/\dot{Q}$. In general, the pattern of the dispersion of perfusion is bimodal (Fig. 37-12).[35,62] These functional findings are consistent with the main pathologic findings, namely extensive consolidation of areas of the lungs, with alveoli completely or partially filled with edema, leukocytes and other cells, causative bacteria, and fibrin.[63] Dead space is by and large slightly increased, and some patients can exhibit areas wherein ventilation is diverted to high $\dot{V}A/\dot{Q}$ ratios. The latter findings may reflect the use of PEEP, which is commonly used in these patients. There is good agreement between predicted Pa_{O_2} and measured Pa_{O_2}, suggesting therefore that additional intrapulmonary factors determining hypoxemia (diffusion limitation to O_2,

FIGURE 37-12 Ventilation-perfusion distributions in a patient with severe pneumonia requiring mechanical ventilation with PEEP. Note that shunt and dead space are markedly increased; likewise, a considerable amount of blood flow is distributed to a zone with low $\dot{V}A/\dot{Q}$ ratios (below 0.1). Compared with patients with ARDS (Fig. 37-5), the bimodal pattern of pulmonary perfusion is more accentuated. (*Reproduced, with permission, from Gea et al.[35]*)

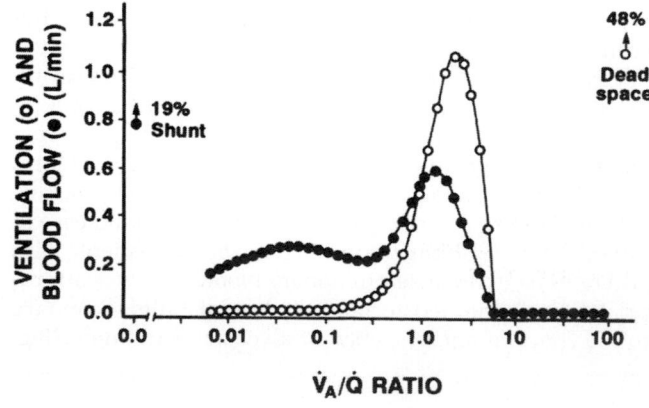

increased intrapulmonary O_2 uptake, and postpulmonary shunt), other than shunt and $\dot{V}_A/\dot{Q}$ mismatch, can be ruled out.[35,62] The coexistence of increased intrapulmonary O_2 consumption within the parenchyma[36] and increased postpulmonary shunt,[64] previously suggested as an additional mechanism contributing to hypoxemia, was not observed in patients with severe pneumonia.[35]

Breathing 100% Oxygen

Breathing 100% O_2 induced no changes in inert-gas shunt or in venous admixture ratio, as might be expected, at least theoretically, in patients whose lungs contain abundant critical alveolar units at risk of undergoing collapse, thereby developing reabsorption atelectasis.[7,38] This suggests that, in lungs with more localized lung injury, low $\dot{V}_A/\dot{Q}$ areas are less liable to collapse during oxygen breathing, probably because of the efficiency of collateral ventilation and the interaction between mechanical forces within the lung. Nevertheless, there was further $\dot{V}_A/\dot{Q}$ deterioration, as assessed by the marked increase in the dispersion of blood flow, indicating release of hypoxic pulmonary vasoconstriction. This finding indicates a considerable hypoxic vascular response of the lung, which may play a protective role against further worsening of gas exchange. In contrast, the dispersion of ventilation tended to decrease (improve) and dead space remained unaltered (Table 37-1). Conceivably, this mild reduction in the dispersion of alveolar ventilation might reflect blood flow redistribution from high- to low-$\dot{V}_A/\dot{Q}$ regions, where hypoxic vasoconstriction takes place.

Postural Changes

Ventilation-perfusion distributions have been studied in a few patients with unilateral lung disease (presence of infiltrates) needing mechanical ventilation.[65] Two patients displayed a predominant decrease in intrapulmonary shunt and two other patients showed an improvement in $\dot{V}_A/\dot{Q}$ distributions when the uninvolved lung side was dependent. Although this difference in response may be related to the lack of clinical uniformity in the small number of patients studied, both responses resulted in increases in Pa_{O_2} when the healthy lung was dependent.

Head Trauma

Patients with head trauma with normal chest radiology and without clinical neurogenic pulmonary edema show mild-to-severe $\dot{V}_A/\dot{Q}$ mismatch, essentially characterized by the presence of areas of low $\dot{V}_A/\dot{Q}$ ratios and mild shunt (less

than 10% of cardiac output) (without PEEP). Although no satisfactory explanation has been given for such gas exchange abnormalities,[66] subclinical pulmonary edema on days before admission, atelectasis, and/or decreased lung compliance have been suggested as potential mechanisms.

When mechanical ventilation was discontinued, shunt remained almost unchanged, while $\dot{V}_A/\dot{Q}$ distributions were less homogeneous and less unimodal, with a substantial increase in perfusion to regions of low $\dot{V}_A/\dot{Q}$. Functional residual capacity, minute ventilation, and cardiac output were no different between both conditions, but pulmonary arterial pressures increased significantly when patients were removed from the ventilator. Two patients improved dramatically in a few days with considerable, although incomplete, restoration of $\dot{V}_A/\dot{Q}$ mismatch to normal. This suggested the return of normal hypoxic pulmonary vasoconstriction.

Cardiac Surgery

Gas exchange has been studied in patients on the day after coronary bypass surgery for myocardial revascularization[67–69] or aortic valvular replacement.[70] Overall, shunt was mildly to moderately increased (less than 15–20% of cardiac output) and $\dot{V}_A/\dot{Q}$ distributions showed a variable degree of severity, in general akin to preoperative findings, with variable patterns (broadly unimodal or clearly bimodal) of $\dot{V}_A/\dot{Q}$ abnormalities. The presence of relatively abundant shunt was also consistent with the presumed underlying multifactorial pathology in these patients. Shunt has been attributed to noncardiogenic pulmonary edema related to cardiopulmonary bypass, reduced functional residual capacity, surfactant alterations, increased closing volume secondary to retained secretions, abnormal hypoxic pulmonary vasoconstriction, and reabsorption atelectasis from a high $F_{I_{O_2}}$.

Breathing 100% O_2 increased the dispersion of blood flow, but neither intrapulmonary shunt nor dispersion of alveolar ventilation increased.[68] These findings were interpreted as release of hypoxic pulmonary vasoconstriction.

In one of the studies,[70] measurements were repeated while the uninvolved (good) right lung was down. Gas-exchange abnormalities in these patients had been previously reported to be more common in the left lung.[70] The improvement of Pa_{O_2} on moving the patient from supine to the right lateral decubitus position was associated with an improvement in $\dot{V}_A/\dot{Q}$ relationships but not in shunt, although a beneficial effect on overall gas exchange, secondary to

TABLE 37-1   Characteristics of Pulmonary Gas Exchange in Acute Lung Injury "Wet Lung"

	ALI/ARDS	Pneumonia
Principal mechanisms		
Shunt	Severe≥20%	Severe≥20%
$\dot{V}_A/\dot{Q}$ mismatch	Absent/mild	Mild/moderate
O_2 diffusion limitation	Absent	Absent
100% Oxygen effects		
Increase in Pa_{O_2}	Mild/moderate ($\leq$300 mmHg)	Marked ($\geq$300 mmHg)
Increase in shunt	Mild/moderate	Absent
Hypoxic vascular response	Absent	Increased

a simultaneous increase of cardiac output, could not be ruled out. These results are at variance with those in patients with unilateral lung disease, in whom either intrapulmonary shunting or $\dot{V}_A/\dot{Q}$ mismatch improved when the uninvolved (good) lung was down.[65]

CHRONIC AIRFLOW LIMITATION ("DRY LUNG")

Although exacerbations of COPD and acute severe asthma have a common functional hallmark, chronic airflow obstruction with or without associated reversibility, they show substantial pathophysiologic differences. A contrasting feature of pulmonary gas exchange in patients with "dry lung" and in patients with "wet lung" is that the functional findings observed during exacerbations can be better interpreted in the light of the findings observed during the stable state.

CHRONIC OBSTRUCTIVE PULMONARY DISEASE EXACERBATIONS

Patients with COPD show up to four different patterns of $\dot{V}_A/\dot{Q}$ distributions (Fig. 37-13). One pattern may be characterized by a mode including a substantial amount of blood flow diverted to lung units with very low $\dot{V}_A/\dot{Q}$ regions, known as "low $\dot{V}_A/\dot{Q}$ mode" (type L).[71,72] Another profile may include alveolar units with high $\dot{V}_A/\dot{Q}$ regions, named "high $\dot{V}_A/\dot{Q}$ mode" (type H). This pattern likely suggests that most of the alveolar ventilation is distributed to zones with higher $\dot{V}_A/\dot{Q}$ ratios. A third profile is a mixed high-low $\dot{V}_A/\dot{Q}$ mode (type H-L), which consists of additional modes above and below the main body of $\dot{V}_A/\dot{Q}$ ratios. A fourth pattern has only two broadly unimodal dispersions. All in all, the dispersions of blood flow or ventilation, or both, tend to be severely increased. Intrapulmonary shunting is slightly elevated and dead space is mildly to moderately increased. The minimal amount of shunt suggests that the efficiency of collateral ventilation is very active or that complete airway obstruction does not occur functionally except in a few airways that are completely occluded, possibly by inspissated bronchial secretions.

An important concept is that patients with a COPD exacerbation, whether requiring or not requiring ventilator support, exhibit mild amounts of shunt (usually less than 10% of cardiac output) although quantitatively more severe $\dot{V}_A/\dot{Q}$ patterns than do patients with stable COPD.[71,72] If a patient with an exacerbation of COPD shows moderate-to-severe amounts of shunt (i.e., 20% of cardiac output) despite normal chest radiology–which excludes collapse, consolidation, or edema within the lung–then the possibility of a reopening of the foramen ovale should be considered.[73,74]

Breathing 100% Oxygen

During COPD exacerbations, administration of 100% O_2 rapidly produces full nitrogen washout of alveolar units, even in patients with low or very low $\dot{V}_A/\dot{Q}$ ratios. A steady state is reached by approximately half an hour, resulting in Pa_{O_2} values close to 500 mmHg.[38,75] These data indicate that shunt is trivial (less than 10% of cardiac output) or negligible.

Breathing 100% O_2 always worsens $\dot{V}_A/\dot{Q}$ relationships, as assessed by a significant increase in the dispersion of blood flow (Log SD Q). In addition, there is a discrete decrease of the dispersion of alveolar ventilation, and dead space tends to increase (Fig. 37-14). As discussed above, the further worsening in $\dot{V}_A/\dot{Q}$ relationships suggests attenuation of hypoxic pulmonary vasoconstriction, even though both pulmonary arterial pressure and vascular resistance remain essentially unaltered. This $\dot{V}_A/\dot{Q}$ deterioration results in a slight but significant increase in Pa_{CO_2}, which also can be influenced by the Haldane effect. The latter was more strongly demonstrated in patients with COPD exacerbations while spontaneously breathing 100% O_2.[76] Alternatively, the slight decrease in the ventilation dispersion could reflect some redistribution of blood flow, from areas

FIGURE 37-13 (*Left panel*) Typical bimodal patterns of both blood flow and alveolar ventilation in a representative patient with COPD needing mechanical ventilation. Both shunt and dead space are modestly increased. For further explanation, see text. (*Reproduced, with permission, from Rodriguez-Roisin.*[32])

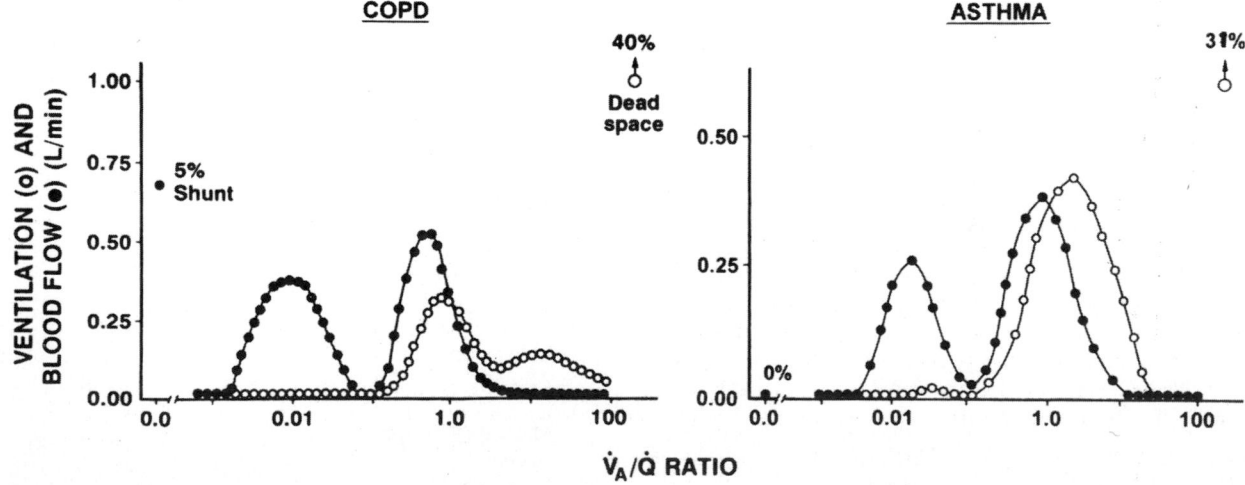

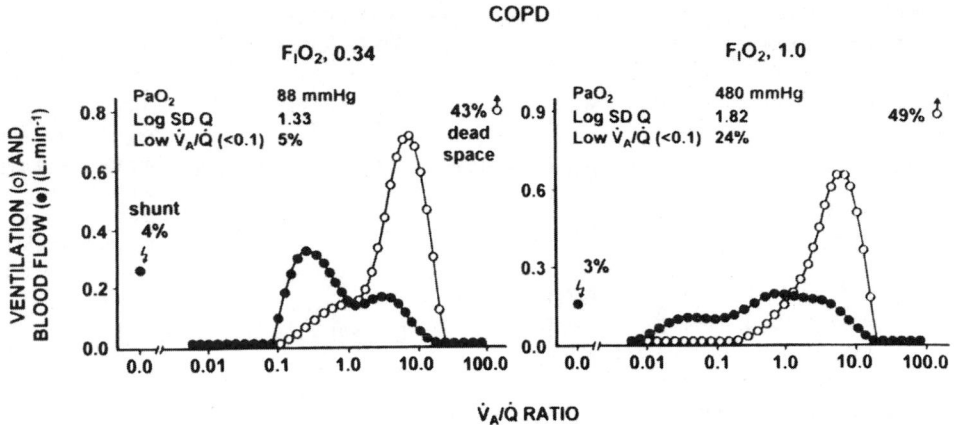

FIGURE 37-14 Effects of breathing 100% oxygen (*right panel*) in a representative patient with COPD. Compared with low F_{IO_2} (*left panel*), Pa_{O_2} increased substantially ($\geq$400 mmHg) but intrapulmonary shunt remained unaltered; in contrast, the dispersion of blood flow (Log SD $\dot{Q}$) and the amount of blood flow distributed to areas with low $\dot{V}A/\dot{Q}$ ratios increased markedly. This suggests release of hypoxic vasoconstriction without developing reabsorption atelectasis. Dead space tended to increase. Compare these data with those in patients with ARDS (Fig. 35-7).

of high to areas of low $\dot{V}A/\dot{Q}$, induced by the accentuated hypoxic vascular response. The lack of increase of shunt in patients with COPD, unlike in patients with ALI/ARDS, indicates that reabsorption atelectasis does not take place. This suggests that either collateral ventilation is very efficient or regional airway occlusion is never functionally complete.

Another striking finding is that when maintenance F_{IO_2} is resumed, Pa_{O_2} rapidly (in less than half an hour) regains the values observed before the institution of breathing 100% O_2.[38] This indicates that nitrogen washout of alveolar units rapidly ceases, even in patients with severe airflow limitation, an observation at variance with ARDS[38] (see Fig. 37-8).

Effects of PEEP

The potential effects of $PEEP_i$ (auto-PEEP)[77] on gas exchange should be kept in mind in patients with COPD requiring mechanical ventilation. In these patients, alveolar pressure can remain positive throughout the respiratory cycle despite the absence of PEEP set on the ventilator.[77]

Because low levels of external PEEP may offset the deleterious effects of $PEEP_i$, investigators assessed the effects of both PEEP and $PEEP_i$ on $\dot{V}A/\dot{Q}$ relationships in patients with chronic airflow obstruction (all but one patient with acute severe asthma had COPD).[78] At low levels of external PEEP (about 50% of $PEEP_i$), arterial blood gases improved secondary to an overall optimization of $\dot{V}A/\dot{Q}$ relationships without changes in pulmonary mechanics or hemodynamics. With further increases in external PEEP so that PEEP was equal to $PEEP_i$, airway pressures slightly increased without further $\dot{V}A/\dot{Q}$ improvement. The investigators also showed that the use of "permissive" or "controlled" hypoventilation[79] to deliberately reduce $PEEP_i$ (by 50%) optimized O_2 delivery secondary to a simultaneous increase in cardiac output. Accordingly, the use of low levels of external PEEP together with "permissive" hypoventilation may be advantageous in patients with COPD needing ventilator support. PEEP may improve gas exchange with less risk of barotrauma. These findings have been strengthened by a study[80] in patients with expiratory flow limitation and

$PEEP_i$ that showed that application of external PEEP below measured $PEEP_1$ did not cause hyperinflation or increased intrathoracic pressure, and resulted in no alteration in lung mechanics, hemodynamics, or gas exchange.

Weaning

$\dot{V}A/\dot{Q}$ relationships in patients with COPD during weaning from mechanical ventilation has been investigated (Fig. 37-15).[75] No major differences in pulmonary and systemic hemodynamics were shown between mechanical and spontaneous breathing, although cardiac output increased significantly when patients were removed from the ventilator. Arterial P_{O_2} and O_2 consumption did not change between the two conditions, but mixed venous P_{O_2} and O_2 delivery increased significantly when patients were weaned from the ventilator. During spontaneous breathing, minute ventilation remained essentially unchanged, but respiratory frequency increased and tidal volume fell, resulting in rapid shallow breathing, increased Pa_{CO_2}, and decreased pH.

A considerable increase in the percentage of blood flow to areas of low $\dot{V}A/\dot{Q}$ was observed during spontaneous ventilation. In contrast, shunt, dispersion of blood flow, and dead space did not change. Therefore, there was further $\dot{V}A/\dot{Q}$ worsening during spontaneous ventilation after removal of ventilator support. This worsening can be explained by alterations in the breathing pattern and also by changes in cardiac output. Yet, Pa_{O_2} did not undergo major changes, indicating that arterial blood gases were not sufficiently sensitive to detect $\dot{V}A/\dot{Q}$ changes because other factors, such as minute ventilation and cardiac output, were modulating pulmonary gas exchange. Indeed, cardiac output increased substantially after cessation of mechanical ventilation because of a simultaneous abrupt increase in venous return. Similarly, there were increases in mixed venous P_{O_2} and O_2 delivery secondary to the increased cardiac output. Nevertheless, the resulting beneficial effect of the increased cardiac output on Pa_{O_2} was counterbalanced by the simultaneous $\dot{V}A/\dot{Q}$ worsening, induced in turn by a less efficient

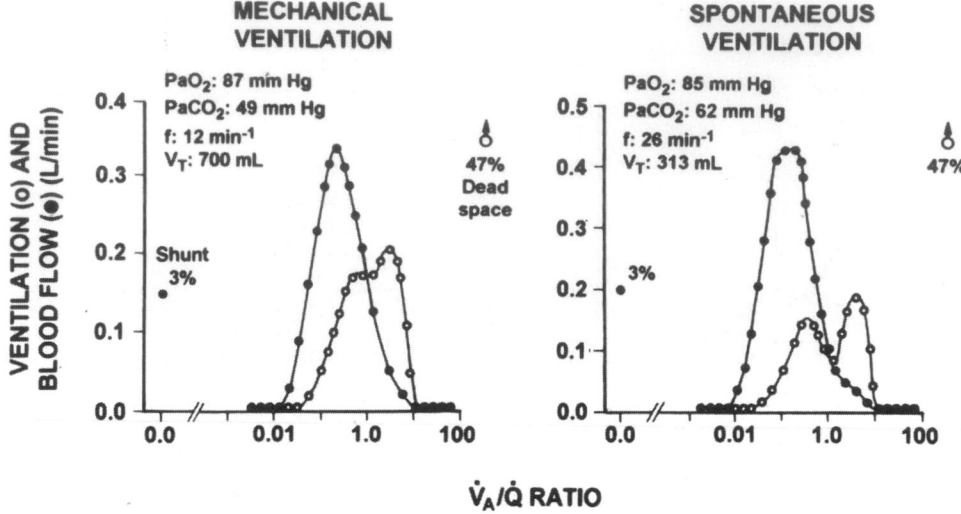

FIGURE 37-15 Effect of ventilator weaning in a representative patient with COPD. Compared with mechanical ventilation (*left panel*), weaning (*right panel*) induced rapid and shallow breathing resulting in increased Pa_{CO_2}. Arterial P_{O_2} did not decrease because the simultaneous increase in cardiac output (not shown) when mechanical ventilation was removed tended to improve Pa_{O_2}, the final result being an unaltered Pa_{O_2}. (*Reproduced, with permission, from Torres et al.[75]*)

breathing pattern and an increased overall blood flow. Further, the use of pressure-support ventilation during weaning in patients with exacerbations of COPD prevent worsening of $\dot{V}_A/\dot{Q}$ relationships during the transition from positive-pressure ventilation to spontaneous breathing.[81] Gas exchange and hemodynamic abnormalities were no different between assist-control and pressure-controlled ventilation when both strategies provided similar levels of ventilator assistance.

Similar results, although without further $\dot{V}_A/\dot{Q}$ worsening, were observed during weaning from mechanical ventilation in patients following coronary artery bypass (half of whom had chronic airflow limitation).[82] Patients with head trauma[63] showed a similar gas-exchange response upon discontinuation of mechanical ventilation, although without associated changes in ventilation and cardiac output.

The key role played by hemodynamic changes has been emphasized during unsuccessful weaning in patients with COPD.[82] Additional factors contributing to weaning failure include preexisting cardiovascular disease, which may be aggravated by dramatic changes in venous return. An increase of gastric pressure during spontaneous ventilation with subsequent increased splanchnic flow could be an additional mechanism.[83] Oxygen consumption also increases significantly. Inert gas and isotopic studies subsequently revealed that the critical alteration of the ventilation during weaning caused the development of basal regions with very low $\dot{V}_A/\dot{Q}$ ratios.[84]

The increased metabolic demands in these patients could have further negatively influenced the final Pa_{O_2}, thus offsetting the positive effects of the increased cardiac output. In patients with COPD, switching mechanical ventilation to either continuous positive pressure ventilation or pressure support, increased O_2 consumption and decreased minute ventilation, with marked increments Pa_{CO_2} and no change in Pa_{O_2}.[18] Conceivably, the simultaneous increase in cardiac output (not measured) prevented a fall in Pa_{O_2}. Subsequently, it was observed that patients needing mechanical ventilation (mostly with COPD and cardiac disorders) who failed a trial of spontaneous breathing developed a progressive reduction of mixed venous O_2 saturation secondary to the combined effect of a relative decrease in O_2 transport, possibly related to a decreased right- and left-ventricular afterload, and an increase in O_2 extraction by the tissues.[85]

Noninvasive Ventilation

The short-term effect of noninvasive ventilation for an exacerbation of COPD has been investigated by our group.[86] The beneficial effect on pulmonary gas exchange–decreased Pa_{CO_2}, and increased Pa_{O_2} and pH–was essentially achieved by a more efficient ventilatory pattern (slower and deeper breathing) without a favorable influence on $\dot{V}_A/\dot{Q}$ imbalance. A significant decrease in cardiac output during mechanical support, because of increased intrathoracic pressure, did not decrease Pa_{O_2}. The combined use of long-term O_2 therapy and nocturnal noninvasive ventilation in patients with advanced COPD and hypercapnic respiratory failure was recently shown to produce substantial improvement in respiratory gases.[46] The usual abnormal $\dot{V}_A/\dot{Q}$ pattern improved remarkably tending towards normalcy. These findings suggest that improvement in $\dot{V}_A/\dot{Q}$ relationships may reflect structure-function remodeling under some special circumstances.

ACUTE SEVERE ASTHMA

In postmortem studies in patients with sudden fatal asthma, bronchioles reveal increased amounts of luminal occlusion, increased smooth-muscle thickness, and inflammatory infiltrate with both mononuclear cells and eosinophils. Muscular pulmonary arteries adjacent to occluded and inflamed peripheral airways showed a marked inflammatory process in their walls more noticeably when close to airways.[87]

MECHANISMS OF HYPOXEMIA

Patients with life-threatening status asthmaticus who need mechanical ventilation show the most abnormal $\dot{V}_A/\dot{Q}$ pattern in patients with asthma: a marked bimodal blood flow profile that may include 50% or more of cardiac output (Fig. 37-16).[88,89] Severe airways obstruction produces

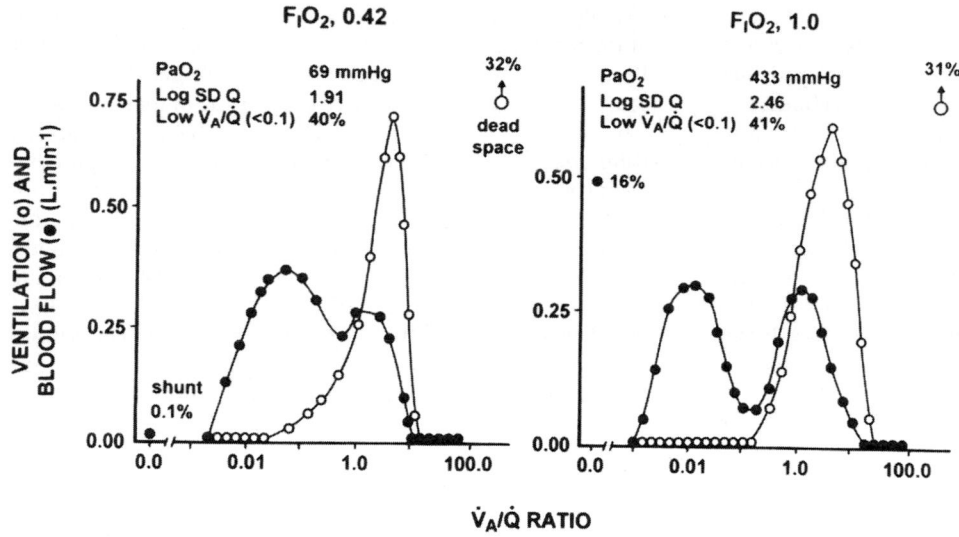

FIGURE 37-16 Effect of breathing 100% O_2 (*right panel*) in a representative patient with acute severe asthma. Compared with low F_{IO_2} (*left panel*), Pa_{O_2} increased substantially ($\geq$400 mmHg) associated with increases in intrapulmonary shunt, the dispersion of blood flow (Log SD Q), and the amount of blood flow distributed to areas of low $\dot{V}_A/\dot{Q}$ ratios. This suggests the development of reabsorption atelectasis (or selective redistribution of pulmonary blood flow) accompanied with the release of hypoxic vasoconstriction. Compare these data with those seen in patients with COPD (Fig. 37-14).

regions of low $\dot{V}_A/\dot{Q}$ that remain perfused but poorly ventilated. This must increase blood flow dispersion more than ventilation dispersion. Conceivably, the high F_{IO_2}, together with high doses of bronchodilators with potential vasodilating effects, may attenuate hypoxic pulmonary vasoconstriction, hence contributing to the increase in perfusion of areas with low $\dot{V}_A/\dot{Q}$ ratios. The relatively well preserved Pa_{O_2} in the presence of such severe $\dot{V}_A/\dot{Q}$ mismatch is noteworthy. This can be attributed to the inordinately high levels of both cardiac output and overall ventilation, which reinforce the major role played by the extrapulmonary determinants of Pa_{O_2} in modulating gas exchange.[16,24,32]

Unexpectedly, shunt was negligible or trivial in these patients. Given the presence of abundant, tenacious, and viscous secretions, one would expect alveolar units distal to narrowed airways to be collapsed. This, however, need not be the case. Collateral ventilation and hypoxic pulmonary vasoconstriction are exceptionally efficient. Moreover, airway occlusion is never functionally complete. Another unexpected finding was the presence of normal dead space, the mechanism of which remains unsettled. The coexistence of diffusion limitation for O_2 was also ruled out (Table 37-2).

BREATHING 100% OXYGEN

Breathing 100% O_2 induced mild amounts of shunt (less than 10% of cardiac output) in patients with asthma (see Fig. 37-16), suggesting either the presence of critical alveolar units leading to reabsorption atelectasis, or redistribution of pulmonary blood flow of preexisting small shunts, or both.[88] In addition, $\dot{V}_A/\dot{Q}$ mismatch substantially deteriorated, as shown by a considerable increase of the dispersion of pulmonary blood flow. This suggests that hypoxic pulmonary vasoconstriction was decreased. These data are consistent with the morphologic postmortem findings[87] showing that muscular pulmonary arteries adjacent to occluded peripheral airways had marked inflammatory wall involvement that was not characteristic of that associated with chronic hypoxia. Conceivably, these structural abnormalities may reflect pulmonary vascular leakage related to the release of inflammatory mediators.[90] In contrast, the dispersion of alveolar ventilation decreased significantly. A redistribution of blood flow from areas with units of high to areas with units of low $\dot{V}_A/\dot{Q}$ ratio is a potential explanation. A tendency towards an increase in dead space, also shown during 100% O_2 breathing, could reflect hyperoxic bronchodilation.

TABLE 37-2 Characteristics of Pulmonary Gas Exchange in Chronic Airflow Limitation ("Dry Lung")

	COPD	Asthma
Principal mechanisms		
Shunt	Mild ($<$10% of Q_T)	Absent
$\dot{V}_A/\dot{Q}$ mismatch	Severe (non-uniform pattern)	Severe (uniform pattern)
O_2 Diffusion limitation	Absent	Absent
100% Oxygen effects		
Increase in Pa_{O_2}	Marked ($\geq$500 mmHg)	Marked ($\geq$500 mmHg)
Increase in shunt	Absent	Mild/moderate
Hypoxic vascular response	Increased	Increased

EFFECTS OF PEEP

The use of PEEP in patients with severe asthma is controversial. Anecdotal reports in patients with life-threatening asthma show conflicting results. While some studies showed improvement in gas exchange and lung mechanics,[91,92] others found marked increases in Pa_{O_2} associated with gas trapping and increased airway and intrathoracic pressures with decreased cardiac output.[93] From a therapeutic viewpoint, a study of our group[78] in patients with COPD and acute respiratory failure suggests that low levels of PEEP, combined with some degree of "permissive" hypoventilation, might help in optimizing gas exchange in patients with acute severe asthma needing mechanical ventilation.

Effect of Special Modes of Ventilation

HIGH FREQUENCY VENTILATION

During the 1980s there was much interest in mechanical ventilation using small tidal volumes combined with very high frequencies. Few techniques of mechanical ventilation have stimulated as much excitement in the minds of investigators as high-frequency ventilation (HFV), resulting in hundreds of research studies. A reduction in complications such as hemodynamic depression and barotrauma associated with conventional modes was invoked as one of the major advantages.[94]

A comparison of HFV and controlled mechanical ventilation (CMV) in a canine model showed that the efficiency of Pa_{O_2} was no different, but the amount of areas of high $\dot{V}_A/\dot{Q}$ was increased.[95,96] Additional experiments showed that there was an enhanced transport of high-solubility inert gases (approximately twice that for other inert gases) along the airways during HFV. It was suggested that this enhanced transport was dependent on the wet luminal surface of conducting airways.[96]

Although the mechanism of gas delivery by HFV remains to be elucidated, one of the hypotheses is based on augmented dispersion.[97] The theory posits that augmented dispersion during HFV should be less dependent on airway resistance and pulmonary compliance than during CMV. Accordingly, regions of low $\dot{V}_A/\dot{Q}$ might be better ventilated than during CMV. In a canine model of extensive areas of low $\dot{V}_A/\dot{Q}$ but little shunt associated with bronchoconstriction and mucus secretion, HFV was no more effective in delivering fresh gas to such areas than was CMV.[98]

CONTINUOUS-FLOW VENTILATION

Continuous-flow ventilation (CFV) is achieved by delivering continuous streams of gas through cannulas directed down the two main bronchi, in the absence of tidal excursions in lung volume. When CFV was compared to CMV in an animal model,[99] CFV caused significant deterioration in $\dot{V}_A/\dot{Q}$ matching secondary to an increase in the amount of dispersion of pulmonary blood flow. This suggested that CFV induced a nonuniform ventilation distribution and a redistribution of pulmonary perfusion.

In supine dogs, CO_2 elimination was more efficient with endotracheal insufflation than with tracheal insufflation, but the alveolar-arterial P_{O_2} difference was larger during CFV than during CMV irrespective of the type of insufflation.[100] Conversely, elimination of CO_2 and alveolar-arterial P_{O_2} difference was lower when prone than when supine. In the prone position, gas distribution was uniform with both modes of ventilation. The increased alveolar-arterial P_{O_2} difference when supine during CFV was negatively correlated with the decreased ventilation of the dependent zones of the lung, suggesting further $\dot{V}_A/\dot{Q}$ inequalities. The improved gas exchange during CFV in dogs lying prone reflects a more efficient $\dot{V}_A/\dot{Q}$ matching, presumably because the distribution of pulmonary blood flow is nearly uniform.

Conclusion

Arterial P_{O_2} and P_{CO_2} are the end-point outcomes of the gas-exchange state and are governed by the interplay of several intrapulmonary and extrapulmonary components. The most remarkable intrapulmonary factors are $\dot{V}_A/\dot{Q}$ mismatching and intrapulmonary shunt; in contrast, diffusion limitation to O_2 plays a marginal role. Among the extrapulmonary factors, inspired P_{O_2}, overall ventilation, cardiac output, and O_2 consumption are viewed as the most influential.

While breathing 100% O_2, despite substantial Pa_{O_2} improvements, $\dot{V}_A/\dot{Q}$ relationships worsen characteristically according to the underlying nature of acute respiratory insufficiency. In patients with "wet lung" (ALI/ARDS), shunt increases secondary to the development of reabsorption atelectasis without release of hypoxic pulmonary vasoconstriction. In patients with "dry lung" (COPD/asthma), hypoxic vasoconstriction is ultimately released while shunt remains unchanged. Gas-exchange abnormalities may be influenced by changes in cardiac output depending on different ventilator modalities, in particular during weaning from mechanical ventilation.

References

1. West JB. Causes of carbon dioxide retention in lung disease. N Engl J Med 1971; 284:1232–36.
2. West JB. State of the art: ventilation-perfusion relationships. Am Rev Respir Dis 1977; 116:919–43.
3. West JB. Ventilation-perfusion inequality and overall gas exchange in computer models of the lung. Respir Physiol 1969; 7:88–110.
4. Dantzker DR. Gas exchange in the adult respiratory distress syndrome. Clin Chest Med 1982; 3:57–67.
5. Von Euler US, Liljestrand G. Observations on the pulmonary arterial pressure in the cat. Acta Physiol Scand 1946; 12:301–20.
6. Voelkel NF. Mechanisms of hypoxic pulmonary vasoconstriction. Am Rev Respir Dis 1986; 133:1186–95.
7. Dantzker DR, Wagner PD, West JB. Instability of lung units with low $\dot{V}_A/\dot{Q}$ ratios during O_2 breathing. J Appl Physiol 1975; 38:886–95.
8. Astin TW. The relationships between arterial blood oxygen saturation, carbon dioxide tension, and pH and airway resistance during 30 per cent oxygen breathing in patients with chronic

bronchitis with airway obstruction. Am Rev Respir Dis 1970; 102:382–7.

9. Libby DM, Briscoe WA, King TK. Relief of hypoxia-related bronchoconstriction by breathing 30 per cent oxygen. Am Rev Respir Dis 1981; 123:171–5.

10. Inoue H, Inoue C, Okayama M, et al. Breathing 30 per cent oxygen attenuates bronchial responsiveness to methacholine in asthmatic patients. Eur Respir J 1989; 2:506–12.

11. Wetzel RC, Herold CJ, Zerhouni EA, Robotham JL. Hypoxic bronchodilation. J Appl Physiol 1992; 73:1202–6.

12. Kato M, Staub NC. Response of small pulmonary arteries to unilobar hypoxia and hypercapnia. Circ Res 1966; 19:426–40.

13. Barer GR, Howard P, Shaw JW. Stimulus-response curves for the pulmonary vascular bed to hypoxia and hypercapnia. J Physiol 1970; 211:139–55.

14. Briscoe WA, Cree EM, Filler J, Houssay HEJ, Cournand A. Lung volume, alveolar ventilation and perfusion interrelationships in chronic pulmonary emphysema. J Appl Physiol 1960; 15: 785–795.

15. Mead J. Mechanical properties of lungs. Physiol Rev 1961; 41:281–330.

16. Rodriguez-Roisin R, Wagner PD. Clinical relevance of ventilation-perfusion inequality determined by inert gas elimination. Eur Respir J 1990; 3:469–82.

17. Wagner PD. Ventilation-perfusion inequality in catastrophic lung disease. In: Prakash O, editor. Applied physiology in clinical respiratory care. The Hague: Martinus Nijhoff, 1982: 363–79.

18. Annat GJ, Viale JP, Dereymez CP, et al. Oxygen cost of breathing and diaphragmatic pressure-time index. Measurement in patients with COPD during weaning with pressure support ventilation. Chest 1990; 98:411–4.

19. Dantzker DR. The influence of cardiovascular function on gas exchange. Clin Chest Med 1983; 4:149–59.

20. Agusti AG, Roca J, Gea J, et al. Mechanisms of gas-exchange impairment in idiopathic pulmonary fibrosis. Am Rev Respir Dis 1991; 143:219–25.

21. Torre-Bueno JR, Wagner PD, Saltzman HA, et al. Diffusion limitation in normal humans during exercise at sea level and simulated altitude. J Appl Physiol 1985; 58:989–95.

22. Lynch JP, Mhyre JG, Dantzker DR. Influence of cardiac output on intrapulmonary shunt. J Appl Physiol 1979; 46:315–21.

23. Dantzker DR, Lynch JP, Weg JG. Depression of cardiac output is a mechanism of shunt reduction in the therapy of acute respiratory failure. Chest 1980; 77:636–42.

24. Wagner PD, Rodriguez-Roisin R. Clinical advances in pulmonary gas exchange. Am Rev Respir Dis 1991; 143:883–8.

25. Laver MB, Morgan J, Bendixen HH, et al. Lung volume, compliance, and arterial oxygen tensions during controlled ventilation. J Appl Physiol 1964; 19:725–33.

26. Wagner PD, Schaffartzik W, Prediletto R, et al. Relationship among cardiac output, shunt, and inspired O_2 concentration. J Appl Physiol 1991; 71:2191–7.

27. Wagner PD, Saltzman HA, West JB. Measurement of continuous distributions of ventilation-perfusion ratios: theory. J Appl Physiol 1974; 36:588–99.

28. Wagner PD, Naumann PF, Laravuso RB. Simultaneous measurement of eight foreign gases in blood by gas chromatography. J Appl Physiol 1974; 36:600–5.

29. Evans JW, Wagner PD. Limits on $\dot{V}A/\dot{Q}$ distributions from analysis of experimental inert gas elimination. J Appl Physiol 1977; 42:889–98.

30. Roca J, Wagner PD. Contribution of multiple inert gas elimination technique to pulmonary medicine. 1. Principles and information content of the multiple inert gas elimination technique. Thorax 1994; 49:815–24.

31. Bernard GR, Artigas A, Brigham KL, et al. The American-European Consensus Conference on ARDS. Definitions, mechanisms, relevant outcomes, and clinical trial coordination. Am J Respir Crit Care Med 1994; 149:818–24.

32. Rodriguez-Roisin R. Ventilation-perfusion relationships. In: Pinsky MR, Dhainaut JF, eds. Pathophysiologic foundations of critical care. Baltimore: Williams & Wilkins, 1993: 389–413.

33. Reyes A, Roca J, Rodriguez-Roisin R, et al. Effect of almitrine on ventilation-perfusion distribution in adult respiratory distress syndrome. Am Rev Respir Dis 1988; 137:1062–7.

34. Dantzker DR, Brook CJ, Dehart P, et al. Ventilation-perfusion distributions in the adult respiratory distress syndrome. Am Rev Respir Dis 1979; 120:1039–52.

35. Gea J, Roca J, Torres A, et al. Mechanisms of abnormal gas exchange in patients with pneumonia. Anesthesiology 1991; 75:782–9.

36. Light RB. Intrapulmonary oxygen consumption in experimental pneumococcal pneumonia. J Appl Physiol 1988; 64:2490–5.

37. Suter PM, Fairley HB, Schlobohm RM. Shunt, lung volume and perfusion during short periods of ventilation with oxygen. Anesthesiology 1975; 43:617–27.

38. Santos C, Ferrer M, Roca J, et al. Pulmonary gas exchange response to oxygen breathing in acute lung injury. Am J Respir Crit Care Med 2000; 161:26–31.

39. Matamis D, Lemaire F, Harf A, et al. Redistribution of pulmonary blood flow induced by positive end-expiratory pressure and dopamine infusion in acute respiratory failure. Am Rev Respir Dis 1984; 129:39–44.

40. Hopewell PC, Murray JF. Effects of continuous positive-pressure ventilation in experimental pulmonary edema. J Appl Physiol 1976; 40:568–74.

41. Ralph DD, Robertson HT, Weaver LJ, et al. Distribution of ventilation and perfusion during positive end-expiratory pressure in the adult respiratory distress syndrome. Am Rev Respir Dis 1985; 131:54–60.

42. Coffey RL, Albert RK, Robertson HT. Mechanisms of physiological dead space response to PEEP after acute oleic acid lung injury. J Appl Physiol 1983; 55:1550–7.

43. Lemaire F, Teisseire B, Harf A. Oxygen exchange across the acutely injured lung. In: Zapol WM, Falke KJ, editors. Acute respiratory failure. New York: Marcel Dekker, 1985: 521–53.

44. Dantzker DR, Foresman B, Gutierrez G. Oxygen supply and utilization relationships. A reevaluation. Am Rev Respir Dis 1991; 143:675–9.

45. Hedenstierna G, White FC, Mazzone R, et al. Redistribution of pulmonary blood flow in the dog with PEEP ventilation. J Appl Physiol 1979; 46:278–87.

46. American Thoracic Society. Medical Section of the American Lung Association. International Consensus Conferences in Intensive Care Medicine: Ventilator-associated Lung Injury in ARDS. Am J Respir Crit Care Med 1999; 160:2118–24.

47. Stewart TE, Meade MO, Cook DJ, et al. Evaluation of a ventilation strategy to prevent barotrauma in patients at high risk for acute respiratory distress syndrome. Pressure- and Volume-Limited Ventilation Strategy Group. N Engl J Med 1998; 338: 355–61.

48. Brochard L, Roudot-Thoraval F, Roupie E, et al. Tidal volume reduction for prevention of ventilator-induced lung injury in acute respiratory distress syndrome. The Multicenter Trial Group on Tidal Volume reduction in ARDS. Am J Respir Crit Care Med 1998; 158:1831–8.

49. Brower RG, Shanholtz CB, Fessler HE, et al. Prospective, randomized, controlled clinical trial comparing traditional versus reduced tidal volume ventilation in acute respiratory distress syndrome patients. Crit Care Med 1999; 27:1492–8.

50. Acute Respiratory Distress Syndrome Network. Ventilation with lower tidal volumes as compared with traditional tidal volumes for acute lung injury and the acute respiratory distress syndrome. N Engl J Med 2000; 342:1301–8.

51. Feihl F, Eckert P, Brimioulle S, et al. Permissive hypercapnia impairs pulmonary gas exchange in the acute respiratory distress syndrome. Am J Respir Crit Care Med 2000; 162:209–15.

52. Pfeiffer B, Hachenberg T, Wendt M, et al. Mechanical ventilation with permissive hypercapnia increases intrapulmonary shunt in septic and nonseptic patients with acute respiratory distress syndrome. Crit Care Med 2002; 30:285–9.

53. Amato MB, Barbas CS, Medeiros DM, et al. Effect of a protective-ventilation strategy on mortality in the acute respiratory distress syndrome. N Engl J Med 1998; 338:347–54.

54. Carvalho CR, Barbas CS, Medeiros DM, et al. Temporal hemodynamic effects of permissive hypercapnia associated with ideal PEEP in ARDS. Am J Respir Crit Care Med 1997; 156:1458–66.

55. Mancini M, Zavala E, Mancebo J, et al. Mechanisms of pulmonary gas exchange improvement during a protective ventilatory strategy in acute respiratory distress syndrome. Am J Respir Crit Care Med 2001; 164:1448–53.

56. Laffey JG, Tanaka M, Engelberts D, et al. Therapeutic hypercapnia reduces pulmonary and systemic injury following in vivo lung reperfusion. Am J Respir Crit Care Med 2000; 162:2287–94.

57. Hickling KG. Lung-protective ventilation in acute respiratory distress syndrome: protection by reduced lung stress or by therapeutic hypercapnia? Am J Respir Crit Care Med 2000; 162: 2021–2.

58. Zavala E, Ferrer M, Polese G, et al. Effect of inverse I:E ratio ventilation on pulmonary gas exchange in acute respiratory distress syndrome. Anesthesiology 1998; 88:35–42.

59. Pappert D, Rossaint R, Slama K, et al. Influence of positioning on ventilation-perfusion relationships in severe adult respiratory distress syndrome. Chest 1994; 106:1511–6.

60. Bein T, Reber A, Metz C, et al. Acute effects of continuous rotational therapy on ventilation-perfusion inequality in lung injury. Intensive Care Med 1998; 24:132–7.

61. Putensen C, Mutz NJ, Putensen-Himmer G, et al. Spontaneous breathing during ventilatory support improves ventilation-perfusion distributions in patients with acute respiratory distress syndrome. Am J Respir Crit Care Med 1999; 159:1241–8.

62. Lampron N, Lemaire F, Teisseire B, et al. Mechanical ventilation with 100% oxygen does not increase intrapulmonary shunt in patients with severe bacterial pneumonia. Am Rev Respir Dis 1985; 131:409–13.

63. Wagner PD, Laravuso RB, Goldzimmer E, et al. Distribution of ventilation-perfusion ratios in dogs with normal and abnormal lungs. J Appl Physiol 1975; 38:1099–109.

64. Alexander JK, Takezawa H, Abu-Nassar HJ, et al. Studies on pulmonary blood flow in pneumococcal pneumonia. Cardiovasc Res Cent Bull 1963; 1:86–92.

65. Gillespie DJ, Rehder K. Body position and ventilation-perfusion relationships in unilateral pulmonary disease. Chest 1987; 91:75–9.

66. Schumacker PT, Rhodes GR, Newell JC, et al. Ventilation-perfusion imbalance after head trauma. Am Rev Respir Dis 1979; 119:33–43.

67. Dantzker DR, Cowenhaven WM, Willoughby WJ, et al. Gas exchange alterations associated with weaning from mechanical ventilation following coronary artery bypass grafting. Chest 1982; 82:674–7.

68. Anjou-Lindskog E, Broman L, Broman M, et al. Effects of oxygen on central haemodynamics and $\dot{V}_A/\dot{Q}$ distribution after coronary bypass surgery. Acta Anaesthesiol Scand 1983; 27: 378–84.

69. Valentine DD, Hammond MD, Downs JB, et al. Distribution of ventilation and perfusion with different modes of mechanical ventilation. Am Rev Respir Dis 1991; 143:1262–6.

70. Gillespie DJ, Didier EP, Rehder K. Ventilation-perfusion distribution after aortic valve replacement. Crit Care Med 1990; 18:136–40.

71. Wagner PD, Dantzker DR, Dueck R, et al. Ventilation-perfusion inequality in chronic obstructive pulmonary disease. J Clin Invest 1977; 59:203–16.

72. Rodríguez-Roisin R, Barbera JA, Roca J. Pulmonary gas exchange. In: Calverley PMA, MacNee W, Pride NB, et al, editors. Chronic obstructive pulmonary disease. London: Arnold, 2003: 175–93.

73. Herve P, Petitpretz P, Simonneau G, et al. The mechanisms of abnormal gas exchange in acute massive pulmonary embolism. Am Rev Respir Dis 1983; 128:1101–2.

74. Glauser FL, Polatty RC, Sessler CN. Worsening oxygenation in the mechanically ventilated patient. Causes, mechanisms, and early detection. Am Rev Respir Dis 1988; 138:458–65.

75. Torres A, Reyes A, Roca J, et al. Ventilation-perfusion mismatching in chronic obstructive pulmonary disease during ventilator weaning. Am Rev Respir Dis 1989; 140:1246–50.

76. Aubier M, Murciano D, Milic-Emili J, et al. Effects of the administration of O_2 on ventilation and blood gases in patients with chronic obstructive pulmonary disease during acute respiratory failure. Am Rev Respir Dis 1980; 122:747–54.

77. Pepe PE, Marini JJ. Occult positive end-expiratory pressure in mechanically ventilated patients with airflow obstruction: the auto-PEEP effect. Am Rev Respir Dis 1982; 126: 166–70.

78. Rossi A, Santos C, Roca J, et al. Effects of PEEP on $\dot{V}_A/\dot{Q}$ mismatching in ventilated patients with chronic airflow obstruction. Am J Respir Crit Care Med 1994; 149:1077–84.

79. Darioli R, Perret C. Mechanical controlled hypoventilation in status asthmaticus. Am Rev Respir Dis 1984; 129:385–7.

80. Ranieri VM, Giuliani R, Cinnella G, et al. Physiologic effects of positive end-expiratory pressure in patients with chronic obstructive pulmonary disease during acute ventilatory failure and controlled mechanical ventilation. Am Rev Respir Dis 1993; 147:5–13.

81. Ferrer M, Iglesia R, Roca J, et al. Pulmonary gas exchange response to weaning with pressure-support ventilation in exacerbated chronic obstructive pulmonary disease patients. Intensive Care Med 2002; 28:1595–9.

82. Lemaire F, Teboul JL, Cinotti L, et al. Acute left ventricular dysfunction during unsuccessful weaning from mechanical ventilation. Anesthesiology 1988; 69:171–9.

83. Permutt S. Circulatory effects of weaning from mechanical ventilation: the importance of transdiaphragmatic pressure. Anesthesiology 1988; 69:157–60.

84. Beydon L, Cinotti L, Rekik N, et al. Changes in the distribution of ventilation and perfusion associated with separation from mechanical ventilation in patients with obstructive pulmonary disease. Anesthesiology 1991; 75:730–8.

85. Jubran A, Mathru M, Dries D, et al. Continuous recordings of mixed venous oxygen saturation during weaning from mechanical ventilation and the ramifications thereof. Am J Respir Crit Care Med 1998; 158:1763–9.

86. Diaz O, Iglesia R, Ferrer M, et al. Effects of noninvasive ventilation on pulmonary gas exchange and hemodynamics during acute hypercapnic exacerbations of chronic obstructive pulmonary disease. Am J Respir Crit Care Med 1997; 156: 1840–1845.

87. Saetta M, Di Stefano A, Rosina C, et al. Quantitative structural analysis of peripheral airways and arteries in sudden fatal asthma. Am Rev Respir Dis 1991; 143:138–43.

88. Rodriguez-Roisin R, Ballester E, Roca J, et al. Mechanisms of hypoxemia in patients with status asthmaticus requiring mechanical ventilation. Am Rev Respir Dis 1989; 139:732–9.

89. Rodriguez-Roisin R, Roca J. Contributions of multiple inert gas elimination technique to pulmonary medicine.3. Bronchial asthma. Thorax 1994; 49:1027–33.

90. Barnes PJ, Baraniuk JN, Belvisi MG. Neuropeptides in the respiratory tract. Part I. Am Rev Respir Dis 1991; 144:1187–98.

91. Qvist J, Andersen JB, Pemberton M, et al. High-level PEEP in severe asthma. N Engl J Med 1982; 307:1347–8.

92. Tenaillon A, Salmona JP, Burdin M, et al. Continuous positive airway pressure in asthma (letter). Am Rev Respir Dis 1983; 127: 658.

93. Tuxen DV. Detrimental effects of positive end-expiratory pressure during controlled mechanical ventilation of patients with severe airflow obstruction. Am Rev Respir Dis 1989; 140: 5–9.

94. Kirby RR, Larson CPJ. Practical and ethical considerations. In: Carlon GC, Howland WS, editors. High-frequency ventilation in intensive care and during surgery. New York: Marcel Dekker, 1985: 7–23.

95. Robertson HT, Coffey RL, Standaert TA, et al. Respiratory and inert gas exchange during high-frequency ventilation. J Appl Physiol 1982; 52:683–9.

96. McEvoy RD, Davies NJ, Mannino FL, et al. Pulmonary gas exchange during high-frequency ventilation. J Appl Physiol 1982; 52:1278–87.

97. Fredberg JJ. Augmented diffusion in the airways can support pulmonary gas exchange. J Appl Physiol 1980; 49:232–8.

98. Kaiser KG, Davies NJ, Rodriguez-Roisin R, et al. Efficacy of high-frequency ventilation in presence of extensive ventilation-perfusion mismatch. J Appl Physiol 1985; 58:996–1004.

99. Schumacker PT, Sznajder JI, Nahum A, et al. Ventilation-perfusion inequality during constant-flow ventilation. J Appl Physiol 1987; 62:1255–63.

100. Vettermann J, Brusasco V, Rehder K. Gas exchange and intrapulmonary distribution of ventilation during continuous-flow ventilation. J Appl Physiol 1988; 64:1864–9.

PART X
ARTIFICIAL AIRWAYS AND MANAGEMENT

Chapter 38
AIRWAY MANAGEMENT

STEVEN DEEM
MICHAEL J. BISHOP

Airway management implies the provision of assistance to a patient in maintaining a patent airway. This chapter will review basic airway management techniques, in addition to reviewing airway anatomy and the physiologic effects of tracheal intubation.

Airway Anatomy

THE NOSE AND NASOPHARYNX

The nose is lined with vessel-rich mucosa designed to warm and humidify the air; during placement of transnasal tubes, the mucosa is easily damaged with consequent bleeding. Bypassing the nose causes dry gases to reach the respiratory tract and necessitates warming and humidification of gases during mechanical ventilation.

The two nares are divided by a nasal septum that is often not midline. In preparation for nasal intubation, the patient should sniff through each nare to demonstrate which one will more readily accept the nasal tube. In each nare are three turbinates (Fig. 38-1) that help to condition the inspired gases. Underneath each turbinate lies the opening of a perinasal sinus. When these openings are occluded, fluid tends to accumulate in the sinuses. Thus, long-term nasal intubation is associated with a high incidence of radiographic sinus opacification and bacterial sinusitis.[1]

The floor of the nose leading to the nasopharynx is in the same plane as the nasal orifices. When a tube is introduced into the nose, it should be directed straight back rather than caudad (Fig. 38-2), and advanced carefully to avoid injuring the turbinates.

THE MOUTH

Oral structures relevant to airway management include the mouth aperture, teeth, and tongue. Introduction of a laryngoscope through the mouth can be impeded by temporomandibular joint fixation, leading to the inability to open the mouth, or mandibular hypo- or hyperplasia. Prominent incisors may also interfere with direct laryngoscopy, and loose or carious teeth may be dislodged or broken during laryngoscopy. An enlarged tongue (e.g., secondary to angioedema or venous congestion) can also interfere with airway patency and impede laryngoscopy.

THE PHARYNX

The pharynx is shaped like a cone (Fig. 38-3) and includes the nasopharynx and the oropharynx, which join to form the hypopharynx. The walls of the pharynx are relatively soft and compliant and thus can become substantially inflamed from infectious or traumatic processes. Substantial increases in pharyngeal soft tissue can make visualization of the larynx extremely difficult.

The digestive and respiratory tracts share a common lumen in the pharynx. The posterior portion of the pharynx continues to form the esophagus whereas the anterior portion ends in a series of pouches or fossae surrounding the larynx. The epiglottis forms the posterior wall of the anterior pouch. The region anterior to the epiglottis is called the *vallecula* and is an important landmark for endotracheal intubation because the tip of a curved laryngoscope blade is typically placed in this fossa.

The epiglottic cartilage is shaped like a leaf and is attached to the posterior surface of the thyroid cartilage. Functionally,

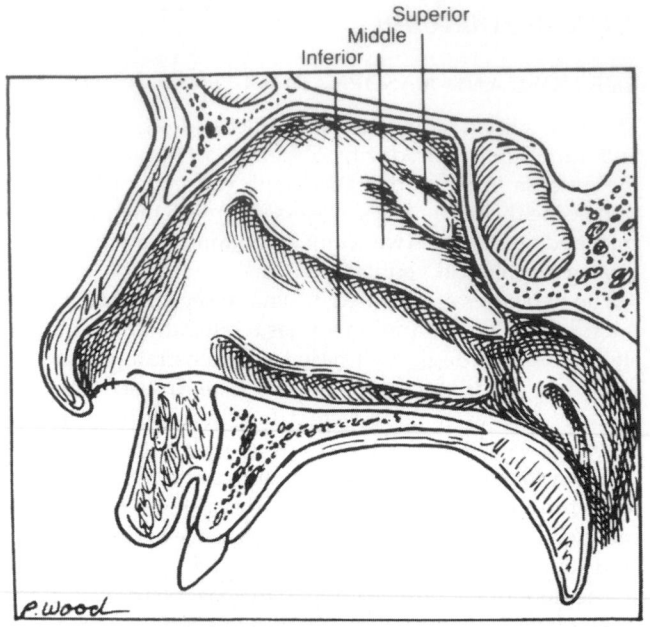

FIGURE 38-1 The nasal turbinates. Note that these are easily traumatized during nasal instrumentation. (*Reproduced, with permission, from Pierson et al, editors: Foundations of respiratory care. New York: Churchill Livingstone, 1992.*)

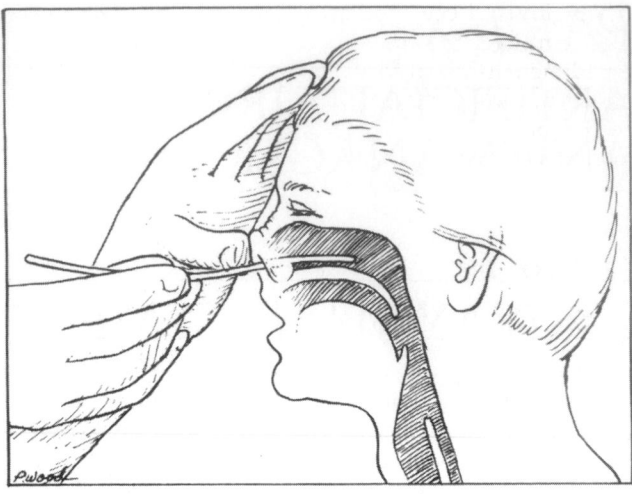

FIGURE 38-2 Insertion of a catheter into the nose. The catheter should be directed in parallel with the floor of the nose. (*Reproduced, with permission, from Pierson et al, editors: Foundations of respiratory care. New York: Churchill Livingstone, 1992.*)

FIGURE 38-3 Lateral (*A*) and posterior oblique (*B*) views of the pharynx and larynx, including the laryngeal skeleton. (*Reproduced, with permission, from Pierson et al, editors: Foundations of respiratory care. New York: Churchill Livingstone, 1992.*)

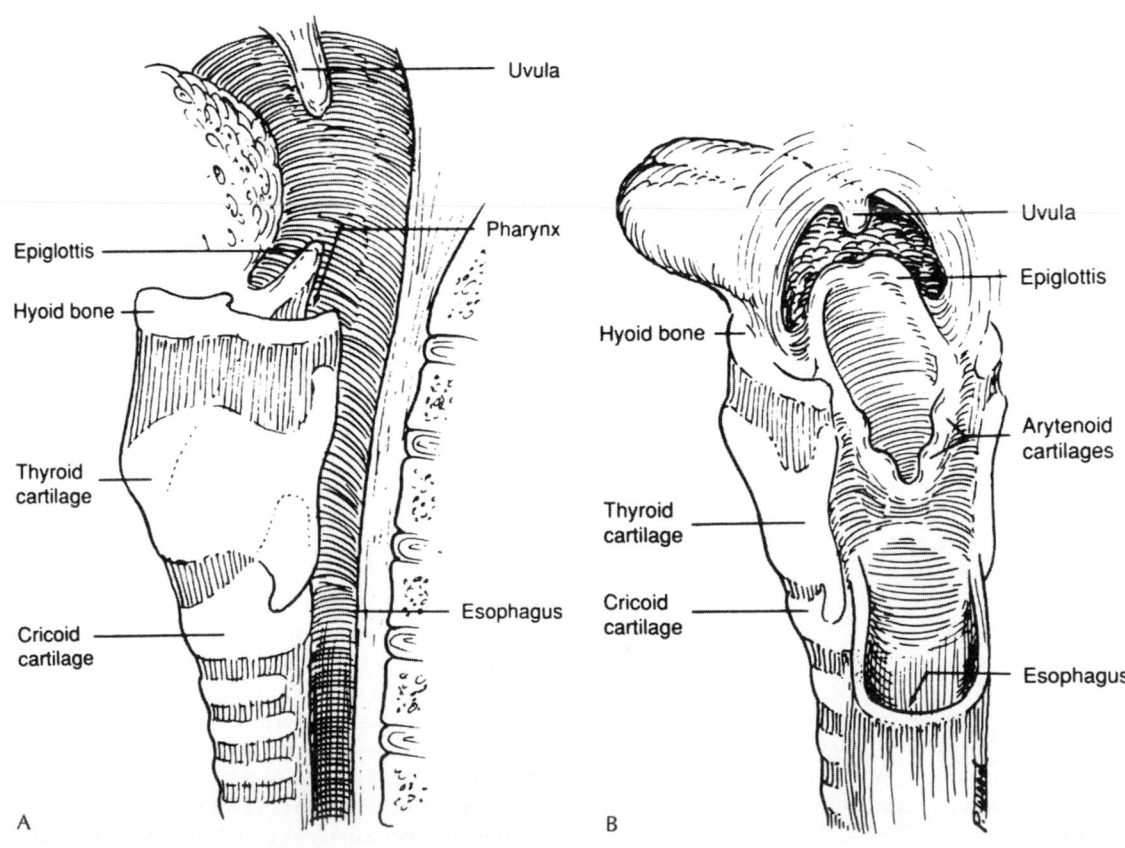

the epiglottis directs food away from the larynx by sitting like a tent over the epiglottic opening. This represents an impediment to visualization of the laryngeal aperture. During laryngoscopy, the epiglottis is lifted out of the way by traction on the hyo-epiglottic ligament, which attaches the epiglottis to the hyoid bone.

THE LARYNX

The laryngeal skeleton consists of a group of cartilages extending between the fourth and sixth cervical vertebrae. The major portion of the laryngeal body consists of the thyroid cartilage anteriorly and the cricoid cartilage posteriorly. The cricoid cartilage is actually a complete ring with a wide posterior portion and a narrow anterior portion that is palpable just inferior to the thyroid cartilage. Between the two cartilages is a small depression that represents the cricothyroid membrane. It is through this membrane that emergency surgical access to the airway is most easily obtained. The space is more than ample to permit placement of a small catheter that can deliver oxygen in case of a difficult intubation, and will accommodate a tracheal tube of up to 5–6 millimeters.

The arytenoid cartilages sit posteriorly atop the cricoid cartilage. These small paired cartilages provide support to the posterior portions of the true vocal cords. The mucosa of the vocal cords covers these cartilages and movement of the cartilages occurs during respiration. Damage to the cricoarytenoid joint can result in glottic stenosis and consequent respiratory difficulties.[2] Care must be taken not to damage the arytenoids during intubation. In some patients, the arytenoids are the only portion of the glottic inlet that is visible during attempted laryngoscopy.

Airway Management without Intubation

Manual airway management without intubation requires a significant level of skill, best mastered in a controlled setting such as the operating room before attempting to do so in an emergent situation. Facemask positive-pressure ventilation is a critical skill as an initial resuscitative measure, when the need for ventilation is very brief, or when tracheal intubation proves difficult or impossible. In addition, in select patients with acute respiratory failure noninvasive positive-pressure mechanical ventilation via a tight-fitting face mask can be administered for hours or days (see Chapter 19 for details). Facemask ventilation, either manual or via a mechanical ventilator, may not be possible if anatomic features preclude a tight mask fit, and is contraindicated for even brief periods in the face of vomiting or bleeding that could cause massive aspiration, except as a rescue technique when severe hypoxemia is present. In these situations, a cuffed endotracheal tube (ETT) should be placed as rapidly as possible.

The following section discusses the technical aspects of manual facemask ventilation.

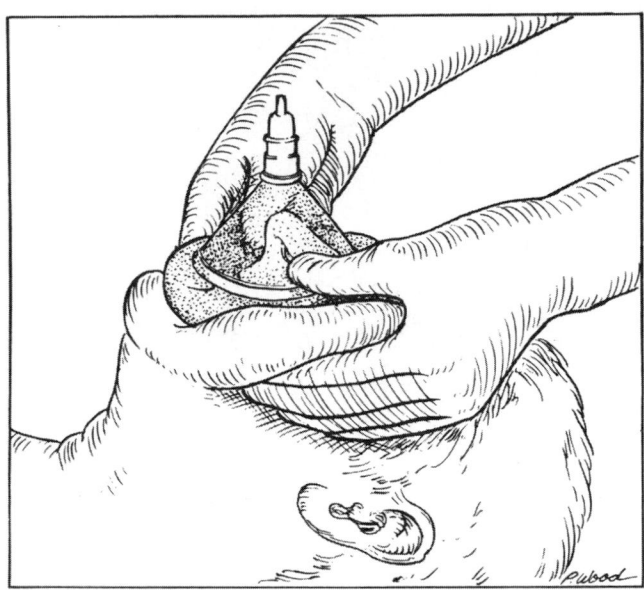

FIGURE 38-4 Pulling the cheeks to meet the rim of the mask helps to create a seal during positive pressure ventilation. (*Reproduced, with permission, from Pierson et al, editors: Foundations of respiratory care. New York: Churchill Livingstone, 1992.*)

MASK FIT

Modern face masks are made of clear plastic with large, highly compliant, inflatable borders that conform to a wide variety of faces. A tight seal between the mask and the patient's face is critical to achieve adequate ventilation, especially in the presence of increased airway resistance or decreased thoracic compliance. A significant leak is more likely in the presence of morbid obesity, bronchoconstriction, or pulmonary edema. Mask fit may also be difficult to achieve in the edentulous patient; the fit may be improved by pulling the cheeks up on either side of the mask (Fig. 38-4), leaving dentures in place during mask ventilation, or placing gauze pads between the alveolar ridge and the cheek.

Other factors that predict difficult mask ventilation include obesity, presence of a beard, age >55 years, and a history of snoring.[3] In the event of difficult facemask ventilation, better ventilation may be achieved if two people participate, with one person securing the mask and the second providing ventilation by squeezing the bag. This technique has been shown to increase delivered tidal volume by 250 ml in a test lung.[4,5]

HEAD POSITION

As consciousness is lost, the base of the tongue and the epiglottis fall posteriorly and compromise the lumen of the airway. Extension of the neck places traction on the hyoid bone and pulls the epiglottis and tongue away from the posterior pharynx. If this maneuver is inadequate, placing traction on the mandible with three fingers positioned behind the posterior mandibular rami will usually open the airway. The thumb and index finger can then be used to keep the mask tightly on the face (Fig. 38-5).

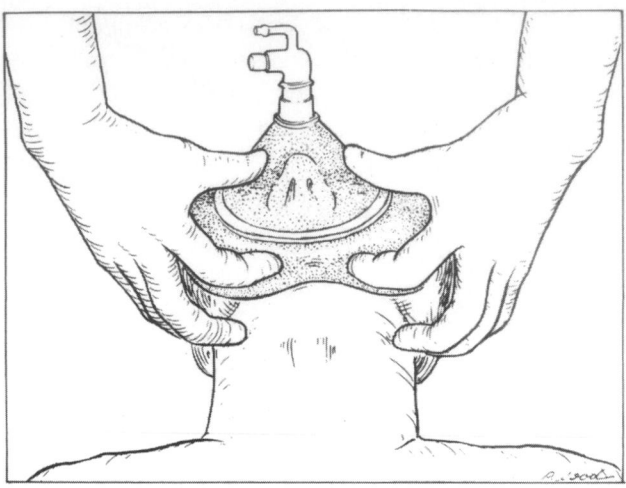

FIGURE 38-5 Traction underneath the mandible helps to pull the soft tissues of the anterior larynx and pharynx forward and thus create an open airway. (*Reproduced, with permission, from Pierson et al, editors: Foundations of respiratory care. New York: Churchill Livingstone, 1992.*)

NASOPHARYNGEAL AND ORAL AIRWAYS

In some patients, including those with obesity and/or obstructive sleep apnea, obstruction will persist despite anterior mandibular traction. Inserting a pharyngeal airway separates the tongue and epiglottis from the posterior pharyngeal wall (Fig. 38-6). Deeply comatose or anesthetized patients tolerate oropharyngeal airways but other patients will bite down or gag on them, in which case a nasopharyngeal airway is better tolerated. The major hazards of inserting a nasopharyngeal airway are bleeding or fracture of a turbinate. In nonemergent situations, prior application of a topical vasoconstrictor will ease insertion and prevent bleeding. Thrombocytopenia or a coagulation disorder contraindicates insertion of a nasal airway.

FIGURE 38-6 Nasal (*A*) and oral (*B*) airways in place. These improve the airway by separating the tongue and epiglottis from the posterior pharyngeal wall. (*Reproduced, with permission, from Pierson DJ, Kacmarek R, editors: Foundations of Respiratory Care. New York: Churchill Livingstone, 1992.*)

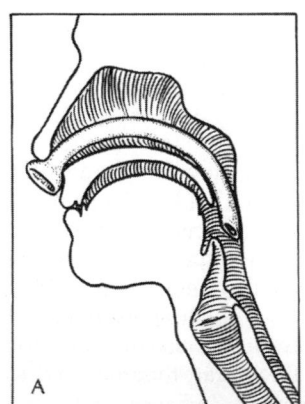
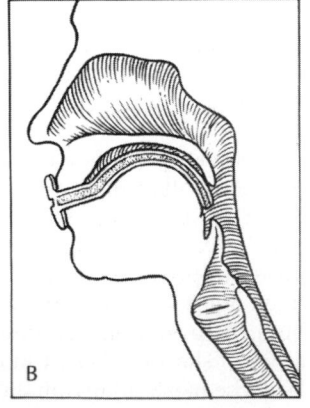

Tracheal Intubation: Indications and Physiology

INDICATIONS FOR TRACHEAL INTUBATION

1. *Maintenance and protection of the airway.* Airway patency may be compromised by reduced mental status (neurologic injury, sedation, or general anesthesia); pharyngeal/laryngeal dysfunction (bulbar palsy or neuromuscular blocking agents); trauma to the face, pharynx, or larynx; or edema secondary to angioedema, anaphylaxis, or postsurgical swelling. In these settings, the rigid walls of an ETT prevent occlusion of the airway.

   The above conditions can produce not only occlusion of the airway but also the inability to close the glottis appropriately. The latter can result in tracheal aspiration of small quantities of oral secretions, orally ingested solids or liquids, or regurgitated gastric contents. The inflated cuff of the tracheal tube provides significant protection against massive aspiration, although microaspiration may occur even when the cuff is properly inflated.[6,7]

   Patients with copious secretions and/or a weak cough who require frequent suctioning of the trachea may require an ETT to minimize the trauma of repeatedly catheterizing the trachea via the nose or mouth.

2. *Use of high oxygen concentrations.* Delivery of oxygen at high concentrations (>60%) is best facilitated by a sealed system. While high oxygen concentrations can be delivered via a mask using high flows or a reservoir system, the failure rate is high without constant observation to ensure that the mask remains in place.

3. *Application of positive pressure to the airway.* Positive pressure is applied to the airway either as continuous positive airway pressure (CPAP) or cyclically (mechanical ventilation) to support oxygenation and/or ventilation. Positive pressure can be applied to the airway via a tight-fitting full-face or nasal mask; this approach is commonly used to treat patients with chronic obstructive sleep apnea, whereby the positive pressure maintains upper airway patency during sleep. In addition, both CPAP and noninvasive positive-pressure ventilation can be applied to select patients with acute respiratory failure for at least limited periods of time (see Chapter 19), thus obviating the need for tracheal intubation. Tracheal intubation, however, is necessary in patients who are at risk for significant tracheal aspiration of secretions or gastric contents, or in those with more severe forms of respiratory failure that require high levels of positive pressure or prolonged ventilation (e.g., acute respiratory distress syndrome), or in those that do not accommodate or tolerate the tight-fitting face mask required for noninvasive ventilation.

PHYSIOLOGIC EFFECTS OF INTUBATION

CARDIOVASCULAR EFFECTS

The upper airway is richly innervated, resulting in a series of physiologic responses during intubation, including activation of both the sympathetic and parasympathetic nervous systems.[8] Bradycardia occasionally will result, most commonly in children. In unanesthetized adults, blood pressure following intubation may reach levels as high as 250/150 mmHg and the pulse will frequently rise to near maximal heart rates. Appropriate anesthesia will generally prevent these responses.

EFFECTS ON INTRACRANIAL PRESSURE

Direct laryngoscopy causes mechanical obstruction of cerebral venous flow, and increases cerebral blood flow secondary to increased cerebral metabolic rate and transient increases in P_{CO_2}.[9,10] In the presence of preexisting intracranial pathology, these factors can lead to a rapid rise in intracranial pressure and carry a risk of herniation of brain contents. The increase in intracranial pressure can be blunted by the prior administration of anesthetic agents.

RESPIRATORY PHYSIOLOGY

Dead Space

The ETT replaces the normal extrathoracic anatomic dead space of 75 ml with a smaller volume of dead space.[11] The exact volume of the ETT is calculated as the volume (V) of a cylinder using the formula $V = \pi r^2 l$, where r is the radius and l is the length of the tube. Thus, an 8-mm inner diameter ETT that is 25 cm in length will have a volume of 12.6 ml; intubation will thus reduce dead space by approximately 60 ml. Tracheostomy tubes are generally shorter and thus have an even smaller dead space, although the difference as a proportion of tidal volume is negligible.

The decreased anatomic dead space represents only the physical effect of intubation. The addition of connecting tubing between the ETT and ventilator tubing (apparatus dead space) may return the dead space to preintubation levels. Moreover, positive pressure ventilation results in an increase in alveolar dead space secondary to maldistribution of ventilation. Thus, total dead space is commonly increased in intubated patients receiving positive pressure ventilation.

Airway Resistance

Tracheal intubation, whether oral, nasal, or via tracheotomy, results in an increase in resistance compared with the normal upper airway. The apparent resistance of an ETT is influenced by the size and shape of the tube, inspiratory flow, and by friction among the gas molecules and friction between the tube wall and the gas molecules.[12,13] Irregular surfaces created by secretions or by ridges from wire reinforcement may create greater friction and greater resistance.[14]

In an ETT, turbulent flow predominates. During laminar flow, the pressure required to move the gas through an ETT is directly proportional to flow, whereas during turbulent flow this pressure is proportional to the square of the flow; thus, the pressure becomes markedly higher at high flow rates (Fig. 38-7). The slope of the pressure-flow graph is the apparent resistance. The apparent resistance of a tube is inversely proportional to the fourth power of the radius during laminar flow (Poiseuille's law), but the fifth power during turbulent flow.

Assuming turbulent flow, the relative resistance of an 8-mm diameter ETT compared with the normal airway (average glottic diameter of approximately 12 mm) is $6^5/4^5$, or

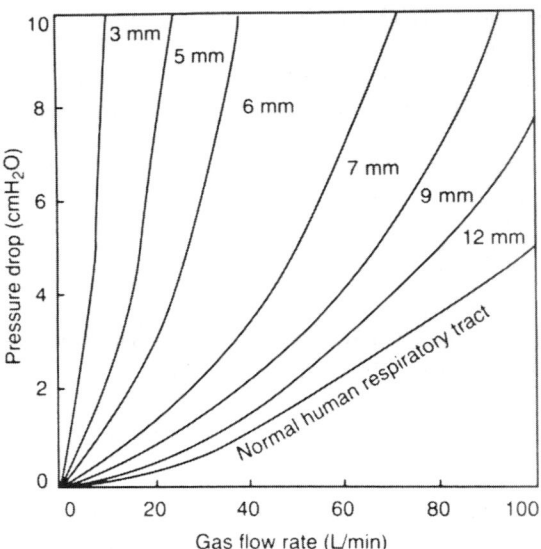

FIGURE 38-7 The pressure drop across various sized endotracheal tubes versus the gas flow rate in liters per minute. (*Adapted, with permission, from Nunn JF: Applied respiratory physiology, 3d ed. London: Butterworths, 1987.*)

7.6-fold greater. Likewise, the relative resistance of a 6-mm ETT versus an 8-mm ETT is $4^5/3^5$, or 4.2-fold greater. Because flow patterns, however, are not entirely predictable, exact respiratory pressure-flow relationships may not be predictable without empiric determination. In addition, changes in tube conformation and secretion and biofilm accretion in the tube after prolonged intubation increase resistance in comparison to fresh, *ex vivo* tubes.[15,16]

The increased resistance imparted by an ETT compared to the normal airway is of relatively little consequence at low minute ventilation. During normal tidal ventilation, about 10% of the work of breathing is performed to overcome the resistance of the upper airway. Even a doubling or tripling of that resistance does not result in an inordinate increase in the total work of breathing. At normal peak flows of 20–30 L/min, a tube as small as 6.5 mm in diameter will not result in extraordinary difficulty in breathing (see Fig. 38-7). At the higher flows found in patients in respiratory failure, however, the resistance of smaller tubes may become a substantial factor in the work of breathing. This factor may become a particular concern during attempts to wean patients from mechanical ventilation. In some cases, replacement of small tubes (<7 mm) with larger tubes may facilitate trials of spontaneous breathing. Alternatively, pressure-support ventilation can be used to compensate for the added work of breathing through the smaller tube until extubation is warranted.[17]

Theoretically, the patient's native airway should have less resistance than any size ETT, and work of breathing should fall after extubation. Some evidence, however, suggests that work of breathing may actually increase after extubation, perhaps secondary to high upper airway resistance.[18–20] The latter may be secondary to airway dysfunction or edema caused by trauma from the indwelling tube. In one study, however, direct visualization of the upper airway at the time of extubation did not reveal gross abnormalities to explain the increased work of breathing observed following extubation.[19]

Tracheal tubes inserted through a tracheotomy have a higher resistance than the normal upper respiratory tract,[21,22] but have lower resistance than oral or nasal endotracheal tubes of comparable diameters because they are shorter. There is, however, little if any difference in the work of breathing imposed by fresh tracheostomy tubes and ETTs of comparable internal diameter.[23] On the other hand, tracheostomy does appear to decrease the work of breathing in patients who have undergone prolonged intubation and mechanical ventilation, perhaps because inspissated secretions or conformational changes increase the resistance in indwelling tubes (tracheostomy tubes have removable internal cannulae that can be replaced or cleaned, whereas conventional ETTs do not).[16,20,24] The latter fact may explain the observation that liberation from mechanical ventilation often occurs more rapidly after a tracheotomy is performed.[24]

Normal subjects develop a mild, clinically insignificant increase in lower airway resistance following tracheal intubation,[25] and patients with reactive airways may develop marked bronchoconstriction. Bronchospasm following induction of general anesthesia accounts for a small but significant proportion of perioperative morbidity; notably, many cases of severe intraoperative bronchospasm occur in patients without previously diagnosed reactive airways disease.[26-29] Ideally, tracheal intubation of patients with known asthma or other reactive airways disease should be preceded by administration of inhaled bronchodilators, in addition to anesthetic drugs with bronchodilating properties (e.g., propofol or ketamine).

Expiratory flow may also be retarded by tracheal intubation, although this appears to be of consequence only at extremely high minute ventilations (30 to 40 L/min). The functional consequence of expiratory flow limitation is air trapping and auto–positive end-expiratory pressure (auto-PEEP). Experimentally, the magnitude of the auto-PEEP correlates directly with the resistance of the ETT.[30]

Cough

Effective coughing requires the ability both to generate a high expiratory flow in the trachea and bronchi and the ability to collapse the airways so that the force of the flow is imparted to the secretions to be expectorated. In awake intubated volunteers, peak airway expiratory flow is reduced, but still adequate to enable secretion clearance.[31] The presence of a tracheal tube, however, prevents collapse of the trachea by acting as a stent. Thus, while secretions can be moved to the central airways, the ETT prevents maximum efficiency of expectoration.

Functional Residual Capacity

The effect of tracheal intubation on functional residual capacity (FRC) is controversial. The debate centers around the principle of "physiologic PEEP," which is theoretically a small positive pressure created by the normal glottis, which, in turn, leads to breathing at a higher lung volume. The existence of positive intratracheal pressure in normal subjects has never been demonstrated. In volunteers who under-

went awake intubation, no consistent change in FRC could be measured.[5,32,33] In contrast, in patients with respiratory failure FRC increased following extubation.[34] Experimentally, rabbits with normal lungs did not demonstrate a difference in oxygenation or tracheal pressure following intubation but, after oleic acid–induced acute lung injury, tracheal intubation worsened oxygenation.[35] These results suggest that during acute lung injury, a glottic closure mechanism is invoked to maintain a positive intratracheal pressure and protect FRC, and that this effect is impeded by tracheal intubation.

Tracheal Intubation: Preparation and Standard Techniques

AIRWAY EVALUATION

The primary objective of airway evaluation before attempted tracheal intubation is to identify patients who may be difficult to facemask ventilate and/or intubate. A substantial body of research has been directed towards identification of patients with "difficult airways"; the unfortunate reality is that all of the described anatomy-based predictors of the difficult airway are notoriously insensitive and have only moderate specificity.[36,37] Nonetheless, a basic history should be obtained and an airway examination performed to the extent possible in all patients to identify risk factors for difficult ventilation/intubation (e.g., previous history, morbid obesity,[38,39] or obstructive sleep apnea[40,41]), and gross physical abnormalities including marked prognathia or retrognathia, other congenital deformities, marked overbite, facial swelling, postradiation fibrosis, or facial dressings that may lead to difficulties. This basic examination includes a view of the patient's facial anatomy from the frontal and lateral perspectives, an oral examination with the mouth maximally open and tongue extended, an assessment of neck extension, and measurement of the distance from the tip of the mandible to the thyroid cartilage.

Based on oral examination, Mallampati et al devised a classification scheme to predict difficult intubation (Table 38-1).[42] In general, the likelihood of difficult intubation increases from Class I to Class IV, although the test has only about 50% sensitivity at identifying difficult airways, and is most useful as a positive predictor at the extreme (Class IV).[42,43] In addition, this test is often impractical in emergency settings, where patient cooperation with the examination is not possible.

The size of the mandible provides some measure of the space available to displace the tongue during laryngoscopy. Mandibular size can be assessed by measurement

TABLE 38-1 Mallampati Airway Classification[42]

Class I:	Soft palate, fauces, uvula and anterior and posterior tonsillar pillars visible
Class II:	Soft palate, fauces, uvula visible
Class III:	Soft palate, base of uvula visible
Class IV:	Soft palate not visible

of the distance between the tip of the mandible and the thyroid cartilage (thyromental distance) using either a ruler or fingerbreadths that have previously been calibrated against a ruler. A thyromental distance of <6-7 cm has a specificity of approximately 90% in identifying the difficult airway, but the test has very poor sensitivity (approximately 30%).[37]

Extension of the head on the neck is necessary to bring the pharyngeal and laryngeal axes into alignment during direct laryngoscopy. Head and neck mobility can be assessed by simple examination, or quantitated by measuring the distance from the sternum to the tip of the mandible (sternomental distance) at maximum neck extension.[44] A sternomental distance of ≤13.5 cm has greater than 50% sensitivity and specificity at predicting difficult intubation, although this test has not been studied as extensively as either the Mallampati classification or the thyromental distance.

Common sense dictates that a combination of the above tests may prove more useful at predicting the difficult airway than the individual tests. There is some literature to support this notion, although the predictive value of these tests remains modest even when used in combination.[45,46]

Other factors that may complicate intubation and require special consideration include:

1. Risk factors for regurgitation and tracheal aspiration of gastric contents, including oral intake within 6 hours, gastroparesis secondary to drugs, intra-abdominal infection, trauma, diabetic neuropathy, increased intra-abdominal pressure (pregnancy or ascites), and bowel obstruction. Most critically ill patients should be considered at risk for aspiration during intubation.
2. Hypovolemia and/or shock predisposes to severe hemodynamic depression during tracheal intubation, secondary to sedative-hypnotic drugs and the initiation of positive-pressure ventilation. Means of vascular access, drugs, fluids, and equipment for resuscitation should be nearby.
3. Increased intracranial pressure, as discussed earlier.
4. Acute trauma poses multiple problems during attempted intubation, including possible airway injury, head injury, cervical spine injury, and hypovolemia. Intubation in the presence of known or possible cervical spine injury must proceed without movement of the spine (inline manual spine stabilization).
5. Hypoxemia reduces the time available for laryngoscopy and intubation before severe oxygen desaturation occurs.

EQUIPMENT AND SETUP

Table 38-2 lists supplies that should be at hand when performing tracheal intubation. In addition, a list of suggested equipment for difficult airways is provided. The latter can be packaged as an emergency airway kit, to be opened only when needed.

Essential pre-intubation equipment includes a working large-bore rigid suction device ("tonsil tip sucker") and a bag and mask (connected to 100% oxygen) that can be used

TABLE 38-2   Supplies for Adult Tracheal Intubation

Routine supplies
Two laryngoscope handles
Laryngoscope blades of varying size and shape
Face mask with inflatable rim
Oro- and nasopharyngeal airways
Bag for positive pressure ventilation
Suction with rigid tip
Endotracheal tubes (7–8 mm) and stylets
Cardiac resuscitation drugs and defibrillator
Carbon dioxide detector and esophageal detection device
   (e.g., self-inflating bulb) for verification of intubation
Drugs
Sedative-hypnotics
Neuromuscular blocking drugs
Additional difficult intubation equipment
Woven (Eschmann) stylet
Laryngeal mask airway and/or esophageal-tracheal
   Combitube
13 to 16-Gauge catheters for percutaneous cricothyrotomy
High-flow injector for transtracheal ventilation
Guidewire for retrograde intubation
#11 or #20 scalpel for cricothyrotomy

to provide positive-pressure ventilation. Additional routine equipment includes a variety of tracheal tubes with appropriate sized stylets, a laryngoscope handle, and a variety of blades. The laryngoscope handle and blades should be checked to ensure that the batteries and light source are in working order.

In emergent situations utilizing direct laryngoscopy and oral intubation, the ETT should be prefitted with a stylet, and a slight anterior hook placed in the tip of the tube. This added rigidity and curvature facilitates placement, particularly if the laryngeal view is suboptimal. In addition, the ETT cuff should be checked for patency.

STANDARD INTUBATION TECHNIQUES

ORAL VERSUS NASAL INTUBATION

The decision to place an oral or nasal tracheal tube is based on a variety of considerations. In general, the oral route is preferred for several reasons. A larger tube is easier to insert orally than nasally, making this route preferable in patients with high minute ventilation, copious secretions, or a need to undergo fiberoptic bronchoscopy. Nasal tubes have a higher resistance than oral tubes because of their smaller lumen rather than differences in the radius of curvature.[14] As discussed earlier, nasal tubes also have the disadvantage of occluding the sinus ostia, leading to a higher incidence of radiographic and possibly bacterial sinusitis as compared with oral tubes.[1,47] Nasal intubation is contraindicated in the presence of coagulopathy or anticoagulation, basilar skull fracture, or significant nasal or sinus deformity.

Nasal intubation is often easier to perform than oral intubation in awake subjects, and may be the route of choice for awake intubation, either by blind technique or with fiberoptic bronchoscopic guidance. Nasal tubes may also be less likely to either cause laryngeal injury or to lead to self-extubation.[48,49] Nasal tubes are often touted as being more

TABLE 38-3 Steps for Rapid-Sequence Induction of Anesthesia and Trachea Intubation

1. Prepare equipment and position patient; use a styletted ETT to optimize likelihood of tracheal intubation on first attempt
2. Preoxygenation for 3–5 minutes with a tight-sealing facemask
3. Application of cricoid pressure by an assistant
4. Rapid administration of a sedative-hypnotic followed by a NMBD (succinylcholine or rocuronium, 1 mg/kg)
5. Wait 60 seconds for the full effect of the NMBD; avoid facemask positive pressure ventilation to avoid gastric insufflation with air
6. Perform rapid direct laryngoscopy and tracheal intubation by an experienced provider
7. Verify intratracheal placement of the tube before releasing cricoid pressure

ABBREVIATIONS: ETT, endotracheal tube; NMBD, neuromuscular blocking drug.

conducive to patient comfort and oral hygiene, although the evidence is anecdotal.

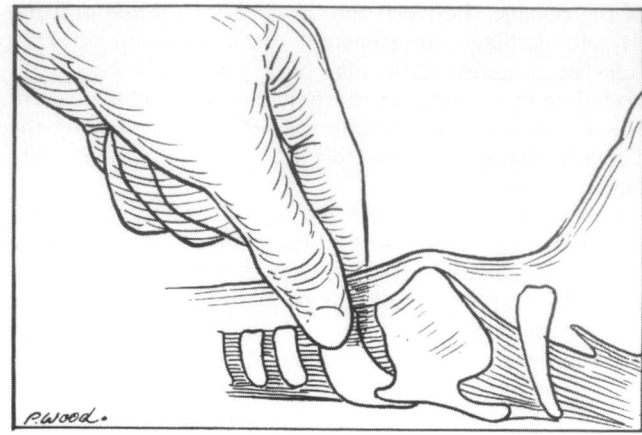

FIGURE 38-8 Application of cricoid pressure during tracheal intubation. Firm pressure must be applied to occlude the esophagus. (*Reproduced, with permission, from Pierson et al, editors: Foundations of respiratory care. New York: Churchill Livingstone, 1992.*)

PATIENT PREPARATION: RAPID-SEQUENCE INDUCTION OF ANESTHESIA

In most cases, the most rapid way to secure the airway is to induce general anesthesia with a sedative-hypnotic, followed by administration of a neuromuscular blocking drug, followed by direct laryngoscopy with tracheal intubation. In situations, however, in which providers are unskilled at direct laryngoscopy, and/or the airway is predicted to pose particular difficulties, alternate approaches should be considered, as discussed in the section on the difficult airway. The remainder of this section will focus on intubation after induction of anesthesia.

If intubation is to be facilitated by a sedative-hypnotic and a neuromuscular blocking agent, and if the patient has risk factors for regurgitation and tracheal aspiration of gastric contents as described earlier, a *rapid-sequence induction* of anesthesia should be used (Table 38-3). This approach, when combined with the application of forceful downward pressure on the cricoid cartilage to occlude the esophagus (Fig. 38-8), minimizes the chances of massive aspiration. *Preoxygenation,* or *denitrogenation,* consists of allowing the patient to breathe 100% oxygen for 3–5 minutes before induction of anesthesia. Preoxygenation uses the FRC as an oxygen reservoir. When FRC and oxygen consumption are normal, preoxygenation allows 8 or more minutes of apnea before oxyhemoglobin desaturation, and greatly increases the margin of safety should there be difficulties in managing the airway.[50] Preoxygenation should be attempted in all emergency intubations, recognizing that it may be neither possible nor effective in some circumstances. If rapid-sequence induction of anesthesia is not indicated, induction may proceed at a more measured pace, without application of cricoid pressure.

DIRECT LARYNGOSCOPY

Intubation using direct laryngoscopy is generally the fastest and surest way of securing an airway. This important life-saving skill, however, can result in great harm if per-

formed incorrectly. The major, feared complications are failure to ventilate and intubate the trachea, and unrecognized esophageal intubation, both of which can lead to severe neurologic injury and death. The likelihood of successful intubation is increased with experience, in addition to the use of proper equipment and suitable pharmacologic adjuncts. Gaining expertise in manual facemask ventilation and direct laryngoscopy in a controlled setting cannot be overemphasized; the operating room provides a controlled environment for focusing on airway management skills, in contrast to the hectic atmosphere of the emergency department or intensive care unit. On average, 45–60 intubations are necessary to achieve a 90% success rate at direct laryngoscopy. Mannequin-based practice does not appear to have a significant effect on acquisition of skill in performing intubation.[51,52]

The variations on techniques of direct laryngoscopy and intubation are many and beyond the scope of this chapter. A brief description, however, of the basic technique follows.

Numerous laryngoscope blades have been devised for various special situations but most intubations are performed using one of two types of blades: (1) blades intended to be used to lift the epiglottis directly ("straight" blades); (2) blades designed to lift the epiglottis indirectly by placing anterior traction on the hyo-epiglottic ligament in the vallecula ("curved" blades) (Fig. 38-9). In the authors' experience, the curved laryngoscope blade is more easily mastered and more commonly used than the straight blade, although facility with both is ideal because each has distinct advantages. Laryngoscope blades are most commonly designed to be held by the left hand (for right-handed individuals), although right-handed blades are available.

Before starting, the patient's head should be positioned near the top of the bed so the laryngoscopist's arms are not fully extended. The force applied during the average intubation is 25 N,[53] the equivalent of lifting a mass of approximately 2.5 kg. This force is most easily applied when the

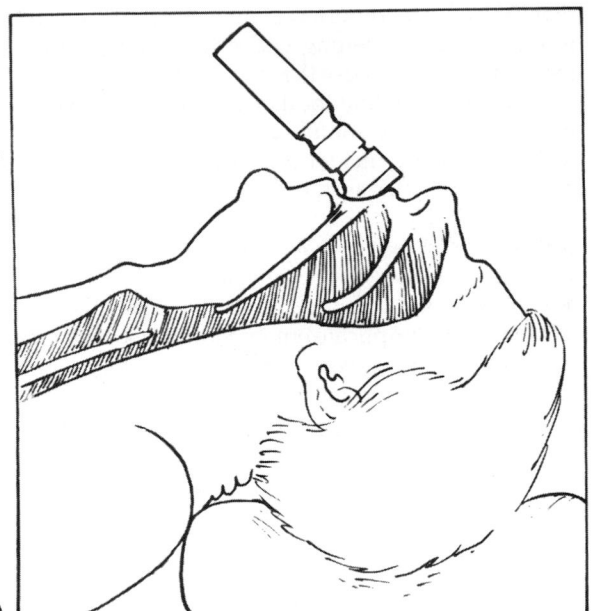
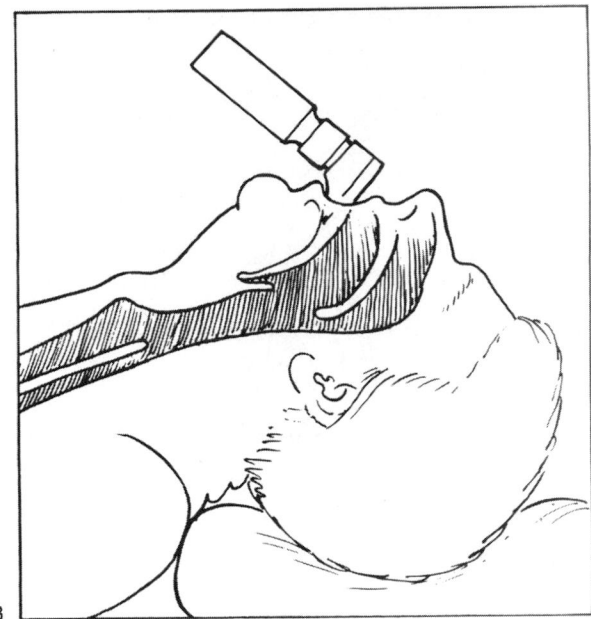

FIGURE 38-9 *A.* A number of straight laryngoscope blades are available, including the Miller. Straight blades directly lift the epiglottis. Though this often provides a clear view of the glottis, the room available for inserting the endotracheal tube into the mouth is limited compared to the use of a curved blade. *B.* The curved blade, the most common variant of which is the Macintosh, is directed into the vallecula and then pulled forward. This lifts the epiglottis away from the glottis. (*Reproduced, with permission, from Pierson et al, editors: Foundations of respiratory care. New York: Churchill Livingstone, 1992.*)

elbow is flexed and relatively close to the laryngoscopist's body.

Classic teaching is that laryngoscopy is facilitated by flexion of the neck at the cervical-thoracic junction and extension of the neck at the atlanto-occipital joint ("sniffing position"); this position brings the laryngeal and pharyngeal axes into alignment. The sniffing position is accomplished by raising the occiput with a firm pillow, folded towels, or other support. Recent studies, however, suggest that cervical extension is the most important component of this maneuver, and that the addition of neck flexion on the thorax improves the laryngoscopic view only in patients with limited neck extension and/or morbid obesity.[54,55]

Laryngoscopy proper begins by positioning the blade in the right side of the patient's mouth; mouth opening can be facilitated with the right hand. The right hand can then move to the occiput to extend or flex the neck into optimal position. The blade is then slowly advanced and the tongue swept to the left. The uvula and then the epiglottis should be identified, and are useful landmarks for maintaining a midline position. The blade should be advanced either into the vallecula (curved blade), or beyond the epiglottis toward the glottis (straight blade), and traction then applied at a 45° angle with floor. The wrist should remain firm, because flexing the wrist may cause pressure on the upper incisors and will push the epiglottis in front of the larynx. Traction at a 45° angle pulls the epiglottis forward to reveal the glottic opening. If the glottis is still not visible, external application of backward (towards the spine), upward (towards the head), or rightward (towards the patient's right side) pressure on the thyroid cartilage ("BURP" maneuver) may push the larynx into view; an assistant can then hold

the larynx in this position.[56] Once the laryngeal aperture is visualized, the ETT can be advanced through the glottis, the stylet removed, and the cuff inflated; correct position should be verified as described below.

If the nasal route is used, application of a topical vasoconstrictor before intubation is of critical importance in increasing the size of the nasal passage and minimizing bleeding. Topical 4% cocaine is effective and provides both vasoconstriction and anesthesia but may be toxic at doses greater than 3–4 mg/kg. An effective alternative is to use a phenylephrine or oxymetazoline nasal spray several minutes before instrumenting the nose, particularly if topical anesthesia is not necessary. Both nostrils should be sprayed in case one side is partially obstructed. The nasal passage can be prelubricated by inserting a nasopharyngeal airway coated with either 2% lidocaine gel (for awake intubations) or water-soluble gel. In addition, briefly warming the ETT in 37°C water will make it much more pliable and less likely to injure the mucosa. Nasal tubes (without a stylet) should be inserted with gentle pressure, directed posteriorly (Fig. 38-10), and advanced into the pharynx. Direct laryngoscopy is then performed, and the tube is guided into the larynx by manipulating the end extending out of the nose. Frequently, the tube tip must be guided with a Magill forceps (see Fig. 38-10) while an assistant advances the tube.

The Difficult Airway

While tracheal intubation is generally a simple and safe procedure, the consequences of a failed intubation can be

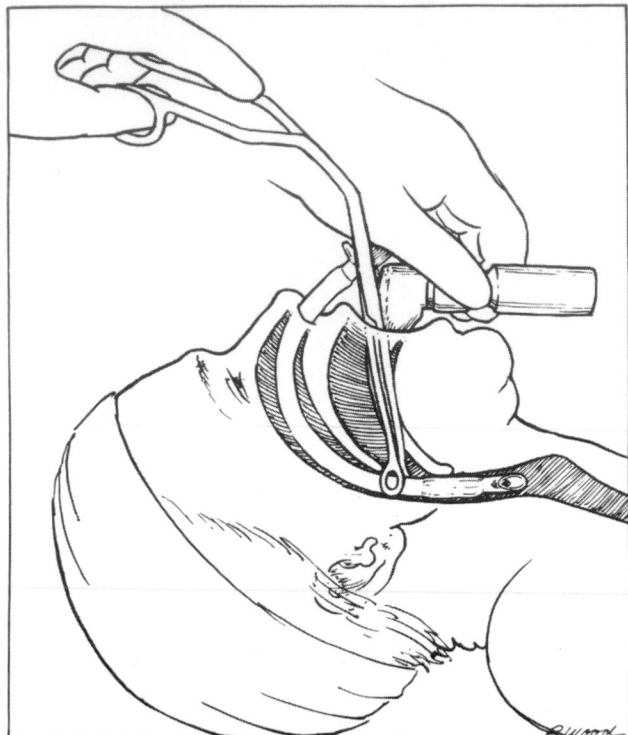

FIGURE 38-10 Use of the Magill forceps to assist in the advancement of a nasal tube through the laryngeal aperture. (*Reproduced, with permission, from Pierson et al, editors: Foundations of respiratory care. New York: Churchill Livingstone, 1992.*)

devastating. Before 1990, 34% of liability claims against anesthesiologists were secondary to adverse respiratory events, and 17% of these were related to difficult airway management.[26] Of these events, 74% resulted in death, brain injury, or other permanent injury. Thus, considerable attention has been directed towards difficult airway management over the past 15 years.

The term "difficult airway" has been defined in a number of ways, with the most clinically relevant being the development of any airway management problem that requires an escalation of interventions (beyond the routine discussed previously) to establish mask ventilation and/or tracheal intubation. For purposes of standardization in studies, difficult intubation is often defined as that requiring more than two attempts at laryngoscopy, or by a grade 3 or 4 laryngoscopic view as described by Cormack and Lehane (Table 38-4), although considerable subjectivity exists for all definitions.[57] "Failed" intubation implies that either attempts were aborted, or that the airway was secured surgically. The estimated incidence of difficult tracheal intubation in the operating room is about 5%, and failed intubation less

TABLE 38-4   Laryngoscopy Grade[57]

Grade 1: Entire glottis can be visualized
Grade 2: Only the posterior glottis can be visualized
Grade 3: Only the epiglottis is visualized
Grade 4: No recognizable structures are visible

than 0.5%.[37] The reported incidence of difficult intubation in the emergency setting varies widely, depending on the locale and experience of the airway providers, but on the average is similar to that for the operating room. The reported incidence, however, of failed intubation is much higher (up to 5%), as is the incidence of other intubation-associated complications such as hypoxemia, aspiration, cardiac arrest, and death.[58–61]

It is not surprising that difficulties in managing the airway are more likely to occur during emergency intubation as compared with elective intubation given the comorbidities that may complicate emergency intubation. Emergency intubation also poses an additional problem, in that the elective surgery patient can be awakened and the surgery postponed while further evaluation is performed or alternate techniques pursued. Critically ill patients are often intubated because they can no longer maintain adequate oxygenation and/or ventilation, and postponement of intubation is not an option.

Guidelines for management of the difficult airway based on available literature and expert opinion have been developed locally (at the hospital or practice level) and regionally or nationally.[37,62–66] The American Society of Anesthesiologists (ASA) was the first organization to publish such guidelines (including an accompanying algorithm), and recently published an update.[62,64] It is the general perception that difficult-airway guidelines and algorithms have resulted in fewer airway mishaps, and preliminary evidence suggests that the ASA guidelines may decrease complications related to emergency airway management.[67] Anesthesiology liability claims related to difficult-airway management, however, did not decrease in the U.S. in the 1990s as compared with the 1980s (pre–airway guidelines).[68] The ASA difficult-airway algorithm has also been criticized for offering too many choices at various branch points, making it relatively unhelpful for real-time application. Thus, other groups have developed guidelines that are more prescriptive.[66] In addition, none of the published guidelines explicitly deal with emergency situations, in which abandoning attempts to intubate is not an option.

Despite the lack of hard supporting evidence, common sense dictates that all airway providers should gain expertise in difficult airway management skills, and should have an algorithm for dealing with the difficult airway. Whether a published algorithm iteration is used is likely not as important as the act of learning and implementing it. Difficult airway algorithms based on those developed by the Difficult Airway Society of the United Kingdom,[66] and modified for use in the emergency setting, are presented in Figs. 38-11 and 38-12.

PREDICTED DIFFICULT AIRWAY: AWAKE INTUBATION

If the patient has a recognized difficult airway and is not combative or uncooperative, an awake intubation is generally preferable. This intubation can be accomplished by one of several techniques, including blindly placing a nasotracheal tube, placing an oral or nasal tube using fiberoptic

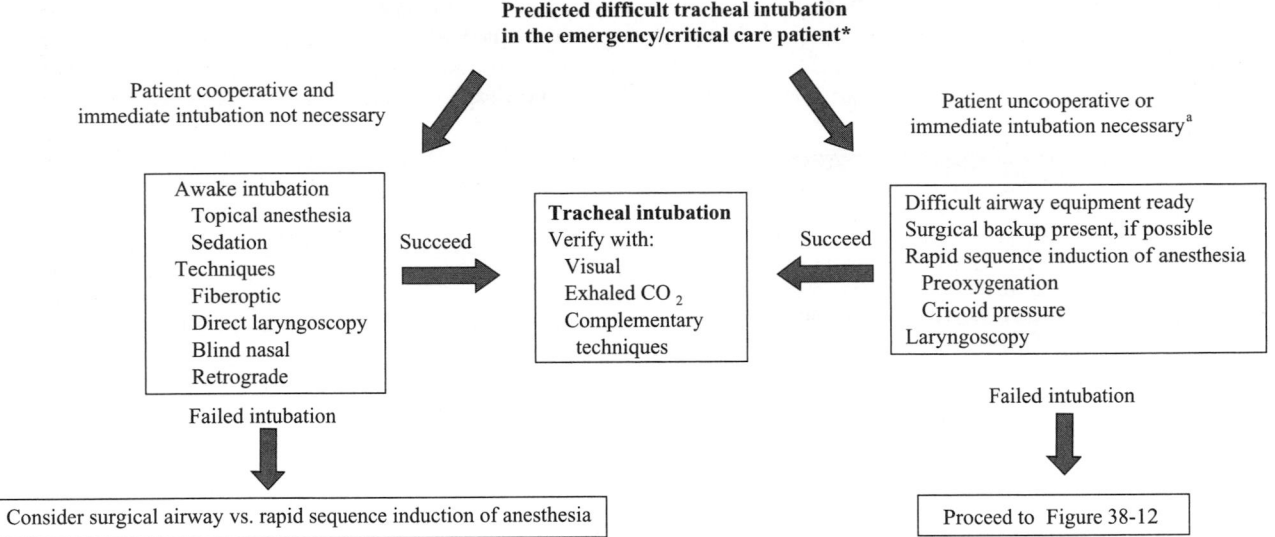

FIGURE 38-11 Algorithm for managing patients with predicted difficult intubation. [a]Risk of delay outweighs the risk of proceeding with immediate intubation.

guidance, using awake direct laryngoscopy, or using a retrograde tube-over-guide technique. Alternatively, the airway may be surgically secured primarily by an awake tracheotomy or, in emergent situations, by an emergency cricothyrotomy. Preparation of the patient and some awake intubation techniques are outlined below.

PATIENT PREPARATION FOR AWAKE INTUBATION

Awake intubation can be performed with surprisingly little discomfort to the patient if topical anesthesia is first applied. Administration of an antisialagogue, such as atropine, glycopyrrolate, or scopolamine, facilitates intubation by decreasing secretions that impair visibility and by improving access of local anesthetics to the mucous membranes. Unfortunately, because intubation of the patient for mechanical ventilation is generally emergent or urgent, there is often insufficient time for the antisialagogue to take effect.

Topical anesthesia of the soft palate, pharynx, and larynx can be obtained by administration of atomized or nebulized lidocaine (2–4%) or benzocaine spray, and/or by asking the patient to gargle with viscous lidocaine solution. Caution is warranted regarding the use of benzocaine, because methemoglobinemia has been reported with this agent, and toxicity is not necessarily related to the administered dose.[69,70] Patients receiving benzocaine should be monitored for the development of cyanosis; arterial saturation estimated by pulse oximetry may fall, but this device underestimates the true oxyhemoglobin saturation.[71] A high level of suspicion is necessary, and methemoglobinemia can be confirmed by co-oximetry. If lidocaine is used, the total dose should be limited to less than 300 mg because absorption via the mucosa is significant and can lead to central nervous system toxicity.[72]

Anesthesia of the trachea can be achieved by nebulization of lidocaine, by spraying lidocaine through a fiberoptic bronchoscope, or via transtracheal injection of lidocaine, with the transtracheal approach providing the best

anesthesia.[73] This can be accomplished by rapid injection of 2–3 ml of 4% lidocaine with a 22-gauge needle at end-exhalation; the subsequent cough helps distribute the anesthetic.

Direct laryngoscopy can be performed in awake patients, provided that adequate topical anesthesia has been applied and is supplemented with judicious administration of sedative agents. Additional techniques that are particularly suited to the awake approach are discussed below.

AWAKE BLIND NASAL INTUBATION

The widespread availability of fiberoptic bronchoscopes has decreased the frequency with which blind nasal intubation is performed. Blind nasal intubation, however, has the advantages of not requiring a laryngoscope (or bronchoscope), it can be performed even when blood or secretions are present in the airway, and it can be performed on a patient in the sitting position. The technique is especially suited to dyspneic patients, because they breathe more comfortably when sitting, have easily-heard breath sounds, and tend to keep their glottis open. Once the tube is in the nasopharynx, it should be directed caudad, using breath sounds as a guide, and advanced through the glottis during inspiration. The course of the tube can sometimes be determined by external palpation of the neck. The larynx can often be pushed gently towards one side if the tube is slightly misaligned. Rotation of the tube and flexion or extension of the neck may also be useful if the tube does not initially enter the trachea. A tube specially designed for nasal intubation (Endotrol) has a filament incorporated into the tube wall that allows the tip to be flexed, which may also assist passing through the glottis. The overall success rate for blind nasal intubation is about 90% in experienced hands.[74]

FIBEROPTIC TRACHEAL INTUBATION

Fiberoptic tracheal intubation provides the advantage of direct visual guidance, and is particularly valuable for elective

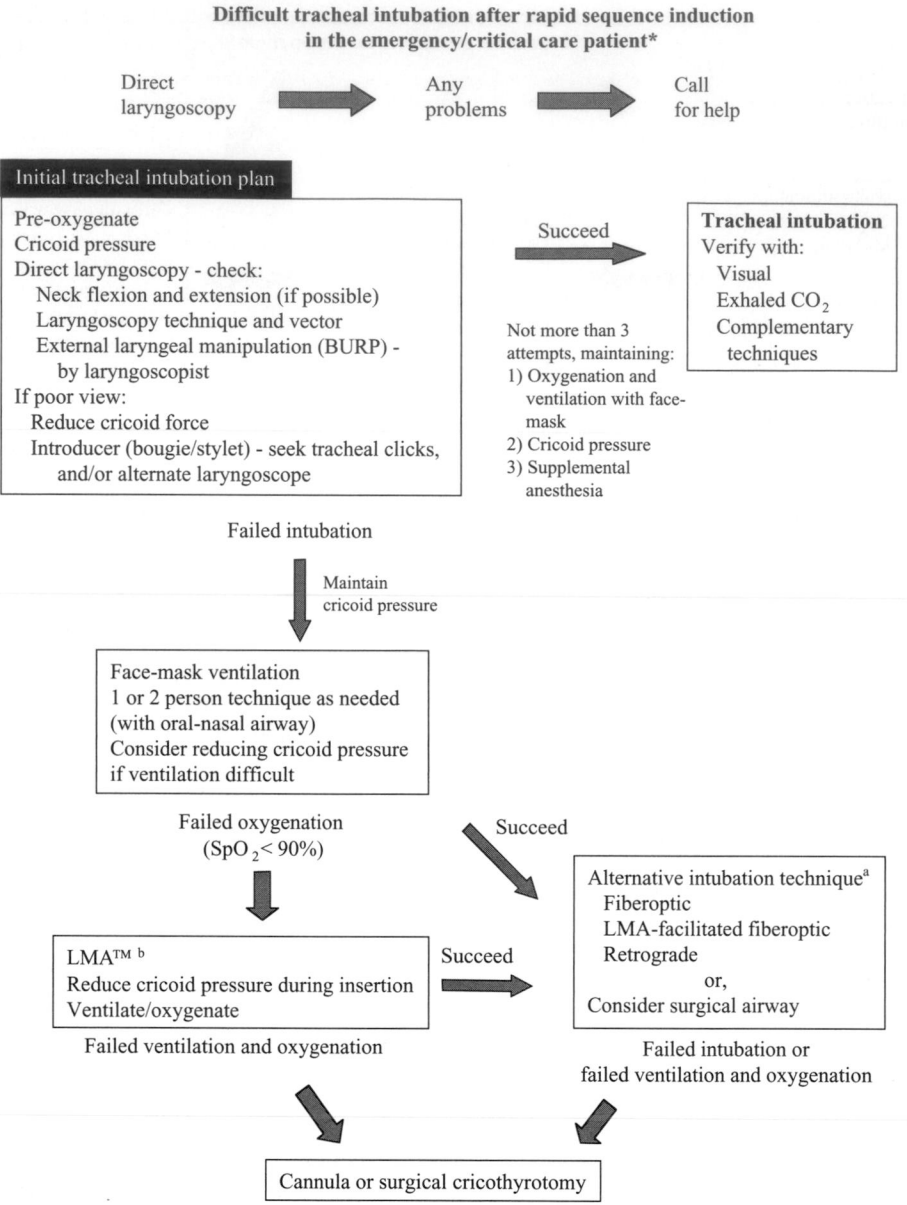

Difficult tracheal intubation after rapid sequence induction in the emergency/critical care patient*

Direct laryngoscopy → Any problems → Call for help

Initial tracheal intubation plan

Pre-oxygenate
Cricoid pressure
Direct laryngoscopy - check:
 Neck flexion and extension (if possible)
 Laryngoscopy technique and vector
 External laryngeal manipulation (BURP) -
  by laryngoscopist
If poor view:
 Reduce cricoid force
 Introducer (bougie/stylet) - seek tracheal clicks,
  and/or alternate laryngoscope

Succeed →

Not more than 3 attempts, maintaining:
1) Oxygenation and ventilation with face-mask
2) Cricoid pressure
3) Supplemental anesthesia

Tracheal intubation
Verify with:
 Visual
 Exhaled CO_2
 Complementary techniques

Failed intubation

Maintain cricoid pressure

Face-mask ventilation
1 or 2 person technique as needed
(with oral-nasal airway)
Consider reducing cricoid pressure
if ventilation difficult

Failed oxygenation
($SpO_2 < 90\%$)

Succeed →

LMA™ [b]
Reduce cricoid pressure during insertion
Ventilate/oxygenate

Succeed →

Alternative intubation technique[a]
 Fiberoptic
 LMA-facilitated fiberoptic
 Retrograde
  or,
 Consider surgical airway

Failed ventilation and oxygenation

Failed intubation or
failed ventilation and oxygenation

Cannula or surgical cricothyrotomy

FIGURE 38-12 Algorithm for managing the identified difficult airway. LMA, laryngeal-mask airway. [a]The choice of technique will depend on local practice, expertise, and equipment availability. [b]The esophageal tracheal Combitube can substitute for the LMA if preferred.

management of the difficult airway. Fiberoptic intubation can be easily accomplished in the awake patient via either the nasal or oral route, and is less stimulating than direct laryngoscopy. In emergency situations, however, when blood, vomitus, or copious secretions are present, it may be quite difficult. Like direct laryngoscopy, proficiency with this technique can only be gained by practice under direct supervision.

Preparation of the patient for awake fiberoptic intubation is described above; the neck should be neutral or slightly extended. Before commencing with intubation, the scope and light source should be verified to be in working order, the bronchoscope lubricated, and the tube passed over it

to ensure proper fit. Oxygen can be insufflated through the suction port of the scope, or directly through the patient's nose or mouth, depending on what intubation route is used. The nasal route may provide the best angle for viewing and entering the larynx. The ETT can be passed into the nose and advanced into the nasopharynx, and the bronchoscope then introduced. If the oral route is chosen, an oral intubating airway may facilitate passage of the scope through the mouth and pharynx. Alternatively, an assistant can grasp and gently pull the patient's tongue with a gauze pad. This opens the pharynx and facilitates visualization of the larynx. If the patient is sedated or uncooperative, a bite block should be inserted to prevent biting of the scope. After the scope enters the trachea, the ETT can be advanced, and its position relative to the carina confirmed before withdrawing the scope. If the tube does not easily pass through the glottis, a 90° clockwise rotation may allow passage beyond the right vocal cord.

RETROGRADE INTUBATION

Retrograde intubation consists of puncturing the cricothyroid membrane with a needle directed cephalad, feeding a guidewire through the needle until the wire emerges from the nose or mouth, and then passing the ETT over the wire into the trachea. Retrograde intubation can be performed under topical anesthesia, or used as a rescue technique in patients under general anesthesia who can be facemask ventilated but not intubated. This procedure may be especially valuable in the presence of severe facial trauma, upper airway masses, or trismus. A number of techniques have been described.[75–79] In the authors' experience, however, this technique is rarely used, and the interested reader is referred to other reviews of airway management for technical details.

VIDEO LARYNGOSCOPY

The GlideScope is a commercially available laryngoscope with a curved blade; a video camera is embedded in the blade, and a view of the larynx is obtainable with this device without having a direct line of sight. The video laryngoscope appears to improve the view of the larynx when compared to conventional laryngoscopes, and may be useful in cases of difficult intubation.[80–82] Published experience, however, with this device in difficult airway management is currently limited.[83] Intubation with the GlideScope is usually done after induction of general anesthesia, but it has been successfully used in awake patients after application of topical anesthesia and sedation.[84]

THE UNRECOGNIZED DIFFICULT AIRWAY

As mentioned previously, prediction of difficult intubation is an inexact science, and it is not uncommon to have unexpected difficulties with tracheal intubation after induction of anesthesia and paralysis. Moreover, in the critically ill patient, awake intubation or postponement of intubation are frequently not options either because of patient combativeness or the immediate need for control of the airway or severe hypoxemia. Thus, perhaps the most essential component of airway management skill is the ability to rapidly and systematically respond to difficulties with intubation and/or facemask ventilation. At the first sign of airway difficulties, help should be summoned, difficult airway equipment obtained if not already present, and a difficult airway algorithm followed (see Fig. 38-12).

If direct laryngoscopy and intubation prove unexpectedly difficult, subsequent attempts should be done with modification of the initial technique; repetition is rarely successful. Potential technique modifications include adjustment of head and neck position, the "BURP" maneuver, or the use of an alternate laryngoscope blade. For example, in large patients for whom the blade is not long enough to reach the vallecula, a longer blade (i.e., a Macintosh #4 instead of a Macintosh #3 blade) may be useful; in patients with a long, floppy epiglottis, switching from a curved to a straight blade may be helpful. If initial intubation attempts fail but mask ventilation is adequate, the situation remains controlled. In general, however, no more than three attempts at laryngoscopy should be made before choosing an alternate technique, because multiple laryngoscopies are associated with increased morbidity.

If the larynx cannot be clearly visualized beyond the epiglottis, a woven stylet (Eschmann introducer or bougie) may be passed blindly into the trachea; the stylet is then used as a guide to feed in an ETT. Entry into the trachea is suggested by the sensation of "clicking" on the tracheal rings as the stylet is advanced distally. Success rates with this technique near 100%, with practice.[85] If this is unsuccessful and mask ventilation remains effective, other alternate techniques to consider are fiberoptic intubation, video laryngoscopy, retrograde intubation, or laryngeal mask–facilitated intubation (see below). If these techniques are not practical for any reason, remaining options are limited, and include a surgical airway and awakening the patient. Awakening the patient, however, is rarely an option in the emergency setting, as discussed above.

DIFFICULT INTUBATION AND DIFFICULT FACEMASK VENTILATION

If initial intubation attempts fail and facemask ventilation becomes inadequate, an alternate airway should be used; the two main choices are the laryngeal-mask airway (LMA) and the esophageal-tracheal Combitube (ETC). The decision to use one or the other of these devices depends on clinical experience and availability of the devices, but one or both should be included in difficult airway storage units.

The LMA was developed to provide an airway for surgical anesthesia and consists of a tube connected to an oval mask with an inflatable rim that fits into the supraglottic area. It has been used quite successfully to provide rescue ventilation in patients in whom facemask ventilation has failed.[86] Although practice with this device is recommended before use in an emergency, the insertion and ventilation success rates are high even in unskilled hands.[87–89] The LMA-supraglottic seal is poor compared with that of an ETT, and a significant air leak commonly develops at ventilation pressures above 20 cmH_2O; this may result in gastric insufflation and compromised ventilation in patients with high airway resistance or poor compliance.[90] In addition, the LMA will not necessarily prevent aspiration of gastric contents, although this has not been a common problem during elective use,[91] nor is it commonly reported in the limited studies that have used the LMA for emergency ventilation. The LMA comes in a variety of sizes, with size 3 appropriate for most adult women and size 5 appropriate for most men; the correct size is important to obtain an optimal seal and ventilation.

Besides its simplicity, ease of insertion, and effectiveness, a major advantage of the LMA is that it can provide a direct route to the larynx and trachea. When the LMA is correctly seated in the supraglottis, its ventilation aperture sits directly opposite the laryngeal opening. Intubation of the trachea through the LMA has been described using several techniques, including: (1) blind passage of an ETT through the LMA lumen into the trachea; (2) passage of a stylet through the LMA into the trachea, followed by withdrawal of the LMA and passage of an ETT over the stylet into the trachea; and (3) passage of a pediatric fiberoptic bronchoscope through the LMA into the trachea, followed by tracheal intubation over the bronchoscope. The clear advantage of the latter technique is that it allows direct visual guidance and confirmation of intratracheal placement, and reported success rates are higher for fiberoptic versus blind intubation.[66,92] The lumen of the originally designed, or "classic" size 3 LMA is only large enough to accept a 6-mm ETT, whereas the size 5 LMA will accept a 7-mm ETT.

An LMA specifically designed for intubation, the LMA-Fastrack is modified to include a lumen large enough to accept an 8-mm ETT, a rigid structure to allow easier tube placement, and a bar to lift the epiglottis away from the laryngeal aperture. Like the classic LMA, placement and ventilation success rates are high with the intubating LMA, even for novice users.[93,94] Intubation can be done blindly or using fiberoptic guidance; although blind intubation is usually successful, multiple attempts may be necessary.[94] Fiberoptic guidance results in a higher success rate on the first attempt. The major disadvantage of the intubating LMA is higher cost as compared with the classic LMA.

The ETC has a large, occlusive pharyngeal cuff, two lumens, perforations in the esophageal lumen, and a distal cuff. The distal cuff seals either the esophagus or trachea (depending on where it is placed). If the ETC is placed in the esophagus either blindly or with the aid of a laryngoscope, the lungs can be ventilated using the esophageal lumen perforations. If the ETC is in the trachea, the lungs can be ventilated via the tracheal lumen. The ETC was initially marketed as an airway resuscitation device for out-of-hospital emergencies, and has a relatively long and successful track record in this regard.[95] It has also been used successfully for difficult airway management,[95,96] and has an advantage over the LMA in that when the tube is placed in the esophagus, the distal balloon can be inflated and the distal lumen connected to suction; this may limit the likelihood of aspiration of gastric contents. In addition, the ETC can provide effective ventilation to patients with compromised pulmonary mechanics, in contrast to the LMA.[97] The major disadvantage of the ETC is an associated risk of esophageal laceration or rupture, which is an uncommon but potentially devastating complication.[98,99] In addition, in contrast to the LMA, the ETC cannot be used as a direct portal to the larynx and trachea.

FAILED INTUBATION AND VENTILATION: CRICOTHYROTOMY

If intubation has been unsuccessful and ventilation via facemask, LMA, or ETC is compromised, particularly if hypoxemia is present, more invasive airway management techniques must be employed. An important skill in airway management is the ability to recognize the need for a surgical airway *before* the development of injury-inducing, severe hypoxemia. The trachea can be accessed either percutaneously or surgically via the cricothyroid membrane; the approach used depends on the skill of the airway practitioner, and surgeon and equipment availability. Percutaneous placement of a large-bore needle or catheter (13–16 gauge) permits transtracheal jet ventilation (TTJV), and generally will provide adequate oxygenation and ventilation before a definitive surgical tracheotomy.[100] In order to carry out TTJV, however, a high-pressure oxygen source and an adjustable, high-pressure device (jet injector) must be available; attempted manual ventilation through a catheter is largely ineffective. In addition, the potential complications associated with TTJV are severe, particularly if the catheter is inadvertently positioned outside the trachea, and include barotrauma, arterial perforation, and gas trapping secondary to airway obstruction or insufficient expiratory time.[101] The correct position of the cannula should be verified by syringe aspiration of air before initiating ventilation, and care must be taken to avoid kinking of the catheter at the insertion site. Practice with percutaneous cricothyrotomy and TTJV on a model is recommended before using it as an airway rescue technique.

Surgical cricothyrotomy is an effective and relatively safe and rapid way to secure the airway in experienced hands.[102,103] The standard surgical cricothyrotomy technique utilizes a #11 scalpel to penetrate the skin, subcutaneous tissue, and cricothyroid membrane, followed by hemostat-aided dilatation of the cricothyroid space before tube insertion. The "rapid four-step technique" uses a #20 scalpel to penetrate the cricothyroid membrane in one move, followed by caudal retraction of the cricoid cartilage and introduction of the tracheal tube.[104] The latter technique appears to be faster with a comparable complication rate. Ideally, these techniques should be reviewed and practiced on a model before use in the emergency setting.

Verification of Intratracheal Tube Placement and Position

A disastrous complication of endotracheal intubation is the unrecognized placement of the ETT in the esophagus.[26] Placement of the tube into a main-stem bronchus is less likely to result in death or severe neurologic injury, but is still a risk for significant morbidity. Although misplacement might seem simple to avoid or to detect, even experienced clinicians are sometime fooled, especially following a difficult intubation. At one time, airway management failures, including unrecognized esophageal intubation, were a small but significant cause of intraoperative mortality, morbidity, and liability claims. Minimum standards for monitoring established by the ASA in 1986 included a directive that all tracheal intubations be confirmed by the measurement of carbon dioxide in the exhaled gas (capnometry). This standard, likely complemented by the additional standard that ventilation be continuously monitored by capnometry during general anesthesia, has been associated with a reduction in the incidence of respiratory-related anesthesiology legal claims, and a more than 50% relative reduction in claims related to esophageal intubation.[68] It is assumed that the incidence of esophageal intubation has also decreased, although this is not directly proven.

CONFIRMATION OF INTRATRACHEAL PLACEMENT

Clinical signs of intratracheal placement include direct observation of the tube entering the glottis, condensation in the ETT with exhalation, and observation and auscultation of the chest. Unfortunately, all clinical methods can and have failed. Inflation of the stomach results in some movement of the chest wall, creating sounds of air movement and some return of gas during the expiratory phase. Experimentally, placing a tube in the esophagus and attempting positive pressure ventilation actually results in some gas exchange because of diaphragmatic movement with consequent lung ventilation. This mechanism is thought to account for cases in which a patient survives for many minutes following an intubation that eventually proves to be esophageal. The latter occurrence is clearly the exception, however, and esophageal intubation that is unrecognized for more that a few minutes generally leads to adverse consequences.

Although observation of the tube entering the glottis would seem a fail-safe test, there are numerous reported cases of esophageal intubation in which the clinician stated that the cords were seen. This may occur because the tube itself obscures the view during placement and the tube may then enter the esophagus.

Multiple methods should be used to confirm intratracheal tube placement for each intubation attempt. These methods should include capnometry, which is now considered the gold standard for confirmation of intratracheal placement. Capnometry may fail to detect esophageal intubation if intubation follows a period of mask ventilation because of exhaled gas that has entered the stomach,[105–107] or if carbonated beverages are ingested shortly before intubation.[108] In these instances, however, the "exhaled" CO_2 levels will decrease to near zero as the gastric gas becomes diluted, whereas CO_2 will persist if the ETT is in the trachea. False-negatives can occur if there is no CO_2 production or pulmonary blood flow, for example during cardiac arrest, after massive pulmonary embolism,[109] or after marked hyperventilation.[110]

Capnography, which refers to the graphical depiction of the exhaled CO_2 waveform, has become standard in operating rooms in the U.S. and much of the rest of the world. Lack of portability and high cost have limited the use of capnography in areas where tracheal intubation is performed less frequently. Alternatives to capnography include portable capnometry using hand-held devices, or colorimetric CO_2 detectors. The latter contain an indicator (metacresol purple) that changes color from purple to yellow when it is exposed to CO_2. Colorimetric capnometry is comparable to capnography in differentiating tracheal from esophageal intubation.[111,112]

An alternative to exhaled CO_2 detection is to apply gentle suction to the in situ tube; if the tube is in the esophagus, the suction causes the pliable esophageal tissue to occlude the tube and no air can be aspirated. If the tube is in trachea, however, the semi-rigid walls prevent tube oc-

clusion when suction is applied, and air can be obtained. Suction can be applied manually with a syringe, or more commonly with a self-inflating bulb ("bulb syringe"). This technique has good sensitivity for detecting esophageal intubation in elective and emergency settings,[113–117] but failures have been reported, particularly in pregnant women.[118] In addition, this technique has a relatively low specificity in detecting esophageal intubation as compared with CO_2 detection, and incorrect identification of correct tube placement (the bulb does not reinflate or air cannot be aspirated) has been reported in patients with morbid obesity, obstructive lung disease, copious secretions, and endobronchial intubation.[115,119,120] Thus, this technique cannot be advocated as a replacement for CO_2 detection, although it appears to have particular value in patients in whom CO_2 detection may fail, particularly during cardiac arrest.[115] Self-inflating bulbs are commercially available and should be considered as a supplement to CO_2 detection and clinical signs for detection of esophageal intubation, and as a routine piece of airway management equipment.

ASSESSING DEPTH OF INTRATRACHEAL PLACEMENT

The ETT tube can move as much as 5 cm during maximal cervical range of motion from flexion through extension; the tube moves cephalad as the neck extends.[121] The average distance from larynx to tracheal carina is 12–14 cm, and the top of the cuff of tracheal tubes in wide use begins approximately 5 cm above the tip of the tube. Thus, the ETT should ideally be placed 5 ± 2 cm above the carina to ensure that the tip does not migrate endobronchially during neck flexion, or that the cuff does not herniate through the glottis with cervical extension.[122]

Endobronchial placement can result in atelectasis and hypoxemia,[123] and inadequate depth of placement has several possible adverse consequences. If the cuff is between the cords the seal will be inadequate, risking both aspiration and inadequate ventilation. Adding more air to the cuff usually will not improve the seal because the cuff has a circular profile and the pentagonal shape of the glottic opening leaves the corners open. Inadequate depth of placement also may lead to serious long-term problems with subglottic stenosis. If the cuff is overinflated in the immediate subglottic region, mucosal ischemia may result. As this heals, scarring will lead to narrowing in the region of the cricoid. This problem is extremely difficult and not readily surgically correctable.

Although auscultation of breath sounds is a reasonable adjunctive test for confirmation of ETT depth, the incidence of missed endobronchial intubation using auscultation alone may approach 10%.[123] In addition, auscultation does not detect ETTs that are either dangerously close to the carina, or positioned too high in the trachea.

The risk of endobronchial intubation can be minimized by: (1) observation of the ETT as it passes through the glottis (insert the tube no more than 3–4 cm after the upper end of the ETT cuff passes the glottis; (2) insertion of the tube no deeper than 21 cm at the teeth in women and 23 cm in men;[124] and (3) palpation of the ETT cuff in the sternal notch.[125] These benchmarks will result in good placement in a high proportion of adults, but may fail at the extremes of stature, and are more likely to fail in women.[126]

Other methods for detecting endobronchial placement include chest radiology and fiberoptic bronchoscopy. Chest radiology confirms the position of the tube relative to the carina. Even if the carina is not visible, a tube tip overlying the third or fourth thoracic vertebral body with the head in the neutral position means the tube is in good position.[122] Fiberoptic bronchoscopy is as reliable as chest radiology and may be less expensive, but is not readily available at all intubation centers. Chest radiology has the added advantage of providing information about the lung fields as well.

Pharmacologic Adjuncts to Tracheal Intubation

Except in cases of cardiac arrest, coma, or extreme neuromuscular weakness, tracheal intubation is facilitated by administration of pharmacologic agents, particularly if direct laryngoscopy is used. The goals of the administered drugs are threefold: (1) to provide optimal intubating conditions by minimizing muscular tone, (2) to ensure patient comfort during the procedure, and (3) to minimize cardiovascular, airway, and intracranial pressure responses to intubation. In addition to topical anesthetics (discussed earlier), the typical drugs administered to facilitate tracheal intubation are sedative-hypnotics, intravenous lidocaine, and neuromuscular blocking drugs ("muscle relaxants").

SEDATIVE-HYPNOTICS

The most common sedative-hypnotics used as adjuncts to tracheal intubation are the short-acting barbiturates, propofol, etomidate, ketamine, and the benzodiazepines. With the exception of ketamine, these drugs are all gamma-aminobutyrate–receptor agonists. They all have dose-dependent cardiovascular and/or respiratory depressant effects of varying degrees, and will result in loss of airway control at higher doses. Barbiturates, propofol, and etomidate are all very effective at reducing intracranial pressure; benzodiazepines are less potent in this regard, and ketamine can increase intracranial pressure.

SHORT-ACTING BARBITURATES

Sodium thiopental, the prototypical intravenous induction agent, is highly lipid soluble and thus rapidly enters the brain to produce unconsciousness. The return of consciousness is also rapid because of rapid redistribution of the drug. There is marked respiratory depression following injection with transient apnea the rule. Barbiturates cause vasodilation and myocardial depression, making them a poor choice for the hypovolemic patient. The typical induction dose of sodium thiopental is 3–5 mg/kg intravenously, with reduced doses given in the presence of cardiovascular instability, hypovolemia, and advanced age. Higher doses may be necessary if there is a history of heavy alcohol or tranquilizer use.

PROPOFOL

Propofol produces rapid loss of consciousness after bolus intravenous administration, with recovery beginning within 1–2 minutes. Propofol has cardiovascular depressant effects that are similar in magnitude to those seen with barbiturates, and its potency appears to be increased during hemorrhagic shock.[127] Thus, large doses of propofol should be avoided in patients with hypovolemia or significant cardiovascular depression secondary to any cause. Propofol profoundly suppresses respiratory drive and airway reflexes, and has bronchodilating properties; thus, it is a useful agent for intubation of patients without concomitant administration of a neuromuscular blocking drug, or for intubation of patients with bronchospasm or reactive airways.[128] Propofol rarely causes myoclonus after bolus administration. Propofol is mixed in a lipid-based solution that supports bacterial growth; thus, propofol-containing syringes must be handled carefully and doses administered within a few hours of opening. Typical induction doses of propofol are 1–2.5 mg/kg intravenously, depending on age and cardiovascular stability.

ETOMIDATE

Etomidate has a rapid onset of action and a rapid recovery, has little effect on myocardial function, and has mild respiratory depressant effects. For one-time use for intubation, this is an extremely safe drug, and it may be the sedative-hypnotic of choice for emergency intubation. Infusions of etomidate in ICU patients, however, have resulted in severe suppression of adrenal cortical function.[129] Etomidate causes self-limited myoclonus relatively frequently. The latter may not be seen if etomidate is given in conjunction with a neuromuscular blocking drug. The typical induction dose is 0.1–0.3 mg/kg intravenously; doses of 4–8 mg in an adult patient will typically produce deep sedation with maintenance of spontaneous ventilation.

KETAMINE

Ketamine is an N-methyl-D-aspartate–receptor antagonist, which gives it a different sedation and side-effect profile than the other agents discussed here. Ketamine produces rapid loss of consciousness, although patients often appear awake because their eyes commonly remain open. Recovery from an intravenous dose of 2 mg/kg may take 10–15 minutes. Ketamine is a direct myocardial depressant[130,131] but clinically produces cardiovascular stimulation via release of catecholamines.[132] This sympathomimetic effect also gives ketamine bronchodilating properties.[133,134] Ketamine's major adverse effects include the potential for myocardial ischemia resulting from cardiovascular stimulation, increased intracranial pressure, and unpleasant dreams or hallucinations during the recovery phase. The typical induction dose of ketamine is 0.5–1 mg/kg, intravenously.

BENZODIAZEPINES

Midazolam is the benzodiazepine most widely used for hypnosis during intubation because of its rapid onset and short duration of action. It and the other benzodiazepines are better suited for use as sedative agents than for full induction of anesthesia, because the large doses of these drugs necessary to produce loss of consciousness result in prolonged sedation. In critically ill patients, however, smaller doses can result in loss of the airway, respiratory depression, and apnea; thus, titrated and closely monitored administration is recommended. Typical doses of midazolam for sedation during awake intubation are 0.5–2 mg intravenously.

INTRAVENOUS LIDOCAINE

High-dose intravenous lidocaine has general anesthetic effects, including a reduction of cerebral metabolic rate and a blunting of the hemodynamic response to intubation. Lidocaine 1.5 mg/kg given intravenously (before laryngoscopy) blunts the increase in intracranial pressure typically seen during intubation of patients with intracranial pathology.[135] Intravenous lidocaine also suppresses cough and bronchoconstriction during laryngoscopy, but only when given at doses of 1.5 mg/kg or greater and approximately 3 minutes before intubation.[136]

NEUROMUSCULAR BLOCKING DRUGS

Although a wide variety of neuromuscular blocking drugs (NMBDs) are available, only two, succinylcholine and rocuronium, are sufficiently rapid in onset to be of value for emergency tracheal intubation. Succinylcholine's pharmacokinetic profile makes it the ideal drug for emergency tracheal intubation. Succinylcholine binds to the nicotinic receptor at the neuromuscular junction to cause depolarization of the endplate, and eventually, of surrounding fibers. This effect persists for several minutes, thus causing the muscle membrane to remain depolarized and refractory to further impulses. The diffuse depolarization of the muscles can be seen as generalized fasciculations. The usual intubating dose of 1 mg/kg of succinylcholine results in adequate intubating conditions in 90% of patients at 1 minute. The termination of drug action results from the metabolism of circulating succinylcholine by pseudocholinesterase with return of muscle strength in 3–5 minutes in most patients. Pseudocholinesterase deficiency occurs rarely, and results in prolonged action of succinylcholine.

Succinylcholine has a number of side effects, some of which are potentially lethal. Succinylcholine is a trigger agent for malignant hyperthermia, and should not be administered to susceptible patients. Administration of succinylcholine results in an efflux of intracellular potassium resulting in a clinically insignificant transient rise in serum potassium in most patients. In patients with central neurologic deficits, however, such as stroke, traumatic brain injury, encephalopathy, spinal cord injury, or after peripheral denervation, succinylcholine administration can lead to massive release of potassium; levels may exceed 10 mEq/L.[137,138] Similar responses are seen in patients with burns (beginning after several days), myopathies, rhabdomyolysis, and after crush injuries.[137] The mechanism of hyperkalemia is in part related to extrajunctional proliferation of nicotinic receptors, but may also be related to direct muscle membrane damage during criti-

cal illness. The reported mortality with succinylcholine-induced hyperkalemia is over 10%.[137] Succinylcholine is thus absolutely contraindicated for at least several days to a week following a burn or new neurologic deficit. In addition, given the high incidence of critical illness–induced myopathy and neuropathy, succinylcholine should be avoided in patients who have been critically ill for a week or more.[139] Given the potential lethality of the hyperkalemic response after succinylcholine, an alternate agent should be used if there is any potential contraindication to succinylcholine.

Succinylcholine may also result in a transient increase in intracranial pressure, although this is probably not clinically significant and should not prevent the use of succinylcholine if rapid control of the airway is necessary.[140]

Rocuronium is a competitive antagonist of acetylcholine at the neuromuscular junction. Rocuronium is nondepolarizing, and does not result in potassium release, and neither does it act as a trigger for malignant hyperthermia. Rocuronium at an intubating dose of approximately 1 mg/kg results in acceptable intubating conditions at 1 minute after administration, although intubation conditions are generally inferior to those achieved after succinylcholine.[141] Rocuronium's major drawback is that its duration of action is determined by hepatic and renal clearance, and has a variable range of 30–90 minutes. This makes rocuronium less than ideal for patients with difficult airways, because the option of allowing return of spontaneous ventilation should intubation and facemask ventilation fail is not available, as it is for succinylcholine. Nonetheless, rocuronium is a valuable substitute for succinylcholine in patients who are at risk for complications from the latter agent.

References

1. Rouby JJ, Laurent P, Gosnach M, et al. Risk factors and clinical relevance of nosocomial maxillary sinusitis in the critically ill. Am J Respir Crit Care Med 1994; 150:776–83.
2. Castella X, Gilabert J, Perez C. Arytenoid dislocation after tracheal intubation: an unusual cause of acute respiratory failure? Anesthesiology 1991; 74:613–5.
3. Langeron O, Masso E, Huraux C, et al. Prediction of difficult mask ventilation. Anesthesiology 2000; 92:1229–36.
4. Hess D, Goff G, Johnson K. The effect of hand size, resuscitator brand, and the use of two hands on volumes delivered during adult bag-valve ventilation. Respir Care 1989; 34:805-10.
5. Hess D, Goff G. The effects of two-hand versus one-hand ventilation on volumes delivered during bag-valve ventilation at various resistances and compliances. Respir Care 1987; 32: 1025–8.
6. Pavlin EG, VanNimwegan D, Hornbein TF. Failure of a high-compliance low-pressure cuff to prevent aspiration. Anesthesiology 1975; 42:216–9.
7. Blunt MC, Young PJ, Patil A, Haddock A. Gel lubrication of the tracheal tube cuff reduces pulmonary aspiration. Anesthesiology 2001; 95:377–81.
8. Fox EJ, Sklar GS, Hill CH, Villanueva R, King BD. Complications related to the pressor response to endotracheal intubation. Anesthesiology 1977; 47:524–5.
9. Shapiro HM, Wyte SR, Harris AB, Galindo A. Acute intraoperative intracranial hypertension in neurosurgical patients:

mechanical and pharmacologic factors. Anesthesiology 1972; 37:399–405.

10. Mi WD, Sakai T, Takahashi S, Matsuki A. Haemodynamic and electroencephalograph responses to intubation during induction with propofol or propofol/fentanyl. Can J Anaesth 1998; 45:19–22.

11. Nunn J, Campbell E, Peckett B. Anatomical subdivisions of the volume of respiratory dead space and effect of position of the jaw. J Appl Physiol 1959; 14:174–6.

12. Hirshman C, Bergman M. Factors influencing intrapulmonary airway calibre during anaesthesia. Br J Anaesth 1990; 65: 30–42.

13. Habib M. Physiologic implications of artificial airways. In: Artificial airways in patients receiving mechanical ventilation (Consensus conference). Chest 1989; 96:180–4.

14. Kil HK, Bishop MJ. Head position and oral vs. nasal route as factors determining endotracheal tube resistance. Chest 1994; 105:1794–7.

15. Wright PE, Marini JJ, Bernard GR. In vitro versus in vivo comparison of endotracheal tube airflow resistance. Am Rev Respir Dis 1989; 140:10–6.

16. Shah C, Kollef MH. Endotracheal tube intraluminal volume loss among mechanically ventilated patients. Crit Care Med 2004; 32:120–5.

17. Brochard L, Rua F, Lorino H, Lemaire F, Harf A. Inspiratory pressure support compensates for the additional work of breathing caused by the endotracheal tube. Anesthesiology 1991; 75:739–45.

18. Nathan SD, Ishaaya AM, Koerner SK, Belman MJ. Prediction of minimal pressure support during weaning from mechanical ventilation. Chest 1993; 103:1215–9.

19. Ishaaya AM, Nathan SD, Belman MJ. Work of breathing after extubation. Chest 1995; 107:204–9.

20. Davis K Jr., Campbell RS, Johannigman JA, Valente JF, Branson RD. Changes in respiratory mechanics after tracheostomy. Arch Surg 1999; 134:59–62.

21. Cavo J, Ogura JH, Sessions DG, Nelson JR. Flow resistance in tracheotomy tubes. Ann Otol Rhinol Laryngol 1973; 82: 827–30.

22. Yung M, Snowdon S. Respiratory resistance of tracheostomy tubes. Arch Otolaryngol 1984; 110:591–5.

23. Vines D, Peters J, Merritt J, Casey H, Shelledy D. A comparison of total patient work of breathing (TPWOB) between 8.0 endotracheal tubes (ETT) and tracheostomy tubes (TT) during spontaneous breathing in a lung model. Am J Respir Crit Care Med 2003; 167:A460.

24. Diehl JL, El Atrous S, Touchard D, Lemaire F, Brochard L. Changes in the work of breathing induced by tracheotomy in ventilator-dependent patients. Am J Respir Crit Care Med 1999; 159:383–8.

25. Gal T, Suratt P. Resistance to breathing in healthy subjects after endotracheal intubation under topical anesthesia. Anesthesiology 1980; 59:270–4.

26. Caplan RA, Posner KL, Ward RJ, Cheney FW. Adverse respiratory events in anesthesia: a closed claims analysis. Anesthesiology 1990; 72:828–33.

27. Cheney FW, Posner KL, Caplan RA. Adverse respiratory events infrequently leading to malpractice suits. A closed claims analysis. Anesthesiology 1991; 75:932–9.

28. Olsson G. Bronchospasm during anaesthesia. A computer - aided incidence study of 136,929 patients. Acta Anaesthesiol Scand 1987; 31:244–52.

29. Tiret L, Desmonts JM, Hatton F, Vourc'h G. Complications associated with anaesthesia—a prospective survey in France. Can Anaesth Soc J 1986; 33:336–44.

30. Scott L, Benson M, Bishop M. Relationship of endotracheal tube size to auto-PEEP at high minute ventilation. Respir Care 1986; 31:1080–1082.

31. Gal T. Effects of endotracheal intubation on normal cough performance. Anesthesiology 1980; 52:324–29.

32. Gal T, Arora N. Respiratory mechanics in supine subjects during progressive partial curarization. J Appl Physiol 1982;52:57–63.

33. Rodenstein D, Stanescue D, Francis C. Demonstration of failure of body plethysmography in airway obstruction. Appl Physiol 1982; 52:949–54.

34. Quan S, Falltrick R, Schlobohm R. Extubation from ambient or expiratory positive airway pressure in adults. Anesthesiology 1984; 55:53–6.

35. Smith RA, Venus B, Johnson MT, Carter C. Influence of glottic mechanism on pulmonary function after acute lung injury. Chest 1990; 98:206–8.

36. Yentis SM. Predicting difficult intubation—worthwhile exercise or pointless ritual? Anaesthesia 2002; 57:105–9.

37. Crosby ET, Cooper RM, Douglas MJ, et al. The unanticipated difficult airway with recommendations for management. Can J Anaesth 1998; 45:757–76.

38. Voyagis GS, Kyriakis KP, Dimitriou V, Vrettou I. Value of oropharyngeal Mallampati classification in predicting difficult laryngoscopy among obese patients. Eur J Anaesthesiol 1998; 15:330–4.

39. Juvin P, Lavaut E, Dupont H, et al. Difficult tracheal intubation is more common in obese than in lean patients. Anesth Analg 2003; 97:595–600, table of contents.

40. Riley RW, Powell NB, Guilleminault C, et al. Obstructive sleep apnea surgery: risk management and complications. Otolaryngol Head Neck Surg 1997; 117:648–52.

41. Siyam MA, Benhamou D. Difficult endotracheal intubation in patients with sleep apnea syndrome. Anesth Analg 2002; 95:1098–102, table of contents.

42. Mallampati SR, Gatt SP, Gugino LD, et al. A clinical sign to predict difficult tracheal intubation: a prospective study. Can Anaesth Soc J 1985; 32:429–34.

43. el-Ganzouri AR, McCarthy RJ, Tuman KJ, Tanck EN, Ivankovich AD. Preoperative airway assessment: predictive value of a multivariate risk index. Anesth Analg 1996; 82:1197–204.

44. Al Ramadhani S, Mohamed LA, Rocke DA, Gouws E. Sternomental distance as the sole predictor of difficult laryngoscopy in obstetric anaesthesia. Br J Anaesth 1996; 77:312–6.

45. Frerk CM. Predicting difficult intubation. Anaesthesia 1991; 46:1005–8.

46. Wilson ME, Spiegelhalter D, Robertson JA, Lesser P. Predicting difficult intubation. Br J Anaesth 1988; 61:211–6.

47. Michelson A, Schuster B, Kamp HD. Paranasal sinusitis associated with nasotracheal and orotracheal long-term intubation. Arch Otolaryngol Head Neck Surg 1992; 118:937–9.

48. Dubick MN, Wright BD. Comparison of laryngeal pathology following long-term oral and nasal endotracheal intubations. Anesth Analg 1978; 57:663–8.

49. Coppolo DP, May JJ. Self-extubations. A 12-month experience. Chest 1990; 98:165–9.

50. Farmery AD, Roe PG. A model to describe the rate of oxyhaemoglobin desaturation during apnoea. Br J Anaesth 1996; 76:284–91.

51. Bradley JS, Billows GL, Olinger ML, et al. Prehospital oral endotracheal intubation by rural basic emergency medical technicians. Ann Emerg Med 1998; 32:26–32.

52. Sayre MR, Sakles JC, Mistler AF, et al. Field trial of endotracheal intubation by basic EMTs. Ann Emerg Med 1998; 31:228–33.

53. Bishop MJ, Harrington RM, Tencer AF. Force applied during tracheal intubation. Anesth Analg 1992; 74:411–4.

54. Adnet F, Borron SW, Dumas JL, et al. Study of the "sniffing position" by magnetic resonance imaging. Anesthesiology 2001; 94:83–6.

55. Adnet F, Baillard C, Borron SW, et al. Randomized study comparing the "sniffing position" with simple head extension for laryngoscopic view in elective surgery patients. Anesthesiology 2001; 95:836–41.

56. Takahata O, Kubota M, Mamiya K, et al. The efficacy of the "BURP" maneuver during a difficult laryngoscopy. Anesth Analg 1997; 84:419–21.

57. Cormack R, Lehane J. Difficult tracheal intubation in obstetrics. Anaesthesia 1984; 39:1105–11.

58. Schwartz DE, Matthay MA, Cohen NH. Death and other complications of emergency airway management in critically ill adults. A prospective investigation of 297 tracheal intubations. Anesthesiology 1995; 82:367–76.

59. Mort TC. Emergency tracheal intubation: complications associated with repeated laryngoscopic attempts. Anesth Analg 2004; 99:607–13, table of contents.

60. Mort TC. The incidence and risk factors for cardiac arrest during emergency tracheal intubation: a justification for incorporating the ASA Guidelines in the remote location. J Clin Anesth 2004; 16:508–16.

61. Peterson GN, Posner KL, Domino KB, Lee L, Cheney FW. Management of the difficult airway in closed malpractice claims. Anesthesiology 2003; 99:A1252.

62. Practice guidelines for management of the difficult airway. A report by the American Society of Anesthesiologists Task Force on Management of the Difficult Airway. Anesthesiology 1993; 78:597–602.

63. Barron FA, Ball DR, Jefferson P, Norrie J. 'Airway Alerts'. How UK anaesthetists organise, document and communicate difficult airway management. Anaesthesia 2003; 58:73–7.

64. Practice guidelines for management of the difficult airway: an updated report by the American Society of Anesthesiologists Task Force on Management of the Difficult Airway. Anesthesiology 2003; 98:1269–77.

65. Combes X, Le Roux B, Suen P, et al. Unanticipated difficult airway in anesthetized patients: prospective validation of a management algorithm. Anesthesiology 2004; 100:1146–50.

66. Henderson JJ, Popat MT, Latto IP, Pearce AC. Difficult Airway Society guidelines for management of the unanticipated difficult intubation. Anaesthesia 2004; 59:675–94.

67. Shaw KM, Mort TC. Emergency airway management in the remote location: incorporating the ASA guidelines can improve patient safety. Anesthesiology 2003; 99:A1249.

68. Cheney FW. Changing trends in anesthesia-related death and permanent brain damage. ASA Newsletter 2002; 66: 6–8.

69. Moore TJ, Walsh CS, Cohen MR. Reported adverse event cases of methemoglobinemia associated with benzocaine products. Arch Intern Med 2004; 164:1192–6.

70. Novaro GM, Aronow HD, Militello MA, Garcia MJ, Sabik EM. Benzocaine-induced methemoglobinemia: experience from a high-volume transesophageal echocardiography laboratory. J Am Soc Echocardiogr 2003; 16:170–5.

71. Barker SJ, Tremper KK, Hyatt J. Effects of methemoglobinemia on pulse oximetry and mixed venous oximetry. Anesthesiology 1989; 70:112–7.

72. Liu SS, Hodgson PS. Local anesthetics. In: Barash PG, Cullen BF, Stoelting RK, editors. Clinical anesthesia. Philadelphia: Lippincott Williams & Wilkins, 2001:449–69.

73. Graham DR, Hay JG, Clague J, Nisar M, Earis JE. Comparison of three different methods used to achieve local anesthesia for fiberoptic bronchoscopy. Chest 1992; 102:704–7.

74. Dauphinee K. Nasotracheal intubation. Emerg Med Clin North Am 1988; 6:715–23.

75. Barriot P, Riou B. Retrograde technique for tracheal intubation in trauma patients. Crit Care Med 1988; 16:712–3.

76. Bourke D, Levesque PR. Modification of retrograde guide for endotracheal intubation. Anesth Analg 1974; 53:1013–4.

77. Hines MH, Meredith JW. Modified retrograde intubation technique for rapid airway access. Am J Surg 1990; 159: 597–9.

78. Lechman MJ, Donahoo JS, Macvaugh H 3rd. Endotracheal intubation using percutaneous retrograde guidewire insertion followed by antegrade fiberoptic bronchoscopy. Crit Care Med 1986; 14:589–90.

79. Waters DJ. Guided blind endotracheal intubation. For patients with deformities of the upper airway. Anaesthesia 1963; 18: 158–62.

80. Sun DA, Warriner CB, Parsons DG, et al. The GlideScope Video Laryngoscope: randomized clinical trial in 200 patients. Br J Anaesth 2004; 94:381–4.

81. Lim TJ, Lim Y, Liu EH. Evaluation of ease of intubation with the GlideScope or Macintosh laryngoscope by anaesthetists in simulated easy and difficult laryngoscopy. Anaesthesia 2005; 60:180–3.

82. Cooper RM, Pacey JA, Bishop MJ, McCluskey SA. Early clinical experience with a new videolaryngoscope (GlidesScope) in 728 patients. Can J Anaesth 2005; 52:191–8.

83. Cooper RM. Use of a new videolaryngoscope (GlideScope) in the management of a difficult airway. Can J Anaesth 2003; 50:611–3.

84. Doyle DJ. Awake intubation using the GlideScope video laryngoscope: initial experience in four cases. Can J Anaesth 2004; 51:520–1.

85. Latto IP, Stacey M, Mecklenburgh J, Vaughan RS. Survey of the use of the gum elastic bougie in clinical practice. Anaesthesia 2002; 57:379–84.

86. Parmet JL, Colonna-Romano P, Horrow JC, et al. The laryngeal mask airway reliably provides rescue ventilation in cases of unanticipated difficult tracheal intubation along with difficult mask ventilation. Anesth Analg 1998; 87:661–5.

87. Tolley P, Watts A, Hickman J. Comparison of the use of the laryngeal mask and face mask by inexperienced personnel. Br J Anaesth 1992; 69:320–1.

88. Choyce A, Avidan MS, Harvey A, et al. The cardiovascular response to insertion of the intubating laryngeal mask airway. Anaesthesia 2002; 57:330–3.

89. Davies P, Tighe S, Greenslade G, Evans G. Laryngeal mask airway and tracheal tube insertion by unskilled personnel. Lancet 1990; 336:977–9.

90. Devitt JH, Wenstone R, Noel AG, O'Donnell MP. The laryngeal mask airway and positive-pressure ventilation. Anesthesiology 1994; 80:550–5.

91. Brimacombe JR, Berry A. The incidence of aspiration associated with the laryngeal mask airway: a meta-analysis of published literature. J Clin Anesth 1995; 7:297–305.

92. Silk JM, Hill HM, Calder I. Difficult intubation and the Laryngeal Mask. Eur J Anaesthesiol Suppl 1991; 4:47–51.

93. Choyce A, Avidan MS, Patel C, et al. Comparison of laryngeal mask and intubating laryngeal mask insertion by the naive intubator. Br J Anaesth 2000; 84:103–5.

94. Baskett PJ, Parr MJ, Nolan JP. The intubating laryngeal mask. Results of a multicentre trial with experience of 500 cases. Anaesthesia 1998; 53:1174–9.

95. Agro F, Frass M, Benumof J, et al. The esophageal tracheal combitube as a non-invasive alternative to endotracheal intubation. A review. Minerva Anestesiol 2001; 67:863–74.

96. Bigenzahn W, Pesau B, Frass M. Emergency ventilation using the Combitube in cases of difficult intubation. Eur Arch Otorhinolaryngol 1991; 248:129–31.

97. Frass M, Frenzer R, Mayer G, Popovic R, Leithner C. Mechanical ventilation with the esophageal tracheal combitube (ETC) in the intensive care unit. Arch Emerg Med 1987; 4:219–25.

98. Klein H, Williamson M, Sue-Ling HM, Vucevic M, Quinn AC. Esophageal rupture associated with the use of the Combitube. Anesth Analg 1997; 85:937–9.

99. Vezina D, Lessard MR, Bussieres J, Topping C, Trepanier CA. Complications associated with the use of the Esophageal-Tracheal Combitube. Can J Anaesth 1998; 45:76–80.

100. Benumof JL, Scheller MS. The importance of transtracheal jet ventilation in the management of the difficult airway. Anesthesiology 1989; 71:769–78.

101. Smith RB, Babinski M, Klain M, Pfaeffle H. Percutaneous transtracheal ventilation. JACEP 1976; 5:765–70.

102. Gillespie MB, Eisele DW. Outcomes of emergency surgical airway procedures in a hospital-wide setting. Laryngoscope 1999; 109:1766–9.

103. Bair AE, Panacek EA, Wisner DH, Bales R, Sakles JC. Cricothyrotomy: a 5-year experience at one institution. J Emerg Med 2003; 24:151–6.

104. Holmes JF, Panacek EA, Sakles JC, Brofeldt BT. Comparison of 2 cricothyrotomy techniques: standard method versus rapid 4-step technique. Ann Emerg Med 1998; 32:442–6.

105. Puntervoll SA, Soreide E, Jacewicz W, Bjelland E. Rapid detection of oesophageal intubation: take care when using colorimetric capnometry. Acta Anaesthesiol Scand 2002; 46:455–7.

106. Murray IP, Modell JH. Early detection of endotracheal tube accidents by monitoring carbon dioxide concentration in respiratory gas. Anesthesiology 1983; 59:344–6.

107. Linko K, Paloheimo M, Tammisto T. Capnography for detection of accidental oesophageal intubation. Acta Anaesthesiol Scand 1983; 27:199–202.

108. Sum Ping ST, Mehta MP, Symreng T. Reliability of capnography in identifying esophageal intubation with carbonated beverage or antacid in the stomach. Anesth Analg 1991; 73:333–7.

109. Ornato JP, Shipley JB, Racht EM, et al. Multicenter study of a portable, hand-size, colorimetric end-tidal carbon dioxide detection device. Ann Emerg Med 1992; 21:518–23.

110. Bhende MS, Thompson AE, Orr RA. Utility of an end-tidal carbon dioxide detector during stabilization and transport of critically ill children. Pediatrics 1992; 89:1042–4.

111. Grmec S. Comparison of three different methods to confirm tracheal tube placement in emergency intubation. Intensive Care Med 2002; 28:701–4.

112. Goldberg JS, Rawle PR, Zehnder JL, Sladen RN. Colorimetric end-tidal carbon dioxide monitoring for tracheal intubation. Anesth Analg 1990; 70:191–4.

113. Wee MY. The oesophageal detector device. Assessment of a new method to distinguish oesophageal from tracheal intubation. Anaesthesia 1988; 43:27–9.

114. Tanigawa K, Takeda T, Goto E, Tanaka K. Accuracy and reliability of the self-inflating bulb to verify tracheal intubation in out-of-hospital cardiac arrest patients. Anesthesiology 2000; 93:1432–6.

115. Kasper CL, Deem S. The self-inflating bulb to detect esophageal intubation during emergency airway management. Anesthesiology 1998; 88:898–902.

116. Zaleski L, Abello D, Gold MI. The esophageal detector device. Does it work? Anesthesiology 1993; 79:244–7.

117. Tanigawa K, Takeda T, Goto E, Tanaka K. The efficacy of esophageal detector devices in verifying tracheal tube placement: a randomized cross-over study of out-of-hospital cardiac arrest patients. Anesth Analg 2001; 92:375–8.

118. Baraka A, Khoury PJ, Siddik SS, Salem MR, Joseph NJ. Efficacy of the self-inflating bulb in differentiating esophageal from tracheal intubation in the parturient undergoing cesarean section. Anesth Analg 1997; 84:533–7.

119. Cardoso MM, Banner MJ, Melker RJ, Bjoraker DG. Portable devices used to detect endotracheal intubation during emergency situations: a review. Crit Care Med 1998; 26: 957–64.

120. Lang DJ, Wafai Y, Salem MR, et al. Efficacy of the self-inflating bulb in confirming tracheal intubation in the morbidly obese. Anesthesiology 1996; 85:246–53.

121. Conrardy PA, Goodman LR, Lainge F, Singer MM. Alteration of endotracheal tube position. Flexion and extension of the neck. Crit Care Med 1976; 4:7–12.

122. Goodman LR, Conrardy PA, Laing F, Singer MM. Radiographic evaluation of endotracheal tube position. AJR Am J Roentgenol 1976; 127:433–4.

123. Bissinger U, Lenz G, Kuhn W. Unrecognized endobronchial intubation of emergency patients. Ann Emerg Med 1989; 18: 853–5.

124. Owen R, Cheney F. Endobronchial intubation: a preventable complication. Anesthesiology 1987; 67:255–7.

125. Goldman JM, Armstrong JP, Vaught LE, Daniel LC. A new method for identifying the depth of insertion of tracheal tubes. Biomed Sci Instrum 1995; 31:225–8.

126. Schwartz DE, Lieberman JA, Cohen NH. Women are at greater risk than men for malpositioning of the endotracheal tube after emergent intubation. Crit Care Med 1994; 22:1127–31.

127. Johnson KB, Egan TD, Kern SE, et al. Influence of hemorrhagic shock followed by crystalloid resuscitation on propofol: a pharmacokinetic and pharmacodynamic analysis. Anesthesiology 2004; 101:647–59.

128. Eames WO, Rooke GA, Wu RS, Bishop MJ. Comparison of the effects of etomidate, propofol, and thiopental on respiratory resistance after tracheal intubation. Anesthesiology 1996; 84: 1307–11.

129. Wagner RL, White PF, Kan PB, Rosenthal MH, Feldman D. Inhibition of adrenal steroidogenesis by the anesthetic etomidate. N Engl J Med 1984; 310:1415–21.

130. Gelissen HP, Epema AH, Henning RH, et al. Inotropic effects of propofol, thiopental, midazolam, etomidate, and ketamine on isolated human atrial muscle. Anesthesiology 1996; 84: 397–403.

131. Pagel PS, Kampine JP, Schmeling WT, Warltier DC. Ketamine depresses myocardial contractility as evaluated by the preload recruitable stroke work relationship in chronically instrumented dogs with autonomic nervous system blockade. Anesthesiology 1992; 76:564–72.

132. Chernow B, Lake CR, Cruess D, et al. Plasma, urine, and CSF catecholamine concentrations during and after ketamine anesthesia. Crit Care Med 1982; 10:600–3.

133. Hemmingsen C, Nielsen PK, Odorico J. Ketamine in the treatment of bronchospasm during mechanical ventilation. Am J Emerg Med 1994; 12:417–20.

134. Hirshman CA, Downes H, Farbood A, Bergman NA. Ketamine block of bronchospasm in experimental canine asthma. Br J Anaesth 1979; 51:713–8.

135. Bedford RF, Persing JA, Pobereskin L, Butler A. Lidocaine or thiopental for rapid control of intracranial hypertension? Anesth Analg 1980; 59:435–7.

136. Yukioka H, et al. Intravenous lidocaine as a suppressant of coughing during tracheal intubation in elderly patients. Anesth Analg 1993; 77:309–12.

137. Gronert GA. Cardiac arrest after succinylcholine: mortality greater with rhabdomyolysis than receptor upregulation. Anesthesiology 2001; 94:523–9.

138. Cooperman LH, Strobel GE Jr., Kennell EM. Massive hyperkalemia after administration of succinylcholine. Anesthesiology 1970; 32:161–4.

139. Matthews JM. Succinylcholine-induced hyperkalemia and rhabdomyolysis in a patient with necrotizing pancreatitis. Anesth Analg 2000; 91:1552–4, table of contents.

140. Kovarik WD, Mayberg TS, Lam AM, Mathisen TL, Winn HR. Succinylcholine does not change intracranial pressure, cerebral blood flow velocity, or the electroencephalogram in patients with neurologic injury. Anesth Analg 1994; 78: 469–73.

141. Perry J, Lee J, Wells G. Rocuronium versus succinylcholine for rapid sequence induction intubation. Cochrane Database Syst Rev 2003:CD002788.

COMPLICATIONS OF TRANSLARYNGEAL INTUBATION

JOHN L. STAUFFER

The term *endotracheal intubation,* or *tracheal intubation,* means the insertion of a definitive artificial airway into the trachea by either the translaryngeal or transtracheal route. This chapter uses the more specific term, *translaryngeal intubation* (TLI), to refer to transoral or transnasal intubation of the airway through the larynx. The term *endotracheal tube* (ETT), which was originally used to describe any artificial airway inserted into the tracheal lumen,[1] is now used to refer to a tube passed via the mouth or nose into the trachea. This chapter uses the term *endotracheal tube,* although *tracheal tube* is recommended by some authorities.[2]

Although TLI was used in resuscitation attempts in the eighteenth century,[3] Macewen is usually given credit for the first successful intubation. In a landmark paper in 1880, he described TLI in four patients for as long as 35 hours and dutifully reported complications, including cough, discomfort, tracheal mucosal congestion, and thickening of the vocal cords and posterior rim of the glottis.[4] In the first half of the twentieth century, TLI was almost exclusively the domain of anesthesiologists, and its use outside of the operating room was uncommon.

The modern era of TLI began in the 1950s when it was reintroduced for the treatment of respiratory failure from drug overdose[5,6] and polio.[1] By the mid-1950s TLI offered a satisfactory alternative to immediate tracheotomy for treatment of respiratory failure, and it was commonly used as a predecessor to tracheotomy when patients required prolonged ventilator support.[1] As experience with TLI grew after the 1950s, so did knowledge of its complications and limitations.[7,8] The monumental literature on complications of TLI includes many anecdotal observations, case reports, and retrospective series, but relatively few prospective studies have been performed. Comprehensive reviews of this subject appeared first in 1950[7] and frequently thereafter.[8–18]

The purposes of this chapter are to provide a practical review of complications of translaryngeal intubation in critically ill adult patients, to help the reader understand the mechanisms underlying these adverse events, and to illustrate how awareness of these complications may lead to their earlier recognition, successful management, and prevention. The chapter reviews important complications and consequences of TLI that are encountered in or are relevant to the practice of adult critical care medicine. They are arranged according to the outline in Table 39-1.

The scope of the chapter includes common and unusual complications of TLI with standard ETTs, whether short-term or prolonged, emergency or elective.

TABLE 39-1 Classification of Complications of Translaryngeal Intubation

Temporal classification
    Complications during endotracheal tube (ETT) placement
    Complications while the ETT is in place
    Complications during and after extubation
Anatomic-physiologic classification
    Facial
    Nasal and paranasal
    Oral
    Pharyngeal
    Laryngeal
    Tracheal
    Bronchial
    Pulmonary
    Miscellaneous
        General
        Esophageal
        Gastric
        Musculoskeletal
        Neurologic
        Physiologic
            Cardiovascular
            Other

TABLE 39-2 Early Complications of Translaryngeal Intubation after 226 Intubations in 143 Adults

Clinical Problem	No.	Percentage
Excessive cuff pressure to achieve seal by minimal occluding pressure technique[a]	42	19
Self-extubation	29	13
Inability to seal airway[b]	24	11
Right mainstem bronchus intubation	21	9
Aspiration[c]	17	8
Lip ulceration or cellulitis	16	7
Pharyngeal injury or bleeding	15	7
Mechanical problems with the ETT[d]	14	6
Difficulty suctioning via the ETT	12	5
Pain in nose, mouth, pharynx, or chest related to the ETT	8	4
Glottic edema	5	2
Oral mucous membrane injury	5	2
Tooth avulsion	4	2
Laryngospasm at the time of extubation	3	1
Pneumothorax	2	1
Esophageal intubation	2	1
Miscellaneous[e]	49	22
Total number of patients: 268		

[a]Defined arbitrarily as >25 mmHg.
[b]Defined as leakage of air around the cuff due to a defect in the cuff or inadequate seal with cuff pressure <60 mmHg.
[c]Defined as aspiration apparent clinically as an immediate result of the intubation attempt or after successful intubation.
[d]Includes partial dislodgment of the tube, length too short or too long, cuff laceration, and biting and occluding the tube.
[e]Includes nasal bleeding, which was recorded 22 times.
SOURCE: Modified, with permission, from Stauffer et al.[23]

Frequency of Complications

The complication rate of TLI varies with the setting, the urgency of the procedure, the type of anesthesia used, the skill of the intubator, and other factors. In the prehospital setting, the rate of complications of TLI ranges from 9.5[19] to 12.2%.[20] In the emergency department setting, Taryle et al prospectively observed one or more complications in 24 (56%) of 43 patients.[21] In a larger and more recent series of emergency department intubations, most of which were facilitated by rapid-sequence intubation, Sakles et al observed complications in 49 (8%) of 610 patients.[22]

In the setting of adult critical care, we reported that 62% of all TLIs had one or more associated adverse events during intubation or while the tube was in place.[23] The mean number of complications per patient was 1.2. The most common early clinical problems were, in descending order of frequency, excessive cuff pressure required to seal the airway, self-extubation, inability to seal the airway, right mainstem bronchus intubation, and aspiration (Table 39-2). Astrachan et al reported very similar results from a retrospective review of 75 TLIs—a complication rate of 57%, with cuff leak and self-extubation being the most common early problems.[24]

Complications during Endotracheal Tube Placement

FACIAL

Lacerations and soft tissue trauma of the face are very rare during placement of an ETT.

NASAL AND PARANASAL

Nasal trauma often occurs when nasal intubation is performed urgently or without adequate premedication. A retrospective study of 105 nasotracheal intubations in the emergency department revealed a 26% rate of immediate complications, including epistaxis, emesis, and mainstem bronchus intubation, and a 23% rate of late complications, including pneumonia, sinusitis, and sepsis.[25] Nasal bleeding complicated 54% of attempts at nasal intubation in an adult ICU.[23] Dislodgment of nasal turbinates[26] and nasal polyps[27] is rare. Intracranial placement of nasotracheal tubes, particularly in the setting of facial trauma, has also been reported.[28]

ORAL

Overall, dental injury from TLI is uncommon, occurring in about 0.9% of prehospital TLIs,[20] 0.1% of anesthesia TLIs,[29] and 2% of critical care unit TLIs.[23] In about 1.1 million TLIs for general anesthesia, the most common types of dental injuries were dislodgment of loose or mobile teeth (47% of cases), chipping or fracture of natural teeth (39% of cases), and damage to dental prostheses (12% of cases).[29] Dental injury is the most common reason for anesthesia-related malpractice claims.[29] Dental trauma during TLI is more likely if the intubator is inexperienced.[29,30] Oral mucous membrane injury has been observed in 1–2% of attempts at oral intubation.[23,24] Lip injury occasionally occurs from pressure exerted by the laryngoscope blade.

PHARYNGEAL

Lacerations, bleeding, contusions, excoriations, submucosal hemorrhage, and edema may result from intubation trauma to the nasopharynx, oropharynx, or hypopharynx. These injuries result from trauma from the laryngoscope blade, ETT, or stylet. Pharyngeal bleeding was detected in 1% of TLIs in one series.[24] Analysis of claims for airway injury from anesthesia reveals that pharyngeal injuries are the second most common site of injury, and half of pharyngeal injuries occur with difficult intubation.[31]

Perforation of the posterior pharyngeal wall or hypopharynx is a particularly serious complication. It may result in mediastinal and subcutaneous emphysema, hematoma, upper airway obstruction, abscess formation,[32,33] mediastinitis, pneumothorax, pneumoperitoneum,[34] and even cardiac arrest.[10,35,36]

Hypopharyngeal injury from TLI has been the subject of a number of reports in both adults[10,35–41] and children.[42] Like oral injury, pharyngeal trauma from TLI occurs mainly in emergency settings and in the hands of inexperienced intubators. Piriform sinus laceration by forceful blind intubation may result in severe barotrauma with bilateral pneumothorax, pneumomediastinum, mediastinal abscess, and cardiac arrest.[37] Figure 39-1 illustrates hypopharyngeal trauma

from repeated unsuccessful attempts at oral intubation by an inexperienced intubator.

LARYNGEAL

The larynx is the most common site of airway injury in anesthesia claims analysis.[31] Laryngeal trauma occurs in about 6% of short-term anesthetic intubations.[43,44] Laryngeal injuries during ETT placement include glottic contusion, vocal cord hematoma and laceration, and arytenoid dislocation. Vocal cord hematoma is reported to be the most common sign of laryngeal injury after short-term anesthetic intubation, occurring in 4–5% of these intubations.[43,44] Vocal cord hematomas are more common on the left true vocal cord,[44,45] a finding attributed to the fact that most intubators are right-handed.[13] The frequency of vocal cord laceration in anesthetic intubation ranges from 0.6[44]–3%.[46] Epiglottic hematoma from TLI is considered very rare.[47,48] Arytenoid dislocation from traumatic intubation occurs in 0.1[43]–1.7%[49] of anesthetic intubations, leading to complications such as hoarseness and aspiration[49] and acute respiratory failure.[50] Colice et al observed no cases of this complication in critical care intubations.[51]

TRACHEAL

Tracheal perforation,[10] laceration,[52] and rupture[53–55] are rare complications of TLI. The large majority of cases occur in women and in patients over 50 years of age,[56] and involve the posterior membranous portion of the trachea at or near the carina.[57] Causes of tracheal tears include forceful

FIGURE 39-1 Autopsy specimen of larynx, hypopharynx, and upper esophagus opened posteriorly. The patient was an older man with COPD and acute respiratory failure in whom repeated forceful attempts at oral intubation by an inexperienced physician were not successful. The tip of the ETT traumatized the airway. Multiple areas of submucosal hemorrhage in the piriform sinuses and hypopharynx are evident (*arrows*).

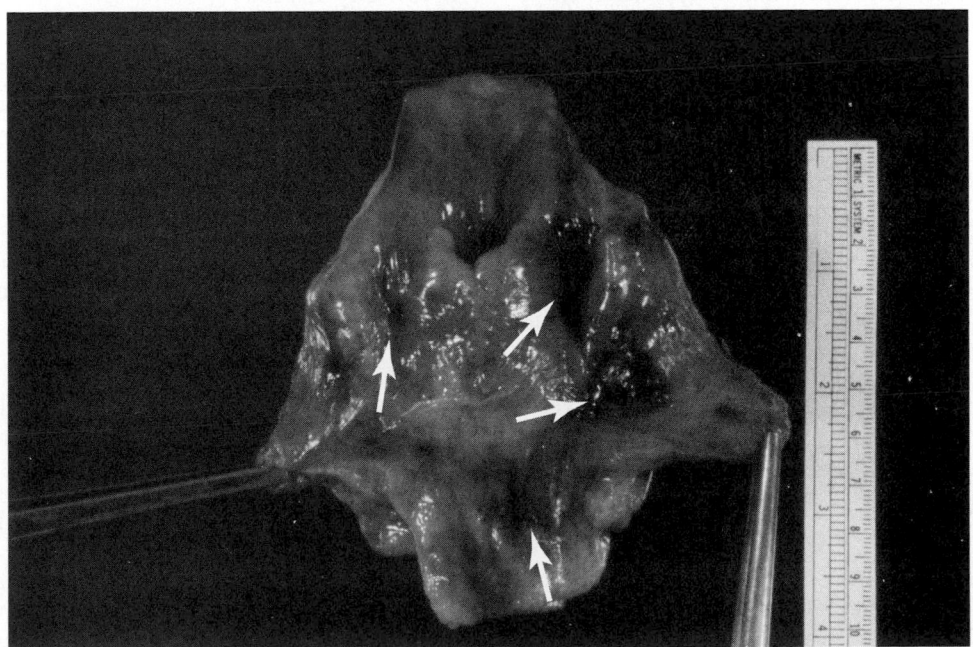

intubation, damage of the posterior membranous trachea by a stylet,[55] overinflation of the cuff,[42,55] excessive coughing or movement during intubation, and pre-existing anatomic abnormalities of the trachea such as tracheomalacia.[52–54,56,58] Subcutaneous emphysema, pneumomediastinum, and respiratory distress are commonly seen after this type of tracheal injury.[52,54,55]

Malpositioning of the ETT in the trachea is a frequent consequence of emergency TLI. In a prospective series of 271 emergency TLIs in critically ill adults, Schwartz et al observed 9 (3.3%) cases in which the ETT tip was too high (>6 cm above the carina) and 23 (8.5%) cases in which it was too low (<2 cm from the carina), in addition to 10 cases (3.7%) of right mainstem bronchus intubation.[59] Malpositioning of the ETT was significantly more common in women than in men.

BRONCHIAL

Intubation of a mainstem bronchus is a potentially serious complication of intubation.[23,24,60,61] It usually occurs in nonanesthetic intubations and is almost always on the right side. Left mainstem bronchus intubation is very rare. Potential complications of right mainstem bronchus intubation include hyperinflation of the right lung, right pneumothorax, atelectasis of part or the entire left lung, and impaired gas exchange. Mainstem bronchus intubation was reported in 3% of cases in a retrospective series[24] and in 3.7[59] and 9.6%[60] of cases in prospective series of critical care intubations.

PULMONARY

Pulmonary complications during attempts to place an ETT include pulmonary aspiration (reported in 4–19% of adult nonanesthetic intubations),[21,23,62] multiple forms of barotrauma, pulmonary edema, and bronchospasm. Also, failed intubation attempts may lead to worsening gas exchange, including severe hypoxemia.[63] Hypoxemia (oxyhemoglobin saturation <90%) has been reported in 18[63]– 21%[64] of emergency TLIs.

The prospective investigation of 297 TLIs in critically ill adults reported by Schwartz et al revealed 12 cases (4%) of new unexplained lung infiltrates (probably related to aspiration) and 2 cases of pneumothorax (1%).[62] Aspiration complicated 5.6% of prehospital TLIs in non–cardiac arrest cases in a large series.[20] Pulmonary edema may follow upper airway obstruction, and postoperative laryngospasm complicating anesthetic intubation is a known cause of this phenomenon.[65] Laryngospasm-induced pulmonary edema occurs with a frequency of 0.05–0.1% of all anesthetics.[66] Bronchospasm was reported in 3 (0.8%) of 358 prehospital TLIs.[20] The bronchospasm response to TLI is rarely severe. Patients with asthma are at the highest risk.

MISCELLANEOUS
GENERAL
Without adequate premedication, critically ill patients may experience pain in the upper airway, generalized discomfort, and anxiety during intubation. These important complications are difficult to assess objectively and are usually overlooked in large case reviews in the literature.

Bacteremia complicating nasotracheal intubation occurs with a frequency of 5.5[67]–16%.[68] The frequency of transient bacteremia following orotracheal intubation ranged from 3.2%[69] in elective TLI for anesthesia to 9% in urgent TLI performed in ICU patients.[70] In the latter series, only *Streptococcus* species were isolated immediately after TLI, and no patient had streptococcal bacteremia before or 1 hour after TLI.

ESOPHAGEAL
An analysis of claims for airway injury from anesthesia showed that the esophagus was the third most common site of injury, and esophageal injuries were more severe than all other types of airway injury combined.[31] Wolff et al reported 3 cases of pharyngeal-esophageal perforation from TLI, emphasizing that this complication occurs during emergency intubations by inexperienced personnel.[39] Difficult intubation has been implicated in other case reports.[71,72] O'Neill et al described two cases of esophageal and pharyngeal perforation from elective anesthetic intubation, noting that this severe complication is not always limited to emergency or difficult intubations.[40] Esophageal perforation during intubation typically occurs when the tip of the ETT lacerates the posterior wall of the cervical esophagus. Subcutaneous emphysema is the most common physical finding of TLI-induced esophageal perforation.[72] Anterior esophageal perforation has not been reported.[72]

Esophageal intubation is a common complication of both emergency and elective TLI, and it carries the risk of severe hypoxemia with irreversible brain injury.[73,74] In one report, 4 (15%) of 27 cardiac arrests during TLI were attributed to esophageal intubation.[75] Esophageal intubation occurred in 37 (5.4%) of 691 patients intubated in the prehospital setting in France,[20] 33 (5.5%) of 603 patients intubated in an emergency department,[22] and in 25 (8%) of 297 emergency TLIs in critically ill adults.[62]

GASTRIC
Gastric distention may result from esophageal intubation. Swallowing of foreign material such as dental appliances and teeth may also occur.[76] TLI may stimulate the gag reflex, leading to vomiting.

MUSCULOSKELETAL
Musculoskeletal complications during intubation are uncommon. Injury to the cervical spine during orotracheal intubation has been reported.[77]

NEUROLOGIC
Neurologic complications of TLI include hypoxic brain injury, injury to the cervical spinal cord,[13] and increased intracranial pressure.[78,79] Hypoxic brain injury may result from ineffective ventilation, oxygenation, or circulation during difficult TLI. Patients with cervical spine injuries or underlying diseases are at greatest risk for traumatic injury to the cervical spinal cord during intubation.[13] Transient increases in intracranial pressure occur with TLI, putting patients with head injury at risk for secondary brain injury.[79]

PHYSIOLOGIC

Cardiovascular

The cardiovascular response to laryngoscopy and TLI includes transient increases in heart rate and both systolic and diastolic blood pressure, a phenomenon known as the "pressor response." This occurs in most patients undergoing uncomplicated TLI, and in healthy individuals it is usually inconsequential. Complications may result when these physiologic responses are exaggerated.[80–82] In patients with hypertension the hemodynamic response to TLI is greater than in normotensive patients.[83] Tachycardia and hypertension represent transient and variable sympathetic reflex responses to TLI provoked by stimulation of the pharynx.[80,84] Some, but not all, studies have documented a rise in plasma epinephrine and norepinephrine levels with TLI.[83,85–87]

The hypertensive response to nasotracheal intubation is greater than that to orotracheal intubation.[88] The hemodynamic response to orotracheal intubation is greater than that to insertion of the Laryngeal Mask Airway (LMA North America, San Diego, CA),[83,85] but less than that to insertion of the esophageal-tracheal Combitube (Tyco Healthcare).[85]

Hypotension also occurs in some patients during TLI. Khan et al reported that hypotension was the most common complication during TLI in a prospective series of 126 critically ill patients.[89] Franklin et al observed that 24 (29%) of 84 patients requiring TLI in an emergency department developed life-threatening hypotension, which was significantly associated with the presence of chronic obstructive pulmonary disease (COPD) and hypercapnia and hypoxemic respiratory failure but not with the administration of sedatives or paralyzing medications.[90]

MacKenzie et al reported cardiac arrhythmias in 58% and 32% of nasal and oral anesthetic intubations, respectively.[91] Bradycardia[63,89] and bradyarrhythmias also occur during TLI.

Other

Increased intraocular pressure[10] may occur during TLI. Stimulation of laryngovagal reflexes may lead to laryngospasm, and stimulation of laryngospinal reflexes may produce vomiting, bucking, and coughing.[10]

CARDIAC ARREST AND MORTALITY RATE OF TRANSLARYNGEAL INTUBATION

Biboulet et al prospectively recorded 11 anesthesia-related cardiac arrests in a series of 101,769 anesthetics performed from 1989 to 1995 (frequency 1.1 per 10,000), and the mortality rate was 0.6 per 10,000.[92] All the cardiac arrests were considered avoidable.

Adnet reported cardiac arrest as a complication of TLI in 4 (1.1%) of 358 patients with initial conditions other than cardiac arrest who required intubation in the prehospital setting.[20] In emergency department practice, none of 43 patients reported by Taryle et al[21] and 3 (0.5%) of 610 patients reported by Sakles et al[22] experienced cardiac arrest from TLI. In the latter series, 2 of the 3 patients had agonal cardiac rhythms before TLI. We reported cardiac arrest in 1 (0.4%) of 226 intubations performed in ICUs, resulting

from prolonged intubation attempts by an inexperienced physician.[23]

Death as a result of TLI is extremely rare. Schwartz et al reported a mortality rate of 0.85% during or within 30 minutes of emergency TLI in critical care patients without pre-existing hypotension.[62] No deaths from TLI were reported in 3 other series.[20,23,93]

Complications While the Endotracheal Tube Is in Place

FACIAL

Skin reactions to adhesive tape and secretions and pressure ulcers from ETT holders may develop.

NASAL AND PARANASAL

NASAL COMPLICATIONS

In a prospective series of 379 patients with nasotracheal intubation, Holdgaard et al found inflammation and ulceration of the nostrils or nasal septum in 110 patients (29%) within 5 days of extubation.[94] Nasal bleeding occurred in 19% of patients and conchae fractures in 11%. Necrosis of the nasal alae may occur at the site of constant pressure on the nose by an upturned nasotracheal tube (Fig. 39-2).[95] This injury was seen in 4% of nasotracheal intubations,[24] and it may be accompanied by bacterial invasion with cellulitis.[14] Nasal septal ulceration is uncommon.[23]

PARANASAL COMPLICATIONS

Sinus Effusions
Nasotracheal intubation for more than a few days commonly results in accumulation of fluid in the paranasal

FIGURE 39-2 Hemorrhagic ulceration of the left ala nasi (*arrow*) as a result of pressure exerted by a previously upturned nasotracheal tube. This type of injury can be prevented by positioning the ETT so that its proximal end points straight down from the anterior naris. (*Modified, with permission, from Zwillich and Pierson.*[95])

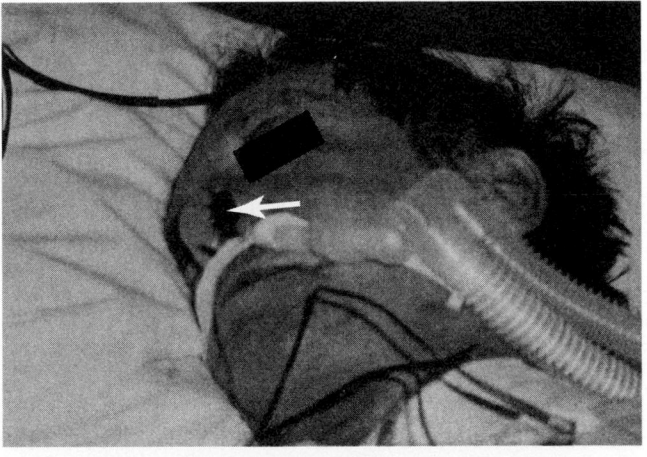

sinuses.[14,96–99] Fassoulaki and Pamouktsoglou found computed tomographic (CT) scan evidence of paranasal sinus fluid accumulation, opacification, or mucosal thickening in all of 16 adult patients studied prospectively by the eighth day of nasotracheal intubation.[98] The maxillary and sphenoid sinuses each were affected in 87% of cases, followed by the ethmoid (50%) and frontal (12.5%) sinuses. Sinus effusions were unilateral and on the same side as the nasotracheal tube. Involvement of more than one sinus at a time was common.[98] Ultrasound evaluation has demonstrated sinus effusions in 30% of patients with nasotracheal intubation[14] and 63% of patients with orotracheal intubation.[99]

Sinusitis

In 1982, Knodel and Beekman called attention to nasotracheal intubation as a cause of maxillary sinusitis with fever in mechanically ventilated patients.[100] Sinusitis has subsequently been recognized as a common and potentially serious complication of TLI, particularly nasotracheal intubation (see Chapter 47).[24,96,97,99,101–111] Infectious sinusitis complicates roughly one-quarter to one-half of prolonged nasotracheal intubations.[96,103,105] Sinusitis may also occur with nasogastric intubation.[110]

Deutschman et al studied 27 nasally intubated patients who developed paranasal sinusitis.[97] Seven patients in that series developed pneumonia and two became septic. Successful treatment required antibiotics and switching from nasal intubation to oral intubation or tracheotomy. In a prospective study of 30 patients requiring nasotracheal intubation and mechanical ventilation for 6–9 days, Guerin et al found CT scan evidence of sinus effusions in 28 (93%).[102] Purulent fluid was aspirated from the maxillary sinuses in 25 (83%) of these patients, all of whom were febrile. Gram-negative infections predominated and 8 patients (27%) had bacteremia. Only one-third of the patients with sinusitis had purulent sinus drainage.[102]

Severe complications of TLI-associated sinusitis include fever, bacteremia, pneumonia, sepsis, and meningitis. Gram-negative bacteria such as *Klebsiella* and *Enterobacter* species are commonly isolated from sinus aspirates in patients with sinusitis complicating nasotracheal intubation. Gram-positive bacteria, particularly *Staphylococcus aureus*, and fungi are also frequently isolated. Anaerobic infection, particularly with *Bacteroides* species, also occurs. Polymicrobial infections are common.

Otitis and Middle Ear Effusions

In neonates and children, nasotracheal intubation is considered a possible risk factor for impaired tympanic membrane mobility, otitis media, and middle ear effusion.[112–114] In adults, however, otitis and middle ear effusions are little known paranasal complications of TLI.

We noted otoscopic evidence of otitis in 9% of intubated adult patients.[23] Cavaliere et al observed that 80% of 35 unconscious ICU patients had middle ear effusion, and there was a significant association with TLI and mechanical ventilation.[115] Lucks et al reported evidence of middle ear effusions in 23 (29%) of 78 adults with prolonged TLI, most of whom were intubated orally.[116] Tympanocentesis revealed organisms in 22% of patients with middle ear effu-

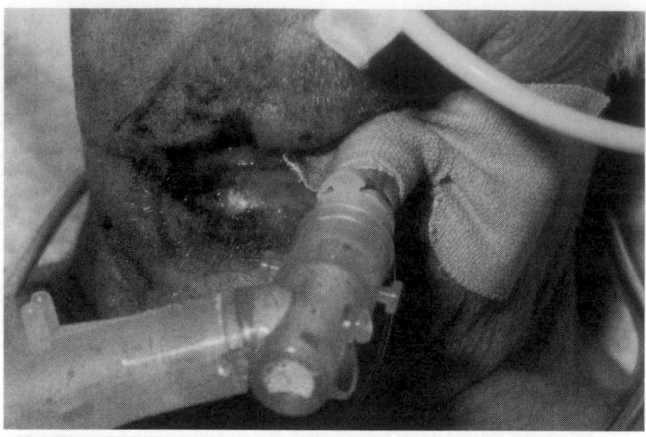

FIGURE 39-3 Ulceration of the right side of the upper and lower lip in a patient with prolonged orotracheal intubation. This type of injury can be prevented by proper securing of the ETT, minimizing the direct pressure transmitted to the mouth from the ETT and ventilator tubing, and regular oral examination during the period of TLI. (*Modified, with permission, from Stauffer.[118]*)

sion, particularly *Pseudomonas aeruginosa*, *Klebsiella oxytoca*, and *Enterobacter cloacae*, typical of the gram-negative organisms colonizing the airway in patients with TLI.[116] Christensen et al found otitis in 11 (16%) of 67 adult trauma patients with TLI for 3 or more days.[117]

ORAL

Ulceration or cellulitis of the lips complicates 7% of TLIs in critically ill adults.[23] Lip edema, bleeding, and hemorrhagic crusts are very common during TLI as a result of pressure injury and abrasion by the orotracheal tube, oropharyngeal airway, tape, orogastric tube, or ETT holder.[23,118] Figure 39-3 illustrates lip injury from prolonged orotracheal intubation.[118] Hanley et al reported reactivation of herpes simplex virus infections in 53% of patients with oral TLI longer than 48 hours, but clinical findings were noted in only half of these cases.[119] Dental injury, stomatitis, erosion of the hard palate, and soft tissue injury to the tongue and oral mucosa may develop during TLI, and in some cases these complications are severe (Fig. 39-4).[23,120] They are more likely to occur in patients with concurrent use of oropharyngeal airways or those with rigid contracture of the jaw or propulsive movements of the tongue.[120]

PHARYNGEAL

Pharyngeal complications while an ETT is in place are uncommon. Pharyngeal inflammation, ulceration, edema, and occasional bleeding have been found in less than 10% of cases.[23]

LARYNGEAL

Laryngeal injury is the most common and potentially the most severe complication of TLI,[12,43,51,121–134] and fear of late laryngeal complications of TLI is cited as the primary reason for performing tracheotomy for long-term airway

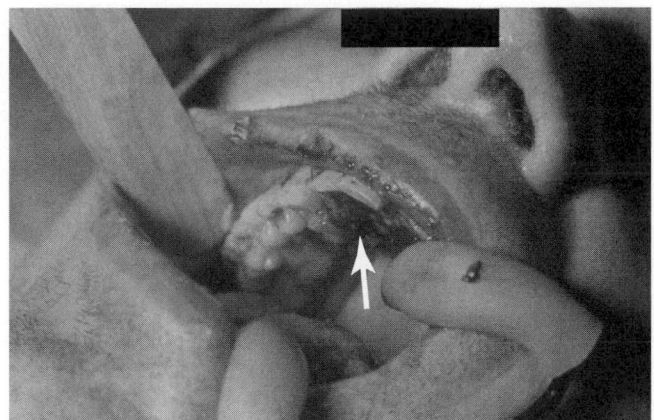
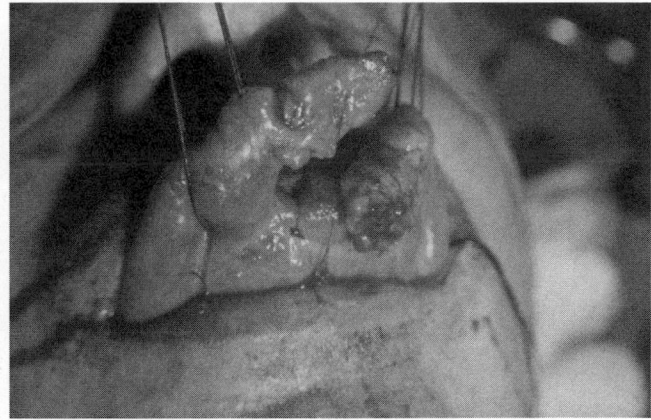

FIGURE 39-4 Severe injury to the mouth may occur during TLI because of pressure-induced necrosis. This patient was a young man who was intubated because of status epilepticus and need to control the airway. Rigid contracture of the jaw occurred repeatedly while an oral pharyngeal airway was in place to prevent occlusion of the ETT by biting. Evidence of oral injury included erosion of the hard palate (*arrow*) by the oropharyngeal airway (*left*), and complete transection of the tongue, photographed at the time of surgical repair (*right*). (*Modified, with permission, from Stauffer and Petty.*[120])

maintenance. The most common postmortem findings in the larynx after prolonged TLI are mucosal ulceration, edema, and submucosal hemorrhage (Table 39-3).[23,135] Figure 39-5 presents a schematic drawing and illustrations of common TLI-induced laryngotracheal lesions. Figure 39-6 presents endoscopic views of selected cases of glottic injury from TLI in Lindholm's comprehensive study.[127]

Experience with prolonged TLI in the 1970s showed moderate to severe laryngeal injury in 4.2[136]–7.2%[130] of cases. Kambic and Radsel found severe laryngeal injury in 62 (6.2%) of 1000 patients after anesthetic intubations, indicating that TLI for short periods and in a controlled setting was not without risk.[43] Most prospective studies reveal that serious permanent laryngeal injury from TLI is very uncommon.[23,125,137] Nearly all TLI-induced laryngeal injuries tend to heal within 6–8 weeks and leave no permanent sequelae.[51,124,137,138]

SUPRAGLOTTIC INJURY

Mucosal ulceration, significant inflammation or edema, and submucosal hemorrhage at autopsy have been noted in 12, 7, and 5%, respectively, of patients with prolonged TLI

TABLE 39-3   Common Autopsy Findings after Prolonged Translaryngeal Intubation in 41 Patients

| | MUCOSAL | | | | | |
| | Mucosal Ulceration | | Inflammation and/or Edema | | Submucosal Hemorrhage | |
Site	No.	%	No.	%	No.	%
Epiglottis	5	12	3	7	2	5
Glottis	21	51	12	29	5	12
Subglottis	5	12	1	2	3	7
Trachea, cuff site	6	15	16	39	3	7
Trachea, other site	2	5	20	49	3	7
Total	39		52		16	

SOURCE: Modified, with permission, from Stauffer et al.[23]

(see Table 39-3).[23] Astrachan et al found severe supraglottic edema in 1% of TLIs.[24]

GLOTTIC INJURY

Laryngeal Ulceration

Ulceration of the posterior aspect of the true vocal cords and arytenoids occurred in 51[23]–79%[127] of TLIs, representing the most common significant complication of TLI.[14,49,128,131–133,136,138–141] Investigators first reported posterior laryngeal ulcers from TLI in the early 1950s.[142,143] Lindholm observed postmortem macroscopic ulceration or necrosis in the interarytenoid area, the medial side of the arytenoids, and the inner posterolateral area of the cricoid cartilage in 9, 79, and 68% of adults, respectively.[127] Laryngeal ulcers from TLI are symmetrical, triangular-shaped erosions of the posterior and medial aspects of the vocal processes (Fig. 39-7) and arytenoids and the posterolateral area of the cricoid cartilages.[49] They are typically 4–12 mm in diameter and 1–5 mm in depth, and they may penetrate into the cartilage[128] and the cricoarytenoid joints. The areas most vulnerable to ulceration by pressure from the shaft of the ETT are the posterior endolarynx, the arytenoids, the cricoarytenoid joints, and the interarytenoid space.[122] Using telelaryngoscopy, Deeb et al examined 142 adults who required tracheotomy because of failed extubation.[144] They observed that mucosal erosions and ulcerations, often with exposed cartilage, were common, and the most severe ulcers affected the intercartilaginous glottis and posterior subglottis, often with extensive granulation tissue. In some cases, the paired posterior ulcers may be large enough to join each other, producing a "horseshoe lesion."[14]

Glottic Edema and Inflammation

Varying degrees of hyperemia, edema, and inflammation of the glottic mucosa occur in practically all patients during TLI.[23,46,51,121,127,138,141] We found severe edema and inflammation at autopsy in 29% of patients following TLI, particularly in the posterior commissure area.[23]

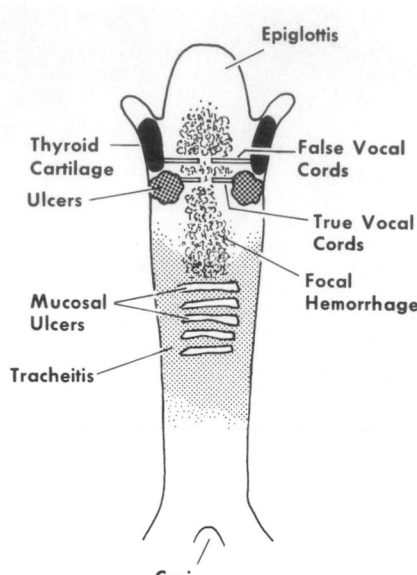
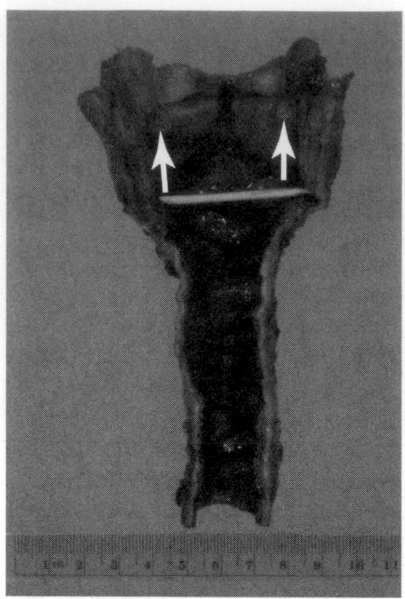
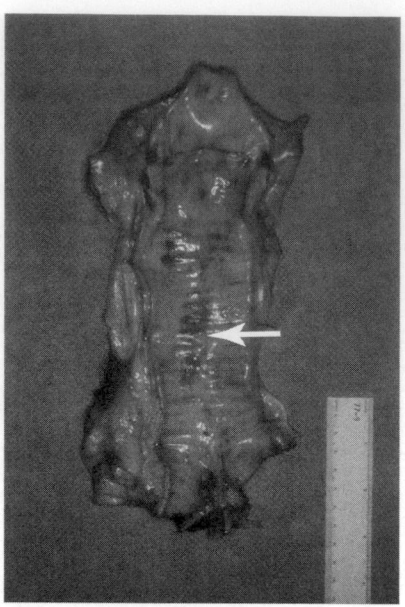

FIGURE 39-5 Schematic drawing of the larynx and trachea opened posteriorly, illustrating common laryngotracheal lesions following TLI in the critical care setting (*left*). Autopsy specimen of larynx and trachea (with the epiglottis trimmed away) showing typical TLI-induced ulcers on the posterior aspect of the true vocal cords (*arrows*) (*center*). An autopsy specimen of larynx and trachea from another patient showing superficial tracheal cuff site ulcer (*arrow*) and focal tracheal mucosal hemorrhage (*right*). (*Left panel modified, with permission, from Stauffer.*[135])

Vocal Cord Paresis and Paralysis

This complication during TLI presents after extubation and is discussed below.

Glottic Hemorrhage

The incidence of glottic hemorrhage developing after intubation is not known. We found evidence of submucosal hemorrhage in the glottis in 12% of TLI cases at autopsy (see Table 39-3).[23]

Granuloma Formation

When used in the context of airway injury from artificial airways, the term *granuloma* refers to growths of granulation tissue at the site of mucosal injury as a result of abnormal tissue healing. Laryngeal granulomas during TLI have been observed in 2.4[23]–16%[124] of patients during TLI. While usually associated with prolonged TLI, they may also occur after intubation for several hours.[145] This topic is discussed below in the section on late complications after extubation.

SUBGLOTTIC INJURY

Cricoid cartilage abscess results from bacterial invasion of the cricoid cartilage after pressure ulceration by the ETT.[13,14] Cricoid cartilage abscess may appear as long as 8 weeks after extubation and predispose to posterior glottic stenosis.[13]

TRACHEAL

Tracheal injury during TLI (Table 39-4) may occur at the site of the inflated cuff, at the level of the tip of the tracheal tube, and at the site of injury by suction catheters. Cuff-site injuries are the most common.[23]

EDEMA AND INFLAMMATION

Mucosal edema or inflammation is found at autopsy in 39% of TLI patients at the cuff site and in 49% at other levels of the trachea (see Table 39-3).[23] Infiltrates of neutrophils and mononuclear cells are found in the mucosa and submucosa at the cuff site.[146,147]

TRACHEAL ULCERATION

The use of high-volume, low-pressure cuffs on ETTs has greatly reduced the frequency of cuff-site ulceration. Figure 39-5 (right panel) illustrates a small cuff-site ulcer with exposed cartilage on the anterior tracheal wall. Severe cuff-site ulcers that were common in the era of hard-cuff ETTs[148,149] are now rarely seen. Modern soft cuff ETTs, however, do not completely protect the mucosa from injury. We reported tracheal mucosal ulceration at autopsy in 15% of patients with prolonged TLI with soft-cuff ETTs at the cuff site and in 5% at other tracheal sites (see Table 39-3).[23] Soft cuffs apply lateral pressure over a longer segment than hard cuffs, and pressure from overlapping folds of the fabric of soft cuffs may create channels in the tracheal mucosa.[150]

GRANULOMA FORMATION

Granulomas in the trachea are much less common than in the larynx following prolonged TLI, because tracheal ulceration is now much less common than laryngeal ulceration. All of the laryngotracheal granulomas observed by Lindholm were in the larynx.[127] Astrachan et al observed tracheal granulomas in only 1% of patients.[24]

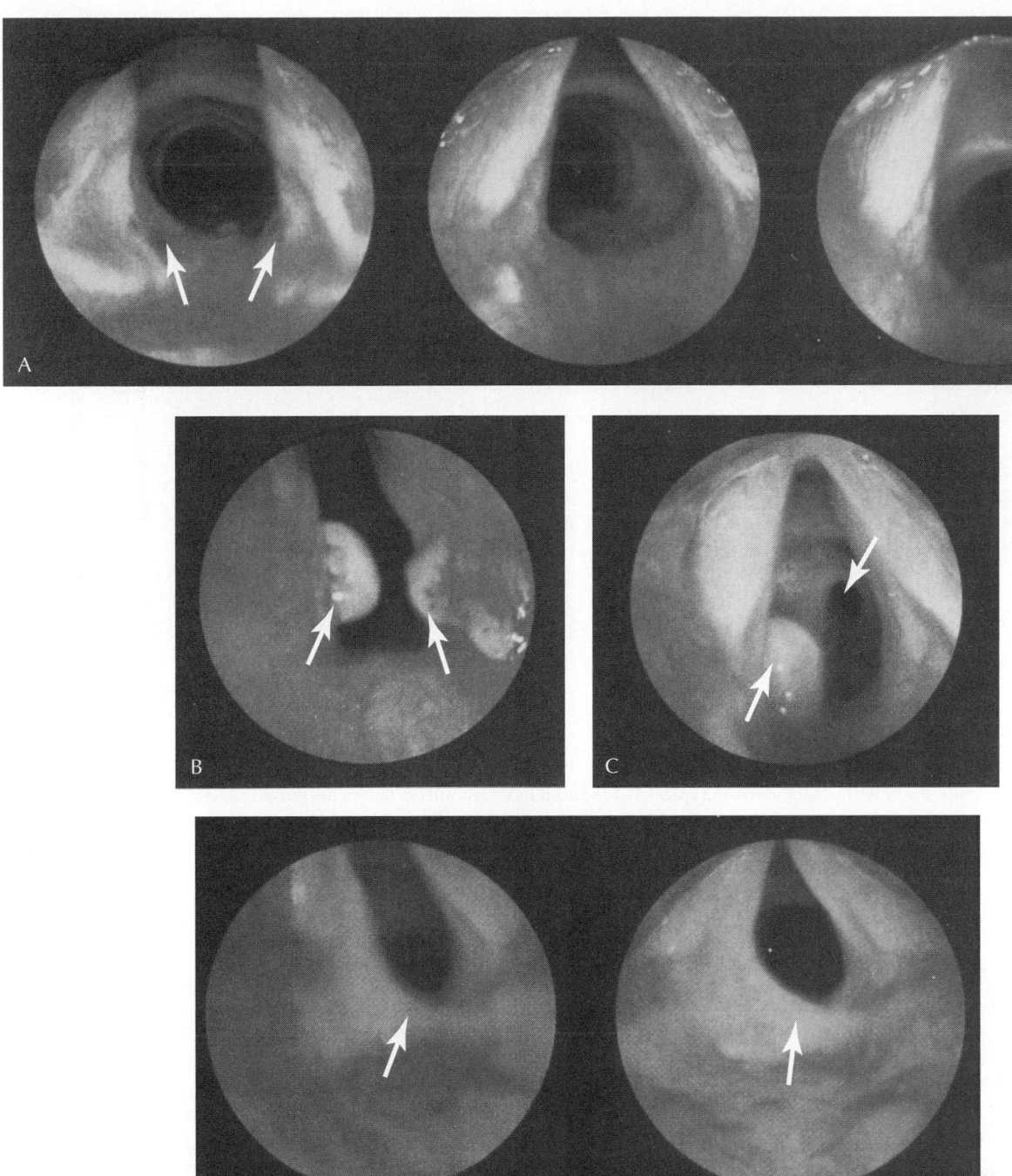

FIGURE 39-6 Endoscopic views representing types of TLI-induced laryngeal injury observed by Lindholm in his prospective study of complications of endotracheal intubation.[127] *A.* Superficial posterior glottic ulcers (*left*) (*arrows*) with healing over 18 days (*center*) and 32 days (*right*). *B.* Bilateral granulomas (*arrows*) that were absent at extubation but appeared by 44 days after extubation. *C.* Left subglottic granuloma (*arrow 1*) 14 months after TLI and tracheotomy. Tracheal stenosis (*arrow 2*) attributed to the tracheotomy is also evident. *D.* Fibrous scar at the left arytenoid region (*arrows*) 15 months (*left*) and 32 months (*right*) after TLI. (*Modified, with permission, from Lindholm.*[127])

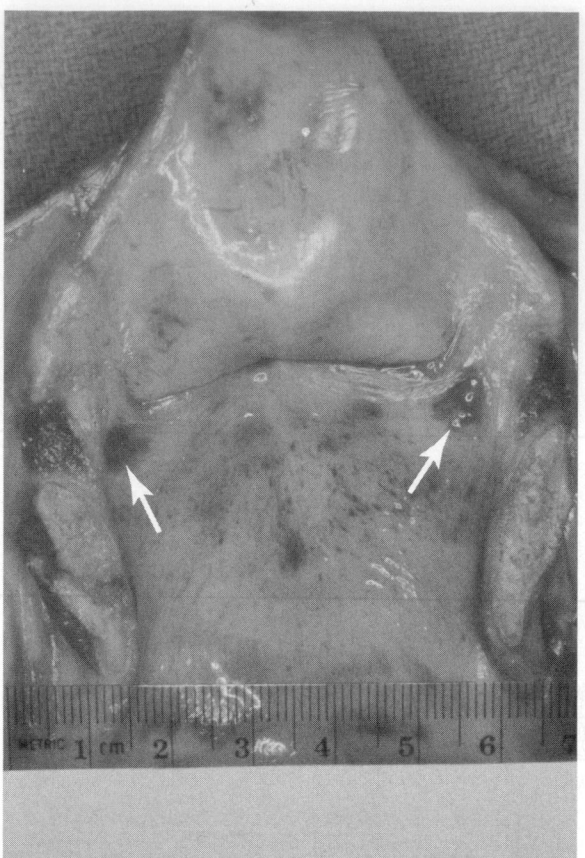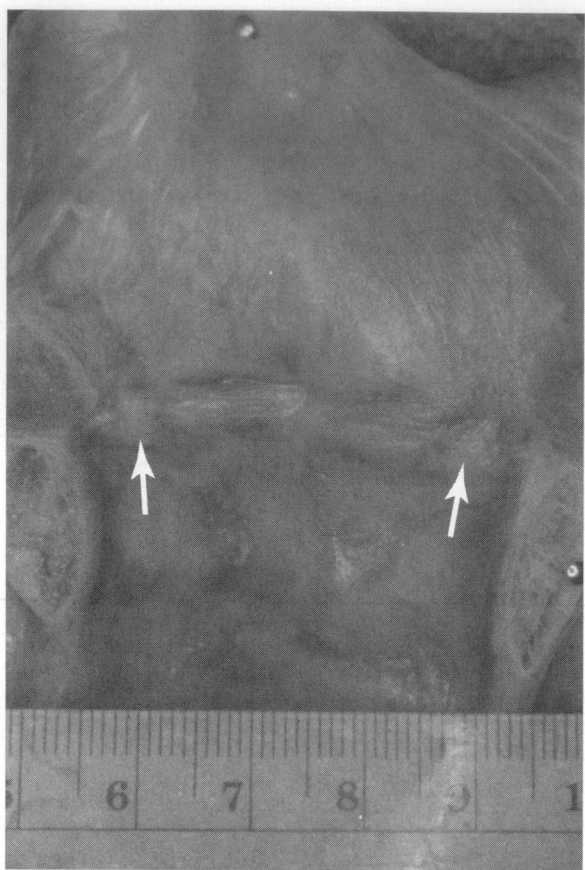

FIGURE 39-7 Autopsy specimens with closer views of typical TLI-induced laryngeal ulcers on the posterior true vocal cords. *Left:* Superficial hemorrhagic ulcers (*arrows*). Focal mucosal hemorrhage is also seen. *Right:* Deeper ulcers to the level of cartilage (*arrows*).

TABLE 39-4   Tracheal Complications While the Endotracheal Tube Is in Place

Edema and inflammation
Ulceration of the mucosa and tracheal wall
Granuloma formation
Submucosal hemorrhage
Necrosis
Destruction of cartilage
Tracheal rupture and tracheal laceration
Tracheal dilation
Tracheomalacia
Tracheoesophageal fistula
Tracheoarterial fistula
Epithelial damage
Squamous metaplasia of tracheal epithelium
Reduction in mucociliary clearance
Airway colonization with bacteria
Pseudomembranous tracheitis
Miscellaneous
   Too high or too low ETT position
   Tracheobronchitis
   Carina irritation, leading to cough and bucking
   Suctioning complications

SUBMUCOSAL HEMORRHAGE

Submucosal hemorrhage site was found at autopsy in 7% of patients at both the cuff and other tracheal sites (see Table 39-3).[23]

TRACHEAL NECROSIS

Abbey et al reported a case of massive tracheal necrosis and suppuration after 10 days of TLI.[151] Possible risk factors included sepsis, hypotension, and elevated cuff pressures.

DESTRUCTION OF TRACHEAL CARTILAGE

Ulceration and eventual destruction of the C-shaped cartilaginous tracheal rings may occur as a result of sustained elevation of cuff pressure,[152] resulting in tracheal dilation, tracheomalacia, and injury to the adjacent great vessels and esophagus.

TRACHEAL RUPTURE AND TRACHEAL LACERATION

Tracheal laceration[52] and tracheal rupture[53] are rare complications of TLI during the period when the ETT is in place.

TRACHEAL DILATION

Dilation of the trachea, a sign of severe tracheal wall damage,[152] may appear even with soft-cuff ETTs during TLI or after extubation (see below),[153] although this complication is mainly related to tracheotomy.[154] When tracheotomy is performed following long-term TLI, it may be difficult to determine whether the cuffed ETT or the cuffed tracheostomy tube was primarily responsible for the injury.[155]

TRACHEOMALACIA
Although tracheomalacia has been reported in patients with tracheotomy following TLI,[156] tracheomalacia after TLI alone is very rare when ETTs with high-volume, low-pressure cuffs are used.

TRACHEOESOPHAGEAL FISTULA
Cuff pressure–induced necrosis and erosion of the posterior membranous portion of the trachea and anterior wall of the esophagus may result in tracheoesophageal fistula.[131,140,157,158] This rare complication of artificial airways has been mainly associated with tracheotomy,[131,159,160] but TLI, even with soft-cuff ETTs, is also a risk factor.[161] The concurrent use of a nasogastric tube may enhance the risk. Tracheoesophageal fistula may be silent or present with the appearance of gastric contents in tracheal secretions or with massive gastric distention.[162] After cuff deflation or extubation, it may present with cough following ingestion of food.[161]

TRACHEOARTERIAL FISTULA
Tracheoarterial fistula is a rare complication of tracheotomy (see Chapter 40). Only a few cases of tracheoarterial fistula during prolonged TLI have been reported.[163–165]

EPITHELIAL DAMAGE
Contact of the tracheal surface with an inflated cuff, ETT tip, or suction catheter results in loss of columnar tracheal epithelium cells and distortion of their cilia.[166–169] Regeneration of the ciliated surface and restoration of ciliary structure and function occurs within 2 weeks after extubation.[167,168]

SQUAMOUS METAPLASIA OF THE TRACHEAL EPITHELIUM
Squamous metaplasia of the tracheal mucosa has been observed in dog models of intubation and in humans[146,147,170,171] and is attributed to abrasion of the mucosa by the inflated cuff or suction catheter. It may involve both surface and glandular epithelium adjacent to necrotic tracheal ulcers following prolonged TLI.[172]

REDUCTION IN MUCOCILIARY CLEARANCE
Tracheal injury at the cuff site depresses mucociliary clearance in both experimental animals and humans. Cuff inflation,[168] squamous metaplasia,[147] and loss of cilia[169] are among the factors that impair the mucociliary transport system during TLI.

AIRWAY COLONIZATION WITH BACTERIA
Colonization of the trachea with bacteria occurs in nearly all patients during TLI,[173–175] mainly from aspiration of secretions above the inflated ETT cuff and from infected ETT biofilm.[176] Gram-negative bacteria, particularly *Pseudomonas* species, have a particular tropism for the tracheobronchial tree. Bacterial colonization of the trachea during TLI is a risk factor for ventilator-associated pneumonia (VAP) (see discussion below).[173,176,177]

PSEUDOMEMBRANOUS TRACHEITIS
Pseudomembranous tracheitis is a rare and little known complication of TLI, which was first reported in 1969.[128] Harbison et al reported a patient who presented with acute stridor from a fibrinous tracheal membrane 3 days after TLI lasting 48 hours.[178] Removal of the membrane by rigid bronchoscopy was curative. Deslee et al described 10 cases of fibrinous tracheal pseudomembrane from TLI, including one fatal case.[179]

MISCELLANEOUS
Tracheobronchitis,[180] protracted coughing, and consequences of ETT suctioning[181] such as chest pain, hypoxemia, and cardiac arrhythmias are sometimes observed.

BRONCHIAL

Mainstem bronchus intubation is mainly a complication during ETT placement, but it may also occur after intubation. In a retrospective series of 278 adult ICU patients with TLI, Kollef et al found that 7 (2.5%) had inadvertent endobronchial ETT placement.[182]

PULMONARY

Pulmonary complications during TLI include aspiration, pneumonia, retained secretions, and atelectasis.

ASPIRATION
Aspiration can be a serious complication while the ETT is in place.[33,183–187] Estimates of the frequency of clinically significant aspiration range from 7[33]–20%.[184]. Silent aspiration of oral secretions, stained with a blue dye marker, was noted in 20% of patients intubated with soft-cuff ETTs.[187] Pavlin et al noted that fluid aspiration may occur by way of channels from overlapping folds of cuff fabric.[185] Aspiration of gastric contents during TLI may be less common than aspiration of oral and pharyngeal secretions, but data are sparse. One study of 30 patients with modern ETTs demonstrated that none aspirated blue dye–stained enteral tube feedings.[183]

PNEUMONIA
Pneumonia (see Chapter 46) is a common and serious threat to patients with artificial airways who require mechanical ventilation.[33,176,177,180,188] Pneumonia occurs in 8–28% of patients during the course of mechanical ventilation.[188] A large, retrospective, matched cohort study showed that VAP developed in 9.3% of adult patients receiving mechanical ventilation for more than 24 hours.[189] The mortality rate of VAP ranges from 24–50%.[188] Mechanisms of pneumonia related to TLI are discussed below.

RETAINED SECRETIONS

TLI may promote retention of bronchopulmonary secretions in the lung because of impaired cough performance.[190,191]

ATELECTASIS

Atelectasis may complicate TLI as a result of retained bronchopulmonary secretions, migration of the ETT into a mainstem bronchus, and other factors operative during mechanical ventilation.

MISCELLANEOUS

GENERAL

Pain, Discomfort, and Psychological Impact

The many discomforts experienced by intubated ICU patients have received relatively little attention in the literature. The immediate and long-term psychological impact of TLI has been the subject of only a few investigations. The psychological health of intubated patients is influenced not only by TLI, but also by noise, light, sleep deprivation, stresses of underlying illness, and other adverse influences in the ICU.[192] Certainly all who have cared for intubated patients recognize that anxiety, depression, feelings of isolation and withdrawal, and frustration with impaired communication are major psychological detriments related to TLI. In a study that was not entirely limited to TLI patients, Swaiss and Badran recorded the following distressing complaints in interviews of adult patients 1 day after discharge from the ICU: anxiety (68%), discomfort from the ETT (60%), fear (54%), pain (52%), discomfort from the nasogastric tube (48%), difficulty in communicating (33%), dreams and hallucinations (31%), discomfort from physiotherapy (24%), noise (15%), insomnia (13%), and thirst (10%).[193]

Unplanned Extubation

"Unplanned extubation" is a broad categorical term that includes self-extubations and other extubations that are variously called "accidental," "deliberate," and "inadvertent" in the literature.[23,24,60,194–196] The frequency of unplanned extubations in critically ill adults ranges from 6%[197]–21%,[24] with a mean of 8.6%.[198] In a prospective epidemiologic study of more than 5000 critically ill adults with TLI, self-extubation was the most common accident related to TLI.[199] Unplanned extubation is more likely to occur with oral than with nasal TLI.[196,200,201] In a large case series, Chevron et al reported that unplanned extubation was usually deliberate (87% of patients) and associated with insufficient sedation.[201] Unplanned extubation may occur from forces applied to the ETT by ventilator tubing, bedrails, patient motion, bucking, coughing, and "tonguing."[196]

Coppolo and May reported a 12-month experience with self-extubation in adult ICU patients and noted self-extubation in 11%, cardiorespiratory sequelae of self-extubation in 31%, and need for reintubation in 31%.[194] Others have documented reintubation rates following self-extubation of 42[197]–74%.[202] Not surprisingly, the need for reintubation is much lower when self-extubation occurs during weaning from mechanical ventilation than during

TABLE 39-5 Mechanical Complications While the Endotracheal Tube Is in Place

Tube dislocation
  Endobronchial intubation
  Self-extubation
Tube obstruction
  From tube and cuff problems
    Kinking of nasotracheal tube
    Overinflation of the cuff
    Herniation of the cuff over the distal end of the tube
  From external compression
    Biting
    Cuff overinflation
  From impaction of the tip of the tube on the tracheal wall
  From internal obstruction
    Retained secretions
    Blood and blood clots
    Foreign body
    Tumor
    Anesthetic jelly
    Nasal turbinate
    Nasal polyp
Disconnection from the ventilator
Difficulty passing suction catheters
Cuff problems
  Leak
  Rupture
  Inability to seal the airway in spite of high cuff inflation pressures
Malfunction of the one-way inflation valve
Severance of the inflation tube or pilot balloon

the period of full ventilator support.[203] Besides the need for reintubation, sequelae of unplanned extubation include longer ICU and hospital stay,[200,204,205] prolongation of mechanical ventilation,[204] and complications of TLI,[205] but not increased hospital mortality.[200,204]

Mechanical Complications

Various mechanical problems with ETTs occur in about 6% of intubations (Table 39-5),[23] and they may place patients at risk for serious complications and need for reintubation. Beckmann and Gillies examined a large database of voluntary incident reports from ICUs in Australia and New Zealand to determine the frequency of reintubations not related to accidental or self-extubation.[206] Among 143 such incidents, the reasons for reintubation included the following mechanical complications: tube malposition (25; 17%), tube securing or taping problems (24; 16%), pilot tube or cuff problem (23; 16%), and blocked or kinked airway (20; 14%), in addition to failed extubation (19; 14%), inadequate preparation for extubation (8; 6%), and other events (24; 17%).[206]

Dislocation or misplacement of an ETT may result in endobronchial intubation (Fig. 39-8), carinal irritation by the ETT tip, high placement at the level of the upper trachea (see Fig. 39-8) or hypopharynx, and self-extubation. If the ETT is positioned too high in the airway, the inflated cuff may injure the larynx and adjacent structures such as the recurrent laryngeal nerves. Other potential complications of high tube placement include inability to seal the airway,

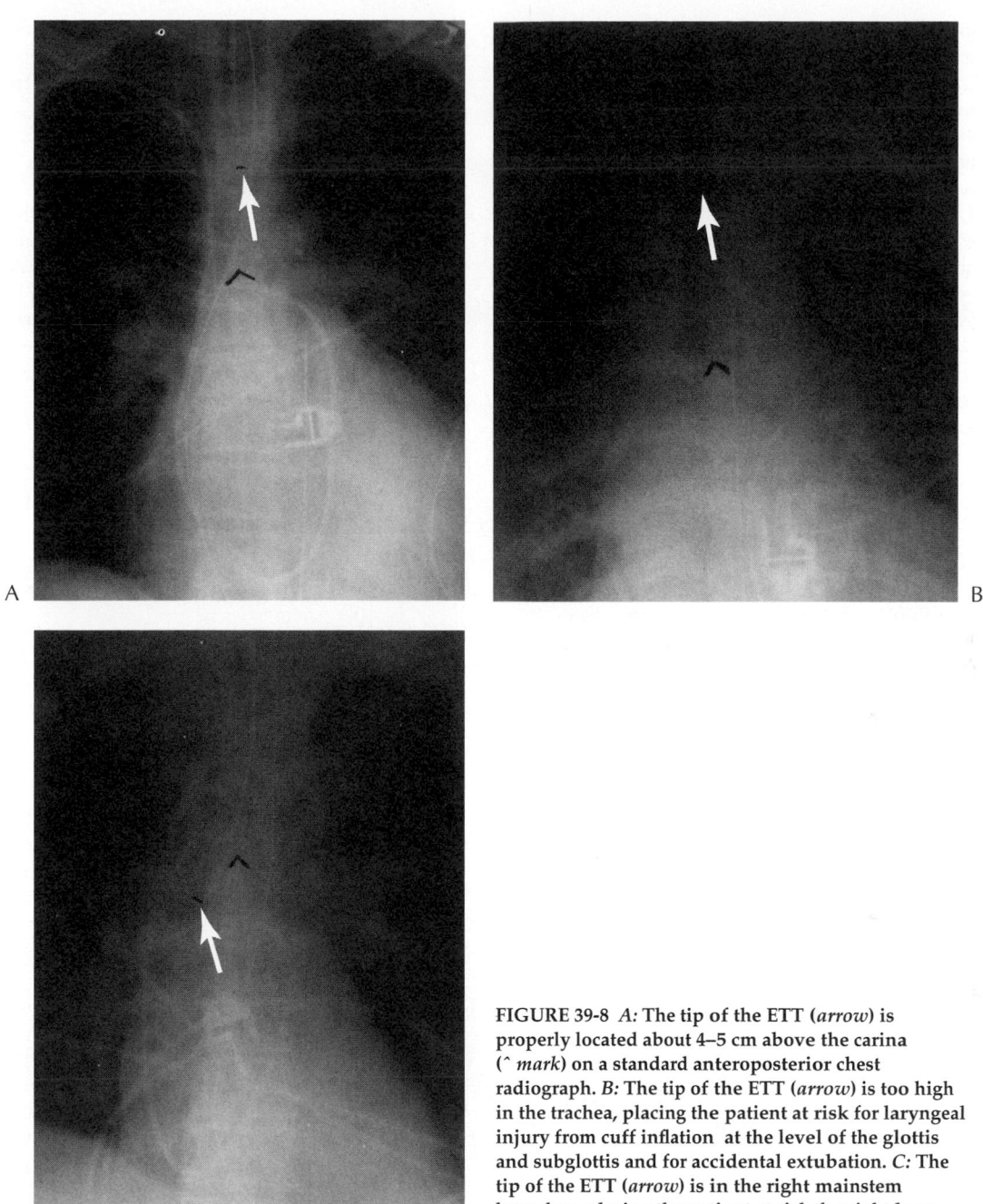

FIGURE 39-8 *A:* The tip of the ETT (*arrow*) is properly located about 4–5 cm above the carina (^ *mark*) on a standard anteroposterior chest radiograph. *B:* The tip of the ETT (*arrow*) is too high in the trachea, placing the patient at risk for laryngeal injury from cuff inflation at the level of the glottis and subglottis and for accidental extubation. *C:* The tip of the ETT (*arrow*) is in the right mainstem bronchus, placing the patient at risk for right lung hyperinflation, right pneumothorax, atelectasis of part or the entire left lung, and impaired gas exchange. (*Modified, with permission, from Stauffer.*[118])

leading to aspiration and inadequate ventilation, and subglottic stenosis. Kollef et al reported that 22 (8%) of 278 adult ICU patients had at least one significant ETT dislocation, with complications such as anoxic encephalopathy, hypoxemia, gastric aspiration, atelectasis, and pneumothorax.[182] Another prospective study revealed ETT malposition in 5 (8.2%) of 61 patients with prolonged TLI.[33]

If an ETT is positioned too low in the trachea, flexion of the neck may allow it to migrate into a mainstem bronchus,

and conversely, if an ETT is positioned too high in the trachea, extension of the neck may allow it to migrate into the pharynx, leading to unplanned extubation.[207] Conrardy et al showed that flexion of the neck moved the tip of the ETT an average of 1.9 cm toward the carina, (range 0–3.1 cm) and extension of the neck moved the ETT an equal distance away from the carina (range 0.2–5.2 cm).[207] The route of intubation (nasal versus oral) and cuff inflation or deflation did not affect tube movement.

The ETT may become partially or completely obstructed during placement or while it is in place,[208] mainly because of patient biting or obstruction of its lumen by retained secretions, blood or blood clots,[209] foreign body,[210] tumor,[211] or other material. Obstruction from tube kinking or external compression by cuff overinflation is very rare. The tip of the ETT may impact on the tracheal mucosa leading to obstruction if the tube lacks a Murphy eye.[212] The use of heat and moisture exchangers (HMEs) in place of heater humidifiers carries an increased risk of ETT occlusion from inspissated secretions.[213–215] Villafane et al observed a progressive decrease in the effective inner diameter of the ETT when HMEs were used, and in four patients ETT occlusion required emergency reintubation.[213]

ETT cuff problems during TLI include leak, rupture, and inability to seal the airway. Rashkin and Davis noted leaky cuffs during TLI in 15 (25%) of their 61 patients.[33] Cuff rupture is rarely observed now with widespread use of low-pressure cuffs. Inability to seal the airway by inflating or overinflating the cuff has been observed in 11–19% of patients during TLI.[23,24] We observed a requirement for more than 25 mmHg cuff pressure in 19% of 226 prospectively studied TLIs with soft-cuff tubes, the most common early clinical problem following TLI.[23] Vyas et al checked cuff pressures in 32 patients intubated with ETTs with high-volume, low-pressure cuffs and found that 62% had elevated cuff pressures, some as high as 100 cmH$_2$O.[216] They performed a telephone survey that revealed that cuff pressure was checked regularly in only 17% of ICUs.

Other mechanical problems seen while the ETT is in place include malfunction of the one-way inflation valve, inadvertent severance of the inflation tube or pilot balloon, disconnection from the ventilator, and difficulty passing a suction catheter through the ETT.

Malnutrition

TLI precludes effective swallowing and necessitates feeding by way of enteric tubes or intravenous lines. Malnutrition in patients with TLI is discussed in Chapter 41.

ESOPHAGEAL

Tracheoesophageal fistula may develop during TLI (see discussion above).

GASTRIC

Gastric distention may occur if a tracheoesophageal fistula develops during TLI.[162]

MUSCULOSKELETAL AND NEUROLOGIC

Musculoskeletal and neurologic complications directly related to TLI while the ETT is in place have not been reported.

PHYSIOLOGIC

Compared with a normal upper airway, an ETT increases the resistance to airflow. Gal and Suratt demonstrated that TLI in healthy men increased total airways resistance from 0.99 cmH$_2$O/L per second to 2.25 cmH$_2$O/L per second, an increase of 178%.[217,218] About half of this increase was attributed to the ETT itself, and the remainder to reflex bronchoconstriction.[217,218] TLI increases lower airway resistance slightly in normals without reactive airways disease by stimulation of irritant receptors, provoking bronchoconstriction,[219] and prophylactic treatment with bronchodilators has a protective effect.[220]

Airflow resistance during TLI increases as the length of the ETT increases or its diameter decreases.[191,221] Because they increase airflow resistance, ETTs increase the patient's work of breathing.[191,222] The work of breathing increases as the patient's minute ventilation increases and as the diameter of the ETT decreases.[222–224] At minute ventilation rates at or below 8 L/min, an ETT has little impact on the work of breathing.[223] Although the extra work of breathing imposed by an ETT is not clinically important in most patients, it may be clinically significant in patients with poor ventilatory function.

Complications During and After Extubation

COMPLICATIONS DURING EXTUBATION

Oral, nasal, pharyngeal, and laryngeal complications that developed while the ETT was in place may, of course, first be detected at extubation. For example, we observed lip ulceration and cellulitis in 15% of patients immediately after extubation.[23] Paresis of the hypoglossal and/or lingual nerves from pressure injury by the laryngoscope blade may appear early in the postextubation period.[10]

New complications occurring in the brief period of extubation are transient and uncommonly reported. Discomfort, pain, and some degree of anxiety are the primary adverse events of extubation.[192] Significant increases in heart rate, blood pressure, and plasma catecholamine levels occur at extubation.[85] The clinical findings we observed at extubation in 81 ICU patients are summarized in Table 39-6. Hoarseness, sore throat, cough, and sputum production were encountered with decreasing frequency. Sore throat and dysphagia are reported by about one-half of patients at extubation.[9,23] Dixon et al reported hoarseness and/or severe sore throat in 20% of patients and observed that these symptoms were more common in women than in men.[93] Nasal bleeding and dental injuries may occur during extubation, but such events are very rare.[29]

Partial laryngeal obstruction at extubation is most often related to laryngeal edema (see discussion below). Laryngeal injury and other complications during self-extubation of an ETT with an inflated cuff have not been adequately studied. Surprisingly, few patients appear to develop laryngeal complications following self-extubation. Pulmonary aspiration may occur with faulty extubation technique. Cardiac arrest has been reported during extubation.[9] The requirement for reintubation soon after extubation is usually caused by laryngeal edema or respiratory failure.

EARLY COMPLICATIONS AFTER EXTUBATION

This section discusses those complications of TLI that appear during roughly the first week after extubation. This

TABLE 39-6   Clinical Findings at Extubation in a Series of 81 Patients

	No.	Percent
History (obtained in 69 patients)		
Symptoms related to TLI	59	86
No symptoms related to TLI	10	14
Specific symptoms		
Hoarseness	49	71
Sore throat	29	42
New cough	18	26
New sputum production	15	22
Hemoptysis	7	10
Other upper airway complaints	9	13
Physical examination (obtained in 78 patients)	42	54
Abnormal, related to TLI		
Normal	36	46
Specific abnormalities		
Auscultatory abnormalities over the trachea	20	26
Lip ulcer or cellulitis	12	15
Pharyngeal bleeding or ulceration	7	9
Ulceration of the palate	6	8
Nasal bleeding	6	8
Oral mucous membrane bleeding, ulceration, or inflammation	5	6
Stridor	4	5
Nasal ulceration	2	3
Tooth avulsion	2	3
Tongue injury	2	3

SOURCE: Modified from Stauffer et al.[23]

period is dominated by symptoms of pharyngeal and laryngeal injury from TLI, including dysphonia, sore throat, cough, dysphagia, and odynophagia.

NASAL, PARANASAL, AND ORAL

There are no specific new complications that develop in this time interval.

PHARYNGEAL

Sore throat has been reported in 22[89]–42%[23] of ICU patients and in 11[44]–56%[225] of anesthesia patients following extubation. Following short-term anesthetic TLI, Rieger et al found same-day complaints of pharyngeal dryness in 75% of patients, dysphonia in 47%, sore throat in 22%, and swallowing discomfort in 13%.[226] Persistent and severe dysphagia after extubation following prolonged TLI should alert the clinician to the possibility of active infection in the posterior larynx, including cricoid abscess.[14]

There may be a temporary loss of the gag reflex after extubation. This was observed in 24% of patients who had direct laryngoscopy within 24 hours of extubation, supporting the notion that some patients have a sensory denervation of the pharynx and larynx from TLI.[51] Loss of upper airway reflexes increases the risk of aspiration.[51] We found pharyngeal bleeding or ulceration in 9% of patients at extubation (see Table 39-6),[23] although Colice et al did not observe this complication after prolonged TLI.[51]

LARYNGEAL

Colice et al performed direct fiberoptic laryngoscopy within 24 hours of extubation in 82 patients who had been intubated for 4 or more days (mean 9.7 ± 0.6 days).[51] Seventy-seven (94%) of their patients had laryngeal injury (42% mild, 29% moderate, and 23% severe). Nearly all patients had posterior true vocal cord ulceration. Laryngeal edema was present in the patients with moderate to severe damage. Two patients had such large ulcers that the vocal cords could not be adducted, permitting free aspiration into the trachea.[51] Most patients who displayed initial laryngeal damage had complete resolution of laryngeal findings on laryngoscopy within 4 weeks after extubation.[51] Kastanos et al reported the following early laryngeal lesions in 19 patients after extubation: true vocal cord granulomas in 8 (42%), true vocal cord ulcerations in 7 (37%), true vocal cord paresis in 1 (5%), and subglottic edema in 1 (5%).[124] Thomas et al performed fiberoptic endoscopy through the ETT just before extubation and found visible laryngeal pathology in 131 (88%) of 150 patients.[227] The important laryngeal complications after TLI are summarized in Table 39-7.

Hoarseness

In 54 adult male patients followed closely by Colice et al after TLI, 30 (56%) had significant hoarseness.[51] Holdgaard et al observed hoarseness in 42% of ICU patients following nasotracheal intubation.[94] Hoarseness following TLI usually resolves within a few days in most patients as laryngeal edema and inflammation subside and normal vocal cord adduction is restored.[121] In some cases, transient postextubation hoarseness requires 7–10 days to resolve. Hoarseness persisting beyond 10–14 days suggests serious laryngeal injury such as granuloma formulation, vocal cord paresis or paralysis, or cricoarytenoid joint dysfunction, and requires the attention of an otolaryngologist-head and neck surgeon.

Edema

Postextubation laryngeal edema, an important complication of TLI, may occur at the supraglottic, glottic, or subglottic levels.[10] It presents with postextubation stridor and dyspnea.

Laryngeal edema is observed immediately after extubation in about 40% of patients after anesthetic intubation[46] and in about half of critical care patients.[51]

TABLE 39-7   Important Early and Late Laryngeal Complications after Extubation

Early
    Hoarseness
    Edema
    Stridor
    Muscle dysfunction
    Vocal cord paresis and paralysis
    Vocal cord hematoma
    Posterior glottic infection and cricoid cartilage abscess
Late
    Glottic and subglottic stenosis
    Granulomas
    Synechiae

Laryngospasm

Postextubation laryngospasm in the recovery from general anesthesia is a well-known phenomenon. Although postextubation stridor in the ICU is sometimes attributed to laryngospasm, this complication after extubation of ICU patients is not well documented. Colice et al reported true laryngospasm in only 1 of 82 ICU patients within 24 hours of extubation.[51] True laryngospasm following extubation of the critically ill patient should be distinguished from laryngeal edema and other more common causes of postextubation stridor.

Stridor

Many studies have investigated postextubation stridor.[23,51,93,228–230] Its reported frequency ranges from 0.1[228]–18%.[230] Stridor occurring after extubation is usually inspiratory, indicating variable extrathoracic airway obstruction. Mackenzie et al observed significant stridor after prolonged TLI in 0.1–0.6% of patients.[228] This complication was found to be caused by vocal cord edema or subglottic stenosis, not laryngospasm. Symptoms of stridor appeared from 5 minutes to 4 hours after extubation.[228] Repeated intubations or tracheotomy were required in the majority of patients. Postextubation stridor should always indicate the possibility of subglottic stenosis at the level of the cricoid cartilage, a level that is particularly vulnerable to airway narrowing in children.

Muscle Dysfunction

Laryngeal incompetence is common after extubation and has been attributed to a sensory impairment or mechanical dysfunction of the larynx.[231] Laryngeal incompetence puts the patient at risk for aspiration. The frequency of aspiration secondary to laryngeal incompetence in postoperative patients ranges from 22–35%.[231,232] Failure of the vocal cords to adduct increases the risk of aspiration.[51,121]

Vocal Cord Paresis and Paralysis

Unilateral or bilateral vocal cord paresis or paralysis is a serious but very uncommon complication of TLI.[44,49,121,233–235] It presents in the early postextubation period as persistent hoarseness or, in the case of bilateral vocal cord paralysis, as severe stridor. Vocal cord paralysis accounted for 34% of laryngeal injury claims in an analysis of all anesthesia claims.[31] Santos et al reported vocal cord immobility in 16 (20%) of 97 patients after extubation, and in half of these cases, a delayed presentation over a period of 1–10 weeks following extubation was observed.[138] Others have reported vocal cord paralysis in less than 1% of cases.[44,49] True bilateral vocal cord paralysis after TLI is very rare.

Whited evaluated 16 patients with vocal cord paresis or paralysis after TLI of 5 days or longer.[121] Common features in these patients were symmetry of vocal cord paresis or paralysis, edema and erythema of the arytenoids and posterior commissure, median or paramedian vocal cord positioning, late return of vocal cord abduction, a tendency for aspiration to occur, and spontaneous recovery in nearly all patients within 4 weeks.[121] Postextubation vocal cord paresis or paralysis may result from traumatic dislocation of the arytenoids, cricoarytenoid joint arthritis, cuff inflation immediately below the vocal cords resulting in compression of the anterior branch of the recurrent laryngeal nerves,[236] or the mechanical effects of laryngeal edema and inflammation.[14] Bilateral vocal cord paralysis from intubation injury may present with hoarseness and recurrent aspiration[236] or with upper airway obstruction requiring immediate tracheotomy.[233–235]

Vocal Cord Hematoma

Hematomas of the vocal cords that occur during placement of an ETT apparently resolve by the time of extubation. They were not seen after extubation in 82 patients studied by Colice et al.[51]

Posterior Glottic Infection and Cricoid Cartilage Abscess

Severe odynophagia or odynophonia after extubation should suggest the possibility of posterior glottic infection or cricoid cartilage abscess.[14] Posterior glottic infection may result in destruction of laryngeal cartilage and predispose to posterior glottic stenosis.[14]

TRACHEAL

In a prospective study of 19 patients, Kastanos et al reported finding tracheal granulomas in 6 patients (31%) and cuff-site tracheitis in 3 (16%).[124]

BRONCHIAL

Bronchial complications of TLI in this time period have not been reported.

PULMONARY

Pulmonary aspiration has been reported in patients with laryngeal incompetence after extubation.[51,121,140,231] Pulmonary aspiration was observed after extubation in 2 (2.4%) of 82 patients after prolonged TLI in the series of Colice et al.[51] This finding was attributed to vocal cord dysfunction and temporary loss of sensorimotor function of the larynx and pharynx.[51] Burgess et al observed aspiration of swallowed contrast material in 33% of surgical patients immediately after extubation.[231] Endoscopic evaluation of swallowing after prolonged TLI has revealed aspiration in 14[237]–45%[238] of patients. The role of vallecular stasis as a risk factor for aspiration is uncertain.

MISCELLANEOUS

There are no significant miscellaneous complications of TLI in the early postextubation period.

LATE COMPLICATIONS AFTER EXTUBATION

Late complications occur weeks to months after extubation. Abnormal mucosal healing with fibrosis or granuloma formation accounts for most of the significant late complications of TLI, of which laryngeal stenosis is the most dreaded.

NASAL AND PARANASAL

Nasal stricture and nasal septal perforation following prolonged nasotracheal intubation are rare.

ORAL

The only late oral complications of TLI are those related to initial dental or oral trauma.

PHARYNGEAL

In some patients, dysphagia may persist for several weeks. Residual problems related to pharyngeal perforation during ETT placement may persist late after extubation.

LARYNGEAL

Fortunately, late laryngeal complications of TLI (see Table 39-7) are uncommon because of the normal healing of laryngeal ulcers and other laryngeal injuries discussed above. Colice et al reported that 10 (19%) of 54 survivors following TLI for longer than 4 days had clinically important laryngeal sequelae, although eventual complete healing was observed.[51] Healing of laryngeal mucosal injury after extubation is usually complete within 8–12 weeks.[137] Nevertheless, abnormal healing may result in serious late laryngeal complications of TLI. Hoarseness that fails to improve for many weeks after extubation suggests abnormal healing with structural deformity of the larynx.[127]

Laryngeal Stenosis

Laryngeal stenosis following TLI may be supraglottic, glottic, or subglottic in location. Supraglottic stenosis is unusual. Glottic or subglottic stenosis is a serious but fortunately uncommon late complication of TLI. Although rarely severe, it represents the most notorious complication of TLI and has received extensive attention in the literature.[14,23,43,51,121–123,127,137,239–243] TLI is the most common cause of posterior glottic laryngeal stenosis.[239]

Most prospective studies of TLI document a very low rate of laryngeal stenosis.[23,124,127,137,244] The reported frequency of this complication ranges from 0–12%. When the results of 7 prospective studies are combined, the overall incidence of laryngeal stenosis is 1.3–2.9% (Table 39-8), depending on whether the disproportionately higher results in the Whited analysis are included. Colice found no cases of laryngeal stenosis in 54 prospectively studied survivors of prolonged TLI.[137] Elliott et al found that 3 (10%) of 30 survivors of the acute respiratory distress syndrome (ARDS) had laryngeal stenosis.[242] Kambic and Radsel reported

TABLE 39-8 Rates of Laryngeal Stenosis after Prolonged Translaryngeal Intubation in Prospective Studies

Year	Reference	Frequency of Laryngeal Stenosis
1969	Lindholm[127]	1/206
1981	Stauffer et al[23]	2/27
1982	Pecora and Seinige[244]	0/21
1983	Kastanos et al[124]	2/19
1983	Whited[122]	12/200
1989	Colice[137]	0/54
1994	Santos et al[138]	0/62
	Total	17/589 (2.9%)[a]

[a]With the exception of the study by Whited, the rate of laryngeal stenosis is 5/389 = 1.3%.

laryngeal scarring in fewer than 1% of patients after brief anesthetic intubations.[43]

Whited found posterior commissure fibrosis with stenosis in 2 (12.5%) of 16 patients with TLI of 5 days or longer who were referred for evaluation of vocal cord paralysis or paresis.[121] Later, he reported frequencies of laryngeal stenosis of 5.5% in 200 patients with prolonged TLI[122] and 14% in 50 patients intubated for 11 days or longer.[123] This rate of laryngeal stenosis is higher than the rates in other prospective studies (see Table 39-8). In Whited's study, duration of TLI was the only independent variable assessed, and other potential risk factors for laryngeal stenosis were not evaluated.[122,123]

Lindholm noted only one case of laryngeal stenosis (subglottic) in 206 adult patients after TLI,[127] but patients in his series had a relatively short duration of intubation (mean 32 hours). We found that 2 (7%) of 27 patients evaluated for airway stenosis with tomograms after extubation had subglottic stenosis, defined as a 10% or greater reduction in transverse diameter of the trachea at the cricoid level.[23] Subglottic stenosis in adults following prolonged TLI appears to be much less common than in neonates and children, in whom this complication occurs with a frequency as high as 8%.[245]

Laryngeal Granuloma Formation

Granuloma formation is an important late complication of TLI, primarily affecting the larynx.[23,127,137,138,246] Laryngeal granulomas (see Fig. 39-6B and C) are usually a few millimeters in diameter and rarely grow large enough to compromise the airway lumen. They may be sessile or pedunculated. As a manifestation of the healing process, albeit abnormal, granulomas may not appear until weeks after extubation. Laryngeal granulomas usually appear at the edges of posterior glottic ulcers, particularly those on the vocal processes and arytenoids.[246] They usually resolve spontaneously, but surgical excision is sometimes required because of persistent hoarseness or airway compromise.[137]

The reported frequency of laryngeal granulomas after TLI is highly variable. After anesthetic intubation, laryngeal granulomas are extremely rare.[246] Colice et al found laryngeal granulomas in 4 (7%) of 54 patients carefully studied after TLI.[51] In that series, all patients with persistent hoarseness after TLI had laryngeal granulomas. Lindholm found postintubation granulomas in about one-third of adults after TLI, but not in any infants or children.[127] In the Lindholm series, only 7 (2.6%) of 265 patients followed after extubation required surgical excision of laryngeal granulomas. The report of Santos et al of 97 patients with prolonged TLI described laryngeal granulomas in 44%, and in 57% of these cases the granulomas developed an average of 4 weeks after extubation.[138]

Synechia Formation

Synechia (membrane or web) formation at the glottis occurs in less than 1% of TLIs.[127,247] Synechia formation may "weld" the vocal cords together, leading to aphonia and airway obstruction.[10]

TRACHEAL

Tracheal Stenosis
Tracheal stenosis in adults surviving prolonged periods of mechanical ventilation is usually attributed to tracheotomy rather than TLI.[248-250] Severe tracheal stenosis following TLI alone is fortunately rare. Santos et al prospectively observed no cases of tracheal stenosis in 62 adults surviving long-term TLI.[138] A retrospective review of laryngotracheal stenosis following TLI, tracheotomy, or both in 315 neurologic patients reported by Richard et al found tracheal stenosis in only 1 patient in the group of 172 patients (0.6%) with TLI only (mean duration 17 days).[243] In contrast, 25 (19%) of 131 patients with TLI followed by tracheotomy had tracheal stenosis.

Brooks et al reported an experience with 9 patients with postintubation tracheal (8 patients) or subglottic (1 patient) stenosis, 8 of whom were intubated for 3–8 days with soft-cuff ETTs.[250] Patients presented with signs of tracheal stenosis 1–6 months after extubation. Subclinical tracheal stenosis following TLI is more common than symptomatic tracheal stenosis.[23]

Tracheal Dilation
Persistent tracheal dilation is caused by cartilaginous injury at the cuff site.[152-154] This complication was reported in 2–5% of patients following use of hard-cuff tracheostomy tubes,[153] and it is rarely seen following TLI with soft-cuff ETTs.

Tracheal Granuloma Formation
Tracheal granulomas occur mainly at the site of tracheal cuff-site ulcers. These are extremely rare in the era of soft-cuff ETTs.

BRONCHIAL
There are no late bronchial complications of TLI.

PULMONARY
There are no late pulmonary complications of TLI.

MISCELLANEOUS
There are no important late miscellaneous complications of TLI other than residual problems related to tracheo-esophageal fistula.

Pathogenesis of Complications of Translaryngeal Intubation

This section reviews the causes and mechanisms of selected complications of TLI. Most of the investigation of mechanisms of complications of TLI has focused on laryngeal injury and tracheal cuff-site injury.

COMPLICATIONS DURING ENDOTRACHEAL TUBE PLACEMENT

Complications during placement of an ETT often occur as a result of suboptimal technique stemming from poor judg-ment or inexperience. Failure to prepare the patient for intubation and equipment malfunction may also lead to complications. For example, during nasal intubation attempts, failure to prepare the nasal mucosa with a topical anesthetic or vasoconstrictor or failure to select the more patent side of the nose for intubation may result in nasal mucosal laceration or turbinate injury.

It is generally taught that complications of intubation are more likely to occur in emergency situations than in elective, controlled intubations, but there are few data to establish this with certainty. Taryle et al noted that emergency TLIs were complicated more often when performed by non-anesthesiologists.[21] Adnet et al found significant associations between the number of intubation attempts and the rate of mechanical and general complications of emergency prehospital TLI,[20] but Schwartz et al did not find this association in critical care intubation.[62]

Incorrect use of the laryngoscope may cause dental injury or pharyngeal laceration. Blind jamming of the ETT into the hypopharynx may cause serious soft tissue injury. Failure to oxygenate and ventilate the patient before intubation may result in hypoxic brain injury. Deep insertion of the ETT far beyond the vocal cords may result in right mainstem bronchus intubation. These are only a few examples of how faulty intubation technique, inexperience, and poor judgment may lead to intubation complications.

COMPLICATIONS WHILE THE ENDOTRACHEAL TUBE IS IN PLACE

Complications of TLI during this time interval depend upon anatomic, physiologic, ETT, and clinical influences.

ANATOMIC AND PHYSIOLOGIC INFLUENCES

Nasal and Paranasal Complications
Necrosis of the nasal alae and ulceration and perforation of the nasal septum result from ischemic necrosis secondary to pressure on these structures from the nasotracheal tube. Sinus effusions and sinusitis are caused by obstruction of the sinus ostia by the adjacent nasotracheal or nasogastric tube, edema, inflammation, or mucus plugging. Otitis and middle ear effusions are related to obstruction of the eustachian tube by the same influences.

Laryngeal and Tracheal Complications
Serious laryngeal and tracheal injury during TLI is generally attributed to ischemic injury of the mucosal surface and deeper tissues by pressure exerted at vulnerable anatomic sites (Fig. 39-9).[251] For example, ischemia occurs when the pressure exerted on the posterolateral wall of the larynx by the ETT or on the tracheal wall by the inflated cuff exceeds the capillary perfusion pressure in these areas. Necrosis, sloughing of the mucosa, and ulceration follow. Microscopically, inflammatory cell infiltrates and bacterial invasion are seen in the devitalized mucosal tissues. Eventually, destruction of soft tissues and cartilage in the wall of the larynx and trachea occur. In severe cases, there is loss of structural integrity of the tracheal wall, producing dilation or softening. If the patient survives, the healing process begins with

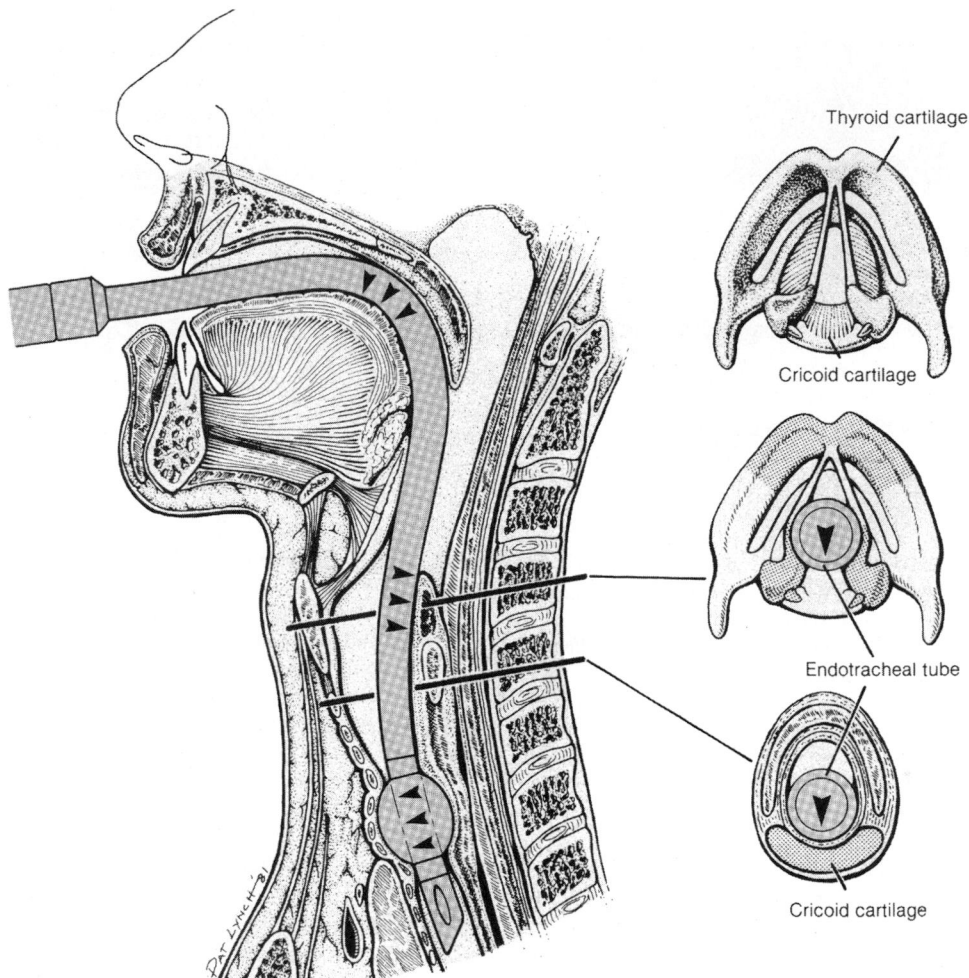

FIGURE 39-9 Pressure exerted on the surface of the airway by the shaft of the ETT and cuff is a major determinant of airway injury during TLI. The arrows and cross-sectional drawings indicate the major pressure points. The posterolateral regions of the glottis and subglottis and the tracheal cuff site are particularly vulnerable to ischemic necrosis and ulceration that may extend beyond the mucosa into underlying structural cartilage. (*Modified, with permission, from Colice and Matthay.[251]*)

one of three eventual outcomes: restoration of normal morphology, development of granulation tissue, or fibrosis. In the larynx, fibrosis results in glottic or subglottic stenosis, synechia formation, or cricoarytenoid joint fixation. In the trachea, fibrosis results in segmental stenosis.

The concept of tracheal mucosal injury by an air-filled cuff was established by studies performed in the 1960s and 1970s. It is outlined in Fig. 39-10. Tracheal mucosal perfusion pressure is a critically important determinant of ischemic injury at the tracheal cuff site.[252–258] In humans, the tracheal capillary perfusion pressure is estimated to be 25 mmHg (range 22–32 mmHg) or 34 cmH$_2$O (range 30–44 cmH$_2$O).[256,257] The role of capillary perfusion pressure in the pathogenesis of tracheal cuff-site injury is discussed below.

Laryngeal and tracheal structures that are vulnerable to ETT pressure are the arytenoids, the posterior rim of the glottis, the subglottis, the cuff site, and the site of the tip of the ETT.[259] The posterior rim of the glottis is a contact point or fulcrum where the ETT abrades and applies

FIGURE 39-10 Outline of pathogenesis of tracheal injury at the site of the air-inflated cuff.

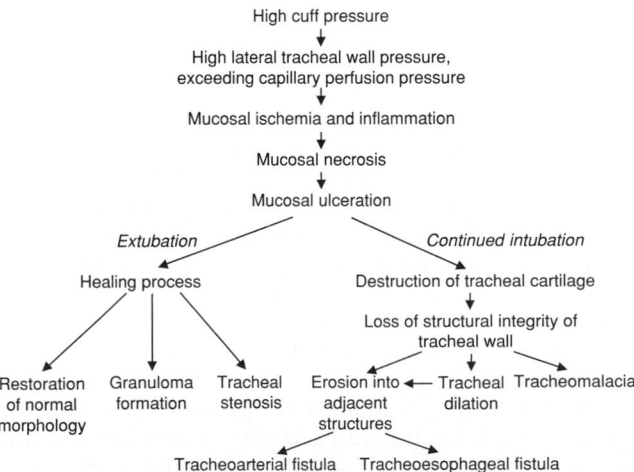

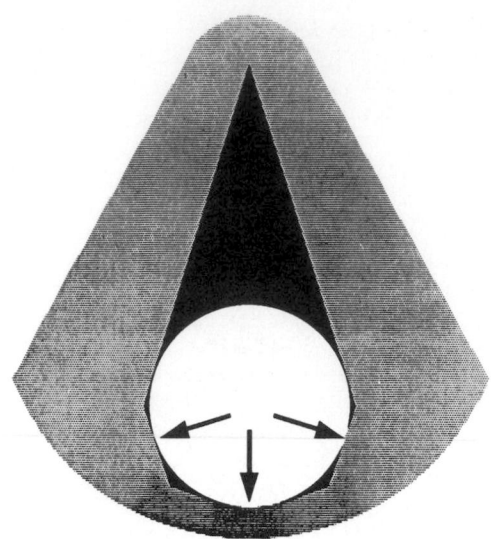

FIGURE 39-11 Schematic drawing of an ETT in the glottis, showing the circular shape of the ETT and the pentagonal shape of the glottis. The arrows indicate the points of maximum pressure on the posterior wall of the glottic opening. (*Modified, with permission, from Quartararo and Bishop.*[45])

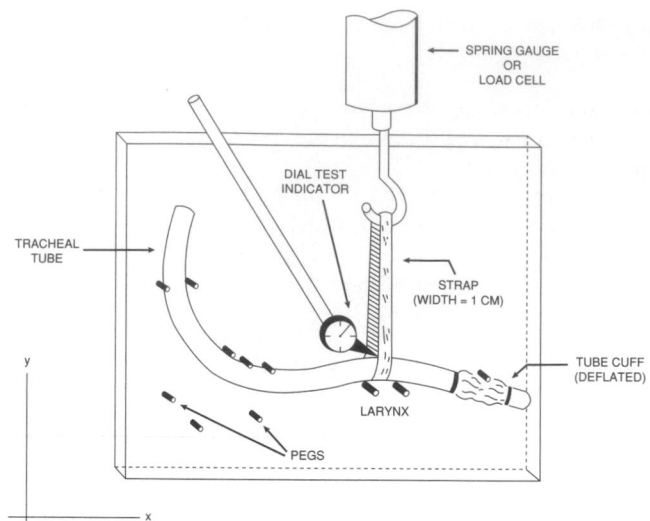

FIGURE 39-12 Method of estimating forces exerted on the posterior larynx by ETTs. A pegboard is used to simulate the shape of the ETT in vivo. A gauge measures the force needed to barely lift the tube at the level of the larynx, thereby estimating pressure on the larynx. Modern polyvinyl chloride and silicone rubber tubes under simulated in vivo conditions exert forces on the larynx in the range of 162–265 grams. (*Modified, with permission, from Steen et al.*[261])

constant pressure to the mucosa, leading to the risk of mucosal ischemia and ulceration.[49,241] Quartararo and Bishop have described the geometric shape of the glottis as a pentagon, which of course does not resemble the circular shape of the ETT.[45] This geometric mismatch creates several points of contact where ulceration is most likely to occur (Fig. 39-11).[45] An experimental ETT has been designed to make the segment of the ETT that rests in the glottis more closely resemble the natural shape of the glottis.[260]

The essential curvature of the ETT necessitates that force be directed posteriorly and laterally at the posterior glottic rim and cricoid ring (see Fig. 39-9). Furthermore, the tongue muscles force the ETT posteriorly. Glottic pressure by the ETT has been estimated in both in vitro[261] (Fig. 39-12) and animal[262] studies to range as high as 200–400 mmHg. In vitro studies of a variety of ETTs indicate that deforming forces from 230–1000 grams are applied to the posterior laryngeal wall.[263] Pressure-induced ischemic injury of the posterior cricoid lamina and vocal processes of the arytenoids is accompanied by cricoid and arytenoid perichondritis and chondritis, which may heal with eventual fibrosis and scar contracture.[239]

Cricoarytenoid joint injury may occur while the ETT is in place but be recognized only after extubation. Postextubation symptoms of hoarseness and odynophagia along with the findings of malposition and no movement of the arytenoids suggest cricoarytenoid joint dysfunction. Paulsen et al reported that laxity of the cricoarytenoid joint capsule and large synovial folds are predisposing factors for cricoarytenoid joint trauma from TLI, including hemarthrosis.[264]

The cricoid ring, a completely circumferential ring that encircles the lower part of the larynx, is an important contact point with an ETT (see Fig. 39-9). Inflammation and edema of the laryngeal mucosa at the level of the cricoid ring narrow the airway lumen, making the subglottic area vulnerable to acute stenosis. Postextubation stridor is a manifestation of this phenomenon.[228] Experiments in dogs have demonstrated clearly that the posterior third of the cricoid cartilage is a major site of deep ulceration from pressure and abrasion by the ETT.[259] Ischemic necrosis in this area may be followed by bacterial invasion and eventual abscess formation.[14] Simultaneous use of a nasogastric tube with an ETT may increase the risk of this complication.

Whited observed that the anterior wall of the trachea is a vulnerable site for tracheal injury from an ETT because of positioning of the cuff and tip of the tube.[259] Surprisingly few complications of TLI, however, are noted in the anterior wall of the trachea in these locations in the modern era of soft-cuff tubes.

ENDOTRACHEAL TUBE INFLUENCES

Physical Characteristics of an Endotracheal Tube

Technical standards for modern ETTs[2,265,266] establish the shape, size, and stiffness of an ETT, all of which influence TLI-induced airway injury. As previously discussed, the curved shape of an ETT invites pressure injury at the contact points with the airway, including the posterior larynx, cricoid cartilage, and tracheal cuff and tip sites.[127,267] The cross-sectional round shape of an ETT is also poorly suited for the shape of the glottis as noted above.[45,268] Large ETTs are more likely than small ones to cause pressure injury to the larynx[127,259,262] and the trachea. Large ETTs also cause more postextubation sore throat and hoarseness than do smaller tubes.[269] Modern ETTs vary considerably in their stiffness and thermolability (ability to become less stiff at body temperature).[270]

Surface Characteristics

Electron microscopic studies of ETTs reveal the deposition of a slimy coating or biofilm on the walls of the tube that may promote the adherence of bacteria.[271–273] The clinical significance of ETT biofilm on the pathogenesis of VAP is discussed below.

Chemical Composition

The manufacture of modern ETTs follows strict guidelines set by Committee F29 on Anesthetic and Respiratory Equipment of the American Society for Testing and Materials.[2,266] Modern ETTs are composed of polyvinyl chloride, which is nontoxic, but chemical additives such as stabilizers, plasticizers, fillers, and pigments may incite inflammatory reactions in tissue.[265] Triandafillu et al reported that the physicochemical characteristics of sections from polyvinyl chloride ETTs influence the adhesion of various strains of *Pseudomonas aeruginosa*.[273]

Cuff Characteristics

The value of cuffs on ETTs to seal the airway became apparent in the 1930s. By the 1940s, it was recognized that high cuff inflation pressures could cause ischemia and sloughing of the tracheal mucosa.[274] Animal studies in the 1960s clarified the mechanisms of cuff-site tracheal injury,[148,275,276] and several groups of investigators established the role of high cuff inflation pressures in producing ischemic necrosis of the tracheal mucosa (see discussion below). Others later implicated high cuff inflation pressures in mucosal inflammation, tracheal dilation, destruction of tracheal cartilage leading to tracheal stenosis and tracheoesophageal fistula, and erosion of the tracheal mucosa and submucosa with loss of submucosal glands.[146] By the early 1970s, it was established clearly that inflating the ETT cuff to pressures that exceeded tracheal capillary perfusion pressure could cause mucosal ischemia. Studies of the microcirculation of the rabbit trachea by Nordin et al revealed that the mucosa overlying the cartilaginous tracheal rings would become ischemic if hard cuffs were inflated to the point where lateral tracheal wall pressure exceeded 30 mmHg.[255]

Besides intracuff pressures, other cuff characteristics may contribute to airway injury. Overlapping folds of cuff fabric may create channels that permit migration of fluid into the lung. This aspiration process is promoted by larger tubes, larger cuff diameters, stiffer cuff fabrics, and spontaneous breathing.[185] Bernhard et al demonstrated that modern ETTs display considerable variability in cuff characteristics such as diameter, thickness, compliance, shape, resting volume, and just-seal volume.[270,277] These various factors, as well as the size and shape of the trachea,[278] may affect the pressure-volume relationship of a given ETT cuff in vivo.[207,277]

CLINICAL INFLUENCES IN LARYNGEAL INJURY

Clinical factors that affect the pathogenesis of complications during TLI will be discussed with respect to laryngeal injury and tracheal cuff-site injury. It is important to recognize that multiple factors may be important in the pathogenesis of

laryngeal and tracheal cuff-site injury during TLI. Clinical investigation of the pathogenesis of airway injury from TLI has been complicated by the inability of investigators to control these many factors while examining the effect of one variable on airway injury. Accordingly, the role of many of the specific clinical influences on laryngeal or tracheal injury discussed below remains unsettled.

Tube Size Relative to Laryngeal Size

Colice et al found no association between the severity of laryngeal injury following extubation and the ratio of tube size to laryngeal size.[51] We were unable to find a relationship between ETT diameter and laryngeal injury at autopsy.[23] Lindholm, however, concluded that large ETT size with respect to laryngeal size is an important determinant of laryngeal injury,[127] and Santos et al observed that laryngeal erythema, ulceration, and delayed true vocal cord immobility were related to ETT size.[138]

Laryngeal Abrasion

Abrasion of the laryngeal mucosa by movement at the interface between the ETT and the surface of the larynx would intuitively seem to be of great importance in the pathogenesis of laryngeal ulceration. This concept, however, has been difficult to prove. Some degree of abrasion of the laryngeal mucosa likely occurs whenever there is movement of the ETT or movement of the larynx. Breathing, swallowing, coughing, yawning, hiccupping, attempted phonation, and head and neck movements[207] are all plausible contributors to the abrasive action of the ETT. ETT movement with cycling of the ventilator, suctioning the airway, and nursing care interventions may further contribute to mucosal abrasion.[122]

The role of laryngeal mucosal abrasion by movement of the ETT has been evaluated by a number of investigators.[23,51,122,125,127,276,279] The findings of El-Naggar et al suggested that friction between the ETT and laryngeal mucosa is an important factor in the pathogenesis of laryngeal injury.[125] Colice et al reported that the severity of laryngeal injury following extubation was significantly associated with neuromotor activity while the ETT was in place.[51] Patients with flaccid paralysis had milder degrees of injury.[51] Conversely, Dunham and LaMonica found more laryngotracheal injury in patients with head and neck rigidity than in those with a nonrigid posture.[279]

Duration of Intubation

Since the early 1950s, clinicians and investigators have speculated that the duration of TLI may be an important determinant of complications of TLI. This relationship obviously has an important influence on decisions about performing tracheotomy for long-term airway maintenance. It would seem intuitively straightforward that a longer duration of TLI increases the risk of laryngeal (or tracheal) injury. This relationship, however, remains controversial because of conflicting data from a number of studies.

Early reports suggested that duration of TLI is important in the pathogenesis of laryngeal injury.[128,140,280,281] Donnelly observed that the severity of histopathologic injury to the larynx at autopsy was related to the duration of TLI.[128] A retrospective study by Hedden et al came to the same conclusion.[140] Later observations by Whited[122,123] and by Supance et al[245] suggested that longer periods of TLI increased the risk of laryngeal stenosis. Santos et al found significant relationships between duration of TLI and aspiration, laryngeal granulomas, and vocal cord immobility, but not laryngeal ulceration.[138] Two more recent prospective studies reported a significant relationship between duration of TLI and postextubation stridor or requirement for reintubation.[229,282]

A number of prospective studies, however, have not been able to establish that duration of TLI is an important determinant of overall laryngeal injury.[23,33,44,51,124,137,279] We found no statistical association between duration of TLI and laryngotracheal injury at autopsy.[23] One patient had laryngeal ulceration after only 7 hours of TLI.[23] Rashkin and Davis found no correlation between acute laryngotracheal injury and duration of TLI in 61 adult patients intubated for more than 3 days,[33] and Kastanos et al found no such relationship in 19 patients intubated longer than 1 day.[124] In a prospective study of trauma patients, Dunham and LaMonica found no difference in laryngotracheal pathology between those patients undergoing early tracheotomy and those with 2 weeks of TLI.[279] Colice et al noted that serious laryngeal injuries could develop after only 1–3 days of TLI.[51] In 54 patients surviving after TLI, they found no relationship between the frequency of nonstenotic laryngeal complications and the duration of intubation.[51] Subsequently, Colice reported that prolonged TLI (>10 days) did not influence the rate of resolution of laryngeal injury.[137]

Some animal studies support the absence of a relationship between duration of TLI and laryngeal complications. Weymuller reported that length of intubation was not related to the severity of laryngeal injury in dogs.[283,284] In that dog model, TLI caused mucosal inflammation and erythema by 24 hours and loss of mucosal architecture within 1 week, but laryngeal damage remained relatively stable after 1 week of TLI.[283]

It can be concluded that studies in both animals and man fail to provide convincing evidence of an association between duration of TLI and laryngeal complications. Most prospective clinical studies have not been able to prove that duration of TLI by itself is an important determinant of laryngeal injury.

Age

Clinical and autopsy findings in prospective studies suggest that age is not a significant determinant of overall laryngeal injury from TLI.[23,51,138]

Gender

The role of gender in laryngeal injury from TLI is unclear. Hedden et al reported in a retrospective study that laryngeal injury at autopsy following TLI was more severe in women than in men.[140] This observation was not confirmed by postmortem observation.[23,128] Clinical studies have suggested that laryngeal stenosis following TLI is more common in women than in men.[239,267] Lindholm interpreted his observations to suggest that tube size relative to laryngeal size is an important determinant of laryngeal injury,[127] but this could not be confirmed by the findings of Colice et al.[51]

Hypotension

The pivotal role of laryngeal and tracheal capillary perfusion pressure in the pathogenesis of ETT-induced airway injury has led investigators to speculate that hypotension is an important risk factor for laryngeal injury during TLI. There are no convincing data, however, to support this concept.[51]

Route of Intubation

Two studies suggest that posterior laryngeal ulcers are more common with oral intubation than nasal intubation.[23,133] Possible reasons for this observation are that nasotracheal tubes are generally smaller than orotracheal tubes, they move less because they are stabilized by the walls of the nasal cavity, and they enter the glottis at a straighter angle of entry, thereby decreasing pressure on the posterior glottis. Another study, however, did not find less laryngeal injury with nasal intubation than oral intubation.[244]

Miscellaneous Factors

Underlying disease state, infection, corticosteroid therapy, head position, state of consciousness, gastric acid reflux, and many other factors have all been considered as possible determinants of laryngeal injury during TLI, but none of these factors have been proven to have a contributing role. Several studies have suggested that laryngeal injury following TLI is more common in patients with diabetes mellitus.[144,267,285] Bacterial invasion of subglottic tissue injured by TLI may have a role in the pathogenesis of subglottic stenosis. In a rabbit model of subglottic ischemic injury from ETT cuff overinflation, Kil et al observed diffuse mucosal and submucosal inflammation, necrosis, and loss of surface epithelium.[286] Treatment with high-dose dexamethasone 1 hour before extubation and 6 hours after extubation had no effect on the histologic pattern of injury.

Posterior glottic stenosis may be more likely if TLI is followed by tracheotomy.[123,287] This association might occur because tracheotomy results in non-use of the larynx, which might promote the formation of adhesions across ulcerated laryngeal surfaces.[239] Whited referred to a high statistical association between posterior laryngeal stenosis after TLI and subsequent tracheotomy, but cautioned that this might reflect selection bias rather than a true cause-and-effect relationship.[122,123] Colice et al also reported in their prospective study that the severity of laryngeal injury after TLI was associated with subsequent tracheotomy.[51] Sasaki et al have implicated contamination of tracheotomy wounds in the pathogenesis of subglottic stenosis attributed to TLI.[288]

In summary, it is likely that many factors contribute to laryngeal injury from TLI. Available data suggest that the mechanical force applied to the posterior larynx by the ETT is the most important risk factor for laryngeal injury. It is intuitive that abrasion of the laryngeal mucosa by movement at the interface with the ETT is an important risk factor, but supportive data are limited. Duration of TLI by itself has an uncertain role in the pathogenesis of laryngeal injury.

CLINICAL INFLUENCES IN LARYNGEAL GRANULOMA FORMATION

The prospective study of 97 patients by Santos et al found significant associations between the early appearance of true vocal cord granulomas after extubation and (1) duration of TLI, (2) subsequent tracheotomy, (3) use of a larger ETT in those patients who required tracheotomy, and (4) use of a nasogastric tube.[138] The delayed appearance of true vocal cord granulomas 2–10 weeks after extubation was significantly associated with subsequent tracheotomy and with use of a nasogastric tube. Lindholm also found a positive correlation between ETT diameter and the subsequent development of laryngeal granulomas.[127]

CLINICAL INFLUENCES IN TRACHEAL CUFF-SITE INJURY

Cuff Pressure

The important role of high cuff inflation pressures in the pathogenesis of tracheal cuff-site injury is now well established, based on studies of both TLI and tracheotomy.[148–150,252,254,256,258,275,276,289–297] The pioneering studies of Cooper, Grillo, et al,[148,149,275,276] Ching, Nealon, et al,[289,290] and Nordin et al[255,257,292] established conclusively in both animal models and in humans that hard cuffs were more injurious to the tracheal mucosa than soft cuffs. These observations were confirmed by other investigators.[252,254,258,298] Figure 39-13 shows the critical role of cuff pressure in causing tracheal cuff-site injury in animal experiments performed by Cooper and Grillo.[148]

Intracuff pressure is transmitted laterally against the wall of the trachea (see Fig. 39-10). The intracuff pressure exceeds the pressure exerted against the tracheal wall (the lateral tracheal wall pressure) by a small amount in soft cuffs and by a greater amount in hard cuffs. Ischemia and eventual necrosis occur when the lateral tracheal wall pressure exceeds the capillary perfusion pressure of about 25 mmHg,[256–258,292,295] as illustrated in Fig. 39-14. Ischemia of the tracheal mucosa occurs in rabbits when the cuff inflation pressure exceeds 30 mmHg.[299] Necrosis of the tracheal mucosa leads to sloughing and ulceration of the mucous membrane, exposing tracheal cartilage. Continued ischemia may be followed by partial or complete destruction of cartilaginous tracheal rings and loss of the structural integrity of the affected tracheal segment, leading to tracheal dilation (see Fig. 39-10).[153,154] Healing of the injured tracheal segment during any stage of this process may lead to a tight fibrous stricture (tracheal stenosis).

Modern soft-cuff ETTs transmit intracuff pressure to the tracheal wall, but not to the extent that hard-cuff ETTs do. Overinflation of soft cuffs, however, may cause high lateral tracheal wall pressures to develop, even to the point at which capillary perfusion pressure is exceeded.[256] The amount of lateral tracheal wall pressure appears to be more important than the duration of intubation in producing tracheal damage.[257,297] We were unable to show a significant association between duration of cuff inflation pressures in excess of 20 or 25 mmHg during TLI and tracheal cuff-site injury at autopsy.[23]

Cuff Design and Shape

The geometric shape of the cuff relative to the shape of the tracheal lumen has been implicated in tracheal cuff-site damage.[290,300–302] In one study, asymmetric inflation of hard cuffs resulted in focal areas of very high lateral tracheal wall pressure and tracheal mucosal injury.[303] With modern

FIGURE 39-13 An experiment in dogs indicated the critical role of high cuff-inflation pressure in causing severe tracheal cuff-site injury. Shown here are severe tracheal ulceration with exposed tracheal cartilage (*left*) and tracheomalacia (*center*) from prolonged intubation with ETTs with low-volume, high-pressure cuffs. The panel on the right shows a normal tracheal surface after prolonged intubation with an ETT with a high-volume, low-pressure cuff. (*Modified, with permission, from Cooper and Grillo.[148]*)

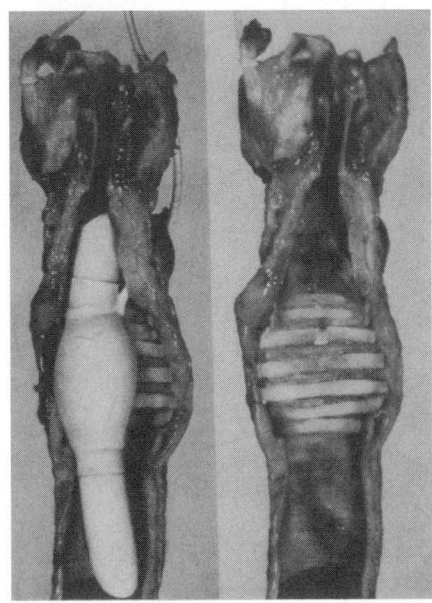
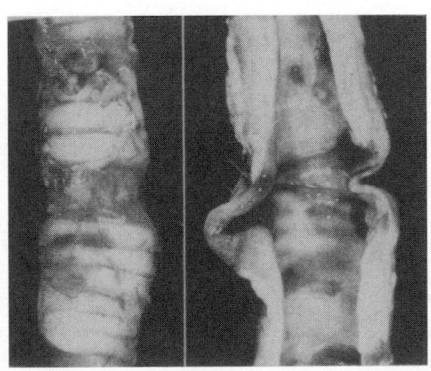
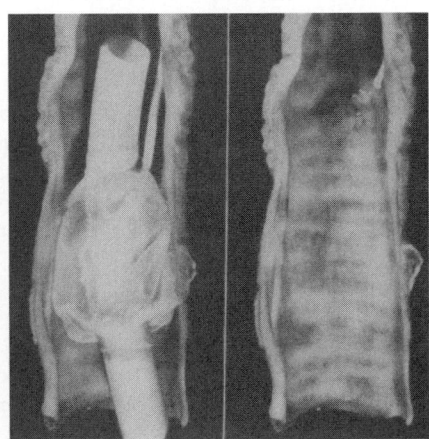

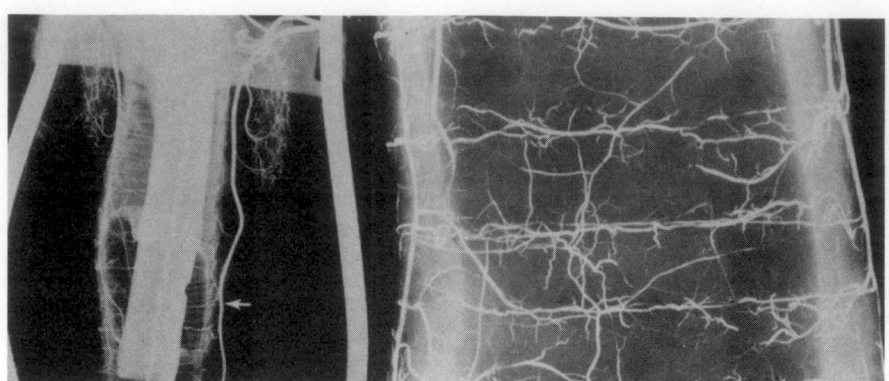

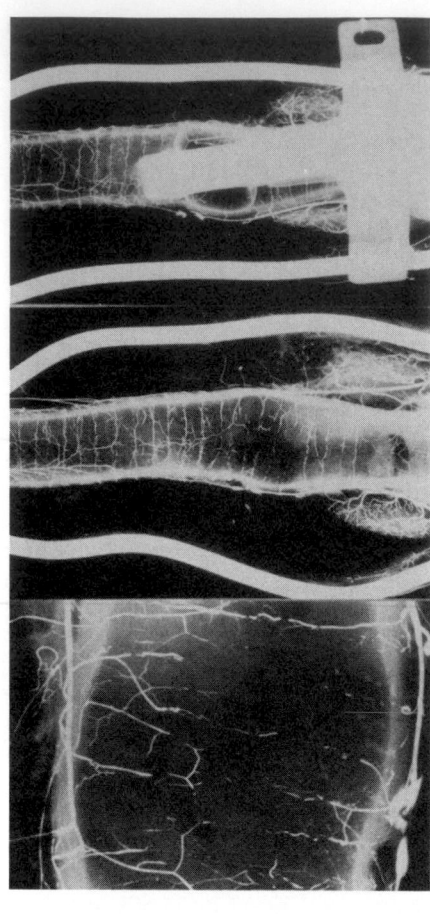

FIGURE 39-14 Radiographs of the tracheal arteries in dogs were performed to investigate the effect of cuff pressure on blood flow from the tracheal arteries to the wall of the trachea at the cuff site. The panel with 3 images on the left shows a marked reduction in small arteries at the cuff site when a low-volume, high-pressure cuff of a tracheostomy tube was inflated for 18 hours to just-seal volume (*top:* cuffed tube in place; *center:* tube removed; *bottom:* magnified view of cuff site). The panel with 2 images on the right shows intact small arteries when a pre-stretched cuff having pressure-volume characteristics of a high-volume, low-pressure cuff was inflated in the same fashion (*left:* cuffed tube in place; *right:* magnified view of cuff site with tube removed). (*Modified, with permission, from Dunn et al.*[295])

soft-cuff tubes that inflate evenly, this phenomenon is no longer observed. Because modern soft-cuff tubes, however, do have quite variable physical characteristics, including inflation diameter, fabric thickness, compliance, and geometric shape, all are not the same in their pressure-volume relationship and potential for mucosal injury.[252,270,277,296,303]

Age
Few studies have examined the influence of age on tracheal cuff-site injury during TLI. We found a relationship between age and cuff-site injury at autopsy of borderline statistical significance.[23] In prospective studies, others have found no relationship between total tracheal injury from TLI and age.[124,125]

Gender
The role of gender in cuff-site tracheal injury from TLI is controversial. We reported that tracheal cuff site injury at autopsy was significantly more common in women than in men.[23] The prospective studies of Kastanos[124] and El-Naggar,[125] however, did not find a relationship of tracheal injury and gender.

Duration of Translaryngeal Intubation
The relationship between duration of TLI and tracheal cuff-site injury is controversial for both hard-cuff and soft-cuff ETTs. We found no statistical association between tracheal cuff-site injury at autopsy and duration of TLI or duration of TLI and tracheotomy together.[23] Similarly, other studies have failed to find a significant relationship between duration of tracheotomy and cuff-site injury.[23,125,304,305] Only one prospective study found that tracheal cuff-site injury was significantly associated with the duration of TLI.[124] There is one report of severe tracheal stenosis following TLI for less than 72 hours.[306]

Hypotension
Few studies have examined the relationship between hypotension and tracheal cuff-site injury in humans. We found no relationship between hypotension and tracheal cuff-site injury at autopsy.[23] In an experimental study of dogs with cuffed tracheostomy tubes, Dunn et al found that intercurrent periods of hypotension did not affect the extent of tracheal injury from tracheostomy tube cuffs.[295]

Corticosteroid Therapy
Two prospective studies reported no association between corticosteroid therapy and tracheal cuff-site injury from TLI.[23,124]

Airway Infection
Nordin found that bacterial invasion of tracheal mucosa damaged by high cuff inflation pressures begins to occur about 4 hours after the onset of cuff inflation.[257] There is, however, no convincing evidence from clinical or

experimental studies that airway infection increases the risk of cuff-site complications.[125,275]

Miscellaneous Factors

Kastanos found statistically significant associations between tracheal injury from TLI and high alveolar-arterial oxygen tension gradient, duration of administration of high concentrations of oxygen, and use of positive end-expiratory pressure (PEEP).[124] Excessive motion between the inflated cuff and the trachea was implicated by the studies of Lindholm.[127]

Siobal et al reported a case of tracheoinnominate artery fistula in a burn patient who was intubated for 40 days with an 8.0-mm internal diameter ETT, which was equipped with a subglottic suction port and held in position by a wire suture to a molar tooth.[165] Erosion of the left anterior wall of the trachea by the tube tip was attributed to the prolonged period of intubation, fixed position of the tube, and decreased flexibility of the tube as a result of the suction channel feature.[165]

CLINICAL INFLUENCES IN PULMONARY COMPLICATIONS

Pneumonia

A myriad of factors predispose to VAP while an ETT is in place (see Chapter 46).[176,188,307–309] These factors include the underlying disease(s), impaired host defenses, antibiotic exposure, aspiration, enteral feeding tubes, sinusitis, impaired mucociliary function, ineffective cough, respiratory equipment, hospital transport out of the ICU, and increased binding of bacteria to the tracheobronchial epithelium. During intubation, the lower airways of ICU patients are heavily colonized with a variety of organisms. Those isolated most frequently as pathogens in VAP are aerobic gram-negative bacilli (especially *Pseudomonas aeruginosa*, Enterobacteriaceae, and *Acinetobacter* species) and *Staphylococcus aureus*.[188] Polymicrobial infections in VAP are common. Anaerobic organisms may also be isolated in cultures of lower respiratory tract secretions in patients with VAP,[310] but their significance in the pathophysiology of VAP remains controversial.[311,312]

An indwelling ETT is by itself a risk factor for VAP, because it is a foreign body and it bypasses protective upper airway defenses. Aspiration of contaminated upper airway secretions and leakage of bacteria-laden fluid that pools above the inflated ETT cuff are important mechanisms of entry of pathogens into the lung.[173,176,183,313–316] The ETT also serves as a reservoir for microorganisms.[272,317] Bacteria adhere to the ETT inner surface in a slimy coat or biofilm,[271,273] fragments of which may be dislodged into the lung. Suctioning may promote this phenomenon. Accordingly, ETT biofilm has been implicated in the pathogenesis of VAP.[176] Adair et al found a significant correlation between cultures of tracheal secretions and cultures of the ETT biofilm in adults with VAP, but not in intubated patients without VAP.[272]

The nasal route of TLI is considered a risk factor for the development of VAP as well as sinusitis.[177] Holzapfel et al found that nosocomial sinusitis increased the risk of VAP by a factor of 3.8.[111] Reintubation may be a separate but important risk factor for VAP.[318]

Aspiration

Aspiration of gastric and upper airway secretions into the lower airway while an ETT is in place may occur for a variety of reasons.[186] TLI per se invites aspiration of secretions because of stenting of the larynx in an open position, prevention of glottic closure, esophageal compression by the inflated cuff, pooling of secretions above the cuff, creation of channels along folds of cuff fabric,[185] and desensitization of protective upper airway reflexes. Elpern et al, in a prospective study of aspiration in intubated adults, observed that cuff inflation to occlusion does not prevent aspiration, nor does a head-up position in bed.[186] They also noted that nasogastric tubes increased the risk of aspiration, whereas level of consciousness and feeding status did not.

COMPLICATIONS DURING AND AFTER EXTUBATION

Sore throat after anesthetic intubation is not related to tube cuff design[319] and is not prevented by lubrication of the ETT before insertion.[320] In a prospective study of critically ill adults, Jaber et al found that postextubation stridor was associated with traumatic or difficult intubation, prior self-extubation, increased cuff pressure at the time of ICU admission, and duration of TLI.[229] Efferen and Elsakr reported that postextubation stridor was associated with cuff pressure, corticosteroid therapy at the time of extubation, and a neurologic disorder necessitating TLI.[230]

The pathogenesis of laryngeal and tracheal stenosis following TLI is related to the healing process of airway injury incurred during TLI. Why some ulcerative lesions heal normally, others with granuloma formation, and others with cicatrix or scar formation is obscure. Table 39-9 summarizes important or potentially important mechanisms of laryngotracheal injury from TLI.

Important Prospective Studies of Complications of Translaryngeal Intubation

Because the literature on complications of artificial airways is largely based on retrospective and anecdotal observations, study of this topic is especially prone to potential bias and faulty conclusions. Few techniques of airway management satisfy the criteria of evidence-based medicine.[321] Fortunately, however, a growing number of prospective studies of complications of TLI, tracheotomy, or both are now available. Large prospective studies of complications of TLI are difficult to perform but they provide valuable information.

Several studies comparing complications of TLI with those of tracheotomy or complications of delayed versus early tracheotomy have had a randomized design.[125,279,322–324] Prospective studies attempting to randomize patients to early tracheotomy have been difficult

TABLE 39-9 Important Mechanisms of Laryngotracheal Injury from Translaryngeal Intubation

Laryngeal ulceration
  High pressure on the posterior endolarynx
    Curvature of the ETT
    Round shape of the ETT
    Stiffness of the ETT
  Abrasion (excessive movement at the tube-mucosa interface)
  Large diameter of the ETT
  Female gender
  Oral route of intubation
Laryngeal granuloma formation
  Laryngeal ulceration
  Nasogastric tube
  Large diameter of the ETT
  Increasing age
Laryngeal stenosis
  Laryngeal ulceration
  Subsequent tracheotomy
    Laryngeal inactivity
    Bacterial invasion
Tracheal cuff-site ulceration
  High lateral tracheal wall pressure

to carry out because of physician bias against this intervention.[23,322] Only a few prospective studies have directly compared complications of TLI with those of tracheotomy.[23,125,127,279] Others have compared early tracheotomy with late tracheotomy but did not directly compare tracheotomy with prolonged TLI alone.[322,323,325,326]

Rumbak et al randomized 120 adult medical ICU patients to early percutaneous tracheotomy within 48 hours or delayed tracheotomy after 10–14 days of TLI.[323] The early tracheotomy group experienced significantly lower mortality, less frequent pneumonia, fewer days in the ICU, fewer days of mechanical ventilation, and fewer days of sedation. Sugerman et al, however, using a similar study design, found no significant differences between the early and the delayed tracheotomy groups with regard to mortality rate, days in the ICU, or frequency of pneumonia.[322] This section will review selected prospective clinical studies of laryngeal or tracheal complications of TLI in adults (Table 39-10).

Lindholm's study represents the most comprehensive study of complications of TLI ever performed.[127] He investigated 457 patients for acute and late complications of in-

TABLE 39-10 Selected Prospective Studies of Complications of TLI

Year	References	No. of Patients
1969	Lindholm[127]	457
1981	Stauffer et al.[23]	150
1984	Whited[123]	200
1989	Colice et al.[51]	82
1994	Santos et al.[138]	97
1995	Schwartz et al.[62]	238
2004	Bouderka et al.[324]	62

tubation. Very few late severe complications and no deaths were attributed to TLI. Large ETT size, ETT stiffness, and excessive laryngeal motion were identified as important risk factors for laryngeal injury. Because, however, the patients were intubated in large part with red rubber and latex tubes with hard cuffs, and the duration of intubation was less than 3 days, the results of the study are not entirely applicable to modern critical care.

Stauffer et al compared complications of TLI with those of tracheotomy in 150 critically ill adults in two large teaching hospitals.[23] Survivors were studied for late complications and nonsurvivors were evaluated at autopsy. An attempt to randomize patients into early tracheotomy and prolonged TLI groups was only partially successful. About two-thirds of TLI and two-thirds of tracheotomies had one or more complications, but the complications were judged to be more severe in the tracheotomy group. Laryngotracheal injury at autopsy did not correlate with the duration of TLI. A few patients appeared to tolerate TLI well for up to 3 weeks.

Whited described his personal experience as an otolaryngologist-head and neck surgeon with 200 patients from the critical care units of two teaching hospitals who had TLI from 2–24 days.[123] Mirror or fiberoptic laryngoscopy-tracheoscopy was performed at extubation and serially thereafter. Fifty survivors (group I) had TLI for 2–5 days, 100 (group II) had TLI for 6–10 days, and 50 (group III) had TLI for 11–24 days. The severity of posterior laryngotracheal injury appeared to increase with the duration of TLI, but statistical analysis was not provided. Chronic posterior commissure stenosis progressing inferiorly to the level of the cricoid ring and into the trachea occurred in 14% of group III patients. Chronic stenosis was more common in patients with TLI followed by tracheotomy than in those with TLI alone. Other variables that might have affected the outcome were not described. The author concluded that TLI for less than 7 days is safe and that TLI beyond 10 days is unacceptable as a routine policy.

Colice et al examined 82 adult patients intubated more than 4 days for laryngeal complications of TLI using direct fiberoptic laryngoscopy and careful follow-up.[51] Nonlaryngeal complications were not evaluated. Ulceration and edema of the posteromedial aspects of the vocal cords were observed in 94% of the patients at extubation. Neuromotor activity and performance of a tracheotomy, but not duration of TLI, were associated with increased laryngeal complications. Initial findings at laryngoscopy did not predict the late development of adverse effects.

Santos et al reported risk factors for laryngeal injury from prolonged TLI in critically ill adult men in an initial report in 1989[327] and updated their findings with a second report in 1994.[138] The latter study described prospective observations in 97 adult men with orotracheal TLI (mean duration 9 days). Postextubation endoscopic findings in 79 survivors included laryngeal erythema (94%), laryngeal ulceration (76% with resolution within 6 weeks), and laryngeal granulomas (44%). True vocal cord (TVC) immobility was seen in 16 (20%) patients and was delayed in onset in half the cases. Duration of TLI was significantly associated with TVC granuloma formation and early and delayed

TVC immobility but not with TVC ulceration. The use of a larger ETT (size 8.0 mm internal diameter as compared with size 7.5), was significantly associated with TVC erythema, ulceration, granuloma formation, and delayed immobility. None of 62 patients with TLI alone developed laryngotracheal stenosis.

Schwartz et al prospectively studied 297 consecutive TLIs in 238 critically ill adults in medical and surgical critical care units of a large teaching hospital in order to assess immediate complications of TLI.[62] The most common indications for TLI were respiratory failure (50%), airway protection (17%), ETT change (13%), and cardiac and/or respiratory arrest (10%). Eleven percent of TLIs required three or more attempts at ETT placement. Eight percent were classified as difficult, but none of these were associated with adverse outcomes. Esophageal intubation occurred during 25 (8%) of the 297 intubation procedures and was not accompanied by any adverse sequelae. A new infiltrate on the postintubation chest radiograph was observed in 8% of cases, and in half of these (4%) aspiration was suspected as the cause.

Bouderka et al reported results of a prospective, randomized trial of early tracheotomy (day 5–6) versus prolonged TLI in 62 adults with severe head injury.[324] The two groups were similar in terms of age, gender, and simplified acute physiology score. Clinical symptoms of laryngotracheal complications did not differ between the two groups, but routine endoscopy to evaluate patients for these complications was unfortunately not performed. The early tracheotomy group experienced fewer days of mechanical ventilation both overall and after pneumonia was diagnosed. No differences in ICU stay, frequency of pneumonia, or mortality were observed.

Recognition and Management of Complications of Translaryngeal Intubation

RECOGNITION OF SELECTED COMPLICATIONS

COMPLICATIONS DURING ENDOTRACHEAL TUBE PLACEMENT

Right Mainstem Bronchus Intubation

The classic physical examination findings of a patient with right mainstem bronchus intubation are greater intensity of breath sounds and expansion of the right hemithorax compared with the left. Right mainstem intubation, however, may be difficult to recognize in many patients, especially those with emphysema, because of distant breath sounds on auscultation and chest hyperinflation.[328] Schwartz et al observed that neither physical examination nor referencing the centimeter markings on the ETT shaft indicated malpositioning of the ETT after emergency TLI.[59] Women are at greater risk than men for malpositioning of the ETT in critical care intubations.[59] Right mainstem bronchus intubation may lead to early hypoxemia and cyanosis, particularly if the patient has underlying lung disease.

Esophageal Intubation

Inadvertent intubation of the esophagus should be recognized immediately by capnography (see below and Chapter 38), although this method is not foolproof. Esophageal intubation may be recognized when manual ventilation after intubation produces poor chest expansion and gurgling sounds on auscultation over the stomach. In some cases, esophageal intubation may be very difficult to detect on physical examination. The patient with an ETT placed in the esophagus may display some degree of chest expansion, and "pseudo" breath sounds may be auscultated as gas enters the stomach. Esophageal intubation should be recognized before a postintubation chest radiograph is obtained. If a radiograph is obtained, however, it may reveal displacement of the ETT slightly away from the tracheal air column. Caution is necessary, however, because slight rotation of the patient may superimpose the tracheal air column over the ETT positioned in the esophagus.

COMPLICATIONS WHILE THE ENDOTRACHEAL TUBE IS IN PLACE

Sinusitis and Otitis

A high index of suspicion is critical to establishing the diagnosis of TLI-associated sinusitis and initiating effective therapy. Sinusitis may present as sinus pain and tenderness, or purulent nasal sinus drainage in an intubated patient, but it is important to emphasize that these findings may be minimal or absent.[96,102] Sinusitis complicating nasotracheal intubation or use of nasogastric tubes typically presents with fever, or in some patients, with bacteremia and sepsis syndrome.

Most reports have emphasized the value of CT scanning for accurate diagnosis of intubation-associated sinusitis, because physical examination is generally unreliable and standard sinus radiographs often fail to establish the diagnosis, especially when there is involvement of the ethmoid or sphenoid sinuses.[96,97,102,329] Radiographic maxillary sinusitis is defined as the presence on CT scanning of an air-fluid level or opacification of the maxillary sinus. Opacification of the other sinuses is common in intubated patients. B-mode ultrasound compares favorably with CT scanning in evaluation of suspected intubation-associated sinusitis and has the advantage of being a quick bedside technique that does not require transport of the ICU patient to the radiology suite.[330] Otitis is detected by routine otoscopic examination, which should also be performed in evaluation of fever of unknown origin in the intubated patient.

Nasal and Oral Injury

Nasal and oral complications during TLI are recognized by daily careful examination of the nose and mouth.

Laryngeal Injury

Recognition of laryngeal injury during TLI is rarely successful, because the ETT hides the injured areas from observation. Posterior ulceration of the larynx is hidden from view during fiberoptic endoscopy unless the ETT is removed, which is dangerous and impractical. Supraglottic and glottic edema is sometimes assessed by direct or indirect laryngoscopy during TLI. There are conflicting reports about the value of laryngoscopy in assessing laryngeal injury during TLI.[141,144] Routine endoscopy of the pharynx and larynx during TLI is not currently advised. Furthermore, endoscopic findings in the larynx during TLI do not clearly guide the timing of tracheotomy or predict long-term laryngeal sequelae of TLI.[51,247]

Tracheal Injury

Tracheal cuff-site injury cannot be detected during TLI unless fiberoptic bronchoscopy is performed while the ETT is retracted upward. This practice has no proven value, however, and is not indicated in decision making about extubation or conversion to tracheotomy. When the ratio of cuff-site diameter to tracheal transverse diameter on a chest radiograph exceeds 1.5, severe damage to the tracheal wall is present.[152] Eighteen (13.5%) of 135 intubated adult patients developed this complication as a result of cartilaginous destruction, and those who survived eventually developed tracheal stenosis or tracheoesophageal fistula.[152] Therefore, patients in whom tracheal dilation develops during TLI should be followed closely for months because of the potential for tracheal stenosis.

COMPLICATIONS DURING AND AFTER EXTUBATION

Laryngeal Injury

Persistent hoarseness, stridor, or dyspnea after extubation should always raise the question of serious laryngeal complications of TLI, including granuloma formation, laryngeal muscle paresis or paralysis, severe ulceration, laryngeal stenosis, cricoarytenoid ankylosis, or synechia formation.[121,127,129,239] The physician should also be aware that dyspnea, hoarseness, and stridor appearing weeks to months after extubation may indicate serious laryngeal (or tracheal) stenosis and should not be dismissed as simply being related to the underlying lung disease.[242] Glottic or subglottic stenosis may take weeks or months to develop after seemingly uneventful TLI and extubation.[287]

The evaluation of patients with suspected serious laryngeal injury after TLI should include physical examination and laryngoscopy. Physical examination may reveal prolonged inspiratory phase, harsh tracheal sounds and palpable thrill over the larynx on inspiration, and inspiratory intercostal retractions. Upper airway stridor transmitted to the thorax should not be misinterpreted as a sign of bronchoconstriction.

Laryngoscopy is necessary in all cases. Vocal cord movement may be evaluated initially by mirror laryngoscopy. If any abnormalities are detected, direct laryngoscopy should be performed. The finding of bilateral vocal cord abduction could be related to cricoarytenoid arthritis or recurrent laryngeal nerve injury.[239] Recurrent laryngeal nerve injury is suggested by absence of vocal cord motion, while in posterior glottic stenosis there is some motion of the cords on inspiration and phonation.[239] Glottic synechiae and laryngeal granulomas are usually readily apparent at the time of direct laryngoscopy.

Imaging the larynx is very helpful in the diagnosis of TLI-induced laryngeal injury. Older imaging techniques such as soft-tissue radiographs and linear tomography have largely been replaced by CT scanning with multiplanar reconstruction capability to create coronal and sagittal reformatted images.[331] MRI plays a lesser role than CT imaging. Radiographic studies and fiberoptic laryngoscopy are more sensitive than the history and physical examination in detecting laryngeal injury from TLI.[23,124]

The maximal expiratory/inspiratory flow-volume loop is sometimes performed in the evaluation of patients with suspected laryngeal (or tracheal) injury from TLI. The classic feature of unilateral vocal cord paralysis on a flow-volume loop is attenuation of inspiratory flow rates. The classic feature of bilateral vocal cord paralysis or laryngeal (or tracheal) fixed stenosis is attenuation of both inspiratory and expiratory flow rates with a "boxed-off" appearance to the flow-volume loop. Classic patterns of these types of injury are not always seen, however, because the flow-volume loop is neither sensitive nor specific. A completely normal flow-volume loop, on the other hand, makes functionally significant laryngeal (or tracheal) disease unlikely.

Tracheal Stenosis

Symptomatic tracheal stenosis after extubation is very uncommon in the modern era of soft-cuff ETTs. Tracheal stenosis, however, is more likely to be encountered if TLI is followed by tracheotomy.[23] Like laryngeal stenosis, tracheal stenosis may not become apparent for weeks to months after extubation.[156,249,332] Typical symptoms of tracheal stenosis include progressive dyspnea on exertion, cough, difficulty clearing sputum, and in some cases, stridor. Unfortunately, these findings are commonly attributed to underlying disorders such as bronchitis, asthma, COPD, or resolving ARDS.[242]

The diagnosis of tracheal stenosis requires an alert physician with a high degree of clinical suspicion based on a history of TLI (or tracheotomy) weeks to months earlier. Initial symptoms of cough, hoarseness, and difficulty clearing lower airway secretions are followed by dyspnea and stridor. Stridor and progressive respiratory distress, however, may not occur until the tracheal diameter is reduced to around 5 mm or less in adults.[248,333] Physical examination may be normal in patients with mild to moderate degrees of tracheal stenosis. In severe cases, stridor is the key finding. Flow-volume loops demonstrate fixed airway obstruction if there is a tight fibrous ring at the stenotic segment. A 50% reduction in tracheal caliber (<8 mm diameter), however, may be needed in order to produce an abnormal flow-volume relationship.[334,335]

Confirmation of the diagnosis of tracheal stenosis is possible with multi-detector CT scanning, including axial imaging, multiplanar reconstruction, and creation of "virtual bronchoscopy" images, all of which are more than 95% accurate in comparison with fiberoptic bronchoscopy.[336,337] Multi-slice three-dimensional CT imaging offers remarkably clear images of tracheal stenosis.[338]

Fiberoptic bronchoscopy, the traditional gold standard for diagnosis of tracheal stenosis, is usually necessary to examine the airway for detail not seen on CT scanning, but caution must be exercised if the stenosis is tight. Rigid bronchoscopy and the use of dilators may be necessary in some cases.[333]

MANAGEMENT OF SELECTED COMPLICATIONS

COMPLICATIONS WHILE THE ENDOTRACHEAL TUBE IS IN PLACE

Sinusitis

Effective management of sinusitis during TLI requires early recognition, appropriate radiographic studies (see above), and culture and sensitivity of aspirated sinus fluid.[105] Nasotracheal and nasogastric tubes should be removed. Consultation with an otolaryngologist-head and neck surgeon is advised. Aspiration of maxillary sinus fluid yields fluid for Gram's stain and cultures for bacteria (aerobic and anaerobic) and fungi, allowing selection of appropriate antimicrobial therapy. Repeated aspiration may be necessary in some patients. Sinus irrigation or lavage via an indwelling catheter is sometimes required.[106] If sinusitis does not resolve after the aforementioned measures and switching to orotracheal intubation, tracheotomy should be considered.[97,105] Treatment with nasal decongestants for short periods is commonly employed.

COMPLICATIONS DURING AND AFTER EXTUBATION

Paranasal Complications

In survivors of prolonged TLI, Cavaliere and Masieri advise otology evaluation after hospital discharge to avert complications related to chronic middle ear effusion.[339]

Laryngeal Complications

Management of stridor occurring immediately after extubation requires careful bedside management by the ICU team. Supplemental oxygen is administered and vital signs and pulse oximetry are monitored carefully. Arterial blood gas measurements may be necessary. Physical examination of the upper airway, neck, and chest is essential, as is suctioning of secretions and removal of any foreign material from the mouth and pharynx. The head and neck are positioned to optimize airway patency. The patient should be reassured and anxiety managed appropriately. Because most cases of postextubation stridor are caused by laryngeal edema, management should be directed with this in mind. A racemic epinephrine aerosol directed to the larynx may quickly decrease laryngeal edema. In this setting, helium-oxygen gas mixtures may help reduce the patient's work of breathing.[340] Helium-oxygen mixtures with more than 40% oxygen are generally not effective. Prevention of recurrent postextubation stridor is discussed below.

The cuff-leak test is valuable in planning for extubation, because little or no leak around the deflated cuff helps to predict the presence of laryngeal edema and postextubation stridor.[341] Jaber et al observed that a cuff-leak volume of less than 130 ml (or less than 12% of tidal volume set at 10–12 ml/kg) was useful in identifying critically ill adult patients at risk for stridor after extubation.[229] Others have reported that cuff leaks of less than 10[282] or 15.5%[342] of tidal volume help to identify patients at risk for reintubation from laryngeal edema.

As stated earlier, limited motion of the vocal cords long after extubation reflects posterior glottic fibrosis or ankylosis of the cricoarytenoid joint.[14] The goal of management is restoration of the voice, prevention of aspiration, and provision of adequate airflow. Management by an experienced otolaryngologist-head and neck surgeon is essential. Surgical and nonsurgical techniques to improve laryngeal function in patients with vocal cord paresis/paralysis are available.[14,343–345] Patients with bilateral vocal cord paralysis may require emergent tracheotomy if there is obstruction to airflow.[14]

Treatments for laryngeal granulomas are directed at their causes, which include vocal abuse and gastroesophageal reflux disease as well as TLI. Granulomas from TLI are usually managed with fiberoptic laryngeal surgery[346] or surgical resection with very good results. Other therapeutic approaches for laryngeal granulomas have been described, including inhaled corticosteroids,[347] injection of corticosteroids,[14] injection of botulinum toxin,[348,349] and radiation.[350]

Laryngeal stenosis requires surgical intervention. Surgical options depend upon the location of the stenotic lesion and include laser therapy, dilation procedures, stenting, laryngofissure, scar resection, keel insertion, and other reconstructive procedures.[351–353] Posterior commissure scarring is difficult to treat surgically.[239,240] Repeated surgical operations for laryngeal stenosis may be required. In many cases, permanent tracheostomy is necessary.[14] Czigner et al treated 29 patients with subglottic stenosis, which was related to TLI or tracheotomy in most cases, with resection of the stenotic segment and end-to-end anastomosis, achieving a success rate of 96%.[354] Pena et al reported very similar results.[352]

Tracheal Complications

Tracheal granulomas are managed by endoscopic removal. Small granulomas may resolve spontaneously. Management of tracheal stenosis depends upon its severity. Patients with mild degrees of tracheal stenosis (arbitrarily defined as <25% reduction in airway diameter) and no symptoms require only periodic follow-up to look for progressive stenosis. Those with greater degrees of airway narrowing and symptoms require more aggressive management. In severe cases with 50–75% narrowing of the trachea, emergent medical and surgical intervention is necessary.

Surgical options in patients with severe tracheal stenosis include dilation procedures,[249,250,355,356] stent placement, electrocautery, laser photoablation,[357,358] and resection of the stenotic segment with re-anastomosis.[248,249,351,359–363] Satisfactory-to-good (and occasionally excellent) results are obtained in most cases of tracheal stenosis requiring tracheal reconstruction.[250] Grillo and Donahue reported good or satisfactory results with surgery in 94% of 503 patients with postintubation tracheal stenosis.[362] If the stenotic segment is long, additional procedures are required to release the trachea from the pulmonary ligaments and the airway above.[14,240,359] The critical role of an experienced surgeon in managing severe tracheal stenosis has been emphasized.[362] Figure 39-15 illustrates linear tomograms of the trachea in a

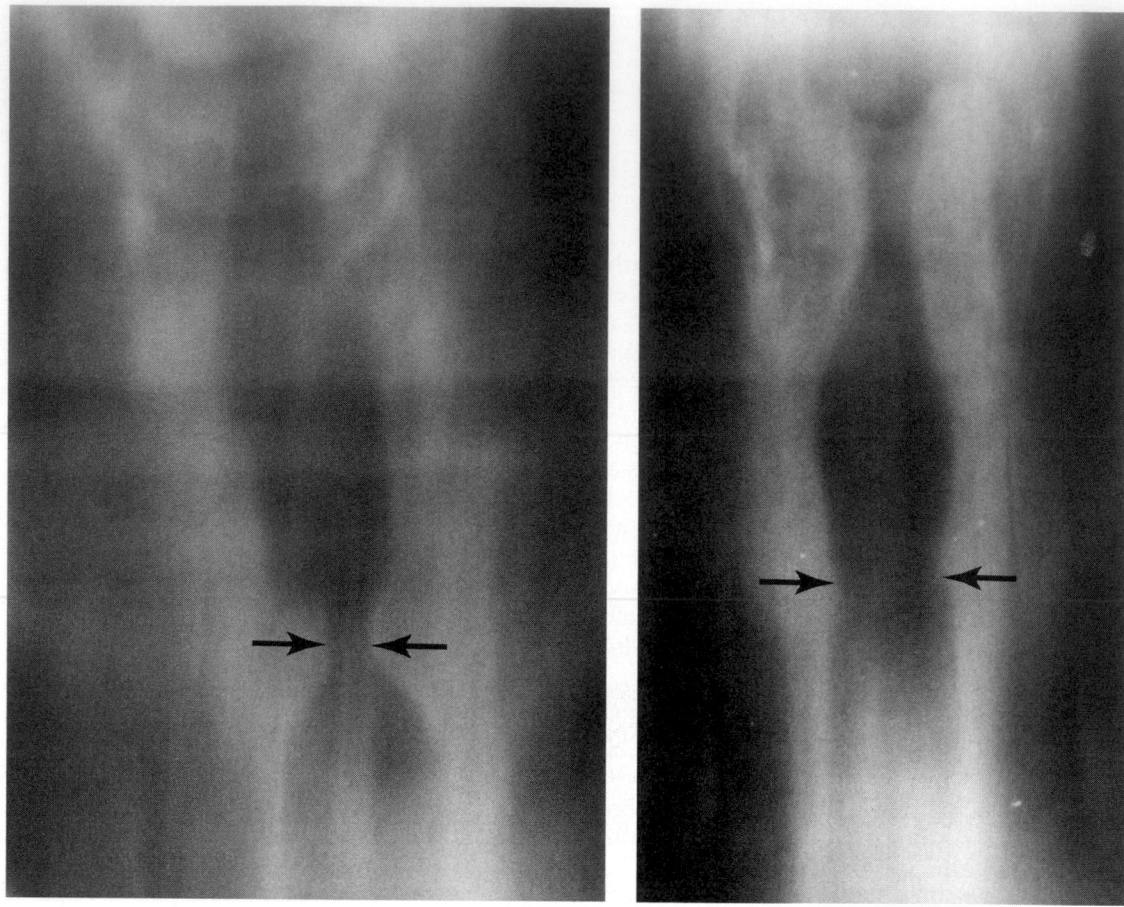

FIGURE 39-15 Linear tomograms of the trachea in a patient with tracheal stenosis (*arrows*) before (*left*) and after (*right*) surgical resection of a short stenotic segment of trachea with re-anastomosis. This type of tracheal injury from TLI alone is rare.

patient with tracheal stenosis before and after resection of a short stenotic segment of trachea with re-anastomosis.

Prevention of Complications of Translaryngeal Intubation

Most of the complications of TLI are preventable. Skilled intubation technique, seasoned clinical judgment, and meticulous care and monitoring of the intubated patient are the key elements in avoidance of TLI complications. Because intubation and reintubation put a patient at risk for airway injury, noninvasive alternatives to TLI, such as use of the Laryngeal Mask Airway (LMA North America, San Diego, CA) or the esophageal-tracheal Combitube (Tyco Healthcare), should always be considered, particularly in difficult and emergency airway management situations.[176,364–367] In patients with respiratory failure from acute exacerbation of COPD, noninvasive positive-pressure ventilation decreases the need for TLI and has advantages such as decreased mortality, rate of complications, and length of hospital stay.[368] An early important step is choosing the appropriate route of TLI for each patient with awareness of the advantages and disadvantages of each.[369] Principles of airway management

to prevent complications of artificial airways have been described elsewhere.[118,181,364,370–373]

COMPLICATIONS DURING ENDOTRACHEAL TUBE PLACEMENT

Complications that occur during ETT placement are particularly preventable. The intubator should be aware of common pitfalls in attempting to place an ETT in proper position (Table 39-11).

SELECTING THE CORRECT ENDOTRACHEAL TUBE
The ETT selected should have a high-volume, low-pressure soft cuff. All ETTs used in modern critical care should meet standards required by the F-29 Committee on Anesthetic and Respiratory Equipment, American Society for Testing and Materials.[2] The ideal ETT should be compliant at body temperature to help conform to the anatomic shape of the patient's airway, thereby reducing force on the posterior larynx. It also should be kink resistant and have a soft cuff that seals the airway and prevents aspiration at minimal lateral tracheal wall pressures.[261,277]

For anesthetic intubation, Stenqvist et al have advocated the use of size 6 or 7 (i.e., the size of the internal diameter in millimeters) ETTs in order to reduce pressure on the

TABLE 39-11   Common Pitfalls in Performing TLI

Inadequate training, practice, and experience in intubation

Failure to assemble necessary intubation equipment and drugs before starting the procedure

Selection of the incorrect route of intubation

Inadequate sedation, muscle relaxation, or topical anesthesia

Failure to prepare the nose with vasoconstrictors, analgesics, and/or decongestants before nasal intubation

Failure to oxygenate and ventilate the patient with bag-and-mask ventilation before intubation

Improper positioning of the head and neck

Use of the laryngoscope blade as a lever to pry the airway open

Use of the teeth as a fulcrum to turn the laryngoscope

Failure to visualize the vocal cords

Forcing the ETT forward against tissue resistance

Prolonged intubation attempts without regard for progressive hypoxemia and acidosis

Advancing the ETT deep into the airway after successfully passing the tube through the larynx

Equipment malfunction

SOURCE: Modified from Stauffer.[181]

laryngeal contact points.[374] For use in the patient with respiratory failure in the ICU, however, small tubes have obvious disadvantages, including difficulty in suctioning and increased airflow resistance that may increase the work of breathing and delay weaning from mechanical ventilation.[375] A size 8.0–8.5 mm tube in men or a size 7.5–8.0 mm tube in women is usually selected for oral intubation. A tube that is 0.5–1.0 mm smaller is selected for nasal intubation in most circumstances.[181] Specific formulas for selecting appropriate ETT size have also been recommended.[376]

PREVENTING INTUBATION TRAUMA

Intubation trauma may be avoided by skilled airway management strategies. These include the initial use of bag-and-mask technique to oxygenate and ventilate the patient, thereby avoiding the necessity for "crash" intubation.[181] Attempts to visualize the glottis with the laryngoscope should be brief and limited in number. Mort reported that the relative risk of airway complications was significantly higher when three or more laryngoscopic attempts were made.[63] Eleven percent of the 297 TLIs in critically ill adults prospectively studied by Schwartz et al required this number of attempts.[62]

Intubation after rapid and nearly simultaneous sedation and paralysis, known as rapid-sequence intubation, has become the preferred technique to facilitate emergency oral intubation of critically ill patients.[377,378] Compared with intubation without paralysis, rapid-sequence intubation was shown to reduce airway complications and the number of attempts required to intubate the trachea in a prospective study of adults.[379]

The value of skill and experience in intubation cannot be overemphasized. For example, nearly all reports of pharyngeal perforation from TLI emphasize that this complication occurs in emergency intubations performed by inexperienced intubators. Skill in intubation may be gained by mannequin or simulation training.[380–383] Bishop et al compared intubation by experienced intubators and novices,

observing that novices required twice as long to intubate and had significantly higher intubation "impulses" (force of intubation multiplied by duration of effort) than experienced intubators.[380] These observations demonstrate the benefits of training, skill, and experience in intubation.

Appropriate management strategies for the difficult intubation are discussed in Chapter 38. Recognition of the potentially difficult intubation requires seasoned clinical judgment that may help to avoid serious intubation complications.[384–386] Critical care providers should be familiar with current clinical practice guidelines to manage the patient with a difficult airway.[387]

Preventing Nasal Bleeding

Nasal intubation should be avoided in patients with coagulation disorders, thrombocytopenia, or platelet dysfunction. Careful examination of the nasal passage before intubation is essential. Softening the nasal ETT with warm water before intubation may make it more compliant, decreasing the frequency and severity of nasal hemorrhage.[388] The more patent side of the nose should always be selected for intubation, and a relatively small ETT selected. Application of a topical decongestant-vasoconstrictor and a topical anesthetic before nasotracheal intubation is advised.[181]

PREVENTING HYPOVENTILATION AND HYPOXEMIA

Monitoring of ventilation and oxygenation after intubation is critical (see Chapter 38). Unrecognized hypoventilation is among the most common preventable complications of intraoperative anesthesia.[30] Recent guidelines emphasize the importance of preventing hypoventilation by confirming proper ETT placement (see discussion below)[367] and by appropriately monitoring ventilation and oxygenation in the sedated patient.[389] Guidelines of the American Society of Anesthesiologists indicate that all patients undergoing sedation/analgesia should be monitored with pulse oximetry and with observation or auscultation of ventilatory function.[389] Monitoring of exhaled carbon dioxide should be considered for all deeply sedated patients and for moderately sedated patients whose ventilation cannot be directly observed.[389]

PREVENTING CARDIOVASCULAR REACTIONS TO TRANSLARYNGEAL INTUBATION

The tachycardic-hypertensive response and cardiac arrhythmias that may accompany laryngoscopy and TLI are potentially preventable.[81,84] The routine use of drugs to prevent these cardiovascular reactions to TLI is not advised, but prophylactic treatment should be considered in patients with hypertension, cardiac disease, or cerebrovascular disease.[390] A wide variety of drug classes and specific drugs are available for this purpose.[84,390]

AVOIDING ESOPHAGEAL INTUBATION

Esophageal intubation represents a misadventure in intubation with potentially disastrous consequences. A number of strategies have been described to avoid and to recognize this complication.[13,391–398] McCulloch and Bishop reviewed the efficacy of 15 different methods to determine correct ETT placement and avoid esophageal intubation.[13] Pulse oximetry to assure adequate oxygenation and quantitative monitoring of carbon dioxide levels of expired gas are now standards of care in the operating room (see Chapter 38). None of the methods to detect esophageal intubation are absolutely foolproof, but capnography comes closest to the mark.[391] It is superior to chest auscultation[397,399] and methods that employ a self-inflating bulb[400,401] or a lighted stylet.[397] Monitoring of end-tidal CO_2 levels after intubation gives a characteristic repeated waveform if the ETT is properly located in the trachea. Failure of capnography to detect esophageal intubation is very rare.[402] Although colorimetric CO_2 indicators are helpful in detecting esophageal placement of an ETT,[395,396] they have the potential for indicating tracheal placement even though the ETT is in the esophagus.[403]

Recent international guidelines for emergency cardiovascular care call for both primary confirmation of correct tracheal placement of the ETT by physical examination and secondary confirmation by an end-tidal CO_2 detector or an esophageal detector device.[367] These steps are followed by careful chest auscultation and a chest radiograph. Use of an ETT holder to prevent subsequent dislodgment is also advised in these guidelines.[367]

AVOIDING RIGHT MAINSTEM BRONCHUS INTUBATION

Physical examination of the chest is not reliable in determining proper positioning of the ETT. Brunel et al reported that 60% of patients with mainstem bronchus intubations had equal breath sounds on chest physical examination.[328] Therefore, in general it is always desirable to obtain a chest radiograph after intubation.[13,181,328,404] An exception is the patient who has had fiberoptic bronchoscopy to facilitate intubation when the bronchoscopy confirms adequate ETT positioning in the trachea. By chest radiograph (or bronchoscopy) the tip of the ETT should be about 4–5 cm above the carina in adults, or at about the level of the third or fourth thoracic vertebra on the chest radiograph (see Fig. 39-8).[398,405,406] When the tip of the ETT is about 4 cm above the carina, the upper end of the ETT cuff is about 2 cm below the vocal cords.[398]

Endobronchial intubation is preventable.[61,398] Intubators must resist the impulse to thrust the ETT too deeply into the trachea after the tube enters the glottis. Insertion to a depth of 21 cm in women or 23 cm in men from the upper incisor teeth or gums is a reasonable first step to avoid endobronchial intubation.[61] This approach will probably avoid endobronchial intubation, but in some patients it may result in positioning the ETT too high in the trachea, risking laryngeal compression or accidental extubation. Cherng et al reported that the correct oral ETT length in adults with the head in a neutral position was correlated with body height.[406] They advocated estimating the length of the tube (in centimeters) from 5 cm above the carina to the angle at the right side of the mouth with this equation: (body height in centimeters/5) – 13.[406] After a chest radiograph confirms proper positioning of an ETT, the tube should be marked with indelible ink at the level of the lip or nasal alae to avoid subsequent inadvertent tube dislocation.

COMPLICATIONS WHILE THE ENDOTRACHEAL TUBE IS IN PLACE

A number of practices may be helpful in preventing complications during TLI (Table 39-12). A careful physical examination of the patient should be performed by the physician at least daily, including examination of the mouth, nose, ears, sinuses, neck, and chest. The entry site of the ETT

TABLE 39-12   Selected Measures to Reduce the Risk of Complications While the Endotracheal Tube Is in Place

Perform a careful bedside examination daily
    Include mouth, nose, ears, and sinuses
Avoid nasal ulceration
    Position the nasotracheal tube so that it points downward
    Avoid too large a nasotracheal tube
    Avoid taping the ETT tightly to the nose
Avoid oral ulceration
    Minimize direct pressure on the lips and soft tissues of the oral cavity from the shaft of the ETT
    Support the weight of the attached ventilator tubing
    Use oropharyngeal airways only if necessary
Select the best ETT for the patient
    Use high-volume low-pressure soft cuffs only
    Avoid very large ETTs (size ≥9.0 mm) to reduce the risk of laryngeal injury
Manage cuff inflation carefully
    Limit intracuff pressure to ≤20 mmHg, 25 mmHg at the maximum
    Consider a trial of a foam cuff ETT if higher inflation pressures are required
    Check and record intracuff pressures every 8 hours
    Check for high cuff pressures after general anesthesia with nitrous oxide and other anesthetic gases
    Use the minimal occluding pressure technique for cuff inflation
    Avoid overinflation of soft cuffs
    Watch the chest radiograph for tracheal cuff-site dilation
Avoid deliberate or inadvertent self-extubation
    Use extremity restraints and sedate the patient if necessary
    Reassure the patient to allay anxiety
    Be certain the ETT is properly located in the trachea, with the tip about 4–5 cm above the carina (for an adult of average height)
Suction the airway carefully
    Avoid excessive movement of the ETT
    Use sterile gloved technique
    Oxygenate and ventilate the patient adequately during suctioning
    Limit suctioning to a maximum of 10–15 seconds at a time
    Suction secretions when necessary, not routinely
Avoid transmission of mechanical forces directly to the patient
    Use elastic connectors and swivels
    Support the weight of ventilator tubing
    Do not tie ventilator tubing to the bedrails
Minimize abrasion of the laryngeal and tracheal mucosa
    Minimize attempts to talk, swallow, and move the head and neck
    Control coughing and aggressively treat agitation, seizures, and rigid posturing
    Sedate the patient if necessary
Use nasogastric tubes judiciously and only if necessary
    Avoid large nasogastric tubes
Attach the ETT to a source of warm, humidified gas
Give the patient reassurance and emotional support
    Facilitate and encourage written communication
Remove the ETT as soon as possible

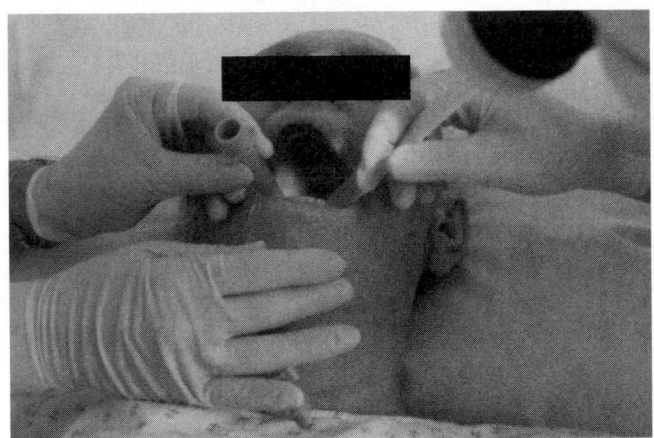

FIGURE 39-16 During translaryngeal intubation the nose and mouth should be inspected carefully every day in order to detect evidence of nasal or oral injury from the ETT.

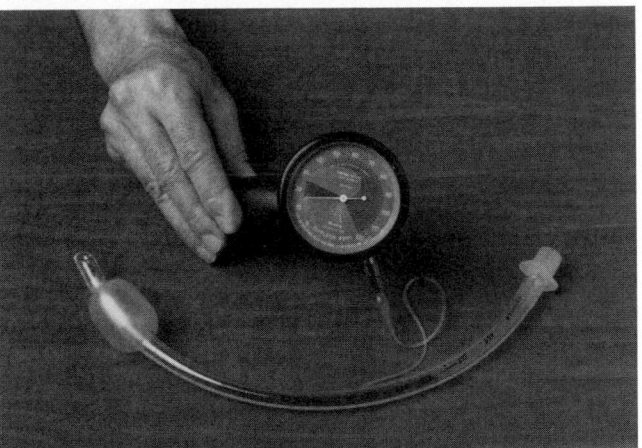

FIGURE 39-17 The pressure in the ETT cuff should be set and checked every nursing shift to help avoid tracheal cuff-site injury. Cuff inflation pressure should be limited to less than 20 mmHg (27 cmH₂O) if possible. The cuff pressure monitoring system shown here (Posey Cufflator, Posey Company, Arcadia, CA) records the pressure in the cuff and aneroid manometer simultaneously.

should be inspected carefully after removing adhesive tape or ETT holders as necessary (Fig. 39-16).

Nasal ulceration (see Fig. 39-2) may be avoided by positioning the ETT so that it points downward straight out of the nose, by avoiding tight taping of the tube to the nose, and by selecting a nasotracheal tube that is not too large for the patient. Oral ulceration (see Fig. 39-3) may be avoided by minimizing the direct pressure transmitted to the lips and soft tissues of the oral cavity from the shaft of the ETT and ventilator tubing. Oropharyngeal airways should not be used routinely.

MANAGING CUFF PRESSURE

Hard-cuff ETTs should not be used in critical care. Hard-cuff tubes are still marketed, however, and are occasionally encountered in patients arriving in the ICU. If a hard-cuff tube is detected by the requirement for very high cuff inflation pressures, it should be removed and replaced with a soft-cuff ETT.[118] The cuff inflation pressure should be limited to less than 20 mmHg (27 cmH₂O) if possible. If higher cuff pressures are required, the cuff pressure should certainly not be allowed to exceed 25 mmHg (34 cmH₂O). If this goal cannot be achieved, consideration should be given to replacing the ETT with a foam-cuff tube. A cuff pressure monitoring system that records the pressure in the cuff and manometer simultaneously should be used (see Fig. 39-17).

Critical care practitioners should be aware that it is necessary to check the ETT cuff for excessive pressure after general anesthesia with nitrous oxide (N₂O) and other anesthetic gases, because these gases diffuse into the cuff.[407–409] In patients undergoing surgery with general anesthesia that included 50% N₂O, Tu et al noted that ETT soft-cuff pressures exceeded 80 cmH₂O.[409] These investigators observed that tracheal cuff-site injury correlated with cuff pressure. Preinflation of the cuff with a 50% N₂O/oxygen mixture, rather than with air, prevented the build-up of excessive cuff pressures and significantly reduced cuff-site injury.[409] Tracheal cuff-site injury correlated with cuff pressure. The cuff pressure should be checked at least every 20–30 minutes during and after anesthesia with N₂O.

The "minimal occluding pressure" technique[270] is advised for maintaining cuff inflation, although some practitioners prefer the "minimal leak" technique.[410] Regardless of the technique of cuff inflation that is used, overinflation of soft cuffs should be avoided. The addition of only a few extra milliliters of air to the soft cuff may raise intracuff pressures sharply, increasing lateral tracheal wall pressure and risking tracheal mucosal injury.[256,289,290,296] Cuff pressures should be recorded at least every 8 hours or once every nursing shift. Routine monitoring of intracuff pressures is desirable, despite the shortcoming that it always overestimates lateral tracheal wall pressure.[411,412] Unfortunately, routine cuff pressure monitoring is not universally performed.[216]

High cuff inflation pressures should be taken seriously. The patient should be watched carefully for signs of excessive cuff pressure, including widening of the tracheal air column on the standard chest radiograph.[152] Rising peak airway pressures during mechanical ventilation require higher cuff inflation pressures in order to prevent cuff air leak. A prospective study of 15 patients undergoing mechanical ventilation for surgery revealed a linear relationship between peak airway pressure and minimal occluding cuff pressure, and in this series a cuff pressure of 25 mmHg corresponded with a peak inflation pressure of 35.3 mmHg (48 cmH₂O).[413]

AVOIDING UNPLANNED EXTUBATION

The patient should be constantly reassured to reduce anxiety. Extremity restraints should be applied if necessary and the patient sedated if it appears that self-extubation is likely. Mechanically ventilated patients who are severely agitated are significantly more likely to self-extubate than those who are not agitated.[414] Tung et al observed in a retrospective case-control study that ICU patients who self-extubated were more than twice as likely as controls to be agitated.[202] Atkins et al reported that patients who deliberately self-extubated were significantly more likely than controls to be restless or agitated and more likely to be physically restrained.[205]

Self-extubation tends to be repetitive, so constant vigilance is necessary. Staff awareness of the potential for self-extubation and the appropriate use of restraints and sedation reduce the risk of its occurrence.[197] Proper positioning of the tip of the ETT about 4–5 cm above the carina also reduces the risk of inadvertent self-extubation such as during movement, patient transport, or extension of the head and neck.[207]

USING SKILLED SUCTIONING TECHNIQUES

Complications of tracheal suctioning during TLI include pain, coughing, hypoxemia, cardiac arrhythmias, bronchoconstriction, and mucosal damage.[415,416] It is therefore important to suction the trachea carefully and never routinely.

Multiuse closed-system tracheal suction catheters save time, eliminate the need to disconnect the patient from the ventilator, and are preferable to open suctioning in patients with severe hypoxemia.[417] There is, however, no consensus that they should be used to prevent VAP.[314]

Open suctioning of the trachea should be performed with clean or sterile gloves, a sterile, single-use catheter, and sterile fluid.[314] Tracheal suctioning should ideally be performed by two attendants in order to avoid excessive movement of the ETT during suctioning and to maintain adequate oxygenation and ventilation. The patient should be adequately oxygenated and ventilated and suctioning intervals limited to a maximum of 10–15 seconds.

AVOIDING TRANSMISSION OF MECHANICAL FORCES FROM THE ENDOTRACHEAL TUBE DIRECTLY TO THE PATIENT

Elastic connectors and swivels between ventilator tubing and the ETT should be used. The weight of ventilator tubing should be supported by a folded towel on the patient's chest or by overhead supports. The ventilator tubing should not be tied to the bedrails. An ETT holder with integrated bite-block can help secure the position of the ETT and prevent the patient from biting and occluding the tube.[418]

MINIMIZING ABRASION OF THE LARYNGEAL AND TRACHEAL MUCOSA

Any motion of the ETT during TLI applies shearing forces to the mucous membranes of the mouth, and more importantly, the glottis and trachea, promoting airway injury. Attempts at talking, swallowing, and moving by the patient should be discouraged. Coughing should be controlled and aggressive measures taken to manage agitation, seizures, and rigid posturing. The ventilator tubing, ETT, and patient should be thought of as one unit and moved together in order to minimize movement at the interface between the ETT and the patient's airway. Nasogastric tubes should be used only if necessary.

REDUCING THE RISK OF VENTILATOR-ASSOCIATED PNEUMONIA

Guidelines to reduce the risk of health care–associated pneumonia and VAP should be followed as much as possible.[176,314] Preventive strategies that are specifically related to TLI include (1) using noninvasive positive-pressure ventilation as an alternative to TLI when feasible, (2) using orotracheal and orogastric tubes as opposed to nasotracheal and nasogastric tubes, (3) continuous or frequent intermittent aspiration of subglottic secretions with a special ETT that has a separate lumen above the cuff, (4) maintaining ETT cuff pressure above 20 cmH2O, (5) avoiding repeat intubation if possible, and (6) shortening the duration of TLI with appropriate sedation, ventilation, and weaning protocols.

MISCELLANEOUS PREVENTIVE STRATEGIES

The ETT should be attached to a source of warm, fully humidified gas to promote clearing of airway secretions and to avoid desiccation of the tracheobronchial mucosa. If a heat and moisture exchanger is used, especially for prolonged periods of time, close observation of ETT patency and airway resistance is necessary because of the risk of tube occlusion. The patient should be reassured and given emotional support throughout the period of TLI. This may help avoid complications such as self-extubation and those caused by excessive motion and agitation. Because ventilated patients experience a high level of frustration and stress related to their difficulty in communication,[419] care providers need to be especially attentive to patients' communication needs. Finally, the ETT should of course be removed as quickly as possible.

MODIFYING THE DESIGN OF THE ENDOTRACHEAL TUBE

Investigators have attempted to reduce the rate of complications of TLI by modifying the design of the ETT. Such innovations have led to the introduction into clinical practice of devices such as the foam-cuff ETT and the ETT with a suctioning lumen above the cuff. The foam-cuff tube described by Kamen and Wilkinson reduces lateral tracheal wall pressure to less than 15 mmHg.[420,421] Experimental innovations have included shaping the ETT to match the anatomic contour of the airway,[422] using a balloon on the shaft of the ETT,[122,259] covering the ETT shaft with foam,[327] lengthening the cuff to provide a larger contact area on the tracheal mucosa,[423] using two cuffs,[424] and adjusting the cuff design to prevent leakage of fluid into the lungs.[316,425] Several authors have advocated the use of self-regulating devices to control cuff pressure.[253,296,303] Limitations of these devices, however, have been described,[412] and they have not gained widespread acceptance.

COMPLICATIONS DURING AND AFTER EXTUBATION

Respiratory care techniques to avoid complications of extubation have been reviewed elsewhere.[181,364] The patient should be adequately oxygenated and ventilated before extubation. The cuff should be fully deflated before the ETT is removed, and the pool of secretions above the cuff should be suctioned from the trachea immediately upon cuff deflation. The rate of failed extubations was reduced by a quality improvement program that addressed risk factors for failed extubation.[426]

AVOIDING STRIDOR

Significant stridor after extubation is so uncommon[228] that routine prophylaxis against postextubation stridor is unwarranted. Routine pre-extubation treatment with topical epinephrine solution is not recommended. A Cochrane Database review concluded that prophylactic treatment of adults with parenteral corticosteroids before extubation had no effect on the occurrence of postextubation stridor or reintubation rates.[427] Meade et al reviewed randomized and nonrandomized controlled clinical trials and concluded that reintubation of critically ill adults was uncommon and not affected by pretreatment with parenteral corticosteroids.[428]

Patients who have displayed one episode of postextubation stridor requiring reintubation represent a serious therapeutic challenge for subsequent attempts at extubation. In this situation, because no particular therapeutic regimen has been studied carefully in adults and proven to be of benefit, all measures are empiric. No matter what measures are employed, experience indicates the need for repeated intubation of such patients. In one study, such patients required a mean of 2.9 intubations.[228] Weymuller et al[14] proposed a rigorous regimen in anticipation of a second episode of postextubation stridor, including general anesthesia in the operating room, followed by direct laryngoscopy. Deeb et al recommended immediate telelaryngoscopy for all patients who appear to require tracheotomy because of failed extubation.[144]

If extubation is attempted in the ICU after one failed extubation because of laryngeal edema, an empiric trial of topical epinephrine solution directed to the hypopharynx in an attempt to reduce laryngeal edema is reasonable. In this setting, therapy with a helium gas mixture should be available on standby, and personnel should be ready to reintubate the patient immediately. After extubation, there is no effective way of preventing early and late complications of TLI because there is no effective way to alter the course of the healing of airway injury.

Important Unknowns

In spite of more than a half century of accumulated experience in airway management of critically ill patients, there is still much that is unknown about complications of TLI and their avoidance. Considering the major advances of the last few decades, it is reasonable to expect even more advances in the decades ahead. It is likely that some of the following questions will be addressed:

1. Are there better techniques to assure correct ETT placement into the trachea?
2. Is there optimal timing of tracheotomy in patients with prolonged need for an artificial airway, and will computerized decision making play a role in timing of tracheotomy?
3. Is there an optimal size of ETT for individual patients based on gender and height?
4. Is there a better shape for the ETT to avoid posterior laryngeal injury?
5. Is abrasion of the mucosa as a result of motion between the patient and the ETT at the level of the posterior glottis an important risk factor for posterior glottis injury?
6. Would reducing ETT shaft stiffness decrease the risk of posterior glottis injury?
7. Is there a better cuff design to minimize tracheal surface injury?
8. What is the appropriate relationship between cuff inflation pressure and airway peak inflation pressure, considering the competing needs of preventing tracheal mucosal ischemic injury and reducing leakage of secretions from above the cuff?
9. What is the optimal composition of the ETT shaft in relationship to its wall thickness, compliance, inner diameter, pressure-flow relationship, and biofilm accumulation?
10. What is the appropriate level of training and experience permissible to perform TLI?

The Future

Extensive experience with TLI over the last five decades has provided a massive list of publications regarding ETT-related complications, mechanisms of airway injury, recommendations for management of the intubated patient, and strategies for prevention, early recognition, and treatment of the complications. Large prospective studies of complications of TLI are challenging to perform. Accordingly, relatively few have been reported, but they provide special insight into the true frequency of complications and the related risk factors. Retrospective observations, individual case reports, and small case series, however, have also added to our growing knowledge about airway complications of TLI. The expanding literature has allowed us to record and classify seemingly countless examples of airway injury from TLI as well as tracheotomy. Since the development of high-volume, low-pressure ETT cuffs more than 30 years ago, however, major advances to prevent ETT injury have not occurred.

Despite the depth and breadth of current knowledge and experience with TLI, there are still a number of challenges to face as we attempt to reduce the impact of complications of artificial airways in the years ahead. These challenges include the following:

1. Perform large multicenter prospective studies of complications of TLI in critically ill adults and children in order to evaluate the need for and timing of tracheotomy for long-term airway management, and to determine what risk factors contribute to that need.
2. Promote credentialing and expand training in advanced airway management, including management of the

difficult airway, for personnel involved in critical care at all levels—paramedical personnel, emergency department staff, and critical care unit practitioners.

3. Support research in new design and composition of artificial airways, including research to make ETTs more compliant, especially at the level of the posterior larynx, to design new and safer cuffs, and to reduce biofilm on tube surfaces.

4. Perform prospective studies of the use, in specific clinical settings, of alternatives to TLI, including the tracheal-esophageal Combitube, the Laryngeal Mask Airway, and noninvasive positive airway pressure devices.

5. Develop national clinical practice guidelines for managing TLI in critically ill patients.

Summary and Conclusions

Complications of TLI in critically ill adults are reviewed and classified according to the time period in which they occur: during ETT placement, while the ETT is in place, and during and after extubation. The chapter reviews mechanisms of these adverse events and describes steps to recognize, manage, and prevent complications of TLI. As the literature on complications of TLI expands, new insights to improve airway management of the critically ill patient continue to develop and evolve.

References

1. Ibsen B. The anesthetist's viewpoint on the treatment of respiratory complications in poliomyelitis during the epidemic in Copenhagen, 1952. Proc R Soc Med 1954; 47:72–74.
2. American Society for Testing and Materials. Anaesthetic and Respiratory Equipment—Tracheal tubes and connectors (ASTM/ANS/ISO 5361-99). Philadelphia: American Society for Testing and Materials, 1999.
3. Morch ET. History of mechanical ventilation. In: Kirby RR, Smith RA, Desautels DA, editors. Mechanical ventilation. New York: Churchill Livingstone, 1985.
4. Macewen W. Introduction of tracheal tubes by the mouth instead of performing tracheotomy or laryngotomy. BMJ 1880; 2:122–24, 163–65.
5. Nilsson E. On treatment of barbiturate poisoning. Acta Med Scand Suppl 1951; 253:7–127.
6. Clemmesen C, Nilsson E. Therapeutic trends in the treatment of barbiturate poisoning. The Scandinavian method. Clin Pharmacol Ther 1961; 2:220–29.
7. Wylie WD. Hazards of intubation. Anaesthesia 1950; 5:143–48.
8. Fields JA. Injuries and sequelae associated with endotracheal anesthesia. Laryngoscope 1959; 69:509–18.
9. Lewis RN, Swerdlow M. Hazards of endotracheal anesthesia. Br J Anaesth 1964; 36:504–15.
10. Blanc VF, Tremblay NAG. The complications of tracheal intubation: a new classification with a review of the literature. Anesth Analg 1974; 53:285–96.
11. Keane WM, Denneny JC, Rowe LD, et al. Complications of intubation. Ann Otol Rhinol Laryngol 1982; 91:584–87.
12. Stauffer JL, Silvestri RC. Complications of endotracheal intubation, tracheostomy, and artificial airways. Respir Care 1982; 27:417–34.
13. McCulloch TM, Bishop MJ. Complications of translaryngeal intubation. Clin Chest Med 1991; 12:507–21.
14. Weymuller EA Jr, Bishop MJ, Santos PM. Problems associated with prolonged intubation in the geriatric patient. Otolaryngol Clin North Am 1990; 23:1057–74. [published erratum in Otolaryngol Clin North Am 1991; 24(6):xi]
15. Stauffer JL. Complications of endotracheal intubation and tracheotomy. Respir Care 1999; 44:828–43.
16. Loh KS, Irish JC. Traumatic complications of intubation and other airway management techniques. Anesthesiol Clin North Am 2002; 20:953–69.
17. Weber S. Traumatic complications of airway management. Anesthesiol Clin North Am 2002; 20:503–12.
18. Sue RD, Susanto I. Long-term complications of artificial airways. Clin Chest Med 2003; 24:457–71.
19. Stewart RD, Paris PM, Winter PM, et al. Field endotracheal intubation by paramedical personnel. Success rates and complications. Chest 1984; 85:341–45.
20. Adnet F, Jouriles NJ, LeToumelin P, et al. Survey of out-of-hospital emergency intubations in the French prehospital medical system: a multicenter study. Ann Emerg Med 1998; 32:454–60.
21. Taryle DA, Chandler JE, Good JT Jr, et al. Emergency room intubations—complications and survival. Chest 1979; 75:541–43.
22. Sakles JC, Laurin EG, Rantapaa AA, et al. Airway management in the emergency department: a one-year study of 610 tracheal intubations. Ann Emerg Med 1998; 31:325–32.
23. Stauffer JL, Olson DE, Petty TL. Complications and consequences of endotracheal intubation and tracheotomy: a prospective study of 150 critically ill adults. Am J Med 1981; 70: 65–76.
24. Astrachan DI, Kirchner JC, Goodwin WJ Jr. Prolonged intubation vs. tracheotomy: complications, practical and psychological considerations. Laryngoscope 1988; 98:1165–69.
25. Roppolo LP, Vilke GM, Chan TC, et al. Nasotracheal intubation in the emergency department, revisited. J Emerg Med 1999; 17:791–99.
26. Knuth TE, Richards JR. Mainstem bronchial obstruction secondary to nasotracheal intubation: a case report and review of the literature. Anesth Analg 1991; 73:487–89.
27. Binning R. A hazard of blind nasal intubation. Anaesthesia 1974; 29:366–67.
28. Marlow TJ, Goltra DJ Jr, Schabel SI. Intracranial placement of a nasotracheal tube after facial fracture: a rare complication. J Emerg Med 1997; 15:187–91.
29. Lockhart PB, Feldbau EV, Gabel RA, et al. Dental complications during and after tracheal intubation. J Am Dent Assoc 1986; 112:480–83.
30. Eichhorn JH. Prevention of intraoperative anesthesia accidents and related severe injury through safety monitoring. Anesthesiology 1989; 70:572–77.
31. Domino KB, Posner KL, Caplan RA, et al. Airway injury during anesthesia. A closed claims analysis. Anesthesiology 1999; 91:1703–11.
32. Majumdar B, Stevens RW, Obara LG. Retropharyngeal abscess following tracheal intubation. Anaesthesia 1982; 37: 67–70.
33. Rashkin MC, Davis T. Acute complications of endotracheal intubation: relationship to reintubation, route, urgency, and duration. Chest 1986; 89:165–67.
34. Woodcock SAA, Bird H, Siriwardena AK, et al. Hypopharyngeal perforation: an uncommon cause of pneumoperitoneum. Emerg Med J 2001; 18:396–98.
35. Myers EM. Hypopharyngeal perforation: a complication of endotracheal intubation. Laryngoscope 1982; 92:583–85.

36. Levine PA. Hypopharyngeal perforation: an untoward complication of endotracheal intubation. Arch Otolaryngol 1980; 106:578–80.

37. Stauffer JL, Petty TL. Accidental intubation of the pyriform sinus: a complication of "roadside" resuscitation. JAMA 1977; 237:2324–25.

38. Hawkins DB, Seltzer DC, Barnett TE, et al. Endotracheal tube perforation of the hypopharynx. West J Med 1974; 120:282–86.

39. Wolff AP, Kuhn FA, Ogura JH. Pharyngeal-esophageal perforations associated with rapid oral endotracheal intubation. Ann Otol Rhinol Laryngol 1972; 81:258–61.

40. O'Neill JE, Giffin JP, Cottrell JP. Pharyngeal and esophageal perforation following endotracheal intubation. Anesthesiology 1984; 60:487–88.

41. Lee T, Jordan J. Pyriform sinus perforation secondary to traumatic intubation in a difficult airway patient. J Clin Anesth 1996; 6:152–55.

42. Pena MT, Aujla PK, Choi SS, et al. Acute airway distress from endotracheal intubation injury in the pediatric aerodigestive tract. Otolaryngol Head Neck Surg 2004; 130:575–78.

43. Kambic V, Radsel Z. Intubation lesions of the larynx. Br J Anaesth 1978; 50:587–90.

44. Peppard SB, Dickens JH. Laryngeal injury following short-term intubation. Ann Otol Rhinol Laryngol 1983; 92:327–30.

45. Quartararo C, Bishop MJ. Complications of tracheal intubation: prevention and treatment. Semin Anesth 1990; 9:119–27.

46. Donnelly WA, Grossman AA, Grem FM. Local sequela of endotracheal anesthesia as observed by examination of one hundred patients. Anesthesiology 1948; 9:490–97.

47. Cheng KS, Li HY. Epiglottic hematoma secondary to endotracheal intubation. Acta Anaesthesiol Sinica 1999; 37:49–52.

48. Brown I, Kleinman B. Epiglottic hematoma leading to airway obstruction after general anesthesia. J Clin Anesth 2002; 14:34–35.

49. Burns HP, Dayal VS, Scott A, et al. Laryngotracheal trauma: observations on its pathogenesis and its prevention following prolonged orotracheal intubation in the adult. Laryngoscope 1979; 89:1316–25.

50. Castella X, Gilabert J, Perez C. Arytenoid dislocation after tracheal intubation: an unusual cause of acute respiratory failure? Anesthesiology 1991; 75:613–15.

51. Colice GL, Stukel TA, Dain B. Laryngeal complications of prolonged intubation. Chest 1989; 96:877–84.

52. Orta DA, Cousar JE III, Yergin BM, et al. Tracheal laceration with massive subcutaneous emphysema: a rare complication of endotracheal intubation. Thorax 1979; 34:665–69.

53. Thompson DS, Read RC. Rupture of the trachea following endotracheal intubation. JAMA 1968; 204:137–39.

54. Sternfeld D, Wright S. Tracheal rupture and the creation of a false passage after emergency intubation. Ann Emerg Med 2003; 42:88–92.

55. Fan C-M, Ko PC-I, Tsai K-C, et al. Tracheal rupture complicating emergent endotracheal intubation. Am J Emerg Med 2004; 22:289–93.

56. Chen EH, Logman ZM, Glass PSA, et al. A case of tracheal injury after emergent endotracheal intubation: a review of the literature and causalities. Anesth Analg 2001; 93:1270–71.

57. Meyer M. Iatrogenic tracheobronchial lesions—a report on 13 cases. Thorac Cardiovasc Surg 2001; 49:115–19.

58. Harris R, Joseph A. Acute tracheal rupture related to endotracheal intubation: case report. J Emerg Med 2000; 18:35–39.

59. Schwartz DE, Lieberman JA, Cohen NH. Women are at greater risk than men for malpositioning of the endotracheal tube after emergent intubation. Crit Care Med 1994; 23:1306–8.

60. Zwillich CW, Pierson DJ, Creagh CE, et al. Complications of assisted ventilation: a prospective study of 354 consecutive episodes. Am J Med 1974; 57:161–70.

61. Owen RL, Cheney FW. Endobronchial intubation: a preventable complication. Anesthesiology 1987; 67:255–57.

62. Schwartz DE, Matthay MA, Cohen NH. Death and other complications of emergency airway management in critically ill adults. Anesthesiology 1995; 82:367–76.

63. Mort TC. Emergency tracheal intubation: complications associated with repeated laryngoscopic attempts. Anesth Analg 2004; 99:607–13.

64. Mateer JR, Olson DW, Stueven HA, et al. Continuous pulse oximetry during emergency endotracheal intubation. Ann Emerg Med 1993; 22:675–79.

65. Scarbrough FE, Wittenberg JM, Smith BR, et al. Pulmonary edema following postoperative laryngospasm: case reports and review of the literature. Anesth Prog 1997; 44:110–16.

66. McConkey PP. Postobstructive pulmonary oedema—a case series and review. Anaesth Intensive Care 2000; 28:72–76.

67. Dinner M, Tjeuw M, Atrusio JF Jr. Bacteremia as a complication of nasotracheal intubation. Anesth Analg 1987; 66:460–62.

68. Berry FA Jr, Blankenbaker WL, Ball CG. A comparison of bacteremia occurring with nasotracheal and orotracheal intubation. Anesth Analg 1973; 52:873–76.

69. Goldstein S, Wolf GL, Kim SJ, et al. Bacteraemia during direct laryngoscopy and endotracheal intubation: a study using a multiple culture, large volume technique. Anaesth Intensive Care 1997; 25:239–44.

70. Rijinders BJ, Wilmer A, Van Eldere J, et al. Frequency of transient streptococcal bacteremia following urgent orotracheal intubation in critically ill patients. Intensive Care Med 2001; 27:434–37.

71. Pillay SP, Ward M, Cowen A, et al. Oesophageal ruptures and perforations—a review. Med J Aust 1989; 150:246–52.

72. Hilmi IA, Sullivan E, Quinlan J, et al. Esophageal tear: an unusual complication after difficult endotracheal intubation. Anesth Analg 2003; 97:911–14.

73. Caplan RA, Posner KL, Ward RJ, et al. Adverse respiratory events in anesthesia: a closed claims analysis. Anesthesiology 1990; 72:48–53.

74. Williamson JA, Webb RK, Szekely S, et al. The Australian Incident Monitoring Study. Difficult intubation: an analysis of 2000 incident reports. Anaesth Intensive Care 1993; 21:602–607.

75. Keenan RL, Boyan CP. Cardiac arrest due to anesthesia: a study of incidence and causes. JAMA 1985; 253:2373–77.

76. Kroesen GA, Haid BC. Fatal complication from swallowed denture following prolonged endotracheal intubation: a case report. Anesth Analg 1976; 55:438–39.

77. Majernick TG, Bieniek R, Houston JB, et al. Cervical spine movement during orotracheal intubation. Ann Emerg Med 1986; 15:417–20.

78. Shapiro HM, Wyte SR, Harris AB, et al. Acute intraoperative intracranial hypertension in neurosurgical patients. Anesthesiology 1972; 37:399–405.

79. Robinson N, Clancy M. In patients with head injury undergoing rapid sequence intubation, does pretreatment with intravenous lignocaine/lidocaine lead to an improved neurological outcome? A review of the literature. Emerg Med J 2001; 18:453–57.

80. Fox EJ, Sklar GS, Hill CH, et al. Complications related to the pressor response to endotracheal intubation. Anesthesiology 1977; 47:524–25.

81. Kaplan JD, Schuster DP. Physiologic consequences of tracheal intubation. Clin Chest Med 1991; 12:425–32.

82. Derbyshire DR, Chmielewski A, Fell D, et al. Plasma catecholamine responses to tracheal intubation. Br J Anaesth 1983; 55:855–60.

83. Fugii Y, Tanaka H, Toyooka H. Circulatory responses to laryngeal mask airway insertion or tracheal intubation in normotensive and hypertensive patients. Can J Anaesth 1995; 42:32–36.

84. Abou-Madi MN, Keszler H, Yacoub JM. Cardiovascular reactions to laryngoscopy and tracheal intubation following small and large intravenous doses of lidocaine. Can Anaesth Soc J 1977; 24:12–19.

85. Oczenski W, Krenn H, Dahaba AA, et al. Hemodynamic and catecholamine stress responses to insertion of the Combitube, laryngeal mask airway or tracheal intubation. Anesth Analg 1999; 88:1389–94.

86. Barak M, Ziser A, Greenberg A, et al. Hemodynamic and catecholamine response to tracheal intubation: direct laryngoscopy compared with fiberoptic intubation. J Clin Anesth 2003; 15:132–36.

87. Pernerstorfer T, Krafft P, Fitzgerald RD, et al. Stress response to tracheal intubation: direct laryngoscopy compared with blind oral intubation. Anaesthesia 1995; 50:17–22.

88. Singh S, Smith JE. Cardiovascular changes after the three stages of nasotracheal intubation. Br J Anaesth 2003; 91:667–71.

89. Khan FH, Khan FA, Irshad R, et al. Complications of endotracheal intubation in mechanically ventilated patients in a general intensive care unit. J Pak Med Assoc 1996; 46:195–98.

90. Franklin C, Samuel J, Hu TC. Life-threatening hypotension associated with emergency intubation and the initiation of mechanical ventilation. Am J Emerg Med 1994; 12:425–28.

91. MacKenzie RA, Gould AB Jr, Bardsley WT. Cardiac arrhythmias with endotracheal intubation. Anesthesiology 1980; 53:S102.

92. Biboulet P, Aubas P, Dubourdieu J, et al. Fatal and nonfatal cardiac arrests related to anesthesia. Can J Anaesth 2001; 48: 326–32.

93. Dixon TC, Sando MJW, Bolton JM, et al. A report of 342 cases of prolonged endotracheal intubation. Med J Aust 1968; 2:529–33.

94. Holdgaard HO, Pedersen J, Schurizek BA, et al. Complications and late sequelae following nasotracheal intubation. Acta Anaesth Scand 1993; 37:475–80.

95. Zwillich CW, Pierson DJ. Nasal necrosis: a complication of nasotracheal intubation. Chest 1973; 64:376–77.

96. O'Reilly MJ, Reddick EJ, Black W, et al. Sepsis from sinusitis in nasotracheally intubated patients: a diagnostic dilemma. Am J Surg 1984; 147:601–4.

97. Deutschman CS, Wilton P, Sinow J, et al. Paranasal sinusitis associated with nasotracheal intubation: a frequently unrecognized and treatable source of sepsis. Crit Care Med 1986; 14:111–14.

98. Fassoulaki A, Pamouktsoglou P. Prolonged nasotracheal intubation and its association with inflammation of paranasal sinuses. Anesth Analg 1989; 69:50–52.

99. Michelson A, Kamp H-D, Schuster B. Sinusitis in intensive care patients: nasal versus oral intubation. Anaesthetist 1991; 40:100–4.

100. Knodel AR, Beekman JF. Unexplained fevers in patients with nasotracheal intubation. JAMA 1982; 248:868–70.

101. Pope TL Jr, Stelling CB, Leitner YB. Maxillary sinusitis after nasotracheal intubation. South Med J 1981; 74:610–12.

102. Guerin JM, Meyer P, Habib Y, et al. Purulent rhinosinusitis is also a cause of sepsis in critically ill patients. Chest 1988; 93:893–94.

103. Grindlinger GA, Niehoff J, Hughes SL, et al. Acute paranasal sinusitis related to nasotracheal intubation of head-injured patients. Crit Care Med 1987; 15:214–17.

104. Gregory GA. Respiratory care of the child. Crit Care Med 1980; 8:582–87.

105. Bach A, Boehrer H, Schmidt H, et al. Nosocomial sinusitis in ventilated patients. Nasotracheal versus orotracheal intubation. Anaesthesia 1992; 47:335–39.

106. Linden BE, Aguilar EA, Allen SJ. Sinusitis in the nasotracheally intubated patient. Arch Otolaryngol Head Neck Surg 1988; 114:860–61.

107. Bert F, Lambert-Zechovsky N. Sinusitis in mechanically ventilated patients and its role in the pathogenesis of nosocomial pneumonia. Eur J Clin Microbiol Infect Dis 1996; 15:533–44.

108. Salord FP, Gaussorgues P, Marti-Flich J, et al. Nosocomial maxillary sinusitis during mechanical ventilation: a prospective comparison of orotracheal versus the nasotracheal route for intubation. Intensive Care Med 1990; 16:390–93.

109. Rouby JJ, Laurent P, Gosnach M, et al. Risk factors and clinical relevance of nosocomial maxillary sinusitis in the critically ill. Am J Respir Crit Care Med 1994; 150:776–83.

110. Lew HL, Han J, Robinson LR, et al. Occult maxillary sinusitis as a cause of fever in tetraplegia: 2 case reports. Arch Phys Med Rehabil 2002; 83:430–32.

111. Holzapfel L, Chevret S, Madinier G, et al. Influence of long-term oro- or nasotracheal intubation on nosocomial maxillary sinusitis and pneumonia: results of a prospective, randomized, clinical trial. Crit Care Med 1993; 21:1132–38.

112. Berman SA, Balkany TJ, Simmons MA. Otitis media in the neonatal intensive care unit. Pediatrics 1978; 62:198–201.

113. Persico M, Barker GA, Mitchell DP. Purulent otitis media—a "silent" source of sepsis in the pediatric intensive care unit. Otolaryngol Head Neck Surg 1985; 93:330–34.

114. Engel J, Mahler E, Anteunis L, et al. Why are NICU infants at risk for chronic otitis media with effusion? Int J Pediatr Otorhinolaryngol 2001; 57:137–44.

115. Cavaliere F, Masieri S, Liberini L, et al. Tympanometry for middle-ear effusion in unconscious ICU patients. Eur J Anaesthesiol 1992; 9:71–75.

116. Lucks D, Consiglio A, Stankiewicz J, et al. Incidence and microbiologic etiology of middle ear effusion complicating endotracheal intubation and mechanical ventilation. J Infect Dis 1988; 157:368–69.

117. Christensen L, Schaffer S, Ross SE. Otitis media in adult trauma patients: incidence and clinical significance. J Trauma 1991; 31:1543–45.

118. Stauffer JL. Monitoring the use of tracheal tubes. In: Tobin MJ, editor. Principles and practice of intensive care monitoring. New York: McGraw-Hill, 1998: 667–82.

119. Hanley PJ, Conaway MM, Halstead DC, et al. Nosocomial herpes simplex virus infection associated with oral endotracheal intubation. Am J Infect Control 1993; 21:310–16.

120. Stauffer JL, Petty TL. Cleft tongue and ulceration of the hard palate: complications of oral intubation. Chest 1978; 74: 317–18.

121. Whited RE. Laryngeal dysfunction following prolonged intubation. Ann Otol Rhinol Laryngol 1979; 88:474–78.

122. Whited RE. Posterior commissure stenosis post long-term intubation. Laryngoscope 1983; 93:1314–18.

123. Whited RE. A prospective study of laryngotracheal sequelae in long-term intubation. Laryngoscope 1984; 94:367–77.

124. Kastanos N, Miro RE, Perez AM, et al. Laryngotracheal injury due to endotracheal intubation: incidence, evolution, and predisposing factors. A prospective long-term study. Crit Care Med 1983; 11:362–67.

125. El-Naggar M, Sadagopan S, Levine H, et al. Factors influencing choice between tracheostomy and prolonged translaryngeal intubation in acute respiratory failure. Anesth Analg 1976; 55:195–201.

126. Deane RS, Shinozaki T, Morgan JG. An evaluation of the cuff characteristics and incidence of laryngeal complications using a new nasotracheal tube in prolonged intubations. J Trauma 1977; 17:311–14.

127. Lindholm C-E. Prolonged endotracheal intubation. Acta Anaesthesiol Scand Suppl 1969; 33:1–131.

128. Donnelly WH. Histopathology of endotracheal intubation: an autopsy study of 99 cases. Arch Pathol 1969; 88:511–20.

129. Sellery GR, Worth A, Greenway RE. Late complications of prolonged tracheal intubation. Can Anaesth Soc J 1978; 25:140–43.

130. Deane RS, Mills EL. Prolonged nasotracheal intubation in adults: a successor and adjunct to tracheostomy. Anesth Analg 1970; 49:89–97.

131. Harley HRS. Ulcerative tracheo-oesophageal fistula during treatment by tracheostomy and intermittent positive pressure ventilation. Thorax 1972; 27:338–52.

132. Dubick MN, Wright BD. Comparison of laryngeal pathology following long-term oral and nasal endotracheal intubations. Anesth Analg 1978; 57:663–68.

133. Dubick MN, Wright BD. Problems with prolonged endotracheal intubations. Chest 1978; 74:479–80.

134. Baron SH, Kohlmoos HW. Laryngeal sequelae of endotracheal anesthesia. Anesth Analg 1975; 54:767–72.

135. Stauffer JL. Establishment and care of the airway. In: Petty TL, editor. Intensive and rehabilitative respiratory care. Philadelphia: Lea & Febiger, 1982: 22–73.

136. Tonkin JP, Harrison GA. The surgical management of the laryngeal complications of prolonged intubation. Laryngoscope 1977; 87:339–46.

137. Colice GL. Resolution of laryngeal injury following translaryngeal intubation. Am Rev Respir Dis 1992; 145:361–64.

138. Santos PM, Afrassiabi A, Weymuller EA Jr. Risk factors associated with prolonged intubation and laryngeal injury. Otolaryngol Head Neck Surg 1994; 111:453–59.

139. Bergstrom J, Moberg A, Orell SR. On the pathogenesis of laryngeal injuries following prolonged intubation. Acta Otolaryngol 1962; 55:342–46.

140. Hedden M, Ersoz CJ, Donnelly WH, et al. Laryngotracheal damage after prolonged use of orotracheal tubes in adults. JAMA 1969; 207:703–8.

141. Vila J, Bosque MD, Garcia M, et al. Endoscopic evolution of laryngeal injuries caused by translaryngeal intubation. Eur Arch Otorhinolaryngol 1997; 254(Suppl 1):S97–S100.

142. Briggs BD. Prolonged endotracheal intubation. Anesthesiology 1950; 11:129–31.

143. Jackson C. Contact ulcer granuloma and other laryngeal complications of endotracheal anesthesia. Anesthesiology 1953; 14:425–36.

144. Deeb ZE, William JB, Campbell TE. Early diagnosis and treatment of laryngeal injuries from prolonged intubation in adults. Otolaryngol Head Neck Surg 1999; 120:25–29.

145. Kaneda N, Goto R, Ishijima S, et al. Laryngeal granuloma caused by short-term endotracheal intubation. Anesthesiology 1999; 90:1482–83.

146. Paegle RD, Bernhard WN. Squamous metaplasia of tracheal epithelium associated with high-volume, low-pressure airway cuffs. Anesth Analg 1975; 54:340–44.

147. Belson TP. Cuff induced tracheal injury in dogs following prolonged intubation. Laryngoscope 1983; 93:549–55.

148. Cooper JD, Grillo HC. Experimental production and prevention of injury due to cuffed tracheal tubes. Surg Gynecol Obstet 1969; 129:1235–41.

149. Grillo HC, Cooper JD, Geffin B, et al. A low-pressure cuff for tracheostomy tubes to minimize tracheal injury: a comparative clinical trial. J Thorac Cardiovasc Surg 1971; 62:898–907.

150. Loeser EA, Hodges M, Gliedman J, et al. Tracheal pathology following short term intubation with low- and high-pressure endotracheal tube cuffs. Anesth Analg 1978; 57:577–79.

151. Abbey NC, Green DE, Cicale MJ. Massive tracheal necrosis complicating endotracheal intubation. Chest 1989; 95:459–60.

152. Khan F, Reddy NC. Enlarging intratracheal tube cuff diameter: A quantitative roentgenographic study of its value in the early prediction of serious tracheal damage. Ann Thorac Surg 1977; 24:49–53.

153. Honig EG, Francis PB. Persistent tracheal dilatation: onset after brief mechanical ventilation with a "soft-cuff" endotracheal tube. South Med J 1979; 72:487–89.

154. Fryer ME, Marshall RD. Tracheal dilatation. Anaesthesia 1976; 31:470–78.

155. Rhodes A, Lamb FJ, Grounds RM, et al. Tracheal dilatation complicating prolonged tracheal intubation. Anaesthesia 1997; 52:70–72.

156. Feist JH, Johnson TH, Wilson RJ. Acquired tracheomalacia: Etiology and differential diagnosis. Chest 1975; 68:340–45.

157. Geha AS, Seegers JV, Kodner IJ, et al. Tracheoesophageal fistula caused by cuffed tracheal tube: successful treatment by tracheal resection and primary repair with four-year follow-up. Arch Surg 1978; 113:338–40.

158. Reed MF, Mathisen DJ. Tracheoesophageal fistula. Chest Surg Clin N Am 2003; 13:271–89.

159. Payne DK, Anderson WM, Romero MD, et al. Tracheoesophageal fistula formation in intubated patients. Risk factors and treatment with high-frequency jet ventilation. Chest 1990; 98:161–64.

160. Bugge-Asperheim B, Birkeland S, Storen G. Tracheo-oesophageal fistula caused by cuffed tracheal tubes. Scand J Thorac Cardiovasc Surg 1981; 15:315–19.

161. Wolf M, Yellin A, Talmi YP, et al. Acquired tracheoesophageal fistula in critically ill patients. Ann Otol Rhinol Laryngol 2000; 109:731–35.

162. Tessler S, Kupfer Y, Lerman A, et al. Massive gastric distention in the intubated patient. A marker for a defective airway. Arch Intern Med 1990; 150:318–20.

163. Rinecker H, Schvetz T. Arterio-tracheal fistula during long-term intubation of an awake patient. Case report. Anaesthetist 1979; 28:180–81.

164. LoCicero J 3rd. Tracheo-carotid artery erosion following endotracheal intubation. J Trauma 1984; 24:907–09.

165. Siobal M, Kallet RH, Kraemer R, et al. Tracheal-innominate artery fistula caused by the endotracheal tube tip: case report and investigation of a fatal complication of prolonged intubation. Respir Care 2001; 46:1012–18.

166. Hilding AC. Laryngotracheal damage during intratracheal anesthesia. Ann Otol Rhinol Laryngol 1971; 80:565–81.

167. Klainer AS, Turndorf H, Wu W, et al. Surface alterations due to endotracheal intubation. Am J Med 1975; 58:674–83.

168. Sanada Y, Kojima Y, Fonkalsrud EW. Injury of cilia induced by tracheal tube cuffs. Surg Gynecol Obstet 1982; 154:648–52.

169. Konrad F, Scheiner R, Marx T, et al. Ultrastructure and mucociliary transport of bronchial respiratory epithelium in intubated patients. Intensive Care Med 1995; 21:482–89.

170. Severson JM, Ketter GW, Belson TP, et al. Experimental induction of squamous metaplasia in the dog trachea with cuffed endotracheal tubes. Otolaryngol Head Neck Surg 1982; 90:555–60.

171. Paegle RD, Ayres SM, Davis S. Rapid tracheal injury by cuffed airways and healing with loss of ciliated epithelium. Arch Surg 1973; 106:31–34.

172. Ben-Izhak O, Ben-Arieh Y. Necrotizing squamous metaplasia in herpetic tracheitis following prolonged intubation: a lesion similar to necrotizing sialometaplasia. Histopathology 1993; 22:265–69.

173. Pingleton SK, Hinthorn DR, Liu C. Enteral nutrition in patients receiving mechanical ventilation: multiple sources of tracheal colonization include the stomach. Am J Med 1986; 80:827–32.

174. Schwartz SN, Dowling JN, Benkovic C, et al. Sources of gram-negative bacilli colonizing the tracheae of intubated patients. J Infect Dis 1978; 138:227–31.

175. Niederman MS, Mantovani R, Schoch P, et al. Patterns and routes of tracheobronchial colonization in mechanically ventilated patients. The role of nutritional status in colonization

of the lower airway by *Pseudomonas* species. Chest 1989; 95: 155–61.

176. American Thoracic Society. Guidelines for the management of adults with hospital-acquired, ventilator-associated, and healthcare-associated pneumonia. Am J Respir Crit Care Med 2005; 171:388–416.

177. Kollef MH. Prevention of hospital-associated pneumonia and ventilator-associated pneumonia. Crit Care Med 2004; 32:1396–405.

178. Harbison J, Collins D, Lynch V, et al. Acute stridor due to an upper tracheal membrane following endotracheal intubation. Eur Respir J 1999; 14:1238.

179. Deslee G, Brichet A, Lebuffe G, et al. Obstructive fibrinous tracheal pseudomembrane. A potentially fatal complication of tracheal intubation. Am J Respir Crit Care Med 2000; 162:1169–71.

180. Bryant LR, Trinkle JK, Mobin-Uddin K, et al. Bacterial colonization profile with tracheal intubation and mechanical ventilation. Arch Surg 1972; 104:647–51.

181. Stauffer JL. Medical management of the airway. Clin Chest Med 1991; 12:449–82.

182. Kollef MH, Legare EJ, Damiano M. Endotracheal tube misplacement: Incidence, risk factors, and impact of a quality improvement program. South Med J 1994; 87:248–54.

183. Treloar DM, Stechmiller J. Pulmonary aspiration in tube-fed patients with artificial airways. Heart Lung 1984; 13:667–71.

184. Bernhard WN, Cottrell JE, Sivakumaran C, et al. Adjustment of intracuff pressure to prevent aspiration. Anesthesiology 1979; 50:363–66.

185. Pavlin EG, VanNimwegan D, Hornbein TF. Failure of a high-compliance low-pressure cuff to prevent aspiration. Anesthesiology 1975; 42:216–19.

186. Elpern EH, Jacobs ER, Bone RC. Incidence of aspiration in tracheally intubated patients. Heart Lung 1987; 16:527–31.

187. Spray SB, Zuidema GD, Cameron JL. Aspiration pneumonia. Incidence of aspiration with endotracheal tubes. Am J Surg 1976; 131:701–3.

188. Chastre J, Fagon J-Y. Ventilator-associated pneumonia. Am J Respir Crit Care Med 2002; 165:867–903.

189. Rello J, Ollendorf DA, Oster G, et al. Epidemiology and outcomes of ventilator-associated pneumonia in a large US database. Chest 2002; 122:2115–21.

190. Gal TJ. Effects of endotracheal intubation on normal cough performance. Anesthesiology 1980; 52:324–29.

191. Habib MP. Physiologic implications of artificial airways. Chest 1989; 96:180–84.

192. Bergbom-Engberg I, Haljamae H. Assessment of patients' experience of discomforts during respirator therapy. Crit Care Med 1989; 17:1068–72.

193. Swaiss IG, Badran I. Discomfort, awareness and recall in the intensive care—still a problem? Middle East J Anesthesiol 2004; 17:951–58.

194. Coppolo DP, May JJ. Self-extubations: a 12-month experience. Chest 1990; 98:165–69.

195. Jayamanne D, Nandipati R, Patel D. Self-extubation: a prospective study. Chest 1988; 94:3S (abstract).

196. Ripoll I, Lindholm C-E, Carroll R, et al. Spontaneous dislocation of endotracheal tubes. Anesthesiology 1978; 49:50–52.

197. Frezza EE, Carleton GL, Valenziano CP, et al. A quality improvement and risk management initiative for surgical ICU patients: a study of the effects of physical restraints and sedation on the incidence of self-extubation. Am J Med Qual 2000; 15:221–25.

198. Listello D, Sessler CN. Unplanned extubation. Clinical predictors for reintubation. Chest 1994; 105:1496–503.

199. Kapadia FN, Bajan KB, Raje KV. Airway accidents in intubated intensive care unit patients: an epidemiological study. Crit Care Med 2000; 28:659–64.

200. Epstein SK, Nevins ML, Chung J. Effect of unplanned extubation on outcome of mechanical ventilation. Am J Respir Crit Care Med 2000; 161:1912–16.

201. Chevron V, Menard JF, Richard JC, et al. Unplanned extubation: risk factors of development and predictive criteria for reintubation. Crit Care Med 1998; 26:1049–53.

202. Tung A, Tadimeti L, Caruana-Montaldo B, et al. The relationship of sedation to deliberate self-extubation. J Clin Anesth 2001; 13:24–29.

203. Betbese A-J, Perez M, Bak E, et al. A prospective study of unplanned endotracheal extubation in intensive care unit patients. Crit Care Med 1998; 26:1180–86.

204. de Lassence A, Alberti C, Azoulay E, et al. Impact of unplanned extubation and reintubation after weaning on nosocomial pneumonia risk in the intensive care unit. Anesthesiology 2002; 97:148–56.

205. Atkins PM, Mion LC, Mendelsom W, et al. Characteristics and outcomes of patients who self-extubate from ventilatory support. A case control study. Chest 1997; 112:1317–23.

206. Beckmann U, Gillies DM. Factors associated with reintubation in intensive care. An analysis of causes and outcomes. Chest 2001; 120:538–42.

207. Conrardy PA, Goodman LR, Laing F, et al. Alteration of endotracheal tube position. Flexion and extension of the neck. Crit Care Med 1976; 4:8–12.

208. Job CA, Betcher AM, Pearson WT, et al. Intraoperative obstruction of endobronchial tubes. Anesthesiology 1979; 51:550–53.

209. Hitchen JE, Wiener AP. Unexpected obstruction of a nasotracheal tube: a case report. J Oral Surg 1973; 31:722–24.

210. Kemmotsu O. Six cases of endotracheal tube obstructions. Masui 1971; 20:259–64.

211. Barat G, Ascorve A, Avello F. Unusual airway obstruction during pneumonectomy. Anaesthesia 1976; 31:1290–91.

212. Glinsman D, Pavlin EG. Airway obstruction after nasal-tracheal intubation. Anesthesiology 1982; 56:229–30.

213. Villafane MC, Cinnella G, Lofaso F, et al. Gradual reduction of endotracheal tube diameter during mechanical ventilation via different humidification devices. Anesthesiology 1996; 85:1341–49.

214. Cohen IL, Weinberg PF, Fein IA, et al. Endotracheal tube occlusion associated with the use of heat and moisture exchangers in the intensive care unit. Crit Care Med 1988; 16: 277–79.

215. Thiery G, Boyer A, Pigne E, et al. Heat and moisture exchangers in mechanically ventilated intensive care unit patients: a plea for independent assessment of their performance. Crit Care Med 2003; 31:699–704.

216. Vyas D, Inweregbu K, Pitard A. Measurement of tracheal tube cuff pressure in critical care. Anaesthesia 2002; 57:275–77.

217. Gal TJ, Suratt PM. Resistance to breathing in healthy subjects following endotracheal intubation under topical anesthesia. Anesth Analg 1980; 59:270–74.

218. Gal TJ. Pulmonary mechanics in normal subjects following endotracheal intubation. Anesthesiology 1980; 52:27–35.

219. Kim ES, Bishop MJ. Endotracheal intubation, but not laryngeal mask airway insertion, produces reversible bronchoconstriction. Anesthesiology 1999; 90:391–94.

220. Kil HK, Rooke GA, Ryan-Dykes MA, et al. Effect of prophylactic bronchodilator treatment on lung resistance after tracheal intubation. Anesthesiology 1994; 81:43–48.

221. Bock KR, Silver P, Rom M, et al. Reduction in tracheal lumen due to endotracheal intubation and its calculated clinical significance. Chest 2000; 118:468–72.

222. Bolder PM, Healy TEJ, Bolder AR, et al. The extra work of breathing through adult endotracheal tubes. Anesth Analg 1986; 65:853–59.

223. Plost J, Campbell SC. The non-elastic work of breathing through endotracheal tubes of various sizes. Am Rev Respir Dis 1984; 129:A106 (abstract).

224. Shapiro M, Wilson K, Casar G, et al. Work of breathing through different sized endotracheal tubes. Crit Care Med 1986; 14:1028–31.

225. Jones GOM, Hale DE, Wasmuth CE, et al. A survey of acute complications associated with endotracheal intubation. Cleve Clin Q 1968; 35:23–31.

226. Rieger A, Brunne B, Hass I, et al. Laryngo-pharyngeal complaints following laryngeal mask airway and endotracheal intubation. J Clin Anesth 1997; 9:42–47.

227. Thomas R, Kumar EV, Kameswaran M, et al. Post intubation laryngeal sequelae in an intensive care unit. J Laryngol Otol 1995; 109:313–16.

228. Mackenzie CF, Shin B, McAslan TC, et al. Severe stridor after prolonged endotracheal intubation using high-volume cuffs. Anesthesiology 1979; 50:235–39.

229. Jaber S, Chanques G, Matecki S, et al. Post-extubation stridor in intensive care unit patients. Risk factors evaluation and importance of the cuff-leak test. Intensive Care Med 2003; 29:69–74.

230. Efferen LS, Elsakr A. Post-extubation stridor: risk factors and outcome. J Assoc Acad Minor Phys 1998; 9:65–68.

231. Burgess GE, Cooper JR Jr, Marino RJ, et al. Laryngeal competence after tracheal extubation. Anesthesiology 1979; 51:73–77.

232. Tomlin PJ, Howarth FH, Robinson JS. Postoperative atelectasis and laryngeal incompetence. Lancet 1968; 1:1402–05.

233. Brandwein M, Abramson AL, Shilkowitz MJ. Bilateral vocal cord paralysis following endotracheal intubation. Arch Otolaryngol Head Neck Surg 1986; 112:877–82.

234. Hahn FW, Martin JT, Lillie JC. Vocal cord paralysis with endotracheal intubation. Arch Otolaryngol 1970; 92:226–29.

235. Holley HS, Gildea JE. Vocal cord paralysis after tracheal intubation. JAMA 1971; 215:281–84.

236. Wason R, Gupta P, Gogia AR. Bilateral adductor vocal cord paresis following endotracheal intubation for general anesthesia. Anaesth Intensive Care 2004; 32:417–18.

237. Barquist E, Brown M, Cohn S, et al. Postextubation fiberoptic endoscopic evaluation of swallowing after prolonged endotracheal intubation: A randomized, prospective trial. Crit Care Med 2001; 29:1710–13.

238. Leder SB, Cohn SM, Moller BA. Fiberoptic endoscopic documentation of the high incidence of aspiration following extubation in critically ill trauma patients. Dysphagia 1998; 13:208–12.

239. Bogdasarian RS, Olson NR. Posterior glottic laryngeal stenosis. Otolaryngol Head Neck Surg 1980; 88:765–72.

240. Streitz JM Jr, Shapshay SM. Airway injury after tracheotomy and endotracheal intubation. Surg Clin North Am 1991; 71:1211–30.

241. Bishop MJ, Weymuller EA Jr, Fink BR. Laryngeal effects of prolonged intubation. Anesth Analg 1984; 63:335–42.

242. Elliott CG, Rasmusson BY, Crapo RO. Upper airway obstruction following adult respiratory distress syndrome: an analysis of 30 survivors. Chest 1988; 94:526–30.

243. Richard I, Giraud M, Perrouin-Verbe B, et al. Laryngotracheal stenosis after intubation or tracheostomy in patients with neurological disease. Arch Phys Med Rehabil 1996;77:493–96.

244. Pecora DV, Seinige U. Prolonged endotracheal intubation. Chest 1982; 82:130.

245. Supance JS, Reilly JS, Doyle WJ, et al. Acquired subglottic stenosis following prolonged endotracheal intubation. Arch Otolaryngol 1982; 108:727–31.

246. Balestrieri F, Watson CB. Intubation granuloma. Otolaryngol Clin North Am 1982; 15:567–69.

247. Panda NK, Mann SB, Raja BA, et al. Fibreoptic assessment of post intubation laryngotracheal injuries. Indian J Chest Dis Allied Sci 1996; 38:241–47.

248. Weber AL, Grillo HC. Tracheal stenosis. An analysis of 151 cases. Radiol Clin North Am 1978; 16:291–308.

249. Arola MK, Inberg MV, Puhakka H. Tracheal stenosis after tracheostomy and after orotracheal cuffed intubation. Acta Chir Scand 1981; 147:183–92.

250. Brooks R, Bartlett RH, Gazzaniga AB. Management of acute and chronic disorders of the trachea and subglottis. Am J Surg 1985; 150:24–31.

251. Colice G, Matthay RA. Current guidelines for doing tracheal intubation. J Respir Dis 1982; 3:43–60.

252. Dobrin P, Canfield T. Cuffed endotracheal tubes: mucosal pressures and tracheal wall blood flow. Am J Surg 1977; 133:562–68.

253. Leigh JM, Maynard JP. Pressure on the tracheal mucosa from cuffed tubes. BMJ 1979; 1:1173–74.

254. Dobrin PB, Goldberg EM, Canfield TR. The endotracheal cuff: A comparative study. Anesth Analg 1974; 53:456–60.

255. Nordin U, Lindholm C-E, Wolgast M. Blood flow in the rabbit tracheal mucosa under normal conditions and under the influence of tracheal intubation. Acta Anaesthesiol Scand 1977; 21:81–94.

256. Seegobin RD, van Hasselt GL. Endotracheal cuff pressure and tracheal mucosal blood flow: endoscopic study of effects of four large volume cuffs. BMJ 1984; 288:965–68.

257. Nordin U. The trachea and cuff-induced tracheal injury. An experimental study on causative factors and prevention. Acta Otolaryngol 1977; Suppl 345:1–71.

258. Knowlson GTG, Bassett HFM. The pressures exerted on the trachea by endotracheal inflatable cuffs. Br J Anaesth 1970; 42:834–37.

259. Whited RE. A study of endotracheal tube injury to the subglottis. Laryngoscope 1985; 95:1216–19.

260. Reali-Forster C, Kolobow T, Giacomini M, et al. New ultrathin-walled endotracheal tube with a novel laryngeal seal design: long-term evaluation in sheep. Anesthesiology 1996; 84: 162–72.

261. Steen JA, Lindholm C-E, Brdlik GC, et al. Tracheal tube forces on the posterior larynx: index of laryngeal loading. Crit Care Med 1982; 10:186–89.

262. Weymuller EA Jr, Bishop MJ, Fink BR, et al. Quantification of intralaryngeal pressure exerted by endotracheal tubes. Ann Otol Rhinol Laryngol 1983; 92:444–47.

263. Lindholm C-E, Carroll RG. Evaluation of tube deformation pressure in vitro. Crit Care Med 1975; 3:196–99.

264. Paulsen FP, Jungmann K, Tillmann BN. The cricoarytenoid joint capsule and its relevance to endotracheal intubation. Anesth Analg 2000; 90:180–85.

265. Colice GL. Technical standards for tracheal tubes. Clin Chest Med 1991; 12:433–48.

266. Jaeger JM, Durbin CG Jr. Specialized endotracheal tubes. Clin Pulm Med 2001; 8:166–76.

267. Gaynor EB, Greenberg SB. Untoward sequelae of prolonged intubation. Laryngoscope 1985; 95:1461–67.

268. Bishop MJ. Mechanisms of laryngotracheal injury following prolonged tracheal intubation. Chest 1989; 96:185–86.

269. Stout DM, Bishop MJ, Dwersteg JF, et al. Correlation of endotracheal tube size with sore throat and hoarseness following general anesthesia. Anesthesiology 1987; 67:419–21.

270. Bernhard WN, Yost L, Joynes D, et al. Intracuff pressures in endotracheal and tracheostomy tubes: related cuff physical characteristics. Chest 1985; 87:720–25.

271. Poisson DM, Arbeille B, Laugier J. Electron microscopic studies of endotracheal tubes used in neonates: do microbes adhere to the polymer? Res Microbiol 1991; 142:1019–21.

272. Adair CG, Gorman SP, Feron BM, et al. Implications of endotracheal tube biofilm for ventilator-associated pneumonia. Intensive Care Med 1999; 25:1072–76.

273. Triandafillu K, Balazs DJ, Aronsson BO, et al. Adhesion of *Pseudomonas aeruginosa* strains of untreated and oxygen-plasma treated poly(vinyl chloride) (PVC) from endotracheal intubation devices. Biomaterials 2003; 24:1507–18.

274. Grimm JE, Knight RT. An improved intratracheal technique. Anesthesiology 1943; 4:6–11.

275. Cooper JD, Grillo HC. The evolution of tracheal injury due to ventilatory assistance through cuffed tubes: A pathologic study. Ann Surg 1969; 169:334–48.

276. Cooper JD, Grillo HC. Analysis of problems related to cuffs on intratracheal tubes. Chest 1972; 62:21S–27S.

277. Bernhard WN, Yost LC, Turndorf H, et al. Cuffed tracheal tubes—physical and behavioral characteristics. Anesth Analg 1982; 61:36–41.

278. Lee T-S, Hsu D. Ischemic damage to the trachea: lateral wall pressure versus intracuff pressure. Crit Care Med 1991; 19:1328.

279. Dunham CM, LaMonica C. Prolonged tracheal intubation in the trauma patient. J Trauma 1984; 24:120–24.

280. Tonkin JP, Harrison GA. The effect on the larynx of prolonged endotracheal intubation. Med J Aust 1966; 2:581–87.

281. Kuner J, Goldman A. Prolonged nasotracheal intubation in adults versus tracheostomy. Dis Chest 1967; 51:270.

282. Sandhu RS, Pasquale MD, Miller K, et al. Measurement of endotracheal tube cuff leak to predict postextubation stridor and need for reintubation. J Am Coll Surg 2000;190:682–87.

283. Bishop MJ, Hibbard AJ, Fink BR, et al. Laryngeal injury in a dog model of prolonged endotracheal intubation. Anesthesiology 1985; 62:770–73.

284. Weymuller EA Jr. Laryngeal injury from prolonged endotracheal intubation. Laryngoscope 1988; 98(Suppl 45):1–15.

285. Volpi D, Lin PT, Kuriloff DB, et al. Risk factors for intubation injury of the larynx. Ann Otol Rhinol Laryngol 1987; 96: 684–86.

286. Kil HK, Alberts M, Liggitt HD, et al. Dexamethasone treatment does not ameliorate subglottic ischemic injury in rabbits. Chest 1997; 111:1356–60.

287. Hawkins DB. Glottic and subglottic stenosis from endotracheal intubation. Laryngoscope 1977; 87:339–46.

288. Sasaki CT, Horiuchi M, Koss N. Tracheostomy-related subglottic stenosis: bacteriologic pathogenesis. Laryngoscope 1979; 89:857–65.

289. Ching NPH, Nealon TB Jr. Clinical experience with new low-pressure high-volume tracheostomy cuffs: Importance of limiting intracuff pressure. NY State J Med 1974; 74:2379–84.

290. Ching NP, Ayres SM, Paegle RP, et al. The contribution of cuff volume and pressure in tracheostomy tube damage. J Thorac Cardiovasc Surg 1971; 62:402–8.

291. Grillo HC. The management of tracheal stenosis following assisted respiration. J Thorac Cardiovasc Surg 1969; 57:52–71.

292. Nordin U, Lyttkens L. New self-adjusting cuff for tracheal tubes. Acta Otolaryngol 1976; 82:455–56.

293. Shelly WM, Dawson RB, May IA. Cuffed tubes as a cause of tracheal stenosis. J Thorac Cardiovasc Surg 1969; 57:623–27.

294. Adriana J, Phillips M. Use of the endotracheal cuff: some data pro and con. Anesthesiology 1957; 18:1–14.

295. Dunn CR, Dunn DL, Moser KM. Determinants of tracheal injury by cuffed tracheostomy tubes. Chest 1974; 65:128–35.

296. Lewis FR Jr, Schlobohm RM, Thomas AN. Prevention of complications from prolonged tracheal intubation. Am J Surg 1978; 135:452–57.

297. Mathias DB, Wedley JR. The effects of cuffed endotracheal tubes on the tracheal wall. Br J Anaesth 1974; 46:849–52.

298. Honeybourne D, Costello JC, Barham C. Tracheal damage after endotracheal intubation: comparison of two types of endotracheal tubes. Thorax 1982; 37:500–2.

299. Perel A, Katzenelson R, Klein E, et al. Collapse of endotracheal

300. Crawley BE, Cross DE. Tracheal cuffs: a review and dynamic pressure study. Anaesthesia 1975; 30:4–11.

301. Carroll RG. Evaluation of tracheal tube cuff designs. Crit Care Med 1973; 1:45–46.

302. Miller DR, Sethi G. Tracheal stenosis following prolonged cuffed intubation: cause and prevention. Ann Surg 1970; 171:283–93.

303. McGinnis GE, Shively JG, Patterson RL, et al. An engineering analysis of intratracheal tube cuffs. Anesth Analg 1971; 50:557–64.

304. Dane TEB, King EG. A prospective study of complications after tracheostomy for assisted ventilation. Chest 1975; 67:398–404.

305. Friman L, Hedenstierna G, Schildt B. Stenosis following tracheostomy: a quantitative study of long-term results. Anaesthesia 1976; 31:479-93.

306. Rubio PA, Farrell EM, Bautista EM. Severe tracheal stenosis after brief endotracheal intubation. South Med J 1979; 72:1628–29.

307. Levine SA, Niederman MS. The impact of tracheal intubation on host defenses and risks for nosocomial pneumonia. Clin Chest Med 1991; 12:523–43.

308. Craven DE, Steger KA. Nosocomial pneumonia in the intubated patient. New concepts on pathogenesis and prevention. Infect Dis Clin North Am 1989; 3:843–66.

309. Craven DE, Daschner FD. Nosocomial pneumonia in the intubated patient: role of gastric colonization. Eur J Clin Microbiol Infect Dis 1989; 8:40–50.

310. Agvald-Ohman C, Wernerman J, Nord CE, et al. Anaerobic bacteria commonly colonize the lower airways of intubated ICU patients. Clin Microbiol Infect 2003; 9:397–405.

311. Robert R, Grollier G, Frat J-P, et al. Colonization of lower respiratory tract with anaerobic bacteria in mechanically ventilated patients. Intensive Care Med 2003; 29:1062–68.

312. Marik PE, Careau P. The role of anaerobes in patients with ventilator-associated pneumonia and aspiration pneumonia. Chest 1999; 115:178–83.

313. Johanson WG Jr, Pierce AK, Sanford JP, et al. Nosocomial respiratory infections with gram-negative bacilli—the significance of colonization of the respiratory tract. Ann Intern Med 1972; 77:701–6.

314. Centers for Disease Control and Prevention. Guidelines for preventing health-care-associated pneumonia, 2003: recommendations of CDC and the Healthcare Infection Control Practices Advisory Committee. MMWR Morb Mortal Wkly Rep 2004; 53(No. RR-3):3–9.

315. Rello J, Diaz E, Roque M, et al. Risk factors for developing pneumonia within 48 hours of intubation. Am J Respir Crit Care Med 1999; 159:1742–46.

316. Young PJ, Ridley SA, Downward G. Evaluation of a new design of tracheal tube cuff to prevent leakage of fluid into the lungs. Br J Anaesth 1998; 80:796–99.

317. Koerner RJ. Contribution of endotracheal tubes to the pathogenesis of ventilator-associated pneumonia. J Hosp Infect 1997; 35:83–89.

318. Torres A, Gatell JM, Aznar E, et al. Re-intubation increases the risk of nosocomial pneumonia in patients needing mechanical ventilation. Am J Respir Crit Care Med 1995; 152:137–41.

319. Stenqvist O, Nilsson K. Postoperative sore throat related to tracheal tube cuff design. Can Anaesth Soc J 1982; 29:384–86.

320. Stock MC, Downs JB. Lubrication of tracheal tubes to prevent sore throat from intubation. Anesthesiology 1982; 57:418–20.

321. Littlewood K, Durbin CG Jr. Evidence-based airway management. Respir Care 2001; 46:1392–405.

322. Sugerman HJ, Wolfe L, Pasquale MD, et al. Multicenter, randomized, prospective trial of early tracheostomy. J Trauma 1997; 43:741–47.

tubes due to overinflation of high-compliance cuffs. Anesth Analg 1977; 56:731–33.

323. Rumbak MJ, Newton M, Truncale T, et al. A prospective, randomized, study comparing early percutaneous dilational tracheotomy to prolonged translaryngeal intubation (delayed tracheotomy) in critically ill medical patients. Crit Care Med 2004; 32:1689–94.

324. Bouderka MA, Fakhir B, Bouaggad A, et al. Early tracheostomy versus prolonged endotracheal intubation in severe head injury. J Trauma 2004; 57:251–54.

325. Kollef MH, Ahrens TS, Shannon W. Clinical predictors and outcomes for patients requiring tracheostomy in the intensive care unit. Crit Care Med 1999; 27:1714–20.

326. Brook AD, Sherman G, Malen J, et al. Early versus late tracheostomy in patients who require prolonged mechanical ventilation. Am J Crit Care 2000; 9:352–59.

327. Santos PM, Afrassiabi A, Weymuller EA Jr. Prospective studies evaluating the standard endotracheal tube and a prototype endotracheal tube. Ann Otol Rhinol Laryngol 1989; 98: 935–40.

328. Brunel W, Coleman DL, Schwartz DE, et al. Assessment of routine chest roentgenograms and the physical examination to confirm endotracheal tube position. Chest 1989; 96:1043–45.

329. Holzapfel L, Chastang C, Demingeon G, et al. A randomized study assessing the systematic search for maxillary sinusitis in nasotracheally mechanically ventilated patients. Am J Respir Crit Care Med 1999; 159:695–701.

330. Hilbert G, Vargas F, Valentino R, et al. Comparison of B-mode ultrasound and computed tomography in the diagnosis of maxillary sinusitis in mechanically ventilated patients. Crit Care Med 2001; 29:1337–42.

331. Salvolini L, Bichi Secchi E, Costarelli L, et al. Clinical applications of 2D and 3D CT imaging of the airways—a review. Eur J Radiol 2000; 34:9–25.

332. Geffin B, Grillo HC, Cooper JD, et al. Stenosis following tracheostomy for respiratory care. JAMA 1971; 216:1984–88.

333. Raghuraman G, Rajan S, Marzouk JK, et al. Is tracheal stenosis caused by percutaneous tracheostomy different from that by surgical tracheostomy? Chest 2005; 127:879–85.

334. Miller RD, Hyatt RE. Obstructing lesions of the larynx and trachea: clinical and physiologic characteristics. Mayo Clin Proc 1969; 44:145–60.

335. Miller RD, Hyatt RE. Evaluation of obstructing lesions of the trachea and larynx by flow-volume loops. Am Rev Respir Dis 1973; 108:475–81.

336. Hoppe H, Walder B, Sonnenschein M, et al. Multidetector CT virtual bronchoscopy to grade tracheobronchial stenosis. AJR Am J Roentgenol 2002; 178:1195–200.

337. Hoppe H, Dinkel H-P, Walder B, et al. Grading airway stenosis down to the segmental level using virtual bronchoscopy. Chest 2004; 125:704–11.

338. Toyota K, Uchida H, Ozasa H, et al. Preoperative airway evaluation using multi-slice three-dimensional computed tomography for a patient with severe tracheal stenosis. Br J Anaesth 2004; 93:865–67.

339. Cavaliere F, Masieri S. Chronic middle ear effusion after prolonged intubation. Anaesthesia 1994; 49:641–42.

340. Curtis JL, Mahlmeister M, Fink JB, et al. Helium-oxygen gas therapy. Use and availability for the emergency treatment of inoperable airway obstruction. Chest 1986; 90:455–57.

341. Miller RL, Cole RP. Association between reduced cuff leak volume and postextubation stridor. Chest 1996; 110:1035–40.

342. De Bast Y, De Backer D, Moraine J-J, et al. The cuff leak test to predict failure of tracheal extubation for laryngeal edema. Intensive Care Med 2002; 28:1267–72.

343. Kwon TK, Buckmire R. Injection laryngoplasty for management of unilateral vocal fold paralysis. Curr Opin Otolaryngol Head Neck Surg 2004; 12:538–42.

344. Zeitels SM, Casiano RR, Gardner GM, et al. Management of common voice problems: Committee report. Otolaryngol Head Neck Surg 2002; 126:333–48.

345. Ludlow CL. Recent advances in laryngeal sensorimotor control for voice, speech and swallowing. Curr Opin Otolaryngol Head Neck Surg 2004; 12:160–65.

346. Hirano S, Kojima H, Tateya I, et al. Fiberoptic laryngeal surgery for vocal process granuloma. Ann Otol Rhinol Laryngol 2002; 111:789–93.

347. Roh HJ, Goh EK, Chon KM, et al. Topical inhalant steroid (budesonide nasal) therapy in intubation granuloma. J Laryngol Otol 1999; 113:427–32.

348. Orloff LA, Goldman SN. Vocal cord granuloma: successful treatment with botulinum toxin. Otolaryngol Head Neck Surg 1999; 121:410–13.

349. de Lima Pontes PA, De Biase NG, Gadelha EC. Clinical evolution of laryngeal granulomas: treatment and prognosis. Laryngoscope 1999; 109:189–294.

350. Harari PM, Blatchford SJ, Coulthard SW, et al. Intubation granuloma of the larynx: successful eradication with low-dose radiotherapy. Head Neck 1991; 13:230–33.

351. Duncavage JA, Koriwchak MJ. Open surgical techniques for laryngotracheal stenosis. Otolaryngol Clin North Am 1995; 28:785–95.

352. Pena J, Cicero R, Marin J, et al. Laryngotracheal reconstruction in subglottic stenosis: an ancient problem still present. Otolaryngol Head Neck Surg 2001;125:397–400.

353. Hoasjoe DK, Franklin SW, Aarstad RF, et al. Posterior glottic mechanism and surgical management. Laryngoscope 1997; 107:675–79.

354. Czigner J, Rovo L, Brzozka M. Circumferential resection of crico-tracheal stenosis with primary end-to-end anastomosis. Otolaryngol Pol 2004; 58:149–55.

355. Chhajed PN, Malouf MA, Glanville AR. Bronchoscopic dilatation in the management of benign (non-transplant) tracheobronchial stenosis. Intern Med J 2001; 31:512–16.

356. Sheski FD, Mathur PN. Long-term results of fibreoptic bronchoscopic balloon dilatation in the management of benign tracheobronchial stenosis. Chest 1998; 114:796–800.

357. Friedman EM, Healy GB, McGill TJI. Carbon dioxide laser management of subglottic and tracheal stenosis. Otolaryngol Clin North Am 1983; 16:871–77.

358. Gelb AF, Epstein JD. Nd-Yag laser treatment of tracheal stenosis. West J Med 1984; 141:472–75.

359. Grillo HC. Surgical treatment of postintubation tracheal injuries. J Thorac Cardiovasc Surg 1979; 78:860–75.

360. Grillo HC, Mathisen DJ. Surgical management of tracheal strictures. Surg Clin North Am 1988; 68:511–24.

361. Zietek E, Matyja G, Kawczynski M. Stenosis of the larynx and trachea: diagnostics and treatment. Otolaryngol Pol 2001; 55:515–20.

362. Grillo HC, Donahue DM. Post intubation tracheal stenosis. Semin Thorac Cardiovasc Surg 1996; 8:370–80.

363. Laccourreye O, Brasnu D, Seckin S, et al. Cricotracheal anastomosis for assisted ventilation-induced stenosis. Arch Otolaryngol Head Neck Surg 1997; 123:1074–77.

364. Blosser SA, Stauffer JL. Intubation of critically ill patients. Clin Chest Med 1996; 17:355–78.

365. Agro F, Frass M, Benumof J, et al. The esophageal tracheal combitube as a non-invasive alternative to endotracheal intubation. Minerva Anestesiol 2001; 67:863–74.

366. Gaitini LA, Vaida SJ, Agro F. The Esophageal-Tracheal Combitube. Anesthesiol Clin North America 2002; 20:893–906.

367. American Heart Association. Guidelines 2000 for cardiopulmonary resuscitation and emergency cardiovascular care. Circulation 2000; 102(Suppl):I1–1384.

368. Ram FS, Lightowler JV, Wedzicha JA. Non-invasive positive pressure ventilation for treatment of respiratory failure due to exacerbations of chronic obstructive pulmonary disease. Cochrane Database Syst Rev 2003; 1:CD004104.

369. Holzapfel L. Nasal vs oral intubation. Minerva Anestesiol 2003; 69:348–52.

370. Weymuller EA Jr. Prevention and management of intubation injury of the larynx and trachea. Am J Otolaryngol 1992; 13:139–44.

371. Heffner JE. Airway management in the critically ill patient. Crit Care Clin 1990; 6:533–50.

372. Dauphinee K. Orotracheal intubation. Emerg Med Clin North Am 1988; 6:699–713.

373. Stone DJ, Bogdonoff DL. Airway considerations in the management of patients requiring long-term endotracheal intubation. Anesth Analg 1992; 74:276–87.

374. Stenqvist O, Sonander H, Nilsson K. Small endotracheal tubes: ventilator and intratracheal pressures during controlled ventilation. Br J Anaesth 1979; 51:375–81.

375. Wright PE, Marini JJ, Bernard GR. In vitro versus in vivo comparison of endotracheal tube airflow resistance. Am Rev Respir Dis 1989; 140:10–16.

376. Victor LD: Endotracheal intubation. In: Victor LD, editor. Manual of critical care procedures. Rockville, MD: Aspen Publishers, 1989: 1–32.

377. Reynolds SF, Heffner J. Airway management of the critically ill patient. Rapid-sequence intubation. Chest 2005; 127:1397–412.

378. Bair AE, Filbin MR, Kulkarni RG, et al. The failed intubation attempt in the emergency department: analysis of prevalence, rescue techniques, and personnel. J Emerg Med 2002; 23:131–40.

379. Li J, Murphy-Lavoie H, Bugas C, et al. Complications of emergency intubation with and without paralysis. Am J Emerg Med 1999; 17:141–44.

380. Bishop MJ, Harrington RM, Tencer AF. Force applied during tracheal intubation. Anesth Analg 1992; 74:411–14.

381. Mayrose J, Kesavadas T, Chugh K, et al. Utilization of virtual reality for endotracheal intubation training. Resuscitation 2003; 59:133–38.

382. Rowe R, Cohen RA. An evaluation of a virtual reality airway simulator. Anesth Analg 2002; 95:62–66.

383. Schwid HA, Rooke GA, Carline J, et al. Evaluation of anesthesia residents using mannequin-based simulation: a multiinstitutional study. Anesthesiology 2002; 97:1434–44.

384. Benumof JL. Management of the difficult adult airway. With special emphasis on awake tracheal intubation. Anesthesiology 1991; 75:1087–1110.

385. Wilson ME, Spiegelhalter D, Robertson JA, et al. Predicting difficult intubation. Br J Anaesth 1988; 61:211–16.

386. Deem S, Bishop MJ. Evaluation and management of the difficult airway. Crit Care Clin 1995; 11:1–27.

387. American Society of Anesthesiologists. Practice guidelines for management of the difficult airway. An updated report by the American Society of Anesthesiologists Task Force on Management of the Difficult Airway. Anesthesiology 2003; 98:1269–77.

388. Lu PP, Liu HP, Shyr MH, et al. Softened endotracheal tube reduces the incidence and severity of epistaxis following nasotracheal intubation. Acta Anesth Sinica 1998; 36:193–97.

389. American Society of Anesthesiologists. Practice guidelines for sedation and analgesia by non-anesthesiologists. An updated report by the American Society of Anesthesiologists Task Force on Sedation and Analgesia by Non-anesthesiologists. Anesthesiology 2002; 96:1004–17.

390. Kovac AL. Controlling the hemodynamic response to laryngoscopy and endotracheal intubation. J Clin Anesth 1996; 8:63–79.

391. Birmingham PK, Cheney FW, Ward RJ. Esophageal intubation: a review of detection techniques. Anesth Analg 1986; 65: 886–91.

392. Goldberg JS, Rawle PR, Zehnder JL, et al. Colorimetric end-tidal carbon dioxide monitoring for tracheal intubation. Anesth Analg 1990; 70:191–94.

393. Linko K, Paloheimo M, Tammisto T. Capnography for detection of accidental oesophageal intubation. Acta Anaesthesiol Scand 1983; 27:199–202.

394. Murray IP, Modell JH. Early detection of endotracheal tube accidents by monitoring carbon dioxide concentration in respiratory gas. Anesthesiology 1983; 59:344–46.

395. Ornato JP, Shipley JB, Racht EM, et al. Multicenter study of a portable, hand-size, colorimetric end-tidal carbon dioxide detection device. Ann Emerg Med 1992; 21:518–23.

396. Anton WR, Gordon RW, Jordan TM, et al. A disposable end-tidal CO_2 detector to verify endotracheal intubation. Ann Emerg Med 1991; 20:271–75.

397. Knapp S, Kofler J, Stoiser B, et al. The assessment of four different methods to verify tracheal tube placement in the critical care setting. Anesth Analg 1999; 88:766–70.

398. Salem MR. Verification of endotracheal tube position. Anesthesiol Clin North America 2001; 19:813–39.

399. Grmec S. Comparison of three different methods to confirm tracheal tube placement. Intensive Care Med 2002; 28:701–4.

400. Kasper CL, Deem S. The self-inflating bulb to detect esophageal intubation during emergency airway management. Anesthesiology 1998; 88:898–902.

401. Tanigawa K, Takeda T, Goto E, et al. Accuracy and reliability of the self-inflating bulb to verify tracheal intubation in out-of-hospital cardiac arrest patients. Anesthesiology 2000; 93:1432–36.

402. Asai T, Shingu K. Case report: a normal capnogram despite esophageal intubation. Can J Anaesth 2001; 48:1025–28.

403. Puntervoll SA, Soreide E, Jacewicz W, et al. Rapid detection of oesophageal intubation: take care when using colorimetric capnometry. Acta Anaesthesiol Scand 2002; 46:455–57.

404. Lotano R, Gerber D, Aseron C, et al. Utility of postintubation chest radiographs in the intensive care unit. Crit Care 2000; 4:50–53.

405. Goodman LR, Conrardy PA, Laing F, et al. Radiographic evaluation of endotracheal tube position. AJR Am J Roentgenol 1976; 127:433–34.

406. Cherng C-H, Wong C-S, Hsu C-H, et al. Airway length in adults: estimation of the optimal endotracheal tube length for orotracheal intubation. J Clin Anesth 2002;14:271–74.

407. Bernhard WN, Yost LC, Turndorf H, et al. Physical characteristics of and rates of nitrous oxide diffusion into tracheal tube cuffs. Anesthesiology 1978; 48:413–17.

408. Stanley TH. Nitrous oxide and pressures and volumes of high- and low-pressure endotracheal-tube cuffs in intubated patients. Anesthesiology 1975; 42:637–40.

409. Tu HN, Saidi N, Lieutaud T, et al. Nitrous oxide increases endotracheal cuff pressure and the incidence of tracheal lesions in anesthetized patients. Anesth Analg 1999; 89:187–90.

410. Off D, Braun SR, Tompkins B, et al. Efficacy of the minimal leak technique of cuff inflation in maintaining proper intracuff pressures for patients with cuffed artificial airways. Respir Care 1983; 28:1115–20.

411. Lee T-S. Routine monitoring of intracuff pressure. Chest 1992; 102:1309.

412. Burns SM, Shasby DM, Burke PA. Controlled pressure cuffed endotracheal tubes may not be controlled. Chest 1983; 83:158–59.

413. Guyton DC, Barlow MR, Besselievre TR. Influence of airway pressure on minimum occlusive endotracheal tube cuff pressure. Crit Care Med 1997; 25:91–94.

414. Woods JC, Mion LC, Connor JT, et al. Severe agitation among ventilated medical intensive care unit patients: frequency, characteristics and outcomes. Intensive Care Med 2004; 30:1066–72.

415. Demers RR. Complications of endotracheal suctioning procedures. Respir Care 1982; 27:453–57.

416. Guglielminotti J, Alzieu M, Maury E, et al. Bedside detection of retained tracheobronchial secretions in patients receiving mechanical ventilation. Is it time for tracheal suctioning? Chest 2000; 118:1095–99.

417. Lorente L, Lecuona M, Martin MM, et al. Ventilator-associated pneumonia using a closed versus an open tracheal suction system. Crit Care Med 2005; 33:115–19.

418. King HK. A new device: Tube Securer. An endotracheal tube holder with integrated bite block. Acta Anesth Sinica 1997; 35:257–59.

419. Patak L, Gawlinski A, Fung NI, et al. Patients' reports of health care practitioner interventions that are related to communication during mechanical ventilation. Heart Lung 2004; 33:308–20.

420. Kamen JM, Wilkinson CJ. A new low-pressure cuff for endotracheal tubes. Anesthesiology 1971; 34:482–85.

421. King K, Mandava B, Kamen JM. Tracheal tube cuffs and tracheal dilatation. Chest 1975; 67:458–62.

422. Lindholm C-E. Experience with a new orotracheal tube. Acta Otolaryngol 1973; 75:389–90.

423. Deane RS, Shinozaki T, Morgan JG. An evaluation of the cuff characteristics and incidence of laryngeal complications using a new nasotracheal tube in prolonged intubations. J Trauma 1977; 17:311–14.

424. Hatcher CR, Calvert JR, Logan WD, et al. Endotracheal tube with double balloon. Surg Gynecol Obstet 1968; 127:759–62.

425. Dullenkopf A, Gerber A, Weiss M. Fluid leakage past tracheal cuffs: evaluation of the new Microcuff endotracheal tube. Intensive Care Med 2003; 29:1849–53.

426. Pronovost PJ, Jenckes M, To M, et al. Reducing failed extubations in the intensive care unit. Jt Comm J Qual Improvement 2002; 28:595–604.

427. Markovitz BP, Randolph AG. Corticosteroids for the prevention and treatment of post-extubation stridor in neonates, children and adults. Cochrane Database Syst Rev 2000; 2:CD001000.

428. Meade MO, Guyatt GH, Cook DJ, et al. Trials of corticosteroids to prevent postextubation airway complications. Chest 2001; 120:464S–68S.

CARE OF THE MECHANICALLY-VENTILATED PATIENT WITH A TRACHEOSTOMY

JOHN E. HEFFNER
BONNIE MARTIN-HARRIS

Although ancient Hindus and Egyptian writings refer to the use of tracheotomy for medical applications nearly 4000 years ago,[1,2] initial descriptions of the procedure in Western literature—then termed "bronchotomy"—did not appear until the middle of the 16th century.[3] By 1718, "tracheotomy" became accepted terminology for the surgical technique that was then primarily used for relief of airway obstruction and removal of aspirated foreign bodies.[4] Typically gruesome clinical results relegated tracheotomy to a reviled role in airway management and gained it a designation as the "scandal of surgery."[5] The diphtheria epidemics of the 19th century popularized tracheotomy, which dramatically decreased the nearly universal lethality of upper airway obstruction in diphtheria. Tracheotomy did not become a widely accepted procedure, however, until 1909 when Chevalier Jackson standardized tracheolaryngeal surgical techniques and decreased the operative mortality of tracheotomy from 25% to the modern-day standard of less than 1%.[6]

Advances in tube design during the 1960s and 1970s and improved understanding of patient management techniques have further contributed to the recognition that tracheotomy is a well-tolerated method of long-term airway access for critically ill, ventilator-dependent patients. The recent advent of percutaneous dilatational tracheostomy (PDT) has further widened the application of tracheotomy for critically ill patients allowing the procedure to be performed by the bedside in the intensive care unit (ICU) by non-surgeons, which has increased the frequency of its use.[7] Up to 10–24% of patients undergoing mechanical ventilation have a tracheostomy performed.[7–9] Acceptable outcomes from tracheotomy, however, remain dependent on the skill of the operator who performs the procedure and the management expertise of the critical care team charged with minimizing complications and promoting patient tolerance of the procedure.

Techniques of Surgical Airway Access

OPEN SURGICAL TRACHEOTOMY

An *open surgical tracheotomy* is a surgical procedure that provides tracheal access through an incisional tracheostoma that enters the trachea between cartilaginous rings (Fig. 40-1). The temporary stoma tract spontaneously closes after removal of the cannulating tube.

Four indications exist for performing a standard tracheotomy in critically ill patients: (1) maintenance of airway patency for patients with functional or mechanical upper airway obstruction, (2) provision of airway access for suctioning retained airway secretions for patients with poor tracheobronchial clearance mechanisms, (3) prevention or limitation of aspiration in patients with glottic dysfunction, and (4) management of patients who require long-term airway access for ventilatory support.[10]

Open surgical tracheotomy is a well-tolerated procedure with an operative mortality less than 1% when performed in stable, ventilator-dependent patients who have a translaryngeal endotracheal tube in place. In contrast, an emergency tracheotomy has a complication rate 5 times higher than the elective procedure and has been supplanted by specialized endotracheal intubation techniques to secure a difficult airway,[11] emergency cricothyroidotomy,[12] and emergency percutaneous techniques.[13–19]

PERCUTANEOUS TRACHEOSTOMY

Percutaneous tracheostomy refers to several techniques that insert a standard or modified tracheal airway with a Seldinger technique below the first or second tracheal rings using a device to cut and spread the trachea[20] or a forceps or dilator technique to cannulate and dilate tracheal tissue between cartilaginous rings[21–23] (see Fig. 40-1). The first percutaneous tracheostomy using a cutting device was

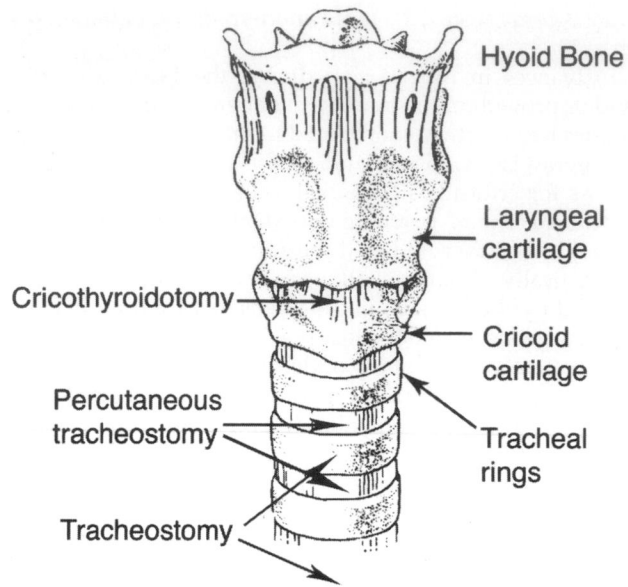

Hyoid Bone

Laryngeal cartilage

Cricothyroidotomy

Cricoid cartilage

Percutaneous tracheostomy

Tracheal rings

Tracheostomy

FIGURE 40-1 Anatomic location of tracheostoma placement for different forms of surgical airway access.

performed by Shelden in 1957[24] followed by Toye et al in 1969 who adopted a Seldinger technique.[20]

Ciaglia first described percutaneous dilatational tracheostomy (PDT) wherein a Seldinger technique allowed the insertion of dilators to insert a tracheostomy tube without cutting tracheal tissue.[22] The Ciaglia technique originally inserted tubes below the cricoid cartilage using multiple dilators of progressively increasing caliber. The procedure later evolved to the insertion of a tracheostomy tube between tracheal rings using a single dilator that increases in caliber from its tip to its base where it matches the diameter of a tracheostomy tube (Ciaglia Blue Rhino technique)[25] (Fig. 40-2).

Multiple studies have demonstrated the safety, speed, and utility of PDT with both the Ciaglia multiple-dilator and Blue Rhino single-dilator techniques as compared to standard tracheostomy in critically ill patients (Table 40-1).[19,25–39] It has a similar mortality rate to surgical tracheostomy.[40] The Ciaglia PDT technique has become the most commonly performed percutaneous tracheostomy procedure in the United States for critically ill patients and is commonly used in Europe.[41,42]

Other techniques for percutaneous tracheostomy include a specialized Guide Wire Guiding Forceps (GWDF) with a groove that allows loading of a guide wire onto the forceps, which are used to dilate the trachea, thread the wire, and insert a tracheostomy tube by a Seldinger technique (Portex GWDF kit, Sims, Inc, Philadelphia, PA).[43] The GWDF technique has been observed to be quick, safe, and effective in critically ill patients.[44–47] Although the forceps technique is faster than the Ciaglia multiple-dilator technique,[48] it has similar time to completion compared with the Ciaglia single-dilator method.[49,50] Comparative studies have shown either higher[51] or similar[44,49,50] complication rates with the GWDF as compared with the Ciaglia Blue Rhino technique with each procedure having unique

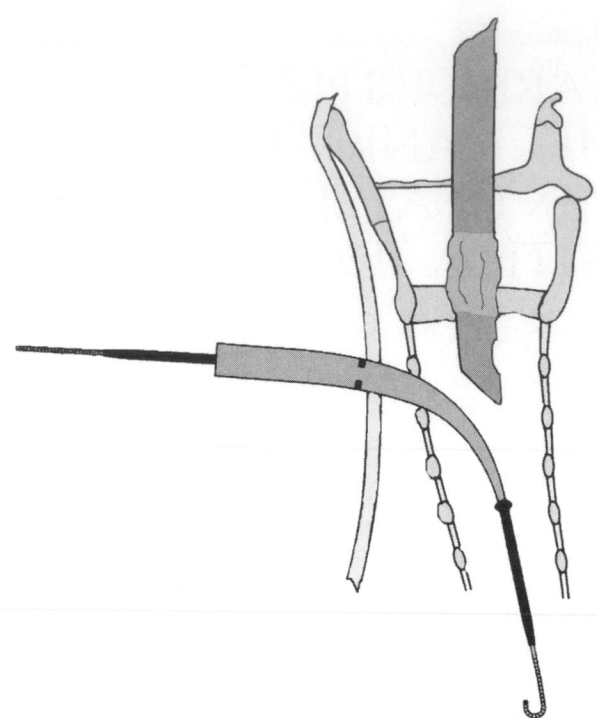

FIGURE 40-2 Insertion of a stoma dilator for percutaneous dilational tracheostomy (Ciaglia Blue Rhino, Cook Critical Care, Bloomington, IN).

complications.[52] Long-term follow-up studies demonstrate acceptable rates of tracheal stenosis and other chronic airway complications with the GWDF technique,[53–56] although one study of 208 patients observed a 38% incidence of a changed voice and a 12% incidence of persistent, severe cough.

The Rapitrac is a dilating forceps device with a metal conus and cutting edge that is designed to advance forcibly over a wire into the airway.[57] Because of a high rate of complications (overall across studies, 23%),[58–60] it is no longer on the United States market.

Frova et al recently described a single-step dilator (PercuTwist, Rusch, Kernen, Germany) that threads a screw-type dilator between tracheal rings.[61] Limited experience exists with the PercuTwist technique to date, but existing trials report variable success with difficulties in learning the procedure and problems with damage to tracheal structures.[27,62–65]

TABLE 40-1 Comparison of Percutaneous Dilatational Tracheostomy with Surgical Tracheostomy in Critically Ill Patients

	Surgical	Percutaneous
Procedure time (minutes)	13.5–33.9	4.3–15.4
Operative bleeding (%)	11–87	13–20
Postoperative complications (%)	36–100	12–25
Stomal infection (%)	4–63	0–10

Summary of five prospective, comparative studies as reported by Freeman et al.[408]

Fantoni described translaryngeal tracheostomy (TT) as a unique procedure that places a tracheostomy tube in a reverse direction from within the airway through the tracheostomy tract.[66] The operator places a needle into the trachea between the second and third tracheal rings. With bronchoscopic guidance, a guidewire is passed retrograde through the needle into a cuffed, rigid bronchoscope, which is then removed from the airway. A tracheostomy tube with a tapered proximal end is loaded onto the cephalad end of the guidewire and pulled through the airway and the needle tract. Comparative studies suggest that it is equally effective and less traumatic than the Ciaglia PDT technique.[67−69]

The various techniques for percutaneous tracheostomy all require a learning curve to gain the requisite skills to complete the procedures quickly and safely.[70−72] Because PDT is the primary technique used in most ICUs, it will be the technique of percutaneous tracheostomy discussed in the remainder of this chapter.

Contraindications to PDT have decreased with increasing experience with the procedure. Conservative recommendations have considered age less than 16 years, bleeding diatheses, severely calcified tracheal rings, and anatomic abnormalities such as obesity and thyromegaly that obscure landmarks,[73] to be relative contraindications.[74,75] The use of careful technique, however, has allowed the safe completion of PDT in patients with body mass indices ≥ 27 kg/m^2.[76] Preoperative ultrasonography may allow selection of patients with anatomic abnormalities of the neck for successful PDT.[77] Trauma patients with known or suspected cervical injury have also undergone successful PDT.[78,79] Some experts recommend avoiding PDT for patients for whom inadvertent decannulation would present extreme difficulty in replacing the tracheostomy tube and loss of an airway would be immediately catastrophic.[80] Recent studies have reported the utility and safety of PDT for patients with thrombocytopenia.[81]

PDT has been performed successfully in patients with severe respiratory failure with dependence on high levels of positive end-expiratory pressure (PEEP). Beiderlinden et al performed bronchoscopically-guided PDT in patients with mean PEEP levels of 16.6 cmH$_2$O (range 12–20 cmH$_2$O) and found no deterioration of arterial oxygen at 1 and 24 hours after the procedure as compared with patients with lower PEEP levels (mean 7.6 cmH$_2$O; range 5.4–9.8 cmH$_2$O).[82] The procedure can also be performed in selected patients who had a previous PDT.[83]

Purported advantages of PDT as compared with open surgical tracheostomy in ventilator-dependent patients include the speed of the procedure (<6 minutes), the ability to place the airway in the ICU without patient transfer to an operating room, avoidance of general anesthesia, decreased cost, reduced operating room use, and limited personnel requirements that include a single operator, a bronchoscopist if bronchoscopy is used, nurse, and respiratory therapist.[22,26,43,58,84−91] Such simplifications decrease costs[88] and avoid complications from intra-institutional transport of critically ill, ventilator-dependent patients to the operating room (OR). They also eliminate dependency on the OR schedule and decrease the time interval from the decision to perform tracheostomy by PDT to when it is actually performed.[36] In regard to the risks of patient transport, Smith et al prospectively analyzed 125 patients transported from the ICU and observed that one-third had at least one mishap that ranged from telemetry lead failure to disruption of vasoactive drug infusions.[92] Fradis et al, however, observed no complications related to transport of critically ill, intubated patients to the operating room for tracheostomy when an experienced anesthesiologist and otolaryngologist accompanied the patient.[93]

Benefits from eliminating patient transport and thereby decreasing costs, however, are contradicted by experiences from several institutions wherein open surgical tracheotomy is performed at the bedside with similar outcomes as reported for PDT.[1,94−101] No randomized studies exist comparing surgical tracheostomy performed in the ICU with that performed in the operating room, but a single-armed study reported a low early postoperative complication rate of 4% for surgical tracheostomy performed on 200 patients in the ICU.[101]

Percutaneous tracheotomy has an additional advantage in dilating rather than incising the subcutaneous tissue and trachea thereby producing a tracheostoma that fits snugly around the tracheotomy tube.[102] This close fit may improve anchoring of the tracheotomy tube, decreasing the incidence of inadvertent extubation, compress blood vessels in the stoma tract thus lessening the risk of postoperative bleeding, and diminish the incidence of wound infections observed with conventionally placed surgical stomas. If inadvertent decannulation occurs, however, the absence of a surgical stoma tract may complicate reinsertion of the percutaneous tracheostomy tube. The smaller skin incision may also result in a better cosmetic appearance after extubation.[80] Some physicians prefer a PDT to a surgical tracheostomy for patients with a fresh sternal incision because of the smaller stoma and lower incidence of infection with a PDT, which may decrease the risk of mediastinitis.[103]

Outcomes studies are beginning to examine these potential advantages of percutaneous tracheotomy[36,87,90,91,98,104−107] of which three are randomized controlled trials.[91,98,107] Most trials of PDT as compared with surgical tracheostomy demonstrate equal or better patient outcomes with PDT. These trials, however, are small, often employ varying techniques, have considerable spectrum bias, and measure heterogenous outcomes with differing definitions between studies.[72] No large, randomized controlled trial exists to clearly establish the superiority of one procedure over the other. Meta-analyses establish that both PDT and surgical tracheostomy have acceptable outcomes and can be employed in institutions with available technical skills.[37,108]

CRICOTHYROIDOTOMY

Cricothyroidotomy is a surgical technique for placing an airway through the cricothyroid space (see Fig. 40-1). Because of the superficial location of airway anatomy at this level and the simplicity of surgical technique, cricothyroidotomy has become a preferred procedure for placement of an emergency airway in patients who cannot undergo translaryngeal intubation.[12] Some centers, however, prefer percutaneous dilatational tracheotomy for emergency airway access after failed intubation attempts.[13-19] Caution is required in performing emergency cricothyroidotomy because as many as 62% of patients have vertically oriented arteries and veins overlying the cricothyroid membrane within the surgical field.[109]

Most surgeons do not employ cricothyroidotomy for elective, long-term airway access in critically ill patients because of concern for delayed airway damage. Chevalier Jackson, the father of otolaryngology, proscribed "high tracheotomies," such as cricothyroidotomies, because of their associated risk of subglottic stenosis.[110]

Brantigan et al, however, popularized routine use of cricothyroidotomy with a report in 1976 of 655 patients who underwent elective cricothyroidotomy for airway access.[111] Although the low 6.1% incidence of complications did not include any instances of subglottic stenosis, patient follow-up was incomplete and the average time of pre-existing translaryngeal intubation, although unstated, appeared to be short. Subsequent investigators determined that subglottic stenosis was a complication of the procedure but the risk of airway injury was diminished if pre-existing translaryngeal intubation was limited to less than 6–7 days.[112,113] The incidence of subglottic stenosis increased to as high as 40–53%, however, if the procedure followed longer periods of translaryngeal intubation.[114,115]

Brantigan et al subsequently reported that 10 of 17 patients with subglottic stenosis after cricothyroidotomy had laryngeal pathology noted at the time of the surgical procedure.[116] They revised their recommendations for the procedure on the basis of this experience, suggesting that cricothyroidotomy be avoided in patients with long-term translaryngeal intubation because of the association of pre-existing laryngeal trauma with subglottic stenosis. More recent reports in patients undergoing mechanical ventilation argue that cricothyroidotomy has a low complication rate and is a reasonable, technically less demanding option in critically ill patients with challenging neck anatomy who require a surgical airway.[100,117,118] These studies were retrospective, however, and did not have systematic patient follow-up to detect long-term airway complications.

Cricothyroidotomy presents additional long-term risks to vocalization after patients undergo extubation. The cricothyroidotomy tube inserted through the cricothyroid membrane lies within 1 cm of the true vocal cords[113] and can produce hoarseness by directly scarring the glottis. Moreover, cicatrization of the cricothyroid membrane after decannulation may prevent anterior pivoting of the laryngeal cartilage, which is required to stretch the vocal cords and increase voice pitch.[119,120] The combined effects on laryngeal function may cause hoarseness in up to 40–78% of patients treated with a cricothyroidotomy.[119-123] Further risks of cricothyroidotomy include esophageal perforation.[124]

Currently, elective cricothyroidotomy remains a secondary technique for providing long-term airway access in most centers in ventilator-dependent patients.[125] It is of value in patients who cannot undergo a standard tracheotomy because of local abnormalities of cervical or airway anatomy.[118] The procedure is contraindicated in patients with pre-existing laryngeal pathology,[116] such as infection or tumor, and in pediatric age groups. Most[113,115,121] but not all[117,118] clinicians reserve the procedure for patients intubated less than 3–7 days. Cricothyroidotomy should also be avoided if possible in patients who depend occupationally on their voice, such as singers or actors.[123]

Although a cricothyroidotomy may offer theoretical advantages for patients with recent sternotomy incisions, no data exist to indicate that a standard tracheotomy is associated with an increased risk of wound or mediastinal infections in this patient population.[114,126] The advent of percutaneous dilatational tracheotomy further decreases concern regarding contamination of fresh sternal infections.[126,127] Common wisdom has recommended conversion of cricothyroidotomies to a tracheostomies at the first opportunity,[12,125] but no data support the necessity of this practice.[117,118,128]

MINITRACHEOTOMY

A *minitracheotomy* is a percutaneous technique first described by Matthews et al in 1984 for inserting through the cricothyroid membrane a specialized 4-mm tube that accommodates a 10F suction catheter[129-131] (see Fig. 40-1). Performed at the patient's bedside, minitracheotomy provides direct access to the airway for suctioning tracheal secretions without interfering with the patient's cough or speech. The catheter can be capped when not needed for airway suctioning. Because of the tube's small caliber (4-mm inner diameter), minitracheotomy has not gained wide application in patients requiring airway access for mechanical ventilation, although it has been used during elective otolaryngologic procedures,[132] in patients undergoing jet ventilation,[133] and in the management of sleep apnea.[134]

The procedure is indicated for patients with or at risk of sputum retention who maintain adequate spontaneous respirations but appear at risk for secretion-related deterioration of lung function.[131,135-141] Patients at high risk for pulmonary complications after thoracic or upper abdominal surgery may benefit from the prophylactic placement of a minitracheostomy at the end of the operative procedure.[135] It is a valuable adjunct for recently extubated patients recovering from respiratory failure if retained secretions compromise recovery and portend a need for reintubation. For this indication, early placement of a minitracheostomy before respiratory compromise occurs can improve outcome.[130] It has also been used as a transition from PDT for patients who have weaned from mechanical ventilation but who cannot manage secretions.[38] Minitracheotomy has also been used to enhance airway clearance in patients with chronic obstructive lung disease undergoing lung resection.[142] It is not indicated when airway secretions can be adequately controlled with physiotherapy or occasional nasotracheal suctioning.

Minitracheotomy is usually well tolerated although some patients may develop temporary discomfort, voice changes while the tube is in place, subcutaneous emphysema, bleeding, and stridor.[143-145] Bleeding is the most common complication, which should be approached initially by the application of pressure followed by exploration of the incision with ligation of the bleeding vessel if necessary.[130] Rare reports exist of pneumothorax subsequent to incorrect placement into a paratracheal position.[146-148] Long-term studies with up to 4 years of follow-up have not detected complications such as subglottic stenosis in patients treated with minitracheotomy.[3,131,136] Operator inexperience, however, can cause major immediate surgical complications such as pneumothorax, profuse bleeding from anterior jugular veins, and esophageal puncture.[124,146,148] Wright has recently described the stepwise technique of minitracheostomy.[130]

Surgical Techniques for Tracheal Cannulation

OPEN SURGICAL TRACHEOTOMY

Elective standard tracheotomy is performed in an operating room under general anesthesia.[149] It may be performed in an ICU room for patients who cannot be transferred if adequate lighting, personnel, and equipment can provide the resources available in an operating room. Circumstances are never ideal, however, in the ICU. The patient's neck is hyperextended with a rolled towel or sheet placed between the shoulder blades to bring the trachea and larynx into a superficial and elevated position. This maneuver may elevate up to 50% of the trachea above the thoracic inlet. The surgeon identifies anatomic landmarks by palpating the cricoid cartilage, tracheal rings, and thyroid cartilage.

Unless the patient has a vertical scar from a previous tracheotomy, most surgeons will perform a 2- to 3-cm transverse incision 2 cm above the suprasternal notch with subsequent electrocautery dissection of the subcutaneous tissues and platysma. A vertical incision then separates the sternohyoid and sternothyroid muscles from the midline allowing retraction of the strap muscles to reveal the thyroid isthmus. The thyroid isthmus can be pulled upward out of the surgical field in most patients, but may rarely need to be divided and oversewn to allow visualization of tracheal rings. The anterior jugular veins lie lateral to the incisional plane but communicating venous branches may need to be divided.

The trachea is elevated and stabilized by placing a tracheal hook under the cricoid cartilage or first tracheal ring or using lateral traction sutures around the second or third tracheal rings. A vertical incision between the second and fourth tracheal rings is made with a scalpel, avoiding electrocautery because of the risks for a flash fire. The translaryngeal endotracheal tube is pulled back above the tracheal incision, which is gently dilated laterally just sufficiently to allow insertion of a tracheostomy tube. The tube size is selected on the basis of airway inspection, choosing a tube that is approximately two-thirds the diameter of the tracheal lumen at the level of the stoma. After inflation of the tracheostomy cuff and confirmation of adequate ventilation, the translaryngeal endotracheal tube is removed. The tracheal traction sutures are also removed because they serve little value in

facilitating recannulation of the trachea if the tracheostomy tube is inadvertently removed.

Specialized techniques and tubes are required for patients with obesity, short necks, or other anatomic variations.[75]

PERCUTANEOUS DILATATIONAL TRACHEOTOMY

The Seldinger technique of Ciaglia utilizes a kit that contains a J-wire guide, Teflon catheter with introducer needle, a Teflon introducer dilator, a translucent Teflon guiding catheter, and a single curved dilator. Some operators first examine the neck after the application of PEEP with the patient in the horizontal position with the neck slightly extended to detect aberrant jugular veins that traverse the operative field.[38] Others examine the neck by ultrasonography to both detect aberrant vessels and select an insertion site (see below). The patient is positioned with the head extended as for a standard tracheostomy. A 2-cm transverse skin incision is made over the first and second tracheal interspaces. Blunt dissection through the incision identifies the anterior tracheal wall.

A video bronchoscope is inserted through the endotracheal tube to visualize the puncture site to ensure its midline position and avoidance of the posterior tracheal wall.[38,89,150-152] After withdrawal of the endotracheal tube above the first tracheal ring, a syringe with the catheter-introducer needle is advanced through the first and second or second and third tracheal rings. Some operators use the bronchoscope to transilluminate the needle insertion site or depress the insertion site with mosquito forceps under bronchoscopic visualization to ensure that the endotracheal tube is above where the needle will be inserted.[153] After air is aspirated through the needle, the J-wire is passed into the trachea toward the carina and the needle is removed. The curved dilator is passed over the wire until the trachea has been dilated sufficiently to receive the tracheostomy tube, which is loaded onto an introducer and inserted over the guide wire. The single, Blue Rhino dilator approach has been observed to result in faster insertion times (3–6 minutes versus 6–10 minutes) as compared with the originally described Ciaglia technique that employed multiple dilators of increasing gauge.[19,27,28] Johnson et al observe that the single curved dilator results in less risk of posterior tracheal injury because it is softer, more flexible, and more easily passed into position with less force required because of its hydrophilic coating.[19]

Not all operators visualize the airway with a bronchoscope during PDT.[154] Bronchoscopy, however, provides several advantages as compared with blind insertion of the needle and dilators.[155] Visualization of the airway ensures withdrawal of the endotracheal tube above the surgical site to prevent interference with insertion of the needle and J-wire.[156] It also decreases the risk of puncture or laceration of the posterior membranous portion of the trachea.[157,158] This complication may be underrecognized if bronchoscopy is not performed.[158]

Winkler et al found that bronchoscopy detected an initial paramedian puncture in 18% (13/72) of patients undergoing PDT by the Ciaglia technique.[38] Reports have observed subcutaneous emphysema, pneumothorax, and paratracheal tube insertion in 12% of patients undergoing PDT.[57,58,84,85] Other studies that use endoscopic guidance of PDT have not reported these complications.[38,151] No prospective randomized trials, however, have demonstrated improved outcomes with bronchoscopy as opposed to PDT without airway visualization when performed by skilled operators. Patients require careful monitoring to avoid partial obstruction of the airway by the bronchoscope with resulting acute hypercapnia.[159] Some experts ensure intratracheal placement of the needle and dilators by capnographic monitoring of exhaled CO_2, which has been reported in a randomized trial of 55 patients to have similar outcomes as compared to bronchoscopy.[160] Insertion of a light wand into the trachea has also been used to guide PDT by transilluminating the pretracheal tissue.[161] Transillumination of pretracheal tissue with a bronchoscope has been recommended for selection of the puncture site for PDT.[162]

The airway becomes unstable when the endotracheal tube cuff is withdrawn into the endolarynx. An additional variation of technique employs withdrawal of the endotracheal tube and insertion of a laryngeal mask airway (LMA) to better stabilize the airway. Recent reports have observed similar outcomes with LMA as compared to performance of PDT with partial withdrawal of the endotracheal tube.[163–165] Ambesh et al, however, reported poor airway control during PDT with an LMA.[166] Another approach inserts a microlaryngeal tube to ventilate the patient during performance of the PDT.[167] Ferraro and colleagues reported the use of a 4-mm internal diameter pediatric endotracheal tube during PDT with ventilator adjustments to maintain adequate gas exchange.[168]

Ultrasonography has been recommended as a preparatory examination to ensure proper placement of a PDT, avoidance of vascular structures, and detection of a deep lying trachea that would indicate a need for surgical tracheostomy.[169,170] Kollig et al performed preprocedure ultrasonography in 72 patients visualizing the thyroid gland and the subcutaneous vessels.[171] The place of tracheal puncture was altered in 24% of the patients because the originally selected site would have penetrated vascular structures. Muhammad et al have emphasized the benefit of preoperative ultrasonography to prevent damage to vascular structures.[172,173] Most portable ultrasonographic devices, however, have limited tissue penetration so deep vascular structures may not be detected.[174] Sustic et al noted a lower incidence of improper placement of PDT tubes between the cricoid cartilage and first tracheal ring when patients were first assessed by ultrasound.[175] Ultrasonography has also been suggested to be of value to assist PDT in patients with obesity or short bull necks.[77] Although the cost effectiveness of routine ultrasonography is unknown, it may be used more often in the future now that portable ultrasonographic equipment is becoming more common in the ICU.

Johnson et al reported the performance of tracheostomy using the Ciaglia Blue Rhino single dilator technique using a modified open approach without bronchoscopy.[19] A 1–3 cm anterior cervical skin incision was followed by limited soft tissue dissection bluntly performed using hemostats to expose the pretracheal fascia. The operator palpated the exposed trachea to verify withdrawal of the endotracheal tube

above the tracheal puncture site. Direct observation of the insertion of needle, guide wire, dilator, and tracheostomy tube avoided misplacement. This approach was stated to decrease the cost of the procedure by avoiding bronchoscopy, although a bronchoscope was kept by the bedside.

Existing data suggest that post-PDT chest radiographs are unnecessary if the procedure is performed under bronchoscopic visualization.[176]

CRICOTHYROIDOTOMY

The cricothyroid membrane lies 2–3 cm below the thyroid notch and is located by palpation of the prominence of the cricoid cartilage. The membrane itself is typically 9–10 mm in height and trapezoidal in shape with a surface area of 3 cm^2. At its most superior margin, it lies 9–10 mm beneath the true vocal cords.[177]

After positioning the patient as for a standard tracheotomy, a sterile field is prepared.[12,178] A horizontal 2-cm skin incision is carried through the subcutaneous tissue to the thyroid cartilage. In the emergency setting, a vertical skin incision avoids severing the anterior jugular veins.[75] The lower border of the cricothyroid membrane is incised transversely and a tracheal hook is placed under the thyroid cartilage. A Trousseau dilator is inserted through the membrane with gentle vertical dilation to allow passage of a 6 or 7 mm tracheostomy tube. The outside diameter of the tube is limited by the height of the cricothyroid membrane (usually 9 mm).

MINITRACHEOTOMY

Minitracheotomy can be performed either by a scalpel or Seldinger technique.[130,137] The scalpel technique employs a kit that contains a scalpel, introducer, a specially adapted 4-mm tracheal cannula with an external flange, and tracheotomy tape. The scalpel has a blade that protrudes 1.4 cm from a plastic guard limiting the depth of insertion through the cricothyroid membrane. After positioning the patient as for standard tracheotomy, the cricothyroid membrane is located and marked by palpating the cricoid cartilage. After tissue infiltration with local anesthetic, the guarded scalpel is inserted through the midline of the cricothyroid membrane into the trachea to produce a 1-cm stab incision. The lubricated curved introducer is gently passed into the trachea through the stab incision. The tracheotomy cannula is then passed over the introducer, which is then removed from the airway. The airway is suctioned immediately through the minitracheotomy cannula to remove any blood or secretions.

The Seldinger dilatation technique uses a 16-gauge needle that is passed through the cricothyroid membrane into the tracheal lumen. After confirmation of correct placement by aspiration of air, the needle tip is angled caudally and a guide wire is passed through it. The needle is then removed and a minitracheotomy tube loaded over a vein dilator is passed over the guide wire into the trachea. The dilator and guide wire are then removed.

Once in place (Fig. 40-3), the minitracheotomy tube should be plugged when not in use for suctioning to prevent

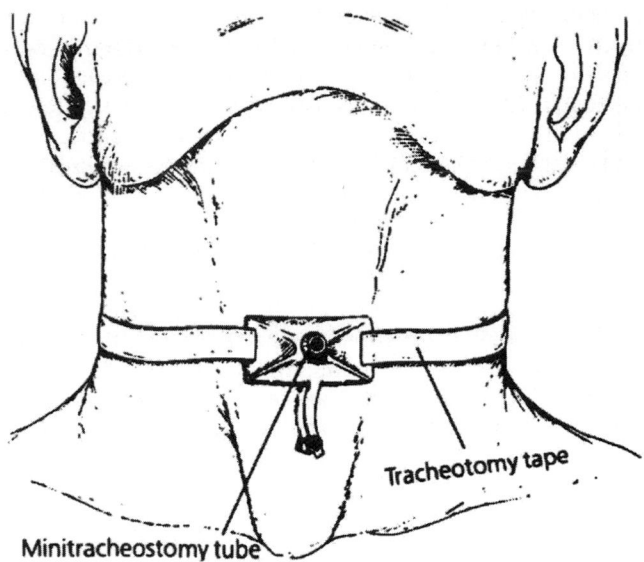

FIGURE 40-3 Minitracheotomy tube positioned to allow tracheal access for suctioning airway secretions. (*Reproduced, with permission, from Heffner: J Crit Illn 6:1249–55, 1991.*)

TABLE 40-2 Complications of Tracheostomy

Aspiration pneumonia
Cardiopulmonary arrest during the procedure
Herniation and fracture of tracheal rings
Inadvertent decannulation
Mediastinitis
Peristomal cellulitis
Pneumomediastinum and pneumothorax
Poor stoma healing after decannulation with scar, keloid, or
   tracheocutaneous fistula
Posterior tracheal wall perforation
Stomal erosion or breakdown
Stoma site infection
Stomal hemorrhage
Subglottic stenosis or atresia
Surgical emphysema
Tracheal dilatation
Tracheal granulomas with obstruction
Tracheal ring rupture
Tracheal stenosis
Tracheoesophageal fistula
Tracheoinnominate fistula
Tracheomalacia

the inhalation of dry ambient air and resultant inspissation of bronchial secretions and dilution of inspired supplemental oxygen.

Complications of Tracheotomy

Techniques and tube designs are sufficiently advanced to allow the safe application of tracheotomy in most ventilator-dependent patients. A 1% mortality rate and varying risks of perioperative and long-term delayed complications persist (Table 40-2), however, and correlate with an institution's expertise in airway management.[101,179]

INTRAOPERATIVE COMPLICATIONS

CARDIORESPIRATORY ARREST
Sudden cardiorespiratory arrest is the most feared immediate complication of surgical tracheotomy, occurring in less than 1% of patients. Underlying etiologies include vasovagal reactions in patients with underlying metabolic or cardiac disturbances, misplacement of the tracheotomy tube, tension pneumothorax, and pulmonary edema after relief of transient upper airway obstruction occurring during the operative procedure. Postobstructive pulmonary edema may also occur in up to 12% of patients undergoing tracheotomy (or translaryngeal intubation) for relief of severe airway obstruction.[180] Pulmonary edema may occur immediately or hours after the completion of the tracheotomy procedure.

HEMORRHAGE
Major hemorrhage is a rare early complication of tracheotomy if the anterior jugular veins, vascular anomalies (such as the thyroid ima artery or a high innominate artery) and thyroid isthmus are correctly identified to avoid inadvertent transection. Tracheotomies performed below

the fourth tracheal ring can risk injury to the innominate artery.

Minor hemorrhage occurs in 1–40% of tracheotomies and appears to depend on operator experience and the presence of a bleeding diathesis.[1] Minor hemorrhage can produce major intraoperative complications by obscuring the surgical field and promoting misplacement of the tracheotomy tube.

PNEUMOTHORAX AND PNEUMOMEDIASTINUM
The reported incidences of pneumothorax and pneumomediastinum after surgical tracheotomy or PDT ranges from 0–4%.[1,88,101,181,182] These complications may occur as a result of dissection of air through the incision and into the mediastinum, rupture of a bleb during hyperinflation related to transient airway obstruction, or direct injury to the apical pleura. Massive insufflation of the mediastinum can result from tracheotomy tube misplacement into soft tissue.

RECURRENT LARYNGEAL NERVE INJURY
The recurrent laryngeal nerves lie along the tracheoesophageal recesses on both sides of the neck. A properly placed midline surgical tracheotomy incision and dissection during a routine tracheotomy should not injure the nerves in their deep positions. Complicated surgical tracheostomy procedures in patients with altered cervical anatomy, however, may result in unilateral or bilateral nerve transection.

TRACHEOESOPHAGEAL FISTULA
Improper technique either with surgical tracheostomy or PDT can lacerate the posterior wall of the trachea, which is membranous at the level of the tracheotomy stoma, and cause a tracheoesophageal fistula. This complication can be avoided with surgical tracheostomy by incising the trachea against the endotracheal tube or carefully extending the tracheal stoma incision with scissors rather than

a scalpel. During placement of tracheal traction sutures, care must be taken not to puncture the posterior tracheal wall, which can then fistulize into the esophagus. Bronchoscopy during PDT assists the prevention of damaging the posterior tracheal wall with the insertion needle and dilators. Trottier et al reported a 12.5% incidence of posterior tracheal wall perforation with PDT[158] but other studies have reported an incidence less than 1% with bronchoscopic guidance.[34,84,157,183]

Significant laceration injuries to the posterior wall of the trachea should be immediately repaired during the initial tracheotomy procedure to avoid the risk of bacterial mediastinitis. The tracheotomy neck incision is extended laterally and the trachea and esophagus are repaired individually with placement of a muscle flap between each structure.[184]

Patients with a tracheoesophageal fistula present with increased secretions, pneumonia, and evidence of aspiration of gastric contents while on mechanical ventilation. When diagnosed after extubation, the most frequent sign of tracheoesophageal fistula is coughing after swallowing. A high index of suspicion is required for critically ill patients who have similar symptoms from other etiologies. The diagnosis is made by tracheoscopy and esophagoscopy. The immediate goal is to minimize tracheal soilage by positioning the cuff of the tracheal tube distal to the fistula. A gastric tube is placed to drain the stomach and nutrition is provided through a jejunostomy tube. The fistula should be surgically repaired after the patient weans from positive-pressure ventilation.[185]

EARLY POSTOPERATIVE COMPLICATIONS

HEMORRHAGE

Onset of wound hemorrhage may be delayed into the early postoperative period when an uncontrolled blood vessel opens during patient coughing or movement. Resolution of hypotension or dissipation of epinephrine may also underlie wound hemorrhage after the patient leaves the operating room. Prolonged oozing that persists for longer than 2–3 days is usually attributable to coagulopathy. The first onset of hemorrhage later than 48 hours after surgery should suggest the possibility of a tracheoinnominate fistula[186,187] (see below). Immediate airway hemorrhage may be less common with PDT as compared with surgical tracheostomy, although instances of massive, fatal airway hemorrhage with PDT have been reported.[174,188]

SUBCUTANEOUS EMPHYSEMA

Subcutaneous emphysema occurs in less than 10% of patients undergoing surgical tracheotomy who are mechanically ventilated.[189] Positive pressure escapes from the airway around an inadequately sealed tracheotomy tube cuff and decompresses into cervical tissue planes. Avoiding gauze packing in the tracheotomy wound decreases the risk of subcutaneous emphysema. The subcutaneous air usually reabsorbs spontaneously, but a chest radiograph should be performed to exclude an accompanying pneumomediastinum or pneumothorax. Pneumoperitoneum has also been reported with tracheostomy.[190]

INADVERTENT DECANNULATION

Inadvertent extubation is a potentially life-threatening complication in mechanically ventilated patients, particularly in the first 72 hours of tracheotomy placement. During this period, the stoma tract has not fully developed and parastomal tissue can obscure the tracheal window and complicate recannulation. Furthermore, blind attempts to replace the tracheotomy tube may result in misplacement into the pretracheal fascia and external compression of the airway.

Ventilator-dependent patients undergoing early extubation should be reintubated through the translaryngeal route if upper airway obstruction is not a factor and if the managing physician is not highly skilled in surgical airway anatomy. The tracheotomy tube can then be reinserted under more controlled conditions. If emergent recannulation of the stoma tract is to be attempted, the patient should be positioned as for surgical tracheotomy with a hyperextended neck. If tracheal traction sutures are present, they can be pulled to bring the anterior wall of the trachea as near to the skin as possible to close the pretracheal fascial planes and allow visualization of the tracheal window. The tracheotomy tube can be replaced if the tracheal window is clearly seen; initial insertion of a smaller sized cannula or placement of a guide catheter, such as a nasogastric tube, over which a tracheotomy tube is inserted may assist in reintubation.

If the tracheal lumen is not clearly seen, a pediatric laryngoscope blade with a light source may assist exploration of the wound and airway visualization. In thick-necked individuals, initial placement of a cuffless pediatric translaryngeal endotracheal tube to rapidly secure the airway followed by delayed recannulation with a tracheotomy tube may be required. A fiberoptic bronchoscope or laryngoscope may serve as a guiding stylet to assist tracheotomy tube reinsertion if the equipment can be quickly available.

The 1–7% incidence of inadvertent decannulation during the first 72 hours can be decreased by careful technique in securing the surgical airway.[1] Tracheotomy tape should wrap closely around the neck allowing sufficient space for insertion of a single finger. Tape should not be secured over gauze dressings that may later shift and loosen tube support. Although avoided by some surgeons, suturing the tracheotomy plate to the skin may decrease the risks of early decannulation.

WOUND INFECTION

Although rapidly contaminated with nosocomial pathogens,[191] a tracheostoma has a low rate of infection because it is left open and drains secretions. Antibiotic therapy of colonizing bacterial flora breeds resistant strains creating a reservoir for nosocomial pneumonia[5] and should be avoided. Patients with more purulent wound drainage usually respond to local tracheostoma care measures. Systemic antibiotic therapy is reserved for patients with a surrounding cellulitis or clinical evidence for breakdown of the tracheal stoma from deep tissue bacterial invasion. Necrotizing tracheostomal infections with paratracheal abscess formation can dissect into cartilaginous tracheal structures, adjacent major blood vessels, and the mediastinum.[192] This complication requires drainage, débridement, and replacement of the tracheotomy tube with a translaryngeal endotracheal tube.[193]

PNEUMONIA

All ventilator-dependent patients are at risk for nosocomial pneumonia. Although observational studies indicate that nosocomial pneumonia occurs more often in tracheostomy patients as compared with patients intubated through the translaryngeal route,[194] the former patient populations were selected on the basis of more protracted and severe clinical courses.[195] Up to 35% of patients in the ICU with a tracheostomy experience aspiration,[196–198] which is most often silent.[198] No evidence exists that aspiration occurs more commonly in ventilator-dependent patients after conversion to a tracheostomy.[199]

TUBE OBSTRUCTION

Partial obstruction of tracheotomy tubes decreases airflow and increases work of breathing for patients receiving partial assist modes of mechanical ventilation (intermittent mechanical ventilation or pressure support). Obstruction usually results from inspissated secretions or clotted blood, but may occur with incorrect selection of cannula size that places the tip of the tracheotomy tube against the tracheal wall or carina. Tracheotomy tubes with an inner cannula that can be removed for cleaning or replacement decrease the incidence of partial obstruction by airway secretions.[200] Obstruction can also occur when the tip of the tube causes traumatic swelling of the posterior tracheal wall with invagination of mucosal tissue into the tracheostomy lumen.[152]

LATE COMPLICATIONS

TRACHEAL STENOSIS

Tracheal stenosis related to tracheotomy can develop at the level of the cuff or at the tracheostoma site. Cuff site stenosis was the more common form of stenosis when tubes were fitted with high pressure–low volume cuffs.[201,202] High intracuff pressures necessary to maintain an airway seal transmit to the tracheal mucosa in the form of high cuff tensions that generate pressure necrosis. Resultant mucosal ulcerations become confluent and expose cartilaginous rings that become infected and disrupted. Ongoing necrosis generates fibrous scar formation and transmural airway narrowing.[203] Nontransmural tracheal stenosis can also develop when cartilaginous structures remain undamaged but proliferative scar formation narrows the intraluminal caliber of the airway. The greatest area of scar formation is usually within 3.5 cm of the stoma and ranges from 0.5–4 cm in length.

After the advent of low pressure–high volume cuffs, the incidence of tracheal stenosis at the cuff site has markedly decreased although it remains a clinical problem.[204] Inappropriate cuff overinflation or use of too small a tracheotomy tube that requires cuff overinflation to maintain an airway seal (see below) can convert a low-pressure to a high-pressure tube system.

The tracheostoma has become the more common site for the development of tracheal stenosis in patients undergoing surgical tracheostomy. The airway is narrowed in an anterolateral dimension with relative preservation of the posterior wall.[205] Factors that contribute to stoma site stenosis include an overly large surgical tracheal incision and excessive movement of the tracheotomy tube against the tracheal opening caused by poorly supported ventilator tubing and uncontrolled patient movement.[201] The trachea may also develop a fixed stenosis from cicatrization or a functional obstruction from tracheomalacia that becomes apparent during coughing or forced expiration.[205]

Case reports exist of severe tracheal stenosis at or above the stoma site after PDT.[206–209] A prospective randomized study comparing 6-month complications after PDT or surgical tracheostomy observed no significant differences in the incidence of tracheal stenosis (0 of 25 surgical tracheostomies versus 2 of 25 PDTs).[105] Other observational studies of airway complications of PDT are limited by small sample sizes and incomplete follow-up. The cumulative data, however, indicate a risk of tracheal stenosis after PDT that is similar to surgical tracheostomy.[59,85,87,208–214]

Clinical manifestations of tracheal stenosis may develop while the tracheotomy tube is still in place but more commonly occur 2–6 weeks after airway decannulation. Delayed onset as late as 4 months after extubation may also occur. Patients with compromised pulmonary function or neuromuscular disease may not manifest symptoms of tracheal stenosis until an episode of bronchitis when increased airway secretions produce respiratory compromise.

The symptoms and signs of tracheal stenosis may be obscured by the patient's underlying disease, but typically include difficulty clearing secretions, exertion-related dyspnea, and cough. Patients with normal underlying lung function may be relatively asymptomatic until a 5-mm critical stenosis develops that causes inspiratory stridor. Because of the nonspecific nature of the clinical manifestations of tracheal stenosis, patients with deteriorating respiratory function and a history of previous intubation should undergo evaluation for airway narrowing.[215]

The diagnostic evaluation of tracheal stenosis depends on imaging and endoscopic studies to detect airway narrowing, which may be fixed or dynamic.[216] Because pulmonary function tests are insensitive and nonspecific indicators of upper airway obstruction, becoming abnormal only after loss of 80% of the tracheal lumen, they do not provide important benefits in patient management.[215]

TRACHEOESOPHAGEAL FISTULA

A tracheoesophageal fistula occurs as a late complication in less than 1% of patients with a tracheotomy from pressure necrosis of the tracheal and esophageal mucosa.[217–219] Risk factors include high cuff pressures, high airway pressures, excessive tube movement, prolonged intubation, presence of a nasogastric tube, and diabetes mellitus.[185,220] During the course of intubation or after extubation, patients demonstrate increased cough or tracheal secretions. Symptoms may occur after eating or swallowing fluids. Patients undergoing positive-pressure mechanical ventilation may experience gastric distension or frequent belching. Recurrent aspiration of esophageal secretions may manifest as a nosocomial pneumonia.[221]

Diagnosis depends on a high clinical suspicion since many of the clinical features of tracheoesophageal fistula simulate exacerbations or complications of the underlying pulmonary disease. Chest radiographs of ventilated patients may demonstrate an air filled esophagus or gastric distension. Patients require bronchoscopy and esophagoscopy to adequately exclude the diagnosis.[185]

Unless surgically repaired, tracheoesophageal fistulae are universally fatal.[185] A single-stage repair of the fistula after weaning from mechanical ventilation is successful in most patients.[184,185,222] Specialized tubes with adjustable flanges exist that allow placement of the tracheostomy tube cuff at or below the level of the fistula track to prevent aspiration (Fig. 40-4).

TRACHEOINNOMINATE FISTULA

A tracheoinnominate fistula occurs in less than 1% of patients with a tracheostomy but is a major, potentially life-threatening complication of both surgical tracheostomy and PDT.[223-225] The innominate artery lies 9–12 tracheal rings below the cricoid cartilage within reach of the tip or cuff of the tracheostomy tube. It can traverse the midline just below the tracheostomy stoma in some patients where the "elbow" of a tracheostomy tube just above the cuff can induce pressure necrosis.[226] Improper traction on the tracheotomy tube by ventilator tubing, placement of the tracheal window below the fourth tracheal ring, sepsis, malnutrition, and corticosteroid therapy increase the risks for this complication.[186,227,228] Patients with head injury and repeated opisthotonic posturing may also be at increased risk.[229]

Pulsations of the tracheotomy tube with cardiac systole and "spotty" herald hemorrhages from the airway may portend a major hemorrhage from a tracheoinnominate fistula. Massive hemorrhage can result from fistula formation from the trachea to other vascular structures including the common carotid artery, inferior thyroid artery, the thyroid ima artery, the innominate vein, and the aortic arch.[230]

Airway hemorrhage can occur as early as several days or as late as 7 months after the initial tracheotomy with the peak incidence between the first and third week.[186,187,224,231] Up to 50% of patients who experience an episode of airway hemorrhage later than 72 hours after a tracheotomy have an underlying tracheoinnominate fistula.[186] The peak incidence of TIF occurs between the first and second week of tracheostomy[232] with 72% of patients presenting within the first 3 weeks of the procedure.[186]

When a herald hemorrhage suggests the existence of a tracheoinnominate fistula, the patient should undergo fiberoptic endoscopic evaluation in an operating room in case airway manipulation precipitates a major hemorrhage.[224] Patients who present with massive hemoptysis should be managed with overinflation of the tracheotomy tube cuff or insertion of a translaryngeal tube with positioning of the cuff over the fistula in an effort to tamponade the hemorrhage. A finger inserted into the stoma tract can attempt to compress the innominate artery anteriorly against the sternum[186,227] (Fig. 40-5). All patients with a tracheoinnominate fistula require a sternotomy with ligation and resection of the artery

FIGURE 40-4 Flexible tracheostomy tubes with adjustable flanges allow customization of a tube for fitting patients with difficult anatomy or a special need to place the cuff over a specific segment of the airway. (*Bivona TTS Adjustable Neck Flange Hyperflex Tracheostomy Tube, Portex, Inc, Keene, NH*).

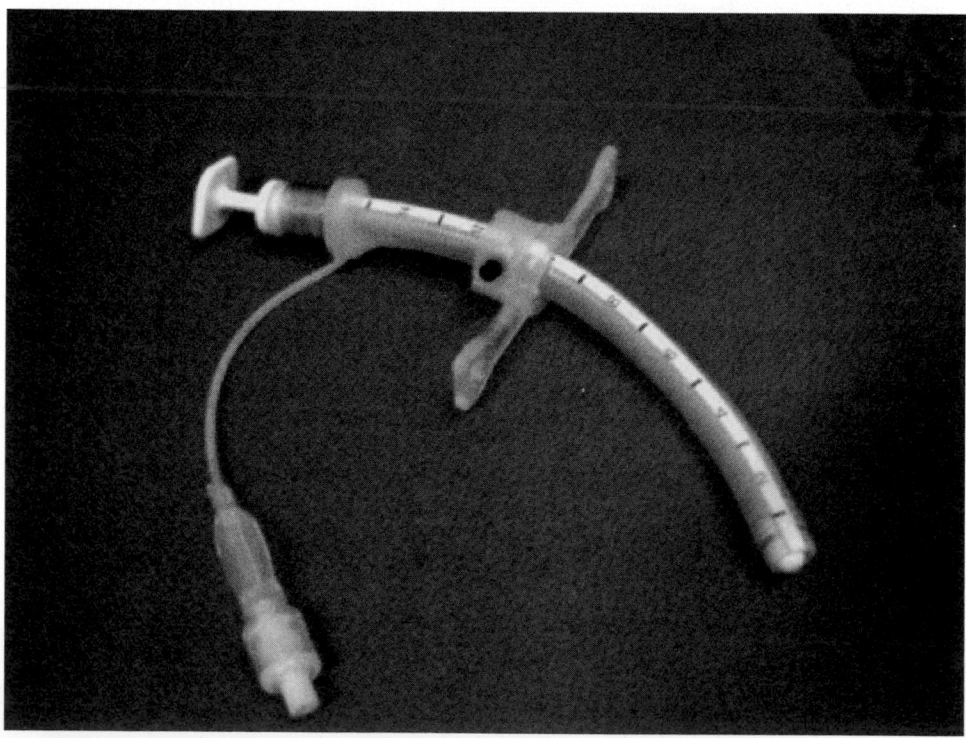

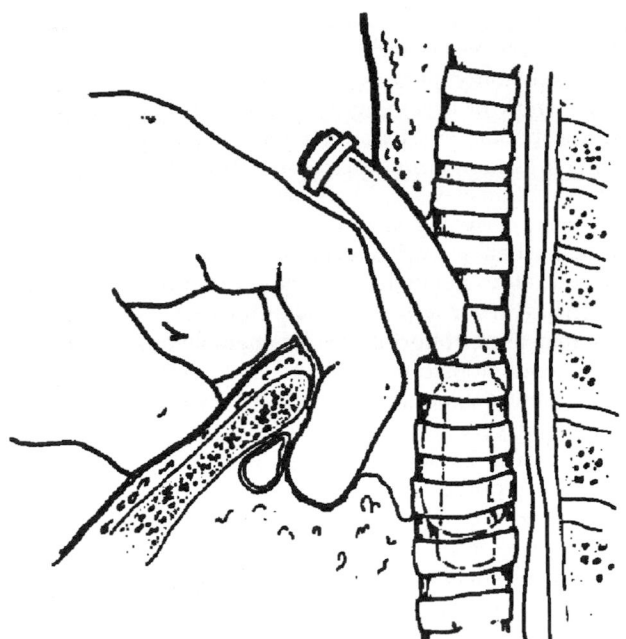

FIGURE 40-5 Hand position for finger tamponade of the innominate artery in a patient with a bleeding tracheoinnominate fistula. (*Reproduced, with permission, from Myers et al.[5]*).

since tissue infection obviates vascular repair.[224,230,233] Interruption of the innominate artery is tolerated in most patients without neurologic sequelae.[224,230,233] The immediacy of the complication usually does not allow sufficient time for angiographic confirmation of the diagnosis,[205,234] although one center has described intravascular tamponade of the fistula with a Fogarty catheter followed by definitive surgery.[235]

TRACHEOCUTANEOUS FISTULA
Failure of a tracheal stoma to spontaneously close after decannulation results from epithelialization of the stoma tract. Surgical closure requires a skin flap inversion to create an epithelialized anterior tracheal wall. The parastomal platysma or a sternohyoid muscle flap can then be pulled over the tracheal repair, followed by skin closure.[236–238] Stanton et al have recommended placement of a dermal interpositional fat graft.[239]

TRACHEAL RING FRACTURE AND HERNIATION
PDT risks fracture and herniation of tracheal rings because the technique dilates rather than incises intercartilaginous tissue.[240–242] Damaged rings can protrude into the airway causing tracheal narrowing.[243] The long-term impact of acute damage to tracheal rings by PDT is not well defined.

Timing of Tracheotomy during Mechanical Ventilation

Advances in tube design during the last 30 years have allowed translaryngeal endotracheal tubes to remain in place

TABLE 40-3   Advantages of Tracheostomy as Compared with Prolonged Translaryngeal Intubation

Decreased airway resistance for promoting weaning from
    mechanical ventilation
Decreases risk of nosocomial pneumonia in patient subgroups
Earlier transfer of ventilator-dependent patients from the ICU
Enhanced oral nutrition
Enhanced phonation and communication
Improved airway suctioning
Increased comfort
Increased patient mobility
Less direct endolaryngeal injury
More secure airway and decreaed risk of inadvertent decannulation

for longer durations without causing tracheolaryngeal injury. Tracheostomy, however, provides multiple advantages for patients who require long-term ventilator support[244,245] (Table 40-3). Determination of the precise timing of tracheostomy for an individual patient to achieve these benefits is complicated by the absence of sufficient clinical trials that assess the impact of timing of tracheostomy on outcomes for patients in specific clinical settings. Most existing trials have small and heterogenous study populations, incomplete follow-up, absence of blinding, and lack of standardization of ventilator and weaning decisions.[195,246] Only one trial has performed tracheostomy with PDT rather than surgical tracheostomy.[247] Moreover, studies have not examined the comfort-related value of tracheostomy from the patient's and family's perspectives.

The decision for timing a tracheostomy for a critically ill patient, therefore, remains a complex challenge that requires individualization of care. No data exist to establish a standard time when tracheostomy must be performed to avoid airway injury from continuing translaryngeal intubation. Moreover, the risks of tracheostomy are acceptably low so that it can be applied when patients appear likely to benefit from the procedure. Recommendations to "calendar watch" and avoid tracheostomy if at all possible for at least 14–21 days because of its attendant risks have become obsolete.[244,248] Accumulating evidence encourages clinicians to perform "earlier" tracheostomy than traditionally recommended in the 1980s.[247] It is unclear, however, whether an "early" procedure should be performed on the second, seventh, tenth, or some other day and what clinical factors should drive the timing decision.[249] Should elderly patients with pneumonia be managed differently than young patients with burns or trauma? In the absence of sufficient data to constrain the decision, patients should be selected for tracheostomy by considering the unique circumstances of the patient and the likelihood that the benefits of tracheostomy will outweigh its inherent risks and the risks of prolonging translaryngeal intubation (Table 40-4).

Benefits of tracheostomy are listed in Table 40-3. For awake patients receiving long-term ventilatory support, conversion to a tracheostomy provides opportunities to improve comfort by allowing oral hygiene, oral nutrition, and transfer to chairs.[250] Patients express an improved sense of well being after conversion to tracheostomy.[251] Moreover,

TABLE 40-4 Complications and Disadvantages of Prolonged Translaryngeal Intubation

Airway perforation
Aspiration pneumonia
Cricoid cartilage abscess
Damage to intrinsic laryngeal muscles
Dislocation or subluxation of the arytenoid
Granulation tissue forming interarytenoid adhesion
Healed fibrous glottic nodules
Inadvertent extubation
Mucosal ulceration
Nasal septal fractures with nasotracheal intubation
Nosocomial sinusitis
Otitis media
Oversedation
Patient discomfort
Posterior glottic stenosis
Subglottic stenosis
Tracheal stenosis
Ulcerative lesions of the nares and pharynx
Vocal cord fixation from fibrosis of the cricoarytenoid joint
Vocal cord laceration
Vocal cord paralysis
Web formation

McGeehin et al surveyed the perceptions of 72 intensive care nurses regarding the comfort of patients after 7 days of mechanical ventilation.[252] Over 90% noted improved patient comfort and 67% observed less family concern about patient comfort after tracheostomy was performed. Seventy-two percent of nurses stated a preference for tracheostomy if they ever required mechanical ventilation longer than 7 days.

Improved patient comfort allows weaning of sedation, which increases the risk of nosocomial pneumonia in ventilated patients and delays weaning.[253] Tracheostomy allows transfer from the ICU to more comfortable and family-centered settings for patients who remain ventilator dependent.[254] Patients also achieve after tracheostomy a capacity for articulated speech, which improves their sense of well being and personal control.[255-258]

The shorter length and rigid structure of tracheostomy tubes have been stated to decrease airway resistance and promote weaning from mechanical ventilation.[259,260] The resistance to airflow of translaryngeal endotracheal tubes in situ increases beyond in vitro predictions because thermolabile tubes assume angulated configurations and become inspissated with secretions, both of which promote turbulent airflow.[261,262] Studies conflict, however, about whether the lower measured resistance of tracheostomy as compared to endotracheal tubes produces meaningful benefits to patients. Lin et al noted no clinically important differences in pulmonary mechanics before and after tracheostomy in ventilator-dependent patients.[263] Three studies, however, have noted small decreases in work of breathing after tracheostomy that became more significant with increasing respiratory rates, in addition to decreases in airway resistance, pressure-time product, and auto-PEEP.[264-266] No

changes in tidal volume, respiratory rate, or dead space ventilation were observed.[264-267]

Tracheostomy provides an opportunity to further decrease work of breathing by removing the inner cannula during spontaneous breathing weaning trials.[268] Enhanced ability to suction through a tracheostomy tube may promote removal of airway secretions, which increase airway resistance of translaryngeal endotracheal tubes.[265,269] It remains unclear whether tracheostomy accelerates weaning for all patients, although benefits of the procedure for individual patients with borderline ventilator function most likely provide increased opportunities for spontaneous breathing. It has been demonstrated, however, that PDT after 48 hours of mechanical ventilation as compared with 14–16 days decreases duration of ventilator dependency (7.6 ±2.0 [SD] versus 17.4 ± 5.3 days).[247]

Studies conflict on the benefits of tracheostomy for decreasing risk of ventilator-associated pneumonia. Rodriguez et al observed a relative risk of 81% for pneumonia in trauma patients who underwent early ($\leq$7 days of ventilation) as opposed to late (>7 days) tracheostomy (254). Kluger et al observed a similar effect on pneumonia among 118 trauma patients converted to a tracheostomy during the first week of mechanical ventilation.[270] Sugerman et al, however, noted no decreased risk of pneumonia among trauma patients with early tracheostomy.[271] The combined data from 289 patients enrolled in prospective studies of early versus late tracheostomy[254,271,272] showed an aggregate relative risk for pneumonia with early tracheotomy of 0.88 (95% confidence interval 0.70–1.10).[195] A quality review of these studies noted multiple design flaws, which further weaken their conclusions.[195] More recently, Rumbak et al compared early PDT (2 days of ventilation) with delayed PDT (14–16 days) and observed a lower incidence of pneumonia in the early-PDT group (5% versus 25%).[247] Although the benefits of early tracheostomy for decreasing the risk of pneumonia remain incompletely defined, existing studies favor earlier tracheostomy.[195,246,249]

Inadvertent extubation occurs in 8.5–21% of ventilator-dependent patients.[217,251,273,274] and exposes patients to risks of adverse cardiopulmonary events that include nosocomial pneumonia.[273,275-277] Tracheostomy provides a more secure airway and decreases the risk of self-extubation.[217,247,273,278]

In considering the potential benefits offered by tracheostomy, clinicians timing conversion to tracheostomy must weigh the competing risks of the procedure discussed in this chapter with the risks of continuing translaryngeal intubation. Risks of prolonged translaryngeal intubation include injury to the larynx resulting in subglottic stenosis, requirements for continued sedation, nosocomial sinusitis, inability to speak, and inability to have oral nutrition.[279,280] The decision to perform tracheostomy would be simplified if the risk of laryngotracheal injury rapidly increased after a specific duration of endotracheal intubation. Aggregate data indicate that some degree of clinically important laryngeal injury occurs in 10–19% of patients managed with prolonged translaryngeal intubation.[179] It is not clear, however, that laryngeal injury can be predicted by the duration of endotracheal intubation or the detection of acute airway lesions in intubated patients.[281–284] "Calendar watching" with the performance of tracheostomy for all patients after a specific interval of translaryngeal intubation in order to prevent long-term airway injury does not, therefore, have sufficient data to support its application in the ICU.

In contrast to calendar watching, many clinicians now endorse "the anticipatory approach" to timing tracheostomy that tailors the decision to perform a tracheostomy to an individual patient's unique needs and avoids delaying the procedure unnecessarily.[179,245,285,286] Patients with respiratory failure first receive necessary critical care to allow stabilization. Patients who appear likely to achieve extubation within the first several days of mechanical ventilation do not require consideration for tracheostomy. If patients remain ventilator dependent after the first several days and appear likely to require ventilation for 14 or more days, a tracheotomy can be *considered*. The actual decision to perform the procedure, however, depends on the multiple patient-dependent factors that determine whether the patient will likely experience the benefits associated with tracheostomy.

Examples of the application of these decision-making guides are as follows. Comatose, quiescent patients who remain clinically unstable and unlikely to self-extubate would not experience the immediate comfort or mobility-enhancing benefits of tracheostomy. The decision to perform the procedure could be delayed until the patient would benefit from tracheostomy for reasons such as transfer from the ICU, improved airway suctioning, or weaning from ventilator support. In contrast, a mentally alert patient who requires sedation for comfort and appears unlikely to undergo successful extubation within 14 days may benefit from early conversion to a tracheostomy if contraindications do not exist. A patient with severe emphysema and pneumonia with excessive airway secretions who remains on high concentrations of inspired oxygen after 48 hours of care would exemplify such a patient. As a final example, patients with progressive causes of respiratory failure, such as amyotrophic lateral sclerosis or high cervical injuries,[287] who have failed noninvasive ventilation do not benefit from a trial of weaning after translaryngeal intubation. These patients benefit from tracheotomy as soon as stabilization occurs after initiation of mechanical ventilation.

The anticipatory approach requires clinicians to have some ability to estimate the anticipated duration of mechanical ventilation. Several studies indicate that clinicians can use clinical features apparent in patients intubated for a variety of pulmonary conditions to estimate within 2–7 days of initial intubation the likelihood of prolonged need for ventilator support.[7,287–296]

The decision to time tracheostomy in a more standardized manner awaits future studies and clinical evidence that performance of the procedure on a specific day of ventilation improves clinical outcome. The study by Rumbak et al is the first to examine PDT performed after 48 hours and show decreased mortality, risk of pneumonia, and inadvertent decannulations, in addition to shorter ICU stays in contrast to late PDT in patients managed in a medical ICU.[247] Additional studies that examine a broader range of patients at other time intervals will advance the evidence base for our timing decisions.

Special Patient Care Considerations

After conversion to tracheotomy, ventilator-dependent patients benefit from a well-organized management plan and an interdisciplinary critical care team experienced in the specialized techniques of surgical airway management. Skills in evaluating patients for oral communication and nutrition, avoiding airway-related complications, initiating an airway weaning protocol, and recognizing complications postextubation improve patient outcome.

MANAGEMENT OF TUBE CUFF PRESSURE

Tracheostomy tube cuff pressures should ideally be managed between 18 and 25 mmHg. Inappropriately high cuff pressures are transmitted to the tracheal mucosa as extreme wall tension that can tamponade mucosal capillaries and cause mucosal ischemia leading to tracheal stenosis. Intracuff pressures below 15 mmHg have been associated with increased microaspiration around the cuff and an increased risk of nosocomial pneumonia.[297,298] Various techniques exist to estimate cuff pressure, such as finger palpation of the external inflation bulb, minimal occlusive volume, and the tension on an inflating syringe. None, however, reliably substitutes for direct measurements of intracuff pressure with a pressure gauge.[299–303] In the absence of routine cuff pressure monitoring, up to 45% of critically ill patients have overly high endotracheal tube cuff pressures.[304] Chest radiographs are an additional safeguard in mechanically ventilated patients since overdistension of the tracheal lumen by a hyperinflated cuff can be detected.[305] Tube cuffs from different manufacturers may seal airways at different pressures.[306]

Several factors can contribute to inadvertent increases in tracheal cuff pressure. High peak airway pressure associated with acute respiratory failure externally compresses the inferior cuff surface raising intracuff pressure and tracheal wall tension.[307] Patients undergoing general anesthesia experience a rapid increase in cuff pressure as anesthetic gases infuse into the air-filled cuff.[308] An inappropriately small tracheotomy tube can also cause increased tracheal wall tension with resultant delayed airway stenosis by necessitating cuff overinflation to cause airway seal during mechanical ventilation.

SWALLOWING

Normal swallowing is a complex physiologic event comprised of simultaneous and sequential contractions of muscles of the oral-facial region, pharynx, larynx, and esophagus. To initiate swallowing, upward and backward motion of the tongue moves a food bolus to the posterior oral cavity or oropharynx,[309–311] where stimulation of neuroreceptors triggers pharyngeal swallowing and halts respiration, typically in the expiratory phase.[312–314] The pharyngeal swallow comprises five overlapping events that protect the airway and clear the pharynx of ingested material. These events are (1) elevation and retraction of the soft palate, (2) elevation and anterior displacement of the hyoid bone and larynx, (3) laryngeal closure, (4) pharyngeal contraction, and (5) opening of the pharyngoesophageal region.[309–311,315–323]

Contraction of the pharyngeal constrictors occurs coincident with forceful retraction of the tongue, which propels the bolus posteriorly to assist pharyngeal clearance.[316,322,323] Contractions of the thyrohyoid and submental extrinsic tongue muscle group elevate and move forward the hyoid bone and larynx as a functional unit. This hyolaryngeal complex movement closes the larynx to prevent aspiration and pulls the cricoid cartilage anteriorly and away from the posterior pharyngeal wall, thereby opening the pharyngoesophageal segment (PES) region to permit entry of the bolus into the cervical esophagus.[316–324] The PES becomes compliant by synchronized relaxation of the cricopharyngeal muscle.[317,320,322] The larynx then descends toward its resting position and respiration resumes characterized by a small expiratory airflow.[312–314] Once in the cervical esophagus, the bolus is propelled by primary and secondary esophageal peristaltic muscle contractions.[325,326] These contractions continue until the bolus progresses into the stomach through the passively relaxed lower esophageal sphincter (LES).

Controversy exists regarding the effects of tracheostomy on swallowing and its contribution to aspiration.[327–331] Clinical evidence suggests, however, that a tracheostomy tube or inflated cuff may interfere with the mechanics of swallowing (Fig. 40-6a and b). A tube can anchor the hyolaryngeal complex and prevent its normal excursion during swallowing causing incomplete airway closure and penetration of liquid and food into the laryngeal vestibule with aspiration below the vocal folds.[332,333] Prevention of the normal upward and forward mobility of the hyolaryngeal complex impedes anterior displacement of the cricoid cartilage leading to incomplete opening of the cervical esophagus and retained pharyngeal contents, which may be aspirated into the open airway after completion of the swallow. An inflated tube cuff may disturb esophageal motility and slow esophageal clearance causing retrograde flow of ingested material into the pharynx with aspiration. Coexisting gastroesophageal reflux disease with esophageal refluxate increases the risk for aspiration.[334] Tracheostomized patients at risk for aspiration should undergo a systematic assessment to determine the nature of any swallowing disorder to prevent aspiration and facilitate weaning to decannulation.

NUTRITION

Feeding patients with a tracheotomy through a nasoenteric tube increases the risk of aspiration and nosocomial pneumonia. Up to 20–69% of patients with a tracheotomy aspirate at least once every 48 hours regardless of mental status.[298,335] A third of ventilated patients with a new tracheostomy experience aspiration, which is usually silent in nature and more common in patients older than 70 years.[196,198] The risk of aspiration is greater with patients managed with a cricothyroidotomy as compared with a tracheostomy.[336] A small-bore feeding tube, continuous infusion rather than bolus instillation of feeding formulas, and patient

FIGURE 40-6 a. Superior and anterior displacement of the hyoid (*H*) and larynx (*L*) results in approximation of the arytenoid cartilages (*A*) and epiglottic petiole (*E*), and release of the posterior cricoid area from the posterior pharyngeal wall. b. The hyoid (*H*) and larynx (*L*) are anchored by the inflated tracheostomy tube cuff leading to incomplete approximation of the arytenoid cartilages (*E*) to the epiglottic petiole (*E*) with resultant penetration, aspiration, and incomplete opening of the cervical esophagus.

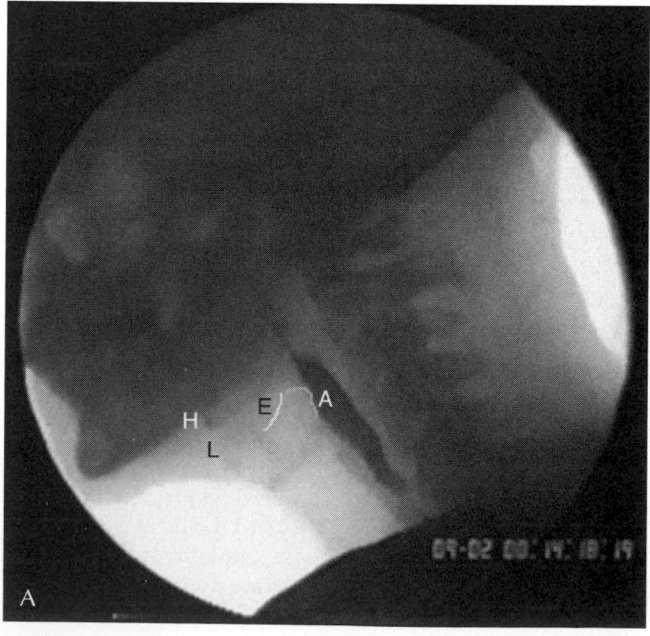
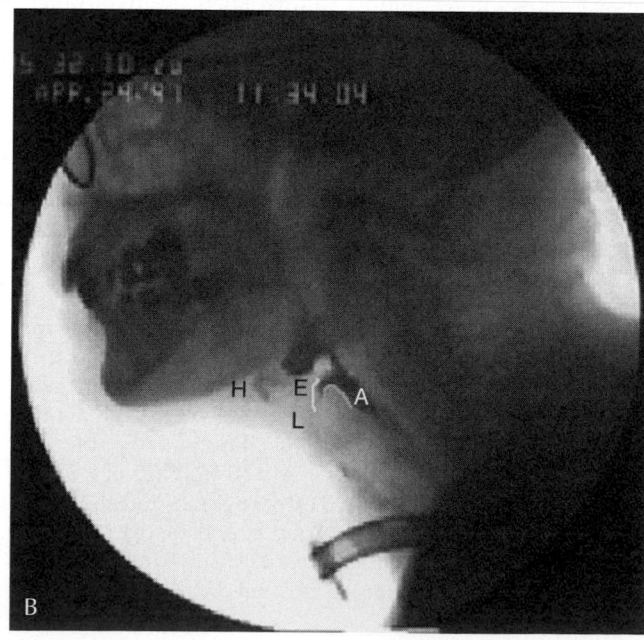

positioning in a 30–45° upright position appear to decrease intragastric pressure and lessen the risks of aspiration and pneumonia.[337,338]

Although a tracheostomy offers opportunities to resume an oral diet, patients recovering from critical illness with a tracheostomy in place commonly have severe swallowing dysfunction,[198,339,340] either from underlying disease or effects of the tube itself.[341] Before resuming oral feeding, patients should undergo evaluation by an interdisciplinary team that includes a speech-language pathologist trained in swallowing assessment.[342]

Bedside examinations serve poorly as screening evaluations because of their unreliability in excluding swallowing dysfunction and aspiration.[309,343,344] Most patients recovering from critical illnesses with a tracheostomy tube require a modified barium swallowing study to assess swallowing fully.[310,311,345] The bedside evaluation includes general observation of the patient's communication-cognitive status, upper extremity movement and manual dexterity, oromotor function, gag reflex, and, when appropriate, results of a swallowing trial with small amounts of food or liquid. The presence of a gag reflex does not exclude the possibility of aspiration.[339,346–349] Signs associated with swallowing impairment and aspiration are listed in Table 40-5.

Adding a colorizing agent to food or the patient's saliva has a 100% specificity but a low sensitivity for detecting aspiration.[350] Many clinicians prefer colored foods, such as grape juice, rather than blue dye (FD&C blue no. 1) because the latter has been associated with systemic absorption and profound metabolic acidosis.[351] Auscultating over the neck may detect sounds of secretions as evidence signaling aspiration.[352]

Flexible endoscopic evaluation of swallowing can assist the evaluation of the functional events that occur early and late in the pharyngeal swallow.[353,354] Endoscopic signs of swallowing dysfunction include persistence of pharyngeal or laryngeal residue after completion of swallowing and evidence of tracheal aspiration. Accumulation of endoscopically visible oropharyngeal secretions located within the laryngeal vestibule is highly predictive of aspiration of food or liquid.[355] Endoscopy cannot assess functional events at the height of the swallow because opposition of pharyngeal structures during hyolaryngeal excursion obscures viewing.[353] Endoscopy also cannot observe the oral cavity during swallowing to assess its normal functioning.[353]

TABLE 40-5 Clinical Warning Signs Suggestive of Swallowing Impairment and Aspiration

• Orofacial weakness	• Delayed cough
• Articulatory imprecision	• Wet vocal quality
• Decreased orofacial sensation	• Hoarse vocal quality
• Drooling	• Harsh vocal quality
• Labored chewing	• Breathy vocal quality
• Labored oral transport	• Strained vocal quality
• Decreased frequency of swallow	• Impaired resonance
• Lung sounds	• Gas-induced cough
• Laryngeal elevation	• Decreased laryngeal sensation
• Sounds of swallow	• Reduced O_2 saturation
• Immediate cough	

The modified barium swallowing study done with videofluoroscopic recording is the preferred evaluative technique because it visualizes bolus flow in relation to structural movement throughout the upper aerodigestive tract in real time.[309–311,315,345] The study also allows detection and timing of aspiration in addition to its pathophysiologic etiology.[310,311,345] Findings on the study can differentiate between swallowing dysfunction due to generalized deconditioning, stroke, or neuromuscular disorders from dysfunction due to effects of the tracheostomy tube. Candidates for a modified barium swallowing study should first undergo oral and tracheal suctioning and deflation of the tube cuff to remove its contribution to swallowing dysfunction (see Fig. 40-6a and b).

In preparation for the introduction of an oral diet, the patient should be adequately oxygenated with low inspired oxygen concentrations and have adequate ventilatory reserve in case aspiration occurs. The gag reflex is evaluated along with the adequacy of volitional and reflex coughing, swallowing, and oral motor strength. Initial attempts at feeding introduce small ice chips followed by soft foods, such as gelatins, which do not present a problem if aspirated.[356] It is unclear whether the tracheostomy tube cuff should be routinely inflated or deflated during initial refeeding to prevent aspiration.[298,335,357] Tippett et al demonstrated in five ventilator-dependent patients with neuromuscular disease that cuff deflation allowed inspiratory ventilator gas to exsufflate from the trachea into the pharynx thereby sweeping airway contaminants into the mouth where they could be swallowed.[357] Conversely, an inflated cuff can bulge posteriorly compressing the esophagus and producing dysphagia. The decision for cuff deflation should be individualized based on a patient's clinical response.

COMMUNICATION: VOICE, SPEECH, AND LANGUAGE

The primary subsystems of voice and speech include: respiration, phonation (i.e., generation of sound produced at the level of the vocal folds), resonance (i.e., created by the filter function of the pharynx), and articulation (i.e., the shaping of the voice airstream via movement of the lips, tongue, and palate). These subsystems are highly interdependent for audible, aesthetic, and intelligible oral communication. Any disruption to one or more of these subsystems will result in an impaired functional compensation of the remaining systems.

As compared to normal physiology, the presence of an indwelling tracheostomy tube disrupts normal voice and speech production. For patients previously intubated with an endotracheal tube, however, a tracheostomy may improve patient well being by increasing options for patient communication.[251,286,358,359] Personal isolation and an inability to communicate during mechanical ventilation are important factors in increasing anxiety in patients, families, and health care providers alike.[359–362] Interruption of spoken communication by a translaryngeal endotracheal tube represents one of the most important determinants in causing feelings of insecurity, fear, agony, and panic in intubated patients.[257,258]

Several techniques for promoting verbal communication with a tracheostomy can be tailored to the individual patient's ability to participate in speech therapy. Patients may also graduate through increasingly more complex techniques as their medical conditions allow. The clinical features and applications of these techniques are outlined in Table 40-6.

Patients undergoing positive-pressure ventilation with moderate to low minute ventilation requirements may be able to whisper during brief periods of partial cuff deflation. Patients mechanically ventilated because of neuromuscular disease can be managed by a cuffless or fenestrated tracheostomy tube during positive-pressure ventilation and retain the ability to speak.[363-365] A portion of the ventilator-delivered tidal volume enters the lower trachea and flows around the tracheostomy tube toward the upper airway during inspiration allowing the patient to talk.

In preparation for speaking sessions for patients with cuffed tracheostomy tubes, the patient's airway is first suctioned through the tracheotomy tube and above the cuff to prevent aspiration. The respiratory therapist slowly deflates the tube cuff until sufficient gas leaks through the mouth to allow short phrases. After a period of practice, speaking sessions are initiated during family visits, physician rounds, and intermittent nursing interactions. Because competition may occur between the airflow needed to produce speech and the airflow needed to maintain gas exchange,[366] patients are observed for signs of hypoventilation and the cuff is reinflated when the respiratory therapist leaves the bedside.[367,368]

The above approach limits speech to inspiration and a short portion of expiration as opposed to normal speech, which occurs during expiration.[366,369-372] Speech throughout the respiratory cycle can be promoted by partial cuff deflation as described above, prolongation of the ventilator's inspiratory phase, and application of low levels of positive end-expiratory pressure.[358,368,372] The resultant continuous air leak around the cuff allows more spontaneous speech because the patient does not have to coordinate speaking efforts with the ventilator respiratory cycle.[373] Pressure-support ventilation in the presence of a leak around a tracheostomy tube causes an increase in inspiratory time and volume,[374-376] both of which may theoretically assist speech production. The addition of PEEP to pressure support represents bilevel positive-pressure ventilation, which has been shown to improve the quality of speech as compared with assist-control ventilation with PEEP for patients with neuromuscular disease.[377]

Specialized tracheotomy tubes, termed "pneumatic speaking tubes" or "talking tubes," promote speech by supplying pressurized gas mixtures to the trachea above the inflated tube cuff.[378-380] The gas escapes through the glottis and pharynx allowing whispered or vocalized speech. A pressurized gas source is connected to a cannula that travels through the wall of the tracheotomy tube and exits at its greater curvature. A gas flow rate of 1.5–10 L/minute successfully produces intelligible speech in 75% of properly selected patients.[381,382] One to five days of careful pa-

tient training is required, however, before adaptation to this method is achieved. Patients or bedside personnel can occlude an external Y connector during speaking efforts to initiate the flow of gas through the airway. Prognostic indicators for successful use of pneumatic speaking tubes include adequate mental status, availability of a well-trained speech-language pathologist for training and positive reinforcement, absence of laryngeal pathology such as vocal fold paralysis, patient motivation, and encouragement from the critical care staff and patient's family.[383]

Pneumatic speaking tubes may fail because the pressurized gas may flow retrograde through the tracheostoma around the tube. Because this retrograde flow can cause subcutaneous emphysema in patients with recent tracheotomies, pneumatic tubes are contraindicated during the first 5–7 days after surgery.[10] Pneumatic tubes may also fail because secretions or granulation tissue above the cuff may occlude the exit port for gas flow.[384] Tubes with single air vents along their greater curvature, such as the Portex "Talk" tubes (Portex, Inc, Wilmington, MA), are easier for learning speaking techniques and are less likely to become occluded because of the high gas flow that is concentrated at the single exit port.

Other complications of pneumatic speaking tubes include desiccation and inflammation of laryngeal mucosal structures caused by the drying effect of the gas flow. Warming and humidification of the gas source along with intermittent use of the technique can prevent the onset of laryngitis. An air mixture rather than pure oxygen should be used to avoid further airway injury from hyperoxia.[367] Careful patient screening is required to determine likelihood of benefit from speaking tracheostomy tubes because of the high incidence of air leaks and need for assistance for coordinating use of the device.[379]

The "electrolarynx" is a valuable device for promoting speech that has a high rate of success in critically ill patients with a tracheotomy.[385,386] These devices consist of a vibrator unit with an attached hand-held battery pack that generates a vibratory tone with variable loudness and pitch. Held firmly against the patient's neck midway between the mandibular angle and the notch of the thyroid cartilage, the electrolarynx substitutes for the vocal cords as an amplifier for speech. Over 90% of mentally alert patients with a tracheotomy can learn to use the electrolarynx successfully.[385] Critical care team members may require frequent inservicing on correct application of the device because of the loss of enthusiasm that develops when patients do not quickly learn the technique.

Patients weaning from mechanical ventilation who have achieved periods of spontaneous ventilation can speak with the assistance of a fenestrated tracheotomy tube.[373] Fenestrated tubes with an inner cannula can provide airway access for mechanical ventilation and a system for speech when the inner cannula is removed. Occlusion of the tracheotomy tube with a gloved finger or plug can divert airflow through the upper airway allowing whispered or vocalized speech. Deflation of the tube cuff can further improve expiratory airflow through the larynx.

A fenestrated tracheotomy tube can also be combined with a one-way valve (Passy-Muir valve, Passy and Passy,

TABLE 40-6   Methods of Communication for Intubated Patients

Communication Option	Advantages	Disadvantages	Considerations	Select Patient Use
Lip reading, mouthing	• Follows a natural communication style • Closely resembles normal speech movement • Limited training required • Makes use of oral motor functions • Allows for natural production of facial expression • Communication letter board assists communication	• Decreased understanding of mouthed messages • May result in patient frustration • Unnatural for patient to decrease rate and length of message • Very limited for orally intubated patients	• Patient should be alert • Requires intact motor functioning • Works best for nasally intubated patients • Requires proper tube taping technique in orally intubated patients for maximal oral movement • Patient at times requires encouragement to mouth words • Patients often require cueing to decrease rate and length of messages	• Can be used with a variety of nonparalyzed patients • Can be used with patients who are unable to use other alternatives for communication
Gestural language (yes–no [Y–N] responses, facial expressions, hand gestures)	• Y–N responses result in effective and rapid communication of basic needs • Appropriate facial expressions can greatly enhance communication and emotion • Message intent is usually understood	• Limited interpretation • Difficulty expressing complex or lengthy messages • Requires coordination and dexterity	• Establish Y–N response mode and communicate to staff and family (strive for natural Y–N responses with head nods) • Patients may require encouragement to use consistently	• Especially helpful for patients with oral intubation and/or oral motor dysfunction
Written communication	• Can be used for effective expression of basic needs and wants	• Timely method of communication • Requires significant patient endurance and alertness • Limited expression of complex ideas and emotion • Often difficult to read patient writings • May require staff assistance • Requires interpretation (language, writing style, etc.) by receiver	• Requires: motor coordination, strength of upper extremity, use of arm free from medical restraints, adequate visual acuity and perception, and supplies at bedside • May require prepositioning for writing comfort and visibility • Use a felt tip marker or other antigravity dark marking device • Provide a clipboard for firm writing surface • Provide glasses before writing attempts	• Can be used as an alternative to other communication options
Communication boards (picture, alphabet, and word boards)	• Effective communication of basic needs	• Timely communication process • Communication limited to items on board • High degree of frustration with alphabet use • Requires coordination for pointing response • Requires intact visual acuity/perception • Potential source of contamination when board used from room to room • Requires immediate accessibility, patient training, and staff patience	• Provide glasses to prescription lons wearers • Board should be kept at bedside • Position board and size of characters to meet patients needs	• Can be used with a variety of nonparalyzed patients • Can be used with patients who are unable to use other alternatives for communication

(continued)

TABLE 40-6 Methods of Communication for Intubated Patients (*Continued*)

Communication Option	Advantages	Disadvantages	Considerations	Select Patient Use
Augmentative communication devices ("parrot," "voice-aided," direct selection, and scanning devices)	• Effective communication of *basic* needs • Provides a programmed speaking voice when selected • Communication programs can be highly individualized to the patient • Easy access to provide complete phrases • Provides a means for more sophisticated, complex communication • Requires minimal energy once patient is familiar with device • Timely communication process	• Must be programmed • Communications limited to items on the board • May be frustrating due to limited options • Requires operator training • Requires concentration for selection of appropriate phrases • Requires coordination for pointing response • Potential source of contamination if board is used from room to room • Requires visual acuity • Requires maintenance (electrical safety, repairs) • May be costly to the patient (equipment, support of speech therapy)	• Patient and family need to be included in programming and selection of communication choices • Provide glasses to prescription lens wearers • Device should be kept at the bedside	• Can be used with a variety of nonparalyzed patients • Can be used with patients who are unable to use other alternatives for communication
Electrolarynx (Servox, Western Electric)	• Provides a voice without using vocal cords • Provides auditory component to speech productions for better understanding • Allows verbal communication of basic needs and emotions • Makes use of oral motor functioning • Useful when trach cuff cannot be deflated for other speaking techniques	• Poor mechanical quality of voice (monotonal) • Requires: assistance from staff, significant patient and staff training dexterity and hand coordination, and intact oral and motor functioning • Patient must be alert and cooperative • Patient must have energy reserve to use effectively • Oral adapter may be uncomfortable and awkward	• Dentures should be in place • Mouth and lips should be moist • Demonstrated technique to patient and family and allow for return demonstration • Allow time for experimentation for this and other options (including oral adapter)	• To be used with nasally intubated or tracheotomy patients (free use of mouth for motion)
Deflated/cuff leak methods (cuff leak on ventilator, T-piece)	• Allows use of own voice through vocal cords' natural communication styles • Results in efficient communication • Requires minimal staff assistance if patient can tolerate deflation • No cost requirements	• May be limited to use for short periods depending on tolerance level of patient • Requires staff assistance to deflate and monitor cuff • Methods contraindicated for acute or medically unstable patients • Requires intact oral motor functioning and respiratory reserve • Requires staff training (to monitor cuff pressures and exhaled volumes)	• Patients must be alert • Patients with copious secretions should be suctioned prior to deflation • Procedure must be fully explained to the patient • Ventilator-dependent patients require cueing for proper voice initiation • T-piece users must have T-piece occluded for voice to be audible • Ventilator adjustments often needed	• For use with ventilator patients who are stable with cuff leak/deflation and who have complex communication needs • Excellent for chronic/long-term vent/trach patients (especially. nonventilator-dependent patients) • Nasotracheal or T-piece patients (stable respiratory status)
Trach valves (Olympic, Passy-Muir, Montgomery)	• Allows for phonation and production of patient's own voice • Natural communication method • Passy-Muir can be used for ventilated patients	• May be limited to use for short periods • Requires staff assistance to plug in most patients • Requires intact oral and motor functioning • Patients without respiratory reserve may not tolerate • Works poorly on patients with stiff lungs or with copious secretions	• Provide support and encouragement during initial plugging periods • Close observation is required • Valve is routinely removed when not in use in acute setting	• For use in long-term/chronic tracheotomy patients • Passy-Muir may be used on ventilated patients

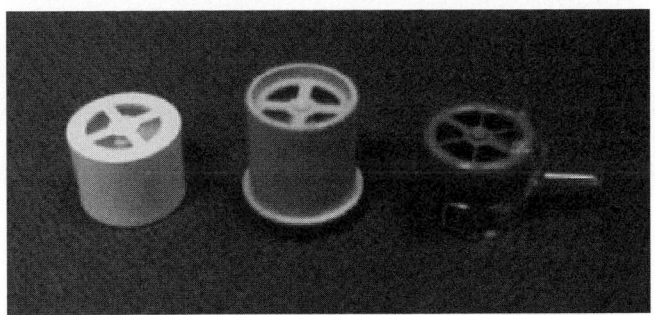

FIGURE 40-7 Passy-Muir one-way valves that allow articulated speech through the native airway for spontaneously breathing patients with a tracheostomy or patients undergoing mechanical ventilation through a tracheostomy tube. (*Passy-Muir Tracheostomy Valves, Passy-Muir Inc, Irvine, CA*).

Inc, Irvine, CA) that allows inspiratory airflow through the tube but closes during expiration diverting airflow through the larynx[387] (Fig. 40-7). One-way valves can be applied to the tracheostomy tube of spontaneously breathing patients and patients undergoing positive-pressure ventilation. The latter circuit includes a pressure popoff feature that allows exhalation through the tracheostomy tube if upper airway obstruction occurs. Commercially available one-way valves vary in their airflow resistive properties[388] and effectiveness for promoting understandable speech.[389] One-way speaking valves have been shown to either improve[390,391] or have no deleterious effects[199] on aspiration for patients with tracheostomies with pre-existing inclinations for aspiration. Contraindications include tracheal or laryngeal obstruction, excessive pulmonary secretions, unconsciousness, gross aspiration, and bilateral vocal cord paralysis.

Difficulties with fenestrated tubes include malpositioning of the fenestrations within the tracheal wall that prevents adequate airflow. Granulation tissue can obstruct the fenestrations, interfering with speech and causing hemorrhage during removal of the tube.[392] Newer tube designs with multiple small rather than single large fenestrations partially resolve these limitations. The increased airway resistance of breathing through a plugged fenestrated tube even with the cuff deflated may interfere with weaning from mechanical ventilation by excessively loading the respiratory muscles and limiting muscle performance.[393] Many centers avoid the use of fenestrated tubes for these reasons.

Recent innovations of tube designs allow inflation of the tracheostomy tube cuff during inspiration and deflation during expiration, which allows exhaled gas to flow through the larynx, promoting speech.[394]

WEANING FROM TRACHEOSTOMY AND DECANNULATION

Patients recovering from prolonged respiratory failure may either tolerate rapid decannulation of the tracheotomy tube or require a stepwise weaning program. The presence of underlying cardiorespiratory disease that persists despite resolution of the respiratory failure increases the likelihood that a period of weaning will be required.

Evaluation for decannulation begins after the patient demonstrates success with spontaneous ventilation off a ventilator for 48 hours. The ability to protect the airway is assessed by deflating the tube cuff and observing the patient for aspiration.[395] A rapid onset of moderate to severe degrees of saliva aspiration warrants indirect laryngoscopy to exclude glottic abnormalities such as vocal cord paralysis. The presence of upper airway obstruction is evaluated by transiently occluding a fenestrated tracheostomy tube with the cuff deflated. Respiratory distress warrants bronchoscopy to evaluate for airway narrowing or collapse during coughing.[396]

Patients who pass the above evaluation after 48 hours of spontaneous breathing can be observed for 30 minutes with the tracheostomy tube occluded. If they remain comfortable with breathing, further consideration of decannulation can occur. Patients who fail the 30-minute test have a high risk of upper airway obstruction.[396]

Several methods exist for weaning once patients tolerate cuff deflation and tube obstruction.[358] Patients with adequate ventilatory capacity who pass the 30-minute breathing trial with the tube obstructed may tolerate immediate decannulation.[396]

Patients with compromised ventilatory function or moderate secretions may benefit from an algorithmic approach that downsizes the tracheostomy tube caliber progressively to a #6 tube with conversion of some patients to a mini-tracheostomy tube for a week before cannulation.[397] This approach is successful in 80% of previously ventilated patients.[397]

Patients with moderate airway secretions and severely compromised lung function may not tolerate spontaneous breathing with partial obstruction of their airway with a tracheostomy tube. Such patients may benefit from a tracheostomy plug or a stoma stent that frees the airway but allows airway suctioning and maintenance of the stoma track for reinsertion of a tracheostomy tube if needed[398] (Fig. 40-8).

Regardless of the weaning method used, adopting a standardized approach improves clinical outcome.[397] Educating patients and families regarding the nature of the tracheostomy tube upon transfer from the ICU improves patient acceptance.[399]

Patient Prognosis after Tracheostomy

Patients who require tracheostomy for respiratory failure have a high cost of care and represent the most resource-consuming diagnostic categories for many acute care hospitals.[400,401] The mortality rate is high for ventilator-dependent patients who undergo tracheostomy in the ICU. Hospital survival is 49–78%.[7,402–404] Patients who undergo tracheostomy for respiratory failure due to surgical problems have a higher hospital survival as compared with patients undergoing mechanical ventilation for medical illnesses.[402] Among those who survive hospitalization, 24%, 30%, and 42% are no longer alive at 100 days, 6 months, and 2 years after discharge, respectively.[402] If decannulation

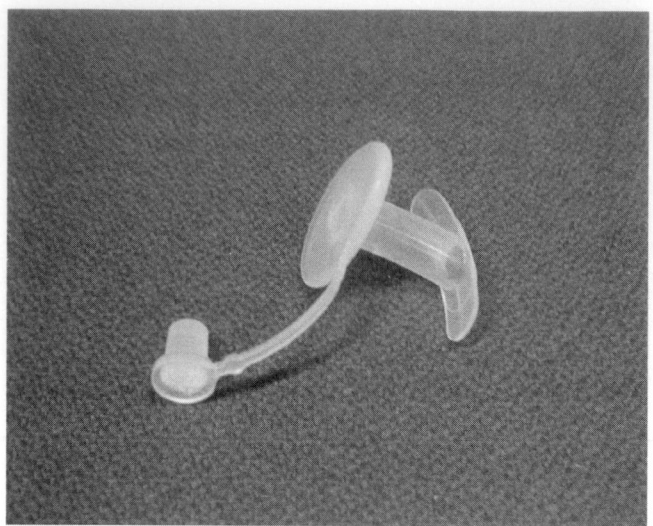

FIGURE 40-8 A stoma stent can maintain patency of the stoma after cannulation for patients who require ongoing airway access for suctioning or replacement of a tracheostomy tube if failure of decannulation occurs. (*Hood Stoma Stent, Hood Laboratories, Pembroke, MA*).

occurs before hospital discharge, 92% of patients are alive 1 year later.[402,405–407] Among mixed medical and surgical patients who survive acute hospitalization after tracheostomy for respiratory failure, 57% are successfully weaned and 30% decannulated before hospital discharge.[402]

References

1. Goldstein SI, Breda SD, Schneider KL. Surgical complications of bedside tracheotomy in an otolaryngology residency program. Laryngoscope 1987; 97:1407–9.
2. Alberti P. Tracheotomy versus intubation: a 19th century controversy. Ann Otol Rhinol Laryngol 1984; 93:333–7.
3. Campbell JB, Watson MG, Povey L, et al. Minitracheotomy and laryngeal function. J Laryngol Otol 1988; 102:49–51.
4. Watts JM. Tracheotomy in modern practice. Br J Surg 1963; 50:954–8.
5. Myers EN, Carrau RL. Early complications of tracheotomy. Incidence and management. Clin Chest Med 1991; 12:589–95.
6. Jackson C. Tracheostomy. Laryngoscope 1909; 19:285–90.
7. Kollef MH, Ahrens TS, Shannon W. Clinical predictors and outcomes for patients requiring tracheostomy in the intensive care unit. Crit Care Med 1999; 27:1714–20.
8. Fischler L, Erhart S, Kleger GR, Frutiger A. Prevalence of tracheostomy in ICU patients. A nation-wide survey in Switzerland. Intensive Care Med 2000; 26):1428–33.
9. Esteban A, Anzueto A, Alia I, et al. How is mechanical ventilation employed in the intensive care unit? An international utilization review. Am J Respir Crit Care Med 2000; 161:1450–8.
10. Heffner JE, Miller KS, Sahn SA. Tracheostomy in the intensive care unit. Part 1: Indications, technique, management. Chest 1986; 90:269–74.
11. Watson CB. Prediction of a difficult intubation: methods for successful intubation. Respir Care 1999; 44:777–98.
12. Walls RM. Cricothyroidotomy. Emerg Med Clinic North Am 1988; 6:725–36.
13. McLure HA, Dob DP, Mannan MM, Soni N. A laboratory comparison of two techniques of emergency percutaneous tracheostomy. Anaesthesia 1997; 52:1199–201.
14. Dob DP, McLure HA, Soni N. Failed intubation and emergency percutaneous tracheostomy. Anaesthesia 1998; 53:72–4.
15. Ault MJ, Ault B, Ng PK. Percutaneous dilatational tracheostomy for emergent airway access. J Intensive Care Med 2003; 18:222–6.
16. Ben-Nun A, Altman E, Best LA. Emergency percutaneous tracheostomy in trauma patients: an early experience. Ann Thorac Surg 2004; 77:1045–7.
17. Klein M, Weksler N, Kaplan DM, et al. Emergency percutaneous tracheostomy is feasable in experienced hands. Eur J Emerg Med 2004; 11:108–12.
18. L'Her E, Goetghebeur D, Boumedienne A, Renault A, Boles JM. Use of the Blue Rhino tracheostomy set for emergency airway management. Intensive Care Med 2001; 27:322.
19. Johnson JL, Cheatham ML, Sagraves SG, Block EF, Nelson LD. Percutaneous dilational tracheostomy: a comparison of single-versus multiple-dilator techniques. Crit Care Med 2001; 29:1251–4.
20. Toye FJ, Weinstein JD. A percutaneous tracheostomy device. 1969; 65:384–9.
21. Ciaglia P. Defining percutaneous dilational tracheostomy. Chest 1994; 106:983.
22. Ciaglia P, Firsching R, Syniec C. Elective percutaneous dilatational tracheostomy. A new simple bedside procedure: preliminary report. Chest 1985; 87:715–9.
23. Griggs WM, Worthley LI, Myburgh JA. Percutaneous tracheostomy. Anaesth Intensive Care 1991; 19:131–2.
24. Shelden C, Pudenz R, Tichy F. Percutaneous tracheostomy. JAMA 1957; 165:2068–70.
25. Bewsher MS, Adams AM, Clarke CW, McConachie I, Kelly DR. Evaluation of a new percutaneous dilatational tracheostomy set apparatus. Anaesthesia 2001; 56:859–64.
26. Fernandez L, Norwood S, Roettger R, Gass D, Wilkins H 3rd. Bedside percutaneous tracheostomy with bronchoscopic guidance in critically ill patients. Arch Surg 1996; 131:129–32.
27. Byhahn C, Westphal K, Meininger D, et al. Single-dilator percutaneous tracheostomy: a comparison of PercuTwist and Ciaglia Blue Rhino techniques. Intensive Care Med 2002; 28: 1262–6.
28. Byhahn C, Wilke HJ, Halbig S, Lischke V, Westphal K. Percutaneous tracheostomy: ciaglia blue rhino versus the basic ciaglia technique of percutaneous dilatational tracheostomy. Anesth Analg 2000; 91:882–6.
29. Cothren C, Offner PJ, Moore EE, et al. Evaluation of a new technique for bedside percutaneous tracheostomy. Am J Surg 2002; 183:280–2.
30. Beiderlinden M, Karl Walz M, Sander A, Groeben H, Peters J. Complications of bronchoscopically guided percutaneous dilational tracheostomy: beyond the learning curve. Intensive Care Med 2002; 28:59–62.
31. Carrillo EH, Spain DA, Bumpous JM, et al. Percutaneous dilational tracheostomy for airway control. Am J Surg 1997; 174: 469–73.
32. McHenry CR, Raeburn CD, Lange RL, Priebe PP. Percutaneous tracheostomy: a cost-effective alternative to standard open tracheostomy [see comments]. Am Surg 1997; 63:646–51; discussion 51–2.
33. Cobean R, Beals M, Moss C, Bredenberg CE. Percutaneous dilatational tracheostomy. A safe, cost-effective bedside procedure. Arch Surg 1996; 131:265–71.
34. Hill BB, Zweng TN, Maley RH, et al. Percutaneous dilational tracheostomy: report of 356 cases. J Trauma 1996; 41:238–43; discussion 43–4.

35. Friedman Y. Experience with percutaneous dilational tracheostomy. Ann Otol Rhinol Laryngol 2001; 110:799.

36. Friedman Y, Fildes J, Mizock B, et al. Comparison of percutaneous and surgical tracheostomies. Chest 1996; 110: 480–5.

37. Friedman Y, Mizock BA. Percutaneous versus surgical tracheostomy: procedure of choice or choice of the procedure. Crit Care Med 1999; 76:1684–5.

38. Winkler WB, Karnik R, Seelmann O, Havlicek J, Slany J. Bedside percutaneous dilational tracheostomy with endoscopic guidance: experience with 71 ICU patients [see comments]. Intensive Care Med 1994; 20:476–9.

39. Toursarkissian B, Zweng TN, Kearney PA, et al. Percutaneous dilational tracheostomy: report of 141 cases. Ann Thorac Surg 1994; 57:862–7.

40. Heikkinen M, Aarnio P, Hannukainen J. Percutaneous dilational tracheostomy or conventional surgical tracheostomy? Crit Care Med 2000; 28:1399–402.

41. Anon JM, Escuela MP, Gomez V, et al. Use of percutaneous tracheostomy in intensive care units in Spain. Results of a national survey. Intensive Care Med 2004; 30:1212–15.

42. Fikkers BG, Fransen GA, van der Hoeven JG, Briede IS, van den Hoogen FJ. Tracheostomy for long-term ventilated patients: a postal survey of ICU practice in The Netherlands. Intensive Care Med 2003; 29:1390–3.

43. Griggs WM, Worthley LIG, Gilligan JE, Thomas PD, Myburg JA. A simple percutaneous tracheostomy technique. Surg Gynecol Obstet 1990; 170:543–5.

44. Borm W, Gleixner M. Experience with two different techniques of percutaneous dilational tracheostomy in 54 neurosurgical patients. Neurosurg Rev 2003; 26:188–91.

45. Byhahn C, Wilke HJ, Lischke V, Rinne T, Westphal K. Bedside percutaneous tracheostomy: clinical comparison of Griggs and Fantoni techniques. World J Surg 2001; 25:296–301.

46. Cantais E, Kaiser E, Le-Goff Y, Palmier B. Percutaneous tracheostomy: prospective comparison of the translaryngeal technique versus the forceps-dilational technique in 100 critically ill adults. Crit Care Med 2002; 30:815–9.

47. Kahveci SF, Goren S, Kutlay O, Ozcan B, Korfali G. Bedside percutaneous tracheostomy experience with 72 critically ill patients. Eur J Anaesthesiol 2000; 17:688–91.

48. Anon JM, Gomez V, Escuela MP, et al. Percutaneous tracheostomy: comparison of Ciaglia and Griggs techniques. Crit Care 2000; 4:124–8.

49. Anon JM, Escuela MP, Gomez V, et al. Percutaneous tracheostomy: Ciaglia Blue Rhino versus Griggs' Guide Wire Dilating Forceps. A prospective randomized trial. Acta Anaesthesiol Scand 2004; 48:451–6.

50. Kost KM. Percutaneous tracheostomy: comparison of Ciaglia and Griggs techniques. Crit Care 2000; 4:143–6.

51. Nates NL, Cooper DJ, Myles PS, Scheinkestel CD, Tuxen DV. Percutaneous tracheostomy in critically ill patients: a prospective, randomized comparison of two techniques. Crit Care Med 2000; 28:3734–9.

52. Ambesh SP, Pandey CK, Srivastava S, Agarwal A, Singh DK. Percutaneous tracheostomy with single dilatation technique: a prospective, randomized comparison of Ciaglia blue rhino versus Griggs' guidewire dilating forceps. Anesth Analg 2002; 95:1739–45.

53. Dollner R, Verch M, Schweiger P, et al. Laryngotracheoscopic findings in long-term follow-up after Griggs tracheostomy. Chest 2002; 122:206–12.

54. Dollner R, Verch M, Schweiger P, Graf B, Wallner F. Long-term outcome after Griggs tracheostomy. J Otolaryngol 2002; 31: 386–9.

55. Steele AP, Evans HW, Afaq MA, et al. Long-term follow-up of Griggs percutaneous tracheostomy with spiral CT and questionnaire. Chest 2000; 117:1430–3.

56. Sviri S, Samie R, Roberts BL, van Heerden PV. Long-term outcomes following percutaneous tracheostomy using the Griggs technique. Anaesth Intensive Care 2003; 31:401–7.

57. Schachner A, Ovil Y, Sidi J, et al. Percutaneous tracheostomy—a new method. Crit Care Med 1989; 17:1052–6.

58. Leinhardt DJ, Mughal M, Bowles B, et al. Appraisal of percutaneous tracheostomy. Br J Surg 1992; 79:255–8.

59. Powell DM, Price PD, Forrest LA. Review of percutaneous tracheostomy. Laryngoscope 1998; 108:170–7.

60. Brathwaite CE. Rapid percutaneous tracheostomy. Chest 1991; 100:1475–6.

61. Frova G, Quintel M. A new simple method for percutaneous tracheostomy: controlled rotating dilation. A preliminary report. Intensive Care Med 2002; 28:299–303.

62. Grundling M, Kuhn SO, Nees J, et al. [PercuTwist dilational tracheostomy: Prospective evaluation of 54 consecutive patients]. Anaesthesist 2004; 53:434–40.

63. Westphal K, Maeser D, Scheifler G, Lischke V, Byhahn C. PercuTwist: a new single-dilator technique for percutaneous tracheostomy. Anesth Analg 2003; 96:229–32.

64. Fikkers BG, Venwiel JM, Tillmans RJ. Percutaneous tracheostomy with the PercuTwist technique not so easy. Anaesthesia 2002; 57:935–6.

65. Thant M, Samuel T. Posterior tracheal wall tear with PercuTwist. Anaesthesia 2002; 57:507–8.

66. Fantoni A. A breakthrough in tracheostomy techniques: translaryngeal tracheostomy. A new era? Minerva Anestesiol 1995; 62:313–25.

67. Westphal K, Byhahn C, Wilke HJ, Lischke V. Percutaneous tracheostomy: a clinical comparison of dilational (Ciaglia) and translaryngeal (Fantoni) techniques. Anesth Analg 1999; 89: 938–43.

68. Sharpe MD, Parnes LS, Drover JW, Harris C. Translaryngeal tracheostomy: experience of 340 cases. Laryngoscope 2003; 113:530–6.

69. MacCallum PL, Parnes LS, Sharpe MD, Harris C. Comparison of open, percutaneous, and translaryngeal tracheostomies. Otolaryngol Head Neck Surg 2000; 122:686–90.

70. Petros S. Percutaneous tracheostomy. Crit Care 1999; 3:R5–R10.

71. Massick DD, Powell DM, Price PD, et al. Quantification of the learning curve for percutaneous dilational tracheotomy. Laryngoscope 2000; 110(2 Pt 1):222–8.

72. Heffner JE. Percutaneous dilational vs standard tracheotomy: a meta-analysis but not the final analysis. Chest 2000; 118: 1236–1.

73. Kumar M, Jaffery A, Jones M. Short-term complications of percutaneous tracheostomy: experience of a district general hospital—otolaryngology department. J Laryngol Otol 2002; 116:1025–7.

74. Heffner JE, Sahn SA. Tracheostomy in critically ill patients: techniques and complications. J Crit Illness 1987; 2:74–81.

75. Walts PA, Murthy SC, DeCamp MM. Techniques of surgical tracheostomy. Clin Chest Med 2003; 24:413–22.

76. Mansharamani NG, Koziel H, Garland R, et al. Safety of bedside percutaneous dilatational tracheostomy in obese patients in the ICU. Chest 2000; 117:1426–9.

77. Sustic A, Zupan Z, Antoncic II. Ultrasound-guided percutaneous dilatational tracheostomy with laryngeal mask airway control in a morbidly obese patient. J Clin Anesth 2004; 16: 121–3.

78. Mayberry JC, Wu IC, Goldman RK, Chesnut RM. Cervical spine clearance and neck extension during percutaneous

tracheostomy in trauma patients. Crit Care Med 2000; 28:3436–40.

79. Sustic A, Krstulovic B, Eskinja N, et al. Surgical tracheostomy versus percutaneous dilational tracheostomy in patients with anterior cervical spine fixation: preliminary report. Spine 2002; 27:1942–5.

80. Gysin C, Dulguerov P, Guyot JP, et al. Percutaneous versus surgical tracheostomy: a double-blind randomized trial. Ann Surg 1999; 230:708–14.

81. Kluge S, Meyer A, Kuhnelt P, Baumann HJ, Kreymann G. Percutaneous tracheostomy is safe in patients with severe thrombocytopenia. Chest 2004; 126:547–51.

82. Beiderlinden M, Groeben H, Peters J. Safety of percutaneous dilational tracheostomy in patients ventilated with high positive end-expiratory pressure (PEEP). Intensive Care Med 2003; 29:944–8.

83. Meyer M, Critchlow J, Mansharamani N, et al. Repeat bedside percutaneous dilational tracheostomy is a safe procedure. Crit Care Med 2002; 30:986–8.

84. Hazard PB, Garrett HEJ, Adams JW, Robbins ET, Aguillard R. Bedside percutaneous tracheotomy: experience with 55 elective procedures. Ann Thorac Surg 1988; 46:63–7.

85. Ciaglia P, Graniero KD. Percutaneous dilational tracheostomy. Results and long-term follow-up. Chest 1992; 101:464–67.

86. Ciaglia P, Graniero KD. Percutaneous dilational subcricoid tracheostomy. Chest 1990; 98:10S.

87. Hazard P, Jones C, Benitone J. Comparative clinical trial of standard operative tracheostomy with percutaneous tracheostomy. Crit Care Med 1991; 19:1018–24.

88. Van Natta TL, Morris JA Jr, Eddy VA, et al. Elective bedside surgery in critically injured patients is safe and cost-effective. Ann Surg 1998; 227:618–24; discussion 24–6.

89. Barba CA, Angood PB, Kauder DR, et al. Bronchoscopic guidance makes percutaneous tracheostomy a safe, cost-effective, and easy-to-teach procedure. Surgery 1995; 118:879–83.

90. Freeman BD, Isabella K, Cobb JP, et al. A prospective, randomized study comparing percutaneous with surgical tracheostomy in critically ill patients. Crit Care Med 2001; 29:926–30.

91. Wu JJ, Huang MS, Tang GJ, et al. Percutaneous dilatational tracheostomy versus open tracheostomy—a prospective, randomized, controlled trial. J Chin Med Assoc 2003; 66:467–73.

92. Smith I, Fleming S, Cernaianu A. Mishaps during transport from the intensive care unit. Crit Care Med 1990; 18:278–81.

93. Fradis M, Malatskey S, Dor I, et al. Early complications of tracheostomy performed in the operating room. J Otolaryngol 2003; 32:55–7.

94. Wenig BL, Applebaum EL. Indications for and techniques of tracheotomy. Clin Chest Med 1991; 12:545–53.

95. Hawkins ML, Burrus EP, Treat RC, Mansberger AR. Tracheostomy in the intensive care unit a safe alternative to the operating room. South Med J 1989; 82:1096–8.

96. Upadhyay A, Maurer J, Turner J, Tiszenkel H, Rosengart T. Elective bedside tracheostomy in the intensive care unit. J Am Coll Surg 1996; 183:51–5.

97. Wease GL, Frikker M, Villalba M, Glover J. Bedside tracheostomy in the intensive care unit. Arch Surg 1996; 131:552–4; discussion 4–5.

98. Massick DD, Yao S, Powell DM, et al. Bedside tracheostomy in the intensive care unit: a prospective randomized trial comparing open surgical tracheostomy with endoscopically guided percutaneous dilational tracheotomy. Laryngoscope 2001; 111:494–500.

99. Grover A, Robbins J, Bendick P, Gibson M, Villalba M. Open versus percutaneous dilatational tracheostomy: effi-cacy and cost analysis. Am Surg 2001; 67:297–301; discussion 301–2.

100. Francois B, Clavel M, Desachy A, et al. Complications of tracheostomy performed in the ICU: subthyroid tracheostomy vs surgical cricothyroidotomy. Chest 2003; 123:151–8.

101. Wang SJ, Sercarz JA, Blackwell KE, Aghamohammadi M, Wang MB. Open bedside tracheotomy in the intensive care unit. Laryngoscope 1999; 109:891–3.

102. Angel LF, Simpson CB. Comparison of surgical and percutaneous dilational tracheostomy. Clin Chest Med 2003; 24:423–9.

103. Gatti G, Cardu G, Bentini C, Pacilli P, Pugliese P. Weaning from ventilator after cardiac operation using the Ciaglia percutaneous tracheostomy. Eur J Cardiothorac Surg 2004; 25:541–7.

104. Holdgaard HO, Pedersen J, Jensen RH, et al. Percutaneous dilatational tracheostomy versus conventional surgical tracheostomy. A clinical randomised study. Acta Anaesthesiol Scand 1998; 42:545–50.

105. Melloni G, Muttini S, Gallioli G, et al. Surgical tracheostomy versus percutaneous dilatational tracheostomy. A prospective-randomized study with long-term follow-up. J Cardiovasc Surg (Torino) 2002; 43:113–21.

106. Stoeckli SJ, Breitbach T, Schmid S. A clinical and histologic comparison of percutaneous dilational versus conventional surgical tracheostomy. Laryngoscope 1997; 107(12 Pt 1):1643–6.

107. Muttini S, Melloni G, Gemma M, et al. [Percutaneous or surgical tracheotomy. Prospective, randomized comparison of the incidence of early and late complications]. Minerva Anestesiol 1999; 65:521–7.

108. Dulguerov P, Gysin C, Perneger TV, Chevrolet JC. Percutaneous or surgical tracheostomy: a meta-analysis. Crit Care Med 1999; 27:1617–25.

109. Little CM, Parker MG, Tarnopolsky R. The incidence of vasculature at risk during cricothyroidotomy. Ann Emerg Med 1986; 15:805–7.

110. Jackson C. High tracheotomy and other errors the chief causes of chronic laryngeal stenosis. Surg Gynecol Obstet 1921; 327:392–8.

111. Brantigan CO, Grow JB. Cricothyroidotomy: elective use in respiratory problems requiring tracheotomy. J Thorac Cardiovasc Surg 1976; 71:72–81.

112. Boyd AD, Romita MC, Conlan AA, Fink SD, Spencer FC. A clinical evaluation of cricothyroidotomy. Surg Gynecol Obstet 1979; 149:365–8.

113. Greisz H, Qvarnstorm O, Willen R. Elective cricothyroidotomy: a clinical and histopathological study. Crit Care Med 1982; 10:387–9.

114. Kuriloff DB, Setzen M, Portnoy W, et al. Laryngotracheal injury following cricothyroidotomy. Laryngoscope 1989; 99:125–30.

115. Weymuller EA, Cummings CW. Cricothyroidotomy: the impact of antecedent endotracheal intubation. Ann Otol Rhinol Laryngol 1982; 91:437–41.

116. Brantigan CO, Grow JB. Subglottic stenosis after cricothyroidotomy. Surgery 1982; 91:217–21.

117. Wright MJ, Greenberg DE, Hunt JP, Madan AK, McSwain NE Jr. Surgical cricothyroidotomy in trauma patients. South Med J 2003; 96:465–7.

118. Rehm CG, Wanek SM, Gagnon EB, Pearson SK, Mullins RJ. Cricothyroidotomy for elective airway management in critically ill trauma patients with technically challenging neck anatomy. Crit Care 2002; 6:531–5.

119. Holst M, Hertegard S, Persson A. Vocal dysfunction following cricothyroidotomy: a prospective study. Laryngoscope 1990; 100:749–55.

120. Holst M, Hedenstierna G, Kumlien JA, Schiratzki H. Five years experience of coniotomy. Intensive Care Med 1985; 11:202–6.

121. Sise MJ, Shackford SR, Cruickshank JC, Murphy G, Fridlund PH. Cricothyroidotomy for long-term tracheal access. A prospective analysis of morbidity and mortality in 76 patients. Ann Surg 1984; 200:13.

122. Jakobsson J, Andersson G, Wiklund PE. Experience with elective coniotomy. Acta Chir Scand Suppl 1984; 520:101–3.

123. Gleeson MJ, Pearson RC, Armistead S, Yates AK. Voice changes following cricothyroidotomy. J Laryngol Otol 1984; 98:1015–9.

124. Claffey LP, Phelan DM. A complication of cricothyroid "minitracheotomy"—oesophageal perforation. Intensive Care Med 1989; 15:140–1.

125. Burkey B, Esclamado R, Morganroth M. The role of cricothyroidotomy in airway management. Clin Chest Med 1991; 12: 561–71.

126. Stamenkovic SA, Morgan IS, Pontefract DR, Campanella C. Is early tracheostomy safe in cardiac patients with median sternotomy incisions? Ann Thorac Surg 2000; 69:1152–4.

127. Byhahn C, Rinne T, Halbig S, et al. Early percutaneous tracheostomy after median sternotomy. J Thorac Cardiovasc Surg 2000; 120:329–34.

128. Gillespie MB, Eisele DW. Outcomes of emergency surgical airway procedures in a hospital-wide setting. Laryngoscope 1999; 109:1766–9.

129. Matthews HR, Hopkinson RB. Treatment of sputum retention by minitracheotomy. Br J Surg 1984; 71:147–50.

130. Wright CD. Minitracheostomy. Clin Chest Med 2003; 24:431–5.

131. van Heurn LW, van Geffen GJ, Brink PR. Percutaneous subcricoid minitracheostomy: report of 50 procedures. Ann Thorac Surg 1995; 59:707–9.

132. Casas JI, Ferrandiz M, Correa J, et al. Minitracheostomy in elective surgery of the larynx: an alternative to formal tracheostomy. Can J Anaesth 1991; 38:761–3.

133. Matthews HR, Ficher BJ, Smith BE, Hopkinson RB. Minitracheostomy: a new delivery system for jet ventilation. J Thorac Cardiovasc Surg 1986; 92:673–5.

134. Hasan A, McGuigan J, Morgan MDL, Matthews HR. Minitracheotomy: a simple alternative to tracheostomy in obstructive sleep apnoea. Thorax 1989; 44:224–5.

135. Bonde P, Papachristos I, McCraith A, et al. Sputum retention after lung operation: prospective, randomized trial shows superiority of prophylactic minitracheostomy in high-risk patients. Ann Thorac Surg 2002; 74:196–202.

136. Ophir D, Konichezky S. Minicricothyrotomy for tracheobronchial toilet. Ann Otol Rhinol Laryngol 1990; 99:337–9.

137. Corke C, Cranswick P. A Seldinger technique for minitracheostomy insertion. Anaesth Intensive Care 1988; 16:206–7.

138. Lewis GA, Hopkinson RB, Matthews HR. Minitracheotomy. A report of its use in intensive care. Anaesthesia 1986; 41: 931–5.

139. Pedersen J, Schurizek BA, Melsen NC, Juhl B. Is minitracheotomy a simple and safe procedure? A prospective investigation in the intensive care unit. Intensive Care Med 1991; 17:333–5.

140. Randell TT, Tierala EK, Lepantalo MJ, Lindgren L. Prophylactic minitracheostomy after thoracotomy: a prospective, random control, clinical trial. Eur J Surg 1991; 157:501–4.

141. Issa MM, Healy DM, Maghur HA, Luke DA. Prophylactic minitracheotomy in lung resections. A randomized controlled study. J Thorac Cardiovasc Surg 1991; 101:895–900.

142. Issa MM, Healy DM, Maghur HA, Luke DA. Prophylactic mini tracheotomy in lung resections. J Thorac Cardiovasc Surg 1991; 101:895–900.

143. Parry GW, Batrick NC, Lau OJ, Cameron CR. Modification of minitracheostomy technique to limit bleeding complications. Eur J Cardiothorac Surg 1995; 9:659–60.

144. Wain JC, Wilson DJ, Mathisen DJ. Clinical experience with minitracheostomy. Ann Thorac Surg 1990; 49:881–5.

145. Choong RK, Solano T. Minitracheostomy—a cautionary tale of late bleeding. Anaesth Intensive Care 2001; 29:552–3.

146. Silk JM, Marsh AM. Pneumothorax caused by minitracheotomy. Anaesthesia 1989; 44:663–4.

147. Randell T, Kalli I, Lindgren L. Mini tracheotomy: complications and follow-up with fiberoptic tracheoscopy. Anesthesia 1990; 45:875–9.

148. Vernon JW. Pneumothorax caused by minitracheostomy. Anaesthesia 1990; 45:172.

149. Wood DE. Tracheostomy. Chest Surg Clin North Am 1996; 6: 749–64.

150. Paul A, Marelli D, Chiu C-J, Vestweber KH, Mulder DS. Percutaneous endoscopic tracheostomy. Ann Thorac Surg 1989; 47:314–5.

151. Marelli D, Paul A, Manolidis S, et al. Endoscopic guided percutaneous tracheostomy: early results of a consecutive trial. J Trauma 1990; 30:433–5.

152. Polderman KH, Spijkstra JJ, de Bree R, et al. Percutaneous dilatational tracheostomy in the ICU: optimal organization, low complication rates, and description of a new complication. Chest 2003; 123:1595–602.

153. deBoisblanc BP. Percutaneous dilational tracheostomy techniques. Clin Chest Med 2003; 24:399–407.

154. Ernst A, Critchlow J. Percutaneous tracheostomy—special considerations. Clin Chest Med 2003; 24:409–12.

155. Hinerman R, Alvarez F, Keller CA. Outcome of bedside percutaneous tracheostomy with bronchoscopic guidance. Intensive Care Med 2000; 26:1850–6.

156. Hill SA. An unusual complication of percutaneous tracheostomy. Anaesthesia 1995; 50:469–70.

157. Berrouschot J, Oeken J, Steiniger L, Schneider D. Perioperative complications of percutaneous dilational tracheostomy. Laryngoscope 1997; 107(11 Pt 1):1538–44.

158. Trottier SJ, Hazard PB, Sakabu SA, et al. Posterior tracheal wall perforation during percutaneous dilational tracheostomy: an investigation into its mechanism and prevention [see comments]. Chest 1999; 115:1383–9.

159. Reilly PM, Sing RF, Giberson FA, et al. Hypercarbia during tracheostomy: a comparison of percutaneous endoscopic, percutaneous Doppler, and standard surgical tracheostomy [see comments]. Intensive Care Med 1997; 23: 859–64.

160. Mallick A, Venkatanath D, Elliot SC, Hollins T, Nanda Kumar CG. A prospective randomised controlled trial of capnography vs. bronchoscopy for Blue Rhino percutaneous tracheostomy. Anaesthesia 2003; 58:864–8.

161. Addas BM, Howes WJ, Hung OR. Light-guided tracheal puncture for percutaneous tracheostomy. Can J Anaesth 2000; 47: 919–22.

162. Imperatore F, Diurno F, Passannanti T, et al. Bronchoscopic transillumination guidance for open standard surgical tracheostomy. MedGenMed 2003; 5:31.

163. Craven RM, Laver SR, Cook TM, Nolan JP. Use of the Pro-Seal LMA facilitates percutaneous dilational tracheostomy. Can J Anaesth 2003; 50:718–20.

164. Cook TM, Taylor M, McKinstry C, Laver SR, Nolan JP. Use of the ProSeal Laryngeal Mask Airway to initiate ventilation during intensive care and subsequent percutaneous tracheostomy. Anesth Analg 2003; 97:848–50.

165. Dosemeci L, Yilmaz M, Gurpinar F, Ramazanoglu A. The use of the laryngeal mask airway as an alternative to the endotracheal

tube during percutaneous dilatational tracheostomy. Intensive Care Med 2002; 28:63–7.

166. Ambesh SP, Sinha PK, Tripathi M, Matreja P. Laryngeal mask airway vs endotracheal tube to facilitate bedside percutaneous tracheostomy in critically ill patients: a prospective comparative study. J Postgrad Med 2002; 48:11–5.

167. Fisher L, Duane D, Lafreniere L, Read D. Percutaneous dilational tracheostomy: a safer technique of airway management using a microlaryngeal tube. Anaesthesia 2002; 57:253–5.

168. Ferraro F, Capasso A, Troise E, et al. Assessment of ventilation during the performance of elective endoscopic-guided percutaneous tracheostomy: clinical evaluation of a new method. Chest 2004; 126:159–64.

169. Hatfield A, Bodenham A. Portable ultrasonic scanning of the anterior neck before percutaneous dilatational tracheostomy. Anaesthesia 1999; 54:660–3.

170. Muhammad JK, Major E, Patton DW. Evaluating the neck for percutaneous dilatational tracheostomy. J Maxillofac Surg 2000; 28:336–42.

171. Kollig E, Heydenreich U, Roetman B, Hopf F, Muhr G. Ultrasound and bronchoscopic controlled percutaneous tracheostomy on trauma ICU. Injury 2000; 31:663–8.

172. Muhammad JK, Patton DW, Evans RM, Major E. Percutaneous dilatational tracheostomy under ultrasound guidance. Br J Oral Maxillofac Surg 1999; 37:309–11.

173. Muhammad JK, Major E, Wood A, Patton DW. Percutaneous dilatational tracheostomy: haemorrhagic complications and the vascular anatomy of the anterior neck. A review based on 497 cases. Int J Oral Maxillofac Surg 2000; 29:217–22.

174. Shlugman D, Satya-Krishna R, Loh L. Acute fatal haemorrhage during percutaneous dilatational tracheostomy. Br J Anaesth 2003; 90:517–20.

175. Sustic A, Kovac D, Zgaljardic Z, Zupan Z, Krstulovic B. Ultrasound-guided percutaneous dilatational tracheostomy: a safe method to avoid cranial misplacement of the tracheostomy tube. Intensive Care Med 2000; 26:1379–81.

176. Datta D, Onyirimba F, McNamee MJ. The utility of chest radiographs following percutaneous dilatational tracheostomy. Chest 2003; 123:1603–6.

177. Goumas P, Kokkinis K, Petrocheilos J, Naxakis S, Mochloulis G. Cricothyroidotomy and the anatomy of the cricothyroid space. An autopsy study. J Laryngol Otol 1997; 111:354–6.

178. Feinberg SE, Peterson LJ. Use of cricothyroidotomy in oral and maxillofacial surgery. J Oral Maxillofac Surg 1987; 45:873–8.

179. Heffner JE. Timing of tracheotomy in ventilator-dependent patients. Clin Chest Med 1991; 12:611–25.

180. Willms D, Shure D. Pulmonary edema due to upper airway obstruction in adults. Chest 1988; 94:1090–3.

181. Crofts SL, Alzeer A, McGuire GP, Wong DT, Charles D. A comparison of percutaneous and operative tracheostomies in intensive care patients. Can J Anaesth 1995; 42:775–9.

182. Fikkers BG, van Veen JA, Kooloos JG, et al. Emphysema and pneumothorax after percutaneous tracheostomy: case reports and an anatomic study. Chest 2004; 125:1805–14.

183. Lin JC, Maley RH Jr, Landreneau RJ. Extensive posterior-lateral tracheal laceration complicating percutaneous dilational tracheostomy. Ann Thorac Surg 2000; 70:1194–6.

184. Grillo HC, Moncure AC, McEnany MT. Repair of inflammatory tracheoesophageal fistula. Ann Thorac Surg 1976; 22:112–6.

185. Reed MF, Mathisen DJ. Tracheoesophageal fistula. Chest Surg Clin North Am 2003; 13:271–89.

186. Jones JW, Reynolds M, Hewitt RL, Drapanas T. Tracheo-innominate artery erosion: successful surgical management of a devastating complication. Ann Surg 1976; 184:194–204.

187. Ross CB, Morris JA. Tracheoinnominate artery fistula: A potentially fatal complication of tracheostomy. J Tenn Med Assoc 1988; 81:446–9.

188. Gwilyn S, Cooney A. Acute fatal haemorrhage during percutaneous dilatational tracheostomy. Br J Anaesth 2004; 92:298.

189. Stock MC, Woodward CG, Shapiro BA, et al. Perioperative complications of elective tracheostomy in critically ill patients. Crit Care Med 1986; 14:861–63.

190. Fraipont V, Lambermont B, Ghaye B, et al. Unusual complication after percutaneous dilatational tracheostomy: pneumoperitoneum with abdominal compartment syndrome. Intensive Care Med 1999; 25:1334–5.

191. Teoh WH, Goh KY, Chan C. The role of early tracheostomy in critically ill neurosurgical patients. Ann Acad Med Singapore 2001; 30:234–8.

192. Watanakunakorn C. Successful novel drainage treatment of mediastinal abscess complicating tracheostomy. Chest 1989; 96:946–8.

193. Snow N, Richardson JD, Flint LM. Management of necrotizing tracheostomy infections. J Thorac Cardiovasc Surg 1981; 82:341–4.

194. Ibrahim EH, Tracy L, Hill C, Fraser VJ, Kollef MH. The occurrence of ventilator-associated pneumonia in a community hospital: risk factors and clinical outcomes. Chest 2001; 120:555–61.

195. Heffner JE. The role of tracheotomy in weaning. Chest 2001; 120(6 Suppl):477S–81S.

196. Leder SB. Incidence and type of aspiration in acute care patients requiring mechanical ventilation via a new tracheotomy. Chest 2002; 122:1721–6.

197. Elpern EH, Jacobs ER, Bone RC. Incidence of aspiration in tracheally intubated adults. Heart Lung 1987; 16:527–31.

198. Elpern EH, Scott MG, Petro L, Ries MH. Pulmonary aspiration in mechanically ventilated patients with tracheostomies. Chest 1994; 105:563–6.

199. Leder SB, Ross DA. Investigation of the causal relationship between tracheotomy and aspiration in the acute care setting. Laryngoscope 2000; 110:641–4.

200. Johnson JT, Wagner RL, Sigler BA. Disposable inner cannula tracheotomy tube: a prospective clinical trial. Otolaryngol Head Neck Surg 1988; 99:83–4.

201. Andrews MJ, Pearson FG. Incidence and pathogenesis of tracheal injury following cuffed tube tracheostomy with assisted ventilation: analysis of a two-year prospective study. Ann Surg 1971; 173:249–63.

202. Cooper JD, Grillo HC. The evolution of tracheal injury due to ventilatory assistance through cuffed tubes. A pathologic study. Ann Surg 1969; 169:334–48.

203. Cooper JD, Grillo HC. Experimental production and prevention of injury due to cuffed tracheal tubes. Surg Gynecol Obstet 1969; 129:1235–41.

204. Wain JC. Postintubation tracheal stenosis. Chest Surg Clin North Am 2003; 13:231–46.

205. Wood DE, Mathisen DJ. Late complications of tracheotomy. Clin Chest Med 1991; 12:597–609.

206. Koitschev A, Graumueller S, Zenner HP, Dommerich S, Simon C. Tracheal stenosis and obliteration above the tracheostoma after percutaneous dilational tracheostomy. Crit Care Med 2003; 31:1574–6.

207. Briche T, Le Manach Y, Pats B. Complications of percutaneous tracheostomy. Chest 2001; 119:1282–3.

208. Norwood S, Vallina VL, Short K, et al. Incidence of tracheal stenosis and other late complications after percutaneous tracheostomy. Ann Surg 2000; 232:233–41.

209. Gambale G, Cancellieri F, Baldini U, et al. Ciaglia percutaneous dilational tracheostomy. Early and late complications and follow-up. Minerva Anestesiol 2003; 69:825–30; 30–3.

210. Callanan V, Gillmore K, Field S, Beaumont A. The use of magnetic resonance imaging to assess tracheal stenosis following percutaneous dilatational tracheostomy. J Laryngol Otol 1997; 111:953–7.

211. van Heurn LW, Goei R, de Ploeg I, Ramsay G, Brink PR. Late complications of percutaneous dilatational tracheotomy. Chest 1996; 110:1572–6.

212. Law RC, Carney AS, Manara AR. Long-term outcome after percutaneous dilational tracheostomy. Endoscopic and spirometry findings. Anaesthesia 1997; 52:51–6.

213. Rosenbower TJ, Morris JA Jr, Eddy VA, Ries WR. The long-term complications of percutaneous dilatational tracheostomy. Am Surg 1998; 64:82–6.

214. Fischler MP, Kuhn M, Cantieni R, Frutiger A. Late outcome of percutaneous dilatational tracheostomy in intensive care patients. Intensive Care Med 1995; 21:475–81.

215. Grillo HC, Mathisen D. Surgical management of tracheal strictures. J Cardiothorac Surg 1988; 68:511–24.

216. Lorenz RR. Adult laryngotracheal stenosis: etiology and surgical management. Curr Opin Otolaryngol Head Neck Surg 2003; 11:467–72.

217. Stauffer JL, Olson DE, Petty TL. Complications and consequences of endotracheal intubation and tracheostomy. A prospective study of 150 critically ill adult patients. Am J Med 1981; 70:65–76.

218. Dayal VS, el Masri W. Tracheostomy in intensive care setting. Laryngoscope 1986; 96:58–60.

219. Louis JS, Antok E, Charretier PA, Winer A, Ocquidant P. [Tracheo-oesophageal fistula. A rare complication of percutaneous tracheostomy]. Ann Fr Anesth Reanim 2003; 22:349–52.

220. Payne DK, Anderson WM, Romero MD, Wissing DR, Fowler M. Tracheoesophageal fistula formation in intubated patients. Risk factors and treatment with high-frequency jet ventilation. Chest 1990; 98:161–4.

221. Grillo HC. Acquired tracheo-esophageal fistula. In: Grillo HC, Austin WG, editors. Current therapy in cardiothoracic surgery. Philadelphia: Decker, 1989: 54–5.

222. Mathisen DJ, Grillo HC, Wain JC, Hilgenberg AD. Management of acquired nonmalignant fistula. Ann Thorac Surg 1991; 52: 759–65.

223. Braidy J, Breton G, Clément L. Effect of corticosteroids on postintubation tracheal stenosis. Thorax 1989; 44:753–5.

224. Allan JS, Wright CD. Tracheoinnominate fistula: diagnosis and management. Chest Surg Clin North Am 2003; 13:331–41.

225. Cokis C, Towler S. Tracheo-innominate fistula after initial percutaneous tracheostomy. Anaesth Intensive Care 2000; 28: 566–9.

226. Dyer RK, Fisher SR. Tracheal-innominate and tracheal-esophageal fistula. In: Wolfe WG, editor. Complications in thoracic surgery. St. Louis: Mosby-Year Book, 1992: 294.

227. Cooper JD. Tracheo-innominate artery fistula: successful management of 3 consecutive patients. Ann Thorac Surg 1977; 24:439–47.

228. Nelms B. Tracheoarterial fistula. In: Grillo HC, Eschapasse H, editors. International trends in general thoracic surgery: Major challenges. Philadelphia: Saunders, 1987: 69–73.

229. Mehalic TF, Farhat SM. Tracheoarterial fistula: a complication of tracheostomy in patients with brain stem injury. J Trauma 1972; 12:140–3.

230. Gelman JJ, Aro M, Weiss SM. Tracheo-innominate artery fistula. J Am Coll Surg 1994; 179:626–34.

231. Oshinsky AE, Rubin JS, Gwozoz CS. The anatomical basis for post-tracheotomy innominate artery rupture. Laryngoscope 1988; 98:1061–3.

232. Grillo HC, Donahue DM, Mathisen DJ, Wain JC, Wright CD. Postintubation tracheal stenosis. Treatment and results. J Thorac Cardiovasc Surg 1995; 109:486–92; discussion 92–3.

233. Yang FY, Criado E, Schwartz JA, Keagy BA, Wilcox BR. Trachea-innominate artery fistula retrospective comparison of treatment methods. South Med J 1988; 81:701–6.

234. Hafez A, Courand L, Velly JF, Bruneteau A. Late cataclysmic hemorrhage from the innominate artery after tracheotomy. Thorac Cardiovasc Surg 1984; 32:315–8.

235. Takano H, Ihara K, Sato S, et al. Tracheo-innominate artery fistula following tracheostomy. J Cardiovasc Surg 1989; 60:860–3.

236. Lawson DW, Grillo HC. Closure of persistent tracheal stomas. Surg Gynecol Obstet 1970; 130:995–6.

237. Berenholz LP, Vail S, Berlet A. Management of tracheo cutaneous fistula. Arch Otolaryngol Head Neck Surg 1992; 118: 869–71.

238. Shen KR, Mathisen DJ. Management of persistent tracheal stoma. Chest Surg Clin North Am 2003; 13:369–73.

239. Stanton DC, Kademani D, Patel C, Foote JW. Management of post-tracheotomy scars and persistent tracheocutaneous fistulas with dermal interpositional fat graft. J Oral Maxillofac Surg 2004; 62:514–7.

240. Thomas A, Subramani K, Mitra S, Subramani S. Tracheal ring fracture—dislodgement after Blue Rhino percutaneous tracheostomy. Anaesthesia 2003; 58:1241.

241. Osborne JE, Osman EZ, Cuddihy P, Ranta M. Tracheal ring herniation following percutaneous dilatational tracheostomy and its resection under endoscopic control. J Laryngol Otol 1999; 113:1116–8.

242. Frosh A, Thomas ML, Weinbren J, Djazaeri B, Richards A. Tracheal ring rupture and herniation during percutaneous dilatational tracheostomy identified by fibreoptic bronchoscopy. Rev Laryngol Otol Rhinol 1997; 118:179–80.

243. van Heurn LW, Theunissen PH, Ramsay G, Brink PR. Pathologic changes of the trachea after percutaneous dilatational tracheotomy. Chest 1996; 109:1466–9.

244. Heffner JE. Timing tracheotomy. Calendar watching or individualization of care? Chest 1998; 114:361–3.

245. Heffner JE. Timing of tracheotomy in mechanically ventilated patients. Am Rev Respir Dis 1993; 147:768–71.

246. Maziak DE, Meade MO, Todd TR. The timing of tracheotomy: a systematic review. Chest 1998; 114:605–9.

247. Rumbak MJ, Newton M, Truncale T, et al. A prospective, randomized, study comparing early percutaneous dilational tracheotomy to prolonged translaryngeal intubation (delayed tracheotomy) in critically ill medical patients. Crit Care Med 2004; 32:1689–94.

248. Marsh HM, Gillespie DJ, Baumgartner AE. Timing of tracheostomy in the critically ill patient. Chest 1989; 96:190–3.

249. Ahrens T, Kollef MH. Early tracheostomy—has its time arrived? Crit Care Med 2004; 32:1796–7.

250. Heffner JE, Hess D. Tracheostomy management in the chronically ventilated patient. Clin Chest Med 2001; 22: 55–69.

251. Astrachan DI, Kirchner JC, Goodwin WJJ. Prolonged intubation vs tracheotomy: complications, practical and psychological considerations. Laryngoscope 1988; 98:1165–9.

252. McGeehin WH, Scoma R, Igidbashian L, Smink RDJ. Tracheostomy versus endotracheal intubation: the ICU nurse's perspective. Crit Care Med 1990; 18:S224.

253. Kollef MH, Levy NT, Ahrens TS, et al. The use of continuous i.v. sedation is associated with prolongation of mechanical ventilation. Chest 1998; 114:541–8.

254. Rodriguez JL, Steinberg SM, Luchetti FA, et al. Early tracheostomy for primary airway management in the surgical critical care setting. Surgery 1990; 108:655–9.

255. Manzano JL, Lubillo S, Henriquez D, et al. Verbal communication of ventilator-dependent patients. Crit Care Med 1993; 21:512–7.

256. Heffner JE, Casey K, Hoffman C. Care of the mechanically ventilated patient with a tracheotomy. In: Tobin MJ, editor. Principles and practice of mechanical ventilation. New York: McGraw Hill, 1994: 749–74.

257. Bergbom-Engbert I, Haljamae H. Assessment of patients' experience of discomforts during respirator therapy. Crit Care Med 1989; 17:1068–72.

258. Fitch M. Patient perceptions: being unable to speak on a ventilator. T: The Canadian Journal of Respiratory Therapy 1987; 23:21–3.

259. Bersten AD, Rutten AJ, Vedig AE, Skowronski GA. Additional work of breathing imposed by endotracheal tubes, breathing circuits, and intensive care ventilators. Crit Care Med 1989; 17:671–7.

260. Jaeger JM, Littlewood KA, Durbin CG Jr. The role of tracheostomy in weaning from mechanical ventilation. Respir Care 2002; 47:469–80; discussion 81–2.

261. Banner MJ, Blanch PB, Kirby RR. Imposed work of breathing and methods of triggering demand-flow, continuous positive airway pressure system. Crit Care Med 1993; 21:183–90.

262. Wright PE, Marini JJ, Bernard GR. In vitro versus in vivo comparison of endotracheal tube airflow resistance. Am Rev Respir Dis 1989; 140:10–6.

263. Lin MC, Huang CC, Yang CT, Tsai YH, Tsao TC. Pulmonary mechanics in patients with prolonged mechanical ventilation requiring tracheostomy. Anaesth Intensive Care 1999; 27: 581–5.

264. Davis K Jr, Campbell RS, Johannigman JA, Valente JF, Branson RD. Changes in respiratory mechanics after tracheostomy. Arch Surg 1999; 134:59–62.

265. Diehl JL, El Atrous S, Touchard D, Lemaire F, Brochard L. Changes in the work of breathing induced by tracheotomy in ventilator-dependent patients. Am J Respir Crit Care Med 1999; 159:383–8.

266. Moscovici da Cruz V, Demarzo SE, Sobrinho JB, et al. Effects of tracheotomy on respiratory mechanics in spontaneously breathing patients. Eur Respir J 2002; 20:112–7.

267. Mohr AM, Rutherford EJ, Cairns BA, Boysen PG. The role of dead space ventilation in predicting outcome of successful weaning from mechanical ventilation. J Trauma 2001; 51: 843–8.

268. Cowan T, Op't Holt TB, Gegenheimer C, Izenberg S, Kulkarni P. Effect of inner cannula removal on the work of breathing imposed by tracheostomy tubes: a bench study. Respir Care 2001; 46:460–5.

269. Villafene MC, Cinnella G, Lofaso F, et al. Gradual reduction of endotracheal tube diameter during mechanical ventilation via different humidification devices. Anesthesiology 1996; 85: 1341–9.

270. Kluger Y, Paul DB, Lucke J, et al. Early tracheostomy in trauma patients. Eur J Emerg Med 1996; 3:95–101.

271. Sugerman HJ, Wolfe L, Pasquale MD, et al. Multicenter, randomized, prospective trial of early tracheostomy. J Trauma 1997; 43:741–7.

272. Dunham MC, LaMonica C. Prolonged tracheal intubation in the trauma patient. Trauma 1984; 24:120–4.

273. Coppolo DP, May JJ. Self-extubations. A 12-month experience. Chest 1990; 98:165–9.

274. Jayamanne D, Nandipati R, Patel D. Self-extubation: a prospective study. Chest 1988; 94:3S.

275. Mort TC. Unplanned tracheal extubation outside the operating room: a quality improvement audit of hemodynamic and tracheal airway complications associated with emergency tracheal reintubation. Anesth Analg 1998; 86: 1171–6.

276. Torres A, Gatell JM, Aznar E, et al. Re-intubation increases the risk of nosocomial pneumonia in patients needing mechanical ventilation. Am J Respir Crit Care Med 1995; 152:137–41.

277. Campbell RS. Extubation and the consequences of reintubation. Respir Care 1999; 44:799–803.

278. Listello D, Sessler CN. Unplanned extubation. Clinical predictors for reintubation. Chest 1994; 105:1496–503.

279. Holzapfel L, Chastang C, Demingeon G, et al. A randomized study assessing the systematic search for maxillary sinusitis in nasotracheally mechanically ventilated patients. Influence of nosocomial maxillary sinusitis on the occurrence of ventilator-associated pneumonia. Am J Respir Crit Care Med 1999; 159:695–701.

280. Heffner JE. Upper airway dysfunction. In: Marini JJ, Slutsky AS, editors. Physiological basis of ventilatory support. New York: Marcel Dekker, 1998: 533–74.

281. Colice GL. Resolution of laryngeal injury following translaryngeal intubation. Am Rev Respir Dis 1992; 145:361–4.

282. Whited RE. A prospective study of laryngotracheal sequelae in long-term intubation. Laryngoscope 1984; 94:367–77.

283. Elliott CG, Rasmussen BY, Crapo RO. Upper airway obstruction following adult respiratory distress syndrome. An analysis of 30 survivors. Chest 1988; 94:526–30.

284. Colice GL, Stukel TA, Dain B. Laryngeal complications of prolonged intubation. Chest 1989; 96:877–84.

285. Plummer AL, Gracey DR. Consensus conference on artificial airways in patients receiving mechanical ventilation. Chest 1989; 96:178–84.

286. Heffner JE. Medical indications for tracheotomy. Chest 1989; 96:186–90.

287. Harrop JS, Sharan AD, Scheid EH Jr, Vaccaro AR, Przybylski GJ. Tracheostomy placement in patients with complete cervical spinal cord injuries: American Spinal Injury Association Grade A. J Neurosurg 2004; 100(1 Suppl):20–3.

288. Sellers BJ, Davis BL, Larkin PW, Morris SE, Saffle JR. Early prediction of prolonged ventilator dependence in thermally injured patients. J Trauma 1997; 43:899–903.

289. Seneff MG, Zimmerman JE, Knaus WA, Wagner DP, Draper EA. Predicting the duration of mechanical ventilation. The importance of disease and patient characteristics. Chest 1996; 110: 469–79.

290. Heffner JE, Zamora CA. Clinical predictors of prolonged translaryngeal intubation in patients with the adult respiratory distress syndrome. Chest 1990; 97:447–52.

291. Johnson SB, Kearney PA, Barker DE. Early criteria predictive of prolonged mechanical ventilation. J Trauma 1992; 33:95–100.

292. Heffner JE, Brown LK, Barbieri C. Prospective validation of an acute respiratory distress syndrome predictive score. Am J Respir Crit Care Med 1995; 162:1518–26.

293. Gurkin SA, Parikshak M, Kralovich KA, et al. Indicators for tracheostomy in patients with traumatic brain injury. Am Surg 2002; 68:324–8; discussion 8–9.

294. Ross BJ, Barker DE, Russell WL, Burns RP. Prediction of long-term ventilatory support in trauma patients. Am Surg 1996; 62:19–25.

295. Major KM, Hui T, Wilson MT, et al. Objective indications for early tracheostomy after blunt head trauma. Am J Surg 2003; 186:615–9; discussion 9.

296. Qureshi AI, Suarez JI, Parekh PD, Bhardwaj A. Prediction and timing of tracheostomy in patients with infratentorial lesions

requiring mechanical ventilatory support. Crit Care Med 2000; 28:1383–7.

297. Rello J, Sonora R, Jubert P, et al. Pneumonia in intubated patients: role of respiratory airway care. Am J Respir Crit Care Med 1996; 154:111–5.

298. Bernhard WN, Cottrell JE, Sivakumaran C, et al. Adjustment of intracuff pressure to prevent aspiration. Anesthesiology 1979; 50:363.

299. Fernandez R, Blanch L, Mancebo J, Bonsoms N, Artigas A. Endotracheal tube cuff pressure assessment: pitfalls of finger estimation and need for objective measurement. Crit Care Med 1990; 18:1423–6.

300. Stewart SL, Secrest JA, Norwood BR, Zachary R. A comparison of endotracheal tube cuff pressures using estimation techniques and direct intracuff measurement. AANA J 2003; 71:443–7.

301. Badenhorst C. Changes in tracheal cuff pressure during respiratory support. Crit Care Med 1987; 15:300–2.

302. Lee TS, Hsu D. Ischemic damage to the trachea: lateral wall pressure versus intracuff pressure. Crit Care Med 1991; 19:1328.

303. Ganner C. The accurate measurement of endotracheal tube cuff pressures. Br J Nurs 2001; 10:1127–34.

304. Braz JR, Navarro LH, Takata IH, Nascimento Junior P. Endotracheal tube cuff pressure: need for precise measurement. Sao Paulo Med J 1999; 117:243–7.

305. Arola MK, Inberg MV, Puhakka H. Tracheal stenosis after tracheostomy and after orotracheal cuffed intubation. Acta Chir Scand 1981; 147:183–92.

306. Asai T, Shingu K. Leakage of fluid around high-volume, low-pressure cuffs apparatus A comparison of four tracheal tubes. Anaesthesia 2001; 56:38–42.

307. Guyton D, Banner MJ, Kirby RR. High-volume, low-pressure cuffs. Are they always low-pressure? Chest 1991; 100:1076–81.

308. Karasawa F, Mori T, Kawatani Y, Ohshima T, Satoh T. Deflationary phenomenon of the nitrous oxide-filled endotracheal tube cuff after cessation of nitrous oxide administration. Anesth Analg 2001; 92:145–8.

309. Dodds WJ, Stewart ET, Logemann JA. Physiology and radiology of the normal oral and pharyngeal phases of swallowing. Am J Roentgenol 1990; 154:953–63.

310. Logemann JA. Manual for the videofluorographic study of swallowing. Austin: ProEd, 1993.

311. Logemann JA. Evaluation and treatment of swallowing disorders, 2nd ed. Austin: ProEd, 1998.

312. Klahn MS, Perlman AL. Temporal and durational patterns associating respiration and swallowing. Dysphagia 1999; 14:131–8.

313. Martin BJ, Logemann JA, Shaker R, Dodds WJ. Coordination between respiration and swallowing: respiratory phase relationships and temporal integration. J Appl Physiol 1994; 76: 714–23.

314. Martin-Harris B, Brodsky MB, Price CC, Michel Y, Walters B. Temporal coordination of pharyngeal and laryngeal dynamics with breathing during swallowing: single liquid swallows. J Appl Physiol 2003; 94:1735–43.

315. Dodds WJ, Logemann JA, Stewart ET. Radiologic assessment of abnormal oral and pharyngeal phases of swallowing. Am J Roentgenol 1990; 154:965–74.

316. Atkinson M, Kramer P, Wyman S, Ingelfinger F. The dynamics of swallow. I. Normal pharyngeal mechanisms. J Clin Invest 1957; 36:581–98.

317. Cook IJ, Dodds WJ, Dantas RO, et al. Timing of videofluoroscopic, manometric events, and bolus transit during the oral and pharyngeal phases of swallowing. Dysphagia 1989;4:8–15.

318. Ekberg O, Sigurjonsson SV. Movement of the epiglottis during deglutition. A cineradiographic study. Gastrointest Radiol 1982; 7:101–7.

319. Jacob P, Kahrilas PJ, Logemann JA, Shah V, Ha T. Upper esophageal sphincter opening and modulation during swallowing. Gastroenterology 1989; 97:1469–78.

320. Kahrilas PJ, Dodds WJ, Dent J, Logemann JA, Shaker R. Upper esophageal sphincter function during deglutition. Gastroenterology 1988; 95:52–62.

321. Logemann J, Kahrilas PJ, Cheng J, et al. Closure mechanism of laryngeal vestibule during swallowing. Gastrointest Liver Physiol 1992; 21:G338–G44.

322. McConnel FM, Cerenko D, Mendelsohn MS. Manofluorographic analysis of swallowing. Otolaryngol Clin North Am 1988; 21:625–35.

323. Sokol EM, Heitmann P, Wolf BS, Cohen B. Simultaneous cineradiographic and manometric study of the pharynx, hypopharynx, and cervical esophagus. Gastroenterology 1966; 51: 960–74.

324. Martin BJW, Robbins J. Physiology of swallowing: protection of the airway. Semin Respir Crit Care Med 1995; 16:448–58.

325. Castell DA, Diederrich LL, Castell JA. Esophageal motility and pH testing, 3rd ed. Highlands Ranch, CO: Sandhill Scientific, Inc, 2000.

326. Levine MS. Radiology of the esophagus. Philadelphia: WB Saunders Co, 1989.

327. Bonanno PC. Swallowing dysfunction after tracheostomy. Ann Surg 1971; 174:29–33.

328. Dikeman KJ, Kazandjian MS. Communication and swallowing management of tracheostomized and ventilator-dependent adults. Clifton Park, NY: Thomson Delmar Learning, 2003.

329. Gross RD, Mahlmann J, Grayhack JP. Physiologic effects of open and closed tracheostomy tubes on the pharyngeal swallow. Ann Otol Rhinol Laryngol 2003; 112:143–52.

330. Leder SB. Effect of a one-way tracheotomy speaking valve on the incidence of aspiration in previously aspirating patients with tracheotomy. Dysphagia 1999; 14:73–7.

331. Logemann JA, Pauloski BR, Rademaker AW, Colangelo LA. Speech and swallowing rehabilitation for head and neck cancer patients. Oncology (Huntingt) 1997; 11:651–6.

332. Martin-Harris B. Swallowing disorders following medical and surgical treatments for head and neck cancer. Support for People with Oral and Neck Cancer 2000; 10:1–6.

333. Martin-Harris B, McMahon S, Haynes R. Aspiration and dysphagia: pathophysiology and outcome. Phonoscope 1998; 2:125–32.

334. Mendell DA, Logemann JA. A retrospective analysis of the pharyngeal swallow in patients with a clinical diagnosis of GERD compared with normal controls: a pilot study. Dysphagia 2002; 17:220–6.

335. Cameron JL, Reynolds J, Zuidema GD. Aspiration in patients with tracheostomies. Surg Gynecol Obstet 1973; 136: 68–70.

336. Lim JW, Lerner PK, Rothstein SG. Epiglottic position after cricothyroidotomy: a comparison with tracheotomy. Ann Otol Rhinol Laryngol 1997; 106(7 Pt 1):560–2.

337. Treloar DM, Stechmiller J. Pulmonary aspiration in tube-fed patients with artificial airways. Heart Lung 1984; 13:667–71.

338. Torres A, Serra-Batlles J, Ros E, et al. Pulmonary aspiration of gastric contents in patients receiving mechanical ventilation: the effect of body position. Ann Intern Med 1992; 116: 540–3.

339. DeVita MA, Spierer-Rundback L. Swallowing disorders in patients with prolonged orotracheal intubation or tracheostomy tubes. Crit Care Med 1990; 18:1328–30.

340. Pannunzio TG. Aspiration of oral feedings in patients with tracheostomies. AACN Clin Issues 1996; 7:560–9.

341. Dikeman KJ, Kazandjjan MS. Managing adults with tracheostomies and ventilator dependence. The ASHA leader 2004; 9:6–7,19–20. Also available online: Dikeman KJ, Kazandjjan MS. Title. http://www.asha.org/about/publications/leader_online/archives/2004/041019/f041019a.htm. Accessed 2/1/06.

342. Higgins DM, Maclean JC. Dysphagia in the patient with a tracheostomy: six cases of inappropriate cuff deflation or removal [see comments]. Heart Lung 1997; 26:215–20.

343. Logemann JA, Veis S, Colangelo L. A screening procedure for oropharyngeal dysphagia. Dysphagia 1999; 14:44–51.

344. McCullough GH, Wertz RT, Rosenbek JC, et al. Inter- and intrajudge reliability of a clinical examination of swallowing in adults. Dysphagia 2000; 15:58–67.

345. Martin-Harris B, Logemann JA, McMahon S, Schleicher M, Sandidge J. Clinical utility of the modified barium swallow. Dysphagia 2000; 15:136–41.

346. Daniels SK, Ballo LA, Mahoney MC, Foundas AL. Clinical predictors of dysphagia and aspiration risk: outcome measures in acute stroke patients. Arch Phys Med Rehabil 2000; 81: 1030–3.

347. Daniels SK, Brailey K, Priestly DH, et al. Aspiration in patients with acute stroke. Arch Phys Med Rehabil 1998; 79:14–9.

348. Horner J, Massey EW, Riski JE, Lathrop DL, Chase KN. Aspiration following stroke: clinical correlates and outcome. Neurology 1988; 38:1359–62.

349. Leder SB. Videofluoroscopic evaluation of aspiration with visual examination of the gag reflex and velar movement. Dysphagia 1997; 12:21–3.

350. Donzelli J, Brady S, Wesling M, Craney M. Simultaneous modified Evans blue dye procedure and video nasal endoscopic evaluation of the swallow. Laryngoscope 2001; 111:1746–50.

351. Lucarelli MR, Shirk MB, Julian MW, Crouser ED. Toxicity of food drug and cosmetic blue no. 1 dye in critically ill patients. Chest 2004; 125:793–5.

352. Zenner PM, Losinski DS, Mills RH. Using cervical auscultation in the clinical dysphagia examination in long-term care. Dysphagia 1995; 10:27–31.

353. Kidder TM, Langmore SE, Martin BJ. Indications and techniques of endoscopy in evaluation of cervical dysphagia: comparison with radiographic techniques. Dysphagia 1994; 9:256–61.

354. Langmore SE, Schatz K, Olsen N. Fiberoptic endoscopic examination of swallowing safety: a new procedure. Dysphagia 1988; 2:216–9.

355. Murray J, Langmore SE, Ginsberg S, Dostie A. The significance of accumulated oropharyngeal secretions and swallowing frequency in predicting aspiration. Dysphagia 1996; 11:99–103.

356. Furiel AE, Putnam JS. Patients with tracheostomies. Prim Care 1978; 5:557–67.

357. Tippett DC, Siebens AA. Using ventilators for speaking and swallowing. Dysphagia 1991; 6:94–9.

358. Godwin JE, Heffner JE. Special critical care considerations in tracheostomy management. Clin Chest Med 1991; 12:573–83.

359. Leder SB. Importance of verbal communication for the ventilation dependent patient. Chest 1990; 98:792–3.

360. Obier K, Haywood LJ. Enhancing therapeutic communications with acutely ill patients. Heart Lung 1973; 2:49–53.

361. Catala JC, Garcia Pedrajas F, Carrera J, et al. Placement of an endotracheal device via the laryngeal mask airway in a patient with tracheal stenosis [letter]. Anesthesiology 1996; 84: 239–40.

362. Albarran AW. A review of communication with intubated patients and those with tracheostomies within an intensive care environment. Intensive Care Nurs 1991; 7:179–86.

363. Bach JR, Alba AS. Tracheostomy ventilation. A study of efficacy with deflated cuffs and cuffless tubes. Chest 1990; 97:679–83.

364. Nomori H, Horio H, Suemasu K. Assisted pressure control ventilation via a mini-tracheostomy tube for postoperative respiratory management of lung cancer patients. Respir Med 2000; 94:214–20.

365. Bach JR. A comparison of long-term ventilatory support alternatives from the perspective of the patient and care giver. Chest 1993; 104:1702–6.

366. Shea SA, Hoit JD, Banzett RB. Competition between gas exchange and speech production in ventilated subjects. Biol Psychol 1998; 49:9–27.

367. Blom ED. Alternative methods of communication for intubated patients in critical care. Indiana Med 1988; 81:398–400.

368. Heffner JE. Care of the intensive care unit patient with a tracheotomy. Problems in Anesthesia 1988; 2:269–77.

369. Bunn JC, Mead J. Control of ventilation during speech. J Appl Physiol 1971; 31:870–2.

370. Hoit JD, Lohmeier HL. Influence of continuous speaking on ventilation. J Speech Lang Hear Res 2000; 43:1240–51.

371. Hoit JD, Shea SA, Banzett RB. Speech production during mechanical ventilation in tracheostomized individuals. J Speech Hear Res 1994; 37:53–63.

372. Hoit JD, Banzett R. Simple adjustments can improve ventilator-supported speech. Am J Speech-Lang Pathol 1997; 6:87–96.

373. Heffner JE. Tracheal intubation in mechanically ventilated patients. Clin Chest Med 1988; 9:23–35.

374. Black JW, Grover BS. A hazard of pressure support ventilation. Chest 1988; 93:333–5.

375. Calderini E, Confalonieri M, Puccio PG, et al. Patient-ventilator asynchrony during noninvasive ventilation: the role of expiratory trigger. Intensive Care Med 1999; 25:662–7.

376. Highcock MP, Shneerson JM, Smith IE. Functional differences in bi-level pressure preset ventilators. Eur Respir J 2001; 17: 268–73.

377. Prigent H, Samuel C, Louis B, et al. Comparative effects of two ventilatory modes on speech in tracheostomized patients with neuromuscular disease. Am J Respir Crit Care Med 2003; 167:114–9.

378. Levine SP, Koester DJ, Kett RL. Independently activated talking tracheostomy systems for quadriplegic patients. Arch Phys Med Rehabil 1987; 68:571–3.

379. Sparker AW, Robbins KT, Nevlud GN, Watkins CN, Jahrsdoerfer RA. A prospective evaluation of speaking tracheostomy tubes for ventilator dependent patients. Laryngoscope 1987; 97:89–92.

380. Leder SB, Traquina DN. Voice intensity of patients using a Communi-Trach I cuffed speaking tracheostomy tube. Laryngoscope 1989; 99(7 Pt 1):744–7.

381. Hansen A, Niemala JR, Olsen GJ. Vocalization via a cuffed tracheostomy tube. Anaesthesia 1975; 30:78–9.

382. Kluin KJ, Maynard F, Bogdasarian RS. The patient requiring mechanical ventilatory support use of the cuffed tracheostomy "talk" tube to establish phonation. Otolaryngol Head Neck Surg 1984; 92:625–7.

383. Leder SB. Prognostic indicators for successful use of "talking" tracheostomy tubes. Perceptl Mot Skills 1991; 73:441–2.

384. Leder SB. Verbal communication for the ventilator-dependent patient: voice intensity with the Portex "Talk" tracheostomy tube. Laryngoscope 1990; 100(10 Pt 1):1116–21.

385. Adler JJ, Zeides J. Evaluation of the electrolarynx in the short-term hospital setting. Chest 1986; 89:407–9.

386. Wu WH, Suh CW, Turndorf H. Use of the artificial larynx during airway intubation. Crit Care Med 1974; 2:152–4.

387. Passy V. Passy-Muir tracheostomy speaking valve. Otolaryngol Head Neck Surg 1986; 95:247–8.

388. Fornataro-Clerici L, Zajac DJ. Aerodynamic characteristics of tracheostomy speaking valves. J Speech Hear Res 1993; 36: 529–32.

389. Leder SB. Perceptual rankings of speech quality produced with one-way tracheostomy speaking valves. J Speech Hear Res 1994; 37:1308–12.

390. Dettelbach MA, Gross RD, Mahlmann J, Eibling DE. Effect of the Passy-Muir Valve on aspiration in patients with tracheostomy. Head Neck 1995; 17:297–302.

391. Elpern EH, Borkgren Okonek M, Bacon M, Gerstung C, Skrzynski M. Effect of the Passy-Muir tracheostomy speaking valve on pulmonary aspiration in adults. Heart Lung 2000; 29: 287–93.

392. Siddarth P, Mazzarella L. Granuloma associated with fenestrated tracheostomy tubes. Am J Surg 1985; 150:279–80.

393. Criner G, Make B, Celli B. Respiratory muscle dysfunction secondary to chronic tracheostomy tube placement. Chest 1987; 91:139–41.

394. Nomori H. Tracheostomy tube enabling speech during mechanical ventilation. Chest 2004; 125:1046–51.

395. Greenbaum DM. Decannulation of the tracheostomized patient. Heart Lung 1976; 5:119–23.

396. Rumbak MJ, Graves AE, Scott MP, et al. Tracheostomy tube occlusion protocol predicts significant tracheal obstruction to air flow in patients requiring prolonged mechanical ventilation. Crit Care Med 1997; 25:413–7.

397. Ceriana P, Carlucci A, Navalesi P, et al. Weaning from tracheotomy in long-term mechanically ventilated patients: feasibility of a decisional flowchart and clinical outcome. Intensive Care Med 2003; 29:845–8.

398. Heffner JE. The technique of weaning from tracheostomy. Criteria for weaning: practical measures to prevent failure. J Crit Illness 1995; 10:729–31.

399. Paul F, Hendry C, Cabrelli L. Meeting patient and relatives' information needs upon transfer from an intensive care unit: the development and evaluation of an information booklet. J Clin Nurs 2004; 13:396–405.

400. Dewar DM, Kurek CJ, Lambrinos J, Cohen IL, Zhong Y. Patterns in costs and outcomes for patients with prolonged mechanical ventilation undergoing tracheostomy: an analysis of discharges under diagnosis-related group 483 in New York State from 1992 to 1996. Crit Care Med 1999; 27:2640–7.

401. Gracey DR. The problem with diagnosis related group 475. Chest 2002; 122:299–301.

402. Engoren M, Arslanian-Engoren C, Fenn-Buderer N. Hospital and long-term outcome after tracheostomy for respiratory failure. Chest 2004; 125:220–7.

403. Kurek CJ, Cohen IL, Lambrinos J, et al. Clinical and economic outcome of patients undergoing tracheostomy for prolonged mechanical ventilation in New York state during 1993: analysis of 6,353 cases under diagnosis-related group 483. Crit Care Med 1997; 25:983–8.

404. Leung R, MacGregor L, Campbell D, Berkowitz RG. Decannulation and survival following tracheostomy in an intensive care unit. Ann Otol Rhinol Laryngol 2003; 112:853–8.

405. Seneff MG, Wagner D, Thompson D, Honeycutt C, Silver MR. The impact of long-term acute-care facilities on the outcome and cost of care for patients undergoing prolonged mechanical ventilation. Crit Care Med 2000; 28:342–50.

406. Engoren M, Buderer NF, Zacharias A. Long-term survival and health status after prolonged mechanical ventilation after cardiac surgery. Crit Care Med 2000; 28:2742–9.

407. Douglas SL, Daly BJ, Brennan PF, et al. Outcomes of long-term ventilator patients: a descriptive study. Am J Crit Care 1997; 6:99–105.

408. Freeman BD, Isabella K, Lin N, Buchman TG. A meta-analysis of prospective trials comparing percutaneous and surgical tracheostomy in critically ill patients. Chest 2000; 118:1412–8.

PART XI

COMPLICATIONS IN VENTILATOR-SUPPORTED PATIENTS

Chapter 41

COMPLICATIONS ASSOCIATED WITH MECHANICAL VENTILATION

SCOTT K. EPSTEIN

Mechanical ventilation can be life saving but it is also associated with numerous complications. The incidence of some complications increases with duration of mechanical ventilation. This together with the observation that complications increase length of stay, increase mortality, and increase costs provides a compelling rationale for efforts to reduce the duration of mechanical ventilation. Indeed, efforts to identify the best approach to weaning and the application of protocols are justified by their capacity to reduce complications of mechanical ventilation.[1–4]

There are numerous mechanisms underlying the development of complications in the ventilated patient. Complications may result from the endotracheal tube or tracheotomy tube (or with noninvasive ventilation, the mask), or from the effects of positive-pressure ventilation. Indeed, an endotracheal tube increases the risk for sinusitis and ventilator-associated pneumonia (see Chapters 46 and 47). Some complications (barotrauma and volutrauma) can result from either the underlying lung disease or the effects of lung overdistension produced by positive-pressure ventilation (see Chapter 44). Complications may result from therapies or the process of care required by most invasively ventilated patients (e.g., immobility and risk of thromboembolism). Other complications may occur as a manifestation of critical illness or underlying comorbid conditions.

Gastrointestinal Complications

Numerous gastrointestinal complications associated with mechanical ventilation have been reported[5] (Table 41-1). These complications may be a direct consequence of mechanical ventilation, a direct result of critical illness, or a complication of therapies delivered in the intensive care unit (ICU). Even when the latter explanations predominate, mechanical ventilation may cause further gastrointestinal injury.

PNEUMOPERITONEUM

Pneumoperitoneum, or radiographically detectable free air in the peritoneal space, is of considerable relevance though it occurs infrequently.[6,7] Free air is most often detected as a radiolucency below the diaphragm on an upright chest radiograph. Pneumoperitoneum reflects perforation of an abdominal visceral structure in about 90% of cases.[8] In the remaining cases, pneumoperitoneum occurs as a consequence of various nonsurgical causes. Pneumoperitoneum can complicate conditions leading to ICU admission such as an overdose of crack cocaine.[9] Alternatively, it can result from a commonly performed ICU procedure, percutaneous endoscopic gastrostomy (PEG).[10] Pseudopneumoperitoneum refers to a condition in which an abnormally radiographic lucency falsely gives the appearance of free intraperitoneal air[8] (Table 41-2). Failure of the radiolucency to migrate in the most superior position and a failure to change with shifting position suggests this diagnosis.[8] Computed tomography can disclose that air seen on plain films is actually within the extraperitoneal space or represents air in a normal structure.[11]

TABLE 41-1 Gastrointestinal Complications Associated with Mechanical Ventilation

Pneumoperitoneum
Effect of mechanical ventilation on splanchnic perfusion
Alteration in gastrointestinal motility
Stress-related mucosal damage
    Asymptomatic
    Clinically significant (gastrointestinal hemorrhage)
Other
    Diarrhea (secondary to enteral nutrition, medications, or *Clostridium difficile*)
    Esophagitis
    Acalculous cholecystitis
    Pancreatitis

In ventilated patients, pneumoperitoneum may represent a manifestation of barotrauma.[8,12] Pneumoperitoneum occurs in up to 3% of ventilated preterm infants, though the prevalence in ventilated adults has not been well established.[8] When a manifestation of barotrauma, pneumoperitoneum usually coexists with pneumothorax, pneumomediastinum, or subcutaneous emphysema. Yet, on occasion pneumoperitoneum may be the initial expression of barotrauma.[13,14] Two pathophysiologic mechanisms have been proposed to explain the movement of air from thorax to peritoneal space. In the first, air passes directly through defects present in the diaphragm and pleura. Alternatively, air may track from the mediastinum along perivascular connections or major diaphragmatic openings into the retroperitoneum and then the peritoneum.[8] When pneumoperitoneum is a manifestation of barotrauma, it is unusual for the patient to have associated gastrointestinal symptoms and signs. Patients with a ruptured viscus typically have fever, abdominal pain and distension, and peritoneal signs. This may not be the case in patients who are heavily sedated, comatose, or those receiving neuromuscular blocking agents. Therefore, it may be extremely challenging to define the etiology of pneumoperitoneum. The implications are crucial because if intraperitoneal air cannot be proven to be a result of barotrauma, consideration should be given to surgical exploration to seek life-threatening intestinal perforation. Computed tomography may help define the etiology by disclosing other evidence of barotrauma or disease localized to a hollow abdominal structure. Water-soluble contrast given via nasogastric tube or rectally can be used to exclude a perforation.[15,16] Other approaches to define the etiology of pneumoperitoneum include aspiration and analysis of the P_{O_2} of the intraperitoneal free gas.[17,18]

TABLE 41-2 Causes of Pseudopneumoperitoneum

Basal pulmonary atelectasis suggesting subphrenic air
Basal lung bulla
Gas trapped in a wound or within the abdominal wall
Subphrenic abscess
Pyonephrosis
Subdiaphragmatic extraperitoneal fat
Chilaiditi syndrome (interposition of the colonic hepatic flexure between the liver and the diaphragm)

When pneumoperitoneum results from barotrauma, pleural air should be evacuated and tidal volume reduced to prevent further alveolar overdistension. On rare occasions, direct evacuation of air from the peritoneum may be necessary if the resulting abdominal distension is compromising mechanical ventilation or causing vascular collapse or tension pneumoperitoneum.[15,19–23]

EFFECT OF MECHANICAL VENTILATION ON SPLANCHNIC PERFUSION

Mechanical ventilation may cause gastrointestinal complications by reducing splanchnic perfusion (Fig. 41-1). In so doing, gastric mucosal hypoperfusion may result followed by stress-related mucosal damage or abnormal gut motility. The reduction in splanchnic perfusion can be secondary to reduced mean arterial pressure or increased gastrointestinal arterial resistance. The splanchnic circulation is prone to hypoperfusion because it lacks the capacity to autoregulate blood flow in instances of reduced blood pressure, persistence of splanchnic vasoconstriction after restoration of perfusion, and the fact that the vascular configuration predisposes the distal component of villi to hypoxia.[5] Furthermore, neurohumoral effects of positive-pressure ventilation and the use of exogenous catecholamines as vasopressors can cause vasoconstriction and redistribution of blood from splanchnic to other vascular beds.[24–29] Agents such as dopexamine may reverse the decrease in splanchnic perfusion seen with positive end-expiratory pressure (PEEP).[30] With the reestablishment of blood flow, reperfusion injury can further harm the gastrointestinal epithelium.[5] Positive airway pressure, particularly PEEP, can additionally decrease splanchnic perfusion, as a result of decreased cardiac output.[31–33] An extreme example is reduced splanchnic blood flow during a recruitment maneuver of 40 cmH$_2$O delivered for 20 seconds.[34] In contrast, placing hemodynamically stable patients with acute lung injury in the prone position altered neither hepatosplanchnic perfusion nor gastric mucosal energy balance.[35] Strategies resulting in an acute increase in Pa$_{CO_2}$ appear to have no major effect on splanchnic blood flow.[36,37] The effects of mechanical ventilation on splanchnic perfusion are influenced by other factors, including intravascular volume and hemodynamic status.[38] In a study of six patients with acute lung injury, PEEP did not consistently affect splanchnic perfusion when cardiac index was stable and ventilation occurred on the linear portion of the pressure-volume curve.[36] Reductions in splanchnic perfusion can also adversely affect gut barrier function, predisposing to translocation of bacteria and bacterial products.[39]

Mechanical ventilation may also adversely affect portal hemodynamics, though studies examining the issue have reached divergent results.[5] Nevertheless, it is reasonable to expect that high levels of positive-pressure ventilation may exacerbate hepatic injury that can result from shock and hypoxemia.

ALTERATIONS IN GASTROINTESTINAL MOTILITY

Abnormal upper and lower gastrointestinal motility (hypomotility) is common in ventilated patients (Table 41-3).

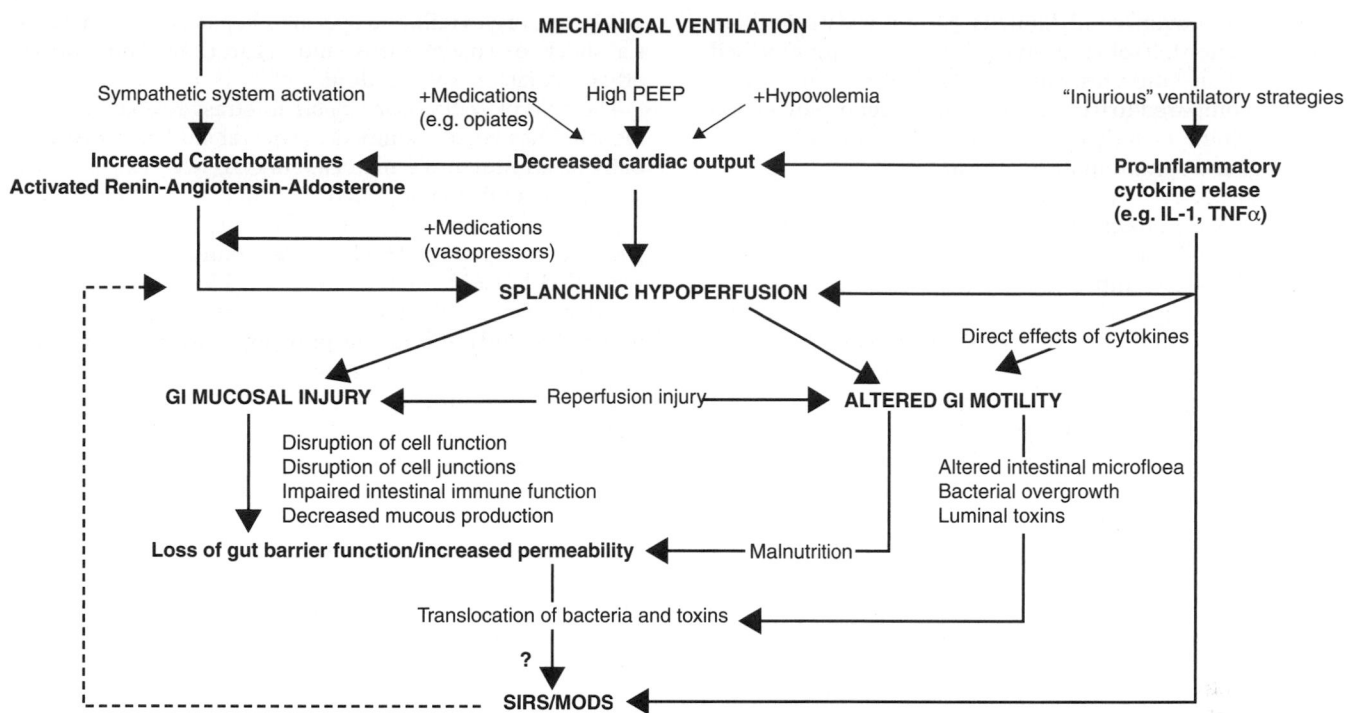

FIGURE 41-1 Proposed mechanism for the development of gastrointestinal complications during mechanical ventilation. (*Reproduced, with permission, from Mutlu et al.*[5])

Major risk factors include the use of opiates, other medications (e.g., dopamine, diltiazem, verapamil, anticholinergics, and phenothiazines), and electrolyte disorders (e.g., hypokalemia and hypomagnesemia).[29,40] Opiates have been shown to impair antroduodenal motility in ventilated patients.[41] Reduced motility may result from splanchnic hypoperfusion and mucosal injury. In addition, increased cytokines may impair intestinal smooth muscle contractility.[42–44] Systemic cytokine elevations are ubiquitous during the systemic inflammatory response syndrome, but also may be seen when injurious ventilator strategies are employed in acute lung injury.[45]

In the setting of critical illness, esophageal motility may be impaired. For example, sedated, ventilated patients have significantly reduced anterograde (propulsive) esophageal motility.[46] This is of clinical relevance because resulting gastroesophageal reflux could contribute to ventilator-associated pneumonia.

Ileus can occur in the postoperative state or may be secondary to medications, electrolyte abnormalities, trauma, shock, or sepsis.[47] Endotoxemia can cause abnormalities in gastrointestinal motility, via a number of mechanisms in-

cluding the effect of cytokines, prostaglandins, inducible nitric oxide synthase, leukocytes within the intestinal muscularis, and superoxide radicals.[44,47–50] Ileus is typically manifested by abdominal distension, diminished bowel sounds, and inability to tolerate enteral feedings. Dive et al simultaneously measured pressure changes in the gastric antrum, proximal duodenum, and distal duodenum, and found gastroduodenal motility severely impaired in 12 ventilated patients.[51] Withholding offending medications and assiduous correction of electrolyte disturbances represent first-line therapy for gastrointestinal hypomotility. For patients who cannot discontinue opiates, one approach is the simultaneous administration of enteral naloxone, allowing for selective blockade of intestinal opioid receptors. Indeed, when 84 ventilated patients who were receiving fentanyl were randomized to enteral naloxone or placebo, the former experienced a reduction in median gastric tube reflux volume and frequency of pneumonia.[52]

Placebo-controlled trials demonstrate that metoclopramide and cisapride improve gastric motility in critically ill patients. In a head-to-head randomized trial, both agents enhanced gastric motility and tolerance for intragastric enteral nutrition, while metoclopramide was superior in reducing gastric residual volume.[53] Cisapride is no longer routinely available because of multiple reports of related life-threatening arrhythmias. Using acetaminophen absorption kinetics to assess gastric motility, Dive et al showed that a single dose of intravenous erythromycin (200 mg over 30 minutes) increases antral motility and accelerates gastric emptying.[54] When these approaches fail or true intestinal pseudo-obstruction occurs, neostigmine can be effective.[55] In a randomized trial of 21 patients with acute colonic

TABLE 41-3 Abnormalities of Gastrointestinal Motility in Ventilated Patients

Decreased esophageal motility
Decreased gastric motility
Ileus
Colonic pseudo-obstruction (Oglivie's syndrome)
Constipation

pseudo-obstruction (cecal diameter ≥10 cm and no mechanical obstruction), 10 of 11 receiving 2 mg of neostigmine had rapid (median 4 minutes, range 3–30 minutes) colonic compression compared to 0 of 10 receiving placebo. Side effects of neostigmine include abdominal pain, excess salivation, vomiting, and symptomatic bradycardia.

In a prospective single-center study, 83% of ICU patients had constipation defined as failure to defecate for 3 consecutive days.[56] Of constipated patients, 43% experienced weaning failure (compared to none of those without constipation), perhaps related to distension, discomfort, and restlessness. In addition, constipation is associated with delayed enteral feeding and, rarely, visceral perforation. One multicenter trial described constipation in 16% of critically ill patients.[57] Constipation is likely related to the use of opiates and sedatives, immobility, dehydration, and the absence of dietary fiber.

GASTROINTESTINAL HEMORRHAGE

Gastrointestinal bleeding in ventilated patients most often results from stress-related mucosal damage. Within 24 hours of ICU admission, endoscopy reveals mucosal erosions in 75–100% of patients.[5] Fortunately, the vast majority of these lesions are asymptomatic and do not cause substantial bleeding. Clinically significant gastrointestinal hemorrhage (need of transfusion or hemodynamic instability) occurs in up to 4% of ventilated patients. Although clinically significant gastrointestinal hemorrhage (as a complication) is relatively uncommon, it leads to increased ICU mortality (relative risk of death, 1–4) and ICU length of stay (excess length of stay 4–8 days).[58,59] Cook et al studied 1666 critically ill (ventilated for at least 48 hours) patients in 16 Canadian university-affiliated ICUs. Fifty-nine patients (3.5%) had clinically important gastrointestinal bleeding and the risk of death was increased in these patients.[59]

The risk of significant bleeding related to stress ulceration varies across populations. For example, in one study of 167 medical-surgical ICU patients, ventilated for >2 days, only one patient (0.6%) experienced stress ulceration–related bleeding despite the absence of stress ulcer prophylaxis.[60] In contrast, Schuster et al found a 14% rate of either overt or occult bleeding with risk highest for those on mechanical ventilation or with coagulopathy.[58] A prospective multicenter study of >2000 critically ill patients identified mechanical ventilation (odds ratio 16) and coagulopathy (odds ratio 4) as major risk factors for significant hemorrhage. Only two of 1405 patients (0.1%) without those two risk factors had clinically relevant bleeding.[61] Subsequently, these investigators examined 1077 critically ill patients who were ventilated for >48 hours who were receiving either intravenous ranitidine or nasogastric sucralfate.[62] Using a logistic-regression model, the only independent predictor of increased risk for bleeding was the maximum serum creatinine. In contrast, enteral nutrition and intravenous ranitidine were associated with decreased risk for bleeding. Other investigators have also suggested that enteral nutrition, perhaps by repleting gastric epithelial energy stores, may decrease the risk of significant stress-related mucosal damage.[63] Smaller investigations have suggested that multiple trauma (including spine

and head), organ failure (especially hepatic and renal), sepsis, shock, extensive burns, and organ transplantation are other risk factors for bleeding.[64–68]

The role of *Helicobacter pylori* in stress-related mucosal bleeding has been examined in several studies. Among 50 patients admitted to a medical-surgical ICU, *H. pylori* was associated with major mucosal injury.[69] In contrast, in a study of 2570 cardiac surgical patients, 1.6% experienced stress ulcer bleeding; *H. pylori* was found in 45% of those who bled but 62% of those without bleeding.[70] If *H. pylori* does play a role, the risk may actually decrease over time. One study found the prevalence of active *H. pylori* infection was 38% on admission but dropped to zero by day seven, presumably because of widespread antibiotic use.[71]

The pathophysiology of stress-related mucosal damage is complex and entails mucosal ischemia, damaging gastric luminal factors, decreased intramucosal pH, and impaired local defense mechanisms[5,72] (Fig. 41-2). Therefore, prophylactic treatment is best aimed at correcting these factors. Improvements in ICU care with an emphasis on maintaining cardiac output, oxygen delivery, and therefore splanchnic blood flow may be effective prophylaxis.[60] More commonly, efforts have focused on reducing gastric acid or improving gastric mucosal protection (Table 41-4). Overall, it is estimated that prophylactic agents reduce the risk of clinically important hemorrhage by 50%.[5] Much work has focused on determining whether intravenous administration is superior to enteral delivery. For example, although continuous infusion of an H_2 blocker more effectively raises gastric pH, it appears no more effective than bolus dosing in preventing significant bleeding.[73,74] Agents used for gastrointestinal prophylaxis are associated with increased risk for ventilator-associated pneumonia, especially antacids and H_2 blockers when compared to sucralfate.[75–78]

A recent nationwide survey found that most critical care physicians in the U.S. correctly estimate the incidence of clinically important bleeding to be 2% or less. Yet, 28.6% of surveyed physicians initiated stress ulcer prophylaxis in all ICU patients independent of bleeding risk.[79] Approximately two-thirds used H_2-receptor blockers as first-line therapy (64%), while a smaller number used proton pump inhibitors (23%) or sucralfate (12%).

A number of meta-analyses have compared the leading prophylactic strategies and reached conflicting results.[69,76,80–82] Cook et al in a multicenter randomized trial of 1200 ventilated patients, comparing sucralfate to ranitidine, carried out the most rigorous comparison. Ranitidine was associated with a lower risk of significant bleeding (1.7% versus 3.8%), while no difference in risk for pneumonia was noted.[82a] A small, randomized controlled trial found omeprazole superior to ranitidine, but the 31% rate of bleeding in the latter arm raises concerns about study design.[83] More recently, a single-center study of 287 patients (with either >48 hours of mechanical ventilation or coagulopathy) found no difference in the incidence of clinically significant upper gastrointestinal bleeding when comparing patients treated with omeprazole, famotidine, sucralfate, or placebo (1%, 3%, 4%, and 1%, respectively).[84] The rate of nosocomial pneumonia was the same for the four groups.

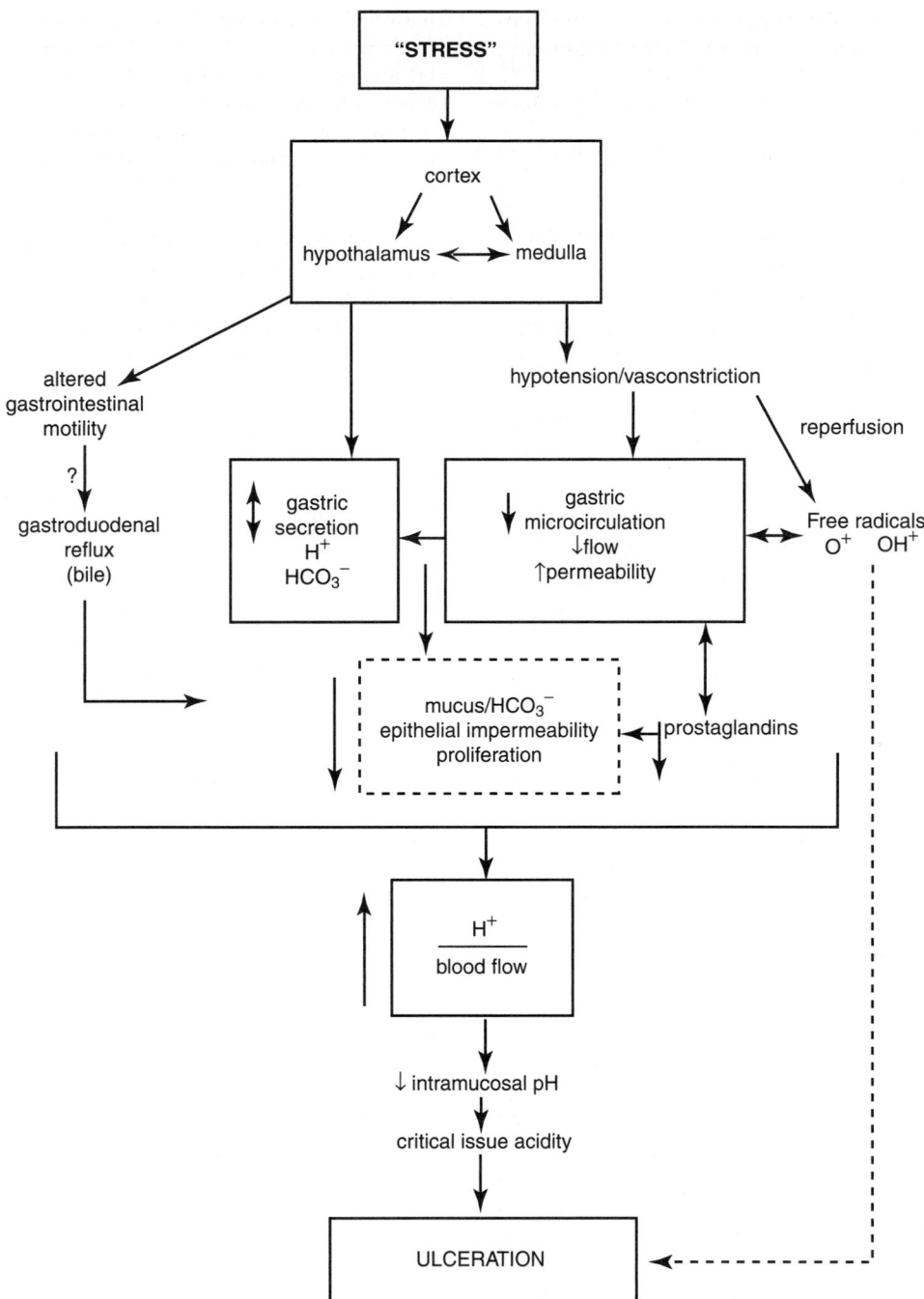

FIGURE 41-2 Proposed mechanism for stress-related mucosal damage. (*Reproduced, with permission, from Bresalier.*[72])

TABLE 41-4   Prevention of Stress-Related Mucosal Damage

Antacids
Histamine$_2$ blockers (e.g., ranitidine)
Sucralfate
Proton pump inhibitors (e.g., omeprazole)
Anticholinergic agents (e.g., pirenzapine)
Prostaglandin analogues
Enteral nutrition

OTHER GASTROINTESTINAL COMPLICATIONS

ACUTE ABDOMEN

Patients in the ICU may develop an acute abdomen resulting from many different processes. In a retrospective study of medical ICU patients, 76 patients (1.3%) developed an acute abdomen with ischemic bowel most common (other causes: perforated ulcer, bowel obstruction, and cholecystitis).[85] Survival was 56% in those undergoing surgery, while none of 26 patients not undergoing surgery survived. Indeed, patients on mechanical ventilation (and those receiving opiates, without peritoneal signs, and with an abnormal mental status) were more likely to experience surgical delay.

DIARRHEA

As many as 50% of critically ill patients develop diarrhea, and respiratory failure is a risk factor.[5,86] Causes of diarrhea include enteral nutrition (related to high infusion rate or hyperosmolar content), *Clostridium difficile*, bowel edema (related to hypoalbuminemia), and medications.

ESOPHAGEAL DISEASE

Approximately 50% of ventilated patients develop esophageal mucosal injury or erosive esophagitis. The latter may account for nearly 25% of cases of upper gastrointestinal bleeding.[87,88] Mechanisms leading to esophageal injury include bile reflux, supine positioning, nasogastric tubes, gastroesophageal reflux, and abnormal gastric emptying.[5,88–90]

ACALCULOUS CHOLECYSTITIS AND PANCREATITIS

Up to 3% of critically ill patients develop acute gallbladder inflammation despite the absence of gallstones (acalculous cholecystitis).[5] Mechanical ventilation for more than 72 hours has been identified as a potential risk factor. Other risk factors include medications (opiates and vasopressors), shock, sepsis, multiple transfusions, total parenteral nutrition, prolonged absence of enteral nutrition, and dehydration. The underlying mechanism of acalculous cholecystitis is likely to be multifactorial, combining inadequate perfusion, chemical injury, and abnormal gallbladder wall contractility. Current approaches to diagnosis include right upper quadrant ultrasonography, abdominal computed tomography, and hepatobiliary scintigraphy (HIDA scan), though the latter is associated with a high false-positive rate.[91] In this critically ill population, percutaneous cholecystostomy is often favored for therapy rather than surgical cholecystectomy.

Severe pancreatitis often leads to multiple organ failure, ICU admission, and the need for ventilator support. The incidence of pancreatitis acquired in the ICU is not well known. Manjuck et al studied 245 critically ill patients (without admission diagnosis of pancreatitis); 40% developed an elevated lipase level during their ICU stay. In a multivariate analysis, mechanical ventilation was an independent risk factor for developing an elevated lipase level. Moreover, those with elevated lipase suffered a longer duration of mechanical ventilation. Yet, pancreatitis could be confirmed in only eleven patients (approximately 10% of those with elevated lipase).[92] One potential cause of pancreatitis in ventilated patients is that resulting from hypertriglyceridemia that can be seen with propofol administration.[93]

Nutritional Complications

ADVERSE EFFECTS OF MALNUTRITION

Evidence indicates that medical patients with malnutrition have higher levels of morbidity and mortality than those with adequate nutrition.[94,95] Malnutrition has been associated with abnormal control of breathing, with a blunted ventilatory response to hypoxia.[96–98] Patients with significant malnutrition can have atrophy of respiratory muscles that can limit respiratory reserve.[99–102] This breakdown of skeletal muscle protein is exacerbated by the catabolic state of critical illness.[103] Respiratory muscle dysfunction is thought to limit weaning from mechanical ventilation. Several retrospective studies suggest that nutritional repletion can improve weaning success.[104,105] Malnutrition is also associated with lymphocyte dysfunction and impaired cell-mediated immunity and thus the risk of infection is increased.[106,107] Classically, malnourished patients have a decreased basal metabolic rate, while it is increased in critically ill patients. The latter is attributable to an elevated catabolic rate, a process that likely contributes to the high morbidity and mortality in critical illness, and one not easily reversed by nutritional repletion.[103,108]

COMPLICATIONS OF NUTRITIONAL SUPPORT

There are few data to show that outcomes for ventilated patients improve with aggressive nutritional repletion.[109] Yet, most experts concur that nutritional repletion is necessary (clearly when pre-existing malnutrition exists), though its timing, magnitude, and route of administration remain controversial.[94,110,111] In a prospective controlled trial, 150 mechanically ventilated medical ICU patients were randomized to early feeding (estimated total daily enteral nutritional requirement on day 1) or late feeding (total requirements on day 5). The late feeding group received 20% of their estimated daily nutritional requirement during the initial 4 days. The early feeding group was more likely to develop ventilator-associated pneumonia (VAP), diarrhea associated with *C. difficile*, and had longer ICU and hospital stay.[112] Other studies suggest no difference in outcome when early nutrition is emphasized.[94]

When gut function is abnormal (as is commonly the case in ventilated patients), clinicians often opt for total parenteral nutrition (TPN). Meta-analyses of recent trials suggest that compared to enteral nutrition, TPN may be associated with increased complication rates and morbidity[111,113,114] (Table 41-5). In a review of 13 studies comparing enteral and parenteral nutrition, the former was associated with fewer infectious complications and less hyperglycemia.[115] Increasing emphasis therefore is placed on delivering enteral nutrition, especially to critically ill ventilated patients. Experimental data show that intestinal villous atrophy occurs in the absence of enteral feeding, and this predisposes to the gut translocation of bacteria and bacterial products, the substrate that drives multiorgan failure. Indeed, randomized trials in patients with pancreatitis

TABLE 41-5 Complications Associated with Total Parenteral Nutrition

Mechanical complications associated with central line placement
Increased risk for catheter-related infection
Increased risk for catheter-related thrombosis
Metabolic complications
    Hyperglycemia
    Hypophosphatemia
    Hypernatremia
    Hyperchloremic metabolic acidosis
Hepatobiliary dysfunction

indicate that outcomes can improve with enteral nutrition.[116,117] Animal data indicate that this approach restores intestinal integrity, reduces gut translocation, and reduces infected pancreatic necrosis.

Issues remain about the optimal manner for administering enteral nutrition. For one, body position appears very important. A study comparing enteral nutrition in supine and prone patients, found that the latter was associated with higher gastric volumes, more emesis, and lower daily caloric intake. The latter likely resulted from the fact that enteral nutrition had to be stopped in 82% of prone patients compared to 49% of supine patients.[118] Frequent interruptions in enteral feeding are common in routine ICU care and can lead to underfeeding.[119,120] In one study, the mean duration of interruption was >5 hours per day; reasons included tests/procedures, positioning, unstable hemodynamics, increased gastric residuals, and nausea and vomiting; the latter two reasons accounted for 20% of all interruptions.[120] Increased gastric residual volumes are often the trigger for suspending tube feedings because of a concern for aspiration, though the practice has recently been questioned. In a prospective study of 40 patients, residual volume (ranging from 0 to >400 ml) did not accurately predict risk for aspiration or regurgitation.[121]

Despite the potential physiologic benefits of enteral nutrition, multiple gastrointestinal complications have been reported in critically ill patients.[57] In a prospective study of 37 ICUs in Spain, one or more gastrointestinal complications occurred in 63% of enterally fed patients, including high gastric residuals (39%), constipation (16%), diarrhea (15%), abdominal distension (13%), vomiting (12%), and regurgitation (6%).[57] Patients suffering complications received a lower percentage of desired nutritional support, and had longer lengths of stay and higher mortality. Receiving inadequate caloric intake may be important because in one study this was associated with an increased risk for nosocomial bloodstream infection.[122] In an effort to enhance tolerance for enteral feeds, improve nutritional delivery, and reduce complications, investigators have examined the efficacy of placing tubes in the small bowel. Nasojejunal tubes are more labor-intensive to place (often requiring endoscopic or fluoroscopic methods) than nasogastric tubes, but they have potential benefits including reduced gastric residuals, improved tolerance for enteral feeding, better caloric intake, earlier attainment of nutritional goals, and perhaps, less risk for nosocomial pneumonia.[123–126] In a review of 10 studies, small bowel feeding was associated with decreased gastroesophageal regurgitation, increased nutritional delivery, shorter time to reach the targeted rate of nutrition, and less VAP.[127] In contrast, a review of medical and neurosurgical trauma studies found no difference in gastric and postpyloric tubes in terms of pneumonia or length of stay; gastric delivery could be initiated sooner.[128] Promotility agents (e.g., single-dose erythromycin) can facilitate nasojejunal tube placement.[129] More significantly, adding a promotility agent (erythromycin or metoclopramide) can improve motility, improve tolerance for enteral feeds, decrease the time needed to meet nutritional goals, and overcome many of the deficiencies associated with gastric placement.[129,130]

Pneumonia is a major complication of mechanical ventilation. Though the explanation is likely multifactorial, gastric colonization followed by aspiration may be one mechanism. Therefore, avoiding the supine position in enterally fed patients is likely to be important. Indeed, one study randomized 86 ventilated patients to supine versus semirecumbent positioning, finding a lower risk for VAP in the latter.[131] With multivariate analysis, supine positioning and enteral feeding were independently associated with the development of VAP. Adding metoclopramide may delay the onset of VAP.[132] Using a small bore feeding tube (compared to large bore) may decrease gastroesophageal reflux and decrease the likelihood of pulmonary aspiration of gastric contents.[90]

Although enteral feeding appears to have fewer complications than TPN there are several unique manifestations to be considered. In heavily sedated patients, small bore, soft feeding tubes (Dobhoff) may be mistakenly placed in the airway and rarely may perforate the visceral pleura.[133] This results in tube feeds being delivered directly in the airway or the creation of an iatrogenic pleural fluid collection. To avoid this complication, some experts prefer to use a standard large bore nasogastric tube, because such a tube is more likely to cause tracheal irritation and cough, thereby signaling its erroneous positioning. Insufflating the tube with air and listening with a stethoscope over the left upper quadrant does not guarantee intragastric positioning; left lower lobe or left pleural placement will mimic the correct positioning. Tubes can be placed under endoscopic or bronchoscopic guidance, though this seems undesirable given the low incidence of this complication. The best approach is radiographic confirmation of tube placement before the initiation of enteral feeding.

Overfeeding, irrespective of the route, may have adverse ventilatory effects. Depending on the nutrient mix, the typical respiratory quotient (the amount of CO_2 produced for the amount of O_2 consumed) ranges from 0.7–1.0. With overfeeding, CO_2 production can increase dramatically, with a respiratory quotient of 4–8. Minute ventilation would need to increase four- to eightfold to maintain a normal Pa_{CO_2}. Such an increase in ventilatory demand may cause ventilator dependency and failure to wean.[134–136] Fortunately, overfeeding may be avoided by using relatively simple maneuvers. Total energy requirements can be determined by using the Harris-Benedict equation, a metabolic cart, data from a pulmonary artery catheter, or a simple estimate of energy needs, 25–35 kcal/kg per day.

Renal Complications

Acute renal failure and abnormal fluid retention can be manifestations of critical illness unrelated to mechanical ventilation. Alternatively, positive-pressure ventilation may directly and adversely affect renal function. Over the last three decades, numerous animal and human studies have sought to define the underlying mechanisms. Proposed mechanisms include a reduction in cardiac output leading to reduced renal blood flow, a redistribution of intrarenal blood flow, stimulation of hormonal and sympathetic systems, and the adverse effects of systemic inflammatory mediators released as an outcome of ventilator-induced lung injury.[137]

ACUTE RENAL FAILURE

Acute renal failure is common in ICU patients, with acute tubular necrosis and prerenal azotemia the most likely mechanisms.[138] Of 487 consecutive patients admitted to a medical ICU, 78 (16%) developed acute renal failure, 63% of whom required renal replacement therapy.[139] Acute renal failure significantly increases ICU mortality, especially among patients with sepsis, with reported rates as high as 50–80%.[140–143] Several studies found mechanical ventilation (respiratory failure) to be an independent risk factor for the development of acute renal failure.[139,144,145] A prospective investigation of patients with acute tubular necrosis found mechanical ventilation to be independently associated with need for dialysis.[144] In addition, mechanical ventilation is associated with increased risk for ICU mortality in patients with renal failure.[146–149] Acute renal failure is associated with poor weaning outcome in patients undergoing prolonged ventilation. In 52 patients with prolonged ventilation and hemodialysis, none were successfully weaned and only three survived.[150] In another investigation, patients with severe renal dysfunction were less likely to be successfully weaned (13 versus 56%).[151] Although therapies such as dopamine, theophylline, atrial natriuretic peptide, captopril, and prostaglandin E_1 have been investigated, none has been shown to prevent the development of acute renal failure.[138]

Mechanical ventilation has the potential to contribute to several pathophysiologic causes of acute renal dysfunction. The ventilation method may also influence the risk. In a study of trauma patients mechanical ventilation increased the odds ratio for acute renal failure, especially if PEEP was >6 cmH$_2$O (odds ratio 3.6 when PEEP was < 6, 17.5 when PEEP was >6).[145] Similarly, two studies found that a lung protective strategy in patients with acute lung injury was associated with a lower incidence of renal failure than the use of higher tidal volumes.[45,152] Ranieri et al[45] found that higher tidal volumes were associated with increased plasma levels of tumor necrosis factor-α, interleukin-1B, interleukin-8, and soluble tumor necrosis factor-α receptor in 44 patients with ARDS. It is hypothesized that systemic increases in cytokines lead to organ dysfunction, including renal failure. Another potential cause for renal failure in ventilated patients is dysregulation of apoptosis. In a rabbit model of acute lung injury, plasma from animals ventilated with 15–17 ml/kg and low PEEP (0–3 cmH$_2$O) resulted in increased rates of epithelial apoptosis in kidney tissue culture.[153]

Acute renal failure is an independent predictor for ICU mortality, but effective preventive strategies have not been convincingly demonstrated. Once acute renal failure becomes manifest, most patients are treated using renal replacement therapy. The latter may be delivered by intermittent hemodialysis or by continuous approaches (continuous renal replacement therapy; CRRT), especially when hemodynamic instability is present.[141]

POSITIVE FLUID BALANCE

Patients with chronic hypercapnic respiratory failure often acutely decompensate and require mechanical ventilation. This disease process may manifest complex renal hormonal effects resulting in sodium and water retention (and possibly volume overload) secondary to catecholamine-induced decreased renal blood flow, increased sodium/proton exchange, and activation of the renin-angiotensin-aldosterone and antidiuretic hormone (ADH) systems.[154–157] Hypercapnia causes renal tubular exchange of hydrogen ions for sodium and bicarbonate; the result is sodium and water retention. Hypoxia and hypercapnia further reduce renal blood flow and activate the renin-angiotensin-aldosterone system.[137,158]

Positive-pressure ventilation itself is thought to be a principal cause of edema in the ICU.[137] More than 50 years ago, continuous positive airway pressure (CPAP) was demonstrated to decrease renal blood flow, glomerular filtration rate, and urine output. Subsequent studies conducted in animals, healthy subjects, and patients with respiratory failure, with CPAP or intermittent mandatory ventilation (IMV), consistently demonstrated that positive-pressure ventilation decreases urine output.[137] These studies did not uniformly demonstrate reductions in renal blood flow, glomerular filtration rate, or free water clearance. Animal and human studies demonstrate that PEEP, from 5–20 cmH$_2$O, consistently decreases urine output; many, but not all, studies demonstrate parallel decreases in cardiac output, cardiac index, renal blood flow, glomerular filtration rate, and fractional excretion of sodium.[137] Indeed, studies in ICU patients show such reductions within 30–60 minutes after the institution of PEEP, changes that reverse when PEEP is discontinued.[159,160] When positive-pressure ventilation causes a reduction in cardiac output, renal perfusion is decreased, causing renin-angiotensin system stimulation, decreased atrial natriuretic peptide, and increased ADH.[137,160–162] These changes cause sodium and fluid retention, often manifested as peripheral edema, decreased urine output, and reduced renal sodium excretion. Other mechanisms may be at work because fluid retention can still occur even if cardiac output and hormonal activation is prevented.[163,164]

Noninvasive, nasal positive-pressure ventilation (NIV), a modality used with increasing frequency in critical care, may exert similar effects. Carlone et al found that after 30 minutes of CPAP, urinary sodium concentration decreased while plasma atrial natriuretic peptide increased. No changes in free water clearance or plasma levels of renin, ADH, and aldosterone were observed.[165] The implication is that NIV mediates changes in sodium and water excretion via renal hemodynamic mechanisms rather than direct hormonal changes. In contrast, Tanaka et al found that NIV (1 hour of 15 cmH$_2$O CPAP) results in an acute neurohumoral response (increase in plasma ADH and norepinephrine) and is associated with decreased urine output, sodium excretion, and free water clearance.[25]

Based on the pathophysiologic cascade delineated above, adverse effects of positive-pressure ventilation on renal function can best be averted by avoiding excessive tidal volume and high levels of PEEP, and carefully maintaining adequate intravascular volume and oxygen delivery. Treatment of unfavorable fluid balance includes diuretics, dopamine (natriuretic), or agents to improve renal perfusion (inotropes). When these mechanisms prove ineffective, ultrafiltration (intermittent or continuous) helps in establishing more favorable fluid balance. Indeed, such an approach may be crucial for reducing elastic work of breathing and aiding weaning. One preliminary report noted that successful diuresis and weight loss were associated with successful weaning from prolonged ventilation.[166]

Endocrinologic Complications

In critically ill patients, increasing severity of illness, sepsis, and multiple organ failure are associated with numerous endocrinologic abnormalities. Importantly, endocrinologic disease can have specific adverse affects on ventilated patients.

THYROID DISEASE

Most critically ill patients with clinically significant thyroid disorders have those entities at the time of admission to the ICU. In contrast, critically ill patients often manifest abnormal thyroid function tests in the absence of true disease (Table 41-6).[167–180] In the ICU, abnormal thyroid function tests may often be present in the absence of true thyroidal illness, a condition referred to as sick euthyroid syndrome or nonthyroidal illness syndrome (NTIS).[181,182] Although the extent of thyroid hormone abnormality correlates both with severity of illness and with mortality, it is uncertain whether this condition is a physiologic (e.g., to reduce unnecessary energy utilization) or a maladaptive response to stress (e.g., compromising tissue function).[167,176,183,184] Several patterns of thyroid hormone test abnormalities have been noted in NTIS, including, (1) low T_3, normal TSH (most common), (2) low T_3, low T_4 (normal free T_4), normal TSH, and (3) low T_3, low T_4, and low TSH.[167] In a study of 32 patients with acute-on-chronic respiratory failure, a low free T_3 was associated with reduced survival.[185] Given the relationship between NTIS and increased ICU mortality, investigators have tested the benefit of T_3 therapy. While conflicting results have been seen in the setting of cardiac surgery, one study conducted in medical ICU patients revealed no clinical benefit.[186–189] Therefore, at present thyroid hormone replacement cannot be recommended for patients with NTIS.

When T_3 and T_4 are low but TSH is elevated (especially when >20 mU/L) primary hypothyroidism is likely. The prevalence of true hypothyroidism is likely to be low, but can still have important implications for the ventilated patient. Specifically, hypothyroidism is associated with reduced ventilatory response to hypoxia and hypercapnia, hypoventilation, and respiratory muscle dysfunction, which can contribute to weaning failure. Although hy-

TABLE 41-6   Factors Associated with Abnormal Thyroid Function Tests in Critically Ill Patients

Malnutrition
Medications (e.g., dopamine, amiodarone, corticosteroids, iodinated contrast agents)
Sepsis
Malignancy
Major surgery
Myocardial infarction
Human immunodeficiency virus

pothyroidism is an unusual cause of weaning failure, it is easily treatable and should be sought in difficult-to-wean patients.[190–192]

Although hyperthyroidism is not a complication of critical illness, its presence can have adverse consequences for the ventilated patient. Thyroid storm is associated with a dramatic increase in metabolic rate, excess carbon dioxide production, and consequent hypercapnia in patients unable to increase minute ventilation appropriately. Hyperthyroidism may also adversely affect respiratory muscle function.[193]

ADRENAL INSUFFICIENCY

Both high and low cortisol levels are associated with increased mortality in critically ill patients.[194,195] In the former, high cortisol levels likely serve as a marker of severity of illness. In the latter, low cortisol levels reflect an inadequate response to life-threatening stress. Ventilated patients may experience adrenal insufficiency for several reasons, most commonly, acute adrenal insufficiency (addisonian crisis) in a patient with chronic adrenal insufficiency, or rarely secondary to an acute adrenal (or rarely pituitary) insult.[196] Severe sepsis is associated with a state of relative adrenal insufficiency. Making a diagnosis of adrenal insufficiency can be particularly challenging in the critical care setting. Acute adrenal insufficiency typically presents with rapid clinical worsening, manifested as fever, abdominal pain, mental status changes, unexplained hypothermia, hypoglycemia, and hypotension.[197] This may result from the superimposed stress of critical illness or the interruption of steroid therapy in a patient with chronic adrenal insufficiency. Alternatively, adrenal insufficiency can be a manifestation of sepsis, shock, adrenal hemorrhage, or secondary to medications (e.g., heparin, rifampin, or ketoconazole).[196] Although few robust data are available, it is likely that adrenal insufficiency may adversely affect weaning from mechanical ventilation.

The diagnosis of adrenal insufficiency is controversial, especially regarding the normal cortisol response to stress and interpretation of corticotropin stimulation (adrenocorticotropic hormone; ACTH) testing. Critically ill patients do not manifest the typical diurnal variation in cortisol production. Thus, early morning levels are not required; random cortisol can be assessed at any time. During critical illness, cortisol values often exceed 45 μg/dl and fewer than 10% of patients manifest values <25 /mug/dL.[167,198,199] Yet, others have argued that values >34 /mug/dL make adrenal insufficiency unlikely.[200] Testing with ACTH (cosyntropin) has been advocated because "elevated" cortisol values can be associated with adrenal insufficiency. An increase in cortisol of <9 /mug/dL in response to 250 /mug of cosyntropin indicates adrenal insufficiency. Although some advocate using a "low-dose" ACTH stimulation test (1 /mug/dl) to improve sensitivity, insufficient data in critically ill patients exists to recommend this approach.[167,196,200]

Treatment of acute adrenal insufficiency consists of hydrocortisone (or equivalent) 100 mg intravenously every 6 to 8 hours. For the relative adrenal insufficiency of severe sepsis, 50 mg every 6 hours is combined with 50 μg of fludrocortisone daily and given for a total of 7 days.[201] Treatment with physiologic doses of corticosteroids appears to be safe, and has not been associated with the myopathy and delayed weaning observed when higher doses are combined with neuromuscular blocking agents.[202,203]

STRESS HORMONES AND WEANING FROM MECHANICAL VENTILATION

A number of older studies, examining principally postoperative patients (and those ventilated <48 hours), suggested that mechanical ventilation had little impact (at least during weaning) on catecholamines and stress hormone response.[204,205] In contrast, Koksal et al recently studied 60 patients and found that patients weaning on a T-piece experienced a greater endocrine stress response than patients weaning on CPAP or pressure support.[206] Specifically, T-piece weaning was associated with higher plasma insulin, cortisol, blood glucose, and urinary vanillylmandelic acid. This study differs from previous work in examining patients not receiving sedative infusions and requiring at least 48 hours of mechanical ventilation. It is possible that patients receiving inadequate ventilator support (or experiencing patient-ventilator dyssynchrony) may experience the same stress response.

STRESS HYPERGLYCEMIA

Stress hyperglycemia is common in critically ill patients even among those without known diabetes mellitus.[207,208] Hyperglycemia in critically ill patients arises from increased hepatic gluconeogenesis, peripheral insulin resistance, and increased circulating free fatty acids.[208] Hyperglycemia is associated with numerous negative effects in critically ill patients, including abnormal tissue function, osmotic diuresis, impaired immunoglobulin and complement function, abnormal leukocyte chemotaxis, and impaired phagocytosis.[208–212] These abnormalities of leukocyte function likely account for increased risk of infection. Hyperglycemia is associated with increased mortality in patients with either acute myocardial infarction or acute stroke.[213–215] Ventilated patients are often infected or have respiratory illnesses for which corticosteroids are administered, therefore increasing the risk for hyperglycemia.

In a randomized trial, van den Berghe et al found that tight glucose control (goal: 80–110 mg/dl), achieved with insulin infusion, was associated with improved outcomes in a cohort of 1548 surgical ICU patients (primarily cardiovascular). Patients with tight control had lower all-cause mortality, reduced duration of mechanical ventilation, less need for renal replacement therapy, and fewer bloodstream infections.[216] In a study in a medical-surgical ICU, a protocol to keep glucose <140 mg/dl resulted in a reduction in the development of new renal insufficiency, and decreased ICU length of stay and hospital mortality when compared to historic controls.[217] A recent meta-analysis of 35 trials found that insulin therapy decreased short-term mortality by 15% in critically ill patients. Insulin therapy decreased mortality in surgical ICU patients with diabetes mellitus, when the goal was glucose control.[218] Randomized trials of insulin therapy in medical ICU patients have not been reported.

To address whether benefits derive from glycemic control or the administration of insulin, van den Berghe et al reanalyzed the data from their trial. Multivariate analysis showed that lowered blood glucose, rather than insulin dose, was associated with reduced mortality.[219] Indeed, Finney et al using a multiple logistic regression model demonstrated that increased insulin administration was actually associated with increased ICU mortality.[220]

Hematologic Complications

ANEMIA

Anemia is common in critically ill ventilated patients, and can result from overt hemorrhage, occult bleeding, bone marrow suppression from overwhelming infection or malignancy, and rarely from hemolytic states.[221–225] Losses from daily phlebotomy can be substantial, and may account for nearly half the blood transfused in ICU patients.[222,226] The number of patients requiring transfusion and the total number of units of packed red blood cells transfused in the ICU can be staggering. In a prospective observational study in 284 ICUs, 44% of patients required a blood transfusion (63% of patients with ICU stay ≥7 days); those transfused received a mean of 4.6 units of packed red blood cells.[225]

Because hemoglobin is crucial for adequate oxygen-carrying capacity, anemia may limit oxygen delivery. Reductions in oxygen transport may be particularly detrimental in ventilated patients, especially when the stress of weaning increases respiratory muscle oxygen consumption.[227,228] Small physiologic studies suggest that blood transfusion given to anemic, ventilated patients with COPD may reduce minute ventilation and work of breathing and increase the likelihood of weaning.[229,230] Hebert et al randomized critically ill patients to two different transfusion goals: hemoglobin of 7–9 g/dl or 10–12 g/dl. Overall the liberal transfusion strategy was not associated with an improvement in outcome, though less severely ill (Acute Physiology, Age, and Chronic Health Evaluation [APACHE] II score <20) and younger patients (age <55) had increased 30-day mortality.[231] In a retrospective analysis of 713 ventilated patients, no differences were found in average duration of mechanical ventilation (8.3 days) or in weaning and extubation success (82% restrictive versus 78% liberal).[232]

The presence of anemia often triggers a blood transfusion of packed red blood cells that may adversely affect the ventilated patient. Transfusions can cause intravascular volume overload and pulmonary edema. Transfusion reactions can cause fever, thereby increasing oxygen consumption and carbon dioxide production. Lastly, transfusion related acute lung injury (TRALI) could result in worsening compliance and oxygenation. Although treatment of anemic ICU patients with erythropoietin modestly decreases transfusion requirements, clinically relevant outcomes, such as survival or decreased duration of mechanical ventilation, were not observed.[233]

THROMBOCYTOPENIA

Thrombocytopenia is common among critically ill patients, though its presence is typically not directly related to mechanical ventilation. Defined as a platelet count $<100,000/\mu l$, thrombocytopenia is seen in 20–40% of medical-surgical ICU patients.[234–236] Severe thrombocytopenia, platelet count $<50,000/\mu l$, is found in 10–20% of such patients. Thrombocytopenia is of considerable clinical relevance. In a prospective observational study, 44% of medical ICU patients had a platelet count $<150,000/\mu l$; the nadir count was an independent risk factor for development of major bleeding.[237] In 40 ICU patients, platelet counts were lower in nonsurvivors and failed to increase over time to the same degree as in survivors.[238] In another study, 41% of patients had at least one platelet count $<150,000/\mu l$, and these patients had longer ICU stay and higher ICU mortality. Bleeding increased from 4% in nonthrombocytopenic patients to 21% in patients with platelet counts between 100,000 and $150,000/\mu l$, and to 53% when platelet counts were $<100,000/\mu l$.[239] Thrombocytopenia may adversely affect outcome by increasing the danger of hemorrhage and the risks associated with performing invasive procedures.[240]

Thrombocytopenia is typically a result of sepsis, disseminated intravascular coagulation (DIC), medications (e.g., antibiotics or heparin), or dilution from massive blood transfusions. Four principal mechanisms have been elucidated: increased platelet destruction, decreased platelet production, dilutional or distributional etiologies, and spurious causes (e.g., platelet clumping on a peripheral blood smear).[235] Though most causes of thrombocytopenia increase the risk for hemorrhage, the most common form of heparin-induced thrombocytopenia (HIT) is associated with increased risk of thrombosis (type II HIT). In a prospective study of 267 heparin-exposed intensive and coronary care unit patients, 15% met the clinical criteria for HIT.[241] Among patients with type II HIT who require anticoagulation, lepirudin (a direct thrombin inhibitor) or danaparoid (heparinoid) can be used, while platelet transfusions are contraindicated.

Infectious Complications

Infection commonly complicates critical illness, especially among ventilated patients, and is a major contributor to ICU length of stay and mortality.[242–244] Most studies report that 20–25% of critically ill patients experience one or more ICU-related nosocomial infections.[245,246] Yet, depending on the population, the risk may be as high as 50%.[247,248] Invasive ventilation is a major risk factor. In a single center study, 26% of 434 critically ill patients had a nosocomial infection; in logistic regression analysis, mechanical ventilation was an independent predictor (odds ratio 16.4) for acquiring infection.[249]

Intubated, ventilated patients are at increased risk for VAP and sinusitis (see Chapters 46 and 47). Other infections complicate critical illness consequent to ubiquitous invasive devices, such as central lines and urinary catheters. Girou et al found that patients treated with NIV for acute respiratory failure were not only less likely to develop nosocomial pneumonia, but also experienced fewer urinary tract infections and bloodstream infections compared to invasive ventilation[250] (Fig. 41-3).

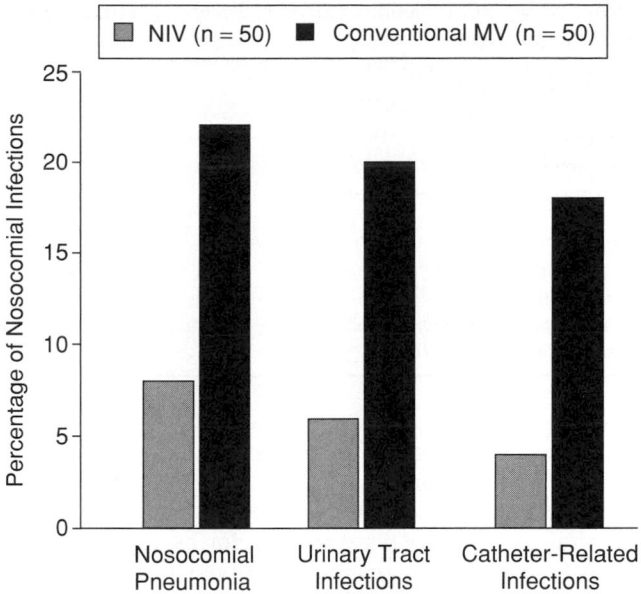

FIGURE 41-3 **Reduction in infectious complications in patients undergoing noninvasive ventilation compared to invasive mechanical ventilation.** (*Reproduced, with permission, from Girou et al.[250]*)

Fever in the ventilated patient is a major diagnostic challenge.[91] Fever and sepsis increase metabolic rate, increase oxygen consumption, raise carbon dioxide production, and may contribute to patient-ventilator dyssynchrony or weaning failure by increasing ventilatory demand. Sepsis is associated with respiratory muscle dysfunction and may contribute to the rapid and shallow breathing often exhibited by weaning failure patients.[251,252]

The most common infections in ventilated patients are VAP, sinusitis, catheter-related infection, *Clostridium difficile* diarrhea, urinary tract infection, abdominal sepsis, and wound infection.[91] The National Nosocomial Infection Surveillance System collected data from nearly 500,000 patients in 205 medical-surgical ICUs across the United States.[253] The most common sites of infection were nosocomial pneumonia (31%), urinary tract infection (UTI) (23%), and primary bloodstream infections (14%). In patients with UTIs, *Escherichia coli* (19%) was the most commonly isolated organism, while fungal isolates were present in 31% of cases. Of the primary bloodstream infections, 87% occurred in patients with central lines; the most frequently isolated organisms were coagulase-negative staphylococci (39%), *Staphylococcus aureus* (12%), and enterococci (12%). Among 180,000 medical ICU patients, the most common sites of infection were UTI (31%), pneumonia (27%), and primary bloodstream infection (19%). Of blood stream infections, 87% were associated with central lines with coagulase-negative staphylococci (36%), enterococci (16%), *Staphylococcus aureus* (13%), and fungi (12%). Nearly all UTIs were associated with urinary catheters and the most commonly isolated organism was *Candida albicans*.[254]

In a study of multidisciplinary ICUs, 51 (4.4%) of 1017 patients acquired bloodstream infection (first positive blood culture ≥ 48 hours after ICU admission).[255] Ventilated

TABLE 41-7 Noninfectious Causes of Fever in Mechanically Ventilated Patients

Adrenal insufficiency
Alcohol withdrawal
Cerebral hemorrhage
Drug fever
Fibroproliferative phase of acute lung injury
Hematoma
Myocardial infarction
Neuroleptic malignant syndrome
Pancreatitis
Transfusion reaction
Venous thromboembolism

patients are at increased risk for bacteremia because of central venous catheters. Up to 5% of patients with central catheters develop bloodstream infection. Injurious ventilator strategies also increase the risk for bacteremia. When animals were randomized to an injurious strategy (tidal volume 21 ml/kg, zero PEEP) or a protective approach (tidal volume 7 ml/kg, PEEP 5 cmH2O) and had tracheal instillation of *Pseudomonas aeruginosa*, the former group had more positive blood cultures (33% versus 11%).[256]

Fever is extraordinarily common in critically ill ventilated patients. Yet, fever may result from both infectious and noninfectious processes (Table 41-7). In a study of 100 patients with nosocomial fever, 25% had noninfectious causes.[257] Among 2419 patients with surgical critical illness, fever developed in 26%. Though only 46% of fevers were infectious in origin, peak temperature was still strongly predictive of increased mortality.[258]

Traditionally clinicians have relied on Gram's stain, stool assay for toxins of *C. difficile*, or culture material from blood, respiratory secretions, and urine to confirm the presence of infection. In cases where data are nondiagnostic, extensive imaging using computed tomography or ultrasonography have been employed, and can be used to direct diagnostic aspiration of fluid collections. For example, pleural effusions are common in critically ill ventilated patients. In a study of 94 such patients with temperature >38°C for at least 8 hours, thoracentesis demonstrated infection in 62%; most were parapneumonic, while one-quarter were empyema. This study also confirmed the safety of ultrasound-guided thoracentesis in ventilated patients.[259] When the diagnosis remains elusive, clinicians often obtain gallium or indium-111 scans to localize sources of infection. These techniques are expensive, time consuming, and necessitate transporting the patient from the ICU. Povoa et al found that C-reactive protein (CRP) was useful in detecting sepsis, and more sensitive than temperature or white cell count.[260] They subsequently found that combining CRP and body temperature yielded the highest area under a ROC curve and a specificity of 100%.[260] Elevated CRP levels have been used to follow the response to therapy.[261] In a study of medical-surgical ICU patients, procalcitonin was more accurate than CRP; areas under the ROC curve were 0.76 versus 0.5.[262] The clinical role of these measurements remains controversial; some studies have found neither test to be sufficiently accurate in the setting of the systemic inflammatory response syndrome.[263] A systematic approach to evaluating the febrile patient on mechanical ventilation is recommended (Fig. 41-4).

Cardiovascular Complications

ARRHYTHMIAS

Arrhythmias are common in ventilated patients, though few studies have examined prevalence, type, and outcomes.[264–266] In a prospective observational study in a multidisciplinary ICU, 133 patients experienced 310 episodes of new-onset, sustained ($\geq$30 seconds) arrhythmia, or 2.9 episodes per patient. Tachyarrhythmias were present 90% of the time, and bradyarrhythmias in 10%.[267] Among the tachyarrhythmias, 30% were atrial fibrillation and 49% were ventricular tachycardia (principally monomorphic); less common were supraventricular tachycardia (8%), atrial flutter (4%), and torsade de pointes (5%). In 596 surgical ICU patients, 89 (14.8%) developed tachyarrhythmias, and 61% of these were atrial fibrillation.[268] Using a case-control design, the authors found that systemic inflammatory response syndrome (SIRS) (or sepsis), high admission Simplified Acute Physiologic Scores (SAPS), and low Pa$_{O_2}$ were significant predictors for tachyarrhythmia. In another SICU study, 5.3% of patients developed atrial fibrillation; multivariate analysis identified five independent predictors, including advanced age, blunt thoracic trauma, shock, pulmonary artery catheter, and previous therapy with calcium channel blockers.[269] Artucio et al found that 78% of 2820 critically ill patients experienced cardiac arrhythmias, with a range of 44% in patients with trauma to 90% in patients with primary cardiovascular disease.[264] Importantly, the presence of arrhythmia increased the relative risk of death, especially among patients with sepsis or neurologic disorders. Arrhythmias may be a marker for severity of illness or could directly contribute to increased mortality. In a study of 23 critically ill patients, recurrent or refractory supraventricular arrhythmias were associated with increased pulmonary artery wedge pressure, decreased cardiac output, and worsening respiratory failure.[270] Control of the ventricular response using intravenous verapamil led to clinical stability. Most patients were eventually stabilized on a long-term intravenous infusion of verapamil. Koh et al examined 68 patients using Holter monitoring and echocardiography within 24 hours of initiation of mechanical ventilation; 18 (26.5%) developed hemodynamically significant arrhythmias. With multiple regression analysis, hemodynamically significant arrhythmias were directly associated with tachycardia ($\geq$120/min), initial mean arterial pressure (<70 mmHg) and, inversely, with use of pressure-controlled ventilation.[271]

Arrhythmias may occur because of underlying cardiac disease or as a complication of acute illness and its related therapies, including mechanical ventilation. Episodic right bundle-branch block has been directly associated with positive-pressure breathing.[272] Critically ill patients frequently experience hypokalemia, hypocalcemia, and hypomagnesemia, metabolic disturbances that can precipitate

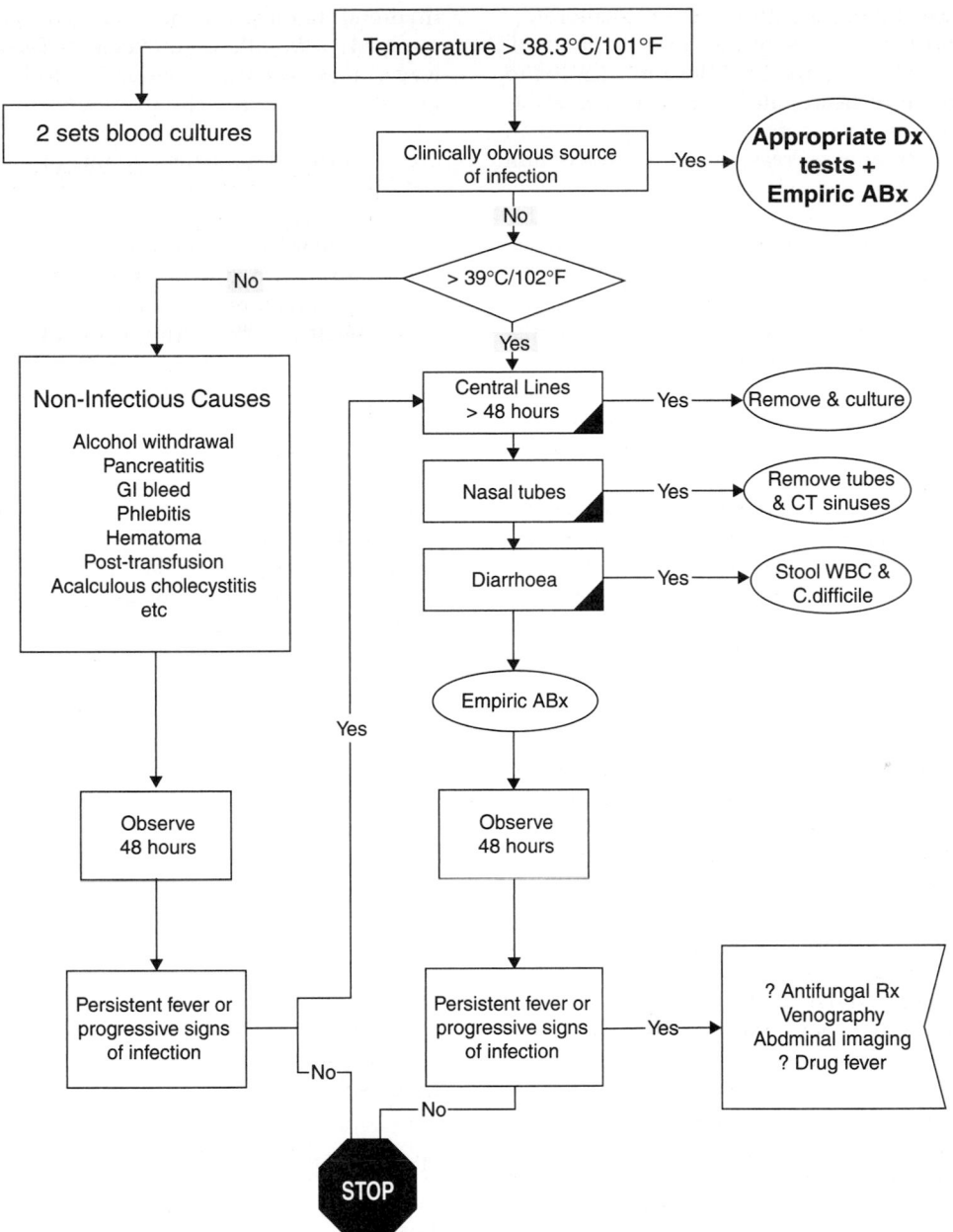

FIGURE 41-4 Diagnostic algorithm for evaluating fever in a patient on mechanical ventilation. (*Reproduced, with permission, from Marik.[91]*)

arrhythmia. These electrolyte abnormalities cause prolongation of the QT interval and predispose to polymorphic ventricular tachycardia, torsade de pointes. Patients with renal failure, especially those needing hemodialysis, are more likely to develop cardiac arrhythmias in the ICU, especially idioventricular rhythm, sustained ventricular tachycardia, ventricular fibrillation, and complete heart block.[273] Ventilated patients often experience hypoxia and disturbances of pH, conditions that contribute to arrhythmia. Patients with COPD in acute-on-chronic respiratory failure may experience significant alkalemia if the machine-delivered minute ventilation is set to normalize the Pa_{CO_2}.[274] Other conditions leading to critical illness have been tied to

increased risk for arrhythmia. Of patients admitted with antidepressant overdose (tricyclic and/or selective serotonin reuptake inhibitor), 15% experienced clinically significant arrhythmia.[275] Of patients with acute subarachnoid hemorrhage, 90% had cardiac arrhythmias on Holter monitoring, including some instances of life-threatening ventricular tachycardia and fibrillation.[276]

Medications administered to critically ill ventilated patients can cause arrhythmias. Systemically administered catecholamines (e.g., dopamine and norepinephrine) can cause sinus tachycardia, atrial or ventricular ectopy, or ventricular tachycardia. High-dose inhaled β agonists may precipitate or aggravate tachycardia.[277] Recurrent supraventricular tachycardia has been reported with nebulized albuterol.[278] Dhand et al found that increasing the dose of albuterol, from 4 to 8 to 16 puffs via a metered-dose inhaler, led to a significant increase in heart rate.[279] In a meta-analysis of 13 randomized trials, single-dose β agonists caused an increase in heart rate and decrease in serum potassium in patients with obstructive lung disease. When β agonists were used for 3 days to 1 year, the relative risk for sinus tachycardia increased; there was also a trend for increased relative risk for other complications (ventricular tachycardia, syncope, atrial fibrillation, and myocardial infarction.).[280] This increase in heart rate may be particularly undesirable in the setting of concomitant cardiac ischemia. Although definitive data are lacking, presumably high-dose inhaled bronchodilators would make preexisting tachyarrhythmias more difficult to control. Under these circumstances, the clinician may try substituting levalbuterol for racemic albuterol. That said, one study found no difference in heart rate when equipotent doses of racemic albuterol and levalbuterol were compared.[281] Alternatively, a meta-analysis has shown that ipratropium bromide alone is as effective as either albuterol alone or the combination of an anticholinergic and albuterol in patients with acute exacerbations of COPD.[282] Although use has diminished over the last decade, theophylline is still occasionally used. Theophylline toxicity is commonly associated with sinus tachycardia and atrial and ventricular ectopy; sustained ventricular or supraventricular (including multifocal atrial tachycardia) tachyarrhythmias are relatively uncommon.[283] Even serum levels in the upper therapeutic range may be associated with atrial or ventricular tachyarrhythmias.

Once tachyarrhythmias occur, therapy is usually indicated with the potential that some agents may have adverse effects in patients ventilated for respiratory failure. When the patient is hemodynamically unstable, emergency cardioversion is indicated though it may be less effective than in non–critically ill patients. In a prospective investigation of new-onset supraventricular tachyarrhythmias, direct-current cardioversion using a monophasic, damped sinus-wave defibrillator restored sinus rhythm in only 13 of 37 SICU patients.[284] Intravenous β-blockade is often first-line pharmacotherapy for acute supraventricular tachyarrhythmias. Concern has been raised that these agents, though selective for the β_1 receptor, still run the risk of exacerbating bronchospasm. In a meta-analysis, Salpeter et al found that cardioselective β-blockers caused no significant short-term adverse effect on forced expiratory volume (FEV$_1$) in patients with mild-to-moderate reactive airway disease.[285] Nevertheless, individual patients may experience a significant decline in FEV$_1$. When concern is high, the short-acting cardioselective agent esmolol may be used.[286]

Procedures performed in the ICU may precipitate arrhythmias. Placement of a pulmonary artery catheter may result in atrial or ventricular tachyarrhythmias or complete heart block.[287,288] Fortunately, such events are transient, occurring during catheter insertion, and are unusual once the catheter is in place. Iberti et al noted advanced arrhythmias in 7 of 56 patients undergoing placement of a pulmonary artery catheter; the longest arrhythmia was a run of seven consecutive premature ventricular contractions.[289] Antiar-

rhythmic therapy was not required and all arrhythmias resolved with catheter movement. Suctioning of the airway can increase vagal tone and contribute to bradycardia. In a study of 72 critically ill patients undergoing postural drainage and chest percussion, 8 developed major arrhythmias and 18 had minor arrhythmias.[290] Patients with major arrhythmias experienced a significant fall in blood pressure. An older study evaluated cardiac output during positive-pressure ventilation after the investigators observed sudden death in two patients during chest physiotherapy.[291] These investigators noted that cardiac output decreased by as much as 50% during chest physiotherapy. In contrast, Mackenzie and Shin could not document significant arrhythmias in 19 ventilated patients undergoing chest physiotherapy.[292]

The optimal medication to treat atrial fibrillation in critically ill patients is unclear. In a prospective randomized trial, Delle Karth et al treated 60 critically ill patients with atrial tachyarrhythmias (57 with atrial fibrillation) with diltiazem (25-mg bolus, then an infusion of 20 mg/h for 24 hours), a 300-mg bolus of amiodarone, or an amiodarone infusion (300-mg bolus then 45 mg/h for 24 hours).[293] There was no difference between groups in achieving the primary endpoint of a >30% reduction in heart rate within 4 hours. Although diltiazem resulted in better rate reduction among patients meeting the primary endpoint, it was more often stopped for significant hypotension. Of note, uncontrolled tachyarrhythmia was seen most often when amiodarone was given only as a bolus. In a study of 131 surgical ICU patients with moderate-to-severe multiple organ dysfunction and narrow-complex non-sinus tachyarrhythmias, high-dose continuous amiodarone infusion for 48 hours resulted in restoration of sinus rhythm in 75%.[294] Caution is necessary if amiodarone is used in patients receiving a high oxygen concentration because acute lung toxicity has been reported.[295] Ibutilide is another effective agent for rapid termination of atrial fibrillation or atrial flutter in critically ill patients.[296]

MYOCARDIAL ISCHEMIA

Patients with acute myocardial infarction who require endotracheal intubation and mechanical ventilation are at markedly increased risk for dying. Indeed, in one retrospective investigation, the mortality rate exceeded 50% and was highest for those with Pa_{O_2} / Fi_{O_2} <200 at admission.[297] Many patients admitted to the ICU for other reasons have risk factors for coronary artery disease and are at risk for acute myocardial ischemia. In addition, positive-pressure ventilation and elevated PEEP have been associated with reduced coronary blood flow.[298] Positive-pressure ventilation can also reduce left ventricular systolic function in the absence of overt ischemia.[299] Furthermore, therapies used to treat acute respiratory failure may induce myocardial ischemia or infarction.[300] Yet, detecting active myocardial disease in this population can be challenging. Previous studies noted that patients with status asthmaticus may have elevated CPK-MB suggestive of myocardial injury.[301] Lovis et al studied 15 patients admitted to the ICU with status asthmaticus. One-third had elevated CPK-MB, but all had normal serum troponin levels, suggesting a nonmyocardial origin for the CPK.[302] Troponin-I was found to be elevated in 58 of 235 patients with acute exacerbations of COPD, but only 7 were eventually diagnosed with acute coronary syndromes.[303] In another study, troponin-I was elevated in 18% of patients admitted to the ICU for severe exacerbations of COPD, and was independently associated with increased risk of death.[304] Importantly, troponin elevations may result from right ventricular injury that occurs when acute respiratory failure is associated with elevated pulmonary vascular resistance. Alternatively, troponin levels may be falsely elevated in the setting of renal insufficiency.

Patients undergoing weaning trials can develop ischemia because of an associated increase in systemic oxygen consumption. Jubran et al[305] found that patients failing T-piece trials failed to adequately increase oxygen transport, partly as a result of increased right and left ventricular afterload. Oxygen extraction increased and mixed venous oxygen saturation fell, resulting in rapid arterial desaturation and deceased tissue oxygen delivery.[305] This series of events can precipitate myocardial ischemia. Ischemia can be detected by either continuous electrocardiographic monitoring or nuclear cardiac scan.[306–310] In a study of 93 patients in a medical/cardiac ICU, 6 (5 with a history of coronary artery disease) developed electrocardiographic evidence of ischemia during weaning.[307] In a follow-up study, 10% of patients with coronary artery disease developed ECG evidence of ischemia.[310] Similarly, a study of surgical ICU patients found ECG evidence of silent myocardial ischemia in 19% of patients weaning after undergoing noncardiac surgery.[306] Of note, these patients infrequently complain of chest discomfort. Indeed, routine ICU monitoring of the electrocardiogram has a low sensitivity for detecting myocardial ischemia.[311] Importantly, such patients are more likely to fail weaning attempts. Presumably, myocardial ischemia can also occur in patients during "full" ventilator support when the degree of support is inadequate.

Treatment of myocardial ischemia during mechanical ventilation is similar to that at other times. The mainstays are aspirin, heparin, nitrates, and β-blockade to reduce myocardial oxygen consumption.

Venous Thromboembolism

INCIDENCE AND RISK FACTORS

Critically ill patients, especially those ventilated for respiratory failure, are at increased risk for venous thromboembolism (VTE).[312–314] The result can be substantial morbidity and mortality when pulmonary embolism results in this cohort of patients with limited pulmonary and hemodynamic reserve. Indeed, up to 60% of deep venous thrombosis (DVT) episodes in ICU patients are found above the knee, increasing the risk for pulmonary embolization.[315,316] Even when DVT alone is present, both mortality and ICU length of stay increase.[317] Making a diagnosis of VTE can be exceedingly challenging in this population. Using autopsy as the gold standard, pulmonary embolism may go undetected in >80% of patients.[318] Pulmonary embolism was found

at autopsy in 14.6% of hospitalized patients and was unsuspected in 70% of patients dying from pulmonary embolism.[319] In another study, 38% of ICU patients with known DVT had a ventilation-perfusion defect consistent with pulmonary embolism despite the absence of symptoms.[320]

The elevated risk for VTE in the ICU derives from the systemic inflammatory state often present (and activation of the coagulation cascade), frequently prolonged immobility (worsened by sedation and paralysis), underlying chronic health problems associated with hypercoagulability (e.g., malignancy), and central venous catheters (vascular injury and nidus of thrombosis).[313,321] Use of femoral venous catheterization is associated with a marked increase in the risk of VTE. In a study in which compression and duplex doppler ultrasound studies of femoral veins were systematically performed in 124 patients, 14 (11.3%) developed iliofemoral vein DVTs (frequently asymptomatic).[322] In a study of 80 patients with femoral catheters, bilateral phlebography performed at the time of catheter removal revealed lower extremity DVT in 24 (34%) patients; one-quarter of these were femoral DVTs, while the remainder were popliteal or posterior tibial vein thrombosis.[323] In a prospective trial of patients undergoing axillary vein catheterization, 8.3% developed partial and 3.3% complete axillary vein thrombosis (all occurred after 6 days of catheterization).[324] Although in the past upper extremity DVTs were thought to be benign, recent studies suggest a pulmonary embolization rate as high as 36%.[325–327]

The role of hereditary thrombophilia in the ICU, and the interaction with acquired factors, is as yet undefined. In a study of 51 critically ill patients, 53% developed a lupus anticoagulant, with sepsis and catecholamine use as major risk factors. Yet, this resolved spontaneously in 63% of patients and no thromboembolic events were observed.[328]

A number of predictors for VTE have been defined for medical-surgical ICU patients, including prior VTE, female gender, duration of pre-ICU hospital stay, mechanical ventilation, central venous catheters, and absence of prophylaxis.[313–316,321,329–333]

The reported incidence of VTE in critically ill ventilated patients depends on the ICU population under investigation, whether prophylaxis is consistently applied, and the diligence with which the clinician seeks the disease[112,313,315,317,329,334–338] (Fig. 41-5). An observational study, in which no imaging screening was performed, found an incidence of clinically relevant VTE of only 5.4%.[313] In a systematic review, 10–30% of medical and surgical ICU patients, 22–35% of neurosurgical patients, 60% of trauma patients, and 50–80% of acute spinal cord injury patients developed DVT during the initial weeks of ICU care.[312] In contrast, studies rigorously employing screening duplex ultrasound detect a much higher incidence of VTE. Hirsch et al found DVT detected by ultrasonography with color doppler imaging performed twice weekly in 33 of 100 patients in a medical ICU, 61 of whom were receiving prophylaxis (half of which were in a proximal lower extremity and 15% of which were in an upper extremity related to a central line).[315] Another study of screening ultrasound in trauma patients not receiving prophylaxis found that 58%

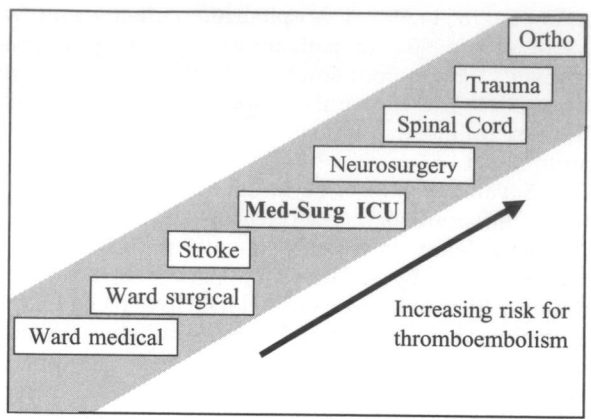

FIGURE 41-5 Risk for venous thromboembolism. (*Reproduced, with permission, from Cook et al: In: Esteban A, et al, editors: Evidence-based management of patients with respiratory failure. Berlin: Springer, 45–50, 2004.***)**

of patients had a DVT detected between days 14 and 21. Of note, one-third of these DVTs were proximal, that is, those with highest risk for pulmonary embolization.[338]

DIAGNOSIS

The clinical diagnosis of VTE is challenging in the ICU. Validated clinical models using symptoms and signs are predictive of VTE in outpatients and non–critically ill inpatients, but this approach is unlikely to be similarly robust in critically-ill ventilated patients.[339] Pulmonary embolism should be suspected when worsening hypoxemia, hemodynamic instability, unexplained tachypnea or tachycardia, or increasing pulmonary artery pressures are noted. Although uncommon, VTE may also present as fever.

Semiquantitative assays for D-dimer have proved useful in outpatient and general inpatient algorithms used to evaluate patients for possible VTE, principally because of a very high negative-predictive value.[339,340] Kollef et al used D-dimer in 239 medical ICU patients suspected of thromboembolic disease and found a sensitivity of 96%, specificity of 20%, negative-predictive value of 92%, and positive-predictive value of 27%.[341] The poor positive-predictive value is explained by the association of elevated D-dimer levels with proinflammatory cytokine levels, a common state in critically ill patients.[342] Interestingly, elevated D-dimer levels have been consistently associated with increased mortality in ICU patients, even in the absence of disseminated intravascular coagulation and VTE.[332,342,343]

Although lower extremity venography is considered the reference standard for detecting lower extremity DVT, it is rarely performed in critically ill patients.[344] This observation is expected, because expertise in performing the procedure has waned in an era when most patients undergo noninvasive lower extremity studies. In addition, the risk of transporting patients out of the ICU can be considerable.[345,346] In a recent survey of Canadian critical care units, bilateral compression doppler ultrasound was the most frequently used test.[344] Although this test is highly sensitive (97%) in symptomatic patients, its accuracy in critically ill patients has not

been investigated. Indeed, accuracy is likely to be reduced because a recent meta-analysis showed a sensitivity of only 62% in asymptomatic, non–critically ill patients.[347]

Diagnosing pulmonary embolism in ventilated patients is particularly challenging (Fig. 41-6). Echocardiography can disclose signs of pulmonary hypertension and right ventricular strain, suggesting a potentially hemodynamically significant pulmonary embolism. Ventilation-perfusion scanning has been widely used to assess patients with possible pulmonary embolism. Of the 46 mechanically ventilated patients in the PIOPED study (total n = 850), most had intermediate-probability scans.[348] In the PISA-PED study, a positive perfusion scan (one or more segmental perfusion defects) had a positive-predictive value of 95%; a negative scan had a negative-predictive value of 81%.[349] Spiral computed tomography has been extensively studied, though few ICU patients have been reported. Velmahos et al noted a sensitivity of 45% (60% for central emboli) in 22 critically ill surgical patients.[350] At present, pulmonary angiography remains the gold standard for ICU patients.[314]

PREVENTION

The risk for VTE is reduced by the use of prophylaxis, yet this modality may be underused in some critically ill patients.[321,351–354] Recently a survey of Canadian and French ICUs (n = 1222 patients, 64% ventilated) found that 92% of patients (without contraindications) received appropriate prophylaxis with either low-dose unfractionated heparin (UFH) or low-molecular-weight heparin (LMWH).[355] In a review, UFH reduced the risk of DVT by 50% in MICU-SICU patients and by 20% in trauma patients.[312] LMWH reduced the incidence by another 30% in the latter group. In neurosurgical patients, mechanical prophylaxis reduced the incidence of DVT when used alone (pooled odds ratio from 5 studies, 0.28) or when combined with LMWH (pooled odds ratio, 0.59). In a regional spinal cord injury center, LMWH and early mobilization initiated within 72 hours of trauma was associated with a reduction in incidence of DVT from 26% to 2%.[356]

The best method for prophylaxis in ventilated medical patients is undefined. Ibrahim et al used duplex ultrasonography of upper and lower extremities every 7 days in a cohort of ventilated medical ICU patients. DVT was detected in 23.6% despite all patients receiving prophylaxis with either subcutaneous UFH or pneumatic compression boots (but not both). Those with DVT were more likely to have malignancy, longer duration of central venous catheterization, and to develop pulmonary embolism.[330] Marik et al found that 5 of 26 patients (19%) with pneumatic compression boots developed DVT compared to 5 of 68 patients with subcutaneous UFH.[329] In a multicenter trial of patients with acute exacerbations of COPD, a low-molecular-weight heparin (nadroparin) was associated with a 45% risk reduction of VTE when compared to placebo.[331] In patients with acute medical illness, higher-dose enoxaparin was more effective in preventing DVT than either low-dose LMWH or placebo.[357] Based on these studies it appears that both forms of heparin are effective agents for preventing VTE, but good head-to-head comparison studies are needed. For

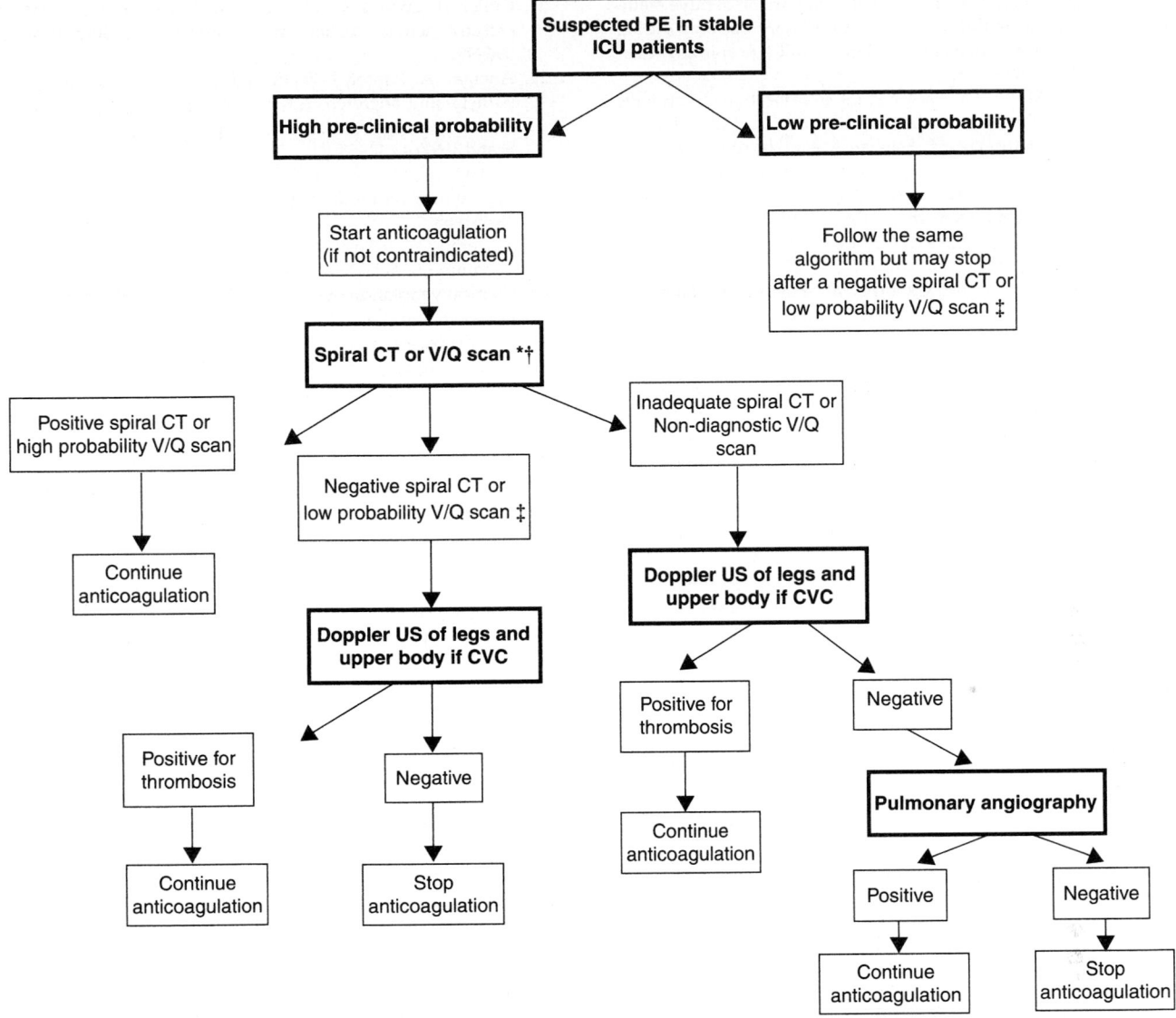

FIGURE 41-6 Diagnostic algorithm for suspected pulmonary embolism in a hemodynamically stable patient. (*Reproduced, with permission, from Rocha et al.[314]*)

VTE associated with central catheters, the best approach is to use heparin-bonded catheters and minimize the duration of catheterization.

Conclusions

Patients undergoing mechanical ventilation are at increased risk for numerous complications affecting many different organ systems. Many of these complications can be prevented by utilizing evidence-based recommendations, including the administration of stress ulcer prophylaxis, thromboembolism prophylaxis, and avoiding the use of excessive tidal volumes. Although strong evidence is lacking, additional measures such as maintaining adequate intravascular volume to maintain renal perfusion are likely to be effective. Because these measures reduce the incidence of complications but do not eliminate them, early detection and monitoring is crucial. This is especially true given that most complications discussed in this chapter are associated with increased mortality.

References

1. Ely EW, Baker AM, Dunagan DP, et al. Effect on the duration of mechanical ventilation of identifying patients capable of breathing spontaneously. N Engl J Med 1996; 335:1864–69.
2. Esteban A, Frutos F, Tobin MJ, et al. A comparison of four methods of weaning patients from mechanical ventilation. Spanish Lung Failure Collaborative Group. N Engl J Med 1995; 332: 345–50.
3. Kollef MH, Shapiro SD, Silver P, et al. A randomized, controlled trial of protocol-directed versus physician-directed weaning from mechanical ventilation. Crit Care Med 1997; 25:567–74.

4. Brochard L, Rauss A, Benito S, et al. Comparison of three methods of gradual withdrawal from ventilatory support during weaning from mechanical ventilation. Am J Respir Crit Care Med 1994; 150:896–903.

5. Mutlu GM, Mutlu EA, Factor P. GI complications in patients receiving mechanical ventilation. Chest 2001; 119:1222–41.

6. Anzueto A, Frutos-Vivar F, Esteban A, et al. Incidence, risk factors and outcome of barotrauma in mechanically ventilated patients. Intensive Care Med 2004; 30:612–19.

7. Benjamin PK, Thompson JE, O'Rourke PP. Complications of mechanical ventilation in a children's hospital multidisciplinary intensive care unit. Respir Care 1990; 35:873–78.

8. Mularski RA, Sippel JM, Osborne ML. Pneumoperitoneum: a review of nonsurgical causes. Crit Care Med 2000; 28:2638–44.

9. Chan YC, Camprodon RA, Kane PA, et al. Abdominal complications from crack cocaine. Ann R Coll Surg Engl 2004; 86:47–50.

10. Nath GD, Goodgame R, Saeed ZA, et al. Pneumoperitoneum: a preventable complication of PEG in mechanically ventilated patients. Gastrointest Endosc 1991; 37:84–85.

11. Balthazar EJ, Moore SL. CT evaluation of infradiaphragmatic air in patients treated with mechanically assisted ventilation: a potential source of error. AJR Am J Roentgenol 1996; 167:731–34.

12. Hillman KM. Pneumoperitoneum—a review. Crit Care Med 1982; 10:476–81.

13. Beilin B, Shulman DL, Weiss AT, et al. Pneumoperitoneum as the presenting sign of pulmonary barotrauma during artificial ventilation. Intensive Care Med 1986; 12:49–51.

14. Keidar S, Freud M, Rothfeld H, et al. Pneumoperitoneum after mechanical ventilation without pneumothorax or pneumomediastinum. Int Surg 1982; 67:275–76.

15. Cameron PA, Rosengarten PL, Johnson WR, et al. Tension pneumoperitoneum after cardiopulmonary resuscitation. Med J Aust 1991; 155:44–47.

16. Rowe NM, Kahn FB, Acinapura AJ, et al. Nonsurgical pneumoperitoneum: a case report and a review. Am Surg 1998; 64:313–22.

17. Murdoch IA, Huggon IC. Rapid diagnosis of the cause of pneumoperitoneum in ventilated asthmatic children. Acta Paediatr 1993; 82:108–10.

18. Vanhaesebrouck P, Leroy JG, De Praeter C, et al. Simple test to distinguish between surgical and non-surgical pneumoperitoneum in ventilated neonates. Arch Dis Child 1989; 64:48–49.

19. Chan SY, Kirsch CM, Jensen WA, et al. Tension pneumoperitoneum. West J Med 1996; 165:61–64.

20. Canivet JL, Yans T, Piret S, et al. Barotrauma-induced tension pneumoperitoneum. Acta Anaesthesiol Belg 2003; 54:233–36.

21. Lellouche N, Bruneel F, Mignon F, et al. Pneumomediastinum causing pneumoperitoneum during mechanical ventilation. J Crit Care 2003; 18:68–69.

22. Bothma PA, Lipman J, Moyes DG, et al. Tension pneumoperitoneum aggravating respiratory failure. A case report. S Afr J Surg 1994; 32:31–32.

23. Stein AL, Lane E. A new treatment modality for pneumoperitoneum associated with mechanical ventilation. Chest 1982; 81:519–20.

24. Sellden H, Sjovall H, Ricksten SE. Sympathetic nerve activity and central haemodynamics during mechanical ventilation with positive end-expiratory pressure in rats. Acta Physiol Scand 1986; 127:51–60.

25. Tanaka S, Sagawa S, Miki K, et al. Changes in muscle sympathetic nerve activity and renal function during positive-pressure breathing in humans. Am J Physiol 1994; 266:R1220–28.

26. Chernow B, Soldano S, Cook D, et al. Positive end-expiratory pressure increases plasma catecholamine levels in non-volume loaded dogs. Anaesth Intensive Care 1986; 14:421–25.

27. Cullen JJ, Ephgrave KS, Caropreso DK. Gastrointestinal myoelectric activity during endotoxemia. Am J Surg 1996; 171:596–99.

28. Aneman A, Ponten J, Fandriks L, et al. Hemodynamic, sympathetic and angiotensin II responses to PEEP ventilation before and during administration of isoflurane. Acta Anaesthesiol Scand 1997; 41:41–48.

29. Debaveye YA, Van den Berghe GH. Is there still a place for dopamine in the modern intensive care unit? Anesth Analg 2004; 98:461–68.

30. Scheeren TW, Schwarte LA, Loer SA, et al. Dopexamine but not dopamine increases gastric mucosal oxygenation during mechanical ventilation in dogs. Crit Care Med 2002; 30:881–87.

31. Love R, Choe E, Lippton H, et al. Positive end-expiratory pressure decreases mesenteric blood flow despite normalization of cardiac output. J Trauma 1995; 39:195–99.

32. Berendes E, Lippert G, Loick HM, et al. Effects of positive end-expiratory pressure ventilation on splanchnic oxygenation in humans. J Cardiothorac Vasc Anesth 1996; 10:598–602.

33. De Backer D. The effects of positive end-expiratory pressure on the splanchnic circulation. Intensive Care Med 2000; 26:361–63.

34. Nunes S, Rothen HU, Brander L, et al. Changes in splanchnic circulation during an alveolar recruitment maneuver in healthy porcine lungs. Anesth Analg 2004; 98:1432–38, table of contents.

35. Matejovic M, Rokyta R Jr, Radermacher P, et al. Effect of prone position on hepato-splanchnic hemodynamics in acute lung injury. Intensive Care Med 2002; 28:1750–55.

36. Kiefer P, Nunes S, Kosonen P, et al. Effect of positive end-expiratory pressure on splanchnic perfusion in acute lung injury. Intensive Care Med 2000; 26:376–83.

37. Mas A, Saura P, Joseph D, et al. Effect of acute moderate changes in PaCO2 on global hemodynamics and gastric perfusion. Crit Care Med 2000; 28:360–65.

38. Lisbon A. Dopexamine, dobutamine, and dopamine increase splanchnic blood flow: what is the evidence? Chest 2003; 123:460S–63S.

39. Spain DA, Kawabe T, Keelan PC, et al. Decreased alpha-adrenergic response in the intestinal microcirculation after "two-hit" hemorrhage/resuscitation and bacteremia. J Surg Res 1999; 84:180–85.

40. Dive A, Foret F, Jamart J, et al. Effect of dopamine on gastrointestinal motility during critical illness. Intensive Care Med 2000; 26:901–7.

41. Bosscha K, Nieuwenhuijs VB, Vos A, et al. Gastrointestinal motility and gastric tube feeding in mechanically ventilated patients. Crit Care Med 1998; 26:1510–17.

42. Cullen JJ, Caropreso DK, Hemann LL, et al. Pathophysiology of adynamic ileus. Dig Dis Sci 1997; 42:731–37.

43. Cullen JJ, Caropreso DK, Ephgrave KS, et al. The effect of endotoxin on canine jejunal motility and transit. J Surg Res 1997; 67:54–57.

44. Lodato RF, Khan AR, Zembowicz MJ, et al. Roles of IL-1 and TNF in the decreased ileal muscle contractility induced by lipopolysaccharide. Am J Physiol 1999; 276:G1356–62.

45. Ranieri VM, Suter PM, Tortorella C, et al. Effect of mechanical ventilation on inflammatory mediators in patients with acute respiratory distress syndrome: a randomized controlled trial. JAMA 1999; 282:54–61.

46. Kolbel CB, Rippel K, Klar H, et al. Esophageal motility disorders in critically ill patients: a 24-hour manometric study. Intensive Care Med 2000; 26:1421–27.

47. Bauer AJ, Schwarz NT, Moore BA, et al. Ileus in critical illness: mechanisms and management. Curr Opin Crit Care 2002; 8:152–57.

48. Eskandari MK, Kalff JC, Billiar TR, et al. Lipopolysaccharide activates the muscularis macrophage network and suppresses circular smooth muscle activity. Am J Physiol 1997;273:G727–34.

49. Eskandari MK, Kalff JC, Billiar TR, et al. LPS-induced muscularis macrophage nitric oxide suppresses rat jejunal circular muscle activity. Am J Physiol 1999; 277:G478–86.

50. Granger DN. Role of xanthine oxidase and granulocytes in ischemia-reperfusion injury. Am J Physiol 1988; 255:H1269–75.

51. Dive A, Moulart M, Jonard P, et al. Gastroduodenal motility in mechanically ventilated critically ill patients: a manometric study. Crit Care Med 1994; 22:441–47.

52. Meissner W, Dohrn B, Reinhart K. Enteral naloxone reduces gastric tube reflux and frequency of pneumonia in critical care patients during opioid analgesia. Crit Care Med 2003; 31:776–80.

53. MacLaren R, Patrick WD, Hall RI, et al. Comparison of cisapride and metoclopramide for facilitating gastric emptying and improving tolerance to intragastric enteral nutrition in critically ill, mechanically ventilated adults. Clin Ther 2001; 23:1855–66.

54. Dive A, Miesse C, Galanti L, et al. Effect of erythromycin on gastric motility in mechanically ventilated critically ill patients: a double-blind, randomized, placebo-controlled study. Crit Care Med 1995; 23:1356–62.

55. Ponec RJ, Saunders MD, Kimmey MB. Neostigmine for the treatment of acute colonic pseudo-obstruction. N Engl J Med 1999; 341:137–41.

56. Mostafa SM, Bhandari S, Ritchie G, et al. Constipation and its implications in the critically ill patient. Br J Anaesth 2003;91:815–19.

57. Montejo JC. Enteral nutrition-related gastrointestinal complications in critically ill patients: a multicenter study. The Nutritional and Metabolic Working Group of the Spanish Society of Intensive Care Medicine and Coronary Units. Crit Care Med 1999; 27:1447–53.

58. Schuster DP, Rowley H, Feinstein S, et al. Prospective evaluation of the risk of upper gastrointestinal bleeding after admission to a medical intensive care unit. Am J Med 1984; 76:623–30.

59. Cook DJ, Griffith LE, Walter SD, et al. The attributable mortality and length of intensive care unit stay of clinically important gastrointestinal bleeding in critically ill patients. Crit Care 2001; 5:368–75.

60. Zandstra DF, Stoutenbeek CP. The virtual absence of stress-ulceration related bleeding in ICU patients receiving prolonged mechanical ventilation without any prophylaxis. A prospective cohort study. Intensive Care Med 1994; 20:335–40.

61. Cook DJ, Fuller HD, Guyatt GH, et al. Risk factors for gastrointestinal bleeding in critically ill patients. Canadian Critical Care Trials Group. N Engl J Med 1994; 330:377–81.

62. Cook D, Heyland D, Griffith L, et al. Risk factors for clinically important upper gastrointestinal bleeding in patients requiring mechanical ventilation. Canadian Critical Care Trials Group. Crit Care Med 1999; 27:2812–17.

63. Raff T, Germann G, Hartmann B. The value of early enteral nutrition in the prophylaxis of stress ulceration in the severely burned patient. Burns 1997; 23:313–18.

64. McBride DQ, Rodts GE. Intensive care of patients with spinal trauma. Neurosurg Clin North Am 1994; 5:755–66.

65. Cook DJ. Stress ulcer prophylaxis: gastrointestinal bleeding and nosocomial pneumonia. Best evidence synthesis. Scand J Gastroenterol Suppl 1995; 210:48–52.

66. Hatton J, Lu WY, Rhoney DH, et al. A step-wise protocol for stress ulcer prophylaxis in the neurosurgical intensive care unit. Surg Neurol 1996; 46:493–99.

67. Martin LF, Booth FV, Reines HD, et al. Stress ulcers and organ failure in intubated patients in surgical intensive care units. Ann Surg 1992; 215:332–37.

68. Shuman RB, Schuster DP, Zuckerman GR. Prophylactic therapy for stress ulcer bleeding: a reappraisal. Ann Intern Med 1987; 106:562–67.

69. van der Voort PH, van der Hulst RW, Zandstra DF, et al. Prevalence of *Helicobacter pylori* infection in stress-induced gastric mucosal injury. Intensive Care Med 2001; 27:68–73.

70. Schilling D, Haisch G, Sloot N, et al. Low seroprevalence of *Helicobacter pylori* infection in patients with stress ulcer bleeding—a prospective evaluation of patients on a cardiosurgical intensive care unit. Intensive Care Med 2000; 26:1832–36.

71. van der Voort PH, van der Hulst RW, Zandstra DF, et al. Suppression of *Helicobacter pylori* infection during intensive care stay: related to stress ulcer bleeding incidence? J Crit Care 2001; 16:182–87.

72. Bresalier RS. The clinical significance and pathophysiology of stress-related gastric mucosal hemorrhage. J Clin Gastroenterol 1991; 13(Suppl 2):S35–43.

73. Ballesteros MA, Hogan DL, Koss MA, et al. Bolus or intravenous infusion of ranitidine: effects on gastric pH and acid secretion. A comparison of relative efficacy and cost. Ann Intern Med 1990; 112:334–39.

74. Baghaie AA, Mojtahedzadeh M, Levine RL, et al. Comparison of the effect of intermittent administration and continuous infusion of famotidine on gastric pH in critically ill patients: results of a prospective, randomized, crossover study. Crit Care Med 1995; 23:687–91.

75. Driks MR, Craven DE, Celli BR, et al. Nosocomial pneumonia in intubated patients given sucralfate as compared with antacids or histamine type 2 blockers. The role of gastric colonization. N Engl J Med 1987; 317:1376–82.

76. Cook DJ, Reeve BK, Guyatt GH, et al. Stress ulcer prophylaxis in critically ill patients. Resolving discordant meta-analyses. JAMA 1996; 275:308–14.

77. Messori A, Trippoli S, Vaiani M, et al. Bleeding and pneumonia in intensive care patients given ranitidine and sucralfate for prevention of stress ulcer: meta-analysis of randomised controlled trials. BMJ 2000; 321:1103–6.

78. Prod'hom G, Leuenberger P, Koerfer J, et al. Nosocomial pneumonia in mechanically ventilated patients receiving antacid, ranitidine, or sucralfate as prophylaxis for stress ulcer. A randomized controlled trial. Ann Intern Med 1994; 120:653–62.

79. Daley RJ, Rebuck JA, Welage LS, et al. Prevention of stress ulceration: current trends in critical care. Crit Care Med 2004; 32:2008–13.

80. Tryba M. Sucralfate versus antacids or H2-antagonists for stress ulcer prophylaxis: a meta-analysis on efficacy and pneumonia rate. Crit Care Med 1991; 19:942–49.

81. Lacroix J, Infante-Rivard C, Jenicek M, et al. Prophylaxis of upper gastrointestinal bleeding in intensive care units: a meta-analysis. Crit Care Med 1989; 17:862–69.

82. Cook DJ, Witt LG, Cook RJ, et al. Stress ulcer prophylaxis in the critically ill: a meta-analysis. Am J Med 1991; 91:519–27.

82a. Cook D, Guyatt G, Marshall J, et al. A comparison of sucralfate and ranitidine for the prevention of upper gastrointestinal bleeding in patients requiring mechanical ventilation. Canadian Critical Care Trials Groups. N Engl J Med 1998 Mar 19;338:791–7.

83. Levy MJ, Seelig CB, Robinson NJ, et al. Comparison of omeprazole and ranitidine for stress ulcer prophylaxis. Dig Dis Sci 1997; 42:1255–59.

84. Kantorova I, Svoboda P, Scheer P, et al. Stress ulcer prophylaxis in critically ill patients: a randomized controlled trial. Hepatogastroenterology 2004; 51:757–61.

85. Gajic O, Urrutia LE, Sewani H, et al. Acute abdomen in the medical intensive care unit. Crit Care Med 2002; 30:1187–90.

86. Ringel AF, Jameson GL, Foster ES. Diarrhea in the intensive care patient. Crit Care Clin 1995; 11:465–77.

87. Plaisier PW, van Buuren HR, Bruining HA. An analysis of upper GI endoscopy done for patients in surgical intensive care: high incidence of, and morbidity from reflux oesophagitis. Eur J Surg 1997; 163:903–7.

88. Wilmer A, Tack J, Frans E, et al. Duodenogastroesophageal reflux and esophageal mucosal injury in mechanically ventilated patients. Gastroenterology 1999; 116:1293–99.

89. Orozco-Levi M, Torres A, Ferrer M, et al. Semirecumbent position protects from pulmonary aspiration but not completely from gastroesophageal reflux in mechanically ventilated patients. Am J Respir Crit Care Med 1995; 152:1387–90.

90. Ibanez J, Penafiel A, Raurich JM, et al. Gastroesophageal reflux in intubated patients receiving enteral nutrition: effect of supine and semirecumbent positions. JPEN J Parenter Enteral Nutr 1992; 16:419–22.

91. Marik PE. Fever in the ICU. Chest 2000; 117:855–69.

92. Manjuck J, Zein J, Carpati C, et al. Clinical significance of increased lipase levels on admission to the ICU. Chest 2005; 127:246–50.

93. Marik PE. Propofol: therapeutic indications and side-effects. Curr Pharm Des 2004; 10:3639–49.

94. Baudouin SV, Evans TW. Nutritional support in critical care. Clin Chest Med 2003; 24:633–44.

95. Corish CA, Kennedy NP. Protein-energy undernutrition in hospital in-patients. Br J Nutr 2000; 83:575–91.

96. Doekel RC Jr, Zwillich CW, Scoggin CH, et al. Clinical semi-starvation: depression of hypoxic ventilatory response. N Engl J Med 1976; 295:358–61.

97. Driver AG, McAlevy MT, Smith JL. Nutritional assessment of patients with chronic obstructive pulmonary disease and acute respiratory failure. Chest 1982; 82:568–71.

98. Rochester DF, Esau SA. Malnutrition and the respiratory system. Chest 1984; 85:411–15.

99. Kelsen SG, Ference M, Kapoor S. Effects of prolonged undernutrition on structure and function of the diaphragm. J Appl Physiol 1985; 58:1354–59.

100. Thurlbeck WM. Diaphragm and body weight in emphysema. Thorax 1978; 33:483–87.

101. Long CL, Birkhahn RH, Geiger JW, et al. Contribution of skeletal muscle protein in elevated rates of whole body protein catabolism in trauma patients. Am J Clin Nutr 1981; 34:1087–93.

102. Arora NS, Rochester DF. Respiratory muscle strength and maximal voluntary ventilation in undernourished patients. Am Rev Respir Dis 1982; 126:5–8.

103. Wernerman J, Hammarqvist F, Gamrin L, et al. Protein metabolism in critical illness. Baillieres Clin Endocrinol Metab 1996; 10:603–15.

104. Bassili HR, Deitel M. Effect of nutritional support on weaning patients off mechanical ventilators. JPEN J Parenter Enteral Nutr 1981; 5:161–63.

105. Larca L, Greenbaum DM. Effectiveness of intensive nutritional regimes in patients who fail to wean from mechanical ventilation. Crit Care Med 1982; 10:297–300.

106. McMurray DN, Loomis SA, Casazza LJ, et al. Development of impaired cell-mediated immunity in mild and moderate malnutrition. Am J Clin Nutr 1981; 34:68–77.

107. Wilson DO, Rogers RM, Sanders MH, et al. Nutritional intervention in malnourished patients with emphysema. Am Rev Respir Dis 1986; 134:672–77.

108. Ziegler TR, Gatzen C, Wilmore DW. Strategies for attenuating protein-catabolic responses in the critically ill. Annu Rev Med 1994; 45:459–80.

109. Koretz RL. Nutritional supplementation in the ICU. How critical is nutrition for the critically ill? Am J Respir Crit Care Med 1995; 151:570–73.

110. Heyland DK, Konopad E, Noseworthy TW, et al. Is it 'worth-while' to continue treating patients with a prolonged stay (>14 days) in the ICU? An economic evaluation. Chest 1998; 114:192–98.

111. Heyland DK. Nutritional support in the critically ill patients. A critical review of the evidence. Crit Care Clin 1998; 14: 423–40.

112. Ibrahim EH, Mehringer L, Prentice D, et al. Early versus late enteral feeding of mechanically ventilated patients: results of a clinical trial. JPEN J Parenter Enteral Nutr 2002; 26:174–81.

113. Heyland DK. Enteral and parenteral nutrition in the seriously ill, hospitalized patient: a critical review of the evidence. J Nutr Health Aging 2000; 4:31–41.

114. Heyland DK, MacDonald S, Keefe L, et al. Total parenteral nutrition in the critically ill patient: a meta-analysis. JAMA 1998; 280:2013–19.

115. Gramlich L, Kichian K, Pinilla J, et al. Does enteral nutrition compared to parenteral nutrition result in better outcomes in critically ill adult patients? A systematic review of the literature. Nutrition 2004; 20:843–48.

116. Abou-Assi S, O'Keefe SJ. Nutrition support during acute pancreatitis. Nutrition 2002; 18:938–43.

117. Avgerinos C, Delis S, Rizos S, et al. Nutritional support in acute pancreatitis. Dig Dis 2003; 21:214–19.

118. Reignier J, Thenoz-Jost N, Fiancette M, et al. Early enteral nutrition in mechanically ventilated patients in the prone position. Crit Care Med 2004; 32:94–99.

119. McClave SA, Sexton LK, Spain DA, et al. Enteral tube feeding in the intensive care unit: factors impeding adequate delivery. Crit Care Med 1999; 27:1252–56.

120. Elpern EH, Stutz L, Peterson S, et al. Outcomes associated with enteral tube feedings in a medical intensive care unit. Am J Crit Care 2004; 13:221–27.

121. McClave SA, Lukan JK, Stefater JA, et al. Poor validity of residual volumes as a marker for risk of aspiration in critically ill patients. Crit Care Med 2005; 33:324–30.

122. Rubinson L, Diette GB, Song X, et al. Low caloric intake is associated with nosocomial bloodstream infections in patients in the medical intensive care unit. Crit Care Med 2004; 32: 350–57.

123. Davies AR, Froomes PR, French CJ, et al. Randomized comparison of nasojejunal and nasogastric feeding in critically ill patients. Crit Care Med 2002; 30:586–90.

124. Montejo JC, Grau T, Acosta J, et al. Multicenter, prospective, randomized, single-blind study comparing the efficacy and gastrointestinal complications of early jejunal feeding with early gastric feeding in critically ill patients. Crit Care Med 2002; 30:796–800.

125. Neumann DA, DeLegge MH. Gastric versus small-bowel tube feeding in the intensive care unit: a prospective comparison of efficacy. Crit Care Med 2002; 30:1436–38.

126. Montecalvo MA, Steger KA, Farber HW, et al. Nutritional outcome and pneumonia in critical care patients randomized to gastric versus jejunal tube feedings. The Critical Care Research Team. Crit Care Med 1992; 20:1377–87.

127. Heyland DK, Drover JW, Dhaliwal R, et al. Optimizing the benefits and minimizing the risks of enteral nutrition in the critically ill: role of small bowel feeding. JPEN J Parenter Enteral Nutr 2002; 26:S51–55; discussion S56–57.

128. Marik PE, Zaloga GP. Gastric versus post-pyloric feeding: a systematic review. Crit Care 2003; 7:R46–51.

129. Booth CM, Heyland DK, Paterson WG. Gastrointestinal promotility drugs in the critical care setting: a systematic review of the evidence. Crit Care Med 2002; 30:1429–35.

130. Boivin MA, Levy H. Gastric feeding with erythromycin is equivalent to transpyloric feeding in the critically ill. Crit Care Med 2001; 29:1916–19.
131. Drakulovic MB, Torres A, Bauer TT, et al. Supine body position as a risk factor for nosocomial pneumonia in mechanically ventilated patients: a randomised trial. Lancet 1999; 354:1851–58.
132. Yavagal DR, Karnad DR, Oak JL. Metoclopramide for preventing pneumonia in critically ill patients receiving enteral tube feeding: a randomized controlled trial. Crit Care Med 2000; 28:1408–11.
133. Hendry PJ, Akyurekli Y, McIntyre R, et al. Bronchopleural complications of nasogastric feeding tubes. Crit Care Med 1986; 14:892–94.
134. Talpers SS, Romberger DJ, Bunce SB, et al. Nutritionally associated increased carbon dioxide production. Excess total calories vs. high proportion of carbohydrate calories. Chest 1992; 102:551–55.
135. Dark DS, Pingleton SK, Kerby GR. Hypercapnia during weaning. A complication of nutritional support. Chest 1985; 88: 141–43.
136. Covelli HD, Black JW, Olsen MS, et al. Respiratory failure precipitated by high carbohydrate loads. Ann Intern Med 1981; 95:579–81.
137. Pannu N, Mehta RL. Effect of mechanical ventilation on the kidney. Best Pract Res Clin Anaesthesiol 2004; 18:189–203.
138. Block CA, Manning HL. Prevention of acute renal failure in the critically ill. Am J Respir Crit Care Med 2002; 165:320–24.
139. Groeneveld AB, Tran DD, van der Meulen J, et al. Acute renal failure in the medical intensive care unit: predisposing, complicating factors and outcome. Nephron 1991; 59:602–10.
140. Neveu H, Kleinknecht D, Brivet F, et al. Prognostic factors in acute renal failure due to sepsis. Results of a prospective multicentre study. The French Study Group on Acute Renal Failure. Nephrol Dial Transplant 1996; 11:293–99.
141. Murray P, Hall J. Renal replacement therapy for acute renal failure. Am J Respir Crit Care Med 2000; 162:777–81.
142. Levy EM, Viscoli CM, Horwitz RI. The effect of acute renal failure on mortality. A cohort analysis. JAMA 1996; 275:1489–94.
143. Briglia A, Paganini EP. Acute renal failure in the intensive care unit. Therapy overview, patient risk stratification, complications of renal replacement, and special circumstances. Clin Chest Med 1999; 20:347–66, viii.
144. Chertow GM, Lazarus JM, Paganini EP, et al. Predictors of mortality and the provision of dialysis in patients with acute tubular necrosis. The Auriculin Anaritide Acute Renal Failure Study Group. J Am Soc Nephrol 1998; 9:692–98.
145. Vivino G, Antonelli M, Moro ML, et al. Risk factors for acute renal failure in trauma patients. Intensive Care Med 1998; 24:808–14.
146. Metnitz PG, Krenn CG, Steltzer H, et al. Effect of acute renal failure requiring renal replacement therapy on outcome in critically ill patients. Crit Care Med 2002; 30:2051–58.
147. Cantarovich F, Verho MT. A simple prognostic index for patients with acute renal failure requiring dialysis. French Multicentric Prospective Study on Furosemide in Acute Renal Failure Requiring Dialysis. Ren Fail 1996; 18:585–92.
148. Paganini EP, Halstenberg WK, Goormastic M. Risk modeling in acute renal failure requiring dialysis: the introduction of a new model. Clin Nephrol 1996; 46:206–11.
149. Yuasa S, Takahashi N, Shoji T, et al. A simple and early prognostic index for acute renal failure patients requiring renal replacement therapy. Artif Organs 1998; 22:273–78.
150. Tafreshi M, Schneider R, Rosen M. Outcome of patients who require long-term mechanical ventilation and hemodialysis (abstract). Chest 1995; 108(suppl):134S.
151. Chao DC, Scheinhorn DJ, Stearn-Hassenpflug M. Impact of renal dysfunction on weaning from prolonged mechanical ventilation. Crit Care (Lond) 1997; 1:101–4.
152. Ventilation with lower tidal volumes as compared with traditional tidal volumes for acute lung injury and the acute respiratory distress syndrome. The Acute Respiratory Distress Syndrome Network. N Engl J Med 2000; 342:1301–8.
153. Imai Y, Parodo J, Kajikawa O, et al. Injurious mechanical ventilation and end-organ epithelial cell apoptosis and organ dysfunction in an experimental model of acute respiratory distress syndrome. JAMA 2003; 289:2104–12.
154. Szatalowicz VL, Goldberg JP, Anderson RJ. Plasma antidiuretic hormone in acute respiratory failure. Am J Med 1982; 72:583–87.
155. Farber MO, Roberts LR, Weinberger MH, et al. Abnormalities of sodium and H_2O handling in chronic obstructive lung disease. Arch Intern Med 1982; 142:1326–30.
156. Anand IS, Chandrashekhar Y, Ferrari R, et al. Pathogenesis of congestive state in chronic obstructive pulmonary disease. Studies of body water and sodium, renal function, hemodynamics, and plasma hormones during edema and after recovery. Circulation 1992; 86:12–21.
157. Adnot S, Andrivet P, Chabrier PE, et al. Plasma levels of atrial natriuretic factor, renin activity, and aldosterone in patients with chronic obstructive pulmonary disease. Response to O2 removal and to hyperoxia. Am Rev Respir Dis 1990; 141:1178–84.
158. Kilburn KH, Dowell AR. Renal function in respiratory failure. Effects of hypoxia, hyperoxia, and hypercapnia. Arch Intern Med 1971; 127:754–62.
159. Hemmer M, Suter PM. Treatment of cardiac and renal effects of PEEP with dopamine in patients with acute respiratory failure. Anesthesiology 1979; 50:399–403.
160. Annat G, Viale JP, Bui Xuan B, et al. Effect of PEEP ventilation on renal function, plasma renin, aldosterone, neurophysins and urinary ADH, and prostaglandins. Anesthesiology 1983; 58: 136–41.
161. Ramamoorthy C, Rooney MW, Dries DJ, et al. Aggressive hydration during continuous positive-pressure ventilation restores atrial transmural pressure, plasma atrial natriuretic peptide concentrations, and renal function. Crit Care Med 1992; 20: 1014–19.
162. Christensen G, Bugge JF, Ostensen J, et al. Atrial natriuretic factor and renal sodium excretion during ventilation with PEEP in hypervolemic dogs. J Appl Physiol 1992; 72:993–97.
163. Rossaint R, Jorres D, Nienhaus M, et al. Positive end-expiratory pressure reduces renal excretion without hormonal activation after volume expansion in dogs. Anesthesiology 1992; 77:700–8.
164. Qvist J, Pontoppidan H, Wilson RS, et al. Hemodynamic responses to mechanical ventilation with PEEP: the effect of hypervolemia. Anesthesiology 1975; 42:45–55.
165. Carlone S, Palange P, Mannix ET, et al. Effect of positive and negative pressure breathing on sodium and water excretion. J Lab Clin Med 1990; 116:298–304.
166. Scheinhorn D. Increase in serum albumin and decrease in body weight correlate with weaning from prolonged mechanical ventilation (abstract). Am Rev Respir Dis 1992; 145:A522.
167. Goldberg PA, Inzucchi SE. Critical issues in endocrinology. Clin Chest Med 2003; 24:583–606, vi.
168. Suda AK, Pittman CS, Shimizu T, et al. The production and metabolism of 3,5,3'-triiodothyronine and 3,3',5-triiodothyronine in normal and fasting subjects. J Clin Endocrinol Metab 1978; 47:1311–19.
169. Spalter AR, Gwirtsman HE, Demitrack MA, et al. Thyroid function in bulimia nervosa. Biol Psychiatry 1993; 33:408–14.
170. Richmand DA, Molitch ME, O'Donnell TF. Altered thyroid hormone levels in bacterial sepsis: the role of nutritional adequacy. Metabolism 1980; 29:936–42.

171. Meinhold H, Gramm HJ, Meissner W, et al. Elevated serum diiodotyrosine (DIT) in severe infections and sepsis: DIT, a possible new marker of leukocyte activity. J Clin Endocrinol Metab 1991; 72:945–53.

172. LoPresti JS, Fried JC, Spencer CA, et al. Unique alterations of thyroid hormone indices in the acquired immunodeficiency syndrome (AIDS). Ann Intern Med 1989; 110:970–75.

173. Grunfeld C, Pang M, Doerrler W, et al. Indices of thyroid function and weight loss in human immunodeficiency virus infection and the acquired immunodeficiency syndrome. Metabolism 1993; 42:1270–76.

174. Adami HO, Rimsten A, Thoren L, et al. Thyroid disease and function in breast cancer patients and non-hospitalized controls evaluated by determination of TSH, T3, rT3 and T4 levels in serum. Acta Chir Scand 1978; 144:89–97.

175. Wehmann RE, Gregerman RI, Burns WH, et al. Suppression of thyrotropin in the low-thyroxine state of severe nonthyroidal illness. N Engl J Med 1985; 312:546–52.

176. Vardarli I, Schmidt R, Wdowinski JM, et al. [The hypothalamo-hypophyseal thyroid axis, plasma protein concentrations and the hypophyseo-gonadal axis in low T3 syndrome following acute myocardial infarct.] Klin Wochenschr 1987; 65:129–33.

177. Holland FW 2nd, Brown PS Jr, Weintraub BD, et al. Cardiopulmonary bypass and thyroid function: a "euthyroid sick syndrome". Ann Thorac Surg 1991; 52:46–50.

178. Faglia G, Ferrari C, Beck-Peccoz P, et al. Reduced plasma thyrotropin response to thyrotropin releasing hormone after dexamethasone administration in normal subjects. Horm Metab Res 1973; 5:289–92.

179. Martino E, Bartalena L, Bogazzi F, et al. The effects of amiodarone on the thyroid. Endocr Rev 2001; 22:240–54.

180. Van den Berghe G, de Zegher F, Lauwers P. Dopamine and the sick euthyroid syndrome in critical illness. Clin Endocrinol (Oxf) 1994; 41:731–37.

181. Wartofsky L, Burman KD. Alterations in thyroid function in patients with systemic illness: the "euthyroid sick syndrome". Endocr Rev 1982; 3:164–217.

182. Chopra IJ. Clinical review 86: Euthyroid sick syndrome: is it a misnomer? J Clin Endocrinol Metab 1997; 82:329–34.

183. Maldonado LS, Murata GH, Hershman JM, et al. Do thyroid function tests independently predict survival in the critically ill? Thyroid 1992; 2:119–23.

184. Slag MF, Morley JE, Elson MK, et al. Hypothyroxinemia in critically ill patients as a predictor of high mortality. JAMA 1981; 245:43–45.

185. Scoscia E, Baglioni S, Eslami A, et al. Low triiodothyronine (T3) state: a predictor of outcome in respiratory failure? Results of a clinical pilot study. Eur J Endocrinol 2004; 151:557–60.

186. Bennett-Guerrero E, Jimenez JL, White WD, et al. Cardiovascular effects of intravenous triiodothyronine in patients undergoing coronary artery bypass graft surgery. A randomized, double-blind, placebo-controlled trial. Duke T3 study group. JAMA 1996; 275:687–92.

187. Klemperer JD, Klein I, Gomez M, et al. Thyroid hormone treatment after coronary-artery bypass surgery. N Engl J Med 1995; 333:1522–27.

188. Mullis-Jansson SL, Argenziano M, Corwin S, et al. A randomized double-blind study of the effect of triiodothyronine on cardiac function and morbidity after coronary bypass surgery. J Thorac Cardiovasc Surg 1999; 117:1128–34.

189. Brent GA, Hershman JM. Thyroxine therapy in patients with severe nonthyroidal illnesses and low serum thyroxine concentration. J Clin Endocrinol Metab 1986; 63:1–8.

190. Behnia M, Clay AS, Farber MO. Management of myxedematous respiratory failure: review of ventilation and weaning principles. Am J Med Sci 2000; 320:368–73.

191. Datta D, Scalise P. Hypothyroidism and failure to wean in patients receiving prolonged mechanical ventilation at a regional weaning center. Chest 2004; 126:1307–12.

192. Pandya K, Lal C, Scheinhorn D, et al. Hypothyroidism and ventilator dependency. Arch Intern Med 1989; 149:2115–16.

193. Goswami R, Guleria R, Gupta AK, et al. Prevalence of diaphragmatic muscle weakness and dyspnoea in Graves' disease and their reversibility with carbimazole therapy. Eur J Endocrinol 2002; 147:299–303.

194. Annane D, Sebille V, Troche G, et al. A 3-level prognostic classification in septic shock based on cortisol levels and cortisol response to corticotropin. JAMA 2000; 283:1038–45.

195. Sibbald WJ, Short A, Cohen MP, et al. Variations in adrenocortical responsiveness during severe bacterial infections. Unrecognized adrenocortical insufficiency in severe bacterial infections. Ann Surg 1977; 186:29–33.

196. Shenker Y, Skatrud JB. Adrenal insufficiency in critically ill patients. Am J Respir Crit Care Med 2001; 163:1520–23.

197. Rao RH. Bilateral massive adrenal hemorrhage. Med Clin North Am 1995; 79:107–129.

198. Marik PE, Zaloga GP. Adrenal insufficiency in the critically ill: a new look at an old problem. Chest 2002; 122:1784–96.

199. Streeten DH, Anderson GH Jr, Dalakos TG, et al. Normal and abnormal function of the hypothalamic-pituitary-adrenocortical system in man. Endocr Rev 1984; 5:371–94.

200. Cooper MS, Stewart PM. Corticosteroid insufficiency in acutely ill patients. N Engl J Med 2003; 348:727–34.

201. Annane D, Sebille V, Charpentier C, et al. Effect of treatment with low doses of hydrocortisone and fludrocortisone on mortality in patients with septic shock. JAMA 2002; 288:862–71.

202. Leatherman JW, Fluegel WL, David WS, et al. Muscle weakness in mechanically ventilated patients with severe asthma. Am J Respir Crit Care Med 1996; 153:1686–90.

203. Amaya-Villar R, Garnacho-Montero J, Garcia-Garmendia JL, et al. Steroid-induced myopathy in patients intubated due to exacerbation of chronic obstructive pulmonary disease. Intensive Care Med 2005; 31:157–61.

204. Quinn MW, de Boer RC, Ansari N, et al. Stress response and mode of ventilation in preterm infants. Arch Dis Child Fetal Neonatal Ed 1998; 78:F195–98.

205. Calzia E, Koch M, Stahl W, et al. Stress response during weaning after cardiac surgery. Br J Anaesth 2001; 87:490–93.

206. Koksal GM, Sayilgan C, Sen O, et al. The effects of different weaning modes on the endocrine stress response. Crit Care 2004; 8:R31–34.

207. McCowen KC, Malhotra A, Bistrian BR. Stress-induced hyperglycemia. Crit Care Clin 2001; 17:107–24.

208. Mizock BA. Alterations in fuel metabolism in critical illness: hyperglycaemia. Best Pract Res Clin Endocrinol Metab 2001; 15:533–51.

209. Black CT, Hennessey PJ, Andrassy RJ. Short-term hyperglycemia depresses immunity through nonenzymatic glycosylation of circulating immunoglobulin. J Trauma 1990; 30:830–32; discussion 832–33.

210. Bagdade JD, Root RK, Bulger RJ. Impaired leukocyte function in patients with poorly controlled diabetes. Diabetes 1974; 23:9–15.

211. Mowat A, Baum J. Chemotaxis of polymorphonuclear leukocytes from patients with diabetes mellitus. N Engl J Med 1971; 284:621–27.

212. Nolan CM, Beaty HN, Bagdade JD. Further characterization of the impaired bactericidal function of granulocytes in patients with poorly controlled diabetes. Diabetes 1978; 27:889–94.

213. Malmberg K, Norhammar A, Wedel H, et al. Glycometabolic state at admission: important risk marker of mortality in conventionally treated patients with diabetes mellitus and acute myocardial infarction: long-term results from the Diabetes and Insulin-Glucose Infusion in Acute Myocardial Infarction (DIGAMI) study. Circulation 1999; 99:2626–32.

214. Gray CS, Taylor R, French JM, et al. The prognostic value of stress hyperglycaemia and previously unrecognized diabetes in acute stroke. Diabet Med 1987; 4:237–40.

215. Capes SE, Hunt D, Malmberg K, et al. Stress hyperglycaemia and increased risk of death after myocardial infarction in patients with and without diabetes: a systematic overview. Lancet 2000; 355:773–78.

216. van den Berghe G, Wouters P, Weekers F, et al. Intensive insulin therapy in the critically ill patients. N Engl J Med 2001; 345: 1359–67.

217. Krinsley JS. Effect of an intensive glucose management protocol on the mortality of critically ill adult patients. Mayo Clin Proc 2004; 79:992–1000.

218. Pittas AG, Siegel RD, Lau J. Insulin therapy for critically ill hospitalized patients: a meta-analysis of randomized controlled trials. Arch Intern Med 2004; 164:2005–11.

219. Van den Berghe G, Wouters PJ, Bouillon R, et al. Outcome benefit of intensive insulin therapy in the critically ill: Insulin dose versus glycemic control. Crit Care Med 2003; 31:359–66.

220. Finney SJ, Zekveld C, Elia A, et al. Glucose control and mortality in critically ill patients. JAMA 2003; 290:2041–47.

221. Napolitano LM. Scope of the problem: epidemiology of anemia and use of blood transfusions in critical care. Crit Care 2004; 8(Suppl 2):S1–8.

222. Vincent JL, Baron JF, Reinhart K, et al. Anemia and blood transfusion in critically ill patients. JAMA 2002; 288:1499–507.

223. Shapiro MJ, Gettinger A, Corwin HL, et al. Anemia and blood transfusion in trauma patients admitted to the intensive care unit. J Trauma 2003; 55:269–73; discussion 273–4.

224. Rao MP, Boralessa H, Morgan C, et al. Blood component use in critically ill patients. Anaesthesia 2002; 57:530–34.

225. Corwin HL, Gettinger A, Pearl RG, et al. The CRIT Study: Anemia and blood transfusion in the critically ill—current clinical practice in the United States. Crit Care Med 2004; 32:39–52.

226. Corwin HL, Parsonnet KC, Gettinger A. RBC transfusion in the ICU. Is there a reason? Chest 1995; 108:767–71.

227. Shikora SA, Benotti PN, Johannigman JA. The oxygen cost of breathing may predict weaning from mechanical ventilation better than the respiratory rate to tidal volume ratio. Arch Surg 1994; 129:269–74.

228. Hubmayr RD, Loosbrock LM, Gillespie DJ, et al. Oxygen uptake during weaning from mechanical ventilation. Chest 1988; 94:1148–55.

229. Schonhofer B, Wenzel M, Geibel M, et al. Blood transfusion and lung function in chronically anemic patients with severe chronic obstructive pulmonary disease. Crit Care Med 1998; 26:1824–28.

230. Schonhofer B, Bohrer H, Kohler D. Blood transfusion facilitating difficult weaning from the ventilator. Anaesthesia 1998; 53:181–84.

231. Hebert PC, Wells G, Blajchman MA, et al. A multicenter, randomized, controlled clinical trial of transfusion requirements in critical care. Transfusion Requirements in Critical Care Investigators, Canadian Critical Care Trials Group. N Engl J Med 1999; 340:409–17.

232. Hebert PC, Blajchman MA, Cook DJ, et al. Do blood transfusions improve outcomes related to mechanical ventilation? Chest 2001; 119:1850–57.

233. Corwin HL, Gettinger A, Pearl RG, et al. Efficacy of recombinant human erythropoietin in critically ill patients: a randomized controlled trial. JAMA 2002; 288:2827–35.

234. Stephan F, Hollande J, Richard O, et al. Thrombocytopenia in a surgical ICU. Chest 1999; 115:1363–70.

235. Drews RE, Weinberger SE. Thrombocytopenic disorders in critically ill patients. Am J Respir Crit Care Med 2000; 162:347–51.

236. Chakraverty R, Davidson S, Peggs K, et al. The incidence and cause of coagulopathies in an intensive care population. Br J Haematol 1996; 93:460–63.

237. Strauss R, Wehler M, Mehler K, et al. Thrombocytopenia in patients in the medical intensive care unit: bleeding prevalence, transfusion requirements, and outcome. Crit Care Med 2002; 30:1765–71.

238. Akca S, Haji-Michael P, de Mendonca A, et al. Time course of platelet counts in critically ill patients. Crit Care Med 2002; 30:753–56.

239. Vanderschueren S, De Weerdt A, Malbrain M, et al. Thrombocytopenia and prognosis in intensive care. Crit Care Med 2000; 28:1871–76.

240. Oppenheim-Eden A, Glantz L, Eidelman LA, et al. Spontaneous intracerebral hemorrhage in critically ill patients: incidence over six years and associated factors. Intensive Care Med 1999; 25: 63–67.

241. Verma AK, Levine M, Shalansky SJ, et al. Frequency of heparin-induced thrombocytopenia in critical care patients. Pharmacotherapy 2003; 23:745–53.

242. Girou E, Stephan F, Novara A, et al. Risk factors and outcome of nosocomial infections: results of a matched case-control study of ICU patients. Am J Respir Crit Care Med 1998; 157:1151–58.

243. Laupland KB, Kirkpatrick AW, Church DL, et al. Intensive-care-unit-acquired bloodstream infections in a regional critically ill population. J Hosp Infect 2004; 58:137–45.

244. Pittet D, Tarara D, Wenzel RP. Nosocomial bloodstream infection in critically ill patients. Excess length of stay, extra costs, and attributable mortality. JAMA 1994; 271:1598–601.

245. Vincent JL, Bihari DJ, Suter PM, et al. The prevalence of nosocomial infection in intensive care units in Europe. Results of the European Prevalence of Infection in Intensive Care (EPIC) Study. EPIC International Advisory Committee. JAMA 1995; 274:639–44.

246. Legras A, Malvy D, Quinioux AI, et al. Nosocomial infections: prospective survey of incidence in five French intensive care units. Intensive Care Med 1998; 24:1040–46.

247. Velasco E, Thuler LC, Martins CA, et al. Nosocomial infections in an oncology intensive care unit. Am J Infect Control 1997; 25:458–62.

248. Esen S, Leblebicioglu H. Prevalence of nosocomial infections at intensive care units in Turkey: a multicentre 1-day point prevalence study. Scand J Infect Dis 2004; 36:144–48.

249. Erbay H, Yalcin AN, Serin S, et al. Nosocomial infections in intensive care unit in a Turkish university hospital: a 2-year survey. Intensive Care Med 2003; 29:1482–88.

250. Girou E, Schortgen F, Delclaux C, et al. Association of noninvasive ventilation with nosocomial infections and survival in critically ill patients. JAMA 2000; 284:2361–67.

251. Hussain SN. Respiratory muscle dysfunction in sepsis. Mol Cell Biochem 1998; 179:125–34.

252. Amoateng-Adjepong Y, Jacob BK, Ahmad M, et al. The effect of sepsis on breathing pattern and weaning outcomes in patients recovering from respiratory failure. Chest 1997; 112:472–77.

253. Richards MJ, Edwards JR, Culver DH, et al. Nosocomial infections in combined medical-surgical intensive care units in the United States. Infect Control Hosp Epidemiol 2000; 21:510–15.

254. Richards MJ, Edwards JR, Culver DH, et al. Nosocomial infections in medical intensive care units in the United States.

National Nosocomial Infections Surveillance System. Crit Care Med 1999; 27:887–92.

255. Laupland KB, Zygun DA, Davies HD, et al. Population-based assessment of intensive care unit-acquired bloodstream infections in adults: Incidence, risk factors, and associated mortality rate. Crit Care Med 2002; 30:2462–67.

256. Lin CY, Zhang H, Cheng KC, et al. Mechanical ventilation may increase susceptibility to the development of bacteremia. Crit Care Med 2003; 31:1429–34.

257. Arbo MJ, Fine MJ, Hanusa BH, et al. Fever of nosocomial origin: etiology, risk factors, and outcomes. Am J Med 1993; 95:505–12.

258. Barie PS, Hydo LJ, Eachempati SR. Causes and consequences of fever complicating critical surgical illness. Surg Infect (Larchmt) 2004; 5:145–59.

259. Tu CY, Hsu WH, Hsia TC, et al. Pleural effusions in febrile medical ICU patients: chest ultrasound study. Chest 2004; 126:1274–80.

260. Povoa P, Coelho L, Almeida E, et al. C-reactive protein as a marker of infection in critically ill patients. Clin Microbiol Infect 2005; 11:101–8.

261. Reny JL, Vuagnat A, Ract C, et al. Diagnosis and follow-up of infections in intensive care patients: value of C-reactive protein compared with other clinical and biological variables. Crit Care Med 2002; 30:529–35.

262. Luzzani A, Polati E, Dorizzi R, et al. Comparison of procalcitonin and C-reactive protein as markers of sepsis. Crit Care Med 2003; 31:1737–41.

263. Suprin E, Camus C, Gacouin A, et al. Procalcitonin: a valuable indicator of infection in a medical ICU? Intensive Care Med 2000; 26:1232–38.

264. Artucio H, Pereira M. Cardiac arrhythmias in critically ill patients: epidemiologic study. Crit Care Med 1990; 18:1383–88.

265. Brathwaite D, Weissman C. The new onset of atrial arrhythmias following major noncardiothoracic surgery is associated with increased mortality. Chest 1998; 114:462–68.

266. Trappe HJ, Brandts B, Weismueller P. Arrhythmias in the intensive care patient. Curr Opin Crit Care 2003; 9:345–55.

267. Reinelt P, Karth GD, Geppert A, et al. Incidence and type of cardiac arrhythmias in critically ill patients: a single center experience in a medical-cardiological ICU. Intensive Care Med 2001; 27:1466–73.

268. Knotzer H, Mayr A, Ulmer H, et al. Tachyarrhythmias in a surgical intensive care unit: a case-controlled epidemiologic study. Intensive Care Med 2000; 26:908–14.

269. Seguin P, Signouret T, Laviolle B, et al. Incidence and risk factors of atrial fibrillation in a surgical intensive care unit. Crit Care Med 2004; 32:722–26.

270. Edwards JD, Kishen R. Significance and management of intractable supraventricular arrhythmias in critically ill patients. Crit Care Med 1986; 14:280–82.

271. Koh Y, Kim TH, Lim CM, et al. Risk factors for the development of hemodynamically significant cardiac arrhythmias in patients with mechanical ventilation. J Crit Care 2000; 15:46–51.

272. Parker JS, deBoisblanc BP. Case report: intermittent, positive pressure ventilation-dependent right bundle branch block. Am J Med Sci 1991; 302:380–81.

273. Soman SS, Sandberg KR, Borzak S, et al. The independent association of renal dysfunction and arrhythmias in critically ill patients. Chest 2002; 122:669–77.

274. Schumaker GL, Epstein SK. Managing acute respiratory failure during exacerbation of chronic obstructive pulmonary disease. Respir Care 2004; 49:766–82.

275. Arranto CA, Mueller C, Hunziker PR, et al. Adverse cardiac events in ICU patients with presumptive antidepressant overdose. Swiss Med Wkly 2003; 133:479–83.

276. Di Pasquale G, Pinelli G, Andreoli A, et al. Holter detection of cardiac arrhythmias in intracranial subarachnoid hemorrhage. Am J Cardiol 1987; 59:596–600.

277. Lin RY, Smith AJ, Hergenroeder P. High serum albuterol levels and tachycardia in adult asthmatics treated with high-dose continuously aerosolized albuterol. Chest 1993; 103:221–25.

278. Duane M, Chandran L, Morelli PJ. Recurrent supraventricular tachycardia as a complication of nebulized albuterol treatment. Clin Pediatr (Phila) 2000; 39:673–77.

279. Dhand R, Duarte AG, Jubran A, et al. Dose-response to bronchodilator delivered by metered-dose inhaler in ventilator-supported patients. Am J Respir Crit Care Med 1996; 154:388–93.

280. Salpeter SR, Ormiston TM, Salpeter EE. Cardiovascular effects of beta-agonists in patients with asthma and COPD: a meta-analysis. Chest 2004; 125:2309–21.

281. Lam S, Chen J. Changes in heart rate associated with nebulized racemic albuterol and levalbuterol in intensive care patients. Am J Health Syst Pharm 2003; 60:1971–75.

282. Bach PB, Brown C, Gelfand SE, et al. Management of acute exacerbations of chronic obstructive pulmonary disease: a summary and appraisal of published evidence. Ann Intern Med 2001; 134:600–20.

283. Sessler CN, Cohen MD. Cardiac arrhythmias during theophylline toxicity. A prospective continuous electrocardiographic study. Chest 1990; 98:672–78.

284. Mayr A, Ritsch N, Knotzer H, et al. Effectiveness of direct-current cardioversion for treatment of supraventricular tachyarrhythmias, in particular atrial fibrillation, in surgical intensive care patients. Crit Care Med 2003; 31:401–5.

285. Salpeter SR, Ormiston TM, Salpeter EE. Cardioselective beta-blockers in patients with reactive airway disease: a meta-analysis. Ann Intern Med 2002; 137:715–25.

286. Sheppard D, DiStefano S, Byrd RC, et al. Effects of esmolol on airway function in patients with asthma. J Clin Pharmacol 1986; 26:169–74.

287. Sprung CL, Elser B, Schein RM, et al. Risk of right bundle-branch block and complete heart block during pulmonary artery catheterization. Crit Care Med 1989; 17:1–3.

288. Sprung CL, Pozen RG, Rozanski JJ, et al. Advanced ventricular arrhythmias during bedside pulmonary artery catheterization. Am J Med 1982; 72:203–8.

289. Iberti TJ, Benjamin E, Gruppi L, et al. Ventricular arrhythmias during pulmonary artery catheterization in the intensive care unit. Prospective study. Am J Med 1985; 78:451–54.

290. Hammon WE, Connors AF Jr, McCaffree DR. Cardiac arrhythmias during postural drainage and chest percussion of critically ill patients. Chest 1992; 102:1836–41.

291. Laws AK, McIntyre RW. Chest physiotherapy: a physiological assessment during intermittent positive pressure ventilation in respiratory failure. Can Anaesth Soc J 1969; 16:487–93.

292. Mackenzie CF, Shin B. Cardiorespiratory function before and after chest physiotherapy in mechanically ventilated patients with post-traumatic respiratory failure. Crit Care Med 1985; 13:483–86.

293. Delle Karth G, Geppert A, Neunteufl T, et al. Amiodarone versus diltiazem for rate control in critically ill patients with atrial tachyarrhythmias. Crit Care Med 2001; 29:1149–53.

294. Mayr AJ, Dunser MW, Ritsch N, et al. High-dosage continuous amiodarone therapy to treat new-onset supraventricular tachyarrhythmias in surgical intensive care patients: an observational study. Wien Klin Wochenschr 2004; 116:310–17.

295. Donaldson L, Grant IS, Naysmith MR, et al. Acute amiodarone-induced lung toxicity. Intensive Care Med 1998; 24:626–30.

296. Varriale P, Sedighi A. Acute management of atrial fibrillation and atrial flutter in the critical care unit: should it be ibutilide? Clin Cardiol 2000; 23:265–68.

297. Lesage A, Ramakers M, Daubin C, et al. Complicated acute myocardial infarction requiring mechanical ventilation in the intensive care unit: prognostic factors of clinical outcome in a series of 157 patients. Crit Care Med 2004; 32:100–5.

298. Ben-Haim SA, Amar R, Shofty R, et al. The effect of positive end-expiratory pressure on the coronary blood flow. Cardiology 1989; 76:193–200.

299. Richard C, Teboul JL, Archambaud F, et al. Left ventricular function during weaning of patients with chronic obstructive pulmonary disease. Intensive Care Med 1994; 20:181–86.

300. Fisher AA, Davis MW, McGill DA. Acute myocardial infarction associated with albuterol. Ann Pharmacother 2004; 38: 2045–49.

301. Alberts WM, Williams JH, Ramsdell JW. Clinical implications of serum creatine kinase levels in acute asthma. West J Med 1986; 144:321–23.

302. Lovis C, Mach F, Unger PF, et al. Elevation of creatine kinase in acute severe asthma is not of cardiac origin. Intensive Care Med 2001; 27:528–33.

303. Harvey MG, Hancox RJ. Elevation of cardiac troponins in exacerbation of chronic obstructive pulmonary disease. Emerg Med Australas 2004; 16:212–15.

304. Baillard C, Boussarsar M, Fosse JP, et al. Cardiac troponin I in patients with severe exacerbation of chronic obstructive pulmonary disease. Intensive Care Med 2003; 29:584–89.

305. Jubran A, Mathru M, Dries D, et al. Continuous recordings of mixed venous oxygen saturation during weaning from mechanical ventilation and the ramifications thereof. Am J Respir Crit Care Med 1998; 158:1763–69.

306. Abalos A, Leibowitz AB, Distefano D, et al. Myocardial ischemia during the weaning period. Am J Crit Care 1992; 1:32–36.

307. Chatila W, Ani S, Guaglianone D, et al. Cardiac ischemia during weaning from mechanical ventilation. Chest 1996; 109:1577–83.

308. Hurford WE, Favorito F. Association of myocardial ischemia with failure to wean from mechanical ventilation. Crit Care Med 1995; 23:1475–80.

309. Hurford WE, Lynch KE, Strauss HW, et al. Myocardial perfusion as assessed by thallium-201 scintigraphy during the discontinuation of mechanical ventilation in ventilator-dependent patients. Anesthesiology 1991; 74:1007–16.

310. Srivastava S, Chatila W, Amoateng-Adjepong Y, et al. Myocardial ischemia and weaning failure in patients with coronary artery disease: an update. Crit Care Med 1999; 27: 2109–12.

311. Martinez EA, Kim LJ, Faraday N, et al. Sensitivity of routine intensive care unit surveillance for detecting myocardial ischemia. Crit Care Med 2003; 31:2302–8.

312. Attia J, Ray JG, Cook DJ, et al. Deep vein thrombosis and its prevention in critically ill adults. Arch Intern Med 2001; 161: 1268–79.

313. Cook D, Attia J, Weaver B, et al. Venous thromboembolic disease: an observational study in medical-surgical intensive care unit patients. J Crit Care 2000; 15:127–32.

314. Rocha AT, Tapson VF. Venous thromboembolism in intensive care patients. Clin Chest Med 2003; 24:103–22.

315. Hirsch DR, Ingenito EP, Goldhaber SZ. Prevalence of deep venous thrombosis among patients in medical intensive care. JAMA 1995; 274:335–37.

316. Ibarra-Perez C, Lau-Cortes E, Colmenero-Zubiate S, et al. Prevalence and prevention of deep venous thrombosis of the lower extremities in high-risk pulmonary patients. Angiology 1988; 39:505–13.

317. Velmahos GC, Nigro J, Tatevossian R, et al. Inability of an aggressive policy of thromboprophylaxis to prevent deep venous thrombosis (DVT) in critically injured patients: are current methods of DVT prophylaxis insufficient? J Am Coll Surg 1998; 187:529–33.

318. Karwinski B, Svendsen E. Comparison of clinical and post-mortem diagnosis of pulmonary embolism. J Clin Pathol 1989; 42:135–39.

319. Stein PD, Henry JW. Prevalence of acute pulmonary embolism among patients in a general hospital and at autopsy. Chest 1995; 108:978–81.

320. Moser KM, Fedullo PF, LitteJohn JK, et al. Frequent asymptomatic pulmonary embolism in patients with deep venous thrombosis. JAMA 1994; 271:223–25.

321. Cade JF. High risk of the critically ill for venous thromboembolism. Crit Care Med 1982; 10:448–50.

322. Joynt GM, Kew J, Gomersall CD, et al. Deep venous thrombosis caused by femoral venous catheters in critically ill adult patients. Chest 2000; 117:178–83.

323. Durbec O, Viviand X, Potie F, et al. A prospective evaluation of the use of femoral venous catheters in critically ill adults. Crit Care Med 1997; 25:1986–89.

324. Martin C, Viviand X, Saux P, et al. Upper-extremity deep vein thrombosis after central venous catheterization via the axillary vein. Crit Care Med 1999; 27:2626–29.

325. Monreal M, Raventos A, Lerma R, et al. Pulmonary embolism in patients with upper extremity DVT associated to venous central lines—a prospective study. Thromb Haemost 1994; 72:548–50.

326. Prandoni P, Polistena P, Bernardi E, et al. Upper-extremity deep vein thrombosis. Risk factors, diagnosis, and complications. Arch Intern Med 1997; 157:57–62.

327. Becker DM, Philbrick JT, Walker FBT. Axillary and subclavian venous thrombosis. Prognosis and treatment. Arch Intern Med 1991; 151:1934–43.

328. Wenzel C, Stoiser B, Locker GJ, et al. Frequent development of lupus anticoagulants in critically ill patients treated under intensive care conditions. Crit Care Med 2002; 30:763–70.

329. Marik PE, Andrews L, Maini B. The incidence of deep venous thrombosis in ICU patients. Chest 1997; 111:661–64.

330. Ibrahim EH, Iregui M, Prentice D, et al. Deep vein thrombosis during prolonged mechanical ventilation despite prophylaxis. Crit Care Med 2002; 30:771–74.

331. Fraisse F, Holzapfel L, Couland JM, et al. Nadroparin in the prevention of deep vein thrombosis in acute decompensated COPD. The Association of Non-University Affiliated Intensive Care Specialist Physicians of France. Am J Respir Crit Care Med 2000; 161:1109–14.

332. Kollef MH, Eisenberg PR, Shannon W. A rapid assay for the detection of circulating D-dimer is associated with clinical outcomes among critically ill patients. Crit Care Med 1998;26: 1054–60.

333. Moser KM, LeMoine JR, Nachtwey FJ, et al. Deep venous thrombosis and pulmonary embolism. Frequency in a respiratory intensive care unit. JAMA 1981; 246:1422–24.

334. Major KM, Wilson M, Nishi GK, et al. The incidence of thromboembolism in the surgical intensive care unit. Am Surg 2003; 69:857–61.

335. Wibbenmeyer LA, Hoballah JJ, Amelon MJ, et al. The prevalence of venous thromboembolism of the lower extremity among thermally injured patients determined by duplex sonography. J Trauma 2003; 55:1162–67.

336. Harrington DT, Mozingo DW, Cancio L, et al. Thermally injured patients are at significant risk for thromboembolic complications. J Trauma 2001; 50:495–99.

337. Harris LM, Curl GR, Booth FV, et al. Screening for asymptomatic deep vein thrombosis in surgical intensive care patients. J Vasc Surg 1997; 26:764–69.

338. Geerts WH, Code KI, Jay RM, et al. A prospective study of venous thromboembolism after major trauma. N Engl J Med 1994; 331:1601–6.

339. Wells PS, Anderson DR, Bormanis J, et al. Application of a diagnostic clinical model for the management of hospitalized patients with suspected deep-vein thrombosis. Thromb Haemost 1999; 81:493–97.

340. Diamond S, Goldbweber R, Katz S. Use of D-dimer to aid in excluding deep venous thrombosis in ambulatory patients. Am J Surg 2005; 189:23–26.

341. Kollef MH, Zahid M, Eisenberg PR. Predictive value of a rapid semiquantitative D-dimer assay in critically ill patients with suspected venous thromboembolic disease. Crit Care Med 2000; 28:414–20.

342. Shorr AF, Thomas SJ, Alkins SA, et al. D-dimer correlates with proinflammatory cytokine levels and outcomes in critically ill patients. Chest 2002; 121:1262–68.

343. Shorr AF, Trotta RF, Alkins SA, et al. D-dimer assay predicts mortality in critically ill patients without disseminated intravascular coagulation or venous thromboembolic disease. Intensive Care Med 1999; 25:207–10.

344. Cook D, McMullin J, Hodder R, et al. Prevention and diagnosis of venous thromboembolism in critically ill patients: a Canadian survey. Crit Care 2001; 5:336–42.

345. Kollef MH, Von Harz B, Prentice D, et al. Patient transport from intensive care increases the risk of developing ventilator-associated pneumonia. Chest 1997; 112:765–73.

346. Braman SS, Dunn SM, Amico CA, et al. Complications of intrahospital transport in critically ill patients. Ann Intern Med 1987; 107:469–73.

347. Kearon C, Julian JA, Newman TE, et al. Noninvasive diagnosis of deep venous thrombosis. McMaster Diagnostic Imaging Practice Guidelines Initiative. Ann Intern Med 1998; 128:663–77.

348. Henry JW, Stein PD, Gottschalk A, et al. Scintigraphic lung scans and clinical assessment in critically ill patients with suspected acute pulmonary embolism. Chest 1996; 109:462–66.

349. Invasive and noninvasive diagnosis of pulmonary embolism. Preliminary results of the Prospective Investigative Study of Acute Pulmonary Embolism Diagnosis (PISA-PED). Chest 1995; 107:33S–38S.

350. Velmahos GC, Vassiliu P, Wilcox A, et al. Spiral computed tomography for the diagnosis of pulmonary embolism in critically ill surgical patients: a comparison with pulmonary angiography. Arch Surg 2001; 136:505–11.

351. Goldhaber SZ. Venous thromboembolism in the intensive care unit: the last frontier for prophylaxis. Chest 1998; 113:5–7.

352. Hull RD, Pineo GF. Intermittent pneumatic compression for the prevention of venous thromboembolism. Chest 1996; 109:6–9.

353. Keane MG, Ingenito EP, Goldhaber SZ. Utilization of venous thromboembolism prophylaxis in the medical intensive care unit. Chest 1994; 106:13–14.

354. Geerts WH, Heit JA, Clagett GP, et al. Prevention of venous thromboembolism. Chest 2001; 119:132S–75S.

355. Lacherade JC, Cook D, Heyland D, et al. Prevention of venous thromboembolism in critically ill medical patients: a Franco-Canadian cross-sectional study. J Crit Care 2003; 18:228–37.

356. Aito S, Pieri A, D'Andrea M, et al. Primary prevention of deep venous thrombosis and pulmonary embolism in acute spinal cord injured patients. Spinal Cord 2002; 40:300–3.

357. Samama MM, Cohen AT, Darmon JY, et al. A comparison of enoxaparin with placebo for the prevention of venous thromboembolism in acutely ill medical patients. Prophylaxis in Medical Patients with Enoxaparin Study Group. N Engl J Med 1999; 341:793–800.

Chapter 42

VENTILATOR-INDUCED LUNG INJURY

DIDIER DREYFUSS
JEAN-DAMIEN RICARD
GEORGES SAUMON

The deleterious effects of mechanical ventilation on the lungs have been long referred to as barotrauma. For many years, clinicians defined barotrauma as the occurrence of air leaks resulting in the accumulation of extra-alveolar air responsible for a number of manifestations, of which the most threatening is tension pneumothorax. In addition to these macroscopic events, whose adverse consequences are usually immediately obvious, mechanical ventilation may produce more subtle physiologic and morphologic alterations, especially when it results in high airway pressures. Our knowledge of such alterations has stemmed mainly from experimental studies and has expanded considerably over recent years. Indeed, alterations in alveolo-capillary barrier integrity and release of both inflammatory and anti-inflammatory mediators have been reported in animals ventilated with modalities resulting in high lung stretching. Tissue damage may also occur during mechanical ventilation when distal airways close and open repeatedly because of the movement of foam in the airway lumen or rupture of liquid menisci. The clinical relevance of these experimental findings received resounding confirmation with the results of the ARDS Network study, which showed a 22% reduction in mortality in patients with the acute respiratory distress syndrome through a simple reduction in tidal volume.[1]

The safety of mechanical ventilation for the treatment of patients with acute respiratory failure was questioned soon after its introduction into medical practice. Greenfield et al[2] raised this fundamental concern by showing atelectasis and increased surface tension of lung extracts in dogs that had been ventilated at 26–32 cmH$_2$O peak inspiratory pressure for 2 hours. In 1968, Sladen et al[3] reported that patients treated for long periods with mechanical ventilation exhibited an increase in alveolo-arterial oxygen gradient and a fall in quasi-static compliance. The potential role of mechanical ventilation in causing lung injury has nevertheless been controversial. Indeed, in an experimental study published in 1971, Nash et al[4] claimed that the term *respirator lung* was a misnomer. They ventilated goats with a peak airway pressure of 13 cmH$_2$O, using either 100% fractional inspired oxygen concentration (F$_{IO_2}$) or room air. Animals subjected to high F$_{IO_2}$ did not survive for more than 4 days because of severe pulmonary edema. In contrast, animals ventilated with room air remained stable for up to 2 weeks, and their lungs were normal. Nash et al concluded that prolonged mechanical ventilation does not cause lung damage. They rightly pointed out, however, that they used only low peak inspiratory pressures. Subsequent studies performed using higher peak inspiratory pressures (PIP) or plateau (end-inspiratory) pressures in the same range conclusively demonstrated that respirator lung is a valid concept. Many studies have sought to determine whether or not mechanical ventilation causes lung injury, to identify risk factors for potential adverse effects of mechanical ventilation, and to develop strategies for preventing ventilator-induced lung damage.

The first comprehensive work demonstrating that mechanical ventilation may be unsafe in intact animals was performed by Webb et al[5] Rats ventilated with 30 or 45 cmH$_2$O PIP displayed pulmonary edema within 20 minutes to 1 hour, depending on the pressure level. Microscopic examination of the lungs disclosed moderate interstitial edema in animals ventilated with the lower peak pressure, contrasting with profuse edema and alveolar flooding in animals ventilated with the highest PIP. Other studies subsequently documented the occurrence of pulmonary edema and lung ultrastructural abnormalities[6,7] after even very short periods of intermittent positive-inspiratory pressure with high PIP.

Findings consistent with the data outlined above were reported in larger animals, albeit after longer periods of ventilation. John et al ventilated rabbits with 20 cmH$_2$O PIP for 6 hours and found that some, but not all, animals had interstitial and alveolar edema upon light microscopic examination[8] and ultrastructural alterations consisting mainly of loss of alveolar type I cell continuity.[9] Kolobow et al[10] reported progressive lung injury in sheep ventilated with 50 cmH$_2$O PIP over 48 hours, manifesting as decreased pulmonary compliance and deterioration in blood oxygenation. Some of the animals died before the 48-hour endpoint. At autopsy, lungs exhibited congestion and severe atelectasis. Lung hemorrhage and inflammatory cell infiltration were observed after long-lasting ventilation with high PIP.[11]

The mechanisms underlying this ventilator-induced lung injury (VILI) have been for the most part elucidated. Two main factors explain its development: the magnitude of lung overdistension and its duration. Ventilation with very high peak transalveolar pressure results in acute, rapidly fatal, permeability pulmonary edema, whereas more protracted ventilation involving alveolar distension of lesser magnitude produces a lung injury in which inflammatory phenomena may play a role. These two situations will be described separately and termed "acute" and "subacute" VILI for the sake of simplicity, although it is easy to imagine that they may overlap.

Acute Ventilator-Induced Lung Injury

Ventilation modalities with very high distending pressures (typically >30 cmH$_2$O, depending on the species) result in pulmonary edema. Both increased filtration and alteration in capillary permeability participate in edema formation. The reason for these abnormalities has been in part elucidated.

EVIDENCE IN SUPPORT OF INCREASED FILTRATION

The first hypothesis put forward to account for ventilator-induced edema involved hydrostatic alterations.[5,12] Increased filtration may result from an increase of pulmonary capillary pressure, a decrease in lung interstitial pressure, or both. Surfactant inactivation and increased lung volume participate in the decrease in lung interstitial pressure.

CAPILLARY PRESSURE
Parker et al[12] calculated that mean lung microvascular pressure increased by 12.5 cmH$_2$O during ventilation of open-chest dogs at 64 cmH$_2$O PIP. Whether these findings apply to intact animals is unclear because pulmonary blood flow decreases more during high-airway-pressure ventilation when the chest is open, suggesting that pulmonary vascular pressures and filtration rates may be lower in closed-chest animals.[12] Lung perfusion, and thus filtration pressure, indeed contributes to VILI in isolated lungs.[13] In a study of the mechanisms of lung injury produced by ventilating closed-chest lambs with 58 cmH$_2$O PIP, Carlton et al[14] found that mean pulmonary arterial transmural pressure increased by no more than 7 cmH$_2$O.

SURFACTANT INACTIVATION
The increase in alveolar surface tension resulting from surfactant inactivation would be expected to further decrease the negative pressures surrounding alveolar vessels, thereby increasing vascular transmural pressure and enhancing fluid filtration. Faridy et al[15] showed that ventilat-

ing excised dog lungs altered pulmonary pressure-volume curves and increased surface tension of lung extracts commensurately with the magnitude of tidal volume and duration of ventilation. Comparable findings were reported in excised rat lungs.[16,17] These anomalies were ascribed to depletion or alteration of surfactant. Several studies[17–20] demonstrated that ventilation in fact increases surfactant release, suggesting that the observed decrease in surface activity was secondary, not to surfactant depletion, but to surfactant inactivation,[17,18] as the result of lower amounts of organized lipid-protein structures,[21] or of a loss of surface-active material in the airways.[22] Surface tension abnormalities proved reversible when lung volume was held constant, probably because of de novo surfactant production, because recovery did not occur in cold lungs or in the absence of oxygen.[15,16] It is interesting to note that surfactant alterations failed to occur when positive end-expiratory pressure (PEEP) was used.[15,16,18,22]

Pattle[23] and Clements[24] suggested that an increase in alveolar surface tension might increase filtration. Albert et al[25] found that the isogravimetric pressure (the vascular pressure at which net fluid flux from pulmonary vessels is zero) decreased when alveolar surface tension was increased by cooling and ventilating lungs at a low resting volume in open-chest dogs. The authors interpreted this fall in isogravimetric pressure as indicative of a fall in perimicrovascular pressure, although they could not definitely rule out changes in microvascular permeability and reflection coefficient. In a study in dogs, Bredenberg et al[26] demonstrated that vascular permeability and reflection coefficient for proteins were not affected when pulmonary edema was produced by increasing alveolar surface tension with an aerosol of detergent. They did not exclude, however, more subtle alterations in endothelial barrier properties, which are discussed below.

Aerosolized ^{99m}Tc-DTPA (diethylenetriamine pentaacetic acid) clearance was found to increase following detergent aerosolization in rabbits[27] and dogs.[28] This finding was ascribed to regional overexpansion secondary to uneven lung inflation during mechanical ventilation of alveoli with altered surface tension rather than to elimination of peculiar barrier properties of surfactant.[28]

ROLE OF INCREASED LUNG VOLUME
Increased filtration during mechanical ventilation probably also occurs at the extra-alveolar level. During lung inflation, because of "pulmonary interdependence," the pressure in the perivascular space surrounding extra-alveolar vessels decreases, and this in turn increases transmural pressure. This effect of lung volume on pulmonary vessels is well documented.[29] Pressure-volume characteristics of the vascular bed have been determined in isolated lung lobes in dogs.[30] Inflating the lungs dilates the extra-alveolar vessels. During inflation from a low transpulmonary pressure, the increase in vessel diameter is such that an effective outward-acting pressure in excess of pleural pressure (1–2 cmH$_2$O for each centimeter of water increase in transpulmonary pressure) expands the vessels.[31] The potential importance of fluid leakage through extra-alveolar vessels has been established in both excised lungs[32] and in-situ lungs of open-chest animals.[33] Moreover, inflation of in-situ lobes under

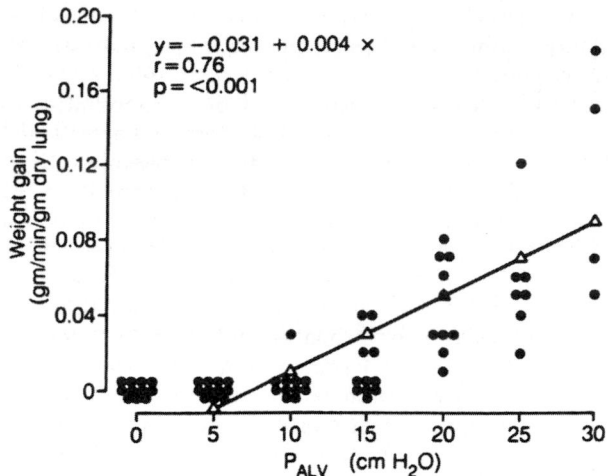

FIGURE 42-1 Relationship between alveolar pressure and rate of hydrostatic edema formation in in-situ lobes of open-chest dogs. Pulmonary arterial and venous pressures were kept at 1 cmH$_2$O. When lung volume was low (alveolar pressure 10 cmH$_2$O), no edema occurred, whereas greater distensions produced a linear increase in lung weight gain, indicating edema formation. (*Reproduced, with permission, from Albert et al.[34]*)

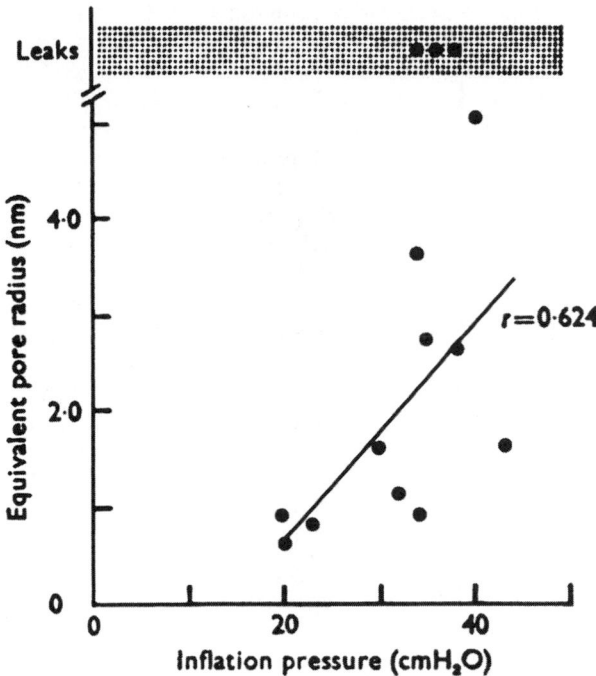

FIGURE 42-2 Effect of inflation pressure on the epithelial permeability of fluid-filled in-situ lobes of sheep lung. Permeability is characterized by an equivalent pore radius. A linear relationship was observed between inflation pressure and pore radius. At the highest levels of inflation, free diffusion of albumin was sometimes observed, indicating the presence of large leaks. (*Reproduced, with permission, from Egan et al.[39]*)

zone 1 conditions was found to precipitate hydrostatic pulmonary edema in dogs.[34] Because there is no flow in capillaries under zone 1 conditions, it is likely that the edema fluid leaked from distended extra-alveolar vessels. The rate of edema formation was significantly correlated with the level of alveolar pressure and, therefore, the magnitude of distension (Fig. 42-1).

The effects of decreased perimicrovascular pressure and surfactant alterations probably combine with increased intravascular pressure to augment transmural microvascular pressure during overinflation. Although the magnitude of these changes is difficult to evaluate with precision, however, the increase in vascular pressure seems relatively modest and is unlikely to explain per se the rapid development of profuse edema (especially in small animals) observed after ventilation at high peak inspiratory pressures.

EVIDENCE IN SUPPORT OF PERMEABILITY ALTERATIONS

Many experimental studies in isolated lungs as well as in open-chest or intact animals have demonstrated permeability alterations (in response to high airway pressures) in the epithelium and, more unexpectedly, the endothelium.

EPITHELIAL PERMEABILITY CHANGES IN RESPONSE TO HIGH AIRWAY PRESSURE

The increase in alveolar epithelial permeability to small hydrophilic solutes observed when lung volume increases is a physiologic phenomenon. Elevation of functional residual capacity (FRC) in sheep, obtained by increasing the level of PEEP during mechanical ventilation[35] or spontaneous ventilation,[36] was associated with an increase in aerosolized DTPA clearance. Clearance augmentation was larger than expected from the changes in alveolar exchange surface area. Increase of epithelial permeability in

response to increased lung volume was also reported in humans.[37,38] Marks et al[37] demonstrated that DTPA clearance increased regardless of whether lung inflation was obtained by positive-pressure breathing or voluntary hyperinflation in humans.

Effects of overinflation on epithelial permeability were studied extensively by Egan et al during static inflation of fluid-filled in-situ lobes.[39,40] The equivalent-pore approach was used to describe the permeability of the epithelium to hydrophilic solutes of various sizes. Equivalent-pore radii increased from about 1 nm at 20 cmH$_2$O inflating pressure to 5 nm at 40 cmH$_2$O alveolar pressure. In some instances, free diffusion of albumin across the epithelium was observed, indicating the presence of large leaks (Fig. 42-2). Permeability alterations persisted or even increased after cessation of inflation, suggesting irreversible epithelial injury. High airway pressures applied to in-situ lobes, however, resulted in supraphysiologic overinflation because of the compression of adjacent parenchyma. Egan[41] performed experiments under less extreme conditions in rabbits, in which both in-situ lobes and entire lungs were distended with 40 cmH$_2$O airway pressure. Static segmental inflation resulted in a 6- to 12-fold increase in lung volume from FRC and in an epithelium permeable to solutes such as albumin, cytochrome c, and cyanocobalamin. In contrast, whole lung inflation resulted in only a three- to fourfold increase in lung volume and a lesser rate of escape of the smaller solutes from the alveolar spaces. The increase in albumin permeability resulting from whole lung

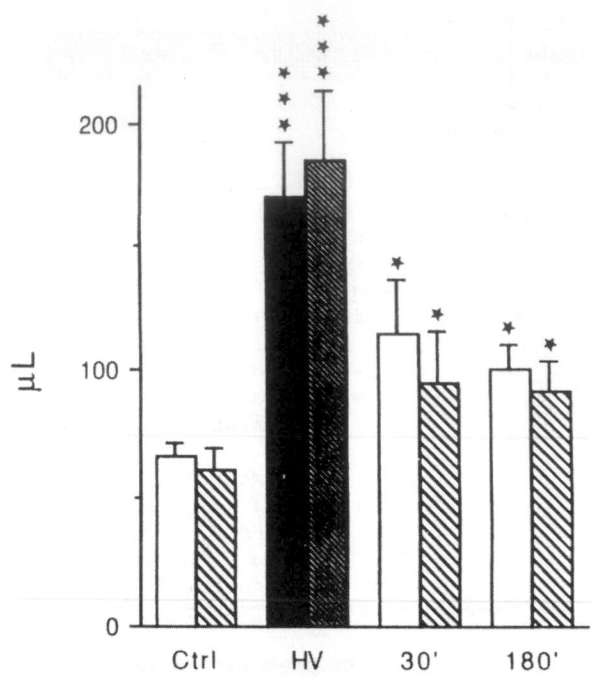

FIGURE 42-3 Estimates of epithelial lining fluid (ELF) volume by bronchoalveolar lavage after ventilation with 45 cmH$_2$O peak airway pressure for 2 minutes (*HV*) and recovery. Two successive lavages were performed (*open and filled bars,* first lavage; *hatched bars,* second lavage). ELF volume increased significantly after HV and then decreased during recovery, but remained higher than in control subjects (*Ctrl*). (*Reproduced, with permission, from Dreyfuss et al.*[7])

ing that epithelium permeability was not modified by static inflation within the physiologic range but increased after overinflation.

Although less well documented on a quantitative basis, epithelial alveolar permeability alterations are probably present in varying degrees during ventilator-induced pulmonary edema. During positive-pressure ventilation with 41 cmH$_2$O PIP, increases in alveolar permeability to small (DTPA), but not large (albumin), solutes were observed after 8 hours by Ramanathan et al in lambs.[43] After 2 minutes of high-pressure ventilation, epithelial lining fluid (ELF) volume calculated from bronchoalveolar lavage fluid increased by 180%[7] (Fig. 42-3). ELF protein content increased by 76% (Fig. 42-4B), whereas protein concentration decreased (Fig. 42-4A); this suggests that most of the excess fluid entered the alveolar-airway lumen through increased convection. In contrast to the severely altered sieving properties of microvessels after only 2 minutes of overinflation, epithelial permeability appears to be better preserved. This speculation is consistent with the scarcity of epithelial cell alterations on electron microscopic examination, contrasting with the widespread endothelial abnormalities.[7] The presence of blood cells in the alveoli, however, suggested a few large endothelial and epithelial tears. During longer (2 hours) ventilation periods with a lower tidal volume (V$_T$) (19 ml/kg in rats, resulting in a PIP of 19 cmH$_2$O), the presence of secretory Clara-cell protein (a protein found in airway lumen) in the vasculature, contrasting with a decrease in its concentration in bronchoalveolar lavage fluid, further suggests an increase in alveolar-barrier permeability.[44] Secretory Clara-cell protein was also found in the plasma of mice ventilated with 35 cmH$_2$O PIP for 2 hours and even earlier (30 minutes) when PIP was 55 cmH$_2$O.[45] Resorption of alveolar liquid by distal airway epithelium is decreased during VILI because of depressed sodium transport mechanisms.[46] It can be restored by β-adrenergic

overinflation was negligible. Hence, only major increases in lung volume produce significant changes in permeability to large molecules. Support for this concept was provided by a study by Kim et al[42] in isolated bullfrog lungs, show-

FIGURE 42-4 Protein concentration (*A*) and protein content (*B*) in epithelial lining fluid (see Fig. 42-3 for details on the lavages). Protein content (expressed as the equivalent plasma volume) increased after high-pressure ventilation (*HV*) and then remained unchanged during recovery. Protein concentration (as a percentage of plasma protein concentration) decreased after HV and returned to normal during recovery (see text for details). (*Reproduced, with permission, from Dreyfuss et al.*[7])

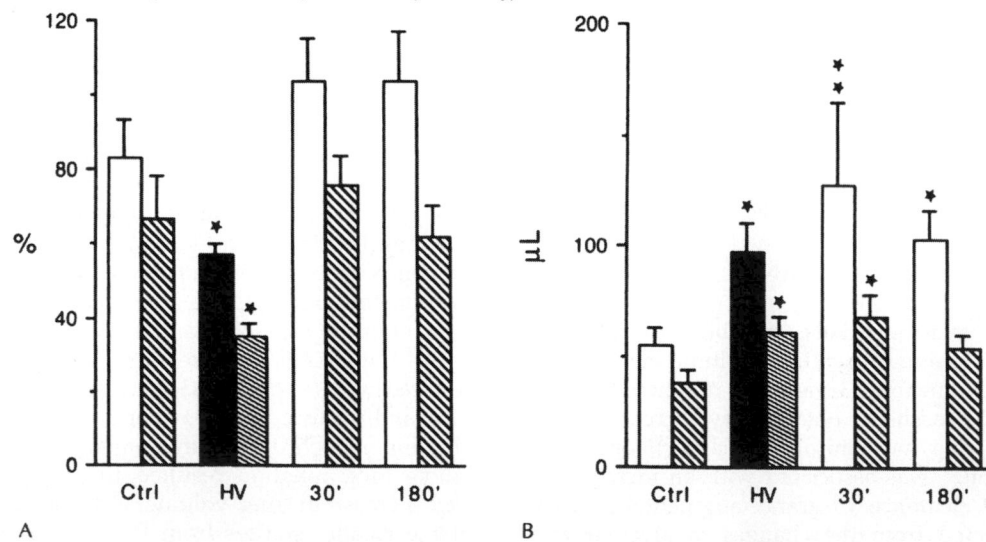

A   B

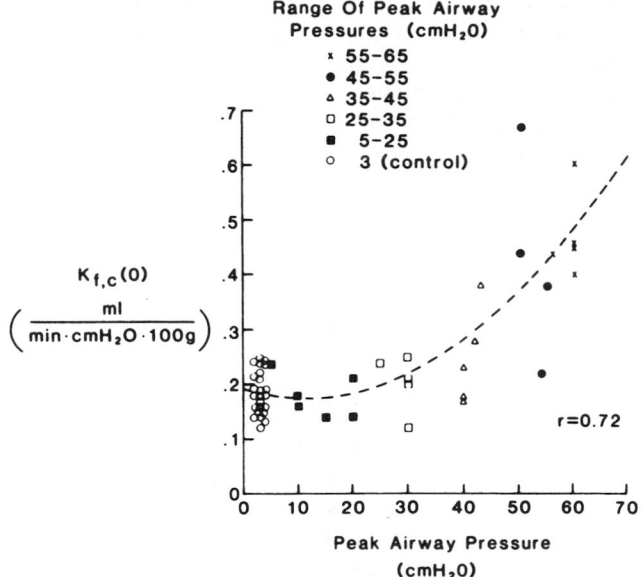

FIGURE 42-5 Effect of peak airway pressure on the capillary filtration coefficient ($K_{f,c}$) of isolated, blood-perfused lobes of dog lungs receiving 20 minutes of intermittent positive-pressure ventilation. Moderate (up to 30 cmH$_2$O) increases in peak pressure did not affect $K_{f,c}$, whereas higher levels of peak pressure resulted in a very steep increase in $K_{f,c}$. (*Reproduced, with permission, from Parker et al.[49]*)

stimulation that recruits ion-transporting proteins to the plasma membrane of alveolar epithelial cells or by β-1 sodium-potassium ATPase subunit gene transfer.[47,48]

MICROVASCULAR PERMEABILITY ALTERATIONS DURING MECHANICAL VENTILATION–INDUCED PULMONARY EDEMA

In a study in isolated blood-perfused lobes from dogs, Parker et al[49] demonstrated that ventilation for 20 minutes with graded increases in PIP did not affect microvascular

permeability up to 30 cmH$_2$O. Higher PIP (45–65 cmH$_2$O) was associated with increases in the capillary filtration coefficient (Fig. 42-5) and decreases in isogravimetric capillary pressure, suggesting the existence of an airway pressure threshold. Similarly, the estimated protein reflection coefficient was decreased only at the highest airway pressures. It is interesting to note that, with airway pressures above the threshold, the increase in capillary filtration coefficient occurred immediately and continued in some lobes after cessation of distension.

In order to evaluate permeability alterations in intact animals, extravascular lung water and bloodless dry-lung weight and the distribution space in lungs of ^{125}I-labeled albumin injected into the systemic circulation were measured in intact rats subjected to 45-cmH$_2$O PIP ventilation.[6] Pulmonary edema developed very rapidly and was easily demonstrable after only 5–10 minutes of high-pressure ventilation (Fig. 42-6). Light microscopic examination revealed that, at this stage, edema fluid remained confined to interstitial spaces, where it accumulated in the large peri-bronchovascular cuffs. No alveolar flooding was apparent. The presence of permeability alterations was indicated by a significant increase in dry-lung weight and of albumin distribution space (see Fig. 42-6). After 10 minutes of high-PIP ventilation, pulmonary edema was more abundant but still involved only the interstitial spaces. After 20 minutes of ventilation, findings were strikingly different, with tracheal flooding in all animals. Widespread alveolar flooding was obvious upon light microscopic examination. The severity of the permeability alterations was such that the ratio of ^{125}I-albumin activity in tracheal fluid versus plasma was close to unity, indicating the loss of permselectivity of the capillary barrier. The severity of the permeability defect was indicated by the relationship between dry-lung weight and extravascular lung water (Fig. 42-7), which indicated that the concentration of protein in extravasated fluid was high, suggesting the presence of numerous large capillary leaks. Similar findings relating the duration of high-PIP

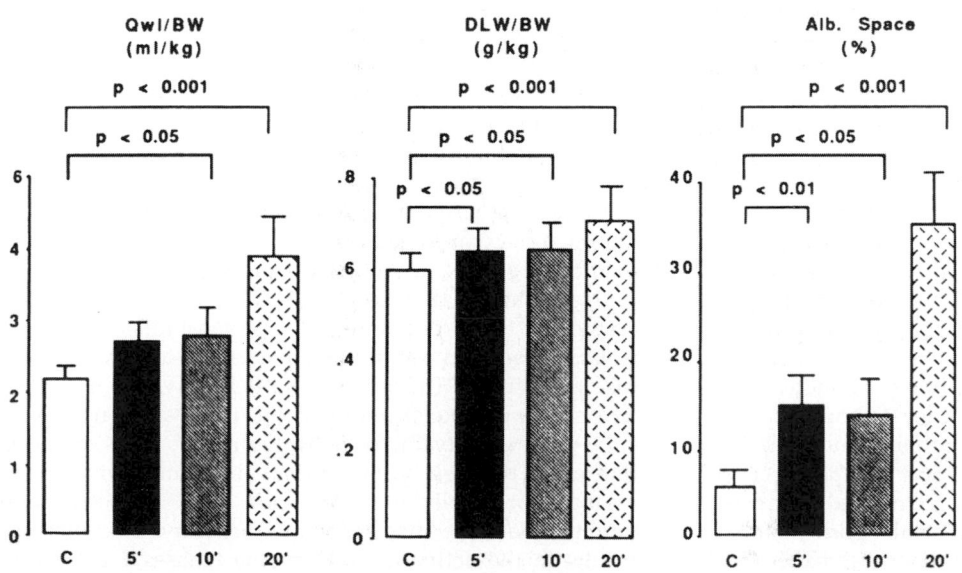

FIGURE 42-6 Effect of 45-cmH$_2$O peak airway pressure ventilation in intact rats. Pulmonary edema was assessed by the determination of extravascular lung water content (*Qwl/BW*) and permeability alterations by the determination of bloodless dry-lung weight (*DLW/BW*) and of the distribution space in the lungs of ^{125}I-labeled albumin (*Alb. Space*). Permeability pulmonary edema developed rapidly (5 minutes). After 20 minutes of mechanical ventilation, there was a dramatic increase in all indexes ($p < .01$ versus other groups). (*Adapted, with permission, from Dreyfuss et al.[6]*)

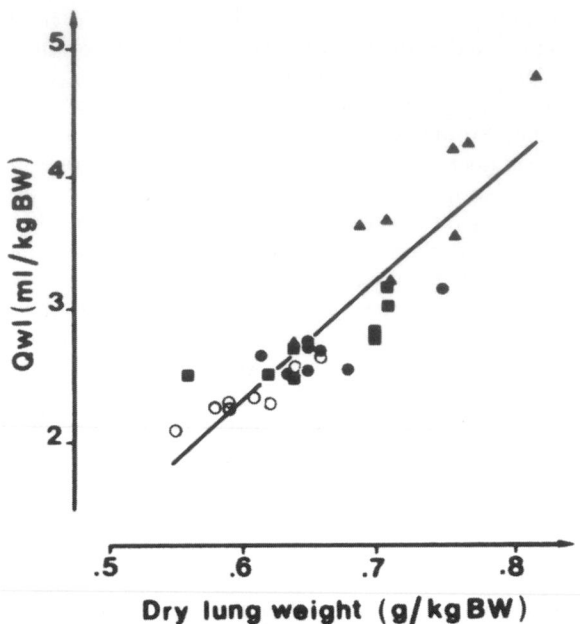

FIGURE 42-7 Relationship between extravascular lung water content [Qwl(ml/kg BW)] and dry-lung weight during mechanical ventilation with peak airway pressure 45 cmH$_2$O. The concentration of proteins in the edema fluid estimated from this relationship was consistent with the outpouring of protein-rich edema fluid, reflecting severe permeability alterations. *Open circles,* control conditions; *closed circles,* 5 minutes of ventilation; *closed squares,* 10 minutes of ventilation; *closed triangles,* 20 minutes of ventilation. (*Reproduced, with permission, from Dreyfuss et al.[6]*)

ventilation and alterations in capillary permeability have been made in mice.[45] This increase in endothelium permeability occurs both at the alveolar and extra-alveolar level.[50]

The time course of edema development depends on the size of the species: in rats, high-PIP ventilation for as little as 2 minutes is sufficient to produce permeability edema,[7] although alterations are minor and result in fairly mild edema. The increase in the ratio of extravascular lung water to blood-free dry-lung weight was increased by only 17% after 2 minutes[7] versus 90% when the duration of the challenge was increased to 20 minutes.[51] In larger animals, considerably longer durations of high-PIP ventilation are required to produce significant alterations. For instance, in lambs mechanically ventilated at 58 cmH$_2$O PIP for 6 hours, Carlton et al[14] found an increase in the ratio of extravascular lung water to dry-lung weight of only 19%. Results of histologic lung studies were either normal or showed only mild perivascular edema with no alveolar edema. In a study by Borelli et al,[52] sheep mechanically ventilated for 18 hours with a PIP of 50 cmH$_2$O developed both interstitial and alveolar edema. Wet-lung weight normalized for body weight increased by 89% compared to normal lungs.[53] After 27 hours of ventilation, pathologic abnormalities were much more marked, and lung weight was increased by 136% compared to normal lungs. Clearly, the ventilation time needed to produce severe edema is less than 1 hour in small species but over 24 hours in large animals. Blood–gas barrier thickness is an important component of capillary resistance to mechanical stretch, and is more important in larger animals.[54] Thus, one reason why permeability alterations were not consistently found is that they may become detectable only after longer ventilation times, in contrast to the immediate occurrence of microvascular pressure anomalies.

In summary, increased microvascular filtration pressure and altered microvascular permeability probably compound their effects to produce high-PIP pulmonary edema. Although the hydrostatic component seems to be moderate on a quantitative basis, at least in closed-chest animals, it may nevertheless have a substantial impact. Indeed, in the face of a microvascular barrier with altered sieving properties, any increase in driving pressure will have a dramatic effect on edema formation.[55–57] The synergistic action of increased hydrostatic forces and severe permeability alterations may explain the occurrence of fulminating pulmonary edema in some instances.

MECHANISMS OF ACUTE INCREASE IN ALVEOLO-CAPILLARY PERMEABILITY DURING LUNG OVERINFLATION

Interest has increasingly focused on the cellular response to mechanical strain and this subject has been comprehensively reviewed.[58] Tschumperlin et al[59] observed increased cell death when alveolar epithelial cells are submitted in vitro to deformation. Cyclic deformation led to significantly greater cell death than did static deformation. The percentage of dead cells after 1 day ranged from 0.5–72% depending on the changes in surface area (up to 50%). In cyclically deformed cells, injury occurred rapidly, with most of cell death occurring during the first 5 minutes of deformation.[60] These authors showed that basement-membrane surface area increased about 40% when lung volume was varied from FRC to total lung capacity.[61] These increases suggest that epithelial cells undergo significant stretch during large inflations. Vlahakis et al[62,63] labeled membrane lipids to study deformation-induced lipid trafficking and studied in a direct manner (laser confocal microscopy) the response of epithelial cells of the alveolar basement membrane to forces. A 25% stretch deformation resulted in lipid transport to the plasma membrane that allowed maintenance of its integrity and an increase in epithelial-cell surface area. Such lipid trafficking occurred in all cells, whereas plasma breaks were seen in only a small percentage of cells. The authors concluded that deformation-induced lipid trafficking serves, in part, to repair plasma breaks in order to maintain plasma-membrane integrity and cell viability, and that this could be viewed as a cytoprotective mechanism against the plasma-membrane stress failure seen during VILI.[51,64]

Overinflating the lungs results in the increase in epithelial[39] and endothelial[6,49] permeability. Using an isolated perfused rat model, Parker et al have shown that gadolinium (that blocks stretch-activated nonselective cation channels) annulled the increase in microvascular permeability induced by high PIP.[65] This suggests that entry through stretch-activated channels and an increase in intracellular calcium ion (Ca^{2+}) concentration might initiate the increase in permeability. This increase results in the activation of tyrosine kinases,[66] activation

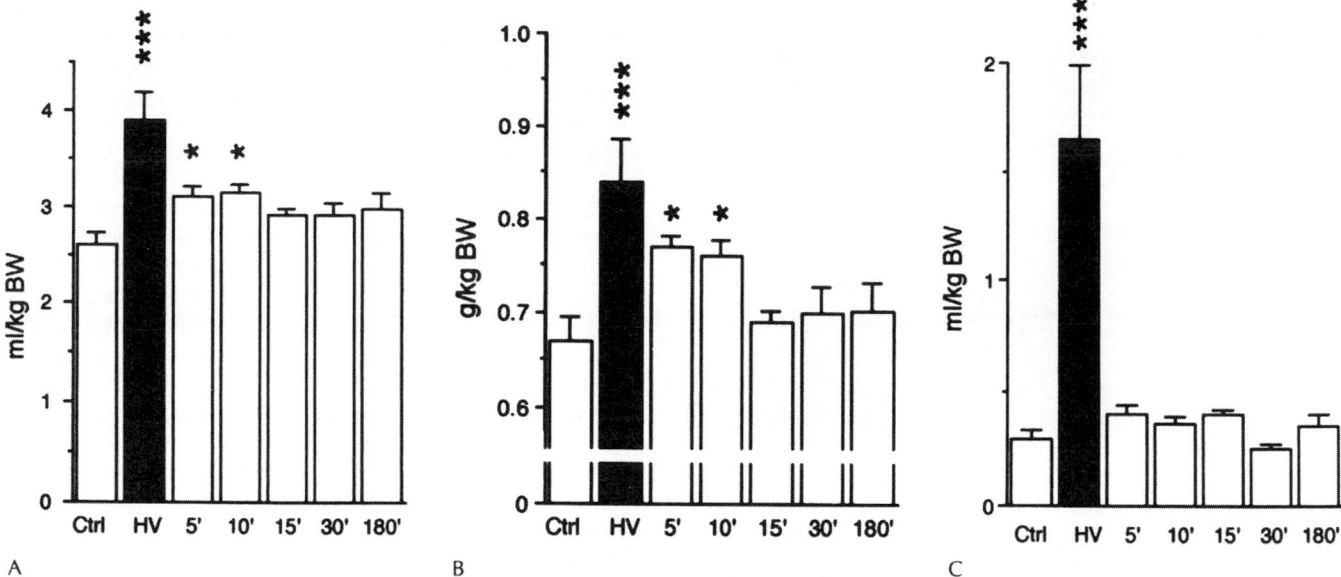

FIGURE 42-8 Effect of 45 cmH$_2$O peak airway pressure ventilation for 2 minutes (*HV*) and followed by recovery for various lengths of time in intact rats. *A.* Extravascular lung water. *B.* Dry lung weight. *C.* Albumin distribution space. Permeability edema already present after 2 minutes cleared rapidly after cessation of ventilation. (*Reproduced, with permission, from Dreyfuss et al.[7]*)

of the Ca^{2+}/calmodulin pathway, and phosphorylation of myosin light chain kinase.[67] Taken together, these results suggest that the increase in microvascular permeability below the cell-rupture point, which occurs under extreme stretch conditions ("stress failure"[64,68]), is not simply a passive physical phenomenon, but the result of biochemical reactions. In vitro studies have shown that cell plasticity and deformation-induced lipid trafficking protect against strain injury. Interventions that impair deformation-induced lipid trafficking reduce the likelihood of plasma membrane resealing[63,69] and increase cell death. It may help explain why the breaks seen across endothelial cells, after short periods of high transmural capillary pressure[70] or overinflation,[7] are transient. In this latter study, rats were subjected to mechanical ventilation with 45 cmH$_2$O PIP for only 2 minutes and allowed to recover for graded periods of up to 3 hours. The animals that were killed immediately after the challenge exhibited mild pulmonary edema with, however, severe permeability alterations, as attested by increases in dry-lung weight and albumin space (Fig. 42-8A, B, and C). The very rapid occurrence of microvascular injury was ascertained by the ultrastructural study, which disclosed changes identical with those previously described after longer periods of ventilation. These data strongly suggest that, at least in small animals, vascular leakage after overinflation is almost immediate and extensive. During recovery, both extravascular lung water and dry-lung weight promptly returned to normal (see Fig. 42-8A and B), indicating that resorption of edema can be very rapid. Edema resorption does not necessarily indicate restoration of the alveolo-capillary barrier. The 30-minute distribution space of ^{125}I-albumin in lungs, however, was found to be normal, indicating that no albumin permeability defect was present after the time of tracer injection (see Fig. 42-8C). Because the tracer was injected during the recovery period (i.e., after

cessation of overinflation), this finding demonstrated reversal of the alterations in permeability. ELF volume decreased after cessation of overinflation (see Fig. 42-3), reflecting resorption of the excess alveolar fluid concomitantly with the decrease in extravascular lung water. Even after 3 hours of recovery, however, ELF volume remained higher than in control animals. No marked changes in epithelial fluid protein content were observed (see Fig. 42-4B), reflecting the slower-than-water clearance of protein in alveolar edema fluid.[71] The absence of notable protein resorption explains why the protein concentration in ELF increased during recovery (see Fig. 42-4A).

ULTRASTRUCTURAL FINDINGS

Electron microscopic studies have confirmed that permeability alterations are prominent in the genesis of ventilator-associated pulmonary edema. Both endothelial and epithelial alterations have been observed.[6,7,45,51]

After short durations (5–10 minutes) of 45-cmH$_2$O PIP mechanical ventilation in rats, striking capillary abnormalities consistent with pulmonary edema of the nonhydrostatic type were observed. Some endothelial cells were detached from their basement membrane, resulting in the formation of intracapillary blebs filled with plasma-like material (Fig. 42-9A). Endothelial cells exhibited focal disruptions (Fig. 42-9B). Bleb formation has been reported in experimental high-permeability edema, regardless of the nature of the causative agent, and in the acute respiratory distress syndrome (ARDS),[72–75] but not in experimental hydrostatic pulmonary edema.[72,73,76] Longer durations (20 minutes) of high-PIP ventilation in rats resulted in alveolar flooding and obvious permeability alterations. Pathologic studies showed that this severe edema was accompanied by diffuse damage to the alveolo-capillary barrier. In addition to the capillary lesions, ultrastructural studies disclosed profound

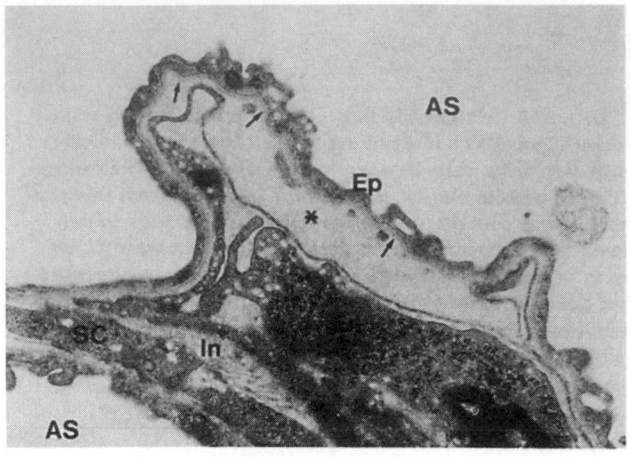

A

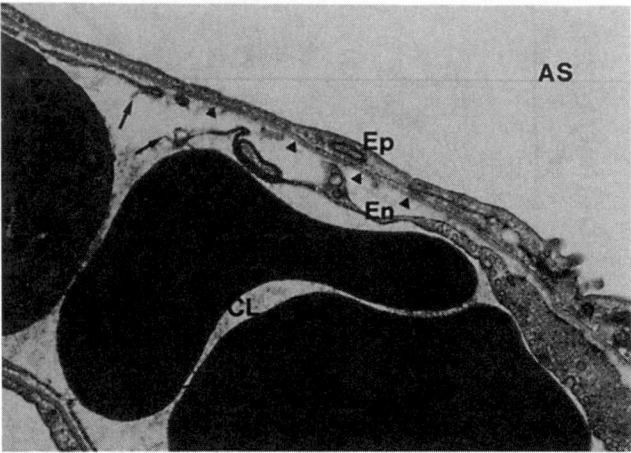

B

FIGURE 42-9 Ultrastructural features of the blood-air barrier after 5 minutes of 45-cmH$_2$O peak airway pressure in a closed chest rat. *A.* The most striking change is the formation of an endothelial bleb secondary to detachment of the thin part of the endothelial cell (*En*) from the basement membrane (*arrows*). This bleb is filled with electron-dense material (*asterisk*) of the same density as plasma. At this stage, epithelial type I cells (*Ep*) are intact. Note interstitial edema (*In*). AS, alveolar space; SC, septal cell. *B.* Arrows indicate a disruption of the thin part of the endothelial cell detached from the basement membrane (*arrowheads*). CL, capillary lumen. (*Panel A reproduced, with permission, from Dreyfuss et al.*[6] *Panel B courtesy of Paul Soler, Ph.D.*)

alterations in the epithelial layer. The severity of alterations varied. In some sites, the epithelial lining appeared intact. In many areas, however, findings included discontinuities (Fig. 42-10A and B) and sometimes almost complete destruction of type I cells, leaving a denuded basement membrane (Fig. 42-10B and C). In contrast, type II cells appeared preserved. Hyaline membranes filled the alveolar spaces in many of the sections examined (Fig. 42-10C). Similar to the endothelial abnormalities, these lesions are not specific and occur in toxic injuries as well as in ARDS.[72–75] In contrast, when pressures remain in the 30- to 40-mmHg range, hydrostatic edema does not affect epithelial integrity.[72,73,77]

Studies using both transmission and scanning electron microscopy have demonstrated ultrastructural breaks in endothelial and epithelial cells when capillary transmural pressure was raised to 40 mmHg or more.[68,78,79] This phenomenon, called capillary stress failure, occurs when capillary wall radial stress is roughly equivalent to that of the aorta in the presence of a 100-mmHg transmural pressure.[68] These breaks are the morphologic correlates of the increased microvascular permeability reported with very high microvascular pressures,[80,81] and described as the stretched-pore phenomenon.[82,83] The similarities between capillary stress failure and VILI are quite remarkable. First, the electron microscopic appearance of endothelial and epithelial cell lesions exhibit similarities (Fig. 42-11).[68,78] Second, both types of damage are partly reversible. Albumin leakage from capillaries during high-volume ventilation ceased almost immediately after discontinuation of ventilation.[7] When capillary pressures were lowered to normal after elevation to a level causing stress failure, the number of endothelial and epithelial breaks fell compared with control experiments in which pressure remained elevated.[70] More importantly, capillary stress failure is influenced by lung inflation: at a capillary transmural pressure of 32.5 cmH$_2$O, increasing lung volume from a transpulmonary pressure of 5 to 20 cmH$_2$O resulted in a significant increase in the number of capillary endothelium and alveolar epithelium breaks (Fig. 42-12).[64] Thus, vascular pressures that are too low to affect microvascular permeability when lung volume is normal may produce permeability alterations when combined with a sufficiently marked increase in lung volume. Furthermore, the increase in the number of breaks was roughly the same for comparable rises in transpulmonary pressure on the one hand and capillary transmural pressure on the other, suggesting that "increases in transpulmonary pressure and capillary transmural pressure are approximately equivalent in terms of their effect on capillary wall stress."[64]

Subacute Ventilator-Induced Lung Injury during Protracted High-Volume Ventilation

The endothelial cell disruptions that have been observed during overinflation edema in small animals may allow direct contact between polymorphonuclear cells and basement membrane (see Fig. 42-10B) and promote leukocyte activation. Proinflammatory mediators may also be released by cells undergoing necrosis. Infiltration of inflammatory cells into the interstitial and alveolar spaces is not seen before several hours of injurious ventilation. In mice subjected to high-PIP ventilation, leukocyte sequestration in lungs (as attested by their myeloperoxidase content) progressively increased with time.[84] In one of the earliest studies on this subject, Woo et al[85] observed that overinflation produced edema in open-chest dogs, and that leukocytes accumulated in the vasculature and macrophages in the alveoli. Further studies have confirmed these results[11] and shown that high transpulmonary pressure increased

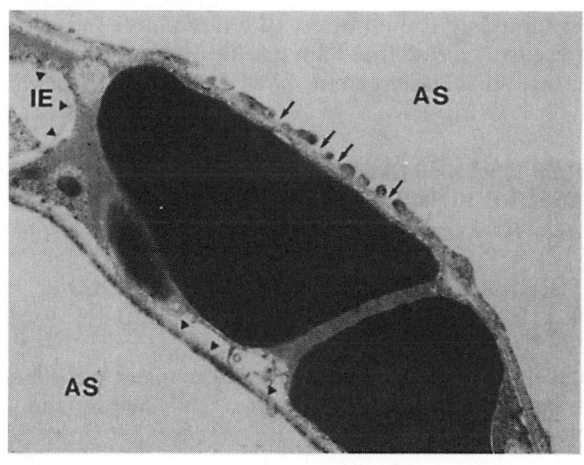

A

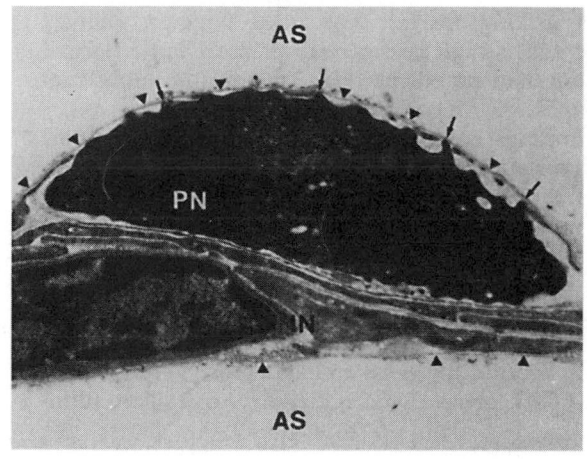

B

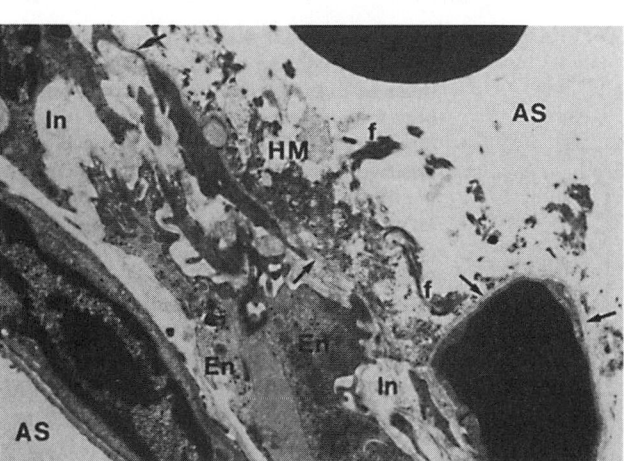

C

FIGURE 42-10 Ultrastructural features of the blood-air barrier after 20 minutes of 45-cmH$_2$O peak airway pressure in a closed chest rat. *A.* Type I cells show numerous gaps (*arrows*). Arrowheads point at the basement membrane from which the endothelial cell is detached. AS, alveolar space; IE, interstitial edema. *B.* Epithelial and endothelial cells are almost completely destroyed, resulting in denuded basement membranes (*arrowheads*). A polymorphonuclear neutrophil (*PN*) inside the capillary lumen exhibits cytoplasmic processes, protruding through gaps in the capillary endothelium. IN, interstitium.*C.* Very severe alteration of the alveolar capillary barrier. Complete lysis of the epithelial layer (upper right quadrant) results in denudation of the basement membrane (*arrows*). Alveolar space is occupied by hyaline membranes (*HM*) composed of cell debris and fibrin (*f*). En, endothelial cells; In, interstitial edema. (*Panels A and B courtesy of Dr. Paul Soler, Ph.D. Panel C reproduced, with permission, from Dreyfuss et al.[6]*)

the transit time of leukocytes in the lungs of rabbits.[86] Lung neutrophil recruitment during high-tidal-volume ventilation is more important in hyperoxic conditions.[87] Conversely, when animals are depleted of neutrophils, high-volume pulmonary edema is less severe. Kawano et al[88] observed that neutrophil-depleted rabbits had preserved gas exchange, little lung albumin leakage, and no hyaline membranes after 4 hours of mechanical ventilation, by contrast to nondepleted animals in a saline-lavage model. Whereas it is predictable that healing of wounded tissue would involve inflammation, several authors have suggested that lung tissue stretching might result in lung damage solely through the release of inflammatory mediators and leukocyte recruitment, the so-called biotrauma hypothesis.

ROLE OF INFLAMMATORY MEDIATORS

Tremblay et al[89] examined the effects of different ventilator strategies on the level of several cytokines in bronchoalveolar lavage fluid of ex-vivo, unperfused rat lungs ventilated with different end-expiratory pressures and tidal volumes. High-tidal-volume ventilation (40 ml/kg BW) with zero end-expiratory pressure resulted in the release of considerable amounts of tumor necrosis factor-α (TNF-α), interleukin-1β, and interleukin-6, and in macrophage inflammatory protein-2 (MIP-2, a potent neutrophil chemoattractant and the rodent functional homolog of human interleukin-8) (Fig. 42-13). These results have not, however, been replicated by other groups using either the same ex vivo lung model or in vivo.[90,91] The release of TNF-α in the perfusate of isolated mouse lungs[92,93] is variable, depending on the mouse strain.[93]

In vivo studies of intact animals show that high-volume mechanical ventilation, which produces a very severe pulmonary edema, does not induce lung release of TNF-α in rats.[90,94] Similarly, TNF-α release was not found in mice ventilated with a high PIP in vivo, although it was found in the perfusate of isolated lungs from the same strain.[93] Studies on TNF-α mRNA also yield conflicting results. Takata et al[95] showed large increases in TNF-α mRNA in the intraalveolar cells of surfactant-depleted rabbits after 1 hour of conventional mechanical ventilation with peak inspiratory and end-expiratory pressures of 28 and 5 cmH$_2$O (resulting in a mean airway pressure of 13 cmH$_2$O). Conversely, Imanaka et al found no increase in lung tissue TNF-α mRNA of rats ventilated with 45 cmH$_2$O PIP.[96]

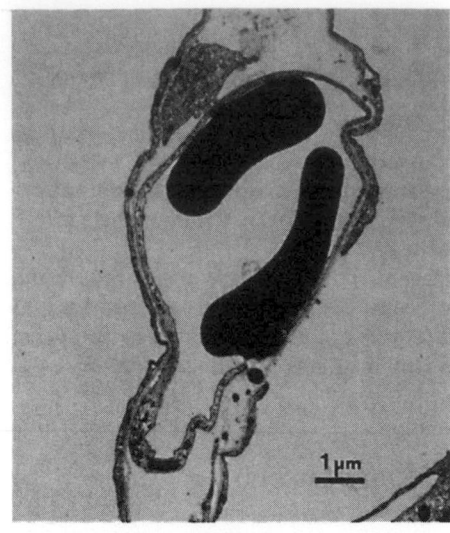

A

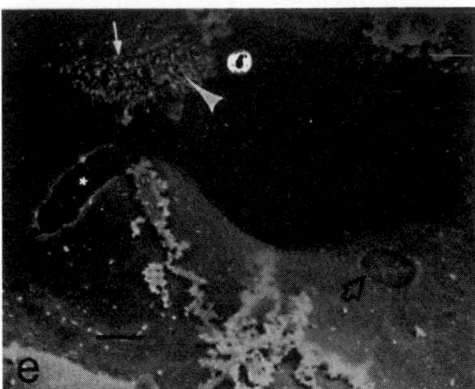

B

FIGURE 42-11 Examples of disruptions of the blood-gas barrier in in-situ rabbit lungs perfused at 72.5 cmH$_2$O capillary transmural pressure. *A*. Transmission electron microscopy. The alveolar epithelium and capillary endothelium are disrupted, but the basement membrane is intact. *B*. Scanning electron microscopy. Circular rupture involving only the epithelial layer (*open arrow*) and complete disruption of the blood-gas barrier (*closed arrow*) showing red blood cells in the opening (*asterisk*). A large amount of proteinaceous material is present in the alveolar lumen. The arrowhead indicates a type II cell with an intercellular junction (*white arrow*). (*Reproduced, with permission, from West et al.[68] and Costello et al.[79]*)

The only mediator that was consistently released by lungs subjected to high-volume ventilation[89,90,92,93,97] or in vitro in stretched lung cells, such as human alveolar macrophages.[98] or cell lines such as A549 epithelial cells,[99] was the chemokine interleukin-8 or its rodent equivalent MIP-2. The release of MIP-2 may explain the recruitment of neutrophils that occurs during subacute VILI.[11,100,101] Leukocyte sequestration during injurious ventilation strategies seems to be the result of polymorphonuclear stiffening and mediated by L-selectin–dependent but CD18 (β_2-integrin)-independent mechanisms.[102] Leukocyte migration across the lung endothelial layer in response to interleukin-8 probably does

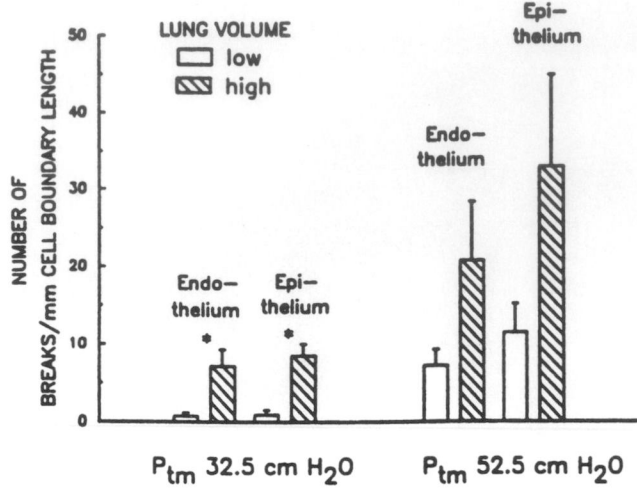

P_{tm} 32.5 cm H$_2$O P_{tm} 52.5 cm H$_2$O

FIGURE 42-12 Effect of lung inflation on capillary stress failure. In-situ rabbit lungs subjected to a capillary transmural pressure of 32.5 cmH$_2$O had more endothelial and epithelial breaks at high lung volume (transpulmonary pressure of 20 cmH$_2$O) than at low lung volume (transpulmonary pressure of 5 cmH$_2$O). (*Reproduced, with permission, from Fu et al.[64]*)

not involve the integrin route.[103] Belperio et al[97] have shown that inhibition of the chemokine interaction with the CXCR2 receptor attenuates neutrophil sequestration and lung injury after 6 hours of high-volume ventilation in mice. Residual abnormalities may thus result from direct mechanical injury, the release of yet unidentified mediators, or the involvement of other receptors. Studies in Clara-cell-protein–deficient mice and the use of calcium-dependent phospholipase A2 (cPLA2) inhibitor suggest that cPLA2 activation is implicated during VILI development, and that Clara cell protein may have a protective effect through inhibition of the enzyme activity.[84] Release of nitric oxide may also be involved because inhibition of nitric oxide synthase by N(G)-nitro-L-arginine methyl ester (L-NAME) reduced the microvascular leak in isolated rabbit lungs subjected to high-PIP ventilation.[104] It is worth noting that the ultrastructural abnormalities observed after high-volume ventilation[6] are similar to those seen during increased endothelial nitric oxide production.[105]

Whether neutrophil recruitment alone is sufficient to produce VILI or it merely accompanies mechanical injury and is a participant is still a subject of debate[91] because of the poor reproducibility of experimental observations. Leukocyte activation, however, is an unlikely explanation for the major vascular leakage observed during high-inflation edema because the speed with which permeability and ultrastructural alterations develop[7] is not consistent with such a mechanism. Besides, the potent proinflammatory mediators, TNF-α and MIP-2, are unlikely to be involved in the acute lung injury consecutive to high-volume ventilation[93] for two reasons. First, there was no correlation between the flux of albumin in alveolar spaces (as reflected by its concentration in bronchoalveolar lavage fluid) and MIP-2 (or interleukin-6) concentration in this fluid. Second, authors did not detect TNF-α in bronchoalveolar lavage fluid in any

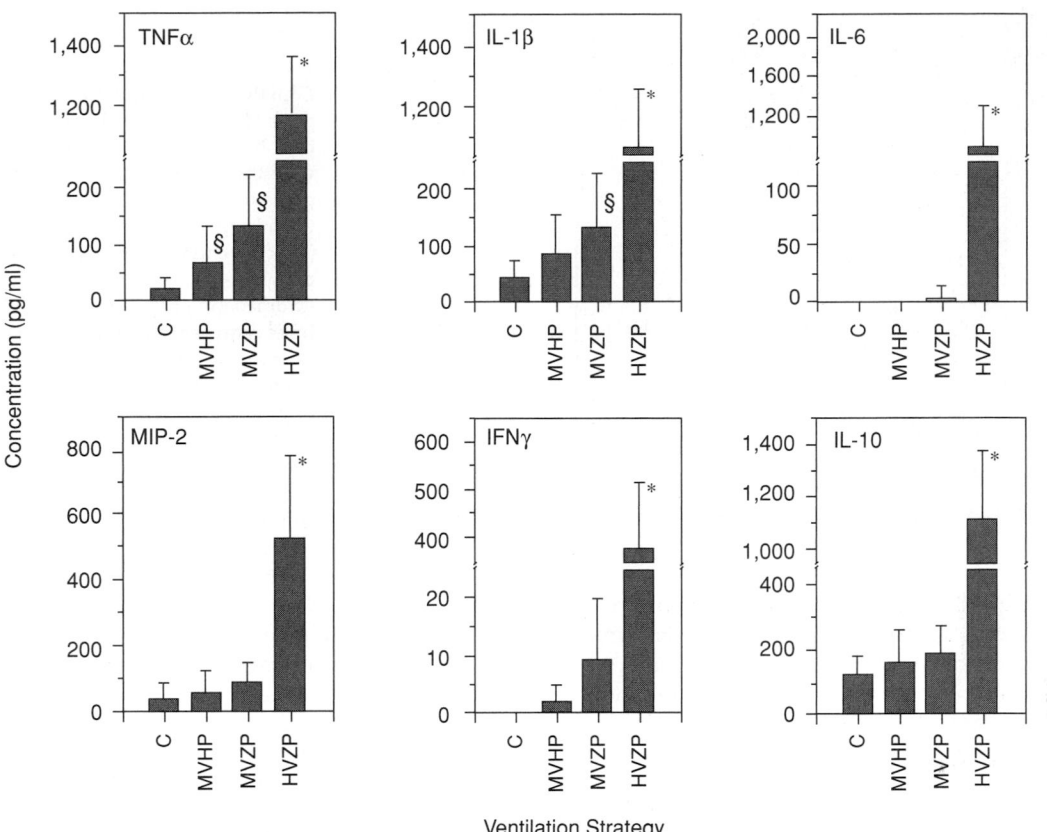

FIGURE 42-13 Effect of different ventilator strategies on cytokine concentrations in lung lavage of isolated unperfused rat lungs. Four ventilator settings were used: controls (*C*, normal tidal volume), moderate tidal volume + high PEEP (*MVHP*), moderate tidal volume + zero PEEP (*MVZP*), high tidal volume + zero PEEP (*HVZP*) resulting in the same end-inspiratory distension as MVHP. Major increases in cytokine concentrations were observed with HVZP. (*Reproduced, with permission, from Tremblay et al.*[89])

intact mouse model that developed pulmonary edema after lung overinflation, and the absence of TNF-α receptors did not preclude the development of acute VILI.[93] These observations confirm that two different types of VILI exist: acute VILI that follows marked overexpansion, and subacute VILI in which inflammatory phenomena prevail.

In addition to increasing the amount of cytokines in the lung, it has been suspected that overinflation during mechanical ventilation may promote the release of cytokines[92,106] or bacteria[107–109] into the blood, thus suggesting that mechanical ventilation plays a causative role in multiorgan dysfunction.[110,111] This hypothesis, however, remains to be proven.[112] The possibility that a pulmonary or systemic inflammatory state might modulate the release of lung mediators during high-PIP ventilation has been put forward to try to explain the discrepancy between observations made in different laboratories under the same experimental conditions.[91] Higher levels of proinflammatory cytokines (TNF-α, interleukin-1β, and MIP-2) were found in lung homogenates of rats ventilated for 2 hours with high PIP when they were previously subjected to mesenteric ischemia-reperfusion.[113] This suggests the validity of the "two-hit" hypothesis, which is that a pre-existing inflammatory state would augment cytokine release during VILI. The combination, however, of intratracheal instillation of endotoxin and high-volume ventilation ex vivo resulted

in less cytokine (TNF-α and MIP-2) release by the lung than did endotoxin alone.[114]

Finally, independently of the occurrence of acute pulmonary edema, activation of several genes involved in inflammatory response was observed during protracted lung stretch[115] or in alveolar epithelial cells.[116]

Determinants of Ventilator-Induced Injury

RESPECTIVE ROLES OF INCREASED AIRWAY PRESSURE AND INCREASED LUNG VOLUME

High inspiratory pressures consistently result in high lung volumes in normal animals. They, however, induce well-documented hemodynamic changes in the systemic circulation[117] and may potentially affect blood flow distribution in the lungs because parts of the lungs are placed under zone 1 condition over the ventilatory cycle. Another possibility is that high pressures per se produce regional distortions that may result in specific deleterious effects. Several studies have been conducted to determine the relative roles of intrathoracic pressure increases and lung distension in the genesis of pulmonary edema.

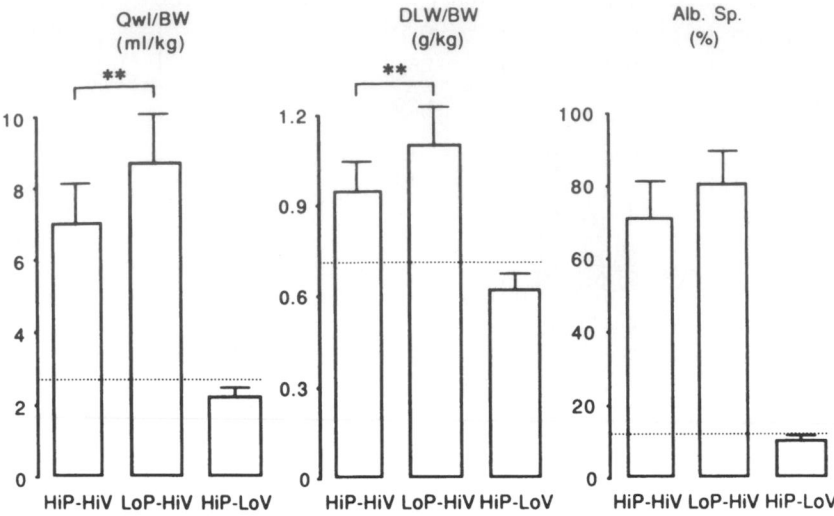

FIGURE 42-14 Comparison of the effects of high peak (45 cmH$_2$O) positive inspiratory pressure plus high-tidal-volume ventilation (HiP-HiV) with the effects of negative inspiratory airway pressure plus high-tidal-volume ventilation (iron lung ventilation; LoP-HiV) and of high peak (45 cmH$_2$O) positive inspiratory pressure plus low-tidal-volume ventilation (thoracoabdominal strapping; HiP-LoV). Dotted lines represent the upper 95% confidence limit for control values. See Fig. 42–6 for details on edema indexes. Permeability edema occurred in both groups receiving high-tidal-volume ventilation. Animals ventilated with a high peak pressure and a normal tidal volume had no edema. (*Reproduced, with permission, from Dreyfuss et al.*[51])

High-volume ventilation with low airway pressures was obtained by ventilating closed-chest rats with intermittent negative perithoracic pressures (using an iron lung). Ventilation with high airway pressures but low tidal volumes was obtained with thoracoabdominal strapping to limit thoracic movements. The effects of high PIP plus high-tidal-volume ventilation were compared with those of intermittent negative airway pressure plus high-tidal-volume ventilation and intermittently positive high PIP plus low-tidal-volume ventilation.[51] Pulmonary edema of the permeability type occurred in both groups of rats that received high-tidal-volume ventilation, irrespective of inspiratory pressure (i.e., positive or negative; Fig. 42-14). In both groups, electron microscopic examination disclosed the same abnormalities as those described above. In striking contrast with these findings, animals ventilated with a high PIP but a normal tidal volume had no edema (see Fig. 42-14) and no ultrastructural changes. These findings have been replicated in rabbits[118] and lambs.[14]

ROLES OF THE MAGNITUDE OF PRESSURE-VOLUME CHANGES AND OF DURATION OF THE CHALLENGE

IS THERE A PRESSURE-VOLUME THRESHOLD FOR THE OCCURRENCE OF EDEMA AND PERMEABILITY ALTERATIONS?

A threshold volume for permeability changes as the lung is overexpanded was suggested by Carlton et al[14] These authors studied the effects of graded increases in tidal volume on lymph flow and protein concentrations in lambs. Peak inspiratory pressure (and therefore tidal volume) was increased in three successive steps (each lasting 4 hours) from baseline (16 cmH$_2$O) to 61 cmH$_2$O. During the first two steps (33 and 43 cmH$_2$O PIP), no changes in lymph flow or protein composition were observed. In contrast, when the highest PIP was reached (corresponding to a tidal volume of 57 ml/kg), lung lymph flow increased four- to sixfold compared with baseline. Similarly, the lymph–plasma protein concentration ratio did not change until the high-

est PIP was reached, at which time it increased significantly compared with controls. The investigators concluded that microvascular alterations in response to overinflation occurred beyond a pressure threshold rather than gradually as pressure increased. They pointed out, however, that the albumin-globulin ratio in lymph versus plasma decreased before maximum PIP was reached, suggesting altered protein sieving and probably abnormal microvascular permeability. Although not specifically discussed in the report, this finding may indicate either that the pressure threshold was lower than the maximum value studied or that no threshold existed. In smaller species, such as rats, in which (as discussed above) VILI occurs more rapidly, edema was demonstrated with a PIP as low as 30 cmH$_2$O, provided ventilation was sufficiently prolonged.[5] Tsuno et al[53] demonstrated that ventilation of sheep with a PIP of 30 cmH$_2$O (corresponding to a tidal volume of 30 ml/kg, roughly comparable to the conditions used by Carlton et al[14]) for more than 40 hours invariably resulted in gross pathologic alterations and an increase in wet-lung weight, findings consistent with the absence of a true pressure threshold.

These studies further emphasize that, in addition to the degree of distension, duration of lung overexpansion is crucial in determining the severity of pulmonary edema (but perhaps not the type, as discussed below). Interestingly, the possibility of a potential pressure-volume threshold for additional lung injury during mechanical ventilation of patients with acute lung injury is also debated. This will be discussed in the section devoted to the clinical relevance of experimental findings.

RESPECTIVE CONTRIBUTIONS OF SUSTAINED INFLATION (POSITIVE END-EXPIRATORY PRESSURE) AND LARGE PRESSURE-VOLUME SWINGS

For the same level of overall lung inflation, increasing FRC by PEEP (and thus reducing tidal volume) results in less severe alterations, the reasons for which may be reduction

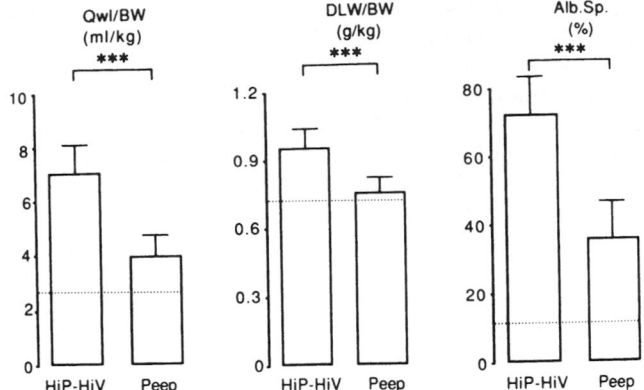

FIGURE 42-15 Effect of 10 cmH$_2$O PEEP during high peak (45 cmH$_2$O) positive inspiratory pressure plus high-tidal-volume ventilation. Dotted lines represent the upper 95% confidence limits for control values. See Fig. 42-6 for details on edema indexes. With PEEP, edema was less marked. (*Reproduced, with permission, from Dreyfuss et al.[51]*)

of V$_T$ at the same respiratory rate, and hence of peak inspiratory flow, or stabilization of terminal units.

It has been proposed that high gas flow rates during inspiration may per se have deleterious effects.[119] The effect of varying peak inspiratory flow was studied in rabbits ventilated with 30 ml/kg tidal volume for 6 hours at 20 breaths/minute and the same plateau pressure. Animals with the highest peak inspiratory flow rate had significantly more gas-exchange deterioration, fall in respiratory system compliance, and macroscopic and microscopic lung injury.[120] Similarly, reduction of inspiratory flow resulted in less lung injury[121] in a model of high-PIP (50 cmH$_2$O) ventilation in sheep. High inflationary flow rate may also worsen inflammation during VILI when no PEEP is applied in open-chest rabbits (that collapse below normal FRC at end-expiration); this effect has been ascribed to increased shear stress during the cyclic opening and closing of peripheral airways.[122]

Webb et al showed that, for a given level of teleinspiratory pressure (i.e., overall level of pressure), edema was less severe when a 10-cmH$_2$O PEEP was applied.[5] It was subsequently shown[51] that, although the amount of edema fluid was smaller (Fig. 42-15) with PEEP, permeability alterations were similar to those observed with zero end-expiratory pressure (ZEEP). When rats were ventilated with PEEP, however, less edema occurred and, in particular, no alveolar flooding was observed on light microscopy.[5,51] More strikingly, whereas diffuse alveolar damage was present in the animals ventilated with ZEEP, no epithelial-cell lining alterations were observed on electron microscopic examination of the lungs of animals ventilated with PEEP. The only ultrastructural alterations consisted of endothelial blebbing. It is worth noting that PEEP decreases lung capillary blood volume,[123] which in turn may lessen the capillary permeability alterations caused by high-PIP ventilation.[124]

This preservation of the alveolar-epithelial layer has received no satisfactory explanation. It may be that PEEP eliminated repetitive opening and closing of terminal airways, thereby decreasing shear stress at this level. Alternatively,

avoidance of alveolar flooding by PEEP[125,126] may have protected the epithelial lining from injury through the effects of yet unidentified humoral mediators.

One of the effects of PEEP is to reduce tidal volume for a given end-inspiratory pressure. It is interesting to note that studies using in-situ perfused canine lobes[127] found that, for equivalent perfusion-flow rates and microvascular hydrostatic pressures, the rate of hydrostatic edema formation increased with tidal volume. When an identical increase in mean airway pressure was achieved either by applying PEEP or by increasing tidal volume, edema was less marked under the former condition, suggesting that large cyclic changes in lung volume promote the development of edema. This explanation was also put forward by Corbridge et al,[128] who observed in hydrochloric acid–injured dog lungs that ventilation with a large tidal volume and a low PEEP resulted in more severe edema than did ventilation with a small tidal volume and a high PEEP. Finally, the potential role of hemodynamic alterations during PEEP ventilation should also be considered. For instance, rats ventilated with 45 cmH$_2$O PIP and 10 cmH$_2$O PEEP had more edema when PEEP-induced hemodynamic alterations were corrected by dopamine administration (Fig. 42-16).[129]

FIGURE 42-16 Effect of hemodynamic support with dopamine during 45-cmH$_2$O peak pressure ventilation with 10-cmH$_2$O PEEP on the amount of edema as evaluated by extravascular lung water. Compared with animals ventilated with 45 cmH$_2$O peak pressure and ZEEP, animals ventilated with 45 cmH$_2$O peak pressure ventilation with 10 cmH$_2$O PEEP had less edema. This reduction of edema associated with PEEP was partly abolished when dopamine was administered. ** $= p < .01$. (*Adapted, with permission, from Dreyfuss et al.[129]*)

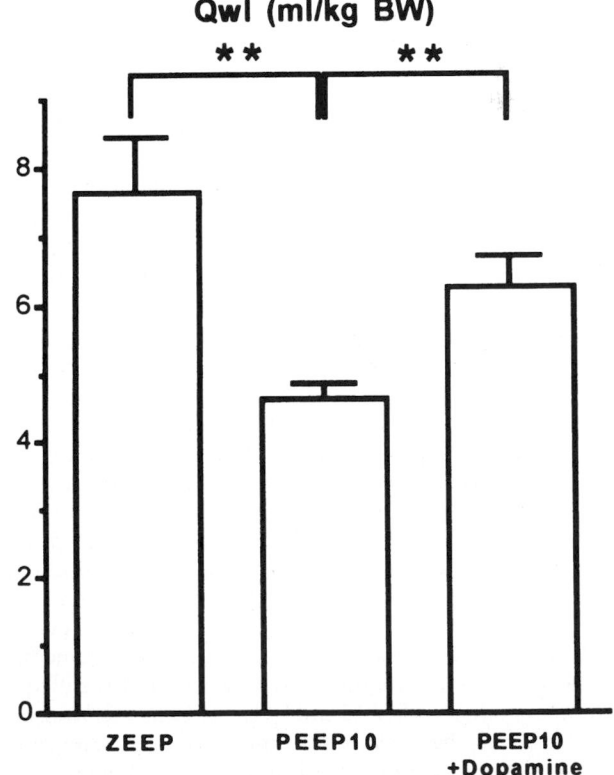

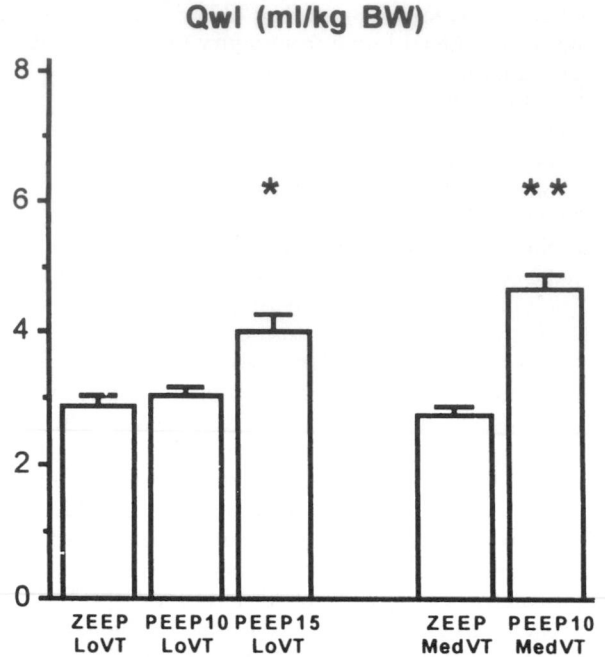

FIGURE 42-17 Effect of increasing PEEP from 0 to 15 cmH$_2$O during ventilation with two levels of tidal volume (7 ml/kg of body weight = LoVT; 14 ml/kg of body weight = MedVT). When PEEP was increased, pulmonary edema (as evaluated by extravascular lung water increases) occurred. The level of PEEP required to produce edema varied with tidal volume; 15 cmH$_2$O PEEP during ventilation with a low tidal volume produced less edema than 10 cmH$_2$O PEEP during ventilation with a moderately increased tidal volume. * = $p < .05$; ** = $p < .01$ versus ZEEP and the same VT. (*Reproduced, with permission, from Dreyfuss et al.*[129])

Moreover, arterial blood pressure was found to be significantly correlated with the amount of pulmonary edema under such conditions. The reason why use of PEEP during ventilation with high PIP is associated with reductions in both the amount of edema and the severity of cell damage may be a combination of hemodynamic alterations, shear stress reduction, and surfactant modifications. It should be borne in mind that this beneficial effect of PEEP during overinflation edema contrasts with the usual lack of reduction or even increase in edema reported with PEEP in most forms of experimental pulmonary edema.[130] Moreover, prophylactic application of expiratory positive airway pressure (a form of PEEP) did not reduce edema formation during oleic acid injury.[131] It would be inappropriate to conclude from the data summarized above that tidal volume, which governs opening and closing of terminal units, is the sole determinant of VILI. On the contrary, the overall degree of lung distension (i.e., teleinspiratory volume) is probably the crucial factor. Hence, rats ventilated with a tidal volume within the physiologic range at two levels of PEEP (10 and 15 cmH$_2$O) developed pulmonary edema only at the higher level of PEEP (Fig. 42-17).[129] Similarly, doubling tidal volume had no effect in animals ventilated with ZEEP, but resulted in pulmonary edema when 10 cmH$_2$O PEEP was used (see Fig. 42-17).[129] Thus, the safety of small tidal volumes depends on whether or not FRC is increased, and raising end-inspiratory

volume by increasing FRC may cause lung injury independently of tidal volume.[129]

It is now clear that VILI occurs whenever a certain degree of lung overinflation is reached, by whatever means. For a given level of teleinspiratory pressure (and volume), adjunct use of PEEP seems to slow the development or diminish the severity of alterations[132] but does not prevent the occurrence of permeability pulmonary edema.[51,129]

Effects of Ventilation on Previously Injured Lungs

This chapter does not consider lung prematurity, which is discussed in Chapter 25.

COMBINATION OF HIGH-VOLUME HIGH-PRESSURE VENTILATION AND PREVIOUS INJURY

THE ROLE OF LUNG MECHANICAL PROPERTIES ON SUSCEPTIBILITY TO VENTILATOR-INDUCED LUNG INJURY

The aforementioned studies were conducted on animals with healthy lungs. It is conceivable, however, that diseased lungs may be more susceptible than healthy lungs to the deleterious effects of mechanical ventilation. Diseased lungs with a patchy distribution of lesions may be subjected to considerably greater regional stress than homogeneously inflated lungs. As stressed by Mead et al, the pressure tending to expand an atelectatic region surrounded by a fully expanded lung is approximately 140 cmH$_2$O at a transpulmonary pressure of 30 cmH$_2$O.[133]

Bowton et al[134] showed that oleic acid–injured, isolated rabbit lungs ventilated with a high tidal volume of 18 ml/kg had a significantly greater weight gain than lungs ventilated with a small tidal volume of 6 ml/kg. Hernandez et al[135] showed that whereas low doses of oleic acid or 25-cmH$_2$O PIP mechanical ventilation did not affect filtration coefficient and wet-dry ratio, the combination of the two did (Fig. 42-18). The same group also reported that the filtration coefficient increase observed during high-PIP (30 to 45 cmH$_2$O) ventilation of isolated perfused rabbit lungs was more marked following inactivation of surfactant by dioctyl succinate instillation.[136] Moreover, whereas light microscopic examination showed only mild abnormalities (minimal hemorrhage and vascular congestion) in the animals subjected to ventilation only or surfactant inactivation only, the combination of surfactant inactivation and ventilation caused severe damage (extensive hemorrhage, pulmonary edema, and hyaline membranes). Thus, ventilator-induced lung edema seems to develop at lower airway pressures in lungs with pre-existing injury. These studies were performed in isolated lungs in which chemical and ventilator results may not have the same consequences as in intact animals. Lung injury is usually inhomogenous. The more compliant zones will thus receive the bulk of ventilation, which may favor their overinflation, a localized "baby lung effect." Analysis of the pressure-volume curve may help understand how pre-existing lung injury may interact with ventilator-induced injury. Before

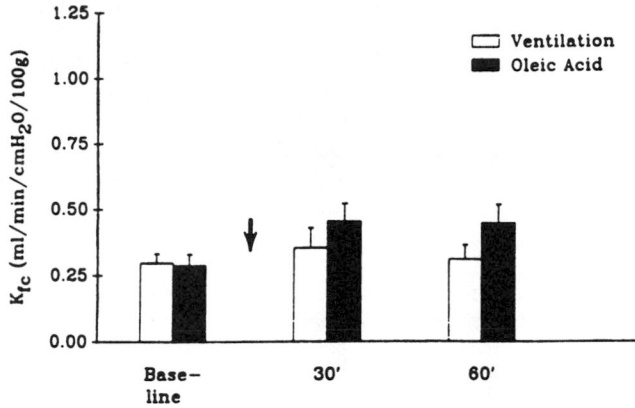

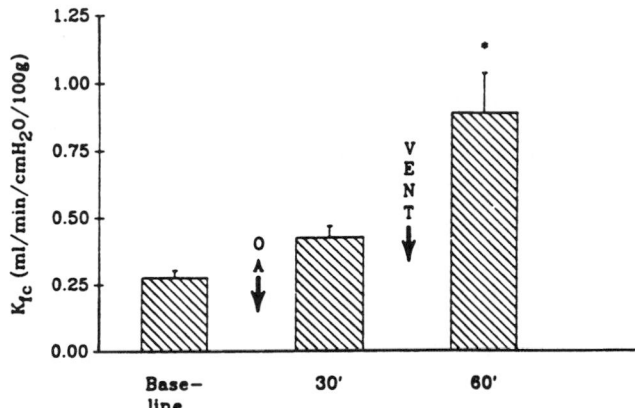

FIGURE 42-18 Effect of single and combined insults on the filtration coefficient of isolated rabbit lungs. A low dose of oleic acid or a moderately high peak pressure (24 cmH$_2$O) alone failed to induce capillary filtration coefficient (K$_{fc}$) changes, whereas the combination of both insults was responsible for a significant increase in K$_{fc}$. (*Reproduced, with permission, from Hernandez et al.[135]*)

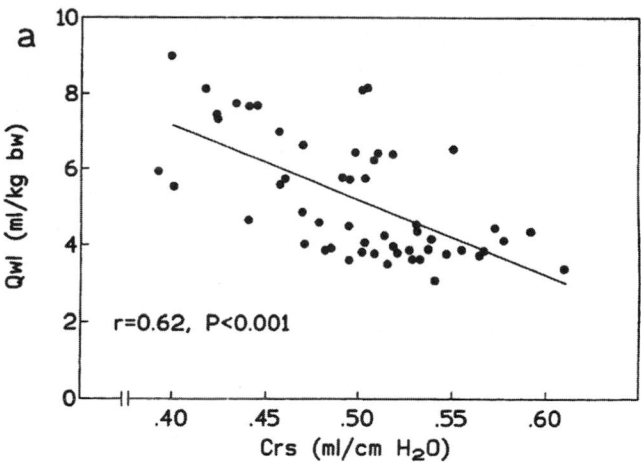

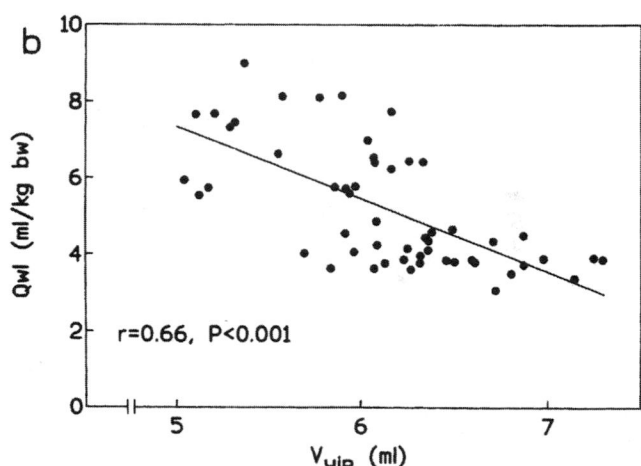

FIGURE 42-19 *a*. Correlation between the amount of edema (extravascular lung water, *Qwl*) produced by high-volume ventilation and the respiratory system compliance (*Crs*) measured before high-volume ventilation. *b*. Correlation between Qwl and the volume at the upper inflection point on the pressure-volume curve (*Vuip*) measured before high-volume ventilation. (*Reproduced, with permission, from Martin-Lefevre et al.[141]*).

examining this interaction, it is important to understand how lung mechanical properties are modified by lung injury.

The upper inflection point (UIP) often seen on the respiratory system inspiratory pressure-volume curve in patients with ARDS has been interpreted as reflecting the beginning of overinflation,[137,138] or the end of recruitment.[139,140] Whether ventilation, however, that results in pressure-volume excursions above the UIP is deleterious is unsettled. Better understanding of UIP significance is required before it can be used to set tidal volume in patients. A recent experimental study examined the hypothesis that pulmonary edema development alters the pressure-volume curve of the respiratory system mainly because of distal airway obstruction,[141] and this reduction in ventilatable lung volume (the baby lung effect) may not only decrease compliance,[142,143] but also affects UIP position. When the distal airways of rats were obstructed by instilling a viscous liquid, the changes in the shape of the pressure-volume

curve (gradual decrease in compliance, the volume at which UIP was seen, and progressive increase in end-inspiratory pressure) were very similar to the changes seen during the development of pulmonary edema. The higher the compliance and volume of the UIP, the lesser was the edema observed after high-PIP ventilation (Fig. 42-19). Taken together, these results suggest that the position of the UIP is a marker of the amount of ventilatable lung volume, and it is both influenced by, and predictive of, the development of edema during mechanical ventilation.

The effect of high-PIP ventilation on injured lungs in intact animals was investigated by comparing different degrees of lung distension in rats whose lungs had been injured by α-naphthylthiourea (ANTU).[144] ANTU infusion alone caused moderate interstitial pulmonary edema of the permeability type. Mechanical ventilation resulted in a permeability edema, the severity of which depended on the tidal volume amplitude. It was possible to calculate the extent to which mechanical ventilation theoretically injures lungs

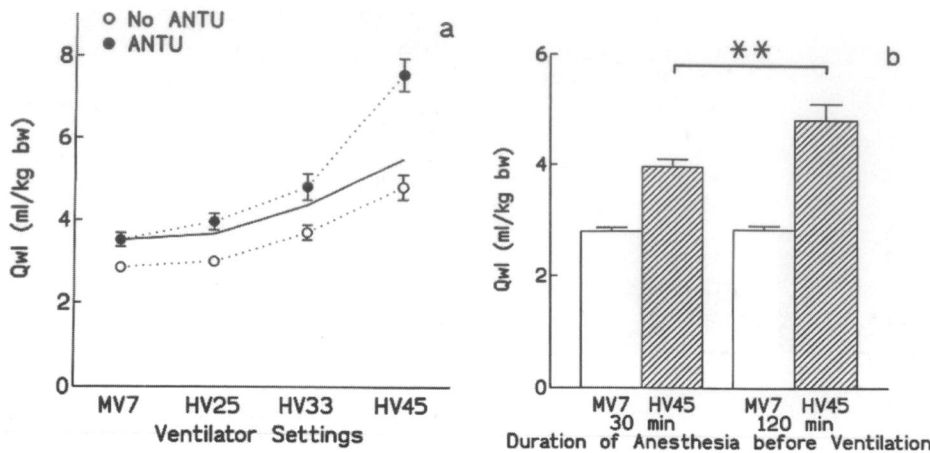

FIGURE 42-20 Interaction between previous lung alterations and mechanical ventilation on pulmonary edema. *a.* Effect of previous toxic lung injury. Extravascular lung water (*Qwl*) after mechanical ventilation in normal rats (*open circles*) and in rats with mild lung injury produced by α-naphthylthiourea (ANTU) (*closed circles*). Tidal volume (V_T) varied from 7 to 45 ml/kg body weight. The solid line represents the Qwl value expected for the aggravating effect of ANTU on edema caused by ventilation, assuming additivity. ANTU did not potentiate the effect of ventilation with V_T up to 33 ml/kg body weight. In contrast, V_T 45 ml/kg body weight produced an increase in edema that greatly exceeded additivity, indicating synergy between the two insults. *b.* Effect of lung functional alteration by prolonged anesthesia. Intact rats were anesthetized and breathed spontaneously for 30 to 120 minutes before ventilation with V_T 7 ml/kg body weight (*open bars*) or 45 ml/kg body weight (*shaded bars*). Qwl of animals ventilated with a high V_T was significantly higher than in animals ventilated with a normal V_T. Qwl was not affected by the duration of anesthesia in animals ventilated with a normal V_T. In contrast, 120 minutes of anesthesia before high-V_T ventilation resulted in a larger increase in Qwl than did 30 minutes of anesthesia (** $p < 0.01$). (*Reproduced, with permission, from Dreyfuss et al.[144]*).

diseased by ANTU by adding the separate effect of mechanical ventilation alone or ANTU alone on edema severity (Fig. 42-20). The lungs of the animals injured by ANTU ventilated at high PIP (45 ml/kg body weight) had more severe permeability edema than predicted (see Fig. 42-20), indicating synergy between the two insults. Even minor alterations, such as those produced by spontaneous ventilation during prolonged anesthesia (which degrades surfactant activity and promotes focal atelectasis), were sufficient to synergistically increase the harmful effects of high-volume ventilation.[144] The extent to which lung mechanical properties deteriorate before ventilation is a key factor in this synergy. The amount of pulmonary edema produced by high-volume ventilation in animals given ANTU, or that had undergone prolonged anesthesia, was inversely proportional to the respiratory system compliance measured at the very beginning of mechanical ventilation.[141,144] The same conclusions were reached about the volume of UIP.[141]

The reason for this synergy requires clarification. Local alveolar flooding in animals subjected to the most harmful ventilation protocol was the most striking difference from animals ventilated with lower, less harmful, tidal volumes.[144] It is conceivable that edema foam in airways reduced the number of alveoli that received the tidal volume, exposing them to overinflation and rendering them more susceptible to injury, further reducing the aerated lung volume. The result is a positive feedback loop. The same reasoning applies to prolonged anesthesia, during which the aerated lung volume was probably gradually reduced by atelectasis. To explore this possibility, alveolar flooding was produced by instilling saline into the tracheas of rats that were immediately ventilated with tidal volumes of up

to 33 ml/kg.[145] Flooding with saline did not significantly affect microvascular permeability when tidal volume was low. As tidal volume was increased, capillary permeability alterations were larger in flooded than in intact animals, reflecting further impairment of their endothelial barrier (Fig. 42-21). There was also a correlation between end-inspiratory airway pressure and capillary permeability alterations in flooded animals ventilated with a high tidal volume. Thus, the less compliant and recruitable the lung was after saline flooding, the more severe were the changes in permeability caused by lung distension.

These studies support the conclusion that the risk of overinflation is more significant in diseased than in healthy lungs. Strategies to prevent VILI should oppose the synergy between ventilation and previous lung injury.

DOES VENTILATION WITHOUT OVERINFLATION AGGRAVATE PREVIOUS LUNG INJURY?

EFFECT OF POSITIVE END-EXPIRATORY PRESSURE
It has been suggested that mechanical ventilation may worsen lung injury because of increased shear stress in distal airspaces secondary to their repeated closing, either because of obstruction by liquid menisci or collapse and reopening. Coker et al[136] reported that the capillary filtration coefficient of isolated perfused rabbit lungs was not modified by either ventilation at 15 cmH$_2$O PIP (which results in much larger tidal volumes in isolated lungs than in intact animals) or surfactant inactivation, but doubled the coefficient when the two insults were combined. Several studies have investigated the effects of conventional ventilation on acutely

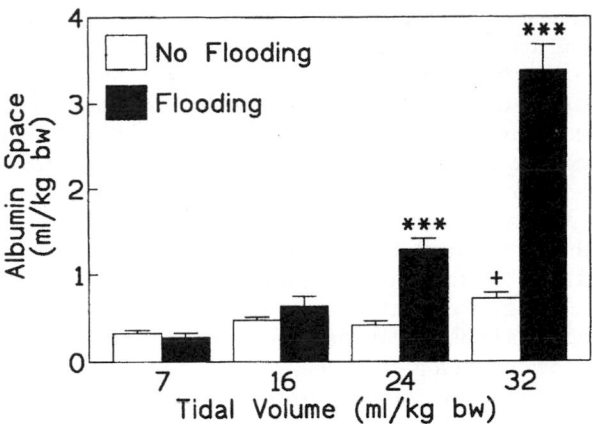

FIGURE 42-21 Effect of increasing tidal volume (VT) during mechanical ventilation for 10 minutes on lung capillary permeability (i.e., extravascular albumin distribution space in lungs) of rats with intact lungs (*open bars*) or with alveolar flooding (*closed bars*) produced by saline instillation. There was a moderate increase in albumin space in intact rats at the larger VT. Lung flooding did not produce significant increases of albumin space when VT was normal or moderately increased. Albumin space was significantly increased with a VT of 24 and 32 ml/kg body weight. The increase in albumin space greatly exceeded additivity, indicating a positive interaction between the two insults. (***$p < 0.001$ as compared with intact animals). (*Reproduced, with permission, from Dreyfuss et al.[145]*).

injured lungs by using sufficiently high PEEP levels to keep the small airways open throughout the entire ventilatory cycle, thereby avoiding repeated closure and reopening.

Most of the available data on this issue were generated by Sykes et al,[146,147] who studied the effect of ventilation in rabbits with surfactant-depleted lungs. The animals were ventilated with a PIP ranging from 15 mmHg at the beginning of the experiment to 25 mmHg at the end (5 hours later) because of the fall in lung compliance (tidal volume was not stated); PEEP was adjusted to position the FRC either above or below the lower inflection point (LIP). Mortality rate was not influenced by PEEP level, although partial arterial oxygen tension (Pa$_{O_2}$) was better preserved in the high-PEEP group.[146,147] There was less hyaline membrane formation in animals ventilated with high PEEP than in animals ventilated with low PEEP. This lessening of pathologic alterations was observed even with ventilator settings that achieved identical mean airway pressures in the low- and high-PEEP groups.[147] Comparable results were reported in isolated, nonperfused, lavaged rabbit lungs ventilated with a low tidal volume and with a level of PEEP set either below or above the LIP.[148] It is noteworthy that Sykes et al could not replicate the same findings in hydrochloric acid–injured rabbit lungs using the same ventilator settings.[149] Thus, it is conceivable that the protective effect of PEEP, when set above the LIP of the pressure-volume curve, is observed only in the very special setting of surfactant deficiency and not during severe alveolar edema, because lung instability and airspace collapse is observed only during the former.

Using in-vivo videomicroscopy, Nieman et al[150–154] directly observed and quantified the dynamic changes in alveolar size, throughout the ventilatory cycle during tidal ventilation, in normal lungs and in lungs in which surfactant had been deactivated by Tween. These injuries occurred independently of the presence of neutrophils.[150] In normal lungs, alveoli never collapsed. These findings agree with the previous findings of Bachofen et al, who showed that alveoli do not change volume appreciably during ventilation.[155] Collapse, and reopening and increase in the alveolar size at end-inspiration were observed in surfactant-deactivated lungs. In a subsequent study, the same authors documented the effect of increasing end-expiratory pressure.[154] The application of PEEP to a surfactant-deactivated lung reversed the observed increase in alveolar size, returning it to control levels .

The reality of the repetitive opening and closure of terminal units and the significance of the LIP on the pressure-volume curve have been recently challenged by Martynowicz et al[156] They studied the regional expansion of oleic acid–injured lungs using a parenchymal marker technique. The gravitational distribution of volume at FRC was not affected by oleic acid injury, and the injury was not associated with decreased parenchymal volume of dependent regions. In addition, temporal inhomogeneity of regional tidal expansion did not increase with oleic acid injury. These findings do not support the hypothesis that a superimposed gravitational pressure gradient during VILI produces compression atelectasis of dependent lung, which in turn produces shear injury from cyclic recruitment and collapse.[156] They propose that the occurrence of a LIP on the pressure-volume curve represents the transition from the liquid-filled state to the air-filled state, then the lung is initially filled with a liquid with constant surface tension properties.[157] Thus, abrupt expansion of distal lung units is unlikely to occur at the LIP.

The protective effect of PEEP, however, is not restricted to the particular setting of surfactant depletion.[5,6,132] Distal airspace damage during tidal ventilation may occur because of repeated airway opening and closing secondary to the movement of foam with increased surface tension[158] or the rupture of liquid menisci. PEEP may prevent diffuse lung damage during prolonged ventilation by stabilizing these units.[159] The beneficial effect of PEEP, however, is variable in different models of lung injury.[160] The difficulty in proving whether or not PEEP exerts a protective effect on VILI may be explained by taking into account the distinction between atelectatic and fluid-filled distal airways when interpreting LIP. In the case of diffuse filling of distal airways with liquid, VILI may be caused by overdistension of already aerated zones rather than by shear stress secondary to opening of collapsed zones.[161] With this scenario, it would be difficult to expect any reduction of injury by PEEP.

This uncertainty about the actual occurrence of injury at low lung volumes contrasts with the unambiguous demonstration of high-volume (overdistension) injury. This uncertainty has a clinical counterpart. A reduction in tidal volume was associated with improved ARDS survival,[1] but it was not possible to demonstrate the superiority of high PEEP over more conventional PEEP during mechanical ventilation of ARDS.[162] This will be further discussed in the section devoted to the clinical relevance of experimental findings.

Effect on Remote Organs

The observation that long-lasting injurious ventilation results in lung inflammation in vivo[11] led to the hypothesis that it might promote or aggravate a systemic inflammatory state and predispose to multiple organ failure through the release of inflammatory mediators in the circulation.[110] The effects of injurious ventilation on inflammatory mediator release by the lungs and the possible systemic diffusion of mediators from lungs to systemic circulation are discussed above.

A few experimental studies have evaluated the consequences of injurious ventilation on peripheral organs. Choi et al[163] found that rats ventilated with high PIP for 2 hours had increased expression of endothelial nitric oxide synthase in lung and kidney tissue and increased microvascular permeability in both organs. Nitric oxide was probably involved in these abnormalities, because N-nitro-L-arginine methyl ester administration attenuated the microvascular leak of lung and kidney and the proteinuria. An increase in gut permeability was also observed during a similarly long-lasting ventilation, albeit with larger tidal volume (30 instead of 20 ml/kg), that was attenuated by anti-TNF-α antibody administration.[164] Injurious ventilation of rabbits with hydrochloric acid–induced lung injury resulted in increased rates of epithelial cell apoptosis in the kidney and small intestine villi.[165]

Protection from Ventilation-Induced Lung Injury

STRATEGIES THAT AIM AT IMPROVING LUNG MECHANICS

DOES LUNG REST IMPROVE LUNG INJURY AS COMPARED WITH CONVENTIONAL VENTILATION?
Because mechanical ventilation may be deleterious to injured lungs, techniques have been developed to achieve lung rest either by not ventilating the lungs at all or by using very low-frequency ventilation, as in extracorporeal membrane oxygenation[166] and extracorporeal CO_2 removal.[167] The search for means of avoiding the large pressure-volume swings generated by conventional ventilation led to the development of high-frequency oscillatory ventilation (HFOV) with or without previous "lung conditioning" to open the greatest possible number of lung units by a sigh maneuver.[168] Because other chapters in this book are specially devoted to these ventilator techniques, we discuss them only briefly.

Borelli et al[52] compared continuous positive airway pressure and extracorporeal CO_2 removal with conventional ventilation in sheep following moderate lung injury with high-PIP (50 cmH₂O) ventilation. Animals ventilated with nonconventional means had better outcomes, but no reduction of wet-lung weight was observed. Prevention of hyaline membrane disease in premature lambs has been achieved using apneic ventilation with extracorporeal CO_2 removal.[169] Similarly, Dorrington et al[170] compared apneic

oxygenation combined with total extracorporeal CO_2 removal and conventional ventilation on the 6-hour survival rate of rabbits with saline lavage–induced respiratory failure. Only one out of six rabbits receiving conventional ventilation survived, compared to five of six rabbits in the CO_2 removal group. Because of the small sample size, this difference was not statistically significant. Nevertheless, histological abnormalities seemed less severe in the animals treated with CO_2 removal. In contrast, Yanos et al[171] did not find that such "resting" reduced pulmonary edema. They compared isogravimetric or extravascular thermal water measurements in oleic acid–induced pulmonary edema in dogs after 5 hours of low-frequency reduced tidal volume ventilation with extracorporeal membrane oxygenation or conventional ventilation. Hypopnea had no beneficial effects on edema.

Results with HFOV were also conflicting. Using rabbits with lavage-induced surfactant deficiency, Hamilton et al[172] showed that HFOV, applied after a short period of sustained inflation to recruit alveolar volume, improved gas exchange compared to conventional ventilation and prevented hyaline membrane formation. The same group, however, found that HFOV was not associated with reductions in the severity of microvascular permeability alterations and did not prevent epithelial necrosis or hyaline membrane formation in premature lambs.[173] The authors attributed this failure to the inability of premature lungs to secrete enough surfactant; in contrast, saline lavage may stimulate surfactant synthesis in adult lungs. It has been proposed that HFOV may be associated with reduced barotrauma only if applied after "opening the lungs" by a successful recruitment maneuver (a prolonged "sigh").[168,174]

USE OF PRESSURE-VOLUME CURVES
The importance of lung mechanics in determining susceptibility to VILI is discussed in detail above. Taking the presence and value of a LIP on the pressure-volume curve into account when setting the level of PEEP may lessen VILI in some[146–148] but not all instances.[149] The concept of lung protection against VILI with the setting of a PEEP above the LIP, however, relies on a putative stabilizing effect of PEEP which would abolish the tendency of distal airways to collapse at end-expiration and reopen during the next inspiration. As discussed above, serious criticisms have been raised against this opening and closing theory.[161] This casts doubt on the usefulness of measuring LIP in order to prevent VILI.

The overall degree of lung distension resulting from the settings of both PEEP and tidal volume is a fundamental determinant of VILI, as previously discussed. Although the exact physiologic significance of UIP is debated (see above), it may indicate lung overstretching. Ventilation that takes place above the UIP was found to be markedly deleterious (see Fig. 42-19),[141] as discussed above. Thus, determination of the volume at which the UIP is observed may help reduce the risk of VILI, because it indicates the maximum stretch that the lung can sustain without noticeable damage.[141] Analysis of the airway pressure-time curve during mechanical ventilation with constant flow has also proven useful in determining the stress applied to lungs. Indeed, an upward concavity of the pressure-time curve suggests that compliance decreases as tidal volume is delivered, with resulting high-volume stress.[175] Such a ventilation pattern was associated with histologic lung injury in an isolated, nonperfused, lavaged model of acute lung injury[175] and with overdistension, as attested by CT-scan analysis, of the lungs of intact animals with saline lavage-induced lung injury.[176]

SURFACTANT

Numerous studies have been conducted on the effect of surfactant administration on gas exchange in experimental models of lung injury. In contrast, few experimental studies have specifically addressed the effect of surfactant administration during VILI. Verbrugge et al studied the effect of surfactant administration on lung function and alveolar permeability during high-PIP ventilation in rats.[177] Rats were ventilated for 20 minutes with 45-cmH$_2$O PIP, and received either exogenous surfactant at increasing doses (50, 100, or 200 ml/kg) or an equivalent volume of saline. Lung function was assessed by the Gruenwald index, the amount of active surfactant in bronchoalveolar lavage fluid, and the minimal surface tension of the crude lavage fluid. Lung function was better preserved in rats that received 200 ml/kg exogenous surfactant than in all other ventilated animals. Alveolar permeability, assessed by the Evans blue dye influx, was significantly reduced in animals receiving the highest doses of surfactant.[177] Exogenous surfactant prevented high-volume (20 ml/kg) lung injury in isolated rat lungs, but it did not affect the release of inflammatory cytokines by these lungs during ventilation.[178] In rats receiving lipopolysaccharide by tracheal instillation, however, surfactant pretreatment reduced decompartmentalization of TNF-α from the lungs to the systemic circulation during injurious mechanical ventilation.[179]

PERFLUOROCARBONS

Partial liquid ventilation[180] with perfluorocarbons has been developed during the last decade as an alternative to conventional gas ventilation for the treatment of acute respiratory failure. Several investigators using different models of acute respiratory failure (surfactant depletion, oleic acid, hydrochloric acid, and prematurity) have reported improvement in gas exchange, lung mechanics, and lung histology.[181] Although some investigators have shown a dose-dependent improvement in gas exchange with perflubron (LiquiVent) in a rabbit model of surfactant depletion,[182] others have highlighted the risk of barotrauma (namely pneumothorax) with the use of large volumes of perfluorocarbon combined with high PEEP or increased tidal volume.[183] Until recently, the effect of partial liquid ventilation on VILI has received little attention. Mechanical nonuniformity of diseased lungs may predispose lungs to VILI by overinflation of the more compliant (ventilatable), aerated zones.[144] Perfluorocarbon may reduce this nonuniformity by suppressing air-liquid interfaces and allowing reopening of collapsed or liquid-filled areas.

The effect of perfluorocarbon instillation on hyperinflation-induced lung injury during alveolar flooding was investigated in rats.[145] Saline was instilled into the trachea to mimic alveolar edema and reduce aerated lung volume.

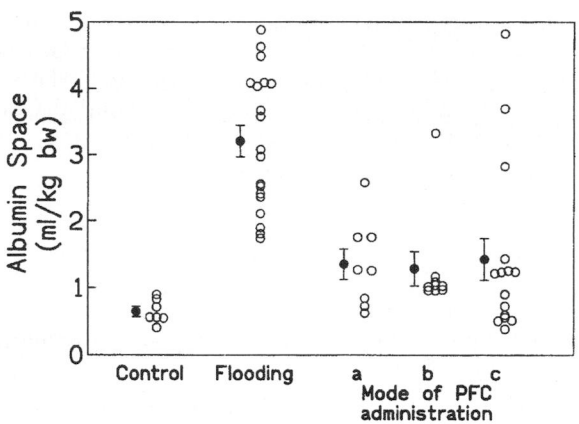

FIGURE 42-22 **Effect of perflubron instillation on permeability pulmonary edema as assessed by the extravascular albumin distribution space in the lungs of rats ventilated with a tidal volume of 33 ml/kg body weight. Flooding significantly increased albumin space ($p < 0.001$). Perflubron given as a bolus (*a*), by slow infusion before flooding (*b*), or as a bolus dose after flooding (*c*) resulted in a significant decrease in albumin space, the values of which remained higher than in controls ($p < 0.05$). Closed circles with error bar indicate means $\pm$ SEM.** (*Reproduced, with permission, from Dreyfuss et al.[145]*).

Alveolar flooding significantly aggravated VILI, as attested by an increase in capillary permeability alterations. Tracheal instillation of a low dose (3.3 ml/kg) of perflubron in these flooded lungs considerably reduced VILI and decreased permeability alterations (Fig. 42-22). Whereas instillation of saline alone raised LIP pressure to values as high as 25 cmH$_2$O, and produced a significant increase in the end-inspiratory pressure, administration of perflubron significantly reduced LIP pressure and normalized end-inspiratory pressure. These decreases were correlated with the lessening of capillary permeability alterations. In some instances, however, perflubron instillation failed to reduce these alterations. Animals in which this occurred had pressures similar to those of animals given saline alone, suggesting that perflubron administration was unable to recruit the flooded areas. Thus in this setting, administration of small doses of perflubron considerably reduced the harmful effects of mechanical ventilation.[145] Nevertheless, the appropriate dose of perfluorocarbon during partial liquid ventilation remains to be determined.

To further investigate the effect of partial liquid ventilation on VILI with respect to the dosage of perfluorocarbon, intact animals received increasing doses of perflubron (from 6 to 20 ml/kg).[184] Hyperinflation-induced pulmonary edema tended to decrease with doses of perflubron lower than 10 ml/kg as compared with animals not given perflubron. By contrast, ventilator-induced pulmonary edema was aggravated in animals given 13 and 16 ml/kg, and even more in animals given 20 ml/kg perflubron. End-inspiratory pressure was significantly correlated with the capillary permeability alterations. In this setting, administration of small doses of perflubron (<10 ml/kg) tended to decrease hyperinflation edema and thus protected lungs against volutrauma.[145] Large doses worsened volutrauma because they increased FRC, thus increasing end-inspiratory volume for the same tidal volume, and because they favored gas trapping in the distal lung. Gas trapping was indeed demonstrated by CT imaging.[184] These observations suggest that monitoring of end-inspiratory pressure might help detect the risk of volutrauma during partial liquid ventilation.

PRONE POSITION

Prone position lessened the deleterious effect of high-PIP ventilation with PEEP in dogs with previous oleic acid lung injury;[185] similar benefit was shown in rabbits[186] and rats.[187] Prone position resulted in a more homogenous distribution of lung injury,[188] an observation that was not confirmed in other studies in rabbits or rats. These differences are probably due to differences in lung size, with a larger lung increasing the influence of gravity. Indeed, CT scans in rats did not disclose a gradient of lung inflation at end-expiration as in humans.[187] In rats, the beneficial effect of prone position was ascribed to a more homogenous distribution of tidal volume and thus of strain, because of the downward displacement of the diaphragm.[187]

PHARMACOLOGIC INTERVENTIONS

Blocking stretch-activated cation channels,[65] inhibiting phosphotyrosine kinase,[67] phosphodiesterase,[67] and calcium-dependent phospholipase A_2[84] reduced the pulmonary capillary permeability alterations caused by high-PIP ventilation. These inhibitions suggest that stretch-induced calcium entry into lung cells and intracellular calcium signaling play an important role in the early response to high-PIP ventilation. Inhibition of nitric oxide synthase[104,163] also lessened ventilator-induced capillary permeability abnormalities.

Ventilation with high tidal volume of isolated mouse lungs for 1 hour resulted in nuclear factor-κB (NF-κB) activation.[189] The amount of cytokines/chemokines, such as TNF-α, interleukin-6, MIP-2, monocyte chemoattractant protein-1, and macrophage inflammatory protein-1α, released in the perfusate was similar to that observed after endotoxin challenge. This early response differed from that caused by endotoxin because it did not implicate toll-like receptor 4. High-PIP ventilation, but not endotoxin caused activation of NF-κB and release of MIP-2 in endotoxin-resistant mice.[189] NF-κB activation was inhibited by dexamethasone.[189] Inhaled carbon monoxide was found to exert anti-inflammatory effects during VILI, via the p38 mitogen-activated protein kinase pathway, but independent of activator protein-1 and NF-κB pathways.[190] Administration of an interleukin-1 receptor antagonist reduced lung albumin, elastase, and neutrophil count; surprisingly, it failed to reduce lung lesions in surfactant-depleted rabbits ventilated with hyperoxia and a high tidal volume.[191] In contrast, administration of an anti-TNF-α antibody via the trachea, but not via the systemic circulation, lessened inflammation in lungs of mice subjected to high-PIP ventilation.[164,192,193] Other pathways are likely to be implicated because VILI can occur independently of TNF-α. Mice with knockout of the TNF receptor had less lung inflammation, but no less release of CXC chemokines (MIP-

2 and keratinocyte-derived chemokine) in bronchoalveolar lavage fluid.[93] Inhibition of MIP-2 activity, by specific antibodies[87] or of the MIP-2 receptor,[97] reduced neutrophil infiltration and lung injury caused by high-PIP ventilation. These observations show that different pathways are involved in VILI development; it is illusory to believe that a single pharmacologic intervention might be beneficial in patients.[91]

HYPERCAPNIA

Ventilator strategies consisting of a low tidal volume to lower the risk of VILI have a positive impact on survival in ARDS.[1] It has been proposed that the hypercapnic acidosis that accompanies a tidal volume reduction may reduce VILI.[194]

Extreme hypoventilation (with Pa_{CO_2} between 150 and 250 mmHg) lessened lung injury in surfactant-depleted rabbits, suggesting a therapeutic role for high Pa_{CO_2}.[195] Studies on isolated rabbit lungs[194] found that hypercapnia lessened the acute (within 30 minutes) increase in endothelial permeability produced by high-PIP ventilation. Other studies in rabbits ventilated for 4 hours showed that hypercapic acidosis lessened neutrophil infiltration and lung injury when tidal volume was high,[196] and also reduced the increases in alveolar-arterial oxygen gradient and airway pressure at a clinically relevant tidal volume.[197] Two other in vivo studies, however, were unable to demonstrate a reduction by hypercapnia of the acute capillary permeability alterations caused by high-tidal-volume ventilation in a rabbit model of surfactant depletion[198] or in intact rats.[199] The latter investigators concluded that hypercapnia probably has a greater influence on late inflammation-dependent phenomena than on acute stress failure.

Studies in isolated rat lungs, however, have shown that hypercapnia lessened lung weight gain and the decrease in compliance during high-tidal-volume ventilation,[200] but the number of subpleural damaged cells, evaluated by confocal microscopy with a membrane impermeant fluorescent tracer, did not differ between normocapnic and hypercapnic lungs. Further, compared to normocapnia, hypercapnia significantly reduced the probability of wound repair in A549 cell cultures.[200] These observations suggest that there is no strong correspondence between the occurrence of cell lesions and the physiologic response of the lung to stretch. They also suggest that the benefit from hypercapnia, if any, may be offset by alterations in the cellular reparation process.[63]

Clinical Relevance

It is clear that microvascular lung injury and pulmonary edema during mechanical ventilation are not the consequences of "barotrauma," but rather of "volutrauma."[51] The main determinant of volutrauma seems to be end-inspiratory volume (the overall lung distension) rather than tidal volume or FRC (which is dependent on the level of PEEP).[129]

It is fascinating to see how the experimental concept of VILI was rapidly translated into a preoccupation of clinicians, as exemplified by the term "ventilator-associated lung injury."[201] Although the validity of this concept could not be directly demonstrated in patients, it formed the rationale beneath all lung protective strategies that aimed to reduce the risk of lung overinflation during ventilation of patients with ARDS. That the lungs in ARDS exhibit significant heterogeneity is well documented,[142,202] and ARDS is a condition that results in uneven distribution of ventilation. Gattinoni et al[142] demonstrated that ARDS lungs include healthy tissue, recruitable tissue, and diseased tissue unresponsive to pressure changes. Healthy units represent as little as 20–30% of total units.[142] These units can be viewed as "baby lung," another term for the "shrunken lung" described by Gibson et al in patients with lung fibrosis.[143] Thus, during conventional ventilator treatment in ARDS, the bulk of ventilation may be directed to healthy units, resulting in regional overdistension, especially when high PIP is required.

Ventilator strategies aimed at reducing the risk of overinflation, such as extracorporeal membrane oxygenation,[166] extracorporeal CO_2 removal,[167] and HFOV[168] were proposed (see Chapters 10, 21 and 22). These techniques are merely experimental (at least in adults) and require special devices and highly trained physicians and nurses. In addition, the lack of demonstrable benefit with extracorporeal CO_2 removal,[203] and the scarcity of data on HFOV in adults[204] preclude their acceptance in many centers. This is in striking contrast to the extraordinarily simple lung protective strategies that accompany permissive hypercapnia.[205] Although caution should be exercised when extrapolating experimental data to clinical situations as complex as infant respiratory distress syndrome or ARDS, the clinical relevance of available experimental data received resounding support with the publication of the ARDS Network study.[1] This study showed that simply reducing tidal volume from 12 ml/kg to 6 ml/kg resulted in a 22% reduction of mortality. The effectiveness of this strategy was attributed to a reduction of lung stress, as attested by markedly decreased airway plateau pressure.[206] The demonstration, however, of a technique to prevent overdistension is difficult. Airway pressure monitoring is easy to perform but cannot completely eliminate the risk of VILI. For instance, application of a continuous distending pressure during HFOV or extracorporeal CO_2 removal may be associated with a gradual increase in lung volume. If the increase in volume is the result of recruitment of previously closed lung units, it is likely to be beneficial, at least in terms of gas exchange, and will probably not cause additional lung damage. On the contrary, failure to recruit closed alveoli may result in overdistension of open alveoli.[207]

Because of the study protocol, the same reduction in tidal volume was employed in all patients allocated to the low-tidal-volume group in the ARDS Network trial.[1] It has, however, been shown repeatedly that the pressure and volume considered safe for some patients with ARDS may cause lung overdistension in others.[137,138,142,208] Conversely, arbitrary settings may result in an unnecessary reduction in tidal volume. As discussed above, information from the inspiratory pressure-volume curve of the respiratory system may be used to tailor ventilator settings, especially when the significance of its particular characteristics (LIP and UIP) are better understood.[141]

Another question that cannot be answered at present is whether or not a threshold tidal volume exists below which experimental VILI or ventilator-associated lung injury in patients does not occur in previously injured lungs. If such a threshold exists, it is unnecessary to drastically reduce tidal volume in all patients as was done in the ARDS Network study,[1] especially in view of possible adverse effects that occur with too great a reduction in tidal volume.[209] In such conditions, staying within the so-called safe limits of plateau pressure[201,206] will be sufficient. In contrast, the absence of such a safe threshold was suggested in the ARDS Network study:[1] mortality was lower in patients with reduced tidal volume independently of static compliance of the respiratory system at baseline. This observation suggests that low tidal volume was advantageous regardless of lung compliance.[1] Notwithstanding, the reduction of mortality by simply reducing end-inspiratory lung stress lends credence to the possibility that end-inspiratory lung volume is the main determinant of volutrauma (as contended at the beginning of this section). Indeed, it was recently suggested that higher tidal volume may be associated with the onset of acute lung injury[210] or ARDS[211] in patients ventilated for other causes of respiratory failure.

In contrast with the experimental and clinical demonstration of the importance of reducing lung stretch by reducing tidal volume, the clinical relevance of the concept of low-lung-volume injury (discussed above) is less obvious. Indeed, there was no difference in survival of patients with ARDS ventilated with higher or lower PEEP levels.[162] The best level of PEEP to apply when ventilating ARDS patients is still unknown.[212]

Improving lung mechanical properties in order to decrease the risk of ventilator-associated lung injury is another option that may combine with protective lung strategies. Two treatments were tested during clinical trials: surfactant administration and partial liquid ventilation. The failure of both strategies could have been predicted on physiologic and experimental grounds.

Administration of surfactant by aerosol[213] or tracheal instillation[214] was not associated with any survival advantage in the treatment of adult patients with ARDS. These treatments failed to improve oxygenation in one study[213] and achieved only mild improvement in another study[214] and were not associated with changes in lung mechanics.[214] It has been suggested that the treatments were not effective in preventing damage caused by lung overstretching or oxygen toxicity, either because the mode of administration was not optimal or because the particular type of surfactant was not physiologically effective in diseased lungs. In contrast, administration of a natural surfactant containing high levels of surfactant-specific protein B in a pediatric population with acute lung injury (premature infants were not included) was associated with increased survival.[215] Moreover, the oxygenation index (which takes into account both lung mechanical properties and oxygenation) was markedly improved.

The recent failure of a multicenter clinical trial of partial liquid ventilation with perflubron (a perfluorocarbon) during mechanical ventilation of adult patients with acute lung injury illustrates the clinical relevance of VILI.[216] The amount of perflubron administered was high and was associated with a high level of PEEP (>13 cmH$_2$O). Consequently, inspiratory pressure was higher in the patients who received perflubron than in controls. Not only was mortality higher (although not significantly) in patients receiving liquid ventilation, but the incidence of macroscopic barotrauma was also particularly high, more than double that in the controls (17% versus 6%, p <0.05). All these results were predictable from careful analysis of experimental studies, which showed increased incidence of barotrauma[183] and worsening of VILI[145,184] when both the amount of instilled perfluorocarbon and the pressures delivered by the respirator were high.

As already discussed, the literature on possible cytokine involvement during VILI contains many contradictions and inconsistencies.[91] Indeed, it is not surprising that the clinical correlate of such experimental findings is very vague. Ranieri et al[217] reported significant decreases in bronchoalveolar fluid and plasma concentrations of many inflammatory and anti-inflammatory mediators in patients ventilated with a so-called lung protective strategy (low tidal volume plus high PEEP). They suggested that nonprotective ventilation (high tidal volume plus low PEEP) was responsible for the inflammatory state. In contrast, Stuber et al[218] reported the release of mainly anti-inflammatory mediators in the bronchoalveolar fluid and plasma of patients ventilated with a nonprotective modality.[112] Finally, very modest although significant decreases of plasma inflammatory cytokines were reported in patients of the low-tidal-volume arm of the ARDS Network study[1] compared with patients of the high-tidal-volume arm.[219] The decrease, however, was trivial and very unlikely to have any clinical consequence. Thus, developing possible anti-inflammatory therapy to prevent ventilator-associated lung injury, based on these findings, is speculative at best. It is important to recognize that tidal volume reduction in patients with ARDS and the resulting improvement of ARDS mortality over time[1,220] was proposed based on physiologic premises that totally ignored cytokine biology.[91,221] The recent negative results (and increased mortality with some new approaches in some instances) with anti-cytokine therapy in sepsis[222,223] should discourage physicians from acting as the sorcerer's apprentice.

Conclusion

Considerable clinical progress has accrued from the extensive physiologic experimental research on VILI. There is now widespread consensus on the need to ease the stress on diseased lungs during mechanical ventilation. The extent, however, to which tidal volume should be decreased, the level of PEEP that should be used, and how to identify lung overdistension in an individual patient remain largely unknown. Further minimization of volutrauma during mechanical ventilation will require the ability to monitor lung volume[224] as well as airway pressures. In particular, the development of a simple tool for determining regional volumes during ventilation would represent a major step forward in the search for safer treatments.

Acknowledgments

The authors gratefully acknowledge Paul Soler, Ph.D., for performing electron microscopy studies and express appreciation to Odile Mathieu-Costello, Ph.D., and John B. West, M.D., for providing EM photomicrographs.

References

1. The Acute Respiratory Distress Syndrome Network. Ventilation with lower tidal volumes as compared with traditional tidal volumes for acute lung injury and the acute respiratory distress syndrome. N Engl J Med 2000; 342:1301–8.
2. Greenfield LJ, Ebert PA, Benson DW. Effect of positive pressure ventilation on surface tension properties of lung extracts. Anesthesiology 1964; 25:312–16.
3. Sladen A, Laver MB, Pontoppidan H. Pulmonary complications and water retention in prolonged mechanical ventilation. N Engl J Med 1968; 279:448–53.
4. Nash G, Bowen JA, Langlinais PC. Respirator lung: a misnomer. Arch Pathol 1971; 21:234–40.
5. Webb HH, Tierney DF. Experimental pulmonary edema due to intermittent positive pressure ventilation with high inflation pressures. Protection by positive end-expiratory pressure. Am Rev Respir Dis 1974; 110:556–65.
6. Dreyfuss D, Basset G, Soler P, Saumon G. Intermittent positive-pressure hyperventilation with high inflation pressures produces pulmonary microvascular injury in rats. Am Rev Respir Dis 1985; 132:880–84.
7. Dreyfuss D, Soler P, Saumon G. Spontaneous resolution of pulmonary edema caused by short periods of cyclic overinflation. J Appl Physiol 1992; 72:2081–89.
8. John E, Ermocilla R, Golden J, McDevitt M, Cassady G. Effects of intermittent positive-pressure ventilation on lungs of normal rabbits. Br J Exp Pathol 1980; 61:315–23.
9. John E, McDevitt M, Wilborn W, Cassady G. Ultrastructure of the lung after ventilation. Br J Exp Pathol 1982; 63:401–7.
10. Kolobow T, Moretti MP, Fumagalli R, et al. Severe impairment in lung function induced by high peak airway pressure during mechanical ventilation. Am Rev Respir Dis 1987; 135:312–15.
11. Tsuno K, Miura K, Takey M, Kolobow T, Morioka T. Histopathologic pulmonary changes from mechanical ventilation at high peak airway pressures. Am Rev Respir Dis 1991; 143:1115–20.
12. Parker JC, Hernandez LA, Longenecker GL, Peevy K, Johnson W. Lung edema caused by high peak inspiratory pressures in dogs. Role of increased microvascular filtration pressure and permeability. Am Rev Respir Dis 1990; 142:321–28.
13. Broccard AF, Hotchkiss JR, Kuwayama N, et al. Consequences of vascular flow on lung injury induced by mechanical ventilation. Am J Respir Crit Care Med 1998; 157:1935–42.
14. Carlton DP, Cummings JJ, Scheerer RG, Poulain FR, Bland RD. Lung overexpansion increases pulmonary microvascular protein permeability in young lambs. J Appl Physiol 1990; 69:577–83.

15. Faridy EE, Permutt S, Riley RL. Effect of ventilation on surface forces in excised dogs' lungs. J Appl Physiol 1966; 21: 1453–62.

16. McClenahan JB, Urtnowski A. Effect of ventilation on surfactant, and its turnover rate. J Appl Physiol 1967; 23:215–20.

17. Veldhuizen RA, Tremblay LN, Govindarajan A, et al. Pulmonary surfactant is altered during mechanical ventilation of isolated rat lung. Crit Care Med 2000; 28:2545–51.

18. Wyszogrodski I, Kyei Aboagye K, Tauecsh Jr HW, Avery ME. Surfactant inactivation by hyperventilation: conservation by end-expiratory pressure. J Appl Physiol 1975; 38:461–66.

19. Oyarzun MJ, Clements JA. Control of lung surfactant by ventilation, adrenergic mediators, and prostaglandins in the rabbit. Am Rev Respir Dis 1978; 117:879–91.

20. Nicholas TE, Barr HA. The release of surfactant in rat lung by brief periods of hyperventilation. Resp Physiol 1983; 52:69–83.

21. Veldhuizen RA, Welk B, Harbottle R, et al. Mechanical ventilation of isolated rat lungs changes the structure and biophysical properties of surfactant. J Appl Physiol 2002; 92:1169–75.

22. Faridy EE. Effect of ventilation on movement of surfactant in airways. Respir Physiol 1976; 27:323–34.

23. Pattle RE. Properties, function and origin of the alveolar lining layer. Nature (Lond) 1955; 175:1125–26.

24. Clements JA. Pulmonary edema and permeability of alveolar membranes. Arch Environ Health 1961; 2:280–83.

25. Albert RK, Lakshminarayan S, Hildebrandt J, Kirk W, Butler J. Increased surface tension favors pulmonary edema formation in anesthetized dogs' lungs. J Clin Invest 1979; 63: 1015–18.

26. Bredenberg CE, Nieman GF, Paskanik AM, Hart KE. Microvascular membrane permeability in high surface tension pulmonary edema. J Appl Physiol 1986; 60:253–59.

27. Jefferies AL, Kawano T, Mori S, Burger R. Effect of increased surface tension and assisted ventilation on 99mTc-DTPA clearance. J Appl Physiol 1988; 64:562–68.

28. Nieman G, Ritter-Hrncirik C, Grossman Z, et al. High alveolar surface tension increases clearance of technetium 99m diethylenetriamine-pentaacetic acid. J Thorac Cardiovasc Surg 1990; 100:129–33.

29. Permutt S. Mechanical influences on water accumulation in the lungs. In: Fishman AP, Renkin EM, editors. Pulmonary edema. Clinical Physiology Series. Bethesda, MD: American Physiological Society, 1979: 175–93.

30. Howell JBL, Permutt S, Proctor DF, Riley RL. Effect of inflation of the lung on different parts of pulmonary vascular bed. J Appl Physiol 1961; 16:71–76.

31. Benjamin JJ, Murtagh PS, Proctor DF, Menkes HA, Permutt S. Pulmonary vascular interdependence in excised dog lobes. J Appl Physiol 1974; 37:887–94.

32. Iliff LD. Extra-alveolar vessels and edema development in excised dog lungs. Circ Res 1971; 28:524–32.

33. Albert RK, Lakshminarayan AS, Huang TW, Butler J. Fluid leaks from extra-alveolar vessels in living dog lungs. J Appl Physiol 1978; 44:759–62.

34. Albert RK, Lakshminarayan S, Kirk W, Butler J. Lung inflation can cause pulmonary edema in zone I of in situ dog lungs. J Appl Physiol 1980; 49:815–19.

35. Cooper JA, Van Der Zee H, Line BR, Malik AB. Relationship of end-expiratory pressure, lung volume, and ^{99m}Tc-DTPA clearance. J Appl Physiol 1987; 63:1586–90.

36. O'Brodovich H, Coates G, Marrin M. Effect of inspiratory resistance and PEEP on ^{99m}Tc-DTPA clearance. J Appl Physiol 1986; 60:1461–65.

37. Marks JD, Luce JM, Lazar NM, et al. Effect of increases in lung volume on clearance of aerosolized solute from human lungs. J Appl Physiol 1985; 59:1242–48.

38. Nolop KB, Maxwell DL, Royston D, Hughes JMB. Effect of raised thoracic pressure and volume on ^{99m}Tc-DTPA clearance in humans. J Appl Physiol 1986; 60:1493–97.

39. Egan EA, Nelson RM, Olver RE. Lung inflation and alveolar permeability to non-electrolytes in the adult sheep in vivo. J Physiol (Lond) 1976; 260:409–24.

40. Egan EA. Response of alveolar epithelial solute permeability to changes in lung inflation. J Appl Physiol 1980; 49: 1032–36.

41. Egan EA. Lung inflation, lung solute permeability, and alveolar edema. J Appl Physiol 1982; 53:121–25.

42. Kim KJ, Crandall ED. Effects of lung inflation on alveolar epithelial solute and water transport properties. J Appl Physiol 1982; 52:1498–505.

43. Ramanathan R, Mason GR, Raj JU. Effect of mechanical ventilation and barotrauma on pulmonary clearance of ^{99m}Technetium diethylenetriamine pentaacetate in lambs. Pediatr Res 1990; 27:70–74.

44. Lesur O, Hermans C, Chalifour JF, et al. Mechanical ventilation-induced pneumoprotein CC-16 vascular transfer in rats: effect of KGF pretreatment. Am J Physiol Lung Cell Mol Physiol 2003; 284:L410–9. Epub 2002 Oct 25.

45. Yoshikawa S, King JA, Reynolds SD, Stripp BR, Parker JC. Time and pressure dependence of transvascular Clara cell protein, albumin, and IgG transport during ventilator-induced lung injury in mice. Am J Physiol Lung Cell Mol Physiol 2004; 286: L604–12.

46. Lecuona E, Saldias F, Comellas A, et al. Ventilator-associated lung injury decreases lung ability to clear edema in rats. Am J Respir Crit Care Med 1999; 159:603–9.

47. Saldias FJ, Lecuona E, Comellas AP, et al. Beta-adrenergic stimulation restores rat lung ability to clear edema in ventilator-associated lung injury. Am J Respir Crit Care Med 2000; 162: 282–7.

48. Adir Y, Factor P, Dumasius V, Ridge KM, Sznajder JI. Na,K-ATPase gene transfer increases liquid clearance during ventilation-induced lung injury. Am J Respir Crit Care Med 2003; 168:1445–8.

49. Parker JC, Townsley MI, Rippe B, Taylor AE, Thigpen J. Increased microvascular permeability in dog lungs due to high airway pressures. J Appl Physiol 1984; 57:1809–16.

50. Parker JC, Yoshikawa S. Vascular segmental permeabilities at high peak inflation pressure in isolated rat lungs. Am J Physiol Lung Cell Mol Physiol 2002; 283:L1203–9.

51. Dreyfuss D, Soler P, Basset G, Saumon G. High inflation pressure pulmonary edema. Respective effects of high airway pressure, high tidal volume, and positive end-expiratory pressure. Am Rev Respir Dis 1988; 137:1159–64.

52. Borelli M, Kolobow T, Spatola R, Prato P, Tsuno K. Severe acute respiratory failure managed with continuous positive airway pressure and partial extracorporeal carbon dioxide removal by an artificial membrane lung. Am Rev Respir Dis 1988; 138: 1480–87.

53. Tsuno K, Prato P, Kolobow T. Acute lung injury from mechanical ventilation at moderately high airway pressures. J Appl Physiol 1990; 69:956–61.

54. Birks EK, Mathieu-Costello O, Fu Z, Tyler WS, West JB. Comparative aspects of the strength of pulmonary capillaries in rabbit, dog, and horse. Respir Physiol 1994; 97:235–46.

55. Prewitt RM, McCarthy J, Wood LDH. Treatment of acute low pressure pulmonary edema in dogs. Relative effects of hydrostatic and oncotic pressure, nitroprusside and positive end-expiratory pressure. J Clin Invest 1981; 67:409–18.

56. Huchon GJ, Hopewell PC, Murray JF. Interactions between permeability and hydrostatic pressure in perfused dogs' lungs. J Appl Physiol 1981; 50:905–11.

57. Guyton AC, Lindsey AW. Effect of elevated left atrial pressure and decreased plasma protein concentration on the development of pulmonary edema. Circ Res 1959; 7:649–53.

58. Dos Santos CC, Slutsky AS. Invited review: mechanisms of ventilator-induced lung injury: a perspective. J Appl Physiol 2000; 89:1645–55.

59. Tschumperlin DJ, Margulies SS. Equibiaxial deformation-induced injury of alveolar epithelial cells in vitro. Am J Physiol 1998; 275:L1173–83.

60. Tschumperlin DJ, Oswari J, Margulies AS. Deformation-induced injury of alveolar epithelial cells. Effect of frequency, duration, and amplitude. Am J Respir Crit Care Med 2000; 162:357–62.

61. Tschumperlin DJ, Margulies SS. Alveolar epithelial surface area-volume relationship in isolated rat lungs. J Appl Physiol 1999; 86:2026–33.

62. Vlahakis NE, Schroeder MA, Pagano RE, Hubmayr RD. Deformation-induced lipid trafficking in alveolar epithelial cells. Am J Physiol Lung Cell Mol Physiol 2001; 280: L938–46.

63. Vlahakis NE, Hubmayr RD. Cellular stress failure in ventilator injured lungs. Am J Respir Crit Care Med 2005; 171:1328–42.

64. Fu Z, Costello ML, Tsukimoto K, et al. High lung volume increases stress failure in pulmonary capillaries. J Appl Physiol 1992; 73:123–33.

65. Parker JC, Ivey CL, Tucker JA. Gadolinium prevents high airway pressure-induced permeability increases in isolated rat lungs. J Appl Physiol 1998; 84:1113–18.

66. Parker JC, Ivey CL, Tucker A. Phosphotyrosine phosphatase and tyrosine kinase inhibition modulate airway pressure-induced lung injury. J Appl Physiol 1998; 85:1753–61.

67. Parker JC. Inhibitors of myosin light chain kinase and phosphodiesterase reduce ventilator-induced lung injury. J Appl Physiol 2000; 89:2241–8.

68. West JB, Tsukimoto K, Mathieu-Costello O, Prediletto R. Stress failure in pulmonary capillaries. J Appl Physiol 1991; 70:1731–42.

69. Vlahakis NE, Schroeder MA, Pagano RE, Hubmayr RD. Role of deformation-induced lipid trafficking in the prevention of plasma membrane stress failure. Am J Respir Crit Care Med 2002; 166:1282–9.

70. Elliott AR, Fu Z, Tsukimoto K, Prediletto R, Mathieu-Costello O, West JB. Short-term reversibility of ultrastructural changes in pulmonary capillaries caused by stress failure. J Appl Physiol 1992; 73:1150–58.

71. Matthay MA, Landolt CA, Staub NC. Differential liquid and protein clearance from alveoli of anesthetized sheep. J Appl Physiol 1982; 53:96–104.

72. Cottrell TS, Levine OR, Senior RM, et al. Electron microscopic alterations at the alveolar level in pulmonary edema. Circ Res 1967; 21:783–97.

73. Teplitz C. Pulmonary cellular and interstitial edema. In: Fishman AP, Renkin EM, editors. Pulmonary edema. Clinical Physiology Series. Bethesda, MD: American Physiological Society, 1979: 97-111.

74. Hurley JV. Types of pulmonary microvascular injury. Ann NY Acad Sci 1982; 384:269–86.

75. Bachofen M, Weibel ER. Structural alterations of lung parenchyma in the adult respiratory distress syndrome. Clinics Chest Med 1982; 3:35–56.

76. DeFouw DO, Berendsen PB. Morphological changes in isolated perfused dog lungs after acute hydrostatic edema. Circ Res 1978; 43:72–82.

77. Montaner JSG, Tsang J, Evans KG, et al. Alveolar epithelial damage. A critical difference between high pressure and oleic acid-induced low pressure pulmonary edema. J Clin Invest 1986; 77:1786–96.

78. Tsukimoto K, Mathieu-Costello O, Prediletto R, Elliott AR, West JB. Ultrastructural appearances of pulmonary capillaries at high transmural pressures. J Appl Physiol 1991; 71:573–82.

79. Costello ML, Mathieu-Costello O, West JB. Stress failure of alveolar epithelial cells studied by scanning electron microscopy. Am Rev Respir Dis 1992; 145:1446–55.

80. Nycolaysen G, Waaler BA, Aarseth P. On the existence of stretchable pores in the exchange vessels of the isolated rabbit lung preparation. Lymphology 1979; 12:201–7.

81. Rippe B, Townsley M, Thigpen J, et al. Effects of vascular pressure on the pulmonary microvasculature in isolated dog lungs. J Appl Physiol 1984; 57:233–39.

82. Shirley HH, Wolfram CG, Wasserman K, Mayerson HS. Capillary permeability to macromolecules: stretched pore phenomenon. Am J Physiol 1957; 190:189–93.

83. Fishman AP, Pietra GG. Hemodynamic pulmonary edema. In: Fishman AP, Renkin EM, editors. Pulmonary edema. Clinical Physiology Series. Bethesda, MD: American Physiological Society, 1979: 79–96.

84. Yoshikawa S, Miyahara T, Reynolds SD, et al. Clara cell secretory protein and phospholipase A2 activity modulate acute ventilator-induced lung injury in mice. J Appl Physiol 2005; 98:1264–71.

85. Woo SW, Hedley-Whyte J. Macrophage accumulation and pulmonary edema due to thoracotomy and lung overinflation. J Appl Physiol 1972; 33:14-21.

86. Markos J, Doerschuk CM, English D, Wiggs BR, Hogg JC. Effect of positive end-expiratory pressure on leukocyte transit in rabbit lungs. J Appl Physiol 1993; 74:2627–33.

87. Quinn DA, Moufarrej RK, Volokhov A, Hales CA. Interactions of lung stretch, hyperoxia, and MIP-2 production in ventilator-induced lung injury. J Appl Physiol 2002; 93:517–25.

88. Kawano T, Mori S, Cybulsky M, et al. Effect of granulocyte depletion in a ventilated surfactant-depleted lung. J Appl Physiol 1987; 62:27–33.

89. Tremblay L, Valenza F, Ribeiro SP, Li J, Slutsky AS. Injurious ventilatory strategies increase cytokines and c-*fos* m-RNA expression in an isolated rat lung model. J Clin Invest 1997; 99: 944–52.

90. Ricard JD, Dreyfuss D, Saumon G. Production of inflammatory cytokines in ventilator-induced lung injury: a reappraisal. Am J Respir Crit Care Med 2001; 163:1176–80.

91. Dreyfuss D, Ricard JD, Saumon G. On the physiologic and clinical relevance of lung-borne cytokines during ventilator-induced lung injury. Am J Respir Crit Care Med 2003; 167:1467–71.

92. von Bethmann A, Brasch F, Nüsing R, et al. Hyperventilation induces release of cytokines from perfused mouse lung. Am J Respir Crit Care Med 1998; 157:263–72.

93. Yoshikawa S, King JA, Lausch RN, et al. Acute ventilator-induced vascular permeability and cytokine responses in isolated and in situ mouse lungs. J Appl Physiol 2004; 97:2190–9.

94. Verbrugge SJ, Uhlig S, Neggers SJ, et al. Different ventilation strategies affect lung function but do not increase tumor necrosis factor-alpha and prostacyclin production in lavaged rat lungs in vivo. Anesthesiology 1999; 91:1834–43.

95. Takata M, Abe J, Tanaka H, et al. Intraalveolar expression of tumor necrosis factor-alpha gene during conventional and high-frequency ventilation. Am J Respir Crit Care Med 1997; 156: 272–79.

96. Imanaka H, Shimaoka M, Matsuura N, et al. Ventilator-induced lung injury is associated with neutrophil infiltration, macrophage activation, and TGF-beta 1 mRNA upregulation in rat lungs. Anesth Analg 2001; 92:428–36.

97. Belperio JA, Keane MP, Burdick MD, et al. Critical role for CXCR2 and CXCR2 ligands during the pathogenesis of ventilator-induced lung injury. J Clin Invest 2002; 110:1703–16.

98. Pugin J, Dunn I, Jolliet P, et al. Activation of human macrophages by mechanical ventilation in vitro. Am J Physiol 1998; 275:L1040–50.

99. Vlahakis NE, Schroeder MA, Limper AH, Hubmayr RD. Stretch induces cytokine release by alveolar epithelial cells in vitro. Am J Physiol 1999; 277:L167–73.

100. Matsuoka T, Kawano T, Miyasaka K. Role of high-frequency ventilation in surfactant-depleted lung injury as measured by granulocytes. J Appl Physiol 1994; 76:539–44.

101. Imai Y, Kawano T, Miyasaka K, et al. Inflammatory chemical mediators during conventional ventilation and during high frequency oscillatory ventilation. Am J Respir Crit Care Med 1994; 150:1550–54.

102. Choudhury S, Wilson MR, Goddard ME, O'Dea KP, Takata M. Mechanisms of early pulmonary neutrophil sequestration in ventilator-induced lung injury in mice. Am J Physiol Lung Cell Mol Physiol 2004; 287:L902–10.

103. Mackarel AJ, Russell KJ, Brady CS, FitzGerald MX, O'Connor CM. Interleukin-8 and leukotriene-B(4), but not formylmethionyl leucylphenylalanine, stimulate CD18-independent migration of neutrophils across human pulmonary endothelial cells in vitro. Am J Respir Cell Mol Biol 2000; 23:154–61.

104. Broccard AF, Feihl F, Vannay C, et al. Effects of L-NAME and inhaled nitric oxide on ventilator-induced lung injury in isolated, perfused rabbit lungs. Crit Care Med 2004; 32:1872–78.

105. Schubert W, Frank PG, Woodman SE, et al. Microvascular hyperpermeability in caveolin-1 (-/-) knock-out mice. Treatment with a specific nitric-oxide synthase inhibitor, L-name, restores normal microvascular permeability in Cav-1 null mice. J Biol Chem 2002; 277:40091–98.

106. Chiumello D, Pristine G, Slutsky AS. Mechanical ventilation affects local and systemic cytokines in an animal model of acute respiratory distress syndrome. Am J Respir Crit Care Med 1999; 160:109–16.

107. Nahum A, Hoyt J, Schmitz L, et al. Effect of mechanical ventilation strategy on dissemination of intratracheally instilled Escherichia coli in dogs. Crit Care Med 1997; 25:1733–43.

108. Verbrugge S, Sorm V, van't Veen A, et al. Lung overinflation without positive end-expiratory pressure promotes bacteremia after experimental Klebsiella pneumoniae inoculation. Intensive Care Med 1998; 24:172–77.

109. Schortgen F, Bouadma L, Joly-Guillou ML, et al. Infectious and inflammatory dissemination are affected by ventilation strategy in rats with unilateral pneumonia. Intensive Care Med 2004; 30:693–701.

110. Slutsky AS, Tremblay LN. Multiple system organ failure: is mechanical ventilation a contributing factor? Am J Respir Crit Care Med 1998; 157:1721–25.

111. Dreyfuss D, Saumon G. From ventilator-induced lung injury to multiple organ dysfunction? Intensive Care Med 1998; 24:102–4.

112. Pugin J. Is the ventilator responsible for lung and systemic inflammation? Intensive Care Med 2002; 28:817–9.

113. Bouadma L, Schortgen F, Ricard J, et al. Ventilation strategy affects cytokine release after mesenteric ischemia-reperfusion in rats. Crit Care Med 2004; 32:1563–69.

114. Whitehead TC, Zhang H, Mullen B, Slutsky AS. Effect of mechanical ventilation on cytokine response to intratracheal lipopolysaccharide. Anesthesiology 2004; 101:52–8.

115. Copland IB, Kavanagh BP, Engelberts D, et al. Early changes in lung gene expression due to high tidal volume. Am J Respir Crit Care Med 2003; 168:1051–9.

116. dos Santos CC, Han B, Andrade CF, et al. DNA microarray analysis of gene expression in alveolar epithelial cells in response to TNFalpha, LPS, and cyclic stretch. Physiol Genomics 2004; 19:331–42.

117. Luce JM. The cardiovascular effects of mechanical ventilation and positive end-expiratory pressure. JAMA 1984; 252:807–11.

118. Hernandez LA, Peevy KJ, Moise AA, Parker JC. Chest wall restriction limits high airway pressure-induced lung injury in young rabbits. J Appl Physiol 1989; 66:2364–68.

119. Peevy KJ, Hernandez LA, Moise AA, Parker JC. Barotrauma and microvascular injury in lungs of nonadult rabbits: effect of ventilation pattern. Crit Care Med 1990; 18:634–37.

120. Maeda Y, Fujino Y, Uchiyama A, et al. Effects of peak inspiratory flow on development of ventilator-induced lung injury in rabbits. Anesthesiology 2004; 101:722–8.

121. Rich PB, Reickert CA, Sawada S, et al. Effect of rate and inspiratory flow on ventilator-induced lung injury. J Trauma 2000; 49:903–11.

122. D'Angelo E, Pecchiari M, Saetta M, Balestro E, Milic-Emili J. Dependence of lung injury on inflation rate during low-volume ventilation in normal open-chest rabbits. J Appl Physiol 2004; 97:260–8.

123. Macnaughton PD, Morgan CJ, Denison DM, Evans TW. Measurement of carbon monoxide transfer and lung volume in ventilated subjects. Eur Respir J 1993; 6:231–6.

124. Broccard AF, Vannay C, Feihl F, Schaller MD. Impact of low pulmonary vascular pressure on ventilator-induced lung injury. Crit Care Med 2002; 30:2183–90.

125. Malo J, Ali J, Wood LDH. How does positive end-expiratory pressure reduce intrapulmonary shunt in canine pulmonary edema? J Appl Physiol 1984; 57:1002–10.

126. Paré PD, Warriner B, Baile EM, Hogg JC. Redistribution of pulmonary extravascular water with positive end-expiratory pressure in canine pulmonary edema. Am Rev Respir Dis 1983; 127:590–93.

127. Bshouty Z, Ali J, Younes M. Effect of tidal volume and PEEP on rate of edema formation in in situ perfused canine lobes. J Appl Physiol 1988; 64:1900–7.

128. Corbridge TC, Wood LDH, Crawford GP, et al. Adverse effects of large tidal volume and low PEEP in canine acid aspiration. Am Rev Respir Dis 1990; 142:311–15.

129. Dreyfuss D, Saumon G. Role of tidal volume, FRC and end-inspiratory volume in the development of pulmonary edema following mechanical ventilation. Am Rev Respir Dis 1993; 148:1194–203.

130. Rizk NW, Murray JF. PEEP and pulmonary edema. Am J Med 1982; 72:381–83.

131. Luce JM, Huang TW, Robertson HT, et al. The effects of prophylactic expiratory positive airway pressure on the resolution of oleic acid-induced lung injury in dogs. Ann Surg 1983; 197:327–36.

132. Valenza F, Guglielmi M, Irace M, et al. Positive end-expiratory pressure delays the progression of lung injury during ventilator strategies involving high airway pressure and lung overdistention. Crit Care Med 2003; 31:1993–8.

133. Mead J, Takishima T, Leith D. Stress distribution in lungs: a model of pulmonary elasticity. J Appl Physiol 1970; 28:596–608.

134. Bowton DL, Kong DL. High tidal volume ventilation produces increased lung water in oleic acid-injured rabbit lungs. Crit Care Med 1989; 17:908–11.

135. Hernandez LA, Coker PJ, May S, Thompson AL, Parker JC. Mechanical ventilation increases microvascular permeability in oleic injured lungs. J Appl Physiol 1990; 69:2057–61.

136. Coker PJ, Hernandez LA, Peevy KJ, Adkins K, Parker JC. Increased sensitivity to mechanical ventilation after surfactant inactivation in young rabbit lungs. Crit Care Med 1992; 20: 635–40.

137. Roupie E, Dambrosio M, Servillo G, et al. Titration of tidal volume and induced hypercapnia in acute respiratory distress syndrome. Am J Respir Crit Care Med 1995; 152:121–28.

138. Dambrosio M, Roupie E, Mollet J-J, et al. Effects of PEEP and different tidal volumes on alveolar recruitment and hyperinflation. Anesthesiology 1997; 87:497–503.

139. Hickling KG. The pressure-volume curve is greatly modified by recruitment. A mathematical model of ARDS lungs. Am J Respir Crit Care Med 1998; 158:194–202.

140. Jonson B, Richard JC, Straus C, et al. Pressure-volume curves and compliance in acute lung injury: evidence of recruitment above the lower inflection point. Am J Respir Crit Care Med 1999; 159:1172–8.

141. Martin-Lefevre L, Ricard JD, Roupie E, Dreyfuss D, Saumon G. Significance of the changes in the respiratory system pressure-volume curve during acute lung injury in rats. Am J Respir Crit Care Med 2001; 164:627–32.

142. Gattinoni L, Pesanti A, Avalli L, Rossi F, Bombino M. Pressure-volume curves of total respiratory system in acute respiratory failure. Computed tomographic scan study. Am Rev Respir Dis 1987; 136:730–36.

143. Gibson GJ, Pride NB. Pulmonary mechanics in fibrosing alveolitis. Am Rev Respir Dis 1977; 116:637–47.

144. Dreyfuss D, Soler P, Saumon G. Mechanical ventilation-induced pulmonary edema. Interaction with previous lung alterations. Am J Respir Crit Care Med 1995; 151:1568–75.

145. Dreyfuss D, Martin-Lefevre L, Saumon G. Hyperinflation-induced lung injury during alveolar flooding in rats: effect of perfluorocarbon instillation. Am J Respir Crit Care Med 1999; 159:1752–7.

146. Argiras EP, Blakeley CR, Dunnill MS, Otremski S, Sykes MK. High peep decreases hyaline membrane formation in surfactant deficient lungs. Br J Anaesth 1987; 59:1278–85.

147. Sandhar BK, Niblett DJ, Argiras EP, Dunnill MS, Sykes MK. Effects of positive end-expiratory pressure on hyaline membrane formation in a rabbit model of the neonatal respiratory distress syndrome. Intensive Care Med 1988; 14:538–46.

148. Muscedere JG, Mullen JBM, Gan K, Bryan AC, Slutsky AS. Tidal ventilation at low airway pressures can augment lung injury. Am J Respir Crit Care Med 1994; 149:1327–34.

149. Sohma A, Brampton WJ, Dunnill MS, Sykes MK. Effect of ventilation with positive end-expiratory pressure on the development of lung damage in experimental acid aspiration pneumonia in the rabbit. Intensive Care Med 1992; 18:112–17.

150. Steinberg JM, Schiller HJ, Halter JM, et al. Alveolar instability causes early ventilator-induced lung injury independent of neutrophils. Am J Respir Crit Care Med 2004; 169:57–63.

151. Schiller HJ, McCann UG 2nd, Carney DE, et al. Altered alveolar mechanics in the acutely injured lung. Crit Care Med 2001; 29:1049–55.

152. Halter JM, Steinberg JM, Schiller HJ, et al. Positive end-expiratory pressure after a recruitment maneuver prevents both alveolar collapse and recruitment/derecruitment. Am J Respir Crit Care Med 2003; 167:1620–6.

153. Steinberg J, Schiller HJ, Halter JM, et al. Tidal volume increases do not affect alveolar mechanics in normal lung but cause alveolar overdistension and exacerbate alveolar instability after surfactant deactivation. Crit Care Med 2002; 30:2675–83.

154. McCann UG 2nd, Schiller HJ, Carney DE, et al. Visual validation of the mechanical stabilizing effects of positive end-expiratory pressure at the alveolar level. J Surg Res 2001; 99:335–42.

155. Wilson TA, Bachofen H. A model for mechanical structure of the alveolar duct. J Appl Physiol 1982; 52:1064–70.

156. Martynowicz MA, Minor TA, Walters BJ, Hubmayr RD. Regional expansion of oleic acid-injured lungs. Am J Respir Crit Care Med 1999; 160:250–8.

157. Wilson TA, Anafi RC, Hubmayr RD. Mechanics of edematous lungs. J Appl Physiol 2001; 90:2088–93.

158. Bilek AM, Dee KC, Gaver DP 3rd. Mechanisms of surface-tension-induced epithelial cell damage in a model of pulmonary airway reopening. J Appl Physiol 2003; 94:770–83.

159. D'Angelo E, Pecchiari M, Baraggia P, et al. Low-volume ventilation causes peripheral airway injury and increased airway resistance in normal rabbits. J Appl Physiol 2002; 92:949–56.

160. Kloot TE, Blanch L, Melynne Youngblood A, et al. Recruitment maneuvers in three experimental models of acute lung injury. Effect on lung volume and gas exchange. Am J Respir Crit Care Med 2000; 161:1485–94.

161. Hubmayr RD. Perspective on lung injury and recruitment: a skeptical look at the opening and collapse story. Am J Respir Crit Care Med 2002; 165:1647–53.

162. Brower RG, Lanken PN, MacIntyre N, et al. Higher versus lower positive end-expiratory pressures in patients with the acute respiratory distress syndrome. N Engl J Med 2004; 351:327–36.

163. Choi WI, Quinn DA, Park KM, et al. Systemic microvascular leak in an in vivo rat model of ventilator-induced lung injury. Am J Respir Crit Care Med 2003; 167:1627–32.

164. Guery BP, Welsh DA, Viget NB, et al. Ventilation-induced lung injury is associated with an increase in gut permeability. Shock 2003; 19:559–63.

165. Imai Y, Parodo J, Kajikawa O, et al. Injurious mechanical ventilation and end-organ epithelial cell apoptosis and organ dysfunction in an experimental model of acute respiratory distress syndrome. JAMA 2003; 289:2104–12.

166. Zapol WM, Snider MT, Hill JD, et al. Extracorporeal membrane oxygenation in severe acute respiratory failure. JAMA 1979; 242:2193–96.

167. Gattinoni L, Pesanti A, Mascheroni D, et al. Low frequency positive pressure ventilation with extracorporeal CO2 removal in severe acute respiratory failure. JAMA 1986; 256:881–86.

168. Froese AB, Bryan AC. High frequency ventilation. Am Rev Respir Dis 1987; 135:1363–74.

169. Pesenti A, Kolobow T, Buckhold DK, et al. Prevention of hyaline membrane disease in premature lambs by apneic oxygenation and extracorporeal carbon dioxide removal. Intensive Care Med 1982; 8:11–17.

170. Dorrington KL, McRae KM, Gardaz JP, et al. A randomized comparison of total extracorporeal CO2 removal with conventional mechanical ventilation in experimental hyaline membrane disease. Intensive Care Med 1989; 15:184–191.

171. Yanos J, Presberg K, Crawford G, et al. The effect of hypopnea on low-pressure pulmonary edema. Am Rev Respir Dis 1990; 142:316–20.

172. Hamilton PP, Onayemi A, Smyth JA, et al. Comparison of conventional and high-frequency ventilation: oxygenation and lung pathology. J Appl Physiol 1983; 55:131–38.

173. Solimano A, Bryan AC, Jobe A, Ikegami M, Jacobs H. Effects of high-frequency and conventional ventilation on the premature lamb lung. J Appl Physiol 1985; 59:1571–77.

174. McCulloch PR, Forkert PG, Froese AB. Lung volume maintenance prevents lung injury during high frequency oscillatory ventilation in surfactant-deficient rabbits. Am Rev Respir Dis 1988; 137:1185–92.

175. Ranieri VM, Zhang H, Mascia L, et al. Pressure-time curve predicts minimally injurious ventilatory strategy in an isolated rat lung model. Anesthesiology 2000; 93:1320–8.

176. Grasso S, Terragni P, Mascia L, et al. Airway pressure-time curve profile (stress index) detects tidal recruitment/hyperinflation in experimental acute lung injury. Crit Care Med 2004; 32: 1018–27.

177. Verbrugge SJ, Vazquez de Anda G, Gommers D, et al. Exogenous surfactant preserves lung function and reduces alveolar Evans blue dye influx in a rat model of ventilation-induced lung injury. Anesthesiology 1998; 89:467–74.

178. Welk B, Malloy JL, Joseph M, Yao LJ, Veldhuizen AW. Surfactant treatment for ventilation-induced lung injury in rats: effects on lung compliance and cytokines. Exp Lung Res 2001; 27:505–20.

179. Haitsma JJ, Uhlig S, Lachmann U, et al. Exogenous surfactant reduces ventilator-induced decompartmentalization of tumor necrosis factor alpha in absence of positive end-expiratory pressure. Intensive Care Med 2002; 28:1131–7.

180. Fuhrman BP, Paczan PR, DeFrancisis M. Perfluorocarbon-associated gas exchange. Crit Care Med 1991; 19:712–22.

181. Lachmann B, Fraterman A, Verbrugge SJC. Liquid ventilation. Physiological basis of mechanical ventilation. New York: Marcel Dekker, 1998.

182. Tütüncü AS, Akpir K, Mulder P, Erdmann W, Lachmann B. Intratracheal perfluorocarbon administration as an aid in the ventilatory management of respiratory distress syndrome. Anesthesiology 1993; 79:1083–93.

183. Cox PN, Frndova H, Tan PS, et al. Concealed air leak associated with large tidal volumes in partial liquid ventilation. Am J Respir Crit Care Med 1997; 156:992–97.

184. Ricard JD, Dreyfuss D, Laissy JP, Saumon G. Dose-response effect of perfluorocarbon administration on lung microvascular permeability in rats. Am J Respir Crit Care Med 2003; 168:1378–82.

185. Broccard AF, Shapiro RS, Schmitz LL, Ravenscraft SA, Marini JJ. Influence of prone position on the extent and distribution of lung injury in a high tidal volume oleic acid model of acute respiratory distress syndrome. Crit Care Med 1997; 25:16–27.

186. Nishimura M, Honda O, Tomiyama N, et al. Body position does not influence the location of ventilator-induced lung injury. Intensive Care Med 2000; 26:1664–9.

187. Valenza F, Guglielmi M, Maffioletti M, et al. Prone position delays the progression of ventilator-induced lung injury in rats: does lung strain distribution play a role? Crit Care Med 2005; 33:361–7.

188. Broccard A, Shapiro RS, Schmitz LL, et al. Prone positioning attenuates and redistributes ventilator-induced lung injury in dogs. Crit Care Med 2000; 28:295–303.

189. Held HD, Boettcher S, Hamann L, Uhlig S. Ventilation-induced chemokine and cytokine release is associated with activation of nuclear factor-kappaB and is blocked by steroids. Am J Respir Crit Care Med 2001; 163:711–6.

190. Dolinay T, Szilasi M, Liu M, Choi AM. Inhaled carbon monoxide confers antiinflammatory effects against ventilator-induced lung injury. Am J Respir Crit Care Med 2004; 170:613–20.

191. Narimanbekov IO, Rozycki HJ. Effect of IL-1 blockade on inflammatory manifestations of acute ventilator-induced lung injury in a rabbit model. Exp Lung Res 1995; 21:239–54.

192. Wilson MR, Choudhury S, Takata M. Pulmonary inflammation induced by high stretch ventilation is mediated by tumor necrosis factor signalling in mice. Am J Physiol Lung Cell Mol Physiol 2005; 288:L599–607.

193. Imai Y, Kawano T, Iwamoto S, et al. Intratracheal anti-tumor necrosis factor-alpha antibody attenuates ventilator-induced lung injury in rabbits. J Appl Physiol 1999; 87:510–5.

194. Broccard AF, Hotchkiss JR, Vannay C, et al. Protective effects of hypercapnic acidosis on ventilator-induced lung injury. Am J Respir Crit Care Med 2001; 164:802–6.

195. Hickling KG, Wright T, Laubscher K, et al. Extreme hypoventilation reduces ventilator-induced lung injury during ventilation with low positive end-expiratory pressure in saline-lavaged rabbits. Crit Care Med 1998; 26:1690–7.

196. Sinclair SE, Kregenow DA, Lamm WJ, et al. Hypercapnic acidosis is protective in an in vivo model of ventilator-induced lung injury. Am J Respir Crit Care Med 2002; 166:403–8.

197. Laffey JG, Engelberts D, Duggan M, et al. Carbon dioxide attenuates pulmonary impairment resulting from hyperventilation. Crit Care Med 2003; 31:2634–40.

198. Rai S, Engelberts D, Laffey JG, et al. Therapeutic hypercapnia is not protective in the in vivo surfactant-depleted rabbit lung. Pediatr Res 2004; 55:42–9.

199. Bouvet F, Dreyfuss D, Lebtahi R, et al. Noninvasive evaluation of acute capillary permeability changes during high-volume ventilation in rats with and without hypercapnic acidosis. Crit Care Med 2005; 33:155–60.

200. Doerr CH, Gajic O, Berrios JC, et al. Hypercapnic acidosis impairs plasma membrane wound resealing in ventilator injured lungs. Am J Respir Crit Care Med 2005; 171:1371–7.

201. International consensus conferences in intensive care medicine. Ventilator-associated lung injury in ARDS. American Thoracic Society, European Society of Intensive Care Medicine, Societe de Reanimation Langue Francaise. Intensive Care Med 1999; 25:1444–52.

202. Maunder RJ, Shuman WP, McHugh JW, Marglin SI, Butler J. Preservation of normal lung regions in the adult respiratory distress syndrome. Analysis by computed tomography. JAMA 1986; 255:2463–65.

203. Morris AH, Wallace CJ, Menlove RL, et al. Randomized clinical trial of pressure-controlled inverse ratio ventilation and extracorporeal CO2 removal for adult respiratory distress syndrome. Am J Respir Crit Care Med 1994; 149:295–305.

204. Ferguson ND, Chiche JD, Kacmarek RM, et al. Combining high-frequency oscillatory ventilation and recruitment maneuvers in adults with early acute respiratory distress syndrome: the Treatment with Oscillation and an Open Lung Strategy (TOOLS) Trial pilot study. Crit Care Med 2005; 33:479–86.

205. Hickling KG, Henderson SJ, Jackson R. Low mortality associated with low volume pressure limited ventilation with permissive hypercapnia in severe adult respiratory distress syndrome. Intensive Care Med 1990; 16:372–77.

206. Tobin MJ. Culmination of an era in research on the acute respiratory distress syndrome. N Engl J Med 2000; 342: 1360–1.

207. Dreyfuss D, Saumon G. Should the lung be rested or recruited? The Charybdis and Scylla of ventilator management. Am J Respir Crit Care Med 1994; 149:1066–68.

208. Gattinoni L, Pelosi P, Crotti S, Valenza F. Effects of positive end-expiratory pressure on regional distribution of tidal volume and recruitment in adult respiratory distress syndrome. Am J Respir Crit Care Med 1995; 151:1807–14.

209. Eichacker PQ, Gerstenberger EP, Banks SM, Cui X, Natanson C. Meta-analysis of acute lung injury and acute respiratory distress syndrome trials testing low tidal volumes. Am J Respir Crit Care Med 2002; 166:1510–4.

210. Gajic O, Dara SI, Mendez JL, et al. Ventilator-associated lung injury in patients without acute lung injury at the onset of mechanical ventilation. Crit Care Med 2004; 32:1817–24.

211. Gajic O, Frutos-Vivar F, Esteban A, Hubmayr RD, Anzueto A. Ventilator settings as a risk factor for acute respiratory distress syndrome in mechanically ventilated patients. Intensive Care Med 2005; 26:26.

212. Dreyfuss D, Saumon G. Pressure-volume curves: searching for the grail or laying patients with adult respiratory distress

syndrome on procrustes' bed? Am J Respir Crit Care Med 2001; 163:2–3.

213. Anzuetto A, Baughman R, Guntupalli KK, et al. Aerosolized surfactant in adults with sepsis-induced acute respiratory distress syndrome. N Engl J Med 1996; 334:1417–21.

214. Spragg RG, Lewis JF, Walmrath HD, et al. Effect of recombinant surfactant protein C-based surfactant on the acute respiratory distress syndrome. N Engl J Med 2004; 351:884–92.

215. Willson DF, Thomas NJ, Markovitz BP, et al. Effect of exogenous surfactant (calfactant) in pediatric acute lung injury: a randomized controlled trial. JAMA 2005; 293:470–6.

216. Kacmarek RM, Wiedemann HP, Lavin PT, Wedel MK, Tutuncu AS, Slutsky AS. Partial Liquid Ventilation in Adult Patients with the Acute Respiratory Distress Syndrome. Am J Respir Crit Care Med 2005 Oct 27; [Epub ahead of print]

217. Ranieri VM, Giunta F, Suter PM, Slutsky AS. Mechanical ventilation as a mediator of multisystem organ failure in acute respiratory distress syndrome. JAMA 2000; 284:43–4.

218. Stuber F, Wrigge H, Schroeder S, et al. Kinetic and reversibility of mechanical ventilation-associated pulmonary and systemic inflammatory response in patients with acute lung injury. Intensive Care Med 2002; 28:834–41.

219. Parsons PE, Eisner MD, Thompson BT, et al. Lower tidal volume ventilation and plasma cytokine markers of inflammation in patients with acute lung injury. Crit Care Med 2005; 33: 1–6.

220. Milberg J, Davis D, Steinberg K, Hudson L. Improved survival of patients with acute respiratory distress syndrome (ARDS): 1983–1993. JAMA 1995; 273:306–9.

221. Dreyfuss D, Saumon G. Ventilator-induced lung injury: Lessons from experimental studies (State of the Art). Am J Respir Crit Care Med 1998; 157:1–30.

222. Abraham E. Why immunomodulatory therapies have not worked in sepsis. Intensive Care Med 1999; 25:556–66.

223. Fisher CJ Jr, Agosti JM, Opal SM, et al. Treatment of septic shock with the tumor necrosis factor receptor:Fc fusion protein. The Soluble TNF Receptor Sepsis Study Group. N Engl J Med 1996; 334:1697–702.

224. Dall'ava-Santucci J, Armaganidis A, Brunet F, et al. Mechanical effects of PEEP in patients with adult respiratory distress syndrome. J Appl Physiol 1990; 68:843–8.

_____

Chapter 43

VENTILATOR-INDUCED DIAPHRAGM DYSFUNCTION

THEODOROS VASSILAKOPOULOS

Mechanical ventilation is a life-saving treatment for respiratory failure. Apart from support of gas exchange, animal models have revealed additional benefits of mechanical ventilation: reversal of respiratory muscle fatigue, prevention of muscle fiber injury during sepsis,[1] and restoration of perfusion to vital organs in shock states[2] when blood flow is "stolen" by the intensely working respiratory muscles.[3] Mechanical ventilation, however, is associated with complications, including infection, barotrauma, cardiovascular compromise, tracheal injuries, oxygen toxicity, and in injured lungs ventilator-induced lung injury (VILI).[4]

Accumulating evidence suggests that mechanical ventilation can also induce dysfunction of the diaphragm, resulting in decreased diaphragmatic force-generating capacity, diaphragmatic atrophy, and diaphragmatic injury, which has been called *ventilator-induced diaphragmatic dysfunction* (VIDD).[5,6]

Evidence Supporting the Existence of Ventilation-Induced Diaphragmatic Dysfunction

Animal studies have documented that controlled mechanical ventilation (CMV) leads to decreased diaphragmatic force-generating capacity. In the intact diaphragm of various animal species (including primates) studied in vivo, transdiaphragmatic pressure generation caused by phrenic nerve stimulation declines at both submaximal and maximal stimulation frequencies (20–100 Hz),[7–9] in a time-dependent manner. The decline is evident early (1 day in rabbits [9] and 3 days in piglets[8]), and worsens as mechanical ventilation is prolonged. Within a few days (3 days in rabbits, 5 days in piglets, and 11 days in baboons), the pressure-generating capacity of the diaphragm declines by 40–50%. Not only is force-generating capacity depressed, but endurance of the diaphragm is also significantly compromised, as suggested by the reduced ability of animals to sustain an inspiratory resistive load.[7]

What is the cause of the decreased force-generating capacity and endurance? The decreased force-generating capacity is not secondary to changes in lung volume because transpulmonary pressure or dynamic lung compliance do not change.[8] Moreover, it is not caused by changes in abdominal compliance, which would affect diaphragmatic afterload and thus diaphragmatic-pressure development, given the nearly stable abdominal pressure over the observation period,[8] and the similar results obtained with abdominal wrapping that prevents changes in abdominal compliance.[7,8]

Neural or neuromuscular transmission remains intact as reflected by the lack of changes in phrenic nerve conduction (latency) and the stable response to repetitive stimulation of the phrenic nerve[8] (Fig. 43-1). In contrast, the decrease in the compound muscle action potential (CMAP) suggests that excitation-contraction coupling or membrane depolarization may be involved in the dysfunction (see Fig. 43-1).[8] Thus, ventilator-induced impairment in force-generating capacity appears to reside within the myofibers.

In vitro results of isometric (both twitch and tetanic)-tension development in isolated diaphragmatic strips[8,10–13] confirm the in vivo findings, and suggest that the decline in contractility is an early (12 hours) and progressive phenomenon (Fig. 43-2);[11] isometric-force development declines by 30–50% after 1–3 days of CMV in rats.

Increased fatigability of the diaphragmatic strips has been documented after CMV in vitro,[9,13] although at an early stage (18 hours) fatigue resistance is improved.[14] Some investigators, however, have failed to document alterations of in vitro fatigability.[12]

Do we have evidence for VIDD in humans? Although conclusive data do not exist, several intriguing observations suggest that VIDD may occur in patients. The twitch transdiaphragmatic pressure elicited by magnetic stimulation of

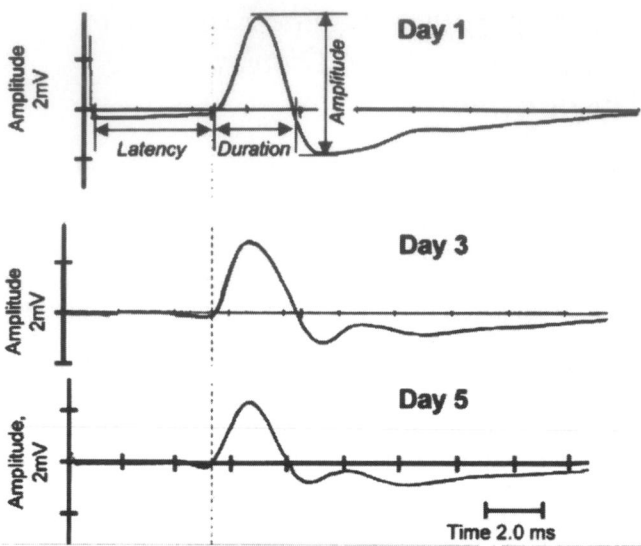

FIGURE 43-1 The evoked compound muscle action potential (CMAP) tracings from one piglet on day 1, day 3, and day 5, respectively, after the institution of controlled mechanical ventilation (CMV). The latency (time from stimulus to onset of CMAP) is constant on the different days after institution of CMV, indicating intact neural and neuromuscular transmission. In contrast, the decrease in the CMAP suggests that excitation-contraction coupling or membrane depolarization may be involved in the dysfunction. (*Reproduced, with permission, from Radell et al.*[8])

the phrenic nerves is reduced in ventilated patients compared with normal subjects,[15] and twitch transdiaphragmatic pressures were reduced in ventilated patients about to undergo weaning trials.[16] Diaphragmatic atrophy was documented (by ultrasound) in a tetraplegic patient after prolonged CMV;[17] the time course of atrophy, however, was not established. Furthermore, denervation atrophy removes

substances originating within the nerve that are trophic for the muscle, which is not the case for VIDD because neural and neuromuscular function remain intact. The presence of confounding factors, such as disease state (e.g., sepsis) and drug therapy (e.g., corticosteroids and neuromuscular blocking agents), makes documentation of VIDD difficult in a clinical setting. Nevertheless, retrospective analysis of postmortem data from neonates who received ventilator assistance for 12 days or more immediately before death revealed diffuse diaphragmatic myofiber atrophy (small myofibers with rounded outlines), which were not present in extradiaphragmatic muscles.[18]

Mechanisms of Dysfunction

MUSCLE ATROPHY

Most evidence shows that CMV leads to diaphragmatic wasting in rats (10).[10,12,19] Ventilator-induced cachexia[20] develops rapidly (as early as 18 hours after instituting CMV[19]). It is more pronounced in the diaphragm, which atrophies earlier than peripheral skeletal muscles, which are also inactive during mechanical ventilation. Within 18 hours of CMV, the diaphragm but not the soleus is affected.[19] By 48 hours, however, both the diaphragm and the peripheral muscles exhibit atrophy.[10,12] Two days of CMV with positive end-expiratory pressure (PEEP) (2 cmH_2O) induced atrophy in rabbits,[13] whereas 3 days of CMV without PEEP did not induce atrophy.[9] These findings suggest that the rapidity of atrophy might be augmented with use of PEEP.

Atrophy can result from decreased protein synthesis, increased proteolysis, or both. Six hours of CMV in rats resulted in a 30% decrease in the in vivo rate of mixed muscle protein synthesis and a 65% decrease in the rate of myosin-heavy-chain protein synthesis, both of which persisted throughout 18 hours of CMV (Fig. 43-3).[21] In addition,

FIGURE 43-2 Effects of prolonged CMV on the in vitro diaphragmatic force-frequency response in rats. Compared with control, CMV (all durations) resulted in a significant (* $P < 0.05$) reduction in diaphragmatic-specific force production at all stimulation frequencies. Values are means ± SE. (*Reproduced, with permission, from Yang et al.*[11])

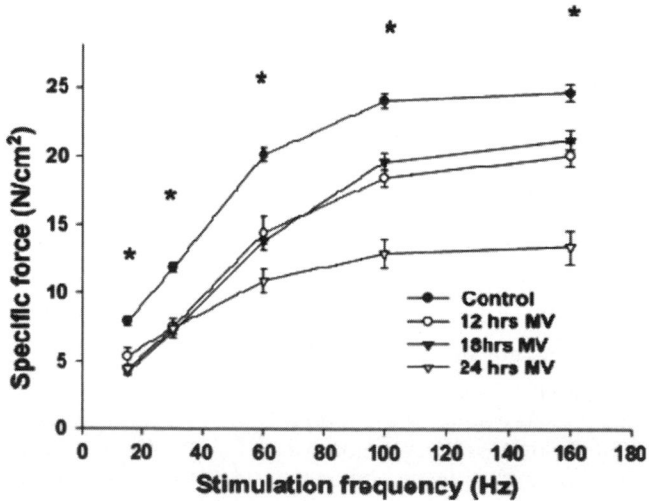

FIGURE 43-3 Fractional synthetic rates of myosin heavy chain (MHC) protein by calculation with tissue fluid [^{13}C]leucine as a surrogate measure of the [^{13}C]leucyl-tRNA precursor pool. Values are expressed as percent per hour. MV, mechanically ventilated animals; SB, spontaneously breathing animals. *Significantly different ($p < 0.05$) from time-matched SB group; ‡significantly different ($p < 0.05$) from SB for 6 hours (SB6). (*Reproduced, with permission, from Shanely et al.*[21])

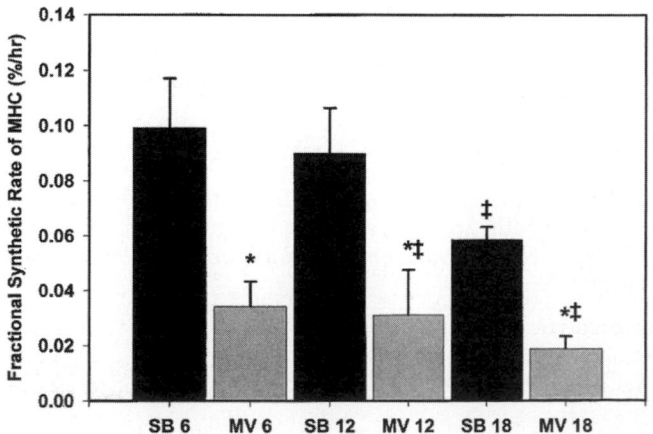

UBIQUITIN CONJUGATION

PROTEIN DEGRADATION

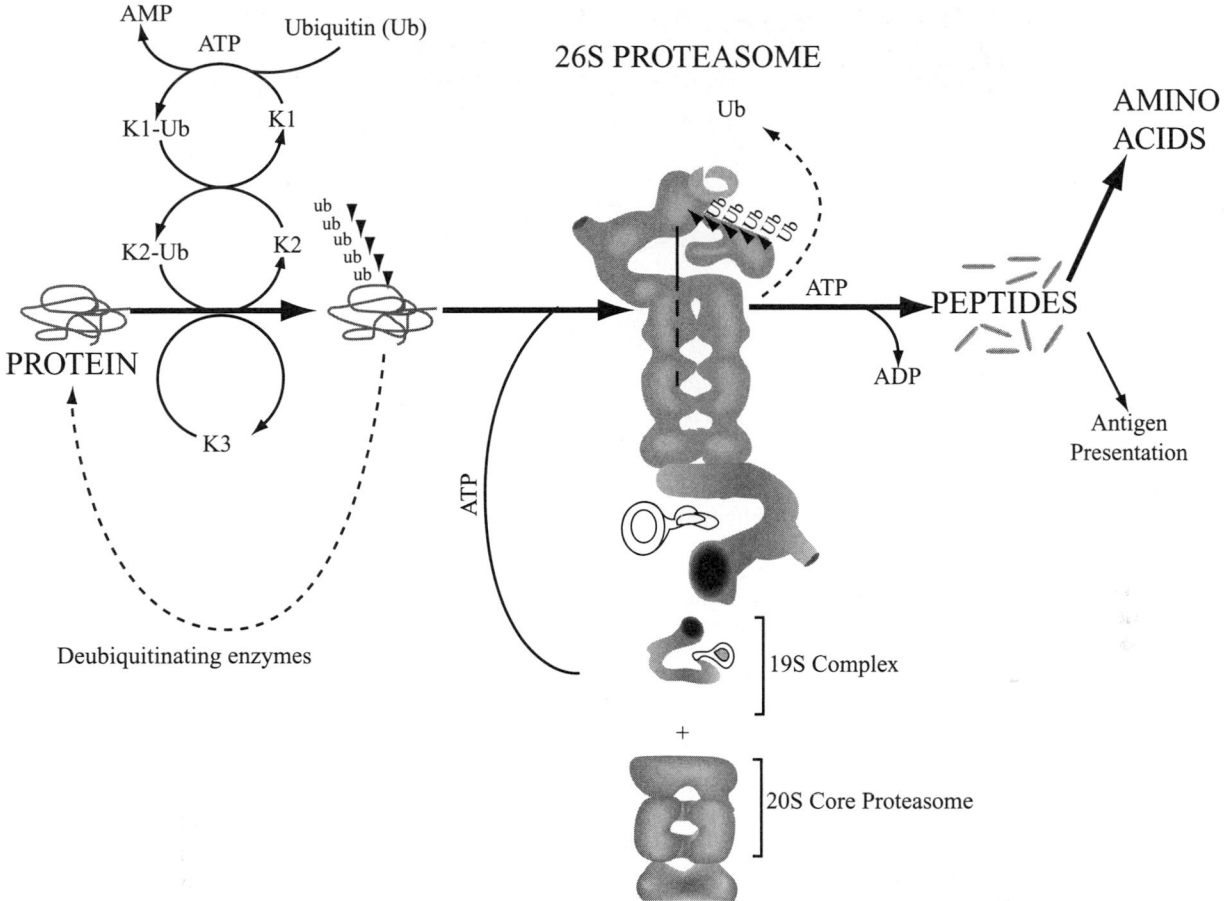

FIGURE 43-4 The ubiquitin–proteasome pathway of proteolysis. Proteins degraded by the ubiquitin–proteasome pathway are first conjugated to ubiquitin (*Ub*). The process of linking ubiquitin to lysine residues in proteins destined for degradation involves the activation of ubiquitin by the E1 enzyme in an ATP-dependent reaction. Activated ubiquitin is transferred to an E2 carrier protein and then to the substrate protein, a reaction catalyzed by an E3 enzyme. This process is repeated as multiple ubiquitin molecules are added to form a ubiquitin chain.

In ATP-dependent reactions, ubiquitin-conjugated proteins are recognized and bound by the 19S complex, which releases the ubiquitin chain and catalyzes the entry of the protein into the 20S core proteasome. Degradation occurs in the 26S core proteasome, which contains multiple proteolytic sites within its two central rings. Peptides produced by the proteasome are released and rapidly degraded to amino acids by peptidases in the cytoplasm or transported to the endoplasmic reticulum and used in the presentation of class I antigens. The ubiquitin is not degraded, but is released and reused. ATP, ADP, and AMP denote adenosine tri-, di-, and monophosphate. (*Reproduced, with permission, from Lecker et al.[24]*)

24 hours of CMV led to decreased levels of insulin-like growth factor (IGF)-1, which stimulates protein synthesis.[22] Thus, CMV decreases protein synthesis in the diaphragm.

Increased proteolysis has been documented in diaphragmatic strips from animals subjected to 18 hours of CMV.[19] Mammalian cells have three systems of proteases for intracellular proteolysis: lysosomal proteases, calpains, and the proteasome system. Both the calpains and the proteasome system are activated after 18 hours of CMV.[19] Calpains do not fully degrade, but only partially cleave proteins in vivo. This renders the proteins susceptible to the third proteolytic system, the proteasome.[20] Using the proteasome inhibitor, lactacystin, Shanely et al[19] showed that the proteasome contributes to the augmented proteolysis in diaphragmatic strips from animals subjected to CMV. The proteasome is a multisubunit multicatalytic complex that exists in two major forms: the core 20S proteasome can be free or bound to a pair of 19S regulators to form the 26S proteasome. Although the 26S proteasome might be activated in ventilator-induced cachexia, this has not been directly documented. CMV, however, increases the level of ubiquitin-protein conjugates of both the cytosolic and myofibrillar fractions of the diaphragm,[23] which are the substrates of the 26S proteasome (Fig. 43-4).[24] Furthermore, key enzymes involved in the function of the ubiquitin-proteasome pathway are upregulated in the diaphragm, such as the ubiquitin ligases muscle atrophy F-box (MAFbx/Atrogin-1),[23,25] and muscle ring finger-1 (MuRF1).[23] Not all mRNAs of the ubiquitin-proteasome pathway, however, are upregulated in the diaphragm, because the ubiquitin-conjugating

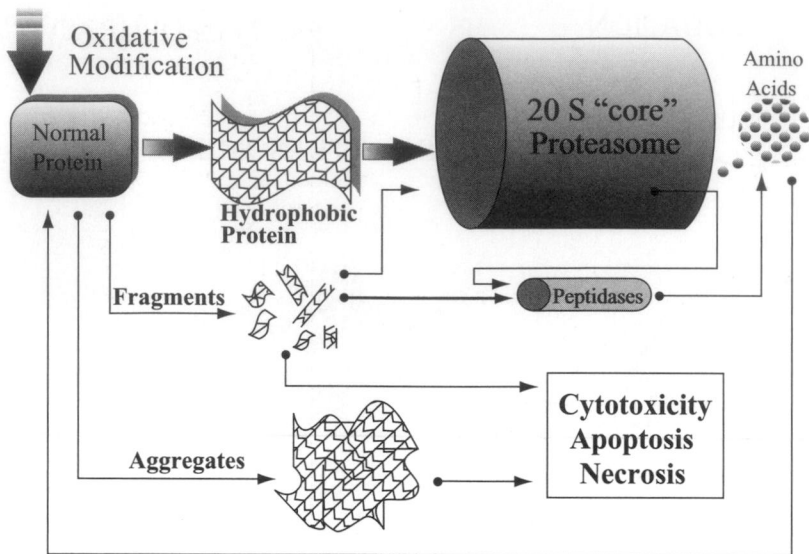

FIGURE 43-5 Proposed scheme for oxidation-induced protein degradation by the 20S proteasome, or fragmentation and aggregation. Mild oxidative stress modifies cellular proteins, generating hydrophobic protein "patches" that bind to the 20S proteasome and ensure rapid degradation. Because most oxidatively modified proteins are efficiently degraded, there is little chance for further oxidation reactions to cause protein fragmentation or aggregation. Under conditions of severe oxidative stress, however, or if proteasome activity declines during aging or disease, the production of protein fragments and cross-linked and oxidized protein aggregates increases. Some of the fragments are still degraded by the 20S proteasome (alone or in cooperation with cellular peptidases) but some may have cytotoxic biomimetic effects. Cross-linked and oxidized protein aggregates still tend to bind to the proteasome, which they then irreversibly inhibit. This process can cause a progressively worsening cycle of protein oxidation and increasing accumulation, which is ultimately cytotoxic. (*Reproduced, with permission, from Davies.*[27])

enzyme $E2_{14k}$, and polyubiquitin did not change after 12 hours of CMV.[23] Interestingly, Shanely et al[19] showed that CMV resulted in a fivefold increase in 20S proteasome activity, which is specialized in degrading proteins oxidized by reactive oxygen species (ROS). Oxidative damage to a protein results in its partial unfolding, exposing hidden hydrophobic residues (Fig. 43-5).[27] Therefore, an oxidized protein does not need to be further modified by ubiquitin conjugation to confer a hydrophobic patch, nor does it require energy from ATP hydrolysis to unfold.[28] This result is in concert with the evidence for oxidative stress–induced modification of proteins obtained from the diaphragms of animals subjected to CMV.[19,26,29]

OXIDATIVE STRESS

CMV is associated with augmented oxidative stress in the diaphragm, as indicated by the rise in both protein oxidation (Fig. 43-6) and lipid peroxidation.[19] The onset of oxidative injury is rapid, occurring within 6 hours of instituting CMV.[26] Activity of antioxidant enzymes (superoxide dismutase) is also augmented,[14] probably as a defense to limit oxidative stress–mediated injury. Oxidative stress has been documented in limb-muscle disuse-atrophy models. The immobilization period, however, was significantly longer (>4 days), and the oxidative stress was documented only after 8 days of disuse.[30] The basis of the different time course is not clear. CMV is a special form of disuse, because the diaphragm is not only inactive but also passively shortened by lung inflation. Passive muscle shortening increases blood flow and affects muscle metabolism,[31] which might partly

explain the different time course of oxidative stress generation. Blood flow to the respiratory muscles, however, is actually reduced during CMV.[32,33] The mechanisms of oxidative-stress generation secondary to CMV are unclear. Immobilization models in limb muscles have shown up-regulation of the superoxide-generating enzyme, xanthine oxidase, and elevated levels of transition metals, such as iron, calcium, copper, and manganese.[30] The increase in ferrous cations (Fe^{2+}) may facilitate the generation of hydroxyl radicals from superoxide and hydrogen peroxide; both copper and manganese may catalyze the oxidation of glutathione, thus reducing the overall antioxidant capacity. Whether such a mechanism occurs in the diaphragm needs experimental confirmation, although decreased glutathione levels have been documented.[19]

Oxidative stress can modify many critical proteins involved in energetics, excitation-contraction coupling, and force generation.[34] Accordingly, CMV-induced diaphragmatic protein oxidation was evident in insoluble (but not soluble) proteins with molecular masses of about 200, 128, 85, and 40 kD (see Fig. 43-6).[26] These findings raise the possibility that actin (40 kD) and/or myosin (200 kD) undergo oxidative modification during CMV (Fig. 43-7). This intriguing possibility awaits confirmation by more specific identification of the modified proteins.

STRUCTURAL INJURY

Structural abnormalities of different subcellular components of diaphragmatic fibers have been found after CMV.[9,35,36] The changes consist of disrupted myofibrils,

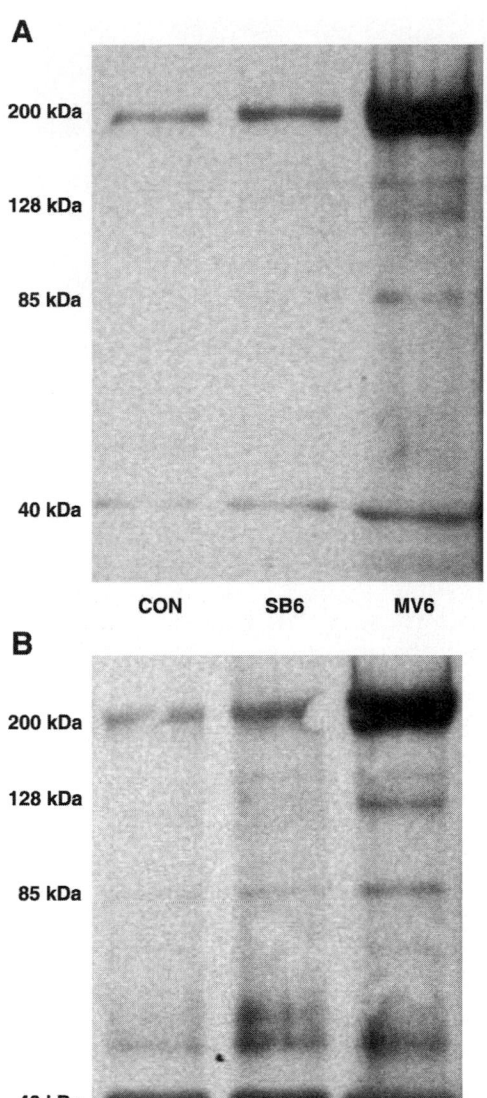

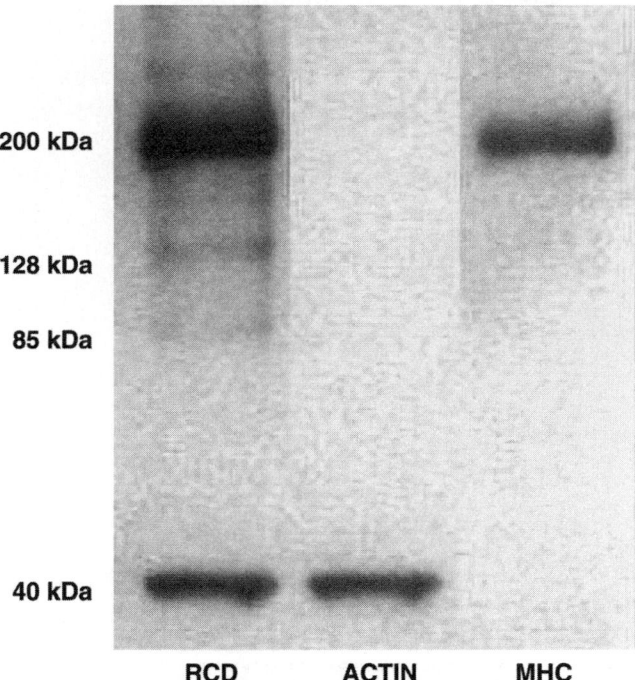

FIGURE 43-7 Illustration of Western blots using monoclonal antibodies to identify oxidized proteins with molecular masses of ~200 to 40 kDa. *Left lane:* Reactive carbonyl derivatives (RCD) in insoluble proteins isolated from the diaphragm of an animal exposed to CMV for 18 hours. *Middle and right lanes:* The same membrane stripped of the 2,4-dinitrophenylhydrazone antibody against RCDs, and then sequentially reprobed with monoclonal antibodies specific for rat skeletal muscle actin and all myosin-heavy-chain (MHC) isoforms. (*Reproduced, with permission, from Zegeroglu et al.*[26])

FIGURE 43-6 Representative Western blots illustrating the level of reactive carbonyl derivatives (RCD), which are the footprints of protein modifications induced by oxidative stress in diaphragmatic insoluble proteins with molecular masses ranging between 200 and 40 kilodaltons (kDa). *A*. Levels of RCD in diaphragmatic insoluble proteins in control animals (*Con*), animals spontaneously breathing for 6 hours (*SB6*), and animals subjected to CMV for 6 hours (*MV6*). *B*. Levels of RCD in diaphragmatic insoluble proteins in control animals (*Con*), animals spontaneously breathing for 18 hours (*SB 18*), and animals subjected to CMV for 18 hours (*MV18*). (*Reproduced, with permission, from Zegeroglu et al.*[26])

increased numbers of lipid vacuoles in the sarcoplasm, and abnormally small mitochondria containing focal membrane disruptions (Fig. 43-8). Similar alterations were observed in the external intercostal muscles of ventilated animals (see Fig. 43-8),[35] but not in the hindlimb muscle.[9] The structural alterations in the myofibrils have detrimental effects on diaphragmatic force-generating capacity, the number of abnormal myofibrils being inversely related to the force output of the diaphragm[9] (Fig. 43-9). The mechanisms of injury have not been elucidated, but may involve activation of calpains, which have the ability to degrade several sarcomeric proteins, and direct cellular injury secondary to augmented oxidative stress.[6] Furthermore, episodes of breakthrough diaphragmatic activity during CMV may (when present) also contribute to the injurious process,[9] given that, after a sustained period of muscle unloading, resumption of muscle activity is associated with an increased vulnerability to contraction-induced muscle fiber injury.[6]

MUSCLE FIBER REMODELING

At the molecular level, the heavy-chain component of the myosin molecule constitutes the primary basis for the traditional classification of muscle fibers into either slow-twitch (type I) or fast-twitch (type II). There are two ways in which muscles can modify their overall myosin heavy-chain (MHC) phenotype: preferential atrophy/hypertrophy of fibers containing a specific MHC isoform, and actual transformation from one fiber type to the other. Both short-term,[19,37] and long-term CMV[12] cause significant modifications of the MHC phenotype. Within 18 hours of CMV,

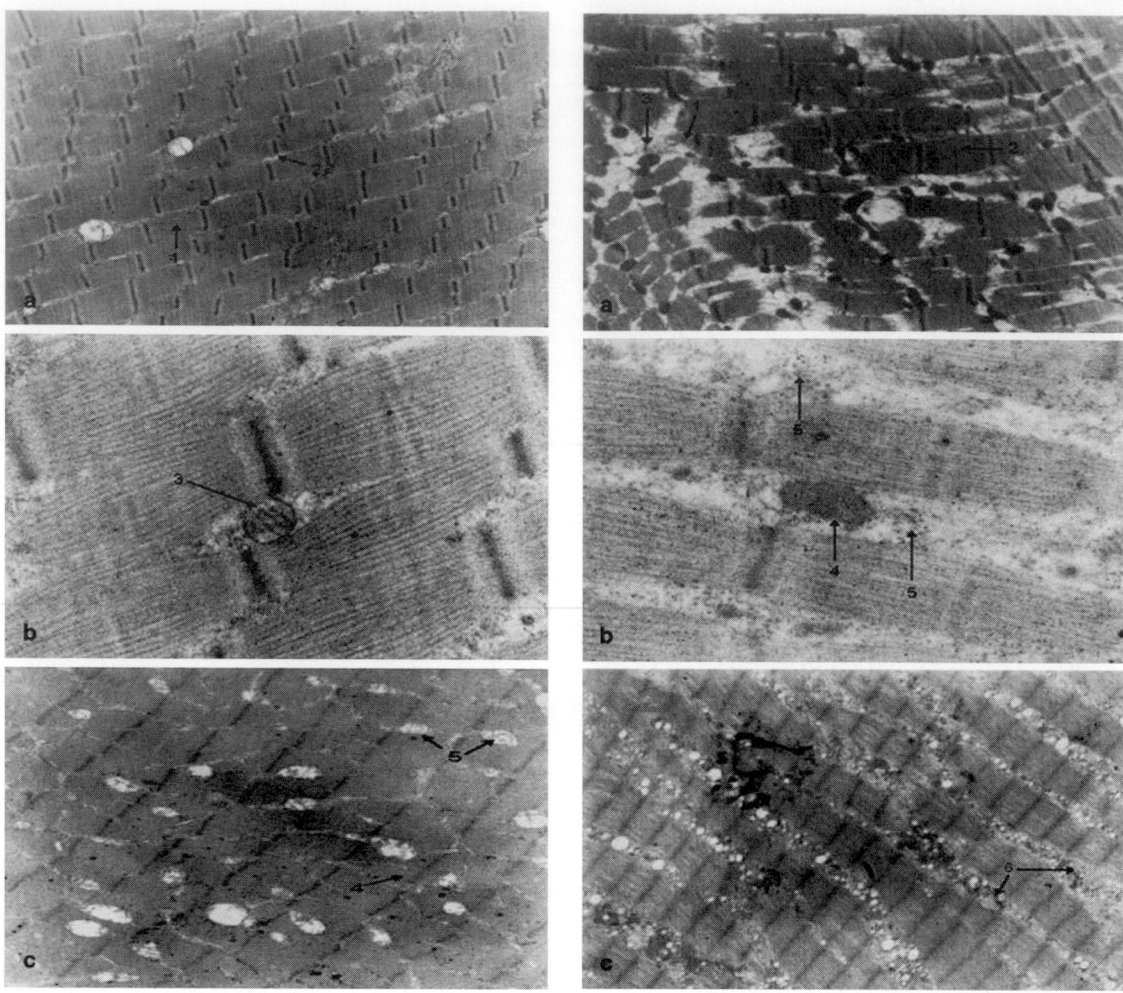

FIGURE 43-8 *A.* Control rabbit respiratory muscle ultrastructure as assessed by electron microscopy. Longitudinal sections. a. Diaphragm of control rabbit ($\times$ 6000). Normal ultrastructure of myofibrils. 1, Normal sarcomeric structure; 1, small band of sarcoplasm. *b.* Diaphragm of control rabbit ($\times$ 30,000). 3, The mitochondrial architecture is normal. *c.* External intercostal muscles of a control rabbit ($\times$ 6000). 4, Normal myofibrillar ultrastructure; 5, normal mitochondria. *B.* Ventilated rabbit respiratory muscle ultrastructure: longitudinal sections. *a.* Diaphragm of ventilated rabbit ($\times$ 6000). Disruption and fragmentation of myofibrils, with large interfibrillar space. 1, Disintegrated sarcomere; 2, preserved sarcomere; 3, sarcoplasmic disorganization. *b.* Diaphragm of ventilated rabbit ($\times$ 40,000). 1, Smaller mitochondria, disruption of outer membranes; 5, increase in sarcoplasmic granular material and cytoplasmic lipid vacuoles. *c.* External intercostal muscle of ventilated rabbit ($\times$ 6000). 6, Increase in sarcoplasm lipid vacuoles and in connective tissue. (*Reproduced, with permission, from Bernard et al.[35]*)

both type I and II fibers are reduced, yet type II fibers exhibit much greater reduction.[19] Within 24 hours of CMV, the transcript levels of the fast 2A and 2B MHC isoforms are decreased by ~20%,[37] consistent with the preferential atrophy observed in the above-mentioned studies. This modification of the MHC phenotype could contribute to the force decline of the diaphragm, because the force produced by slow fibers is less than the force produced by fast fibers.[38] Prolonged (44–93 hours) CMV, however, results in a different pattern of MHC phenotype modification: a decreased number of type I fibers, and increases in fast MHC isoforms mainly within hybrid fibers (fibers co-expressing both slow and fast isoforms).[12] This slow-to-fast transformation does not compromise diaphragmatic contractility per se, but reduces diaphragmatic endurance, because fewer slow-twitch fatigue-resistant fibers are available.

What is the basis of this different response? The ventilator strategy was different in these two studies. Despite similar respiratory rates, tidal volume and thus the degree of phasic diaphragmatic shortening was twice as high in the study of Shanely et al[19] (1 ml/100 g body weight) than in the study of Yang et al[12] (0.5 ml/100 g body weight). In contrast, the degree of tonic diaphragmatic shortening imposed by PEEP was much greater in the study of Yang et al[12] (PEEP = 4 cmH$_2$O) than in the study of Shanely et al[19] (PEEP = 1 cmH$_2$O).

Whether different ventilator patterns result in different fiber type transformations is not known. Interestingly, limb muscle inactivity models have shown that the duration of inactivity is very influential for the fiber type transformation observed. Whereas short-term inactivity results in fast-to-slow transformation (similar to short-term mechanical

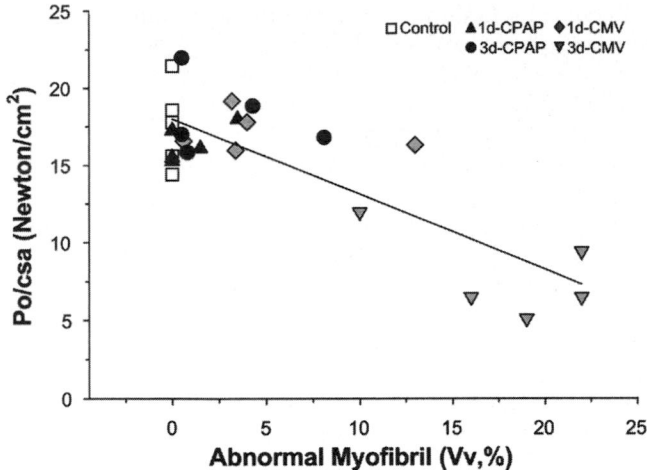

FIGURE 43-9 Correlation between the maximum tetanic force (P_o) developed by the diaphragm and the percentage of abnormal myofibrils in the control state, after 1 day of CPAP, after 3 days of CPAP, after 1 day of CMV, and after 3 days of CMV. $y = -0.5 \times + 18.0$, ($r = 0.82$, $P < 0.01$). CPAP, continuous positive airway pressure of 0 cmH_2O; CMV, controlled mechanical ventilation. (*Reproduced, with permission, from Sassoon et al.*[9])

ventilation), longer inactivity results in slow-to-fast transformation. Although the duration of inactivity was much longer (6 weeks) in limb muscles, the diaphragm might exhibit much faster adaptation to inactivity, because it is continuously contracting throughout life with much higher duty cycles (duration of contraction relative to relaxation) than the limb muscles. In rabbits, two days of CMV resulted in atrophy of the respiratory muscles and in decreased cross-sectional area of type IIa and IIb fibers but not of type I fibers (fast-to-slow transformation) and no change in their proportion.[13] Three days of CMV, however, did not affect the percentage and cross-sectional areas of slow and fast fibers and resulted in rather reciprocal changes in fast MHC isoform expression, with increased percentage of MHC2A and decreased expression of MHC2X.[9] The differences might be attributed to the presence of PEEP (2 cmH_2O in Capdevila et al[13] and 0 cmH_2O in Sassoon et al[9]), or to episodes of breakthrough diaphragmatic activity.[9] In piglets, 5 days of CMV resulted in increased type IIbx fibers compared with controls, with a decrease in type I and IIa fiber proportions that did not reach statistical significance.[36] Thus, fiber type transformations might be dependent on the time spent on CMV, the ventilator settings used, and the species.

Interestingly, 24 hours of CMV resulted in changes in the mRNA expression of the myogenic regulatory transcription factors, myoD (myogenic determination gene D) (decrease) and myogenin (increase), with a consequent decrease in the myoD/myogenin ratio.[37] These factors are driving myoblast determination and differentiation during embryogenesis, but may also influence fiber type transformation in the adult muscle. In fact, the levels of myoD are significantly greater in fast than in slow muscle fibers, and myogenin is preferentially located in slow fibers, and their ratio

is highly correlated with muscle-fiber phenotype. Whether this correlation is causal is debated.[39] The relationship between the myoD/myogenin ratio and muscle fiber phenotype is complex and overridden by other regulatory factors (under some conditions).[39]

The remodeling of the diaphragm is not limited to fibertype transformations. Whereas 24 hours of CMV do not affect the optimal length of the diaphragm,[11] more than 48 hours causes significant decreases in length,[10,12] suggesting that the diaphragm is dropping out sarcomeres. Moreover, a significant number of regenerative fibers is present in the diaphragm secondary to CMV.[36]

METABOLIC ENZYMES

Changes in myofiber enzymes (either content or activity), which are implicated in metabolic pathways and thus could contribute to VIDD (citrate synthase, lactate dehydrogenase, and succinate dehydrogenase), have not been documented.[9,10] Quite early (18 hours), however, citrate synthase activity is increased.[14] Furthermore, only minor changes in oxidative phosphorylation coupling have been found.[35] Taken together, these results suggest that changes in metabolism do not play a significant role in the development of VIDD.

DRUGS

To achieve diaphragmatic inactivity, anesthetics and/or neuromuscular blockers have been used, which can decrease diaphragmatic force-generating capacity in the clinical setting.[40] Neuromuscular blockers[7,12] cannot account for the decreased contractility, because similar results were obtained in studies that did not use these drugs.[9,11] Anesthetics can also be excluded; studies that used appropriate controls (to the extent feasible; i.e., a group of anesthetized spontaneously breathing animals) concluded that the decreased contractility was secondary to the effects of mechanical ventilation per se (and not to the anesthetic).[9]

In summary, diaphragmatic atrophy, oxidative stress, structural injury, and diaphragmatic remodeling are proven mechanisms that contribute to VIDD.

Role of Ventilator Mode and Ventilator Settings

VENTILATOR MODE

Evidence for VIDD comes from studies in which CMV was exclusively used; few data exist about other ventilator modes. Assisted (flow-triggered, pressure-limited) ventilation, from the onset of ventilator support, resulted in attenuation of the force loss induced by CMV (Fig. 43-10).[25] Tetanic and twitch force decreased by 14% and 9%, respectively, with assisted ventilation relative to control animals, which tended toward, but did not reach, statistical significance. In contrast, the changes with CMV were respectively 48% and 47%.[25] Thus, it stands to reason that preserving

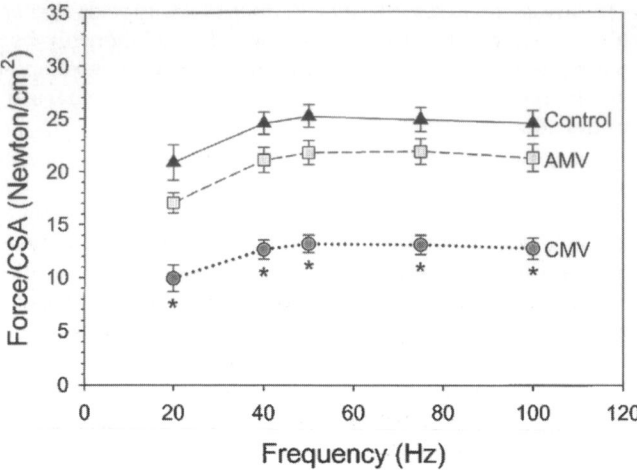

FIGURE 43-10 Diaphragmatic tetanic force at various stimulation frequencies in the control state, with assisted-controlled ventilation (AMV), and with controlled mechanical ventilation (CMV). Values are mean ± SE. *p <0.01, CMV versus control and AMV. CSA, cross-sectional area. (*Reproduced, with permission, from Sassoon et al.[25]*)

diaphragmatic contractions during mechanical ventilation should attenuate the force loss induced by CMV. Other forms of partial ventilator support, such as pressure-support and synchronized intermittent mechanical ventilation, have not been experimentally tested.

VENTILATOR SETTINGS

The role of ventilator settings in the development of VIDD is not clear. During mechanical ventilation, the diaphragm is intermittently and repetitively shortened by cyclical lung inflation. Therefore, changes in the respiratory rate and tidal volume applied during mechanical ventilation necessarily alter the speed and extent of diaphragmatic shortening. The use of PEEP, by contrast, leads to baseline shortening of the diaphragm at functional residual capacity. It has long been known that the adverse effects of disuse on limb muscle structure are exacerbated by muscle shortening.[41] In addition, maintaining skeletal muscles (including the diaphragm) in a shortened position causes a loss of sarcomeres in series.[42] Interestingly, two studies that employed PEEP[10,12] found that CMV (48 hours or more) resulted in significantly decreased optimal length of the diaphragm, a finding that strongly suggests the presence of such sarcomere loss. Differences in myosin isoform expression patterns and the degree of atrophy observed in certain studies may be at least partly related to the extent of diaphragmatic shortening imposed by the particular ventilator settings in these investigations.

Reversibility

There is no information on the time course of reversal of VIDD once it has been established. Based on peripheral skeletal muscle studies, however, the time course of recovery is expected to be slow.[43,44]

Clinical Relevance

The typical clinical scenario in which to suspect VIDD is a patient who fails to wean after a period of CMV, because weaning failure is commonly related to respiratory muscle dysfunction. Other known causes of respiratory muscle weakness such as shock, ongoing sepsis, major malnutrition, electrolyte disturbances, and neuromuscular disorders, must be ruled out.[45] For example, prolonged neuromuscular blockade can be excluded by the lack of an abnormal response to train-of-four stimulation, critical illness polyneuropathy by the absence of neuropathic changes on electrophysiological testing, and acute quadriplegic myopathy by the lack of corticosteroid exposure history (or by muscle biopsy in indeterminate cases).[45]

Preventive Countermeasures

VENTILATOR STRATEGY

Presently, it is prudent to curtail the period of CMV as much as possible, especially in older individuals. Animal studies suggest that the effects of aging and mechanical ventilation are additive.[46] Although CMV induced similar losses (24%) in diaphragmatic isometric tension in both young and old animals, the combination of aging and CMV resulted in a 34% decrement in diaphragmatic isometric tension compared to young control animals.

When feasible, partial support modes that allow diaphragmatic contractions should be used. Recent studies raise the possibility that partial support modes can be used in situations traditionally considered as indications for CMV, such as acute lung injury/acute respiratory distress syndrome (ALI/ARDS).[47,48]

Noninvasive ventilation can be an alternative strategy in patients who experience weaning failure and are traditionally ventilated using CMV, a strategy based on the premise that respiratory muscle fatigue (requiring rest to recover) is the cause of weaning failure. Recent evidence does not support the existence of fatigue in patients who fail to wean,[16] thus no reason exists to completely unload the respiratory muscles with CMV.

In patients in whom use of CMV is inevitable, short periods of diaphragmatic activity have been suggested as a potentially preventive countermeasure.[6] This could be achieved with phrenic nerve stimulation.[17,49] During prolonged CMV in a tetraplegic patient, only 30 minutes of pacing of one hemidiaphragm each day was adequate to attenuate atrophy in that hemidiaphragm compared to the non-paced hemidiaphragm.[17] In VIDD, however, trophic influences from the nerve are present, and thus the situation might be different. Short periods of diaphragmatic activity can also be achieved by allowing periods of intermittent spontaneous breathing between the periods of CMV. Neither 5 nor 60 minutes of spontaneous breathing every

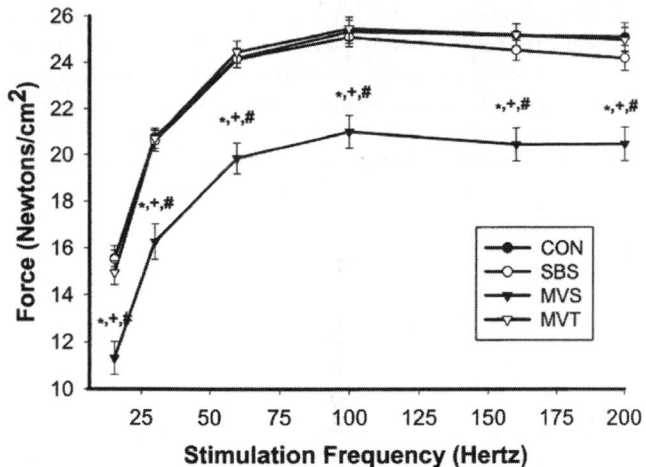

FIGURE 43-11 Force–frequency curves of in vitro diaphragm strips from control (*CON*), spontaneously breathing (*SBS*), mechanical ventilation (*MVS*), and mechanical ventilation in animals receiving Trolox (*MVT*). Values represent means ± SEM. *Significantly different from CON group, $p < 0.05$; +significantly different from SBS group, $p < 0.05$; #significantly different from MVT group, $p < 0.05$. (*Reproduced, with permission, from Betters et al.*[29])

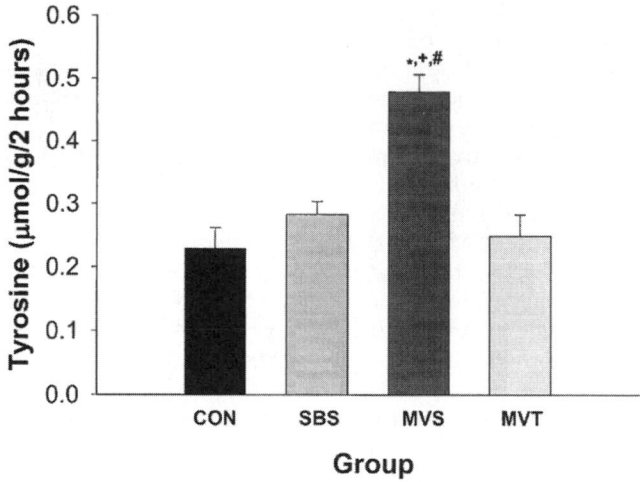

FIGURE 43-12 Effect of mechanical ventilation and Trolox supplementation on total in vitro protein degradation as measured by the rate of tyrosine release from diaphragmatic strips per wet weight of muscle in 2 hours. CON, control; MVS, mechanical ventilation; MVT, mechanical ventilation in animals receiving Trolox; SBS, spontaneously breathing. Values represent means ± SEM. *Significantly different from CON group, $p < 0.05$; +significantly different from SBS group, $p < 0.05$; #significantly different from MVT group, $p < 0.05$. (*Reproduced, with permission, from Betters et al.*[29])

6 hours during CMV in rats were able to significantly attenuate the decrease in diaphragmatic force production induced by CMV, despite being able to prevent atrophy.[50] Whether more frequent intervals of spontaneous breathing might be more effective awaits experimental proof.

NONVENTILATORY COUNTERMEASURES

Antioxidant supplementation can decrease the oxidative stress and thus might attenuate VIDD. When rats were administered the antioxidant Trolox (an analogue of vitamin E), from the onset of CMV, its detrimental effects on contractility (Fig. 43-11) and proteolysis (Fig. 43-12) were prevented.[29]

A similar approach is adopted by nature itself. Various dormant animals immobilized for prolonged periods avoid muscle atrophy through a decrease in metabolic rate, which reduces formation of ROS, and a concomitant rise in antioxidant enzymes.[51,52] A combination of vitamins E and C administered to critically ill (mostly trauma) patients was effective in reducing the duration of mechanical ventilation as compared to nonsupplemented patients.[53] It is tempting to suggest that some of this beneficial effect was mediated by preventing VIDD. Until antioxidant therapy is shown to be beneficial and feasible, meticulous nutritional support is mandatory because the effects of disuse and malnutrition are synergistic.[54]

Important Unknowns

Several important and clinically relevant questions need to be addressed in the future. One, how is the susceptibility to VIDD influenced by alterations in the baseline state of the diaphragm? All animal studies of VIDD to date have been performed in previously normal diaphragms. We do not know to what extent the response to CMV might be modified by various conditions. For instance, oxidative stress is implicated in the loss of diaphragmatic force-generating capacity associated with sepsis[55] and mechanical ventilation.[29] Short-term CMV, however, actually improves force-generating capacity of the diaphragm in sepsis, and it does not appear to alter the level of oxidative stress in this situation.[1] Along these lines, the response to mechanical ventilation might be different in a diaphragm previously loaded to the point of injury and/or fatigue, both of which are also associated with increased oxidative stress.[56,57] Under these circumstances, would mechanical ventilation favor or prevent the development of further oxidative stress, injury, and contractile dysfunction? Once diaphragmatic injury has occurred, would mechanical ventilation facilitate or impair the subsequent muscle repair process, particularly if it alters the expression of myogenic transcription factors involved in muscle regeneration?[58] The answers await further study.

Two, does diaphragmatic disuse associated with CMV increase the susceptibility to subsequent contraction-induced injury, once respiratory efforts are resumed? Preliminary data suggest that subjecting rats to 24 hours of CMV produced a 26% decrement in diaphragmatic maximal specific force, with no apparent injury to the cell membrane or evidence of inflammation. Subjecting the rats to two further hours of reloading did not exacerbate CMV-induced contractile dysfunction or induce membrane injury or macrophage invasion.[59] Nonetheless, reloading was associated with increased myeloperoxidase activity and neutrophil infiltration, which might be injurious for the diaphragm at a later time, if reloading were continued.

Three, what is the optimal degree of respiratory muscle effort that should be targeted during mechanical ventilation in order to promote diaphragmatic fiber repair, once injury has occurred, and to prevent the onset of contraction-induced muscle fiber injury when reattempting spontaneous breathing? The best method to condition or train the respiratory muscles after CMV has to be determined.

Four, what is the time course for development of VIDD in humans? Animal studies suggest that VIDD secondary to CMV develops rapidly. The rate of muscle atrophy declines as the body-mass–specific metabolic rate decreases, and thus is much smaller in large animals than in smaller animals.[52] Consequently, onset of VIDD is expected to be less rapid in patients than in rodents. Organ donors with brain death could provide a useful clinical model to study the time course of VIDD development in humans, because they are maintained on CMV for variable periods and are usually free of comorbidities.

Five, how is VIDD modified by the presence of other factors (corticosteroid use, neuromuscular blockade, or ICU-acquired neuromuscular disorders)? What are the potential countermeasures to VIDD under these conditions? Unfortunately, findings from models of limb muscle disuse are not directly applicable to VIDD because not only does the diaphragm differ from limb muscles, but the pattern of disuse is different: (1) in hindlimb suspension, the muscle is unloaded but EMG activity is largely unaffected; (2) in denervation studies, the muscle is unloaded and EMG activity is eliminated, but there is interruption of trophic influences from the nerve; and (3) responses to muscle disuse are greatly affected by the degree of muscle shortening and lengthening that are present. Therefore, CMV imposes a unique form of skeletal muscle disuse: the diaphragm is simultaneously unloaded, electrically quiescent, and phasically shortened, by cyclical lung inflation, or tonically shortened, when PEEP is used. Intense research is needed on this specific form of disuse atrophy.

The Future

Future development of tissue-specific proteasome and calpain inhibitors might ameliorate ventilator-induced cachexia[60] and thus possibly VIDD. Furthermore, newer methods of ventilator triggering[61] might provide fine titration of respiratory muscle loading/unloading during mechanical ventilation, which would prevent VIDD or promote its reversal.

Summary and Conclusion

In the last few years, clinicians and scientists have become aware that mechanical ventilation can damage previously injured lungs. The knowledge acquired about ventilator-induced lung injury[4] led to clinical trials resulting in improved outcome of ALI/ARDS patients.[62,63] Mechanical

ventilation can also damage previously normal respiratory muscles. Intense research is required to unravel the mechanisms of VIDD, and to develop ways of translating this knowledge into clinical benefit. The respiratory muscles are not an inert pump that can casually be substituted by the ventilator. The vital pump is active, plastic, and vulnerable.

References

1. Ebihara S, Hussain SN, Danialou G, et al. Mechanical ventilation protects against diaphragm injury in sepsis: interaction of oxidative and mechanical stresses. Am J Respir Crit Care Med 2002; 165:221–8.
2. Viires N, Sillye G, Aubier M, Rassidakis A, Roussos C. Regional blood flow distribution in dog during induced hypotension and low cardiac output. Spontaneous breathing versus artificial ventilation. J Clin Invest 1983; 72:935–47.
3. Vassilakopoulos T, Zakynthinos S, Roussos C. Respiratory muscles and weaning failure. Eur Respir J 1996; 9:2383–400.
4. International consensus conferences in intensive care medicine: ventilator-associated lung injury in ARDS. This official conference report was cosponsored by the American Thoracic Society, The European Society of Intensive Care Medicine, and The Societe de Reanimation de Langue Francaise, and was approved by the ATS Board of Directors, July 1999. Am J Respir Crit Care Med 1999; 160:2118–24.
5. Sassoon CS. Ventilator-associated diaphragmatic dysfunction. Am J Respir Crit Care Med 2002; 166:1017–8.
6. Vassilakopoulos T, Petrof BJ. Ventilator-induced diaphragmatic dysfunction. Am J Respir Crit Care Med 2004; 169:336–41.
7. Anzueto A, Peters JI, Tobin MJ, et al. Effects of prolonged controlled mechanical ventilation on diaphragmatic function in healthy adult baboons. Crit Care Med 1997; 25:1187–90.
8. Radell PJ, Remahl S, Nichols DG, Eriksson LI. Effects of prolonged mechanical ventilation and inactivity on piglet diaphragm function. Intensive Care Med 2002; 28:358–64.
9. Sassoon CS, Caiozzo VJ, Manka A, Sieck GC. Altered diaphragm contractile properties with controlled mechanical ventilation. J Appl Physiol 2002; 92:2585–95.
10. Le Bourdelles G, Viires N, Boczkowski J, et al. Effects of mechanical ventilation on diaphragmatic contractile properties in rats. Am J Respir Crit Care Med 1994; 149:1539–44.
11. Powers SK, Shanely RA, Coombes JS, et al. Mechanical ventilation results in progressive contractile dysfunction in the diaphragm. J Appl Physiol 2002; 92:1851–8.
12. Yang L, Luo J, Bourdon J, et al. Controlled mechanical ventilation leads to remodeling of the rat diaphragm. Am J Respir Crit Care Med 2002; 166:1135–40.
13. Capdevila X, Lopez S, Bernard N, et al. Effects of controlled mechanical ventilation on respiratory muscle contractile properties in rabbits. Intensive Care Med 2003; 29:103–10.
14. Shanely RA, Coombes JS, Zergeroglu AM, Webb AI, Powers SK. Short-duration mechanical ventilation enhances diaphragmatic fatigue resistance but impairs force production. Chest 2003; 123:195–201.
15. Watson AC, Hughes PD, Louise HM, et al. Measurement of twitch transdiaphragmatic, esophageal, and endotracheal tube pressure with bilateral anterolateral magnetic phrenic nerve stimulation in patients in the intensive care unit. Crit Care Med 2001; 29:1325–31.
16. Laghi F, Cattapan SE, Jubran A, et al. Is weaning failure caused by low-frequency fatigue of the diaphragm? Am J Respir Crit Care Med 2003; 167:120–7.

17. Ayas NT, McCool FD, Gore R, Lieberman SL, Brown R. Prevention of human diaphragm atrophy with short periods of electrical stimulation. Am J Respir Crit Care Med 1999; 159:2018–20.

18. Knisely AS, Leal SM, Singer DB. Abnormalities of diaphragmatic muscle in neonates with ventilated lungs. J Pediatr 1988; 113:1074–7.

19. Shanely RA, Zergeroglu MA, Lennon SL, et al. Mechanical ventilation-induced diaphragmatic atrophy is associated with oxidative injury and increased proteolytic activity. Am J Respir Crit Care Med 2002; 166:1369–74.

20. Hussain SN, Vassilakopoulos T. Ventilator-induced cachexia. Am J Respir Crit Care Med 2002; 166:1307–8.

21. Shanely RA, Van Gammeren D, Deruisseau KC, et al. Mechanical ventilation depresses protein synthesis in the rat diaphragm. Am J Respir Crit Care Med 2004; 170:994–9.

22. Gayan-Ramirez G, De Paepe K, Cadot P, Decramer M. Detrimental effects of short-term mechanical ventilation on diaphragm function and IGF-I mRNA in rats. Intensive Care Med 2003; 29:825–33.

23. Deruisseau KC, Kavazis AN, Deering MA, et al. Mechanical ventilation induces alterations of the ubiquitin-proteasome pathway in the diaphragm. J Appl Physiol 2004; 98:1314–21.

24. Lecker SH, Solomon V, Mitch WE, Goldberg AL. Muscle protein breakdown and the critical role of the ubiquitin-proteasome pathway in normal and disease states. J Nutr 1999; 129(1S Suppl):227S–37S.

25. Sassoon CS, Zhu E, Caiozzo VJ. Assist-control mechanical ventilation attenuates ventilator-induced diaphragmatic dysfunction. Am J Respir Crit Care Med 2004; 170:626–32.

26. Zergeroglu MA, McKenzie MJ, Shanely RA, et al. Mechanical ventilation–induced oxidative stress in the diaphragm. J Appl Physiol 2003; 95:1116–1124.

27. Davies KJ. Degradation of oxidized proteins by the 20S proteasome. Biochimie 2001; 83:301–10.

28. Shringarpure R, Grune T, Mehlhase J, Davies KJ. Ubiquitin-conjugation is not required for the degradation of oxidized proteins by the proteasome. J Biol Chem 2003;278:311–18.

29. Betters JL, Criswell DS, Shanely RA, et al. Trolox attenuates mechanical ventilation–induced diaphragmatic dysfunction and proteolysis. Am J Respir Crit Care Med 2004; 170:1179–84.

30. Kondo H, Miura M, Nakagaki I, Sasaki S, Itokawa Y. Trace element movement and oxidative stress in skeletal muscle atrophied by immobilization. Am J Physiol 1992; 262(5 Pt 1):E583–E590.

31. Holmang A, Mimura K, Lonnroth P. Involuntary leg movements affect interstitial nutrient gradients and blood flow in rat skeletal muscle. J Appl Physiol 2002; 92:982–8.

32. Hering R, Viehofer A, Berg A, et al. Weight loss of respiratory muscles during mechanical ventilation. Intensive Care Med 2003; 29:1612.

33. Magder S, Erian R, Roussos C. Respiratory muscle blood flow in oleic acid–induced pulmonary edema. J Appl Physiol 1986; 60:1849–56.

34. Reid MB. Invited review: redox modulation of skeletal muscle contraction: what we know and what we don't. J Appl Physiol 2001; 90:724–31.

35. Bernard N, Matecki S, Py G, et al. Effects of prolonged mechanical ventilation on respiratory muscle ultrastructure and mitochondrial respiration in rabbits. Intensive Care Med 2003; 29: 111–8.

36. Radell P, Edstrom L, Stibler H, Eriksson LI, Ansved T. Changes in diaphragm structure following prolonged mechanical ventilation in piglets. Acta Anaesthesiol Scand 2004; 48:430–7.

37. Racz G, Gayan-Ramirez G, De Paepe K, et al. Early changes in rat diaphragm biology with mechanical ventilation. Am J Respir Crit Care Med 2003; 168:297–304.

38. Geiger PC, Cody MJ, Macken RL, Sieck GC. Maximum specific force depends on myosin heavy chain content in rat diaphragm muscle fibers. J Appl Physiol 2000; 89:695–703.

39. Talmadge RJ. Myosin heavy chain isoform expression following reduced neuromuscular activity: potential regulatory mechanisms. Muscle Nerve 2000; 23:661–79.

40. Vassilakopoulos T, Roussos C, Zakynthinos S. Weaning from mechanical ventilation. J Crit Care 1999; 14:39–62.

41. Goldspink DF, Morton AJ, Loughna P, Goldspink G. The effect of hypokinesia and hypodynamia on protein turnover and the growth of four skeletal muscles of the rat. Pflugers Arch 1986; 407:333–40.

42. Farkas GA, Roussos C. Diaphragm in emphysematous hamsters: sarcomere adaptability. J Appl Physiol 1983; 54:1635–40.

43. Itai Y, Kariya Y, Hoshino Y. Morphological changes in rat hindlimb muscle fibres during recovery from disuse atrophy. Acta Physiologica Scandinavica 2004; 181:217–24.

44. Vandenborne K, Elliott MA, Walter GA, et al. Longitudinal study of skeletal muscle adaptations during immobilization and rehabilitation. Muscle Nerve 1998; 21:1006–12.

45. Deem S, Lee CM, Curtis JR. Acquired neuromuscular disorders in the intensive care unit. Am J Respir Crit Care Med 2003; 168:735–9.

46. Criswell DS, Shanely RA, Betters JJ, et al. Cumulative effects of aging and mechanical ventilation on in vitro diaphragm function. Chest 2003; 124:2302–8.

47. Zakynthinos SG, Vassilakopoulos T, Daniil Z, et al. Pressure support ventilation in adult respiratory distress syndrome: short-term effects of a servocontrolled mode. J Crit Care 1997; 12: 161–72.

48. Putensen C, Zech S, Wrigge H, et al. Long-term effects of spontaneous breathing during ventilatory support in patients with acute lung injury. Am J Respir Crit Care Med 2001; 164: 43–9.

49. Pavlovic D, Wendt M. Diaphragm pacing during prolonged mechanical ventilation of the lungs could prevent from respiratory muscle fatigue. Med Hypotheses 2003; 60: 398–403.

50. Gayan-Ramirez G, Testelmans D, Racz G, et al. Intermittent spontaneous breathing protects the rat diaphragm from the detrimental effects of mechanical ventilation. Am J Respir Crit Care Med 2004; 169:A123.

51. Grundy JE, Storey KB. Antioxidant defenses and lipid peroxidation damage in estivating toads, Scaphiopus couchii. J Comp Physiol [B] 1998; 168:132–42.

52. Hudson NJ, Franklin CE. Maintaining muscle mass during extended disuse: aestivating frogs as a model species. J Exp Biol 2002; 205(Pt 15):2297–303.

53. Nathens AB, Neff MJ, Jurkovich GJ, et al. Randomized, prospective trial of antioxidant supplementation in critically ill surgical patients. Ann Surg 2002; 236:814–822.

54. Lewis MI, Lorusso TJ, Zhan WZ, Sieck GC. Interactive effects of denervation and malnutrition on diaphragm structure and function. J Appl Physiol 1996; 81:2165–2172.

55. Supinski G, Nethery D, DiMarco A. Effect of free radical scavengers on endotoxin-induced respiratory muscle dysfunction. Am Rev Respir Dis 1993; 148:1318–24.

56. Anzueto A, Andrade FH, Maxwell LC, et al. Resistive breathing activates the glutathione redox cycle and impairs performance of rat diaphragm. J Appl Physiol 1992; 72:529–34.

57. Jiang TX, Reid WD, Road JD. Free radical scavengers and diaphragm injury following inspiratory resistive loading. Am J Respir Crit Care Med 2001; 164:1288–94.

58. Belcastro AN, Shewchuk LD, Raj DA. Exercise-induced muscle injury: a calpain hypothesis. Mol Cell Biochem 1998; 179(1-2): 135–45.

59. Van Gammeren D, Falk D, Deruisseau KC, et al. Diaphragm reloading following prolonged mechanical ventilation does not exacerbate injury. Am J Respir Crit Care Med 2004;169:A443.

60. Goldberg AL, Rock K. Not just research tools—proteasome inhibitors offer therapeutic promise. Nat Med 2002; 8:338–40.

61. Sinderby C, Navalesi P, Beck J, et al. Neural control of mechanical ventilation in respiratory failure. Nat Med 1999; 5:1433–6.

62. Amato MB, Barbas CS, Medeiros DM, et al. Effect of a protective-ventilation strategy on mortality in the acute respiratory distress syndrome. N Engl J Med 1998; 338:347–54.

63. Ventilation with lower tidal volumes as compared with traditional tidal volumes for acute lung injury and the acute respiratory distress syndrome. The Acute Respiratory Distress Syndrome Network. N Engl J Med 2000; 342:1301–8.

Chapter 44

BAROTRAUMA AND BRONCHOPLEURAL FISTULA

DAVID J PIERSON

Pneumothorax, subcutaneous emphysema, and other clinical forms of extra-alveolar air occurring in association with mechanical ventilation are commonly referred to as *barotrauma*. This term is doubly unfortunate, *-trauma* connoting iatrogenic injury and *baro-* implying that it is pressure, rather than volume, shear force, or some other factor that produces it. In fact, these implications of both roots of the word are probably incorrect, and the expression *ventilator-associated extra-alveolar air* would be technically more appropriate. Similarly, the term *bronchopleural air leak*

would be more accurate than *bronchopleural fistula*, because of the implications of inflammation and suppuration associated with the word *fistula* in surgical and other settings. Like *barotrauma*, however, the latter is so ingrained in clinical usage that change is unlikely, and the more familiar terms are used in this chapter, as elsewhere in this book.

Although extra-alveolar air appearing during ventilator support may not be caused by the ventilator itself, the expression *ventilator-induced lung injury* would seem as applicable to clinical barotrauma as to parenchymal damage associated with mechanical stretch and overdistension. Again, however, owing more to convention than to logical etymology, the term *ventilator-induced lung injury* is generally reserved for the latter, in this book and in the broader literature.

Usually, barotrauma in mechanically ventilated patients is automatically assumed to be a complication of mechanical ventilation. As with nosocomial pneumonia, however, ventilatory muscle dysfunction, and most of the other adverse developments to which ventilated patients are prone, whether the ventilator per se is responsible is usually unclear, because patients ill enough to require endotracheal intubation, supplemental oxygen, positive pressure ventilation, and management in an intensive care unit (ICU) tend to have numerous other predispositions to such complications. Each of these things would be better thought of as complications *associated with*, rather than *of*, mechanical ventilation.[1–4]

This chapter considers the possible origins of extra-alveolar air in ventilated patients and then reviews the manifestations and most frequent clinical settings of its various forms. After a discussion of general principles of management and a review of reported therapeutic approaches, it presents logical steps for prevention in susceptible patients and points out important gaps in the existing evidence base pertaining to this important topic. Although all the clinical forms of barotrauma are touched upon, most attention is devoted to those that pose a threat to life.

Only overt extra-alveolar air is covered in this chapter. The reader is referred to Chapter 42 for a discussion of lung damage at the tissue or subcellular level related to mechanical lung distension and the application of positive pressure to the airways. Because data from laboratory studies are covered extensively in that discussion, this chapter deals primarily with barotrauma as a complication in patients, referring mainly to the clinical literature. As will be apparent, although the latter is replete with anecdotes and observational reports, this focus primarily on human data means that the evidence base in terms of prospective studies and "hard data" available to the clinician is remarkably limited. Spontaneous pneumothorax and other forms of extra-alveolar air encountered in patients who are not intubated or receiving mechanical ventilation are not dealt with extensively here, nor is decompression-related barotrauma or bronchopleural fistula complicating lung resection.

Pathophysiology

POSSIBLE SOURCES OF EXTRA-ALVEOLAR AIR

Although clinical barotrauma as a direct complication of mechanical ventilation is most likely caused by alveolar rupture, as discussed below, it is important to be cognizant of other possible sources (Table 44-1).[5,6] Air originating in the upper respiratory tract can dissect downward from the head and neck and produce subcutaneous emphysema, pneumomediastinum, and conceivably even pneumothorax. During mechanical ventilation, this could occur in the presence of negative intrathoracic pressure, as with vigorous efforts against a partially occluded airway or in severe patient-ventilator dyssynchrony. Reported causes of pneumomediastinum from air dissection from above include facial or mandibular fractures,[7] retropharyngeal abscess,[8] and dental extractions, particularly if these involve the lower molar teeth and air-turbine drilling.[9]

Mediastinal air and other barotrauma can also originate in the intrathoracic airways, as after blunt or penetrating chest trauma,[10,11] as a complication of bronchoscopic procedures, during percutaneous dilatational tracheotomy,[12] or from perforation by a foreign body. Injury to the upper airway or laceration of the posterior membranous trachea may occur during attempted endotracheal intubation, particularly when a stylet is used, and this has been associated with clinical barotrauma in numerous reports.[13-20] Endoscopic procedures[21-23] and other interventions may rupture or perforate the esophagus, providing access for air into the mediastinum. In many instances, but not always, signs of mediastinitis accompany the appearance of pneumomediastinum following esophageal procedures.[6] Air in the mediastinum is also a characteristic feature of Boerhaave's syndrome,[24] and the typical history of vigorous retching after a large meal may be absent.

Most often the origin of clinical barotrauma is the lung parenchyma, but even then the mechanism may be other than "spontaneous" alveolar rupture. Other possibilities include penetrating trauma that lacerates pulmonary tissue, surgical procedures involving the intrathoracic structures, bronchoscopic procedures, and transthoracic needle aspiration. When acute mediastinitis or pleural empyema involves gas-producing organisms, palpable or radiographically detectable extra-alveolar air may result; gas arising from soft-tissue infections such as clostridial gangrene may also be confused with barotrauma.

Finally, exogenous air may find its way into the pleural space, subcutaneous tissues, or mediastinum. Most commonly this occurs during or following thoracentesis, chest tube insertion, tracheotomy,[25] or mediastinoscopy. Rarely, air may enter the soft tissues following cutaneous injury to an extremity[26] or elsewhere in the body, producing subcutaneous emphysema that could be confused with barotrauma.

MECHANISM OF ALVEOLAR DISRUPTION

Barotrauma in a patient receiving positive pressure ventilation has a number of potential causes[5] (Table 44-2). Pneumothorax appearing within the first few hours following initiation of mechanical ventilation may be the result of previous trauma, or of overinflation during manual ventilation. Attempts at central-line placement or some other procedure before intubation may have lacerated the visceral pleura. Even in patients already receiving ventilator support, the appearance of extra-alveolar air may

---

TABLE 44-1   Possible Origins of Extra-Alveolar Air

Upper respiratory Aract
  Fractures of facial bones, mandible, etc.
  Other traumatic mucosal disruption
  Dental extractions and other oral surgical procedures
Intrathoracic airways
  Airway rupture or laceration in blunt or penetrating chest trauma
  Complications of intubation or airway instrumentation
  Foreign body in upper or lower airways
  Bronchoscopy-related procedures (e.g., transbronchial biopsy, bronchial brushing, or transbronchial needle aspiration)
Lung parenchyma
  Penetrating trauma
  Surgical procedures
  Diagnostic procedures as above
  Thoracentesis
  Percutaneous needle aspiration or biopsy
  Alveolar rupture
Gastrointestinal tract
  Perforation of esophagus or abdominal viscus
Infection with gas-producing organisms
  Pleural empyema
  Acute mediastinitis
  Necrotizing fasciitis or other soft-tissue infection
Exogenous source (air from outside the body)
  Penetrating trauma
  Thoracentesis or closed pleural biopsy
  Surgical procedures (e.g., chest tube insertion, tracheotomy, or mediastinoscopy)

TABLE 44-2   Possible Mechanisms for "Barotrauma" in Mechanically Ventilated Patients

Airway disruption or alveolar rupture prior to initiation of ventilatory support
  Trauma (penetrating or blunt)
  Resuscitation (mouth-to-mouth or manual ventilation)
  Airway laceration or perforation during intubation attempts
  Attempted central line placement (e.g., via the internal jugular or subclavian route)
  Biopsy or surgical procedure
Direct laceration of visceral pleura or airway during mechanical ventilation ("pseudobarotrauma")
  Central line placement
  Thoracentesis or chest tube placement
  Transbronchial biopsy or bronchial brushing
"Spontaneous" alveolar rupture
  Manifestation of a primary disease process
  Complication of ventilator-associated pneumonia or sepsis
  Inadvertent alveolar overdistension (e.g., right main bronchus intubation or manual ventilation)
  Related to ventilator management per se (e.g., tidal volume, positive end-expiratory pressure, recruitment maneuvers, or breath-stacking)

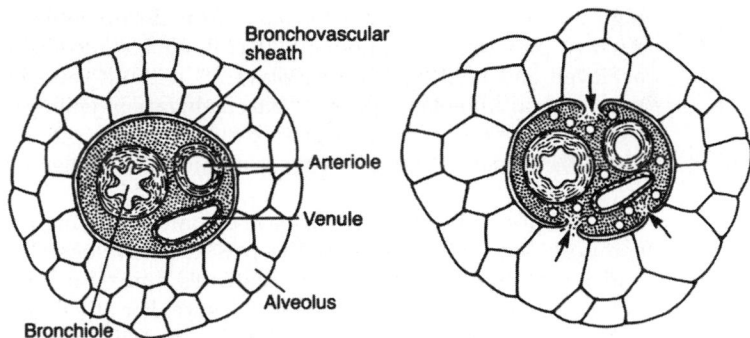

FIGURE 44-1 Mechanism of alveolar rupture during mechanical ventilation. Pressures between adjacent alveoli equalize rapidly, but, especially in the presence of high alveolar volume, increased alveolar pressure in comparison with that in the adjacent bronchovascular sheath establishes a pressure gradient that may result in rupture of the alveolar wall, allowing passage of air into the interstitial tissue of the bronchovascular sheath. (*Reproduced, with permission, from Maunder et al.[27]*)

represent "pseudobarotrauma"—external trauma to the lung from attempts to obtain venous access via internal jugular or subclavian routes, or transbronchial injury during bronchoscopic procedures—rather than "spontaneous" alveolar rupture.

Most often, however, extra-alveolar air during mechanical ventilation results from overdistension of alveoli and rupture of their walls down a pressure gradient from airspace into bronchovascular sheath, as illustrated in Fig. 44-1.[27] This mechanism was worked out many years ago in elegant animal experiments by C.C. and M.T. Macklin:[28,29] ". . . pulmonic interstitial emphysema and its sequelae— air in the mediastinum, peritoneal cavity, subcutaneous tissues, and pleural cavity—are present in many conditions; differing widely in their cause, their clinical manifestations and their seriousness. All of these conditions, however, have a single common factor, a gradient of pressure between the alveoli and vessel sheath, and hence an opportunity for air to gain access to the interstitial tissues of the lung."[29]

According to the work of the Macklins,[28,29] the basic requirement for alveolar rupture is the presence of a pressure gradient between the alveoli and their surrounding structures. Interalveolar walls are probably not susceptible to such pressure gradients, as they are very thin and the pressures between adjacent alveoli are probably equal. Any sudden increase in alveolar pressure (or presumably a fall in perivascular interstitial pressure), however, may establish a gradient sufficiently large to disrupt alveolar walls at their bases (see Fig. 44-1), introducing air into the pulmonary interstitium. Alveolar overdistension would tend to thin and stretch the alveolar membranes, facilitating rupture once the pressure gradient was established. This mechanism can readily be understood in the case of extra-alveolar air following sudden deceleration injury, such as falling into water from a height,[30] but it likely is the main means of alveolar rupture in the majority of other clinical settings as well.[5,6,27]

Spread of extra-alveolar air via bronchovascular sheaths after alveolar rupture was dramatically demonstrated by Jamadar et al when pneumomediastinum developed in a patient undergoing liquid ventilation.[31] After the liquid medium was removed from the bronchial tree and alveoli, computed tomography of the chest demonstrated persistence of the radiopaque perfluorocarbon fluid in the bronchovascular sheaths, confirming the mechanism elucidated a half century earlier by the Macklins.

AIRWAY PRESSURE VERSUS ALVEOLAR DISTENSION

For many years, a primary goal of mechanical ventilation was to limit peak airway pressures, based on the belief that high peak airway pressures were a primary mediator of barotrauma.[32–36] The desire to avoid high peak airway pressures was a main driver in the introduction of pressure-targeted modes of ventilation and the different forms of high-frequency ventilation.[5] As discussed in Chapter 42, however, a large body of evidence now supports the conclusion that it is excessive volume, not airway pressure per se, and especially not peak airway pressure measured outside the patient, that primarily determines the occurrence and severity of ventilator-induced lung injury.

Peak airway pressure during mechanical ventilation can be influenced by a number of factors (Table 44-3), most of which do not affect (or reflect) alveolar volume. This can readily be understood by envisioning the various potential sources for high peak airway pressure as sensed at the ventilator's manometer (Fig. 44-2). Increased resistance to

TABLE 44-3 Possible Causes of High Peak Airway Pressure during Mechanical Ventilation

High inspiratory flow (increases proximally-measured peak airway
    pressure at any given total airway resistance)
High resistance in the ventilator circuit or endotracheal tube
    Inspissated secretions
    Smaller-than-usual endotracheal or tracheostomy tube
    Kinking
    Obstructed distal orifice
High resistance in the patient's airways
    Bronchospasm
    Secretions
    Airway edema
    Neoplasm, stenosis, or foreign body in trachea or main bronchus
Alveolar overdistension
High pleural or transthoracic pressure
    Coughing
    Agitation, shivering, or seizures
    Splinting due to chest wall pain
    Pneumothorax or pleural effusion
    Ascites or abdominal packs or binding
    Head-down position
    Bandages, casts, or restraints

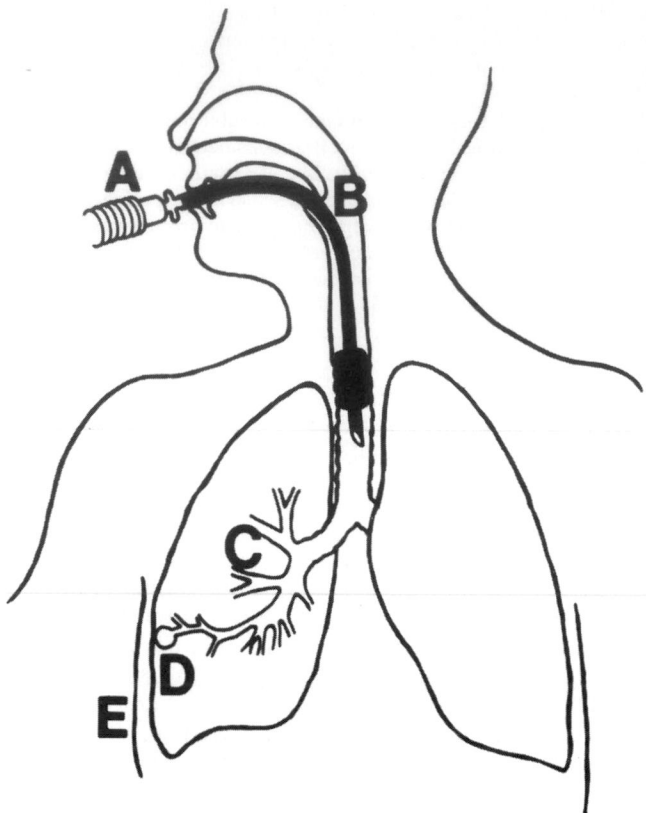

FIGURE 44-2 Possible sources for high peak inspiratory airway pressure as detected at the ventilator's pressure manometer. High pressures due to resistance or obstruction in the ventilator circuit (*A*), endotracheal tube (*B*), or proximal airways (*C*) have different clinical implications than those arising from alveolar distension (*D*). Splinting the chest wall (*E*), as in coughing or from tight bandages, will raise peak pressures throughout the system but do not imply a high transalveolar distending pressure.

airflow in the ventilator circuit or endotracheal tube, or in the patient's conducting airways, will be reflected in an increased peak inspiratory airway pressure. Likewise, an increase in chest-wall pressure, as with coughing, chest strapping, or massive generalized edema, will increase peak airway pressure without increasing transalveolar pressure or alveolar volume. Even increased pressure at the alveolar level should not cause disruption of alveolar walls unless this pressure is unevenly distributed between adjacent alveoli or between alveoli and the adjoining bronchovascular sheath.

This conclusion becomes obvious when one considers the common activities that markedly raise peak airway pressure without causing alveolar rupture.[5] Normal persons routinely generate peak airway pressures up to 200 cmH$_2$O or more during a cough or sneeze.[37] In a study of 56 normal male subjects ranging in age from 6 to 64 years, Cook et al[38] found their mean individual maximum peak expiratory airway pressures to be 237 ± 45 cm H$_2$O. In that study, the subjects sustained these pressures for at least 1–2 seconds, and even longer periods of sustained high peak airway pressures can be maintained during the Valsalva maneuver, during which pressures as

high as 200 torr (286 cmH$_2$O) have been documented.[39] Airway pressures well above 100 cmH$_2$O are routinely achieved and held by trumpet players[40] without causing barotrauma. Alveolar rupture is extremely rare in wind instrument players, as it is in glass blowers, weight lifters, and other healthy people after coughing, sneezing, or straining.[5,41]

In addition, for any given airway resistance, varying inspiratory flow will also vary the pressure developed as a given volume is delivered to a patient's lungs, but will not affect end-inspiratory alveolar pressure. For any given volume-targeted inspiratory waveform, shortening inspiratory time will increase peak airway pressure but will not affect overall lung distension if the set tidal volume is unchanged; in fact, higher proximal airway pressures will decrease delivered alveolar volume because of increased compressed volume in the tubing. Conversely, increasing inspiratory time will lower peak airway pressure but could even increase alveolar distension over a series of breaths if insufficient time were provided for complete exhalation, resulting in air-trapping and endogenous positive end-expiratory pressure (auto-PEEP).

THE IMPORTANCE OF VENTILATOR MODE AND OTHER SETTINGS

If excessive alveolar distension causes barotrauma, it might be expected that widespread implementation of lung-protective ventilation in the management of acute lung injury and other conditions would reduce the incidence of clinical barotrauma as well as of ventilator-induced lung injury. No studies, however, have directly demonstrated this. In 6 large series published between 1974 and 1983, including data from 2980 mechanically ventilated patients, the incidence of detectable extra-alveolar air ranged from 4–11%, with most in the range of 5–7%.[34,36,42–45] While some patients with acute lung injury (ALI) and acute respiratory distress syndrome (ARDS) were included in these series, barotrauma was not specifically examined in those conditions.

More recently, several studies have examined the incidence of barotrauma in patients with ALI and ARDS who were managed with different ventilation strategies.[46–50] Data from a prospective trial of two ventilation strategies in 116 patients with ARDS,[51] examined retrospectively,[46] found an incidence of pneumothorax of 12.3% but no correlation with tidal volume or airway pressure. Weg et al,[49] examining a large database of ARDS patients enrolled in a pharmaceutical trial, similarly found no relationship between ventilator settings and the development of barotrauma. A multicenter Canadian study of two pressure and volume strategies in managing 120 patients with ARDS found no difference in barotrauma incidence in the two groups.[48] In the ARDS Network trial of 6- versus 12-ml/kg tidal volumes based on predicted body weight, no differences in barotrauma were observed despite a marked difference in mortality.[50] When data from 718 patients enrolled in the ARDS Network clinical trials were further examined by Eisner et al,[47] the use of higher levels of PEEP correlated with increased likelihood of developing clinical barotrauma during the first 4 days (relative hazard 1.5), although the 95% confidence interval included 1 (0.98–2.3).[47] This finding could be interpreted in two ways: either higher levels of PEEP predispose to barotrauma, or sicker patients (who require higher levels of PEEP) are more likely to develop barotrauma.

Boussarsar et al[46] reviewed the findings of 11 studies (2270 patients) that reported the incidence of barotrauma in patients with ARDS. These studies varied with respect to patient population and ventilator management, and reported incidences of barotrauma that varied from zero to 76%. In the analysis of the results of Boussarsar et al, however, end-inspiratory plateau pressure was the only ventilator management–related variable that correlated statistically with the occurrence of barotrauma.[46] There were no significant correlations with tidal volume (either absolute or expressed in milliliters per kilogram), PEEP, or peak inspiratory pressure. In their international study of 5183 mechanically ventilated adult patients with a wide variety of diagnoses, discussed below, Anzueto et al[52] found no correlation between any ventilator setting or pressure measurement and the development of barotrauma.

A circumstance in which tidal volumes and airway pressures substantially in excess of what is desirable may be delivered to patients is manual (bag) ventilation, an adjunctive ventilation method used immediately following intubation, during cardiopulmonary resuscitation, in association with airway suctioning, for chest physiotherapy, and during patient transport.[53] The volumes delivered and the pressures generated during manual ventilation are typically not monitored and can vary substantially depending on the size of the operator's hands, whether one hand or two is used, and other factors. Tidal volumes during manual ventilation ranged between 838 and 1674 mL in one study, with a mean value of 170% of the ventilator's set tidal volume.[54] In a recent bench study, in which experienced respiratory therapists performed manual ventilation on a lung model to simulate ventilating a 70-kg patient, delivered tidal volumes varied from 400 to more than 1000 mL, with airway pressures sometimes exceeding 100 cmH$_2$O.[55] Indeed, the development of clinical barotrauma during manual ventilation has been reported several times.[56–58]

THE IMPORTANCE OF THE UNDERLYING DISEASE PROCESS

The occurrence of alveolar rupture during mechanical ventilation is influenced markedly by the presence and nature of underlying lung pathology. Barotrauma is rare in patients with normal lungs—for example, in routine postoperative ventilation[45] or in paralytic states such as high cervical spinal cord injury or Guillain-Barré syndrome. In contrast, barotrauma has been shown to be more common in patients with underlying obstructive or restrictive lung disease.[52,59] In an observational cohort study of 5183 patients who underwent mechanical ventilation for more than 12 hours in 361 ICUs in 20 countries,[60] barotrauma was observed in 154 patients (2.9%).[52] In this study, barotrauma included pulmonary interstitial emphysema, pneumotho-rax, pneumomediastinum, pneumoperitoneum, or subcutaneous emphysema. Its incidence was 2.9% in patients with chronic obstructive pulmonary disease (COPD), 4.2% in pneumonia, 6.3% in asthma, 6.5% in ARDS, and 10.0% in chronic interstitial lung disease.[52] Logistic regression analysis identified the last three of these conditions as independent risk factors for development of barotrauma. An earlier analysis by Gammon et al[61] of 168 consecutive patients who underwent mechanical ventilation at one center found with multivariate analysis that of all variables examined, only the presence of ARDS correlated with development of pneumothorax.

THE SPREAD OF EXTRA-ALVEOLAR AIR ONCE ALVEOLAR RUPTURE OCCURS

Because pressures in the interstitium and bronchovascular sheath tend to be slightly less than those in the alveoli at peak lung inflation, there is a tendency for air to move into these areas once the alveolar walls are disrupted.[27–29] While this is also accepted as the mechanism of the spread of extra-alveolar air in spontaneously breathing patients, it is particularly facilitated by positive pressure ventilation, especially when large tidal volumes are used. Figure 44-3 depicts the possible routes of spread once air leaves the alveolus. Except for systemic air embolism, which is uncommon, and pulmonary interstitial emphysema, the common pathway for all the clinical forms of barotrauma is pneumomediastinum.[6] Once in the mediastinum, air follows the path of least resistance and may rupture through the delicate mediastinal fascia and overlying pleura into the pleural space. Why this occurs in some patients and not in others may be determined by local pleural scarring in some cases but is usually not readily apparent.

The spread of extra-alveolar air to a wide variety of locations in the body can be understood through reference to the fascial planes of the neck, mediastinum, and retroperitoneum, as shown in Fig. 44-4. (27) Three distinct cervical compartments exist—a previsceral space lying between the deep cervical fascia and the pretracheal fascia, a visceral space lying between the pretracheal fascia and the prevertebral fascia, and a prevertebral space situated behind the prevertebral fascia. These cervical compartments continue via the mediastinum through the thorax and trunk, providing the potential for the spread of air into the retroperitoneal space, and from there to the peritoneal cavity.

Air may continue to leave the airways as shown in Fig. 44-3 so long as the alveolar rent is large enough and a sufficient pressure gradient exists. If this path of least resistance leads up the mediastinum and into the soft tissues of the neck and upper chest, subcutaneous emphysema may become massive, spreading extensively over the body. Occasionally the pressure gradient and local anatomy favor passage of air into the retroperitoneal space, from which it decompresses into the peritoneum,[62–66] causing massive abdominal distension. When the extra-alveolar air has reached the pleural cavity, the resultant pneumothorax may rapidly increase with successive positive-pressure breaths. Air readily leaves the torn alveolus and passes into

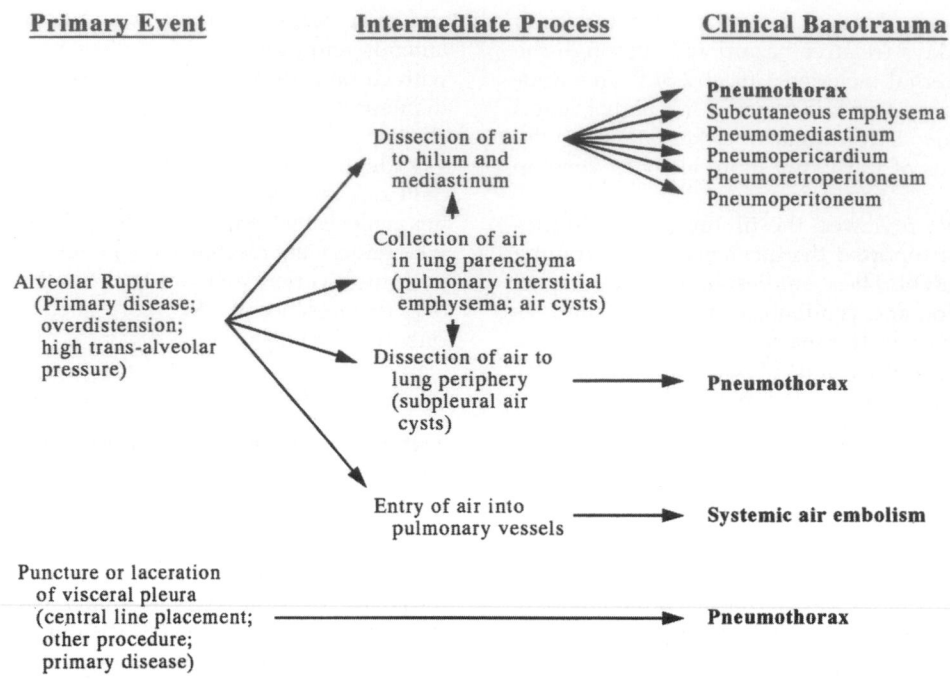

FIGURE 44-3 Pathogenesis of the various forms of barotrauma, with those of greatest clinical importance in bold type.

the pleural space, but cannot return between inspirations because of the collapsability of the lung and mediastinum. A ball-valve mechanism is created and fatal tension pneumothorax can rapidly result.

BRONCHOPLEURAL FISTULA

After evacuation of a pneumothorax via tube thoracostomy, air may continue to leak into the pleural space and via external suction into the pleural collection device. Such a bronchopleural air leak tends to be perpetuated by the very measures often required to reinflate the collapsed lung and to maintain gas exchange in patients with severe acute respiratory failure. As depicted in Fig. 44-5, once a rent exists at either the alveolar or visceral pleural level, the higher the pressure gradient between airways and pleural space, the greater will be the tendency of the bronchopleural fistula to leak. It therefore stands to reason that management should focus on decreasing airway pressure and minimizing pleural suction. As discussed later, however, little experimental evidence is at hand to support this hypothesis, and the management needs of critically ill patients often prevent the realization of these goals.

Clinical Manifestations

The different clinical forms of barotrauma shown in the right-hand column in Fig. 44-3 vary considerably in their clinical manifestations, relative frequency, and potential for doing harm to the patient. Table 44-4 lists the nine categories of extra-alveolar air to be discussed in the remainder of this chapter, and shows their relative frequency in ventilated

patients along with their relative seriousness and potential threat to life. With few data from prospective studies of the incidence of the different forms of barotrauma across the broad range of patients managed on mechanical ventilation, the frequencies listed in the table are based on the author's clinical experience and what little information can be gleaned from the literature. Tension pneumothorax and systemic air embolism are always potentially fatal events. Beyond these, however, the effects of barotrauma on survival, organ dysfunction, ICU stay, and other outcomes, separate from those of the underlying disease, are largely unknown.

PULMONARY INTERSTITIAL EMPHYSEMA AND CYSTIC DILATATION

Air in the interstitium of the lung can be identified at autopsy in patients who die with clinical barotrauma associated with positive pressure ventilation, and is easily demonstrated using computed tomography (CT) scanning.[67–69] With appropriate technique pulmonary interstitial emphysema may also be detected on plain radiology of the chest, and be present without other signs of extra-alveolar air.[70,71] A variety of patterns have been described.[70] Parenchymal stippling, thought to represent multiple small pulmonary vessels and their air-distended vascular sheaths in cross-section, has been referred to as a "salt and pepper" pattern.[71] Air dissection within the pulmonary interstitium is believed responsible for lucent mottling (Fig. 44-6),[70] with small cyst-like lucencies that can sometimes be observed to increase progressively in size on successive films. Other signs of pulmonary interstitial emphysema include lucent streaks, believed to be produced by air dissecting toward the hilum along the course of larger pulmonary vessels, and

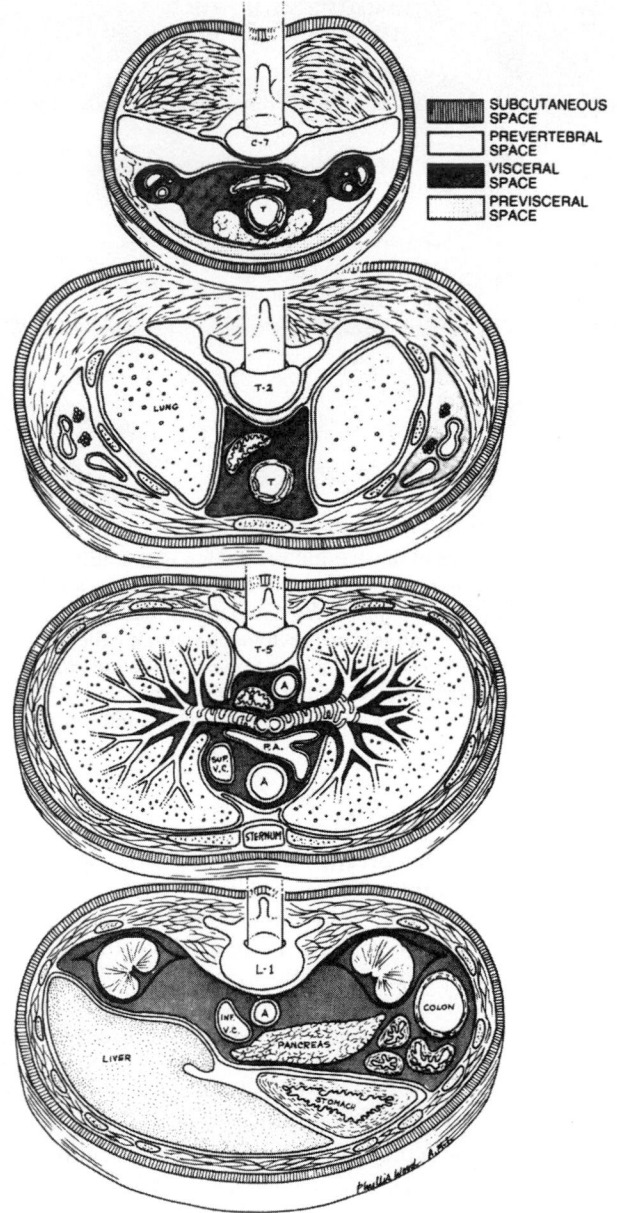

FIGURE 44-4 Fascial planes of the neck, mediastinum, and retroperitoneum, as depicted at the levels of C-7, T-2, T-5, and L-1, respectively. Because the soft-tissue compartments are continuous, air can dissect into a wide variety of anatomic locations. (*Reproduced, with permission, from Maunder et al.[27]*)

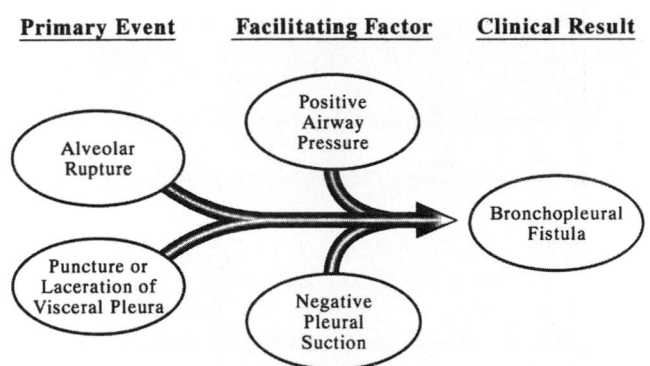

FIGURE 44-5 Pathogenesis of bronchopleural fistula during positive pressure ventilation. The magnitudes of both positive airway pressure and negative pleural suction via the chest tube would be expected to contribute to the size of the air leak.

perivascular halos in the perihilar regions of the lung, representing such air collections seen end-on. All these signs are most readily seen in the presence of diffuse pulmonary consolidation or atelectasis, which increases the radiographic contrast between parenchyma and extra-alveolar air.

Although it is well-defined pathophysiologically (see Figs. 44-1 and 44-3), pulmonary interstitial emphysema in mechanically ventilated adult patients has doubtful practical clinical importance, primarily because of the realities of bedside imaging in the ICU. Several older studies described pulmonary interstitial emphysema in critically ill patients,[35,36,72-74] and in some instances it has been shown

to precede the development of pneumothorax. The subtle changes identifying this entity, however, are beyond the resolution of most bedside radiologic tools. In one study attempting to elucidate the patterns and risk factors for barotrauma in ventilated patients, the investigators abandoned their initial plan to determine whether pulmonary interstitial emphysema precedes pneumothorax because they could not reliably or reproducibly detect the former.[75] In this author's experience, the degree of resolution and inter-exposure consistency required to detect and follow this radiographic finding are beyond the capabilities of most portable x-ray units, that must frequently shoot through bandages and bedding, with suboptimal positioning and patients who cannot hold still or take a deep breath.

Intrapulmonary cyst-like air collections in patients with ARDS have been recognized with increased frequency since the use of CT in such patients became commonplace. The early studies of Maunder et al[76] and Gattinoni et al[77] demonstrated the heterogeneous nature of lung involvement in ARDS, and especially late in the course of this disorder large collections of free air within the pulmonary parenchyma are common (Fig. 44-7). Pneumothorax also seems to be common in this setting, although no study published to date has documented this observation objectively.

TABLE 44-4 Clinical Forms of Barotrauma during Mechanical Ventilation

Form	Relative Frequency	Potential Threat to Life
Pulmonary interstitial emphysema	?	+
Intraparenchymal air cysts	++	++
Pneumomediastinum	++++	++
Pneumopericardium	+	+++
Subcutaneous emphysema	+++	+
Pneumoperitoneum	+	++
Systemic air embolism	+	++++
Pneumothorax	+++	++++
Bronchopleural fistula	++	+++

A

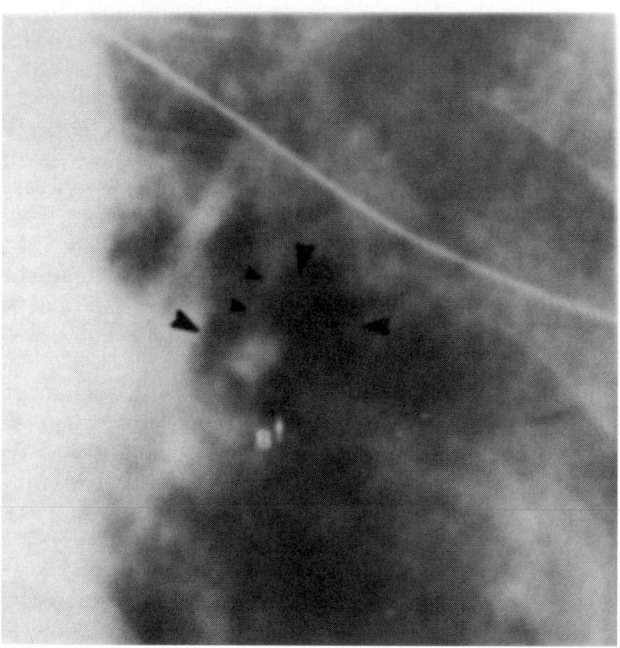

B

FIGURE 44-6 Radiographic signs of pulmonary interstitial emphysema during positive pressure ventilation. *A.* Lucent mottling in the right lung base. Irregular and circular collections of air are contrasted by the adjacent opacified lung parenchyma. *B.* Collection of air around a bronchus (*B*) near the left hilum, seen in cross-section. Large arrows indicate expansion of the vascular sheath; small arrows indicate a streaky density consistent with fibrous stranding of pulmonary interstitial tissue. (*Reproduced, with permission, from Unger et al.[70]*)

Small subpleural air collections, also identified on CT scans (see Fig. 44-7), occur frequently during the course of ARDS.[78] These collections probably represent centrifugal dissection of air through the interstitium to the visceral pleura, and they are likely the source for pleural air in some patients.

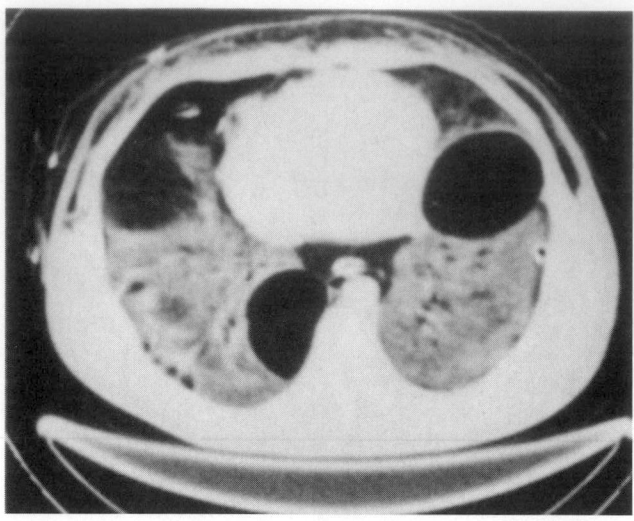

FIGURE 44-7 CT image through the mid-chest in a patient with ARDS after 3 weeks of mechanical ventilation with PEEP. Parenchymal involvement is markedly inhomogeneous, with relatively normal areas (*upper left*), dense consolidation (*posterior areas on both sides*), and intraparenchymal cystic air collections. Several small subpleural air cysts can be seen in the lower left portion of the image. Subcutaneous emphysema, pneumomediastinum, and a loculated anterior pneumothorax are present.

PNEUMOMEDIASTINUM

The mechanisms for alveolar rupture and the spread of air to the mediastinum illustrated in Figs. 44-1 and 44-3 apply to spontaneously breathing, nonintubated patients as well as to those receiving mechanical ventilation.[6] In the former, symptoms referable to pneumomediastinum are frequent and characteristic. Stabbing precordial chest pain is the most common complaint,[79–82] occurring in 80–90% of patients.[27,83] "Hamman's crunch," a crunching or clicking sound best heard over the retrosternal area synchronous with cardiac systole,[84] can be detected in many patients who present with spontaneous pneumomediastinum. It is not specific, however, and may occur in patients with spontaneous pneumothorax without evidence of pneumomediastinum.[85]

Symptoms may be unobtainable from an intubated, critically ill patient, however, and the physical findings characteristic of pneumomediastinum may be hard to detect amid the hubbub of the ICU. Most often, pneumomediastinum is first detected radiologically, usually on routine morning chest radiology. The most common finding is a radiolucent area paralleling the left heart border. This is readily detected in the presence of fluid density in the adjacent lung tissue, as with pneumonia or pulmonary edema. A thin, vertically oriented white line representing the mediastinal pleura may be seen when the pneumomediastinum is bordered by normal lung parenchyma. Once detected, a pneumomediastinum can often be traced cephalad beyond the hilum and into the neck. Other radiographic findings include highlighting of the aortic knob, which is surrounded by more lucent gas density than usual, and the "continuous diaphragm sign" described by Levin[86] (Fig. 44-8). Many

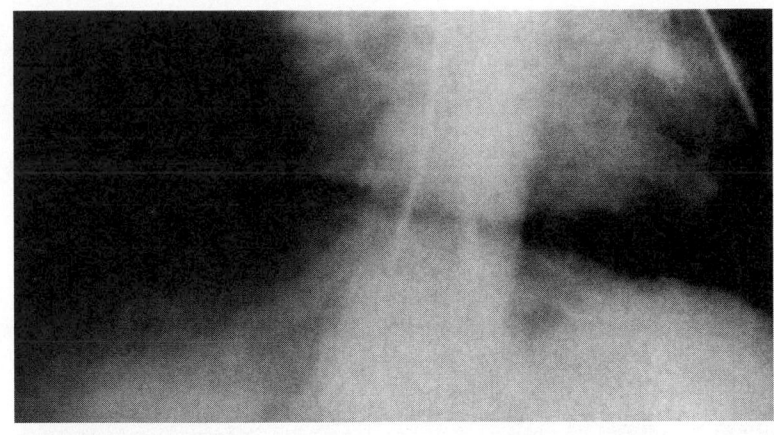

FIGURE 44-8 The "continuous diaphragm sign" of pneumomediastinum in a patient with barotrauma complicating ARDS. An unbroken radiolucent line extends from one hemidiaphragm to the other, rendering the inferior heart border clearly visible. (*Reproduced, with permission, from Pierson: In: Murray JF, Nadel JA, editors: Textbook of respiratory medicine. Philadelphia: WB Saunders, 1782–808, 1988.*)

patients with ventilator-associated pneumomediastinum also develop subcutaneous emphysema, which is typically more obvious radiographically.

Pneumomediastinum is frequently the first sign of barotrauma, and a substantial number of cases go on to development of pneumothorax. In one retrospective study,[75] 34 of 139 intubated patients had radiographic signs of barotrauma at some point in their ICU course. Pneumomediastinum was the initial manifestation in 24 of the 34 patients, and in 10 (42%) a pneumothorax was subsequently diagnosed.

PNEUMOPERICARDIUM

Dissection of air into the pericardium can follow alveolar rupture, and pneumopericardium may occasionally be the only sign of barotrauma. Long known as a complication of respiratory distress syndrome in neonates, it has been reported in adults as well,[87,88] particularly following blunt chest trauma,[89,90] and complicating severe bacterial pneumonia.[91–93] Although hemodynamically significant pneumopericardium in ventilated adults is not generally considered likely, presumably because the adult pericardium communicates less readily with the rest of the mediastinum than is the case in neonates, one group[88] reviewed 81 previously published cases and found 37% of them to have been hemodynamically significant. Several patients in this series were said to have required emergency pericardiocentesis. Adding to the uncertainty about the frequency and clinical importance of pneumopericardium in ventilated adult patients is the difficulty often encountered by portable radiographic devices to distinguish air in the pericardium from the much more common finding of pneumomediastinum.

SUBCUTANEOUS EMPHYSEMA

Although subcutaneous emphysema is commonly observed both radiographically and on physical examination around chest-tube insertion sites, most often this form of barotrauma is encountered in the neck and upper anterior chest as it is vented from the superior mediastinum. When present in only small amounts, subcutaneous air produces the typical findings of crepitations on palpation. If the leak con-

tinues, as may be seen in severe ARDS when large tidal volumes and high inflation pressures are used, obvious distortion of the neck and anterior chest wall can be seen, and palpation shows a characteristic "pneumatic sponginess" as the skin and subcutaneous tissues are depressed to touch the underlying ribs. Air is commonly noted outlining the pectoralis musculature on routine chest radiology; chest CT reveals the spread of air throughout the soft tissues and in all fascial planes (Fig. 44-9*A* and 44-9*B*).

From the neck and chest wall the air can spread literally everywhere in the body, collecting especially in areas with loose subcutaneous tissue such as the upper arms and axillae and the abdominal wall. Periorbital accumulation may become extensive enough to force the eyelids shut. Radiographic studies obtained for other reasons in patients with widespread subcutaneous emphysema may reveal air in a variety of unexpected locations (Fig. 44-9*C*).

Although it may be uncomfortable for the patient and distressing to the caregivers at the bedside, subcutaneous emphysema is nearly always clinically benign. Air in the subcutaneous tissues or dissecting along deeper fascial planes poses little if any direct threat to the adjacent tissues. The air tends to collect in areas with loose connecting tissue, whose blood supply is not compromised by the stretching and other distortion. Like pneumomediastinum, this form of barotrauma serves mainly as an indicator rather than constituting a management problem per se. It signifies the presence of a substantial air leak, and should alert the clinician to the possibility of pneumothorax, but therapy for the subcutaneous air itself is seldom indicated. Airway compromise[94] and hemodynamic collapse,[95] however, have been reported in the context of large airway disruptions and the use of high inflation pressures. In a recent case of the author's experience, tracheal laceration during multiple attempts at intubation was followed by massive subcutaneous emphysema with hemodynamic compromise and abdominal compartment syndrome when high inflation pressures were applied during mechanical ventilation (Fig. 44-10).

PNEUMOPERITONEUM

Figure 44-4 shows how air from the lung that reaches the mediastinum can spread to the retroperitoneal space and thence into the peritoneum itself. The appearance of free air

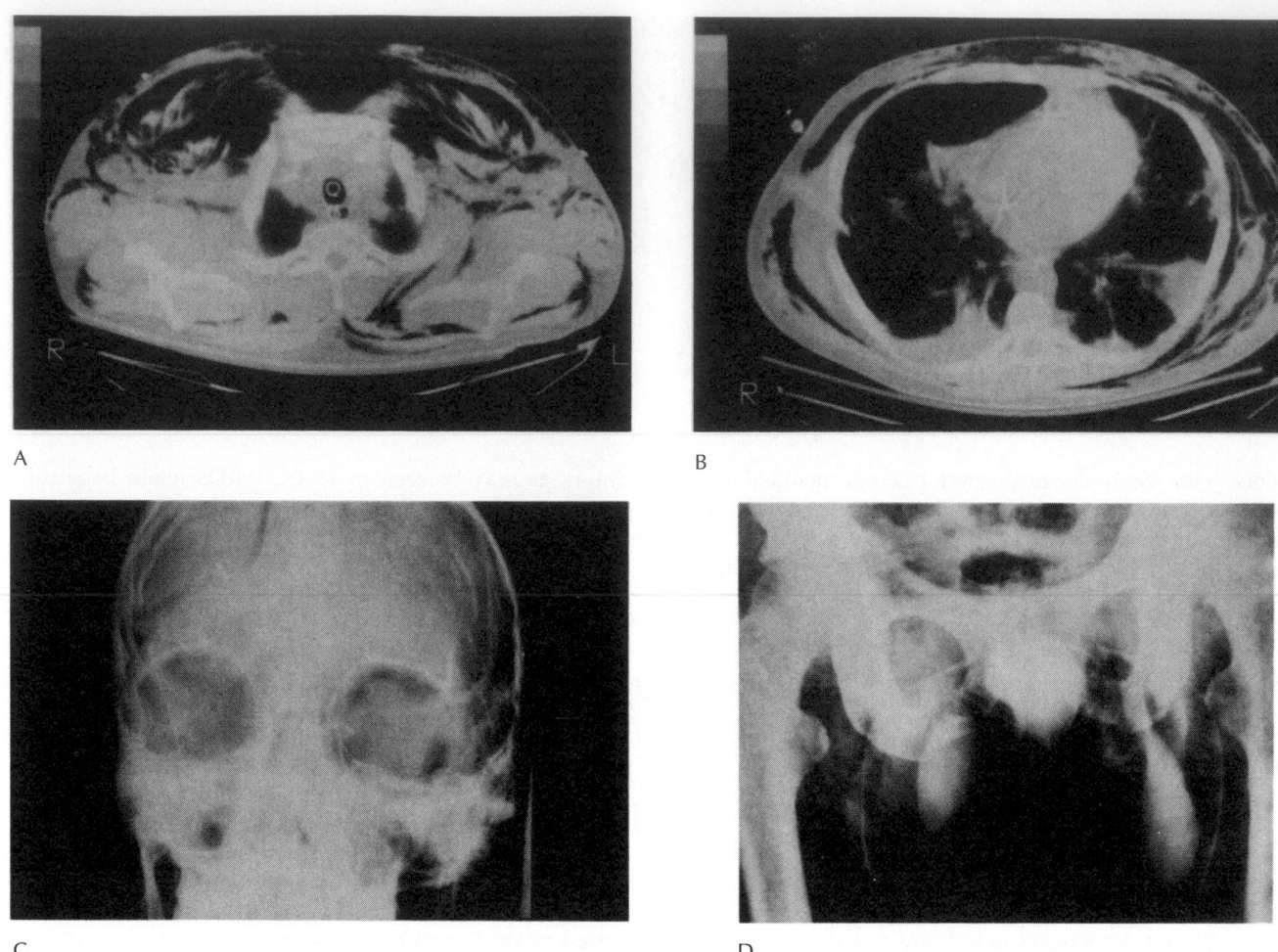

FIGURE 44-9 Examples of widespread subcutaneous emphysema in patients with barotrauma complicating ventilatory management in severe ARDS. *A.* CT image through the shoulders at the most cephalad extension of the lung apices, showing air widely dispersed in and under the skin and outlining the musculature. *B.* CT image farther caudad in the same patient, showing extensive subcutaneous and soft-tissue emphysema. Air has dissected to the periosteal surfaces of the ribs. A loculated anterior pneumothorax is present on the right, because a chest tube is entering the chest wall at this level. This patient survived and made a full recovery. *C.* Bedside skull film in the same patient as in *A* and *B*, showing air beneath the scalp on the left and in the orbit surrounding the ocular globe. A craniotomy defect can be seen on the right. *D.* Tension pneumoscrotum, in a different patient with widespread extra-alveolar air including pneumoperitoneum and extensive subcutaneous emphysema.

in the peritoneal cavity in a patient receiving mechanical ventilation poses a diagnostic dilemma, even when subcutaneous emphysema and other signs of the wide spread of extra-alveolar air are present. Avoidance of an exploratory laparotomy or other invasive procedure may be exceedingly difficult in such circumstances. Determining the P_{O_2} of aspirated peritoneal gas has been reported as a means of differentiating pneumoperitoneum from a ruptured abdominal viscus from air dissecting into the peritoneum under positive pressure ventilation after alveolar rupture,[96] although the accuracy of this procedure has not been validated by others.

Air in the retroperitoneal and peritoneal spaces poses no intrinsic threat to health, and produces no physical signs other than subcutaneous emphysema and abdominal distension. In rare instances, air from ventilator-associated barotrauma can even dissect into the scrotum (Fig. 44-9*D*), presumably via the peritoneum; here again, no threat to tissue viability is posed and the distension will resolve once the leak stops.

SYSTEMIC AIR EMBOLISM

Systemic air embolism may occur more commonly as a manifestation of barotrauma during mechanical ventilation than has previously been believed. Marini and Culver[97] describe the cases of two young adult patients with ARDS, necrotizing pneumonia, and prior pneumothoraces, in whom enlarging intraparenchymal air cysts and pulmonary interstitial emphysema were noted. While in a semi-upright position, each of these patients developed sudden neurologic events (facial twitching, hemiparesis, and seizures),

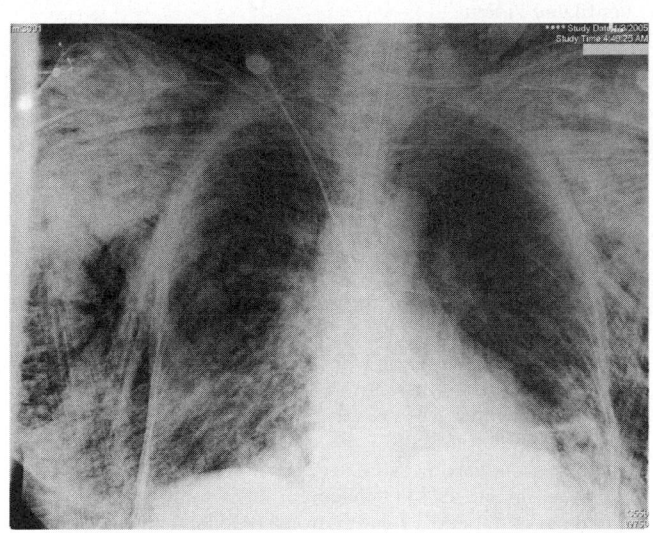

A

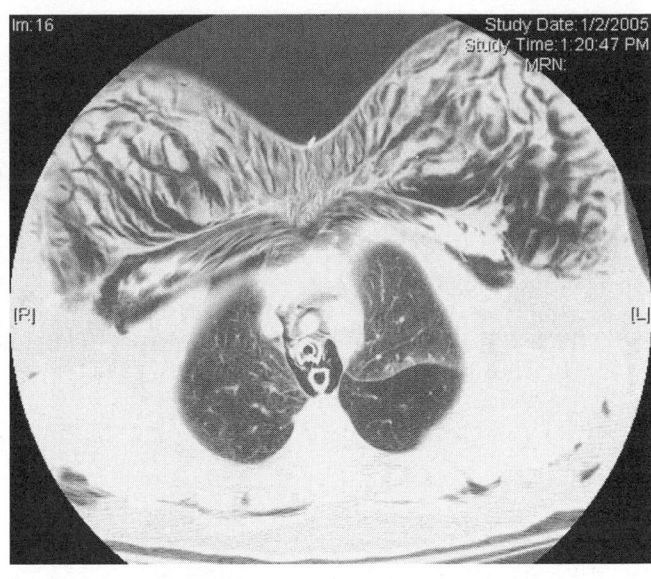

B

FIGURE 44-10 *A.* Supine anteroposterior portable chest radiograph showing pneumomediastinum and extensive subcutaneous emphysema during mechanical ventilation. Air is seen throughout all soft tissues included on the film, and can be seen outlining the pectoral muscles bilaterally. *B.* Computed tomographic image in the same patient at the level of the upper lobes showing pneumomediastinum and dramatic subcutaneous emphysema but no pneumothorax. An endotracheal tube is visible in the trachea, whose posterior membranous portion is bowed inward. Mediastinal gas outlines both the trachea and the esophagus directly posterior to it. Large quantities of air are seen outlining the pectoral muscles and dissecting diffusely throughout the breasts and subcutaneous tissues. Smaller amounts of air are seen in the posterior chest wall. In this patient with an intubation-related tracheal tear as the source for pneumomediastinum and subcutaneous emphysema, tense soft-tissue air in the setting of high-pressure mechanical ventilation produced severe circulatory compromise and findings of abdominal compartment syndrome.

evidence of acute myocardial injury, and focal livedo reticularis over the shoulder and anterior chest. Focal angioedema of the face subsequently developed. No other explanation for these events could be found, and in each patient there was evidence for recurrent episodes of air embolism. One patient survived without long-term sequelae; the other died of refractory hypoxemia and hypotension. Other cases of fatal air embolism as a manifestation of barotrauma have been reported.[98,99] In one instance, a patient being ventilated with PEEP for ARDS was found at postmortem examination to have air in the coronary and cerebral circulations, as well as in the pulmonary veins.[98]

Morris et al[100] reported the occurrence of venous air embolism via the inferior vena cava (IVC), as detected with transesophageal echocardiography (TEE), in three surgical patients, two with ARDS and one with multiple trauma. One 26-year-old patient developed an acute myocardial infarction on the 13th day of ARDS, while on 30 cmH$_2$O of PEEP, and TEE revealed continuous bubbling of air in the IVC. In the other two patients TEE revealed IVC bubbles without prior clinical signs of systemic air embolism. Each of these patients had had previous evidence for extra-alveolar air, and the authors postulated that the bubbling originated from subcutaneous or intraperitoneal air that gained entry into the splanchnic venous system.

Several cases of cerebral air embolism have been seen in association with mechanical ventilation in patients with traumatic lung contusion.[101,102] In several reports, gas bubbling has been observed in the left atrium and left ventricle (but not on the right side) during ventilation with large tidal volumes and PEEP, with cessation during apnea and disappearance or diminution when lower tidal volumes and PEEP were used.[101,103] Cerebral air embolism has also been reported as a feature of barotrauma in patients receiving noninvasive ventilation via face mask.[104]

In some patients, once alveolar rupture occurs during mechanical ventilation, decompression into the bronchovascular sheath by the mechanism described by Macklin[28,29] may fail to occur, allowing pulmonary interstitial air to accumulate under pressure as tension air cysts.[78] Development of such cysts has been observed to precede the appearance of tension pneumothorax in several instances.[78,105] In ARDS, Marini and Culver[97] postulate that, in the presence of such intraparenchymal air collections, the strong retractive tendency of the infiltrated parenchyma may tether open vascular channels that have been disrupted by inflammation or shear stress, allowing entry of air.

Systemic air embolism should be considered when patients receiving positive pressure ventilation (especially for ARDS or with high levels of PEEP) develop unexplained agitation, changed mental status, focal neurologic findings, seizures, or disturbances in cardiac rhythm. The finding of focal livedo reticularis, particularly over the neck, shoulder, or anterior chest wall, should raise the strong suspicion of this complication, as should the occurrence of focal angioedema of the face or neck.

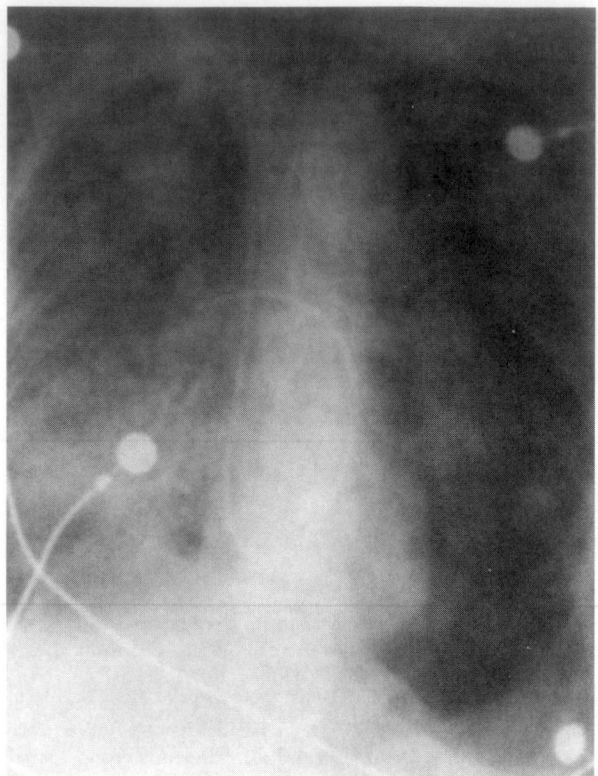

FIGURE 44-11 Loculated left-sided anterior pneumothorax in a patient with ARDS. Lung markings are present throughout the left hemithorax and there is no visible air laterally between the parietal and visceral pleurae. With anterior pneumothorax the only signs may be an increase in overall lucency in one hemithorax, typically confined to the lower lung field, and an increase in the clarity of the left heart border. In this example the epicardial fat pad can also be seen inferior to the heart border. There is displacement of the mediastinum to the right (note the positions of the trachea and the pulmonary artery catheter), suggesting that tension pneumothorax is present, although the latter is a clinical rather than a radiographic diagnosis.

PNEUMOTHORAX

Pneumothorax in patients receiving positive pressure ventilation manifests in three ways. Commonly it is first detected on a routine chest radiograph without clinical signs. The findings may be subtle. Typical radiographic signs of pneumothorax, such as a rim of lucency without lung markings completely surrounding the lung, demarcated by the visceral pleura and more dense lung tissue, may be absent. Often the only indication of free pleural air is an increase in overall lucency in one hemithorax or one area of the lung, particularly the lower zone (Fig. 44-11). In some cases the deep sulcus sign is the only clue to the presence of the pneumothorax. Physical signs of pneumothorax (diminished chest wall excursion, increased percussion resonance, and diminished breath sounds) can rarely if ever be detected in a patient who does not have a tension pneumothorax.

The second presentation for pneumothorax in the ventilated patient is with a change in laboratory or bedside monitoring findings, but without an obvious change in the patient's clinical state. Worsening oxygenation,[106] an increase

TABLE 44-5 When to Suspect a Pneumothorax in the Ventilated Patient

Clinical change in patient's status
  Sudden or progressive increase in inspiratory peak or plateau airway pressure
  Hypotension or cardiovascular collapse
  Sudden onset of agitation and respiratory distress ("fighting the ventilator")
Chest radiographic findings
  General increase in volume of one hemithorax
  Deep sulcus sign: downward displacement of costophrenic angle and/or hemidiaphragm
  Increase in relative radiolucency of one lung or part of one lung
Clinical settings suggesting high risk for pneumothorax
  Use of large tidal Volumes (e.g., >8–10 ml/kg) in patients with acute lung injury or underlying chronic pulmonary disease
  Use of high levels of PEEP (e.g., >15 cmH$_2$O)
  High peak airway pressure (e.g., >50–60 cmH$_2$O), especially if increasing on the same inspiratory flow settings
  Acute respiratory distress syndrome (ARDS), especially late in its course (e.g., 2–3 weeks)
  Severe underlying obstructive lung disease
  Pulmonary infection complicating ARDS

in peak inspiratory airway pressure, or a fall in lung-chest wall compliance may signal the development of a pneumothorax that has affected pulmonary function but has not yet become hemodynamically significant.

Tension pneumothorax is the third presentation. This is primarily a bedside diagnosis, in that this complication is defined better by its adverse effects on cardiovascular function than by its radiographic characteristics. The latter include mediastinal displacement away from the pneumothorax, reversal of the diaphragmatic curve, and overall enlargement of the affected hemithorax, but these signs can occur in the absence of adverse physiologic effects, and the physiologic effects of pleural tension may be present without them. Most commonly the patient with tension pneumothorax presents with agitation and respiratory distress, hypotension, and other signs of cardiovascular collapse. While tension pneumothorax is uncommon in spontaneously breathing patients, even in the presence of total lung collapse, the clinician should assume that every radiographically detected pneumothorax can rapidly accumulate under tension.

Table 44-5 lists a number of clinical settings in which acute pneumothorax should be suspected or anticipated in the ventilated patient.

BRONCHOPLEURAL FISTULA

The presence of a bronchopleural air leak following insertion of a chest tube could potentially create several important clinical problems (Table 44-6). Unfortunately, relatively little is known about the natural history of this entity, and few data exist to substantiate the individual points in the table.

Bronchopleural fistula is a relatively uncommon complication, even in institutions managing large numbers of patients with ARDS and other forms of acute respiratory

TABLE 44-6   Potential Adverse Effects of Bronchopleural Fistula in the Ventilated Patient

Effect	Problems	Comment
Incomplete lung expansion	Atelectasis Worsened ventilation-perfusion mismatching ?Failure of leak to close	Occurs mainly with very large leaks (e.g., tracheobronchial injury) or with underlying restrictive lung disease
Loss of effective tidal volume	Incomplete expansion of other lung areas Worsened ventilation-perfusion mismatching	Attempts to compensate with increased delivered V_T may increase leak and exacerbate problem
Inability to remove CO_2	Acute respiratory acidosis	Unusual; life-threatening acidemia rare
Loss of positive end-expiratory pressure	Incomplete lung expansion Hypoxemia	May not be correctable in presence of large or multiple leaks
Pleural space infection	Infected secretions from airways pass through pleural space	Increases morbidity and ?mortality rates; ?additional source for sepsis
Factitious ventilator triggering	Ineffective ventilation	Due to transmission of negative pressure from chest tube to central airways

failure. Of 1700 patients ventilated during a 4-year period at a major trauma center in the early 1980s, 39 (2%) developed a bronchopleural air leak that persisted at least 24 hours after chest tube insertion.[107] Postsurgical leaks such as bronchial stump breakdown were not included in this series. The leak varied in size in these patients from only intermittent bubbling into the chest drainage device to 900 ml/breath. Despite this, refractory hypercapnia causing arterial pH <7.30 occurred in only two patients, suggesting that inability to excrete CO_2 is very uncommon when bronchopleural fistula occurs as a complication during ventilator management.

Bronchopleural fistula occurred in two distinct settings in this study.[107] It was either the result of direct lung injury (e.g., blunt chest trauma or instrumentation) occurring within 24 hours of the onset of mechanical ventilation, or a manifestation of spontaneous alveolar rupture considerably later in the clinical course. In the latter circumstance, most often seen in patients with ARDS, bronchopleural fistula first developed a mean of 13 days after the onset of positive pressure ventilation.

At the time of this writing, the series just discussed,[107] reported in the context of ventilator management 25 years ago, remains the only published study of the incidence of persistent bronchopleural air leak as a feature of barotrauma. As discussed earlier for barotrauma in general, whether bronchopleural fistula as a complication of ventilator support has become less common in the era of lung-protective ventilation is unknown. Similarly, the possible effect of this complication on patient outcomes remains unknown. Development of a bronchopleural fistula appears to identify patients as having a poor prognosis, but whether the fistula plays any independent role in this remains to be established.[107,108]

Management

GENERAL PRINCIPLES

Of the clinical forms of barotrauma (see Table 44-4), pneumothorax and systemic air embolism present a threat to the life of the patient and thus require immediate treatment. All of the others should be considered primarily as signs, either of the severity of the pulmonary disease or of the possibility of inappropriate ventilator management. Because extra-alveolar air is easily recognized and readily apparent at the bedside, there is a temptation to initiate therapy directed at the barotrauma itself. More important, however, is therapy of the underlying primary disease. Certain ventilator adjustments, though, are appropriate in order to reduce the likelihood of further damage. These should include reducing PEEP, tidal volume, and minute ventilation to the lowest values compatible with acceptable patient support, and consideration of lung-protective ventilation and permissive hypercapnia as discussed elsewhere in this volume for reducing the likelihood of lung damage.

PULMONARY INTERSTITIAL EMPHYSEMA AND CYSTIC DILATATION

As mentioned earlier, although pulmonary interstitial emphysema is an important intermediate step between alveolar disruption and clinical barotrauma, it is difficult to detect reliably on portable radiography obtained in the ICU. With the increasing use of CT in patients with ARDS and other settings of acute respiratory failure, however, these forms of barotrauma are increasingly recognized. Along with intraparenchymal air cyst formation, pulmonary interstitial emphysema is an important sign that alveolar overdistension is occurring, and that tension pneumothorax and other forms of barotrauma are likely to occur. Their recognition is an indication to monitor the patient closely, and to modify the ventilator settings to reduce alveolar overdistension if this is clinically feasible. Aside from these measures, however, there is no specific treatment for these phenomena. Although CT-guided percutaneous catheter drainage of intraparenchymal air cysts has been reported,[109] documentation of the clinical necessity of this is scant.

SUBCUTANEOUS EMPHYSEMA

In the great majority of cases, subcutaneous emphysema requires no treatment other than to treat the underlying lung pathology so that the leak will cease. Rarely, accumulation of massive amounts of air in the chest and abdominal walls can be physiologically important and require surgical decompression.[110,111] Most accounts of such intervention provide little to convince the reader that the air was compromising vital organ function. If the air leak is massive and continuous, however, as can be seen in tracheal perforation as a complication of attempted intubation, urgent intervention may be warranted. In such instances, circulatory compromise, oliguria, and other manifestations of the abdominal compartment syndrome (such as increased bladder pressure) should be evident, and should improve dramatically upon release of the subcutaneous air.

PNEUMOPERITONEUM

Continued air leak resulting in massive spread of extra-alveolar air during positive pressure ventilation can lead to accumulation of air in many soft tissue spaces, as shown in Fig. 44-9. This air poses no threat to the tissues themselves, although in the case of pneumoperitoneum it can cause diagnostic confusion. Critically ill patients with barotrauma are also susceptible to perforating stress ulcers, mesenteric ischemia, and other potential causes of free air in the peritoneal cavity, particularly if they have experienced a period of hypotension. Even in the presence of widespread subcutaneous emphysema and other forms of extra-alveolar air, it may not be possible to exclude a surgical abdomen without laparotomy. One recent report, however, of the use of measured oxygen tension in the gas aspirated from the peritoneal cavity,[96] if confirmed by other investigators, may prove useful in this regard. Aside from the need to exclude an abdominal emergency unrelated to barotrauma, the presence of free air in the retroperitoneal tissue planes or peritoneal cavity generally poses no danger to the patient, and will be resorbed once the need for positive pressure ventilation diminishes.

SYSTEMIC AIR EMBOLISM

The diagnosis of systemic air embolism is based on the clinical setting rather than on any specific test. Demonstration of air bubbles in the left atrium or left ventricle by echocardiography is highly suggestive of ongoing extra-alveolar air entry, but CT and magnetic resonance imaging have not proven to be helpful in this condition.

No therapy has been shown convincingly to be effective. Although hyperbaric oxygen therapy is often recommended, its efficacy has not been shown in controlled trials. Conventional therapy includes placing the patient in the left lateral decubitus position to prevent air remaining in the heart from embolizing to the brain, and administration of high concentrations of oxygen in order to raise Pa_{O_2} and hasten bubble absorption.[112] Reductions in PEEP, tidal volume, and minute ventilation should be carried out if feasible, in order to reduce the likelihood of further air entry into the vasculature.

PNEUMOTHORAX

Because of the threat of tension pneumothorax, chest tube drainage is advisable anytime free pleural air is detected during positive pressure ventilation. There is little reported experience in this setting with the small catheter drainage sets often used for treating uncomplicated primary spontaneous pneumothorax, and the use of a larger, standard chest tube and drainage system is advisable. The routine application of suction (e.g., 20 cmH$_2$O) is customary in the U.S., although this is not the case in all areas of the world; chest tube suction should be applied or increased if the lung does not fully reinflate. Once the lung is fully inflated and there is no residual air leak, the tube is placed to water seal and removed, usually after an additional day. No evidence supports the use of "prophylactic" thoracostomy tubes in patients at high risk for pneumothorax.

BRONCHOPLEURAL FISTULA

DIAGNOSIS AND QUANTITATION OF AIR LEAK

In pneumothorax, once a chest tube is inserted and external suction applied, air is evacuated from the pleural space, as shown by bubbling through the water seal of the chest-drainage device. If there is no persistent communication between the airways and the pleural space this bubbling will cease once the lung is fully reinflated. Air may continue to leak into the pleural space for minutes to a few hours, but in most instances this soon stops. When it does not, and the bubbling continues for 24 hours or more, a bronchopleural air leak (bronchopleural fistula) is present. Most such leaks are small—a few bubbles through the water seal in synchrony with the inspiratory phase of the ventilator—although they may reach several hundred milliliters per breath.

Although precise quantitation of the air leak is rarely needed for clinical management, several methods for doing this have been described. The leaked volume can be estimated by subtracting the expired from the inspired tidal volume as long as the leak exceeds 100–200 ml per breath and the measurements are made at the same point in the ventilator circuit to avoid error secondary to compression in the inspiratory limb. For smaller leaks, or if more precision is desired for research purposes, two accurate methods are available.[113] The first of these is to connect the distal port of the chest drainage unit to a 120-liter water-seal (Tissot-type) spirometer, and to collect the leaked gas while manually creating the same suction as applied to the chest tube by pulling down on the suspension chain, as described by Ritz et al.[114] This technique is accurate but cumbersome. The other valid method is to place a sterile, heated pneumotachometer of appropriate diameter in line between the chest tube and the pleural drainage unit, although this requires breaking the circuit and the possibility of contamination.[113] Hand-held electronic spirometers and mechanical spinning-vane-type (Wright's) spirometers may substantially under- or overestimate the actual leaked volume.[113]

While it is seldom necessary to quantitate the leak precisely for patient management, it is sometimes useful to determine whether the gas leaking into the pleural drainage unit originates in the patient's airways or from the room, as may occur around the chest tube insertion site or with breaks in the circuit between the patient and the drainage unit. Removal of the chest tube is unwise in the presence of a bronchopleural air leak, but may be indicated if there is an external leak, because the same circuit break that introduces air may also permit ingress of contaminating organisms. Most leaks from the patient's airways vary with the respiratory cycle, and stop or diminish during exhalation when intrathoracic pressure is lower. A more definitive test is to withdraw a sample of leaked gas from the connecting tubing under sterile conditions and to pass it through a capnometer; except in cases of proximal bronchial disruption, gas from the patient's airways will contain CO_2, whereas air from the room will not.

Bishop et al[115] collected leaked gas in 9 patients with bronchopleural fistulas complicating ARDS. Total delivered minute ventilation in these patients ranged from 16.6 to 42.6 L/min (mean 23.9 L/min), with 4–53% of each tidal volume lost through the fistula (mean 25%). As the proportion of total minute ventilation lost through the leak increased, so did the fraction of the patients' total CO_2 production that exited through the chest tube (Fig. 44-12). (115) In several patients, more CO_2 was excreted through the chest tube than through the endotracheal tube. Thus, at least in ARDS, gas leaked through a bronchopleural fistula has participated in gas exchange and is similar to gas exiting via the trachea (Fig. 44-13).[115] This observation is consistent with the finding that unmanageable CO_2 retention is unusual in bronchopleural fistula,[107] and suggests that respiratory acidosis in most patients with such a fistula is a manifestation of the severity of their underlying lung disease rather than of the air leak per se.

Measurements of oxygen consumption, CO_2 production, respiratory quotient, and resting energy expenditure can be erroneous in patients with significant bronchopleural air leaks because of the CO_2 lost through the chest tube.[116]

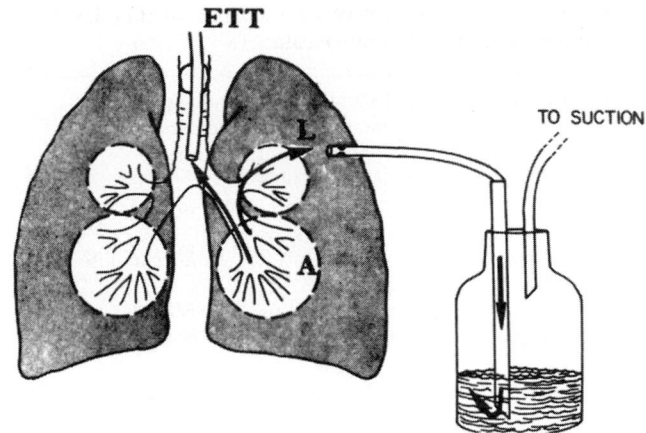

FIGURE 44-13 Schematic representation of CO_2 excretion in ARDS complicated by bronchopleural fistula. Gas delivered to area *A* participates in gas exchange; having given up oxygen and accumulated CO_2, it leaves the lung either through the endotracheal tube (*ETT*) or through the leak (*L*), depending on the pressure at *A*, the relative resistances in the two paths, and the level of suction applied to the chest tube. (*Reproduced, with permission, from Bishop et al.[115]*)

Accurate measurement of CO_2 production in patients with ARDS requires collection of the leaked gas, although dead space-to-tidal volume ratio can be determined using the usual technique of endotracheally expired gas collection, because the proportion of CO_2 excreted via trachea and fistula are approximately equal.[116]

GENERAL MEASURES

In general, management of the patient with a bronchopleural fistula is the same as if the fistula were not there, provided that a functioning chest tube and pleural-drainage system are in place. Table 44-7 lists a number of common-sense measures that should be taken to diminish the magnitude of the leak and the probability of further pulmonary parenchymal damage.

Weaning the patient from positive pressure ventilation altogether would be optimal from the standpoint of decreasing the leak. When this is not feasible, a ventilator strategy should be selected that minimizes both minute ventilation and mean intrathoracic pressure. Respiratory alkalosis should be avoided, and consideration should be given to permissive hypercapnia in patients with very low lung–chest wall compliance and high minute ventilation requirements. Because the "lost" volume participates in gas exchange, delivered tidal volume should not be increased beyond a certain point to "chase" the air leak.

Positive end-expiratory pressure (both dialed-in and endogenous) and pulmonary hyperinflation should be minimized. The use of high inspiratory flows and low-compressible-volume, low-compliance ventilator tubing can independently and additively decrease auto-PEEP,[117] and these measures should be taken when the latter is detected or suspected in a patient with a bronchopleural fistula. Vigorous therapy for bronchospasm and obstructing airway secretions should be pursued.

FIGURE 44-12 Proportion of total CO_2 production that passed out through the chest tube, in relation to the proportion of total minute ventilation lost through the leak, in 9 patients with bronchopleural fistula complicating ARDS. The solid line corresponds to the least squares regression line for the data, and the dashed line represents the line of identity. Several patients excreted more CO_2 through the chest tube than via the trachea. (*Reproduced, with permission, from Bishop et al.[115]*)

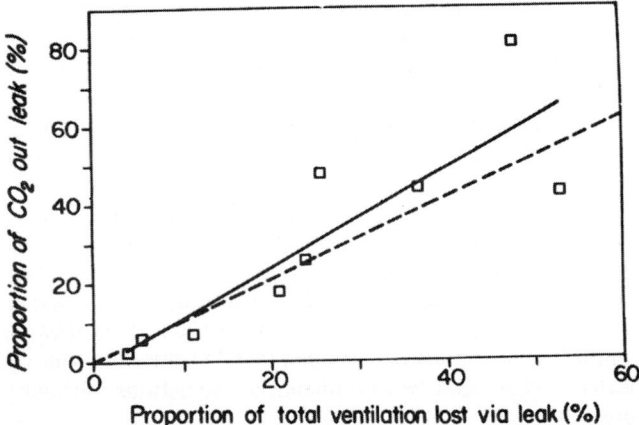

TABLE 44-7 Principles of Ventilator Management in the Patient with a Bronchopleural Fistula

Use the lowest number of mechanical breaths that permits acceptable alveolar ventilation (reduce both mean airway pressure and number of high-pressure breaths)

Wean the patient completely if possible

Partial ventilatory support may be preferable to total ventilatory support (e.g., pressure-support ventilation)

Avoid or correct respiratory alkalosis (to minimize minute ventilation)

Unless contraindicated, consider the use of permissive hypercapnia to reduce minute ventilation by allowing Pa_{CO_2} to rise

Limit effective (returned) tidal volume to <6–8 ml/kg

Minimize inspiratory time

  Keep inspiration:expiration ratio low (e.g., 1:2)

  Use high inspiratory flow (e.g., 70–100 L/min)

  Avoid end-inspiratory pause and inverse-ratio ventilation

  Use low-compressible-volume ventilator circuit, to minimize delivered tidal volume

Minimize both dialed-in and endogenous positive end-expiratory pressure

Use the least amount of chest tube suction that maintains lung inflation

Explore positional differences; avoid placing the patient in positions that exacerbate leak

Treat bronchospasm and other causes of expiratory airflow obstruction

Consider specific or unconventional measures (e.g., independent lung ventilation, endobronchial measures) if the patient remains unstable or develops clinically harmful, uncorrectable respiratory acidosis despite the above measures

Treat the underlying cause of respiratory failure, maintaining nutritional and other support, with the goal of discontinuing mechanical ventilation as soon as possible

SPECIFIC MEASURES

As stated previously, the role of a bronchopleural fistula in the overall prognosis of acute respiratory failure has not been established, and available data suggest that the great majority of such fistulae have little impact on gas exchange. Of all the clinical forms of barotrauma, however, this is the one that has been the subject of the most published reports of novel approaches to therapy. Most of the literature consists of descriptions of techniques for decreasing the size of the leak, and available clinical reports consist almost exclusively of anecdotal descriptions of immediate and short-term physiological changes that lack both longer-term outcome data and convincing evidence that "conventional" ventilator management had been inadequate. The subjects of most of these reports have been critically ill patients, many of whom died in spite of the short-term physiologic improvements documented under the reported intervention.

Several reports have described the use of independent lung ventilation via double-lumen endotracheal tube and two ventilators in patients with bronchopleural fistula.[118–121] As with the use of this ventilator technique in other settings, improved gas exchange has generally been achieved. The reported experience is with fewer than 10 patients, although this technique has no doubt been used in

others. As with the other reported approaches discussed below, in nearly all cases described, the necessity of switching to this complicated and expensive technique is unconvincingly described. Placement and maintenance of a double-lumen endotracheal tube in a critically ill patient require considerable expertise, and the small lumens of these tubes make bronchial hygiene difficult in patients with significant secretions.

Bronchopleural fistula is one of the primary clinical settings in which high-frequency jet ventilation (HFJV) has been used.[122–128] Enthusiasm has waned, however, and there have been few new reports of the use of this technique in the last 20 years.[129,130] Clinical experience with HFJV in patients without underlying lung disease, as in traumatic bronchial disruption or during tracheobronchial surgery, has generally been positive.[124,131] When bronchopleural fistula occurs as a manifestation of barotrauma complicating severe diffuse pulmonary disease, however, as in ARDS, both short-term and outcome results have been discouraging. In one study of 7 patients with severe ARDS and large air leaks, when HFJV was adjusted to provide the same mean airway pressures as resulted from conventional ventilation, oxygenation and/or effective alveolar ventilation deteriorated in every patient, and the size of the leak increased in 5 of 7 patients.[132] Because of this experience, the use of HFJV as treatment for bronchopleural fistula complicating severe acute respiratory failure has been abandoned in the author's institution. High-frequency oscillatory ventilation has been reported in one case of bronchopleural fistula,[133] but whether this technique offers any advantage over adjustments in conventional ventilation remains to be seen.

Several approaches have been reported for decreasing the size of the air leak through manipulation of the pleural drainage system.[134–137] The total patient population in which these approaches have been reported is very small. Their application becomes progressively more difficult as the number of chest tubes increases in a given patient, and incomplete lung expansion on the side of the leak is a common problem.

Commercial chest drainage units vary considerably in their ability to handle air leaks. In one bench study, the maximum leak flow that four widely used commercial chest drainage units could accommodate varied from 5.8 to 35.5 L/min.[138] In a subsequent study using an animal model of bronchopleural fistula, two commonly used devices became ineffective at leak flows as low as 4–5 L/min because of increased resistance.[139] A freestanding suction pump independent of wall suction (Emerson suction pump) consistently demonstrated the highest capacity to evacuate leaked air in these studies, and when flow through a bronchopleural fistula exceeds 4–5 L/min the use of such a device is recommended.

Several approaches have been reported for plugging or otherwise sealing bronchopleural air leaks using the flexible or rigid bronchoscope.[129,140–150] Only about 10% of the patients comprising these case reports and small series, however, have had bronchopleural fistulas in the setting of ventilator-associated barotrauma.[141,142,148] Most of the reported experience is with bronchopleural fistulas following lung resection.

Although it is tempting to think that the ultimate therapy for bronchopleural fistula would be direct surgical closure, this is seldom possible for technical reasons in settings other than acute traumatic tracheobronchial disruption. If the fistula is localized and associated with a necrotizing pneumonia, resection of the affected lobe may be feasible. A bronchopleural air leak following lung biopsy or other procedure, in a patient without pneumonia or acute respiratory failure, may be amenable to surgical repair by thoracoscopy or thoracotomy. In most instances of barotrauma, however, the air leak is a manifestation of the severity of the underlying pulmonary disease, and direct suture or cautery of the leak or leaks is simply not technically possible.

The clinician seeking the best way to manage a patient with bronchopleural fistula complicating positive pressure ventilation is poorly served by the existing experimental literature, which consists largely of technical descriptions and anecdotal reports of immediate changes in leak size and arterial blood gas values, and is virtually devoid of evidence that the therapies described affect patient outcome. There is an understandable desire to intervene when something so obvious as a bronchopleural fistula develops during the course of ARDS or other form of severe acute respiratory failure. Yet except for the unusual circumstance of inability to reinflate the affected lung, evidence for harm by the air leak per se is strikingly lacking, and all the reported techniques for diminishing it have the potential for serious harm to the patient.

The clinician should approach any unconventional therapeutic measure with caution, realizing that it constitutes experimental, unproven, and potentially harmful therapy for a condition that may be more a sign of an adverse prognosis than its mechanism. Table 44-8 summarizes a number of general principles for the approach to managing patients with bronchopleural fistula complicating severe acute respiratory failure, taken mainly from clinical experience in an area whose scientific basis remains woefully inadequate.

Prevention

The degree to which all forms of clinical barotrauma are iatrogenic, as a result of how ventilator support is used in severe respiratory failure rather than primarily of the underlying pathology, remains unclear. Nonetheless, from the material discussed in this chapter several general principles emerge that are reasonable if not scientifically proven to reduce the likelihood of barotrauma during mechanical ventilation. These principles are summarized in Table 44-9.

The large (e.g., 12 ml/kg) tidal volumes traditionally used in ventilating adult patients originated many years ago in studies of individuals with normal lungs who were undergoing anesthesia. These tidal volumes are inappropriate for patients with diffuse lung disease, either restrictive (e.g., ARDS) or obstructive (e.g., COPD or severe asthma). For such patients considerably smaller tidal volumes (e.g., 6 ml/kg, proportioned to predicted body weight) should be used, especially when PEEP is present with its attendant risk for local or overall pulmonary hyperinflation.

PEEP, whether externally applied or endogenous, increases the likelihood of pulmonary hyperinflation, particularly when the lungs are heterogeneously involved, as is now recognized to be the case in ARDS. Insofar as

---

TABLE 44-8 Eight General Observations about Managing Bronchopleural Fistula in the Patients with ARDS

1. BPF in the patient with ARDS is a manifestation of the severty of the underlying disease, perhaps initiated or exacerbated by its management, that will not resolve until the ARDS resolves or improves
2. BPF in ARDS is physiologically significant in only a minority of cases (perhaps 10%), even in the presence of hypercapnia
3. Reducing the leak size per se typically has little effect on gas exchange as measured by arterial blood gases
4. Measures directed at decreasing the size of the leak will generally prove unsuccessful until the underlying lung injury improves
5. When the ARDS improves, the BPF will nearly always improve without specific therapy
6. None of the specific measures (e.g., high-frequency ventilation, bronchoscopic interventions, etc) discussed in the text has been shown to affect patient outcome
7. Patients almost never die *of* BPF. They die *with* BPF, usually *of* multiple organ failure and occasionally of gas exchange failure due to ARDS
8. Careful attention to general management principles (Table 46-7) is more important than any specific measure to decrease the leak

ARDS, acute respiratory distress syndrome; BPF, bronchopleural fistula.

TABLE 44-9 Practical Measures to Reduce the Likelihood of Barotrauma during Mechanical Ventilation

- Use small tidal volumes (6 ml or less per kilogram predicted body weight) and other aspects of lung-protective ventilation in patients with ARDS or obstructive lung disease, particularly in the presence of PEEP (dialed-in or endogenous)
- Avoid hyperventilation except where deliberately employed for specific indications
- Use PEEP cautiously in patients at increased risk for alveolar rupture, including those with: ARDS

    Any unilateral, patchy, or cavitary lung disease
    Nosocomial pneumonia or sepsis
    Obstructive lung disease (e.g., COPD or asthma)

- Monitor respiratory system compliance as PEEP is applied or increased; decrease PEEP if compliance falls with increasing levels
- Monitor all ventilated patients for auto-PEEP; take specific measures to reduce auto-PEEP if its presence could be harmful to the patient:

    Reduced minute ventilation, with normo- or hypercapnia
    High inspiratory flow (e.g., 70–100 L/min)
    Low-compressible-volume, low-compliance ventilator circuit

- Use extreme care in high-risk patients when placing subclavian or internal jugular lines or performing thoracentesis
- Take special care to avoid nosocomial pneumonia:

    Practice good hand cleansing and other infection control techniques
    Avoid circuit interruption
    Employ scrupulous suctioning and other airway care procedures

ARDS, acute respiratory distress syndrome; COPD, chronic obstructive pulmonary disease; PEEP, positive end-expiratory pressure.

hyperinflation predisposes to alveolar disruption, PEEP should be used cautiously in ARDS, and auto-PEEP should be sought in all ventilated patients and minimized when present. Because of the increased propensity of patients with ARDS to develop barotrauma late in the course of this disorder, and the apparent association of alveolar rupture with ongoing pulmonary infection and inflammation, scrupulous attention to infection control measures in all aspects of the care of such patients seems especially important.

Important Unknowns

Surprisingly little is known about barotrauma complicating mechanical ventilation in terms of pathogenesis, clinical implications, optimum management, and prevention. The literature on this topic consists mainly of anecdotal observations and reports of interventions, the latter generally incompletely documented and at best with short-term physiologic endpoints. While tension pneumothorax, air embolism—and, rarely, pneumomediastinum and subcutaneous emphysema—produce potential threats to life, whether the other forms of barotrauma discussed in this chapter exert independent effects on morbidity, mortality, or the natural history of acute respiratory failure is not known. Even bronchopleural fistula, one of the more dramatic forms of clinical barotrauma, has not been shown to affect any patient-relevant outcome. The trend toward use of smaller tidal volumes, particularly in patients with acute lung injury or obstructive lung disease, would be expected to reduce the incidence of barotrauma, although to date no studies have demonstrated whether this is indeed the case.

The Future

If the use of lower inflating pressures and distending volumes during mechanical ventilation, which is becoming widespread largely as a result of the demonstration that such measures reduce mortality in patients with acute lung injury, also reduces the risk of alveolar disruption, then clinical barotrauma should become less frequent. The lack of evidence that special devices or unconventional approaches to ventilator support reduce the incidence of barotrauma or hasten its resolution once present may lead to their being used less often in patient management, which may lessen costs and the risk for attendant complications. In view of the lack of evidence that specific measures impact the severity or natural course of barotrauma, focusing on prevention through less injurious ventilatory support and better general care during critical illness is likely to be more beneficial than the continued search for specific interventions for its management.

Summary and Conclusion

Part of a spectrum of complications occurring during mechanical ventilation that includes ventilator-induced lung injury, extra-alveolar air can be the result of alveolar disruption from overdistension or be caused by several other mechanisms. As a possible result of the ventilator settings being used, barotrauma is always of clinical concern. Among its several clinical forms, however, those of greatest importance are systemic gas embolism and pneumothorax, as these can be fatal. Rarely, pneumopericardium and subcutaneous emphysema can also create a threat to life, and pneumoperitoneum poses a dilemma with respect to the possibility of a ruptured abdominal viscus. Bronchopleural fistula is an indicator of pathology that needs attention, but is usually not physiologically important and seldom requires specific measures targeted at the leak site. Barotrauma from alveolar rupture tends to occur in severely ill patients, and whether this complication independently contributes to mortality or morbidity remains unknown. Prevention of barotrauma, and management once it occurs, consist primarily of practicing sound general ventilator management, including limiting distending volumes and static airway pressures, to stop or reduce the passage of air into the bronchovascular sheaths and elsewhere.

References

1. Strieter RM, Lynch JP 3rd. Complications in the ventilated patient. Clin Chest Med 1988; 9:127–39.
2. Pierson DJ. Complications associated with mechanical ventilation. Crit Care Clin 1990; 6:711–24.
3. Mutlu GM, Factor P. Complications of mechanical ventilation. Respir Care Clin North Am 2000; 6:213–52, v.
4. Chatila WM, Criner GJ. Complications of long-term mechanical ventilation. Respir Care Clin North Am 2002; 8:631–47.
5. Pierson DJ. Alveolar rupture during mechanical ventilation: Role of PEEP, peak airway pressure, and distending volume. Respir Care 1988; 33:472–84.
6. Park DR, Vallieres E. Pneumomediastinum and mediastinitis. In: Murray JF, Nadel JA, Mason RJ, Broaddus VC, editors. Textbook of respiratory medicine, 4th ed. Philadelphia: Saunders, 2005:2039–2068.
7. Henry CH, Ellis EC. Traumatic emphysema of the head, neck, and mediastinum associated with maxillofacial trauma. J Oral Maxillofac Surg 1989; 47:876–82.
8. Moncada R, Warpeha R, Pickleman J, et al. Mediastinitis from odontogenic and deep cervical infection: Anatomic pathways of propagation. Chest 1978; 73:497–500.
9. Nahlieli O, Neder A. Iatrogenic pneumomediastinum after endodontic therapy. Oral Surg Oral Med Oral Pathol 1991; 71:618–19.
10. Bertelson S, Howitz P. Injuries of the trachea and bronchi. Thorax 1972; 27:188–94.
11. Wiot JF. Tracheobronchial trauma. Semin Roentgenol 1983; 18:15–22.
12. Lin JC, Maley RH Jr, Landreneau RJ. Extensive posterior-lateral tracheal laceration complicating percutaneous dilational tracheostomy. Ann Thorac Surg 2000; 70:1194–6.
13. Orta DA, Cousar JE 3rd, Yergin BM, et al. Tracheal laceration with massive subcutaneous emphysema: a rare complication of endotracheal intubation. Thorax 1979; 34:665–9.
14. Marty-Ane CH, Picard E, Jonquet O, et al. Membranous tracheal rupture after endotracheal intubation. Ann Thorac Surg 1995; 60:1367–71.
15. Borasio P, Ardissone F, Chiampo G. Post-intubation tracheal rupture. A report on ten cases. Eur J Cardiothorac Surg 1997; 12:98–100.

16. Evagelopoulos N, Tossios P, Wanke W, et al. Tracheobronchial rupture after emergency intubation. Thorac Cardiovasc Surg 1999; 47:395–7.

17. Chen EH, Logman ZM, Glass PS, et al. A case of tracheal injury after emergent endotracheal intubation: a review of the literature and causalities. Anesth Analg 2001; 93:1270–1.

18. Hofmann HS, Rettig G, Radke J, et al. Iatrogenic ruptures of the tracheobronchial tree. Eur J Cardiothorac Surg 2002; 21:649–52.

19. Stannard K, Wells J, Cokis C. Tracheal rupture following endotracheal intubation. Anaesth Intensive Care 2003; 31:588–91.

20. Fan CM, Ko PC, Tsai KC, et al. Tracheal rupture complicating emergent endotracheal intubation. Am J Emerg Med 2004; 22:289–93.

21. Edling JE, Bacon BR. Pleuropulmonary complications of endoscopic variceal sclerotherapy. Chest 1991; 99:1252–57.

22. Schuman BM, Beckman JW, Tedesco FJ, et al. Complications of endoscopic injection sclerotherapy: A review. Am J Gastroenterol 1987; 82:823–30.

23. Baydur A, Korula J. Cardiorespiratory effects of endoscopic esophageal variceal sclerotherapy. Am J Med 1990; 89:477–82.

24. Henderson JAM, Peloquin AJM. Boerhaave revisited: Spontaneous esophageal perforation as a diagnostic masquerader. Am J Med 1989; 86:559–67.

25. Durbin CG Jr. Early complications of tracheostomy. Respir Care 2005; 50:511–5.

26. Winshall JS, Weissman BN: Benign subcutaneous emphysema of the upper extremity. N Engl J Med 2005; 352:1357.

27. Maunder RJ, Pierson DJ, Hudson LD. Subcutaneous and mediastinal emphysema: Pathophysiology, diagnosis, and management. Arch Intern Med 1984; 144:1447–53.

28. Macklin CC. Transport of air along sheaths of blood vessels from alveoli to mediastinum: Clinical implications. Arch Intern Med 1939; 64:913–26.

29. Macklin MT, Macklin CC. Malignant interstitial emphysema of the lungs and mediastinum as an important occult complication in many respiratory diseases and other conditions: An interpretation of the clinical literature in the light of laboratory experiment. Medicine 1944; 23:281–52.

30. Robertson HT, Lakshminarayan S, Hudson LD. Lung injury following a 50-metre fall into water. Thorax 1978; 33:175–80.

31. Jamadar DA, Kazerooni EA, Hirschl RB. Pneumomediastinum: elucidation of the anatomic pathway by liquid ventilation. J Comput Assist Tomogr 1996; 20:309–11.

32. Powner DJ, Grenvik A. Ventilatory management of life-threatening bronchopleural fistulae: A summary. Crit Care Med 1981; 9:54–8.

33. Haake R, Schlichtig R, Ulstad DR, et al. Barotrauma. Pathophysiology, risk factors, and prevention. Chest 1987; 91:608–13.

34. Petersen HP, Baier H. Incidence of pulmonary barotrauma in a medical ICU. Crit Care Med 1983; 11:67–9.

35. Woodring JH. Pulmonary interstitial emphysema in the adult respiratory distress syndrome. Crit Care Med 1985; 13:786–91.

36. Rohlfing BM, Webb WR, Schlobohm RM. Ventilator-related extra-alveolar air in adults. Radiology 1976; 121:25–31.

37. Ross BB, Gromiak R, Rahn H. Physical dynamics of the cough mechanism. J Appl Physiol 1955; 8:264–68.

38. Cook CD, Mead J, Orzalesi MM. Static volume-pressure characteristics of the respiratory system during maximal efforts. J Appl Physiol 1964; 19:1016–22.

39. Comroe JH Jr. Physiology of respiration. Chicago: Year Book Medical Publishers, 1965: 188.

40. Bouhuys A. Physiology and musical instruments. Nature 1969; 221:1199–204.

41. Sound production in man. Ann NY Acad Sci 1968; 155:1–381.

42. Carlon CG, Howland WS, Ray C, et al. High-frequency jet ventilation: a prospective randomized evaluation. Chest 1983; 84:551–59.

43. de Latorre FJ, Tomasa A, Klamburg J, et al. Incidence of pneumothorax and pneumomediastinum in patients with aspiration pneumonia requiring ventilatory support. Chest 1977; 72:141–44.

44. Zwillich CW, Pierson DJ, Creagh CE, et al. Complications of assisted ventilation: A prospective study of 354 consecutive episodes. Am J Med 1974; 57:161–70.

45. Cullen DJ, Caldera DL. The incidence of ventilator-induced pulmonary barotrauma in critically ill patients. Anesthesiology 1979; 50:185–90.

46. Boussarsar M, Thierry G, Jaber S, et al. Relationship between ventilatory settings and barotrauma in the acute respiratory distress syndrome. Intensive Care Med 2002; 28:406–13.

47. Eisner MD, Thompson BT, Schoenfeld D, et al. Acute Respiratory Distress Syndrome Network. Airway pressures and early barotrauma in patients with acute lung injury and acute respiratory distress syndrome. Am J Respir Crit Care Med 2002; 165:978–82.

48. Stewart TE, Meade MO, Cook DJ, et al. Evaluation of a ventilation strategy to prevent barotrauma in patients at high risk for acute respiratory distress syndrome. Pressure- and Volume-Limited Ventilation Strategy Group. N Engl J Med 1998; 338:355–61.

49. Weg JG, Anzueto A, Balk RA, et al. The relation of pneumothorax and other air leaks to mortality in the acute respiratory distress syndrome. N Engl J Med 1998; 338:341–6.

50. The Acute Respiratory Distress Syndrome Network. Ventilation with lower tidal volumes as compared with traditional tidal volumes for acute lung injury and the acute respiratory distress syndrome. N Engl J Med 2000; 342:1301–8.

51. Brochard L, Roudot-Thoraval F, Roupie E, et al. Tidal volume reduction for prevention of ventilator-induced lung injury in acute respiratory distress syndrome. The Multicenter Trial Group on Tidal Volume Reduction in ARDS. Am J Respir Crit Care Med 1998; 158:1831–8.

52. Anzueto A, Frutos-Vivar F, Esteban A, et al. Incidence, risk factors and outcome of barotrauma in mechanically ventilated patients. Intensive Care Med 2004; 30:612–9.

53. Ricard JD. Manual ventilation and risk of barotrauma: *primum non nocere*. Respir Care 2005; 50:338–9.

54. Clarke RC, Kelly BE, Convery PN, et al. Ventilatory characteristics in mechanically ventilated patients during manual hyperventilation for chest physiotherapy. Anaesthesia 1999; 54:936–40.

55. Turki M, Young MP, Waters SS, et al. Peak pressures during manual ventilation. Respir Care 2005; 50:340–44.

56. Silbergleit R, Lee DC, Blank-Reid C, et al. Sudden severe barotrauma from self-inflating bag-valve devices. J Trauma 1996; 40:320–22.

57. Reid-Nicholson MD, Escoffery CT. Severe pulmonary barotrauma. West Indian Med J 2000; 49:344–46.

58. Lopez Rodriguez A, Lopez Sanchez L, Julia JA. Pneumoperitoneum associated with manual ventilation using a bag-valve device. Acad Emerg Med 1995; 2:944.

59. Ricard JD. Barotrauma during mechanical ventilation: why aren't we seeing any more? Intensive Care Med 2004; 30:533–5.

60. Esteban A, Anzueto A, Frutos F, et al. Mechanical Ventilation International Study Group. A 28-day international study of the characteristics and outcomes in patients receiving mechanical ventilation. JAMA 2002; 287:345–55.

61. Gammon RB, Shin MS, Groves RH Jr, et al. Clinical risk factors for pulmonary barotrauma: a multivariate analysis. Am J Respir Crit Care Med 1995; 152(4 Pt 1):1235–40.

62. Ralston lC, Clutton-Brock TH, Hutton P. Tension pneumoperitoneum. Intensive Care Med 1989; 15:532–3.

63. Winer-Muram HT, Rumbak MJ, Bain RS Jr. Tension pneumoperitoneum as a complication of barotrauma. Crit Care Med 1993; 21:941–3.

64. Chan SY, Kirsch CM, Jensen WA, et al. Tension pneumoperitoneum. West J Med 1996; 165(1–2):61–4.

65. Canivet JL, Yans T, Piret S, et al. Barotrauma-induced tension pneumoperitoneum. Acta Anaesthesiol Belg 2003; 54:233–6.

66. Lellouche N, Bruneel F, Mignon F, et al. Pneumomediastinum causing pneumoperitoneum during mechanical ventilation. J Crit Care 2003; 18:68–9.

67. Satoh K, Kobayashi T, Kawase Y, et al. CT appearance of interstitial pulmonary emphysema. J Thorac Imaging 1996; 1:153–4.

68. Kemper AC, Steinberg KP, Stern EJ. Pulmonary interstitial emphysema: CT findings. AJR Am J Roentgenol 1999; 172:1642.

69. Thoongsuwan N, Stern EJ. Pulmonary interstitial emphysema. Curr Probl Diagn Radiol 2002; 31:63–4.

70. Unger JM, England DM, Bogust GA. Interstitial emphysema in adults: recognition and prognostic implications. J Thorac Imag 1989; 4:86–94.

71. Milne ENC. A physiological approach to reading critical care unit films. J Thorac Imag 1986; 1:60–90.

72. McLoud TC, Barash PG, Ravin CE. PEEP: Radiographic features and associated complications. Am J Roentgenol 1977; 129:209–13.

73. Altman AR, Johnson TH. Roentgenographic findings in PEEP therapy. Indicators of pulmonary complications. JAMA 1979; 242:727–30.

74. Aberle DR, Brown K. Radiologic considerations in the adult respiratory distress syndrome. Clin Chest Med 1990; 11:737–54.

75. Gammon RB, Shin MS, Buchalter SE. Pulmonary barotrauma in mechanical ventilation. Patterns and risk factors. Chest 1992; 102:568–72.

76. Maunder RJ, Shuman WP, McHugh JW, et al. Preservation of normal lung regions in the adult respiratory distress syndrome. JAMA 1986; 255:2463–65.

77. Gattinoni L, Pelosi P, Pesenti A, et al. CT scan in ARDS: clinical and physiopathological insights. Acta Anaesthesiol Scand 1991; 35(Suppl 95):87–96.

78. Albelda SM, Gefter WB, Kelley MA, et al. Ventilator-induced subpleural air cysts: Clinical, radiographic, and pathologic significance. Am Rev Respir Dis 1983; 127:360–5.

79. Jougon JB, Ballester M, Delcambre F, et al. Assessment of spontaneous pneumomediastinum: experience with 12 patients. Ann Thorac Surg 2003; 75:1711–4.

80. Panacek EA, Singer AJ, Sherman BW, et al. Spontaneous pneumomediastinum: clinical and natural history. Ann Emerg Med 1992; 21:1222–7.

81. Holmes KD, McGuirt WF. Spontaneous pneumomediastinum: Evaluation and treatment. J Fam Pract 1990; 31:422–6.

82. Yellin A, Gapany-Gapanavicius M, Lieberman Y. Spontaneous pneumomediastinum: Is it a rare cause of chest pain? Thorax 1983; 38:383–5.

83. Munsell WP. Pneumomediastinum. JAMA 1967; 202:129–33.

84. Hamman L. Mediastinal emphysema. JAMA 1945; 128:1–6.

85. Baumann MH, Sahn SA. Hamman's sign revisited. Pneumothorax or pneumomediastinum? Chest 1992; 102:1281–2.

86. Levin B. The continuous diaphragm sign. Radiology 1973; 24:337–8.

87. Hurd TE, Novak R, Gallagher TJ. Tension pneumopericardium: A complication of mechanical ventilation. Crit Care Med 1984; 12:200–1.

88. Cummings RG, Wesly RL, Adams DH, et al. Pneumopericardium resulting in cardiac tamponade. Ann Thorac Surg 1984; 37:511–8.

89. Gould JC, Schurr MA. Tension pneumopericardium after blunt chest trauma. Ann Thorac Surg 2001; 72:1728–30.

90. Ladurner R, Qvick LM, Hohenbleicher F, et al. Pneumopericardium in blunt chest trauma after high-speed motor vehicle accidents. Am J Emerg Med 2005; 23:83–6.

91. Maki DD, Sehgal M, Kricun ME, et al. Spontaneous tension pneumopericardium complicating staphylococcal pneumonia. J Thorac Imaging 1999; 14:215–7.

92. Bleeker-Rovers CP, van den Elshout FJ, Bloemen TI, et al. Tension pneumopericardium caused by positive pressure ventilation complicating anaerobic pneumonia. Neth J Med 2003; 61:54–6.

93. Barquero Romero J, Izquierdo Hidalgo J, Macia Botejara E, et al. Spontaneous pneumopericardium in a patient with community-acquired pneumonia. Rev Esp Cardiol 2005; 58:227–9.

94. Schumann R, Polaner DM. Massive subcutaneous emphysema and sudden airway compromise after postoperative vomiting. Anesth Analg 1999; 89:796–7.

95. Reiche-Fischel O, Helfrick JF. Intraoperative life-threatening emphysema associated with endotracheal intubation and air insufflation devices: report of two cases. J Oral Maxillofac Surg 1995; 53:1103–7.

96. Murdoch IA, Huggon IC. Rapid diagnosis of the cause of pneumoperitoneum in ventilated asthmatic children. Acta Paediatr 1993; 82:108–10.

97. Marini JJ, Culver BH. Systemic gas embolism complicating mechanical ventilation in the adult respiratory distress syndrome. Ann Intern Med 1989; 110:699–703.

98. Weaver LK, Morris A. Venous and arterial gas embolism associated with positive pressure ventilation. Chest 1998; 113:1132–4.

99. Ibrahim AE, Stanwood PL, Freund PR. Pneumothorax and systemic air embolism during positive-pressure ventilation. Anesthesiology 1999; 90:1479–81.

100. Morris WP, Butler BD, Tonnesen AS, et al. Continuous venous air embolism in patients receiving positive end-expiratory pressure. Am Rev Respir Dis 1993; 147:1034–7.

101. Saada M, Goarin JP, Riou B, et al. Systemic gas embolism complicating pulmonary contusion. Diagnosis and management using transesophageal echocardiography. Am J Respir Crit Care Med 1995; 152:812–5.

102. Brownlow HA, Edibam C. Systemic air embolism after intercostal chest drain insertion and positive pressure ventilation in chest trauma. Anaesth Intensive Care 2002; 30:660–4.

103. Avanzas P, Garcia-Fernandez MA, Quiles J. Echocardiographic detection of systemic air embolism during positive pressure ventilation. Heart 2003; 89:1321.

104. Hung SC, Hsu HC, Chang SC. Cerebral air embolism complicating bilevel positive airway pressure therapy. Eur Respir J 1998; 12:235–7.

105. Westcott JL, Cole SR. Interstitial pulmonary emphysema in children and adults: Roentgenographic features. Radiology 1974; 111:367–8.

106. Glauser FL, Polatty RC, Sessler CN. Worsening oxygenation in the mechanically ventilated patient: Causes, mechanisms, and early detection. Am Rev Respir Dis 1988; 138:458–65.

107. Pierson DJ, Horton CA, Bates PW. Persistent bronchopleural air leak during mechanical ventilation: A review of 39 cases. Chest 1986; 90:321–3.

108. Pierson DJ. Persistent bronchopleural air leak during mechanical ventilation: A review. Respir Care 1982; 27:408–16.

109. Chon KS, vanSonnenberg E, D'Agostino HB, et al. CT-guided catheter drainage of loculated thoracic air collections in mechanically ventilated patients with acute respiratory distress syndrome. AJR Am J Roentgenol 1999; 173:1345–50.

110. Tonnesen AS, Wagner W, Mackey-Hargadine J. Tension subcutaneous emphysema. Anesthesiology 1985; 62:90–2.

111. Herlan DB, Landreneau RJ, Ferson PF. Massive spontaneous subcutaneous emphysema: Acute management with infraclavicular "blow holes." Chest 1992; 102:503–5.

112. O'Quin RJ, Lakshminarayan S. Venous air embolism. Arch Intern Med 1982; 142:2173–6.

113. Larson RP, Capps JS, Pierson DJ: A comparison of three devices used for quantitating bronchopleural air leak. Respir Care 1986; 31:1065–1068.

114. Ritz R, Benson M, Bishop MJ. Measuring gas leakage from bronchopleural fistulas during high-frequency jet ventilation. Crit Care Med 1984; 12:836–7.

115. Bishop MJ, Benson MS, Pierson DJ: Carbon dioxide excretion via bronchopleural fistulas in adult respiratory distress syndrome. Chest 1987; 91:400–2.

116. Benson MS, Bishop MJ, Pierson DJ. Determination of dead-space ventilation and CO_2 production in the presence of gas leak from bronchopleural fistula complicating ARDS. Respir Care 1986; 31:398–401.

117. Scott LR, Benson MS, Pierson DJ. Effect of inspiratory flowrate and circuit compressible volume on auto-PEEP during mechanical ventilation. Respir Care 1986; 31:1075–9.

118. Rafferty TD, Palma J, Motoyama EK, et al. Management of a bronchopleural fistula with differential lung ventilation and positive end-expiratory pressure. Respir Care 1980; 25:654–7.

119. Dodds CP, Hillman KM. Management of massive air leak with asynchronous independent lung ventilation. Intensive Care Med 1982; 8:287–90.

120. Crimi G, Candiani A, Conti G, et al. Clinical applications of independent lung ventilation with unilateral high-frequency jet ventilation (ILV-UHFJV). Intensive Care Med 1986; 12: 90–4.

121. Feeley TW, Keating D, Nishimura T. Independent lung ventilation using high-frequency ventilation in the management of a bronchopleural fistula. Anesthesiology 1988; 69:420–2.

122. Carlon GC, Ray C, Klain M, et al. High-frequency positive-pressure ventilation in management of a patient with bronchopleural fistula. Anesthesiology 1980; 50:160–2.

123. Carlon GC, Kahn RC, Howland WS, et al. Clinical experience with high frequency jet ventilation. Crit Care Med 1981; 9:1–6.

124. Turnbull AD, Carlon GC, Howland WS, et al. High-frequency jet ventilation in major airway or pulmonary disruption. Ann Thorac Surg 1981; 32:468–4.

125. Derderian SS, Rajagopal KR, Abbrecht PH, et al. High frequency positive pressure jet ventilation in bilateral bronchopleural fistulae. Crit Care Med 1982; 10:119–21.

126. Mendez M, Pratt DS, May JJ. Prolonged high-frequency jet ventilation. Crit Care Med 1984; 12:838–9.

127. Rubio JJ, Algora-Weber A, Dominguez-de Villota E, et al. Prolonged high-frequency jet ventilation in a patient with bilateral bronchopleural fistula: An alternative mode of ventilation. Intensive Care Med 1986; 12:161–3.

128. Baumann MH, Sahn SA. Medical management and therapy of bronchopleural fistulas in the mechanically ventilated patient. Chest 1990; 97:721–8.

129. Bartels HE, Stein HJ, Siewert JR. Respiratory management and outcome of non-malignant tracheo-bronchial fistula following esophagectomy. Dis Esophagus 1998; 11:125–9.

130. Campbell D, Steinmann M, Porayko L. Nitric oxide and high frequency jet ventilation in a patient with bilateral bronchopleural fistulae and ARDS. Can J Anaesth 2000; 47:53–7.

131. Carlon GC, Ray C, Pierri MK, et al. High frequency jet ventilation: Theoretical considerations and clinical observations. Chest 1982; 81:350–4.

132. Bishop MJ, Benson MS, Sato P, et al. Comparison of high-frequency jet ventilation with conventional mechanical ventilation for bronchopleural fistula. Anesth Analg 1987; 66:833–8.

133. Ha DV, Johnson D. High frequency oscillatory ventilation in the management of a high output bronchopleural fistula: a case report. Can J Anaesth 2004; 51:78–83.

134. Gallagher TJ, Smith RA, Kirby RR, et al. Intermittent inspiratory chest tube occlusion to limit bronchopleural cutaneous air leaks. Crit Care Med 1976; 4:328–30.

135. Phillips YY, Lonigan RM, Joyner LR. A simple technique for managing a bronchopleural fistula while maintaining positive pressure ventilation. Crit Care Med 1979; 7:351–3.

136. Bevelaqua FA, Kay S. A modified technique for the management of bronchopleural fistula in ventilator-dependent patients: a report of two cases. Respiratory Care 1986; 31:904–8.

137. Blanch PB, Koens JC, Layon AJ. A new device that allows synchronous intermittent inspiratory chest tube occlusion with any mechanical ventilator. Chest 1990; 97:1426–30.

138. Capps JS, Tyler ML, Rusch VW, et al. Potential of chest drainage units to evacuate broncho-pleural air leaks (abstract). Chest 1985; 88:57s.

139. Rusch VW, Capps JS, Tyler ML, et al. The performance of four pleural drainage systems in an animal model of bronchopleural fistula. Chest 1988; 93:859–63.

140. Cant WF, Tinker JH, Tarhan S. Bronchial blockade in a child with a bronchopleural cutaneous fistula using a balloon-tipped catheter. Anesth Analg 1976; 55:874–5.

141. Ratliff JL, Hill JD, Tucker H, Fallat R. Endobronchial control of bronchopleural fistulae. Chest 1977; 71:98–9.

142. Ellis JH, Sequeira FW, Weber TR, et al. Balloon catheter occlusion of bronchopleural fistulae. AJR Am J Roentgenol 1982; 138:157–9.

143. Roksvaag H, Skalleberg L, Nordberg C, et al. Endoscopic closure of bronchial fistula. Thorax 1983; 38:696–7.

144. Jones DP, David I. Gelfoam occlusion of peripheral bronchopleural fistulas. Ann Thorac Surg 1986; 42:334–5.

145. Lan R, Lee C, Tsai Y, et al. Fiberoptic bronchial blockade in a small bronchopleural fistula. Chest 1987; 92:944–6.

146. Glover W, Chavis TV, Daniel TM, et al. Fibrin glue application through the flexible fiberoptic bronchoscope: closure of bronchopleural fistulas. J Thorac Cardiovasc Surg 1987; 93: 470–2.

147. Torre M, Chiesa G, Ravini M, et al. Endoscopic gluing of bronchopleural fistula. Ann Thorac Surg 1987; 43:295–7.

148. Regal G, Sturm JA, Neumann C, et al. Occlusion of bronchopleural fistula after lung injury—a new treatment by bronchoscopy. J Trauma 1989; 29:223–6.

149. York EL, Lewall DB, Hirji M, et al. Endoscopic diagnosis and treatment of postoperative bronchopleural fistula. Chest 1990; 97:1390–2.

150. McCormick BA, Wilson IH, Berrisford RG. Bronchopleural fistula complicating group A beta-haemolytic streptococcal pneumonia. Use of a Fogarty embolectomy catheter for selective bronchial blockade. Intensive Care Med 1999; 25:535–7.

OXYGEN TOXICITY

ROBERT F. LODATO

The importance of the physiology and toxicology of oxygen (O_2) breathing have increased in recent years. The past two decades have witnessed a remarkable upsurge of knowledge and interest in "oxidative stress" throughout all of biology. The use of O_2 continues to grow, from critically ill to ambulatory patients and even to recreational use at "oxygen bars." Recent advances in patient care have refocused attention on the optimum use of O_2. For example, currently, strategies to protect the lung from mechanical injury during mechanical ventilation emphasize the use of lower tidal volumes. But such strategies may impair gas exchange, resulting in higher requirements for inspired O_2 fraction (F_{IO_2}).[1]

Lavoisier initially characterized O_2 as "highly respirable air"[2] and "vital air" before eventually giving it the name "principe oxygine" (acidifying principle) in 1777. He took the name from the Greek roots "oxy" (acid) and "gen" (to

form), because initially oxygen was incorrectly believed to be the essential principle in the formation of acids.[3] Normobaric hyperoxia may be defined as an inspired O_2 tension, P_{IO_2}, between 160 and 760 torr (i.e., between 0.21 and 1.0 atmosphere [atm]) of pressure, whereas hyperbaric hyperoxia denotes that $P_{IO_2} > 760$ torr.

J.B.S. Haldane[4] and others[5] speculated, and it is now generally accepted, that life on earth began anaerobically when the earth's atmosphere was virtually devoid of O_2. Gilbert[5] postulated that in this primordial reducing atmosphere, the first living cells used hydrogen, diffusing into the cell from the environment, as an energy source (e.g., metabolizing carbohydrates to methane and water). Gilbert[5] speculated further that because hydrogen would also reduce essential cellular constituents and thereby poison the cell, these early cells also had to develop antihydrogen defenses and actively transport hydrogen ions out of the cell. As the atmosphere was transformed from a reducing to an oxidizing one, O_2 replaced hydrogen as an energy source. Therefore, to avoid O_2 poisoning, cells then had to develop antioxygen/antioxidant defenses. These observations emphasize that as an energy source for cells, O_2 has a dual effect: it is both life promoting and life destroying. This dual nature of O_2 (Fig. 45-1) was noted by Priestley in 1775 shortly after his discovery of O_2: "though pure [oxygen] might be very useful as a medicine, ... as a candle burns out much faster in [oxygen] ... so we might ... *live out too fast.*"[6] Indeed, even at ambient concentrations, O_2 is now considered to play a role in the natural process of aging.[7,8] In 1777, Scheele, who independently discovered O_2, noted along with Priestley that O_2 is toxic to plants. In 1785, Lavoisier, who first recognized the vital role of O_2 in the equivalent processes of respiration and combustion, commented explicitly on the dual nature of O_2: "when there is an excess of vital air [oxygen], the animal only undergoes a severe illness; when it is lacking, death is almost instantaneous."[5] In experiments carried out with Laplace, he described right heart and pulmonary congestion in guinea pigs that died in O_2 under a bell jar before the O_2 was used up.[9,10]

In 1873, Paul Bert became the first to systematically study O_2 toxicity.[9] He documented the toxicity of O_2, particularly the lethality of hyperbaric hyperoxia, in all forms of life from mammals to viruses. He concluded that "no living thing is exempt from damage that can be produced by oxygen."[11] Grand mal seizures are the most notorious toxic effect of hyperbaric hyperoxia and have been referred to as the "Paul Bert effect."[9] J.B.S. Haldane experienced such seizures himself.[9] The pathophysiologic effects of hyperbaric hyperoxia have been reviewed elsewhere.[9,11–15] This chapter focuses on the effects of normobaric hyperoxia.

Respiratory Effects of Oxygen Breathing

The best known and most studied effects of normobaric hyperoxia concern the respiratory system. Lavoisier was the first to note changes in the lungs of animals that died from hyperoxia: ". . . the lung was very flaccid, but bright red, even on the outside, and highly congested with blood . . ."[16]

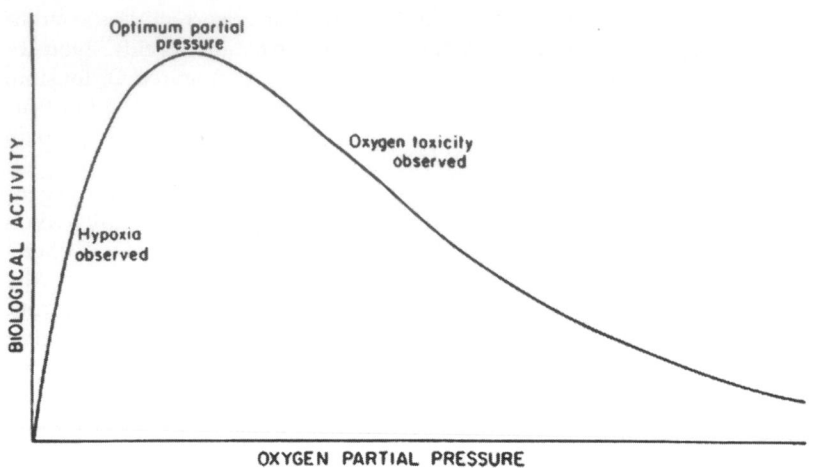

FIGURE 45-1 Dual effect of oxygen (O_2) on biological activity. (*Reproduced, with permission, from Gilbert.*[7])

In 1899, J. Lorrain Smith became the first to systematically study the pulmonary pathology of normobaric hyperoxia, specifically, a 4-day exposure to a fractional concentration of inspired O_2, $F_{I_{O_2}}$, of 0.74 to 0.80 in mammals. The diffuse intense lung damage from O_2 toxicity described by Smith, and many others since, has been named the "Lorrain Smith effect."[9]

The symptoms and physiologic changes in healthy human volunteers associated with normobaric hyperoxia have been the subject of several reviews.[9,11,14,15,17–26] The respiratory effects of O_2 breathing are listed in Table 45-1.

RESPIRATORY DEPRESSION AND STIMULATION, PULMONARY VASODILATION, AND HYPERCAPNIA

The depression in respiratory drive is primarily related to decreased stimulation of the hypoxia-sensitive chemoreceptors in the carotid and aortic bodies. These chemoreceptors are the only known O_2 sensors that initiate chemoreflexes.[27] Dejours et al showed that the O_2 chemoreceptor drive of respiration, which may account for 10–15% of resting ventilation, disappears above an alveolar P_{O_2} of 170 torr, corresponding to a $P_{I_{O_2}}$ of 230 torr, or an $F_{I_{O_2}}$ of 0.30.[14] When O_2 breathing is suddenly initiated, the normal response is twofold.[18,28,29] First, there is a nearly immediate, precipitous decrease in ventilation, whose nadir occurs within 20–30 seconds (Fig. 45-2), followed by a gradual return to and slightly above baseline (see Fig. 45-2). The acute transient depression is mediated by the arterial chemoreceptor

TABLE 45-1 Respiratory Effects of Oxygen Breathing (Normobaric Hyperoxia)

- Depression of respiration
- Stimulation of respiration
- Pulmonary vasodilation; ventilation/perfusion mismatching
- Hypercapnia
- Absorption atelectasis
- Acute tracheobronchitis; decreased mucociliary clearance
- Diffuse alveolar damage; acute respiratory distress syndrome
- Bronchopulmonary dysplasia

reflexes and may be taken as an index of the level of chemoreceptor activity present during normoxia.[28,30] The subacute mild sustained ventilatory stimulation appears to be secondary to an indirect effect of hyperoxia on the respiratory centers in the brainstem. That is, hyperoxia causes an increase in tissue carbon dioxide tension (P_{CO_2}) secondary to the Haldane effect, or Christian-Douglas-Haldane effect[31] (the increase in blood P_{CO_2}, at a fixed CO_2 content, caused by the release of hemoglobin-bound hydrogen ions and CO_2, bound as carbamino compounds, that occurs on the oxygenation of hemoglobin). Ironically, in one of the earliest reports (1921) of this hyperoxia-induced mild hyperventilation, Dautrebande et al[32] proposed that hyperoxic vasoconstriction of the central nervous system vasculature produces tissue hypercapnia, which in turn directly stimulates the respiratory center.

In normal subjects the mild respiratory stimulation induced in the steady state by hyperoxia results in a mild hyperventilation and a mild decrease in Pa_{CO_2} by a few millimeters of mercury, which in turn limits the degree of hyperventilation. But in the presence of inspired CO_2, the paradoxical respiratory stimulant effect of O_2 is much more obvious, as noted as early as 1918 by Yamada.[33] When the normally modest fall in Pa_{CO_2} is prevented, (isocapnic) hyperoxia produces a dramatic increase in ventilation (Fig. 45-3),[34–36] by 21% at $F_{I_{O_2}} = 0.30$ and by a remarkable 115% at $F_{I_{O_2}} = 0.75$.[34,35] Becker et al[35] showed that in both poikilocapnic (non-isocapnic) and isocapnic hyperoxia, the Haldane effect is the most important mechanism of the respiratory stimulant effect of hyperoxia in normals. Rucker et al[36] used these observations and showed in normal subjects that, compared with poikilocapnic hyperoxia, isocapnic hyperoxia more rapidly eliminates carbon monoxide and improves cerebral blood flow and O_2 delivery (secondary to the vasodilator effect of the higher level of Pa_{CO_2}) (see Fig. 45-3).

In contrast to the steady-state respiratory stimulant effect of hyperoxia in normals, hyperoxia may instead cause severe respiratory depression in patients with severe chronic obstructive pulmonary disease (COPD). The relative importance of the various mechanisms remains controversial. The conventional view is that hyperoxic hypercapnia is

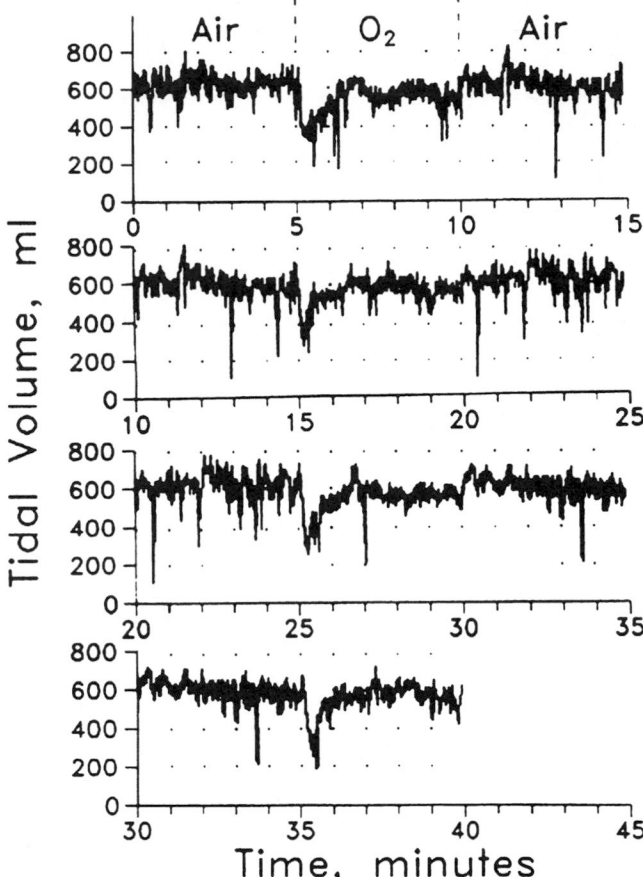

FIGURE 45-2 Acute depression of respiration by normobaric hyperoxia illustrated in a healthy conscious dog breathing from a mask as the inspired gas was alternated between air and O_2 every 5 minutes for 40 minutes. At the onset of each period of O_2 breathing, the continuous record of tidal volume shows a precipitous fall to a mean value of 54% of the normoxia baseline. This decrease in tidal volume is evident by 10 seconds and reaches a nadir at about 18 seconds. It is transient, and despite continued hyperoxia, it has returned nearly to baseline by 1.5 minutes. The record is plotted such that the normoxia data at the end of each 15-minute period are repeated on the next line as the beginning of the next 15-minute period to emphasize the repeating, cyclic nature of the alterations in inspired gas and to demonstrate more clearly the response pattern of tidal volume to hyperoxia. (*Reproduced, with permission, from Lodato et al.*[28])

caused by alveolar hypoventilation resulting from reduced hypoxic ventilatory drive secondary to the rise in arterial P_{O_2} (Pa_{O_2}),[37] analogous to "oxygen apnea" in patients recovering from general anesthesia.[15] Other mechanisms include the Haldane effect, deterioration of ventilation/perfusion ($\dot{V}/\dot{Q}$) matching in the lung secondary to hyperoxic release of hypoxic pulmonary vasoconstriction, and development of atelectasis (true shunt). O_2 may also impair $\dot{V}/\dot{Q}$ matching by release of hypoxia-induced bronchoconstriction.[38,39]

The data in both acutely decompensated[40] and stable[41–43] patients with COPD, however, indicate that deterioration of $\dot{V}/\dot{Q}$ matching is the predominant mechanism. Using the multiple inert gas elimination technique in patients with COPD, Wagner et al[44] found no systematic changes in the distribution of $\dot{V}/\dot{Q}$ ratios with 100% O_2. But they did not report attempts to correlate individual changes in Pa_{CO_2} and changes in $\dot{V}/\dot{Q}$ distribution. In mechanically ventilated patients Dunn et al[45] reported that hyperoxia both worsened $\dot{V}/\dot{Q}$ matching and depressed respiratory drive. For an informative interchange, see Stradling[46] and Aubier et al.[47]

In a more recent study of patients with exacerbations of COPD, Robinson et al[39] used the multiple inert gas elimination technique to compare those patients who retained CO_2 with O_2 with those who did not. In both groups, hyperoxia worsened $\dot{V}/\dot{Q}$ matching by increasing perfusion to relatively poorly ventilated lung units (release of hypoxic vasoconstriction). In only the group who retained CO_2, however, hyperoxia decreased minute ventilation (by 20%) and increased ventilation to overventilated units (increased alveolar dead space). Later, they[48] concluded that in the group who retained CO_2, the largest contribution (46%) was from a decrease in minute ventilation, followed closely (43%) by an increase in alveolar dead space, with a much smaller contribution from the Haldane effect. They also showed that the risk of hyperoxic hypercapnia is better predicted by a low baseline Pa_{O_2} than by the baseline Pa_{CO_2}.[39]

Neff et al[49] showed that severe *chronic* respiratory acidosis (mean P_{CO_2} of 90 torr, mean pH of 7.32) in patients with COPD is well tolerated. Acute hyperoxic respiratory depression can be avoided by using controlled low-flow O_2 administration.[50,51] Hyperoxic hypercapnia may also occur in neuromuscular disease[52] and near-fatal asthma.[53,54]

In a prospective trial[55] of resuscitation of asphyxiated newborn human infants, those resuscitated with room air had better outcomes (Apgar scores, time to first breath, and first cry) than those resuscitated with 100% O_2. These results were attributed to the respiratory depressant effect of O_2[55] and have prompted review of existing guidelines for newborn resuscitation.[56]

ABSORPTION ATELECTASIS

Absorption atelectasis during O_2 breathing occurs in lung units with sufficiently low $\dot{V}/\dot{Q}$ ratios.[57] In such units the rate of capillary absorption of O_2 exceeds the rate of replenishment of alveolar gas during inspiration. This effect depends on the $\dot{V}/\dot{Q}$ ratio, the pattern of ventilation (e.g., the presence of sighs), the $F_{I_{O_2}}$, the duration of the O_2 exposure, the intrinsic stability of the lung units (e.g., tissue and surfactant factors), and the sensitivity of the local hypoxic pulmonary vasoconstriction to hyperoxic release (which acts synergistically by further lowering the $\dot{V}/\dot{Q}$ ratio). Using the inert gas elimination technique in healthy nonsmoking subjects, Wagner et al[57] showed that within 30 minutes of breathing 100% O_2, 8 of the 9 subjects had developed small shunts, averaging 0.5–3.2%, with the largest at 10.7% (Fig. 45-4). Theoretically, only about 6 minutes is required for the development of such shunts.[58] Clearly, when 100% O_2 breathing is used to quantify a shunt, its magnitude might be overestimated compared to that present during air breathing.

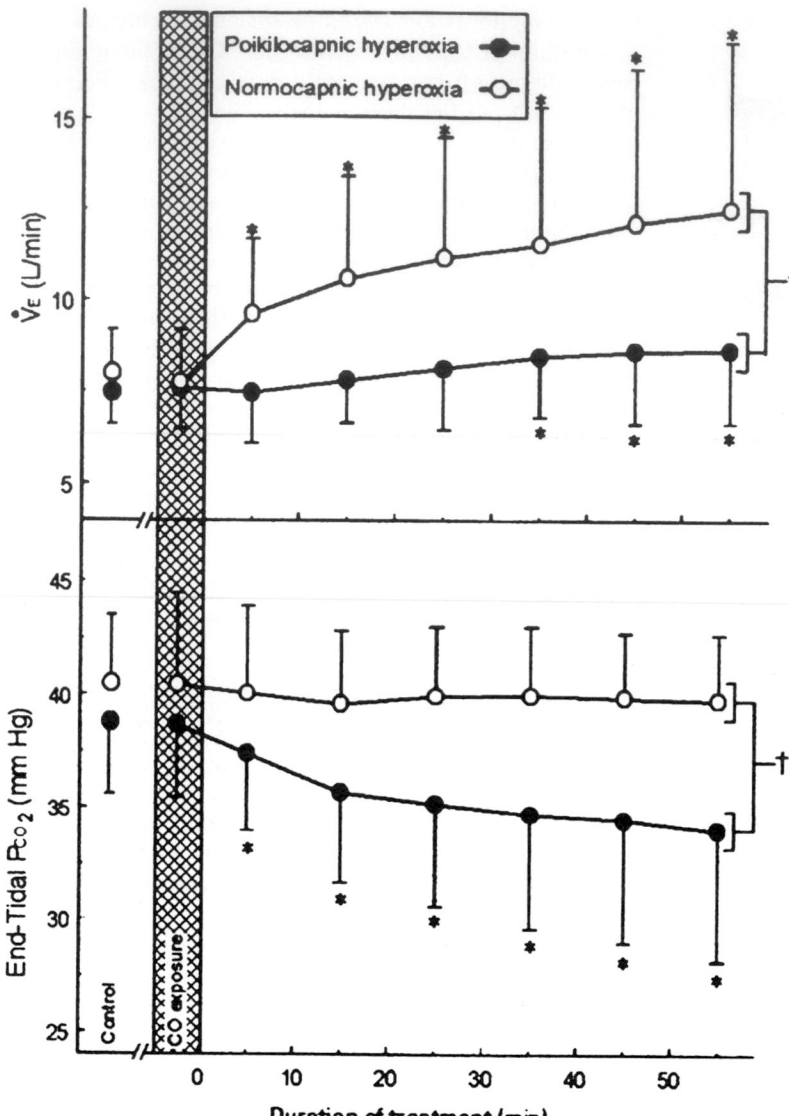

FIGURE 45-3 Steady-state responses of minute ventilation (V_E) and end-tidal P_{CO_2} to breathing 100% O_2 (hyperoxia) in healthy human subjects (mean ± SD; n = 14). Poikilocapnic hyperoxia (end-tidal P_{CO_2} was not controlled) produced a mild increase in minute ventilation and a small (4-mmHg) decrease in end-tidal P_{CO_2}. Normocapnic hyperoxia (CO_2 was added to the inspirate to maintain constant end-tidal P_{CO_2}) produced a marked and progressive increase in minute ventilation. These respiratory stimulant effects of hyperoxia are due largely to the Haldane effect, which results in increased P_{CO_2} in the brain. Note: Before time = 0, subjects were exposed to carbon monoxide in this study of CO elimination. (*Reproduced, with permission, from Rucker et al.[36]*)

Hyperoxia also enhances absorption from other gas spaces: middle ear and sinuses (causing headache), and therapeutically in pneumothorax, bowel obstruction or ileus, and subcutaneous emphysema.[15]

Hyperoxia may also cause atelectasis by interfering with the pulmonary surfactant system,[59] both by injury to the alveolar type II pneumocyte, which synthesizes, secretes, and recycles surfactant, and by injury to the alveolar-capillary interface, resulting in the influx of plasma proteins, which inhibit surfactant function. Hyperoxia-induced atelectasis has also been demonstrated in patients with acute lung injury[60] using the multiple inert gas elimination technique.

ACUTE TRACHEOBRONCHITIS

Acute tracheobronchitis was described in 1945 by Comroe et al.[61] Normal subjects breathing 100% O_2 for 24 hours noted: substernal distress, cough, sore throat, nasal conges-

tion, eye irritation, ear discomfort, fatigue, and paresthesias, and had a reduction in vital capacity. Symptoms began within 4–22 hours. Substernal distress was also noted while breathing 75% O_2, but not 50% O_2, for 24 hours. Substernal distress is generally the first symptom noted in normal subjects. It is thought to represent acute tracheobronchitis,[23] but it may also be the result of atelectasis alone.[62] Using fiberoptic bronchoscopy, Sackner et al[63] directly observed evidence of such tracheobronchial inflammation (focal areas of redness, edema, and injection of small vessels of the trachea, and depression of mucus velocity) in healthy human subjects after 6 hours of breathing 90–95% O_2.

A decrease in vital capacity[61] is considered the best index of O_2 toxicity. In humans this decrease in vital capacity probably results from the inspiratory pain of the acute tracheobronchitis and from absorption atelectasis. In animals it is more clearly related to parenchymal lung injury. By impairing an important host defense mechanism, acute tracheobronchitis could predispose to nosocomial pneumonia,[63,64]

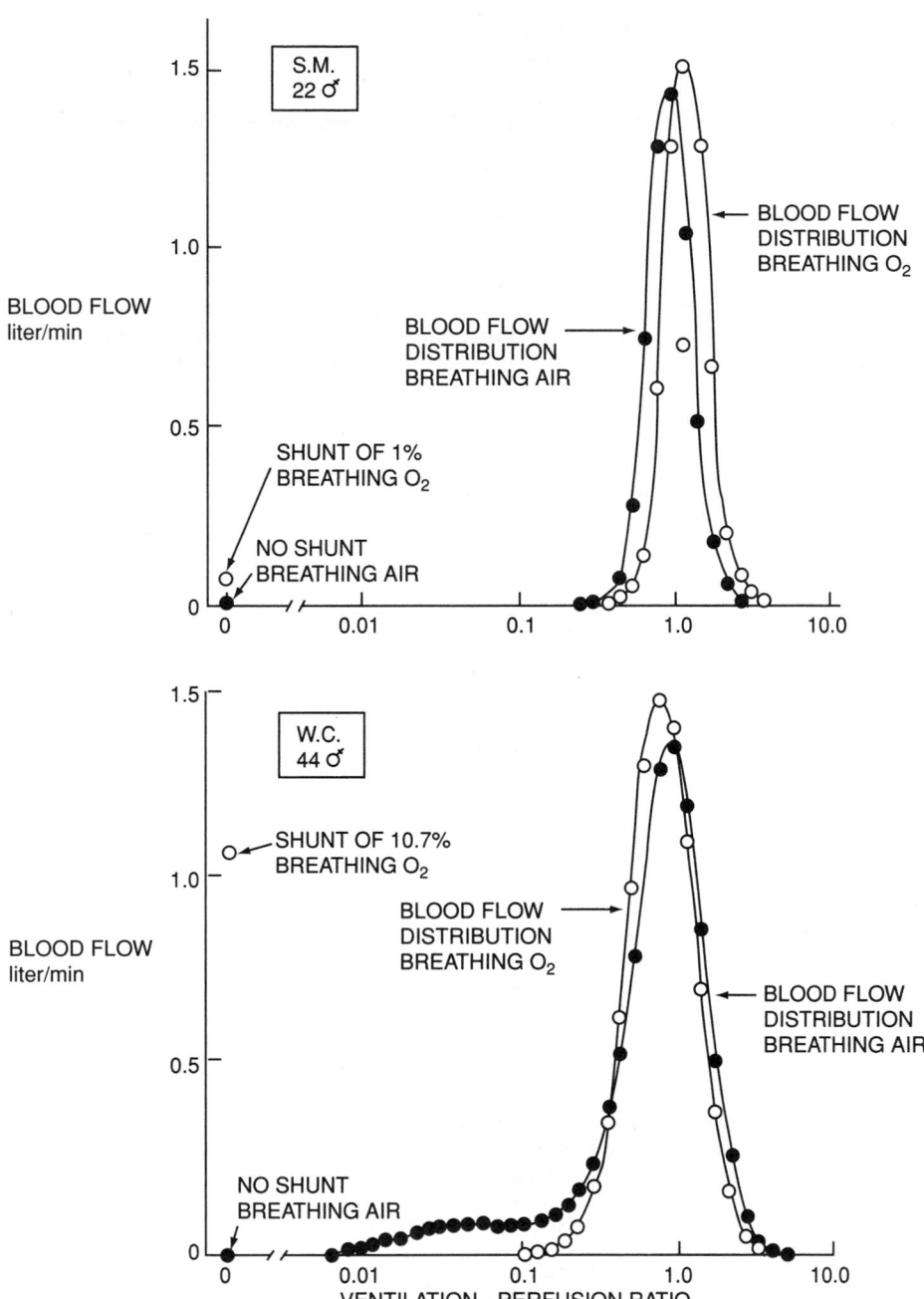

FIGURE 45-4 Distributions of blood flow with respect to ventilation/ perfusion ($\dot{V}_A/\dot{Q}$) ratios in two normal subjects while breathing air (normoxia) and after 30 minutes of breathing 100% O_2 (normobaric hyperoxia). *Upper panel:* In the younger subject hyperoxia produced: (1) a 1% shunt, indicating a minor degree of hyperoxia-induced atelectasis, and (2) an overall shift of the main body of the distribution to the right to higher $\dot{V}_A/\dot{Q}$ ratios, indicating mild hyperoxia-induced hyperventilation in the steady state. *Lower panel:* In the older subject hyperoxia produced more dramatic changes: the left "shoulder" of the normoxic blood flow distribution (i.e., the blood flow distributed to lung units with low $\dot{V}_A/\dot{Q}$ ratios) was converted by hyperoxia to a 10.7% shunt, indicating substantial amounts of hyperoxia-induced atelectasis, but the main body of the distribution was little altered. (*Reproduced, with permission, from Wagner et al.[57]*)

but this has not been well studied. In rats hyperoxia also impairs alveolar macrophage function,[65] perhaps adding to the risk of ventilator-associated pneumonia. In healthy subjects with moderate responsiveness to methacholine at baseline, breathing 95% O_2 for 12 hours produced no change in methacholine responsiveness, despite signs and symptoms of acute tracheobronchitis.[66]

THRESHOLD OXYGEN TENSION FOR THE DEVELOPMENT OF OXYGEN TOXICITY

Like other toxic drugs, the effects of O_2 can be viewed in terms of a classic pharmacologic dose-response curve.[11] The dose of O_2 can be expressed as the product of P_{IO_2} and the duration of the exposure (i.e., dose = P_{IO_2} × time). When plotted, this relationship is a rectangular hyperbola (Fig. 45-5), which expresses the dose response in terms of vital capacity decrements. The horizontal asymptote of 50% O_2, or 0.5 atm, assumes that at that level of hyperoxia, individuals can be exposed safely for prolonged periods of time.

The validity of setting at 0.5 atm the threshold P_{IO_2} for the development of O_2 toxicity, as reflected by a decrease in vital capacity, for exposures of indefinite duration has been carefully discussed by Clark et al[18] and Clark.[19] Earlier these authors had suggested a less conservative threshold of

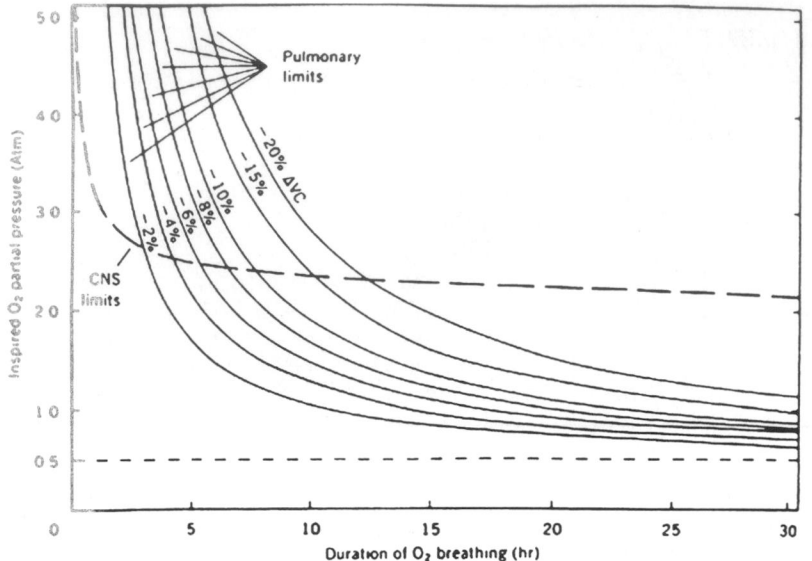

FIGURE 45-5 Oxygen tolerance or dose-response curves for pulmonary and central nervous system (CNS) toxicity in healthy human subjects. Each curve in the family of curves for pulmonary O_2 toxicity is a rectangular hyperbola and represents equivalent O_2 partial pressure-duration "doses" of O_2 exposures. These curves are based on the development of the indicated changes in vital capacity in 50% of the individuals subjected to the indicated O_2 partial pressure-duration exposures. The horizontal asymptote for the lowest pulmonary toxicity curve is at an O_2 partial pressure of about 0.6 atmospheres (atm), indicating that O_2 partial pressures below 0.6 atm appear to be safe for exposures of indefinite duration. (*Reproduced, with permission, from Lambertsen CL: In: Mountcastle VB, et al, editors: Medical physiology, 14th ed. St. Louis: CV Mosby, 1901–44, 1980.*)

0.6 atm.[67] The rationale for the 0.5-atm P_{IO_2} threshold is based largely on the responses of vital capacity to prolonged hyperoxia in healthy men in the three studies of Comroe et al,[61] Helvey et al,[68] and Michel et al.[69] Fig. 45-6 summarizes these exposures and those of two subsequent studies in healthy men.[70,71] Comroe et al[61] exposed 9 normal men to a P_{IO_2} of 0.75 atm for 24 hours, with return to air breathing for 15 minutes every 3 hours. They found that 5 of the 9 had chest symptoms and that the group had a modest decrease in vital capacity (mean decrease <300 ml). None of 6 subjects exposed to P_{IO_2} = 0.5 atm for 24 hours had chest symptoms, and the mean decrease in vital capacity was even less (only about 210 ml). They concluded that the safe limit of P_{IO_2} lies between 0.5 and 0.75 atm, probably close to 0.6 atm.[61] Similar findings were reported by Ohlsson[72] (not plotted in Fig. 45-6) in 6 men exposed to a P_{IO_2} of 0.78–0.88 atm for 53–57 hours. Helvey et al[68] found no change in vital capacity, Pa_{O_2}, or chest radiographs after 14 days of exposure to 0.49 atm. Michel et al[69] reported no net change in vital capacity during a 7-day exposure of 6 normal U.S. Navy men to P_{IO_2} = 0.55 atm. Fife et al[70] studied 3 subjects at P_{IO_2} of 0.47 atm for 7 days; none developed chest symptoms or a change in vital capacity.

At P_{IO_2} = 0.50 atm for 45 hours, Griffith et al[73] found increased pulmonary clearance of an inhaled tracer and increased albumin in bronchoalveolar lavage fluid, suggesting the possibility of injury to the alveolar-capillary barrier, or alternatively, only inflamed airways.[74]

Data from the U.S. Navy's Shallow Habitat Air Diving (SHAD) program support 0.60 atm P_{IO_2} as safe for prolonged O_2 exposure.[14] Men tolerated well exposures of 0.51 and 0.57 atm P_{IO_2} for 29.5 and 28 days, without changes in pulmonary functiong.[14,71,75] With 9-day exposures to mean P_{IO_2} of 0.61 atm (each day, 16 hours at P_{IO_2} = 0.51 atm and 8 hours at P_{IO_2} = 0.81 atm), only 1 of the 3 men showed decreased vital capacity (9.7%) and chest discomfort, both coinciding with the daily 8-hour excursions to P_{IO_2} = 0.81 atm.[14,71,75]

TOXICITY OF OXYGEN NEAR 1 ATMOSPHERE IN NORMAL SUBJECTS

Several studies examining physiologic parameters and other indices of lung injury have also been carried out in humans with exposures at or near a P_{IO_2} = 1.0 atm (Fig. 45-7). Burger et al[62] reported chest pain and tightness and

FIGURE 45-6 A summary of studies of prolonged exposure of normal human subjects to an inspired O_2 tension (P_{IO_2}) near 0.5 atm. The points indicate the P_{IO_2} and duration of exposure for the respective studies. The name associated with each point indicates the original reference. Each of these studies reported that the hyperoxic exposure was generally well tolerated, with little or no symptoms of chest tightness, little or no decrease in vital capacity or other pulmonary function tests, and no long-term sequelae. See text for details. (*Data from Comroe et al,[61] Helvey et al,[68] Michel et al,[69] Fife et al,[70] and Dougherty et al.[71]*)

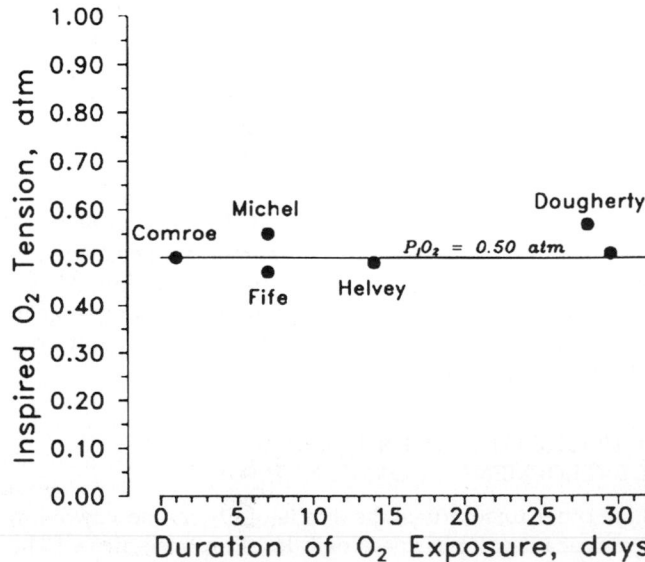

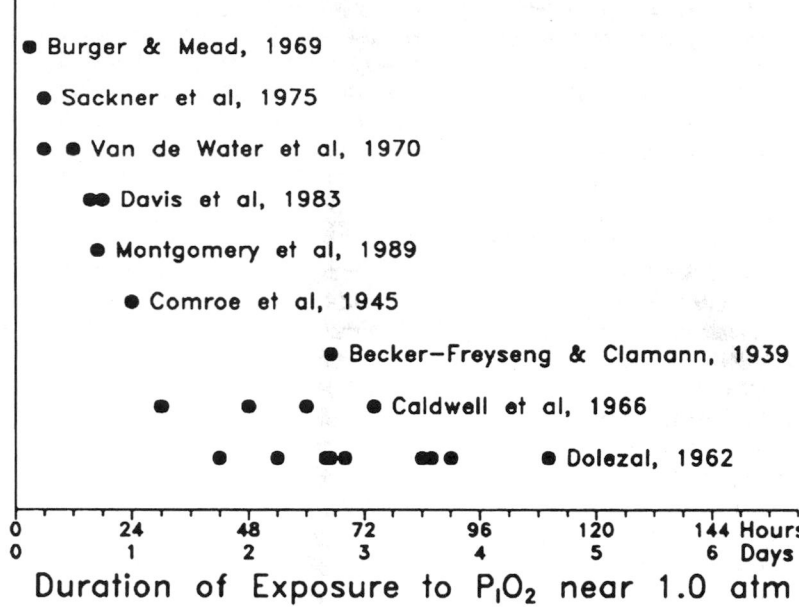

FIGURE 45-7 A summary of studies of prolonged exposure of normal human subjects to an inspired O_2 tension (P_{IO_2}) near 1.0 atm. The horizontal arrays of points indicate the various durations of exposure within a given study. The names associated with each horizontal array of points indicate the original references. See text for details. (*Data from Comroe et al,[61] Burger et al,[62] Sackner et al,[63] Montgomery et al,[74] van de Water et al,[76] Davis et al,[77] Becker-Freyseng et al,[78] Caldwell et al,[79] and Dolezal.[82]*)

decreases in pulmonary compliance after only 3 hours of breathing pure O_2 at various ambient pressures including 1.0 atm. The subjects were instructed to refrain from taking deep breaths, yawning, or sighing during the exposure. Postexposure the decrease in compliance and the chest symptoms readily resolved on deep breathing or sighing, suggesting to them that atelectasis rather than direct O_2 toxicity was the etiology. Remarkably, in this study[62] breathing pure O_2 at only 0.39 atm ambient pressure (P_{IO_2} of only 0.39 atm) produced symptoms that were qualitatively and quantitatively no different from breathing pure O_2 at 1.0 atm ambient pressure ($P_{IO_2} = 1.0$). Yet, breathing with a P_{IO_2} of 1.0 atm, but in the presence of an equal amount of nitrogen ($P_{IN_2} = 1.0$ atm, and total ambient pressure = $P_{IO_2} + P_{IN_2} = 2.0$ atm) was virtually no different from control (air breathing at 1.0 atm ambient pressure). These findings further convinced these investigators that atelectasis, promoted by the lack of nitrogen, was the mechanism of both the chest symptoms and the compliance changes.

As already noted, Sackner et al[63] found bronchoscopic evidence of tracheitis in each of 10 normal subjects inspiring a P_{IO_2} of 0.90–0.95 atm for 6 hours. None had substernal distress or changes in pulmonary function tests. Tracheal mucus velocity was depressed at 3 hours but was restored by a β_2-adrenergic agonist. They speculated that the effect on mucus velocity could predispose to bacterial superinfection.[63] In men exposed to 6–12 hours of $P_{IO_2} = 1.0$ atm and taking a deep breath every 20 minutes, van de Water et al[76] found no chest symptoms or changes in pulmonary function or oxygenation.

In 14 subjects exposed to a P_{IO_2} of 0.95 atm for a mean of 17 hours, Davis et al[77] found that 9 had substernal discomfort and 6 had mild erythema on bronchoscopy. Bronchoalveolar lavage fluid showed increased albumin, transferrin, and total protein, consistent with alveolar-capillary leak, but no change in inflammatory cells. In contrast, despite chest pain in subjects breathing $P_{IO_2} = 1.0$ atm for 17 hours, Montgomery et al[74] found no changes in pulmonary function tests, solute permeability, or systemic or pulmonary endothelial injury (as reflected by plasma fibronectin and factor VIII). They suggested that the increased albumin and transferrin in the bronchoalveolar lavage fluid seen by Davis et al[77] and Griffith et al[73] may not indicate lung parenchymal injury, but may instead have come from the inflamed airways.

Comroe et al[61] studied men exposed to $P_{IO_2} = 0.99$ atm for 24 hours and found no changes in chest radiographs or oxygenation. Burger et al[62] found that breathing pure O_2 at ambient pressure of 0.5 atm, such that $P_{IO_2} = 0.50$ atm and $P_{IN_2} = 0$, produced no symptoms but decreased vital capacity.

In 1939 Becker-Freyseng et al[78] reported exposures of 2 men to a P_{IO_2} of 0.9 atm for 65 hours, or 2.7 days. Both had decreased vital capacity. One developed nausea, vomiting, tachycardia, a febrile tracheobronchitis, dyspnea, and pain in the elbows and knees. The etiology of nausea and vomiting is not clear but could be related to the absorption of bowel gas owing to the absence of nitrogen.[15]

Caldwell et al[79] studied 4 subjects exposed to $P_{IO_2} = 0.98$ atm for, respectively, 30, 48, 60, and 74 hours (i.e., 1.25, 2.0, 2.5, and 3.1 days). They were instructed to take five deep breaths and a cough every 2 hours throughout the day but not at night. In addition to chest pain and cough, 3 of the 4 had paresthesias, and 3 had anorexia. They noted decreases in lung volumes and diffusing capacity, but not in forced expiratory volume in 1 second/forced vital capacity (FEV_1/FVC) ratio, and a modest increase in alveolar-arterial (A-a) P_{O_2} gradient (89 torr). Chest radiographs were clear. The authors could not exclude atelectasis as the etiology of the decreased vital capacity. However, the subject with the longest (74 hours) exposure was hospitalized for 2 days postexposure "until his sense of well being and appetite returned." This subject had dyspnea on exertion for 3–4 days postexposure, and his vital capacity did not return to baseline until 24 weeks postexposure.[79] In humans normobaric hyperoxia does not produce airway obstruction[66] but may do so in dogs[9,80] and primates[81] Hyperbaric hyperoxia may produce airway obstruction in humans.[22]

The longest voluntary human exposures to 100% O_2 are by Dolezal.[82] Twelve subjects were exposed to the limit of tolerance. The mean exposure was 74 hours (3.1 days), with a range from 42 hours (1.75 days) to a remarkable 110 hours (4.6 days). P_{CO_2} of the exposure chamber remained high, about 7–8 torr (1%). In addition to retrosternal pain and cough, the subjects eventually experienced dyspnea, loss of gustatory sensation, anorexia, nausea (after 48–60 hours) and vomiting, general weakness, and vertigo (beyond 60–72 hours). Three developed fevers of 38.5–39.3°C. As evidence of additional systemic (nonrespiratory) toxicity, 9 of the 12 noted paresthesias and hypesthesias of the tips of fingers and toes, which did not resolve until 14–21 days postexposure. Vital capacity decreased by 17%, minute ventilation progressively increased by 39% throughout the exposure, and a mild respiratory alkalosis developed. Remarkably, arterial O_2 saturation remained at or near 100% throughout the exposure and was normal postexposure. Dolezal interpreted this intact oxygenation as evidence that pulmonary edema and "hepatization foci," as seen in animal studies, had not developed.[82]

Thus, taken together, these reports seem to imply that evidence for major sustained parenchymal lung injury, or the equivalent of acute respiratory distress syndrome (ARDS), has been much more readily observed in animals than in normal humans.

TOXICITY OF OXYGEN NEAR 1 ATMOSPHERE IN PATIENTS

Most patients who receive prolonged high F_{IO_2} have severe parenchymal lung injury (e.g., ARDS). Intriguing data are available, however, from human patients without major lung disease. In 18 patients postoperative from cardiac surgery, Singer et al[83] confirmed that short exposures of 24 hours mean (range 15–48 hours) to 100% O_2 have no demonstrable adverse effects. They found no change in shunt, compliance, dead space, radiologic atelectasis, or clinical course compared to a group who received only the F_{IO_2} (mean 0.32) required for adequate oxygenation. Singer et al[83] also reported two additional patients who were ventilated with 100% O_2 for 5 and 7 days, respectively. Throughout the 5- and 7-day periods, these patients showed progressive improvement in Pa_{O_2}, from 368 to 430 torr and from 155 to 404 torr, respectively. The first patient was extubated on the fifth day and subsequently discharged from the hospital. The second patient died on the seventh day of massive pulmonary hemorrhage related to a greatly prolonged bleeding time on anticoagulants.

In a companion paper by the same group, Barber et al[84] reported the effects of ventilating patients with massive cerebral trauma and resultant irreversible, ultimately fatal brain damage, with either 100% O_2 (n = 5) or air (n = 5). Ventilation with the respective gases continued until death, which occurred within 31 to 72 hours, or 1.3 to 3 days (mean 2.2 days), in the O_2 group and within 50 to 216 hours, or 2.1 to 9 days (mean 4.3 days), in the air group. None had preexisting lung disease. None had spontaneous respirations. All received tidal volumes greater than 800 ml, periodic tracheal suctioning, frequent changes in body position, and treatment with corticosteroids. After 2 days, the O_2 group had a lower mean Pa_{O_2} (120 versus >400 torr, tested on 100% O_2 in both groups), greater shunt and dead space, but no difference in compliance. The O_2 group also had greater worsening of chest radiographs, progressing to multilobar infiltrates, consolidation, or collapse. At autopsy the O_2 group also had greater lung weights. Perhaps the most striking finding was that at autopsy no histologic differences between the groups were apparent. Both had varying degrees of bronchopneumonia, intra-alveolar and interstitial edema, atelectasis, congestion, hemorrhage, and intravascular coagulation. Hyaline membranes, however, were "conspicuously absent" in both groups. It seems likely that hyperoxia-induced atelectasis (and perhaps ventilator-induced lung injury, with 800 ml tidal volume) could explain many if not all of their findings, especially in such patients with no spontaneous respiratory effort.

Hyde and Rawson[85] reported the effects of inadvertent exposure to 83–91% O_2 for 12–32 days in 5 intubated patients with neuromuscular disease. The authors made a presumptive diagnosis of hyperoxic pneumonitis based on scattered patchy infiltrates on chest radiographs, fever, and leukocytosis. The postmortem examination of the one patient who died (a depressed patient who was found dead with the respirator disconnected) showed "thickening of the alveolar septa by edema and fibroblastic proliferation ... fibrin deposition and increased numbers of lining cells in the alveolar lumina." No hyaline membranes were described. Interpretation of their findings, however, is confounded by the fact that these patients also had copious secretions, "a major degree of atelectasis" (4 of the 5 patients), and pneumonia (4 of 5), which are common complications of such patients even in the absence of hyperoxia. Furthermore, unlike ARDS, these patients responded rapidly to minimizing the F_{IO_2}, "vigorous tracheal aspiration (and) meticulous tracheal toilet," and antibiotics. In fact, after these changes in management, all 4 were weaned from mechanical ventilation within only 2–5 days.

Perhaps the longest reported exposure of a patient to hyperoxia was that of a 32-year-old man with myasthenia gravis, who was ventilated with 80% O_2 (which could not be lowered for technical reasons) for 150 days, at which time he developed blindness bilaterally with retinal artery constriction and retinal atrophy.[86] Hyperoxia constricts retinal arteries in adults as well as neonates.[87] During the exposure his Pa_{O_2} remained 250–300 torr. He remained another 130 days on 60% O_2 (Pa_{O_2} 120–160 torr) before weaning from mechanical ventilation on day 280, after which his Pa_{O_2} remained normal (80–100 torr). Except for the elevated A-a P_{O_2} gradient, consistent with atelectasis, inadequate control of secretions, or pneumonia, no signs or symptoms of pulmonary O_2 toxicity were reported.

In a brief communication Smith et al[88] reported the absence of any evidence of O_2 toxicity, as determined by radiographs, pulmonary function, bronchoscopy, or histopathology, in 41 patients treated with high-frequency jet ventilation using a mean F_{IO_2} of 0.92 (range 0.80–0.95) for a mean of 4.1 days (range 8 hours to 12 days). They suggested that their lack of O_2 toxicity may be secondary to the lack of "stretching and shearing forces" encountered in conventional mechanical ventilation.

More recently, Capellier et al[89] retrospectively studied 74 patients with $F_{IO_2} \geq 0.90$ continuously for at least 48 hours. They found that the duration of this exposure in the 17 survivors was surprisingly long (mean 5.6 days) and no different from the 57 nonsurvivors (5.9 days). One of the survivors had exposure to $F_{IO_2} \geq 0.90$ for 15 days and was eventually discharged, breathing spontaneously with a normal Pa_{O_2} on room air. The majority of deaths were related to sepsis and multiorgan failure rather than to progressive hypoxemic respiratory failure. Of the 37 patients exposed to $F_{IO_2} \geq 0.90$ for at least 4 days, only 5 (14%) died with hypoxemia. These authors concluded that the lungs of patients with acute respiratory failure appear relatively resistant to prolonged hyperoxia, that high plateau pressures may be more injurious than high F_{IO_2}, and that a prospective trial may be helpful in clarifying the optimum management of F_{IO_2} for such patients.[89]

PATHOLOGY OF PULMONARY OXYGEN TOXICITY: DIFFUSE ALVEOLAR DAMAGE

In 1958 Pratt[90] was the first to note in patients pathological changes attributed to hyperoxia. The pathology of pulmonary O_2 toxicity has been reviewed by a number of authors[11,14,17,20–23,25,91,92] and is the subject of a monograph[9] Because of preexisting lung disease in most human studies, the most persuasive data come from animals. A few studies, however, of hyperoxic pulmonary pathology in humans without preexisting lung disease are available,[93–95] and the findings are consistent with those in animals. The histologic pathology of hyperoxia-induced acute lung injury is that of diffuse alveolar damage, or DAD.[92] DAD is a descriptive term for the predictable but nonspecific features of acute lung injury from a variety of toxins, including infectious agents, other inhalants, pharmaceutical agents and other ingestants, radiation, and the multiple causes of ARDS including trauma and sepsis[92] Hyperoxia has in common with all other causes of DAD an initial injury to both the alveolar endothelial and epithelial cells.

DAD can be divided into two stages, as first defined by Nash et al,.[96] and detailed in Table 45-2.[91] The first is an early acute or exudative stage within the first week, characterized by interstitial and intra-alveolar edema, intra-alveolar hemorrhage and fibrin deposition, sloughing of the alveolar lining cells (type I pneumocytes) with denudation of the alveolar basement membrane, and hyaline membranes, which represent cytoplasmic and nuclear debris from sloughed cells mixed with fibrin.[92] Late in the first week an inflammatory cell infiltrate into the interstitium is evident. The small pulmonary arterioles and alveolar capillaries may show fibrin thrombi. Also by the end of the first week, proliferation of type II pneumocytes appears along the alveolar lining, representing a reparative phase; the type II pneumocytes can later differentiate into type I pneumocytes.[92]

The second stage of DAD[92] is a proliferative or organizing stage and is noted beyond the first week. Fibroblastic proliferation in the interstitium and focal intra-alveolar fibrosis appear. Whereas the edema and hyaline membranes have largely resolved, the interstitial inflammatory infiltrate and the alveolar lining cell hyperplasia are still present. A striking interstitial fibrosis develops in association with extensive interstitial deposition of collagen.

The issue of just how sensitive the human lung is to hyperoxic lung injury is still somewhat open to question. Remarkably, as noted above, in patients without prior lung injury who received 100% O_2 for up to 7 days, typical histologic lesions were not found.[83,84] These observations prompted Katzenstein[92] to suggest that humans may be susceptible to significant hyperoxic lung injury only after their lungs are first damaged by other insults. Other authors have concluded simply that no consistent evidence shows that hyperoxia ($F_{IO_2} > 0.60$) is dangerous in acute lung injury or ARDS.[97]

BRONCHOPULMONARY DYSPLASIA

Bronchopulmonary dysplasia was initially described in 1967[98] and has been reviewed in detail by Balentine[9] and Truog.[99] It is a form of chronic lung disease that follows therapy for idiopathic respiratory distress syndrome (IRDS) of the newborn, or hyaline membrane disease. Bronchopulmonary dysplasia develops in very-low-birth weight infants ($\leq$1500 g at birth). Its incidence and prevalence have

TABLE 45-2 Diffuse Alveolar Damage in Humans at 0.8–1 Atmosphere of Oxygen

Changes	Time of Occurrence
Exudative	
1. Capillary congestion, focal intra-alveolar edema, a few cases with fibrin thrombi in capillaries and small arteries	Less than 3 days
2. Interstitial edema	After 3 days
3. Hyaline membranes lining alveolar septa	22 Hours to 7 days, decreasing or focal thereafter
4. Interstitial mononuclear cell infiltrates (lymphocytes, plasma cells, unclassified cells)	Less than 1 week
Proliferative	
1. Alveolar lining cell hyperplasia	Focal at 3 days, diffuse at 1 week
2. Interstitial fibrosis	Focal at 3 days, diffuse at 8 days, severe by 2 weeks

Derived from light microscopic data of Katzenstein et al.[94]
SOURCE: Modified, with permission, from Balentine.[9]

risen dramatically in recent years because of the markedly increased survival of these infants.[99] It has become the most common cause of chronic lung disease in infants.[100] Its pathologic features include fibrosis and destruction of acinar structures with a resultant combination of scarring and emphysematous changes. It appears to have three contributing mechanisms: (1) barotrauma from mechanical ventilation (ventilator-induced lung injury), (2) hyperoxia, with increased O_2 radicals in the presence of an immature antioxidant defense system, and (3) peribronchial pulmonary edema secondary to the birth-related increased pulmonary blood flow through an immature and injured pulmonary microcirculation.[99] Because high levels of both mechanical ventilation and hyperoxia virtually always occur together in patients with IRDS, the relative roles of these two etiologic factors is unclear. Churg et al[101] have described the equivalent of bronchopulmonary dysplasia, including "honeycombing," in three adult patients who also had received the combination of high ventilator pressures and high F_{IO_2} for 3–7 weeks. Baboon and other animal models for bronchopulmonary dysplasia exist.[102,103]

Management of bronchopulmonary dysplasia includes (1) adequate but not excessive O_2, especially until the retinas are fully vascularized, (2) mechanical ventilation as needed, (3) diuretics for pulmonary edema, (4) nutritional support, (5) bronchodilators, and (6) airway anti-inflammatory agents, cromolyn sodium, and corticosteroids.[99]

Nonrespiratory Effects of Oxygen Breathing

The nonrespiratory effects of hyperoxia have been extensively reviewed elsewhere.[9,11,25,104] The best-recognized effects include hemodynamic changes, suppression of erythropoiesis and serum erythropoietin,[105] the Haldane effect (see above), retinopathy of prematurity (previously called retrolental fibroplasia), and, only at O_2 pressures exceeding 2 atm, seizures.

Retinopathy of prematurity results from hyperoxic vasoconstriction and injury to the exquisitely susceptible, growing retinal capillaries of premature neonates (<26 weeks' gestation).[9,106,107] The resulting paradoxical "hyperoxic hypoxia" and tissue ischemia induces neovascularization within the retina and adjacent vitreous. This retinovitreal neovascularization eventually results in retinal detachment and blindness,[107] a process similar to that seen in diabetic and sickle cell retinopathies.[106] The incidence and severity of retinopathy of prematurity correlates with the duration of exposure to Pa_{O_2} >80 torr.[108]

ACUTE HEMODYNAMIC EFFECTS

The acute hemodynamic effects of normobaric hyperoxia in healthy humans have been studied by a number of investigators[104,109–121] and recently summarized by Lodato,[25,104,117] who also found virtually identical responses

TABLE 45-3   Acute Hemodynamic Effects of Oxygen Breathing (Normobaric Hyperoxia)

Parameter	Effect
Heart rate	Decreased
Cardiac output	Decreased
Right ventricular stroke work	Decreased
Left ventricular stroke work	Unchanged
Right and left ventricular work rates	Decreased
Systemic arterial pressure	Variably increased, decreased, or unchanged
Pulmonary artery pressure	Decreased
Pulmonary arterial wedge pressure	Unchanged
Right atrial pressure	Increased
Systemic vascular resistance	Increased
Pulmonary vascular resistance	Decreased

SOURCE: Derived from Lodato.[104]

in conscious dogs[104,117] These results are summarized in Table 45-3. The decrease in heart rate is vagally mediated[28,110] The decrease in cardiac output is primarily the result of the relative bradycardia, but some studies have also shown an independent contribution from a decrease in stroke volume or diastolic dysfunction.[122] The decrease in cardiac work[104] is primarily the result of the bradycardia, but right ventricular afterload is reduced by pulmonary vasodilation.[123]

Systemic vasoconstriction is one of the most consistent findings and occurs independently of any changes in P_{CO_2}.[124,125] Virtually all systemic beds constrict during hyperoxia, but in rats the splanchnic circulation vasodilates.[126] The central nervous system vasoconstrictive effect has been used to treat vascular headaches.[15] The mechanisms are not fully understood and appear quite diverse among various vascular beds. Hyperoxic vasoconstriction may be a continuum of the mechanism of hypoxic vasodilatation.[127] That is, red blood cells can regulate vasomotor tone depending on their degree of oxyhemoglobin saturation: as saturation rises with hyperoxia (or falls with hypoxia), the red blood cell releases less (or more, respectively) of the vasodilators adenosine 5' triphosphate (ATP)[128] and nitric oxide from S-nitroso-hemoglobin.[129] In the central nervous system[130,131] and in the human forearm,[132] hyperoxia vasoconstricts by inactivation of endothelium-derived relaxing factor/nitric oxide by superoxide anion.[127,133] In the coronary bed, hyperoxia constricts by closure of ATP-sensitive potassium channels.[134] In the human retinal artery the reported mechanisms include release of endothelin-1[135] and prostanoids,[136] in addition to the mechanisms above.[125] The human umbilical vein vasoconstricts to hyperoxia via local release of norepinephrine.[137]

Despite the systemic vasoconstriction, systemic arterial pressure is variably affected, owing to the concurrent decrease in cardiac output. Jubran et al[138] showed that the bradycardia is independent of the arterial baroreceptor reflex.

The hemodynamic changes induced by hyperoxia have also been documented in patients with a wide variety of conditions, including general anesthesia,[139] during cardiopulmonary bypass,[140] immediately following coronary bypass surgery,[141] with cardiac risk,[142] congestive heart failure,[122,143,144] sepsis,[145,146] cirrhosis,[147] and children with acyanotic congenital heart disease.[148]

In patients with pulmonary hypertension from a variety of causes (primary, portal, human immunodeficiency virus, atrial septal defect, ventricular septal defect, and scleroderma) with mean baseline $Pa_{O_2} = 64$ mmHg, breathing 100% O_2 has been reported to decrease pulmonary vascular resistance by 24%.[149] A limitation of this study is that cardiac output was calculated from the Fick principle, assuming that hyperoxia did not change O_2 consumption, an invalid assumption.[104]

OXYGEN CONSUMPTION

Contrary to Priestley's speculation, which he based on his observations of a candle burning more vigorously in O_2 (see above), that hyperoxia may enhance metabolic rate, recent evidence indicates that hyperoxia can actually decrease metabolic rate as measured by O_2 consumption. Chapler et al[150] showed that under certain experimental conditions (e.g., acute anemia or autonomic inhibition) in anesthetized dogs, hyperoxia paradoxically decreased O_2 consumption. Lodato.[104] showed under more general physiologic conditions in unsedated, intact healthy conscious dogs, that hyperoxia (mean $Pa_{O_2} = 475$ torr) decreased whole body O_2 consumption by nearly 20% (Fig. 45-8). Unexpectedly, in this study the arteriovenous difference in O_2 content decreased along with the decrease in cardiac output (both by about 10%). Paradoxically, O_2 delivery (cardiac output × arterial O_2 content) did not change, and O_2 extraction (O_2 consumption/O_2 delivery) decreased. Subsequently, Lodato.[117] reported that when O_2 consumption and O_2 delivery were plotted in the conventional way, as ordinate and abscissa, respectively, hyperoxia produced a unique parallel shift downward in the O_2 consumption–O_2 delivery relationship (Fig. 45-9). Hyperoxia-induced decreases in O_2 consumption have also been reported in children with acyanotic congenital heart disease,[148] patients with sepsis,[145,146] cardiac-risk patients,[142] and patients during cardiopulmonary bypass.[140]

The mechanisms by which hyperoxia could induce such a decrease in O_2 consumption are obscure. The possibilities include[104] that hyperoxia may produce (1) systemic cellular O_2 toxicity, (2) a paradoxically inadequate O_2 supply ("hyperoxic hypoxia") at the microcirculatory level, owing to the diffuse systemic vasoconstriction;[151–154] or (3) a facultative decrease in O_2 demand, as has been demonstrated in mammals under certain physiologic challenges unrelated to hyperoxia.[155] Reinhart et al[146] investigated the second possibility. In patients with sepsis[146] and in stable patients with cardiac risk,[142] they infused the antioxidant N-acetylcysteine. They found that N-acetylcysteine attenuated the hyperoxia-induced decreases in both O_2 consumption (from 34% to only 11%) and gastric intramucosal pH

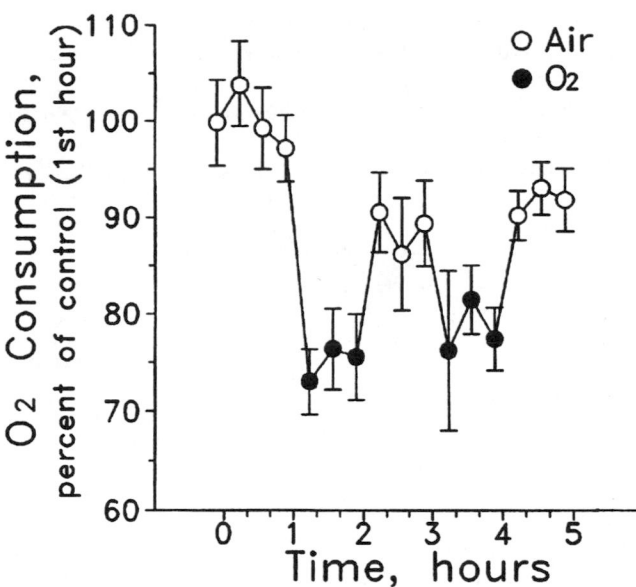

FIGURE 45-8 **Time course of resting whole body O_2 consumption as the inspired gas was alternated hourly between air (*open circles*) and O_2 breathing (hyperoxia; mean $Pa_{O_2} = 475$ torr) (*closed circles*) in six conscious dogs. Each point is expressed as percentage of mean O_2 consumption (6.19 ± 0.65 ml $O_2 \cdot min^{-1} \cdot kg^{-1}$) during the control period (first hour). Paradoxical decrease in O_2 consumption during hyperoxia was fully developed by 20 minutes, was maintained for at least 1 hour, and was both reversible and reproducible. The mean of each 1-hour period was statistically significantly different from the mean of its adjacent 1-hour periods. (*Reproduced, with permission, from Lodato.[104]*)**

(by tonometry, used as a marker of the adequacy of gastric O_2 supply).[146]

PULMONARY VERSUS SYSTEMIC CAUSE OF DEATH FROM HYPEROXIA

Death in experimental animals exposed to prolonged hyperoxia is usually attributable to ARDS-like acute lung injury.[156,157] Hypoxemia, however, is generally absent. Matalon et al[157] found in sheep a terminal severe acute respiratory acidosis but supranormal $Pa_{O_2} = 200$ torr at death. Harabin et al[158] provided intriguing evidence that *systemic*, rather than pulmonary, O_2 toxicity may be the predominant cause of death. Dogs exposed continuously to 100% O_2 lived for a mean of 88 hours (3.7 days), but surprisingly, they maintained Pa_{O_2} at about 500 torr until shortly before death. Their brief preterminal course was characterized by a precipitous decrease in cardiac output and blood pressure accompanied by metabolic acidosis, all of which preceded the terminal deterioration in gas exchange. In fact, the acidosis (presumably lactic as seen terminally in hyperoxemic rabbits[159]) occurred in the face of supranormal Pa_{O_2} of 200–400 torr, indicating a systemic, or cardiovascular, rather than a pulmonary (hypoxemic) mechanism of their terminal deterioration.[158] Thus, these animals

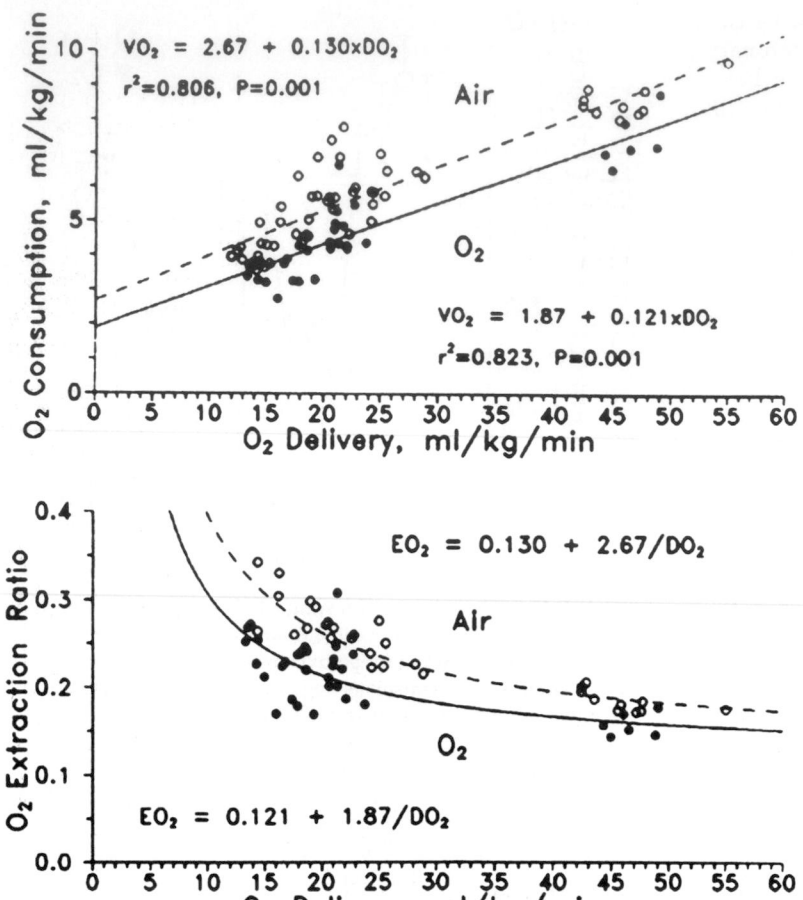

FIGURE 45-9 *Upper panel:* Relationship between O_2 consumption and O_2 delivery in 6 healthy resting conscious dogs for air (*open circles*) versus O_2 breathing (normobaric hyperoxia; *closed circles*). Each dog is represented by 10 independent determinations during air breathing and by 6 independent determinations during hyperoxia. Hyperoxia produced a unique parallel shift downward in the O_2 consumption–O_2 delivery relationship (see text). *Lower panel:* Oxygen extraction ratios corresponding to the data points in upper panel. (*Reproduced, with permission, from Lodato.[117]*)

died clearly *with* lung injury but not so clearly *from* lung injury.

Further evidence of primary cardiovascular O_2 toxicity has been provided by Busing et al[160] (and others[9]), who described disseminated microscopic foci of myocardial necrosis (Fig. 45-10), especially in the subendocardium of the left ventricle, occurring in rabbits subjected to 60 hours (2.5 days) of 100% O_2. Hypoxemia from hyperoxic lung injury was excluded as the mechanism because the cardiac necrosis developed while the Pa_{O_2} was 300–400 torr, and, in fact, it preceded any morphologic pulmonary changes. Fracica et al[81,161] reported that baboons exposed to 100% O_2 for >80 hours (>3.3 days) had substantial deterioration in cardiac function without significant deterioration in oxygenation (mean Pa_{O_2} = 437 torr). These animals also showed focal areas of myocardial necrosis.[161] Robinson et al[162] studied several species of primates exposed to 100% O_2 for up to 14 days. Pa_{O_2} remained high (400–500 torr) until near death when it fell sharply and Pa_{CO_2} rose. The baboons did, however, have other clinical (increased respiratory effort) and pathologic evidence of severe lung injury. In contrast, the squirrel monkeys were surprisingly insensitive to pulmonary O_2 toxicity. They too died from the hyperoxic environment but of undetermined cause. Cardiac histopathologic examination was not reported.

Thus, it appears that experimental animals exposed to hyperoxia die primarily from systemic rather than pulmonary O_2 toxicity.

Mechanisms of Oxygen Toxicity

FORMATION OF REACTIVE OXYGEN SPECIES

It is now generally accepted that the toxic effects of hyperoxia are the direct result of increased concentrations of highly reactive O_2-derived free radicals.[17,163–167] This extensive topic is now the subject of two recent monographs.[168,169] The "O_2 radical hypothesis" was first proposed in 1954 by Gerschman et al,[170] who suggested that hyperoxia-induced tissue injury and x-irradiation–induced tissue injury have as a common mechanism the production of reactive O_2 species in excess of the antioxidant defenses. Gerschman[171] pointed out that O_2 at 20% is potentially toxic and that its gradual accumulation in the atmosphere induced the evolution of cellular-defense mechanisms.

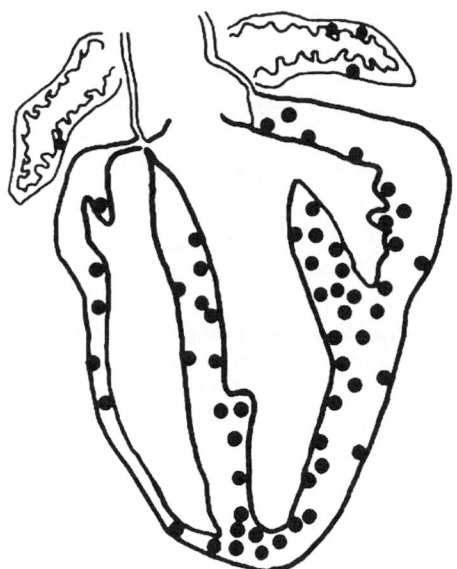

FIGURE 45-10 Distribution of disseminated microscopic foci of myocardial necrosis seen in rabbits exposed to 100% O_2 (normobaric hyperoxia) for >60 hours, as illustrated by a schematic longitudinal section through all chambers of the heart. All four chambers were affected, but the subendocardium of the left ventricle, including the papillary muscle and the septum, were the most vulnerable. The arterial O_2 tension was consistently >300 torr, indicating that hypoxemia (from possible hyperoxic lung injury) was not the mechanism of the necrotizing cardiomyopathy. (*Reproduced, with permission, from Busing et al.*[160])

The basic chemistry of reactive O_2 species has been recently extensively reviewed.[172–176] Molecular O_2 itself is generally nontoxic and only modestly reactive. However, when it is chemically reduced by the sequential addition of electrons (e^-), it forms partially reduced reactive O_2 species (ROS), as follows:

$$O_2 \xrightarrow{e^-} O_2^- \xrightarrow{e^- + 2H} H_2O_2 \xrightarrow{e^- + H} OH \cdot \xrightarrow{e^- + H} H_2O$$

where O_2^- is superoxide anion radical, H_2O_2 is hydrogen peroxide, and $OH \cdot$ is the hydroxyl radical. Superoxide is only modestly reactive. It can, however, yield the very highly reactive hydroxyl radical. Alternatively, superoxide can react with nitric oxide, $NO\cdot$, also a free radical, forming the very highly reactive peroxynitrite anion, $ONOO^-$. Of the ROS, the hydroxyl radical is by far the most reactive, reacting with all known biomolecules so rapidly that it acts only locally where it is produced.[173] In contrast, O_2^- and H_2O_2 can travel some distance and enter cells, H_2O_2 by simple diffusion across the cell membrane and O_2^- via anion channels.[175,177] The high reactivities of ROS and reactive nitrogen species (RNS) such as NO and peroxynitrite are the result of their very high affinity for additional electrons. This extreme electron affinity causes these agents to rapidly pull an electron from the nearest available molecule, resulting in oxidative damage to nearby lipids, proteins, and DNA.

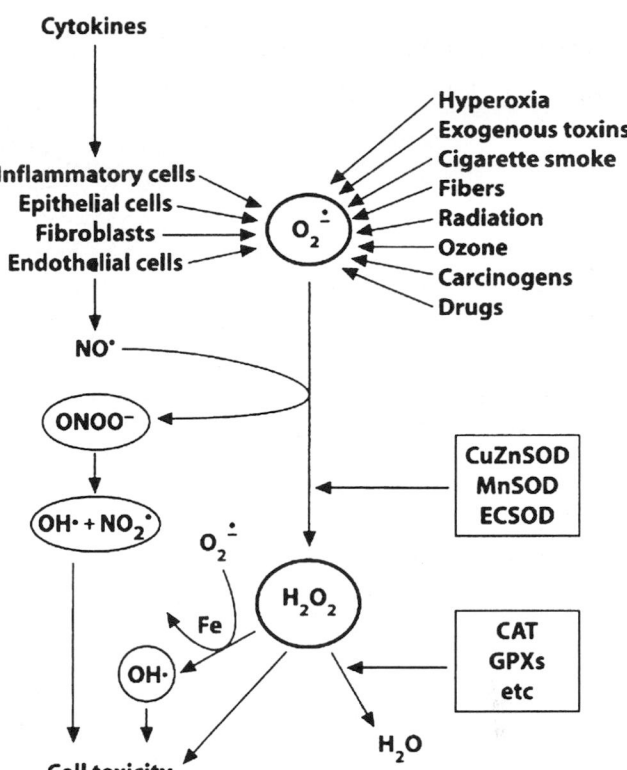

FIGURE 45-11 Sources of reactive oxygen species (ROS) and reactive nitrogen species (RNS) in the lung. Both inflammation (*upper left*) and exogenous toxins (*upper right*), including hyperoxia, produce superoxide (O_2^-), which can react with nitric oxide (NO) to produce peroxynitrite ($ONOO^-$) and other toxic RNS and ROS. Or, superoxide may be metabolized to hydrogen peroxide (H_2O_2), which may yield water (H_2O) or the toxic hydroxyl radical ($OH\cdot$). See text for details. CAT, catalase; GPx, glutathione peroxidase; SOD, superoxide dismutase. (*Reproduced, with permission, from Kinnula et al.*[172])

This oxidant damage is manifested by lipid peroxidation, enzyme inhibition, and DNA strand breakage, which can lead ultimately to loss of cell integrity and cell death.

The sources of ROS are many (Fig. 45-11). In the normal processes of cellular metabolism, ROS are produced at basal rates. Superoxide radical can be generated by both enzymatic and nonenzymatic (auto-oxidation) reactions. The major source of ROS in the lung is the mitochondrial electron-transport chain, during the production of ATP via oxidative phosphorylation.[176] The fate of nearly all O_2 taken up by the body is 4-electron catalytic reduction by mitochondrial cytochrome c oxidase to form water. Normally, a tiny fraction (0.1–2%[175,178]) of the electron flow along this chain "leaks" off upstream of cytochrome oxidase, principally at NADH dehydrogenase and ubiquinone (Fig. 45-12), and partially reduces O_2 to yield O_2^-.[164,179] Other sources of intracellular superoxide and hydrogen peroxide exist.[180]

Under pathologic conditions, such as hyperoxia or inflammation, which may itself result from hyperoxic injury or from invading microorganisms, or other exogenous toxins (ozone, cigarette smoke, fibrogenic material, ionizing

MITOCHONDRIAL ELECTRON TRANSPORT

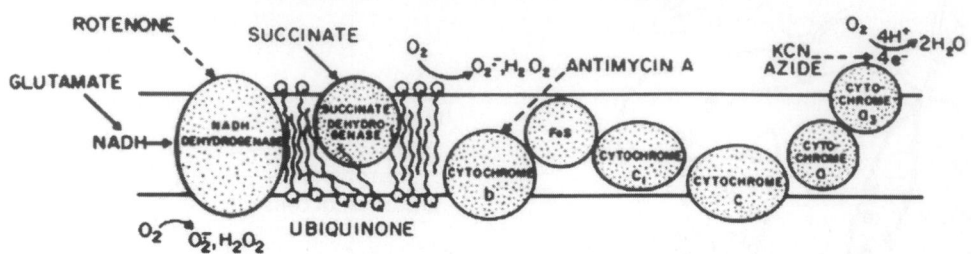

FIGURE 45-12 Generation of reactive oxygen species (ROS) in the mitochondria. The major source of mitochondrial ROS is the electron transport chain located on the inner mitochondrial membrane. Ubiquinone is reduced in a one-electron transfer to form the ubisemiquinone radical, which is reoxidized by molecular oxygen (auto-oxidation) to form the superoxide radical (O_2^-); this reaction is the major source of mitochondrial superoxide radical, which serves as a precursor to hydrogen peroxide (H_2O_2) and the hydroxyl radical (OH·), as shown. The auto-oxidation of the reduced form of NADH dehydrogenase (a member of the class of flavoproteins) by molecular O_2 is an additional but quantitatively less important source of mitochondrial superoxide radical and thus, hydrogen peroxide and the hydroxyl radical. Also shown are various electron transport inhibitors (*dashed arrows*) used to study mitochondrial sources of superoxide radical. (*Reproduced, with permission, from Freeman et al.[166]*)

radiation, paraquat, or cytotoxic drugs), the production of both ROS and RNS is increased (see Fig. 45-11).[165,172–176] One-hundred percent O_2 results in a 10- to 15-fold increase in mitochondrial H_2O_2 production.[181,182]

Inflammation results in increased production of ROS and RNS by release of proinflammatory chemokines and cytokines, which recruit neutrophils and other inflammatory cells (see Fig. 45-11). These proinflammatory stimuli also activate the membrane-bound NADPH-oxidase complex, which generates large amounts of superoxide,[175] manifested as the "respiratory burst" of neutrophils and macrophages (Fig. 45-13). Inflammation also upregulates inducible nitric oxide synthase (NOS), which produces great quantities of NO from L-arginine.[183] Thus, as above, su-

peroxide and NO may react to yield the very highly reactive peroxynitrite anion, ONOO⁻, which may be the most important species responsible for the incapacitation of microorganisms.[173] Inducible NOS can also generate superoxide.[184] An additional enzymatic pathway to increased ROS and RNS, particularly following ischemia, is via xanthine dehydrogenase.[175]

Superoxide radical, produced by any of the several pathways above, is converted to hydrogen peroxide by both spontaneous and enzymatic dismutation. Hydrogen peroxide, in turn, can be further reduced by transition metals to generate the hydroxyl radical. The metal ion–dependent formation of OH· from H_2O_2 is accelerated by O_2^- according to the metal-catalyzed Haber-Weiss reaction, which is referred

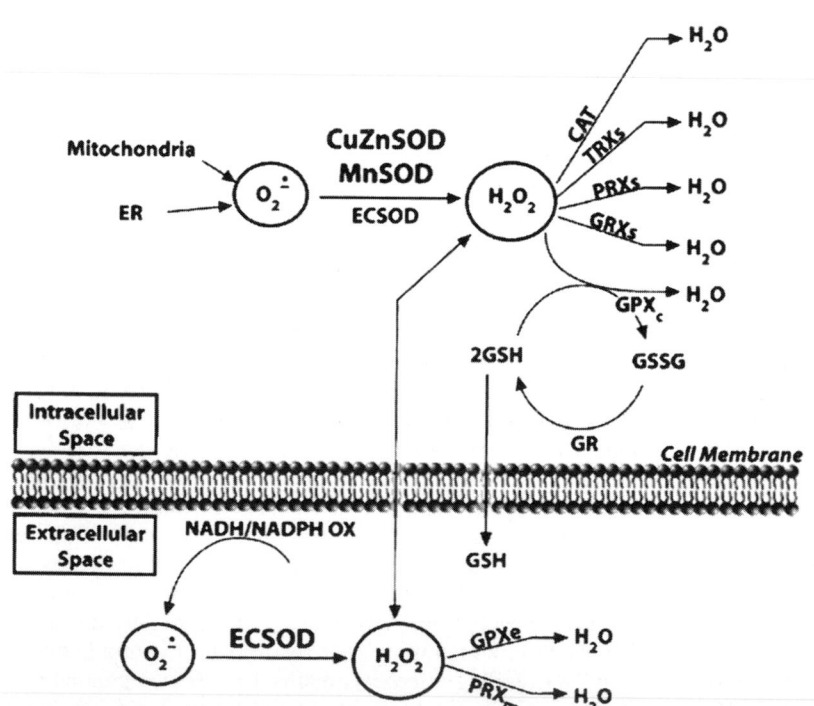

FIGURE 45-13 Major antioxidant pathways in the lung, intracellular and extracellular, scavenging superoxide (O_2^-) and hydrogen peroxide (H_2O_2). See text for details. CAT, catalase; ER, endoplasmic reticulum; GPXc, intracellular glutathione peroxidase; GPXe, extracellular glutathione peroxidase; GR, glutathione reductase; GRXs, glutaredoxins; GSH, reduced glutathione; GSSG, oxidized glutathione; PRXs, peroxiredoxins; SOD, superoxide dismutase; TRXs, thioredoxins. (*Reproduced, with permission, from Kinnula et al.[172]*)

to as the Fenton reaction if the metal is iron:[185]

$$O_2^- + Fe^{3+} \longrightarrow O_2 + Fe^{2+}$$

$$H_2O_2 + Fe^{2+} \longrightarrow OH^{\cdot} + OH^- + Fe^{3+}$$

ANTIOXIDANT DEFENSE MECHANISMS

Four antioxidant defense mechanisms exist in the cell:[186] (1) prevention of the formation of free radicals, (2) conversion of ROS to less toxic species, (3) compartmentalization of ROS away from vital cellular structures (e.g., the binding of intracellular iron to ferritin to prevent its participation in the Haber-Weiss reaction), and (4) repair of molecular injury induced by ROS.

The primary cellular defense against ROS are enzymes that catalyze the removal of superoxide and hydrogen peroxide, namely, superoxide dismutase (SOD), catalase, and the enzymes of the glutathione redox cycle (see Fig. 45-13).[172,186] No enzyme scavenging system exists for the hydroxyl radical.[175] Superoxide radical is converted by dismutation to hydrogen peroxide by SOD:

$$2O_2^- + 2H^+ \xrightarrow{\text{superoxide dismutase}} H_2O_2 + O_2$$

The lung contains three forms of SOD. These have been recently reviewed in detail.[172,174] The cytosolic form of SOD contains copper and zinc (CuZnSOD). The mitochondrial form contains manganese (MnSOD). An extracellular form (ECSOD) is concentrated in airway and vessel walls.[187]

Hydrogen peroxide is converted to water by the enzymes catalase (a hemoprotein) and glutathione peroxidase:[173]

$$2H_2O_2 \xrightarrow{\text{catalase}} 2H_2O + O_2$$

Glutathione peroxidase is a selenium-dependent enzyme that inactivates both hydrogen peroxide and lipid peroxides. It is the key enzyme in the glutathione redox cycle (Fig. 45-14),[186] and requires the sulfhydryl-containing tripeptide glutathione (GSH; L-gamma-glutamyl-L-cysteinyl-glycine) as a cosubstrate. The enzyme catalyzes the reaction that forms oxidized glutathione,[188] or glutathione disulfide (GSSG), according to,

$$H_2O_2 + 2GSH \xrightarrow{\text{glutathione peroxidase}} GSSG + 2H_2O$$

or, in the case of lipid hydroperoxides,[186]

$$L\text{-OOH} + 2GSH \xrightarrow{\text{glutathione peroxidase}} GSSG + L\text{-OH} + H_2O$$

GSSG is rapidly reduced back to GSH by the NADPH-dependent enzyme glutathione reductase. NADPH is in turn restored from NADP$^+$ by the hexose monophosphate shunt[188] (see Fig. 45-12). The glutathione redox cycle is apparently more important than catalase in reducing and eliminating intracellular H_2O_2.[186]

Within the cell are several other antioxidants.[172,174] These include water-soluble cytoplasmic antioxidants (e.g, ascorbate [vitamin C]), and fat-soluble membrane-associated antioxidants (e.g., alpha-tocopherol [vitamin E]), beta-carotene, and ubiquinol. Vitamin E, one of the most important of the nonenzymatic antioxidants, partitions into and protects lipid membranes.[186] Vitamin E is particularly effective against O_2^- and OH$^{\cdot}$, and blocks propagation of lipid peroxidation by scavenging peroxy free radicals.[174]

The human lung has recently been shown to express several other enzymes capable of inactivating H_2O_2.[172] These include the thioredoxin–thioredoxin reductase system, thioredoxin peroxidases (peroxiredoxins), and glutaredoxins.[189–191]

Other nonenzymatic antioxidants include glutathione, surfactant protein D, albumin, and proteins that bind iron and copper (powerful promoters of oxidative damage) such as transferrin, ferritin, ceruloplasmin, and lactoferrin.[172] Others include urate and bilirubin.[176]

Diagnosis and Management of Pulmonary Oxygen Toxicity

DIAGNOSIS

At present, there is no clinically useful means of diagnosing pulmonary O_2 toxicity in patients. Such a diagnostic capability would be most useful in ARDS. Physiologic indexes of pulmonary function (e.g., decrements in vital capacity), require patient cooperation and specialized equipment. But their greatest limitation is that in patients with ARDS such tests cannot distinguish between progressive O_2 toxicity and progression of the underlying cardiopulmonary condition. Chest radiographs also share this diagnostic limitation. Indexes of the lung's ability to metabolize biogenic amines (e.g., serotonin), polypeptides (e.g., by angiotensin-converting enzyme), and prostaglandins have been shown to be sensitive in experimental animals but their use in critically ill patients is limited by their lack of specificity, dependence on capillary surface area and transit time, and the production by the injured lung of related compounds.[22] The pathology of pulmonary O_2 toxicity, diffuse alveolar damage, is a nonspecific (albeit clearly identifiable) pattern seen in ARDS from any cause. The sophisticated study by Montgomery et al,[74] which examined solute permeability of the lung, indexes of systemic toxicity, and pulmonary function, demonstrated that there is no better index of O_2 toxicity than the individual's subjective symptoms of retrosternal pain suggestive of acute tracheobronchitis. Studies such as theirs suggest that critical care physicians should maintain a heightened awareness and seek out such symptoms in patients on high levels of O_2 and include the possibility of pulmonary O_2 toxicity in the differential diagnosis of chest pain in such patients.

EXOGENOUS ANTIOXIDANT THERAPY FOR THE LUNG

The many approaches that have been taken in efforts to increase pulmonary antioxidant capacity have been recently

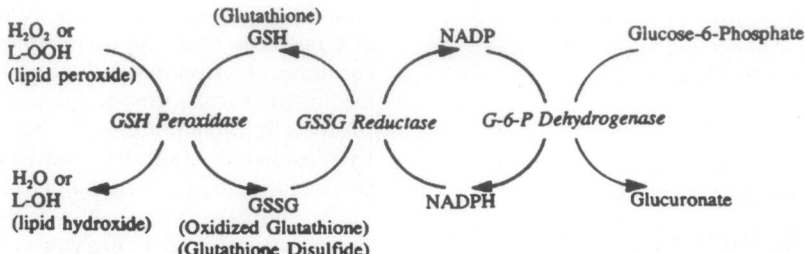

FIGURE 45-14 The glutathione (GSH) redox cycle and its pivotal role in the reduction of toxic intracellular hydroperoxides, including hydrogen peroxide and lipid peroxides. The key enzyme in the GSH redox cycle is GSH peroxidase, a predominantly cytosolic enzyme that requires reduced GSH as a substrate. Regeneration of reduced GSH by GSSG reductase, which is tightly bound to GSH peroxidase, requires NADPH, which is supplied by glucose-6-phosphate (G6P) dehydrogenase in the hexose monophosphate shunt.

reviewed.[174–176,192] The major antioxidant strategies that have been evaluated for the lung include: (1) exogenous administration of normal intracellular enzymatic antioxidants, such as SOD, catalase, and GSH; (2) administration of synthetic antioxidant mimetics; (3) pharmacologic inhibition of free radical–generating systems, such as by the iron chelator deferoxamine; (4) supplementation with nonenzyme antioxidants, such as vitamin E, N-acetylcysteine, or dietary supplementation with polyunsaturated fatty acid; and (5) agents to prevent the neutrophil-mediated amplification of the hyperoxic injury. All these approaches have been tried in vitro or in animal models, but only a few have been tried in human patients.

In transgenic mice the overexpression of either CuZnSOD or MnSOD alone was not sufficient to prevent hyperoxic lung injury,[193] but overexpressing ECSOD increased tolerance to hyperoxia.[194,195] In adult baboons exposed to 96 hours of 100% O_2, aerosolized recombinant human (rh) MnSOD improved oxygenation and alveolar epithelial histology, and decreased lung edema.[196,197] Because in these latter reports the MnSOD was found extracellularly, Asikainen et al[176] speculated that the beneficial effect of rhMnSOD may have been scavenging ROS generated by activated inflammatory cells. In premature human infants, intratracheal rhCuZnSOD did not change the 28-day mortality or the incidence of bronchopulmonary dysplasia.[198,199] Among the surviving infants, however, those who had been treated with rhCuZnSOD had less frequent acute respiratory events (asthma medication requirements, emergency department visits, and hospitalizations) over the first year of life.[199]

Synthetic SOD-mimetic (catalytic) antioxidants appear promising,[174,176] particularly the metalloporphyrins. They are highly active, stable, potentially nontoxic, and protect against ROS-mediated lung injury in experimental models.[176] They scavenge superoxide, hydrogen peroxide, and peroxynitrite, and inhibit lipid peroxidation.[200] In a fetal baboon model of bronchopulmonary dysplasia, the catalytic antioxidant metalloporphyrin AEOL 10113, given by continuous intravenous infusion, improved histology and proinflammatory mediators, but not oxygenation.[103]

A number of studies have been carried out in an effort to enhance the GSH-dependent antioxidant capacity of the lung. N-acetylcysteine readily crosses into cells and, by undergoing deacetylation, forms cysteine, the rate-limiting amino acid in GSH biosynthesis. N-acetylcysteine acts both by directly reducing O_2^-, H_2O_2, OH^-, and HOCl (hypochlorous acid), and by supporting GSH synthesis.[201] Its clinical use is well established in the treatment of acetaminophen-induced hepatotoxicity.[202] In animal studies[203–208] N-acetylcysteine protects against oxidant lung injury. In human studies, however, disappointingly, a half dozen clinical trials of N-acetylcysteine in critically ill patients with acute lung injury, ARDS, or multiple organ failure have failed to show benefit in survival or oxygenation.[209–213] In 1998 a clinical trial with procysteine in patients with acute lung injury or ARDS was stopped for lack of efficacy.[214] In very-low-birth weight infants, supplementation of selenium (required for glutathione peroxidase) also failed to improve outcome.[215]

Clinical trials of vitamin E supplementation failed to prevent bronchopulmonary dysplasia in premature newborns[216] or hyperoxic lung injury in neonates.[217] In contrast, vitamin A supplementation slightly decreased the incidence of bronchopulmonary dysplasia in extremely-low-birth weight infants.[218] In adult critically ill surgical patients, the combination of vitamins E and C reduced the incidence of organ failure and length of stay in the intensive care unit.[219]

Newborn rats have increased survival during hyperoxic challenge after dietary supplementation with polyunsaturated fatty acid (PUFA), including n-6 PUFA (linoleic and arachidonic acid, from safflower oil),[220] n-3 PUFA (eicosapentaenoic and docosahexaenoic acid, from fish oil),[221] or enteral Intralipid (commercial combination n-6 and n-3 PUFA, from soybean oil).[222] In ARDS, the combination of vitamins E and C plus fish oil (eicosapentaenoic acid) and borage oil (gamma-linolenic acid) improved pulmonary neutrophil recruitment, gas exchange, requirement for mechanical ventilation, length of ICU stay, and number of new organ failures.[223] A retrospective analysis of a subset of only 43 of these patients[224] reported that the 21 treated patients had decreased levels of interleukin-8, leukotriene B_4, and neutrophils in bronchoalveolar lavage fluid and decreased alveolar capillary membrane permeability.

In premature baboons, use of the iron chelator deferoxamine to prevent hyperoxic lung injury (by inhibiting iron-catalyzed ROS generation) resulted in rapid cardiovascular collapse and death (<42 hours) in all animals.[225]

Another approach to lung protection from hyperoxic injury is to block neutrophil accumulation in the lung and thereby block further amplification and propagation of ROS-mediated injury.[174] Such blockade can be achieved by antibodies directed against cytokine-induced neutrophil chemoattractant-1 (CINC-1), which is the major rat neutrophil chemoattractant cytokine, or chemokine.[226] This antibody, given intraperitoneally in a newborn-rat model of bronchopulmonary dysplasia, prevented neutrophil influx and preserved lung compliance, alveolar development, and lung cell proliferation.[226] Neutrophil influx can also be prevented by blocking the receptor, CXCR2, through which the chemokines act. In the same rat model Auten et al[227] showed that a competitive antagonist (SB-265610, a nonpeptide) of this chemokine receptor also prevented hyperoxia-induced neutrophil accumulation. Recent studies have also shown that other chemokines, including interleukin-8 and monocyte chemoattractant protein-1, play important roles in neutrophil attraction to the lung[174,228] and are potential therapeutic targets. Mercer et al[174] have pointed out that the neutrophil-blocking approach and the ECSOD-enhancement approach appear mutually complementary. That is, ECSOD enhancement protects against direct oxidant injury and neutrophil blockade prevents injury in areas not well protected by the enhanced ECSOD.

Several other experimental approaches have been investigated and reviewed in detail by Asikainen et al[176] These include catalytic antibodies, lazaroids, and novel approaches involving transcription factors, signaling pathways, DNA repair mechanisms, and growth factors. Despite their promise, none has yet been investigated in humans.

INDUCTION OF TOLERANCE TO HYPEROXIA

In 1978, Frank et al[229] made the fortuitous discovery that endotoxin fully protected rats from hyperoxic morbidity and mortality. Similar results had been reported earlier following other toxic insults to the lung, including oleic acid,[230] alpha naphthylthiourea,[231] and diphosgene,[72] all of which were reported to increase survival on subsequent exposure to hyperoxia. Frank et al[229] also showed that endotoxin induced lung SOD, catalase, and glutathione peroxidase. They speculated that in patients with acute respiratory failure ("for example . . . hyaline membrane disease", or infant respiratory distress syndrome), coincident gram-negative infection may modulate the toxic effects of therapeutic hyperoxia.[229]

In animals, other challenges that are protective against the lethality of subsequent exposure to hyperoxia include: sublethal hyperoxia,[232,233] hypoxia (in the absence of hypercarbia),[234,235] and the combination of tumor necrosis factor-α plus interleukin-1.[236] Tumor necrosis factor and interleukin-1 are proinflammatory cytokines that mediate much of the pathophysiology of endotoxin.[183,237,238] In rats, the protective effects of each of these pretreatments can be explained by the induction of SOD, catalase, and glutathione peroxidase.[229,232,235,239] The protective effect, however, may also occur in the absence of antioxidant enzyme induction. In the study by White et al,[239] the induction of the antioxidant enzymes induced by pretreatment with tumor necrosis factor plus interleukin-1, occurred relatively late (after 72 hours), after all control rats had already died. These authors suggested that the mechanisms of the lung protection may include, in addition to enzyme induction, the recruitment to the lung of more resistant cell lines.[239] Baker et al[233] showed that the protective effect of preexposure to sublethal hyperoxia in adult rabbits, unlike that in neonatal rabbits[240] and rats, is not accompanied by an increase in antioxidant enzymes; it may be explained, instead, by the observed increase in endogenous surfactant induced by the preexposure to hyperoxia.[233]

The clinical relevance of these observations is obvious. Critically ill patients with acute respiratory failure are commonly exposed to such "pretreatments," namely, hyperoxia, hypoxia, endotoxin, tumor necrosis factor, and interleukin-1. Additionally, as part of routine nutritional support, these patients commonly receive supplementation with polyunsaturated fatty acid (e.g., Intralipid), as discussed above.

EXOGENOUS SURFACTANT ADMINISTRATION

Surfactant is discussed in detail in Chapter 60 of the present text and has been recently reviewed elsewhere.[241,242] Endogenous surfactant is a complex mixture of about 85–90% phospholipids, 7–10% apoproteins (surfactant proteins A, B, C, and D), and 4–7% neutral lipids.[241] Its primary function is to reduce the otherwise high liquid-gas surface tension within the alveoli and thereby decrease their tendency to collapse. Hyperoxia impairs surfactant function.[243] Both ROS and RNS degrade surfactant, particularly the surfactant proteins, but the damage from RNS, especially peroxynitrite, appears more important.[241] In most species, despite its impairment of surfactant function, hyperoxia also induces surfactant synthesis.[233,244,245] Endogenous surfactant has intrinsic antioxidant activity,[246,247] can enhance intracellular antioxidant enzyme content,[246] and in animal models, protects from hyperoxic lung injury and death.[59,246,248]

Exogenous surfactants vary significantly in their composition.[242] They also have antioxidant activity[249] and in animal models, protect against hyperoxic lung injury and death.[249–252] After administration of exogenous surfactant (Curosurf), human preterm infants with respiratory distress syndrome show enhanced SOD and catalase activity in their tracheobronchial secretions.[253]

Exogenous surfactant therapy is now standard in neonatal intensive care units.[242] A number of clinical trials in young patients have reported beneficial outcomes: in newborns with respiratory distress syndrome,[254–256] in infants with acute respiratory failure due to respiratory syncytial virus,[257] and in children with hypoxemic acute respiratory failure.[258] In contrast, in adult patients with ARDS, the results have been disappointing.[242] The largest clinical trial to date using surfactant (Exosurf) found no benefit in adult patients with sepsis-induced ARDS.[259,260] The failure of this trial may be related in part to differences in both the surfactant constitutions and the delivery systems, between the neonatal-pediatric trials and the adult trials.[242]

MINIMIZATION OF OXYGEN TXOICITY IN THE INTENSIVE CARE UNIT

Ironically, in several ways the disease process of ARDS itself would seem to provide some degree of protection against hyperoxic injury. First, the alveolar epithelial and endothelial cells in the areas of shunt (presumably the areas of greatest injury) have, by definition, relatively low values of P_{O_2}, similar to the P_{O_2} of the mixed venous blood, and thus are not directly exposed to hyperoxia. Second, in ARDS the systemic circulation is also protected from hyperoxia because, by definition, this syndrome is characterized by systemic arterial hypoxemia. Third, the pathophysiology of ARDS and its management include exposure to hyperoxia, hypoxia, tumor necrosis factor,[261] and interleukin-1,[261,262] and commonly endotoxin.[261,262] As discussed above, however, prior exposure to each of these agents has been shown in animals to induce tolerance and protection against future exposure to hyperoxia. Thus, patients who survive the initial insult of ARDS may be better able to withstand ongoing hyperoxic exposure. Fourth, the intra-alveolar hemorrhage and exudation of plasma that is characteristic of ARDS (see discussion of pathology, above) provides erythrocytes rich in antioxidant enzyme capacity, as noted above, and plasma proteins with substantial antioxidant activities. In fact, bronchoalveolar lavage fluid from ARDS patients has been shown to possess greater antioxidant activity than lavage fluid from normal subjects, secondary largely to the plasma proteins transferrin and ceruloplasmin.[263]

Once the possibility of pulmonary O_2 toxicity is considered (generally in a patient with ARDS requiring $F_{I_{O_2}} \geq 0.60$ for >24–48 hours), the only accepted treatment clinically at present is to reduce the $F_{I_{O_2}}$ to the lowest level consistent with adequate systemic oxygenation. This goal should be approached by first minimizing excess O_2 demand (e.g., secondary to fever, infection, or "fighting the ventilator") while optimizing all other determinants of systemic oxygenation, such as hemoglobin concentration and overall respiratory and cardiovascular status.[264] As discussed in detail elsewhere in this text, the best principles and practice of mechanical ventilation should be applied. These would include: optimizing positive end-expiratory pressure (PEEP), consideration of alternative modes of ventilation (e.g., high-frequency ventilation), prone positioning, inhaled nitric oxide, extracorporeal membrane oxygenation, and so on. Complicating conditions interfering with oxygenation should be meticulously sought out and treated. These conditions may include superimposed nosocomial pneumonia, excessive secretions, bronchospasm, occult pneumothorax and other parenchymal ventilatory-induced lung injury, inadvertent intubation of a mainstem bronchus, large pleural effusions, hydrostatic-pressure pulmonary edema (elevated pulmonary arterial wedge pressure), cardiopulmonary shunts unrelated to parenchymal lung injury (e.g., patent foramen ovale[265]), pulmonary emboli, low cardiac output, and cor pulmonale. Inotropic agents (e.g., dobutamine) should be considered as a possible means of decreasing the pulmonary arterial wedge pressure (and thus the hydrostatic gradient for pulmonary edema formation) while maintaining or increasing cardiac output.

After these concerns have been adequately addressed, the $F_{I_{O_2}}$ should be adjusted to the lowest value required to maintain the arterial saturation within an acceptable range (e.g., 88–95%[1]). (Mountain climbers tolerate $Pa_{O_2} = 28$ torr[266] and $Sa_{O_2} = 62\%$ at exercise.[267]) Although the treatment of ARDS is largely supportive, treatment should, of course, be given for the underlying disease that may have produced the ARDS, particularly if it is infection.

In especially difficult patients with ARDS and refractory hypoxemia requiring sustained high levels of inspired O_2, the clinician may be faced with the very difficult task of choosing among: (1) accepting a lower level of arterial oxygenation, (2) increasing the already high airway pressures and risking ventilator-induced lung injury, or (3) continuing or even increasing the already high $F_{I_{O_2}}$. In these very difficult cases it seems prudent to keep in mind that, based on information to date, the known immediate risks of systemic hypoxia or ventilator-induced lung injury are clearly more established and devastating than the potential future risk of hyperoxia-induced lung injury.

Important Unknowns and the Future

The most important unknown is the optimum inspired O_2 fraction to use in ARDS. Remarkably, the answer is still unknown nearly four decades after ARDS was defined.[268] Other unknowns concern the relationship between O_2 toxicity and ventilator-induced lung injury. They have in common that both are a concern in acute respiratory failure, both share mechanisms of injury, both initiate their injury in the lung, but both may cause death from systemic multiorgan organ failure more than from their pulmonary injury. Future work should resolve their relative importance in acute lung injury: Are they independent or synergistic forces? Will therapy for one also be therapeutic for the other? Future research should resolve how optimally to trade off the risks of hypoxemia, ventilator-induced lung injury, and O_2 toxicity. This tradeoff will be facilitated when more specific markers of O_2 toxicity become available. The degree to which patients with ARDS have induction of tolerance to hyperoxia (by preexisting hyperoxia, hypoxia, endotoxin, and cytokines) is unknown. This induction could be manipulated to optimize a patient's antioxidant defenses. The potential benefit of combining two or more complementary therapies (e.g., neutrophil blocking plus ECSOD enhancement[174]) are yet to be explored. Novel therapies, like activated protein C, which has been successful in severe sepsis,[269] give hope that similar results can be achieved in ARDS and O_2 toxicity. Other proposed novel approaches involve transcription factors, signaling pathways, DNA repair mechanisms, and growth factors.[176]

Summary and Conclusion

More than two centuries after his discovery of O_2, Priestley seems remarkably prescient regarding its medical and toxic potential. O_2 is now recognized as life saving in patient conditions ranging from ambulatory to critically ill. The enormous expansion of knowledge about its biochemistry, physiology, and toxicology has relevance throughout all of biology. Continuing growth in our understanding of this "vital air" of Lavoisier is vital to continuing improvement in the care and safety of patients.

References

1. The Acute Respiratory Distress Syndrome Network. Ventilation with lower tidal volumes as compared with traditional tidal volumes for acute lung injury and the acute respiratory distress syndrome. The Acute Respiratory Distress Syndrome Network. N Engl J Med 2000; 342:1301–8.

2. Lavoisier A. On the burning of phosphorus and the formation of its acid, 1775. In: Comroe JH, editor. Pulmonary and respiratory physiology, Part I. Stroudsburg, PA: Dowden, Hutchinson, & Ross, Inc., 1976.

3. Oxford Dictionary. The compact edition of the Oxford english dictionary, 1971:2047.

4. Haldane JBS. The origin of life: The rationalist annual, 1929.

5. Gilbert DL. Oxygen: Evolution and history. In: Gottlieb SF, Longmuir IS, Trotter JR, editors. Oxygen: An in-depth study of its pathophysiology. Bethesda, MD: The Twenty-Eighth Undersea Medical Society Workshop, 1984.

6. Priestley J. The discovery of oxygen, Part I, 1775. In: Alembic Club Reprints, no 7. Edinburgh: William F. Clay, 1894.

7. Gilbert DL. Oxygen: An overall biological view. In: Gilbert DL, editor. Oxygen and living processes. New York: Springer-Verlag, 1981: 376–92.

8. Cutler RG. Aging and oxygen radicals. In: Taylor AE, Matalon S, Ward P, editors. Physiology of oxygen radicals. Bethesda, MD: American Physiological Society, 1986: 251–86.

9. Balentine JD. Pathology of oxygen toxicity. New York: Academic Press, 1982.

10. Duveen DI. Lavoisier. In: Gingerich O, editor. Scientific genius and creativity readings from scientific american. New York: W.H. Freeman and Co., 1982: 35–9.

11. Lambertsen CJ. Effects of hyperoxia on organs and their tissues. In: Robin ED, editor. Extrapulmonary manifestations of respiratory disease. New York: Marcel Dekker, 1978: 239–303.

12. Fife CE, Piantadosi CA. Oxygen toxicity. Prob Respir Care 1991; 4:150–71.

13. Fagraeus L. Cardiorespiratory and metabolic functions during exercise in the hyperbaric environment. Acta Physiol Scand Suppl 1974; 414:1–40.

14. Schaefer KE. Hyperbaria-O_2 toxicity. In: Loeppky JA, Riedesel ML, editors. Oxygen transport to human tissues. New York: Elsevier North Holland, 1982: 291–304.

15. Comroe JH Jr, Dripps RD. The physiological basis for oxygen therapy. Springfield, IL: Charles C. Thomas, 1950.

16. Astrup P, Severinghaus JW. The history of blood gases, acids and bases. Copenhagen: Munksgaard, 1986.

17. Bryan CL, Jenkinson SG. Oxygen toxicity. Clin Chest Med 1988; 9:141–52.

18. Clark JM, Lambertsen CJ. Pulmonary oxygen toxicity: a review. Pharmacol Rev 1971; 23:37–133.

19. Clark JM. Oxygen toxicity. In: Bennet PB, Elliot DH, editors. The physiology and medicine of diving, 3rd ed. London: Bailliere Tindall, 1982: 200–38.

20. Duane P. Pulmonary insults due to transfusions, radiation, and hyperoxia. Semin Respir Infect 1988; 3:240–6.

21. Fisher AB. Oxygen therapy. Side effects and toxicity. Am Rev Respir Dis 1980; 122:61–9.

22. Jackson RM. Pulmonary oxygen toxicity. Chest 1985; 88:900–5.

23. Sackner MA. Oxygen therapy. A history of oxygen usage in chronic obstructive pulmonary disease. Am Rev Respir Dis 1974; 110:25–34.

24. Klein J. Normobaric pulmonary oxygen toxicity. Anesthesiol Analg 1990; 70:195–207.

25. Lodato RF. Oxygen toxicity. Crit Care Clin 1990; 6:749–65.

26. Winter PM, Smith G. The toxicity of oxygen. Anesthesiology 1972; 37:210–41.

27. Lahiri S. Physiological responses: Peripheral chemoreceptors and chemoreflexes. In: Crystal R, West JB, Barnes P, Weibel E, editors. The lung: Scientific foundations, 2nd ed. Philadelphia: Lippincott-Raven, 1997: 1747–56.

28. Lodato RF, Jubran A. Response time, autonomic mediation, and reversibility of hyperoxic bradycardia in conscious dogs. J Appl Physiol 1993; 74:634–42.

29. Karetzky MS, Keighley JF, Mithoefer JC. The effect of oxygen administration on gas exchange and cardiopulmonary function in normal subjects. Respir Physiol 1971; 12:361–70.

30. Stockley RA. The estimation of the resting reflex hypoxic drive to respiration in normal man. Respir Physiol 1977; 31:217– 30.

31. Christiansen J, Douglas C, Haldane J. The absorbtion and dissociation of carbon dioxide by human blood. J Physiol Lond 1914; 48:244–71.

32. Dautrebande L, Haldane JS. The effects of respiration of oxygen on breathing and circulation. J Physiol 1921; 55:296–9.

33. Yamada M. Methodische Untersuchungen uber das Haldane-Hendersonsche Verfahren der Bestimmung der alveolaren CO_2-Spannung und uber den Einfluss von Sauerstoff auf die Erregbarkeit des Atemzentrums. Biochemische Zeitschrift 1918; 89:27–47.

34. Becker H, Polo O, McNamara SG, Berthon-Jones M, Sullivan CE. Ventilatory response to isocapnic hyperoxia. J Appl Physiol 1995; 78:696–701.

35. Becker HF, Polo O, McNamara SG, Berthon-Jones M, Sullivan CE. Effect of different levels of hyperoxia on breathing in healthy subjects. J Appl Physiol 1996; 81:1683–90.

36. Rucker J, Tesler J, Fedorko L, et al. Normocapnia improves cerebral oxygen delivery during conventional oxygen therapy in carbon monoxide-exposed research subjects. Ann Emerg Med 2002; 40:611–8.

37. Stradling JR. Hypercapnia during oxygen therapy in airways obstruction: a reappraisal. Thorax 1986; 41:897–902.

38. Libby DM, Briscoe WA, King TKC. Relief of hypoxia-related bronchoconstriction by breathing 30 per cent oxygen. Am Rev Respir Dis 1981; 123:171–5.

39. Robinson TD, Freiberg DB, Regnis JA, Young IH. The role of hypoventilation and ventilation-perfusion redistribution in oxygen-induced hypercapnia during acute exacerbations of chronic obstructive pulmonary disease. Am J Respir Crit Care Med 2000; 161:1524–9.

40. Aubier M, Murciano D, Milic-Emili J, et al. Effects of the administration of O_2 on ventilation and blood gases in patients with chronic obstructive pulmonary disease during acute respiratory failure. Am Rev Respir Dis 1980; 122:747–54.

41. Gasparini S, Sanguinetti CM, De Luca S, Massei V. Interindividual variability of the response to oxygen administration in hypercapnic patients. Eur J Respir Dis 1986; 69(Suppl 146): 427–34.

42. Sassoon CSH, Hassell KT, Mahutte CK. Hyperoxic-induced hypercapnia in stable chronic obstructive pulmonary disease. Am Rev Respir Dis 1987; 135:907–11.

43. Dick CR, Liu Z, Sassoon CS, Berry RB, Mahutte CK. O_2-induced change in ventilation and ventilatory drive in COPD. Am J Respir Crit Care Med 1997; 155:609–14.

44. Wagner PD, Dantzker DR, Dueck R, Clausen JL, West JB. Ventilation-perfusion inequality in chronic obstructive pulmonary disease. J Clin Invest 1977; 59:203–16.

45. Dunn WF, Nelson SB, Hubmayr RD. Oxygen-induced hypercarbia in obstructive pulmonary disease. Am Rev Respir Dis 1991; 144:526–30.

46. Stradling J. Effects of the administration of O_2 on ventilation and blood gases in patients with chronic obstructive pulmonary disease during acute respiratory failure. Letter. Am Rev Respir Dis 1987; 135:274.

47. Aubier M, Murciano D, Milic-Emili J, et al. Effects of the administration of O_2 on ventilation and blood gases in patients with chronic obstructive pulmonary disease during acute respiratory failure. Letter. Am Rev Respir Dis 1987; 135:274.

48. Robinson T, Young I. Letter to the Editor: The role of hypoventilation and ventilation-perfusion redistribution in oxygen-induced hypercapnia during acute exacerbations of chronic obstructive pulmonary disease. Am J Respir Crit Care Med 2001; 163:1755.

49. Neff TA, Petty TL. Tolerance and survival in severe chronic hypercapnia. Arch Intern Med 1972; 129:591–6.

50. Campbell EJM. Respiratory failure, the relation between oxygen concentrations of inspired air and arterial blood. Lancet 1960; 2:10.

51. Campbell EJM. A method of controlled oxygen administration which reduces the risk of carbon-dioxide retention. Lancet 1960; 2:12.

52. Gay PC, Edmonds LC. Severe hypercapnia after low-flow oxygen therapy in patients with neuromuscular disease and diaphragmatic dysfunction. Mayo Clin Proc 1995; 70:327–30.

53. Molfino NA, Nannini LJ, Martelli AN, Slutsky AS. Respiratory arrest in near-fatal asthma. N Engl J Med 1991; 324:285–8.

54. McFadden ER Jr. Fatal and near-fatal asthma. Editorial. N Engl J Med 1991; 324:409–11.

55. Saugstad OD, Rootwelt T, Aalen O. Resuscitation of asphyxiated newborn infants with room air or oxygen: an international controlled trial: the Resair 2 study. Pediatrics 1998; 102:e1.

56. Saugstad OD. Resuscitation with room-air or oxygen supplementation. Clin Perinatol 1998; 25:741–56, xi.

57. Wagner PD, Laravuso RB, Uhl RR, West JB. Continuous distributions of ventilation-perfusion ratios in normal subjects breathing air and 100% O_2. J Clin Invest 1974; 54:54–68.

58. West JB, Wagner PD. Pulmonary gas exchange. In: West JB, editor. Bioengineering aspects of the lung. New York: Marcel Dekker, Inc, 1977: 361–457.

59. Matalon S, Baker RR, Engstrom PC. Mechanisms and modifications of hyperoxic injury to the mammalian pulmonary surfactant system. In: Reinhart K, Eyrich K, editors. Clinical aspects of O_2 transport and tissue oxygenation. New York: Springer-Verlag, 1989: 115–32.

60. Santos C, Ferrer M, Roca J, et al. Pulmonary gas exchange response to oxygen breathing in acute lung injury. Am J Respir Crit Care Med 2000; 161:26–31.

61. Comroe JH, Dripps RD, Dumke PR, Deming M. The effect of inhalation of high concentrations of oxygen for 24 hours on normal men at sea level and at a simulated altitude of 18,000. JAMA 1945; 128:710–7.

62. Burger EJ, Mead J. Static properties of lungs after oxygen exposure. J Appl Physiol 1969; 27:191–7.

63. Sackner MA, Landa J, Hirsch J, Zapata A. Pulmonary effects of oxygen breathing: A 6-hour study in normal men. Ann Intern Med 1975; 82:40–3.

64. Rothan-Tondeur M, Meaume S, Girard L, et al. Risk factors for nosocomial pneumonia in a geriatric hospital: a control-case one-center study. J Am Geriatr Soc 2003; 51:997–1001.

65. Baleeiro CE, Wilcoxen SE, Morris SB, Standiford TJ, Paine R 3rd. Sublethal hyperoxia impairs pulmonary innate immunity. J Immunol 2003; 171:955–63.

66. Beckett WS, Wong ND. Effect of normobaric hyperoxia on airways of normal subjects. J Appl Physiol 1988;64:1683–7.

67. Clark JM, Lambertsen CJ. Pulmonary oxygen tolerance and the rate of development of pulmonary oxygen toxicity in man at two atmospheres inspired oxygen tension. In: Lambertsen CJ, editor. Underwater Physiology Proceedings of the Third Symposium on Underwater Physiology. Baltimore: Williams & Wilkins, 1967: 439–51.

68. Helvey WM, Albright GA, Benjamin FB, et al. Effects of prolonged exposure to pure oxygen on human performance: Republic Aviation Corporation, Report 393-1, NASA Contr. NASr-92; 1962.

69. Michel EL, Langevin RW, Gell CF. Effect of continuous human exposure to oxygen tension of 418 mm Hg for 168 hours. Aerospace Med 1960; 31:138–44.

70. Fife WP, Edwards ML, Schroeder WW, Ferrari FD, Freeberg LR. Effect of the hydro-lab environment on pulmonary function. Hydro-Lab J 1973; 2:73–80.

71. Dougherty JJH, Frayre RL, Miller DA, Schaefer KE. Pulmonary function during shallow habitat air dives (Shad I, II, III). In: Schilling CW, Beckett MW, editors. Underwater Physiology VI: Proceedings of the Sixth Symposium on Underwater Physiology. Bethesda, MD: FASEB, 1978: 193–204.

72. Ohlsson WTL. A study on oxygen toxicity at atmospheric pressure. Acta Med Scand 1947; 128:1–93.

73. Griffith DE, Holden WE, Morris JF, Min LK, Krishnamurthy GT. Effect of common therapeutic concentrations of oxygen on lung clearance of ^{99m}Tc-DTPA and bronchoalveolar lavage albumin concentration. Am Rev Respir Dis 1986; 134:233–7.

74. Montgomery AB, Luce JM, Murray JF. Retrosternal pain is an early indicator of oxygen toxicity. Am Rev Respir Dis 1989; 139:1548–50.

75. Adams G, Williamson R, Harvey C, Murray R, Hester R. Shallow habitat air diving with excursions between 5 and 250 FSWG: a review of four simulated dives. In: Shilling CW, Beckett MW, editors. Underwater Physiology VI: Proceedings of the Sixth Symposium on Underwater Physiology. Bethesda: FASEB, 1978: 423–34.

76. Van de Water JM, Kagey KS, Miller IT, et al. Response of the lung to six to twelve hours of 100 per cent oxygen inhalation in normal man. N Engl J Med 1970; 283:621–6.

77. Davis WB, Rennard SI, Bitterman PB, Crystal RB. Pulmonary oxygen toxicity. Early reversible changes in human alveolar structures induced by hyperoxia. N Engl J Med 1983; 309: 878–83.

78. Becker-Freyseng H, Clamann HG. Zur Frage der Sauerstoffvergiftung. Klin Wchnschr 1939; 18:1382–5.

79. Caldwell PRB, Lee WL, Schildkraut HS, Archibald ER. Changes in lung volume, diffusing capacity, and blood gases in men breathing oxygen. J Appl Physiol 1966; 21:1477–83.

80. Paine JR, Lynn D, Keys A. Observations on the effects of prolonged administration of high oxygen concentrations to dogs. J Thorac Cardiovasc Surg 1941; 11:151–68.

81. Fracica PJ, Knapp MJ, Piantadosi CA, et al. Responses of baboons to prolonged hyperoxia: physiology and qualitative pathology. J Appl Physiol 1991; 71:2352–62.

82. Dolezal V. The effect of long-lasting oxygen inhalation upon respiratory parameters in man. Physiologia Bohemoslovenica 1962; 11:149–58.

83. Singer M, Wright F, Stanley L, Roe B, Hamilton W. Oxygen toxicity in man. A prospective study in patients after open heart surgery. N Engl J Med 1970; 283:1473–8.

84. Barber R, Lee J, Hamilton W. Oxygen toxicity in man. A prospective study in patients with irreversible brain damage. N Engl J Med 1970; 283:1478–84.

85. Hyde RW, Rawson AJ. Unintentional iatrogenic oxygen pneumonitis—Response to therapy. Ann Intern Med 1969; 71:517–31.

86. Kobayashi T, Murakami S. Blindness of an adult caused by oxygen. JAMA 1972; 219:741–2.

87. Nicholos CW, Lambertsen CJ. Effects of high oxygen pressures on the eye. N Engl J Med 1969; 281:25–30.

88. Smith BE, Scott PV, Fischer HBJ, Johnston P. Absence of pulmonary oxygen toxicity in association with high-frequency jet ventilation. Letter. Lancet 1984; 1(8375):505.

89. Capellier G, Beuret P, Clement G, et al. Oxygen tolerance in patients with acute respiratory failure. Intensive Care Med 1998; 24:422–8.

90. Pratt PC. Pulmonary capillary proliferation induced by oxygen inhalation. Am J Pathol 1958; 34:1033–49.

91. Katzenstein A-LA, Askin FB, editors. Surgical pathology of non-neoplastic lung disease. Philadelphia: W.B. Sanders, 1990.

92. Katzenstein A-LA. Acute lung injury patterns: Diffuse alveolar damage and bronchiolitis obliterans-organizing pneumonia. In: Katzenstein A-LA, editor. Katzenstein and Askin's surgical pathology of non-neoplastic lung disease, 3rd ed. Philadelphia: W.B. Saunders, 1997: 14–47.

93. Gould VE, Tosco R, Wheelis RF, Gould NS, Kapanci Y. Oxygen pneumonitis in man. Ultrastructural observations on the development of alveolar lesions. Lab Invest 1972; 26:499–508.

94. Katzenstein AL, Bloor CM, Leibow AA. Diffuse alveolar damage—the role of oxygen, shock and related factors. Am J Pathol 1976; 85:210–29.

95. Kapanci Y, Tosco R, Eggermann J, Gould VE. Oxygen pneumonitis in man. Light and electron-microscopic morphometric studies. Chest 1972; 62:162–9.

96. Nash G, Blennerhassett JB, Pontoppidan H. Pulmonary lesions associated with oxygen therapy and artificial ventilation. N Engl J Med 1967; 276:368–74.

97. Gattinoni L, Pelosi P, Brazzi L, Valenza F. Acute respiratory distress syndrome. In: Albert R, Spiro S, Jett J, editors. Clinical respiratory medicine, 2nd ed. Philadelphia: Mosby, 2004: 743–58.

98. Northway WH, Rosan RC, Porter DY. Pulmonary disease following respirator therapy of hyaline membrane disease. N Engl J Med 1967; 267:357–68.

99. Truog WE. Bronchopulmonary dysplasia: issues in long-term management. J Respir Dis 1993; 14:130–47.

100. Northway WH Jr. Bronchopulmonary dysplasia: twenty-five years later. Pediatrics 1992; 89(5 Pt 1):969–73.

101. Churg A, Golden J, Fligiel S, Hogg JC. Bronchopulmonary dysplasia in the adult. Am Rev Respir Dis 1983; 127:117–20.

102. Coalson JJ, Winter VT, Gerstmann DR, et al. Pathophysiologic, morphometric, and biochemical studies of the premature baboon with bronchopulmonary dysplasia. Am Rev Respir Dis 1992; 145(4 Pt 1):872–81.

103. Chang LY, Subramaniam M, Yoder BA, et al. A catalytic antioxidant attenuates alveolar structural remodeling in bronchopulmonary dysplasia. Am J Respir Crit Care Med 2003; 167: 57–64.

104. Lodato RF. Decreased O_2 consumption and cardiac output during normobaric hyperoxia in conscious dogs. J Appl Physiol 1989; 67:1551–9.

105. Strom K, Odeberg H, Andersson AC, et al. S-erythropoietin levels decrease in patients with chronic hypoxia starting domiciliary oxygen therapy. Eur Respir J 1991; 4:820–3.

106. Phelps DL. Retinopathy of prematurity. N Engl J Med 1992; 326:1078–80.

107. Bossi E, Koerner F. Retinopathy of prematurity. Intensive Care Med 1995; 21:241–6.

108. Flynn JT, Bancalari E, Snyder ES, et al. A cohort study of transcutaneous oxygen tension and the incidence and severity of retinopathy of prematurity. N Engl J Med 1992; 326: 1050–4.

109. Anderson A, Hillestad L. Hemodynamic responses to oxygen breathing and the effect of pharmacological blockade. Acta Med Scand 1970; 188:419–24.

110. Daly WJ, Bondurant S. Effects of oxygen breathing on the heart rate, blood pressure, and cardiac index of normal men—resting, with reactive hyperemia, and after atropine. J Clin Invest 1962; 41:126–32.

111. Dripps RD, Comroe JH Jr. The effect of the inhalation of high and low oxygen concentrations on respiration, pulse rate, ballistocardiogram and arterial oxygen saturation (oximeter) of normal individuals. Am J Physiol 1947; 149:277–91.

112. Eggers GWN Jr, Paley HW, Leonard JJ, Warren JV. Hemodynamic responses to oxygen breathing in man. J Appl Physiol 1962; 17:75–9.

113. Ganz W, Donoso R, Marcus H, Swan HJC. Coronary hemodynamics and myocardial oxygen metabolism during oxygen breathing in patients with and without coronary artery disease. Circulation 1972; 45:763–8.

114. Kenmure ACF, Murdoch WR, Hutton I, Cameron AJV. Hemodynamic effects of oxygen at 1 and 2 Ata pressure in healthy subjects. J Appl Physiol 1972; 32:223–6.

115. Reinhart K, Specht M, Fohring U, Mayr O, Eyrich K. Einfluss der Praoxygenierung auf Hamodynamik und Sauerstoffverbrauch. Anaesthesist 1989; 38:233–7.

116. Whitehorn WV, Edelmann A, Hitchcock FA. The cardiovascular responses to the breathing of 100 percent oxygen at normal barometric pressure. Am J Physiol 1946; 146:61–5.

117. Lodato RF. Effects of normobaric hyperoxia on hemodynamics and O_2 utilization in conscious dogs. In: Piiper J, Goldstick TK, Meyer M, editors. Adv Exp Med Biol, Vol 277: Oxygen transport to tissue XII. New York: Plenum Press, 1990: 807–15.

118. Waring WS, Thomson AJ, Adwani SH, et al. Cardiovascular effects of acute oxygen administration in healthy adults. J Cardiovasc Pharmacol 2003; 42:245–50.

119. Harten JM, Anderson KJ, Angerson WJ, Booth MG, Kinsella J. The effect of normobaric hyperoxia on cardiac index in healthy awake volunteers. Anaesthesia 2003; 58:885–8.

120. Rossi P, Boussuges A. Hyperoxia-induced arterial compliance decrease in healthy man. Clin Physiol Funct Imaging 2005; 25:10–5.

121. Rousseau A, Bak Z, Janerot-Sjoberg B, Sjoberg F. Acute hyperoxaemia-induced effects on regional blood flow, oxygen consumption and central circulation in man. Acta Physiol Scand 2005; 183:231–40.

122. Mak S, Azevedo ER, Liu PP, Newton GE. Effect of hyperoxia on left ventricular function and filling pressures in patients with and without congestive heart failure. Chest 2001; 120: 467–73.

123. Lodato RF, Michael JR, Murray PA. Multipoint pulmonary vascular pressure-cardiac output plots in conscious dogs. Am J Physiol 1985; 249(2 Pt 2):H351–7.

124. Floyd TF, Clark JM, Gelfand R, et al. Independent cerebral vasoconstrictive effects of hyperoxia and accompanying arterial hypocapnia at 1 ATA. J Appl Physiol 2003; 95:2453–61.

125. Gilmore ED, Hudson C, Preiss D, Fisher J. Retinal arteriolar diameter, blood velocity, and blood flow response to an isocapnic hyperoxic provocation. Am J Physiol Heart Circ Physiol 2005; 288:H2912–7.

126. Hughes SJ, Yang W, Juszczak M, et al. Effect of inspired oxygen on portal and hepatic oxygenation: effective arterialization of portal blood by hyperoxia. Cell Transplant 2004; 13(7–8):801–8.

127. Lodato RF. The control of cardiac output. In: Dantzker DR, editor. Cardiopulmonary critical care, 2nd ed. Philadelphia: W.B. Saunders, 1991: 71–85.

128. Ellsworth ML. The red blood cell as an oxygen sensor: what is the evidence? Acta Physiol Scand 2000; 168:551–9.

129. McMahon TJ, Moon RE, Luschinger BP, et al. Nitric oxide in the human respiratory cycle. Nat Med 2002; 8:711–7.

130. Demchenko IT, Oury TD, Crapo JD, Piantadosi CA. Regulation of the brain's vascular responses to oxygen. Circ Res 2002; 91:1031–7.

131. Zhilyaev SY, Moskvin AN, Platonova TF, et al. Hyperoxic vasoconstriction in the brain is mediated by inactivation of nitric oxide by superoxide anions. Neurosci Behav Physiol 2003; 33:783–7.

132. Mak S, Egri Z, Tanna G, Colman R, Newton GE. Vitamin C prevents hyperoxia-mediated vasoconstriction and impairment of endothelium-dependent vasodilation. Am J Physiol Heart Circ Physiol 2002; 282:H2414–21.

133. Rubanyi GM, Vanhoutte PM. Superoxide anions and hyperoxia inactivate endothelium-derived relaxing factor. Am J Physiol 1986; 250(5 Pt 2):H822–7.

134. Mouren S, Souktani R, Beaussier M, et al. Mechanisms of coronary vasoconstriction induced by high arterial oxygen tension. Am J Physiol 1997; 272(1 Pt 2):H67–75.

135. Dallinger S, Dorner GT, Wenzel R, et al. Endothelin-1 contributes to hyperoxia-induced vasoconstriction in the human retina. Invest Ophthalmol Vis Sci 2000; 41:864–9.

136. Yu DY, Su EN, Cringle SJ, et al. Comparison of the vasoactive effects of the docosanoid unoprostone and selected prostanoids on isolated perfused retinal arterioles. Invest Ophthalmol Vis Sci 2001; 42:1499–504.

137. Mildenberger E, Siegel G, Versmold HT. Locally released norepinephrine in the oxygen-dependent regulation of vascular tone of human umbilical vein. Pediatr Res 2004; 55:267–72.

138. Jubran A, Lodato RF. Role of baroreceptors in hyperoxia-induced decrease in heart rate in conscious dogs. FASEB J 1990; 4:A427.

139. Anderson KJ, Harten JM, Booth MG, Kinsella J. The cardiovascular effects of inspired oxygen fraction in anaesthetized patients. Eur J Anaesthesiol 2005; 22:420–5.

140. Joachimsson PO, Sjoberg F, Forsman M, et al. Adverse effects of hyperoxemia during cardiopulmonary bypass. J Thorac Cardiovasc Surg 1996; 112:812–9.

141. Harten JM, Anderson KJ, Kinsella J, Higgins MJ. Normobaric hyperoxia reduces cardiac index in patients after coronary artery bypass surgery. J Cardiothorac Vasc Anesth 2005; 19:173–5.

142. Spies C, Giese C, Meier-Hellmann A, et al. [The effect of prophylactically administered N-acetylcysteine on clinical indicators for tissue oxygenation during hyperoxic ventilation in cardiac risk patients.] Anaesthesist 1996; 45:343–50.

143. Haque WA, Boehmer J, Clemson BS, et al. Hemodynamic effects of supplemental oxygen administration in congestive heart failure. J Am Coll Cardiol 1996; 27:353–7.

144. Saadjian A, Paganelli F, Levy S. Hemodynamic response to oxygen administration in chronic heart failure: role of chemoreflexes. J Cardiovasc Pharmacol 1999; 33:144–50.

145. Reinhart K, Bloos F, Konig F, Bredle D, Hannemann L. Reversible decrease of oxygen consumption by hyperoxia. Chest 1991; 99:690–4.

146. Reinhart K, Spies CD, Meier-Hellmann A, et al. N-acetylcysteine preserves oxygen consumption and gastric mucosal pH during hyperoxic ventilation. Am J Respir Crit Care Med 1995; 151(3 Pt 1):773–9.

147. Moller S, Becker U, Schifter S, Abrahamsen J, Henriksen JH. Effect of oxygen inhalation on systemic, central, and splanchnic haemodynamics in cirrhosis. J Hepatol 1996; 25:316–28.

148. Beekman RH, Rocchini AP, Rosenthal A. Cardiovascular effects of breathing 95 percent oxygen in children with congenital heart disease. Am J Cardiol 1983; 52:106–11.

149. Roberts DH, Lepore JJ, Maroo A, Semigran MJ, Ginns LC. Oxygen therapy improves cardiac index and pulmonary vascular resistance in patients with pulmonary hypertension. Chest 2001; 120:1547–55.

150. Chapler CK, Cain SM, Stainsby WN. The effects of hyperoxia on oxygen uptake during acute anemia. Can J Physiol Pharmacol 1984; 62:806–14.

151. Bourdeau-Martini J, Odoroff CL, Honig CR. Dual effect of oxygen on magnitude and uniformity of coronary intercapillary distance. Am J Physiol 1974; 226:800–10.

152. Lund N, Jorfeldt L, Lewis DH. Skeletal muscle oxygen pressure fields in healthy human volunteers. Acta Anaesthesiol Scand 1980; 24:272–8.

153. Thorborg P, Gustafsson U, Sjoberg F, Harrison DK, Lewis DH. Effect of hyperoxemia and ritanserin on skeletal muscle microflow. J Appl Physiol 1990; 68:1494–500.

154. Tsai AG, Cabrales P, Winslow RM, Intaglietta M. Microvascular oxygen distribution in awake hamster window chamber model during hyperoxia. Am J Physiol Heart Circ Physiol 2003; 285:H1537–45.

155. Cain SM. Gas exchange in hypoxia, apnea, and hyperoxia. In: Handbook of physiology, Sect 3: Respiration, Vol IV, Gas exchange. Bethesda, MD: Am Physiol Soc, 1987: 403–22.

156. Smith CW, Lehan PH, Monks JJ. Cardiopulmonary manifestations with high O_2 tensions at atmospheric pressure. J Appl Physiol 1963; 18:849–53.

157. Matalon S, Nesarajah MS, Farhi LE. Pulmonary and circulatory changes in conscious sheep exposed to 100% O_2 at 1 ATA. J Appl Physiol 1982; 53:110–6.

158. Harabin AL, Homer LD, Bradley ME. Pulmonary oxygen toxicity in awake dogs: metabolic and physiological effects. J Appl Physiol 1984; 57:1480–8.

159. Cassuto Y, Farhi LE. Circulatory response to arterial hyperoxia. J Appl Physiol 1979; 46:973–7.

160. Busing CM, Kreinsen U, Buhler F, Bleyl U. Light and electron microscopic examinations of experimentally produced heart muscle necroses following normobaric hyperoxia. Virchows Arch A Pathol Anat Histol 1975; 366: 137–47.

161. Fracica PJ, Knapp MJ, Jafri A, et al. Hyperoxic cardiac dysfunction in primates. Surg Forum 1987; 38:246–8.

162. Robinson FR, Sopher RL, Witchett CE, Carter VL Jr. Pathology of normobaric oxygen toxicity in primates. Aerospace Med 1969; 40:879–84.

163. Denison DM, editor. Oxygen supply and uses in tissues. New York: Springer-Verlag, 1989.

164. Fisher AB. Intracellular production of oxygen-derived free radicals. In: Halliwell B, editor. Oxygen radicals and tissue injury. Bethesda, MD: FASEB (Upjohn Symposium), 1988: 34–9.

165. Freeman BA, Crapo JD. Hyperoxia increases oxygen radical production in rat lungs and lung mitochondria. J Biological Chem 1981; 256:10986–92.

166. Freeman BA, Crapo JD. Biology of disease. Free radicals and tissue injury. Lab Invest 1982; 47:412–26.

167. Massaro D. Tolerance to hyperoxia. Curr Pulmonol 1987; 8:115–26.

168. Vallyathan V, Shi X, Castranova V, editors. Oxygen/nitrogen radicals: Lung injury and disease. New York: Marcel Dekker, Inc, 2004.

169. Notter RH, Finkelstein JN, Holm BA, eds. Lung injury: Mechanisms, pathophysiology, and therapy. New York: Marcel Dekker, Inc, 2005.

170. Gerschman R, Gilbert DL, Nye SW, Dwyer P, Fenn WO. Oxygen poisoning and x-irradiation: a mechanism in common. Science 1954; 119:623–6.

171. Gerschman R. Biological effects of oxygen. In: Dickens F, Neil E, editors. Oxygen in the animal organism. New York: Macmillan, 1964: 475–94.

172. Kinnula VL, Crapo JD. Superoxide dismutases in the lung and human lung diseases. Am J Respir Crit Care Med 2003; 167:1600–19.

173. Aust AE. Reactive oxygen/nitrogen species. In: Vallyathan V, Castranova V, Shi X, editors. Oxygen/nitrogen radicals lung injury and disease. New York: Marcel Dekker, 2004: 1–34.

174. Mercer RR, Crapo JD. Cellular responses of the lungs to hyperoxia. In: Lenfant C, editor. Oxygen/nitrogen radicals lung injury and disease. New York: Marcel Dekker, 2004: 445–73.

175. Davis IC, Lang JD, Matalon S. Roles of reactive oxygen and nitrogen species in lung injury. In: Notter R, Finkelstein J, Holm B, editors. Lung injury mechanisms, pathophysiology, and therapy. New York: Taylor & Francis Group, 2005: 227–68.

176. Asikainen TM, White CW. Antioxidant therapy for lung injury. In: Notter RH, Finkelstein JN, Holm BA, editors. Lung injury mechanisms, pathophysiology, and therapy. New York: Taylor & Francis, 2005: 665–703.

177. Fridovich I. Fundamental aspects of reactive oxygen species, or what's the matter with oxygen? Ann NY Acad Sci 1999; 893:13–8.

178. Fridovich I. Mitochondria: are they the seat of senescence? Aging Cell 2004; 3:13–6.

179. Grisham MB, Granger DN. Metabolic sources of reactive oxygen metabolites during oxidant stress and ischemia with reperfusion. Clin Chest Med 1989; 10:71–81.

180. Yusa T, Beckman JS, Crapo JD, Freeman BA. Hyperoxia increases H_2O_2 production by brain in vivo. J Appl Physiol 1987; 63: 353–8.

181. Turrens JF, Freeman BA, Crapo JD. Hyperoxia increases H_2O_2 release by lung mitochondria and microsomes. Arch Biochem Biophys 1982; 217:411–21.

182. Turrens JF. Superoxide production by the mitochondrial respiratory chain. Biosci Rep 1997; 17:3–8.

183. Kilbourn RG, Gross SS, Jubran A, et al. NG-methyl-L-arginine inhibits tumor necrosis factor–induced hypotension: implications for the involvement of nitric oxide. Proc Natl Acad Sci USA 1990; 87:3629–32.

184. Xia Y, Roman LJ, Masters BS, Zweier JL. Inducible nitric-oxide synthase generates superoxide from the reductase domain. J Biol Chem 1998; 273:22635–9.

185. Halliwell B. A radical approach to human disease. In: Halliwell B, editor. Oxygen radicals and tissue injury. Bethesda, MD: FASEB (Upjohn Symposium), 1988: 139–43.

186. Heffner JE, Repine JE. Pulmonary strategies of antioxidant defense. State of the art. Am Rev Respir Dis 1989; 140:531–54.

187. Oury TD, Chang LY, Marklund SL, Day BJ, Crapo JD. Immunocytochemical localization of extracellular superoxide dismutase in human lung. Lab Invest 1994; 70:889–98.

188. Risberg B, Smith L, Ortenwall P. Oxygen radicals and lung injury. Acta Anaesthesiol Scand 1991; 35(Suppl 95):106–18.

189. Rhee SG, Kang SW, Netto LE, Seo MS, Stadtman ER. A family of novel peroxidases, peroxiredoxins. Biofactors 1999; 10(2–3):207–9.

190. Holmgren A. Antioxidant function of thioredoxin and glutaredoxin systems. Antioxid Redox Signal 2000; 2:811–20.

191. Powis G, Mustacich D, Coon A. The role of the redox protein thioredoxin in cell growth and cancer. Free Radic Biol Med 2000; 29(3–4):312–22.

192. Pryhuber GS, D'Angio CT, Finkelstein JN, Notter RH. Combination therapies for lung injury. In: Notter RH, Finkelstein JN, Holm BA, editors. Lung injury mechanisms, pathophysiology, and therapy. New York: Taylor & Francis, 2005: 779–838.

193. Ho YS. Transgenic and knockout models for studying the role of lung antioxidant enzymes in defense against hyperoxia. Am J Respir Crit Care Med 2002; 166(12 Pt 2):S51–6.

194. Folz RJ, Abushamaa AM, Suliman HB. Extracellular superoxide dismutase in the airways of transgenic mice reduces inflammation and attenuates lung toxicity following hyperoxia. J Clin Invest 1999; 103:1055–66.

195. Ahmed MN, Suliman HB, Folz RJ, et al. Extracellular superoxide dismutase protects lung development in hyperoxia-exposed newborn mice. Am J Respir Crit Care Med 2003; 167:400–5.

196. Simonson SG, Welty-Wolf KE, Huang YC, et al. Aerosolized manganese SOD decreases hyperoxic pulmonary injury in primates. I. Physiology and biochemistry. J Appl Physiol 1997; 83:550–8.

197. Welty-Wolf KE, Simonson SG, Huang YC, et al. Aerosolized manganese SOD decreases hyperoxic pulmonary injury in primates. II. Morphometric analysis. J Appl Physiol 1997; 83:559–68.

198. Rosenfeld WN, Davis JM, Parton L, et al. Safety and pharmacokinetics of recombinant human superoxide dismutase administered intratracheally to premature neonates with respiratory distress syndrome. Pediatrics 1996; 97(6 Pt 1):811–7.

199. Davis JM, Parad RB, Michele T, et al. Pulmonary outcome at 1 year corrected age in premature infants treated at birth with recombinant human CuZn superoxide dismutase. Pediatrics 2003; 111:469–76.

200. Patel M, Day BJ. Metalloporphyrin class of therapeutic catalytic antioxidants. Trends Pharmacol Sci 1999; 20:359–64.

201. Gillissen A, Nowak D. Characterization of N-acetylcysteine and ambroxol in anti-oxidant therapy. Respir Med 1998; 92:609–23.

202. Vale JA, Proudfoot AT. Paracetamol (acetaminophen) poisoning. Lancet 1995; 346:547–52.

203. Bernard GR, Lucht WD, Niedermeyer ME, et al. Effect of N-acetylcysteine on the pulmonary response to endotoxin in the awake sheep and upon in vitro granulocyte function. J Clin Invest 1984; 73:1772–84.

204. Wagner PD, Mathieu-Costello O, Bebout DE, et al. Protection against pulmonary O_2 toxicity by N-acetylcysteine. Eur Respir J 1989; 2:116–26.

205. Langley SC, Kelly FJ. N-acetylcysteine ameliorates hyperoxic lung injury in the preterm guinea pig. Biochem Pharmacol 1993; 45:841–6.

206. Leff JA, Wilke CP, Hybertson BM, et al. Postinsult treatment with N-acetyl-L-cysteine decreases IL-1-induced neutrophil influx and lung leak in rats. Am J Physiol 1993; 265(5 Pt 1): L501–6.

207. Sastre J, Asensi M, Rodrigo F, et al. Antioxidant administration to the mother prevents oxidative stress associated with birth in the neonatal rat. Life Sci 1994; 54:2055–9.

208. Davreux CJ, Soric I, Nathens AB, et al. N-acetyl cysteine attenuates acute lung injury in the rat. Shock 1997; 8:432–8.

209. Jepsen S, Herlevsen P, Knudsen P, Bud MI, Klausen NO. Antioxidant treatment with N-acetylcysteine during adult respiratory distress syndrome: a prospective, randomized, placebo-controlled study. Crit Care Med 1992; 20:918–23.

210. Suter PM, Domenighetti G, Schaller MD, et al. N-acetylcysteine enhances recovery from acute lung injury in man. A randomized, double-blind, placebo-controlled clinical study. Chest 1994; 105:190–4.

211. Domenighetti G, Suter PM, Schaller MD, Ritz R, Perret C. Treatment with N-acetylcysteine during acute respiratory distress

syndrome: a randomized, double-blind, placebo-controlled clinical study. J Crit Care 1997; 12:177–82.

212. Bernard GR, Wheeler AP, Arons MM, et al. A trial of antioxidants N-acetylcysteine and procysteine in ARDS. The Antioxidant in ARDS Study Group. Chest 1997; 112:164–72.

213. Molnar Z, Shearer E, Lowe D. N-Acetylcysteine treatment to prevent the progression of multisystem organ failure: a prospective, randomized, placebo-controlled study. Crit Care Med 1999; 27:1100–4.

214. Ware LB, Matthay MA. The acute respiratory distress syndrome. N Engl J Med 2000; 342:1334–49.

215. Darlow BA, Winterbourn CC, Inder TE, et al. The effect of selenium supplementation on outcome in very low birth weight infants: a randomized controlled trial. The New Zealand Neonatal Study Group. J Pediatr 2000; 136:473–80.

216. Watts JL, Milner R, Zipursky A, et al. Failure of supplementation with vitamin E to prevent bronchopulmonary dysplasia in infants less than 1500 g birth weight. Eur Respir J 1991; 4:188–90.

217. Ehrenkranz RA, Ablow RC, Warshaw JB. Effect of vitamin E on the development of oxygen-induced lung injury in neonates. Ann NY Acad Sci 1982; 393:452–66.

218. Tyson JE, Wright LL, Oh W, et al. Vitamin A supplementation for extremely-low-birth-weight infants. National Institute of Child Health and Human Development Neonatal Research Network. N Engl J Med 1999; 340:1962–8.

219. Nathens AB, Neff MJ, Jurkovich GJ, et al. Randomized, prospective trial of antioxidant supplementation in critically ill surgical patients. Ann Surg 2002; 236:814–22.

220. Sosenko IR, Innis SM, Frank L. Polyunsaturated fatty acids and protection of newborn rats from oxygen toxicity. J Pediatr 1988; 112:630–7.

221. Sosenko IR, Innis SM, Frank L. Menhaden fish oil, n-3 polyunsaturated fatty acids, and protection of newborn rats from oxygen toxicity. Pediatr Res 1989; 25:399–404.

222. Sosenko IR, Innis SM, Frank L. Intralipid increases lung polyunsaturated fatty acids and protects newborn rats from oxygen toxicity. Pediatr Res 1991; 30:413–7.

223. Gadek JE, DeMichele SJ, Karlstad MD, et al. Effect of enteral feeding with eicosapentaenoic acid, gamma-linolenic acid, and antioxidants in patients with acute respiratory distress syndrome. Enteral Nutrition in ARDS Study Group. Crit Care Med 1999; 27:1409–20.

224. Pacht ER, DeMichele SJ, Nelson JL, et al. Enteral nutrition with eicosapentaenoic acid, gamma-linolenic acid, and antioxidants reduces alveolar inflammatory mediators and protein influx in patients with acute respiratory distress syndrome. Crit Care Med 2003; 31:491–500.

225. deLemos RA, Roberts RJ, Coalson JJ, et al. Toxic effects associated with the administration of deferoxamine in the premature baboon with hyaline membrane disease. Am J Dis Child 1990; 144:915–9.

226. Auten RL Jr, Mason SN, Tanaka DT, Welty-Wolf K, Whorton MH. Anti-neutrophil chemokine preserves alveolar development in hyperoxia-exposed newborn rats. Am J Physiol Lung Cell Mol Physiol 2001; 281:L336–44.

227. Auten RL, Richardson RM, White JR, et al. Nonpeptide CXCR2 antagonist prevents neutrophil accumulation in hyperoxia-exposed newborn rats. J Pharmacol Exp Ther 2001; 299:90–5.

228. Hay DW, Sarau HM. Interleukin-8 receptor antagonists in pulmonary diseases. Curr Opin Pharmacol 2001; 1:242–7.

229. Frank L, Yam J, Roberts RJ. The role of endotoxin in protection of adult rats from oxygen-induced lung toxicity. J Clin Invest 1978; 61:269–75.

230. Smith G, Winter PM, Wheelis RF. Increased normobaric oxygen tolerance of rabbits following oleic acid-induced lung damage. J Appl Physiol 1973; 35:395–400.

231. Huber GL, Finder E, LaForce FM. Prevention of oxygen toxicity in the lung. Chest 1972; 62(Suppl):365S.

232. Crapo JD, Barry BE, Foscue HA, Shelburne J. Structural and biochemical changes in rat lungs occurring during exposures to lethal and adaptive doses of oxygen. Am Rev Respir Dis 1980; 122:123–43.

233. Baker RR, Holm BA, Panus PC, Matalon S. Development of O_2 tolerance in rabbits with no increase in antioxidant enzymes. J Appl Physiol 1989; 66:1679–84.

234. Clark JM. Interacting effects of hypoxia adaptation and acute hypercapnia on oxygen tolerance in rats. J Appl Physiol 1984;56:1191–8.

235. Frank L. Protection from O_2 toxicity by preexposure to hypoxia: lung antioxidant enzyme role. J Appl Physiol 1982; 53:475–82.

236. White CW, Ghezzi P, Dinarello CA, et al. Recombinant tumor necrosis factor/cachectin and interleukin 1 pretreatment decreases lung oxidized glutathione accumulation, lung injury, and mortality in rats exposed to hyperoxia. J Clin Invest 1987; 79:1868–73.

237. Kilbourn RG, Gross SS, Lodato RF, et al. Inhibition of interleukin-1-alpha–induced nitric oxide synthase in vascular smooth muscle and full reversal of interleukin-1-alpha–induced hypotension by N omega-amino-L-arginine. J Natl Cancer Inst 1992; 84:1008–16.

238. Kilbourn RG, Jubran A, Gross SS, et al. Reversal of endotoxin-mediated shock by NG-methyl-L-arginine, an inhibitor of nitric oxide synthesis. Biochem Biophys Res Commun 1990; 172: 1132–8.

239. White CW, Ghezzi P, McMahon S, Dinarello CA, Repine JE. Cytokines increase rat lung antioxidant enzymes during exposure to hyperoxia. J Appl Physiol 1989; 66:1003–7.

240. Frank L, Bucher JR, Roberts RJ. Oxygen toxicity in neonatal and adult animals of various species. J Appl Physiol 1978; 45:699–704.

241. Wang Z, Holm BA, Matalon S, Notter RH. Surfactant activity and dysfunction in lung injury. In: Notter RH, Finkelstein JN, Holm BA, editors. Lung injury mechanisms, pathophysiology, and therapy. New York: Taylor & Francis, 2005: 297–352.

242. Chess PR, Finkelstein JN, Holm BA, Notter RH. Surfactant replacement therapy in lung injury. In: Notter RH, Finkelstein JN, Holm BA, editors. Lung injury mechanisms, pathophysiology, and therapy. New York: Taylor & Francis, 2005: 617–63.

243. Zenri H, Rodriquez-Capote K, McCaig L, et al. Hyperoxia exposure impairs surfactant function and metabolism. Crit Care Med 2004; 32:1155–60.

244. White CW, Greene KE, Allen CB, Shannon JM. Elevated expression of surfactant proteins in newborn rats during adaptation to hyperoxia. Am J Respir Cell Mol Biol 2001; 25:51–9.

245. Boggaram V. Regulation of surfactant protein gene expression by hyperoxia in the lung. Antioxid Redox Signal 2004; 6:185–90.

246. Matalon S, Holm BA, Baker RR, Whitfield MK, Freeman BA. Characterization of antioxidant activities of pulmonary surfactant mixtures. Biochim Biophys Acta 1990; 1035:121–7.

247. Bridges JP, Davis HW, Damodarasamy M, et al. Pulmonary surfactant proteins A and D are potent endogenous inhibitors of lipid peroxidation and oxidative cellular injury. J Biol Chem 2000; 275:38848–55.

248. Tokieda K, Ikegami M, Wert SE, et al. Surfactant protein B corrects oxygen-induced pulmonary dysfunction in heterozygous surfactant protein B–deficient mice. Pediatr Res 1999; 46:708–14.

249. Ghio AJ, Fracica PJ, Young SL, Piantadosi CA. Synthetic surfactant scavenges oxidants and protects against hyperoxic lung injury. J Appl Physiol 1994; 77:1217–23.

250. Lewis JF, Jobe AH. Surfactant and the adult respiratory distress syndrome. State of the art. Am Rev Respir Dis 1993; 147:218–33.

251. Sachs S, Ghio AJ, Young SL. Tyloxapol confers durable protection against hyperoxic lung injury in the rat. Exp Lung Res 1999; 25:543–59.

252. Piantadosi CA, Fracica PJ, Duhaylongsod FG, et al. Artificial surfactant attenuates hyperoxic lung injury in primates. II. Morphometric analysis. J Appl Physiol 1995; 78:1823–31.

253. Schroder A, Herting E, Speer CP. [Superoxide dismutase and catalase activity in tracheobronchial secretions after surfactant treatment of newborn infants with respiratory distress syndrome.] Z Geburtshilfe Neonatol 1999; 203:201–6.

254. Auten RL, Notter RH, Kendig JW, Davis JM, Shapiro DL. Surfactant treatment of full-term newborns with respiratory failure. Pediatrics 1991; 87:101–7.

255. Findlay RD, Taeusch HW, Walther FJ. Surfactant replacement therapy for meconium aspiration syndrome. Pediatrics 1996; 97:48–52.

256. Lotze A, Mitchell BR, Bulas DI, et al. Multicenter study of surfactant (beractant) use in the treatment of term infants with severe respiratory failure. Survanta in Term Infants Study Group. J Pediatr 1998; 132:40–7.

257. Luchetti M, Ferrero F, Gallini C, et al. Multicenter, randomized, controlled study of porcine surfactant in severe respiratory syncytial virus-induced respiratory failure. Pediatr Crit Care Med 2002; 3:261–8.

258. Willson DF, Zaritsky A, Bauman LA, et al. Instillation of calf lung surfactant extract (calfactant) is beneficial in pediatric acute hypoxemic respiratory failure. Members of the Mid-Atlantic Pediatric Critical Care Network. Crit Care Med 1999; 27:188–95.

259. Anzueto A, Baughman RP, Guntupalli KK, et al. Aerosolized surfactant in adults with sepsis-induced acute respiratory distress syndrome. Exosurf Acute Respiratory Distress Syndrome Sepsis Study Group. N Engl J Med 1996; 334:1417–21.

260. Matthay MA. The acute respiratory distress syndrome. N Engl J Med 1996; 334:1469–70.

261. Rinaldo JE, Christman JW. Mechanisms and mediators of the adult respiratory distress syndrome. Clin Chest Med 1990; 11:621–32.

262. Niederman MS, Fein AM. Sepsis syndrome, the adult respiratory distress syndrome, and nosocomial pneumonia: a common clinical sequence. Clin Chest Med 1990; 11:633–56.

263. Lykens MG, Davis WB, Pacht ER. Antioxidant activity of bronchoalveolar lavage fluid in the adult respiratory distress syndrome. Am J Physiol (Lung Cell Mol Physiol) 1992; 262:L169–75.

264. Rivers E, Nguyen B, Havstad S, et al. Early goal-directed therapy in the treatment of severe sepsis and septic shock. N Engl J Med 2001; 345:1368–77.

265. Lodato RF, Barasch E, Thandroyen FT, Schroth G. Prevalence of patent foramen ovale (PFO) in the adult respiratory distress syndrome (ARDS). Am J Respir Crit Care Med 1998; 157: A679.

266. West JB. Human physiology at extreme altitudes on Mount Everest. Science 1984; 223:784–8.

267. Richalet JP, Bittel J, Herry JP, et al. Use of a hypobaric chamber for pre-acclimatization before climbing Mount Everest. Int J Sports Med 1992; 13(Suppl 1):S216–20.

268. Ashbaugh DG, Bigelow DB, Petty TL, Levine BE. Acute respiratory distress in adults. Lancet 1967; 2:319–23.

269. Bernard GR, Vincent JL, Laterre PF, et al. Efficacy and safety of recombinant human activated protein C for severe sepsis. N Engl J Med 2001; 344:699–709.

Chapter 46

PNEUMONIA IN THE VENTILATOR-DEPENDENT PATIENT

JEAN CHASTRE
JEAN-YVES FAGON

Ventilator-associated pneumonia (VAP) is the most frequent ICU-acquired infection among patients receiving mechanical ventilation.[1] In contrast to infections of other frequently involved organs (e.g., urinary tract and skin), for which mortality is low, ranging from 1–4%, the mortality rate for VAP, defined as pneumonia occurring >48 hours after endotracheal intubation and initiation of mechanical ventilation, ranges from 24–50% and can reach 76% in some specific settings or when lung infection is caused by high-risk pathogens.[1-3] Although the attributable mortality rate for VAP is still debated, it has been shown that these infections prolong both the duration of ventilation and the duration of intensive care unit (ICU) stay.[1,2] Approximately 50% of all antibiotics prescribed in an ICU are administered for respiratory tract infections.[4] Because several studies have shown that appropriate antimicrobial treatment of patients with VAP significantly improves outcome, more rapid identification of infected patients and accurate selection of antimicrobial agents represent important clinical goals.[2] Consensus, however, on appropriate diagnostic, therapeutic, and preventive strategies for VAP has yet to be reached. In this chapter, we summarize published studies on epidemiology, diagnosis, treatment, and prevention of nosocomial pulmonary infection in critically ill patients mechanically ventilated in the ICU, and present our experience with these infections.

Epidemiology

Accurate data on the epidemiology of VAP are limited by the lack of standardized criteria for its diagnosis. Conceptually, VAP is defined as an inflammation of the lung parenchyma caused by infectious agents not present or incubating at the time mechanical ventilation was started. Despite the clarity of this conception, the past three decades have witnessed the appearance of numerous operational definitions, none of which is universally accepted. Even definitions based on histopathologic findings at autopsy may fail to find consensus or provide certainty. Pneumonia in focal areas of a lobe may be missed, microbiologic studies may be negative despite of presence of inflammation in the lung, and pathologists may disagree on the findings.[5] The absence of a gold standard continues to fuel controversy about the adequacy and relevance of many studies in this field.

INCIDENCE OF VENTILATOR-ASSOCIATED PNEUMONIA

A large-scale 1-day point-prevalence study of pneumonia arising in the ICU was conducted on April 29, 1992, in 1417 ICUs.[6] A total of 10,038 patients were evaluated: 2064 (21%) had ICU-acquired infections, including pneumonia in 967 (47%) patients, for an overall nosocomial pneumonia prevalence of 10%. In that study, logistic regression analysis identified mechanical ventilation as one of the 7 risk factors for ICU-acquired infections. Based on their analyses of overall rates of nosocomial pneumonia, Cross et al reported tenfold higher frequencies for ventilated patients than those without respiratory assistance.[7] Similarly, in a nationwide American study, the pneumonia rate was 21-fold higher for patients receiving continuous ventilator support than for those not requiring mechanical ventilation,[8] in agreement with a multivariate analysis of 120 consecutive VAP episodes and 120 controls that had shown intubation to independently increase the risk of nosocomial pneumonia approximately sevenfold.[9] These data confirmed the considerably higher risk of VAP observed in the subset of ICU patients treated with mechanical ventilation.

When quantitative cultures of specimens obtained with a protected specimen brush (PSB) during fiberoptic bronchoscopy were used to define pneumonia in 567 ventilated patients, the VAP rate was 9%.[10] According to an actuarial method, the cumulative risk of pneumonia in that context was estimated to be 7% at 10 days and 19% at 20 days after the institution of mechanical ventilation. Furthermore, in that study, the incremental risk of pneumonia was virtually constant throughout the entire ventilation period, with a mean rate of about 1% per day. In contrast, Cook et al demonstrated in a large series of 1014 mechanically ventilated patients that, although the cumulative risk for developing VAP increased over time, the daily hazard rate decreased after day 5.[11] The risk per day was evaluated at 3% on day 5, 2% on day 10, and 1% on day 15. Independent predictors of VAP as determined by multivariate analysis were a primary admitting diagnosis of burns (risk ratio [RR], 5.1; 95% confidence interval [CI], 1.5–17.0), trauma (RR, 5.0; 95% CI, 1.9–13.1), central nervous system disease (RR, 3.4; 95% CI, 1.3–8.8), respiratory disease (RR, 2.8; 95% CI, 1.1–7.5), cardiac disease (RR, 2.7; 95% CI, 1.1–7.0), mechanical ventilation during the preceding 24 hours (RR, 2.3; 95% CI, 1.1–4.7), witnessed aspiration (RR, 3.2; 95% CI, 1.6–6.5), and paralytic agents (RR, 1.6; 95% CI, 1.1–2.4). Exposure to antibiotics conferred protection (RR, 0.4; 95% CI, 0.3–0.5), but this effect was attenuated over time. Thus, the daily risk for developing VAP is highly dependent on the population being studied and also on many other factors, particularly the number of patients in the given population who received antibiotics immediately after admission to the ICU.

VAP is thought to be a common complication of the acute respiratory distress syndrome (ARDS). Most clinical studies have found that pulmonary infection affects between 34 and >70% of patients with ARDS, often leading to the development of sepsis, multiple organ failure, and death. When the lungs of patients who died of ARDS were examined histologically at autopsy, pneumonia could be demonstrated in as many as 73%.[12] The diagnosis of pulmonary infection in patients with ARDS, however, is often difficult. Several studies have clearly demonstrated the inability of physicians to accurately diagnose nosocomial pneumonia in this setting based on clinical criteria alone.[13,14] According to four studies, the VAP rate was higher in patients with ARDS than other ventilated patients.[15–18] In one study of 56 patients with ARDS, PSB and bronchoalveolar lavage (BAL) were used to define pneumonia; the VAP rate was 55%, whereas it was only 28% for 187 patients without ARDS, diagnosed by the same criteria during the same period.[15] It was specified that early-onset VAP (occurring before day 7) was relatively rare in patients with ARDS: only 10% of the first VAP episodes were in ARDS patients, as opposed to 40% of patients without ARDS. Those observations were confirmed in 30 patients with ARDS in whom repeated quantitative culture results of specimens obtained with a plugged catheter were available and in 94 patients with ARDS and suspected VAP who underwent 172 bronchoscopies; the VAP rates were 60% (incidence density, 4.2/100 ventilator-days) and 43%, respectively.[16] In another prospective multicenter study, VAP was bacteriologically confirmed in 49

(37%) out of 134 patients with ARDS, versus 23% of ventilated patients without ARDS (p <0.002).[17]

MORTALITY

Crude ICU mortality rates of 24–76% have been reported for VAP at a variety of institutions.[1,2,19] ICU ventilated patients with VAP appear to have a two- to tenfold higher risk of death compared to patients without pneumonia. Although these statistics indicate that VAP is a severe disease, previous studies have not clearly demonstrated that pneumonia is indeed responsible for the higher mortality rate of these patients. Two independent factors make it difficult to assign responsibility unambiguously. The first is, once again, the difficulty in establishing a firm diagnosis (i.e., to clearly identify patients with VAP); thus, the widely diverging VAP mortality rates reported might reflect not only differences in the populations studied, but also differences in the diagnostic criteria used. Second, numerous studies have demonstrated that severe underlying illness predisposes ICU patients to the development of pneumonia, and their mortality rates are, consequently, high.[6,20,21] Therefore, it is difficult to determine whether such patients would have survived if VAP had not occurred. Nosocomial pneumonia, however, has been recognized in several case-controlled studies or studies using multivariate analysis as an important prognostic factor for different groups of critically ill patients.[6,21–25] Other factors beyond the simple development of VAP, such as the severity of the disease or the responsible pathogens, may be more important determinants of outcome for patients in whom VAP as well as other nosocomial infections develop. Indeed, it may well be that VAP increases mortality only in the subset of patients with intermediate severity[25] and/or in patients with VAP caused by high-risk pathogens, as indicated below. Patients with very low severity and early-onset pneumonia caused by organisms such as *Haemophilus influenzae* or *Streptococcus pneumoniae* have excellent prognoses with or without VAP, whereas very ill patients with late-onset VAP occurring while they are in a quasi-terminal state would die anyway.

The prognosis for aerobic, gram-negative bacilli (GNB) VAP is considerably worse than that for infection with gram-positive pathogens, when these organisms are fully susceptible to antibiotics.[22,26–28] Concerning gram-positive pathogens, in a study comparing VAP secondary to methicillin-resistant *Staphylococcus aureus* (MRSA) or methicillin-sensitive *S. aureus* (MSSA), mortality was found to be directly attributable to pneumonia for 86% of the former cases versus 12% of the latter, with a relative risk of death equal to 20.7 for MRSA pneumonia.[29] The important prognostic role played by the adequacy of the initial empiric antimicrobial therapy was also analyzed by several other investigators.[30–37]

Thus, considering many different kinds of evidence, VAP seems indeed associated with a 20–30% higher risk of death than that secondary to the underlying disease alone, at least in several subgroups of patients requiring mechanical ventilation, which indicates the need for new approaches to improve the management of ventilator-dependent patients, including more effective prophylactic measures, and earlier diagnosis and treatment.

MORBIDITY AND COST

It is impossible to evaluate precisely the morbidity and excess costs associated with VAP. With respect, however, to morbidity measures, the prolonged hospital stay as a direct consequence of VAP has been estimated in several studies.[19,23,38,39] Recently, Heyland et al[40] compared 177 VAP patients with matched patients who did not develop VAP, and showed that VAP patients stayed in the ICU 4.3 days longer than controls; the attributable ICU length of stay was longer for medical than surgical patients (6.5 versus 0.7 days), and for patients infected with "high-risk" as opposed to "low-risk" organisms (9.1 versus 2.9 days). In ARDS patients, all studies clearly identified prolonged duration of mechanical ventilation and lengthened ICU and hospital stays for patients with VAP compared to those without.[15,17,18] Thus, summarizing available data, VAP likely extended the ICU stay by at least 4 days.

These prolonged hospitalizations underscore the considerable financial burden imposed by the development of VAP. A precise and universal evaluation, however, of such overcosts is very difficult. Cost analysis is, indeed, dependent on a wide variety of factors that differ from one country to another, including health-care system, organization of the hospital and the ICU, the possibility of patients being treated by private practitioners, cost of antibiotics, and so on. Recently, the extra hospital charges attributed to nosocomial pneumonia occurring in trauma patients were evaluated to be US$40,000.[41]

ETIOLOGIC AGENTS

Microorganisms responsible for VAP may differ according to the population of ICU patients, the durations of hospital and ICU stays, and the specific diagnostic method(s) used. The high rate of respiratory infections secondary to GNB in this setting has been repeatedly documented.[1,2] Several studies have reported that >60% of cases of VAP are caused by aerobic GNB. More recently, however, some investigators have reported that gram-positive bacteria have become increasingly more common in this setting, with *S. aureus* being the predominant gram-positive isolate. For example, *S. aureus* was responsible for most episodes of nosocomial pneumonia in the EPIC study, accounting for 31% of the 836 cases with identified responsible pathogens.[42] The data from 24 investigations conducted on ventilated patients, for whom bacteriologic studies were restricted to uncontaminated specimens, confirmed those results: GNB represented 58% of recovered organisms (Table 46-1). The predominant GNB were *P. aeruginosa* and *Acinetobacter* spp., followed by *Proteus* spp., *Escherichia coli, Klebsiella* spp., and *H. influenzae*. A relatively high rate of gram-positive pneumonias was also reported in those studies, with *S. aureus* involved in 20% of the cases.

The high rate of polymicrobial infection in VAP has been emphasized repeatedly. In a study on 172 episodes of bacteremic nosocomial pneumonia, 13% of lung infections were

TABLE 46-1 Etiology of Ventilator-Associated Pneumonia as Documented by Bronchoscopic Techniques in 24 Studies for a Total of 1689 Episodes and 2490 Pathogens

Pathogen	Frequency (%)
Pseudomonas aeruginosa	24.4
Acinetobacter spp.	7.9
Stenotrophomonas maltophilia	1.7
Enterobacteriaceae[a]	14.1
Haemophilus spp.	9.8
Staphylococcus aureus[b]	20.4
Streptococcus spp.	8.0
Streptococcus pneumoniae	4.1
Coagulase-negative staphylococci	1.4
Neisseria spp.	2.6
Anaerobes	0.9
Fungi	0.9
Others (<1% each)[c]	3.8

[a]Distribution when specified: *Klebsiella* spp., 15.6%; *Escherichia coli*, 24.1%; *Proteus* spp., 22.3%; *Enterobacter* spp., 18.8%; *Serratia* spp., 12.1%; *Citrobacter* spp., 5.0%; *Hafnia alvei*, 2.1%.
[b]Distribution when specified: MRSA, 55.7%; MSSA, 44.3%.
[c]Including *Corynebacterium* spp., *Moraxella* spp., and *Enterococcus* spp.
SOURCE: Adapted, with permission, from Chastre et al.[1]

caused by multiple pathogens.[43] Findings were also similar for patients with ARDS: 58% of the 106 VAP episodes were polymicrobial, of which, 55% and 60%, respectively, occurred in patients with and without ARDS.[15]

Underlying diseases may predispose patients to infection with specific organisms. Patients with chronic obstructive pulmonary disease (COPD) are, for example, at increased risk for *H. influenzae, Moraxella catarrhalis,* or *S. pneumoniae* infections; cystic fibrosis increases the risk of *P. aeruginosa* and/or *S. aureus* infections, while trauma and neurologic patients are at increased risk for *S. aureus* infection. Furthermore, the causative agent for pneumonia differs among ICU surgical populations, with 18% of the nosocomial pneumonias being caused by *Haemophilus* or pneumococci, particularly in trauma patients, but not in patients with malignancy, transplantation, or abdominal or cardiovascular surgery.[44]

Despite somewhat different definitions of early-onset pneumonia, varying from <3 to <7 days, high rates of *H. influenzae, S. pneumoniae,* MSSA, or susceptible Enterobacteriaceae were constantly found in early-onset VAP, whereas *P. aeruginosa, Acinetobacter* spp., MRSA, and multiresistant GNB were significantly more frequent in late-onset VAP.[2,45,46] This different distribution pattern of etiologic agents between early- and late-onset VAP is also linked to the frequent administration of prior antimicrobial therapy in many patients with late-onset VAP. In a prospective study which included 129 episodes of nosocomial pneumonia documented by PSB specimens, the distributions of responsible pathogens were compared according to whether or not the patients had received antimicrobial therapy before pneumonia onset.[30] The most striking finding was that the rate of pneumonia caused by gram-positive cocci or *H. influenzae* was significantly lower (*p* <0.05) in patients who had received antibiotics, whereas the rate of pneumonia caused by *P. aeruginosa* was significantly higher (p <0.01). A stepwise logistic regression analysis retained only prior antibiotic use (OR, 9.2; p <0.0001) as significantly influencing the risk of death from pneumonia.[30] Very similar results were obtained when multivariate analysis was used to determine risk factors for VAP caused by potentially drug-resistant bacteria such as MRSA, *P. aeruginosa*, *A. baumannii*, and/or *S. maltophilia* in 135 consecutive episodes of VAP.[47] Only three variables remained significant: duration of MV before VAP onset ≥7 days (OR, 6.0), prior antibiotic use (OR, 13.5), and prior use of broad-spectrum drugs (a third-generation cephalosporin, fluoroquinolone, and/or imipenem) (OR, 4.1).[47] Not all studies, however, have confirmed this distribution pattern. For example, one recent study found that the most common pathogens associated with early-onset VAP were *P. aeruginosa* (25%), MRSA (18%), and *Enterobacter* spp. (10%), with similar pathogens being associated with late-onset VAP.[48] Their finding may, in part, be caused by the prior hospitalization and use of antibiotics in many patients developing early-onset VAP before their transfer to the ICU.

The incidence of multiresistant pathogens is also closely linked to local factors and varies widely from one institution to another. Consequently, each ICU has to continuously collect meticulous epidemiologic data.[49] Clinicians must clearly be aware of the common microorganisms associated with both early-onset and late-onset VAP in their own hospitals in order to avoid the administration of initial inadequate antimicrobial therapy.

Legionella spp., anaerobes, fungi, viruses, and even *Pneumocystis carinii* should be mentioned as potential causative agents but are not considered to be common in the context of pneumonia acquired during mechanical ventilation. Several of these causative agents, however, may be more common and potentially underreported because of difficulties involved with the diagnostic techniques used to identify them, including anaerobic bacteria and viruses.[50,51] By examining currently available data, the clinical significance of anaerobes in the pathogenesis and outcome of VAP remains unclear, except as etiologic agents in patients with necrotizing pneumonitis, lung abscess, or pleuropulmonary infections. Anaerobic infection and coverage with antibiotics, such as clindamycin or metronidazole, should probably also be considered for patients with gram-positive respiratory secretions documenting numerous extra- and intracellular microorganisms in the absence of positive cultures for aerobic pathogens.

Isolation of fungi, most frequently *Candida* species, at significant concentrations poses interpretative problems. Invasive disease has been reported in VAP but, more frequently, yeasts are isolated from respiratory tract specimens in the apparent absence of disease. One prospective study examined the relevance of isolating *Candida* spp. from 25 nonneutropenic patients who had been mechanically ventilated for at least 72 hours.[52] Just after death, multiple culture and biopsy specimens were obtained with bronchoscopic techniques. Although ten patients had at least one biopsy specimen positive for *Candida* spp., only two had evidence of invasive pneumonia as demonstrated by histologic examination. Many of the endotracheal aspirates, PSB speci-

mens, and BAL specimens also yielded positive cultures for *Candida* spp., sometimes in high concentrations, but they did not contribute to diagnosing invasive disease. Based on these data and other studies,[53] the use of the commonly available respiratory sampling methods (bronchoscopic or nonbronchoscopic) in ventilated patients appears insufficient for the diagnosis of *Candida* pneumonia. At present, the only sure method to establish that *Candida* is the primary lung pathogen is to demonstrate yeast or pseudohyphae in a lung biopsy.

Pathogenesis and Predisposing Factors

Pneumonia results from microbial invasion of the normally sterile lower respiratory tract and lung parenchyma caused by either a defect in host defenses, challenge by a particularly virulent microorganism, or an overwhelming inoculum. The normal human respiratory tract possesses a variety of defense mechanisms that protect the lung from infection. Examples include: anatomic barriers, such as the glottis and larynx; cough reflexes; tracheobronchial secretions; mucociliary lining; cell-mediated and humoral immunity; and a dual phagocytic system that involves both alveolar macrophages and neutrophils.[1] When these coordinated components function properly, invading microbes are eliminated and clinical disease is avoided. When these defenses are impaired, however, or if they are overcome by virtue of a high inoculum of organisms or organisms of unusual virulence, pneumonitis results.

As suggested by the infrequent association of VAP with bacteremia, most of these infections appear to result from aspiration of potential pathogens that have colonized the mucosal surfaces of the oropharyngeal airways. Intubation of the patient not only compromises the natural barrier between the oropharynx and trachea, but may also facilitate the entry of bacteria into the lung by pooling and leakage of contaminated secretions around the endotracheal tube cuff.[54] This phenomenon occurs in most intubated patients, whose supine position may facilitate its occurrence. In previously healthy, newly hospitalized patients, normal mouth flora or pathogens associated with community-acquired pneumonia may predominate. In sicker patients who have been hospitalized more than 5 days, GNB and *S. aureus* frequently colonize the upper airway.[55]

Uncommonly, VAP may arise in other ways. Observed "macroaspirations" of gastric material initiate the process in some patients. Allowing condensates in ventilator tubing to drain into the patient's airway may have the same effect. Fiberoptic bronchoscopy, tracheal suctioning or manual ventilation with contaminated equipment may also bring pathogens to the lower respiratory tract. More recently, concerns have focused on the potential role of contaminated in-line medication nebulizers, but these devices are infrequently associated with VAP.

Although tracheal colonization by potentially pathogenic microorganisms occurs before lung infection in a majority of ventilated patients, its relationship with VAP development remains controversial. In 1972, Johanson et al established that upper airway colonization is a frequent occurrence in ventilated patients and that it can act as a harbinger of nosocomial pneumonia in this setting.[55] Those authors demonstrated that 45% of 213 patients admitted to a medical ICU became colonized with aerobic GNB by the end of 1 week in the hospital. Among the 95 colonized patients, 22 (23%) subsequently developed nosocomial pneumonia. By comparison, only 4 of the 118 (3.4%) noncolonized patients developed pneumonia. As determined in that study and several others, the tracheobronchial tree as well as the oropharynx of ventilated patients is frequently colonized by enteric GNB.[55–57] Risk factors for tracheobronchial colonization with GNB appear to be the same as those that favor pneumonia and include more severe illness, longer hospitalization, prior or concomitant use of antibiotics, malnutrition, intubation, azotemia, and underlying pulmonary disease.[57] Experimental investigations have linked some of these risk factors to changes in adherence of GNB to respiratory epithelial cells. Although formerly attributed to losses of cell-surface fibronectin, these changes in adherence more likely reflect alterations of cell-surface carbohydrates. Bacterial adhesins and prior antimicrobial therapy appear to facilitate the process. Interestingly, Enterobacteriaceae usually appear in the oropharynx first, whereas *P. aeruginosa* more often appears first in the trachea.[58]

Other sources of pathogens causing VAP include the paranasal sinuses, dental plaque, and the subglottic area between the true vocal cords and the endotracheal tube cuff. Not all authors agree that the gastropulmonary route of infection is truly operative in ICU patients.[59] Colonization from the stomach to the upper respiratory tract eventually leading to 14 VAP episodes could not be clearly demonstrated in one study.[59] Similarly, de Latorre et al[60] demonstrated that only 19 of 72 patients developed tracheal colonization after pharyngeal or gastric colonization by the same organisms; moreover, among the 12 patients who developed VAP, the microorganism(s) responsible had already colonized the trachea in 10 of them, but only 10 of the 21 responsible microorganisms isolated from VAP had previously colonized the pharynx or stomach. Lastly, efforts to eliminate the gastric reservoir with antimicrobial therapy without decontaminating the oropharyngeal cavity have generally failed to prevent VAP.[61] In fact, there is more than one potential pathway for colonization of the oropharynx and trachea in such a setting, including fecal-oral cross-infection on the hands of health care personnel, and contaminated respiratory therapy equipment. Patient care activities, such as bathing, oral care, tracheal suctioning, enteral feeding, and the tube manipulations, provide ample opportunities for transmission of pathogens when infection-control practices are substandard.[62]

In summary, the relationship between VAP, tracheal, pharyngeal, and/or gastric colonizations remains to be elucidated for patients with an endotracheal tube. To date, these findings lead to the following conclusions: (1) tracheal colonization precedes VAP in most, but not all, patients; (2) only a minority of patients with tracheal colonization develop VAP; (3) and the stomach can be a reservoir for pneumonia pathogens, although this is not the case in many ICU patients requiring mechanical ventilation.

TABLE 46-2 Independent Factors for Ventilator-Associated Pneumonia Identified by Multivariate Analysis

Host Factors	Intervention Factors
Serum albumin <2.2 g/dl	H$_2$-blockers ± antacids
Age ≥60 years	Paralytic agents and continuous intravenous
Acute respiratory distress syndrome	Sedation
COPD or other pulmonary disease	>4 Units of blood products
Coma or impaired consciousness	Intracranial pressure monitoring
Burns and trauma	Mechanical ventilation >2 days
Organ failure	Positive end-expiratory pressure
More severe illness	Frequent ventilator circuit changes
Large-volume gastric aspiration	Reintubation
Gastric colonization and pH	Nasogastric tube
Upper respiratory tract colonization	Supine head position
Sinusitis	Transport out of the ICU
	Prior antibiotic or no antibiotic therapy[a]
	Other factor: Season: fall and winter

[a]See text for explanations.

PREDISPOSING FACTORS

Risk factors provide information on the probability of lung infection developing in individuals and populations. Thus, they may contribute to the elaboration of effective preventive strategies by indicating which patients might be most likely to benefit from prophylaxis against pneumonia. Independent factors for VAP that were identified by multivariate analyses in selected studies are summarized in Table 46-2.[9,11,20,30,41,63–68]

SURGERY

Postsurgical patients are at increased risk for VAP. In a 1981 report, the pneumonia rate during the postoperative period was 17%.[69] Those authors stated that the development of pneumonia was closely associated with preoperative markers of severity of the underlying disease, such as low serum albumin concentration and a high score on the American Society of Anesthesiologists preanesthesia physical status classification. A history of smoking, longer preoperative stays, longer surgical procedures, and thoracic or upper abdominal surgery were also significant risk factors for postsurgical pneumonia. Another study comparing adult ICU populations demonstrated that postoperative patients had consistently higher rates of nosocomial pneumonia than did medical ICU patients, with a risk ratio of 2.2.[67] Multiple regression analysis was performed to identify independent predictors of nosocomial pneumonia in the two groups; for surgical ICU patients, mechanical ventilation (>2 days) and Acute Physiology, Age, and Chronic Health Evaluation (APACHE) score were retained by the model; for the medical ICU population, only MV (>2 days) remained significant. It has been suggested that different surgical ICU patient populations may have different risks for nosocomial pneumonia: cardiothoracic surgery and trauma (particularly the head) patients were more likely to develop VAP than medical or other types of surgical patients.[11]

ANTIMICROBIAL AGENTS

The use of antibiotics in the hospital setting has been associated with an increased risk of nosocomial pneumonia and selection of resistant pathogens.[21,30,42,47,55,70-72] In a cohort study of 320 patients, prior antibiotic administration was identified by logistic regression analysis to be one of the four variables independently associated with VAP along with organ failure, age >60 years, and the patient's head positioning (i.e., flat on the back or supine versus head and thorax raised 30–40° or semirecumbent).[21] Other investigators, however, found that antibiotic administration during the first 8 days was associated with a lower risk of early-onset VAP.[73] For example, Sirvent et al showed that a single dose of a first-generation cephalosporin given prophylactically was associated with a lower rate of early-onset VAP in patients with structural coma.[74] Moreover, multiple logistic regression analysis of risk factors for VAP in 358 medical ICU patients identified the absence of antimicrobial therapy as one of the factors independently associated with VAP onset.[75] Finally, the results of the multicenter Canadian study on the incidence of and risk factors for VAP indicated that antibiotic treatment conferred protection against VAP.[11] This apparent protective effect of antibiotics disappears after 2–3 weeks, suggesting that a higher risk of VAP cannot be excluded beyond this point. Thus, risk factors for VAP change over time, thereby explaining why they differ from one series to another.

STRESS-ULCER PROPHYLAXIS

In theory, patients receiving stress-ulcer prophylaxis that does not change gastric acidity, such as sucralfate, should have lower rates of gastric bacterial colonization and, consequently, a lower risk for nosocomial pneumonia, than those receiving antacids or H_2-blockers.[76,77]

According to meta-analyses of the efficacy of stress-ulcer prophylaxis in ICU patients, respiratory tract infections were significantly less frequent in patients treated with sucralfate than those receiving antacids or H_2-blockers.[78,79] This conclusion, however, was not fully confirmed in a very large, multicenter, randomized, blinded, placebo-controlled trial that compared sucralfate suspension (1 g every 6 hours) with the H_2-receptor antagonist ranitidine (50 mg every 8 hours) for the prevention of upper gastrointestinal bleeding in 1200 ventilated patients.[80] Clinically relevant gastrointestinal bleeding developed in 10 of the 596 (1.7%) patients receiving ranitidine, as compared with 23 of the 604 (3.8%) receiving sucralfate (RR, 0.44; 95% CI, 0.21–0.92; $p = 0.02$). In the ranitidine group, 114 of 596 (19.1%) patients had VAP, as diagnosed by an adjudication committee using a modified version of the CDC criteria, versus 98 of 604 (16.2%) in the sucralfate group (RR, 1.18; 95% CI, 0.92–1.51; $p = 0.19$). Thus, although pneumonia rates were similar for the two groups, the relative risks suggest a trend towards a lower pneumonia rate for patients receiving sucralfate. Furthermore, VAP occurred significantly less frequently in patients receiving sucralfate when the diagnosis of pneumonia was based on Memphis VAP Consensus Conference criteria (if there was radiographic evidence of abscess and a positive needle aspirate, or histologic proof of pneumonia at biopsy or autopsy) ($p = 0.03$).[80]

Sucralfate appears to have a small protective effect against VAP because stress-ulcer prophylactic medications that raise the gastric pH might themselves increase the incidence of pneumonia. This contention is supported by direct comparisons of trials of H_2-receptor antagonists versus no prophylaxis, which showed a trend towards higher pneumonia rates among the patients receiving H_2-receptor antagonists (OR, 1.25; 95% CI, 0.78–2.00).[78] Furthermore, the comparative effects of sucralfate and no prophylaxis are unclear. Among 226 patients enrolled in two randomized trials, those receiving sucralfate tended to develop pneumonia more frequently than those given no prophylaxis (OR, 2.11; 95% CI, 0.82–5.44).[81,82]

ENDOTRACHEAL TUBE, REINTUBATION, AND TRACHEOTOMY

The presence of an endotracheal tube by itself circumvents host defenses, causes local trauma and inflammation, and increases the probability of aspiration of nosocomial pathogens from the oropharynx around the cuff. Scanning electron microscopy of 25 endotracheal tubes revealed that 96% had partial bacterial colonization and 84% were completely coated with bacteria in a biofilm or glycocalyx.[83] The authors hypothesized that bacterial aggregates in biofilm dislodged during suctioning might not be killed by antibiotics or effectively cleared by host immune defenses. Clearly, the type of endotracheal tube may also influence the likelihood of aspiration. Use of low-volume, high-pressure endotracheal cuffs reduced the rate to 56% and the advent of high-volume, low-pressure cuffs further lowered it to 20%.[84] Leakage around the cuff allows secretions pooled above the cuff to enter the trachea; this mechanism, recently confirmed, underlines the importance of maintaining adequate intracuff pressure for preventing VAP.[85]

In addition to the presence of endotracheal tubes, reintubation is, per se, a risk factor for VAP.[86] This finding probably reflects an increased risk of aspiration of colonized oropharyngeal secretions into the lower airways by patients with subglottic dysfunction or impaired consciousness after several days of intubation. Another explanation is direct aspiration of gastric contents into the lower airways, particularly when a nasogastric tube is kept in place after extubation.

The role of early tracheotomy in VAP prevention remains controversial, with only a few studies that examined this issue.[87-92] While some studies found a reduction in the rate of VAP in patients with early tracheotomy,[91] others could not demonstrate any benefit. In the absence of any meaningful data, practice patterns are influenced and guided by strong assumptions and quasi-religious dogma. Until a properly constructed randomized trial is performed to define the timing and utility of tracheotomy in the ICU, its true impact on decreasing VAP will remain merely speculative.[93]

NASOGASTRIC TUBE, ENTERAL FEEDING, AND POSITION OF THE PATIENT

Almost all ventilated patients have a nasogastric tube inserted to evacuate gastric and enteral secretions, prevent gastric distention, and/or provide nutritional support. The nasogastric tube is not generally considered to be a potential risk factor for VAP, but it may increase oropharyngeal colonization, cause stagnation of oropharyngeal secretions, and increase reflux and the risk of aspiration. A multivariate analysis retained the presence of a nasogastric tube as one of the three independent risk factors for nosocomial pneumonia based on a series of 203 patients admitted to the ICU for 72 hours or more.[65]

Early initiation of enteral feeding is generally regarded as beneficial in critically ill patients, but it may increase the risk of gastric colonization, gastroesophageal reflux, aspiration, and pneumonia.[94,95] The aspiration rate generally varies as a function of differences in the patient population, neurologic function, type of feeding tube, location of the feeding port and method of evaluating aspiration. Clinical impressions and preliminary data suggest that postpyloric or jejunal feeding entails less risk of aspiration and may therefore be associated with fewer infectious complications than gastric feeding, although this point remains controversial.[96] Nonetheless, aspiration can easily occur should the feeding tube be inadvertently dislodged. A retrospective study of non-critically ill adult patients showed a 40% rate of accidental feeding-tube dislodgment, but all the patients whose tube was dislodged were confused, disoriented, or had altered awareness, as is frequently observed in ICU patients.[97]

Maintaining ventilated patients with a nasogastric tube in place in a supine position is also a risk factor for aspiration of gastric contents into the lower airways. When radioactive material was injected through a nasogastric tube directly into the stomach of 19 ventilated patients, the mean radioactive counts in endobronchial secretions were higher in a time-dependent fashion in samples obtained from patients in a supine position than in those obtained from patients in a semirecumbent position.[98] The same microorganisms were isolated from the stomach, pharynx, and endobronchial samples of 32% of the specimens taken while patients were lying supine. The same investigators conducted a randomized trial comparing semirecumbent and supine positions.[99] The trial, which included 86 intubated and ventilated patients, was stopped after the planned interim analysis because the frequency and the risk of VAP were significantly lower for the semirecumbent group. These findings were indirectly confirmed by the demonstration that the head position of the supine patient during the first 24 hours of mechanical ventilation was an independent risk factor for acquiring VAP.[21]

RESPIRATORY EQUIPMENT

Ventilators with humidifying cascades often have high levels of tubing colonization and condensate formation that may also be risk factors for pneumonia. The rate of condensate formation in the ventilator circuit is linked to the temperature difference between the inspiratory-phase gas and the ambient temperature, and may be as high as 20–40 ml/hour.[100,101] Examination of condensate coloniza-

tion in 20 circuits detected a median level of 2.0×10^5 organisms/ml, and 73% of the 52 gram-negative isolates present in the patients' sputum samples were subsequently isolated from condensates.[101] Because most of the tubing colonization was derived from the patients' secretions, the highest bacterial counts were present near the endotracheal tube. Simple procedures, such as turning the patient or raising the bed rail, may accidentally spill contaminated condensate directly into the patient's tracheobronchial tree.[102] Inoculation of large amounts of fluid with high bacterial concentrations is an excellent way to overwhelm pulmonary defense mechanisms and cause pneumonia. Heating ventilator tubing markedly lowers the rate of condensate formation, but heated circuits are often nondisposable and expensive. In-line devices with one-way valves to collect the condensate are probably the easiest way to handle this problem; they must be correctly positioned in disposable circuits and emptied regularly.

To decrease condensation and moisture accumulation in ventilator circuits, several studies have investigated the use of heat-moisture exchangers (HMEs) in place of conventional heated-water humidification systems. Slightly lower VAP rates were observed in four studies and a significant difference in a fifth study, suggesting that HMEs are at least comparable to heated humidifiers and may be associated with lower VAP rates than heated humidifiers.[103–107] Changing the HME every 48 hours did not affect ventilator-circuit colonization and the authors concluded that the cost of mechanical ventilation might be substantially reduced without any detriment to the patient by prolonging the time between HME changes from 24 to 48 hours.[108] Furthermore, using HMEs may decrease the nurses' workload (no need to refill cascades, to void water traps on circuits, and so on), decrease the number of septic procedures (it was clearly shown that respiratory tubing condensates must be handled as an infectious waste product), and reduce the cost of mechanical ventilation, especially when used for prolonged periods without change. Because some observational studies, however, have documented an increased resistive load and a larger dead space associated with exchangers,[109,110] their use should be discouraged in patients with ARDS ventilated with a low tidal volume and in patients with COPD during the weaning period, if pressure support, and not T-piece trials, are used.

There is no apparent advantage to changing ventilator circuits frequently for VAP prevention. This holds true whether circuits are changed every 2 days or every 7 days compared with no change at all, and whether they are changed weekly as opposed to 3 times per week.[111–113] A policy of no circuit changes or infrequent circuit changes is simple to implement and the costs are likely lower than those generated by regular, frequent circuit changes; thus, such a policy is strongly recommended by the 1997 CDC guidelines.[114]

SINUSITIS

While many studies have compared the risk of nosocomial sinusitis as a function of the intubation method used and the associated risk of VAP, only a few were adequately powered to give a clear answer. In one study of 300 patients who required mechanical ventilation for at least 7 days and were randomly assigned to undergo nasotracheal or orotracheal intubation, computed tomographic evidence of sinusitis was observed slightly more frequently in the nasal than the oral endotracheal group ($p = 0.08$), but this difference disappeared when only bacteriologically confirmed sinusitis was considered.[115] The rate of infectious maxillary sinusitis and its clinical relevance were also prospectively studied in 162 consecutive critically ill patients, who had been intubated and ventilated for 1 hour to 12 days before enrollment.[116] All had a paranasal computed tomography scan within 48 hours of admission which was used to divide them into three groups (no, moderate, or severe sinusitis), according to the radiologic appearance of the maxillary sinuses. Patients who had no sinusitis at admission (n = 40) were randomized to receive endotracheal and gastric tubes via the nasal or oral route and, based on radiologic images, respective sinusitis rates were 96% and 23% ($p < 0.03$); yet, no differences in the rates of infectious sinusitis were documented according to the intubation route. VAP, however, was more common in patients with infectious sinusitis, with 67% of them developing lung infection in the days following the diagnosis of sinusitis.[116] Therefore, whereas it seems clear that infectious sinusitis is a risk factor for VAP, no studies have yet been able to definitively demonstrate that orotracheal intubation decreases the infectious sinusitis rate compared to nasotracheal intubation. Thus no firm recommendations on the best route of intubation to prevent VAP can be advanced.

INTRAHOSPITAL PATIENT TRANSPORT

A prospective cohort study conducted in 531 ventilated patients evaluated the impact of transporting the patient out of the ICU to other sites within the hospital.[117] Results showed that 52% of the patients had to be moved at least once for a total of 993 transports, and that 24% of the transported patients developed VAP compared with 4% of the patients confined to the ICU ($p < 0.001$). Multiple logistic regression analysis confirmed that transport out of the ICU was independently associated with VAP (OR, 3.8; $p < 0.001$).

Diagnosis

Two diagnostic algorithms can be used in cases of suspected VAP. One option is to treat every patient clinically suspected of having a pulmonary infection with new antibiotics, even when the likelihood of infection is low, arguing that several studies showed that immediate initiation of appropriate antibiotics was associated with reduced mortality.[35,118,119] In this option, the selection of appropriate empiric therapy is based on risk factors, local resistance patterns, and involves qualitative testing to identify possible pathogens, antimicrobial therapy being adjusted according to culture results or clinical response (Fig. 46-1). This "clinical" approach has two potential advantages: first, no specialized microbiologic techniques are requested, and second, the risk of missing a patient who needs antimicrobial treatment is minimal, at

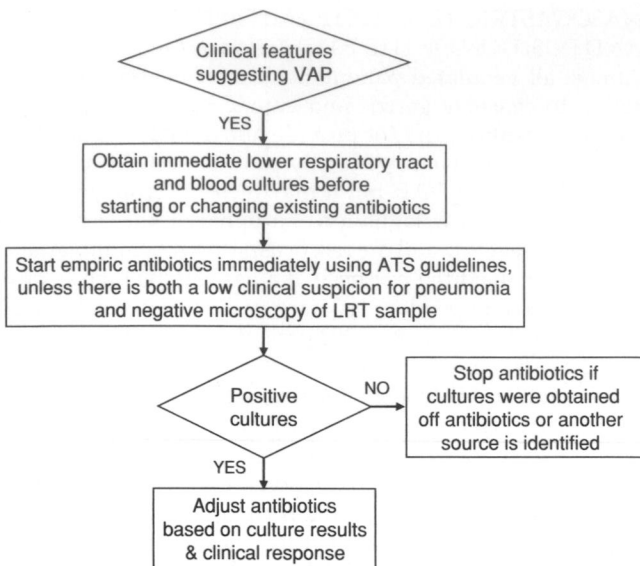

FIGURE 46-1 A diagnostic and therapeutic strategy applied to patients managed with the "clinical" strategy. LRT, lower respiratory tract; VAP, ventilator-associated pneumonia.

least when all suspected patients are treated with new antibiotics. Such a strategy, however, leads to overestimation of the incidence of VAP because tracheobronchial colonization and noninfectious processes mimicking it are included. Qualitative endotracheal aspirate cultures contribute indisputably to the diagnosis of VAP only when they are completely negative for a patient with no modification of prior antimicrobial treatment. In such a case, the negative predictive value is very high and the probability of the patient having pneumonia is close to zero.[5]

Concern about the inaccuracy of clinical approaches to VAP recognition and the impossibility of using such a strategy to avoid overprescription of antibiotics in the ICU had led numerous investigators to postulate that specialized diagnostic methods, including quantitative cultures of endotracheal aspirates or specimens obtained with bronchoscopic or nonbronchoscopic techniques including bronchoalveolar lavage (BAL) and/or protected specimen brush (PSB), could improve identification of patients with true VAP, and facilitate decisions whether or not to treat, and thus also improve clinical outcome.[1,120,121] Using such a strategy, the decision algorithm is similar to the one described in Fig. 46-1, except that therapeutic decisions are taken based on results of direct examination of distal pulmonary samples and results of quantitative cultures (Fig. 46-2).

BRONCHOSCOPIC VERSUS NONBRONCHOSCOPIC TECHNIQUES

Bronchoscopy provides direct access to the lower airways for sampling bronchial and parenchymal tissues directly at the site of lung inflammation. One major technical problem with all bronchoscopic techniques is proper selection of the sampling area in the tracheobronchial tree. Almost

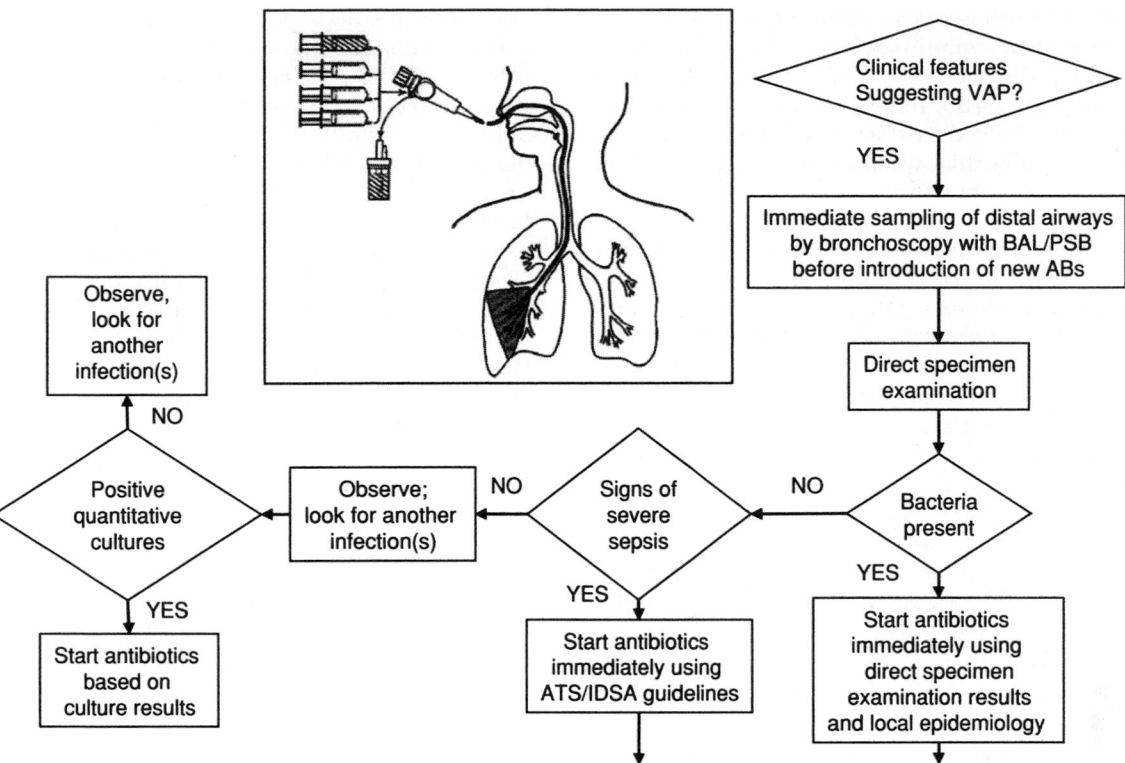

FIGURE 46-2 A diagnostic and therapeutic strategy applied to patients managed with the "invasive" strategy. AB, antibiotic; BAL, bronchoalveolar lavage; PSB, protected specimen brush.

all intubated patients have purulent-looking secretions and the secretions first seen may represent those aspirated from another site into gravity-dependent airways or from upper-airway secretions aspirated around the endotracheal tube. Usually, the sampling area is selected based on the location of infiltrate on chest radiograph or the segment visualized during bronchoscopy as having purulent secretions.[122] Collection of secretions in the lower trachea or main-stem bronchi, which may represent secretions that were recently aspirated around the endotracheal tube cuff, should be avoided. In patients with diffuse pulmonary infiltrates or minimal changes in a previously abnormal chest radiograph, determining the correct airway to sample may be difficult. In these cases, sampling should be directed to the area where endobronchial abnormalities are maximal. In case of doubt, and because autopsy studies indicate that VAP frequently involves the posterior portion of the right lower lobe, this area should probably be sampled as a first priority.[123] While in the immunosuppressed host with diffuse infiltrates bilateral sampling has been advocated, there is no convincing evidence that multiple specimens are more accurate than single specimens for diagnosing nosocomial bacterial pneumonia in ventilated patients.

The risk inherent in bronchoscopy appears slight, even in critically-ill ventilated patients, although cardiac arrhythmias, hypoxemia, or bronchospasm are not unusual. A study conducted by Trouillet et al in 107 ventilated patients has shown that fiberoptic bronchoscopy under midazolam is practical in this setting.[124] No death or cardiac arrest occurred during or within the 2 hours immediately following

the procedure. Patients in the ICU, however, are at risk of relative hypoxemia during bronchoscopy, even when high levels of oxygen are provided to the ventilator and gas leaks around the endoscope are minimized by a special adaptor. An average decline in mean arterial oxygen tension (Pa_{O_2}) of 26% was observed at the end of the procedure (compared to the baseline), associated with a mild increase in Pa_{CO_2}. The degree of hypoxemia induced by bronchoscopy was linked to the severity of pulmonary dysfunction and the decrease in alveolar ventilation. Multivariate analysis showed that clinical hypoxemia, as defined by Pa_{O_2} lower than 60 mmHg, was more frequent in patients with ARDS and in those who "fought" the ventilator during the procedure. Careful attention to the anesthetic protocol with addition of a short-acting neuromuscular blocking agent, and monitoring of patients should permit rapid correction and more frequent prevention of hypoxemia in this setting, and therefore should further decrease the morbidity of bronchoscopy. In another study, conducted in a large series of patients with ARDS, only 5% had arterial oxygen desaturation to <90% during bronchoscopy despite severe hypoxemia in many patients prebronchoscopy.[125]

Certain procedures, however, increase the risk of complications, particularly in some subsets of patients. Risk of bleeding with PSB sampling is particularly significant in patients with thrombocytopenia or a coagulopathy. Pneumothorax is principally a complication of PSB, although it can occur after BAL alone, in ventilated patients. The risk with bronchoscopy is paradoxically more important in nonventilated patients than in ventilated patients, because performance of bronchoscopy in a critically-ill patient with impending respiratory failure may lead to profound hypoxemia and rapid decompensation. While bacteremia does not appear to occur after PSB, release of the cytokine tumor necrosis factor has been documented in patients undergoing BAL.[126] Transbronchial spread of infection is also an extremely remote possibility.[122]

At least 15 studies have described a variety of nonbronchoscopic techniques using various types of endobronchial catheters for sampling distal lower respiratory tract secretions; results have been similar to those obtained with bronchoscopy.[127] Compared to conventional PSB and/or BAL, nonbronchoscopic techniques are less invasive, can be performed by clinicians not qualified to perform bronchoscopy, have lower initial costs than bronchoscopy, avoid potential contamination by the bronchoscopic channel, are associated with less compromise of gas exchange during the procedure, and can be performed even in patients intubated with small endotracheal tubes. Disadvantages include the potential sampling errors inherent in a blind technique and the lack of airway visualization. Although autopsy studies indicate that pneumonia in ventilator-dependent patients has often spread into every pulmonary lobe and predominantly involves the posterior portion of the lower lobes, several clinical studies on ventilated patients with pneumonia contradict those findings, because some patients had sterile cultures of PSB specimens from the noninvolved lung.[18,128] Furthermore, although the authors of most studies concluded that the sensitivities of nonbronchoscopic and bronchoscopic techniques were comparable, the overall concordance was only approximately 80%, emphasizing that, in some patients, the diagnosis could be missed by a blind technique, especially in the case of pneumonia involving the left lung, as demonstrated by Meduri et al.[18]

Simple qualitative culture of endotracheal aspirates is a technique with a high percentage of false-positive results caused by bacterial colonization of the proximal airways that is seen in most ICU patients. Some recent studies using quantitative culture techniques, however, suggest that endotracheal aspirate cultures may have an acceptable overall diagnostic accuracy, similar to that of several other more invasive techniques.[129] To assess the reliability of that method, bronchoscopy with PSB and BAL was used to study 57 episodes of suspected lung infection in 39 ventilator-dependent patients with no recent changes of antimicrobial therapy.[130] The operating characteristics of endotracheal aspirate cultures were calculated over a range of cutoff values (from 10^3–10^7 colony-forming units (cfu)/ml); the threshold of 10^6 cfu/ml appeared to be the most accurate, with a sensitivity of 68% and a specificity of 84%. When this threshold was applied to the study population, however, almost one-third of the patients with pneumonia were not identified. Furthermore, only 40% of microorganisms cultured in endotracheal aspirate samples coincided with those obtained from PSB specimens. Other authors have emphasized that, although quantitative endotracheal aspirate cultures can correctly identify patients with pneumonia, microbiologic results cannot be used to infer which microorganisms present in the trachea are really present in the lungs. In a study comparing quantitative endotracheal aspi-

rate culture results to postmortem quantitative lung-biopsy cultures, only 53% of the microorganisms isolated from the former samples at concentrations $>10^7$ cfu/ml were also found in the latter cultures.[131] Therefore, quantitative endotracheal aspirate cultures may be an adequate tool for diagnosing pneumonia when no fiberoptic techniques are available, but it must be kept in mind that this technique has several potential pitfalls. First, many patients may not be identified using the cutoff value of 10^6 cfu/ml. Second, as soon as a lower threshold is used, specificity declines sharply and overtreatment becomes a problem. Finally, selecting antimicrobial therapy solely on the basis of endotracheal aspirate culture results can lead to either unnecessary antibiotic therapy or overtreatment with broad-spectrum antimicrobial agents.

SPECIMEN TYPES AND LABORATORY METHODS

The methodology for PSB sampling was originally described by Wimberley et al.[132] This method is in fact based on a combination of four different techniques: (1) use of bronchoscopy to directly sample the site of inflammation in the lung; (2) use of a double-lumen catheter brush system with a distal occluding plug to prevent secretions from entering the catheter during passage through the bronchoscope channel; (3) use of a brush to calibrate the volume of secretions retrieved; and (4) use of quantitative culture techniques to aid in distinguishing between airway colonization and serious underlying infection, with a cutoff point of 10^3 cfu/ml for making this distinction. In an in vitro study, this system proved to be the most effective among seven different types tested as follows. Catheters containing a protected brush were passed through a bronchoscope heavily contaminated with saliva to reach the distal sample (i.e., a Petri dish containing a known number of organisms).[132] Single-sheathed catheter brushes and telescoping plugged catheter tips with or without distal plugs are, however, also available, and have been used for the diagnosis of pneumonia, even though neither has been subjected to the rigorous evaluation reported for the PSB.[133]

BAL requires careful wedging of the tip of the bronchoscope into an airway lumen, isolating that airway from the rest of the central airways. Infusion of at least 120 ml of saline in several (3–6) aliquots is needed to sample fluids and secretions in the distal respiratory bronchioles and alveoli.[1,122,134] It is estimated that the alveolar surface area distal to the wedged bronchoscope is 100 times greater than that of the peripheral airway, and that approximately 1 million alveoli (1% of the lung surface) are sampled, with approximately 1 ml of actual lung secretions retrieved in the total lavage fluid. The fluid return on BAL varies greatly and may affect the validity of results. In patients with emphysema, collapse of airways with the negative pressure needed to aspirate fluid may limit the amount of fluid retrieved. A very small return may contain only diluted material from the bronchial rather than alveolar level and results in false-negative results.

Regardless of the technique used, rapid processing of specimens for culture is desirable to prevent loss of viability of pathogens or overgrowth of contaminants. For PSB, it is recommended that the brush be aseptically cut into a measured volume (1 ml) of sterile diluent, most commonly, nonbacteriostatic saline or lactated Ringer's solution.[134] For BAL, transport in a sterile, leakproof, nonadherent glass container is recommended to avoid loss of cells for cytologic assessment. The initial aliquot, which is usually considered as essentially representative of distal bronchi, should be either discarded or transported separately from the remaining pooled fractions.[122,134] Excessive delays in transport to the laboratory should be avoided.[135] Although no absolute guideline exists, it is generally accepted that no more than 30 minutes should elapse before specimens are processed for microbiologic analysis. According to some investigators, refrigeration to prolong transport time may be used, but this technique remains controversial.[136,137]

Once specimens are received in the laboratory, they should be processed according to clearly defined procedures (see references 134 and 135 for a complete description). Because of inevitable oropharyngeal bacterial contamination that occurs in the collection of all respiratory secretion samples, quantitative culture techniques are always needed to differentiate infecting organisms from oropharyngeal contaminants present at low concentrations. Pathogens are present in lower respiratory tract inflammatory secretions at concentrations of at least 10^5–10^6 cfu/ml, whereas contaminants are generally present at $<10^4$ cfu/ml.[138] The diagnostic thresholds proposed for PSB and BAL are based on this concept. Because PSB collects between 0.001 and 0.01 ml of secretions, the presence of $>10^3$ bacteria in the originally diluted sample (1 ml) actually represents 10^5–10^6 cfu/ml of pulmonary secretions. Similarly, 10^4 cfu/ml for BAL, which collects 1 ml of secretions in 10–100 ml of effluent, represents actual levels of 10^5–10^6 cfu/ml.[135]

Although PSB samples can be subjected to direct microscopy, the optimal method for smear preparation has not yet been established. For BAL, it is recommended that a total cell count be performed to assess adequacy and a differential count be performed to assess cellularity. For quality assessment, the percentages of squamous and bronchial epithelial cells may be used to predict heavy upper respiratory contamination. Although only a few studies have directly assessed this point, it is proposed that the sample be rejected if more than 1% of the total cells are squamous or bronchial epithelial cells.[139] Modified Giemsa staining (e.g., Diff-Quik, American Scientific Products, McGraw Park, IL) is recommended, because it offers a number of advantages over Gram's staining, including better visualization of host-cell morphology, improved detection of bacteria, particularly intracellular bacteria, and detection of some protozoan and fungal pathogens (e.g., *Histoplasma, Pneumocystis, Toxoplasma,* and *Candida* spp.).[135] Because BAL harvests of cells and secretions from a large area of the lung and specimens can be microscopically examined immediately after the procedure to detect the presence or absence of intracellular or extracellular bacteria in the lower respiratory tract, it is particularly well suited to provide rapid identification of patients with pneumonia (Figs. 46-3 and 46-4).[140–146] Assessment of the degree of qualitative agreement between Gram's stains of BAL fluid and PSB quantitative cultures for a series

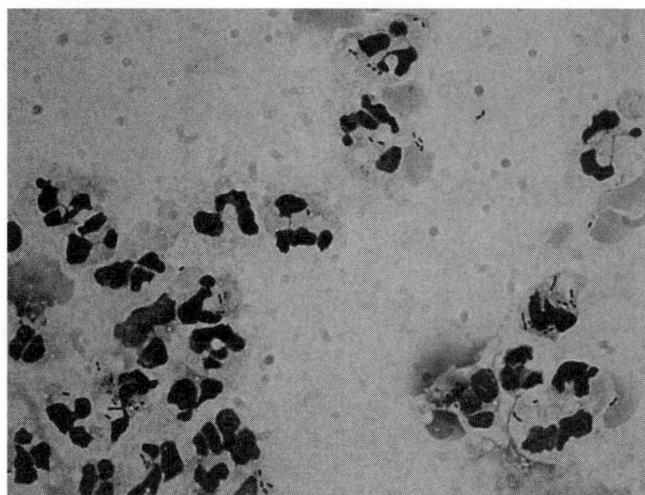

FIGURE 46-3 Light photomicrograph of cells recovered by BAL from a patient with *Pseudomonas aeruginosa* pneumonia.

of 51 patients with VAP, however, showed correspondence to be complete for 51%, partial for 39%, and nonexistent for 10% of the cases.[143].

DIAGNOSTIC ACCURACY OF PROTECTED SPECIMEN BRUSH AND BRONCHOALVEOLAR LAVAGE TECHNIQUES

The contribution of the PSB technique in evaluating ICU patients suspected of VAP has been extensively investigated in both human and animal studies. The studies include eight investigations in which the accuracy of this culture technique was determined by comparison with both histologic features and quantitative cultures from the same area of the lung.[142,147–153] Despite the need for cautious interpretation, the studies show that the PSB technique offers a sensitive and specific approach to identifying the microorganisms involved in pneumonia in critically ill patients, and differentiating between colonization of the upper respiratory tract and distal lung infection. Pooling the results of the

FIGURE 46-4 Light photomicrograph of cells recovered by BAL from a patient with *Staphylococcus aureus* pneumonia.

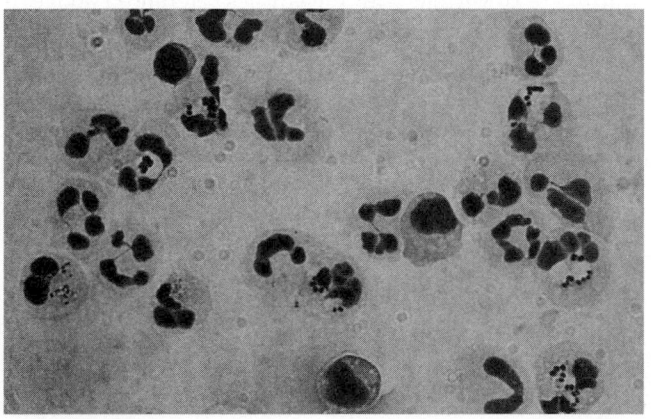

18 studies evaluating the PSB technique in a total of 795 critically ill patients shows that the overall accuracy for diagnosing pneumonia is high: sensitivity 89% (95% CI, 87–93%), specificity 94% (95% CI, 92–97%).[154,155].

Although providing a broader assessment of lung content than PSB, BAL is subject to the same risk of contamination as protected bronchial brushings. Many groups have now investigated the value of quantitative BAL culture for the diagnosis of pneumonia in ICU patients.[142,154,156] Some investigators have concluded that BAL provides the best reflection of the lung's bacterial burden, both quantitatively and qualitatively. Others have reported mixed results, with poor specificity of BAL fluid cultures in patients with high tracheobronchial colonization. When the results of the 11 studies evaluating BAL fluids from a total of 435 ICU patients with nosocomial pneumonia were pooled, overall accuracy was very close to that of PSB: the Q value was 0.84 (Q represents the intersection between the summary receiver operating characteristics [ROC] curve and a diagonal from the upper left corner to the lower right corner of the ROC space).[154] Similar conclusions were drawn in another meta-analysis, which pooled the results of 23 studies: sensitivity and specificity of BAL were $73 \pm 18\%$ and $82 \pm 19\%$, respectively.[156]

PATIENTS ALREADY RECEIVING ANTIMICROBIAL THERAPY

Performing microbiologic cultures of pulmonary secretions for diagnostic purposes after initiation of new antibiotic therapy in patients suspected of having developed nosocomial pneumonia leads to a high rate of false-negative results, regardless of the method of obtaining the secretions. In fact, all microbiologic techniques are of limited value in patients with a recent infiltrate who have received new antibiotics, even for less than 24 hours. A negative finding could indicate that the patient has been successfully treated for pneumonia and the bacteria are eradicated, or that the patient had no lung infection to begin with. Using both PSB and BAL, Souweine et al prospectively investigated 63 episodes of suspected VAP.[157] Based on prior antibiotic treatment, three groups were defined: no previous antibiotic treatments (n = 12); antibiotic treatment initiated >72 hours earlier (n = 31); and a new antibiotic treatment class started within the preceding 24 hours (n = 20). Results were consistent with the studies referenced above. If patients had been treated with antibiotics but did not have a recent change in antibiotic class, sensitivity of PSB and BAL culture (83% and 77%, respectively) were similar to the sensitivities achieved in patients not being treated with antibiotics. In other words, prior therapy did not reduce the yield of diagnostic testing among patients receiving current antibiotics given to treat a prior infection. Conversely, if therapy was recent, sensitivity of invasive diagnostic methods, using traditional thresholds, was only 38% with BAL and 40% with PSB.[157–159] These two clinical situations should be clearly distinguished before interpreting the results of pulmonary secretion cultures, irrespective of how they were obtained. In the second situation, when the patient receives new antibiotics after the appearance of signs suggesting pulmonary infection, no conclusion concerning the presence or absence of pneumonia can be drawn if culture results are negative. Pulmonary secretions therefore need to be obtained before starting new antibiotics, as is the case for all types of microbiologic samples.

POTENTIAL LIMITATIONS OF BRONCHOSCOPIC TECHNIQUES

Four studies involving postmortem lung biopsies have suggested that, in the presence of prior antibiotic treatment, many patients with histopathologic signs of pneumonia have no or only minimal growth from lung and bronchoscopic specimen cultures.[5,123,153,160]

It should be remembered, however, that several constraints specific to the evaluation of any procedure used in the diagnosis of bacterial pneumonia must be respected, even when using a model in which the gold standard includes both histologic features and quantitative cultures of lung tissue. First, diagnostic methods based on microbiologic techniques can only document, both qualitatively and quantitatively, the bacterial burden present in lung tissue. In no cases can these techniques retrospectively identify a resolving pneumonia, at a time when antimicrobial treatment and lung antibacterial defenses might have been successful in suppressing microbial growth in lung tissue. Therefore, to evaluate the accuracy of any technique that uses lung cultures as the gold standard, it is imperative that no new antibiotics were introduced during this time interval. Second, using histologic criteria as a reference implies that the patient had not developed a lung infection before the episode under evaluation; otherwise, it would be difficult (if not impossible) to distinguish a recent infection from the sequelae of a previous infection, and thus correctly interpret the results of the diagnostic tool(s) under evaluation. Finally, lesions of bronchopneumonia in patients with VAP may be confined to certain locations in the lungs.[123,160] Therefore, if postmortem tissue samples are too small, the histologic diagnosis of pneumonia can be underestimated. Conversely a technique based on peripheral samplings can provide information only on the lung segment from which specimens had been taken, and so-called "false-negative" results of PSB or BAL, as defined by examination of the entire lung, can be explained by the absence of pneumonia at the exact location of sampling.

When analysis in these studies was restricted to patients without prior antibiotics or when only lung tissue cultures were used as the gold standard, results of bronchoscopic techniques used to detect pneumonia were much better: sensitivity was always >80%. Other studies have confirmed the accuracy of bronchoscopic techniques for diagnosing nosocomial pneumonia. In a study evaluating spontaneous lung infections occurring in ventilated baboons with permeability pulmonary edema, Johanson et al found excellent correlation between the bacterial content of lung tissue and results of quantitative culture of lavage fluid and PSB specimens.[147] BAL recovered 74% of all species present in lung tissue, including 100% of species present at a concentration $\geq 10^4$ cfu/g of tissue. In this study, PSB specimens identified only 41% of all species recovered from lung tissue. Only microorganisms present at low concentrations in the lung were missed, because 78% of species present at concentrations $>10^4$ cfu/g of tissue were correctly isolated. Similarly, in 20 ventilated patients who had not developed pneumonia before the terminal phase of disease and who had no recent changes in antimicrobial therapy, Chastre et al found that bronchoscopic PSB and BAL specimens obtained just after death identified 80% of all species present in the lung, with a strong correlation between the results of quantitative cultures of both specimens.[142] These findings confirm that bronchoscopic PSB and/or BAL samples very reliably identify, both qualitatively and quantitatively, microorganisms present in lung segments, even when the pneumonia develops as a superinfection in a patient already receiving antimicrobial treatment for several days.

Values within 1 $\log_{10}$ of the cutoff must, however, be interpreted cautiously, and bronchoscopy should be repeated in symptomatic patients with a negative ($<10^3$ cfu/ml) result.[161] Many technical factors, including medium and adequacy of incubation, and antibiotic or other toxic components may influence results. Reproducibility of PSB sampling has recently been evaluated by three groups. Although in vitro repeatability was excellent and in vivo qualitative recovery 100%, quantitative results were more variable. In 14–17% of patients, results of replicate samples fell on both sides of the 10^3-cfu/ml threshold, and results varied by more than 1 $\log_{10}$ in 59–67% of samples.[162–164] This variability is presumably related to both the irregular distribution of organisms in secretions and the very small volume actually sampled by PSB. In conclusion, as with all diagnostic tests, borderline PSB and/or BAL quantitative culture results should be interpreted cautiously, and the clinical circumstances should be considered before reaching any therapeutic decision.

ARGUMENTS FOR QUANTITATIVE TECHNIQUE IN THE DIAGNOSIS OF VENTILATOR-ASSOCIATED PNEUMONIA

Invasive techniques, such as fiberoptic bronchoscopy coupled with quantitative cultures of PSB or BAL specimens, help direct initial antibiotic therapy in addition to confirming the actual diagnosis of nosocomial pneumonia. When culture results are available, they facilitate precise identification of the offending organisms and their susceptibility patterns. Such data are invaluable for optimal antibiotic selection. They also increase the confidence and comfort level of health care workers in managing patients with suspected nosocomial pneumonia.[165]

The second most compelling argument for invasive techniques is that they can reduce excessive antibiotic use. There is little disagreement that the clinical diagnosis of nosocomial pneumonia is overly sensitive and leads to the unnecessary use of broad-spectrum antibiotics. Because bronchoscopic techniques may be more specific, their use would reduce antibiotic pressure in the ICU, thereby limiting the emergence of drug-resistant strains and the attendant increased risks of superinfection.[21,166] Most epidemiologic investigations have clearly demonstrated that indiscrimi-

nant use of antimicrobial agents in ICU patients may have immediate and long-term consequences, which contribute to emergence of multiresistant pathogens and increase the risk of serious superinfections.[167] This risk is not limited to one patient. Instead, the risk of colonization or infection by multidrug-resistant strains is increased in patients throughout the ICU and even the entire hospital. Virtually all reports emphasize that better antibiotic control programs to limit bacterial resistance are urgently needed in ICUs, and that patients without true infection should not receive antimicrobial treatment.[167]

The more targeted use of antibiotics also could reduce overall costs, despite the expense of bronchoscopy and quantitative cultures, and minimize antibiotic-related toxicity. This is particularly true in patients who have late-onset VAP, in whom expensive combination therapy is commonly recommended. A conservative cost analysis in a trauma ICU suggested that the discontinuation of antibiotics upon the return of negative bronchoscopic quantitative culture results could lead to a savings of more than $1700 per patient suspected of VAP.[168]

Finally, the most important risk of not performing bronchoscopy is that another site of infection may be missed. A major benefit of a negative bronchoscopy is to direct attention away from the lungs as the source of fever. Many hospitalized patients with negative bronchoscopic cultures have other potential sites of infection that can be identified via a simple diagnostic protocol. In 50 patients with suspected VAP who underwent a systematic diagnostic protocol designed to identify all potential causes of fever and pulmonary densities, Meduri et al confirmed that lung infection was present in only 42% of cases; the frequent occurrence of multiple infectious and noninfectious processes justifies a systematic search for the source of fever in this setting.[169] Delay in diagnosis or definitive treatment of the true site of infection may lead to prolonged antibiotic therapy, more antibiotic-associated complications, and induction of further organ dysfunction.[170]

Other than decision-analysis studies.[171–173] and one retrospective study,[165] only four trials assessed the impact of a diagnostic strategy on antibiotic use and outcome of patients suspected of hospital-acquired pneumonia using a randomized scheme[32,33,121,174] One of the first studies to clearly demonstrate a benefit of the bacteriologic strategy was a prospective cohort study conducted in 10 Canadian ICUs.[165] The authors compared 92 patients with suspected pneumonia who underwent fiberoptic bronchoscopy and 49 patients who did not. Mortality among bronchoscopy patients was 19% versus 35% for controls ($p = 0.03$). Patients managed with a bacteriologic strategy received fewer antibiotics and more patients had all antibiotics discontinued compared to the control group.

No differences in mortality and morbidity were found when either invasive (PSB and/or BAL) or noninvasive (quantitative endotracheal aspirate cultures) techniques were used to diagnose VAP in three Spanish randomized studies.[32,33,174] Those studies, however, were based on relatively few patients (51, 76, and 88, respectively). Antibiotics were continued in all patients despite negative cultures, thereby neutralizing one potential advantage of any diagnostic test in patients with suspected VAP. Concerning the latter, several prospective studies have concluded that antibiotics can be stopped in patients with negative quantitative cultures, without adversely affecting the recurrence of pneumonia and mortality.[120,140]

A large, prospective, randomized trial compared clinical versus bacteriologic strategy for the management of 413 patients suspected of having VAP.[121] The clinical strategy included empiric antimicrobial therapy, based on clinical evaluation and the presence of bacteria on direct examination of tracheal aspirates, and possible subsequent adjustment or discontinuation according to the results of qualitative cultures of endotracheal aspirates. The bacteriologic strategy consisted of fiberoptic bronchoscopy with direct examination of BAL and/or PSB samples, and empiric therapy initiated only when results were positive. Definitive diagnosis, based on quantitative culture results of samples obtained with PSB or BAL, was awaited before adjusting, discontinuing, or, for some patients with negative direct examination (no bacteria identified on cytocentrifuge preparation of BAL fluid or PSB samples) and positive quantitative cultures ($>10^3$ cfu/ml for PSB and $>10^4$ cfu/ml for BAL), starting therapy (see Fig. 46-2). Empirical antimicrobial therapy was initiated in 91% of patients in the clinical strategy group and in only 52% of those in the bacteriologic strategy group. Compared with patients managed clinically, those receiving bacteriologic management had a lower mortality rate on day 14 (25% and 16%; $p = 0.02$), lower sepsis-related organ failure assessment scores on days 3 and 7 ($p = 0.04$), and less antibiotic use (mean number of antibiotic-free days, 2 ± 3 and 5 ± 5; $p < 0.001$). Multivariate analysis showed a significant difference in mortality on day 28 in favor of bacteriologic management, associated with a significant reduction in antibiotic consumption. Pertinently, 22 nonpulmonary infections were diagnosed in the bacteriologic strategy group and only 5 in the clinical strategy group, suggesting that overdiagnosis of VAP may lead to missed nonpulmonary infections. The possible consequences of delayed treatment or definitive diagnosis secondary to antibiotic interference are prolonged antibiotic therapy, more antibiotic-associated complications, and induction of additional organ dysfunctions.

Our personal bias is that use of bronchoscopic techniques to obtain PSB and BAL specimens from an affected area of the lung in ventilated patients with signs suggestive of pneumonia enables the formulation of a therapeutic strategy that is superior to that based exclusively on clinical evaluation. Bronchoscopic techniques, when performed before the introduction of new antibiotics, enable physicians to identify most patients who need immediate treatment, and help select optimal therapy that is safe and well-tolerated. These techniques also avoid resorting to broad-spectrum coverage of all patients with a clinical suspicion of infection.[175] The full impact of this decision tree on patient outcome remains controversial. Yet, being able to withhold antimicrobial treatment from some patients without infection may constitute a distinct advantage in the long term, by minimizing the emergence of resistant microorganisms in the ICU and redirecting the search toward the actual infection site.

In patients with clinical evidence of severe sepsis and rapidly worsening organ dysfunction, hypoperfusion, or hypotension, or patients with a very high pretest probability of disease, the initiation of antibiotic therapy should not be delayed while awaiting the results of bronchoscopy. These patients should be given immediate antibiotics. In this situation, simple nonbronchoscopic procedures find their best justification, allowing distal pulmonary secretions to be obtained on a 24-hour basis, just before starting new antimicrobial therapy.

Despite broad experience with both PSB and BAL, it remains unclear which should be used. Most investigators prefer BAL over PSB to diagnose bacterial pneumonia, because BAL: (1) has a slightly higher sensitivity to identify VAP-causative microorganisms, (2) enables better selection of an empiric antimicrobial treatment regimen before culture results are available, (3) is less dangerous for many critically ill patients, (4) is less costly, and (5) may provide useful clues for the diagnosis of other types of infections. Nevertheless, a very small return on BAL may contain only diluted material from the bronchial rather than alveolar level, and thus give rise to false-negative results, particularly in patients with very severe COPD. In these patients, the value of BAL is greatly diminished and PSB is preferred.[134]

When bronchoscopy is not available, we recommend replacing bronchoscopy in the algorithm in Fig. 46-2 with one of the simplified nonbronchoscopic diagnostic techniques, or following the strategy described by Singh et al,[184] in which decisions regarding antibiotic therapy are based on a score constructed from seven variables, known as the clinical pulmonary infection score (CPIS). Patients with a CPIS >6 are treated as having VAP, with antibiotics for 10–21 days (Fig. 46-5); antibiotics are discontinued if the CPIS is ≤6 at 3 days. Such an approach avoids prolonged treatment of patients with a low likelihood of infection, while allowing immediate treatment of patients with VAP. Two conditions, however, must be rigorously adhered to when implementing this strategy. First, selection of initial

FIGURE 46-5 A diagnostic and therapeutic strategy applied to patients managed with the strategy proposed by Singh et al. (*shape Reproduced, with permission, from Singh et al.[184]*)

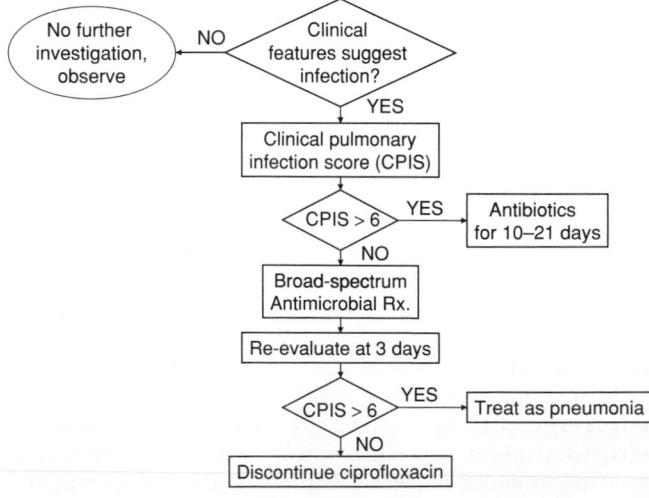

antimicrobial therapy should be based on the flora responsible for most cases of VAP at each institution. Ciprofloxacin is unlikely to be the right choice in numerous institutions that have a high prevalence of MRSA infections.[176] Second, physicians should re-evaluate antimicrobial treatment on day 3, when susceptibility patterns of the microorganism(s) considered to be VAP-causative are available, in order to select treatment with a narrower spectrum antibiotic.

Treatment

INITIAL THERAPY

Failure to initiate prompt appropriate and adequate therapy (the etiologic organism is sensitive to the therapeutic agent, the dose is optimal, and the correct route of administration is used) has been a consistent factor associated with increased mortality.[118,177,178] Because pathogens associated with inappropriate initial empiric antimicrobial therapy mostly include antibiotic-resistant microorganisms, such as *P. aeruginosa*, *Acinetobacter* spp., *K. pneumoniae*, *Enterobacter* spp., and MRSA, patients at risk for infection with these organisms should initially receive a combination of agents that can provide a very broad spectrum of coverage (Table 46-3).[2,179] The choice of agents should be based on local patterns of antimicrobial susceptibility and anticipated side effects. The choice should also take into account which therapies patients have recently received (within the past 2 weeks), striving not to repeat the same antimicrobial class, if possible.[180] Having a current and frequently-updated knowledge base of local bacteriologic patterns can increase the likelihood that the appropriate antibiotic treatment will be initially prescribed.[49] Only patients with early-onset infection and no specific risk factors, such as prolonged duration of hospitalization (≥5 days), admission from a health care–related facility, and recent prolonged antibiotic therapy, can be treated with a narrow-spectrum drug, such as a nonpseudomonal third-generation cephalosporin.[1,2,181]

STOPPING THERAPY WHEN THE DIAGNOSIS OF INFECTION BECOMES UNLIKELY

Because clinical signs of infection are nonspecific and can be caused by any condition associated with an inflammatory response, many more patients than necessary are treated with antibiotics. Thus, it is important to use serial clinical evaluations and microbiologic data to re-evaluate therapy after 48–72 hours, whenever possible.[2]

All diagnostic strategies for managing suspicion of VAP should include a statement that treatment be re-evaluated after 48–72 hours. The decision tree should contain an explicit statement that patients with a low probability of infection will be identified and therapy stopped when infection appears unlikely. The algorithm cannot be exactly the same for a "clinical" or an "invasive" strategy, depending on the general principles and microbiologic techniques on which the diagnostic strategy is constructed. Using a "clinical strategy" in which all patients with clinically suspected pulmonary infection are treated with new antibiotics, even when the likelihood of infection is low, the decision whether to continue antibiotics or not on day 3 will be based essentially on a combination of clinical signs (see Fig. 46-1; Table 46-4).[182] Briefly, antibiotics are discontinued if and only if the following three criteria are fulfilled: (1) clinical diagnosis of VAP is unlikely (there are no definite infiltrates found on chest radiography at follow-up and no more than one of the three following findings: temperature >38.3°C, leukocytosis or leukopenia, and purulent tracheobronchial secretions) or an alternative noninfectious diagnosis is confirmed, (2) tracheobronchial aspirate culture results are nonsignificant, and (3) there is no severe sepsis or shock.

This clinical approach of avoiding overprescription of antibiotics in the ICU may be inaccurate. Accordingly, several

TABLE 46-3 Initial Empiric Therapy for Ventilator-Associated Pneumonia in Patients with Late-Onset Disease or Risk Factors for Multidrug-Resistant (MDR) Pathogens

Potential Pathogens	Combination Antibiotic Therapy
MDR pathogens	Antipseudomonal cephalosporin (cefepime, ceftazidime)
Pseudomonas aeruginosa	
Klebsiella pneumoniae (ESBL)	**or**
Enterobacter spp.	Antipseudomonal carbapenem (imipenem or meropenem)
Serratia marcescens	
Acinetobacter spp.	**or**
Methiciilin-resistant	β-Lactam, β-lactamase inhibitor (piperacillintazobactam)
Staphylococcus aureus (MRSA)	
	plus
	Antipseudomonal fluoroquinolone (ciprofloxacin or high-dose levofloxacin)
	or
	Aminoglycoside (amikacin, gentamicin, or tobramycin)
	plus
	Linezolid or vancomycin (if MRSA risk factors are present or there is a high incidence locally)

ABBREVIATIONS: ESBL, extended-spectrum β-lactamase; MRSA, methicillin-resistant *Staphylococcus aureus*.
SOURCE: Modified, with permission, from American Thoracic Society.[2]

TABLE 46-4 Proposed Strategy for Management of Suspected Ventilator–Associated Pneumonia When a Clinical Strategy is Used

Clinical Condition	Management Strategy	Rationale
Step 1: Initial evaluation		
Clinical suspicion of VAP (based on classic criteria)[a]	Retrieval of respiratory secretions for quantitative or semi–quantitative cultures of tracheobronchial aspirate; immediate initiation of antimicrobial treatment	Risk of delayed or inappropriate antimicrobial treatment outweighs risks associated with antimicrobial overuse
Step 2: Re-evaluation at 48–72 hours		
Clinical suspicion of VAP confirmed (clinically, microbiologically, or both)	Continuation of antimicrobial treatment (with adjustment according to culture results)	Therapeutic benefit in terms of outcome evident
Clinical diagnosis likely, culture results nonsignificant, and no servere sepsis or shock[b]	No firm general recommendation; individual decision (usually to continue antimicrobial treatment)[c]	Risks of both selection pressure and lack of treatment should be considered; culture results must not be the only criterion for decision making, given 10–40% false–negative rate
Nonpulmonary site of infection identified (or unexplained severe sepsis or shock)	Adjustment of antimicrobial treatment according to the site of infection and culture results	Therapeutic benefit in terms of outcome evident
Clinical diagnosis of VAP unlikely and culture results nonsignificant (low risk of VAP) or alternative (noninfectious) diagnosis confirmed; no severe sepsis or shock[d]	Discontinuation of antimicrobial treatment	No harm to patient; reduces antimicrobial selection pressure

[a]The clinical criteria are the presence of new and persistent infiltrates plus two of the following (or one in patients with the acute respiratory distress syndrome): a body temperature of more than 38.3°C, leukocytosis or leukopenia, and purulent tracheobronchical secretions.
[b]Nonsignificant culture results are defined as colony counts below the predefined thresholds for microbiologic diagnosis of VAP.
[c]Antimicrobial treatment can be stopped if there has been no previous antimicrobial treatment and if the cultures are completely negative.
[d]Low risk of VAP: there are no define infiltrates found on chest radiography at follow-up and two of the three clinical criteria are absent.
SOURCE: Modified, with permission, from Torres et al.[182]

investigators have tried to modify the approach by using the clinical pulmonary infection score (CPIS), as originally described by Pugin et al[183] for stopping antibiotics at day 3.[184] Using this algorithm (see Fig. 46-5), patients with CPIS >6 are treated as having VAP with a full course of antibiotics; therapy is discontinued when CPIS is ≤6 at day 3. Such an approach avoids prolonged treatment of patients with a low likelihood of infection, while still allowing immediate treatment of patients with hospital-acquired pneumonia and/or VAP. Other decision trees for stopping antibiotics at 3 days can be constructed, for example, by incorporating results of serial levels of procalcitonin in the blood or soluble triggering receptor expressed on myeloid cells in bronchial secretions, but still require validation.[185–187]

The decision algorithm for withholding or withdrawing antibiotics using the "invasive strategy" is based on results of direct examination of distal pulmonary samples obtained by bronchoscopic or nonbronchoscopic BAL and results of quantitative cultures (see Fig. 46-2). Briefly, antibiotics are withheld in patients with no bacteria on gram-stained cytocentrifuged preparations and no signs of severe sepsis or septic shock, and discontinued when quantitative culture results are below the cutoff defining a positive result, except in patients with proven extrapulmonary infection and/or severe sepsis.[121] As demonstrated by several studies, patients managed with such a bacteriologic strategy receive fewer antibiotics, and more patients have all their antibiotics discontinued compared to the those in the clinical strategy group, thereby confirming that the two strategies actually differed.[120,121,146,165,175] Future studies should,

however, compare bronchoscopy against and in addition to a clinical strategy incorporating an explicit statement for stopping antibiotics in patients with a low probability of infection, for example using the algorithm described in Table 46-4 or the CPIS score, as proposed by Singh et al.[184,188,189] Formal economic analysis is also required because prevention of resistance and better antibiotic control may result in cost savings. Whatever the diagnostic strategy used, each ICU team should monitor the adherence of their physicians to it and implement corrective measures, as needed.

FOCUSING THERAPY ONCE THE INFECTING AGENT IS IDENTIFIED

Once the results of respiratory tract and blood cultures become available, therapy can often be focused or narrowed, based on the identity of specific pathogens and their susceptibility to specific antibiotics, in order to avoid prolonged use of a broader spectrum of antibiotic therapy than is justified by the available information. For many patients, including those with late-onset infection, therapy can be narrowed because an anticipated organism (such as *P. aeruginosa*, *Acinetobacter* species, or MRSA) was not recovered or because the organism isolated is sensitive to a more narrow-spectrum antibiotic than that used in the initial regimen. For example, vancomycin and linezolid should be stopped if no MRSA is identified, unless the patient is allergic to β-lactams and has developed an infection caused by a gram-positive microorganism. Very broad-spectrum agents, such as carbapenems, piperacillin-tazobactam, and/or cefepime should also be restricted to patients with infections caused by pathogens only susceptible to these agents. In case of infection caused by a piperacillin-susceptible *P. aeruginosa* strain, antimicrobial treatment should be streamlined to this specific drug. Similarly, in the absence of an infection caused by a nonfermenting GNB or an extended-spectrum β-lactamase–producing member of the Enterobacteriaceae, the β-lactam should be changed to a nonantipseudomonal antibiotic, such as ceftriaxone or cefotaxime. Clinicians must be aware, however, that emergence of stable derepressed resistant mutants may lead to treatment failure when third-generation cephalosporins are chosen in the case of infections caused by *Enterobacter, Citrobacter, Morganella morganii*, indole-positive *Proteus*, and *Serratia* spp., even if the isolate appears susceptible on initial testing.

OPTIMIZING ANTIMICROBIAL THERAPY

Several published reports have demonstrated a relationship among serum concentrations of β-lactams or other antibiotics, the minimal inhibitory concentration (MIC) of the infecting organism, and the rate of bacterial eradication from respiratory secretions in patients with lung infection. Consequently, clinical and bacteriologic outcomes can be improved by optimizing a therapeutic regimen according to pharmacokinetic properties of the agent(s) selected for treatment.[190–196] Most investigators distinguish between antimicrobial agents that kill by a concentration-dependent mechanism (e.g., aminoglycosides and fluoroquinolones) from those that kill by a time-dependent mechanism (e.g., β-lactams and vancomycin). Multivariate analyses based on 74 acutely ill, mostly VAP patients, who were treated with intravenous ciprofloxacin (200 mg bid to 400 mg tid), demonstrated that the most important independent factor for probability of cure was a pharmacodynamic variable (i.e., the 24-hour area under the concentration-time curve divided by the MIC [AUIC]).[190] For AUIC <125, the probabilities of clinical and microbiologic cures were 42 and 26%, respectively; with AUIC >125, the probabilities were 80 and 82%, respectively.

Pharmacokinetic–pharmacodynamic models have also been used to optimize aminoglycoside therapy for VAP caused by GNB, using the first measured maximum concentration of drug in serum (C_{max}).[191] Seventy-eight patients with VAP were analyzed, and the investigators reported an 89% success rate for temperature normalization by day 7 of therapy for C_{max}/MIC >4.7, and an 86% success rate for leukocyte count normalization by day 7 of therapy for C_{max}/MIC >4.5. Logistic regression analysis predicted a 90% probability of temperature and leukocyte count normalizations by day 7 if a C_{max}/MIC >10 was achieved within the first 48 hours of aminoglycoside administration. Aggressive aminoglycoside doses immediately followed by pharmacokinetic monitoring for each patient would ensure that C_{max}/MIC target ratios are achieved early during therapy.

These findings confirm the need to adjust the target dose of antimicrobial agents (used in treating severe pulmonary infection) to an individual patient's pharmacokinetics and putative bacterial pathogens' susceptibilities. Development

of a priori dosing algorithms based on MIC, patient creatinine clearance and weight, and the clinician-specified AUIC target might be a valid way to improve treatment of these patients, leading to a more precise approach than current guidelines for use of antimicrobial agents.[192–196]

SWITCHING TO MONOTHERAPY AT DAYS 3–5

The commonly cited reason to use combination therapy is to achieve synergy in the therapy of *P. aeruginosa* or other difficult-to-treat GNB infections. Synergy, however, has only been clearly documented to be valuable in vitro and in patients with neutropenia[197] or bacteremic infection,[198,199] which is uncommon in hospital-acquired pneumonia or VAP.[1] The in vitro finding of synergy has been inconsistently demonstrated, and has been difficult to show as being clinically relevant, especially in randomized controlled studies.[200–204] Combination regimens have also been recommended as a method to prevent the emergence of resistance during therapy, a common phenomenon when *P. aeruginosa* is treated with a variety of single agents and when *Enterobacter* is treated with third-generation cephalosporins.[205] Prevention of this type of antibiotic resistance by combination therapy, however, has not been well documented, particularly if a carbapenem or a fourth-generation cephalosporin is used.[200–202,206] A recent meta-analysis has evaluated all prospective randomized trials of β-lactam monotherapy compared to β-lactam-aminoglycoside combination regimens in patients with sepsis, of which at least 1200 of the reported 7586 patients had either hospital-acquired pneumonia or VAP.[207] Clinical failure was more common with combination therapy, and there was no advantage in the therapy of *P. aeruginosa* infections compared to monotherapy. Combination therapy did not prevent the emergence of resistance during therapy, but did lead to a significantly higher rate of nephrotoxicity. In a recent retrospective analysis of 115 episodes of *P. aeruginosa* bacteremia, the use of adequate combination antimicrobial therapy as empiric treatment until receipt of the sensitivity was associated with a better rate of survival at 30 days than the use of monotherapy.[208] Adequate combination antimicrobial therapy given as definitive treatment for *P. aeruginosa* bacteremia, however, did not improve the rate of survival compared to adequate definitive monotherapy.

Based on these data, therapy could be switched to monotherapy in most patients after 3–5 days, provided that initial therapy was appropriate, the clinical course appears favorable, and provided that microbiologic data do not suggest a very difficult-to-treat microorganism, with a very high in vitro minimal inhibitory concentration, as can be observed with some nonfermenting-GNB infections.

SHORTENING DURATION OF THERAPY

Efforts to reduce the duration of therapy for VAP are justified by studies of the natural history of the response to therapy. Dennesen et al demonstrated that when VAP was adequately treated, significant improvements were observed for all clinical parameters, generally within the first 6 days of antibiotic use.[209] The consequence of prolonged therapy to 14 days or more was newly acquired colonization, especially with *P. aeruginosa* and Enterobacteriaceae, generally during the second week of therapy. These data support the premise that most patients with VAP, who receive appropriate antimicrobial therapy, have a good clinical response within the first 6 days.[209–211] Prolonged therapy simply leads to colonization with antibiotic-resistant bacteria, which may precede a recurrent episode of VAP.

Reducing duration of therapy in patients with VAP has led to good outcomes with less antibiotic use with a variety of different strategies. Singh et al used a modification of the CPIS scoring system to identify low-risk patients (CPIS ≤6) with suspected VAP who could be treated with 3 days of antibiotics as opposed to the conventional practice of 10–21 days of antibiotic therapy.[184] Patients receiving the shorter course of antibiotic therapy had better clinical outcomes than the patients receiving longer therapy, with fewer subsequent superinfections attributed to antibiotic-resistant pathogens, although many of these patients may not have had pneumonia. A recent multicenter, randomized, controlled trial demonstrated in a large series of 413 patients with microbiologically-proven VAP that patients who received appropriate, initial empiric therapy for 8 days had similar outcomes to patients who received therapy for 15 days.[212] A trend towards greater rates of relapse for short-duration therapy was seen if the etiologic agent was *P. aeruginosa* or *Acinetobacter* spp., but clinical outcomes were exactly the same. These results were recently confirmed by two other studies, including a prospective, randomized trial of 290 patients evaluating an antibiotic discontinuation policy.[176,188]

Based on these data, an 8-day regimen can probably be standard for patients with VAP. Possible exceptions to this recommendation include immunosuppressed patients, those whose initial antimicrobial treatment was not appropriate for the causative microorganism(s), and patients whose infection was caused by very difficult-to-treat microorganisms and had no improvement in clinical signs of infection.

In summary, antimicrobial therapy of patients with VAP is a two-stage process. The first stage involves administering broad-spectrum antibiotics to avoid inappropriate treatment in patients with true bacterial pneumonia.[2] The second stage focuses on trying to achieve this objective without overusing and abusing antibiotics. In general, the first goal can be accomplished by identifying patients with pneumonia in a rapid fashion and starting therapy with an empiric regimen that is likely to be accurate. This requires that the choice be driven by anticipation of the likely etiologic pathogens, modified by knowledge of local patterns of antimicrobial resistance and local microbiology. The second goal involves combining a number of different steps, including stopping therapy in patients with a low probability of the disease, commitment to focus and narrow treatment once the etiologic agent is known, switching to monotherapy after day 3, and shortening duration of therapy to 7–8 days in most patients, as dictated by the patient's clinical response and information about the bacteriology.

Prevention

Because VAP is associated with increased morbidity, longer hospital stay, increased health care costs, and higher mortality rates, prevention is a major challenge for intensive care medicine.[2,213,214] A number of recommendations for the prevention of nosocomial pneumonia are empiric rather than based on controlled observations, which make evaluation of the impact of such interventions difficult in this setting for several reasons: (1) the difficulty in obtaining an accurate diagnosis of VAP (i.e., to distinguish patients with true infection from patients with tracheal colonization and/or other pathologic processes because only patients who develop true VAP are likely to benefit from preventive measures); (2) the difficulty of precisely determining the impact of prophylactic measures on the overall mortality of a general ICU population (i.e., to identify preventable deaths, directly attributable to VAP, among all deaths occurring in a population of ventilated ICU patients); and (3) the difficulty of evaluating the consequences of a preventive measure on a potentially pathogenic mechanism, for example, to evaluate the exact role played by prevention or reduction of tracheal colonization in modifying the development of VAP.

CONVENTIONAL INFECTION-CONTROL APPROACHES

The measures outlined here should be the first step taken in any prevention program.[215] The design of the ICU has a direct effect on the potential for development of nosocomial infections. Adequate space and lighting, proper functioning of ventilation systems, and ready access to facilities for handwashing lead to lower infection rates.[216] It should, however, be kept in mind that physical upgrading of the environment does not per se reduce the infection rate unless the attitude and practices of personnel are also improved. In any ICU, one of the most important factors is the team that staffs it: the number, quality, and motivation of medical, nursing, and ancillary members. The team should include a sufficient number of nurses so they do not have to move rapidly from one patient to another, and to avoid having them work under constant pressure.[217–220] The importance of personal cleanliness and attention to aseptic procedures must be emphasized at every possible opportunity. At the same time, unnecessarily rigid restrictions should be avoided. It is clear that careful monitoring, decontamination, and compliance with the guidelines for use of respiratory equipment decrease the incidence of nosocomial pneumonia.[219] In any case, handwashing and rubbing hands with alcohol-based solutions remain uncontested as the most important infection-control practices.[114,219,221]

A bacterial monitoring policy facilitates the early recognition of colonization and infection, and has been associated with significant reductions in nosocomial infection rates.[222] The focal point for infection-control activities in the ICU is a surveillance system designed to establish and maintain a database that describes endemic rates of nosocomial infection. Awareness of the endemic rates enables the recognition of the onset of an epidemic when infection rates rise above a calculated threshold.

Preventing infection by modifying host risk factors has focused on treatment of underlying diseases and complications and control of antibiotic use. Adoption of an antibiotic policy restricting the prescription of broad-spectrum agents and useless antibiotics is of major importance.[223] Simple, safe, inexpensive, logical, but unproven measures including the use of physiotherapy, the judicious use and prompt removal of a useless nasogastric tube, and removal of tubing condensate, may have tremendous impact on the frequency of nosocomial pneumonia in ventilated patients.

SPECIFIC PROPHYLAXIS AGAINST VENTILATOR-ASSOCIATED PNEUMONIA

Because invasive ventilation is a risk factor for VAP, strategies that reduce its duration might reduce its incidence. Optimization of sedation and weaning protocols is a first way to reduce the duration of exposure to risk.[224–229] Noninvasive ventilation is an alternative approach to the use of artificial airways to avoid infectious complications and injury of the trachea in patients with acute respiratory failure. Many observational studies and seven randomized trials suggest that patients who tolerate noninvasive ventilation have a lower incidence of pneumonia than those tracheally intubated.[224,230–238]

Apart from these protocols aimed at reducing the duration of mechanical ventilation, seven prophylactic approaches have been studied: semi-recumbent positioning, oscillating and rotating beds, continuous or intermittent aspiration of subglottic secretions, ventilator circuit management, methods of enteral feeding, stress ulcer prophylaxis, and antibiotic use including selective digestive decontamination.

SEMI-RECUMBENT POSITIONING

Supine positioning is independently associated with the development of VAP.[21] Placing ventilated patients in a semi-recumbent position to minimize reflux and aspiration of gastric contents is a simple measure, although some practical problems can occur in unstable patients. Three trials have evaluated the efficacy of semi-recumbent positioning.[98,99,239] Only one measured the incidence of VAP: Drakulovic et al observed lower rates of both clinically suspected and bacteriologically confirmed VAP, and identified supine positioning as an independent risk factor for VAP along with enteral nutrition, ventilation for ≥7 days, and a Glasgow Coma Scale score of <9 points. These results explained the higher risk of VAP in patients receiving enteral nutrition in the supine position.[99]

OSCILLATING AND ROTATING BED

Immobility in critically ill patients treated with mechanical ventilation results in atelectasis, impaired drainage of secretions, and potentially predisposes to pulmonary complications including VAP. Oscillating and rotating beds may help in preventing pneumonia.[213] Six randomized trials, including mostly surgical and trauma patients, ventilated or not,

summarized in a meta-analysis by Choi et al.[240] have compared continuous lateral rotational therapy with standard beds. The meta-analysis found a significant reduction in the risk for pneumonia, principally concerning early-onset (<5 days) pneumonia and a decreased duration of ICU stay. Notably, the only randomized, controlled trial—not included in the meta-analysis—conducted on a general ICU population did not show any differences in pneumonia rates but showed a significantly shorter length of ICU stay.[241] Some adverse events have been described with these beds including disconnection of catheters or pressure ulceration; in addition, nursing care is potentially complicated by oscillating beds. Finally, despite the cost of such beds, cost-benefit analyses suggested favorable results, mainly caused by the reduction of ICU length of stay.

ASPIRATION OF SUBGLOTTIC SECRETIONS

Repeated micro-inhalations of colonized oro-pharyngeal (subglottic) secretions are the major mechanism of VAP. Continuous or intermittent suctioning of oropharyngeal secretions has been proposed as a means to avoid chronic aspiration of secretions through the tracheal cuff of intubated patients. Aspiration of subglottic secretions requires the use of a specially designed endotracheal tube with a separate lumen that opens into the subglottic region. Five randomized controlled trials have studied aspiration of subglottic secretions for the prevention of VAP.[242–247] Mahul et al found that pneumonia was significantly less frequent in patients with an endotracheal tube having a separate dorsal lumen for hourly suctioning of stagnant secretions above the cuff than in others, and that VAP development was delayed.[242] Similarly, in a 3-year prospective, randomized, controlled study, Valles et al documented a lower VAP rate when continuous subglottic aspiration was performed.[243] This difference, however, was fully explained by VAP episodes during the first week, whereas late-onset pneumonias were more frequent in the aspiration group. Furthermore, detailed microbiologic analysis demonstrated that this reduction concerned only pneumonia caused by *H. influenzae* or gram-positive cocci. The incidence of VAP caused by *P. aeruginosa* or Enterobacteriaceae did not differ between the two groups. Kollef et al performed a randomized trial on 343 post–cardiac surgery patients, comparing continuous subglottic aspiration and standard postoperative medical care.[244] Although rates of VAP were similar in both groups, VAP episodes occurred significantly later in patients receiving subglottic aspiration than those treated conventionally. No difference in mortality rates was observed in these three studies. No adverse events were reported with aspiration of subglottic secretions, although experimental data suggest the possibility of tracheal damage in sheep intubated with this type of tube.[248]

VENTILATOR CIRCUIT MANAGEMENT

Decreased frequency of ventilator circuit change, replacement of heated humidifiers by heat and moisture exchangers, decreased frequency of heat and moisture exchanger change, and closed suctioning systems have been tested for preventing VAP.[2,213,214] Four randomized trials of decreased frequency of ventilator circuit changes have been published. Changes every 2 days, every 7 days, and no scheduled change did not show any significant difference in the rate of VAP as summarized in a recent meta-analysis.[249] One meta-analysis summarized the results of five randomized, controlled trials which compared the effects of heated humidifiers and heat and moisture exchangers on the risk of VAP.[214] Only one out of these five studies found a significant reduction of VAP rate with the use of heat and moisture exchangers.[107] Efficacy of both humidification strategies seems comparable. Two studies, however, reported increased rates of endotracheal tube occlusion with the use of heat and moisture exchangers; the increased resistive load can cause difficulties in ventilation and weaning in patients with severe acute respiratory distress syndrome, related to larger dead space. No other adverse effects were observed. No effect on mortality was reported. Finally, one study has evaluated the impact of less frequent changes (daily versus every 5 days) in heat and moisture exchangers on the development of VAP.[250] No difference in the VAP rates was observed.

To avoid hypoxia, hypotension, and contamination of suction catheters entering the tracheal tube, investigators have examined closed suctioning systems.[251,252] They either found an insignificantly lower prevalence of VAP for patients managed with the closed system compared to the open system, without any adverse effect,[252] or they found that its use was associated with an increased frequency of endotracheal colonization.[251]

METHODS OF ENTERAL FEEDING

Nearly all ventilated patients have a nasogastric tube inserted to manage gastric and enteral secretions, prevent gastric distention, or provide nutritional support. A nasogastric tube may increase the risk for gastroesophageal reflux, aspiration, and VAP.[65] Four randomized, controlled trials have evaluated methods of enteral feeding aimed at preventing VAP: postpyloric or jejunal feeding (versus gastric feeding), the use of motility agents (metoclopramide versus placebo), acidification of feeding (with addition of hydrochloric acid), and intermittent (versus continuous) feeding.[95,253,254] These studies did not find differences in incidence of VAP and/or mortality rates. Potentially serious adverse effects have been observed in patients receiving acidified feeding (gastrointestinal bleeding) or intermittent enteral feeding (increased gastric volume and lower volumes of feeding). Thus, to date, methods of enteral feeding aimed at reducing the incidence of VAP cannot be recommended for routine use.

STRESS ULCER PROPHYLAXIS

Gastric colonization by potentially pathogenic organisms has been shown to increase with decreasing gastric acidity.[255] Thus, medications that decrease gastric acidity (antacids and H_2-blockers) may increase organism counts and increase the risk of VAP. In contrast, medications that do not affect gastric acidity (sucralfate) may not increase this risk. Several meta-analyses of more than 20 randomized trials have evaluated the risk of VAP associated with the methods used to prevent gastrointestinal bleeding in critically ill patients.[78,79] Because the largest randomized trial comparing ranitidine to sucralfate showed that ranitidine

was superior in preventing gastrointestinal bleeding and did not increase the risk of VAP,[80] clinicians must weigh the potential benefit of sucralfate (with potentially less VAP and more gastrointestinal bleeding) versus H_2-blockers (with potentially more VAP and less gastrointestinal bleeding), and probably should limit stress ulcer prophylaxis to high-risk patients.

SELECTIVE DIGESTIVE DECONTAMINATION

Several groups have used topical prophylactic antibiotics for selective decontamination of the oropharynx and digestive tract (SDD) in patients at high risk for nosocomial pneumonia. The SDD regimen usually includes a short course of systemic antibiotic therapy, such as cefotaxime, trimethoprim or a fluoroquinolone, and non-absorbable local antibiotic prophylaxis consisting of a combination of an aminoglycoside, polymyxin B, and amphotericin.[256] Since the original study published by Stoutenbeck et al in 1984,[257] which demonstrated a decrease in the overall infection rate in patients receiving the SDD regimen, more than 40 randomized, controlled trials, and 7 meta-analyses have been published. All seven meta-analyses reported a significant reduction in the risk of VAP, and four reported a significant reduction in mortality.[73,258-260] No mortality benefit occurred with topical prophylaxis alone. A clear consensus as to the effectiveness of SDD has not been established, however, because of discordances among the meta-analyses related to limitations and methodologic deficiencies of the analyzed studies. Particular problems include: the use of clinical diagnosis of pneumonia as a study endpoint; the heterogeneity of the populations studied; the wide variety of oral regimens; inconsistent addition of systemic administration of antibiotics (cefotaxime or ceftazidime); and differences in analytic methods.[213,214,261] Recently, de Jonge et al were able to demonstrate in a large, prospective, randomised, unblinded clinical trial of 934 patients that SDD can decrease ICU and hospital mortality and colonization with resistant aerobic GNB in a setting with a low prevalence of vancomycin-resistant enterococci and methicillin-resistant *S. aureus*.[262]

The influence of rotating antibiotics (generally associated with restrictive use) in the ICU on VAP prevalence was recently investigated by comparing successive periods during which one antibiotic was used in place of another for the empiric treatment of suspected GNB infections. Some investigators found that VAP occurred significantly less frequently during the after period compared with the before period,[263,264] but the efficacy of such measures remains controversial.[265]

Conclusion

Ventilator-associated pneumonia is an entity that should be viewed as a subcategory of health care–associated pneumonia. Health care–associated pneumonia includes any patient who was recently hospitalized in an acute care hospital for two or more days within 90 days of the infection; resided in a nursing home or long-term care facility; received recent antibiotic therapy, chemotherapy, or wound care within the previous 30 days of the current infection; or attended a hospital or hemodialysis clinic.[2] The high level of bacterial resistance observed in such a setting limits the treatment options available to clinicians and demands the use of antibiotic regimens combining several broad-spectrum drugs, even if the pretest probability of the disease is low, because initial inappropriate antimicrobial therapy has been documented to be associated with a poor prognosis. Besides its economic impact, this practice of "spiraling empiricism" increasingly leads to the unnecessary administration of antibiotics in many ICU patients without true infection, paradoxically resulting in the emergence of infections caused by more antibiotic-resistant microorganisms that are in turn associated with increased rates of patient morbidity and mortality. Antimicrobial therapy of patients with VAP should, therefore, follow a two-stage process. The first stage involves administering broad-spectrum antibiotics to avoid inappropriate treatment in patients with true bacterial pneumonia. The second stage focuses on trying to achieve this objective without overusing and abusing antibiotics by combining a number of different steps, such as stopping therapy in patients with a low probability of disease, streamlining treatment once the etiologic agent is known, switching to monotherapy after 3–5 days, and shortening duration of therapy to 7–8 days, as dictated by the patient's clinical response and bacteriology results. In the event that one or several specific etiologic agents are identified by a reliable diagnostic technique, the choice of antimicrobial drugs is much easier, because the optimal treatment can be selected in light of the susceptibility pattern of the causative pathogens without resorting to broad-spectrum drugs or risking inappropriate treatment. Every possible effort should therefore be made to obtain—before new antibiotics are administered—reliable pulmonary specimens for direct microscopic examination and cultures from each patient clinically suspected of having developed VAP. Because respiratory tract colonization of ICU patients is generally very complex, corresponding to a mix of self-colonization and cross-transmission, only a multifaceted and multidisciplinary preventive program can be effective.

References

1. Chastre J, Fagon JY. Ventilator-associated pneumonia. Am J Respir Crit Care Med 2002; 165:867–903.
2. American Thoracic Society; Infectious Diseases Society of America. Guidelines for the Management of adults with hospital-acquired, ventilator-associated, and healthcare-associated pneumonia. Am J Respir Crit Care Med 2005; 171:388–416.
3. National Nosocomial Infections Surveillance (NNIS) System report, data summary from January 1990–May 1999, issued June 1999. Am J Infect Control 1999; 27:520–32.
4. Bergmans DC, Bonten MJ, Gaillard CA, et al. Indications for antibiotic use in ICU patients: a one-year prospective surveillance. J Antimicrob Chemother 1997; 39:527–35.
5. Kirtland SH, Corley DE, Winterbauer RH, et al. The diagnosis of ventilator-associated pneumonia: a comparison of histologic, microbiologic, and clinical criteria. Chest 1997; 112:445–57.
6. Vincent JL, Bihari DJ, Suter PM, et al. The prevalence of nosocomial infection in intensive care units in Europe. Results of the European Prevalence of Infection in Intensive Care (EPIC) Study. EPIC International Advisory Committee [see comments]. JAMA 1995; 274:639–44.
7. Cross AS, Roup B. Role of respiratory assistance devices in endemic nosocomial pneumonia. Am J Med 1981; 70:681–5.
8. Horan TC, Culver DH, Gaynes RP, et al. Nosocomial infections in surgical patients in the United States, January 1986–June 1992. National Nosocomial Infections Surveillance (NNIS) System. Infect Control Hosp Epidemiol 1993; 14:73–80.
9. Celis R, Torres A, Gatell JM, et al. Nosocomial pneumonia. A multivariate analysis of risk and prognosis. Chest 1988; 93:318–24.
10. Fagon JY, Chastre J, Domart Y, et al. Nosocomial pneumonia in patients receiving continuous mechanical ventilation. Prospective analysis of 52 episodes with use of a protected specimen brush and quantitative culture techniques. Am Rev Respir Dis 1989; 139:877–84.
11. Cook DJ, Walter SD, Cook RJ, et al. Incidence of and risk factors for ventilator-associated pneumonia in critically ill patients [see comments]. Ann Intern Med 1998; 129:433–40.
12. Bell RC, Coalson JJ, Smith JD, Johanson WG. Multiple organ system failure and infection in adult respiratory distress syndrome. Ann Intern Med 1983; 99:293–8.
13. Andrews CP, Coalson JJ, Smith JD, Johanson WG. Diagnosis of nosocomial bacterial pneumonia in acute, diffuse lung injury. Chest 1981; 80:254–8.
14. Sutherland KR, Steinberg KP, Maunder RJ, et al. Pulmonary infection during the acute respiratory distress syndrome. Am J Respir Crit Care Med 1995; 152:550–6.
15. Chastre J, Trouillet JL, Vuagnat A, et al. Nosocomial pneumonia in patients with acute respiratory distress syndrome. Am J Respir Crit Care Med 1998; 157:1165–72.
16. Delclaux C, Roupie E, Blot F, et al. Lower respiratory tract colonization and infection during severe acute respiratory distress syndrome: incidence and diagnosis. Am J Respir Crit Care Med 1997; 156:1092–8.
17. Markowicz P, Wolff M, Djedaini K, et al. Multicenter prospective study of ventilator-associated pneumonia during acute respiratory distress syndrome. Incidence, prognosis, and risk factors. ARDS Study Group. Am J Respir Crit Care Med 2000; 161:1942–8.
18. Meduri GU, Reddy RC, Stanley T, El-Zeky F. Pneumonia in acute respiratory distress syndrome. A prospective evaluation of bilateral bronchoscopic sampling. Am J Respir Crit Care Med 1998; 158:870–5.
19. Rello J, Ollendorf DA, Oster G, et al. Epidemiology and outcomes of ventilator-associated pneumonia in a large U.S. database. Chest 2002; 122:2115–21.
20. Chevret S, Hemmer M, Carlet J, Langer M. Incidence and risk factors of pneumonia acquired in intensive care units. Results from a multicenter prospective study on 996 patients. European Cooperative Group on Nosocomial Pneumonia. Intensive Care Med 1993; 19:256–64.
21. Kollef MH. Ventilator-associated pneumonia. A multivariate analysis. JAMA 1993; 270:1965–70.
22. Fagon JY, Chastre J, Hance AJ, et al. Nosocomial pneumonia in ventilated patients: a cohort study evaluating attributable mortality and hospital stay. Am J Med 1993; 94:281–8.
23. Fagon JY, Chastre J, Vuagnat A, et al. Nosocomial pneumonia and mortality among patients in intensive care units. JAMA 1996; 275:866–9.
24. Gross PA, Neu HC, Aswapokee P, Van Antwerpen C, Aswapokee N. Deaths from nosocomial infections: experience in a

university hospital and a community hospital. Am J Med 1980; 68:219–23.

25. Bueno-Cavanillas A, Delgado-Rodriguez M, Lopez-Luque A, Schaffino-Cano S, Galvez-Vargas R. Influence of nosocomial infection on mortality rate in an intensive care unit. Crit Care Med 1994; 22:55–60.

26. Fagon JY, Chastre J, Domart Y, Trouillet JL, Gibert C. Mortality due to ventilator-associated pneumonia or colonization with *Pseudomonas* or *Acinetobacter* species: assessment by quantitative culture of samples obtained by a protected specimen brush. Clin Infect Dis 1996; 23:538–42.

27. Kollef MH, Silver P, Murphy DM, Trovillion E. The effect of late-onset ventilator-associated pneumonia in determining patient mortality. Chest 1995; 108:1655–62.

28. Rello J, Jubert P, Valles J, et al. Evaluation of outcome for intubated patients with pneumonia due to *Pseudomonas aeruginosa*. Clin Infect Dis 1996; 23:973–8.

29. Rello J, Torres A, Ricart M, et al. Ventilator-associated pneumonia by *Staphylococcus aureus*. Comparison of methicillin-resistant and methicillin-sensitive episodes. Am J Respir Crit Care Med 1994; 150:1545–9.

30. Rello J, Ausina V, Ricart M, Castella J, Prats G. Impact of previous antimicrobial therapy on the etiology and outcome of ventilator-associated pneumonia. Chest 1993; 104:1230–5.

31. Luna CM, Vujacich P, Niederman MS, et al. Impact of BAL data on the therapy and outcome of ventilator-associated pneumonia. Chest 1997; 111:676–85.

32. Sanchez-Nieto JM, Torres A, Garcia-Cordoba F, et al. Impact of invasive and noninvasive quantitative culture sampling on outcome of ventilator-associated pneumonia: a pilot study [see comments] [published erratum appears in Am J Respir Crit Care Med 1998; 157(3 Pt 1):1005]. Am J Respir Crit Care Med 1998; 157:371–6.

33. Ruiz M, Torres A, Ewig S, et al. Noninvasive versus invasive microbial investigation in ventilator-associated pneumonia: evaluation of outcome. Am J Respir Crit Care Med 2000; 162:119–25.

34. Kollef MH, Sherman G, Ward S, Fraser VJ. Inadequate antimicrobial treatment of infections: a risk factor for hospital mortality among critically ill patients. Chest 1999; 115:462–74.

35. Alvarez-Lerma F. Modification of empiric antibiotic treatment in patients with pneumonia acquired in the intensive care unit. ICU-Acquired Pneumonia Study Group. Intensive Care Med 1996; 22:387–94.

36. Dupont H, Mentec H, Sollet JP, Bleichner G. Impact of appropriateness of initial antibiotic therapy on the outcome of ventilator-associated pneumonia. Intensive Care Med 2001; 27:355–62.

37. Kollef MH. Antimicrobial therapy of ventilator-associated pneumonia: how to select an appropriate drug regimen [editorial; comment]. Chest 1999; 115:8–11.

38. Timsit JF, Chevret S, Valcke J, et al. Mortality of nosocomial pneumonia in ventilated patients: influence of diagnostic tools. Am J Respir Crit Care Med 1996; 154:116–23.

39. Jimenez P, Torres A, Rodriguez-Roisin R, et al. Incidence and etiology of pneumonia acquired during mechanical ventilation. Crit Care Med 1989; 17:882–5.

40. Heyland DK, Cook DJ, Griffith L, Keenan SP, Brun-Buisson C. The attributable morbidity and mortality of ventilator-associated pneumonia in the critically ill patient. The Canadian Critical Trials Group. Am J Respir Crit Care Med 1999; 159:1249–56.

41. Baker AM, Meredith JW, Haponik EF. Pneumonia in intubated trauma patients. Microbiology and outcomes. Am J Respir Crit Care Med 1996; 153:343–9.

42. Spencer RC. Predominant pathogens found in the European Prevalence of Infection in Intensive Care Study. Eur J Clin Microbiol Infect Dis 1996; 15:281–5.

43. Combes A, Figliolini C, Trouillet JL, et al. Incidence and outcome of polymicrobial ventilator-associated pneumonia. Chest 2002; 121:1618–23.

44. Singh N, Falestiny MN, Rogers P, et al. Pulmonary infiltrates in the surgical ICU: prospective assessment of predictors of etiology and mortality. Chest 1998; 114:1129–36.

45. Langer M, Mosconi P, Cigada M, Mandelli M. Long-term respiratory support and risk of pneumonia in critically ill patients. Intensive Care Unit Group of Infection Control. Am Rev Respir Dis 1989; 140:302–5.

46. Langer M, Cigada M, Mandelli M, Mosconi P, Tognoni G. Early onset pneumonia: a multicenter study in intensive care units. Intensive Care Med 1987; 13:342–6.

47. Trouillet JL, Chastre J, Vuagnat A, et al. Ventilator-associated pneumonia caused by potentially drug-resistant bacteria. Am J Respir Crit Care Med 1998; 157:531–9.

48. Ibrahim EH, Ward S, Sherman G, Kollef MH. A comparative analysis of patients with early-onset vs. late-onset nosocomial pneumonia in the ICU setting. Chest 2000; 117:1434–42.

49. Rello J, Sa-Borges M, Correa H, Leal SR, Baraibar J. Variations in etiology of ventilator-associated pneumonia across four treatment sites: implications for antimicrobial prescribing practices. Am J Respir Crit Care Med 1999; 160: 608–13.

50. Dore P, Robert R, Grollier G, et al. Incidence of anaerobes in ventilator-associated pneumonia with use of a protected specimen brush. Am J Respir Crit Care Med 1996; 153:1292–8.

51. Bruynseels P, Jorens PG, Demey HE, et al. Herpes simplex virus in the respiratory tract of critical care patients: a prospective study. Lancet 2003; 362:1536–41.

52. el-Ebiary M, Torres A, Fabregas N, et al. Significance of the isolation of *Candida* species from respiratory samples in critically ill, non-neutropenic patients. An immediate postmortem histologic study. Am J Respir Crit Care Med 1997; 156:583–90.

53. Rello J, Esandi ME, Diaz E, et al. The role of *Candida* spp isolated from bronchoscopic samples in nonneutropenic patients. Chest 1998; 114:146–9.

54. Craven DE, De Rosa FG, Thornton D. Nosocomial pneumonia: emerging concepts in diagnosis, management, and prophylaxis. Curr Opin Crit Care 2002; 8:421–9.

55. Johanson WG, Pierce AK, Sanford JP, Thomas GD. Nosocomial respiratory infections with gram-negative bacilli. The significance of colonization of the respiratory tract. Ann Intern Med 1972; 77:701–6.

56. Garrouste-Orgeas M, Chevret S, Arlet G, et al. Oropharyngeal or gastric colonization and nosocomial pneumonia in adult intensive care unit patients. A prospective study based on genomic DNA analysis. Am J Respir Crit Care Med 1997; 156:1647–55.

57. Bonten MJ, Gaillard CA, de Leeuw PW, Stobberingh EE. Role of colonization of the upper intestinal tract in the pathogenesis of ventilator-associated pneumonia [see comments]. Clin Infect Dis 1997; 24:309–19.

58. Bonten MJ, Bergmans DC, Speijer H, Stobberingh EE. Characteristics of polyclonal endemicity of *Pseudomonas aeruginosa* colonization in intensive care units. Implications for infection control. Am J Respir Crit Care Med 1999; 160:1212–9.

59. Bonten MJ, Gaillard CA, van Tiel FH, et al. The stomach is not a source for colonization of the upper respiratory tract and pneumonia in ICU patients [see comments]. Chest 1994; 105:878–84.

60. de Latorre FJ, Pont T, Ferrer A, et al. Pattern of tracheal colonization during mechanical ventilation. Am J Respir Crit Care Med 1995; 152:1028–33.

61. Bonten MJ, Kullberg BJ, van Dalen R, et al. Selective digestive decontamination in patients in intensive care. J Antimicrob Chemother 2000; 46:351–62.

62. Bonten MJ. Controversies on diagnosis and prevention of ventilator-associated pneumonia. Diagn Microbiol Infect Dis 1999; 34:199–204.

63. Torres A, Aznar R, Gatell JM, et al. Incidence, risk, and prognosis factors of nosocomial pneumonia in mechanically ventilated patients. Am Rev Respir Dis 1990; 142:523–8.

64. Craven DE, Kunches LM, Kilinsky V, et al. Risk factors for pneumonia and fatality in patients receiving continuous mechanical ventilation. Am Rev Respir Dis 1986; 133:792–6.

65. Joshi N, Localio AR, Hamory BH. A predictive risk index for nosocomial pneumonia in the intensive care unit. Am J Med 1992; 93:135–42.

66. Antonelli M, Moro ML, Capelli O, et al. Risk factors for early onset pneumonia in trauma patients. Chest 1994; 105:224–8.

67. Cunnion KM, Weber DJ, Broadhead WE, et al. Risk factors for nosocomial pneumonia: comparing adult critical-care populations. Am J Respir Crit Care Med 1996; 153:158–62.

68. Daschner F, Kappstein I, Engels I, et al. Stress ulcer prophylaxis and ventilation pneumonia: prevention by antibacterial cytoprotective agents? Infect Control Hosp Epidemiol 1988; 9:59–65.

69. Garibaldi RA, Britt MR, Coleman ML, Reading JC, Pace NL. Risk factors for postoperative pneumonia. Am J Med 1981; 70:677–80.

70. Tillotson JR, Finland M. Secondary pulmonary infections following antibiotic therapy for primary bacterial pneumonia. Antimicrobial Agents Chemother 1968; 8:326–30.

71. Rello J, Ausina V, Ricart M, et al. Risk factors for infection by *Pseudomonas aeruginosa* in patients with ventilator-associated pneumonia. Intensive Care Med 1994; 20:193–8.

72. Jarvis WR, Edwards JR, Culver DH, et al. Nosocomial infection rates in adult and pediatric intensive care units in the United States. National Nosocomial Infections Surveillance System. Am J Med 1991; 91:185S–191S.

73. D'Amico R, Pifferi S, Leonetti C, et al. Effectiveness of antibiotic prophylaxis in critically ill adult patients: systematic review of randomised controlled trials. BMJ 1998; 316:1275–85.

74. Sirvent JM, Torres A, El-Ebiary M, et al. Protective effect of intravenously administered cefuroxime against nosocomial pneumonia in patients with structural coma. Am J Respir Crit Care Med 1997; 155:1729–34.

75. George DL, Falk PS, Wunderink RG, et al. Epidemiology of ventilator-acquired pneumonia based on protected bronchoscopic sampling. Am J Respir Crit Care Med 1998; 158:1839–47.

76. Atherton ST, White DJ. Stomach as source of bacteria colonising respiratory tract during artificial ventilation. Lancet 1978; 2:968–9.

77. du Moulin GC, Paterson DG, Hedley-Whyte J, Lisbon A. Aspiration of gastric bacteria in antacid-treated patients: a frequent cause of postoperative colonisation of the airway. Lancet 1982; 1:242–5.

78. Cook DJ, Reeve BK, Guyatt GH, et al. Stress ulcer prophylaxis in critically ill patients. Resolving discordant meta-analyses. JAMA 1996; 275:308–14.

79. Messori A, Trippoli S, Vaiani M, Gorini M, Corrado A. Bleeding and pneumonia in intensive care patients given ranitidine and sucralfate for prevention of stress ulcer: meta-analysis of randomised controlled trials. BMJ 2000; 321:1103–6.

80. Cook D, Guyatt G, Marshall J, et al. A comparison of sucralfate and ranitidine for the prevention of upper gastrointestinal bleeding in patients requiring mechanical ventilation. Canadian Critical Care Trials Group [see comments]. N Engl J Med 1998; 338:791–7.

81. Ben-Menachem T, Fogel R, Patel RV, et al. Prophylaxis for stress-related gastric hemorrhage in the medical intensive care unit. A randomized, controlled, single-blind study. Ann Intern Med 1994; 121:568–75.

82. Eddleston JM, Pearson RC, Holland J, et al. Prospective endoscopic study of stress erosions and ulcers in critically ill adult patients treated with either sucralfate or placebo. Crit Care Med 1994; 22:1949–54.

83. Sottile FD, Marrie TJ, Prough DS, et al. Nosocomial pulmonary infection: possible etiologic significance of bacterial adhesion to endotracheal tubes. Crit Care Med 1986; 14:265–70.

84. Spray SB, Zuidema GD, Cameron JL. Aspiration pneumonia; incidence of aspiration with endotracheal tubes. Am J Surg 1976; 131:701–3.

85. Rello J, Diaz E, Roque M, Valles J. Risk factors for developing pneumonia within 48 hours of intubation. Am J Respir Crit Care Med 1999; 159:1742–6.

86. Torres A, Gatell JM, Aznar E, et al. Re-intubation increases the risk of nosocomial pneumonia in patients needing mechanical ventilation. Am J Respir Crit Care Med 1995; 152:137–41.

87. Brook AD, Sherman G, Malen J, Kollef MH. Early versus late tracheostomy in patients who require prolonged mechanical ventilation. Am J Crit Care 2000; 9:352–9.

88. Lesnik I, Rappaport W, Fulginiti J, Witzke D. The role of early tracheostomy in blunt, multiple organ trauma. Am Surg 1992; 58:346–9.

89. Rodriguez JL, Steinberg SM, Luchetti FA, et al. Early tracheostomy for primary airway management in the surgical critical care setting. Surgery 1990; 108:655–9.

90. Sugerman HJ, Wolfe L, Pasquale MD, et al. Multicenter, randomized, prospective trial of early tracheostomy. J Trauma 1997; 43:741–7.

91. Rumbak MJ, Newton M, Truncale T, et al. A prospective, randomized, study comparing early percutaneous dilational tracheotomy to prolonged translaryngeal intubation (delayed tracheotomy) in critically ill medical patients. Crit Care Med 2004; 32:1689–94.

92. Frutos-Vivar F, Esteban A, Apezteguia C, et al. Outcome of mechanically ventilated patients who require a tracheostomy. Crit Care Med 2005; 33:290–8.

93. Livingston DH. Prevention of ventilator-associated pneumonia. Am J Surg 2000; 179:12S–17S.

94. Moore FA, Moore EE, Jones TN, McCroskey BL, Peterson VM. TEN versus TPN following major abdominal trauma—reduced septic morbidity. J Trauma 1989; 29:916–22; discussion 922–3.

95. Heyland DK, Cook DJ, Schoenfeld PS, et al. The effect of acidified enteral feeds on gastric colonization in critically ill patients: results of a multicenter randomized trial. Canadian Critical Care Trials Group. Crit Care Med 1999; 27:2399–406.

96. Montecalvo MA, Steger KA, Farber HW, et al. Nutritional outcome and pneumonia in critical care patients randomized to gastric versus jejunal tube feedings. The Critical Care Research Team. Crit Care Med 1992; 20:1377–87.

97. Meer JA. Inadvertent dislodgement of nasoenteral feeding tubes: incidence and prevention. JPEN J Parenter Enteral Nutr 1987; 11:187–9.

98. Torres A, Serra-Batlles J, Ros E, et al. Pulmonary aspiration of gastric contents in patients receiving mechanical ventilation: the effect of body position. Ann Intern Med 1992; 116:540–3.

99. Drakulovic MB, Torres A, Bauer TT, et al. Supine body position as a risk factor for nosocomial pneumonia in mechanically ventilated patients: a randomised trial. Lancet 1999; 354:1851–8.

100. Goularte TA, Manning M, Craven DE. Bacterial colonization in humidifying cascade reservoirs after 24 and 48 hours of continuous mechanical ventilation. Infect Control 1987; 8:200–3.

101. Craven DE, Goularte TA, Make BJ. Contaminated condensate in mechanical ventilator circuits. A risk factor for nosocomial pneumonia? Am Rev Respir Dis 1984; 129:625–8.

102. Craven DE, Steger KA, Barber TW. Preventing nosocomial pneumonia: state of the art and perspectives for the 1990s. Am J Med 1991; 91:44S–53S.

103. Martin C, Perrin G, Gevaudan MJ, Saux P, Gouin F. Heat and moisture exchangers and vaporizing humidifiers in the intensive care unit. Chest 1990; 97:144–9.

104. Roustan JP, Kienlen J, Aubas P, Aubas S, du Cailar J. Comparison of hydrophobic heat and moisture exchangers with heated humidifier during prolonged mechanical ventilation. Intensive Care Med 1992; 18:97–100.

105. Dreyfuss D, Djedaini K, Gros I, et al. Mechanical ventilation with heated humidifiers or heat and moisture exchangers: effects on patient colonization and incidence of nosocomial pneumonia. Am J Respir Crit Care Med 1995; 151:986–92.

106. Hurni JM, Feihl F, Lazor R, Leuenberger P, Perret C. Safety of combined heat and moisture exchanger filters in long-term mechanical ventilation. Chest 1997; 111:686–91.

107. Kirton OC, DeHaven B, Morgan J, Morejon O, Civetta J. A prospective, randomized comparison of an in-line heat moisture exchange filter and heated wire humidifiers: rates of ventilator-associated early-onset (community-acquired) or late-onset (hospital-acquired) pneumonia and incidence of endotracheal tube occlusion. Chest 1997; 112:1055–9.

108. Djedaini K, Billiard M, Mier L, et al. Changing heat and moisture exchangers every 48 hours rather than 24 hours does not affect their efficacy and the incidence of nosocomial pneumonia. Am J Respir Crit Care Med 1995; 152:1562–9.

109. Conti G, De Blasi RA, Rocco M, et al. Effects of the heat-moisture exchangers on dynamic hyperinflation of mechanically ventilated COPD patients. Intensive Care Med 1990; 16:441–3.

110. Ploysongsang Y, Branson R, Rashkin MC, Hurst JM. Pressure flow characteristics of commonly used heat-moisture exchangers. Am Rev Respir Dis 1988; 138:675–8.

111. Dreyfuss D, Djedaini K, Weber P, et al. Prospective study of nosocomial pneumonia and of patient and circuit colonization during mechanical ventilation with circuit changes every 48 hours versus no change. Am Rev Respir Dis 1991; 143:738–43.

112. Kollef MH, Shapiro SD, Fraser VJ, et al. Mechanical ventilation with or without 7-day circuit changes. A randomized controlled trial [see comments]. Ann Intern Med 1995; 123:168–74.

113. Long MN, Wickstrom G, Grimes A, et al. Prospective, randomized study of ventilator-associated pneumonia in patients with one versus three ventilator circuit changes per week. Infect Control Hosp Epidemiol 1996; 17:14–9.

114. Guidelines for prevention of nosocomial pneumonia. Centers for Disease Control and Prevention. MMWR Morb Mortal Wkly Rep 1997; 46:1–79.

115. Holzapfel L, Chastang C, Demingeon G, et al. A randomized study assessing the systematic search for maxillary sinusitis in nasotracheally mechanically ventilated patients. Influence of nosocomial maxillary sinusitis on the occurrence of ventilator-associated pneumonia. Am J Respir Crit Care Med 1999; 159:695–701.

116. Rouby JJ, Laurent P, Gosnach M, et al. Risk factors and clinical relevance of nosocomial maxillary sinusitis in the critically ill. Am J Respir Crit Care Med 1994; 150:776–83.

117. Kollef MH, Von Harz B, Prentice D, et al. Patient transport from intensive care increases the risk of developing ventilator-associated pneumonia. Chest 1997; 112:765–73.

118. Iregui M, Ward S, Sherman G, Fraser VJ, Kollef MH. Clinical importance of delays in the initiation of appropriate antibiotic treatment for ventilator-associated pneumonia. Chest 2002; 122:262–8.

119. Rello J, Gallego M, Mariscal D, Sonora R, Valles J. The value of routine microbial investigation in ventilator-associated pneumonia. Am J Respir Crit Care Med 1997; 156:196–200.

120. Bonten MJ, Bergmans DC, Stobberingh EE, et al. Implementation of bronchoscopic techniques in the diagnosis of ventilator-associated pneumonia to reduce antibiotic use. Am J Respir Crit Care Med 1997; 156:1820–4.

121. Fagon JY, Chastre J, Wolff M, et al. Invasive and noninvasive strategies for management of suspected ventilator-associated pneumonia. A randomized trial. Ann Intern Med 2000; 132:621–30.

122. Meduri GU, Chastre J. The standardization of bronchoscopic techniques for ventilator- associated pneumonia. Chest 1992; 102:557S–564S.

123. Rouby JJ. Histology and microbiology of ventilator-associated pneumonias. Semin Respir Infect 1996; 11:54–61.

124. Trouillet JL, Guiguet M, Gibert C, et al. Fiberoptic bronchoscopy in ventilated patients. Evaluation of cardiopulmonary risk under midazolam sedation. Chest 1990; 97:927–33.

125. Steinberg KP, Mitchell DR, Maunder RJ, et al. Safety of bronchoalveolar lavage in patients with adult respiratory distress syndrome. Am Rev Respir Dis 1993; 148:556–61.

126. Pugin J, Suter PM. Diagnostic bronchoalveolar lavage in patients with pneumonia produces sepsis-like systemic effects. Intensive Care Med 1992; 18:6–10.

127. Baughman RP. Nonbronchoscopic evaluation of ventilator-associated pneumonia. Semin Respir Infect 2003; 18:95–102.

128. Jorda R, Parras F, Ibanez J, et al. Diagnosis of nosocomial pneumonia in mechanically ventilated patients by the blind protected telescoping catheter [see comments]. Intensive Care Med 1993; 19:377–82.

129. Cook D, Mandell L. Endotracheal aspiration in the diagnosis of ventilator-associated pneumonia. Chest 2000; 117:195S–197S.

130. Jourdain B, Novara A, Joly-Guillou ML, et al. Role of quantitative cultures of endotracheal aspirates in the diagnosis of nosocomial pneumonia. Am J Respir Crit Care Med 1995; 152:241–6.

131. Borderon E, Leprince A, Gueveler C, Borderon JC. [The diagnostic value of quantitative bacteriology in tracheal aspirates compared to lung biopsy (author's transl.)]. Rev Fr Mal Respir 1981; 9:229–39.

132. Wimberley N, Faling LJ, Bartlett JG. A fiberoptic bronchoscopy technique to obtain uncontaminated lower airway secretions for bacterial culture. Am Rev Respir Dis 1979; 119:337–43.

133. Pham LH, Brun-Buisson C, Legrand P, et al. Diagnosis of nosocomial pneumonia in mechanically ventilated patients. Comparison of a plugged telescoping catheter with the protected specimen brush. Am Rev Respir Dis 1991; 143:1055–61.

134. Baselski VS, Wunderink RG. Bronchoscopic diagnosis of pneumonia. Clin Microbiol Rev 1994; 7:533–58.

135. Baselski V. Microbiologic diagnosis of ventilator-associated pneumonia. Infect Dis Clin North Am 1993; 7:331–57.

136. de Lassence A, Joly-Guillou ML, Martin-Lefevre L, et al. Accuracy of delayed cultures of plugged telescoping catheter samples for diagnosing bacterial pneumonia. Crit Care Med 2001; 29:1311–7.

137. Forceville X, Fiacre A, Faibis F, et al. Reproducibility of protected specimen brush and bronchoalveolar lavage conserved at 4 degrees C for 48 hours. Intensive Care Med 2002; 28:857–63.

138. Bartlett JG, Finegold SM. Bacteriology of expectorated sputum with quantitative culture and wash technique compared to transtracheal aspirates. Am Rev Respir Dis 1978; 117:1019–27.

139. Kahn FW, Jones JM. Diagnosing bacterial respiratory infection by bronchoalveolar lavage. J Infect Dis 1987; 155:862–9.

140. Croce MA, Fabian TC, Waddle-Smith L, et al. Utility of Gram's stain and efficacy of quantitative cultures for posttraumatic pneumonia: a prospective study. Ann Surg 1998; 227:743–51; discussion 751–5.

141. Chastre J, Fagon JY, Soler P, et al. Diagnosis of nosocomial bacterial pneumonia in intubated patients undergoing ventilation:

comparison of the usefulness of bronchoalveolar lavage and the protected specimen brush [published erratum appears in Am J Med 1989; 86:258]. Am J Med 1988; 85:499–506.

142. Chastre J, Fagon JY, Bornet-Lecso M, et al. Evaluation of bronchoscopic techniques for the diagnosis of nosocomial pneumonia. Am J Respir Crit Care Med 1995; 152:231–40.

143. Allaouchiche B, Jaumain H, Chassard D, Bouletreau P. Gram stain of bronchoalveolar lavage fluid in the early diagnosis of ventilator-associated pneumonia. Br J Anaesth 1999; 83:845–9.

144. Torres A, El-Ebiary M, Fabregas N, et al. Value of intracellular bacteria detection in the diagnosis of ventilator associated pneumonia. Thorax 1996; 51:378–84.

145. Veber B, Souweine B, Gachot B, et al. Comparison of direct examination of three types of bronchoscopy specimens used to diagnose nosocomial pneumonia. Crit Care Med 2000; 28:962–8.

146. Timsit JF, Cheval C, Gachot B, et al. Usefulness of a strategy based on bronchoscopy with direct examination of bronchoalveolar lavage fluid in the initial antibiotic therapy of suspected ventilator-associated pneumonia. Intensive Care Med 2001; 27:640–7.

147. Johanson WG Jr, Seidenfeld JJ, Gomez P, de los Santos R, Coalson JJ. Bacteriologic diagnosis of nosocomial pneumonia following prolonged mechanical ventilation. Am Rev Respir Dis 1988; 137:259–64.

148. Moser KM, Maurer J, Jassy L, et al. Sensitivity, specificity, and risk of diagnostic procedures in a canine model of *Streptococcus pneumoniae* pneumonia. Am Rev Respir Dis 1982; 125:436–42.

149. Higuchi JH, Coalson JJ, Johanson WG. Bacteriologic diagnosis of nosocomial pneumonia in primates. Usefulness of the protected specimen brush. Am Rev Respir Dis 1982; 125:53–7.

150. Chastre J, Viau F, Brun P, et al. Prospective evaluation of the protected specimen brush for the diagnosis of pulmonary infections in ventilated patients. Am Rev Respir Dis 1984; 130:924–9.

151. Rouby JJ, Martin De Lassale E, et al. Nosocomial bronchopneumonia in the critically ill. Histologic and bacteriologic aspects [see comments]. Am Rev Respir Dis 1992; 146:1059–66.

152. Marquette CH, Copin MC, Wallet F, et al. Diagnostic tests for pneumonia in ventilated patients: prospective evaluation of diagnostic accuracy using histology as a diagnostic gold standard. Am J Respir Crit Care Med 1995; 151:1878–88.

153. Torres A, Fabregas N, Ewig S, et al. Sampling methods for ventilator-associated pneumonia: validation using different histologic and microbiological references. Crit Care Med 2000; 28:2799–804.

154. de Jaeger A, Litalien C, Lacroix J, Guertin MC, Infante-Rivard C. Protected specimen brush or bronchoalveolar lavage to diagnose bacterial nosocomial pneumonia in ventilated adults: a meta-analysis. Crit Care Med 1999; 27:2548–60.

155. Baughman RP. Protected-specimen brush technique in the diagnosis of ventilator-associated pneumonia. Chest 2000; 117:203S–206S.

156. Torres A, El-Ebiary M. Bronchoscopic BAL in the diagnosis of ventilator-associated pneumonia. Chest 2000; 117:198S–202S.

157. Souweine B, Veber B, Bedos JP, et al. Diagnostic accuracy of protected specimen brush and bronchoalveolar lavage in nosocomial pneumonia: impact of previous antimicrobial treatments [see comments]. Crit Care Med 1998; 26:236–44.

158. Prats E, Dorca J, Pujol M, et al. Effects of antibiotics on protected specimen brush sampling in ventilator-associated pneumonia. Eur Respir J 2002; 19:944–51.

159. Montravers P, Fagon JY, Chastre J, et al. Follow-up protected specimen brushes to assess treatment in nosocomial pneumonia. Am Rev Respir Dis 1993; 147:38–44.

160. Marquette CH, Wallet F, Copin MC, et al. Relationship between microbiologic and histologic features in bacterial pneumonia. Am J Respir Crit Care Med 1996; 154:1784–7.

161. Dreyfuss D, Mier L, Le Bourdelles G, et al. Clinical significance of borderline quantitative protected brush specimen culture results. Am Rev Respir Dis 1993; 147:946–51.

162. Marquette CH, Herengt F, Mathieu D, et al. Diagnosis of pneumonia in mechanically ventilated patients. Repeatability of the protected specimen brush. Am Rev Respir Dis 1993; 147:211–4.

163. Timsit JF, Misset B, Francoual S, et al. Is protected specimen brush a reproducible method to diagnose ICU-acquired pneumonia? Chest 1993; 104:104–8.

164. Gerbeaux P, Ledoray V, Boussuges A, et al. Diagnosis of nosocomial pneumonia in mechanically ventilated patients: repeatability of the bronchoalveolar lavage. Am J Respir Crit Care Med 1998; 157:76–80.

165. Heyland DK, Cook DJ, Marshall J, et al. The clinical utility of invasive diagnostic techniques in the setting of ventilator-associated pneumonia. Canadian Critical Care Trials Group. Chest 1999; 115:1076–84.

166. McGowan JE. Antimicrobial resistance in hospital organisms and its relation to antibiotic use. Rev Infect Dis 1983; 5:1033–48.

167. Kollef MH, Fraser VJ. Antibiotic resistance in the intensive care unit. Ann Intern Med 2001; 134:298–314.

168. Croce MA, Fabian TC, Shaw B, et al. Analysis of charges associated with diagnosis of nosocomial pneumonia: can routine bronchoscopy be justified? J Trauma 1994; 37:721–7.

169. Meduri GU, Mauldin GL, Wunderink RG, et al. Causes of fever and pulmonary densities in patients with clinical manifestations of ventilator-associated pneumonia. Chest 1994; 106: 221–35.

170. Liu YC, Huang WK, Huang TS, Kunin CM. Inappropriate use of antibiotics and the risk for delayed admission and masked diagnosis of infectious diseases: a lesson from Taiwan. Arch Intern Med 2001; 161:2366–70.

171. Baker AM, Bowton DL, Haponik EF. Decision making in nosocomial pneumonia. An analytic approach to the interpretation of quantitative bronchoscopic cultures. Chest 1995; 107:85–95.

172. Sterling TR, Ho EJ, Brehm WT, Kirkpatrick MB. Diagnosis and treatment of ventilator-associated pneumonia—impact on survival. A decision analysis. Chest 1996; 110:1025–34.

173. Babcock HM, Zack JE, Garrison T, et al. Ventilator-associated pneumonia in a multi-hospital system: differences in microbiology by location. Infect Control Hosp Epidemiol 2003; 24:853–8.

174. Sole Violan J, Fernandez JA, Benitez AB, Cardenosa Cendrero JA, Rodriguez de Castro F. Impact of quantitative invasive diagnostic techniques in the management and outcome of mechanically ventilated patients with suspected pneumonia. Crit Care Med 2000; 28:2737–41.

175. Shorr AF, Sherner JH, Jackson WL, Kollef MH. Invasive approaches to the diagnosis of ventilator-associated pneumonia: A meta-analysis. Crit Care Med 2005; 33:46–53.

176. Ibrahim EH, Ward S, Sherman G, et al. Experience with a clinical guideline for the treatment of ventilator-associated pneumonia. Crit Care Med 2001; 29:1109–15.

177. Niederman MS. Appropriate use of antimicrobial agents: Challenges and strategies for improvement. Crit Care Med 2003; 31:608–16.

178. Kolleff MH. Appropriate antibiotic therapy for ventilator-associated pneumonia and sepsis: a necessity, not an issue for debate. Intensive Care Med 2003; 29:147–9.

179. Kollef MH, Ward S, Sherman G, et al. Inadequate treatment of nosocomial infections is associated with certain empiric antibiotic choices. Crit Care Med 2000; 28:3456–64.

180. Trouillet JL, Vuagnat A, Combes A, et al. *Pseudomonas aeruginosa* ventilator-associated pneumonia: comparison of episodes

due to piperacillin-resistant versus piperacillin-susceptible organisms. Clin Infect Dis 2002; 34:1047–54.

181. Hospital-acquired pneumonia in adults: diagnosis, assessment of severity, initial antimicrobial therapy, and preventive strategies. A consensus statement, American Thoracic Society, November 1995. Am J Respir Crit Care Med 1996; 153:1711–25.

182. Torres A, Ewig S. Diagnosing ventilator-associated pneumonia. N Engl J Med 2004; 350:433–5.

183. Pugin J, Auckenthaler R, Mili N, et al. Diagnosis of ventilator-associated pneumonia by bacteriologic analysis of bronchoscopic and nonbronchoscopic "blind" bronchoalveolar lavage fluid. Am Rev Respir Dis 1991; 143:1121–9.

184. Singh N, Rogers P, Atwood CW, Wagener MM, Yu VL. Short-course empiric antibiotic therapy for patients with pulmonary infiltrates in the intensive care unit. A proposed solution for indiscriminate antibiotic prescription. Am J Respir Crit Care Med 2000; 162:505–11.

185. Muller B. Procalcitonin and ventilator-associated pneumonia: yet another breath of fresh air. Am J Respir Crit Care Med 2005; 171:2–3.

186. Luyt CE, Guerin V, Combes A, et al. Procalcitonin kinetics as a prognostic marker of ventilator-associated pneumonia. Am J Respir Crit Care Med 2005; 171:48–53.

187. Gibot S, Cravoisy A, Levy B, et al. Soluble triggering receptor expressed on myeloid cells and the diagnosis of pneumonia. N Engl J Med 2004; 350:451–8.

188. Micek ST, Ward S, Fraser VJ, Kollef MH. A randomized controlled trial of an antibiotic discontinuation policy for clinically suspected ventilator-associated pneumonia. Chest 2004; 125:1791–9.

189. Luyt CE, Chastre J, Fagon JY. Value of the clinical pulmonary infection score for the identification and management of ventilator-associated pneumonia. Intensive Care Med 2004; 30:844–52.

190. Forrest A, Nix DE, Ballow CH, et al. Pharmacodynamics of intravenous ciprofloxacin in seriously ill patients. Antimicrob Agents Chemother 1993; 37:1073–81.

191. Kashuba AD, Nafziger AN, Drusano GL, Bertino JS Jr. Optimizing aminoglycoside therapy for nosocomial pneumonia caused by gram-negative bacteria. Antimicrob Agents Chemother 1999; 43:623–9.

192. Peloquin CA, Cumbo TJ, Nix DE, Sands MF, Schentag JJ. Evaluation of intravenous ciprofloxacin in patients with nosocomial lower respiratory tract infections. Impact of plasma concentrations, organism, minimum inhibitory concentration, and clinical condition on bacterial eradication. Arch Intern Med 1989; 149:2269–73.

193. Schentag JJ, Birmingham MC, Paladino JA, et al. In nosocomial pneumonia, optimizing antibiotics other than aminoglycosides is a more important determinant of successful clinical outcome, and a better means of avoiding resistance. Semin Respir Infect 1997; 12:278–93.

194. Schentag JJ, Strenkoski-Nix LC, Nix DE, Forrest A. Pharmacodynamic interactions of antibiotics alone and in combination. Clin Infect Dis 1998; 27:40–6.

195. Schentag JJ. Antimicrobial action and pharmacokinetics/pharmacodynamics: the use of AUIC to improve efficacy and avoid resistance. J Chemother 1999; 11:426–39.

196. Schentag JJ. Pharmacokinetic and pharmacodynamic surrogate markers: studies with fluoroquinolones in patients. Am J Health Syst Pharm 1999; 56:S21–4.

197. Ceftazidime combined with a short or long course of amikacin for empirical therapy of gram-negative bacteremia in cancer patients with granulocytopenia. The EORTC International Antimicrobial Therapy Cooperative Group. N Engl J Med 1987; 317:1692–8.

198. Hilf M, Yu VL, Sharp J, et al. Antibiotic therapy for *Pseudomonas aeruginosa* bacteremia: outcome correlations in a prospective study of 200 patients [see comments]. Am J Med 1989; 87:540–6.

199. Korvick JA, Bryan CS, Farber B, et al. Prospective observational study of *Klebsiella* bacteremia in 230 patients: outcome for antibiotic combinations versus monotherapy. Antimicrob Agents Chemother 1992; 36:2639–44.

200. Cometta A, Baumgartner JD, Lew D, et al. Prospective randomized comparison of imipenem monotherapy with imipenem plus netilmicin for treatment of severe infections in non-neutropenic patients. Antimicrob Agents Chemother 1994;38:1309–13.

201. Cometta A, Calandra T, Gaya H, et al. Monotherapy with meropenem versus combination therapy with ceftazidime plus amikacin as empiric therapy for fever in granulocytopenic patients with cancer. The International Antimicrobial Therapy Cooperative Group of the European Organization for Research and Treatment of Cancer and the Gruppo Italiano Malattie Ematologiche Maligne dell'Adulto Infection Program. Antimicrob Agents Chemother 1996; 40:1108–15.

202. Cometta A, Zinner S, de Bock R, et al. Piperacillin-tazobactam plus amikacin versus ceftazidime plus amikacin as empiric therapy for fever in granulocytopenic patients with cancer. The International Antimicrobial Therapy Cooperative Group of the European Organization for Research and Treatment of Cancer. Antimicrob Agents Chemother 1995; 39:445–52.

203. Dupont H, Carbon C, Carlet J. Monotherapy with a broad-spectrum beta-lactam is as effective as its combination with an aminoglycoside in treatment of severe generalized peritonitis: a multicenter randomized controlled trial. The Severe Generalized Peritonitis Study Group. Antimicrob Agents Chemother 2000; 44:2028–33.

204. Bochud PY, Glauser MP, Calandra T. Antibiotics in sepsis. Intensive Care Med 2001; 27:S33–48.

205. Thomas JK, Forrest A, Bhavnani SM, et al. Pharmacodynamic evaluation of factors associated with the development of bacterial resistance in acutely ill patients during therapy. Antimicrob Agents Chemother 1998; 42:521–7.

206. Leibovici L, Paul M, Poznanski O, et al. Monotherapy versus beta-lactam-aminoglycoside combination treatment for gram-negative bacteremia: a prospective, observational study. Antimicrob Agents Chemother 1997; 41:1127–33.

207. Paul M, Soares-Weiser K, Leibovici L. Beta lactam monotherapy versus beta lactam-aminoglycoside combination therapy for fever with neutropenia: systematic review and meta-analysis. BMJ 2003; 326:1111.

208. Chamot E, Boffi El Amari E, Rohner P, Van Delden C. Effectiveness of combination antimicrobial therapy for *Pseudomonas aeruginosa* bacteremia. Antimicrob Agents Chemother 2003; 47:2756–64.

209. Dennesen PJ, van der Ven AJ, Kessels AG, Ramsay G, Bonten MJ. Resolution of infectious parameters after antimicrobial therapy in patients with ventilator-associated pneumonia. Am J Respir Crit Care Med 2001; 163:1371–5.

210. Luna CM, Blanzaco D, Niederman MS, et al. Resolution of ventilator-associated pneumonia: Prospective evaluation of the clinical pulmonary infection score as an early clinical predictor of outcome. Crit Care Med 2003; 31:676–82.

211. Combes A, Figliolini C, Trouillet JL, et al. Factors predicting ventilator-associated pneumonia recurrence. Crit Care Med 2003; 31:1102–7.

212. Chastre J, Wolff M, Fagon JY, et al. Comparison of 8 vs 15 days of antibiotic therapy for ventilator-associated pneumonia in adults: a randomized trial. JAMA 2003; 290:2588–98.

213. Dodek P, Keenan S, Cook D, et al. Evidence-based clinical practice guideline for the prevention of ventilator-associated pneumonia. Ann Intern Med 2004; 141:305–13.

214. Collard HR, Saint S, Matthay MA. Prevention of ventilator-associated pneumonia: An evidence-based systematic review. Ann Intern Med 2003; 138:494–501.

215. Flaherty JP, Weinstein RA. Infection control and pneumonia prophylaxis strategies in the intensive care unit. Semin Respir Infect 1990; 5:191–203.

216. du Moulin G. Minimizing the potential for nosocomial pneumonia: architectural, engineering, and environmental considerations for the intensive care unit. Eur J Clin Microbiol Infect Dis 1989; 8:69–74.

217. Needleman J, Buerhaus P, Mattke S, Stewart M, Zelevinsky K. Nurse-staffing levels and the quality of care in hospitals. N Engl J Med 2002; 346:1715–22.

218. Aiken LH, Clarke SP, Cheung RB, Sloane DM, Silber JH. Educational levels of hospital nurses and surgical patient mortality. JAMA 2003; 290:1617–23.

219. Pittet D, Mourouga P, Perneger TV. Compliance with handwashing in a teaching hospital. Infection Control Program. Ann Intern Med 1999; 130:126–30.

220. Pittet D. Improving compliance with hand hygiene in hospitals. Infect Control Hosp Epidemiol 2000; 21:381–6.

221. Girou E, Loyeau S, Legrand P, Oppein F, Brun-Buisson C. Efficacy of handrubbing with alcohol based solution versus standard handwashing with antiseptic soap: randomised clinical trial. BMJ 2002; 325:362.

222. Haley RW, Culver DH, White JW, et al. The efficacy of infection surveillance and control programs in preventing nosocomial infections in US hospitals. Am J Epidemiol 1985; 121:182–205.

223. Gruson D, Hilbert G, Vargas F, et al. Rotation and restricted use of antibiotics in a medical intensive care unit. Impact on the incidence of ventilator-associated pneumonia caused by antibiotic-resistant gram-negative bacteria. Am J Respir Crit Care Med 2000; 162:837–43.

224. Nava S, Ambrosino N, Clini E, et al. Noninvasive mechanical ventilation in the weaning of patients with respiratory failure due to chronic obstructive pulmonary disease. A randomized, controlled trial. Ann Intern Med 1998; 128:721–8.

225. Kress JP, Pohlman AS, O'Connor MF, Hall JB. Daily interruption of sedative infusions in critically ill patients undergoing mechanical ventilation. N Engl J Med 2000; 342:1471–7.

226. Krishnan JA, Moore D, Robeson C, Rand CS, Fessler HE. A prospective, controlled trial of a protocol-based strategy to discontinue mechanical ventilation. Am J Respir Crit Care Med 2004; 169:673–8.

227. Brook AD, Ahrens TS, Schaiff R, et al. Effect of a nursing-implemented sedation protocol on the duration of mechanical ventilation. Crit Care Med 1999; 27:2609–15.

228. Barrientos-Vega R, Mar Sanchez-Soria M, Morales-Garcia C, et al. Prolonged sedation of critically ill patients with midazolam or propofol: impact on weaning and costs. Crit Care Med 1997; 25:33–40.

229. Kollef MH, Shapiro SD, Silver P, et al. A randomized, controlled trial of protocol-directed versus physician-directed weaning from mechanical ventilation. Crit Care Med 1997; 25:567–74.

230. Girou E, Schortgen F, Delclaux C, et al. Association of noninvasive ventilation with nosocomial infections and survival in critically ill patients. JAMA 2000; 284:2361–7.

231. Kagramanov V, Lyman A. Noninvasive ventilation and nosocomial infection. JAMA 2001; 285:881.

232. Carlucci A, Richard JC, Wysocki M, Lepage E, Brochard L. Noninvasive versus conventional mechanical ventilation. An epidemiologic survey. Am J Respir Crit Care Med 2001; 163:874–80.

233. Nourdine K, Combes P, Carton MJ, et al. Does noninvasive ventilation reduce the ICU nosocomial infection risk? A prospective clinical survey. Intensive Care Med 1999; 25:567–73.

234. Brochard L, Mancebo J, Wysocki M, et al. Noninvasive ventilation for acute exacerbations of chronic obstructive pulmonary disease. N Engl J Med 1995; 333:817–22.

235. Confalonieri M, Parigi P, Scartabellati A, et al. Noninvasive mechanical ventilation improves the immediate and long-term outcome of COPD patients with acute respiratory failure. Eur Respir J 1996; 9:422–30.

236. Wood KA, Lewis L, Von Harz B, Kollef MH. The use of noninvasive positive pressure ventilation in the emergency department: results of a randomized clinical trial. Chest 1998; 113:1339–46.

237. Antonelli M, Conti G. Noninvasive positive pressure ventilation as treatment for acute respiratory failure in critically ill patients. Crit Care 2000; 4:15–22.

238. Antonelli M, Conti G, Rocco M, et al. A comparison of noninvasive positive-pressure ventilation and conventional mechanical ventilation in patients with acute respiratory failure. N Engl J Med 1998; 339:429–35.

239. Orozco-Levi M, Torres A, Ferrer M, et al. Semirecumbent position protects from pulmonary aspiration but not completely from gastroesophageal reflux in mechanically ventilated patients. Am J Respir Crit Care Med 1995; 152:1387–90.

240. Choi SC, Nelson LD. Kinetic therapy in critically ill patients: combined results based on meta-analysis. J Crit Care 1992; 7:57–62.

241. Traver GA, Tyler ML, Hudson LD, Sherrill DL, Quan SF. Continuous oscillation: outcome in critically ill patients. J Crit Care 1995; 10:97–103.

242. Mahul P, Auboyer C, Jospe R, et al. Prevention of nosocomial pneumonia in intubated patients: respective role of mechanical subglottic secretions drainage and stress ulcer prophylaxis. Intensive Care Med 1992; 18:20–5.

243. Valles J, Artigas A, Rello J, et al. Continuous aspiration of subglottic secretions in preventing ventilator-associated pneumonia. Ann Intern Med 1995; 122:179–86.

244. Kollef MH, Skubas NJ, Sundt TM. A randomized clinical trial of continuous aspiration of subglottic secretions in cardiac surgery patients [see comments]. Chest 1999; 116:1339–46.

245. Bo H, He L, Qu J. [Influence of the subglottic secretion drainage on the morbidity of ventilator associated pneumonia in mechanically ventilated patients]. Zhonghua Jie He He Hu Xi Za Zhi 2000; 23:472–4.

246. Smulders K, van Der Hoeven H, Weers-Pothoff I, Vandenbroucke-Grauls C. A randomized clinical trial of intermittent subglottic secretion drainage in patients receiving mechanical ventilation. Chest 2002; 121:858–62.

247. Dezfulian C, Shojania K, Collard HR, et al. Subglottic secretion drainage for preventing ventilator-associated pneumonia: A meta-analysis. Am J Med 2005; 118:11–8.

248. Berra L, De Marchi L, Panigada M, et al. Evaluation of continuous aspiration of subglottic secretion in an in vivo study. Crit Care Med 2004; 32:2071–8.

249. Stamm AM. Ventilator-associated pneumonia and frequency of circuit changes. Am J Infect Control 1998; 26:71–3.

250. Davis K Jr, Evans SL, Campbell RS, et al. Prolonged use of heat and moisture exchangers does not affect device efficiency or frequency rate of nosocomial pneumonia [see comments]. Crit Care Med 2000; 28:1412–8.

251. Deppe SA, Kelly JW, Thoi LL, et al. Incidence of colonization, nosocomial pneumonia, and mortality in critically ill patients using a Trach Care closed-suction system versus an open-suction system: prospective, randomized study. Crit Care Med 1990; 18:1389–93.

252. Combes P, Fauvage B, Oleyer C. Nosocomial pneumonia in mechanically ventilated patients, a prospective randomised evaluation of the Stericath closed suctioning system. Intensive Care Med 2000; 26:878–82.

253. Yavagal DR, Karnad DR, Oak JL. Metoclopramide for preventing pneumonia in critically ill patients receiving enteral tube feeding: a randomized controlled trial. Crit Care Med 2000; 28:1408–11.

254. Kearns PJ, Chin D, Mueller L, et al. The incidence of ventilator-associated pneumonia and success in nutrient delivery with gastric versus small intestinal feeding: a randomized clinical trial. Crit Care Med 2000; 28:1742–6.

255. Donowitz LG, Page MC, Mileur BL, Guenthner SH. Alteration of normal gastric flora in critical care patients receiving antacid and cimetidine therapy. Infect Control 1986; 7:23–6.

256. van Saene HK, Stoutenbeek CC, Stoller JK. Selective decontamination of the digestive tract in the intensive care unit: current status and future prospects. Crit Care Med 1992; 20: 691–703.

257. Stoutenbeek CP, van Saene HK, Miranda DR, Zandstra DF. The effect of selective decontamination of the digestive tract on colonisation and infection rate in multiple trauma patients. Intensive Care Med 1984; 10:185–92.

258. Heyland DK, Cook DJ, Jaeschke R, et al. Selective decontamination of the digestive tract. An overview. Chest 1994; 105:1221–9.

259. Hurley JC. Prophylaxis with enteral antibiotics in ventilated patients: selective decontamination or selective cross-infection? Antimicrob Agents Chemother 1995; 39:941–7.

260. Nathens AB, Marshall JC. Selective decontamination of the digestive tract in surgical patients: a systematic review of the evidence [see comments]. Arch Surg 1999; 134:170–6.

261. Bonten MJ. Prevention of infection in the intensive care unit. Curr Opin Crit Care 2004; 10:364–8.

262. de Jonge E, Schultz MJ, Spanjaard L, et al. Effects of selective decontamination of digestive tract on mortality and acquisition of resistant bacteria in intensive care: a randomised controlled trial. Lancet 2003; 362:1011–6.

263. Gruson D, Hilbert G, Vargas F, et al. Strategy of antibiotic rotation: long-term effect on incidence and susceptibilities of Gram-negative bacilli responsible for ventilator-associated pneumonia. Crit Care Med 2003; 31:1908–14.

264. Raymond DP, Pelletier SJ, Crabtree TD, et al. Impact of a rotating empiric antibiotic schedule on infectious mortality in an intensive care unit. Crit Care Med 2001; 29:1101–8.

265. Bergstrom CT, Lo M, Lipsitch M. Ecological theory suggests that antimicrobial cycling will not reduce antimicrobial resistance in hospitals. Proc Natl Acad Sci USA 2004; 101:13285–90.

Chapter 47

SINUS INFECTIONS IN THE VENTILATED PATIENT

JEAN-JACQUES ROUBY
QIN LU

PHYSIOLOGY OF PARANASAL SINUSES
    Classical Hypotheses
    Recent Hypothesis: The Role of the Regional
        Production of Nitric Oxide
PATHOGENESIS AND PREDISPOSING FACTORS
    Experimental Models
    Macroscopic and Microscopic Aspects of Sinusitis
        Complicating Mechanical Ventilation
    Predisposing Factors
EPIDEMIOLOGY AND COMPLICATIONS
    Incidence
    Nosocomial Sinusitis and Ventilator-Associated
        Pneumonia
DIAGNOSIS
    Clinical Diagnosis
    Radiographic Diagnosis
    Microbiologic Diagnosis
TREATMENT
    Prevention of Ventilator-Associated Sinusitis
    Treatment of Infectious Maxillary Sinusitis
IMPORTANT UNKNOWNS
    Clinical Relevance of Frontal, Ethmoid,
        and Sphenoid Sinusitis
    Role of Antibiotics in the Therapy of
        Ventilator-Associated Maxillary Sinusitis
CONCLUSIONS AND FUTURE PROSPECTS

Infection of paranasal sinus cavities is a well-recognized cause of fever in mechanically ventilated patients.[1–7] Easy to detect in maxillary sinuses, the infectious process also frequently involves ethmoid, frontal, and sphenoid sinuses[8] where the diagnosis is more difficult to establish.[9] Infectious sinusitis represents an important reservoir of bacteria[10] which may disseminate into the respiratory tract[11] and intracranially.[12] In contrast to community-acquired sinusitis, ventilator-associated sinusitis is often clinically silent in sedated critically ill patients and may be underdiagnosed if not systematically screened for in the presence of fever of unknown origin. In the absence of diagnosis and appropriate treatment, bacteremia,[2,5] ventilator-associated pneumonia,[13] and life-threatening complications, such as orbital infection,[14] meningitis, mastoiditis, cerebral abscess, or thrombosis of the sinus cavernosus, may result.[12] Early detection and treatment of infectious maxillary sinusitis

have been shown to significantly reduce the incidence of ventilator-associated pneumonia and may decrease intensive care mortality.[11]

Physiology of Paranasal Sinuses

CLASSICAL HYPOTHESES

Located at the entry of the respiratory system, paranasal sinuses and the nose serve to humidify, filter, warm, and sense inspiratory gas.[15,16] A number of other presupposed physiologic roles have not yet received firm scientific confirmation.[17] Among them, the most popular are that paranasal sinuses help lighten the bones of the skull, improve the resonance of the voice, serve as a sound box for opera singers, increase the surface area of the olfactory membrane, serve as shock absorbers in mechanical impacts, protect against high pressure in the nasal region when sneezing, act as thermal insulators of the brain, and promote facial growth and architecture. More simply, paranasal sinuses might be considered as evolutionary relics or faults, whose form results from the influence of the forces created during the act of chewing.

RECENT HYPOTHESIS: THE ROLE OF THE REGIONAL PRODUCTION OF NITRIC OXIDE

Large amounts of nitric oxide are produced in human paranasal sinuses[18,19] and permanently released in the upper airways through the different ostia that link antral cavities to the nostrils.[20] As shown in Fig. 47-1, an inducible form of nitric oxide synthetase is present in cilia and microvilli of the maxillary sinus epithelium of healthy volunteers.[18,19] Significant nitric oxide concentrations are also found in the exhaled gas of guinea pigs, pigs, rhesus monkeys, rats, rabbits, horses, and Asian elephants, all species possessing open paranasal sinuses.[20–24] Interestingly, seals and baboons, which do not have open paranasal sinuses, do not exhale nitric oxide,[25,26] thus confirming that pneumatic facial cavities play a critical role in the nasal production of nitric oxide in mammals. Humming, by accelerating gas exchange in sinus cavities, markedly increases exhaled nasal nitric oxide[27] whereas moderate exercise has an opposite effect.[28] Nitric oxide produced in the paranasal sinuses likely has an important role in host defense against inhaled pathogens, in the optimization of ventilation:perfusion ratios during normal breathing,[29] and in the regulation of ciliary motility.[30,31]

Each paranasal sinus communicates with the corresponding nostril by an ostium, which provides aeration of the antral cavity. Bacteria are present in nasal secretions covering the mucociliary epithelium and on the gingival mucosa and its crevices. Microorganisms may enter the maxillary cavity by the canine fossa and the inferior meatus. Paranasal sinuses, however, are normally sterile[32] as a result of two different protective mechanisms. First, the antral mucosa is covered with a protective mucus layer produced by goblet cells. Bacteria penetrating into the maxillary cavity are immediately enveloped by mucus and moved rapidly to the sinus ostium by respiratory cilia. Second, the antral

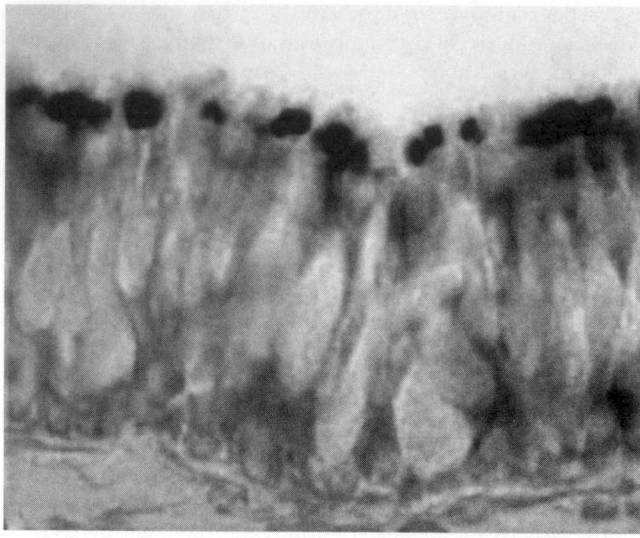

A

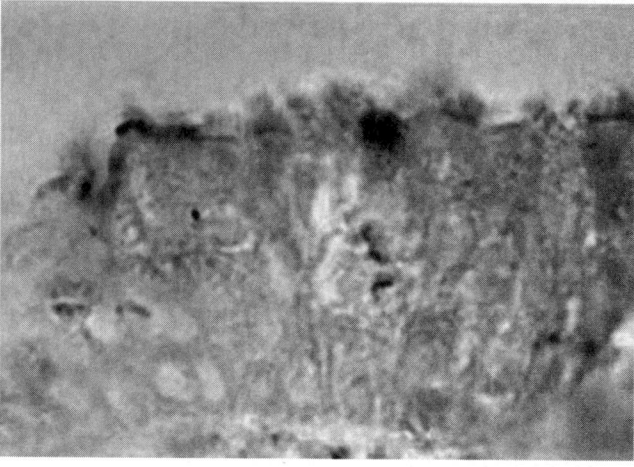

B

FIGURE 47-1 Immunoreactive sinus inducible nitric oxide synthetase distribution is represented in black on biopsy samples from maxillary sinus epithelium. In a healthy subject (*A*), a strong immunoreactivity is detected in the apical part of the ciliated epithelial cells near the surface. In a patient with radiographic maxillary sinusitis (*B*), the signal is weaker or absent. (*Reproduced, with permission, from Deja et al.[19]*)

concentrations of nitric oxide exert a bacteriostatic effect. Many pathogens are sensitive to nitric oxide in concentrations less than 1 part per million.[33–36] The antral concentrations of nitric oxide, produced by the maxillary epithelium, are ≥2 parts per million and likely contribute to antral sterility.[32]

Pathogenesis and Predisposing Factors

Pathogenesis of radiographic sinusitis diagnosed in intubated and tracheostomized patients is incompletely un-

derstood. Either nonspecific inflammation or infection of paranasal sinuses can be observed and several predisposing factors have been identified.

EXPERIMENTAL MODELS

If relevant to human disease, animal models are useful for understanding pathogenesis and assessing the efficacy of treatment. Rabbits have large and accessible nostrils and their sinuses show anatomical similarities to those of humans. In this species, sinuses consist of a number of cavities connected to each other and can be considered as one, called the maxillary sinus.[37] Historically, a surgical model was the first to be set-up in rabbits:[38] the maxillary sinus was opened through an anterior-wall antrostomy, the natural ostium was glued and closed and bacterial strains were directly injected into the maxillary cavity. Although the model is extremely reliable for producing purulent sinusitis, it causes a traumatic injury that questions its relevance for human sinusitis. As a consequence, a rhinogenic model was proposed in the late 1990s and remains to date the reference:[39,40] a foreign body—an endotracheal tube,[41] a catheter,[42] or a sponge impregnated or not with bacteria[43]—is implanted into nostrils for a period of time ranging from several days to several weeks. In the rhinogenic rabbit model, computed tomographic evidence of maxillary sinusitis is detected at the sixth day following foreign body nasal placement.[43]

A number of lessons can be drawn from experimental studies. Direct or indirect obstruction of the ostia rapidly induces an acute sinus inflammation. The intranasal placement of a foreign body over several days results in purulent sinusitis, characterized by the accumulation of a thick and purulent discharge within the sinus cavity.[43] Initial histological lesions are made of inflammation and exudation of maxillary mucosa: the number of goblet cells increases, augmenting mucus production and causing fluid accumulation within the cavity. Then, inflammatory polyp formation is observed,[41,43,44] associated with permanent loss of cilia, squamous metaplasia, and fibrosis.[43,45] The risk of sinusitis increases with the nasal catheterization period and the size of the intranasal catheter.[41,42] Relief of ostial obstruction promotes resolution of radiographic sinusitis within a few days,[46] whereas sinus inflammation persists for several weeks.[43] Over time, the fluid-filled maxillary cavity is contaminated[41] or infected[43] by streptococci, staphylococci, *Pseudomonas* and *Acinetobacter* species, and *Escherichia coli* and *Proteus* species present in the adjacent nostril.[41] Surprisingly, bacteria impregnating the intranasal sponge are rarely found in the nasal cavity and are often replaced by bacteria belonging to the normal flora of the rabbit nostrils.[43,47]

Finally, the following sequence may lead to bacterial sinusitis. First, the presence of a nasal foreign body induces an ipsilateral inflammatory antral disease. Second, mucus accumulates within the antral cavity because of goblet cell proliferation, impairment of mucociliary clearance, and ostial obstruction. Third, the antral contents are contaminated and infected by microorganisms issued from the nostrils whose proliferation into the sinus cavity is facilitated by the lack of regional nitric oxide production.

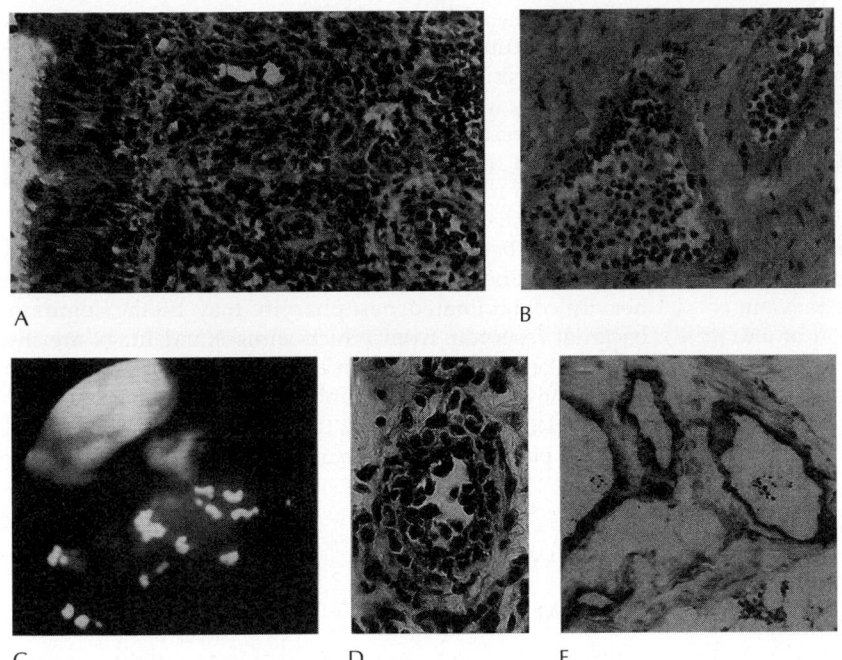

A   B   C   D   E

FIGURE 47-2 *a*. Photomicrograph of left maxillary sinus mucosa showing pronounced inflammation consisting of massive infiltration by polymorphonuclear neutrophils, eosinophils, monocytes, macrophages, and lymphocytes in a patient with bacterial sinusitis caused by anaerobes. *b*. Photomicrograph of two vessels with numerous inflammatory cells (polymorphonuclear neutrophils, eosinophils, and lymphocytes) in a patient with left bacterial maxillary sinusitis caused by *Peptostreptococcus anaerobius* and *Eubacterium*. *c*. Corresponding sinoscopic view after removal of foul-smelling pus. An intensive and red edematous mucosa (*left*) and some pus (*right*) are seen at the medial wall of the maxillary sinus. *d*. In the same patient, a vessel is shown with adhesion of inflammatory cells as well as penetration through the vessel. *e*. Photomicrograph of two vessels showing a strong expression of P-selectin, a key factor facilitating activation and recruitment of leukocytes in inflammatory maxillary sinusitis. (*Reproduced, with permission, from Westergren et al.*[48])

MACROSCOPIC AND MICROSCOPIC ASPECTS OF SINUSITIS COMPLICATING MECHANICAL VENTILATION

Only a few studies have reported macroscopic and histologic disorders characterizing radiographic maxillary sinusitis in critically ill patients.[19,48–50] In 33 neurosurgical patients receiving prolonged mechanical ventilation with radiographic maxillary sinusitis, antroscopies were performed by the canine-fossa route.[49] Most of radiographic maxillary sinusitis corresponded to "inflammatory" sinusitis, with the antral cavity filled with thin and transparent secretions and/or gelatinous and transparent mucus with a neutral smell. In a minority of patients, bacterial sinusitis was diagnosed as the presence of viscous and opaque pus with a foul smell. Both types of sinusitis were associated with varying mucosal reactions, ranging from pallid to vermilion edema with different degrees of transparency. Interestingly, in two patients with "inflammatory" sinusitis and one patient with bacterial sinusitis, maxillary mucosa was macroscopically normal. When present, mucosal edema always included the medial side with the ostial region.[49] Biopsy specimens of antral mucosa revealed various grades of inflammation. As shown in Fig. 47-2, acute inflammation involving the maxillary epithelium, the connective tissue, and the vessels with a massive infiltration by polymorphonuclear neutrophils was observed in patients with bacterial maxillary sinusitis. In patients with "inflammatory" sinusitis, mild inflammation was observed, characterized by a moderate cellular infiltration of the connective tissue with a massive infiltration of vessels by eosinophils.[48]

PREDISPOSING FACTORS

A number of factors predisposing to nosocomial sinusitis have been identified in ventilated critically ill patients.

FOREIGN BODIES WITHIN THE NOSTRILS

Several prospective and retrospective studies have shown that the occurrence of radiographic sinusitis has a higher incidence in the antrum adjacent to nasotracheal and nasogastric tubes than in the nonadjacent sinus.[3,4,6,7,51–62] The presence of a nasogastric tube for enteral feeding appears as an independent risk factor.[63] As in experimental sinusitis, the presence of a foreign body within the nostrils creates an ostial obstruction that initiates sinus inflammation and mucus accumulation within the sinus cavity. Confirming experimental data,[42] a large endotracheal tube induces radiographic sinusitis more frequently and faster than a small nasogastric tube.[55,58] In addition, the plastic nasotracheal tube is the site of biofilm formation for bacteria with adhesive capacity and enhanced pathogenicity:[64–66] microorganisms adhere to the internal and external surfaces of the endotracheal tube and some species exude an exopolysaccharide that acts as a slime-like adhesive.[67] Bacteria encased in this biofilm become partially resistant to the action of antimicrobials and host defences.[68,69] The bacterial proliferation around nasal foreign bodies forms a reservoir from which microorganisms penetrate into the antral cavity.[41]

SIZE OF THE MEATUS INFERIOR AND BODY POSITION

Ostial size, upon which drainage and ventilation of the sinus cavities depends, can markedly vary from one patient to another.[70] In humans, supine position is known to reduce ostial patency[71] by inducing swelling of the ostiomeatal complex.[72] A functional ostial area <5 mm^2 induces hypoventilation of the maxillary cavity, local hypoxia, decrease in mucosal blood flow, and predispose to maxillary sinusitis by impairing mucociliary clearance.[73]

SEPSIS

Generalized sepsis, well known for stimulating numerous tissue-inducible nitric oxide synthetases, inhibits the nitric oxide metabolic pathway at the maxillary level.[19] Autoinhaled nitric oxide plays an important anti-inflammatory and antiviral role in colds.[74] Community-acquired, as well as ventilator-associated, sinusitis decreases exhaled nasal nitric oxide[19,75,76] by reducing its antral production (see Fig. 47-1). Sepsis originating in other organs also markedly inhibits the antral production of nitric oxide through a downregulation of inducible nitric oxide synthetase messenger ribonucleic acid.[19] The sepsis-induced reduction of antral nitric oxide concentrations contributes to impaired mucociliary clearance and decreased perfusion of the maxillary epithelium, both factors that facilitate infection of the maxillary cavity by impairing bacterial cleansing.[77]

Epidemiology and Complications

INCIDENCE

In critically ill patients, the reported incidence of radiographic sinusitis varies from 25–75%.[78] More than 80% of radiographic abnormalities of the maxillary sinuses are associated with radiographic abnormalities of the ethmoid, sphenoid, and frontal sinuses.[8,79] Variability in the estimated incidence stems from the many radiographic techniques used for diagnosis: conventional radiography is much less accurate than computed tomography or maxillary ultrasound. After 12 hours of nasal endotracheal intubation and/or nasogastric tube placement, 38% of critically ill patients have computed tomographic evidence of radiographic maxillary sinusitis.[8] In orally intubated patients with an oral gastric tube, the incidence of radiographic maxillary sinusitis decreases to 34%, confirming that factors other than the presence of a foreign body in the nostrils contribute to antral disease.[8] Among these, the supine position, head[63] and/or facial trauma,[51,53,80] allergy, and sepsis have been incriminated.[81] After 7 days, the incidence of radiographic maxillary sinusitis increases to 80%.[8] Infectious sinusitis is less frequent than radiographic sinusitis, occurring only in 20–30% of patients intubated longer than 7 days.[79] Its incidence is higher in nasotracheally than in orotracheally intubated patients.[8]

NOSOCOMIAL SINUSITIS AND VENTILATOR-ASSOCIATED PNEUMONIA

A link between infectious maxillary sinusitis and bronchopneumonia has been established experimentally.[47,82] In critically ill patients, nosocomial sinusitis is considered a major cause of ventilator-associated pneumonia.[8,13,56,62] In a randomized study assessing a systematic search for sinusitis in nasotracheally ventilated patients, the incidence of ventilator-associated pneumonia was significantly higher in the control group than in the study group, where infectious maxillary sinusitis was systematically sought and treated, when confirmed, by sinus drainage and intravenous antibiotics.[11] In addition, the mortality rate significantly decreased from 46% in the control group to 36% in the study group. Although the association between nosocomial sinusitis and ventilator-associated pneumonia appears highly likely, the frequent discordance between microbiologic results from sinus and lower airway cultures[8,11] suggest that these two infections may also arise simultaneously and independently because of shared risk factors and diminished host defense for infection.[83] The nature of the link between nosocomial sinusitis and ventilator-associated pneumonia is complex and multifactorial. A heavily contaminated nasopharynx may be the common bacterial reservoir from which sinuses and lungs are infected. Conversely, antral infection, characterized by high concentrations of microorganisms,[8] can also be a reservoir from which the oropharynx, the tracheobronchial tree, and the lung parenchyma are secondarily infected.

Diagnosis

CLINICAL DIAGNOSIS

Unlike clinical symptomatology of community-acquired maxillary sinusitis, clinical signs of ventilator-associated maxillary sinusitis are scarce and of limited specificity.[78] Critically ill patients are rarely able to communicate, and any complaint related to sinusitis will go unnoticed by the physician. General signs of infection such as fever and leukocytosis have poor specificity. Mucopurulent nasal discharge is evocative but of limited sensitivity.[51] Frontal headache is often blunted by sedative drugs aimed at facilitating mechanical ventilation. As a consequence, ventilator-associated maxillary sinusitis cannot be reliably detected on clinical signs alone and should be systematically sought in the presence of fever of unknown origin.[11,83,84]

RADIOGRAPHIC DIAGNOSIS

SINUS RADIOGRAPHY

In ambulatory and spontaneously breathing patients, standard sinus radiography using the Blondeau's view and performed in the upright position, is the classic diagnostic tool for demonstrating community-acquired acute maxillary sinusitis. Ultrasound, which was introduced in the 1980s, is also very accurate for establishing the diagnosis.[85,86] In ventilated patients lying in the supine position, sinus radiography is cumbersome and appropriate radiographic projections are difficult to obtain. Many factors related to the intensive care environment, contribute to the poor quality of sinus radiography: the difficulty of placing the patient in the upright position, the use of portable equipment, the negative impact of nasogastric and nasotracheal tubes on radiographic resolution, and the variability of exposure.

COMPUTED TOMOGRAPHY SCAN

Paranasal computed tomography is the reference technique for establishing the diagnosis of radiographic sinusitis.[8,87–91] A thin-section, low-dose computed tomography examination is preferred to the classic spiral technique in order to avoid excessive radiation exposure.[91] Ten

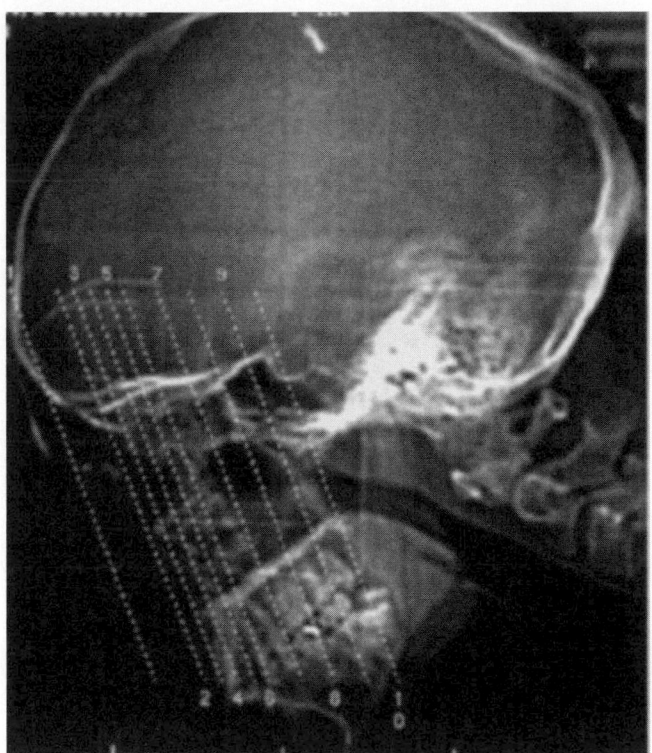

FIGURE 47-3 Scout view with different interslice gap between the 10 slices of the low-dose computed tomography protocol recommended for diagnosis of radiographic sinusitis. (*Reproduced, with permission, from Hagtvedt et al.[91]*)

thin noncontiguous computed tomography sections, using an initial interslice gap of 15 mm aimed at avoiding direct radiation to the eye lens (Fig. 47-3), should be performed. Such a technique decreases radiation exposure by more than 90% without seriously affecting the quality of the images (Fig. 47-4).

In ventilated patients, the computed tomographic image of a given paranasal sinus can be classified into three categories:[8] normal (Fig. 47-5), mucosal thickening (Fig. 47-6), and radiographic maxillary sinusitis, characterized by a liquid content within the sinus cavity (Fig. 47-7). Very often, these categories coexist in the different paranasal sinuses of critically ill patients. More than 80% of patients with radiographic abnormalities of maxillary sinuses have also abnormal frontal, ethmoid, and sphenoid sinuses. Conversely, only half of ventilated patients with normally aerated maxillary sinuses have radiographic abnormalities of frontal, ethmoid, and sphenoid sinuses.[8] An air-fluid level in the sinus cavity or the complete sinus opacification are evocative of infectious sinusitis and call for a bacteriologic confirmation. The significance of mucosal thickening in ventilated patients is incompletely understood. Very frequently, it represents an early stage of radiographic sinusitis.[8]

Although considered the gold standard, several limitations preclude the routine use of computed tomography for diagnosing ventilator-associated sinusitis. It requires transportation of ventilated patients outside the intensive care unit, a risky procedure.[92] It is costly and not easily repeatable. As a consequence, ultrasound techniques have been developed over the last 15 years and are currently considered an attractive alternative diagnostic tool.[61,88–90,93]

ULTRASOUND EXAMINATION OF MAXILLARY SINUSES

A-mode sinus ultrasound was proposed in the early 1990s for diagnosing radiographic maxillary sinusitis in ventilated patients.[61] In the late 1990s, it was demonstrated that maxillary sinus A-mode ultrasound examination correlated well with sinuscopic findings in a series of neurosurgical critically ill patients receiving prolonged mechanical ventilation.[93] It is difficult, however, to discriminate polyps from mucosal thickening and the absence of direct imaging of the sinus cavity complicates the interpretation for the clinician. Therefore, bedside B-mode ultrasound was proposed as an attractive alternative.[88,89] The patient should be examined at the bedside in a semi-recumbent position with a 3.5-MHz probe. The ultrasonic procedure should be performed in a transversal plane using different probe angulations, at the level of the front maxillary sinus wall, delineated by the lower orbital border, the nose, the upper maxilla, and the external cheekbone.[89] Image formation

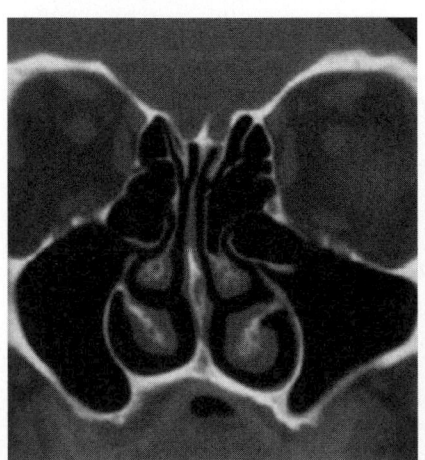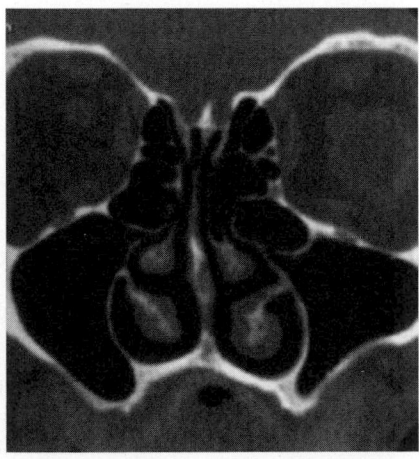

A

B

FIGURE 47-4 Standard-dose (*a*) compared to low-dose (*b*) computed tomography images of normal ethmoid and maxillary sinuses obtained in a coronal plane through the ostiomeatal complex. (*Reproduced, with permission, from Hagtvedt et al.[91]*)

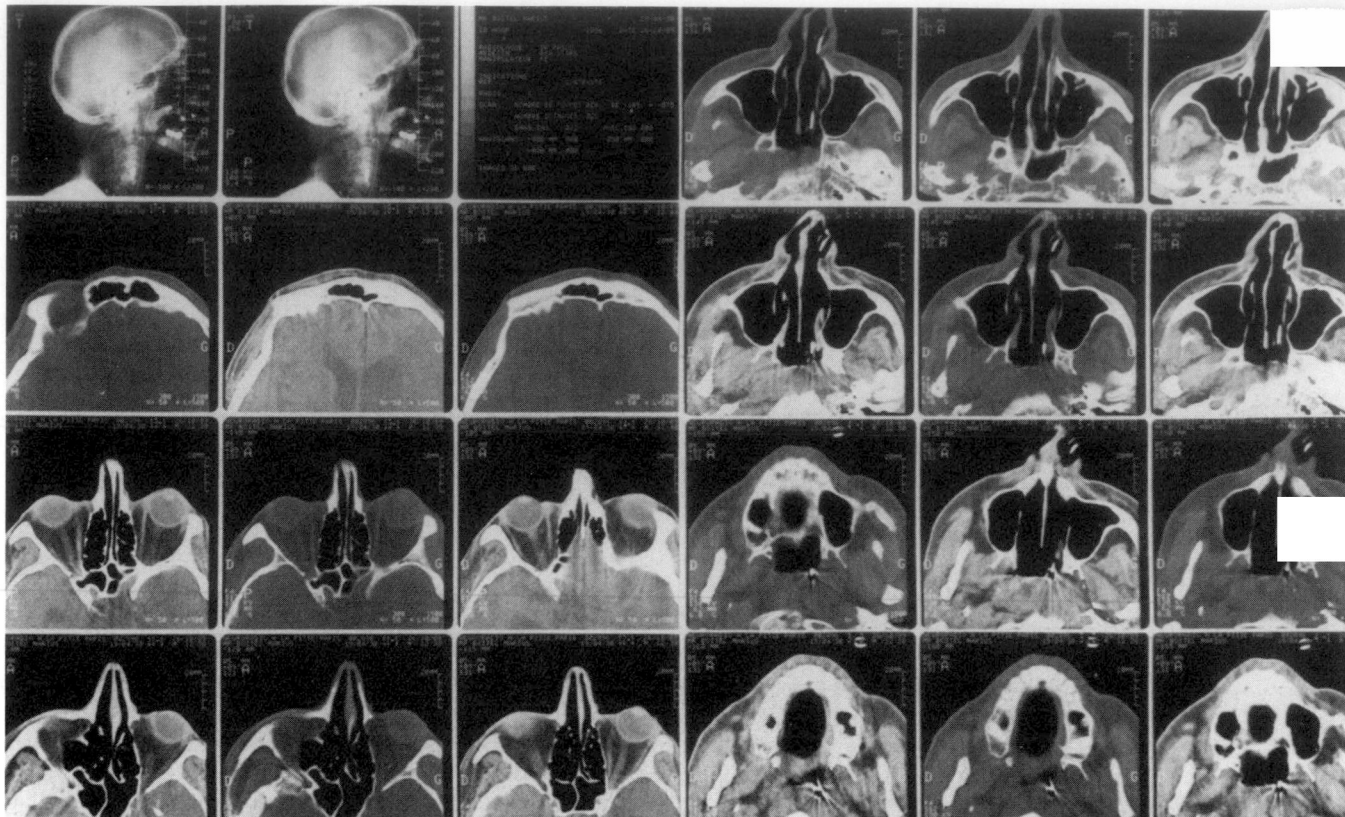

FIGURE 47-5 Normally aerated maxillary, ethmoid, sphenoid, and frontal sinuses in a ventilated patient with orotracheal intubation and the gastric tube positioned in the left nostril. (*Reproduced, with permission, from Rouby et al.*[8])

depends on the presence of fluid or mucosal thickening within the sinus cavity that transmits the ultrasonic beam to deep anatomic structures. When the posterior bony wall of the maxillary sinus becomes visible in part or completely, depending on the amount of gas present in the sinus cavity, a "sinusogram" is observed (Fig. 47-8).

In ventilated patients, the ultrasound image of the maxillary sinus can be classified into three categories:[89] absence of "sinusogram," partial "sinusogram," and complete "sinusogram" (Fig. 47-9). As shown in Figs. 47-8 and 47-9, the absence of a "sinusogram" in a ventilated patient lying in the supine position may correspond either to an air-fluid level or to a normally aerated sinus. Repeating the ultrasound procedure in the half-sitting position, however, may reveal an incomplete "sinusogram," thereby asserting the diagnosis of radiographic maxillary sinusitis.[90,93] A partial "sinusogram" may indicate either mucosal thickening, simple inflammation of the sinus mucosa, or an air-fluid level. Note that in half the patients with complete opacification of the maxillary cavity on computed tomography exhibit a partial "sinusogram," resulting from the presence of small bubbles within the collection.[89] Repeating ultrasound in the supine position may facilitate the differentiation between mucosal thickening and true maxillary sinusitis.[93] The apparition of a complete "sinusogram" in the supine position is evocative of the presence of bubbles within a fluid collection filling the antral cavity. The disappearance of the partial "sinusogram"

in the supine position is evocative of an air-fluid level, characteristic of radiographic maxillary sinusitis. In contrast, the persistence of a partial "sinusogram" in the supine position is strongly suggestive of mucosal thickening.

If radiographic doubt persists and clinical signs are evocative of infectious maxillary sinusitis—purulent nasal discharge associated with fever of unknown origin—then a paranasal computed tomography scan should be performed. A complete "sinusogram" is always related to a true radiographic maxillary sinusitis and requires antral puncture in the presence of fever of unknown origin. Based on these recommendations, bedside maxillary ultrasound has a sensitivity of 100% and a specificity of 97% for diagnosing radiographic maxillary sinusitis in intubated patients undergoing mechanical ventilation.[90] An important limitation of bedside maxillary ultrasound is that it does not provide any reliable information on frontal, ethmoid, and sphenoid sinuses.

MICROBIOLOGIC DIAGNOSIS

DIAGNOSTIC CRITERIA FOR INFECTIOUS MAXILLARY SINUSITIS

Infectious maxillary sinusitis has to be clearly differentiated from radiographic maxillary sinusitis. The latter corresponds to fluid accumulation within the antral cavity, the liquid being either mucus or pus. Infectious sinusitis is

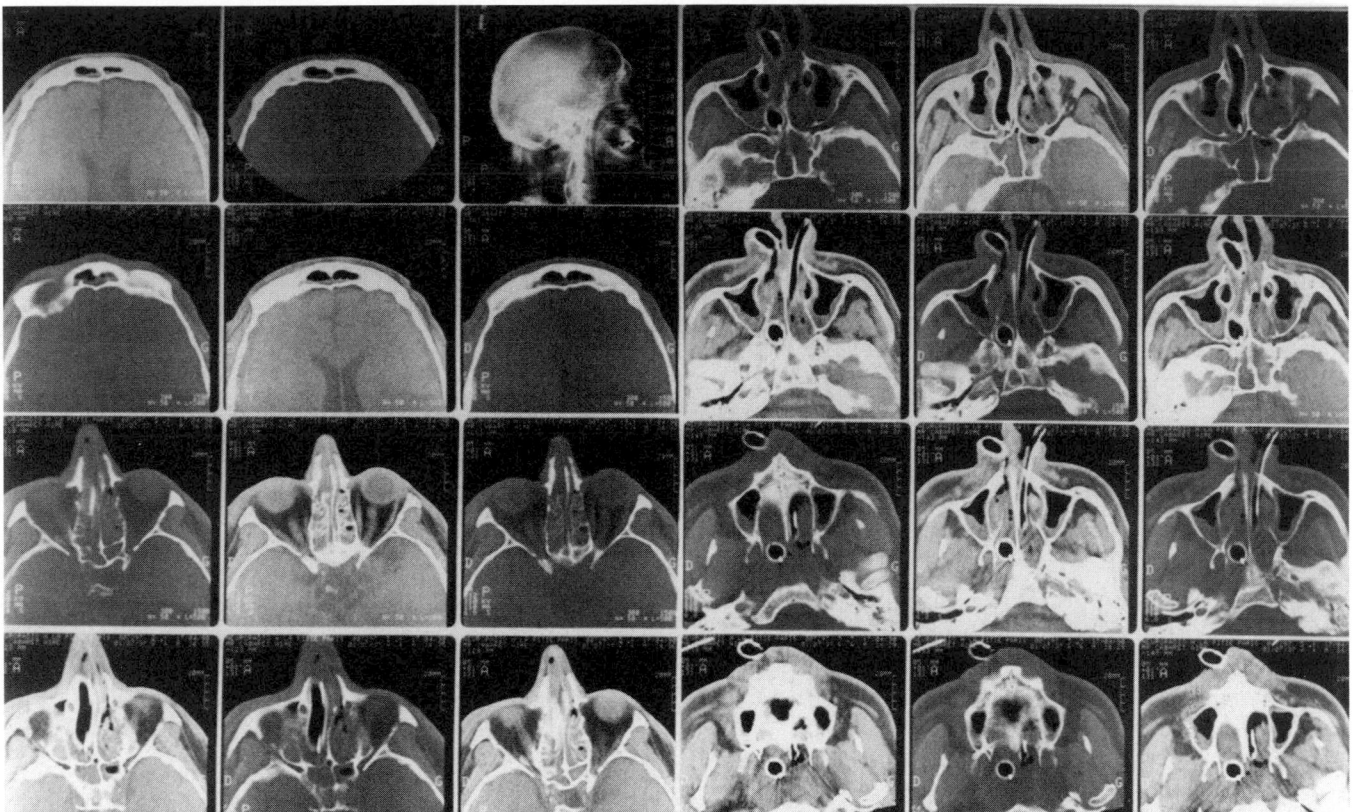

FIGURE 47-6 Computed tomography scan showing mucosal thickening of the right and left maxillary and frontal sinuses, and of the left ethmoid and sphenoid sinuses, associated with complete opacification of the right ethmoid and sphenoid sinuses in a ventilated patient with right nasotracheal intubation and a gastric tube positioned in the left nostril. On a second paranasal computed tomography scan, performed 1 week later without changing the initial position of the endotracheal and gastric tubes, complete opacification of the maxillary, ethmoid, and sphenoid sinuses was observed with a persistent mucosal thickening of both frontal sinuses. (*Reproduced, with permission, from Rouby et al.[8]*)

defined by the presence of pus in the maxillary cavity and requires cellular and bacterial analysis of the sinus contents. Therefore, antral puncture is indispensable for an accurate diagnosis. Examination of the sinus contents is impossible for frontal and ethmoid sinuses. It requires an easy-to-perform antral puncture for the maxillary sinus and a highly-specialized endoscopic puncture for the sphenoid sinus. Maxillary puncture can be performed either by the transnasal or the canine fossa routes.[94]

The transnasal and canine fossa approaches are exposed to massive bacterial contamination issued from the nostrils and gingiva, which are heavily contaminated by nosocomial microorganisms in critically ill patients. The presence of a foreign body in the nose further increases the bacterial burden and seriously complicates the process of nasal decontamination.[8] After a meticulous and time-consuming disinfection of the nasal cavities, only 50% of the nostrils are sterile and 11% remain heavily contaminated.[8] As a result, transnasal puncture of the maxillary sinus carries a significant risk of introducing bacteria into the antral cavity and overestimating the likelihood of infectious sinusitis.[81] As a consequence, a rigid protocol should be followed when performing a transnasal puncture and strict diagnostic criteria

required for establishing the diagnosis. After a careful and prolonged disinfection of the nasal cavity using a povidone-iodine or a chlorhexidine alcoholic solution,[8,95] a nasal swab is performed in order to assess the efficacy of nasal disinfection. Then, transnasal puncture is performed using an Albertini trocar placed below the inferior turbinate and sinus contents are directly aspirated before any lavage. The recovered fluid is then examined, using cell and quantitative bacterial analysis preceded by a Gram's stain. In addition, the nasal swab is analyzed using a semiquantitative bacteriologic analysis. The diagnosis of infectious sinusitis requires fulfillment of the following criteria: more than 5 altered polymorphonuclear leukocytes per oil immersion field and a positive culture with a bacterial concentration $\geq 10^3$ colony-forming units (CFU)/ml in the case of negative nasal swab, or $\geq 10^4$ CFU/ml in the case of positive nasal swab.[8]

MICROBIOLOGY OF VENTILATOR-ASSOCIATED MAXILLARY SINUSITIS

Community-acquired maxillary sinusitis is predominantly caused by *Streptococcus pneumoniae, Moraxella catarrhalis,* and *Haemophilus influenzae.* In contrast, the most frequent

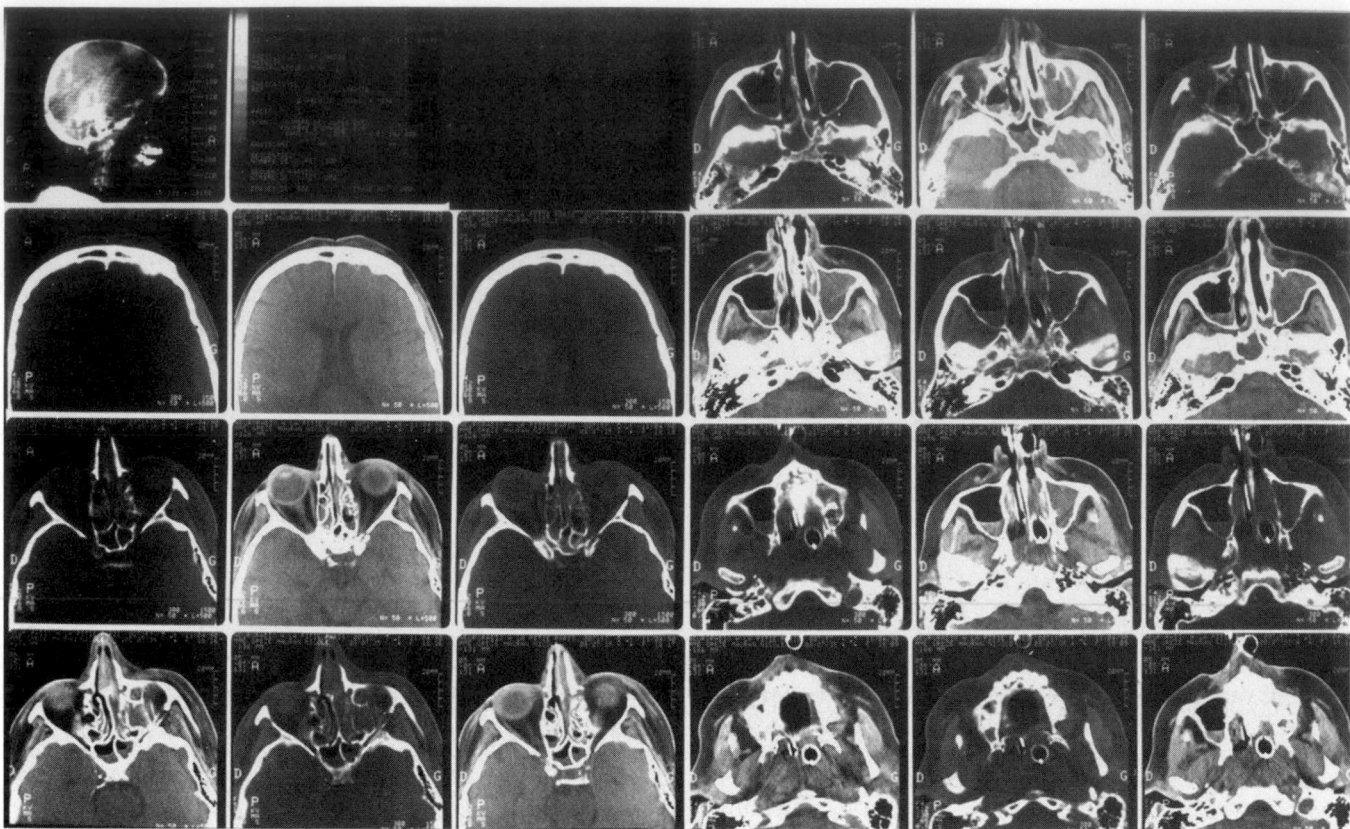

FIGURE 47-7 Typical aspect of radiographic maxillary sinusitis in a ventilated patient with left nasotracheal intubation and a right nasogastric tube. The left maxillary sinus exhibits complete opacification, whereas the right maxillary sinus exhibits a characteristic air-fluid level. Mucosal thickening can be seen in both ethmoid sinuses and the left frontal sinus. Both sphenoid sinuses exhibit air-fluid levels, whereas the right frontal sinus is normally aerated. (*Reproduced, with permission, from Rouby et al.[8]*)

microorganisms recovered in ventilated adult patients with infectious maxillary sinusitis, are gram-negative bacteria such as Enterobacteriaceae species, gram-positive cocci such as staphylococci or streptococci, anaerobes, and yeasts.[8,11,81,95–97] Very frequently, infection of the antral cavity is polymicrobial.[8,62,79,84] Anaerobes are the causative pathogens in more than 60% of cases of infectious maxillary sinusitis, either in association with aerobic species or alone.[98]

In adult patients, the most common anaerobes infecting the antral cavity are *Prevotella* species and *Fusobacterium nucleatum*, all bacteria which belong to the commensal nasal flora and are known to produce β-lactamases, which reduces their sensitivity to antibiotics.[98] Similar findings have been reported in ventilated children with nosocomial sinusitis: aerobes were present in only 40% of the patients, anaerobes in only 25% of the patients, and mixed aerobic and anaerobic flora in 35% of the patients.[97] The predominant aerobes were *Pseudomonas aeruginosa, Staphylococcus aureus, Escherichia coli,* and *Klebsiella pneumoniae.* The predominant anaerobes were *Peptostreptococcus* species, *Prevotella* species, and *Fusobacterium* species.

Anaerobes are more commonly isolated from sinus aspirate samples obtained after prolonged mechanical ventilation.[97] The high incidence of anaerobes and their

underestimation by classic means of bacterial examination probably explain the high number of purulent antral secretions remaining sterile on culture.[84] Bacteria infecting the antral cavity stem either from the gingival mucosa and its mucosal crevices using the canine fossa, or from the nasal cavity, using the inferior meatus. The presence of a nasal foreign body (endotracheal or gastric tube) markedly increases bacterial colonization of the ipsilateral middle meatus.[84] In Fig. 47-10, a logical approach, including diagnostic criteria, is proposed for establishing the diagnosis of infectious maxillary sinusitis.

Treatment

PREVENTION OF VENTILATOR-ASSOCIATED SINUSITIS

Although some of the published data on the prevention of sinus infection in ventilated patients are conflicting,[8,56,61,62,99] the following measures can be recommended for reducing the incidence of ventilator-associated sinusitis. First, nasotracheal intubation and nasogastric tubes should be avoided. Most prospective studies that have examined the influence of nasotracheal intubation on

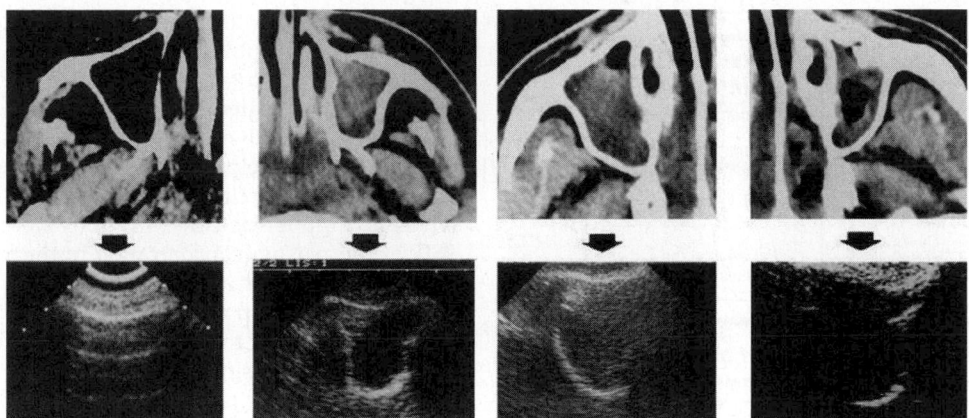

FIGURE 47-8 Normal versus pathologic ultrasound pattern. Computed tomography sections of maxillary sinuses are in the upper row with their corresponding ultrasound pattern in the lower row. From left to right: normal pattern—total opacity of the left maxillary sinus (the internal, posterior, and external walls of the sinus are visible, giving a complete "sinusogram"); 90% air-fluid level of the right maxillary sinus (the internal wall is not visualized, giving an incomplete "sinusogram"); and mucosal thickening of the left maxillary sinus (the internal wall is not visible and the external wall is ill-defined, giving a partial "sinusogram"). (*Reproduced, with permission, from Lichtenstein et al.[89]*)

ventilator-associated sinusitis have shown an increased incidence of maxillary sinusitis in nasotracheally intubated patients.[8,56,61,99] On the other hand, in a randomized single-center study that included 300 ventilated patients, there was no statistically significant difference in the occurrence of ventilator-associated sinusitis between patients intubated via the nasal versus the oral route. A trend ($p = 0.08$), however, suggested less sinusitis in the orotracheal group.[62] Second, the nostrils should remain free of foreign bodies and be regularly cleaned of nasal secretions that tend to accumulate. Third, the patient should be kept preferentially in the semi-recumbent position to ensure patency of the different ostia. The observance of these preventive measures does not, however, fully protect against ventilator-associated si-

nusitis. General sepsis, restrictions in regional blood flow resulting from circulatory shock, as well as allergy and systemic inflammation, all factors encountered in the critical care environment, certainly contribute to antral disease and secondary infection of sinus cavities.

TREATMENT OF INFECTIOUS MAXILLARY SINUSITIS

Classically, sinus infection diagnosed in ventilated patients requires the administration of intravenous antibiotics.[11,62,78] Removal of nasal foreign bodies, semi-recumbent positioning, sinus drainage, topical decongestants, and serum

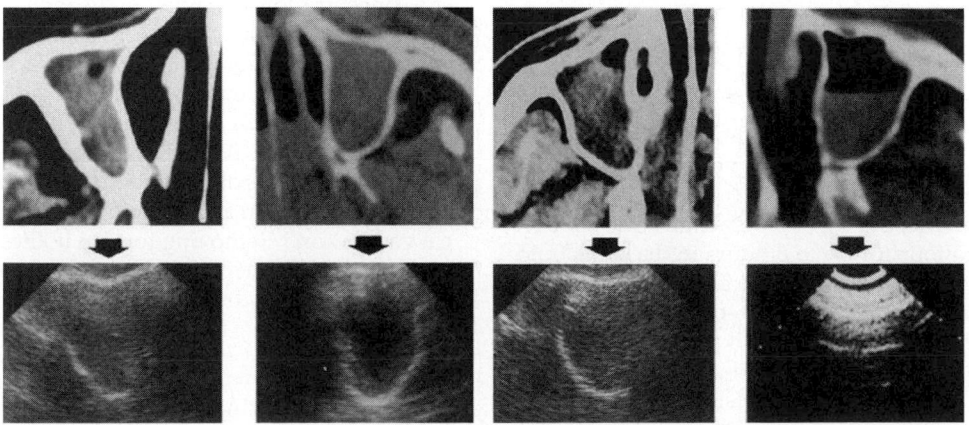

FIGURE 47-9 Different abnormal ultrasound patterns. Computed tomography sections of maxillary sinuses are in the upper row with their corresponding ultrasound pattern in the lower row. From the left to the right: total opacity of the right maxillary sinus with a small anterior air bubble (the external wall is visible and the internal wall is not visible, giving an incomplete "sinusogram"); total opacity of the left maxillary sinus (the internal, posterior, and external walls of the sinus are visible, giving a complete "sinusogram"); 90% air-fluid level of the right maxillary sinus (the internal wall is not visualized, giving an incomplete "sinusogram"); and 50% air-fluid level of the left maxillary sinus (the walls are not visible, giving an acoustic barrier, and thus no "sinusogram"). (*Reproduced, with permission, from Lichtenstein et al.[89]*)

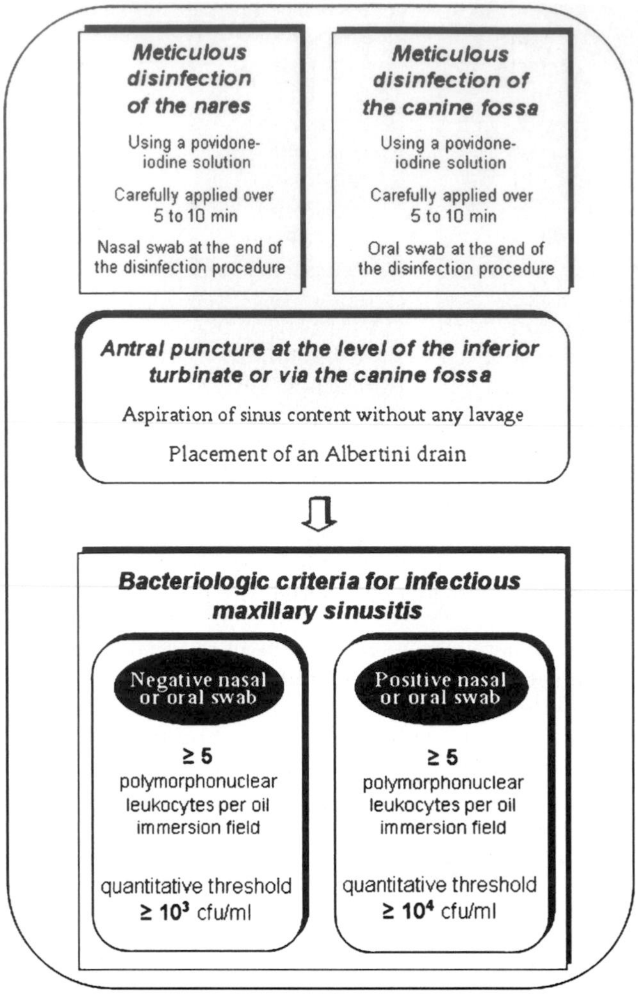

FIGURE 47-10 Chart summarizing a logical diagnostic approach and proposing criteria for infectious maxillary sinusitis.

lavage of the antral cavity through the drains are useful adjunctive therapies.

PENETRATION OF ANTIBIOTICS INTO ANTRAL MUCOSA

Two studies have shown adequate sinus deposition of intravenous antibiotics in patients with ventilator-associated maxillary sinusitis.[100,101] In a series of 6 ventilated patients, a single intravenous dose of 4 g of piperacillin achieved bactericidal concentrations for up to 8 hours in the sinus fluid obtained by maxillary drainage.[100] In a series of 20 ventilated patients with ventilator-associated sinusitis, a single intravenous dose of 15 mg/kg of amikacin achieved high peak concentrations in the sinus fluid obtained by maxillary drainage.[101] These encouraging results, however, were challenged by a subsequent study performed in 7 critically ill patients with inflammatory and bacterial maxillary sinusitis.[102] In all patients, extracellular tissue concentrations of cefuroxime, ampicillin, and vancomycin measured on biopsy samples obtained by sinuscopy were lower than the corresponding plasma concentrations. In patients with noninfectious maxillary sinusitis, the ratio between tissue and plasma concentrations varied from 10–73%. In one patient treated with intravenous cefuroxime for a nasogastric tube–induced purulent maxillary sinusitis, very low plasma concentrations with no measurable mucosal concentrations were found. In one patient treated with intravenous ampicillin for a nasotracheal tube–induced purulent maxillary sinusitis, high tissue concentrations were found, reaching 95% of the plasma concentration in the left antral mucosa and 53% in the right antral mucosa. In one tracheostomized patient treated with vancomycin for a left purulent maxillary sinusitis, high mucosal concentrations of vancomycin were found. Surprisingly, in the three patients with purulent maxillary sinusitis, bacterial cultures of the sinus biopsies were positive, irrespective of the antibiotic tissue concentrations.

SINUS DRAINAGE AND ANTIBIOTIC THERAPY

In critically ill patients, infectious maxillary sinusitis frequently emerges despite prior antibiotic administration to which the causative microorganisms are sensitive,[95,102] suggesting that antibiotics may not be a sufficient therapy for ventilator-associated bacterial maxillary sinusitis. Several hypotheses have been proposed for explaining the persistence of bacteria within the antral cavity despite the intravenous administration of appropriate antibiotics. As demonstrated in a small number of patients, antral penetration of systemic antibiotics is very variable and mucosal concentrations may remain below minimal inhibitory concentrations.[102] In patients on long-term mechanical ventilation, the presence of a chronic anaerobic infection might be associated with biofilm formation protecting the bacteria against the bactericidal effects of antibiotics.[102] Measurements of antral antibiotic concentrations requires sinuscopy and/or the insertion of drains into the sinus cavity.[94,100–102] Such invasive procedures may create a regional inflammatory reaction responsible for increased antral antibiotic concentrations that may no longer be representative of true tissue concentrations obtained in the intact sinus cavity.

The logical implication of these clinical findings and hypotheses is that sinus drainage should be adopted as a first-line therapy for ventilator-associated maxillary sinusitis, together with daily sinus lavage and topical antibiotic administration.[8,95] To avoid recurrence of infectious maxillary sinusitis, sinus drains should be left in place until endotracheal extubation and definitive weaning from mechanical ventilation.[8] Removing foreign bodies from the nostrils and positioning the patient in the semi-recumbent position may help recovery from antral disease.

Important Unknowns

CLINICAL RELEVANCE OF FRONTAL, ETHMOID, AND SPHENOID SINUSITIS

Radiographic abnormalities of the ethmoid and sphenoid sinuses are found in more than 80% of ventilated patients.[8] In ventilated patients with computed tomography–delineated abnormalities of maxillary sinuses, more than 95% have radiographic ethmoid and sphenoid sinusitis. Half of ventilated patients with normal maxillary sinuses have computed tomography–delineated abnormalities (mucosal thickening or complete opacification of the sinus cavities) of the ethmoid and sphenoid sinuses.[8] The meaning and clinical impact of these abnormalities remain unknown. Despite sinus drainage associated with topical administration of appropriate antibiotics and the absence of other sites of infection, more than 10% of ventilated patients with documented infectious maxillary sinusitis remain febrile with persistent signs of sepsis, raising the possibility of a residual infection within the ethmoid and sphenoid cavities.[8] Although community-acquired infectious sphenoid sinusitis remains a rare entity,[103,104] further studies are required for assessing the exact incidence of infectious ethmoid and sphenoid sinusitis as a cause of occult fever in ventilated patients.

ROLE OF ANTIBIOTICS IN THE THERAPY OF VENTILATOR-ASSOCIATED MAXILLARY SINUSITIS

To date, there is an ongoing controversy as to whether intravenous or topical antibiotics should be administered to ventilated patients with documented infectious maxillary sinusitis. Available data on the penetration of systemic antibiotics into the diseased antral mucosa of ventilated patients are scarce and are based on very few critically ill patients.[100–102] In addition, the role of viruses in the infection of sinus cavities remains unknown. As with community-acquired acute maxillary sinusitis, the clinical course of which is not influenced by antibiotic treatment,[105] ventilator-associated infectious maxillary sinusitis might be caused by viruses and require specific antiviral therapy rather than intravenous antibiotics. Clinical data support the concept that radiographic maxillary sinusitis is the first step along the path to an established sinus infection[8] and raise the issue of whether removal of nasal foreign bodies and placement of sinus drainage catheters should not be undertaken before frank infection and sepsis occur.[10] Further studies are required to assess factors influencing the penetration of antibacterial agents into the sinus cavities and to clarify many uncertainties concerning treatment optimization of ventilator-associated sinusitis.

Conclusions and Future Prospects

Infection of paranasal sinuses is an important cause of occult sepsis in critically ill patients receiving mechanical ventilation. It is a typical nosocomial infection resulting mainly from the presence of nasal foreign bodies. Mechanical and edematous obstruction of the sinus ostia, suppression of the normal sinus ventilation, inhibition of the maxillary production of nitric oxide, and cessation of the normal sinus mucociliary clearance are different factors causing an inflammatory antral disease, that becomes rapidly superinfected by pathogens proliferating around nasotracheal and naso-

gastric tubes. Like any nosocomial infection that may weigh heavily against patients' chances of survival, an active policy of detection and prevention should be undertaken and not lead to antibiotic overuse. Faced with an unknown cause of sepsis, the clinician should systematically perform maxillary sinus ultrasonography at the bedside, searching for radiographic maxillary sinusitis. When present, maxillary sinus puncture should be performed with careful attention to avoid nasal contamination of sinus contents. Once confirmed by quantitative bacteriology and cell analysis, infectious maxillary sinusitis should be treated by prolonged sinus drainage, removal of nasal foreign bodies, positioning in the semi-recumbent position, and administration of intravenous or topical antibiotics. If applied early after initiation of mechanical ventilation, orotracheal intubation, oral placement of gastric tubes, and semi-recumbent positioning may decrease the incidence of ventilator-associated maxillary sinusitis. A large multicenter randomized study should be undertaken to assess whether these preventive measures are associated with a decrease in the incidence of ventilator-associated pneumonia and mortality.

References

1. Arens JF, LeJeune FE Jr, Webre DR. Maxillary sinusitis, a complication of nasotracheal intubation. Anesthesiology 1974; 40:415–6.
2. O'Reilly MJ, Reddick EJ, Black W, et al. Sepsis from sinusitis in nasotracheally intubated patients. A diagnostic dilemma. Am J Surg 1984; 147:601–4.
3. Kronberg FG, Goodwin WJ Jr. Sinusitis in intensive care unit patients. Laryngoscope 1985; 95:936–8.
4. Deutschman CS, Wilton PB, Sinow J, et al. Paranasal sinusitis: a common complication of nasotracheal intubation in neurosurgical patients. Neurosurgery 1985; 17:296–9.
5. Deutschman CS, Wilton P, Sinow J, et al. Paranasal sinusitis associated with nasotracheal intubation: a frequently unrecognized and treatable source of sepsis. Crit Care Med 1986; 14:111–4.
6. Aebert H, Hunefeld G, Regel G. Paranasal sinusitis and sepsis in ICU patients with nasotracheal intubation. Intensive Care Med 1988; 15:27–30.
7. Bos AP, Tibboel D, Hazebroek FW, et al. Sinusitis: hidden source of sepsis in postoperative pediatric intensive care patients. Crit Care Med 1989; 17:886–8.
8. Rouby JJ, Laurent P, Gosnach M, et al. Risk factors and clinical relevance of nosocomial maxillary sinusitis in the critically ill. Am J Respir Crit Care Med 1994; 150:776–83.
9. Aalokken TM, Hagtvedt T, Dalen I, Kolbenstvedt A. Conventional sinus radiography compared with CT in the diagnosis of acute sinusitis. Dentomaxillofac Radiol 2003; 32:60–2.
10. Heffner JE. Nosocomial sinusitis. Den of multiresistant thieves? Am J Respir Crit Care Med 1994; 150:608–9.
11. Holzapfel L, Chastang C, Demingeon G, et al. A randomized study assessing the systematic search for maxillary sinusitis in nasotracheally mechanically ventilated patients. Influence of nosocomial maxillary sinusitis on the occurrence of ventilator-associated pneumonia. Am J Respir Crit Care Med 1999; 159:695–701.
12. Carter BL, Bankoff MS, Fisk JD. Computed tomographic detection of sinusitis responsible for intracranial and extracranial infections. Radiology 1983; 147:739–42.

13. Meyer P, Guerin JM, Habib Y, Levy C. [Secondary lung diseases in patients with nasotracheal intubation. Role of nosocomial sinusitis.] Ann Fr Anesth Reanim 1988; 7:26–30.

14. Goodwin WJ Jr. Orbital complications of ethmoiditis. Otolaryngol Clin North Am 1985; 18:139–47.

15. Jones N: The nose and paranasal sinuses physiology and anatomy. Adv Drug Deliv Rev 2001; 51:5–19.

16. Van Cauwenberge P, Sys L, De Belder T, Watelet JB. Anatomy and physiology of the nose and the paranasal sinuses. Immunol Allergy Clin North Am 2004; 24:1–17.

17. Bergler W, Eberius K, Petroianu G, Hormann K. [Paranasal sinuses: only one of nature's games?] Laryngorhinootologie 1998; 77:454–61.

18. Lundberg JO, Farkas-Szallasi T, Weitzberg E, et al. High nitric oxide production in human paranasal sinuses. Nat Med 1995; 1:370–3.

19. Deja M, Busch T, Bachmann S, et al. Reduced nitric oxide in sinus epithelium of patients with radiologic maxillary sinusitis and sepsis. Am J Respir Crit Care Med 2003; 168:281–6.

20. Gustafsson LE, Leone AM, Persson MG, Wiklund NP, Moncada S. Endogenous nitric oxide is present in the exhaled air of rabbits, guinea pigs and humans. Biochem Biophys Res Commun 1991; 181:852–7.

21. Schedin U, Frostell C, Gustafsson LE. Nitric oxide occurs in high concentrations in monkey upper airways. Acta Physiol Scand 1995; 155:473–4.

22. Stewart TE, Valenza F, Ribeiro SP, et al. Increased nitric oxide in exhaled gas as an early marker of lung inflammation in a model of sepsis. Am J Respir Crit Care Med 1995; 151:713–8.

23. Mills PC, Marlin DJ, Demoncheaux E, et al. Nitric oxide and exercise in the horse. J Physiol 1996; 495(Pt 3):863–74.

24. Lewandowski K, Busch T, Lewandowski M, et al. Evidence of nitric oxide in the exhaled gas of Asian elephants (*Elephas maximus*). Respir Physiol 1996; 106:91–8.

25. Stanek K, Roberts J, Zapol W, et al. Thoracic circumference and nitric oxide activity in the free diving Weddell seal. Antarctic J 1995; 29:172–4.

26. Lewandowski K, Busch T, Lohbrunner H, et al. Low nitric oxide concentrations in exhaled gas and nasal airways of mammals without paranasal sinuses. J Appl Physiol 1998; 85:405–10.

27. Maniscalco M, Weitzberg E, Sundberg J, Sofia M, Lundberg JO. Assessment of nasal and sinus nitric oxide output using single-breath humming exhalations. Eur Respir J 2003; 22:323–9.

28. Busch T, Kuhlen R, Knorr M, et al. Nasal, pulmonary and autoinhaled nitric oxide at rest and during moderate exercise. Intensive Care Med 2000; 26:391–9.

29. Settergren G, Angdin M, Astudillo R, et al. Decreased pulmonary vascular resistance during nasal breathing: modulation by endogenous nitric oxide from the paranasal sinuses. Acta Physiol Scand 1998; 163:235–9.

30. Lundberg JO, Weitzberg E. Nasal nitric oxide in man. Thorax 1999; 54:947–52.

31. Djupesland PG, Chatkin JM, Qian W, Haight JS. Nitric oxide in the nasal airway: a new dimension in otorhinolaryngology. Am J Otolaryngol 2001; 22:19–32.

32. Sobin J, Engquist S, Nord CE. Bacteriology of the maxillary sinus in healthy volunteers. Scand J Infect Dis 1992; 24:633–5.

33. Malawista SE, Montgomery RR, van Blaricom G. Evidence for reactive nitrogen intermediates in killing of staphylococci by human neutrophil cytoplasts. A new microbicidal pathway for polymorphonuclear leukocytes. J Clin Invest 1992; 90:631–6.

34. Karupiah G, Harris N. Inhibition of viral replication by nitric oxide and its reversal by ferrous sulfate and tricarboxylic acid cycle metabolites. J Exp Med 1995; 181:2171–9.

35. Long R, Light B, Talbot JA. Mycobacteriocidal action of exogenous nitric oxide. Antimicrob Agents Chemother 1999; 43:403–5.

36. Lowenstein CJ, Padalko E. iNOS (NOS2) at a glance. J Cell Sci 2004; 117:2865–7.

37. Kelemen G. The nasal and paranasal cavities of the rabbit in experimental work. AMA Arch Otolaryngol 1955; 61:497–512.

38. Johansson P, Kumlien J, Carlsoo B, Drettner B, Nord CE. Experimental acute sinusitis in rabbits. A bacteriological and histological study. Acta Otolaryngol 1988; 105:357–66.

39. Marks SC. Acute sinusitis in the rabbit: a new rhinogenic model. Laryngoscope 1997; 107:1579–85.

40. Kara CO, Cetin CB, Colakoglu N, Sengul M, Pakdemirli E. Experimentally induced rhinosinusitis in rabbits. J Otolaryngol 2002; 31:294–8.

41. Westergren V, Otori N, Stierna P. Experimental nasal intubation: a study of changes in nasoantral mucosa and bacterial flora. Laryngoscope 1999; 109:1068–73.

42. Cetin CB, Kara CO, Colakoglu N, Sengul M, Pinar HS. Experimental sinusitis in nasally catheterised rabbits. Rhinology 2002; 40:154–8.

43. Kara CO, Cetin CB, Demirkan N, et al. Experimental sinusitis in a rhinogenic model. Laryngoscope 2004; 114:273–8.

44. Norlander T, Westrin KM, Fukami M, Stierna P, Carlsoo B. Experimentally induced polyps in the sinus mucosa: a structural analysis of the initial stages. Laryngoscope 1996; 106:196–203.

45. Toskala E, Westrin KM, Stierna P, Rautiainen M. Ciliary ultrastructure in experimental sinusitis. Acta Otolaryngol Suppl 1997; 529:137–9.

46. Beste DJ, Capper DT, Shaffer K, Kehl KS, Kajdacsy-Balla A. Antimicrobial effect on rabbit sinusitis after temporary ostial occlusion. Am J Rhinol 1997; 11:485–9.

47. Kara CO. Animal models of sinusitis: relevance to human disease. Curr Allergy Asthma Rep 2004; 4:496–9.

48. Westergren V, Viale G, Dell'Orto P, Pellegrini C, Hellquist HB. RANTES is more prevalent in bacterial than in nonbacterial maxillary sinusitis: and P-selectin is preferentially up-regulated in diseased mucosae. Arch Otolaryngol Head Neck Surg 1997; 123:1103–10.

49. Westergren V, Lundblad L, Forsum U. Ventilator-associated sinusitis: antroscopic findings and bacteriology when excluding contaminants. Acta Otolaryngol 1998; 118:574–80.

50. Westergren V, Lundblad L, Timpka T. Interobserver variations in assessment of antral disease from direct sinoscopic observations compared to video recordings. Am J Rhinol 1998; 12:159–65.

51. Caplan ES, Hoyt NJ. Nosocomial sinusitis. JAMA 1982; 247:639–41.

52. Guerin JM, Meyer P, Segrestaa JM, Reizine D, Levy C. [Nosocomial sinusitis and nasotracheal intubation. Prospective study of 53 patients.] Ann Med Interne (Paris) 1989; 140:106–7.

53. Bell RM, Page GV, Bynoe RP, Dunham ME, Brill AH. Posttraumatic sinusitis. J Trauma 1988; 28:923–30.

54. Linden BE, Aguilar EA, Allen SJ. Sinusitis in the nasotracheally intubated patient. Arch Otolaryngol Head Neck Surg 1988; 114:860–1.

55. Fassoulaki A, Pamouktsoglou P. Prolonged nasotracheal intubation and its association with inflammation of paranasal sinuses. Anesth Analg 1989; 69:50–2.

56. Salord F, Gaussorgues P, Marti-Flich J, et al. Nosocomial maxillary sinusitis during mechanical ventilation: a prospective comparison of orotracheal versus the nasotracheal route for intubation. Intensive Care Med 1990; 16:390–3.

57. Desmond P, Raman R, Idikula J. Effect of nasogastric tubes on the nose and maxillary sinus. Crit Care Med 1991; 19:509–11.

58. Pedersen J, Schurizek BA, Melsen NC, Juhl B. The effect of nasotracheal intubation on the paranasal sinuses. A prospective study of 434 intensive care patients. Acta Anaesthesiol Scand 1991; 35:11–3.

59. Bach A, Boehrer H, Schmidt H, Geiss HK. Nosocomial sinusitis in ventilated patients. Nasotracheal versus orotracheal intubation. Anaesthesia 1992; 47:335–9.

60. Borman KR, Brown PM, Mezera KK, Jhaveri H. Occult fever in surgical intensive care unit patients is seldom caused by sinusitis. Am J Surg 1992; 164:412–5, discussion 415–6.

61. Michelson A, Schuster B, Kamp HD. Paranasal sinusitis associated with nasotracheal and orotracheal long-term intubation. Arch Otolaryngol Head Neck Surg 1992; 118:937–9.

62. Holzapfel L, Chevret S, Madinier G, et al. Influence of long-term oro- or nasotracheal intubation on nosocomial maxillary sinusitis and pneumonia: results of a prospective, randomized, clinical trial. Crit Care Med 1993; 21:1132–8.

63. George DL, Falk PS, Umberto Meduri G, et al. Nosocomial sinusitis in patients in the medical intensive care unit: a prospective epidemiological study. Clin Infect Dis 1998; 27:463–70.

64. Sottile FD, Marrie TJ, Prough DS, et al. Nosocomial pulmonary infection: possible etiologic significance of bacterial adhesion to endotracheal tubes. Crit Care Med 1986; 14:265–70.

65. Poisson DM, Touquet S, Bercault N, Arbeille B. Electron microscopic description of accretions occurring in endotracheal tubes used in adults. Pathol Biol (Paris) 1993; 41:537–41.

66. Gristina AG, Giridhar G, Gabriel BL, Naylor PT, Myrvik QN. Cell biology and molecular mechanisms in artificial device infections. Int J Artif Organs 1993; 16:755–63.

67. Adair CG, Gorman SP, Feron BM, et al. Implications of endotracheal tube biofilm for ventilator-associated pneumonia. Intensive Care Med 1999; 25:1072–6.

68. Inglis TJ, Millar MR, Jones JG, Robinson DA. Tracheal tube biofilm as a source of bacterial colonization of the lung. J Clin Microbiol 1989; 27:2014–8.

69. Koerner RJ. Contribution of endotracheal tubes to the pathogenesis of ventilator-associated pneumonia. J Hosp Infect 1997; 35:83–9.

70. Aust R, Drettner B. The functional size of the human maxillary ostium in vivo. Acta Otolaryngol 1974; 78:432–5.

71. Aust R, Drettner B. The patency of the maxillary ostium in relation to body posture. Acta Otolaryngol 1975; 80:443–6.

72. Rundcrantz H. Postural variations of nasal patency. Acta Otolaryngol 1969; 68:435–43.

73. Aust R, Stierna P, Drettner B. Basic experimental studies of ostial patency and local metabolic environment of the maxillary sinus. Acta Otolaryngol Suppl 1994; 515:7–10, discussion 11.

74. Sanders SP, Siekierski ES, Porter JD, Richards SM, Proud D. Nitric oxide inhibits rhinovirus-induced cytokine production and viral replication in a human respiratory epithelial cell line. J Virol 1998; 72:934–42.

75. Lindberg S, Cervin A, Runer T. Nitric oxide (NO) production in the upper airways is decreased in chronic sinusitis. Acta Otolaryngol 1997; 117:113–7.

76. Baraldi E, Azzolin NM, Biban P, Zacchello F. Effect of antibiotic therapy on nasal nitric oxide concentration in children with acute sinusitis. Am J Respir Crit Care Med 1997; 155:1680–3.

77. Rouby JJ. The nose, nitric oxide, and paranasal sinuses: the outpost of pulmonary antiinfective defenses? Am J Respir Crit Care Med 2003; 168:265–6.

78. Talmor M, Li P, Barie PS. Acute paranasal sinusitis in critically ill patients: guidelines for prevention, diagnosis, and treatment. Clin Infect Dis 1997; 25:1441–6.

79. Bert F, Lambert-Zechovsky N. Sinusitis in mechanically ventilated patients and its role in the pathogenesis of nosocomial pneumonia. Eur J Clin Microbiol Infect Dis 1996; 15:533–44.

80. Eistert B, Furch B, Glanz H. [The pathogenesis of sinusitis in intensive care patients.] HNO 1993; 41:480–4.

81. Westergren V, Lundblad L, Hellquist HB, Forsum U. Ventilator-associated sinusitis: a review. Clin Infect Dis 1998; 27:851–64.

82. Berglof A, Norlander T, Feinstein R, et al. Association of bronchopneumonia with sinusitis due to *Bordetella bronchiseptica* in an experimental rabbit model. Am J Rhinol 2000; 14:125–30.

83. Hall J. Assessment of fever in the intensive care unit. Is the answer just beyond the tip of our nose? Am J Respir Crit Care Med 1999; 159:693–4.

84. Vandenbussche T, De Moor S, Bachert C, Van Cauwenberge P. Value of antral puncture in the intensive care patient with fever of unknown origin. Laryngoscope 2000; 110:1702–6.

85. Bockmann P, Andreasson L, Holmer NG, Jannert M, Lorinc P. Ultrasonic versus radiologic investigation of the paranasal sinuses. Rhinology 1982; 20:111–9.

86. Varonen H, Makela M, Savolainen S, Laara E, Hilden J. Comparison of ultrasound, radiography, and clinical examination in the diagnosis of acute maxillary sinusitis: a systematic review. J Clin Epidemiol 2000; 53:940–8.

87. Zinreich SJ. Rhinosinusitis: radiologic diagnosis. Otolaryngol Head Neck Surg 1997; 117:S27–S34.

88. Puidupin M, Guiavarch M, Paris A, et al. B-mode ultrasound in the diagnosis of maxillary sinusitis in intensive care unit. Intensive Care Med 1997; 23:1174–5.

89. Lichtenstein D, Biderman P, Meziere G, Gepner A. The "sinusogram", a real-time ultrasound sign of maxillary sinusitis. Intensive Care Med 1998; 24:1057–61.

90. Hilbert G, Vargas F, Valentino R, et al. Comparison of B-mode ultrasound and computed tomography in the diagnosis of maxillary sinusitis in mechanically ventilated patients. Crit Care Med 2001; 29:1337–42.

91. Hagtvedt T, Aalokken TM, Notthellen J, Kolbenstvedt A. A new low-dose CT examination compared with standard-dose CT in the diagnosis of acute sinusitis. Eur Radiol 2003; 13:976–80.

92. Beckmann U, Gillies DM, Berenholtz SM, Wu AW, Pronovost P. Incidents relating to the intra-hospital transfer of critically ill patients. An analysis of the reports submitted to the Australian Incident Monitoring Study in Intensive Care. Intensive Care Med 2004; 30:1579–85.

93. Westergren V, Berg S, Lundgren J. Ultrasonographic bedside evaluation of maxillary sinus disease in mechanically ventilated patients. Intensive Care Med 1997; 23:393–8.

94. Westergren V, Forsum U, Lundgren J. Possible errors in diagnosis of bacterial sinusitis in tracheal intubated patients. Acta Anaesthesiol Scand 1994; 38:699–703.

95. Souweine B, Mom T, Traore O, et al. Ventilator-associated sinusitis: microbiological results of sinus aspirates in patients on antibiotics. Anesthesiology 2000; 93:1255–60.

96. Bert F, Lambert-Zechovsky N. Microbiology of nosocomial sinusitis in intensive care unit patients. J Infect 1995; 31:5–8.

97. Brook I. Microbiology of nosocomial sinusitis in mechanically ventilated children. Arch Otolaryngol Head Neck Surg 1998; 124:35–8.

98. Le Moal G, Lemerre D, Grollier G, et al. Nosocomial sinusitis with isolation of anaerobic bacteria in ICU patients. Intensive Care Med 1999; 25:1066–71.

99. Michelson A, Kamp HD, Schuster B. [Sinusitis in long-term intubated, intensive care patients: nasal versus oral intubation.] Anaesthesist 1991; 40:100–4.

100. Holzapfel L, Jehl F, Miranda P, et al. [Diffusion of piperacillin into the sinuses of patients with nosocomial sinusitis.] Presse Med 1991; 20:1889–91.

101. Holzapfel L, Villette P, Ohen F, et al. [Diffusion of amikacin into the sinuses in patients with nosocomial sinusitis. Administration of a single dose per day.] Presse Med 1992; 21:1612–5.

102. Westergren V, Nilsson M, Forsum U. Penetration of antibiotics in diseased antral mucosa. Arch Otolaryngol Head Neck Surg 1996; 122:1390–4.

103. Erminy M, Bonfils P. [Acute and chronic sphenoid sinusitis. Review of the literature.] Ann Otolaryngol Chir Cervicofac 1998; 115:106–16, quiz 117.

104. Mra Z, Roach JC, Brook AL. Infectious and neoplastic diseases of the sphenoid sinus—a report of 10 cases. Rhinology 2002; 40:34–40.

105. van Buchem FL, Knottnerus JA, Schrijnemaekers VJ, Peeters MF. Primary-care-based randomised placebo-controlled trial of antibiotic treatment in acute maxillary sinusitis. Lancet 1997; 349:683–7.

Chapter 48

IMAGING OF THE MECHANICALLY VENTILATED PATIENT

The mechanically ventilated patient presents difficult diagnostic challenges for both the clinician and the radiologist. The lungs often reflect a combination of acute problems (atelectasis, edema, or pneumonia) superimposed upon chronic structural problems, such as chronic obstructive pulmonary disease (COPD) or left-heart failure. Systemic disorders such as the acute respiratory distress syndrome (ARDS), pulmonary embolus (PE), or renal failure may further cloud the radiographic appearance. In addition, mechanical ventilation and its problems can alter the radiograph.[1]

The purpose of this chapter is to present the radiographic appearance of the ventilated patient and the complications of mechanical ventilation. Many of the pathophysiologic and clinical aspects of topics such as endotracheal intubation, tracheostomy, and mechanical ventilation are covered in other chapters. Rather than duplicating much of the background material, I will concentrate on the imaging of the critically-ill ventilated patient. Although the anteroposterior (AP) portable chest radiograph remains the mainstay of imaging, other radiographic views and the use of cross-sectional imaging modalities, such as computed tomogra-

phy (CT), magnetic resonance imaging (MRI), and sonography, can be very helpful and cost-effective when used in a judicious and purposeful manner.

Every attempt should be made to *obtain erect radiographs*. This facilitates the diagnosis of pneumothorax, pleural effusion, and vascular congestion. Even with a cooperative patient sitting erect, the depth of inspiration does not approach that of a conventional chest radiograph. For portable radiography, the distance between the x-ray tube and the cassette is usually 40–48 inches, which causes image unsharpness compared to a conventional PA radiograph made at 6 feet. In the supine position, the heart and mediastinum are magnified, the upper-lobe vessels distend, pleural effusions layer posteriorly, and pneumothorax collects anteriorly and inferiorly.[1]

Portable radiographs are by nature inferior images. Over the last decade, two new developments have greatly enhanced their value. Conventional x-ray film is being replaced by computed radiography. This filmless system utilizes a phosphor plate similar to an x-ray plate, which is placed behind the patient. When the x-ray beam penetrates the patient, a latent image is formed on the plate. This is subsequently read by a laser scanner that produces a digitized image. This system has wider latitude (i.e., is more forgiving) and the digitized image can be displayed on a video monitor.[2] The window and level, and other imaging parameters, can be adjusted to optimize the image. The addition of a low-resolution grid, during the imaging procedure, cleans up much of the scattered radiation that degrades the image, especially in larger patients. This is highly recommended.

Picture archiving and communications systems (PACS) are now available in many hospitals. Computed radiographs are already in digital format and can be distributed instantaneously throughout the hospital.[2] Images still done on x-ray film can be digitized and distributed in a similar manner. PACS have led to marked improvement in the quality of the final image, in the timely distribution of images, and in potential shortening of patient stays. Kundel et al[3] found that faster access to images shortened the time to initiation of actions, whereas Watkins et al[4] found no effect. The benefits in the post-PACS environment are, at least in part, dependent upon the efficiency of the pre-PACS environment. It has been an almost universal finding that the availability of images in the ICU has diminished interaction between the radiologist and the clinician.

Successful and meaningful diagnostic examinations are most often achieved when there is good communication between the clinical team and the radiologist. Clinicians or radiologists working in isolation will derive considerably less information from the radiograph than when there is a cooperative give-and-take discussion. Daily morning conferences between the two services provide ideal milieux for pooling information and optimizing diagnosis. It is especially valuable in determining which additional diagnostic imaging tests are likely to clarify diagnostic problems. The yield of additional imaging increases while decreasing the number of examinations in the critically ill.[5]

Are daily portable radiographs worth the effort and expense? Some have concluded "yes" and others, "no."[6–11] An American College of Radiology (ACR) Expert Panel[12] has

TABLE 48-1 American College of Radiology Appropriateness Criteria for Routine Daily Portable X-Ray 1999

Endotracheal tubes: recommendation

Endotracheal tubes are significantly malpositioned in approximately 15% of patients. The vast majority of malpositioned tubes are not detected by physical examination. Consequences of malpositioning are potentially high. Routine radiographs are indicated.

CVP catheters: recommendation

There is good evidence to support obtaining a chest radiograph after insertion of a central venous pressure catheter. Beyond the initial insertion, follow-up radiographs have a low yield. Follow-up radiographs are suggested only when complications are suspected clinically.

Swan-Ganz catheters: recommendation

Approximately 10% of Swan-Ganz catheters have been found to be misplaced on the initial radiograph and 5% of patients were found to have pneumothorax. Portable radiography is suggested after catheter insertion. Once pneumothorax has been excluded and proper positioning has been assured, follow-up radiographs are not required except for specific clinical indications.

Nasogastric tubes: recommendation

Should every tube insertion be documented to be in satisfactory position with a chest radiograph? Based on limited evidence and our experience, small-bore feeding tubes may, in a small but significant number of patients, be inadvertently placed in the lungs. This error is not always detectable clinically and may lead to injection of feeding material down the tube, or penetration of the lung, with subsequent pneumothorax. These are both very significant complications with high morbidity and potential mortality. The chest radiograph is warranted in these patients, after initial insertion but before the first feeding. In patients with routine nasogastric tube insertion, the yield from radiography is probably lower depending on clinical judgment, the experience of the operator, the auscultation of left upper quadrant gas on injecting the tube, and the return of gastric contents upon suctioning the tube. In either event, beyond the initial radiograph, follow-up radiographs are not required.

Chest tubes: recommendation

There is not enough evidence to make a strong recommendation. Immediately after insertion, the film will show the position of the tube, the success of the drainage, and complications of the intubation. Thus, obtaining a film after insertion appears warranted. Beyond this point, follow-up films simply to evaluate the tube position are not warranted. Many of these patients will have serial radiographs taken anyway, because of complex pleural and parenchymal lung disease.

SOURCE: Reprinted with permission of the American College of Radiology. No other representation of this material is authorized without expressed, written permission from the American College of Radiology.

concluded that in ICU patients with acute cardiopulmonary disease, and in those receiving mechanical ventilation, daily radiographs serve a useful purpose. When additional tubes and catheters are placed, postprocedure radiographs are valuable to assure proper position, and to exclude complications such as a pneumothorax. Routine chest x-rays have been shown to be of little value in stable cardiac patients and in patients after abdominal surgery that have no clinical reason to suspect cardiopulmonary disease. The ACR recommendations are summarized in Table 48-1.

Computed tomography, ultrasonography, to a lesser extent magnetic resonance imaging, and nuclear medicine are playing an increasing role in diagnosis and management. Although this is not within the purview of this chapter, images will be included where appropriate.

Tubes and Catheters

ENDOTRACHEAL INTUBATION

A properly positioned endotracheal tube sits in the mid-trachea several centimeters above the carina and several centimeters below the vocal cords. After intubation, clinical evaluation fails to detect the majority of malpositioned tubes.[13] The reported incidence of endotracheal malpositioning on the initial radiograph varies between 10 and 25%.[6,7,13] Henschke et al[8] reported a 12% incidence of endotracheal tube malpositioning on serial radiographs.

Endotracheal tube position is not static. It changes considerably with flexion and extension of the head and neck. Con-

rardy et al[14] demonstrated that, when the head and neck are flexed from the neutral position, the endotracheal tube descends approximately 2 cm (range 0.0–3.1 cm) and, when the head and neck are extended from the neutral position, the tube tip ascends approximately 2 cm (range 0.2–5.2 cm).[15] Thus, the average excursion from full flexion to full extension is approximately 4 cm in the average 12-cm trachea. Frequently, the position of the head and neck can be assessed on the portable radiograph. In neutral position, the lower chin projects over the lower cervical vertebra (C5 or C6), whereas in flexion, the chin is over the upper thoracic vertebra, and in extension, the chin is above C4. Thus, in the neutral position, an endotracheal tube 5–7 cm above the carina should remain within the mid-trachea in the flexion, extension, or neutral positioning (Fig. 48-1).[15]

In a significant minority of patients, the carina is not visible on the radiograph. Its position may be estimated from previous portable radiographs or its position can be estimated relative to the vertebral bodies. In the vast majority of portable radiographs, the carina is at the level of the T6 ± 1 vertebral body.[15] Alternatively, if the endotracheal tube tip is at the top of the aortic knob, it is at approximately the mid-tracheal level.[16] The inflated cuff should fill the tracheal lumen but not bulge the lateral tracheal walls (Fig. 48-2).

Inadvertent main-stem bronchus intubation leads to contralateral lung collapse. The speed at which the lung collapses depends on the presence or absence of a side hole in the endotracheal tube, the elasticity of the excluded lung, and the composition of the gas administered. The richer the oxygen mixture, the faster the absorption and the more rapid and total the pulmonary collapse. Deep intubation

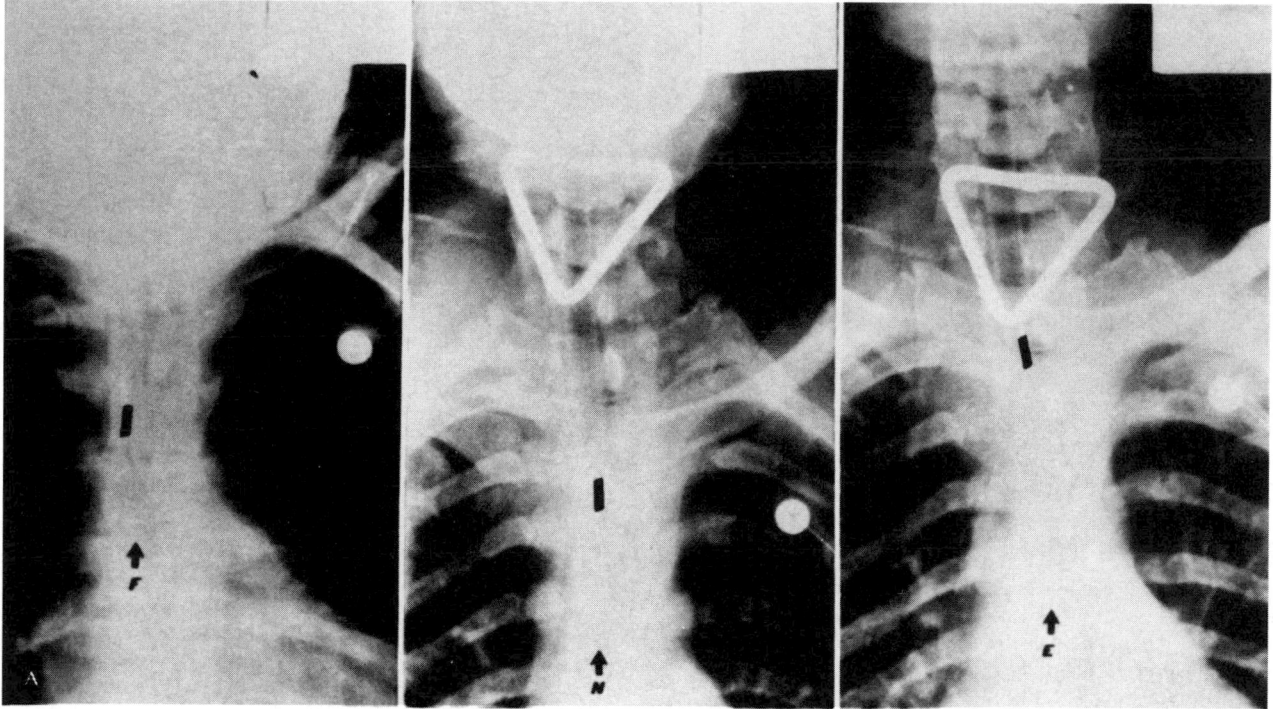

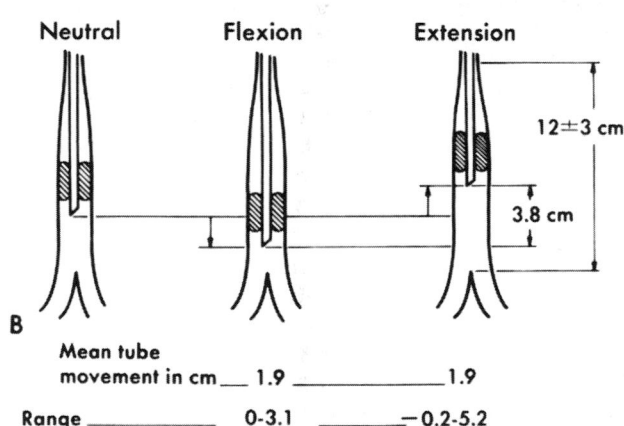

FIGURE 48-1 *A.* Effects of flexion and extension of the head and neck on endotracheal tube position (*arrows indicate the carina*). The tube descends approximately 2 cm when the neck is flexed (*F*), and it ascends approximately 3 cm when the neck is extended (*E*). In the neutral position (*N*), the mandible is over the lower cervical spine. When the neck is flexed, the mandible is over the upper thoracic spine. When the neck is extended, the mandible is above C4, often off the film. *B.* Mean endotracheal tube movement with flexion and extension of the neck from the neutral position (in 20 patients). The mean tube movement is approximately 4 cm, one-third the length of the normal adult trachea. (*Panel A reproduced, with permission, from Goodman et al.[1] Panel B reproduced, with permission, from Conrardy et al.[14]*)

of the right main-stem bronchus may bypass the takeoff of the right upper lobe bronchus, leading to right upper lobe collapse as well.

When differential ventilation of the two lungs is required, a double-lumen tube is used. The long arm of the tube enters the main bronchus to be ventilated (Fig. 48-3). When kinking of the endotracheal tube is a concern, an armored tube with wire reinforcement of the walls is used (Fig. 48-4). The wire terminates several centimeters short of the tube tip. The distal portion, without the wire, may be difficult to see on the radiograph.

If the endotracheal tube is positioned too high, there may be inadvertent extubation or cuff-induced injury of the vocal cords. This may be due to extension of the neck, coughing, or tension on the endotracheal tube from ventilator tubing or at the time of suctioning. If airway continuity is lost, patients tend to regurgitate and aspirate and the reintubation may be difficult.

Inadvertent insertion of the endotracheal tube into the esophagus is a potentially dangerous and often underdiagnosed complication. On the radiograph, the endotracheal tube projects to the left of the tracheal air column, an inflated cuff may displace the trachea to the right or appear to extend beyond the trachea, and the stomach and/or esophagus may be dilated with air (Figs. 48-5 and 48-6). If the radiographic signs are not clear-cut, a right posterior oblique (RPO) radiograph should project the trachea to the right and the esophagus to the left, thus confirming or refuting the possibility of an esophageal intubation.[17]

TRACHEOSTOMY

A well-placed tracheostomy tube should be parallel to the long axis of the trachea, be approximately one-half to two-thirds the diameter of the trachea, and end several centimeters above the carina (Fig. 48-7). Because the tube is affected

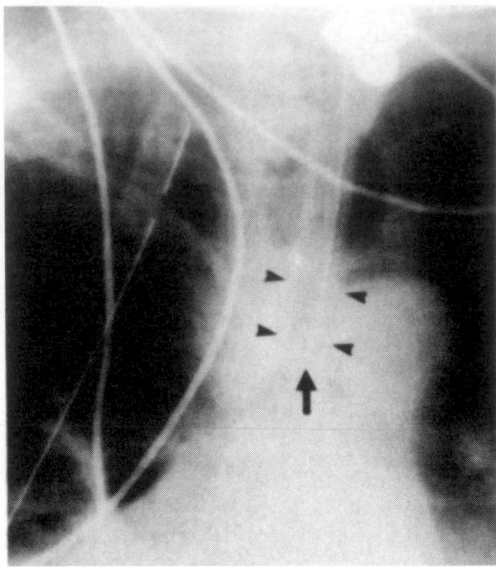

FIGURE 48-2 Overinflated endotracheal balloon. Note that the diameter of the cuff is approximately twice that of the trachea (*arrowheads*). Also, the tip of the endotracheal tube is at the level of the carina (*arrow*). The carina is hardly visible, but the tip is several centimeters below the top of the aortic arch.

FIGURE 48-3 Double-lumen endotracheal tube. Ventilation of the left lung is performed through the tube in the left main-stem bronchus (*arrowheads*). Ventilation of the right lung takes place through the lumen in the trachea (*arrow*). This patient had a right-sided bronchopleural fistula, and it was hoped that ventilation of the right lung, with lower pressures, would help close the fistula.

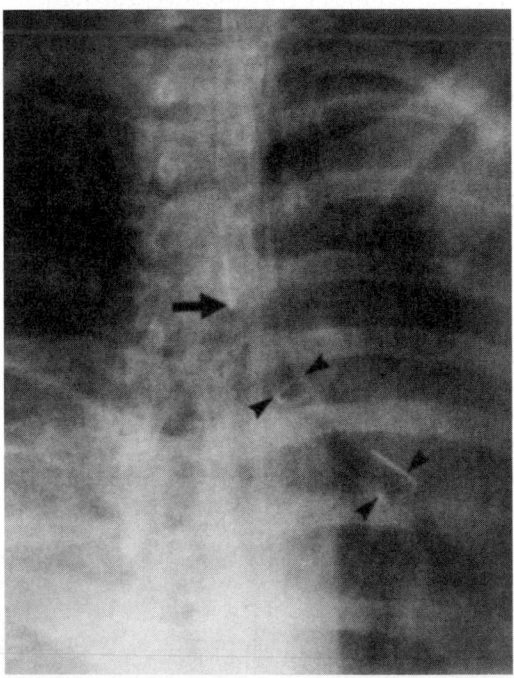

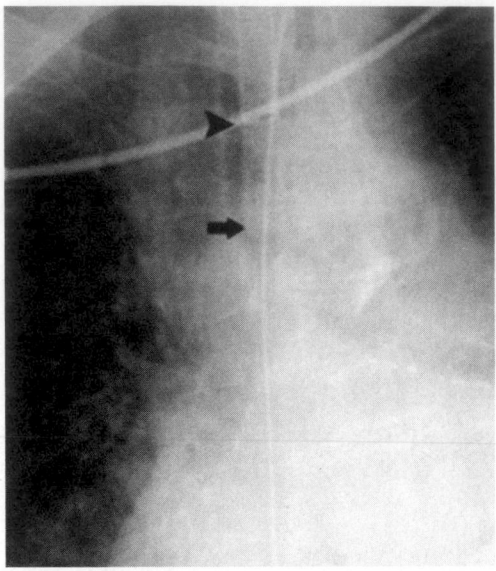

FIGURE 48-4 Armored tube. The wire (*arrowhead*) in the tube stops several centimeters before the tip of the catheter (*arrow*). The tip is several centimeters above the carina.

little by head or neck movement, a tube closer to the carina is usually well tolerated. If, on the anteroposterior radiograph, the tube appears parallel to the x-ray beam ("looking down the barrel"), it is likely that the tube is not well seated within the tracheal lumen. A radiograph taken with caudal angulation of the beam or in a severely kyphotic patient will have a similar appearance. If in doubt, a lateral radiograph is extremely helpful.[18]

FIGURE 48-5 Esophageal intubation. Note the eccentric position of the inflated cuff (*arrows*) relative to the trachea (*arrowheads*), with the endotracheal tube and cuff projected to the left of the trachea.

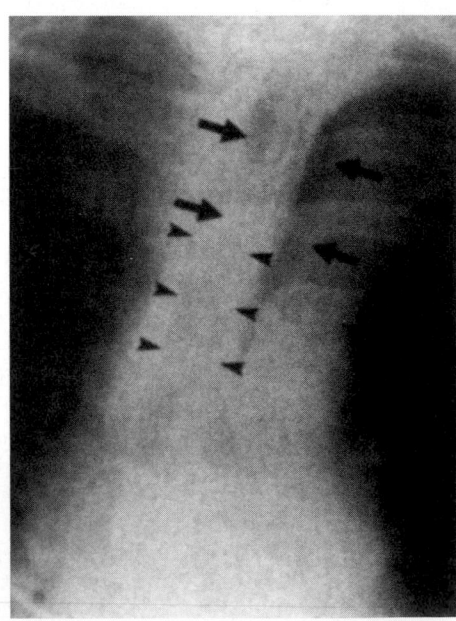

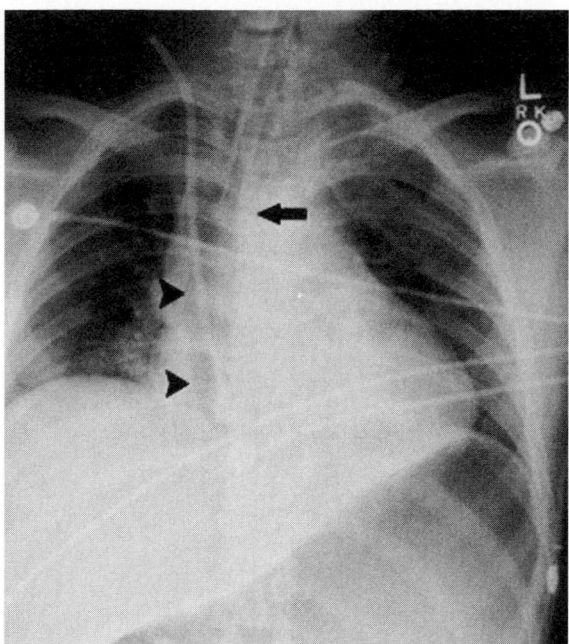

FIGURE 48-6 The endotracheal tube *appears* to be in the distal trachea (*arrow*). Overdistension of the esophagus (*arrowhead*) and stomach suggest, correctly, that this is an endoesophageal intubation.

An eccentric tracheostomy stoma or an inappropriately fitted or curved tube may cause the tube to be constantly angled in one direction on serial radiographs. Such tubes are more likely to cause tracheal mucosal ulceration and ultimately tracheal stenosis, malacia, or perforation. Especially worrisome is the tube that points consistently anteriorly and to the right (10 o'clock position), the region where the innominate artery crosses the anterior tracheal wall. This may lead to the uncommon, but often fatal, complication of tracheal-innominate fistula.[17]

Injury to the trachea, mediastinum, and lung are infrequent but potentially serious complications of tracheostomy tube insertion. A small amount of air in the subcutaneous tissue and upper mediastinum following tracheostomy is common and is merely a consequence of the blunt dissection. Progressive subcutaneous emphysema or pneumomediastinum suggests the possibility of tracheal perforation, extratracheal location of the tube, rupture of the trachea, or tight packing around the tracheal stoma, which prevents air leaking through the stoma from escaping into the atmosphere. Pneumothorax following tracheostomy is usually secondary to injury to the apical pleural space at the time of surgery. Because this is often not detected clinically, every patient should have an erect radiograph following tracheostomy.[12,18]

Following nasotracheal intubation or nasogastric tube insertion, nasal mucosal edema and fluid retention in the ipsilateral paranasal sinuses are frequent. The presence of fluid does not necessarily indicate a significant sinus infection. If one routinely undertakes CT scanning in patients several days after nasotracheal intubation, most patients have

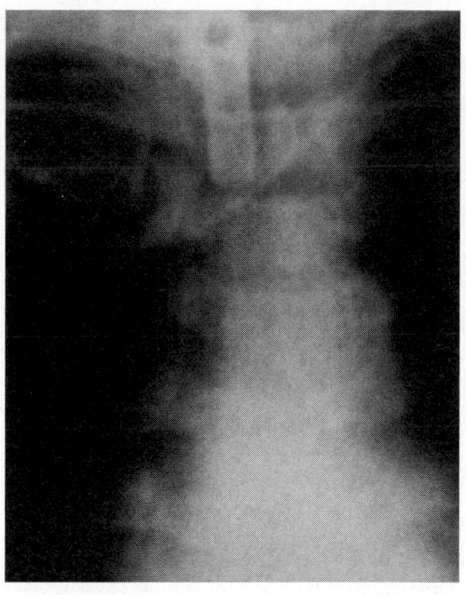

A

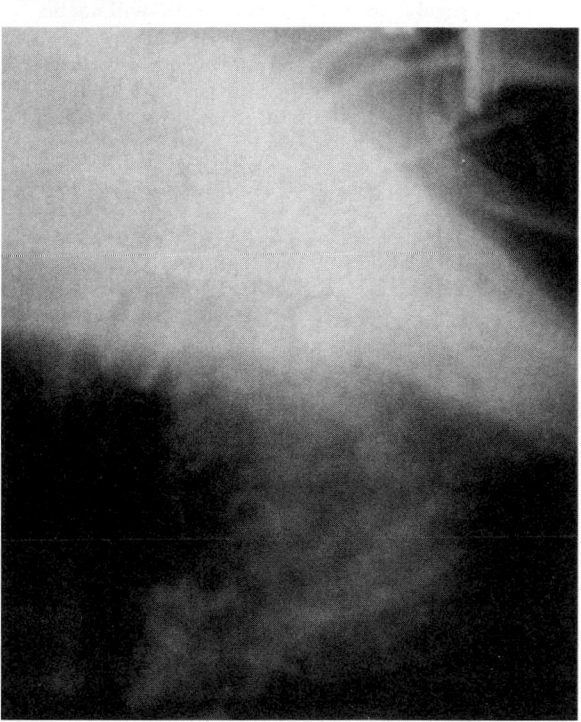

B

FIGURE 48-7 *A.* Well-positioned tracheostomy tube, the walls of which are parallel to the trachea. *B.* Lateral view in a different patient showing a relatively short endotracheal course (inferiorly from arrow) and posterior obliquity. Such a tube could cause complications due to impingement on the posterior tracheal wall.

ipsilateral mucosal thickening or fluid. This fluid usually clears with extubation without antibiotic administration.[19] If sinusitis is suspected as the source of the patient's fever, the fluid from the sinus must be sampled for bacteriologic confirmation.

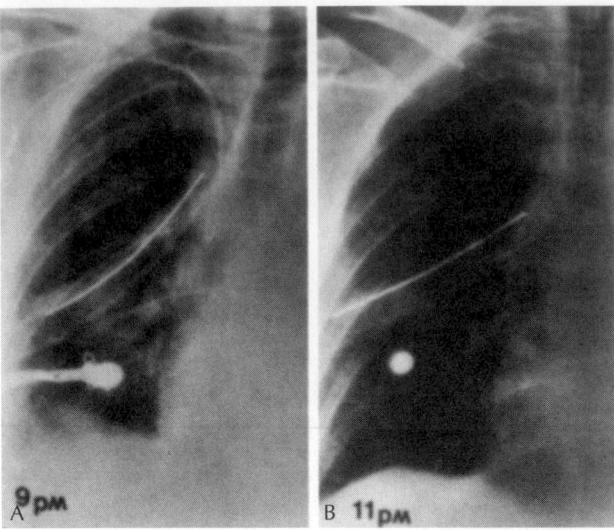

FIGURE 48-8 *A*. Focal pulmonary consolidation is noted in the right middle and lower zones. The central venous pressure (CVP) line is coiled within the superior vena cava with its tip probably in the anterior jugular venous arch, where CVP will not be measured accurately. The chest tube is well positioned. *B*. Two hours later, the CVP line has been removed, an endotracheal tube has been inserted, and positive pressure ventilation with PEEP has been instituted. Note the improved lung expansion, the resolution of the middle- and lower-zone atelectasis, and the better definition of the diaphragm. (*Reproduced, with permission, from Goodman et al.[1]*)

MONITORING AND THERAPEUTIC CATHETERS

Intravenous catheters may be placed to administer fluids, measure physiologic parameters, or provide access for dialysis.[20,21] For central venous fluid administration or physiologic monitoring, the tip is ideally located within the superior vena cava, beyond the valves of the innominate and subclavian veins. If the tip is beyond the costal cartilage of the first rib on the right, the catheter is usually well situated. For long-dwelling catheters, especially for the infusion of sclerosing medications, positioning the catheter tip in the proximal right atrium is beneficial.[22,23] Even when perfectly placed initially, catheters may migrate with time and change position between supine and erect. Myocardial penetration and catheter-induced arrhythmias are potential problems of the right atrial position.

The complication rate for catheter insertion varies widely (1–15%).[20,24–27] Catheter malpositioning into a secondary vein, or in an unintended direction, are the most common complications and should be checked on the initial and subsequent radiographs (Figs. 48-8*A* and *B* and 48-9). Pneumothorax may complicate as many as 6% of subclavian insertions and 1% of jugular insertions. Erect radiographs are mandatory to exclude pneumothorax after insertion (Fig. 48-10).

Extravascular fluid infusion or bleeding secondary to perivascular placement, or vascular injury, may give rise to mediastinal widening or pleural effusion. Imminent or actual catheter-tip perforation through the vein wall may be indicated by an acutely angulated catheter tip on the chest

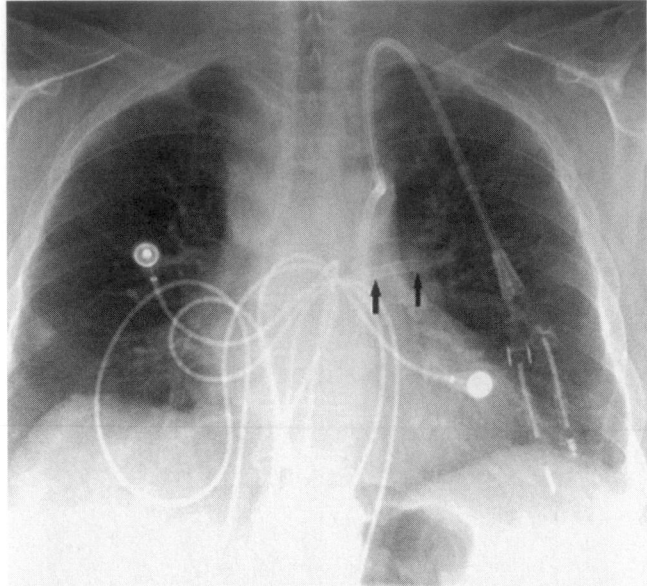

FIGURE 48-9 A large-bore jugular catheter is seen to the left of the spine. This is most likely in the accessory hemiazygos system. A catheter in the left superior vena cava would also project to the left of the spine. A broken piece of catheter is seen in the left pulmonary artery (*arrows*).

FIGURE 48-10 Pneumothorax in a ventilated patient after insertion of a right subclavian CVP catheter (*arrowheads*). The lung edge is clearly seen as a white line. Note also the air within the horizontal fissure (*straight arrow*).

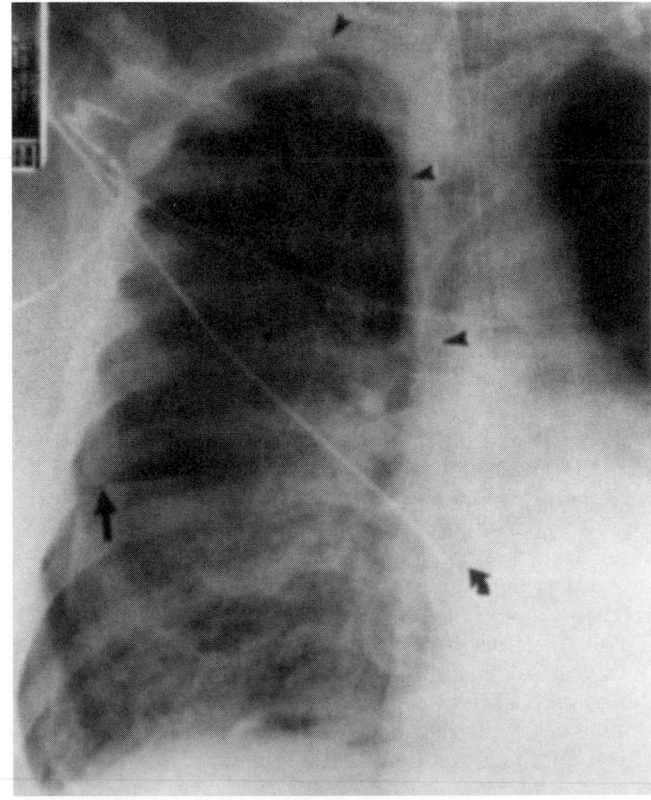

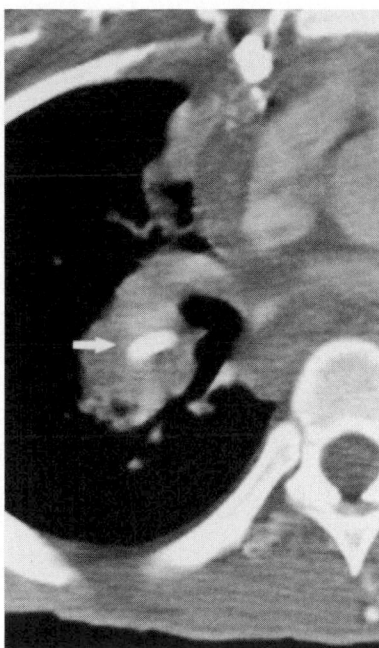

FIGURE 48-11 A catheter fragment is seen in the right main pulmonary artery on CT scan (*arrow*).

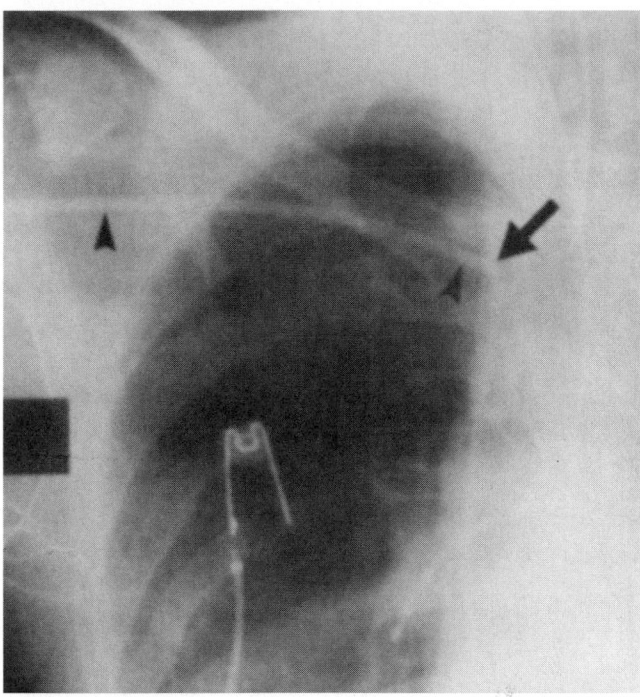

FIGURE 48-12 Kinked Swan-Ganz catheter at the origin of the right brachiocephalic vein. Note that the thin radiopaque line of the sheath (*arrowheads*), through which the catheter is passing, extends to the point at which the kink occurs. Withdrawing the sheath a little may be sufficient to straighten the kink.

radiograph.[28,29] Additional complications include venous thrombosis, catheter embolization (see Fig. 48-9; Fig. 48-11), air embolism, and catheter sepsis.[21,25]

Peripherally inserted central catheters (PICC) are small-bore catheters that may be inserted into the forearm veins. These are increasingly being placed by nurses and/or interventional radiology teams. Interventional radiologists are performing an increasing number of tunneled catheter procedures using a percutaneous, ultrasound-guided approach. These teams have increased the successful catheterization rate, decreased short- and long-term complication rates, and decreased infection rates.[30,31]

Contrast-enhanced CTs are being performed with great frequency now in ICU patients. The injection rate may be as high as 4–6 ml per second for systemic and pulmonary vascular studies. Catheters used in the ICU vary considerably in their ability to accommodate these injections. If CT studies are anticipated, one should assure that appropriate catheters are used initially. Unfortunately, there are no clear-cut guidelines on power injections through intravenous routine catheters.[23,32–34] In general, most central PICC lines will withstand 1.25- to 2-ml-per-second injections. This is barely adequate for some routine CT studies, and inadequate for vascular studies. Recently developed PICC catheters will withstand high-volume injections. Injections into access chemotherapy ports are best avoided.

Ideally, the tip of pulmonary artery catheters should be placed in the right or left main pulmonary artery. When the balloon is inflated, it can then migrate peripherally to wedge in a small lower pulmonary artery, from which it returns on deflation. The inflated balloon should never be visible on the radiograph. When the catheter tip is in the upper or middle lobe, it is anterior to the left atrium in the supine patient and therefore wedge-pressure readings are unreliable. If the

balloon fails to deflate or if the catheter is positioned in a segmental or subsegmental pulmonary artery, then occlusion of the vessel may lead to pulmonary infarction.[35] Pulmonary artery perforation and pulmonary artery pseudoaneurysm formation are rare but serious complications of peripheral balloon placement.[36] Cardiac arrhythmias may be caused by placement within the right ventricle or by the presence of a redundant loop within this chamber. Intracardiac knotting of the catheter may occasionally occur. Kinking at the origin of the right brachiocephalic vein is often secondary to the catheter bending as it exits the sheath (Fig. 48-12).

Any catheter or wire passing between the clavicle and the anterior first rib may be pinched by the subclavius muscle or the costoclavicular ligament as the arm raises and lowers (Fig. 48-13).[37] Pinching may lead to catheter obstruction or, ultimately, catheter or wire fatigue. It may shear and embolize to the heart or pulmonary artery (see Fig. 48-11). Shearing may also occur at the sites of suture fixation. Pinched catheters should be replaced.

Intra-aortic balloon pumps (IABPs) improve cardiac function by decreasing cardiac workload and increasing perfusion of the coronary arteries. The catheter tip should be positioned just distal to the origin of the left subclavian artery (Fig. 48-14). Positioning within the arch of the aorta predisposes to cerebral embolism. A middle or distal descending aorta location results in less effective counterpulsation or the balloon may obstruct the celiac, superior mesenteric, and renal artery origins and embolization or thrombosis to these vessels has been reported (Fig. 48-15).[38] Aortic dissection can occur during placement of the catheter, and this may

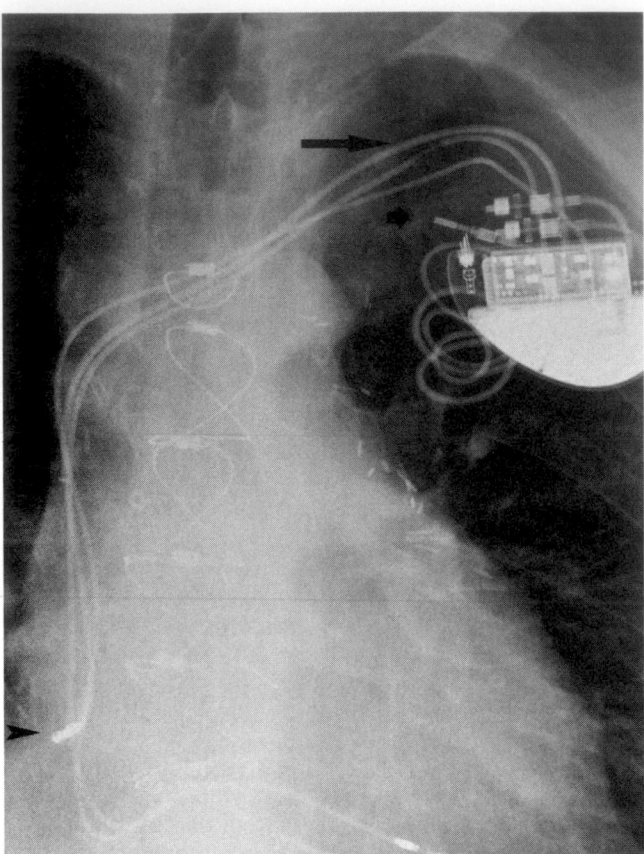

FIGURE 48-13 AV pacer in place. There are two leads in the right ventricle and one lead in the right atrium (*arrowhead*). The original lead wire is fractured just beneath the clavicle (*large arrow*). That lead is detached from the pacer (*small arrow*).

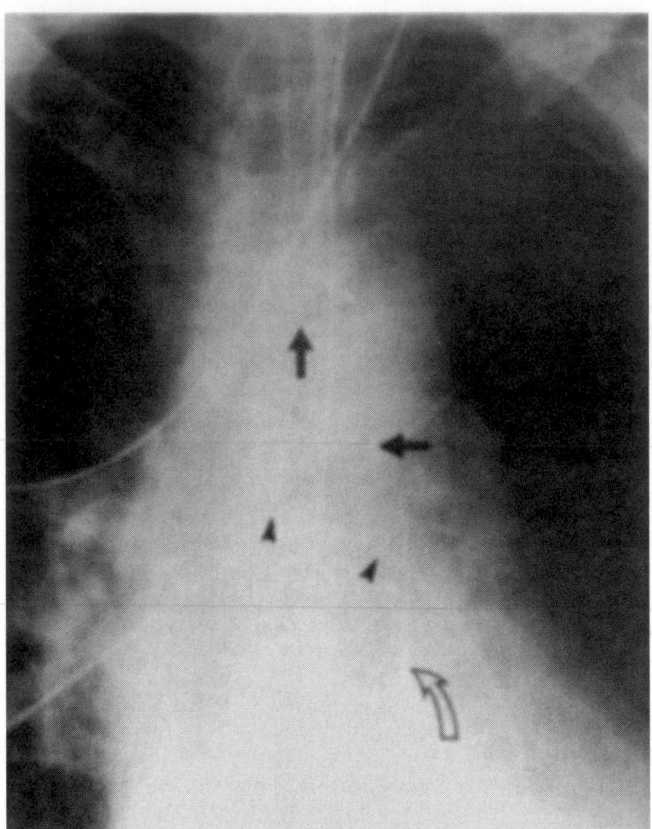

FIGURE 48-14 The rectangular radiopaque tip of an intra-aortic balloon pump is projected over the inferior border of the aortic arch (*closed arrow*). The tip of a femorally placed Swan-Ganz catheter is well positioned within the right pulmonary artery (*arrowheads*). A mediastinal drain (*open arrow*), nasogastric tube, and well-positioned endotracheal tube (*arrow*) are also seen.

occasionally be recognized by loss of the descending aorta contour on the chest radiograph. Vascular insufficiency in the catheterized lower limb is a well-known complication.[39]

There has been a rapid proliferation of transvenous pacemakers and defibrillators and appearances differ from manufacturer to manufacturer. Ideally, the right ventricular lead points anteriorly and inferiorly in the right ventricle. On the AP film, it often appears to be pointed toward the left ventricular apex. Atrial pacing is accomplished by a catheter that curves anteriorly and superiorly in the upper right heart (see Fig. 48-13). Lateral films are often required to ensure proper positioning. Coronary sinus pacing and transseptal pacing are less frequent positions. Myocardial perforation is rare. The tip of the catheter may appear at the cardiac surface. Hemopericardium and tamponade is an infrequent complication. The great variety of pacemakers, defibrillators, stents, intra-cardiac devices, and external bypass devices are beyond the scope of this text. The reader is referred to pictorial reviews by Hunter et al and Landay et al.[16,40]

Chest tubes are frequently employed in ventilated patients for the drainage of air or fluid collections. Because these patients spend much of their time in a supine position, it would seem logical that an anteriorly and superiorly placed tube would be ideal for pneumothorax drainage and a posteroinferiorly placed tube would be ideal for drainage

of fluid collections (see Fig. 48-8)[41] Curtin et al[42] found that initial location may be less important than previously thought. Tubes often function adequately when located within a fissure.[42,43] Tubes should not be replaced simply because the radiograph shows an interfissural location. Precise tube positioning is essential for drainage of loculated effusions or empyema and sonographic or CT guidance is invaluable in this situation. Tubes that abut mediastinal structures may lead to compression or injury of these structures and should be repositioned. Tubes that are not sufficiently far advanced have their side holes within the subcutaneous tissues, may results in inefficient drainage and subcutaneous emphysema (see Fig. 48-26). A tube placed within the parenchyma causes laceration and may lead to bronchopleural fistula formation. CT is often required to make this diagnosis.

After the placement of a nasogastric tube or a feeding tube, radiographs should be obtained to check tube position (Fig 48-16). Clinical signs suggesting correct gastrointestinal location are not always reliable. The ideal nasogastric tube should be coiled in the stomach with its side hole beyond the gastroesophageal junction. The ideal feeding tube tip should traverse the pylorus and the duodenal sweep and rest at the ligament of Treitz. Tubes may inadvertently

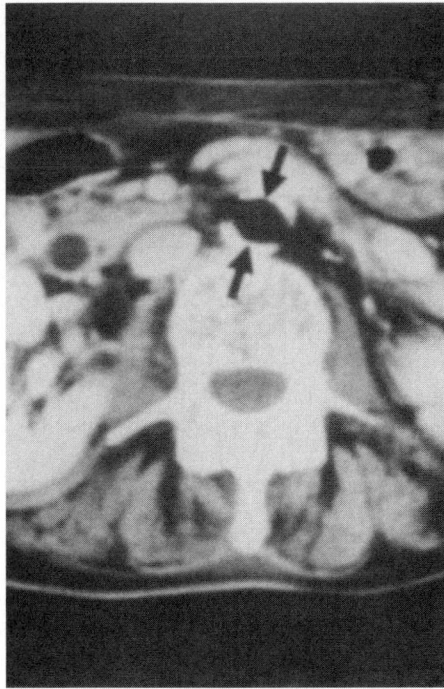

FIGURE 48-15 CT scan at the level of the renal hilum in a patient with an intra-aortic balloon pump in situ. Note the air lucency within the aorta (*arrows*) secondary to the inflated balloon, which extends below the celiac, superior mesenteric, and renal artery origins. The patient has had a left nephrectomy.

be placed in the bronchial tree and lead to chemical pneumonitis if tube feeding is initiated. The tube may penetrate the pleura and lead to hydropneumothorax delayed. Pneumothorax may occur after withdrawal of the tube, when the hole is no longer plugged by the tube (Fig. 48-17).[44,45]

FIGURE 48-16 Nasogastric tube in the lung, probably in the lingula (*arrow*). There is no pneumothorax.

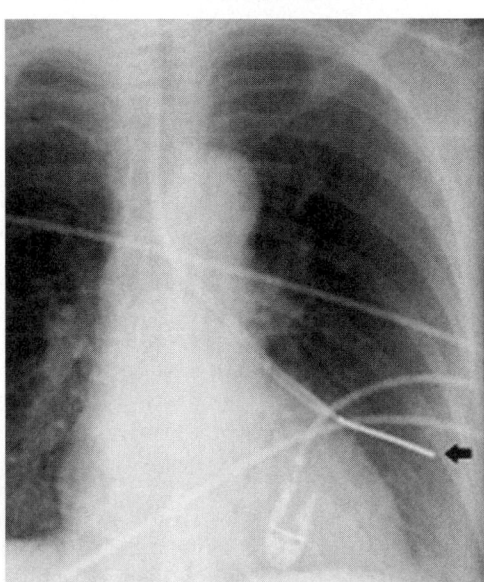

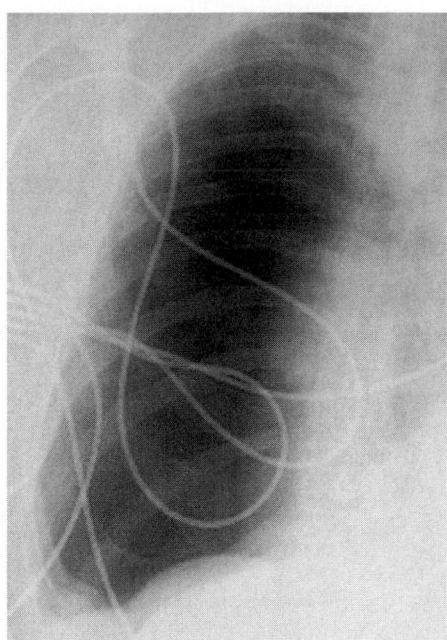

FIGURE 48-17 A prior chest x-ray showed a feeding tube in the right lung or pleural space. There was no pneumothorax. Immediately after removal of the tube, the patient experienced marked shortness of breath. Chest x-ray shows tension pneumothorax with a depressed diaphragm and deviation of the mediastinum to the opposite side.

Mechanical Ventilation

Under most circumstances, patients receiving mechanical ventilation receive daily chest x-rays, initially to detect new disease but, more importantly, to follow the progression of known disease and to prevent or detect potential complications. To make valid comparisons about disease progression, radiographs must be made at the same degree of inspiration (mechanical ventilation settings) (Fig. 48-18).[46,47] Zimmerman et al[47] and McLoud et al[46] showed that PEEP markedly alters the appearance of the radiograph. Zimmermann et al[47] radiographed 12 mechanically ventilated patients, 4 times each, within 15 minutes. The initial baseline radiograph (V_{T1}) was at "ideal" calculated tidal volume (550–1000 ml), the second radiograph ("sigh") at 1.5–2 times the initial tidal volume (900–1800 ml), the third radiograph (PEEP) at tidal volume plus PEEP (12–20 cmH$_2$O), and the fourth radiograph (V_{T2}) at the original tidal volume. In every patient, PEEP changed the appearance of the pulmonary consolidation. In 10 of the 12 patients, when PEEP was applied, there was less radiographic evidence of consolidation than on the other 3 radiographs in the set. In 7 of the 12 radiographs, the "sigh" setting also diminished the visible disease (Fig. 48-19). The final radiograph (V_{T2}), taken several minutes after discontinuing PEEP, returned to the appearance of the V_{T1} film in 7 patients. In three patients, the V_{T2} film demonstrated slightly less consolidation than the V_{T1} film. If only the PEEP film had been available, readers subjectively estimated that their diagnosis would have

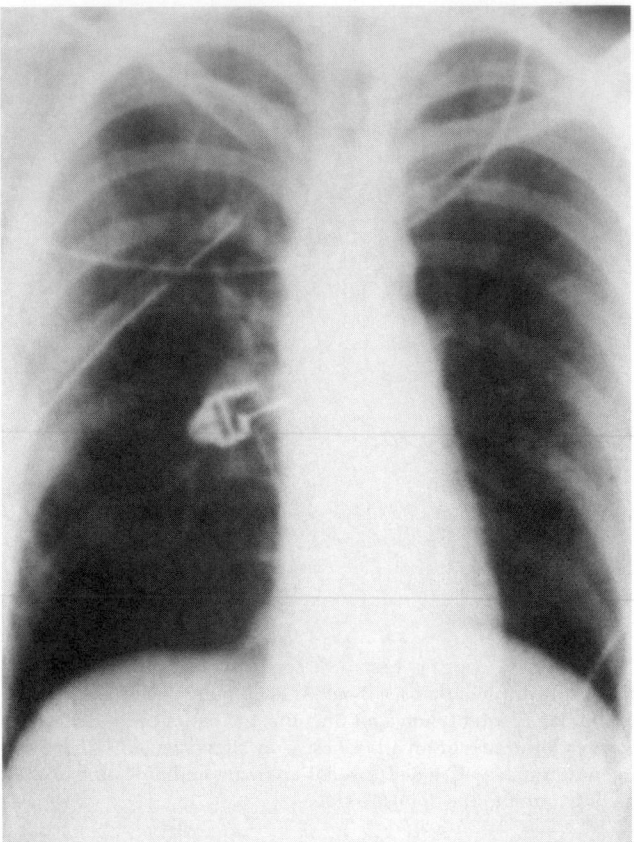

A

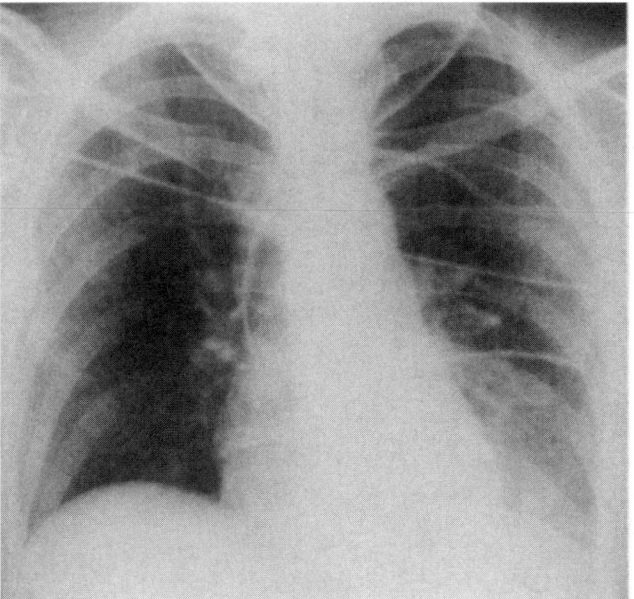

B

FIGURE 48-18 *A.* Ventilated patient who is receiving excessive tidal volume, similar to a "sigh" tidal volume, demonstrating hyperinflated lungs and an elongated, narrow cardiac silhouette. A right chest tube is in position for treatment of a pneumothorax, and subcutaneous emphysema is seen in the right axillary region. *B.* The same patient 1 week later, after insertion of a tracheostomy tube. The lungs and heart have returned to their normal volumes and shapes. There is left lower lobe consolidation. A double-lumen catheter tip is in the proximal right atrium.

been changed in 4 patients and the severity of the disease underestimated in 3.

Those crude radiographic observations have been elegantly expanded by CT scanning. CT scanning of normal and critically-ill patients is adding new insight into normal respiratory mechanics, the distribution of disease, and the mechanisms by which patient physiology and radiography are affected by both mechanical ventilation and gravity. In the normal supine patient, during full inspiration, there is an x-ray attenuation gradient in the lung that is gravity dependent (i.e., ventral to dorsal) (Fig. 48-20). When the patient is turned prone, the gradient reverses within minutes. In addition, there is a density gradient from apex to base. Expiration accentuates the density gradient (Fig. 48-21). ARDS is inhomogeneous, and has a dorsal-ventral gradient and a cranio-caudal gradient.[48-53] The physiologic results of these observations are discussed in other chapters.

In another study, Zimmerman et al[54] demonstrated that, when patients with pulmonary edema lie in the decubitus position for 2 hours and then are radiographed sitting erect, the dependent side shows more consolidation, while the other side improves. Patients with other types of consolidation showed little or no gravity-dependent shift. They attributed the shift to increased edema in the dependent lung and decreased edema on the other side secondary to altered hydrostatic pressure relationships. Gattinoni et al[55], using CT, demonstrated that the consolidation shifts in a matter of minutes, not hours. It is likely, therefore, that the rapid shift is again caused by shifting atelectasis rather than shifting edema. It is possible that some of the 2-hour shift is secondary to shifting hydrostatic edema.

Therefore, the effects of mechanical ventilation and gravity should be considered when interpreting the radiograph. One should anticipate an apparent decrease in pulmonary consolidation with the initiation of assisted ventilation and an apparent increase of the consolidation when the patient is weaned (see Figs. 48-18 and 48-19), and that these changes may not be clinically significant. These changes will be most pronounced when the increased lung density is caused by hypoventilation atelectasis or edema rather than pulmonary consolidation.

COMPLICATIONS OF MECHANICAL VENTILATION

Barotrauma is a frequent and potentially lethal complication of mechanical ventilation. Once a major problem in ventilated patients, sophisticated ventilator management has markedly decreased the incidence and severity. Barotrauma develops from positive pressure ventilation when the alveolar pressure exceeds the interstitial pressure. There is distal airway rupture, and air enters the adjacent bronchovascular connective tissue.[18,56-59] The air may dissect centrally toward the hilum or peripherally toward the pleura. The centripetal air eventually enters the mediastinum, where it can decompress cephalad into the visceral compartment of the neck or caudally into the retroperitoneum and root of the mesentery. If these routes do not adequately decompress the mediastinum, air ruptures through the mediastinal pleura into the pleural space or peritoneal cavity.

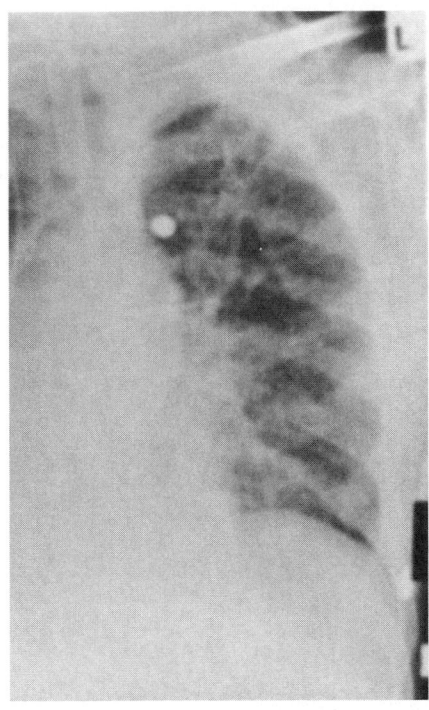
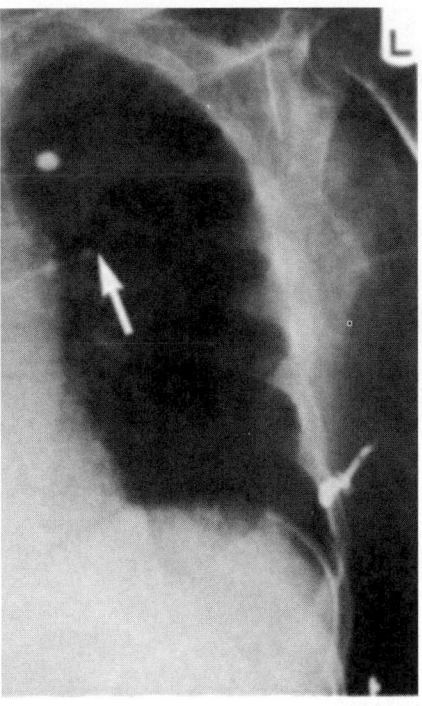

A

B

FIGURE 48-19 *A.* Chest radiograph with tracheostomy tube in situ. The pulmonary vessels are enlarged, and there is interstitial and alveolar opacification consistent with pulmonary edema. There are also areas of atelectasis at both bases. *B.* After institution of positive pressure ventilation with PEEP of 10 cmH$_2$O. Even allowing for the difference in penetration, there has been significant improvement in the edema and atelectasis with a reduction in the pulmonary vessel size. Note that the tip of the Swan-Ganz catheter (*arrow*) is in a left upper lobe vessel. (*Reproduced, with permission, from Zimmerman et al.[47]*)

Assuming this sequence of events, the earliest radiographic finding of barotrauma should be air in the lung along the bronchovascular sheaths as it tracks medially and air in the subpleural space as it tracks laterally. Interstitial emphysema is only discerned radiographically when there is moderate-to-severe consolidation of the lung to provide contrast between the normal bronchial and the abnormal peribronchial air.[36,60,61]

The most frequent radiographic appearance is mottled radiolucencies in the medial two-thirds of the lung or multiple streaky lucencies simulating an air bronchogram. These lucencies are very numerous and do not branch and taper smoothly, as one would expect with true air bronchograms. They may have a "string of beads" appearance or appear as multiple tiny lucencies in a focal area (Fig. 48-22). A specific but uncommon sign of interstitial emphysema is the so-called "halo sign." This represents air in the interstitium around a pulmonary artery or vein, seen end-on.

Peripheral air within the interlobular septa may give a striated appearance to the lateral lung, corresponding to the radiographic negative of Kerley lines. The centrifugal air may lodge in the subpleural connective tissue and form round or oval subpleural cysts. These cysts are seen most frequently in the anterior basal or medial aspects of the lung or along the fissures.[59] The cysts often develop rapidly, change rapidly, are thin-walled, and may appear in areas previously relatively free of disease. These cysts may at times be difficult to separate from basilar areas of pneumothorax, abscesses, bullae, or enlarging pulmonary lacerations. In any event, progressive enlargement of air-containing lung structures in a ventilated patient indicates a potential area of rupture and should lead to the reassessment for the need for positive pressure ventilation. On occasion, cysts stabilize and persist for days to weeks (Fig. 48-23).

Interstitial emphysema is often suspected on the radiograph but difficult to prove. On CT scan, one may see lines of air parallel to bronchi, air surrounding vessels, and subpleural cysts. CT is especially helpful in distinguishing basilar subpleural cysts from subpneumonic pneumothorax in the supine patient (see Fig. 48-22).[61,62]

In the majority of patients, interstitial emphysema is not visible. The first sign of barotrauma may then be pneumomediastinum or subcutaneous emphysema in the base of the neck. The radiographic signs of pneumomediastinum may be subtle. A small pneumomediastinum is most often visualized along the aortic knob or the aortopulmonary window, where the pleura is elevated and seen as a sharp line and a thin lucency outlining the left margin of the mediastinum. Mediastinal air may outline other mediastinal structures, such as the superior vena cava, the subclavian arteries, or the great vessels in the neck (see Figs. 48-22 and 48-23). Air in the lower mediastinum may outline the central portion of the diaphragm under the cardiac silhouette (the "continuous diaphragm sign"), outline the descending aorta, or dissect between the parietal pleura and the diaphragm, causing lucent streaks between the slips of the diaphragm. Subcutaneous air in the base of the neck or in the muscles over the upper thorax may be the first radiographic or clinical sign of pneumomediastinum and is a presumptive indicator of barotrauma if there has been no recent instrumentation.

The presence of air in the interstitium, mediastinum, neck, or retroperitoneum should provoke a search for the pneumothorax. Every effort should be made to obtain an erect radiograph. In addition to the absence of pulmonary markings at the apex, the radiodense pleural stripe must be visualized. The simple absence of markings at the apex is unreliable, because many patients without pneumothorax have vague apical markings on portable radiographs. Unfortunately, many patients cannot be sat erect. A lateral decubitus

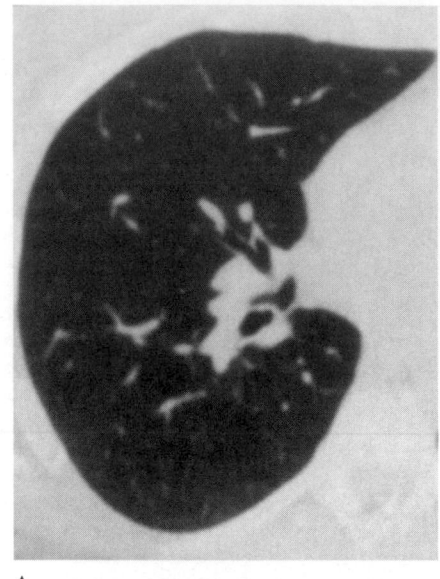

A

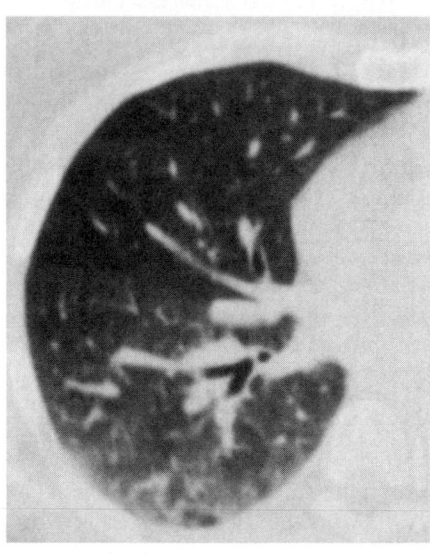

B

FIGURE 48-20 *A.* CT section taken on full inspiration. The density gradient from anterior to posterior is subtle but definite. *B.* CT section at the same level taken at expiration, showing a marked increase in density, especially posteriorly, resulting in a very obvious anterior-to-posterior gradient. Note focal areas of air trapping posteriorly.

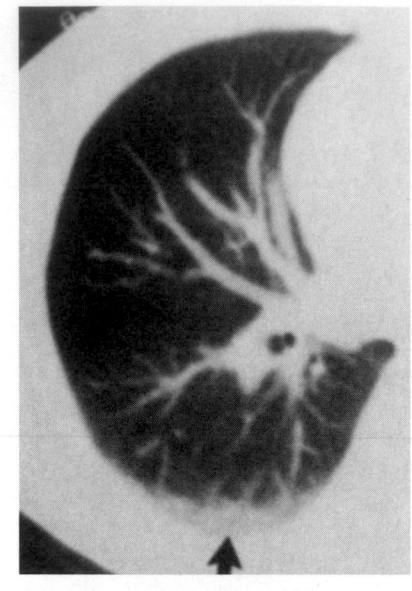

A

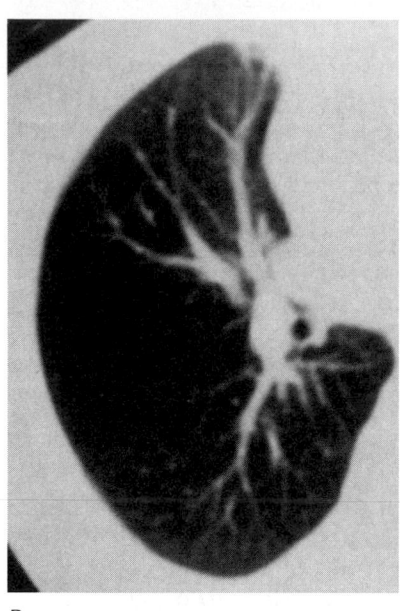

B

FIGURE 48-21 *A.* Supine section through lower zones, showing normal density gradient from anterior to posterior. In addition, areas of atelectasis (*arrows*) are present posteriorly. *B.* Prone CT section at a similar level (the image has been inverted for ease of comparison) in the same patient showing increasing density from posterior to anterior and resolution of the posterior areas of atelectasis.

radiograph, with the side in question elevated, offers an adequate but not foolproof substitute. The diagnosis of pneumothorax is slightly less accurate on decubitus than on erect radiographs.[63]

Unequivocally, the least reliable radiograph for diagnosing a pneumothorax is the supine radiograph. Air will rise anteriorly in the thorax unless impeded by pleural adhesions or attracted by decreased transpleural pressure secondary to adjacent atelectasis. In a study of 88 supine ICU patients with pneumothorax, Tocino[62] found that most air collections were anteromedial or subpulmonic in location. If air is present when there are pleural adhesions or dif-

fusely consolidated lung, lung collapse is incomplete, even in the presence of tension pneumothorax. Other signs of tension pneumothorax, depressed diaphragm and shifted mediastinum, should be sought.

In an anterior medial pneumothorax, air accumulates in front of the lung and highlights the anterior mediastinal structures.[62] Superiorly, air outlines the superior vena cava and azygos vein on the right or the subclavian artery on the left. Inferiorly, the pneumothorax will outline the heart

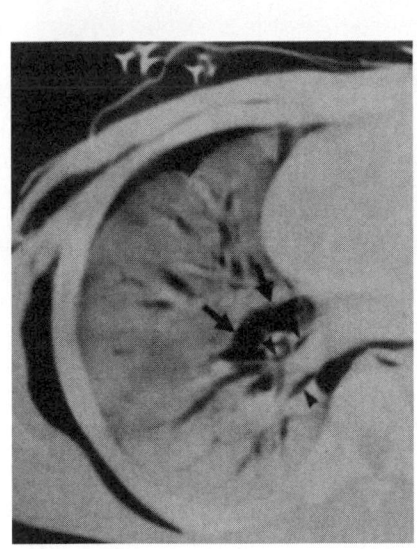

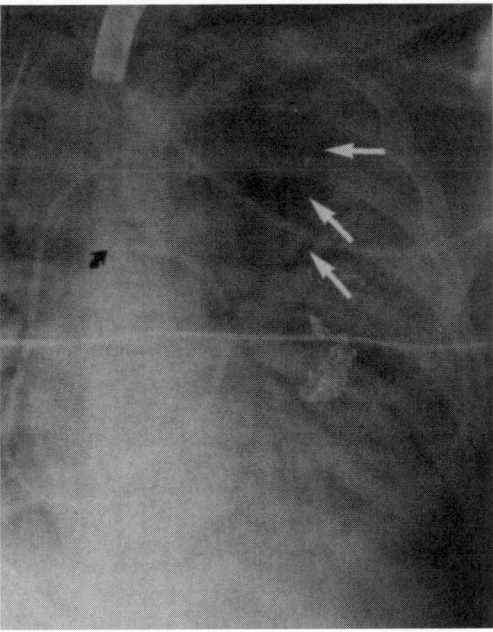

A   B

FIGURE 48-22 *A.* Supine chest radiograph showing bilateral homogeneous consolidation with air bronchograms. A pneumomediastinum is visible outlining the left and inferior heart borders. The tip of the tracheostomy tube is impinging on the right lateral tracheal wall. *B.* CT through the lower lung, (different patient). There is subcutaneous emphysema laterally, and pneumomediastinum centrally (between the heart and spine). There is a small right pneumothorax not apparent on the supine chest x-ray. Mediastinal air extends along the right inferior pulmonary vein. Multiple linear lucencies are seen in the left lung. Although some may be bronchograms, several relatively large nontapering lucencies in the left upper lobe (*arrows*) probably represent interstitial emphysema.

border, outline the cardiac fat pad, or cause the costophrenic angle and the upper liver or spleen to appear more lucent than normal ("deep sulcus sign"; see Fig. 48-23; Fig. 48-25). If air collects along the lateral heart border and is not seen elsewhere, differentiation between a medial pneumothorax, pneumomediastinum, and pneumopericardium may not be possible. In the adult, however, pneumopericardium is extremely rare following barotrauma (Fig. 48-26).

Additional signs of pneumothorax elsewhere in the chest include air within the minor fissure (see Fig. 48-10), a minor fissure that does not contact the lateral chest wall, a generalized increased lucency over one hemithorax without

FIGURE 48-23 *A.* Chest radiograph of a patient who had sustained injuries in a motor vehicle accident and subsequently developed ARDS. Bilateral pneumothoraces persist despite the presence of two chest tubes. In fact, there is a mediastinal shift to the right and depression of the left hemidiaphragm, indicating that the left pneumothorax is under tension. Patchy consolidation is present in both lungs, but is more marked on the right. An oval 4 × 3-cm lucency is seen in the right lower zone. The tip of the CVP line is in the right atrium (*arrowheads*). *B.* Cross-section showing the bilateral pneumothorax, diffuse right lung consolidation, and patchy left lung consolidation. The large oval lucency visible on the chest radiograph is seen as a cyst in the right lung, and another cyst is seen in the left lung laterally (*arrows*). Subcutaneous emphysema is present over the chest wall bilaterally.

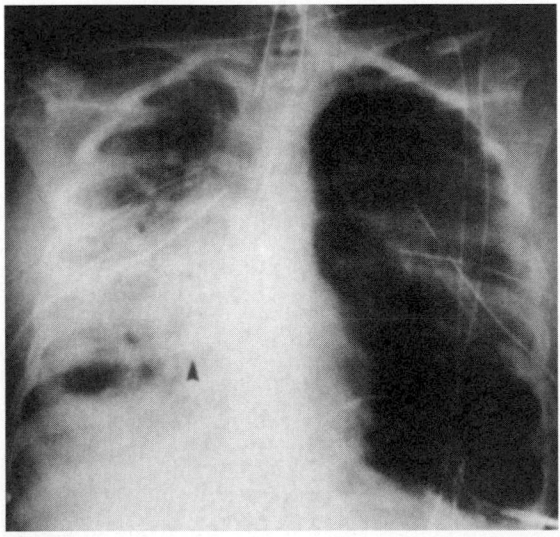

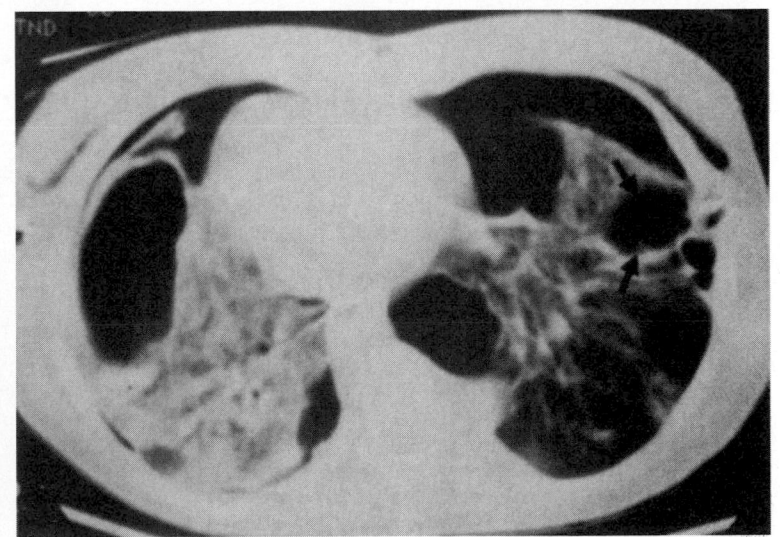

A   B

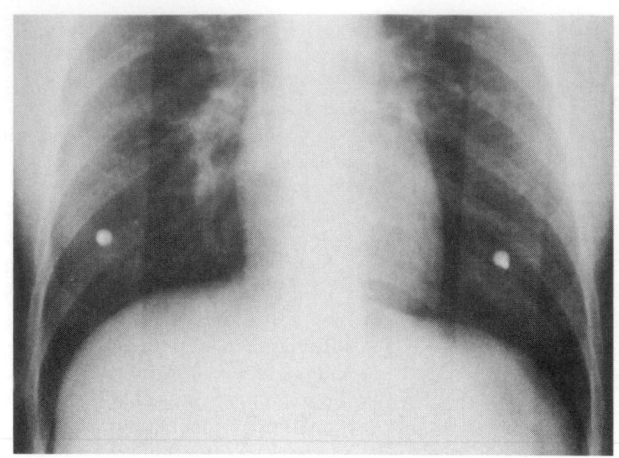
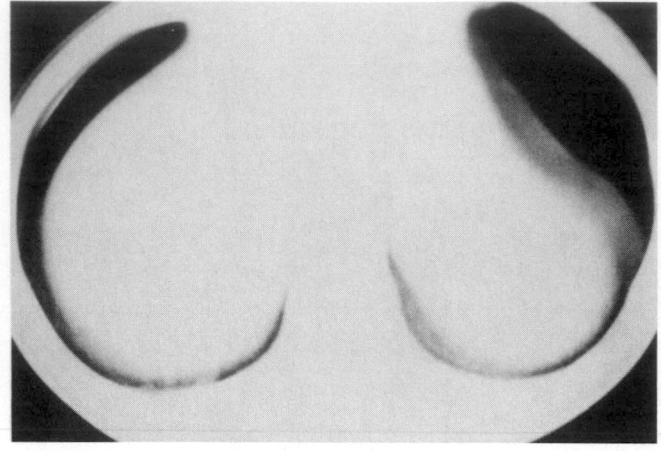

A   B

FIGURE 48-24 *A.* Supine radiograph showing increased lucency and depth of the costophrenic angles, the "deep sulcus sign" of pneumothorax in the supine position. A definite lung edge is not visible. *B.* CT section through the lower thorax in the same patient, confirming bilateral pneumothoraces.

FIGURE 48-25 Patient with ARDS. Patchy consolidation is present throughout the right lung. This supine radiograph demonstrates a subpulmonic pneumothorax as a band of lucency superior to the diaphragm and inferior to the inferior visceral pleura (*arrows*). Note also the subcutaneous emphysema and the poorly positioned chest tube, the tip of which appears to lie barely within the pleural space (*arrowheads*).

FIGURE 48-26 Supine chest radiograph of a patient with a large pneumopericardium. There is increased lucency over the left side of the heart and displacement of the parietal pericardium from the cardiac surface (*white arrows*). The resulting white line, however, does not extend above the level of the aortic pulmonary window, unlike pneumomediastinum. The endotracheal tube (*black arrow*) is several centimeters above the carina (*arrowhead*).

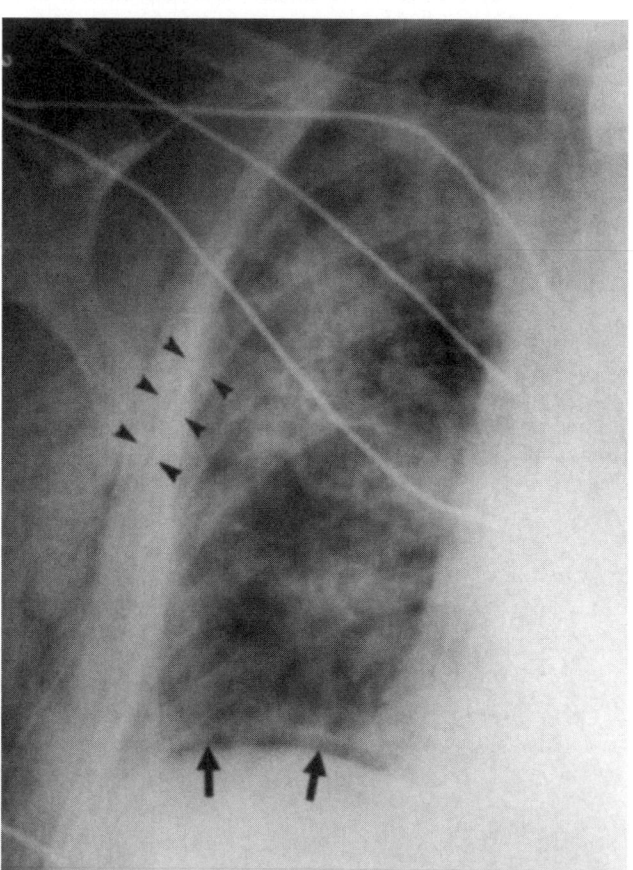

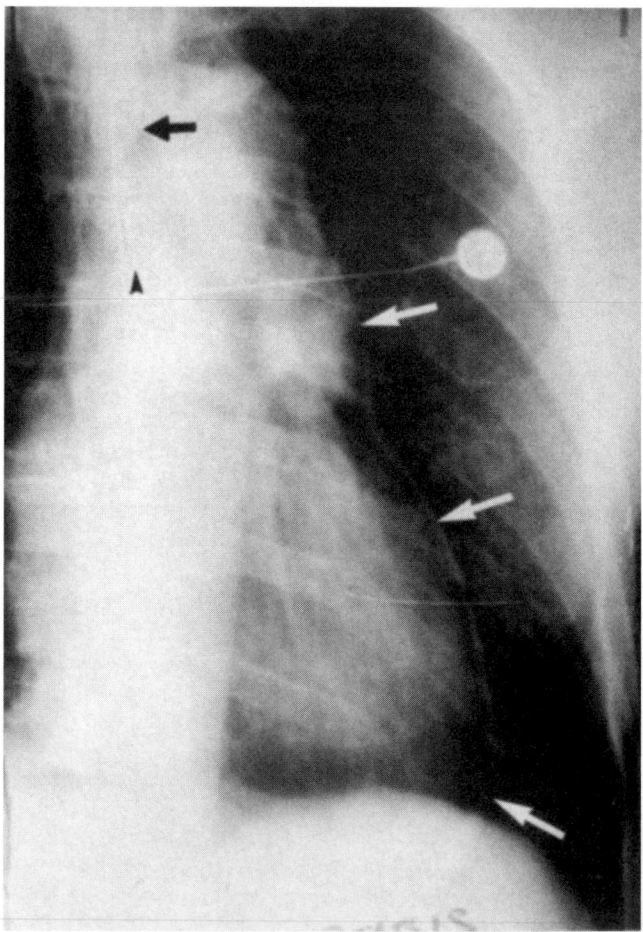

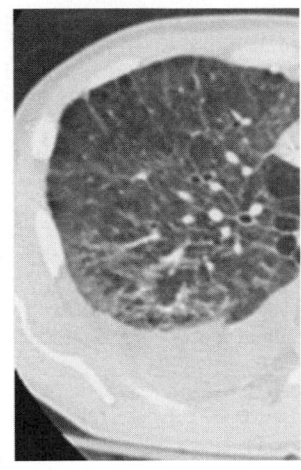
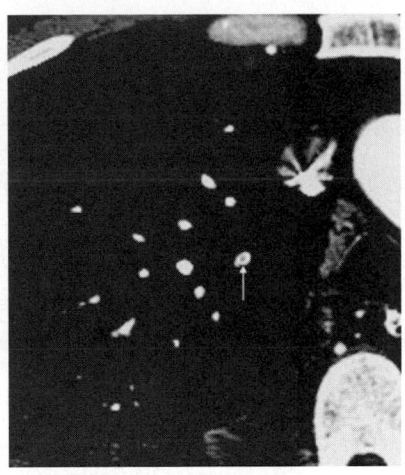

A   B

FIGURE 48-27   *A.* ARDS in fibrotic stage. *B.* Segmental pulmonary embolus (*arrow*).

visualization of the pleural reflection, or air collecting posteromedially outlining posterior mediastinal structures, such as the paraspinal line, the descending aorta, the medial inferior diaphragmatic vertebral angle, the inferior vena cava, or the azygoesophageal recess.

IMAGING ALTERNATIVES IN THE VENTILATED PATIENT

With increasing understanding of the limitations of the portable radiograph and the increased availability of more sophisticated alternative imaging modalities, alternative imaging is now a daily event in the ICU.

A trip to the CT scanner, once an exotic voyage to a far-off place, is now a daily occurrence.[64] With the current generation of high-end multislice scanners, chest studies that often took 20–60 seconds to complete can now be completed in 5 seconds or less. Individual images can now be performed in 0.5 seconds or less and cardiac motion can stopped with ECG gating. Considerably less contrast medium is required and newer non-ionic contrast agents are less toxic and have little or no effect on water and electrolyte balance.

CT can rapidly diagnose complications of lung disease and respiratory therapy, such as infection, abscess formation, bronchopleural fistula, unsuspected pneumothoraces, and unsuspected pulmonary emboli (Fig. 48-27).[65,66] CT has largely replaced scintigraphy for the diagnosis of PE, because scintigraphy is usually not diagnostic in the face of parenchymal disease. CT can also evaluate for deep venous thrombosis. Withholding CT, because of the perceived problems of transportation alone, is a mistake, given the potential wealth of information available in well-selected patients.

Sonographic studies are also very useful for early detection of pleural or pericardial effusion or air and for guiding intervention in the pleural space or pericardial space.[67] The success rate of pleural interventions improves and the complication rate decreases with ultrasonic guidance.

Angiography and MRI, like CT, require the patient to be transported from the ICU to the appropriate imaging suite. MRI does not offer significant advantages over CT in the investigation of most chest pathology in the ventilated patient, although it is very useful for the imaging of the heart, arteries, veins, brain, and spine. An appropriate ventilator, however, must be available that can be used safely in the vicinity of a strong magnetic field.[68] Multidetector CT has replaced conventional angiography, and to a certain extent MRI, for the evaluation of both systemic and pulmonary vessels.

PARENCHYMAL DISEASE IN THE VENTILATED PATIENT

It is beyond the scope of this chapter to discuss the various cardiopulmonary diseases affecting the ICU patient. Many will be reviewed elsewhere in this text. The current generation of high-end CT scanners can provide previously unimagined imaging and help unravel the complex intricacies of cardiopulmonary disease in the ICU. Imaginative and judicious use of these scanners should be highly beneficial to both patient and physician.[69,70]

References

1. Goodman LR, Putman CE. A radiologist's perspective of critical care imaging. In: Goodman LR, Putman CE, editors. Critical care imaging. Philadelphia: Saunders, 1992.
2. MacMahon H, Giger M. Portable chest radiography techniques and teleradiology. Radiol Clin North Am 1996; 34:1–20.
3. Kundel HL, Seshadri SB, Langlotz CP. Prospective study of a PACS: information flow and clinical action in a medical intensive care unit. Radiology 1996; 199:143–9.
4. Watkins J, Weatherburn G, Bryan S. The impact of picture archiving and communication system (PACS) upon an intensive care unit. J Vasc Intervent Radiol 2000; 34:3–8.
5. Baker SR, Stein HD. Radiologic consultation: its application to an acute care surgical ward. AJR Am J Roentgenol 1986; 147:637–40.
6. Gray P, Sullivan G, Ostryamiuk P. Value of postprocedural chest radiographs in the adult intensive care unit. Crit Care Med 1992; 20:1513–8.
7. Lotano R, Gerber D, Aseron C. Utility of postintubation chest radiographs in the intensive care unit. Crit Care 2000; 4: 50–3.
8. Henschke CI, Yankelevitz DF, Wand A, et al. Accuracy and efficacy of chest radiography in the intensive care unit. Radiol Clin North Am 1996; 34:21–31.

9. Chang TC, Funaki B, Szymski GX. Are routine chest radiographs necessary after image-guided placement of internal jugular central access devices? AJR Am J Roentgenol 1998; 170:335–7.

10. Bekemeyer WB, Crapo RO, Calhoon S, et al. Efficacy of chest radiography in a respiratory intensive care unit: A prospective study. Chest 1985; 88:691–6.

11. Hall JB, White SR, Karrison T. Efficacy of daily routine chest radiographs in intubated, mechanically ventilated patients. Crit Care Med 1991; 19:689–92.

12. American College of Radiology. ACR Appropriateness Criteria - "Routine Daily Portable X-Rays," 1999.

13. Brunel W, Colemna DL, Schwartz DE, et al. Assessment of routine chest roentgenograms and the physical examination to confirm endotracheal tube position. Chest 1989; 96:1043–5.

14. Conrardy PA, Goodman LR, Lainge R, et al. Alteration of endotracheal tube position: Flexion and extension of the neck. Crit Care Med 1976; 4:7–12.

15. Goodman LR, Conrardy PA, Laing F, et al. Radiographic evaluation of endotracheal tube position. AJR Am J Roentgenol 1976; 127:433–4.

16. Hunter TB, Taljanovic MS, Tsau PH, et al. Medical devices of the chest. RadioGraphics 2004; 24:1725–46.

17. Smith GM, Reed JC, Chaplin RH. Radiographic detection of esophageal malpositioning of endotracheal tubes. AJR Am J Roentgenol 1990; 154:23–6.

18. Goodman LR. Pulmonary support and monitoring apparatus. In: Goodman LR, Putman CE, editors. Critical care imaging. Philadelphia: Saunders, 1992:35–59.

19. Fassoulaki A, Pamouktsoglou P. Prolonged nasotracheal intubation and its association with inflammation of paranasal sinuses. Anesth Analg 1989; 69:50–2.

20. Maffessanti M, Berlot G, Bortolotto P. Chest roentgenology in the intensive care unit: an overview. Eur Radiol 1998; 8:69–78.

21. Trotman-Dickenson B. Radiology in the intensive care unit (Part I). J Intensive Care Med 2003; 18:198–210.

22. Vesely TM. Central venous catheter tip position: a continuing controversy. J Vasc Intervent Radiol 2003; 6:35–41.

23. Funaki B. Central venous access: a primer for the diagnostic radiologist. AJR Am J Roentgenol 2002; 179:309–18.

24. Sitzmann JV, Townsend TR, Siler MC, et al. Septic and technical complications of central venous catheterization: A prospective study of 200 consecutive patients. Ann Surg 1985; 202:766–70.

25. Knutstad K, Hager B, Hauser M. Radiologic diagnosis and management of complications related to central venous access. Acta Radiol 2003; 44:508–16.

26. Bailey SH, Shapiro SB, Mone MC, et al. Is immediate chest radiograph necessary after central venous catheter placement in a surgical intensive care unit? Am J Surg 2000; 180:517–21.

27. Kattan KR. Migration of central venous catheters. AJR Am J Roentgenol 1985; 145:727–8.

28. Tocino IM, Watanabe A. Impending catheter perforation of the superior vena cava: Radiographic recognition. AJR Am J Roentgenol 1986; 146:487–90.

29. Duntley P, Siever J, Korwes ML. Vascular erosion by central venous catheters. Chest 1992; 101:1633–8.

30. Reeves AR, Shashadri R, Trerotolai SO. Recent trends in central venous catheter placement: a comparison of interventional radiology with other specialties. J Vasc Intervent Radiol 2001; 12:1211–4.

31. McBride KD, Fisher R, Warnock N, et al. A comparative analysis of radiological and surgical placement of central venous catheters. Cardiovasc Intervent Radiol 1997; 20:17–22.

32. Herts BR, O'Malley CM, Wirth SL, et al. Power injection of contrast media using central venous catheters: feasibility, safety, and efficacy. AJR Am J Roentgenol 2001; 176:447–53.

33. Rivitz SM, Drucker EA. Power injection of peripherally inserted central catheters. J Vasc Intervent Radiol 1997; 8:857–63.

34. Ruess L, Bulas DI, Rivera O, et al. In-line pressures generated in small-bore central venous catheters during power injection of CT contrast media. Radiology 1997; 203:625–9.

35. McLoud TC, Putman CE. Radiology of the Swan-Ganz catheter and associated pulmonary complications. Radiology 1975; 116:19–22.

36. Dieden JD, Friloux LA 3rd, Renner JW. Pulmonary artery false aneurysms secondary to Swan-Ganz pulmonary artery catheters. AJR Am J Roentgenol 1987; 149:901–6.

37. Hinke DH, Zandt-Stastny DA, Goodman LR, et al. Pinch off syndrome: a complication of implantable subclavian venous access devices. Radiology 1990; 177:353–6.

38. Jannolowski CR, Poirier RL. Small bowel infarction complicating intra-aortic balloon counter pulsation via the descending aorta. J Thorac Cardiovasc Surg 1980; 79:735–7.

39. Alderman JD, Gabliani GI, McCage CR, et al. Incidence and management of limb ischaemia with percutaneous wire-guided intra-aortic balloon catheter. J Am Coll Cardiol 1987; 9: 526–30.

40. Landay MJ, Estrera AS, Bordlee RP. Cardiac valve reconstruction and replacement: a brief review. RadioGraphics 1992; 12:659–71.

41. Laws D, Neville E, Duffy J. BTS guidelines for the insertion of a chest drain. Thorax 2003; 58(Suppl 2):ii53–9.

42. Curtin JJ, Goodman LR, Quebbeman EJ, et al. Thoracostomy tubes after acute chest injury: Relationship between location in a pleural fissure and function. AJR Am J Roentgenol 1994; 163:1339–42.

43. Maurer JR, Friedman PJ, Wing VW. Thoracostomy tube in an interlobar fissure: radiologic recognition of a potential problem. AJR Am J Roentgenol 1982; 139:1155–61.

44. Woodall BH, Winfield DF, Bisset GS 3rd. Inadvertent tracheobronchial placement of feeding tubes. Radiology 1987; 165:727–9.

45. Metheny NA, Eisenberg P, Spies M. Aspiration pneumonia in patients fed through nasoantral tubes. Heart Lung 1986; 15:256–61.

46. McLoud TC, Barash PG, Ravin CE. PEEP: radiographic features and associated complications. AJR Am J Roentgenol 1977; 129:209–13.

47. Zimmerman JE, Goodman LR, Shahvari MB. Effect of mechanical ventilation and positive end-expiratory pressure (PEEP) on chest radiograph. AJR Am J Roentgenol 1979; 133:811–5.

48. Webb WR, Stern EJ, Kanth N, et al. Dynamic pulmonary CT: findings in healthy adult men. Radiology 1993; 186:117–24.

49. Gattinoni L, Caironi P, Pelosi P, et al. What has computed tomography taught us about the acute respiratory distress syndrome? Am J Respir Crit Care Med 2001; 164:1701–11.

50. Gattinoni L, Pesenti A, Bombino M, et al. Relationships between lung computed tomographic density, gas exchange, and PEEP in acute respiratory failure. Anesthesiology 1988; 69:824–32.

51. Maunder RJ, Shuman WP, McHugh JW, et al. Preservation of normal lung regions in the adult respiratory distress syndrome. Analysis by computed tomography. JAMA 1986; 255:2463–5.

52. Malbouisson LM, Muller JC, Constantin JM, et al. Computed tomography assessment of positive end-expiratory pressure–induced alveolar recruitment in patients with acute respiratory distress syndrome. Am J Respir Crit Care Med 2001; 163:1444–50.

53. Puybasset L, Cluzel P, Chao N, et al. A computed tomography scan assessment of regional lung volume in acute lung injury. Am J Respir Crit Care Med 1998; 158:1644–55.

54. Zimmerman JE, Goodman LR, St Andre AC, et al. Radiographic detection of mobilizable lung water: the gravitational shift test. AJR Am J Roentgenol 1982; 138:59–64.

55. Gattinoni L, Pelosi P, Vitale G, et al. Body position changes redistribute lung computed-tomographic density in patients with acute respiratory failure. Anesthesiology 1991; 74:15–23.

56. Haake R, Schlichtig R, Ulstad DR, et al. Barotrauma. Pathophysiology, risk factors, and prevention. Chest 1987; 91:608–13.
57. Macklin MR, Macklin CE. Malignant interstitial emphysema of the lungs and mediastinum as an important occult complication in many respiratory diseases and other conditions: An interpretation of the clinical literature in the light of laboratory experiment. Medicine 1944; 23: 281–358.
58. Maunder RJ, Pierson DJ, Hudson LD. Subcutaneous and mediastinal emphysema. Arch Intern Med 1984; 144:1447–53.
59. Tocino I, Westcott JL. Barotrauma. Radiol Clin North Am 1996; 34:59–81.
60. Altman AR, Johnson TH. Roentgenographic findings in PEEP therapy. Indicators of pulmonary complications. JAMA 1979; 242:727–30.
61. Unger JM, England DM, Bogust GA. Interstitial emphysema in adults: recognition and prognostic implications. J Thoracic Imaging 1989; 4:86–94.
62. Tocino IM. Abnormal air and pleural fluid collections. In: Goodman LR, Putman CE, editors. Critical care imaging. Philadelphia: Saunders, 1992:137–60.
63. Beres RA, Goodman LR. Pneumothorax: detection with upright versus decubitus radiography. Radiology 1993; 186:19–22.
64. Weg JG, Haas CF. Safe intrahospital transport of critically ill ventilator-dependent patients. Chest 1989; 96:631–5.
65. Miller WT Jr, Tino G, Friedburg JS. Thoracic CT in the intensive care unit: assessment of clinical usefulness. Radiology 1998; 209:491–8.
66. Barkhausen J, Stoblen F, Dominguez-Fernandez E, et al. Impact of CT in patients with sepsis of unknown origin. Acta Radiologica 1999; 40:552–5.
67. O'Moore PV, Mueller PR, Simeone JF, et al. Sonographic guidance in diagnostic and therapeutic interventions in the pleural space. AJR Am J Roentgenol 1987; 149:1–5.
68. Krapf R, Loiacono J, Pesola GR, et al. Ventilatory support during magnetic resonance imaging. Chest 1992; 102:632–3.
69. Goodman LR, Kuzo R. Radiologic Clinics of North America. In: Goodman LR, Kuzo R, editors. Intensive care radiology, Vol. 34. Philadelphia: Saunders, 1996.
70. Trotman-Dickenson B. Radiology in the intensive care unit (Part II). J Intensive Care Med 2003; 18:239–52.

Chapter 49

MONITORING DURING MECHANICAL VENTILATION

AMAL JUBRAN
MARTIN J. TOBIN

Patients are admitted to an intensive care unit (ICU) for two main reasons. One is for delivery of mechanical ventilation, the varied aspects of which are the subject of this book. The second is to observe a patient more closely than is possible on a hospital ward. That is, to avail of specialized devices used for the monitoring of vital functions (and of staff who have expertise in their operation).

The literature published on these two subjects constitutes the unique corpus of knowledge required for the expert practice of intensive care medicine. Management of some critically ill patients is based on knowledge outside these two areas, such as patients with acute gastrointestinal bleeding or acute renal failure. The principles for managing such conditions have been developed by physician-investigators within the relevant subspecialties rather than by intensive care physicians. Beyond the areas of mechanical ventilation and monitoring, an intensivist seeking the most authoritative writing on a subject must turn to articles and texts published by non-intensivists.

Patients receiving mechanical ventilation are exposed to the full range of monitoring devices. An in-depth discussion of each device would require as much space as the rest of this book. For such discussions the reader is referred to the companion text, *Principles and Practice of Intensive Care Monitoring*.[1] Rather than attempting a synopsis of each individual monitoring technique, we provide in this chapter a bird's eye view of the subject. We map out the territory of monitoring through discussion of its goals, the principles of measurement, usefulness of monitoring in various settings, the forms of clinical reasoning used in interpreting generated data, evaluation of the benefit of monitors, and the problems in designing studies that attempt such evaluations. To give a sense of the detailed contours of the terrain being traversed, we offer specific examples of how the general topics relate to the everyday use of monitors.

What Is Monitoring?

An unsatisfactory—and embarrassing—aspect of writing about monitoring is the absence of a generally accepted definition. A definition tries to set criteria that demarcate the boundaries between concepts (or things) so as to prevent overlapping or confusion, and has the goal of providing order or a clear understanding.

The word "monitor" comes from the Latin *monere*, which means, "to warn." This meaning connotes one goal of monitoring, to provide an alert, an alarm. But monitors serve other functions. Monitors replicate many of the characteristics of diagnostic testing, and interpretation of the generated data must comply with the scientific principles developed for use of diagnostic tests. Thus, it might seem reasonable to define monitoring as the serial performance of diagnostic tests at frequent intervals. But how should we demarcate the frequency at which measurements are repeated? Certain signals have such a high frequency content that obtaining 50 measurements in a second is not sufficient to capture a critical data point.

Having struggled long and hard in trying to formulate a meaningful but precise definition of monitoring, we admit defeat. We can do no better than offer a naturalist's definition: monitoring refers to what physicians and allied health personnel do with monitors.

Goals of Monitoring

The major goals of monitoring are: to continuously measure key variables that enhance understanding of a patient's underlying disease state, to aid with diagnosis, and to guide management.[2] To accomplish these goals, the monitor should measure a variable that is pertinent to the disease process, be technically accurate, provide interpretable data, be practical for use, and not cause harm.[2,3] The ability of today's monitors to meet these goals depends largely on two factors: whether a monitor is capable of accurately measuring the function or disease manifestation in question, and whether the recorded information will help improve patient outcome. Inextricably linked to these two factors is the caregiver's ability to interpret data, integrate data from multiple sources, discard data that are not important, and then, make a wise judgment about diagnosis and therapy.

Accuracy of Measurements

Advances in electronic and computer technology over the last 30 years have generated several monitoring systems that are accurate and easy to use. To know how to operate a machine and interpret the provided data, a physician needs much more than a manufacturer's manual. The physician needs to know the principles of the monitoring device, how to operate it, the reliability of the measurements, indications and contraindications, complications with use of the device, and how to troubleshoot problems as they arise.

To determine whether the data generated by a monitor are valid, a physician needs to have a basic understanding of measurement theory and its applications. For an extensive review of the science of measurement, the reader is referred to the chapter by Chatburn[4] in the companion book, *Principles and Practice of Intensive Care Monitoring.*[1]

FUNDAMENTALS OF MEASUREMENT THEORY

Every measurement has errors. Errors can be systematic or random. Systematic errors occur in a predictable manner; they cause measurements to *either* consistently underestimate or consistently overestimate the true value. Systematic error (also termed bias) is the difference between the mean value of repeated measurements and the true value. Random errors occur in an unpredictable manner because of uncontrollable factors; they cause measurements to *both* under- and overestimate the true value. Random errors are a measure of the imprecision of a measurement (Fig. 49-1). Accordingly, the measured value is the sum of the true value and the error.[4]

ACCURACY

Accuracy is the ability of a measuring device (or monitoring technique) to capture the true value of a quantity. Accuracy is usually expressed as a percentage of the full scale. In today's ventilators, pressure-measuring systems have an accuracy of ± 2 cmH$_2$O plus 4% of the signal. In other words, if the true pressure is 25 cmH$_2$O, the displayed pressure could be anything between 22 and 28 cmH$_2$O.[5] In contrast, the accuracy of flow sensors within ventilators varies much more: from ± 1% to ± 20% of the setting, depending on the ventilator.[6] Despite their common use, remarkably little information on the accuracy of flow- and pressure-measuring devices has been published in peer-reviewed journals; in general, users must resort to data on accuracy provided by the manufacturers.

The monitoring device that has been studied the most in critically-ill patients is the pulse oximeter. Compared with the measurement standard (a multiwavelength CO-

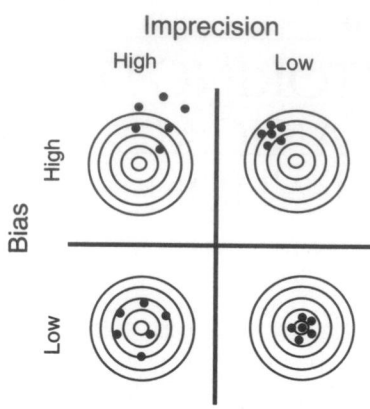

FIGURE 49-1 The effects of bias and imprecision (systematic and random errors) on measurements using the analogy of target practice at a rifle range. When bias is low, measurements (bullet holes) group around the true value (bull's-eye). When imprecision is low, the cluster of measurements is tight: the random error of repeated measurements (rifle shots) is small. Ideally both bias and imprecision are low, resulting in a small total error for repeated measurements. (*Reprinted, with permission, from Chatburn.*[4])

oximeter), pulse oximeters have a mean difference (bias) of <1% and a standard deviation (precision) of <2% when arterial oxygen saturation (Sa$_{O_2}$) is 90% or above (Fig. 49-2).[7-9]

PRECISION

Precision is the ability of a monitor to display the same value repeatedly assuming that the actual quantity has not changed; that is, the degree of consistency between repeated results. Precision is usually expressed in terms of variance, standard deviation, or confidence intervals. In ventilated patients, the precision (quantified as standard deviation) of pulse oximetry in measuring oxygen saturation (Sp$_{O_2}$) is <1.2% when Sa$_{O_2}$ is above 90%, and it increases to 2.7% when Sa$_{O_2}$ drops to 90% or less (Fig. 49-3).[10,11]

Reproducibility is the ability of the monitoring technique (or device) to maintain its precision during long-term use. Knowing the reproducibility of a measurement is important for judging whether a change is truly of clinical significance. The reproducibility of thermodilution technique in measuring cardiac output, quantified as the ratio of standard error to average cardiac output (SEM), varied between 2 and 5% when measurements were repeated (an average of three times), and varied between 2.5 and 8.7% for single measurements.[12] Thus, before concluding that a change in cardiac output is clinically significant, a clinician would need to observe a 12–15% difference between repeated determinations (3 measurements per determination). Repeat measurements of static respiratory compliance (using the airway occlusion method) have a reproducibility no better than 10%, and a 20–30% difference between breaths may be observed.[2,13,14] As such, it is recommended that compliance measurements should be based on at least 3 breaths.

A technique may yield reproducible measurements at one sitting, but be unreliable when employed by a different investigator or on a different day. In ventilated patients, a single investigator obtained highly reproducible measurement

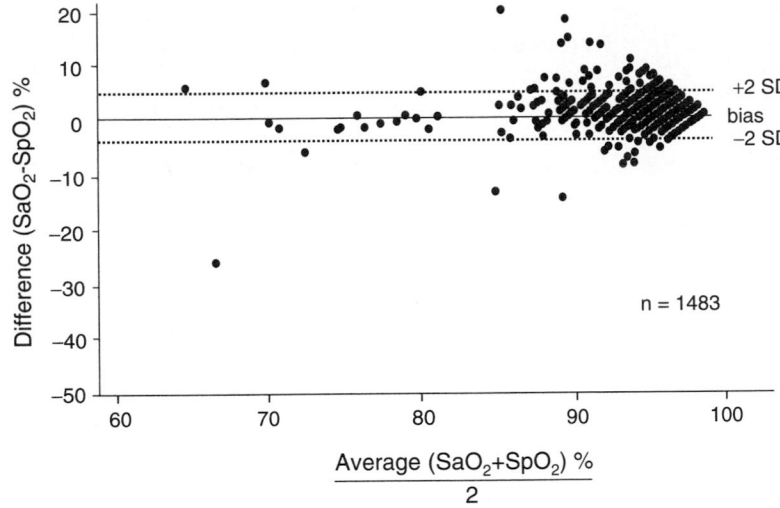

FIGURE 49-2 Differences between arterial oxygen saturation (Sa_{O_2}) measured by hematoxymeter and oxygen saturation measured by pulse oximetry (Sp_{O_2}) plotted against the average O_2 saturation in 102 critically-ill patients. The solid line is the bias and the dashed lines are 95% confidence intervals. Mean difference (bias) between the two measurements is small. (*Reproduced, with permission, from van de Louw et al.*[7])

of maximal inspiratory pressure at a single sitting: the co-efficient of variation for triplicate efforts was 11%.[15] When different investigators undertook the measurements, however, the coefficient of variation was $32 \pm 4\%$, despite the measurements being obtained in the same patient and on the same day.

LINEARITY

A device is considered linear when a plot of output data from the device (the measured values) versus the input data (the known values) can be fitted with a straight line. Occasionally, a system measures pressure accurately only over

part rather than the entire range of pressures; that is, the system is alinear (Fig. 49-4). Alinearity may occur because the given transducer is not designed for use over the entire range or because it is not functioning properly.

CALIBRATION

Calibration is the process of adjusting the output of a device to match a known input value. Thus, systematic error is minimized. Calibration is considered static when pressure is changed in steps and each step is maintained long enough to achieve a stable signal output. For a linear measurement system, calibration is a simple two-step procedure. First, the readout is set at zero while no input signal is applied to the instrument. If an offset error occurs, it is adjusted. For a flow-sensing device, the flow sensor is occluded and a reading of no flow should result. If some flow is registered, the readout is adjusted to zero to correct for the offset error. Next, sensitivity (gain or slope) is set by applying an input signal of known value (say 12 L/second from a rotameter), preferably at the upper end of the output range; the readout on the flow sensor is then adjusted to read 12 (Fig. 49-5). If the system is linear, the readouts for all input values between these two calibration points will be accurate.

The dynamic response of a measurement system, such as a pressure transducer, is typically tested using a

FIGURE 49-3 Arterial O_2 saturation (Sa_{O_2}) versus O_2 saturation measured by pulse oximetry (Sp_{O_2}) in patients receiving mechanical ventilation. The solid line is the line of identity and the dashed lines are isopleths of different levels of bias. Accuracy of pulse oximetry deteriorates when Sa_{O_2} is less than 90%. (*Reproduced, with permission, from Jubran et al.*[10])

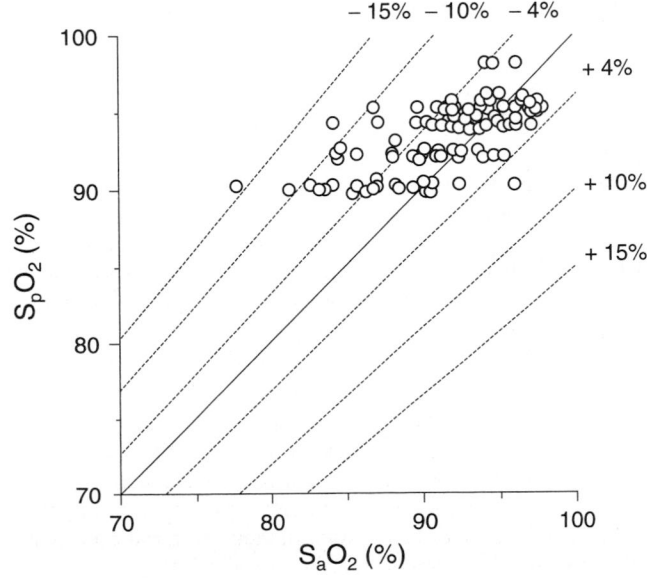

FIGURE 49-4 Measured pressure plotted against the true pressure in a linear (*left panel*) and an alinear (*right panel*) pressure-measuring system. (*Reproduced, with permission, from Gallagher.*[5])

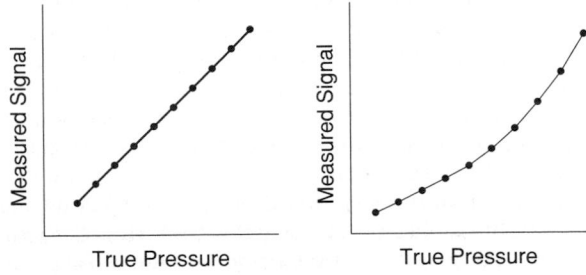

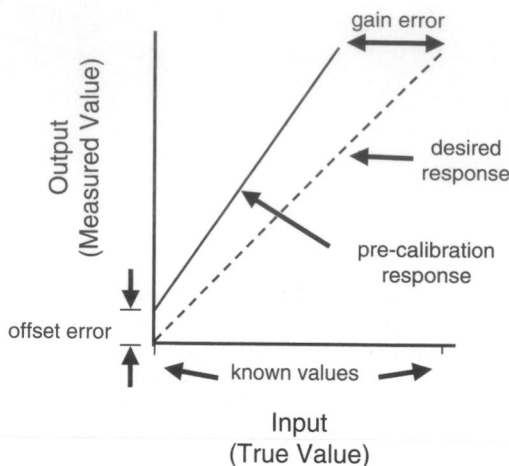

FIGURE 49-5 The two-point calibration procedure. First the readout on the instrument is adjusted to read zero to overcome offset error. Then the gain is adjusted to read the desired response. See text for details. (*Reproduced, with permission, from Chatburn.*[4])

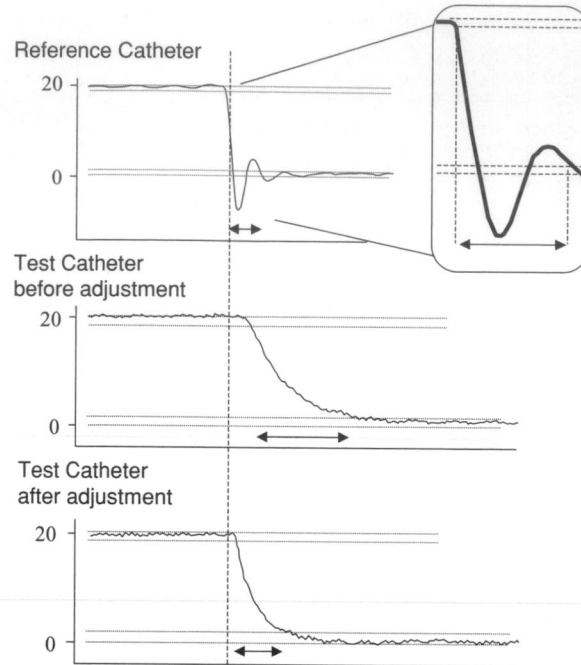

FIGURE 49-6 *Upper panel:* The 95% response (settling time) of the reference catheter was 12.5 ms. *Inset:* The points used in making this measurement. The uppermost dashed horizontal line is 100% of starting pressure (20 cmH$_2$O), the next horizontal line represents a 5% decrease in pressure, the bottom horizontal line is 0 cmH$_2$O, and the horizontal line above it represents a 95% drop from starting pressure. The right-hand vertical dashed line denotes the point at which the oscillation in the pressure signal last crossed the horizontal line, which represents a 95% drop in pressure. *Middle panel:* The 10% to 90% fall time for the test balloon catheter was 35.1 ms. *Lower panel:* After shortening the catheter length and increasing the size of holes in the portion of the catheter within the esophageal balloon, the 10% to 90% fall time decreased to 20 ms, which is satisfactory for the monitoring of respiratory mechanics. (*Reproduced, with permission, from Tobin.*[19])

square-wave (or sinusoidal) pressure generator. A step change in pressure is followed by a brief delay before the measured pressure begins to change.[16–19] (When the system is underdamped, the measured pressure overshoots the true value and then oscillates around it. When the system is overdamped, the measured signal gradually approaches the true value.) The 90% response time is the time from the step change in pressure until the measured signal settles within 10% of its final value (Fig. 49-6). The amplitude of the test should be within ±5% of the amplitude of the reference system at the highest frequency tested. The phase lag is the temporal difference between the two systems (Fig. 49-7).

SOURCES OF MEASUREMENT ERROR DURING MONITORING

One of the major challenges in interpreting data from monitors is to determine which data constitute truth and which constitute artifact. Both systematic and random errors can cause artifact.

SYSTEMATIC ERROR

Zero offset error occurs when the zero point is not correctly set during calibration but the gain is correct. Consequently, the instrument will read consistently either an inaccurately low or an inaccurately high value over the entire scale. The zero point can also change secondary to patient movement without staff being aware. The pressure recorded by a pulmonary artery catheter develops a large systematic error when a patient sits up.

Response time is the time that a monitoring device takes to respond to a step change in a recorded physiologic variable. The response time for a pulse oximeter probe varies with its location. Probes placed on the ear respond more rapidly than probes on the finger.[20–22] During calibration of a monitoring device, a slow response time causes error if

the user does not allow sufficient time for the instrument to stabilize at the known value.

Frequency response is an instrument's ability to accurately measure an oscillating signal. When the frequency of a signal increases, a measurement system will generate either an underestimate (attenuation) or overestimate (amplification)

FIGURE 49-7 The dynamic calibration using sinusoidal forcing. The ratio of the amplitude of the output signal to the amplitude of the input signal is the amplitude ratio. The phase lag is the temporal difference between the two signals and is expressed as a fraction of duration of one sinusoid and expressed in degrees. The phase lag in the figure is one-tenth of the cycle duration: 10% of 360°, or 36°. (*Reproduced, with permission, from Gallagher.*[5])

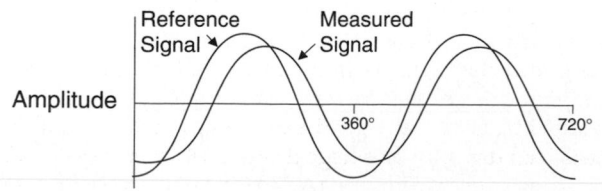

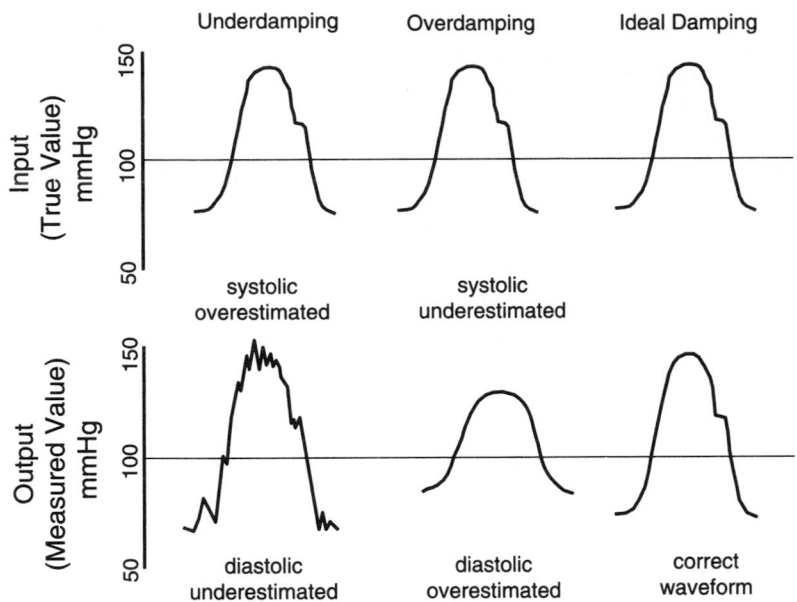

FIGURE 49-8 Effect of three different blood pressure transducers with different damping characteristics on the measurement of blood pressure. (*Reproduced, with permission, from Chatburn.*[4])

of the true amplitude of the signal. An optimally damped system will measure all signal frequencies within the working range with equal amplitude (Fig. 49-8).

A system is considered damped when some of the signal-component frequencies are attenuated. Overdamping causes systolic pressure to decrease and diastolic pressure to increase. In a system for measuring vascular pressure, sources of overdamping include air bubbles in the transducer or pressure tubing, clot or fibrin at the catheter tip, and a kinked or partially occluded catheter. Underdamping amplifies the higher harmonics, producing oscillations, which obscure systolic and diastolic values. As such, underdamping causes systolic pressure to increase and diastolic pressure to decrease. Common sources of underdamping include an increase in heart rate interfering with the natural frequency of the pressure-transducer system; a "catheter whip," commonly observed with a pulmonary artery (PA) catheter, can produce an underdamped signal.

Pulmonary artery waveforms generally contain more high-frequency information than do systemic arterial waveforms, and small errors in pressure assume more clinical significance. Poor dynamic frequency response and overdamped pressure tracings accounted for over half the technical problems encountered in measuring PA wedge pressure.[23] A simple test for assessing the dynamic response of a vascular pressure catheter system is the rapid-flush test (Fig. 49-9).[24]

Alignment of Signals

When employing two different signals to quantify lung mechanics (flow and pressure), it is important to ensure the absence of a phase lag between the two signals. A lag can induce large errors in measurement of resistance and compliance.[5] Phase lags also cause major errors when dynamic intrinsic positive end-expiratory pressure (PEEPi) is measured using an esophageal balloon-catheter system. If a phase lag causes the esophageal signal to occur before flow,

PEEPi will be overestimated or considered present when it is truly absent. If a phase lag causes the esophageal signal to occur after flow, PEEPi may be underestimated (Fig. 49-10).

Variable Conditions Between Calibration and Data Collection

If a measurement system is used under conditions that differ from the conditions of calibration, and no correction is made, systematic errors may result. Flow or volume readings on a ventilator are inaccurate if the temperature or humidity during the recording differs from those present during calibration.[25,26] During calibration, volume may be measured under conditions of ambient temperature, with gas fully saturated with water vapor. If appropriate corrections are not made, subsequent readings of volume, under conditions of normal body temperature and with pressure saturated with water vapor, will underestimate the true volume of gas moving through the lungs. A mass of gas that is 1000 mL at 21°C can become 1095 mL at 37°C.

FIGURE 49-9 Rapid-flush test. *A.* Appropriately damped system. *B.* Overdamped systems. When the flush device is pinched open to connect the high-pressure flush system to the transducer, the catheter results in the generation of very high pressures near the transducer. Upon closure of the flushing device, there should be a rapid fall in pressure, with an "overshoot" if the system is properly damped. In a properly functioning recording system, the pressure system should reverberate one or two times and then decay back to the underlying pressure (*A*). In contrast, a slow return to baseline without an overshoot suggests that the system is overdamped (*B*). (*Reproduced, with permission, from Leatherman et al.*[24])

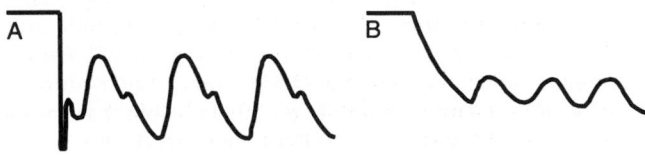

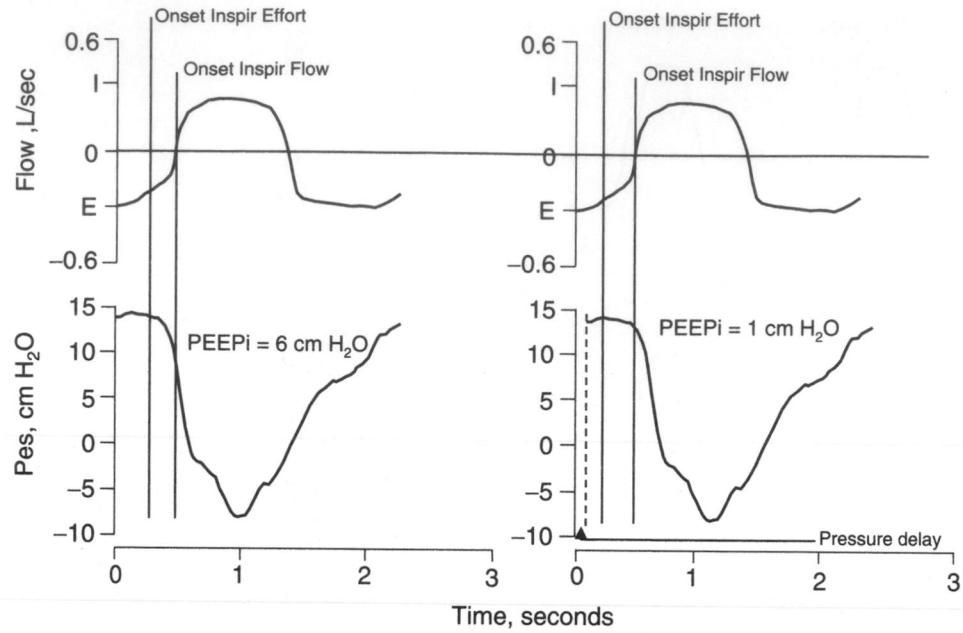

FIGURE 49-10 *Left panel:* Flow and esophageal pressure (Pes) signals are properly aligned. Intrinsic PEEP (PEEPi), measured as the difference between the onset of inspiratory effort and onset of inspiratory flow, is 6 cmH$_2$O. *Right panel:* Poor phase alignment of flow and Pes signals: flow precedes Pes, causing underestimation of PEEPi.

Pneumotachographic measurements during mechanical ventilation will become inaccurate if the dimensions of the ventilator tubing during data recording differ from the dimensions used during calibration. The differences in air turbulence and the distribution of flow through the resistive element under the two conditions can lead to measurement errors. When a pneumotachograph was initially calibrated under ideal conditions (with tubing that provided optimized flow characteristics) and then subsequently attached to commonly used ventilator tubing, flow was underestimated by as much as 10% and volume by as much as 15% (Fig. 49-11).[27]

RANDOM ERROR

Noise

All measurements are subject to some degree of rapidly changing interference, termed noise or artifact (Fig. 49-12).[11] The source of noise can be difficult to trace. Noise distortions occur randomly, so their effects are lessened if measurements are repeated sufficiently. The distortions are not reduced by calibration. The efficiency with which the signal can be distinguished from background noise is defined as the signal-to-noise ratio.[28] Unless the ratio exceeds 1, the signal will be undetectable.

Noise is particularly troublesome when weak signals are highly amplified. Noise is then amplified along with the signal, which eventually limits the sensitivity of the measurement. Cardiac contractions can distort an esophageal pressure signal such that pressure swings appear greater than they truly are (Fig. 49-13). As a signal is being transmitted to an amplifier, it is subjected to electrostatic and electromagnetic noise from nearby power lines.[29] Radio-frequency noise may also be added from cellular phones. Finally, physical movement of the catheter cable changes its capacitance and may add low-frequency noise.

Physical factors are major sources of noise in ICU monitors. A pulse oximeter probe slipping off the patient's skin accounted for 35% of false alarms recorded in an ICU (Fig. 49-14).[30] Patient movement disturbs the electrode-skin interface and causes electrocardiogram (ECG) noise.[31] Patient movement produces erroneous pulse oximetry readings;[32] interference from fluorescent and xenon arc surgical lamps

FIGURE 49-11 Relationship between true and measured flows with the Fleisch No. 2 pneumotachograph connected to an ideal tube configuration (*closed squares*) and to ventilator tubing with either plastic connectors (*open squares*) or diffuse cones (*crosses*). Measured flow was falsely low when the pneumotachographs were adapted to ventilator tubing with either plastic connectors or diffuse cones; the underestimate became more pronounced as flow increased. (*Reproduced, with permission, from Kreit et al.[27]*)

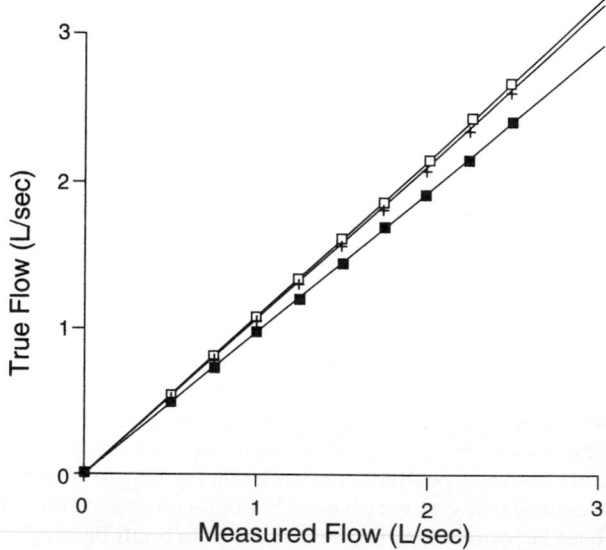

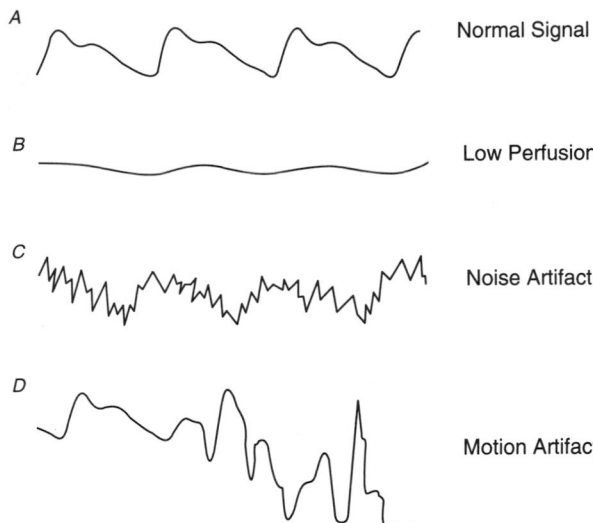

FIGURE 49-12 **Common pulsatile signals of a pulse oximeter.**
A. **Normal signal showing the sharp waveform with a clear
dicrotic notch.** *B.* **Pulsatile signal during low perfusion showing a
typical sine wave.** *C.* **Pulsatile signal with superimposed noise
artifact giving a jagged appearance.** *D.* **Pulsatile signal during
motion artifact showing an erratic waveform.** (*Reproduced, with
permission, from Jubran.*[11])

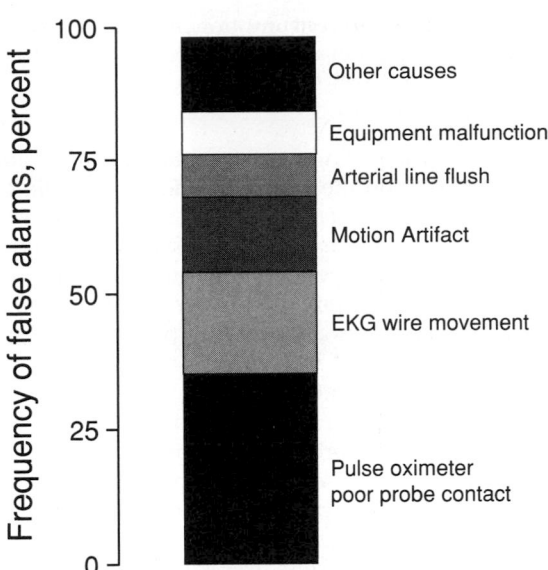

FIGURE 49-14 **Causes of false alarms reported in an ICU. The
slipping off of the finger probe of a pulse oximeter is the most
common cause of false alarms.** (*Data source from Tsien et al.*[30])

also cause inaccurate readings.[33–35] "Ringing" after flushing an arterial catheter can interfere with the blood pressure
signal and cause faulty readings.[36]

A particularly annoying consequence of signal noise is
false alarms.[37–39] Investigators prospectively waited at the
bedside for 298 hours in an adult ICU. Of 2942 alarms, 2525
(86%) were false.[30] In a pediatric ICU, 68% of alarms were

false.[38] A high rate of false alarms causes noise pollution,
wastes nursing time, and contributes to staff burnout.[40]

Nonlinearity

Nonlinearity introduces unpredictable error that varies over
the operating range. With measurements of O_2 consumption, nonlinearity of the O_2-sensing system causes a progressive increase in error as fractional inspired oxygen concentration (F_{IO_2}) is increased from 0.21 to 1.0.[41,42] Thus, error

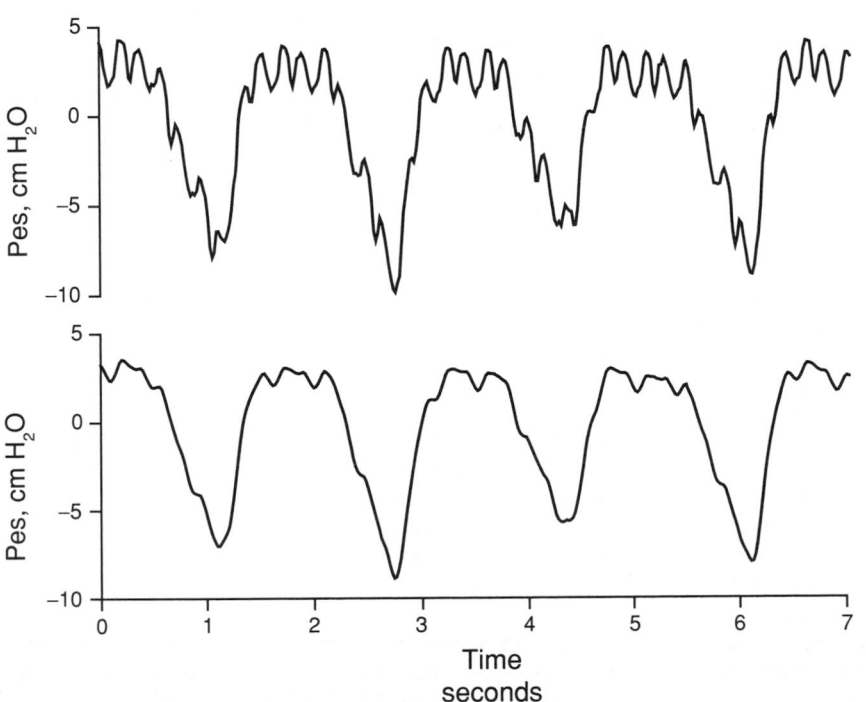

FIGURE 49-13 *Top panel:* **Esophageal pressure
(Pes) tracing in a patient during a T-piece trial.
The oscillations in the Pes tracing represent
cardiac artifacts.** *Bottom panel:* **Applying
moving average function to the Pes signal
reduced the cardiac artifact.**

in measurements of O_2 consumption increases from 2.6% at room air to 17% at an F_{IO_2} of 0.80.[41]

Human Error

Human error in acquiring data is another source of random error. Depending on the angle at which the needle on an analog scale is read, different people can perceive different values for the same actual plateau pressure. Measurements that require patient cooperation introduce another source of error. Use of the end-expiratory airway occlusion method to measure PEEPi requires a cooperative patient who does not resist the occlusion.[43] Of 283 attempts in ventilated patients, Kress et al[44] could quantify PEEPi in only 86 (30%); most of time PEEPi could not be quantified because the patient made an expiratory effort during the occlusion maneuvers. Patient cooperation is also needed for reliable measurement of maximal inspiratory pressure, a measure of respiratory muscle strength.[45] In patients with low respiratory drive, coaching patients to make vigorous inspiratory efforts led to a 28% increase in pressure.[46]

Other Barriers to Accurate Data Gathering

Factors other than accuracy of the measurement can lead to faulty interpretation by the clinician.

PHYSIOLOGIC VARIATION

Even when a patient is in a steady state, variables monitored in the ICU may not be consistent. To know if a new measurement is a true difference from an earlier measurement, it is necessary to know the normal physiologic variation of the variable (Fig. 49-15).[23] Arterial pressure varies throughout the respiratory cycle. Minute-to-minute variation in systolic pressure (quantified as standard deviation) is about 4 mmHg, and diastolic pressure varies 2–3 mmHg. In healthy subjects, arterial pressure differs by as much as 20 mmHg between the two arms.[47] Thus, a difference of 20 mmHg between the two arms does not necessarily indicate an underlying disorder such as aortic dissection. Arterial blood gas recordings vary by as much as 5% (in terms of coefficient of variation) for arterial O_2 tension (Pa_{O_2}) and 3% for arterial carbon dioxide tension (Pa_{CO_2}) in stable ICU patients (Fig. 49-16).[48,49]

INHERENT LIMITATIONS OF MONITORS

No machine, including a monitor, is 100% reliable. Despite its undisputed popularity, pulse oximetry fails to provide valid measurements of Sa_{O_2} in a variety of settings.[50] The incidence of overall failure (defined as at least one continuous gap in data that exceeded 10 minutes) in anesthetized patients in an operating room was 9%.[51] Risk factors for pulse oximetry failure include patient status, type of surgery, and intraoperative events.

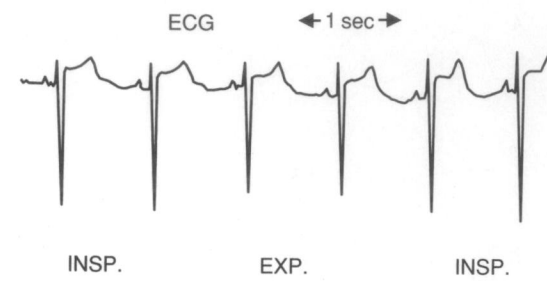

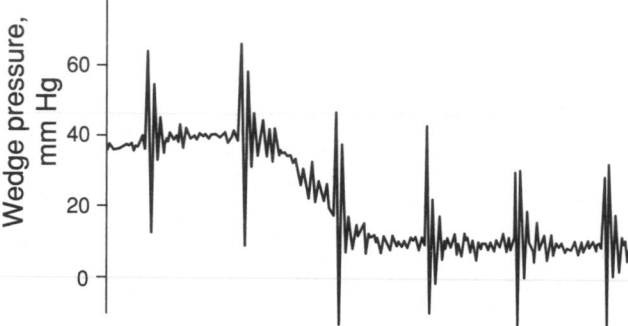

FIGURE 49-15 Tracings of ECG (*upper panel*) and pulmonary artery wedge pressure (*bottom panel*). The change in wedge pressure from 40 to 10 mmHg did not result from changes in the respiratory cycle; it represents an unexplained spontaneous variation. (*Reproduced, with permission, from Morris et al.*[23])

COMPLEXITY OF MEASUREMENTS

Many users of monitors have a limited understanding of how a machine functions and the implications of its measurements. In one survey, 30% of physicians (and 93% of nurses) thought that a pulse oximeter measured Pa_{O_2}.[52] Some clinicians have limited knowledge of the O_2-dissociation curve. They do not realize that Sp_{O_2} values in the high 80s represent seriously low values of Pa_{O_2}. In the above-mentioned survey, some physicians and nurses were not especially worried about Sp_{O_2} values as low as 80% (equivalent to $Pa_{O_2} \leq 45$ torr).

Iberti et al[53] found that 47% of physicians (77% of whom were in training) were unable to interpret a straightforward recording of a PA wedge pressure. On average, physicians incorrectly answered 10 of 31 questions dealing with insertion and complications, cardiac physiology, and interpretation and application of data. More respondents had difficulty with questions regarding data interpretation and patient treatment than with questions related to catheter insertion or cardiac physiology (Table 49-1). Similar results were obtained in studies evaluating ICU nurses' knowledge of PA catheters: the mean score of correct answers was 57%.[54] In both studies, the amount of formal training, frequency of exposure to the catheter, and professional certification (in critical care) correlated with higher scores.

Modern ventilators provide a continuous on-line display of physiologic signals (such as flow, volume, and airway pressure) and numeric computations (resistance, compliance, and work of breathing). The complexity of the physiologic principles that underpin respiratory mechanics, however, has impeded the use of the measurements in

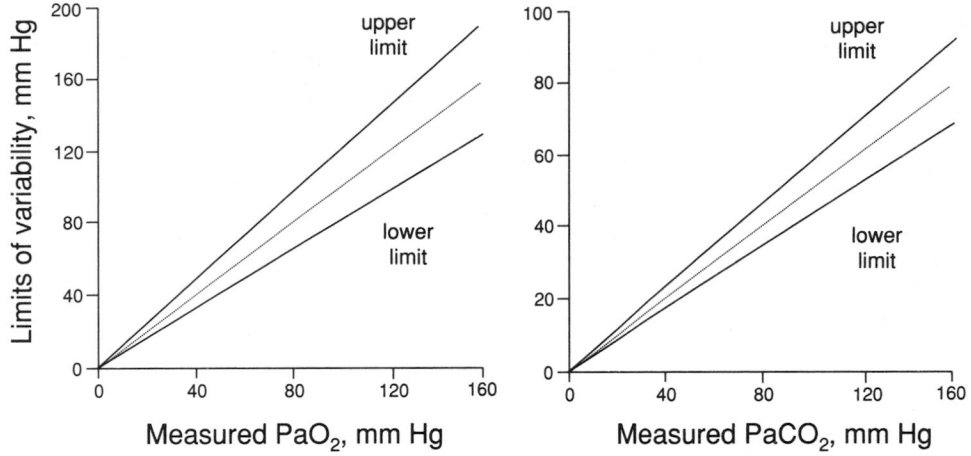

FIGURE 49-16 *Left panel:* Upper and lower limits of spontaneous variability of arterial oxygen tension (Pa$_{O_2}$) based on a coefficient of variation of 9.8%, which represent the 95th percentile. If a patient has a reported Pa$_{O_2}$ of 80 mmHg, the true Pa$_{O_2}$ could be as low as 64 mmHg or as high as 96 mmHg secondary to spontaneous variability. *Right panel:* Upper and lower limits of spontaneous variability of arterial carbon dioxide tension (Pa$_{CO_2}$) based on a coefficient of variation of 7.4%, which represent the 95th percentile. If a patient has a reported Pa$_{CO_2}$ of 40 mmHg, the true Pa$_{CO_2}$ could be as low as 34 mmHg or as high as 46 mmHg secondary to spontaneous variability. (*Reproduced, with permission, from Hess et al.*[49])

clinical practice. The poor understanding of lung mechanics by medicine residents was highlighted in the recent survey.[55] Some 35% of residents were unable to select a ventilator setting that would decrease PEEPi in a patient with chronic obstructive pulmonary disease (COPD) who had become hypotensive immediately after intubation.

The mountains of data generated by monitors make it extremely difficult to differentiate relevant from irrelevant information. More than 230 new data points may be available for review in a single patient on morning ICU rounds.[56] Psychologists have shown that the human mind is capable of assimilating no more than seven variables simultaneously.[57] When the same variable is measured by more than one machine (heart rate recorded by an ECG monitor and a pulse oximeter), the problem is compounded.

MONITORING THE RIGHT PHYSIOLOGIC PHENOMENON

A major purpose of monitoring is to measure key variables that enhance understanding of underlying pathophysiology. Because of technical limitations, however, we tend to monitor that which we can rather than seeking the information we need.[3,58]

The primary goal of mechanical ventilation is to rest the respiratory muscles. Thus, activity of the respiratory muscles is the single variable most needed when monitoring a ventilated patient. Ventilator settings, however, are usually adjusted on the basis of arterial blood gases. Yet, arterial blood gases provide zero information about whether the respiratory muscles are being adequately rested. Consider synchronized intermittent mandatory ventilation (SIMV), which has always been adjusted according to arterial blood gases. The failure of arterial blood gases to provide insight into work of breathing probably accounts for the gap of 20 years between the introduction of this mode and recognition of its harmful effects.[59–61]

Thinking in terms of ventricular preload, a patient's end-diastolic volume is pivotal for logical assessment of hemodynamic performance in a critically-ill patient.[62] No simple method is available, however, to measure end-diastolic volume. Many clinicians use central venous pressure to assess preload despite numerous studies showing that central venous pressure is extremely unreliable in estimating end-diastolic volume in critically-ill patients.[63–68]

TABLE 49-1   Physician Knowledge of the Pulmonary Artery Catheter

Subject Area	No. of Questions	Mean Score	SD	% Correct
Overall	31	20.7	5.4	66.8
Insertion and complication	6	3.9	1.4	65.0
Cardiac physiology	3	2.1	0.9	70.0
Interpretation[a]	14	9.1	2.7	65.0
Application of data	8	5.7	1.7	71.2

[a]Of waveforms, pulmonary artery catheter data, and pressure volume relationships.

DIFFERENT TECHNIQUES FOR MEASURING THE SAME PHYSIOLOGIC PROCESS

In the ICU, different techniques can be used to measure the same physiologic function. The resulting differing numbers, however, may suggest different clinical states. Arterial oxygenation can be assessed by measuring O$_2$ saturation with a pulse oximeter or P$_{O_2}$ by blood gas analysis. In a study of patients with acute respiratory distress syndrome, change in Sp$_{O_2}$ moved in an opposite direction to the change in Pa$_{O_2}$ in 25% of the measurements. In some patients, a decrease in Pa$_{O_2}$ of 20 mmHg was accompanied by a simultaneous

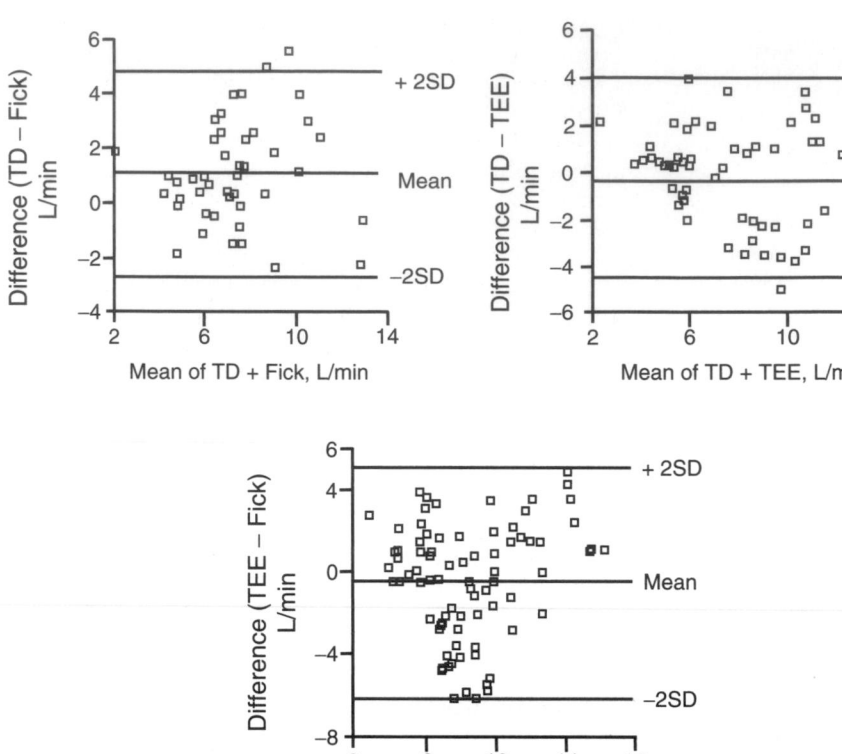

FIGURE 49-17 Bland-Altman comparison of measurements of cardiac output obtained by three techniques: thermodilution (TD), the Fick method, and transesophageal echocardiography (TEE). The mean differences between any two techniques are small (<1 L/min), but the wide confidence intervals indicate poor agreement among the three techniques. (*Reproduced, with permission, from Axler et al.[70]*)

increase in SpO$_2$ of 20%.[69] Therapeutic decisions based on SpO$_2$ alone differed from decisions based on PaO$_2$ on 16% of occasions.

Cardiac output can be measured with three techniques: thermodilution, the Fick method, and transesophageal echocardiography. A comparison of these three techniques in 13 critically-ill patients revealed widely scattered results. In some patients, the 95% confidence intervals for agreement between any two of the methods exceeded 4 L/min (Fig. 49-17).[70]

Clinical Applications

The range of options for monitoring a ventilated patient is enormous and beyond the scope of this chapter. A few examples are provided. For a comprehensive review of the clinical applications of ICU monitoring, the reader is referred to the companion book, *Principles and Practice of Intensive Care Monitoring*.[1]

ENHANCE UNDERSTANDING OF PATHOPHYSIOLOGY

To properly interpret information—medical or nonmedical—a person must take into account the relevant context. To properly understand the results of a diagnostic test, a clinician requires a good understanding of pertinent pathophysiology.

Measuring pressure, flow, and volume during mechanical ventilation assists in the differential diagnosis of respiratory failure. The airway occlusion technique makes it possible to carefully characterize the mechanics of the lung, the chest wall, and the total respiratory system.[71-74] In patients with acute respiratory distress syndrome (ARDS), static elastance of the respiratory system was found to be equivalent irrespective of whether the ARDS was caused by pulmonary conditions or nonpulmonary conditions.[75] Elastance of the lung, however, was higher with pulmonary ARDS, indicating a stiffer lung. Elastance of the chest wall was twice as high in nonpulmonary ARDS, indicating a stiffer chest wall. The different distributions of elastance between the two subgroups suggest that patients with ARDS of pulmonary origin are at greater risk for ventilator-induced lung injury than are patients with ARDS of nonpulmonary origin.

Recording expiratory muscle activity during spontaneous breathing helps differentiate PEEPi caused by dynamic hyperinflation from that caused by expiratory muscle activity (Fig. 49-18).[76-78] If PEEPi is mostly caused by dynamic hyperinflation, addition of external PEEP is likely to decrease work of inspiration.[79,80] If, however, an increase in PEEPi is caused by increased activity of the expiratory muscles,[81] addition of external PEEP will impose an additional elastic load. More importantly, it will also increase the operating lung volume.[80,82]

During a weaning trial, esophageal pressure and flow measurements can be used to partition patient effort into its resistive, elastic, and PEEPi components.[83] All three components are increased in weaning failure patients, with PEEPi increasing the most. Thus, therapy to decrease these abnormalities (such as bronchodilators or diuretics) may help expedite weaning outcome.

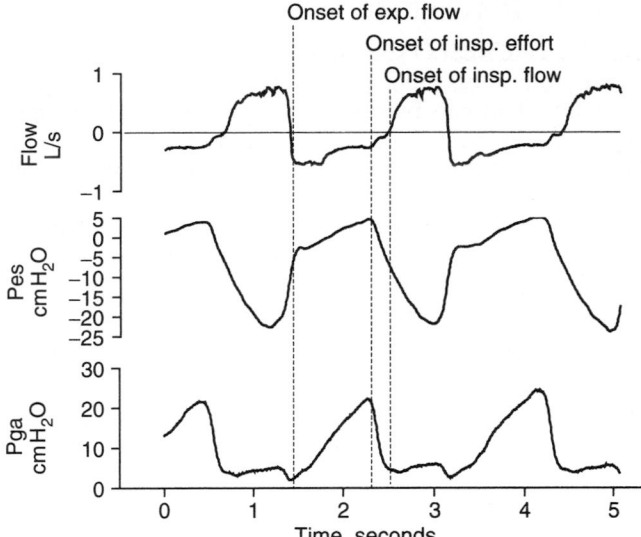

FIGURE 49-18 Flow, esophageal pressure (Pes), and gastric (Pga) pressure in a patient during a trial of spontaneous breathing. Dynamic intrinsic PEEP (PEEPi) is estimated as the decrease in Pes between the onset of inspiratory effort (*second vertical line*) and the onset of inspiratory flow (*third vertical line*). Estimation of the expiratory muscle contribution to swings in Pes and dynamic PEEPi is obtained by measuring the increase in Pga between the onset of expiratory flow (*first vertical line*) and the onset of inspiratory effort (*second vertical line*).

AID WITH DIAGNOSIS

Capnometry helps in detecting esophageal intubation.[84–86] The use of end-tidal CO_2 monitoring is based on the premise that CO_2 recorded at the end of a tidal breath reflects arterial P_{CO_2}. When the trachea of a patient with an intact pul-

monary circulation is intubated, end-tidal CO_2 is recorded. When, however, the endotracheal tube is erroneously placed in the esophagus, end-tidal CO_2 will be zero. Monitoring of end-tidal CO_2 has been compared with three other methods (auscultation, a negative pressure test using a self-inflating bulb, and transillumination) for verifying tracheal tube placement.[87] (The second approach, the negative pressure test, uses a self-inflating bulb: if the endotracheal tube is in the esophagus, suction on the bulb causes the pliable esophageal wall to collapse and no air can be aspirated; if the tube is in the trachea, the semi-rigid walls prevent tube occlusion when suction is applied and air can be aspirated.) Monitoring of end-tidal CO_2 was found to be the most reliable (Fig. 49-19).

Monitoring flow-volume curves helps in detecting the need for endotracheal suctioning. A sawtooth pattern during spontaneous breathing indicates the presence of secretions, with a positive predictive value of 94%. Absence of a sawtooth pattern indicates the absence of secretions, with a negative predictive value of 77%.[88] Clinical examination had much higher false-positive and false-negative rates (42% and 43%, respectively) than the flow-volume curves (12% and 14%, respectively). Accordingly, reliance on clinical examination leads to unnecessary suctioning in patients who do not have secretions and inadequate suctioning in patients who do.

Persistence of expiratory flow throughout expiration, without return to zero, suggests PEEPi (Fig. 49-20); this suspicion can be verified by occluding the expiratory port of the ventilator immediately before the onset of the next breath.[89] Occlusion causes pressure in the lungs and ventilator circuit to equilibrate. The pressure displayed on the ventilator manometer is PEEPi.[90] The presence of PEEPi can help explain an unexpected drop in cardiac output or electromechanical dissociation (during cardiopulmonary

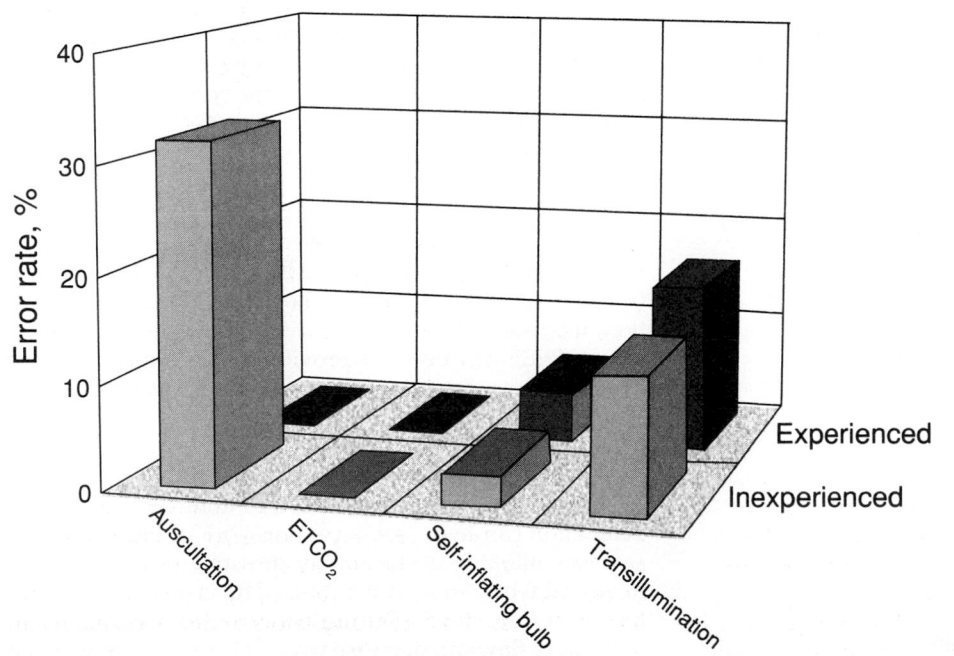

FIGURE 49-19 Error rates of experienced and inexperienced examiners in verifying the placement of a tracheal tube using four methods: auscultation, capnographic determination of end-tidal CO_2 (ET_{CO_2}), negative pressure test using a self-inflating bulb, and transillumination using a lighted stylet. Capnography was the most reliable method regardless of the examiner's experience. (*Reproduced, with permission, from Knapp et al.*[87])

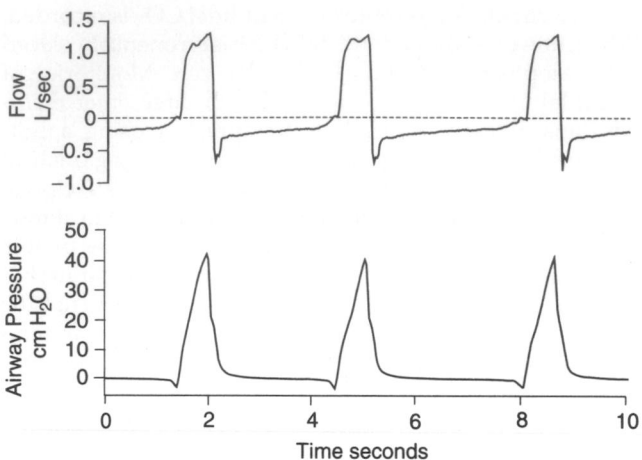

FIGURE 49-20 Flow and airway pressure in a patient being ventilated using assist-control ventilation. The failure of expiratory flow to return to zero at the onset of the successive mechanical breaths indicates the presence of intrinsic PEEP (PEEPi).

resuscitation).[91] Steps to overcome PEEPi can decrease patient work of breathing and improve triggering of the ventilator (Fig. 49-21).[90,92,93]

Monitoring physiologic variables, such as the ratio of respiratory frequency to tidal volume (f/VT), helps in deciding whether a patient has a reasonable likelihood to tolerate discontinuation of mechanical ventilation. A f/VT of 80, which has a likelihood ratio of 7.5, is associated with almost a 95% posttest probability of successful weaning. If the f/VT is higher than 100, the likelihood ratio is 0.04 and the posttest probability of successful weaning is less than 5%.[94]

FIGURE 49-21 Airway pressure (Paw) and esophageal pressure (Pes) in a patient receiving mechanical ventilation at PEEP 0 (*left panel*) and PEEP of 8 cmH2O (*right panel*). Addition of PEEP decreased Pes swings, indicating a decrease in patient effort.

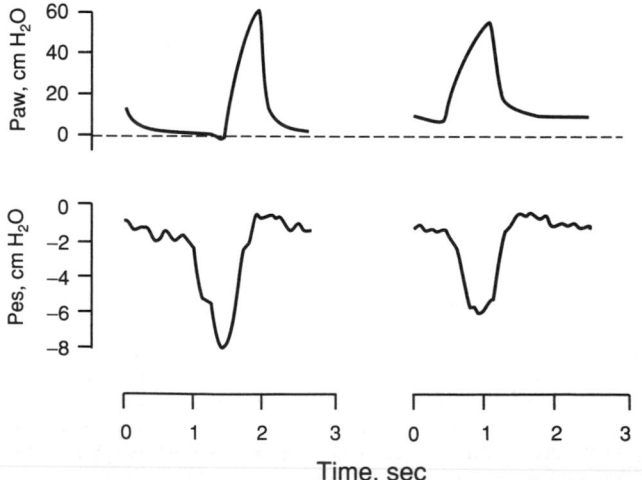

GUIDE MANAGEMENT

ASSESS THE RESPONSE OF DRUGS

Monitoring is essential with administration of therapeutic agents that can produce rapid and dramatic changes in a patient's condition. A physician would not dream of administering a potent, rapid-acting intravenous vasoactive agent (vasodilator, vasopressor, or inotropic agent) without monitoring arterial pressure. It would be unconscionable to perform cardiac resuscitation without ECG monitoring.

Measurement of airway resistance helps in assessing the response to bronchodilator therapy. In ventilator-dependent patients with COPD, delivery of albuterol from a metered-dose inhaler produces a decrease in airway resistance within 5 minutes; the effect is sustained for at least 60 minutes.[95,96]

OPTIMIZE VENTILATOR SETTING

Titrating F_{IO_2}
Pulse oximetry is commonly used when titrating F_{IO_2} in ventilated patients. A Sp_{O_2} of 92% is a reliable target in white patients. In black patients, however, an Sp_{O_2} of 92% is associated with significant hypoxemia, and a higher target, 95%, is required.[10]

Adjusting Pressure Support
Tidal volume and respiratory rate are commonly used to set pressure-support ventilation.[97–101] A reasonable level of inspiratory effort is an inspiratory pressure-time product <125 cmH2O·sec/minute. Using this target, a respiratory rate of 30 breaths/minute and tidal volume of 600 mL resulted in the fewest false classifications (Fig. 49-22).[101]

Setting Peep
In a patient with acute lung injury, the right level of PEEP is that which optimizes arterial oxygenation without causing O2 toxicity or ventilator-induced lung injury.[102–105] Balancing the benefit of keeping the lung open (during tidal ventilation) against the risks of lung overinflation may require monitoring of the pressure-volume curve, lung morphology, and gas exchange (Fig. 49-23).[106–111] When loss of aeration has a focal distribution (atelectatic lower lobes coexisting with aerated upper lobes), a high level of PEEP can cause overinflation of already aerated areas and only partial recruitment of atelectatic areas.[112] In such patients, some experts recommend limiting PEEP to low levels (~10 cmH2O).[102] In patients who have diffuse loss of aeration, the risk of overinflation with PEEP is low.[113] Thus, a higher PEEP can be used provided it does not cause the plateau pressure to rise above the upper inflection point (Fig. 49-24).[102,114]

Assessing Patient Work of Breathing
Inspection of the airway pressure contour during assisted ventilation can help assess patient work of breathing. Excessive scalloping of the airway pressure tracing indicates increased work, such as that caused by insufficient inspiratory flow (Fig. 49-25). During assist-control ventilation, an increase in flow can decrease work of breathing by as much

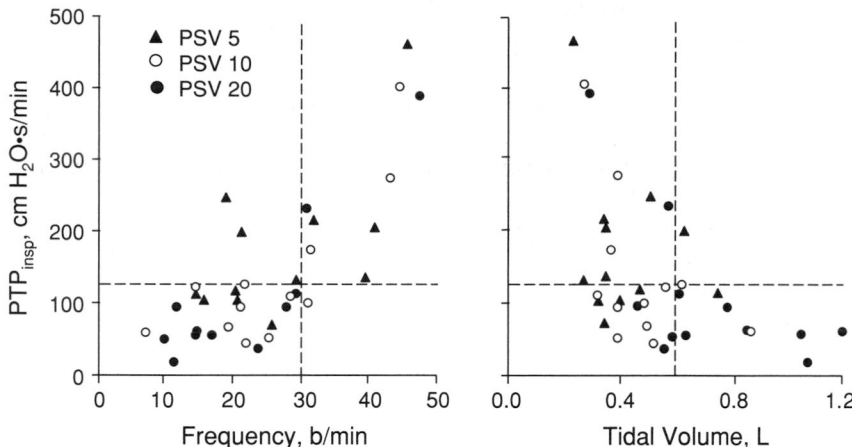

FIGURE 49-22 A four-quadrant diagram of inspiratory pressure-time product (PTPinsp), respiratory frequency (*left panel*), and tidal volume (*right panel*) at different levels of pressure-support ventilation (PSV). PTPinsp values below the horizontal dashed line of 125 cmH$_2$O·sec/minute are considered to represent a desirable level of patient effort. The vertical dashed line at a frequency of 30 breaths/minute and at a tidal volume of 0.6 L resulted in the fewest misclassifications. Of the 24 values with a PTPinsp <125 cmH$_2$O·sec/minute, 23 (96%) were associated with a frequency of ≤30 breaths/minute, whereas only 10 (42%) had a tidal volume >0.6 L. (*Reproduced, with permission, from Jubran et al.[101]*)

as 60% in patients with acute respiratory failure. Higher flow rates can also decrease inspiratory effort in stable patients with COPD.[115,116]

Continuous displays of pressure and flow have led to increased awareness that patient effort is frequently insufficient to trigger the ventilator.[76,92] During pressure support or assist-control ventilation, up to a third of patient efforts may fail to trigger the machine (Fig. 49-26). Such nontriggering has been shown to result from premature inspiratory efforts that are not sufficient to overcome the elastic recoil associated with dynamic hyperinflation.[92] To trigger the ventilator, patient effort has to first generate a negative intrathoracic pressure to counterbalance the elastic recoil and then overcome the set sensitivity. The full consequences of wasted inspiratory efforts are not known. They certainly place an unnecessary burden on patients whose inspiratory muscles are already under

stress. Such added stress can interfere with subsequent weaning.[117,118]

AVOID COMPLICATIONS

The heterogeneous lung involvement in ARDS puts some regions at risk of developing alveolar overdistension when a ventilator breath is delivered.[119–121] Plateau pressure is monitored as a surrogate for end-inspiratory alveolar pressure, and may help to minimize lung injury.[122] Studies have shown that patients with ARDS who had plateau pressures greater than 32 cmH$_2$O had higher mortality.[114,123,124]

Daily radiographs in ventilated patients can reveal unsuspected or significant abnormalities.[125,126] Malpositioning of devices (endotracheal tubes, nasogastric tubes, and central venous pressure lines) and pneumothorax or pleural effusions are detected in 20% of patients (Fig. 49-27).[127]

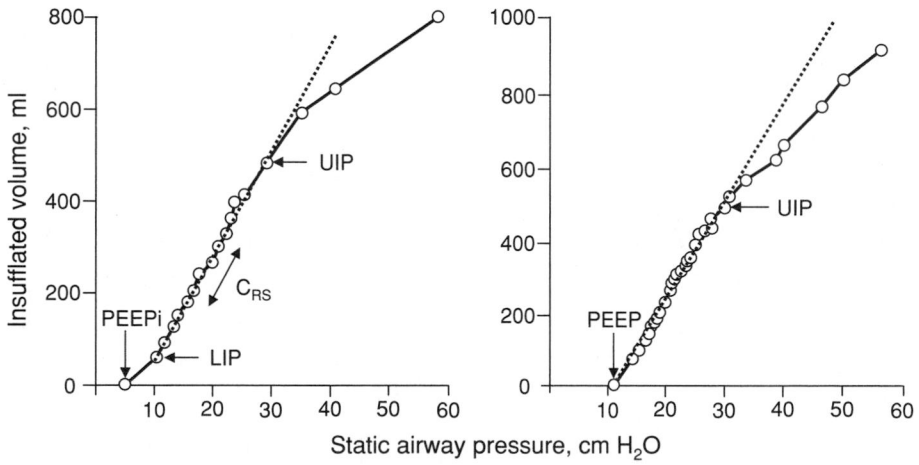

FIGURE 49-23 A pressure-volume curve recorded at zero end-expiratory pressure (ZEEP) (*left panel*) and PEEP 12 cmH$_2$O (*right panel*) in a patient with ARDS using the "ventilator technique" to achieve different insufflation volumes. The dashed line represents the linear part of the curve. At ZEEP, a lower inflection point (LIP) and an upper inflection point (UIP) can be identified as the two points where the curve starts to separate consistently from the straight line. Compliance (Crs) is usually measured on the linear part of the curve. The intercept of the pressure-volume curve with the x-axis corresponds to intrinsic PEEP (PEEPi). At a PEEP of 12 cmH$_2$O (*right panel*), the lower inflection point is absent, whereas the upper inflection point (UIP) is still present. (*Reproduced, with permission, from Brochard.[106]*)

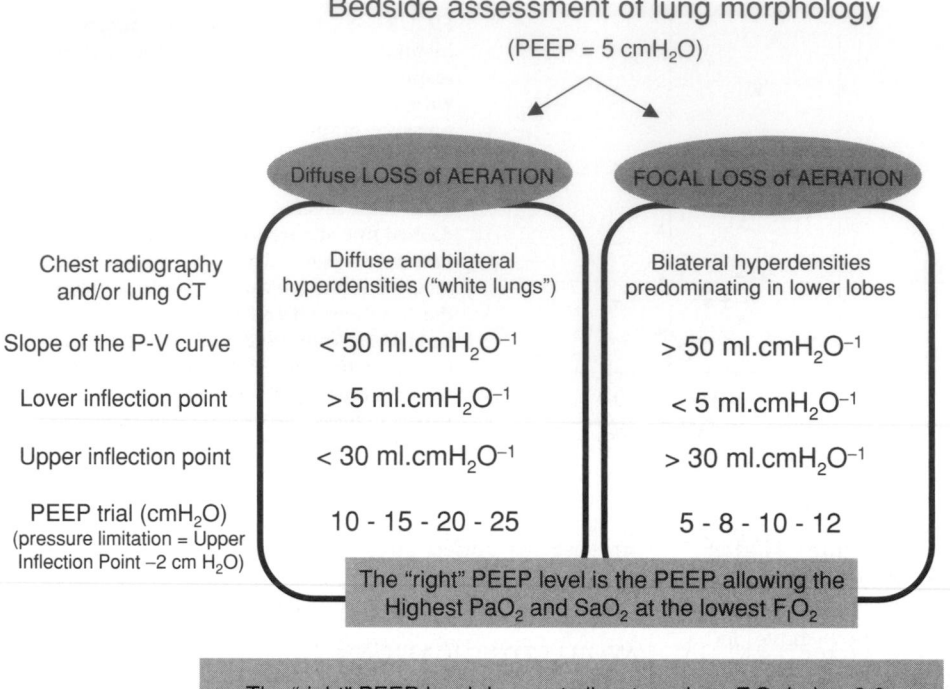

Bedside assessment of lung morphology
(PEEP = 5 cmH₂O)

	Diffuse LOSS of AERATION	FOCAL LOSS of AERATION
Chest radiography and/or lung CT	Diffuse and bilateral hyperdensities ("white lungs")	Bilateral hyperdensities predominating in lower lobes
Slope of the P-V curve	< 50 ml.cmH₂O⁻¹	> 50 ml.cmH₂O⁻¹
Lover inflection point	> 5 ml.cmH₂O⁻¹	< 5 ml.cmH₂O⁻¹
Upper inflection point	< 30 ml.cmH₂O⁻¹	> 30 ml.cmH₂O⁻¹
PEEP trial (cmH₂O) (pressure limitation = Upper Inflection Point –2 cm H₂O)	10 - 15 - 20 - 25	5 - 8 - 10 - 12

The "right" PEEP level is the PEEP allowing the Highest PaO₂ and SaO₂ at the lowest F₁O₂

The "right" PEEP level does not allow to reduce F₁O₂ below 0.6

FIGURE 49-24 Sequence of steps in selecting the right level of PEEP for a given patient. The right level is defined as the PEEP level that allows optimization of arterial oxygenation without causing oxygen toxicity and ventilator-induced lung injury. (*Reproduced, with permission, from Rouby et al.[102]*)

Physicians had not anticipated these findings. The importance of early detection of abnormalities was underscored in a study by Steier et al.[128] Mortality was 7% when pneumothorax was diagnosed immediately. Mortality quadrupled when diagnosis (and treatment) was delayed.

PROVIDE ALARMS

Pulse oximetry can provide an early warning of hypoxemia. In 20,802 surgical patients, use of pulse oximetry resulted in 19-fold greater detection of hypoxemia (defined as an SpO₂ <90%) as compared with patients in whom an oximeter was not used.[129] Myocardial ischemia was less common in the oximetry group than in the control group, 12 and 26 patients, respectively. The anesthesiologists reported that oximetry led to a change in therapy on one or more occasions in 10.5% of patients in the operating room and in 17% in the postanesthesia care unit.

An alarm on a ventilator may sound (or flash) because of a change in ventilator performance or patient clinical status.

FIGURE 49-25 Flow and airway pressure (Paw) during assist-control ventilation at a flow of 60 L/minute (*A*) and a flow of 30 L/minute (*B*). In panel *A*, the small negative phase and smooth rise and convex appearance of the Paw waveform indicate that the patient is making a slight inspiratory effort to breathe. In panel *B*, the more pronounced negative phase together with excessive scalloping of the Paw waveform indicates that the patient is making a strenuous effort to breathe as a result of the inadequate flow setting.

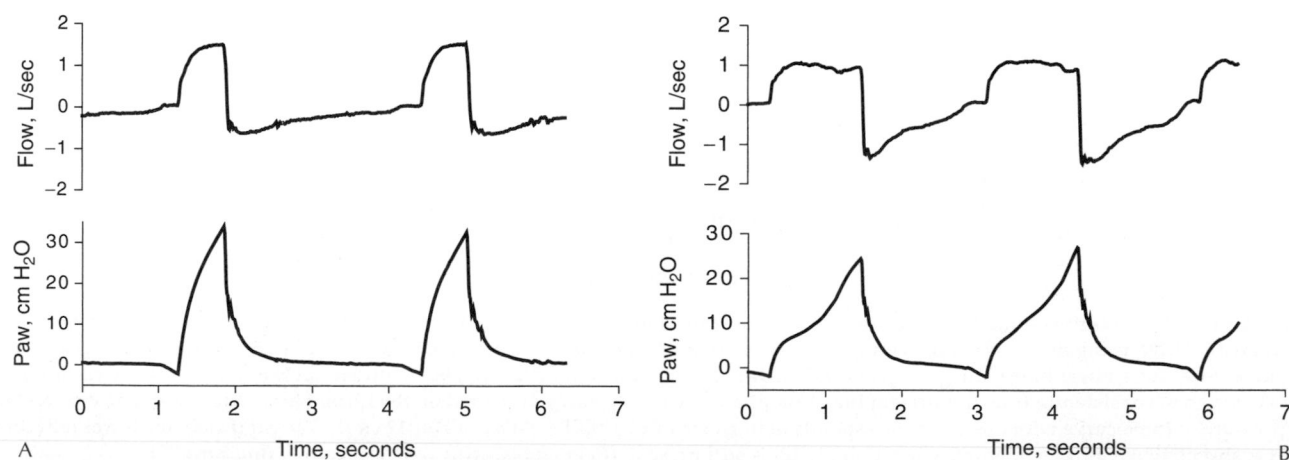

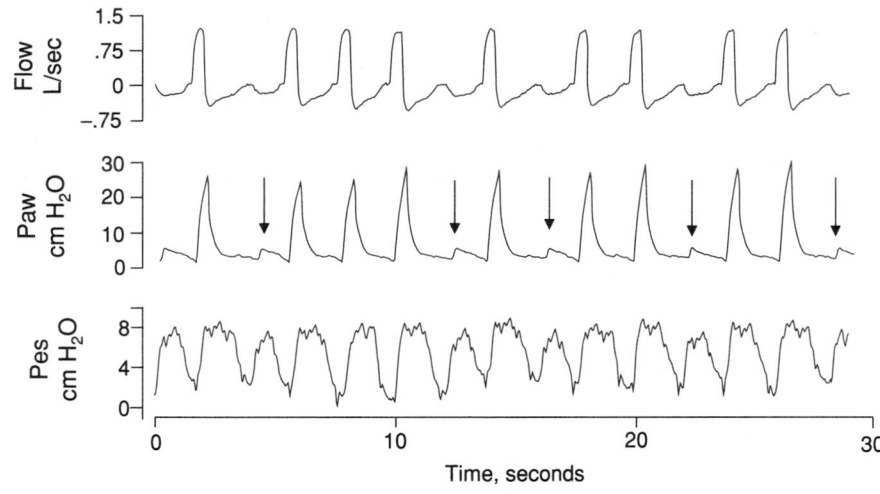

FIGURE 49-26 Flow, airway pressure (Paw), and esophageal pressure (Pes) in a patient receiving assist-control ventilation. The arrows indicate inspiratory attempts that failed to trigger the opening of the ventilator valve.

An abrupt increase in peak airway pressure can arise with endotracheal obstruction or ventilator malfunction. A decrease in peak pressure can arise with a leak in the circuit. An increase in the baseline airway pressure can signal malfunction of the exhalation valve (or inadvertent PEEP).[130,131]

Continuous monitoring of cardiac rhythm can be life saving in patients with a recent myocardial infarction. Early recognition of sustained ventricular tachycardia in the periinfarction period can lead to immediate therapeutic intervention in an attempt to prevent further myocardial ischemia, ventricular fibrillation, or both (Fig. 49-28).[132,133]

The role of monitoring as a warning sign was highlighted in a study of anesthesia-related malpractice claims.[134] Of 1097 cases reviewed, negative outcomes were prevented in 32% by the use of additional monitors. The authors estimated that use of a pulse oximeter and capnometer would have prevented 93% of the mishaps.[134]

FIGURE 49-27 Distribution of new major findings detected by daily chest radiography and missed by clinical assessment in ventilated patients. Malposition of endotracheal tubes and nasogastric tubes accounted for most of the findings. (*Reproduced, with permission, from Hall et al.*[127])

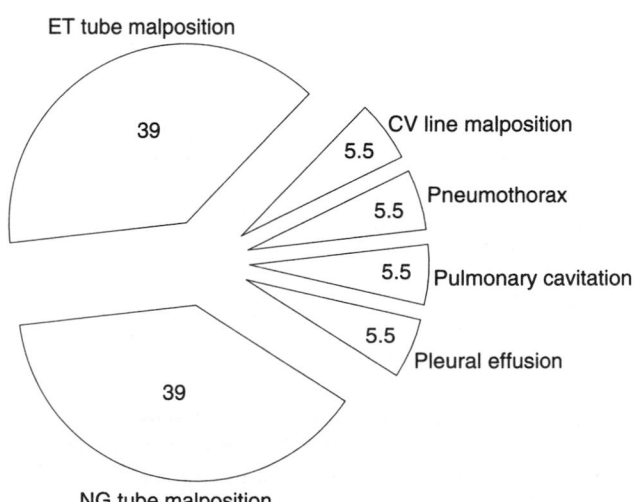

ASSESSMENT OF TRENDS

Monitoring of physiologic variables over time helps in assessing a therapeutic response.[135] When vasopressor therapy is being titrated, continuous monitoring of arterial pressure is essential. Monitoring the motor response to peripheral nerve stimulation helps avoid the accumulation of neuromuscular blocking agents (with risk of prolonged paralysis).[136,137] Train-of-four stimulation uses a series of four supramaximal stimuli delivered at a frequency of two stimuli per second (Fig. 49-29). The dose of a neuromuscular blocking agent is usually titrated to obtain no more than two visible muscle twitches in response to each train-of-four. If the patient fails to demonstrate any response with the train-of-four stimulation, the blocking agent should be discontinued temporarily or the dosage reduced.[137-139]

Checking for trends assists in following the course of a disease. Severe ischemic hepatitis, secondary to hypovolemic shock, causes dramatic increases in transaminases by 24–36 hours. A sharp decrease follows within a week. Thereafter, bilirubin may rise and prothrombin time may become prolonged (Fig. 49-30).[140] If a physician first sees a patient late in the clinical course, severe jaundice and coagulopathy may be evident. Without having witnessed the earlier changes in transaminases, the physician may fail to recognize that the patient is suffering from progression of an ischemic event. When evaluating a patient suffering from acetaminophen overdose, monitoring the plasma concentration over the first 24 hours helps predict the risk of hepatotoxicity (Fig. 49-31).[141,142] If the level is 200 mg/L at 4 hours after ingestion, the patient is at risk

FIGURE 49-28 Rhythm strip in a critically ill patient showing the development of ventricular tachycardia.

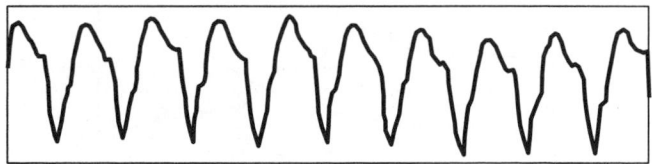

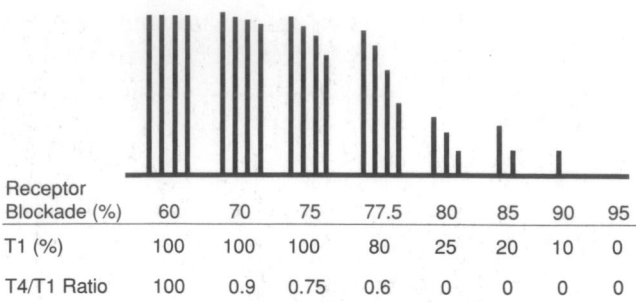

Receptor Blockade (%)	60	70	75	77.5	80	85	90	95
T1 (%)	100	100	100	80	25	20	10	0
T4/T1 Ratio	100	0.9	0.75	0.6	0	0	0	0

FIGURE 49-29 Train-of-four (TOF) stimulation consists of a series (train) of four electrical impulses delivered at a frequency of two stimuli per second. When neuromuscular blocking agents are not being used, the response to TOF stimulation is four strong twitches. As the receptors begin to load up with the neuromuscular blocking agent, four twitches are still present, although the response is weaker and a decrease is evident between the first and the fourth twitch. Comparison of muscular movement on the first (T1) and fourth twitch (T4) enables the calculation of a T4/T1 ratio; this ratio can detect an earlier stage of receptor blockade than twitch loss. (*Reproduced, with permission, from Strange.*[139])

for hepatotoxicity; a level of 25 mg/L at 16 hours indicates continued risk.

Monitoring patient effort can guide patient management during a weaning trial (Fig. 49-32).[83,143] Changes in esophageal pressure over the first 9 minutes of a trial, quantified as a trend index, revealed sensitivity 0.91, specificity 0.89, positive predictive value 0.83, and negative predictive value 0.94 (Fig. 49-33).[143] The area under a receiver-operating characteristic (ROC) curve for the trend index (0.94) was greater than for first-minute measurement of esophageal pressure (0.44, $p < 0.05$) and tended to be greater than that for frequency-to-tidal volume (0.78, $p = 0.13$). Likelihood ratio was highest for the trend index (8.2, $p < 0.05$).

Continuous monitoring of ST segments in patients with unstable angina or non–Q wave myocardial infarction can identify patients with silent ischemia; ischemia in such

FIGURE 49-30 Severe insults to the liver result in an abrupt, severe but transient increase in transaminases (serum glutamate oxaloacetate transaminase; SGOT). Several days later, increases in prothrombin time and total bilirubin are observed. (*Reproduced, with permission, from Kramer.*[140])

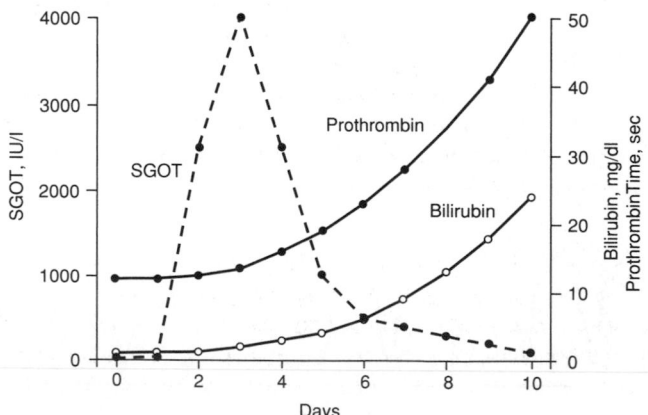

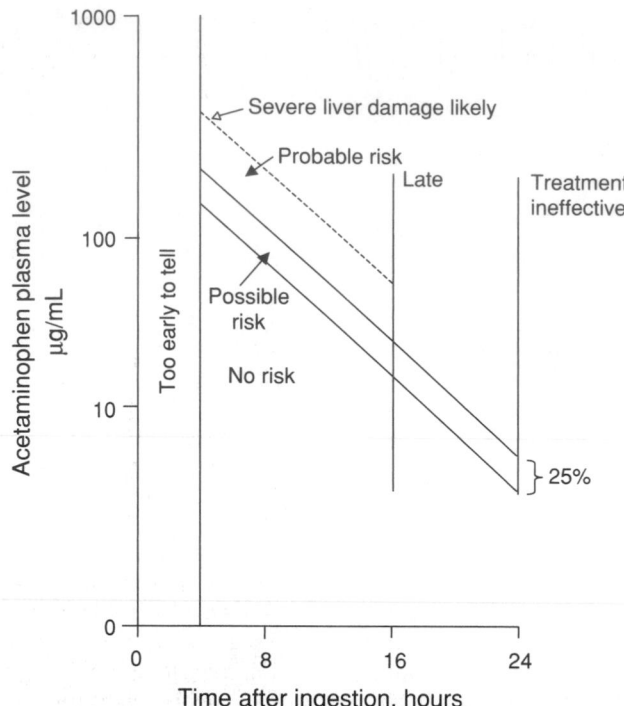

FIGURE 49-31 Nomogram for predicting the risk of hepatotoxicity based on elapsed time from the point of acetaminophen ingestion. The upper solid diagonal line is the standard nomogram line. The lower solid diagonal line represents plasma levels 25% below the standard nomogram line, which are used to allow for possible errors in acetaminophen plasma assay and estimated time from ingestion. Patients who fall between the two diagonal lines are at risk for hepatotoxicity. (*Reproduced, with permission, from Susla.*[142])

patients places them at risk for subsequent death and new myocardial infarctions (Fig. 49-34).[144–147] In a meta-analysis of 995 patients from three randomized trials, a direct relationship was observed between the number of ischemic episodes (per 24 hours) and the risk of a cardiac event (death or myocardial infarction) at 5 and 30 days after enrollment.[146,148–150] The incidence of cardiac events was 3.3% among patients without ST episodes and 15.5% in patients with more than five ST episodes. At 30 days, these figures were 5.7% and 19.7%, respectively.[151]

Changes in lactate levels can predict the development and severity of cardiogenic and other forms of shock.[152–156] After admission to the ICU, serial lactate levels decreased in shock survivors, whereas nonsurvivors showed little change.[154] A change in lactate level over the first 3 hours of resuscitation was a better predictor of outcome than a single measurement (Fig. 49-35).

Effect of Monitoring on Patient Outcome

Because of expectation of improvement in patient outcome, monitoring is subjected to closer scrutiny than most diagnostic tests.[58] Although complications derived from use of a monitor are relatively easy to evaluate, few monitoring devices have been subjected to studies of their effect on

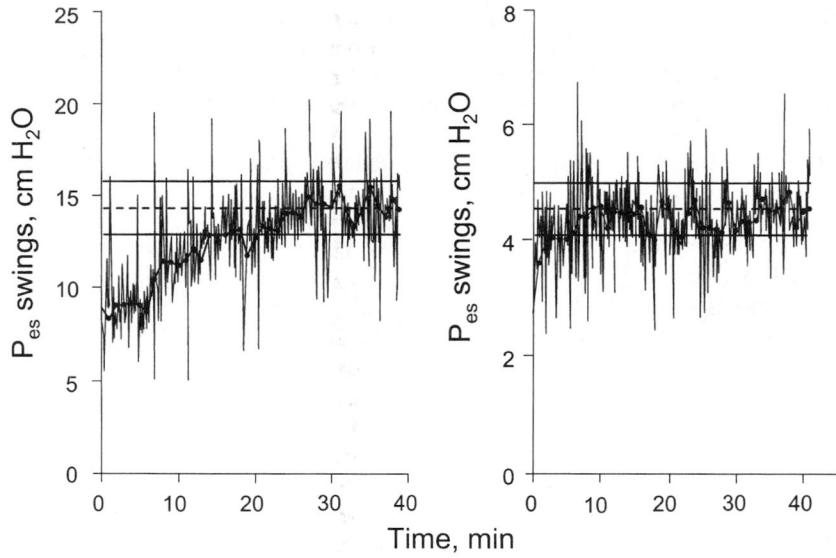

FIGURE 49-32 Time-series plot of swings in esophageal pressure (Pes) in a weaning failure patient (*left panel*) and a weaning success patient (*right panel*) during a trial of spontaneous breathing. Black dots represent 1-minute averages. The solid line indicates the average value of Pes swings of the final minute of the trial. The dashed lines indicate ±10% of the final minute values of Pes swings. The time taken to reach ±10% of the final value for Pes swings was 14 minutes for the failed patient and 6 minutes for the successful patient. (*Reproduced, with permission, from Jubran et al.*[143])

mortality or other clinical outcomes. Those few studies have not revealed clear-cut benefits. Three recently conducted randomized trials of the PA catheter (in 2714 patients and 120 ICUs) did not reveal improved outcome (Fig. 49-36).[157–159] In 20,802 surgical patients, Moller et al[129] found that pulse oximetry had no demonstrable benefit on the rate of postoperative complications. Accordingly, it is reasonable to ask whether monitoring has any role in the management of a critically-ill patient. At first glance, the studies say no. Before reaching that conclusion, however, we need to scrutinize the data.

FIGURE 49-33 Esophageal pressure swings (Pes) in weaning failure (*solid line*) and weaning success groups (*dashed lines*) that were generated by the multiple adaptive swings in the failure patients occurred during the first minute. The greatest difference in Pes swings between the failure (14.5 cmH$_2$O, 95% confidence intervals 18.9–11.2) and success groups (7.9 cmH$_2$O, 95% confidence intervals 11.8–0.8) was at the transition between the ninth and tenth minute. (*Reproduced, with permission, from Jubran et al.*[143])

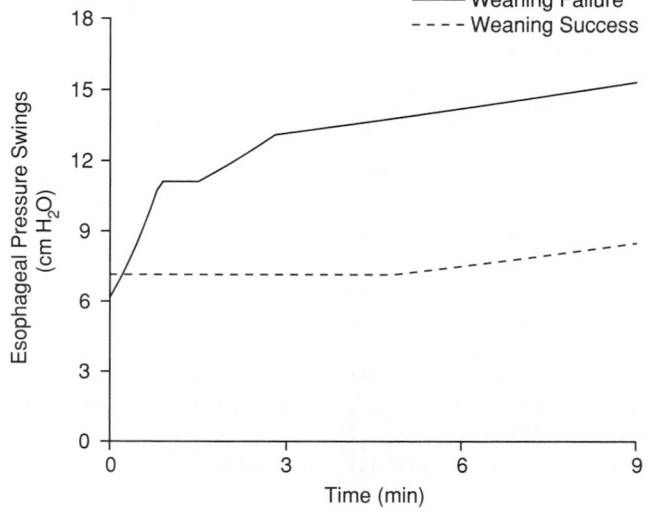

The gold standard for evaluating outcome is a randomized controlled trial. In a typical trial, the effect of some intervention on outcome is assessed in a well-defined patient population. Such trial designs are mostly used to assess the risks and benefits of a therapeutic agent. Using a randomized trial to assess the benefits of a monitor can be problematic because of poorly defined patient populations, complexity of the therapeutic intervention, and choice of the primary outcome.

FAILURE TO PRECISELY DEFINE DISEASE STATES

The first step in evaluating the effect of an intervention is to ensure a well-defined study population. Definition and categorization of disease states—the discipline of nosology—is especially difficult in critically ill patients.[160] (The reader is referred to a detailed discussion of nosology in Chapter 5.) The most precise way to define a disease is in etiologic terms (e.g., Legionnaire's disease). Most randomized trials of monitoring techniques have been conducted in groups of patients identified in terms of a syndrome—that is, a condition defined on the basis of a constellation of symptoms and signs. A typical definition of sepsis is the following: temperature >38°C or <36°C, respiratory rate >20breaths/minute or PCO$_2$ <32 mmHg, and signs of hypoperfusion, among others.[158] (Note that the respiratory rate commonly listed as a criterion for sepsis falls in the middle of the normal range.) When a disease is defined in an imprecise manner, very different types of patients may be assigned to the two arms of a trial. This factor could be a major contributor to negative outcome of a study of a monitoring technique.

COMPLEXITY OF EVALUATING THE INTERVENTION

Evaluating the benefit and risk of any intervention in the ICU is challenging. The huge number of procedures and treatments typically used in any single ICU constitute confounding variables. These covariates contribute to

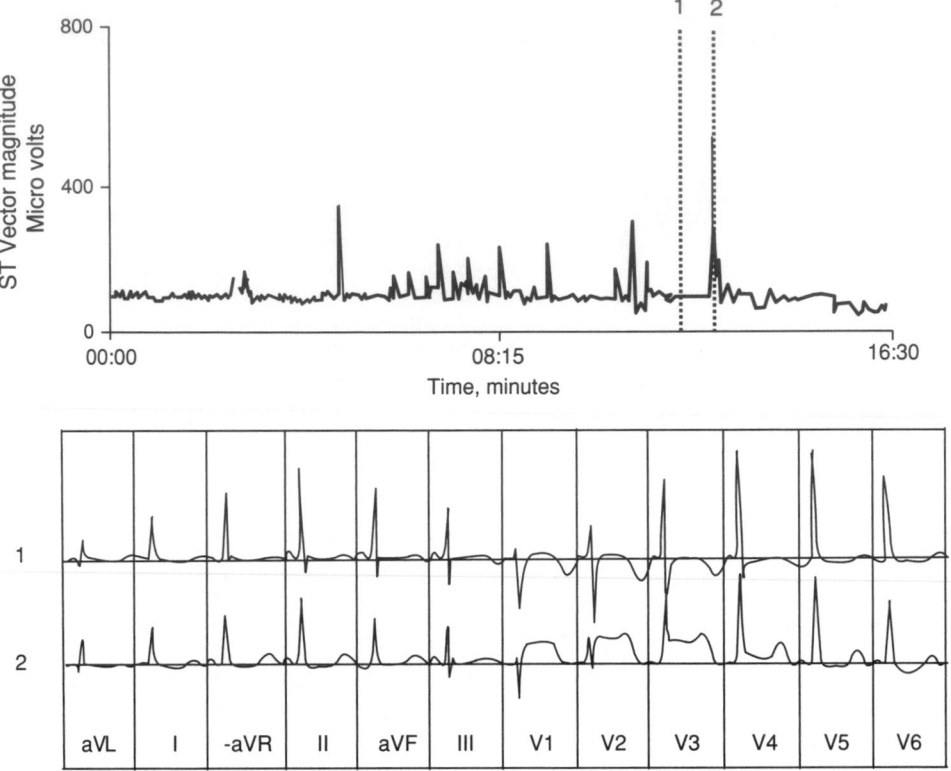

FIGURE 49-34 *Top panel:* Trend curve of ST vector magnitude in a patient with unstable angina as displayed by a vectorcardiography monitoring system. Transient increases of ST vector >50 μV from baseline for more than 1 minute indicate an episode of myocardial ischemia. The vertical line 1 represents the baseline ECG tracing without any abnormalities, and vertical line 2 represents an episode of transient ischemia. *Bottom panel:* Corresponding 12-lead ECG tracings recorded at baseline (*vertical line 1*) and during an episode of transient ischemia (*vertical line 2*). (*Reproduced, with permission, from Norgaard et al.[145]*)

considerable experimental noise in a trial, masking benefits that are truly present.

To illustrate these considerations, we discuss a hypothetical study designed to determine whether PA catheter monitoring improves survival in septic shock. In designing such a trial, the covariables shown in Fig. 49-37 must be controlled for or taken into account.

FIGURE 49-35 Lactate levels over time in patients who survived (*open circles*) and who did not survive (*closed circles*) an episode of shock. Serial lactate levels decreased after admission in the survivors but little change was seen in the nonsurvivors. A change in the lactate level during the first 3 hours of resuscitation was a better predictor of outcome than a single measurement. (*Reproduced, with permission, from Kost.[152]*)

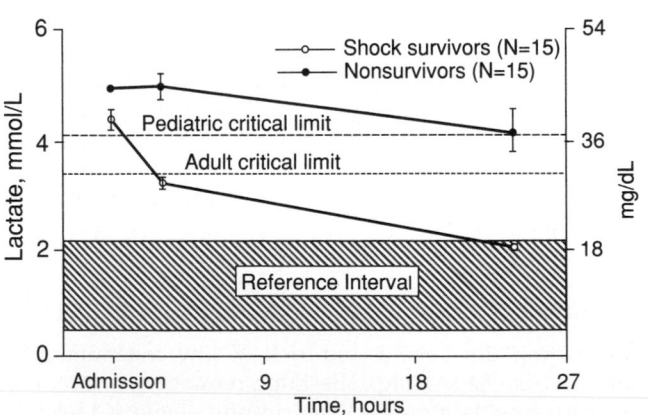

PATIENT SELECTION: DISTINCTION BETWEEN TRUE INDICATIONS VERSUS STUDY INCLUSION CRITERIA

The choice of the most appropriate monitoring device is dictated by a patient's condition. To decide whether a monitor is indicated in a particular patient, the physician must balance potential benefits and risks. When wondering whether to insert a PA catheter in a patient with septic shock who is unresponsive to fluid and vasopressor therapy, a physician should consider three factors. One, will end-organ dysfunction proceed and become irreversible if therapy is not changed? Two, will large volumes of fluids, administered empirically but on an incorrect assumption that intravascular volume is depleted, predispose to hypoxemia should acute lung injury be present? Three, if a PA catheter is inserted, will the physician withhold fluids if the wedge pressure is normal?

The uncertain probability of organ dysfunction and its time course, the risks of monitoring, and the variable efficacy of therapy highlights the complexity of clinical decision making, even when the clinician is highly skilled and experienced. The above three questions, and other factors that impinge on the decision of whether a PA catheter is indicated in a particular patient, are omitted from the design of a randomized clinical trial. Instead, patients are selected on the basis of carefully defined eligibility criteria. The study is thus focused on a narrowly defined spectrum of patients, who poorly reflect the more heterogeneous range of disease seen in everyday practice. As a result, the patients receiving a PA catheter in a randomized trial may bear little relationship to what an experienced and cautious physician does in everyday practice. A skilled physician is unlikely to insert a

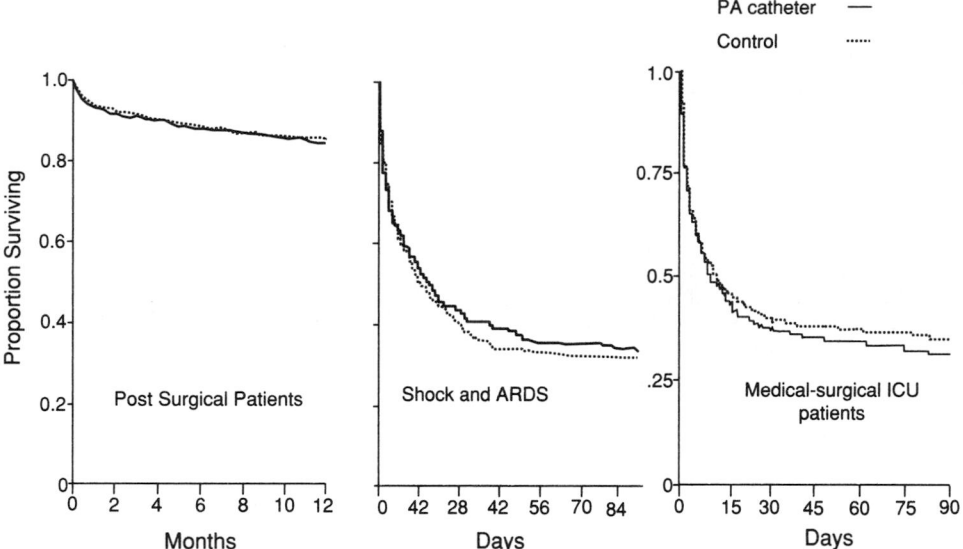

FIGURE 49-36 Probability of survival in patients monitored with (*solid line*) and without (*dotted line*) a pulmonary artery (PA) catheter. The left panel represents data from postsurgical patients, the middle panel data from patients with shock and ARDS, and the right panel from medical-surgical ICU patients. Use of the PA catheter was not associated with an increase in mortality in any of the patient groups. (*Reproduced, with permission, from Sandham et al,[157] Richard et al,[158] and Harvey et al.[159]*)

PA catheter in many of the patients assigned to the intervention arm of a trial, believing that the resulting information would have little likelihood of influencing patient management. If patients are entered into a trial and are randomized to the PA catheter arm, although a judicious physician would not insert a catheter in the same patients, the consequence will be to dilute any likely benefit from the catheter but at the same time increase the risk of complications.

In a study of a mixed group of medical and surgical patients, Connors et al[161] found that a PA catheter was more likely to be used in patients who were sicker and more likely to die. Richard et al[158] studied the benefit of a PA catheter in patients with shock and ARDS. Patients were eligible for monitoring with a PA catheter if their systolic blood pressure was $\geq$95 mmHg (on 3 μg/kg per minute of dopamine), heart rate $\geq$92 beats/minute, Pa_{CO_2} $\leq$32 mmHg while breathing spontaneously, and an elevated lactate

FIGURE 49-37 Factors that can influence the effect of a monitoring device on patient outcome, such as survival. See text for details.

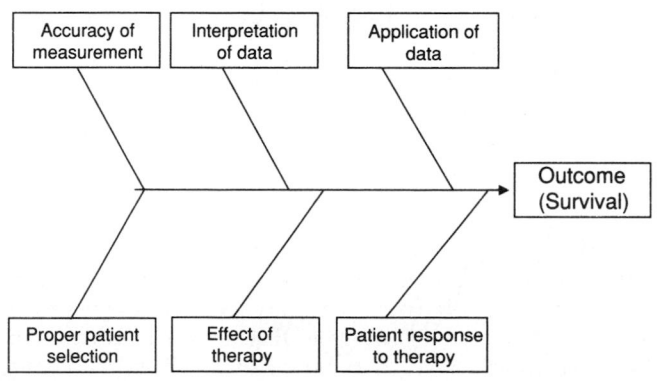

level. We suspect most physicians would not insert a PA catheter in all (or even most) patients who meet these four criteria. In the study of Sandham et al[157] in high-risk surgical patients, 87% of patients who had a PA catheter inserted were not at high risk for death (as identified by New York Heart Association or American Society of Anesthesiologists classifications). In the most recent study, by Harvey et al[159] in 1041 medical and surgical ICU patients, patients were randomized to the PA catheter arm if the primary physician considered the patient as someone who "should" be managed with a PA catheter; precise criteria of what constitutes "should" were not given. Again, this latest study did not demonstrate a benefit from a PA catheter. But if a PA catheter is inserted in a patient in whom there is no clear indication for its use, would you expect the catheter to improve outcome? We expect all readers to answer no. Thus, the outcomes in the randomized trials by Richard et al,[158] Sandham et al,[157] and Harvey et al[159] were all pre-ordained as negative before the first patient was enrolled.

ACCURACY OF THE MONITORS

Studies evaluating the impact of monitoring devices on outcome are predicated on the assumption that the clinical staff are employing the monitor in a knowledgeable manner and obtaining reliable readings. A PA catheter system has been shown to provide accurate and reproducible measurements of pressure when used by experienced staff.[162–165] Reliability of PA catheter readings, however, is highly dependent on catheter placement, calibration of the transducers, and interpretation of the data. Of 282 measurements of PA wedge pressure, Morris et al[166] found that 103 (36%) of the readings were inaccurate. Of 103 erroneous readings, 89 were associated with technical problems, such as damped tracings, poor dynamic response, overinflation of the balloon

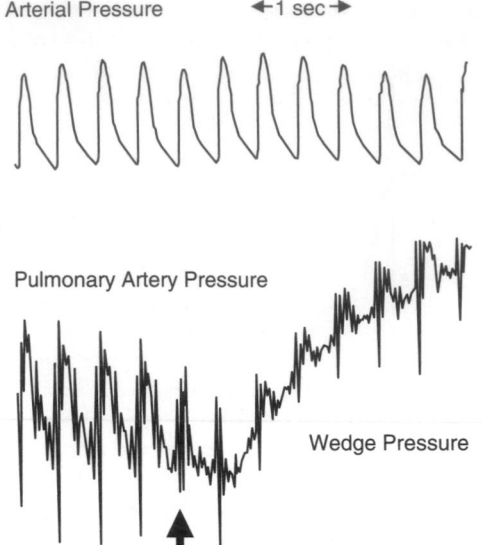

Arterial Pressure   ←1 sec→

Pulmonary Artery Pressure

Wedge Pressure

FIGURE 49-38 Simultaneous recordings of systemic arterial pressure (*top panel*) and pulmonary artery pressure (*bottom panel*). Arrow indicates time of balloon inflation. A steadily increasing wedge pressure after balloon inflation that exceeds the phasic pulmonary artery pressure suggests overinflation of the balloon. (*Reproduced, with permission, from Morris et al.[23]*)

(Fig. 49-38), or incomplete wedging (Fig. 49-39). Errors in wedge pressure as great as 23 mmHg have been reported.[23] Technical problems with use of the PA catheter, or steps taken to correct them, were not taken into account in the randomized trials conducted by Richard et al[158] and Sandham et al.[157] Specifically, Harvey et al[159] state, "we did not assess the quality of use." Even with great care, these technical problems cannot be eliminated completely. For a simple device, such as a pulse oximeter, overall instrument failure (because of poor peripheral perfusion, patient restlessness, interference by electrocautery, battery failure, finger probe failure, difficulty in probe application, or tremor)

was 7.2% among the sicker patients in the study of Moller et all.[129] Such operational problems are commonly not listed in reports of clinical trials.

INTERPRETATION OF THE DATA

Several studies reveal that many clinicians have limited skills in the accurate interpretation of data generated by a PA catheter.[53,54,167,168] In their survey, Iberti et al[53] found that almost half of physicians incorrectly interpreted a straightforward recording of wedge pressure. Another study revealed that physicians arrived at a wide range of wedge pressures for the same tracing.[169] If the wedge pressure is incorrectly and repeatedly read as low in a patient with ARDS, then continued administration of fluids is likely to result in an unfavorable outcome.

APPLICATION OF DATA IN CLINICAL DECISION MAKING

Even if data are accurate and properly interpreted, benefit will occur only if the physician applies the information logically in the management of patients. Some monitoring decisions can be made by simple rules of thumb (heuristics); these are easy to incorporate into an algorithm.[170,171] Simple rules take the if-then form. If serum glucose in a patient with insulin-dependent diabetes is high, then insulin should be administered. This strategy is straightforward because the probability of hyperglycemia is high, the consequences of untreated hyperglycemia are great, the risk of monitoring (drawing a blood sample) is low, the benefit of treatment is high, and the risks when insulin is properly administered are small.

The monitoring dilemmas that arise in most critically ill patients are complex and cannot be captured in an algorithm. Intensivists frequently have to make rapid decisions under conditions of considerable uncertainty, involving substantial risks and unpredictable benefit. To combine, integrate, and interpret diagnostic data in their

FIGURE 49-39 Simultaneous recordings of electrocardiogram (ECG) and pulmonary artery (PA) pressure to illustrate incomplete wedge pressure (Ppw). *Left panel:* With balloon inflation, there is a fall in wedge pressure to a value that approximates pulmonary artery diastolic pressure (Ppad). After balloon inflation, a single positive wave coincides with the T wave on the ECG—a pattern inconsistent with a left atrial waveform. *Right panel:* Waveforms after the catheter has been retracted and the balloon reinflated. A large Ppad-Ppw gradient is evident and the tracing is consistent with a left atrial waveform. Scale is in millimeters of mercury. (*Reproduced, with permission, from Leatherman et al.[24]*)

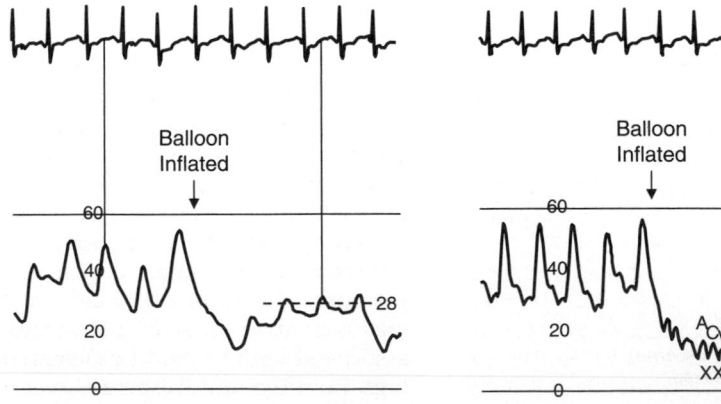
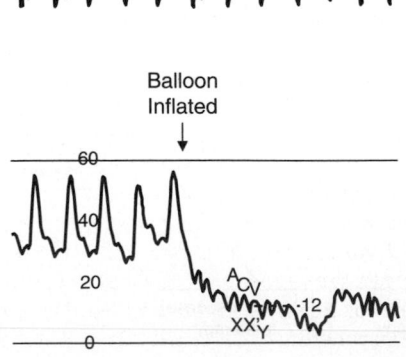

decision-making process, intensivists employ a number of strategies of clinical reasoning.

Probabilistic Reasoning

Diagnostic uncertainty arises because data are insufficient or because the relationship between the data and the disease process is poorly understood.[171] To cope with uncertainty, physicians may use probabilities if available.[172] Probabilistic reasoning is based on the known sensitivity and specificity of a diagnostic (or monitoring) test. A physician forms an initial gestalt as to the likelihood of some condition, which is the pretest probability. Then, based on the known sensitivity and specificity of the test, he or she forms a new estimate of likelihood, the posttest probability. Take a physician who has no inkling as to whether a patient can (or cannot) tolerate a weaning trial. The pretest probability will be 50%. The physician then measures f/V_T and obtains a reading of 80. This reading has a likelihood ratio of 7.5 (that the patient will tolerate a weaning trial). Based on the nomogram of Fagan,[173] a likelihood ratio of 7.5 is associated with a posttest probability of 95% (if pretest probability is 50%). This means that when physicians are in complete doubt (50-50) as to whether a patient can be weaned, obtaining an f/V_T value of less than 80 will substantially decrease their doubt.

Unfortunately, the published data necessary for precise application of probabilistic reasoning are available for few diagnostic (or monitoring) techniques in the ICU. Because physicians cannot communicate in precise quantitative terms, they use expressions such as "most likely," "unlikely," and "rare." Consider a patient in septic shock that remains hypotensive despite fluid resuscitation and a moderate dose of a vasoactive agent (dopamine >10 μg/kg per minute). A common cause of hypotension in such a patient is left ventricular dysfunction. To determine whether left ventricular dysfunction is present or absent, the physician measures the patient's cardiac index. Before measuring cardiac index, the physician forms a gestalt of the patient's likelihood of left ventricular dysfunction (based on previous experience of patients with similar clinical characteristics). After inserting a PA catheter, measuring cardiac index, and based on the reported sensitivity and specificity of cardiac index, the clinician revises his or her assessment of the patient's likelihood of left ventricular dysfunction. This scenario is idealistic, not realistic, because sensitivity and specificity of cardiac index for detecting left ventricular dysfunction in patients with septic shock have not been studied.[174,175]

Another problem arises with use of monitored data. Although data are generally recorded as continuous variables, clinicians typically view data in dichotomous terms. What is the breakpoint in cardiac index below which a patient is classified as having left ventricular dysfunction? Reports on cardiac index as a diagnostic criterion of left ventricular dysfunction usually present a range of possible values, such as 1.6–2.3 L/minute per meter square, rather than a discrete value.[176] The threshold value of cardiac index that is best in distinguishing between the presence and absence of left ventricular dysfunction has never been determined. Is it an index of 2.2 L/minute per meter square? Is it 2.0 L/minute

per meter square? Without a defined threshold value, one cannot attempt to measure the sensitivity and specificity of a diagnostic test.

A further layer of complexity arises with the choice of gold standard. All tests are inaccurate to varying degrees. Thus, the degree of accuracy of a diagnostic (or monitoring) test is measured against a reference test (gold standard). Ideally, the gold standard should be measurable in concrete terms: histology or precise level of narrowing on angiography. For left ventricular dysfunction, however, the gold standard is based on clinical criteria. Studies suggest that a cardiac index of 2.2 L/minute per meter square is an important threshold in predicting the outcome of patients with acute myocardial infarction.[176] Will the physician use the same cardiac index threshold in deciding whether to start treatment with dobutamine in the above-described patient with sepsis who has failed dopamine therapy? Moreover, in making decisions in a particular patient, a clinician may decide to raise or lower the threshold value, taking into account aspects unique to a particular patient's condition. Because of dobutamine's chronotropic action on the heart, a physician may decide to withhold this drug in a patient with underlying coronary artery disease until the cardiac index falls to 1.8 L/minute per meter square.

There is a deeper, more fundamental problem with probabilistic reasoning. This relates to its epistemologic grounding. (Epistemology is the branch of philosophy concerned with the study of the very foundation on which our knowledge rests.) On their own, data derived from randomized trials are unable to explain *why* a particular relationship exists. In contrast, research in physiology, molecular biology, and many other fields, has as its objective the elucidation of underlying mechanisms (explanations for why relationships occur). Tanenbaum[177] undertook an ethnographic study of the reasoning employed by physicians as they made clinical decisions. She found that the clinicians were primarily realists (or determinists): they based decisions on a mental picture of a world of real relationships, real events. Data from mechanistic research enrich this mental picture, offering explanations (meaning) on which physicians can base clinical decisions. When physicians operate as realists, they conduct themselves as if they know what is really happening to a sick person. Data from a randomized trial simply show that some relationship was observed, but provide no epistemologic basis for its occurrence, no understanding of cause and effect. In clinical decision making, realists image a disease process; probabilists play the odds.

Physiologic Reasoning

To attain greater confidence in diagnosis, clinicians employ physiologic (or causal) reasoning. As discussed immediately above, the hope is to form a more coherent picture of cause-and-effect relationships in a given patient. This type of reasoning is particularly suited to the ICU, because monitoring is geared towards detecting changes in pathophysiology. Causal reasoning involves testing and validating (or refuting) apparent cause-and-effect connections.

Take a patient with COPD and congestive heart failure who is being ventilated. A PA catheter is inserted and reveals a wedge pressure of 28 mmHg. Based on probabilistic considerations, the likelihood of pulmonary edema is great. Using causal (physiologic) reasoning, wedge pressure is viewed as a reliable estimate of preload (left ventricular end-diastolic volume). In this patient, the clinician judges the elevated wedge pressure to signify hypervolemia. The true advantage of causal reasoning becomes more clear when we learn that a 60-second interruption of positive-pressure ventilation caused this patient's wedge pressure to fall to 15 mmHg. Probabilistic reasoning would steer us toward diagnoses such as hypervolemia or cardiac dysfunction. Physiologic (or causal) reasoning leads us to suspect that the high wedge pressure (28 mmHg) is caused by PEEPi rather than hypervolemia or cardiac dysfunction.

Causal reasoning forms the bedrock for many diagnostic decisions made outside the ICU. Our understanding of the pathophysiology of critical illnesses, however, is too rudimentary to apply it when managing most ICU patients. The above example highlights the need for much more research into pathophysiologic mechanisms in critically ill patients. Data generated by randomized controlled trials can never provide the information needed for causal reasoning—the type of reasoning that is dominant in the decisions made by physicians in their everyday practice.[177]

Deterministic Reasoning

Deterministic or categorical reasoning is used to reduce information overload. Deterministic reasoning applies a set of rules that take the form of "if-then" statements. For example, *if* a ventilated patient with COPD develops a sudden and equivalent increase in peak and plateau pressures, *then* a non-airway problem, such as a pneumothorax, should be considered. If a patient develops acute renal failure without proteinuria and the fractional excretion of sodium is less than 1%, then the renal failure is prerenal in origin.

Such if-then rules look simple and attractive. The difficult part is figuring out if the antecedent condition (the "if" part of the rule) has been met. When the developers of clinical protocols incorporate such rules into an algorithm, they deliberately eliminate contingencies that can influence the application of the rule. The elimination of such ambiguities means that the rule can be more precisely and concisely expressed on paper. But the elimination of context means that the rule is artificial and cannot be applied in a consistent manner during routine clinical practice.

An algorithm is available for treating hypokalemia in an ICU patient receiving diuretics. If serum potassium is 3.5 mEq/L and the patient is asymptomatic, the algorithm dictates not to give a potassium supplement. The context of everyday ICU practice, however, is more complex. If the patient has heart disease and is taking digitalis or undergoing cardiac surgery, most clinicians would administer potassium if serum potassium is 3.5 mEq/L in order to prevent life-threatening arrhythmias. Likewise, if a patient has cirrhosis, physicians would treat a potassium of 3.5 mEq/L to minimize the risk of hepatic coma. The problem of hypokalemia is further complicated if there is concurrent hypomagnesemia, which promotes potassium wasting. It would be difficult if not impossible to capture all such nuances in the few steps of an algorithm.

Research studies of monitoring devices have included algorithms in an attempt to control for variations in clinical practice. These attempts did not achieve their desired goals. Gattinoni et al[178] undertook a study to evaluate the benefit of directing fluid and pharmacotherapy to achieve a supranormal cardiac index (guided by a PA catheter). Survival was equivalent in the groups with supranormal and normal

FIGURE 49-40 Box plots of maximal attained values for cardiac index (*white boxes*) and O_2-delivery index (*gray boxes*) at baseline and during preoperative, intraoperative, and postoperative periods in patients assigned to pulmonary artery (PA) catheters. Lower and upper limits of boxes indicate the 25th and 75th percentile values; dots inside boxes indicate median values. The lines extending from the boxes indicate the range of non-outlying values. Outliers are plotted separately (*open circles*). The portion of the box plots above the dotted horizontal line corresponds to the subgroup of patients in whom the defined goals were met. The cardiac index target was reached in 19% of patients at study entry and 79% after surgery; the respective values for the O_2-delivery target were 21% at study entry and 63% after surgery. (*Reproduced, with permission, from Sandham et al.*[157])

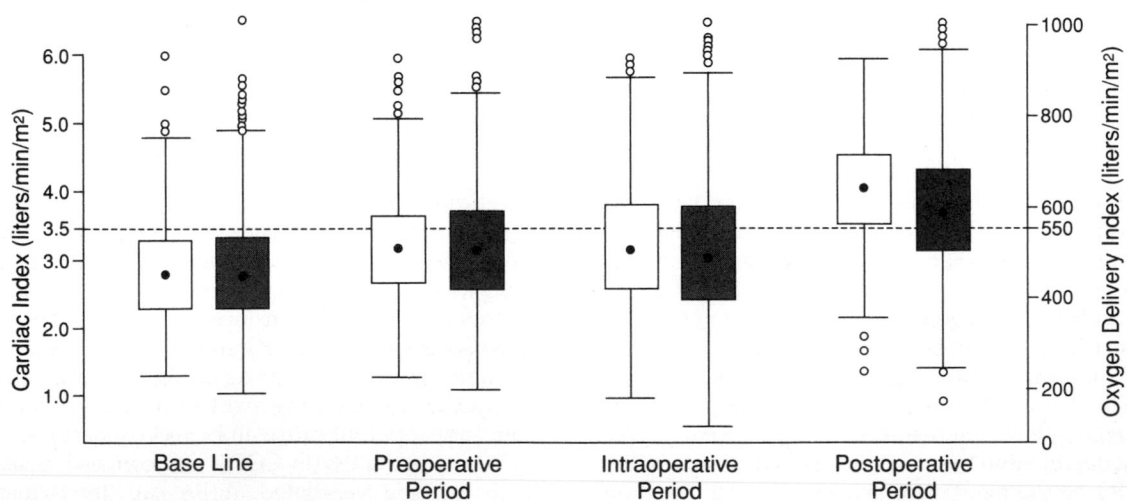

cardiac index. At first sight, the findings suggest that targeting therapy to a supranormal cardiac index does not improve outcome. Perhaps that is true. But such a conclusion cannot be rationally defended based on the presented data. The target of supranormal cardiac index was reached in only 46% of patients in that study arm. Canadian researchers strove for a similar goal.[157] They compared therapy based on predefined physiologic targets (guided by a PA catheter) versus therapy based on usual care (without a PA catheter). The O_2-delivery target in the experimental arm was reached in only 21% of patients at study entry and in 63% of patients after surgery (Fig. 49-40). These two studies provide a vivid illustration of the problems that investigators face in achieving the physiologic objectives that are the true focus of their randomized trial. If the target is not being achieved, what exactly is being studied in these clinical experiments?

Casuistry

Physicians face many, many decisions that have never been subjected to a randomized controlled trial. A physician with many years of experience will relate a current patient to previously similar cases that he or she has handled, paying close attention to how the present patient is similar to, or differs from, the previously managed cases. The physician may also draw on knowledge gained from case reports and observational studies—the only type of literature that pertains to many problems in the ICU. Few randomized controlled trials have specifically addressed fluid management of patients with ARDS. A number of observational studies have been conducted,[179,180] and knowledge gained from such reports combined with previous experience guide decisions on fluid management in this setting.

Reasoning along these lines, primarily in terms of analogy, is referred to as casuistry. Casuistry literally means being concerned with concrete individual cases, as opposed to abstract generalities.[181,182] Casuistry involves reasoning based on precedent (previous example). It is the type of reasoning used in case law, and is the main foundation of the legal system. In deciding how best to manage a particular patient, a physician also needs to take into account a patient's personal preferences.

Tacit or Implicit Knowledge

Physicians make many decisions using tacit knowledge: the type of unexpressable knowledge in *knowing how* versus *knowing what*. Tacit knowledge is knowledge that cannot be articulated. It is implicit knowledge based in actions rather than in conscious thoughts. For more than 80% of complex situations, cognitive psychologists have found that experts such as intensive care staff did not employ an analytical approach to decisions. Instead, they relied on tacit knowledge.[183]

The term *tacit knowledge* was introduced by Michael Polanyi, who pointed out that human beings know more than they can impart.[184] Tacit knowledge is acquired without the intervention of explicit reasoning. It suggests an activity that takes place below the level of conscious reasoning, whether by habit, by being deeply ingrained, or by instinct. By definition, its content is indefinable.

Examples of tacit knowledge include the surgeon's knowledge of the right amount of tension to place on a suture, knowing when to intubate a patient in respiratory distress, and knowing when to extubate a patient after completion of a weaning trial. The skill in performing bronchoscopy is another example. The physician knows how to position the bronchoscope spatially as if it were an extension of his or her fingertips, and how to serially weave the instrument to enter the posterior segment of right lower lobe bronchus. An added dimension is knowing how much pressure to exert, and sensing resistance, when performing a transbronchial biopsy. The physician cannot communicate this knowledge in explicit terms. Instead, the knowledge is something the physician feels and shows while performing the procedure.

The failure of the possessor of tacit knowledge to identify and communicate its content is often attributed to poor power of introspection. When a physician is asked to recount the mental steps involved in solving a complex problem, the reconstruction often sounds unconvincing, even naïve. An attending physician may decide not to extubate a patient who is breathing at a rate of 28 breaths per minute and who has reasonable arterial blood gas values. The fellow may appear puzzled by this decision. To explain his (or her) decision, the attending may use words such as "intuition" or "gut feeling." The word *intuition* is loaded with negative connotations. It is equated with random guessing, confused superstition, mystical thought, weird unfathomable emotion, and an excuse for prejudice. Yet, intuition, not explicit logical reasoning, lies at the heart of originality in science.

People are not born with some free-floating gift of intuition. Instead, the unconscious decisions and automatic actions that reflect tacit knowledge stem from years and years of experience and reflection in a particular field. Intuition is needed to know *when* is the right time to adapt (to judge when is a plan falling apart); to know *how* to adapt (hatching a scheme on the hoof); and in *evaluating* adaptive steps (spotting new steps that may cause problems subsequently). Tacit knowledge is exemplified by an experienced clinician who knows at what juncture it is prudent to insert a PA catheter in a patient who is septic, who remains hypotensive despite 20 $\mu g/kg$ per minute of dopamine, and who has started to exhibit a decrease in urine output. Improvisation in patient care requires considerable expertise; it is the antithesis of following a protocol.

Experts do not use guidelines or analytical reasoning when faced with familiar problems. Instead, they generate a single course of action—they do what normally works. An expert sees the world differently than does a novice. An expert spots things that other people miss: how things usually work, patterns, anomalies, fine details but at the same time the big picture, and soft underbellies for attack. The expert is not using tacit knowledge as a substitute for the explicit analytical method, but as an improvement over it.[183]

Take the case of a patient who is admitted to the ICU with fever, respiratory distress, and hypotension. The resident examines the patient, but is unable to find an obvious source for the fever. Chest radiography and urinalysis are negative. The resident makes a presumptive diagnosis of septic shock. He begins therapy with vasopressors, fluids, and broad-spectrum antibiotics. The patient remains hypotensive. The next day, the attending physician hears a crunching sound over the apex, and suspects a Hamman's crunch. At first, she is not convinced it is present, because the crunch is obscured by the noise of the ventilator. On closer listening, the crunch is synchronous with the heartbeat. The attending physician infers that the patient has an esophageal perforation, which is causing the sepsis. Surgical repair is successfully undertaken. The resident asks the attending physician, "How did you know what to look for?" "I don't know why," she replies, "I just sensed it." This is an example of tacit knowledge used by the attending physician. The attending answers, "I don't know why," because she is not able to recall the precise train of thought that inspired her to suspect mediastinal emphysema. In part, the attending physician's thinking is based on extensive experience, and the many similar cases she has seen in the past—an example of casuistry. Her inspired guess, diagnostic acumen, does not stem solely from tacit knowledge. It is also based on explicit knowledge. Hearing a crunching sound in the precordium is of no value without the book learning that tells the physician what the sound signifies. The case exemplifies the intermingling of tacit and explicit knowledge.

The skills of an outstanding diagnostician are like those of the connoisseur, a refined ability to discern between nuances governed by a heightened sensibility (good taste). It is a mistake to imagine that the listing of a series of explicit steps in a protocol can substitute for the skills of a connoisseur.

CLINICAL JUDGMENT

To understand the contribution of the above five forms of reasoning, it is useful to consider each on its own. Expert clinicians, however, call on all these forms of reasoning, and blend them together without using each on an independent basis. The amalgam of these forms of reasoning constitute clinical judgment—a term widely used but rarely explicated.

Clinical judgment refers to the totality of mental resources and cognitive processes that a physician uses in deciding what to do for a particular patient. A good judge is someone who examines different pieces of evidence; he or she compares critically and impartially the merits of each, and makes a decision as to where the truth lies. An experienced clinician blends tacit and explicit knowledge in the process of making clinical decisions. Such blending of knowledge cannot be reduced to, or captured in, a mathematical model that would apply universally in all critically ill patients. It is obviously impossible to control or standardize tacit knowledge and clinical judgment among the clinicians participating in a randomized controlled trial. The marked variation in degree of skill among participating physicians is an important unmeasurable factor that can confound the outcome of a trial. Recognition of this factor has led to calls for the inclusion of an extra arm in a clinical trial that reflects the usual care of the participating physicians.

CONFLATION OF THERAPY AND MONITORING

The fundamental goal of monitoring is to guide a clinician in management decisions. Thus, monitoring is inextricably linked to treatment. A monitoring device on its own never cured anyone. It can improve outcome only if it leads to more effective therapy. This link is not always recognized. Yet it hovers over all assessments of a monitoring device. The conflation of monitoring with therapy differs from the evaluation of diagnostic techniques in other areas of medicine; a test is judged by its diagnostic accuracy, not on the expectation that it will improve outcome.

Consider the use of hemodynamic monitoring in an unstable patient with septic shock. Therapeutic options include fluids, vasopressors, or inotropic agents. None of these agents directly correct the underlying problem. Each may also cause harm. When a supranormal cardiac index was used as a target for hemodynamic management in 762 critically ill patients, survival was no better than with usual care.[178] When high-dose dobutamine was used to achieve a high cardiac index, Hayes et al[185] found that treated patients had a higher mortality than the usual care group: 54% versus 34%. In a complex patient with septic shock, when initial hemodynamic therapy is not successful, it is common to undertake invasive monitoring (often involving a PA catheter) to guide more aggressive therapy. An unsuccessful outcome in such patients may be the result of ineffective pharmacologic agents or complications caused by them. Yet, the results of such trials are commonly interpreted as evidence that hemodynamic monitoring is not effective.

PATIENT RESPONSE TO THERAPY

In medicine, we treat patients, not diseases. Patients have varying responses to therapy depending on their disease. Although the right therapy may be chosen (cefotaxime for meningococcemia), a patient may have an undesired response to the therapy, which worsens outcome. A PA catheter may be inserted in a patient in septic shock to guide therapy. The patient may develop cardiogenic pulmonary edema (with fluid resuscitation), a life-threatening arrhythmia (with dobutamine), or digital ischemia (with norepinephrine). These adverse reactions can outweigh beneficial effects of the monitoring device (the PA catheter) itself. No monitoring modality is likely to improve outcome unless it is combined with a therapeutic intervention that has a good benefit-risk ratio.

FINAL OUTCOME

An outcome event is an occurrence (such as death) that may be modified after implementing some intervention (monitoring wedge pressure with a PA catheter). Outcomes research is defined by the statistical analysis of clinical data to determine whether particular interventions are associated with particular results. To discriminate between benefits and risks of an intervention, an adequate sample size is necessary. Sample size is calculated on the basis of baseline event rate, expected benefit, level of significance (α) and the power to detect a difference $(1-\beta)$.[186] Studies evaluating the effect of monitoring on patient outcome often lack statistical power. Statistical power is especially important when complications are rare and the expected impact (of an intervention) is small. If the outcome under evaluation occurs frequently, fewer patients will be needed than if the outcome occurs infrequently. Moller et al[129,187] conducted a prospective, randomized trial of the effect of pulse oximetry on the rate of postoperative complications in 20,802 surgical patients. Hypoxemia (defined as a Sp_{O_2} <90%) was detected 19 times more often in the oximeter group than in the control group (p <0.0001). The primary goal of the study, however, was to determine whether the rate of postoperative complications was decreased. For this goal, statistical significance was not reached. The investigators concluded that it would take at least 500,000 patients to show a reduction in a rare event such as myocardial infarction and 1,900,000 patients to show a reduction in anesthesia-related deaths.

The American Society of Anesthesiologists introduced monitoring standards that mandated use of pulse oximetry in every patient undergoing anesthesia. Subsequently, Eichhorn[188] observed a threefold reduction in the incidence of major preventable intraoperative injury (10 in 757,000 versus 1 in 244,000 anesthetics), yet the reduction did not reach statistical significance. Because the incidence of serious adverse events is low, it is estimated that an additional 6,545,605 cases would be needed to detect a significant reduction in major preventable intraoperative injury.[11,189] Given the necessary effort, would anyone suggest that it makes sense to undertake such a study to find out if pulse oximetry is helpful during anesthesia? If the study were negative, would anesthesiologists stop using this monitoring device? Unlikely.

When anesthesiologists were surveyed in the study of Moller et al,[129,187] 80% of them felt more secure when they used a pulse oximeter. Of 104 anesthesiologists, 19 believed that the pulse oximeter helped them avoid serious complications (such as esophageal intubation, tracheal tube disconnection or displacement, anesthesia machine failure, and respiratory problems immediately after extubation). It is this mindset that has established pulse oximetry as an essential component of the standard of care despite a failure to achieve a p <0.05 level of proven efficacy. The lack of concurrence between proof of efficacy in randomized trials of pulse oximetry and its requirement as part of the standard of care has major ramifications for all monitoring techniques.

When researchers evaluate the usefulness of a monitoring device, the selected outcome measure (mortality or complication rates) may be unrealistic. If benefit is expected to be small, an outcome based on mortality may not be sufficiently sensitive to detect it. Undertaking inappropriately designed studies may cause valuable tools to be discarded. At face value, the outcome of the study of Moller et al[129] should lead physicians to stop using pulse oximetry—at least in the operating room.

Authors commonly cite examples where intermediate outcomes (prevention of hypertension, hypoxemia, or ischemia; or suppressing premature ventricular contractions following myocardial infarction) were misleading. A widely cited study is the CAST (Cardiac Arrhythmia Suppression Trial) study. This consisted of a randomized trial, which tested the hypothesis that suppression of asymptomatic or mildly symptomatic premature ventricular contractions (PVCs) with antiarrhythmic agents in patients who have suffered a myocardial infarction improves survival.[190–193] It was believed that suppression of PVCs would prevent ventricular tachycardia and ventricular fibrillation and thus decrease mortality. Patients treated with antiarrhythmic

agents (flecainide, encainide, or moricizine), however, had a higher mortality (8.0%, 63/755) than patients receiving placebo (3.5%, 26/743).

The increased mortality in the intervention arm of the CAST study is often interpreted as evidence that physiologic reasoning is unreliable, and that mortality is the only study outcome that reliably captures truth of efficacy.[56] Before accepting that conclusion, the data need to be closely scrutinized. A number of concerns arise. Mortality in the placebo group (3.5%) was much lower than expected.[194] The low mortality was partly a consequence of study design.[195,196] Only patients whose ventricular arrhythmias were suppressed during an open-label titration phase of the study were randomized to the active drug or placebo. Patients whose ventricular arrhythmias were not suppressed or who did not tolerate the pharmacologic agent were not randomized to either arm.[190,193] Thus, patients randomized into the study had a low risk for death for two reasons: the exclusion of patients who had died and exclusion of patients in whom arrhythmias could not be suppressed (with drugs) during the open-label titration (prerandomization) phase.[196] Of patients in the placebo arm, 80% had PVCs alone without having nonsustained ventricular tachycardia; moreover, more than half had a near-normal ejection fraction (above 40%).[193] There is further evidence that mortality in the placebo group is not generalizable. The CAST investigators undertook a subsequent analysis in the 318 patients who survived the open-label titration phase but who were not randomized to either arm of the study and the 942 patients who were randomized to the placebo arm.[197] Occurrence of death or a resuscitated cardiac arrest was higher in the nonrandomized patients (8.5%, 27/318) than in the placebo group (4%, 38/942).[197] In summary, the adverse effects of the antiarrhythmic agents in the CAST study may largely reflect the failure of the investigators to recruit representative patients into the placebo arm, insofar as the investigators excluded patients in whom they could not suppress their arrhythmias (a marker of increased mortality).[192,198–200] Certainly, it is inappropriate to use data from the CAST study to conclude that therapy guided by ECG monitoring (that is, physiologic reasoning) is not helpful.

Conclusion

Does the failure of research studies to show that monitoring devices improve patient outcome mean that monitoring has no place in modern critical care medicine? No. As discussed above, a critically ill patient is subjected to numerous insults, which change rapidly and unpredictably. Thus, it is almost impossible to undertake a randomized controlled trial that will demonstrate that a monitoring device improves outcome. This consideration, however, will not stop investigators from undertaking further studies. And negative results will be taken to mean that the monitoring device is not beneficial (and should be discarded). Most monitors in common use were introduced in the absence of data demonstrating a benefit on outcome. Ethical concerns arise when designing a study to evaluate a technology that is already in use. When physicians already believe a procedure is beneficial, they are reluctant to enter patients into a trial to test its efficacy. If a substantial number of physicians are unwilling to randomize patients, it becomes impossible to achieve an adequate study sample.

Should we advocate the undertaking of randomized trials before introducing all new technologies into the ICU? To pursue that line of reasoning with logical consistency would mean that we discard many techniques that physicians believe help their patients—not only in the ICU but elsewhere. And what would be the basis for such an action? Because a device has not been proven to be of benefit in a randomized controlled trial? When such an ideology guides our actions, a trialist's pursuit of certainty becomes harmful to patients.

Acknowledgments

This work was supported by a Merit Review grant from the Veterans Administration Research Service.

References

1. Tobin, MJ. Principles and practice of intensive care monitoring. New York: McGraw-Hill, 1998.
2. Tobin MJ. State of the art: Respiratory monitoring in the intensive care unit. Am Rev Respir Dis 1988; 138:1625–42.
3. Pierson DJ. Goals and indications for monitoring. In: Tobin MJ, editor. Principles and practice of intensive care monitoring. New York: McGraw-Hill, 1998: 33–44.
4. Chatburn RL. Principles of measurement. In: Tobin MJ, editor. Principles and practice of intensive care monitoring. New York: McGraw-Hill, 1998: 45–61.
5. Gallagher CG. Measurement of respiratory pressures. In: Tobin MJ, editor. Principles and practice of intensive care monitoring. New York: McGraw-Hill, 1998: 81–90.
6. O'Donnell D, Webb K. Measurement of respired flow and volume. In: Tobin MJ, editor. Principles and practice of intensive care monitoring. New York: McGraw-Hill, 1998: 63–80.
7. Van de Louw A, Cracco C, Cerf C, et al. Accuracy of pulse oximetry in the intensive care unit. Intensive Care Med 2001; 27: 1606–13.
8. Emergency Care Research Institute. Next-generation pulse oximetry. Health Devices 2003; 32:49–103.
9. Jubran A. Pulse oximetry. Intensive Care Med 2004; 30:2017–20.
10. Jubran A, Tobin MJ. Reliability of pulse oximetry in titrating supplemental oxygen therapy in ventilator-dependent patients. Chest 1990; 97:1420–25.
11. Jubran A. Pulse oximetry. In: Tobin MJ, editor. Principles and practice of intensive care monitoring. New York: McGraw-Hill, 1998: 261–87.
12. Stetz CW, Miller RG, Kelly GE, Raffin TA. Reliability of the thermodilution method in the determination of cardiac output in clinical practice. Am Rev Respir Dis 1982; 126:1001–4.
13. Fallat R, McQuitty J. Bedside testing and intensive care monitoring of pulmonary function. In: Clausen JL, editor. Pulmonary function testing, guidelines and controversies. Orlando, FL: Grune and Stratton, 1982: 294–310.
14. Jubran A, Tobin MJ. Monitoring during mechanical ventilation. In: Marini JJ, Nahum A, editors. Clinics in Chest Medicine 1996; 17:453–73.
15. Multz AS, Aldrich TK, Prezant DJ, Karpel JP, Hendler JM. Maximal inspiratory pressure is not a reliable test of inspiratory muscle strength in mechanically ventilated patients. Am Rev Respir Dis 1990; 142:529–32.
16. Proulx PA, Harf A, Lorino H, Atlan G, Laurent D. Dynamic characteristics of air-filled differential pressure transducers. J Appl Physiol 1979; 46:608–14.
17. Gabe I. Pressure measurement in experimental physiology. In: Bergek D, editor. Cardiovascular fluid dynamics. London: Academic Press, 1972.
18. Fry D, Stead W, Ebert R, Lubin R, Wells H. The measurement of intraesophageal pressure and its relationship to intrathoracic pressure. J Lab Clin Med 1952; 40:664–73.
19. Tobin MJ. Monitoring respiratory mechanics in spontaneously breathing patients. In: Tobin MJ, editor. Principles and practice of intensive care monitoring. New York: McGraw-Hill, 1998: 617–53.
20. Severinghaus JW, Naifeh KH. Accuracy of response of six pulse oximeters to profound hypoxia. Anesthesiology 1987; 67:551–8.
21. Kagle DM, Alexander CM, Berko RS, Giuffre M, Gross JB. Evaluation of the Ohmeda 3700 pulse oximeter: steady-state and transient response characteristics. Anesthesiology 1987; 66: 376–80.
22. Young D, Jewkes C, Spittal M, et al. Response time of pulse oximeters assessed using acute decompression. Anesth Analg 1992; 74:189–95.
23. Morris AH, Chapman RH, Gardner RM. Frequency of technical problems encountered in the measurement of pulmonary artery wedge pressure. Crit Care Med 1984; 12:164–70.
24. Leatherman JW, Marini JJ. Pulmonary artery catheterization: interpretation of pressure recordings. In: Tobin MJ, editor. Principles and practice of intensive care monitoring. New York: McGraw-Hill, 1998: 821–37.
25. Sullivan W, Peters GM, Enright P. Pneumotachographs: theory and clinical application. Respir Care 1984; 736–49.
26. Standardization of Spirometry, 1994 Update. American Thoracic Society. Am J Respir Crit Care Med 1995; 152:1107–36.
27. Kreit JW, Sciurba FC. The accuracy of pneumotachograph measurements during mechanical ventilation. Am J Respir Crit Care Med 1996; 154:913–17.
28. Tyson N. Signal versus noise. Nat Hist 1996; 105:72–76.
29. Gardner RM. Fidelity of recording: improving the signal-to-noise ratio. In: Tobin MJ, editor. Principles and practice of intensive care monitoring. New York: McGraw-Hill, 1998: 123–32.
30. Tsien CL, Fackler JC. Poor prognosis for existing monitors in the intensive care unit. Crit Care Med 1997; 25:614–19.
31. Gardner RM, Hollingsworth KW. Optimizing the electrocardiogram and pressure monitoring. Crit Care Med 1986; 14:651–8.
32. Dumas C, Wahr JA, Tremper KK. Clinical evaluation of a prototype motion artifact resistant pulse oximeter in the recovery room. Anesth Analg 1996; 83:269–72.
33. Amar D, Neidzwski J, Wald A, Finck AD. Fluorescent light interferes with pulse oximetry. J Clin Monit 1989; 5:135–6.
34. Levy H, Servilla M, Simpson SQ. Oximeter malfunction (letter). Chest 1995; 105:975.
35. Munley AJ, Sik MJ. An unpredictable and possibly dangerous artefact affecting a pulse oximeter. Anaesthesia 1988; 43:334.
36. Gardner R, Monis S, Oehler P. Monitoring direct blood pressure: algorithm enhancements. IEEE Comput Cardiol 1986; 13:607–10.
37. Chambrin MC, Ravaux P, Calvelo-Aros D, et al. Multicentric study of monitoring alarms in the adult intensive care unit (ICU): a descriptive analysis. Intensive Care Med 1999; 25:1360–6.
38. Lawless ST. Crying wolf: False alarms in a pediatric intensive care unit. Crit Care Med 1994; 22:981–5.
39. Wiklund L, Hok B, Stahl K, Jordeby-Jonsson A. Postanesthesia monitoring revisited: Frequency of true and false alarms from different monitoring devices. J Clin Anesth 1994; 6:182–188.

40. Topf M, Dillon E. Noise-induced stress as a predictor of burnout in critical care nurses. Heart Lung 1988; 17:567–73.

41. Eccles RC, Swinamer DL, Jones RL, King EG. Validation of a compact system for measuring gas exchange. Crit Care Med 1986; 14:807–11.

42. Westenskow DR, Cutler CA, Wallace WD. Instrumentation for monitoring gas exchange and metabolic rate in critically ill patients. Crit Care Med 1984; 12:183–7.

43. Rossi A, Gottfried SB, Zocchi L, et al. Measurement of static compliance of the total respiratory system in patients with acute respiratory failure during mechanical ventilation: the effect of intrinsic PEEP. Am Rev Respir Dis 1985; 131:672–7.

44. Kress JP, O'Connor MF, Schmidt GA. Clinical examination reliably detects intrinsic positive end-expiratory pressure in critically ill, mechanically ventilated patients. Am J Respir Crit Care Med 1999; 159:290–4.

45. Larson JL, Covey MK, Vitalo CA, et al. Maximal inspiratory pressure: learning effect and test-retest reliability in patients with chronic obstructive pulmonary disease. Chest 1993; 104:448–53.

46. Truwit JD, Marini JJ. Validation of a technique to assess maximal inspiratory pressure in poorly cooperative patients. Chest 1992; 102:1216–9.

47. Singer AJ, Hollander JE. Blood pressure. Assessment of interarm differences. Arch Intern Med 1996; 156:2005–8.

48. Thorson SH, Marini JJ, Pierson DJ, Hudson LD. Variability of arterial blood gas values in stable patients in the ICU. Chest 1983; 84:14–18.

49. Hess D, Agarwal NN. Variability of blood gases, pulse oximeter saturation, and end-tidal carbon dioxide pressure in stable, mechanically ventilated trauma patients. J Clin Monit 1992; 8: 111–5.

50. Freund PR, Overand PT, Cooper J, et al. A prospective study of intraoperative pulse oximetry failure. J Clin Monit 1991; 7:253–8.

51. Reich DL, Timcenko A, Bodian CA, et al. Predictors of pulse oximetry data failure. Anesthesiology 1996; 84:859–64.

52. Stoneham MD, Saville GM, Wilson IH. Knowledge about pulse oximetry among medical and nursing staff. Lancet 1994; 344:1339–42.

53. Iberti TJ, Fischer EP, Leibowitz AB, et al. A multicenter study of physicians' knowledge of the pulmonary artery catheter. Pulmonary Artery Catheter Study Group. JAMA 1990; 264:2928–32.

54. Burns D, Burns D, Shively M. Critical care nurses' knowledge of pulmonary artery catheters. Am J Crit Care 1996; 5:49–54.

55. Cox CE, Carson SS, Ely EW, et al. Effectiveness of medical resident education in mechanical ventilation. Am J Respir Crit Care Med 2003; 167:32–38.

56. Morris AH. Algorithm-based decision making. In: Tobin MJ, editor. Principles and practice of intensive care monitoring. New York: McGraw-Hill, 1998: 1355–82.

57. Miller GA. The magical number seven, plus or minus two: some limits on our capacity for processing information. Psychol Rev 1956; 63:81–97.

58. Tobin MJ. Preface. In: Tobin MJ, editor. Principles and practice of intensive care monitoring. McGraw-Hill, 1998: xix–xv.

59. Marini JJ, Smith TC, Lamb VJ. External work output and force generation during synchronized intermittent mechanical ventilation: effect of machine assistance on breathing effort. Am Rev Respir Dis 1988; 138:1169–79.

60. Brochard L, Rauss A, Benito S, et al. Comparison of three methods of gradual withdrawing from ventilatory support during weaning from mechanical ventilation. Am J Respir Crit Care Med 1994; 150:896–903.

61. Esteban A, Frutos F, Tobin MJ, et al. A comparison of four methods of weaning patients from mechanical ventilation. N Engl J Med 1995; 332:345–50.

62. Rajacich N, Burchard KW, Hasan FM, Singh AK. Central venous pressure and pulmonary capillary wedge pressure as estimates of left atrial pressure: effects of positive end-expiratory pressure and catheter tip malposition. Crit Care Med 1989; 17:7–11.

63. Calvin JE, Driedger AA, Sibbald WJ. Does the pulmonary capillary wedge pressure predict left ventricular preload in critically ill patients? Crit Care Med 1981; 9:437–43.

64. Ishida T, Lee T, Shimabukuro T, Niinami H. Right ventricular end-diastolic volume monitoring after cardiac surgery. Ann Thorac Cardiovasc Surg 2004; 10:167–70.

65. Lichtwarck-Aschoff M, Zeravik J, Pfeiffer UJ. Intrathoracic blood volume accurately reflects circulatory volume status in critically ill patients with mechanical ventilation. Intensive Care Med 1992; 18:142–7.

66. Buhre W, Weyland A, Schorn B, et al. Changes in central venous pressure and pulmonary capillary wedge pressure do not indicate changes in right and left heart volume in patients undergoing coronary artery bypass surgery. Eur J Anaesthesiol 1999; 16:11–17.

67. Reuse C, Vincent JL, Pinsky MR. Measurements of right ventricular volumes during fluid challenge. Chest 1990; 98:1450–54.

68. Calvin JE, Driedger AA, Sibbald WJ. The hemodynamic effect of rapid fluid infusion in critically ill patients. Surgery 1981; 90:61–76.

69. East T, Morris A, Wallace J, et al. Can pulse oximetry be used reliably to predict arterial oxygenation? Crit Care Med 1995; 23:A27.

70. Axler O, Tousignant C, Thompson CR, et al. Comparison of transesophageal echocardiographic, fick, and thermodilution cardiac output in critically ill patients. J Crit Care 1996; 11:109–16.

71. Bates JHT, Rossi A, Milic-Emili J. Analysis of the behaviour of the respiratory system with constant inspiratory flow. J Appl Physiol 1985; 58:1840–48.

72. Polese G, Rossi A, Appendini L, et al. Partitioning of respiratory mechanics in mechanically ventilated patients. J Appl Physiol 1991; 71:2425–33.

73. Guerin C, Coussa ML, Eissa NT, et al. Lung and chest wall mechanics in mechanically ventilated COPD patients. J Appl Physiol 1993; 74:1570–80.

74. Jubran A, Tobin MJ. Passive mechanics of lung and chest wall in patients who failed and succeeded in trials of weaning. Am J Respir Crit Care Med 1997; 155:916–21.

75. Gattinoni L, Pelosi P, Suter PM, et al. Acute respiratory distress syndrome caused by pulmonary and extrapulmonary disease. Different syndromes? Am J Respir Crit Care Med 1998; 158:3–11.

76. Tobin MJ, Jubran A, Laghi F. Patient-ventilator interaction. Am J Respir Crit Care Med 2001; 163:1059–63.

77. Parthasarathy S, Jubran A, Tobin MJ. Cycling of inspiratory and expiratory muscle groups with the ventilator in airflow limitation. Am J Respir Crit Care Med 1998; 158:1471–78.

78. Lessard MR, Lofaso F, Brochard L. Expiratory muscle activity increases intrinsic positive end-expiratory pressure independently of dynamic hyperinflation in mechanically ventilated patients. Am J Respir Crit Care Med 1995; 151:562–69.

79. Smith TC, Marini JJ. Impact of PEEP on lung mechanics and work of breathing in severe airflow obstruction. J Appl Physiol 1988; 65:1488–99.

80. Petrof BJ, Legaré M, Goldberg P, Milic-Emili J, Gottfried SB. Continuous positive airway pressure reduces work of breathing and dyspnea during weaning from mechanical ventilation in severe chronic obstructive pulmonary disease. Am Rev Respir Dis 1990; 141:281–89.

81. Ninane V, Yernault JC, DeTroyer A. Intrinsic PEEP in patients with chronic obstructive pulmonary disease: role of expiratory muscles. Am Rev Respir Dis 1993; 148:1037–42.

82. Ranieri VM, Guiliani R, Cinnella G, et al. Physiologic effects of positive end-expiratory pressure in patients with chronic obstructive pulmonary disease during acute ventilatory failure and controlled mechanical ventilation. Am Rev Respir Dis 1993; 147:5–13.

83. Jubran A, Tobin MJ. Pathophysiological basis of acute respiratory distress in patients who fail a trial of weaning from mechanical ventilation. Am J Respir Crit Care Med 1997; 155:906–15.

84. Birmingham PK, Cheney FW, Ward RJ. Esophageal intubation: a review of detection techniques. Anesth Analg 1986; 65: 886–91.

85. Vaghadia H, Jenkins LC, Ford RW. Comparison of end-tidal carbon dioxide, oxygen saturation and clinical signs for the detection of oesophageal intubation. Can J Anaesth 1989; 36:560–64.

86. Linko K, Paloheimo M, Tammisto T. Capnography for detection of accidental oesophageal intubation. Acta Anaesthesiol Scand 1983; 27:199–202.

87. Knapp S, Kofler J, Stoiser B, et al. The assessment of four different methods to verify tracheal tube placement in the critical care setting. Anesth Analg 1999; 88:766–70.

88. Jubran A, Tobin MJ. Use of flow-volume curves in detecting secretions in ventilator-dependent patients. Am J Respir Crit Care Med 1994; 150:766–69.

89. Rossi A, Polese G, Brandi G, Conti G. The intrinsic positive end expiratory pressure (PEEPi): physiology, implications, measurement, and treatment. Intensive Care Med 1995; 21:522–36.

90. Pepe PE, Marini JJ. Occult positive end-expiratory pressure in mechanically ventilated patients with airflow obstruction. Am Rev Respir Dis 1982; 126:166–70.

91. Lapinsky SE, Leung RS. Auto-PEEP and electromechanical dissociation. N Engl J Med 1996; 335:674(letter).

92. Leung P, Jubran A, Tobin MJ. Comparison of assisted ventilator modes on triggering, patient effort, and dyspnea. Am J Respir Crit Care Med 1997; 155:1940–48.

93. Coussa ML, Guerin C, Eissa NT, et al. Partitioning of work of breathing in mechanically ventilated COPD patients. J Appl Physiol 1993; 75:1711–19.

94. Yang K, Tobin MJ. A prospective study of indexes predicting outcome of trials of weaning from mechanical ventilation. N Engl J Med 1991; 324:1445–50.

95. Dhand R, Jubran A, Tobin MJ. Efficacy of bronchodilator delivered by metered-dose inhaler in ventilator-supported patients with COPD. Am J Respir Crit Care Med 1995; 152:129–36.

96. Dhand R, Duarte AG, Jubran A, et al. Dose response to bronchodilator delivered by metered-dose inhaler in ventilator-supported patients. Am J Respir Crit Care Med 1996; 154: 388–93.

97. MacIntyre NR. Respiratory function during pressure support ventilation. Chest 1986; 89:677–83.

98. Brochard L, Harf A, Lorino H, Lemaire F. Inspiratory pressure support prevents diaphragmatic fatigue during weaning from mechanical ventilation. Am Rev Respir Dis 1989; 139:513–21.

99. Kimura T, Takezawa J, Nishiwaki K, Shimada Y. Determination of the optimal pressure support level evaluated by measuring transdiaphragmatic pressure. Chest 1991; 100:112–17.

100. MacIntyre NR, Ho L. Effects of initial flow rate and breath termination criteria on pressure support ventilation. Chest 1991; 99:134–38.

101. Jubran A, Van de Graaff WB, Tobin MJ. Variability of patient-ventilator interaction with pressure-support ventilation in patients with COPD. Am J Respir Crit Care Med 1995; 152: 129–36.

102. Rouby JJ, Lu Q, Goldstein I. Selecting the right level of positive end-expiratory pressure in patients with acute respiratory distress syndrome. Am J Respir Crit Care Med 2002; 165:1182–86.

103. Richard JC, Maggiore SM, Jonson B, et al. Influence of tidal volume on alveolar recruitment. Respective role of PEEP and a recruitment maneuver. Am J Respir Crit Care Med 2001; 163: 1609–13.

104. Suter PM, Fairley B, Isenberg MD. Optimum end-expiratory airway pressure in patients with acute pulmonary failure. N Engl J Med 1975; 292:284–89.

105. Lachmann B. Open up the lung and keep the lung open. Intensive Care Med 1992; 18:319–21.

106. Brochard L. Respiratory pressure-volume curves. In: Tobin MJ, editor. Principles and practice of intensive care monitoring. New York: McGraw-Hill, 1998: 597–616.

107. Goldstein I, Bughalo MT, Marquette CH, et al. Mechanical ventilation-induced air-space enlargement during experimental pneumonia in piglets. Am J Respir Crit Care Med 2001; 163: 958–64.

108. Rouby JJ, Lherm T, Martin DL, et al. Histologic aspects of pulmonary barotrauma in critically ill patients with acute respiratory failure. Intensive Care Med 1993; 19:383–89.

109. Roupie E, Dambrosio M, Servillo G, et al. Titration of tidal volume and induced hypercapnia in acute respiratory distress syndrome. Am J Respir Crit Care Med 1995; 152:121–28.

110. Matamis D, Lemaire F, Harf A, et al. Total respiratory pressure-volume curves in the adult respiratory distress syndrome. Chest 1984; 86:58–66.

111. Tobin MJ. Advances in mechanical ventilation. N Engl J Med 2001; 344:1986–96.

112. Vieira SR, Puybasset L, Lu Q, et al. A scanographic assessment of pulmonary morphology in acute lung injury. Significance of the lower inflection point detected on the lung pressure-volume curve. Am J Respir Crit Care Med 1999; 159:1612–23.

113. Puybasset L, Gusman P, Muller JC, et al. Regional distribution of gas and tissue in acute respiratory distress syndrome. III. Consequences for the effects of positive end-expiratory pressure. CT Scan ARDS Study Group. Adult Respiratory Distress Syndrome. Intensive Care Med 2000; 26:1215–27.

114. Amato MBP, Barbas CSV, Medeiros D, et al. Effect of a protective-ventilation strategy on mortality in the acute respiratory distress syndrome. N Engl J Med 1998; 338:347–54.

115. Laghi F, Segal J, Choe WK, Tobin MJ. Effect of imposed inflation time on respiratory frequency and hyperinflation in patients with chronic obstructive pulmonary disease. Am J Respir Crit Care Med 2001; 163:1365–70.

116. Ward ME, Corbeil C, Gibbons W, Newman S, Macklem PT. Optimization of respiratory muscle relaxation during mechanical ventilation. Anesthesiology 1988; 69:29–35.

117. Chao DC, Scheinhorn DJ, Stearn-Hassenpflug M. Patient-ventilator trigger asynchrony in prolonged mechanical ventilation. Chest 1997; 112:1592–99.

118. Purro A, Appendini L, De Gaetano A, et al. Physiologic determinants of ventilator dependence in long-term mechanically ventilated patients. Am J Respir Crit Care Med 2000; 161: 1115–23.

119. Gattinoni L, Pesenti A, Avalli L, Rossi F, Bombino M. Pressure-volume curve of total respiratory system in acute respiratory failure: computed tomographic scan study. Am Rev Respir Dis 1987; 136:730–36.

120. Slutsky AS. Mechanical ventilation. Chest 1993; 104:1833–59.

121. Dreyfuss D, Saumon G. Ventilator-induced lung injury: lessons from experimental studies. Am J Respir Crit Care Med 1998; 157:294–323.

122. Tobin MJ. Mechanical ventilation. N Engl J Med 1994; 330: 1056–61.

123. Ventilation with lower tidal volumes as compared with traditional tidal volumes for acute lung injury and the acute

respiratory distress syndrome. The Acute Respiratory Distress Syndrome Network. N Engl J Med 2000; 342:1301–8.

124. Tobin MJ. Culmination of an era in research on the acute respiratory distress syndrome [editorial]. N Engl J Med 2000; 342: 1360–61.

125. Henschke CI, Pasternack GS, Schroeder S, Hart KK, Herman PG. Bedside chest radiography: diagnostic efficacy. Radiology 1983; 149:23–26.

126. Fong Y, Whalen GF, Hariri RJ, Barie PS. Utility of routine chest radiographs in the surgical intensive care unit. A prospective study. Arch Surg 1995; 130:764–68.

127. Hall JB, White SR, Karrison T. Efficacy of daily routine chest radiographs in intubated, mechanically ventilated patients. Crit Care Med 1991; 19:689–93.

128. Steier M, Ching N, Roberts EB, Nealon TF Jr. Pneumothorax complicating continuous ventilatory support. J Thorac Cardiovasc Surg 1974; 67:17–23.

129. Moller JT, Johannessen NW, Espersen K, et al. Randomized evaluation of pulse oximetry in 20,802 patients: II. Perioperative events and postoperative complications. Anesthesiology 1993; 78:445–53.

130. Marsh RH, Weir PM, Marshall RD. Faults in expiratory valves. Anaesthesia 1985; 40:505–6.

131. Johnson T. A sticking valve. Anaesthesia 1993; 48:89.

132. Ryan TJ, Antman EM, Brooks NH, et al. 1999 update: ACC/AHA Guidelines for the Management of Patients with Acute Myocardial Infarction: Executive Summary and Recommendations: A report of the American College of Cardiology/American Heart Association Task Force on Practice Guidelines (Committee on Management of Acute Myocardial Infarction). Circulation 1999; 100:1016–30.

133. Antman EM, Anbe DT, Armstrong PW, et al. ACC/AHA guidelines for the management of patients with ST-elevation myocardial infarction—executive summary: a report of the American College of Cardiology/American Heart Association Task Force on Practice Guidelines (Writing Committee to Revise the 1999 Guidelines for the Management of Patients with Acute Myocardial Infarction). Circulation 2004; 110:588–636.

134. Tinker JH, Dull DL, Caplan RA, Ward RJ, Cheney FW. Role of monitoring devices in prevention of anesthetic mishaps: a closed claims analysis. Anesthesiology 1989; 71:541–46.

135. Weil M. Patient evaluation, "vital signs", and initial care. In: Shoemaker W, Thompson W, editors. Critical care, state of the art. Fullerton, CA: Society of Critical Care Medicine, 1980: 1–31.

136. Shapiro BA, Warren J, Egol AB, et al. Practice parameters for sustained neuromuscular blockade in the adult critically ill patient: an executive summary. Society of Critical Care Medicine. Crit Care Med 1995; 23:1601–5.

137. Rudis MI, Sikora CA, Angus E, et al. A prospective, randomized, controlled evaluation of peripheral nerve stimulation versus standard clinical dosing of neuromuscular blocking agents in critically ill patients. Crit Care Med 1997; 25:575–83.

138. Strange C, Vaughan L, Franklin C, Johnson J. Comparison of train-of-four and best clinical assessment during continuous paralysis. Am J Respir Crit Care Med 1997; 156:1556–61.

139. Strange C. Peripheral neuromuscular function. In: Tobin MJ, editor. Principles and practice of intensive care monitoring. New York: McGraw-Hill, 1998: 1047–55.

140. Kramer DJ. Liver function monitoring in the critically ill patient. In: Tobin MJ, editor. Principles and practice of intensive care monitoring. New York: McGraw-Hill, 1998: 1085–98.

141. Rumack BH, Peterson RC, Koch GG, Amara IA. Acetaminophen overdose. 662 cases with evaluation of oral acetylcysteine treatment. Arch Intern Med 1981; 141:380–85.

142. Susla G. Therapeutic drug monitoring in intensive care. In: Tobin MJ, editor. Principles and practice of intensive care monitoring. New York: McGraw-Hill, 1998: 1162–91.

143. Jubran A, Grant BJ, Laghi F, Parthasarathy S, Tobin MJ. Weaning prediction: esophageal pressure monitoring complements readiness testing. Am J Respir Crit Care Med 2005; 171:1252–59.

144. Gottlieb SO, Weisfeldt ML, Ouyang P, Mellits ED, Gerstenblith G. Silent ischemia as a marker for early unfavorable outcomes in patients with unstable angina. N Engl J Med 1986; 314:1214–19.

145. Norgaard BL, Andersen K, Dellborg M, et al. Admission risk assessment by cardiac troponin T in unstable coronary artery disease: additional prognostic information from continuous ST segment monitoring. TRIM study group. Thrombin Inhibition in Myocardial Ischemia. J Am Coll Cardiol 1999; 33: 1519–27.

146. Akkerhuis KM, Maas AC, Klootwijk PA, et al. Recurrent ischemia during continuous 12-lead ECG-ischemia monitoring in patients with acute coronary syndromes treated with eptifibatide: relation with death and myocardial infarction. PURSUIT ECG-Ischemia Monitoring Substudy Investigators. Platelet glycoprotein IIb/IIIa in unstable angina: Receptor Suppression Using Integrilin Therapy. J Electrocardiol 2000; 33:127–36.

147. Andersen K, Eriksson P, Dellborg M. Non-invasive risk stratification within 48 h of hospital admission in patients with unstable coronary disease. Eur Heart J 1997; 18:780–88.

148. Klootwijk P, Meij S, Melkert R, Lenderink T, Simoons ML. Reduction of recurrent ischemia with abciximab during continuous ECG-ischemia monitoring in patients with unstable angina refractory to standard treatment (CAPTURE). Circulation 1998; 98:1358–64.

149. Randomised placebo-controlled trial of abciximab before and during coronary intervention in refractory unstable angina: the CAPTURE Study. Lancet 1997; 349:1429–35.

150. Akkerhuis KM, Neuhaus KL, Wilcox RG, et al. Safety and preliminary efficacy of one month glycoprotein IIb/IIIa inhibition with lefradafiban in patients with acute coronary syndromes without ST-elevation; a phase II study. Eur Heart J 2000; 21: 2042–55.

151. Akkerhuis KM, Klootwijk PA, Lindeboom W, et al. Recurrent ischaemia during continuous multilead ST-segment monitoring identifies patients with acute coronary syndromes at high risk of adverse cardiac events; meta-analysis of three studies involving 995 patients. Eur Heart J 2001; 22:1997–2006.

152. Kost GJ. Point-of-care testing in intensive care. In: Tobin MJ, editor. Principles and practice of intensive care monitoring. New York: McGraw-Hill, 1998: 1267–96.

153. Kost GJ. New whole blood analyzers and their impact on cardiac and critical care. Crit Rev Clin Lab Sci 1993; 30:153–202.

154. Cowan BN, Burns HJ, Boyle P, Ledingham IM. The relative prognostic value of lactate and haemodynamic measurements in early shock. Anaesthesia 1984; 39:750–55.

155. Broder G, Weil M. Excess lactate: An index of reversibility of shock in human patients. Science 1964; 143:1457–59.

156. Mavric Z, Zaputovic L, Zagar D, Matana A, Smokvina D. Usefulness of blood lactate as a predictor of shock development in acute myocardial infarction. Am J Cardiol 1991; 67:565–68.

157. Sandham JD, Hull RD, Brant RF, et al. A randomized, controlled trial of the use of pulmonary-artery catheters in high-risk surgical patients. N Engl J Med 2003; 348:5–14.

158. Richard C, Warszawski J, Anguel N, et al. Early use of the pulmonary artery catheter and outcomes in patients with shock and acute respiratory distress syndrome: a randomized controlled trial. JAMA 2003; 290:2713–20.

159. Harvey S, Harrison DA, Singer M, et al. Assessment of the clinical effectiveness of pulmonary artery catheters in management

of patients in intensive care (PAC-Man): a randomised controlled trial. Lancet 2005; 366:472–77.

160. Scadding J. Principles of definition in medicine with special reference to chronic bronchitis and emphysema. Lancet 1954; I:323–25.

161. Connors AF Jr, Speroff T, Dawson NV, et al. The effectiveness of right heart catheterization in the initial care of critically ill patients. SUPPORT Investigators. JAMA 1996; 276:889–97.

162. Connors AF Jr, McCaffree DR, Gray BA. Evaluation of right-heart catheterization in the critically ill patient without acute myocardial infarction. N Engl J Med 1983; 308:263–67.

163. Eisenberg PR, Jaffe AS, Schuster DP. Clinical evaluation compared to pulmonary artery catheterization in the hemodynamic assessment of critically ill patients. Crit Care Med 1984; 12:549–53.

164. Connolly D, Kirklin J, Wood E. The relationship between pulmonary artery wedge pressure and left atrial pressure in man. Circ Res 1954; 2:434–40.

165. Lappas D, Lell WA, Gabel JC, Civetta JM, Lowenstein E. Indirect measurement of left-atrial pressure in surgical patients—pulmonary-capillary wedge and pulmonary-artery diastolic pressures compared with left-atrial pressure. Anesthesiology 1973; 38:394–97.

166. Morris AH, Chapman RH, Gardner RM. Frequency of wedge pressure errors in the ICU. Crit Care Med 1985; 13:705–8.

167. Iberti TJ, Daily EK, Leibowitz AB, et al. Assessment of critical care nurses' knowledge of the pulmonary artery catheter. The Pulmonary Artery Catheter Study Group. Crit Care Med 1994; 22:1674–78.

168. Gnaegi A, Feihl F, Perret C. Intensive care physicians' insufficient knowledge of right-heart catheterization at the bedside: time to act? Crit Care Med 1997; 25:213–20.

169. Komadina KH, Schenk DA, LaVeau P, Duncan CA, Chambers SL. Interobserver variability in the interpretation of pulmonary artery catheter pressure tracings. Chest 1991; 100:1647–54.

170. Epstein SK, Pauker SG. Principles of clinical decision making. In: Tobin MJ, editor. Principles and practice of intensive care monitoring. New York: McGraw-Hill, 1998: 149–72.

171. Kassirer JP. Diagnostic reasoning. Ann Intern Med 1989; 110:893–900.

172. Sox HC. Probability theory in the use of diagnostic tests: application to critical study of the literature. In: Sox HC Jr, editor. Common diagnostic tests: Use and interpretation. Philadelphia: American College of Physicians, 1987: 1–17.

173. Fagan T. Nomogram for Bayes' theorem. N Engl J Med 1975; 293:257.

174. Magder S. Cardiac output. In: Tobin MJ, editor. Principles and practice of intensive care monitoring. New York: McGraw-Hill, 1998: 797–810.

175. Connors AF Jr. Pulmonary artery catheterization: role in clinical decision making. In: Tobin MJ, editor. Principles and practice of intensive care monitoring. New York: McGraw-Hill, 1998: 839–54.

176. Forrester JS, Diamond GA, Swan HJ. Correlative classification of clinical and hemodynamic function after acute myocardial infarction. Am J Cardiol 1977; 39:137–45.

177. Tanenbaum SJ. Knowing and acting in medical practice: the epistemological politics of outcomes research. J Health Polit Policy Law 1994; 19:27–44.

178. Gattinoni L, Brazzi L, Pelosi P, et al. A trial of goal-oriented hemodynamic therapy in critically ill patients. SvO2 Collaborative Group. N Engl J Med 1995; 333:1025–32.

179. Mitchell JP, Schuller D, Calandrino FS, Schuster DP. Improved outcome based on fluid management in critically ill patients requiring pulmonary artery catheterization. Am Rev Respir Dis 1992; 145:990–98.

180. Eisenberg PR, Hansbrough JR, Anderson D, Schuster DP. A prospective study of lung water measurements during patient management in an intensive care unit. Am Rev Respir Dis 1987; 136:662–68.

181. Beauchamp T, Childress J. Principles of biomedical ethics, 5th ed. New York: Oxford University Press, 2001.

182. Tonelli MR. The philosophical limits of evidence-based medicine. Acad Med 1998; 73:1234–40.

183. Klein G. Sources of power: How people make decisions. Cambridge: The MIT Press, 1999.

184. Polanyi M. Personal knowledge: Towards a post-critical philosophy. London: Routledge and Kegan Paul, 1958.

185. Hayes MA, Timmins AC, Yau EH, et al. Elevation of systemic oxygen delivery in the treatment of critically ill patients. N Engl J Med 1994; 330:1717–22.

186. Hebert PC, Cook DJ, Wells G, Marshall J. The design of randomized clinical trials in critically ill patients. Chest 2002; 121:1290–300.

187. Moller JT, Pedersen T, Rasmussen LS, et al. Randomized evaluation of pulse oximetry in 20,802 patients: I. Design, demography, pulse oximetry failure rate and overall complication rate. Anesthesiology 1993; 78:436–44.

188. Eichhorn JH. Effect of monitoring standards on anesthesia outcome. Int Anesthesiol Clin 1993; 31:181–90.

189. Orkin FK. Practice standards: the Midas touch or the emperor's new clothes? Anesthesiology 1989; 70:567–71.

190. Echt DS, Liebson PR, Mitchell LB, et al. Mortality and morbidity in patients receiving encainide, flecainide, or placebo. The Cardiac Arrhythmia Suppression Trial. N Engl J Med 1991; 324:781–88.

191. Effect of the antiarrhythmic agent moricizine on survival after myocardial infarction. The Cardiac Arrhythmia Suppression Trial II Investigators. N Engl J Med 1992; 327:227–33.

192. Epstein AE, Hallstrom AP, Rogers WJ, et al. Mortality following ventricular arrhythmia suppression by encainide, flecainide, and moricizine after myocardial infarction. The original design concept of the Cardiac Arrhythmia Suppression Trial (CAST). JAMA 1993; 270:2451–55.

193. Preliminary report: effect of encainide and flecainide on mortality in a randomized trial of arrhythmia suppression after myocardial infarction. The Cardiac Arrhythmia Suppression Trial (CAST) Investigators. N Engl J Med 1989; 321:406–12.

194. The cardiac arrhythmia suppression trial. N Engl J Med 1989; 321:1754–56.

195. Epstein AE, Bigger JT Jr, Wyse DG, et al. Events in the Cardiac Arrhythmia Suppression Trial (CAST): mortality in the entire population enrolled. J Am Coll Cardiol 1991; 18:14–19.

196. Ruskin JN. The cardiac arrhythmia suppression trial (CAST). N Engl J Med 1989; 321:386–88.

197. Wyse DG, Hallstrom A, McBride R, et al. Events in the Cardiac Arrhythmia Suppression Trial (CAST): mortality in patients surviving open label titration but not randomized to double-blind therapy. J Am Coll Cardiol 1991; 18:20–28.

198. Goldstein S, Brooks MM, Ledingham R, et al. Association between ease of suppression of ventricular arrhythmia and survival. Circulation 1995; 91:79–83.

199. Hallstrom AP, Greene HL, Huther ML. The healthy responder phenomenon in non-randomized clinical trials. CAST Investigators. Stat Med 1991; 10:1621–31.

200. Steinbeck G, Andresen D, Bach P, et al. A comparison of electrophysiologically guided antiarrhythmic drug therapy with beta-blocker therapy in patients with symptomatic, sustained ventricular tachyarrhythmias. N Engl J Med 1992; 327:987–92.

PART XIII

MANAGEMENT OF THE VENTILATOR-SUPPORTED PATIENT

Chapter 50

PRONE POSITIONING IN ACUTE RESPIRATORY FAILURE

LUCIANO GATTINONI
FRANCO VALENZA
PAOLO PELOSI
DANIELE MASCHERONI

EFFECTS OF PRONE POSITIONING
ON GAS EXCHANGE
   Regional Lung Inflation
   Distribution of Ventilation
   Distribution of Perfusion
   Ventilation-Perfusion Matching
CLINICAL APPLICATION OF PRONE POSITIONING
IN ACUTE RESPIRATORY FAILURE
   Effects on Arterial Oxygenation
   The Role of Prone Positioning in Treating Acute
      Respiratory Failure

About 30 years ago, the use of the prone position was proposed to improve the arterial oxygenation in patients with acute respiratory failure (ARF).[1-3] The prone position, however, may have variable effects on gas exchange. Moreover, it has been suggested that, independent of gas exchange, the prone position may decrease the harm of mechanical ventilation, making it safer. In this chapter, we discuss the mechanisms responsible for the changes in gas exchange consequent to the prone position in patients with ARF, and the clinical relevance of prone positioning in adult critically ill patients.

Effects of Prone Positioning on Gas Exchange

The effects of prone positioning on gas exchange may result from a combination of the following mechanisms:

(1) changes in regional lung inflation, (2) redistribution of ventilation, and (3) redistribution of perfusion. These three mechanisms apply to both the normal and diseased lung. In the diseased lung, however, these mechanisms are also affected by the underlying pathology. Moreover, because the underlying pathology is an evolving process, it is likely that the effects of positioning on arterial oxygenation will vary with time.

REGIONAL LUNG INFLATION

METHODS OF INVESTIGATION

Most of the studies dealing with regional lung inflation in normal subjects were performed with radioactive xenon.[4,5] We used computed tomography (CT) to quantify regional lung.[6,7] The CT scan provides a computer-reconstructed image that is composed of several hundred elementary units (voxels). Each voxel ($1.5 \times 1.5 \times 9$ mm) is characterized by a given level of absorption of x-rays, which mainly reflects the density of the material being studied. The density is usually expressed in CT numbers or Hounsfield units (H).[8] A density equal to 0 H characterizes a voxel composed of water, while a voxel with a density of -1000 H is composed of gas. A voxel with a CT number equal to -500 H has a composition of 50% gas and 50% tissue. By analysis of the CT numbers, we quantitatively describe the regional lung inflation of a single CT section, at the level of the lung base, that is representative of the entire lung.[6] The CT section was divided into 10 levels along the vertical axis, each one including approximately 300–400 voxels (Fig. 50-1). The gas/tissue ratio (g/t), which is our index of regional lung inflation, was computed from the average CT number at each lung level.

NORMAL LUNGS

Regional Inflation in Supine Position
As shown in Fig. 50-2, the regional inflation, expressed as the g/t ratio, decreases along the vertical axis (from ventral to dorsal). The decrease is exponential; thus, the rate of change of regional lung inflation with height may be characterized by a constant (K_d). The lower the value of K_d, the higher the rate of the decrease of regional lung inflation along the vertical axis. The K_d in normal subjects is 13.6 ± 2.5 cm. At this distance from the ventral surface, the g/t ratio is 37% of the g/t value computed at the ventral surface. In other words, the alveolar dimensions, in the dorsal regions, should be approximately one-third of those at the ventral surface.

Regional Inflation in Prone Position
When a normal subject is shifted from supine to prone, the regional inflation distribution changes, increasing in the dorsal regions and decreasing in the ventral regions (see Fig. 50-2). The regional inflation decreases exponentially from dorsal to ventral for both supine and prone positions; however, the K_d is higher in the prone position compared with the supine position (K_d prone, 26.2 ± 2.2 cm; K_d supine, 13.6 ± 2.5 cm). This indicates that the regional inflation distribution is more homogeneous in the prone than in the supine position, and therefore the prone position does not

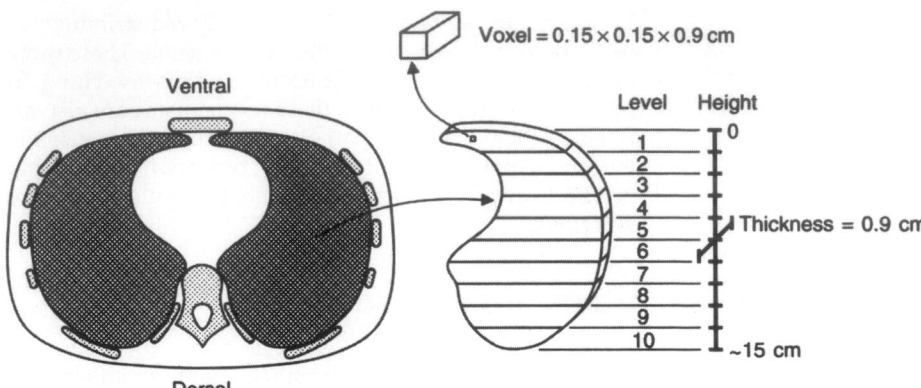

FIGURE 50-1 Regional analysis of the CT scan image. The vertical distance from ventral to dorsal surface (height) is divided into 10 equal intervals. Ten lung levels are then obtained. Each level is composed of 300–400 elementary units (voxels), each characterized by a given CT number expressed in Hounsfield units (H). (*Reproduced, with permission, from Pelosi et al.[16]*)

simply reverse the regional inflation distribution. We recently confirmed these concepts in animal studies by means of CT scan.[9]

Mechanism of Vertical Inflation Gradient

The regional inflation is believed to depend on the local transpulmonary pressure (i.e., the absolute difference between pressure in the alveoli and pressure at the pleural surface [Ppl]). At functional residual capacity, alveolar pressure equals atmospheric pressure; thus, changes in transpulmonary pressure are caused by regional differences in Ppl. The Ppl gradient in normal subjects is approximately 0.2–0.3 cmH_2O/cm.[10] The nature of this pressure gradient, however, is still controversial and is mainly attributed to the following factors: (1) lung weight, (2) shape and mechanical properties of the chest wall, and (3) shape and mechanical properties of the lung.

The role of lung weight in normal subjects is considered a predominant mechanism by some investigators.[11–14] It was first stressed by Krueger et al,[15] who found that the normal Ppl gradient was very similar to the normal density

FIGURE 50-2 The gas/tissue ratio (g/t) as a function of lung height in the supine (*diamonds*) and prone (*circles*) positions. The white symbols refer to normal lungs (N = 14) and the black symbols refer to lungs of patients with acute respiratory distress syndrome (ARDS) (N = 20). It is important to note that the height = 0 refers to the ventral surface in the supine position and to the dorsal surface in the prone position. The height scale direction is from nondependent (0) to dependent (100).

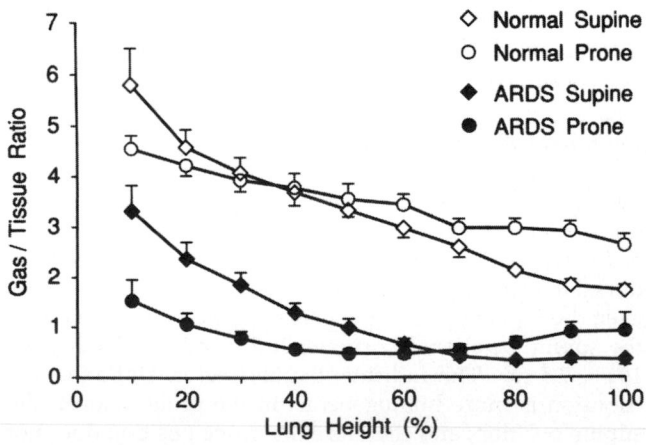

of the lung (0.22 g/L). The lung-weight theory assumes that the lung behaves as a fluid and that the hydrostatic pressures are transmitted through the lung parenchyma as in a liquid (i.e., at a given lung height, the superimposed pressure [SPL] is equal to the product of the height of the lung column and density). Estimating the SPL with the CT scan, in normal subjects, we found an average SPL gradient of 0.23 cmH_2O/cm,[16] which is similar to the Ppl gradient classically reported in physiology. Factors other than lung weight, however, may play a substantial role in determining Ppl. In fact, in the prone position, the decay of the regional inflation with height is less than in the supine position (i.e., the Ppl gradient is probably lower in the prone than in the supine position) (see Fig. 50-2). If the SPL was the only determinant of Ppl, the decay of the regional lung inflation would be similar in prone and supine positions. As shown in Fig. 50-2, however, the regional inflation distribution, along the vertical axis, was different in the supine and prone positions. Our findings are in keeping with those of Mutoh et al[17] in normal dogs, in which the Ppl gradient was directly measured. Factors such as the thoracic lung shape and compliance should then be involved in determining the regional inflation changes with positioning. In addition, the prone position eliminates the compression of the lungs by the heart, which also contributes to a more homogeneous distribution of lung inflation.[18,19]

LUNGS IN ACUTE RESPIRATORY FAILURE

Anatomic Changes During ARF

The early phases of ARF are characterized by lung edema. The edema causes a large increase in lung tissue and therefore in lung weight. In ARF patients, we found that lung weight, as measured by the CT scan technique, was two to three times greater than normal,[20] and this is consistent with the lung weight values reported in autopsy series.[21] We also found that edema (i.e., the amount of tissue mass in excess of normal [excess tissue mass]) does not accumulate preferentially in the dependent regions, and it is quite evenly distributed at each lung level (Fig. 50-3). The nongravitational distribution of edema has been reported in a series of animal experiments using different techniques.[22,23] This homogeneous increase in lung edema has two important consequences for regional inflation. First, although ARF is characterized by a marked decrease in lung gas volume,[20]

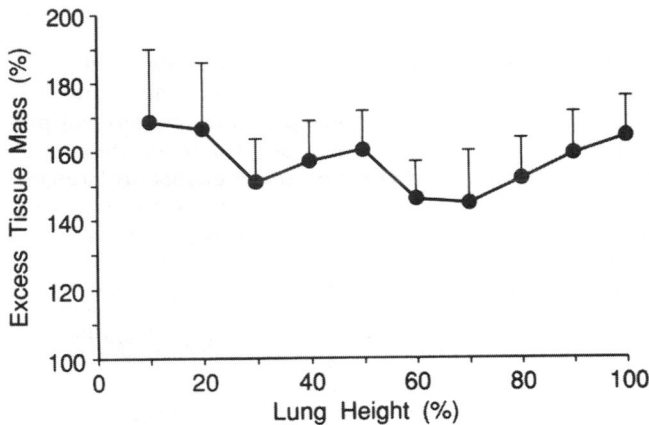

FIGURE 50-3 The distribution of excess tissue mass (i.e., the mass in excess of the expected normal mass) as a function of lung height. Data refer to 34 ARF lungs studied in the supine position. Zero on the abscissa refers to the ventral lung surface. (*Reproduced, with permission, from Gattinoni et al.*[51])

the total lung dimensions are similar to normal secondary to the increase in lung tissue mass (edema).[16] Second, the increased lung tissue mass leads to a dramatic increase in SP_L, which may be as high as 10–15 cmH$_2$O in the most dependent regions.[6,7,16]

Regional Inflation in the Supine Position

The behavior of regional inflation in patients with ARF in the supine position is shown in Fig. 50-2. As in the normal lung, the regional inflation decreases exponentially along the ventral-dorsal axis.[16] Two important differences, however, must be stressed. First, the regional inflation at the ventral surface is only half that of the normal lung. Second, the decay in the regional inflation with height (K_d) is almost half that of normal; that is, the rate of the decrease of regional inflation from the ventral to dorsal region is double that of the normal lung (K_d ARF = 6.9 ± 1.2 cm versus K_d normal = 13.6 ± 2.5 cm). This suggests that in supine ARF patients at 0 cmH$_2$O positive end-expiratory pressure (PEEP), there is almost total alveolar collapse in the posterior half of their lungs, as confirmed by the CT scan image (Fig. 50-4).

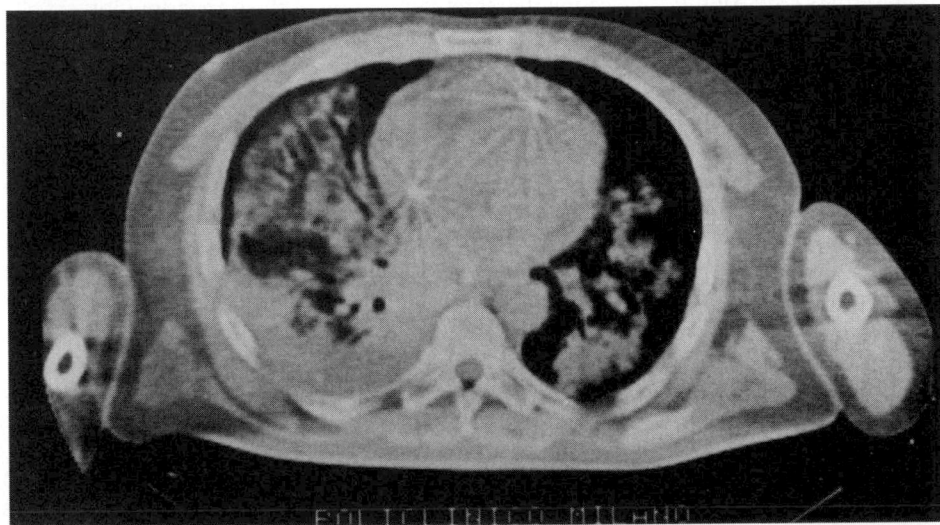

A

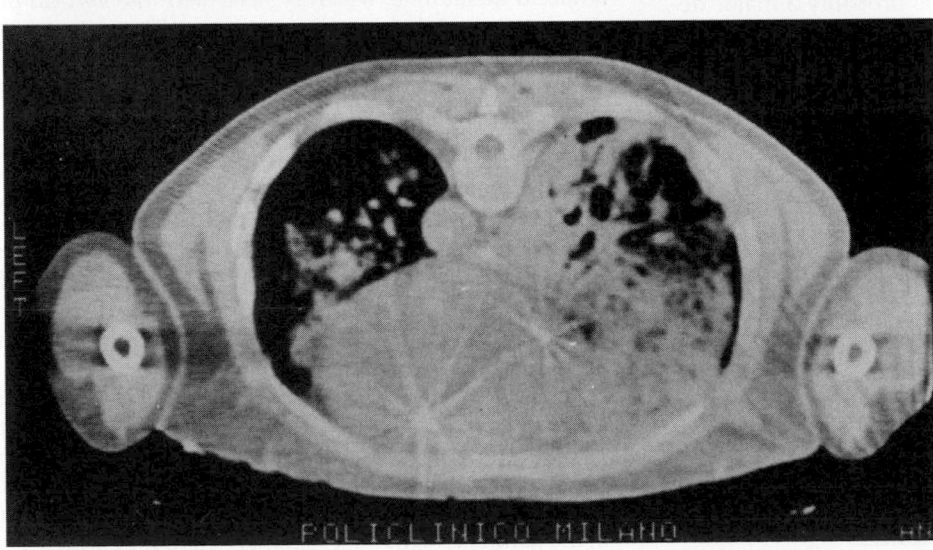

B

FIGURE 50-4 A representative CT scan image in supine (*A*) and in prone (*B*) positions. Note the typical redistribution of lung densities. Images taken 10 minutes apart, and at end-expiration apnea, with 10 cmH$_2$O PEEP. (*Reproduced, with permission, from Gattinoni et al.*[6])

Regional Inflation in the Prone Position

The behavior of regional inflation in the prone position is shown in Fig. 50-2. As with normal subjects, the inflation gradient is reversed, and the regional inflation is greater in dorsal regions and lower in ventral regions. Once again, the dependent lung regions (ventral) are collapsed (see Fig. 50-4). As with normal subjects, regional inflation is more homogeneously distributed than in the supine position; however, exponential fitting of the experimental data did not reach a level of significance in all patients.

Mechanism of Vertical Inflation Gradient

The main difference in regional inflation between normal subjects and patients with ARF is the greater rate of decrease of regional inflation along the vertical axis in ARF lungs. This suggests that the Ppl gradient is higher in patients with ARF than in normal individuals.[16] The most likely explanation of the increased Ppl in ARF is increased lung weight; the overall lung shape, in fact, is no different between normal individuals and patients with ARF.[16] The thoracic-lung shape modifications when the patients are turned prone, however, probably change the Ppl gradient (i.e., the modifications of the lung and the chest-wall shape may redistribute the forces acting at the pleural surface).

The relationships between lung shape modifications and distribution of regional lung inflation in ARF patients will be discussed in Mechanisms Involved in Arterial Oxygenation Changes in the Prone Position, below.

SUMMARY

In patients with ARF, lung densities redistribute from the dorsal to the ventral region when turned prone. Regional inflation decreases exponentially from the nondependent to the dependent lung region in both the supine and prone positions. The decay in regional inflation, both in normal individuals and in patients with ARF, is greater in the supine than in the prone position. This indicates that regional inflation is usually more homogeneously distributed in the prone position. The regional inflation gradient is secondary to the Ppl gradient. Lung weight is probably a major determinant in increasing the Ppl gradient in ARF. Thoracic-lung shape modifications from supine to prone, however, may produce a more homogeneous distribution of regional inflation in the prone position.

DISTRIBUTION OF VENTILATION

As a general rule, ventilation relates to applied pressures, flows, and resistances according to the following equation:

$$DV = C \times (DP_L - \dot{V} \times R)$$

where DV is variation in volume, C is compliance, DP_L is transpulmonary pressure, $\dot{V}$ is flow, and R is resistance. It follows that regional ventilation depends on regional compliances, regional transpulmonary pressure swings, regional flow rates, and regional resistances.

NORMAL LUNGS

Distribution of Ventilation in the Supine Position

When a bolus of radioactive gas is inhaled by spontaneously breathing subjects in the supine position, ventilation is predominantly distributed to the dependent lung regions.[24] From available data, the major determinants of the distribution of ventilation appear to be: (1) the regional inflation distribution and (2) the pattern of diaphragmatic movement (active or passive).

Mead et al,[25] Otis et al,[26] and Pedley et al[27] proposed a lung model divided into two compartments: upper and lower. Regional inflation is greater in the upper (ventral) compartment and smaller in the lower (dorsal) compartment. The upper lung regions are closer to the flat portion of their pressure-volume curve, while the lower regions are on the steeper portion of the curve. Consequently, for a given applied pressure, ventilation is greater in the lower lung regions than in the upper regions.

In the supine position, a large portion of the lung is close to the diaphragm, which may vary its tension, shape, and position. During tidal spontaneous breathing, there is a greater displacement of the dependent hemidiaphragm, with consequent greater ventilation of the dependent lung.[28–30] Accordingly, in spontaneously breathing subjects, both regional inflation and diaphragmatic movement cooperate to distribute ventilation preferentially to the dependent lung. There are, however, three major conditions in which the ventilation is greater in the nondependent lung: (1) ventilation at low lung volume, (2) ventilation at high inspiratory flow rate, and (3) mechanical ventilation. The preferential ventilation of the upper compartment at a low lung volume is easily explained by the work of Otis et al[26] (i.e., at a low lung volume, the upper lung regions are probably shifted on the steeper part of the pressure-volume curve). At a high inspiratory flow rate, the accessory respiratory muscles appear to play a determining role in the redistribution of ventilation to the upper compartment.[31–32] During mechanical ventilation, particularly during anesthesia and paralysis, the diaphragm appears to play a major role in the distribution of ventilation.[33–35] In this situation, the diaphragm behaves as a flaccid membrane, which is faced with the vertical pressure gradient of the abdominal contents. The upper, nondependent part of the diaphragm moves passively and faces a lower abdominal pressure; thus, ventilation is greater in the nondependent lung regions.

Distribution of Ventilation in the Prone Position

Distribution of ventilation in prone position is still controversial. Indeed, some authors found a uniform vertical distribution of ventilation in spontaneously breathing subjects,[36] while others found a vertical gradient with either greater ventilation in the dependent (ventral) regions[4] or in the nondependent lung regions.[37]

No data are available concerning ventilation at low lung volumes or at a high inspiratory flow rate in the prone position. During mechanical ventilation in anesthetized paralyzed normal individuals in the prone position, Rehder et al[37] found that the distribution of ventilation was greater in the nondependent lung regions, where the passive upper position of the diaphragm faced a lower abdominal pressure.

Recently, in an animal study, we confirmed that the distribution of ventilation in the prone position is more homogeneous than in the supine position, and that in the prone position there is less lung strain once tidal volume is delivered.[38]

LUNGS IN ACUTE RESPIRATORY FAILURE

Distribution of Ventilation in the Supine Position

CT scan studies in patients with ARF have shown that ventilation is distributed preferentially to the nondependent lung because the dependent lung is usually collapsed and/or consolidated (see Fig. 50-4). We obtained CT scans at both end-expiration and end-inspiration in 10 patients during the early phase of ARF (unpublished observations). In these patients, we indeed found that "ventilation" was preferentially distributed to the nondependent (ventral) lung regions. The pattern was in part modified by application of PEEP. With an increase in PEEP and reopening of the dependent lung regions, "ventilation" was more uniformly distributed (gas could reach the recruited dependent regions).

Distribution of Ventilation in the Prone Position

Few data have been published on the distribution of ventilation in patients with ARF placed in the prone position. Because regional inflation is more uniform in the prone position, similarly to the pattern in normal lungs, however, one would expect that ventilation should be more uniform in this posture. Recently, Vieillard-Baron et al showed that the prone position does indeed improve homogenization of tidal ventilation by reducing time-constant inequalities.[39]

SUMMARY

In spontaneously breathing normal subjects, when supine, ventilation is preferentially distributed to the dependent lung regions, while prone position data are controversial. During mechanical ventilation, this pattern is reversed with preferential distribution of ventilation to the nondependent lung in both supine and prone positions. Accordingly, the main determinant of ventilation distribution is the regional inflation gradient and transdiaphragmatic pressures. In mechanically ventilated patients with ARF, ventilation is preferentially distributed to the nondependent lung regions, because the dependent regions are collapsed and/or consolidated. In the prone position, we expect a similar pattern of ventilation distribution, because the collapsed areas move from the dorsal to the ventral regions. Tidal volume, however, is more homogeneously distributed in the prone position, because of a reduction in the slow compartment zones of the lung and possibly a more homogeneous distribution of regional inflation.

DISTRIBUTION OF PERFUSION

NORMAL LUNGS

Distribution of Perfusion in the Supine Position

The most widely accepted model that describes the pulmonary perfusion pattern is that described by West et al.[40] According to these investigators, the relationship between blood flow and pulmonary artery pressure, alveolar pressure, and venous pressure can be modeled as in a Starling resistor, where a collapsible tube traverses a closed chamber (the gas compartment) in which pressure (the alveolar pressure) may be varied at will. When the inflow pressure (pulmonary artery pressure) is lower than the chamber pressure (alveolar pressure), blood flow stops (zone 1). When the inflow pressure is higher than the chamber pressure, the flow through the system is governed by either the difference between pulmonary artery pressure and alveolar pressure (zone 2) or the difference between pulmonary artery pressure and venous pressure, when the outflow pressure (venous pressure) exceeds the chamber pressure (zone 3).

According to this "gravitational" view, perfusion should progressively increase down the lung. In the supine position, the lung should be characterized by perfusion in zone 2 and zone 3, increasing from ventral (zone 2) to dorsal (zone 3), because zone 1 conditions do not occur. Several authors, suggesting that factors other than gravity can determine the perfusion heterogeneity, have challenged the model of West et al.[41–45]

Distribution of Perfusion in the Prone Position

According to the "gravitational" theory, a perfusion gradient should exist from dorsal to ventral. Few data confirm this pattern in human subjects.[4] A perfusion gradient, however, could not be observed in the prone position in dogs;[44,46] in the supine posture, regional blood flow was positively correlated with flow to the same regions as in the prone position (and not negatively, as expected according to the "gravitational" theory).

LUNGS IN ACUTE RESPIRATORY FAILURE

Distribution of Perfusion in the Supine Position

Whatever the determinants of perfusion in the normal lung, several physiologic and anatomic factors are likely to alter the perfusion distribution in ARF. Among these are: (1) hypoxic vasoconstriction, (2) vessel obliteration, and (3) extrinsic vessel compression.

The effects of hypoxic vasoconstriction were evaluated in the lateral position using separate lung ventilation.[47] The inspiration of a hypoxic gas mixture by the dependent lung failed to redirect blood flow toward the nondependent lung, whereas diversion occurred in the supine position. This suggests that hypoxic vasoconstriction alone is not able to counteract the effects of posture on pulmonary blood flow.

Both macro- and microthrombi have been found at various stages of ARF.[48] These anatomic alterations were associated with the appearance of filling defects when selective angiography was performed.[49] Unfortunately, data are not available regarding the distribution of these defects (homogeneous, dependent, or nondependent?), but obviously the presence of vessel obliteration will alter perfusion distribution. Nonthrombotic obliterative vascular disease may also occur in the early stage of ARF secondary to congestion or compression of vessels, and in the intermediate or late stages of ARF secondary to focal obstruction of small arteries and veins as a result of fibrosis.

Increased SPL in ARF could also cause extrinsic vessel compression: the radiologic equivalent would be the "pruning" of vessels on selective angiography. In early ARF, we found (unpublished observation) that selective angiography was usually positive (filling defects and/or pruning) when the tip of the catheter was positioned in the dependent lung regions (dense on CT scan), and negative when it was in the nondependent lung regions. Moreover, we occasionally found changes in the selective angiography findings (from positive to negative) when the patients were turned from supine to prone, and the angiography was repeated in the same lung region.

All these data suggest that the pulmonary flow distribution is altered in ARF. If the compression mechanism and hypoxic vasoconstriction were operating, both should act mainly in the dependent lung regions (less aeration and higher SPL), and the blood flow should in part be diverted toward the nondependent regions, as observed in cardiogenic pulmonary edema.[50] This would partly protect against hypoxemia. In fact, it is not unusual to find 60–70% of airless lung (in the dependent regions) with a shunt fraction of 30–40%.[51] This indirectly proves that, in the supine position, part of the pulmonary blood flow is redistributed to the nondependent lung.

Distribution of Perfusion in the Prone Position

Few data are available, to our knowledge, on the distribution of pulmonary blood flow in patients with ARF mechanically ventilated in the prone position. Experimental evidence in dogs suggests that perfusion to the dorsal regions is greater than to the ventral regions in the prone position.[46] This occurrence might lead to a more even distribution of blood flow;[52] diversion of blood flow from the hypoxic lung is greater in the supine position than in the prone position.[53] Endogenous nitric oxide plays a role in the regulation of regional pulmonary perfusion. In fact, after the inhibition of nitric oxide synthase by N(G)-monomethyl-L-arginine infusion, nitric oxide synthase mRNA expression and nitric oxide production were significantly higher in dorsal as compared with ventral lung regions. In the supine position, lung perfusion was shifted to ventral regions during nitric oxide synthase inhibition, whereas in the prone position lung perfusion remained unchanged.[54] Moreover, acute changes of oxygenation consequent to positioning in patients with ARDS do not induce any short-term effect on pulmonary endothelin-1 net clearance or angiotensin-II net formation.[55] These data suggest that mechanisms other than gravity or hypoxic pulmonary vasoconstriction operate in the prone position to distribute blood flow.

SUMMARY

In the normal lung, blood flow is distributed according to gravity. Factors other than gravity, however, may play a role in governing regional perfusion. These factors seem prevalent in the prone position, where the vertical perfusion gradient may disappear. In the edematous ARF lung, available data suggest that pulmonary blood flow is partly diverted toward the nondependent, more aerated, regions. Vessel compression and hypoxic vasoconstriction may play a role in this pattern of blood flow distribution. In the prone position, during ARF, the nondependent, dorsal regions seem more perfused than the ventral regions. In ARF, perfusion seems, therefore, less dependent on gravity than in normal conditions.

VENTILATION-PERFUSION MATCHING

While few studies deal with the distribution of regional perfusion and ventilation, a number of investigators have used the multiple inert gas technique to study ventilation-perfusion ($\dot{V}_A/\dot{Q}$) relationships in different forms of ARF.[56–58] The general conclusions of these studies can be summarized as follows: ventilation and perfusion are usually well matched in ARF lungs; however, a consistent portion of pulmonary flow traverses airless regions (true shunt), and low $\dot{V}_A/\dot{Q}$ compartments are scarcely represented.

From the available data, we may then infer the following model: in the supine position in spontaneously breathing normal individuals, ventilation and perfusion are distributed along the vertical axis, and both are greater in the dependent regions. In the prone position, the ventilation and perfusion gradient along the vertical axis is decreased or abolished; consequently, perfusion and ventilation should be distributed more homogeneously.

During mechanical ventilation in normal subjects, ventilation is preferentially distributed to the nondependent lung regions, in both the supine and prone positions, while perfusion is probably greater in the dependent lung regions, causing some $\dot{V}_A/\dot{Q}$ mismatch. During ARF in the supine position, ventilation is diverted to the nondependent lung regions because the dependent regions are usually collapsed or consolidated. Perfusion of the dependent regions is probably decreased secondary to hypoxic vasoconstriction and/or vessel compression and/or obliteration. The few experimental data available regarding the prone position suggest that ventilation is more evenly distributed, and that perfusion is less gravity dependent, than in the supine position.

Clinical Application of Prone Positioning in Acute Respiratory Failure

EFFECTS ON ARTERIAL OXYGENATION

Over the last 25 years a series of reports appeared in the literature dealing with the use of the prone position as a tool to improve arterial oxygenation in patients with ARF. Over the years, early and late studies have been conducted, including many randomized trials,[59–61] prospective studies,[6,39,62–77] retrospective studies,[2,3,78–81] case reports,[82] and letters.[70,83]

From the published data and from our own personal experience, some generalizations may be made.

1. The prone position in most reported studies improves arterial oxygenation. It must be pointed out, however, that (a) the degree of improvement is highly variable (from a few to hundreds of millimeters of mercury change in

Pa_{O_2}, (b) a variable fraction of patients (from 0–80% in the reported series) do not show any improvement or even show a deterioration in arterial oxygenation while prone, and (c) the particular response to the prone position is hard to predict.

2. In the patients who respond, the improvement in gas exchange is progressive, and it may take hours to appear; moreover, some of these patients show a progressive decrease in arterial oxygenation if the prone position is maintained for long periods of time. Thus, the response to the prone position ranges from deterioration to great improvement, and it may be time dependent (slow improvement and slow deterioration).

3. The issue is further complicated when analyzing the effects of returning the patients to the supine position after they have been prone. Three different responses have been observed in patients who improved oxygenation in the prone position: (1) *some* patients return to basal supine oxygenation values when returned to the supine position (these patients are then considered "prone dependent"); (2) some patients display better oxygenation than in the original supine position, although the values are lower than in the prone position; and (3) some patients display improved oxygenation compared to both the previous supine and prone values.

4. When the same patient is turned several times, the effects of the maneuver may change in time (no improvement, whereas previous positioning in the prone position produced marked improvement or the reverse).

From the above description, it is obvious that the effects of positioning depend on the individual patient (i.e., the underlying pathology and pathophysiologic status, which may vary over time). Over the years, several authors have described the response to prone position in specific categories of ARDS[68,76] and patients without ARDS[77,84] and the improvement in oxygenation induced by inhaled nitric oxide.[62,63,65,66,71,75] The predictability of the oxygenation response to prone positioning, however, remains uncertain.[72]

MECHANISMS INVOLVED IN ARTERIAL OXYGENATION CHANGES IN THE PRONE POSITION

We can attempt to infer the mechanisms involved in arterial oxygenation changes when patients are turned to the prone position. We first discuss the mechanisms that may operate in the early period after positioning and then the mechanisms that are possibly time related.

Early Effects

An increase or decrease in Pa_{O_2} is caused by changes in regional lung inflation, ventilation distribution, and perfusion distribution. The effects on oxygenation (improvement or deterioration) are likely explained by a varying interaction between the mentioned factors in the different postures.

As previously discussed, regional inflation decreases from ventral to dorsal in the supine position, and from dorsal to ventral in the prone position. The rate of decrease in regional inflation, however, is steeper in the supine position than in the prone position (see Fig. 50-2). Because the decrease in inflation may be expressed in exponential form,

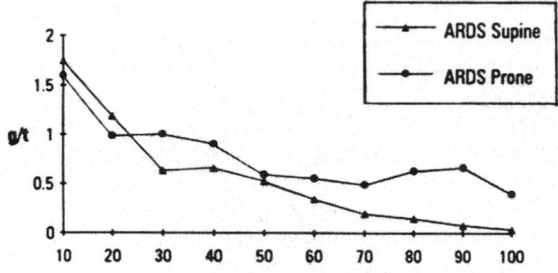
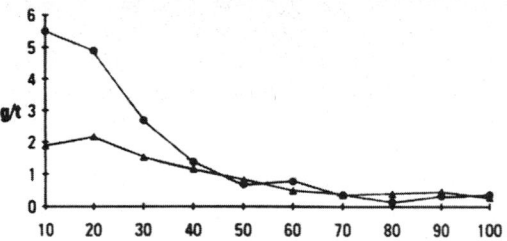
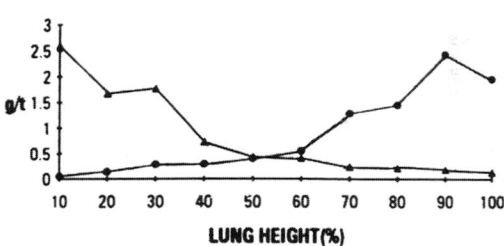

FIGURE 50-5 Different behaviors of regional inflation (g/t) as a function of lung height in the supine (*triangles*) and prone (*circles*) positions in three patients. Zero on the height scale refers to the ventral lung surface in the supine position and to the dorsal lung surface in the prone position. As such, the direction of the lung scale is always from the nondependent to dependent lung region (see text for further explanation).

this is equivalent to saying that the decay rate of regional inflation along the vertical axis (K_d) is lower in the supine position than in the prone position. This, however, refers to average values. In an individual patient, the pattern may be substantially different.

In Fig. 50-5, we report three patients who showed different patterns of regional inflation in the supine and prone positions. In the first patient (upper panel), regional inflation behaves as for the average population (see Fig. 50-2). The exponential fitting of the decay of regional inflation ($r = 0.91$) showed a K_d of 4.2 cm in the supine position. In the prone position, the decay of regional inflation was smoother, as reflected by the higher value of K_d, 14 cm (exponential fitting, $r = 0.97$). In this patient, Pa_{O_2} improved by 65 mmHg on moving from the supine to the prone position.

The middle panel in Fig. 50-5 shows the regional inflation pattern of a patient in which the decay of regional inflation was significant in both the supine and prone positions ($r = 0.96$ and $r = 0.98$, respectively). In this case, however, K_d was lower in the prone position than in the supine position (4.3 and 9.4 cm, respectively). In this case, Pa_{O_2} deteriorated when the patient was turned from supine to prone (101 mmHg when supine and 71.5 mmHg when prone).

The third panel in Fig. 50-5 refers to a very unusual patient. In this case, the low regional inflation areas in the supine position did not redistribute on switching to the prone position, and the pattern of regional inflation remained the same in the two positions. In this case, Pa_{O_2} did not change with alteration in position (61 mmHg when supine and 68 mmHg when prone).

We then tested the hypothesis that, in the individual patient, improvement in Pa_{O_2} on switching from supine to prone occurs when the decay in regional inflation is smoother (i.e., a higher K_d) in the prone position, whereas a deterioration in Pa_{O_2} occurs on switching from the supine to the prone position when the decay in regional lung inflation is steeper in the prone position (lower K_d). Plotting the individual K_d differences between prone and supine positions (DK_d,) and the individual changes in Pa_{O_2} (DPa_{O_2}) we found a significant correlation between DK_d and DPa_{O_2} (Fig. 50-6). This suggests that the response in Pa_{O_2} is associated with a change in regional inflation: the position in which regional inflation is more homogeneous (higher K_d) is associated with a better Pa_{O_2}. When the regional inflation gradient along the vertical axis does not differ between the prone and supine positions (i.e., equal decrease from nondependent to dependent lung regions, whatever position is assumed), the Pa_{O_2} does not change. To state that the Pa_{O_2} changes are caused by regional inflation changes and not simply associated with them, however, we must assume that (1) ventilation behaves like regional inflation (i.e., it is more homogeneously distributed when inflation is more homogeneously distributed), and (2) perfusion is not changed when the position is changed (i.e., the relative perfusion of the dorsal and ventral regions does not change with position).

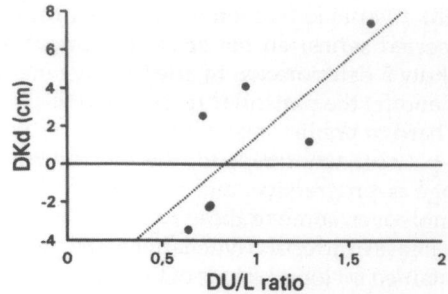

FIGURE 50-7 Changes in the regional lung inflation decay constants (dK_d) as a function of the changes of upper/lower lung ratio (dU/L ratio) between the prone and supine positions. ($dK_d = -7 + 8.3 \times$ dU/L ratio; r = 0.77; P <.05).

The question remains as to why in some patients regional inflation is more homogeneous in the prone position (and oxygenation improves in this position), while in other patients regional inflation is more homogeneous in the supine position (and oxygenation is better in this position). As previously discussed, regional inflation is dictated by Ppl, and this may in turn be influenced by SPL and lung shape. Because SPL is similar in the supine and prone positions,[6] it is possible that the postural changes in regional inflation are caused by the associated lung-shape variations. We attempted to quantify the variation in lung shape on switching from the supine to the prone position by dividing the lung area into two compartments (at 50% of the ventral-dorsal distance), the upper (U) and the lower (L) compartment, and calculating the U/L ratio in the prone and supine positions. The difference in U/L ratio between the prone and supine positions (DU/L ratio) gives a quantitative estimate of lung-shape change. For example, when the DU/L ratio is zero, lung shape is unmodified, and the greater the dU/L ratio, the greater the U compartment is in the prone position. We found that the DU/L ratio significantly correlated with both dK_d (Fig. 50-7) and DPa_{O_2} (Fig. 50-8).

This indicates that, when the U/L ratio is much lower in the supine position and much higher in the prone position, oxygenation will improve in the prone position. We then suggest that, according to these data, lung-shape modifications, as well as the modifications in regional inflation, may be predictive, in individual patients, of the early effects of positioning on arterial oxygenation.

FIGURE 50-6 Relationship between changes in Pa_{O_2} (dPa_{O_2}) and changes in the regional lung decay constants (dK_d) between the prone and supine positions. Data are from seven patients with ARF (regional inflation was computed as weighted mean of the two lungs). Positive values of dPa_{O_2} indicate that the Pa_{O_2} is higher in the prone position, while negative dPa_{O_2} values indicate that Pa_{O_2} is higher in the supine position. When dK_d is close to zero (i.e., the decrease of regional inflation is similar in the prone and supine positions), the dPa_{O_2} is close to zero ($dPa_{O_2} = -1.7 + 6.6 \times dK_d$; r = 0.86; P <.05).

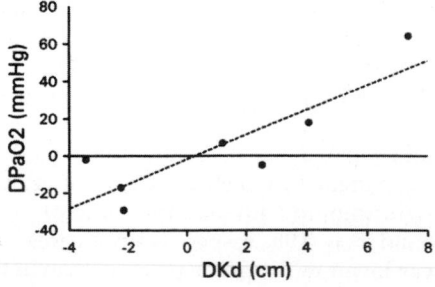

FIGURE 50-8 dPa_{O_2} as a function of the changes in upper/lower lung ratio (dU/L ratio) between the prone and supine positions ($dPa_{O_2} = -63 + 71.2 \times$ dU/L ratio; r = 0.85; P <.05).

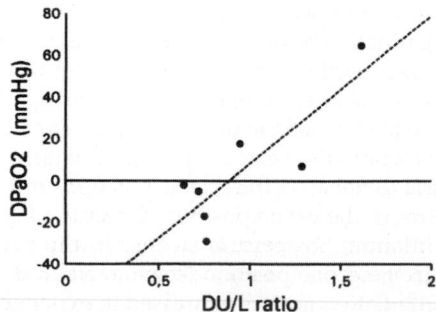

Late Effects

When the positioning maneuvers are prolonged over time or are repeated several times during the course of ARF, the oxygenation response may be highly variable. No data are available with which to speculate on the possible mechanisms. We know, however, that with time edema may redistribute, lung pathology may progress from edema to fibrosis, and vascular characteristics may change. Further studies are needed to understand the time-related effects of positioning on arterial oxygenation.

Effects on Arterial CO_2

Recently there has been a paradigmatic shift of attention from changes in Pa_{O_2} to changes in Pa_{CO_2} consequent to prone positioning in patients with ARF. According to Pa_{CO_2} change, patients may be divided into two categories: those who show a decrease of Pa_{CO_2} secondary to prone position, and those whose Pa_{CO_2} does not change or even increases.

Before discussing the meaning of Pa_{CO_2} change it is worth remembering that expected changes in Pa_{CO_2} are relatively smaller than changes in Pa_{O_2} because of the different slopes of the content/tension relationship. For a similar change in content, the change in tension of CO_2 (partial pressure of the gas) is expected to be approximately 12% of the change in Pa_{O_2}. This would result, for instance, in a change in P_{CO_2} of 5 mmHg versus a change in P_{O_2} of 40 mmHg, implying not only more controlled measurements, but also greater accuracy.

The fact that Pa_{CO_2} increases during the course of ARDS, in association with structural changes of the lung, was known for many years.[60,61] Recently Kallet et al found that an increase in dead space is a prognostic marker of ARDS mortality.[85]

We recently found that patients who display a decrease in Pa_{CO_2} in the prone position experience a greater survival (dose dependent) than do patients who do not show a decrease, or even show an increase in Pa_{CO_2}.[86] This response to Pa_{CO_2} likely reflects different underlying pathology: predominant recruitment in Pa_{CO_2} responders (secondary to increased alveolar ventilation in the prone position) versus blood-flow diversion in nonresponders. Interestingly, only the changes in Pa_{CO_2} were associated with survival, not the changes in Pa_{O_2}.

THE ROLE OF PRONE POSITIONING IN TREATING ACUTE RESPIRATORY FAILURE

RATIONALE

Since the first report dating back to the 1970s,[1-3] the prone position has been proposed and used to improve oxygenation. The progressive recognition of the mechanism underlying this effect, however, led to the hypothesis that the prone position may decrease the danger associated with mechanical ventilation (ventilator-induced lung injury).[87,88] The hypothesis is based primarily on the observation that in the prone position there is a more homogeneous distribution of inflation, suggesting indirectly a more homogeneous distribution of stress and strain, which are likely the first triggers of ventilator-induced lung injury. In fact, in several animal models, it has been shown that the prone position decreases ventilator-induced lung injury or at least delays its progression.[9,89,90] CT scan studies in animals documented a decrease in regional strain in the prone as compared with the supine position.[9] Indeed, the possible favorable effects of prone positioning on outcome of patients with ARF should not be related to oxygenation changes, which were not found to be associated with outcome, but, instead, to changes in regional lung mechanics, by which forces applied by the ventilator should be more evenly distributed throughout the lung parenchyma.

RANDOMIZED CLINICAL TRIALS OF PRONE POSITION

Three major trials have addressed outcome in relation to prone position,[59-61] one of which is published only as an abstract.[59] All studies demonstrated no beneficial outcome and some concerns with the safety of the maneuver. A post hoc analysis, however, showed that the survival of sicker patients was higher with the prone position in the group of patients from the trial of Gattinoni et al.[61] Moreover, the study by Guerin et al showed that prone positioning may lower the incidence of ventilator-associated pneumonia.[60]

Compliance with prone positioning treatment was somewhat poor in both the studies of Gattinoni et al and Guerin et al; the time in the prone position was only 7–8 hours per day. Those few hours may have contributed to significantly improved oxygenation. But as described above, oxygenation improvement does not predict outcome, whereas changes in Pa_{CO_2} do.[86] Perhaps patients who display decreases in Pa_{CO_2} and behave as lung recruiters may be more protected against ventilator-induced lung injury by the prone position. If this holds true, however, the time spent in the prone position may influence outcome. This is the rationale for an ongoing study, being carried out by our institution, in which patients are treated in the prone position at least 20 hours a day. The results of this study will enhance our knowledge of the use of prone positioning in critically ill patients.

One may ask: What is the true place of prone positioning in the treatment of patients with ARDS? No doubt, the prone position is indicated as a rescue maneuver during severe hypoxemia. Its routine use, however, did not improve outcome despite the solid rationale behind its use.[91]

References

1. Bryan AC. Conference on the scientific basis of respiratory therapy. Pulmonary physiotherapy in the pediatric age group. Comments of a devil's advocate. Am Rev Respir Dis 1974; 110:143–4.
2. Piehl MA, Brown RS. Use of extreme position changes in acute respiratory failure. Crit Care Med 1976; 4:13–4.
3. Douglas WW, Rehder K, Beynen FM, Sessler AD, Marsh HM. Improved oxygenation in patients with acute respiratory failure: the prone position. Am Rev Respir Dis 1977; 115:559–66.
4. Kaneko K, Milic-Emili J, Dolovich MB, Dawson A, Bates DV. Regional distribution of ventilation and perfusion as a function of body position. J Appl Physiol 1966; 21:767–77.

5. Rehder K, Sessler AD, Rodarte JR. Regional intrapulmonary gas distribution in awake and anesthetized-paralyzed man. J Appl Physiol 1977; 42:391–402.

6. Gattinoni L, Pelosi P, Vitale G, et al. Body position changes redistribute lung computed-tomographic density in patients with acute respiratory failure. Anesthesiology 1991; 74:15–23.

7. Gattinoni L, D'Andrea L, Pelosi P, et al. Regional effects and mechanism of positive end-expiratory pressure in early adult respiratory distress syndrome. JAMA 1993; 269:2122–7.

8. Gattinoni L, Pesenti A, Torresin A, et al. Adult respiratory distress syndrome profiles by computed tomography. J Thorac Imaging 1986; 1:25–30.

9. Valenza F, Guglielmi M, Maffioletti M, et al. Prone position delays the progression of ventilator-induced lung injury in rats: Does lung strain play a role? Crit Care Med 2005; 33:361–7.

10. Milic-Emili J. Pulmonary statics. In: Widdicombe JG, editor. Respiratory physiology I, Vol. 2. Baltimore: University Park Press, 1974: 105–37.

11. Bryan AC, Milic-Emili J, Pengelly D. Effect of gravity on the distribution of pulmonary ventilation. J Appl Physiol 1966; 21:778–84.

12. Milic-Emili J, Henderson JA, Dolovich MB, Trop D, Kaneko K. Regional distribution of inspired gas in the lung. J Appl Physiol 1966; 21:749–59.

13. Glaister DH. Distribution of pulmonary blood flow and ventilation during forward (plus Gx) acceleration. J Appl Physiol 1970; 29:432–9.

14. Michels DB, West JB. Distribution of pulmonary ventilation and perfusion during short periods of weightlessness. J Appl Physiol 1978; 45:987–98.

15. Krueger JJ, Bain T, Patterson JL Jr. Elevation gradient of intrathoracic pressure. J Appl Physiol 1961; 16:465–8.

16. Pelosi P, D'Andrea L, Vitale G, Pesenti A, Gattinoni L. Vertical gradient of regional lung inflation in adult respiratory distress syndrome. Am J Respir Crit Care Med 1994; 149:8–13.

17. Mutoh T, Guest RJ, Lamm WJ, Albert RK. Prone position alters the effect of volume overload on regional pleural pressures and improves hypoxemia in pigs in vivo. Am Rev Respir Dis 1992; 146:300–6.

18. Albert RK, Hubmayr RD. The prone position eliminates compression of the lungs by the heart. Am J Respir Crit Care Med 2000; 161:1660–5.

19. Malbouisson LM, Busch CJ, Puybasset L, et al. Role of the heart in the loss of aeration characterizing lower lobes in acute respiratory distress syndrome. CT Scan ARDS Study Group. Am J Respir Crit Care Med 2000; 161:2005–12.

20. Gattinoni L, Pesenti A, Bombino M, et al. Relationships between lung computed tomographic density, gas exchange, and PEEP in acute respiratory failure. Anesthesiology 1988; 69:824–32.

21. Teplitz C. The core pathobiology and integrated medical science of adult acute respiratory insufficiency. Surg Clin North Am 1976; 56:1091–133.

22. Jones T, Jones HA, Rhodes CG, Buckingham PD, Hughes JM. Distribution of extravascular fluid volumes in isolated perfused lungs measured with H2¹⁵O. J Clin Invest 1976; 57:706–13.

23. Hales CA, Kanarek DJ, Ahluwalia B, et al. Regional edema formation in isolated perfused dog lungs. Circ Res 1981; 48:121–7.

24. Engel LA, Utz G, Wood LD, Macklem PT. Ventilation distribution in anatomical lung units. J Appl Physiol 1974; 37:194–200.

25. Mead J, Lindgren I, Gaensler EA. The mechanical properties of the lungs in emphysema. J Clin Invest 1955; 34:1005–16.

26. Otis AB, McKernow CB, Bartlett RA, McKernow CB. Mechanical factors in distribution of pulmonary ventilation. J Appl Physiol 1956; 8:427–43.

27. Pedley TJ, Sudlow MF, Milic-Emili J. A non-linear theory of the distribution of pulmonary ventilation. Respir Physiol 1972; 15:1–38.

28. Froese AB, Bryan AC. Effects of anesthesia and paralysis on diaphragmatic mechanics in man. Anesthesiology 1974; 41:242–55.

29. Chevrolet JC, Emrich J, Martin RR, Engel LA. Voluntary changes in ventilation distribution in the lateral posture. Respir Physiol 1979; 38:313–23.

30. Chevrolet JC, Martin JG, Flood R, Martin RR, Engel LA. Topographical ventilation and perfusion distribution during IPPB in the lateral posture. Am Rev Respir Dis 1978; 118:847–54.

31. D'Angelo E. Cranio-caudal rib cage distortion with increasing inspiratory airflow in man. Respir Physiol 1981; 44:215–37.

32. Fixley MS, Roussos CS, Murphy B, Martin RR, Engel LA. Flow dependence of gas distribution and the pattern of inspiratory muscle contraction. J Appl Physiol 1978; 45:733–41.

33. Potgieter AV. Atelectasis: its evolution during upper urinary tract surgery. Br J Anaesth 1959; 31:472–83.

34. Nunn JF. The distribution of inspired gas during thoracic surgery. Ann R Coll Surg Engl 1961; 28:223–37.

35. Rehder K, Hatch DJ, Sessler AD, Fowler WS. The function of each lung of anesthetized and paralyzed man during mechanical ventilation. Anesthesiology 1972; 37:16–26.

36. Amis TC. Regional lung function in man and in dog. London: University of London, 1979.

37. Rehder K, Knopp TJ, Sessler AD. Regional intrapulmonary gas distribution in awake and anesthetized-paralyzed prone man. J Appl Physiol 1978; 45:528–35.

38. Gattinoni L, Carlesso E, Valenza F, Chiumello D, Caspani ML. Acute respiratory distress syndrome, the critical care paradigm: what we learned and what we forgot. Curr Opin Crit Care 2004; 10:272–8.

39. Vieillard-Baron A, Rabiller A, Chergui K, et al. Prone position improves mechanics and alveolar ventilation in acute respiratory distress syndrome. Intensive Care Med 2005; 31:220–6.

40. West JB, Dollery CT, Naimark A. Distribution of blood flow in isolated lung; relation to vascular and alveolar pressures. J Appl Physiol 1964; 19:713–24.

41. Amis TC, Jones HA, Hughes JM. Effect of posture on interregional distribution of pulmonary perfusion and VA/Q ratios in man. Respir Physiol 1984; 56:169–82.

42. Orphanidou D, Hughes JM, Myers MJ, Al-Suhali AR, Henderson B. Tomography of regional ventilation and perfusion using krypton 81m in normal subjects and asthmatic patients. Thorax 1986; 41:542–51.

43. Reed JHJ, Wood EH. Effect of body position on vertical distribution of pulmonary blood flow. J Appl Physiol 1970; 28:303–11.

44. Wiener CM, Kirk W, Albert RK. Prone position reverses gravitational distribution of perfusion in dog lungs with oleic acid–induced injury. J Appl Physiol 1990; 68:1386–92.

45. Glenny RW, Robertson HT. Fractal properties of pulmonary blood flow: characterization of spatial heterogeneity. J Appl Physiol 1990; 69:532–45.

46. Glenny RW, Lamm WJ, Albert RK, Robertson HT. Gravity is a minor determinant of pulmonary blood flow distribution. J Appl Physiol 1991; 71:620–9.

47. Arborelius MJ, Lundin G, Svanberg L, Defares JG. Influence of unilateral hypoxia on blood flow through the lungs in man in lateral position. J Appl Physiol 1960; 15:595–7.

48. Jones R, Reid LM, Zapol WM, Tomashefski JF, Kirton OC, Kobayashi K. Pulmonary vascular pathology: human and experimental studies. In: Zapol WM, Falke KJ, editors. Acute respiratory failure, Vol. 24. New York: Marcel Dekker, 1985:23–160.

49. Greene R, Zapol WM, Snider MT, et al. Early bedside detection of pulmonary vascular occlusion during acute respiratory failure. Am Rev Respir Dis 1981; 124:593–601.

50. Wollmer P, Rhodes CG, Deanfield J, et al. Regional extravascular density of the lung in patients with acute pulmonary edema. J Appl Physiol 1987; 63:1890–5.

51. Gattinoni L, Pelosi P, Pesenti A, et al. CT scan in ARDS: clinical and physiopathological insights. Acta Anaesthesiol Scand Suppl 1991; 95:87–94.

52. Schuster DP, Haller J. Effects of body position on regional pulmonary perfusion blood flow during acute pulmonary edema in dogs: a positron emission tomography study. J Crit Care 1991; 6:19–28.

53. Walther SM, Domino KB, Hlastala MP. Effects of posture on blood flow diversion by hypoxic pulmonary vasoconstriction in dogs. Br J Anaesth 1998; 81:425–9.

54. Rimeika D, Nyren S, Wiklund NP, et al. Regulation of regional lung perfusion by nitric oxide. Am J Respir Crit Care Med 2004; 170:450–5.

55. Wenz M, Hoffmann B, Bohlender J, Kaczmarczyk G. Angiotensin II formation and endothelin clearance in ARDS patients in supine and prone positions. Intensive Care Med 2000; 26:292–8.

56. Dantzker DR, Brook CJ, Dehart P, Lynch JP, Weg JG. Ventilation-perfusion distributions in the adult respiratory distress syndrome. Am Rev Respir Dis 1979; 120:1039–52.

57. Ralph DD, Robertson HT, Weaver LJ, et al. Distribution of ventilation and perfusion during positive end-expiratory pressure in the adult respiratory distress syndrome. Am Rev Respir Dis 1985; 131:54–60.

58. Wagner PD, Rodriguez-Roisin R. Clinical advances in pulmonary gas exchange. Am Rev Respir Dis 1991; 143:883–8.

59. Mancebo J, Rialp G, Fernandez R. Randomized multicenter trial in ARDS: supine versus prone position. Intensive Care Med 2003; 29:S64.

60. Guerin C, Gaillard S, Lemasson S, et al. Effects of systematic prone positioning in hypoxemic acute respiratory failure: a randomized controlled trial. JAMA 2004; 292:2379–87.

61. Gattinoni L, Tognoni G, Pesenti A, et al. Effect of prone positioning on the survival of patients with acute respiratory failure. N Engl J Med 2001; 345:568–73.

62. Borelli M, Lampati L, Vascotto E, Fumagalli R, Pesenti A. Hemodynamic and gas exchange response to inhaled nitric oxide and prone positioning in acute respiratory distress syndrome patients. Crit Care Med 2000; 28:2707–12.

63. Dupont H, Mentec H, Cheval C, et al. Short-term effect of inhaled nitric oxide and prone positioning on gas exchange in patients with severe acute respiratory distress syndrome. Crit Care Med 2000; 28:304–8.

64. Gillart T, Bazin JE, Cosserant B, et al. Combined nitric oxide inhalation, prone positioning and almitrine infusion improve oxygenation in severe ARDS. Can J Anaesth 1998; 45:402–9.

65. Johannigman JA, Davis K Jr, Miller SL, et al. Prone positioning and inhaled nitric oxide: synergistic therapies for acute respiratory distress syndrome. J Trauma 2001; 50:589–95.

66. Jolliet P, Bulpa P, Ritz M, et al. Additive beneficial effects of the prone position, nitric oxide, and almitrine bismesylate on gas exchange and oxygen transport in acute respiratory distress syndrome. Crit Care Med 1997; 25:786–94.

67. Langer M, Mascheroni D, Marcolin R, Gattinoni L. The prone position in ARDS patients. A clinical study. Chest 1988; 94:103–7.

68. Lee DL, Chiang HT, Lin SL, et al. Prone-position ventilation induces sustained improvement in oxygenation in patients with acute respiratory distress syndrome who have a large shunt. Crit Care Med 2002; 30:1446–52.

69. Lim CM, Kim EK, Lee JS, et al. Comparison of the response to the prone position between pulmonary and extrapulmonary acute respiratory distress syndrome. Intensive Care Med 2001; 27:477–85.

70. Manara AR, Fromant SM, Canter C, Park GR. Improving oxygenation using the prone position. Intensive Care Med 1987; 13:218–9.

71. Papazian L, Bregeon F, Gaillat F, et al. Respective and combined effects of prone position and inhaled nitric oxide in patients with acute respiratory distress syndrome. Am J Respir Crit Care Med 1998; 157:580–5.

72. Papazian L, Paladini MH, Bregeon F, et al. Can the tomographic aspect characteristics of patients presenting with acute respiratory distress syndrome predict improvement in oxygenation-related response to the prone position? Anesthesiology 2002; 97:599–607.

73. Pappert D, Rossaint R, Slama K, Gruning T, Falke KJ. Influence of positioning on ventilation-perfusion relationships in severe adult respiratory distress syndrome. Chest 1994; 106:1511–6.

74. Rialp G, Betbese AJ, Perez-Marquez M, Mancebo J. Short-term effects of inhaled nitric oxide and prone position in pulmonary and extrapulmonary acute respiratory distress syndrome. Am J Respir Crit Care Med 2001; 164:243–9.

75. Richard JC, Janier M, Lavenne F, et al. Effect of position, nitric oxide, and almitrine on lung perfusion in a porcine model of acute lung injury. J Appl Physiol 2002; 93:2181–91.

76. Venet C, Guyomarc'h S, Migeot C, et al. The oxygenation variations related to prone positioning during mechanical ventilation: a clinical comparison between ARDS and non-ARDS hypoxemic patients. Intensive Care Med 2001; 27:1352–9.

77. Voggenreiter G, Neudeck F, Aufmkolk M, et al. Intermittent prone positioning in the treatment of severe and moderate posttraumatic lung injury. Crit Care Med 1999; 27:2375–82.

78. Walz M, Muhr G. [Continuously alternating prone and supine positioning in acute lung failure.] Chirurg 1992; 63:931–7.

79. Shichinohe Y, Ujike Y, Kurihara M, et al. [Respiratory care with prone position for diffuse atelectasis in critically ill patients.] Kokyu To Junkan 1991; 39:51–5.

80. Albert RK. New ideas in treatment of ARDS. Yearbook of intensive care and emergency medicine. In: Vincent JL, editor. Berlin: Springer-Verlag, 1993: 135–47.

81. DuBois JM, Gaussorgues Ph, Sirodot M, et al. Prone position dependency in severely hypoxic patients. Intensive Care Med. 1992; 18(suppl):A18.

82. Thulig B, Hachenberg T, Wendt M, Wiesmann W, Sulkowski U. [Artificial respiration in the prone position in a case of acute respiratory distress syndrome.] Anasthesiol Intensivmed Notfallmed Schmerzther 1991; 26:196–8.

83. Faller JP, Feissel M, Kara A, Camelot R, Simon G. [Ventilation in prone position in acute respiratory distress syndrome of severe course. 3 cases.] Presse Med 1988; 17:1154.

84. Mentzelopoulos SD, Roussos C, Zakynthinos SG. Prone position improves expiratory airway mechanics in severe chronic bronchitis. Eur Respir J 2005; 25:259–68.

85. Kallet RH, Alonso JA, Pittet JF, Matthay MA. Prognostic value of the pulmonary dead-space fraction during the first 6 days of acute respiratory distress syndrome. Respir Care 2004; 49:1008–14.

86. Gattinoni L, Vagginelli F, Carlesso E, et al. Decrease in $PaCO_2$ with prone position is predictive of improved outcome in acute respiratory distress syndrome. Crit Care Med 2003; 31:2727–33.

87. Slutsky AS. The acute respiratory distress syndrome, mechanical ventilation, and the prone position. N Engl J Med 2001; 345:610–2.

88. Reignier J. Prone position: Can we move from better oxygenation to better survival? Crit Care Med 2005; 33: 453–4.

89. Broccard A, Shapiro RS, Schmitz LL, et al. Prone positioning attenuates and redistributes ventilator-induced lung injury in dogs. Crit Care Med 2000; 28:295–303.

90. Nishimura M, Honda O, Tomiyama N, et al. Body position does not influence the location of ventilator-induced lung injury. Intensive Care Med 2000; 26: 1664–9.

91. Dellinger RP, Carlet JM, Masur H, et al. Surviving Sepsis Campaign guidelines for management of severe sepsis and septic shock. Crit Care Med 2004; 32:858–73.

Chapter 51

PAIN CONTROL, SEDATION, AND NEUROMUSCULAR BLOCKADE

JOHN P. KRESS
JESSE B. HALL

Mechanically ventilated patients often require sedatives and analgesics. The myriad disease processes causing respiratory failure frequently elicit a sense of respiratory distress in these patients. In addition, therapies such as endotracheal intubation and positive pressure ventilation bring about discomfort to a significant number of patients in the intensive care unit (ICU), and patients often receive these life support treatments after surgical interventions or medical conditions that themselves carry a burden of pain. Accordingly, most patients receive analgesics and/or sedatives while undergoing mechanical ventilation. Though there are many drugs available to carry out the goals of pain control and, if necessary, sedation, studies of the impact of the use of these agents in ICU patients were limited until recently. Instead, most information came from experiences in other settings such as the operating room or procedure suite. With accumulation of evidence directed at ICU patient outcomes, a growing awareness of the complex pharmacology of sedatives and analgesics has emerged. At the same time, heightened awareness of the complications associated with the use of neuromuscular blocking agents has relegated their use to mostly short-term indications such as general anesthesia in the operating room, with ICU use now relatively rare. The drugs used to achieve analgesia and sedation of mechanically ventilated patients are potent—a property important for addressing distress during mechanical ventilation. Awareness, however, of the potential for enduring effects when these drugs are used without discretion has impacted strategies for their administration.

Rationale

Recognition of the fundamental pathophysiologies of respiratory failure, and the institution of mechanical ventilation as a supportive therapy, will allow goals of pain control, sedation, and neuromuscular blockade to complement the supportive goals of mechanical ventilation. An individualized strategy can then be executed, recognizing goals unique to each patient. This chapter will discuss principles and goals of pain control, sedation, and the rarely employed neuromuscular blockade in mechanically ventilated patients, as well as review the drugs currently available to achieve these goals.

Pain Control

We begin our discussion with the analgesic agents because most patients experience pain to some degree, because inadequate control of pain is unfortunately a memory patients may have after ICU management, and the ability of the patient to clearly indicate and quantify pain may be significantly impaired by respiratory failure and the devices employed to treat it. This last fact can lead to the unfortunate circumstance of pain in the mechanically ventilated patient presenting as agitation, which, if treated with sedatives alone is often inadequately treated and leads to excessive drug administration.

INDICATIONS

The indications for analgesia during mechanical ventilation come directly from the multiple reasons for pain in these patients. Pain from surgical incisions or trauma is self-evident, but other indications for pain control are more subtle. These include endotracheal suctioning or placement of invasive catheters such as arterial or venous lines. Preexisting problems such as skeletal fractures from metastatic cancer and prolonged immobility during bed rest[1,2] should be considered as other potential causes of pain. The mere presence of an endotracheal tube causes pain in many patients. Failure to recognize these common, but covert, indications for pain control frequently leads to discomfort in mechanically ventilated patients.

Pain may cause many adverse effects including increased endogenous catecholamine activity, myocardial ischemia, hypercoagulability, hypermetabolic states, sleep deprivation, anxiety, and delirium.[3] Treating pain has been shown to diminish some of these detrimental effects.[4]

ASSESSING ADEQUACY

It is undeniable that pain is a common experience for most mechanically ventilated patients.[1,5,6] Failure to recognize that pain can cause agitation may lead to inappropriate administration of nonanalgesic sedatives. Accordingly, an aggressive approach to managing pain has been strongly recommended by consensus opinions regarding sedation of mechanically ventilated patients.[7,8] Indeed, it is prudent to actively inquire for the presence of pain and begin the assessment of mechanically ventilated patients by postulating that pain is present as a symptom. The ability to accurately discern pain may be difficult because many ventilated patients are unable to convey its presence and clinical parameters such as changes in vital signs are often not reliable indicators. As such, a high level of vigilance toward analgesia is essential in mechanically ventilated patients.

In spite of such recommendations and vigilance, the management of pain in ventilated patients is often inadequate.[9–11] Ineffective communication with patients may be at the root of this problem, because delirium in the ICU is common.[12] Concern over addiction to opiates,[13] adverse cardiopulmonary effects of analgesics, and arbitrary limits placed on drug doses are other reasons for inadequate analgesia in ventilated patients.

Tools to categorize pain, such as scales or scoring systems, may be beneficial. In general, simpler scales are more effective because communication for many ventilated patients is limited. The visual analog scale (VAS), though not specifically evaluated in critically ill, mechanically ventilated patients, has very good reliability and validity.[14,15] This scale uses a self-reported measure of pain intensity that consists of a 10-cm line on paper with verbal anchors ("no pain" and "severe pain") on the ends. A similar scale is the numeric rating scale. This scale also consists of a horizontal line with numeric markings 1 and 10 anchoring either extreme of the pain-intensity scale.[16,17] It may be preferred because it can be completed by writing, speaking, or using hand gestures and may have better performance across various age groups.[7]

Previous studies have shown that benzodiazepines may enhance the analgesic effects of opiates[18,19] and that opiate requirements are decreased in patients sedated with benzodiazepines compared with propofol.[20,21] Notwithstanding this interesting observation, it is imperative that sedative agents are not used in the place of analgesics.

SELECTION OF AGENT

Nonpharmacologic analgesic strategies are worth considering. For example, malpositioning of invasive catheters (e.g., an endotracheal tube impinging on the main carina) is a problem that may be easily remedied. Likewise, optimal patient positioning in bed may at least partially relieve low back pain, pain from chest tubes, and so on. In spite of appropriate attention to nonpharmacologic approaches, most patients require administration of pharmacologic agents. Opiates are given in most circumstances and are discussed below.

OPIATES

Opiate receptors are ubiquitous, being found in the central nervous system as well as peripheral tissues. The two most clinically important opiate receptors are μ and κ. There are two subtypes of μ receptors, μ_1 and μ_2. Of these subtypes μ_1 receptors mediate analgesia, while μ_2 receptors mediate respiratory depression, nausea, vomiting, constipation, and euphoria. The κ receptors are responsible for such effects as sedation, miosis, and spinal analgesia. Several opiate drugs are available for clinical use and are discussed in detail below.

Morphine

Morphine is the most commonly used opiate agent and is the drug with which all other opiates are typically compared. When given intravenously, it has a relatively slow onset of action (typically 5–10 minutes); this is due to its low lipid solubility, which delays movement of the drug across the blood–brain barrier. The duration of action after a single dose of morphine is approximately 4 hours. When given repeatedly, accumulation in tissue stores may prolong the effect. It is metabolized in the liver, undergoing glucuronide conjugation, and its active metabolite, morphine-6-glucuronide, may accumulate, particularly in renal failure. Elimination occurs in the kidney, so effects may be prolonged in renal failure. The primary central effect of all opiates is analgesia, which is mediated through the μ and κ receptors. Opiates have some anxiolytic properties, but no reliable amnesia.

Fentanyl

Fentanyl is a synthetic opiate. It has a very high lipid solubility, unlike morphine, leading to rapid movement across the blood–brain barrier and rapid onset of action. Redistribution into peripheral tissues leads to short duration of action after a single dose (0.5–1 hour). When fentanyl is given repeatedly and tissue stores become saturated, its clinical effect can be prolonged. Fentanyl has no active metabolites and does not release histamine.[22]

Hydromorphone

Hydromorphone has similar pharmacologic properties as morphine with regard to onset of action. Because it has no active metabolites, however, the duration of action after long periods of hydromorphone administration may be less than that of morphine.

Meperidine

Meperidine is a lipid soluble opiate with rapid movement across the blood–brain barrier and a rapid onset of action (3–5 minutes). The higher lipid solubility leads to peripheral redistribution so that duration after a single dose may be shorter as compared with morphine (1–4 hours). Meperidine undergoes hepatic metabolism and renal elimination. Because metabolites of meperidine may accumulate secondary to the common organ dysfunctions that accrue in critically ill patients, and because these metabolites have neurotoxic effects that may cause seizures, this agent should be used with extreme caution if at all in the patient with respiratory failure (see below).

Remifentanil

Remifentanil is another synthetic, lipid soluble drug with a rapid onset of action. It is quickly metabolized via hydrolysis by nonspecific blood and tissue esterases. As such, its pharmacokinetic profile is not affected by hepatic or renal insufficiency. It is given by continuous infusion because of its rapid metabolism and recovery time. To date, the drug has not been studied for long term use in the critical care setting, with most studies reporting short-term use in neurosurgical and cardiac surgical ICU settings. When remifentanil is used during general anesthesia, available data suggest that postoperative respiratory failure is reduced, presumably because patients wake up more rapidly. This action can reduce the need for ICU admissions by allowing extubation in the operating room and preventing the need for postoperative intensive care.[23,24]

METHODS OF DELIVERY

For most patients, intravenous injection of opiate analgesics is the preferred route. Intramuscular injections are discouraged because of pain related to the injection itself and unpredictable absorption in critically ill patients. Dosing strategies for intravenous administration of opiates include continuous infusions and intermittent dosing strategies. Intermittent dosing can be further divided into scheduled administration, administration on an *as needed* or *prn* basis, and patient-controlled analgesia (PCA). Dosing given as needed may lead to fluctuations between inadequate and excessive analgesia. Patients alert enough to respond to their own pain needs may benefit from PCA strategies, though most ventilated patients are not alert enough to utilize a PCA device. Transdermal opiates may be continued in patients who are chronically receiving such medications, although transcutaneous absorption is unpredictable during critical illness. Certainly, this route should not be used for treating acute pain in mechanically ventilated patients.

TOXICITY

All opiates induce respiratory depression, which is centrally mediated and dose dependent. Depression is mediated by the mu-2 receptors in the brainstem medulla; the typical pattern is one of reduced respiratory rate but preserved tidal volume. The response to hypercapnia is decreased and the ventilatory response to hypoxia is obliterated. The depressed respiratory property of these drugs can be exploited in ventilated patients suffering from subjective dyspnea or coughing.

The hemodynamic effects of opiates in euvolemic patients are typically minimal. Hypovolemic patients with blood pressure sustained by sympathetic hyperactivity may suffer hypotension after the administration of opiates. Most opiates cause a decrease in heart rate because of decreased sympathetic activity. Though morphine causes histamine release, this does not usually cause hemodynamic com-

promise. Remifentanil may cause bradycardia and hypotension, particularly when administered concurrently with drugs having vasodilating properties, such as propofol. Hypertension after remifentanil, though described, is uncommon.

Gastrointestinal dysfunction in the form of pharmacologic ileus is common with the use of opiates in mechanically ventilated patients. Methylnaltrexone, a specific antagonist of mu-2 receptors in the gut, has been reported to attenuate opiate-induced gastrointestinal ileus in humans.[25] The utility of methylnaltrexone in critically ill, mechanically ventilated patients has not been tested.

Seizures are a toxicity unique to meperidine and occur as a result of its metabolite normeperidine, which is a central nervous system stimulant. Patients with renal failure and/or with prolonged use are especially prone to normeperidine accumulation. Because meperidine offers no significant advantage over other available opiates, its side-effect profile should largely preclude its use in critically ill patients.

Muscle rigidity occasionally occurs with synthetic opiates such as fentanyl and remifentanil. It is not seen with naturally occurring opiates like morphine. It is usually seen when high doses of these drugs are injected rapidly and may affect chest-wall muscles. The mechanism of opiate-induced skeletal muscle rigidity, though not fully understood, is thought to involve supraspinal activity of the drugs in the striata and substantia nigra. In the most extreme cases, respiratory-muscle rigidity makes ventilation impossible. Neuromuscular blockade, typically with succinylcholine, reverses this problem. Fortunately, this problem is extremely rare with the doses of opiates used in the management of ventilated patients in the ICU.

Dependence and withdrawal can be seen in patients receiving opiates for extended time periods when the drugs are discontinued. Patients who abuse opiates are at risk for this when hospitalized during critical illness. The signs and symptoms seen in withdrawal syndromes are mostly nonspecific and include pupillary dilation, sweating, lacrimation, rhinorrhea, piloerection, tachycardia, vomiting, diarrhea, hypertension, yawning, fever, tachypnea, restlessness, irritability, increased sensitivity to pain, nausea, cramps, muscle aches, dysphoria, insomnia, symptoms of opioid craving, and anxiety. Patients without previous illicit drug use may also experience opiate withdrawal when pharmacologically administered opiates given for extended time periods are suddenly stopped. Whether any preemptive strategies, such as downward titration or regular interruption of dosing, will attenuate or prevent opiate withdrawal is not known. One study of trauma patients reported a 32% incidence of withdrawal in patients receiving opiates and/or sedatives who were in the ICU for more than 1 week.[26] Those manifesting withdrawal received higher opiate and benzodiazepine drug doses than their counterparts without withdrawal. The role of long-acting opiates such as methadone to overcome this problem has not been studied in the ICU. Table 51-1 summarizes the pharmacologic properties of commonly used opiates.

TABLE 51-1 Properties of Commonly Used Opiates

	Morphine	Meperidine	Fentanyl	Methadone
Typical starting dose	2–5mg	20–50mg	25–50 μg	5–10 mg
Onset	10 minutes	3–5 minutes	0.5–1 minute	10–20 minutes
Duration after single dose	4 hours	1–4 hours	0.5–1 hour	6–24 hours
Metabolism	Hepatic	Hepatic	Hepatic	Hepatic
Elimination	Renal	Renal	Renal	Renal
Anxiolysis	+	++	++	+
Analgesia	++++	++++	++++	++++
Hypnosis	No reliable effect	No reliable effect	No reliable effect	No reliable effect
Amnesia	No reliable effect	No reliable effect	No reliable effect	No reliable effect
Seizure threshold	No effect	May decrease	No effect	No effect
Reducing dyspnea	++++	++++	++++	++++
Cardiovascular effect	Venodilation	Venodilation	Venodilation	Venodilation
Respiratory effect	Hypoventilation	Hypoventilation	Hypoventilation	Hypoventilation
Common side-effects	Nausea and vomiting, ileus, itching	Seizure, nausea and vomiting, ileus, itching	Nausea and vomiting, ileus, itching	Nausea and vomiting, ileus, itching

+, minimal effect; ++, mild effect; +++, moderate effect; ++++, large effect.

Sedation

INDICATIONS

Sedation needs vary widely in mechanically ventilated patients. Though nonpharmacologic approaches such as comfortable positioning in bed and verbal reassurance are reasonable initial considerations, treatment with sedative and analgesic agents is frequently needed. Effective use of sedatives and analgesics in critically ill patients begins with an understanding of their various indications. Effective *analgesia* (discussed above) is extremely important and should be considered concurrently with sedation. *Anxiety* occurs frequently in ventilated patients and is one of the most common indications for sedation. Anxiety may result from: (1) uncertainty of one's surroundings, diagnosis, or prognosis; (2) uncomfortable experiences such as the presence of an endotracheal tube or invasive diagnostic or therapeutic procedures; and (3) isolation from family and friends. Sedatives may be required to facilitate routine nursing care of mechanically ventilated patients. Procedures such as endotracheal suctioning, dressing changes, and repositioning regularly elicit distress requiring sedatives. *Dyspnea* is common in ventilated patients and may be a source of distress requiring sedation. Excessive coughing may contribute to patient-ventilator dyssynchrony in some patients. Many patients requiring mechanical ventilation suffer from cardiopulmonary instability and impaired gas exchange. Abnormal elevations in oxygen consumption and carbon dioxide production may compromise such patients. Reduction of oxygen consumption can stabilize the balance between oxygen supply and demand.[20] Such a reduction may be critical in ventilated patients with shock or severe hypoxemic respiratory failure. Autonomic instability and elevated endogenous catecholamine activity are common in ventilated patients and may lead to hemodynamic changes (e.g., tachycardia or hypertension) that may elicit myocardial ischemia in some patients, particularly those at risk for coronary artery disease.[27] Sedatives may be administered to counter such autonomic hyperactivity. *Amnesia* is often cited as an indication for sedation of ventilated patients. Certainly, for those patients mechanically ventilated during surgical procedures, the importance of amnesia is indisputable.[28] On the contrary, in patients ventilated during critical illness, the necessity of continuous amnesia is far less certain. Although amnesia for certain portions of critical illness requiring mechanical ventilation may seem logical (e.g., during invasive procedures), complete amnesia for extended periods during mechanical ventilation in the ICU has never been proven to confer benefit. Indeed, some data suggest that prolonged ICU amnesia may be detrimental to long-term neuropsychiatric recovery from critical illness.[29–31] It is clear, however, that complete amnesia is mandatory whenever neuromuscular blocking agents are administered. The relationship between *delirium* and sedation is indisputable. Delirium—defined as an acutely changing or fluctuating mental state, inattention, disorganized thinking, and an altered level of consciousness that may or may not be accompanied by agitation—has been reported in most critically ill patients.[12,32] Hyperactive or agitated delirium may occur with anxiety as well as sepsis, fevers, encephalopathy (e.g., hepatic or renal), withdrawal syndromes (alcohol, tobacco, or other illicit drugs), or medications. Such hyperactive delirium is frequently treated with neuroleptic medications such as haloperidol.[7] A substantial fraction, however, of ventilated ICU patients exhibit an insidious, hypoactive form of delirium. It is unclear whether this form of delirium is an indication for any pharmacologic therapy; on the contrary, it appears that currently available sedative medications are more likely to exacerbate rather than alleviate this type of delirium.

ASSESSING ADEQUACY

The assessment of sedation adequacy requires a thorough awareness of the indications for sedation. Even when indications are clear, adequacy assessment is challenging because of its subjective nature. As such, a reliable instrument to categorize level of sedation is an important initial step. In view of that, several sedation scales such as the Ramsay Sedation Score,[33] the Sedation Agitation Scale (SAS),[34] and the Richmond Agitation-Sedation Scale (RASS)[35] have been developed. The Ramsay scale, described over 30 years ago, is by far the most frequently referenced in clinical investigations of sedation. While it has the benefit of simplicity, it does not effectively measure quality or degree of sedation with regard to the indications outlined above.[36] Moreover, it has never been objectively validated.[37] More recently, other sedation scales such as the SAS and RASS have been tested extensively for validity and reliability.[34,35,38] The RASS is perhaps the most extensively evaluated scale. It has been validated for ability to detect changes in sedation status over consecutive days of ICU care, as well as against constructs of level of consciousness and delirium. Furthermore, this scale has been shown to correlate with doses of sedative and analgesic medications administered to critically ill patients. Because of their more precise scientific evaluations, the RASS and SAS should be viewed as preferable compared to the traditional Ramsay scale.

Ultimately, the evaluation of sedation adequacy is an individualized bedside maneuver. Guidance from nurses is useful, because changes in level of sedation are often first noticed by these omnipresent care providers. In practice, most schemas for administration of sedatives must take into account the fact that they will be titrated the vast majority of the time by the bedside nurse. Theoretically, the optimal level of sedation would result in a state in which all indications for sedation are attended to, and the patient is fully communicative with bedside caregivers. This state of being awake and communicative while sedatives are being administered is ideal, and is possible in some patients. Unfortunately, for many, the stresses of respiratory failure and mechanical ventilation do not permit such a state. Rather, many patients requiring mechanical ventilation require sedation to a point at which constant communication is impossible.

Objective monitors of sedation level would be attractive tools for ventilated patients. The bispectral index monitor processes raw EEG signals into a discrete scaled number from 0 (absence of cortical activity) to 100 (fully awake). This monitor has been shown to track the level of consciousness under general anesthesia.[39] Preliminary data suggest a good correlation between the bispectral index and the sedation agitation scale[40] as well as the RASS;[38] however, this device has not been extensively evaluated in the ICU and awaits more extensive validation before its role in the critical care setting is established.[7]

SELECTION OF AGENT

After indications for sedation are established, the clinician must choose one or more agents to administer. This section outlines the various agents currently available and discusses the pharmacologic properties of each agent.

BENZODIAZEPINES

Benzodiazepines act by potentiating GABA (γ-aminobutyric acid)-receptor mediated inhibition of the central nervous system. The GABA receptor complex regulates a chloride channel on the cell membrane, and, by increasing the intracellular flow of chloride ions, neurons become hyperpolarized, with a higher threshold for excitability. The GABA receptor can be competitively antagonized with the synthetic agent flumazenil, thereby reversing the pharmacologic effects of benzodiazepines. Midazolam, lorazepam, and diazepam are the three available parenteral benzodiazepines.

The onset of action of midazolam is rapid (0.5–5 minutes) and the duration following a single dose is short (~2 hours). All parenteral benzodiazepines, including midazolam, are lipid soluble with a large volume of distribution, and are therefore widely distributed throughout body tissues. For all benzodiazepines, the duration of action after a single bolus depends mainly on the rate of redistribution to peripheral tissues, especially adipose tissue. Midazolam undergoes hepatic metabolism and renal excretion. One metabolite of midazolam (α-hydroxymidazolam) has active pharmacologic properties. In the presence of normal renal function, α-hydroxymidazolam has a half-life of 1 hour. The pharmacokinetics of midazolam are very different when it is administered to critically ill patients, especially when given by continuous infusion for prolonged periods. Under these circumstances, preferential accumulation of the drug in peripheral tissues, where metabolism is not possible, is the rule. When drug infusions are stopped, the peripheral tissue stores release midazolam back into the bloodstream, leading to prolongation of clinical effect.[41] Obese patients with larger volumes of distribution and elderly patients with decreased hepatic and renal function may be even more prone to prolonged effects.

Intravenous lorazepam has a slower onset of action when compared to midazolam (5 minutes). This is due to a lower lipid solubility of lorazepam, which slows the drug's ability to cross the blood–brain barrier. The duration of action following a single dose is long (6–10 hours) and is proportional to the dose given. Because these data refer to healthy volunteers, applicability to critically ill patients is difficult. Lorazepam's longer duration of action is caused by lower lipid solubility with decreased peripheral tissue redistribution.

Intravenous diazepam has a rapid onset of action (1–3 minutes) and a limited duration of action following a single dose (30–60 minutes). Like midazolam, these pharmacologic properties are caused by the high lipid solubility, which leads to rapid peripheral redistribution of diazepam. After the peripheral tissues become saturated, prolonged recovery lasting days may be seen. The fact that diazepam has several active metabolites exacerbates recovery time. Diazepam metabolism requires intact hepatic function and is therefore prolonged in patients with liver disease. The above properties make diazepam a poor choice for sedation during mechanical ventilation. Accordingly, it is rarely given by continuous infusion in the ICU.

The parenteral benzodiazepines have similar pharmacodynamic effects. All cause dose-dependent suppression of awareness along a spectrum from mild depression of responsiveness to obtundation. They are potent anxiolytic drugs and reliably produce amnesia;[42,43] lorazepam appears to produce the longest duration of antegrade amnesia. Another common feature of these drugs is their reliable anticonvulsant effect.[44] Rarely, benzodiazepines cause agitation. This paradoxical response typically accelerates as additional benzodiazepine is given; though rare, it has a propensity to affect elderly patients. All benzodiazepines induce dose-dependent depression of respiratory drive. This ventilatory depression, while less extreme than that seen with opiates, behaves in a synergistic manner with opiate-induced respiratory depression. Distinguishing benzodiazepine-from opiate-induced respiratory depression may be difficult. A pattern of reduced tidal volume and slightly increased respiratory rate, however, may help to discern a benzodiazepine effect from the pattern of slow, deep breathing typically seen with opiates. Benzodiazepines, like opiates, can obliterate the hypoxic ventilatory drive. They have minimal effects on the cardiovascular system of euvolemic patients, typically causing slight decreases in blood pressure without a significant change in heart rate. The effect is exacerbated in the presence of relative hypovolemia. In patients with elevated endogenous sympathetic drive, more profound decreases in blood pressure can be seen. Table 51-2 summarizes the pharmacologic properties of the parenteral benzodiazepines.

PROPOFOL

Propofol is an intravenous anesthetic with an alkylphenol molecular structure. Like benzodiazepines, it appears to act on the GABA receptor, though not at the same site as the benzodiazepines. The drug is hydrophobic and is prepared as a lipid emulsion. Because of the drug's lipid solubility, it rapidly crosses the blood–brain barrier, leading to a rapid onset of sedation, particularly when a loading dose is given. The high lipid solubility allows for rapid redistribution of the drug to the peripheral tissues with a duration of only a few minutes.[45,46] With prolonged continuous infusions,

duration may be increased slightly, although it is rare for the effect to last beyond 60 minutes from the time of infusion discontinuation. When the infusion is stopped, the peripheral tissue stores redistribute the drug back into the plasma, but usually not to clinically significant levels because of the drug's high lipid affinity. Propofol is ultimately metabolized predominantly in the liver. It has an elimination half-life of 4–7 hours and no active metabolites.

Propofol has predictable pharmacodynamic effects on the central nervous system, acting as a hypnotic agent causing a dose-dependent depression of responsiveness and awareness. It is also a potent anxiolytic and amnestic agent.[47] Indeed, at high infusion rates, propofol is commonly used for general anesthesia. Though preliminary reports of propofol's impact on seizure threshold were conflicting, it is currently viewed by most authorities as an effective anticonvulsant.[48] Propofol has no detectable analgesic activity and is not recommended as a sole agent for the management of mechanically ventilated patients, because pain control is important in most of these patients.[7] The drug causes ventilatory depression and even apnea in some patients. Because apnea with propofol is unpredictable and not always dose dependent, it should not be used without readiness to secure the airway. The typical respiratory pattern with propofol is a decrease in tidal volume and a slight increase in respiratory rate. Propofol can cause significant decreases in blood pressure, especially in hypovolemic patients. Hypotension is mainly due to preload reduction from dilation of venous capacitance vessels. Deep sedation produced by any agent tends to have its primary effect upon blood pressure by this mechanism, and is associated with a generalized blunting of autonomic tone; propofol may be particularly potent in this regard. There is mild myocardial depression that also contributes to hypotension seen with propofol.[49,50] The hemodynamic effect is generally more pronounced than with the benzodiazepines and it should be given cautiously to patients with cardiac disease. Hyperlipidemia is a unique side effect of propofol.[51,52]

TABLE 51-2 Properties of Commonly Used Benzodiazepines

	Midazolam	Lorazepam	Diazepam
Typical starting dose	1–2 mg	0.5–1 mg	5–10 mg
Onset	0.5–2 minutes	3–5 minutes	1–3 minutes
Duration after single dose	2 hours	6–10 hours	1–6 hours
Metabolism	Hepatic	Hepatic (less influenced by age and liver disease)	Hepatic
Elimination	Renal	Renal	Renal
Anxiolysis	++++	++++	++++
Analgesia	No effect	No effect	No effect
Hypnosis	++++	++++	++++
Amnesia	++++	++++	++++
Seizure threshold	+++	++++	+++
Reducing dyspnea	+	+	+
Cardiovascular effect	Venodilation	Venodilation	Venodilation
Respiratory effect	Hypoventilation	Hypoventilation	Hypoventilation
Common side-effects	Paradoxical agitation	Paradoxical agitation	Paradoxical agitation

+, minimal effect; ++, mild effect; +++, moderate effect; ++++, large effect.

As noted above, the drug is delivered in an intralipid carrier, and propofol 1% solution has 1.1 kcal/ml.[53] Therefore, parenteral lipid feedings must be adjusted according to the propofol infusion rate to account for the calories administered with this drug. Triglyceride levels should be checked frequently and the drug stopped if hypertriglyceridemia is noted. Strict aseptic technique and frequent changing of infusion tubing is essential to prevent iatrogenic transmission of bacteria and fungi because propofol can support their growth.[54] A "propofol infusion syndrome," manifest as dysrhythmias, heart failure, metabolic acidosis, hyperkalemia, and rhabdomyolysis, is a rare complication. It appears to be more likely to occur when high doses (>80 μg/kg/min) and/or higher concentrations (2% versus 1%) of propofol are used.[55] An unpublished randomized, controlled trial of propofol in 327 pediatric patients reviewed by the Food and Drug Administration described a concentration-dependent increase in 28-day mortality in propofol-treated patients versus patients treated with other sedatives (4% mortality with sedatives other than propofol, 8% mortality with 1% propofol, and 11% mortality with 2% propofol).[56,57]

BUTYROPHENONES

Butyrophenones such as haloperidol are sometimes used for sedation of mechanically ventilated patients. These drugs induce a state of tranquility, and patients often behave with a detached affect. Butyrophenones appear to antagonize dopamine, especially in the basal ganglia, though their exact site of action is not known.

The onset time of intravenous haloperidol is 2–5 minutes and the half-life is 2 hours. Starting doses of 1–10 mg are typically used with titration depending on the desired end point. The drug is metabolized in the liver.

As mentioned above, patients receiving haloperidol respond with a calm, detached appearance. These drugs are typically reserved for patients who are acutely agitated and hyperactive. Patients may exhibit an appearance of indifference to their surroundings[58] and a state of cataleptic immobility is occasionally seen. Haloperidol provides no amnesia, no effect on seizure activity, and minimal analgesia. Butyrophenones such as haloperidol are the drugs of choice for agitated delirium. Recent data have implicated an association between the use of haloperidol in ventilated patients and a reduction in mortality, although these data are preliminary and retrospective in nature.[59]

Haloperidol has no significant effect on the respiratory system when used alone and there is little attenuation of respiratory depression when used in conjunction with opiates. Butyrophenones appear to preserve hypoxic pulmonary drive.[60] Reliable maintenance of respiratory function is an attractive feature of haloperidol, because most sedative or analgesic drugs cause respiratory depression.

Potential cardiovascular side effects of haloperidol are one reason for relatively limited use as a sedative in critically ill patients. Haloperidol is known to prolong the QT interval in some patients; it has been reported to result in torsades de pointes.[61] Even though this problem is rare, concern for its potential occurrence may limit its attractiveness to some clinicians. The drug also mildly antagonizes the α_1

receptor and may decrease the neurotransmitter function of dopamine, resulting in mild hypotension.

Extrapyramidal effects are occasionally seen with these drugs, but are much less common with intravenous than with oral butyrophenones. When these complications occur, treatment with diphenhydramine or benztropine may be necessary. This is an extremely rare problem with intravenous use in mechanically ventilated patients. The neuroleptic malignant syndrome is another extremely rare problem, thought to result from central dopaminergic blockade leading to extrapyramidal side effects, muscle rigidity, and excess heat generation. It is a life-threatening complication, manifested by "lead pipe" muscle rigidity, fever, and mental status changes. Bromocriptine, dantrolene, and pancuronium have all been used as successful therapies.[62]

DEXMEDETOMIDINE

Dexmedetomidine is a selective α_2 agonist with both sedative and analgesic properties.[63–65] Patients receiving this drug are sedated when undisturbed, but they arouse easily with minimal stimulation. Dexmedetomidine is unique in that patients transition from sedated to awake states quickly and easily without needing to discontinue the drug infusion, which permits frequent neurologic examinations. The drug is approved for short-term use (<24 hours) in patients initially receiving mechanical ventilation. Dexmedetomidine has been shown to be analgesic sparing in postoperative patients.[66] It causes no respiratory depression and therefore can be continued after discontinuation of mechanical ventilation and extubation. Side effects include bradycardia and hypotension,[67] especially with hypovolemia or high endogenous sympathetic tone. Vasoconstriction and hypertension with increasing doses of dexmedetomidine has also been described.[68,69] To date, most studies with dexmedetomidine have evaluated postoperative ICU patients.[70,71] Unfortunately, dexmedetomidine has not been extensively studied as an agent for long-term administration in critically ill, mechanically ventilated patients. Table 51-3 summarizes the pharmacologic properties of the other commonly used sedative agents: propofol, haloperidol, and dexmedetomidine.

KETAMINE

Ketamine is a dissociative anesthetic with a molecular structure similar to phencyclidine. Patients experience a state of mind in which perception is separated from sensation, a "detached from surroundings" or so-called "dissociative" state. Patients, while appearing unaware of their surroundings, keep eyes open and maintain a protective cough reflex. They may behave with coordinated movements that appear to be without purpose. The drug has profound analgesic properties without producing respiratory depression. The circulatory effects of hypertension and tachycardia, typically seen, reflect increased activity of the sympathetic nervous system. Some, but not all patients, experience amnesia after receiving ketamine. The common side effects of emergence delirium and severe hallucinations greatly limit its utility for sedation and analgesia in mechanically ventilated

TABLE 51-3 Properties of Other Sedative Agents

	Propofol	Haloperidol	Dexmedetomidine
Typical starting dose	1–2 mg/kg	0.5–1 mg	0.5–1.0 μg/kg over 10 minutes; 0.2–0.7 μg/kg/hour infusion
Onset	0.5–1 minute	2–5 minutes	5–10 minutes
Duration after single dose	2–8 minutes	2 hours	30–60 minutes
Metabolism	Hepatic, renal, lungs?	Hepatic	Hepatic
Elimination	Renal	Renal	Renal
Anxiolysis	++++	+++	+++
Analgesia	No effect	No effect	++
Hypnosis	++++	++	+++
Amnesia	++++	No effect	+
Seizure threshold	??	No effect	No effect
Reducing dyspnea	+	No effect	No effect
Cardiovascular effect	Venodilation, arteriolar dilation, myocardial depression	Venodilation, arteriolar dilation	Venodilation arteriolar dilation, bradycardia, occasional hypertension
Respiratory effect	Hypoventilation	No effect	No effect
Common side-effects	Increased triglycerides	Neuroleptic malignant syndrome (rare), extrapyramidal effects (rare)	Hypotension, bradycardia

+, minimal effect; ++, mild effect; +++, moderate effect; ++++, large effect.

patients. Indeed, this phencyclidine derivative has recently gained popularity as an illicit drug of abuse.

BARBITURATES
Barbiturates such as thiopental and pentobarbital are potent agents that cause amnesia and unconsciousness. They have no role as sedatives in mechanically ventilated patients because of a propensity to cause hemodynamic instability and accumulation in peripheral tissues secondary to lipid solubility, leading to prolonged effect. Thiopental is sometimes used to induce anesthesia to facilitate endotracheal intubation. These drugs may be used to induce a pharmacologic coma in patients with severe brain injury.

INHALATIONAL ANESTHETICS
Inhalational anesthetics are used widely in the operating room to maintain general anesthesia in mechanically ventilated patients. These exhaled gases must be effectively scavenged because they are not metabolized to any significant degree. The delivery and scavenging of inhaled anesthetics is a technically challenging problem, which has limited greatly the use of these agents outside of the operating room. Some authors, however, have reported that use of such inhaled anesthetics can be successful in mechanically ventilated, critically ill patients. For example, isoflurane, which has analgesic, amnestic, and hypnotic properties, has been described as an effective single agent for mechanically ventilated patients in the ICU.[72]

STRATEGIES FOR DELIVERY OF SEDATIVES IN CRITICALLY ILL MECHANICALLY VENTILATED PATIENTS

Because no single drug can achieve all of the indications for sedation and pain control in the ICU, a combination of drugs, each titrated to specific end points, may be more ef-

fective. This strategy can allow lower doses of individual drugs and reduce problems of drug accumulation. In the ICU, sedatives and analgesics are almost always administered via the intravenous route. Both continuous infusion and intermittent bolus techniques have been advocated. Intermittent administration of sedatives and analgesics may lead to fluctuations in level of sedation and increase demands on nursing time, potentially distracting attention away from other patient-care issues. The perceived benefits of continuous sedative infusions include a more consistent level of sedation with better patient comfort. The convenience of the continuous infusion strategy for both patients and caregivers is likely the greatest reason for its popularity.

Ideally, strategies for sedation and analgesia in critically ill patients should adhere to pharmacokinetic and pharmacodynamic principles. Unfortunately, ICU patients frequently exhibit unpredictable alterations in pharmacology[73] so that precise guidelines for drug administration are not possible. For instance, when short-acting benzodiazepines[74,75] such as midazolam and lorazepam are administered in the ICU, these drugs accumulate in tissue stores with consequent prolonged clinical effect.[76–79] Other circumstances that confound prediction of pharmacologic behavior of sedatives and analgesics include altered hepatic and/or renal function,[80] polypharmacy in the ICU with complex drug-drug interactions, altered protein binding, and circulatory instability. The multicompartmental pharmacokinetics typical in critically ill patients defy simple bedside pharmacokinetic profiling. As such, titration of sedatives and analgesics against discernible clinical end points, while imprecise, is the most commonly utilized tool. Further confounding administration of sedatives in the ICU is the dramatic difference between extremes of sedation. Because oversedated patients are easier to manage than undersedated patients, clinicians may be heavy handed when sedating agitated patients. In the initial stages of critical illness, this is appropriate; however, maintaining deep levels of sedation after patients are stabilized on mechanical ventilation can lead to the problems of prolonged sedation alluded to above.

It is not uncommon for some critically ill patients to require extraordinarily high doses of sedatives to achieve tranquility; such doses may be much greater than those quoted in the literature and recommended by drug manufacturers.[81] Indeed, as discussed below in the section on neuromuscular blocking drugs, occasional patients may even require pharmacologic paralysis to achieve synchrony with mechanical ventilation.[82]

Recently, evidence-based treatment strategies for many common conditions seen in critical illness have emerged. In the last decade, improved outcomes for critically ill patients with acute respiratory distress syndrome (ARDS),[83] sepsis,[84,85] acute renal failure,[86] status asthmaticus,[87] and cancer[88] have all been reported. As sicker patients continue to demonstrate improved outcomes in the ICU, more aggressive levels of sedation and analgesia may be necessary. This is particularly likely for patients managed with unconventional ventilator strategies (e.g., permissive hypercapnia, low tidal volumes, prone positioning, and pressure-controlled ventilation), because these strategies may be inherently distressing to many patients. For selected patients, deep sedation may be the only practical option.

The use of deep sedation, however, may carry a high price, because the neurologic examination is severely limited. Ideally, a head-to-toe daily assessment for the presence of organ failures should be routine for every critically ill patient. This is particularly so during resuscitative phases of care, when assessing the adequacy of end-organ perfusion and function is vital. The mental status examination is an important gauge of brain perfusion. Because brain injury is a devastating complication of critical illness, acute cerebral dysfunction must be detected quickly and corrected if possible before permanent injury takes place. The veil of sedation severely handicaps clinicians' ability to serially follow a patient's neurologic condition. Communication and thorough physical examination may detect problems quickly and obviate urgent diagnostic studies and therapeutic interventions after a problem has advanced.

A protocol-driven approach to sedation has been shown to alleviate many of the problems mentioned above. A protocol directed by bedside nurses can shorten duration of mechanical ventilation, ICU and hospital length of stay, and the need for tracheostomy[89] (Fig. 51-1). Such protocols assure adequate analgesia and sedation using frequent assessments of patient needs with goal-directed titration of analgesics and sedatives. Alternatively, a routine protocol of daily interruption of continuous sedative infusions can reduce many of the complications of sedation in the ICU setting, including duration of mechanical ventilation and ICU length of stay[21] (Figs. 51-2 and 51-3). Such a strategy allows patients to spend some of their ICU time awake and interactive, potentially reducing the amount of sedative and opiate given, as well as reducing the need for diagnostic studies (e.g., brain CT scan) to evaluate unexplained alterations in mental status. Such protocol-driven sedation strategies al-

low a focused downward titration of sedative infusion rates over time, streamlining administration of these drugs and minimizing the tendency for accumulation.

Protocol-driven sedation may allow the depth of sedation to be decreased without compromising the stated goals of sedation. Initially, the thought of decreasing or stopping sedatives in a critically ill patient who has been agitated may be unsettling. As such, clinicians may aggressively sedate patients early in their ICU course, and maintain the same level of deep sedation indefinitely. A daily holiday from sedatives can eliminate the tendency to "lock in" to a high sedative infusion rate, which—while appropriate early in ICU care—may be unnecessary on subsequent days. When sedative infusions are decreased or stopped, tissue stores can redistribute drug back into the circulation. Sometimes, interruption of sedative infusions may lead to abrupt awakening and agitation. This must be anticipated by the ICU team to avoid complications such as patient self-extubation; if excessive agitation is noted, sedatives should be restarted. Though the attempt at waking and communication may fail on a given day, this does not portend inevitable failure on all subsequent days. When awakening patients from sedation, reaching the brink of consciousness, without precipitating excessive agitation may be ideal for some. Once objective signs of consciousness are demonstrated, restarting sedatives *as needed* is reasonable. Restarting the sedative infusion at half of the previous dose is reasonable. Adjustments from this starting point can be individualized to patient needs.

It is clear that sedatives may impact the duration of mechanical ventilation.[21,89] Protocolized sedation strategies may reduce duration of mechanical ventilation by allowing earlier recognition of patient readiness to undergo a spontaneous breathing trial. Others have previously reported an important link between a successful spontaneous breathing trial and subsequent liberation from mechanical ventilation.[90,91]

Literature evaluating long-term consequences of recovery from respiratory failure and sedation is limited. Available data suggest that post-ICU depression is common in patients who require mechanical ventilation during critical illness.[92] Posttraumatic stress disorder following recovery has been reported as well.[31,93] Some data suggest that lack of awareness related to sedation and/or underlying illness is associated with development of this disorder, and that preservation of awareness during mechanical ventilation may reduce this problem.[29–31]

Neuromuscular Blocking Agents

INDICATIONS

The use of neuromuscular blocking agents (NMBs) during mechanical ventilation has decreased considerably in the last decade. These agents remain a common tool to facilitate endotracheal intubation and assure immobility during mechanical ventilation for surgical procedures. The role of these drugs, however, in the ICU has changed dramatically. Neuromuscular blockade was previously proposed as a strategy to facilitate mechanical ventilation of intubated

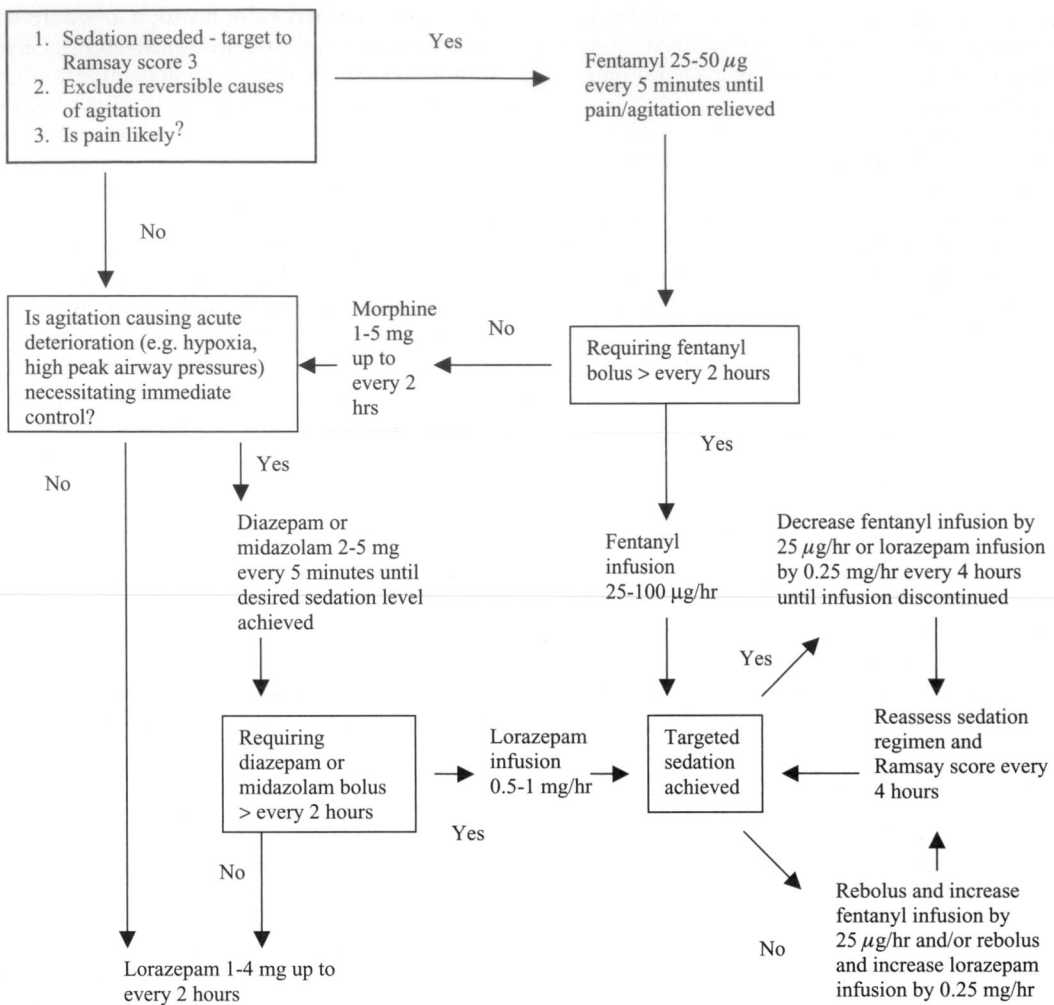

FIGURE 51-1 Protocol for nursing management of sedation during mechanical ventilation. (*Reproduced, with permission, from Brook et al.[89]*)

patients. Certainly, absence of skeletal-muscle activity assures that mechanical ventilation is completely controlled by the clinician, with no patient-ventilator dyssynchrony. Complications, however, related to the sustained use of NMBs during critical illness have relegated these agents to use as a last resort, usually only for extreme derangements in cardiopulmonary physiology.

Indications for neuromuscular blockade include facilitation of mechanical ventilation in the rare patient who continues to have *ventilator dyssynchrony* despite aggressive administration of sedatives and analgesics. Occasionally, a patient remains so dyssynchronous with the ventilator that effective ventilation is not possible and severe derangements in gas exchange ensue. If adjustments of ventilator settings (e.g., changing the mode to improve synchrony) and deepening of sedation and analgesia are not effective, neuromuscular blockade may be necessary. Patients with *tetanus* may require neuromuscular blockade because of chest-wall rigidity, which may prohibit effective chest-wall excursion and ventilation. As mentioned above in the discussion of opiate toxicities, the rare occurrence of *skeletal muscle rigidity with high-dose synthetic opiates* may require

neuromuscular blockade to permit ventilation. This problem is rare and muscle rigidity short-lived, so that neuromuscular blockade is necessary for only a short time. Lastly, circulation in patients with *severe hemodynamic instability* may become more compromised when respiratory distress demands even greater blood flow to the respiratory muscles from a circulation that cannot accommodate such demands. In such cases, cessation of respiratory-muscle activity facilitates redistribution of blood flow (away from respiratory muscles) to more vital organs such as the brain, heart, and kidneys. It is mandatory that patients given NMBs receive drugs to assure amnesia while they are pharmacologically paralyzed.

ASSESSING LEVEL OF BLOCKADE

Normally, at the neuromuscular junction, acetylcholine is released from synaptic vesicles at the terminal end of the motor nerve. Acetylcholine binds to the postsynaptic end plate, propagating an electrical signal through the muscle and leading to muscle contraction. Pharmacologic NMBs bind to the acetylcholine receptor at the terminal end of the

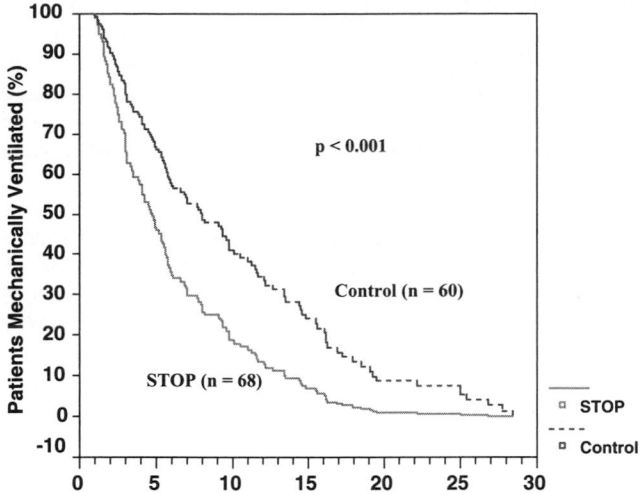

FIGURE 51-2 Kaplan-Meier analysis of the duration of mechanical ventilation. After adjustment for baseline variables (age, sex, weight, APACHE II score, and type of respiratory failure), a Cox proportional-hazards analysis showed mechanical ventilation was discontinued more quickly in the STOP group compared to the control group (relative risk of extubation 1.88; 95% confidence interval 1.30–2.73; $p <0.001$). (*Reproduced, with permission, from Kress et al.[21]*)

motor nerve. These agents can activate the acetylcholine receptor (depolarizing agents) or competitively inhibit the receptor without activating it (nondepolarizing agents). The depth of neuromuscular blockade from nondepolarizing agents is most accurately monitored with the use of

FIGURE 51-3 Kaplan-Meier analysis of the ICU length of stay. After adjustment for baseline variables (age, sex, weight, APACHE II score, and type of respiratory failure), a Cox proportional-hazards analysis showed ICU discharge occurred more quickly in the STOP group compared to the control group (relative risk of ICU discharge 1.56; 95% confidence interval 1.08–2.25; $p = 0.02$). (*Reproduced, with permission, from Kress et al.[21]*)

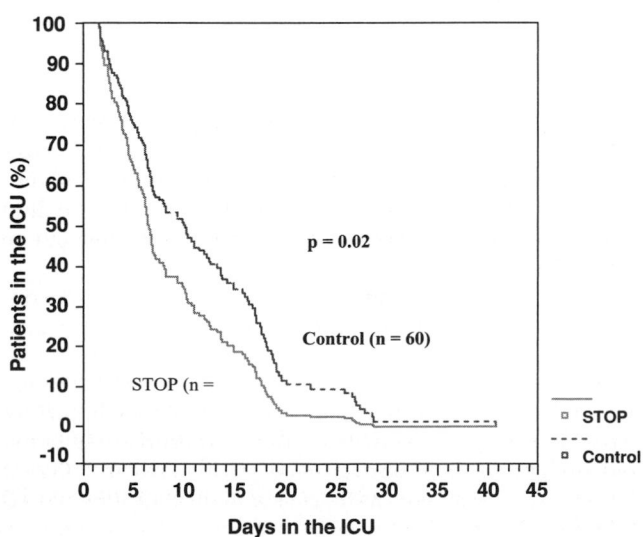

a peripheral nerve stimulator. This device sends a current between electrodes placed on the skin along the course of a peripheral nerve, most commonly the ulnar nerve. With this set-up, the twitches of the adductor pollicis muscle are evaluated to assess depth of neuromuscular blockade. The peripheral nerve stimulator is programmed to deliver four sequential stimuli at 2 Hz, referred to as a "train-of-four." Each electrical stimulus causes release of acetylcholine from synaptic vesicles at the neuromuscular junction. In the absence of pharmacologic neuromuscular blockade, the fourth twitch of the adductor pollicis muscle will be as strong as the first twitch. When neuromuscular receptors, however, are occupied by nondepolarizing NMBs, the strength of the fourth twitch is less than the first, until eventually the muscle does not twitch with the fourth stimulus. This phenomenon is known as *fade*. When 85–90% of the neuromuscular receptors are occupied by NMBs, only the first twitch in the train-of-four is visible. With 70–85% occupation, between two to four twitches are typically visible. Usually, two or three out of four twitches are sought and dosing of NMBs is titrated to this goal. Peripheral nerve stimulator use in the ICU has been shown to reduce the amount of NMB drug used and shorten recovery of neuromuscular function and spontaneous ventilation.[94] Another study showed a reduction in the incidence of persistent neuromuscular weakness.[95]

SELECTION OF AGENT

DEPOLARIZING NEUROMUSCULAR BLOCKING AGENTS

Succinylcholine
Succinylcholine is the only available depolarizing NMB. It has the most rapid and reliable onset of neuromuscular blockade, with paralysis sufficient to permit endotracheal intubation within 60 seconds of dosing. As such, succinylcholine is used only to facilitate endotracheal intubation but is not indicated for ongoing neuromuscular blockade in critically ill patients.

NONDEPOLARIZING NEUROMUSCULAR BLOCKING AGENTS
A number of nondepolarizing NMBs are currently available. The pharmacology of the drugs commonly used during mechanical ventilation in the ICU is discussed below.

Pancuronium
Pancuronium is an older NMB used during general anesthesia as well as in the ICU. It has an aminosteroidal molecular structure. The drug has a long half-life, with a duration of action between 60 and 90 minutes after a single intravenous bolus dose of 0.1 mg/kg. Its vagolytic side effect (typically results in a heart rate increase of ~10 beats/min), active metabolite (3-hydroxypancuronium), and reliance on renal clearance limit its attractiveness in critically ill patients.

Vecuronium
Vecuronium also has an aminosteroidal molecular structure, but a shorter half-life than pancuronium. After a bolus

of 0.1 mg/kg, this drug typically lasts 30 minutes. Half of the drug is excreted in bile, so prolonged action may be seen in patients with liver dysfunction. In addition, one-third of the drug is excreted in the kidneys, so that accumulation in the setting of renal insufficiency may be seen. The active metabolite 3-desacetylvecuronium may lead to prolongation of effect with repeated dosing, particularly in patients with renal failure.[96]

Rocuronium

Rocuronium also has an aminosteroidal molecular structure. Unlike the other aminosteroidal nondepolarizing NMBs, rocuronium has a rapid onset of action, typically within 60–90 seconds. It may be used to facilitate endotracheal intubation, as a substitute for succinylcholine, when the latter is contraindicated (e.g., burns, muscle tissue injury, and upper motor neuron lesions). The usual bolus dose is 0.6–1.0 mg/kg, with a duration of effect of 30–45 minutes, similar to vecuronium. The metabolite, 17-desacetylrocuronium, has minimal neuromuscular blocking activity.

Doxacurium

Doxacurium is a benzylisoquinolinium agent with a long half-life, 60–90 minutes. The usual bolus dose is 0.5–1.0 mg/kg. The drug is eliminated by renal excretion and has no hemodynamic effects.

Atracurium

Atracurium is a benzylisoquinolinium compound with a duration of action between 20 and 45 minutes. The initial loading dose is 0.4–0.5 mg/kg. The drug is usually given by continuous infusion in critically ill, mechanically ventilated patients at a dose of 10–20 μg/kg/min. Atracurium is inactivated in plasma by ester hydrolysis and Hofmann elimination so that renal or hepatic dysfunction do not impact its duration of blockade. This feature has made it attractive for use in ICU patients, since those requiring NMBs often suffer from renal or hepatic dysfunction or are at high risk for developing these organ failures. Atracurium may cause histamine release, and its breakdown product, laudanosine, has been associated with central nervous system excitation and seizures in animal models.

Cisatracurium

An isomer of atracurium is cisatracurium, which has a similar pharmacologic profile to atracurium. The initial loading dose is 0.1–0.2 mg/kg and the duration of action is approximately 25 minutes. Like atracurium, this drug is inactivated in plasma by ester hydrolysis and Hofmann elimination. Cisatracurium does not cause histamine release. Because of its short half-life, it requires administration by continuous infusion. The usual dose is 2.5–3 μg/kg/min. This drug is currently one of the most frequently used for neuromuscular blockade in mechanically ventilated ICU patients.

TOXICITY

In normal individuals, depolarization of skeletal muscle beds after administration of depolarizing neuromuscular blocking agents such as succinylcholine leads to release of intracellular potassium, typically resulting in an increase in serum potassium of approximately 0.5 mEq/L. Denervation of skeletal muscle from tissue injury, such as with burns or upper motor neuron lesions, may result in more dramatic rises in serum potassium with administration of succinylcholine, which may precipitate malignant cardiac dysrhythmias.

The major toxicity with nondepolarizing NMBs is prolonged weakness, which occurs by two separate mechanisms. The accumulation of NMB parent drug or its metabolites is seen with some agents (e.g., pancuronium and vecuronium), especially in patients with renal and/or hepatic dysfunction.[97] The use of drugs such as atracurium and cisatracurium has significantly reduced the incidence of prolonged weakness secondary to NMB parent drug or metabolite accumulation. The second cause of weakness associated with NMBs is known as acute quadriplegic myopathy syndrome and is currently a more significant problem. Patients with this syndrome manifest acute paresis, myonecrosis with increased creatine phosphokinase concentration, and abnormal electromyography. Electromyographic findings are consistent with denervation of skeletal muscle (decreased compound motor action potential amplitudes). Denervation may progress to muscle atrophy and occasionally even muscle necrosis.

Concerns over complications of NMBs have led to a dramatic decrease in their use in the ICU.[94] This is particularly noteworthy when corticosteroids are used in conjunction with NMBs. Several studies have suggested this combination is associated with a significant incidence of myopathy.[98,99] Table 51-4 summarizes the pharmacologic properties of commonly used neuromuscular blocking agents.

Important Unknowns and the Future

Currently available drugs for pain control, sedation, and neuromuscular blockade in mechanically ventilated patients all have important limitations. The newer agents have not undergone adequate evaluation in critically ill, mechanically ventilated patients. It is tempting to expect that a drug with less tendency to accumulate over time (e.g., propofol, dexmedetomidine, or remifentanil) may result in fewer residual effects. These newer drugs need to be studied in patients receiving them for prolonged periods, in order to evaluate potential benefits and limitations. Whether differences in sedative pharmacology can translate into widespread differences in patient outcomes remains to be determined.

Protocol-driven management of sedation and pain control can clearly improve patient outcomes. More experience with protocols and better understanding of potential limitations is needed in order to continue to optimize patient outcomes, both short and long term. As such, further expansion of protocol-driven administration of sedation and analgesia should be evaluated, particularly in different ICU environments such as trauma or neurologically injured patients.

TABLE 51-4 Properties of Commonly Used Neuromuscular Blocking Agents

	Succinylcholine	Pancuronium	Vecuronium	Rocuronium	Atracurium	Cisatracurium
Type	Depolarizing	Nondepolarizing	Nondepolarizing	Nondepolarizing	Nondepolarizing	Nondepolarizing
Typical loading/intubation dose	1.0–1.5 mg/kg	0.1 mg/kg	0.1 mg/kg	0.6–1.0 mg/kg	0.5 mg/kg	0.1–0.2 mg/kg
Continuous infusion (dose)	No	No	No	No	Yes (10–20 μg/kg/min)	Yes (2–3 μg/kg/min)
Onset	60 seconds	3–5 minutes	3–5 minutes	1–2 minutes	3–5 minutes	3–5 minutes
Duration after loading dose	7–9 minutes	60–90 minutes	30–40 minutes	30–45 minutes	20–45 minutes	25 minutes
Metabolism	Plasma cholinesterase	Hepatic	Hepatic/Biliary	Hepatic	Ester hydrolysis/Hofmann elimination	Ester hydrolysis/Hofmann elimination
Elimination		Renal	Renal/biliary	Biliary clearance of parent molecule from palsma		
Active metabolite	No	Yes	Yes	Yes (minimal)	No	No
Cardiovascular effect	Supraventricular and ventricular rhythm disturbances with hyperkalemia	Vagolytic—tachycardia	None	None	Histamine release	No histamine release
Common side-effects	Hyperkalemia	None	None	None	Histamine release	None

1105

Widespread use of scales describing sedation level and titration of drugs based upon goals described by these objective scales should allow optimization of sedation and analgesia. The impact of sedation and analgesia on delirium during critical illness must be further studied, given the magnitude of this problem in terms of prevalence and associated morbidity. The impact of neuromuscular blockade, sedation, and pain control on recovery following respiratory failure is poorly understood. Patients who require mechanical ventilation during critical illness suffer numerous psychological as well as physical complications and recovery may be slow and often incomplete.[100,101] With recognition of psychological maladjustment, a few strategies achieving improved outcomes have been reported,[31,102] but more studies in this area are needed. Physical debilitation after respiratory failure and critical illness is well described, with most studies focusing on recovery from ARDS.[100,103–105] Many of these patients suffer from critical illness–related polyneuropathy and myopathy.[106–108] Whether sedation strategies during respiratory failure impact critical illness polyneuropathy and myopathy is not known; although prolonged immobility and deconditioning should be considered as potentially contributing to these neuromyopathies.[109]

Summary and Conclusion

Pain control, sedation, and neuromuscular blockade are important components of the treatment of patients who require mechanical ventilation. Directing treatment to specific and individualized goals will assure that patient needs are met. All currently available agents for use in ventilated patients have limitations and complications related to their use. Rather than seeking an ideal drug, strategies of drug administration that focus attention on principles of sedative pharmacology in critical illness should be utilized. When these drugs are given to individual patients, recognition of specific goals will allow rational administration strategies to be implemented, which should lead to improvement in both short- and long-term outcomes.

References

1. Novaes MA, Knobel E, Bork AM, et al. Stressors in the ICU: perception of the patient, relatives and healthcare team. Intensive Care Med 1999; 25:1421–6.
2. Desbiens NA, Wu AW, Broste SK, et al. Pain and satisfaction with pain control in seriously ill hospitalized adults: Findings from the SUPPORT research investigators. Crit Care Med 1996; 24:1953–61.
3. Epstein J, Breslow MJ. The stress response of critical illness. Crit Care Clin 1999; 15:17–33.
4. Lewis KS, Whipple JK, Michael KA, et al. Effect of analgesic treatment on the physiological consequences of acute pain. Am J Hosp Pharm 1994; 51:1539–54.
5. Puntillo KA. Pain experiences of intensive care unit patients. Heart Lung 1990; 19:526–33.
6. Turner JS, Briggs SJ, Springhorn HE, et al. Patients' recollection of intensive care unit experience. Crit Care Med 1990; 18:966–8.
7. Jacobi J, Fraser GL, Coursin DB, et al. Clinical practice guidelines for the sustained use of sedatives and analgesics in the critically ill adult. Crit Care Med 2002; 30:119–41.
8. Shapiro BA, Warren J, Egol AB, et al. Practice parameters for intravenous analgesia and sedation for adult patients in the intensive care unit: an executive summary. Crit Care Med 1995; 23:1596–600.
9. World Health Organization Expert Committee Report. Cancer pain relief and palliative care. Technical report series 804. Geneva: World Health Organization, 1990.
10. Carroll KC, Atkins PJ, Herold GR, et al. Pain assessment and management in critically ill postoperative and trauma patients: a multicenter study. Am J Crit Care 1999; 8:105–17.
11. Ferguson J, Gilroy D, Puntillo K. Dimensions of pain and analgesic administration associated with coronary artery bypass in an Australian intensive care unit. J Adv Nurs 1997; 26:1065–72.
12. Ely EW, Inouye SK, Bernard GR, et al. Delirium in mechanically ventilated patients: validity and reliability of the confusion assessment method for the intensive care unit [CAM-ICU]. JAMA 2001; 286:2703–10.
13. Sun X, Weissman C. The use of analgesics and sedatives in critically ill patients: physicians' orders versus medications administered. Heart Lung 1994; 23:169–76.
14. Price DD, Bush FM, Long S, et al. A comparison of pain measurement characteristics of mechanical visual analogue and simple numerical rating scales. Pain 1994; 56:217–26.
15. Price DD, McGrath PA, Rafii A, et al. The validation of visual analogue scales as ratio scale measures for chronic and experimental pain. Pain 1983; 17:45–56.
16. Jensen MP, Karoly P, Braver S. The measurement of clinical pain intensity: a comparison of six methods. Pain 1986; 27:117–26.
17. Meehan DA, RcRae ME, Rourke DA, et al. Analgesia administration, pain intensity, and patient satisfaction in cardiac surgical patients. Am J Crit Care 1995; 4:435–42.
18. Bianchi M, Mantegazza P, Tammiso R, et al. Peripherally administered benzodiazepines increase morphine-induced analgesia in the rat. Effect of RO 15-3505 and FG 7142. Arch Int Pharmacodyn Ther 1993; 322:5–13.
19. Sivam SP, Ho IK. GABA in morphine analgesia and tolerance. Life Sci 1985; 37:199–208.
20. Kress JP, O'Connor MF, Pohlman AS, et al. Sedation of critically ill patients during mechanical ventilation. A comparison of propofol and midazolam. Am J Respir Crit Care Med 1996; 153:1012–18.
21. Kress JP, Pohlman A, O'Connor MF, et al. Daily interruption of sedative infusions in critically ill patients undergoing mechanical ventilation. N Engl J Med 2000; 342:1471–77.
22. Rosow CE, Moss J, Philbin DM, et al. Histamine release during morphine and fentanyl anesthesia. Anesthesiology 1982; 56:93.
23. Park GR, Evans TN, Hutchins J, et al. Reducing the demand for admission to intensive care after major abdominal surgery by a change in anesthetic practice and the use of remifentanil. Eur J Anesthesiol 2000; 17:111–19.
24. Cohen J, Royston D. Remifentanil. Curr Opin Crit Care 2001; 7:227–31.
25. Yuan CS, Foss JF, O'Connor MF, et al. Methylnaltrexone for reversal of constipation due to chronic methadone use: a randomized controlled trial. JAMA 2000; 283:367–72.
26. Cammarano WB, Pittet JF, Weitz S, et al. Acute withdrawal syndrome related to the administration of analgesic and sedative medications in adult intensive care unit patients. Crit Care Med 1998; 26:676–84.

27. Srivastava S, Chatila W, Amoateng-Adjepong Y, et al. Myocardial ischemia and weaning failure in patients with coronary artery disease: an update. Crit Care Med 1999; 27:2109–12.

28. Jones JG. Perception and memory during general anaesthesia. Br J Anaesth 1994; 73:31–7.

29. Jones C, Griffiths RD. Disturbed memory and amnesia related to intensive care. Memory 2000; 8:79–94.

30. Jones C, Griffiths RD, Humphris G, et al. Memory, delusions, and the development of acute posttraumatic stress disorder–related symptoms after intensive care. Crit Care Med 2001; 29: 573–80.

31. Kress JP, Lacy M, Pliskin N, et al. The long term psychological effects of daily sedative interruption in critically ill patients. Am J Respir Crit Care Med 2003; 168:1457–61.

32. Ely EW, Shintani A, Truman B, et al. Delirium as a predictor of mortality in mechanically ventilated patients in the intensive care unit. JAMA 2004; 291:1753–62.

33. Ramsay MAE, Savege TM, Simpson BRJ, et al. Controlled sedation with alphalaxone-alphadolone. BMJ 1974; 2:656–9.

34. Riker RR, Picard JT, Fraser GL. Prospective evaluation of the sedation-agitation scale for adult critically ill patients. Crit Care Med 1999; 27:1325–9.

35. Sessler CN, Gosnell MS, Grap MJ, et al. The Richmond agitation-sedation scale: validity and reliability in adult intensive care unit patients. Am J Respir Crit Care Med 2002; 166:1338–44.

36. Crippen DW. Neurologic monitoring in the intensive care unit. New Horizons 1994; 2:107–20.

37. Hansen-Flaschen J, Cowen J, Polomano RC. Beyond the Ramsay scale: need for a validated measure of sedating drug efficacy in the intensive care unit. Crit Care Med 1994; 22:732–3.

38. Ely EW, Truman B, Shintani A, et al. Monitoring sedation status over time in ICU patients: reliability and validity of the Richmond agitation-sedation scale (RASS). JAMA 2003; 289:2983–91.

39. Glass PS, Bloom M, Kearse L, et al. Bispectral analysis measures sedation and memory effects of propofol, midazolam, isoflurane, and alfentanil in healthy volunteers. Anesthesiology 1997; 86:836–47.

40. Simmons LE, Riker RR, Prato BS, et al. Assessing sedation during intensive care unit mechanical ventilation with the bispectral index and the sedation-agitation scale. Crit Care Med 1999; 27:1499–504.

41. Byatt CM, Lewis LD, Dawling S, et al. Accumulation of midazolam after repeated dosage in patients receiving mechanical ventilation in an intensive care unit. BMJ 1984; 289:799–800.

42. Dundee JW, Wilson DB. Amnesic action of midazolam. Anaesthesia 1980; 35:459–61.

43. George KA, Dundee JW. Relative amnesiac actions of diazepam, flunitrazepam and lorazepam in man. Br J Clin Pharm 1977; 4:45–50.

44. Treiman DM. The role of benzodiazepines in the management of status epilepticus. Neurology 1990; 40:32–42.

45. Shafer SL. Advances in propofol pharmacokinetics and pharmacodynamics. J Clin Anesth 1993; 5:14S–21S.

46. Bailie GR, Cockshott ID, Douglas EJ, et al. Pharmacokinetics of propofol during and after long term continuous infusion for maintenance of sedation on ICU patients. Br J Anesth 1992; 68:486–91.

47. Veselis RA, Reinsel RA, Marino P, et al. Propofol in sedative doses is an amnestic agent. Anesthesiology 1991; 75:A1023.

48. Marik PE, Varon J. The management of status epilepticus. Chest 2004; 126:582–91.

49. Goodchild CS. Cardiovascular effects of propofol and relevance to use in patients with compromised cardiovascular function. Semin Anesth 1992; 11:S37–8.

50. Mouren S, Baron J, Albo C. Effects of propofol and thiopental on coronary blood flow and myocardial performance in an isolated rabbit heart. Anesthesiology 1994; 80:634–41.

51. Gottardis M, Khuenl-Brady KS, Koller W, et al. Effect of prolonged sedation with propofol on serum triglyceride and cholesterol concentrations. Br J Anesth 1989; 62:393–6.

52. Barrientos-Vega R, Mar Sanchez-Soria M, Morales-Garcia C, et al. Prolonged sedation of critically ill patients with midazolam or propofol: impact on weaning and costs. Crit Care Med 1997; 25:33–40.

53. Roth MS, Martin AB, Katz JA. Nutritional implications of prolonged propofol use. Am J Health-Syst Pharm 1997; 54:694–5.

54. Bennett SN, McNeil MM, Bland LA, et al. Postoperative infections traced to contamination of an intravenous anesthetic, propofol. N Engl J Med 1995; 333:147–54.

55. Cremer OL, Moons KGM, Bouman EAC, et al. Long-term propofol infusion and cardiac failure in adult head-injured patients. Lancet 2001; 357:117–8.

56. http://www.fda.gov/safety/2001/diprivan_deardoc.pdf

57. Felmet K, Nguyen T, Clark RS, et al. The FDA warning against prolonged sedation with propofol in children remains warranted. Pediatrics 2003; 112:1002–3.

58. Riker RR, Fraser GL, Cox PM. Continuous infusion of haloperidol controls agitation in critically ill patients. Crit Care Med 1994; 22:433–40.

59. Millbrandt EB, Kersten A, Kong L, et al. Haloperidol use is associated with lower hospital mortality in mechanically ventilated patients. Crit Care Med 2005; 33:226–30.

60. Ward DS. Stimulation of the hypoxic pulmonary drive by droperidol. Anesth Analg 1984; 63:106–10.

61. Zee-Cheng CS, Mueller CE, Seifert CF, et al. Haloperidol and torsades de pointes. Ann Intern Med 1985; 102:418.

62. Burke C, Fulda GJ, Castellano J. Neuroleptic malignant syndrome in a trauma patient. J Trauma 1995; 39:796–8.

63. Peden CJ, Cloote AH, Stratford N, et al. The effect of intravenous dexmedetomidine premedication on the dose requirement of propofol to induce loss of consciousness in patients receiving alfentanil. Anaesthesia 2001; 56:408–13.

64. Venn RM, Bradshaw CJ, Spencer R, et al. Preliminary UK experience of dexmedetomidine, a novel agent for postoperative sedation in the intensive care unit. Anaesthesia 1999; 54:1136–42.

65. Venn RM, Newman PJ, Grounds RM. A phase II study to evaluate the efficacy of dexmedetomidine for sedation in the medical intensive care unit. Intensive Care Med; 2003:201–7.

66. Venn RM, Grounds RM. Comparison between dexmedetomidine and propofol for sedation in the intensive care unit: patient and clinician perceptions. Br J Anaesth 2001; 87: 684–90.

67. Dasta JF, Kane-Gill SL, Durtschi AJ. Comparing dexmedetomidine prescribing patterns and safety in the naturalistic setting versus published data. Ann Pharmacother 2004; 38:1130–5.

68. Ebert TJ, Hall JE, Barney JA, et al. The effects of increasing plasma concentrations of dexmedetomidine in humans. Anesthesiology 2000; 93:382–94.

69. Talke P, Lobo E, Brown B. Systemically administered alpha-agonist-induced peripheral vasoconstriction in humans. Anesthesiology 2003; 99:65–70.

70. Martin E, Ramsay G, Mantz J, et al. The role of the alpha2-adrenoceptor agonist dexmedetomidine in postsurgical sedation in the intensive care unit. J Intensive Care Med 2003; 18:29–41.

71. Herr DL, Sum-Ping ST, England M. ICU sedation after coronary artery bypass graft surgery: dexmedetomidine-based versus propofol-based sedation regimens. J Cardiothorac Vasc Anesth 2003; 17:576–84.

72. Spencer EM, Willatts SM. Isoflurane for prolonged sedation in the intensive care unit: efficacy and safety. Intensive Care Med 1992; 18:415–21.

73. Bodenham A, Shelly MP, Park GR. The altered pharmacokinetics and pharmacodynamics of drugs commonly used in critically ill patients. Clin Pharmacokinet 1988; 14:347–73.

74. Wagner BKJ, O'Hara DA. Pharmacokinetics and pharmacodynamics of sedatives and analgesics in the treatment of agitated critically ill patients. Clin Pharmacokinet 1997; 33:426–53.

75. Michalk S, Moncorge C, Fichelle A, et al. Midazolam infusion for basal sedation in intensive care: absence of accumulation. Intensive Care Med 1988; 15:37–41.

76. Kollef MH, Levy NT, Ahrens TS, et al. The use of continuous IV sedation is associated with prolongation of mechanical ventilation. Chest 1998; 114:541–8.

77. Shelly MP, Mendel L, Park GR. Failure of critically ill patients to metabolise midazolam. Anaesthesia 1987; 42:619–26.

78. Malacrida R, Fritz ME, Suter PM, et al. Pharmacokinetics of midazolam administered by continuous intravenous infusion to intensive care patients. Crit Care Med 1992; 20:1123–6.

79. Ostermann ME, Keenan SP, Seiferling RA, et al. Sedation in the intensive care unit: a systematic review. JAMA 2000; 283: 1451–9.

80. Bertz RJ, Granneman GR. Use of in vitro and in vivo data to estimate the likelihood of metabolic pharmacokinetic interactions. Clin Pharmacokinet 1997; 32:210–58.

81. Oldenhof H, de Jong M, Steenhoek A, et al. Clinical pharmacokinetics of midazolam in intensive care patients, a wide interpatient variability? Clin Pharmacol Ther 1988; 43:263–9.

82. Gottlieb JE, Park P, Girod A, et al. Comparison of neuromuscular blocker and sedative use among patients with ARDS treated with low versus high tidal volume. Am J Respir Crit Care Med 2000; 161:A506.

83. The Acute Respiratory Distress Syndrome Network. Ventilation with lower tidal volumes as compared with traditional tidal volumes for acute lung injury and the acute respiratory distress syndrome. N Engl J Med 2000; 342:1301–8.

84. Bernard GR, Vincent JL, Laterre PF, et al. Recombinant human protein C Worldwide Evaluation in Severe Sepsis (PROWESS) study group. Efficacy and safety of recombinant human activated protein C for severe sepsis. N Engl J Med 2001; 344:699–709.

85. Rivers E, Nguyen B, Havstad S, et al. Early goal-directed therapy in the treatment of severe sepsis and septic shock. N Engl J Med 2001; 345:1368–77.

86. Schiffl H, Lang SM, Fischer R. Daily hemodialysis and the outcome of acute renal failure. N Engl J Med 2002; 346:305–10.

87. Tuxen DV, Williams T, Scheinkestel C. Limiting dynamic hyperinflation in mechanically ventilated patients with severe asthma reduces complications. Anaesth Intensive Care 1993; 21:718.

88. Rubenfeld GD, Crawford SW: Withdrawing life support from mechanically ventilated recipients of bone marrow transplants: a case for evidence-based guidelines. Ann Intern Med 1996; 125:625–33.

89. Brook AD, Ahrens TS, Schaiff R, et al. Effect of a nursing-implemented sedation protocol on the duration of mechanical ventilation. Crit Care Med 1999; 27:2609–15.

90. Ely EW, Baker AM, Dunagan DP, et al. Effect on the duration of mechanical ventilation of identifying patients capable of breathing spontaneously. N Engl J Med 1996; 335:1864–9.

91. Kollef MH, Shapiro SD, Silver P, et al. A randomized, controlled trial of protocol-directed versus physician-directed weaning from mechanical ventilation. Crit Care Med 1997; 25:567–74.

92. Schelling G, Stoll G, Haller C, et al. Health-related quality of life and PTSD in survivors of ARDS. Crit Care Med 1998; 26:651–9.

93. Nelson BJ, Weinert CR, Bury CL, et al. Intensive care unit drug use and subsequent quality of life in acute lung injury. Crit Care Med 2000; 28:3626–30.

94. Frankel H, Jeng J, Tilly E, et al. The impact of implementation of neuromuscular blockade monitoring standards in a surgical intensive care unit. Am Surg 1996; 62:503–6.

95. Tavernier B, Rannou JJ, Vallet B. Peripheral nerve stimulation and clinical assessment for dosing of neuromuscular blocking agents in critically ill patients. Crit Care Med 1998; 26:804–5.

96. Segredo V, Caldwell JE, Matthay MA, et al. Persistent paralysis in critically ill patients after long-term administration of vecuronium. N Engl J Med 1992; 327:524–8.

97. Murray M, Cowen J, DeBlock H, et al. Clinical practice guidelines for sustained neuromuscular blockade in the adult critically ill patient. Crit Care Med 2002; 30:142–56.

98. Leatherman JW, Fluegel WL, David WS, et al. Muscle weakness in mechanically ventilated patients with severe asthma. Am J Respir Crit Care Med 1996; 153:1686–90.

99. Behbehani NA, Al-Mane F, D'yachkova Y, et al. Myopathy following mechanical ventilation for acute severe asthma: the role of muscle relaxants and corticosteroids. Chest 1999; 115:1627–31.

100. Herridge MS, Cheung AM, Tansey CM, et al. One-year outcomes in survivors of the acute respiratory distress syndrome. N Engl J Med 2003; 348:683–93.

101. Hopkins RO, Weaver LK, Pope D, et al. Neuropsychological sequelae and impaired health status in survivors of severe acute respiratory distress syndrome. Am J Respir Crit Care Med 1999; 160:50–6.

102. Jones C, Skirrow P, Griffiths RD, et al. Rehabilitation after critical illness: a randomized, controlled trial. Crit Care Med 2003; 31:2456-61.

103. McHugh LG, Milberg JA, Whitcomb ME, et al. Recovery of function in survivors of the acute respiratory distress syndrome. Am J Respir Crit Care Med 1994; 150:90–4.

104. Weinert CR, Gross CR, Kangas JR, et al. Health-related quality of life after acute lung injury. Am J Respir Crit Care Med 1997; 156:1120–8;

105. Davidson TA, Caldwell ES, Curtis JR, et al. Reduced quality of life in survivors of acute respiratory distress syndrome compared with critically ill control patients JAMA 1999; 281:354–60.

106. Bolton CF, Gilbert JJ, Hahn AF, et al. Polyneuropathy in critically ill patients. J Neurol Neurosurg Psychiatry 1984; 47:1223–31.

107. Leijten FSS, DeWeerd AW, Poortvliet DCJ, et al. Critical illness polyneuropathy in multiple organ dysfunction syndrome and weaning from the ventilator. Intensive Care Med 1996; 22:856–61.

108. de Letter MA, Schmitz PM, Visser LH, et al. Risk factors for the development of polyneuropathy and myopathy in critically ill patients. Crit Care Med 2001; 29:2281–6.

109. Herridge MS. Long-term outcomes after critical illness. Curr Opin Crit Care 2002; 8:331–6.

HUMIDIFICATION

JEAN-DAMIEN RICARD

Humidification issues are overlooked by many clinicians in the ICU. Because the need to heat and humidify inspired gases during mechanical ventilation is unanimously accepted, this process is considered the basic, supportive standard of care, about which there is no real debate. Yet, considerable controversy has surrounded central issues concerning humidification such as the level of adequate humidification and how to provide it, the influence of humidification devices on the incidence of ventilator-associated pneumonia, and certain patients and clinical situations and their requirements, such as the need for humidification during noninvasive ventilation. This may account for important differences in the practice of humidification between countries.[1] Fortunately, renewed interest has emerged over the past decade, as indicated by several clinical studies that have helped settle some controversies. This chapter will review the reasons for conditioning inspired gases by recalling the normal process of heating and humidifying air during spontaneous breathing, the physical principles of humidification, and the consequences of inappropriate conditioning. Devices to achieve this conditioning will be covered and their advantages and potential drawbacks discussed. Finally, practical guidelines will be provided.

Rationale

As mentioned below, the upper respiratory tract is responsible for most of the conditioning of the inspired gases. Important features of this conditioning (reviewed by Irlbeck[2]) include heat, humidification, and filtration, in order to deliver to the lower respiratory tract a warm (32°C), humid (95% relative humidity), and pathogen- and particle-free gas. The last step is achieved in the lower respiratory tract. During invasive mechanical ventilation, the endotracheal tube bypasses the upper respiratory tract. This places the burden of supplying heat and humidity to the cold and dry medical gases on the lower respiratory tract, a task for which it is poorly suited.[3]

Anatomy and Physiology of the Upper Airway

The upper respiratory tract (nose, mouth, nasopharynx, oropharynx, laryngopharynx, and larynx, but mainly the nose) is responsible for most of the conditioning of inspired gas. Anatomic structure and physiologic function of the nose are intimately linked. The highly vascular mucosa of the nose is ciliated and rich in mucosal glands and goblet cells. Three curved bony plates on the lateral side of each nasal cavity (the superior, middle, and inferior concha or turbinate bones), covered with a mucous membrane, ensure the important function of satisfactorily conditioning inspired gases. Their large surface area and position in relationship with the air current enable sufficient contact with the inspired gas. This mucous membrane also lines the paranasal sinuses, trachea, and bronchi but not the pharynx, which does not take part in the air-conditioning process.

Physical Principles of Humidification

Humidity can be defined as the moisture content of the atmosphere and by extension, water present as vapor in a gas mixture. Vaporization indicates the change of a liquid (or a solid) to a gas or vapor. There is no strict difference between the terms *gas* and *vapor*, although gas is generally used to describe a substance that appears in the gaseous state under standard conditions of pressure and temperature, and vapor to describe the gaseous state of a substance that appears ordinarily as a liquid or solid. Such a change of state requires a certain amount of energy or heat to overcome van der Waals' forces that bind the molecules together in the liquid state. They then escape the liquid as individual molecules of vapor. This amount of heat, specific for each substance, is known as the latent heat of vaporization of the substance.

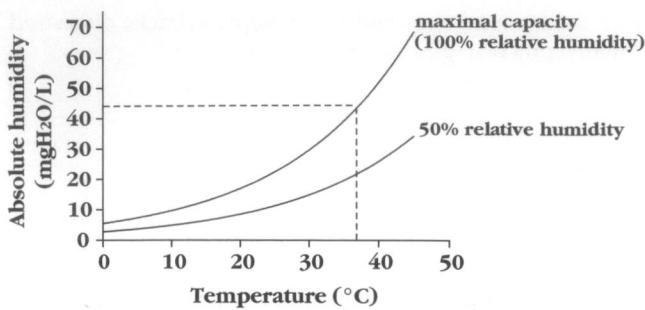

FIGURE 52-1 Absolute humidity (mass of water vapor) of air as a function of temperature at two relative humidities (100% and 50%). The dotted lines indicate the value of absolute humidity (44 mgH$_2$O/L) at core body temperature (37°C) when air is fully saturated (100% relative humidity).

Importantly, liquids can change to gases at temperatures below their boiling points. Vaporization of a liquid below its boiling point is called evaporation, and can occur at any temperature when the surface of a liquid is exposed in an unconfined space. Molecules of liquid that leave the surface of the liquid (because of sufficient kinetic energy) turn to vapor. They do so with their latent heat; the loss of heat causes the liquid's temperature to decrease. These molecules of vapor exert a certain amount of pressure known as vapor pressure. Vapor pressure is substance- and temperature-specific (i.e., each substance has a specific vapor pressure for each given temperature). At its boiling point, the vapor pressure of a liquid is equal to the atmospheric pressure. Therefore, vapor pressure of water at 100°C is 760 mmHg.

Measurements of humidity include absolute humidity and relative humidity. Absolute humidity is the mass of water vapor per unit volume of the gas mixture and is measured in milligrams of water per liter of gas (mgH$_2$O/L). Importantly, at any given temperature, a gas may contain only up to a certain amount of water vapor, corresponding to its maximal capacity at that temperature. Any extra water vapor will condense back into a liquid state. Relative humidity indicates the ratio of the actual water-vapor content of the gas mixture to its total capacity at the given temperature. The amount of water vapor a gas can contain is directly proportional to the temperature of the gas (Fig. 52-1). For example, air with 50% relative humidity contains 22 mg of H$_2$O at 37°C, but only 8.5 mg of H$_2$O at 20°C.

Physiologic Principles of Humidification

Physiologic humidification delivers inspired air at 37°C and saturated with water vapor (100% relative humidity) to the lungs. Figure 52-1 indicates that in these conditions, the gas mixture contains 44 mg of H$_2$O per liter. The principle of humidification lies in the heat and humidity gradient that exists between the inspired gas and the respiratory tract.

As indicated above, humidification occurs first and mainly in the nose, then in the trachea and up to the second-generation bronchi. The large surface area of the turbinates, in combination with their irregular shape and protrusion into the nasal cavity that create a turbulent flow, enables a rapid transfer of heat from the mucosa to the inspired air. This heat gain is sufficient to allow water to evaporate from the mucosa into the inspired gas, enabling its humidification. As a result, inspired gas is warmed and humidified and nasal mucosal temperature decreases from 37°C to 31°C.

During expiration, the opposite occurs. The gas leaves the alveolus at 37°C with 44 mg/L of H$_2$O, and transfers heat to the cooler upper airway. As its temperature decreases, so does its maximal water content capacity. Condensation on the mucosa then occurs. At the end of expiration, approximately one-third of the heat and humidity has been transferred back to the mucosa.

Until the inspired gas has reached 37°C with 44 mg/L water content, heat and water are lost from the respiratory tract. The point at which inspired gas reaches core temperature and 100% relative humidity is called the isothermic saturation boundary. It is usually situated in the second-generation bronchi. After this point, temperature and humidity of inspired gas remain constant, in order to ensure adequate gas exchange in the alveolus. Depending on climatic conditions, the isothermic saturation boundary may move up or down the respiratory tract.

Pathophysiology of the Upper Airway

UNDERHUMIDIFICATION

Underhumidification results from the bypassing of the upper airway that follows tracheal intubation and from the absence or inadequacy of conditioning of the dry, compressed, medical gas. Delivery to the lower respiratory tract of insufficiently warmed and humidified gas displaces the isothermic saturation boundary further down the bronchial tree. Moisture and heat loss ensues, inducing structural damages of the respiratory tract that may lead to physiologic and functional impairments with clinical repercussions.

EFFECTS OF MOISTURE LOSS

Moisture loss from the respiratory tract is, under normal conditions, a physiologic phenomenon (approximately 150 ml water) and contributes to the body's insensible water loss. The loss may be much greater if minute ventilation is increased, or if the gradient between the water content of inspired and expired air is large or both. This situation is encountered during mechanical ventilation and was first described during general anesthesia. In one of the first comprehensive studies on this topic, Burton described the reduction of mucociliary function after several hours of dry gas ventilation. When heat and humidity were added, mucociliary function was restored.[4] Numerous studies have been performed subsequently, and exhaustively reviewed.[3] The adverse effects of inadequate humidification comprise structural damages such as loss of ciliary function, cilia destruction, damage to mucus glands, cytoplasmic and nuclear degeneration, cellular desquamation, mucosal ulceration, changes in tracheal cytology, and loss of surfactant. Such structural damage has functional repercussions: destruction of the mucociliary escalator, increase in sputum viscosity, increased airway resistance, decreased pulmonary compliance, reduced functional capacity, and increased pulmonary shunting. Clinical consequences include retained secretions, mucus plugging, atelectasis, increased work of breathing, hypothermia, and hypoxemia.[2] In clinical practice, the worst and most feared adverse effect of underhumidification is life-threatening endotracheal tube occlusion, which requires urgent endotracheal tube replacement (see section on effectiveness and outcome, below).

EFFECT OF HEAT LOSS

During general anesthesia, the amount of heat loss through the respiratory tract is very small in comparison with that of other sources (e.g., the operative field and skin). Two mechanisms may account for this loss. Heat is transferred from the respiratory mucosa to the inspired gases, and the amount will depend on the patient's minute ventilation, the temperature gradient between the respiratory tract and the inspired gas, and the latter's specific heat. Given the very low specific heat of air, minimal heat is required to raise its temperature. The second and major mechanism by which heat is lost is vaporization (change of liquid water of the respiratory mucosa into vapor and its transfer to the inspired gas). Given the high specific heat of water, a significant amount of heat is required to raise the relative humidity of inspired gases. The amount of heat is further increased when the relative humidity of the inspired gas is very low (i.e., dry medical gas). These considerations may be important during prolonged surgery in infants and young children, keeping in mind that skin, operative site, and fluid administration are the major contributors to the heat loss.

OVERHUMIDIFICATION

Because heat and moisture exchangers (HMEs) act passively (see below), they cannot deliver excessive heat or water to the respiratory tract. Consequently, the adverse effects described below are only possible with heated humidifiers and aerosol humidifiers and are now seldom encountered.[5]

EXCESS WATER

The volume of water that can be added to the airway mucosa depends on the state it is in. With heating and humidifying devices, water is in a molecular form (vapor) and is therefore unlikely to result in overhumidification, given the amount of water vapor contained in inspired gases. To significantly increase this amount would require excessive heating of the inspired gas (way above body temperature), thus causing thermal injury before overhydration. Effects of excess water have been reported in the past with the use of aerosol humidifiers[6] but clinicians are now well aware of these side effects.

EXCESS HEAT

Reports of lung injury secondary to excessive heat are rare[5] and are related to the misuse of heated humidifiers.[7]

Methods of Humidification

Although many different types of humidifiers have been developed in the past, clinicians mainly use two types of devices to condition inspired gas during mechanical ventilation: heated humidifiers and HMEs.

HEATED HUMIDIFIERS

The general working principle of heated humidifiers is to heat water contained in a humidification chamber that humidifies inspired gas passing through it[8] (Fig. 52-2). Heating the water enables evaporation to occur, and the gas leaves the chamber saturated with water vapor. Evaporation depends on the surface area over which it occurs, the temperature of the liquid water, and the magnitude of the vapor pressure above the water surface. It can therefore be increased by augmenting the contact of inspired gas and water (larger humidification chamber), by raising the temperature of the liquid water, and by increasing the mass flow of gas above the water surface in order to decrease the vapor pressure. Once the inspired gas has left the humidifier, it cools along the breathing circuit before reaching the patient. Thus the temperature one wished to achieve at the patient's level will not be reached. There are two ways to help overcome this problem. Inspired gas can be heated in the chamber to above the temperature one wishes to deliver to a patient, to take into account the heat loss across the circuit. Abundant condensation, however, will occur inside the tubing, providing an ideal reservoir for bacterial colonization[9,10] and will need to be drained, exposing health-care workers to

FIGURE 52-2 Heated humidifier with a heated breathing circuit. Two temperature probes monitor gas temperature at the exit of the humidifier chamber and at the Y-piece before the endotracheal tube (*black arrows*).

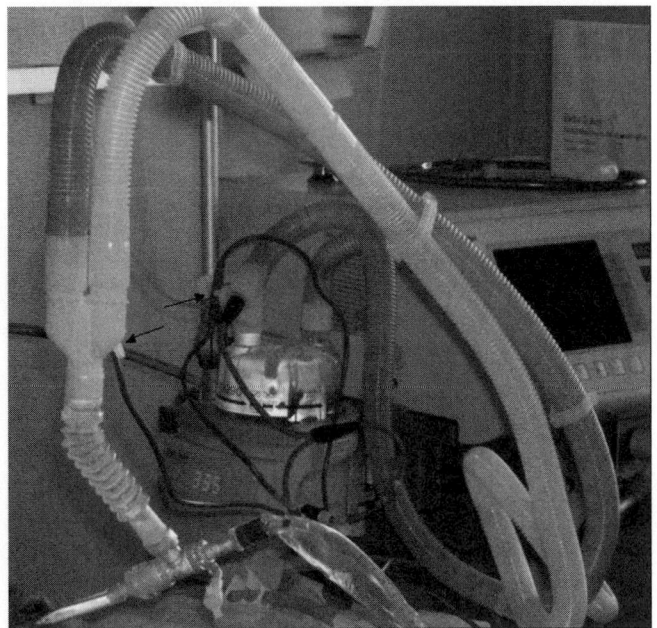

contaminated fluids and placing other patients at risk of cross-contamination.[11] To prevent this condensation (that results from the decrease in the temperature of the gas whose maximum vapor-carrying capacity is therefore reduced), breathing circuits can be heated by placing electric heater wires either in the wall or in the lumen of the circuit.

New devices are now servo-controlled by means of temperature sensors placed at the exit of the humidification chamber and just before the catheter mount (or flex tube). Because only the temperature is monitored (and not the humidity), however, these devices may become faulty in certain circumstances (see below).[12,13]

HEAT AND MOISTURE EXCHANGERS

HMEs were first described in the mid-1950s[14] and the early 1960s[15] and have undergone considerable development since the beginning of the 1970s.[16] The basic principle of all HMEs lies in their capacity to retain heat and moisture during expiration and deliver these to the incoming dry medical gas during subsequent inspiration[17] (Fig. 52-3). This passive function may be achieved by different mechanisms. The first HMEs were simple condensers, made with metal elements with a large surface area such as rolled wire gauze[14] or stainless steel tubes.[15] Because of the high density and thermal conductivity of metal, no effective temperature gradient was achieved across the device. Metal elements of the

condenser were then replaced by disposable foam, plastic, or paper. Increased moisture output was further achieved by coating the condenser element with a hygroscopic chemical (calcium or lithium chloride), which chemically adsorbs expired water vapor that is then returned to the inspired gas. These HMEs were called hygroscopic condensers. Derived from the field of filtration, hydrophobic HMEs were also used to heat and humidify inspired gas. The very large surface area of pleated, water-repellent ceramic of the first hydrophobic HMEs along with its low thermal conductivity enabled an important temperature gradient to develop within the HME that favored heat and moisture retention. Finally hygroscopic and hydrophobic elements were used in a single HME to create a "combined" HME. Hygrometric performance of these various HMEs differ considerably,[18] with hydrophobic HMEs exhibiting the lowest humidity outputs (with the attendant risk of endotracheal tube occlusion) and combined HMEs the highest, although recent measurements indicate that some purely hygroscopic HMEs provide levels of absolute humidity comparable to those of combined HMEs.[19,20]

ACTIVE HEAT AND MOISTURE EXCHANGERS
New devices have been designed to boost the humidifying performance of HMEs.[21] Briefly, these devices, which are added to the circuit between the HME and the endotracheal tube, consist of a ceramic heating element fed by an electrical energy source that vaporizes water (fed into the system by a side port) into the airway. They enable a 3- to 4-mgH$_2$O/L increase in absolute humidity delivered by the HME,[21] although the actual clinical benefit of this increase is uncertain.

Application

Based on the above principles, supplying heat and humidity to inspired gases is mandatory when the upper airway is bypassed during tracheal intubation. This supply must be provided as soon as the patient is connected to the ventilator, either by an HME or by a heated humidifier. Apart from certain specific situations (see section on practical steps, below), both HMEs or heated humidifiers serve equally well. Despite this, practices differ considerably among countries.[1,22] A recent survey found that HMEs were used for all patients in 63% of French ICUs, whereas this was the case in only 13% of Canadian ICUs.[1] Conversely, heated humidifiers were primarily used in 60% of Canadian ICUs and in only 20% of French ICUs. These results may account for some of the difference in cost of mechanical ventilation between the two countries.[22] Rationalizing the choice of a given humidifying device should help decrease costs in mechanical ventilation without impeding quality of care.

Effectiveness and Outcome

Several important aspects must be taken into account when analyzing the effectiveness and outcomes of inspired gas conditioning. These include:

FIGURE 52-3 A combined (hydrophobic and hygroscopic) heat and moisture exchanger. Dark arrows indicate the presence of dripping wet condensation in the flexible tubing (the bright reflection seen on the wall of the tubing) suggesting that adequate humidity is being delivered by the heat and moisture exchanger (see text for details). Note that the heat and moisture exchanger is positioned vertically above the endotracheal tube, thus limiting the amount of secretions refluxing from the tube to the heat and moisture exchanger.

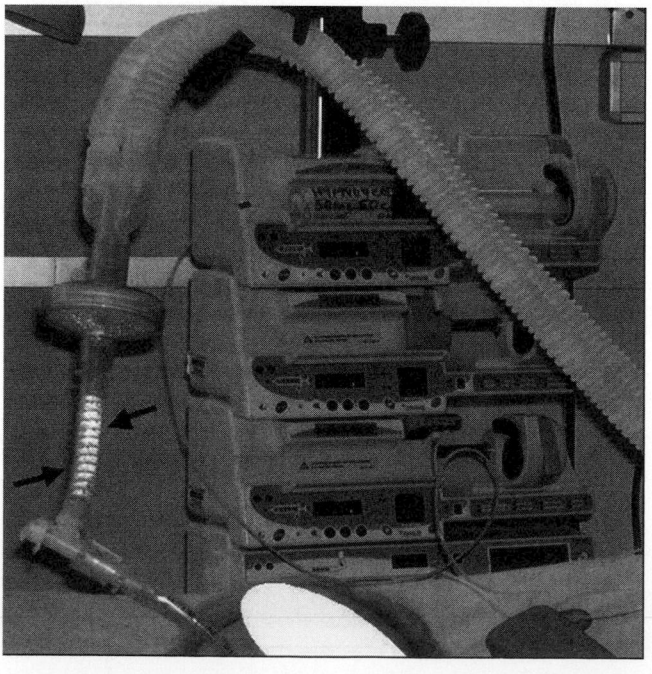

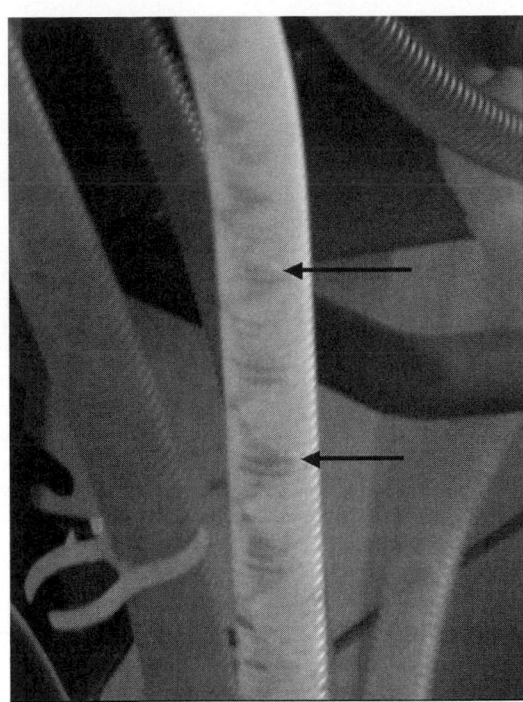

FIGURE 52-4 A heavily contaminated breathing circuit.

- The avoidance of endotracheal tube occlusion (which is the worst and most feared complication of inadequate gas conditioning), and this aspect is directly linked to the performance of the humidifying device in terms of heat and humidity delivery;
- The avoidance of spreading microorganisms (and in particular multi–drug-resistant organisms), and this is directly linked to the humidifying device's capacity to prevent contamination of the respiratory tubing (Fig. 52-4);
- The addition of minimal resistance and dead space;
- The practicability of use of the device;
- The minimal maintenance necessary to ensure optimal use of the device; and
- The minimal cost associated with the purchase and the long-term use of the device.

Using this list, one can define the characteristics of the ideal humidifier: a device that provides adequate levels of humidification whatever the ventilator and patient conditions; one that does so automatically; one that is safe to operate (i.e., is electric-shock free, with no or a limited number of connections that can become faulty); one that protects the environment from the patient's pathogens; one that is easy to use; and one that requires low maintenance and is inexpensive.

ENSURING ADEQUATE HUMIDIFICATION

The adequate level of humidification can be defined as a level at which there is no excessive heat or water loss by the respiratory tract. The difficulty arises when one tries to set the minimum value of absolute humidity a device should deliver. This may be useful when selecting and comparing different devices. Although ranges as wide as 25–35 mgH_2O/L have been suggested in the past,[23] the figure of 30 mgH_2O/L is recommended today.[24] That is, a clinician wishing to select an appropriate humidifying device should make sure that the device delivers at least 30 mgH_2O/L of absolute humidity. Another definition of adequate humidification is the one that avoids endotracheal tube occlusion. Some may argue that restricting adequate humidification to minimize the risk of endotracheal occlusion is oversimplistic. One must bear in mind, however, that it is the worst and most feared side effect of insufficient humidity, and it may be sometimes fatal.[25]

There is no doubt that 20 years ago, HMEs and heated humidifiers were not equivalent in terms of humidity output. In 1988, Cohen et al alerted clinicians to the risk of endotracheal tube occlusions associated with the use of HMEs.[26] Two years later, Martin et al reported a fatal case of endotracheal tube occlusion with an HME.[25] Two other publications confirmed the increase in endotracheal tube occlusion risk with HMEs in comparison with heated humidifiers.[27,28] These studies, however, all used purely hydrophobic HMEs, whose measured performance displayed low values of absolute humidity.[18,19,29,30]

It has been shown that endotracheal tube occlusion occurs after a gradual reduction in the tube's inner diameter caused by clots of secretions that collect on the inner surface of the tube.[31] This reduction was found to be significantly greater with a purely hydrophobic HME than with a heated humidifier or a combined (hydrophobic and hygroscopic) HME.[31] Although hygrometric measurements were not performed simultaneously in this study,[31] it seems evident that inner diameter reduction (and thus ultimately endotracheal tube occlusion) is dependent on the amount of humidity delivered by the humidifying device. Indeed, humidity measurements of the devices used by Villafane et al[31] have been made by others and the results are consistent with their findings (i.e., the hydrophobic HMEs that suffered the greatest inner diameter reduction displayed the poorest humidity output[18,29,30]) (Fig. 52-5). This leads to the question of hygrometric and clinical performance.

Although heated humidifiers indisputably deliver greater values of absolute humidity than HMEs[18,29,30] (see Fig. 52-5), there is to date no evidence of any benefit of these greater values in terms of clinical outcome, including endotracheal tube occlusion. Table 52-1 displays the incidence of endotracheal tube occlusion reported in recently published studies. It is important to note that: (1) endotracheal tube occlusion rates have drastically dropped in comparison with earlier studies;[26–28] (2) endotracheal tube occlusion is also reported with the use of heated humidifiers; and (3) the incidence of endotracheal tube occlusion no longer appears to be greater with HMEs than with heated humidifiers. In one study, the incidence was greater with heated humidifiers than with HMEs.[32]

The reasons for this unusually high rate of endotracheal occlusions deserve particular attention. As indicated above (see section on methods of humidification), new heated humidifiers are servo-controlled. Because the temperature of the incoming gas mixture has a direct effect on the heating mechanism of the plate that warms the humidification chamber, if the temperature is too high, the plate no longer heats, resulting in very low levels of absolute humidity,[12,13]

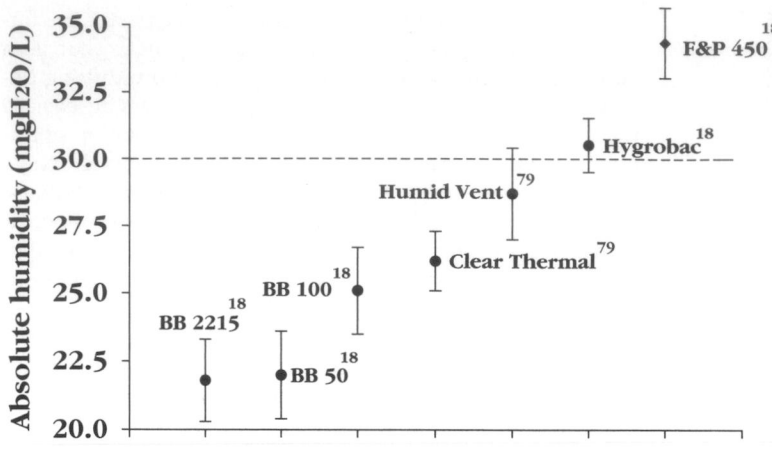

Figures in superscript indicates study reference number

FIGURE 52-5 Values of absolute humidity delivered by several heat and moisture exchangers and one heated humidifier. The dotted horizontal line delineates the minimum value of humidity (30 mgH2O/L) a device should deliver. Note the discrepancies that exist among heat and moisture exchangers (*black circles*). The HMEs exhibiting the lowest values of absolute humidity are those most strongly associated with endotracheal tube occlusions. The heated humidifier (*black diamond*) exhibited the highest value for absolute humidity.

sometimes below 20 mgH2O/L.[13] These very low values, well below the 44 mgH2O/L expected with these devices, are encountered when the temperature of the gas exiting the ventilator is high and/or when the ambient temperature is high.[12,13] It is notable that depending on the type of ICU ventilator, the output ventilator temperature may vary from 26–35°C.[13] An automatic compensation system has been designed that seems to be effective in overcoming this worrisome problem.[13,33] This system is available on some, but not all, heated humidifiers. If not, HMEs should be used.

RESISTANCE

Both types of humidifying devices (HMEs and heated humidifiers) marginally increase resistance to flow in the respiratory circuit[34–37] with no impact on auto–positive end-expiratory pressure (auto-PEEP), even in patients with chronic obstructive pulmonary disease (COPD).[38] Thus, resistance to flow of humidifying devices during invasive mechanical ventilation is not a major problem clinically.

DEAD SPACE

Because of their internal volume, HMEs increase dead space in the ventilator circuit.[37,39,40] This increase is directly proportional to the internal volume of the HME, which may vary between 30 and 95 ml.[40] The impact of dead space on work of breathing and arterial CO2 depends on the mode of ventilation and tidal volume used. During volume-assist control ventilation, internal dead space will only influence Pa_{CO_2} and pH: the smaller the tidal volume used (in combination with an HME with a large internal volume), the greater the impact on arterial CO2 and pH.[41,42] During invasive and noninvasive pressure-support ventilation, use of HMEs may increase work of breathing in COPD and in difficult-to-wean patients.[36,43–47] This increase in work of breathing, however, is easily overcome by increasing the level of pressure support by 5–10 cmH2O.[36,43,45,46]

MICROBIOLOGIC OUTCOME

NOSOCOMIAL PNEUMONIA
The problem of nosocomial infection related to respiratory equipment is not new, and older inhalation therapy equipment posed a considerable challenge in ICUs in the past.[48–51] Similarly, it has been suggested that contamination of respiratory tubing used with heated humidifiers may be a risk factor for ventilator-associated pneumonia.[9,52] This hypothesis stemmed from the rapid and considerable bacterial colonization of respiratory tubing encountered with use of heated humidifiers.[9–11,53] Because HMEs prevent bacterial contamination of respiratory tubing,[54,55] the question arose as to whether, or not, the incidence of ventilator-associated pneumonia was greater with heated humidifiers.[56] There is now overwhelming evidence that the method of humidification does not influence occurrence of ventilator-associated pneumonia.[32,54,57–60] This is not very surprising considering

TABLE 52-1 Endotracheal Tube Occlusion Rates in Studies Comparing Heated Humidifier and Heat and Moisture Exchangers

Reference	No. of Patients	NO. OF ETT[1] OBSTRUCTIONS HH[2]	HME[3]
Branson et al 1993[75]	120	0	0
Dreyfuss et al 1995[54]	131	0	1
Branson et al 1996[76]	200	0	0
Villafane et al 1996[31]	23	1	0
Boots et al 1997[57]	116	0	0
Hurni et al 1997[78]	115	1	0
Kollef et al 1998[58]	310	0	0
Thomachot et al 1998[74]	29	0	0
Kirton et al 1998[56]	280	1	0
Lacherade et al 2002[32]	370	5	1
Jaber et al 2004[93]	60	2	1

ABBREVIATIONS: ETT, endotracheal tube; HH, heated humidifier; HME, heat and moisture exchanger.

the pathogenesis, mainly the silent aspiration of contaminated gastric and oropharyngeal secretions.[61] Consistent with this reasoning, the incidence of ventilator-associated pneumonia is not affected by the duration of use of HMEs, whether changed every 48 hours,[62] 72 hours,[19] or only once a week.[63] Similarly, the type of HME does not influence the rate of ventilator-associated pneumonia.[64,65] Despite these facts, some have recently recommended they be preferred to heated humidifiers to prevent nosocomial pneumonia.[66]

CROSS CONTAMINATION

Although use of heated humidifiers is not associated with a greater incidence of ventilator-associated pneumonia, these devices do have the potential for cross infection.[11] Craven et al studied ventilator-circuit colonization during the first 24 hours after a circuit change. They found a rapid colonization: 33% of circuits were colonized at 2 hours, 64% at 12 hours and 80% at 24 hours. The median level of colonization at 24 hours was 7×10^4 organisms/ml.[9] Bacteria isolated in respiratory tubing condensates correlate with the microorganisms found in patients' tracheobronchial secretions.[9,53,67] These highly contaminated condensates should therefore be handled as infectious waste and regularly emptied.[9] Repeating these septic maneuvers several times a day increases the risk of cross infection, especially when patients are colonized with multi–drug-resistant bacteria.[67]

Preventing respiratory tubing contamination confers on HMEs a great advantage over heated humidifiers.[20,54,57] Attempts have been made to reduce formation of condensation in the circuits by heating both the inspiratory and the expiratory limb of the circuit. Such new equipment needs to be evaluated in the clinical setting. A preliminary report found that condensation still occurred in up to 50% of patients ventilated with these heated circuits,[67] leading to substantial bacterial colonization (see Fig. 52-4).

PRACTICABILITY AND MAINTENANCE

For obvious reasons, HMEs are far easier to handle than heated humidifiers. They require no maintenance and several studies indicate that they reduce staff work load.[54,58,68] Several technical improvements brought to the new heated humidifiers (servo control, automatic water filling system, heated respiratory circuits, and so on) have considerably reduced the time required to check and operate them.

SAFETY

Clinicians are well aware of the hazards associated with HMEs (mainly endotracheal tube occlusion),[1] but may be less aware of the hazards associated with heated humidifiers. Some recently described hazards deserve particular attention. Burns to the patients and breathing circuit meltdowns have occurred in the past because of heated wires.[24,69,70] More frequent and more recent is the risk of ventilator shutdown because of rain out from heated humidifiers.[71–73]

COSTS

Several studies have compared the costs of humidification with HMEs with those of heated humidifiers.[54,56–58,68,74,75] All conclude that considerable cost savings can be achieved by using HMEs, not only because heated humidifiers are expensive to buy, but also because they are expensive to run (especially because of the price of heated respiratory tubing). Costs can be further reduced by extending the use of HMEs; several studies indicate that these devices may be used without change for up to a week (see below).[55,58,63]

Practical Steps

INVASIVE MECHANICAL VENTILATION

WHICH DEVICE FOR WHICH PATIENTS
There are very few and rare contraindications to the use of HMEs. Because they act passively, the amount of heat and moisture they deliver to the inspired gases depends on the amount of heat and moisture they retain during expiration. Therefore, patients with profound hypothermia or important bronchopleural fistulas should preferably be ventilated with a heated humidifier. In addition, a heated humidifier may be preferable in patients ventilated for acute asthma or acute respiratory distress syndrome, in whom a drastic decrease in tidal volume induces extreme respiratory acidosis (to avoid increased dead space with HMEs).[41,42] A heated humidifier can be used until the patient's respiratory condition improves sufficiently to enable the use of an HME. Apart from these specific situations, HMEs should be considered first to heat and humidify inspired gases of all ventilated patients. They are as effective as heated humidifiers, and are much cheaper and much easier to use. Importantly, medical as well as surgical patients can benefit from them.

Despite the former practice of restricting their use to patients without a history of respiratory disease and only for the first 5 days of mechanical ventilation,[75,76] several studies have clearly shown that they may be used in any ventilated patient, even in patients with COPD and for any length of mechanical ventilation. Because patients with COPD represent the most important subgroup of ventilated patients in the United States,[77] and because their duration of ventilation is longer than that of other patients,[77] adequate humidification is probably more critical in such patients than in patients ventilated for shorter periods. Numerous studies have shown that long-term mechanical ventilation can be safely conducted in such patients with HMEs.[20,55,57,58,78–80] Three studies have specifically compared humidity output of HMEs in patients with and without COPD and consistently found that the measured values for absolute humidity were very similar (Fig. 52-6).[20,55,80]

FREQUENCY OF HME REPLACEMENT
There is now considerable evidence that HMEs may be used for longer than the 24 hours recommended by manufacturers.[19,20,58,62,63,74,79–83] Compelling results stem from rigorous clinical evaluation[58,62] or extensive bedside

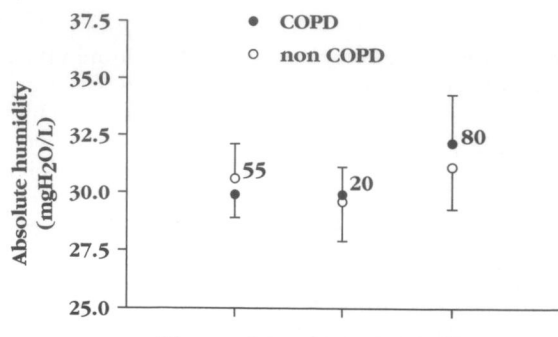

Figures in superscript indicate study reference number

FIGURE 52-6 Comparison of the absolute humidity delivered by heat and moisture exchangers in patients with and without COPD. Values are similar, indicating that these devices are suitable for patients with COPD undergoing mechanical ventilation.

measurement of humidity delivery.[19,20,55,63,79–81] Figure 52-7 shows that humidity delivery of a combined HME (Hygrobac, DAR, Mirandola, Italy) used for 7 days without change was remarkably stable throughout this period. Progressive clogging of the device with tracheal secretions (that seriously increase resistance to airflow) could have been a drawback. Repeated measurements of the resistance of the HME over 7 days indicate that this phenomenon did not occur.[55] (see Fig. 52-7).

Keeping the HME vertically above the tracheal tube (see Fig. 52-3) (and having nurses and doctors repeatedly check the position of the HME) prevents secretions from refluxing from the tracheal tube and obstructing the HME.[20,55] Use of HMEs may be extended in both medical patients (including those with COPD[20,55,79,80]) and surgical patients.[19,63,74,82] This practice is now widely accepted,[84] and recommendations have been made to change HMEs only once a week.[66] In our own published[55,80] and unpublished experience, we

FIGURE 52-7 Absolute humidity (*left Y axis*) and resistance (*right Y axis*) measured over time in combined heat and moisture exchangers used for 7 days without change. Note the perfect stability of the humidity output and the lack of increase in resistance over time. (*Adapted, with permission, from Ricard et al.*[55])

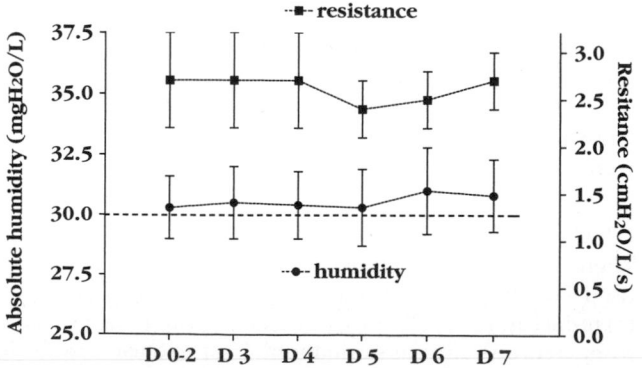

have been changing HMEs only once a week since 1997, and have not encountered endotracheal tube occlusions.

NONINVASIVE MECHANICAL VENTILATION

The question of heat and humidification requirements during noninvasive ventilation has gone unanswered until very recently. The last international consensus conference on noninvasive ventilation made no recommendation as to whether a humidifying device should be used or not.[85] A recent exhaustive review on noninvasive ventilation stated that "humidification is usually unnecessary for short-term (i.e., <1 day) applications, unless there is excessive air leaking, because normal air conditioning functions of the upper airway are left intact."[86] Recent physiologic studies have provided conflicting results of the influence of the humidifying device on respiratory variables. In a randomized cross-over study in nine patients receiving noninvasive ventilation for moderate to severe acute hypercapnic respiratory failure, a significant increase in work of breathing was found with HMEs in comparison with heated humidifiers (11.3 ± 5.7 versus 7.3 ± 3.8 J/min, respectively), although this did not significantly impact Pa_{CO_2} (60 ± 16 versus 57 ± 16 mmHg, respectively).[46] In a larger number of patients (n = 29) studied in a similar manner (cross-over study), there was a modest increase in Pa_{CO_2} (43.4 ± 8.9 versus 40.8 ± 8.2 mmHg; p <0.005).[47] The dead space of HMEs is obviously responsible for these observations. A recent preliminary study suggests that use of an HME with a very small dead space does not alter respiratory variables, compared with heated humidifiers.[87]

The question that arises is whether the negative effects of HMEs during noninvasive ventilation affect outcome, especially the intubation rate. To address this issue, given the increasing use of noninvasive ventilation as a first-line therapy,[88] a large multicenter randomized trial tested the hypothesis that the use of HMEs would increase intubation rates.[89] During 13 months, 247 patients were randomized to noninvasive ventilation either with an HME or a heated humidifier. The intubation rate (failure of noninvasive ventilation) was higher with a heated humidifier than with an HME, although the difference did not reach statistical significance (37.6% versus 30.6%; p = 0.31). Mortality tended to be higher in the heated humidifier group (21.5% versus 14.1%; p = 0.18). Pa_{CO_2} tended to be lower in the heated humidifier group (66 versus 72 mmHg; p = 0.08).[89] These preliminary results suggest that the observed increases in work of breathing, minute ventilation, and Pa_{CO_2} in carefully conducted physiologic studies (but on a small number of selected patients) may only play a marginal role in the clinical setting.

ADJUSTMENTS AT THE BEDSIDE AND TROUBLESHOOTING

Assessing humidification at the bedside is desirable, if not essential, for at least two reasons: (1) a life-threatening tracheal tube occlusion[25] may occur without any precursory clinical signs of insufficient humidification; and (2) devices may not deliver, in some instances, the heat and humidity that is expected of them, because they are either malfunctioning[13] or performance in the clinical setting does not attain that stated by the manufacturer.[13,80]

Such assessment raises two questions: (1) Is the device delivering enough heat and humidity (according to the standards)? (2) Is the amount of heat and moisture delivered appropriate for a given patient?

ASSESSING HMES AND HEATED HUMIDIFIERS AT THE BEDSIDE

A simple means of evaluating the humidity delivered by a given device is to assess the amount of condensation seen in the flexible tubing that connects either the Y-piece (when using a heated humidifier) or the HME to the endotracheal tube.[13,18,90] Indeed, the amount of condensation seen in the flexible tubing is positively correlated with the absolute humidity measured at the bedside.[13,18] If the tubing remains constantly dry over time, or only very few droplets of water are seen, then absolute humidity delivered by a device is probably below 25 mgH$_2$O/L, and the patient is at risk of endotracheal tube occlusion. When numerous droplets are seen in the tubing or if it is dripping wet, the device is probably delivering sufficient absolute humidity to prevent endotracheal tube occlusion.[18]

ASSESSING ADEQUACY OF INSPIRED GAS CONDITIONING

Although it is conceivable that some patients have special humidification needs, the prevailing literature indicates that heated humidifiers and HMEs equally meet humidification requirements in the vast majority of ventilated patients. Therefore, monitoring the characteristics of secretions (thick and tenacious, or watery and abundant) as a guide to insufficient or excessive humidification may be of limited value, because changes in mucus characteristics may be entirely caused by the patient's condition (respiratory status, fluid balance, and so on), and not a consequence of the humidifying device. It has been shown that air humidification with either an HME or a heated humidifier has similar effects on mucus rheologic properties, contact angle, and transportability by cilia in patients undergoing mechanical ventilation.[91]

Important Unknowns

The preliminary results showing a trend toward higher intubation and mortality rates following noninvasive ventilation with a heated humidifier[89] strongly bring into question the use of these devices during noninvasive ventilation, at least in patients for whom Pa$_{CO_2}$ is not the main problem. An unanswered question is whether a humidification device is necessary in every single patient undergoing noninvasive ventilation. Because noninvasive ventilation is usually delivered intermittently, my opinion is that only patients ventilated continuously or for very long periods require additional heat and moisture. Future studies are needed to determine whether these patients, who are heavily dependent on noninvasive ventilation and suffer more often from hy-

poxemic than hypercapnic acute respiratory failure, should be managed preferably with HMEs or not.

The Future

In the field of airway management, underhumidification is no longer the main threat associated with invasive mechanical ventilation. The challenge now facing clinicians is the increasing proportion of ventilator-associated pneumonias caused by multiresistant pathogens.[92] Some recommend the use of HMEs to prevent ventilator-associated pneumonia.[66] We, however, believe the real difference between HMEs and heated humidifiers in this area lies in their respective risks of cross contamination.[11,54] Because the hands of health-care workers are the principal source of cross contamination, reducing the handling of the humidifying device and respiratory circuits will reduce the risk of infection with multiresistant pathogens. In this respect, HMEs offer an undisputable advantage over heated humidifiers. Given the remarkable stability of the humidifying performance measured over time of some HMEs (even after a whole week of continuous use),[19,63,83] one can question the systematic and scheduled replacement of these devices.[84] Conceivably, they could be changed only if they are visibly soiled, thus further reducing the number of maneuvers.

Summary and Conclusion

Adding heat and moisture to the inspired gas during invasive mechanical ventilation is mandatory. This can be efficiently achieved either by heated humidifiers or by HMEs. Although hygrometric performance of combined HMEs is slightly lower than that of heated humidifiers, they are clinically as efficient and do not cause more endotracheal tube occlusions. They may be used in the vast majority of medical (including COPD) and surgical ICU patients and for the entire duration of mechanical ventilation. Specific situations, however, such as menacing respiratory acidosis during mechanical ventilation of patients with acute asthma or very severe acute respiratory distress syndrome, require the use of a heated humidifier until the respiratory condition improves sufficiently to enable the use of an HME. Use of heated humidifiers does not increase the risk of ventilator-associated pneumonia, nor does prolonged use of HMEs. Because circuits, however, get rapidly contaminated with heated humidifiers (unlike HMEs), they carry the potential for cross contamination. Finally, costs of mechanical ventilation are greatly reduced with the use of HMEs.

References

1. Ricard JD, Cook D, Griffith L, Brochard L, Dreyfuss D. Physicians' attitude to use heat and moisture exchangers or heated humidifiers: a Franco-Canadian survey. Intensive Care Med 2002; 28:719–25.

2. Irlbeck D. Normal mechanisms of heat and moisture exchange in the respiratory tract. Respir Care Clin North Am 1998; 4:189–98.

3. Branson RD. The effects of inadequate humidity. Respir Care Clin North Am 1998; 4:199–214.

4. Burton J. Effects of dry anaesthetic gases on the respiratory membrane. Lancet 1962; 1:235–8.

5. Williams R. The effects of excessive humidity. Respir Care Clin North Am 1998; 4:215–228.

6. Sladen A, Laver MB, Pontoppidan H. Pulmonary complications and water retention in prolonged mechanical ventilation. N Engl J Med 1968; 279:448–53.

7. Klein EF Jr, Graves SA. "Hot pot" tracheitis. Chest 1974; 65:225–6.

8. Peterson B. Heated humidifiers: structure and function. Respir Care Clin North Am 1998; 4:243–259.

9. Craven DE, Goularte TA, Make BJ. Contaminated condensate in mechanical ventilator circuits. A risk factor for nosocomial pneumonia. Am Rev Respir Dis 1984; 129:625–8.

10. Craven DE, Connolly MG Jr, Lichtenberg DA, Primeau PJ, McCabe WR. Contamination of mechanical ventilators with tubing changes every 24 or 48 hours. N Engl J Med 1982; 306:1505–9.

11. Christopher KL, Saravolatz LD, Bush TL, Conway WA. The potential role of respiratory therapy equipment in cross infection. A study using a canine model for pneumonia. Am Rev Respir Dis 1983; 128:271–5.

12. Carter BG, Whittington N, Hochmann M, Osborne A. The effect of inlet gas temperatures on heated humidifier performance. J Aerosol Med 2002; 15:7–13.

13. Lellouche F, Taille S, Maggiore SM, et al. Influence of ambient and ventilator output temperatures on performance of heated-wire humidifiers. Am J Respir Crit Care Med 2004; 170:1073–9.

14. Walley R. Humidifier for use with tracheotomy and positive pressure respiration. Lancet 1956; 270:781–2.

15. Toremalm NG. A heat and moisture exchanger for post tracheotomy care. An experimental study. Acta Otolaryngology (Stockholm) 1960; 52:461.

16. Weeks D. Humidification with an inexpensive condenser-humidifier in the semi-closed circle. Anesthesiology 1974; 41:601–604.

17. Wilkes A. Heat and moisture exchanger: structure and function. Respir Care Clin North Am 1998; 4:261–279.

18. Ricard J-D, Markowicz P, Djedaïni K, et al. Bedside evaluation of efficient airway humidification during mechanical ventilation of the critically ill. Chest 1999; 115:1646–52.

19. Davis K Jr, Evans SL, Campbell RS, et al. Prolonged use of heat and moisture exchangers does not affect device efficiency or frequency rate of nosocomial pneumonia. Crit Care Med 2000; 28:1412–8.

20. Boyer A, Thiery G, Lasry S, et al. Long-term mechanical ventilation with hygroscopic heat and moisture exchangers used for 48 hours: a prospective, clinical, hygrometric and bacteriologic study. Crit Care Med 2003; 31:823–9.

21. Thomachot L, Viviand X, Boyadjiev I, Vialet R, Martin C. The combination of a heat and moisture exchanger and a Booster (TM): a clinical and bacteriological evaluation over 96 h. Intensive Care Med 2002; 28:147–53.

22. Cook D, Ricard JD, Reeve B, et al. Ventilator circuit and secretion management strategies: a Franco-Canadian survey. Crit Care Med 2000; 28:3547–54.

23. Branson R, Brougher P, Chatburn R, et al. Consensus statement on the essentials of mechanical ventilators. Respir Care 1992; 37:1000–8.

24. AARC clinical practice guideline. Humidification during mechanical ventilation. American Association for Respiratory Care. Respir Care 1992; 37:887–90.

25. Martin C, Perrin G, Gevaudan MJ, Saux P, Gouin F. Heat and moisture exchangers and vaporizing humidifiers in the intensive care unit. Chest 1990; 97:144–9.

26. Cohen IL, Weinberg PF, Fein IA, Rowinski GS. Endotracheal tube occlusion associated with the use of heat and moisture exchangers in the intensive care unit. Crit Care Med 1988; 16:277–9.

27. Misset B, Escudier B, Rivara D, Leclercq B, Nitenberg G. Heat and moisture exchanger vs heated humidifier during long-term mechanical ventilation. A prospective randomized study. Chest 1991; 100:160–3.

28. Roustan JP, Kienlen J, Aubas P, Aubas S, du Cailar J. Comparison of hydrophobic heat and moisture exchangers with heated humidifier during prolonged mechanical ventilation. Intensive Care Med 1992; 18:97–100.

29. Martin C, Papazian L, Perrin G, Bantz P, Gouin F. Performance evaluation of three vaporizing humidifiers and two heat and moisture exchangers in patients with minute ventilation >10 L/min. Chest 1992; 102:1347–50.

30. Martin C, Thomachot L, Quinio B, Viviand X, Albanese J. Comparing two heat and moisture exchangers with one vaporizing humidifier in patients with minute ventilation greater than 10 L/min. Chest 1995; 107:1411–5.

31. Villafane MC, Cinnella G, Lofaso F, et al. Gradual reduction of endotracheal tube diameter during mechanical ventilation via different humidification devices. Anesthesiology 1996; 85:1341–9.

32. Lacherade JC, Auburtin M, Ceif C, et al. Impact of humidification systems on ventilator-associated pneumonia: a randomized multicenter study. Am J Respir Crit Care Med 2005; 172:1276–82.

33. Carter BG, Kemp T, Mynard J, Hochmann M, Osborne A. Compensating for the effect of inlet gas temperature on heated humidifier performance. Anaesth Intensive Care 2003; 31:54–7.

34. Oh TE, Lin ES, Bhatt S. Resistance of humidifiers, and inspiratory work imposed by a ventilator-humidifier circuit. Br J Anaesth 1991; 66:258–63.

35. Chiaranda M, Verona L, Pinamonti O, et al. Use of heat and moisture exchanging (HME) filters in mechanically ventilated ICU patients: influence on airway flow-resistance. Intensive Care Med 1993; 19:462–6.

36. Iotti GA, Olivei MC, Palo A, et al. Unfavorable mechanical effects of heat and moisture exchangers in ventilated patients. Intensive Care Med 1997; 23:399–405.

37. Campbell RS, Davis K Jr, Johannigman JA, Branson RD. The effects of passive humidifier dead space on respiratory variables in paralyzed and spontaneously breathing patients. Respir Care 2000; 45:306–12.

38. Conti G, de Blasi RA, Rocco M, et al. Effects of heat-moisture exchangers on dynamic hyperinflation of mechanically ventilated COPD patients. Intensive Care Med 1990; 16:441–3.

39. Richecoeur J, Lu Q, Vieira SR, et al. Expiratory washout versus optimization of mechanical ventilation during permissive hypercapnia in patients with severe acute respiratory distress syndrome. Am J Respir Crit Care Med 1999; 160:77–5.

40. Branson RD, Davis KJ. Evaluation of 21 passive humidifiers according to the ISO 9360 standard: moisture output, dead space, and flow resistance. Respir Care 1996; 41:736–743.

41. Prin S, Chergui K, Augarde R, et al. Ability and safety of a heated humidifier to control hypercapnic acidosis in severe ARDS. Intensive Care Med 2002; 28:1756–60.

42. Prat G, Renault A, Tonnelier JM, et al. Influence of the humidification device during acute respiratory distress syndrome. Intensive Care Med 2003; 29:2211–5.

43. Pelosi P, Solca M, Ravagnan I, et al. Effects of heat and moisture exchangers on minute ventilation, ventilatory drive, and work of

breathing during pressure-support ventilation in acute respiratory failure. Crit Care Med 1996; 24:1184–8.

44. Le Bourdelles G, Mier L, Fiquet B, et al. Comparison of the effects of heat and moisture exchangers and heated humidifiers on ventilation and gas exchange during weaning trials from mechanical ventilation. Chest 1996; 110:1294–8.

45. Girault C, Breton L, Richard J, et al. Effects of airway humidification devices during difficult weaning from mechanical ventilation [abstract]. Am J Respir Crit Care Med 2000; 161:A560.

46. Lellouche F, Maggiore SM, Deye N, et al. Effect of the humidification device on the work of breathing during noninvasive ventilation. Intensive Care Med 2002; 28:1582–9.

47. Jaber S, Chanques G, Matecki S, et al. Comparison of the effects of heat and moisture exchangers and heated humidifiers on ventilation and gas exchange during non-invasive ventilation. Intensive Care Med 2002; 28:1590–4.

48. Mertz JJ, Scharer L, McClement JH. A hospital outbreak of *Klebsiella* pneumonia from inhalation therapy with contaminated aerosol solutions. Am Rev Respir Dis 1967; 95:454–60.

49. Grieble HG, Colton FR, Bird TJ, Toigo A, Griffith LG. Fine-particle humidifiers. Source of *Pseudomonas aeruginosa* infections in a respiratory-disease unit. N Engl J Med 1970; 282: 531–5.

50. Pierce AK, Sanford JP. Bacterial contamination of aerosols. Arch Intern Med 1973; 131:156–9.

51. Reinarz JA, Pierce AK, Mays BB, Sanford JP. The potential role of inhalation therapy equipment in nosocomial pulmonary infection. J Clin Invest 1965; 44:831–9.

52. Craven DE, Kunches LM, Kilinsky V, et al. Risk factors for pneumonia and fatality in patients receiving continuous mechanical ventilation. Am Rev Respir Dis 1986; 133:792–6.

53. Comhaire A, Lamy M. Contamination rate of sterilized ventilators in an ICU. Crit Care Med 1981; 9:546–8.

54. Dreyfuss D, Djedaini K, Gros I, et al. Mechanical ventilation with heated humidifiers or heat and moisture exchangers: effects on patient colonization and incidence of nosocomial pneumonia. Am J Respir Crit Care Med 1995; 151:986–92.

55. Ricard J-D, Le Mière E, Markowicz P, et al. Efficiency and safety of mechanical ventilation with a heat and moisture exchanger changed only once a week. Am J Respir Crit Care Med 2000; 161:104–109.

56. Kirton O, DeHaven B, Morgan J, Civetta J. A prospective, randomized comparison of an in-line heat and moisture exchange filter and heated wire humidifiers: rates of ventilator-associated early-onset (community-acquired) or late-onset (hospital-acquired) pneumonia and incidence of endotracheal tube occlusion. Chest 1998; 112:1055–1059.

57. Boots RJ, Howe S, George N, Harris FM, Faoagali J. Clinical utility of hygroscopic heat and moisture exchangers in intensive care patients. Crit Care Med 1997; 25:1707–12.

58. Kollef M, Shapiro S, Boyd V, et al. A randomized clinical trial comparing an extended-use hygroscopic condenser humidifier with heated-water humidification in mechanically ventilated patients. Chest 1998; 113:759–767.

59. Richards G. The role of filtration during humidification. Respir Care Clin North Am 1998; 4:329–39.

60. Memish ZA, Oni GA, Djazmati W, Cunningham G, Mah MW. A randomized clinical trial to compare the effects of a heat and moisture exchanger with a heated humidifying system on the occurrence rate of ventilator-associated pneumonia. Am J Infect Control 2001; 29:301–5.

61. Kollef M. The prevention of ventilator-associated pneumonia. N Engl J Med 1999; 340:627–34.

62. Djedaïni K, Billiard M, Mier L, et al. Changing heat and moisture exchangers every 48 hours rather than 24 hours does not affect their efficacy and the incidence of nosocomial pneumonia. Am J Respir Crit Care Med 1995; 152:1562–9.

63. Thomachot L, Leone M, Razzouk K, et al. Randomized clinical trial of extended use of a hydrophobic condenser humidifier: 1 vs. 7 days. Crit Care Med 2002; 30:232–7.

64. Thomachot L, Viviand X, Arnaud S, Boisson C, Martin CD. Comparing two heat and moisture exchangers, one hydrophobic and one hygroscopic, on humidifying efficacy and the rate of nosocomial pneumonia. Chest 1998; 114:1383–9.

65. Thomachot L, Vialet R, Arnaud S, et al. Do the components of heat and moisture exchanger filters affect their humidifying efficacy and the incidence of nosocomial pneumonia? Crit Care Med 1999; 27:923–8.

66. Dodek P, Keenan S, Cook D, et al. Evidence-based clinical practice guideline for the prevention of ventilator-associated pneumonia. Ann Intern Med 2004; 141:305–13.

67. Ricard J-D, Hidri N, Blivet A, et al. New heated breathing circuits do not prevent condensation and contamination of ventilator circuits with heated humidifiers [abstract]. Am J Respir Crit Care Med 2003; 167:A861.

68. Tenaillon A, Cholley G, Boiteau R, Perrin-Gachadoat D, Burdin M. Filtres échangeurs de chaleur et d'humidité versus humidificateurs chauffant en ventilation mécanique. Réanim Soins Intens Méd Urg 1989; 5:5–10.

69. Heated wires can melt disposable breathing circuits. Health Devices 1989; 18:174–5.

70. Inappropriate Fisher & Paykel heater-wire adapter melts allegiance breathing circuit. Health Devices 2000; 29:86–7.

71. Rainout from a Fisher & Paykel heated humidification system can shut down certain ventilators. Health Devices 2002; 31: 114–5.

72. Rainout puts ventilator-dependent patients at risk. Health Devices 2002; 31:461–3.

73. Rainout from Fisher & Paykel's 850 humidification system shuts down Respironics Esprit and adversely affects other ventilators. Health Devices 2005; 34:46–8.

74. Thomachot L, Vialet R, Viguier JM, et al. Efficacy of heat and moisture exchangers after changing every 48 hours rather than 24 hours. Crit Care Med 1998; 26:477–81.

75. Branson RD, Davis KJ, Campbell RS, Johnson DJ, Porembka DT. Humidification in the intensive care unit. Prospective study of a new protocol utilizing heated humidification and a hygroscopic condenser humidifier. Chest 1993; 104:1800–5.

76. Branson RD, Davis KJ, Brown R, Rashkin M. Comparison of three humidification techniques during mechanical ventilation: patient selection, cost, and infection considerations. Respir Care 1996; 41:809–16.

77. Esteban A, Anzueto A, Alia I, et al. How is mechanical ventilation employed in the intensive care unit? Am J Respir Crit Care Med 2000; 161:1450–8.

78. Hurni JM, Feihl F, Lazor R, Leuenberger P, Perret C. Safety of combined heat and moisture exchanger filters in long-term mechanical ventilation. Chest 1997; 111:686–91.

79. Markowicz P, Ricard J-D, Dreyfuss D, et al. Safety, efficacy and cost effectiveness of mechanical ventilation with humidifying filters changed every 48 hours: a prospective, randomized study. Crit Care Med 2000; 28:665–71.

80. Thiéry G, Boyer A, Pigné E, et al. Heat and moisture exchangers in mechanically ventilated intensive care unit patients: A plea for an independent assessment of their performance. Crit Care Med 2003; 31:699–704.

81. Boisson C, Viviand X, Arnaud S, et al. Changing a hydrophobic heat and moisture exchanger after 48 hours rather than 24 hours: a clinical and microbiological evaluation. Intensive Care Med 1999; 25:1237–43.

82. Thomachot L, Boisson C, Arnaud S, et al. Changing heat and moisture exchangers after 96 hours rather than after 24 hours: a clinical and microbiological evaluation. Crit Care Med 2000; 28:714–20.

83. Ricard J-D, Dreyfuss D. Efficiency and safety of mechanical ventilation with a heat and moisture exchanger changed once a week [letter to the editor]. Am J Respir Crit Care Med 2001; 164:1999–2000.

84. Hess D. Prolonged use of heat and moisture exchangers: why do we keep changing things? Crit Care Med 2000; 28:1667–8.

85. International consensus conferences in intensive care medicine: noninvasive positive pressure ventilation in acute respiratory failure. Am J Respir Crit Care Med 2001; 163:283–91.

86. Mehta S, Hill N. Noninvasive ventilation. Am J Respir Crit Care Med 2003; 163:540–577.

87. Boyer A, Vargas F, Mousset-Hovaere M, et al. Prospective study of the influence of humidification mode on ventilation parameters and arterial blood gases during non invasive ventilation [abstract]. Am J Respir Crit Care Med 2004; 169:A522.

88. Carlucci A, Richard J-C, Wysocki M, et al. Noninvasive versus conventional mechanical ventilation. An epidemiologic survey. Am J Respir Crit Care Med 2001; 163:874–80.

89. Lellouche F, L'Her E, Abrouk F, et al. Impact of the humidifying device on intubation rate during NIV: results of a multicenter RCT [abstract]. Intensive Care Med 2005; 31:S266.

90. Beydon L, Tong D, Jackson N, Dreyfuss D. Correlation between simple clinical parameters and the in vitro humidification characteristics of filter heat and moisture exchangers. Groupe de Travail sur les Respirateurs [see comments]. Chest 1997; 112:739–44.

91. Nakagawa NK, Macchione M, Petrolino HM, et al. Effects of a heat and moisture exchanger and a heated humidifier on respiratory mucus in patients undergoing mechanical ventilation. Crit Care Med 2000; 28:312–7.

92. Chastre J, Fagon J. Ventilator-associated pneumonia. Am J Respir Crit Care Med 2002; 165:867–903.

93. Jaber S, Pigeot J, Fodil R, et al. Long-term effects of different humidification systems on endotracheal tube patency: evaluation by the acoustic reflection method. Anesthesiology 2004; 100:782–8.

Chapter 53

FIGHTING THE VENTILATOR

MARTIN J TOBIN
CHARLES G. ALEX
PATRICK J. FAHEY

INITIAL ASSESSMENT
SPECIFIC PROBLEMS
   Artificial Airway Problems
   Other Problems
   Ventilator Malfunction
PHARMACOTHERAPY
SUMMARY

A patient is connected to the ventilator. His eyes are closed and he appears calm. The ventilator is making soft rhythmic noises, and the patient's chest is expanding and receding in unison with the ventilator. A sweep of signals is gently traversing the monitor screen. This peaceful scene erupts suddenly. The patient bolts upright. His eyelids retract. His nostrils flare. Sweat drips from his brow. His skin turns blue. His sternocleidomastoids contract vigorously. His rib spaces retract. One or more alarms sound loudly.

A patient fighting (or bucking) the ventilator is frightening not only to the patient but to staff. If the physician cannot find the source of the problem and fix it, the patient may die in minutes. The physician must immediately diagnose and manage the problem, and do both concurrently. The physician quickly scans the monitors for clues. Sometimes the problem is immediately spotted and solved, such as disconnected ventilator tubing. If the cause is not immediately obvious, the physician's primary responsibility is to ensure adequate ventilation. This requirement takes precedence over diagnosis. After disconnecting the patient from the ventilator, the physician (or staff) starts to ventilate the patient manually with a self-inflating bag containing 100% oxygen (O_2). This step is both therapeutic and diagnostic (Fig. 53-1).[1,2] If the distress resolves, it indicates that the problem originated in the ventilator. If the distress continues, it indicates the problem is within the patient.

Initial Assessment

Where a physician begins the assessment varies with the particulars of the patient's presentation. The following sequence will not be appropriate for all patients.

Because hypoxia can be rapidly lethal, the pulse oximeter reading is noted. Although several factors can give rise to erroneous readings, the displayed saturation generally bears a close relationship to the O_2 saturation on an arterial blood gas test.[3]

If the high-airway-pressure alarm is sounding, the physician should, if possible, measure the plateau pressure. An increase in peak airway pressure without a proportional increase in plateau pressure indicates narrowing of the airway.[4] Narrowing may arise from bronchoconstriction, an increase in secretions, a collection of fluid in the inspiratory limb of the ventilator circuit, kinking of the tubing, a foreign body, or herniation of the cuff of the endotracheal tube over its distal tip.

An increase in peak airway pressure accompanied by a proportional increase in plateau pressure indicates a decrease in thoracic compliance, which may arise within the lung or from extrinsic compression. A decrease in lung compliance may arise from pulmonary edema, early stages of the acute respiratory distress syndrome (ARDS), dynamic hyperinflation associated with intrinsic positive end-expiratory pressure (PEEPi), and atelectasis. Extrinsic compression may be caused by rapid collection of pleural fluid (hemothorax, parapneumonic effusion, or transudative effusion) or a pneumothorax. If a tension pneumothorax is suspected and death appears imminent, the physician should insert a small-gauge needle attached to a fluid-filled syringe in the intercostal space between the second and third ribs anteriorly; if air bubbles through the syringe, a thoracostomy tube is inserted. Gastric distension, ileus, ascites, or extensive eschar formation can also cause a decrease in thoracic compliance.

A major obstruction of the airway will commonly cause O_2 desaturation and an increase in peak airway pressure. If obstruction is suspected, the clinician should pass a suction catheter through the airway to determine if the airway is patent, and to remove secretions or other material that is causing a blockage.

The alarm may signal a low tidal volume (VT). This can arise because of movement of the endotracheal tube into the hypopharynx or esophagus. It can also arise because of a disconnection in the ventilator circuit or a leak in the system. Many conditions can cause an increase in respiratory rate. Accordingly, a high rate is a very sensitive marker of an important change in a patient's condition. Because it is influenced by so many factors, it is not helpful in directing the clinician to the cause of the new change.

The patient's pattern of breathing may signal a marked increase in work of breathing. Important signs include tracheal tug (how much the larynx descends with each inspiration); palpable activity of the sternocleidomastoid muscles; recession in the suprasternal notch, supraclavicular space, and intercostal spaces; and paradoxical movement of the rib cage and abdomen.

Auscultation of the chest may suggest a pneumothorax or movement of the endotracheal tube into the right main-stem bronchus. Cardiac auscultation may reveal a Hamman's crunch, signaling the presence of pneumomediastinum. A new murmur may signal the development of a ventricular septal defect or other cardiac source of acute distress.

The pressure and flow tracings on the ventilator screen may provide clues to the sudden change in patient status. The contour of the airway pressure tracing may exhibit

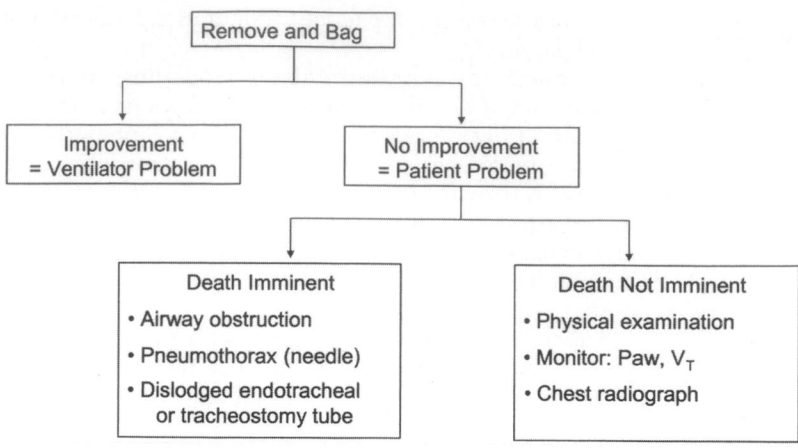

FIGURE 53-1 Removing the patient from the ventilator and providing manual ventilation with a bag (100% oxygen) is both therapeutic and diagnostic. Patient improvement indicates that the ventilator is the cause of the distress. Lack of improvement indicates that the problem is within the patient. If death appears imminent, the physician rapidly checks for airway obstruction (by passing a suction catheter), a dislodged endotracheal or tracheostomy tube, and a pneumothorax (if deemed likely, a small-gauge needle is inserted). If death is not imminent, the physician undertakes a more detailed physical examination and assessment of monitored variables. A chest radiograph may also be obtained.

excessive scooping, indicating increased inspiratory effort; this pattern is seen when the delivered inspiratory flow no longer meets patient demand (Fig. 53-2).[5] The flow tracing may not return to the zero-flow line in the period immediately before the next inspiration, indicating PEEPi.[4] The flow tracing may exhibit a sawtooth pattern, indicating excessive secretions.[6]

A decrease in end-tidal carbon dioxide tension (P_{CO_2}) can be helpful. A sudden decrease in end-tidal P_{CO2} may arise with pulmonary embolism or air embolism. Esophageal intubation also causes end-tidal P_{CO_2} to fall to zero. Unfortunately, end-tidal CO_2 readings do not reliably reflect arterial CO_2 tension ($PaCO_2$) in patients with underlying lung disease.

The blood pressure reading may signal a hypertensive crisis. The differential diagnosis of a fall in arterial pressure is wide, and influenced by clinical context. In a patient with a myocardial infarction, a fall in arterial pressure may signal the onset of cardiogenic shock. A pulmonary artery catheter can provide important clues. A new onset of large v (ventricular) waves in the pulmonary artery wedge tracing suggests the development of acute mitral regurgitation secondary to ruptured chordae tendineae cordis.[7] The ECG may reveal arrhythmias or ST segment elevation.

In contrast to the average patient, communication with an intubated patient is very difficult. A nonintubated patient who develops acute distress consequent to an acute myocardial infarction is able to relay the onset of crushing chest pain to staff. The presence of a tracheal tube prohibits speech. Nevertheless, clinicians can obtain a considerable amount of information about the nature of symptoms. Nurses are frequently more patient and skilled than physicians in achieving an ongoing dialogue with a patient.

The sequence of the above steps will vary with the clinical context. The approach is also incomplete. For example, sudden distress may have no cardiopulmonary cause. Instead, it may originate in a blocked Foley catheter leading to an overdistended bladder.

Specific Problems

Based on the initial assessment, a clinician diagnoses the most likely cause of a change in a patient's condition. The most common causes of sudden respiratory distress in a ventilated patient are listed in Table 53-1.

ARTIFICIAL AIRWAY PROBLEMS

Several different problems with artificial airways can produce acute respiratory distress in the ventilated patient.

MOVEMENT OF THE ENDOTRACHEAL TUBE

An endotracheal or tracheostomy tube that is initially properly positioned may subsequently move up or down in a patient's airway. Downward movement into a main-stem bronchus (endobronchial intubation) is estimated to occur in about 10% of ventilated patients.[8–10] It is usually caused by inadequate external fixation of the endotracheal tube, excessive neck movement, or both.[11] In a study of adult patients with ventilatory failure, Conrardy et al[11] found that neck flexion caused an endotracheal tube to move an average of 1.9 cm (range, 0–3.1 cm) towards the carina.

Main-stem intubation occurs more often on the right side, probably because the right main-stem bronchus forms a less acute angle with the trachea than does the left main-stem

FIGURE 53-2 Airway-pressure waveforms recorded during assist-control ventilation. The tracings represent changes in airway pressure during inspiration in a completely relaxed patient and in patients making a slight and a strenuous effort to breathe. The distance between the *dashed line* (representing controlled ventilation) and the *solid line* (representing spontaneous breathing) is proportional to the patient's work of breathing. (*Reproduced, with permission, from Tobin.*[5])

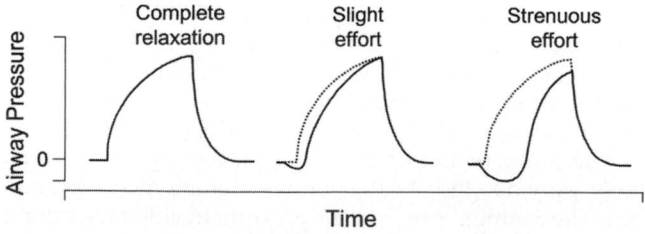

TABLE 53-1   Causes of Sudden Respiratory Distress in a Patient Receiving Mechanical Ventilation

Patient-related causes
  Artificial airway problems
    Movement of the endotracheal tube
    Cuff herniation
    Cuff leak
    Endotracheal tube kinking
    Foreign body
    Tracheoesophageal fistula
    Innominate artery rupture
    Malpositioning of the nasogastric tube
    Build-up of secretions
    Bronchospasm
    Pneumothorax
    Pulmonary edema
    Pulmonary embolism
    Acute hypoxemia
    Blood in the endotracheal tube
    Dynamic hyperinflation
    Abnormal respiratory drive
    Alteration in body posture
    Drug-induced problems
    Abdominal distension
    Agitation
Ventilator-related causes
  Ventilator malfunction
  External ventilator circuit
  Leaks or disconnects
  Condensate
  In-line nebulizers
  Inadequate ventilator support
  Patient-ventilator dyssynchrony

bronchus.[10] The lack of ventilation to the contralateral lung produces atelectasis, which, in turn, causes shunting of blood and hypoxemia. The delivery of a high volume to the intubated lung predisposes to the development of a pneumothorax.[4]

Clues to the development of endobronchial intubation include an increase in peak airway pressure accompanied by a proportional increase in plateau pressure, asymmetric expansion of each hemithorax, and a decrease in breath sounds over the contralateral lung. In a prospective study, however, Brunel et al[9] found that clinicians considered breath sounds equal over both lung fields in 60% of patients with an endobronchial intubation.

If endobronchial intubation is suspected, the endotracheal tube should be pulled back a few centimeters, the chest auscultated again, and the position of the tube confirmed by radiography. The problem can be prevented by securing the tip of the tube at least 3-4 cm from the carina, and obtaining a radiograph at the time of intubation.[11] In addition, centimeter markings on an endotracheal tube are helpful as a reference, although not completely reliable.[9] In general, an endotracheal tube should be secured at reference markings of 23 cm in men and 21 cm in women.[9] On the chest radiograph, the tip of the endotracheal tube should be located at a level corresponding to the top of the aortic knob when the head is in a neutral position.[12]

An endotracheal tube may also migrate above the vocal cords, or get dislodged into the esophagus.[10] Esophageal intubation may arise as a result of attempts to blindly reposition an endotracheal tube. Malpositioning causes sudden distress accompanied by phonation, audible escape of air through the nose and mouth, absence of tube condensation, decrease in VT, decrease (or increase) in peak airway pressure, and abdominal distension. Chest radiography can be misleading because the trachea overlays the esophagus, making it difficult to tell whether the tube is located in the esophagus or trachea. A reading of zero on an end-tidal CO_2 monitor helps in detecting esophageal intubation. Upward movement of an endotracheal tube usually results from excessive neck movement and/or inadequate tube fixation. Conrardy et al[11] found that neck extension caused an endotracheal tube to move an average of 1.9 cm away from the carina, but movement was as much as 5.2 cm in some patients. This observation may explain why patients who are carefully restrained can still self-extubate.

CUFF HERNIATION
Herniation of the cuff of an endotracheal tube over its distal tip can cause complete airway obstruction.[10] This problem most commonly occurs after changes in position of the tube or changes in the posture of the head and neck. Clues to cuff herniation include an increase in peak airway pressure, resistance during manual ventilation, a decrease in VT, difficulty in passing a suction catheter, and an abnormal musical sound during inspiration.[2] Deflation of the cuff produces immediate relief. In a stable patient with an unclear source of airway obstruction, the diagnosis may not be made without bronchoscopy.

CUFF LEAK
The failure of the cuff on an endotracheal tube to form a seal with the wall of the trachea leads to gas leakage, which may or may not be of clinical consequence.[10] A large leak may cause the ventilator alarms to sound, signaling a low peak airway pressure and low exhaled VT, and cause alveolar hypoventilation. Other clues include ability to phonate, frothy secretions in the patient's mouth, hearing a gurgle over the trachea or larynx on auscultation, a discrepancy between expired and inspired VT, and failure to maintain a set level of PEEP.[10] The most common cause of cuff leak is malposition of the endotracheal tube. Consequently, the development of a cuff leak should cause the physician to re-evaluate tube position. The cuff may be deflated not only because of a leak in the cuff itself, but also because of a leak in the pilot balloon or in the external valve assembly.[12] A clamp placed on the cuff inflation tubing proximal to the valve and pilot balloon can temporarily correct this problem (without having to immediately replace the endotracheal tube). Complete rupture of a cuff can lead to aspiration of saliva, vomit, or food; the entire endotracheal tube needs to be replaced.

ENDOTRACHEAL TUBE KINKING
The endotracheal tube can become kinked as a result of changes in the position of the head and neck, and the use of soft rubber nasotracheal tubes.[10] It may also arise when the tube is warmed by heated humidified gas,[12] or when the

patient bites the tube. This uncommon problem is usually corrected by slight manipulation of the head, neck, or tube.

FOREIGN BODY

The endotracheal tube can become occluded with a variety of foreign bodies, including dried lubricant,[13] surgical tape,[13] a broken stylet sheath,[14] plastic debris retained from the time of manufacturing the Murphy eye in the tube,[15] and nasal turbinates avulsed during nasotracheal intubation.[16]

TRACHEOESOPHAGEAL FISTULA

Tracheoesophageal fistula is a rare complication that is primarily caused by ischemia of the tracheal wall secondary to pressure from an overinflated cuff or by movement of a tracheal tube or its tip.[17] Patients with this complication typically have had both a tracheal tube and a nasogastric tube in place for a long time.[10,18] Clues to the presence of a tracheoesophageal fistula include the inability to deliver a preset V_T despite a functional cuff, gastric distension, audible leak of air through the mouth, copious airway secretions, the suctioning of gastric contents from the lower respiratory tract, and clinical deterioration and coughing on deflation of the cuff.[12] Diagnosis needs to be verified by bronchoscopy with direct visualization of the esophagus or by cine-esophagography or cinetracheography.[12] Most experts believe that closure of the fistula demands operative repair; opinions vary as to optimal timing.[12]

INNOMINATE ARTERY RUPTURE

Erosion of the innominate artery has been reported to occur in 0.4–4.5% of tracheostomies.[19] Most ruptures occur at some point during the first 3 weeks after a tracheotomy.[19] The underside of the tracheal tube, the tracheal cuff, or the tip of the tube erode through the anterolateral tracheal wall, at the point where the innominate artery crosses the trachea. Risk factors include placing the tracheostomy tube below the third tracheal ring, excessive movement of the tube, and overinflation of the cuff.

The clinical presentation may be quite dramatic, with blood gushing from the tracheal tube. It may be heralded by a pulsation of the tracheal cannula or a "sentinel bleed." If this sign is recognized, the cuff should be overinflated in an attempt to achieve tamponade. Manual compression of the artery should be attempted: an index finger should be inserted into the stoma to compress the artery against the sternum.[19] If this is successful, a blood transfusion should be administered while the patient is being transported to the operating room for sternotomy and ligation of the vessel. Mortality is extremely high: >85% in a review of the world literature.[20]

OTHER PROBLEMS

MALPOSITION OF THE NASOGASTRIC TUBE

A stiff nasogastric tube can easily bypass the cuff of an endotracheal tube and enter the airway. If the nasogastric tube is connected to suction, the continuous negative pressure will create a constant flow of gas out of the airways.[21] Consequently, the low V_T alarm will sound. The negative pressure can also cause triggering of the ventilator. In particular, ventilator triggering in a patient who is receiving a paralytic agent suggests that a nasogastric tube is misplaced in the airway. Other complications of nasogastric tubes include passage of the tube through the tracheobronchial tree into the pleural space, causing the formation of a bronchopleural fistula; infusion of nutritional solutions through the misplaced nasogastric tube can cause an empyema. A nasogastric tube can also cause esophageal perforation leading to pneumomediastinum, pneumothorax, and tracheoesophageal fistula.

SECRETIONS

Airway secretions can cause problems by being too copious or too dry. Excessive secretions can lead to mucus plugging and atelectasis. To avoid this problem, careful bronchial toilet and frequent suctioning are necessary in patients with copious secretions. If atelectasis occurs and fails to resolve with conservative measures, bronchoscopy should be undertaken.

A helpful clue to the presence of excessive secretions is the presence of a sawtooth pattern on the flow tracing.[6] In a study of 50 intubated patients, Jubran and Tobin[6] found that the presence of a sawtooth pattern was about 6–8 times more likely in patients who had secretions than in patients without secretions. Conversely, a smooth flow-volume curve was about one-quarter as likely to be found in patients with secretions as in patients without secretions. Clinical examination had much higher false-positive and false-negative rates (42 and 43%, respectively) than the flow-volume curves (12 and 14%, respectively). The usefulness of a sawtooth pattern for detecting secretions was confirmed by Guglielminotti et al[22] in a study of 62 patients who were receiving pressure-support or assist-control ventilation.

A tracheal tube bypasses the upper airway, which normally heats and humidifies inspired gas. Consequently, secretions may become excessively dry and encrusted. Inspissated secretions can cause significant blockage of the tracheal tube over a relatively short period.[18] Clues to this problem include an increase in peak airway pressure without an associated increase in plateau pressure, and difficulty in passing a suction catheter. Obstruction appears to be a greater problem when heat and moisture exchangers are employed, as opposed to hot water humidifiers (see Chapter 52).

When secretions dry and accumulate, they can cause complete obstruction or ball-valve obstruction of the endotracheal tube. When this occurs at the distal tip of the tube, positive pressure during inspiration will cause the mass to move away from the tip, permitting the flow of gas. During expiration, expiratory pressure will push the mass of dried secretions into the distal port producing occlusion and cessation of airflow. The ball-valve obstruction causes pulmonary hyperinflation and may produce a tension pneumothorax.[23]

BRONCHOSPASM

Bronchoconstriction is a common cause of sudden respiratory distress. Clues to its development include an increase in peak airway pressure with little or no change in plateau pressure. Clinical manifestations include wheezes, pulsus paradoxus, and evidence of increased work of breathing (recession of the suprasternal space, supraclavicular fossae, and intercostal spaces; heightened activity of the accessory muscles; tracheal tug; and paradoxic motion of the rib cage and abdomen). Management includes bronchodilator therapy.

PNEUMOTHORAX

Sudden respiratory distress in a ventilator-supported patient should always arouse suspicion of a pneumothorax, because 60–90% of such pneumothoraces are reported to be under tension.[24] A full discussion of barotrauma and its pathogenesis is available in Chapter 44. A pneumothorax is typically associated with an increase in peak airway pressure and a proportional increase in plateau pressure. Other manifestations include hyperresonance, tracheal deviation to the contralateral side, decreased breath sounds, and cardiovascular collapse. If a pneumothorax is suspected and death is imminent, a 14- to 16-gauge needle attached to a liquid-filled syringe should be inserted into a second intercostal space; if air bubbles through the syringe, a thoracostomy tube is inserted. If the patient is stable, however, a chest radiograph should first be performed to verify the diagnosis before inserting a chest tube.

PULMONARY EDEMA

Pulmonary edema can cause sudden distress associated with an increase in plateau pressure and a smaller increase in the gradient between the peak and plateau pressures. When present, pink frothy secretions and an increase in pulmonary artery wedge pressure are particularly helpful.

PULMONARY EMBOLISM

Acute pulmonary embolism is an uncommon cause of sudden respiratory distress in a ventilated patient. Typical manifestations include dyspnea, tachypnea, chest pain, fever, hemoptysis, pleural rub, and features of deep vein thrombosis. An important clue, when it occurs, is sudden hypoxemia with no change in peak airway pressure—a unique combination. The risks associated with transporting a critically ill patient alter the approach to diagnosis. Bedside duplex ultrasonography of the leg veins is a reasonable initial test.[25] Although ventilation-perfusion scans are difficult to perform in a ventilated patient, they have reasonable diagnostic reliability.[26] Helical computed tomographic scanning is worthwhile, although doubts have been raised about its accuracy in this setting.[27]

ACUTE HYPOXEMIA

Some ventilated patients present with acute hypoxemia, which may or may not be accompanied by acute distress. The differential diagnosis for new onset of hypoxemia can be considered in terms of ventilator-related problems, progression of the underlying disease, onset of a new medical problem, effects of interventions and procedures, and medications.[28] Causes of each are listed in Table 53–2.

BLOOD FROM THE ENDOTRACHEAL TUBE

The return of bright red blood from a tracheal tube is alarming.[29] It is most commonly caused by trauma from a suction catheter, especially in patients with inflamed air-

TABLE 53-2 Causes of Worsening Oxygenation in the Ventilated Patient

Ventilator-related problems
  Airway malfunction
  External circuit malfunction
  Ventilator malfunction
  Inappropriate ventilator settings
Progression of an underlying disease process
  Acute respiratory distress syndrome
  Cardiogenic pulmonary edema
  Pneumonia
  Sepsis
  Acute exacerbation of asthma or chronic obstructive
    pulmonary disease
Onset of a new problem
  Pneumothorax
  Atelectasis
  Aspiration (gastric or oropharyngeal)
  Ventilator-associated pneumonia
  Sepsis
  Pulmonary thromboembolism
  Fluid overload
  Bronchospasm
  Retained secretions
  Shock
  Seizure
Effects of interventions and procedures
  Endotracheal suctioning
  Changes in body position
  Chest physiotheraphy
  Bronchoscopy
  Thoracentesis
  Peritoneal dialysis
  Hemodialysis
Medications
  Bronchodilators
  Vasodilators
    β-Blockers

SOURCE: Adapted, with permission, from Glauser et al.[28]

ways. Trauma secondary to the cuff also causes bleeding: the most dramatic form is innominate artery fistula. Airway bleeding may arise with infection, such as necrotizing pneumonia or tracheobronchitis. Pulmonary hemorrhage may be part of the underlying disease, such as Goodpasture's syndrome, Wegener's granulomatosis, neoplasm, or disseminated intravascular coagulation. Blood mixed with pink frothy secretions suggests pulmonary edema. Pulmonary embolism accounts for a small proportion of patients with hemoptysis.

Pulmonary artery rupture can arise as a complication of pulmonary artery catheterization.[30] Rupture usually results from inflating the balloon when the catheter is too far distal. Risk factors include advancing the catheter with the balloon deflated, failure to observe the pulmonary artery pressure while the balloon is being inflated (inflation should cease immediately when a wedged tracing is obtained), hand flushing of the catheter while it is wedged, and pulmonary hypertension. If pulmonary artery rupture is suspected, the patient should be placed in a lateral decubitus position with the affected lung down, a double-lumen endotracheal tube inserted (to protect the contralateral lung), and arrangements made for surgical intervention.

DYNAMIC HYPERINFLATION

Ventilator-supported patients commonly display tachypnea and an increased time constant (secondary to increased respiratory resistance and/or low pulmonary compliance), which predisposes to the development of dynamic hyperinflation.[31] This hyperinflation is associated with the presence of a positive recoil pressure at the end of expiration, termed *intrinsic PEEP (PEEPi)* or *auto-PEEP*.[32,33] Hyperinflation may cause significant patient discomfort for at least two reasons. One, it decreases the efficiency of force generation by the respiratory muscles. Two, it increases work of breathing because inspiration occurs at the upper, less compliant portion of the pressure-volume curve of the lung, where inwardly directed elastic recoil of the chest wall poses an additional elastic load.[34,35] To initiate inspiratory gas flow, a patient has to generate a negative pressure equal in magnitude to the opposing elastic recoil pressure (level of PEEPi). Likewise, if a patient with PEEPi is triggering a ventilator, he or she has to generate a negative pressure equal in magnitude to the level of PEEPi in addition to the set minimum circuit pressure drop before a ventilator-assisted breath is initiated. This is one factor that accounts for the common occurrence of failure to trigger the ventilator despite obvious respiratory effort[36] (Fig. 53-3).

Therapeutic measures to decrease PEEPi include bronchodilator agents, employment of a large-bore endotracheal tube; decreasing the minute ventilation by controlling fever or pain; and minimizing the ratio of inspiratory time to expiratory time by increasing inspiratory flow rate, or using nondistensible tubing in the ventilator circuit. Addition of external PEEP can also decrease work secondary to the inspiratory threshold load effect of PEEPi.[33,37] To initiate inspiratory flow, alveolar pressure must be decreased below ambient pressure. During normal spontaneous breathing, this is accomplished by only a small decrease in pleural pressure. For alveolar pressure to fall below ambient pressure in the presence of hyperinflation, however, a much greater decrease in pleural pressure is required. If ambient pressure is elevated by the application of external PEEP, inspiration is more easily accomplished because alveolar pressure needs to be decreased only below the level of external PEEP (rather than below zero). This may seem paradoxical: external PEEP, which is commonly used to induce hyperinflation in patients with microatelectasis, is being used to decrease the work of breathing induced by hyperinflation. This paradox can be understood by considering the analogy of a waterfall over a dam.[35] The height of the waterfall represents the critical closing pressure of airways in patients with PEEPi and chronic obstructive pulmonary disease (COPD) (Fig. 53-4). Thus, elevating downstream pressure, as with external PEEP, has no influence on either expiratory airflow or the pressure upstream (PEEPi) from the site of critical closure (upper panel of Fig. 53-4). This situation exists until downstream pressure is elevated to a value equal to the critical closing pressure (middle panel of Fig. 53-4). Once downstream pressure is elevated above the critical closing pressure (the height of the waterfall), however, the pres-

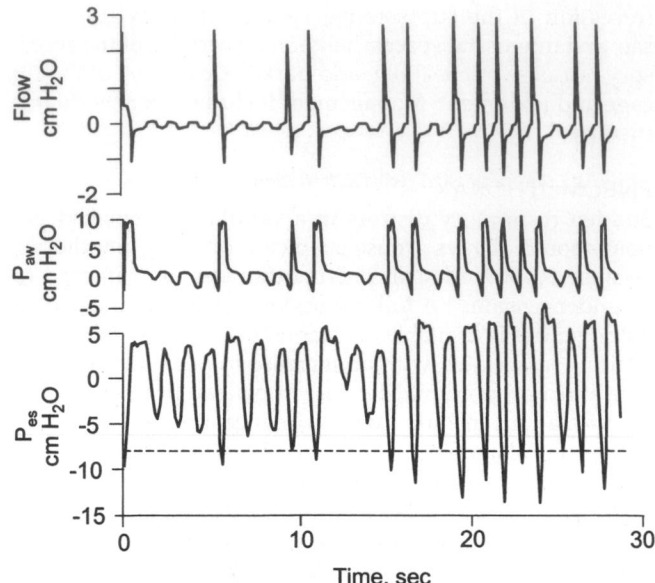

FIGURE 53-3 Recordings of tidal volume, flow, airway pressure (P_{aw}) and esophageal pressure (P_{es}) in a patient with chronic obstructive pulmonary disease receiving pressure-support ventilation. About half of the inspiratory efforts fail to trigger the ventilator. Triggering occurred only when the patient generated a P_{es} more negative than -8 cmH$_2$O (indicated by the interrupted horizontal line), which was equal in magnitude to the opposing elastic recoil pressure. Each ineffective triggering attempt is signaled by a braking of expiratory flow, whereby flow returns to zero secondary to inspiratory muscle action. Thus, monitoring of expiratory flow provides a more accurate measurement of the patient's intrinsic respiratory rate than the number of machine cycles displayed on the bedside monitor. (*Reproduced, with permission, from Tobin et al.[36]*)

sure upstream increases immediately, and hyperinflation is exacerbated (lower panel of Fig. 53-4).

The counteracting effect of external PEEP operates only in the setting of airflow limitation. In the absence of airflow limitation, or when PEEPi results from expiratory muscle activity, the addition of external PEEP is a hindrance and adds to work of expiration. It is important to keep in mind that while external PEEP can help decrease inspiratory work, it does nothing to relieve the accompanying hyperinflation, which has other detrimental effects.[34] Another caveat is the heterogenous distribution of lung units in patients with airflow limitation, each with its own critical closing pressure.[38] Given the regional inhomogeneities among lung units, the average level of PEEPi must exceed the lowest regional alveolar pressure. Thus, external PEEP equal to PEEPi could cause hyperinflation in the faster-emptying lung units.[39–41] To minimize this risk, it is prudent to limit the level of external PEEP to about 70% of the level of PEEPi.

The importance of PEEPi as a cause of electromechanical dissociation during cardiopulmonary resuscitation is now well recognized.[42,43] Rosengarten et al[42] reported a dramatic example. A young woman with acute severe asthma was intubated 25 minutes after initial presentation. Ventilation was commenced with V$_T$ 8–10 ml/kg and respiratory rate 10–14 breaths/minute. O$_2$ saturation increased

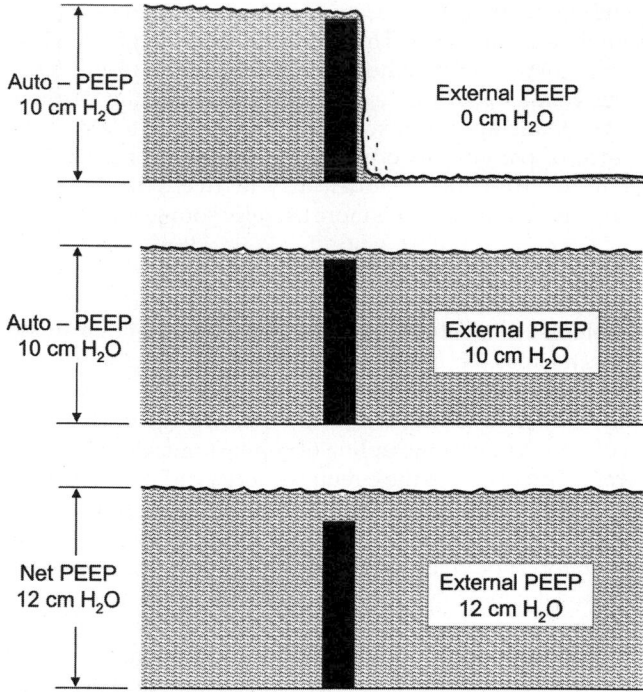

FIGURE 53-4 The analogy of a waterfall over a dam (indicated by the solid block) is used to explain the effect of external PEEP (downstream pressure) on PEEPi (upstream pressure) during expiration. Elevation of downstream pressure with external PEEP has no influence on either expiratory flow or upstream pressure (PEEPi) until it is equal to the critical closing pressure. When downstream pressure exceeds the critical closing pressure, the pressure upstream increases and hyperinflation is exacerbated. (*Reproduced, with permission, from Tobin and Lodato.[35]*)

momentarily. Five minutes after intubation, blood pressure could not be recorded. External cardiac massage was instituted, but the patient remained in electromechanical dissociation. Twenty-five minutes after intubation, the situation was considered irretrievable. All resuscitation was stopped. Three minutes later, the patient returned to sinus rhythm, and the pulses became palpable. Ventilation was recommenced at 15 breaths/minute. Within 15 seconds, the pulse disappeared. Ventilation was reduced to 6–8 breaths/min, and the pulse returned. Ventilation was transiently increased on three more occasions, and blood pressure disappeared each time. Seventy-five minutes after commencing resuscitation, the patient's blood pressure was 165/80 mm Hg. The patient suffered initial ischemic brain damage, but eventually made a close to complete recovery. In retrospect, it is clear that this patient suffered repeated episodes of circulatory arrest as a result of unrecognized ventilator-induced hyperinflation.

If faced with persistent hypotension in a patient with airflow limitation who is undergoing cardiopulmonary resuscitation, elevated PEEPi should be suspected. In such instances, the patient should be subjected to an apnea trial (after first ventilating the patient with 100% oxygen).[12] Ventilation is stopped for 1 minute, and blood pressure measured. If blood pressure improves, ventilation is resumed, but aiming to achieve a lower minute ventilation.

INADEQUATE RESPIRATORY DRIVE

Decreased respiratory neuromuscular output may cause sudden deterioration in a patient's respiratory status. Decreased drive, however, is not typically accompanied by respiratory distress. Respiratory drive may be decreased as a result of acute neurologic disorders, heavy sedation, or neuromuscular blocking agents.[44] A normal, or even elevated, drive may be insufficient to maintain alveolar ventilation if ventilatory demands or the mechanical load suddenly increase.

ELEVATED RESPIRATORY DRIVE

Excessive respiratory drive may cause severe respiratory alkalosis, which, in turn, may cause arrhythmias, hypotension, cerebral vasoconstriction, and seizures.[45,46] Ventilation can be stimulated by many physiologic, psychologic, and pathologic factors.[44] Extreme anxiety and panic cause dyspnea, fear, tachycardia, and palpitations, and when a patient misinterprets the basis of these symptoms, hyperventilation commonly develops.[47,48] A patient's likelihood of hyperventilating in response to stress probably depends on biologic vulnerability, personality, and cognitive variables.[48]

Several respiratory and nonrespiratory organic disorders stimulate breathing. The best known example is asthma, and even mild or moderate airway obstruction may be accompanied by a fall in Pa_{CO_2} to below 25 mmHg.[49] The mechanism of the hyperventilation is uncertain: it is probably related to hyperinflation[50] and stimulation of vagal afferents,[51] and it is not reversed by bronchodilation.[52] The reduction in Pa_{CO_2} is quantitatively consistent with hypoxic stimulation of the peripheral chemoreceptors, although supplemental O_2 does not restore ventilation to normal.[53] Respiratory stimulation also occurs in patients with COPD,[54] pulmonary fibrosis,[54,55] pneumonia,[56] pulmonary embolism,[57] pulmonary hypertension,[54,58] and heart failure.[59] In asthma, the most profound hyperventilation occurs with relatively mild disease,[49,60] and the same may apply with the other causes of respiratory stimulation. Pain stimulates breathing,[61] whereas hyperventilation increases the pain threshold.[62] Hyperventilation can be severe with certain drug overdoses, such as aspirin,[63] and it is a striking feature of sepsis[64] and major organ system failure,[65] although it does not occur in thyrotoxicosis. Acute diabetic ketoacidosis stimulates the peripheral chemoreceptors to produce deep rapid breathing and hypocapnia.[66]

Plum et al[67] coined the term *central neurogenic hyperventilation* to describe nine patients with tachypnea, of metronomic regularity, which persisted for hours or days at a time. Plum et al[68] subsequently revised their opinion, and attributed the heightened ventilation to stimulation of afferent peripheral reflexes arising in the lung and chest wall. It has not been possible to reproduce central neurogenic hyperventilation in animals. In their own clinical practice, Plum et al[68] are convinced of having seen only three patients with the condition, although brain histology was obtained in none of these cases. A few patients have been reported who displayed profound respiratory alkalosis, persisting during sleep or after administration of morphine, with normal oxygenation, normal chest radiography, and who had histologic evidence of pathology in the pons or some other area of the brain.[69–74] The rarity of this disorder is supported by the data of North et al.[75] Of 227 patients admitted to a neurosurgical unit, 57 had a respiratory rate >25 breaths/minute and 9 of these had a Pa_{CO_2} <30 mmHg. In all but one patient, however, the tachypnea and hypocapnia could be explained by hypoxemia associated with a pulmonary abnormality or metabolic acidosis. While hyperventilation in critically ill patients with an acute neurologic disorder is rarely neurogenic in nature, it nevertheless carries a poor prognosis.[75–78]

BODY POSTURE

An alteration in body posture can cause a significant fall in Pa_{CO_2}, as much as 30%,[28,79] especially in patients with unilateral lung disease. The hypoxemia is secondary to the effect of gravity on blood flow, as blood is shunted through the diseased dependent lung.

DRUG-INDUCED DETERIORATION

Hypoxemia may result from worsening of ventilation-perfusion relationships secondary to bronchodilators or vasodilators (e.g., nitroglycerin or nitroprusside). Administration of intravenous lipid compounds can also produce hypoxemia.[28] Aminoglycoside antibiotics can provoke or aggravate neuromuscular blockade and produce respiratory embarrassment.[80] High levels of theophylline may produce agitation and/or seizures.

ABDOMINAL DISTENSION

Abdominal distension can cause elevation of the diaphragm, basilar atelectasis, and deterioration in ventilation-perfusion relationships. Abdominal distension may result from gastric distension, ascites, peritoneal dialysis, or bowel perforation. Gastric distension may result from: a prolonged or difficult attempt at intubation; elevation of mouth pressure above the lower esophageal sphincter pressure during the delivery of manual ventilation; or tracheal pressure exceeding the cuff pressure and lower esophageal sphincter pressure and the mouth remaining closed during mechanical ventilation.[81,82] Massive distension, "meteorism," can produce gastric rupture. Insertion of a small-bore nasogastric tube helps prevent or alleviate this complication.

Massive colonic distension without small intestinal dilation or distal obstruction (Ogilvie's syndrome) has been described in patients receiving mechanical ventilation.[83] The mechanism is not known, but exaggerated aerophagia may be an important factor. Perforation of an overdistended cecum is often the first evidence of this complication. Accordingly, abdominal radiographs should be obtained in patients with abdominal distension, and cecostomy should be considered when the cecal diameter exceeds 9 cm.

AGITATION

Ventilated patients develop agitation as a result of four major factors: pain, anxiety, delirium, and dyspnea. Innumerable factors can cause pain in a critically ill patient, ranging from simple factors such as poorly applied adhesive tape to the pain of a major surgical procedure. Feelings of anxiety, insecurity, fear, and panic are very common in ventilator-dependent patients,[84,85] including a fear of impending death. Untreated pain and anxiety can lead to insomnia and delirium. These problems are aggravated by the discomfort of dyspnea, which may result from injudicious ventilator settings (see below). It is important to follow a systematic approach when evaluating a patient for the source of pain or anxiety, because simple problems, such as an overdistended bladder, may be overlooked while a search is conducted for a more esoteric source of distress.

VENTILATOR MALFUNCTION

Resolution of a patient's distress with the onset of bagging indicates that the problem lies within the ventilator or its external circuit (see Fig. 53-1). Malfunction of the ventilator may arise from tubing connected to a wrong outlet; a poor fit of connections; uncoupling of connections; defective material; obstruction of the circuit secondary to kinks, intraluminal fluids, or a malfunctioning valve; or malfunction of microprocessor controls. If malfunction is suspected, the ventilator should be replaced while each component is checked against the schematic circuit diagram. When a patient's delivered V_T is adequate and distress is relieved by manual ventilation, a fault in the setting of the fractional inspired O_2 concentration (FI_{O_2}) should be suspected. This problem can be verified by obtaining an independent direct measurement of FI_{O_2}.

EXTERNAL VENTILATOR CIRCUIT

The ventilator circuit primarily consists of the tubing and connectors that form inspiratory and exhalation limbs; the humidifier; the exhalation valve assembly and flow measuring devices; adaptors placed within the circuit for monitoring or delivering medications; and in-line filters.[12] Problems within this circuit that can cause patient distress include leaks, disconnects, accumulation of condensate, and in-line nebulizers.

Leaks or Disconnects

A leak may arise in parts of the circuit assembly that screw together. Leaks or uncoupling of connections will cause sounding of the low pressure and low V_T alarms. The Y-connection to the tracheal tube is the most common site of a disconnection. Other locations of disconnections and leaks include the humidifier system, an incompetent exhalation valve assembly, disconnection of the proximal line that connects the pressure tap at the Y-piece to the ventilator manometer, or small ruptures in the tubing.

In patients ventilated with pressure support, a leak at any location in the circuit, including at the cuff of the endotracheal tube, predisposes to a unique problem.[86] During pressure support, the ventilator strives to maintain a preset level of pressure throughout inspiration. A leak, however, will tend to cause the airway pressure to fall. To prevent the fall in airway pressure, the ventilator increases inspiratory flow. The algorithm employed by many ventilators for terminating the time of lung inflation is a fall in inspiratory flow to an absolute value of 5 liters per minute (or a fall in flow of 75% from the peak value). The increase in flow being delivered by the ventilator means that inspiratory flow never falls to the threshold required for termination of inflation.

This phenomenon results in the unremitting application of positive pressure, which is relieved by correcting the leak.

Condensate

Gas supplied to the inspiratory limb is typically warmed to 32–34°C and fully saturated with water vapor. The gas cools as it passes through the inspiratory tubing, causing condensate to form. The condensate accumulates in a U-loop of the circuit. If enough condensate accumulates, movement of the water can cause the ventilator to trigger. During assist-control ventilation, excessive triggering can lead to barotrauma or hemodynamic compromise. During pressure-support or pressure-controlled ventilation, the resistance caused by the condensate may cause a decrease in achieved V_T for a set airway pressure.

In-Line Nebulizers

The insertion of a continuous-flow nebulizer between the patient and the pressure sensor within the ventilator can lead to hypoventilation during pressure-support or intermittent mandatory ventilation (IMV).[87] When a patient's mean inspiratory flow rate is less than the flow of gas used to power the nebulizer (6–10 liters per minute), airway pressure will not fall sufficiently to trigger the ventilator. Moreover, the continuous flow from the nebulizer creates a bias flow, which the ventilator interprets as forming part of the patient's minute ventilation. Consequently, the low minute volume alarm will not sound.

PATIENT-VENTILATOR DYSSYNCHRONY

Patient-ventilator dyssynchrony can lead to considerable patient distress, and it also impedes the effectiveness of the ventilator in decreasing respiratory work. For the most effective unloading of the inspiratory muscles, the ventilator should cycle in synchrony with the patient's central respiratory rhythm. For perfect synchronization, the period of mechanical inflation must match the period of neural inspiratory time (the duration of inspiratory effort), and the period of mechanical inactivity must match the neural expiratory time.[88,89] The interplay between the ventilator and the respiratory neuromuscular apparatus is complex, and problems can arise at several points in the respiratory cycle: the onset of ventilator triggering, the remainder of inspiration after triggering, the switch from inspiration to expiration, and the end of expiration.

Triggering of the Ventilator

Patients reach the set sensitivity by activating their inspiratory muscles. But when the threshold is reached, inspiratory neurons do not simply switch off.[90] Consequently, the patient may expend considerable inspiratory effort throughout the machine-cycled inflation.[90] The level of patient effort during this post-trigger phase is closely related to a patient's respiratory drive at the point of triggering ($r = 0.78$).[91] As such, measures that decrease respiratory drive may enhance respiratory muscle rest during mechanical ventilation.

If respiratory drive at the point of triggering is important, one might expect that effort during the time of triggering would determine patient effort during the remainder of inspiration.[92] To investigate this issue, Leung et al[91] applied graded levels of pressure support in 11 critically ill patients. They achieved a fourfold reduction in overall patient effort. Yet patient effort during the time of triggering did not change. The constancy of effort during the trigger phase was probably secondary to different factors becoming operational as the level of ventilator assistance was varied (Fig. 53-5). Thus, increases in the level of ventilator

FIGURE 53-5 Graded increases in pressure support produced a decrease in total pressure-time product (PTP) per breath (*closed symbols*), although PTP during the trigger phase (*open symbols*) did not change (*left panel*). The constancy of PTP during triggering probably resulted from different factors becoming operational at different levels of assistance (*right panel*). At low levels of pressure support, respiratory drive (dP/dt) and intrinsic positive end-expiratory pressure (PEEPi) were high but triggering time was short, resulting in a large change in pleural pressure over a brief interval. At high levels of pressure support, dP/dt and PEEPi were low but triggering time was long, resulting in a smaller change in pleural pressure over a longer time. (*Based on data from Leung et al.[91]*)

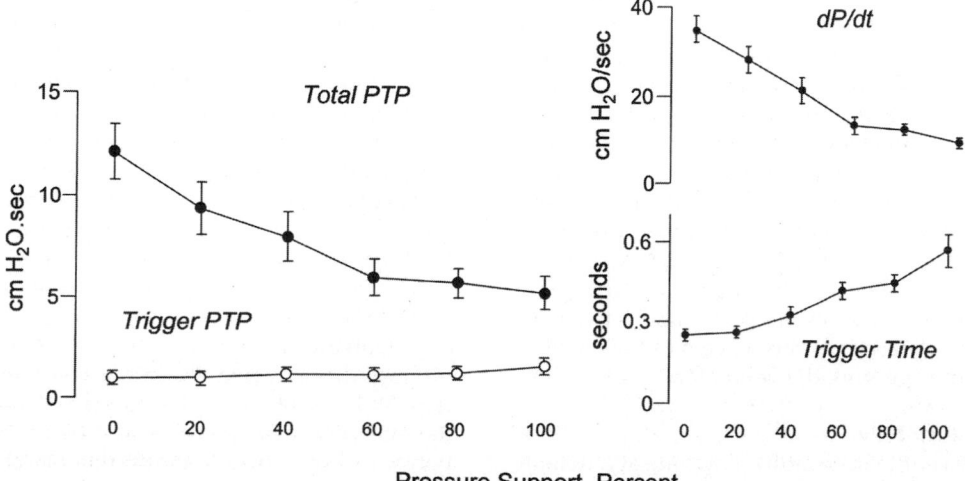

assistance do not substantially decrease patient effort during the time of triggering.

Ineffective Triggering

At high levels of mechanical assistance, up to one-third of a patient's inspiratory efforts may fail to trigger the machine (see Fig. 53-3).[91,93,94] The number of ineffective triggering attempts increases in direct proportion to the level of ventilator assistance.[91] Surprisingly, unsuccessful triggering is not the result of poor inspiratory effort. In a study of factors contributing to ineffective triggering, Leung et al[91] found that effort is more than a third greater when the threshold for triggering the ventilator is not reached than when it is reached. Significant differences, however, were noted in the characteristics of the breaths before the triggering and nontriggering attempts. Breaths before nontriggering attempts had a higher V_T than did the breaths before triggering attempts, 486 ± 19 and 444 ± 16 ml, respectively, and a shorter expiratory time, 1.02 ± 0.04 and 1.24 ± 0.03 seconds, respectively. An abbreviated expiratory time does not allow the lung to return to its relaxation volume, leading to an increase in elastic recoil pressure. Indeed, PEEPi was higher at the onset of nontriggering attempts than at the onset of triggering attempts: 4.22 ± 0.26 versus 3.25 ± 0.23 cmH$_2$O. Thus, nontriggering results from premature inspiratory efforts that are not sufficient to overcome the increased elastic recoil associated with dynamic hyperinflation.[91]

An elevated PEEPi may result from an increase in elastic recoil pressure or expiratory muscle activity. Parthasarathy et al[89] investigated the relative contributions of these two factors to ineffective triggering in healthy subjects receiving pressure support and in whom they induced airflow limitation with a Starling resistor. Nontriggering was linked to the fraction of PEEPi caused by elastic recoil but not to the fraction caused by expiratory effort. This observation suggests that external PEEP might be clinically useful in reducing ineffective triggering.

Although the magnitude of expiratory effort does not appear to influence the success of triggering attempts, the time that expiratory efforts commence in relation to the cycling of the ventilator is an important factor. Parthasarathy et al[89] quantified the relationship between the onset of expiratory muscle activity, measured with a wire electrode in the subject's transversus abdominis, and the termination of mechanical inflation by the ventilator. At pressure support of 20 cmH$_2$O, mechanical inflation was found to continue for a longer time into neural expiration in the breaths preceding nontriggering attempts. Continuation of mechanical inflation into neural expiration counters expiratory flow, and also decreases the time available for unopposed exhalation. Consequently, elastic recoil increases. In turn, a greater inspiratory effort will be needed to achieve effective triggering. In this way, the time that a patient commences an expiratory effort (in relation to cycling-off of mechanical inflation) partly determines the success of the ensuing inspiratory effort in triggering the ventilator.

Setting of Inspiratory Flow

Clinicians initially set the inspiratory flow rate at a default value, such as 60 liters per minute. Many critically ill patients, however, have an elevated respiratory drive and the initial flow setting may be insufficient to meet flow demands. As a result, patients will struggle against their own respiratory impedance and that of the ventilator. Consequently, work of breathing increases. Clinicians sometimes increase flow in order to shorten the inspiratory time and increase the expiratory time. But an increase in flow causes immediate and persistent tachypnea; as a result, expiratory time may be shortened.[95] In healthy subjects, Laghi et al[96] found that increases in inspiratory flow from 30 liters per minute to 60 and 90 liters per minute caused increases in the respiratory rate of 20 and 41%, respectively.

One of the main reasons that clinicians increase inspiratory flow is to decrease inspiratory time, in the hope of allowing more time for expiration and thus decrease PEEPi, especially in patients with COPD. Because increased flow usually leads to an increase in rate, the expected shortening of expiratory time might actually increase PEEPi. Laghi et al[97] studied this phenomenon in 10 patients with COPD (Fig. 53-6). As with healthy subjects, an increase in flow from 30 to 90 L/min caused the respiratory rate to increase from 16.1 ± 1.0 to 20.8 ± 1.5 breaths per minute. Despite the increase in rate, PEEPi fell from 7.0 ± 1.3 to 6.4 ± 1.1 cmH$_2$O. The decrease in PEEPi arose because of an increase in expiratory time, 2.1 ± 0.2 to 2.3 ± 0.2 seconds, which allowed more time for lung deflation. Why did expiratory time increase? An increase in inspiratory flow is usually achieved by shortening mechanical inspiratory time. The shortened inspiratory time combined with time-constant inhomogeneity of COPD will cause overinflation of some lung units to persist into neural expiration. Continued inflation during neural expiration causes stimulation of the vagus nerve, which prolongs expiratory time.[98,99]

MODE-SPECIFIC EFFECTS OF INSPIRATORY UNLOADING

Pressure support and IMV are sometimes combined in a given patient. In an international survey of mechanical ventilation,[100] this combination tied with assist-control ventilation as the most commonly used mode of ventilation in North America (34% for each). The rationale for combining the two modes is unclear. Presumably, clinicians use pressure support to overcome the work imposed by the endotracheal tube and demand valve during the non-mandatory breaths.

Examining the response of the respiratory centers to this combination of modes provides useful insight into patient-ventilator interaction. A decrease in the number of mandatory breaths produces a decrease in the average V_T,[91] with inevitable increase in the ratio of dead space to V_T. To avoid a decrease in alveolar ventilation, the patients increased respiratory drive, inspiratory effort, and rate. Adding pressure support of 10 cmH$_2$O caused a decrease in effort at any given IMV rate. The decrease in effort during the mandatory ventilator breaths was related to the decrease in respiratory drive during the intervening breaths ($r = 0.67$)[91] (Fig. 53-7). In other words, the reduction in drive during the intervening breaths achieved by adding pressure support was carried over to the mandatory breaths, facilitating greater unloading. Combining IMV and pressure support

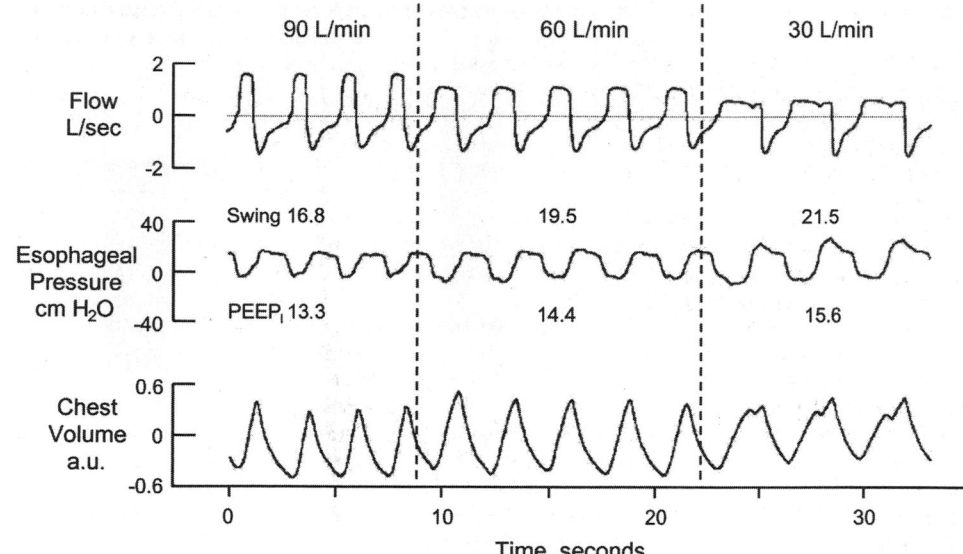

FIGURE 53-6 Continuous recordings of flow, esophageal pressure (P_{es}), and the sum of rib-cage and abdominal motion, in a patient with COPD receiving assist-control ventilation at a constant tidal volume. As flow increased from 30 to 60 and 90 L/min (from right to left), frequency increased (from 18 to 23 and 26 breaths/minute, respectively), PEEPi decreased (from 15.6 to 14.4 and 13.3 cmH$_2$O, respectively), and end-expiratory lung volume also fell. Increases in flow from 30 L/min to 60 and 90 L/min also led to decreases in the swings in P_{es} from 21.5 to 19.5 and 16.8 cmH$_2$O, respectively. (*Reproduced, with permission, from Laghi et al.[97]*)

provides a sometimes useful means of achieving a high level of assistance; the combination has a clinical advantage when it is difficult to achieve a high inspiratory flow in the assist-control mode, as with the Siemens 900C ventilator (Siemens Corporation, New York, NY).

FIGURE 53-7 The change in pressure-time product per breath (PTP/breath) during mandatory breaths (of IMV) consequent to the addition of pressure support of 10 cmH$_2$O to a given level of IMV was related to the change in respiratory drive (dP/dt) effected by pressure support during the intervening breaths (r = 0.67; $p < 0.0001$). The more that pressure support decreased respiratory drive during the intervening breaths, the greater was the reduction in patient work during the mandatory ventilator breaths delivered during IMV. (*Reproduced, with permission, from Leung et al.[91]*)

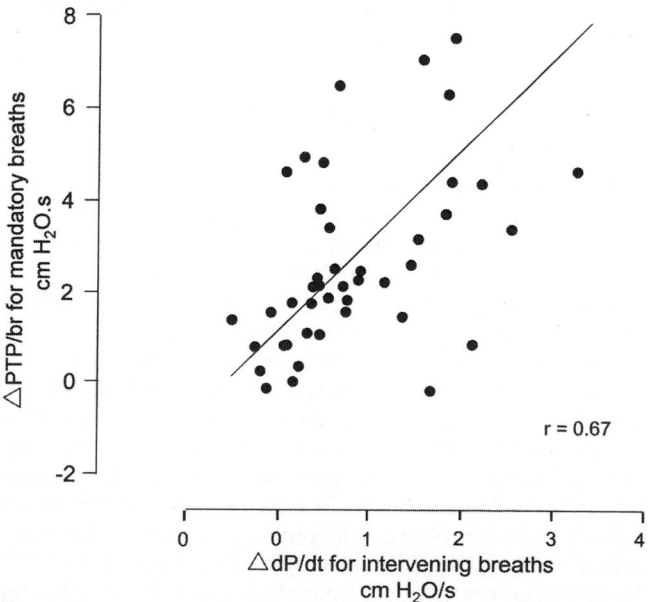

INSPIRATION-EXPIRATION SWITCHING

In studies of interactions between patient effort and mechanical ventilation, remarkably little attention has been paid to the switch between inspiration and expiration. The most common mode of ventilation is some form of volume assistance,[100] such as assist control or IMV. "Cycling-off" of mechanical inflation, however, may be based only indirectly on volume. Instead, inspiratory flow is commonly preset and the ventilator adjusts inspiratory time to achieve a given V_T. This system is more precisely termed *time-cycled ventilation*. Inflation time is constant with a time-cycled machine, but patients invariably display considerable breath-to-breath variability in inspiratory time.[101] Accordingly, a patient's neural inspiratory time may be shorter or longer than the inflation time of the machine. If the machine delivers the set V_T before the end of a patient's neural inspiratory time, ventilator assistance will cease while the patient continues to make an inspiratory effort—with double triggering (two ventilator breaths for a single effort) a likely consequence.[102]

With the use of pressure support, ventilator assistance ceases when patient inspiratory flow falls by a preset amount (such as to 25% of the peak flow; see Chapter 9). The algorithm for cycling-off of mechanical inflation causes problems in patients with COPD, because increases in resistance and compliance produce a slow time constant (of the respiratory system). The longer time needed for flow to fall to the threshold value can cause mechanical inflation to persist into neural expiration. In 12 patients with COPD receiving pressure support of 20 cmH$_2$O, Jubran et al[103] found that 5 recruited their expiratory muscles while the machine was still inflating the thorax (Fig. 53-8). Interestingly, the patients who recruited their expiratory muscles during mechanical inflation had an average time constant of 0.54 second, compared with an average of 0.38 second in the patients who did not exhibit expiratory muscle activity. The persistence of mechanical inflation into neural expiration is very uncomfortable, as is well recognized with the use of inverse-ratio

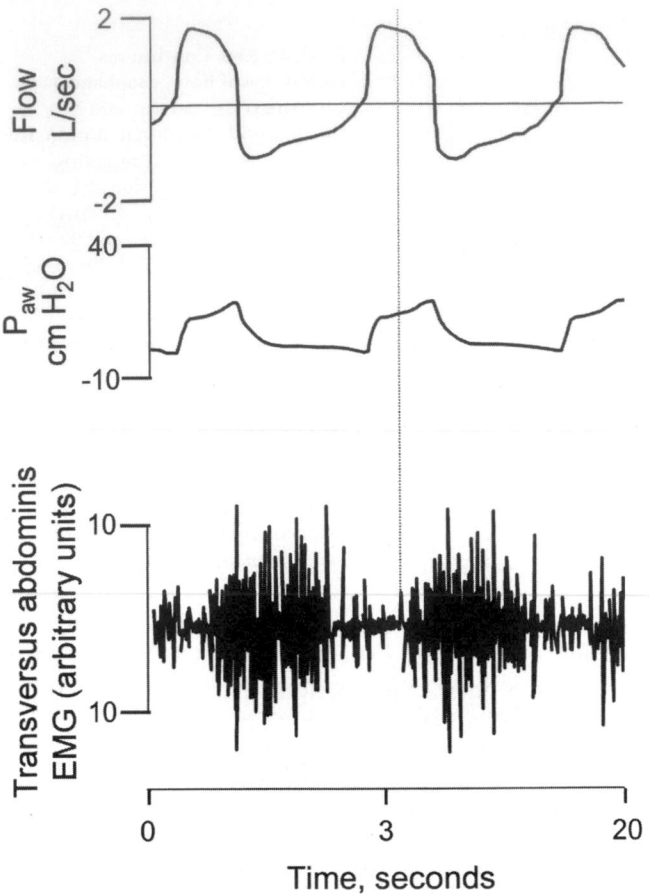

FIGURE 53-8 Recordings of flow, airway pressure (P_{aw}), and transversus abdominis electromyography in a critically ill patient with COPD receiving pressure support of 20 cmH$_2$O. The onset of expiratory muscle activity (*vertical dotted line*) occurred when mechanical inflation was only partly completed. (*Reproduced, with permission, from Parthasarathy et al.[89]*)

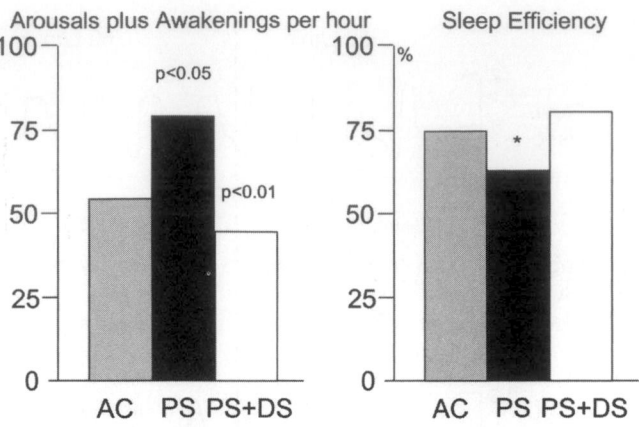

FIGURE 53-9 Sleep fragmentation (*left panel*) and sleep efficiency (*right panel*) during assist-control ventilation and pressure support with and without dead space. Sleep fragmentation, measured as the number of arousals and awakenings, was greater during pressure support (*solid bars*) than during assist-control ventilation (*hatched bars*) or pressure support with dead space (*open bars*). Sleep efficiency (*right panel*) was also lower during pressure support (*solid bars*) than during assist-control ventilation (*hatched bars*) or pressure support with dead space (*open bars*). (*Modified, with permission, from Parthasarathy and Tobin.[109]*)

ventilation (see Chapter 10). Other investigators have also demonstrated a relationship between unsatisfactory selection of the criteria used for terminating inflation and patient work of breathing[104] and patient discomfort.[105]

SLEEP-WAKE STATE

The transition between sleep and wakefulness can lead to respiratory distress in the ventilated patient. More surprisingly, the transition between wakefulness and sleep can also cause distress. Specifically, the selection of ventilator mode and settings can provoke sleep disruption. Ventilated patients experience considerable sleep disruption, with as many as 20–63 arousals and awakenings per hour.[106,107] Sleep disruption can adversely affect patient outcome.[108]

In 11 critically ill patients, Parthasarathy and Tobin[109] studied the interaction between ventilator mode and sleep. Sleep fragmentation was greater during pressure support than during assist-control ventilation: 79 versus 54 arousals and awakenings per hour (Fig. 53-9). Six of the eleven patients developed central apneas during pressure support, but not during assist-control ventilation. V_T was 8 ml per kg during assist-control; pressure support was titrated to

achieve the same V_T. The level of pressure support was 16.8 ± 1.5 cmH$_2$O in patients with apneas and 19.6 ± 2.6 cmH$_2$O in patients without apneas; thus, apneas did result simply from a higher level of pressure support.

Total sleep fragmentation, measured as the sum of arousals (at least 3 seconds) and awakenings (more than half of a 30-second epoch), was greater during pressure support than during assist-control ventilation: 79 ± 7 versus 54 ± 7 arousals and awakenings/hour.[109] Sleep efficiency (the time a patient was asleep divided by the duration of the study; 2 hours) was 75 ± 5% during assist-control ventilation and 63 ± 5% during pressure support. The more disturbed sleep during pressure support was related to the development of central apneas.

The most important determinant of apneas was the difference between P_{CO_2} during resting breathing and the patient's apnea threshold. When a patient's resting P_{CO_2} was close to the apnea threshold, central apneas were more likely to develop.[109] The addition of dead space caused a further increase in resting P_{CO_2} above the apnea threshold and decreased the sum of arousals and awakenings from 83 to 44 events per hour (in the patients who developed central apneas during pressure support). Sleep efficiency (time asleep as a percentage of study duration) increased from 63 to 81% with the addition of dead space (see Fig. 53-9).

The alterations in breathing pattern and gas exchange induced by sleep have important implications for the selection of ventilator settings. Physicians typically adjust ventilator settings during the daytime and often do not know whether a patient is asleep or awake. During pressure support, sleep induced a 23% increase in inspiratory time and a 126% increase in expiratory time, as compared with wakefulness.[109] Sleep caused the respiratory rate to decrease by 33% during

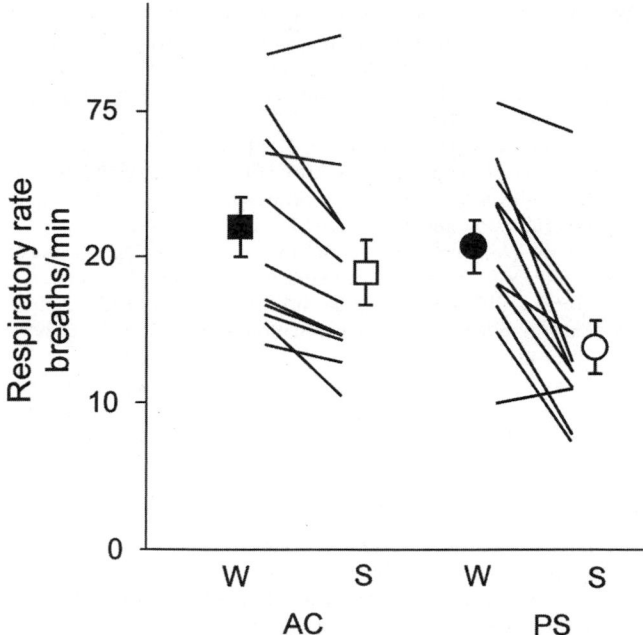

FIGURE 53-10 Respiratory rate during assist-control ventilation (*AC*) and pressure support (*PS*) in 11 critically ill patients. For each mode, the lines connect the mean value for each patient during wakefulness (*W, left*) and sleep (*S, right*). Compared with wakefulness, group mean respiratory rate was lower during sleep (*closed symbols*) than during wakefulness (*open symbols*). The difference between sleep and wakefulness was greater for pressure support than for assist-control ventilation. (*Modified, with permission, from Parthasarathy and Tobin.[109]*)

pressure support and by 15% during assist-control ventilation (Fig. 53-10). The level of pressure support is commonly titrated to respiratory rate, which provides a reasonable guide to patient effort.[103,110] A patient may be asleep at the point that a physician uses respiratory rate to select a suitable level of pressure support (the respiratory rate will be relatively low during sleep). Then, on awakening, patient rate typically increases and may be accompanied by considerable increase in effort.

Pharmacotherapy

If a specific cause of acute distress cannot be detected and corrected (see Table 53-1) and reassurance provides no relief, pharmacologic agents are commonly employed. The agents most often used are derived from the following primary classes: opiate analgesics, benzodiazepines, and neuromuscular blocking agents. A complete discussion of these agents is found in Chapter 51.

In managing the patient who is fighting the ventilator, neuromuscular blocking agents have several disadvantages: they mask a patient's complaints and physical findings; unrecognized disconnection of the ventilator circuit can produce apnea with catastrophic hypoxemia; elimination of cough predisposes to the development of atelectasis; and prolonged paralysis or weakness may persist after their use.

Summary

Sudden distress in a ventilator-supported patient is a medical emergency. The first rule is to ensure adequate ventilation. The patient should be disconnected from the ventilator and manually ventilated with 100% O_2. While this is being performed, a systematic effort should be made to try to determine the cause of distress and correct it. If the distress is the result of poor coordination of a patient's respiratory efforts with the rhythm of the ventilator, this can usually be resolved by careful adjustment of the ventilator settings and the administration of analgesic or sedative agents, or both.

References

1. Tobin MJ. What should a clinician do when a patient "fights the ventilator"? Respiratory Care 1991; 36:395–406.
2. Hudson LD. Diagnosis and management of acute respiratory distress in patients on mechanical ventilators. In: Moser KM, Spragg RG, editors. Respiratory emergencies. St. Louis: Mosby, 1982: 201–213.
3. Jubran A. Pulse oximetry. In: Tobin MJ, editor. Principles and practice of intensive care monitoring. New York: McGraw-Hill, 1998: 261–287.
4. Rossi A. Monitoring respiratory mechanics in ventilator-dependent patients. In: Tobin MJ, editor. Principles and practice of intensive care monitoring. New York: McGraw-Hill, 1998: 553–596.
5. Tobin MJ. Mechanical ventilation. N Engl J Med 1994; 330: 1056–61.
6. Jubran A, Tobin MJ. Use of flow-volume curves in detecting secretions in ventilator-dependent patients. Am J Respir Crit Care Med 1994; 150:766–9.
7. Leatherman J. Pulmonary artery catheterization: Interpretation of pressure recordings. In: Tobin MJ, editor. Principles and practice of intensive care monitoring. New York: McGraw-Hill, 1998: 821–37.
8. Zwillich CW, Pierson DJ, Creagh CE, et al. Complications of assisted ventilation. A prospective study of 354 consecutive episodes. Am J Med 1974; 57:161–70.
9. Brunel W, Coleman DL, Schwartz DE, Peper E, Cohen NH. Assessment of routine chest roentgenograms and the physical examination to confirm endotracheal tube position. Chest 1989; 96:1043–5.
10. Stauffer J. Monitoring the use of tracheal tubes. In: Tobin MJ, editor. Principles and practice of intensive care monitoring. New York: McGraw-Hill, 1998: 667–82.
11. Conrardy PA, Goodman LR, Lainge F, Singer MM. Alteration of endotracheal tube position. Flexion and extension of the neck. Crit Care Med 1976; 4:7–12.
12. Marcy TW, Marini JJ. Respiratory distress in the ventilated patient. Clin Chest Med 1994; 15:55–73.
13. Hosking MP, Lennon RL, Warner MA, et al. Endotracheal tube obstruction: recognition and management. Mil Med 1989; 154:489–91.
14. Zmyslowski WP, Kam D, Simpson GT. An unusual cause of endotracheal tube obstruction. Anesthesiology 1989; 70:883.
15. Harrington JF. An unusual cause of endotracheal tube obstruction. Anesthesiology 1984; 61:116–17.
16. Sprung J, Bourke DL, Harrison C, Barnas GM. Endotracheal tube and tracheobronchial obstruction as causes of hypoventilation with high inspiratory pressures. Chest 1994; 105:550–52.

17. Harley HR. Ulcerative tracheo-oesophageal fistula during treatment by tracheostomy and intermittent positive pressure ventilation. Thorax 1972; 27:338–52.

18. Wood DE, Mathisen DJ. Late complications of tracheotomy. Clin Chest Med 1991; 12:597–609.

19. Myers EN, Carrau RL. Early complications of tracheotomy. Incidence and management. Clin Chest Med 1991; 12:589–95.

20. Nelems B. Tracheoarterial fistula. In: Grillo HC, Eschapasse H, editors. International trends in general thoracic surgery, Vol 2: Major challenges. Philadelphia: Saunders, 1987: 69–73.

21. Tenholder MF, Erwin WA, Nelson HS. "Lost" tidal volumes in a 71-year-old ventilated patient. Chest 1994; 106:1869–71.

22. Guglielminotti J, Alzieu M, Maury E, Guidet B, Offenstadt G. Bedside detection of retained tracheobronchial secretions in patients receiving mechanical ventilation: is it time for tracheal suctioning? Chest 2000; 118:1095–99.

23. Russomanno JH, Brown LK. Pneumothorax due to ball-valve obstruction of an endotracheal tube in a mechanically ventilated patient. Chest 1992; 101:1444–45.

24. Albelda SM, Gefter WB, Kelley MA, Epstein DM, Miller WT. Ventilator-induced subpleural air cysts: clinical, radiographic, and pathologic significance. Am Rev Respir Dis 1983; 127: 360–5.

25. Fedullo PF, Tapson VF. Clinical practice. The evaluation of suspected pulmonary embolism. N Engl J Med 2003; 349:1247–56.

26. Henry JW, Stein PD, Gottschalk A, Relyea B, Leeper KV Jr. Scintigraphic lung scans and clinical assessment in critically ill patients with suspected acute pulmonary embolism. Chest 1996; 109:462–66.

27. Velmahos GC, Vassiliu P, Wilcox A, et al. Spiral computed tomography for the diagnosis of pulmonary embolism in critically ill surgical patients: a comparison with pulmonary angiography. Arch Surg 2001; 136:505–11.

28. Glauser FL, Polatty RC, Sessler CN. Worsening oxygenation in the mechanically ventilated patient. Causes, mechanisms, and early detection. Am Rev Respir Dis 1988; 138:458–65.

29. Keith RL, Pierson DJ. Complications of mechanical ventilation. A bedside approach. Clin Chest Med 1996; 17:439–51.

30. DePietro M. Complications of pulmonary artery catheterization. In: Tobin MJ, editor. Principles and practice of intensive care monitoring. New York: McGraw-Hill, 1998: 855–70.

31. Tobin MJ. Noninvasive monitoring of ventilation. In: Tobin MJ, editor. Principles and practice of intensive care monitoring. New York: McGraw-Hill, 1998: 465–95.

32. Pepe PE, Marini JJ. Occult positive end-expiratory pressure in mechanically ventilated patients with airflow obstruction: the auto-PEEP effect. Am Rev Respir Dis 1982; 126: 166–70.

33. Rossi A, Gottfried SB, Zocchi L, et al. Measurement of static compliance of the total respiratory system in patients with acute respiratory failure during mechanical ventilation. The effect of intrinsic positive end-expiratory pressure. Am Rev Respir Dis 1985; 131:672–77.

34. Laghi F, Tobin MJ. Disorders of the respiratory muscles. Am J Respir Crit Care Med 2003; 168:10–48.

35. Tobin MJ, Lodato RF. PEEP, auto-PEEP, and waterfalls. Chest 1989; 96:449–51.

36. Tobin MJ, Jubran A. Pathophysiology of failure to wean from mechanical ventilation. Schweiz Med Wochenschr 1994; 124:2139–145.

37. Smith TC, Marini JJ. Impact of PEEP on lung mechanics and work of breathing in severe airflow obstruction. J Appl Physiol 1988; 65:1488–499.

38. Lodato RF, Tobin MJ. Estimation of auto-PEEP. Chest 1991; 99:520–22.

39. Petrof BJ, Legare M, Goldberg P, Milic-Emili J, Gottfried SB. Continuous positive airway pressure reduces work of breathing and dyspnea during weaning from mechanical ventilation in severe chronic obstructive pulmonary disease. Am Rev Respir Dis 1990; 141:281–89.

40. Georgopoulos D, Giannouli E, Patakas D. Effects of extrinsic positive end-expiratory pressure on mechanically ventilated patients with chronic obstructive pulmonary disease and dynamic hyperinflation. Intensive Care Med 1993; 19:197–203.

41. Ranieri VM, Giuliani R, Cinnella G, et al. Physiologic effects of positive end-expiratory pressure in patients with chronic obstructive pulmonary disease during acute ventilatory failure and controlled mechanical ventilation. Am Rev Respir Dis 1993; 147:5–13.

42. Rosengarten PL, Tuxen DV, Dziukas L, et al. Circulatory arrest induced by intermittent positive pressure ventilation in a patient with severe asthma. Anaesth Intensive Care 1991; 19:118–21.

43. Rogers PL, Schlichtig R, Miro A, Pinsky M. Auto-PEEP during CPR. An "occult" cause of electromechanical dissociation? Chest 1991; 99:492–93.

44. Tobin MJ, Gardner WN. Monitoring of the control of breathing. In: Tobin MJ, editor. Principles and practice of intensive care monitoring. New York: McGraw-Hill, 1998: 415–64.

45. Rotheram EB Jr, Safar P, Robin E. CNS disorder during mechanical ventilation in chronic pulmonary disease. JAMA 1964; 189:993–96.

46. Kilburn KH. Shock, seizures, and coma with alkalosis during mechanical ventilation. Ann Intern Med 1966; 65:977–84.

47. Tobin MJ. Dyspnea. Pathophysiologic basis, clinical presentation, and management. Arch Intern Med 1990; 150:1604–13.

48. Gardner WN. The pathophysiology of hyperventilation disorders. Chest 1996; 109:516–34.

49. McFadden ER Jr, Lyons HA. Arterial-blood gas tension in asthma. N Engl J Med 1968; 278:1027–32.

50. Muller N, Bryan AC, Zamel N. Tonic inspiratory muscle activity as a cause of hyperinflation in asthma. J Appl Physiol 1981; 50:279–82.

51. Cotton DJ, Bleecker ER, Fischer SP, et al. Rapid, shallow breathing after *Ascaris suum* antigen inhalation: role of vagus nerves. J Appl Physiol 1977; 42:101–106.

52. Tobin MJ, Birch S, Jenouri G, Sackner MA. Acute effects of aerosolized metaproterenol on breathing pattern of patients with symptomatic bronchial asthma. J Allergy Clin Immunol 1985; 76:166–72.

53. Kesten S, Maleki-Yazdi R, Sanders BR, et al. Respiratory rate during acute asthma. Chest 1990; 97:58–62.

54. Tobin MJ, Chadha TS, Jenouri G, et al. Breathing patterns. 2. Diseased subjects. Chest 1983; 84:286–94.

55. Javaheri S, Sicilian L. Lung function, breathing pattern, and gas exchange in interstitial lung disease. Thorax 1992; 47: 93–97.

56. Kassabian J, Miller KD, Lavietes MH. Respiratory center output and ventilatory timing in patients with acute airway (asthma) and alveolar (pneumonia) disease. Chest 1982; 81:536–43.

57. Szucs MM Jr, Brooks HL, Grossman W, et al. Diagnostic sensitivity of laboratory findings in acute pulmonary embolism. Ann Intern Med 1971; 74:161–66.

58. Sietsema KE, Simon JI, Wasserman K. Pulmonary hypertension presenting as a panic disorder. Chest 1987; 91:910–12.

59. Avery WG, Samet P, Sackner MA. The acidosis of pulmonary edema. Am J Med 1970; 48:320–24.

60. Gardner WN, Bass C, Moxham J. Recurrent hyperventilation tetany due to mild asthma. Respir Med 1992; 86:349–51.

61. Glynn CJ, Lloyd JW, Folkhard S. Ventilatory response to intractable pain. Pain 1981; 11:201–11.

62. Geddes IC, Gray TC. Hyperventilation for the maintenance of anaesthesia. Lancet 1959; 2:4–6.
63. Temple AR. Acute and chronic effects of aspirin toxicity and their treatment. Arch Intern Med 1981; 141:364–69.
64. Kasnitz P, Druger GL, Yorra F, Simmons DH. Mixed venous oxygen tension and hyperlactatemia. Survival in severe cardiopulmonary disease. JAMA 1976; 236:570–74.
65. Vanamee P, Poppell JW, Glicksman AS, Randall HT, Roberts KE. Respiratory alkalosis in hepatic coma. AMA Arch Intern Med 1956; 97:762–67.
66. Kaufmann P, Smolle KH, Fleck S, Lueger A. Ketoacidotic diabetic metabolic dysregulation: pathophysiology, clinical aspects, diagnosis and therapy. Wien Klin Wochenschr 1994; 106:119–27.
67. Plum F, Swanson AG. Central neurogenic hyperventilation in man. AMA Arch Neurol Psychiatry 1959; 81:535–49.
68. Plum F, Posner JB. The diagnosis of stupor and coma, 3rd ed. Philadelphia: FA Davis, 1980.
69. Lange LS, Laszlo G. Cerebral tumour presenting with hyperventilation. J Neurol Neurosurg Psychiatry 1965; 28:3 17–19.
70. Rodriguez M, Baele PL, Marsh HM, Okazaki H. Central neurogenic hyperventilation in an awake patient with brainstem astrocytoma. Ann Neurol 1982; 11:625–28.
71. Sunderrajan EV, Passamonte PM. Lymphomatoid granulomatosis presenting as central neurogenic hyperventilation. Chest 1984; 86:634–36.
72. Bateman DE, Gibson GJ, Hudgson P, Tomlinson BE. Central neurogenic hyperventilation in a conscious patient with a primary cerebral lymphoma. Ann Neurol 1985; 17:402–405.
73. Gottlieb D, Michowitz SD, Steiner I, Wald U. Central neurogenic hyperventilation in a patient with medulloblastoma. Eur Neurol 1987; 27:51–54.
74. Pauzner R, Mouallem M, Sadeh M, Tadmor R, Farfel Z. High incidence of primary cerebral lymphoma in tumor-induced central neurogenic hyperventilation. Arch Neurol 1989; 46: 510–12.
75. North JB, Jennett S. Abnormal breathing patterns associated with acute brain damage. Arch Neurol 1974; 31:338–44.
76. Rout MW, Lane DJ, Wollner L. Prognosis in acute cerebrovascular accidents in relation to respiratory pattern and blood gas tensions. Br Med J 1971; 3:7–9.
77. Leigh RJ, Shaw DA. Rapid regular respiration in unconscious patients. Arch Neurol 1976; 33:356–61.
78. Lee MC, Klassen AC, Resch JA. Respiratory pattern disturbances in ischemic cerebral vascular disease. Stroke 1974; 5:612–16.
79. Langer M, Mascheroni D, Marcolin R, Gattinoni L. The prone position in ARDS patients. A clinical study. Chest 1988; 94: 103–107.
80. Argov Z, Mastaglia FL. Drug therapy: Disorders of neuromuscular transmission caused by drugs. N Engl J Med 1979; 301: 409–13.
81. Barker SJ, Karagianes T. Gastric barotrauma: a case report and theoretical considerations. Anesth Analg 1985; 64:1026–28.
82. Tessler S, Kupfer Y, Lerman A, Arsura EL. Massive gastric distention in the intubated patient. A marker for a defective airway. Arch Intern Med 1990; 150:318–20.
83. Golden GT, Chandler JG. Colonic ileus and cecal perforation in patients requiring mechanical ventilatory support. Chest 1975; 68:661–64.
84. Misak CJ. The critical care experience: a patient's view. Am J Respir Crit Care Med 2004; 170:357–59.
85. Bergbom-Engberg I, Haljamae H. Assessment of patients' experience of discomforts during respirator therapy. Crit Care Med 1989; 17:1068–72.
86. Black JW, Grover BS. A hazard of pressure support ventilation. Chest 1988; 93:333–35.
87. Beaty CD, Ritz RH, Benson MS. Continuous in-line nebulizers complicate pressure support ventilation. Chest 1989; 96: 1360–63.
88. Simon PM, Zurob AS, Wies WM, Leiter JC, Hubmayr RD. Entrainment of respiration in humans by periodic lung inflations. Effect of state and CO(2). Am J Respir Crit Care Med 1999; 160:950–60.
89. Parthasarathy S, Jubran A, Tobin MJ. Cycling of inspiratory and expiratory muscle groups with the ventilator in airflow limitation. Am J Respir Crit Care Med 1998; 158:1471–78.
90. Marini JJ, Capps JS, Culver BH. The inspiratory work of breathing during assisted mechanical ventilation. Chest 1985; 87: 612–18.
91. Leung P, Jubran A, Tobin MJ. Comparison of assisted ventilator modes on triggering, patient effort, and dyspnea. Am J Respir Crit Care Med 1997; 155:1940–48.
92. Giuliani R, Mascia L, Recchia F, et al. Patient-ventilator interaction during synchronized intermittent mandatory ventilation. Effects of flow triggering. Am J Respir Crit Care Med 1995; 151: 1–9.
93. Giannouli E, Webster K, Roberts D, Younes M. Response of ventilator-dependent patients to different levels of pressure support and proportional assist. Am J Respir Crit Care Med 1999; 159:1716–25.
94. Sinderby C, Navalesi P, Beck J, et al. Neural control of mechanical ventilation in respiratory failure. Nat Med 1999; 5:1433–36.
95. Puddy A, Younes M. Effect of inspiratory flow rate on respiratory output in normal subjects. Am Rev Respir Dis 1992; 146: 787–89.
96. Laghi F, Karamchandani K, Tobin MJ. Influence of ventilator settings in determining respiratory frequency during mechanical ventilation. Am J Respir Crit Care Med 1999; 160:1766–70.
97. Laghi F, Segal J, Choe WK, Tobin MJ. Effect of imposed inflation time on respiratory frequency and hyperinflation in patients with chronic obstructive pulmonary disease. Am J Respir Crit Care Med 2001; 163:1365–70.
98. Younes M, Vaillancourt P, Milic-Emili J. Interaction between chemical factors and duration of apnea following lung inflation. J Appl Physiol 1974; 36:190–201.
99. Zuperku EJ, Hopp FA, Kampine JP. Central integration of pulmonary stretch receptor input in the control of expiration. J Appl Physiol 1982; 52:1296–315.
100. Esteban A, Anzueto A, Alia I, et al. How is mechanical ventilation employed in the intensive care unit? An international utilization review. Am J Respir Crit Care Med 2000; 161: 1450–58.
101. Tobin MJ, Yang KL, Jubran A, Lodato RF. Interrelationship of breath components in neighboring breaths of normal eupneic subjects. Am J Respir Crit Care Med 1995; 152(6 Pt 1):1967–76.
102. Younes M. Interactions between patients and ventilators. In: Roussos C, editor. The thorax. New York: Marcel Dekker, 1995: 2367–420.
103. Jubran A, Van de Graaff WB, Tobin MJ. Variability of patient-ventilator interaction with pressure support ventilation in patients with chronic obstructive pulmonary disease. Am J Respir Crit Care Med 1995; 152:129–36.
104. Tokioka H, Tanaka T, Ishizu T, et al. The effect of breath termination criterion on breathing patterns and the work of breathing during pressure support ventilation. Anesth Analg 2001; 92: 161–65.
105. Calderini E, Confalonieri M, Puccio PG, et al. Patient-ventilator asynchrony during noninvasive ventilation: the role of expiratory trigger. Intensive Care Med 1999; 25:662–67.

106. Cooper AB, Thornley KS, Young GB, et al. Sleep in critically ill patients requiring mechanical ventilation. Chest 2000; 117: 809–18.
107. Gabor JY, Cooper AB, Crombach SA, et al. Contribution of the intensive care unit environment to sleep disruption in mechanically ventilated patients and healthy subjects. Am J Respir Crit Care Med 2003; 167:708–15.
108. Parthasarathy S, Tobin MJ. Sleep in the intensive care unit. Intensive Care Med 2004; 30:197–206.
109. Parthasarathy S, Tobin MJ. Effect of ventilator mode on sleep quality in critically ill patients. Am J Respir Crit Care Med 2002; 166:1423–29.
110. Tobin MJ, Jubran A, Laghi F. Patient-ventilator interaction. Am J Respir Crit Care Med 2001; 163:1059–63.

Chapter 54 _____

PSYCHOLOGICAL PROBLEMS IN THE VENTILATED PATIENT

UBALDO J. MARTIN
GERARD J. CRINER

Psychological problems are commonly reported in chronic illnesses,[1] after general surgery,[2] after cardiac surgery,[3,4] in the intensive care unit (ICU) setting,[5] and in mechanically ventilated patients.[6,7] Our ability to improve survival in patients with devastating medical or surgical illnesses, who require prolonged ventilation, has given rise to a population of patients at risk for long-term physical and psychological problems. Although psychological disorders are reported to affect weaning from mechanical ventilation,[8] data examining psychological function in ventilated patients is limited.[9] Delirium and agitation significantly affect outcomes in ventilated patients,[7,10] and new attempts are being made to diagnose and categorize these problems.[6,11–13] Multiple questions, however, such as prevention of psychological problems and their treatment, remain largely unanswered. This is surprising, because many factors reported to cause psychological dysfunction (severe illness, chronic illness, sleep deprivation, inability to speak, and immobility) are commonly present in ventilated patients (Fig. 54-1). Despite the lack of psychological information in ventilated patients, over the past decade we have witnessed a significant increase in the number of studies examining the incidence and outcomes of psychological problems in the ICU, and these have provided insight into the psychological issues affecting ventilated patients.

In this chapter, we integrate and summarize current evidence regarding the incidence, prevalence, outcomes, and diagnosis of psychological disturbances in the ICU, with special emphasis on the ventilated patient. We also discuss current options for evaluation and treatment.

Magnitude of the Problem

INCIDENCE OF PSYCHOLOGICAL DISTURBANCES

Most patients who undergo mechanical ventilation receive at least a part of their care in the ICU. Psychological problems occur in 14–72% of ICU patients compared with <1% of non-ICU hospitalized patients.[14,15] This wide range likely reflects methodological discrepancies between studies,[12] and up to now, the absence of operational definitions and diagnostic tools. Various psychological problems may arise in ICU patients (Table 54-1), including anxiety, agitation, apathy, depression, and delirium. Agitated behavior is common in the ICU; its differential diagnosis is extensive, with delirium being the most disconcerting problem because of its associated high morbidity and mortality.[6,16,17] Dubois et al reported a 20% incidence of delirium in ICU patients with a mean Acute Physiology and Chronic Health Evaluation (APACHE) II score of 15 ± 8.[17] In 48 ICU patients, 24 of whom received mechanical ventilation with a mean APACHE II score of 17, Ely et al reported a 60% incidence of delirium.[16] In a study confined to ventilated patients, 32% were delirious at enrollment and 82% developed delirium at some point during their ICU stay.[7] In our ventilator rehabilitation unit, which treats patients with chronic mechanical ventilation (mean duration of mechanical ventilation >21 days), Repetz et al reported delirium in 52% of patients.[18]

Anxiety is common in ventilated patients. Moderate to high levels of anxiety as assessed by a version of the State Anxiety Inventory (SAI) were reported in patients receiving ventilation for various surgical or medical conditions.[19,20] In the absence of delirium, Sessler et al reported mild, moderate, and severe agitation in medical ICU patients, with an incidence of 32%, 20%, and 5%, respectively.[21]

Despite the high incidence and prevalence of neuropsychological disorders in ventilated ICU patients, awareness of psychological dysfunction among health providers is limited. In a recent study of 912 health care professionals, only 40% reported routine screening for delirium, and only 16% reported using a specific tool to assess delirium. This practice occurred despite 68% of the interviewees thinking that delirium occurred in >25% of all ICU patients.[22]

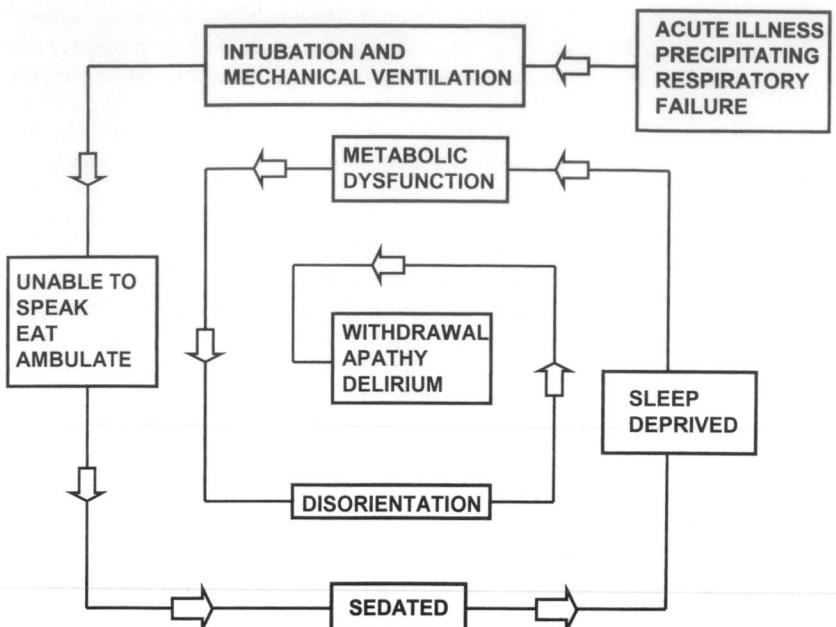

FIGURE 54-1 Cascade of factors contributing to psychological dysfunction in ventilated patients.

IMPACT ON COGNITIVE OUTCOMES AND SURVIVAL

Although technological and medical advances have markedly improved outcomes and survival of ICU patients, survivors frequently do not return to their prior baseline level of health and report an overall decreased quality of life.[23,24] The strong relationship between critical illness, mechanical ventilation, and cognitive outcomes is becoming increasingly clear.[25–28] Hopkins et al reported that all ARDS survivors exhibited cognitive and affective impairments at the time of discharge; after 1 year, 30% still displayed generalized impaired cognition.[29] Of 55 patients, 43 had impaired memory, concentration, and/or speed of mental processing.[29] Rothenhausler et al reported that 24% of ARDS survivors had cognitive defects at 6 years (median) following discharge.[30] These studies suggest that patients with critical illness and respiratory failure who require prolonged mechanical ventilation exhibit long-term neuropsychological impairment.

A relationship also appears to exist between neuropsychological disorders, particularly delirium, and greater morbidity and mortality in ICU patients. Delirium is associated with complications, such as self-extubation and removal of catheters,[17] and an increased hospital stay.[16] In a study of 224 ventilated patients, more than 80% developed delirium at

some point during their ICU stay.[7] Six-month mortality was higher in delirious patients than in nondelirious patients (34% versus 15%; $p = 0.03$); also, hospital stay was longer, with fewer ventilator-free days.[7] The cumulative dose of lorazepam was also higher in patients exhibiting delirium, an important factor that precipitates prolonged hospitalization, unwarranted neurological work-ups, and prolonged duration of ventilation, and may increase mortality.[10,32] Among 40 patients receiving prolonged ventilation in a ventilator rehabilitation unit, delirium was associated with increased mortality at 1 year ($p < 0.01$), and associated with greater likelihood of discharge to a nursing home or long-term-care institution.[18]

Forms of Psychological Disturbance

DELIRIUM

The most common psychiatric disorder in the ICU is delirium. Depressed mood and anxiety occur as discrete disorders, but frequently arise secondary to delirium. As underscored by Lipowski,[32] the many terms used to denote delirium impede communication, education, and research. Acute confusional state, encephalopathy, ICU psychosis, and ICU syndrome are all used to describe delirium; the terms inappropriately suggest that onset of delirium is solely related to the environment. Such attribution may harm patients, by inadvertently hindering the search for potentially reversible metabolic, pharmacologic, or organic causes.

CLINICAL FEATURES

Several clinical features help distinguish delirium from other mental disorders. Delirium generally develops over hours to days, with marked fluctuation of its clinical

TABLE 54-1 Forms of Psychological Dysfunction in the ICU Patient

- Anxiety
- Agitation
- Apathy
- Depression
- Posttraumatic stress disorder
- Delirium

features. Sometimes, the state of flux is extremely rapid. Delirious patients have disturbed consciousness, manifested by reduced clarity, sleepiness, and lethargy, and difficulty in focusing, sustaining, and shifting attention. Cognition, including memory, orientation, language, and executive function is also impaired.[33] Cognition defects frequently result in alterations in mood, behavior, and perception. In its early stages, delirium is frequently manifested as anxiety and restlessness. As the syndrome worsens, agitation may ensue, followed by visual and auditory hallucinations. The perceptual changes may interfere with a patient's understanding of treatment, the intentions of health care professionals, and ability to consent for procedures.[33]

Two subtypes of delirium have been recognized: hyperactive and hypoactive forms. The hyperactive form, also called agitated or hypervigilant delirium, is characterized by increased alertness, agitation, loud speech, restlessness, aggressiveness, hallucinations, and delusions. The hypoactive form is marked by apathy and lethargy.[34] The hypoactive form appears to be more common in elderly and severely ill patients[16,33] and may be mistaken for depression.[35] In a recent study of ventilated ICU patients, 94% of delirious patients were hypoactive and 6% were hyperactive.[7]

DIAGNOSIS

Inattentiveness and inability to provide a reliable history are clues to delirium. Psychiatrists use criteria from the *Diagnostic and Statistical Manual of Mental Disorders* of the American Psychiatric Association (DSM-IV).[36] The Confusion Assessment Method (CAM) is the most widely used and validated instrument used by others.[33] Ely et al[6] modified CAM for use in ventilated patients. Using a simple algorithm, CAM-ICU diagnoses delirium in the presence of acute changes in mental status and inattention, plus either disorganized thinking or altered consciousness (Table 54-2). Hart et al[38] developed the Cognitive Test for Delirium, specifically for ICU patients. This test is short, can be administered to intubated and immobilized patients, and differentiates delirium from dementia and other major psychiatric disorders. A commonly used test of cognition in the hospital is the 30-item Folstein Mini-Mental State Examination (MMSE).[39] Up to 42% of ICU patients, however, cannot reliably complete the MMSE; this instrument does not differentiate dementia from delirium.[37]

PREVALENCE AND INCIDENCE

Delirium appears to increase with severity of illness. Delirium is found in 14–24% of elderly patients in a general ward.[33] Dyer et al[2] reviewed 80 studies evaluating postoperative delirium and calculated an average incidence of 40%. Ely et al reported an 80% incidence of delirium in ventilated ICU patients, occurring after 2.7 ± 1.7 days and lasting 3.4 ± 1.9 days.

PREDISPOSING AND PRECIPITATING FACTORS

Age and severe critical illness are two key precipitants of delirium.[40] Other precipitating factors include brain injury, cognitive impairment, hypoalbuminemia, alcohol abuse, and depression.[2,32,40,41]

Age may be a marker for other factors because elderly patients have greater cognitive, sensory, and functional impairments; chronic illnesses; malnutrition; abnormal liver, renal, and metabolic function; and use more medications. Most cases of delirium are multifactorial. Francis et al[42] reported that patients with ≥3 risk factors had a 60% risk of delirium. In ventilated patients, Ely et al[16] found that use of benzodiazepines or narcotics were the most common risk factors for delirium (present in 98% of those with delirium). Other risk factors included rectal or bladder catheters (79%), visual or hearing impairment (69%), and central venous catheters.

Anticholinergic medications, opioids,[43] and benzodiazepines[42] are the drugs most often associated with delirium. Other drugs include corticosteroids, dopaminergic agonists, antibiotics, anticonvulsants, antiarrhythmic agents, digoxin, and histamine-2 antagonists.[32] Nicotine patches helped in resolving delirium in five critically ill heavy smokers.[44]

Metabolic factors, such as hypercalcemia, hyperglycemia, hypoglycemia, and thyroid disorders may cause

TABLE 54-2 Features, Description, and Assessment of Confusion

Feature	Description	Methods
Acute onset and fluctuating course	Is there evidence of an acute change in mental status based on family or nurse observations? Did it fluctuate during the day, come and go, or increase or decrease in severity?	Baseline assessment (MBDRS or IQCODE); information from nurses and family members; direct observation
Inattention	Did the patient have difficulty focusing attention, was easily distractible, or had difficulty keeping track of what was said?	Attention screening; examinations; picture recognition test; vigilance; a random letter test
Disorganized thinking	Was there disorganized thinking; incoherence; rambling, irrelevant conversation; unclear or illogical flow of ideas; or unpredictable switching of ideas?	Yes/no logic questions; simple commands; conversation if verbal
Altered level of consciousness	Was the level of consciousness other than alert and awake (i.e., vigilant, lethargic, stuporous, or comatose)?	Glasgow Coma Scale or Richmond Agitation-Sedation Scale

ABBREVIATIONS: IQCODE, Informant Questionnaire on Cognitive Decline in the Elderly; MBDRS, Modified Blessed Dementia Rating Scale.
SOURCE: Adapted, with permission, from Ely et al.[6]

confusion.[33] Dehydration, hypernatremia, and hyponatremia may also increase confusion.[2,40,42] Delirium frequently occurs in the context of infection. Diffuse neuropsychological deficits occur in toxic shock syndrome.[45] Up to 70% of patients with sepsis develop significant cognitive alterations.[46]

MANAGEMENT

The most important step in managing delirium is to identify and treat the causative factors. Its multifactorial nature in a ventilated patient[16,42] makes this a formidable task. The history should be reviewed for alcohol, opiate, and/or benzodiazepine dependence, considering overdose or withdrawal as possible causes. Patients should be evaluated for infection, electrolyte and metabolic abnormalities, and end-organ damage. Drugs that can induce delirium should be discontinued. General measures should be taken to reorient patients, provide safety, and aid them to effectively communicate concerns to the staff (*vide infra*).

In a prospective controlled study, Inouye et al[47] compared interventions aimed at reducing risk factors that cause delirium in 870 patients >70 years old. The intervention consisted of six standardized protocols for six risk factors (cognitive impairment, hearing impairment, visual impairment, dehydration, immobility, and sleep deprivation). The intervention group experienced less delirium (9.9% versus 15%; odds ratio 0.6), fewer days with delirium (105 versus 161; $p = 0.02$), and fewer delirium episodes (62 versus 90; $p = 0.03$).[47] Although these findings are important, it is difficult to extrapolate the results to the ICU setting where it is more difficult to control the environment. To date, multicomponent interventions to prevent delirium have not been studied in the ICU or in ventilated patients.

POSTTRAUMATIC STRESS DISORDER

Posttraumatic stress disorder (PTSD) is a complex, chronic and severe disorder with high rates of psychiatric comorbidity.[48] In patients admitted to the ICU with burns, the incidence varies between 8 and 45%.[49] Cuthbertson et al[26] prospectively studied the incidence and severity of PTSD in 111 ICU patients using the Davidson Trauma Scale. At 3 months after discharge, the overall score correlated with the duration of mechanical ventilation, but not with gender, ICU length of stay, or APACHE II score. Full diagnostic criteria for PTSD were fulfilled by 14% of patients. In a study of patients who had daily interruptions of sedative agents, instead of a continuous infusion, Kress et al demonstrated a trend towards a lower incidence of PTSD (0 versus 32%; $p = 0.06$);[50] these patients also displayed a trend towards fewer days of mechanical ventilation. Thus, length of mechanical ventilation, use of sedative agents, and the presence and severity of PTSD appear causally linked, and may influence duration of mechanical ventilation and psychological function after discharge.

DEPRESSION

In critically ill patients, depression presents with low mood, sadness, inability to experience pleasure, and changes in sleep, energy, and appetite. Diagnoses seen in medical patients include major depressive disorder, adjustment disorder, and depression secondary to medications or substances. Major depressive disorder is the most important to recognize because of its morbidity, need for specialized treatment, and impact of refusal of treatment. ICU patients may develop a depressed mood but often do not meet criteria for major depressive disorder because of transience of symptoms, or because somatic symptoms, such as poor appetite, weight loss, and sleep disturbances are attributed to the underlying disease.[51] Anxiety, discomfort, anger, and depression are counterproductive to weaning.[52] Little information, however, exists on the incidence and prevalence of depressive illness in ICU or ventilated patients. Prevalence of major depression in medical elderly patients is 10–14%.[53]

EPIDEMIOLOGY AND RISK FACTORS

Depressive disorders in elderly ICU patients is around 40%; the figure may be an overestimate because of inclusion of patients with adjustment disorders, depression secondary to medications or substances, and failure of authors to exclude delirious patients.[53] Ventilated patients experience several risk factors for depression, including disability and inability to pursue pleasant activities. Stressors, such as hospitalization, isolation, physical disabilities, mental disabilities, and having to face one's own death can result in adjustment disorders, and should be considered.

DIAGNOSIS AND TREATMENT

When evaluating depressed patients, the most important step is to exclude delirium. Mood symptoms in patients with delirium will improve with correction of the underlying disorder; addition of an antidepressant may worsen symptoms and cause agitation. Depression-rating instruments, such as the Geriatric Depression Scale, are useful for scoring the severity of the problem,[53] thereby elevating the priority for treating depression in a patient in light of other problems, or escalating treatment intensity. Treatment includes supportive measures, such as education about medical problems and procedures. Medical causes (hypothyroidism, metabolic derangements, and medications) should be excluded. Psychopharmacotherapy is used in more severe cases. Selective serotonin reuptake inhibitors have few adverse effects and are useful in the ICU setting. Glassman et al, in a double-blind trial, reported that sertraline was safe and more effective than placebo in patients admitted for myocardial infarction or angina.[54] Only a few studies have included psychological factors as independent variables affecting a patient's ability to wean: anxiety, fatigue, depression, and perception of dyspnea were linked to weaning success.[55,56] Methylphenidate, a stimulant with rapid effects on mood and few side effects, was found to be useful in difficult-to-wean patients.[57,58] Methylphenidate was used in seven patients receiving chronic ventilation (median 30 days) with clear evidence of severe depression (DSM-IV criteria). Five patients had a moderate to marked response in depressive symptoms, mood, activity, and respiratory symptoms within 4 days. These patients weaned in 8–14 days.[58] Although only case reports, the findings suggest that certain patients may benefit from aggressive treatment of depression, which may in turn increase the likelihood of weaning from prolonged ventilation.

ANXIETY

In the ICU, anxiety is commonly attributable to situational stressors. Clinical features include excessive fears or worries, cognitive changes such as hypervigilance, diaphoresis, palpitations, and motor abnormalities such as restlessness.[51]

Using a stressful-experiences questionnaire on discharge in 100 patients who received mechanical ventilation for >48 hours, Rotondi et al reported that pain from the endotracheal tube, intubation, and inability to communicate were major sources of significant distress.[59] Pochard et al[60] administered a questionnaire 48–96 hours postextubation to 54 patients who had been intubated and ventilated for a mean of 14 days. Almost 40% reported diffuse anxiety and 30% reported an intense fear of dying at least once during the ventilation period.[60] Twenty-five patients felt an inability to communicate, 18 were bothered by noise and 16 by light, and 9 felt abandoned by staff.[60] In a study using the Faces Anxiety Scale, some degree of anxiety was reported by nearly 85% of patients receiving mechanical ventilation.[61] As with other disorders, anxiety is diagnosed after careful exclusion of delirium.

AGITATION

Despite its frequency in the ICU, there is no clear, concise definition of agitation. Overall, agitated patients exhibit continual movement, and remain disoriented in several spheres, frequently exhibiting abnormal vital signs. A detailed discussion of the etiology of agitation is beyond the scope of this chapter; the reader is referred to Chapter 55.

Etiologies and Risk Factors

ETIOLOGIES OF PSYCHOLOGICAL DISTURBANCES

SEVERITY OF ILLNESS

Severity of underlying illness is closely associated with the onset of psychological disturbances (Table 54-3). Blachy et al[62] found that patients with American Heart Association class I heart failure had a 29% incidence of delirium, whereas the incidence was 100% in patients with class IV heart fail-

TABLE 54-3 Etiologies of Psychological Dysfunction in the Ventilator-Dependent Patient

- Severity of illness
- Sleep deprivation
- Sensory deprivation
- Medication side effects
- The process of mechanical ventilation

ure. Duration of cardiopulmonary bypass and complexity of the procedure increases the risk of perioperative delirium. An illness severe enough to necessitate admission to the ICU is among the most important predictors for the development of delirium.[40] Delirium also parallels disease severity and shock in predicting mortality among ventilated patients.[7,63] More frequent psychological disturbances in severely ill patients may be related to a greater incidence of precipitating factors in this group, such as hypoxemia, subclinical infection, and electrolyte and metabolic disturbances.

SLEEP DEPRIVATION

Both organic and environmental factors are implicated in the development of psychological problems in ICU patients. Frequent patient assessment and medical intervention, coupled with sophisticated hemodynamic and respiratory monitoring, create an environment that fosters sleep and sensory deprivation and an exposure to continuous monotonous sensory input.

Baker[64] and Kahn et al[65] suggested that noise levels below 35 A-weighted decibels [dB(A)] are needed for sleep to occur. Reported ICU noise levels, however, are between 45 and 85 dB(A), with the highest levels occurring between 12:00 PM and 6:00 PM.[65] A ventilator constantly generates between 60 and 65 dB(A). Aaron et al[66] measured sound peaks >80 dB(A) while continuously monitoring electroencephalogram tracings for 24–48 hours in 6 nonventilated ICU patients. The number of arousals were correlated with the number of sound peaks >80 dB(A).

Several polysomnographic studies have demonstrated sleep deprivation, sleep fragmentation, and altered sleep architecture[67–72] in the ICU setting. Environmental factors that affect sleep include noise related to monitor and ventilator alarms, and conversation among staff.[66,73–77] Repeated interruptions by nurses, physicians, and lab and x-ray technicians can lead to sleep deprivation.[75,76] Loss of the normal day-night and light-dark cycle, and the type of room also contribute to disturbed sleep.[76] In a study that monitored noise levels and patient arousals in an ICU setting (21 of 22 patients on mechanical ventilation), 12% of arousals and 17% of awakenings were solely caused by noise.[74] This study did not take into account other factors. Gabor et al noted that less than 30% of arousals and awakenings in ventilated patients were explained by noise and patient-care activities.[76] They suggested that patient-ventilator dyssynchrony, or mode-specific interactions, were responsible for at least some of the arousals. Ventilator-induced sleep disturbance is an important problem because about 40% of ICU patients receive mechanical ventilation.[78] Factors that may contribute to disordered sleep include discomfort caused by the endotracheal tube and suctioning, underlying illness, and mode of ventilation.[79,80] Meza et al demonstrated that normal individuals receiving pressure support develop central apneas when Pa_{CO_2} falls below the apnea threshold.[79] Parthasarathy et al evaluated the effect of pressure-support assist-control ventilation on sleep disordered breathing in 11 patients.[80] Six patients developed central apneas during pressure-support, but not during assist-control ventilation. Sleep fragmentation, the sum of arousals and awakenings,

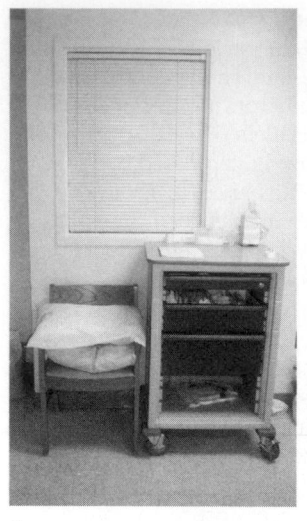 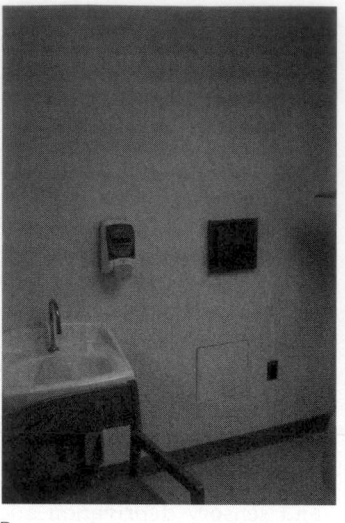 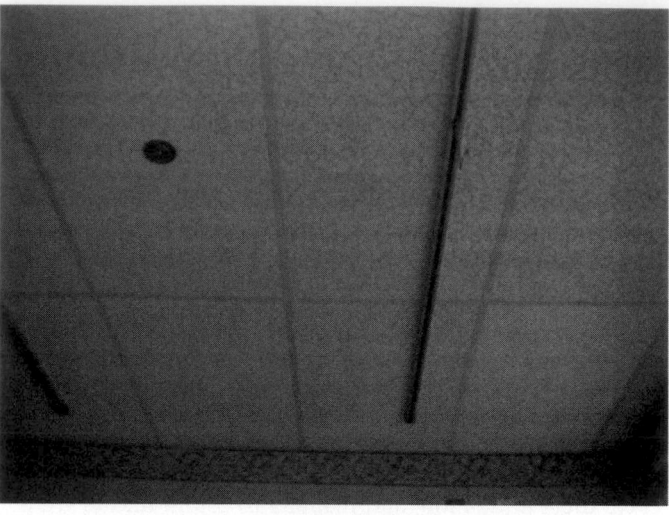

A   B   C

FIGURE 54-2 Sensory deprivation in the intensive care unit is fostered by the lack of windows with a view (*A*), and the monotony of the ceiling and empty walls (*B and C*).

was greater during pressure-support than during assist-control ventilation (79 versus 54; $p = 0.002$). Helton et al[81] found that 24% of ICU patients developed severe sleep deprivation (>50% sleep loss) and 16% moderate sleep deprivation (<50% sleep loss) during the first 5 days following admission. Severity of sleep deprivation was correlated with development of psychological abnormalities (delirium; 33% of severely and 10% of moderately sleep-deprived patients demonstrated mental status changes).

SENSORY DEPRIVATION

Sensory deprivation may foster psychological disturbances (Fig. 54-2). Wilson[5] compared the incidence of delirium in 50 surgical patients treated for 3 days or longer in an ICU without windows and in 50 patients treated in an ICU with windows (that faced outside). Although the groups were similar in age, type of surgery, and nursing care, the patients treated in the windowless ICU experienced two to three times more postoperative delirium. Wilson surmised that the absence of a window limited the ability of patients to orient themselves to time of day, and season, and fostered a sense of isolation and disconnection. In a study of 216 ICU patients, Dubois et al reported that windows protected against the development of delirium; their absence roughly doubled the risk for delirium.[17]

Davis et al[82] reported that uniform and meaningless stimuli may induce hallucinations and disordered thoughts. Apart from brief visiting hours and limited interactions with ICU staff, a patient's visual stimuli tend to be restricted. Acoustic stimulation is limited, largely consisting of the monotonous sounds of monitors, mechanical ventilators, feeding pumps, and oxygen outlets. Neher[83] reported that intermittent auditory stimulation may produce visual and auditory isolation in normal subjects. Sensory deprivation is aggravated by the patient's own visual and hearing impairments. Ely et al[16] found that visual and hearing impairment were present in almost 70% of patients devel-

oping delirium, constituting the third most common risk factor for delirium in these patients. Allowing patients to use their glasses and hearing aids may help prevent or ameliorate delirium in the ICU.

PHARMACOLOGIC AGENTS

Multiple drugs are associated with psychological disturbances. Particular drugs, however, such as sedative agents, have a greater association with delirium, and directly impact outcome in ventilated patients.[10,31,50]

Sedative agents, particularly benzodiazepines, are associated with delirium in postoperative patients[84] and elderly hospitalized patients.[42] High doses of benzodiazepines roughly tripled the risk of delirium in ICU patients, while low doses did not increase the risk.[17] Kress et al[10] studied the effects of daily interruption of sedative agents in ventilated patients. The control group received continuous sedation. The intervention group had a once-daily reduction in sedative agents, aiming for a patient capable of following simple commands. Ventilation was discontinued earlier in the intervention group, resulting in fewer ventilator days and total ICU days. The incidence of psychological disturbances was not reported, but fewer diagnostic tests to evaluate mental status were documented in the intervention group. In a follow-up study, Kress et al[50] found that patients subjected to daily interruptions of their sedative agents showed a better PTSD profile by three different tests. Six patients in the continuous sedation group had overt PTSD, but no cases occurred in the interruption group.

Medications with anticholinergic properties are frequently implicated in the development of delirium. Indeed, elevated serum anticholinergic activity has been reported during illness.[85]

Opioids are associated with delirium, particularly after surgery.[84] On univariate analysis, morphine at low and high doses was associated with a high risk of delirium; morphine was one of only five factors retained in the multivariate analysis (odds ratio 6–9.2).[17]

SPECIAL CONSIDERATIONS IN THE VENTILATOR-DEPENDENT PATIENT

In addition to the stresses facing critically ill patients, ventilated patients experience the additional stress of dependence on a machine. Riggio et al[86] studied perceptions of ventilated patients about sources of psychological stress, and found that inability to communicate, disorientation, memory loss, pain, and discomfort were all perceived as significant problems. Bergbom-Engberg et al[87] assessed retrospective recall of emotional reactions to mechanical ventilation after discharge. They found that 47% of patients felt anxious or fearful during their period of ventilation and 90% recalled the experience as stressful or unpleasant up to 4 years later. Ventilator support involves a loss of independence and control over the most vital voluntary life-sustaining activity: breathing. Patients are usually most concerned with fears of death and abandonment by family or staff, which may provoke symptoms of anxiety, depression, or overly dependent behavior.[9]

Adjustment to the ventilator and other apparatus is an important source of psychological stress. The inability to communicate secondary to intubation is reported by many patients as the predominant reason for perceived stress[87] and decreased sense of control[86] during mechanical ventilation. Patients' decreased ability to interact while ventilated has been characterized as communicator isolation.[88] Gale et al[88] pointed out that not only are patients unable to talk while intubated, but they also cannot sigh, gasp, sneeze, or produce other emotional expressions that are part of the usual respiratory vocabulary. The inability of ventilated patients to fully communicate their physical and emotional needs to others creates further isolation and feelings of abandonment by family and staff.[9]

Most patients have described suctioning as uncomfortable, and many compare suctioning to gagging[89] or suffocating.[90] The noise emitted by a ventilator is monotonous and unnatural, contributing to sensory overload and sleep disturbance.[88] Patients are usually limited in the distance they can move (i.e., by the typical 6 feet of ventilator tubing), which increases a sense of isolation from others.

Thus, the stresses facing ventilated patients are similar to those encountered by critically-ill patients, but include the added stress of dependency on a machine for life-sustaining ventilation, and the associated problems of immobility, isolation, and impaired communication.

Assessment of the Patient

GENERAL APPROACH

A comprehensive medical history and physical examination are critical in the initial assessment of the ventilated patient with psychological dysfunction. As previously stated, various medical and physiologic conditions, and medications can contribute.

PSYCHOLOGICAL ASSESSMENT

Psychosocial assessment includes questions about education, childhood learning and behavioral problems, marital discord, family support structure, work history, socioeconomic status, living arrangements, legal and military history, and drug and alcohol use. A history of previous psychological or psychiatric symptoms in the patient or family members should be solicited as well as an assessment of the patient's history of coping strategies for prior life stresses, illness, or death.

Assessment includes observation of a patient's interaction with family and treatment staff. Among the most sensitive indicators of anxiety and depression are somatic symptoms (e.g., decreased appetite, sleep disturbance, tiredness, or loss of libido), change in mood (e.g., sad, anxious, or nervous), decreased motivation, lack of independence to perform simple tasks, decreased self-esteem, and decreased cognition.

There should also be an assessment of whether the patient is experiencing frank psychiatric problems (hallucinations, illusions, or delusions) and an evaluation of their mental status and cognitive function using standard assessment tools. Specific areas include: orientation to person, place and time; capacity for sustained attention; immediate and delayed memory; and reasoning ability. Other skills that can be assessed include: visual skills, motor function, long-term memory, expressive language function, reading ability, and abstract and logical thinking skills.

In our center, a psychologist performs a complete assessment of neuropsychological function that complements the physician, nursing, physical therapist, and social work assessments. Integration of all evaluations is then used to develop a comprehensive and individualized treatment plan geared towards restoration of functional status and improvement of quality of life.

COGNITIVE ASSESSMENT IN THE VENTILATED PATIENT

The impact of delirium in ventilated patients cannot be overemphasized. Guidelines from the Society of Critical Care Medicine recommend screening for delirium in all ICU patients.[91] Key to the assessment is defining a baseline cognitive status and then recognizing the development of a new cognitive impairment or delirium.

Determining a baseline cognitive status is the first step (Fig. 54-3). Direct assessment of pre-existing cognitive function is often not possible and is performed with standardized proxy measures. The prevalence of pre-existing cognitive impairment was found to be 31–42%[92] in a study using previously validated proxy measures, the Blessed Dementia Rating Scale[93] and Informant Questionnaire on Cognitive Decline.[94]

The second step is to establish the level of consciousness. The Glasgow Coma Scale does not assess agitation, which is frequently present in delirium.[95] The Richmond Agitation-Sedation Scale assesses agitation and sedation,[96] and correlates with sedation, and bispectral electroencephalography.[97]

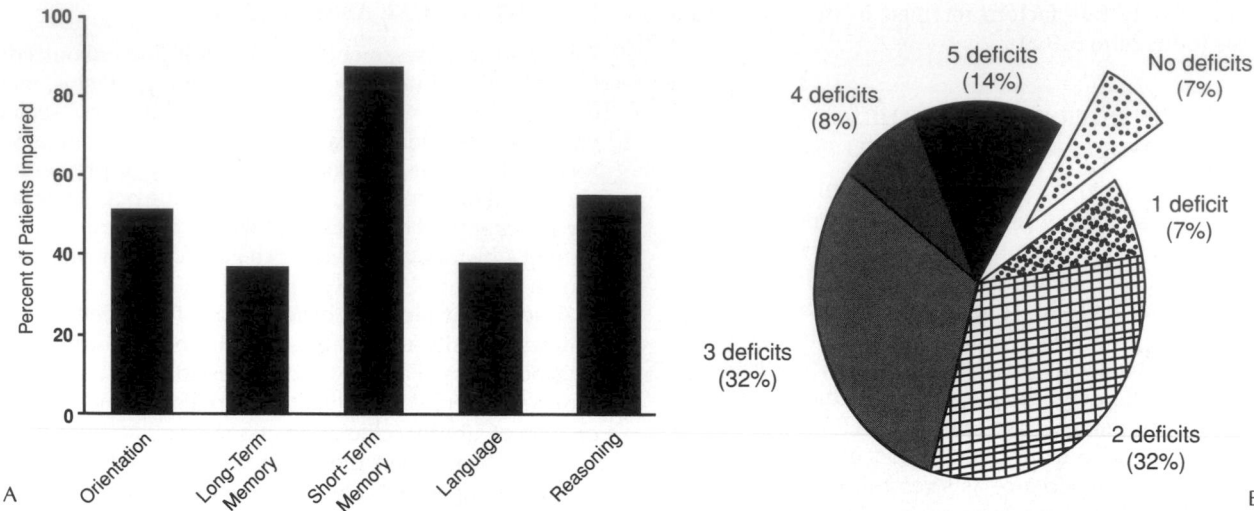

FIGURE 54-3 *A.* **Presence of cognitive defects in 28 patients receiving prolonged mechanical ventilation. Memory was the most frequently impaired function. Disorientation and impaired reasoning were observed in half of the patients.** *B.* **Only 7% of patients were normal when tested for cognitive function. Most patients showed multiple cognitive defects.**

The third step is formal cognitive assessment. The Cognitive Test for Delirium developed by Hart et al[38] and the CAM-ICU[6] have been validated in ventilated patients. The CAM-ICU uses four key features to detect delirium: acute change or fluctuation in mental status, inattention, disorganized thinking, and altered level of consciousness (see Table 54-2). Each feature is tested; a diagnosis of delirium is based on finding the first two features, and one of the other two features.

Treatment of Psychological Disturbances in Ventilated Patients

GENERAL MEASURES

The overall approach includes the basic tenets used for treating psychological problems in patients with chronic lung diseases and critical illnesses coupled with a treatment plan directed at special problems created by mechanical ventilation (Table 54-4). The physician and other caregivers must establish themselves as people the patient can trust and work with to achieve realistic and achievable goals. Factors contributing to an abnormal psychological state (the ICU

TABLE 54-4   Treatment of Psychological Dysfunction in the Ventilator-Dependent Patient

- Establish a relationship between caregivers and patients
- Create an environment that minimizes patient seclusion and enhances interaction with others
- Restore normal bodily function (speaking, eating, ambulating, breathing)
- Selectively use psychotropic medications
- Implement comprehensive multidisciplinary rehabilitation
- Teach biofeedback
- Decrease dyspnea

environment, limited mobility, and impaired communication) should be identified and systematically dealt with to improve the patient's sense of control and ability to interact appropriately with the medical staff.

THE ENVIRONMENT

One of the first steps is to minimize patient seclusion and enhance interaction with staff and family. Kornfeld[98] proposed: (1) placing patients in individual rooms; (2) minimizing nocturnal interventions to maximize uninterrupted sleep; (3) reducing monotonous sensory input by placing monitoring equipment outside of the room; (4) increasing patient mobility; (5) equipping patient rooms with orientation aids such as clocks, calendars, and family artifacts; and (6) making an outside window visible to each patient (Fig. 54-4).

COMMUNICATION

An important step is to enhance communication.[9] Improved communication between ventilated patients and families or staff decreases stress, improves decision making, and decreases the likelihood of patient isolation and withdrawal. Several different modalities (e.g., Passy-Muir valves, cuffless tracheostomy tubes, fenestrated tracheostomy tubes, electrolarynx, buccal resonators, "magic slates," and "talking-trachs") are available to facilitate verbal or written communication in ventilated patients (see Chapter 56).

PSYCHOTROPIC MEDICATIONS

In some patients, the selective use of psychotropic medications may be warranted in addition to behavioral techniques and supportive psychotherapy.[99] Short-acting anxiolytics (benzodiazepines) can be useful in treating extreme anxiety. Small doses of neuroleptic agents (butyrophenones

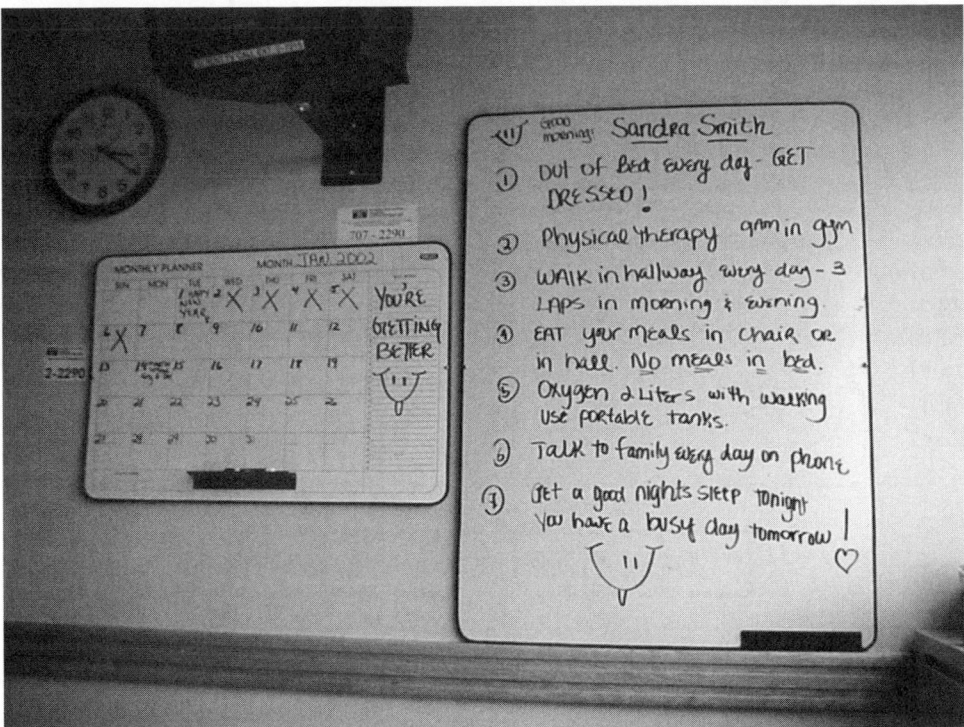

FIGURE 54-4 Orientation techniques in chronic ventilated patients should include a wall clock, calendar, and a bulletin board that provides details of daily goals.

such as haloperidol) help in controlling agitated or restless ventilated patients. Antidepressant agents are required in some patients with intractable fatigue and apathy.

COMPREHENSIVE MULTIDISCIPLINARY TREATMENT PLANS

Studies in patients with COPD[100] and those receiving chronic ventilation[101] reveal that involvement of patients and family in a comprehensive rehabilitation program can improve physical and psychological status. Programs include a multidisciplinary team of physical and occupational therapists, respiratory therapists, psychologists, nutritionists, speech therapists, social workers, nurses, and physicians (Fig. 54-5). These programs have been shown to reduce costs of care.[102] Noninvasive respiratory care units may also modify psychological problems by decreasing sensory and sleep deprivation as compared with an ICU environment.

We investigated the effect of a comprehensive multidisciplinary rehabilitation program in a noninvasive respiratory care unit on cognitive function and affective disorders in 25 patients and their families.[103] Patients and their families reported fewer affective disorders and less impaired cognition in the rehabilitation unit as compared to the ICU (Fig. 54-6). The reduction in cognitive problems probably resulted from specific strategies to minimize disorientation and compensate for memory disturbances. Patients in the unit were provided with clocks and calendars to maintain orientation, patients were encouraged to dress themselves and get out of bed, and bulletin boards were used to inform patients of the weaning schedule, rehabilitation exercises,

and to chart progress in learning home mechanical ventilation and respiratory care activities (see Fig. 54-4). Active ongoing psychological support may have enhanced weaning by minimizing emotional stress, and providing supportive counseling and encouragement. Total immobility is no longer a prerequisite for mechanical ventilation. Patients are mostly managed with portable ventilators that facilitate patient mobility and whole body reconditioning (Fig. 54-7). In selected patients, portable volume ventilators allow for successful home discharge.[104] These findings suggest that well-structured multidisciplinary noninvasive respiratory care units can benefit psychological function in ventilated patients and decrease cost of care.[102,106-107]

PSYCHOLOGICAL TREATMENTS TO FACILITATE WEANING

BIOFEEDBACK TRAINING
Biofeedback or relaxation techniques can reduce anxiety and dyspnea. Biofeedback encourages a patient to control a physiologic response (e.g., heart rate, respiratory rate, and blood pressure) through use of relaxation techniques and monitoring of visual or auditory signals to achieve targeted training goals.

Corson et al[108] used biofeedback in an uncontrolled fashion to wean two paralyzed ventilated patients by increasing tidal volume and reducing respiratory rate. Sessions were conducted for 40 minutes a day, 3 or 4 times a week, for 3 months. Patients were provided with visual feedback on an oscilloscope of tidal volume and respiratory rate, which provided targets during biofeedback sessions.

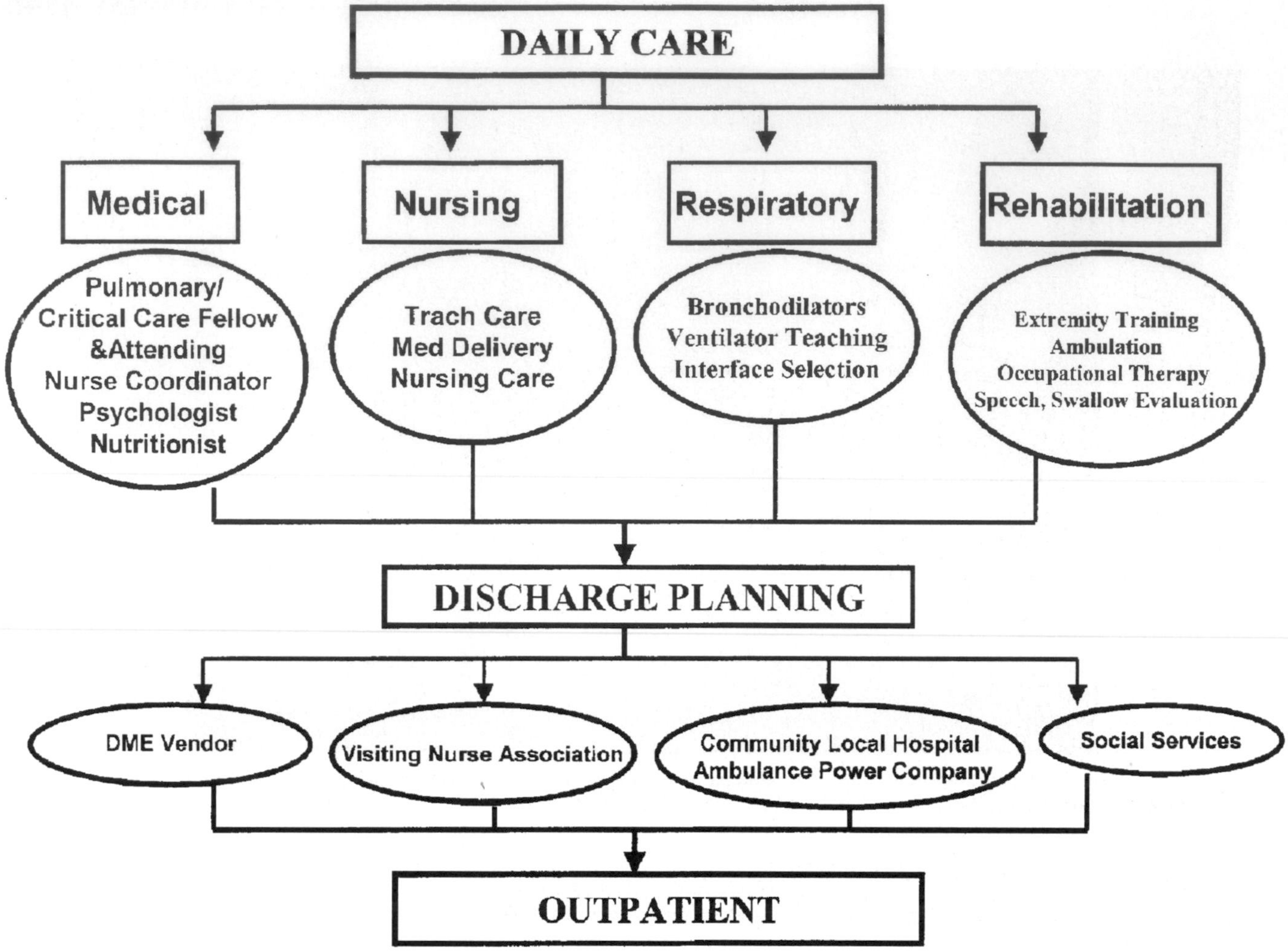

DAILY CARE
Medical
Nursing
Respiratory
Rehabilitation
Pulmonary/
Critical Care Fellow
&Attending
Nurse Coordinator
Psychologist
Nutritionist
Trach Care
Med Delivery
Nursing Care
Bronchodilators
Ventilator Teaching
Interface Selection
Extremity Training
Ambulation
Occupational Therapy
Speech, Swallow Evaluation
DISCHARGE PLANNING
DME Vendor
Visiting Nurse Association
Community Local Hospital
Ambulance Power Company
Social Services
OUTPATIENT

FIGURE 54-5 Organizational scheme of a multidisciplinary ventilator rehabilitation unit that combines delivery of ventilator care with a comprehensive rehabilitation program.

Patients
Families
Frequency
0
1
2
3
4
VSDU
ICU
Staff Attentiveness
Staff Availability
Affective Problems
Cognitive Impairment
Encouragement
Weaning

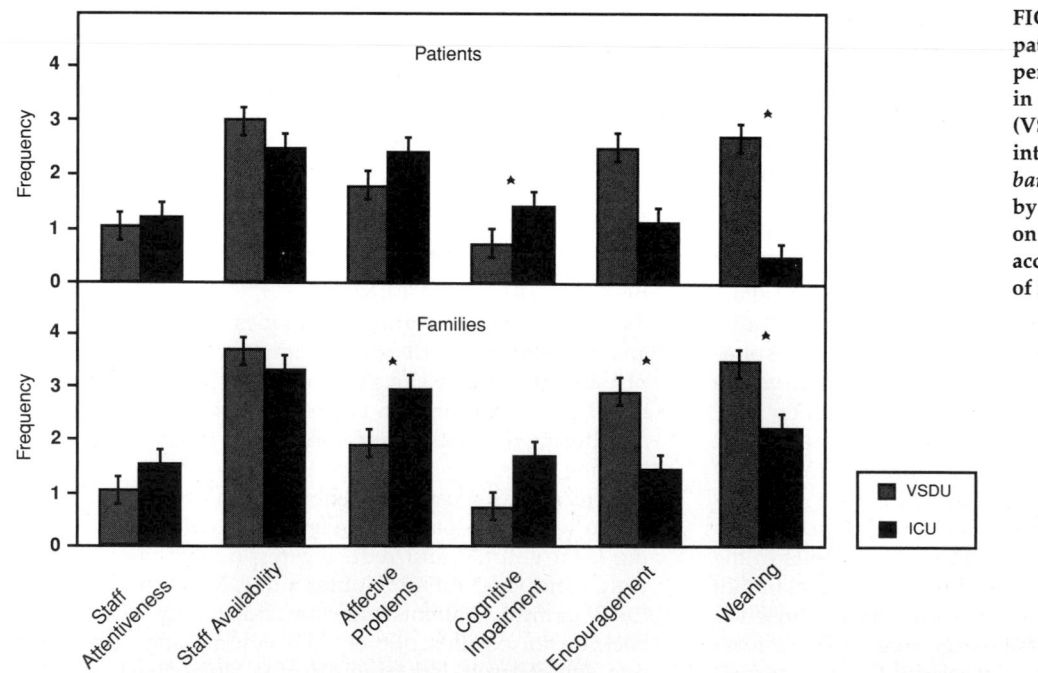

FIGURE 54-6 Mean ratings by patients and families for perceptions of overall experience in the ventilator rehabilitation unit (VSDU) (*shaded bars*) and an intensive care unit (ICU) (*black bars*) settings. Each item was rated by the patients or family members on five-point interval scales according to the perceived extent of frequency of each criterion.

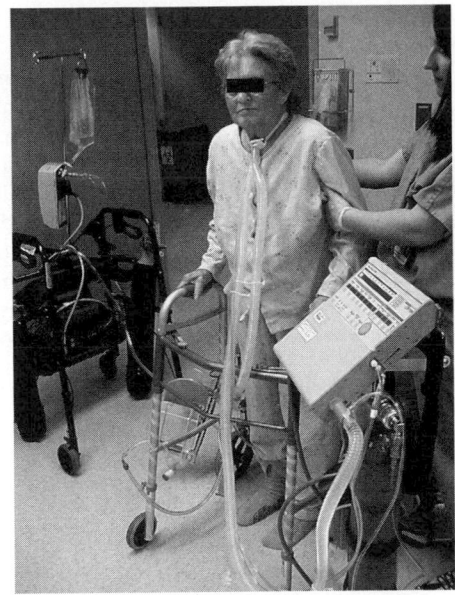
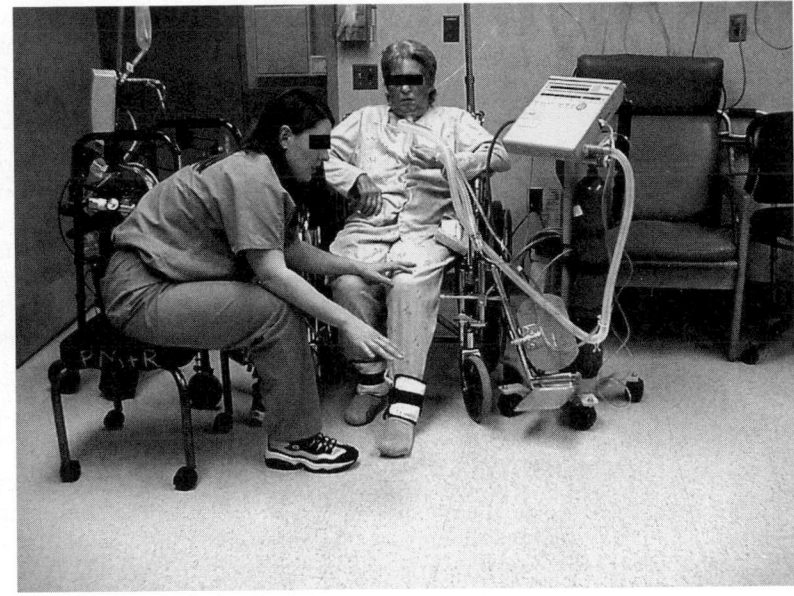

A

B

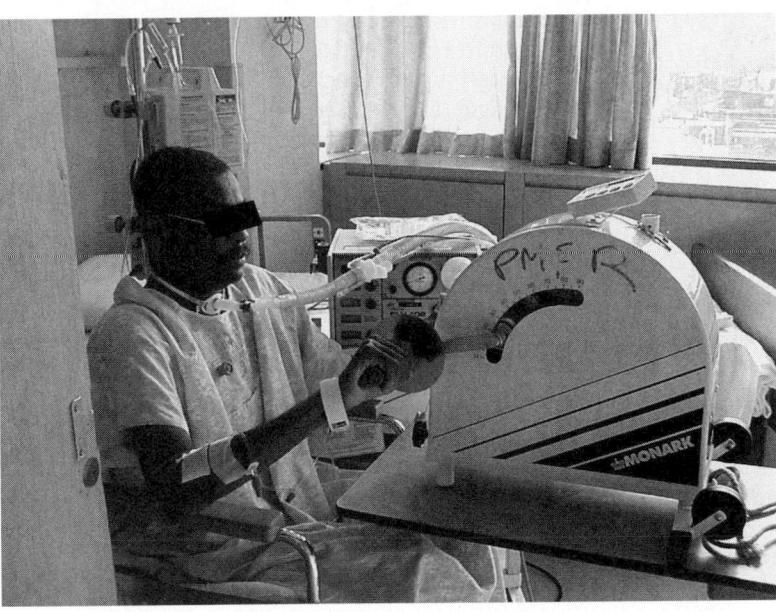

C

FIGURE 54-7 Mechanical ventilation via portable ventilators facilitates patient mobility and whole body reconditioning.

LaRiccia et al[109] used biofeedback from chest-wall movements, recorded by magnetometry, to wean a patient with multiple sclerosis who had failed several previous attempts.

In a prospective, randomized controlled study, Holliday et al[110] used biofeedback to improve weaning outcome in 40 patients ventilated for ≥7 days. Patients received visual and auditory feedback from rib-cage and abdominal movement; a display of frontalis muscle EMG activity was used to control anxiety through muscle relaxation (Fig. 54-8). The biofeedback group received 30–50 minute training sessions 5 days per week until extubation. The biofeedback group showed a reduction in ventilator days compared to the control group (20.6 ± 8.9 versus 32.6 ± 17.6 [SD] days) asso-

ciated with an increase in tidal volume (415 ± 45 versus 295 ± 41 ml), mean inspiratory flow (560 ± 66 versus 361 ± 40 ml/sec) and tidal volume-to-diaphragmatic EMG ratio (0.94 ± 0.21 versus 0.33 ± 0.09 L/mV). The latter was used as an index of respiratory muscle efficiency. Patients receiving biofeedback reported less anxiety, and they felt more relaxed during the biofeedback sessions. The requirement for special equipment and trained personnel limits the broad application of the methods reported by Holliday et al. Yarnal et al[111] used the numerical display of expired tidal volume and respiratory rate on the ventilator as visual feedback to successfully wean difficult patients. The true role of biofeedback and relaxation techniques awaits further study.

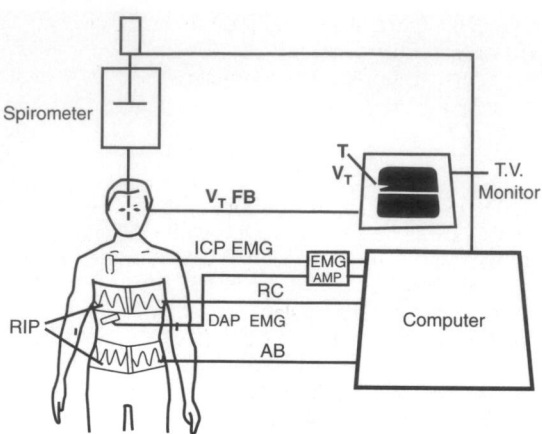

$$V_T = RC + AB$$

FIGURE 54-8 Schematic representation of apparatus used by Holliday et al to provide visual and auditory feedback to patients being weaned from mechanical ventilation. Respiratory inductive plethysmograph (RIP) bands were placed around the ribcage (*RC*) and abdomen (*AB*). Patients were given visual and auditory feedback (*FB*) from rib-cage and abdominal contributions to tidal volume (V_T) generation. A display of frontalis muscle EMG activity was used to control anxiety by muscle relaxation. EMG activity was recorded from the diaphragm (*DAP EMG*) and related to tidal volume (*VT/DAP*) as a measure of respiratory muscle efficacy. (*Reproduced, with permission, from Holliday et al.[110]*)

COLD FACIAL STIMULATION

Patients with extreme breathlessness often note relief when cool air is directed on the face by a fan or open window. Studies in animals[112–114] and man[115–117] have shown that application of airflow or cold solutions to the pharynx, nasal mucosa, or face can decrease total ventilation[112,113,115–117] or alter breathing patterns.[114] Schwarzenstein et al[118] found that cold air directed to the face produced a significant reduction in dyspnea in 16 healthy subjects who breathed against an inspiratory load. Other investigators[119] have confirmed this observation. Marchetti et al[120] showed that directing cold air to the face during exercise resulted in increased exercise time, decreased dyspnea, and decreased central respiratory drive in normal individuals and COPD patients.

MUSIC

In nonventilated patients, music was shown to decrease respiratory rate and heart rate more than 45 years ago, and these results have been replicated more recently.[121–122] Chlan[19] randomized 54 ventilated patients to music (n = 27) or to rest in a quiet, dark environment, each for 30 minutes. Patients had received 7 days of mechanical ventilation at enrollment, and 70% received intermittent mandatory ventilation during the trial. Patients exposed to music experienced a greater decrease in anxiety, respiratory rate, and heart rate.[19] Wong et al[20] reproduced these findings and also observed a decrease in blood pressure.

EFFECT OF PSYCHOTROPIC MEDICATIONS ON DYSPNEA

Dyspnea is frequent despite full ventilator support.[123–125] In 22 ventilated patients, dyspnea exhibited a moderate correlation with total mood disturbance scores, but did not predict weaning success.[123]

Acute administration of opiates can reduce dyspnea and increase exercise tolerance without affecting lung function.[126–131] Studies of aerosolized morphine have yielded inconsistent results.[132–136] Despite early anecdotal reports of anxiolytic therapy in dyspnea,[137] data are limited and inconclusive.[138,139] Although opiates can decrease dyspnea and increase exercise capacity, side effects of sedation and hypercapnia may limit their usefulness for weaning. At present, use of opiates for weaning cannot be routinely advocated (see Chapter 61).

Summary and Conclusions

Psychological disturbances are frequent in ventilated patients. Treatment plans should focus on identifying and reversing factors contributing to the patient's medical condition, need for mechanical ventilation, and psychological dysfunction. Integrating this treatment strategy with a comprehensive multidisciplinary rehabilitation program that focuses on restoring normal body functions (ambulation, eating, performance of daily hygiene chores, and spontaneous breathing) and social interaction (speaking and social interchange), has the best chance of reversing psychological problems that result from critical illness and the need for mechanical ventilation.

References

1. Cassileth BR, Lush FJ, Strouse TB, et al. Psychosocial status in chronic illness: comparative analysis of six diagnostic groups. N Engl J Med 1984; 311:506–11.
2. Dyer CB, Ashton CM, Teasdale CA. Postoperative delirium. A review of 80 primary data collection studies. Arch Intern Med 1995; 155:461–5.
3. Kornfeld DS, Zimbers S, Malm JR. Psychiatric complications of open heart surgery. N Engl J Med 1965; 273:287–92.
4. Egerton N, Kay JH. Psychological disturbances associated with open heart surgery. Br J Psych 1964; 110:433–439.
5. Wilson M. Intensive care delirium. Arch Intern Med 1972; 130:225–6.
6. Ely EW, Inouye SK, Bernard GR, et al. Delirium in mechanically ventilated patients: validity and reliability of the confusion assessment method for the intensive care unit (CAM-ICU). JAMA 2001; 286:2703–10.
7. Ely EW, Shintani A, Francis J, et al. Delirium as a predictor of mortality in mechanically ventilated patients in the intensive care unit. JAMA 2004; 291:1756–64.
8. Tobin MJ, Yang K. Weaning from mechanical ventilation. Crit Care Clin 1990; 6:725–47.
9. LaFond L, Horner J. Psychosocial issues related to long-term ventilatory support. Problems in Resp Care 1988; 1:241–56.
10. Kress JP, Pohlman AS, O'Connor MF, Hall JB. Daily interruption of sedative infusions in critically ill patients undergoing mechanical ventilation. N Engl J Med 2000; 342:1471–7.
11. De Jonghe B, Cook D, Appere-De-Vecchi C, Guyatt G, et al. Using and understanding sedation scoring systems: a systematic review. Intensive Care Med 2000; 26:275–85.
12. Sessler CN, Gosnell M, Grap MJ, et al. The Richmond agitation-sedation scale: validity and reliability in adult intensive care patients. Am J Respir Crit Care Med 2002; 166:1338–44.

13. Ely EW, Truman B, Shintani A, et al. Monitoring sedation status over time in ICU patients: the reliability and validity of the Richmond agitation sedation scale (RASS). JAMA 2003; 289:2983–91.

14. Dubin WR, Field HL, Gastfriend DR. Postcardiotomy delirium: a critical review. J Thorac Cardiovasc Surg 1979; 77:586–91.

15. Wilson VS. Identification of stressors related to patients' psychologic responses to the surgical intensive care unit. Heart Lung 1987; 16:267–73.

16. Ely EW, Gautam S, Margolin R, et al. The impact of delirium in the intensive care unit on hospital length of stay. Intensive Care Med 2001; 27:1892–900.

17. Dubois MJ, Bergeron N, Dumont M, et al. Delirium in an intensive care unit: a study of risk factors. Intensive Care Med 2001; 27:1297–1304.

18. Repetz N, Ciccolella DE, Criner GJ. Long-term outcome of patients with delirium on admission to a multidisciplinary ventilator rehabilitation unit (VRU). Am J Respir Crit Care Med 2001; 163:A889.

19. Chlan L. Effectiveness of a music therapy intervention on relaxation and anxiety for patients receiving ventilatory assistance. Heart Lung 1998; 27:169–76.

20. Wong H, Lopez-Nahas V, Molassiotis A. Effects of music therapy on anxiety in ventilator-dependent patients. Heart Lung 2001; 30:376–87.

21. Sessler CN, Rutherford L, Best A, et al. Agitation in a medical intensive care unit: prospective analysis of incidence and risk factors. Chest 1992; 102:191S.

22. Ely EW, Stephens RK, Jackson JC, et al. Current opinions regarding the importance, diagnosis, and management of delirium in the intensive care unit: A survey of 912 healthcare professionals. Crit Care Med 2004; 32:106–12.

23. Hurel D, Loirat P, Saulnier F, et al. Qualify of life 6 months after intensive care: Results of a prospective multicenter study using a generic health status scale and a satisfaction scale. Intensive Care Med 1997; 23:331–7.

24. Davidson TA, Caldwell ES, Curtis JR, et al. Reduced quality of life in survivors of acute respiratory distress syndrome compared with critically ill control patients. JAMA 1999; 281: 354–60.

25. Stoll C, Schelling G, Goetz AE, et al. Health-related quality of life and post-traumatic stress disorder in patients after cardiac surgery and intensive care treatment. J Thorac Cardiovasc Surg 2000; 120:505–12.

26. Cuthbertson BH, Hull A, Strachan M, et al. Post-traumatic stress disorder after critical illness requiring general intensive care. Intensive Care Med 2004; 30:450–55.

27. Jones C, Griffiths RD, Humphris G, et al. Memory, delusions, and the development of acute posttraumatic stress disorder–related symptoms after intensive care. Crit Care Med 2001; 29:573–7.

28. Scragg P, Jones A, Fauvel N. Psychological problems following ICU treatment. Anaesthesia 2001; 56:9–14.

29. Hopkins RO, Weaver LK, Pope D, et al. Neuropsychological sequelae and impaired health status in survivors of severe acute respiratory distress syndrome. Am J Respir Crit Care Med 1999; 160:50–6.

30. Rothenhausler HB, Ehrentraut S, Stoll C, et al. The relationship between cognitive performance and employment and health status in long-term survivors of the acute respiratory distress syndrome: Results of an exploratory study. Gen Hosp Psychiatry 2001; 23:90–6.

31. Kolleff MH, Levy MT, Ahrens TS, et al. The use of continuous IV sedation is associated with prolongation of mechanical ventilation. Chest 1998; 114:541–8.

32. Lipowski ZJ. Delirium: acute confusional states. New York: Oxford University Press, 1990.

33. Inouye SK. Delirium in hospitalized older patients. Clin Geriatr Med 1998; 14:745–64.

34. Liptzin B, Levkoff SE. An empirical study of delirium subtypes. Br J Psychiatry 1992; 161:843–5.

35. Farrell KR, Ganzini L. Misdiagnosing delirium as depression in medically ill elderly patients. Arch Intern Med 1995; 155: 2459–64.

36. American Psychiatric Association. Diagnostic and statistical manual of mental disorders: DSM-IV, 4th edition. Washington: American Psychiatric Association, 1994.

37. Inouye SK, van Dyck CH, Alessi CA, et al. Clarifying confusion: the confusion assessment method. A new method for detection of delirium. Ann Intern Med 1990; 113:941–8.

38. Hart RP, Levenson JL, Sessler CN, et al. Validation of a cognitive test for delirium in medical ICU patients. Psychosomatics 1996; 37:533–46.

39. Folstein MF, Folstein SE, McHugh PR. Mini-mental state. A practical method for grading the cognitive state of patients for the clinician. J Psychiatr Res 1975; 12:189–98.

40. Inouye SK, Viscoli CM, Horwitz RI, et al. A predictive model for delirium in hospitalized elderly medical patients based on admission characteristics. Ann Intern Med 1993; 119:474–81.

41. Ostermann ME, Keenan SP, Seiferling RA, Sibbald WJ. Sedation in the intensive care unit: a systematic review. JAMA 2000; 283:1451–9.

42. Francis J, Martin D, Kapoor WN. A prospective study of delirium in hospitalized elderly. JAMA 1990; 263:1097–101

43. Schor JD, Levkoff SE, Lipsitz LA, et al. Risk factors for delirium in the hospitalized elderly. JAMA 1992; 267:827–31.

44. Mayer SA, Chong JY, Ridgway E, et al. Delirium from nicotine withdrawal in neuro-ICU patients. Neurology 2001; 57: 551–3.

45. Rosene KA, Copass MK, Kastner LS, et al. Persistent neuropsychological sequelae of toxic shock. Ann Intern Med 2002; 96: 865–70.

46. Eidelman LA, Putterman D, Putterman C, et al. The spectrum of septic encephalopathy: Definitions, etiologies, and mortalities. JAMA 1996; 275:470–3.

47. Inouye SK, Bogardus ST, Charpentier PA, et al. A multicomponent intervention to prevent delirium in hospitalized older patients. N Engl J Med 1999; 340:669–76.

48. Kessler RC. Post-traumatic stress disorder: the burden to the individual and to society. J Clin Psychiatry 2000; 61:4–12.

49. Yu BH, Dimsdale JE. Posttraumatic stress disorder in patients with burn injuries. J Burn Care Rehabil 1999; 20:426–33.

50. Kress JP, Gehlbach B, Lacy M, et al. The long-term psychological effects of daily sedative interruption on critically ill patients. Am J Respir Crit Care Med 2003; 168:1457–61.

51. Misra S, Ganzini L. Delirium, depression, and anxiety. Crit Care Clin 2003; 19:771–87.

52. Burns SM, Clochesy JM, Hannemann SK, et al. Weaning from long-term ventilation. Am J Crit Care 1995; 4:4–22.

53. Koenig HG, Cohen HJ, Blazer DG, et al. Profile of depressive symptoms in young and older medical inpatients with major depression. J Am Geriatr Soc 1993; 41:1169–73.

54. Glassman AH, O'Connor CM, Califf RM, et al. Sertraline treatment of major depression in patients with acute MI or unstable angina. JAMA 2002; 288:701–9.

55. Higgins PA. Patient perception of fatigue while undergoing long-term mechanical ventilation: incidence and associated factors. Heart Lung 1998; 27:177–83.

56. Bouley GH, Froman R, Shah H. The experience of dyspnea during weaning. Heart Lung 1992; 21:471–6.

57. Johnson CJ, Auger WR, Fedullo PF. Methylphenidate in the "hard to wean" patient. J Psychosom Res 1995; 39:63–8.

58. Rothenhausler HB, Ehrentraut S, Degenfeld GV, et al. Treatment of depression with methylphenidate in patients difficult to wean from mechanical ventilation in the intensive care unit. J Clin Psychiatry 2000; 61:750–755.

59. Rotondi AJ, Chelluri L, Sirio C, et al. Patients' recollections of stressful experiences while receiving prolonged mechanical ventilation in an intensive care unit. Crit Care Med 2002; 30: 746–52.

60. Pochard F, Lanore JJ, Bellivier FF, et al. Subjective psychological status of severely ill patients discharged from mechanical ventilation. Clin Intensive Care 1995; 6:57–61.

61. McKinley S, Stein-Parbury J, Chehelnaby A, et al. Assessment of anxiety in intensive care patients by using the faces anxiety scale. Am J Crit Care 2004; 13:146–52.

62. Blachy PH, Starr A. Post-cardiotomy delirium. Am J Psychiatry 1964; 121:371–5.

63. Lin S-M, Liu C-Y, Wang C-H, et al. The impact of delirium on the survival of mechanically ventilated patients. Crit Care Med 2004; 32:2254–9.

64. Baker CF. Sensory overload and noise in the ICU: sources of environmental stress. Crit Care Q 1984; 6:66–80.

65. Kahn DM, Cook TE, Carlisle CC, et al. Identification and modification of environmental noise in an ICU setting. Chest 1998; 114:535–40.

66. Aaron JC, Carlisle M, Carskadon T, et al. Environmental noise as a cause of sleep disruption in an intermediate respiratory care unit. Sleep 2002; 19:707–10.

67. Aurell J, Elmquist D. Sleep in the surgical intensive care unit: continuous polygraphic recording in nine patients receiving postoperative care. BMJ 1985; 190:1029–32.

68. Broughton R, Baron R. Sleep patterns in the intensive care unit and on the ward after acute myocardial infarction. Electroencephalogr Clin Neurophysiol 1998; 45:348–60.

69. Buckle P, Pouliot Z, Millar T, Kerr P, Kryger M. Polysomnography in acutely ill intensive care unit patients. Chest 1992; 102:288–91.

70. Fontaine D. Measurement of nocturnal sleep patterns in trauma patients. Heart Lung 1989; 18:402–10.

71. Hilton B. Quantity and quality of patient's sleep and sleep disturbing factors in a respiratory intensive care unit. J Adv Nurs 1986; 1:453–68.

72. Richards K, Bairnsfather L. A description of night sleep patterns in the critical care unit. Heart Lung 1988; 17:35–42.

73. Bentley S, Murphy F, Dudley H. Perceived noise in surgical wards and an intensive care area: an objective analysis. Br Med J 1977; 2:1503–6.

74. Freedman NS, Gazendam J, Levan L, et al. Abnormal sleep/wake cycles and the effect of environmental noise on sleep disruption in the intensive care unit. Am J Respir Crit Care Med 2001; 163:451–7.

75. Freedman NS, Kotzer N, Schwab RJ. Patient perception of sleep quality and etiology of sleep disruption in the intensive care unit. Am J Respir Crit Care Med 1999; 159:1155–62.

76. Gabor JY, Cooper AB, Crombach SA, et al. Contribution of intensive care unit environment to sleep disruption in mechanically ventilated patients and healthy subjects. Am J Respir Crit Care Med 2003; 167:708–5.

77. Meyers TJ, Eveloff SE, Bauer MS, et al. Adverse environmental conditions in the respiratory and medical ICU settings. Chest 1994; 105:1211–6.

78. Esteban A, Anzueto A, Alia I, et al. How is mechanical ventilation employed in the intensive care unit? An international utilization review. Am J Respir Crit Care Med 2002; 161: 1450–8.

79. Meza S, Mendez M, Ostrowski M, Younes M. Susceptibility to periodic breathing with assisted ventilation during sleep in normal subjects. J Appl Physiol 1998; 85:1929–40.

80. Parthasarathy S, Tobin MJ. Effect of ventilator mode on sleep quality in critically ill patients. Am J Respir Crit Care Med 2002; 166:1423–9.

81. Helton MC, Gordon SH, Nunnery SL. The correlation between sleep deprivation and the intensive care unit syndrome. Heart Lung 1980; 9:464–8.

82. Davis JM, McCourt WF, Solomon P. The effect of visual stimulation of hallucinations and other mental experiences during sensory deprivation. Am J Psychiatry 1960; 116:889–92.

83. Neher A. Auditory driving observed with scalp electrodes in normal subjects. Electroencephalograph Clin Neurophysiol 1961; 13:449–51.

84. Marcantonio ER, Juarez G, Goldman L, et al. The relationship of postoperative delirium with psychoactive medications. JAMA 1994; 272:1518–22.

85. Flacker JM, Lipsitz LA. Serum anticholinergic activity changes with acute illness in elderly medical patients. J Gerontol Med Sci 1999; 54A:M12.

86. Riggio RE, Singer RD, Hartaran K, Sneider R. Psychological issues in the care of critically ill respirator patients: Differential perceptions of patient's relatives and staff. Psychol Rep 1982; 51:363–9.

87. Bergbom-Engberg I, Haljamae H. Assessment of patient's experience of discomforts during respirator therapy. Crit Care Med 1989; 17:1068–72.

88. Gale J, O'Shannick GJ. Psychiatric aspects of respirator treatment and pulmonary intensive care. Adv Psychosom Med 1985; 14:93–108.

89. Heaton RK, Grant I, McSweeny AJ, Adams KM, Petty TL. Psychologic effects of continuous and nocturnal oxygen therapy in hypoxemic chronic obstructive pulmonary disease. Arch Intern Med 1983; 143:1941–7.

90. Isaac L, Hungerpillar J, Criner G. Neuropsychologic deficits in chronic ventilator-dependent patients. Chest 1989; 96:255S.

91. Jacobi J, Fraser GL, Coursin DB, et al. Clinical practice guidelines for the sustained use of sedatives and analgesics in the critically ill adult. Crit Care Med 2002; 30:119–41.

92. Pisani M, Inouye SK, McNicoll L, et al. Screening for pre-existing cognitive impairment in older intensive care unit. Journal of the American Geriatrics Society 2003; 51:591–8.

93. Blessed G, Tomlinson BE, Roth M. The association of between quantitative measures of dementia and of senile change in the cerebral gray matter of elderly subjects. Br J Psychiatry 1968; 114:797–811.

94. Jorm AF. A short form of the Informant Questionnaire on Cognitive Decline in the Elderly (IQCODE): development and cross-validation. Psychol Med 1994; 24:145–53.

95. Teasdale G, Jennet B. Assessment of coma and impaired consciousness: A practical scale. Lancet 1974; 2:81–4.

96. Sessler CN, Gosnell MS, Grap MJ, et al. The Richmond Agitation-Sedation Scale: validity and reliability in adult intensive care unit patients. Am J Respir Crit Care 2002; 166:1338–44.

97. Ely EW, Truman B, Shintani A, et al. Monitoring sedation status of time in ICU patients. Reliability and validity of the Richmond agitation-sedation scale (RASS). JAMA 2003; 289:2983–9.

98. Kornfeld DS. Psychiatric view of the intensive care unit. Br Med J 1969; 1:108–10.

99. Sandhu HS. Psychosocial issues in chronic obstructive pulmonary disease. Clin Chest Med 1986; 7:629–42.

100. Fishman DB, Petty TL. Physical, symptomatic and psychological improvement in patients receiving comprehensive care for chronic airway obstruction. J Chronic Dis 1971; 24: 775–85.

101. Make B, Gilmartin M. Rehabilitation and home care for ventilator assisted individuals. Clin Chest Med 1986; 7:679–91.

102. Elpern EM, Silver MR, Rosen RL, Bone RC. The noninvasive respiratory care unit. Patterns of use and financial implications. Chest 1991; 99:205–8.

103. Isaac L, Criner G. Patient and family perceptions on weaning

from mechanical ventilation in a specialized rehabilitation unit. Am Rev Resp Dis 1990; 141:A411.

104. Make BJ, Gilmartin M. Mechanical ventilation in the home. Crit Care Clinics 1990; 693:785–96.

105. O'Donohue WJ. Chronic ventilator-dependent units in hospitals: Attacking the front end of a long term problem. Mayo Clin Proc 1992; 67:198–200.

106. Gracey DR, Viggiano RW, Nawssens JM, et al. Outcomes of patients admitted to a chronic ventilator-dependent unit in an acute care hospital. Mayo Clin Proc 1992; 67:131–6.

107. Kreiger BP, Ershowsky P, Spivack D, Thorstenson J, Sackner MA. Initial experience with a central respiratory monitoring unit as a cost-saving alternative to the intensive care unit for Medicare patients who require long-term ventilator support. Chest 1988; 93:395–7.

108. Corson JA, Grant JL, Moulton DP, Green RL, Dunkel PT. Use of biofeedback in weaning paralyzed patients from respirators. Chest 1979; 76:543–5.

109. LaRiccia PJ, Katz RH, Peters JW, Atkinson GW, Weiss T. Biofeedback and hypnosis in weaning from mechanical ventilators. Chest 1985; 87:267–9.

110. Holliday JE, Hyers TM. The reduction of weaning time from mechanical ventilation using tidal volume and relaxation biofeedback. Am Rev Respir Dis 1990; 141:1214–20.

111. Yarnal J, Herrell D, Sivak E. Routine use of biofeedback in weaning patients from mechanical ventilation. Chest 1981; 79:127–8.

112. Sant'Ambrogio G, Mathew OP, Sant'Ambrogio FB, Fisher JT. Laryngeal cold receptors. Respir Physiol 1985; 59:35–44.

113. Mortola JP, Al-Shway S, Noworaj A. Importance of upper airway airflow in the ventilatory depression of laryngeal origin. Pediatr Res 1983; 17:550–2.

114. Sessle BJ, Greenwood LF, Lund JP, Lucier GE. Effects of upper respiratory tract stimuli on respiration and single respiratory neurons in the adult cat. Exp Neurol 1978; 61:245–59.

115. McBride B, Whitelaw WA. A physiological stimulus to upper airway receptors in humans. J Appl Physiol 1981; 51:1189–97.

116. Burgess KR, Whitelaw WA. Reducing ventilatory response to carbon dioxide by breathing cold air. Am Rev Respir Dis 1984; 129:687–90.

117. Folgering H, Olivier O. The diving response depresses ventilation in man. Bull Eur Physiolpathol Respir 1985; 21:143–7.

118. Schwartzstein RM, Lahive K, Pope A, Weinberger SE, Weiss JW. Cold facial stimulation reduces breathlessness induced in normal subjects. Am Rev Respir Dis 1987; 136:58–61.

119. Freedman S. Cold facial stimulation reduces breathlessness induced in normal subjects. Am Rev Respir Dis 1988; 137:492–3.

120. Marchetti N, Travaline JM, Criner GJ. Air current applied to the face of COPD patients enhances leg ergometry performance. Am J Resp Crit Care Med 2004; 169:A773.

121. Ellis DS, Bringhouse G. Effects of music on respiration and heart rate. Am J Psychol 1952; 65:39.

122. Bolwerk CA. Effects of relaxing music on state of anxiety in myocardial infarction patients. Crit Care Nurs Q 1990; 13:63–72.

123. Connelly B, Gunzerath L, Knebel A. A pilot study exploring mood state and dyspnea in mechanically ventilated patients. Heart Lung 2000; 29:173–9.

124. Nelson JE, Meier DE, Oei EJ, et al. Self-reported symptom experience of critically ill cancer patients receiving intensive care. Crit Care Med 2001; 29:277–82.

125. Knebel A, Janson-Bjerklie S, Malley JD, et al. Comparison of breathing comfort during weaning with two ventilatory modes. Am J Respir Crit Care Med 1994; 149:14–8.

126. Woodcock AA, Gross ER, Gellert A, et al. Effects of dihydrocodeine, alcohol, and caffeine on breathlessness and exercise tolerance in patients with chronic obstructive lung disease and normal blood gases. N Engl J Med 1981; 305:1611–6.

127. Light RW, Muro JR, Sato RI, et al. Effects of oral morphine on breathlessness and exercise tolerance in patients with chronic obstructive pulmonary disease. Am Rev Respir Dis 1989; 139:126–33.

128. Light RW, Stansbury DW, Webster JS. Effect of 30 mg of morphine alone or with promethazine or prochlorperazine on the exercise capacity of patients with COPD. Chest 1996; 109:975–81.

129. Santiago TV, Johnson J, Riley DJ, Edelman NH. Effects of morphine on ventilatory response to exercise. J Appl Physiol: Respir Environ Exercise Physiol 1979; 47:112–8.

130. Weil JV, McCullough RF, Kline JS, Sodal IE. Diminished ventilatory response to hypoxia and hypercapnia after morphine in normal man. N Engl J Med 1975; 292:1103–6.

131. Jennings AL, Davies AN, Higgins JP, Gibbs JS, Broadley KE. A systematic review of the use of opioids in the management of dyspnoea. Thorax 2002; 57:922–3.

132. Harris-Eze AO, Sridar G, Clemens RE, et al. Low-dose nebulized morphine does not improve exercise in interstitial lung disease. Am J Respir Crit Care Med 1995; 152:1940–5.

133. Masood AR, Reed JW, Thomas SHL. Lack of effect of inhaled morphine on exercise-induced breathlessness in chronic obstructive pulmonary disease. Thorax 1995; 50:629–34.

134. Masood AR, Subhan MMF, Reed JW, et al. Effects of inhaled nebulized morphine on ventilation and breathlessness during exercise in healthy man. Clin Sci 1995; 88:447–52.

135. Young IH, Daviskas E, Keena VA. Effect of low dose nebulized morphine on exercise endurance in patients with chronic lung disease. Thorax 1989; 44:387–90.

136. Zeppetella G. Nebulized morphine in the palliation of dyspnea. Palliat Med 1997; 11:267–75.

137. Mitchell-Heggs P, Murphy K, Minty K, et al. Diazepam in the treatment of dyspnoea in the "pink puffer" syndrome. Q J Med 1980; 49:9–20.

138. Man GCW, Hsu K, Sproule BJ. Effect of alprazolam on exercise and dyspnea in patients with chronic obstructive pulmonary disease. Chest 1986; 90:832–836.

139. Argyropoulou P, Patakas D, Koukou A, et al. Buspirone effect on breathlessness and exercise performance in patients with chronic obstructive pulmonary disease. Respiration 1993; 60:216–20.

ADDRESSING RESPIRATORY DISCOMFORT IN THE VENTILATED PATIENT

ROBERT B. BANZETT
ROBERT BROWN

Although respiratory discomfort (dyspnea) is as common as pain in hospitalized patients,[1] there is no formal requirement to assess and manage it, such as the "fifth vital sign" requirement for pain assessment and management. Ventilated patients do experience respiratory discomfort, they can report and quantify it, and there are strategies to address it. In this chapter we (1) propose that respiratory discomfort be routinely assessed in ventilated patients, and (2) suggest some approaches to managing this discomfort with minimal sedation. Together, these could be termed "patient-centered ventilation."[2] Although there is evidence to support both the need for and the potential of this approach, there is a paucity of studies directly addressing prevalence, outcomes, and mechanisms of dyspnea and its relief in acutely ventilated patients.

Occurrence and Sequelae of Respiratory Discomfort in Ventilated Patients

Although we lack large scale studies on the prevalence of dyspnea in mechanical ventilation, there have been a few studies in which a small sample of acutely ventilated patients have been asked to rate dyspnea.[3-6] Estimates of the prevalence of dyspnea range from 11-50%, with a significant number of patients reporting moderate to severe discomfort. Many patients, however, were too heavily sedated to respond; some of these latter patients had probably been sedated to alleviate respiratory discomfort. Dyspnea is frequently assessed indirectly from physical signs (see assessment section, below). For instance, dyssynchrony between patient and ventilator is very common (see Chapter 6), and it is widely thought (though seldom explicitly stated) that dyssynchrony indicates dyspnea.

There is a clear association between anxiety and dyspnea in patients.[7-9] Emotional reactions such as panic, anxiety, and fear in critically ill patients are significantly correlated with patient-ventilator dyssynchrony.[10] Dyspnea can cause anxiety, even in healthy subjects who experience dyspnea in a safe laboratory situation.[11,12] On the other hand, anxiety can cause dyspnea even in the absence of cardiopulmonary pathology; for example, dyspnea is the most common symptom in anxiety and panic disorders.[13] Because of this reciprocal causation, the possibility of positive feedback exists in ventilated patients, with dyspnea causing anxiety, which then exacerbates the dyspnea. Posttraumatic stress disorder (PTSD) is now recognized as a common sequela of the intensive care unit (ICU) experience.[14-16] PTSD symptom scores in the post-ICU population are significantly correlated with duration of mechanical ventilation,[15] and with recalled memories of respiratory distress.[14] A number of reasons for these connections can be postulated, but the possibility cannot be ignored that inescapable dyspnea is one of the traumatizing events leading to PTSD in this population.

Assessment of Discomfort in the Ventilated Patient

ASK THE PATIENT

The first step in addressing dyspnea is to determine how much and what kind of discomfort the patient is experiencing. A full assessment requires that the patient be alert enough to respond to simple direct questions regarding the intensity and quality of discomfort. In heavily sedated patients, the daily wake-up practiced in many ICUs[17] provides an opportunity to assess the intensity of dyspnea and attempt to reduce it with nonpharmacologic approaches before evaluating the need for further sedation.

Several rating methods have been shown to be feasible in intubated and ventilated patients. Patients who are alert enough to respond but who cannot speak can provide

TABLE 55-1 Sample Patient Assessment Questionnaire

Please indicate on this 10 point scale how your breathing feels:
10 EXTREMELY SHORT OF BREATH
9
8
7
6
5
4
3
2
1
0 BREATHING IS COMFORTABLE

Which of the following phrases describes the way you feel?
1. Not getting enough air (if yes, ask a and b and skip 2; if no, ask 2)
   a. Breaths are not deep enough
   b. Breaths are not fast enough
2. Getting too much air (if yes, ask a and b)
   a. Breaths are too deep
   b. Breaths are too fast
3. Too much effort to breathe
4. Chest feels tight or constricted

---

information through simple number, word, or visual analog scales, similar to those routinely used in clinical pain assessment.[5,6,18] Patients can point to the appropriate responses but in some cases the interviewer will need to say or point to responses in succession and stop when the patient indicates with a blink or other sign. The intensity scale may be combined ad hoc with a list of descriptors from which the subject can choose; descriptor lists often make the process easier for patients who find it difficult to describe unfamiliar internal sensations.[19] A brief sample assessment procedure is shown in Table 55-1. More extensive and sophisticated assessment may be required for research purposes.[20]

PHYSICAL SIGNS MAY CORRELATE POORLY WITH DISCOMFORT LEVEL

Many caregivers rely on physical signs such as respiratory rate, heart rate, use of accessory muscles, synchrony with mechanical ventilation, diaphoresis, and facial expression. These signs can be very useful when patients are unable to communicate, but they can be misleading.[5] Patients vary widely in their behavioral responses to discomfort; thus, as with pain, physical signs may either overestimate or underestimate the degree of discomfort, and they give little information regarding its cause. Reliance on inconsistent physical signs was also a problem in pain assessment until accrediting organizations, such as JCAHO, began to require more direct assessment and management of pain.[21]

DISCOMFORT CAN BE CAUSED BY DYSPNEA COMBINED WITH OTHER SENSATIONS

A particular patient's discomfort may be caused by a mix of respiratory discomfort and nonrespiratory sensations such as pain and nausea. The limited data available suggest that simultaneous dyspnea and pain can be separately scaled, and that the presence of one does not strongly affect the

other, at least under controlled circumstances.[22] Sensations of respiratory discomfort other than dyspnea (e.g., due to cough or irritation from the endotracheal tube) may also be present. Different forms of dyspnea such as air hunger and excessive work of breathing may be simultaneously present (see below). The problems of ventilator patients are therefore varied and complex; there is no single approach that will work in all patients. Information from the patient may be useful in guiding interventions.

Primer on Dyspnea

DIFFERENT FORMS OF DYSPNEA

Several different mechanisms give rise to respiratory discomfort; the mechanism(s) operating in an individual patient will guide the treatment approach selected. The quality of discomfort is one guide to understanding which mechanisms are in play; other clues come from physical examination and measurement of ventilatory variables (see the section below on approach). There are at least three distinct qualities of uncomfortable breathing sensations: *air hunger*, *effort* or *work*, and *tightness*. These different forms of dyspnea are caused by different afferent mechanisms and are evoked by different physiologic stimuli.

Theories developed in the late 1960s and early 1970s attributed all dyspnea to excessive work or effort of breathing.[23] Although work of breathing has since been disproved as the sole origin of dyspnea,[24-26] this model still dominates thinking in the realm of clinical mechanical ventilation.[27,28] Attempts to understand a patient's discomfort based only on work of breathing will not be fully effective; in fact, extremely unpleasant dyspnea can be evoked in the absence of any respiratory work.

AIR HUNGER

Air hunger is the conscious perception of the need for more air that is typically described by subjects as "not getting enough air," "uncomfortable urge to breathe." This is the sensation felt by normal subjects at the end of a long breath hold.[12,25] Subjects comment that air hunger is a threatening or frightening sensation. Healthy subjects exposed briefly to air hunger in our laboratory have reported that "it's a feeling ... you're going to die because you're not getting enough air." Even moderate air hunger is highly aversive if prolonged, with one subject commenting that "if I felt I had to live my life feeling like that I would jump out the window [commit suicide]." Quotes from patients with dyspnea can be remarkably similar: "When the shortness of breath was at its extreme I thought I was going to die," and "... wouldn't want to live if it continued."[29]

Air hunger arises from stimulation of arterial chemoreceptors and from other drives to breathe; a rise in Pa_{CO_2} or a fall in Pa_{O_2} will evoke air hunger.[24,30-33] Air hunger is not related to contraction of respiratory muscles; complete respiratory paralysis does not abolish or even diminish the air hunger response to CO_2.[24-26] It is hypothesized that air hunger is transmitted to the cerebral cortex by a corollary discharge of medullary respiratory center activity (also known as *ventilatory drive*). Such a corollary discharge has been described in the midbrain and thalamus of decorticate cats, presumably en route to the cortex.[34-36] Although air hunger is stimulated by medullary drive, the two are not equivalent; other processes modify the translation of drive into the perception of air hunger in the cerebral cortex. Air hunger is associated with activation of the paralimbic cortex in humans, in areas associated with several other unpleasant sensations, such as pain, thirst, and hunger.[37,38] Air hunger also activates the amygdala, which is implicated in the perception of fear.

EFFECT OF BLOOD GASES ON AIR HUNGER

There is a substantial amount of information on the interaction of blood gas levels, level of minute ventilation, and air hunger during mechanical ventilation in normal subjects and in patients who are ventilator-dependent secondary to neuromuscular paralysis. In a typical study of 16 healthy subjects ventilated at 10 L/min, which acutely raised end-tidal carbon dioxide tension (PET_{CO_2}) by 10 torr, this produced a level of respiratory discomfort that subjects could not tolerate even for a few minutes[12] (Fig. 55-1). This occurred despite a background of high oxygen and with minute ventilation ($\dot{V}_E$) >150% of the normal resting level. In practical terms, this implies that modest acute increases in P_{CO_2} that may seem clinically unimportant, can be a source of profound discomfort.

An acute rise in Pa_{CO_2} evokes severely uncomfortable air hunger during volume-control ventilation in both healthy subjects and in alert patients ventilated for respiratory muscle paralysis.[18,25,26] Partial neuromuscular block in spontaneously breathing healthy subjects increases sensations of air hunger and work/effort, even at PET_{CO_2} and $\dot{V}_E$ levels similar to those present before the block.[39,40] This may

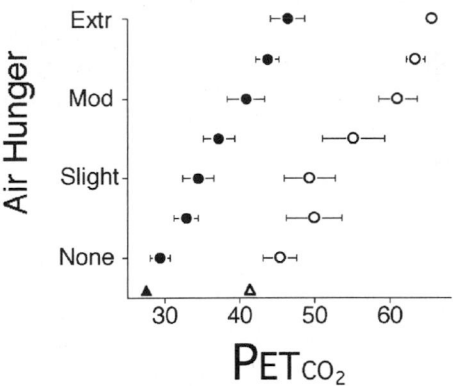

FIGURE 55-2 Adaptation of air-hunger response to prevailing chronic level of PET_{CO_2} (*triangles*) in four ventilator-dependent patients. Response to acute hypercapnia (*circles*) is shown at baseline chronic level of PET_{CO_2} (*filled symbols*; mean of 27 torr in these chronically overventilated patients), and after adaptation for several days to a mean PET_{CO_2} of 41 torr (*open symbols*). The increase in chronic P_{CO_2} was effected by adding inspired CO_2 at the same $\dot{V}_E$. (*Data re-plotted from Bloch-Salisbury et al.[18]*)

explain why dyspnea occurs in patients with profound neuromuscular weakness.

How do responses to chronically altered blood gases compare to the acute stimulus-response relationships for air hunger detailed above (which were obtained in exposures of 10 minutes or less)? Common clinical experience leads to the hypothesis that there is adaptation to chronic changes in blood gases; for instance, the common observation that some patients with COPD do not report dyspnea at resting P_{CO_2} in excess of 50 torr, a level that is intolerable to normal subjects at comparable ventilation levels. A direct test of the hypothesis was obtained in mechanically ventilated patients who adapted to a slow 15-torr rise in Pa_{CO_2} produced by raising inspired P_{CO_2} while holding ventilation and Pa_{O_2} constant.[18] The air-hunger response to acute hypercapnia was tested before and after the adaptation period. Within 2-3 days, the acute response to hypercapnia had also shifted by 15 torr, essentially complete adaptation (Fig. 55-2). The authors attributed this shift to neural adaptation, rather than acid-base compensation; thus it may apply to other stimuli such as hypoxia.

Subjects report little or no difference between the quality of air hunger evoked by hypoxia versus that evoked by hypercapnia. If P_{CO_2} and ventilation are near normal, pronounced hypoxia is required to evoke air hunger; in healthy subjects an arterial P_{O_2} of 40-50 torr produces only mild air hunger.[33] The effects of hypoxia are enhanced by hypercapnia.

EFFECT OF LUNG INFLATION ON AIR HUNGER

Mechanoreceptor input arising from breathing can dramatically reduce air hunger, as demonstrated by the classic experiment in which subjects held their breath until breakpoint and then breathed from a bag containing gas with alveolar concentrations of CO_2 and O_2, preventing improvement of arterial blood gases.[11,41] Subjects reported immediate relief and could even continue with another breathhold.

FIGURE 55-1 Air hunger response to an acute rise in end-tidal carbon dioxide tension (PET_{CO_2}) produced by inspired CO_2 in normal healthy men and women (*closed circles*). The prevailing chronic level of PET_{CO_2} is indicated by triangles. Bars indicate standard error of the mean. Volume-control ventilation was delivered via a mouthpiece at 0.16 L · min^{-1} · kg^{-1}. Subjects in these experiments were instructed to rate "discomfort due to your urge to breathe." "Extreme" on the rating scale was defined to the subjects as an intolerable level, and "moderate" was defined as a level that could be tolerated for several minutes. (*Data were re-plotted from Banzett et al.[12]*)

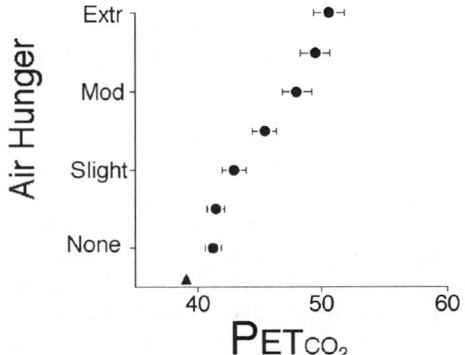

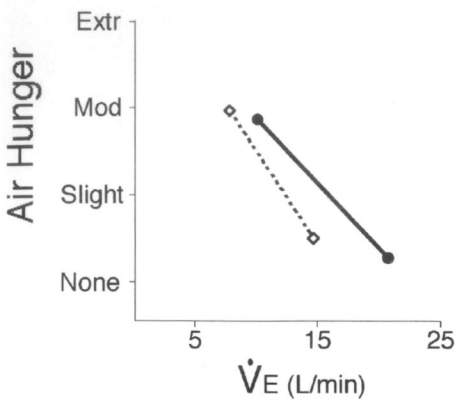

FIGURE 55-3 Relief of air hunger by increased minute ventilation at constant PET_{CO_2} in normal subjects (*solid line, closed symbols*) and patients with high cervical quadriplegia (*dotted line, open symbols*). In all cases, air hunger was generated by adding inspired CO_2 to increase PET_{CO_2} above the subjects' baseline PET_{CO_2}. (Mean PET_{CO_2} in normal subjects was 44 torr and in quadriplegic patients 34 torr, owing to their lower baseline P_{CO_2}.) PET_{CO_2} and respiratory frequency were held constant as ventilator tidal volume was varied. (*Data for normal subjects combined from Harty et al*[43] *and Banzett et al,*[37] *data for quadriplegic patients combined from Manning et al*[44] *and Bloch-Salisbury et al.*[18])

This phenomenon is manifested during mechanical ventilation as a decrease in dyspnea when tidal volume is increased, as was initially shown in polio patients.[42] Subsequently, mechanoreceptor relief of air hunger has been shown in normal subjects.[37,38,43,44] Studies of healthy subjects on volume-control ventilation, who have been initially made uncomfortable with mildly elevated P_{CO_2}, show that there is a decline in discomfort (air hunger) as $\dot{V}_E$ is increased with constant blood gas levels (the solid line in Fig. 55-3). In these subjects, zero discomfort can be achieved, and further increases have no effect, or produce a different form of discomfort, "too much pressure." In normal subjects, the relationship between ventilation and air hunger is linear (A.P. Binks, personal communication). This relief is undiminished in C1–C2 quadriplegic patients who have no motor or sensory innervation of the rib cage and diaphragm, showing that pulmonary stretch receptors that send impulses via the vagus nerve, are able to produce the full response[44] (dotted line in Fig. 55-3). It is not clear, however, whether chest-wall receptors form a fully redundant pathway capable of providing relief. Tidal volume provided somewhat less relief in double lung transplant patients than in normal subjects;[43] however, even the diminished response present in these transplant patients may have been caused by re-innervation of the transplanted lung, because the patients were studied 1–9 years posttransplant.[45]

WORK OR EFFORT OF BREATHING
The sense of breathing work or effort arises both from muscle receptors and from corollary discharge arising from cerebral motor cortex activation during volitional respiratory efforts.[46] (Corollary discharge from medullary respiratory

centers probably does not give rise to increased work or effort of breathing.) Although some studies of well-trained subjects have shown a distinction between effort and work, most normal subjects and patients do not distinguish the two; thus, we will use work/effort to denote the sensation. Work/effort of breathing is perceived when the physical work of breathing is increased by loading the respiratory muscles with high $\dot{V}_E$ or increased impedance, or when increased cortical motor drive is necessitated by respiratory muscle weakness.[40,47–49] Breathing at high lung volume both weakens the muscles (by placing them at a disadvantageous point in the length-tension curve) and loads them by increasing preload and system elastance; this is thought to be an important source of dyspnea in obstructive pulmonary disease.[50–52] In normal subjects, high levels of respiratory work/effort unaccompanied by blood gas derangements are not as unpleasant or threatening as air hunger.[47,49]

In theory, the ventilated patient need not do any respiratory work; ventilators have ample power to assume all work of breathing. Two sources of work, however, commonly arise in ventilated patients. The first we will term "wasted work," (i.e., work that does not result in air movement); this includes respiratory efforts that are ineffective because they are out of synchrony with the ventilator, or efforts (although in synchrony) that do not alter airflow (e.g., inspiratory efforts during volume-control inspirations). The second, "productive work" is performed to lower airway pressure to trigger inspiration during assist control, or to trigger and prolong inspiratory flow during pressure support. Productive work may still be excessive, if for instance the trigger pressure or flow thresholds are set too high (see below). A common cause of high trigger threshold is the presence of intrinsic PEEP: in this case the patient must generate inspiratory muscle pressure to overcome the difference between ventilator PEEP and intrinsic PEEP before the ventilator can be triggered. Thus, the effort required to trigger the ventilator can give rise to excessive work/effort and, depending on the ventilator setting, can cause inadequate ventilation, giving rise to air hunger.

DYSPNEA ARISING FROM PULMONARY AFFERENTS
There are several diseases in which dyspnea seems to arise from derangements of pulmonary afferent traffic; less is known about the neurophysiology of these forms of dyspnea. *Tightness* is specific to asthmatic bronchoconstriction.[53,54] Tightness is undiminished by mechanical ventilation, and preliminary evidence suggests that it is present during bronchoconstriction in quadriplegic patients with denervated chest walls, suggesting that it arises from pulmonary afferents.[55,56] Pulmonary embolism, pulmonary hypertension, and congestive heart failure all give rise to dyspnea that is disproportional to blood gas changes or to increased work of breathing. All directly impinge on the lung or its vasculature. It has thus been speculated that these conditions give rise to dyspnea via pulmonary receptors, and there is some evidence implicating vagal afferents, perhaps unmyelinated J-receptors.[57–59]

Approach to the Ventilated Patient With Dyspnea

If the ventilated patient is experiencing dyspnea, steps should be taken to establish the reason for the dyspnea and corrective measures should be attempted. It may be useful to establish a routine protocol to suit the needs of the unit. If diagnosis and corrective measures are expected to take more than a few minutes, interim relief can usually be obtained by increasing the level of ventilator support (see section on ventilator settings, below). Sedation should be used as a last resort because of the related risks (see section on sedation, below). There are several avenues to pursue before resorting to sedation: assess and remedy problems with obstructed airways, a stiff respiratory system, or weak respiratory muscles; improve ventilator settings; and address neuropsychiatric problems.

Essential information can be obtained from the physical examination (e.g., onset of wheezing, absence of breath sounds, new crackles, use of accessory muscles of ventilation, or pulsus paradoxus) and by measuring airways resistance (R_{AW}), intrinsic PEEP, spontaneous and ventilator-assisted tidal volume, maximal inspiratory and expiratory pressures, and compliance of the respiratory system (sometimes with the use of an esophageal balloon-catheter system to obtain compliance of the lung and chest wall separately).

INCREASED RESPIRATORY IMPEDANCE

Increased resistive or elastic impedance may give rise to air hunger in the ventilated patient by reducing ventilation, either by causing patient triggering efforts to fail, or by reducing tidal volumes delivered by pressure-targeted ventilators. Increased impedance may also give rise to a sense of excessive effort by increasing both wasted and productive work.

EXCESSIVE RESISTANCE

Airways obstruction as reflected by R_{AW} values greater than about 10 cmH$_2$O/L/sec is a frequent cause of dyspnea. Common causes of high R_{AW} are listed in Table 55-2.

In addition to resistance and compliance measures, the pressure and flow waveforms from the ventilator can provide useful diagnostic clues: a saw-toothed pattern is usu-

TABLE 55-2   Common Causes of High Airways Resistance

- Bronchoconstriction
- Inspissated debris in the endotracheal or tracheostomy tube
- Retained secretions in the trachea or bronchi
- Obstruction of the orifice of the endotracheal or tracheostomy tube by the posterior membranous sheath of the trachea secondary to tracheomalacia or a poorly fitting tube
- Granulation tissue (most often at the site of the cuff or tip of the tube or at the anastomosis site of a transplanted lung or lobe)
- Dislodged tracheostomy tube (most common in obese patients in whom selection of the proper size and shape of the tracheostomy tube can be difficult)

ally caused by retained secretions. Interruption of exhalation by a new inhalation before flow reaches zero indicates the presence of intrinsic PEEP, the magnitude of which should then be measured (see Chapter 3). Intrinsic PEEP secondary to flow limitation can be distinguished by pressing on the patient's abdomen during expiration. If there is flow limitation, the expiratory waveform will not change. Many of the causes of high R_{AW} listed in Table 55-2 can be identified easily by bronchoscopy. In other instances, the quality of dyspnea reported by the patient can provide important diagnostic clues. For example, our experience is that when bronchoconstriction is the cause, patients complain of chest tightness, whereas other causes of obstruction are usually associated with a sense of increased effort or work to breathe.

The goal is to reduce or eliminate excessive R_{AW} if possible, for instance by suctioning (with a bronchoscope if necessary), replacement of the endotracheal or tracheostomy tube, administration of bronchodilators or corticosteroids, or removal of granulation tissue. Until these measures are successful in alleviating intrinsic PEEP, however, an important step in achieving relief is to set the PEEP to equal the intrinsic PEEP (which reduces the preload the patient must overcome before triggering inspiration).[60] An alternative is to switch to mandatory volume-control ventilation, in which intrinsic PEEP does not affect delivery of tidal volume.

LOW COMPLIANCE

Stiffness of the respiratory system, as reflected by compliance (C_{RS}) values less than about 40 ml/cmH$_2$O, is also a common cause of dyspnea. Common causes of low C_{RS} are disorders involving the parenchyma (airspace diseases, fibrosis, and pulmonary edema), pleura (large pleural effusions, pleural thickening secondary to empyema, fibrosis, and tumor), or chest wall (kyphoscoliosis, ankylosing spondylitis, thoracoplasty, or obesity, especially in supine patients). These problems tend to be associated with a sense of effort to breathe, and with air hunger if hypoxemia or hypercapnia occurs. Many of the causes can be identified by chest CT scan. Relief is obtained by reversal of the problem when possible.

FIGHTING THE VENTILATOR

Respiratory efforts out of phase with the ventilator often reduce its effectiveness (see Chapter 53). These counterproductive efforts can be both an effect of dyspnea and resultant anxiety, and conversely, the efforts and consequent reduction in ventilation can be a cause of further dyspnea.

DYSPNEA ASSOCIATED WITH CARE ACTIVITIES

Dyspnea is frequently associated with normal care activities such as planned turns, transfers, bathing, and suctioning.[5] Good oxygenation should be assured before the activity, and it may be desirable to administer a pre-emptive dose of a very short-acting sedative or narcotic agent before commencing. A hazard of using even short-acting drugs repeatedly is that the drug will accumulate and produce prolonged sedation (see section on sedation, below).

VENTILATOR SETTINGS

Very few research papers have reported measures of dyspnea in patients during mechanical ventilation,[2] and fewer still report the effect of systematic manipulations designed to reduce dyspnea. In most of these studies, respiratory discomfort was not the primary outcome measure, and ventilator settings were optimized according to the investigators' criteria, not according to subjects' reports of comfort.[27,28,61,62] A few studies in normal subjects and none in patients have systematically examined independent variables such as flow rate while holding other known stimuli for dyspnea constant. Usually several mechanoreceptor stimuli changed simultaneously; for instance, in one study when flow rate was changed, tidal volume also changed. In other cases, important physiologic variables secondary to ventilation were not controlled, and were often not even measured. For instance, although it is well known that Pa_{CO_2} and Pa_{O_2} have a powerful effect on air hunger, these variables are frequently not controlled or reported. Despite these limitations, it is clear from these studies that changing ventilator settings can reduce dyspnea, and that patients can report these changes in dyspnea—the two essential features to enable patient-centered ventilation.

LEVEL OF VENTILATOR SUPPORT

Major relief of dyspnea in ventilated patients can be obtained by altering the level of ventilator support provided by the ventilator. There is, however, very little systematic information on this phenomenon; we are aware of only one study in which ventilatory variables, work of breathing, and dyspnea were measured at different levels of support by invasive ventilation.[28] This study of patients with COPD presents data on respiratory sensation at graded levels of assistance. Increasing the percentage of respiratory work done each minute by the ventilator proportionally decreased ratings of "difficulty breathing" (Fig. 55-4). The effect was large, with breathing difficulty ratings falling from 60% of scale with no support to 30% of scale with 80% support (ratings were not reported for full support). There were equally good correlations when ratings were re-plotted against a number of relevant physiologic indices (average tidal volume, frequency, minute ventilation, and work of breathing), so the afferent mechanism cannot be deduced from this experiment alone.

There are several mechanisms that could account for the relief achieved by increasing support. When support was increased in the above study, tidal volume also increased, as it would in most clinical situations. Relief correlated with tidal volume equally well as with percentage of support, and it is well known that increasing tidal volume can profoundly decrease air hunger (see above). Alveolar ventilation also increased with ventilator support in this study, presumably causing an improvement in blood gases, although these were not measured. Lowering Pa_{CO_2} has also been shown to have a profound effect on air hunger (see sec-

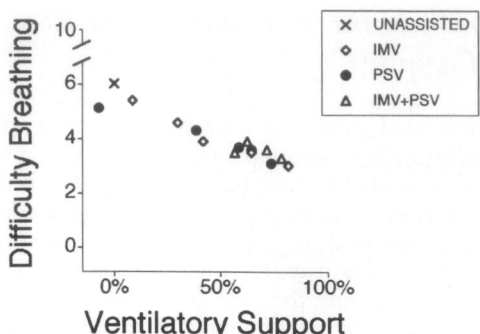

FIGURE 55-4 Effect of ventilator support on dyspnea. Subjects were instructed to rate "difficulty breathing" on a 10-point scale. Work of breathing was measured as the pressure-time product of inspiratory muscles, including all breaths, spontaneous and mandatory. Ventilator support is calculated as the difference from work of breathing in the unassisted control state. Data are shown for unassisted breathing, pressure-support ventilation, intermittent mandatory volume ventilation, and a combination of modes. (*Data re-analyzed and redrawn from Leung et al.*[28])

tion on air hunger, above), providing another possible relief mechanism (not mutually exclusive).

OTHER ASPECTS OF VENTILATOR SETTINGS

Rate of inflation has been shown to have an effect on comfort. In healthy subjects on volume control ventilation, inflation rates higher or lower than an optimum rate were less comfortable; there was, however, a broad range of comfortable inspiratory flow rates.[63] At inflation rates below the optimum, subjects reported air hunger. At inflation rates above the optimum, subjects reported sensations of too much pressure. Optimal flow rate has also been shown in patients on pressure-support ventilation for conditions ranging from pneumonia to stroke; discomfort increased above and below the preferred setting.[27] In this latter study, however, there were concomitant changes in tidal volume, which may have contributed to changes in discomfort ratings.

There is also evidence that PEEP level affects comfort via two distinctly different mechanisms: triggering effort and mean lung volume. The first, and best understood, arises from the interaction between ventilator PEEP and intrinsic PEEP in determining the effective trigger threshold (see Chapters 3, 11, and 56). In this case, dyspnea can be reduced with little or no change in tidal volume by adjusting PEEP to minimize inspiratory muscle preload. The second effect is through the effect of lung volume on comfort. There is some evidence that chronic ventilator patients are more comfortable (or require less tidal volume to achieve comfort) when end-expiratory lung volume is raised with PEEP,[64] possibly secondary to increased pulmonary mechanoreceptor activity.

EFFECT OF VENTILATOR CONTROL MODE

Most comparisons of sensation during different ventilator modes have not controlled the relevant physiologic variables. Leung et al[28] compared respiratory sensation during graded levels of support in two ventilator modes, pressure-support and intermittent mandatory ventilation, allowing meaningful comparisons of the two modes. The ratings of dyspnea ("difficulty breathing") depended only on the amount of assistance, not on the mode of ventilation (see Fig. 55-4). Both modes provided equivalent relief of dyspnea when ratings were re-plotted against a number of relevant physiologic indices. We conclude that judicious setting of volume-control ventilation parameters (see below) is likely to reduce dyspnea as effectively as subject-controlled ventilation when ventilatory demand is relatively constant.

A great deal of attention is paid to allowing patients to control the inspiration delivered by the ventilator; several clever schemes have been devised to perfect this control (see Chapters 6 through 13). It is thought by many that patient control of the ventilator is more comfortable, either because it ensures coincident timing of lung inflation with neural inspiration, or because it provides a sense of control to the patient. There is, however, no direct evidence that patient-triggered ventilation is inherently more comfortable than the same ventilator parameters set externally; differences appear to be more dependent on the parameter values chosen, and perhaps on the preference and familiarity of the operator for one mode versus another.

If timing ventilator inflation to coincide with neural inspiration were crucial, spontaneous breathing in healthy subjects would be more comfortable than volume-control; this is not the case. During hypercapnia in healthy subjects, spontaneous breathing was no more comfortable than volume-control mechanical ventilation at the same $\dot{V}_E$.[65] This may be because timing is irrelevant, or because neural timing adapts quickly to reasonable ventilator timing.[66,67]

If a psychological sense of control were important, giving the patient direct control of ventilator parameters would improve comfort; this is not the case, at least in chronically ventilated patients. When paralyzed patients on volume-control ventilation were allowed to control the tidal volume setting of the ventilator using a "sip/puff switch," they obtained no more relief from hypercapnia-induced discomfort than when the experimenter surreptitiously increased the volume.[68]

Patient-controlled ventilation may, however, have important advantages when ventilatory demand is highly variable. Two such instances are ambulatory patients assisted with noninvasive positive-pressure ventilation, whose ventilatory demand changes with physical activity,[61] and patients who use ventilator-delivered air to generate speech (see Chapter 56).

THE EXAMPLE OF CHRONICALLY VENTILATOR-DEPENDENT PATIENTS

An illustrative case is that of the chronically ventilator-dependent neuromuscular patient. These patients are nearly always comfortable with their usual ventilator settings. The reason for this is that they are not sedated, and thus clearly and insistently communicate their ventilatory desires to caregivers. In response, the caregivers set the ventilator to satisfy the patient. In our experience, this always results in high tidal volumes, frequencies of 10 to 15 breaths per minute, and very low PET_{CO_2}. In general, nearly all breaths are delivered by the ventilator as manda-

tory breaths, even when triggering is possible. Presumably this is because ventilation is high enough to suppress spontaneous efforts. Studies in which PET_{CO_2} is slowly raised show that complete comfort is maintained at normal PET_{CO_2}, leading us to conclude that the factor suppressing dyspnea and spontaneous efforts is large tidal volume, rather than low P_{CO_2}. Patients with lung and heart disease present additional constraints that complicate the issue, but the general principle of obtaining feedback from the patient as part of the ventilator-setting process can probably be applied to most awake patients.

UNWANTED EFFECTS OF VENTILATOR ADJUSTMENTS

Ventilator-induced lung injury can be caused by overly high tidal volumes in vulnerable patients (see Chapter 42). It may not be necessary to give excessively high tidal volumes to achieve patient comfort. Although one observational study suggests that the tidal volume limit should be reduced in all patients, the study design limits the strength of the conclusions.[69] We also note that chronically ventilator-dependent neuromuscular patients are routinely maintained for years with much larger tidal volumes without experiencing ventilator-induced lung injury.[18,44,64,70] More restrictive limits should be observed in patients at risk for the acute respiratory distress syndrome, in which case other means must be used to avoid dyspnea. Clinicians should be sure to apprise themselves of the current state of the art for tidal volume limits, as this is a rapidly changing field.

Some clinicians become concerned if arterial P_{CO_2} falls below normal values. Again we note the experience of chronically ventilator-dependent neuromuscular patients, who invariably have arterial P_{CO_2} 10–20 torr lower than normal for many years without apparent ill effect. It is important, however, to avoid acute increases in Pa_{CO_2} that give rise to dyspnea. Thus, for instance, if a patient is preparing to wean and is unlikely to have the ventilatory capacity to sustain low P_{CO_2}, the P_{CO_2} should be slowly raised over the course of a day or more to a level the patient is likely to be able to sustain with spontaneous breathing.

SEDATION

Mild sedation that does not obtund consciousness is often desirable in the ICU setting. Low doses of opiates can be effective in reducing dyspnea. If the nonpharmacologic measures proposed above fail to alleviate dyspnea, heavy sedation may be the only recourse (see Chapter 51). Prolonged sedation and neuromuscular blockade have serious drawbacks themselves, such as hemodynamic disturbances, lack of communication with loved ones, gastrointestinal stasis, delayed weaning from the ventilator, and cost.[71–73]

Important Unknowns and the Future

EPIDEMIOLOGY

There are only a few small studies of the prevalence of dyspnea in mechanically ventilated patients. These pilot studies strongly suggest there is a reason for concern, but studies defining the extent of the problem and its variation in different categories of patients and in different care settings are needed. In addition, the connection between dyspnea in ICU patients and poor psychological outcomes needs to be more carefully studied. Having defined the extent of the problem, it will be necessary to study the effectiveness of patient-centered ventilation strategies on both immediate comfort and long-term medical and psychological outcomes.

RESPIRATORY INTERVENTIONS

Systematic studies of the effect of each of the multitude of ventilator setting modes on patient comfort are needed. These should be accomplished with state-of-the-art methods for dyspnea measurement, and with proper measurement and control of interrelated physiologic variables that may change. Further investigation is also needed to determine whether obtaining descriptions of the nature of discomfort will be a useful and practical guide to treatment of the mechanically ventilated patient, or whether feedback on intensity of discomfort will suffice. On the basis of this mechanistic knowledge, a more systematic approach to achieving comfort can be devised.

NONRESPIRATORY INTERVENTIONS

There are several potential schemes for altering afferent input without actually altering ventilatory variables, in a sense "fooling" the system to reduce perception of dyspnea. These have not been studied in the context of mechanical ventilation. Cool air directed over the face has a significant effect on dyspnea.[74] In some studies, phasic vibration of intercostal spaces has been shown to have an effect on work/effort dyspnea,[75–77] but no effect on air hunger.[78] Aerosolized furosemide has also been shown to reduce air hunger dyspnea.[79–81]

Summary and Conclusion

Substantial respiratory discomfort is common in mechanically ventilated patients and is likely responsible for important emotional reactions, such as anxiety, fear, and PTSD. Although it is not common current practice, we have recommended that, in ventilator units, there be routine formal assessment of the quality and intensity of the discomfort, for example, when vital signs are obtained. The cause(s) of the dyspnea should be sought and corrective measures attempted. The patient's description of the discomfort, the physical examination, and physiologic measurements, such as airways resistance and respiratory system compliance, provide important clues about the cause of the dyspnea. Increasing the level of mechanical support usually provides relief, but the best method for this is not yet known and may vary with the cause. Heavy sedation should be used only when necessary because it is associated with an increase in days requiring mechanical ventilation, occurrence

of pneumonia, and length of stay in the hospital. Whether the patient-centered ventilation approach that we have recommended will yield beneficial outcomes remains to be determined and should be the subject of future research.

Acknowledgements

The authors wish to thank Dean R. Hess and Robert W. Lansing for their helpful input. Supported in part by National Institutes of Health grant HL46690.

References

1. Desbiens NA, Mueller-Rizner N, Connors AF, et al. The relationship of nausea and dyspnea to pain in seriously ill patients. Pain 1997; 71:149–56.
2. Hansen-Flaschen JH. Dyspnea in the ventilated patient: a call for patient-centered mechanical ventilation. Respir Care 2000; 45:1460–4, discussion 1464–7.
3. Powers J, Bennett SJ. Measurement of dyspnea in patients treated with mechanical ventilation. Am J Crit Care 1999; 8:254–61.
4. Knebel AR, Janson-Bjerklie SL, Malley JD, et al. Comparison of breathing comfort during weaning with two ventilatory modes [see comment]. Am J Respir Crit Care Med 1994; 149:14–8.
5. Lush MT, Janson-Bjerklie S, Carrieri VK, et al. Dyspnea in the ventilator-assisted patient. Heart Lung 1988; 17:528–35.
6. Karampela I, Hansen-Flaschen J, Smith S, et al. A dyspnea evaluation protocol for respiratory therapists: a feasibility study. Respir Care 2002; 47:1158–61.
7. Carrieri-Kohlman V, Gormley JM, Douglas MK, et al. Exercise training decreases dyspnea and the distress and anxiety associated with it. Monitoring alone may be as effective as coaching. Chest 1996; 110:1526–35.
8. Gift AG. Psychologic and physiologic aspects of acute dyspnea in asthmatics. Nurs Res 1991; 40:196–9.
9. De Peuter S, Van Diest I, Lemaigre V, et al. Dyspnea: the role of psychological processes. Clin Psychol Rev 2004; 24:557–81.
10. Bergbom-Engberg I, Haljamae H. Assessment of patients' experience of discomforts during respirator therapy. Crit Care Med 1989; 17:1068–72.
11. Hill L, Flack F. The effect of excess of carbon dioxide and of want of oxygen upon the respiration and the circulation. J Physiol (Lond) 1908; 37:77–111.
12. Banzett R, Lansing R, Evans K, et al. Stimulus-response characteristics of CO_2-induced air hunger in normal subjects. Respir Physiol 1996; 103:19–31.
13. Smoller JW, Pollack MH, Otto MW, et al. Panic anxiety, dyspnea, and respiratory disease. Theoretical and clinical considerations. Am J Respir Crit Care Med 1996; 154:6–17.
14. Schelling G. Effects of stress hormones on traumatic memory formation and the development of posttraumatic stress disorder in critically ill patients. Neurobiol Learn Mem 2002; 78:596–609.
15. Cuthbertson BH, Hull A, Strachan M, et al. Post-traumatic stress disorder after critical illness requiring general intensive care. Intensive Care Med 2004; 30:450–5.
16. Scragg P, Jones A, Fauvel N. Psychological problems following ICU treatment. Anaesthesia 2001; 56:9–14.
17. Schweickert WD, Gehlbach BK, Pohlman AS, et al. Daily interruption of sedative infusions and complications of critical illness in mechanically ventilated patients. Crit Care Med 2004; 32:1272–6.

18. Bloch-Salisbury E, Shea SA, Brown R, et al. Air hunger induced by acute increase in PCO_2 adapts to chronic elevation of PCO_2 in ventilated humans. J Appl Physiol 1996; 81:949–56.

19. Schwartzstein R. The language of dyspnea: using verbal clues to diagnose. J Crit Illness 1999; 14:435–41.

20. Lansing R, Banzett R. Psychophysical methods in the study of respiratory sensation. In: Adams L, Guz A, editors. Respiratory sensation. New York: Marcel Dekker, 1996: 69–100.

21. Phillips DM. JCAHO pain management standards are unveiled. Joint Commission on Accreditation of Healthcare Organizations. JAMA 2000; 284:428–9.

22. Nishino T, Shimoyama N, Ide T, et al. Experimental pain augments experimental dyspnea, but not vice versa in human volunteers. Anesthesiology 1999; 91:1633–8.

23. Cherniack NS, Altose MD. Mechanisms of dyspnea. Clin Chest Med 1987; 8:207–14.

24. Banzett RB, Lansing RW, Reid MB, et al. 'Air hunger' arising from increased PCO_2 in mechanically ventilated quadriplegics. Respir Physiol 1989; 76:53–67.

25. Banzett RB, Lansing RW, Brown R, et al. 'Air hunger' from increased PCO_2 persists after complete neuromuscular block in humans. Respir Physiol 1990; 81:1–17.

26. Gandevia SC, Killian K, McKenzie DK, et al. Respiratory sensations, cardiovascular control, kinaesthesia and transcranial stimulation during paralysis in humans. J Physiol (Lond) 1993; 470: 85–107.

27. Chiumello D, Pelosi P, Croci M, et al. The effects of pressurization rate on breathing pattern, work of breathing, gas exchange and patient comfort in pressure support ventilation. Eur Respir J 2001; 18:107–14.

28. Leung P, Jubran A, Tobin MJ. Comparison of assisted ventilator modes on triggering, patient effort, and dyspnea. Am J Respir Crit Care Med 1997; 155:1940–8.

29. O'Driscoll M, Corner J, Bailey C. The experience of breathlessness in lung cancer. Eur J Cancer Care (Engl) 1999; 8:37–43.

30. Adams L, Lane R, Shea SA, et al. Breathlessness during different forms of ventilatory stimulation: a study of mechanisms in normal subjects and respiratory patients. Clin Sci 1985; 69:663–72.

31. Davidson JT, Whipp BJ, Wasserman K, et al. Role of the carotid bodies in breath-holding. N Engl J Med 1974; 290:819–22.

32. Wright GW, Branscomb BV. The origin of the sensations of dyspnea? Trans Am Clin Clin Assn 1954; 66:116–25.

33. Moosavi SH, Golestanian E, Binks AP, et al. Hypoxic and hypercapnic drives to breathe generate equivalent levels of air hunger in humans. J Appl Physiol 2003; 94:141–54.

34. Chen Z, Eldridge FL, Wagner PG. Respiratory-associated rhythmic firing of midbrain neurones in cats: relation to level of respiratory drive. J Physiol (Lond) 1991; 437:305–25.

35. Chen Z, Eldridge FL, Wagner PG. Respiratory-associated thalamic activity is related to level of respiratory drive. Respir Physiol 1992; 90:99–113.

36. Eldridge FL, Chen Z. Respiratory-associated rhythmic firing of midbrain neurons is modulated by vagal input. Respir Physiol 1992; 90:31–46.

37. Banzett RB, Mulnier HE, Murphy K, et al. Breathlessness in humans activates insular cortex. Neuroreport 2000; 11:2117–20.

38. Evans KC, Banzett RB, Adams L, et al. BOLD fMRI identifies limbic, paralimbic, and cerebellar activation during air hunger. J Neurophysiol 2002; 88:1500–11.

39. Campbell EJM, Gandevia SC, Killian KJ, et al. Changes in the perception of inspiratory resistive loads during partial curarization. J Physiol (Lond) 1980; 309:93–100.

40. Moosavi SH, Topulos GP, Hafer A, et al. Acute partial paralysis alters perceptions of air hunger, work and effort at constant PCO_2 and V_E. Respir Physiol 2000; 122:45–60.

41. Fowler WS. Breaking point of breath holding. J Appl Physiol 1954; 6:539–545.

42. Opie L, Smith A, Spalding J. Conscious appreciation of the effects produced by independent changes of ventilation volume and of end-tidal PCO_2 in paralysed patients. J Physiol (Lond) 1959; 149:494–9.

43. Harty HR, Mummery CJ, Adams L, et al. Ventilatory relief of the sensation of the urge to breathe in humans: are pulmonary receptors important? J Physiol (Lond) 1996; 490:805–15.

44. Manning HL, Shea SA, Schwartzstein RM, et al. Reduced tidal volume increases 'air hunger' at fixed PCO_2 in ventilated quadriplegics. Respir Physiol 1992; 90:19–30.

45. Butler JE, Anand A, Crawford MR, et al. Changes in respiratory sensations induced by lobeline after human bilateral lung transplantation. J Physiol 2001; 534:583–93.

46. Killian KJ, Gandevia SC. Sense of effort and dyspnea. In: Adams L, Guz A, editors. Respiratory sensation, 1st ed. New York: Marcel Dekker, 1996: 181–99.

47. Lansing RW, Im BS, Thwing JI, et al. The perception of respiratory work and effort can be independent of the perception of air hunger. Am J Respir Crit Care Med 2000; 162:1690–6.

48. Killian KJ, Gandevia SC, Summers E, et al. Effect of increased lung volume on perception of breathlessness, effort, and tension. J Appl Physiol 1984; 57:686–91.

49. Chonan T, Mulholland MB, Altose MD, et al. Effects of changes in level and pattern of breathing on the sensation of dyspnea. J Appl Physiol 1990; 69:1290–5.

50. O'Donnell DE, Revill SM, Webb KA. Dynamic hyperinflation and exercise intolerance in chronic obstructive pulmonary disease. Am J Respir Crit Care Med 2001; 164:770–7.

51. O'Donnell DE, Lam M, Webb KA. Measurement of symptoms, lung hyperinflation, and endurance during exercise in chronic obstructive pulmonary disease. Am J Respir Crit Care Med 1998; 158:1557–65.

52. O'Donnell DE. Dyspnea in advanced chronic obstructive pulmonary disease. J Heart Lung Transplant 1998; 17:544–54.

53. Moy ML, Weiss JW, Sparrow D, et al. Quality of dyspnea in bronchoconstriction differs from external resistive loads. Am J Respir Crit Care Med 2000; 162:451–5.

54. Simon PM, Schwartzstein RM, Weiss JW, et al. Distinguishable types of dyspnea in patients with shortness of breath. Am Rev Respir Dis 1990; 142:1009–14.

55. Cristiano L, Klenz J, Shao A, et al. Rib cage innervation is not necessary for perception of chest tightness during methacholine-induced bronchoconstriction. Am J Resp Crit Care Med 1994; 149:52–9.

56. Binks AP, Moosavi SH, Banzett RB, et al. "Tightness" sensation of asthma does not arise from the work of breathing. Am J Respir Crit Care Med 2002; 165:78–82.

57. Davies SF, McQuaid KR, Iber C, et al. Extreme dyspnea from unilateral pulmonary venous obstruction. Demonstration of a vagal mechanism and relief by right vagotomy. Am Rev Respir Dis 1987; 136:184–8.

58. Guz A, Noble M, Eisele J, et al. Experimental results of vagal block in cardiopulmonary disease. In: Porter R, editor. Breathing: Hering-Breuer centenary symposium. London: Churchill, 1970: 315–36.

59. Dehghani GA, Parvizi MR, Sharif-Kazemi MB, et al. Presence of lobeline-like sensations in exercising patients with left ventricular dysfunction. Respir Physiol Neurobiol 2004; 143:9–20.

60. MacIntyre NR, Cheng KC, McConnell R. Applied PEEP during pressure support reduces the inspiratory threshold load of intrinsic PEEP. Chest 1997; 111:188–93.

61. Gay PC, Hess DR, Hill NS. Noninvasive proportional assist ventilation for acute respiratory insufficiency. Comparison with

pressure support ventilation. Am J Respir Crit Care Med 2001; 164:1606–11.

62. Guttmann J, Bernhard H, Mols G, et al. Respiratory comfort of automatic tube compensation and inspiratory pressure support in conscious humans. Intensive Care Med 1997; 23:1119–24.

63. Manning HL, Molinary EJ, Leiter JC. Effect of inspiratory flow rate on respiratory sensation and pattern of breathing. Am J Respir Crit Care Med 1995; 151:751–7.

64. Hoit JD, Banzett RB, Lohmeier HL, et al. Clinical ventilator adjustments that improve speech. Chest 2003; 124:1512–21.

65. Shea SA, Harty HR, Banzett RB. Self-control of level of mechanical ventilation to minimize CO_2 induced air hunger. Respir Physiol 1996; 103:113–25.

66. Simon PM, Zurob AS, Wies WM, et al. Entrainment of respiration in humans by periodic lung inflations. Effect of state and CO_2. Am J Respir Crit Care Med 1999; 160:950–60.

67. Simon PM, Habel AM, Daubenspeck JA, et al. Vagal feedback in the entrainment of respiration to mechanical ventilation in sleeping humans. J Appl Physiol 2000; 89:760–9.

68. Bloch-Salisbury E, Spengler CM, Brown R, et al. Self-control and external control of mechanical ventilation give equal air hunger relief. Am J Respir Crit Care Med 1998; 157:415–20.

69. Gajic O, Dara SI, Mendez JL, et al. Ventilator-associated lung injury in patients without acute lung injury at the onset of mechanical ventilation. Crit Care Med 2004; 32:1817–24.

70. Banzett RB, Lansing RW, Brown R. High-level quadriplegics perceive lung volume change. J Appl Physiol 1987; 62:567–73.

71. Kollef MH, Levy NT, Ahrens TS, et al. The use of continuous i.v. sedation is associated with prolongation of mechanical ventilation. Chest 1998; 114:541–8.

72. Stannard C, Jones J. Neuromuscular blockade, sedation, and pain control. In: Tobin MJ, editor. Principles and practice of mechanical ventilation. New York: McGraw-Hill, 1994: 1125–47.

73. Kress JP, Pohlman AS, O'Connor MF, et al. Daily interruption of sedative infusions in critically ill patients undergoing mechanical ventilation. N Engl J Med 2000; 342:1471–7.

74. Schwartzstein RM, Lahive K, Pope A, et al. Cold facial stimulation reduces breathlessness induced in normal subjects. Am Rev Respir Dis 1987; 136:58–61.

75. Manning HL, Basner R, Ringler J, et al. Effect of chest wall vibration on breathlessness in normal subjects. J Appl Physiol 1991; 71:175–81.

76. Edo H, Kimura H, Niijima M, et al. Effects of chest wall vibration on breathlessness during hypercapnic ventilatory response. J Appl Physiol 1998; 84:1487–91.

77. Cristiano LM, Schwartzstein RM. Effect of chest wall vibration on dyspnea during hypercapnia and exercise in chronic obstructive pulmonary disease. Am J Respir Crit Care Med 1997; 155:1552–9.

78. Bloch-Salisbury E, Binks AP, Banzett RB, et al. Mechanical chest-wall vibration does not relieve air hunger. Respir Physiol Neurobiol 2003; 134:177–90.

79. Moosavi S, Binks A, Lansing R, et al. Furosemide inhalation reduces air hunger sensitivity in healthy individuals. Am J Respir Crit Care Med 2002; 165:B20.

80. Nishino T, Ide T, Sudo T, et al. Inhaled furosemide greatly alleviates the sensation of experimentally induced dyspnea. Am J Respir Crit Care Med 2000; 161:1963–7.

81. Kohara H, Ueoka H, Aoe K, et al. Effect of nebulized furosemide in terminally ill cancer patients with dyspnea. J Pain Symptom Manage 2003; 26:962–7.

Chapter 56

VENTILATOR-SUPPORTED SPEECH

JEANNETTE D. HOIT
ROBERT B. BANZETT
ROBERT BROWN

Under normal circumstances, the respiratory system supplies the aeromechanical drive that allows the vocal folds, tongue, lips, and other structures to create the sounds of speech. Although a simplification, this drive can be understood as the tracheal pressure. Usually this pressure is exquisitely and actively controlled by muscles of the chest wall. When speech is produced with ventilator support, however, the ventilator and the respiratory system must work together to produce the pressure that drives speech production. In most cases, this pressure is markedly different from that of normal speech production. As a result, the act of speaking can be challenging for patients, and they often require assistance from their pulmonologist, respiratory therapist, and speech-language pathologist. The views presented here are that patients should be enabled to speak whenever possible, and that ventilator-supported speech

can often be improved by using interventions such as those described in this chapter.

The Importance of Speech

Communication is critical to maintaining good quality of life. Communication is the key to being able to express needs, participate in social activities, and retain control over important life decisions.[1-3] It can be especially important in intensive care or during end-of-life care.[4] There are many ways to communicate, but of these, speech is the fastest and most convenient. It works in the dark and across telephone lines, and it conveys meaning and emotions through words and tone of voice (i.e., pitch, loudness, quality, and timing).

Patients who are ventilator-supported often complain of speech problems, especially unwanted pauses and inadequate loudness.[5] This is illustrated in the following quotation,[6] which comes from a patient who was asked, "Do you have any problems with your speech?" Note that the pauses between phrases were 3 to 4 seconds (• = 1 second), and that some words were produced without voice (shown in parentheses). To appreciate the severity of the speech problem, this quotation should be read aloud with timed pauses:

"Yes •••• Um, getting cut (off) •••• people interfering with me ••• trying to finish my sentences (for me) •••• that's the most frustrating (part)."

Fortunately, it is nearly always possible to improve ventilator-supported speech. The following quotation comes from the same patient, after she received speech interventions. Pauses were reduced to approximately 1 second, and the amount of speech per breath increased by about 50%.

"Since I've been able to talk better • I've par- participated in talking with more people and • and in conversation instead of just doing the listening • and talking as little as possible • I've joined in and, and • I don't know, I've just been part of a group more • Very few people try to finish my sentences now and • second guess what I'm going to say • It's, it's helped a lot."

Fundamentals of Speech Breathing

Speech comprises the tones, hisses, pops, and buzzes that are the acoustic representation of language.[7] Speech is usually produced by the coordinated efforts of more than 100 muscles spanning the chest wall, larynx, and upper airway structures (pharynx, velum, jaw, lips, and tongue). Speech breathing is the process by which the driving forces are supplied to downstream structures to generate speech, and it is tailored to simultaneously serve speech-related functions and meet gas exchange requirements.[8]

The normal speech breathing cycle has an inspiratory phase ranging from 0.5–0.7 seconds.[9-13] These inspirations are so short that the pauses they create are hardly noticeable. The longer, more variable expiratory phase of the cycle is the speaking phase. Its duration averages 3–5 seconds, but varies substantially as a function of linguistic factors, cognitive variables, mechanical constraints, and ventilatory needs.[10,11,13–15] Speech is usually produced throughout most of the expiratory phase, although nonspeech expirations are likely to occur in senescent subjects,[16] with high cognitive-linguistic demands,[17] and under conditions of elevated ventilatory drive.[13,18,19] The tidal volumes used in speech breathing are typically about twice as large as those of resting tidal breathing.[20]

The normal speech breathing cycle has a characteristic tracheal pressure profile. During inspiration, pressure is substantially and briefly negative, and during expiration (speaking) it is moderately positive and relatively steady. For speech of conversational loudness, pressure is generally in the range of 5–10 cmH_2O.[21,22] Pressure usually remains relatively constant throughout expiration so that loudness and voice quality remain relatively constant.[23,24] An increase in pressure generally causes an increase in loudness. To produce voiced speech sounds (such as vowels), the vocal folds must oscillate, which requires a minimum pressure of approximately 2 cmH_2O.[25,26] When voiced sounds are produced with a constricted oral airway (such as the plosive /d/ or the fricative /v/), slightly higher pressures are needed.

The pressures of normal speech breathing are controlled actively throughout the cycle by muscles of the chest wall.[24] Inspiration is driven by the diaphragm, and expiration (speaking) is driven by both expiratory rib cage and abdominal muscular pressures (with the latter predominating) when in upright body positions, and by expiratory rib cage muscular pressure alone when in the supine body position. These muscular pressures are usually supplemented by positive recoil pressure, because most conversational speech is produced above the resting expiratory level. On rare occasions, when speech is initiated at a very large lung volume (i.e., near total lung capacity), positive recoil force may be so great that inspiratory muscular pressure must be called into play to counteract (i.e., "brake") the high positive pressure.

A Framework for Understanding Ventilator-Supported Speech

During ventilator-supported speech breathing, tracheal pressure is seldom as constant as it is during normal speaking. Rather, tracheal pressure takes on a temporal pattern that reflects the combined contributions of the patient's prevailing respiratory recoil pressure, active muscular pressures (if the patient is able to activate chest wall muscles), and inspiratory and/or expiratory drive from the ventilator, among other factors. A useful framework for understanding, evaluating, and managing ventilator-supported speech is to relate speech to tracheal pressure.[6,8,27]

Speech with Invasive Positive-Pressure Ventilation

Invasive positive-pressure ventilation (InPPV) is used here to mean intermittent positive-pressure ventilation via tra-

cheostomy. Because an endotracheal tube prohibits vocalizing and can damage the vocal folds, speech is one of several factors to consider when deciding whether and when to tracheostomize (see Chapter 40). Speaking with InPPV is substantially different from speaking with other forms of ventilation, but it can be very successful. The primary differences stem from the fact that the ventilator-delivered air enters below the larynx.

DEFLATE THE TRACHEOSTOMY TUBE CUFF

For a patient to speak, the first and most critical step is to configure the tracheostomy tube so that flow (and thus pressure) can reach the larynx. This means that the cuff on the tube must be deflated (and/or the tube must contain a fenestration). If cuff deflation or use of a fenestrated tube is deemed inadvisable, alternative forms of speech or communication must be sought (see Chapter 40, and the section below on alternatives to ventilator-supported speech).

Cuff deflation is feasible in most chronically ventilated patients[28,29] and in acutely ventilated patients who are otherwise stable. Indeed, in some patients, the cuff can be deflated and speech training initiated on the first day after the tracheotomy has been performed. Unfortunately, cuff deflation and speech training are often delayed (or not performed at all) because of unfamiliarity with the procedure, concerns about aspiration, and fear of causing hypoventilation and hypoxemia. Hypoventilation and hypoxemia can be avoided by increasing the ventilator-delivered tidal volume. In many stable patients, the cuff can remain deflated all day (and inflated only for sleep). In less stable patients, cuff deflation may need to be brief (to allow communication with family members or caregivers) and performed only in the presence of a pulmonologist or respiratory therapist. The recommended procedure for initial cuff deflation is described in the section titled "important cautions," below.

After cuff deflation, the patient's voice should be assessed. If voice problems are noted, the resistance to "bypass" gas flow around the cuff should be estimated to determine if it is sufficiently low to allow good vocalizing. Bypass resistance can be estimated by blocking expiratory flow where it exits the ventilator and observing tracheal pressure during expiration. When the resistive pressure drop is less than 5 cmH_2O, cuff deflation is generally successful, but when pressure exceeds 10 cmH_2O, cuff deflation often fails. Bypass resistance can usually be reduced by downsizing the tracheostomy tube. If the patient still cannot vocalize, the upper airway and larynx should be viewed via nasendoscopy to rule out conditions such as excessive secretions, laryngeal edema, granulation tissue, tracheal scar formation, or vocal fold paralysis.

Figure 56-1 illustrates the flow routes for inspiration and expiration with an inflated cuff (closed system) and deflated cuff (open system). When the cuff is inflated, no flow reaches the larynx. When the cuff is deflated, flow reaches the larynx during inspiration and expiration, making it theoretically possible to produce speech during both phases of the ventilator's cycle. The ventilator's settings, however, are strong determinants of when within the cycle speech can be produced. Speech produced with InPPV is often plagued by long pauses, short phrases, variable loudness,

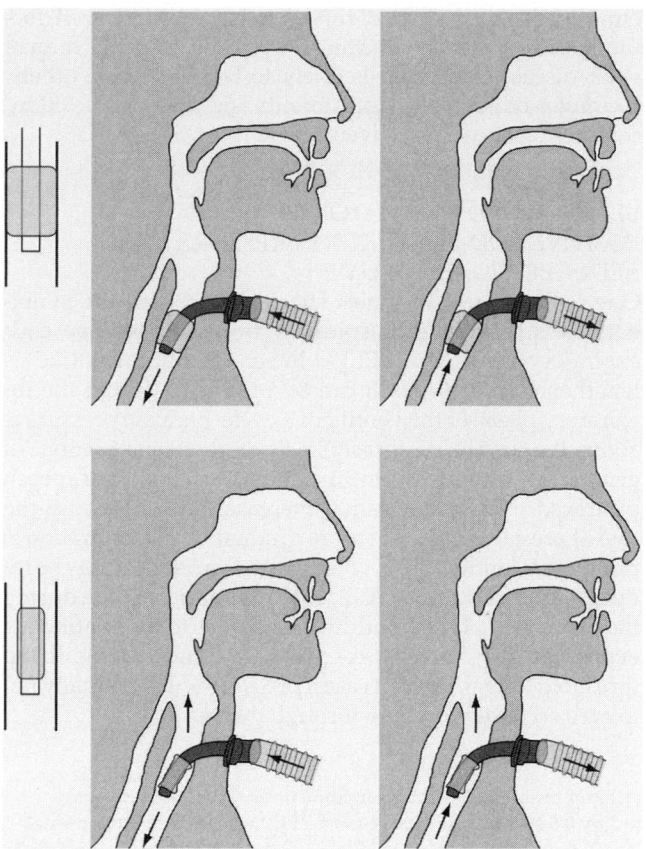

FIGURE 56-1 Inflated and deflated tracheostomy tube cuff during inspiration (*left*) and expiration (*right*). When the cuff is inflated, no flow reaches the larynx, and when the cuff is deflated, flow reaches the larynx during both inspiration and expiration. (*Adapted and reprinted, with permission, from Hixon and Hoit.*[8])

and variable voice quality.[27,30,31] These speech features are most easily explained by relating them to the tracheal pressure.

Clinical Scenario 1

Mrs. Z was a 52-year-old woman with breast cancer that had metastasized to her lungs, causing her to be very short of breath and unable to breathe on her own. She obtained relief from assisted ventilation via a tracheostomy and could not be weaned from the ventilator. She was frustrated by not being able to speak to her caregivers, husband, and daughters about the nature and intensity of the care she wished to receive and about her impending death. Communication by writing was tedious. She was advised that the cuff of her tracheostomy tube could be deflated so that she could speak, but that she would likely experience periods of breathlessness at first while ventilator adjustments were being made. She was very fearful of this, but with encouragement and reassurance the procedure was successful. For several minutes at a time, with only slight shortness of breath, she was able to speak and communicate her wishes to her family. She went home on the ventilator and died peacefully there.

SPEECH PRODUCTION WITH VOLUME-CONTROLLED VENTILATION

Figure 56-2 illustrates tracheal pressure with volume-controlled ventilation compared with that of normal speech production. A glance is sufficient to see that these pressures differ markedly. Pressure during normal speaking is low and constant. This steady pressure allows vocal fold oscillations to be relatively constant in amplitude and waveform, translating to relatively constant loudness and voice quality. Also, pressure remains above the vocalizing threshold throughout expiration during normal speech production.

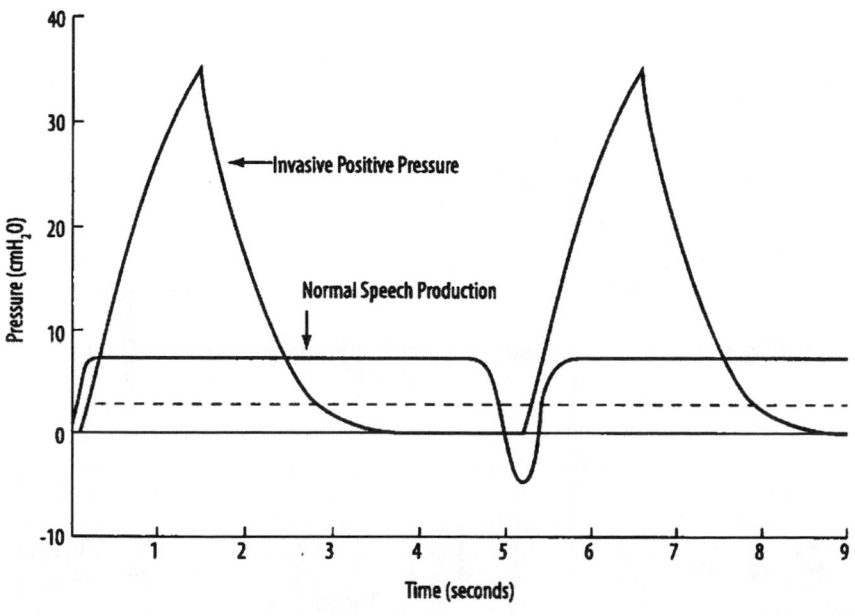

FIGURE 56-2 Tracheal pressure during volume-controlled InPPV and during normal speech production. The dashed line shows the minimum pressure needed for vocalizing. (*Reprinted, with permission, from Hixon and Hoit.*[8])

By contrast, pressure during volume-controlled InPPV rises quickly during inspiration, falls sharply when the expiration valve opens, and then remains below the vocalizing threshold for a substantial portion of the cycle. The rapidly changing pressure is the primary cause of loudness and voice quality problems, and the periods of low pressure (below the vocalizing threshold) explain the long pauses and the short phrases.

VENTILATOR ADJUSTMENTS THAT CAN IMPROVE SPEECH

Abnormal magnitude and time course of tracheal pressure are at the root of the speech problems associated with volume-controlled InPPV. Therefore, the unifying principle for improving speech is to adjust the ventilator so as to generate a pressure that is better suited for speech production, while accommodating the patient's cardiopulmonary needs and comfort. Ventilator adjustments to improve speech are designed to: (1) increase the portion of the cycle during which pressure remains above the vocalizing threshold (i.e., at least 2 cmH$_2$O); and (2) reduce the rate and magnitude of pressure changes during the period in which speech is produced. Many adjustments are possible, and the optimal combination for a given patient must be determined empirically. The success of this approach has been well documented in patients with spinal cord injury and neuromuscular disease,[27,31,32] and is likely to be effective in others. Examples of ventilator adjustments and their predicted influences on speech are given below.

LENGTHENED INSPIRATORY TIME, POSITIVE END-EXPIRATORY PRESSURE, AND REDUCED TIDAL VOLUME

One of the easiest and most successful adjustment combinations is lengthened inspiratory time and positive end-expiratory pressure (PEEP). When inspiratory time is lengthened, more speech can be produced during the inspiratory phase of the ventilator's cycle, because pressure is above the vocalizing threshold throughout inspiration. In general, as inspiratory time increases, the amount of speech produced during inspiration increases. Also, because the rate of pressure change is more gradual when inspiration is prolonged, loudness and voice quality variability may be reduced. The addition of PEEP extends speaking time during the expiratory phase by adding resistance to the ventilator's expiratory line, which keeps pressure above the vocalizing threshold longer. In most cases, pressure will eventually fall to zero secondary to flow through the larynx.

FIGURE 56-3 The tracheal pressure and speech signal under the usual (*left*) and best (*right*) ventilator conditions. The best settings represented the following adjustments: (a) inspiratory time was lengthened by 0.5 second; (b) 4 cmH$_2$O of PEEP was added; (c) and tidal volume was reduced by about 0.3 L. (*Adapted and reprinted, with permission, from Hoit and Banzett.*[27])

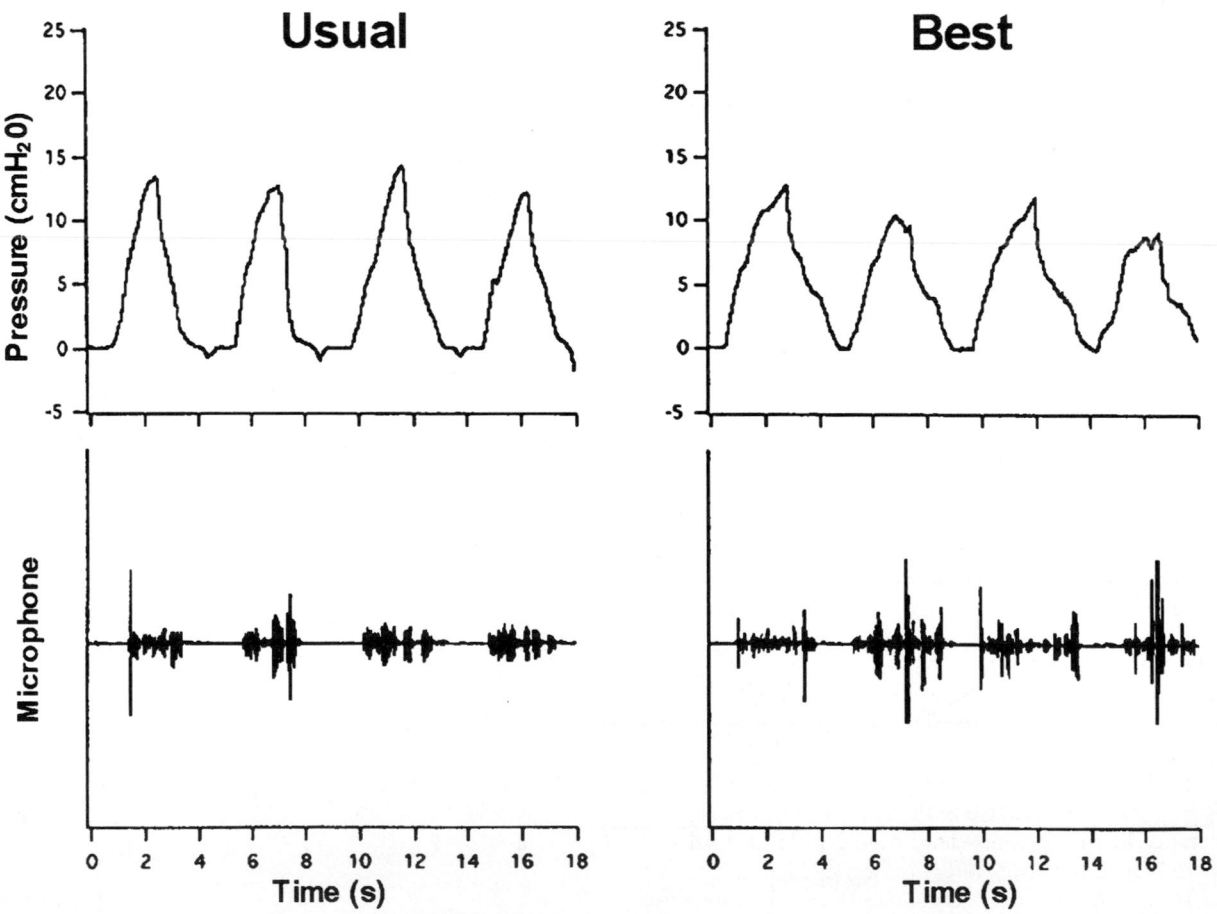

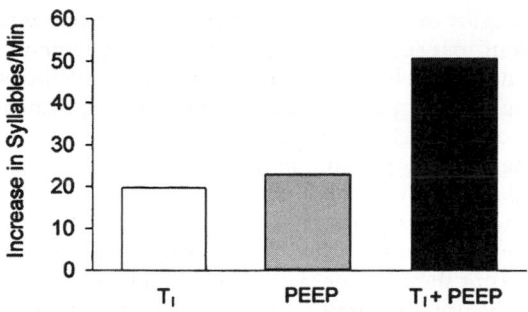

FIGURE 56-4 Changes (from usual) in speaking rate for lengthened inspiratory time, PEEP, and combined lengthened inspiratory time and PEEP. (*Adapted and reprinted, with permission, from Hoit et al.*[31])

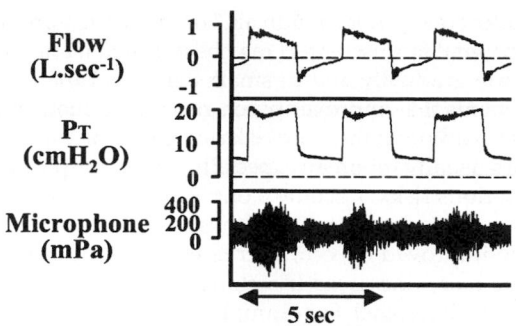

FIGURE 56-5 Flow, pressure, and speech signal during sustained vowel production with pressure-targeted ventilation and PEEP. (*Adapted and reprinted, with permission, from Prigent et al.*[32])

Sometimes it is physiologically appropriate to also reduce the ventilator-delivered tidal volume in patients whose tidal volumes are too large. When tidal volume is reduced, peak pressure is lowered, which helps to smooth out loudness and voice quality. A smaller tidal volume can also benefit patients who are chronically hyperventilated. Although patients are usually uncomfortable when tidal volume is reduced, they are often comfortable if PEEP is added first.

An example of the effect of these adjustments on tracheal pressure and the acoustic speech signal is shown in Fig. 56-3 as a comparison of a patient's "usual" and "best" ventilator settings. Although the ventilator adjustments resulted in only subtle changes in the pressure waveform, the changes in speech were substantial and easily perceptible to listeners.[27] On average, an increase in inspiratory time of 17–25% combined with PEEP of 5–10 cmH$_2$O results in an increase in speaking time of 55% per cycle.[31] As shown in Fig. 56-4, the increase in speaking time for lengthened inspiratory time and the PEEP adjustment is additive.

PRESSURE-CONTROLLED VENTILATION AND POSITIVE END-EXPIRATORY PRESSURE

Pressure-controlled ventilation (and its variants, such as pressure-support ventilation) target a given airway pressure (rather than a volume). Thus, inspiration may be associated with a relatively steady pressure, somewhat similar to that associated with normal speech production (except higher). With this form of ventilation, pressure remains above the vocalizing threshold throughout inspiration. And, when pressure is steady, loudness and voice quality are more apt to be constant. When PEEP is added, pressure is maintained above the vocalizing threshold longer during expiration. Figure 56-5 shows that vocalizing can continue throughout the entire ventilator cycle (as it can with appropriate volume-controlled adjustments).

POSITIVE END-EXPIRATORY PRESSURE REPLACES A ONE-WAY VALVE

A one-way valve can improve speech in a patient with a tracheostomy who breathes spontaneously (see Chapter 40). Such a valve can also improve speech in a patient with InPPV; however, its use with InPPV can be dangerous. For instance, if the tracheostomy tube cuff is inflated and the valve is inadvertently left in place, the patient cannot expire. This can be lethal by causing asphyxia, by impeding

venous return, or, if the pressure-limit device fails, by rupturing the lungs. A safer approach is to add PEEP.[33] When PEEP is adequately high (Fig. 56-6), speech is indistinguishable from that produced with a one-way valve.[31]

RISKS AND BENEFITS OF VENTILATOR ADJUSTMENTS

Ventilator adjustments can have adverse effects if not properly chosen and implemented. For instance, when inspiratory time is lengthened with volume-controlled ventilation, the patient may hypoventilate while speaking, because there is more time for inspiratory flow to "bleed off." If this happens, most patients experience air hunger and intuitively stop speaking to catch their breath,[34,35] but patients with diminished chemosensitivity may be at risk. If too much of the total cycle is devoted to inspiration, the shortened expiratory time may lead to dynamic hyperinflation, especially in patients with severe obstructive airways disease. Any adjustment that excessively increases intrathoracic pressure may reduce cardiac output and impede venous return. To minimize this risk, the lowest level of PEEP adjustment that reaps adequate speech improvement should be used, and dynamic hyperinflation (intrinsic PEEP) should be assessed following any changes to the ventilator. Also, ventilator adjustments can cause patient

FIGURE 56-6 Tracheal pressure during speaking with a one-way valve and with PEEP set to 15 cmH$_2$O. (*Adapted and reprinted, with permission, from Hoit et al.*[31])

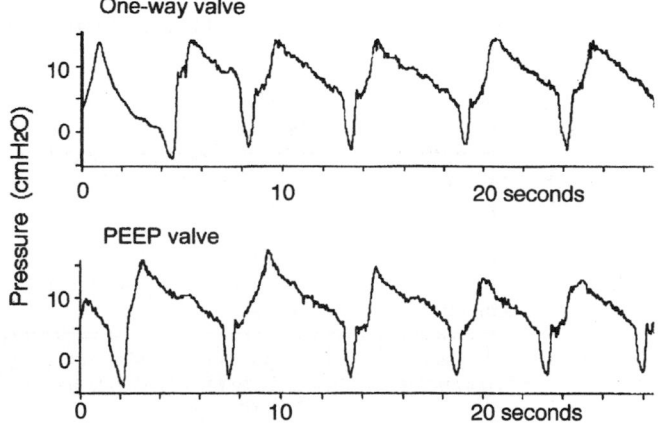

discomfort (e.g., "not enough air," or "too much pressure"). The potential for discomfort may be lessened if adjustments are made gradually and in small steps. Fortunately, most adjustments that improve speech also fortuitously improve comfort. Although there are risks to ventilator adjustments, they are usually minimal, especially when compared to the more serious risks posed by a one-way valve.

The most obvious benefits of these ventilator adjustments include improved speech, decreased speaking effort, and, in some cases, increased breathing comfort. There may be other benefits as well. For example, if a patient is chronically hyperventilated,[36] speech adjustments may move ventilation toward normal (e.g., because the patient is comfortable with a smaller tidal volume if PEEP is applied).

Clinical Scenario 2

JT, a man with a C2 spinal cord injury and InPPV, was referred to the speech-language pathologist for a speech evaluation. The evaluation revealed that JT spoke in short phrases (3–4 syllables per breath) with excessively long pauses (up to 5 seconds), and he complained that he was "interrupted all the time." The speech-language pathologist recommended to JT's pulmonologist that ventilator adjustments be tested to improve his speech. The pulmonologist agreed and wrote the order, adding that "if the ventilator adjustments can also reduce his ventilation, that would be a bonus." Ventilator adjustments were tested (with the pulmonologist, respiratory therapist, and speech-language pathologist present) and it was found that lengthened inspiratory time, a PEEP adjustment, and reduced tidal volume improved his speech dramatically. Pre- and postadjustment measures revealed a moderate increase in arterial P_{CO_2} (from 22 to 29 torr) and greater breathing comfort. The patient, his speech-language pathologist, his pulmonologist, and his family and friends were delighted with the outcome.

BEHAVIORAL INTERVENTIONS THAT CAN IMPROVE SPEECH

Once appropriate ventilator adjustments have been made, behavioral interventions, guided by a speech-language pathologist, may further improve speech (see reference 8 for extensive discussion of this topic). For example, linguis-

tic strategies may be helpful for patients who continue to have long pauses between phrases despite ventilator adjustments. These linguistic strategies might take the form of pausing at appropriate linguistic junctures (e.g., at phrase, clause, or sentence boundaries) when speaking didactically, but intentionally pausing at *in*appropriate linguistic junctures (e.g., within a phrase or following a conjunction) when speaking conversationally. When a pause occurs at an inappropriate point in conversation, the listener is less apt to interrupt the speaker (a common problem among those who are ventilator-supported). It may also be useful to teach buccal speech (i.e., "Donald Duck"-type speech) as a compensatory strategy. Such speech, which is produced entirely within the upper airway and requires no drive from chest-wall muscles,[37] can be used to add a syllable or two after the pressure has fallen below the vocalizing threshold. These are just two examples of the many behavioral strategies that a speech-language pathologist can offer a patient.

Speech with Other Forms of Ventilator Support

Whereas speech is produced during both inspiration and expiration with InPPV, it is produced only during expiration with other forms of ventilator support (see Table 56-1 and Chapters 17, 18, 19, and 62). Although research is sparse, ventilator adjustments and behavioral interventions have strong potential to improve speech produced with these other forms of ventilator support. Noninvasive positive-pressure ventilation (NPPV) and phrenic nerve pacer ventilation are discussed below as illustrations of how this might be done.

NONINVASIVE POSITIVE-PRESSURE VENTILATION

An important speech consideration when using NPPV is selection of the patient-ventilator interface. Choices for interfaces include mouthpieces, nasal pillows, nasal masks, and facemasks. Of these, the clear choice for speech breathing is a mouthpiece that is not secured to the patient's mouth. To use this interface, the patient places his lips around the mouthpiece during inspiration and pulls his lips away during expiration. Thus, the patient's face is completely unencumbered during speech production. The next best interface options are nasal interfaces, because they allow the lips and jaw to

TABLE 56-1 Summary of Speech Produced Using Different Types of Ventilator Support

Type of Ventilator Support	Speech Production	Can Ventilator Adjustments Improve Speech?	Can Behavioral Interventions Improve Speech?
Invasive positive pressure	Inspiration/expiration	Yes	Yes
Noninvasive positive pressure	Expiration	Yes	Yes
Negative pressure	Expiration	Yes	Yes
Phrenic nerve pacer	Expiration	Yes	Yes
Rocking bed	Expiration	No	Yes
Abdominal pneumobelt	Expiration	Yes	Yes

Included here are the phase(s) of the ventilator cycle during which speech is produced and whether or not ventilator adjustments and behavioral interventions have potential to improve speech.

move freely during speaking. Nevertheless, they encumber the nasal airway and can distort nasal consonants (m, n, and ng, in English). By far the least desirable interface is the facemask, because it encumbers both the oral and nasal airways. A facemask dampens and distorts the speech signal and removes essentially all of the visual cues that a listener might want to use to help compensate for reduced intelligibility.

For many patients who use NPPV, one of the best strategies for improving speech is to increase inspiratory volume. In the case of the patient with neurologically complete chest-wall paralysis, pressure (and loudness) at the beginning of expiration is determined primarily by inspiratory volume and respiratory system elastance, and the rate at which pressure drops (and loudness decreases) is determined by the rate at which volume is expended during speaking. By increasing inspiratory volume, speech can be louder (at least at the beginning of expiration) and last longer.

One way to increase inspiratory volume is to adjust the ventilator's tidal volume. Another way is to train the patient to use glossopharygneal breathing. Glossopharyngeal breathing can be effective, not only for increasing tidal volume, but also for replenishing volume (and pressure) while speaking.[38]

PHRENIC NERVE PACER VENTILATION

Speech with phrenic nerve pacer ventilation may be characterized by low loudness, fading loudness, short breath groups, and long inspiratory pauses in patients with paralysis from high cervical spinal cord injury.[39] Phrenic nerve pacers can be adjusted, within limits, to alter tidal volume, breathing frequency, and inspiratory time.[40] Such adjustments have the potential to improve speech. For example, a larger tidal volume can increase speech loudness and duration (as discussed above) and a shorter inspiratory time can reduce the degree to which speech is interrupted by inspiratory pauses.

Another way to increase tidal volume is to apply an abdominal binder.[41,42] Use of an abdominal binder or truss has been shown to improve speech in patients with chest-wall paralysis who use phrenic nerve pacers[43] as well as in those who can breathe on their own.[44,45] Speech improvements include louder speech, longer breath groups, and better voice quality. Glossopharyngeal breathing is another good strategy for increasing tidal volume in patients who use phrenic nerve pacers.

Which Patients Are Candidates for Speech Interventions?

Many of the speech interventions described in this chapter have been tested systematically in patients with neuromotor impairments who were chronically ventilated. Nevertheless, acutely ventilated patients, including those with other medical conditions, are also candidates for these interventions, especially cuff deflation. Cuff deflation and speech training are performed routinely in the post-critical respiratory care stepdown unit at Massachusetts General Hospital.

There are several issues to consider when determining if a patient is a candidate for ventilator adjustments. Most importantly, ventilator adjustments must be deemed medically safe and should not be attempted if the pulmonologist, cardiologist, or other physician judges them to be unsafe for a given patient. The patient should also have motivation to speak, functional cognitive and language skills, and adequate laryngeal and upper airway control to benefit from such adjustments.

Behavioral interventions can be even more broadly applied than ventilator adjustments. There is a vast repertoire of behavioral interventions that include strategies for improving speech intelligibility, use of augmented communication, and many others.

Important Cautions

The initial deflation of the tracheostomy tube cuff should be done in a cautious and organized manner. To begin, the patient should be advised to expect flow of air through the mouth (as many are surprised by the sensation). Before deflating the cuff, the patient's oropharynx should be suctioned thoroughly and adequate oxygen saturation should be assured. An anesthesia bag supplied by oxygen should be attached to the tracheostomy tube and, at the moment of cuff deflation, a positive-pressure breath should be given to propel secretions that lie between the larynx and cuff into the pharynx for further suctioning. This technique minimizes aspiration of the retained secretions. Patients who have had endotracheal intubation before tracheostomy are at increased risk for aspiration secondary to laryngeal dysfunction and should be evaluated by a speech-language pathologist before more than brief cuff deflation.

Although dynamic hyperinflation and intrinsic PEEP are observed rarely when inspiratory time is lengthened, it is nevertheless a risk in patients with obstructive lung disease. Positive end-expiratory intrathoracic pressure can lead to decreased cardiac output and hypotension. Cardiovascular reflexes usually compensate, but may be impaired in patients with autonomic dysfunction. These include patients with diabetes or with neurologically complete cervical spinal cord injury (particularly during the phase of spinal shock).

To help ensure patient safety, ventilator adjustments to improve speech should only be made with the approval and oversight of a pulmonologist. Furthermore, while adjustments are being made, cardiopulmonary variables should be monitored (e.g., O_2 saturation, end-tidal P_{CO_2}, heart rate, blood pressure, and intrinsic PEEP), and the patient should be systematically asked about comfort (see Chapter 55).

Alternatives to Ventilator-Supported Speech

Sometimes it is impossible for a patient to speak. When this results from severe laryngeal and/or upper airway impairment, it is usually necessary to provide the patient with augmentative and alternative communication

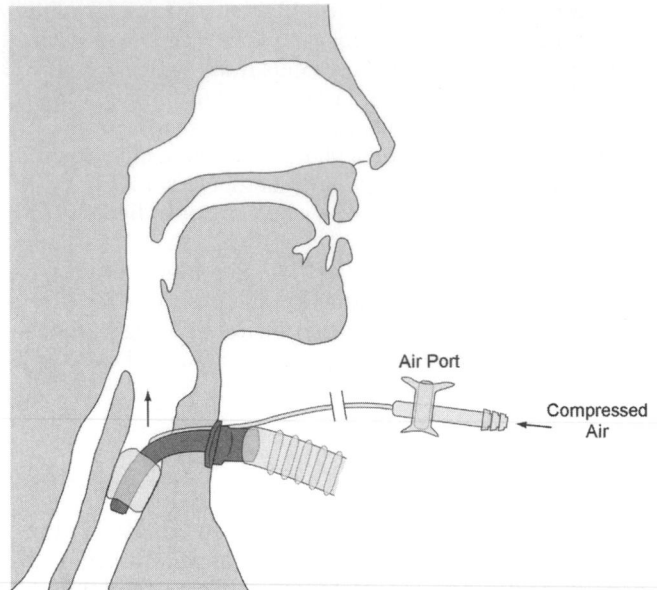

FIGURE 56-7 Talking tracheostomy tube. The air port is occluded to route flow from a compressed air source to the larynx for speaking. (*Reprinted, with permission, from Hixon and Hoit.*[8])

(see Chapter 40). Some patients, with good laryngeal and upper airway function however can benefit from a talking tracheostomy tube,[5,46,47] which provides a separate air source to produce speech while the tracheostomy tube cuff is inflated (Fig. 56-7). Flow is adjusted to determine what produces the best voice quality and is comfortable for the patient.[46,48,49] Common problems include discomfort from drying of the mucosa, crimping of the tubing, inability to vocalize, and inability to turn the air source on or off independently.[50]

Another device is called a voice tracheostomy tube.[51] The cuff on this specially constructed tracheostomy tube inflates during inspiration (preventing speech production) and deflates during expiration. Thus, nearly all of the ventilator-delivered inspiration reaches the patient's lungs, whereas some of the expired air can be used for speaking. This device may be useful for patients with poor laryngeal control, but most patients can speak using a conventional tracheostomy tube with a deflated cuff and some form of volume compensation.

Roles of Health Care Professionals

Speech management for patients who are ventilator-supported requires a team of health care professionals. Pulmonary/critical care physicians and respiratory therapists operating under them can make substantial improvements in speech. Speech-language pathologists can further optimize speech by evaluating speech, language, and communication, and recommending a management plan to the medical team. If evaluation or management includes ventilator adjustments, it is important for a physician or suitable proxy to be present to assess cardiopulmonary effects of the ad-justments as they are made. The physician in charge must decide whether such adjustments should be made permanently or only when essential for communication. Behavioral interventions (such as glossopharyngeal breathing and linguistic strategies) can be offered by the speech-language pathologist.

Important Unknowns and Future Research

Research on ventilator-supported speech has largely been limited to patients with spinal cord injury and neuromuscular disease. Much needs to be learned about the influence of ventilator adjustments on speech in other patients, especially those with obstructive airways disease. The speech effects of ventilator adjustments with certain forms of ventilator support (such as NPPV) and various behavioral interventions also have yet to be studied systematically.

Summary and Conclusions

For most people, speech is an important requisite to good quality of life. Thus, a patient should be given the opportunity to speak, if medically possible. For the patient who is ventilated invasively, this means deflating the tracheostomy tube cuff. For the patient who is already able to speak, there are often ways to improve speech by modifying the tracheal pressure. Ventilation requirements always have primacy over speech improvements, but these are often complementary, rather than competing, goals. A patient's speech can be optimized through the collaborative efforts of competent and creative physicians, respiratory therapists, and speech-language pathologists.

Acknowledgments

This chapter is dedicated to the late Susan Kropoff, who used a ventilator for nearly 40 years, and who has taught us more about ventilator-supported speech than anyone else we know. We are grateful to Thomas J. Hixon and Robert W. Lansing for their helpful suggestions on this chapter.

References

1. Bach JR. Amyotrophic lateral sclerosis: Communication status and survival with ventilatory support. Am J Phys Med Rehabil 1982; 72:343–9.
2. Silverstein MD, Stocking CB, Antel JP, et al. Amyotrophic lateral sclerosis and life-sustaining therapy: Patients' desires for information, participation in decision making, and life-sustaining therapy. Mayo Clin Proc 1991; 66:906–13.
3. Wang TG, Bach JR, Avilla C, et al. Survival of individuals with spinal muscular atrophy on ventilatory support. Am J Phys Med Rehabil 1994; 73:207–11.

4. Nelson JE, Meier DE, Oei EJ, et al. Self-reported symptom experience of critically ill cancer patients receiving intensive care. Crit Care Med 2001; 29:277–82.

5. Lohmeier HL, Hoit JD. Ventilator-supported communication: A survey of ventilator users. J Med Speech-Lang Pathol 2003; 11:61–72.

6. Hoit JD, Banzett RB, Brown R. Improving Ventilator-Supported Speech. TELEROUNDS #39 Live Satellite Transmission. National Center for Communication Disorders, Tucson, AZ, December 10, 1997 (videotape available).

7. Hixon TJ, Abbs JH. Normal speech production. In: Hixon TJ, Shriberg LD, Saxman JH, editors. Introduction to communication disorders. Englewood Cliffs, NJ: Prentice-Hall, 1980:42–87.

8. Hixon TJ, Hoit JD. Evaluation and management of speech breathing disorders: Principles and Methods. Tucson, AZ: Redington Brown, 2005.

9. Louden RG, Lee L, Holcomb BJ. Volumes and breathing patterns during speech in healthy and asthmatic subjects. J Speech Hear Res 1988; 31:219–27.

10. Lee L, Louden RG, Jacobson BH, et al. Speech breathing in patients with lung disease. Am Rev Respir Dis 1993; 147:1199–206.

11. Solomon NP, Hixon TJ. Speech breathing in Parkinson's disease. J Speech Hear Res 1993; 36:294–310.

12. McFarland DH. Respiratory markers of conversational interaction. J Speech Lang Hear Res 2001; 44:128–43.

13. Bailey EF, Hoit JD. Speaking and breathing in high respiratory drive. J Speech Lang Hear Res 2002; 45:89–99.

14. Winkworth AL, Davis PJ, Ellis E, et al. Variability and consistency in speech breathing during reading: Lung volumes, speech intensity, and linguistic factors. J Speech Hear Res 1994; 37:535–56.

15. Winkworth AL, Davis PJ, Adams RD, et al. Breathing patterns during spontaneous speech. J Speech Hear Res 1995; 38:124–44.

16. Sperry EE, Klich RJ. Speech breathing in senescent and younger women during oral reading. J Speech Hear Res 1992; 35:1246–55.

17. Mitchell HL, Hoit JD, Watson PJ. Cognitive-linguistic demands and speech breathing. J Speech Hear Res 1996; 39:93–104.

18. Bunn JC, Mead J. Control of ventilation during speech. J Appl Physiol 1971; 31:870–2.

19. Doust JH, Patrick JM. The limitation of exercise ventilation during speech. Respir Physiol 1981; 46:137–47.

20. Hixon TJ, Goldman MD, Mead J. Kinematics of the chest wall during speech production: Volume displacements of the rib cage, abdomen, and lung. J Speech Hear Res 1973; 16:78–115.

21. Netsell RW. Subglottal and intraoral air pressures during the intervocalic contrast of /t/ and /d/. Phonetica 1969; 20:68–73.

22. Murry T, Brown WS. Subglottal air pressure during two types of vocal activity: Vocal fry and modal phonation. Folia Phoniatrica 1971; 23:440–9.

23. Bouhuys A, Proctor DF, Mead J. Kinetic aspects of singing. J Appl Physiol 1966; 21:483–96.

24. Hixon TJ, Mead J, Goldman MD. Dynamics of the chest wall during speech production: Function of the thorax, rib cage, diaphragm, and abdomen. J Speech Hear Res 1976; 19:297–356.

25. Draper MH, Ladefoged P, Whitteridge D. Expiratory pressures and air flow during speech. British Med J 1960; 1:1837–43.

26. Lieberman P, Knudson R, Mead J. Determination of the rate of change of fundamental frequency with respect to subglottal pressure during sustained phonation. J Acoust Soc Am 1969; 45:1537–43.

27. Hoit JD, Banzett RB. Simple adjustments can improve ventilator-supported speech. Am J Speech-Lang Pathol 1997; 6:87–96.

28. Bach JR, Alba AS. Trachestomy ventilation: A study of efficacy with deflated cuffs and cuffless tubes. Chest 1990; 97:679–83.

29. Tippett DC, Siebens AA. Preserving oral communication in individuals with tracheostomy and ventilator dependency. Am J Speech-Lang Pathol 1995; 4:55–61.

30. Hoit JD, Shea SA, Banzett RB. Speech production during mechanical ventilation in tracheostomized individuals. J Speech Hearing Res 1994; 37:53–63.

31. Hoit JD, Banzett RB, Lohmeier HL, et al. Clinical ventilator adjustments that improve speech. Chest 2003; 124:1512–21.

32. Prigent H, Samuel C, Louis B, et al. Comparative effects of two ventilatory modes on speech in tracheostomized patients with neuromuscular disease. Am J Respir Crit Care Med 2003; 167:114–9.

33. Hoit JD, Banzett RB. Je peux parler! Am J Respir Crit Care Med 2003; 167:101–2.

34. Banzett RB, Lansing RW, Reid MB, et al. 'Air hunger' arising from increased PCO_2 in mechanically ventilated quadriplegics. Respir Physiol 1989; 76:53–67.

35. Shea SA, Hoit JD, Banzett RB. Competition between gas exchange and speech production in ventilated patients. Bio Psychol 1998; 49:9–27.

36. Bach JR, Haber II, Wang TG, et al. Alveolar ventilation as a function of ventilatory support method. Eur J Phys Med Rehabil 1995; 5:80–4.

37. Weinberg B, Westerhouse J. A study of buccal speech. J Speech Hear Res 1971; 14:652–8.

38. Hixon TJ, Putnam AHB, Sharp JT. Speech production with flaccid paralysis of the rib cage, diaphragm, and abdomen. J Speech Hear Dis 1983; 48:315–27.

39. Hoit JD, Shea SA. Speech production and speech with a phrenic nerve pacer. Am J Speech-Lang Pathol 1996; 5:53–60.

40. Creasy G, Elefteriades J, DiMarco A, et al. Electrical stimulation to restore respiration. J Rehabil Res Dev 1996; 33:123–32.

41. Danon J, Druz WS, Goldberg NB, et al. Function of the isolated paced diaphragm and the cervical accessory muscles in C1 quadriplegics. Am Rev Respir Dis 1979; 119:909–19.

42. Strohl KP, Mead J, Banzett RB, et al. Effect of posture on upper and lower rib cage motion and tidal volume during diaphragm pacing. Am Rev Respir Dis 1984; 130:320–1.

43. Hoit JD, Banzett RB, Brown R. Binding the abdomen can improve speech in men with phrenic nerve pacers. Am J Speech-Lang Pathol 2002; 11:71–6.

44. Sataloff RT, Heur RJ, O'Connor M. Rehabilitation of a quadriplegic professional singer. Arch Otolaryngol 1984; 110:682–5.

45. Watson PJ, Hixon TJ. Effects of abdominal trussing on breathing and speech in men with cervical spinal cord injury. J Speech Lang Hear Res 2001; 44:751–62.

46. Kluin KJ, Maynard F, Bogdasarian RS. The patient requiring mechanical ventilatory support: Use of the cuffed tracheostomy "talk" tube to establish phonation. Otolaryngol Head Neck Surg 1984; 92:625–7.

47. Sparker AW, Robbins KT, Nevlud GN, et al. A prospective evaluation of speaking tracheostomy tubes for ventilator dependent patients. Laryngoscope 1987; 97:89–92.

48. Safer P, Grenvik A. Speaking cuffed tracheostomy tube. Crit Care Med 1975; 3:23–6.

49. Leder SB, Traquina DN: Voice intensity of patients using a Communi-Trach I® cuffed speaking tracheostomy tube. Laryngoscope 1989; 99:744–7.

50. Tippett DC, Vogelman L. Communication, tracheostomy and ventilator dependency. In: Tippett DC, editor. Tracheostomy and ventilator dependency: Management of breathing, speaking, and swallowing. New York: Thieme, 2000: 93–142.

51. Nomori H. Tracheostomy tube enabling speech during mechanical ventilation. Chest 2004; 125:1046–51.

SLEEP IN THE VENTILATED PATIENT

PATRICK J. HANLY

It is well recognized that sleep is abnormal in mechanically ventilated patients in the intensive care unit (ICU). Although this has been described for decades, there is still no consensus on the underlying pathogenesis and the best way to manage it. Moreover, the assumption that abnormal sleep is not good for patients who are critically ill is based primarily on extrapolation from models of sleep loss and sleep disruption in other patient populations and not on evidence that abnormal sleep affects the clinical outcomes of patients in the ICU. Nevertheless, there is growing interest in this topic as the technology to measure sleep evolves and new ways are sought to improve patients' ability to recover from their critical illness. This chapter outlines the current understanding of the causes and potential consequences of sleep disruption in ventilated patients and how this may be further researched and treated.

Normal Sleep

Sleep is objectively assessed by means of polysomnography, the simultaneous recording of several electroencephalographic and physiologic parameters.[1] Sleep periods are classified as non–rapid eye movement (NREM) and rapid eye movement (REM) sleep. NREM sleep is further subdivided into four stages, with stages 3 and 4 also referred to as slow-wave sleep (SWS). Each sleep stage is recognized by characteristic changes on the electroencephalogram and, in addition, REM sleep has distinctive, intermittent rapid eye movements. During normal sleep, periods of NREM and REM alternate throughout the night in a recognizable pattern, so that most SWS occurs during the first half of the night and most REM sleep occurs during the second half (Fig. 57-1). The "normal" duration of sleep required and the proportion of time spent in each stage of sleep depends on many factors including age and genotype.[2] In healthy, middle-aged individuals, however, nocturnal sleep lasts 7–8 hours, and 5–10% of that time is spent in stage 1 NREM sleep, 50% in stage 2 NREM sleep, 15–20% in SWS, and 25% in REM sleep.[1] There are also standardized electroencephalographic criteria for identifying arousals and awakenings on the polysomnograph;[3,4] up to 10 arousals per hour of sleep is considered to be within normal limits.[5] The term *sleep architecture* refers to the amount of time spent in each sleep stage and *sleep disruption* is reflected by an increased frequency of arousals and awakenings.

Sleep in the Intensive Care Unit

PATIENT PERCEPTION

When questioned after discharge from the ICU, patients consistently report sleep disruption during their stay.[6–10] In one study,[10] 200 patients from four different ICUs received questionnaires that evaluated the quality of their sleep at home and in the ICU and the effect of noise and a variety of activities (such as nursing interventions, phlebotomy, and diagnostic procedures) on their sleep quality. Sleep quality in the ICU was perceived as significantly poorer than sleep quality at home. In addition, sleep quality did not change significantly over the course of the ICU admission, and no differences were reported between ICUs or between ventilated and nonventilated patients. Ventilated patients, however, reported greater daytime sleepiness, perhaps because of the greater administration of sedatives or more severe illness. Patients selected the recording of vital signs and phlebotomy as the most sleep-disrupting environmental factors. Noise was not rated as the primary cause of sleep disruption; of the many forms of environmental noise stimuli, however, communication between staff members and telemetry alarms were perceived as the most disruptive. Although very thorough in design and statistical analysis, the study was limited by potential recall bias, lack of objective sleep assessment by polysomnography, and the absence of a control group.

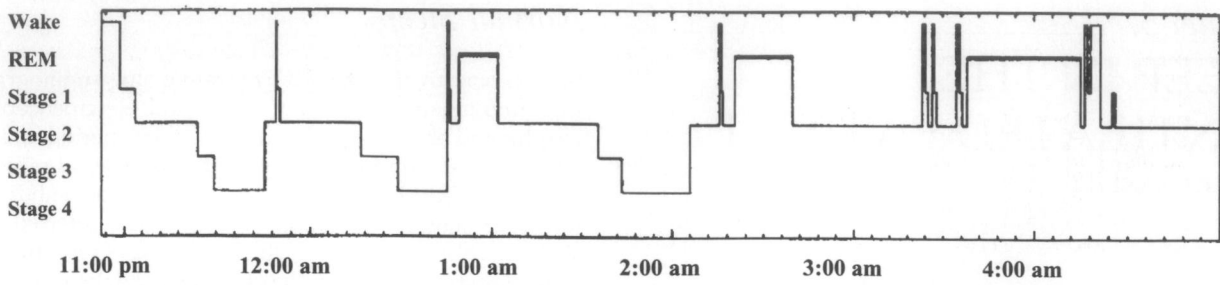

FIGURE 57-1 Normal sleep (nocturnal hypnogram). *Vertical axis: REM*, rapid eye movement sleep; *NREM*, non–rapid eye movement sleep stages 1, 2, 3 and 4. *Horizontal axis:* time in hours.

POLYSOMNOGRAPHY

Since the mid-1970s, numerous polysomnographic studies in ICU patients have consistently revealed both sleep fragmentation and sleep loss.[6,11–18] Hilton[6] studied nonventilated patients by 24-hour polysomnography and found a decreased total sleep time, an increase in stage 1 NREM sleep, and a concomitant decrease in SWS and REM sleep. Hilton also observed an apparent uncoupling of sleep from the day-night circadian pattern: only 50–60% of sleep occurred at night.[6] These characteristic sleep patterns have

also been observed in subsequent 24-hour polysomnography studies.[11,15]

Cooper et al investigated sleep in ventilated patients in the ICU and categorized patients into three groups based on polysomnographic findings: disrupted sleep, atypical sleep, and coma.[11] As seen in other ICU cohorts, patients in the disrupted sleep group (Fig. 57-2) showed the abnormal temporal distribution of sleep described earlier as well as reduced amounts of SWS and REM sleep and an increased frequency of arousals and awakenings. Patients in the atypical sleep group had EEG features intermediate between

FIGURE 57-2 Disrupted sleep in the ICU (24-hour hypnograms in 8 patients). *Vertical axis: REM*, rapid eye movement sleep; *NREM*, non–rapid eye movement sleep stages 1, 2, 3 and 4. *Horizontal axis:* time in hours. Note (1) sleep was distributed throughout the 24-hour period in all patients except patient 8, in whom sleep was predominantly nocturnal; (2) frequent awakenings; and (3) prolonged wakefulness, especially patients 4, 5, and 6. (*Reproduced, with permission, from Cooper et al.[11]*)

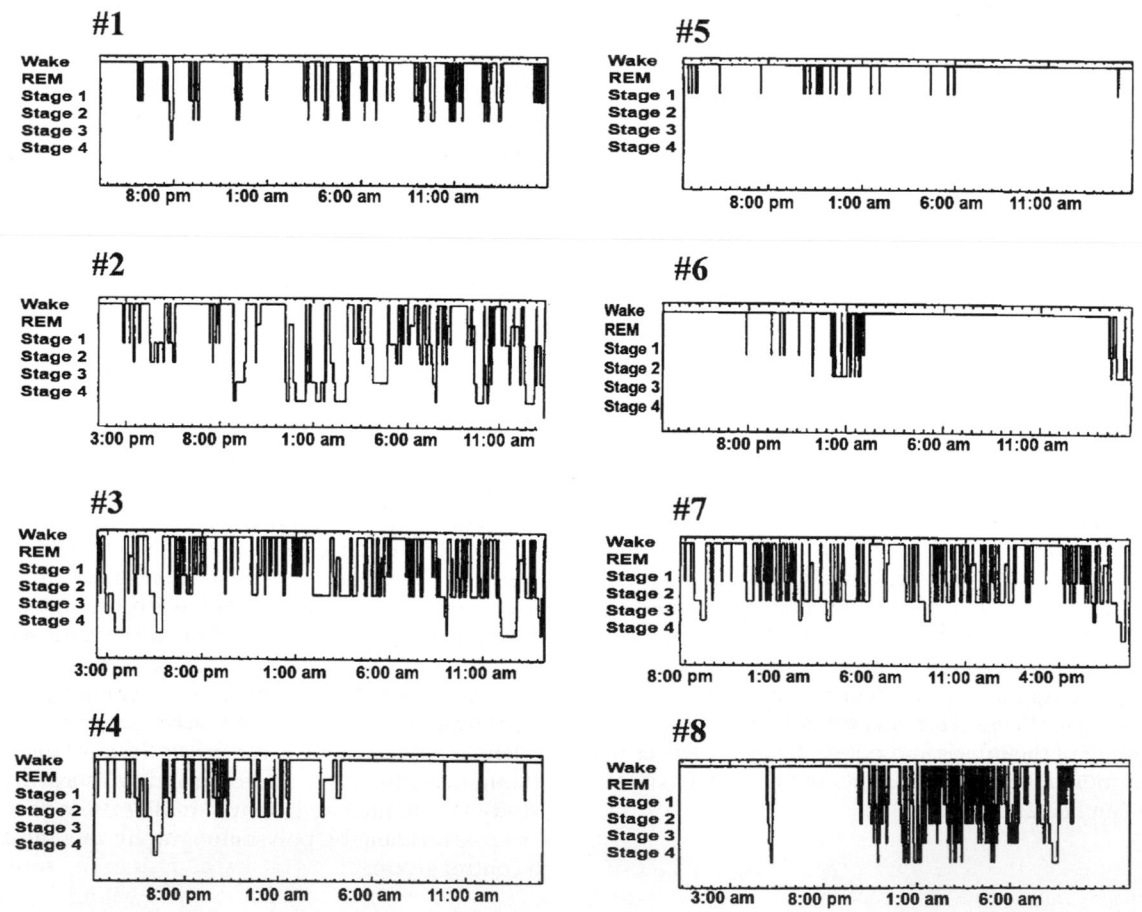

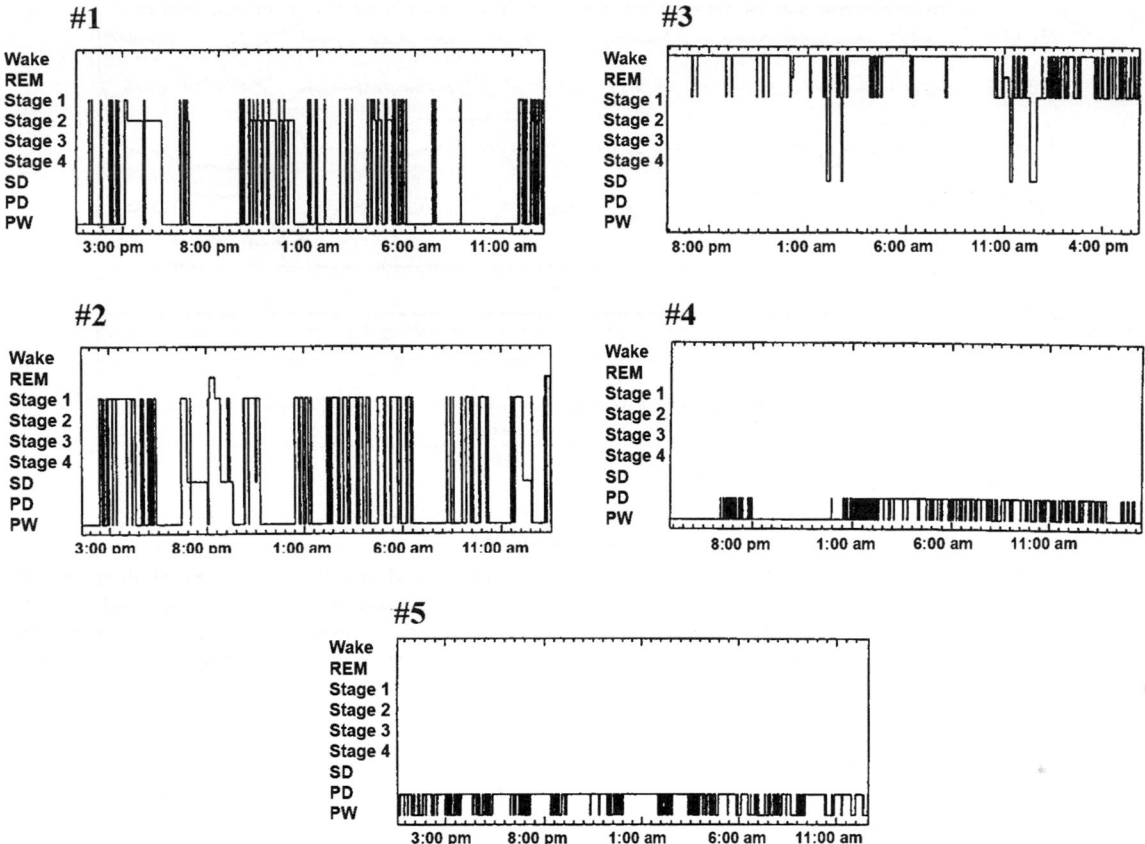

FIGURE 57-3 Atypical sleep in the ICU (24-hour hypnograms in 5 patients). *Vertical axis: REM,* rapid eye movement sleep; *NREM,* non–rapid eye movement sleep stages 1, 2, 3, and 4; sleep delta (*SD*); pathological delta (*PW*); and pathological wakefulness (*PW*). *Horizontal axis:* time in hours. (*Reproduced, with permission, from Cooper et al.*[11])

sleep and coma, characterized by a virtual absence of stage 2 NREM sleep and REM sleep (Fig. 57-3). In addition, patients displayed "pathological wakefulness," where behavioral correlates of wakefulness (such as saccadic eye movements and sustained chin muscle activity) coincided with EEG features of SWS (Fig. 57-4). The coma group was characterized by EEG features of coma according to the classification of Young et al.[19] The authors concluded that sleep could not be identified by polysomnography in all critically ill patients. They proposed the following criteria to select ICU patients in whom sleep can be reliably measured by polysomnography: acute physiology score <13, Glasgow Coma Scale score >10, and sedative doses of lorazepam equivalents and morphine equivalents <10 μg/kg per hour. These cutoffs approximated the point estimate of the atypical sleep group. Subsequent data suggest that sleep disruption can be measured by polysomnography in approximately 50% of patients in a general ICU.[20]

Causes of Sleep Disruption in the Intensive Care Unit

MEDICAL DISORDERS

Patients may enter the ICU with pre-existing medical or sleep disorders, such as asthma or sleep apnea, which cause disruption of sleep if inadequately controlled. More importantly, the acute illness that precipitated the ICU admission, such as major surgery, can disrupt sleep. A very consistent finding in surgical patients is the reduction or absence of both SWS and REM sleep in the immediate postoperative period. This is characteristically followed by "REM rebound," an increase in both the number of phasic eye movements and the overall amount of REM sleep.[12,14,17,18] REM rebound may result from the withdrawal of REM-suppressing medications, such as narcotics,[17] analgesics, and benzodiazepines,[21] and/or a decrease in illness-related sleep disruptors such as pain.

MEDICATIONS

Several medications can alter sleep. A comprehensive review of this topic has been published.[21,22] Table 57-1 summarizes the effects of some medications that are commonly used in the ICU. Although benzodiazepines can increase total sleep time, they are known to reduce both SWS and REM sleep and are associated with rebound insomnia once they are stopped.[23] Opiates also decrease SWS and REM sleep, increase the amount of wakefulness after sleep onset, and are associated with withdrawal hypersomnolence.[21,23,24] Glucocorticoids are often associated with insomnia[22] and many selective serotonin reuptake inhibitors increase alertness and restlessness, in addition to exacerbating sleep disorders

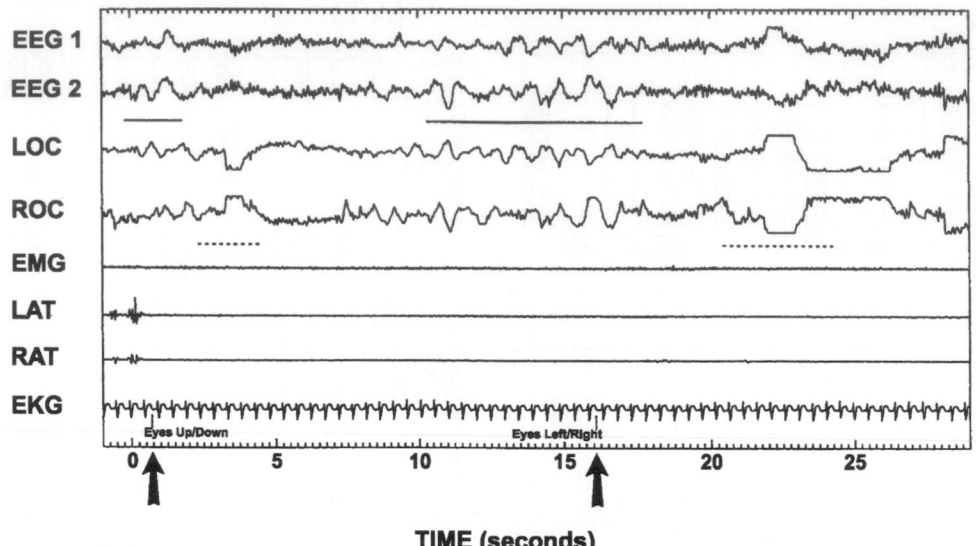

TIME (seconds)

FIGURE 57-4 Pathological wakefulness during atypical sleep (30-second epoch). *Vertical axis: EEG,* electroencephalogram; *LOC,* left oculogram; *ROC,* right oculogram; *EMG,* submental electromyogram; *LAT,* left anterior tibialis EMG; *RAT,* right anterior tibialis EMG; *EKG,* electrocardiogram. *Horizontal axis:* time in seconds. Note the slow-wave EEG activity (indicated by the solid horizontal bar) during the patient's responses (eye movements, indicated by broken horizontal lines) to biocalibration (indicated by a bold arrow). (*Reproduced, with permission, from Cooper et al.[11]*)

such as restless legs syndrome and periodic limb movement disorder.[25]

ALTERED CIRCADIAN RHYTHM

Almost all biological functions have a circadian rhythm, which synchronizes interactions both among themselves and with the external environment. Alteration of the circa-

dian rhythm that regulates sleep and wakefulness is a recognized cause of insomnia in patients who are not critically ill[26] and may contribute to sleep disruption in the ICU. The circadian clock has been evaluated in critically ill patients by measuring either core body temperature or melatonin levels in the blood or urine. Two retrospective studies, which measured core body temperature, found that circadian

TABLE 57-1 Effects of Medications on Sleep

Medication	Clinical Effects	Changes on Polysomnography
CNS medications		
Narcotics	Varies with agent; withdrawal hypersomnolence	Acute: ↑WASO, ↓SWS, ↓REM
Benzodiazepines	Sedation, withdrawal insomnia	↑TST, ↓SL, ↓W, ↓SWS, ↓REM
Tricyclic antidepressants	Improve sleep; may be sedating	Generally ↑TST, ↓W, ↓REM
Selective serotonin reuptake inhibitors	May worsen sleep; few daytime complaints	Generally ↓TST, ↑W, ↓REM
Barbiturates	Sedation, withdrawal insomnia	↑TST, ↓W, ↑↓SWS, ↓REM
Phenytoin	Sedation	↓SL
Carbamazepine	Sedation	?↓SL and ↑TST
Cardiac medications		
β-Antagonists	Insomnia, nightmares	↑W, ↓REM
α₂-Agonists (clonidine, methyldopa)	Insomnia, nightmares, sedation	↑TST, ↑↓REM
α-β-Antagonists	Insomnia, fatigue, somnolence	No studies
Diltiazem	Insomnia, abnormal dreams, sleepiness	No studies
Amiodarone	Insomnia, nightmares	No studies
Other medications		
Aspirin	—	Acute: ↓SWS
Glucocorticoids	Insomnia	↑W, ↓REM
Theophylline	Insomnia	↑W, ↓TST

ABBREVIATIONS: REM, rapid eye movement sleep; SL, sleep latency; SWS, slow wave sleep; TST, total sleep time; W, wakefulness; WASO, wakefulness after sleep onset.
SOURCE: Adapted, with permission, from Wooten[21] and Schweitzer.[22]

rhythm was absent in 20–80% of patients.[27,28] More recently, Gazendam et al[29] recorded core body temperature in 21 patients and reported that a 24-hour rhythm was detectable in all patients. The rhythm, however, was advanced or delayed by several hours compared with control subjects, and the degree of displacement was correlated with the severity of illness, reflected by Acute Physiology, Age, and Chronic Health Evaluation (APACHE) 3 scores. Several studies have measured melatonin levels in ICU patients.[30–34] Melatonin is secreted by the pineal gland and its release is closely synchronized with sleep in healthy individuals;[35] it starts to rise between 9 and 11 PM, peaks between 1 and 3 AM, and falls to low baseline values between 7 and 9 AM. The characteristic nocturnal rise in melatonin is absent in critically ill patients and this has been correlated with the use of mechanical ventilation,[33,34] sepsis,[32] and the postoperative period.[31] Although altered circadian rhythm may contribute to sleep disruption in the ICU, this has yet to be proven. Moreover, the extent of its role is likely to vary among individual patients depending on factors such as the ICU environment, illness severity, the length of stay, and the impact of competing sources of sleep disruption.

INTENSIVE CARE UNIT ENVIRONMENT

Several studies have examined the role of light, patient-care activities, and noise in causing sleep disruption in the ICU.[36–42] Meyer et al[40] found that circadian light levels were maintained in the ICU, and modern ICUs minimize light intensity at nighttime. Consequently, light does not appear to be a significant source of sleep disruption. Nursing interventions occur at least hourly in the ICU[40] (Fig. 57-5), and have been associated with arousals.[12] The presence of excessive noise in the ICU has been thoroughly documented.[36,39–42] Aaron et al observed a strong correlation between the number of sound peaks of >80 A-weighted decibels and arousals from sleep in a group of ICU patients.[41] Balogh et al reported that alarms were the most irritating noise, and observed that even during the night, the longest "quiet" interval was only 22 minutes.[39]

Another investigative approach has been to simulate the noisy ICU environment in a controlled setting such as a sleep laboratory. Exposure of healthy subjects in a sleep laboratory to recorded ICU noise induced sleep disruption similar to that observed in patients in the ICU.[37,37,38,42] These studies in the ICU and sleep research laboratory led to the assumption that sleep disruption in the ICU was predominantly caused by noise and patient-care activities. The ICU studies, however, did not include simultaneous monitoring of noise and arousals. Consequently, the association was, at best, indirect. Furthermore, the simulated ICU environment is limited by the fact that it evaluates the impact of noise in isolation without the interaction of other competing sleep disruptors that are found in the ICU. Consequently, the role of the ICU environment, specifically noise and patient-care activities, were reassessed. Freedman et al,[43] using polysomnography and time-synchronized recording of environmental noise, directly linked noise to arousals. They determined that noise was responsible for only 15% of all

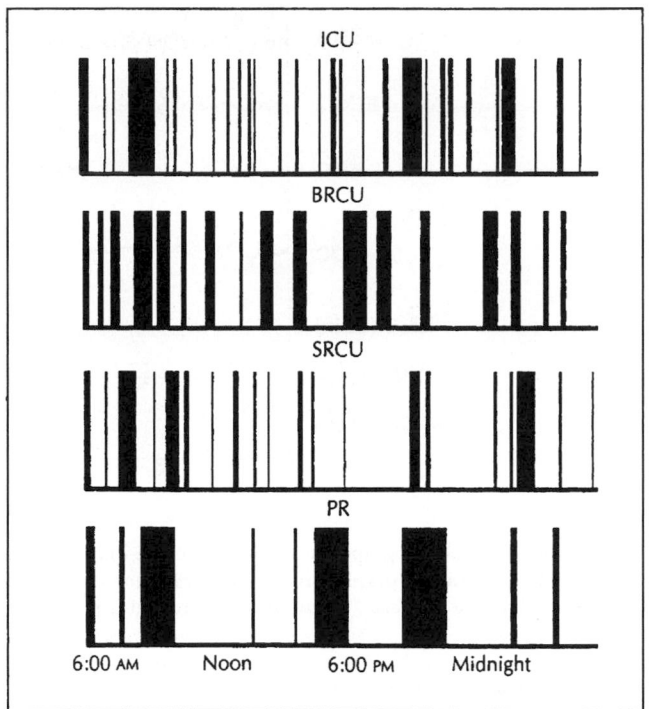

FIGURE 57-5 Patient interruptions by staff over 24 hours in four areas: a three-bed medical ICU, a three-bed respiratory care unit (*BRCU*), a single respiratory care unit room (*SRCU*), and a private room (*PR*) on a general medical floor. The dark areas represent interruptions and the clear areas represent time available for sleep. (*Reproduced, with permission, from Meyer et al.[40]*)

arousals and awakenings. Although it was the first study to demonstrate that common noise elevations directly cause arousals in ICU patients, other environmental factors such as patient-care activities were not assessed.

Gabor et al subsequently evaluated the contribution of the ICU environment to sleep disruption in both ventilated patients and healthy subjects, and also evaluated the effectiveness of a noise-reduction strategy (moving the subject from the open ICU to a single room).[44] They performed comprehensive, synchronized monitoring of sleep polysomnography, noise (calibrated sound meter), and all patient-care activities (audio-visual recording) for 24 hours. Although loud noise and frequent patient-care activities were prevalent in the ICU environment, they were only responsible for <30% of the observed sleep disruption (Fig. 57-6). Healthy individuals slept relatively well in this potentially disruptive environment. Although noise accounted for a significant proportion of sleep disruption in this group, its extent was not pathologic. A quantitative improvement in sleep quality was observed as a result of noise reduction; however, there was no change in sleep architecture. The cause of 68% of arousals and awakenings in these mechanically ventilated patients could not be attributed to noise or any patient-care activity (Table 57-2).

MECHANICAL VENTILATION

In addition to the noise associated with ventilators and their alarms, mechanical ventilation can disrupt sleep by

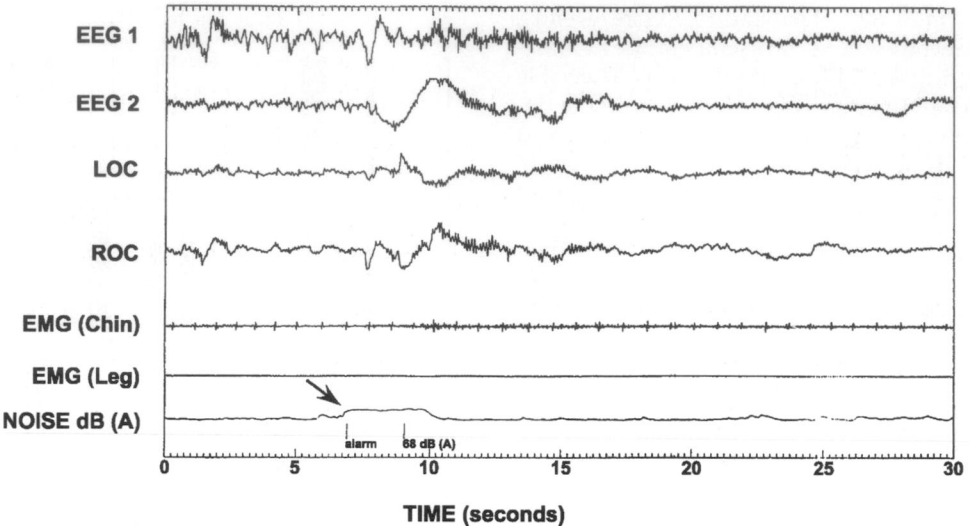

FIGURE 57-6 Polysomnographic example of a noise-induced arousal. *Vertical axis: EEG,* electroencephalogram; *LOC,* left oculogram; *ROC,* right oculogram; *EMG,* electromyogram. *Horizontal axis:* time in seconds. Arrow indicates abrupt increase in noise (68 A-weighted decibels) caused by an alarm, followed by an arousal from stage 2 non-REM sleep. *(Reproduced, with permission, from Gabor et al.[44])*

producing periodic breathing with recurrent central apneas, or through the development of patient-ventilator dyssynchrony. Recurrent central apneas occur when the ventilator assist is excessive relative to the patient's ventilatory demand.[45] This is most likely to occur during sleep when demand is lowest.

Dyssynchrony occurs when cycling of the ventilator is not in phase with the patient's efforts. Thus the ventilator may be delivering gas when the patient wants to exhale, and vice versa. This dyssynchrony is common during conventional mechanical ventilation. Leung et al found that 28% of patients' inspiratory efforts occur during the ventilator's expiratory phase (ineffective efforts).[46] When one considers that ineffective efforts are the most extreme form of dyssynchrony, the incidence of less extreme forms of dyssynchrony (e.g., excessive delay in triggering or in cycling off the ventilator) may be even more common. In awake individuals, such dyssynchrony is very uncomfortable. It would, therefore, seem reasonable to expect dyssynchrony to result in arousals from sleep. The investigation of patient-ventilator dyssynchrony as a source of sleep disruption has received scant attention. Subjectively, 30% of patients in an ICU reported "agony/panic" during mechanical ventilation, which was associated with difficulties to synchronize the patients' breathing with the ventilator.[47]

A recent study that investigated the impact of ventilator mode on sleep in the ICU[48] reported a higher frequency of arousals and awakenings during pressure-support ventilation versus assist-control ventilation (79 ± 7 versus 54 ± 7 per hour) in 11 critically ill patients (Fig. 57-7). Six patients, with underlying heart failure, had a high frequency of central apnea (53 ± 8 per hour) during pressure-support ventilation, which was reduced (to 4 ± 2) by the addition of dead space (which eliminated the central apneas by increasing ventilatory demand). The decrease in central apneas was accompanied by a fall in the frequency of arousals and awakenings (83 ± 12 to 44 ± 6 per hour). The very high frequency of arousals and awakenings, particularly during pressure-support ventilation, supports the notion that patient-ventilator dyssynchrony is an important source of sleep disruption in the ICU, and that it can be influenced by the mode of mechanical ventilation.

Potential Consequences of Sleep Disruption

Sleep is a biological requirement for survival, which has been well documented in laboratory animals.[49,50] Prolonged sleep-deprivation experiments (5–9 days) in healthy

TABLE 57-2 Impact of Noise and Patient-Care Activities on Sleep Disruption

Event Type	Number per Hour of Sleep	Percentage Causing Disruption	Percentage of Total Disruption
Sound	36.5 ± 20.1	11.7 ± 8.3	20.9 ± 11.3
Family visits	0.7 ± 0.7	38.6 ± 39.3	1.0 ± 1.3
RT/physio	0.4 ± 0.5	30.7 ± 32.6	0.5 ± 0.7
Suctioning	0.2 ± 0.8	62.5 ± 47.9	0.6 ± 0.8
RN visits	3.5 ± 1.8	21.7 ± 11.6	4.1 ± 3.5
Assess vitals	0.3 ± 0.4	51.4 ± 34.4	0.7 ± 0.9
Med admin	2.7 ± 3.1	49.4 ± 25.6	0.9 ± 1.0
All medical care	7.8 ± 4.2	17.7 ± 5.4	7.1 ± 4.4
Apparatus/tech	1.1 ± 1.0	21.6 ± 26.3	1.4 ± 1.8
Unidentifiable	—	—	68.1 ± 9.7

ABBREVIATIONS: Apparatus/tech, noise from the sleep/environmental monitoring equipment or actions by the attending research assistant; Med admin, administering medication to a patient; RT/physio, any care provided by a respiratory therapist or physiotherapist; RN visits, any care provided by a nurse; Sound, sound peaks.
SOURCE: Reproduced, with permission, from Gabor et al.[44]

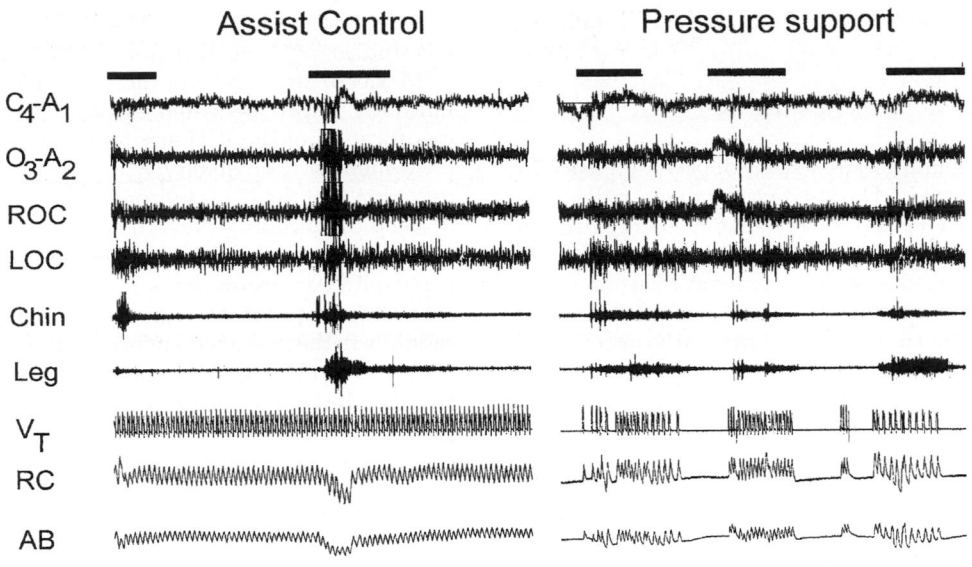

FIGURE 57-7 Sleep disruption during mechanical ventilation. Polysomnographic tracings during assist-control ventilation and pressure-support ventilation in a single patient. Electroencephalogram (*C4 − A1, O3 − A2*), electro-oculogram (*ROC, LOC*), electromyograms (chin and leg), integrated tidal volume (*VT*), rib-cage (*RC*) and abdominal (*AB*) excursions on respiratory inductance plethysmography. Arousals and awakenings, indicated by horizontal bars, were more numerous during pressure-support than during assist-control ventilation. (*Reproduced, with permission, from Parthasarathy et al.[48]*)

subjects have produced marked cognitive impairment,[51] some objective neurologic signs,[52,53] and collapse requiring hospitalization.[54] In addition, there are four specific areas in which sleep disruption can adversely affect the clinical outcome of patients in the ICU.

INTENSIVE CARE UNIT PSYCHOSIS

This refers to a state of delirium that characteristically starts after admission to the ICU.[55,56] Delirium is estimated to occur in 19% of patients in the ICU.[55] The pathogenesis is multifactorial, but includes sleep disruption associated with the patient's acute illness.[57] In addition, the rebound of REM sleep referred to earlier can be associated with delirium and nightmares. Persistence of this altered mental state impairs the ability of patients to interact with their caregivers, and can increase morbidity and delay weaning from the ventilator and discharge from the ICU.[56–58]

REBOUND OF RAPID EYE MOVEMENT SLEEP

During REM sleep, heart rate, respiration, and blood pressure are highly variable[1] and can exhibit transient irregularities, making REM sleep, and more specifically REM rebound, potentially dangerous to a recuperating critically ill patient. It has been hypothesized that REM rebound, with associated episodes of hypoxemia, variable blood pressure, and cardiac arrhythmias, may play a role in the etiology of postoperative myocardial ischemia and

infarction.[14,17,18] This is supported by the observation that REM rebound peaks at approximately the same time that these delayed complications of anesthesia and surgery occur most frequently.[17] This cardiovascular instability has particular relevance in patients who have significant vascular comorbidities.

DELAYED LIBERATION FROM MECHANICAL VENTILATION

Studies in healthy volunteers and animal models have shown that sleep deprivation can cause negative nitrogen balance,[49,59] decreased respiratory muscle endurance,[60] and a blunted genioglossus electromyogram response to carbon dioxide, which became more severe with advancing age.[61] Other investigators have reported decreased ventilatory responsiveness to hypoxemia and hypercapnia[62–64] and increased upper airway compliance[65] following sleep deprivation. The combination of decreased central drive and reduced respiratory muscle endurance can be further aggravated by the fact that sleep deprivation is associated with increased oxygen consumption and carbon dioxide production.[66] Weaning difficulty is related to inability of respiratory muscles to cope with the demands imposed by ventilatory requirements and mechanical load.[67–69] Consequently, the consequences of sleep disruption (decreased respiratory muscle endurance and increased metabolic rate, and hence, ventilatory requirements) may delay weaning, particularly in patients who have limited respiratory reserve.

HOST DEFENSE

Studies in animals indicate that sleep deprivation leads to failure of host defense.[70] During 3 weeks of sleep deprivation, rats developed a progressive negative energy balance and sympathetic activation.[50,71] This culminated in host-defense failure manifested by bloodstream infection and a cachectic-like moribund state.[70] More recently, sleep deprivation in rats has been associated with early infection of the mesenteric lymph nodes by both aerobic and facultative anaerobic intestinal bacteria with migration to major organs.[72] The translocation of bacteria and endotoxin from the intestinal mucosa and their dissemination to extraintestinal sites is thought to drive a systemic inflammatory state and multiple organ failure in critically ill patients.[73–76] The contribution of sleep disruption to this syndrome in patients has not been determined, although sleep loss in humans has been associated with changes in some parameters of host defense.[77]

Strategies to Improve Sleep in the Intensive Care Unit

No studies have systematically evaluated strategies to improve sleep in the ICU. Nevertheless, several options can be considered based on our current, albeit limited, understanding of the pathogenesis of sleep disruption in this patient population and on anecdotal experience.

TREATMENT OF THE UNDERLYING ILLNESS

All sources of sleep disruption related to a patient's underlying medical condition should be reduced as much as possible. This includes management of the acute illness, such as optimal control of postoperative pain, as well as maintaining pre-existing treatment for chronic medical disorders such as chronic cough associated with chronic obstructive pulmonary disease or restless legs syndrome. Detailed management of all such conditions is beyond the scope of this chapter.

OPTIMIZATION OF THE INTENSIVE CARE UNIT ENVIRONMENT

Although this has the greatest intuitive appeal to improve sleep in the ICU, it has not been shown to have a dramatic effect. Studies that have minimized disruption from light, noise, and nursing interventions did not decrease sleep disruption.[15] Successful reduction of ICU noise and light levels was not associated with improved sleep quality as assessed by the nursing staff.[78] The use of earplugs subjectively improved sleep in a group of acutely ill patients compared to a control group.[79] When healthy volunteers were exposed to recorded ICU noise in a sleep laboratory,[80] subjects without earplugs displayed an increased number

of awakenings and decreased REM sleep, similar to previous studies.[37,38,42] Furthermore, REM latency (time to enter REM sleep) and the duration of REM sleep were significantly improved when earplugs were worn. Overall, modification of the ICU environment yielded modest improvement in sleep quality, which is consistent with the observation that the ICU environment is not the major source of sleep disruption.[44] Nevertheless, it is important that all reasonable measures be taken to avoid an excessively disruptive ICU environment.

Several nonpharmacologic therapies have been used successfully in the management of chronic insomnia.[81,82] These therapies can be applied to patients in the ICU, despite the fact they have not been evaluated in this population. Reestablishment of a regular sleep schedule and avoidance of excessive sleep during the day may be feasible in ventilated patients once they have recovered from their acute illness and are being weaned from the ventilator.

MEDICATION

Patients in the ICU receive multiple medications that should be reviewed for their potential to cause sleep disruption or sleep loss (see Table 57-1). Medication can also be used to consolidate sleep, either a pure hypnotic, such as zopiclone, or medication that treats the underlying cause of sleep disruption such as anxiety, depression, or delirium. Few studies have addressed the impact of such interventions on sleep in critically ill patients. One study randomized ICU patients to nocturnal infusions of either midazolam or propofol.[83] Although sleep was not assessed objectively by polysomnography, daily self-assessment questionnaires showed improved sleep with both agents. An alternative approach by Shilo et al[30] found that patients on the hospital ward had the typical nocturnal peak in melatonin levels, whereas nocturnal secretion was blunted in ICU patients. Administration of melatonin to nonventilated ICU patients improved the duration and continuity of sleep, as assessed indirectly by actigraphy.[84] It is possible that other strategies to re-synchronize circadian rhythm such as bright-light therapy, which has been used successfully in ambulatory patients,[35] may improve sleep in some ICU patients.

MODE OF MECHANICAL VENTILATION

As outlined above, the study by Parthasarathy et al[48] supports the notion that some modes of mechanical ventilation are more "sleep-friendly" than others. They found that sleep fragmentation was less during assist-control ventilation than with pressure-support ventilation, predominantly because of a reduction in the frequency of central apnea. The assist-control mode, however, is not itself free of dyssynchrony,[46] which may have contributed to the persistent sleep fragmentation that was seen. It is possible that newer modes, such as proportional assist ventilation,[85] which corrects patient-ventilator dyssynchrony, will further improve sleep quality. If sleep fragmentation is proven to be ventilator-mode specific, appropriate adjustments might consolidate nocturnal sleep, either in isolation or in conjunction with other therapies such as hypnotic medication.

Important Unknowns

Despite increasing interest and research on sleep disruption in ventilated patients, there is much that we do not know. We do not have a comprehensive understanding of the pathogenesis of sleep disruption in this patient population and the relative contribution of all of the potential sources of sleep disruption discussed above. We also do not know how sleep disruption changes over time in the ICU. Second, we do not know the impact of sleep disruption on outcomes such as weaning, length of stay in the ICU, and hospital morbidity and mortality. Third, it is not clear how much sleep can be improved in ICU patients and what treatment strategies work best. Finally, we do not know whether sleep disruption associated with mechanical ventilation leads to long-term sleep disorders such as chronic insomnia.

The Future

Two issues need to be addressed to facilitate further research on this topic. First, the methodology to monitor sleep needs modification. Although attended polysomnography is the gold standard for monitoring sleep, it is labor-intensive, costly, cumbersome for staff and patients, and not suited to repeated measurement, especially in the ICU environment. Alternative methodologies that address these limitations and are validated in mechanically ventilated patients are required. Secondly, larger studies are needed. To date, most studies have consisted of small numbers of patients from a single academic center. Although they have provided new and valuable data, their small sample size raises concern about how applicable these findings are to the broad ICU population. These concerns could be addressed by multi-center studies that recruit patients both from academic and community-based ICUs.

Summary and Conclusions

There is strong evidence that sleep is severely disrupted in mechanically ventilated patients in the ICU, which has the potential to increase their morbidity and mortality through its effect on neurocognitive, cardiorespiratory, and immune function. Although sleep disruption has been attributed predominantly to the noisy ICU environment, recent evidence indicates that noise and patient-care activities account for less than 30% of sleep disruption. Further research is required to provide a comprehensive understanding of the causes of sleep disruption in this patient population, which will form the basis for the evaluation of therapeutic strategies and their impact on both short- and long-term clinical outcomes.

Acknowledgement

The author thanks Ms. Patty Nielsen for her clerical assistance.

References

1. Chokroverty S. Sleep disorders medicine: Basic science, technical considerations, and clinical aspects. Boston: Butterworth-Heinemann, 1999: 7–16, 95–126, 151.
2. Carskadon MA, Dement WC. Normal human sleep: An overview. In: Kryger MH, Roth T, Dement WC, editors. Principles and practice of sleep medicine, 3rd ed. Philadelphia: WB Saunders, 2000: 20.
3. American Sleep Disorders Association. EEG arousals: scoring rules and examples. Sleep 1992; 15:174–84.
4. Rechtschaffen A, Kales A, University of California at Los Angeles, et al. A manual of standardized terminology, techniques and scoring system for sleep stages in human subjects, no. 204 ed. Bethesda, MD: U.S. Dept. of Health, Education, and Welfare, Public Health Service-National Institutes of Health, National Institute of Neurological Diseases and Blindness, Neurological Information Network, 1968.
5. Mathur R, Douglas NJ. Frequency of EEG arousals from nocturnal sleep in normal subjects. Sleep 1995; 18:330–3.
6. Hilton BA. Quantity and quality of patients' sleep and sleep-disturbing factors in a respiratory intensive care unit. J Adv Nurs 1976; 1:453–68.
7. Jones J, Hoggart B, Withey J, et al. What the patients say: A study of reactions to an intensive care unit. Intensive Care Med 1979; 5:89–92.
8. Simini B. Patients' perceptions of intensive care. Lancet 1999; 354:571–2.
9. Russell S. An exploratory study of patients' perceptions, memories and experiences of an intensive care unit. J Adv Nurs 1999; 29:783–91.
10. Freedman NS, Kotzer N, Schwab RJ. Patient perception of sleep quality and etiology of sleep disruption in the intensive care unit. Am J Respir Crit Care Med 1999; 159:1155–62.
11. Cooper AB, Thornley KS, Young GB, et al. Sleep in critically ill patients requiring mechanical ventilation. Chest 2000; 117: 809–18.
12. Orr WC, Stahl ML. Sleep disturbances after open heart surgery. Am J Cardiology 1977; 39:196–201.
13. Broughton R, Baron R. Sleep patterns in the intensive care unit and on the ward after acute myocardial infarction. Electroenceph Clin Neurophysiol 1978; 45:348–60.
14. Kavey NB, Ahshuler KZ. Sleep in herniorrhaphy patients. Am J Surg 1979; 138:683–7.
15. Aurell J, Elmqvist D. Sleep in the surgical intensive care unit: continuous polygraphic recording of sleep in nine patients receiving postoperative care. Br Med J Clin Res Ed 1985; 290:1029–32.
16. Richards KC, Bairnsfather L. A description of night sleep patterns in the critical care unit. Heart Lung: J Acute Crit Care 1988; 17:35–42.
17. Knill RL, Moote CA, Skinner MI, et al. Anesthesia with abdominal surgery leads to intense REM sleep during the first postoperative week. Anesthesiology 1990; 73:52–61.
18. Rosenberg J, Wildschiodtz G, Pedersen MH, et al. Late postoperative nocturnal episodic hypoxaemia and associated sleep pattern. Br J Anaesth 1994; 72:145–50.
19. Young GB, McLachlan RS, Kreeft JH, et al. An electroencephalographic classification for coma. Can J Neurol Sci 1997; 24:320–5.
20. Cooper AB, Gabor JY, Hanly P. Sleep in the ICU: Estimated prevalence of reliable polysomnography. Critical Care Med 2000; 28:A194.
21. Wooten V. Sleep disorders in psychiatric illness. In: Chokroverty S, editor. Sleep disorders medicine. Boston: Butterworth-Heinemann, 1999: 337–47.
22. Schweitzer PK. Drugs that disturb sleep and wakefulness. In: Kryger MH, Roth T, Dement WC, editors. Principles and

practice of sleep medicine, 3rd ed. Philadelphia: WB Saunders, 2000: 441–61.

23. Gaillard JM, Blois R. Effect of the benzodiazepine antagonist Ro 15-1788 on flunitrazepam-induced sleep changes. Br J Clin Pharmacol 1983; 15:529–36.

24. Bradley CM, Nicholson AN, Viveash JP. Opioids and non-opioids. In: Klepper ID, Sanders LD, Rosen M, editors. Ambulatory anaesthesia and sedation: impairment and recovery. Boston: Blackwell Scientific Publications, 1991: 218–34.

25. Bakshi R. Fluoxetine and restless legs syndrome. J Neurol Sci 1996; 142:151–2.

26. Baker SK, Zee PC. Circadian disorders of the sleep-wake cycle. In: Kryger MH, Roth T, Dement WC, editors. Principles and practice of sleep medicine, 3rd ed. Philadelphia: WB Saunders, 2000: 606–14.

27. Dauch WA, Bauer S. Circadian rhythms in the body temperatures of intensive care patients with brain lesions. J Neurol Neurosurg Psychiatry 1990; 53:345–7.

28. Tweedie IE, Bell CF, Clegg A, et al. Retrospective study of temperature rhythms of intensive care patients. Critical Care Med 1989; 17:1159–65.

29. Gazendam JAC, Van Dongen HPA, Freedman NS, et al. The circadian rhythm of core body temperature in the intensive care unit. Intensive Care Med 2002; 28:S153–S153.

30. Shilo L, Dagan Y, Smorjik Y, et al. Patients in the intensive care unit suffer from severe lack of sleep associated with loss of normal melatonin secretion pattern. Am J Med Sci 1999; 317:278–81.

31. Cronin AJ, Keifer JC, Davies MF, et al. Melatonin secretion after surgery. Lancet 2000; 356:1244–5.

32. Mundigler G, le-Karth G, Koreny M, et al. Impaired circadian rhythm of melatonin secretion in sedated critically ill patients with severe sepsis 2. Crit Care Med 2002; 30:536–40.

33. Olofsson K, Alling C, Lundberg D, et al. Abolished circadian rhythm of melatonin secretion in sedated and artificially ventilated intensive care patients. Acta Anaesthesiol Scand 2004; 48:679–84.

34. Frisk U, Olsson J, Nylen P, et al. Low melatonin excretion during mechanical ventilation in the intensive care unit. Clin Sci (Lond) 2004; 107:47–53.

35. Czeisler CA, Cajochen C, Turek F. Melatonin in the regulation of sleep and circadian rhythms. In: Kryger MH, Roth T, Dement WC, editors. Principles and practice of sleep medicine, 3rd ed. Philadelphia: WB Saunders, 2000: 606–14.

36. Bentley S, Murphy F, Dudley H. Perceived noise in surgical wards and an intensive care area: an objective analysis. Br Med J 1977; 2:1503–6.

37. Topf M. Effects of personal control over hospital noise on sleep. Res Nurs Health 1992; 15:19–28.

38. Topf M, Davis JE. Critical care unit noise and rapid eye movement (REM) sleep. Heart Lung 1993; 22:252–8.

39. Balogh D, Kittinger E, Benzer A, et al. Noise in the ICU. Intensive Care Med 1919; 6:343–6.

40. Meyer TJ, Eveloff SE, Bauer MS, et al. Adverse environmental conditions in the respiratory and medical ICU settings. Chest 1994; 105:1211–6.

41. Aaron JN, Carlisle CC, Carskadon MA, et al. Environmental noise as a cause of sleep disruption in an intermediate respiratory care unit. Sleep 1996; 19:707–10.

42. Topf M, Bookman M, Arand D. Effects of critical care unit noise on the subjective quality of sleep. J Adv Nurs 1996; 24:545–51.

43. Freedman NS, Gazendam J, Levan L, et al. Abnormal sleep/wake cycles and the effect of environmental noise on sleep disruption in the intensive care unit. Am J Respir Crit Care Med 2001; 163: 451–7.

44. Gabor JY, Cooper AB, Crombach SA, et al. Contribution of the intensive care unit environment to sleep disruption in mechanically ventilated patients and healthy subjects. Am J Respir Crit Care Med 2003; 167:708–15.

45. Younes M. Patient-ventilator interaction with pressure-assisted modalities of ventilatory support. Semin Respir Med 1993; 14:299–322.

46. Leung P, Jubran A, Tobin MJ. Comparison of assisted ventilator modes on triggering, patient effort, and dyspnea. Am J Respir Crit Care Med 1997; 155:1940–48.

47. Bergbom-Engberg I, Haljamae H. Assessment of patients' experience of discomforts during respirator therapy. Crit Care Med 1989; 17:1068–72.

48. Parthasarathy S, Tobin MJ. Effect of ventilator mode on sleep quality in critically ill patients. Am J Respir Crit Care Med 2002; 166:1423–9.

49. Rechtschaffen A, Gilliland MA, Bergmann BM, et al. Physiological correlates of prolonged sleep deprivation in rats. Science 1983; 221:182–4.

50. Everson CA, Bergmann BM, Rechtschaffen A. Sleep deprivation in the rat: III. Total sleep deprivation. Sleep 1989; 12:13–21.

51. Horne JA. Why we sleep: The functions of sleep in humans and other mammals. Oxford: Oxford University Press, 1998: 13–103.

52. Kollar EJ, Pasnau RO, Rubin RT, et al. Psychological, psychophysiological, and biochemical correlates of prolonged sleep deprivation. Am J Psych 1969; 126:488–97.

53. Naitoh P, Kelly TL, Englund C. Health effects of sleep deprivation. Occup Med 1990; 5:209–37.

54. Luby E, Frohman C, Grisell J, et al. Sleep deprivation: effects on behaviour, thinking, motor performance, and biological energy transfer systems. Psychosomatic Med 1960; 22:182–92.

55. Dubois MJ, Bergeron N, Dumont M, et al. Delirium in an intensive care unit: a study of risk factors. Intensive Care Med 2001; 27:1297–304.

56. McGuire BE, Basten CJ, Ryan CJ, et al. Intensive care unit syndrome: a dangerous misnomer. Arch Intern Med 2000; 160:906–9.

57. Hansell HN. The behavioral effects of noise on man: the patient with "intensive care unit psychosis." Heart Lung 1984; 13:59–65.

58. Ely EW, Gautam S, Margolin R, et al. The impact of delirium in the intensive care unit on hospital length of stay. Intensive Care Med 2001; 27:1892–900.

59. Scrimshaw NS, Habicht JP, Pellet P, et al. Effects of sleep deprivation and reversal of diurnal activity on protein metabolism of young men. Am J Clin Nutr 1919; 5:313–9.

60. Chen HI, Tang YR. Sleep loss impairs inspiratory muscle endurance. Am Rev Respir Dis 1989; 140:907–9.

61. Leiter JC, Knuth SL, Bartlett D Jr. The effect of sleep deprivation on activity of the genioglossus muscle. Am Rev Respir Dis 1985; 132:1242–5.

62. Cooper KR, Phillips BA. Effect of short-term sleep loss on breathing. J Appl Physiol 1982; 53:855–8.

63. White DP, Douglas NJ, Pickett CK, et al. Sleep deprivation and the control of ventilation. Am Rev Respir Dis 1983; 128:984–6.

64. Schiffman PL, Trontell MC, Mazar MF, et al. Sleep deprivation decreases ventilatory response to CO_2 but not load compensation. Chest 1983; 84:695–8.

65. Series F, Roy N, Marc I. Effects of sleep deprivation and sleep fragmentation on upper airway collapsibility in normal subjects. Am J Respir Crit Care Med 1994; 150:481–5.

66. Bonnet MH, Berry RB, Arand DL. Metabolism during normal, fragmented, and recovery sleep. J Appl Physiol 1991; 71:1112–8.

67. Purro A, Appendini L, De GA, et al. Physiologic determinants of ventilator dependence in long-term mechanically ventilated patients. Am J Respir Crit Care Med 2000; 161:1115–23.

68. Vassilakopoulos T, Zakynthinos S, Roussos C. The tension-time index and the frequency/tidal volume ratio are the major pathophysiologic determinants of weaning failure and success. Am J Respir Crit Care Med 1998; 158:378–85.

69. Zakynthinos SG, Vassilakopoulos T, Roussos C. The load of inspiratory muscles in patients needing mechanical ventilation. Am J Respir Crit Care Med 1995; 152:1248–55.

70. Everson CA. Sustained sleep deprivation impairs host defense. Am J Physiol 1993; 265:R1148–54.

71. Bergmann BM, Everson CA, Kushida CA, et al. Sleep deprivation in the rat: V. Energy use and mediation. Sleep 1989; 12:31–41.

72. Everson CA, Toth LA. Systemic bacterial invasion induced by sleep deprivation. Am J Physiol 2000; 278:R905–16.

73. Carrico CJ, Meakins JL, Marshall JC, et al. Multiple-organ-failure syndrome. Arch Surg 1986; 121:196–208.

74. Garrison RN, Fry DE, Berberich S, et al. Enterococcal bacteremia: clinical implications and determinants of death. Ann Surg 1982; 1:43–7.

75. O'Boyle CJ, MacFie J, Mitchell CJ, et al. Microbiology of bacterial translocation in humans. Gut 1998; 42:29–35.

76. Tani T, Hanasawa K, Endo Y, et al. Bacterial translocation as a cause of septic shock in humans: a report of two cases. Surg Today 1997; 27:447–9.

77. Benca RM, Quintas J. Sleep and host defenses: a review. Sleep 1920; 11:1027–37.

78. Walder B, Francioli D, Meyer JJ, et al. Effects of guidelines implementation in a surgical intensive care unit to control nighttime light and noise levels. Crit Care Med 2000; 28:2242–7.

79. Haddock J. Reducing the effects of noise in hospital. Nurs Stand 1994; 8:25–8.

80. Wallace CJ, Robins J, Alvord LS, et al. The effect of earplugs on sleep measures during exposure to simulated intensive care unit noise. Am J Critical Care 1999; 8:210–9.

81. Stepanski E. Behavioral therapy for insomnia. In: Kryger MH, Roth T, Dement WC, editors. Principles and practice of sleep medicine, 3rd ed. Philadelphia: WB Saunders, 2000: 647–56.

82. Zarcone V. Sleep hygiene. In: Kryger MH, Roth T, Dement WC, editors. Principles and practice of sleep medicine, 3rd ed. Philadelphia: WB Saunders, 2000: 657–61.

83. Treggiari-Venzi M, Borgeat A, Fuchs-Buder T, et al. Overnight sedation with midazolam or propofol in the ICU: effects on sleep quality, anxiety, and depression. Intensive Care Med 1996; 22:1186–90.

84. Shilo L, Dagan Y, Smorjik Y, et al. Effect of melatonin on sleep quality of COPD intensive care patients: a pilot study. Chronobiol Int 2000; 17:71–6.

85. Grasso S, Puntillo F, Mascia L, et al. Compensation for increase in respiratory workload during mechanical ventilation. Pressure-support versus proportional-assist ventilation. Am J Respir Crit Care Med 2000; 161:819–826.

Chapter 58

WEANING FROM MECHANICAL VENTILATION

MARTIN J. TOBIN
AMAL JUBRAN

Twenty-five years ago, the weaning of patients from the ventilator was relegated to nurses and respiratory therapists. It aroused little interest among physicians. It certainly wasn't thought worthy of serious scientific inquiry. All this has changed. No other area of critical care has undergone so great a transformation. But the illumination has also cast shadows. In particular, discussion of weaning is now bedeviled by imprecise language. This can be seen as just deserts insofar as few clinicians use the term "weaning" in the strict literal sense—a gradual reduction in the level of ventilator support. Instead, most patients today are taken off the ventilator cold turkey. It would be fine if the confused language stopped there. But this is only one small example of how fundamental scientific misunderstanding has arisen from imprecise word choices.

Under the cloak of imprecise language, much muddled thinking, flawed logic, and misinterpretation has crept into the field. These language problems are not just pedantic quirks. Instead, they impede the rigor of research in this area, as well as interpretation of the findings. Communication is also hindered by the lumping together of many distinct components of this complex process. To enhance clarity, we shall divide weaning into seven stages.

Seven Stages of Weaning

We divide weaning into seven stages to draw attention to areas that receive minimal attention (Fig. 58-1). Stage 1 is pre-weaning, when no attempt at weaning is desirable. For example, when a patient is receiving 80% oxygen (O_2) and positive end-expiratory pressure (PEEP) of 15 cmH$_2$O, performing any disconnect from the ventilator (for measurement of weaning predictors) is inappropriate and may even be dangerous. Every ventilated patient begins at stage 1, and some patients never get beyond that stage. For example, in a prospective study of 249 ventilated patients,[1] 65 patients (26%) died during mechanical ventilation without any attempt at weaning. In another report of 357 patients entered into a trial of weaning techniques,[2] 12.9% never reached the stage of any active weaning attempt. We identify this pre-weaning stage to emphasize the importance of the transition between it and the next stage of a patient's clinical course.

Stage 2 is the period during which the clinician contemplates the possibility that the patient is ready for weaning. This statement may seem obvious to the point of banality. But the point at which this thought first enters the mind of a physician managing a complex patient is not so straightforward. In such a patient, the key act is for a physician to *think* that the patient just *might* come off the ventilator successfully. Except for self-extubations, this decision is not made by the patient. The idea has to *begin* in the doctor's brain. Several large studies have documented that many patients are ventilated for a week or more and the ventilator is then successfully discontinued on the first day that weaning predictor tests are measured.[3,4] A physician has to ask him- or herself whether the patient might have tolerated extubation a day or so earlier. Failure to recognize this second stage may be the greatest obstacle to expeditious weaning.

Psychologists have extensively studied how people perceive, process, and evaluate the probabilities of uncertain events.[5,6] These studies have repeatedly shown that people tend to be overconfident in their judgments. Psychologists have traced such extreme responses to the use of simple, but inappropriate, best-guess strategies. To minimize this likelihood, physicians need to repeatedly revise their estimate that a patient can breathe on his or her own as new information becomes available.

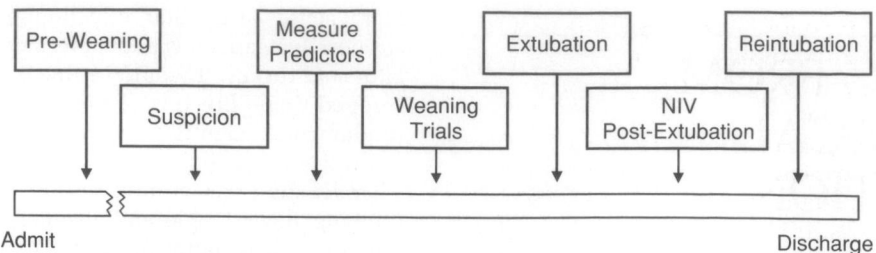

FIGURE 58-1 Seven stages of weaning. Stage 1 is pre-weaning, a stage that many patients never get beyond. Stage 2 is the period of diagnostic triggering, the time when a physician begins to think that the patient might be ready come off the ventilator. Stage 3 is the time of measuring and interpreting weaning predictors. Stage 4 is the time of decreasing ventilator support (abruptly or gradually). Stage 5 is either extubation (of a weaning success patient) or reinstitution of mechanical ventilation (in a weaning failure patient). Stage 6 is use of noninvasive ventilation after extubation. Stage 7 is reintubation. Failure to appreciate stage 2 probably leads to the greatest delays in weaning.

Stage 3 is the time of obtaining physiologic measurements that serve as predictors, and interpreting the data appropriately in the context of each patient's unique clinical condition. The critical word here is *interpretation*. It is imperative to be clear about why these predictor tests are being performed, the influence of a patient's pre-existing condition on the interpretation of the results, what action to take based on the results, and when is it prudent to adjust the thresholds for taking action. These points may seem self-evident, but the literature is replete with evidence of cloudy thinking on each point.

Stage 4 is to decrease ventilator support. Support is either removed abruptly and completely (T-tube trial) or gradually decreased over hours or days. Stage 5 is extubation of a patient who tolerated stage 4 or reinstitution of mechanical ventilation in a patient who failed the weaning trial. Stage 6 is continued ventilator support after extubation using noninvasive ventilation; this stage applies to only a minority of patients. Stage 7 is reintubation, usually accompanied by the reinstitution of mechanical ventilation.

Pathophysiology of Weaning Failure

Over the last twenty years, understanding of the mechanisms that cause patients to fail their first attempt to recommence spontaneous breathing has increased considerably. Advances in this aspect of weaning research have been enormously greater than change in clinical management. Greater understanding of pathophysiology has led to new approaches to the timing of the weaning process, prediction of outcome, and techniques used for weaning. Delineation of pathophysiologic principles led to the undertaking of clinical trials. The trials, in contrast, have contributed little to our understanding of the pathophysiology of weaning failure.

Research on pathophysiology has been limited to failure of attempts at spontaneous breathing when a still-intubated patient is first disconnected from the ventilator. Virtually no pathophysiologic research has been conducted in patients who develop acute respiratory failure in the hours immediately after extubation. Likewise, very little research has been conducted in patients who fail repeated weaning attempts, and, as a consequence, may be transferred to centers that specialize in the delivery of mechanical ventilation in the post–intensive care setting.

When intubated patients are disconnected from the ventilator and left to breathe on their own, about a fifth are not able to sustain spontaneous ventilation. If the trial is extended, these weaning failure patients will develop hypercapnia unless severe hypoxemia first intervenes. The pathophysiologic mechanisms that cause weaning failure can be divided into those occurring at the level of control of breathing, mechanics of the lung and chest wall, the respiratory muscles, the cardiovascular system, and gas-exchange properties of the lung.

CONTROL OF BREATHING

The physiologic processes that fall under the heading of control of breathing primarily include afferent and efferent signals, and the processing of these signals in the brainstem. Clinical research on control of breathing has primarily focused on the overall level of respiratory motor output, termed respiratory drive. In human research, it is not realistic to obtain electrode recordings from the respiratory centers, and it is extremely difficult to measure phrenic nerve traffic. Consequently, a number of indirect methods have been used to assess respiratory drive. Measurement of the ventilatory response to hypercapnia or hypoxia is used in ambulatory patients, but difficult to apply in weaning failure patients. Electromyographic (EMG) recordings from the diaphragm reflect phrenic nerve traffic, but are difficult to standardize among patients.

Most data on respiratory drive in weaning failure patients has been obtained with two techniques: the airway occlusion method ($P_{0.1}$) and mean inspiratory flow (V_T/T_I) of breathing pattern analysis. In a spontaneously breathing patient, it is not possible to measure $P_{0.1}$ on every breath or even at frequent intervals. If $P_{0.1}$ is measured repeatedly, the act of measurement will alter respiratory drive.[7] As such, continuous measurements of respiratory drive over the evolution of weaning failure have been limited to V_T/T_I. V_T/T_I suffers from the limitation that oral airflow is far removed from the brainstem. Any intervening impediment, such as abnormal lung mechanics, can cause a decrease in V_T/T_I. Thus, there is always the possibility that V_T/T_I is providing an underestimate of respiratory drive. An advantage, however, of breathing pattern analysis over other methods of measuring respiratory drive is that it also provides information on respiratory timing.

Tobin et al[8] studied 17 patients who underwent a T-tube trial of weaning. Seven patients developed severe distress, and arterial carbon dioxide tension (Pa_{CO_2}) rose from 42 to 56 mmHg, and pH fell from 7.43 to 7.35. Between the beginning and end of the trial, which lasted 40 ± 11 minutes, the patients developed an increase in V_T/T_I: 265 ± 27 to 328 ± 32 ml per second. These findings were surprising. At that time, it was expected that acute hypoventilation—the physiologic terminology for an increase in Pa_{CO_2}—would have been accompanied by a decrease in drive. Yet, not one patient had a value of V_T/T_I below the 95% confidence limits of normal subjects. Although V_T/T_I was not depressed in the weaning failure patients, it was not higher than in the weaning success patients. Subsequent studies, using $P_{0.1}$, revealed that respiratory drive is higher in weaning failure patients than in weaning success patients.[9–13]

The patients also showed marked changes in respiratory timing (Fig. 58-2). Upon resumption of spontaneous breathing, the weaning failure patients exhibited immediate and marked shortening of inspiratory time (T_I): 0.81 ± 0.11 versus 1.41 ± 0.27 seconds in weaning success patients. Within the respiratory centers, expiratory time (T_E) is strongly coupled to T_I. Consequently, T_E was also shorter in the weaning failure patients than in the weaning success patients: 1.24 ± 0.27 versus 2.48 ± 0.47 seconds. The combined changes in T_I and T_E led to a marked increase in respiratory frequency (f): 32.3 ± 2.3 versus 20.9 ± 2.8 breaths per minute. Because the rate of inspiratory flow (V_T/T_I) was equivalent in the two

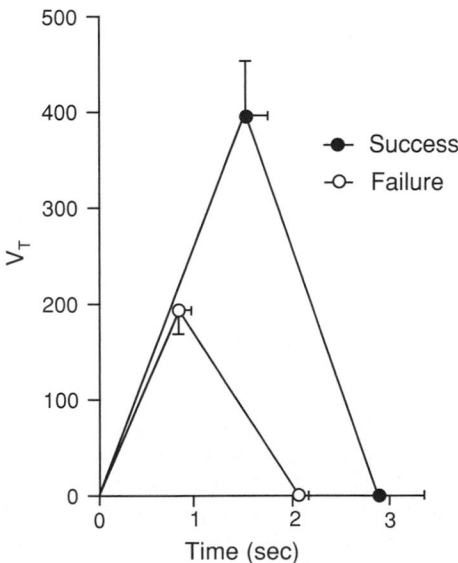

FIGURE 58-2 The mean respiratory cycle during spontaneous breathing in 7 weaning failure and 10 weaning success patients. The early termination of inspiratory time in the weaning failure patients leads to a decrease in tidal volume. The decrease in inspiratory time, coupled with a decrease in expiratory time, results in a faster respiratory frequency. Bars represent 1 SE. (*Reproduced, with permission, from Tobin et al.[8]*)

patient groups, the short T_I resulted in a lower tidal volume (V_T) in the weaning failure patients: 194 ± 23 versus 398 ± 56 ml. The decrease in V_T was balanced by the increase in f, and thus minute ventilation ($\dot{V}_E$) was equivalent in the two groups. A decrease in V_T without an increase in $\dot{V}_E$ must result in higher overall dead space ventilation (V_D/V_T). Indeed, the combined changes in V_T and f accounted for 81% of the increase in Pa_{CO_2} observed in the weaning failure patients. From the above discussion, it is evident that the fundamental abnormality in control of breathing in weaning failure is a shortening of T_I.

Several groups of investigators have shown that the combination of increased f and low V_T is a characteristic abnormality in weaning failure patients. Vassilakopoulos et al[14] studied 30 patients at two points in time. Measurements were first obtained shortly after the patients failed a T-tube trial. Measurements were repeated about 9 days later, shortly before the patients were successfully extubated. The investigators found that an index of rapid shallow breathing, frequency-to-tidal volume ratio (f/V_T), was lower in weaning failure than in weaning success patients: 62 ± 21 versus 98 ± 38. They obtained additional detailed measurements of lung mechanics and respiratory muscle function, and found that only two variables, tension-time index and f/V_T, were significant determinants of weaning failure.

Research indicates that most weaning failure patients develop an increase in respiratory drive as they experience progressive ventilatory failure. Clinical experience, however, suggests that at least some patients have depressed respiratory drive. Jubran and Tobin[15] observed that 2 of 17 (11.8%) weaning failure patients developed Pa_{CO_2} values of >70 mmHg during a T-tube trial, and yet detailed measurements of their lung mechanics and respiratory muscle function were within the range of the weaning success patients. These limited data suggest that perhaps 10% of patients who develop hypercapnia during a failed weaning trial may do so primarily because of respiratory center depression.

RESPIRATORY MECHANICS

Many physiologic variables are available for quantifying different aspects of lung mechanics, but all can be grouped under three major headings: resistance, elastance (the inverse of compliance), and gas trapping. The most detailed study of respiratory mechanics during weaning trials was carried out by Jubran and Tobin.[15] They studied 17 patients with chronic obstructive pulmonary disease (COPD) who developed distress during a T-tube trial that lasted 45 ± 8 minutes, at which point mechanical ventilation was reinstituted. These patients had developed an increase in Pa_{CO_2} (from 45 to 58 mmHg) and a decrease in pH (from 7.43 to 7.36) by the end of the trial. Another group of 14 patients with COPD, who tolerated a T-tube trial (also lasting 45 minutes) and were successfully extubated, served as a control group.

At the start of the trial, inspiratory lung resistance was equivalent in the weaning failure and weaning success patients: 9.0 ± 1.7 versus 5.3 ± 1.1 cmH$_2$O per liter per second[15] (Fig. 58-3). By the end of the trial, resistance increased to

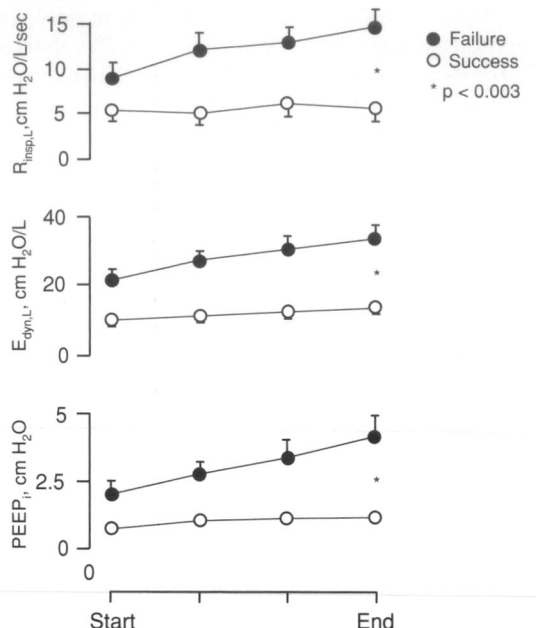

FIGURE 58-3 Inspiratory resistance of the lung ($R_{insp,L}$), dynamic lung elastance ($E_{dyn,L}$), and intrinsic positive end-expiratory pressure (*PEEPi*) in 17 weaning failure patients and 14 weaning success patients. Data displayed were obtained during the second and last minute of a T-tube trial, and at one-third and two-thirds of the trial duration. Between the onset and end of the trial, the failure group developed increases in $R_{insp,L}$ ($p < 0.009$), $E_{dyn,L}$ ($p < 0.0001$), and PEEPi ($p < 0.0001$) and the success group developed increases in $E_{dyn,L}$ ($p < 0.006$) and PEEPi ($p < 0.02$). Over the course of the trial, the failure group had higher values of $R_{insp,L}$ ($p < 0.003$), $E_{dyn,L}$ ($p < 0.006$), and PEEPi ($p < 0.009$) than the success group. (Reproduced, with permission, from Jubran and Tobin.[15])

14.8 ± 2.0 cmH$_2$O per liter per second in the failure patients, but it did not change in the success patients. Four factors may account for the increase in resistance: (1) an increase in inspiratory flow (unlikely because the increase in flow was no higher in failure patients than in success patients); (2) a decrease in lung volume (unlikely because all patients also developed gas trapping); (3) accumulation of secretions (unlikely because all patients had been suctioned before the trial, and secretions were no different in the two groups); and (4) bronchoconstriction. Bronchoconstriction appears to be the most likely explanation in that patients with COPD have heightened airway reactivity—although it is not clear why this should be greater in weaning failure than in weaning success patients.

Dynamic lung elastance was higher in weaning failure patients than in weaning success patients at the start of the trial: 21.2 ± 3.4 versus 9.9 ± 1.7 cmH$_2$O per liter[15] (see Fig. 58-3). At the end of the trial, elastance increased to 34.1 ± 4.0 cmH$_2$O per liter in the failure patients and to 14.0 ± 2.0 cmH$_2$O per liter in the success patients. The elevated elastance at the start of the trial was probably secondary to frequency-dependence of elastance. Three factors may account for the increase in elastance over the course of the trial: (1) dynamic hyperinflation (this possibility is supported by

a twofold increase in intrinsic PEEP [PEEPi] by the end of the trial); (2) development of subclinical pulmonary edema secondary to increased left ventricular afterload; and (3) microatelectasis (a possibility supported by the marked decrease in VT).

PEEPi was higher in the failure patients than in the success patients at the onset of the trial: 2.0 ± 0.5 versus 0.7 ± 0.1 cmH$_2$O. By the end of the trial, PEEPi increased to 4.1 ± 0.8 cmH$_2$O in the failure patients and to 1.1 ± 0.2 cmH$_2$O in the success patients[15] (see Fig. 58-3). The increase in PEEPi in the failure patients suggests the development of dynamic hyperinflation, although a contribution from expiratory muscle contraction cannot be excluded. Over the course of the T-tube trial, the levels of resistance, elastance, and PEEPi were higher in the failure patients than in the success patients. Moreover, the increases between the beginning and end of the trial for these three variables were greater in the failure patients than in the success patients.

Other investigators have also reported a worsening of lung mechanics in weaning failure patients. An innovative approach was employed by Vassilakopoulos et al.[14] They first studied patients at the end of a T-tube trial. Then they reinstituted ventilation in the assist-control mode, sedated the patients, and hyperventilated them to abolish spontaneous respiratory muscle activity. Next they adjusted the ventilator settings to simulate a patient's pattern of spontaneous breathing, and measured lung mechanics under passive conditions. The investigators studied patients at two points in time: shortly after they first failed a T-tube trial, and about 9 days later, shortly before they were successfully extubated. Between the time of weaning failure and weaning success, airway resistance decreased from 9.6 ± 3.4 to 7.9 ± 3.3 cmH$_2$O per liter per second, static PEEPi decreased from 6.1 ± 2.5 to 3.8 ± 2.7 cmH$_2$O, and static respiratory compliance did not change. The investigators also disconnected the patients from the ventilator (after first delivering some breaths simulating spontaneous breathing), and allowed them to exhale freely until zero expiratory flow was reached. This point was taken as the elastic equilibrium volume of the respiratory system, and the increase in functional residual capacity secondary to gas trapping (PEEPi) was taken as the difference between inspired and expired volume. This volume was 327 ± 180 ml during weaning failure, and it fell to 213 ± 175 at the time of weaning success.

The observation that weaning failure patients display more severely deranged lung mechanics than do weaning success patients raises the question of whether the derangements might be detectable even before patients reattempt spontaneous breathing (that is, while patients are still receiving full ventilator support). Jubran and Tobin[16] studied lung and chest wall mechanics of patients before the onset of a T-tube trial. They measured airway pressure, transpulmonary pressure, and esophageal pressure, and used the end-inspiratory occlusion method to characterize the mechanics of the total respiratory system, the lung itself, and the chest wall. Inspiratory resistance was equivalent in the weaning failure and weaning success patients: 13.9 and 13.0 cmH$_2$O per liter per second, respectively (Fig. 58-4). These values are about 14 times higher

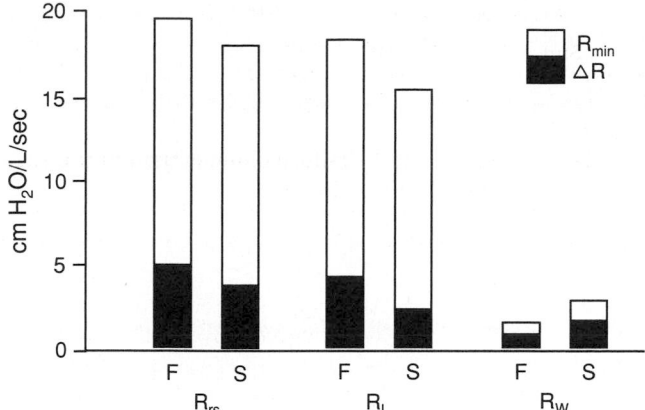

FIGURE 58-4 Maximal resistance (overall column height) of the respiratory system ($R_{max,rs}$), lung ($R_{max,L}$), and chest wall ($R_{max,w}$) in weaning failure (F) and weaning success (S) patients during passive ventilation; the clear portions of the columns represent minimum resistance ($R_{min,rs}$) while the shaded portions represent additional resistance (ΔR_{rs}). No differences in $R_{max,rs}$, $R_{min,rs}$, or ΔR_{rs} were observed between the groups, nor between the lung and chest wall components. (*Reproduced, with permission, from Jubran and Tobin.[16]*)

than those seen in healthy subjects. The resistances are also much higher than those observed in the same patients while they were breathing spontaneously. The difference is explained by the markedly higher flow during mechanical ventilation and the nonlinear pressure-flow characteristics of the respiratory system. The increase in resistance originated almost totally in the lungs, with minimal contribution from the chest wall. In turn, the lung resistance originated predominantly within the airways, with a small contribution from time-constant inhomogeneities and viscoelastic pressure dissipations (stress relaxation) within the lungs.

Dynamic elastance of the lung was higher in the failure patients than in the success patients: 28 ± 3 versus 17.8 ± 2 cmH$_2$O/L[16] (see Fig. 58-4). Indeed, this was the only measurement of lung mechanics measured under passive conditions that differentiated the two groups of patients. Considerable overlap, however, was evident among individual patients in the two groups. The static elastance of the lung and the chest wall elastance were similar in the two groups. The value of dynamic lung elastance in the success patients was similar to values reported in other studies of patients with COPD.[17,18] In both patient groups, dynamic elastance was much higher during passive ventilation than in the same patients during spontaneous breathing. The difference is explained in part because the passive measurements were recorded at a higher lung volume, and also by the nonlinear pressure-volume relationships of the respiratory system.

Dynamic PEEPi during passive ventilation did not differ between the failure and success patients: 3.4 ± 0.5 versus 2.5 ± 0.4 cmH$_2$O.[16] These values are lower than the values of PEEPi commonly reported in ventilated patients with COPD.[17–19] The higher values in these other studies arise because investigators measured static PEEPi, which is about

two to three times higher than dynamic PEEPi because of time-constant inequalities.

Apart from the slightly higher dynamic lung elastance in weaning failure patients, overall lung resistance, static elastance, and PEEPi during passive ventilation (before the onset of spontaneous breathing) in weaning failure patients were no different than in the success patients. This picture contrasts with the more severely deranged mechanics in failure patients during a T-tube trial. The difference indicates that something in the act of spontaneous breathing, rather than an intrinsic abnormality in respiratory mechanics, is responsible for the marked difference between failure and success patients during a weaning trial.

PATIENT EFFORT

Deterioration in lung mechanics causes an increase in the work of breathing, which has been studied by several groups of investigators. Fiastro et al[20] studied 11 weaning success and 6 weaning failure patients. Work of breathing per minute was >15.7 Joules/minute in all 6 ventilator-dependent patients and 4 had work per liter values >1.37 Joules/Liter. The measurements were confined to assessment of work performed on the lungs (ignoring work on the chest wall). Henning et al,[21] also measuring work performed only on the lungs, noted that patients remained ventilator-dependent when the work rate was >16.66 Joules/minute, and spontaneous ventilation could usually be sustained if the work rate was ≤9.80 Joules/minute.

To cope with an increase in work of breathing, patients have to make a greater inspiratory effort, as reflected by greater swings in esophageal pressure (Fig. 58-5). Measurement of work of breathing, however, can substantially underestimate the full effort made by a patient because the measurement is totally insensitive to isometric respiratory muscle contractions, and it also fails to take into account the duration of a muscle contraction.[22] Measurement of pressure-time product overcomes these problems and provides a closer estimate of O$_2$ consumption by the respiratory muscles.

Jubran and Tobin[15] found that pressure-time product was no different in weaning failure and weaning success patients at the onset of a T-tube trial: 255 ± 59 and 158 ± 23 cmH$_2$O* second per minute (normal, 94 ± 12). At the end of the trial, pressure-time product increased more in the failure patients than in the success patients: 388 ± 68 versus 205 ± 25 cm H$_2$O* second per minute. Partitioning of the increase in pressure-time product at end of trial in the failure patients revealed that the influence of the three fundamental components of lung mechanics differed. The fraction of pressure-time product caused by PEEPi increased by 111%, the fraction caused by the non-PEEPi elastic component increased by 33%, and the fraction caused by the resistive component increased by 42%.

RESPIRATORY MUSCLES

The respiratory muscles alone shoulder the entire burden of the increase in respiratory work that occurs in weaning failure patients. Aware of this fact, researchers have studied

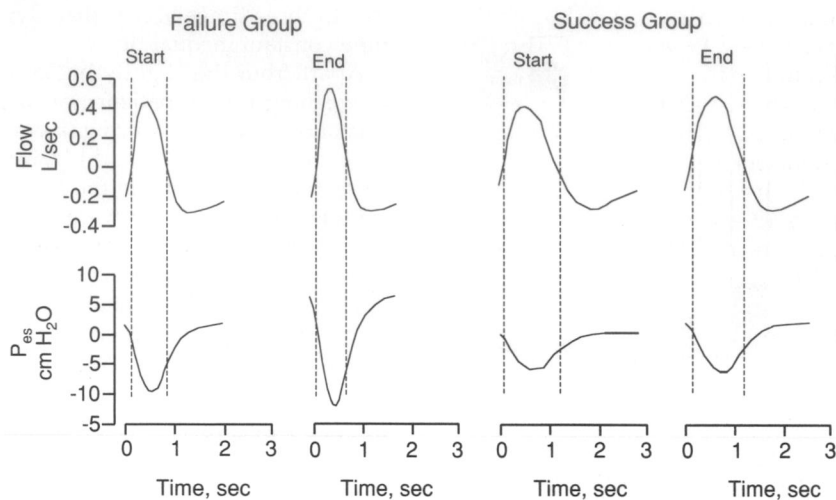

FIGURE 58-5 Ensemble average plots of flow and esophageal pressure (P_{es}) at the start and end of a T-tube trial in 17 weaning failure patients and 14 weaning success patients. At the start of the trial, the inspiratory excursion in P_{es} was greater in the failure patients, and it increased further by the end of the trial. To generate these plots, flow and P_{es} tracings were divided into 25 equal time intervals over a single respiratory cycle for each of the 5 breaths for each patient in the two groups. For a given patient, the 5 breaths from the start of the trial were then superimposed and aligned with respect to time, and the average at each time point was calculated. The group mean tracings were then generated by ensemble averaging of the individual mean from each patient. The same procedure was performed for breaths at the end of the trial. (*Reproduced, with permission, from Jubran and Tobin.[15]*)

respiratory muscle performance in weaning failure patients. In reviewing this research, it is useful to distinguish between respiratory muscle strength and endurance (the inverse of fatigue).

Overall strength of the inspiratory muscles is usually assessed by measuring the pressure generated during a maximal inspiratory effort against an occluded airway.[23] Early investigators reported that maximal inspiratory pressure (P_{I}max) was lower in weaning failure patients than in weaning success patients. Indeed, the difference was considered so marked and reproducible that P_{I}max became a primary weaning predictor.[24] Many investigators have since demonstrated that P_{I}max is no lower in weaning failure patients than in weaning success patients.[12,20,25,26] The equivalence of inspiratory strength in the two groups has caused researchers to believe that muscle endurance must be more important than muscle strength in determining weaning outcome.

A fundamental limitation of the method for measuring P_{I}max is its total dependence on patient motivation and cooperation. (This limitation is even greater in critically ill patients.) By employing the twitch interpolation technique, however, it is possible to spot when a patient is failing to make a maximal effort.[23,27] At the point of apparent maximal voluntary effort, the investigator stimulates the phrenic nerves externally (electrically or magnetically). If the stimulus fails to produce an additional increase in inspiratory pressure, one concludes that the patient is making maximal effort. If the stimulus produces a superimposed spike on the pressure tracing, it means that the patient is not making a maximal effort. Laghi et al[28] applied this technique in 7 weaning patients. It was possible to detect a superimposed spike at the point of apparent maximal voluntary effort in every patient. These data highlight that the usual method

of assessing inspiratory effort underestimates inspiratory strength.

The pressure generated by a muscle in response to neural stimulation reflects contractility, and provides a measure of muscle strength that is independent of patient volition. In a study of weaning failure patients, Laghi et al[28] found that 6 had twitch transdiaphragmatic pressure (Pdi) values below 10 cmH$_2$O. Healthy subjects have twitch Pdi values of 35–39 cmH$_2$O, and stable patients with COPD have values of 17–20 cmH$_2$O. Contrary to recent thinking, these data indicate that weaning failure patents may have marked muscle weakness.

For years, researchers and clinicians have believed that most if not all weaning failure patients develop respiratory muscle fatigue by the time a failed weaning trial is stopped. This belief has been largely based on observations made by Cohen et al.[29] These investigators studied 12 patients who exhibited difficulties during weaning. Seven patients developed a shift in the power spectrum of the EMG signal recorded from the diaphragm, a finding judged to signify muscle fatigue. Six of the seven patients also exhibited paradoxical motion of the abdomen (inward displacement of the abdomen during inspiration) and four exhibited respiratory alternans (phasic alternation between the contribution of the rib cage and abdominal compartments to VT). The changes in rib cage–abdominal motion were not observed in the five patients who did not develop EMG changes. The investigators concluded that respiratory muscle fatigue was a common cause of weaning failure, and that its presence could be detected by finding paradoxical motion of the abdomen.

Subsequent detailed recordings of rib cage–abdominal motion revealed that when paradoxical motion of the abdomen occurs in weaning failure patients, it occurs immediately upon discontinuation of the ventilator and displays no progression over time.[30] When quantified objectively, the extent of abdominal paradox was no greater in weaning failure patients than in weaning success patients. In studies of healthy volunteers, fatigue was found to be neither necessary nor sufficient to induce abnormal rib cage–abdominal motion.[31] These data indicated that rib cage–abdominal motion could not be used for detecting respiratory muscle fatigue. The studies, however, did not exclude the possibility that fatigue is common in weaning failure patients.

Investigators also evaluated a more complex measure of fatigability, tension–time index. Tension–time index is the product of two fractions: (mean pressure per breath/$P_I$max) $\times$ (T_I/T_{TOT}). Studies in healthy volunteers have shown that respiratory muscle fatigue becomes inevitable when subjects breathe against an inspiratory load that causes tension–time index to rise above a threshold of 0.15. In a number of studies,[14,15,32] many more weaning failure patients than weaning success patients were found to exhibit tension–time index values above 0.15. As such, weaning failure patients experience workloads that are sufficient to induce respiratory muscle fatigue.

The EMG power spectrum and tension–time index provide only indirect evidence of fatigue, and do not provide direct proof of its occurrence. In neurophysiologic terms, fatigue means that a muscle is generating less force in response to a given neural stimulus than it had generated in the past. The most direct method for detecting fatigue in patients is to stimulate the phrenic nerves in the neck and measure the resulting change in transdiaphragmatic pressure (Pdi). The challenge with use of phrenic nerve stimulation in critically ill patients is to ensure that successive twitches are all generated at the same end-expiratory lung volume, a constant degree of neural depolarization is achieved by the stimulator, and twitch potentiation (the increase in pressure that occurs with a recent forceful contraction) is avoided. Laghi et al[28] measured twitch Pdi using phrenic stimulation in 11 weaning failure patients and 8 weaning success patients before and after a T-tube trial. Twitch Pdi was 8.9 $\pm$ 2.2 cmH_2O before the trial and 9.4 $\pm$ 2.4 cmH_2O after the trial in the weaning failure patients (Fig. 58-6). The respective values in the weaning success patients were 10.3 $\pm$ 1.5 and 11.2 $\pm$ 1.8 cmH_2O. No patient in either group exhibited a fall in twitch Pdi. The failure to develop fatigue was surprising because 7 of the 8 weaning failure patients had a tension–time index above 0.15.

The most likely reason that patients did not develop fatigue is because physicians reinstituted mechanical ventilation before there was enough time for its development. The relationship between tension–time index and the length of time that a load can be sustained until task failure follows an inverse-power function. Bellemare and Grassino[33] expressed the relationship as: time to task failure = 0.1 (tension–time index)$^{-3.6}$. The increase in tension–time index over the course of the weaning trial[28] and predicted time to task failure[33] are shown in Fig. 58-7. At the point that the physician reinstituted mechanical ventilation, patients were predicted to be able to sustain an additional 13 minutes of spontaneous breathing before developing task

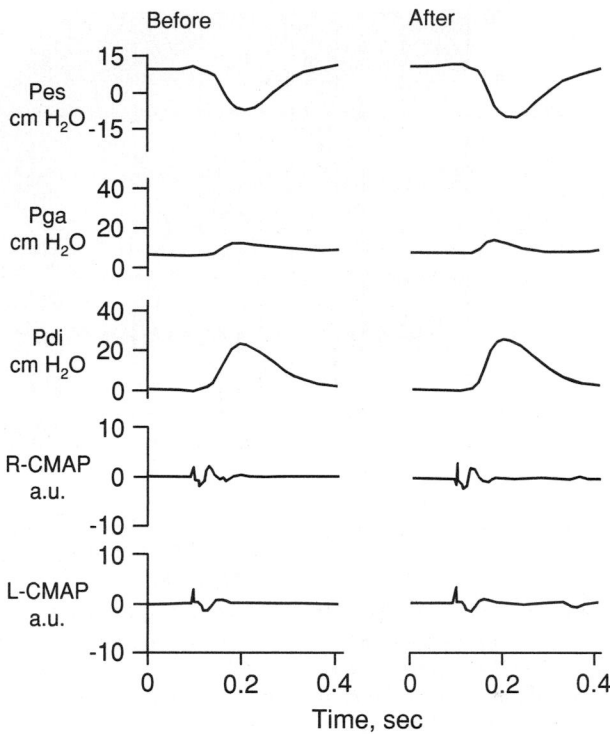

FIGURE 58-6 Esophageal pressure (*Pes*), gastric pressure (*Pga*), transdiaphragmatic pressure (*Pdi*), and compound motor action potentials (*CAMP*) of the right and left hemidiaphragms after phrenic nerve stimulation before (*left*) and after (*right*) a T-tube trial in a weaning failure patient. The end-expiratory value of Pes and the amplitude of the right and left CAMPs were the same before and after the trial, indicating that the stimulations were delivered at the same lung volume and that the stimulations achieved the same extent of diaphragmatic recruitment. The amplitude of twitch Pdi elicited by phrenic nerve stimulation was the same before and after weaning. (*Reproduced, with permission, from Laghi et al.[28]*)

failure. In other words, clinical manifestations of severe respiratory distress were evident for a substantial time before the patients were predicted to develop fatigue. In an intensive care setting, these clinical signs will lead attendants to reinstitute mechanical ventilation before fatigue has time to develop.

CARDIOVASCULAR PERFORMANCE

Although the respiratory muscles do not develop fatigue, they perform a huge workload. Thus, they depend on an efficient transport of O_2 by the cardiovascular system. Aware of this fact, several researchers have examined cardiovascular performance during weaning. Lemaire et al[34] studied 15 patients with COPD, 7 of whom had documented ischemic heart disease. The patients had previously failed at least two weaning attempts (lasting >30 minutes). After 10 minutes of breathing (through the ventilator without PEEP), the patients developed increases in transmural pulmonary artery wedge pressure (8 to 25 mmHg), cardiac index (3.2 to 4.3 L/min/m^2), left ventricular end-diastolic volume index (65 to 83 ml/m^2), and right ventricular end-diastolic volume

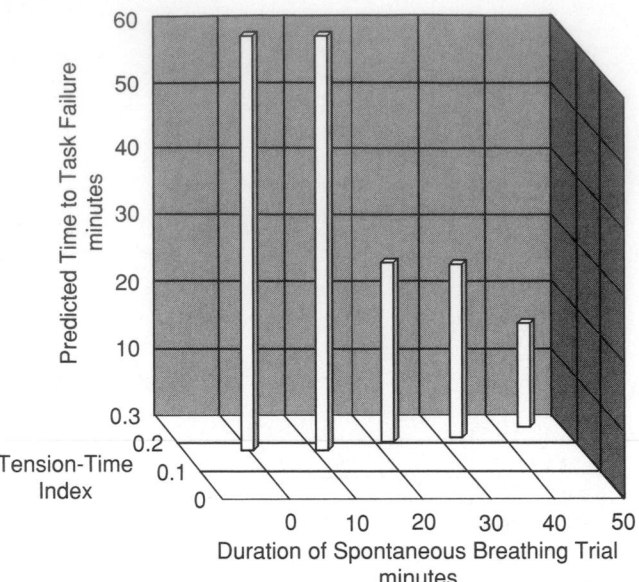

FIGURE 58-7 Interrelationship between the duration of a spontaneous breathing trial, tension–time index of the diaphragm, and predicted time to task failure in 9 patients who failed a trial of weaning from mechanical ventilation. The patients breathed spontaneously for an average of 44 minutes before a physician terminated the trial. At the start of the trial, the tension–time index was 0.17, and the formula of Bellemare and Grassino[33] (see text for details) predicted that patients could sustain spontaneous breathing for another 59 minutes before developing task failure. As the trial progressed, the tension–time index increased and the predicted time to development of task failure decreased. At the end of the trial, the tension–time index reached 0.26. That patients were predicted to sustain spontaneous breathing for another 13 minutes before developing task failure clarifies why patients did not develop a decrease in diaphragmatic twitch pressure. In other words, physicians interrupted the trial on the basis of clinical manifestations of respiratory distress, before patients had sufficient time to develop contractile fatigue. (*Reproduced, with permission, from Laghi and Tobin.[27]*)

index (83 to 103 ml/m²). The investigators attributed the increase in left ventricular end-diastolic volume to augmentation of venous return (secondary to low pleural pressure during spontaneous breathing and central translocation of blood volume secondary to peripheral vasoconstriction) and increased left ventricular afterload (secondary to markedly negative pleural pressure swings and increased catecholamine release). Nine of the 15 patients were weaned after 10 days of diuretic therapy, at which time wedge pressure had fallen to 9 mmHg.

Hurford et al[35] measured myocardial perfusion during a weaning trial in 15 ventilator-dependent patients using ^{201}thallium myocardial scintigraphy. Seven patients had documented coronary artery disease, and 10 had COPD. The initial scan during mechanical ventilation revealed fixed defects in 93% (13/14) of the patients. After 10 minutes of spontaneous breathing, 47% (7/15) of the patients developed significant alterations in their scans: either myocar-

dial redistribution of thallium or transient left ventricular dilatation (both attributed to transient ischemia).

Unlike the preceding investigators, Richard et al[36] studied a group of 12 patients with COPD who did not have documented coronary artery disease. All of the patients tolerated at least two 30-minute T-tube trials. (This finding suggests that they were weaning success patients, although it is not stated that they tolerated extubation.) Ejection fraction, measured by technetium^{99m} radionuclide angiography, was 54.5 ± 12.4% during mechanical ventilation. Spontaneous breathing resulted in a fall in ejection fraction to 47 ± 13%. The fall was homogenous and not accompanied by regional wall abnormalities that occur with myocardial ischemia. Moreover, thallium imaging performed 15 minutes after the weaning trial revealed normal myocardial perfusion. The investigators attributed the decrease in ejection fraction to increased left ventricular afterload.

Chatila et al[37] obtained continuous electrocardiographic recordings in 93 patients undergoing a weaning trial (some by T-tube trials, some by pressure support plus PEEP). Six patients (6.4%) developed a greater than 1-mm elevation of the ST segment and four of the patients failed the trial. The product of heart rate and systolic blood pressure increased during weaning, 12.0 to 13.4 mmHg*bpm*10³. A subsequent study by the same group[38] confirmed these observations.

Jubran et al[39] continuously recorded mixed venous O_2 saturation ($S\bar{v}_{O_2}$) in 8 weaning failure and 11 weaning success patients over the course of T-tube trials that lasted about 40 minutes. Immediately before the trial, $S\bar{v}_{O_2}$ was equivalent in the two groups. On discontinuation of the ventilator, $S\bar{v}_{O_2}$ fell progressively in the failure patients (to 51.5 ± 7.9% at the end of the trial), whereas it did not change in the success patients (Fig. 58-8). O_2 demand ($\dot{V}_{O_2}$) was similar in the two groups during the weaning trial, although it differed in the manner with which it was met.

The success patients demonstrated an increase in cardiac index between mechanical ventilation and the end of the trial, 3.07 to 3.51 L/m/m², which was accompanied by an increase in O_2 transport (Fig. 58-9). The failure group did not experience an increase in O_2 transport (partly because of elevations in right and left ventricular afterload); instead, they experienced an increase in O_2 extraction ratio, which, in turn, contributed to the fall in $S\bar{v}_{O_2}$. The failure patients also had more impaired pulmonary gas exchange ($\dot{Q}_{VA}/\dot{Q}_T$ was 0.32 at the start of the trial). The combination of greater venous admixture and low $S\bar{v}_{O_2}$ led to rapid arterial desaturation and a relative decrease in O_2 being supplied to the tissues.

Although the failure patients developed an increase in O_2 extraction ratio, the ratio at the end of the trial (0.37) did not reach the value associated with the onset of anaerobic metabolism (0.60). The failure patients developed a fall in pH (to 7.35), but the acidosis was completely explained by hypoventilation, further indicating that energy requirements were met solely by aerobic pathways. That the failure patients dealt with respiratory muscle energy demands through aerobic pathways is explained by the capacity of the diaphragm to achieve higher blood flow than most other

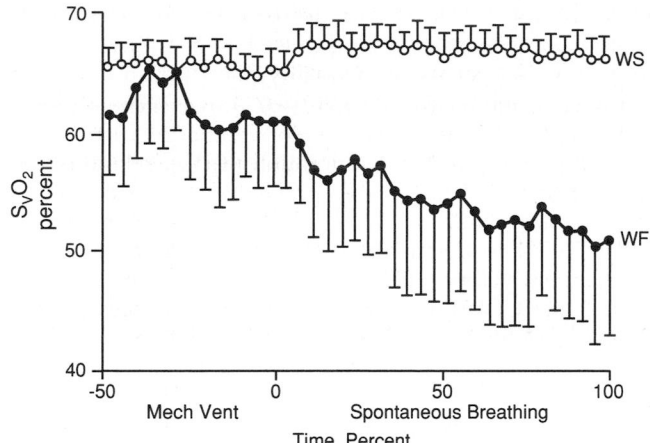

FIGURE 58-8 Ensemble averages of the interpolated values of mixed venous oxygen saturation ($S\bar{v}_{O_2}$) during mechanical ventilation and a trial of spontaneous breathing in weaning success patients (*open symbols*) and weaning failure patients (*closed symbols*). During mechanical ventilation, $S\bar{v}_{O_2}$ was similar in the two groups ($p = 0.28$). Between the onset and the end of the trial, $S\bar{v}_{O_2}$ decreased in the failure patients ($p <0.01$), whereas it did not change in the success patients ($p = 0.48$). Over the course of the trial, $S\bar{v}_{O_2}$ was lower in the failure patients than in the success patients ($p <0.02$). (Bars represent SE.) (*Reproduced, with permission, from Jubran et al.[39]*)

skeletal muscles.[40] The lowest partial mixed venous oxygen pressure ($P\bar{v}_{O_2}$) in the failure patients was 26 mmHg, which is above the threshold for onset of diaphragmatic lactate production.

Mean pulmonary artery pressure was higher in the failure patients than in the success patients during mechanical ventilation (Fig. 58-10). The pressure increased further over the course of the trial in the failure patients, whereas the success patients showed no change. Several factors account for the increase in pulmonary artery pressure. Hypoxemia and acidosis are potent vasoconstrictors. Pulmonary artery pressure can also be increased by alveolar vessel compression secondary to the increase in alveolar pressure that accompanies the dynamic hyperinflation and deterioration in pulmonary mechanics in weaning failure. During mechanical ventilation, the two groups had an equivalent mean arterial pressure, which increased in the failure patients by the end of the trial. The increase in mean arterial pressure combined with no change in cardiac index indicates an increase in left ventricular afterload.

De Backer et al[41] studied the hemodynamic response during a successful T-tube trial in 80 postoperative patients. The increase in $\dot{V}_{O_2}$ was similar in 52 patients after cardiac surgery, 17 patients after cardiac transplantation, and 11 patients after abdominal aortic surgery. The cardiovascular responses, however, differed among the groups. The increase in $\dot{V}_{O_2}$ was achieved by combined increases in cardiac output and O_2 extraction in the patients who underwent cardiac surgery or cardiac transplantation, and by an increase in cardiac output alone in the patients who underwent abdominal aortic surgery.

GAS EXCHANGE

A primary goal of mechanical ventilation is to improve gas exchange, and accordingly one expects some deterioration in gas exchange with the resumption of spontaneous breathing. The most detailed study of gas exchange during weaning is that conducted by Beydon et al.[42] They studied 8 patients with COPD who were considered ventilator

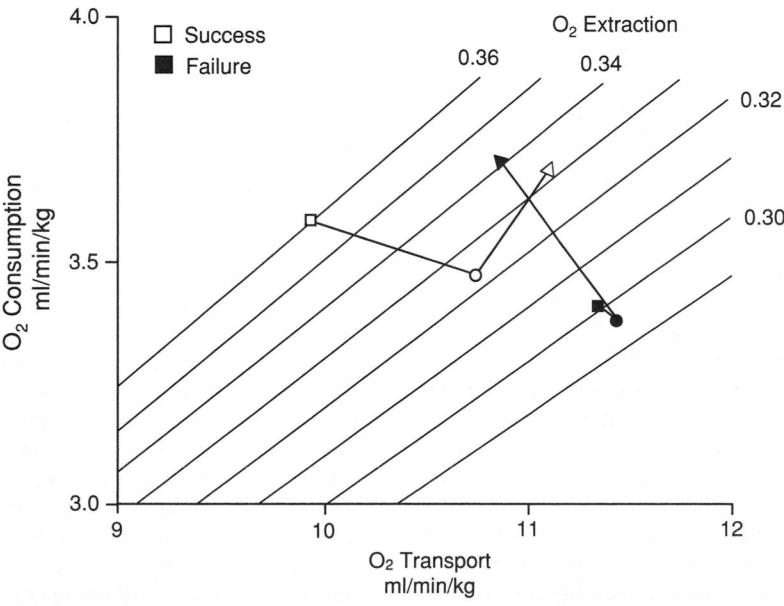

FIGURE 58-9 Oxygen transport, oxygen consumption, and isopleths of oxygen extraction ratio in weaning success (*open symbols*) and weaning failure patients (*closed symbols*) during mechanical ventilation (*squares*) and at the onset (*circles*) and end (*triangles*) of a T-tube trial. (*Reproduced, with permission, from Jubran et al.[39]*)

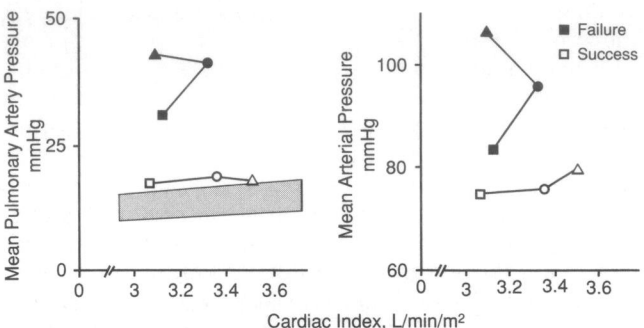

FIGURE 58-10 Mean pulmonary artery pressure and mean arterial pressure versus cardiac index during mechanical ventilation (*squares*) and at the onset (*circles*) and end (*triangles*) of a T-tube trial in weaning success (*open symbols*) and weaning failure patients (*closed symbols*). The shaded area represents the normal range of increase in mean pulmonary artery pressure with cardiac index. In the success patients, cardiac index increased between mechanical ventilation and the end of the trial, mean pulmonary artery pressure remained slightly above the normal range, and mean arterial pressure did not change. Conversely, in the failure patients, cardiac index was similar during mechanical ventilation and at the end of the T-tube trial, but both mean pulmonary artery pressure and mean arterial pressure were higher by the end of the trial (*p* <0.025 and *p* <0.05, respectively). The increases in these vascular pressures, together with the lack of change in cardiac index, indicate increases in right and left ventricular afterload in the failure patients. (*Reproduced, with permission, from Jubran et al.[39]*)

dependent (although the patients were able to sustain at least 1- to 3-hour periods of spontaneous breathing). When switched from controlled ventilation, patients developed an increase in frequency, fall in V_T (without change in $\dot{V}_E$), and an increase in P_{CO_2} (41 to 49 mmHg). Using the multiple inert gas technique, the investigators found that the distribution of ventilation to regions of ventilation-perfusion ($\dot{V}_A/\dot{Q}$) relationships above 100 (i.e., V_D/V_T) increased from $39 \pm 8\%$ during controlled ventilation to $46 \pm 7\%$ during spontaneous breathing. Perfusion of low-$\dot{V}_A/\dot{Q}$ regions was higher during spontaneous breathing than during controlled ventilation (15 ± 11 versus $6 \pm 8\%$). The investigators also performed isotope scans, which revealed a decrease in $\dot{V}_A/\dot{Q}$ ratios between the apex and the base of the lungs. This observation indicated that the low-$\dot{V}_A/\dot{Q}$ units identified by the inert gas technique were located at the lung bases. The major determinant of the $\dot{V}_A/\dot{Q}$ abnormalities was the size of V_T: it correlated with perfusion in the low-$\dot{V}_A/\dot{Q}$ range, the decrease of $\dot{V}_A/\dot{Q}$ ratios in the bases, and widening of the isotopic craniocaudal gradient. The maldistribution of $\dot{V}_A/\dot{Q}$ ratios during spontaneous breathing were improved by controlled ventilation but not by pressure support of 10 cmH_2O.

Torres et al[43] used the multiple inert gas technique to study 8 patients with COPD who were apparently successfully weaned. Measurements were first obtained during assist-control ventilation (V_T 700 ml, rate 12 breaths/min, and $F_{IO_2} \leq 0.40$). On discontinuation of the ventilator, the patients developed rapid shallow breathing (relative to ventilator settings) and acute respiratory acidosis (increase in

P_{CO_2} from 49 to 59 mmHg, decrease in pH from 7.42 to 7.36). Spontaneous breathing caused an overall worsening of ventilation-perfusion inequality: the fraction of cardiac output distributed to low-$\dot{V}_A/\dot{Q}$ (<0.1) areas increased from 9.4 to 19.6%; and the dispersion of ventilation distribution increased. Despite the deterioration in P_{CO_2} relationships, the expected fall in P_{O_2} was prevented by an increase in cardiac output (4.7 to 6.7 L/min) and increase in mixed venous P_{O_2} (37 to 42 mmHg). A largely similar pattern of gas exchange was reported by Ferrer et al,[44] who studied 7 patients with COPD that were not yet ready to tolerate complete discontinuation of mechanical ventilation.

Predicting Outcomes

GENERAL PRINCIPLES OF MEDICAL DECISION ANALYSIS

Research on prediction of weaning outcome employs the tools of medical decision analysis. To understand this literature, the reader has to cope with a huge number of specialized terms, many of which are not intuitive. Specificity, for example, measures the fraction of patients who are correctly identified as not having the disease under consideration. In regular everyday speech, specificity means that something is "clearly defined and definite" or "possessing properties that characterize a species." These ideas are the opposite of the absence of a property (disease). The terms are also duplicative. Specificity is also known as true-negative rate and as 1 minus false-positive rate. All of the specialized expressions are simply different ways of combining true-positive, true-negative, false-positive, and false-negative results. Life would be easier and make more sense if research on weaning predictors were solely communicated using these four test characteristics, and terms such as specificity were avoided. The reader, however, cannot adopt this minimalist approach and must instead grapple with the many terms because of their widespread use.

A second problem arises when a reader desires a more fundamental understanding and consults a textbook on medical decision analysis. Diagnostic test results are called "positive" (or abnormal) when they diagnose a "disease" (or undesirable condition), and "negative" when they indicate a normal or desirable condition.[45] When applying these concepts to weaning, the reader must think of "disease" as "weaning success" and a positive or abnormal test result as one that predicts weaning success. This orientation may seem counterintuitive. But too large a body of research already exists to make a fundamental change.

A third problem for the reader of a textbook on decision analysis is that the discussion is usually in generic terms, covering all possible disease states and all forms of diagnostic testing. This generic or abstract approach makes the discussion long-winded. The reader has to relate abstract concepts to the particular clinical situation that he or she is interested in. To ease discussion, we discuss the fundamental principles of decision analysis in terms of a single diagnostic test. We select a test used for predicting weaning outcome, the frequency-tidal volume ratio (f/V_T), because it has been subjected to the most investigation. And we focus on a single outcome: a patient's ability to tolerate a 30-minute T-tube trial without distress that is followed by extubation. This outcome is weaning success. Thus, a positive diagnostic test result is an index that predicts actual successful weaning outcome without the need for reintubation. The development of distress during a T-tube trial that leads to the reinstitution of mechanical ventilation is weaning failure; extubation followed by reintubation is not a necessary requirement to satisfy the definition of weaning failure. Thus, a negative diagnostic test result is an index that predicts either the development of distress during a T-tube trial (leading to the reinstitution of mechanical ventilation) or the need for reintubation after extubation. The reader can apply the same framework to other diagnostic tests (such as maximum inspiratory pressure) and to other outcomes (such as the prediction of reintubation in a patient who is extubated after a successful weaning trial).

The data generated by most diagnostic tests, including f/V_T, are reported as continuous variables. It is common, however, to focus on a threshold and view the data in dichotomous terms: an f/V_T value ≤ 100 (breaths per minute per liter) is referred to as a positive result (indicating a high likelihood of weaning success). All tests are inaccurate to varying degrees: no diagnostic test has a one-to-one correspondence with a disease state. The degree of error is assessed by comparing a test's performance against a reference test (gold standard). For weaning predictors, the gold standard is a patient's ability to tolerate a weaning trial that leads to extubation. This gold standard gives rise to significant difficulties in interpreting research findings (see below). Its lack of concreteness (necessary if a disorder is to fit an ontological model of disease) contrasts with more rigorous gold standards available for other diagnostic tests (histologic findings for evaluating a cancer marker).

The characteristics of test results are most easily displayed by a fourfold table, often referred to as a "2 × 2" table (Fig. 58-11). For f/V_T, a true-positive result is a reading of ≤ 100 (the test predicts weaning success) in a patient who actually tolerates a T-tube trial that leads to extubation (weaning success). A true-negative result is an f/V_T reading > 100 (the test predicts weaning failure) in a patient who actually develops distress during a T-tube trial and requires the reinstitution of mechanical ventilation (weaning failure). A false-positive result is an f/V_T reading ≤ 100 (the test predicts weaning success) in a patient who actually fails a weaning trial. A false-negative result is an f/V_T reading > 100 (the test predicts weaning failure) in a patient who actually tolerates a weaning trial and is extubated.

Each cell in Fig. 58-11 represents one of the four unique characteristics of a test (true-positive, true-negative, false-positive, and false-negative results). When developing a new weaning predictor, researchers need to undertake the initial evaluation in roughly equal numbers of weaning success and weaning failure patients if the predictor is to prove reliable under future testing.[46] Once the four test characteristics have been determined in a broad spectrum of weaning success and weaning failure patients, the test characteristics

are considered constant and the test can be applied to the evaluation of any given patient. There is, however, one major assumption, which is all too often ignored. *The formulae assume that the prevalence of weaning success and weaning failure in the new groups in which the test is being applied is the same as in the sample from which the four test characteristics were originally developed.*[46–48] If researchers are mindful of this fundamental requirement, much confusion can be avoided.

Sensitivity (also known as true-positive rate, a more intuitive term) answers the question: "In a weaning success patient, what is the likelihood that the predictor index will be positive ($f/V_T \leq 100$)?" Thus, sensitivity measures the proportion of weaning success patients in whom the predictive index is positive ($f/V_T \leq 100$). When clinicians are primarily interested in *screening*, they employ diagnostic tests that have a high sensitivity.[47] The purpose of a screening test is to pick up as many cases of a disease as possible out of the population being tested; screening can also be viewed as an exercise in ruling out disease, and a test for this purpose should have a low number of false-negative results (thus, a high sensitivity).[49] (Mnemonics have been proposed to remember these relationships. *SnNout*: if a test has a sufficiently high Sensitivity, a Negative result rules *out* the target disorder. Also, sensitivity is *PiD*, Positivity *In* Disease.) In the weaning context, this step is equivalent to using a predictor that will identify as many patients as possible who will actually pass a T-tube trial. Screening tests are typically performed in situations in which the pretest probability of the disease in question is very low (< 0.01).[45] Because results are most often negative, the test should be easy to perform. As such, a test that takes 30 minutes or more to conduct, such as a T-tube trial, is not a satisfactory screening test.

Specificity (also known as true-negative rate) answers: "In a weaning failure patient, what is the likelihood that the predictor index will be negative ($f/V_T > 100$)?" Thus, specificity measures the proportion of weaning failure patients in whom the predictive index is negative ($f/V_T > 100$). When clinicians are primarily interested in *confirming* (or ruling in) the presence of a disease, they employ diagnostic tests that have a low number of false-positive results, and thus, a high specificity.[47,49] (A mnemonic to remember this relationship is *SpPin*: if a test has a sufficiently high Specificity, a Positive result rules *in* the target disorder. Also, specificity is seen as *NiH*, Negativity *In* Health.) For example, using the criterion of a forced expiratory volume in 1 second (FEV_1) $< 80\%$ of predicted normal as a positive test is a poor test to *screen* for the presence of COPD because its sensitivity is unacceptably low (20%). But this criterion is adequate to *confirm* the presence of COPD because of its high specificity. Sensitivity of FEV_1 could be improved by relaxing the requirement for a positive test (defining a positive test as $< 90\%$ of predicted, but specificity would decrease because many people without COPD would be falsely identified as having the disorder). Because f/V_T has a relatively low specificity (0.64 in the original study[26]), it alone is not sufficient to confirm the presence of weaning failure. Instead, clinicians should undertake additional diagnostic testing, such as with a T-tube trial.

With rare exceptions, a single diagnostic test will not be both sufficiently sensitive to find all cases of a disease

Gold Standard
Success Fail

		Success	Fail
Test (f/V$_T$)	Positive (≤100)	TP	FP
	Negative (>100)	FN	TN

TP = Test predicts weaning success and patient actually succeeds

TN = Test predicts weaning failure and patient actually fails

FP = Test predicts weaning success and patient actually fails

FN = Test predicts weaning failure and patient actually succeeds

$$\text{Sensitivity} = \frac{TP}{TP + FN} = TPR = [1 - FNR]$$

$$\text{Specificity} = \frac{TN}{TN + FP} = TNR = [1 - FPR]$$

$$PPV = \frac{TP}{TP + FP}$$

$$NPV = \frac{TN}{TN + FN}$$

FN Rate = 1 - Sensitivity

FP Rate = 1 - Specificity

Likelihood ratio for a positive test = TPR / FPR = sensitivity / (1 - specificity)

Likelihood ratio for a negative test = FNR / TNR = (1 − sensitivity) / specificity

Prevalence = TP + FN / (TP + TN + FP + FN)

Diagnostic accuracy = [TP + TN] / [TP + TN + FP + FN]

FIGURE 58-11 A 2 × 2 tabular display of the characteristics of diagnostic tests. The vertical columns represent the results of the gold standard test. The horizontal rows represent the results of the index test. Readings of f/V$_T$ ≤100 are classified as positive test results and readings >100 are classified as negative test results. The relationship of these binary results to the outcome of a T-tube weaning trial forms a decision matrix that has four possible combinations.

(screening) and sufficiently specific to simultaneously avoid false-positive results (confirming).[50] For example, chest radiography is reasonably sensitive (but nonspecific) in detecting lung cancer. Almost all patients with lung cancer will have an abnormal chest radiograph. (The corollary is that a normal chest radiograph is good in ruling out lung cancer.) But not everyone with an abnormal chest radiograph has lung cancer (high false-positive rate). Conversely, a positive histology result on bronchoscopic biopsy is a reasonably specific diagnostic method (false-positive results are uncommon). But it is insensitive (often failing to capture cancers at inaccessible sites). For these reasons, clinicians commonly use diagnostic tests in combination.

Sensitivity and specificity are often regarded as constant properties of a diagnostic test. The characteristics, however, for any diagnostic test are derived from data collected in a selected group of patients. Consequently, sensitivity and specificity of diagnostic tests vary across different parts of the clinical spectrum of the disease they are attempting to identify or exclude.[48,51] Both sensitivity and specificity also perform differently in populations with different distributions of disease severity. For example, the sensitivity and specificity of electrocardiographic stress testing differs between patients with triple-vessel coronary artery disease and patients with mild single-vessel disease.[52]

False-positive rate answers: "What is the likelihood that a weaning failure patient will have a positive test result (f/V$_T$ ≤100)?" Thus, false-positive rate measures the proportion of positive test results (f/V$_T$ ≤100) in all weaning failure patients. In a weaning failure patient, test results are only true-negatives or false-positives. Thus, false-positive rate is the complement of true-negative rate (false-positive rate = 1 minus true-negative rate).

False-negative rate answers: "What is the likelihood that a weaning success patient will have a negative test result (f/VT >100)?" Thus, false-negative rate measures the proportion of negative test results (f/VT >100) in all weaning success patients. In a weaning success patient, test results are only true-positives or false-negatives. Thus, false-negative rate is the complement of true-positive rate (false-negative rate = 1 minus true-positive rate).

Sensitivity and specificity are calculated in patients in whom a diagnosis is already known. Clinicians, however, are faced with positive and negative results in patients whose diagnosis is not yet established. When contemplating a diagnosis, a clinician is not oriented down the vertical columns of the 2 × 2 table, but across the horizontal rows (see Fig. 58-11). Thus, clinicians think more in terms of positive- and negative-predictive values than in terms of sensitivity and specificity.[52] *Positive-predictive value* answers: "What is the likelihood of weaning success in a patient who has an f/VT ≤100?" Thus, positive-predictive value measures the fraction of patients with positive test results (f/VT ≤100) who are successfully weaned. *Negative-predictive value* answers: "What is the likelihood of weaning failure in a patient who has an f/VT >100?" Thus, negative-predictive value measures the fraction of patients with negative test results (f/VT >100) who fail a weaning trial. The positive- and negative-predictive values of a diagnostic test are particularly susceptible to variation in the prevalence of the condition under consideration (see below).

Likelihood ratio combines sensitivity and specificity into a single number. The likelihood ratio for a positive test relates the likelihood that a weaning success patient will have a positive test result (f/VT ≤100) to the likelihood that a weaning failure patient will have a positive test result. In other words, it is the probability of a positive test result (f/VT ≤100) in weaning success patients divided by probability of the same test result in weaning failure patients. It is calculated as true-positive rate/false-positive rate [or, sensitivity/(1 minus specificity)]. The likelihood ratio for a negative test relates the likelihood that a weaning success patient will have a negative test result (f/VT >100) to the likelihood that a weaning failure patient will have a negative test result. In other words, it is the probability of a negative test result (f/VT >100) in weaning success patients divided by probability of the same test result in weaning failure patients. It is calculated as false-negative rate/true-negative rate [or, (1 minus sensitivity)/specificity].

BAYES' THEOREM

Before clinicians perform a diagnostic test, they formulate a pretest (or prior) probability of disease. In the context of weaning, clinicians form an initial gestalt of a patient's likelihood of passing a T-tube trial based on their previous experience of patients with similar clinical characteristics. After measuring a weaning predictor test, and knowing its test characteristics (sensitivity and specificity), the clinician formulates a new probability statement (of whether the patient is likely to pass the T-tube trial). The new statement is the posttest (or posterior) probability. Bayes' theorem is an equation that describes the relationship between pretest probability and posttest probability. It is used to estimate how much the uncertainty of weaning outcome changes from before measurement of a predictor test (the pretest probability) to after obtaining the new information (the conditional probability).

Conditional probability is the probability that some event will occur given that some other event has occurred.[48] In the weaning context, it addresses, "What is the probability of a positive f/VT result (<100) conditional upon the patient's passing (or failing) a weaning trial?" A clinician can calculate the posttest probability of weaning success if he or she has three pieces of information: (1) the pretest probability of weaning success (typically, the prevalence); (2) the probability of a positive f/VT result (≤100) conditional upon the patient's passing a weaning trial (true-positive rate, or sensitivity); and (3) the probability of a positive f/VT result (≤100) conditional upon the patient's failing a weaning trial (false-positive rate, or 1 minus specificity). A useful weaning index has a high conditional probability (a high likelihood ratio), and thus markedly alters the posttest probability of weaning success. Bayes' theorem is employed to convert the vertical indices in the 2 × 2 table (sensitivity and specificity) into the desired horizontal indices of disease prediction, which indicate posttest probability.[50] The posttest probability of weaning success after obtaining a positive test result (f/VT ≤100) is the positive-predictive value. The posttest probability of weaning failure after obtaining a negative test result (f/VT >100) is the negative-predictive value.

Bayes' theorem operates on the assumption that the sensitivity and specificity of a test are constant irrespective of the pretest probability of disease. But "In the few instances in which this assumption has been checked," notes Feinstein,[50] "it was found to be erroneous." In a study of exercise electrocardiography for the diagnosis of coronary artery disease, Hlatky et al[53] found sensitivity was 0.80 in patients with typical angina and 0.53 in patients with atypical chest pain; sensitivity was 0.85 in patients with triple-vessel disease and 0.48 in patients with single-vessel disease. Specificity was 0.85 when left-ventricular ejection fraction was ≥50% and 0.73 when ejection fraction was 30–49%. In a study of patients being evaluated for urinary tract infection, Lachs et al[51] found that sensitivity of the dipstick test was 0.92 in patients with a high (>0.50) pretest probability of infection (patients with dysuria, urgency, and hematuria), and sensitivity was 0.56 in patients with a low pretest probability (≤0.50). Conversely, specificity was 0.42 in patients with a high pretest probability for infection, and 0.78 in patients with a low pretest probability. Indeed, for any condition, history and physical examination is likely to be more abnormal when a disease is extensive, and thus, the clinician will assign a high pretest probability.[54] In many studies of weaning predictors, researchers have assumed that reported values for sensitivity and specificity apply in all circumstances. This assumption can give rise to errors when Bayes' theorem is applied.[48,50,55]

PRETEST PROBABILITY OF SUCCESSFUL OUTCOME

In evaluating the performance of weaning predictors, probably no aspect is ignored more often—and the source of greater confusion—than recognizing the fundamental importance of pretest probability (the anticipated prevalence of a disorder). The pretest probability is the fraction of weaning success patients out of an entire weaning population (both success and failure patients). This pretest probability markedly affects the interpretation of new test information. In their book on medical decision analysis, Sox and colleagues[45] state, "Perhaps the most important idea in this book is the following: *The interpretation of a test result depends on the pretest probability of disease.*" That is, a clinician's interpretation of new diagnostic information depends on what he or she believed before doing the test. As a clinician's estimate of pretest probability of weaning success increases, so also does the posttest probability of weaning success.

The pretest probability has an enormous influence over the ability of the results of any diagnostic test to alter the posttest probability of disease. When the pretest probability of weaning success is high, a positive test result ($f/V_T \leq 100$) has little effect. (The probability cannot increase much after a positive test because of a ceiling effect.) A negative test result ($f/V_T > 100$) will drop the probability considerably, but only into the large middle range of probability that is diagnostically inconclusive.[55] Conversely, when the pretest probability of weaning success is low, a negative test result ($f/V_T > 100$) has little effect. (The probability does not have anywhere to drop after a negative test. A positive test result [$f/V_T \leq 100$] has a large effect, but it only brings the clinician into the large middle range of probability.) Thus, when the pretest probability is already close to diagnostic certainty (high or low), a test that does not confirm the diagnostic suspicion can produce substantial changes in posttest probability. The above description is not unique to weaning predictors, but applies to all diagnostic tests in medicine. The only exception to this relationship between pretest probability and postprobability is an imaginary test with 100% sensitivity and 100% specificity.

A clinician gains the maximum increase in posttest probability for a positive test when pretest probability is 40%, and gains the maximum increase for a negative test when the pretest probability is 60%.[47] That is, physicians have most to gain from diagnostic testing when the pretest probability of a condition is close to 50%.[47] For a weaning predictor test to influence decision making, it needs to be measured early in a patient's course (expediting the transition between weaning stage 2 and stage 3). If a clinician observes that half or more of his or her measurements of weaning predictors generate positive results (indicating that a patient is ready for a weaning trial), that clinician is not measuring the predictor test early enough in the patient's course. A clinician who is measuring predictor tests early in a patient's course will obtain negative test results (indicating that a patient is not ready for a weaning trial) at least as often as positive results. (In a trial of weaning techniques, for example, Ely et al[56] obtained positive results in 113 of 149 tested patients [76%]; many of the 113 patients would likely have satisfied the same criteria and tolerated extubation a day or more sooner than actually happened.) Given the above, it is obvious that measuring weaning predictors in patients who have already passed a weaning trial is a futile undertaking.

Unfortunately, most studies of weaning predictors have been conducted in patients who had a pretest probability of weaning success of 75% or higher (Table 58-1).

SEQUENTIAL DIAGNOSTIC TESTING

The implications of pretest probability are greater for weaning than for many clinical situations because weaning almost invariably involves a sequence of diagnostic tests: measurement of predictors, followed by a weaning trial, followed by a trial of extubation. Bayes' theorem assumes that the conditional probability of a test result is independent of pretest (prior) information—the *assumption of conditional independence*. The idea of independence is one of the most important concepts in probability theory.[57]

Two events are judged *independent* if the knowledge that one event has occurred tells you nothing about whether the second event will occur. The events "the patient has a skull fracture" and "the patient has cholecystitis" are independent. That is, conditioning on one event does not change the probability of the other event. In contrast, the events "the patient has cholecystitis" and "the patient has abdominal pain" are not independent. The conditioning probability of abdominal pain, given cholecystitis, is much higher than the nonconditional probability of abdominal pain (the proportion of all patients in the world with abdominal pain). When both an exercise electrocardiogram and a radionuclide myocardial scan are performed before coronary arteriography, the false-positive rate of each test depends on the results of the other test.[45] That is, the assumption of conditional independence of the two tests is invalid. Likewise, the conditioning probability that a T-tube trial will be successful and lead to extubation is much higher given a positive f/V_T test result (≤ 100). The two events, a positive f/V_T test result (≤ 100) and a successful T-tube trial, are not conditionally independent.

Because the assumption of conditional independence has not been verified for most combinations of two or more tests, experts recommend that the posttest probability of the first test be used as the pretest probability of the second test.[45] Figure 58-12 shows typical changes in pretest probability of successful extubation and posttest probability of successful extubation with the sequential performance of f/V_T measurement, a T-tube trial, and a trial of extubation.

SPECTRUM BIAS AND TEST-REFERRAL BIAS

The term *spectrum* denotes the range of disease presentation and severity found in patients used to challenge the sensitivity and specificity of a diagnostic test.[49] *Spectrum bias* occurs when a diagnostic test performs differently in different groups of patients.[51] The first form of spectrum bias occurs when the new study population contains more sick patients than the population in which a diagnostic test was originally developed. A second form of spectrum bias, *test-referral bias*, occurs when the results of a test under evaluation (f/V_T) are used to select patients for the gold standard test (T-tube trial).

To illustrate both forms of bias, we discuss the evaluation of a hypothetical new liver scan for diagnosing metastases

TABLE 58-1   Accuracy of Frequency-to-Tidal Volume Ratio (f/V$_T$) in Predicting Weaning Outcome

Threshold	Sensitivity	Specificity	PPV	NPV	No. of Patients	PPS	Author
≤105	0.97	0.64	0.78	0.95	64	0.56	Yang and Tobin[26]
<96	0.89	0.83	0.93	0.77	40	0.7	Gandia and Blanco[11]
≤100	0.97	0.40	0.85	0.80	45	0.78	Sassoon and Mahutte[12]
≤100	0.94	0.73	0.79	0.92	31	0.52	Yang[26]
≤105 (PS 7–8)	1.00	0.27	0.69	1.00	29	0.62	Mohsenifar et al[72]
≤105 (PS ?)	0.72	0.11	0.79	0.08	52	0.83	Lee et al[79]
60	0.73	0.75	0.92	0.36	67	0.82	Capdevila et al[13]
<100	0.92	0.22	0.83	0.40	94	0.81	Epstein[1]
≤100	0.89	0.41	0.72	0.68	100	0.63	Chatila et al[104]
≤100	0.98	0.59	0.83	0.94	100	0.63	Chatila et al[104]
<100	0.94	0.81	0.80	0.94	38	0.45	Dojat et al[74]
≤100 (PS 7)	0.96	0.00	0.98	0.00	163	0.982	Leitch et al[59]
<105	0.65	0.58	0.60	0.63	75	0.49	Mergoni et al[80]
≤105	1.00	0.40	0.77	1.00	15	0.67	Bouachour et al[114]
≤11 bpm/ml/kg	0.79	0.78	0.94	0.47	47 Ped	0.81	Baumeister[77]
Not stated	0.84	0.83	0.80	0.86	127	–	Гологорский et al[149]
100	0.97	0.33	0.94	0.50	183	0.92	Jacob et al[75]
100	0.96	0.31	0.94	0.40	183	0.92	Jacob et al[75]
≤105	0.74	0.73	0.90	0.44	49	0.78	Krieger et al[81]
≤130 at 3 h	0.93	0.89	0.97	0.80	49	0.78	Krieger et al[81]
65 (PS 5)	0.90	0.80	0.90	0.70	40	0.7	Rivera and Weissman[73]
65 (PS + IMV)	1.00	0.82	0.84	1.00	40	0.7	Rivera and Weissman[73]
≤11 bpm/ml/kg	0.48	0.86	0.53	0.83	84 Ped	0.75	Farias et al[70]
≤100	0.90	0.36	0.66	0.73	217	0.58	Vallverdu et al[61]
≤8 bpm/ml/kg	0.74	0.74	0.97	0.22	227 Ped	0.89	Thiagarajan et al[150]
<88	0.77	0.79	0.68	0.86	101	0.63	Zeggwagh et al[78]
≤105	0.93	0.75	0.83	0.89	27	0.56	Maldonado et al[76]
<100 (PS 5)	0.96	0.18	0.78	0.60	68	0.75	Uusaro et al[62]
≤105	0.84	0.17	0.82	0.19	100	0.82	Khamiees et al[63]
<100	0.90	0.42	0.92	0.36	115	0.89	Smina et al[65]
≤100	0.81	0.14	0.71	0.22	51	0.73	Conti et al[71]
<50	0.35	0.56	0.81	0.14	57	0.84	Fernandez et al[66]
≤105	0.81	0.57	NR	NR	55	0.58	Jiang et al[83]

ABBREVIATIONS: bpm, breaths per minute; IMV, intermittent mandatory ventilation; NPV, negative predictive value; PPS, pretest probability of success; PPV, positive predictive value; PS, pressure support.
The listed studies are those that reported data on the accuracy of f/V$_T$ as a predictor of weaning outcome. Three groups of investigators, Chatila et al,[104] Jacob et al,[75] and Krieger et al,[81] report data under two different conditions in their articles; both sets of data are presented. Pretest probability of success in a study is the fraction of patients with a successful outcome of the total population (both success and failure patients) included in that study.

to the liver, which is compared against liver histology as the gold standard. (A true-positive test result is the presence of opacities [positive scan] in a patient who is found to have evidence of cancer on liver biopsy.) Importantly, the clinicians in this study are using the results of the scan to select the patients they refer for a liver biopsy. This step has two effects on the true-positive rate of the study population. One, the complete or partial exclusion of patients who have negative scans causes the study population to become weighted towards patients who may on average be sicker, which predisposes to overestimation of the true-positive rate (spectrum bias). Two, fewer patients with negative scans undergo a liver biopsy (test-referral bias; also termed work-up bias or verification bias).Inevitably, the denominator in the equation for true-positive rate [true-positives/(true-positives + false-negatives)] gets smaller. (A false-negative test result is the absence of opacities [negative scan] in a patient who is found to have evidence of cancer on liver biopsy.) Referral

of patients with positive scans does not change. Thus, the numerator in the equation for true-positive rate is unaffected. Both spectrum bias (caused by the skewing of the study population towards patients who tend to be sicker on average) and test-referral bias (the complete or partial exclusion of patients with negative scans) produce an increase in the true-positive rate. The false-positive rate is also affected. The complete or partial exclusion of patients who have negative scans lowers the number of true-negative results in the denominator [false-positive rate = false-positives/(true-negatives + false positives)]. (A false-positive test result is the presence of a positive scan in a patient who does not have evidence of cancer on liver biopsy.) Because referral of patients with positive scans does not change, there is a disproportionate increase in false-positive results, and thus an inflated false-positive rate. In some studies, the effect of test-referral bias has resulted in as few as 3% of a clinically relevant population being included in a study population.[45]

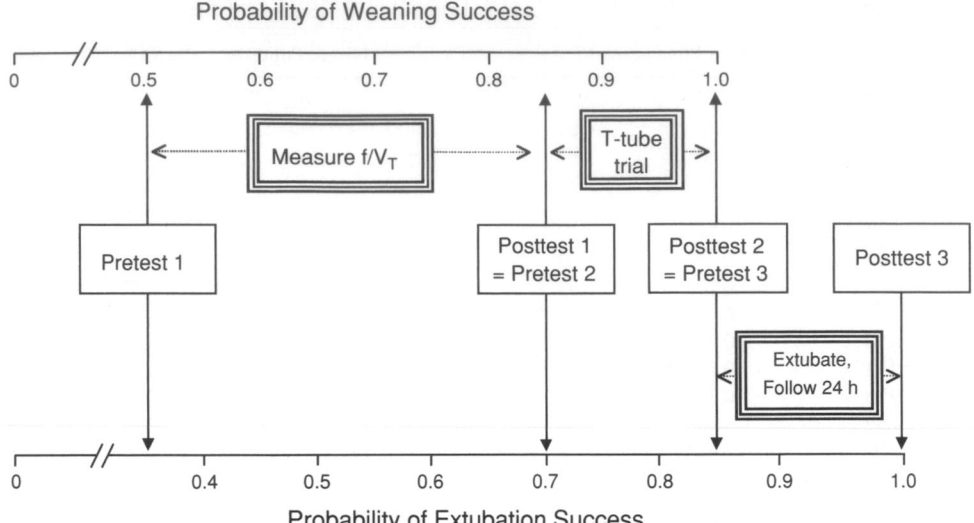

FIGURE 58-12 Interpreting the sequence of diagnostic testing in a patient who is weaned from mechanical ventilation and then extubated, with successful outcome defined as the ability to breathe spontaneously without ventilator assistance for 24 hours after extubation. Pretest 1 is the pretest probability of extubation success before measurement of f/V_T. The f/V_T reading constitutes the posttest results of the first diagnostic test, and also pretest probability of extubation success for the second diagnostic test, a T-tube trial. The outcome of the T-tube trial constitutes the posttest results of the second diagnostic test, and also the pretest probability of extubation success for the third diagnostic test, a trial of extubation. The outcome of the trial of extubation constitutes the posttest result of the third diagnostic test. In this hypothetical example, pretest probability of weaning success for the first diagnostic test is set arbitrarily at 0.50; the extent of the change for each subsequent step is based on average changes reported in published studies.

When statistical evaluation of a diagnostic test is based only on data obtained in patients who had both the initial diagnostic test (liver scan in the above example) and the definitive diagnostic procedure (liver biopsy), many patients who have negative test results will be omitted from the 2×2 diagnostic table.[50] Consequently, the numbers in the top two horizontal cells (true-positives and false-positives), where results of the first diagnostic test are positive, will be excessive. Thus, sensitivity will be falsely elevated and specificity falsely reduced.

Spectrum bias and test-referral bias accounts for much confusion in the interpretation of studies of weaning predictor tests. A skilled clinician who measures f/V_T will obtain on average at least as many (if not more) negative test results as positive test results (if he or she is trying to move the transition between stage 2 and stage 3 of weaning [see Fig. 58-1] to an earlier time in a patient's course). Thus, pretest probability of weaning success is 50% or lower. Clinicians commonly use the f/V_T result to decide which patients will progress that day to a weaning trial. They subsequently use the results of the weaning trial to decide which patients will undergo a trial of extubation. If tolerance of extubation is used as the gold standard for evaluating the accuracy of f/V_T, the requirement to pass a weaning trial before extubation (as a criterion for entry into a study) will lead to fewer patients with negative test results ($f/V_T > 100$) and relatively more patients with positive test results ($f/V_T \leq 100$) in the study population (test-referral bias). Thus, the patients in the new study population will have a lower f/V_T on average than the population in which the weaning predictor was originally developed (spectrum bias). Test-referral

bias leads to an increase in both true-positive rate and false-positive rate.

A good illustration of the effect of test-referral bias is provided by the data of Epstein.[1] He evaluated the ability of f/V_T to predict successful toleration of extubation. He measured f/V_T in 94 patients before a trial of spontaneous breathing that resulted in extubation. By the investigator's definition, any patient who failed the spontaneous breathing trial was excluded from the study population. Of 94 patients, 76 breathed without assistance for >72 hours after extubation and 18 patients required reintubation. The test characteristics (the four numbers of a 2×2 table) were: true-positive results 70, false-positive results 14, false-negative results 6, and true-negative results 4. The pretest probability of successful outcome was higher, 0.81, than in the original report of f/V_T.[26] Only 10 of the 94 patients had negative test results ($f/V_T > 100$); this weighting of f/V_T values towards low readings produced spectrum bias. Test-referral bias also occurred because all of the patients had to pass a spontaneous breathing trial to gain entry into the study; consequently, there were fewer true-negative and false-negative test results. The combination of spectrum bias and test-referral bias resulted in different test performance than that originally reported:[26] lower specificity, 0.22 versus 0.64, lower negative-predictive value, 0.40 versus 0.95, and higher positive-predictive value, 0.83 versus 0.78. We discuss this study in detail because Epstein provided all the numbers of a 2×2 table for his study patients. Several other studies of weaning predictors also suffer from the flaws of spectrum bias and test-referral bias.[13,58-66] The misinformation that has resulted from failure to take into account test-referral and other forms of bias brings to mind the comment of the late Alvan Feinstein, the founding father of clinical epidemiology:[43] ". . . the most important issues in biostatistics are not expressed with statistical procedures. The issues are inherently scientific, rather than purely statistical, and relate to the architectural design of research, not to the numbers with which the data are cited and interpreted."

The extreme case of test-referral bias is the situation in which investigators require a positive f/V_T result (value ≤ 100) before subjecting a patient to a T-tube trial. By design, no patient with a negative f/V_T result (value >100) would undergo a T-tube trial. In that instance, all failed T-tube trials would be in patients who had positive f/V_T results. Thus, the false-positive rate of $f/V_T \leq 100$ would tend towards 1.0, and specificity to 0. Investigators who have evaluated the accuracy of f/V_T have not required an $f/V_T \leq 100$ per se before referring patients for a weaning trial (the gold standard test). Vallverdu et al[61] and Fernandez et al,[66] however, did require patients to have a frequency ≤ 35 breaths per minute and $V_T \geq 5$ ml/kg; for an average 70-kg patient, these criteria result in $f/V_T < 100$. Khamiees et al[63] required $f/V_T < 125$ for entry. Not surprisingly, these three groups reported very low specificities for f/V_T (see Table 58-1). (Specificity in the study of Fernandez et al[66] is inflated through use of an f/V_T threshold of 50.)

Test-referral bias has been described in many clinical settings. In an investigation into the dramatic reduction in the specificity of radionuclide ventriculography (shortly after its introduction), Rozanski et al[67] referred to test-referral bias as a "Catch -22." The better the initial reports of sensitivity and specificity, the greater the likelihood that a test will be used as a criterion for referral (for coronary angiography in their case). Then, the more the test is used as a referral criterion, the less well it will appear to perform.

Another feature of test-referral (and spectrum) bias is a study population with an extremely high rate of weaning success. In a study of weaning predictors, Leitch et al[59] reported a weaning success rate of 98%. Extremely high success rates do not indicate that the managing physicians are astute or skilled. Instead, they suggest that many patients judged likely to fail a weaning trial were in reality ready for that step. Such misjudgment translates into patients staying on the ventilator longer than is necessary, with consumption of resources and an increased risk of ventilator-induced complications.

TAILORING A PREDICTOR TO PATIENT NEEDS

The threshold value of a test (the single value that separates positive from negative results) is determined by conducting research in a large number of patients. When applying the test to an individual patient, however, clinicians may decide to raise or lower the threshold value, taking into account unique aspects of a particular patient's condition.

Consider a severely immunocompromised patient in whom the physician believes that the risk of complications with continued ventilation far outweigh the risk of weaning failure or reintubation. With that mindset, the physician wants a weaning predictor test that has a very low rate of

false-negative results. (A false-negative result is a test that predicts failure, $f/V_T > 100$, but the patient succeeds.) False-negative results are reflected in sensitivity (for f/V_T, 0.97[26]) and negative-predictive value (for f/V_T, 0.95[26]). To minimize the likelihood of a false-negative result in this patient, the physician may decide to undertake a T-tube trial even when f/V_T is higher than the usual threshold of 100 (say, 115 or 125). Use of a higher threshold will move borderline patients away from being kept on the ventilator and push them towards a weaning attempt. The clinician must recognize that a lower false-negative likelihood can only be achieved by also accepting a higher false-positive likelihood for the test result.

The second example relates to a patient with a neck deformity in whom the physician is leaning towards keeping the patient on the ventilator for an additional day or longer rather than taking a risk of weaning failure and reintubation. The physician wants a weaning predictor test that has a very low rate of false-positive results. (A false-positive is a test that predicts success, $f/V_T < 100$, but the patient will fail a weaning trial.) False-positive results are reflected in specificity (for f/V_T, 0.64[26]) and positive-predictive value (for f/V_T, 0.78[26]). To minimize the likelihood of a false-positive result in this patient, the physician may decide to undertake a T-tube trial only if the f/V_T threshold is lower than the usual 100 (say, 90 or 80). But, again, the lower false-positive likelihood can be achieved only by accepting a higher false-negative likelihood for the test result.

If the particular group of patients that a clinician manages usually have a high likelihood of weaning success (high prevalence, or pretest probability, of success), the clinician should use an f/V_T threshold higher than 105, and thus accept a higher false-positive rate so as to maintain a high true-positive rate.[68] This new threshold will result in a higher sensitivity and lower specificity.

How much to adjust thresholds in an attempt to minimize false-negative results and false-positive results is an area of active decision-analysis research. In population studies, the threshold of a test is set such that "the burden of false-positive results multiplied by the number of false-positive results" balances "the burden of false-negative results multiplied by the number of false-negative results." When adjusting the threshold value for an individual patient, the clinician needs to do an analogous computation. Reducing the occurrence of one undesirable test result can only be achieved by simultaneously increasing the occurrence of the other undesirable result. In the language of game theory, this balancing action is a zero-sum game (one goal is achieved at the expense of another).

Prediction of Weaning Outcome

FREQUENCY-TO-TIDAL VOLUME RATIO

The introduction of f/V_T as a weaning predictor stemmed from research into the pathophysiology of weaning failure. Patients who failed a T-tube trial exhibited an increase in frequency and a fall in V_T in the first few minutes after removal of ventilator support[8] (Fig. 58-13). In a subsequent

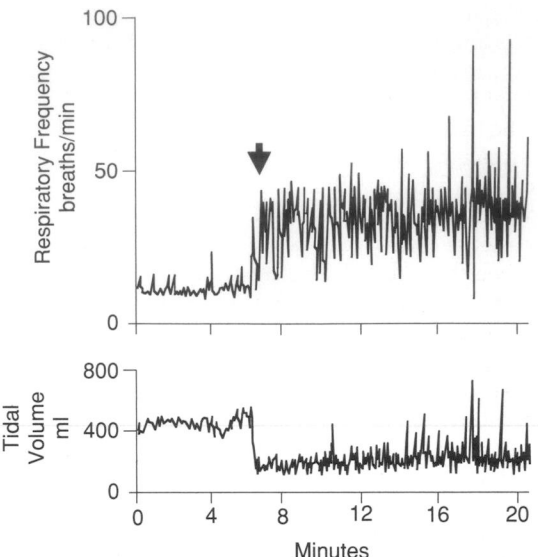

FIGURE 58-13 A time-series, breath-by-breath plot of respiratory frequency and tidal volume in a patient who failed a weaning trial. The arrow indicates the point of resuming spontaneous breathing. Rapid, shallow breathing developed almost immediately after discontinuation of the ventilator. (*Reproduced, with permission, from Tobin et al.[8]*)

study, Yang and Tobin[26] found that f/V_T was superior to nine other weaning predictors. In that initial study, sensitivity was 0.97, specificity 0.64, positive-predictive value 0.78, and negative-predictive value 0.95.

VARIATION IN PERFORMANCE AMONG STUDIES

The accuracy of this predictor has been evaluated in more than 25 subsequent studies, as listed in Table 58-1. As expected, many of the findings are conflicting, and careful examination of each study is required to make sense of the reported information. There was variation in the outcome being studied, the timing of the measurement in relationship to the stage of a patient's clinical course, the conditions under which f/V_T was measured, and availability of f/V_T to clinicians making the decisions under investigation. When these and other aspects are varied and combined in different permutations, it is no surprise that the picture is confusing. We will discuss how these aspects vary among studies.

Different Outcomes

In the original study of f/V_T, a successful study outcome was defined as patients who did not develop distress during a trial of spontaneous breathing, as judged by their primary physician.[26] Because of poor physician judgment, some patients could be classified as weaning success, but then develop distress immediately after extubation and require reintubation. To avoid this problem, the definition of weaning success was broadened to include the requirement that patients sustain spontaneous breathing for ≥24 hours after extubation. All of the remaining patients were classified as an unsuccessful study outcome; that is, the combination of patients who developed clinical distress during a trial of spontaneous breathing or who required reintubation. In

retrospect, it would have minimized subsequent confusion had the two subsets of an unsuccessful outcome—failure of a trial of spontaneous breathing and reintubation—been reported individually.

Subsequent evaluations of the accuracy of f/V_T have focused on its ability to predict either failure of a T-tube trial or the need for reintubation,[61,69–71] failure of a trial of breathing with pressure support (PS, fixed or diminishing levels),[66,72] failure of a trial of weaning achieved by progressively decreasing the level of synchronized intermittent mandatory ventilation,[73] failure of either a weaning trial or the need for reintubation,[74,75] failure of a weaning trial with the exclusion of patients who required reintubation,[76] the need for reintubation in patients who had been extubated after already tolerating a weaning trial,[1,13,58–60,63–66,77] and the need for reintubation in patients who had been extubated without first passing a weaning trial.[78]

Timing of Making Measurement

The original study of f/V_T was undertaken to predict "the earliest time that a patient might resume spontaneous breathing."[26] In other words, the intent was to move the transition between stage 2 and stage 3 of weaning (see Fig. 58-1) to an earlier time in a patient's course. In that study, f/V_T was measured in the first few minutes after disconnection from the ventilator and before a T-tube trial. Subsequent investigators have measured f/V_T after patients had already demonstrated the ability to tolerate 20 minutes of a T-tube trial (a point at which most weaning failure patients will have declared themselves),[13] or, after excluding weaning failure patients, and evaluating the accuracy of f/V_T in predicting successful extubation.[1,58–60,63–66,77]

Prior Use of Frequency-to-Tidal Volume Ratio Before its Evaluation

In the early evaluations of f/V_T, clinicians were using neither frequency nor V_T when making weaning decisions. Instead, decisions were largely based on Pa_{O_2}, P_Imax, $\dot{V}_E$, and vital capacity. Once clinicians start to base clinical decisions on a diagnostic test, it becomes increasingly difficult to evaluate the accuracy of the test in a meaningful manner. The method for quantifying the effect (helpful or unhelpful) of a diagnostic test is to measure the change from pretest probability to posttest probability (see above discussion of Bayes' theorem). If, however, clinicians have already used frequency and V_T for deciding when to begin weaning attempts—and especially if they used the measurements to exclude patients from a weaning attempt—one cannot expect f/V_T to substantially increase the posttest probability because the pretest probability has already been based on the measurements of frequency and V_T.

In many studies, investigators state that f/V_T was available to the clinicians who made the weaning decisions.[1,58,59,61–63,65,66,71,76,79–83] In some evaluations of the accuracy of f/V_T, investigators first excluded patients with rapid shallow breathing. Entry criteria included frequency <35 breaths/minute and V_T >5 ml/kg[61,66,76] (for an average size patient, these criteria result in f/V_T <100). Naturally, such exclusion criteria have a major influence on the evaluation of a weaning predictor (see above discussion on test-referral bias). The skewed study population also means that the findings cannot be generalized to everyday clinical practice where physicians make decisions regarding patients about whom they are equally doubtful as to whether weaning will succeed or fail (pretest probability of success 50%).

Conditions of Making Measurements

The threshold value of f/V_T was derived from measurements made in patients breathing without ventilator assistance. Some researchers, however, have evaluated the accuracy of the same threshold despite measuring f/V_T during PS. This step is surprising in that the most documented physiologic action of PS is that it lowers frequency and increases V_T (see Chapter 9). In ventilator-supported patients, f/V_T during unassisted breathing has been shown to be 23–52% higher than with PS of 5 cmH$_2$O and 46–82% higher than with PS of 10 cmH$_2$O.[84–87] Several investigators, however, have conducted studies in which they measured f/V_T during PS and concluded that a threshold of 100 was unreliable in predicting weaning outcome.[59,72,79,88] In reality, this conclusion could have been reached through a simple thought experiment without ever subjecting patients to the ordeal of a research study. (The assertion that PS of 5–10 cmH$_2$O is simply overcoming the resistance posed by an endotracheal tube has been negated by Strauss et al;[89] see below.)

The measurement of f/V_T while a patient is receiving continuous positive airway pressure (CPAP) suffers from the same flaw. In a patient with auto-PEEP, CPAP of 5 cmH$_2$O or so will decrease mechanical load and alter the breathing pattern. The effect of CPAP on breathing pattern has been studied in detail in healthy subjects.[90] Compared with no CPAP, the addition of CPAP of 5 cmH$_2$O caused f/V_T to decrease by 38% when delivered by a demand valve and by 28% when delivered by a high-flow reservoir. In 33 patients being weaned from mechanical ventilation after coronary bypass surgery, El-Khatib et al[91] found that a 1-minute measurement of f/V_T was 36 ± 14 (SD) when patients received CPAP 5 cmH$_2$O plus F$_{IO_2}$ 0.21; f/V_T did not change when F$_{IO_2}$ was increased to 0.40. When CPAP was removed and the patients breathed room air spontaneously off the ventilator, f/V_T increased (by 97.3%) to 71 ± 23.

Time Lapse Between Measurement and Outcome

In the original study, a T-tube trial was conducted immediately after the measurement of f/V_T. Patients who passed the trial were immediately extubated. Subsequent investigators have evaluated the accuracy of f/V_T several hours after its measurement.[1,81] One group of investigators evaluated the accuracy of f/V_T in predicting the ability to discontinue mechanical ventilation at 3 and 7 days after its measurement.[82]

Variation in Pretest Probability of Weaning Outcome

The performance of f/V_T varies enormously among studies (see Table 58-1). Specificity, for example, ranges from 0.00 to >0.80.[11,59,74] As discussed above, the formulae used for measuring the test characteristics of a weaning predictor

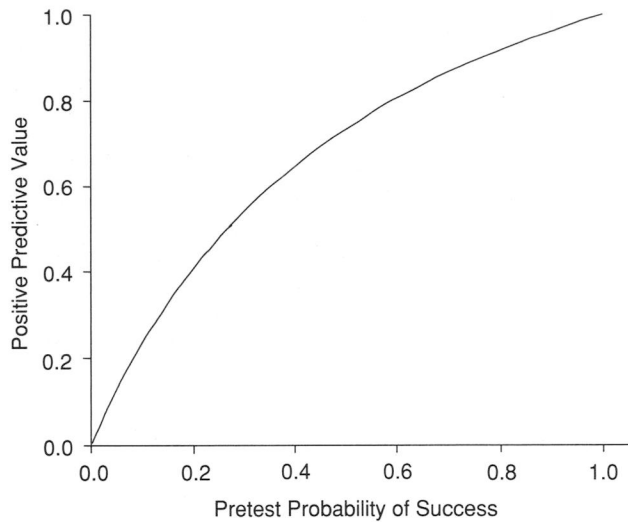

FIGURE 58-14 Positive-predictive value (posttest probability of weaning success) for f/V_T <105 plotted against the pretest probability of weaning success. The curve is based on the sensitivity and specificity originally reported by Yang and Tobin[26] and Bayes' formula.[45]

test assume that the prevalence of weaning success in a new study population is the same as in the population in which the test was originally developed.[46,47] The sequential nature of diagnostic testing during weaning, however, predisposes to spectrum bias and test-referral bias. Consequently, the prevalence of weaning success varies considerably among different study populations.

A useful way to evaluate the influence of prevalence variation on diagnostic testing is to plot positive- and negative-predictive values against the prevalence (or pretest probability) of weaning success.[52] The shape of the resulting plots reflects the sensitivity and specificity of the test. The degree of bowing of a curve reflects the usefulness of a test; a worthless test (sensitivity 0.50, specificity 0.50) produces a diagonal line. When pretest probability exceeds 0.80, negative-predictive value decreases abruptly (all the way to zero) even when sensitivity exceeds 0.90 and specificity 0.90; likewise, positive-predictive value decreases when pretest probability is less than 0.20.[52]

Figures 58-14 and 58-15 show plots of positive- and negative-predictive value of f/V_T against pretest probability of weaning success. The curves were generated by using Bayes' formula and the sensitivity (0.97) and specificity (0.64) originally reported by Yang and Tobin.[26,45] The curves show the expected predictive values (of f/V_T) for varying levels of pretest probability of weaning success as predicted from the original results of Yang and Tobin.[26] As expected, when pretest probability is very high (>0.90), the negative-predictive value of f/V_T shows a dramatic fall. Likewise, when pretest probability is very low (>0.10), the positive-predictive value of f/V_T falls dramatically.

THRESHOLDS OF FREQUENCY-TO-TIDAL VOLUME RATIO

In the original study on f/V_T, the investigators found that a threshold value of ≤ 105 provided the best discrimination

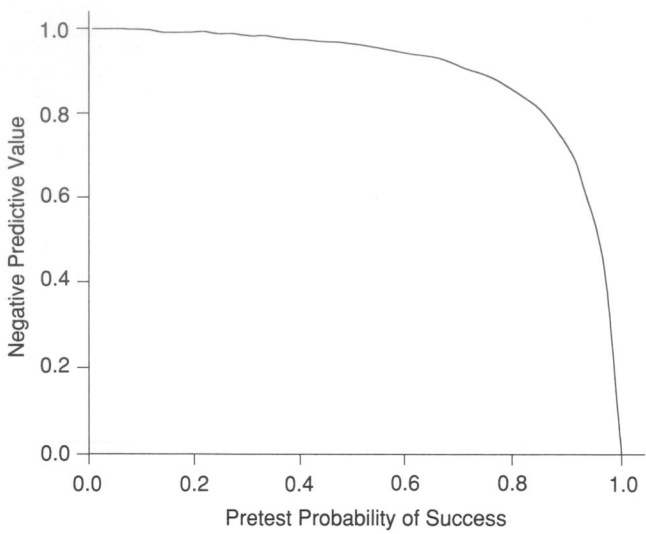

FIGURE 58-15 **Negative-predictive value (posttest probability of weaning failure) for f/VT <105 plotted against the pretest probability of weaning success. The curve is based on the sensitivity and specificity originally reported by Yang and Tobin[26] and Bayes' formula.[45]**

between weaning success and weaning failure patients. This threshold has commonly been rounded to 100. As with any diagnostic test, a clinician should not feel tethered to a threshold of 100 (or 105) in every patient (see earlier discussion of tailoring a predictor to patient needs). In a study of 218 patients, Epstein and Ciubotaru[58] found that f/VT was higher in patients who had endotracheal tubes with internal diameter ≤7 mm than in patients with larger diameter tubes: 86 ± 7 versus 68 ± 6. f/VT was also higher in women than in men: 79 ± 5 versus 56 ± 3. This study was confined to patients who passed a weaning trial, all of whom were extubated. The results suggest that clinicians should not be reluctant to undertake a weaning trial in a woman with a size 7 endotracheal tube simply because her f/VT is 110.

Dichotomizing the readings of a diagnostic test on the basis of a single cut-off value inevitably means that much information is discarded. For example, the positive likelihood ratio for an f/VT <80 is higher than for an f/VT ≤105: 7.53 versus 2.69.[92] That is, f/VT <80 is 7.53 times more likely in weaning success patients than in weaning failure patients. The negative likelihood ratio for f/VT >100 is 0.04, meaning that an f/VT >100 is $^1/_{25}$ as likely to occur in weaning success patients as in weaning failure patients. Based on these considerations, clinicians should tailor the decision to progress to a weaning trial based on the actual reading of f/VT and the characteristics of the patients, rather than feeling constrained by a single cut-off value.

COMPARISON OF FREQUENCY-TO-TIDAL VOLUME RATIO WITH OTHER DIAGNOSTIC TESTS
A detailed evaluation of a diagnostic test, when confined to that test alone, leaves a reader with an incomplete understanding of its usefulness. It is helpful for a reader to compare the performance of the test against other tests in

common use. Table 58-2 provides a listing of true-positive rate (sensitivity), false-positive rate (1 minus specificity), and likelihood ratios for f/VT as a weaning predictor and a number of other tests in common use, as reported by Sox et al.[45]

ARTERIAL BLOOD GAS VALUES

Other than in the course of withdrawing life support, mechanical ventilation is virtually never discontinued in a patient who has severe hypoxemia, such as a Pa_{O_2} <55 mmHg with $F_{I_{O_2}}$ >0.40. Computations such as the $Pa_{O_2}/F_{I_{O_2}}$ ratio or alveolar-arterial P_{O_2} gradient are often used to quantify gas-exchange function. The relationship of these variables to more direct measurements of ventilation-perfusion relationships and shunt is based on many assumptions, and the relationship is variably affected by changes in the concentration of inhaled O_2.[93] Few of these measurements have been rigorously evaluated as predictors of weaning outcome.

Krieger et al[94] found that a $Pa_{O_2}/F_{I_{O_2}}$ ratio of 238 (equivalent to a Pa_{O_2} of 50 with an $F_{I_{O_2}}$ of 0.21) had a positive-predictive value of 90% and a negative-predictive value of 10%. Yang and Tobin[26] found that a Pa_{O_2}/PA_{O_2} ratio of 0.35 provided the best separation between weaning success and weaning failure patients in an initial training data set. When that threshold was evaluated in a subsequent validation data set, the positive-predictive value was 0.59 and negative-predictive value was 0.53. These poor test performances do not mean that measurement of gas exchange is of no value in predicting weaning outcome. All such studies suffer from test-referral bias and patients with severe hypoxia were excluded from the study population. While threshold values of the efficiency of gas exchange cannot be recommended for weaning prediction, weaning attempts are not recommended in patients with borderline hypoxemia.

MINUTE VENTILATION

Normal minute ventilation ($\dot{V}_E$) is about 6 L/min.[95,96] Based on an initial report of Sahn and Lakshminarayan,[24] $\dot{V}_E$ <10 L/min became one of the standard weaning predictors. Subsequent studies with accessible data on the accuracy of $\dot{V}_E$ as a predictor of weaning outcome are summarized in Table 58-3. When interpreting these data, it is essential to recognize the influence of test-referral bias, because clinicians are reluctant to initiate weaning attempts in patients with a high $\dot{V}_E$.

MAXIMUM INSPIRATORY PRESSURE

The airway pressure during a maximum inspiratory effort ($P_I max$) provides a global measure of inspiratory muscle strength. The measurement is usually made at the opening of the endotracheal tube with an aneroid manometer while the patient makes a maximum effort against a closed airway.[97] The use of $P_I max$ as a weaning predictor stems from a study by Sahn and Lakshminarayan.[24] They found that all patients with a $P_I max$ value more negative than

TABLE 58-2   Test Characteristics of Some Common Diagnostic Tests

Test	TPR	FPR	Positive LR	Negative LR
$f/V_T \leq 105$	0.97	0.36	2.72	0.04
f/V_T 100	0.97	0.32	3.03	0.04
f/V_T 80	0.81	0.11	7.52	0.22
Acid phosphatase for prostatic metastases	0.83	0.01–.003	42	0.17
Angiography in abdominal aortic aneurysm	0.70	0.05	14	0.32
Chest x-ray in lung cancer	0.60	0.04	15	0.42
CPK-MB in acute myocardial infarction	0.94	0.10	9.4	0.07
Ventilation-perfusion scan (segmental/larger) in PE	0.76	0.20	3.8	0.30
Pa_{O_2} <90 mmHg in pulmonary embolism	0.95	0.50	1.9	0.10
FEV_1 <80% for COPD				
Young, minimal symptoms, nonsmoker	0.07	0.05	1.4	0.98
Middle age, moderate symptoms, smoker	0.27	0.10	2.7	0.81
Stress ECG for coronary artery disease	0.60	0.17	3.5	0.45
Theophylline >20 $\mu g/ml$ for toxicity	0.60	0.10	6.0	0.44
Ultrasound for endocarditis	0.37	0.04	9.3	0.66
WBC indium scan for abdominal abscess	0.86	0.05	17.2	0.15

COPD, chronic obstructive pulmonary disease; CPK-MB, creatine phosphokinase-MB; ECG, electrocardiogram; FEV_1, forced expiratory volume in 1 second; FPR, false-positive rate (1 – specificity); f/V_T, frequency-to-tidal volume ratio; LR, likelihood ratio; Pa_{O_2}, partial arterial oxygen pressure; PE, pulmonary embolism; TPR, true-positive rate; WBC, white blood cell count.
LR > 10 or < 0.1 = generates large and often conclusive changes in pretest to posttest probability
LR 5–10 or 0.1–0.2 = generates moderate and usually useful shift in pretest to posttest probability
LR 2–5 or 0.5–0.2 = generates a small and sometimes important change in pretest probability
LR 1–2 or 0.5–1.0 = generates a small and rarely important change in pretest probability
SOURCE: Reproduced, with permission, from Sox et al.[45]

–30 cmH$_2$O were successfully weaned, whereas all patients with a P$_I$max less negative than –20 cmH$_2$O failed a weaning trial. Subsequent studies with accessible data on the accuracy of P$_I$max as a predictor of weaning outcome are summarized in Table 58-4.

VITAL CAPACITY

The normal vital capacity is usually between 65 and 75 ml/kg, and a value of 10 ml/kg or more has been suggested to predict a successful weaning outcome. Many investigators have found that vital capacity is often unreliable. For example, Milbern et al[98] found vital capacity of 15 ml/kg to be falsely positive in 15% and falsely negative in 63% of patients. In a study of 10 patients with Guillain-Barré

syndrome, Chevrolet and Deleamont[99] reported that vital capacity was helpful in guiding the weaning process. Patients with a vital capacity of <7 ml/kg were unable to tolerate as few as 15 minutes of spontaneous breathing. As vital capacity increased to >15 ml/kg with recovery from the illness, patients were safely extubated. Apart from unique circumstances, such as patients with Guillain-Barré syndrome, vital capacity is rarely used as a weaning predictor.

AIRWAY OCCLUSION PRESSURE

The pressure generated during the first 0.1 second of an airway occlusion (P$_{0.1}$) is widely used as an index of respiratory center motor output.[100,101] During resting breathing in normal subjects, P$_{0.1}$ is about 0.5–1.5 cmH$_2$O. Several

TABLE 58-3   Accuracy of Minute Ventilation in Predicting Weaning Outcome

Threshold L/min	Sensitivity	Specificity	Positive Predictive Value	Negative Predictive Value	Number of Patients	Probability of Weaning Success	Authors
<9.9	1.00	0.32	0.46	1.00	101	0.63	Zeggwagh et al[78]
10	0.45	0.78	0.89	0.25	47	0.81	Tahvanainen et al[25]
<10	0.79	0.32	0.67	0.48	100	0.63	Chatila et al[104]
	0.50	0.67	0.98	0.20	163	0.988	Leitch et al[59]
	0.31	0.61	0.50	0.40	64	0.56	Yang and Tobin[26]
$\leq$10	0.76	0.07	0.92	0.14	183	0.92	Jacob et al[75]
	0.96	0.47	0.90	0.73	100	0.83	Sahn and Lakshminarayan[24]
<12	0.40	0.50	0.74	0.19	45	0.78	Sassoon and Mahutte[12]
$\leq$12	0.86	0.14	0.72	0.31	92	0.73	Conti et al[71]
>12.5	0.75	0.64	0.45	0.86	40	0.70	Gandia and Blanco[11]
<15	0.97	0.11	0.65	0.67	100	0.63	Chatila et al[104]
	0.78	0.18	0.55	0.38	64	0.56	Yang and Tobin[26]
$\leq$15	0.81	0.20	0.52	0.50	31	0.52	Yang[69]

TABLE 58-4 Accuracy of Maximal Inspiratory Pressure (P_1max) in Predicting Weaning Outcome

P_1max Threshold cm H_2O	Sensitivity	Specificity	Positive Predictive Value	Negative Predictive Value	Number of Patients	Probability of Weaning Success	Authors
≤-30	0.68	0	0.74	0	42	0.81	Tahvanainen et al[25]
≤-30	0.57	0	0.44	0	12	0.58	Sassoon et al[9]
	1	0	0.67	0	17	0.65	Fiastro et al[20]
	NR	NR	0.92	0.21	269	0.9	Krieger et al[94]
	0.67	0.69	0.78	0.55	100	0.63	Chatila et al[104]
	0.86	0.21	0.58	0.55	100	0.56	Yang and Tobin[26]
≤-25	0.59	0.75	0.59	0.79	101	0.63	Zeggwagh et al[78]
≤-20	NR	NR	0.91	0.22	269	0.93	Krieger et al[94]
	1	0.14	0.6	1	100	0.56	Yang and Tobin[26]
	0.91	0.3	0.82	0.55	45	0.78	Sassoon and Mahutte[12]
	0.9	0.26	0.67	0.6	100	0.63	Chatila et al[104]
	0.96	0.07	0.92	0.14	183	0.92	Jacob et al[75]
<-16	0.92	0.07	0.72	0.36	92	0.73	Conti et al[71]
<-15	1	0.11	0.59	1	100	0.56	Yang and Tobin[26]

NR, not reported.

investigators have evaluated the usefulness of $P_{0.1}$ as a predictor of weaning outcome (Table 58-5). In these studies, the threshold value of $P_{0.1}$ discriminating between weaning success and weaning failure ranged from 3.4 to 6.0 cmH_2O.

REPRODUCIBILITY OF STANDARD WEANING PREDICTORS

As with any diagnostic test, it is important to have precise details of the instrumentation used for the measurement, the conditions of the measurement, key steps in making the measurement, and reproducibility of the values. Reproducibility should be assessed in terms of variation in measurements made by one individual on several occasions, and variations in measurements made by several individuals at one point in time. The reproducibility of weaning predictor tests has been assessed to varying extents.

Before worrying about reproducibility, the first requirement for measuring a physiologic variable is to ensure that the patient has achieved a steady state (before the record-

ing is commenced). This requirement can be difficult to satisfy when measuring weaning predictors: the switch between assisted ventilation and autonomous breathing means that there will be some intervening period when a steady state will not be present. For example, if measurement of frequency and V_T commences immediately after disconnecting a patient from the ventilator (say, within 10 seconds of the last ventilator breath and continued over the next 60 seconds), the patient may initially experience apneas (consequent to ventilator-induced neuromechanical inhibition).[102,103] The recorded values of frequency and V_T will be different than if the investigators had waited a minute or so to first ensure that the patient had begun to breathe in a steady manner. Chatila et al[104] reported that measurements of f/V_T at 30 minutes into a weaning trial more accurately predict outcome than measurements in the first minute.[75] While it is true that including data of the first 30 seconds or so may be unrepresentative, this does not mean that it takes 30 minutes to establish a steady state.

TABLE 58-5 Accuracy of Occlusion Pressure in Predicting Weaning Outcome

Threshold cm H_2O	Sensitivity	Specificity	Positive Predictive Value	Negative Predictive Value	Number of Patients	Probability of Weaning Success	Authors
> 2.8	0.67	0.52	0.21	0.89	130	0.88	Fernandez et al[66]
≥ 3.4	0.75	0.61	0.45	0.85	30	0.7	Gandia and Blanco[11]
≤ 4.0	0.83	0.90	0.93	0.78	20	0.6	Fernandez et al[151]
≤ 4.0	0.94	0.07	0.73	0.33	92	0.73	Conti et al[71]
≤ 4.2	0.78	1.00	1.00	0.89	20	0.35	Herrera et al[152]
	0.71	0.43	0.56	0.6	11	0.5	Montgomery et al[10]
≤ 4.5	1.00	1.00	1.00	1.00	13	0.46	Conti et al[153]
	0.75	0.55	0.7	0.62	217	0.58	Vallverdu et al[61]
5.0	0.87	0.91	0.96	0.65	75	0.82	Capdevila et al[13]
< 5.5	0.91	0.36	0.56	0.82	68	0.75	Uusaro et al[62]
≤ 5.5	09.7	0.40	0.85	0.80	45	0.78	Sassoon and Mahutte[12]
≤ 6.0	0.86	0.29	0.55	0.67	11	0.5	Montgomery et al[10]
< 6.0	1.00	1.00	1.00	1.00	12	0.58	Sassoon et al[9]

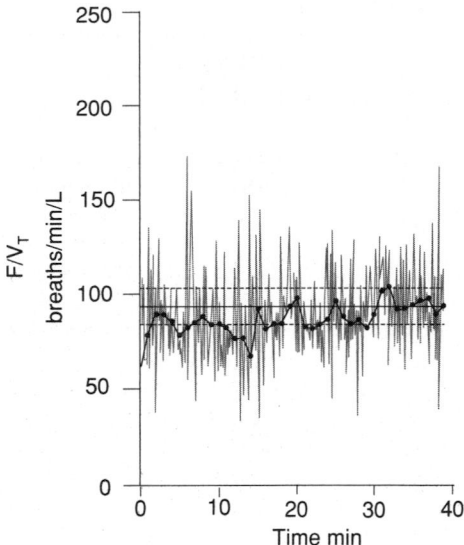

FIGURE 58-16 Time-series plot of frequency-to-tidal volume ratio (f/V_T) during a T-tube trial of spontaneous breathing in a weaning failure patient. Black dots represent 1-minute averages. The solid line indicates the average value of f/V_T of the final minute of the trial. The dashed lines indicate ±10% of the final minute values of f/V_T. The time taken to reach ±10% of the final value of f/V_T was 2 minutes. (*Reproduced, with permission, from Jubran et al.[105]*)

Jubran et al[105] studied the time required for f/V_T to reach a point of equilibration in 17 weaning failure and 14 weaning success patients. The median time (plus interquartile range) to reach ±10% of the final value of f/V_T was 2 (1–2) minutes in both the weaning success and weaning failure patients (Fig. 58-16). Within 2 minutes of the onset of the T-tube trial, 77% of the failure patients and 73% of the success patients had reached ±10% of the final value of f/V_T. The rapid equilibration of f/V_T contrasts with the slower equilibration of swings in esophageal pressure. The median time to reach ±10% of the final value of swings in esophageal pressure was 7.5 (4.2–14.75) minutes in the failure patients and 5 (2–8.5) minutes in the success patients. Based on these data, it is reasonable to usually commence measurement of f/V_T at 60 seconds after removal of the ventilator and then continue the measurement for another 60 seconds.

Yang and Tobin[26] investigated the methods used for measuring $\dot{V}_E$ and its subsets. In a survey of 25 hospitals, the most common condition for the measurement was unassisted breathing while receiving room air (13 hospitals). Ten hospitals made the measurement during assisted breathing while receiving O_2 supplied by three different methods. Two hospitals measured $\dot{V}_E$ during ventilator support. The latter error seemed laughable in 1991, but today it is even more widely made.

Yang and Tobin[106] measured $\dot{V}_E$ and its subsets in 33 patients, who were clinically stable and considered ready to undergo a trial of weaning. $\dot{V}_E$ was 11.9 ± 0.8 L/min while patients spontaneously breathed O_2 through the ventilator circuit (the same F_{IO_2} as patients had received during ventilator support; achieved Pa_{O_2} 89 ± 4 mmHg). When the

patients were switched to room air, $\dot{V}_E$ increased to 13.5 ± 1.1 L/min; frequency also increased from 30.1 ± 11.8 to 33.9 ± 2.2 breaths/min, whereas V_T did not change. Fifteen patients satisfied the $\dot{V}_E$ threshold to progress to a weaning trial ($\dot{V}_E$ <10 L/min) while they breathed O_2, but 7 of them (47%) no longer satisfied this threshold when switched to room air. The study illustrates a wide range of conditions under which $\dot{V}_E$ is measured, and emphasizes the need to control the conditions of the measurement.

Yang[107] examined the reproducibility of predictor measurements in 30 patients about to undergo a weaning trial. Repeat measurements were obtained by a single individual on three trials over 15 minutes. The coefficients of variation for the repeated measurements (during 1 minute of room air breathing) were 10.8 ± 2.1% for $\dot{V}_E$, 6.7 ± 1.2% for frequency, 7.6 ± 1.2% for V_T, and 9.5 ± 1.1% for f/V_T. The coefficient of variation for measurements of $P_{I}max$ (measured with a one-way valve, ensuring a lung volume below functional residual capacity) was 10.6 ± 1.5%. Repeat measurements of vital capacity were the least reproducible, with a coefficient of variation of 19.6 ± 2.8%.

Multz et al[108] undertook a more detailed study of the reproducibility of $P_{I}max$ (measured with an aneroid manometer) in 14 ventilator-dependent patients. Triplicate measurements were obtained by five experienced investigators who encouraged the patients to make vigorous inspiratory efforts. Measurements of $P_{I}max$ at a single sitting by a single investigator showed good reproducibility: coefficient of variation of 12 ± 1%. Much greater variation was observed when $P_{I}max$ was measured in the same patient on the same day by different investigators: coefficient of variation 32 ± 4%.

Measurements of $P_{0.1}$ exhibit the greatest variability, perhaps because the pressures recorded are very small (normal, 0.5–1.5 cmH_2O) and the need for precise timing (0.1 second). The coefficient of variation within individual subjects is about 50%.[109,110] The interindividual coefficient of variation is about 20–33% during a single set of measurements,[110,111] but on repeated measurements (during CO_2 rebreathing trials) it is about 60%.[112]

GASTRIC TONOMETRY

Gastric tonometry is a new monitoring tool that has attracted considerable attention as a predictor of weaning outcome. The rationale for its use is that the gastrointestinal mucosa becomes ischemic early with the development of either hemodynamic compromise or a redistribution of blood flow. One factor that leads to blood flow redistribution is an increase in respiratory muscle effort. Gastric tonometry is based on the principle that P_{CO_2} of fluid in the gastric lumen equilibrates with P_{CO_2} of the mucosal layer, and that the recording of P_{CO_2} in gastric fluid provides a reliable estimate of the pH of the gut mucosa.[113]

In the first evaluation of gastric intramural pH as a weaning predictor, Mohsenifar et al[72] estimated the pH from measurements of the P_{CO_2} of gastric juice. They studied 29 patients undergoing a weaning trial with PS 7–8 cmH_2O. The 11 weaning failure patients developed a decrease in intramural pH from 7.36 during mechanical ventilation to 7.09 after 20 minutes of the weaning trial. No change was observed in 18 weaning success patients (respective readings of 7.45 and 7.46). From these findings, the investigators concluded that patients are likely to fail a weaning trial if they have an initial gastric intramural pHi <7.30 or if it decreases by ≥0.09 during a weaning trial.

Subsequent investigators criticized the methodology of this study. Estimates of intramural pH from measurements of gastric juice acidity are prone to errors caused by enteral feeding or by drugs that alter intraluminal pH (histamine$_2$-receptor blockers). The assumption that P_{CO_2} in the gastric lumen is similar to that in the tissues of the gastric wall may not be true, especially in patients who experience an uneven distribution of gastric blood flow.

To circumvent some of these problems, Bouachour et al[114] used a commercial tonometer in an intragastric latex balloon that indirectly determines intramucosal pH. After inserting the device, its position was confirmed radiologically. The anaerobic balloon was filled with 2.5 ml of saline. After saline loading of the tonometer, the investigators waited 30 minutes before obtaining a sample (the equilibration time was 20 minutes for their third measurement). At the time of obtaining a saline sample, the investigators simultaneously drew an arterial blood gas. From the saline P_{CO_2}, arterial HCO_3, the Henderson-Hasselbalch equation, and an adjustment factor (from the manufacturers), they calculated gastric intramucosal pH. To improve accuracy, they administered histamine$_2$-receptor blockers and stopped enteral feeding.

These investigators[114] undertook a 2-hour T-tube trial in 26 patients with COPD; 20 were successfully weaned and 6 failed the trial. During mechanical ventilation (immediately before the weaning trial), gastric intramucosal pH was lower in the weaning failure patients than in the weaning success patients: 7.26 ± 0.04 versus 7.43 ± 0.08. A threshold intramucosal pH of 7.30 provided perfect discrimination between the two groups: sensitivity of 1.00 and specificity of 1.00. During mechanical ventilation, intramural P_{CO_2} was higher in the weaning failure patients than in the weaning success patients: 74.3 ± 8.0 versus 51.9 ± 6.7 mmHg. A threshold intramural P_{CO_2} of ≤60 mmHg had a sensitivity of 0.95 and specificity of 1.00. After 20 minutes of breathing through the T-tube circuit, the weaning success patients experienced a decrease in intramucosal pH and an increase in intramural P_{CO_2}; the weaning failure patients showed no change from mechanical ventilation. At 20 minutes of the T-tube trial, the area under a receiver operating characteristic (ROC) curve was 0.91 ± 0.06.

The same commercial tonometer was used by Bocquillon et al[115] to study 27 patients with COPD who underwent a 2-hour weaning trial with PS of 8 cmH$_2$O. Sixteen patients tolerated the trial, and eleven failed. During mechanical ventilation, gastric intramucosal pH was equivalent in the two groups. Both groups exhibited decreases in gastric intramucosal pH during the trial, and the values were lower in the failure patients than in the success patients both at 1 hour, 7.32 ± 0.02 versus 7.38 ± 0.02, and at 2 hours, 7.29 ± 0.02 versus 7.38 ± 0.02. Both groups also exhibited in-

creases in gastric intramucosal P_{CO_2}, and at 2 hours the value was higher in the failure patients than in the success patients: 61 ± 2 versus 52 ± 2 mmHg. The investigators used a laser-doppler device to measure gastric mucosal blood flow. Blood flow at 2 hours fell by 22 ± 11% (from baseline) in the failure patients, whereas it rose by 85 ± 27% in the success patients. The investigators did not comment on the sensitivity or specificity of the measurements.

Uusaro et al[62] studied 51 weaning success patients and 17 patients who tolerated a weaning trial but required reintubation (during the weaning trial that preceded extubation, these clinicians did not detect even one patient who required reintubation after extubation). The investigators observed that P_{CO_2} in gastric juice and the gastric-to-arterial P_{CO_2} difference were equivalent in the two patient groups while they were ventilated with a PS of 5 cmH$_2$O. After a 1-hour trial of PS 0 (plus CPAP 5 cmH$_2$O) for 60 minutes, the P_{CO_2} in the gastric juice was 1.8 times higher in the failure patients than in the success patients, and the gastric-to-arterial P_{CO_2} difference was 14 times higher in the failure patients. A gastric-to-arterial P_{CO_2} difference <12 mmHg while breathing at PS 0 had a sensitivity of 0.70, specificity of 0.94, and an area under a ROC curve of 0.80 ± 0.06.

The most recent study is that by Maldonado et al,[76] who used the commercial tonometer used by other investigators.[114,115] They studied 15 successful and 12 failed T-tube trials. During the period between mechanical ventilation and the T-tube trial, weaning failure patients exhibited an increase in intramucosal P_{CO_2}, from 60.4 ± 15.0 to 67.4 ± 21.0 mmHg, and a decrease in intramucosal pH, from 7.32 ± 0.11 to 7.28 ± 0.13. In contrast, the weaning success patients exhibited a decrease in intramucosal P_{CO_2}, 61.5 ± 15.0 to 56.3 ± 16.7 mm Hg, and an increase in intramucosal pH, from 7.29 ± 0.12 to 7.35 ± 0.12, between mechanical ventilation and the T-tube trial. The absolute values, however, for intramucosal P_{CO_2} were no different between the failure and success patients, either during mechanical ventilation, 60.4 ± 15.0 versus 61.5 ± 15.0 mmHg, or a T-tube trial, 67.4 ± 21.0 versus 56.3 ± 16.7 mm Hg. The gastric tonometry measurements were less accurate in predicting weaning outcome than was f/V$_T$. The area under a ROC curve for intramucosal P_{CO_2} was 0.519 ± 0.114, for intramucosal pH 0.561 ± 0.113, and for f/V$_T$ 0.844 ± 0.081.

These five studies differ in methodology, and they also reveal different patterns of abnormality for intramucosal pH and P_{CO_2} in patients undergoing weaning trials. Some investigators found that the measurements discriminated between the weaning success and weaning failure patients during mechanical ventilation,[72,114] whereas others did not.[62,76,115] If the ventilator was set at a level to achieve satisfactory muscle rest, it is difficult to see why gastric intramucosal pH should differ between the groups before the onset of spontaneous breathing. The studies reveal different levels of accuracy in predicting weaning outcome. The reported accuracy represents an overestimate because none of the investigators divided their data sets into training and validation subsets. Several investigators comment that the technique is simple. Yet, it involves inserting a special intragastric tonometer, obtaining a radiograph to confirm location, administration of histamine$_2$-receptor blockers, withholding enteral feeding, waiting sufficient time for satisfactory equilibration, and withdrawing and analyzing a saline sample and an arterial blood gas.

Techniques of Weaning

Researchers who developed weaning predictors never recommended that patients be immediately extubated if a patient passed the predictor test. A one-step approach would be reasonable if the risks associated with the development of postextubation distress and the need for reintubation were trivial. Instead, clinicians decide whether to extubate a patient after performing two diagnostic tests in sequence (measurement of predictors followed by a weaning trial). The importance of this two-step approach is illustrated by the study of Zeggwagh et al.[78] They studied 101 patients, ventilated for >48 hours (mean, 10 ± 10 days; range, 2–60 days), who were considered ready for weaning by the unit team. The unit team then extubated the patients without first undertaking any formal weaning trial. (The extubation decision was based on relatively crude variables, and not the results of more sophisticated weaning predictor tests.) Of the 101 patients, 37 required reintubation. This rate is double (or more) the rate reported in most other studies. These data of Zeggwagh et al[78] emphasize the need for a formal weaning trial before extubation.

The two-step strategy long employed by clinicians is consistent with the theoretical reasoning of the ideal approach to diagnostic testing. Clinicians first contemplate the possibility of a condition (typically a disease, but here it is the possibility of weaning success). At this stage they need a test with very high sensitivity. When the test results are negative (normal), the condition can be confidently ruled out.[47] If the test results are positive (abnormal), the clinician ideally follows the now stronger suspicion (based on the initial very sensitive test) with a second diagnostic test that is very specific. When the result of a very specific test is positive (abnormal), it essentially rules in a disease.[47] Studies of f/V$_T$ have shown it to have a much higher sensitivity than specificity; several investigators have reported sensitivities of 0.90 or higher[1,61,65,69,71,74,76,81] or 0.97 or higher.[12,26,73,75,79,104]

For the second diagnostic test, a T-tube or some other weaning trial, clinicians operate on the assumption that it has a high specificity, although this assumption has never been formally tested. A test with high specificity has a low rate of false-positive results (patients who pass a T-tube trial, are extubated, but require reintubation). The usual rate of reintubation after passing a T-tube trial is 15–20%, although some investigators have reported reintubation rates as high as 29%.[62,64,74,76,116] The true-negative rate is also needed for calculation of specificity. Determination of the true-negative rate for a T-tube trial would require the extubation of all patients who fail the trial and counting how many require reintubation (an experiment that is unethical).

A second rationale for the use of weaning techniques is that they somehow improve the patient's likelihood of tolerating extubation. That is, weaning techniques have some therapeutic action beyond their diagnostic role. This rationale is generally couched in terms of improved reconditioning of the respiratory muscles.

A weaning task force[117,118] has suggested that measuring predictors may inhibit expeditious weaning, and they advocated the bypassing of this step and starting weaning evaluation with a trial of spontaneous breathing. Yet in a study used to support this viewpoint, Ely et al[119] found that physicians refused to order a spontaneous breathing trial in 64–89% of patients who had already demonstrated satisfactory respiratory function on their weaning predictors. Respiratory therapists had demonstrated >95% compliance in measuring f/V$_T$. It is difficult to understand how the demonstration of good physiologic performance on weaning predictors could have resulted in the failure to undertake a trial of spontaneous breathing in up to 90% of patients.

The major techniques that are used include T-tube trial, PS, intermittent mandatory ventilation (IMV), or some combination of these three.

INTERMITTENT MANDATORY VENTILATION

IMV is discussed in detail in Chapter 8. With IMV, the patient receives periodic positive-pressure breaths from the ventilator at a preset volume and rate. In addition, the patient can take spontaneous breaths between these mandatory breaths.

When IMV is used for weaning, the mandatory rate from the ventilator is reduced in steps of 1–3 breaths per minute, and an arterial blood gas is obtained about 30 minutes after each change. Unfortunately, adjusting the number of ventilator breaths in accordance with the results of blood gases can lead to a false sense of security. As little as 2–3 positive-pressure breaths per minute can achieve acceptable blood gases, but these values provide no information about a patient's work of breathing, which may be excessive.

IMV was originally seen as the ideal mode for weaning: the ventilator breaths were expected to provide respiratory muscle rest, and the intervening spontaneous breaths to facilitate reconditioning. Accordingly, it was thought that respiratory muscle rest would be proportional to the number of positive-pressure breaths. Subsequent studies revealed that patients have difficulty in adapting to the intermittent nature of the assistance.[120,121] Studies revealed that inspiratory effort is equivalent for the assisted and unassisted breaths. At IMV rates of 14 breaths per minute or less, tension–time index for both the assisted and unassisted breaths is above the threshold associated with respiratory muscle fatigue. At a moderate level of ventilator assistance (where the ventilator accounts for 20–50% of the total ventilation), electromyographic recordings reveal that activity of the diaphragm and sternomastoid muscles during assisted breaths is no lower than that during unassisted breaths.[121] These findings suggest that respiratory center output is preprogrammed and unable to adapt to breath-by-breath changes in load as occur with IMV. Consequently, IMV may contribute to the development of respiratory muscle fatigue or prevent recovery from it.

PRESSURE SUPPORT

PS is discussed in detail in Chapter 9. Like IMV, PS provides graded assistance, but differs from IMV in that the clinician sets the level of pressure (rather than the volume) to augment every spontaneous respiratory effort. The level of pressure is usually adjusted in accordance with the patient's frequency. The frequency, however, that signals a satisfactory level of respiratory muscle rest has never been well defined, and recommendations range from 16 to 30 breaths per minute.[87,122,123]

When PS is used for weaning, the level of pressure is reduced gradually, in decrements of 3–6 cmH$_2$O, titrated to the patient's frequency. PS is commonly used to counteract the work imposed by breathing through the endotracheal tube and ventilator circuit. Consequently, the notion arose that if a patient was able to sustain ventilation at this "compensatory level" of PS, he or she should be able to breathe without difficulty after extubation. Investigators have estimated this compensatory level of PS to range from 3–13 cmH$_2$O. No method has ever been shown to reliably estimate the compensatory level of PS required by an individual patient.

Individuals who recommended the addition of PS for overcoming resistance of the endotracheal tube failed to recognize that the upper airways become inflamed and edematous after an endotracheal tube has been in place for some time. When the endotracheal tube is removed, the resistance of the upper airway is higher than normal. This subject was investigated rigorously by Straus et al.[89] They studied 14 patients who tolerated a 2-hour T-tube trial and were then extubated. Work of breathing did not change between the start and end of the trial, 20.0 ± 9.1 and 22.1 ± 10.6 Joules per minute, respectively. Importantly, work did not decrease after extubation, 22.6 ± 9.7 Joules per minute. The work dissipated against the supraglottic airway after extubation was almost identical to the work dissipated against the endotracheal tube before extubation (about 11% of total work of breathing). These data indicate that the addition of any level of PS will lead to underestimation of a patient's work of breathing after extubation—the very goal that is being attempted by a weaning trial that uses a low level of PS. Mehta et al[124] measured work of breathing in 22 patients before and 15 minutes after extubation. The work of breathing at PS 5 cmH$_2$O before extubation underestimated the work of breathing performed after extubation by 36%; work of breathing at CPAP 5 cmH$_2$O underestimated the work of breathing performed after extubation by 23%.

Most investigators have focused on the effect of PS on inspiratory muscle effort. The switch between inspiration and expiration can give rise to problems, particularly in patients with COPD. With PS, ventilator assistance ceases when the patient's inspiratory flow falls to a preset amount (such as 25% of the peak flow). Air flow changes more slowly in patients with COPD, and these patients often begin to exhale while the ventilator is still pumping gas into their

chests. In a study of patients with COPD who were receiving PS 20 cmH$_2$O, almost half recruited their expiratory muscles before the ventilator had completed mechanical inflation.

T-TUBE TRIALS

The oldest weaning technique is to undertake trials of spontaneous breathing through a T-tube circuit. In the past, these trials started with a duration of about 3–5 minutes, and were repeated every 30 minutes.[125] The duration of spontaneous breathing was progressively increased according to patient tolerance, as decided by physical examination and arterial blood gas measurements. Patients were not extubated until they tolerated the T-tube trial for several hours: up to 8 hours in the classic study of Sahn and Lakshminarayan,[24] up to 16 hours in a study from the late 1980s,[94] and 12 hours in a study from the mid-1990s.[126] The need for frequent changes to the ventilator circuit (every hour or more often) placed enormous demands on the intensive care staff, and the approach become extremely unpopular. By the late 1980s, T-tube trials had been largely supplanted by IMV.[127]

Today, it is usual to limit a T-tube trial to 2 hours or less. We typically extubate a patient who does not develop distress during a 30-minute T-tube trial. If a patient fails a T-tube trial, we wait 24 hours before we undertake a subsequent trial. Our reasoning is based on the knowledge that most patients who fail a T-tube trial experience considerable stress on the respiratory muscles secondary to marked increases in their work of breathing. The respiratory muscles take 24 hours or longer to recover from this stress[128] (Fig. 58-17). Accordingly, we reinstitute full assistance with assist-control

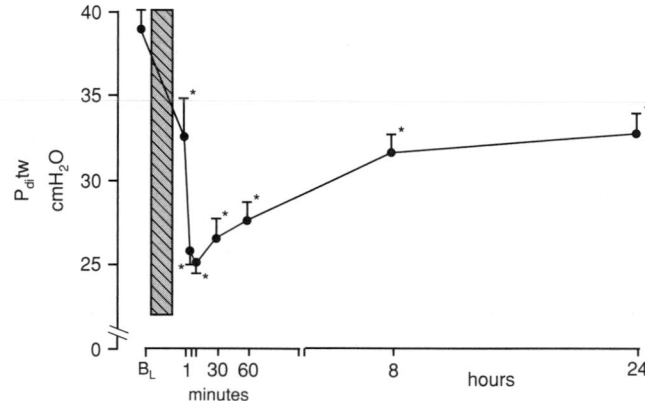

FIGURE 58-17 Induction of diaphragmatic fatigue (*stippled bar*) produced a significant fall in transdiaphragmatic pressure (*P$_{di}$*) elicited by twitch stimulation of both phrenic nerves. Significant recovery of twitch pressure was noted in the first 8 hours after completion of the fatigue protocol; no further change was observed between 8 and 24 hours, and the 24-hour value was significantly lower than baseline. The delay in reaching the nadir of twitch transdiaphragmatic pressure probably results from twitch potentiation, induced by repeated contractions, which was present at the end of the protocol. Values are mean ± SE. *Significant difference compared with baseline value, *p* <0.01. (*Reproduced, with permission, from Laghi et al.*[128])

ventilation for at least 24 hours before reassessing the patient for another T-tube trial.

Optimal plumbing of the T-tube circuit is necessary to avoid imposing respiratory work. Humidified gas is commonly provided in the form of a heated or cool aerosol of water from a large-volume nebulizer. This system can provoke bronchospasm in patients with reactive airways disease. Such patients can be managed with a non-aerosol-generating system, such as a heated passover humidifier.

A T-tube trial serves as a diagnostic test. It is primarily a means of evaluating a patient's ability to sustain spontaneous ventilation. Patients are judged to have failed a T-tube trial when they develop severe tachypnea, increased accessory muscle activity, diaphoresis, facial signs of respiratory distress, O_2 desaturation, tachycardia, arrhythmias, or hypotension. The degree of change in these variables, however, varies from report to report.

A standardized approach to patient monitoring during a T-tube trial does not exist. Indeed, there is no agreement as to whether the monitoring of any variable helps in deciding whether to continue a T-tube trial for an initially planned duration, prolong it, or curtail it. We monitor all such patients with a pulse oximeter. In a report on more than 1000 spontaneous breathing trials, Ely et al[119] observed only 1 transient episode of desaturation—a rate so staggeringly low as to beggar belief. In a study of 17 patients with COPD who failed a T-tube trial, Jubran and Tobin[15] found that severe hypoxemia ($P_{O_2} \leq 46$ mmHg) was the primary cause of failure in two patients. In a study of 100 spontaneous breathing trials in 83 patients, Salam et al[129] observed seven instances in which the results of arterial blood gases caused physicians to defer extubation in patients judged otherwise to have passed the trial. Recent data indicate that patients failing a T-tube trial do not develop low-frequency fatigue.[28] These data, however, do not exclude the possibility of high-frequency fatigue.[27] Moreover, weaning failure patients (on average) experience more than four times the normal level of inspiratory effort (at the end of a T-tube trial), and some patients experience more than six times the normal value.[15] Given the magnitude of these changes, we do not recommend the undertaking of a T-tube trial in a cavalier manner. Such large increases in respiratory effort cause severe dyspnea, and, apart from humanitarian considerations, we do not know what imprint severe dyspnea leaves on a patient's psyche.

Jubran et al[105] investigated whether repeated measurements of esophageal pressure throughout a trial of spontaneous breathing might provide additional guidance over a single measurement obtained during the first minute of the trial. They quantified the change in esophageal pressure over the first 9 minutes of the trial using a multivariate adaptive regression spline procedure. In a study of 60 patients, an esophageal pressure–trend index had a sensitivity of 0.91 and specificity of 0.89. Specifically, an esophageal pressure–trend index reading of ≤ 0.44 was 8.2 times more likely to occur in weaning failure than in weaning success patients. These data suggest that the continuous monitoring of esophageal pressure swings during a T-tube trial may provide additional guidance in patient management over tests used for deciding when to initiate weaning.

An implied goal of techniques that involve a gradual reduction in ventilator assistance—whether with IMV, PS, or T-tube trials of increasing duration—is to recondition the respiratory muscles, which may have been weakened during the period of mechanical ventilation. Theoretically, a once-daily trial of spontaneous breathing and a prolonged period of rest may be the most effective method of eliciting adaptive changes.[130,131] That approach meets the three principal requirements of a conditioning program: overload, particularity, and reversibility.[130] During a T-tube trial, patients breathe against an elevated intrinsic load, thus satisfying the overload requirement. Particularity is also satisfied, in that the trial is an endurance stimulus and the desired objective is enhanced endurance. Finally, the use of a daily trial prevents regression of the adaptive changes. This reasoning, however, is solely based on indirect evidence. The effect of different weaning techniques on respiratory muscle reconditioning has not been investigated.

SPONTANEOUS BREATHING TRIALS

During a T-tube trial, a patient is not connected to the ventilator. To convey the lack of assistance, T-tube trials were also described as trials of spontaneous breathing. The two labels were considered synonymous, and used interchangeably. Subsequently, the term "spontaneous breathing trial" was also used to describe patients who were breathing through the ventilator but not receiving any positive-pressure inspiratory assistance as occurs with use of "flow-by." Flow-by avoided the substantial respiratory work imposed by the demand valves in older ventilators, and became a popular alternative to a T-tube circuit for conducting a trial of spontaneous breathing.

Authors, unfortunately, now use the term "spontaneous breathing trial" to describe weaning trials conducted with a fixed level of PS, ranging from 5 to 10 cmH₂O. It is an oxymoron to label PS as spontaneous breathing. The word "support" is an antonym of "unassisted." The problem is not simply semantic. It is unscientific to regard positive-pressure assistance (of 5–10 cmH₂O) with every inspiratory effort as unassisted breathing. This unscientific thinking has led authors to believe that measurements of breathing pattern at PS of 5–10 cmH₂O is no different than measuring breathing pattern while a patient is disconnected from the ventilator. The argument that PS of 5–10 cmH₂O does no more than compensate for the work imposed by an endotracheal tube is now known to be invalid (see above).

The weaning of a patient from the ventilator boils down to making clinical judgments as to whether a patient will be able to sustain ventilation on his or her own, and, if not, how much ventilator assistance is required. It is unfortunate that the same term "spontaneous breathing" is now used to describe both breathing without any ventilator assistance and breathing with the delivery of positive-pressure assistance with every inspiratory effort. An expression that formerly facilitated meaningful communication has been corrupted such that it misleads not only readers but also the authors themselves.

The sloppiness of communication has reached its apogee in the trials of noninvasive ventilation for management of postextubation distress. Before extubation, patients undergo a trial of "spontaneous breathing" at PS 5–8 cmH$_2$O. After extubation, the major intervention is the delivery of PS (perhaps at a lower level) by facemask. The nonchalant representation of PS 7 cmH$_2$O as "spontaneous breathing" signifies a fundamental misunderstanding of physiology.

ADDITION OF POSITIVE END-EXPIRATORY PRESSURE TO REPLACE PHYSIOLOGIC POSITIVE END-EXPIRATORY PRESSURE

Some clinicians recommend that all patients with an endotracheal tube should receive PEEP of 5 cmH$_2$O, claiming that this level of PEEP is replacing a loss of physiologic PEEP produced by intermittent narrowing of the vocal cords. These claims do not square with long-standing knowledge of pulmonary physiology. Lung volume at end-expiration generally approximates the relaxation volume of the respiratory system (i.e., the lung volume determined by the static balance between the opposing elastic recoil of the lung and chest wall).[132,133] The static recoil pressure of the respiratory system is thus zero at end-expiration in a healthy person.

The addition of PEEP of 5 cmH$_2$O is not without consequence. In 10 ventilated patients who had PEEPi of 6.2 ± 1.0 cmH$_2$O, Smith and Marini[134] found that that the addition of external PEEP of 5 cmH$_2$O decreased work of inspiration by 19%. The addition of PEEP can also substantially increase cardiac output in patients with left ventricular failure. In either circumstance, the rapid removal of PEEP may lead to rapid decompensation at the time of extubation. Thus, the generic order of "5 of PEEP" may cause physicians to underestimate the likely challenges that a patient will face after extubation.

In many patients, it is appropriate to add external PEEP to treat an abnormality such as PEEPi or atelectasis. In such instances, PEEP is being used as a therapy to reverse a pathophysiologic entity. The application of external PEEP cannot be considered as inducing a normal physiologic state.

HEAD-TO-HEAD COMPARISONS

The first randomized controlled trial of the three major weaning techniques was conducted by Brochard et al.[3] They randomized 109 difficult-to-wean patients (defined as failure to tolerate their first 2-hour T-tube trial) to three study arms. At 21 days, there were fewer weaning failure patients among the PS group (2/26, 8%) than among the patients weaned by T-tube trials (10/30, 33%), or IMV (16/41, 39%). Also, less time was taken to wean with PS (5.7 ± 3.7 days) than with T-tube trials (8.5 ± 8.3 days) or IMV (9.9 ± 8.2 days). Statistically, however, the only difference was a shorter weaning time for PS patients (5.7 ± 3.7 days) than for the combined T-tube and IMV patients (9.3 ± 8.2 days; $p < 0.05$).

Esteban et al[4] undertook a randomized controlled trial that had a similar design to that of Brochard et al. They randomized 130 difficult-to-wean patients (again defined as failure to tolerate their first 2-hour T-tube trial) to four study arms: IMV, PS, once daily T-tube trials, and intermittent spontaneous breathing trials (this terminology was used because 6 patients breathed through a circuit providing CPAP 5 cmH$_2$O; the remaining 27 had T-tube trials; the trials were of gradually increasing duration, at least twice daily, with ≥ 1 hour of assist-control ventilation between each trial). At 14 days, mechanical ventilation was still required by 17% of IMV patients, 11% of PS patients, 3% of once-daily T-tube patients, and 3% of patients weaned by intermittent T-tube or CPAP trials. The time taken to wean was a median of 5 days for IMV (quartiles 3 and 11), 4 days for PS (quartiles 2 and 12), 3 days for once-daily T-tube trials (quartiles 1 and 6), and 3 days for intermittent T-tube/CPAP trials (quartiles 2 and 6). The rate of successful weaning with once-daily T-tube trials was about three times faster than with IMV and two times faster than with PS; there was no difference between the speed of weaning with once-daily T-tube trials versus intermittent T-tube/CPAP trials.

These two studies concur in finding that IMV was the least effective method for weaning a difficult patient. The steps taken in setting the IMV rate were largely the same in the two studies: the initial IMV rate was half the respiratory frequency seen during ACV (IMV of about 10 breaths per minute in both studies). Then, IMV rate was decreased by 2–4 breaths per minute twice a day if the patient tolerated it. The point for extubation differed between the studies. In the study of Brochard et al, patients were extubated when they tolerated an IMV of 4 breaths per minute for 24 hours. In the study of Esteban et al, patients were extubated when they tolerated an IMV of 5 breaths per minute for 2 hours. This difference probably accounts for the shorter weaning time with IMV in the study of Esteban et al versus that of Brochard et al: 5 versus 10 days.

The data appear to differ in the relative efficacy of PS and T-tube trials. The reason for the difference can again be understood by examining the two protocols. The initial level of PS was largely similar in the two studies: pressure titrated to respiratory frequency (20–30 breaths/minute;[3] <25 breaths/minute[4]). This resulted in a PS of 18 cmH$_2$O in both studies. PS was decreased by 2–4 cmH$_2$O twice a day in the study of Brochard et al, and by that amount or more in the study of Esteban et al. The point for extubation differed between the studies. In the study of Brochard et al, patients were extubated when they tolerated PS of 8 cmH$_2$O for 24 hours. In the study of Esteban et al, patients were extubated when they tolerated PS of 5 cmH$_2$O for 2 hours. This difference probably accounts for the shorter weaning time with PS in the study of Esteban et al than in the study of Brochard et al: 4 versus 6 days. The approach to T-tube trials also differed. Brochard et al performed trials of increasing duration twice a day. Esteban et al used two approaches to T-tube trials: one arm consisted of T-tube trials once a day, and the second arm consisted of intermittent spontaneous breathing trials. The point for extubation differed between the studies. In the study of Brochard et al, extubation was contemplated when patients tolerated a 2-hour T-tube trial, but there could be as many as three separate 2-hour trials. In the study of Esteban et al, patients were extubated when they first tolerated a 2-hour trial.

The investigators of the two preceding studies[3,4] set the duration of T-tube trials at 2 hours. In a subsequent study, conducted in 526 patients who had received >48 hours of ventilation, Esteban et al[135] found that the rate of weaning failure was equivalent for trials lasting 30 and 120 minutes: 12% (33/270) and 16% (40/256), respectively. The rates of reintubation were virtually identical (13%); about 74% of patients in the two arms were successfully extubated. This study consisted of patients undergoing a first weaning attempt, unlike the two earlier trials that were limited to patients with demonstrable difficulty in being weaned. The findings, however, suggest that most patients can be weaned after a 30-minute trial, which simplifies management by freeing staff time for other patient care tasks. With a similar goal, Perren et al[136] found that the rate of weaning failure was equivalent when 98 patients were randomized to breathe with pressure support of 7 cmH_2O for 30 or 120 minutes: 6.5% (3/46) and 11.5% (6/52). The rates of reintubation did not differ significantly (7% and 4%, respectively).

In a group of 484 patients who had received >48 hours of ventilation, Esteban et al[137] compared weaning trials consisting of a 2-hour T-tube trial versus 2 hours of PS 7 cmH_2O. The rate of trial failure was higher for the T-tube trials than for PS: 22% versus 14%. The rate of reintubation was equivalent (about 19%) in both arms. There was no difference in the rate of patients successfully extubated, nor in length of stay.

Koh et al[138] investigated whether adding a 1-hour T-tube trial would alter outcome in patients who had already undergone progressive decreases in PS (3–5 cmH_2O every hour) to a level estimated to offset imposed respiratory work (by the endotracheal tube and ventilator circuit: mean 7.6 ± 0.4 cmH_2O [SE]; range 4–13 cmH_2O). The rate of weaning failure was not significantly different in patients who were extubated after the additional T-tube trial and those extubated directly, 45% (10/22) and 30% (6/20), respectively, nor did the rates of reintubation differ, 18% (4/22) and 20% (4/20), respectively.

Matic and Majeric-Kogler[139] studied 260 patients who had received mechanical ventilation for >48 hours and who had who satisfied several criteria of readiness for weaning (such as frequency <35 breaths/minute, V_T > 5 ml/kg, f/V_T <100, and P_{O_2} >60 mmHg on F_{IO_2} <0.40). Patients were randomized to a 2-hour T-tube trial or a 2-hour trial of PS 8 cmH_2O. Of the 150 patients in the PS trial group, 120 (80.0%) passed the trial and were extubated. Of the 110 patients in the T-tube trial group, 80 (72.7%) passed the trial and were extubated ($p = 0.06$). The remaining patients who failed the initial weaning trial were returned to assist-control ventilation, and the previously assigned weaning technique was again attempted after 24 hours (or when the patient's condition permitted). The rate of weaning success was higher in the PS group than in the T-tube trial group: 26/30 (86.7%) versus 21/30 (70%); the time for weaning was shorter for the PS group, 54 (quartiles 47 and 88) versus 94 (quartiles 79 and 132) hours, as was total time for mechanical ventilation, 215 hours (quartiles 187 and 259) versus 262 hours (quartiles 216 and 328). The rate of reintubation was equivalent for the PS and T-tube trial groups: 1 (3.5%) versus 2 (6.7%) patients.

Vitacca et al[140] studied 75 patients with COPD who had been transferred to a long-term weaning unit. The patients had required >15 days of mechanical ventilation, and all had a tracheostomy. Of the 75 patients, 23 (31%) tolerated a T-tube trial for 48 hours and were studied no further. The remaining 52 patients failed the T-tube trial after 290 ± 452 minutes, and were randomly assigned to weaning by PS or T-tube trials. Weaning was deemed successful when patients tolerated spontaneous breathing for ≥48 hours. Clinical outcomes were equivalent in the PS and T-tube trial groups: weaning success rate 73% (19/26) versus 77% (20/26); mortality 11.5% (3/26) versus 7.6% (2/26); ventilator duration 181 ± 161 versus 130 ± 106 hours; weaning unit stay 33 ± 12 versus 35 ± 15 days; and hospital stay 49 ± 27 versus 50 ± 32 days. The investigators also retrospectively compared 55 patients managed by the protocols of this study with 62 control patients managed in the same institution during the 2 years preceding the study. The study patients exhibited better outcomes than the historical control group: 30-day weaning success rate 87 versus 70%; ventilator duration 103 ± 144 versus 170 ± 127 hours; weaning unit stay 27 ± 12 versus 38 ± 18 days; and hospital stay 38 ± 17 versus 47 ± 18 days.

WEANING BY PROTOCOL VERSUS USUAL CARE

Several investigators have examined whether formalizing weaning steps into a protocol might alter weaning outcome (Table 58-6). Saura et al[141] compared a subgroup of 51 patients from an earlier randomized trial[4] with a retrospective control group of 50 patients weaned according to usual care (apparently progressive reductions in partial ventilator assistance). The study group underwent a 2-hour T-tube trial as soon as they met a series of clinical criteria (including frequency <35 breaths per minute and V_T >5 ml per kg). Patients who tolerated the T-tube trial without distress were immediately extubated. Such direct extubation occurred in 80% of the protocol group and 10% of the control group. Total duration of mechanical ventilation was shorter in the protocol group: 10.4 ± 11.6 versus 14.4 ± 10 days. Eighty percent of patients in the study group were extubated after their first T-tube trial. If these patients had been returned to the ventilator to enable a gradual reduction in the level of ventilator assistance (before extubation), such a step would

TABLE 58-6 Comparisons of Weaning by protocol versus Usual Care

Authors	Year	No. of Patients	Weaning by Protocol Superior to Usual Care?
Saura et al[141]	1996	101	Yes
Ely et al[56]	1996	300	Yes
Kollef et al[2]	1997	357	Overall, yes; individually significant in only 1 of 4 ICUs
Marelich et al[144]	2000	335	Overall, yes; but not in 1 of the 2 study ICUs
Namen et al[143]	2001	100	No
Randolph et al[145]	2002	182	No
Krishnan et al[146]	2004	199	No

have prolonged the overall duration of ventilation. Saying that it is safe to extubate patients without first gradually decreasing the level of ventilator assistance may sound trite today, but this was not widely accepted in the early 1990s.

Ely et al[56] borrowed two steps from previous studies—measurement of f/V_T (and other predictors) and a 2-hour T-tube trial—and combined them into an algorithm. They randomized 300 patients (dependent on mechanical ventilation for ≥ 2 weeks before entry) into intervention and usual care groups (76% of the patients in the usual care arm were managed by IMV alone or in combination with PS). Patients in the intervention group were screened in the early morning. To pass the screen, patients had to meet all of the following 5 criteria: f/V_T <105; Pa_{O_2}/Fi_{O_2} >200; PEEP ≤ 5 cmH$_2$O; adequate cough during suctioning; and no infusions of vasopressors or sedatives (with the exception of dopamine ≤ 5 μg/kg per minute and intermittent sedative boluses). Patients who passed the screen automatically underwent a trial of spontaneous breathing (a T-tube trial or flow-by and CPAP 5 cmH$_2$O) later that morning (without requiring an order from the primary physician). If the patient tolerated the trial, the primary physician was informed both orally and by a note in the chart. The time taken to wean (from the point of satisfying the predictor criteria until the discontinuation of mechanical ventilation) was shorter in the intervention group than in the usual care group: 1 day (median; quartiles 0–2) versus 3 days (quartiles 2–7). The duration of ventilation was also shorter: 4.5 days (quartiles 2–9) versus 6 days (quartiles 3–11). Reintubation was less common in the intervention group than in the usual care group: 4 versus 10%. This study demonstrates that a two-step approach—systematic measurement of predictors followed by a single daily T-tube (or flow-by/CPAP) trial—was superior to usual care (consisting largely of IMV and PS).

A closer inspection of the data illustrates some important points about weaning. Among the 149 patients in the intervention group, 113 (76%) met the predictor criteria. Of these 113 patients, 88 (78%) passed the spontaneous breathing trial. Yet, extubation was not attempted that day in 45% (40/88) of the patients who passed the trial. In a subsequent analysis of the data, Ely et al[142] noted that 84 of the 300 patients never satisfied the weaning predictor thresholds. Of these 84 patients, 59 (70.2%) were never extubated. The remaining 25 patients (25/300; 8.3%) were successfully extubated despite never satisfying the predictor thresholds. Of these 25 patients, 15 had Pa_{O_2}/Fi_{O_2} ratios <200 (5%) and 10 (3.3%) had f/V_T readings higher than 105. These data highlight that (1) the major source of delay in weaning of patients in the intervention group resulted from the failure of physicians to take action in patients who passed a spontaneous breathing trial (extubation was delayed in 45% of these patients), (2) almost 80% of patients who meet predictor thresholds will tolerate an immediate spontaneous breathing trial, and (3) f/V_T (105) falsely identifies about 3% of patients who can be extubated.

Ely et al[119] subsequently examined the ability to apply a modification of the above two-step protocol in a larger group of patients. The major change from the original algorithm was that patients passing the predictor screen

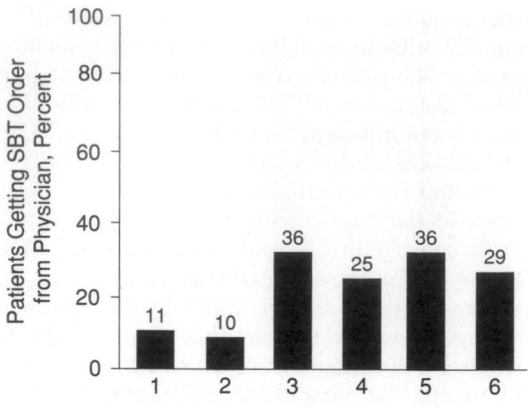

FIGURE 58-18 The percentage of patients with satisfactory weaning predictors who received a spontaneous breathing trial. The data represent six successive 2-month periods. The increase in ordering of trials after 4 months coincided with educational in-service sessions for all members of the groups. The average rate of obtaining a spontaneous breathing trial was 24.5% for the 6 periods. In the earlier study of Ely et al,[56] 100% of patients with satisfactory weaning predictors progressed to a trial that same morning. In the earlier study, an order from the managing physician was not required to undertake a trial, whereas in this study an order was required. (*Reproduced, with permission, from Ely et al.[119]*)

(same weaning predictor criteria as in earlier study: f/V_T, Pa_{O_2}/Fi_{O_2}, PEEP <5 cmH$_2$O, cough, and no vasopressors or sedatives) did not automatically progress to a spontaneous breathing trial. Instead, that step required the permission of the managing physician. Respiratory therapists in this study exhibited a compliance rate of 97% in obtaining the weaning predictors.

Figure 58-18 shows the compliance in obtaining a spontaneous breathing trial in patients who had satisfactory weaning predictors. For six successive 2-month periods, compliance was respectively 11, 10, 36, 25, 36 and 29%. Thus, even for the best period, 64% of patients meeting weaning predictor criteria did not progress to a spontaneous breathing trial (in the worst period, 89% did not progress to a spontaneous breathing trial).

A recent evidence-based medicine task force on weaning[117,118] concluded that clinicians should bypass the measurement of weaning predictors and begin the weaning process with a trial of spontaneous breathing. Given the preceding findings,[119] the conclusion of the task force requires the use of inverse logic. Ely et al[119] found that physicians refused to order a spontaneous breathing trial in 64–89% of patients who had satisfactory weaning predictors. To conclude that use of predictor tests slows weaning would mean that physicians decide to postpone a weaning trial whenever they are informed that the predictor tests reveal a patient's readiness for the trial—a line of reasoning that is contrary to common sense. Instead, these data[119] show that using a weaning trial as the starting point would slow the process because of the demonstrated hesitation of physicians in undertaking such trials. Moreover, in the initial study of Ely et al,[56,142] f/V_T was found to be falsely negative in only

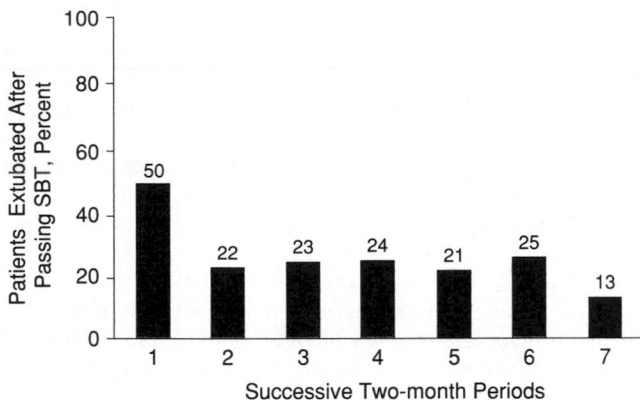

FIGURE 58-19 The percentage of patients who were extubated after passing a spontaneous breathing trial. The data represent seven successive 2-month periods. In the first 2 months, 50% of the patients who passed a trial progressed to extubation. Over the next year, the rate dropped to under 25%. In the first study of Ely et al,[56] 55% of patients who passed a spontaneous breathing trial were extubated that same day. In that study, a patient's success in tolerating a trial was orally communicated to the managing physicians (of the medical and coronary ICUs); that level of communication was not documented for the neurosurgeons. (*Reproduced, with permission, from Namen et al.[143]*)

3.3% of patients (patients who were successfully extubated despite having an f/V_T >105).

The latter study of Ely et al[119] did not have a control group, and it was largely undertaken to detect which elements of a protocol are easy to employ and which pose obstacles. Namen et al[143] of the same research group undertook an additional study of the effectiveness of the two-step weaning algorithm in a neurosurgical ICU. There were 49 patients in the intervention arm and 51 patients in the usual care arm. Once again, patients who satisfied weaning predictors (same criteria as before) did not progress automatically to a spontaneous breathing trial. On this occasion, that step required the permission of the study (not managing) physician. A respiratory therapist undertook a spontaneous breathing trial on 199 of the 201 occasions that patients satisfied the weaning predictors. Figure 58-19 shows the rate of extubation in patients who passed a spontaneous breathing trial. In the first 2 months, 50% of patients who passed a spontaneous breathing trial progressed to extubation. A year later, however, only 13% of patients who passed a spontaneous breathing trial progressed to extubation.

Figure 58-19 conveys the main message of this study. Neurosurgeons did not extubate 75% (on average) of patients who passed a spontaneous breathing trial (and who had also satisfied weaning predictors). Although not mentioned by the authors, the main reason for the disappointing outcome is probably the unfamiliarity of these neurosurgeons with spontaneous breathing trials. This explanation is supported by the fact that only 1% of the patients were managed with assist-control ventilation (74% were managed with IMV alone or in combination with PS). The previous study of Ely et al[119] highlighted that physicians refused to order a spontaneous breathing trial in 64–89% of patients who had satisfactory weaning predictors. This study of

Namen et al[143] emphasizes that the educational challenge is enormous. Even when neurosurgeons were informed of the results of a spontaneous breathing trial (a trial that was ordered by a research physician), they refused to request extubation in 50–87% of the patients who passed the trial. In reality, this study is an assessment of the understanding of respiratory pathophysiology by these managing physicians. Given the managing physicians' (neurosurgeons') apparent limited understanding of the principles of ventilator weaning, it is not logical to use these data[143] to form a judgment on the clinical efficacy of weaning predictors or of spontaneous breathing trials.

An additional component of the study by Namen et al[143] dealt with an evaluation of physiologic variables for predicting extubation outcome. Half of the 44 failed extubation attempts, however, were associated with the withdrawal of life support (all of these patients died). It is a meaningless exercise to interpret data on predictors of extubation when half of the extubation decisions were for the purpose of withdrawing life support.

Kollef et al[2] reasoned that effective weaning depended more on the use of a protocol, and that the precise technique of weaning is less important. They randomized 179 patients to a protocol group (implemented by nurses and respiratory therapists) and 178 patients to usual (physician-directed) care. The study was conducted in four ICUs, and weaning techniques were a mixture of PS, CPAP, and IMV (the use of T-tube trials was not listed). Overall, the duration of mechanical ventilation was shorter for the protocol group than for the usual care group: 35 hours (median; quartiles 15 and 114) versus 44 hours (quartiles 21 and 209). The difference, however, was significant in only one of the four ICUs. Moreover, interpretation of the data for this ICU is not straightforward. Patients in the usual care group were significantly sicker than were the patients in the protocol group: Acute Physiology, Age, and Chronic Health Evaluation (APACHE) II scores were 15.4 versus 13.6. In separate analysis, the investigators found that APACHE II score was at least as important as protocol management as a determinant of the duration of mechanical ventilation. In the other 3 ICUs, there was no difference in duration of mechanical ventilation between the protocol and usual care groups; in one ICU, the trend was in the opposite direction.

Marelich et al[144] undertook a randomized comparison of weaning by protocol (directed by nurses and therapists) versus usual care in 335 patients, about half of whom were in the medical ICU and half in the surgical ICU. They randomized 186 patients to a protocol arm and 189 patients to a usual care arm. Patients in the protocol arm were screened twice a day, and if they satisfied preset criteria, they were advanced to a spontaneous breathing trial (without requiring physician approval). The 30-minute trial consisted of breathing on flow-by with PS <8 cmH$_2$O plus PEEP <8 cmH$_2$O or a T-tube trial. Criteria for stopping the trial were frequency >30 breaths/minute, spontaneous V_T <5 ml/kg, S$_{O2}$ <92%, or respiratory distress. If a patient tolerated the trial, the physician was asked to approve discontinuation of the ventilator. If the patient failed the trial, he or she was returned to the ventilator, and re-screened every 6 hours. (Patients could undergo a maximum of 2 spontaneous breathing trials per day.)

The duration of mechanical ventilation was shorter for the protocol arm than for the usual care arm: 68 hours (quartiles 33 and 164) versus 124 hours (quartiles 54 and 334) ($p = 0.001$).[144] Benefit, however, was confined to the medical ICU. Protocol management achieved no advantage in the surgical ICU. The time of apparent improvement was also inconsistent between the two ICUs. The protocol achieved its greatest effect in the medical ICU between the time of entry and when patients first met criteria for the discontinuation of mechanical ventilation; in the surgical ICU, apparent benefit was greatest from the time of first meeting criteria for discontinuation of the ventilator until its actual discontinuation.

Randolph et al[145] randomized 182 children who had failed to satisfy criteria for extubation (and had been ventilated for >24 hours) to three arms: PS protocol, volume-support ventilation protocol (whereby PS is adjusted to achieve a minimal minute ventilation), and usual care. The rate of weaning failure was equivalent for PS, volume-support ventilation, and usual care, 15%, 24%, and 17%, respectively, as was the median duration of weaning, 1.6, 1.8, and 2.0 days, respectively. The authors concluded that protocols did not shorten the duration of weaning.

Krishnan et al[146] did a randomized trial in 154 patients assigned to weaning by protocol and 145 patients weaned according to usual care. Stable patients in the protocol arm had f/VT measured in the morning by a respiratory therapist; if the ratio was 105 or less, respiratory and nursing staff undertook a spontaneous breathing trial (without physician intervention). If the patient passed the 1-hour trial, the physician was informed. Patients failing the assessment were rested until the following day. In the usual care arm, patients were managed at the discretion of their physicians. Patients did not undergo any scheduled screening, although physicians were free to make measurements at the bedside. The duration of mechanical ventilation was equivalent for protocol weaning and usual care, 60.4 versus 68.0 hours, as was the rate of successful weaning, 74.7% versus 75.2%.

To date, there have been six randomized controlled trials comparing the use of protocols for weaning with usual care. The reports of Namen et al,[143] Randolph et al,[145] and Krishnan et al[146] show no advantage for a protocol approach. The reports of Ely et al,[56] Kollef et al,[2] and Marelich et al[144] are viewed as evidence for the superiority of a protocol approach to weaning. In the trial of Kollef et al, a significant advantage for a protocol approach to weaning was observed in only one of the four study ICUs. The usual care patients were significantly sicker than the protocol patients in that ICU, which markedly weakens (if not destroys) any assertion that protocol weaning was superior. Moreover, no advantage for weaning by protocol was observed in three of the four ICUs in this study.[2] Marelich et al[144] studied weaning by protocol in two ICUs, and found no significant advantage in one ICU. The study of Ely et al[56] does not consist of a straightforward comparison of protocol versus nonprotocol care. All of the patients in the intervention arm were weaned by T-tube or flow-by trials, whereas 76% of the patients in the nonintervention arm were managed by IMV alone or in combination with PS. Physiologic studies and randomized trials have repeatedly shown that IMV is the least effective weaning modality. With this fundamental difference in techniques, it is unscientific to use data from this study to form a judgment about the efficacy of a protocol per se. Instead, the report of Ely et al[56] can be viewed primarily as another study of IMV, confirming the reports of Brochard et al[3] and Esteban et al[4] that IMV slows weaning.

On reflection, it is not surprising that the use of a protocol does not improve weaning outcome. One needs to make a distinction between the use of algorithms in research protocols and their subsequent application in everyday practice. The algorithm in a research protocol is specified with exacting precision.[147] For example, if f/VT ≤ 100 is the nodal point for advancement to a T-tube trial, then patients with an f/VT of 100 will undergo the trial whereas patients with an f/VT of 101 will return to mechanical ventilation for another 24 hours. An experienced clinician, however, would think it daft to slavishly comply with a protocol in which an entire day of ventilator management was totally reliant on a one-unit difference in a single measurement of f/VT (or any other weaning predictor). Instead, an intelligent physician customizes the knowledge generated by research to the particulars of each patient. The intelligent application of physiologic principles is likely to outperform an inflexible application of a protocol. This view is illustrated by the longer time between initiation of a spontaneous breathing trial and extubation in the protocol group versus the usual care group in the study of Krishnan et al:[146] 3.0 versus 1.6 hours.

It would be unfortunate if clinicians were to interpret the results of the three negative trials[143,145,146] of a protocol approach to weaning (versus usual care) as signifying that physiologic principles do not help in the weaning of patients. In the study of Krishnan et al,[146] the question is not what went wrong with weaning by protocol but what was right with usual care.[148] Physicians are adept at extracting principles that emerge from research studies and incorporating them into their everyday practice. Once these principles have crept into a clinician's brain, they cannot be extirpated surgically. To interpret the three studies that have shown no benefit with a protocol approach to weaning[143,145,146] to mean that it is not necessary to undertake weaning in a deliberate manner would be to throw a physiologic baby out with the protocol bathwater.[148]

The attention to protocols is a distraction from the fundamental requirement in weaning. There is no substitute for judgment and clinical wisdom.

Conclusion

The hazards of mechanical ventilation make it imperative to wean patients at the earliest possible time in their clinical course. Premature weaning attempts, however, cause considerable respiratory distress that may set back a patient's course. Premature extubation is also hazardous. To minimize both delayed weaning and premature extubation, a two-step diagnostic strategy is recommended:

measurement of weaning predictors followed by a weaning trial. Because each step constitutes a diagnostic test, clinicians must be mindful of the scientific principles of clinical decision making when interpreting the information generated by each step.

The critical step is for the physician to contemplate the possibility that a patient *just might* be able to tolerate weaning. Such diagnostic triggering is facilitated through use of a screening test, which is the rationale for measurement of weaning predictor tests. It is important not to postpone this first step by waiting for a more complex diagnostic test, such as a T-tube trial. A positive result on a screening test (weaning predictor test) is followed by a confirmatory test (weaning trial), to increase the likelihood that a patient will tolerate extubation.

Many complex facets of pulmonary pathophysiology impinge on weaning management. Thus, weaning requires individualized care at a high level of sophistication. Few other activities undertaken by physicians in the ICU require a greater intellectual input and carry greater potential for improving patient outcome than the application of physiologic principles in the weaning of patients.

References

1. Epstein SK. Etiology of extubation failure and the predictive value of the rapid shallow breathing index. Am J Respir Crit Care Med 1995; 152:545–49.
2. Kollef MH, Shapiro SD, Silver P, et al. A randomized, controlled trial of protocol-directed versus physician-directed weaning from mechanical ventilation. Crit Care Med 1997; 25:567–74.
3. Brochard L, Rauss A, Benito S, et al. Comparison of three methods of gradual withdrawal from ventilatory support during weaning from mechanical ventilation. Am J Respir Crit Care Med 1994; 150:896–903.
4. Esteban A, Frutos F, Tobin MJ, et al. A comparison of four methods of weaning patients from mechanical ventilation. Spanish Lung Failure Collaborative Group. N Engl J Med 1995; 332:345–50.
5. Slovic P, Fischhoff B, Lichtenstein S. Behavioral decision theory. Ann Rev Psychol 1977; 28:1–39.
6. Tversky A, Kahneman D. Judgment under uncertainty: Heuristics and biases. Science 1974; 185:1124–31.
7. Tobin MJ, Mador MJ, Guenther SM, Lodato RF, Sackner MA. Variability of resting respiratory drive and timing in healthy subjects. J Appl Physiol 1988; 65:309–17.
8. Tobin MJ, Perez W, Guenther SM, et al. The pattern of breathing during successful and unsuccessful trials of weaning from mechanical ventilation. Am Rev Respir Dis 1986; 134:1111–18.
9. Sassoon CS, Te TT, Mahutte CK, Light RW. Airway occlusion pressure. An important indicator for successful weaning in patients with chronic obstructive pulmonary disease. Am Rev Respir Dis 1987; 135:107–13.
10. Montgomery AB, Holle RH, Neagley SR, Pierson DJ, Schoene RB. Prediction of successful ventilator weaning using airway occlusion pressure and hypercapnic challenge. Chest 1987; 91:496–99.
11. Gandia F, Blanco J. Evaluation of indexes predicting the outcome of ventilator weaning and value of adding supplemental inspiratory load. Intensive Care Med 1992; 18:327–33.
12. Sassoon CS, Mahutte CK. Airway occlusion pressure and breathing pattern as predictors of weaning outcome. Am Rev Respir Dis 1993; 148:860–66.
13. Capdevila XJ, Perrigault PF, Perey PJ, Roustan JP, d'Athis F. Occlusion pressure and its ratio to maximum inspiratory pressure are useful predictors for successful extubation following T-piece weaning trial. Chest 1995; 108:482–89.
14. Vassilakopoulos T, Zakynthinos S, Roussos C. The tension-time index and the frequency/tidal volume ratio are the major pathophysiologic determinants of weaning failure and success. Am J Respir Crit Care Med 1998; 158:378–85.
15. Jubran A, Tobin MJ. Pathophysiologic basis of acute respiratory distress in patients who fail a trial of weaning from mechanical ventilation. Am J Respir Crit Care Med 1997; 155:906–15.
16. Jubran A, Tobin MJ. Passive mechanics of lung and chest wall in patients who failed or succeeded in trials of weaning. Am J Respir Crit Care Med 1997; 155:916–21.
17. Polese G, Rossi A, Appendini L, et al. Partitioning of respiratory mechanics in mechanically ventilated patients. J Appl Physiol 1991; 71:2425–33.
18. Guerin C, Coussa ML, Eissa NT, et al. Lung and chest wall mechanics in mechanically ventilated COPD patients. J Appl Physiol 1993; 74:1570–80.
19. Tantucci C, Corbeil C, Chasse M, et al. Flow resistance in patients with chronic obstructive pulmonary disease in acute respiratory failure. Effects of flow and volume. Am Rev Respir Dis 1991; 144:384–89.
20. Fiastro JF, Habib MP, Shon BY, Campbell SC. Comparison of standard weaning parameters and the mechanical work of breathing in mechanically ventilated patients. Chest 1988; 94:232–38.
21. Henning RJ, Shubin H, Weil MH. The measurement of the work of breathing for the clinical assessment of ventilator dependence. Crit Care Med 1977; 5:264–68.
22. Tobin MJ. Monitoring respiratory mechanics in spontaneously breathing patients. In: Tobin MJ, editor. Principles and practice of intensive care monitoring. New York: McGraw-Hill, 1998: 617–54.
23. Tobin MJ, Laghi F. Monitoring of respiratory muscle function. In: Tobin MJ, editor. Principles and practice of intensive care monitoring. New York: McGraw-Hill, 1998: 497–544.
24. Sahn SA, Lakshminarayan S. Bedside criteria for discontinuation of mechanical ventilation. Chest 1973; 63:1002–5.
25. Tahvanainen J, Salmenpera M, Nikki P. Extubation criteria after weaning from intermittent mandatory ventilation and continuous positive airway pressure. Crit Care Med 1983; 11:702–7.
26. Yang KL, Tobin MJ. A prospective study of indexes predicting the outcome of trials of weaning from mechanical ventilation. N Engl J Med 1991; 324:1445–50.
27. Laghi F, Tobin MJ. Disorders of the respiratory muscles. Am J Respir Crit Care Med 2003; 168:10–48.
28. Laghi F, Cattapan SE, Jubran A, et al. Is weaning failure caused by low-frequency fatigue of the diaphragm? Am J Respir Crit Care Med 2003; 167:120–27.
29. Cohen CA, Zagelbaum G, Gross D, Roussos C, Macklem PT. Clinical manifestations of inspiratory muscle fatigue. Am J Med 1982; 73:308–16.
30. Tobin MJ, Guenther SM, Perez W, et al. Konno-Mead analysis of ribcage-abdominal motion during successful and unsuccessful trials of weaning from mechanical ventilation. Am Rev Respir Dis 1987; 135:1320–28.
31. Tobin MJ, Perez W, Guenther SM, Lodato RF, Dantzker DR. Does rib cage-abdominal paradox signify respiratory muscle fatigue? J Appl Physiol 1987; 63:851–60.

32. Capdevila X, Perrigault PF, Ramonatxo M, et al. Changes in breathing pattern and respiratory muscle performance parameters during difficult weaning. Crit Care Med 1998; 26: 79–87.

33. Bellemare F, Grassino A. Effect of pressure and timing of contraction on human diaphragm fatigue. J Appl Physiol 1982; 53: 1190–95.

34. Lemaire F, Teboul JL, Cinotti L, et al. Acute left ventricular dysfunction during unsuccessful weaning from mechanical ventilation. Anesthesiology 1988; 69:171–79.

35. Hurford WE, Lynch KE, Strauss HW, Lowenstein E, Zapol WM. Myocardial perfusion as assessed by thallium-201 scintigraphy during the discontinuation of mechanical ventilation in ventilator-dependent patients. Anesthesiology 1991; 74: 1007–16.

36. Richard C, Teboul JL, Archambaud F, et al. Left ventricular function during weaning of patients with chronic obstructive pulmonary disease. Intensive Care Med 1994; 20:181–86.

37. Chatila W, Ani S, Guaglianone D, et al. Cardiac ischemia during weaning from mechanical ventilation. Chest 1996; 109:1577–83.

38. Srivastava S, Chatila W, Amoateng-Adjepong Y, et al. Myocardial ischemia and weaning failure in patients with coronary artery disease: an update. Crit Care Med 1999; 27:2109–12.

39. Jubran A, Mathru M, Dries D, Tobin MJ. Continuous recordings of mixed venous oxygen saturation during weaning from mechanical ventilation and the ramifications thereof. Am J Respir Crit Care Med 1998; 158:1763–69.

40. Reid MB, Johnson RL Jr. Efficiency, maximal blood flow, and aerobic work capacity of canine diaphragm. J Appl Physiol 1983; 54:763–72.

41. De Backer D, El Haddad P, Preiser JC, Vincent JL. Hemodynamic responses to successful weaning from mechanical ventilation after cardiovascular surgery. Intensive Care Med 2000; 26: 1201–6.

42. Beydon L, Cinotti L, Rekik N, et al. Changes in the distribution of ventilation and perfusion associated with separation from mechanical ventilation in patients with obstructive pulmonary disease. Anesthesiology 1991; 75:730–38.

43. Torres A, Reyes A, Roca J, Wagner PD, Rodriguez-Roisin R. Ventilation-perfusion mismatching in chronic obstructive pulmonary disease during ventilator weaning. Am Rev Respir Dis 1989; 140:1246–50.

44. Ferrer M, Iglesia R, Roca J, et al. Pulmonary gas exchange response to weaning with pressure-support ventilation in exacerbated chronic obstructive pulmonary disease patients. Intensive Care Med 2002; 28:1595–99.

45. Sox HC Jr, Clatt MA, Higgins MC, Marton KI. Medical decision making. Boston: Butterworths, 1988.

46. Lang TA. How to report statistics in medicine. Philadelphia: American College of Physicians, 1997.

47. Griner PF, Mayewski RJ, Mushlin AI, Greenland P. Selection and interpretation of diagnostic tests and procedures. Principles and applications. Ann Intern Med 1981; 94:557–92.

48. Diamond GA. Reverend Bayes' silent majority. An alternative factor affecting sensitivity and specificity of exercise electrocardiography. Am J Cardiol 1986; 57:1175–80.

49. Ransohoff DF, Feinstein AR. Problems of spectrum and bias in evaluating the efficacy of diagnostic tests. N Engl J Med 1978; 299:926–30.

50. Feinstein AR. Clinical epidemiology: The architecture of clinical research. Philadelphia: WB Saunders, 1985.

51. Lachs MS, Nachamkin I, Edelstein PH, et al. Spectrum bias in the evaluation of diagnostic tests: lessons from the rapid dipstick test for urinary tract infection. Ann Intern Med 1992; 117:135–40.

52. Eisenberg MJ. Accuracy and predictive values in clinical decision-making. Cleve Clin J Med 1995; 62:311–16.

53. Hlatky MA, Pryor DB, Harrell FE Jr, et al. Factors affecting sensitivity and specificity of exercise electrocardiography. Multivariable analysis. Am J Med 1984; 77:64–71.

54. Sox HC. The evaluation of diagnostic tests: principles, problems, and new developments. Annu Rev Med 1996; 47:463–71.

55. Sox HC Jr. Probability theory in the use of diagnostic tests. An introduction to critical study of the literature. Ann Intern Med 1986; 104:60–66.

56. Ely EW, Baker AM, Dunagan DP, et al. Effect on the duration of mechanical ventilation of identifying patients capable of breathing spontaneously. N Engl J Med 1996; 335:1864–69.

57. Shott S. Statistics for health professionals. Philadelphia: WB Saunders, 1990.

58. Epstein SK, Ciubotaru RL. Influence of gender and endotracheal tube size on preextubation breathing pattern. Am J Respir Crit Care Med 1996; 154:1647–52.

59. Leitch EA, Moran JL, Grealy B. Weaning and extubation in the intensive care unit. Clinical or index-driven approach? Intensive Care Med 1996; 22:752–59.

60. Khan N, Brown A, Venkataraman ST. Predictors of extubation success and failure in mechanically ventilated infants and children. Crit Care Med 1996; 24:1568–79.

61. Vallverdu I, Calaf N, Subirana M, et al. Clinical characteristics, respiratory functional parameters, and outcome of a two-hour T-piece trial in patients weaning from mechanical ventilation. Am J Respir Crit Care Med 1998; 158:1855–62.

62. Uusaro A, Chittock DR, Russell JA, Walley KR. Stress test and gastric-arterial PCO2 measurement improve prediction of successful extubation. Crit Care Med 2000; 28:2313–19.

63. Khamiees M, Raju P, DeGirolamo A, Amoateng-Adjepong Y, Manthous CA. Predictors of extubation outcome in patients who have successfully completed a spontaneous breathing trial. Chest 2001; 120:1262–70.

64. Cohen JD, Shapiro M, Grozovski E, Singer P. Automatic tube compensation-assisted respiratory rate to tidal volume ratio improves the prediction of weaning outcome. Chest 2002; 122: 980–84.

65. Smina M, Salam A, Khamiees M, et al. Cough peak flows and extubation outcomes. Chest 2003; 124:262–68.

66. Fernandez R, Raurich JM, Mut T, et al. Extubation failure: diagnostic value of occlusion pressure (P0.1) and P0.1-derived parameters. Intensive Care Med 2004; 30:234–40.

67. Rozanski A, Diamond GA, Berman D, et al. The declining specificity of exercise radionuclide ventriculography. N Engl J Med 1983; 309:518–22.

68. Metz CE. Basic principles of ROC analysis. Semin Nucl Med 1978; 8:283–98.

69. Yang KL. Inspiratory pressure/maximal inspiratory pressure ratio: a predictive index of weaning outcome. Intensive Care Med 1993; 19:204–8.

70. Farias JA, Alia I, Esteban A, Golubicki AN, Olazarri FA. Weaning from mechanical ventilation in pediatric intensive care patients. Intensive Care Med 1998; 24:1070–75.

71. Conti G, Montini L, Pennisi MA, et al. A prospective, blinded evaluation of indexes proposed to predict weaning from mechanical ventilation. Intensive Care Med 2004; 30:830–36.

72. Mohsenifar Z, Hay A, Hay J, Lewis MI, Koerner SK. Gastric intramural pH as a predictor of success or failure in weaning patients from mechanical ventilation. Ann Intern Med 1993; 119:794–98.

73. Rivera L, Weissman C. Dynamic ventilatory characteristics during weaning in postoperative critically ill patients. Anesth Analg 1997; 84:1250–55.

74. Dojat M, Harf A, Touchard D, et al. Evaluation of a knowledge-based system providing ventilatory management and decision for extubation. Am J Respir Crit Care Med 1996; 153:997–1004.

75. Jacob B, Chatila W, Manthous CA. The unassisted respiratory rate/tidal volume ratio accurately predicts weaning outcome in postoperative patients. Crit Care Med 1997; 25:253–57.

76. Maldonado A, Bauer TT, Ferrer M, et al. Capnometric recirculation gas tonometry and weaning from mechanical ventilation. Am J Respir Crit Care Med 2000; 161:171–76.

77. Baumeister BL, el Khatib M, Smith PG, Blumer JL. Evaluation of predictors of weaning from mechanical ventilation in pediatric patients. Pediatr Pulmonol 1997; 24:344–52.

78. Zeggwagh AA, Abouqal R, Madani N, Zekraoui A, Kerkeb O. Weaning from mechanical ventilation: a model for extubation. Intensive Care Med 1999; 25:1077–83.

79. Lee KH, Hui KP, Chan TB, Tan WC, Lim TK. Rapid shallow breathing (frequency-tidal volume ratio) did not predict extubation outcome. Chest 1994; 105:540–43.

80. Mergoni M, Costa A, Primavera S, et al. Valutazione di alcuni nuovi parametri predittivi dell'esito dello svezzamento dalla ventilazione meccanica. Minerva Anestesiol 1996; 62:153–64.

81. Krieger BP, Isber J, Breitenbucher A, Throop G, Ershowsky P. Serial measurements of the rapid-shallow-breathing index as a predictor of weaning outcome in elderly medical patients. Chest 1997; 112:1029–34.

82. Afessa B, Hogans L, Murphy R. Predicting 3-day and 7-day outcomes of weaning from mechanical ventilation. Chest 1999; 116:456–61.

83. Jiang JR, Tsai TH, Jerng JS, et al. Ultrasonographic evaluation of liver/spleen movements and extubation outcome. Chest 2004; 126:179–85.

84. Brochard L, Pluskwa F, Lemaire F. Improved efficacy of spontaneous breathing with inspiratory pressure support. Am Rev Respir Dis 1987; 136:411–15.

85. Tokioka H, Saito S, Kosaka F. Effect of pressure support ventilation on breathing patterns and respiratory work. Intensive Care Med 1989; 15:491–94.

86. Sassoon CS, Light RW, Lodia R, Sieck GC, Mahutte CK. Pressure-time product during continuous positive airway pressure, pressure support ventilation, and T-piece during weaning from mechanical ventilation. Am Rev Respir Dis 1991; 143:469–75.

87. Jubran A, Van de Graaff WB, Tobin MJ. Variability of patient-ventilator interaction with pressure support ventilation in patients with chronic obstructive pulmonary disease. Am J Respir Crit Care Med 1995; 152:129–36.

88. Razek T, Gracias V, Sullivan D, et al. Assessing the need for reintubation: a prospective evaluation of unplanned endotracheal extubation. J Trauma 2000; 48:466–69.

89. Straus C, Louis B, Isabey D, et al. Contribution of the endotracheal tube and the upper airway to breathing workload. Am J Respir Crit Care Med 1998; 157:23–30.

90. Tobin MJ, Jenouri G, Birch S, et al. Effect of positive end-expiratory pressure on breathing patterns of normal subjects and intubated patients with respiratory failure. Crit Care Med 1983; 11:859–67.

91. El Khatib MF, Jamaleddine GW, Khoury AR, Obeid MY. Effect of continuous positive airway pressure on the rapid shallow breathing index in patients following cardiac surgery. Chest 2002; 121:475–79.

92. Jaeschke RZ, Meade MO, Guyatt GH, Keenan SP, Cook DJ. How to use diagnostic test articles in the intensive care unit: diagnosing weanability using f/Vt. Crit Care Med 1997; 25:1514–21.

93. Kufel TJ, Grant B. Arterial blood-gas monitoring: Respiratory assessment. In: Tobin MJ, editor. Principles and practice of intensive care monitoring. New York: McGraw-Hill, 1998: 197–215.

94. Krieger BP, Ershowsky PF, Becker DA, Gazeroglu HB. Evaluation of conventional criteria for predicting successful weaning from mechanical ventilatory support in elderly patients. Crit Care Med 1989; 17:858–61.

95. Tobin MJ. Noninvasive monitoring of ventilation. In: Tobin MJ, editor. Principles and practice of intensive care monitoring. New York: McGraw-Hill, 1998: 465–95.

96. Tobin MJ, Chadha TS, Jenouri G, et al. Breathing patterns. 1. Normal subjects. Chest 1983; 84:202–5.

97. Marini JJ, Smith TC, Lamb V. Estimation of inspiratory muscle strength in mechanically ventilated patients: The measurement of maximal inspiratory pressure. J Crit Care 1986; 1:32–38.

98. Millbern SM, Downs JB, Jumper LC, Modell JH. Evaluation of criteria for discontinuing mechanical ventilatory support. Arch Surg 1978; 113:1441–43.

99. Chevrolet JC, Deleamont P. Repeated vital capacity measurements as predictive parameters for mechanical ventilation need and weaning success in the Guillain-Barre syndrome. Am Rev Respir Dis 1991; 144:814–18.

100. Whitelaw WA, Derenne JP, Milic-Emili J. Occlusion pressure as a measure of respiratory center output in conscious man. Respir Physiol 1975; 23:181–99.

101. Tobin MJ, Gardner WN. Monitoring of the control of breathing. In: Tobin MJ, editor. Principles and practice of intensive care monitoring. New York: McGraw-Hill, 1998: 415–64.

102. Leevers AM, Simon PM, Dempsey JA. Apnea after normocapnic mechanical ventilation during NREM sleep. J Appl Physiol 1994; 77:2079–85.

103. Rice AJ, Nakayama HC, Haverkamp HC, et al. Controlled versus assisted mechanical ventilation effects on respiratory motor output in sleeping humans. Am J Respir Crit Care Med 2003; 168:92–101.

104. Chatila W, Jacob B, Guaglionone D, Manthous CA. The unassisted respiratory rate-tidal volume ratio accurately predicts weaning outcome. Am J Med 1996; 101:61–67.

105. Jubran A, Grant BJ, Laghi F, Parthasarathy S, Tobin MJ. Weaning prediction: esophageal pressure monitoring complements readiness testing. Am J Respir Crit Care Med 2005; 171:1252–59.

106. Yang KL, Tobin MJ. Measurement of minute ventilation in ventilator-dependent patients: need for standardization. Crit Care Med 1991; 19:49–53.

107. Yang KL. Reproducibility of weaning parameters. A need for standardization. Chest 1992; 102:1829–32.

108. Multz AS, Aldrich TK, Prezant DJ, Karpel JP, Hendler JM. Maximal inspiratory pressure is not a reliable test of inspiratory muscle strength in mechanically ventilated patients. Am Rev Respir Dis 1990; 142:529–32.

109. Brenner M, Mukai DS, Russell JE, Spiritus EM, Wilson AF. A new method for measurement of airway occlusion pressure. Chest 1990; 98:421–27.

110. Burki NK. The effects of changes in functional residual capacity with posture on mouth occlusion pressure and ventilatory pattern. Am Rev Respir Dis 1977; 116:895–900.

111. Mann J, Bradley CA, Anthonisen NR. Occlusion pressure in acute bronchospasm induced by methylcholine. Respir Physiol 1978; 33:339–47.

112. Lederer DH, Altose MD, Kelsen SG, Cherniack NS. Comparison of occlusion pressure and ventilatory responses. Thorax 1977; 32:212–20.

113. Brown SD, Gutierrez G. Gut mucosal pH monitoring. In: Tobin MJ, editor. Principles and practice of intensive care monitoring. New York: McGraw-Hill, 1998: 351–68.

114. Bouachour G, Guiraud MP, Gouello JP, Roy PM, Alquier P. Gastric intramucosal pH: an indicator of weaning outcome from mechanical ventilation in COPD patients. Eur Respir J 1996; 9:1868–73.

115. Bocquillon N, Mathieu D, Neviere R, et al. Gastric mucosal pH and blood flow during weaning from mechanical ventilation in patients with chronic obstructive pulmonary disease. Am J Respir Crit Care Med 1999; 160:1555–61.

116. Torres A, Gatell JM, Aznar E, et al. Re-intubation increases the risk of nosocomial pneumonia in patients needing mechanical ventilation. Am J Respir Crit Care Med 1995; 152: 137–41.

117. MacIntyre NR, Cook DJ, Ely EW Jr, et al. Evidence-based guidelines for weaning and discontinuing ventilatory support: a collective task force facilitated by the American College of Chest Physicians; the American Association for Respiratory Care; and the American College of Critical Care Medicine. Chest 2001; 120:375S–95S.

118. Meade M, Guyatt G, Cook D, et al. Predicting success in weaning from mechanical ventilation. Chest 2001; 120:400S–24S.

119. Ely EW, Bennett PA, Bowton DL, et al. Large scale implementation of a respiratory therapist-driven protocol for ventilator weaning. Am J Respir Crit Care Med 1999; 159:439–46.

120. Marini JJ, Smith TC, Lamb VJ. External work output and force generation during synchronized intermittent mechanical ventilation. Effect of machine assistance on breathing effort. Am Rev Respir Dis 1988; 138:1169–79.

121. Imsand C, Feihl F, Perret C, Fitting JW. Regulation of inspiratory neuromuscular output during synchronized intermittent mechanical ventilation. Anesthesiology 1994; 80:13–22.

122. MacIntyre NR. Respiratory function during pressure support ventilation. Chest 1986; 89:677–83.

123. Brochard L, Harf A, Lorino H, Lemaire F. Inspiratory pressure support prevents diaphragmatic fatigue during weaning from mechanical ventilation. Am Rev Respir Dis 1989; 139: 513–21.

124. Mehta S, Nelson DL, Klinger JR, Buczko GB, Levy MM. Prediction of post-extubation work of breathing. Crit Care Med 2000; 28:1341–46.

125. Sahn SA, Lakshminarayan S, Petty TL. Weaning from mechanical ventilation. JAMA 1976; 235:2208–12.

126. Pichard C, Kyle U, Chevrolet JC, et al. Lack of effects of recombinant growth hormone on muscle function in patients requiring prolonged mechanical ventilation: a prospective, randomized, controlled study. Crit Care Med 1996; 24:403–13.

127. Venus B, Smith RA, Mathru M. National survey of methods and criteria used for weaning from mechanical ventilation. Crit Care Med 1987; 15:530–33.

128. Laghi F, D'Alfonso N, Tobin MJ. Pattern of recovery from diaphragmatic fatigue over 24 hours. J Appl Physiol 1995; 79: 539–46.

129. Salam A, Smina M, Gada P, et al. The effect of arterial blood gas values on extubation decisions. Respir Care 2003; 48: 1033–37.

130. Faulkner JA. Structural and functional adaptations of skeletal muscle. In: Roussos C, Macklem PT, editors. The thorax Part B. Vol. 29 of Lung biology in health and disease. New York: Marcel Dekker, 1985: 1329–51.

131. Rochester DF. Does respiratory muscle rest relieve fatigue or incipient fatigue? Am Rev Respir Dis 1988; 138:516–17.

132. Vinegar A, Sinnett EE, Leith DE. Dynamic mechanisms determine functional residual capacity in mice, *Mus musculus*. J Appl Physiol 1979; 46:867–71.

133. Martin JG, De Troyer A. The thorax and control of functional residual capacity. In: Roussos C, Macklem PT, editors. The thorax Part B. Vol. 29 of Lung biology in health and disease. New York: Marcel Dekker, 1985: 899–921.

134. Smith TC, Marini JJ. Impact of PEEP on lung mechanics and work of breathing in severe airflow obstruction. J Appl Physiol 1988; 65:1488–99.

135. Esteban A, Alia I, Tobin MJ, et al. Effect of spontaneous breathing trial duration on outcome of attempts to discontinue mechanical

136. Perren A, Domenighetti G, Mauri S, Genini F, Vizzardi N. Protocol-directed weaning from mechanical ventilation: clinical outcome in patients randomized for a 30-min or 120-min trial with pressure support ventilation. Intensive Care Med 2002; 28:1058–63.

137. Esteban A, Alia I, Gordo F, et al. Extubation outcome after spontaneous breathing trials with T-tube or pressure support ventilation. The Spanish Lung Failure Collaborative Group. Am J Respir Crit Care Med 1997; 156:459–65.

138. Koh Y, Hong SB, Lim CM, et al. Effect of an additional 1-hour T-piece trial on weaning outcome at minimal pressure support. J Crit Care 2000; 15:41–45.

139. Matic I, Majeric-Kogler V. Comparison of pressure support and T-tube weaning from mechanical ventilation: Randomized prospective study. Croatian Med J 2004; 45:162–66.

140. Vitacca M, Vianello A, Colombo D, et al. Comparison of two methods for weaning patients with chronic obstructive pulmonary disease requiring mechanical ventilation for more than 15 days. Am J Respir Crit Care Med 2001; 164:225–30.

141. Saura P, Blanch L, Mestre J, et al. Clinical consequences of the implementation of a weaning protocol. Intensive Care Med 1996; 22:1052–56.

142. Ely EW, Baker AM, Evans GW, Haponik EF. The prognostic significance of passing a daily screen of weaning parameters. Intensive Care Med 1999; 25:581–87.

143. Namen AM, Ely EW, Tatter SB, et al. Predictors of successful extubation in neurosurgical patients. Am J Respir Crit Care Med 2001; 163:658–64.

144. Marelich GP, Murin S, Battistella F, et al. Protocol weaning of mechanical ventilation in medical and surgical patients by respiratory care practitioners and nurses: effect on weaning time and incidence of ventilator-associated pneumonia. Chest 2000; 118:459–67.

145. Randolph AG, Wypij D, Venkataraman ST, et al. Effect of mechanical ventilator weaning protocols on respiratory outcomes in infants and children: a randomized controlled trial. JAMA 2002; 288:2561–68.

146. Krishnan JA, Moore D, Robeson C, Rand CS, Fessler HE. A prospective, controlled trial of a protocol-based strategy to discontinue mechanical ventilation. Am J Respir Crit Care Med 2004; 169:673–78.

147. Morris AH. Algorithm-based decision making. In: Tobin MJ, editor. Principles and practice of intensive care monitoring. New York: McGraw-Hill, 1998: 1355–81.

148. Tobin MJ. Of principles and protocols and weaning. Am J Respir Crit Care Med 2004; 169:661–62.

149. Гологорский ВА, Гельфанд БР, Стамов ВИ, Лапшина ИЮ, Нистратов С Л. Прекрашение длительной ИВЛ и перевод на спонтанное дыхание хирургических больных. Анестезиология и реаниматология 1997 №1; 4–10.

150. Thiagarajan RR, Bratton SL, Martin LD, Brogan TV, Taylor D. Predictors of successful extubation in children. Am J Respir Crit Care Med 1999; 160:1562–66.

151. Fernandez R, Cabrera J, Calaf N, Benito S. P 0.1/PIMax: an index for assessing respiratory capacity in acute respiratory failure. Intensive Care Med 1990; 16:175–79.

152. Herrera M, Blasco J, Venegas J, et al. Mouth occlusion pressure (P0.1) in acute respiratory failure. Intensive Care Med 1985; 11:134–39.

153. Conti G, De Blasi R, Pelaia P, et al. Early prediction of successful weaning during pressure support ventilation in chronic obstructive pulmonary disease patients. Crit Care Med 1992; 20: 366–71.

EXTUBATION

MARTIN J TOBIN
FRANCO LAGHI

It is easy to merge decisions about extubation with decisions about weaning in everyday practice. Indeed, much patient mismanagement is caused by conflating these two subjects. But the conflation is not confined to clinicians. Many researchers have also merged the two subjects, such as using weaning predictors to predict reintubation in a patient who has already tolerated a weaning trial. The result is scientific confusion.

When a patient tolerates a weaning trial without distress, a clinician feels reasonably confident that the patient will be able to sustain spontaneous ventilation after extubation. But this is not the only consideration. The clinician also has to consider whether the patient will be able to maintain a patent upper airway after extubation.

Removal of an endotracheal tube is typically performed under controlled conditions. The patient has satisfactorily tolerated a weaning trial. Enteral feeding is temporally withheld for about 4 hours. The patient is usually positioned in a sitting posture. The endotracheal tube, mouth, and upper airway are suctioned, paying attention to the collection of secretions above an inflated cuff. Some clinicians recommend keeping a suction catheter in place (aiming for the catheter to barely protrude from the distal end of the endotracheal tube) as the cuff is deflated; this step is taken in an attempt to capture any secretions sitting on top of an inflated cuff, that might fall into the airway after deflating the cuff. Some clinicians forcefully inflate the lungs with an Ambu Bag immediately before pulling out the endotracheal tube, hoping that the larger than usual ensuing exhalation will push secretions upward and outward. After removal of the endotracheal tube, the patient is given supplemental oxygen (O_2), titrated to oxygen saturation (S_{O_2}), being particularly cautious with a patient who is at risk of carbon dioxide (CO_2) retention. Patients may have impaired airway protection reflexes immediately after extubation. If speech is impaired for >24 hours, indirect laryngoscopy should be undertaken to assess vocal cord function. Oral intake should be delayed in patients who have been intubated for a prolonged period.

In the hours following extubation, patients are carefully monitored for ability to protect the upper airway and sustain ventilation. Most patients will display progressive improvement, allowing the discontinuation of supplemental O_2 and ultimate discharge from the intensive care unit (ICU).

Postextubation Distress

Between $2\%^{1,2}$ and $30\%^{3-6}$ of patients experience respiratory distress in the postextubation period (Table 59-1). Many, but not all, require reinsertion of the endotracheal tube and mechanical ventilation. These patients are commonly classified as *extubation failures*, a term popularized by Demling et al.[7] These investigators defined extubation failure as the need for reintubation within 7 days. Unfortunately, the meaning of extubation failure varies among authors, leading to scientific confusion. Even when authors employ it as a synonym for reintubation, the period under study varies: within 24, 48, or 72 hours, or as long as 7 days.

Extubation failure is most often defined as the need for reintubation. The corollary of this definition is that all patients who do not require reintubation should be classified as extubation successes no matter how much difficulty they experience. A number of patients develop stridor after extubation, which resolves with inhalation of racemic epinephrine or other therapy without requiring reintubation. If extubation failure is defined as reintubation, such patients should be excluded. But if the focus is the study of respiratory distress and failure after extubation, all patients with significant postextubation stridor should be included. Much confusion could be avoided if researchers used the term "reintubation" when that is their sole criterion for extubation failure. If researchers use the term "extubation failure," it seems logical to assume that their study population includes some patients with postextubation distress who did not require reintubation. In many reports, however, it is not clear whether (or not) some such cases are being included as extubation failures.

Investigators have variably classified patients who required noninvasive ventilation (NIV) after extubation as satisfying or not satisfying the definition of extubation failure. De Lassence et al[8] specified that they excluded patients who were managed by NIV in a cohort of extubation

TABLE 59-1   Frequency of Reintubation and Mortality

Authors	Number of Patients	Percent Reintubated	Percent Mortality	Time Frame
Tahvanainen et al[67]	47	19.1	22.2	—
DeHaven et al[68]	48	6.3	NR	—
Demling et al[7]	400	4.4	40	7 days
Demling et al[7]	299	3.3	10	7 days
Krieger et al[69]	269	10.4	NR	—
Mohsenifar et al[70]	29	14.3	NR	24 h
Sassoon et al[71]	40	12.5	NR	48 h
Brochard et al[72]	109	11	NR	48 h
Lee et al[73]	52	17	33.3	NR
Capdevila et al[45]	67	17.9	NR	48 h
Esteban et al[74]	530	15.6	NR	48 h
Torres et al[27]	170	23.5	35	—
Chatila et al[75]	100	9.5		<24 h
Dojat et al[3]	38	29.4	40	48 h
Ely et al[76]	300	3.7	NR	48 h
Leitch et al[1]	163	1.8	NR	<24 h
Miller et al[32]	88	17	NR	NR
Epstein et al[12]	289	14.5	42.5	—
Esteban et al[26]	484	18.6	27	48 h
Jacob et al[77]	183	4.5	NR	24 h
Kollef et al[78]	357	11.5	NR	NR
Vallverdu et al[42]	217	15.5	NR	48 h
Esteban et al[15]	526	13.5	32.8	48 h
Zeggwagh et al[30]	101	37	NR	48 h
Coplin et al[41]	136	17.6	NR	NR
Koh et al[79]	36	19	NR	48 h
Maldonado et al[5]	24	26.7	NR	24 h
Khamiees et al[39]	91	12.8	NR	72 h
Namen et al[13]	100	16	NR	NR
Cohen et al[4]	35	28.6	10	48 h
De Bast et al[22]	76	18.4	NR	24 h
Perren et al[80]	98	6.7	33	48 h
Smina et al[16]	95	11.3	—	72
Conti et al[2]	92	1.7	NR	48 h
Fernandez et al[46]	130	18	NR	48 h

failure patients. Maldonado et al[5] included patients managed by NIV among their group of extubation failures, as did Haberthur et al[9] and Jiang et al.[10] Moreover, Haberthur et al[9] extended the term "extubation failure" to include patients experiencing unjustified delay in extubation with one particular weaning technique if that patient tolerated extubation after being switched to an alternative weaning technique.

If patients die from a cardiorespiratory cause without being reintubated, it seems unscientific to classify them as extubation successes. Some authors[11] have specified that their definition of extubation failure included both the need for reintubation or unexpected death within 72 hours. Most authors, however, do not address this issue. Some extubated patients refuse reintubation (as part of a decision for withdrawal of life support) and die. How should these patients be classified? Demling et al[7] classified fatal outcomes as extubation failures, Epstein et al[12] excluded such patients from their group of extubation failures, and Namen et al[13] classified such patients (who died) as extubation successes.

How should patients who experience unplanned extubation followed by reintubation be classified? In a group of

42 extubation failures, Epstein et al[12] included 4 unplanned extubations (who required reintubation within 72 hours) because these occurred while a weaning trial was in progress, but excluded 16 other unplanned extubations (requiring immediate extubation) because these did not occur during weaning trials. If patients are extubated because of a defective endotracheal tube and then reintubated, how should they be classified? Epstein and Ciubotaru[14] excluded such patients, but many authors do not state clearly how such patients are classified.

Some patients may be inappropriately reintubated because of poor clinical judgment. What criteria should be set for judging a reintubation as appropriate? Epstein and Ciubotaru[14] listed the following criteria: increase in arterial carbon dioxide tension (P_{CO_2}) >10 mmHg and decrease in pH of 0.10; arterial oxygen tension (P_{O_2}) <60 mmHg or S_{O_2} <90% with an inspired oxygen concentration ($F_{I_{O_2}}$) >0.50; signs of increased work of breathing (high respiratory rate, accessory muscle use, or paradoxical breathing); and inability to protect the airway (secondary to upper airway obstruction or excess secretions). Many of these criteria are similar to those used for defining weaning failure, but it is more difficult to ensure their rigorous and consistent application as criteria for reintubation. Weaning failure typically occurs under controlled conditions, usually within 1 hour of starting a weaning trial. Reintubation for postextubation distress may not occur until many hours after extubation, and the listing of satisfied criteria may not be entered on a data form until hours after the event.

Causes and Pathophysiology of Postextubation Distress

The listed indications for reintubation vary considerably from study to study. Of these, postextubation stridor has attracted the most attention.

POSTEXTUBATION UPPER AIRWAY OBSTRUCTION

A number of investigators have reported that upper airway obstruction accounts for about 15% of patients requiring reintubation (15% in the study of Epstein and Ciubotaru[14]; 14.7% in that of Esteban et al[15]; and 15.4% in that of Smina et al[16]). These investigators, however, did not report what proportion of patients who developed clinical manifestations of upper airway obstruction did not require reintubation. Upper airway obstruction may result from supraglottic edema, reflex closure of the vocal cords (laryngospasm), or compromise of the tracheal lumen (tracheomalacia or compression by a hematoma). Upper airway obstruction causes stridor only if the patient is capable of generating sufficient airflow; if airflow is insufficient, obstruction may cause hypercapnia, hypoxemia, or paradoxical breathing.

Of 110 extubated patients, Sandhu et al[17] observed that 13 (11.8%) developed stridor, but only 6 (46.2%) required reintubation (no patient required reintubation for any reason other than stridor in this series). Jaber et al[18] observed stridor in 13 of 112 (11.6%) extubated patients, 9 of whom (69.2%) required reintubation (only 2% [2/99] of patients without stridor required reintubation). A much higher rate of stridor was reported by Ho et al:[19] 22% of 77 (17/77) extubated patients, although only 1 patient required reintubation; 39% of the women (7/18) in this series developed stridor. In contrast, Darmon et al[20] observed stridor in only 4.2% of 663 extubations (28/663), and only 1.1% (7/663) required reintubation. An even lower rate of stridor was noted by Engoren:[21] 0.6% (3/531) of extubations.

In the above studies, upper airway obstruction has typically been diagnosed on the basis of clinical manifestations. De Bast et al[22] undertook fiberoptic examination before reintubation or directly inspected the glottis during reintubation to confirm the presence of laryngeal edema. Of 76 patients who had been intubated for at least 12 hours, 14 required reintubation within 24 hours of extubation (reintubation rate, 18.4%). Of these 14 patients, 8 (57.1%) had laryngeal edema. A unique feature of this study is the use of a rigorous method for verifying laryngeal edema; rigorous methodology might be expected to result in a lower incidence of edema. On the contrary, 57% of the patients requiring reintubation had laryngeal edema, whereas other investigators

report laryngeal edema accounting for 15% or fewer of cases requiring reintubation.

When upper airway obstruction occurs, it typically becomes manifest soon after extubation. Of the 28 patients who developed stridor in the series of Darmon et al,[20] 75% (21/28) developed it within 8 hours of extubation. Of the 8 patients in the series of De Bast et al[22] who developed laryngeal edema, 7 developed it within 12 hours. And of the 13 patients with postextubation stridor in the series of Jaber et al,[18] the average time for its development was 3.2 ± 3.3 hours.

Although laryngeal edema can develop as early as 6 hours after intubation,[22] many, but not all,[19] investigators have noted that the rate of postextubation stridor increases in proportion to the duration of ventilation. Jaber et al[18] observed that duration of intubation was longer in 13 patients with stridor than in 99 patients without stridor: 10.9 versus 5.5 days. Sandhu et al[17] likewise observed a longer duration of intubation in 6 patients who developed postextubation stridor than in 97 patients who did not: 6.5 ± 1.9 versus 2.6 ± 2.6 days. Darmon et al[20] observed that stridor was more common among patients intubated for longer than 36 hours than among patients intubated for a shorter time: 7.2% (25/346) versus 0.9% (3/317).

Women are more susceptible to postextubation stridor than men, and the rate may vary with ethnicity. In a series from France, Darmon et al[20] observed stridor in 7.4% (20/284) of women and 2.1% (8/379) of men. In a series from Taiwan, Ho et al[19] observed stridor in 39% (7/18) of women and 17% (10/59) of men.

Other risk factors associated with the development of laryngeal edema include traumatic intubation, excessive tube size, excessive tube mobility secondary to insufficient fixation, a patient fighting against the tube or trying to speak, excessive pressure in the cuff, too frequent or too aggressive tracheal suctioning, occurrence of infections or hypotension, and the presence of a nasogastric tube that predisposes to gastroesophageal reflux.[22] It is also possible that a biochemical reaction between the tube material and the airway mucosa may cause laryngeal edema.[22] Compared with the 99 patients without stridor, the 13 patients who developed stridor in the series of Jaber et al[18] were more likely to have the following: a traumatic and/or difficult intubation (54% versus 7%), a history of self-extubation (38 versus 4%), a higher balloon cuff pressure (83 versus 40 cmH$_2$O), a higher simplified acute physiology score (SAPS) II score (50 versus 38), and a medical rather than a surgical reason for admission (46 versus 18%).

OTHER CAUSES OF POSTEXTUBATION DISTRESS

Conditions other than upper airway obstruction that cause postextubation distress vary from study to study. In a report on reasons for reintubation, Epstein and Ciubotaru[14] noted upper airway obstruction in 15%; other reasons for reintubation included respiratory failure (28%), congestive heart failure (23%), aspiration or excessive secretions (16%), encephalopathy (9%), and other conditions (8%). The frequency of a particular reason differs among studies. For example, cardiac failure accounted for 23% of the cases of Epstein and Ciubotaru,[14] 6.6% (4/61) of the cases of

Esteban et al,[15] but none of the cases of Smina et al[16] or De Bast et al.[22] Because of the limited rigor of these studies, there is little point in attempting a more detailed analysis of the relative incidence of other causes of reintubation.

PATHOPHYSIOLOGY

None of the studies of reasons for postextubation cardiorespiratory distress can be considered as studies of pathophysiologic mechanisms in the same sense as are studies of the pathophysiology of weaning failure. For studies of postextubation distress, investigators filled out case report forms. These forms constitute post-hoc incident reports completed after some event. In many cases, investigators are making a best guess as to what might explain a patient's deterioration. In contrast, research into the pathophysiology of weaning failure is based on the simultaneous recording of several signals, starting before a weaning trial and continuing until after its completion. In this way, it is possible to understand the relative roles of control of breathing, respiratory muscle activity, derangements of lung and chest wall mechanics, gas exchange, and cardiovascular performance in weaning failure. Conducting similar types of studies to delineate the mechanisms of postextubation cardiorespiratory distress will be challenging.

The first challenge will be instrumentation. The recording of swings in intrathoracic pressure, as reflected by esophageal pressure, is relatively easy. But on its own, esophageal pressure is of limited value. Derivation of most indices, such as airway resistance, compliance, and intrinsic positive end-expiratory pressure (PEEPi), require a simultaneous measurement of airflow. It is extremely difficult to obtain a meaningful measure of airflow or tidal volume in a recently extubated patient.[23] The use of a mouthpiece or facemask causes marked distortion of the breathing pattern. Inductive plethysmography provides a means for overcoming this problem. For example, Tobin et al[24] used this technique to study changes in breathing pattern in 10 patients at the point of extubation. During the first 15 minutes after extubation, both minute ventilation and mean inspiratory flow (a measure of respiratory drive) increased, accompanied by a decrease in the degree of abdominal paradox. By the end of the first hour after extubation, respiratory drive and minute ventilation had returned to preextubation levels. No further change in breathing pattern was observed over the subsequent 24 hours. The investigators did not study any patients who developed postextubation distress. When inductive plethysmography is combined with esophageal pressure recordings, great care is required to ensure that the two signals are perfectly aligned. The smallest misalignment will cause major errors in estimates of PEEPi and other measures of lung mechanics. A requirement not faced by researchers studying the pathophysiology of weaning failure is the need to record the development of laryngeal obstruction. As such, additional research instrumentation includes fiberoptic endoscopy.

Perhaps an even greater challenge than the instrumentation is the timing. Weaning failure almost invariably occurs within the first hour of attempted spontaneous breathing.

TABLE 59-2 Association between Reintubation and Mortality

Reference	Mortality in Reintubated Patients	Mortality in Patients Tolerating Extubation
Daley et al[25]	8% (2/24)	6.5% (224/2516)
Epstein et al[12]	43% (17/40)	9.1% (21/232)
Esteban et al[26]	27.0%	2.6%
Esteban et al[15]	32.8% (20/61)	4.6% (1/392)
Perren et al[80]	33%	3.6%

The time course for the development of postextubation cardiorespiratory distress extends over a longer span. In the study of Epstein and Ciubotaru,[14] for example, only 33% of reintubations occurred within the first 12 hours after extubation, and 42% occurred after 24 hours.

Consequences of Postextubation Distress

Many, but not all,[25] investigators have reported that mortality is many times higher in patients who require reintubation than in patients who tolerate extubation (Table 59-2). Three explanations have been offered to account for the increased mortality: complications associated with the act of reintubation itself; development of a new problem in the interval between extubation and reintubation; and that the need for reintubation is simply serving as a marker for a poor prognosis.

Endotracheal intubation is typically performed under elective and controlled conditions. It is more challenging to perform intubation in a patient developing acute distress in the period after extubation. Complications have been reported to occur at the time of reintubation in 15%,[26] 18%,[15] and 28% of patients.[14] In a study of 40 consecutive patients requiring reintubation (for any reason), Torres et al[27] reported that 47% (19/40) developed nosocomial pneumonia after reintubation as compared with 10% of matched control patients (odds ratio, 5.9). In a study of 297 intubations performed under emergency conditions (in 238 adults), Schwartz et al[28] reported 7 deaths (mortality, 2.4%) at the time of or within 30 minutes after intubation; 5 of the deaths were associated with a systolic blood pressure <90 mmHg. In contrast to the experience of Torres et al[27] only 4% of patients developed a radiographic infiltrate compatible with a new aspiration pneumonia.[28] In a study by Esteban et al,[15] mortality was no greater among the 11 patients who developed complications at the time of reintubation than in the remaining 50 patients (45.4% and 30.0%, respectively; $p = 0.53$). Based on the above considerations, it seems unlikely that the higher mortality in reintubated patients is a direct consequence of complications associated with the act of reintubation itself.

A second explanation is the development of a new problem during the interval between extubation and reintubation. In support of this possibility is the observation of Epstein and Cibotaru[14] that mortality increases in proportion to the time between extubation and reintubation: mortality of 69% in patients reintubated between 49 and

72 hours after extubation (17% of the group), 24% in patients reintubated in the first 12 hours after extubation (33% of the group), and 39% in patients reintubated between 13 and 24 hours after extubation (25% of the group).

The third explanation for higher mortality in reintubated patients is that reintubation is simply serving as a marker for a poor prognosis. Sicker patients are more likely to undergo reintubation. Epstein and Ciubotaru[14] have argued against this explanation. They note that reintubation continues to have a strong independent effect on mortality even after controlling for generalized severity of illness at weaning onset, comorbidity, age, and need for acute dialysis. It is, however, possible that the need for reintubation is measuring some additional aspect of disease severity not captured by the above variables.

Consistent with reports of increased mortality, Epstein et al[12] observed that reintubated patients exhibited other features of adverse outcome when compared with patients who tolerate extubation: longer ICU stay (26 versus 9 days), longer hospital stay (36 versus 20 days), and greater need for transfer to a long-term care facility (38 versus 21%). Reintubated patients were also older (64 versus 55 years), had higher Acute Physiology, Age, and Chronic Health Evaluation (APACHE) II scores at the start of weaning trials (12 versus 10), and were more likely to have a cardiac etiology for their cardiorespiratory failure (43 versus 26%).

Predictors of Postextubation Distress

Because reintubation causes serious complications in some patients, attempts are made to predict its likely occurrence. A number of physiologic variables have been evaluated for their ability to predict this likelihood. For some patients, the likelihood of reintubation is considered so high that a clinician may proceed to tracheotomy without first attempting extubation.

ABILITY TO SUSTAIN SPONTANEOUS VENTILATION

It is extremely uncommon to undertake planned extubation without first assessing a patient's ability to sustain spontaneous ventilation. This assessment typically consists of observing a patient breathing through a T-tube circuit or while assisted by a low level of pressure support (PS) or intermittent mandatory ventilation (IMV). A weaning trial serves primarily as an additional diagnostic test, with the aim of predicting whether a patient will develop distress after extubation and need reintubation. The predictive accuracy of a weaning trial as a diagnostic test has never been evaluated in a rigorous scientific manner.

A true-positive result of a T-tube trial is defined as a patient who tolerates the trial without distress, is then extubated, and does not require reintubation. The usual rate of reintubation is 15–20% (sometimes lower), but higher reintubation rates have been reported by some investigators: 23.5%,[27] 25%,[29] 26.7%,[5] 28.6%,[4] and 29.4%.[3] These false-positive test results mean that the positive predictive value and specificity of passing a T-tube trial in predicting that a

patient will not require reintubation is much less than 100%. To measure the false-negative rate would require extubating patients who fail a T-tube trial, and counting how many do not require reintubation. For obvious ethical reasons, we do not know this number. Given the natural caution of physicians, we can confidently assume that it is higher than 0%. As such, sensitivity and negative predictive value will be less than 100%. It is no surprise that the ability of a T-tube trial to predict reintubation has a sensitivity and specificity of less than 100%; no diagnostic test is perfect. But a weaning trial is not solely used as a diagnostic test for predicting the likelihood of reintubation. The outcome of a weaning trial is also used as a gold standard against which the accuracy of weaning predictor tests are measured.

WEANING PREDICTOR TESTS

Several investigators have investigated the ability of weaning predictor tests to predict the development of distress after extubation. The question posed is along these lines, "Does frequency-to-tidal-volume ratio (f/V_T), or some other predictor test, measured before a T-tube trial, predict the likelihood of reintubation?" To answer this question with scientific validity, it is imperative that the investigators take clearly defined steps to ensure that clinicians are *not* taking the results of the T-tube trial into account when deciding whether to extubate the study patients. (In other words, a decision to extubate the patient must be taken before the T-tube trial, and must proceed even if the patient exhibits significant distress during the trial.) If researchers allow clinicians to use results of a T-tube trial (done after measurement of the weaning predictor test) when deciding whether or not to proceed with extubation, the researchers need a different experimental design because they are asking a different research question. The question is now, "In what instances do weaning predictor tests override the results of a subsequently undertaken T-tube trial?"

Before we discuss the findings of studies on the use of tests to predict the likelihood of postextubation distress, we ask the reader to undertake a simple thought experiment. You, as the patient's clinician, record f/V_T, and obtain a reading of 60. You then proceed to a T-tube trial. If the patient develops severe distress during the trial, would you extubate the patient? (Please exclude circumstances in which you believe that the internal diameter of the endotracheal tube is the main cause of distress.) We believe that most experienced clinicians will answer, "no." Consider another scenario: a resident measures f/V_T in your patient, obtains a value of 120 and proceeds to a T-tube trial. If the patient tolerates the trial without significant distress, would you defer extubation? We believe most experienced clinicians would again answer "no," although they might monitor the postextubation period more closely than if the patient had an f/V_T reading of 90 before the trial.

For both of the preceding scenarios, we believe that few if any experienced clinicians would allow a measurement of f/V_T (made before a T-tube trial) to override a judgment based on how well a patient tolerates a T-tube trial. Given the results of the thought experiments, it makes little sense to undertake research studies of the accuracy of weaning predictor tests (measured before a weaning trial) to forecast a patient's likely need for reintubation (in a patient who passes a weaning trial). It makes even less sense when one considers that a clinician's action based on the patient's performance during the weaning trial will have inevitably muddied the experimental waters. Let us consider a patient in whom a weaning predictor test predicts a high likelihood of respiratory distress. A weaning trial is nevertheless undertaken. The patient develops distress, and so is not extubated. By excluding such patients from a study, the investigators are markedly underestimating the true-negative rate of the test for predicting distress after extubation (where the test predicts distress and the patient actually develops distress).

It is difficult to understand why so many investigators have undertaken this type of research. We suspect they have been seduced by affirmative answers to two subsidiary questions. "Do patients with satisfactory weaning predictors usually tolerate a spontaneous breathing trial?" Yes. "Do patients who tolerate a spontaneous breathing trial usually avoid reintubation?" Yes. It might seem logical to conflate these two issues, and ask, "Do patients with satisfactory weaning predictors usually avoid reintubation?" The only way to address this question in a scientific manner is to measure weaning predictors and extubate the patient without an intervening weaning trial. Zeggwagh et al[30] are the only group of investigators to undertake such a study.

The investigators prospectively studied 101 patients (ventilated for 10.4 ± 10.3 days) at the point that their ICU physicians contemplated weaning. They measured a series of physiologic measurements during 2 minutes of spontaneous breathing; the results of these measurements were not communicated to the primary team. The team then extubated the patients without first undertaking any form of weaning trial. The extubation decision was made by the ICU team, based on the following criteria: improvement or resolution of the condition precipitating the need for mechanical ventilation; good level of consciousness with cessation of all sedative agents; temperature $<38°C$; respiratory frequency <35 breaths per minute; $S_{O_2} >90\%$ on $F_{I O_2} \leq 0.40$; hemodynamic stability; and the absence of electrolyte disorders, acid-base disturbance, or hemoglobin <10 g%.

Reintubation was necessary in 37% of the patients. Several variables predicted the need for reintubation with a reasonable degree of accuracy. For example, f/V_T had sensitivity 0.77 and specificity 0.79, with an area under a receiver operating curve (ROC) curve of 0.81 ± 0.06; maximum expiratory pressure had a sensitivity 0.52 and specificity 0.92, with an area under a ROC curve of 0.73 ± 0.07. The investigators developed a model based on three variables: f/V_T, maximum expiratory pressure, and vital capacity. The area under the ROC curve for the model was 0.91 ± 0.04 for a development data series and 0.86 ± 0.06 for a validation data series.

This study by Zeggwagh et al[30] suggests that undertaking a weaning trial before extubation is useful because their rate of reintubation is about double that reported in studies in which weaning trials precede extubation. The clinicians in the study by Zeggwagh et al[30] based their decision for extubation on only the most rudimentary clinical assessment. If the clinicians had made the decision to extubate using more

sophisticated physiologic predictors (but still did not undertake a weaning trial), it is likely that the rate of reintubation would have been lower. The accuracy of weaning predictors in this study contrasts sharply with their accuracy in studies in which the investigators permitted a weaning trial (which altered clinician's extubation decisions) between measurement of the predictors and extubation (see Table 58-1 in Chapter 58).

CUFF-LEAK TEST

Some patients show satisfactory recovery of lung function but develop upper airway obstruction after extubation. The presence of an endotracheal tube, however, makes it extremely difficult to evaluate the structure and function of the airway before extubation. The amount of air leaking around the outside of an endotracheal tube on deflating the balloon cuff has been used by a number of investigators to predict upper airway obstruction after extubation (Fig. 59-1). The idea was first reported by Adderley and Mullins[31] who studied 31 planned extubations in 28 children with croup. After extubation, reintubation was required in 13% (3/23) of children who had an audible leak (on coughing or when plateau pressure was 40 cmH$_2$O), and reintubation was required in 38% (3/8) of children without a leak. The cuff-leak test has since been evaluated with varying degrees of scientific rigor (Table 59-3).

Miller and Cole[32] undertook the first systematic evaluation of the cuff-leak test. They studied 100 intubations in 88 ventilated patients. During assist-control ventilation, they noted that the set inspired tidal volume (V_T) and displayed expired V_T were always within 20 ml of each other (they did not state the volume setting). To measure the leak, they deflated the cuff and recorded expiratory V_T over the subsequent 6 cycles; they used the average of the three lowest values to calculate the leak. After extubation, 17% of patients

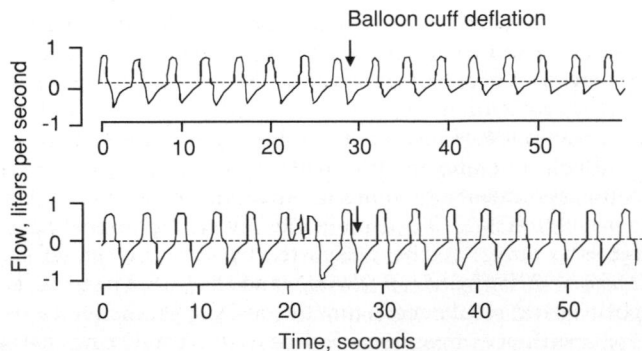

FIGURE 59-1 Tracings of inspiratory flow (*upgoing*) and expiratory flow (*downgoing*) in two patients before and after deflation of the cuff on the endotracheal tube (*arrow*). The patient in the upper panel had a large leak (positive test result): after deflation of the cuff, expiratory flow became substantially smaller than inspiratory flow. The patient in the lower tracing had a small leak (<12% of inspired tidal volume; negative test result): expiratory flow exhibited little if any decrease after cuff deflation. (*Modified, with permission, from Jaber et al.[18]*)

TABLE 59-3   Accuracy of the Cuff-Leak Test

Authors	No[a]	Leak Criterion	Outcome Criterion	Sensitivity	Specificity	PPV	NPV
Adderley et al[31]	31	Audible	Reintubation	0.80	0.50	0.87	0.38
Miller et al[32]	100	<110 ml	Stridor	0.67	0.99	0.80	NR
Engoren[21]	531	<110 ml	Leak <110 ml	0.00	0.96	0.00	1.00
Sandhu et al[17]	110	<10% insp V_T	Stridor or reintubation	NR	0.96	NR	NR
De Bast et al[22]	76	<15.5% insp V_T	Reintubation secondary to laryngeal edema	0.75	0.72	0.25	0.96
Jaber et al[18]	112	<130 ml or <12% insp V_T	Stridor and leak <130 ml or <12% of insp V_T	0.85	0.95	0.69	0.98

[a]Number of extubations.

ABBREVIATIONS: insp, inspiratory; NPV, negative predictive value; NR, not reported; PPV, positive predictive value; V_T, tidal volume.

required reintubation. Of the 6 patients who developed stridor, reintubation was required in 3. The leak (measured during the 24 hours before extubation) was smaller in patients who subsequently developed postextubation stridor than in patients who did not: 180 ± 157 versus 360 ± 157 ml. ROC curve analysis indicated that a leak of <110 ml provided the best threshold for predicting postextubation stridor. A leak of <110 ml had sensitivity 0.67, specificity 0.99, and positive predictive value 0.80 (negative predictive value was not reported).

Engoren[21] studied 531 extubations in 524 cardiac surgery patients using the cuff-leak method of Miller and Cole.[32] Only 3 patients (0.6%) developed postextubation stridor, all of whom had cuff leaks higher than 300 ml; 1 of these patients required reintubation. A leak <110 ml was recorded in 20 patients, and none required reintubation. These data suggest that the cuff-leak test is not helpful in patients who are intubated for a short time. (The average duration of intubation was 12.9 hours in this study, and only 5.1% received mechanical ventilation for >48 hours.)

Sandhu et al[17] measured the cuff leak in 110 trauma patients. To measure cuff leak, they placed the patient on assist-control ventilation (V_T not stated). They measured cuff leak as a percentage: [(Expired V_T with cuff inflated − Expired V_T with cuff deflated)/Expired V_T with cuff inflated] × 100. They obtained six readings with the cuff inflated and six readings with the cuff deflated. The leak was 408 ± 201 ml ($57.2 \pm 23.9\%$) in patients with uneventful extubation. Postextubation stridor developed in 13 patients (11.8%; 13/110), and 6 (5.5%) required reintubation. The leak in these 6 patients was 68 ± 75 ml ($9.2 \pm 9.9\%$); an equivalent leak was found in the 7 patients with stridor who did not require reintubation: 58 ± 74 ml ($8.4 \pm 10.7\%$). A leak of 0 ml was noted in 8 patients: 2 were extubated uneventfully, 2 developed stridor and were reintubated, and 4 others developed stridor. They concluded that a cuff leak of 10% V_T identified stridor or reintubation with a specificity of 0.96, but did not report sensitivity, positive predictive value, or negative predictive value.

Jaber et al[18] evaluated the cuff-leak test in 112 patients. The leak was smaller in 13 patients who developed postextubation stridor than in the 99 patients who did not develop stridor after extubation: 59 ± 92 versus 372 ± 170 ml (with V_T 10–12 ml/kg during assist-control ventilation); expressed in terms of relative volumes, $9 \pm 3\%$ versus $56 \pm 20\%$. Reintubation was required in 69.2% (9/13) of the patients with stridor as compared with 2.0% (2/99) of patients

without stridor. They used ROC curve analysis to find the best threshold; they considered a true-positive test as a leak <130 ml or <12% of inspired V_T and postextubation stridor. At this threshold, sensitivity was 0.85, specificity 0.95, positive predictive value 0.69, and negative predictive value 0.98.

De Bast et al[22] prospectively studied 76 patients who had been intubated ≥12 hours. They measured cuff leak as a percentage: [(Expired V_T with cuff inflated − Expired V_T with cuff deflated)/Expired V_T with cuff inflated] × 100. They took the average of 6 measurements that varied by <30%. The measurements were not available to the staff in charge of patients. If patients developed stridor associated with signs of respiratory distress within 24 hours of extubation and required reintubation, laryngeal edema was confirmed or excluded by fiberoptic examination before the reintubation, or by direct examination of the glottis during reintubation. The investigators excluded patients who were reintubated for reasons other than laryngeal edema.

Within the first 24 hours, 10.5% (8/76) of the patients of De Bast et al[22] required reintubation for laryngeal edema. These patients had smaller leaks than did the other patients: 9% (3, 18; 25th, 75th percentiles) versus 35% (13, 53; 25th, 75th percentiles). (Of the 10 patients who developed postextubation stridor, 8 were reintubated.) ROC curve analysis revealed that the best threshold was a leak of 15.5%. This threshold had a sensitivity 0.75, specificity 0.72, positive predictive value 0.25, and negative predictive value 0.96. The low positive predictive value, 0.25, indicates that 75% of the patients with a leak <15.5% were successfully extubated (without laryngeal edema or requiring reintubation). Thus, a low leak volume should not be used to postpone extubation indefinitely. The negative predictive value of 0.96 means that when patients exhibit a large leak (a negative test result) they are not likely to require reintubation (because of laryngeal edema). A leak >23% excluded all patients who required reintubation because of laryngeal edema.

In summary, the studies of the cuff-leak test are of varying quality. The method for performing the test has not been standardized. In particular, none of the investigators addressed the setting of inspired V_T, which may influence the size of the leak. The method for quantifying the leak varies between absolute units (milliliters) and percentage of inspired V_T. The outcome criterion is not always clearly stated: rate of reintubation for any reason, occurrence of stridor of any severity, or occurrence of stridor that requires reintubation. The rates of stridor vary considerably among studies, suggesting that investigators used different criteria (admittedly, it is not obvious that severity of stridor can be graded in any reproducible manner). Only De Bast et al[22] used an objective method (fiberoptic endoscopy) to verify the presence of laryngeal edema. In some studies, it is not clear whether the investigators carefully excluded reasons for reintubation other than stridor. If a patient is reintubated because of left ventricular failure, it is not logical to expect the cuff-leak test to predict such an event. What is the best gold standard? Should a true-positive test result be restricted to postextubation stridor that requires reintubation? Is it important to predict the development of postextubation stridor that will respond to aerosolized epinephrine? The manner of reporting test performance is not consistent. The thresholds for defining a significant leak vary. All calculations of test performance are inevitably overestimates, because none of the investigators split their data set into training and validation subsets. Admittedly, the latter step would be a challenge because the number of true-positive test results in any study is very low. The rate of reintubation is usually 10–20%, and a much smaller fraction is the result of laryngeal edema.

SECRETIONS AND COUGH

A proportion of patients fail either a weaning attempt or an extubation attempt because of excessive airway secretions. This proportion varies among reports, largely because there is no consistent definition of "excessive secretions" or even how best to quantify secretions. If one quantifies secretions according to the volume obtained by suctioning over a fixed time interval, a patient who coughs and expels secretions without difficulty may get classified as having a greater secretion problem than a patient who has thick viscid secretions that cannot be dislodged from the lower airways.

The act of suctioning per se is associated with a number of serious complications, such as life-threatening hypoxemia, mucosal trauma, hemorrhage, bronchoconstriction, atelectasis, cardiac arrhythmias, and even cardiac arrest.[33–36] Jubran and Tobin[37] investigated the possibility that a sawtooth pattern on the flow-volume curve might provide a noninvasive means of detecting secretions. In 50 intubated patients, the presence of a sawtooth pattern on flow-volume curves recorded during 1 minute of spontaneous breathing was a strong predictor of the presence of secretions (positive predictive value, 94%), and the absence of this pattern suggested that secretions were unlikely to be present (negative predictive value, 77%) (Figs. 59-2 and 59-3). Expressed in terms of likelihood ratios, a sawtooth pattern was about 6–8 times more likely to be found in patients who had secretions than in patients without secretions. Conversely, a smooth flow-volume curve was about one-quarter as likely to be found in patients with secretions as in those without secretions. Clinical examination had much higher false-positive and false-negative rates (42 and 43%, respectively) than the flow-volume curves (12 and 14%, respectively). Accordingly, reliance on clinical examination will lead to unnecessary suctioning in patients without secretions and inadequate suctioning in patients with secretions.

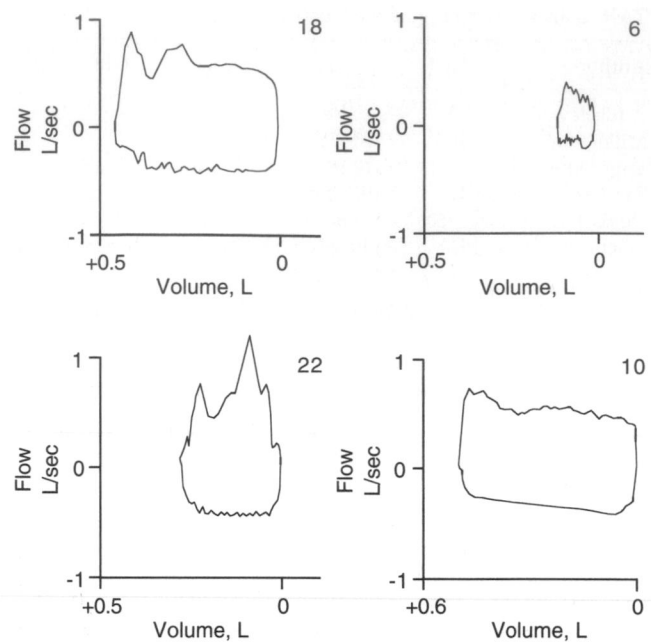

FIGURE 59-2 Flow-volume curves obtained in four patients with secretions. Note the presence of a sawtooth pattern on both the inspiratory and expiratory flow-volume curves. (*Reproduced, with permission, from Jubran and Tobin.*[37])

Guglielminotti et al[38] re-evaluated the usefulness of the sawtooth pattern for detecting secretions in 62 patients who were receiving pressure support or assist-control ventilation. In the earlier study, patients were breathing spontaneously after having been briefly disconnected from the ventilator. Two investigators independently inspected

FIGURE 59-3 Flow-volume curves obtained in four patients without secretions. Note the smooth contour of the curves. (*Reproduced, with permission, from Jubran and Tobin.*[37])

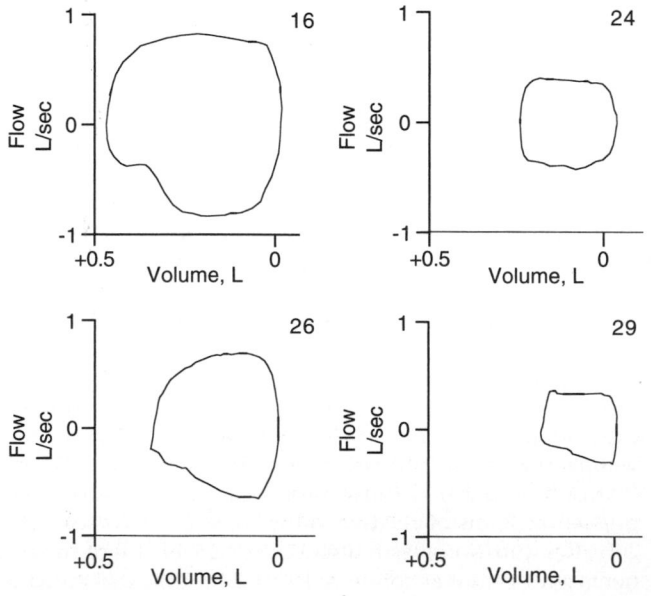

flow-volume loops on the ventilator monitor screen in real time. A sawtooth pattern was observed in 32 of 39 patients (82%) classified as having increased secretions (>0.5 ml found on a second suctioning after the passage of 2 hours; mean volume 2.6 ml) as compared with 8 of 27 patients (30%) classified as having little or no secretions (0.1 ml over 2 hours). In addition, the investigators listened over the trachea. The combination of a sawtooth pattern plus respiratory sounds was found in 58.9% of patients with secretions and in 3.7% of patients with few secretions; the positive likelihood ratio was 14.7, and the negative likelihood ratio was 0.42.

Investigators have recently evaluated measurements of secretions as predictors of postextubation distress. Khamiees et al[39] attempted to quantify cough strength by placing a white card at 1–2 cm from the end of the endotracheal tube and requesting the patient to cough as many as three to four times just before extubation. Any wetness on the card was classified as a positive test (assessment was made by a single observer). This test was seen as a test of cough strength and not of the amount of secretions present. They studied 100 extubations in 91 patients; 18 patients were classified as extubation failures and 11 were reintubated within 72 hours of extubation (the criteria for classifying the other 7 patients as extubation failures are not clear). Extubation failure was three times more likely in patients with a negative white-card test (no secretions coughed onto the card). Three other measures also predicted extubation failure. Extubation failure was four times more likely among patients who had a weak or absent cough than in patients with a moderate or strong cough. Extubation failure was 8 times more likely in patients classified as having moderate or abundant secretions by the nursing staff in the 4–6 hours preceding extubation than in patients with absent or mild secretions. Extubation failure was 16 times more likely among patients whose secretions required suctioning every 2 hours or less.

Smina et al[16] of the same research group studied the ability to predict reintubation after 115 extubations in 95 patients (on this occasion, the investigators specify that extubation failure was synonymous with reintubation). Reintubation within 72 hours was required in 11.3%. The magnitude of secretions was not associated with extubation failure, which contrasts with their previous report that extubation failure was increased 16 times if patients required frequent suctioning. This failure to reproduce an earlier observation illustrates a common problem with all studies of clinical predictors. After the report of findings of an initial study, physicians modify their approach to a particular problem; in statistical terminology, clinicians change their pretest probability (based on the report). When a research team reinvestigates the same phenomenon in a new group of patients, they fail to reproduce the original finding. Many patients in the second study who had secretions were not advanced to extubation, leading to a decrease in the number of true-positive test results. The study of Khamiees et al[39] indicated that frequent suctioning was associated with a high reintubation rate. Smina et al,[16] however, found that only 4% of patients in their follow-up study had >20 ml of secretions per hour before extubation. Clearly, physicians

in the second study had reduced the number of extubations attempted in patients with larger volumes of secretions. The physicians had altered their pretest probability of extubation failure based on the need for frequent suctioning. The physicians refused to advance such patients to extubation (test-referral bias), and thus, the results of the study give an erroneous impression that frequent suctioning is not a good predictor of reintubation.

In this study, Smina et al[16] found that a measure of cough strength predicted likelihood of reintubation. Cough peak expiratory flow (the best of three voluntary attempts) was lower in reintubated patients than in successfully extubated patients: 64 ± 7 versus 82 ± 3 L/minute. ROC curve analysis revealed that a cough flow of <60 L/minute provided the best discrimination: patients with flows below this threshold were 5 times more likely to require reintubation (and 19 times more likely to die). f/V_T also predicted extubation failure: values >100 were 4.1 times more likely to require reintubation.

Salam et al[40] of the same investigation group undertook a further study of predictors of reintubation in 88 patients who underwent 100 extubations (extubation failure was defined as reintubation). Reintubation within 72 hours was required in 15.9% (14/88) of the patients. As in the study by Smina et al,[16] cough peak flow was lower in reintubated patients than in patients successfully extubated: 58.1 ± 4.6 (SE) versus 79.7 ± 4.1 L/minute. A threshold peak flow of ≤ 60 L/minute had a sensitivity 0.77, specificity 0.66, likelihood ratio 2.3, and risk ratio 4.8. The investigators also re-evaluated the white-card test described by Khamiees et al,[39] and found that it did not predict reintubation. (A limitation of the white-card test is that it will be negative in patients with a strong cough who have little or no secretions.) The volume of secretions collected in the 2–3 hours before extubation was equivalent in reintubated and successfully extubated patients: 2.5 ± 0.9 versus 2.3 ± 0.4 ml/hour. A threshold of > 2.5 ml secretions per hour, however, did discriminate between the groups: sensitivity 0.71, specificity 0.62, likelihood ratio 1.9, and risk ratio 3.0.

In a group of 136 ventilated patients with brain injury, Coplin et al[41] found that two measures on an airway care score were associated with successful extubation: spontaneous cough and frequency of suctioning. Vallverdu et al[42] proposed maximum expiratory pressure as an index of cough strength and the ability to clear secretions. Maximum expiratory pressure was lower in 92 patients who failed a weaning trial or required reintubation than in 125 successfully extubated patients: 37 ± 17 versus 53 ± 25 (SD) cmH$_2$O. The investigators did not specify a threshold value nor report on the accuracy of maximum expiratory pressure for predicting reintubation.

NEUROLOGIC ASSESSMENT

Some ventilated patients demonstrate good respiratory function and tolerate a T-tube trial without distress, yet their physicians are reluctant to extubate them because they fear that the patients will not be able to protect their airway after extubation. Although widely used, the term "protecting the airway" is rarely clearly defined. We take it to mean that a patient has unsatisfactory neural control over the airway, such that the tongue (of a recumbent patient) may fall back and occlude the airway lumen (as happens in patients with sleep apnea), or the patient has impaired laryngeal (and other upper airway) reflexes, placing him or her at risk of aspiration of secretions (from the mouth and airways) or ingested food.

Concern about protecting the airway most often arises in a patient with evidence of brain injury. Three groups of investigators have studied the role of brain function in patients being considered for extubation. The most rigorous study is that by Coplin et al,[41] who studied 136 brain-injury patients. They evaluated patients for extubation using a broad screen: absence of neurologic deterioration on physical examination; intracranial pressure <20 mm Hg; satisfactory oxygenation, lung mechanics, f/V_T, blood pressure, and heart rate; and absence of a specific indication for mechanical ventilation (such as surgery planned within the subsequent 72 hours).

Of the 136 patients, 72.8% (99/136) were extubated within 48 hours of meeting the above readiness criteria; the remaining 27.2% (37/136) remained intubated for a median of 3 days (range, 2–19 days). They defined a delay in extubation as the time from meeting readiness criteria to the time of extubation, but subtracted 48 hours (to allow for time needed for communication among caregivers). Neurologic evaluation based on the Glasgow Coma Scale (GCS) score was performed daily. (This scale ranges from 3 to 15, with 15 indicating the best brain function and 5 indicating severe brain dysfunction; a score ≥13 indicates *possible* mild brain injury, 9–12 moderate injury, and ≤8 severe brain injury.)

Sixty patients were judged comatose (score ≤8 on the GCS) on the day of meeting extubation readiness criteria; extubation was delayed in 48.3% (29/60) as compared with 10.5% (8/76) of patients not classified as comatose. The two groups, however, exhibited considerable overlap. Of 60 comatose patients (score ≤8), 51.7% (31/60) were extubated without delay. Indeed, among patients with more severe brain injury, with GCS scores of 4 and lower, 40% (4/10) were extubated without delay. Conversely, 10.5% (8/76) of patients with scores ≥9 experienced delayed extubation. Coplin et al[41] assessed whether the decision to extubate was influenced by change in neurologic status over time: 57% (21/37) of patients improved between the day of meeting the readiness criteria and extubation, but the remaining 43% showed no change or deterioration in neurologic function.

Absence of a gag reflex has been considered a contraindication to extubation in the past. About 20% of healthy people, however, do not have a gag reflex, and aspiration pneumonia may still occur in people who do.[43] The importance of the gag reflex in the extubation period was addressed by Coplin et al:[41] 89% (32/36) of patients with a weak or absent gag reflex were successfully extubated.

One of the major reasons to postpone extubation in a neurologically impaired patient is the fear of aspiration pneumonia. The occurrence of pneumonia, however, was higher in patients experiencing delayed extubation: 38 versus 21%. These patients also had longer stays in the ICU (8.6 versus 3.8 days) and in hospital (19.9 versus 13.2 days). Based on their data, Coplin et al[41] concluded that a depressed level of

consciousness should never be used as the sole indication for prolonged intubation.

In contrast to Coplin et al[41], Namen et al[13] concluded that the Glasgow Coma Scale helps in predicting successful extubation. They studied 100 brain-injury patients, whose mechanical ventilation was managed by neurosurgeons. On ROC curve analysis, a score of ≥8 on the GCS provided the best discrimination of extubation outcome. Extubation was successful in 36% (14/38) of patients with GCS scores ≤7 as compared with 75% (60/80) of patients with a score ≥8. The area under the ROC curve for GCS score, however, was only 0.681. A more fundamental problem with this study is that half of the extubations were part of the withdrawal of life-support therapy (all these patients died). Because these patients were not reintubated, it appears that the authors classified them as extubation successes. Irrespective of how these 22 patients were classified, it is impossible to interpret data on extubation predictors where half of the extubations arose from a decision to withdraw life support.

The studies of Coplin et al and Namen et al were conducted in patients with brain injury, whereas Salam et al[40] studied neurologic function as a predictor of reintubation in 88 medical-cardiac ICU patients who underwent 100 extubations. Neurologic performance was quantified by requesting patients to perform four simple tasks:[44] to open their eyes, to follow an observer with their eyes, to grasp the observer's hand, and stick out their tongue. Reintubation within 72 hours was required in 15.9% (14/88) of the patients. Patients tolerating extubation performed a higher number of tasks than did the reintubated patients: 3.8 ± 0.1 versus 2.9 ± 0.5. Patients who were unable to complete all 4 tasks were 4.3 times more likely to require reintubation than were patients who could complete all 4 tasks. The failure to perform any of the 4 tasks had a sensitivity of 0.42 and specificity of 0.91 in predicting reintubation.

RESPIRATORY DRIVE IN THE POSTEXTUBATION PERIOD

Capdevila et al[45] reported that the measurement of airway occlusion pressure ($P_{0.1}$), an index of respiratory drive, after patients breathed through a T-tube circuit for 20 minutes was accurate in predicting the need for reintubation. The 12 patients who required reintubation had higher readings of $P_{0.1}$ than did the 55 successfully extubated patients: 7.38 ± 2.67 versus 3.62 ± 1.35 cmH$_2$O. A threshold $P_{0.1}$ value of 5 cmH$_2$O had a sensitivity of 0.87 and a specificity of 0.91. Fernandez et al[46] also investigated the ability of $P_{0.1}$ to predict the need for reintubation. Measurements were made before and during a 30-minute weaning trial with pressure support of 7 cmH$_2$O. The 21 patients who required reintubation had higher readings of $P_{0.1}$ than did the 93 successfully extubated patients: 3.0 (2.2, 4.0; 25th, 75th percentiles) versus 2.6 (2.0, 3.8; 25th, 75th percentiles) cmH$_2$O. A threshold $P_{0.1}$ value of 2.8 cmH$_2$O had a sensitivity of 0.52 and a specificity of 0.67.

Hilbert et al[47] took a different approach and focused on measurement of $P_{0.1}$ after extubation. They first measured $P_{0.1}$ before extubating 40 patients with chronic obstructive pulmonary disease (COPD). All patients (irrespective of how well they tolerated extubation) then received NIV (pressure support of 4 cmH_2O) by full facemask to enable measurement of $P_{0.1}$. Of the 40 patients, 13 (32%) developed postextubation respiratory distress (30 breaths/min, P_{CO_2} 74 ± 6 mmHg, pH 7.32 ± 0.04) at 16 ± 14 (SD) hours. These patients were treated with NIV, and 3 (7.5%; 3/40) required reintubation. The patients who developed postextubation distress exhibited an increase in $P_{0.1}$ from before extubation, 2.9 ± 0.7 cmH_2O, to 4.2 ± 0.9 cmH_2O at 30 minutes after extubation. In the 27 patients who did not develop distress, $P_{0.1}$ was 2.4 ± 0.9 cmH_2O before extubation and 1.8 ± 0.8 cmH_2O at 30 minutes after extubation. The investigators did not state whether $P_{0.1}$ discriminated between the 3 reintubated patients and the other 10 with postextubation distress. These findings are interesting from a pathophysiologic viewpoint, but it is doubtful that physicians would be willing to initiate NIV in all extubated patients for the purpose of measuring $P_{0.1}$.

Treatment of Postextubation Laryngeal Edema

Trials of therapies for postextubation respiratory distress have largely been confined to patients with laryngeal edema. For decades, patients with postextubation stridor and other upper airway disorders have been treated with aerosolized racemic epinephrine. Racemic epinephrine consists of equal amounts of the dextro (d)- and levo (l)-isomers. Most of epinephrine's pharmacologic action results from the levo-isomer, which is 30 times more potent than the dextro-isomer.[48] Popularity of the more expensive racemic form is based on the supposition that it produces epinephrine's vasoconstrictor action without rebound vasodilation; thus, less tachycardia, hypertension, and tremor is expected with aerosolized racemic epinephrine than with levo-epinephrine. The stated different actions, however, may have arisen from comparisons of inappropriate dosages.

Nutman et al[49] randomized 28 children with postextubation stridor (average age, 1 year) to receive 0.25 ml of either 2.25% racemic epinephrine or 1% levo-epinephrine, each diluted with 2 ml of isotonic saline. These dosages were selected to reflect the relative potency of the two compounds. Each was delivered over 15 minutes by facemask. Both groups exhibited significant improvement: 71.4% (10/14) of the levo-epinephrine group and 76.9% (10/13) of the racemic group exhibited decreases of 2 points on an 8-point stridor score after 40 minutes. By 8 hours, the stridor score was less than 1 in both groups. These data reveal that levo-epinephrine is as effective as the more expensive racemic epinephrine in children with postextubation stridor, although it is not known how likely the stridor would have resolved without any aerosolized therapy.

The ability of dexamethasone to prevent postextubation stridor in children has been evaluated by two groups of investigators. In both studies, dexamethasone (0.5 mg/kg every 6 hours for 6 doses, beginning 6–12 hours before extubation) was compared against placebo. In their study of 153

children, ranging from under 1 to older than 5 years, Tellez et al[50] observed postextubation stridor requiring therapy in 21.1% (16/76) of the dexamethasone group and 29.9% (23/77) of the control group. Reintubation was required in 11.8% (9/76) of the dexamethasone group and 5.2% (4/77) of the control group. In a study of 66 children under 5 years old, Anene et al[51] observed stridor at 10 minutes in 45.2% (14/31) of the dexamethasone group and 87.5% (28/32) of the control group. Epinephrine aerosol was required in 12.9% (4/31) of the dexamethasone group and 68.8% (22/32) of the control group. Reintubation was required in 0/31 of the dexamethasone group and 21.9% (7/32) of the control group. Apart from the different conclusions on the benefit of dexamethasone, the different outcomes in the two control groups is striking: postextubation stridor requiring therapy was reported in 68.8% of the patients of Anene et al[51] as contrasted with 29.9% of the patients of Tellez et al;[50] the respective rates for reintubation were 21.9% and 5.2%.

Two groups of investigators concluded that administration of glucocorticoids before extubation is of no value in adult patients. Darmon et al[20] randomized 663 patients to a bolus of dexamethasone 8 mg or placebo 1 hour before extubation. The overall incidence of laryngeal edema was 4.2% (28/663), and reintubation was necessary in 1% (7/663). No difference was seen between patients receiving dexamethasone or placebo. Ho et al[19] randomized 77 intubated patients to hydrocortisone 100 mg or placebo, given 60 minutes before extubation. Overall, 22% (17/77) developed stridor within 24 hours, and only 1 patient required reintubation. Outcomes were equivalent for patients receiving hydrocortisone and placebo.

Intervention to Reduce Need for Reintubation

Pronovost et al[52] investigated the effect of a new quality improvement intervention on the frequency of reintubation in their surgical ICU. Their study was undertaken in three phases. In the first phase, they identified risk factors associated with reintubation. In the second phase, ten ICU physicians engaged in a Delphi process, attempting to develop clinical practice guidelines. The physicians could not agree on priorities; they concluded that there were too many conditional probabilities that would require the use of so many decisional nodes, as to render a guideline impractical. This group used data collected in the first phase to develop a pre-extubation worksheet designed to highlight factors associated with reintubation. In discussion with a patient's nurse and respiratory therapist, physicians listed several variables on this form. Variables included: whether intubation had been difficult, ventilator settings, O_2 saturation, arterial blood gas results, f/V_T, frequency of suctioning, and mental status. In the third phase of the study, they studied the effect of implementing the pre-extubation worksheet on physician behavior. Staff was instructed not to extubate a patient if the worksheet had not been filled out.

The rate of reintubation before the quality improvement intervention was 8 per 1000 ventilator days. After the

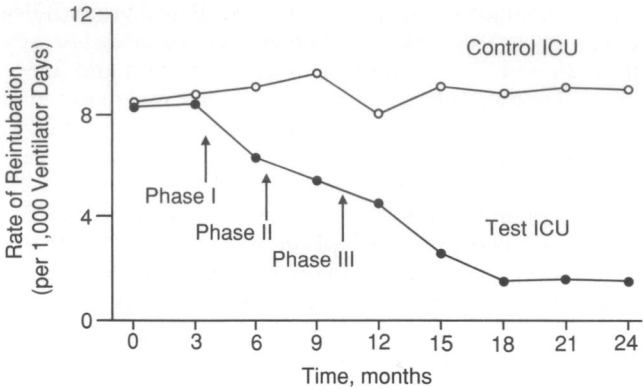

FIGURE 59-4 The rate of reintubation per 1000 ventilator days in a surgical ICU that introduced a new quality improvement intervention and in a control surgical ICU. The intervention was introduced in three phases in the study ICU. The intervention led to a decrease in the rate of reintubation from 8 to 1.5 per 1000 ventilator days. The rate of reintubation did not change in the control ICU. (*Reproduced, with permission, from Pronovost et al.[52]*)

intervention, reintubation decreased to 1.5 per 1000 ventilator days. In another (control) surgical ICU in the same hospital, the rate of reintubation did not change over the same period (Fig. 59-4). The average duration of mechanical ventilation decreased from 4.6 days in the first phase of the study to 3.4 days in the third phase. Three factors were associated with reintubation: suctioning more often than every 4 hours (odds ratio, 11.3); being agitated or sedated versus alert (odds ratio, 4.5); and S_{O_2} <95% on $F_{I_{O_2}}$ 0.40 (odds ratio, 4.0). The accuracy of these and other variables is clearly influenced by test-referral bias. The authors speculate that the pre-extubation worksheet helped to bring directly to the staff's attention the most important factors to consider when deciding to extubate.

Noninvasive Ventilation in Weaning and Extubation

Not long after NIV was shown to be effective in the management of patients in acute respiratory failure, investigators wondered whether NIV could be used to make discontinuation of mechanical ventilation more expeditious and effective. For this subject, we again need to discriminate between weaning and extubation. Is NIV being used as an aid to weaning? Or is NIV being used to prevent or treat respiratory distress in extubated patients? The situations are quite different, yet they are commonly discussed in the same breath. If we think NIV could serve as a weaning aid, this means employing NIV in a patient who is believed to be not quite ready for extubation. If we think NIV could play a role in the management of postextubation distress, we are no longer talking about weaning. And if we are talking about NIV in the postextubation period, we need to discriminate between its role for preventing versus treating respiratory

distress. Six randomized trials have been conducted in this area, dealing with different aspects of the above three issues.

Three trials deal with NIV as a weaning aid. The first trial was conducted by Nava et al.[53] They studied patients with COPD who had severe respiratory acidosis on admission to hospital: P_{CO_2} 94 ± 24 mmHg, pH 7.18 ± 0.06. All patients received assist-control ventilation for the first 12 hours, and then pressure support 21 ± 2 cmH$_2$O for an additional 24–36 hours. All patients then underwent a T-tube trial. Patients who failed this trial were randomized to either extubation immediately followed by NIV or a conventional arm. NIV was delivered by full facemask using pressure support (19 ± 2 cmH$_2$O). It was in place for 20–22 hours a day during the first 48 hours. NIV was weaned by decreasing pressure support by 2–4 cmH$_2$O per day, and at least 2 trials of spontaneous breathing (presumably off NIV) of gradually increasing duration were attempted each day. In the conventional arm, management consisted of the initial reinstitution of mechanical ventilation; weaning was then carried out by a gradual decrease in pressure support followed by intermittent T-tube trials or continuous positive airway pressure (CPAP) trials (of gradually increasing duration) at least twice daily.

Survival at 60 days was higher in the NIV group than in the conventional group: 92 versus 72%. Other features of improved outcome in the NIV group included a higher rate of weaning success at 60 days, 88% (22/25) versus 68% (17/25), a lower rate of nosocomial pneumonia, 0 versus 28% (7/25), fewer days of mechanical ventilation, 10.2 ± 6.8 versus 16.6 ± 11.8 days, and shorter ICU stay, 15 ± 5 versus 24 ± 7 days.

Girault et al[54] also investigated the usefulness of NIV as a weaning aid. Unlike the study of Nava et al,[53] only 51.5% of the 33 patients had COPD. All patients were initially managed by conventional mechanical ventilation. When deemed ready for weaning, all patients underwent a 2-hour T-tube trial. Of the 33 patients failing the T-tube trial, 17 were randomly assigned to extubation followed by NIV and 16 were returned to mechanical ventilation for further conventional weaning. The only difference in outcome was a decrease in the total duration of conventional mechanical ventilation: 4.6 ± 1.9 versus 7.7 ± 3.8 days.

The third randomized trial of the usefulness of NIV as a weaning aid was conducted by Ferrer et al.[55] They enrolled 43 patients who had failed T-tube trials (once daily) for three consecutive days; 44.2% (19/43) had COPD. Twenty-one patients were assigned to extubation followed by immediate NIV (inspiratory positive airway pressure [IPAP], 10 to 20 cmH$_2$O, and expiratory positive airway pressure [EPAP] 4 to 5 cmH$_2$O) and 22 patients were reconnected to the ventilator and underwent conventional weaning (daily T-tube trials). An interim analysis after half the planned number of patients had been studied revealed a superior outcome in the NIV arm, and the study was stopped. Features of the better outcome in the NIV group (versus conventional weaning) included a higher ICU survival, 19.9% versus 13.6%; shorter duration of invasive ventilation, 9.5 versus 20.1 days; shorter ICU stay, 14.1 versus 25.0 days; shorter hospital stay, 27.8 versus 40.8 days; less frequent tracheotomy, 1.5 versus 13.6%; lower incidence of nosocomial pneumonia, 5.2 versus 13.6%; and lower incidence of septic shock, 2.1 versus 9.4%.

The three preceding studies demonstrated that NIV is beneficial if instituted at the point when patients have just failed their first[53,54] or third T-tube trial.[55] In contrast, two groups of investigators have reported that NIV is not beneficial if instituted at a point after patients developed respiratory failure in the 48 hours after extubation. Keenan et al[56] studied patients who had received >48 hours of mechanical ventilation (overall, 4–5 days). All study patients were extubated, and then followed for 48 hours. Of 358 eligible patients, 22.6% (81/358) developed at least one of four criteria of respiratory distress: respiratory frequency >30 breaths/minute, increase in respiratory frequency by >50%, use of accessory muscles, or abdominal paradox. Of the patients with distress, 42 were randomly assigned to standard therapy (supplemental O_2 to maintain $S_{O_2} \geq 95\%$), and 39 to NIV. NIV was delivered by full facemask and only in the ICU. NIV was started with IPAP 9 cmH_2O and EPAP 4 cmH_2O; EPAP was titrated in increments of 2 cmH_2O to achieve $S_{O_2} > 92\%$; IPAP was titrated in increments of 2 cmH_2O according to respiratory frequency and V_T. The goal was to apply NIV continually for first 12 hours, and then intermittently to achieve a satisfactory S_{O_2} and pH >7.35.

The rate of reintubation was equivalent for the two groups: 72% (28/39) for NIV and 69% (29/42) for usual care, as was hospital mortality (31% for both groups). The duration of conventional mechanical ventilation tended to be shorter with NIV: 8.4 ± 7.4 versus 17.5 ± 28.0 days ($p = 0.11$). After the first year of the study, the investigators judged it unethical to withhold NIV in patients with COPD, because of published data indicating the superior performance of patients with COPD with NIV. Thus, only 11.1% (9/81) of the study population had COPD.

Like Keenan et al,[56] Esteban et al[6] also investigated the value of instituting NIV in patients after they have developed postextubation distress. For 48 hours after extubation, patients were observed for the development of respiratory failure defined as at least two of the following: respiratory frequency >25 breaths/minute for 2 consecutive hours; S_{O_2} <90% or P_{O_2} <80 mmHg with $F_{I_{O_2}}$ >0.50; pH <7.35 with P_{CO_2} >45 mmHg; and clinical signs of increased respiratory effort or respiratory muscle fatigue, which included use of accessory muscles, intercostal retraction, or paradoxical motion of the abdomen. (Incidentally, it has been recognized for many years that these signs are neither sensitive nor specific for respiratory muscle fatigue.[57,58]) Of 980 extubated patients, 24.9% (244/980) met the above criteria for respiratory failure. Urgent reintubation was necessary in 23 patients. Of the remaining patients, 114 were randomly assigned to NIV and 107 to usual care. (The time between extubation and randomization was 9 (3, 21) hours.)

NIV was delivered by full facemask in the ICU, using pressure support (the level was not reported) to achieve a V_T >5 ml/kg, frequency <25 breaths/minute, and S_{O_2} >90%; the settings were later adjusted to achieve comfort, adequate S_{O_2}, and pH >7.35. Patients were encouraged to use NIV continuously for 4-hour periods. Mortality in the ICU was higher with NIV, 25% (28/114), than with usual care, 14% (15/107). Reintubation was required in 48.2% (55/114) of

patients in the NIV group, and in 47.7% (51/107) of patients in the usual care group. The difference in mortality was most evident among reintubated patients: 38% (21/55) of the NIV group and 22% (11/51) of the usual care group died ($p = 0.06$). The interval between extubation and reintubation was longer in the NIV group than in the usual care group: 12 versus 2.5 hours ($p = 0.02$).

An important aspect of this study concerns the patients who were randomized to the usual care arm. When these patients developed distress and satisfied criteria for intubation, physicians had a choice to either reintubate them or manage them with NIV. Among the 28 patients who were crossed over to NIV, mortality was 11%. These 28 patients represent a sicker subgroup of the 107 patients in the usual care group, yet they had the lowest mortality of all groups requiring ventilator support. Of all patients receiving NIV in the study, these 28 patients were the only ones in whom it was instituted based on a physician's clinical judgment. Thus, it is possible that instituting NIV based on clinical judgment as opposed to a random allocation at the point of first observing respiratory distress has a major influence on the success of NIV.

Keenan et al[56] excluded patients with COPD after 1 year because of ethical concerns; this consideration was not mentioned in the report of Esteban et al.[6] Yet, the fraction of patients with COPD in that study, 10.4% (23/221), was no higher than that in the study of Keenan et al, 11.1% (9/81). The relatively low number of patients with COPD in both studies may have been a major factor in the failure to demonstrate a benefit with NIV. In the study of Esteban et al, the average time between the institution of NIV (for postextubation distress) and reintubation was 12 hours. A substantial proportion of these patients had a decrease in S_{O_2} to less than 85%. It is perhaps not surprising that patients with significant respiratory failure of this magnitude over a prolonged period would experience a higher mortality after reintubation. Although the role of NIV in the management of postextubation distress in patients with COPD is not resolved by these studies, NIV does not appear to have a role in the treatment of other causes of postextubation distress.

A striking feature of the two negative studies is the limited inspiratory assistance that was provided. Patients received IPAP and EPAP settings of 9 and 4 cmH_2O, respectively, in the study of Keenan et al,[56] which is equivalent to pressure support of 5 cmH_2O. Delivered V_T was as little as 5 ml/kg in the study of Esteban et al[6]—a V_T setting too low for most patients in acute respiratory failure, with the possible exception of patients with acute respiratory distress syndrome (ARDS). The low assistance setting in these two negative studies contrasts with a pressure support setting of 19 ± 2 cmH_2O in the study of Nava et al[53] and the IPAP and EPAP settings of 10 to 20 cmH_2O and 4 to 5 cmH_2O, respectively, in the study of Ferrer et al.[55] Application of a facemask connected to an inadequate level of positive pressure may pose an impediment for patients, and may have contributed to the negative outcomes in these two studies.[6,56]

The only study that has addressed the role of NIV in the prevention of postextubation distress was conducted by Jiang et al.[59] They instituted NIV (initially at IPAP 12 cmH_2O and EPAP 5 cmH_2O) immediately (apparently) after

TABLE 59-4 Frequency of Unplanned Extubation and Subtypes

Author	Total[a] Number[a]	UNPLANNED EXTUBATION		SELF-EXTUBATION		ACCIDENTAL EXTUBATION	
		Percent of Total	Reintubation (%)	Percent of Total	Reintubation (%)	Percent of Total	Reintubation (%)
Zwillich et al[81]	354	8.5	47	30	47		
Stauffer et al[82]	226	12.8	NR				
Whelan et al[83]	319	7.2	78.2	91.3		8.7	
Tindol et al[84]	460	2.8	46.2	92.3		7.7	
Listello et al[85]	NR	NR	48.2				
Tominaga et al[66]		15.2	NR				
Boulain[86]	426	10.8	60.9				
Betbese et al[63]	750	7.3		78			
Chevron et al[87]	414	16	37.0	87			
Jiang et al[59]	97	42	37.8				
Kapadia et al[88]	5046	0.7					
Epstein et al[65]	682	11	56.0	94.7		5.3	
De Lassence et al[8]	750	8	76.7	63.3	63	36.7	100
Esteban et al[89]	5183	3.4	41.3				
Moons et al[61]	627	26	4.2	76.9	45	23.1	100

[a]Total number of ventilated or intubated patients.
ABBREVIATION: NR, not reported.

extubation. Reintubation was required in 13 of the 47 patients (27.7%) randomly assigned to NIV and in 7 of the 46 (15.2%) of patients assigned to usual care. The major problem with this study is that only 52 of the study patients were electively extubated after weaning; the other 37 (39.8%) patients were enrolled after unplanned extubation. Patients who experience unplanned extubation have a substantially higher rate of reintubation than electively extubated patients, yet the investigators did not state whether these patients were evenly distributed between the two arms of the study. They also do not state how many of their patients had COPD.

In summary, three studies have shown that the institution of NIV in certain patients (in particular those with COPD) may expedite the weaning process. In contrast, two studies suggest that NIV is not beneficial in postextubated patients when instituted after they already have clinical manifestations of respiratory distress. It is possible, however, that NIV is beneficial in the subgroup with COPD. In the two negative studies, it is possible that an inadequate level of positive pressure was supplied to properly test its usefulness in postextubated patients. One can also argue that NIV was unlikely to be beneficial when instituted at such a late stage. An attempt has been made to address the question of whether NIV can prevent the development of postextubation distress,[59] but it is not possible to form any conclusion because of the limitations of the study.

Unplanned Extubation

The topic of unplanned extubation is discussed in Chapter 39. The subject is of particular importance for research on weaning because of the insight it may offer into unnecessary delays in the discontinuation of ventilation. The reported frequency of unplanned extubation ranges from less than 1% to 42% of intubated patients; a frequency of 8–12% is most commonly reported (Table 59-4). Unplanned extubation is divided into two major subsets. Self-extubation refers to the deliberate removal of an endotracheal tube by a patient for whom the physician considers intubation beneficial. Accidental extubation refers to inadvertent extubation by a caregiver during a bedside procedure. Both of these situations differ from the usual planned extubation. Between 63 and 95% of unplanned extubations are self-extubations.

The rate of reintubation after unplanned extubation ranges from 15–78%, with many investigators reporting rates of 35–60%. These rates are considerably higher than reintubation rates of 10–20% after planned extubation. The rate of reintubation after accidental extubation is especially high, 83%[60] to 100%.[8,61] That 40% or more of self-extubated patients do not require reintubation is often used as evidence that physicians delay extubation unnecessarily. Extubation is undoubtedly delayed in some patients, but the two groups of patients may not be strictly comparable. Patients who have enough strength—and wit—to self-extubate may be less sick than the average ventilated patient, and thus would be expected to experience a lower reintubation rate. Moreover, it is totally unclear as to what the source of the delay is in these self-extubated patients. Is it caused by clinicians who are not aware of a patient's readiness for extubation because they have yet to measure weaning predictor tests? Is it because the predictor test readings represent false-negative results? Is it because the physician interprets the predictor test results incorrectly? Is it because the physician delays in ordering a weaning trial?[62] Is it because the physician delays extubating a patient who has passed a weaning trial?[62] The recent data of Ely et al[62,13] would suggest that the most likely source of delay is in ordering a weaning trial and extubating a patient who has passed the trial.

The rate of reintubation after unplanned extubation is lower in patients who have already entered the phase of weaning than in patients who are still receiving full ventilator support. Betbese et al[63] reported that 16% of 32 patients who experienced unplanned extubation during weaning required reintubation, as contrasted with 82% of 27 patients who experienced unplanned extubation while receiving full ventilator support. Razek et al[64] reported reintubation after unplanned extubation in 15.2% of 33 weaning patients and 60.7% of 28 patients requiring full ventilator support. And Epstein et al[65] reported reintubation after unplanned extubation in 30% of 33 weaning patients and 76% of 42 patients requiring full ventilator support. Epstein et al[65] noted that patients who tolerated unplanned extubation tended to have shorter time from the onset of weaning to extubation than did a control group, 0.9 versus 2.0 days ($p = 0.06$), although the overall duration of mechanical ventilation did not differ.

Moons et al[61] found that most unplanned extubations occurred on the same day that extubation had been planned (42.9%), or the subsequent (42.9%) or preceding day (14.3%). Compared to a control group of 48 patients that did not experience unplanned extubation, a study group of 26 patients experiencing unplanned extubation had a lower Ramsey Sedation Scale score, 2 (1, 5; 25th, 75th percentiles) versus 5 (3.3, 6; 25th, 75th percentiles), and a higher Glasgow Coma Scale score, 12 (8, 13; 25th, 75th percentiles) versus 4 (3, 7; 25th, 75th percentiles). The difference between the two groups was confined to the subgroup experiencing deliberate self-extubation; patients experiencing accidental extubation were comparable to the control group. In a multiple logistic regression analysis, deliberate self-extubation was associated with a lower sedation score (odds ratio, 2.04) and higher level of consciousness on the GCS (odds ratio, 1.40). The model explained 67.3% of variance of deliberate self-extubation. These data suggest that the weaning period is a high-risk time for deliberate self-extubation because patients are receiving less sedative agents and have a higher level of consciousness.

De Lassence et al[8] undertook a prospective multicenter study of the morbidity and mortality associated with unplanned extubation. Compared with 45 of 690 patients who required reintubation after planned extubation, the 46 (of 60) patients who were reintubated after an unplanned extubation experienced a longer duration of mechanical ventilation, 17 versus 6 days, longer ICU stay, 22 versus 9 days, and longer hospital stay, 34 versus 18 days. The frequency of nosocomial pneumonia was higher after unplanned extubation than after planned extubation: 28% versus 14%; this increase was entirely explained by accidental extubation. ICU mortality was 40.9% in patients with accidental extubation, 21.1% in patients with self-extubation, and 38% in the control group—these rates did not differ statistically.[8] In a retrospective case-control study, Epstein et al[65] also observed no difference in mortality between patients experiencing unplanned extubation, 32%, and a control group, 30%. The mortality in the control groups of both these series[8,65] is considerably higher than the mortality of less than 10% usually reported in successfully extubated patients.

Tominaga et al[66] undertook a prospective study of four interventions designed to influence the frequency of unplanned extubation. At baseline, 15.2% of intubated patients experienced unplanned extubation. When the investigators switched from their usual method of securing the endotracheal tube, cloth or Velcro ties, to the use of waterproof tape around the tube, upper lip, and face, the frequency of unplanned extubations decreased to 4% (8/213). The frequency was not altered by the more liberal use of sedative or paralytic agents. A decrease in the use of hand restraints led to an increase in the rate of unplanned extubations.

Conclusion

The development of severe respiratory distress after removal of an endotracheal tube, if sufficient to require reintubation, is associated with a high mortality rate. Clinicians are accordingly cautious and try to avoid premature extubation. Despite such caution, as many as two of every ten extubated patients require reintubation. To improve accuracy in forecasting extubation outcome, clinicians use diagnostic testing. The major diagnostic test for this purpose is a weaning trial. But unlike weaning predictor diagnostic tests, the diagnostic accuracy of weaning trials in predicting the outcome of a trial of extubation is unknown. Moreover, the accuracy is impossible to determine, because the experiments necessary to measure the sensitivity and specificity of a weaning trial (for predicting extubation outcome) are unethical. The mechanisms of weaning failure have been intensely investigated. Enhanced understanding of the pathophysiology has led to new approaches to the timing of the weaning process, prediction of outcome, and techniques used for weaning. In contrast, understanding of the pathophysiology of severe respiratory distress in the postextubation period is rudimentary to nonexistent. Acquiring such knowledge poses a great research challenge, but holds great promise for significantly advancing patient care.

References

1. Leitch EA, Moran JL, Grealy B. Weaning and extubation in the intensive care unit. Clinical or index-driven approach? Intensive Care Med 1996; 22:752–59.
2. Conti G, Montini L, Pennisi MA, et al. A prospective, blinded evaluation of indexes proposed to predict weaning from mechanical ventilation. Intensive Care Med 2004; 30:830–36.
3. Dojat M, Harf A, Touchard D, et al. Evaluation of a knowledge-based system providing ventilatory management and decision for extubation. Am J Respir Crit Care Med 1996; 153:997–1004.
4. Cohen JD, Shapiro M, Grozovski E, Singer P. Automatic tube compensation-assisted respiratory rate to tidal volume ratio improves the prediction of weaning outcome. Chest 2002; 122: 980–84.
5. Maldonado A, Bauer TT, Ferrer M, et al. Capnometric recirculation gas tonometry and weaning from mechanical ventilation. Am J Respir Crit Care Med 2000; 161: 171–76.
6. Esteban A, Frutos-Vivar F, Ferguson ND, et al. Noninvasive positive-pressure ventilation for respiratory failure after extubation. N Engl J Med 2004; 350:2452–60.
7. Demling RH, Read T, Lind LJ, Flanagan HL. Incidence and morbidity of extubation failure in surgical intensive care patients. Crit Care Med 1988; 16:573–77.

8. de Lassence A, Alberti C, Azoulay E, et al. Impact of unplanned extubation and reintubation after weaning on nosocomial pneumonia risk in the intensive care unit: a prospective multicenter study. Anesthesiology 2002; 97:148–56.

9. Haberthur C, Mols G, Elsasser S, et al. Extubation after breathing trials with automatic tube compensation, T-tube, or pressure support ventilation. Acta Anaesthesiol Scand 2002; 46:973–79.

10. Jiang JR, Tsai TH, Jerng JS, et al. Ultrasonographic evaluation of liver/spleen movements and extubation outcome. Chest 2004; 126:179–85.

11. Epstein SK. Etiology of extubation failure and the predictive value of the rapid shallow breathing index. Am J Respir Crit Care Med 1995; 152:545–49.

12. Epstein SK, Ciubotaru RL, Wong JB. Effect of failed extubation on the outcome of mechanical ventilation. Chest 1997; 112:186–92.

13. Namen AM, Ely EW, Tatter SB, et al. Predictors of successful extubation in neurosurgical patients. Am J Respir Crit Care Med 2001; 163:658–64.

14. Epstein SK, Ciubotaru RL. Independent effects of etiology of failure and time to reintubation on outcome for patients failing extubation. Am J Respir Crit Care Med 1998; 158:489–93.

15. Esteban A, Alia I, Tobin MJ, et al. Effect of spontaneous breathing trial duration on outcome of attempts to discontinue mechanical ventilation. Spanish Lung Failure Collaborative Group. Am J Respir Crit Care Med 1999; 159:512–18.

16. Smina M, Salam A, Khamiees M, et al. Cough peak flows and extubation outcomes. Chest 2003; 124:262–68.

17. Sandhu RS, Pasquale MD, Miller K, Wasser TE. Measurement of endotracheal tube cuff leak to predict postextubation stridor and need for reintubation. J Am Coll Surg 2000; 190:682–87.

18. Jaber S, Chanques G, Matecki S, et al. Post-extubation stridor in intensive care unit patients. Risk factors evaluation and importance of the cuff-leak test. Intensive Care Med 2003; 29: 69–74.

19. Ho LI, Harn HJ, Lien TC, Hu PY, Wang JH. Postextubation laryngeal edema in adults. Risk factor evaluation and prevention by hydrocortisone. Intensive Care Med 1996; 22:933–36.

20. Darmon JY, Rauss A, Dreyfuss D, et al. Evaluation of risk factors for laryngeal edema after tracheal extubation in adults and its prevention by dexamethasone. A placebo-controlled, double-blind, multicenter study. Anesthesiology 1992; 77:245–51.

21. Engoren M. Evaluation of the cuff-leak test in a cardiac surgery population. Chest 1999; 116:1029–31.

22. De Bast Y, De Backer D, Moraine JJ, et al. The cuff leak test to predict failure of tracheal extubation for laryngeal edema. Intensive Care Med 2002; 28:1267–72.

23. Tobin MJ. Noninvasive monitoring of ventilation. In: Tobin MJ, editor. Principles and practice of intensive care monitoring. New York: McGraw-Hill, 1998: 465–95.

24. Tobin MJ, Perez W, Guenther SM, et al. The pattern of breathing during successful and unsuccessful trials of weaning from mechanical ventilation. Am Rev Respir Dis 1986; 134:1111–18.

25. Daley BJ, Garcia-Perez F, Ross SE. Reintubation as an outcome predictor in trauma patients. Chest 1996; 110:1577–80.

26. Esteban A, Alia I, Gordo F, et al. Extubation outcome after spontaneous breathing trials with T-tube or pressure support ventilation. The Spanish Lung Failure Collaborative Group. Am J Respir Crit Care Med 1997; 156:459–65.

27. Torres A, Gatell JM, Aznar E, et al. Re-intubation increases the risk of nosocomial pneumonia in patients needing mechanical ventilation. Am J Respir Crit Care Med 1995; 152:137–41.

28. Schwartz DE, Matthay MA, Cohen NH. Death and other complications of emergency airway management in critically ill adults. A prospective investigation of 297 tracheal intubations. Anesthesiology 1995; 82:367–76.

29. Uusaro A, Chittock DR, Russell JA, Walley KR. Stress test and gastric-arterial PCO2 measurement improve prediction of successful extubation. Crit Care Med 2000; 28:2313–19.

30. Zeggwagh AA, Abouqal R, Madani N, Zekraoui A, Kerkeb O. Weaning from mechanical ventilation: a model for extubation. Intensive Care Med 1999; 25:1077–83.

31. Adderley RJ, Mullins GC. When to extubate the croup patient: the "leak" test. Can J Anaesth 1987; 34:304–306.

32. Miller RL, Cole RP. Association between reduced cuff leak volume and postextubation stridor. Chest 1996; 110:1035–40.

33. Shim C, Fine N, Fernandez R, Williams MH Jr. Cardiac arrhythmias resulting from tracheal suctioning. Ann Intern Med 1969; 71:1149–1153.

34. Boutros AR. Arterial blood oxygenation during and after endotracheal suctioning in the apneic patient. Anesthesiology 1970; 32:114–118.

35. Landa J, Amikan B, Sackner MA. Pathogenesis and prevention of tracheobronchial erosions occurring during suctioning. Am Rev Respir Dis 1971; 103:875–76.

36. Brochard L, Mion G, Isabey D, et al. Constant-flow insufflation prevents arterial oxygen desaturation during endotracheal suctioning. Am Rev Respir Dis 1991; 144:395–400.

37. Jubran A, Tobin MJ. Use of flow-volume curves in detecting secretions in ventilator-dependent patients. Am J Respir Crit Care Med 1994; 150:766–69.

38. Guglielminotti J, Alzieu M, Maury E, Guidet B, Offenstadt G. Bedside detection of retained tracheobronchial secretions in patients receiving mechanical ventilation: is it time for tracheal suctioning? Chest 2000; 118:1095–99.

39. Khamiees M, Raju P, DeGirolamo A, Amoateng-Adjepong Y, Manthous CA. Predictors of extubation outcome in patients who have successfully completed a spontaneous breathing trial. Chest 2001; 120:1262–70.

40. Salam A, Tilluckdharry L, Amoateng-Adjepong Y, Manthous CA. Neurologic status, cough, secretions and extubation outcomes. Intensive Care Med 2004; 30:1334–39.

41. Coplin WM, Pierson DJ, Cooley KD, Newell DW, Rubenfeld GD. Implications of extubation delay in brain-injured patients meeting standard weaning criteria. Am J Respir Crit Care Med 2000; 161:1530–36.

42. Vallverdu I, Calaf N, Subirana M, et al. Clinical characteristics, respiratory functional parameters, and outcome of a two-hour T-piece trial in patients weaning from mechanical ventilation. Am J Respir Crit Care Med 1998; 158:1855–62.

43. Kulig K, Rumack BH, Rosen P. Gag reflex in assessing level of consciousness. Lancet 1982; 1:565.

44. Kress JP, O'Connor MF, Pohlman AS, et al. Sedation of critically ill patients during mechanical ventilation. A comparison of propofol and midazolam. Am J Respir Crit Care Med 1996; 153: 1012–18.

45. Capdevila XJ, Perrigault PF, Perey PJ, Roustan JP, d'Athis F. Occlusion pressure and its ratio to maximum inspiratory pressure are useful predictors for successful extubation following T-piece weaning trial. Chest 1995; 108:482–89.

46. Fernandez R, Raurich JM, Mut T, et al. Extubation failure: diagnostic value of occlusion pressure (P0.1) and P0.1-derived parameters. Intensive Care Med 2004; 30:234–40.

47. Hilbert G, Gruson D, Portel L, et al. Airway occlusion pressure at 0.1 s (P0.1) after extubation: an early indicator of postextubation hypercapnic respiratory insufficiency. Intensive Care Med 1998; 24:1277–1282.

48. Weiner N. Norepinephrine, epinephrine, and the sympathomimetic amines. In: Gilman AG, Goodman LS, Pall WT, editors. Goodman and Gilman. The pharmacologic basis of therapeutics. New York: MacMillan Publishing, 1986: 150–51.

49. Nutman J, Brooks LJ, Deakins KM, et al. Racemic versus l-epinephrine aerosol in the treatment of postextubation laryngeal edema: results from a prospective, randomized, double-blind study. Crit Care Med 1994; 22:1591–94.

50. Tellez DW, Galvis AG, Storgion SA, et al. Dexamethasone in the prevention of postextubation stridor in children. J Pediatr 1991; 118:289–94.

51. Anene O, Meert KL, Uy H, Simpson P, Sarnaik AP. Dexamethasone for the prevention of postextubation airway obstruction: a prospective, randomized, double-blind, placebo-controlled trial. Crit Care Med 1996; 24:1666–69.

52. Pronovost PJ, Jenckes M, To M, et al. Reducing failed extubations in the intensive care unit. Jt Comm J Qual Improv 2002; 28:595–604.

53. Nava S, Ambrosino N, Clini E, et al. Noninvasive mechanical ventilation in the weaning of patients with respiratory failure due to chronic obstructive pulmonary disease. A randomized, controlled trial. Ann Intern Med 1998; 128:721–28.

54. Girault C, Daudenthun I, Chevron V, et al. Noninvasive ventilation as a systematic extubation and weaning technique in acute-on-chronic respiratory failure: a prospective, randomized controlled study. Am J Respir Crit Care Med 1999; 160:86–92.

55. Ferrer M, Esquinas A, Arancibia F, et al. Noninvasive ventilation during persistent weaning failure: a randomized controlled trial. Am J Respir Crit Care Med 2003; 168:70–76.

56. Keenan SP, Powers C, McCormack DG, Block G. Noninvasive positive-pressure ventilation for postextubation respiratory distress: a randomized controlled trial. JAMA 2002; 287:3238–44.

57. Tobin MJ, Perez W, Guenther SM, Lodato RF, Dantzker DR. Does rib cage-abdominal paradox signify respiratory muscle fatigue? J Appl Physiol 1987; 63:851–60.

58. Tobin MJ, Guenther SM, Perez W, et al. Konno-Mead analysis of ribcage-abdominal motion during successful and unsuccessful trials of weaning from mechanical ventilation. Am Rev Respir Dis 1987; 135:1320–28.

59. Jiang JS, Kao SJ, Wang SN. Effect of early application of biphasic positive airway pressure on the outcome of extubation in ventilator weaning. Respirology 1999; 4:161–65.

60. Vassal T, Anh NG, Gabillet JM, et al. Prospective evaluation of self-extubations in a medical intensive care unit. Intensive Care Med 1993; 19:340–42.

61. Moons P, Sels K, De Becker W, De Geest S, Ferdinande P. Development of a risk assessment tool for deliberate self-extubation in intensive care patients. Intensive Care Med 2004; 30:1348–55.

62. Ely EW, Bennett PA, Bowton DL, et al. Large scale implementation of a respiratory therapist-driven protocol for ventilator weaning. Am J Respir Crit Care Med 1999; 159:439–46.

63. Betbese AJ, Perez M, Bak E, Rialp G, Mancebo J. A prospective study of unplanned endotracheal extubation in intensive care unit patients. Crit Care Med 1998; 26:1180–86.

64. Razek T, Gracias V, Sullivan D, et al. Assessing the need for reintubation: a prospective evaluation of unplanned endotracheal extubation. J Trauma 2000; 48:466–69.

65. Epstein SK, Nevins ML, Chung J. Effect of unplanned extubation on outcome of mechanical ventilation. Am J Respir Crit Care Med 2000; 161:1912–16.

66. Tominaga GT, Rudzwick H, Scannell G, Waxman K. Decreasing unplanned extubations in the surgical intensive care unit. Am J Surg 1995; 170:586–89.

67. Tahvanainen J, Salmenpera M, Nikki P. Extubation criteria after weaning from intermittent mandatory ventilation and continuous positive airway pressure. Crit Care Med 1983; 11:702–7.

68. DeHaven CB Jr, Hurst JM, Branson RD. Evaluation of two different extubation criteria: attributes contributing to success. Crit Care Med 1986; 14:92–94.

69. Krieger BP, Ershowsky PF, Becker DA, Gazeroglu HB. Evaluation of conventional criteria for predicting successful weaning from mechanical ventilatory support in elderly patients. Crit Care Med 1989; 17:858–61.

70. Mohsenifar Z, Hay A, Hay J, Lewis MI, Koerner SK. Gastric intramural pH as a predictor of success or failure in weaning patients from mechanical ventilation. Ann Intern Med 1993; 119:794–98.

71. Sassoon CS, Mahutte CK. Airway occlusion pressure and breathing pattern as predictors of weaning outcome. Am Rev Respir Dis 1993; 148:860–66.

72. Brochard L, Rauss A, Benito S, et al. Comparison of three methods of gradual withdrawal from ventilatory support during weaning from mechanical ventilation. Am J Respir Crit Care Med 1994; 150:896–903.

73. Lee KH, Hui KP, Chan TB, Tan WC, Lim TK. Rapid shallow breathing (frequency-tidal volume ratio) did not predict extubation outcome. Chest 1994; 105:540–43.

74. Esteban A, Frutos F, Tobin MJ, et al. A comparison of four methods of weaning patients from mechanical ventilation. Spanish Lung Failure Collaborative Group. N Engl J Med 1995; 332:345–50.

75. Chatila W, Jacob B, Guaglionone D, Manthous CA. The unassisted respiratory rate-tidal volume ratio accurately predicts weaning outcome. Am J Med 1996; 101:61–67.

76. Ely EW, Baker AM, Dunagan DP, et al. Effect on the duration of mechanical ventilation of identifying patients capable of breathing spontaneously. N Engl J Med 1996; 335:1864–69.

77. Jacob B, Chatila W, Manthous CA. The unassisted respiratory rate/tidal volume ratio accurately predicts weaning outcome in postoperative patients. Crit Care Med 1997; 25:253–57.

78. Kollef MH, Shapiro SD, Silver P, et al. A randomized, controlled trial of protocol-directed versus physician-directed weaning from mechanical ventilation. Crit Care Med 1997; 25:567–74.

79. Koh Y, Hong SB, Lim CM, et al. Effect of an additional 1-hour T-piece trial on weaning outcome at minimal pressure support. J Crit Care 2000; 15:41–45.

80. Perren A, Domenighetti G, Mauri S, Genini F, Vizzardi N. Protocol-directed weaning from mechanical ventilation: clinical outcome in patients randomized for a 30-min or 120-min trial with pressure support ventilation. Intensive Care Med 2002; 28:1058–63.

81. Zwillich CW, Pierson DJ, Creagh CE, et al. Complications of assisted ventilation. A prospective study of 354 consecutive episodes. Am J Med 1974; 57:161–70.

82. Stauffer JL, Olson DE, Petty TL. Complications and consequences of endotracheal intubation and tracheotomy. A prospective study of 150 critically ill adult patients. Am J Med 1981; 70:65–76.

83. Whelan J, Simpson SQ, Levy H. Unplanned extubation. Predictors of successful termination of mechanical ventilatory support. Chest 1994; 105:1808–12.

84. Tindol GA Jr, DiBenedetto RJ, Kosciuk L. Unplanned extubations. Chest 1994; 105:1804–07.

85. Listello D, Sessler CN. Unplanned extubation. Clinical predictors for reintubation. Chest 1994; 105:1496–503.

86. Boulain T. Unplanned extubations in the adult intensive care unit: a prospective multicenter study. Association des Reanimateurs du Centre-Ouest. Am J Respir Crit Care Med 1998; 157:1131–37.

87. Chevron V, Menard JF, Richard JC, et al. Unplanned extubation: risk factors of development and predictive criteria for reintubation. Crit Care Med 1998; 26:1049–53.

88. Kapadia FN, Bajan KB, Raje KV. Airway accidents in intubated intensive care unit patients: an epidemiological study. Crit Care Med 2000; 28:659–64.

89. Esteban A, Anzueto A, Frutos F, et al. Characteristics and outcomes in adult patients receiving mechanical ventilation: a 28-day international study. JAMA 2002; 287:345–55.

PART XIV
ADJUNCTIVE THERAPY

Chapter 60 _____
SURFACTANT

JAMES F. LEWIS

Pulmonary surfactant lines the inner layer of the lung and serves to lower surface tension at the air-liquid interface thereby maintaining alveolar stability. In the absence of surfactant, the work of breathing increases markedly, ultimately resulting in respiratory failure secondary to atelectasis, alveolar flooding, and severe hypoxemia. The clinical correlate of surfactant deficiency is the neonatal respiratory distress syndrome (nRDS) in preterm infants, which before the mid-1980s was a devastating and fatal disease. Now, because of the advent of exogenous surfactant replacement therapy, infant mortality from nRDS has decreased dramatically. Alterations of the endogenous surfactant system in the mature lung are not as well understood but currently represent an area of intense investigation. The various surfactant changes that occur in the setting of acute lung injury (ALI) and/or the acute respiratory distress syndrome (ARDS) are more complex than the primary surfactant deficiency of nRDS. This complexity has resulted in inconsistent results of clinical trials evaluating exogenous surfactant administration in this patient population.

The goal of this chapter is to review surfactant metabolism and function in the mature lung and its role in maintaining normal lung homeostasis, including its more recently described host defense functions. The metabolism and function of surfactant in the injured lung will also be outlined, with particular reference to the effects of mechanical ventilation on the alveolar surfactant system. Subsequently, the status of clinical trials evaluating exogenous surfactant administration in patients with ALI/ARDS will be addressed, as will the various factors that may influence a host's response to this therapy. Future research directions relevant to the understanding of the role of surfactant both in ALI/ARDS and other lung diseases will conclude the chapter.

Surfactant Composition and Metabolism

COMPOSITION

The composition of surfactant is remarkably similar among mammalian species, consisting of approximately 90% lipids and 10% surfactant-associated proteins.[1-3] The major phospholipid (PL) component is phosphatidylcholine (PC), half of which is the disaturated species, dipalmitoylphosphatidylcholine (DPPC).[3] This latter molecule is the major surface-active component responsible for lowering surface tension at the air-liquid interface, and is an essential component of all exogenous surfactant preparations currently available for clinical use. Other lipids include phosphatidylglycerol (PG) and a few minor lipid species, which are felt to be important in the generation and maintenance of the surface film. The surfactant-associated proteins have been designated as SP-A, B, C, and D.[4,5] SP-B and C are small, hydrophobic proteins closely associated with the PLs where they play a major role in generating and maintaining the surface tension–reducing surface film.[6-8] SP-B is an 18-kd dimer while SP-C is a 4-kd monomer, the latter being the more hydrophobic of these two proteins.[9,10] The most clinically effective exogenous surfactant preparations currently in use contain at least one of these natural hydrophobic proteins, or similar types of synthetic/recombinant molecules. SP-A is an octodecamer made up of six trimers in a "bouquet" arrangement.[11,12] Under reducing conditions, it is a 28-kd monomer with a 35-kd glycosylated form. SP-D is a large, multimeric cruciform structure, which is 42 kd under reducing conditions. Both proteins are very hydrophilic and belong to the collectin family of proteins. They are not components of any of the available natural exogenous preparations consequent to their removal with purification processes, and are not yet available as synthetic or recombinant molecules. Recent evidence suggests that they play a more important role in host defense rather than biophysical functions, so there has been renewed interest in developing exogenous preparations containing some form of these proteins.[11-14]

INTRACELLULAR METABOLISM

Surfactant is synthesized within alveolar type II cells[15] (Fig. 60-1). Initial assembly occurs in the endoplasmic

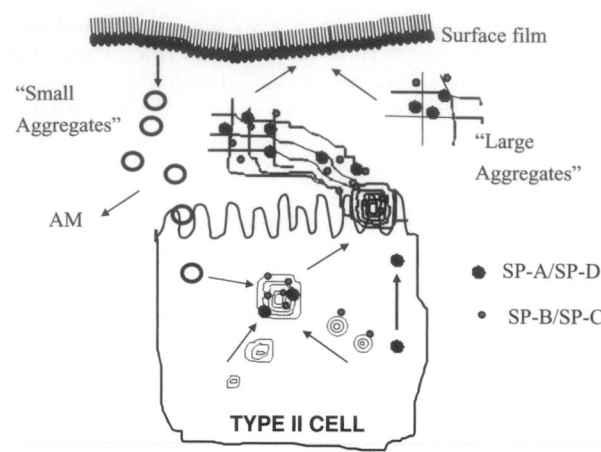

FIGURE 60-1 Surfactant metabolism starts with synthesis within the type II cell, secretion into the airspace as lamellar bodies containing both lipid and protein components, and formation of tubular myelin structures. Large aggregates (*LA*) are composed of tubular myelin and freshly secreted lamellar bodies and represent precursors to the surface film. With respiratory motion, small aggregates are formed, which are taken back up into type II cells or cleared via alveolar macrophages (*AM*).

reticulum with intracellular transport via the Golgi apparatus. Surfactant is stored within lamellar bodies of the type II cell and is secreted into the airspace via exocytosis.[16,17] Studies that have investigated the intracellular metabolic pathways of surfactant lipids and proteins have used radiolabeled precursors injected both intravenously and intratracheally. Basically, these studies have shown that while the hydrophobic proteins are assembled and secreted in conjunction with the lipids, SP-A and D are metabolized separately.[18] For example, the dominant route for SP-A secretion is by direct, constitutive pathways independent of lamellar body exocytosis, although smaller amounts undergo regulated secretion in association with these organelles.[19,20] SP-D is also metabolized independently of surfactant lipids, and, unlike the other surfactant proteins, has been identified in nonpulmonary organs such as the gut.[21,22] Within the healthy lung, various pharmacologic agents, such as β-agonists can stimulate surfactant secretion, as can physical stretch of alveolar type II cells.[23] This latter phenomenon is particularly relevant to specific aspects of mechanical ventilation because higher tidal volumes increase the stretch of the alveolus, leading to immediate surfactant secretion from type II cells. These effects are relatively short-lived, however, and may be quite different within the injured lung, where the health of type II cells may be compromised.

Recent studies have focused more on the extracellular metabolism of pulmonary surfactant, once the material has been secreted from the type II cell into the alveolus (see Fig. 60-1). Within the airspace, mechanical ventilation has been shown to have a significant and immediate impact on the surfactant system by influencing the metabolism of extracellular surfactant aggregate forms. Because this effect may have important clinical consequences in patients with ALI/ARDS, a more detailed discussion of this area is warranted.

EXTRACELLULAR METABOLISM

Once secreted into the airspace, alveolar surfactant undergoes physical rearrangement from the lamellar structures into tubular myelin, a process involving SP-A, SP-B, DPPC, PG, and calcium.[24,25] After differential centrifugation of isolated lung lavage, large lipid structures containing SP-A, B, and C, representing the heavier and functionally active forms of alveolar surfactant form a pellet, and are called large aggregates (LA).[26,27] They adsorb rapidly to the air-liquid interface and are subsequently converted into smaller, vesicular forms called small aggregates (SA) (see Fig. 60-1). These latter subfractions are poorly functioning, contain little surfactant protein, and are thought to represent surfactant forms that have left the surface film and are subsequently available for reuptake via type II cells for resynthesis into new LA, or are cleared entirely from the airspace via catabolism, mainly within alveolar macrophages.[28-30]

The process of conversion of the functionally active LA forms into inactive SA within the airspace is specifically relevant when discussing the effects of mechanical ventilation on surfactant metabolism. In vitro studies using the surface-area cycling technique have shown that this conversion of LA into SA is mediated by two main factors: a carboxylesterase enzyme called convertase and a phasic change in surface area.[27,31-33] The latter factor has been investigated in vivo using different tidal volumes to mechanically ventilate normal rabbits. These studies showed that increasing tidal volume, but not positive end-expiratory pressure (PEEP) resulted in an increased conversion of LA into SA, and that this conversion occurred relatively soon after the onset of ventilation[34] (Fig. 60-2). In normal lungs, these changes did not result in significant alterations in aggregate pool sizes, presumably because of the capabilities of the normal alveolar environment to regulate surfactant metabolism. This does not appear to be the case in the injured lung, however, where alterations in surfactant metabolism occur both intracellularly

FIGURE 60-2 The rate of small aggregate (*SA*) formation increases in direct proportion to the tidal volumes used to ventilate normal adult rabbits. SA formation was determined by measuring ^{3}H-label recovery in the SA fraction of surfactant 1 hour after injection of a trace dose of ^{3}H-labeled large aggregates into the animals' lungs (*Reproduced, with permission, from Ito et al.[35]*)

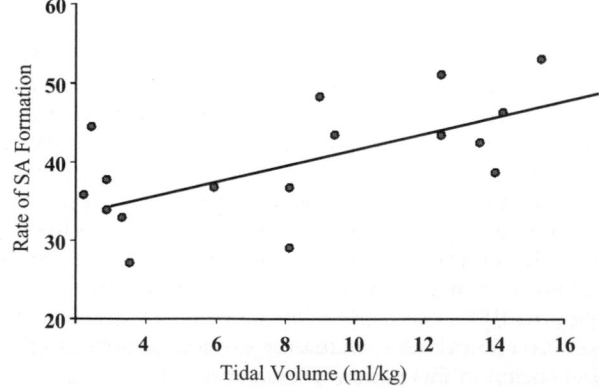

and extracellularly.[35,36] For example, within the lungs of patients with ALI/ARDS, increased aggregate conversion associated with higher tidal volumes is thought to result in increased SA pools, which, together with the associated decrease in functionally active LA pools, may contribute to progressive lung dysfunction. Indeed, these specific changes have been demonstrated in animal models of lung injury and have not only underscored the importance of instituting and maintaining optimal modes of mechanical ventilation within injured lungs, but also in the setting of exogenous surfactant, both during and after administration. This latter situation will be discussed in more detail in subsequent sections.

Surfactant Physiology in the Normal Lung

BIOPHYSICAL FUNCTION

The major role of the surfactant system is related to its biophysical function of lowering surface tension at the air-liquid interface.[2,3,37] This is most evident clinically in preterm infants born deficient in surfactant who quickly die of respiratory failure unless supplemented with an exogenous surfactant preparation.[38–40] As noted previously, the major lipid component contributing to lowering surface tension is DPPC, although the hydrophobic proteins and some other lipids are also essential.[7–10] Full-term babies born deficient in SP-B develop severe lung dysfunction resistant to traditional surfactant therapy and ultimately require lung transplantation for survival.[41] Likewise, mice deficient in this protein suffer a similar outcome and have also been shown to have abnormal processing of SP-C.[42] Mice deficient in SP-C alone, on the other hand, have relatively minor biophysical abnormalities, which predominantly manifest only at low lung volumes, suggesting a potential role for this protein in the surface film stabilization.[43]

From a physiologic perspective, the initial discovery that surface tension was important for lung stability was made by von Neergaard in 1929, when he observed that it took more pressure to inflate air-filled than saline-filled lungs.[44] This was the direct result of the surface tension forces existing at the air-liquid interface. This concept is further advanced by Laplace's law, which states that the pressure gradient across a sphere, which we can roughly extrapolate to an alveolus, is directly related to the surface tension within the sphere divided by the radius of the sphere ($\Delta P = 2\delta/r$), where P is pressure, δ is surface tension, and r is radius. From this equation, it is clear that during exhalation, when the alveolar radius decreases, the tendency for this alveolus to collapse will increase (i.e., ΔP) unless surface tension decreases as well. Because of its strategic location at the air-liquid interface, and the presence of both hydrophobic and hydrophilic regions, a surfactant film lining the air-liquid interface is able to lower surface tension to near zero levels as the film is compressed at low lung volumes. This decrease in surface tension not only serves to maintain alveolar stability and decrease the work of breathing, but also prevents alveolar flooding because high surface tension

tends to draw fluid from the interstitium into the airspace.[45] Finally, because surfactant also lines the conducting airways, its biophysical function serves to maintain the patency and stability of small airways and enhance ciliary clearance of particles (46,47).

HOST DEFENSE FUNCTION

As noted previously, the surfactant proteins SP-A and D are members of the collectin family and, secondary to their molecular composition and structure, can bind to microbial and inflammatory cell walls, thus mediating phagocytosis and the killing of pathogens within the lung.[11,13,48] In addition, these proteins, as well as some of the hydrophobic components of surfactant, can influence production of nitric oxide (NO), oxygen radicals, and inflammatory mediators from activated cells.[49–51] Underscoring the importance of SP-A in host defense functions are in vivo studies demonstrating that mice deficient in this protein (which are phenotypically normal when not stressed) had increased pulmonary inflammation compared to wild-type animals when bacteria, viruses, or lipopolysaccharide (LPS) were instilled into their lungs.[52,53] These changes were mitigated when exogenous SP-A was administered to these animals. Similar, albeit slightly modified functions of SP-D have been shown both in vitro and in vivo; unlike the normal phenotype of the SP-A null mice, however, the phenotype of unstressed SP-D knockout animals is abnormal with enlarged airspaces and significantly altered surfactant pool sizes.[54,55] The host-defense functions of the various surfactant lipids have also been evaluated and in general show that these phospholipids downregulate inflammation, presumably because of their "coating" effects on particles and cells.[56,57] Very little information is available regarding the role of SP-B and C in this setting.

Surfactant Physiology in the Injured Lung

SURFACTANT ALTERATIONS IN ACUTE LUNG INJURY/ACUTE RESPIRATORY DISTRESS SYNDROME

The definition of ALI/ARDS is rather simplistic and is based on physiologic criteria more than specific etiologies. For example, any acute inflammatory insult that ultimately affects the lungs causing decreased lung compliance, hypoxemia, and bilateral infiltrates on chest radiography (not of cardiac origin) essentially fulfills the diagnostic criteria of ALI/ARDS.[58,59] The pathophysiologic changes that occur during this process, including the surfactant alterations reported in numerous studies, are complex and reflect the lack of effective treatments for this disorder.

The first postmortem descriptions of the lungs of patients dying from ARDS suggested that surfactant dysfunction may have played a role in their demise.[60] Subsequently, many studies have reported consistent changes in the surfactant system in lavage samples obtained from these patients, including decreased PC and DPPC levels, decreased PG levels, decreased SP-A, B, C and D levels, and a decrease in the functionally active LA forms relative to SA.[61–63]

Interestingly, in these severely ill patients, serum levels of SP-A and D were shown to be elevated, likely consequent to a marked increase in pulmonary permeability.[64,65] The biophysical consequence of these collective changes in the endogenous surfactant system is an inability to adequately reduce surface tension, resulting in decreased lung compliance, increased permeability with edema formation, and hypoxemia. The next section will address the mechanisms responsible for the surfactant changes observed in these patients. Only with a better understanding of these mechanisms will optimal treatment strategies be developed, aimed at restoring normal surface tension forces within injured lungs, or perhaps, more importantly, preventing the development of these changes.

MECHANISMS RESPONSIBLE FOR SURFACTANT ALTERATIONS

Unlike nRDS, in which the preterm animal represents a reasonable correlate of the clinical condition of nRDS, and is thus suitable for reliable mechanistic studies, no one animal model adequately reflects the complexity of patients with ALI/ARDS. Proposed mechanisms in the latter setting are therefore derived from many different animal models, a factor that needs to be considered when extrapolating results of such studies to the clinical situation.

The observed changes in the PL composition of endogenous surfactant within the injured lung represents a relatively late finding in models of ALI when severe lung dysfunction is present. These changes are likely related to abnormal synthetic and/or secretory pathways within the type II cell, as well as alterations in the degradation process of some lipids within the airspace via increased phospholipase activity[66-69] (Fig. 60-3). A similar mechanism is likely responsible for the decreased surfactant protein levels observed in these lungs, although with the permeability abnormalities demonstrated in these patients, there may also be

transfer of SP-A, B, and D across the alveolar-capillary barrier into the serum.[64,65] Interestingly, clinical studies have shown that serum levels of SP-A and B were inversely related to oxygenation values in patients with ARDS, and serum SP-D levels positively correlated with the survival of these patients.[64,65] In addition to these quantitative changes in surfactant protein levels, there may also be modifications to their composition in the form of nitration and/or oxidation, which would also compromise their function but may not impact measurable levels.[70-72]

The mechanisms responsible for the changes observed in surfactant aggregate forms have been alluded to earlier. Briefly, decreased LA pools may be caused by decreased type II cell synthesis and/or secretion in the severely injured lung, but an increased conversion of LA into SA forms likely occurs at earlier stages of the disease, particularly in patients undergoing mechanical ventilation.[33-36] This was recently investigated in animal studies in which spontaneously breathing septic rats with relatively mild lung dysfunction had unchanged LA pools, whereas SA pools were significantly decreased compared to sham animals.[73] These changes were opposite to those documented in severely injured lungs; it was hypothesized that they may have represented the host's compensatory response aimed at maintaining endogenous surfactant in LA forms. For example, by utilizing smaller tidal volumes (with higher respiratory rates), these animals would decrease LA conversion secondary to the smaller changes in alveolar surface area, thereby attempting to maintain lung function. Indeed, very soon after the onset of mechanical ventilation of these animals, which involved using higher tidal volumes than those associated with spontaneous breathing, conversion of LA into SA increased dramatically and lung function deteriorated rapidly.[74] Of clinical relevance, however, was the ability to mitigate both the aggregate conversion and progressive lung dysfunction observed by using lower tidal volumes from the onset of ventilation. In fact, high-frequency

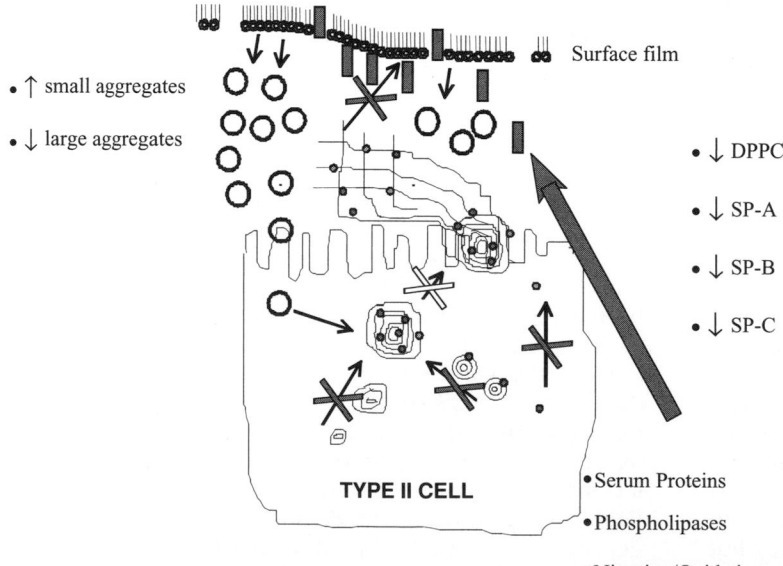

- ↑ small aggregates
- ↓ large aggregates

Surface film

- ↓ DPPC
- ↓ SP-A
- ↓ SP-B
- ↓ SP-C

TYPE II CELL

- Serum Proteins
- Phospholipases
- Nitration/Oxidation

FIGURE 60-3 Mechanisms leading to surfactant alterations in the injured lung include abnormal type II cell metabolism, increased phospholipase activity, nitration and oxidation of surfactant, increased conversion of large aggregates into small aggregates, and inhibition of surfactant by serum proteins leaking into the airspace. See text for details.

oscillation (HFO), a strategy involving extremely small tidal volumes with high respiratory rates, proved to be superior to all other "lung protective" modes of ventilation with respect to aggregate conversion, lung function, and inflammatory changes.[75] Interestingly, these laboratory results are consistent with recent clinical trials evaluating different modes of mechanical ventilation in patients with acute lung injury. One large trial showed that lower tidal volumes resulted in superior outcomes compared to higher tidal volumes in patients with ALI/ARDS.[76]

Finally, within a permeable lung, characteristic of patients with ARDS, serum proteins such as albumin, hemoglobin, and fibrinogen can leak into the airspace and competitively inhibit the function of remaining LA forms.[77] Fortunately, this latter mechanism may be overcome via the administration of large amounts of an effective exogenous surfactant preparation, thus providing important rationale for this therapeutic approach.[78]

Exogenous Surfactant Administration in the Injured Lung

RESULTS OF PHASE II AND III CLINICAL TRIALS

Exogenous surfactant administration has been evaluated in patients with ARDS based on the rationale that surfactant alterations contribute, at least in part, to the lung dysfunction associated with this disorder. Moreover, preclinical studies evaluating the efficacy of exogenous surfactant administration in animal models of acute lung injury have shown promising results. Unfortunately, the outcomes of clinical trials conducted to date have been variable (Table 60-1). For example, the first large, randomized phase III clinical trial, involving over 700 patients, administered aerosolized Exosurf (a preparation with no surfactant proteins) to patients with severe, sepsis-induced ARDS over a 5-day period.[79] Mortality was similar in the treatment (41%) and standard care (41%) groups. A subsequent, albeit smaller trial, with approximately 50 patients, evaluated tracheally-instilled Survanta (a natural bovine preparation) in a relatively similar patient population with good results: a mortality of 19% compared to 44% in the control group.[80] In this study, the surfactant preparation contained both SP-B and C, and much larger quantities of the material reached the airspace compared to the Exosurf trial. Other, relatively small clinical studies include a recent phase II trial

that used a porcine natural surfactant preparation, HL-10, which also contains SP-B and C. This surfactant was instilled in large doses directly into the lungs of patients with severe ALI/ARDS, but was recently terminated because of lack of efficacy. Surfaxin, a synthetic surfactant preparation containing an SP-B–like peptide, was tested in 12 patients with ARDS and administered via a lung-lavage procedure.[81] Preliminary results have been promising, and a larger phase II trial is currently underway.

Results from a large, randomized phase III trial that tested the efficacy of an exogenous surfactant preparation composed of a recombinant SP-C protein with lipids (Venticute) were recently published.[82] The material was instilled into the lungs of patients with severe ARDS of multiple etiologies, and results showed no overall difference in mortality between the surfactant-treated group (36%) and standard therapy (32%). Of note, however, a post-hoc analysis showed a significant interaction between the surfactant treatment and the mechanism of lung injury. Patients with "direct" lung injuries, induced by pneumonia and/or aspiration, had a statistically significantly higher survival rate when treated with surfactant compared to standard therapy; no such relationship existed for patients with "indirect" causes of ARDS, such as sepsis and trauma. The conclusions and recommendations from this study were that a follow-up, prospectively designed clinical trial focused on patients with direct lung injuries was warranted (and is currently underway), and that a more prolonged treatment period involving a larger number of doses may be required in such critically ill patients.

In summary, there is relatively strong physiologic rationale for administering exogenous surfactant to patients with acute lung injury. Although results of clinical trials have been inconsistent, the information gained from these trials, as well as preclinical studies, has been insightful and supports the need for further research in this area. In the next section, the various factors that have been shown to influence a host's response to exogenous surfactant will be reviewed.

FACTORS INFLUENCING THE EFFICACY OF EXOGENOUS SURFACTANT

SURFACTANT PREPARATION

A number of surfactant preparations have been tested in clinical trials involving patients with ARDS, and are generally classified based on their surfactant protein content

TABLE 60-1 Published Phase II/III Clinical Trials Involving Exogenous Surfactant

Surfactant Preparation/ Concentration	Delivery Method	Dose	Mortality (vs Standard Therapy)	Ref.
Exosurf (13.5 mg DPPC/ml)	Aerosolization	112 mg/kg per day × 5 days	41% vs 41%	(79)
Survanta (25 mg DPPC/ml)	Bolus instillation	4 or 8 doses of 50 or 100 mg/kg	19% vs 44%	(80)
Venticute (25 mg DPPC/ml)	Bolus instillation	Up to 4 doses of 50 mg lipid/kg	36% vs 32%	(82)

TABLE 60-2 Exogenous Surfactant Preparations

Brand Name	Source/Composition
Natural Protein-Containing	
Survanta	Bovine-lung tissue extract
BLES	Bovine-lung lavage extract
Infasurf	Bovine-calf lavage extract
Alveofact	Bovine-lung lavage extract
Curosurf	Porcine-lung tissue extract
HL-10	Porcine-lung tissue extract
Synthetic/Recombinant Protein-Containing	
Surfaxin	DPPC[a], POPG[b], PA[c], "SP-B-like peptide"
Venticute	DPPC[a], POPG[b], PA[c], rSP-C[d]
Non Protein-Containing	
ALEC	DPPC[a], PG[e]
Exosurf	DPPC[a], hexadecanol, tyloxepol

[a]DPPC, dipalmitoyl-phosphatidylcholine
[b]POPG, palmitoyloleoylphosphatidyl glycerol
[c]PA, palmitic acid
[d]rSP-C, recombinant human SP-C
[e]PG, phosphatidyl glycerol

(Table 60-2). Natural surfactant products contain various amounts of SP-B and SP-C along with natural lipids. They are derived from either bovine (Survanta, Infasurf, Alveofact, and bovine lipid extract surfactant [BLES]) or porcine (Curosurf and HL-10) sources, and have consistently been shown to have excellent biophysical activity. Currently available synthetic surfactant preparations contain either synthetic or recombinant surfactant-specific proteins combined with commercially available lipids. These preparations include Venticute and Surfaxin. Venticute is composed of a recombinant SP-C protein together with DPPC and smaller amounts of palmitoyloleoylphosphatidyl glycerol (POPG) and palmitic acid.[82] Surfaxin contains a synthetic SP-B-like peptide as well as DPPC, POPG, and palmitic acid.[81] Both have been tested in preclinical studies involving models of acute lung injury and are currently being evaluated in clinical trials as noted above. Two other synthetic surfactant preparations previously used in neonates with nRDS and tested in patients with ARDS include Exosurf (DPPC; hexadecanol, and tyloxepol) and artificial lung-expanding compound (ALEC, DPPC and PG).[83] These preparations contain no surfactant proteins, perhaps explaining the poor results of these latter trials. No further studies are being conducted with these preparations at this time. Animal studies that have directly compared the various surfactant preparations have generally shown that those containing surfactant proteins, either from natural or synthetic/recombinant sources, are superior to those having no proteins.[84,85] Furthermore, meta-analyses of several studies involving neonates with nRDS have also shown that clinical trials utilizing natural products resulted in better outcomes than those using the synthetic preparations with no surfactant proteins.[86]

Based on preclinical data and results of these clinical trials, it is likely that some type of protein-containing surfactant will be required for optimal results in patients with ALI/ARDS. Whether the natural products will be more effective than the protein-containing, synthetic surfactants in

this setting is unknown, and will be difficult to prove in this complex patient population. As a result, other factors may need to be considered when making this decision. For example, although animal-based products may well be as effective or superior to any synthetic products available (or to be developed in the future), they have the theoretical potential of transmitting molecules and/or infectious agents to the host. This, however, has not been demonstrated over the past 20 years of use in neonates. In addition, given the potentially large patient population that would ultimately benefit from this therapy, even if natural products are shown to be superior, availability may be a factor because of resource limitations. These issues do not exist for the recombinant/synthetic preparations, perhaps favoring further development of effective and easily manufactured synthetic products.

SURFACTANT DELIVERY AND DOSING

The various delivery methods that have been utilized for administering exogenous surfactant to patients with acute lung injury include: (1) instillation of a liquid bolus through the endotracheal tube,[82] (2) bronchoscopic instillation of smaller aliquots of surfactant to the various segments of the lung,[87] (3) sequential segmental lavage of lung units with a surfactant preparation via the bronchoscope,[81] and (4) aerosolization of surfactant via a nebulizer.[79] For all methods of delivery, the common goal is to deliver sufficient amounts of material to the distal lung in an optimal distribution pattern. Unfortunately, the lung injury in critically ill patients is often nonuniform and varies over time as lung dysfunction deteriorates. As a result, it is likely that individual treatment strategies may have to be tailored to the specific patient involved. For example, patients with severe lung dysfunction with a nonuniform distribution of injury would not benefit from any aerosolized surfactant preparation, because relatively small quantities of surfactant are deposited within lung tissue and most of the material would be deposited in the most compliant regions of the lung, areas that need it the least.[88] In this situation, delivering large amounts of surfactant as a liquid bolus (50–200 mg lipid per kg body weight), either through the endotracheal tube or in sequential aliquots (with or without segmental lavage) via the bronchoscope, may be superior. The lavage approach may offer the advantage of removing inflammatory cell products and serum proteins, which tend to inhibit surfactant function, while leaving sufficient quantities of surfactant behind in the alveoli to improve lung function.[81,89] Although this latter approach is rather invasive, is more time-consuming, and requires a skilled bronchoscopist to perform when compared to the bolus instillation technique, it may be optimal for specific types of severely ill patients. Currently, there is little doubt that patients with severe lung injury will require relatively large doses of surfactant in order to overcome surface tension–inhibitory forces within the injured lung, the latter being induced either by serum proteins leaking into the airspace or inactivation of surfactant via nitration and/or oxidation, as previously described.[70–72,77] The decision as to whether surfactant should be delivered via a liquid bolus, or by using a segmental lavage approach, will likely depend on the status of the patient and/or the feasibility and preference of the attending physician, assuming of course that the results of the ongoing clinical trials are positive.

Aerosolization would only be applicable to patients with milder disease who require smaller amounts of material and have relatively uniform injuries, a situation in which exogenous surfactant administration has yet to be tested in the clinical setting. In addition, a consistent and cost-effective nebulizer able to deliver reasonable amounts of surfactant over an extended period of time is not yet available. Despite the numerous studies that have evaluated these various delivery methods in animals and humans, it is still not clear which delivery method should be used for specific types of patients, how much surfactant should be delivered per dose for the various delivery methods available, and how many doses will be required over time for each patient to achieve an optimal outcome. More research is certainly required in this area.

EFFECTS OF MECHANICAL VENTILATION

Mechanical ventilation is an important supportive therapy for patients with ALI/ARDS, and has recently been shown to impact the outcome of these patients.[76] Similar to its impact on the endogenous surfactant system, the specific mode of mechanical ventilation used in surfactant-treated lungs can influence the metabolism of the administered material. For example, animal studies have shown that lower tidal volumes resulted in superior physiologic responses compared to higher tidal volumes after exogenous surfactant was delivered as a liquid bolus; this was associated with less conversion of the administered LA forms into dysfunctional SA.[90,91] Clinically, these findings suggest that the mode of mechanical ventilation may have a significant impact on the duration of response to a particular dose of surfactant, which in turn would decrease the number of doses required. It is also important to optimize ventilation during and immediately after surfactant administration in order to optimize the distribution of the material and prevent airway obstruction. PEEP levels must be maintained during instillation to prevent alveolar collapse, and adequate tidal volumes must be delivered immediately after instillation to maintain recruitment and enhance peripheral distribution of the material.[90–92]

Similar to the situation in the non–surfactant treated lung, the use of recruitment maneuvers in conjunction with exogenous surfactant is somewhat controversial, with both beneficial and even harmful effects reported.[93,94] It is likely that the timing and specific nature of the maneuver (i.e., frequency, duration, and so on) will impact its effects in the clinical setting of surfactant administration.

Finally, given the promising, albeit early, results of high-frequency oscillation (HFO) in patients with acute lung injury, some comments regarding its potential in the setting of exogenous surfactant administration are warranted. Very few studies have been performed to date, and results are inconsistent. Froese et al demonstrated that HFO was superior to conventional modes of ventilation after surfactant administration in saline-lavaged adult rabbits, but relatively high mean airway pressures were required to maintain lung recruitment with HFO.[95] On the other hand, a recent study in saline-lavaged adult sheep showed that exogenous surfactant may obstruct conducting airways when delivered in association with HFO; a period of more conventional tidal ventilation during and immediately following administration may be required for optimal distribution before switching over to HFO.[96] Further studies are required to determine how HFO and recruitment maneuvers should be used in conjunction with exogenous surfactant administration in patients with ALI/ARDS.

NATURE OF THE UNDERLYING INJURY

As alluded to in previous sections, the efficacy of a particular surfactant treatment strategy may predominantly depend on the specific type of patient involved, and, in this regard, influence all of the factors previously described (Fig. 60-4). ALI/ARDS can be initiated by several different insults including those directly affecting the lung, such as aspiration and pneumonia, as well as indirect causes, such as systemic sepsis and trauma. The results of the recent phase III clinical trial, involving the synthetic surfactant preparation Venticute administered to patients with various types of ARDS, suggested that patients with direct lung injuries initiating the development of the disease would benefit the most from surfactant therapy.[82] A note of caution is warranted, however, because these results may not necessarily reflect an alternative strategy involving a different surfactant preparation given via a different dosing regimen and delivery technique. Previous studies have shown that each of these factors in and of themselves may influence a host's response to surfactant; thus predicting consistent outcomes can be a problem in this patient population. Unfortunately, animal models that accurately reflect the various types of patients who develop ARDS, and ultimately those who would respond to exogenous surfactant, are lacking. Patients with ARDS have a complex pathophysiology involving various types and severities of insults. As a result, we are left with the challenge of pursuing large, expensive,

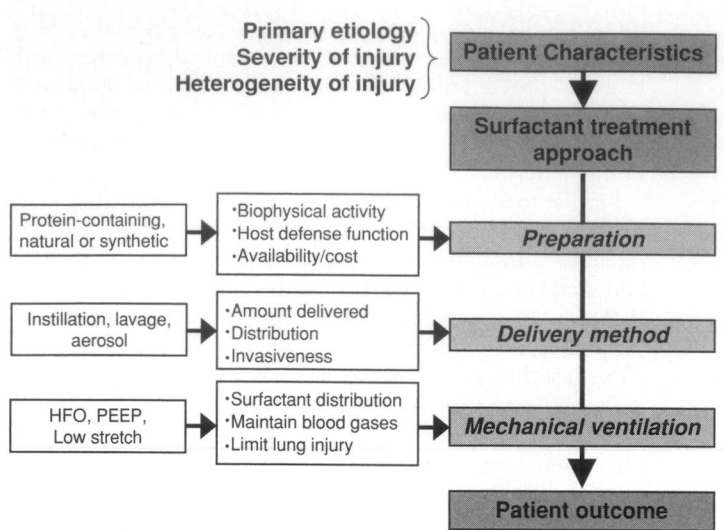

FIGURE 60-4 Various factors may influence a host's response to exogenous surfactant, including specific surfactant preparation, dosing and delivery method, mode of mechanical ventilation implemented during and after surfactant administration, and nature of the underlying injury. See text for details.

and time-consuming clinical trials with no guarantees that they will demonstrate beneficial results. It is imperative, therefore, that we gain as much insight as possible from the preclinical and clinical studies that have been conducted to date. Based on the information currently available, therefore, a study evaluating Venticute, instilled as a liquid bolus to patients with direct lung injuries induced by pneumonia or aspiration, as well as a study testing Surfaxin, administered via segmental lung lavage in patients with severe ARDS, are underway and should yield interesting results.

Future Research Directions

COMBINATION THERAPIES

The biophysical properties of surfactant make it a suitable candidate for combination therapy involving other agents.[97] For example, an effective surfactant adsorbs readily to the air-liquid interface and spreads rapidly across the alveolar space.[2,3,37] This puts the surfactant, as well as the added agent, in close proximity to alveolar epithelial cells as well as the pulmonary vasculature, ideally with a good distribution pattern. These particular characteristics would result in high local pulmonary concentrations of a therapeutic agent with minimal side effects or toxicity. Indeed, surfactant has been shown to enhance the delivery as well as the expression of an adenoviral vector, and has been shown to improve the peripheral distribution and activity of recombinant superoxide dismutases and antibiotics.[98–100] The combination of exogenous surfactant with other physiologically active compounds, such as nitric oxide and perfluorocarbons, has also been tested and shown to have synergistic effects.[101,102] Future applications for surfactant as a carrier vehicle and/or as part of a cocktail mixture for patients with lung injury require further investigation.

ROLE OF SURFACTANT IN OTHER DISEASES

The vast majority of surfactant research that has focused on the mature lung has involved animal models and/or

patients with ALI/ARDS. Recent evidence would suggest, however, that alterations in the endogenous surfactant system may also be implicated in several other diseases of the lung, which would potentially lead to novel therapeutic approaches to these disorders in the future. One such disease reflecting alterations in endogenous surfactant metabolism is pulmonary alveolar proteinosis.[103] Increased synthesis and secretion together with decreased catabolism of surfactant results in excessive accumulation of surfactant lipids and proteins within the airspace. Removal of this excess material via whole lung lavage has resulted in long-term benefits for most patients.

In addition, given the extensive in vitro and in vivo data showing that the various components of surfactant can affect immune-cell regulation, inflammatory cell responses, and bacterial and viral proliferation/killing, it is likely that surfactant also plays an important role in bacterial and viral pneumonia. Surfactant alterations have been consistently reported in these patients. A clinical trial involving children with respiratory syncytial virus showed improved lung function and shorter hospital stays in those receiving exogenous surfactant compared to non–surfactant treated control subjects.[104,105] It is difficult, however, to separate the biophysical aspects of the improved lung function observed from the immunomodulatory effects of surfactant on the development and progression of the infection itself. More animal studies and clinical trials evaluating early exogenous surfactant administration in this setting are necessary to determine if surfactant plays an important role in pulmonary infections.

Surfactant alterations have also been documented in patients with various interstitial lung diseases. These reports have shown decreased lipid and SP-A levels in the bronchoalveolar lavage fluid of patients with idiopathic pulmonary fibrosis, which in one study predicted 5-year survival.[106,107] SP-A levels were actually increased in the lungs of patients with sarcoidosis and hypersensitivity pneumonitis, suggesting that, similarly to the various types of ARDS, the role of surfactant may vary according to the specific type of interstitial disease and insult involved.[108]

Various studies suggest that surfactant plays an important role in obstructive lung diseases.[109] Surfactant facilitates ciliary function, downregulates some of the inflammatory processes implicated in these diseases (asthma and cystic fibrosis), and has been shown to be important in maintaining the patency of conducting airways.[46,47] Although various studies have reported surfactant alterations in most obstructive diseases, only a few small studies have tested the efficacy of exogenous surfactant administration in this setting.[110] The results of these preliminary studies suggest that surfactant may be effective as therapy in asthma, although further research is required.

Finally, surfactant changes were demonstrated in the ischemia-reperfusion injury associated with lung transplantation. Exogenous surfactant, administered to the donor lung before storage, mitigated this injury, even in the setting of prolonged organ storage.[111] This indication for surfactant administration has not been tested in clinical trials to date.

Summary and Conclusions

Pulmonary surfactant is critical for maintaining alveolar stability and normal lung function. Although the composition of surfactant is relatively consistent among mammalian species, there is still much to be learned regarding the specific functions of the individual components of surfactant, particularly with respect to host defense. Most research to date involving surfactant perturbations in the mature lung have focused on the lung injury associated with ALI/ARDS, and has lead to clinical trials evaluating the efficacy of exogenous surfactant administration in this setting. Unfortunately, results of these trials have been inconsistent. Careful analyses of these results, together with extensive preclinical studies, have provided important insight into the various factors that may influence a host's response to this therapy. This has lead to ongoing, more focused trials tailored to the specific types of patients that would most likely benefit from this intervention. Research conducted over the next few years will not only yield potentially exciting results from these studies, but also provide important insight into the role of the surfactant system in other lung diseases such as pneumonia and obstructive and restrictive disorders.

References

1. Postle AD, Heeley EL, Wilton DC. A comparison of the molecular species compositions of mammalian lung surfactant phospholipids. Comp Biochem Physiol A Mol Integr Physiol 2001; 129:65–73.
2. Clements JA, Nellenbogen J, Traham HJ. Pulmonary surfactant and evolution of the lungs. Science 1970; 169:603–4.
3. Goerke J. Pulmonary surfactant: functions and molecular composition. Biochim Biophys Acta 1998; 1408:79–89.
4. Possmayer F. A proposed nomenclature for pulmonary surfactant-associated proteins. Am Rev Respir Dis 1988; 138:990–8.
5. Kuroki Y, Voelker DR. Pulmonary surfactant proteins. J Biol Chem 1994; 269:25943–6.
6. Weaver T, Conkright J. Function of surfactant proteins B and C. Annu Rev Physiol 2001; 63:555–78.
7. Takahashi A, Waring AJ, Amirkhanian J, Fan B, Taeusch HW. Structure-function relationships of bovine pulmonary surfactant proteins: SP-B and SP-C. Biochim Biophys Acta 1990; 1044:43–9.
8. Veldhuizen EJ, Batenburg JJ, Van Golde LM, Haagsman HP. The role of surfactant proteins in DPPC enrichment of surface films. Biophys J 2000; 79:3164–71.
9. Zaltash S, Palmblad M, Curstedt T, Johansson J, Persson B. Pulmonary surfactant protein B: a structural model and a functional analogue. Biochim Biophys Acta 2000; 1466:179–86.
10. Johansson J. Structure and properties of surfactant protein C. Biochim Biophys Acta 1998; 1408:161–72.
11. Mason RJ, Greene K, Voelker DR. Surfactant protein A and surfactant protein D in health and disease. Am J Physiol 1998; 275:L1–L13.
12. Crouch E, Wright J. Surfactant proteins a and d and pulmonary host defense. Annu Rev Physiol 2001; 63:521–54.
13. McCormack FX, Whitsett JA. The pulmonary collectins, SP-A and SP-D, orchestrate innate immunity in the lung. J Clin Invest 2002; 109:707–12.
14. Pison U, Max M, Neuendank A, Weissbach S, Pietschmann S. Host defence capacities of pulmonary surfactant: Evidence for 'non-surfactant' functions of the surfactant system. Eur J Clin Invest 1994; 24:586–99.
15. Wright JR, Hawgood S. Pulmonary surfactant metabolism. Clin Chest Med 1989; 10:83–93.
16. Wright JR, Dobbs LG. Regulation of pulmonary surfactant secretion and clearance. Annu Rev Physiol 1991; 53:395–414.
17. Rooney SA. Regulation of surfactant secretion. Comp Biochem Physiol A Mol Integr Physiol 2001; 129:233–43.
18. Hawgood S, Poulain F. The pulmonary collectins and surfactant metabolism. Annu Rev Physiol 2001; 63:495–519.
19. McCormack FX. Structure, processing and properties of surfactant protein A. Biochim Biophys Acta 1998; 1408:109–31.
20. Froh D, Bonzales LW, Ballard P. Secretion of surfactant protein A and phosphatidylcholine from type II cells of human fetal lung. Am J Respir Cell Mol Biol 1993; 8:556–61.
21. Crouch E, Parghi D, Kuan S-F, et al. Surfactant protein D: Subcellular localization in nonciliated bronchiolar epithelial cells. Am J Physiol 1992; 263:L60–6.
22. Crouch EC. Structure, biologic properties, and expression of surfactant protein D. Biochim Biophys Acta 1998; 1408:278–89.
23. Wirtz HRW, Dobbs LG. Calcium mobilization and exocytosis after one mechanical stretch of lung epithelial cells. Science 1990; 250:1266–9.
24. Suzuki Y, Fujita Y, Kogishi K. Reconstitution of tubular myelin from synthetic lipids and proteins associated with pig pulmonary surfactant. Am Rev Respir Dis 1989; 140:75–81.
25. Williams MC, Hawgood S, Hamilton RL. Changes in lipid structure produced by surfactant proteins SP-A, SP-B, and SP-C. Am J Respir Cell Mol Biol 1991; 5:41–50.
26. Baritussio A, Bellina L, Carraro R, et al. Heterogeneity of alveolar surfactant in the rabbit: composition, morphology, and labelling of subfractions isolated by centrifugation of lung lavage. Eur J Clin Invest 1984; 14:24–9.
27. Gross NJ, Narine KR. Surfactant subtypes in mice: characterization and quantitation. J Appl Physiol 1989; 66:342–9.
28. Putz G, Goerke J, Clements JA. Surface activity of rabbit pulmonary surfactant subfractions at different concentrations in a captive bubble. J Appl Physiol 1994; 77:597–605.
29. Wright JR. Clearance and recycling of pulmonary surfactant. Am J Physiol 1990; 259:L1–12.

30. Brackenbury AM, Malloy JL, McCaig LA, et al. Evaluation of alveolar surfactant aggregates in vitro and in vivo. Eur Respir J 2002; 19:41–6.

31. Gross NJ, Schultz RM. Requirements for extracellular metabolism of pulmonary surfactant: Tentative identification of serine protease. Am J Physiol 1992; 262:L446–53.

32. Krishnasamy S, Gross NJ, Teng AL, et al. Lung "surfactant convertase" is a member of the carboxylesterase family. Biochem Biophys Res Commun 1997; 235:180–4.

33. Veldhuizen RA, Yao L, Lewis JF. An examination of the different variables affecting surfactant aggregate conversion in vitro. Exp Lung Res 1999; 25:127–41.

34. Veldhuizen RAW, Marcou J, Yao L-J, et al. Alveolar surfactant aggregate conversion in ventilated normal and injured rabbits. Am J Physiol 1996; 270:L152–8.

35. Ito Y, Veldhuizen R, Yao L, et al. Ventilation strategies affect surfactant aggregate conversion in acute lung injury. Am J Respir Crit Care 1997; 155:493–9.

36. Veldhuizen RAW, Ito Y, Marcou J, et al. Effects of lung injury on pulmonary surfactant aggregate conversion in vivo and in vitro. Am J Physiol 1997; 16:L872–8.

37. Pattle RE. Properties, function and origin of the alveolar lining layer. Nature 1955; 175:1125–6.

38. Avery M, Mead J. Surface properties in relation to atelectasis and hyaline membrane disease. Am J Dis Child 1959; 97:517–23.

39. Enhorning G, Shennan A, Possmayer F, et al. Prevention of neonatal respiratory distress syndrome by tracheal instillation of surfactant: a randomized clinical trial. Pediatrics 1985; 76:145–53.

40. Dunn MS, Shennan AT, Possmayer F. Single- versus multiple-dose surfactant replacement therapy in neonates of 30 to 36 weeks' gestation with respiratory distress syndrome. Pediatrics 1990; 86:564–71.

41. Nogee LM, Garnier G, Dietz HC, et al. A mutation in the surfactant protein B gene responsible for fatal neonatal respiratory disease in multiple kindreds. J Clin Invest 1994; 93:1860–3.

42. Tokieda K, Whitsett JA, Clark JC, et al. Pulmonary dysfunction in neonatal SP-B-deficient mice. Am J Physiol 1997; 273:L875–L882.

43. Glasser SW, Burhans MS, Korfhagen TR, et al. Altered stability of pulmonary surfactant in SP-C-deficient mice. Proc Natl Acad Sci USA 2001; 98:6366–71.

44. von Neergaard K. New interpretations of basic concepts of respiratory mechanisms. A Gesamte Exp Med 1929; 66:373–94.

45. Albert RK, Lakshmirnarayan S, Hildebrandt J, et al. Increased surface tension favors pulmonary edema formation in anesthetized dogs' lungs. J Clin Invest 1979; 63:1015–8.

46. Enhorning G, Holm BA. Disruption of pulmonary surfactant's ability to maintain openness of a narrow tube. J Appl Physiol 1993; 74:2922–7.

47. DeSanctis GT, Tomkiewicz RP, Rubin BK, et al. Exogenous surfactant enhances mucociliary clearance in the anesthetized dog. Eur Respir J 1994; 7:1616–21.

48. van Iwaarden F, Welmers B, Verhoef J, et al. Pulmonary surfactant protein A enhances the host-defense mechanism of rat alveolar macrophages. Am J Respir Cell Mol Biol 1990; 2:91–8.

49. Weissbach S, Neuendan A, Pettersson M, et al. Surfactant protein A modulates release of reactive oxygen species from alveolar macrophages. Am J Physiol 1994; 267:L660–6.

50. van Iwaarden JF, Shimizu H, Van Golde PHM, et al. Rat surfactant protein D enhances the production of oxygen radicals by rat alveolar macrophages. Biochem J 1992; 286:5–8.

51. Zhu S, Ware LB, Geiser T, et al. Increased levels of nitrate and surfactant protein A nitration in the pulmonary edema fluid of patients with acute lung injury. Am J Respir Crit Care Med 2001; 163:166–72.

52. LeVine AM, Whitsett JA, Gwozdz JA, et al. Distinct effects of surfactant protein A or D deficiency during bacterial infection on the lung. J Immunol 2000; 165:3934–40.

53. LeVine AM, Kurak KE, Wright JR, et al. Surfactant protein-A binds group B *Streptococcus*, enhancing phagocytosis and clearance from lungs of surfactant protein-A-deficient mice. Am J Respir Cell Mol Biol 1999; 20:279–86.

54. Hartshorn K, Crouch EC, Ehite MR, et al. Evidence for a protective role of pulmonary surfactant protein D (SP-D) against influenza A viruses. J Clin Invest 1994; 94:311–9.

55. Wert S, Jones T, Korfhagen T, Fisher J, Whitsett J. Spontaneous emphysema in surfactant protein D gene-targeted mice. Chest 2000; 117:248S.

56. Wright JR. Immunomodulatory functions of surfactant. Physiol Rev 1997; 77:931–62.

57. Pison U, Max M, Neudendan A, et al. Host defense capacities of pulmonary surfactant: Evidence for "non-surfactant" functions of the surfactant system. Eur J Clin Invest 1994; 24:586–99.

58. Bernard GR, Artigas A, Brigham KL, et al. The American-European consensus conference on ARDS: definitions, mechanisms, relevant outcomes, and clinical trial coordination. Am J Respir Crit Care Med 1994; 149:818–24.

59. Artigas A, Bernard GR, Carlet J, et al. The American-European Consensus Conference on ARDS, part 2: Ventilatory, pharmacologic, supportive therapy, study design strategies, and issues related to recovery and remodeling. Acute respiratory distress syndrome. Am J Respir Crit Care Med 1998; 157(4 Pt 1):1332–47.

60. Ashbaugh DG, Bigelow DB, Petty TL, Levine BE. Acute respiratory distress in adults. Lancet 1967; 2:319–23.

61. Lewis JF, Jobe A. Surfactant and the adult respiratory distress syndrome. Am Rev Resp Dis 1993; 147:218–33.

62. Gunther A, Siebert C, Schmidt R, et al. Surfactant alterations in severe pneumonia, acute respiratory distress syndrome, and cardiogenic lung edema. Am J Respir Crit Care Med 1996; 153:176–84.

63. Veldhuizen RA, McCaig LA, Akino T, Lewis JF. Pulmonary surfactant subfractions in patients with the acute respiratory distress syndrome. Am J Respir Crit Care Med 1995; 152:1867–71.

64. Doyle IR, Bersten AD, Nicholas TE. Surfactant proteins-A and -B are elevated in plasma of patients with acute respiratory failure. Am J Respir Crit Care Med 1997; 156:1217–29.

65. Greene KE, Ye S, Mason RJ, Parsons PE. Serum surfactant protein-A levels predict development of ARDS in at-risk patients. Chest 1999; 116:90S–1S.

66. Lewis JF, Ikegami M, Jobe AH. Altered surfactant function and metabolism in rabbits with acute lung injury. J Appl Physiol 1990; 69:2303–10.

67. Uhlig S, Brasch F, Wollin L, et al. Functional and fine structural changes in isolated rat lungs challenged with endotoxin ex vivo and in vitro. Am J Pathol 1995; 146:1235–47.

68. Hite RD, Seeds MC, Jacinto RB, et al. Hydrolysis of surfactant-associated phosphatidylcholine by mammalian secretory phospholipases a2. Am J Physiol 1998; 275:L740–7.

69. Lee CT, Fein AM, Lippmann M, et al. Elastolytic activity in pulmonary lavage fluid from patients with adult respiratory-distress syndrome. N Engl J Med 1981; 304:192–6.

70. Haddad IY, Pataki G, Hu P, et al. Quantitation of nitrotyrosine levels in lung sections of patients and animals with acute lung injury. J Clin Invest 1994; 94:2407–13.

71. Haddad IY, Zhu S, Ischiropoulos H, Matalon S. Nitration of surfactant protein A results in decreased ability to aggregate lipids. Am J Physiol 1996; 270:L281–8.

72. Zhu S, Kachel DL, Martin WJ, Matalon S. Nitrated SP-A does not enhance adherence of *Pneumocystis carinii* to alveolar macrophages. Am J Physiol 1998; 275:L1031–9.

73. Malloy J, McCaig L, Veldhuizen R, et al. Alterations of endogenous surfactant system in septic adult rats. Am J Respir Crit Care Med 1997; 156:617–23.

74. Malloy J, Veldhuizen R, Lewis J. Effects of ventilation on the surfactant system in sepsis-induced lung injury. J Appl Physiol 2000; 88:401–8.

75. Kerr C, Veldhuizen R, Lewis J. Effects of high frequency oscillation on alveolar surfactant aggregates in an acute lung injury model. Am J Respir Crit Care Med 2001; 164:237–42.

76. Brower RG, Matthay MA, Morris A, et al. Ventilation with lower tidal volumes as compared with traditional tidal volumes for acute lung injury and the acute respiratory distress syndrome. The Acute Respiratory Distress Syndrome Network. N Engl J Med 2000; 342:1301–8.

77. Seeger W, Grube C, Gunther A, Schmidt R. Surfactant inhibition by plasma proteins: differential sensitivity of various surfactant preparations. Eur Respir J 1993; 6:971–7.

78. Lachmann B, Eijking EP, So KL, Gommers D. In vivo evaluation of the inhibitory capacity of human plasma on exogenous surfactant function. Intensive Care Med 1994; 20:6–11.

79. Anzueto A, Baughman RP, Guntupalli KK, et al. Aerosolized surfactant in adults with sepsis-induced acute respiratory distress syndrome. N Engl J Med 1996; 334:1417–21.

80. Gregory TJ, Steinberg KP, Spragg R, et al. Bovine surfactant therapy for patients with acute respiratory distress syndrome. Am J Respir Crit Care Med 1997; 155:1309–15.

81. Wiswell TE, Smith RM, Katz LB, et al. Bronchopulmonary segmental lavage with Surfaxin (KL(4)-surfactant) for acute respiratory distress syndrome. Am J Respir Crit Care Med 1999; 160:1188–95.

82. Spragg R, Lewis J, Walmrath H, et al. Effect of recombinant surfactant protein C based surfactant on patients with the acute respiratory distress syndrome. N Engl J Med 2004; 351:884–92.

83. Takahashi A, Nemoto T, Fujiwara T. Biophysical properties of protein-free, totally synthetic pulmonary surfactants, ALEC and Exosurf, in comparison with surfactant TA. Acta Paediatr Jpn 1994; 36:613–8.

84. Corcoran JD, Berggren P, Sun B, et al. Comparison of surface properties and physiological effects of a synthetic and a natural surfactant in preterm rabbits. Arch Dis Child Fetal Neonatal Ed 1994; 71:F165–9.

85. Sood SL, Balaraman V, Finn KC, et al. Exogenous surfactants in a piglet model of acute respiratory distress syndrome. Am J Respir Crit Care Med 1996; 153:820–8.

86. Kresch MJ, Clive JM. Meta-analyses of surfactant replacement therapy of infants with birth weights less than 2000 grams. J Perinatol 1998; 18:276–83.

87. Walmrath D, Grimminger F, Pappert D, et al. Bronchoscopic administration of bovine natural surfactant in ARDS and septic shock; impact on gas exchange and haemodynamics. Eur Respir J 2002; 19:805–10.

88. Lewis JF, McCaig LA. Aerosolized versus instilled exogenous surfactant in a nonuniform pattern of lung injury. Am Rev Respir Dis 1993; 148:1187–93.

89. Balaraman V, Meister J, Ku TL, Sood SL, et al. Lavage administration of dilute surfactants after acute lung injury in neonatal piglets. Am J Respir Crit Care Med 1998; 158:12–7.

90. Ito Y, Manwell SEE, Kerr CL, et al. Effect of ventilation strategies on the efficacy of exogenous surfactant therapy in a rabbit model of acute lung injury. Am J Respir Crit Care Med 1998; 157:149–55.

91. Kerr CL, Ito Y, Manwell SE, et al. Effects of surfactant distribution and ventilation strategies on efficacy of exogenous surfactant. J Appl Physiol 1998; 85:676–84.

92. Ikegami M, Ueda T, Absolom D, et al. Changes in exogenous surfactant in ventilated preterm lamb lungs. Am Rev Respir Dis 1993; 148:837–44.

93. Bjorklund LJ, Ingimarsson J, Curstedt T, et al. Lung recruitment at birth does not improve lung function in immature lambs receiving surfactant. Acta Anaesthesiol Scand 2001; 45: 986–93.

94. Krause MF, Jakel C, Haberstroh J, et al. Alveolar recruitment promotes homogeneous surfactant distribution in a piglet model of lung injury. Pediatr Res 2001; 50:34–43.

95. Froese AB, McCulloch PR, Sugiura M, et al. Optimizing alveolar expansion prolongs the effectiveness of exogenous surfactant therapy in the adult rabbit. Am Rev Respir Dis 1993; 148:569–77.

96. Kerr C, McCaig L, Veldhuizen R, Lewis J. High frequency oscillation and exogenous surfactant administration in lung injured adult sheep. Crit Care Med 2003; 164:237–42.

97. Haitsma JJ, Lachmann U, Lachmann B. Exogenous surfactant as a drug delivery agent. Adv Drug Deliv Rev 2001; 47:197–207.

98. Jobe AH, Ikegami M, Yei S, Whitsett JA, Trapnell B. Surfactant effects on aerosolized and instilled adenoviral-mediated gene transfer. Hum Gene Ther 1996; 7:697–704.

99. Katkin JP, Husser RC, Langston C, Welty SE. Exogenous surfactant enhances the delivery of recombinant adenoviral vectors to the lung. Hum Gene Ther 1997; 8:171–6.

100. van't Veen A, Mouton JW, Gommers D, Lachmann B. Pulmonary surfactant as vehicle for intratracheally instilled tobramycin in mice infected with *Klebsiella pneumoniae*. Br J Pharmacol 1996; 119:1145–8.

101. Hartog A, Gommers D, van't Veen A, Erdmann W, Lachmann B. Exogenous surfactant and nitric oxide have a synergistic effect in improving gas exchange in experimental ARDS. Adv Exp Med Biol 1997; 428:277–9.

102. Tarczy-Hornoch P, Hildebrandt J, Mates EA, et al. Effects of exogenous surfactant on lung pressure-volume characteristics during liquid ventilation. J Appl Physiol 1996; 80:1764–71.

103. Doyle IR, Davidson KG, Barr HA, et al. Quantity and structure of surfactant proteins vary among patients with alveolar proteinosis. Am J Respir Crit Care Med 1998; 157:658–64.

104. Van Daal GJ, Bos JA, Eijking EP, et al. Surfactant replacement therapy improves pulmonary mechanics in end-stage influenza A pneumonia in mice. Am Rev Respir Dis 1992; 145:859–63.

105. Tibby SM, Hatherill M, Wright SM, et al. Exogenous surfactant supplementation in infants with respiratory syncytial virus bronchiolitis. Am J Respir Crit Care Med 2000; 162: 1251–6.

106. McCormack FX, King TEJ, Voelker DR, et al. Idiopathic pulmonary fibrosis. Abnormalities in the bronchoalveolar lavage content of surfactant protein A. Am Rev Respir Dis 1991; 144:160–6.

107. McCormack FX, King TE Jr, Bucher BL, et al. Surfactant protein A predicts survival in idiopathic pulmonary fibrosis. Am J Respir Crit Care Med 1995; 152:751–9.

108. Hamm H, Luhrs J, Guzman y Rotaeche J, et al. Elevated surfactant protein A in bronchoalveolar lavage fluids from sarcoidosis and hypersensitivity pneumonitis patients. Chest 1994; 106:1766–70.

109. Hohlfeld J, Fabel H, Hamm H. The role of pulmonary surfactant in obstructive airway disease. Eur Respir J 1997; 10:482–91.

110. Lin M, Wang L, Li E, et al. Pulmonary surfactant given prophylactically alleviates an asthma attack in guinea pigs. Clin Exp Allergy 1996; 26:270–5.

111. Novick RJ, Veldhuizen RAW, Possmayer F, et al. Exogenous surfactant therapy in thirty-eight hour lung graft preservation for transplantation. J Thorac Cardiovasc Surg 1994; 108: 259–68.

Chapter 61

INHALED NITRIC OXIDE

KLAUS LEWANDOWSKI

As the saying goes, unexpected scientific discoveries are often the most important. The "principle of limited sloppiness," a term coined to describe fortuitous or accidental discoveries, hit in the 1970s, when Zawadski, a technician in the laboratories of Robert F. Furchgott, failed to follow his superior's directions correctly and did not remove the endothelium in a rabbit aorta preparation. In this prepara-

tion, acetylcholine caused potent relaxation whereas contraction was expected. Shortly thereafter, it was established that acetylcholine was acting on endothelial cell receptors to produce a substance that could diffuse to the vascular smooth muscle and initiate its relaxation.[1] This substance was called *endothelium derived relaxing factor* (EDRF). It took another 8 years for independent working groups to confirm that the chemical structure of EDRF was identical to that of nitric oxide (NO).[2,3]

The scientific and global community honored the substance itself and its discovery by naming NO "Molecule of the Year" in 1992.[4] The Nobel Prize in Physiology or Medicine for 1998 was awarded jointly to Robert F. Furchgott, Louis J. Ignarro, and Ferid Murad, for their breakthroughs concerning "nitric oxide as a signaling molecule in the cardiovascular system."

NO is a colorless and odorless gas. It is a toxic air pollutant, present in motor vehicle exhaust and power plant effluent. The gas is found in the atmosphere in the range of 10–500 parts per billion (ppb), and locations with heavy vehicular traffic can exceed 1.5 parts per million (ppm). In the hot cone of a glowing cigarette, concentrations of 1000 ppm were measured in a 40-ml puff. NO is a free radical; it quickly reacts with oxygen to form poisonous nitrogen dioxide.

In the 1980s it became evident that NO is an essential molecule that regulates a wide range of human physiologic processes. Early studies revealed that NO is produced in endothelial cells and diffuses to vascular smooth muscle cells, where it mediates relaxation. Further studies demonstrated that the substance controls several other physiologic systems, including the immune system, platelet aggregation, and neurotransmission. The focus of this chapter is the prominent role of NO in respiratory physiology and its therapeutic application by inhalation.

Nitric Oxide Physiology in the Normal Respiratory System

ENDOGENOUS NITRIC OXIDE SYNTHESIS

Endogenous NO is produced by the enzyme system, nitric oxide synthase (NOS). In human subjects, NOS activity can be found in the epithelium of nasal and paranasal mucosa, the bronchial epithelium, type II alveolar epithelial cells, airway nerves, inflammatory cells, airway and vascular smooth muscle cells, and endothelial cells. Three isoforms of the enzyme have been identified: the constitutive neuronal NOS (nNOS), the inducible NOS (iNOS) that is incited by cytokines, and the constitutive endothelial NOS (eNOS). There is evidence that a fourth isoform, mitochondrial NOS (mtNOS) exists, which has important functions in cellular metabolism.

NO generated by nNOS in the peripheral nervous system acts as a neurotransmitter that modulates smooth muscle relaxation in the respiratory tract. Inflammatory cells express iNOS that enhances NO synthesis, thereby mediating anti-inflammatory effects. Concurrently, overproduction of

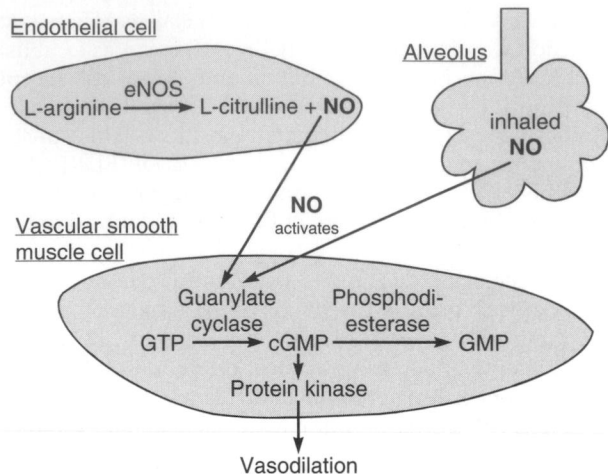

FIGURE 61-1 Endogenous or inhaled NO mediates vasodilation of vascular smooth muscle cells. NO is endogenously produced in endothelial cells of the pulmonary vasculature from the amino acid L-arginine, which is converted to L-citrulline and NO by the enzyme nitric oxide synthase. NO expressed by the endothelial cells, or inhaled NO, diffuses rapidly into the vascular smooth muscle cells, where it activates soluble guanylate cyclase, which converts GTP into cGMP. The high intracellular concentration of cGMP relaxes the smooth muscle via cGMP-dependent protein kinase. cGMP is inactivated by the enzyme phosphodiesterase, which catalyzes the conversion of cGMP to GMP. *NO*, nitric oxide; *iNO*, inhaled nitric oxide; *GTP*, guanosine triphosphate; *cGMP*, cyclic guanosine monophosphate; *eNOS*, endothelial nitric oxide synthase.

NO is also associated with the worsening of certain infectious diseases. NO formed by eNOS in vascular endothelial cells regulates pulmonary and systemic vascular tone. The schematic pathway of NO signal transduction is shown in Fig. 61-1.

ENDOGENOUS NITRIC OXIDE CONCENTRATIONS IN THE AIRWAYS

The concentrations of NO in healthy human airways differ depending on the measurement site. About 100 ppb were measured in the nasopharynx of healthy nonsmoking volunteers during nose breathing. During mouth breathing, even higher concentrations of 650 ppb were seen in the nasopharynx. The highest NO concentrations (1–30 ppm) were detected in the paranasal sinuses.[5] In the trachea of intubated patients the NO concentrations were markedly lower; they ranged between 5 and 10 ppb. Recently, it was demonstrated that the cilia of the epithelial cells of the maxillary sinuses contain high amounts of iNOS and can be viewed as a major production site of NO in the respiratory tract.[6]

FUNCTION OF ENDOGENOUS NITRIC OXIDE IN THE RESPIRATORY SYSTEM

Endogenous NO was suggested to be an important signaling molecule in numerous physiologic processes. Autoinhaled NO from the paranasal sinuses is able to induce selec-

tive pulmonary vasodilation in ventilated areas. The blood flow through well-aerated lung areas with higher intra-alveolar oxygen concentrations increases and ventilation-perfusion mismatch is antagonized. Endogenous NO is also involved in host defense and has direct microbicidal effects. Other findings substantiate that endogenous NO increases airway mucus secretion. Ciliary beat frequency, responsible for microbial clearance, is also enhanced by iNOS stimulators. Bronchodilation is suppressed by NOS inhibitors, indicating that endogenous NO modulates basal bronchial tone. Furthermore, endogenous NO possibly regulates the coagulation system. Formation of endogenous NO also seems to be involved in mediating pulmonary vasodilation during transition of the pulmonary circulation at birth.

Nitric Oxide Physiology in the Diseased Respiratory System

NITRIC OXIDE AND IMMUNE RESPONSES

Cytokines are produced and released in the lung during inflammatory processes. It has been shown that some cytokines induce the production of NO; others, however, inhibit the expression of iNOS. NO, in turn, is able to suppress lipopolysaccharide-stimulated cytokine production by macrophages. The gas seems to play a modulatory role in pro inflammatory cytokine secretion.[7]

T-helper 1 (Th1) cells are stimulated by antigens to express cytokines and large amounts of NO. The cytokines are also able to activate macrophages to express NO. NO, on the other hand, suppresses the cytokine secretion of Th1 cells. It is supposed that NO plays a self-regulatory role in host defense and inflammatory processes mediated by Th1 cells.

ASTHMA

In asthma, endogenous NO originates in airway epithelial cells, macrophages, and Th1 cells. Cytokines expressed by macrophages and Th1 cells are also able to activate iNOS in epithelial cells. In exhaled air of patients with asthma, high levels of NO can be measured. The question, however, of whether NO is beneficial or harmful in asthma remains unanswered. There is evidence that endogenous NO may protect the airways of asthmatic patients from bronchoconstriction.[8] This beneficial response seems to be mainly mediated by activation of eNOS. The high concentrations of NO in the airways of patients with asthma, however, are believed to mirror the stimulation of iNOS by proinflammatory cytokines and seem to have harmful effects, such as inflammation and increased vascular permeability.

CELL PROLIFERATION

NO was shown in vitro to suppress proliferation of human airway smooth muscle cells. Hypertrophy of airway smooth muscle cells can be found in asthma. In lung-transplant patients with chronic graft rejection, NO, synthesized by iNOS, is assumed to promote epithelial destruction and stimulate fibroproliferation.

CANCER

NO is genotoxic. It may initiate deoxyribonucleic acid mutations, strand breaks, and inhibit deoxyribonucleic acid repair systems either directly or by its oxides. NO and its oxides are suspected to initiate lung cancer. On the other hand, NO was found to have cytostatic and tumoricidal effects. In patients with lung cancer, increased exhaled NO levels can be measured, reflecting the high NO production rate of iNOS by macrophages.

PARANASAL SINUSES

NO concentrations are typically very high in the presence of infections. Astonishingly, the nasal concentration of NO is very low in sinusitis. This finding was traced back to significant inhibition of the expression of the paranasal NOS.[6] Low levels of endogenous NO in the paranasal sinuses may impair local host defense against bacterial or viral invaders; they may result in vasoconstriction of local blood vessels, intravascular platelet aggregation, and reduced ciliary-beat frequency and coordination.

Rationale for the Use of Exogenous Nitric Oxide

Inhaled nitric oxide (iNO) acts as a selective pulmonary vasodilator. As a gas, it reaches only ventilated alveoli and produces relaxation of the accompanying pulmonary blood vessels. iNO acts by producing vasodilation in well-ventilated lung units and redistributing pulmonary blood flow from unventilated to ventilated regions of the lung. The activity of iNO is limited to the area of deposition because NO is instantly inactivated by binding to hemoglobin at the moment it diffuses into the blood vessel. This explains why NO has no deleterious systemic side effects and acts almost exclusively in the pulmonary circulation (Fig. 61-2).

Indications and Outcome of Inhaled Nitric Oxide Therapy

ADULTS AND CHILDREN

Inhaling low concentrations of NO causes rapid and safe reduction of an elevated pulmonary artery pressure (PAP), and improves the impaired oxygenation in many patients without causing systemic hypotension. Additionally, the immunomodulatory effect of NO may be beneficial.

In patients with acute respiratory distress syndrome (ARDS), the improvement of oxygenation and reduction of PAP is an important therapeutic goal. iNO selectively enhances perfusion in ventilated lung areas and counteracts the ventilation-perfusion mismatch typical of this condition. Because NO works only in aerated lung tissue, mea-

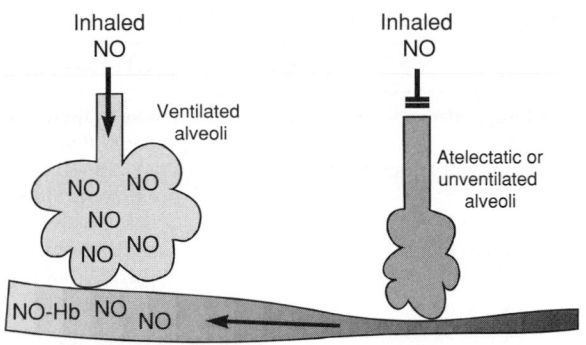

FIGURE 61-2 Inhaled NO selectively produces vasodilation in ventilated alveoli. iNO produces vasodilation in well-ventilated lung units and redistributes pulmonary blood flow from unventilated to ventilated lung regions. In patients with ventilation-perfusion mismatch (e.g., patients with ARDS), this leads to improvement in oxygenation and reduction of intrapulmonary right-to-left shunt. Selective vasodilation in the pulmonary circulation causes significant reduction of elevated pulmonary artery pressure; thus iNO is a valuable therapy in patients with all kinds of pulmonary hypertension. Systemic vasodilation does not occur because NO rapidly binds to hemoglobin and is thereby inactivated. *ARDS*, acute respiratory distress syndrome; *NO*, nitric oxide; *iNO*, inhaled nitric oxide; *Hb*, hemoglobin; *PAP*, pulmonary arterial pressure; $\dot{Q}_S/\dot{Q}_T$, intrapulmonary right-to-left shunt; Pa_{O_2}, arterial partial pressure of oxygen.

sures that recruit previously collapsed alveoli can enhance the beneficial effect of NO. The overall effect of iNO is often an impressively increased arterial partial pressure of oxygen (Pa_{O_2}) and a reduction of the elevated PAP. Several enthusiastic reports encouraged the hope that iNO would prove to be the promising new therapy that would ultimately improve the low survival rates in ARDS. Disappointingly, no randomized controlled trial has shown improved outcome.[9–14] In the results of one large[12] and one small[14] study, NO was found to lower the frequency of extracorporeal membrane oxygenation (ECMO). Follow-up investigations conducted after 8–38 months in acute lung injury or ARDS survivors who had been treated with iNO for longer than 4 hours revealed that their impairment in pulmonary function did not differ from the results of other published studies in comparable patient groups who had not received iNO therapy.[15]

The significant improvements in oxygenation and elevated PAP by iNO, however, could not be denied, and prompted scientists to study the effect of iNO in other diseases associated with pulmonary hypertension. Tables 61-1 and 61-2 present several conditions that can be treated with iNO. In most cases of high PAP, iNO is effective.

One-third of all patients with primary pulmonary hypertension benefit from iNO. In chronic pulmonary hypertension, the response to iNO predicts the efficacy of long-term therapy with oral vasodilators. Effects of iNO in patients with chronic obstructive pulmonary disease are not

TABLE 61-1 Applications for Inhaled Nitric Oxide Treatment in Adults and Children

Diagnosis	Effect of NO Inhalation
Acute lung injury	iNO was found to improve oxygenation during the first 48 hours after study entry. Mortality and days off MV were no different in the iNO group and the control group.[13]
Acute respiratory distress syndrome	iNO reduced elevated PAP, improved oxygenation, and decreased intrapulmonary right-to-left shunt during the first days of treatment.[34] No difference in ventilator-free days and mortality between iNO groups and placebo groups was seen.[55]
Primary pulmonary hypertension	Only 37% of patients responded with a marked decrease in total pulmonary resistance after iNO therapy. iNO did not induce a systemic effect.[56] In an experimental study, prolonged inhalation of NO protected against pulmonary hypertension and pulmonary vascular remodeling in response to chronic hypoxia.[57]
High-altitude pulmonary edema	In mountaineers prone to high-altitude pulmonary edema, iNO produced a marked decrease in PAP. In subjects with radiographic evidence of pulmonary edema, iNO improved oxygenation.[58]
Chronic pulmonary hypertension	The acute decrease of PAP with iNO is the best predictor of the long-term response to oral vasodilator treatment.[59]
Chronic obstructive pulmonary disease	Effects of iNO in patients with chronic obstructive pulmonary disease are contradictory. In one study, iNO improved oxygenation and reduced PAP while right ventricular ejection fraction increased.[60] In another study, iNO reduced PAP but did not improve right ventricular ejection fraction or arterial oxygenation in patients with acute respiratory failure caused by acute exacerbation.[61] In a third study, however, addition of iNO to inhaled oxygen did not improve or worsen arterial partial oxygen pressure, but caused a significant decrease in mean PAP. Cardiac output increased. Long-term use of iNO was effective.[62]
Asthma	Inhalation of NO results only in a minor relaxation of airway tone in adults.[63,64] In children with asthma, iNO has no apparent bronchodilatory effect.[65] In five children with life-threatening status asthmaticus who required MV and did not respond to maximal medical management, however, iNO decreased Pa_{CO_2} significantly. Four children survived.[66]
Bronchopulmonary dysplasia	Hyperoxia plus iNO caused marked pulmonary vasodilation in patients with bronchopulmonary dysplasia.[67]
Portopulmonary hypertension	In patients with pulmonary artery hypertension in association with liver failure, iNO reduced PAP and pulmonary vascular resistance.[68] It remains unclear whether iNO could improve the outcome in these severely ill patients.
Thoracic surgery	In patients with pulmonary hypertension during single-lung ventilation, iNO caused a significant reduction of mean PAP and improved oxygenation in patients with hypoxemia.[69]
Lung transplantation	Some studies in the 1990s reported that iNO reduced reperfusion injury in transplanted lungs. A recent study, however, showed that prophylactic iNO does not prevent reperfusion injury.[70] Contrary to earlier studies, a large randomized controlled trial could also not detect a significant effect on physiologic variables or outcomes in the group of iNO-treated patients, in whom iNO was initiated 10 minutes after reperfusion.[71] The occurrence of acute graft rejection, however, was less frequent in the iNO group in comparison with historical controls.[72] In an experimental study, therapy with iNO immediately after lung transplantation worsened arterial oxygenation and was deleterious for the surfactant system.[73]
Acute pulmonary embolism	iNO decreased the elevated PAP by 10–20% in different animal models of pulmonary embolism. Pulmonary gas exchange-did not improve. iNO may improve hemodynamics during acute pulmonary embolism.[74]
Congenital and acquired heart disease with PH	Inhalation of NO induced pulmonary vasodilation in 29% of patients.[75] Responders to iNO had a significantly higher 5-year survival than nonresponders.[76]
Myocardial infarction and cardiogenic shock	iNO improved hemodynamic function. Mean right atrial pressure decreased; mean PAP was reduced and cardiac index increased by 24%.[77]
Cardiac surgery	In patients undergoing cardiac surgery requiring cardiopulmonary bypass, PAP decreased before and after cardiopulmonary bypass with iNO. Systemic hemodynamics were unaffected during NO breathing.[78] iNO decreased the elevated mean PAP in patients undergoing cardiac surgery for different reasons. A significant increase in cardiac index and in the ratio of arterial partial pressure of oxygen to fraction of inspired oxygen was observed.[79] Inhalation of NO during and after cardiopulmonary bypass for aortic valve replacement diminishes the release of markers of myocardial injury. Left ventricular dysfunction during and immediately after cardiopulmonary bypass is antagonized.[80]
Heart transplantation	In heart transplant recipients with pulmonary hypertension, iNO given in the postoperative period selectively reduced PVR and enhanced right ventricular stroke work.[81]
Sickle cell disease	In severe vaso-occlusive crisis, inhalation of 80 ppm NO decreased pain scores and morphine use.[82]

ABBREVIATIONS: iNO, inhaled nitric oxide; NO, nitric oxide; MV, mechanical ventilation; Pa_{CO_2}, arterial partial pressure of carbon dioxide; PAP, pulmonary artery pressure; PH, pulmonary hypertension; ppm, parts per million; PVR, pulmonary vascular resistance.

TABLE 61-2 Applications for Inhaled Nitric Oxide in Preterm and Term Neonates

Diagnosis	Effect of NO Inhalation
Premature infants	Five infants of very low birth weight with severe respiratory failure and PPHN who did not respond to surfactant received iNO. All infants responded strikingly, survived, and appeared normal in follow-up.[83] INO improved oxygenation rapidly and consistently in very low birth weight infants with pulmonary hyperplasia. All iNO-treated infants survived longer than 28 days, while 50% of the control infants died.[84] In 207 premature infants with respiratory distress syndrome, the use of iNO decreased the incidence of chronic lung disease and death.[22] Preterm infants were followed-up for 30 months. No significant differences were found in long-term mortality or neurodevelopmental outcome between iNO-treated and control infants.[85]
Persistent pulmonary hypertension of the newborn	iNO in nine infants with severe PPHN resulted in improvement in oxygenation without systemic hypotension.[86] In a randomized controlled trial, iNO successfully doubled systemic oxygenation in 53% of the infants. Additionally, the frequency of ECMO was significantly lower in the iNO group (40%) than in the control group (71%). The number of deaths was similar in both groups.[18] In another randomized controlled trial, infants with moderate PPHN were studied; 58% of the control patients developed severe PPHN, while only 15% of the iNO-treated patients developed severe PPHN. iNO improved arterial P_{O_2} significantly and reduced the amount of ventilator support required.[87] Fifteen infants with PPHN were treated with iNO immediately after birth and survived. In a 3-year follow-up, frequency of survival with normal neurodevelopmental outcome was significantly higher in the group that showed early response to iNO.[88]
Congenital diaphragmatic hernia	Early surgery and iNO improves the outcome and reduces the requirement for ECMO in the treatment of antenatally diagnosed congenital diaphragmatic hernia.[89]

ABBREVIATIONS: iNO, inhaled nitric oxide; NO, nitric oxide; P_{O_2}, partial oxygen pressure; PPHN, persistent pulmonary hypertension of the newborn; ECMO, extracorporeal membrane oxygenation.

uniform, although elevated PAP decreased in almost every study. In asthma, however, the bronchodilator effect of iNO is only minor.

In lung transplantation, the rationale for inhalation of NO was not simply to decrease elevated PAP and improve oxygenation, but also to provide a possible immunomodulatory effect that might decrease reperfusion injury and graft rejection. Several studies have addressed these issues, but the results are controversial (see Table 61-1).

Cardiac surgery is a another promising field for iNO therapy. iNO can lower elevated PAP in patients undergoing cardiac surgery. An increase in oxygenation and cardiac index may accompany this change. Especially before and after cardiopulmonary bypass, iNO is able to lower PAP and it can antagonize left ventricular dysfunction immediately after extracorporeal circulation. A relatively new indication for iNO may be myocardial infarction with cardiogenic shock. In these patients, NO can relieve the right heart and increase cardiac index significantly.

Other possible indications of iNO and their appraisal are described in Table 61-1. When considering iNO as therapy in adult patients, it is important to recognize that certain pathophysiologic variables may significantly improve, although in no instance was survival clearly enhanced.

What indications for the use of iNO in adult patients still remain? It may be indicated in patients with ARDS, who are in a phase of severely impaired gas exchange unresponsive to maximal medical therapy. In such settings, application of iNO can significantly enhance pulmonary gas exchange and thereby prevent hypoxic organ damage. Moreover, iNO can be tried in all patients suffering from pulmonary hypertension. In most cases, elevated PAP drops and relieves the right heart. In cardiac patients, even left heart function can benefit. In lung transplantation, chronic obstructive pulmonary disease, and asthma, the use of iNO is

disputed, and further studies are warranted to define particular indications.

INFANTS

Application of iNO yielded the best results in critically ill infants (see Table 61-2). In neonates with respiratory failure, persistent pulmonary hypertension of the newborn (PPHN) is common. PPHN is characterized by elevated pulmonary resistance, pulmonary vasoconstriction, and altered vascular reactivity. Desaturated blood circulates partly through an extrapulmonary right-to-left shunt, across the foramen ovale and ductus arteriosus. Since 1970, ECMO has been the treatment of choice if PPHN is present. Survival rates of up to 80%[16] were achieved with ECMO therapy whereas survival with conservative therapy was about 50%.[17] In hypoxemic newborns with PPHN, clinical studies indicate that iNO increases systemic oxygen levels, decreases PAP, and mitigates ventilation-perfusion mismatch. Randomized, placebo-controlled trials of iNO in neonates with PPHN, however, failed to show a significant decrease in mortality rates in the iNO group; iNO therapy did, however, cut down the requirement for ECMO.[18] In newborns with PPHN, the frequencies of abnormalities (medication for pulmonary disease, need for supplemental oxygen, abnormal neurologic findings, or developmental delay) were no different in the iNO and control groups 1 year after the disease.[19,20] Another study in neonates revealed that iNO therapy is not associated with an increase in neurodevelopmental, behavioral, or medical abnormalities at 2 years of age.[21]

In premature infants with lung failure and hypoxemia, iNO also improves oxygenation. If premature infants do not respond to iNO, it may help to administer surfactant before starting the iNO therapy. The effectiveness of iNO was recently documented in a large randomized controlled trial; its use decreased the incidence of chronic lung disease and death in preterm infants.[22]

Physicians caring for infants with hypoxic respiratory failure and PPHN should be familiar with the use of iNO. In newborns it should be used liberally if these indications are present because ECMO therapy can be avoided in many cases. In preterm infants, higher survival rates can probably be expected when iNO is used.

Technique of Nitric Oxide Inhalation

NO is manufactured from the reaction of liquid sulfuric acid and liquid sodium nitrite. A gas mixture of 95% NO and 5% nitrogen dioxide (NO_2) is diluted in inert carrier gases, nitrogen(preferred) or helium. The minimum purity of NO needs to be 99.0%. The gas is typically filled in 10-liter cylinders made of aluminum alloy, supplying NO concentrations from 100–1000 ppm.

The delivery device for iNO should allow for synchronized application, a very low production of NO_2 (<1 ppm is possible), and easy operation. It is recommended to have a manual NO supply device for emergency or transport reasons near the ventilator.

NO may be administered continuously or pulsed into the inspiratory limb of the respiratory circuit. The former technique may lead to significant variations in inspiratory NO concentrations, which can be avoided by establishing an additional mixing chamber. Using the latter technique, the physician can determine exactly in which phase of the inspiratory cycle a given NO concentration is delivered. It was shown that administering NO in early inspiration (first 60% of inspiration) leads to optimal oxygenation and reduction of intrapulmonary right-to-left shunt in anesthetized horses.[23]

For scavenging of NO_2 from the inspiratory limb of the ventilator circuit, researchers and clinicians previously evaluated soda lime and charcoal absorbers. Scavenging of NO_2 is possible to varying extents (0–100%) depending on the absorber product, the applied iNO concentration, and the duration of exposure. Several types of absorber scavenge a variable proportion of the iNO applied.

Monitoring of Inhaled Nitric Oxide Concentration

Concentrations of NO and oxides of nitrogen should be monitored continuously during therapy with iNO. At the bedside, electrochemical measurement and the chemiluminescence technique have been used. Electrochemical devices make use of a simple electrochemical principle for the detection of NO. The gas of interest passes through a plastic membrane into a liquid acid electrode. The electrolyte solution contains the sensing electrode (anode), a counter electrode (cathode), and a reference electrode. The voltage between the two poles is maintained and the electric current that flows through the anode reflects the concentration of NO. The chemiluminescence technique is based on a gas-phase chemiluminescence reaction between NO and ozone

that produces nitrogen dioxide and light. The emitted light has a wavelength of 640–3000 nm with a maximum at 1200 nm and is detected by a red-sensitive photomultiplier tube.

At present, fast-reacting chemiluminescence analyzers represent the gold standard for monitoring concentrations of NO and oxides of nitrogen. In comparison, electrochemical detectors are not so expensive, not so large, and sufficiently sensitive to reliably monitor NO concentrations in the range between 5 and 80 ppm.

Dosage of Inhaled Nitric Oxide

Dose-response studies in patients with ARDS have shown that very low concentrations of iNO, only 10 ppb, are able to enhance oxygenation; higher concentrations are necessary to decrease the elevated PAP. The respective effective doses whereby 50% of individuals will show the expected response to iNO are 100 ppb and 2–3 ppm. Improvement in oxygenation reached a maximum at 10 ppm and deteriorated at higher NO doses; PAP further decreased with higher NO concentrations. Studies were stopped at 100 ppm.[24] Data suggest that higher doses of NO, secondary to a spillover phenomenon, reach blood vessels supplying partially or nonventilated lung areas. For exact dosage, the registration of an individual dose-response curve for each patient is indispensable (Fig. 61-3). Concentrations of >80–100 ppm should not be exceeded. In neonates, dose-response data indicate that maximal benefit of iNO on oxygenation and PAP is observed at concentrations of <30 ppm.[25] In patients with indications other than ARDS, the recording of individual dose-response curves is also recommended. At present, systematic dose-response studies are not available.

Responders and Nonresponders

Regarding oxygenation and PAP, about a third of critically ill patients do not react favorably to NO (i.e., an increase in Pa_{O_2} of ≥10 mmHg or a decrease in PAP of ≥2 mmHg). Reasons include: persistent pulmonary blood flow to dorsal edematous lung areas; physical barriers, such as the presence of exudate or fibrosis; molecular mechanisms, such as increased activity of phosphodiesterase; unfavorable ventilator settings; and, most likely, a number of currently unknown factors. It appears sensible to evaluate a patient's response to iNO on a daily basis because initial nonresponders may convert to responders over time, and vice versa.

Adjunctive Therapy

When the clinician faces a patient in acute respiratory failure who does not respond to iNO at all or the patient's response is very weak, adjunctive measures can positively change the situation.

Re-evaluation of the level of positive end-expiratory pressure represents one of these measures. Recruiting additional

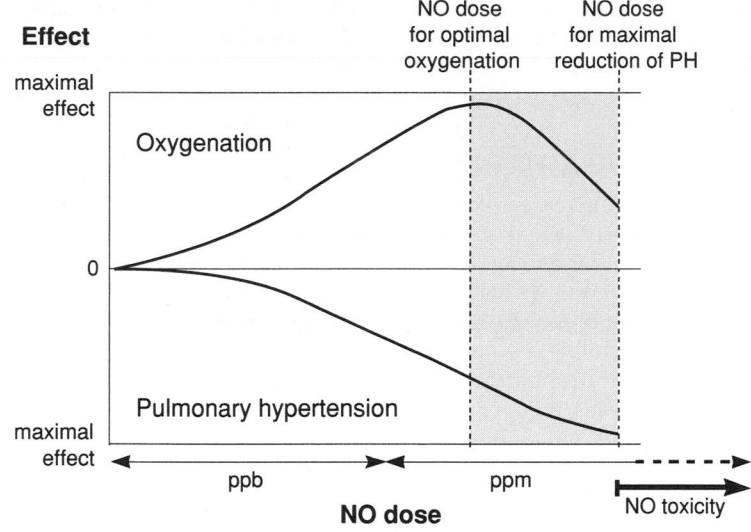

FIGURE 61-3 Schematic dose-response curve for patients with ARDS treated with iNO. Low doses of iNO (in the parts per billion range) are able to improve oxygenation while higher levels of iNO are necessary to significantly decrease the elevated PAP. Oxygenation improves to a maximum and then deteriorates at higher NO concentrations. Maximal reduction of PAP needs even higher doses of NO. It is recommended to verify the dose-response characteristics for each individual patient starting before NO treatment. *PH*, pulmonary hypertension; *NO*, nitric oxide; *iNO*, inhaled nitric oxide; *PAP*, pulmonary arterial pressure; *ppb*, parts per billion; *ppm*, parts per million.

alveoli may increase the number of alveoli, whereby NO can easily flow in and exert its beneficial effects. This idea has been tested in experimental and clinical trials. It was shown that when positive end-expiratory pressure led to alveolar recruitment, a rise in Pa_{O_2} of more than 100 mmHg could be achieved.[26,27]

Ventilating critically ill patients in the prone position may dramatically enhance oxygenation by antagonizing ventilation-perfusion mismatch. Exploiting this mechanism in patients receiving iNO therapy can further enhance oxygenation as compared with iNO in the supine position.[28]

Almitrine bismesylate acts as a pulmonary vasoconstrictor mainly in pulmonary vessels supplying hypoxic lung regions and reduces their perfusion. Theoretically, it was hoped that NO, a selective pulmonary vasodilator, and almitrine, a selective pulmonary vasoconstrictor, would act additively on oxygenation. This effect was later confirmed in patients with ARDS,[29] in hypoxemic patients with focal lung lesions,[30] and during one-lung ventilation in patients undergoing thoracic procedures.[31] Fortunately, the associated rise in PAP was only mild (1–2 mmHg). To date, serious side effects have not been reported after the use of almitrine.

As an alternative to almitrine, phenylephrine has been suggested. This α-receptor agonist has pulmonary as well as systemic vasoconstricting properties. When given intravenously in combination with iNO, an additive effect on oxygenation is observed.

Side Effects and Toxicology

An adage attributed to the physician, astrologer, and theologian, Philippus Theophrastus Bombastus of Hohenheim, better known as Paracelsus (1493–1541), reads: "All substances are poisons; there is none which is not. The right dose differentiates a poison from a remedy." Regarding NO, this is surely true. Only a narrow margin exists between an effective and a toxic dose.

FORMATION OF NITROGEN DIOXIDE

Formation of harmful concentrations of nitrogen dioxide (NO_2) is uncommon, especially when therapeutic doses of NO are inhaled. NO reacts with oxygen and forms toxic NO_2. NO_2 concentrations above 10 ppm may induce pulmonary edema, alveolar hemorrhage, methemoglobinemia, hypoxemia, changes in surfactant activity, hyperplasia of type II alveolar cells, intrapulmonary accumulation of fibrin, neutrophils, and macrophages, and eventually death.[32] Consequently, the U. S. Occupational Safety and Health Administration has prescribed the 8-hour time-weighted average exposure limits for NO at 25 ppm and for NO_2 at 5 ppm.

REBOUND AFTER NITRIC OXIDE WITHDRAWAL

During weaning from NO, its rapid withdrawal can cause marked rebound pulmonary vasospasms,[33] high intrapulmonary right-to-left shunt, and decreased Pa_{O_2}.[34] This phenomenon can be explained by downregulation of nitric oxide synthase activity in the presence of exogenous NO. In pediatric patients after cardiac surgery, longer continuation of iNO and its lower final concentration are factors that contribute to its successful weaning. Consequently, it seems prudent to slowly wean a patient from iNO. Alternatively, the clinician can exchange NO for a different pulmonary vasodilator, or wait until the patient's endogenous production recommences.

PRO- AND ANTIOXIDANT EFFECTS

NO can have both pro- and antioxidant effects in the lung. In rats, high doses of iNO (100 ppm) cause increased vascular permeability to protein during hyperoxia; inhalation of 10 ppm NO had no effect on vascular leakage and improved alveolar liquid clearance. Inhibition of endogenous NO formation with L-NAME (L-NG nitroarginine methyl ester) worsened hyperoxic lung injury and reduced survival, indicating a protective effect of endogenous NO.[35] The antioxidant effects of NO are apparent when low doses of NO are produced or inhaled. Scavenging of reactive oxygen molecules, such as superoxide anion, may be the main antioxidant property of NO. When high NO concentrations are present, toxic pro-oxidant effects may predominate and these are mainly mediated by the synthesis of cytotoxic nitrogen molecules, such as dinitrogen trioxide or peroxynitrite.

SYSTEMIC VASODILATION

For many years, a key characteristic of NO seemed to be its selectivity as a pulmonary vasodilator. This characteristic was explained by its rapid binding to the heme moiety of hemoglobin and its very short duration of action. Indeed, in many clinical trials and animal experiments, substantial effects on arterial blood pressure or other systemic circulation variables have not been observed. In some instances, however, reductions in systemic blood pressure and systemic vascular resistance were documented.[36,37] A new insight helps explain this phenomenon: NO can bind reversibly with albumin and hemoglobin and thereby enter the systemic circulation.[38–40]

METHEMOGLOBINEMIA

iNO can combine with hemoglobin to form nitrosylhemoglobin, which is rapidly oxidized to methemoglobin. In numerous clinical studies, however, severe methemoglobinemia was not observed with inhalation of NO. A review of more than 471 patients, compiled from four large trials, revealed that methemoglobinemia (defined as levels above 5%) occurred in 3% of the patients.

INTERFERENCE WITH SURFACTANT

Analyses of surfactants recovered from experimental animals that had received 80–120 ppm iNO revealed reduced quality, in terms of capacity to lower surface tension. It is unclear whether this is a consequence of the toxic actions of various NO by-products, such as peroxynitrite and NO_2, or if it is mediated by hemoglobin found in the alveoli when there is high-permeability lung edema.[41,42] Fortunately, surfactant in infants with PPHN receiving low NO concentrations of 20 ppm was equivalent to that of control patients with PPHN.

EFFECTS ON COAGULATION

Inhibition of human platelet aggregation by iNO has been reported in several studies. In addition, prolongation of bleeding time and inhibition of P-selectin expression with decreased binding of fibrinogen to the platelet glycoprotein IIb/IIIa receptor was demonstrated.[43–45] In healthy subjects, however, NO may[44] or may not[46] prolong bleeding time and exert effects on various coagulation parameters. In patients with ARDS, inhibition of platelet aggregation was reported, although a prolonged bleeding time was not observed in every study.[43,47] In infants, significantly prolonged bleeding times were documented with iNO therapy;[48] in premature

infants with respiratory distress syndrome, an increased risk of intracranial hemorrhage must be considered.[49]

NITRIC OXIDE AND DEOXYRIBONUCLEIC ACID ALTERATIONS

NO increases the formation of cyclic guanosine monophosphate via activation of the enzyme guanylate cyclase. High intracellular cyclic guanosine monophosphate levels mediate the relaxation of smooth muscle cells, but also contribute to NO toxicity. Cyclic guanosine monophosphate modulates deoxyribonucleic acid synthesis and inhibits cellular proliferation. NO may also decrease the proliferation of cells independently from cyclic guanosine monophosphate. Given in therapeutic doses, iNO suppresses the proliferation of smooth muscle cells in the lung and reduces vascular remodeling in response to hypoxia, thereby preventing obstruction of pulmonary blood vessels and fixed pulmonary hypertension. Toxic effects of iNO include alterations in deoxyribonucleic acid and chromosomal aberrations, which have been shown in in vitro and in vivo experiments. Formation of peroxynitrite may also be deleterious; it can cause changes of deoxyribonucleic acid base sequence or deoxyribonucleic acid strand breaks, resulting in cell death.

OTHER TOXIC SIDE EFFECTS OF INHALED NITRIC OXIDE

In a large randomized controlled trial, patients treated with NO exhibited a higher incidence of renal failure.[12] This observation remains enigmatic and has not received much attention. It is reassuring that volunteers who inhaled 40 ppm NO for 2 hours had increased urinary volumes and no changes in creatinine clearance.[50] Again, no explanation is available for these findings. Nephrotoxicity of iNO in clinically applied doses does not appear likely.

Safe Inhaled Nitric Oxide Therapy and Contraindications

Safe iNO therapy requires continuous analysis of NO and NO_2 concentrations, closely integrated monitoring of the patient, periodic analyses of methemoglobin levels, use of certified NO tanks, and administration of the lowest concentration required.

Contraindications to iNO therapy are based on its toxicology. In clinical practice, methemoglobin formation and bleeding disposition are of interest. In patients with high levels of methemoglobin, additional iNO therapy may not be indicated. Patients with a hemorrhagic diathesis or coagulation or bleeding problems should not receive iNO therapy. Clear-cut recommendations, however, cannot be given because few studies deal with contraindications to NO; most are anecdotal reports or trials that revealed contradictory results.

The Future

What are upcoming scientific challenges in studying this extraordinary substance? Can the application of iNO be made easier and more convenient? What about the development of alternative NO therapies for the respiratory system?

First, more high-quality studies of diseases in which iNO therapy is of benefit are needed. These studies should evaluate not only survival rates with iNO therapy, but also outcome parameters such as quality of life, cognitive impairment, and lung function, which affect the lives of the patients. Dose-response studies for the different indications of iNO therapy are needed, and safety of long-term application of iNO should be investigated. It would be good if manufacturers developed clever, miniaturized iNO application devices to simplify clinical use, transport, and long-term inhalation. The responder/nonresponder problem also needs to be probed.

Basic scientific work is needed to investigate the problem of the physiologic autoinhalation of endogenous NO from the paranasal sinuses, which is excluded in intubated and mechanically ventilated patients. It is assumed that some concentration of autoinhaled NO in the airways is necessary and protective against infection. During intubation and mechanical ventilation, low doses of iNO may restore the physiologic airway concentration of NO and protect against ventilator-associated pneumonia. It is possible that a patient's own nasal NO may be redirected into the inspiratory limb of the ventilatory circuit.

Therapy with iNO (INOmax, INO Therapeutics, Clinton, NJ) is expensive and technically demanding. Future research may yield cheaper, alternative drugs that selectively supply NO in ventilated lung regions. A new approach may be the inhalation of aerosolized sodium nitrite, which acts through conversion to NO. Nitrite may prove to be a simple and inexpensive agent for iNO applications, although experimental and clinical studies are warranted.[51] Moreover, a new generation of aerosolized (DS-1 [linear polyethylenimine-nitric oxide/nucleophile adduct], DETA/NO)[52,53] or microencapsulated (PROLI/NO)[54] nitric oxide donors has recently been developed, which may provide a stable inhalable form of NO. But what scientists are really looking for is an IV or oral vasodilator, possibly an NO donor, which acts selectively in the (ventilated) pulmonary blood vessels.

Summary and Conclusion

NO is an important signaling molecule in the respiratory system. It modulates perfusion of lung units and it can prevent inflammatory processes. Administered by inhalation, low doses of NO selectively dilate pulmonary blood vessels in ventilated lung areas and redistribute blood flow from atelectatic to aerated lung units. Systemic vasodilation does not occur because NO rapidly binds to hemoglobin and is thus inactivated. The overall effect of NO inhalation is a sustained reduction of elevated PAP and improvement in oxygenation if a ventilation-perfusion mismatch of the lung is present. iNO is used to treat several cardiopulmonary disorders that are associated with pulmonary hypertension; its main application, however, is in neonatology. In infants with PPHN, NO significantly reduces the need for extracorporeal membrane oxygenation. In no instance, however, was NO clearly shown to enhance long-term survival. There is no end in sight for the future role of NO inhalation. What we urgently need are more high-quality studies of the diseases in which iNO therapy is effective, and, hopefully, to demonstrate higher survival rates or at least improved quality of life.

Acknowledgments

I thank Dr. Monika Lewandowski for literature research, preparation of tables and figures, and Professor Konrad J. Falke for manuscript review. Part of this work was done during the author's appointment at the Charité, Berlin, Germany.

References

1. Furchgott RF, Zawadzki JV. The obligatory role of endothelial cells in the relaxation of arterial smooth muscle by acetylcholine. Nature (London) 1980; 288:373–6.
2. Ignarro LJ, Byrns RE, Buga GM, et al. Endothelium derived relaxing factor from pulmonary artery and vein possesses pharmacological and chemical properties that are identical to those of nitric oxide radical. Circ Res 1987; 61:866–79.
3. Palmer RMJ, Ferrige AG, Moncada S. Nitric oxide release accounts for the biological activity of endothelium-derived relaxing factor. Nature (London)1987; 327:524–6.
4. Koshland DE. The molecule of the year. Science 1992; 258:1861.
5. Lundberg JON, Farkas-Szallasi T, Weitzberg E, et al. High nitric oxide production in human paranasal sinuses. Nature Medicine 1995; 1:370–3.
6. Deja M, Busch T, Bachmann S, et al. Reduced nitric oxide in sinus epithelium of patients with radiologic maxillary sinusitis and sepsis. Am J Respir Crit Care Med 2003; 168:281–6.
7. Thomassen MJ, Buhrow LT, Connors MJ, et al. Nitric oxide inhibits inflammatory cytokine production by human alveolar macrophages. Am J Respir Cell Mol Biol 1997; 17:279–83.
8. Ricciardolo FL, Gepetti P, Mistretta A, et al. Randomised double-blind placebo-controlled study of the effect of inhibition of nitric oxide synthesis in bradykinin-induced asthma. Lancet 1996; 348:374–7.
9. Dellinger RP, Zimmerman JL, Taylor RW, et al. Effects of inhaled nitric oxide in patients with acute respiratory distress syndrome: results of a randomized phase II trial. Inhaled Nitric Oxide in ARDS Study Group. Crit Care Med 1998; 26: 15–23.
10. Troncy E, Collet JP, Shapiro S, et al. Inhaled nitric oxide in acute respiratory distress syndrome: a pilot randomized controlled study. Am J Respir Crit Care Med 1998; 157:1483–8.
11. Michael JR, Barton RG, Saffle JR, et al. Inhaled nitric oxide versus conventional therapy: effect on oxygenation in ARDS. Am J Respir Crit Care Med 1998; 157:1372–80.
12. Lundin S, Mang H, Smithies M, et al. Inhalation of nitric oxide in acute lung injury: results of a European multicentre study. The European Study Group of Inhaled Nitric Oxide. Intensive Care Med 1999; 25:911–9.
13. Taylor RW, Zimmerman JL, Dellinger RP, et al. Inhaled Nitric Oxide in ARDS Study Group. Low-dose inhaled nitric oxide in

patients with acute lung injury: a randomized controlled trial. JAMA 2004; 291:1603–9.

14. Gerlach H, Keh D, Semmerow A, et al. Dose-response characteristics during long-term inhalation of nitric oxide in patients with severe acute respiratory distress syndrome. A prospective, randomized, controlled study. Am J Respir Crit Care Med 2003; 167:1008–15.

15. Luhr O, Aardal S, Nathorst-Westfelt U, et al. Pulmonary function in adult survivors of severe acute lung injury treated with inhaled nitric oxide. Acta Anaesthesiol Scand 1998; 42: 391–8.

16. Zwischenberger JB, Cox CS. Extracorporeal membrane oxygenation (ECMO) for neonatal respiratory failure. Thorac Cardiovasc Surg 1992; 40:316–22.

17. Weinberger B, Weiss K, Heck DE, et al. Pharmacologic therapy of persistent pulmonary hypertension of the newborn. Pharmacol Ther 2001; 89:67–79.

18. Roberts JD, Fineman JR, Morin FC, et al. Inhaled nitric oxide and persistent pulmonary hypertension of the newborn. The Inhaled Nitric Oxide Study Group. N Engl J Med 1997; 336:605–10.

19. Clark RH, Huckaby JL, Kueser TJ, et al. Low-dose nitric oxide therapy for persistent pulmonary hypertension: 1-year follow-up. J Perinatol 2003; 23:300–3.

20. Lipkin PH, Davidson D, Spivak L, et al. Neurodevelopmental and medical outcomes of persistent pulmonary hypertension in term newborns treated with nitric oxide. J Pediatr 2002; 140:306–10.

21. Neonatal Inhaled Nitric Oxide Study Group. Inhaled nitric oxide in term and near-term infants: neurodevelopmental follow-up of the neonatal inhaled nitric oxide study group (NINOS). J Pediatr 2000; 136:611–7.

22. Schreiber MD, Gin-Mestan K, Marks JD, et al. Inhaled nitric oxide in premature infants with the respiratory distress syndrome. N Engl J Med 2003; 349:2099–107.

23. Heinonen E, Nyman G, Merilainen P, et al. Effect of different pulses of nitric oxide on venous admixture in the anaesthetized horse. Br J Anaesth 2002; 88:394–8.

24. Gerlach H, Rossaint R, Pappert D, et al. Time-course and dose-response of nitric oxide inhalation for systemic oxygenation and pulmonary hypertension in patients with adult respiratory distress syndrome. Eur J Clin Invest 1993; 23:499–502.

25. Macrae DJ, Field D, Mercier J-C, et al. Inhaled nitric oxide therapy in neonates and children: reaching a European consensus. Intensive Care Med 2004; 30:372–80.

26. Puybasset L, Rouby JJ, Mourgeon E, et al. Factors influencing cardiopulmonary effects of inhaled nitric oxide in acute respiratory failure. Am J Respir Crit Care Med 1995; 152:318–28.

27. Putensen C, Rasanen J, Lopez FA, et al. Continuous positive airway pressure modulates effect of inhaled nitric oxide on the ventilation-perfusion distributions in canine lung injury. Chest 1994; 106:1563–9.

28. Rialp G, Betbesé AJ, Péres-Márquez M, et al. Short-term effects of inhaled nitric oxide and prone position in pulmonary and extrapulmonary acute respiratory distress syndrome. Am J Respir Crit Care Med 2001; 164:243–9.

29. Gallart L, Lu Q, Puybasset L, et al. Intravenous almitrine combined with inhaled nitric oxide for acute respiratory distress syndrome. Am J Respir Crit Care Med 1998; 158:1770–7.

30. Payen D, Muret J, Beloucif S, et al. Inhaled nitric oxide, almitrine infusion, or their coadministration as a treatment of severe hypoxemic focal lung lesions. Anesthesiology 1998; 89: 1157–65.

31. Moutafis M, Liu N, Dalibon N, et al. The effect of nitric oxide and its combination with intravenous almitrine on PaO_2 during one-lung ventilation in patients undergoing thoracoscopic procedures. Anesth Analg 1997; 85:1130–5.

32. Greenbaum R, Bay J, Hargreaves MD, et al. Effects of higher oxides of nitrogen on the anaesthetized dog. Br J Anaesth 1967; 39:393–404.

33. Cueto E, Lopez-Herce J, Sanchez A, et al. Life-threatening effects of discontinuing inhaled nitric oxide in children. Acta Paediatr 1997; 86:1337–9.

34. Rossaint R, Falke KJ, Lopez F, et al. Inhaled nitric oxide for the adult respiratory distress syndrome. N Engl J Med 1993; 328:399–405.

35. Garat C, Jayr C, Eddahibi S, et al. Effects of inhaled nitric oxide or inhibition of endogenous nitric oxide formation on hyperoxic lung injury. Am J Respir Crit Care Med 1997; 155:1957–64.

36. Quezado ZM, Natanson C, Karzai W, et al. Cardiopulmonary effects of inhaled nitric oxide in normal dogs and during E. coli pneumonia and sepsis. J Appl Physiol 1998; 84:107–15.

37. Wessel DL, Adatia I, Giglia TM, et al. Use of inhaled nitric oxide and acetylcholine in the evaluation of pulmonary hypertension and endothelial function after cardiopulmonary bypass. Circulation 1993; 88:2128–38.

38. Keaney JFJ, Simon DL, Stamler JS, et al. NO forms an adduct with serum albumin that has endothelium-derived relaxing factor-like properties. J Clin Invest 1993; 91:1582–9.

39. Gow AJ, Luchsinger BP, Pawloski JR, et al. The oxyhemoglobin reaction of nitric oxide. Proc Natl Acad Sci USA 1999; 96:9027–32.

40. Stamler JS, Jia L, Eu JP, et al. Blood flow regulation by S-nitrosohemoglobin in the physiological oxygen gradient. Science 1997; 276:2034–7.

41. Matalon S, DeMarco V, Haddad IY, et al. Inhaled nitric oxide injures the pulmonary surfactant system of lambs in vivo. Am J Physiol 1996; 270:L273–80.

42. Hallman M, Bry K. Nitric oxide and lung surfactant. Semin Perinatol 1996; 20:173–85.

43. Gries A, Bode C, Peter K, et al. Inhaled nitric oxide inhibits human platelet aggregation, P-selectin expression, and fibrinogen binding in vitro and in vivo. Circulation 1998; 97:1481–7.

44. Gries A, Herr A, Motsch J, et al. Randomized, placebo-controlled, blinded and cross-matched study on the antiplatelet effect of inhaled nitric oxide in healthy volunteers. Thromb Haemost 2000; 83:309–15.

45. Beghetti M, Sparling C, Cox PN, et al. Inhaled NO inhibits platelet aggregation and elevates plasma but not intraplatelet cGMP in healthy human volunteers. Am J Physiol Heart Circ Physiol 2003; 285:H637–42.

46. Albert J, Norman M, Wallen NH, et al. Inhaled nitric oxide does not influence bleeding time or platelet function in healthy volunteers. Eur J Clin Invest 1999; 29:953–9.

47. Samama CM, Diaby M, Fellahi JL, et al. Inhibition of platelet aggregation by inhaled nitric oxide in patients with acute respiratory distress syndrome. Anesthesiology 1995; 83:56–65.

48. George TN, Johnson KJ, Bates JN, et al. The effect of inhaled nitric oxide therapy on bleeding time and platelet aggregation in neonates. J Pediatr 1998; 132:731–4.

49. Meurs KP, Rhine WD, Asselin JM, et al. Response of premature infants with severe respiratory failure to inhaled nitric oxide. Preemie NO Collaborative Group. Pediatr Pulmonol 1997; 24:319–23.

50. Wraight WM, Young JD. Renal effects of inhaled nitric oxide in humans. Br J Anaesth 2001; 86:267–9.

51. Hunter CJ, Dejam A, Blood AB, et al. Inhaled nebulized nitrite is a hypoxia-sensitive NO-dependent selective pulmonary vasodilator. Nat Med 2004; 10:1122–7.

52. Kirov MY, Evgenov OV, Kuklin VN, et al. Aerosolized linear polyethylenimine-nitric oxide/nucleophile adduct attenuates endotoxin-induced lung injury in sheep. Am J Respir Crit Care Med 2002; 166:1436–42.

53. Lam CF, Van Heerden PV, Blott J, et al. The selective pulmonary vasodilatory effect of inhaled DETA/NO, a novel nitric oxide donor, in ARDS—a pilot human trial. J Crit Care 2004; 19:48–53.

54. Jeh HS, Lu S, George SC. Encapsulation of PROLI/NO in biodegradable microparticles. J Microencapsul 2004; 21:3–13.

55. Sokol J, Jacobs SE, Bohn D. Inhaled nitric oxide for acute hypoxic respiratory failure in children and adults: a meta-analysis. Anesth Analg 2003; 97:989–98.

56. Sitbon O, Brenot F, Denjean A, et al. Inhaled nitric oxide as a screening vasodilator agent in primary pulmonary hypertension. A dose-response study and comparison with prostacyclin. Am J Respir Crit Care Med 1995; 151:384–89.

57. Kouyoumdjian C, Adnot S, Levame M, et al. Continuous inhalation of nitric oxide protects against development of pulmonary hypertension in chronically hypoxic rats. J Clin Invest 1994; 94:578–84.

58. Scherrer U, Vollenweider L, Delabas A, et al. Inhaled nitric oxide for high-altitude pulmonary edema. N Engl J Med 1996; 334:624–9.

59. Morales-Blanhir J, Santos S, de Jover L, et al. Clinical value of vasodilator test with inhaled nitric oxide for predicting long-term response to oral vasodilators in pulmonary hypertension. Respir Med 2004; 98:225–34.

60. Germann P, Ziesche R, Leitner C, et al. Addition of nitric oxide to oxygen improves cardiopulmonary function in patients with severe COPD. Chest 1998; 114:29–35.

61. Baigorri F, Joseph D, Artigas A, et al. Inhaled nitric oxide does not improve cardiac or pulmonary function in patients with an exacerbation of chronic obstructive pulmonary disease. Crit Care Med 1999; 27:2153–8.

62. Vonbank K, Ziesche R, Higenbottam TW, et al. Controlled prospective randomised trial on the effects on pulmonary haemodynamics of the ambulatory long term use of nitric oxide and oxygen in patients with severe COPD. Thorax 2003; 58:289–93.

63. Kacmarek RM, Ripple R, Cockrill BA, et al. Inhaled nitric oxide. A bronchodilator in mild asthmatics with metacholine-induced bronchospasm. Am J Respir Crit Care Med 1996; 153:128–35.

64. Högman M, Frostell CG, Hedenstrom H, et al. Inhalation of nitric oxide modulates adult human bronchial tone. Am Rev Respir Dis 1993; 148:1474–8.

65. Pfeffer KD, Ellison G, Robertson D, et al. The effect of inhaled nitric oxide in pediatric asthma. Am J Respir Crit Care Med 1996; 153:747–51.

66. Nakagawa TA, Johnston SJ, Falkos SA, et al. Life-threatening status asthmaticus treated with inhaled nitric oxide. J Pediatr 2000; 137:119–22.

67. Mourani PM, Ivy DD, Gao D, et al. Pulmonary vascular effects of inhaled nitric oxide and oxygen tension in bronchopulmonary dysplasia. Am J Respir Crit Care Med 2004; 170:1006–13.

68. Findlay JY, Harrison BA, Plevak DJ, et al. Inhaled nitric oxide reduces pulmonary artery pressures in portopulmonary hypertension. Liver Transpl Surg 1999; 5:381–7.

69. Rocca GD, Passariello M, Coccia C, et al. Inhaled nitric oxide administration during one-lung ventilation in patients undergoing thoracic surgery. J Cardiothorac Vasc Anesth 2001; 15:218–23.

70. Ardehali A, Laks H, Levine M, et al. A prospective trial of inhaled nitric oxide in clinical lung transplantation. Transplantation 2001; 72:112–5.

71. Meade MO, Granton JT, Matte-Martyn A, et al. A randomized trial of inhaled nitric oxide to prevent ischemia-reperfusion injury after lung transplantation. Am J Respir Crit Care Med 2003; 167:1483–9.

72. Cornfield DN, Milla CE, Haddad IY, et al. Safety of inhaled nitric oxide after lung transplantation. J Heart Lung Transplant 2003; 22:903–7.

73. Valino F, Casals C, Guerrero R, et al. Inhaled nitric oxide affects endogenous surfactant in experimental lung transplantation. Transplantation 2004; 77:812–818.

74. Tanus-Santos JE, Theodorakis MJ. Is there a place for inhaled nitric oxide in the therapy of acute pulmonary embolism? Am J Respir Med 2002; 1:167–76.

75. Budts W, Van Pelt N, Gillyns H, et al. Residual pulmonary vasoreactivity to inhaled nitric oxide in patients with severe obstructive pulmonary hypertension and Eisenmenger syndrome. Heart 2001; 86:553–8.

76. Post MC, Janssens S, Van De Werf F, et al. Responsiveness to inhaled nitric oxide is a predictor for mid-term survival in adult patients with congenital heart defects and pulmonary arterial hypertension. Eur Heart J 2004; 25:1651–6.

77. Inglessis I, Shin JT, Lepore JJ, et al. Hemodynamic effects of inhaled nitric oxide in right ventricular myocardial infarction and cardiogenic shock. J Am Coll Cardiol 2004; 44:793–8.

78. Rich GF, Murphy GD, Roos CM, et al. Inhaled nitric oxide: Selective pulmonary vasodilation in cardiac surgical patients. Anesthesiology 1993; 78:1028–35.

79. Maxey TS, Smith CD, Kern JA, et al. Beneficial effects of inhaled nitric oxide in adult cardiac surgical patients. Ann Thorac Surg 2002; 73:529–32.

80. Gianetti J, Del Sarto P, Bevilacqua S, et al. Supplemental nitric oxide and its effect on myocardial injury and function in patients undergoing cardiac surgery with extracorporeal circulation. Thorac Cardiovasc Surg 2004; 127:44–50.

81. Ardehali A, Hughes K, Sadeghi A, et al. Inhaled nitric oxide for pulmonary hypertension after heart transplantation. Transplantation 2001; 72:638–41.

82. Weiner DL, Hibberd PL, Betit P, et al. Preliminary assessment of inhaled nitric oxide for acute vaso-occlusive crisis in pediatric patients with sickle cell disease. JAMA 2003; 289:1136–42.

83. Aikio O, Saarela T, Pokela ML, et al. Nitric oxide treatment and acute pulmonary inflammatory response in very premature infants with intractable respiratory failure shortly after birth. Acta Paediatr 2003; 92:65–9.

84. Uga N, Ishii T, Kawase Y, et al. Nitric oxide inhalation therapy in very low-birthweight infants with hypoplastic lung due to oligohydramnios. Pediatr Int 2004; 46:10–14.

85. Bennett AJ, Shaw NJ, Gregg JE, et al. Neurodevelopmental outcome in high-risk preterm infants treated with inhaled nitric oxide. Acta Paediatr 2001; 90:573–6.

86. Kinsella JP, Neish SR, Shaffer E, et al. Low-dose inhalational nitric oxide in persistent pulmonary hypertension of the newborn. Lancet 1992; 340:819–20.

87. Sadiq HF, Mantych G, Benawra RS, et al. Inhaled nitric oxide in the treatment of moderate persistent pulmonary hypertension of the newborn: a randomized controlled, multicenter trial. J Perinatol 2003; 23:98–103.

88. Ichiba H, Matsunami S, Itoh F, et al. Three-year follow up of term and near term infants treated with inhaled nitric oxide. Pediatr Int 2003; 45:290–3.

89. Okuyama H, Kubota A, Oue T, et al. Inhaled nitric oxide with early surgery improves the outcome of antenatally diagnosed congenital diaphragmatic hernia. J Pediatr Surg 2002; 37:1188–90.

DIAPHRAGMATIC PACING

ANTHONY F. DIMARCO

Chronic respiratory failure requiring ventilator support is usually caused by severe derangements in the function of the lungs, chest wall, and/or respiratory muscles. Mechanical ventilation is the only feasible option for most patients with these disorders. In certain patients, however, the function of the respiratory apparatus is completely intact except for lack of adequate nervous output from the respiratory centers in the medulla (central hypoventilation syndrome; CHS)[1,2] or interruption of electrical signals from the medulla to the nerves innervating the major inspiratory muscles (cervical spinal cord injury). These patients can be offered an alternative means of respiratory support by diaphragmatic pacing (DP), a more natural and physiologic form of breathing.[3–11]

While straightforward in concept, DP required several significant scientific developments before becoming a clinically useful modality. A brief historical perspective provides some insight into the evolution of DP and understanding of its clinical utility.

More than two centuries ago, Caldani[12] observed that diaphragmatic movement could be achieved by electrical stimulation of the phrenic nerve. In the latter 19th century, Duchenne found phrenic nerve stimulation to be the best method of producing natural respiration.[6] The application of moistened sponges over the outer borders of the sternocleidomastoid muscles resulted in activation of the phrenic nerves and became an accepted method of restoring ventilation.[13,14] The technique of phrenic nerve stimulation was supplanted by the development of the more reliable mechanical ventilators in the early 20th century. In the 1940s, however, Sarnoff et al[15,16] demonstrated that ventilation could be maintained in an acute setting in patients with bulbar poliomyelitis utilizing percutaneous electrodes. The lack of implantable devices that were safe and reliable, however, limited the long-term usefulness of this technique.

It was the critically important work of Glenn et al in the 1960s that resolved major technological issues and led to the development and implementation of modern-day pacing systems.[17–19] These investigators defined the appropriate patient selection criteria, preoperative assessment methodology, surgical methods including optimal electrode placement, and appropriate stimulation parameters necessary to achieve full-time ventilatory support.[7–11,19,20] Further refinements to this early design were made by other investigators with regard to improved electrode design[21,22] and less invasive methods of electrode placement.[23–26] As a consequence, DP has evolved into a safe and practical method of providing ventilatory support in select patient groups.

Rationale for Diaphragmatic Pacing

For patients requiring chronic ventilatory support, DP provides several advantages compared to mechanical ventilation (Table 62-1).[4,5,10,27–31] While the realized benefits of DP are subjective and vary between individuals, most patients describe an improved sense of well being and overall health. This could be attributable to one or more factors. Because patients are utilizing their own breathing muscles, patients relate the sensation of more normal breathing. Negative-pressure ventilation also has the potential to reduce the incidence of barotrauma and may have beneficial cardiovascular effects.[32] Because ventilator tubing is unnecessary, tension on the tracheostomy tube by attached tubing is eliminated, improving patient comfort.

Although the volume of speech may be less with DP than with mechanical ventilation, quality of speech is often improved because ventilator interference is eliminated. Speech can be enhanced by use of an abdominal binder.[33] Olfactory sensation is also restored with DP.

A life-support system that requires attachment to a mechanical ventilator by connecting tubing is extremely restrictive. Patient mobility and patient transport therefore are usually enhanced by DP. Simple daily maneuvers such as transfer from bed to chair are less cumbersome and eventful. Transport of patients outside the home is also easier. Improved mobility may allow patients to acquire gainful employment, become eligible for participation in

TABLE 62-1 Potential Benefits of Diaphragmatic Pacing

A. Improved quality of life
  1. Subjective sense of more normal breathing
     a. Utilization of breathing muscles
     b. Negative pressure respiratory support
  2. Improved comfort level
     a. Elimination of pull of ventilator tubing
     b. Negative-pressure breathing
  3. Improved speech
  4. Restoration of olfactory sensation
  5. Increased mobility
     a. Easier transport outside the home
     b. Easier transfer to and from bed
  6. Reduced anxiety and embarrassment
     a. Elimination of ventilator noise
     b. Elimination of fear of ventilator disconnection
     c. Elimination of ventilator tubing
     d. Daytime closure of tracheostomy
B. Reduced overall costs
  1. Reduction or elimination of ventilator supplies
  2. Reduced level of nursing and respiratory therapy services

SOURCE: Reproduced, with permission, from DiMarco.[27]

specific rehabilitation programs, and participate in more social events.[27,30,34–36]

Other concerns for many patients include social embarrassment because of ventilator noise, attached tubing, and being tethered to a machine. Many patients cannot support themselves off the ventilator and live in constant fear of disconnection. By comparison, DP is virtually indistinguishable from normal breathing by observers and the fear of ventilator disconnection is eliminated.

The institution of DP is very expensive and can easily exceed $100,000. Once in place, however, servicing and maintenance costs are minimal.[29,37] Despite the high initial cost, it can be argued that DP is cost effective. Many patients are transferred to less intensive and less expensive care settings.[27,28,38] The high cost of maintenance supplies necessary with mechanical ventilators is reduced. Because most patients who undergo DP are young and require respiratory support for many years, these cost savings can be substantial.[39–41]

Equipment

The basic configuration of commercially available DP pacing systems is very similar, consisting of both implanted materials and external components (Fig. 62-1). The electrodes, radio-frequency receivers, and connecting wiring comprise the surgically implanted components. An external power supply, radio-frequency transmitter, and antenna wires comprise components outside of the body.

With each system, a single stimulating electrode is surgically positioned on each phrenic nerve. With unipolar systems, an indifferent electrode is also implanted subcutaneously.[9] Wires are tunneled subcutaneously to connect each electrode to a radio-frequency receiver that is positioned over the anterior chest wall, usually over the lower rib cage.[9] The external battery-powered transmitter

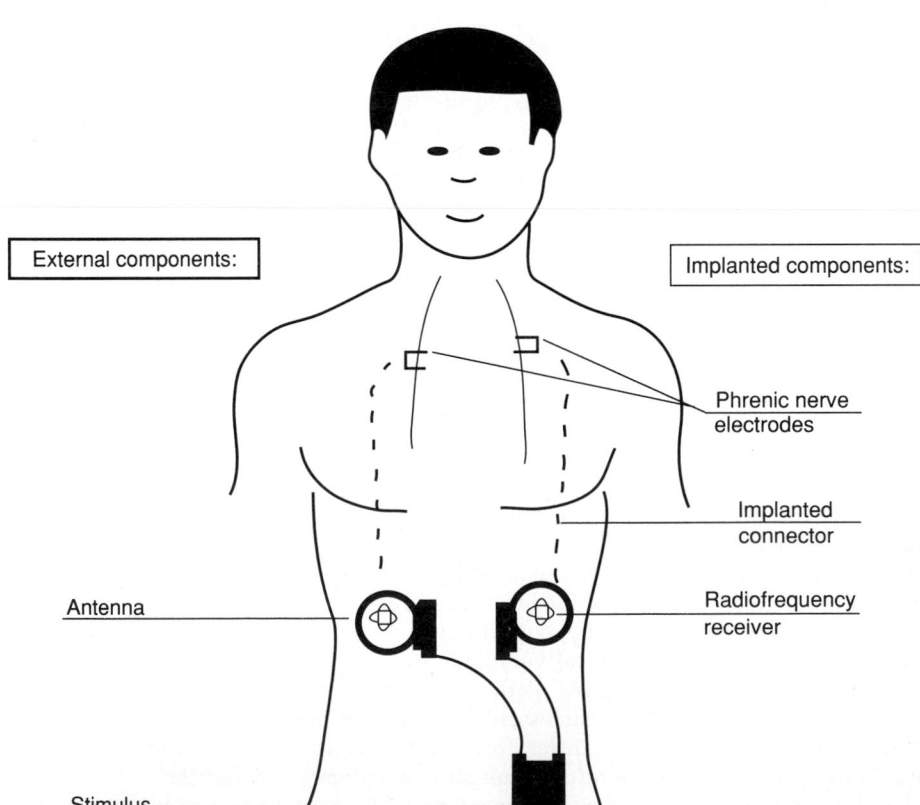

External components:

Implanted components:

Phrenic nerve electrodes

Implanted connector

Antenna

Radiofrequency receiver

Stimulus transmitter

FIGURE 62-1 Basic design of commercially available diaphragmatic pacing systems. The internal components (*left side*) consist of a single electrode implanted on each phrenic nerve in the thorax; each electrode is connected by wires to a subcutaneously implanted radio-frequency receiver. The external components consist of a stimulus transmitter and attached rubberized antennae, which must be positioned over the radio-frequency receivers. The receiver converts radio-frequency signals from the transmitter and converts them to electrical signals, which stimulate the phrenic nerves to activate the diaphragm. (*Reprinted, with permission, from DiMarco.*[28])

TABLE 62-2   Technical Features of Phrenic Nerve Pacing Systems

Manufacturer	Avery Laboratories	Atrotech OY	Medimplant
Transmitter (stimulus generator)	Mark IV[a]	PX 244	Medimplant 8-channel stimulator
Size (mm)	146 × 140 × 25	185 × 88 × 28	170 × 130 × 51
Transmitter/battery weight (kg)	0.54	0.45 + 0.6 (12V) 0.45 + 0.046 (9V)	1.42
Rate (breaths/min)	6–24	8–35	5–60
Amplitude (mA)	0–10	0–6	0–4
Pulse width (μs)	150	200	100–1000
Battery life (hr)	400	160–320 (12V) 8 (9V)	24
Sigh possible	Yes	Yes	Yes
Antenna	902A	TC 27-250/80	RF transmission coil
Receiver	Model I-110A	RX 44-27-2	Implantable receiver
size (mm)	30 (diam) × 8	49 (diam) × 8.5	56 × 53 × 14
Electrodes	Monopolar, bipolar	Quadripolar	Quadripolar
No. of receivers to stimulate both hemidiaphragms	2	2	1

[a]The Mark IV supercedes all earlier versions manufactured by Avery Laboratories. Most patients implanted with earlier models have been upgraded to the Mark IV without surgery.
SOURCE: Reproduced, with permission, from DiMarco.[27]

generates radio-frequency signals, which are inductively coupled to the receivers via circular rubberized antennas. Each antenna must be positioned directly over each receiver and secured in place to ensure proper transmission of the signal. The transmitter signal is demodulated by the receivers, converting the radio-frequency signals to electrical signals, which are transmitted to the electrodes to stimulate the phrenic nerves and activate the diaphragm.[9,16]

The transmitter allows adjustment of stimulus amplitude (milliamperes; mA) and stimulus frequency (Hertz; Hz) to modulate the magnitude of tidal volume. Respiratory rate can be adjusted by altering the train rate. Inspiratory time and inspiratory flow rate can be adjusted, in tandem, by alterations of stimulus on-time. Sigh breaths can also be provided.

Of the three commercially available DP pacing systems, only the Avery system is available world-wide. The technical characteristics of each device are provided in Table 62-2.

AVERY LABORATORIES MARK IV

Glenn et al performed the basic science and clinical studies that led to the commercial application of the Avery system in the 1960s.[42,43] The electrode consists of a semicircular platinum-iridium ribbon embedded in molded silicone rubber. The electrode contains a shallow trough for placement of the phrenic nerve. Monopolar and bipolar electrodes (recommended for patients with cardiac pacemakers) are available.[9] The recent Avery Mark IV transmitter (Commack, NY) is lighter and provides a wider range of stimulus amplitudes than previous models.[29] An optional interface also allows biofeedback control from pulse oximetry and CO_2 monitoring.[29] Trans-telephonic monitoring is available, which allows the electronic output and neuro-

physiologic response of the pacing system to be monitored by telephone.[44]

ATROTECH OY

The unique feature of the Atrotech system (Tampere, Finland) lies in its electrode technology, which consists of a four-pole electrode design.[21,45] The electrode consists of two identical strips of Teflon fabric with two platinum buttons mounted onto each strip. Theoretically, when appropriately placed, the phrenic nerve is divided equally into four stimulation compartments. Each quadrant of the nerve, which supplies a specific set of diaphragm motor units, is stimulated sequentially. During one stimulus sequence, which consists of four current combinations, one pole in turn acts as a cathode and one pole on the opposite side as an anode. The result is four excitation compartments around the nerve. Combined stimulation of all quadrants of the nerve (each at 5–6 Hz) results in activation of the diaphragm near its optimum fusion frequency of 20–25 Hz, resulting in smooth contraction of the diaphragm.[21,45]

By this method, the stimulation frequency of individual axons is less than with monopolar stimulation. The slower stimulus frequency should provide more time for recovery, improve the endurance characteristics of the diaphragm, and shorten the conditioning process, compared to conventional unipolar stimulation.[21,45,46] This technique had been approved by the FDA through an investigational device exemption (IDE). However, as of October 2005, the IDE study has been terminated. Further availability of this device in the USA is unknown.

MEDIMPLANT BIOTECHNISCHES LABOR

The Medimplant Biotechnisches Labor system (Vienna, Austria) is also differentiated by a unique electrode design.[22]

A complex microsurgical technique involving placement of four electrode leads around each phrenic nerve is required. The nerve tissue between each electrode lead comprises different stimulating compartments, only one of which is stimulated during any single inspiration. The various compartments are stimulated in sequence during subsequent inspirations (carousel stimulation).[47] Sixteen different electrode combinations can be adjusted individually for each nerve. Similar to the Atrotech device, only a portion of the nerve is stimulated at any given time, allowing more recovery time and therefore less chance for the development of fatigue compared to the unipolar design. Availability of this system is limited predominantly to Austria and Germany.

DIFFERENT TECHNOLOGICAL METHODOLOGIES

CERVICAL VERSUS THORACIC ELECTRODE PLACEMENT

Surgical techniques have been developed for both cervical and thoracic placement of phrenic nerve electrodes.[7–9,11] While less invasive from a surgical standpoint, the cervical approach has significant disadvantages. First, an accessory branch from a lower segment of the cervical cord may join the main trunk of the phrenic nerve low in the neck or in the upper thorax.[8] Activation of the cervical portion of the phrenic nerve may therefore lead to incomplete activation of the phrenic nerve and reduce the chance of successful pacing. Second, other nerves in close proximity to the phrenic nerve may also be activated, resulting in pain and/or unwanted movement.[35] Finally, neck movement may displace the electrode, resulting in incomplete diaphragmatic activation and/or place significant mechanical stress on the nerve increasing the risk of injury. Consequently, the thoracic approach is the preferred method of stimulation.[22,28,48]

ALTERNATIVE METHODS OF ELECTRODE PLACEMENT

A thoracotomy is associated with significant perioperative morbidity, requiring an inpatient hospital stay and high cost. These disadvantages have limited the number of patients undergoing this procedure, and is a significant obstacle for patients undertaking phrenic nerve pacing.

Two alternative methods of electrode placement have been investigated.

Thoracoscopic Placement of Phrenic Nerve Electrodes

Phrenic nerve electrodes have been successfully placed thoracoscopically.[26,49] This procedure involves placement of trocars in several intercostal spaces and is technically quite demanding. Successful pacing was achieved for 12–14 hours/day while awake in a small group of children, primarily for management of congenital CHS. Moreover, while less invasive than thoracotomy, these patients also developed complications of pneumonia, atelectasis, and pneumothorax postoperatively. Additional studies are necessary to determine the long-term success of this procedure and its applicability to patients with cervical spinal cord injury.

Phrenic Nerve Stimulation Via Intramuscular Diaphragmatic Electrodes

The phrenic nerves can also be activated via placement of electrodes directly into the diaphragm.[23,24,50,51] Conventional laparoscopy is employed for electrode placement.[52] Four laparoscopic ports are required to provide access to the abdominal cavity for visualization, insufflation of the abdominal cavity, diaphragm mapping, and insertion of the implant tool (Fig. 62-2). Specially designed surgical tools and intramuscular electrodes are required for implantation.[23–25,53–55] Two intramuscular electrodes are implanted into each hemidiaphragm near the phrenic nerve motor points.[56,57] A mapping procedure is required for appropriate electrode placement.[23,24] By this method, full-time ventilator support can also be maintained in ventilator-dependent tetraplegic patients with success rates similar to those of direct phrenic nerve stimulation.[15,23,24,30]

The advantages of this technique include the fact that laparoscopy is less invasive[58] compared to thoracotomy, and it can be performed on an outpatient basis or with an overnight observational stay, significantly reducing costs.[23,24] The risk of nerve injury is virtually eliminated because this procedure does not require manipulation of the phrenic nerve. Postoperative pain is less for patients with CHS.

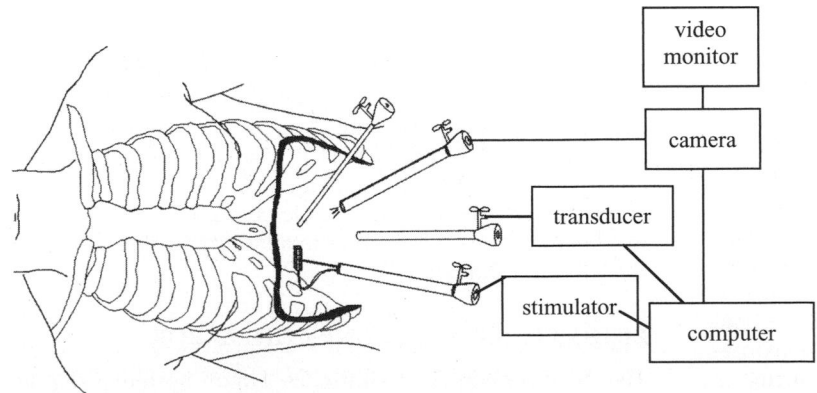

FIGURE 62-2 Schematic illustration of laparoscopic implant materials required for implantation of intramuscular diaphragmatic electrodes. Four laparoscopic ports are necessary to provide access to the abdominal cavity. Ports are necessary for visualization, insufflation of the abdominal cavity, diaphragmatic mapping, and insertion of the electrode implant tool. (*Reproduced, with permission, from DiMarco et al.[24]*)

This technique is not yet commercially available but has received approval by the FDA through an IDE (Synapse Biomedical LLC, Cleveland, OH).

Combined Intercostal and Diaphragmatic Pacing

Many patients with cervical spinal cord injury have damage to one or both phrenic motor neuron pools in the spinal cord and/or phrenic rootlets, and therefore cannot be offered DP.[27,59,60] By placing electrodes epidurally on the ventral surface of the upper thoracic spinal cord, however, the inspiratory intercostal muscles of the upper rib cage can also be stimulated to produce large inspired volumes.[34,61–64] Moreover, gas exchange during intercostal breathing alone is comparable to diaphragmatic breathing.[65]

In initial clinical trials, in patients with absent diaphragmatic function, stimulation of the intercostal muscles alone produced inspired volumes of similar magnitude to those resulting from activation of a single hemidiaphragm.[63] Inspired volume, however, was not sufficient to support ventilation for prolonged periods. In subsequent trials in tetraplegic patients with unilateral diaphragmatic function, however, stimulation of the intercostal muscles in combination with unilateral phrenic nerve stimulation was successful in providing long-term ventilatory support.[64]

Side effects of intercostal muscle stimulation included mild flexion of both hands and contraction of the muscles of the upper torso, which was well tolerated.[63,64] Intercostal pacing may be a useful adjunct to enhance tidal volume in patients whose inspired volume with phrenic nerve pacing alone is suboptimal.

This technique is not yet commercially available but has received approval by the FDA through an IDE.

Patient Selection

As mentioned, DP provides clinical benefit in two patient groups: ventilator-dependent tetraplegics[7,10,30] and patients with CHS.[4,5,66] While phrenic nerve pacing has been tried in patients with chronic obstructive pulmonary disease to prevent ventilatory depression associated with oxygen administration,[67] noninvasive ventilator support is of equal or greater effectiveness.

In all patients, significant lung, chest wall, or primary muscle disease must be excluded because these conditions may preclude successful pacing.[35,48,68] The adequacy of phrenic nerve function must also be established.

VENTILATOR-DEPENDENT TETRAPLEGIA

Respiratory failure is common following acute cervical spinal cord injury.[59,60] Fortunately, most patients achieve significant recovery following their initial presentation and are able to breathe spontaneously. Nonetheless, ~4% require lifelong respiratory support.[58] While the time

course of recovery is variable, the degree of impairment is likely permanent 12–15 months following injury.[60,69] Given the high cost and the invasive procedure required, conventional DP should not be considered before this time.

Vigorous attempts should be made to wean tetraplegic patients from mechanical ventilation. Vital capacity measurements of <10 ml/kg suggest inadequate inspiratory muscle function to maintain spontaneous breathing.[60] In some patients with sufficient inspiratory muscle strength, however, noninvasive ventilator support may be a suitable alternative to DP.[70,71]

Individual psychosocial conditions are important factors in the ultimate success of phrenic nerve pacing.[23,27,30,42] A high level of motivation and cooperation of the patient and family members is imperative. A home situation in which the family unit is anxious to improve the mobility, social interaction, occupational potential, and ability of the patient to function independently is optimal. Consequently, a psychosocial evaluation should be conducted before any technical evaluation. The evaluation process of potential candidates for DP is shown in Fig. 62-3.

CENTRAL HYPOVENTILATION SYNDROMES

Patients with CHS consist mainly of infants and children. Pacing is not instituted before 6–12 months of age to allow time to identify other potential abnormalities and determine the full extent of the ventilatory deficit.[3] CHS can be congenital[1,2] or secondary to brainstem dysfunction from injury, bleeding, tumor, encephalitis, or Arnold-Chiari malformations.[3,10] To assess the presence and degree of hypoventilation, arterial blood gases, nocturnal polysomnograms, and ventilatory responses to hypercarbia and hypoxia should be performed.

The diagnosis of congenital CHS is usually made shortly after birth. Many of these patients have normal wake ventilation and therefore require DP only during sleep.[3,4] Patients who require full-time ventilator support are paced during the day and maintained on mechanical ventilation during sleep. A psychosocial evaluation of these patients should also be performed.

EVALUATION OF PHRENIC NERVE FUNCTION

Before instituting DP, a thorough evaluation of phrenic nerve function is mandatory in all patients.[9,19,23,66] Phrenic nerve function can be assessed by measurements of nerve conduction times.[40,72,73] Diaphragmatic action potentials are monitored by surface electrodes positioned between the seventh and ninth intercostal spaces. The phrenic nerves can be electrically stimulated by surface electrodes or monopolar needle electrodes at the posterior border of the sternocleidomastoid muscle at the level of the cricoid cartilage. Electrical current is applied with single pulses of gradually increasing intensity until a supramaximal M wave is seen. With stimulation, the abdominal wall expands outward. Phrenic nerve conduction time can be determined by measuring the time interval between the applied

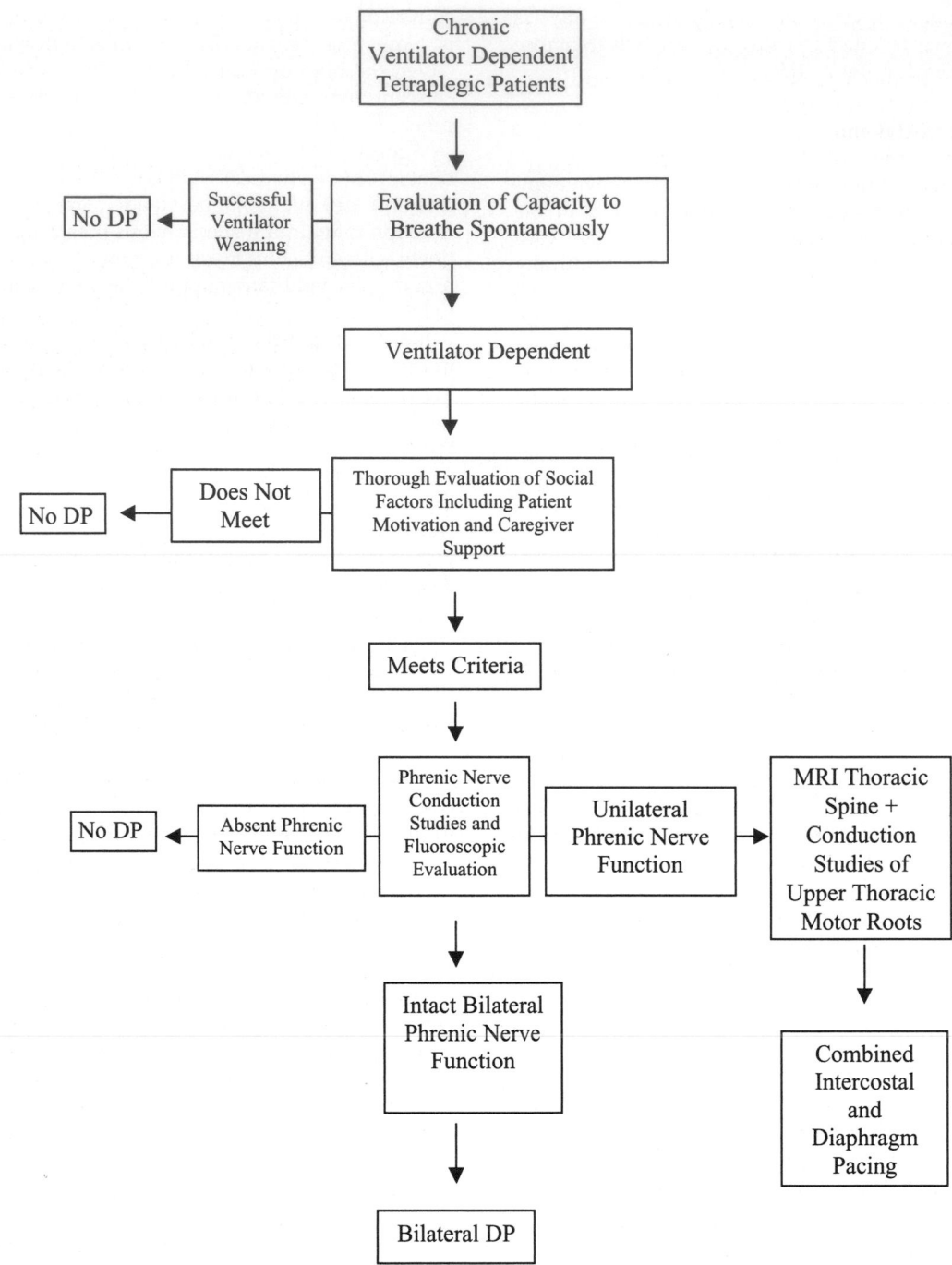

FIGURE 62-3 Evaluation of potential candidates with cervical spinal cord injury for diaphragmatic pacing.

stimulus and onset of the compound muscle action potential (CAP). Phrenic nerve function can also be assessed by cervical magnetic stimulation of the phrenic nerves.[74,75] Mean onset latency is 7–9 ms in normal adults.[40,72,73] Mild prolongation of conduction times (up to14 ms), however, does not preclude successful pacing.[11] In children, latencies are significantly shorter at 2.2 ms at 6 months of age, but increase to 4.2 ms between 5 and 11 years of age.[6,76] The magnitude of the CAP is a less reliable indicator of phrenic nerve function compared to conduction time.[28,72]

Because of false-positives and false-negatives associated with conduction time measurements, fluoroscopy should also be performed (personal observation). The diaphragm should descend at least 3–4 cm following stimulation.[9,27,40] In children with CHS, diaphragm descent of at least 2 rib spaces following spontaneous effort indicates adequate phrenic nerve function.[3] In this population, phrenic nerve stimulation is reserved for patients in whom fluoroscopic results are questionable.

Phrenic nerve function can also be assessed by measurements of transdiaphragmatic pressure (Pdi) (i.e., the pressure difference across the diaphragm).[37] By this method, small balloon-tipped catheters are placed into the esophagus and stomach to determine intrathoracic and intra-abdominal pressures, respectively. Single shock stimulation results in Pdi values of ~10 cmH$_2$O for each side in normal subjects.[77] Because of diaphragmatic atrophy, this value may be reduced significantly in ventilator-dependent patients. In spontaneously breathing individuals, diaphragmatic strength can be assessed by measuring Pdi during a maximal sniff maneuver.[77]

Implementation

The various surgical techniques to implant electrodes necessary for DP have been described previously[8,11,78] and are beyond the scope of this chapter.

DP should not commence until 10–14 days postoperatively to allow resolution of inflammation and edema at the electrode/nerve interface and initial healing of surgical wounds.[9] In patients who have been maintained on mechanical ventilation for prolonged periods, the transition to DP requires a gradual conditioning period, because of diaphragmatic atrophy.[10,19,20,79] Too rapid institution of pacing carries the risk of diaphragmatic fatigue and possible injury.

DETERMINATION OF STIMULUS-OUTPUT VALUES

Several parameters should be determined initially and then monitored regularly.[11,28] These include stimulus threshold values (minimum stimulus amplitude that results in visible or palpable diaphragmatic contraction) and supramaximal amplitudes and frequencies (lowest stimulus parameters that result in maximum inspired volume production). Changes in airway pressure during airway occlusion also provide a useful assessment of diaphragmatic force. The magnitude of inspired volumes and force generation gradually increase during the conditioning phase. Plateaus in these indices over time suggest that the conditioning phase is complete and optimum diaphragmatic function has been achieved. Assessment of diaphragmatic action potentials may also be useful in the determination of maximum stimulus amplitude.[3]

DETERMINATION OF STIMULUS PARAMETERS TO ACHIEVE ADEQUATE VENTILATION

Utilizing supramaximal amplitudes, tidal volume is adjusted by changing stimulus frequency. With respiratory rates (stimulus train rates) between 8 and 14 breaths/min stimulus frequency is adjusted to achieve inspired volumes resulting in P$_{CO_2}$ values in the low normal range. Stimulus frequency should be set at the lowest level possible and should not exceed 20 Hz. Respiratory rate and tidal volume are further adjusted for patient comfort. Inspired volume measurements should be made both in the supine and upright postures. While sitting, spinal cord–injured patients should wear a snugly fitting binder due to the shorter di-

aphragm length and higher resting lung volume associated with this posture. Higher stimulus parameters may be required in this posture.

INSTITUTION OF DIAPHRAGMATIC PACING

The methods of transition from mechanical ventilation to pacing are somewhat arbitrary. With the objective of achieving full-time DP as quickly as possible, but without the development of diaphragmatic fatigue, the following protocol is suggested. Utilizing the above-mentioned stimulus parameters, continuous bilateral DP is initially provided until significant blood gas derangements (reductions in oxygen saturation or elevations in end-tidal P$_{CO_2}$), reductions in inspired volume generation (monitored every 5–10 minutes), or patient discomfort related to air hunger are observed. Pacing is then initiated for a somewhat shorter time period (~5 minutes) every hour during the day, for the first week. This assessment is repeated weekly and a new pacing schedule is applied accordingly. After full-time pacing is achieved during wakefulness, pacing is provided during sleep. Most patients cap the tracheostomy tube while pacing during the day. During sleep, however, airflow through the tracheostomy must be maintained to prevent upper airway obstruction. This occurs secondary to the dyssynchrony between upper airway and diaphragmatic contraction during sleep.[4,19]

Previous studies have demonstrated that chronic diaphragmatic stimulation at high frequencies can be associated with myopathic changes and consequent reductions in force generation.[7,30,80] Consequently, it is important that DP occur at low stimulus frequencies (<20 Hz), which convert the diaphragm from a mixed fiber type population to predominantly high-oxidative, slow-twitch fatigue-resistant type I fibers.[7,81] As the conditioning phase progresses, stimulation frequencies and respiratory rates should be gradually reduced to the lowest values that maintain adequate ventilation and patient comfort. With the Avery system, stimulation frequency can usually be reduced to 7–9 Hz with respiratory rates of 6–12 breaths/min in the supine position.[7] Less adjustment is usually required with the Atrotech device secondary to the initial application of low frequencies via sequential nerve stimulation. With intramuscular stimulation, stimulation is initiated with 4 electrodes at 20 Hz. Stimulation frequency can be reduced to as low as 11 Hz with stimulation of only 2 electrodes.[23] Infants and young children require higher respiratory rates in the range of 20 breaths/min, but can be maintained with lower inspiratory times of 0.6–0.9 second compared to the requirement of 1–1.4 second in adults.[4,82] Conditioning time can vary between 4 weeks and several months. In most instances, however, conditioning is accomplished within 6–10 weeks.

In patients with CHS who employ DP only during sleep, DP should be adjusted in a sleep laboratory.[3] Given the high compliance of the rib cage and higher ventilatory requirements, bilateral pacing is always necessary to support ventilation in infants and young children.[3,4] In patients undergoing daytime pacing, pacing parameters must be re-evaluated because ventilatory requirements are typically higher during wakefulness.

COMBINING PACING WITH MECHANICAL VENTILATION

Full-time pacing is generally not advisable in infants and small children to avoid fatigue and the risk of permanent injury to the diaphragm and phrenic nerves.[3,4,82] Consequently, children with tetraplegia and those with CHS who require full-time ventilator support utilize DP during the day and are maintained on mechanical ventilation at night. Likewise, adult patients who do not achieve inspired volumes sufficient to maintain full-time pacing can be maintained on ventilator support at night. Because the major advantages of DP are realized during the day and most patients still require a tracheostomy, part-time DP does not detract significantly from the benefits of this device.

In some instances, patients cannot tolerate significant time off mechanical ventilation and initial inspired volumes achieved by pacing are insufficient to maintain adequate ventilation for even short periods.[53] In these patients, the initial phase of muscle reconditioning can be performed in conjunction with mechanical ventilation. This can be accomplished by setting the ventilator in the assist mode. The negative inspiratory pressure generated at the tracheal opening by pacing can be used to trigger the ventilator.

Effect of Diaphragmatic Pacing on Patient Outcome

Clinical studies reveal that DP is a feasible and effective means of providing ventilatory support in patients with tetraplegia and CHS. In most patients requiring full-time ventilatory support, DP can be utilized as the sole mode of respiration.[7,10,23,30]

The actual success rate of DP, however, is difficult to ascertain because most patients have undergone this technique at centers where patient numbers are small.[31,35,83] Moreover, previous large series have evaluated the outcome of DP while technology was still in development.[19,84–86] Consequently, these results are not applicable to systems available today.

In a recent report, the clinical outcome of patients whose phrenic nerves were implanted before 1987 was compared to patients implanted between 1981 and 1987.[30] The earlier group underwent high-frequency DP; the success rate in terms of achieving full-time pacing was small because of development of diaphragmatic fatigue. The later group underwent low-frequency stimulation at low respiratory rates; DP was successful in each of the 12 patients, stressing the importance of current pacing regimens. Six patients continued pacing for a mean duration of 14.8 years. The other 6 patients did not achieve sustained long-term pacing because of lack of adequate financial and social support or concomitant medical conditions. The results of this analysis indicate that the long-term success of diaphragmatic pacing

depends heavily on adherence to strict criteria for patient selection. High success rates have also been observed in infants and children in whom a more modest goal of part-time pacing (<15 hours/day) was achieved.[3]

The more recently developed quadripolar electrode design and receiver (Atrotech OY) is associated with high success rates. Based on analysis of 64 patients, successful pacing was achieved in 94% of pediatric and 86% of adult patients.[46] At the time of study, however, the average duration of pacing was only ~2 years.

Complications and Side Effects

Technical developments and clinical experience with DP over the past 20 years have markedly reduced the incidence of complications and side effects. With modern day equipment, appropriate patient selection, proper use of stimulus paradigms, and adequate patient monitoring, complications are few. As with any life-support system, patients must be carefully monitored because pacemaker failure can have catastrophic consequences. For this reason, all patients who are unable to maintain adequate spontaneous ventilation for prolonged periods should have emergency access to mechanical ventilation.

Several technical problems can cause reductions in volume production (Table 62-3). The most common cause of mechanical failure is loss of battery power. With current pacing systems, however, routine maintenance requires regular battery changes and recharging schedules. Low-battery alarms are also present. Breakage of the external antenna wires at stress points, either near the connection to the transmitter or more commonly at the connection to the receivers, can occur.

Concerning the internally implanted components, failure of the radio-frequency receiver was a fairly common problem with older systems secondary to leakage of body fluid through the epoxy encapsulation. Wire breakage within

---

TABLE 62-3 Complications and Side Effects of Phrenic Nerve Pacing

A. Technical malfunction
   1. External components
      a. Battery failure
      b. Breakage of antenna wires
   2. Implanted components
      a. Receiver failure
      b. Electrode malfunction
      c. Breakage of implanted connecting wires
B. Infection
   1. Receiver site
   2. Electrode site
C. Mechanical injury to the phrenic nerve
   1. Iatrogenic injury at the time of surgery
   2. Late injury due to scar formation and/or tension on the nerve
D. Upper airway obstruction after tracheostomy closure
E. Paradoxical movement of the upper rib cage, particularly in children

the receiver can occur.[84] With older systems, this problem often occurred within 5 years of implantation.[19,48,84] With improvement in housing materials, receiver life has been extended significantly and reports of receiver failure are much less common.[46] Electrode wire malfunction or breakage is also much less common but can occur unpredictably at variable time periods following implantation. The most recent analysis of the quadripolar electrode system in patients who had undergone DP for ~2 years, demonstrated an electrode failure rate of 3.1%.[46] Failure rates were similar in tetraplegics and patients with CHS, and in adults and children. Failure of one or more of the four electrode combinations was fairly common, but usually did not interfere with successful pacing.[46]

Iatrogenic injury of the phrenic nerve can occur secondary to mechanical trauma during electrode implantation or secondary to subsequent tissue reaction and fibrosis around the electrode.[10,19,84] When performed at centers, however, by surgeons with expertise in DP and use of monopolar or quadripolar electrodes, rather than the older bipolar cuff electrodes that encircled the nerve, phrenic injury is infrequent.[46,87]

As with any foreign body, implantation of the internal components carries some risk of infection. Since the institution of this technique in the 1970s, infection rates have been relatively constant in the range of 3–5%.[19,46,84] The higher infection rate observed in active children with CHS is thought to occur as a result of the greater likelihood of local trauma in this population.[46] The development of infection usually requires the removal of all implanted materials.

Although there are some reports of successful tracheostomy closure following institution of DP, these are very uncommon. During the day, the state of wakefulness is associated with synchronous activation of the upper airway muscles and diaphragm during DP. During sleep, however, there is reduced activation of the upper airway dilator muscles and a greater tendency toward asynchronous upper airway muscle contraction resulting in upper airway obstruction, a form of obstructive sleep apnea.[4,88,89] With few exceptions, therefore, patients undergoing DP require a patent tracheostomy for nocturnal use. Maintenance of a tracheostomy also facilitates application of mechanical ventilation in the event of pacemaker malfunction or instances of increased respiratory demand such as acute infections.

In young children, paradoxical movement of the rib cage may occur as a result of the high chest-wall compliance, resulting in reduced inspired volume generation. Consequently, bilateral pacing is required because of paradoxical movement of the contralateral diaphragm and chest wall during DP.[3,19]

Finally, strong magnetic fields, such as those that occur with MRI scanning, can override the electronic circuitry of pacing systems. The substantial energy transmission associated with this scanning could be transmitted to the electrode resulting in phrenic nerve injury. The pacing system's internal components would also be attracted to the magnet. Exposure to electrotherapeutic devices that generate strong radio-frequency fields should also be avoided because they may interfere with the pacing system.

Monitoring

Unlike mechanical ventilators, DP systems have no alarm systems that reflect inadequate levels of ventilation. When not receiving direct attendance by caregivers, patients should employ a pulse oximeter as a monitor for possible pacemaker malfunction or inadequate tidal volume generation secondary to patient-related issues.

BEDSIDE EVALUATION

For all patients supported by DP, breathing should be comfortable and effortless. Caregivers should evaluate pacemaker function on a routine basis and also in situations that give rise to dyspnea. On palpation of the chest wall, inspiration should be associated with vigorous lateral expansion of the lower rib cage and anterior abdominal wall, bilaterally. Attachment of a spirometer to the tracheostomy tube allows easy measurement of tidal volume. The transmitter enables separate stimulation of each hemidiaphragm, allowing evaluation of each side independently. Adequacy of ventilation should be assessed with pulse oximetry and end-tidal CO_2 measurements.[27,28,37,66]

Troubleshooting

If inspired volume is inadequate, the function of the external components should be evaluated first. Initially, the batteries should be replaced because this is the most common cause of pacemaker malfunction. Subsequently, the antenna should be replaced. If function is not restored, the back-up transmitter should then be changed.[3]

The occurrence of abnormal lung mechanics can also cause reductions in inspired-volume generation during DP. For example, most tetraplegics have a markedly reduced ability to cough and consequently accumulate airway secretions that require regular evacuation. Retained secretions cause increases in airway resistance and the development of atelectasis with secondary reductions in lung compliance. These mechanical derangements will reduce inspired-volume generation. Removal of secretions usually results in prompt improvement. Likewise, bronchitis and pneumonia also result in reductions in inspired volume. If reductions in inspired volume are persistent, therefore, chest radiography may be necessary. This test is also useful to evaluate for wire breakage and electrode position.

Evaluation of the internal components can be performed according to previously described techniques.[84] Surface electrodes are placed at the costal margin to record the pacemaker stimulus pulse and diaphragmatic action potential. The signals are amplified and recorded on an oscilloscope. A schematic illustration of the signals obtained from the chest leads are shown in Fig. 62-4. The DP system is functioning properly if the radio-frequency signal from the transmitting antenna, stimulus pulse from the phrenic nerve electrode, and diaphragmatic action potential are seen on the oscilloscope. If the radio-frequency signal and stimulus pulse are

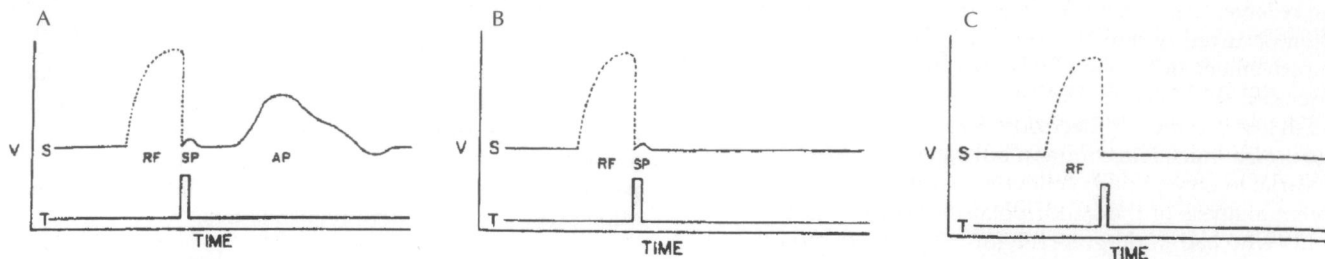

FIGURE 62-4 *A.* Schematic illustration of an oscilloscope tracing showing a properly functioning diaphragmatic pacing system. The lower tracing *T* represents the output from an extra receiver that was used to trigger the oscilloscope sweep. The upper trace (*S*) represents the signal obtained from the percutaneous leads on the chest. Shown in sequence are the radio-frequency signal (*RF*) from the transmitting antenna, the stimulus pulse (*SP*) from the electrode on the phrenic nerve, and the compound action potential (*AP*) from the diaphragm. *B.* Schematic of a malfunctioning pacing system. The tracing is the same except for the absence of the action potential. Breakage of wire insulation, lack of adequate phrenic nerve/electrode contact, or phrenic nerve damage are consistent with this finding. *C.* Schematic of another type of malfunctioning pacing system. In this case, the action potential and radio-frequency signal are absent. This finding suggests receiver malfunction. (*Reproduced, with permission, from Weese-Mayer et al.*[84])

observed without the action potential, this indicates that the wire insulation is no longer intact, the phrenic nerve is not in contact with the electrode, or the phrenic nerve has been damaged. If the stimulus pulse and action potential are both not seen, the receiver is not functional.

Important Unknowns

Prospective studies comparing outcomes between patients on mechanical ventilation versus DP do not exist. Carter et al,[90] however, compared survival rates in a retrospective analysis. Overall survival rates were similar between groups, but the patients on mechanical ventilation expired earlier than did patients maintained on DP. A higher incidence of respiratory tract infections in ventilated patients might account for this difference.

In the absence of depressed mental status and weakness of oropharyngeal muscles, some investigators have demonstrated that direct airway pressure methods, including mouth and nasal intermittent positive-pressure ventilation, can maintain adequate ventilation in tetraplegic patients.[68,69] These modalities offer the significant advantage of tracheostomy closure. Given the high cost and invasive nature of phrenic nerve implantation, these modalities may be better suited for some individuals. Newer methods of electrode placement, however, may swing the advantage in favor of DP.[23,24]

The Future

While existing DP systems provide substantial lifestyle advantages to patients compared to mechanical ventilation, current systems are somewhat cumbersome and have significant disadvantages and limitations. With the ultimate goal of complete restoration of normal respiratory system function, several refinements are needed.

Perhaps most significant is the future development of systems that synchronize upper-airway muscle and diaphragmatic contraction, which would eliminate upper-airway ob-

struction during DP.[88,89] One option would be to use an upper-airway muscle signal to trigger diaphragm activation. Such a device would not only eliminate the need for a tracheostomy but also provide ventilation on demand, allowing for changes in ventilatory requirements. A totally implantable system has not yet been developed, in part secondary to the high energy requirements of phrenic nerve pacing. A totally implantable system, similar to cardiac pacemakers, would eliminate the need for attachment of materials to the body surface, connection to a transmitter box, and battery changes. This development would further improve patient convenience and mobility.

Current DP systems are costly and require invasive procedures for electrode implantation. Early clinical results of thoracoscopic phrenic nerve implantation[26] and use of intramuscular diaphragmatic electrodes, which can be placed laparoscopically,[23,24] hold promise of added convenience, reduced risk, and lower overall costs of DP. DP in tetraplegic patients also requires a long reconditioning program because of disuse atrophy. Implantation of less invasive intramuscular electrodes soon after injury would allow more tetraplegic patients to use DP in place of mechanical ventilation. In patients in whom weaning is possible, electrodes can subsequently be removed without injury. Using this technique, it is also conceivable that ICU patients who require prolonged mechanical ventilation with the expectation of eventual recovery may benefit from DP to prevent diaphragmatic atrophy and consequent difficulty in weaning.

Finally, in patients with bilateral phrenic nerve injury, intercostal to phrenic nerve transfer may restore phrenic nerve viability and provide patients with the option of DP.[91]

Summary and Conclusions

In patients with ventilator-dependent tetraplegia and CHS, DP represents a practical method of ventilatory support with significant health and lifestyle advantages compared to mechanical ventilation. Advantages include increased mobility and level of independence, improved speech, improved sense of smell, and reduced anxiety and embarrassment associated with mechanical ventilation. The DP systems are smaller and more portable than ventilators and require less maintenance. Patients, however, must be carefully screened for social factors, including level of patient motivation and caregiver support, as well as coexisting medical conditions. Adequacy of phrenic nerve function must also be thoroughly evaluated preoperatively. In some patients, other means of support such as noninvasive ventilation may be more appropriate. Clinical studies examining less invasive and less costly means of applying DP and methods of activating the inspiratory intercostal muscles are underway. These new techniques are likely to increase the number of eligible patients and expand the clinical indications for DP.

Acknowledgements

The author wishes to acknowledge the assistance of Ms. Dana Hromyak, RRT for her invaluable assistance in the preparation of this chapter.

References

1. Mellins RB, Balfour HH Jr, Turino GM, Winters RW. Failure of automatic control of ventilation (Odine's curse). Report of an infant born with this syndrome and review of literature. Medicine (Baltimore) 1970; 49:487–504.
2. Deonna T, Arczynska W, Torrado A. Congenital failure of automatic ventilation (Odine's curse). A case report. J Pediatr 1974; 84:710–14.
3. Weese-Mayer DE, Hunt CE, Brouillette RT, Silvestri JM. Diaphragm pacing in infants and children. J Pediatr 1992; 120:1–8.
4. Hunt CE, Brouillette RT, Weese-Mayer DE, Morrow A, Ilbawi MN. Diaphragm pacing in infants and children. Pacing Clin Electrophysiol 1988; 11:2135–41.
5. Ilbawi MN, Idriss FS, Hunt CE, Brouillette RT, DeLeon SY. Diaphragmatic pacing in infants: techniques and results. Ann Thorac Surg 1985; 40:323–9.
6. Brouillette RT, Ilbawi MN, Hunt CE. Phrenic nerve pacing in infants and children: A review of experience and report on the usefulness of phrenic nerve stimulation studies. J Pediatr 1983; 102:32–9.
7. Glenn WW, Hogan JF, Loke JS, et al. Ventilatory support by pacing of the conditioned diaphragm in quadriplegia. N Engl J Med 1984; 310:1150–5.
8. Glenn WW, Hogan JF, Phelps ML. Ventilatory support of the quadriplegic patient with respiratory paralysis by diaphragm pacing. Surg Clin North Am 1980; 60:1055–78.
9. Glenn WW, Phelps ML. Diaphragm pacing by electrical stimulation of the phrenic nerve. Neurosurgery 1985; 17:974–84.
10. Glenn WW, Phelps ML, Elefteriades JA, Dentz B, Hogan JF. Twenty years of experience in phrenic nerve stimulation to pace the diaphragm. Pacing Clin Electrophysiol 1986; 9:780–4.
11. Glenn WW, Sairenji H. Diaphragm pacing in the treatment of chronic ventilatory insufficiency. In: Roussos C, Macklem PT, editors. The thorax: Lung biology in health and disease. New York: Marcel Dekker, 1985; 29:1407–40.
12. Caldani LMA. Institutiones physiologicae, Venezia, 1786. Cited by Schechter DC: Application of electrotherapy to noncardiac thoracic disorders. Bull NY Acad Med 1970; 46:932–51.
13. Beard GM, Rockwell AD. A practical treatise on the medical & surgical uses of electricity, including localized and general faradization; localized and central galvanization: electrolysis and galvano-cautery. New York: William Wood & Co, 1875.
14. Ferguson ??. Cited by Schechter DC: Application of electrotherapy to noncardiac thoracic disorder. Bull NY Acad Med 1970; 46:932–51.
15. Sarnoff SJ, Hardenberg E, Whittenberger JL. Electrophrenic respiration. Am J Physiol 1948; 155:1–9.
16. Whittenberger JL, Sarnoff SJ, Hardenberg E. Electrophrenic respiration. II. Its use in man. J Clin Invest 1949; 28:124–8.
17. Chae J, Triolo RJ, Kilgore KL, Creasey GH, DiMarco AF. Neuromuscular electrical stimulation in spinal cord injury. In: Kirshblum S, Campagnolo DI, DeLisa JA, editors. Spinal cord medicine. Philadelphia: Lippincott Williams & Wilkins, 2002: 360–88.
18. Chen CF, Lien IN. Spinal cord injuries in Taipei, Taiwan, 1978–1981. Paraplegia 1985; 23:364–70.
19. Glenn WW, Brouillette RT, Dentz B, et al. Fundamental considerations in pacing of the diaphragm for chronic ventilatory insufficiency: A multi-center study. Pacing Clin Electrophysiol 1988; 11:2121–7.
20. Oda T, Glenn WWL, Fukuda Y, Hogan JF, Gorfien J. Evaluation of electrical parameters for diaphragm pacing: An experimental study. J Surg Res 1981; 30:142–53.
21. Talonen PP, Baer GA, Hakkinen V, Ojala JK. Neurophysiological and technical considerations for the design of an implantable phrenic nerve stimulator. Med Biol Eng Comput 1990; 28:31–7.
22. Thoma H, Gerner H, Holle J, et al. The phrenic pacemaker: substitution of paralyzed functions in tetraplegia. ASAIO Trans 1987; 33:472–9.
23. DiMarco AF, Onders RP, Ignagni A, et al. Phrenic nerve pacing via intramuscular diaphragm electrodes in tetraplegic subjects. Chest 2005; 127:671–8.
24. DiMarco AF, Onders RP, Kowalski KE, et al. Phrenic nerve pacing in a tetraplegic patient via intramuscular diaphragm electrodes. Am J Respir Crit Care Med 2002; 166:1604–6.
25. Onders RP, DiMarco AF, Ignagni AR, Aiyar H, Mortimer JT. Mapping the phrenic nerve motor point: the key to a successful laparoscopic diaphragm pacing system in the first human series. Surgery 2004; 136:819–26.
26. Shaul DB, Danielson PD, McComb JG, Keens TG. Throacoscopic placement of phrenic nerve electrodes for diaphragmatic pacing in children. J Pediatr Surg 2002; 37:974–8.
27. DiMarco AF. Diaphragm pacing in patients with spinal cord injury. Top Spinal Cord Inj Rehabil 1999; 5:6–20.
28. DiMarco AF. Respiratory muscle stimulation in patients with spinal cord injury. In: Horch KW, Dhillon GS, editors. Neuroprosthetics: Theory and practice. New Jersey: World Scientific, 2004: 951–78.
29. Dobelle WH, D'Angelo MS, Goetz BF, et al. 200 Cases with a new breathing pacemaker dispel myths about diaphragm pacing. ASAIO J 1994; 40:M244–52.
30. Elefteriades JA, Quin JA, Hogan JF, et al. Long-term follow-up of pacing of the conditioned diaphragm in quadriplegia. Pacing Clin Electrophysiol 2002; 25:897–906.
31. Tibballs J. Diaphragmatic pacing: An alternative to long-term mechanical ventilation. Anaesth Intensive Care 1 1991; 19:597–601.
32. Langou RA, Cohen LS, Sheps D, Wolfson S, Glenn WW. Odine's curse: hemodynamic response to diaphragm pacing (electrophrenic respiration). Am Heart J 1978; 95:295–300.
33. Holt JD, Banzett AB, Brown R. Binding the abdomen can improve speech in men with phrenic nerve pacers. Am J Speech Lang Pathol 2002; 11:71–6.
34. DiMarco AF. Neural prostheses in the respiratory system. J Rehabil Res Dev 2001; 38:601–7.

35. Fodstad H. The Swedish experience in phrenic nerve stimulation. Pacing Clin Electrophysiol 1987; 10:246–51.

36. Fodstad H. Pacing of the diaphragm to control breathing in patients with paralysis of central nervous system origin. Stereotact Funct Neurosurg 1989; 53:209–22.

37. Moxham J, Shneerson JM. Diaphragmatic pacing. Am Rev Respir Dis 1993; 148:533–6.

38. DiMarco AF, Supinski G, Petro J, Takaoka Y. Artificial respiration via combined intercostal and diaphragm pacing in a quadriplegic patient. Am Rev Respir Dis 1994; 149:A135.

39. Esclarin A, Bravo P, Arroyo O, et al. Tracheostomy ventilation versus diaphragmatic pacemaker ventilation in high spinal cord injury. Paraplegia 1994; 32:687–93.

40. DeVivo MJ, Ivie CS III. Life expectancy of ventilator-dependent persons with spinal cord injuries. Chest 1995; 108:226–32.

41. Whiteneck GG, Charlifue SW, Frankel HL, et al. Mortality, morbidity, and psychosocial outcomes of persons spinal cord injured more than 20 years ago. Paraplegia 1992; 30:617–30.

42. Glenn WWL, Hageman JH, Mauro A, Eisenberg L, Flanigan S, Harvard M. Electrical stimulation of exciteable tissue by radiofrequency transmission. Ann Surg 1964;160:338–50.

43. Judson JP, Glenn WWL. Radio-frequency electrophrenic respiration: Long-term application to a patient with primary hypoventilation. JAMA 1968; 203:1033–7.

44. Auerbach AA, Dobelle WH. Transtelephonic monitoring of patients with implanted neurostimulators. Lancet 1987; 1:224–5.

45. Baer GA, Talonen PP, Shneerson JM, et al. Phrenic nerve stimulation for central ventilatory failure with bipolar and four-pole electrode systems. Pacing Clin Electrophysiol 1990; 19:1061–72.

46. Weese-Mayer DE, Silvestri JM, Kenny AS, et al. Diaphragm pacing with a quadripolar phrenic nerve electrode: an international study. Pacing Clin Electrophysiol 1996; 19:1311–9.

47. Mayr W, Bijak M, Girsch W, et al. Multichannel stimulation of phrenic nerves by epineural electrodes. ASAIO J 1993; 39:M729–35.

48. Vanderlinden RG, Epstein SW, Hyland RH, Smythe HS, Vanderlinden LD. Management of chronic ventilatory insufficiency with electrical diaphragm pacing. Can J Neuro Sci 1988; 15:63–7.

49. Shoji T, Oku Y, Ishikawa S, Wada H. Thoracoscopic electrode implantation for diaphragm pacing in dogs. Respiration 2002; 69:69–74.

50. Nochomovitz ML, DiMarco AF, Mortimer JT, Cherniack NS. Diaphragm activation with intramuscular stimulation in dogs. Am Rev Respir Dis 1983; 127:325–9.

51. Peterson DK, Nochomovitz M, DiMarco AF, Mortimer JT. Intramuscular electrical activation of the phrenic nerve. IEEE Trans Biomed Eng 1986; 33:342–52.

52. Stellato TA, Peterson DK, Buehner P, Nochomovitz ML. Taking the laparoscope to the laboratory for ventilatory research. Am Surg 1990; 56:131–3.

53. Aiyar H, Stellato TA, Onders RP, Mortimer JT. Laparoscopic implant instrument for the placement of intramuscular electrodes in the diaphragm. IEEE Trans Rehabil Eng 1999; 7:360–71.

54. Peterson DK, Nochomovitz ML, Stellato TA, Mortimer JT. Long-term intramuscular electrical activation of phrenic nerve: safety and reliability. IEEE Trans Biomed Eng 1994; 41:1115–26.

55. Peterson DK, Nochomovitz ML, Stellato TA, Mortimer JT. Long-term intramuscular electrical activation of phrenic nerve: efficacy as a ventilatory prosthesis. IEEE Trans Biomed Eng 1994; 41:1127–35.

56. Schmit BD, Mortimer JT. The effects of epimysial electrode location on phrenic nerve recruitment and the relation between tidal volume and interpulse interval. IEEE Trans Rehabil Eng 1999; 7:150–8.

57. Schmit BD, Stellato TA, Miller ME, Mortimer JM. Laparoscopic placement of electrodes for diaphragm pacing using stimulation to locate the phrenic nerve motor points. IEEE Trans Rehabil Eng 1998; 6:382–90.

58. Paw P, Sackier JM. Complications of laparoscopy and thoracoscopy. J Intensive Care Med 1994; 9:290–304.

59. National Spinal Cord Injury Statistical Center, University of Alabama at Birmingham. Annual Statistical Report 2004. Birmingham: University of Alabama.

60. Oo T, Watt JWH, Soni BM, Sett PK. Delayed diaphragm recovery in 12 patients after high cervical spinal cord injury. A retrospective review of the diaphragm status of 107 patients ventilated after acute spinal cord injury. Spinal Cord 1999; 37:117–22.

61. DiMarco AF, Altose MD, Cropp A, Durand D. Activation of intercostal muscles by electrical stimulation of the spinal cord. Am Rev Respir Dis 1987; 136:1385–90.

62. DiMarco AF, Budzinska K, Supinski GS. Artificial ventilation by means of electrical activation of intercostal/accessory muscles alone in anesthetized dogs. Am Rev Respir Dis 1989; 139: 961–7.

63. DiMarco AF, Supinski GS, Petro J, Takaoka Y. Evaluation of intercostal pacing to provide artificial ventilation in quadriplegics. Am J Respir Crit Care Med 1994; 150:934–40.

64. DiMarco AF, Takaoka Y, Kowalski KE. Combined intercostal and diaphragm pacing to provide artificial ventilation in patients with tetraplegics. Arch Phys Med Rehabil 2005;86:1200–7.

65. DiMarco AF, Connors AF, Kowalski KE. Gas exchange during separate diaphragm and intercostal muscle breathing. J Appl Physiol 2004; 96:2120–4.

66. Flageole H. Central hypoventilation and diaphragmatic eventration: diagnosis and management. Semin Pediatr Surg 2003; 12:38–45.

67. Glenn WW, Gee JBL, Schachter EN. Diaphragm pacing: Application to a patient with chronic obstructive lung disease. J Thorac Cardiovasc Surg 1978; 75:273–81.

68. Oliven A. Electrical stimulation of the respiratory muscles. In: Cherniack NS, Altose MD, Homma I, editors. Rehabilitation of the patient with respiratory disease. New York: McGraw-Hill, 1999: 535–42.

69. Carter RE. Unilateral diaphragmatic paralysis in spinal cord injury patients. Paraplegia 1980; 18:267–74.

70. Bach JR, Alba AS. Noninvasive options for ventilatory support of the traumatic high level tetraplegic patient. Chest 1990; 98:613–9.

71. Bach JR, Alba AS. Management of chronic alveolar hypoventilation by nasal ventilation. Chest 1990; 97:52–7.

72. MacLean IC, Mattioni TA. Phrenic nerve conduction studies: a new technique and its application in quadriplegic patients. Arch Phys Med Rehabil 1981; 62:70–3.

73. McKenzie DK, Gandevia SC. Phrenic nerve conduction times and twitch pressures of the human diaphragm. J Appl Physiol 1985; 58:1496–504.

74. Similowski T, Fleury B, Launois S, et al. Cervical magnetic stimulation: a new painless method for bilateral phrenic nerve stimulation in conscious humans. J Appl Physiol 1989; 67:1311–8.

75. Aquilina R, Wragg S, Moran J, et al. Magnetic stimulation as a simple and reliable method for stimulating the phrenic nerves in the neck. Thorax 1991; 46:754.

76. Moosa A. Phrenic nerve conduction in children. Dev Med Child Neurol 1981; 23:434–48.

77. Miller JM, Moxham J, Green M. The maximal sniff in the assessment of diaphragm function in man. Clin Sci (London) 1985; 69:91–6.

78. Ilbawi MN, Idriss FS, Hunt CE, Brouillette RT, DeLeon SY. Diaphragmatic pacing in infants: techniques and results. Ann Throac Surg 1985; 40:323–9.

79. Nochomovitz ML, Hopkins M, Brodkey J, et al. Conditioning of the diaphragm with phrenic nerve stimulation after prolonged disuse. Am Rev Respir Dis 1984; 130:685–8.

80. Ciesielski TE, Fukuda Y, Glenn WW, et al. Response of the diaphragm muscle to electrical stimulation of the phrenic nerve. A histochemical and ultrastructural study. J Neurosurg 1983; 58:92–100.

81. Salmons S, Henriksson J. The adaptive response of skeletal muscle to increased use. Muscle Nerve 1981; 4:94–105.

82. Brouillette RT, Ilbawi MN, Klemka-Walden L, Hunt CE. Stimulus parameters for phrenic nerve pacing in infants and children. Pediatr Pulmonol 1988; 4:33–8.

83. Hunt CE, Matalon SV, Thompson TR, et al. Central hypoventilation syndrome: Experience with bilateral phrenic nerve pacing in 3 neonates. Am Rev Respir Dis 1978; 118:23–8.

84. Weese-Mayer DE, Morrow AS, Brouillette RT, Ilbawi MN, Hunt CE. Diaphragm pacing in infants and children. A life-table analysis of implanted components. Am Rev Respir Dis 1989; 139:974–9.

85. McMichan JC, Piepgras DG, Gracey DR, Marsh HM, Sittipong R. Electrophrenic respiration. Mayo Clin Proc 1979; 54:662–8.

86. Oakes DD, Wilmot CB, Halverson D, Hamilton RD. Neurogenic respiratory failure: a 5-year experience using implantable phrenic nerve stimulators. Ann Thorac Surg 1980; 30:118–21.

87. Jaeger RJ, Langbein EW, Kralj A. Augmenting cough by FES in tetraplegia: A comparison of results at three clinical centers. Basic Appl Myol 1994; 4:195–200.

88. Glenn WW, Gee JB, Cole DR, et al. Combined central alveolar hypoventilation and upper airway obstruction. Treatment by tracheostomy and diaphragm pacing. Am J Med 1978; 64:50–60.

89. Scharf SM, Feldman NT, Goldman MD, et al. Vocal cord closure. A cause of upper airway obstruction during controlled ventilation. Am Rev Respir Dis 1978; 117:391–7.

90. Carter RE, Dono WH, Halstead L, Wilkerson MA. Comparative study of electrophrenic nerve stimulation and mechanical ventilatory support in traumatic spinal cord injury. Paraplegia 1987; 25:86–91.

91. Krieger LM, Krieger AJ. The intercostal to phrenic nerve transfer: an effective means of reanimating the diaphragm in patients with high cervical spine injury. Plast Reconstr Surg 2000; 105:1255–61.

Chapter 63

BRONCHODILATOR THERAPY

RAJIV DHAND

Bronchodilator therapy is frequently employed in mechanically-ventilated patients with chronic obstructive pulmonary disease (COPD) or asthma. Until recently, many barriers were thought to preclude effective inhalation therapy in ventilated patients. The major problems contributing to this opinion were the poor efficiency of aerosol-generating devices when employed in ventilator circuits, inadequate understanding of the factors influencing delivery of aerosols, and mechanical ventilators that were not designed to optimize aerosol use. There is now greater awareness of the needs of ventilated patients for bronchodilators and optimal techniques have been described for administration of inhaled drugs. In this chapter, bronchodilators employed in mechanically-ventilated patients are discussed with a special emphasis on inhalation therapy.

Rationale

Ventilator-dependent patients with acute exacerbations of COPD and acute severe asthma routinely receive bronchodilators to relieve bronchoconstriction. By reducing airway resistance, bronchodilators reduce the pressure required to ventilate the lung. This reduction in pressure may protect the lung against injury and enhance patient comfort. A general population of ventilated patients in a medical intensive care unit (ICU)[1] and patients with acute respiratory distress syndrome (ARDS)[2,3] showed improvement in expiratory airflow and airway resistance after bronchodilators. Infants with bronchopulmonary dysplasia, asthma, and bronchiolitis also receive bronchodilators on a routine basis.[4–8] In ventilated patients with COPD, elevated airway resistance and intrinsic positive end-expiratory pressure (PEEPi) are major causes for weaning failure.[9] In these patients, bronchodilators may facilitate weaning.[10] Therapy with bronchodilators is, therefore, routinely and commonly employed for many indications in ventilator-dependent patients.[11]

Pharmacologic Agents

$β$-Adrenergic agonists, anticholinergic drugs, and methylxanthines are the three major classes of bronchodilators. $β$-Adrenergic agonists and anticholinergics are usually administered by the inhaled route, whereas methylxanthines can only be administered enterally or parenterally. Inhaled bronchodilator therapy is preferred because the drug is delivered directly to its site of action in the airways, a smaller quantity of drug produces an effect comparable to that observed with systemic administration, onset of effect is rapid, and systemic absorption of the drug is limited, thus minimizing side effects.

ANATOMY OF THE AUTONOMIC INNERVATION TO THE LUNG

The sympathetic and parasympathetic nerves supplying the lung form a plexus at the hilum, and the nerves accompany the bronchovascular bundle. The preganglionic parasympathetic nerve fibers synapse with ganglia in the airway wall. Postganglionic fibers then innervate the smooth muscle and mucus glands. Although innervation proceeds as far as the level of the terminal bronchioles,[12] the greatest effect of cholinergic stimulation is seen in intermediate bronchi (1–5 mm in diameter).[13]

    The sympathetic system arises from the upper thoracic ganglia; sympathetic innervation is distributed through the pulmonary plexus, and is generally sparse. No adrenergic innervation is seen in the trachealis muscle, while a few

TABLE 63-1 Neurotransmitters for the Nonadrenergic Noncholinergic System (NANC) in Lung

Inhibitory NANC (i-NANC)	Vasoactive intestinal polypeptide (VIP), nitric oxide (NO)
Excitatory NANC (e-NANC)	Calcitonin gene-related peptide (CGRP), substance P (SP), neurokinin A

adrenergic fibers are seen in the fourth to seventh order bronchi.[14] The airways, however, have α- and β-adrenergic receptors and these are probably acted upon by circulating catecholamines. Some adrenergic fibers terminate on the parasympathetic system and may modulate the parasympathetic output.[15,16]

The parasympathetic fibers are the anatomic substrate for the bronchodilatory inhibitory nonadrenergic noncholinergic system (i-NANC) (Table 63-1). At least part of the NANC pathway is anatomically co-localized with the classic neurotransmitters. The mediators for i-NANC, such as nitric oxide and vasoactive intestinal polypeptide, are co-released with acetylcholine. Nitric oxide is probably the more important bronchodilator of the two mediators.[17] The excitatory NANC system (e-NANC) is composed of a group of unmyelinated C fibers that release calcitonin gene-related peptide, tachykinins like substance P, and neurokinin A.[18]

BETA AGONISTS

STRUCTURE OF THE β_2-ADRENERGIC RECEPTOR

β_2-Adrenergic receptors are part of a family of G protein coupled receptors. There is a common structural motif to these proteins, with seven transmembrane domains that form a pocket to which the agonist binds.[19] The intracellular domains of the receptor are associated with trimeric proteins consisting of α, β, and γ subunits. The α subunit is mobile, whereas the β and γ subunits are associated and fixed within the membrane. In the inactive state, the α subunit is bound to guanosine diphosphate (GDP). Once the

agonist binds to the receptor, the α subunit binds to guanosine triphosphate (GTP), dissociates from the $\beta\gamma$ complex, and binds to the effector site (Fig. 63-1). The hydrolysis of GTP to GDP results in activation of the effector and dissociation of the α subunit with reconstitution of the inactive $\alpha\beta\gamma$ trimer.[20]

ORGAN DISTRIBUTION AND EXTRAPULMONARY EFFECTS OF β_2-ADRENERGIC RECEPTOR ACTIVATION

The extrapulmonary effects of β_2-agonists, include effects on the cardiovascular system, metabolism, and skeletal muscle.

Cardiovascular System

β_2-Agonists can elicit cardiovascular responses through both direct and indirect actions.[21] In the heart, β_2-receptors comprise 30–40% of the atrial and 20–30% of the ventricular β-receptors,[22] being especially rich in the sinoatrial node.[23] Activation of β_2-receptors results in inotropic and chronotropic responses. Heart rate increases, in part, from direct stimulation of β_2-receptors,[24] especially those located in the sinoatrial node.[25] Albuterol produces a modest increase in heart rate,[26,27] which occurs within 1 hour and returns to baseline within 4 hours.[27] Tachyphylaxis occurs to the chronotropic response after chronic albuterol treatment.[28] Albuterol acts on β_2-receptors in the peripheral vasculature to produce vasodilation and this may reflexly increase heart rate. Inotropic responses to β_2-agonists result from direct stimulation of cardiac receptors or from reflex increase in sympathetic outflow and decrease in parasympathetic outflow accompanying peripheral vasodilation.[25]

Albuterol infusion produces pronounced shortening of refractory period and conduction time in nodal tissue.[29] While the atrial and ventricular myocardial refractory period decreases after albuterol, the ventricular depolarization time and QT dispersion increases.[29] An increase in QT dispersion is associated with increased mortality, possibly from ventricular arrhythmia and sudden cardiac death;[30] this might explain earlier observations of increased

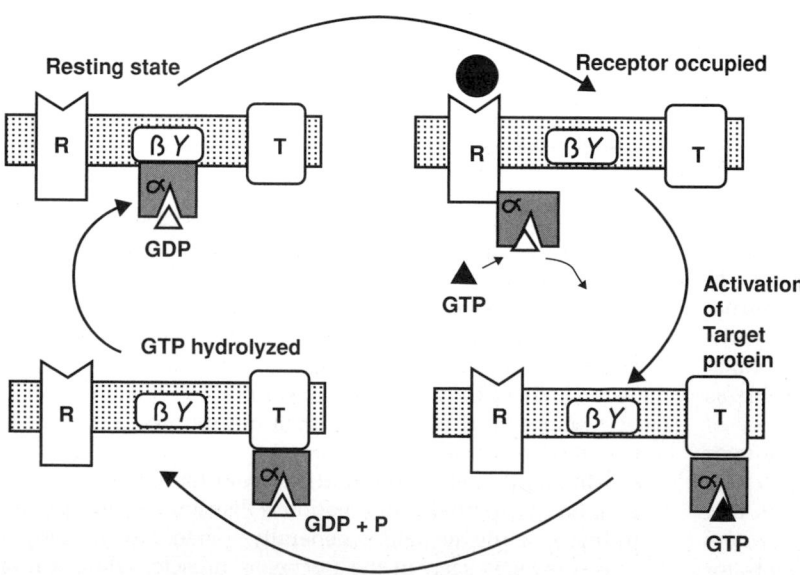

FIGURE 63-1 The intracellular domains of the β-adrenergic receptor are associated with trimeric proteins consisting of α, β, and γ subunits. In the resting state, the α subunit is bound to GDP. When the agonist binds the receptor, the α subunit binds to GTP, dissociates from the $\beta\gamma$ complex and binds to the effector site. Subsequently, the hydrolysis of GTP to GDP results in activation of the receptor and dissociation of the α subunit. The α subunit then binds to the $\beta\gamma$ complex with reconstitution of the $\alpha\beta\gamma$ trimer.

arrhythmogenicity observed after oral albuterol administration in patients with congestive heart failure.[31]

Intravenous albuterol infusion caused a fall in diastolic[29,32,33] and mean arterial pressure,[29] but systolic pressures were unchanged or increased.[32] The increase in stroke volume was not influenced by the dose of albuterol.[29] β_2-Receptor genotype could affect the systemic responses to inhaled salbutamol.[33] Lee et al[33] found that a single dose of inhaled albuterol exhibited a greater decrease in serum potassium and diastolic blood pressure in patients with asthma with the Arg16-Gln27 genotype than in patients with the Gly16-Glu27 genotype.

Metabolic Actions

β_2-Agonists produce hypokalemia.[34,35] The mechanism probably involves activation of the Na-K-ATPase pump, hyperglycemia, and enhanced insulin secretion.[36] Because it lowers serum potassium, albuterol has been used for treatment of hyperkalemia, especially in patients with end-stage renal disease. The fall in serum potassium with albuterol is dose dependent, and lasts for at least 2 hours.[37] An initial transient increase in serum potassium occurs after albuterol,[38] and a sufficient fall in potassium levels is not uniformly seen. Thus, albuterol is not recommended as a first-line therapy for hyperkalemia.[39]

A modest, dose-dependent increase in plasma glucose occurs after albuterol administration.[40] Patients may develop tachyphylaxis to this effect, especially after regular administration of high doses.[28] Tachyphylaxis occurs to the systemic effects of other β-agonists as well.[41,42] The dose-dependent increase in metabolic rate with albuterol[43] is also prone to tachyphylaxis.[44]

Skeletal Muscle

β-Agonists enhance both normal ballistocardiographic tremor (the normal vibration of the entire body in concert with cardiac systole) and normal postural tremor.[45] β-Agonist–induced tremors are probably caused by accentuation of normal postural tremor; this effect is dose related and shows tachyphylaxis with chronic use.[45]

β_2-ADRENERGIC—RECEPTOR ACTIVATION AND AIRWAY SMOOTH MUSCLE RELAXATION

The β_2-adrenergic agonist receptor complex activates multiple effectors.[46,47] Alteration in myosin light chain kinase (MLCK) activity is thought to play a role. MLCK phosphorylates and activates myosin and initiates muscle contraction. β_2-Receptor activation can decrease MLCK activity through cyclic adenosine monophosphate (cAMP)-mediated phosphorylation of MLCK.[48,49] Myosin activation depends on the relative activities of MLCK and myosin light chain phosphatase (MLCP), which dephosphorylates and reduces myosin activity. The role of MLCP in decreasing myosin activity and inducing relaxation in human airway smooth muscle is unclear.[50]

Activation of calcium-activated potassium channels (K_{Ca})[51] leading to hyperpolarization and relaxation, directly or through inhibition of voltage-dependent calcium influx, is another proposed mechanism for β-agonist–induced relaxation of airway smooth muscle. The effect on potassium channel activation, however, is unlikely to be a major mechanism for β-agonist–induced smooth muscle relaxation.[52]

Modulation of intracellular calcium levels may mediate β-agonist–induced smooth muscle relaxation.[53–55] An inhibitor of the sarcoplasmic reticulum calcium pump, however, did not alter the relaxation response induced by isoproterenol in human airway smooth muscle.[50]

In summary, although several mechanisms have been proposed to explain β-agonist–induced smooth muscle relaxation, there is insufficient evidence to conclusively support the role of any one mechanism of action.

BRONCHODILATION AND BRONCHOPROTECTION

A distinction is made between the increase in forced expiratory volume in 1 second (FEV_1) noted after β-agonist use with or without a preceding provocative challenge (bronchodilation) versus the ability of β-agonists to protect against a future bronchoprovocative challenge (bronchoprotection).[56–58] Following β-agonist use, tolerance to bronchoprotection develops faster and more reliably than tolerance to bronchodilation.[58] The methods of measurement, however, also differ and may partially explain the perceived differences.[57] The molecular mechanisms differentiating these characteristics are not known.

Increase in Airway Responsiveness and Tolerance to Bronchoprotection and Bronchodilation

Increase in airway responsiveness refers to the increase in sensitivity to direct[59,60] or indirect[61] stimuli that is demonstrable following cessation of chronic use of β-agonists. Direct stimuli (e.g., histamine and methacholine) act via smooth muscle cell membrane receptors. Indirect stimuli (e.g., cold air or allergens) result in the release of mediators from mast cells that then act on smooth muscle cell membrane receptors. Increase in airway responsiveness has been seen after use of short-acting β-agonists in some studies,[59,60,62] but not in others.[63,64] In contrast, studies done with long-acting β-agonists have not shown such increases in airway responsiveness after cessation of therapy.[65,66] The mechanism of the increased sensitivity to bronchoconstrictor stimuli is not well established, but is thought to involve β-receptor downregulation and desensitization. Other mechanisms (e.g., increased expression in phospholipase c-β) may also be involved.[67] A greater degree of β-receptor downregulation on mast cell membranes may explain increased responsiveness to indirect stimuli but not to methacholine, which acts directly on smooth muscle cells.[68] The clinical significance of the heightened responsiveness after discontinuation of regular β-agonists is not known.[69]

Tolerance to the bronchoprotective effect is rapid, as soon as 12 hours after exposure, does not appear to be progressive,[66] occurs with both short-acting[68,70] and long-acting agents,[64,71,72] and is of unknown clinical significance.[58] Tolerance to bronchoprotection in stable asthma may be less significant because the decreased bronchoprotective effect is still significantly therapeutic.[73] Currently, there are not enough data to caution against use of long-acting β-agonists for fear of losing bronchoprotection.[73] In this regard, it is important to consider that a combination of inhaled corticosteroids and long-acting bronchodilators controls asthma symptoms better than higher doses of inhaled corticosteroids alone.[74]

Tolerance to bronchodilation has been more difficult to prove.[28,75] Tolerance was better demonstrated against a background of provoked bronchoconstriction than in a setting of stable asthma.[76,77] A recent meta-analysis found a decrease in bronchodilator effect and a decrease in bronchoprotective effect after regular use of β-agonists for at least 1 week.[78] Tolerance to the bronchodilator effect may be clinically significant because frequent as-needed use may compromise the bronchodilator effects of β-agonists administered for an acute exacerbation. There is a debate whether regular long-acting β-agonist use without concurrent inhaled corticosteroids decreases the effectiveness of inhaled β-agonists during exacerbations.[79–82] Chronic frequent use of β-agonists, especially when used as the only medication, should be avoided in clinical practice.

The mechanism of tolerance to β-agonists is complex and several factors including uncoupling of receptors from the signal transduction chain, internalization of receptors, and decreased production of new receptors may contribute to its development.[83] The differences in development of tolerance with various β_2-receptor gentotypes[84–87] could be explained by differences in the sensitivity of certain receptor subtypes to downregulation by endogenous catecholamines.[88]

OTHER EFFECTS OF β_2-ADRENERGIC ACTIVATION IN THE LUNGS

Activation of β_2-receptors on the mast cell surface can prevent degranulation and release of mediators from mast cells.[89] β-Agonists decrease vascular permeability while increasing blood flow in animal models.[90,91] Salmeterol reduces allergen-induced vascular permeability during nasal challenge in patients with allergic rhinitis.[92] β-Agonist activation results in an increase in ciliary beat frequency, and an increase in tracheal mucus velocity and whole lung clearance. The effect on mucociliary clearance appears more prominent in healthy persons than in those with obstructive airway disease, and its clinical significance has not been elucidated.[93]

STRUCTURE-FUNCTION RELATIONSHIP FOR β_2-ADRENERGIC AGONISTS

The underlying structure of most drugs active at the adrenergic receptor is a phenylethylamine moiety. Substitution at various sites on this basic molecule can alter the overall efficacy of the drug as well as alter the selectivity for different receptors. In general, the presence of hydroxyl groups on positions 3 and 4 of the benzene ring confers increased activity at adrenergic receptors. Large substituents on the amino group result in increased activity at the β-adrenergic receptors. The presence of hydroxyl groups at positions 3 and 5 confer selectivity for β_2-receptors. Substitution at the α carbon atom blocks breakdown by monoamine oxidase and prolongs action of these drugs.[94] The duration of action of β_2-agonists generally ranges from 3–6 hours. The prolonged duration of action of salmeterol has been attributed to exosite binding, and more recently, to its enhanced lipophilicity.[95]

AGONIST-RECEPTOR INTERACTION

The agonist binding site on the β-adrenergic receptor responds to agonist binding by conformational changes that strengthen the interaction. There may be transiently stable intermediate configurations of the receptor-agonist complex as the transition is made from an unoccupied β-adrenergic receptor to a receptor occupied by an appropriate agonist. There is evidence that the intermediate receptor configurations may be responsible for activating different downstream effectors.[96]

ROUTE OF ADMINISTRATION OF β_2-ADRENERGIC AGONISTS

β-Agonists have been given by oral, subcutaneous, intravenous, and inhaled routes. The inhaled approach is currently preferred; the oral approach has been all but abandoned, and there appears to be no advantage to the intravenous route even in severe asthma with hypercapnia.[97] A meta-analysis found no evidence of benefit for the intravenous use of β-agonists in patients who are refractory to inhaled β-agonists.[98] Thus, clinical assessment should guide therapy with intravenous or subcutaneous routes being reserved for special situations in which inhaled therapy is not effective (e.g., coughing, weak inspiratory effort, or moribund patient). Continuous albuterol nebulization may have an advantage over intermittent delivery in patients with severe asthma.[99,100] The different modes of inhalational delivery and relative advantages and disadvantages of each are discussed later.

DOSE-RESPONSE RELATIONSHIP FOR β_2-ADRENERGIC AGONISTS

The dose-response curve and the rationale for the recommended dosage of albuterol has been reviewed previously.[100,101] Briefly, increase in FEV$_1$ is observed with increasing doses of albuterol, with a plateau in FEV$_1$ improvement occurring in some patients.[102,103] Nelson et al[104] suggested that the increase in FEV$_1$ was linearly related to the log dose of albuterol administered. There is no reliable predictor of the minimum dose required to reach optimum bronchodilation, although some data suggest that patients with low initial FEV$_1$ need higher doses.[36] Doses for individual drugs are listed in Table 63-2. Patients who are admitted to the hospital with acute asthma exacerbations are more likely to have a shallow dose-response curve to albuterol; $\sim$30% of patients do not respond even to high doses of β-agonists.[100] The duration of bronchodilation shortens with continued β-agonist use, and such an effect may be observed as early as the third continuous day of therapy.[105]

SIDE EFFECTS OF β_2-ADRENERGIC RECEPTOR ACTIVATION

Cardiac

Increase in heart rate occurs predictably after administration of β_2-agonists, but the incidence of symptomatic tachycardia is unknown. Occasional occurrences of angina[106] and myocardial infarction[107] suggest that myocardial injury can result. In a group of stable patients with documented coronary artery disease, however, inhaled albuterol did not increase myocardial ischemia, ventricular arrhythmias, or

TABLE 63-2 Doses and Duration of Action of Commonly Used Bronchodilators

Agent	Dose	Time Course (Onset, Peak, (Duration)	Trade Names
Albuterol* (salbutamol)	SVN: 0.5% solution, 0.3 mL (2.5 mg) tid or qid MDI: 90 μg/puff, 2 puffs tid or qid DPI: 200 μg capsule, 1 capsule q4–6h	5–15 minutes, 30–60 minutes, 5–8 hours	Proventil, Proventil HFA, Ventolin
Levalbuterol	SVN: 0.63 mg q6–8h, or 1.25 mg tid	15 minutes, 30–60 minutes, 5–8 hours	Xopenex
Terbutaline	MDI: 200 μg/puff, 2 puffs q4–6h	5–30 minutes, 30–60 minutes, 3–6 hours	Brethine
Formoterol	DPI: 12 μg capsule, 1 capsule q12h	1–3 minutes, 1–3 hours, 8–12 hours	Foradil
Salmeterol	DPI: 50 μg/blister, 1 inhalation bid	10–20 minutes, 3–5 hours, 12 hours	Serevent
Ipratropium*	MDI: 18 μg/puff, 2 puffs bid SVN: 0.02% solution, 2.5 mL (0.5 mg) qid	15 minutes, 90–120 minutes, 6–8 hours	Atrovent
Tiotropium	DPI: 18 μg capsule, 1 capsule q24h	30 minutes, 90–180 minutes, 24 hours	Spiriva

ABBREVIATIONS: DPI, dry-powder inhaler; MDI, metered-dose inhaler; SVN, small-volume nebulizer.
*Combinations of albuterol and ipratropium are available as MDI (Combivent) and nebulizer (Duoneb) formulations.

heart rate variability.[108] The results cannot be extrapolated to unstable or hypoxic patients, as β_2-agonists are known to interact with changes produced by these stimuli.[109,110]

Hypoxia

Arterial oxygen tension (Pa_{O_2}) may decrease transiently after β-agonist inhalation, probably secondary to pulmonary vasodilation mediated by β_2-receptors. This vasodilator effect reverses the pulmonary vasoconstriction that limits blood flow to poorly ventilated areas and the resultant worsening ventilation-perfusion mismatch causes a decrease in overall Pa_{O_2}.[36] In contrast, reduction in Pa_{O_2} was either not seen after inhalation of antimuscarinic agents[111] or was less than the decrement produced by albuterol and salmeterol.[112] The decrease in Pa_{O_2} with albuterol inhalation is transient and small, hence its clinical significance is doubtful.[112] Significant drops in Pa_{O_2}, however, can occur occasionally,[110,113] and close monitoring may be required in patients with marginal oxygenation.

INDIVIDUAL AGENTS

Albuterol

Albuterol is today's standard short-acting bronchodilator. Its pharmacokinetics depend on the dose administered, the formulation of albuterol used (dry powder, MDI, or nebulized) and the clinical situation (mechanically ventilated or ambulatory). (For dosing and schedule of administration, see section on clinical use of bronchodilator drugs.) Although increasing doses of albuterol produce greater bronchodilation, the optimum dose is difficult to predict. Peak bronchodilator response after 10 puffs of albuterol in ven-

tilated patients was seen within 5 minutes and sustained for 60 minutes.[10] Duration of action of 6 puffs of albuterol delivered from an MDI to ventilated patients ranged from less than 2 hours to more than 4 hours.[114] Systemic effects are dose related, usually appearing within an hour of administration with a return to baseline within 4 hours.[27]

Levalbuterol

Commonly available racemic albuterol is a 50/50 mixture of R- and S-albuterol. Levalbuterol, the R-enantiomer, was formulated to avoid possible adverse effects of the S-enantiomer. For doses that produce similar increases in FEV_1, increases in heart rate are less with levalbuterol (2–4 beats/minute) than with albuterol;[115] the clinical significance is, however, questionable. The role of levalbuterol in patients with acute severe asthma or in patients receiving mechanical ventilation is not well defined.

Salmeterol

Salmeterol is a long acting β_2-agonist. Its onset of action is slower than that of albuterol in vitro (mean 6.4 versus 1.9 minutes)[116] and in vivo (mean 10 versus 4 minutes).[117] With salmeterol, peak bronchodilator response was seen at 5 hours versus 1 hour with albuterol, and FEV_1 was higher than pre-dose FEV_1 levels for 12 hours.[117] Systemic effects of salmeterol are dose related, manifest later, and last longer; maximum effects on heart rate occur within 75–135 minutes and are still evident after 4 hours.[27]

Formoterol

Formoterol is a long-acting agent like salmeterol but is distinguished by its relatively quicker onset of action. Duration of effect is about 12 hours. There are concerns about a partial agonist effect and blockade of full agonist action by other β-agonist drugs when these are used concurrently. Pretreatment with formoterol, however, does not inhibit responses to further doses of albuterol[118] or fenoterol (a full agonist).[119]

ANTICHOLINERGICS

The parasympathetic system, in contrast to the sympathetic system, directly innervates the bronchial smooth muscle and is the dominant autonomic arm controlling airway smooth muscle function.[120] The vagus nerve mediates baseline bronchomotor tone.[121,122] An increase in vagal efferent output causes further bronchoconstriction. Anticholinergic bronchodilator drugs competitively inhibit the action of acetylcholine on muscarinic receptors, produce bronchodilation, and confer some bronchoprotection. The bronchodilator effect varies among individuals. Parasympathetic activity is reported to be increased in patients with asthma and COPD.[123]

STRUCTURE AND SUBTYPES OF THE MUSCARINIC RECEPTOR

Muscarinic receptors are G protein linked receptors, and therefore have the general structure described above for β-receptors. The receptors are linked to their intracellular effectors through the $\alpha\beta\gamma$ heterotrimeric protein. Five subtypes are known (M_1–M_5). The M_2 and M_3 subtypes are the most common type of muscarinic receptor in the lung (Fig. 63-2). M_3 receptors mediate contraction of smooth muscle in the airways.[124] M_1, M_3, and M_5 receptors are linked to their effectors through α subunits of the $G_{q/11}$ family.[125] Phospholipase C is one of the downstream effectors activated by this α subunit. Activation of phospholipase C results in the formation of IP_3 and diacylglycerol, which, in turn, results in calcium release and protein kinase C activation, respectively. M_2 receptors are important in the modulation of acetylcholine release. Activation of prejunctional M_2 receptors inhibits acetylcholine release. Loss of M_2 receptor action may underlie airway hyperreactivity in animal models and in asthma.[123] Although muscarinic receptors are widespread in the body, currently used inhaled antimuscarinic agents have few systemic side effects. The quaternary ammonium group in modern antimuscarinic agents (ipratropium and tiotropium) results in poor systemic absorption across mucosal surfaces and also poor penetration into the central nervous system. Administration by inhalation allows higher doses of inhaled quaternary antimuscarinic agents to be used with few systemic effects.

ANTICHOLINERGIC ACTION AND AIRWAY SMOOTH MUSCLE RELAXATION

The principal mechanism of action of muscarinic antagonists is to block vagally mediated bronchoconstriction. In patients with COPD, a greater bronchodilator response occurs after atropine than after albuterol. The bronchodilator response to atropine in patients with COPD is greater than that in normal subjects. These data suggest enhanced parasympathetic activity in COPD.[126,127] Patients with chronic asthma do not show as much benefit with anticholinergic agents, although patients with acute asthma exacerbations benefit from inhaled anticholinergic agents. Enhanced parasympathetic activity is known to occur after viral infections and other triggers responsible for an asthma exacerbation.[128]

OTHER EFFECTS OF ANTICHOLINERGIC ACTION IN THE LUNGS

The quarternary ammonium–containing muscarinic antagonists in current use have no significant effects on mucus secretion or the rheologic properties of mucus,[129] although some reports do suggest a decrease in sputum volume.[130] Mucociliary clearance is unchanged with inhaled ipratropium.[131,132]

Acetylcholine can stimulate alveolar macrophages to release chemotactic factors.[133] Long-acting anticholinergics may thus decrease airway inflammation by blocking the actions of acetylcholine,[134] but further studies are needed to support these preliminary observations.

SIDE EFFECTS OF ANTICHOLINERGICS

Dryness of mouth is the most common side effect. Blurring of vision has been reported in about 1.2% of patients. Unilateral mydriasis is believed to result from direct contact of the nebulized solution with the eyes.[135,136] In the Lung Health Study, Anthonisen et al[137] found a higher incidence of supraventricular arrhythmias as well as significant increases in hospitalization and mortality rates in the ipratropium group as compared to the placebo group.

INDIVIDUAL AGENTS

Ipratropium

The usual dose is 36 μg (2 puffs from an MDI) every 4–6 hours. There is a plateau in the achievable improvement in FEV_1 with increasing doses with no significant improvement beyond a dose of 72 μg.[138] In patients with severe airway obstruction, however, the amount of drug delivered to the site of action may vary and higher doses may be needed. The usual nebulized dose is 500 μg every 6 hours. The onset of action is within 30 minutes of an inhaled dose and

FIGURE 63-2 Muscarinic receptors in the lung. The M_1 and M_3 receptors stimulate the action of acetylcholine, whereas the action of M_2 receptors is autoinhibitory.

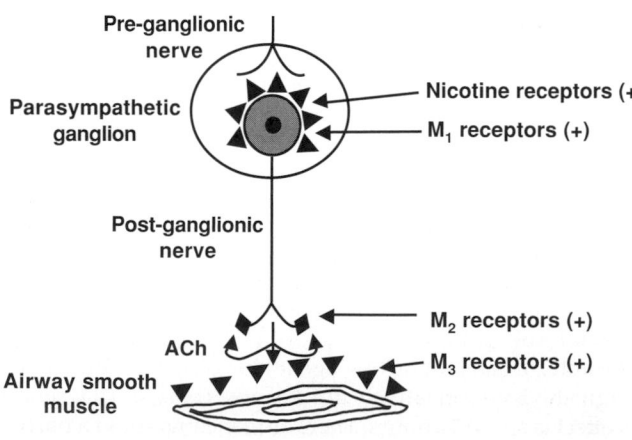

the effects last for about 4–6 hours. Ipratropium blocks all muscarinic receptor subtypes in the lung. Systemic side effects are minimal because of poor absorption across mucosal surfaces of the lung and gastrointestinal tract. The bronchodilation produced is variable, probably because of individual variation in cholinergic tone. Tachyphylaxis to the bronchodilator effects of ipratropium has not been demonstrated.

Tiotropium

Tiotropium is a long-acting bronchodilator, which has equal binding affinity for M_1, M_2, and M_3 receptor subtypes. It dissociates much more slowly from M_3 receptors than from M_2 receptors.[139] In view of the role of M_2 receptors in inhibiting acetylcholine release, this may represent a beneficial aspect of its action. Tiotropium is inhaled once daily. Onset of action is within 30 minutes. An increase in FEV_1 from baseline is present at 24 hours.[140] Tiotropium has not been evaluated for use in acute exacerbations of COPD and in ventilated patients.

CLINICAL USE OF BRONCHODILATOR DRUGS

There is an urgent need for bronchodilation in patients presenting with acute severe asthma and exacerbations of COPD. Appropriate dosing and choice of agents have been explored to a greater extent in ambulatory patients. The findings in ambulatory patients are not applicable to ventilated patients because of interactions between the dose, delivery mechanism, and ventilator set-up (see below).

BETA AGONISTS IN ASTHMA AND CHRONIC OBSTRUCTIVE PULMONARY DISEASE

In general, there is a dose-response relationship with increasing doses of β-agonists resulting in increasing bronchodilation.[104] Newhouse et al[141] administered albuterol or fenoterol up to a maximum of 1600 μg and 3200 μg (4 puffs initially and 2 puffs every 10 minutes). FEV_1 response was greater with the higher doses. A plateau in bronchodilator effect was seen in 62% of patients. Only one patient discontinued treatment because of tremor. Rodrigo and Rodrigo[142] administered 400 μg of albuterol via metered-dose inhaler/holding chamber (MDI/HC) every 10 minutes (2.4 mg per hour) for 3 hours. FEV_1 and peak expiratory flow (PEF) responses were dose dependent with a mean improvement of 90.4% for FEV_1 over the baseline values. Heart rates were reduced and changes in serum potassium were not significant. In a different study, higher doses of albuterol via MDI/HC (600 μg versus 400 μg, each given at 10-minute intervals) were not found to produce significant improvements in FEV_1, but adverse effects were greater than with the 400-μg dose.[143] These data suggest that 2.4 mg of albuterol every hour (400 μg every 10 minutes) delivered via an MDI/HC produces clinically significant bronchodilation and higher doses increase the incidence of adverse effects without enhancing bronchodilation.

A recent review summarized the characteristics of various delivery devices in different clinical scenarios.[144] In adults with acute asthma, bronchodilators are commonly administered via a nebulizer. Lin et al[145] administered albuterol at a dose of 0.4 mg/kg per hour via continuous nebulization. Mean increase in FEV_1 was 36.8%. High serum albuterol and a significant increase in heart rate, however, were also observed. In a separate study, Lin et al[146] compared 30 mg of albuterol over 110 minutes given either continuously or as 5-mg intermittent nebulizations. The mean increase in FEV_1 did not significantly differ; in a subgroup analysis, patients with a baseline FEV_1 <50% showed a significantly higher rate of improvement in FEV_1 with continuous nebulization.[146] Stein et al compared continuous nebulized albuterol at 7.5 mg/hour versus 15 mg/hour. Improvement in PEF at 1 hour did not significantly differ between the low-dose and the high-dose group (44% versus 30%).[147] Shrestha et al[99] studied the effect of 7.5 mg and 2.5 mg of albuterol given either continuously or intermittently every hour for 2 hours. The continuous regimens were better than the intermittent regimens. There were no significant differences between the two doses given continuously. Likewise, Emerman et al[148] found similar increases in FEV_1 after 2.5 mg versus 7.5 mg of albuterol (each given every 20 minutes) in patients with acute severe asthma.

In a prospective sequential design, McFadden et al[149] compared the effects of three doses of 2.5 mg given every 20 minutes (standard nebulized albuterol therapy) to two doses of 5 mg of albuterol given every 20 minutes (high-dose therapy). Increase in PEF was higher with 5 mg than with 2.5 mg after the first and second treatment (55% versus 47% and 63% versus 51%, respectively). There was no significant difference when cumulative doses were compared (i.e., two doses of 2.5 mg produced the same increase in PEF as one dose of 5 mg [51% versus 55%]). The authors concluded that the high-dose therapy was effective and achieved more rapid and greater increases than the standard approach. A further study from the same group indicated that a single dose of 7.5 mg of albuterol given once produced the same increase in FEV_1 as 2.5 mg given every 20 minutes.[150] The incidence of all adverse effects combined, however, was nearly twice as high in the single-dose group.[150] Overall, it appears that the cumulative dose, and not the dosage regimen, influences the bronchodilator response (i.e., the same response was obtained when 5 mg was given as a single dose as when it was given as two doses of 2.5 mg).

The usual dose necessary to produce bronchodilation in severe asthma is between 5 and 10 mg of albuterol. In a study by Colacone et al,[151] 40 patients received albuterol via MDI/HC (400 μg every 30 minutes) and 40 patients received albuterol via intermittent nebulization (2.5 mg every 30 minutes). Maximal bronchodilation was achieved after two doses in 65% of the MDI group and 75% of the nebulizer group; almost all patients had achieved maximal bronchodilation with four doses from either system. McFadden et al[149] found a significant improvement with either single (5 mg given once) or cumulative doses (2.5 mg given twice) of albuterol given via a nebulizer. Additional doses of 5 mg (cumulative dose 10 mg) and 2.5 mg (cumulative dose 7.5 mg), produced an improvement to near normal levels of PEF in both groups with no significant differences between the groups.

Use of higher doses during the initial phase of an acute exacerbation of asthma may have clinical utility. A faster response may be seen, and, because most patients respond to 5–10 mg of albuterol, nonresponders may be identified. Nonresponders, defined as those requiring admission versus discharge from an emergency department, were found to have a flatter dose-response curve to albuterol, with PEF remaining below 45% despite high doses of albuterol.[149,152,153]

The logistical problem in repeatedly administering doses of nebulized albuterol (intermittent therapy) has stimulated interest in continuous nebulization. More data is available in children than in adults. Moler et al[154] continuously nebulized terbutaline at 4 mg/hour for a mean of 15.4 hours in children with severe asthma and impending respiratory failure. Over 8 hours of therapy, clinical asthma score improved and mean Pa_{CO_2} decreased. Lin et al[146] found no difference between 15 mg/hour of albuterol administered either continuously or intermittently. Patients with initial FEV_1 <50% showed a higher rate of increase of FEV_1 with continuous nebulization. Rudnitsky et al[155] also found that patients with initial PEF <200 L/minute displayed a greater improvement in PEF with continuous than with intermittent nebulization. In patients with PEF >200 L/minute, improvement was equivalent with both approaches.[155] In a meta-analysis based on 393 patients in 6 trials, no significant differences were seen between continuous and intermittent nebulization of β-agonists in terms PEF or FEV_1.[156] In a more recent meta-analysis, Camargo et al[157] reached a different conclusion. At 60 minutes, there was no significant difference between continuous and intermittent nebulization in PEF and a small difference in FEV_1. At 2–3 hours, statistically significant differences favored continuous nebulized β-agonist therapy in terms of the hospital admission rates and pulmonary function. These meta-analyses had a large overlap of trials included.

In summary, the severity of an individual episode is better measured as response to bronchodilator therapy rather than by baseline pulmonary function. Continuous nebulization may be employed in patients with acute severe asthma in whom pulmonary function does not improve by the end of the first hour of intensive bronchodilator therapy.

CHOICE OF DELIVERY SYSTEM

In clinical studies evaluating bronchodilator administration through MDI/HC versus nebulizers, equivalent changes in FEV_1 were produced by 6 mg/hour of albuterol given by the nebulized route and 2.4 mg/hour of albuterol given by MDI/HC, an equivalent dose ratio of 2.5:1. A higher incidence of tremor and anxiety and higher serum albuterol was seen in the nebulizer group.[158] Improvement in pulmonary function is similar[151,159,160] or slightly better[161,162] with MDI/HC than with nebulizers, while increases in heart rate are more frequent with nebulizers.[151]

ANTICHOLINERGICS IN ASTHMA AND CHRONIC OBSTRUCTIVE PULMONARY DISEASE

The ideal bronchodilator and optimal regimen for acute exacerbations of COPD have not been established. A pooled analysis comparing the effects of β-agonists (fenoterol and metaproterenol) and anticholinergics (ipratropium) found no significant differences in improvement in FEV_1.[163] Short-

acting β-agonists are generally recommended as first-line therapy. If response is suboptimal or the exacerbation is severe, ipratropium can be added.[164]

In patients with stable COPD, a combination of ipratropium and albuterol administered by MDI[165] or small-volume nebulizer[166,167] produced significant increases in FEV_1 compared to using each drug alone. In a randomized, double-blind study in patients with acute exacerbations of COPD, Shrestha et al[168] found that isoetharine and ipratropium versus isoetharine alone produced equivalent changes in FEV_1 and FVC. Fernandez et al.[169] found an improvement in airway pressures in ventilated patients with the combination of ipratropium and fenoterol in comparison to ipratropium; ipratropium alone achieved no benefit. In patients with acute COPD, Cydulka et al.[170] found a greater increase from pretreatment FEV_1 with a combination of glycopyrrolate and albuterol compared to albuterol and placebo.

Other investigators found no advantage to combination therapy. Moayyedi et al[171] found no significant difference in length of stay or spirometric values between 70 patients randomized to receive either nebulized albuterol or nebulized albuterol and ipratropium. Patrick et al[172] added ipratropium or placebo to "usual therapy" (albuterol, intravenous methylprednisolone, intravenous aminophylline, and antibiotics). Patients with asthma responded to added ipratropium to a greater degree than patients with COPD. Within the COPD group, improvement in FEV_1 did not differ between the placebo and ipratropium group. O'Driscoll et al[166] found similar results in 103 patients presenting with acute airflow obstruction (56 with asthma, 47 with COPD) who were treated with nebulized albuterol and ipratropium or nebulized albuterol alone. Patients with asthma exhibited a greater rise in PEF after treatment with the combination of albuterol and ipratropium, but no difference was seen in the COPD group.[166]

In acute asthma, combined anticholinergic and β-agonist therapy appears to provide additional benefits over β-agonists alone. Karpel et al[173] found an increase in the number of responders (>15% change in FEV_1) with combined albuterol and ipratropium compared to albuterol alone in patients with acute asthma at 45 minutes. There was, however, no difference in hospitalization rates or incidence of adverse effects[173] McFadden et al[174] found no difference in the rates of hospitalization, PEF, or length of stay between albuterol versus albuterol and ipratropium. Other investigators have reached different conclusions. In a randomized, double-blind trial in patients with acute asthma, Lin et al[175] found that the increase in PEF with albuterol alone (2.5 mg at 20-minute intervals for 3 doses) was less than the same dosage of albuterol with ipratropium (0.5 mg with the first dose alone). The admission rate was also lower for the combined therapy. Lanes et al,[176] in a pooled analysis of three randomized double-blind trials, found a small but significant improvement in FEV_1 at 45 minutes in the albuterol and ipratropium group compared to the albuterol group. Weber et al[177] compared continuous nebulization of albuterol with and without the addition of ipratropium in patients with asthma (mean PEF <45% at baseline). The differences were not statistically significant. A meta-analysis by Stoodley et al[178] that compared albuterol alone to albuterol with ipratropium found an overall improvement of 7.3% in FEV_1 and 22.1% in PEF with the combination. Hospitalization rates were reduced for the combination for three studies in which data were available.[178]

A more recent meta-analysis by Rodrigo and Rodrigo[179] found benefit for a combination of anticholinergics with albuterol in severe asthma (FEV_1 <50%). When multiple doses of anticholinergics were used (500 μg of ipratropium every 20 minutes or 4 puffs [80 μg] every 10–20 minutes via MDI/spacer), there was a 30–60% reduction in the number of hospital admissions. Lung function was improved with combination therapy with no increase in adverse effects. Thus, there could be benefit from combining anticholinergics with β-agonists in severe asthma.

METHYLXANTHINES

Clinical use of theophylline has declined in recent years in North America, but in many countries, it remains an inexpensive and commonly employed bronchodilator. Theophylline produces nonselective inhibition of several cyclic AMP phosphodiesterases (PDE III and PDE IV), increases intracellular cyclic AMP and cyclic GMP concentrations, and causes smooth muscle relaxation.[180,181] When concentrations of theophylline are maintained within the recommended therapeutic range (see below), however, only minor degrees of PDE inhibition are achieved.[182] Several other mechanisms have been suggested to explain theophylline's clinical effects. Recently, a synergistic action of theophylline with corticosteroids by activation of histone deacetylases was proposed.[183] Histone deacetylases are induced by corticosteroids to switch off inflammatory gene expression.[183–185] Theophylline also antagonizes adenosine at adenosine receptors, reduces activity of inflammatory cells, reduces airway microvascular leak, promotes interleukin-10 release, promotes apoptosis, and inhibits secretion of tumor necrosis factor.[186–190] At low plasma concentrations, theophylline also reduces eosinophil levels in bronchial biopsies and induced sputum.[191]

The nonbronchodilator actions of theophylline may produce important benefits. Patients with asthma and COPD improve clinically without significant improvement in objective measures of pulmonary function, gas exchange, or exercise capacity.[192,193] These benefits may be mediated by theophylline's action to increase respiratory muscle contractility.[194–196] Patients with concomitant cardiac disease may benefit from the actions of theophylline that lead to increase in cardiac output, decrease in pulmonary vascular resistance, and improved myocardial perfusion to ischemic regions.[197–199]

According to recent recommendations, plasma levels of theophylline should be maintained between 5 and 15 mg/L because of frequent occurrence of adverse effects with higher levels.[200–202] At concentrations <15 mg/L, theophylline is a relatively weak bronchodilator and its beneficial effects are more likely explained by its anti-inflammatory action, particularly in synergy with corticosteroids.[180]

TABLE 63-3 Drugs Affecting Theophylline Clearance

Decrease Clearance	Increase Clearance
Cimetidine	Phenytoin
Ciprofloxacin	Carbamazepine
Erythromycin	Rifampin
Ketoconazole	Phenobarbital
Diltiazem	
Propranolol	
Verapamil	
Amiodarone	
Propafenone	
Allopurinol	
Propofol	
Oral contraceptives	

Theophylline readily distributes into fat tissue in both adults and children. It is metabolized by microsomal cytochrome P450 mixed function oxidases in the liver; the CYP1A2 microenzyme is the most important pathway for metabolism.[203] Renal excretion accounts for 10–15% of the overall excretion in adults,[204] but may be as high as 50% in neonates. Especially in critically ill patients, the half-life of theophylline can vary widely secondary to liver disease, pulmonary edema, febrile reactions, or concurrent drug administration (Table 63-3).[205] Small differences in metabolism produce marked variations in drug clearance. In critically ill patients with impaired liver function due to heart failure, shock, sepsis, or liver disease, theophylline clearance can be markedly depressed initially with subsequent improvement as the patients recover.[206] As a result, serum levels may fluctuate with changes in the patient's condition.

Theophylline administration requires empiric loading and maintenance dosing with frequent measurement of serum levels and dose adjustment.[207] One approach to intravenous dosing is outlined in Table 63-4.

In acute asthma, intravenous aminophylline (80% theophylline by weight) is less effective than nebulized β-agonists. Theophylline does not confer additional bronchodilation in patients receiving intensive therapy with inhaled β-agonists and IV corticosteroids.[208–210] The NIH expert guidelines,[208,211] a Cochrane review,[212] and others[202,213] found no additional benefit from the routine use of theophylline in hospitalized patients with severe asthma. Currently, theophylline is recommended only for patients who fail to respond to β-agonists, those who have paradoxical bronchospasm after inhalation of β-agonists, or those with impending respiratory failure. Likewise, routine use of theophylline in acute exacerbations of COPD is not supported by large, randomized controlled trials.[168] Theophylline may have a role in reducing hospitalization among patients receiving emergency department treatment for asthma and COPD.[214]

Few investigators have reported on the use of theophylline in ventilated patients.[169,215,216] In the neonatal ICU, theophylline is employed to prevent apneas.[217] In adults, loading doses of IV theophylline produced significant bronchodilation, comparable to that achieved with two inhalations of either albuterol or ipratropium

TABLE 63-4   Dosing Guidelines for Intravenous Aminophylline

Patient Not on Theophylline	Patient Receiving Theophylline
Give loading dose	
6 mg/kg ideal body weight over 20 min	Draw blood level
Check levels after 30–60 min	Begin maintenance dose; load as needed
If levels below therapeutic, give additional loading dose	
Each 1 mg/kg body weight of additional aminophylline increases serum level by 2 mg/L	
Maintenance dose[a]	
0.5 mg/kg ideal body weight/hour	Measure serum levels after 12–24 hours
Measure serum levels after 12–24 hours	Thereafter, measure serum levels daily
Thereafter, measure serum levels daily	
Change in maintenance dose	
New infusion rate = $\dfrac{\text{Desired levels}}{\text{Present level}}$ × Present infusion rate	

[a] Maintenance doses required to maintain serum levels in the therapeutic range after giving the loading dose. In patients who are already receiving theophylline, a loading dose may not be required and therapy could be initiated with a maintenance dose. Lower maintenance dose (<0.5 mg/kg body weight) recommended in critically ill patients, and higher dose (0.7 mg/kg body weight) in current smokers.

bromide.[169,215,216] The increased respiratory muscle strength with theophylline[194–196] may help in weaning.

Frequent side effects are a major drawback to theophylline's routine use. Nausea and vomiting are the most frequent. Because side effects are directly related to the serum concentrations (Table 63-5), levels require frequent monitoring. Theophylline is best avoided in patients with hemodynamic instability, sepsis, hepatic dysfunction, neurologic disease, and in those with a history of seizures or serious cardiac arrhythmias. Older patients and those with a low serum albumin are particularly susceptible to serious toxicity, such as cardiac arrhythmias and seizures.[218–220] Likewise, extreme caution is needed when theophylline is employed in morbidly obese patients. Intravenous administration of theophylline requires a slow injection or the use of an infusion pump because rapid intravenous injections

TABLE 63-5   Serum Levels and Side Effects of Theophylline[a]

Serum Levels	Adverse Effects
≤10 mg/L	Nausea, vomiting, diarrhea
>10 mg/L	Tachycardia, tremors, electrolyte abnormalities (hypokalemia, hypomagnesemia, hypophosphatemia), acidosis, hyperglycemia
>30 mg/L	Seizures
	Cardiac arrhythmias,[b] shock, cardiac arrest

[a] Toxicity due to theophylline may differ in patients with acute overdose compared to those with chronic overdosing.
[b] Includes atrial fibrillation, atrial flutter, multifocal atrial tachycardia, ventricular tachycardia, and ventricular fibrillation.

may cause dizziness, palpitations, flushing, hypotension, profound bradycardia, and even cardiac arrest.

In summary, the high frequency of side effects with theophylline, its relatively low efficacy, frequent drug interactions, complicated dosing regimens, and the need for repeated monitoring of serum levels have significantly limited its use in the ICU.

SELECTIVE PHOSPHODIESTERASE E₄ INHIBITORS

Phosphodiesterase E_4 (PDE$_4$) is the predominant isozyme responsible for metabolizing cAMP in airway smooth muscle, and in immune and inflammatory cells.[221,222] Elevation of cAMP by selective PDE$_4$ inhibition has a wide variety of pharmacologic effects. Several selective PDE$_4$ inhibitors are being tested for therapeutic potential in asthma and COPD, but only cilomilast and roflumilast are undergoing phase III clinical trials. Both agents are given orally; the inhaled route remains investigational. Cilomilast is rapidly absorbed after oral administration and has an elimination half-life of 7 hours.[223,224] The drug shows dose-related linear pharmacokinetics that are unaffected by age or food. Roflumilast has an elimination half-life of 10 hours and bioavailability is not affected by food, smoking, diurnal dosing, or renal insufficiency.[225] Unlike theophylline, no significant drug interactions (e.g., with digoxin, warfarin, or erythromycin) have been reported with these agents.[223,224,226] The selective PDE$_4$ inhibitors have significant bronchodilator and anti-inflammatory effects in patients with asthma and COPD.[225,227–230] Side effects, such as nausea and headache, are generally mild to moderate, but could limit use in critically ill patients.

Factors Influencing Aerosol Delivery during Mechanical Ventilation

Several factors influence aerosol delivery during mechanical ventilation, including variables related to the aerosol-generating device, the ventilator and ventilator circuit, the inhaled drug or agent, and the patient (Fig. 63-3). Aerosol delivery during mechanical ventilation depends to a great extent on the type of aerosol-generating device employed.

AEROSOL-GENERATING DEVICES

NEBULIZERS
Nebulizers convert liquids into small droplets that can be inhaled into the lower respiratory tract.[231] Two types of nebulizers, jet and ultrasonic, are employed for inhalation therapy in ventilated patients.

Jet Nebulizers
A jet of compressed air or oxygen under high pressure passes through a narrow opening near the tip of a capillary tube whose base is immersed in the drug solution to be nebulized (Fig. 63-4).[231,232] The low pressure created by the expansion of the jet draws the liquid up the capillary

Ventilator-Related
- Ventilation mode
- Tidal volume
- Respiratory rate
- Duty cycle
- Inspiratory waveform
- Breath-triggering mechanism

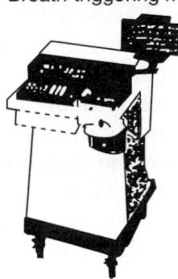

Device-Related - MDI
- Type of spacer or adapter
- Position of spacer in circuit
- Timing of MDI actuation
- Type of MDI

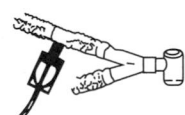

Device-Related - Nebulizer
- Type of nebulizer
- Fill volume
- Gas flow
- Cycling: inspiration vs continuous
- Duration of nebulization
- Position in the circuit

Circuit-Related
- Endotracheal tube size
- Humidity of inhaled gas
- Density of inhaled gas

Drug-Related
- Dose
- Formulation
- Aerosol particle size
- Targeted site for delivery
- Duration of action

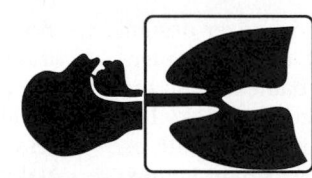

Patient-Related
- Severity of airway obstruction
- Mechanism of airway obstruction
- Presence of dynamic hyperinflation
- Patient-ventilator synchrony

FIGURE 63-3 Factors influencing aerosol delivery in mechanically ventilated patients. MDI, metered-dose inhaler. (*Modified, with permission, from Dhand et al.*[270])

FIGURE 63-4 Several types of nebulizers are available for clinical use, including jet nebulizers (*left*), ultrasonic nebulizers (*upper right*), and vibrating mesh nebulizers (*lower right*). The jet nebulizers employ compressed gas or air to generate an aerosol. In ultrasonic nebulizers, aerosol is generated by vibration of a piezoelectric crystal at ultrasonic frequencies. In the vibrating mesh nebulizers, aerosol is produced by high-frequency vibration of a plate with multiple apertures. Vibration of the aperture plate pushes the liquid to be nebulized through the apertures and generates a fine particle mist.

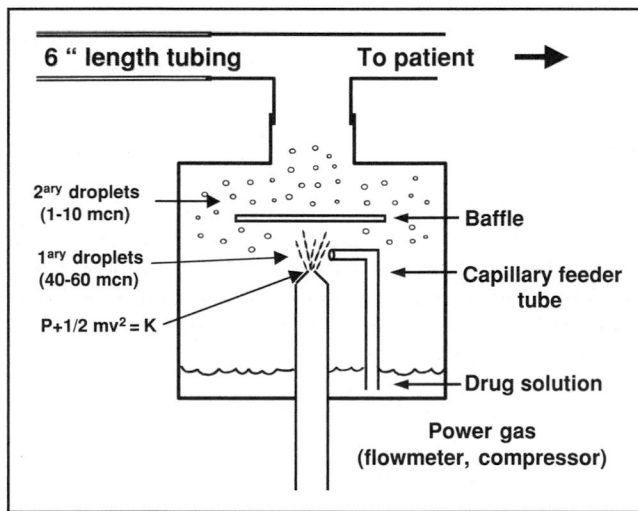

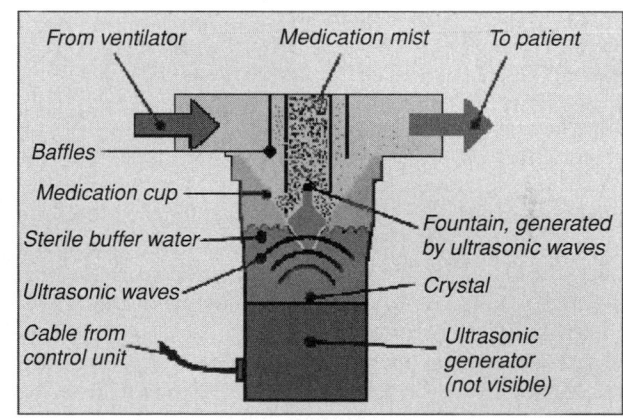

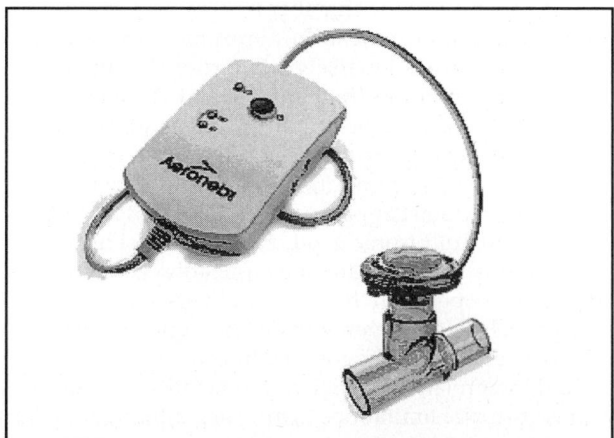

tube. The shearing force of the jet stream produces a liquid film that breaks up into small droplets secondary to surface-tension forces. Larger particles deposit on a baffle placed upstream of the aerosol stream and on the walls of the nebulizer, whereas the smallest droplets leave the nebulizer.

Aerosol particle size is influenced by nebulizer design, solution characteristics (density, viscosity, and surface tension) and volume, gas pressure and flow, baffle design, and ratio of liquid to gas flow.[232-234] Droplet size decreases when gas flow increases, whereas droplet size increases with increase in the ratio of liquid to gas flow. A certain volume of solution (dead or residual volume) cannot be nebulized. Residual volume varies from 1 to 3 ml; it can be reduced by using a nebulizer with a conical shape, improving the wetness of the plastic surfaces, and reducing the internal surface area of the nebulizer.[232,234]

During operation, the solution concentration increases and its temperature decreases secondary to evaporative losses.[235,236] Both increased solution concentration and cooling influence nebulizer output and particle size.[234,237] Moreover, nebulizer drug output markedly decreases after it starts sputtering. Significant disadvantages of jet nebulizers are the requirement for a power source, inconveniently long treatment time, need for equipment setup and cleaning, and significant variations in the performance of various nebulizers, both within the same brand and across different brands.[238-240]

Ultrasonic Nebulizers

These devices transmit sound waves generated by vibrating a piezoelectric crystal at high frequencies (>1 MHz) to the surface of the drug solution. Standing waves are created and droplets breaking free from the crests of these waves produce an aerosol (see Fig. 63-4).[241,242] Baffles remove larger droplets within the aerosol and a fan blows the aerosol to the patient. The source and flow of the gas used to carry the aerosol to the patient can influence droplet size and drug concentration. Low flow rates produce smaller particles and higher concentration of aerosol, whereas high flow rates yield larger droplets and lower aerosol concentrations. The solution to be nebulized is placed directly over the transducer in some ultrasonic nebulizers, whereas in others there is a water couplant chamber between the transducer and the medication chamber. In ultrasonic nebulizers, the aerosol particle size is inversely proportional to the piezoelectric crystal vibration frequency[243] and drug output is directly proportional to the amplitude of crystal vibration. Similarly to jet nebulizers, the drug solution becomes more concentrated during operation; in contrast to jet nebulizers, however, the solution temperature increases by $10°–15°C$ after 10 minutes of ultrasonic nebulization.[235] Most ultrasonic nebulizers have a higher rate of nebulization and require a shorter time of operation than jet nebulizers. Generally, the aerosol particle size is larger with ultrasonic nebulizers compared to jet nebulizers. The cost and bulk of ultrasonic nebulizers and their relative inefficiency in nebulizing drug suspensions are major limitations to their use, although smaller

ultrasonic nebulizers are available and some have been employed during mechanical ventilation.[244-247]

Vibrating Mesh Nebulizers

A newer generation of nebulizers employs a vibrating mesh or plate with multiple apertures to produce an aerosol.[248,249] Because the frequency of vibration of the plates is lower than that in ultrasonic nebulizers, these devices can be operated either with a battery pack or another type of electrical source. As a result, these devices are portable and less noisy. Moreover, these devices have negligible residual volume, and this significantly improves the drug output. The Aeroneb Pro (Aerogen Inc., Mountain View, CA) is specifically designed as an in-line nebulizer (see Fig. 63-4); a breath-synchronized version of the Aeroneb Pro is being evaluated in clinical trials.

The vibrating mesh nebulizers have a high rate of nebulization and drug output is 2–3 times higher than with jet nebulizers.[250] The aerosol particle size can be varied by changing the exit diameter of the apertures in the vibrating plate. Unlike ultrasonic nebulizers, the temperature of the solution does not change during operation of the vibrating mesh nebulizers, and proteins and peptides can be nebulized with minimal risk of denaturation.

Intratracheal Catheter

The intracorporeal nebulizing catheter (Aeroprobe; Trudell Medical International, London, Ontario, Canada) is a novel device that produces an aerosol in the trachea.[251,252] A central lumen transmits the solution to be nebulized and compressed gas is forced under high pressure (100 psi) at a variable flow rate (0.1–3.0 L/minute) through several additional lumens that surround the central lumen (Fig. 63-5). Droplets of drug solution form at the tip of the catheter and aerosol is formed by the pressurized gas breaking up the liquid droplets. The catheter produces an aerosol continuously or intermittently when a pulsed gas flow is employed. The pressure and flow rate of the gas determine the aerosol particle size. Preliminary data suggest that lung deposition is improved with the use of the catheter compared to more conventional forms of aerosol administration.[253,254] The use of the intratracheal catheter is investigational at present.

PRESSURIZED METERED-DOSE INHALERS

The MDI canister contains a pressurized mixture of propellants, surfactants, preservatives, flavoring agents, and active drug, the latter comprising ~1% of the total contents (Fig. 63-6).[255,256] This mixture is released from the canister through a metering valve and stem, which fits into an actuator boot.[255,256] Previously, most pressurized metered-dose inhalers (pMDIs) used chlorofluorocarbon (CFC) propellants, but a newer generation of pMDIs contain hydrofluoroalkane (HFA) propellants.[257] The formulation, metering valve, and actuator design of HFA-pMDIs are different from those of CFC-pMDIs.

The aerosol particle size depends on propellant vapor pressure, ambient temperature, design of the valve stem and actuator orifices, and drug concentration.[257-260] High-vapor-pressure propellants produce finer aerosol sprays,

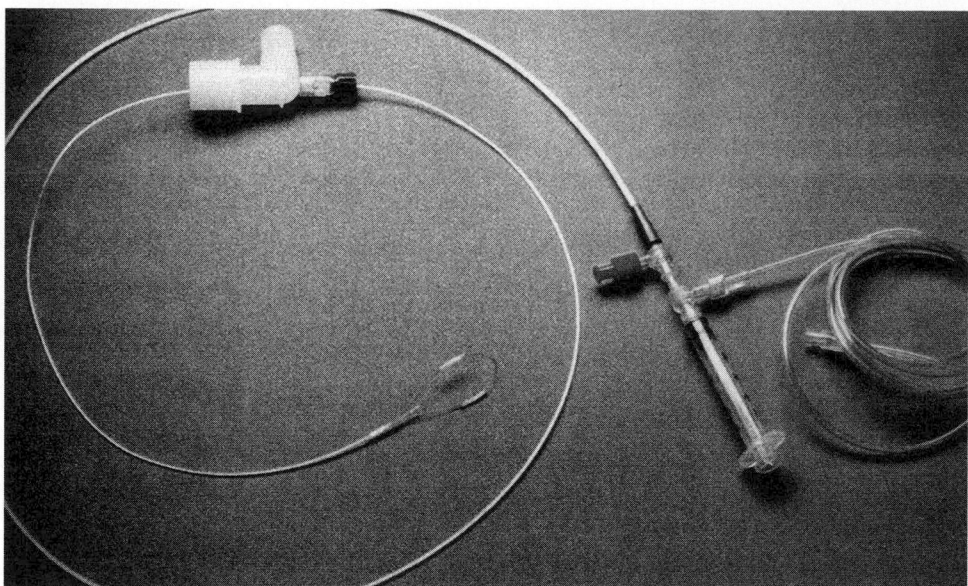

FIGURE 63-5 The intracorporeal nebulizing catheter is a novel device that produces an aerosol in the airways. It can be used to bypass the upper airway or endotracheal tube. The liquid to be nebulized is placed in a syringe connected to the proximal end of the catheter. The liquid passes through a central lumen in the catheter to the distal end. The distal end of the catheter tapers to a fine tip (diameter ∼0.5 mm). At the tip, the central lumen is surrounded by jets of compressed gas coming from apertures surrounding the central lumen. Drops of liquid that form at the tip of the catheter are aerosolized into a fine mist by the jets of compressed gas. (*Reproduced, with permission, from Dhand.*[252])

whereas increasing the drug concentration increases the particle size of the aerosol generated. Initially, drug particles are coated by a mixture of surfactant and propellant as they emerge from the pMDI. Propellant evaporation leads to a decrease in droplet diameter. Because HFA propellants are incompatible with surfactants, many of the agents

FIGURE 63-6 A section through a metered-dose inhaler showing its various components.

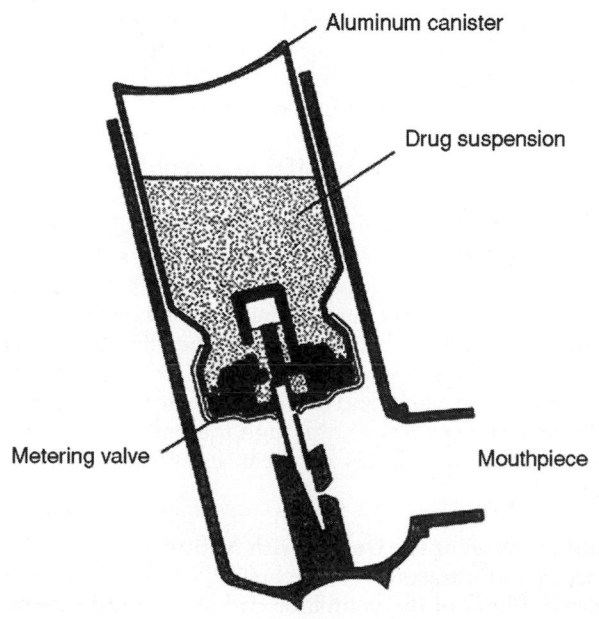

used with HFA-pMDIs have been reformulated as solutions, resulting in a finer aerosol spray with greater peripheral lung deposition and improved efficacy compared to the CFC-pMDIs.[261,262] In bench models of mechanical ventilation, however, HFA-pMDIs provide drug delivery that is lower than that with CFC-pMDIs.[263] To improve drug delivery with HFA-pMDIs during mechanical ventilation, actuators that better fit the stem of the HFA-pMDI canister are required.

DRY POWDER INHALERS

Dry powder inhalers (DPIs) create aerosols by drawing air through a powder that contains aggregates of micronized particles. The micronized particles are either in the form of loose aggregates or they are bound to larger carrier particles (usually lactose or glucose). Each DPI has three essential elements: drug formulation, metering system, and dispersion mechanism. The aerosol performance and characteristics depend on the particle characteristics and processing (formulation), as well as on the aerodynamic and flow properties of the inhaler device.

Most DPIs in current use are passive systems (i.e., they require the energy from inhalation to generate an aerosol). Active DPIs, on the other hand, employ an impeller or other mechanical device to generate inspiratory airflow. DPIs could be employed in-line in ventilator circuits either by employing the ventilator's inspiratory airflow to generate an aerosol or by first producing an aerosol and then entraining the drug particles into the airflow from the ventilator. Everard et al[264] employed a modified Turbuhaler in a dry ventilator circuit (Fig. 63-7), and found that ∼20% of the

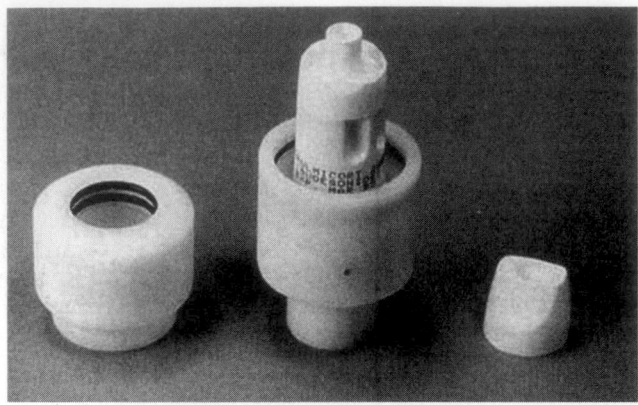 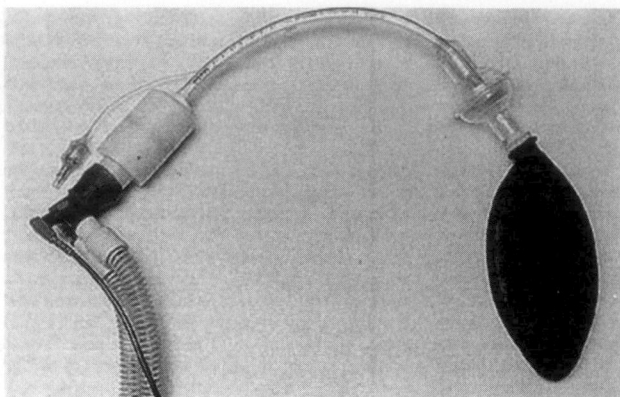

FIGURE 63-7 *Left panel:* A budesonide Turbuhaler was modified by cutting back the outer covering. The Turbuhaler was then enclosed in a chamber, which allowed air to flow through the device and was connected to the proximal end of the endotracheal tube. *Right panel:* The modified Turbuhaler was connected between the circuit Y and endotracheal tube. (*Reproduced, with permission, from Everard.*[264])

nominal dose was delivered to a filter placed at the distal end of the endotracheal tube. Although humidity reduces drug delivery from DPIs,[265] Lindsay et al[266] found no difference in clinical effect between albuterol given by Turbuhaler or the same drug given by a pMDI in a hot and humid region. Because ventilated patients routinely receive warm and humidified gas, the feasibility of administering dry powders in a humid environment needs further evaluation.

METHODS TO ASSESS AEROSOL DELIVERY DURING MECHANICAL VENTILATION

In the past, MDIs and nebulizers[267,268] were shown to have poor efficiency during mechanical ventilation, mainly because of drug deposition in the ventilator circuit and artificial airway.[263,269] Both in-vitro and in-vivo studies have helped in understanding the complex factors governing aerosol delivery during mechanical ventilation.[269–271]

Whereas in-vitro methods measure *drug delivery* to the lower respiratory tract, in-vivo methods measure the amount of *drug deposition* in the lung. This distinction is important because a variable portion of inhaled particles do not deposit in the lung and are exhaled. A "mass balance" technique that matches ventilator circuits and ventilator parameters has been employed to determine the correlation between the results of in-vitro tests and those in ventilator-supported patients.[272,273] With such techniques, it was estimated that ~5% of the nominal dose of albuterol administered by an MDI is exhaled by ventilated patients,[274] compared to <1% exhaled by ambulatory patients.[275] The mean exhaled fraction (7%) with nebulizers in ventilated patients is similar to that with MDIs, but there is considerable variability (coefficient of variation, 74%) among patients.[272]

IN-VITRO STUDIES

Carefully performed in-vitro tests that simulate the conditions of actual clinical use have played an important role in determining the optimal techniques for administering aerosols to ventilated patients.[263,272,273,276–279, 280–282,274,283–285] Table 63-6 shows various bench models that were used. Models that employ a tracheobronchial model

and directly measure the amount of drug deposited on a filter placed distal to the endotracheal tube[263,274,281,282,285,286] have produced the most reproducible results.

For any given aerosol-generating device, the efficiency of drug delivered varies widely; for MDIs, it varies from 0.3–97.5% and for nebulizers from 0–42%. These variations in drug delivery underscore the need for optimizing the techniques of administration with each device. With MDIs, the type of MDI propellant formulation[285] and the drug formulation[284] also influence drug delivery.

Configuration of the Device with Metered-Dose Inhalers

For an MDI to be employed in a ventilator circuit, the canister must be removed from the actuator (supplied by the manufacturer) and connected to the ventilator circuit with another different adapter, thereby making it a unique device with different aerosol characteristics and performance. Several types of adapters, including elbow adapters, in-line devices that may be unidirectional or bi-directional, and chamber or reservoir adapters, are commercially available[252,271] (Fig. 63-8). The adapter efficiency could have a significant influence on the dose required to produce a therapeutic effect.[289] Several investigators have shown that employing a chamber spacer with an MDI in a ventilator circuit results in four- to sixfold greater aerosol drug delivery compared with either an elbow adapter or a unidirectional in-line spacer.[277,283,286,290] An MDI and chamber spacer placed at a distance of approximately 15 cm from the endotracheal tube provides efficient aerosol delivery and elicits a significant bronchodilator response.[291,292] The efficiency of a bi-directional inline spacer was higher than that of a unidirectional in-line spacer[284] and was comparable to that achieved with chamber spacers,[284] although the performance of the bi-directional spacer has not been established in clinical studies.

Configuration of the Device with Nebulizers

Both jet and ultrasonic nebulizers are connected in the inspiratory limb of the ventilator circuit or at the patient Y. Placing a jet nebulizer at a distance from the endotracheal

TABLE 63-6 Determination of Lower Respiratory Tract Deposition of Aerosol Delivered by a Metered-Dose Inhaler Using In Vitro Models

Type of Model and Reference No.	Type of Adapter	Breath Type	Measurement	Results
ETT (6.0, 7.5 and 9.0 mm) in trachea[276]	Swivel adapter	Continuous flow or MDI actuation then flow	Filter weight	Greater efficiency with larger ETT and actuation into continuous flow
ETT and laser spectrometer[277]	Three different adapters in-line or cylindrical spacer	V_T 800 mL; flow 60 L min^{-1}	Particle volume 1–5 μm	Adapters produced lower volume of particles than standard actuator
Ventilator circuit; ETT (8 mm)[286]	Swivel adapter at ETT or cylindrical spacer	V_T 800 mL; flow 48 L min^{-1}	Albuterol assay	Greater deposition with cylindrical spacer
ETT and laser spectrometer[278]	Nine different MDI spacers or adapters	—	Particle volume 0.7–5.0 μm	Chamber spacers delivered greater volume than other adapters
Ventilator circuit[279]	MDI with large chamber or small chamber spacer	V_T 700 mL; flow 50 L min^{-1}	Radioactivity	Similar delivery with both the devices
Plastic syringe and simulated carina[281]	MDI with catheter	—	Albuterol assay	≈ 90% of dose delivered beyond ETT
ETT (6 mm) and swivel adapter[282]	Catheters placed in ETT (13 or 22 cm long)	Flow 30 L min^{-1}	Albuterol assay	Longer catheters delivered greater dose than shorter catheters
Model of trachea and main bronchi[263]	Cylindrical spacer 8 mm ETT	Flow 40 L min^{-1}	Albuterol assay	Decreased deposition with humidification and CMV breaths

ABBREVIATIONS: CMV, controlled mechanical ventilation; ETT, endotracheal tube; MDI, metered-dose inhaler; V_T, tidal volume.

FIGURE 63-8 Commercially available spacers and adapters that are used to connect a metered-dose inhaler canister in the ventilator circuit. *Top left:* collapsible spacer chamber. *Middle left:* aerosol cloud enhancer, wherein the aerosol flume is directed away from the patient. *Bottom left:* Non-collapsible spacer chamber. *Top right:* bi-directional actuator (mini spacer). *Bottom right:* in-line adapter. (*Reproduced, with permission, from Rau et al.[284]*)

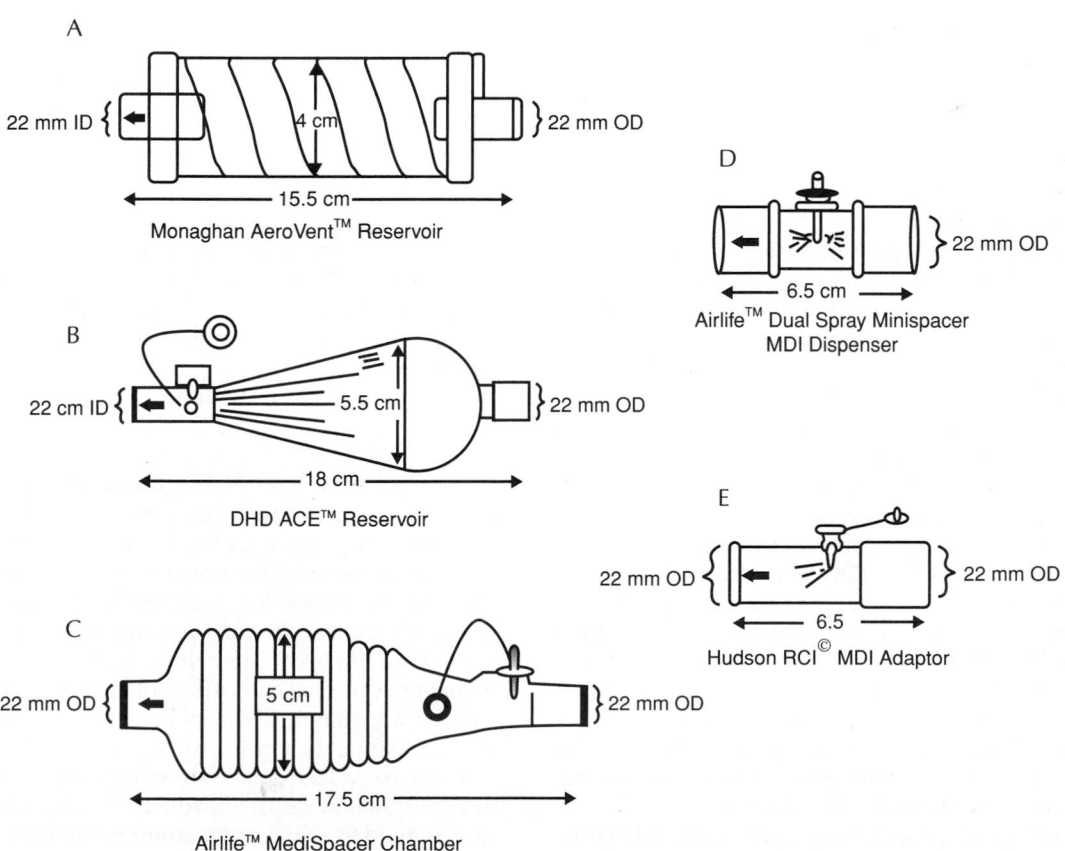

tube improves its efficiency compared with placing it between the patient Y and endotracheal tube.[280,287,293] Addition of a reservoir between the nebulizer and endotracheal tube also modestly increases efficiency of drug delivery.[288] The nebulizer brand,[240,280] diluent volume, operating pressures and flows, and duration of treatment,[231,240] influence the efficiency of aerosol generation.

Ultrasonic nebulizers are infrequently employed for bronchodilator therapy during mechanical ventilation and there is scant published information about drug delivery with these devices.[246] Moreover, the particle size of aerosols produced by ultrasonic nebulizers in ventilator circuits has not been well characterized. Likewise, there are as yet insufficient clinical data with the newer vibrating mesh nebulizers in ventilated patients.

Synchronizing Aerosol Generation with Inspiratory Airflow

The actuation of an MDI must be synchronized with the precise onset of inspiratory airflow from the ventilator.[294,295] As short as a 1- to 1.5-second delay between MDI actuation and a ventilator breath can profoundly reduce the efficiency of drug delivery.[283]

In a ventilator circuit, nebulizers can be operated continuously or intermittently by airflow from the ventilator. Continuous aerosol generation requires a pressurized source of gas (from a wall outlet, pressurized tank, or an air compressor), whereas intermittent operation requires a separate line to conduct inspiratory airflow from the ventilator to the nebulizer. Intermittent operation of the nebulizer is more efficient for aerosol delivery compared with continuous aerosol generation because it minimizes aerosol wastage during the exhalation phase of the breathing cycle.[273,293] The lower driving pressure provided by the ventilator (<15 psi) than that provided by pressurized gas (≥50 psi) could decrease the efficiency of some nebulizers.[296] Aerosol generated by a nebulizer operating at the lower pressure may generate particles whose diameter is larger than the 1–5 μm that is optimal for aerosol deposition. When intermittent nebulizer operation is employed, the specific ventilator and nebulizer brand should be tested to determine the characteristics of the aerosol generated and the efficiency of drug delivery.[273]

Ventilator-Related Factors

The characteristics of the ventilator breath have an important influence on aerosol drug delivery. A tidal volume of 500 ml or more (in an adult),[263] longer inspiratory time, and slower inspiratory flows improve aerosol delivery[263,297] (Fig. 63-9). Drug delivery is linearly correlated with a longer duty cycle (T_I/T_{TOT}) for both MDIs and nebulizers.[263,274,280] Moreover, drug delivery is improved when an MDI is synchronized with a simulated spontaneous breath compared with a controlled ventilator breath of similar tidal volume.

The inspiratory waveform influences drug delivery from nebulizers, but has much less influence on drug delivery from an MDI.[298] Unlike MDIs, nebulizer efficiency could be different during pressure-controlled ventilation than during volume-controlled ventilation (Fig. 63-10).

The breath-triggering mechanism does not significantly influence drug delivery from an MDI, but use of a flow

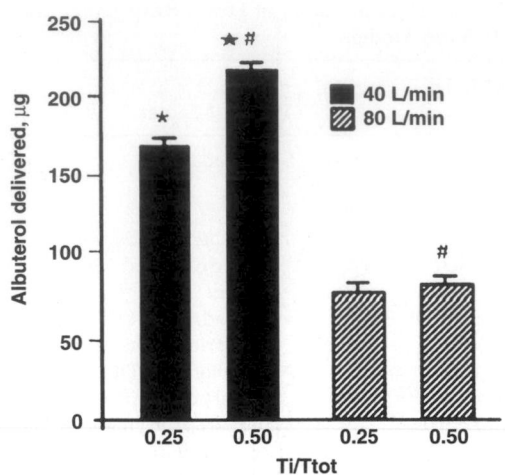

FIGURE 63-9 Comparison of aerosol delivery at different inspiratory airflows and duty cycles (T_I/T_{TOT}) in a bench model of mechanical ventilation. The ventilator delivered a tidal volume of 1000 ml with a constant inspiratory flow of 40 or 80 L/minute, and the frequency of breathing was varied to achieve T_I/T_{TOT} values of 0.25 or 0.50 at each inspiratory flow setting. Albuterol delivery to the bronchi was greater with a T_I/T_{TOT} of 0.50 than of 0.25 at inspiratory flows of 40 L/minute and 80 L/minute. For each value of T_I/T_{TOT}, drug delivery with a slower inspiratory airflow (40 L/minute) was almost twice that at the faster inspiratory airflow (80 L/minute) (*p <0.01, 40 L/minute versus 80 L/minute at T_I/T_{TOT} of 0.25 and T_I/T_{TOT} of 0.50; #p <0.01 T_I/T_{TOT} of 0.5 versus T_I/T_{TOT} of 0.25 at 40 L/minute and 80 L/minute). (*Reproduced, with permission, from Fink et al.*[274])

trigger with a nebulizer could dilute the aerosol and increase the washout of the aerosol into the expiratory limb between breaths.[263]

Circuit-Related Factors

Several investigators have found that drug delivery to the lower respiratory tract from both MDIs and nebulizers is reduced by 40% or more in a humidified compared to a dry circuit (Fig. 63-11).[244,273,274,279,280,283] Circuit humidity increases the size of drug particles generated by a nebulizer[299] When an MDI is employed in a ventilator circuit, humidity probably interferes with propellant evaporation so that drug particles remain of a larger size and impaction losses are increased.[291,300]

The density of the inhaled gas also influences drug delivery. High inspiratory flows employed during mechanical ventilation are associated with turbulence. Inhalation of a less dense gas, such as a helium-oxygen 70/30 mixture, makes airflow less turbulent and more laminar. The use of helium-oxygen mixtures improved drug delivery in a pediatric model of mechanical ventilation.[301] In a bench model of adult mechanical ventilation, drug delivery from an MDI was noted to be 50% higher with a helium-oxygen 80/20 mixture than with oxygen alone[302] (Fig. 63-12A). In contrast, nebulizer operation with helium-oxygen reduced drug output and respirable mass[302,303] (Fig. 63-12B). A practical method to achieve maximum pulmonary deposition of aerosol from a nebulizer during mechanical ventilation is

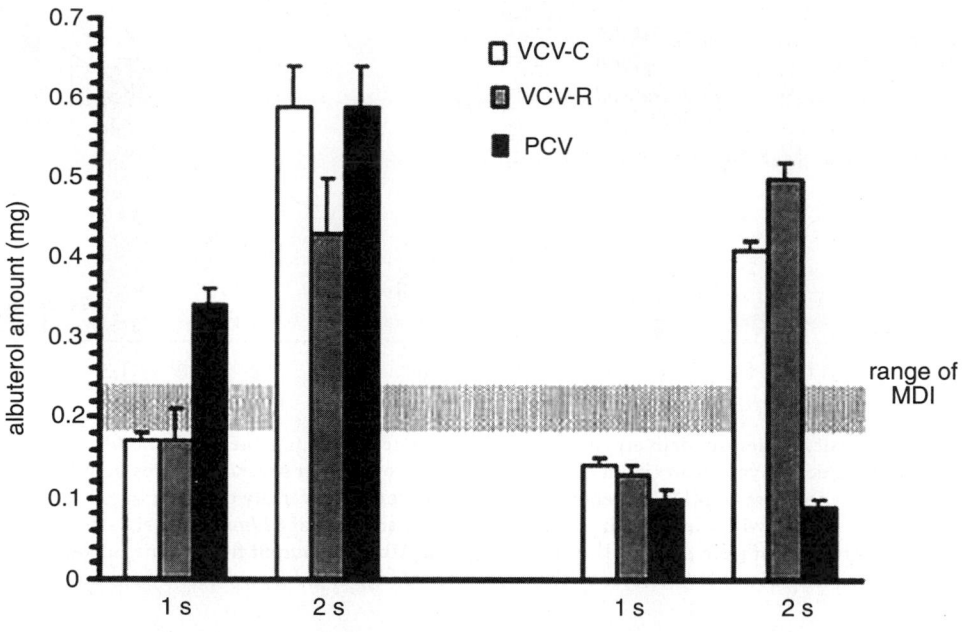

FIGURE 63-10 Comparison of aerosol delivery from metered-dose inhaler and jet nebulizer in bench models of pressure-controlled and volume-controlled ventilation. The lung mechanics were varied by selecting two settings of resistance and compliance to achieve high or low time constants. For each condition, the amounts of aerosol delivered during inspiratory times of 1 second or 2 seconds were measured. Increasing the duration of inspiration from 1 second to 2 seconds improved the nebulizer efficiency . In the high compliance/high resistance setting with 1-second inspiration, nebulizer efficiency was higher during pressure-controlled than during volume-controlled ventilation, whereas the converse occurred in the low compliance/low resistance setting with 2 seconds inspiratory time. In contrast, the efficiency of an MDI (*horizontal stippled area*) remained fairly constant under the various conditions simulated in the bench model. Thus, several factors, such as inspiratory time, pattern of inspiratory flow, and lung mechanics, that could influence drug delivery from a nebulizer, have minimal influence on drug delivery from an MDI. PCV, pressure-controlled ventilation; VCV-C, volume-controlled ventilation with a constant inspiratory flow; VCV-R, volume-controlled ventilation with a descending ramp flow pattern. (*Reproduced, with permission, from Hess et al.[298]*)

to operate the nebulizer with oxygen at a flow rate of 6–8 L/minute and to entrain the aerosol generated into a ventilator circuit containing helium-oxygen[302] (Fig. 63-13).

Aerosol impaction on the endotracheal tube poses a significant barrier to effective drug delivery in infant and pediatric mechanical ventilation (endotracheal tube internal diameter [ID] 3–6 mm).[276,304] In adult mechanical ventilation, there was no difference in nebulizer efficiency with endotracheal tubes of ID 7 mm versus ID 9 mm.[280] Drug losses within the endotracheal tube could be minimized by placing the aerosol generator at a distance from the endotracheal tube instead of being directly connected to it.[269] Some

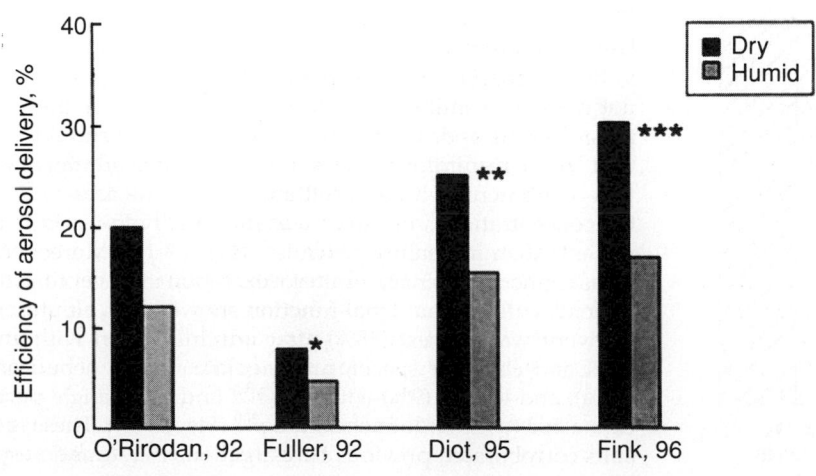

FIGURE 63-11 Effect of humidity on aerosol delivery. The delivery of aerosol to the lower respiratory tract in bench models of mechanical ventilation is reduced by ~40% when the circuit is humidified versus dry. *$p < 0.05$; **$p < 0.01$; ***$p < 0.001$. Studies: O'Riordan et al,[272] Fuller et al,[279] Diot et al,[283] and Fink et al.[263] (*Reproduced, with permission, from Dhand et al.[270]*)

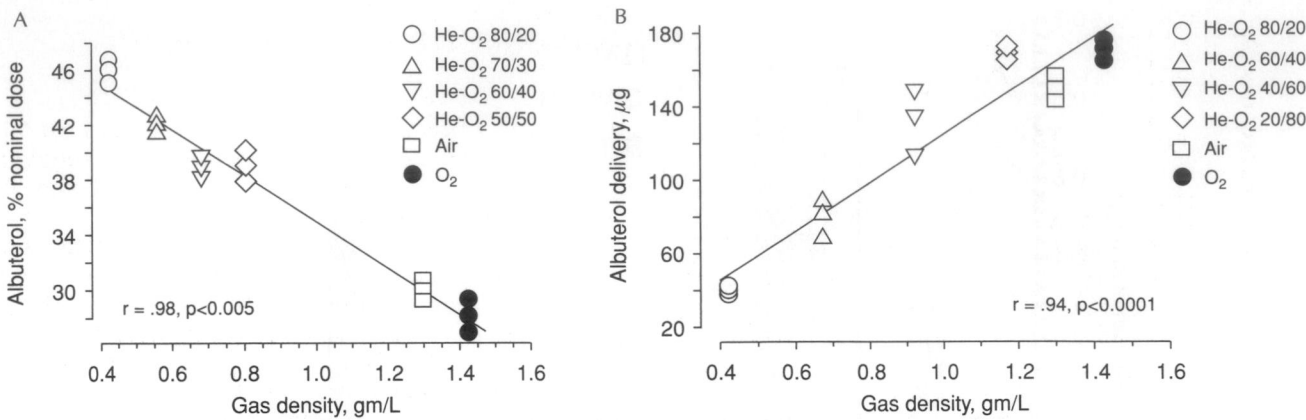

FIGURE 63-12 Effect of gas density on aerosol delivery from an MDI and jet nebulizer. In panel *A*, albuterol was administered via an MDI and chamber spacer in an unheated dry ventilator circuit containing air, 100% oxygen, or several mixtures of helium-oxygen (80/20, 70/30, 60/40, and 50/50). Albuterol delivery from an MDI (percentage of nominal dose) was inversely related (r = −0.98; *p* <0.005) to gas density. In panel *B*, albuterol was administered with a jet nebulizer operated at a constant flow of 6 L/minute of air, 100% oxygen, or helium-oxygen mixtures (as above) and albuterol output from the nebulizer was measured. Albuterol output from the nebulizer was positively correlated (r = 0.94; *p* <0.0001) with the density of gas used to operate the nebulizer. (*Modified, with permission, from Goode et al.*[302])

investigators attached a long catheter to the nozzle of an MDI and delivered aerosol directly into the trachea (i.e., beyond the endotracheal tube).[282] With this delivery system, concerns have been raised about catheter blockage and mucosal damage induced by propellants, surfactant, or other constituents of the MDI formulation.[305]

FIGURE 63-13 Effect of gas density and operating flow on aerosol delivery from a nebulizer. A jet nebulizer was operated with 100% oxygen at 6 L/minute, helium-oxygen (70/30) at 6 L/minute, or helium-oxygen (70/30) at 15 L/minute. Drug delivery on filters was measured with the circuit containing helium-oxygen (*stippled bars*) or oxygen (*hatched bars*). Albuterol delivery was greatest when the nebulizer was operated with oxygen and the ventilator circuit contained helium-oxygen. Bars represent SE. (*Reproduced, with permission, from Goode et al.*[302]).

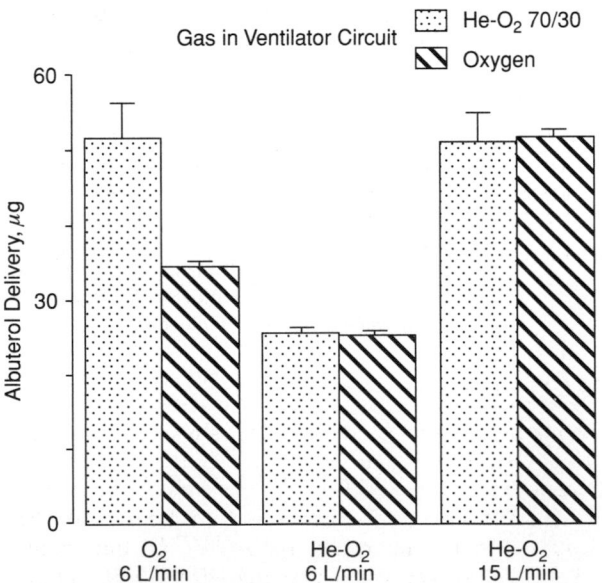

IN-VIVO STUDIES

Several investigators have used radionuclides and measured plasma or urinary drug levels to determine pulmonary deposition of aerosols in ventilated patients.

Radionuclide Studies

In ventilated patients, the pulmonary deposition of nebulized radiolabeled aerosol has been variously reported to be 1.22 ± 0.4%,[268] 2.22 ± 0.8%,[244] 2.9 ± 0.7%,[267] and 15.3 ± 9.5%.[272] Several factors, including type of radiolabel used, nebulizer brand, treatment time, circuit humidity, and methods used to calculate the amount of aerosol deposition,[272,273,280] contribute to the reported variation. With an MDI and spacer chamber, about 6% of the dose was deposited in the lower respiratory tract[268,290] this value was significantly lower than reported values (10–20%) with an MDI and spacer in nonintubated ambulatory patients.[306,307]

Pharmacokinetic Studies

Unlike nonintubated patients, direct deposition of aerosol in the oropharynx and subsequent enteral absorption cannot occur in ventilated patients. Therefore, estimation of plasma levels of drugs administered by an MDI should reflect lower respiratory tract deposition. After administration of albuterol with an MDI and spacer, the area under the concentration-time curve was marginally lower in the patients than in healthy controls[308] (Fig. 63-14). Moreover, measurement of urinary albuterol excretion in 30 ventilated patients with normal renal function showed that albuterol recovery was highest (38%) after administration with an MDI and chamber spacer, intermediate with a nebulizer (16%), and lowest (9%) with an MDI and right angle port connected to the endotracheal tube[309] (Fig. 63-15). These results corroborated previous investigations that found very

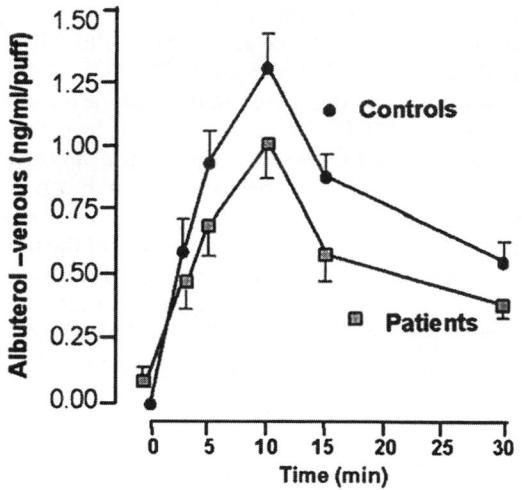

FIGURE 63-14 Comparison of serum albuterol levels in stable mechanically ventilated patients with chronic obstructive pulmonary disease versus controls (normal volunteers using a MDI with holding chamber with an optimal technique). The serum levels of albuterol per dose from the MDI that were achieved in ventilated patients were, for the most part, comparable to those in normal controls. $p < 0.05$ levels in controls versus patients 15 minutes after albuterol. (*Modified, with permission, from Duarte et al.[308]*)

low efficiency of drug delivery with the adapter connected to the endotracheal tube.[283,286,290] Thus, pharmacokinetic studies show that pulmonary drug deposition in ventilated patients is comparable to that achieved in healthy controls.

FIGURE 63-15 Comparison of systemic bioavailability of albuterol administered by MDI and right angle elbow adapter, MDI and chamber spacer, or jet nebulizer. Urine was collected for 6 hours after drug administration and the amounts of albuterol and its sulfate conjugate determined. The efficiency of the delivery device was determined by determining the percentage of drug excreted. The three delivery systems varied in the efficiency of drug delivery. The MDI and elbow adapter had the lowest efficiency, the jet nebulizer was intermediate, and the MDI with chamber spacer had the highest efficiency. (*Reproduced, with permission, from Marik et al.[309]*)

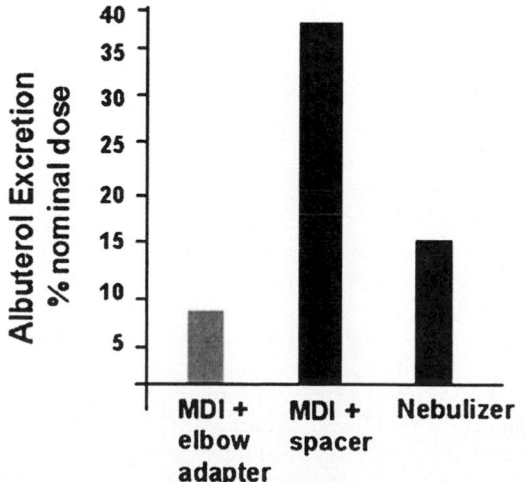

RECONCILING IN-VITRO ESTIMATES OF DRUG DELIVERY WITH IN-VIVO ESTIMATES OF DRUG DEPOSITION

The wide variation between in-vitro[263,279,283,286] and in-vivo estimates[268] of device efficiency can be reconciled by taking into account the effects of humidity in the ventilator circuit,[263] the quantity of exhaled aerosol that is not included in the in vitro measurement,[274] and by correcting for the quenching of radioactivity by the tissues of the chest wall.[290] When these factors are accounted for, in-vitro data obtained with humidified ventilator circuits and in-vivo gamma scintigraphic studies reveal that ~11% of the nominal dose from an MDI and spacer chamber is deposited in the lower respiratory tract of ventilated patients. This value is remarkably close to values observed with the optimal use of an MDI without a spacer (10–14%) in ambulatory patients.[306,307]

Drug delivery from nebulizers also shows discrepancies between values obtained with bench models versus those obtained by gamma scintigraphy.[244,267,268,288] Miller et al[273] found that accounting for circuit humidity and breath-actuated nebulization could reconcile most observed differences.

Thus, in-vitro investigations that accurately simulate the clinical settings could play an important role in determining the performance of various inhalation devices under a variety of conditions encountered during mechanical ventilation.

Clinical Use of Bronchodilators

BRONCHODILATORS USED

Bronchodilators are among the most commonly used drugs in the ICU.[11] In ventilator-supported patients with asthma or COPD, the goals of bronchodilator therapy are to reverse bronchoconstriction, decrease work of breathing, and/or relieve dyspnea. A response has been observed after administration of either aerosolized β-adrenergic[1,7,8,10,114,215,289,292,310–320] or anticholinergic bronchodilators.[215,318,321,322] Inhaled isoproterenol,[310,323] isoetharine,[324] metaproterenol,[1] fenoterol,[311,318] and albuterol[7,8,10,114,289,292,312–317,319,320] produce significant bronchodilation in ventilated patients. The combination of fenoterol and ipratropium bromide was found more effective than ipratropium in ventilated patients with COPD.[169] No long-acting bronchodilator is presently available for use in ventilated patients. Likewise, there are no published clinical studies on the use of levalbuterol in ventilated patients.

SELECTION OF PATIENTS

Ventilated patients with COPD demonstrate a significant decrease in airway resistance after administration of bronchodilators.[10,114,215,292,311,314,316,317,319–322] Bronchodilators have been successfully used to treat acute bronchospasm in the operating room,[310,323,324] and they are widely used in ventilated patients with severe asthma.[325]

In addition, expiratory flow improved after bronchodilator administration in a heterogenous group of ventilated patients.[1] Nebulized metaproterenol reduced elevated levels of airway resistance in patients with acute respiratory distress syndrome.[2,3] Thus, a wide spectrum of patients receiving mechanical ventilation could benefit from bronchodilators.

BRONCHODILATOR EFFICACY

ASSESSMENT OF BRONCHODILATOR RESPONSE

The response to bronchodilators depends on several variables: patient airway geometry, degree of airway responsiveness, severity of disease, quantity of secretions, and counterregulatory effects of airway inflammation and other drugs. Most investigators assess response by measuring inspiratory airway resistance. Airway resistance in ventilated patients is commonly measured by performing rapid airway occlusions at constant flow inflation.[326,327] This technique involves performing a breath-hold at end-inspiration by occluding the expiratory port. Total or maximal inspiratory resistance (Rrs max) can be partitioned into minimal inspiratory resistance (Rrs min), which reflects "ohmic" resistance of the airways, and additional effective resistance (ΔRrs). The latter resistance represents time-constant inhomogeneities within the lung ("pendelluft") and viscoelastic behavior of the pulmonary tissues.[326,327] Similarly, airway occlusion at end-expiration produces an increase in airway pressure to a plateau value, signifying intrinsic positive end-expiratory pressure (PEEPi).[10] Comparisons of airway resistance and intrinsic PEEP before and after drug administration are useful for assessing response.

Most ventilated patients with COPD demonstrate a decrease in airway resistance and intrinsic PEEP following bronchodilator administration.[2,7,10,114,289,292,311,314,316–320] That ΔRrs does not decrease significantly after albuterol delivery with an MDI[10,292] suggests that the bronchodilator effect occurs predominantly in the central airways with little effect on viscoelastic behavior or time-constant inhomogeneities in the lung. Moreover, albuterol does not significantly influence the elastic properties of the lung.[10] In contrast, a greater decline in ΔRrs was noted after nebulizer delivery of albuterol and ipratropium bromide.[318] This difference in response between MDIs and nebulizers could be due to higher drug deposition in peripheral airways with the use of a nebulizer.

DOSE RESPONSE TO BRONCHODILATOR ADMINISTRATION IN VENTILATED PATIENTS

Few investigators have examined the dose response to bronchodilators in ventilated patients.[289,292,314,311,320] Most investigators found that the response with the higher doses was no greater than that observed after the initial dose (Figs. 63-16 and 63-17).[292,311] Dose-response curves in stable, ventilated patients with COPD are shallow; when the technique of administration is carefully executed, most patients achieved near maximal bronchodilation with 4 puffs of albuterol.[292] Mouloudi et al[316,317,319] recently showed that, with an optimal technique of administration, alterations in mechanical ventilator settings do not influence the response to albuterol in stable patients with COPD. Patients with acute exacerbations of asthma or COPD may require higher doses.

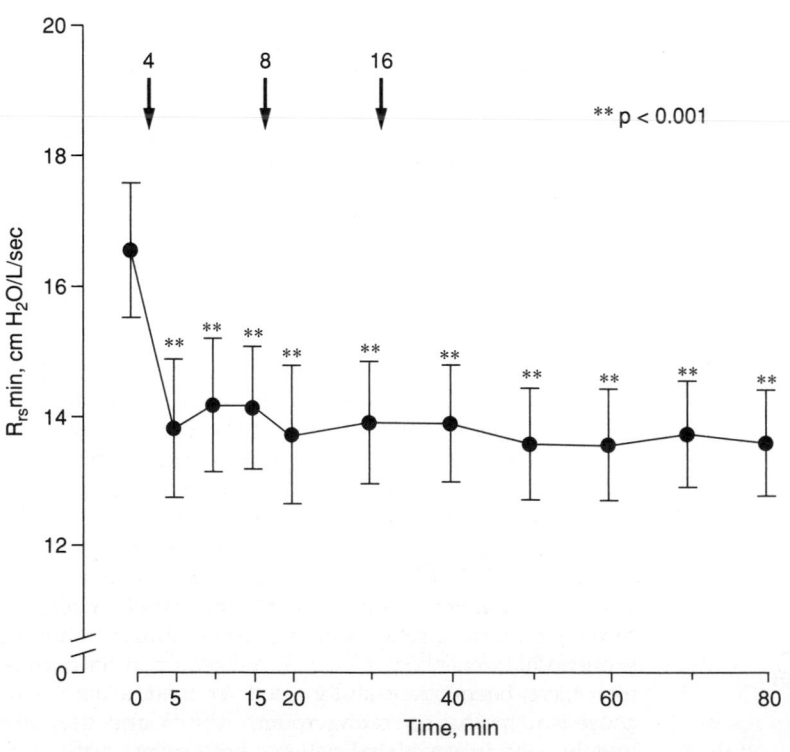

FIGURE 63-16 Effect of albuterol on minimal inspiratory resistance (*Rrs min*) in 12 stable mechanically ventilated patients with COPD. Significant decreases in Rrs min occurred within 5 minutes of administration of 4 puffs of albuterol. The addition of 8 and 16 puffs (cumulative doses of 12 and 28 puffs, respectively) did not achieve a significantly greater effect than that with 4 puffs ($p > 0.05$). Bars represent SE. ** $p < 0.001$. (*Reproduced, with permission, from Dhand et al.*[292])

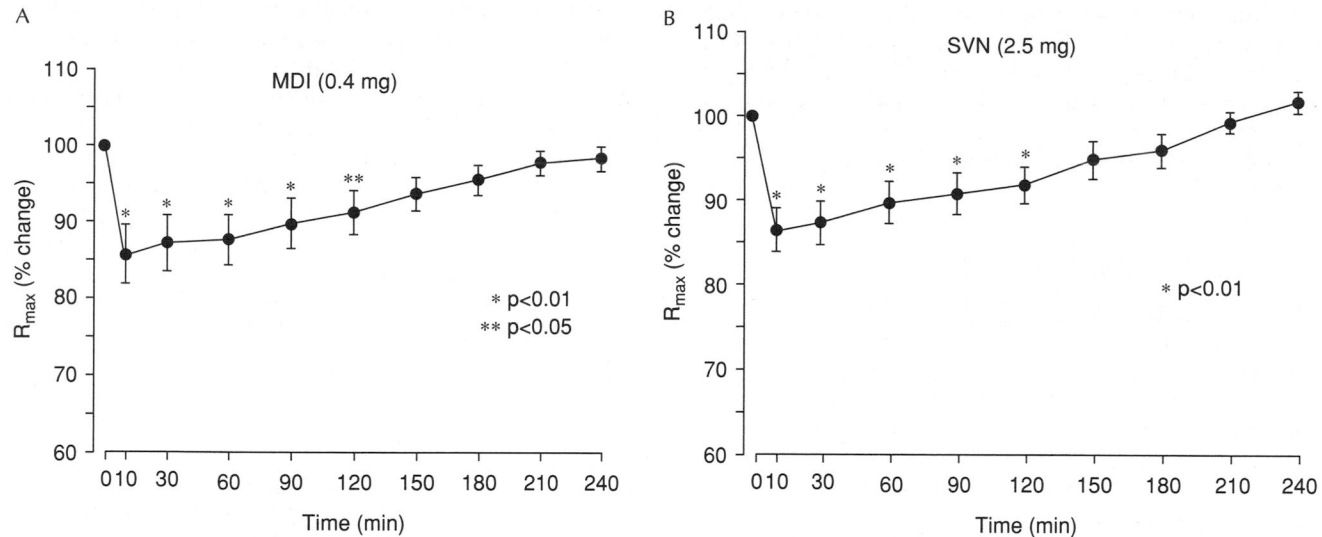

FIGURE 63-17 Effect of albuterol on maximum inspiratory airway resistance (*Rrs max*) in stable, mechanically ventilated patients with COPD. There was a decrease in Rrs max from baseline values within 10 minutes of albuterol administration. *A.* Change in Rrs max from baseline (time 0) after 4 doses of albuterol from a pMDI. *B.* Change in Rrs max from baseline (time 0) after 2.5 mg of albuterol given by nebulizer. Significant reductions in Rrs max were sustained for 2 hours and returned to baseline by 4 hours. The response to albuterol administered by pMDI (0.4 mg) was comparable to that achieved with 2.5 mg administered by nebulizer. Bars represent SEM. (*Reproduced, with permission, from Duarte et al.[320]*)

DURATION OF BRONCHODILATOR RESPONSE

In stable ventilated patients with COPD, the bronchodilator effect of albuterol is sustained for 2–3 hours.[114,320] Thus, in contrast to the four-times-a-day and as-needed albuterol dosing in ambulatory patients, ventilated patients may require dosing every 3–4 hours.

Aerosol Therapy in Mechanically-Ventilated Neonates and Infants

Infants breathe with a high frequency and low tidal volume. This rapid shallow breathing pattern reduces drug deposition in the lung by limiting the time available for particle deposition. In nonintubated, spontaneously breathing infants, pulmonary deposition of radiolabeled aerosols administered via MDI and facemask, or nebulizer and facemask, is as low as 0.3–2.6% of the nominal dose.[328–332] Several investigators have reported similar decreases in aerosol delivery in ventilated neonates and infants because of small-diameter endotracheal tubes and ventilator tubing, and the low tidal volumes employed.[304,333,334] Moreover, ventilator modes differ; pressure-limited and time-cycled modes of ventilation are more common, with continuous flow through the circuit and very short duty cycles. Investigators have performed in-vitro studies to determine the influence of various factors.

IN-VITRO STUDIES OF AEROSOL DRUG DELIVERY IN INFANTS

METERED-DOSE INHALERS

When the MDI was actuated into a prototype spacer chamber, there was a 10-fold variation (from 0.2–2.0% of the nominal dose) in drug delivery to a filter placed beyond the endotracheal tube.[335] Higher values of drug delivery were achieved when the MDI was actuated before inspiration than after inspiration, and when higher tidal volumes and longer inspiratory times (I:E ratio 1:1) were employed. The type of spacer employed to actuate an MDI has a dramatic influence on drug delivery[336–339] (Table 63-7). In a dry infant ventilator circuit, drug delivery as high as 14.2% was achieved when an Aerochamber MV15 (Monaghan Medical Corp., Plattsburgh, NY) was placed between the ventilator Y and endotracheal tube and the MDI was actuated at end-expiration.[336] With an ACE spacer in a humidified circuit during infant mechanical ventilation, an HFA-albuterol MDI formulation gave marginally higher drug delivery than a CFC-albuterol MDI formulation (5.7% versus 4.8%, respectively).[339]

NEBULIZERS

In bench models of infant ventilation, nebulizers have shown uniformly poor efficiency for drug delivery. During simulated infant ventilation, nebulizers deliver <2% of the nominal drug dose.[336,337,340–342] Many factors influence drug delivery with a nebulizer: type of nebulizer[336,340] and its position in the circuit,[339] intermittent versus continuous nebulization,[342] nebulizer flow,[337] inspiratory time,[337] volume-limited versus pressure-limited ventilation,[339] humidity, and size of the endotracheal tube. The very low efficiency of nebulizers during infant mechanical ventilation, however, means that pulmonary drug deposition would be marginally influenced by altering the ventilator conditions. In fact, underdosing is a concern when a nebulizer is employed with settings that have very poor efficiency (as low as ~0.1%) for drug delivery.

TABLE 63-7 Efficiency of Drug Delivery with a Metered-Dose Inhaler and Spacer in Infant Ventilation

Lead Author[a]	Spacer	ET(mm)	VT(ml)	Mode	Efficiency (%)
Everard	Prototype	3.0	11–22	Pressure limited, 30 cmH$_2$O	1.5–2
Coleman	ACE	3.5	55	Pressure 60/5 cmH$_2$O	14.5
	Aerochamber MV				11.9
	Aerovent				6.8
	In-line adapter				6.4
Avent	Aerochamber	3.5	—	Pressure 20/2 cmH$_2$O	2.2
	In-line adapter			Humidified circuit	0.1
Lugo	CFC-MDI with ACE	3.0	7	Pressure 25/4 cmH$_2$O	4.8
	HFA-MDI with ACE			Humidified circuit	5.7

[a]Data from Everard et al,[335] Coleman et al,[337] Avent et al,[338] and Lugo et al.[339]
ET, internal diameter of endotracheal tube; VT, tidal volume.

METERED-DOSE INHALERS VERSUS NEBULIZERS

Few investigators have compared the efficiency of MDIs with that of nebulizers during infant mechanical ventilation.[336,337,339,343] With optimal technique, the efficiency of MDIs (~14%) is considerably higher than that of nebulizers (~2%). Given the poor efficiency of drug delivery with MDIs and nebulizers, it may not be necessary to modify drug doses because the lower patient weight is compensated by the low lung deposition of drug. With a carefully executed technique of administration,[336] one or two doses of albuterol administered by MDI and chamber spacer should be adequate for routine bronchodilator therapy in infants.

IN-VITRO STUDIES OF AEROSOL DRUG DELIVERY IN OLDER CHILDREN

In older children, the efficiency of MDIs and nebulizers improve with increasing age[333,344] and the factors influencing drug delivery are similar to those in adults.

IN-VIVO STUDIES OF DRUG DELIVERY IN INFANTS AND NEONATES

The lung deposition of radiolabeled aerosols in ventilated infants with bronchopulmonary dysplasia was as low as 0.98 ± 0.2% and 0.22 ± 0.1% with an MDI and spacer or a jet nebulizer, respectively.[345] Additional scintigraphic studies are needed to determine the efficiency of drug delivery with an MDI with optimal techniques of administration.

CLINICAL STUDIES

Inhaled bronchodilators (β-adrenergic and anticholinergic drugs)[4–8,346–349] are effective in ventilated neonates and infants with acute, subacute, and chronic lung disease. Response to inhaled albuterol was similar to that seen after intravenous administration.[347] Albuterol administered with an MDI and Aerochamber was found to be more effective than administration with a nebulizer (Fig. 63-18).[8,349] Ultrasonic nebulizers may be as (or more) effective than MDIs for bronchodilator administration in infants (see Fig. 63-18). In addition to monitoring airway resistance and pulmonary compliance, changes in heart rate should be assessed to pre-

vent overdosing. Inhaled corticosteroids have been advocated in infants for prevention[350,351] and treatment of bronchopulmonary dysplasia,[352–354] but their efficacy has not been established.

In summary, during infant mechanical ventilation, MDIs appear to be more efficient than nebulizers; with a careful technique of administration, one or two doses from an albuterol MDI and spacer chamber should suffice for routine therapy.

Techniques of Aerosol Administration

The optimal techniques for administration of inhaled drugs to ventilated patients are based on the various factors discussed above. The technique employed may have to compromise between the optimum operating characteristics of the device and the patient's condition. For example, a higher duty cycle increases aerosol delivery.[263,272] but it may

FIGURE 63-18 Total resistance of the respiratory system (*Rrs*) before and at 15, 30, 60, and 120 minutes after albuterol via metered-dose inhaler (*MDI*), jet nebulizer (*Jet*), and ultrasonic nebulizer (*US*) during infant ventilation. *Posttreatment Rrs was significantly lower than pretreatment Rrs ($p < 0.0001$). The response to albuterol after administration with an MDI was greater than that obtained with a jet nebulizer but was comparable to that obtained with an ultrasonic nebulizer. (*Reproduced with permission, from Fok et al.[349]*)

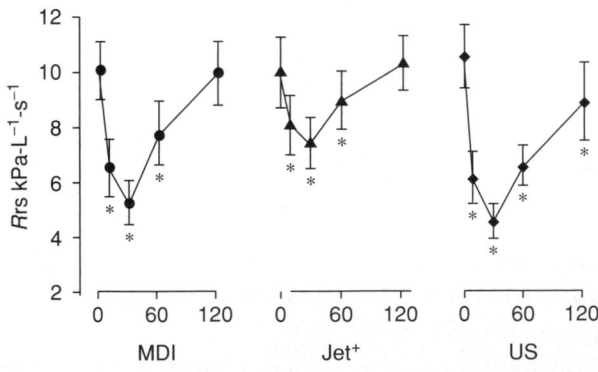

Duration after aerosol treatment min

TABLE 63-8 Optimal Technique for Drug Delivery by Metered-Dose Inhaler in Ventilated Patients

1. Review order, identify patient, and assess need for bronchodilator.
2. Suction endotracheal tube and airway secretions.
3. Shake MDI and warm to hand temperature.
4. Place MDI in space chamber adapter in ventilator circuit.
5. Remove heat and moisture exchanger. Do not disconnect humidifier.
6. Coordinate MDI actuation with beginning of inspiration.
7. Wait at least 15 seconds between actuations; administer total dose.
8. Monitor for adverse response.
9. Reconnect heat and moisture exchanger.
10. Document clinical outcome.

worsen dynamic hyperinflation in patients with airflow limitation. With this caveat in mind, the technique of administration for MDIs in ventilated patients is shown in Table 63-8 and that for nebulizers in Table 63-9. The key aspects of the technique with MDIs are to place an appropriate adapter at a short distance (~15 cm) from the endotracheal tube and to synchronize actuation with inspiratory flow. For nebulizers, it is critical to use the device as recommended by the manufacturer and to place it at a distance from the patient. When these techniques are employed, adequate drug deposition is achieved in the lung[263,273,274] and a significant bronchodilator response is observed[10,114,289,292,314,316–320]

USE OF METERED-DOSE INHALERS OR NEBULIZERS

The characteristics of the aerosol produced by an aerosol generator has a significant influence on drug delivery and deposition in the lower respiratory tract. During mechanical ventilation, larger particles produced by MDIs and nebulizers are trapped in the ventilator circuit and endotra-

TABLE 63-9 Optimal Technique for Drug Delivery by Jet Nebulizer in Ventilated Patients

1. Review order, identify patient, and assess need for bronchodilator.
2. Suction endotracheal and airway secretions.
3. Place drug in nebulizer to fill volume of 4–6 ml.
4. Place nebulizer in the inspiratory line 18 in. (46 cm) from the patient Y connector.
5. Turn off flow-by or continuous flow during nebulizer operation.
6. Remove heat and moisture exchanger from circuit (do not disconnect humidifier).
7. Set gas flow to nebulizer at 6–8 L/minute.
   a. Use a ventilator if it meets the nebulizer flow requirements and cycles on inspiration, or
   b. Use continuous flow from external source.
8. Adjust ventilator volume or pressure limit to compensate for added flow.
9. Tap nebulizer periodically until nebulizer begins to sputter.
10. Remove nebulizer from circuit, rinse with sterile water and run dry, store in a safe place.
11. Reconnect heat and moisture exchanger and return ventilator settings and alarms to their previous values.
12. Monitor patient for adverse response.
13. Assess outcome and document findings.

cheal tube; therefore, devices that produce aerosols with mass median aerodynamic diameter (MMAD) <2 μm are more efficient during mechanical ventilation than devices that produce aerosols with larger particles.[272,283] Nebulizers that produce smaller particle size have been employed, but they require a considerably greater time to deliver a standard dose.[273,283] Similarly, MDIs and nebulizers delivered an equivalent mass of aerosol beyond the endotracheal tube in a ventilator model;[283] in ventilated patients, both devices produced similar therapeutic effects.[312,318,320] When used optimally, MDIs and nebulizers are equally effective in the treatment of patients with obstructive lung disease.[144]

MDIs are preferred in ventilated patients because of several problems associated with the use of nebulizers. The rate of nebulizer aerosol production is highly variable, not only among brands of nebulizers, but even in different batches of the same brand.[238–240] The nature of the aerosol produced, especially particle size, is highly variable among different nebulizers.[240,243] Furthermore, operational efficiency of a nebulizer changes with the pressure of the driving gas and with different fill volumes. Performance of some nebulizers is compromised because the pressure of gas supplied by a ventilator (to drive the nebulizer during inspiration) is lower than that supplied by a tank/air compressor unit. Moreover, ventilator mode (pressure-control versus volume-control ventilation) and lung mechanics can influence drug delivery from a nebulizer.[298] Therefore, before using a nebulizer in a ventilated patient it is imperative to characterize its efficiency in a ventilator circuit, under the typical clinical conditions in which it will be employed.

Unless scrupulously cleaned and disinfected, nebulizers can be a source for aerosolization of bacteria,[355] and thus predispose patients to nosocomial pneumonia.[356] The gas flow driving the nebulizer produces additional airflow in the ventilator circuit. Hypoventilation was reported with older ventilator models secondary to patient inability to trigger the ventilator during pressure-assisted modes because of additional gas flow arising from nebulizer operation.[357] In contrast, MDIs are easy to administer, require less personnel time, provide a reliable dose, and do not pose a risk of bacterial contamination. Moreover, when MDIs are used with a collapsible cylindrical spacer, the circuit need not be disconnected at the time of each treatment, thus reducing the risk of pneumonia.

Cost is another factor influencing the selection of a device.[144] Use of MDIs rather than nebulizers saves cost and time.[358–360] Costs of bronchodilators have a significant impact on overall costs of care.[360]

In summary, MDIs offer several advantages over nebulizers for routine bronchodilator therapy. One survey found that most reporting centers (57%) were using MDIs in neonates and use had steadily increased since 1988.[361] Similar data are not available for adults.

Drug Toxicity

Higher doses of β-agonists delivered by an MDI can cause hypokalemia, and atrial and ventricular arrhythmias.[32,362,363] Manthous et al[289] observed sinus tachycardia or supraventricular ectopy after a cumulative dose of 7.5 mg of albuterol administered by a nebulizer in four of ten patients, and most of the remaining patients developed premature atrial and ventricular contractions with a cumulative dose of 15 mg.[289] Although most investigators have reported no adverse effects following administration of albuterol with an MDI,[10,215,268,289,314] a dose-dependent increase in heart rate occurs with higher doses.[292] No significant arrhythmias or other serious cardiovascular side effects were observed in ambulatory patients in an emergency department who were treated for acute asthma with up to 16 puffs each of albuterol or fenoterol administered with an MDI attached to a holding chamber and facemask.[141] Continuous nebulization of β-agonists is effective and safe in nonintubated children[364] and adults[99] with acute severe asthma; but the efficacy and safety of continuous nebulization has not been established in ventilated patients. A few anecdotal reports have described cardiotoxicity secondary to chlorofluorocarbons (CFCs).[365] Adverse cardiac effects are unlikely to occur with the doses recommended in clinical practice, particularly if there is a short interval between successive doses, because CFCs have a short half-life (<40 seconds) in blood after administration via MDI in healthy volunteers.[366] With a catheter connected to an MDI nozzle, however, a substantial portion of the total mass output of the MDI is delivered directly onto the tracheobronchial mucosa and there is potential for local and systemic toxicity.[305]

Guidelines for Inhaled Therapy

Subtle differences in the method of administration can markedly decrease aerosol deposition in the lower respiratory tract.[263,274,280,283,289,298] Controlled ventilation is not a prerequisite for aerosol administration. In bench studies, aerosol delivery is improved when an aerosol is administered in synchrony with a spontaneous breath.[263] Therefore, routine bronchodilator therapy can be given successfully with assisted modes if aerosol delivery is synchronized with inspiratory flow from the ventilator. Based on the recommendation for use of MDIs in ambulatory patients, some investigators use a postinspiratory breath-hold after aerosol administration.[215,312] With an optimal technique, this maneuver does not influence bronchodilator response in ventilated patients.[316] Mouloudi et al[317,319] have also shown that increasing the tidal volume from 8 ml/kg to 12 ml/kg or using pressure-control (decelerating flow pattern) versus volume-control (constant flow pattern) ventilation did not affect the response to albuterol inhalation with an MDI. These findings are consistent with other studies showing shallow dose-response curves in ventilated patients.[7,215,292,311,320] Thus, there may be little justification for manipulating ventilator settings to enhance drug deposition in the lung provided an optimal MDI technique is employed.

Although humidification of the circuit reduces aerosol deposition by ~40%,[263] bypassing the humidifier is not recommended because it would require disconnection of the ventilator circuit and several minutes would be added to each bronchodilator treatment while waiting for the circuit to become dry. Even with a humidified circuit, a significant effect is observed with as few as 4 puffs.[292] Bypassing the humidifier may be one method to improve pulmonary drug delivery with more expensive, nonbronchodilator agents. Before such a practice can be routinely recommended, however, studies are needed to document the safety of repeatedly administering nonhumidified gases, albeit for limited periods, to ventilated patients.

Bronchodilator Therapy during Noninvasive Ventilation

Noninvasive positive-pressure ventilation (NIPPV) is being increasingly employed for treatment of patients with acute and chronic respiratory failure.[367] Successful application of NIPPV with a nasal or facemask can often obviate the need for endotracheal intubation and improve mortality.[368-371] Patients with acute or acute-on-chronic respiratory failure who are receiving NIPPV often require inhaled bronchodilators for relief of airway obstruction. Initial enthusiasm for administration of bronchodilators with intermittent positive-pressure breathing[372] was dampened by the observation that drug delivery was reduced by this technique.[373] In a bench model, 10-cmH$_2$O continuous positive airway pressure (CPAP) reduced drug delivery from a jet nebulizer.[374] Chatmongkolchart et al[375] found a fivefold variation (between 5 and 25% of the nominal dose) in the amount of albuterol delivered by a jet nebulizer in vitro; delivery was highest (25%) when the nebulizer was close to the patient (between the leak port and patient connection), inspiratory pressure was high (20 cmH$_2$O), and expiratory pressure was low (5 cmH$_2$O).[375] Conversely, Faroux et al[376] found that in children with cystic fibrosis, pulmonary deposition of radiolabeled aerosol was increased by the application of 10 cmH$_2$O inspiratory pressure support. In summary, the optimum settings required for maximum drug delivery with an MDI during NIPPV have not been established. Nevertheless, significant bronchodilator responses occur after albuterol administration with a jet nebulizer or an MDI in stable patients receiving NIPPV with mask.[374,377] Patients with acute asthma exacerbations who received albuterol administered during bi-level positive airway pressure ventilation[378] had greater improvement in PEF than patients receiving a similar dose by nebulizer alone. Both MDIs and nebulizers could be employed during NIPPV, although factors influencing drug delivery during NIPPV are poorly understood.

Important Unknowns

Despite frequent use of bronchodilators in ventilated patients, their effects on clinically relevant outcomes, such as duration of mechanical ventilation, length of ICU stay, development of ventilator-associated pneumonia, and mortality have not been studied. In fact, few randomized controlled studies have been performed in this patient population.[144] Variations in the methods of administration and assessment of response make it difficult to compare results.

The phase-out of CFC-MDIs poses a challenge. Efficiency of albuterol HFA-MDIs is reduced when they are employed with currently available in-line actuators.[274] Device manufacturers should take note of this deficiency and design suitable in-line actuators for HFA-MDIs. Further work is also needed to determine whether DPIs can be successfully adapted for use during mechanical ventilation.

The Future

Ventilated patients present a unique opportunity to exploit the advantages of the inhaled route for drug delivery. The past decade has seen impressive gains in knowledge and understanding of methods to deliver inhaled therapies to ventilated patients. Within the past few years, newer aerosol-generating devices designed for use during mechanical ventilation have become available. These devices are far more efficient than previous devices. In the future, further improvements in device design and efficiency can be expected. The goal will not only be to deliver inhaled drugs with high efficiency, but also to ensure precision, reliability, and consistency of dosing.

Although nebulizers have been an integral part of mechanical ventilation since its inception, aerosol therapy has remained largely unregulated in ventilated patients. Lack of regulation of therapy with nebulizers may be secondary to the perception that bronchodilators, the most commonly employed inhaled drugs, have a low risk for causing harm to ventilated patients. In the near future, aerosol-generating devices will be integrated into modern ventilators. This integration should further improve the characterization of aerosols and consistency of dosing.

NIPPV is being increasingly employed, especially in patients with acute exacerbations of COPD. Further work is needed to improve our understanding of the factors influencing inhaled drug delivery in this setting. Delivery devices that are designed specifically for mask ventilation would be helpful.

Summary and Conclusion

Bronchodilator therapy is commonly employed in ventilated patients. Inhaled β-agonist and anticholinergic bronchodilators are widely used, whereas use of theophylline in the ICU has declined significantly. Optimal techniques for employing MDIs and nebulizers in ventilator circuits have been developed as a result of better understanding of the factors influencing aerosol delivery to the lower respiratory tract of ventilated patients. Important variables that influence aerosol delivery include the type of nebulizer used, actuation of an MDI into an in-line chamber spacer, timing of actuation, ventilator mode, tidal volume, circuit humidification, and duty cycle. With proper technique, drug depo-

sition in the lower respiratory tract of ventilator-dependent patients is comparable to that in ambulatory patients. A somewhat higher dose than that used in ambulatory patients is recommended in ventilated patients, mostly to compensate for the effects of humidity in the ventilator circuit. Typically, dose-response curves to bronchodilators in ventilator-supported patients are shallow and the duration of the drug effect is variable. Although both nebulizers and MDIs are employed for administering bronchodilators in mechanically-ventilated patients, MDIs offer several advantages over nebulizers for routine bronchodilator therapy.

Acknowledgment

The author thanks Anil Gopinath, MD for his support in the preparation of this manuscript.

References

1. Gay PC, Rodarte JR, Tayyab M, et al. Evaluation of bronchodilator responsiveness in mechanically ventilated patients. Am Rev Respir Dis 1987; 136:880–85.
2. Wright PE, Carmichael LC, Bernard GR. Effect of bronchodilators on lung mechanics in the acute respiratory distress syndrome (ARDS). Chest 1994; 106:1517–23.
3. Morina P, Herrera M, Venegas J, et al. Effects of nebulized salbutamol on respiratory mechanics in adult respiratory distress syndrome. Intensive Care Med 1997; 23:58–64.
4. Wilkie RA, Bryan MH. Effect of bronchodilators on airway resistance in ventilator-dependent neonates with chronic lung disease. J Pediatr 1987; 111:278–82.
5. Motoyama EK, Fort MD, Klesh KW, et al. Early onset of airway reactivity in premature infants with bronchopulmonary dysplasia. Am Rev Respir Dis 1987; 136:50–57.
6. Denjean A, Guimaraes H, Migdal M, et al. Dose-related bronchodilator response to aerosolized salbutamol (albuterol) in ventilator-dependent premature infants. J Pediatr 1992; 120:974–79.
7. Torres A Jr, Anders M, Anderson P, et al. Efficacy of metered-dose inhaler administration of albuterol in intubated infants. Chest 1997; 112:484–90.
8. Sivakumar D, Bosque E, Goldman SL. Bronchodilator delivered by metered dose inhaler and spacer improves respiratory system compliance more than nebulizer-delivered bronchodilator in ventilated premature infants. Pediatr Pulmonol 1999; 27:208–12.
9. Jubran A, Tobin MJ. Pathophysiologic basis of acute respiratory distress in patients who fail a trial of weaning from mechanical ventilation. Am J Respir Crit Care Med 1997; 155:906–15.
10. Dhand R, Jubran A, Tobin MJ. Bronchodilator delivery by metered-dose inhaler in ventilator-supported patients. Am J Respir Crit Care Med 1995; 151:1827–33.
11. Boucher BA, Kuhl DA, Coffey BC, et al. Drug use in a trauma intensive-care unit. Am J Hosp Pharm 1990; 47:805–10.
12. Richardson JB. Nerve supply to the lungs. Am Rev Respir Dis 1979; 119:785–802.
13. Nadel JA, Cabezas GA, Austin JH. In vivo roentgenographic examination of parasympathetic innervation of small airways. Use of powdered tantalum and a fine focal spot x-ray tube. Invest Radiol 1971; 6:9–17.

14. Davis C, Kannan MS. Sympathetic innervation of human tracheal and bronchial smooth muscle. Respir Physiol 1987; 68: 53–61.
15. Barnes PJ. Neural control of human airways in health and disease. Am Rev Respir Dis 1986; 134:1289–314.
16. de Jongste JC, Jongejan RC, Kerrebijn KF. Control of airway caliber by autonomic nerves in asthma and in chronic obstructive pulmonary disease. Am Rev Respir Dis 1991; 143:1421–26.
17. Belvisi MG, Ward JK, Mitchell JA, et al. Nitric oxide as a neurotransmitter in human airways. Arch Int Pharmacodyn Ther 1995; 329:97–110.
18. van der Velden VH, Hulsmann AR. Autonomic innervation of human airways: structure, function, and pathophysiology in asthma. Neuroimmunomodulation 1999; 6:145–59.
19. Liggett SB. Update on current concepts of the molecular basis of beta2-adrenergic receptor signaling. J Allergy Clin Immunol 2002; 110:S223–27.
20. Barnes PJ. Respiratory pharmacology: General pharmacologic principles. In: Murray JF, Nadel JA, Mason RJ, et al, editors. Textbook of respiratory medicine. Philadelphia: Saunders, 2000: 231–65.
21. Brodde OE, Michel MC. Adrenergic and muscarinic receptors in the human heart. Pharmacol Rev 1999; 51:651–90.
22. Brodde OE. Beta 1- and beta 2-adrenoceptors in the human heart: properties, function, and alterations in chronic heart failure. Pharmacol Rev 1991; 43:203–42.
23. Rodefeld MD, Beau SL, Schuessler RB, et al. Beta-adrenergic and muscarinic cholinergic receptor densities in the human sinoatrial node: identification of a high beta 2-adrenergic receptor density. J Cardiovasc Electrophysiol 1996; 7:1039–49.
24. Hall JA, Petch MC, Brown MJ. Intracoronary injections of salbutamol demonstrate the presence of functional beta 2-adrenoceptors in the human heart. Circ Res 1989; 65:546–53.
25. Newton GE, Azevedo ER, Parker JD. Inotropic and sympathetic responses to the intracoronary infusion of a beta2-receptor agonist: a human in vivo study. Circulation 1999; 99:2402–7.
26. Wong CS, Pavord ID, Williams J, et al. Bronchodilator, cardiovascular, and hypokalaemic effects of fenoterol, salbutamol, and terbutaline in asthma. Lancet 1990; 336:1396–99.
27. Bennett JA, Tattersfield AE. Time course and relative dose potency of systemic effects from salmeterol and salbutamol in healthy subjects. Thorax 1997; 52:458–64.
28. Lipworth BJ, Struthers AD, McDevitt DG. Tachyphylaxis to systemic but not to airway responses during prolonged therapy with high dose inhaled salbutamol in asthmatics. Am Rev Respir Dis 1989; 140:586–92.
29. Insulander P, Juhlin-Dannfelt A, Freyschuss U, et al. Electrophysiologic effects of salbutamol, a beta2-selective agonist. J Cardiovasc Electrophysiol 2004; 15:316–22.
30. Chen A, Kusumoto FM. QT dispersion: much ado about something? Chest 2004; 125:1974–77.
31. Mettauer B, Rouleau JL, Burgess JH. Detrimental arrhythmogenic and sustained beneficial hemodynamic effects of oral salbutamol in patients with chronic congestive heart failure. Am Heart J 1985; 109:840–47.
32. Kung M, Croley SW, Phillips BA. Systemic cardiovascular and metabolic effects associated with the inhalation of an increased dose of albuterol. Influence of mouth rinsing and gargling. Chest 1987; 91:382–87.
33. Lee DK, Bates CE, Lipworth BJ. Acute systemic effects of inhaled salbutamol in asthmatic subjects expressing common homozygous beta2-adrenoceptor haplotypes at positions 16 and 27. Br J Clin Pharmacol 2004; 57:100–4.
34. Lipworth BJ, Tregaskis BF, McDevitt DG. Comparison of hypokalaemic, electrocardiographic and haemodynamic responses to inhaled isoprenaline and salbutamol in young and elderly subjects. Eur J Clin Pharmacol 1991; 40:255–60.
35. Tveskov C, Djurhuus MS, Klitgaard NA, et al. Potassium and magnesium distribution, ECG changes, and ventricular ectopic beats during beta 2-adrenergic stimulation with terbutaline in healthy subjects. Chest 1994; 106:1654–59.
36. Jenne JW. Physiologic actions of beta-adrenergic agonists. In: Leff AR, editor. Pulmonary and critical care pharmacology and therapeutics. New York: McGraw-Hill Health Professions Division, 1996: 473–82.
37. Allon M, Dunlay R, Copkney C. Nebulized albuterol for acute hyperkalemia in patients on hemodialysis. Ann Intern Med 1989; 110:426–29.
38. Mandelberg A, Krupnik Z, Houri S, et al. Salbutamol metered-dose inhaler with spacer for hyperkalemia: how fast? How safe? Chest 1999; 115:617–22.
39. Kamel KS, Wei C. Controversial issues in the treatment of hyperkalaemia. Nephrol Dial Transplant 2003; 18:2215–18.
40. Allon M, Copkney C. Albuterol and insulin for treatment of hyperkalemia in hemodialysis patients. Kidney Int 1990; 38:869–72.
41. Jenne JW, Chick TW, Strickland RD, et al. Subsensitivity of beta responses during therapy with a long-acting beta-2 preparation. J Allergy Clin Immunol 1977; 59:383–90.
42. Maconochie JG, Minton NA, Chilton JE, et al. Does tachyphylaxis occur to the non-pulmonary effects of salmeterol? Br J Clin Pharmacol 1994; 37:199–204.
43. Amoroso P, Wilson SR, Moxham J, et al. Acute effects of inhaled salbutamol on the metabolic rate of normal subjects. Thorax 1993; 48:882–85.
44. Wilson SR, Amoroso P, Moxham J, et al. Modification of the thermogenic effect of acutely inhaled salbutamol by chronic inhalation in normal subjects. Thorax 1993; 48:886–89.
45. Ahrens RC. Skeletal muscle tremor and the influence of adrenergic drugs. J Asthma 1990; 27:11–20.
46. Thirstrup S. Control of airway smooth muscle tone: II-pharmacology of relaxation. Respir Med 2000; 94:519–28.
47. Hall IP. Second messengers, ion channels and pharmacology of airway smooth muscle. Eur Respir J 2000; 15:1120–27.
48. Conti MA, Adelstein RS. The relationship between calmodulin binding and phosphorylation of smooth muscle myosin kinase by the catalytic subunit of 3′:5′ cAMP-dependent protein kinase. J Biol Chem 1981; 256:3178–81.
49. Stull JT, Hsu LC, Tansey MG, et al. Myosin light chain kinase phosphorylation in tracheal smooth muscle. J Biol Chem 1990; 265:16683–90.
50. Janssen LJ, Tazzeo T, Zuo J. Enhanced myosin phosphatase and Ca(2+)-uptake mediate adrenergic relaxation of airway smooth muscle. Am J Respir Cell Mol Biol 2004; 30:548–54.
51. Kume H, Hall IP, Washabau RJ, et al. Beta-adrenergic agonists regulate KCa channels in airway smooth muscle by cAMP-dependent and -independent mechanisms. J Clin Invest 1994; 93:371–79.
52. Janssen LJ. Ionic mechanisms and Ca(2+) regulation in airway smooth muscle contraction: do the data contradict dogma? Am J Physiol Lung Cell Mol Physiol 2002; 282:L1161–78.
53. Hall IP, Donaldson J, Hill SJ. Inhibition of histamine-stimulated inositol phospholipid hydrolysis by agents which increase cyclic AMP levels in bovine tracheal smooth muscle. Br J Pharmacol 1989; 97:603–13.
54. Chilvers ER, Lynch BJ, Challiss RA. Dissociation between beta-adrenoceptor-mediated cyclic AMP accumulation and inhibition of histamine-stimulated phosphoinositide metabolism in airways smooth muscle. Biochem Pharmacol 1997; 53: 1565–68.
55. Felbel J, Trockur B, Ecker T, et al. Regulation of cytosolic calcium

by cAMP and cGMP in freshly isolated smooth muscle cells from bovine trachea. J Biol Chem 1988; 263:16764–71.

56. Ahrens RC, Bonham AC, Maxwell GA, et al. A method for comparing the peak intensity and duration of action of aerosolized bronchodilators using bronchoprovocation with methacholine. Am Rev Respir Dis 1984; 129:903–6.

57. Cockcroft DW, Swystun VA. Functional antagonism: tolerance produced by inhaled beta 2 agonists. Thorax 1996; 51:1051–56.

58. Abisheganaden J, Boushey HA. Long-acting inhaled beta 2-agonists and the loss of "bronchoprotective" efficacy. Am J Med 1998; 104:494–97.

59. Vathenen AS, Knox AJ, Higgins BG, et al. Rebound increase in bronchial responsiveness after treatment with inhaled terbutaline. Lancet 1988; 1:554–58.

60. Wahedna I, Wong CS, Wisniewski AF, et al. Asthma control during and after cessation of regular beta 2-agonist treatment. Am Rev Respir Dis 1993; 148:707–12.

61. Cockcroft DW, O'Byrne PM, Swystun VA, et al. Regular use of inhaled albuterol and the allergen-induced late asthmatic response. J Allergy Clin Immunol 1995; 96:44–49.

62. van Schayck CP, Graafsma SJ, Visch MB, et al. Increased bronchial hyperresponsiveness after inhaling salbutamol during 1 year is not caused by subsensitization to salbutamol. J Allergy Clin Immunol 1990; 86:793–800.

63. Jokic R, Swystun VA, Davis BE, et al. Regular inhaled salbutamol: effect on airway responsiveness to methacholine and adenosine 5'-monophosphate and tolerance to bronchoprotection. Chest 2001; 119:370–75.

64. Cheung D, Timmers MC, Zwinderman AH, et al. Long-term effects of a long-acting beta 2-adrenoceptor agonist, salmeterol, on airway hyperresponsiveness in patients with mild asthma. N Engl J Med 1992; 327:1198–203.

65. van Schayck CP, Cloosterman SG, Bijl-Hofland ID, et al. Is the increase in bronchial responsiveness or FEV1 shortly after cessation of beta2-agonists reflecting a real deterioration of the disease in allergic asthmatic patients? A comparison between short-acting and long-acting beta2-agonists. Respir Med 2002; 96:155–62.

66. Rosenthal RR, Busse WW, Kemp JP, et al. Effect of long-term salmeterol therapy compared with as-needed albuterol use on airway hyperresponsiveness. Chest 1999; 116:595–602.

67. McGraw DW, Almoosa KF, Paul RJ, et al. Antithetic regulation by beta-adrenergic receptors of Gq receptor signaling via phospholipase C underlies the airway beta-agonist paradox. J Clin Invest 2003; 112:619–26.

68. O'Connor BJ, Aikman SL, Barnes PJ. Tolerance to the nonbronchodilator effects of inhaled beta 2-agonists in asthma. N Engl J Med 1992; 327:1204–8.

69. Larj MJ, Bleecker ER. Effects of beta2-agonists on airway tone and bronchial responsiveness. J Allergy Clin Immunol 2002; 110:S304–12.

70. Cockcroft DW, McParland CP, Britto SA, et al. Regular inhaled salbutamol and airway responsiveness to allergen. Lancet 1993; 342:833–37.

71. Ramage L, Lipworth BJ, Ingram CG, et al. Reduced protection against exercise induced bronchoconstriction after chronic dosing with salmeterol. Respir Med 1994; 88:363–68.

72. Lipworth B, Tan S, Devlin M, et al. Effects of treatment with formoterol on bronchoprotection against methacholine. Am J Med 1998; 104:431–38.

73. Nathan RA. Is the tolerance to the bronchoprotective effect of salmeterol clinically relevant? Ann Allergy Asthma Immunol 1998; 80:1–3; discussion 4.

74. Greening AP, Ind PW, Northfield M, et al. Added salmeterol versus higher-dose corticosteroid in asthma patients with symptoms on existing inhaled corticosteroid. Allen & Hanburys Limited UK Study Group. Lancet 1994; 344:219–24.

75. Larsson S, Svedmyr N, Thiringer G. Lack of bronchial beta adrenoceptor resistance in asthmatics during long-term treatment with terbutaline. J Allergy Clin Immunol 1977; 59:93–100.

76. Hancox RJ, Aldridge RE, Cowan JO, et al. Tolerance to beta-agonists during acute bronchoconstriction. Eur Respir J 1999; 14:283–87.

77. Wraight JM, Hancox RJ, Herbison GP, et al. Bronchodilator tolerance: the impact of increasing bronchoconstriction. Eur Respir J 2003; 21:810–15.

78. Salpeter SR, Ormiston TM, Salpeter EE. Meta-analysis: respiratory tolerance to regular beta2-agonist use in patients with asthma. Ann Intern Med 2004; 140:802–13.

79. Langley SJ, Masterson CM, Batty EP, et al. Bronchodilator response to salbutamol after chronic dosing with salmeterol or placebo. Eur Respir J 1998; 11:1081–85.

80. Nelson HS, Berkowitz RB, Tinkelman DA, et al. Lack of subsensitivity to albuterol after treatment with salmeterol in patients with asthma. Am J Respir Crit Care Med 1999; 159:1556–61.

81. van der Woude HJ, Winter TH, Aalbers R. Decreased bronchodilating effect of salbutamol in relieving methacholine induced moderate to severe bronchoconstriction during high dose treatment with long acting beta2 agonists. Thorax 2001; 56:529–35.

82. Jones SL, Cowan JO, Flannery EM, et al. Reversing acute bronchoconstriction in asthma: the effect of bronchodilator tolerance after treatment with formoterol. Eur Respir J 2001; 17:368–73.

83. Shore SA, Moore PE. Regulation of beta-adrenergic responses in airway smooth muscle. Respir Physiol Neurobiol 2003; 137:179–95.

84. Green SA, Turki J, Bejarano P, et al. Influence of beta 2-adrenergic receptor genotypes on signal transduction in human airway smooth muscle cells. Am J Respir Cell Mol Biol 1995; 13:25–33.

85. Taylor DR, Drazen JM, Herbison GP, et al. Asthma exacerbations during long term beta agonist use: influence of beta(2) adrenoceptor polymorphism. Thorax 2000; 55:762–67.

86. Israel E, Drazen JM, Liggett SB, et al. The effect of polymorphisms of the beta(2)-adrenergic receptor on the response to regular use of albuterol in asthma. Am J Respir Crit Care Med 2000; 162:75–80.

87. Israel E, Chinchilli VM, Ford JG, et al. Use of regularly scheduled albuterol treatment in asthma: genotype-stratified, randomised, placebo-controlled cross-over trial. Lancet 2004; 364:1505–12.

88. Liggett SB. Pharmacogenetics of beta-1- and beta-2-adrenergic receptors. Pharmacology 2000; 61:167–73.

89. Butchers PR, Vardey CJ, Johnson M. Salmeterol: a potent and long-acting inhibitor of inflammatory mediator release from human lung. Br J Pharmacol 1991; 104:672–76.

90. Erjefalt I, Persson CG. Long duration and high potency of antiexudative effects of formoterol in guinea-pig tracheobronchial airways. Am Rev Respir Dis 1991; 144:788–91.

91. Erjefalt I, Persson CG. Pharmacologic control of plasma exudation into tracheobronchial airways. Am Rev Respir Dis 1991; 143:1008–14.

92. Proud D, Reynolds CJ, Lichtenstein LM, et al. Intranasal salmeterol inhibits allergen-induced vascular permeability but not mast cell activation or cellular infiltration. Clin Exp Allergy 1998; 28:868–75.

93. Bennett WD. Effect of beta-adrenergic agonists on mucociliary clearance. J Allergy Clin Immunol 2002; 110:S291–97.

94. Hoffman BB. Catecholamines, sympathomimetic drugs, and adrenergic receptor antagonists. In: Hardman JG, Limbird LE, Gilman AG, editors. Goodman & Gilman's the pharmacological basis of therapeutics. New York: McGraw-Hill, 2001: 215–68.

95. Austin RP, Barton P, Bonnert RV, et al. QSAR and the rational design of long-acting dual D2-receptor/beta 2-adrenoceptor agonists. J Med Chem 2003; 46:3210–20.

96. Kobilka B. Agonist binding: a multistep process. Mol Pharmacol 2004; 65:1060–62.

97. Salmeron S, Brochard L, Mal H, et al. Nebulized versus intravenous albuterol in hypercapnic acute asthma. A multicenter, double-blind, randomized study. Am J Respir Crit Care Med 1994; 149:1466–70.

98. Travers AH, Rowe BH, Barker S, et al. The effectiveness of IV beta-agonists in treating patients with acute asthma in the emergency department: a meta-analysis. Chest 2002; 122:1200–7.

99. Shrestha M, Bidadi K, Gourlay S, et al. Continuous vs. intermittent albuterol, at high and low doses, in the treatment of severe acute asthma in adults. Chest 1996; 110:42–47.

100. Fink J, Dhand R. Bronchodilator resuscitation in the emergency department. Part 2 of 2: dosing strategies. Respir Care 2000; 45:497–512.

101. Clark DJ, Lipworth BJ. Dose-response of inhaled drugs in asthma. An update. Clin Pharmacokinet 1997; 32:58–74.

102. Lipworth BJ, Clark RA, Dhillon DP, et al. Beta-adrenoceptor responses to high doses of inhaled salbutamol in patients with bronchial asthma. Br J Clin Pharmacol 1988; 26:527–33.

103. Barnes PJ, Pride NB. Dose-response curves to inhaled beta-adrenoceptor agonists in normal and asthmatic subjects. Br J Clin Pharmacol 1983; 15:677–82.

104. Nelson HS, Spector SL, Whitsett TL, et al. The bronchodilator response to inhalation of increasing doses of aerosolized albuterol. J Allergy Clin Immunol 1983; 72:371–75.

105. Hancox RJ, Cowan JO, Flannery EM, et al. Bronchodilator tolerance and rebound bronchoconstriction during regular inhaled beta-agonist treatment. Respir Med 2000; 94:767–71.

106. Neville E, Corris PA, Vivian J, et al. Nebulised salbutamol and angina. Br Med J (Clin Res Ed) 1982; 285:796–97.

107. Fisher AA, Davis MW, McGill DA. Acute myocardial infarction associated with albuterol. Ann Pharmacother 2004; 38:2045–49.

108. Rossinen J, Partanen J, Stenius-Aarniala B, et al. Salbutamol inhalation has no effect on myocardial ischaemia, arrhythmias and heart-rate variability in patients with coronary artery disease plus asthma or chronic obstructive pulmonary disease. J Intern Med 1998; 243:361–66.

109. Kiely DG, Cargill RI, Lipworth BJ. Cardiopulmonary interactions of salbutamol and hypoxaemia in healthy young volunteers. Br J Clin Pharmacol 1995; 40:313–18.

110. Burggraaf J, Westendorp RG, in't Veen JC, et al. Cardiovascular side effects of inhaled salbutamol in hypoxic asthmatic patients. Thorax 2001; 56:567–69.

111. Gross NJ, Bankwala Z. Effects of an anticholinergic bronchodilator on arterial blood gases of hypoxemic patients with chronic obstructive pulmonary disease. Comparison with a beta-adrenergic agent. Am Rev Respir Dis 1987; 136:1091–94.

112. Khoukaz G, Gross NJ. Effects of salmeterol on arterial blood gases in patients with stable chronic obstructive pulmonary disease. Comparison with albuterol and ipratropium. Am J Respir Crit Care Med 1999; 160:1028–30.

113. Tal A, Pasterkamp H, Leahy F. Arterial oxygen desaturation following salbutamol inhalation in acute asthma. Chest 1984; 86:868–69.

114. Mouloudi E, Maliotakis C, Kondili E, et al. Duration of salbutamol-induced bronchodilation delivered by metered-dose inhaler in mechanically ventilated COPD patients. Monaldi Arch Chest Dis 2001; 56:189–94.

115. Nelson HS, Bensch G, Pleskow WW, et al. Improved bronchodilation with levalbuterol compared with racemic albuterol in patients with asthma. J Allergy Clin Immunol 1998; 102:943–52.

116. Naline E, Zhang Y, Qian Y, et al. Relaxant effects and durations of action of formoterol and salmeterol on the isolated human bronchus. Eur Respir J 1994; 7:914–20.

117. Cazzola M, Santangelo G, Piccolo A, et al. Effect of salmeterol and formoterol in patients with chronic obstructive pulmonary disease. Pulm Pharmacol 1994; 7:103–7.

118. Cazzola M, Di Perna F, Noschese P, et al. Effects of formoterol, salmeterol or oxitropium bromide on airway responses to salbutamol in COPD. Eur Respir J 1998; 11:1337–41.

119. Grove A, Lipworth BJ. Effects of prior treatment with salmeterol and formoterol on airway and systemic beta 2 responses to fenoterol. Thorax 1996; 51:585–89.

120. Fryer AD. The cholinergic control of the airways. In: Barnes PJ, editor. Autonomic control of the respiratory system. Amsterdam: Harwood Academic Publishers, 1997: 59–86.

121. Severinghaus JW, Stupfel M. Respiratory dead space increase following atropine in man, and atropine, vagal or ganglionic blockade and hypothermia in dogs. J Appl Physiol 1955; 8:81–87.

122. Olsen CR, Colebatch HJH, Mebel PE, Nadel JA, Staub NC. Motor control of pulmonary airways studied by nerve stimulation. J Appl Physiol 1965; 20:202–8.

123. Coulson FR, Fryer AD. Muscarinic acetylcholine receptors and airway diseases. Pharmacol Ther 2003; 98:59–69.

124. Roffel AF, Elzinga CR, Zaagsma J. Muscarinic M3 receptors mediate contraction of human central and peripheral airway smooth muscle. Pulm Pharmacol 1990; 3:47–51.

125. Caulfield MP. Muscarinic receptors—characterization, coupling and function. Pharmacol Ther 1993; 58:319–79.

126. Gross NJ, Skorodin MS. Role of the parasympathetic system in airway obstruction due to emphysema. N Engl J Med 1984; 311:421–25.

127. Gross NJ, Co E, Skorodin MS. Cholinergic bronchomotor tone in COPD. Estimates of its amount in comparison with that in normal subjects. Chest 1989; 96:984–87.

128. Jacoby DB, Fryer AD. Anticholinergic therapy for airway diseases. Life Sci 2001; 68:2565–72.

129. Houtmeyers E, Gosselink R, Gayan-Ramirez G, et al. Effects of drugs on mucus clearance. Eur Respir J 1999; 14:452–67.

130. Tamaoki J, Chiyotani A, Tagaya E, et al. Effect of long term treatment with oxitropium bromide on airway secretion in chronic bronchitis and diffuse panbronchiolitis. Thorax 1994; 49:545–48.

131. Francis RA, Thompson ML, Pavia D, et al. Ipratropium bromide: mucociliary clearance rate and airway resistance in normal subjects. Br J Dis Chest 1977; 71:173–78.

132. Pavia D, Bateman JR, Sheahan NF, et al. Effect of ipratropium bromide on mucociliary clearance and pulmonary function in reversible airways obstruction. Thorax 1979; 34:501–7.

133. Sato E, Koyama S, Okubo Y, et al. Acetylcholine stimulates alveolar macrophages to release inflammatory cell chemotactic activity. Am J Physiol 1998; 274:L970–79.

134. Disse B. Antimuscarinic treatment for lung diseases from research to clinical practice. Life Sci 2001; 68:2557–64.

135. Weir RE, Whitehead DE, Zaidi FH, et al. Pupil blown by a puffer. Lancet 2004; 363:1853.

136. Lust K, Livingstone I. Nebulizer-induced anisocoria. Ann Intern Med 1998; 128:327.

137. Anthonisen NR, Connett JE, Enright PL, et al. Hospitalizations and mortality in the Lung Health Study. Am J Respir Crit Care Med 2002; 166:333–39.

138. Gomm SA, Keaney NP, Hunt LP, et al. Dose-response comparison of ipratropium bromide from a metered-dose inhaler and by jet nebulisation. Thorax 1983; 38:297–301.

139. Barnes PJ, Belvisi MG, Mak JC, et al. Tiotropium bromide (Ba 679 BR), a novel long-acting muscarinic antagonist for the treatment of obstructive airways disease. Life Sci 1995; 56:853–59.

140. Casaburi R, Briggs DD Jr, Donohue JF, et al. The spirometric efficacy of once-daily dosing with tiotropium in stable COPD: a 13-week multicenter trial. The US Tiotropium Study Group. Chest 2000; 118:1294–302.

141. Newhouse MT, Chapman KR, McCallum AL, et al. Cardiovascular safety of high doses of inhaled fenoterol and albuterol in acute severe asthma. Chest 1996; 110:595–603.

142. Rodrigo C, Rodrigo G. High-dose MDI salbutamol treatment of asthma in the ED. Am J Emerg Med 1995; 13:21–26.

143. Rodrigo G, Rodrigo C. Metered dose inhaler salbutamol treatment of asthma in the ED: comparison of two doses with plasma levels. Am J Emerg Med 1996; 14:144–50.

144. Dolovich MB, Ahrens RC, Hess DR, et al. Device selection and outcomes of aerosol therapy: Evidence-based guidelines: American College of Chest Physicians/American College of Asthma, Allergy, and Immunology. Chest 2005; 127:335–71.

145. Lin RY, Smith AJ, Hergenroeder P. High serum albuterol levels and tachycardia in adult asthmatics treated with high-dose continuously aerosolized albuterol. Chest 1993; 103:221–25.

146. Lin RY, Sauter D, Newman T, et al. Continuous versus intermittent albuterol nebulization in the treatment of acute asthma. Ann Emerg Med 1993; 22:1847–53.

147. Stein J, Levitt MA. A randomized, controlled double-blind trial of usual-dose versus high-dose albuterol via continuous nebulization in patients with acute bronchospasm. Acad Emerg Med 2003; 10:31–36.

148. Emerman CL, Cydulka RK, McFadden ER. Comparison of 2.5 vs 7.5 mg of inhaled albuterol in the treatment of acute asthma. Chest 1999; 115:92–96.

149. McFadden ER Jr, Strauss L, Hejal R, et al. Comparison of two dosage regimens of albuterol in acute asthma. Am J Med 1998; 105:12–17.

150. Cydulka RK, McFadden ER, Sarver JH, et al. Comparison of single 7.5-mg dose treatment vs sequential multidose 2.5-mg treatments with nebulized albuterol in the treatment of acute asthma. Chest 2002; 122:1982–87.

151. Colacone A, Afilalo M, Wolkove N, et al. A comparison of albuterol administered by metered dose inhaler (and holding chamber) or wet nebulizer in acute asthma. Chest 1993; 104:835–41.

152. Strauss L, Hejal R, Galan G, et al. Observations on the effects of aerosolized albuterol in acute asthma. Am J Respir Crit Care Med 1997; 155:454–58.

153. Rodrigo C, Rodrigo G. Therapeutic response patterns to high and cumulative doses of salbutamol in acute severe asthma. Chest 1998; 113:593–98.

154. Moler FW, Hurwitz ME, Custer JR. Improvement in clinical asthma score and PaCO2 in children with severe asthma treated with continuously nebulized terbutaline. J Allergy Clin Immunol 1988; 81:1101–9.

155. Rudnitsky GS, Eberlein RS, Schoffstall JM, et al. Comparison of intermittent and continuously nebulized albuterol for treatment of asthma in an urban emergency department. Ann Emerg Med 1993; 22:1842–46.

156. Rodrigo GJ, Rodrigo C. Continuous vs intermittent beta-agonists in the treatment of acute adult asthma: a systematic review with meta-analysis. Chest 2002; 122:160–65.

157. Camargo CA Jr, Spooner CH, Rowe BH. Continuous versus intermittent beta-agonists in the treatment of acute asthma. Cochrane Database Syst Rev 2003:CD001115.

158. Rodrigo C, Rodrigo G. Comparison of salbutamol delivered by nebulizer or metered-dose inhaler with a pear-shaped spacer in acute asthma. Curr Ther Res Clin Exp 1993; 54:797–808.

159. Newman KB, Milne S, Hamilton C, et al. A comparison of albuterol administered by metered-dose inhaler and spacer with albuterol by nebulizer in adults presenting to an urban emergency department with acute asthma. Chest 2002; 121: 1036–41.

160. Cates CJ, Bara A, Crilly JA, et al. Holding chambers versus nebulisers for beta-agonist treatment of acute asthma. Cochrane Database Syst Rev 2004; 4:4.

161. Turner MO, Patel A, Ginsburg S, et al. Bronchodilator delivery in acute airflow obstruction. A meta-analysis. Arch Intern Med 1997; 157:1736–44.

162. Levitt MA, Gambrioli EF, Fink JB. Comparative trial of continuous nebulization versus metered-dose inhaler in the treatment of acute bronchospasm. Ann Emerg Med 1995; 26:273–77.

163. Brown CD, McCrory D, White J. Inhaled short-acting beta2-agonists versus ipratropium for acute exacerbations of chronic obstructive pulmonary disease. Cochrane Database Syst Rev 2005; 1:1.

164. BTS guidelines for the management of chronic obstructive pulmonary disease. The COPD Guidelines Group of the Standards of Care Committee of the BTS. Thorax 1997; 52(Suppl 5):S1–28.

165. In chronic obstructive pulmonary disease, a combination of ipratropium and albuterol is more effective than either agent alone. An 85-day multicenter trial. COMBIVENT Inhalation Aerosol Study Group. Chest 1994; 105:1411–19.

166. O'Driscoll BR, Taylor RJ, Horsley MG, et al. Nebulised salbutamol with and without ipratropium bromide in acute airflow obstruction. Lancet 1989; 1:1418–20.

167. Routine nebulized ipratropium and albuterol together are better than either alone in COPD. The COMBIVENT Inhalation Solution Study Group. Chest 1997; 112:1514–21.

168. Shrestha M, O'Brien T, Haddox R, et al. Decreased duration of emergency department treatment of chronic obstructive pulmonary disease exacerbations with the addition of ipratropium bromide to beta-agonist therapy. Ann Emerg Med 1991; 20:1206–9.

169. Fernandez A, Munoz J, de la Calle B, et al. Comparison of one versus two bronchodilators in ventilated COPD patients. Intensive Care Med 1994; 20:199–202.

170. Cydulka RK, Emerman CL. Effects of combined treatment with glycopyrrolate and albuterol in acute exacerbation of chronic obstructive pulmonary disease. Ann Emerg Med 1995; 25:470–73.

171. Moayyedi P, Congleton J, Page RL, et al. Comparison of nebulised salbutamol and ipratropium bromide with salbutamol alone in the treatment of chronic obstructive pulmonary disease. Thorax 1995; 50:834–37.

172. Patrick DM, Dales RE, Stark RM, et al. Severe exacerbations of COPD and asthma. Incremental benefit of adding ipratropium to usual therapy. Chest 1990; 98:295–97.

173. Karpel JP, Schacter EN, Fanta C, et al. A comparison of ipratropium and albuterol vs albuterol alone for the treatment of acute asthma. Chest 1996; 110:611–16.

174. McFadden ER Jr, elSanadi N, Strauss L, et al. The influence of parasympatholytics on the resolution of acute attacks of asthma. Am J Med 1997; 102:7–13.

175. Lin RY, Pesola GR, Bakalchuk L, et al. Superiority of ipratropium plus albuterol over albuterol alone in the emergency department management of adult asthma: a randomized clinical trial. Ann Emerg Med 1998; 31:208–13.

176. Lanes SF, Garrett JE, Wentworth CE 3rd, et al. The effect of adding ipratropium bromide to salbutamol in the treatment of acute asthma: a pooled analysis of three trials. Chest 1998; 114:365–72.

177. Weber EJ, Levitt MA, Covington JK, et al. Effect of continuously nebulized ipratropium bromide plus albuterol on emergency department length of stay and hospital admission rates in patients with acute bronchospasm. A randomized, controlled trial. Chest 1999; 115:937–44.

178. Stoodley RG, Aaron SD, Dales RE. The role of ipratropium bromide in the emergency management of acute asthma exacerbation: a metaanalysis of randomized clinical trials. Ann Emerg Med 1999; 34:8–18.

179. Rodrigo GJ, Rodrigo C. The role of anticholinergics in acute asthma treatment: an evidence-based evaluation. Chest 2002; 121:1977–87.

180. Barnes PJ. Theophylline: new perspectives for an old drug. Am J Respir Crit Care Med 2003; 167:813–18.

181. Rabe KF, Magnussen H, Dent G. Theophylline and selective PDE inhibitors as bronchodilators and smooth muscle relaxants. Eur Respir J 1995; 8:637–42.

182. Polson JB, Krzanowski JJ, Goldman AL, et al. Inhibition of human pulmonary phosphodiesterase activity by therapeutic levels of theophylline. Clin Exp Pharmacol Physiol 1978; 5: 535–39.

183. Ito K, Lim S, Caramori G, et al. A molecular mechanism of action of theophylline: Induction of histone deacetylase activity to decrease inflammatory gene expression. Proc Natl Acad Sci USA 2002; 99:8921–26.

184. Ito K, Barnes PJ, Adcock IM. Glucocorticoid receptor recruitment of histone deacetylase 2 inhibits interleukin-1beta-induced histone H4 acetylation on lysines 8 and 12. Mol Cell Biol 2000; 20:6891–903.

185. Ito K, Caramori G, Lim S, et al. Expression and activity of histone deacetylases in human asthmatic airways. Am J Respir Crit Care Med 2002; 166:392–96.

186. Pauwels RA, Joos GF. Characterization of the adenosine receptors in the airways. Arch Int Pharmacodyn Ther 1995; 329:151–60.

187. Ward AJ, McKenniff M, Evans JM, et al. Theophylline—an immunomodulatory role in asthma? Am Rev Respir Dis 1993; 147:518–23.

188. Mascali JJ, Cvietusa P, Negri J, et al. Anti-inflammatory effects of theophylline: modulation of cytokine production. Ann Allergy Asthma Immunol 1996; 77:34–38.

189. Jaffar ZH, Sullivan P, Page C, et al. Low-dose theophylline modulates T-lymphocyte activation in allergen-challenged asthmatics. Eur Respir J 1996; 9:456–62.

190. Kidney J, Dominguez M, Taylor PM, et al. Immunomodulation by theophylline in asthma. Demonstration by withdrawal of therapy. Am J Respir Crit Care Med 1995; 151:1907–14.

191. Lim S, Tomita K, Caramori G, et al. Low-dose theophylline reduces eosinophilic inflammation but not exhaled nitric oxide in mild asthma. Am J Respir Crit Care Med 2001; 164:273–76.

192. Supinski GS. Effects of methylxanthines on respiratory skeletal muscle and neural drive. In: Jenne JW, Murphy S, editors. Drug therapy for asthma: research and clinical practice. New York: Marcel Dekker, 1987.

193. Mahler DA, Matthay RA, Snyder PE, et al. Sustained-release theophylline reduces dyspnea in nonreversible obstructive airway disease. Am Rev Respir Dis 1985; 131:22–25.

194. Aubier M, De Troyer A, Sampson M, et al. Aminophylline improves diaphragmatic contractility. N Engl J Med 1981; 305:249–52.

195. Murciano D, Aubier M, Lecocguic Y, et al. Effects of theophylline on diaphragmatic strength and fatigue in patients with chronic obstructive pulmonary disease. N Engl J Med 1984; 311:349–53.

196. Landsberg KF, Vaughan LM, Heffner JE. The effect of theophylline on respiratory muscle contractility and fatigue. Pharmacotherapy 1990; 10:271–79.

197. Vestal RE, Eiriksson CE Jr, Musser B, et al. Effect of intravenous aminophylline on plasma levels of catecholamines and related cardiovascular and metabolic responses in man. Circulation 1983; 67:162–71.

198. Parker JO, Ashekian PB, Di Giorgi S, et al. Hemodynamic effects of aminophylline in chronic obstructive pulmonary disease. Circulation 1967; 35:365–72.

199. Matthay RA, Berger HJ, Davies R, et al. Improvement in cardiac performance by oral long-acting theophylline in chronic obstructive pulmonary disease. Am Heart J 1982; 104: 1022–26.

200. Expert Panel Report 2: Guidelines for the Diagnosis and Management of Asthma, NIH Publication 97-4051. Bethesda, MD: National Institutes of Health, 1997.

201. Self TH, Heilker GM, Alloway RR, et al. Reassessing the therapeutic range for theophylline on laboratory report forms: the importance of 5-15 micrograms/ml. Pharmacotherapy 1993; 13:590–94.

202. Self TH, Redmond AM, Nguyen WT. Reassessment of theophylline use for severe asthma exacerbation: is it justified in critically ill hospitalized patients? J Asthma 2002; 39:677–86.

203. Zhang ZY, Kaminsky LS. Characterization of human cytochromes P450 involved in theophylline 8-hydroxylation. Biochem Pharmacol 1995; 50:205–11.

204. Tang-Liu DD, Williams RL, Riegelman S. Nonlinear theophylline elimination. Clin Pharmacol Ther 1982; 31:358–69.

205. Pea F, Furlanut M. Pharmacokinetic aspects of treating infections in the intensive care unit: focus on drug interactions. Clin Pharmacokinet 2001; 40:833–68.

206. Toft P, Heslet L, Hansen M, et al. Theophylline and ethylenediamine pharmacokinetics following administration of aminophylline to septic patients with multiorgan failure. Intensive Care Med 1991; 17:465–68.

207. Gross NJ, Jenne JW, Hess D. Bronchodilator therapy. In: Tobin MJ, editor. Principles and practice of mechanical ventilation. New York: McGraw Hill, 1994: 1077–123.

208. Littenberg B. Aminophylline treatment in severe, acute asthma. A meta-analysis. JAMA 1988; 259:1678–84.

209. Siegel D, Sheppard D, Gelb A, et al. Aminophylline increases the toxicity but not the efficacy of an inhaled beta-adrenergic agonist in the treatment of acute exacerbations of asthma. Am Rev Respir Dis 1985; 132:283–86.

210. Fanta CH, Rossing TH, McFadden ER Jr. Treatment of acute asthma. Is combination therapy with sympathomimetics and methylxanthines indicated? Am J Med 1986; 80:5–10.

211. Self TH, Abou-Shala N, Burns R, et al. Inhaled albuterol and oral prednisone therapy in hospitalized adult asthmatics. Does aminophylline add any benefit? Chest 1990; 98:1317–21.

212. Parameswaran K, Belda J, Rowe BH. Addition of intravenous aminophylline to beta2-agonists in adults with acute asthma. Cochrane Database Syst Rev 2000:CD002742.

213. Werner HA. Status asthmaticus in children: a review. Chest 2001; 119:1913–29.

214. Wrenn K, Slovis CM, Murphy F, et al. Aminophylline therapy for acute bronchospastic disease in the emergency room. Ann Intern Med 1991; 115:241–47.

215. Fernandez A, Lazaro A, Garcia A, et al. Bronchodilators in patients with chronic obstructive pulmonary disease on mechanical ventilation. Utilization of metered-dose inhalers. Am Rev Respir Dis 1990; 141:164–68.

216. Poggi R, Brandolese R, Bernasconi M, et al. Doxofylline and respiratory mechanics. Short-term effects in mechanically ventilated patients with airflow obstruction and respiratory failure. Chest 1989; 96:772–78.

217. du Preez MJ, Botha JH, McFadyen ML, et al. The effect of theophylline on apnoea and hypoxaemic episodes in the premature neonate during the 1st 3 days after birth. Ann Trop Paediatr 1998; 18:217–24.

218. Shannon M. Life-threatening events after theophylline overdose: a 10-year prospective analysis. Arch Intern Med 1999; 159:989–94.

219. Shannon M, Lovejoy FH Jr. The influence of age vs peak serum concentration on life-threatening events after chronic theophylline intoxication. Arch Intern Med 1990; 150:2045–48.

220. Leopold D, Webb D, Buss DC, et al. The ex vivo plasma protein binding of theophylline in renal disease. Br J Clin Pharmacol 1985; 19:823–25.

221. Torphy TJ. Phosphodiesterase isozymes: molecular targets for novel antiasthma agents. Am J Respir Crit Care Med 1998; 157:351–70.

222. Souness JE, Aldous D, Sargent C. Immunosuppressive and antiinflammatory effects of cyclic AMP phosphodiesterase (PDE) type 4 inhibitors. Immunopharmacology 2000; 47:127–62.

223. Zussman BD, Benincosa LJ, Webber DM, et al. An overview of the pharmacokinetics of cilomilast (Ariflo), a new, orally active phosphodiesterase 4 inhibitor, in healthy young and elderly volunteers. J Clin Pharmacol 2001; 41:950–58.

224. Zussman BD, Kelly J, Murdoch RD, et al. Cilomilast: pharmacokinetic and pharmacodynamic interactions with digoxin. Clin Ther 2001; 23:921–31.

225. Lipworth BJ. Phosphodiesterase-4 inhibitors for asthma and chronic obstructive pulmonary disease. Lancet 2005; 365:167–75.

226. Kelly J, Murdoch RD, Clark DJ, et al. Warfarin pharmacodynamics unaffected by cilomilast. Ann Pharmacother 2001; 35:1535–39.

227. Compton CH, Gubb J, Nieman R, et al. Cilomilast, a selective phosphodiesterase-4 inhibitor for treatment of patients with chronic obstructive pulmonary disease: a randomised, dose-ranging study. Lancet 2001; 358:265–70.

228. Timmer W, Leclerc V, Birraux G, et al. The new phosphodiesterase 4 inhibitor roflumilast is efficacious in exercise-induced asthma and leads to suppression of LPS-stimulated TNF-alpha ex vivo. J Clin Pharmacol 2002; 42:297–303.

229. Gamble E, Grootendorst DC, Brightling CE, et al. Antiinflammatory effects of the phosphodiesterase-4 inhibitor cilomilast (Ariflo) in chronic obstructive pulmonary disease. Am J Respir Crit Care Med 2003; 168:976–82.

230. Spina D. Phosphodiesterase-4 inhibitors in the treatment of inflammatory lung disease. Drugs 2003; 63:2575–94.

231. Rau JL. Design principles of liquid nebulization devices currently in use. Respir Care 2002; 47:1257–75; discussion 1275–78.

232. Dalby RN, Tiano SL, Hickey AJ. Medical devices for the delivery of therapeutic aerosols to the lungs. In: Hickey AJ, editor. Inhalation aerosols: Physical and biological basis for therapy. New York: Marcel Dekker, 1996: 441–73.

233. Nerbrink O, Dahlback M, Hansson HC. Why do medical nebulizers differ in their output and particle size characteristics? J Aerosol Med 1994; 7:259–76.

234. Niven RW. Atomization and nebulizers. In: Hickey AJ, editor. Inhalation aerosols: physical and biological basis for therapy. New York: Marcel Dekker, 1996: 273–312.

235. Phipps PR, Gonda I. Droplets produced by medical nebulizers. Some factors affecting their size and solute concentration. Chest 1990; 97:1327–32.

236. Stapleton KW, Finlay WH. Determining solute concentration within aerosol droplets output by jet nebulizers. J Aerosol Sci 1995;26:137–45.

237. Clay MM, Pavia D, Newman SP, et al. Assessment of jet nebulisers for lung aerosol therapy. Lancet 1983; 2:592–94.

238. Alvine GF, Rodgers P, Fitzsimmons KM, et al. Disposable jet nebulizers. How reliable are they? Chest 1992; 101:316–19.

239. Loffert DT, Ikle D, Nelson HS. A comparison of commercial jet nebulizers. Chest 1994; 106:1788–92.

240. Hess D, Fisher D, Williams P, et al. Medication nebulizer performance. Effects of diluent volume, nebulizer flow, and nebulizer brand. Chest 1996; 110:498–505.

241. Boucher RM, Kreuter J. The fundamentals of the ultrasonic atomization of medicated solutions. Ann Allergy 1968; 26:591–600.

242. Mercer TT, Goddard RF, Flores RL. Output characteristics of three ultrasonic nebulizers. Ann Allergy 1968; 26:18–27.

243. Sterk PJ, Plomp A, van de Vate JF, et al. Physical properties of aerosols produced by several jet- and ultrasonic nebulizers. Bull Eur Physiopathol Respir 1984; 20:65–72.

244. Thomas SHL, O'Doherty MJ, Page CJ, et al. Delivery of ultrasonic nebulized aerosols to a lung model during mechanical ventilation. Am Rev Respir Dis 1993; 148:872–77.

245. Kemming GI, Kreyling W, Habler O, et al. Aerosol production and aerosol droplet size distribution during mechanical ventilation (IPPV) with a new ultrasonic nebulizer. Eur J Med Res 1996; 1:321–27.

246. Harvey CJ, O'Doherty MJ, Page CJ, et al. Comparison of jet and ultrasonic nebulizer pulmonary aerosol deposition during mechanical ventilation. Eur Respir J 1997; 10:905–9.

247. Williams L, Fletcher GC, Daniel M, et al. A simple in vitro method for the evaluation of an ultrasonic nebulizer for drug delivery to intubated, ventilated patients and the effect of nebulizer and ventilator settings on the uptake of fluid from the nebulizer chamber. Eur J Anaesthesiol 1999; 16:479–84.

248. Dhand R. Nebulizers that use a vibrating mesh or plate with multiple apertures to generate aerosol. Respir Care 2002; 47:1406–16; discussion 1416–8.

249. Dennis JH, Nerbrink O. New nebulizer technology. In: Bisgaard H, O'Callaghan C, Smaldone GC, editors. Drug delivery to the lung. New York: Marcel Dekker, 2002: 303–36.

250. Fink JB, Barraza P, Bisgaard J. Aerosol delivery during mechanical ventilation with high frequency oscillation: an in vitro evaluation (abstract). Chest 2001; 120:S277.

251. Tronde A, Baran G, Eirefelt S, et al. Miniaturized nebulization catheters: a new approach for delivery of defined aerosol doses to the rat lung. J Aerosol Med 2002; 15:283–96.

252. Dhand R. New frontiers in aerosol delivery during mechanical ventilation. Respir Care 2004; 49:666–77.

253. Leong BK, Coombs JK, Sabaitis CP, et al. Quantitative morphometric analysis of pulmonary deposition of aerosol particles inhaled via intratracheal nebulization, intratracheal instillation or nose-only inhalation in rats. J Appl Toxicol 1998; 18:149–60.

254. Koping-Hoggard M, Issa MM, Kohler T, et al. A miniaturized nebulization catheter for improved gene delivery to the mouse lung. J Gene Med 2005; 7:1215–22.

255. Moren F. Aerosol dosage forms and formulations. In: Moren F, Dolovich MB, Newhouse MT, et al, editors. Aerosols in medicine. Amsterdam: Elsevier, 1993: 321–50.

256. O'Callaghan C, Wright P. The metered-dose inhaler. In: Bisgaard H, O'Callaghan C, Smaldone GC, editors. Drug delivery to the lung. New York.: Marcel Dekker, 2002: 337–70.

257. Ross DL, Gabrio BJ. Advances in metered dose inhaler technology with the development of a chlorofluorocarbon-free drug delivery system. J Aerosol Med 1999; 12:151–60.

258. Polli GP, Grim WM, Bacher FA, et al. Influence of formulation on aerosol particle size. J Pharm Sci 1969; 58:484–86.

259. Kim CS, Trujillo D, Sackner MA. Size aspects of metered-dose inhaler aerosols. Am Rev Respir Dis 1985; 132:137–42.

260. Dolovich M. Measurement of particle size characteristics of metered dose inhaler (MDI) aerosols. J Aerosol Med 1991; 4:251–63.

261. Leach CL, Davidson PJ, Boudreau RJ. Improved airway targeting with the CFC-free HFA-beclomethasone metered-dose inhaler compared with CFC-beclomethasone. Eur Respir J 1998; 12:1346–53.

262. Gross G, Thompson PJ, Chervinsky P, et al. Hydrofluoroalkane-134a beclomethasone dipropionate, 400 microg, is as effective as chlorofluorocarbon beclomethasone dipropionate, 800 microg, for the treatment of moderate asthma. Chest 1999; 115:343–51.

263. Fink JB, Dhand R, Duarte AG, et al. Aerosol delivery from a metered-dose inhaler during mechanical ventilation. An in vitro model. Am J Respir Crit Care Med 1996; 154:382–87.

264. Everard ML, Devadason SG, Le Souef PN. In vitro assessment of drug delivery through an endotracheal tube using a dry powder inhaler delivery system. Thorax 1996; 51:75–77.

265. Jashnani RN, Byron PR, Dalby RN. Testing of dry powder aerosol formulations in different environmental conditions. Int J Pharm 1995; 113:123–30.

266. Lindsay DA, Russell NL, Thompson JE, et al. A multicentre comparison of the efficacy of terbutaline Turbuhaler and salbutamol pressurized metered dose inhaler in hot, humid regions. Eur Respir J 1994; 7:342–45.

267. MacIntyre NR, Silver RM, Miller CW, et al. Aerosol delivery in intubated, mechanically ventilated patients. Crit Care Med 1985; 13:81–84.

268. Fuller HD, Dolovich MB, Posmituck G, et al. Pressurized aerosol versus jet aerosol delivery to mechanically ventilated patients. Comparison of dose to the lungs. Am Rev Respir Dis 1990; 141:440–44.

269. Dhand R. Special problems in aerosol delivery: artificial airways. Respir Care 2000; 45:636–45.

270. Dhand R, Tobin MJ. Inhaled bronchodilator therapy in mechanically ventilated patients. Am J Respir Crit Care Med 1997; 156:3–10.

271. Dhand R. Basic techniques for aerosol delivery during mechanical ventilation. Respir Care 2004; 49:611–22.

272. O'Riordan TG, Palmer LB, Smaldone GC. Aerosol deposition in mechanically ventilated patients. Optimizing nebulizer delivery. Am J Respir Crit Care Med 1994; 149:214–19.

273. Miller DD, Amin MM, Palmer LB, et al. Aerosol delivery and modern mechanical ventilation: in vitro/in vivo evaluation. Am J Respir Crit Care Med 2003; 168:1205–9.

274. Fink JB, Dhand R, Grychowski J, et al. Reconciling in vitro and in vivo measurements of aerosol delivery from a metered-dose inhaler during mechanical ventilation and defining efficiency-enhancing factors. Am J Respir Crit Care Med 1999; 159:63–68.

275. Moren F, Andersson J. Fraction of dose exhaled after administration of pressurized inhalation aerosols. Int J Pharm 1980; 6:295–300.

276. Crogan SJ, Bishop MJ. Delivery efficiency of metered dose aerosols given via endotracheal tubes. Anesthesiology 1989; 70:1008–10.

277. Bishop MJ, Larson RP, Buschman DL. Metered dose inhaler aerosol characteristics are affected by the endotracheal tube actuator/adapter used. Anesthesiology 1990; 73:1263–65.

278. Ebert J, Adams AB, Green-Eide B. An evaluation of MDI (metered dose inhaler) spacers and adapters: their effect on the respirable volume of medication. Respir Care 1992; 37:862–68.

279. Fuller HD, Dolovich MB, Chambers C, et al. Aerosol delivery during mechanical ventilation: a predictive in vitro lung model. J Aerosol Med 1992; 5:251–59.

280. O'Riordan TG, Greco MJ, Perry RJ, et al. Nebulizer function during mechanical ventilation. Am Rev Respir Dis 1992; 145:1117–22.

281. Niven RW, Kacmarek RM, Brain JD, et al. Small bore nozzle extensions to improve the delivery efficiency of drugs from metered dose inhalers: laboratory evaluation. Am Rev Respir Dis 1993; 147:1590–94.

282. Taylor RH, Lerman J, Chambers C, et al. Dosing efficiency and particle-size characteristics of pressurized metered-dose inhaler aerosols in narrow catheters. Chest 1993; 103:920–24.

283. Diot P, Morra L, Smaldone GC. Albuterol delivery in a model of mechanical ventilation. Comparison of metered-dose inhaler and nebulizer efficiency. Am J Respir Crit Care Med 1995; 152:1391–94.

284. Rau JL, Dunlevy CL, Hill RL. A comparison of inline MDI actuators for delivery of a beta agonist and a corticosteroid with a mechanically-ventilated lung model. Respir Care 1998; 43:705–12.

285. Mitchell JP, Nagel MW, Wiersema KJ, et al. The delivery of chlorofluorocarbon-propelled versus hydrofluoroalkane-propelled beclomethasone dipropionate aerosol to the mechanically ventilated patient: a laboratory study. Respir Care 2003; 48:1025–32.

286. Rau JL, Harwood RJ, Groff JL. Evaluation of a reservoir device for metered-dose bronchodilator delivery to intubated adults. An in vitro study. Chest 1992; 102:924–30.

287. O'Doherty MJ, Thomas SH, Page CJ, et al. Delivery of a nebulized aerosol to a lung model during mechanical ventilation. Effect of ventilator settings and nebulizer type, position, and volume of fill. Am Rev Respir Dis 1992; 146:383–88.

288. Harvey CJ, O'Doherty MJ, Page CJ, et al. Effect of a spacer on pulmonary aerosol deposition from a jet nebuliser during mechanical ventilation. Thorax 1995; 50:50–53.

289. Manthous CA, Hall JB, Schmidt GA, et al. Metered-dose inhaler versus nebulized albuterol in mechanically ventilated patients. Am Rev Respir Dis 1993; 148:1567–70.

290. Fuller HD, Dolovich MB, Turpie FH, et al. Efficiency of bronchodilator aerosol delivery to the lungs from the metered dose inhaler in mechanically ventilated patients. A study comparing four different actuator devices. Chest 1994; 105:214–18.

291. Dhand R, Tobin MJ. Bronchodilator delivery with metered-dose inhalers in mechanically-ventilated patients. Eur Respir J 1996; 9:585–95.

292. Dhand R, Duarte AG, Jubran A, et al. Dose-response to bronchodilator delivered by metered-dose inhaler in ventilator-supported patients. Am J Respir Crit Care Med 1996; 154:388–93.

293. Hughes JM, Saez J. Effects of nebulizer mode and position in a mechanical ventilator circuit on dose efficiency. Respir Care 1987; 32:1131–35.

294. Dhand R. Maximizing aerosol delivery during mechanical ventilation: go with the flow and go slow. Intensive Care Med 2003; 29:1041–42.

295. Dhand R. Aerosol therapy during mechanical ventilation: getting ready for prime time. Am J Respir Crit Care Med 2003; 168:1148–49.

296. McPeck M, O'Riordan TG, Smaldone GC. Predicting aerosol delivery to intubated patients: influence of choice of mechanical ventilator on nebulizer efficiency. Respir Care 1993; 38:887.

297. Dolovich MA. Influence of inspiratory flow rate, particle size, and airway caliber on aerosolized drug delivery to the lung. Respir Care 2000; 45:597–608.

298. Hess DR, Dillman C, Kacmarek RM. In vitro evaluation of aerosol bronchodilator delivery during mechanical ventilation: pressure-control vs. volume control ventilation. Intensive Care Med 2003; 29:1145–50.

299. Ferron GA, Karg E, Peter J. Estimation of deposition of polydisperse hygroscopic aerosols in the human respiratory tract. J Aerosol Sci 1993; 24:655–70.

300. Lange CF, Finlay WH. Overcoming the adverse effect of humidity in aerosol delivery via pressurized metered-dose inhalers during mechanical ventilation. Am J Respir Crit Care Med 2000; 161:1614–18.

301. Habib DM, Garner SS, Brandeburg S. Effect of helium-oxygen on delivery of albuterol in a pediatric, volume-cycled, ventilated lung model. Pharmacotherapy 1999; 19:143–49.

302. Goode ML, Fink JB, Dhand R, et al. Improvement in aerosol delivery with helium-oxygen mixtures during mechanical ventilation. Am J Respir Crit Care Med 2001; 163:109–14.

303. Hess DR, Acosta FL, Ritz RH, et al. The effect of heliox on nebulizer function using a beta-agonist bronchodilator. Chest 1999; 115:184–89.

304. Ahrens RC, Ries RA, Popendorf W, et al. The delivery of therapeutic aerosols through endotracheal tubes. Pediatr Pulmonol 1986; 2:19–26.

305. Spahr-Schopfer IA, Lerman J, Cutz E, et al. Proximate delivery of a large experimental dose from salbutamol MDI induces epithelial airway lesions in intubated rabbits. Am J Respir Crit Care Med 1994; 150:790–94.

306. Newman SP, Pavia D, Moren F, et al. Deposition of pressurised aerosols in the human respiratory tract. Thorax 1981; 36:52–55.

307. Dolovich M, Ruffin RE, Roberts R, et al. Optimal delivery of aerosols from metered dose inhalers. Chest 1981; 80:911–15.

308. Duarte AG, Dhand R, Reid R, et al. Serum albuterol levels in mechanically ventilated patients and healthy subjects after metered-dose inhaler administration. Am J Respir Crit Care Med 1996; 154:1658–63.

309. Marik P, Hogan J, Krikorian J. A comparison of bronchodilator therapy delivered by nebulization and metered-dose inhaler in mechanically ventilated patients. Chest 1999; 115:1653–57.

310. Gold MI. Treatment of bronchospasm during anesthesia. Anesth Analg 1975; 54:783–86.

311. Bernasconi M, Brandolese R, Poggi R, et al. Dose-response effects and time course of effects of inhaled fenoterol on respiratory mechanics and arterial oxygen tension in mechanically ventilated patients with chronic airflow obstruction. Intensive Care Med 1990; 16:108–14.

312. Gay PC, Patel HG, Nelson SB, et al. Metered dose inhalers for bronchodilator delivery in intubated, mechanically ventilated patients. Chest 1991; 99:66–71.

313. Mancebo J, Amaro P, Lorino H, et al. Effects of albuterol inhalation on the work of breathing during weaning from mechanical ventilation. Am Rev Respir Dis 1991; 144:95–100.

314. Manthous CA, Chatila W, Schmidt GA, et al. Treatment of bronchospasm by metered-dose inhaler albuterol in mechanically ventilated patients. Chest 1995; 107:210–13.

315. Waugh JB, Jones DF, Aranson R, et al. Bronchodilator response with use of OptiVent versus Aerosol Cloud Enhancer metered-dose inhaler spacers in patients receiving ventilatory assistance. Heart Lung 1998; 27:418–23.

316. Mouloudi E, Katsanoulas K, Anastasaki M, et al. Bronchodilator delivery by metered-dose inhaler in mechanically ventilated COPD patients: influence of end-inspiratory pause. Eur Respir J 1998; 12:165–69.

317. Mouloudi E, Katsanoulas K, Anastasaki M, et al. Bronchodilator delivery by metered-dose inhaler in mechanically ventilated COPD patients: influence of tidal volume. Intensive Care Med 1999; 25:1215–21.

318. Guerin C, Chevre A, Dessirier P, et al. Inhaled fenoterol-ipratropium bromide in mechanically ventilated patients with chronic obstructive pulmonary disease. Am J Respir Crit Care Med 1999; 159:1036–42.

319. Mouloudi E, Prinianakis G, Kondili E, et al. Bronchodilator delivery by metered-dose inhaler in mechanically ventilated COPD patients: influence of flow pattern. Eur Respir J 2000; 16:263–68.

320. Duarte AG, Momii K, Bidani A. Bronchodilator therapy with metered-dose inhaler and spacer versus nebulizer in mechanically ventilated patients: comparison of magnitude and duration of response. Respir Care 2000; 45:817–23.

321. Wegener T, Wretman S, Sandhagen B, et al. Effect of ipratropium bromide aerosol on respiratory function in patients

under ventilator treatment. Acta Anaesthesiol Scand 1987; 31: 652–54.

322. Yang SC, Yang SP, Lee TS. Nebulized ipratropium bromide in ventilator-assisted patients with chronic bronchitis. Chest 1994; 105:1511–15.

323. Fresoli RP, Smith RM Jr, Young JA, et al. Use of aerosol isoproterenol in an anesthesia circuit. Anesth Analg 1968; 47:127–32.

324. Sprague DH. Treatment of intraoperative bronchospasm with nebulized isoetharine. Anesthesiology 1977; 46:222–24.

325. Corbridge T, Hall JB. Pharmacotherapy of status asthmaticus. In: Leff AR, editor. Pulmonary and critical care pharmacology and therapeutics. New York: McGraw Hill, 1996: 773–81.

326. Bates JH, Rossi A, Milic-Emili J. Analysis of the behavior of the respiratory system with constant inspiratory flow. J Appl Physiol 1985; 58:1840–48.

327. Bates JHT, Milic-Emili J. The flow interruption technique for measuring respiratory resistance. J Crit Care 1991; 6:227–38.

328. Salmon B, Wilson NM, Silverman M. How much aerosol reaches the lungs of wheezy infants and toddlers? Arch Dis Child 1990; 65:401–3.

329. Chua HL, Collis GG, Newbury AM, et al. The influence of age on aerosol deposition in children with cystic fibrosis. Eur Respir J 1994; 7:2185–91.

330. Mallol J, Rattray S, Walker G, et al. Aerosol deposition in infants with cystic fibrosis. Pediatr Pulmonol 1996; 21:276–81.

331. Amirav I, Balanov I, Gorenberg M, et al. Beta-agonist aerosol distribution in respiratory syncytial virus bronchiolitis in infants. J Nucl Med 2002; 43:487–91.

332. Amirav I, Balanov I, Gorenberg M, et al. Nebuliser hood compared to mask in wheezy infants: aerosol therapy without tears! Arch Dis Child 2003; 88:719–23.

333. Garner SS, Wiest DB, Bradley JW. Albuterol delivery by metered-dose inhaler with a pediatric mechanical ventilatory circuit model. Pharmacotherapy 1994; 14:210–14.

334. Cameron D, Clay M, Silverman M. Evaluation of nebulizers for use in neonatal ventilator circuits. Crit Care Med 1990; 18:866–70.

335. Everard ML, Stammers J, Hardy JG, et al. New aerosol delivery system for neonatal ventilator circuits. Arch Dis Child 1992; 67:826–30.

336. Arnon S, Grigg J, Nikander K, et al. Delivery of micronized budesonide suspension by metered dose inhaler and jet nebulizer into a neonatal ventilator circuit. Pediatr Pulmonol 1992; 13:172–75.

337. Coleman DM, Kelly HW, McWilliams BC. Determinants of aerosolized albuterol delivery to mechanically ventilated infants. Chest 1996; 109:1607–13.

338. Avent ML, Gal P, Ransom JL, et al. Comparing the delivery of albuterol metered-dose inhaler via an adapter and spacer device in an in vitro infant ventilator lung model. Ann Pharmacother 1999; 33:141–43.

339. Lugo RA, Kenney JK, Keenan J, et al. Albuterol delivery in a neonatal ventilated lung model: Nebulization versus chlorofluorocarbon- and hydrofluoroalkane-pressurized metered dose inhalers. Pediatr Pulmonol 2001; 31:247–54.

340. Cameron D, Arnot R, Clay M, et al. Aerosol delivery in neonatal ventilator circuits: a rabbit lung model. Pediatr Pulmonol 1991; 10:208–13.

341. Grigg J, Arnon S, Jones T, et al. Delivery of therapeutic aerosols to intubated babies. Arch Dis Child 1992; 67:25–30.

342. Pelkonen AS, Nikander K, Turpeinen M. Jet nebulization of budesonide suspension into a neonatal ventilator circuit: synchronized versus continuous nebulizer flow. Pediatr Pulmonol 1997; 24:282–86.

343. Avent ML, Gal P, Ransom JL, et al. Evaluating the delivery of nebulized and metered-dose inhalers in an in vitro

infant ventilator lung model. Ann Pharmacother 1999; 33: 144–48.

344. Wildhaber JH, Dore ND, Wilson JM, et al. Inhalation therapy in asthma: nebulizer or pressurized metered-dose inhaler with holding chamber? In vivo comparison of lung deposition in children. J Pediatr 1999; 135:28–33.

345. Fok TF, Monkman S, Dolovich M, et al. Efficiency of aerosol medication delivery from a metered dose inhaler versus jet nebulizer in infants with bronchopulmonary dysplasia. Pediatr Pulmonol 1996; 21:301–9.

346. Rotschild A, Solimano A, Puterman M, et al. Increased compliance in response to salbutamol in premature infants with developing bronchopulmonary dysplasia. J Pediatr 1989; 115:984–91.

347. Pfenninger J, Aebi C. Respiratory response to salbutamol (albuterol) in ventilator-dependent infants with chronic lung disease: pressurized aerosol delivery versus intravenous injection. Intensive Care Med 1993; 19:251–55.

348. Holt WJ, Greenspan JS, Antunes MJ, et al. Pulmonary response to an inhaled bronchodilator in chronically ventilated preterm infants with suspected airway reactivity. Respir Care 1995; 40:145–51.

349. Fok TF, Lam K, Ng PC, et al. Delivery of salbutamol to nonventilated preterm infants by metered-dose inhaler, jet nebulizer, and ultrasonic nebulizer. Eur Respir J 1998; 12:159–64.

350. Cole CH, Colton T, Shah BL, et al. Early inhaled glucocorticoid therapy to prevent bronchopulmonary dysplasia. N Engl J Med 1999; 340:1005–10.

351. Jonsson B, Eriksson M, Soder O, et al. Budesonide delivered by dosimetric jet nebulization to preterm very low birthweight infants at high risk for development of chronic lung disease. Acta Paediatr 2000; 89:1449–55.

352. Giep T, Raibble P, Zuerlein T, et al. Trial of beclomethasone dipropionate by metered-dose inhaler in ventilator-dependent neonates less than 1500 grams. Am J Perinatol 1996; 13:5–9.

353. Arnon S, Grigg J, Silverman M. Effectiveness of budesonide aerosol in ventilator-dependent preterm babies: a preliminary report. Pediatr Pulmonol 1996; 21:231–35.

354. Merz U, Kusenbach G, Hausler M, et al. Inhaled budesonide in ventilator-dependent preterm infants: a randomized, double-blind pilot study. Biol Neonate 1999; 75:46–53.

355. Craven DE, Lichtenberg DA, Goularte TA, et al. Contaminated medication nebulizers in mechanical ventilator circuits. Source of bacterial aerosols. Am J Med 1984; 77:834–38.

356. Hamill RJ, Houston ED, Georghiou PR, et al. An outbreak of *Burkholderia* (formerly *Pseudomonas*) *cepacia* respiratory tract colonization and infection associated with nebulized albuterol therapy. Ann Intern Med 1995; 122:762–66.

357. Beaty CD, Ritz RH, Benson MS. Continuous in-line nebulizers complicate pressure support ventilation. Chest 1989; 96:1360–63.

358. Summer W, Elston R, Tharpe L, et al. Aerosol bronchodilator delivery methods. Relative impact on pulmonary function and cost of respiratory care. Arch Intern Med 1989; 149:618–23.

359. Bowton DL, Goldsmith WM, Haponik EF. Substitution of metered-dose inhalers for hand-held nebulizers. Success and cost savings in a large, acute-care hospital. Chest 1992; 101: 305–8.

360. Ely EW, Baker AM, Evans GW, et al. The distribution of costs of care in mechanically ventilated patients with chronic obstructive pulmonary disease. Crit Care Med 2000; 28:408–13.

361. Ballard J, Lugo RA, Salyer JW. A survey of albuterol administration practices in intubated patients in the neonatal intensive care unit. Respir Care 2002; 47:31–38.

362. Higgins RM, Cookson WO, Lane DJ, et al. Cardiac arrhythmias caused by nebulised beta-agonist therapy. Lancet 1987; 2: 863–64.

363. Breeden CC, Safirstein BH. Albuterol and spacer-induced atrial fibrillation. Chest 1990; 98:762–63.

364. Papo MC, Frank J, Thompson AE. A prospective, randomized study of continuous versus intermittent nebulized albuterol for severe status asthmaticus in children. Crit Care Med 1993; 21:1479–86.

365. Silverglade A. Cardiac toxicity of aerosol propellants. JAMA 1972; 222:827–28.

366. Dollery CT, Williams FM, Draffan GH, et al. Arterial blood levels of fluorocarbons in asthmatic patients following use of pressurized aerosols. Clin Pharmacol Ther 1974; 15:59–66.

367. Mehta S, Hill NS. Noninvasive ventilation. Am J Respir Crit Care Med 2001; 163:540–77.

368. Bott J, Carroll MP, Conway JH, et al. Randomised controlled trial of nasal ventilation in acute ventilatory failure due to chronic obstructive airways disease. Lancet 1993; 341:1555–57.

369. Brochard L, Mancebo J, Wysocki M, et al. Noninvasive ventilation for acute exacerbations of chronic obstructive pulmonary disease. N Engl J Med 1995; 333:817–22.

370. Kramer N, Meyer TJ, Meharg J, et al. Randomized, prospective trial of noninvasive positive pressure ventilation in acute respiratory failure. Am J Respir Crit Care Med 1995; 151:1799–806.

371. Ram FSF, Picot J, Lightowler J, et al. Non-invasive positive pressure ventilation for treatment of respiratory failure due to exacerbations of chronic obstructive pulmonary disease. Cochrane Database Syst Rev 2005; 3:CD004360.

372. Shenfield GM, Evans ME, Walker SR, et al. The fate of nebulized salbutamol (albuterol) administered by intermittent positive pressure respiration to asthmatic patients. Am Rev Respir Dis 1973; 108:501–5.

373. Dolovich MB, Killian D, Wolff RK, et al. Pulmonary aerosol deposition in chronic bronchitis: intermittent positive pressure breathing versus quiet breathing. Am Rev Respir Dis 1977; 115:397–402.

374. Parkes SN, Bersten AD. Aerosol kinetics and bronchodilator efficacy during continuous positive airway pressure delivered by face mask. Thorax 1997; 52:171–75.

375. Chatmongkolchart S, Schettino GP, Dillman C, et al. In vitro evaluation of aerosol bronchodilator delivery during noninvasive positive pressure ventilation: effect of ventilator settings and nebulizer position. Crit Care Med 2002; 30:2515–19.

376. Fauroux B, Itti E, Pigeot J, et al. Optimization of aerosol deposition by pressure support in children with cystic fibrosis: an experimental and clinical study. Am J Respir Crit Care Med 2000; 162:2265–71.

377. Nava S, Karakurt S, Rampulla C, et al. Salbutamol delivery during non-invasive mechanical ventilation in patients with chronic obstructive pulmonary disease: a randomized, controlled study. Intensive Care Med 2001; 27:1627–35.

378. Pollack CV Jr, Fleisch KB, Dowsey K. Treatment of acute bronchospasm with beta-adrenergic agonist aerosols delivered by a nasal bilevel positive airway pressure circuit. Ann Emerg Med 1995; 26:552–57.

Chapter 64

INHALED ANTIBIOTIC THERAPY

JEAN-JACQUES ROUBY
IVAN GOLDSTEIN
QIN LU

Ventilator-associated pneumonia is the main cause of nosocomial infection in critically ill patients.[1–3] Its incidence ranges between 8 and 28% in patients receiving mechanical ventilation for more than 48 hours, and between 34 and 70% in patients with acute lung injury or acute respiratory distress syndrome.[4] It prolongs the duration of stay in the intensive care unit and hospital, and increases costs.[5] Associated mortality ranges from 24–76%, and appears far greater than the mortality resulting from other nosocomial infections. It may even exceed 85% when high-risk gram-negative bacteria, such as *Pseudomonas aeruginosa* or *Acinetobacter baumannii*, are the causative pathogens.[6] Many studies have demonstrated that the early intravenous administration of appropriate antibiotics improves the prognosis. Lung deposition of antibiotics, however, administered by the intravenous route is either limited or poorly documented and treatment failure is common, leading to increased dosage and risk of systemic toxicity. Despite antimicrobial therapy and adequate supporting treatment, the mortality rate from ventilator-associated pneumonia remains very high, indicating a need for a more effective route of administration that is associated with less systemic

toxicity. Inhaled antibiotic therapy may represent such an alternative if the technique of nebulization provides antibiotic lung tissue concentrations equal to or greater than the minimal inhibitory concentration for the causative pathogen at the site of infection.

Rationale

At least three major theoretical arguments support the administration of inhaled antibiotics in critically ill patients with ventilator-associated pneumonia: the very pathogenesis of lung infection that originates in the tracheobronchial tree, the possibility of obtaining high lung tissue concentrations by bypassing the alveolar-capillary barrier, and the potential for decreasing systemic toxicity.

DEEP LUNG INFECTION ORIGINATES IN THE UPPER AIRWAYS

The normal human respiratory tract possesses efficient defenses against bacteria colonizing the pharynx. The glottis and larynx serve as natural anatomic barriers. The cough reflex, tracheobronchial secretions, mucociliary clearance, and regional immunity contribute to elimination of invading pathogens and prevention of infection deep in the lungs. Endotracheal and tracheostomy tubes bypass the natural barrier between the oropharynx and tracheobronchial tree. Bacteria penetrate into the trachea by leakage of infected secretions and/or contaminated gastric contents around the low-pressure cuff of an endotracheal tube.[7] In ventilated and deeply sedated patients, many of the mechanisms that protect against the spread of bacteria towards the lung parenchyma are either impaired or suppressed. Of particular importance is the depressed cough reflex, resulting from sedation, and inhibition of the ciliary escalator, caused by endotracheal intubation.[8,9] In addition, the internal wall of the endotracheal tube rapidly becomes coated with an antibiotic-resistant bacterial biofilm, which than can become fragmented and disseminated into the deep lung during tracheal suctioning or fiberoptic procedures.[10,11] Therefore it appears reasonable to hypothesize that antibiotics administered by the inhalational route may not only achieve bactericidal concentrations in the infected lung, but it may also reduce bacterial inoculum by stopping the continuous bacterial seeding from the upper airways.

BYPASSING THE ALVEOLAR-CAPILLARY BARRIER MAY PROVIDE HIGH ANTIBIOTIC TISSUE CONCENTRATIONS

Killing bacteria infecting the lung parenchyma requires that an antibiotic achieve a pulmonary concentration that is at least equal to the minimal inhibitory concentration for the infecting pathogen. Reaching subinhibitory concentrations in the infected parenchyma may trigger the emergence of resistant bacterial strains.[12] When antibiotics are intravenously administered, the alveolar-capillary barrier imposes a difficult-to-cross obstacle, which impairs lung deposition even if lung inflammation increases capillary

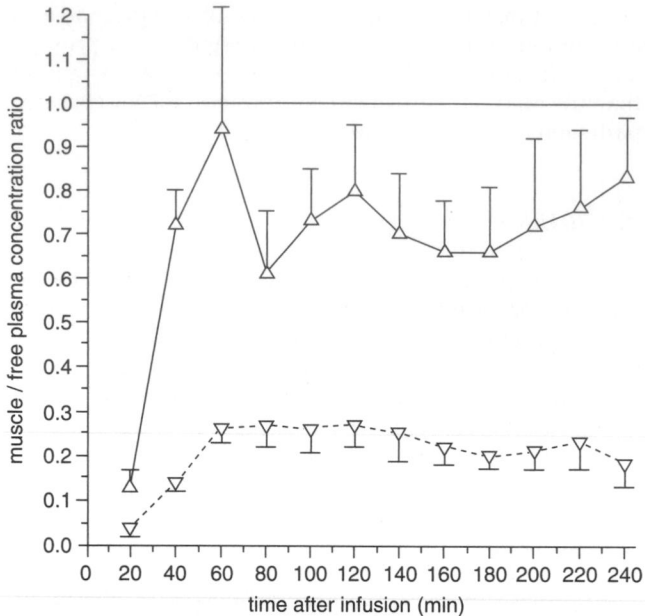

FIGURE 64-1 Time course of the ratio between unbound piperacillin concentrations measured in the interstitial space fluid of skeletal muscle and the concentrations measured in the plasma (mean ± SEM) after administration of a single intravenous dose of 4 g to six septic patients (*inverted triangle dotted line*) and six control healthy volunteers (*triangle solid line*). Piperacillin levels were measured using high-pressure liquid chromatography via microdialysis probes inserted into skeletal muscles. (*Reproduced, with permission, from Joukhadar et al.[15]*)

permeability.[13] Pulmonary vasoconstriction and regional thrombosis, two pathophysiologic abnormalities characterizing severe bronchopneumonia, reduce lung perfusion and tend to impair pulmonary penetration of circulating antibiotics. Major surgery and septic shock are associated with a significant decrease in the ratio between systemic and interstitial antibiotic concentrations (Fig. 64-1). All these factors contribute to markedly reduce the antibiotic concentrations at the site of infection, and may explain failure of intravenous antibacterial treatment.[14,15] During the initial phase of pulmonary infection, some degree of aeration persists within the bronchiolar lumen and alveolar space. Therefore, the early inhalation of antibiotics may represent a unique opportunity to reach bactericidal concentrations at the site of infection. In the presence of severe bronchopneumonia, the existence of the alveolar-capillary barrier and reduced lung perfusion are far from being deleterious; instead, they may be beneficial by limiting systemic absorption and reducing systemic toxicity of nebulized antibiotics.

Factors Influencing Lung Deposition

A number of factors influence lung deposition of nebulized antibiotics during mechanical ventilation: aerosol particle size, type of nebulizer, ventilator settings, grade of bronchopneumonia, and lung aeration. In the 1990s, the mechanical ventilator and associated tubings were considered as impassable obstacles, impairing antibiotic delivery to the deep lung. At present, a better understanding of the conditions regulating lung deposition[16] and the tremendous growth of technological innovations[17] potentially make the nebulization of antibiotics an attractive alternative to the classic intravenous administration.

AEROSOL PARTICLE SIZE

An essential condition for an aerosol particle to reach the deep lung is to ensure that the mass median aerodynamic diameter ranges between 1 and 5 μm.[18] Larger particles tend to impact and attach to ventilator circuits and endotracheal tubes, thereby limiting lung deposition.[19,20] Aerosol-generating devices, such as dry powder inhalers, metered dose inhalers, jet nebulizers, ultrasonic nebulizers, or vibrating plate nebulizers, all produce particles whose mass median aerodynamic diameter is <5 μm. It has to be emphasized that nebulizers that produce the smallest particles require considerably more time to deliver a standard antibiotic dose.[21]

TYPE AND POSITION OF NEBULIZERS

A nebulizer equipped with a large reservoir is needed for delivering sufficient amounts of antibiotics to the respiratory system. As a consequence, metered dose inhalers are not the most appropriate devices for nebulizing antibiotics and should be reserved for inhaled bronchodilators and corticosteroids.[22]

Jet nebulizers produce aerosol particles by superimposing an additional flow on the inspiratory flow that comes from the ventilator. The high-speed turbulent flow that generates the aerosol, however, also promotes particle impaction on ventilator circuits and proximal airways, thereby limiting deposition deep in the lung.

Ultrasonic nebulizers are appropriate for antibiotic nebulization for several reasons: they are generally equipped with a large reservoir; they generate particles whose mass median aerodynamic diameter is <5 μm through quartz vibrations; and the aerosol is entrained into the tracheobronchial tree by a low flow, independent of the inspiratory flow coming from the ventilator. The quartz vibration increases the temperature of the antibiotic solution and may alter the chemical structure of the antibiotic molecule.

Recently, vibrating plate nebulizers have been developed and seem appropriate for inhaled antibiotic therapy.[17] The aerosol is generated by a ceramic vibrational element and a domed aperture plate, which has about 1000 tapered holes that are electroformed in a sheet. The antibiotic is placed in a reservoir above the domed aperture plate. Powered by an alternating current, the vibrational element expands and contracts causing the domed aperture plate to move upward and downward; this action causes a micro-pump effect that produces the aerosol.[23] Particle size depends on the aperture diameter that can be changed by the manufacturer to optimize lung deposition. Vibrating plate nebulizers have several potential advantages over ultrasonic nebulizers: at the end of nebulization, the residual volume in the reservoir is negligible; the temperature of the antibiotic solution in the reservoir does not increase, thereby limiting the risk of altering the chemical structure of the antibiotic; the aerosol generation can be synchronized with inspiration, minimizing aerosol waste during exhalation;[21] and the aerosol can be delivered through an intratracheal catheter that can be inserted into a flexible bronchoscope.[24] Both ultrasonic and vibrating plate nebulizers should be placed in parallel with the inspiratory limb before the Y-piece. The ventilator tubing between the nebulizer and the Y-piece serves as a reservoir containing the aerosol generated during the expiratory phase, which is entrained into the tracheobronchial tree during the next inspiration (bolus effect). Ultrasonic nebulizers should be placed 40 cm before the Y-piece to provide enough flexibility; vibrating plate nebulizers, which are less bulky, can be placed 10 cm before the Y-piece. When aerosol delivery is synchronized with inspiration, the vibrating plate nebulizer can be placed between the Y-piece and the proximal tip of the endotracheal tube, thus limiting extrapulmonary deposition. Limiting the nebulization period to a portion of the inspiratory phase, however, significantly increases the time of nebulization, which, in turn, reduces the maximal dose that can be nebulized.

If the nebulizer is placed distally to the endotracheal tube, instead of being directly connected to it, the inner diameter of the endotracheal tube does not markedly influence the efficiency of aerosol delivery.[25]

VENTILATOR MODES AND SETTINGS

During mechanical ventilation, a laminar inspiratory flow provides better distal lung deposition of aerosol particles than a turbulent flow.[26] Turbulence causes wall impaction of particles in the trachea and proximal bronchioles, thereby limiting antibiotic deposition in the lung parenchyma. As a consequence, specific ventilator settings aimed at limiting inspiratory flow turbulence should be implemented during the nebulization phase. In a patient fully adapted to the ventilator, a volume-controlled mode is preferred with the following settings:[27] constant and low inspiratory flow,[28] a minute ventilation limited to 6 L/min, a respiratory frequency of 12 breaths/min, an inspiratory-to-expiratory ratio of 50%, and an end-inspiratory pause that constitutes 20% of the duty cycle, in order to facilitate settling of aerosol particles in the alveolar spaces. Decelerating flows should be avoided[29] as should patient triggering.[30] Inspiratory-to-expiratory ratios shorter than 50% should not be used because they do not provide enough time for settling of particles in the bronchoalveolar space.[31] These ventilator settings may not provide adequate CO_2 elimination in partially awake patients with acute bronchopneumonia. Consequently, dyssynchrony with the ventilator may result, generating turbulence in the ventilator circuits and the tracheobronchial tree. In order to provide adequate lung deposition, complete adaptation to the ventilator is required and can be achieved through a continuous infusion of propofol limited to the nebulization period.

HEAT, HUMIDITY, AND DENSITY OF THE CARRYING GAS

If the gas coming from the ventilator is heated and humidified, distal lung deposition of aerosol particles is markedly reduced.[21,32] Two factors contribute to this undesirable effect: increase in the mass median aerodynamic diameter of aerosol particles[33] and increased deposition in ventilator circuits.[34] If the period of nebulization does not exceed 30 minutes, it is recommended to simply remove the heat and moisture exchanger; the aerosol will provide partial humidification of the inspired gas coming from the ventilator. If the period of nebulization exceeds 30 minutes, then a conventional humidifier should be inserted in the inspiratory limb to avoid damage to the tracheal and bronchial mucosa caused by prolonged administration of cold, dry inspiratory gas. As a result, the aerosol deposition might be reduced by 40%.[22]

Several in vitro studies have shown that reducing the density of the inspired gas, by replacing nitrogen with helium, increases lung deposition of aerosol particles.[27,35,36] This beneficial effect likely results from helium-induced reduction in flow turbulence, limiting extrapulmonary deposition and tracheobronchial wall impaction of aerosol particles. On the other hand, operating the nebulizer with heliox reduces drug output and disposable mass.[37] Therefore, it is recommended to operate the nebulizer with a nitrogen-oxygen mixture and to entrain aerosol particles with a helium-oxygen mixture in order to maximize lung deposition.[27] These in vitro studies have been confirmed in a recent experimental study performed in mechanically ventilated piglets with healthy lungs: ceftazidime lung tissue concentrations following aerosol administration were 5- to 30-fold higher than after intravenous administration, and increased by 33% when a helium-oxygen (65%/35%) mixture was used as the operating gas of the ventilator.[38] Unfortunately, this beneficial effect was not confirmed in animals with experimental *Pseudomonas aeruginosa* bronchopneumonia; presumably, the loss of alveolar aeration resulting from bronchiolitis predominated over the helium-induced reduction in flow turbulence.[38] At present, the routine use of a helium-oxygen mixture cannot be recommended for nebulizing antibiotics in ventilated patients with infected lungs.

PATIENT-RELATED FACTORS

Experimental studies performed in anesthetized piglets receiving prolonged mechanical ventilation have demonstrated that lung deposition of nebulized amikacin is significantly greater in animals with healthy lungs than in animals with severe *Escherichia coli* bronchopneumonia.[39,40] In addition, amikacin lung tissue concentrations were homogeneously distributed in healthy animals, whereas they were heterogeneously distributed in infected animals. As shown in Fig. 64-2, dependent lung segments that were heavily infected had the lowest amikacin lung tissue concentrations. The loss of lung aeration, the severity and extension of parenchymal infection, and the injury to the alveolar-capillary barrier are the factors that determine lung deposition of nebulized antibiotics.

LUNG AERATION

In patients with ventilator-associated bronchopneumonia, the obstruction of distal bronchioles by purulent plugs.[41]

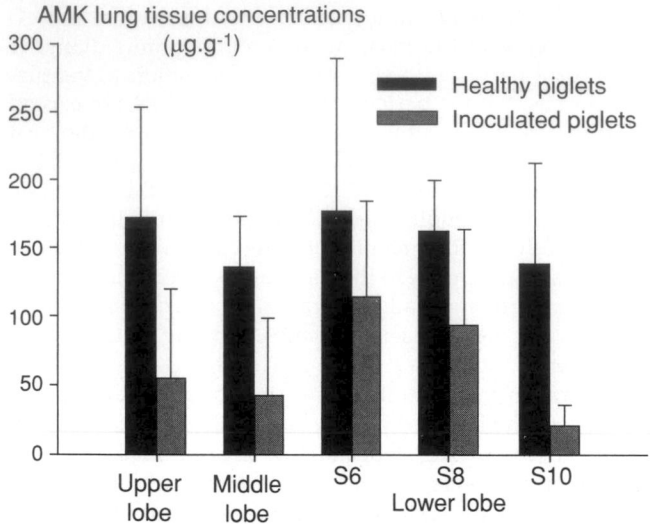

FIGURE 64-2 Amikacin (*AMK*) lung tissue concentrations (mean ± SD) measured in different pulmonary lobes and segments 1 hour after a second daily nebulization of amikacin 45 mg/kg in mechanically ventilated piglets with healthy lungs (*black bars*, n = 5) and in piglets with infected lungs (*gray bars*, n = 8), inoculated 24 hours before the first administration with a solution of *Escherichia coli*. In the lower lobe, postmortem specimens were sampled from dependent (segments 6 and 10) and nondependent (segment 8) lung regions. (*Reproduced, with permission, from Goldstein et al.*[40])

may impair lung deposition of inhaled antibiotics, and result in lower pulmonary concentrations than those obtained in patients with healthy lungs. In anesthetized piglets receiving prolonged mechanical ventilation for a severe experimental *Escherichia coli* bronchopneumonia, amikacin pulmonary tissue concentrations were 3–30 times higher after nebulization than after the intravenous administration of an equivalent dose.[42] As shown in Fig. 64-3, the degree of lung aeration had the opposite effect in animals receiving intravenous amikacin and in animals receiving nebu-

lized amikacin. The loss of lung aeration tended to increase amikacin tissue concentrations in the intravenous group, whereas the opposite effect was observed in the nebulization group. Very likely, the increased permeability of the alveolar-capillary barrier resulting from severe lung infection tends to promote intravenous amikacin penetration into the lung, whereas the multiple purulent plugs obstructing distal bronchioles tend to impair lung deposition of nebulized amikacin. It should be pointed out that despite the increased permeability of the alveolar-capillary barrier, amikacin lung tissue concentrations remained hopelessly low after intravenous injection. From these experimental data, it is reasonable to hypothesize that ventilator settings aimed at recruiting nonaerated lung areas, such as positive end-expiratory pressure or recruitment maneuvers, may increase lung deposition of nebulized antibiotics.

SEVERITY AND EXTENSION OF BRONCHOPNEUMONIA

The extension and severity of human lung infection can be evaluated according to an histologic classification proposed in the early 1990s.[41,43] Bronchiolitis is the immediate stage preceding lung infection. It is characterized by the proliferation of polymorphonuclear leukocytes within the bronchial lumen, forming purulent plugs, necrosis, and disruption of the bronchial mucosa. Neutrophilic infiltrates present in alveolar septa and distal bronchioles are characteristic of interstitial bronchopneumonia. The intense proliferation of polymorphonuclear leukocytes into surrounding alveoli characterizes foci of bronchopneumonia and decreases lung aeration. These foci of lung infection may extend to one or more pulmonary lobules resulting in confluent bronchopneumonia characterized by a severe aeration loss. Pulmonary abscess and purulent bronchopneumonia, the most severe forms of lung infection, are characterized by tissue necrosis, disruption of the normal lung architecture, vascular destruction, consolidation, and complete loss of aeration. In anesthetized piglets receiving prolonged mechanical

FIGURE 64-3 Amikacin (*AMK*) pulmonary concentrations according to aeration of lung segments (each dot represents a single segment) measured in anesthetized piglets mechanically ventilated for a severe *Escherichia coli* bronchopneumonia. In the intravenous group, animals received an intravenous dose of amikacin (15 mg/kg). In the nebulization group, animals received an equivalent dose by the inhalation route (via ultrasonic nebulizer). Lung aeration was quantified on postmortem histologic samples using an image analyzer computerized system coupled to a high-resolution color camera and an optical microscope. (*Reproduced, with permission, from Elman et al.*[42])

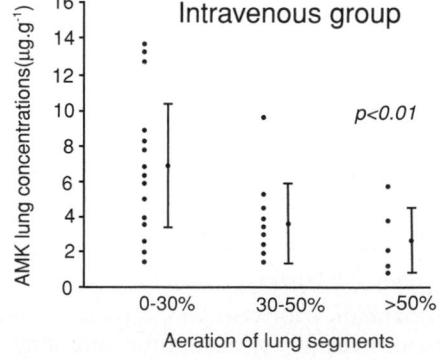
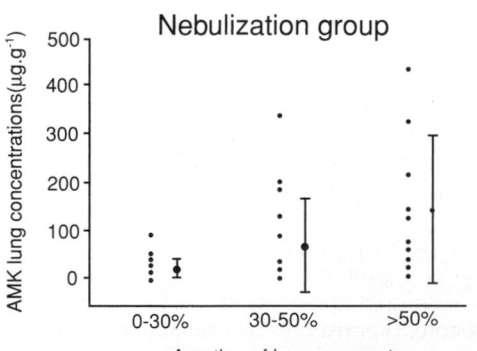

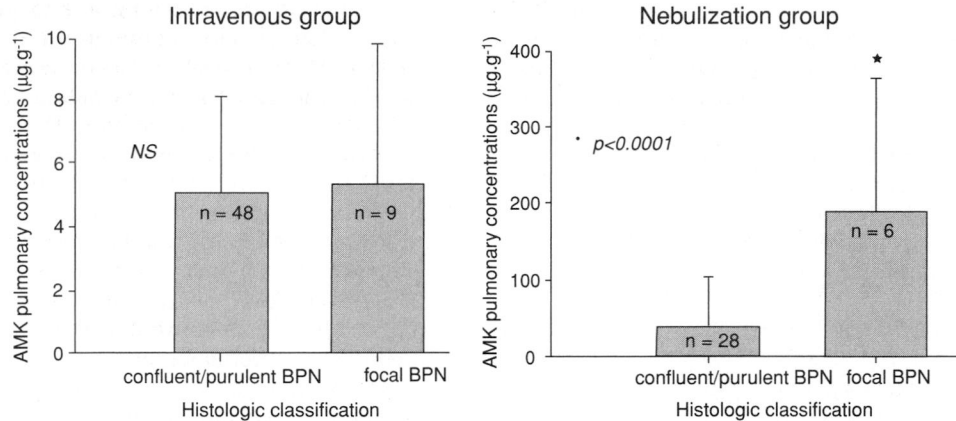

FIGURE 64-4 Amikacin (*AMK*) lung tissue concentrations according to histologic stages of bronchopneumonia (*BPN*) characterizing lung segments (mean ± SD), measured in anesthetized piglets mechanically ventilated for a severe *Escherichia coli* bronchopneumonia. In the intravenous group, animals received an intravenous dose of amikacin (15 mg/kg). In the nebulization group, animals received an equivalent dose by the inhalational route (via ultrasonic nebulizer). (*Reproduced, with permission, from Elman et al.[42]*)

ventilation for severe experimental *Escherichia coli* bronchopneumonia, lung tissue concentrations of nebulized amikacin were markedly higher in pulmonary segments with early stages of bronchopneumonia than in segments with confluent bronchopneumonia and lung abscess.[42] As shown in Fig. 64-4, such differences were not observed when amikacin was intravenously administered. These experimental data clearly support the administration of nebulized antibiotics in the early stages of ventilator-associated pneumonia.

INJURY TO THE ALVEOLAR-CAPILLARY BARRIER

A critical factor influencing antibiotic lung deposition is the diffusion through physiologic barriers, such as the bronchial epithelium or vascular endothelium. The normal alveolar-capillary barrier offers high resistance to lung penetration of intravenous antibiotics and systemic diffusion of nebulized antibiotics.[39] Lung infection, as with any type of lung injury, results in increased permeability of the alveolar-capillary barrier,[13] which, in turn, facilitates the diffusion of nebulized antibiotics into the bloodstream.[40] Experimentally, amikacin plasma concentrations are no different after nebulization or intravenous administration in the presence of severe lung infection. In addition, systemic bioavailability is markedly increased.[40] In other words, damage to the alveolar-capillary barrier, resulting from the infectious process, facilitates leakage of nebulized antibiotics toward the systemic compartment, thereby decreasing the tissue concentration and increasing the risk of systemic toxicity.

EFFICIENCY OF AEROSOL DELIVERY

In the 1980s, lung deposition of aerosolized antibiotics was assessed using radiolabeled aerosols and gamma scintigraphy.[44] In the early studies, mechanical ventilation was considered to limit the aerosol lung deposition to less than 5% of the dose placed in the nebulizer.[45] Over the following 15 years, improvements in aerosol technology, as well as an understanding of factors influencing lung deposition during mechanical ventilation, have increased aerosol delivery efficiency to 30–80%.[20,21,39,40,46,47] Pneumatic jet

nebulizers deliver less than 15% of the initial dose, because of high residual volume, massive deposition of aerosol particles in ventilator circuits and endotracheal tube, and loss to atmosphere by the expiratory limb.[48] Ultrasonic nebulizers

FIGURE 64-5 The mechanisms by which the dose of antibiotic inserted into the nebulizer may differ markedly from the dose delivered to the distal lung. Patient-related factors and medical interventions can interfere with different steps in the nebulization process.

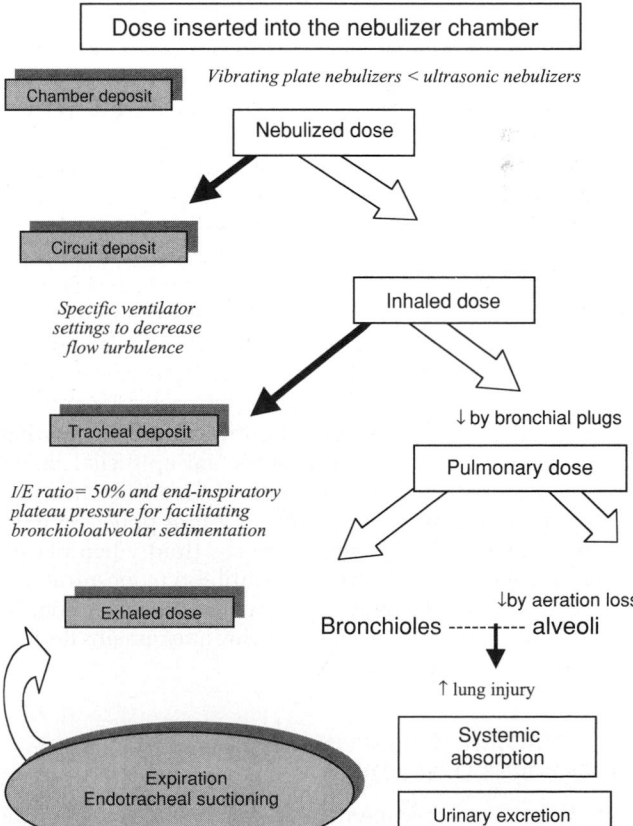

have increased the efficiency of aerosol delivery to 30–40%.[39,40] The recent development of aerosol devices using vibrating plate technology, together with synchronizing aerosol delivery to the inspiratory phase, may even increase aerosol efficiency above 70%.

In conclusion, three factors contribute to reduced antibiotic pulmonary tissue concentrations in the infected lung: bronchiolar plugs, loss of alveolar aeration, and increased systemic diffusion. The multiple factors influencing aerosol efficiency and lung deposition of nebulized antibiotics are illustrated in Fig. 64-5.

Assessment of the Microbiologic Response

METHODS FOR ASSESSING MICROBIOLOGIC RESPONSE

Antibacterial efficiency of nebulized antibiotics can be basically defined as obtaining appropriate lung tissue concentrations that kill pathogens infecting the lung parenchyma. It is directly assessed in experimental animals by measuring antibiotic lung tissue concentrations and assessing quantitative bacteriology of postmortem lung tissue samples.[40] In patients with ventilator-associated pneumonia, it can only be assessed indirectly as the regression of clinical, biologic, and radiologic signs of lung infection, and the disappearance of pathogens initially found in cultures of distal pulmonary samples. In ventilated critically ill patients, a number of confounding factors may hamper the clinical evaluation. The bronchial deposition of nebulized antibiotics may render cultures of distal samples falsely negative although the lung parenchyma is still positive. Critically ill patients frequently have several sites of infection, and persisting fever and biologic signs of infection may be related to a persisting extrapulmonary infection.

Antibiotic concentrations representative of the alveolar space can be assessed from a bronchoalveolar lavage. To obtain the antibiotic concentration representative of the epithelial lining fluid, the concentration measured in the aspirated fluid is corrected by a dilution factor, which is derived from the ratio between urea concentrations simultaneously measured in plasma and the bronchoalveolar lavage.[49,50] Such a measurement cannot be repeatedly performed and dilution errors are always possible. Of particular interest is a bronchoscopic microsampling method for measuring the antibiotic concentration in bronchial epithelial lining fluid.[51] It consists of introducing, through a bronchoscope positioned in the airways, an inner 1.9-mm polyester fiber rod probe, which immediately adsorbs fluid when placed on a bronchial wall for 10 seconds. Antibiotic concentrations are then measured from the probe without any dilution. To date, this attractive but expensive technique remains limited to research studies.

MICROBIOLOGIC RESPONSE IN EXPERIMENTAL STUDIES

In the late 1970s, experimental studies performed in nonventilated mice with *Klebsiella pneumoniae* bronchopneumonia had reported enhanced bacterial killing and higher survival rates when kanamycin was nebulized in comparison to intramuscular administration.[52,53] In spontaneously breathing squirrel monkeys, these investigators demonstrated that nebulized kanamycin efficiently protected against *Klebsiella pneumoniae* bronchopneumonia induced by intratracheal bacterial instillation, whereas the intramuscular administration was not protective.[53] Antibiotic clearance curves indicated that nebulized kanamycin remained longer in the lungs and at higher concentrations than intramuscular kanamycin. In the early 1990s, an experimental study performed in spontaneously breathing guinea pigs demonstrated that a combination of aerosolized and intramuscular tobramycin achieved slightly higher survival and total eradication of *Pseudomonas aeruginosa* compared to nebulized or intramuscular tobramycin alone.[54] Ten years later, an experimental study looked at the antibacterial efficiency of nebulized amikacin in anesthetized piglets ventilated for a severe *Escherichia coli* bronchopneumonia.[40] Twenty-four hours after a massive bacterial inoculation, ventilated animals received equivalent doses of amikacin, either by ultrasonic nebulization or intravenously. Because of a 60% extrapulmonary deposition, 45 mg/kg were nebulized in a single dose and 15 mg/kg administered intravenously. The animals received a second dose after 24 additional hours of mechanical ventilation, were killed 1 hour later, and 5 subpleural specimens were excised from the upper, middle, and lower lobes. Amikacin lung tissue peak concentrations were 3- to 30-fold higher after nebulization than after intravenous administration. As shown in Fig. 64-6, after two nebulizations and 25 hours of treatment, 71% of lung segments were sterile, whereas cultures of lung segments were comparable in nontreated and intravenously

FIGURE 64-6 Lung bacterial burden of *Escherichia coli* (expressed in colony-forming units per gram of lung tissue) in lung segments of anesthetized piglets mechanically ventilated for severe *Escherichia coli* bronchopneumonia. Postmortem tissue samples were collected 1 hour after the second aerosol or intravenous (IV) dose of amikacin, or 48 hours after the bacterial inoculation in the untreated control group. Each triangle refers to a single lung specimen. The lung bacterial burden is significantly lower in the aerosol group as compared with the intravenous or control groups (*Reproduced, with permission, from Goldstein et al.[40]*)

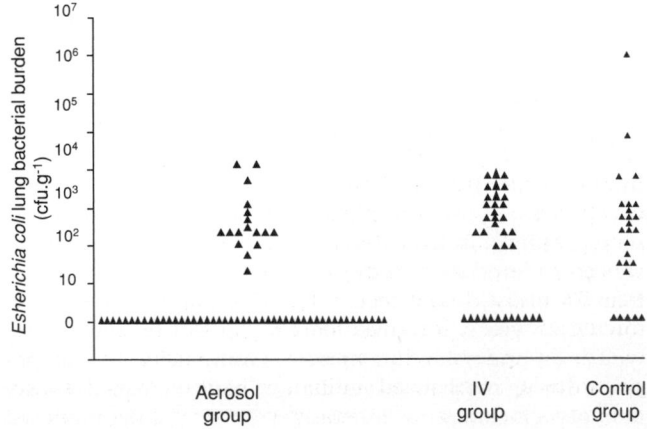

treated animals. Another experimental study looked at the lung tissue concentrations of ceftazidime administered to anesthetized piglets ventilated for a severe *Pseudomonas aeruginosa* bronchopneumonia.[38] Twenty-four hours after a massive bacterial inoculation, animals received equivalent doses of ceftazidime either by ultrasonic nebulization or intravenously. Because of a 30% extrapulmonary deposition, 50 mg/kg were nebulized in a single dose and 33 mg/kg intravenously administered. The animals were sacrificed 1 hour later, and 5 subpleural specimens were excised from the upper, middle, and lower lobes. Ceftazidime lung tissue concentrations following nebulization were 5- to 30-fold higher than after intravenous administration.[38] These experimental studies, performed in different animal species with bronchopneumonia caused by various gram-negative bacteria, clearly suggest that aminoglycosides and cephalosporins have a higher bactericidal efficiency when administered by nebulization than by the parenteral route.

MICROBIOLOGIC RESPONSE IN HUMAN STUDIES

Beneficial effects of nebulization and endotracheal administration of antibiotics have been repeatedly reported in spontaneously breathing patients with cystic fibrosis.[55–61] Several human studies have also demonstrated that the endotracheal administration or nebulization of aminoglycosides and polymyxins may prevent bronchial infection and ventilator-associated pneumonia in ventilated critically ill patients.[62–65] The risk of encouraging resistive strains, however, has limited this prophylactic approach.[66] Two studies performed in ventilated patients treated by intravenous antibiotics have demonstrated that the addition of endotracheal tobramycin is useful for eradicating the pathogens that cause gram-negative pneumonia.[67,68] In 1992, a comparative pharmacokinetic study, performed in ventilated patients with nosocomial pneumonia, reported high antibiotic bronchial concentrations following the nebulization or the endotracheal administration of 1 g of ceftazidime.[69] In addition, the minimal inhibitory concentrations for 90% of the most important pathogens responsible for nosocomial infections were exceeded by concentrations in bronchial secretions for up to 12 hours after intravenous infusion and for up to 24 hours after endotracheal and aerosol administration.[69]

More than 40 years ago, aerosols of colistin were successfully administered to spontaneously breathing patients with pulmonary suppuration.[70] In the early 1970s, two spontaneously breathing patients with *Pseudomonas aeruginosa* pneumonia were treated with inhaled polymyxin B, but aerosols had to be stopped because of airway obstruction.[71] Recent clinical studies reporting a beneficial microbiologic response following nebulization of antibiotics to critically ill patients are scarce, and limited to ventilator-associated pneumonia caused by multiresistant gram-negative bacteria[72,73] and pneumonia complicating the acquired immunodeficiency syndrome.[74] Except for a single case report describing the successful administration of aerosolized tobramycin to a spontaneously breathing patient with resistant *Pseudomonas aeruginosa* pneumonia,[75] nebulized antibiotics have always been delivered as an adjunctive therapy to intravenous antibiotics

administered for multidrug-resistant pneumonia.[72,73] An initial clinical report described two spontaneously breathing and one ventilated patient with nosocomial pneumonia or tracheobronchitis secondary to multiresistant strains of *Pseudomonas aeruginosa* for whom aerosolized colistin proved beneficial as supplemental therapy to intravenous antibiotics.[72] A second retrospective study reported the successful administration of aerosolized colistin to eight ventilated critically ill patients with multidrug-resistant gram-negative pneumonia.[73] Pneumonia was caused by *Pseudomonas aeruginosa* in one patient and *Acinetobacter baumannii* in seven patients. All patients received various combinations of intravenous antibiotics including colistin in six patients with nebulized colistin in doses ranging between 1.5 and 6 million IU/24 hours for 3–19 days. A beneficial clinical effect was observed in seven patients and causative pathogens were eradicated in four of the five patients in whom follow-up cultures were available.[73] Apart from their potential higher bactericidal effect in the infected lung parenchyma, nebulized antibiotics may also prevent microbial biofilm formation on the endotracheal tube internal surface[76] and suppress a reservoir of infecting microorganisms for the deep lung.[10]

Important Unknowns and Issues to be Resolved

The existing literature is not sufficiently definitive to recommend the routine use of nebulized antibiotics for treating ventilated patients with bronchopneumonia. Several major issues must be resolved before nebulized antibiotics can be recommended as an attractive alternative to intravenous anti-infectious therapy in critically ill patients.

CAN NEBULIZATION OF TIME-DEPENDENT ANTIBIOTICS PROVIDE BACTERICIDAL TISSUE CONCENTRATIONS?

Treating ventilator-associated pneumonia by nebulized antibiotics alone requires combined therapy. Analogously to intravenous antibiotics, it seems reasonable to combine a concentration and a time-dependent antibiotic. Most experimental studies of nebulized antibiotics included aminoglycosides, a family of antibiotics exerting a concentration-dependent antibacterial effect.[39,40,42,77] With concentration-dependent antibiotics, a single daily nebulization, ensuring high lung tissue concentrations, is enough to achieve a bactericidal effect at the site of infection for a period of 12–24 hours. The post-antibiotic effect prevents the regrowth of bacterial strains despite the antibiotic lung tissue concentrations falling below the minimal inhibitory concentration. After several consecutive daily nebulizations, there is no time-dependent tissue accumulation.[78] With time-dependent antibiotics, such as cephalosporins, tissue concentrations have to be maintained permanently above minimal inhibitory concentrations to provide a bactericidal effect. Experimental studies are needed to assess whether appropriate tissue concentrations can be maintained when nebulizing time-dependent antibiotics. The number of nebulizations per day has also to be determined.

SIDE EFFECTS OF NEBULIZED ANTIBIOTICS

Very few complications have been described in patients receiving inhaled antibiotics. Bronchoconstriction, chest tightness, and apnea are the main adverse effects of colistin aerosols.[56,79] Hypoxemia may result from aerosol nebulization of any drug, particularly in patients with acute lung injury or acute respiratory distress syndrome. With aminoglycosides, the most common adverse effect is tinnitus.[61] Potential side effects of nebulized cephalosporins or other antibiotics remain unknown.

Another serious potential complication of nebulized antibiotics is the emergence of multiresistant pathogens. Conflicting results have been published. Some old studies reported the emergence of resistant strains complicating the intratracheal administration of gentamycin, sisomycin, or colistin for preventing and treating ventilator-associated pneumonia.[62,66,67,80] More recent experimental[81] and clinical[64] studies did not find any increase in the incidence of resistant pathogens when polymyxin B or colistin were endotracheally administered to prevent ventilator-associated pneumonia. When aminoglycosides are nebulized into the tracheobronchial tree, significant concentrations are found in the serum.[39,40,78] Most often, these concentrations are below the minimal inhibitory concentrations

FIGURE 64-7 Guidelines for inhaled antibiotic therapy in ventilated patients.

Use ultrasonic or vibrating plate nebulizers, producing aerosols whose particles have a mass median aerodynamic diameter < 5 μm.

Remove heat and moisture exchanger and conventional humidifier and stop humidification during the period of nebulization.

Place the nebulizer on the inspiratory limb, 20 cm from the Y piece.

Determine in vitro the extrapulmonary deposition in the ventilator circuits using ventilator settings applied during the nebulization period:

> *The amount of antibiotic deposited into inspiratory and expiratory circuits, should be measured after lavage of each part of the circuit with a known volume of water.*

Determine the daily dose to be placed in the nebulizer chamber:

> *If the aminoglycoside is administered exclusively by nebulization, the dose should be calculated as the intravenous dose x 1/extrapulmonary deposition (%). If the aminoglycoside is concomitantly intravenously administered, then the determination of the appropriate dosage is difficult. Through plasma concentrations should be daily monitored in order to avoid systemic accumulation.*

> *If colistin is administered exclusively by nebulization, the dose should range between 6 and 15 millions International Units / day. If it is also intravenously administered, then the determination of the appropriate dosage is difficult. Through plasma concentrations should be daily monitored in order to avoid systemic accumulation.*

Determine the interval between each nebulization:

> *For aminoglycosides, a single daily nebulization.*
> *For colistin, 3 daily nebulizations (every 8 h).*

Use specific ventilatory settings during the nebulization period which should not exceed 30 minutes (for details see figure 64-8) of gram-negative bacteria, a fact that may promote the emergence of aminoglycoside-resistant strains if an extrapulmonary infection is present. As a consequence, it seems reasonable to limit the administration of nebulized antibiotics to isolated and nonbacteremic ventilator-associated pneumonias.

Guidelines for Inhaled Antibiotic Therapy

In 2005, administration of inhaled antibiotics to ventilated patients should be considered as rescue therapy for treating bronchopneumonia caused by resistant gram-negative bacteria. Nebulized antibiotics should be administered as an adjunctive therapy to intravenous antibiotics for increasing the bactericidal effect at the site of infection: the lung parenchyma. Pending additional experimental studies of other antibiotic families, and according to the existing literature, the nebulization of antibiotics should be limited to aminoglycosides and colistin.[21,39,40,42,72,73,78] It is important to recognize that inhaled antibiotics for treating ventilator-associated pneumonia differ in several ways from inhaled bronchodilator therapy for treating bronchospasm in ventilated patients.[22] Nebulized antibiotics must penetrate into the distal lung, whereas bronchodilators only need to reach the bronchial tree. Because antibiotic tissue concentrations in the infected lung parenchyma should exceed minimal inhibitory concentrations of causative pathogens, optimizing dosage is a more critical issue for inhaled antibiotic therapy than for inhaled bronchodilator therapy. Great attention must be paid to the period of nebulization: specific ventilator settings should be used to limit flow turbulence, and a short-acting sedative may be required to avoid flow triggering and dyssynchrony with the ventilator. Guidelines for delivering nebulized aminoglycosides and colistin during mechanical ventilation are summarized in Figs. 64-7 and 64-8.

Conclusions and the Future

Although inhaled antibiotic therapy has been episodically used in ventilated patients for more than 30 years, convincing clinical data are still unavailable to support its routine use. The recent understanding of physical and physiologic factors influencing lung deposition of aerosolized antibiotics together with an impressive growth of new technologies fuel a renewed interest for treating ventilator-associated pneumonia with nebulized antibiotics. Going too far and too fast, however, would inevitably lead to an underappreciation of this promising technique. Before performing randomized multicenter studies that assess the impact of inhaled versus intravenous antibiotic therapy on morbidity and mortality in ventilated patients with infected lungs, several issues must be addressed. First, experimental studies on the nebulization of antibiotics belonging to families other than aminoglycosides or polymyxins should be performed. Aerosolized time-dependent cephalosporins are of particular interest. Second, well-conducted phase II trials

Use a controlled mode of mechanical ventilation
with the following ventilator settings:

- *Constant inspiratory flow*
- *Tidal volume of 7 – 9 ml/kg*
- *Respiratory frequency 12 bpm*
- *Inspiratory to expiratory ratio 1 / 1*
- *Inspiratory plateau pressure 20%*
- *Remove any humidification system*
  Optimize alveolar recruitment

Avoid assisted modes of mechanical ventilation
Where the patient triggers flow during spontaneous inspiratory efforts

Avoid discoordination of the patient
with the ventilator:

If necessary, provide sedation with a
continuous infusion of propofol during
the nebulization period

FIGURE 64-8 Specific ventilator settings for inhaled antibiotic therapy in ventilated patients.

should be performed in ventilated patients to determine whether the impressive results obtained in experimental animals with severe bronchopneumonia are relevant to human patients. Several factors may limit the efficiency of inhaled antibiotic therapy in humans; critical factors include the different configuration of the human bronchial tree, and the higher inspiratory flow required by adult patients compared with smaller animals. If phase II trials show that inhaled antibiotic therapy is equivalent to intravenous antibiotics, then multicenter randomized studies should be set up to assess the impact of inhaled antibiotic therapy on mortality, morbidity, and costs in ventilated critically ill patients with ventilator-associated pneumonia.

References

1. Rouby JJ. Nosocomial infection in the critically ill: the lung as a target organ. Anesthesiology 1996; 84:757–9.
2. Celis R, Torres A, Gatell JM, et al. Nosocomial pneumonia. A multivariate analysis of risk and prognosis. Chest 1988; 93:318–24.
3. Torres A, Aznar R, Gatell JM, et al. Incidence, risk, and prognosis factors of nosocomial pneumonia in mechanically ventilated patients. Am Rev Respir Dis 1990; 142:523–8.
4. Chastre J, Fagon JY. Ventilator-associated pneumonia. Am J Respir Crit Care Med 2002; 165:867–903.
5. Warren DK, Shukla SJ, Olsen MA, et al. Outcome and attributable cost of ventilator-associated pneumonia among intensive care unit patients in a suburban medical center. Crit Care Med 2003; 31:1312–7.
6. Fagon JY, Chastre J, Domart Y, et al. Nosocomial pneumonia in patients receiving continuous mechanical ventilation. Prospective analysis of 52 episodes with use of a protected specimen

brush and quantitative culture techniques. Am Rev Respir Dis 1989; 139:877–84.

7. Alcon A, Fabregas N, Torres A. Hospital-acquired pneumonia: etiologic considerations. Infect Dis Clin North Am 2003; 17:679–95.

8. Wanner A, Salathe M, O'Riordan TG. Mucociliary clearance in the airways. Am J Respir Crit Care Med 1996; 154:1868–902.

9. Lewis RM. Airway clearance techniques for the patient with an artificial airway. Respir Care 2002; 47:808–17.

10. Adair CG, Gorman SP, Feron BM, et al. Implications of endotracheal tube biofilm for ventilator-associated pneumonia. Intensive Care Med 1999; 25:1072–6.

11. Bauer TT, Torres A, Ferrer R, et al. Biofilm formation in endotracheal tubes. Association between pneumonia and the persistence of pathogens. Monaldi Arch Chest Dis 2002; 57:84–7.

12. Licitra CM, Brooks RG, Sieger BE. Clinical efficacy and levels of ciprofloxacin in tissue in patients with soft tissue infection. Antimicrob Agents Chemother 1987; 31:805–7.

13. Matthay MA. Function of the alveolar epithelial barrier under pathologic conditions. Chest 1994; 105:67S–74S.

14. Brunner M, Pernerstorfer T, Mayer BX, et al. Surgery and intensive care procedures affect the target site distribution of piperacillin. Crit Care Med 2000; 28:1754–9.

15. Joukhadar C, Frossard M, Mayer BX, et al. Impaired target site penetration of beta-lactams may account for therapeutic failure in patients with septic shock. Crit Care Med 2001; 29:385–91.

16. Dhand R. Basic techniques for aerosol delivery during mechanical ventilation. Respir Care 2004; 49:611–22.

17. Dhand R. New frontiers in aerosol delivery during mechanical ventilation. Respir Care 2004; 49:666–77.

18. Brain JD, Valberg PA. Deposition of aerosol in the respiratory tract. Am Rev Respir Dis 1979; 120:1325–73.

19. Crogan SJ, Bishop MJ. Delivery efficiency of metered dose aerosols given via endotracheal tubes. Anesthesiology 1989; 70:1008–10.

20. O'Riordan TG, Palmer LB, Smaldone GC. Aerosol deposition in mechanically ventilated patients. Optimizing nebulizer delivery [see comments]. Am J Respir Crit Care Med 1994; 149:214–219.

21. Miller DD, Amin MM, Palmer LB, et al. Aerosol delivery and modern mechanical ventilation: in vitro/in vivo evaluation. Am J Respir Crit Care Med 2003; 168:1205–9.

22. Dhand R, Tobin MJ. Inhaled bronchodilator therapy in mechanically ventilated patients. Am J Respir Crit Care Med 1997; 156:3–10.

23. Dhand R. Nebulizers that use a vibrating mesh or plate with multiple apertures to generate aerosol. Respir Care 2002; 47:1406–16.

24. Tronde A, Baran G, Eirefelt S, et al. Miniaturized nebulization catheters: a new approach for delivery of defined aerosol doses to the rat lung. J Aerosol Med 2002; 15:283–96.

25. Dhand R. Special problems in aerosol delivery: artificial airways. Respir Care 2000; 45:636–45.

26. Dolovich MA. Influence of inspiratory flow rate, particle size, and airway caliber on aerosolized drug delivery to the lung. Respir Care 2000; 45:597–608.

27. O'Doherty MJ, Thomas SH, Page CJ, et al. Delivery of a nebulized aerosol to a lung model during mechanical ventilation. Effect of ventilator settings and nebulizer type, position, and volume of fill. Am Rev Respir Dis 1992; 146:383–8.

28. Dhand R. Maximizing aerosol delivery during mechanical ventilation: go with the flow and go slow. Intensive Care Med 2003; 29:1041–2.

29. Hess DR, Dillman C, Kacmarek RM. In vitro evaluation of aerosol bronchodilator delivery during mechanical ventilation: pressure-control vs. volume control ventilation. Intensive Care Med 2003; 29:1145–50.

30. Fink JB, Dhand R, Duarte AG, et al. Aerosol delivery from a metered-dose inhaler during mechanical ventilation. An in vitro model. Am J Respir Crit Care Med 1996; 154:382–7.

31. Fink JB, Dhand R, Grychowski J, et al. Reconciling in vitro and in vivo measurements of aerosol delivery from a metered-dose inhaler during mechanical ventilation and defining efficiency-enhancing factors. Am J Respir Crit Care Med 1999; 159:63–68.

32. O'Riordan TG, Greco MJ, Perry RJ, et al. Nebulizer function during mechanical ventilation. Am Rev Respir Dis 1992; 145:1117–22.

33. Ferron GA, Kerrebijn KF, Weber J. Properties of aerosols produced by three nebulizers. Am Rev Respir Dis 1976; 114:899–908.

34. Dhand R, Tobin MJ. Bronchodilator delivery with metered-dose inhalers in mechanically-ventilated patients. Eur Respir J 1996; 9:585–95.

35. Habib DM, Garner SS, Brandeburg S. Effect of helium-oxygen on delivery of albuterol in a pediatric, volume-cycled, ventilated lung model. Pharmacotherapy 1999; 19:143–9.

36. Goode ML, Fink JB, Dhand R, et al. Improvement in aerosol delivery with helium-oxygen mixtures during mechanical ventilation. Am J Respir Crit Care Med 2001; 163:109–14.

37. Hess DR, Acosta FL, Ritz RH, et al. The effect of heliox on nebulizer function using a beta-agonist bronchodilator. Chest 1999; 115:184–9.

38. Tonnellier M, Ferrari F, Goldstein I, Sartorius A, et al. Intravenous versus nebulized ceftazidime in ventilated piglets with and without experimental bronchopneumonia. comparative effects of helium and nitrogen. Anesthesiology 2005; 102:995–1000.

39. Goldstein I, Wallet F, Robert J, et al. Lung tissue concentrations of nebulized amikacin during mechanical ventilation in piglets with healthy lungs. Am J Respir Crit Care Med 2002; 165:171–5.

40. Goldstein I, Wallet F, Nicolas-Robin A, et al. Lung deposition and efficiency of nebulized amikacin during *Escherichia coli* pneumonia in ventilated piglets. Am J Respir Crit Care Med 2002; 166:1375–81.

41. Rouby JJ, Martin De Lassale E, Poete P, et al. Nosocomial bronchopneumonia in the critically ill. Histologic and bacteriologic aspects. Am Rev Respir Dis 1992; 146:1059–66.

42. Elman M, Goldstein I, Marquette CH, et al. Influence of lung aeration on pulmonary concentrations of nebulized and intravenous amikacin in ventilated piglets with severe bronchopneumonia. Anesthesiology 2002; 97:199–206.

43. Fabregas N, Torres A, El-Ebiary M, et al. Histopathologic and microbiologic aspects of ventilator-associated pneumonia. Anesthesiology 1996; 84:760–71.

44. MacIntyre NR, Silver RM, Miller CW, et al. Aerosol delivery in intubated, mechanically ventilated patients. Crit Care Med 1985; 13:81–4.

45. Fuller HD, Dolovich MB, Posmituck G, et al. Pressurized aerosol versus jet aerosol delivery to mechanically ventilated patients. Comparison of dose to the lungs. Am Rev Respir Dis 1990; 141:440–4.

46. Thomas SH, O'Doherty MJ, Page CJ, et al. Delivery of ultrasonic nebulized aerosols to a lung model during mechanical ventilation. Pulmonary deposition of a nebulised aerosol during mechanical ventilation. Am Rev Respir Dis 1993; 148:872–7.

47. Diot P, Morra L, Smaldone GC. Albuterol delivery in a model of mechanical ventilation. Comparison of metered-dose inhaler and nebulizer efficiency. Am J Respir Crit Care Med 1995; 152:1391–4.

48. Duarte AG, Fink JB, Dhand R. Inhalation therapy during mechanical ventilation. Respir Care Clin North Am 2001; 7:233–60.

49. Gotfried MH, Danziger LH, Rodvold KA. Steady-state plasma and bronchopulmonary characteristics of clarithromycin extended-release tablets in normal healthy adult subjects. J Antimicrob Chemother 2003; 52:450–6.

50. Rodvold KA, Danziger LH, Gotfried MH. Steady-state plasma and bronchopulmonary concentrations of intravenous levofloxacin and azithromycin in healthy adults. Antimicrob Agents Chemother 2003; 47:2450–7.

51. Yamazaki K, Ogura S, Ishizaka A, et al. Bronchoscopic microsampling method for measuring drug concentration in epithelial lining fluid. Am J Respir Crit Care Med 2003; 168:1304–7.

52. Berendt RF, Long GG, Walker JS. Treatment of respiratory *Klebsiella pneumoniae* infection in mice with aerosols of kanamycin. Antimicrob Agents Chemother 1975; 8:585–90.

53. Berendt RF, Magruder RD, Frola FR. Treatment of *Klebsiella pneumoniae* respiratory tract infection of squirrel monkeys with aerosol administration of kanamycin. Am J Vet Res 1980; 41:1492–4.

54. Makhoul IR, Merzbach D, Lichtig C, et al. Antibiotic treatment of experimental *Pseudomonas aeruginosa* pneumonia in guinea pigs: comparison of aerosol and systemic administration. J Infect Dis 1993; 168:1296–9.

55. Jensen T, Pedersen SS, Garne S, et al. Colistin inhalation therapy in cystic fibrosis patients with chronic *Pseudomonas aeruginosa* lung infection. J Antimicrob Chemother 1987; 19:831–8.

56. Maddison J, Dodd M, Webb AK. Nebulized colistin causes chest tightness in adults with cystic fibrosis. Respir Med 1994; 88:145–7.

57. Bauldoff GS, Nunley DR, Manzetti JD, et al. Use of aerosolized colistin sodium in cystic fibrosis patients awaiting lung transplantation. Transplantation 1997; 64:748–52.

58. Ramsey BW, Pepe MS, Quan JM, et al. Intermittent administration of inhaled tobramycin in patients with cystic fibrosis. Cystic Fibrosis Inhaled Tobramycin Study Group. N Engl J Med 1999; 340:23–30.

59. Beringer P. The clinical use of colistin in patients with cystic fibrosis. Curr Opin Pulm Med 2001; 7:434–40.

60. Hodson ME, Gallagher CG, Govan JR. A randomised clinical trial of nebulised tobramycin or colistin in cystic fibrosis. Eur Respir J 2002; 20:658–64.

61. Cheer SM, Waugh J, Noble S. Inhaled tobramycin (TOBI): a review of its use in the management of *Pseudomonas aeruginosa* infections in patients with cystic fibrosis. Drugs 2003; 63:2501–20.

62. Klastersky J, Hensgens C, Noterman J, et al. Endotracheal antibiotics for the prevention of tracheobronchial infections in tracheotomized unconscious patients. A comparative study of gentamicin and aminosidin-polymyxin B combination. Chest 1975; 68:302–6.

63. Klick JM, du Moulin GC, Hedley-Whyte J, et al. Prevention of gram-negative bacillary pneumonia using polymyxin aerosol as prophylaxis. II. Effect on the incidence of pneumonia in seriously ill patients. J Clin Invest 1975; 55:514–9.

64. Rouby JJ, Poete P, Martin de Lassale E, et al. Prevention of gram negative nosocomial bronchopneumonia by intratracheal colistin in critically ill patients. Histologic and bacteriologic study. Intensive Care Med 1994; 20:187–92.

65. Zylberberg H, Vargaftig J, Barbieux C, et al. Prolonged efficiency of secondary prophylaxis with colistin aerosols for respiratory infection due to *Pseudomonas aeruginosa* in patients infected with human immunodeficiency virus. Clin Infect Dis 1996; 23:641–3.

66. Feeley TW, Du Moulin GC, Hedley-Whyte J, et al. Aerosol polymyxin and pneumonia in seriously ill patients. N Engl J Med 1975; 293:471–5.

67. Klastersky J, Carpentier-Meunier F, Kahan-Coppens L, et al. Endotracheally administered antibiotics for gram-negative bronchopneumonia. Chest 1979; 75:586–91.

68. Brown RB, Kruse JA, Counts GW, et al. Double-blind study of endotracheal tobramycin in the treatment of gram-negative bacterial pneumonia. The Endotracheal Tobramycin Study Group. Antimicrob Agents Chemother 1990; 34:269–72.

69. Bressolle F, de la Coussaye JE, Ayoub R, et al. Endotracheal and aerosol administrations of ceftazidime in patients with nosocomial pneumonia: pharmacokinetics and absolute bioavailability. Antimicrob Agents Chemother 1992; 36:1404–11.

70. Pino G, Conterno G, Colongo PG. [Clinical observations on the activity of aerosol colimycin and of endobronchial instillations of colimycin in patients with pulmonary suppurations.] Minerva Med 1963; 54:2117–22.

71. Marschke G, Sarauw A. Danger of polymyxin B inhalation. Ann Intern Med 1971; 74:296–7.

72. Hamer DH. Treatment of nosocomial pneumonia and tracheobronchitis caused by multidrug-resistant *Pseudomonas aeruginosa* with aerosolized colistin. Am J Respir Crit Care Med 2000; 162:328–30.

73. Michalopoulos A, Kasiakou SK, Mastora Z, et al. Aerosolized colistin for the treatment of nosocomial pneumonia due to multidrug-resistant Gram-negative bacteria in patients without cystic fibrosis. Critical Care 2005; 9:R53–R59.

74. Green ST, Nathwani D, Gourlay Y, et al. Nebulized colistin (polymyxin E) for AIDS-associated *Pseudomonas aeruginosa* pneumonia. Int J STD AIDS 1992; 3:130–1.

75. McCall CY, Spruill WJ, Wade WE. The use of aerosolized tobramycin in the treatment of a resistant pseudomonal pneumonitis. Ther Drug Monit 1989; 11:692–5.

76. Adair CG, Gorman SP, Byers LM, et al. Eradication of endotracheal tube biofilm by nebulised gentamicin. Intensive Care Med 2002; 28:426–31.

77. Girardi C, Tonnellier M, Sartorius A, et al. Concentrations tissulaires pulmonaires en Ceftazidime après administration par aérosol ou par voie intraveineuse chez le porc ventilé. Ann Francaises Anesthésie Réanimation 2003; 22:333.

78. Ferrari F, Goldstein I, Nieszkowska A, et al. Lack of lung tissue and systemic accumulation after consecutive daily aerosols of amikacin in ventilated piglets with healthy lungs. Anesthesiology 2003; 98:1016–9.

79. Cunningham S, Prasad A, Collyer L, et al. Bronchoconstriction following nebulised colistin in cystic fibrosis. Arch Dis Child 2001; 84:432–3.

80. Klastersky J, Huysmans E, Weerts D, et al. Endotracheally administered gentamicin for the prevention of infections of the respiratory tract in patients with tracheostomy: a double-blind study. Chest 1974; 65:650–4.

81. Johanson WG Jr, Seidenfeld JJ, de los Santos R, et al. Prevention of nosocomial pneumonia using topical and parenteral antimicrobial agents. Am Rev Respir Dis 1988; 137:265–72.

Chapter 65

FLUID MANAGEMENT IN THE VENTILATED PATIENT

ANDREW D. BERSTEN

Fluid management during mechanical ventilation is complicated by both the influence of positive airway pressure on normal homeostatic control of bodily fluids, and the interaction of mechanical ventilation with fluid status. Hypovolemia may lead to hemodynamic intolerance of positive airway pressure, and fluid overload may result in both impaired gas exchange and respiratory mechanics, and deleterious systemic effects. Consequently, fluid management requires an integrated approach to maintenance and resuscitation fluids.

Physiologic Considerations

FLUID COMPARTMENTS[1]

In the normal adult male, total body water accounts for ~60% of body weight. In turn, ~40% of body weight is intracellular water and ~20% is distributed into the extracellular fluid volume, made up of interstitial fluid (~16%), plasma volume (~4%), and usually negligible volumes of lymph and transcellular fluid (cerebrospinal fluid and pericardial, intrapleural, and peritoneal fluid). Tissues such as brain, kidney, liver, and muscle have high water contents (70–80%) but adipose tissue has low water content (~10%). Consequently, women, who tend to have more adipose tissue, have a lower total body water (~50% of body weight). Total body water decreases in the elderly due to a loss of muscle mass.

The extracellular volume is distributed in interstitial fluid and plasma volume, and consists of two compartments.

Seventy percent of the volume is rapidly equilibrating (~20 min), and the remainder slowly equilibrates (~24 hours) in dense connective tissue and bone. Sodium balance regulates the extracellular volume, whereas water balance regulates the intracellular volume.

WATER BALANCE

Water balance is primarily determined by thirst and the renal action of arginine vasopressin, also termed antidiuretic hormone, which is secreted from the posterior pituitary following synthesis in the hypothalamus, in response to a wide variety of stimuli, particularly plasma osmolality. Vasopressin activates V_2 receptors on the basolateral surface of the distal renal tubule and collecting duct, leading to an increase in water permeability, and reabsorption of filtrate, through fusion of aquaporin-2 with the luminal membrane. Vasopressin also reduces water clearance by decreasing renal medullary blood flow, and independently increases the renal medullary concentration gradient by stimulating a urea transporter.[2]

Under normal circumstances, a plasma osmolality of 280 mOsm/kg suppresses vasopressin secretion allowing maximal urinary dilution. As osmolality progressively rises to 295 mOsm/kg so does the secretion of vasopressin, with an associated reduction in free water clearance. The kidney can normally concentrate filtrate up to 1200 mOsm/kg under the influence of vasopressin, although this tends to deteriorate with age and renal dysfunction. Other stimuli that influence vasopressin secretion are listed in Table 65-1. High-pressure stretch receptors in the aortic arch and carotid sinus sense a significant (>10%) fall in blood pressure (BP), leading to an increase in vasopressin release. As vasopressin also causes vasoconstriction through stimulation of V_1 receptors, this is an important homeostatic response in shock,[2] but appears to be reset within 32 hours of sustained hypovolemia.[3] Stimulation of low pressure stretch receptors in the atria primarily results in an increase in both sympathetic tone and renin, and a decrease in atrial natriuretic peptide (ANP), with vasopressin release unaffected until the systemic BP falls.

SODIUM BALANCE

The extracellular volume is primarily regulated through control of sodium balance, which is in turn regulated through control of effective plasma volume and its composition. The total body sodium content is ~4000 mmol; most is found extracellularly, and about half is rapidly exchangeable. While the standard Western diet contains ~150 mmol of sodium per 24 hours, this varies widely and urinary sodium excretion varies between 0.2 and 242 mmol per 24 hours,[4] reflecting a balance between sodium input and output. Although a moderate range of total body sodium content is well tolerated, once effective plasma volume is significantly affected, short- and longer-term homeostatic responses are initiated.

A fall in effective plasma volume leads to activation of baroreceptors with augmentation of myocardial performance and peripheral vascular tone, and defense of plasma volume through shift of fluid from the interstitium. Longer-term responses include reduced sodium loss by the

TABLE 65-1 Factors that Influence Vasopressin Secretion

Increase Vasopressin Secretion	Decrease Vasopressin Secretion
Plasma osmolality >280 mOsm/kg	Ethanol
Hypovolemia	Drugs
Hypotension	Narcotic antagonists
High-pressure baroreceptors	Phenytoin
Low-pressure baroreceptors	Clonidine
Angiotensin II	Atrial natriuretic peptide
Pain	
Nausea	
Drugs	
Nicotine	
Narcotics	
Barbiturates	
Carbamazepine	
Amitriptyline	
Cyclophosphamide	
Vincristine	
Clofibrate	
Hypercapnia	
Hypoxemia	

kidney and sweat glands, through a direct effect of aldosterone. When the baroreceptors are stimulated the increase in sympathetic tone reduces sodium loss through reduced glomerular filtration rate (GFR), and through increased tubular sodium reabsorption, both through a direct effect and through the actions of increased renin, angiotensin II, and aldosterone. In addition, ANP is released from the cardiac atria in response to stretch, and directly increases GFR through afferent arteriolar vasodilation, increases renal medullary blood flow, antagonizes vasoconstriction secondary to angiotensin II, and decreases sodium reabsorption by the collecting duct. Dopamine is produced in the kidney following conversion from L-dopa under the action of the cytosolic enzyme L-amino acid decarboxylase present in the proximal tubules.[5] This is upregulated following a high-salt diet, leading to increased urinary sodium loss as dopamine acts to inhibit sodium reabsorption in the proximal tubule,[6] and contributes to the increase in urine output sometimes seen following administration of low-dose dopamine. The renal synthesis of prostaglandins, such as PGE_2 and PGI_2, tends to maintain renal blood flow and GFR through vasodilation, and directly increase water and sodium excretion. Consequently, in stressed patients cyclooxygenase inhibitors can precipitate renal dysfunction. Dopaminergic renal vasodilation in part acts through release of PGI_2, because administration of dopaminergic antagonists leads to reduced urinary prostaglandins and loss of dopaminergic vasodilation,[7] perhaps explaining why low-dose dopamine appears to be ineffective in septic ICU patients[8] who already have a prostaglandin-driven kidney.

INFLUENCE OF POSITIVE-PRESSURE VENTILATION ON FLUID BALANCE

Positive-pressure ventilation and positive end-expiratory pressure (PEEP) raise intrathoracic pressure, resulting in reduced venous return and transmural pressure (see Chapter 36), with consequent complex neurohumoral responses leading to sodium and water retention. Because assisted, supported, and spontaneous modes of ventilation progressively ameliorate the elevation of intrathoracic pressure and its consequences, different ventilator modes variably reduce venous return. Reductions in stroke volume, cardiac output, and BP then lead to stimulation of high-pressure baroreceptors, and altered regional blood flow. Both low- and high-pressure baroreceptor stimulation lead to increased sympathetic outflow, and release of renin, aldosterone, and ANP. Renal denervation does not prevent sodium and water retention.[9] Angiotensin-converting enzyme inhibitors[10] and deliberate hypervolemia,[9] however, reduce sodium and water retention during positive-pressure ventilation.

Right atrial transmural pressure and stretch are also reduced by PEEP and positive-pressure ventilation, and this leads to reduced secretion of ANP,[11,12] with consequent reduction in water and sodium excretion reversed by restoration of venous return with lower body positive pressure. PEEP levels above 10 cmH$_2$O may lead to an increase in central venous pressure (CVP), and regional venous pressures, which in the kidney contribute to reduced sodium and water excretion, independent of neurohumoral effects.[13]

In summary, various neurohumoral responses to positive-pressure ventilation lead to retention of sodium and water, as a homeostatic response to raised intrathoracic pressure. A major consequence of this response is expanded plasma volume, and a tendency toward systemic and pulmonary edema.

THE STARLING EQUATION

The major difference between plasma volume and interstitial fluid is the lower concentration of plasma proteins in the interstitial fluid, typically 40% of their plasma concentration. Although this concentration difference has little effect on the osmotic pressure between these two compartments, it leads to an important difference in oncotic pressure, and 80% of this is attributed to differences in albumin concentration. The normal plasma osmotic pressure is ~5500–6000 mmHg, with ~20 mmHg contributed by plasma proteins, despite having an osmolality of ~1.2 mOsm/kg.

The Starling equation quantitates the transvascular flux of fluids across the microcirculation (J_v). It is usually written as:

$$J_v = K_{f,c}([P_{cap} - P_{int}] - \sigma[\pi_{cap} - \pi_{int}])$$

where $K_{f,c}$ is the capillary filtration coefficient, P_{cap} is the hydrostatic microvascular pressure, P_{int} is the interstitial pressure (usually taken as –3 mmHg), π_{cap} is the plasma oncotic pressure (usually 28 mmHg), π_{int} is the interstitial oncotic pressure (usually 8 mmHg), and σ is the osmotic reflection coefficient. $K_{f,c}$ is determined by both endothelial hydraulic conductance and endothelial surface area, and σ is a measure of protein selectivity. The osmotic reflection coefficient is thought to be 1 in the cerebral microcirculation where the blood–brain barrier effectively prevents protein flux, and about 0.7–0.8 in the normal pulmonary microcirculation, although this is markedly reduced during lung injury.[14] In a typical systemic microcirculatory bed the arterial end of P_{cap} is 30 mmHg and the venous end is 10 mmHg. Assuming σ equals 1, the net driving pressure out of the capillary at the arterial end of the microcirculation will be ([30 − 3] − [28 − 13]) or 13 mmHg, although the effective π_{int} may be a little lower.[14] At the venous end of the microcirculation the net driving pressure into the capillary will be 7 mmHg, and most of the filtered fluid is reabsorbed, with the lymphatics draining the remainder.

In the healthy lung, P_{cap} is usually assumed to be 7 mmHg, P_{int} as −8 mmHg, and π_{int} as 14 mmHg. Consequently, the driving pressure across the pulmonary circulation is thought to be positive ([7 + 8 + 14]) − (28 mmHg) leading to net filtration of fluid, with lymphatic absorption usually estimated to be ∼20 ml/h. The final filtration rate is determined by the capillary surface area, convective forces, and diffusive forces. When P_{cap} is suddenly raised, the filtration rate may increase more than threefold.[14]

There are a number of safety factors that are thought to help prevent alveolar edema. These include low epithelial permeability (pore size about 10% that of the endothelium), low alveolar surface tension reflecting normal surfactant function, active pumping of sodium out of the alveolus across the basolateral membrane of alveolar type II cells, and favorable interstitial function and lymphatic drainage (edema fluid moves along a negative-pressure gradient centrally away from the alveolus, while an associated reduction in the negative pressure and dilution of interstitial oncotic pressure reduce filtration).[15] Changes in either Starling forces or these safety factors can lead to pulmonary edema. For example, an increase in P_{cap} is the basis for hydrostatic pulmonary edema; a decrease in P_{int}, as might be seen with an obstructed airway and vigorous respiratory efforts, is thought to cause postobstructive pulmonary edema; although a decrease in σ is the basis for permeability pulmonary edema, concurrent surfactant dysfunction leads to an increase in surface tension and a decrease in P_{int}, also favoring the development of edema.[16-18] Remodeling of the lung parenchyma in chronic heart failure and conditions of persistently elevated P_{cap} such as mitral stenosis allow patients to tolerate a relatively high P_{cap} without developing marked pulmonary edema. Careful studies in models of chronic heart failure demonstrate a reduction in $K_{f,c}$, normal lung water despite elevated P_{cap}, and increased dry lung weight with vascular and alveolar remodeling.[19,20]

Fluid Targets

In formulating an approach to fluid management in the ventilated patient, a balance between parsimonious and generous fluid therapy needs to be considered. While this is commonly termed the "dry or wet" approach, and this may be an appropriate general description for particular groups of patients, most clinicians classify fluid therapy as (1) maintenance, (2) replacement, and (3) resuscitation fluids. In general, the tendency of ventilated patients to retain fluids, and the benefits of fluid restriction, argue for the dry approach

provided there is due attention to adequate resuscitation. A recent consensus statement classified fluid restriction as grade IIa evidence in acute lung injury (ALI) and acute respiratory distress syndrome (ARDS).[21]

MAINTENANCE FLUIDS

The volume of appropriate maintenance fluids in a ventilated patient is usually the most contentious of these parameters. As noted in Table 65-2, ∼1350 ml of fluid per day should be adequate maintenance in ventilated patients; this amount is less than in nonventilated subjects because all gases are humidified. In practice, metabolic production of water is usually ignored, allowing a total intake of 1700 ml/day; this represents a baseline volume that needs to be reviewed following clinical and biochemical assessment of plasma volume and total body water. Nevertheless, in balance, this volume should be sufficient to generate a urine output of ∼800 ml per day or 0.5 ml/kg per hour; because the normal daily solute load excreted by the kidney is ∼600 mOsm, this is easily achieved by the normal kidney with this urine volume by concentrating urine to 700–800 mOsm/L. The planned sum of enteral and parenteral maintenance fluids, however, may be less than this because of obligatory fluids given with drug infusions and hydrostatic pressure transducer flush (∼3 ml/h per transducer). Other factors influencing maintenance fluids include the size of the patient, covert losses, such as a diaphoresis, fever that increases fluid loss by ∼10 ml/kg per day for each degree of temperature elevation, and the ease of supplying adequate nutrition. Although 1700 ml is given as an adequate maintenance fluid volume, many centers use greater volumes, and many patients tolerate greater maintenance fluid volumes.

THE DRY APPROACH

The neurohumoral response to positive-pressure ventilation tends to retain sodium and water, and this may lead to both peripheral and pulmonary edema. Daily weights are inconvenient and infrequently performed in ventilated patients, and clinical examination and investigations are

TABLE 65-2 Typical Fluid Balance in Healthy (Nonventilated) Subjects and Ventilated Patients

	Healthy Subjects (ml)	Ventilated Patients (ml)
Typical obligatory fluid (water) losses		
Gastrointestinal fluid	200	200
Insensible skin loss	500	500
Humidification of inhaled air	500	0
Urine output	1000	800
Total	2200	1700
Typical fluid (water) intake		
Metabolically generated water	350	350
Water content of food	750	0
Remaining fluid intake	1100	1350
Total	2200	1700

In practice, many clinicians ignore the metabolic production of water, and prescribe 1700 ml of fluid in a ventilated patient.

relatively insensitive to edema. Peripheral edema needs to be carefully sought, and is often evident in the limbs of bedridden patients, and as a wedge-shaped swelling in the flanks. Pulmonary edema is typically detected as dependent crackles on auscultation, but this is a late sign and requires an appropriately placed stethoscope. Other techniques include chest radiographs and measurement of extravascular lung water. In addition to lack of sensitivity, these methods may be troublesome to interpret in disease states such as ALI.

Moderate hypohydration (mean 4.5% loss in body weight) leads to a reversible improvement in lung volume and airflow resistance in normal subjects.[22] Excess fluids may lead to pulmonary edema which is associated with impaired oxygenation, prolonged ventilation and ICU stay, and difficulty weaning. In both ALI and ARDS,[23] however, and in acute cardiogenic pulmonary edema,[24] extravascular lung water does not correlate with CVP or pulmonary artery occlusion pressure (PaOP). While the PaOP is an important determinant of the pulmonary capillary filtration pressure, the extravascular lung water is also influenced by permeability and temporal effects. In acute pulmonary edema, empiric treatment with diuretics, nitrates, and ventilator support will often lead to marked reduction of CVP and PaOP before resolution of the pulmonary edema.[24] Indeed, there may be transient hypovolemia secondary to extravasation of fluid in the lung, requiring volume loading.

In ALI and ARDS, extravascular lung water is usually elevated despite normal filtration pressure. Excess lung water portends a worse outcome.[25] Patients with ARDS who achieve a significant reduction in PaOP[26] or total body water, as estimated from weight loss or cumulative fluid balance,[27] are more likely to survive. Prospective, randomized studies have reported improved oxygenation in hypoproteinemic patients with ALI when a negative fluid balance was produced using furosemide and concentrated albumin;[28] and management of pulmonary edema according to lung water, as compared to PaOP, can lead to a lower cumulative fluid balance, fewer ventilator days, and shorter ICU stay.[29] Prevention of acute left ventricular failure by diuresis allows weaning in some ventilator-dependent patients with chronic obstructive pulmonary disease.[30] Fluid restriction, leading to significantly less weight gain following colonic resection, reduces both cardiopulmonary and tissue healing complications.[31] Taken together, these data suggest that accumulation of excess fluid is common, often difficult to detect, may be associated with serious adverse events, and ventricular filling pressures require careful clinical interpretation.

REPLACEMENT FLUIDS

There is little argument regarding replacement of excess fluid loss. Once the volume becomes significant or contributes to difficulties with fluid balance, it should be replaced. Typical electrolyte compositions of gastrointestinal fluids are listed in Table 65-3. In the setting of a postobstructive diuresis, it is common to use 0.45% normal saline with 10 mmol KCl per 500-ml flask; however, greater certainty

TABLE 65-3 Composition of Gastrointestinal Losses

	Volume (ml)	Na$^+$ (mmol/L)	K$^+$ (mmol/L)	Cl$^-$ (mmol/L)	HCO$_3^-$ (mmol/L)
Salivary	500–1000	50	20	40	30
Gastric	1500	60–100	10	150	30 (H$^+$)
Pancreatic	400–1000	140	5	75	115
Bile	400–1000	140	5	100	35–60
Ileal	1000–3000	140	5	70–115	30–50
Colon		60	70	15	30

As noted above, gastric fluid is usually acidic with an H$^+$ concentration of ~30 mmol/L; this will be markedly reduced by the use of proton pump inhibitors or H$_2$-antagonists.

regarding composition of excess fluid losses can be gained by measuring the electrolyte composition.

RESUSCITATION FLUIDS

Critically ill ventilated patients commonly require administration of resuscitation fluids to correct hypovolemia. Underpinning the use of resuscitation fluids is the relationship between increased ventricular preload and increased stroke volume. The trigger for a bolus of fluids often appears fairly obvious: for example, hypotension in a patient with overt bleeding. On other occasions, it may be unclear as to whether a patient will be fluid responsive or whether hemodynamic support is indicated. Yet, early recognition of the need for fluid resuscitation with rapid and titrated administration cannot be underestimated.

CHOICE OF RESUSCITATION FLUIDS

A variety of isotonic and hypertonic fluids have been examined for resuscitation, with varied results. This is often simplified as the "crystalloid versus colloid" controversy. Colloids are fluids with oncotically active contents, such as albumin (molecular weight 66 kd), which theoretically should ensure that the fluid primarily expands the plasma volume, with little contribution to interstitial volume and edema. If permeability is increased, however, these oncotic substances may also leak across into the interstitium possibly contributing to edema formation. Typical electrolyte compositions of commonly used crystalloids and colloids are listed in Table 65-4.

Blood and Blood Products

These fluids preferentially expand the plasma volume, and may be indicated for appropriate correction of coagulopathy or maintenance of oxygen carriage and delivery. An important distinction needs to be made between stable and unstable patients when considering transfusion. Data from a large randomized study of stable critically ill patients supports use of a restrictive transfusion policy using a hemoglobin (Hb) threshold of 7 g per deciliter, to aim for a target Hb of 7–9 g per deciliter.[32] Although even mild degrees of anemia can result in angina in patients with severe coronary artery disease, observational data of transfusion practice in acute myocardial infarction do not strongly argue

TABLE 65-4   Composition of Typical Crystalloids and Colloids

	Osmolality	Na+	K+	Cl−	Organic Anion
0.9% Saline[1]	300	150		150	
Hartmann's solution[1]	274	129	5	109	29 (lactate)
Ringer's lactate	272	130	4	109	28 (lactate)
Plasma-Lyte 148	296	140	5	98	50 (acetate, gluconate)
Albumex 4[2]	260	140		128	6.4 (octanoate)
Gelofusine[3]	283	144		120	
Dextran 40 in 0.9% saline	325	150		150	
Dextran 70 in 0.9% saline	306	150		150	
Hetastarch 6% in 0.9% saline	310	154		154	
7.5% saline in 6% dextran 70	2567	1283		1283	

[1]Baxter Healthcare, Toongabbie, Australia.
[2]CSL Limited, Parkville, Australia.
[3]Braun, Bella Vista, Australia.

for a higher transfusion threshold.[33] In unstable patients a different approach should be considered, and recent recommendations for management of severe sepsis and septic shock suggest a transfusion threshold of 100 g/L during the initial 6-hour resuscitation period.[34]

Crystalloid or Colloid Resuscitation

Comparing colloids and crystalloids for fluid resuscitation in critically ill patients, a recent Cochrane review[35] and a mega-trial (total 6997 patients) of saline versus albumin (SAFE)[36] found no difference in outcome. In the SAFE study more than 60% of the patients were ventilated, and the trigger for fluid loading was based on common clinical grounds and clinician judgment (Table 65-5). Although specific groups, such as post–cardiac surgery, post–liver or post–kidney transplantation, and burns were excluded, the data from the SAFE study are widely applicable to critically ill patients.[37] In current European practice,[38] most clinicians use a combination of crystalloids and colloids. Crystalloids offer equivalent efficacy, cost, and fewer adverse effects, while colloids offer more rapid volume correction, longer duration of action, reduced risk of pulmonary and interstitial edema, and they may be more appropriate for the clinical setting. While clinical practice will be influenced by the SAFE study, it seems likely that issues such as patient subgroups, cost and availability, and clinician preference will still influence choice of fluid for volume expansion.

TABLE 65-5   Clinical Signs Used by the SAFE Study that Support Volume Loading

Heart rate >90 beats/min
Systolic blood pressure (BP) <100 mmHg, or a mean BP <75 mmHg, or a 40-mmHg fall in systolic BP or mean
BP from baseline, or requirements for inotropes or vasopressors to maintain BP
Central venous pressure <10 mmHg
Pulmonary artery occlusion pressure <12 mmHg
Respiratory variation in systolic or mean BP >5 mmHg
Capillary refill >1 second
Urine output <0.5 ml/kg for 1 hour

SOURCE: Modified, with permission, from the SAFE Study Investigators.[36]

Albumin

Albumin is usually administered as either an iso-osmotic solution (e.g., 4% albumin which has 40 g/L albumin and sodium 140 mmol/L) or as a more concentrated form (e.g., 20% albumin). It appears to be the safest of the commonly used colloids[39] with a reported serious adverse event rate of ∼1 per 10[6] infusions.[40] Compared to albumin, the anaphylactoid reaction rates of comparable colloids are higher with risk ratios ∼2 for dextran, ∼4.5 for hydroxyethyl starch, and ∼12 for gelatin, with a pooled rate of ∼9 per 10[5] infusions.[39] In normal subjects, albumin has a metabolic half-life of 16–20 days, with a turnover of 12–15 g/day.[41] The normal escape of albumin from plasma occurs at about 10% per hour, which is markedly increased during sepsis with 32% of the initial rise following albumin administration lost by 4 hours.[41] Increased catabolism and reduced production of albumin by the liver also contribute to reduced serum albumin levels in critically ill patients. Albumin binds numerous substances such as fatty acids, calcium, thyroxine, amino acids, and hydrogen ions; in addition, many commonly used drugs such as warfarin, phenytoin, midazolam, and antibiotics are highly protein bound.[21] Consequently, hypoalbuminemia may have important physiologic and pharmacologic effects.

Subgroup analysis of the SAFE study suggested that patients with traumatic brain injury may have a higher mortality rate with albumin resuscitation (relative risk of death 1.62; 95% confidence interval 1.12–2.34), and that patients with severe sepsis may have a reduced mortality rate (relative risk of death 0.87; 95% confidence interval 0.74–1.02); further study, however, is needed. In patients with severe liver disease and spontaneous bacterial peritonitis, albumin reduces renal dysfunction and mortality.[42] Circulatory dysfunction following paracentesis in cirrhotic patients, defined as an increase in plasma renin activity, is reduced with albumin as compared to gelatin, dextran,[43] or saline,[44] and albumin appears preferable to gelatin for reversal of diuretic-induced hepatic encephalopathy, possibly due to a reduction in oxidant stress.[45] Finally, albumin and furosemide may have some benefit in hypoproteinemic patients with ALI.[28]

Hydoxyethyl Starch

Hydroxyethyl starch is available in a variety of molecular weights (high, medium, and low: 450–480, 130–200, and 40–70 kd), C2/C6 ratios (high and low : >8, <8), and molar substitutions (high or low : 0.6–0.7, 0.4–0.5), which alter their breakdown, intravascular half-life, and in vivo molecular weight.[46] Smaller, lower half-life starches and volumes less than 1500 ml tend to be associated with few adverse effects.[46] The bleeding risk after cardiac surgery, however, is increased, and starches have been associated with hepatic dysfunction, pruritus, and renal dysfunction;[39,47] the high in vivo molecular weight[46] is thought to contribute to hyperoncotic renal injury.[48] Starches have also been shown to have both immunosuppressive and immunostimulant effects,[49] although albumin appears to have a protective role, possibly secondary to reduced oxidant stress.[50]

Other Colloids

Dextrans are rarely used as volume expanders in ventilated patients because of increases in both bleeding risk and allergic reaction.[39,49] They are glucose polymers of either average molecular weight 40 or 70 kd, with dextran 70 sometimes used to reduce red cell and platelet sludging. Gelatins are a group of volume expanders with a low molecular weight (35 kd), leading to a half-life of about 2 hours.[49] Again allergic reactions are more common, and the main use of gelatins is outside the ICU or for short-lived periods of volume expansion, such as post–cardiac surgery.

Crystalloids

Crystalloids are usually isotonic solutions (e.g., 0.9% saline), but hypertonic solutions (e.g., 7.5% saline) have been increasingly used, particularly in the prehospital management of trauma where this may correct hypotension and reduce cerebral edema. A recent double-blind, prospective randomized study, however, comparing 7.5% saline with Ringer's lactate solution in 229 prehospital trauma patients, with a systolic BP <100 mmHg and a Glasgow Coma Scale score <9, found similar rates for hospital mortality and 6-month neurologic outcome.[51] Large volumes of 0.9% saline, or colloids that contain this electrolyte composition, may lead to a non–anion gap acidosis. An alternative approach is to use balanced crystalloids, such as Ringer's lactate (or Hartmann's solution), which contain a modest amount of organic anion (e.g., lactate or acetate) that is metabolized to bicarbonate, and tend to maintain a more normal acid-base state. Various adverse effects, such as increased production of nitric oxide, acute lung injury, hypotension, renal dysfunction, impaired gastric perfusion, nausea, abdominal pain, and bleeding have been attributed to this acidosis.[52,53] Apart from the change in acid-base state, however, there is little evidence of improved clinical outcome with a balanced solution.[54]

Isotonic fluids freely distribute into the extracellular space leading to edema and greater volume requirement than colloids. While the ratio of crystalloid to colloid needed to achieve the same effect is expected to be at least 3:1, in the SAFE study it was 1.4:1.[36] This was associated with a small but significantly greater heart rate, however, and both lower CVP and transfused volume in the crystalloid arm. In normal subjects, rapid infusion of 0.9% saline at 30 ml/kg over 20–30 minutes may reduce forced vital capacity, reduce forced expiratory volume in 1 second,[55] and produce premature airway closure and hypoxemia.[56] Maximum oxygen consumption may also be reduced, possibly because of edema of skeletal muscle and impaired O_2 diffusion.[55] A smaller volume of rapidly infused saline (10 ml/kg), however, only leads to adverse effects in patients with left-ventricular dysfunction.[57] Although there are no direct comparisons of crystalloid with colloid loading, these adverse effects, and the benefits of reducing lung water, argue for care with crystalloids. If a choice is available, it also seems sensible to use a balanced electrolyte fluid provided there is adequate hepatic function and perfusion to metabolize the associated organic anion.

Monitoring Fluid Therapy

An excess of body water in relation to sodium is manifest as hyponatremia, and deficiency of water in relation to sodium as hypernatremia, which is often associated with a disproportionate increase of urea relative to plasma creatinine. Factitious results (e.g., hyponatremia in the setting of hyperglycemia) and coexistent disease processes, such as Addison's disease, may result in hyponatremia, while sepsis and gastrointestinal blood are other common causes of a disproportionate rise in urea.

Monitoring of both the trigger and response to volume loading can be very useful because excessive fluid therapy can result in adverse events, and only 40–72% of critically ill patients increase stroke volume or cardiac output with volume loading.[58] The SAFE study[36] used simple triggers for volume loading (see Table 65-5), while recent guidelines for management of severe sepsis and septic shock[34] used a lower mean BP threshold (65 mmHg) and aimed for central or mixed venous oxygen saturation ≥70% based on improved survival and reduced organ dysfunction in a randomized study of early goal-directed therapy.[59] While perioperative mortality may be reduced in high-risk patients with a strategy that targeted increased oxygen delivery,[60] studies in critically ill patients show no benefit[61] or a worse outcome,[62] perhaps reflecting later intervention when organ dysfunction has already been initiated.

MINIMALLY INVASIVE METHODS

CHEST RADIOGRAPHS

In addition to heart size, and the presence of pulmonary infiltrates and pleural effusions, the vascular pedicle width, measured as the horizontal distance between a line dropped from the point where the left subclavian artery leaves the aortic arch to the point where the right main bronchus crosses the superior vena cava, may provide an additional useful measure of volume status. A vascular pedicle width greater than 63–70 mm can help distinguish hydrostatic from permeability pulmonary edema,[63] and it falls with negative fluid balance in ALI.[64] A decrease in vascular pedicle width of 5 mm, however, corresponded to a 3.2-liter negative balance,[64] suggesting that this technique may not be sensitive enough for acute fluid management decisions, and most patients with permeability pulmonary edema have some signs usually ascribed to volume overload.[63]

DYNAMIC MEASURES

Blood Pressure Variation

Significant changes in BP with respiration sensitively predicts an increase in blood flow with volume loading, and are a better discriminator than CVP, PaOP, or left ventricular end-diastolic area.[65–67] Initial studies used the systolic pressure variation, the difference between maximum and minimum systolic pressure, during a respiratory cycle.[66] Some subsequent studies have promoted the use of pulse pressure variation, because both systolic and diastolic pressures are influenced by changes in pleural pressure. Because a positive pressure alters both left-ventricular stroke volume and aortic pressure, pulse pressure variation may better isolate the stroke volume component. Both techniques show strong correlations with change in cardiac index, and have high sensitivity and specificity for fluid responsiveness.[65,67] Nevertheless, there are a number of important caveats: valid conclusions from arterial pressure variation requires the absence of spontaneous respiratory effort and a regular cardiac rhythm. The magnitude will vary with tidal volume, compliance of the lung and chest wall, and heart rate and aortic elastance. Many studies exclude patients with impaired left-ventricular function, and the presence of volume responsiveness is not necessarily an indication for fluid loading.[66] Similar reservations apply to the recently described use of respiratory variations in the pre-ejection period (the time between the Q wave on the ECG and the upstroke of the arterial pressure waveform)[68] and stroke volume[69] as a measure of fluid responsiveness.

Ultrasound

While left-ventricular end-diastolic area is not predictive, echocardiography has been used to assess respiratory variation in the diameter of the vena cava as a measure of fluid responsiveness. In septic patients a threshold of 36% for superior vena cava collapse during inspiration is both sensitive and specific,[70] and is not correlated with the CVP, but is similar to dynamic pulse pressure changes as a measure of fluid responsiveness. Echocardiography, however, offers the advantage of detection of severe right-ventricular failure, which may lead to false-positive results with pulse pressure variation. Respiratory changes in inferior vena cava diameter also appear promising, but may be invalidated by raised intra-abdominal pressure.[71] Because both techniques require similar conditions to those needed for BP variation measures, they may not be widely applicable in the ICU.

Parameters derived from the esophageal doppler, such as the heart-rate corrected time to peak flow (a preload measure) and the descending aortic flow, may be used to predict volume responsiveness. A number of studies have used the esophageal doppler to guide perioperative fluid management; fewer complications and shorter hospital stays were associated with greater fluid administration.[72] The use of this technique, however, appears limited in most ventilated ICU patients; they will not tolerate an esophageal probe without additional sedation, a fixed 70% of the aortic blood flow is assumed to pass to the descending aorta, and patients with irregular cardiac rhythms, an intra-aortic balloon pump, or esophageal disease are usually excluded. Although a recent review[73] found good agreement of esophageal doppler with thermodilution cardiac output, others have found substantial variability.[74,75]

INVASIVE MEASURES

CENTRAL VENOUS CATHETER

The CVP is determined by the venous return and right-heart function. It is increased by many factors, including high levels of PEEP and decreased venous capacitance; it does not correlate particularly well with right or left end-diastolic volume in critically ill patients. Although a number of studies have not found the CVP predictive of volume responsiveness,[58,67] it may still be a useful measure.[76] Above a CVP of 12 mmHg, few patients are volume responsive, and changes in the CVP may be helpful. An unchanged CVP after volume loading is suggestive of volume responsiveness, whereas a large increase is not. Similarly, the absence of a fall in CVP with spontaneous respiratory effort suggests lack of volume response.[76] Rivers et al[59] used a target CVP of 8–12 mmHg, and continuously measured the central venous oxygen saturation in their goal-directed group with a target of $\geq$70%. Under normal conditions, a mixed venous oxygen saturation of 75% corresponds to an intracellular P_{O_2} of 11 mmHg, but this falls to 0.8 mmHg at a saturation of 50%. Consequently, central venous access may be useful in determining fluid responsiveness or the need for other means of augmenting cardiac output.

Transpulmonary thermodilution is a technique that allows intermittent and continuous measurement of cardiac output, and closely agrees with pulmonary artery thermodilution measurement.[77] Additional measures include extravascular lung water and global end-diastolic volume, which is a measure of the total volume of the four heart chambers, and may be a useful preload measure.[78] In addition to central venous access, this technique requires insertion of a thermodilution arterial catheter, which is usually inserted via the femoral artery although it can be inserted via the brachial artery. While it is a promising technique, it does increase the risk of complications, and requires further investigation.

PULMONARY ARTERY CATHETER

Although the PaOP should be a measure of left-ventricular preload, it correlates poorly with left ventricular end-diastolic volume in critically ill patients, and is a poor marker of volume responsiveness. Measurement of the PaOP requires insertion of a pulmonary artery catheter which may allow measurement of a number of variables including cardiac output, pulmonary artery pressure, mixed venous oxygen saturation, and right ventricular volumes; numerous derived variables can be subsequently calculated. The accuracy and interpretation, however, of some of these data have been questioned, and serious complications from the catheter and its insertion are well described.

Retrospective analysis found that use of the pulmonary artery catheter in critically ill patients was associated with increased mortality, hospital stay, and costs despite careful adjustment for severity.[79] A more recent prospective observational study found that there was a marked increase in postoperative events.[80] Nevertheless, data measured by the pulmonary artery catheter can be extremely useful in particular patients, and central venous oxygen saturation,[59] a surrogate for mixed venous oxygen saturation, may be an important endpoint for resuscitation.

Mortality, morbidity, and complications are not influenced by the presence of a pulmonary artery catheter in patients with shock and/or ARDS,[81] although high-risk surgical patients may have a higher rate of pulmonary embolism.[82] Large prospective randomized studies are needed, and underway, with protocolized targets and treatments[59] such as fluid therapy to more fully understand this complex issue.

Conclusions

As both physiologic measures and outcome are influenced by fluid management, an integrated approach is essential to the management of ventilated patients. The tendency to retain sodium and water, and the adverse effects of pulmonary and peripheral edema, argue for a parsimonious approach to maintenance fluids, provided there is adequate resuscitation. While colloids appear as safe as crystalloids, there may be particular circumstances in which one is preferable, while it remains unclear whether balanced salt solutions improve clinical outcomes. Dynamic measures of fluid responsiveness, such as respiratory variations in blood pressure, are superior to static measures, such as an isolated CVP or PaOP reading. It is not clear, however, whether this translates into improved outcome, and resuscitation strategies based upon clinical endpoints and surrogate measures such as venous saturation improve outcome. Perhaps, more important than the choice of fluid, or assessment of fluid responsiveness, is the definition of integrated pathways that can be simply applied to patient care.

References

1. Guyton AC, Hall JE. Textbook of medical physiology, 9th ed. Philadelphia: WB Saunders Company, 1996.
2. Holmes CL, Patel BM, Russell JA, et al. Physiology of vasopressin relevant to management of septic shock. Chest 2001; 120:989–1002.
3. Iwasaki Y, Gaskill MB, Robertson GL. Adaptive resetting of the volume control of vasopressin secretion during sustained hypovolemia. Am J Physiol 1995; 268:R349–57.
4. Intersalt: An international study of electrolyte excretion and blood pressure. Results for 24 hour urinary sodium and potassium excretion. Intersalt Cooperative Research Group. BMJ 1988; 297:319–28.
5. Seri I, Kone BC, Gullans SR, et al. Locally formed dopamine inhibits Na⁺-K⁺-ATPase activity in rat renal cortical tubule cells. Am J Physiol 1988; 255:F666–73.
6. Seri I, Kone BC, Gullans SR, et al. Influence of Na⁺ intake on dopamine-induced inhibition of renal cortical Na(+)-K(+)-ATPase. Am J Physiol 1990; 258:F52–60.
7. Manoogian C, Nadler J, Ehrlich L, et al. The renal vasodilating effect of dopamine is mediated by calcium flux and prostacyclin release in man. J Clin Endocrinol Metab 1988; 66:678–83.
8. Bellomo R, Chapman M, Finfer S, et al. Low-dose dopamine in patients with early renal dysfunction: a placebo-controlled randomised trial. Australian and New Zealand Intensive Care Society (ANZICS) Clinical Trials Group. Lancet 2000; 356:2139–43.
9. Boemke W, Krebs M, Djalali K, et al. Renal nerves are not involved in sodium and water retention during mechanical ventilation in dogs. Anesthesiology 1998; 89:942–53.
10. Kaczmarczyk G, Rossaint R, Altmann C, et al. ACE inhibition facilitates sodium and water excretion during PEEP in conscious volume-expanded dogs. J Appl Physiol 1992; 73:962–7.
11. Wilkins MA, Su X-L, Palayew MD, et al. The effects of posture change and continuous positive airway pressure on cardiac natriuretic peptides in congestive heart failure. Chest 1995; 107: 909–15.
12. Andrivet P, Adnot S, Brun-Buisson C, et al. Involvement of ANF in the acute antidiuresis during PEEP ventilation. J Appl Physiol 1988; 65:1967–74.
13. Rossaint R, Krebs M, Forther J, et al. Inferior vena caval pressure increase contributes to sodium and water retention during PEEP in awake dogs. J Appl Physiol 1993; 75:2484–92.
14. Parker JC, Townsley MI. Evaluation of lung injury in rats and mice. J Appl Physiol 2004; 286:L231–6.
15. Gehlbach BK, Geppert E. The pulmonary manifestations of left heart failure. Chest 2004; 125:669–82.
16. Hilda W, Hildebrandt J. Alveolar surface tension, lung inflation, and hydration affect interstitial pressure [Px(f)]. J Appl Physiol 1984; 57:262–70.
17. Albert RK, Lakshminarayan S, Hildebrandt J, et al. Increased surface tension favors pulmonary edema formation in anesthetized dog's lungs. J Clin Invest 1979; 63:1015–8.
18. Bredenberg CE, Nieman GF, Paskanik AM, et al. Microvascular membrane permeability in high surface tension pulmonary edema. J Appl Physiol 1986; 60:253–9.
19. Townsley MI, Fu Z, Mathieu-Costello O, et al. Pulmonary microvascular permeability: Responses to high vascular pressure after induction of pacing-induced heart failure in dogs. Circ Res 1995; 77:317–25.
20. Huang W, Kingsbury MP, Turner MA, et al. Capillary filtration is reduced in lungs adapted to chronic heart failure: morphological and haemodynamic correlates. Cardiovasc Res 2001; 49:207–17.
21. Evidence-based colloid use in the critically ill: American Thoracic Society consensus statement. Am J Respir Crit Care Med 2004; 170:1247–59.
22. Javaheri S, Bosken CH, Lim SP, et al. Effects of hypohydration on lung function in humans. Am Rev Respir Dis 1987; 135:597–9.
23. Boussat S, Jacques T, Levy B, et al. Intravascular volume monitoring and extravascular lung water in septic patients with pulmonary edema. Intensive Care Med 2002; 28:712–8.
24. Bindels AJGH, van der Hoeven JG, Meinders AE. Pulmonary artery wedge pressure and extravascular lung water in patients with acute cardiogenic pulmonary edema requiring mechanical ventilation. Am J Cardiol 1999; 84:1158–63.
25. Sakka SG, Klein M, Reinhart K, et al. Prognostic value of extravascular lung water in critically ill patients. Chest 2002; 122:2080–6.
26. Humphrey H, Hall J, Sznajder I, et al. Improved survival in ARDS patients associated with a reduction in pulmonary capillary wedge pressure. Chest 1990; 97:1176–80.
27. Simmons RS, Berdine GG, Seidenfeld JJ, et al. Fluid balance and the adult respiratory distress syndrome. Am Rev Respir Dis 1987; 135:924–9.

28. Martin GS, Mangialardi RJ, Wheeler AP, et al. Albumin and furosemide therapy in hypoproteinemic patients with acute lung injury. Crit Care Med 2002; 30:2175–82.

29. Mitchell JP, Schuller D, Calandrino FS, et al. Improved outcome based on fluid management in critically ill patients requiring pulmonary artery catheterization. Am Rev Respir Dis 1992; 145: 990–8.

30. Lemaire F, Teboul JL, Cinotti L, et al. Acute left ventricular dysfunction during unsuccessful weaning from mechanical ventilation. Anesthesiology 1988; 69:171–9.

31. Brandstrup B, Tonnesen H, Beier-Holgersen R, et al. Effects of intravenous fluid restriction on postoperative complications: comparison of two perioperative fluid regimens. A randomized assessor-blinded multicenter trial. Ann Surg 2003; 238:641–8.

32. Hebert PC, Wells G, Blajchman MA, et al. The transfusion requirements in critical care investigators for the Canadian Critical Care Trials Group. A multicenter, randomized controlled clinical trial of transfusion in critical care. N Engl J Med 1999; 340:409–17.

33. Hebert PC, Fergusson DA. Do transfusions get to the heart of the matter? JAMA 2004; 292:1610–2.

34. Dellinger RP, Carlet JM, Masur H, et al for the Surviving Sepsis Campaign Management Guidelines Committee. Crit Care Med 2004; 32:858–73.

35. Roberts I, Alderson P, Bunn F, et al. Colloids versus crystalloids for fluid resuscitation in critically ill patients. Cochrane Database Syst Rev 2004; 4:CD000567.pub2.DOI:DOI 10.1002/14651858.CD000567.pub2.

36. The SAFE Study Investigators. A comparison of albumin and saline for fluid resuscitation in the intensive care unit. N Engl J Med 2004; 350:2247–56.

37. Cook D. Is albumin safe? N Engl J Med 2004; 350:2294–6.

38. Schortgen F, Deye N, Brochard L, for the CRYCO Study Group. Preferred plasma volume expanders for critically ill patients: results of an international survey. Intensive Care Med 2004; 30:2222–9.

39. Barron ME, Wilkes MM, Navickis RJ. A systematic review of the comparative safety of colloids. Arch Surg 2004; 139:552–63.

40. Von Hoegen I, Waller C. Safety of human albumin based on spontaneously reported serious adverse events. Crit Care Med 2001; 29:994–6.

41. Margarson MP, Soni NC. Changes in serum albumin concentration and volume expanding effects of a bolus of albumin 20% in septic patients. Br J Anaesth 2004; 92:821–6.

42. Sort P, Navasa M, Arroyo V, et al. Effect of intravenous albumin on renal impairment and mortality in patients with cirrhosis and spontaneous bacterial peritonitis. N Engl J Med 1999; 341:403–9.

43. Gines A, Fernandez-Esparrach G, Monescillo A, et al. Randomized trial comparing albumin, dextran 70, and polygeline in cirrhotic patients with ascites treated by paracentesis. Gastroenterology 1996; 111:1002–10.

44. Sola-Vera J, Minana J, Ricart E, et al. Randomized trial comparing albumin and saline in the prevention of paracentesis-induced circulatory dysfunction in cirrhotic patients with ascites. Hepatology 2003; 37:1147–53.

45. Jalan R, Kapoor D. Reversal of diuretic-induced hepatic encephalopathy with infusion of albumin but not colloid. Clin Sci 2004; 106:467–74.

46. Treib J, Baron J-F, Grauer MT, et al. An international view of hydroxyethyl starches. Intensive Care Med 1999; 25:258–68.

47. Schortgen F, Lacherade J-C, Bruneel F, et al. Effects of hydroxyethylstarch and gelatin on renal function in severe sepsis: a multicentre randomised trial. Lancet 2001; 357:911–6.

48. Gosling P, Rittoo D, Manji M, et al. Hydroxyethyl starch as a risk factor for acute renal failure in severe sepsis. Lancet 2001; 358:581.

49. Boldt J. Volume therapy in the intensive care patient—we are still confused, but. . . Intensive Care Med 2000; 26:1181–92.

50. Lang JD, Figueroa M, Chumley P, et al. Albumin and hydroxyethyl starch modulate oxidative inflammatory injury to vascular endothelium. Anesthesiology 2004; 100:51–8.

51. Cooper DJ, Myles PS, McDermott FT, et al, for the HTS Study Investigators. Prehospital hypertonic saline resuscitation of patients with hypotension and severe traumatic brain injury. A randomized controlled trial. JAMA 2004; 291:1350–7.

52. Pedoto A, Caruso JE, Nandi J, et al. Acidosis stimulates nitric oxide production and lung damage in rats. Am J Respir Crit Care Med 1999; 159:397–402.

53. Kellum JA, Song M, Venkataraman R. Effects of hyperchloremic acidosis on arterial pressure and circulating molecules in experimental sepsis. Chest 2004; 125:243–8.

54. Waters JH, Gottlieb A, Schoenwald P, et al. Normal saline versus lactated Ringer's solution for intraoperative fluid management in patients undergoing abdominal aortic aneurysm repair: An outcome study. Anesth Analg 2001; 93:817–22.

55. Robertson HT, Pellegrino R, Pini D, et al. Exercise response after rapid intravenous infusion of saline in healthy humans. J Appl Physiol 2004; 97:697–703.

56. Muir AL, Flenley DC, Kirby BJ, et al. Cardiorespiratory effects of rapid saline infusion in normal man. J Appl Physiol 1975; 38:786–93.

57. Puri S, Dutka DP, Baker L, et al. Acute saline infusion reduces alveolar-capillary membrane conductance and increases airflow obstruction in patients with left ventricular dysfunction. Circulation 1999; 99:1190–6.

58. Michard F, Teboul J-L. Predicting fluid responsiveness in ICU patients: A critical analysis of the evidence. Chest 2002; 121: 2000–8.

59. Rivers E, Nguyen B, Havstad S, et al, for the Early Goal-Directed Collaborative Group. Early goal directed therapy in the treatment of severe sepsis and septic shock. N Engl J Med 2001; 345:1368–77.

60. Boyd O, Grounds RM, Bennett ED. A randomized clinical trial of deliberate perioperative increase of oxygen delivery on mortality in high-risk surgical patients. JAMA 1993; 270:2699–707.

61. Gattinoni L, Brazzi L, Pelosi P, et al. A trial of goal-orientated hemodynamic therapy in critically ill patients. SvO2 collaborative group. N Engl J Med 1995; 333:1025–32.

62. Hayes MA, Timmins AC, Yau EHS, et al. Elevation of systemic oxygen delivery in the treatment of critically ill patients. N Engl J Med 1994; 330:1717–22.

63. Thomsaon JWW, Ely EW, Chiles C, et al. Appraising pulmonary edema using supine chest roentgenograms in ventilated patients. Am J Respir Crit Care Med 1998; 157:1600–8.

64. Martin GS, Ely EW, Carroll FE, et al. Findings on the portable chest radiograph correlate with fluid balance in critically ill patients. Chest 2002; 122:2087–95.

65. Kramer A, Zygun D, Hawes H, et al. Pulse pressure variation predicts fluid responsiveness following coronary artery bypass surgery. Chest 2004; 126:1563–8.

66. Magder S. Clinical usefulness of respiratory variations in arterial pressure. Am J Respir Crit Care Med 2004; 169:151–5.

67. Michard F, Boussat S, Chemla D, et al. Relation between respiratory changes in arterial pulse pressure and fluid responsiveness in septic patients with acute circulatory failure. Am J Respir Crit Care Med 2000; 162:134–8.

68. Bendjelid K, Suter PM, Romand JA. The respiratory change in preejection period: a new method to predict fluid responsiveness. J Appl Physiol 2004; 96:337–42.

69. Rex S, Brose S, Metzelder S, et al. Prediction of fluid responsiveness in patients during cardiac surgery. Br J Anaesth 2004; 93:782–8.

70. Viellard-Baron A, Cherugi K, Rabiller A, et al. Superior vena caval collapsibility as a gauge of volume status in ventilated septic patients. Intensive Care Med 2004; 30:1734–9.

71. Vignon P. Evaluation of fluid responsiveness in ventilated septic patients: back to venous return. Intensive Care Med 2004; 30:1699–1701.

72. Singer M. What's in a beat. Intensive Care Med 2003; 29:1617–20.

73. Dark PM, Singer M. The validity of trans-esophageal Doppler ultrasonography as a measure of cardiac output in critically ill adults. Intensive Care Med 2004; 30:2060–6.

74. Roeck M, Jakob SM, Boehlen T, et al. Change in stroke volume in response to fluid challenge: assessment using esophageal Doppler. Intensive Care Med 2003; 29:1729–35.

75. Kim K, Kwok I, Chang H, et al. Comparison of cardiac outputs of major burn patients undergoing extensive early escharectomy: esophageal Doppler monitor versus thermodilution pulmonary artery catheter. J Trauma 2004; 57:1013–7.

76. Magder S. More respect for the CVP. Intensive Care Med 1998; 24:651–3.

77. Della Rocca G, Costa MG, Pompei L, et al. Continuous and intermittent cardiac output measurement: pulmonary artery catheter versus aortic transpulmonary technique. Br J Anaesth 2002; 88:350–6.

78. Michard F, Alaya S, Zarka V, et al. Global end-diastolic volume as an indicator of cardiac preload in patients with septic shock. Chest 2003; 124:1900–8.

79. Connors AF Jr, Speroff T, Dawson NV, et al, for the SUPPORT investigators. The effectiveness of the right heart catheter in the initial care of critically ill patients. JAMA 1996; 276:889–97.

80. Polanczyk CA, Rohde LE, Goldman L, et al. Right heart catheterization and cardiac complications in patients undergoing noncardiac surgery: an observational study. JAMA 1996; 286:309–14.

81. Richard C, Warszawski J, Anguel N, et al, for the French Pulmonary Artery Catheter Study Group. Early use of the pulmonary artery catheter and outcomes in patients with shock and acute respiratory distress syndrome. A randomized controlled trial. JAMA 2003; 290:2713–20.

82. Sandham JD, Hull RD, Brant RF, et al, for the Canadian Critical Care Clinical Trials Group. A randomized, controlled trial of the use of pulmonary-artery catheters in high-risk surgical patients. N Engl J Med 2003; 348:5–14.

PART XV
ETHICS AND ECONOMICS

Chapter 66

THE ETHICS OF WITHHOLDING AND WITHDRAWING MECHANICAL VENTILATION

ÉLIE AZOULAY

Intensivists strive to save the lives of patients with severe conditions involving vital organs and use of sophisticated technologies to support organs until specific treatment reverses the problem. Most patients recover from the acute event, a few die rapidly, and the remainder fail to improve and remain dependent on life-sustaining treatments. In this last group, the chance of recovery changes from one day to the next, and questions often arise about the appropriateness of continuing life support, especially mechanical ventilation.[1]

Over the last half century, health care professionals in intensive care units (ICUs) have been forced to make decisions for patients who remain dependent on mechanical ventilation with death in the short term as the only possible outcome.[2] In these patients, continued treatment in the hope of cure is rarely the best option.[3] Mechanical ventilation may be prolonged beyond the point of beneficence, robbing patients of their dignity and families of their right to honest prognostic information and an opportunity to prepare for bereavement. The best option here is a decision to forego life-sustaining treatment (DFLST).

Because respiratory failure, shock, and coma are common reasons for ICU admission, mechanical ventilation is the most widely used life-sustaining treatment in the ICU.[4] Thus, mechanical ventilation is also the most common target of DFLST.[5-10] Although most patients are successfully weaned off the ventilator, a few die while on the ventilator or immediately after weaning.[11] Ideally, DFLST, which consists of moving from curative care to comfort care, should be based on the patient's wishes.[12,13] When the issue of comfort care arises, however, fewer than 5% of patients are able to participate in decisions, and knowledge of their preferences is usually unavailable.[14,15] Therefore, concern that curative care may be harmful is often voiced first by the ICU team, which then broaches the issue with the family or surrogate decision maker. Thus, barely a few years after the creation of ICUs, intensivists realized that, in addition to fighting death, their duties included the daunting task of accepting and managing death. This task requires (1) identifying situations in which all hope of recovery is lost and life-prolonging treatments become death-prolonging treatments, which should be withdrawn or withheld; (2) promptly initiating a continuous process of family care based on sensitive and straightforward information and communication; and (3) improving the ability to manage death, via epidemiologic studies of practices, interventional studies of end-of-life strategies, and continuing education aimed at honing the information and communication skills of all ICU professionals. Warding off death and restoring self-sufficiency have been the main goals of intensivists for decades; now, ICU professionals are becoming acutely aware that they must develop a professional approach to dying patients, learn what makes a "good death," and provide dying patients and their families with support, reassurance, comfort, dignity, and freedom from guilt.

The literature on end of life in the ICU comprises epidemiologic studies (descriptive, deductive, or quantitative) and qualitative studies of theoretical concepts that allow subtle interpretations of structures, experiences, roles, interactions, and perspectives. This review provides an interpretation of published data on limiting mechanical ventilation and other life-supporting treatments in patients dying in the ICU. Its goal is to help readers understand and organize the decision-making process within an ICU team and to ensure that decisions are implemented in order to give the patient a "good death" and families bereavement support.

Fundamental Issues of Ethics

The field of bioethics, born in the late 1960s, rests on four fundamental ethical principles (beneficence, nonmaleficence,

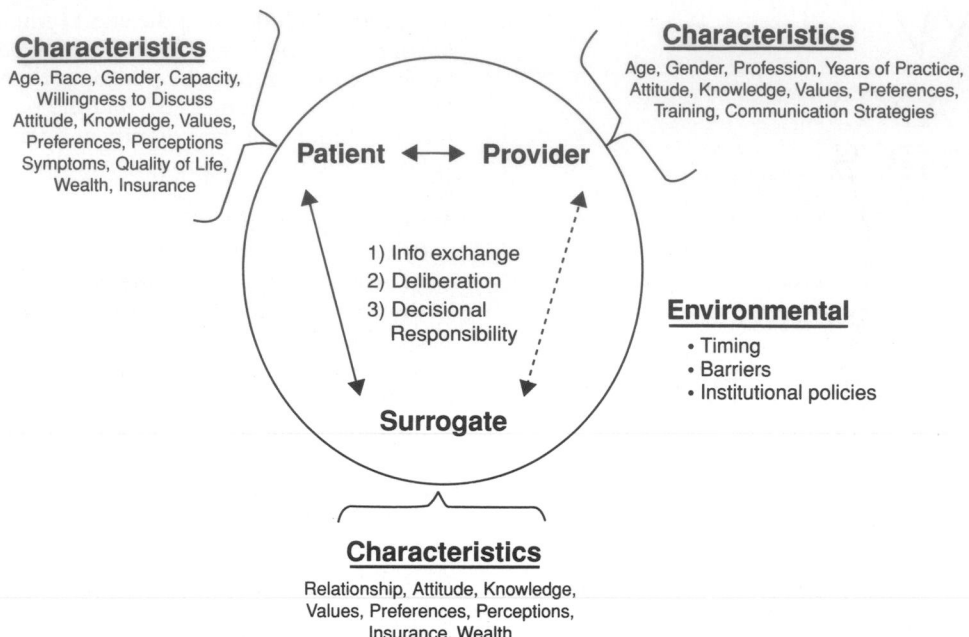

FIGURE 66-1 Conceptual framework of a patient-physician interaction. (*Adapted, with permission, from Heyland et al.*[202])

autonomy, and distributive justice) and describes a spectrum of patient-physician relationship styles ranging from paternalism to autonomy (Fig. 66-1).[16] The four fundamental ethical principles guide decisions in the ICU management of dying patients and their families. Patients are discussed here and families later on in this chapter. Regarding beneficence and nonmaleficence, I will discuss studies that address the specific needs and expectations of dying patients. I will then briefly contrast paternalism and autonomy, and I will argue that the long-standing controversy opposing these two models should give way to emphasis on the shared decision-making model. I will also discuss the principle of double-effect accepted by the U.S. Supreme Court, Society of Critical Care Medicine (SCCM) recommendations, and international consensus in the support of the use of sedation and analgesia to relieve symptoms, provided death is not intended, although it may be foreseen.[17–20] The unresolved debate regarding the relative merits of terminal extubation and terminal weaning for taking dying patients off the ventilator will be mentioned. Regarding justice, I will do my utmost to convince the reader that cost considerations are irrelevant to DFLST.

In a study by Singer et al,[21] patients identified five domains of quality end-of-life care: adequate relief from pain and anxiety,[22] avoiding inappropriate prolongation of dying, achieving a sense of control, relieving burden, and strengthening relationships with loved ones. When a patient is dying, intensivists must make it clear that they are dedicated to providing optimal care throughout the dying process;[23] to treating the patient with respect and dignity; and to relieving pain caused by physical, emotional, social, and spiritual factors.[24,25] Patients fear to be abandoned. They should be assured that the doctor is and will remain on their side, stopping useless interventions, and providing treatments that ensure comfort.[26] Encouraging family

and friends to be present at all times is another component of this effort to ensure beneficence; however, some family members may be unbearably distressed by having to spend long hours with their dying relative. The presence of a chaplain, chosen by the patient and family, and access to religious rites should be encouraged.[27]

After years of heated debate opposing autonomy and paternalism, a model in which decision making is shared with family members is gaining precedence (Fig. 66-2). This model upholds patient autonomy[28] without forcing family members to be involved in decisions they do not want to make[29] or are not ready to make.[30] The shared decision-making model stands in sharp contrast to paternalism, in which the physician shields the patient, making decisions alone in order to protect the patient and family from the potentially harmful effects of making painful decisions.[13] Because most ICU patients are unable to make decisions,[31,32] sharing in DFLST shifts to the family members.[12] Attempting to wake ICU patients so that they can participate in decisions in the name of autonomy clashes violently with the principles of beneficence and nonmaleficence.[33] Beneficence requires that family members be empowered to understand the patient's situation,[34] to identify and meet their expectations,[35,36] and to gain awareness of possible anxiety or depression that might impair their decision-making capabilities.[37] Under no circumstances should anxiety or depression in family members be used to justify benevolent paternalism; on the contrary, communication with families must receive close attention as a means of empowering families to share in decisions.[12] Reports from Canada, Sweden, and the U.S. describe sharing discussions and decisions as rational[38] and as crucial to family satisfaction.[39–42] In addition, studies of family outcomes several weeks or months after the death of a patient in the ICU have

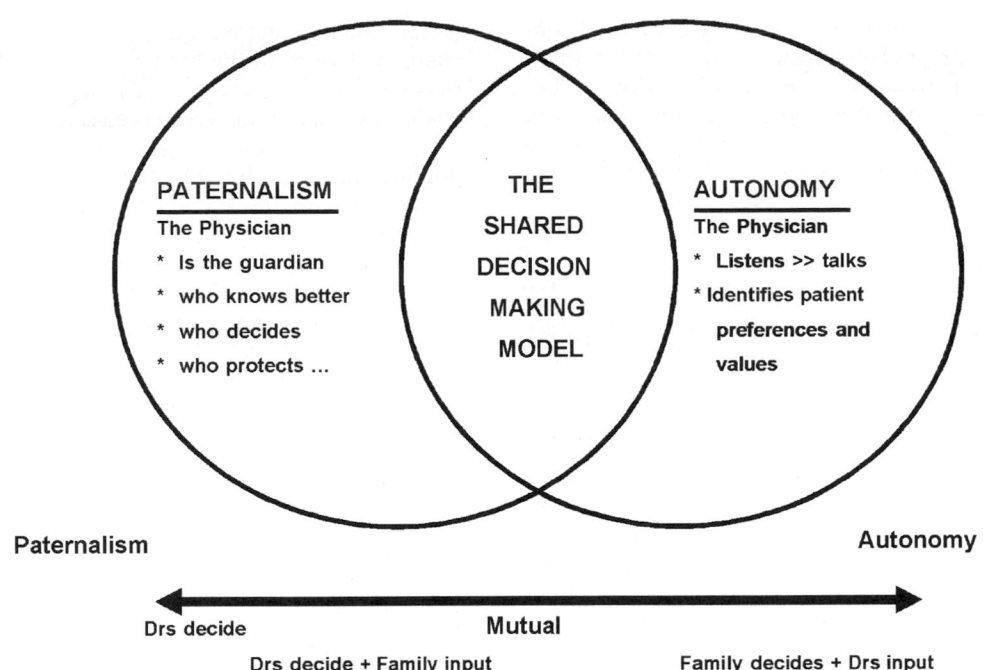

FIGURE 66-2 The shared decision-making model.

highlighted major difficulties and profound inadequacies in information.[27,43–45] Finally, nonmaleficence in this setting requires intensive communication with families if needed; a multidisciplinary approach can be used, or external ethical advice obtained, with the objective of empowering families to achieve their own goal (whether this is sharing in decisions or leaving decisions to the intensivists) and of convincing families that comfort care is preferable over aggressive interventions.[46–48] When family members have not received optimal information, involving them in the decision-making process probably carries a risk of subsequent posttraumatic stress and abnormal grief reactions.[30]

The SUPPORT studies showed a high rate of unacceptable pain in dying patients.[49,50] When withholding or withdrawing mechanical ventilation is in order, clinicians have the duty to emphasize comfort and to relieve pain and anxiety in their patients. Opioids and anxiolytics remain the reference treatment for these symptoms.[17–20] Opioids may hasten death by inducing respiratory depression,[51] but this risk is legally and ethically acceptable.[19,52–54] In contrast, use of high-dose opioids to cause death by a person making the decision alone is not consonant with optimal end-of-life care. This is voluntary euthanasia and is illegal, even in The Netherlands, Belgium, and Oregon, where patients can request and obtain the assistance of a physician to commit suicide.[19,52] Because it is the physician's intention that separates opioid use to relieve pain and anxiety from opioid use to hasten death, the line between the ethical and the unethical, the legal and the illegal, is subjective.[18,55] Although some physicians may tend to use higher doses in order to ensure patient comfort, this practice cannot be likened to euthanasia.[56] Nevertheless, eliminating ambiguity from end-of-life decisions can be extremely difficult.[57]

The optimal method for taking dying patients off the ventilator remains actively debated. The controversy consists of advocates of terminal weaning, in which volumes, respiratory rate, and F_{IO_2} are reduced gradually, versus proponents of terminal extubation with sedation,[58] which restores the normal appearance of the patient but carries a risk of respiratory secretion accumulation with asphyxia and gasping.[59,60] Terminal weaning is perceived as less active and therefore less distressing for health care professionals; furthermore, the family members are spared the ordeal of witnessing gasps, which they interpret as suffering.[61] In addition, extubation may wrongly suggest to the family that the patient is better and no longer needs the ventilator.[61] Opponents of extubation for ventilation withdrawal have pointed out that even patients who survive extubation remember the weaning period as a time of stress, discomfort, loss of hope, and extreme fear.[62]

Cost considerations have been entered into the treatment-limitation debate on the grounds that using ineffective treatments in one patient may deprive another patient of life-saving treatment or ICU admission, thereby violating the principle of distributive justice.[63] Guidelines[64] suggest that elderly patients and patients with chronic conditions (cancer, hematologic malignancies, or chronic obstructive pulmonary disease) should be denied ICU admission or should receive DFLST earlier than other patients. Whether the principle of distributive justice applies to DFLST is controversial, and the relevance of the cost/efficacy concept to ICU management has been challenged.[65] Denying ICU admission to a seriously ill patient for cost-containment reasons makes little sense, because other resources will then be used for the patient elsewhere, sometimes for a longer period and to the detriment of patient comfort.[66] Furthermore, patient-centered care allows the patient to die with dignity, free of pain and anxiety, while placing the family in optimal conditions for preparing the bereavement process.[63,67,68] Interventional studies of intensive communication with families of patients dying in the ICU found cost savings related to conflict prevention[69,70] that diminished the use of ineffective treatments.[46–48]

Terminology

Five mutually exclusive categories of DFLST have been defined. The first category is the do-not-resuscitate order for cardiac arrest. The second category comprises DFLST in patients who are in a chronic vegetative state. Third is the decision to withhold a potentially beneficial treatment (e.g., mechanical ventilation, catecholamine administration, or dialysis). Fourth is withdrawal of life-sustaining treatment. The fifth category involves active induction of death (administration of a treatment that results in death). Do-not-resuscitate orders are not relevant to the present chapter. I will not discuss patients in a chronic vegetative state, because they raise specific issues whose resolution relies on concepts that do not apply to other ICU patients. Neither will I deal with euthanasia (injection of a lethal substance), which has been used in the past but is no longer an acceptable component of end-of-life care in ICU patients. Euthanasia does not constitute care, virtually never involves a rational collegial decision-making process, leaves anxiety and pain unrelieved, and fails to respect the dignity of the patient and family. I believe that euthanasia should be banned from ICUs and all other places where medical care is delivered.

Epidemiology of the Decision to Forego Life-Sustaining Treatment in the ICU: Geographic, Cultural, and Religious Variations

Today, in most countries, most deaths in the ICU are preceded by DFLST.[7,9,40,71–75] In addition, the incidence of DFLST may be increasing over time.[76,77] In patients discharged alive from the ICU, a DFLST taken in the ICU influences hospital survival.[78] In practice, withholding mechanical ventilation precedes or occurs concomitantly with withdrawal of all other life-sustaining treatments.[10,71] Withholding and withdrawal occur within 3 days after ICU admission, and the patient usually dies within the next 24 hours. There is widespread agreement that there is no ethical difference between withholding and withdrawal,[79] although withdrawal has been described as more difficult for intensivists[72] and is not used in some countries.[71]

There are cultural variations regarding the incidence and characteristics of patients who die after DFLST, and the decision-making procedures used for withholding and withdrawing life support. These variations across countries and cultures have been identified in studies comparing practices,[80,81] studies of responses to ethical scenarios,[72,82] and vast descriptive studies.[71] Several studies have described end-of-life practices in ICUs across countries.[7,9–11,71,73,74,76,80,83–92] Table 66-1 reports the variations identified in these studies. Although compassion and respect for the patient are universally recognized as crucial, the role given to the patient's and family's opinion varies widely.[12,13] In the late 1980s the U.S. adopted a model based on patient autonomy and self-determination,[89,93] whereas other countries kept a paternalistic model in which the physician alone determines the appropriate level of treatment intensity.[7,9,72,82,83,94,95] Evidence, however, suggests that variability exists within a given country, with some physicians in traditionally paternalistic countries involving patients and families in the end-of-life decision-making process, and vice versa.[73,76,86,88] For instance, religious beliefs have been reported to influence the attitudes of intensivists toward end-of-life care.[80] The vast Ethicus study identified a number of possible explanations for variations across Europe.[71] The investigators obtained detailed descriptive data on DFLST practices in 37 ICUs in 17 European countries (Table 66-2). In southern Europe, the proportion of deaths after unsuccessful resuscitation was greater than in the rest of Europe. In northern Europe, the time from DFLST to death was shorter. In addition, the Ethicus study identified variations across religions, with Jewish, Greek Orthodox, and Muslim physicians being less likely to make DFLST.[71] These

TABLE 66-1 Variations Across Countries in the Incidence of Decisions to Forego Life-Sustaining Treatments and in Family Involvement in These Decisions

	References	WH/WD in Dying Patients (%)	Involvement of Families in Discussions and Decisions (%)
United States	6, 11, 73, 76, 88	>90	90
Canada	86, 107	80	90
Europe (Ethicus)	71	76	—
Israel	108	91 (no WD)	28
England	109	85	>90
France	7, 9, 30	50	50
Hong Kong	110	23–61	95
Spain	74	34	41
Italy	91	8	58

ABBREVIATIONS: WH, withholding; WD, withdrawal.

TABLE 66-2 Distribution of Categories of Dying Patients in Europe

	Unsuccessful CPR	Brain Death	WH	WD	Active Shortening of the Dying Process
Northern Europe	154 (10.2%)	48 (3.2%)	575 (38.2%)	714 (47.4)	14 (0.9%)
Central Europe	217 (17.9%)	92 (7.6%)	412 (34.1%)	409 (33.8%)	79 (6.5%)
Southern Europe	461 (30.1%)	190 (12.4%)	607 (39.6%)	275 (17.9%)	1 (0.1%)
Whole of Europe	832 (19.6%)	330 (7.8%)	1594 (37.5%)	1398 (32.9%)	94 (2.2%)
Hospital mortality	100%	100%	89%	89%	100%
Total	832 (19.6%)	330 (7.8%)	1594 (37.5%)	1398 (32.9%)	94 (2.2%)

ABBREVIATIONS: CPR, cardiopulmonary resuscitation; WH, withholding; WD, withdrawal.
SOURCE: Adapted, with permission, from Sprung et al.[71]

data confirm the considerable variability in approaches to bioethical issues in Europe.[80,98]

ICU admission policies may influence the incidence of DFLST. For example, the SUPPORT study group found that half the patients with chronic diseases were in the ICU within the 3 days preceding death and that one-third of patients spent at least 10 days in the ICU during the hospitalization that preceded death.[50] Similarly, in 1995, 20% of deaths in the U.S. or Canada occurred in the ICU.[99,100] Most deaths in the ICU are preceded by DFLST.[6,7,9,56,73,74,76,88,101,102] In other countries, ICU admission policies are more restrictive,[103–105] so that comparisons are inherently biased (see Table 66-1). The high incidence of in-hospital deaths, which has emerged over recent decades in industrialized countries, must be considered under the harsh light of data showing poorer quality end-of-life care in hospitals, most notably ICUs, as compared to home hospice care.[106]

Legal Decisions to Date

The courts recognize that withholding or withdrawing life-sustaining treatment and giving palliative care are legal. In the U.S., the ethical principle informing laws that allow DFLST is autonomy, manifesting as informed consent from the patient or family, who can also refuse treatment withholding or withdrawal.[14,19,52,111] Among European countries, The Netherlands was the first to allow euthanasia and physician-assisted suicide.[98] Belgium followed suit in 2002.[112,113] Nevertheless, in neither country does the law deal specifically with patients receiving life support in the ICU.[114] In France, the Senate has recently passed a law authorizing physicians to let patients die if they are kept alive only through artificial means, treatment is futile, and death is imminent.[115]

After the advances in mechanical ventilation achieved in the 1970s and 1980s, the notion that mechanical ventilation should at times be withheld or withdrawn was deeply disturbing to many intensivists. By the 1980s, however, intensivists could no longer deny that life-sustaining treatment merely prolongs the dying process in some patients.[22,79,93]

The confusion that exists between ethical concepts and legal concepts is frequently disconcerting to intensivists. From both the ethical and legal points of view, a DFLST

is acceptable only when it constitutes an expression of the patient's personal autonomy, that is, when it is made with the informed consent of a competent patient or, when the patient is incompetent, based on knowledge of the patient's wishes. All adults have the right to accept or refuse treatment and to define their preferences and values.[28,33,116,117] This right does not end when an ICU patient becomes mentally incompetent, and it can be exercised by the patient's surrogate decision maker.[14,52] In 1990, the U.S. Supreme Court upheld the withdrawal of life-sustaining treatment at a patient's request;[116] more recently, it stated that DFLST in ICUs did not constitute physician-assisted suicide or euthanasia.[118] These rulings apply to all 50 states, in theory at least. Furthermore, the Supreme Court has ruled that physicians cannot use futility as a basis for taking DFLST of their own accord. Nevertheless, the Supreme Court issued detailed recommendations on palliative care, acknowledging that sedatives and analgesics may be given, when needed, to alleviate the symptoms of a dying patient, even when this is expected—but not intended—to hasten death (the doctrine of double effect).[19]

The information above relates to the law. Physicians must comply with the laws of their country. A medical decision, however, may be legal yet unethical. I believe that the confusion between ethical principles and legal obligations that exists in the minds of many physicians can distort the decision-making process. When DFLST are entirely based on standardized criteria, which comply with the law but ignore the specific factors characterizing each individual patient,[119] they may produce deleterious effects, ranging from loss of opportunity to treat to administration of useless treatments. Furthermore, the confusion between ethical and legal obligations may hinder openness in communicating decisions; for instance, physicians may be reluctant to record the nature and implementation modalities of DFLST in the patient's medical record.[120]

When DFLST are taken, fewer than 5% of patients are able to participate in discussions or decisions.[111] In addition, patient preferences are usually not known.[20] Consequently, intensivists have turned to families as the primary partners for initiating a DFLST. The patient may be represented by a surrogate decision maker holding a durable power of attorney for health care; if the patient has not designated a surrogate, the intensivists discuss decisions with family members. The person representing the patient is asked for advice in some countries[96,115] and for decision-making input in others.[19,121]

Whether the information on patient wishes used to make DFLST in patients receiving mechanical ventilation should be obtained from family members has been challenged. Many families do not understand what is at stake;[122] have no knowledge of the patient's wishes;[123] want, but do not have, written instructions from the patient;[124] have opinions that disagree with patient wishes;[125] and, most importantly, suffer a burden of stress and anxiety that may impair their decision-making capacities.[37] Advance directives have been suggested as a means of allowing patients to remain in control of their care, even when they have lost their decision-making capacity, as is the case for intubated patients in the ICU.[126] Unfortunately, a complex set of reasons[127] impairs the effectiveness of advance directives in ensuring that patient wishes are honored[128] and that treatments given in the ICU or wards are changed in accordance with patient instructions.[67,129] In addition, patients may change their minds over time, so that advance directives may no longer reflect their wishes at the time DFLST are taken.[67,127-130] Interestingly, a 1990 survey among members of the American Thoracic Society found that one-third of respondents provided care that contradicted the wishes of patients and surrogates, and that more than 80% unilaterally made and implemented DFLST, at times over the objections of patients and surrogates.[84] Finally, the SUPPORT investigators found that 10% of older inpatients with serious illnesses received care they did not want[49] and that advance directives or families' wishes were often disregarded.[50] Having a specifically trained nurse talk to the patients, families, physicians, and other hospital staff members failed to improve compliance with patients' wishes.[50] I next discuss the role for the surrogate.

The Decision-Making Procedure: High Complexity, High Stakes

Evaluating the prognosis is the key issue: when continuing mechanical ventilation and other aggressive interventions, that may ensure recovery from the acute life-threatening event that prompted ICU admission, full care must be provided, without which the patient may suffer a loss of chance. Therefore, intensivists must be able to identify those patients whose chances of recovery are virtually nonexistent. For these patients, aggressive care, far from inducing benefits, prolongs the dying process, puts the patient's dignity in jeopardy, and hinders the bereavement process for family members. Clearly, the stakes are extraordinarily high for all concerned with the decision, who must achieve a consensus about what to do and how to do it.

Because DFLST force patients, families, and health care professionals to stand very close to the line that separates killing from allowing patients to die, they carry a destructive power that must be acknowledged and kept under control. To this end, intensivists have worked on developing decision-making procedures that maximize objectivity, legitimacy, serenity, and agreement among all those involved. Two main factors govern DFLST: the imminence of death and the patient's wishes regarding life support. The first

factor was investigated by pursuing two avenues concomitantly: one consisted in defining futility, a concept based on clinical experience, and the other in developing mortality-prediction tools, based on physiologic disturbances or organ failures. These efforts were intended to assist in objectively identifying situations that warrant DFLST; however, they failed to reduce the complexity of the decision-making process. The second factor, patient wishes, faced a major obstacle: the inability of most patients to express their wishes at the time DFLST are considered.[10,20,71] To ensure that patient wishes would nevertheless be honored, three approaches were suggested: advance directives, formal designation of a surrogate decision maker holding a durable power of attorney, and family participation in decisions.

I will now discuss data from the literature on mortality prediction and respect for patient wishes. Predicting mortality has relied chiefly on severity scores developed in the U.S. and Europe[131-134] to characterize patients (based on age, chronic morbidities, recruitment type, and severity of each organ involvement) and to constitute homogeneous patient groups (i.e., groups with a similar risk of hospital death). These scores have proved useful for measuring the performance of ICUs (via determination of the standardized mortality ratio [SMR]) and for establishing homogeneous patient groups for inclusion in therapeutic trials. Their poor calibration and discrimination, however, make them unhelpful for predicting the risk of death in the individual patient. Furthermore, because these scores are determined at a single point in time (ICU admission) and developed in a given population, they fail to reflect changes in organ failures over time[135,136] or advances made in the management of a specific condition[137] Therefore, mortality-prediction scores are of no assistance in deciding when treatment withholding or withdrawal is appropriate.

Futility is a concept that was widely used to determine that DFLST were appropriate. The patient benefit–centered view defines futility as use of interventions that are unlikely to benefit the patient.[138] I prefer the definition suggested by Schneiderman et al in 1990: "When physicians conclude (either through personal experience, experiences shared with colleagues, or consideration of published empiric data) that in the last 100 cases a medical treatment has been useless, they should regard that treatment as futile," and "if the likelihood of functional recovery after a proposed course of therapy is less than 1%, then physicians may assert the prerogative to withdraw therapy without the consent of the patient or surrogate decision maker."[139]

The concept of futility has been fiercely criticized. Its opponents argue that the definition of futility is neither clear nor reproducible, the concept is clearly intended to increase the power of the physician while undermining patient autonomy, treatment data do not necessarily apply to an individual patient, the 1% cutoff is not supported by scientific evidence, and the use of futility allows physicians to make decisions unilaterally.[140,141] The futility debate ultimately condenses into a conflict in which patients or families and physicians disagree about the patient's right to receive a treatment that is highly unlikely to succeed. The futility concept fails to acknowledge the huge amount of excellent work done by ICU professionals to involve families in the decision-making process and to recognize the emotional and social problems raised by family participation in decision making.[29,30] Rather than speak of the physician's right to withhold or withdraw treatment, we should speak of the physician's duty to prepare the ICU team and the family for a clearly identifiable shift from curative care to care aimed at optimizing patient comfort and dignity while alleviating distress in the family members.[142,143] ICU teams must move beyond the futility debate toward a position firmly rooted in a care, an ethic which gives a meaningful role to all staff members (physicians, nurses, and other health care professionals) in organizing the decision-making process with the patients and families, while interfacing with health care institutions, third-party payers, and, most importantly, the general public.[144]

Factors Associated with Decisions to Forego Life-Sustaining Treatment

Several studies compared patients with and without decisions to withhold or withdraw mechanical ventilation. The decision to withhold or withdraw mechanical ventilation from an ICU patient usually rests on patient age, previous health status (cognitive function, self-sufficiency, and chronic morbidities), time spent in the ICU, severity at ICU admission, and worsening organ failure despite ICU management.[7,9,11,71] Nevertheless, these factors may be overshadowed by events or perceptions that develop during an ICU stay,[145] such as dependency on catecholamines and intensivists' perceptions that the prognosis is poor and the condition irreversible.[10] Thus, multiple factors exist and may compete with one another, clearly indicating a need for a rigorous and collegial decision-making process based on consensus-building centered on the patient's and family's preferences.[9,94,146,147] Several studies show that intensivists pay close attention to quality of life.[7,9,72,84,86] Nevertheless, there is evidence that intensivists underestimate the quality of life of their patients, and that quality of life does not influence patient preferences regarding the intensity of treatment received in the ICU.[148]

Studies have found that the frequency and nature of DFLST vary with the personal characteristics of physicians and with their experience.[28,149] As pointed out above, religious beliefs and cultural background play a role. In addition, physician gender,[81] specialty,[150] time working in ICUs,[151] working in private versus public institutions,[152] and teaching status of the hospital[88] influence practices regarding end-of-life care.[88,150]

The Decision-Making Procedure: A Response that Adapts Continuously to Unfolding Events

Christakis et al identified four major sources of bias affecting the nature of treatments withdrawn from patients in whom a DFLST had been made.[153] These biases may have clini-

cal, social, and ethical consequences. Intensivists were more likely to withdraw treatments supporting organs that failed for chronic or "natural" reasons than for iatrogenic reasons, treatments started recently, and treatments whose withdrawal would result in immediate death, although when the diagnosis was uncertain, they preferred treatment withdrawals that resulted in delayed death. Similarly, Asch et al found that intensivists preferred to withdraw treatments that were expensive, scarce, and invasive.[154] The incidence of DFLST increases with ICU stay duration, indicating that intensivists respond rationally to persistent or worsening organ failures by adapting their management strategy.[20] Thus, Cook et al identified several time-dependent factors associated with withdrawal of mechanical ventilation: dependency on catecholamines, the physician's prediction of a low likelihood of surviving the ICU stay or a high likelihood of poor cognitive function, and physician perception that the patient did not want life support.[10] Recent data on prolonged mechanical ventilation in ICU patients showed a high rate of major dependency among survivors.[155–157] Asch et al reported that treatment withdrawal in the ICU usually occurs in the following order: blood products, dialysis, catecholamines, mechanical ventilation, parenteral nutrition, antibiotics, infusions, and enteral nutrition.[158] Whereas Cook et al found that mechanical ventilation was often stopped at the same time as dialysis or catecholamines,[10,97] others reported that mechanical ventilation was sometimes continued after the withdrawal of dialysis and catecholamines.[7,9] In France, nutrition and hydration are rarely withdrawn.[7,9] Thus, even when a DFLST is taken, the sequence of withdrawals is influenced by multiple, complex, nonclinical factors that may seem irrelevant. These factors may be ethical, social, religious, or related to family preferences.[86] In one study, the same intensivists made contradictory decisions about the same clinical scenarios at different points in time.[159] Similarly, our group and others have shown that making a DFLST influences survival independently of all other factors known to affect survival, indicating that DFLST depend in part on setting-specific characteristics that are difficult to identify.[160–162]

Who Decides?

For simplicity, I will artificially distinguish two phases in the end-of-life management of ICU patients. The first phase is making the DFLST by building a consensus that treatment must move from curative interventions to palliative (comfort) care.[26] Ideally, this consensus is achieved using the shared decision-making model recommended by SCCM in 2001 and an international consensus conference in 2003.[17,18] In this model, the decision is made by a well-organized team in which physicians and nurses communicate openly, determine a patient's preferences soon after admission, and communicate often with the family to provide information and other components of family care. From the beginning of the decision-making process, the family members participate, either by bearing witness to the patient's wishes or by explaining their own wishes.[12] Most families accept and understand the need for DFLST. When this is not the case, negotiations between the ICU staff and the family may rapidly put an end to the conflict.[69] Nevertheless, a previous conflict, inadequate information, or economic restrictions imposed by managed care may lead families to view DFLST with distrust.[163] The course of action implicitly recommended to physicians is to refrain from implementing their decision over the objections of the family.[164] On the contrary, physicians should intensify communication with families,[3] initiate a process of negotiation,[89,165-167] seek external advice, or show families that the decision is consistent with institutional policies and recommendations issued by learned societies.[111,168] The literature emphasizes strongly that DFLST are clinical procedures,[169] taken by ICU teams that are acutely aware of the complexity of end-of-life care and determined to respect both ethical principles and the dignity of patients and families.[170-172] Also obvious from the literature is that intensivists are aware of the need to continuously improve their communication skills and their ability to support dying patients and their families.[40,171,173-178]

The second phase in the end-of-life management of ICU patients consists in implementing the DFLST. This requires an organized strategy relying on both human and technological resources to meet the expectations of patients and families. ICU teams must learn this approach, if needed with the help of palliative care teams or consulting ethicists, where available.[17,18,20,46,70,146,165,168-170,177,179,180] This phase may last a few hours to a few days. Support must be provided not only to families, but also to ICU staff members, who should be confident at all times that comfort care is preferable over the use of sophisticated technologies that prolong life artificially.[181] The ICU team may need to orchestrate the dying process by adjusting the treatment to the needs of the family (e.g., maintaining mechanical ventilation unchanged until the entire family is ready or a family member arrives from a far-away location).[181,182]

The ICU Health Care Team: A Key Role in Communicating with Families of Dying Patients

Several studies have sought to identify the needs and expectations of families of ICU patients.[35,36,39,41,183] The specific needs of families of dying patients have been investigated in studies of the overall long-term impact on families of the ICU experience and bereavement,[27,43-45,49,184,185] in studies of interventions (the presence of families during resuscitation or involvement of families in decisions),[30,186] and in studies of the impact of family conferences on the DFLST process.[173,187] Families have stated that a pain-free death was a key priority,[49] and that they often perceived information as quantitatively or qualitatively inadequate. For instance, some families complained that they did not know the cause of death. These data have been used to identify specific needs of families of patients dying in the ICU (Tables 66-3 and 66-4).[18,20] Keenan et al found that fami-

TABLE 66-3 Ten Most Important Needs of Families of Critically Ill Dying Patients

1. To be with the person
2. To be helpful to the dying person
3. To be informed of the dying person's changing condition
4. To understand what is being done to the patient and why
5. To be assured of the patient's comfort
6. To be comforted
7. To express emotions
8. To be assured that their decisions were right
9. To find meaning in the dying of their loved one
10. To be fed, hydrated, and rested

SOURCE: Reproduced, with permission, from Truog et al.[18]

lies had seven major needs directly related to the decision-making process: that the process be well explained, that it proceed as expected, that the patient be comfortable, that the discussion be initiated by a member of the ICU team, that the family and friends be prepared for the decision, that the family be allowed privacy during implementation of the DFLST, and the family be given opportunities to voice concerns and to make special requests.[184] Others have emphasized the importance of meeting the spiritual and religious needs of patients and family members.[27,188]

Meeting these needs empowers and motivates families to participate in the process of deciding to forego life-sustaining treatment. Burdens weighing on families should not be construed as reasons to exclude families from decision making.[12] Conversely, involving families at all costs without previously providing them with information and with psychological and social support may lead to severe residual disorders, including severe persistent guilt and abnormal bereavement.[30,186] Thus, sharing decisions with families is intricately linked with a procedure of intensive communication that supports and guides the family at the time of the DFLST.[46-48,168,180] The reasons justifying a DFLST and, subsequently, the specific implementation modalities are discussed, usually during family conferences attended by members of the family and members of the ICU team (physicians, nurses, and social workers).[146] Informal conversations, however, at the bedside or in the hallway or waiting room are also useful and may involve a

TABLE 66-4 A Dozen Needs of the Family in the Setting of Critical Illness

1. To have questions answered honestly
2. To know specific facts about what is wrong with the patient
3. To know the prognosis for recovery
4. To be called at home about changes in the patient's status
5. To receive information from the physician (at least) once daily
6. To receive information in understandable language
7. To believe that hospital personnel care about the patient
8. To be assured of the patient's comfort
9. To be comforted
10. To express emotions
11. To find meaning in the death of their loved one
12. To have the opportunity to eat, drink, and sleep

SOURCE: Reproduced, with permission, from Prendergast et al.[20]

smaller number of people (often the intensivist and the patient's spouse). Nevertheless, formal family conferences are invaluable for strengthening communication between the family and the ICU team. They should be offered as often as needed, and at least once for each family.

During the conferences, the ICU team members are familiar faces for the family members, and the physician leading the conference starts by introducing each person. Each conference is prepared by the ICU team to establish a consensus among staff members[174,189-192] as a prerequisite to the development of a consensus with the family.[20,166,167,190] Regular decision-making meetings of physicians and nurses and debriefing meetings are essential to ensure that physicians and nurses understand one another's points of view.[12] Similarly, because residents receive insufficient training in ethical principles,[193] informal discussions between residents and seniors should be encouraged to improve residents' confidence in withdrawal decisions. Residents should also be encouraged to participate in family meetings.[194] During family conferences, the word "death" should be used and the manner in which the patient will die should be explained to the family members, with emphasis on patient comfort. The ICU staff must allow the family members to speak and to vent their emotions, but they must also anticipate questions the family members cannot bring themselves to ask.[173,187] Studies have shown not only that inadequate information is a source of dissatisfaction among families of patients dying in the ICU, but also that targeted interventions aimed at improving communication may be ineffective.[50] In addition, clinicians lack training in techniques that help families consider decision sharing, express their opinions, and cope with the attendant burden.[170,193,195,196]

A key objective of the family conference is to assure family members that the patient's wishes will be honored, although the patient is incompetent.[170] Neither families nor health care professionals know how to predict patients' wishes regarding DFLST in the ICU.[122,124,130,192,197,198] In practice, the physicians must first ask the family whether the patient has expressed wishes about end-of-life care. If the patient has expressed wishes, then the family members describe them and use substituted judgment to participate in DFLST. When nothing is known about the patient's wishes, the best interests of the patient guide the decision-making process. Placing the patient's wishes at the center of the discussions and negotiations ensures that decision making is of high moral and ethical quality despite the absence of patient participation.[167] Surrogate decision makers should receive active support from the ICU team.[46] Furthermore, by making it clear that families speak for their loved one and not for themselves, this approach should minimize feelings of guilt secondary to involvement in DFLST.[199]

For most DFLST, a consensus is achieved rapidly with the family.[76] In difficult cases, a process of negotiation should be initiated to convince the family that the patient cannot survive and that the patient's best interests govern decisions.[200] It may be possible to continue life support for a few hours in order to convince the family that the patient's condition is irreversible. Compassion and understanding must sustain the relationship with families. Families are often dissatisfied with the level of communication, but are unable to express their dissatisfaction because they do not wish to provoke an open conflict. Intensive communication is the only road leading from a potential battle of diverging opinions to a consensus in which the family accepts, probably with pain and sadness, that the best care available for their loved one is discontinuation of aggressive artificial treatments and continuous painstaking attention to comfort. This awareness that treatments must be withheld or withdrawn is acquired via a multifaceted process whose components are cognitive (understanding the information and trusting the ICU team), emotional (believing that the patient is not being abandoned but has reached the end of his or her life[20]), and interpersonal (protecting the family and friends from long-term harm related to participation in decision making).[185,201] At this stage, lifting restrictions on visiting hours and encouraging participation in patient care (washing, massaging, pain-relief treatment, and so on) provides families with a sense of comfort, intimacy, and utility. Family members have a strong desire for opportunities to communicate with the patient (by touching, speaking, looking at photos, and listening to music). The health care professionals must respect the silence, rituals, emotions, and religious practices of each family. Again, everything must be done to minimize feelings of guilt.

Conclusion

Mechanical ventilation is the life-sustaining treatment most often used in the ICU. Most patients are successfully weaned off the ventilator. A few, however, cannot recover from their disease, remain dependent on the ventilator, and have a very high likelihood of death in the short term. In this situation, intensivists must engage in the complex process of deciding to withdraw mechanical ventilation. These patients must be offered the best possible death. We must remain at their side and on their side, keeping them comfortable at all times, while encouraging family involvement in decisions and care, if they so wish, welcoming family members in the ICU as partners rather than as visitors, alleviating their guilt, and helping them to prepare for the bereavement process.

Over the last 15 years, several descriptive studies have provided detailed epidemiologic data on practices and changes to practices over time, as well as on targets for improvement. Qualitative studies have helped us to understand the complexity of the decision-making process, to recognize that upholding ethical principles requires more than compliance with the law, and to distinguish intentions from practices. The results of these studies indicate a need for major improvements in end-of-life care for ICU patients, most notably regarding our skill in communicating, imparting information, and organizing and implementing treatment withholding and withdrawal. Further knowledge of the decision-making process and of the individuals involved in it will help to improve our end-of-life practices, rest our DFLST on ethical principles, and validate the shared decision-making model by studies of outcomes in family members long after the ICU experience. Serving the principle of autonomy requires not only that a patient's wishes be honored, but also that the family be able to proceed through the bereavement process with the least possible guilt, remorse, and regret. Thus, our end-of-life practice should be tailored to the specific characteristics of each region and culture, each clinical situation, each patient, each family, and each ICU professional.

In the future, intensive multidisciplinary programs and early incorporation of palliative care into ICU management should be encouraged in order to improve information and communication. Multidisciplinary teams could either handle communication with families of dying patients or assist the ICU staff members and teach them palliative care strategies. Data from the literature strongly support a strong emphasis on palliative care.[203,204] By facilitating prognostic information and promoting communication with patients and families, huge efforts on the part of investigators have been successful in identifying patient preferences and wishes regarding treatment intensity. Use of a palliative strategy has reduced medical futility and avoided prolongation of dying. This program of intensive palliative care offered to dying ICU patients holds promise as a means of improving communication at a time when openness is crucial.[47,48,168,203,204] Nevertheless, the generalizability and feasibility of this strategy require evaluation in a range of countries and cultures.[50] A possible obstacle may be a feeling on the part of the ICU staff that they are less useful, because they no longer play a role in end-of-life care. Recognizing this possible obstacle and ensuring open communication between the ICU team and the palliative care team should be a priority.

References

1. Ruark JE, Raffin TA. Initiating and withdrawing life support. Principles and practice in adult medicine. N Engl J Med 1988; 318:25–30.
2. Emanuel EJ. Should physicians withhold life-sustaining care from patients who are not terminally ill? Lancet 1988; 1:106–8.
3. Burns JP, Edwards J, Johnson J, Cassem NH, Truog RD. Do-not-resuscitate order after 25 years. Crit Care Med 2003; 31:1543–50.
4. Tobin MJ. Advances in mechanical ventilation. N Engl J Med 2001; 344:1986–96.
5. Jayes RL, Zimmerman JE, Wagner DP, Draper EA, Knaus WA. Do-not-resuscitate orders in intensive care units. Current practices and recent changes. JAMA 1993; 270:2213–7.
6. Hall RI, Rocker GM. End-of-life care in the ICU: treatments provided when life support was or was not withdrawn. Chest 2000; 118:1424–30.
7. Ferrand E, Robert R, Ingrand P, Lemaire F. Withholding and withdrawal of life support in intensive-care units in France: a prospective survey. French LATAREA Group. Lancet 2001; 357:9–14.
8. Lee DK, Swinburne AJ, Fedullo AJ, Wahl GW. Withdrawing care. Experience in a medical intensive care unit. JAMA 1994; 271:1358–61.
9. Pochard F, Azoulay E, Chevret S, et al. French intensivists do not apply American recommendations regarding decisions to forgo life-sustaining therapy. Crit Care Med 2001; 29:1887–92.
10. Cook D, Rocker G, Marshall J, et al. Withdrawal of mechanical ventilation in anticipation of death in the intensive care unit. N Engl J Med 2003; 349:1123–32.
11. Smedira NG, Evans BH, Grais LS, et al. Withholding and withdrawal of life support from the critically ill. N Engl J Med 1990; 322:309–15.
12. Azoulay E, Sprung CL. Family-physician interactions in the intensive care unit. Crit Care Med 2004; 32:2323–8.
13. Cook D. Patient autonomy versus parentalism. Crit Care Med 2001; 29(2 Suppl):N24–5.
14. Luce JM. New standards for patient rights and medical competence. Crit Care Med 2000; 28:3114–5.
15. Way J, Back AL, Curtis JR. Withdrawing life support and resolution of conflict with families. BMJ 2002; 325:1342–5.
16. Beauchamp TL. Methods and principles in biomedical ethics. J Med Ethics 2003; 29:269–74.
17. Carlet J, Thijs LG, Antonelli M, et al. Challenges in end-of-life care in the ICU. Statement of the 5th International Consensus Conference in Critical Care: Brussels, Belgium, April 2003. Intensive Care Med 2004; 30:770–84. Epub 2004 Apr 20.
18. Truog RD, Cist AF, Brackett SE, et al. Recommendations for end-of-life care in the intensive care unit: The Ethics Committee of the Society of Critical Care Medicine. Crit Care Med 2001; 29:2332–48.
19. Luce JM, Alpers A. End-of-life care: what do the American courts say? Crit Care Med 2001; 29(2 Suppl):N40–5.
20. Prendergast TJ, Puntillo KA. Withdrawal of life support: intensive caring at the end of life. JAMA 2002; 288:2732–40.
21. Singer PA, Lowy FH. Rationing, patient preferences, and cost of care at the end of life. Arch Intern Med 1992; 152:478–80.
22. Good care of the dying patient. Council on Scientific Affairs, American Medical Association. JAMA 1996; 275:474–8.
23. Quill TE. Perspectives on care at the close of life. Initiating end-of-life discussions with seriously ill patients: addressing the "elephant in the room". JAMA 2000; 284:2502–7.
24. Emanuel LL. Facing requests for physician-assisted suicide: toward a practical and principled clinical skill set. JAMA 1998; 280:643–7.
25. Emanuel EJ, Daniels ER, Fairclough DL, Clarridge BR. The practice of euthanasia and physician-assisted suicide in the United States: adherence to proposed safeguards and effects on physicians. JAMA 1998; 280:507–13.
26. Faber-Langendoen K, Lanken PN. Dying patients in the intensive care unit: forgoing treatment, maintaining care. Ann Intern Med 2000; 133:886–93.
27. Abbott KH, Sago JG, Breen CM, Abernethy AP, Tulsky JA. Families looking back: one year after discussion of withdrawal or withholding of life-sustaining support. Crit Care Med 2001; 29:197–201.
28. Quill TE, Brody H. Physician recommendations and patient autonomy: finding a balance between physician power and patient choice. Ann Intern Med 1996; 125:763–9.
29. Azoulay E, Pochard F, Chevret S, et al. Half the family members of intensive care unit patients do not want to share in the decision-making process: a study in 78 French intensive care units. Crit Care Med 2004; 32:1832–8.
30. Azoulay E, Pochard F, Kentish-Barnes N, et al. Risk of posttraumatic stress symptoms in family members of intensive care unit patients. Am J Respir Crit Care Med 2005; 21:21.
31. Sprung CL, Eidelman LA. Worldwide similarities and differences in the foregoing of life-sustaining treatments. Intensive Care Med 1996; 22:1003–5.
32. Campbell ML, Bizek KS, Thill M. Patient responses during rapid terminal weaning from mechanical ventilation: a prospective study. Crit Care Med 1999; 27:73–7.
33. Tonelli MR. Waking the dying: must we always attempt to involve critically ill patients in end-of-life decisions? Chest 2005; 127:637–42.

34. Azoulay E, Chevret S, Leleu G, et al. Half the families of intensive care unit patients experience inadequate communication with physicians. Crit Care Med 2000; 28:3044–9.

35. Johnson D, Wilson M, Cavanaugh B, et al. Measuring the ability to meet family needs in an intensive care unit. Crit Care Med 1998; 26:266–71.

36. Azoulay E, Pochard F, Chevret S, et al. Meeting the needs of intensive care unit patient families: a multicenter study. Am J Respir Crit Care Med 2001; 163:135–9.

37. Pochard F, Azoulay E, Chevret S, et al. Symptoms of anxiety and depression in family members of intensive care unit patients: ethical hypothesis regarding decision-making capacity. Crit Care Med 2001; 29:1893–7.

38. Epstein RM, Alper BS, Quill TE. Communicating evidence for participatory decision making. JAMA 2004; 291:2359–66.

39. Heyland DK, Tranmer JE. Measuring family satisfaction with care in the intensive care unit: the development of a questionnaire and preliminary results. J Crit Care 2001; 16:142–9.

40. Sjokvist P, Nilstun T, Svantesson M, Berggren L. Withdrawal of life support—who should decide? Differences in attitudes among the general public, nurses and physicians. Intensive Care Med 1999; 25:949–54.

41. Wasser T, Pasquale MA, Matchett SC, Bryan Y, Pasquale M. Establishing reliability and validity of the critical care family satisfaction survey. Crit Care Med 2001; 29:192–6.

42. Hanson LC, Danis M, Garrett JM, Mutran E. Who decides? Physicians' willingness to use life-sustaining treatment. Arch Intern Med 1996; 156:785–9.

43. Cuthbertson SJ, Margetts MA, Streat SJ. Bereavement follow-up after critical illness. Crit Care Med 2000; 28:1196–201.

44. Covinsky KE, Goldman L, Cook EF, et al. The impact of serious illness on patients' families. SUPPORT Investigators. Study to Understand Prognoses and Preferences for Outcomes and Risks of Treatment. JAMA 1994; 272:1839–44.

45. Malacrida R, Bettelini CM, Degrate A, et al. Reasons for dissatisfaction: a survey of relatives of intensive care patients who died. Crit Care Med 1998; 26:1187–93.

46. Lilly CM, De Meo DL, Sonna LA, et al. An intensive communication intervention for the critically ill. Am J Med 2000; 109:469–75.

47. Dowdy MD, Robertson C, Bander JA. A study of proactive ethics consultation for critically and terminally ill patients with extended lengths of stay. Crit Care Med 1998; 26:252–9.

48. Schneiderman LJ, Gilmer T, Teetzel HD. Impact of ethics consultations in the intensive care setting: a randomized, controlled trial. Crit Care Med 2000; 28:3920–4.

49. Lynn J, Teno JM, Phillips RS, et al. Perceptions by family members of the dying experience of older and seriously ill patients. SUPPORT Investigators. Study to Understand Prognoses and Preferences for Outcomes and Risks of Treatments. Ann Intern Med 1997; 126:97–106.

50. A controlled trial to improve care for seriously ill hospitalized patients. The study to understand prognoses and preferences for outcomes and risks of treatments (SUPPORT). The SUPPORT Principal Investigators. JAMA 1995; 274:1591–8.

51. Quill TE, Dresser R, Brock DW. The rule of double effect—a critique of its role in end-of-life decision making. N Engl J Med 1997; 337:1768–71.

52. Luce JM, Alpers A. Legal aspects of withholding and withdrawing life support from critically ill patients in the United States and providing palliative care to them. Am J Respir Crit Care Med 2000; 162:2029–32.

53. Sulmasy DP, Pellegrino ED. The rule of double effect: clearing up the double talk. Arch Intern Med 1999; 159:545–50.

54. Sulmasy DP, Sood JR, Ury WA. The quality of care plans for patients with do-not-resuscitate orders. Arch Intern Med 2004; 164:1573–8.

55. Quill TE. The ambiguity of clinical intentions. N Engl J Med 1993; 329:1039–40.

56. Keenan SP, Busche KD, Chen LM, et al. A retrospective review of a large cohort of patients undergoing the process of withholding or withdrawal of life support. Crit Care Med 1997; 25:1324–31.

57. Quill TE. Barbiturates in the care of the terminally ill. N Engl J Med 1993; 328:1350, author reply 1.

58. Holzapfel L, Demingeon G, Piralla B, Biot L, Nallet B. A four-step protocol for limitation of treatment in terminal care. An observational study in 475 intensive care unit patients. Intensive Care Med 2002; 28:1309–15.

59. Brody H, Campbell ML, Faber-Langendoen K, Ogle KS. Withdrawing intensive life-sustaining treatment—recommendations for compassionate clinical management. N Engl J Med 1997; 336:652–7.

60. Krishna G, Raffin TA. Terminal weaning from mechanical ventilation. Crit Care Med 1999; 27:9–10.

61. Faber-Langendoen K. The clinical management of dying patients receiving mechanical ventilation. A survey of physician practice. Chest 1994; 106:880–8.

62. Cook DJ, Meade MO, Perry AG. Qualitative studies on the patient's experience of weaning from mechanical ventilation. Chest 2001; 120(6 Suppl):469S–473S.

63. Pronovost P, Angus DC. Economics of end-of-life care in the intensive care unit. Crit Care Med 2001; 29(2 Suppl):N46–N51.

64. Guidelines for intensive care unit admission, discharge, and triage. Task Force of the American College of Critical Care Medicine, Society of Critical Care Medicine. Crit Care Med 1999; 27:633–8.

65. Understanding Costs and Cost-Effectiveness in Critical Care. Report from the Second American Thoracic Society Workshop on Outcomes Research. Am J Respir Crit Care Med 2002; 165:540–50.

66. Luce JM, Rubenfeld GD. Can health care costs be reduced by limiting intensive care at the end of life? Am J Respir Crit Care Med 2002; 165:750–4.

67. Danis M, Mutran E, Garrett JM, et al. A prospective study of the impact of patient preferences on life-sustaining treatment and hospital cost. Crit Care Med 1996; 24:1811–7.

68. Emanuel EJ. Cost savings at the end of life. What do the data show? JAMA 1996; 275:1907–14.

69. Studdert DM, Mello MM, Burns JP, et al. Conflict in the care of patients with prolonged stay in the ICU: types, sources, and predictors. Intensive Care Med 2003; 29:1489–97. Epub 2003 Jul 19.

70. Burns JP, Mello MM, Studdert DM, et al. Results of a clinical trial on care improvement for the critically ill. Crit Care Med 2003; 31:2107–17.

71. Sprung CL, Cohen SL, Sjokvist P, et al. End-of-life practices in European intensive care units: the Ethicus Study. JAMA 2003; 290:790–7.

72. Vincent JL. Forgoing life support in western European intensive care units: the results of an ethical questionnaire. Crit Care Med 1999; 27:1626–33.

73. Prendergast TJ, Claessens MT, Luce JM. A national survey of end-of-life care for critically ill patients. Am J Respir Crit Care Med 1998; 158:1163–7.

74. Esteban A, Gordo F, Solsona JF, et al. Withdrawing and withholding life support in the intensive care unit: a Spanish prospective multi-centre observational study. Intensive Care Med 2001; 27:1744–9.

75. Eidelman LA, Jakobson DJ, Worner TM, et al. End-of-life intensive care unit decisions, communication, and documentation: an evaluation of physician training. J Crit Care 2003; 18:11–6.

76. Prendergast TJ, Luce JM. Increasing incidence of withholding and withdrawal of life support from the critically ill. Am J Respir Crit Care Med 1997; 155:15–20.

77. Jakobson DJ, Eidelman LA, Worner TM, et al. Evaluation of changes in forgoing life-sustaining treatment in Israeli ICU patients. Chest 2004; 126:1969–73.

78. Azoulay E, Adrie C, De Lassence A, et al. Determinants of postintensive care unit mortality: a prospective multicenter study. Crit Care Med 2003; 31:428–32.

79. Withholding and withdrawing life-sustaining therapy. This Official Statement of the American Thoracic Society was adopted by the ATS Board of Directors, March 1991. Am Rev Respir Dis 1991; 144(3 Pt 1):726–31.

80. Asai A, Fukuhara S, Lo B. Attitudes of Japanese and Japanese-American physicians towards life-sustaining treatment. Lancet 1995; 346:356–9.

81. Mebane EW, Oman RF, Kroonen LT, Goldstein MK. The influence of physician race, age, and gender on physician attitudes toward advance care directives and preferences for end-of-life decision-making. J Am Geriatr Soc 1999; 47:579–91.

82. Vincent JL. Cultural differences in end-of-life care. Crit Care Med 2001; 29(2 Suppl):N52–5.

83. Abizanda R, Almendros Corral L, Balerdi Perez B. [Ethical aspects of intensive medicine. Results of an opinion survey.] Med Clin (Barc) 1994; 102:521–6.

84. Asch DA, Hansen-Flaschen J, Lanken PN. Decisions to limit or continue life-sustaining treatment by critical care physicians in the United States: conflicts between physicians' practices and patients' wishes. Am J Respir Crit Care Med 1995; 151(2 Pt 1):288–92.

85. Asch DA, DeKay ML. Euthanasia among US critical care nurses. Practices, attitudes, and social and professional correlates. Med Care 1997; 35:890–900.

86. Cook DJ, Guyatt GH, Jaeschke R, et al. Determinants in Canadian health care workers of the decision to withdraw life support from the critically ill. Canadian Critical Care Trials Group. JAMA 1995; 273:703–8.

87. Heyland DK, Rocker GM, O'Callaghan CJ, Dodek PM, Cook DJ. Dying in the ICU: perspectives of family members. Chest 2003; 124:392–7.

88. Keenan SP, Busche KD, Chen LM, et al. Withdrawal and withholding of life support in the intensive care unit: a comparison of teaching and community hospitals. The Southwestern Ontario Critical Care Research Network. Crit Care Med 1998; 26:245–51.

89. Teres D. Trends from the United States with end of life decisions in the intensive care unit. Intensive Care Med 1993; 19:316–22.

90. Wenger NS, Pearson ML, Desmond KA, et al. Epidemiology of do-not-resuscitate orders. Disparity by age, diagnosis, gender, race, and functional impairment. Arch Intern Med 1995; 155:2056–62.

91. Giannini A, Pessina A, Tacchi EM. End-of-life decisions in intensive care units: attitudes of physicians in an Italian urban setting. Intensive Care Med 2003; 29:1902–10. Epub 2003 Sep 11.

92. Cardoso T, Fonseca T, Pereira S, Lencastre L. Life-sustaining treatment decisions in Portuguese intensive care units: a national survey of intensive care physicians. Crit Care 2003; 7:R167–75. Epub 2003 Oct 06.

93. Consensus report on the ethics of foregoing life-sustaining treatments in the critically ill. Task Force on Ethics of the Society of Critical Care Medicine. Crit Care Med 1990; 18:1435–9.

94. Vincent JL. Information in the ICU: are we being honest with our patients? The results of a European questionnaire. Intensive Care Med 1998; 24:1251–6.

95. Emanuel EJ, Emanuel LL. Four models of the physician-patient relationship. JAMA 1992; 267:2221–6.

96. Luce JM, Lemaire F. Two transatlantic viewpoints on an ethical quandary. Am J Respir Crit Care Med 2001; 163:818–21.

97. Cook DJ, Guyatt G, Rocker G, et al. Cardiopulmonary resuscitation directives on admission to intensive-care unit: an international observational study. Lancet 2001; 358:1941–5.

98. van der Maas PJ, van der Wal G, Haverkate I, et al. Euthanasia, physician-assisted suicide, and other medical practices involving the end of life in the Netherlands, 1990–1995. N Engl J Med 1996; 335:1699–705.

99. McLean RF, Tarshis J, Mazer CD, Szalai JP. Death in two Canadian intensive care units: institutional difference and changes over time. Crit Care Med 2000; 28:100–3.

100. Angus DC, Barnato AE, Linde-Zwirble WT, et al. Use of intensive care at the end of life in the United States: an epidemiologic study. Crit Care Med 2004; 32:638–43.

101. Faber-Langendoen K, Bartels DM. Process of forgoing life-sustaining treatment in a university hospital: an empirical study. Crit Care Med 1992; 20:570–7.

102. Faber-Langendoen K. A multi-institutional study of care given to patients dying in hospitals. Ethical and practice implications. Arch Intern Med 1996; 156:2130–6.

103. Sprung CL, Geber D, Eidelman LA, et al. Evaluation of triage decisions for intensive care admission. Crit Care Med 1999; 27:1073–9.

104. Azoulay E, Pochard F, Chevret S, et al. Compliance with triage to intensive care recommendations. Crit Care Med 2001; 29:2132–6.

105. Garrouste-Orgeas M, Montuclard L, Timsit JF, et al. Triaging patients to the ICU: a pilot study of factors influencing admission decisions and patient outcomes. Intensive Care Med 2003; 29:774–81. Epub 2003 Apr 02.

106. Teno JM, Clarridge BR, Casey V, et al. Family perspectives on end-of-life care at the last place of care. JAMA 2004; 291:88–93.

107. Heyland DK, Lavery JV, Tranmer JE, Shortt SE, Taylor SJ. Dying in Canada: is it an institutionalized, technologically supported experience? J Palliat Care 2000; 16(Suppl):S10–6.

108. Soudry E, Sprung CL, Levin PD, Grunfeld GB, Einav S. Forgoing life-sustaining treatments: comparison of attitudes between Israeli and North American intensive care healthcare professionals. Isr Med Assoc J 2003; 5:770–4.

109. Turner JS, Michell WL, Morgan CJ, Benatar SR. Limitation of life support: frequency and practice in a London and a Cape Town intensive care unit. Intensive Care Med 1996; 22:1020–5.

110. Buckley TA, Joynt GM. Limitation of life support in the critically ill: the Hong Kong perspective. Ann Acad Med Singapore 2001; 30:281–6.

111. Luce JM. Making decisions about the forgoing of life-sustaining therapy. Am J Respir Crit Care Med 1997; 156:1715–8.

112. The Belgian act on euthanasia of May, 28th 2002. Eur J Health Law 2003; 10:329–35.

113. Nys H. A presentation of the Belgian act on euthanasia against the background of Dutch euthanasia law. Eur J Health Law 2003; 10:239–55.

114. Damas F, Damas P, Lamy M. Euthanasia: a law in Belgium? Intensive Care Med 2001; 27:1683.

115. Lemaire FJ. A law for end of life care in France? Intensive Care Med 2004; 30:2120.

116. Luce JM. Three patients who asked that life support be withheld or withdrawn in the surgical intensive care unit. Crit Care Med 2002; 30:775–80.

117. Meier DE, Morrison RS. Autonomy reconsidered. N Engl J Med 2002; 346:1087–9.

118. Alpers A, Lo B. Does it make clinical sense to equate terminally ill patients who require life-sustaining interventions with those who do not? JAMA 1997; 277:1705–8.

119. Whitney SN, McGuire AL, McCullough LB. A typology of shared decision making, informed consent, and simple consent. Ann Intern Med 2004; 140:54–9.

120. Kirchhoff KT, Anumandla PR, Foth KT, Lues SN, Gilbertson-White SH. Documentation on withdrawal of life support in adult patients in the intensive care unit. Am J Crit Care 2004; 13:328–34.

121. Heyland DK, Cook DJ, Rocker GM, et al. Decision-making in the ICU: perspectives of the substitute decision-maker. Intensive Care Med 2003; 29:75–82.

122. Upadya A, Muralidharan V, Thorevska N, Amoateng-Adjepong Y, Manthous CA. Patient, physician, and family member understanding of living wills. Am J Respir Crit Care Med 2002; 166:1430–5.

123. Rabow MW, Hauser JM, Adams J. Supporting family caregivers at the end of life: "they don't know what they don't know". JAMA 2004; 291:483–91.

124. Hines SC, Glover JJ, Babrow AS, et al. Improving advance care planning by accommodating family preferences. J Palliat Med 2001; 4:481–9.

125. Terry PB, Vettese M, Song J, et al. End-of-life decision making: when patients and surrogates disagree. J Clin Ethics 1999; 10:286–93.

126. Emanuel EJ, Emanuel LL, Orentlicher D. Advance directives. JAMA 1991; 266:2563.

127. Prendergast TJ. Advance care planning: pitfalls, progress, promise. Crit Care Med 2001; 29(2 Suppl):N34–9.

128. Danis M, Southerland LI, Garrett JM, et al. A prospective study of advance directives for life-sustaining care. N Engl J Med 1991; 324:882–8.

129. Goodman MD, Tarnoff M, Slotman GJ. Effect of advance directives on the management of elderly critically ill patients. Crit Care Med 1998; 26:701–4.

130. Sulmasy DP, Terry PB, Weisman CS, et al. The accuracy of substituted judgments in patients with terminal diagnoses. Ann Intern Med 1998; 128:621–9.

131. Knaus WA, Zimmerman JE, Wagner DP, Draper EA, Lawrence DE. APACHE-acute physiology and chronic health evaluation: a physiologically based classification system. Crit Care Med 1981; 9:591–7.

132. Knaus WA, Draper EA, Wagner DP, Zimmerman JE. APACHE II: a severity of disease classification system. Crit Care Med 1985; 13:818–29.

133. Le Gall JR, Lemeshow S, Saulnier F. A new Simplified Acute Physiology Score (SAPS II) based on a European/North American multicenter study. JAMA 1993; 270:2957–63.

134. Le Gall JR, Klar J, Lemeshow S, et al. The Logistic Organ Dysfunction system. A new way to assess organ dysfunction in the intensive care unit. ICU Scoring Group. JAMA 1996; 276:802–10.

135. Timsit JF, Fosse JP, Troche G, et al. Accuracy of a composite score using daily SAPS II and LOD scores for predicting hospital mortality in ICU patients hospitalized for more than 72 h. Intensive Care Med 2001; 27:1012–21.

136. Timsit JF, Fosse JP, Troche G, et al. Calibration and discrimination by daily LOD scoring comparatively with daily SOFA scoring for predicting hospital mortality in critically ill patients. Crit Care Med 2002; 30:2003–13.

137. Sculier JP, Paesmans M, Markiewicz E, Berghmans T. Scoring systems in cancer patients admitted for an acute complication in a medical intensive care unit. Crit Care Med 2000; 28:2786–92.

138. Schneiderman LJ, Spragg RG. Ethical decisions in discontinuing mechanical ventilation. N Engl J Med 1988; 318:984–8.

139. Schneiderman LJ, Jecker NS, Jonsen AR. Medical futility: its meaning and ethical implications. Ann Intern Med 1990; 112:949–54.

140. Schneiderman LJ, Jecker NS, Jonsen AR. Medical futility: response to critiques. Ann Intern Med 1996; 125:669–74.

141. Prendergast TJ. Futility and the common cold. How requests for antibiotics can illuminate care at the end of life. Chest 1995; 107:836–44.

142. Schneiderman LJ, Jecker NS, Jonsen AR. Abuse of futility. Arch Intern Med 2001; 161:128–30.

143. Schneiderman LJ. The rise and fall of the futility movement. N Engl J Med 2000; 343:1575, discussion 6–7.

144. Schneiderman LJ, Faber-Langendoen K, Jecker NS. Beyond futility to an ethic of care. Am J Med 1994; 96:110–4.

145. Rocker G, Cook D, Sjokvist P, et al. Clinician predictions of intensive care unit mortality. Crit Care Med 2004; 32:1149–54.

146. Curtis JR, Patrick DL, Shannon SE, et al. The family conference as a focus to improve communication about end-of-life care in the intensive care unit: opportunities for improvement. Crit Care Med 2001; 29(2 Suppl):N26–33.

147. Ravenscroft AJ, Bell MD. 'End-of-life' decision making within intensive care—objective, consistent, defensible? J Med Ethics 2000; 26:435–40.

148. Uhlmann RF, Pearlman RA. Perceived quality of life and preferences for life-sustaining treatment in older adults. Arch Intern Med 1991; 151:495–7.

149. Kaplan SH, Greenfield S, Gandek B, Rogers WH, Ware JE Jr. Characteristics of physicians with participatory decision-making styles. Ann Intern Med 1996; 124:497–504.

150. Luce JM, Breeling JL. Critical care practices of chest physicians. Chest 1988; 93:163–5.

151. Kelly WF, Eliasson AH, Stocker DJ, Hnatiuk OW. Do specialists differ on do-not-resuscitate decisions? Chest 2002; 121:957–63.

152. Kollef MH. Private attending physician status and the withdrawal of life-sustaining interventions in a medical intensive care unit population. Crit Care Med 1996; 24:968–75.

153. Christakis NA, Asch DA. Biases in how physicians choose to withdraw life support. Lancet 1993; 342:642–6.

154. Asch DA, Christakis NA. Why do physicians prefer to withdraw some forms of life support over others? Intrinsic attributes of life-sustaining treatments are associated with physicians' preferences. Med Care 1996; 34:103–11.

155. Chelluri L, Im KA, Belle SH, et al. Long-term mortality and quality of life after prolonged mechanical ventilation. Crit Care Med 2004; 32:61–9.

156. Herridge MS, Cheung AM, Tansey CM, et al. One-year outcomes in survivors of the acute respiratory distress syndrome. N Engl J Med 2003; 348:683–93.

157. Im K, Belle SH, Schulz R, Mendelsohn AB, Chelluri L. Prevalence and outcomes of caregiving after prolonged mechanical ventilation in the ICU. Chest 2004; 125:597–606.

158. Asch DA, Faber-Langendoen K, Shea JA, Christakis NA. The sequence of withdrawing life-sustaining treatment from patients. Am J Med 1999; 107:153–6.

159. Walter SD, Cook DJ, Guyatt GH, et al. Confidence in life-support decisions in the intensive care unit: a survey of healthcare workers. Canadian Critical Care Trials Group. Crit Care Med 1998; 26:44–9.

160. Azoulay E, Pochard F, Garrouste-Orgeas M, et al. Decisions to forgo life-sustaining therapy in ICU patients independently predict hospital death. Intensive Care Med 2003; 29:1895–901.

161. Shepardson LB, Youngner SJ, Speroff T, Rosenthal GE. Increased risk of death in patients with do-not-resuscitate orders. Med Care 1999; 37:727–37.

162. Sulmasy DP. Do patients die because they have DNR orders, or do they have DNR orders because they are going to die? Med Care 1999; 37:719–21.

163. Luce JM. The art of negotiating. Crit Care Med 2001; 29:1078–9.

164. Rivera S, Kim D, Garone S, Morgenstern L, Mohsenifar Z. Motivating factors in futile clinical interventions. Chest 2001; 119:1944–7.

165. Bowman KW. Communication, negotiation, and mediation: dealing with conflict in end-of-life decisions. J Palliat Care 2000; 16(Suppl):S17–23.

166. Prendergast TJ. Resolving conflicts surrounding end-of-life care. New Horiz 1997; 5:62–71.

167. Miller DK, Coe RM, Hyers TM. Achieving consensus on withdrawing or withholding care for critically ill patients. J Gen Intern Med 1992; 7:475–80.

168. Schneiderman LJ, Gilmer T, Teetzel HD, et al. Effect of ethics consultations on nonbeneficial life-sustaining treatments in the intensive care setting: a randomized controlled trial. JAMA 2003; 290:1166–72.

169. Mularski RA, Bascom P, Osborne ML. Educational agendas for interdisciplinary end-of-life curricula. Crit Care Med 2001; 29(2 Suppl):N16–23.

170. Clarke EB, Curtis JR, Luce JM, et al. Quality indicators for end-of-life care in the intensive care unit. Crit Care Med 2003; 31:2255–62.

171. Curtis JR, Patrick DL, Engelberg RA, et al. A measure of the quality of dying and death. Initial validation using after-death interviews with family members. J Pain Symptom Manage 2002; 24:17–31.

172. Fried TR, Bradley EH, Towle VR, Allore H. Understanding the treatment preferences of seriously ill patients. N Engl J Med 2002; 346:1061–6.

173. Curtis JR, Engelberg RA, Wenrich MD, et al. Missed opportunities during family conferences about end-of-life care in the intensive care unit. Am J Respir Crit Care Med 2005; 171: 844–9.

174. Danis M, Federman D, Fins JJ, et al. Incorporating palliative care into critical care education: principles, challenges, and opportunities. Crit Care Med 1999; 27:2005–13.

175. DeVita MA, Arnold RM, Barnard D. Teaching palliative care to critical care medicine trainees. Crit Care Med 2003; 31:1257–62.

176. Nyman DJ, Sprung CL. End-of-life decision making in the intensive care unit. Intensive Care Med 2000; 26:1414–20.

177. Johnson N, Cook D, Giacomini M, Willms D. Towards a "good" death: end-of-life narratives constructed in an intensive care unit. Cult Med Psychiatry 2000; 24:275–95.

178. Nelson JE, Danis M. End-of-life care in the intensive care unit: where are we now? Crit Care Med 2001; 29(2 Suppl):N2–9.

179. Fins JJ, Solomon MZ. Communication in intensive care settings: the challenge of futility disputes. Crit Care Med 2001; 29(2 Suppl):N10–5.

180. Lilly CM, Sonna LA, Haley KJ, Massaro AF. Intensive communication: four-year follow-up from a clinical practice study. Crit Care Med 2003; 31(5 Suppl):S394–9.

181. Seymour JE. Negotiating natural death in intensive care. Soc Sci Med 2000; 51:1241–52.

182. Cook DJ, Giacomini M, Johnson N, Willms D. Life support in the intensive care unit: a qualitative investigation of technological purposes. Canadian Critical Care Trials Group. CMAJ 1999; 161:1109–13.

183. Curtis JR, Engelberg RA, Wenrich MD, et al. Studying communication about end-of-life care during the ICU family conference: development of a framework. J Crit Care 2002; 17:147–60.

184. Keenan SP, Mawdsley C, Plotkin D, Webster GK, Priestap F. Withdrawal of life support: how the family feels, and why. J Palliat Care 2000; 16(Suppl):S40–4.

185. Steinhauser KE, Christakis NA, Clipp EC, et al. Factors considered important at the end of life by patients, family, physicians, and other care providers. JAMA 2000; 284:2476–82.

186. Robinson SM, Mackenzie-Ross S, Campbell Hewson GL, Egleston CV, Prevost AT. Psychological effect of witnessed resuscitation on bereaved relatives. Lancet 1998; 352:614–7.

187. McDonagh JR, Elliott TB, Engelberg RA, et al. Family satisfaction with family conferences about end-of-life care in the intensive care unit: increased proportion of family speech is associated with increased satisfaction. Crit Care Med 2004; 32:1484–8.

188. Lo B, Ruston D, Kates LW, et al. Discussing religious and spiritual issues at the end of life: a practical guide for physicians. JAMA 2002; 287:749–54.

189. Asch DA. The role of critical care nurses in euthanasia and assisted suicide. N Engl J Med 1996; 334:1374–9.

190. Ferrand E, Lemaire F, Regnier B, et al. Discrepancies between perceptions by physicians and nursing staff of intensive care unit end-of-life decisions. Am J Respir Crit Care Med 2003; 167:1310–5. Epub 2003 Jan 24.

191. Puntillo KA, Benner P, Drought T, et al. End-of-life issues in intensive care units: a national random survey of nurses' knowledge and beliefs. Am J Crit Care 2001; 10:216–29.

192. Kirchhoff KT, Beckstrand RL. Critical care nurses' perceptions of obstacles and helpful behaviors in providing end-of-life care to dying patients. Am J Crit Care 2000; 9:96–105.

193. Stevens L, Cook D, Guyatt G, et al. Education, ethics, and end-of-life decisions in the intensive care unit. Crit Care Med 2002; 30:290–6.

194. Moreau D, Goldgran-Toledano D, Alberti C, et al. Junior versus senior physicians for informing families of intensive care unit patients. Am J Respir Crit Care Med 2003; 4:4.

195. Curtis JR, Patrick DL, Caldwell ES, Collier AC. Why don't patients and physicians talk about end-of-life care? Barriers to communication for patients with acquired immunodeficiency syndrome and their primary care clinicians. Arch Intern Med 2000; 160:1690–6.

196. Hanson LC, Tulsky JA, Danis M. Can clinical interventions change care at the end of life? Ann Intern Med 1997; 126:381–8.

197. Covinsky KE, Fuller JD, Yaffe K, et al. Communication and decision-making in seriously ill patients: findings of the SUPPORT project. The Study to Understand Prognoses and Preferences for Outcomes and Risks of Treatments. J Am Geriatr Soc 2000; 48(5 Suppl):S187–93.

198. Treece PD, Engelberg RA, Crowley L, et al. Evaluation of a standardized order form for the withdrawal of life support in the intensive care unit. Crit Care Med 2004; 32:1141–8.

199. Arnold RM, Kellum J. Moral justifications for surrogate decision making in the intensive care unit: implications and limitations. Crit Care Med 2003; 31(5 Suppl):S347–53.

200. Goold SD, Williams B, Arnold RM. Conflicts regarding decisions to limit treatment: a differential diagnosis. JAMA 2000; 283: 909–14.

201. Hammes BJ, Rooney BL. Death and end-of-life planning in one midwestern community. Arch Intern Med 1998; 158:383–90.

202. Heyland DK, Rocker GM, Dodek PM, et al. Family satisfaction with care in the intensive care unit: results of a multiple center study. Crit Care Med 2002; 30:1413–8.

203. Campbell ML, Guzman JA. A proactive approach to improve end-of-life care in a medical intensive care unit for patients with terminal dementia. Crit Care Med 2004; 32:1839–43.

204. Campbell ML, Guzman JA. Impact of a proactive approach to improve end-of-life care in a medical ICU. Chest 2003; 123: 266–71.

INTERPRETING CLINICAL TRIALS OF MECHANICAL VENTILATION: THE IMPORTANCE OF ROUTINE CARE

KATHERINE J. DEANS
PETER C. MINNECI
XIZHONG CUI
STEVEN M. BANKS
CHARLES NATANSON
PETER Q. EICHACKER

ROUTINE PRACTICE: A RELATIONSHIP BETWEEN SEVERITY OF LUNG INJURY AND TIDAL VOLUME SELECTION
INTERPRETING FIVE LOW-TIDAL-VOLUME TRIALS IN THE CONTEXT OF ROUTINE PRACTICE IN THE 1990S
DOES UNDERSTANDING OF CURRENT PRACTICE HELP EXPLAIN THE DIFFERENCES AMONG LOW-TIDAL-VOLUME TRIALS?
CONCLUSION

Mechanical ventilation has been the primary supportive therapy for the acute respiratory distress syndrome (ARDS) ever since the first description of this lethal condition in the 1960s. Clinical application of mechanical ventilation, however, in patients with ARDS has evolved. Notably, laboratory evidence during the 1980s suggested that tidal volumes should be reduced to prevent lung injury from excessive distention (volutrauma) and pressure (barotrauma).[1–3] Clinical studies employing historical controls in the early 1990s supported this approach.[4,5]

Based on this body of evidence, the suspected benefits associated with reductions in tidal volume and airway pressure were tested in randomized trials. In five trials, initiated between 1992 and 1996, patients with ARDS or acute lung injury (ALI) were randomized to receive either a high or low tidal volume independent of the severity of their underlying lung injury.[6–11] None of these trials included a current-practice control arm, or characterized the relationship between tidal volume adjustment and severity of lung injury before the trial. While three of these trials failed to show significant differences in outcome comparing low and high tidal volumes, two reported significant improvements in survival with low-tidal-volume strategies. At the time, explanations for these disparate results were based on dif-

ferences in the size of the trials or insufficient reductions in tidal volume in the three trials not showing significant effects.[12,13] Proponents of the two beneficial trials believed the results provided strong evidence supporting use of low tidal volumes in all patients with ARDS or ALI; yet, studies have shown that physicians have been reluctant to adopt this practice.[12–19]

In order to make recommendations on how current practice should incorporate the results of these five trials, it is important to understand why these five trials differed and why physicians appear to be reluctant to prescribe low tidal volumes to all patients with ARDS. We believe that such clarification requires an understanding of then-current practice at the time the studies were conducted. In order to reassess the results of the five trials, we will present the results of surveys and a consensus conference as well as retrospective studies of ventilator management in the 1990s.

Routine Practice: A Relationship between Severity of Lung Injury and Tidal Volume Selection

A survey was conducted in 1992 to characterize how intensivists diagnosed and managed patients with ARDS and ALI.[20] The intensivists were asked to choose from one of five tidal volume categories: <5, 5–9, 10–13, 14–17, or 17 ml/kg. Of the more than 1000 respondents to this survey, 93% indicated they would use tidal volumes of 5–9 ml/kg or 10–13 ml/kg. Almost all (96%) also stated that tidal volume selection was influenced by level of airway pressure. A consensus conference 1 year later recommended lowering tidal volumes in patients with ARDS to as low as 5 ml/kg during mechanical ventilation to avoid plateau airway pressures of 35 cmH_2O or greater.[21] Based on these data, existing practice in the 1990s is characterized by the use of lower tidal volumes in patients with more severe ARDS and less compliant lungs and higher volumes in patients with less severe disease and greater lung compliance. These approaches resulted in overall airway pressures that were considered safe in the early 1990s. Although this survey and consensus conference did not provide data to demonstrate such a relationship, recent studies looking back at routine practice in the 1990s are consistent with this relationship.

One retrospective study assessed mechanical ventilation in 398 patients with ARDS or ALI in three teaching hospitals in Minnesota from 1994 to 2001.[18] Combined across all years of the study, tidal volumes were significantly lower in patients with greater lung injury (Fig. 67-1A). Moreover, mean plateau airway pressures were consistently kept close to or below 30 cmH_2O every year of the study (Fig. 67-1B). In an international survey conducted over a 1-month period in 1998, routine ventilator practice was assessed in 467 patients with ARDS from 361 intensive care units in 20 countries.[22,23] Tidal volumes in these patients were normally distributed over a wide range (Fig. 67-2A). Tidal volumes were lowest in patients with the least compliant lungs; tidal volumes increased as the lungs became more compliant (Fig. 67-2B).

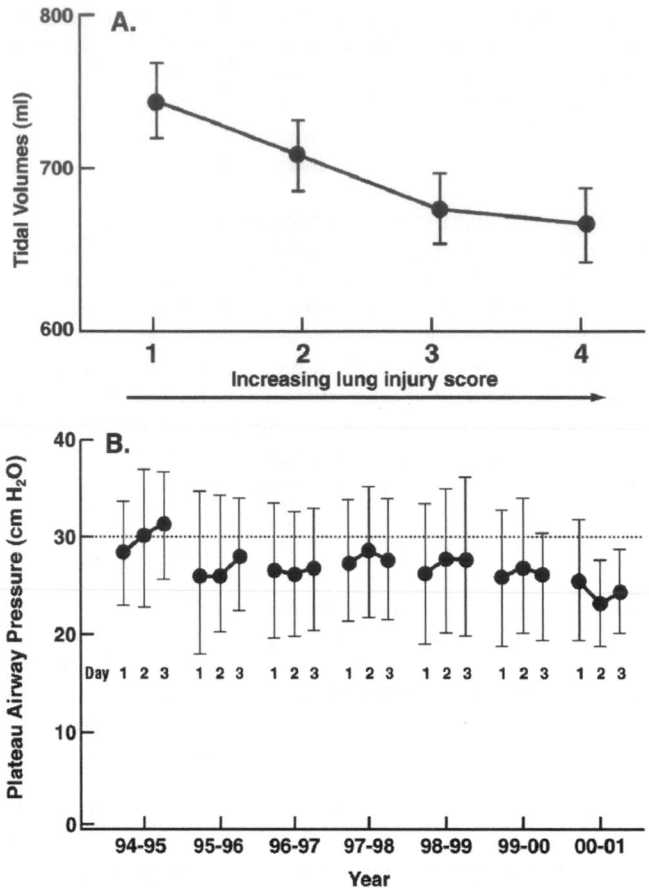

FIGURE 67-1 Relationship between tidal volume and surrogate markers of lung injury in Minnesota hospitals during the 1990s. Data are from 398 patients with ARDS studied between 1994 and 2001 at three Minnesota hospitals. *A.* This panel demonstrates that tidal volumes were decreased with higher lung injury scores. Mean tidal volume over the first 3 days of admission ($\pm$ SD) decreases with increasing lung injury score ($p < 0.001$ for the difference between quartile 1 and quartiles 2, 3, and 4). *B.* This panel demonstrates that mean daily plateau airway pressure ($\pm$ SD) on each of the first 3 days of admission annually was maintained close to 30 cmH$_2$O throughout the period of study. (*Reproduced, with permission, from Weinert et al.[18]*)

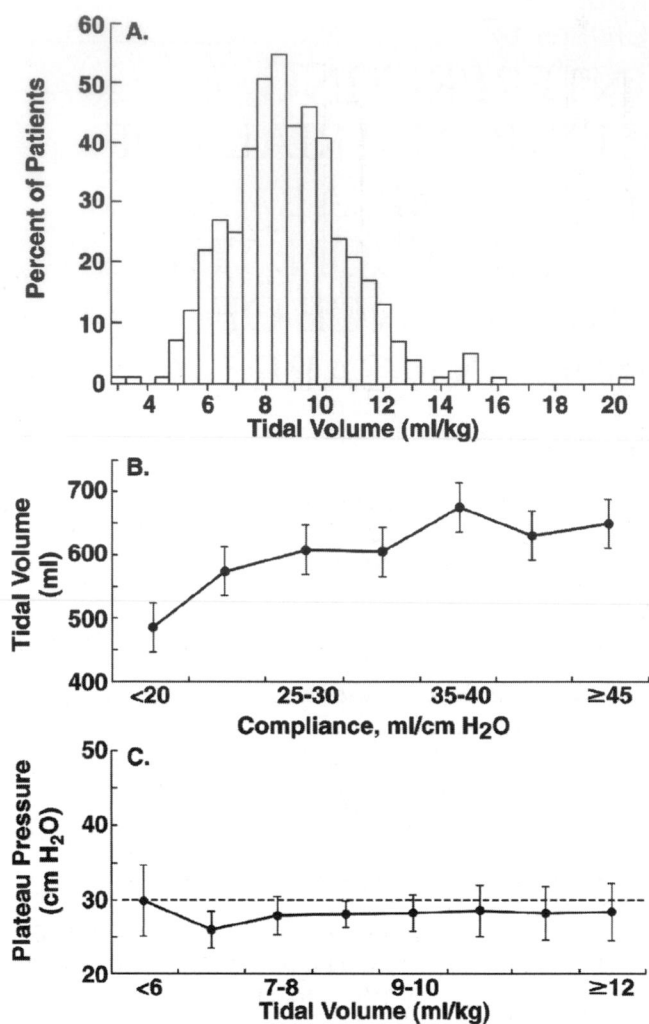

FIGURE 67-2 Relationship between tidal volume and surrogate markers of lung injury in an international survey taken during the 1990s. Data were collected during the first week of admission in an international survey of patients with ARDS from 361 ICUs in 20 countries in March 1998. *A.* This panel demonstrates that prescribed tidal volumes were normally distributed. *B.* This panel demonstrates that mean tidal volumes ($\pm$ SD) decreased as compliance decreased ($p < 0.001$). *C.* This panel demonstrates that plateau pressures (mean $\pm$ SD) were maintained close to 30 cmH$_2$O over a wide range of tidal volumes. (*Reproduced, with permission, from Esteban et al.[22]*)

As a result of adjusting tidal volumes, mean plateau airway pressures were consistently close to or less than 30 cmH$_2$O regardless of the underlying level of lung compliance (Fig. 67-2C).

The ARDSNetwork, a consortium of 10 academic centers in North America, conducted the largest of the five randomized trials of low-tidal-volume ventilation (ARMA trial).[11] The study was initiated in 1996 and was completed in 1999. It included almost three quarters of all the patients studied in the five randomized trials testing low-tidal-volume ventilation. Pre-randomization data from this trial, available both in published correspondence and from the Office of Human Research Protections via the Freedom of Information Act, provides additional information regarding existing ventilator management during the 1990s.[24–27] Similar to the above discussed international survey, pre-randomization

tidal volumes were normally distributed over a wide range (Fig. 67-3A). The relationship between compliance and tidal volume was biphasic (Fig. 67-3B). In patients with less compliant lungs (defined as a compliance <0.6 ml/cmH$_2$O per kilogram predicted body weight [PBW]), there was a direct linear relationship between compliance and tidal volume; in patients with more compliant lungs (defined as compliance $\geq$0.6 ml/cmH$_2$O per kilogram PBW), there was no such relationship. Overall plateau airway pressures, however, at all tidal volumes were maintained on average close to or less than 30 cmH$_2$O in patients before they were enrolled in the ARDSNetwork trial (Fig. 67-3C).

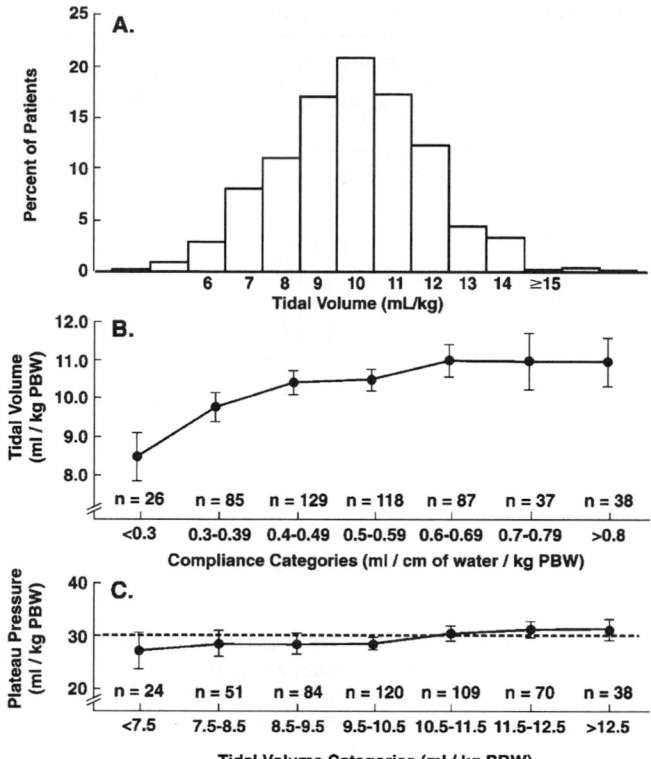

FIGURE 67-3 Relationship between pre-randomization tidal volume and surrogate markers of lung injury in the ARMA trial. Data from 520 patients receiving routine volume-control ventilation before randomization in the ARDSNetwork low-tidal-volume trial. *A.* This panel demonstrates that prescribed tidal volumes were normally distributed. *B.* This panel demonstrates that tidal volumes (mean ± SD) decreased as compliance decreased ($p = 0.008$). *C.* This panel demonstrates a modest reduction in plateau pressure (mean ± SD) as tidal volumes decreased ($p = 0.0002$). Overall, plateau pressures remained close to 30 cmH$_2$O across a wide range of tidal volumes. (*Reproduced, with permission, from Slutsky,[21] Esteban et al,[22] Ferguson et al,[23] and Brower et al.[24]*)

Thus, during the 1990s, ventilation in patients with ARDS and ALI did not consist of a single tidal volume or even a discrete range of tidal volumes. Instead, it consisted of physicians adjusting tidal volumes over a wide range based on the severity of underlying lung injury. This titration maintained plateau airway pressure on average near 30 cmH$_2$O, particularly in patients with less compliant lungs. Although there was variability in practice, the ARDSNetwork pre-randomization data reveals that this variability was not random. Based on our own analysis of the ARDSNetwork data for this chapter, patients with ARDS and ALI with a compliance less than 0.6 ml/cmH$_2$O per kilogram PBW were four times more likely to receive a tidal volume less than 10.5 (median value) ml/kg PBW ($p < 0.0001$). Patients with a compliance greater than 0.6 ml/cmH$_2$O per kilogram PBW were four times more likely to receive a tidal volume greater than 10.5 ml/kg PBW ($p < 0.0001$). By characterizing the relationship between prescribed tidal volume and surrogates of lung injury (such as airway pressure and compliance), we

can better understand why clinicians are reticent to adopt low-tidal-volume ventilation for all patients. It also provides an important framework for understanding the disparate results of the five trials of low tidal volume in patients with ARDS and ALI.

Interpreting Five Low-Tidal-Volume Trials in the Context of Routine Practice in the 1990s

The cause of the different outcomes in these low-tidal-volume trials can be best determined by first dividing the trials into homogenous groups. Two trials demonstrated significant improvement in the odds ratio of survival, while three found a nonsignificant decrease in the odds ratio of survival[28] (Fig. 67-4). The tidal volumes studied are difficult to compare among the five trials because there is no direct conversion for the differing techniques used to standardize volume to body size. In the two beneficial trials, however, patients were randomized to single values of set tidal volume values at the ends of the ranges of current practice. In contrast, the three nonbeneficial trials randomized patients to non-overlapping high or low ranges of tidal volume (Table 67-1).

In the two trials showing benefit, pre-randomization mean plateau pressures were consistent with current practice (29.5 and 30.3 cmH$_2$O)[6,7,11,28,29] (Fig. 67-5). After randomization to a set tidal volume of 12 ml/kg, mean plateau airway pressures were no longer consistent with current practice, and significantly increased over the first 7 days of the study to mean levels of 36.3 and 34.1 cmH$_2$O ($p < 0.001$).[6,7,11,28,29] In contrast, in each of the three nonbeneficial trials, the mean plateau airway pressures in the

FIGURE 67-4 Differences in treatment effects in the low-tidal-volume ventilation trials. Overall odds ratio of survival (± SEM) of low-tidal-volume ventilation compared to high-tidal-volume ventilation based on dividing the trials of low-tidal-volume ventilation into nonbeneficial trials (n = 3) and beneficial trials (n = 2). The individual odds ratios of survival (± SEM) in the three nonbeneficial trials were 0.70 (0.48, 1.02), 0.89 (0.62, 1.28), and 0.85 (0.49, 1.48). The individual odds ratios of survival (± SEM) in the two beneficial trials were 1.47 (1.28, 1.70) and 3.97 (2.20, 7.17). (*Reproduced, with permission, from Eichacker et al,[25] Amato et al,[7] Amato et al,[6] Stewart et al,[8] Brochard et al,[9] and Hickling et al.[5]*)

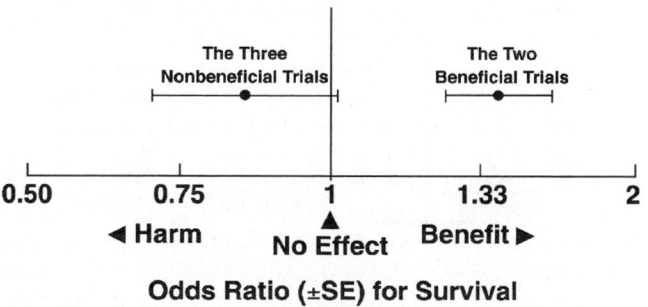

TABLE 67-1 Number of Patients, Tidal Volumes Studied, and Mortality Rates in Five Randomized Clinical Trials

Author (Ref.)	Number of Patients		Tidal Volume		Mortality Rate		Reported Mortality Difference (*p* volume)
	Low Tidal Volume	Control	Low Tidal Volume[a] (ml/kg)	Control (ml/kg)	Low Tidal Volume[a] (%)	Control (%)	
Amato et al,[7]	29	24	$6.1 \pm 0.2^{b,c}$	$11.9 \pm 0.5^{b,c}$	38	71	<0.001
Stewart et al,[8]	60	60	7.2 ± 0.8^{d}	10.6 ± 0.2^{d}	50	47	0.72
Brochard et al,[9]	58	58	7.2 ± 0.2^{e}	10.4 ± 0.2^{e}	47	38	0.38
Brower et al,[10]	26	26	7.3 ± 0.1^{f}	10.2 ± 0.1^{f}	50	46	0.60
ARDSNet[11]	432	429	6.3 ± 0.1^{f}	11.7 ± 0.1^{f}	31	40	0.007

[a]Summary data(means ± SEM)

[b] To estimate the actual mean tidal volume per kilogram body weight administered, we used the fact that 6- and 12-ml/kg tidal volumes were targeted during the first hour and we assumed that weight was constant over the 7 days.

[c] Measured body weight.

[d]Ideal body weight = $25 \times$ [(height in meters)^2].

[e]Dry weight = measured weight minus estimated weight gain from salt and water retention.

[f]Predicted body weight = 50 (for males) or 45.5 (for females) + 2.3 [(height in inches) − 60].

FIGURE 67-5 Plateau airway pressures in the low-tidal-volume ventilation trials. Serial plateau airway pressures (mean ± SEM) before and after randomization to control tidal volumes (*A*) or low tidal volumes (*B*) in the five prospective randomized trials of low-tidal-volume ventilation. All values after initiation of treatment were used to calculate the mean, represented by the clear line between each pair of bars (± SEM), except day 14 values reported in a single study, which did not alter the results when included in a sensitivity analysis. The solid circles represent the individual mean plateau airway pressures reported for each study. After randomization they are connected over time by a solid line. See Table 67-1 for the study references indicated by the lead author names shown above the curves, and for the tidal volumes (mean ± SEM) used in each of these studies, which were calculated in a similar manner to the mean plateau airway pressures. One study provided a mean value over 5 days with individual daily mean values displayed graphically; these have been transposed onto this figure. Finally, only two studies published pre-randomization plateau airway pressures. (*Reproduced, with permission, from Hickling et al,[5] Amato et al,[6] Amato et al,[7] Stewart et al,[8] Brochard et al,[9] and Eichacker et al.[25]*)

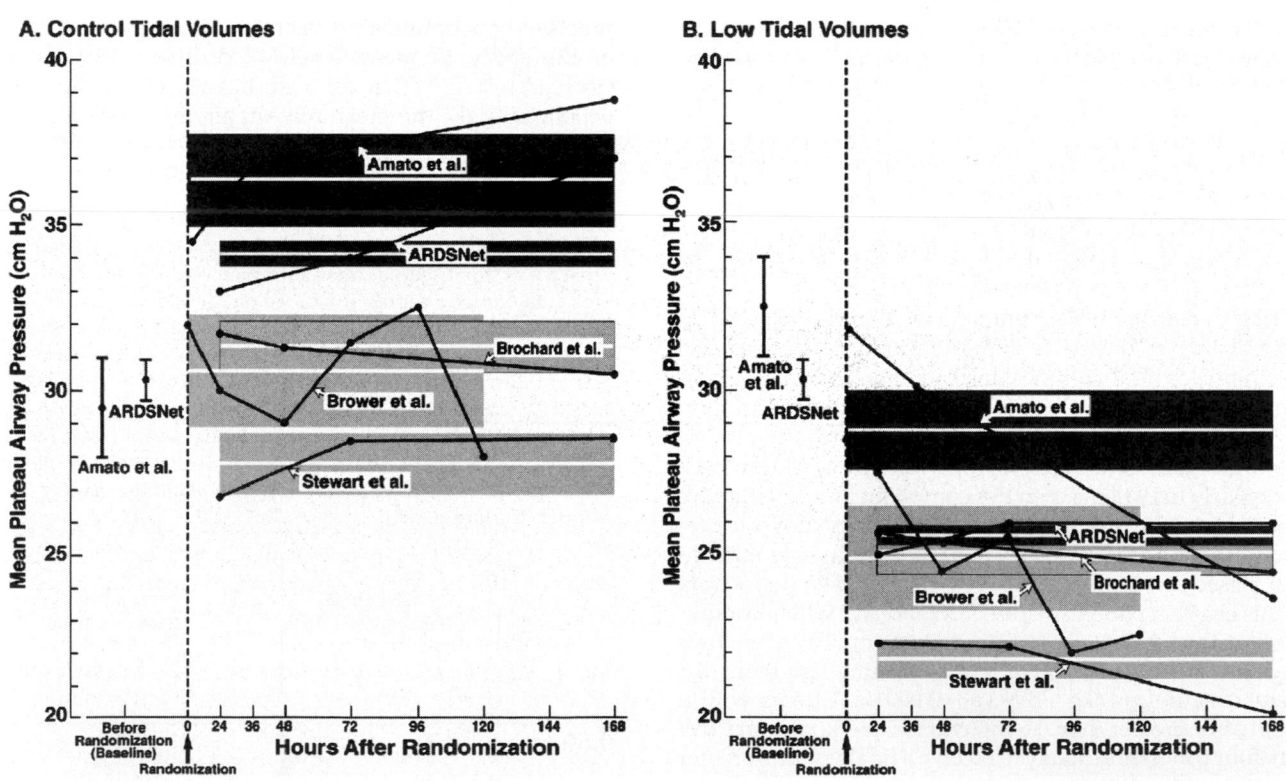

high-tidal-volume arms were 31.6, 27.8, and 30.6.[8–10,28] These values were consistent with current practice (see Fig. 67-5) and were significantly lower than the pressures observed in the high-tidal-volume arms of the two beneficial trials ($p < 0.001$) (see Fig. 67-5). In contrast, comparison of low-tidal-volume arms in all five trials demonstrated that plateau pressures were low and not significantly different (28.8 and 25.6 cmH$_2$O in the two beneficial trials and 21.8, 25.1, and 24.9 cmH$_2$O in the three nonbeneficial trials) (see Fig. 67-5).[6–11,28] This analysis suggests that the disparate results from the five trials were related to differences among the high-tidal-volume arms. Therefore, the apparent benefit in two trials may have resulted from increased plateau pressures in the high-tidal-volume arms causing increases in mortality.

Analysis of baseline pulmonary compliance and mortality data from the ARDSNetwork reveals that mortality was dependent upon pre-randomization compliance in the 6- versus 12-ml/kg tidal volume trial ($p = 0.003$) (Fig. 67-6). In patients with lower pulmonary compliance (<0.6 ml cmH$_2$O per kilogram PBW), raising tidal volumes increased mortality rates (43%) compared to lowering tidal volumes (29%). In contrast, in patients with higher compliance ($\geq$0.6 ml cmH$_2$O per kilogram PBW), the lowering of tidal volume increased mortality rates (35%) compared with the raising of tidal volume (21%). This effect remains highly significant and unchanged ($p = 0.003$) after controlling for differences in age, Acute Physiology, Age, and Chronic Health

FIGURE 67-6 The effect of changing tidal volume on mortality is dependent on pulmonary compliance in the ARMA trial. The effect of changes in tidal volume on mortality in the ARDSNetwork low-tidal-volume trial is significantly influenced by underlying pulmonary compliance ($p = 0.003$). In patients with lower pulmonary compliance, the raising of tidal volume increased mortality compared with the lowering of tidal volume (*filled circles*; 42% versus 29%). In contrast, in patients with higher pulmonary compliance, the raising of tidal volume decreased mortality compared with the lowering of tidal volume (*open circles*; 21% versus 37%). This interaction remained significant after controlling for differences in age, Pa$_{O_2}$/F$_{I_{O_2}}$ ratio, and Acute Physiology, Age, and Chronic Health Evaluation II score in univariable and multivariable analyses. This interaction remained unchanged with multiple sensitivity analyses, such as dividing compliance across the median and excluding patients who had their tidal volumes increased to 6 ml/kg or decreased to 12 ml/kg with randomization. (*Reproduced, with permission, from Brochard et al,[9] Ferguson et al,[23] and Brower et al.[24]*)

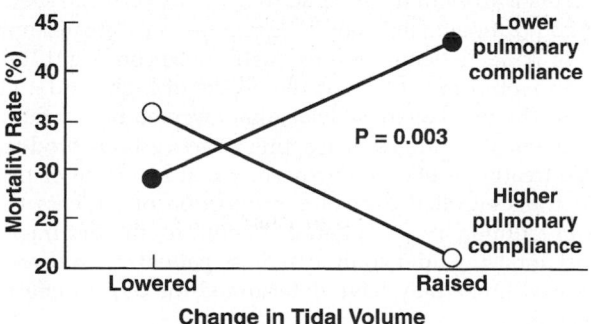

Evaluation (APACHE) II score, and Pa$_{O_2}$/F$_{I_{O_2}}$ (arterial oxygen tension to fractional inspired oxygen concentration) ratio in univariate and multivariate analyses. Furthermore, this interaction is unchanged if patients are stratified based on median compliance rather than a compliance (or a stratification) determined by modeling of the pre-randomization data. It is also unchanged if the small number of patients who had their tidal volumes increased to 6 ml/kg and decreased to 12 ml/kg are excluded.

The interaction between compliance, tidal volume, and outcome in the 6- versus 12-ml/kg tidal volume trial is not unexpected when one considers the magnitude of change in tidal volume that occurred with randomization in many of the study patients. Patients with lower pulmonary compliance (<0.6 ml cmH$_2$O per kilogram PBW) who were receiving tidal volumes of 6–10 ml/kg PBW before randomization, had their tidal volumes increased by 2–6 ml/kg PBW when randomized to the high-tidal-volume arm. In a 70-kg person, this represents an addition of 140–280 ml to the tidal volume he or she was receiving before randomization. The elevations in airway pressure in this group of patients with lower compliance likely exacerbated lung injury. In contrast, patients with higher pulmonary compliance ($\geq$0.6 ml cmH$_2$O per kilogram PBW) who were receiving tidal volumes of 10–15 ml/kg PBW had their tidal volumes decreased by 4–9 ml/kg PBW when randomized to the low-tidal-volume arm. In a 70-kg person, this translates to a reduction in tidal volume of 280–630 ml from what they were receiving before randomization. Worsened mortality in this more compliant group may have been related to lung injury secondary to tidal alveolar collapse, increased sedation requirements caused by greater dyspnea, worsened respiratory acidosis, or some combination of these three.[30–34]

Based on this analysis, it is apparent that changing the proportion of patients with high or low compliance enrolled in such a trial would alter the outcome. A greater number of patients with either high or low compliance would have favored the effects of the 12- or 6-ml/kg targeted tidal volumes, respectively. This relationship between compliance and treatment effect confounds any single interpretation of the findings from the ARDSNetwork trial. The fact that low tidal volumes were beneficial overall in this study most likely reflects the fact that most (close to 70%) of the patients in the trial had poorly compliant lungs at baseline.

Although the ARDSNetwork did not employ a current practice control group in their trial of low-tidal-volume ventilation, an observational cohort of patients who did not enroll in the study were followed simultaneously during the course of the trial at the participating institutions. The ARDSNetwork screened over 6000 patients for enrollment in the trial.[26,27] There were 2587 patients who met enrollment criteria, but were ineligible for six different technical reasons (Fig. 67-7). This ineligible group of patients received routine care during the course of the trial by the same physicians in the same hospitals, and their mortality rate was documented similarly to the study patients. The overall mortality rate in this group of patients was 31.7%. This mortality rate was very consistent across the six different

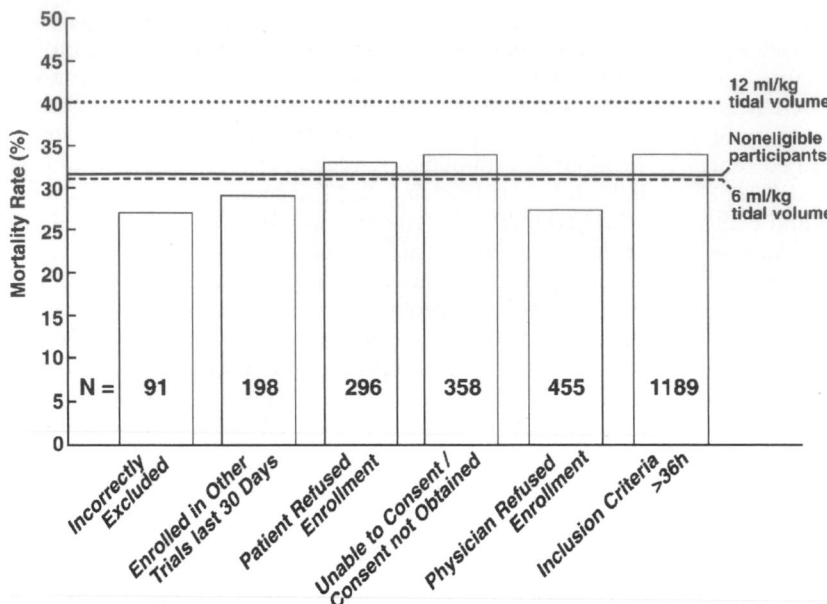

FIGURE 67-7 **Mortality rate in the ARDSNetwork low-tidal-volume trial (9, 23, 24). The overall mortality of non-eligible patients excluded for technical reasons (***solid line***; n = 2567), the 12-ml/kg tidal volume group (***dotted line***; n = 429), and the 6-ml/kg tidal volume group (***dashed line***; n = 432) are shown. Within the group of non-eligible patients, mortality was consistent across the six reasons for technical exclusion (***vertical bars***). (***Reproduced, with permission, from Brochard et al,***[9] ***Ferguson et al,***[23] ***and Brower et al.***[24])**

reasons for technical exclusion. Moreover, it was similar to the mortality rate of the low-tidal-volume arm (31%), and lower than the high-tidal-volume arm of the trial (40%). Importantly, if one only examines patients with lower compliance (<0.6 ml cmH$_2$O per kilogram PBW), low tidal volumes actually appear to have improved survival compared to current practice (27% versus 31.7%). This potential beneficial effect, however, was offset by the relatively harmful effect of low tidal volumes in patients with greater compliance compared to current practice (35% versus 31.7%, respectively).

Of note, a current-practice control group was not made available to the data safety and monitoring boards (DSMB) in the ARDSNetwork or any of the other low-tidal-volume trials. Examination of data, however, from the ARDSNetwork study also provides insight into the potential importance of such a group for the safety of future clinical trials for critically ill patients. Based on data provided to the Office of Human Research Protection in the ARDSNetwork trial, the *p* value for a difference in mortality between the 12- versus the 6-ml/kg-tidal-volume arms was significant after only 183 patients had been effectively enrolled (43% versus 26%; *p* <0.003 uncorrected for multiple looks). The trial was continued to avoid a type 1 error. If mortality rate, however, in patients who had met enrollment criteria, but were ineligible for technical reasons at this first inspection, was consistent or even lower than the final mortality in this group (31% of 2587 patients) and the DSMB was aware of it, a different decision might have been made and the trial stopped earlier. In trials of rapidly lethal diseases with high mortality rates such as ARDS, death and multiple organ injury is expected and treatment-related adverse events may be easily attributed to the disease process itself.[35] Incorporation of a routine care control group allows such trials to be stopped early if the tested intervention has a mortality rate that is significantly greater than such routine care and minimizes risk to the participants.[36] If it had been possible

to stop the ARDSNetwork trial based on the findings from the initial 183 patients that had been enrolled, as many as 30 deaths related to increasing tidal volumes to 12 ml/kg might have been prevented.

Does Understanding of Current Practice Help Explain the Differences Among Low-Tidal-Volume Trials?

The insight gained from examining the ARDSNetwork trial in the context of current practice may help explain the differences in outcome between the two beneficial and three nonbeneficial trials of low-tidal-volume ventilation. In the three nonbeneficial trials in which tidal volumes were chosen from a restricted range, physicians ventilated patients in the high-tidal-volume group at the lower end of the range. The allowance of titration within a range may have caused less disruption of routine care, and therefore produced smaller effects with randomization. It is also possible that each of these three trials enrolled equal numbers of compliant and noncompliant patients, resulting in counteracting risks and benefits in both arms and no overall change in outcome. It is noteworthy that one of these nonbeneficial trials excluded patients with evidence of increased airway pressures before randomization.[8] This may have resulted in a greater number of patients being enrolled with more compliant lungs which would in turn favor the effects of higher tidal volumes. The two beneficial trials that targeted tidal volumes at the ends of ranges of existing practice both produced large treatment effects. Furthermore, at least one of these two trials enrolled a greater proportion of patients with lower pulmonary compliance. Therefore, the detrimental effect of raising tidal volume in these patients with severely diseased lungs may have determined the overall effect of the trial.

Conclusion

Levels of lung injury vary among patients with ALI and ARDS. Reports from studies beginning in the early 1990s showed that physicians adjusted tidal volumes based on surrogates of lung injury. As a result, tidal volumes appeared normally distributed over a wide range in order to maintain plateau airway pressures near 30 cmH$_2$O. In all five trials testing low-tidal-volume ventilation, however, patients were randomized to either high- or low-tidal-volume groups independent of their underlying level of lung injury. Data from these trials showed that such randomization may have had different effects on outcome in patients with ARDS and ALI, depending on severity of lung injury (respiratory compliance). Without controlling for severity of lung injury, randomization exposed subgroups in each treatment arm to increased risk.

It is apparent from these trials that using higher tidal volumes in patients with poorly complaint lungs should be avoided. Moreover, the optimal level to which tidal volumes should be reduced in these patients remains unclear. Additionally, in patients with ARDS and ALI who have more compliant lungs and low airway pressures, very low tidal volumes may be harmful. In light of the analysis of these five trials, it appears important that clinicians continue to adjust tidal volume to avoid injury believed to be associated with plateau pressures greater than 30 cmH$_2$O, but be wary of the potential risks of underventilation in patients with higher compliance.

By incorporating current practice in the design, future trials of mechanical ventilation will be better able to make recommendations on changing current practice and maximize patient safety. This entails the use of a current-practice control group as well as the characterization of current practice before initiating a trial. As a result of a better understanding of current practice, it may be necessary to restrict the range of lung injury studied, stratify patients based on the severity of lung injury before randomization, or employ an adaptive study design that allows for titration within the trial based on a predetermined set of guidelines. Although each one of these designs would require extensive investigation before enrollment and the results of each trial might only be applicable to restricted segments of clinical practice, this process appears critical to improve the interpretability and safety of such studies. Further discussions are needed within the scientific community to develop trial designs that ensure participant safety and provide conclusive insights into the efficacy of current practice.

References

1. Webb HH, Tierney DF. Experimental pulmonary edema due to intermittent positive pressure ventilation with high inflation pressures. Protection by positive end-expiratory pressure. Am Rev Respir Dis 1974; 110:556–65.
2. Kolobow T, Moretti MP, Fumagelli R, et al. Severe impairment in lung function induced by high peak airway pressure during mechanical ventilation: an experimental study. Am Rev Respir Dis 1987; 135:312–15.
3. Dreyfuss D, Soler P, Basset G, Saumon G. High inflation pressure pulmonary edema. Respective effects of high airway pressure, high tidal volume, and positive end-expiratory pressure. Am Rev Respir Dis 1988; 137:1159–64.
4. Hickling KG, Walsh J, Henderson S, et al. Low mortality rate in adult respiratory distress syndrome using low-volume, pressure-limited ventilation with permissive hypercapnia: a prospective study. Crit Care Med 1994; 22:1568–78.
5. Hickling KG, Henderson SJ, Jackson R. Low mortality associated with low pressure limited ventilation with permissive hypercapnia in severe adult respiratory distress syndrome. Intensive Care Med 1990; 16:372–77.
6. Amato MB, Barbas CS, Medeiros DM, et al. Beneficial effects of the "open lung approach" with low distending pressures in acute respiratory distress syndrome. A prospective randomized study on mechanical ventilation. Am J Respir Crit Care Med 1995; 152:1835–46.
7. Amato MB, Barbas CSV, Medeiros DM, et al. Effect of a protective-ventilation strategy on mortality in the acute respiratory distress syndrome. N Engl J Med 1998; 338:347–54.
8. Stewart TE, Meade MO, Cook DJ, et al. Evaluation of a ventilation strategy to prevent barotrauma in patients at high risk for acute respiratory distress syndrome. N Engl J Med 1998; 338:355–61.
9. Brochard L, Roudot-Thorval F, Roupie E, et al. Tidal volume reduction for prevention of ventilator-induced lung injury in acute respiratory distress syndrome. The Multicenter Trial Group on Tidal Volume Reduction in ARDS. Am J Respir Crit Care Med 1998; 158:1831–8.
10. Brower RG, Shanholtz CB, Fessler HF, et al. Prospective, randomized, controlled clinical trial comparing traditional versus reduced tidal volume ventilation in acute respiratory distress syndrome patients. Crit Care Med 1999; 27:1492–8.
11. The Acute Respiratory Distress Syndrome Network. Ventilation with lower tidal volumes compared with traditional tidal volumes for acute lung injury and the acute respiratory distress syndrome. N Engl J Med 2000; 342:1301–8.
12. Ware L, Matthay MA. The acute respiratory distress syndrome. N Engl J Med 2000; 342:1334–49.
13. Brower RG, Ware L, Berthiaume Y, Matthay MA. Treatment of ARDS. Chest 2001; 120:1347–67.
14. Brower RG, Thompson BT, Ancukiewicz M, et al. Clinical trial of mechanical ventilation with traditional versus lower tidal volumes in acute lung injury and the acute respiratory distress syndrome: Effect on physicians' practices. Am J Respir Crit Care Med 2004; 169:A256.
15. Young MP, Manning HL, Wilson DL, et al. Ventilation of patients with acute lung injury and acute respiratory distress syndrome: has new evidence changed clinical practice. Crit Care Med 2004; 32:1260–5.
16. Sakr Y, Vincent JL, Le Gall JR, et al. High tidal volume and positive fluid balance in acute lung injury are associated with worse outcome. Chest 2003; 124:180S-a.
17. Brower RG, Lanken PN, MacIntyre N, et al. Higher versus lower positive end-expiratory pressures in patients with the acute respiratory distress syndrome. N Engl J Med 2004; 351:327–36.
18. Weinert CR, Gross CR, Marinelli WA. Impact of randomized trial results on acute lung injury ventilator therapy in teaching hospitals. Am J Respir Crit Care Med 2003; 167:1304–9.
19. Ricard JD. Are we really reducing tidal volume—and should we? Am J Respir Crit Care Med 2003; 167:1297–8.
20. Carmichael LC , Dorinsky PM, Higgins SB, et al. Diagnosis and treatment of acute respiratory distress syndrome in adults: an international survey. J Crit Care 1996; 11:9–18.
21. Slutsky AS. Mechanical Ventilation. American College of Chest Physicians' Consensus Conference. Chest 1993; 104:1833–59.
22. Esteban A, Anzueto A, Frutos F, et al with the Mechanical

Ventilation International Study Group. Characteristics and outcomes in adult patients receiving mechanical ventilation: a 28-day international study. JAMA 2002; 287:345–55.

23. Ferguson N, Fernando FV, Esteban A, et al. Airway pressures, tidal volumes, and mortality in patients with acute respiratory distress syndrome. Crit Care Med 2005; 33:21–30.

24. Brower RG, Matthay M, Schoenfeld D. Meta-analysis of acute lung injury and acute respiratory distress syndrome trials (letter). Am J Respir Crit Care Med 2002; 166:1515–7.

25. Eichacker PQ, Banks SM, Natanson C. Meta-analysis of tidal volumes in ARDS. Am J Respir Crit Care Med 2003; 167:798–800.

26. Data provided to the Office of Human Research Protections from ARDSNetwork investigators from the ARMA trial for use at the June 9–11, 2003 consultants meeting. Available under the Freedom of Information Act. Requests should be sent to Public Health Service, Freedom of Information Office, Rm. 17A46, 5600 Fishers Lane, Rockville, MD 20857.

27. Deans KJ, Minneci PC, Banks SM, Natanson C, Eichacker PQ. Mechanical ventilation in ARDS: One size does not fit all. Crit Care Med 2005; 33:1141–3.

28. Eichacker PQ, Gerstenberger EP, Banks SM, Cui X, Natanson C. Meta-analysis of acute lung injury and acute respiratory distress syndrome trials testing low tidal volumes. Am J Respir Crit Care Med 2002; 166:1510–4.

29. Thompson BT, Hayden D, Matthay MA, Brower R, Parsons PE.

30. Muscdere JG, Mullen JB, Gan K, Slutsky AS. Tidal ventilation at low airway pressures can augment lung injury. Am J Respir Care Med 1994; 149:1327–34.

31. Kress JP, Pohlman AS, O'Connor MF, Hall JB. Daily interruption of sedative infusions in critically ill patients undergoing mechanical ventilation. N Engl J Med 2000; 342:1471–7.

32. Kollef MH, Levy NT, Ahrens TS, et al. The use of continuous i.v. sedation is associated with prolongation of mechanical ventilation. Chest 1998; 114:541–8.

33. Feihl F, Perret C. Permissive hypercapnia: how permissive should we be? Am J Respir Crit Care Med 1994; 150:1722–37.

34. Thorens JB, Jolliet P, Ritz M, Chevrolet JC. Effects of rapid permissive hypercapnia on hemodynamics, gas exchange, and oxygen transport and consumption during mechanical ventilation for the acute respiratory distress syndrome. Intensive Care Med 1996; 22:182–91.

35. Freeman BD, Danner RL, Banks SM, Natanson C. Safeguarding patients in clinical trials with high mortality rates. Am J Respir Crit Care Med 2001; 164:190–2.

36. Silverman HJ, Miller FG. Control group selection in critical care randomized controlled trials evaluating interventional strategies: An ethical assessment. Crit Care Med 2004; 32:852–7.

Clinicians' approaches to mechanical ventilation in acute lung injury and ARDS. Chest 2001; 120:1622–7.

ECONOMICS OF VENTILATOR CARE

SHANNON S. CARSON

One of the most important targets for improved efficiencies in inpatient hospital care has been critical care services. In 1985, intensive care unit (ICU) beds constituted 7.8% of hospital beds in the United States. By 2002, ICU beds accounted for 13.3% of hospital beds, and critical care medicine accounted for $55.5 billion in national health care costs.[1] Critical care expenditures have increased by 190% since 1985. Patients requiring mechanical ventilation are among the largest consumers of critical care resources, and hospitals often experience financial losses in providing care for them. The demand for ICU services is expected to rise dramatically as a result of the aging population worldwide. This will be particularly relevant to ventilated patients, because the risk of respiratory failure rises exponentially after the age of 65. This chapter reviews the economic implications of mechanical ventilation. Basic principles of health economics are reviewed to provide a framework for interpreting health economic analyses devoted to mechanical ventilation. Actual costs of mechanical ventilation are addressed, followed by a discussion of whether mechanical ventilation is cost effective. Finally, strategies for cost containment are reviewed.

Basic Principles of Health Economics

The goal of *health economics* is to ascertain the highest level of efficiency in providing health care.[2,3] A key assumption in this field is that health resources are a finite commodity. This is never more evident than in health care systems that are tightly controlled by a fixed budget. In that setting, if resources are devoted to a specific intervention or program, another intervention or program will need to be eliminated. If the delivery of a resource-intense service can be optimized so that it can be provided at lower costs, multiple other less costly services can be initiated. In such a system, a series of questions must be answered regarding any new or current medical intervention:

- Is the intervention effective relative to other available therapies?
- How much does it cost relative to other available therapies?
- From whose perspective are the costs being considered?
- How widely will the intervention be utilized?

Measured approaches to answering these questions allow health care systems to select medical therapies based upon evidence rather than assumptions, commercial marketing, or bias. Economic analysis as a component of decision making for health systems has become standard in countries such as Canada or Australia, where health care is centralized on a national level. In countries such as the United States, delivery of health care is much less regulated, and many practitioners have unbounded access to any available therapies. Few physicians in the United States, however, are able to practice without significant awareness of resource implications of their decision making. Encounters with uninsured patients, financially troubled or overburdened hospitals, or tightly controlled health plans can influence medical decision making toward higher efficiency. Rapidly growing health care costs are again resulting in rising copayments and premiums for insured patients. It is highly likely that third party payors will increase efforts to balance available services with more efficient delivery.

Medicare, the largest third party payor in the United States, had a major impact on inpatient care when they adopted the prospective payment system of reimbursement. This system provided a fixed payment for care based on the patient's principal diagnosis (diagnosis-related grouping, or DRG) rather than actual resources that were provided. Therefore hospitals had a clear incentive to provide more efficient care. Length of hospital stay decreased for many diagnoses, often with the help of management protocols or clinical pathways. Drug use was reviewed and restricted, ancillary services were streamlined, and many medical and surgical services were shifted to the outpatient setting. In some cases, the improved efficiencies induced by the DRG system created higher burdens for patients, their families, nurses, and ancillary personnel because discharges occurred earlier, and the general acuity of illness on hospital wards increased. Many of the trends for Medicare patients were mirrored by managed care plans with similar results.

The Medicare prospective payment system is an example of economics influencing health care priorities at the level of a health authority. Similar decision making takes place regularly at the level of the hospital when choices are made about what equipment to purchase or which drugs to make available on a formulary. Individual physicians are increasingly being required to make medical economic decisions on a case-by-case basis as the costs of interventions continue to rise. Health plans are beginning to monitor physicians' practices to improve their economic decision making. Capitated reimbursement systems in which primary physicians are provided a fixed amount of resources with which to provide comprehensive medical care for a group of patients is an extreme example of how daily physician practice might be influenced by practical economic principles. Therefore a basic understanding of how the efficiency of various health care practices is defined is becoming essential to the practicing clinician. The following section will outline some of the common definitions and methodologies employed in health economic analysis.

COSTS

When considering the cost of therapies, the unit price of a drug or piece of equipment is often the basis of discussion in the clinical setting, especially if the analysis is being performed in the interest of the physician or hospital. Payors may have a broader view, especially if they are responsible for health care costs after hospital discharge. Patients and society view the cost of illness from an even larger perspective including a longer time frame. Ideally, economic analyses determine the true costs that are accrued from the beginning of a patient's disease to the ultimate outcome of the patient. These costs are categorized as direct medical costs, direct nonmedical costs, and indirect costs.[2,3]

DIRECT MEDICAL COSTS

Direct medical costs are costs used by the provider in providing a service. These can include *variable costs* such as physician labor, drug costs, or use of diagnostic or therapeutic equipment. Variable costs are not generated unless the service is provided. Nursing labor is usually considered a *fixed cost*, because nurse salaries must be paid regardless of bed occupancy, unless staff are laid off. Other fixed costs include general operations of the hospital or clinic such as utilities, leases, administrative overhead or taxes. Overhead costs are occasionally referred to as indirect costs, although another definition for indirect costs is given below. Overhead costs are generally difficult to measure, but many hospitals are now using standard economic software that factors general operating expenses into the direct costs of various services.

Most hospitals increase the patient charge for many services above acquisition costs and application expenses to help pay for services that are otherwise inadequately reimbursed. Because this practice can vary according to different payment plans, hospital *charges* are an inappropriate surrogate for hospital *costs*. Large studies involving patients under a single payor such as Medicare can adjust charges using a standard cost/charge ratio to gain acceptable estimates of costs, but this is less reliable with more heterogeneous groups of patients and payors.

Direct costs measured in the unique setting of an ICU vary somewhat depending on local staffing and practice patterns, but a rather consistent finding is that nursing time

TABLE 68-1 Costs of Managing ICU Patients by Human and Capital Component

Component	% Component Cost	% Total Cost
Human		63.8
Nursing	64.6	41.2
Medical	15.1	9.6
Professional	14.3	9.1
Support	6.1	3.9
Supplies		11.7
Laboratory		11.4
Chemistry	62.0	7.1
Hematology	23.5	3.3
Microbiology	9.9	1.1
Other	4.6	0.5
Medication		7.4
Diagnostic imaging		4.5
Capital equipment		1.2

SOURCE: Modified, with permission, from Noseworthy et al.[4]

accounts for as much as 50% of direct costs for a critically ill patient[4,5] (Table 68-1). Because nursing time, monitoring costs, physician costs, and certain laboratory and radiology ordering practices are linked to a patient's presence in an ICU, ICU length of stay is a reliable and convenient surrogate for ICU costs.[6] Most studies estimate that a day in the ICU costs two to three times the amount of care on a medical or surgical hospital floor.[1,7] For comparisons between institutions, length of stay can be confounded by differences in ICU admission criteria, nurse/patient ratios, and presence of intermediate care or "stepdown" units. In order to standardize resource use between different ICU settings, instruments such as the Therapeutic Intervention Scoring System[8] (TISS) can be utilized. The TISS instrument assigns weights to 76 ICU interventions based on the severity of illness associated with the need for each intervention. Intensity of ICU care can then be assessed by comparing the added weights or TISS scores between intervention groups, and costs can be standardized by applying a specific cost to each service.

DIRECT NONMEDICAL COSTS

Direct nonmedical costs include costs incurred by the patient that are not related to care provided by the physician or hospital. These costs may include emergency transportation to the hospital, transportation and lodging for the patient's family, and domestic help and rehabilitative services after discharge. While these costs are difficult to measure, they can have an important impact on the patient and his or her perception of the benefits of care.

INDIRECT COSTS

Indirect costs include the overall financial burden of illness to the patient. This can include loss of wages and benefits secondary to missed work or loss of earnings and unpaid care provided by family members. This too is difficult to measure, but it has substantial impact on the well being of the patient. Indirect costs can ultimately affect direct costs for a health care system. If economic burdens on the patient decrease medical compliance or result in incomplete recovery, then recurrence of hospitalization or even critical illness can result.

Cost data for economic evaluations can come from multiple sources, but the most common approach is to collect cost data prospectively during clinical trials.[9] Utilizing cost data from a single large clinical trial has the advantage of uniform methodology, but it may not be generalizable if the trial involved highly selected patients managed in ways that are not standard to the typical clinical setting. Treatment effect from clinical trials can sometimes be overestimated. Economic models can also be generated from meta-analyses. This approach has the advantage of including data from different settings for enhanced generalizability, but if methodologies of the studies are not similar, the comparisons could be invalid. A combined approach that begins with data from a large clinical trial and adds multiple scenarios that account for clinical variability is useful. When clinical trial data are not available, cost and outcome data can be derived from cohort studies. With this approach, sensitivity analyses to account for clinical variability and potential biases in the cohort studies are particularly important.

TYPES OF ECONOMIC ANALYSES

Economic analyses function to provide more than just a description of the costs of a therapy. Their role is to compare costs between therapies relative to the benefits or efficacies of those therapies. The four primary types of economic analyses[2,3,9] are described below and in Table 68-2.

COST-MINIMIZATION ANALYSES

Cost-minimization analyses compare the costs of two therapies that have the same efficacy. The difference in monetary value between the therapies is the primary outcome. These studies are most commonly conducted to justify introducing a new drug in a class that already contains multiple competitors. It is important for a cost-minimization study to demonstrate that the clinical outcomes are indeed equivalent. Often, however, important secondary clinical outcomes such as side effects may be different.

COST-BENEFIT ANALYSES

Cost-benefit analyses attempt to assign a direct monetary value to costs and benefits of therapies for purposes of description or comparison. Although they allow for comparison of interventions that have different outcomes, these studies are complicated because it is difficult to assign monetary value to outcomes such as death or quality of life. Cost-benefit analyses are unusual in the medical literature.

COST-EFFECTIVENESS ANALYSES

Cost-effectiveness analyses use standard clinical measures such as life years gained or quality of life units rather than monetary units to assess benefit. Outcomes are expressed as a ratio of cost to measure of benefit (e.g., cost per life year gained). Cost-effectiveness analyses are easy to understand for clinicians and have the advantage of not having to assign a monetary value to outcomes. Therefore they are the most common type of economic evaluation performed. They can, however, only compare the costs of therapies that have a common clinical outcome.

COST-UTILITY ANALYSES

Cost-utility analyses are performed when therapies are likely to have an impact on quality of life as well as mortality. This is often relevant to interventions in critical care. The level of well being for a given health state (rated from 0 for worst health or death to 1 for best health) is multiplied by the amount of time spent in that health state. The resulting index is called a *quality-adjusted life year* or QALY. For example, a therapy that results in a health state valued at 0.5 for 2 years would yield 1 QALY. The ratings for health states, or *utilities*, can be measured by interviewing participants within a clinical trial, or predetermined values measured in similar groups of patients can be utilized. Results are expressed as cost per QALY. Results of selected cost-utility

TABLE 68-2   Types of Economic Analyses

Type	Comparisons	Result	Advantages and Disadvantages
Cost-minimization	Costs of therapies with similar efficacies	Cost difference	Few therapies have similar efficacies for multiple outcomes
Cost-benefit	Monetary value of costs and benefits of therapies	Cost/monetary benefit	Therapies for different conditions and outcomes can be compared, but it is difficult to place a monetary value on clinical outcomes
Cost-effectiveness	Therapies with efficacies measured using similar clinical outcomes	Cost/clinical outcome (e.g., life years saved)	Utilize clinically relevant outcomes; analyses using different outcomes cannot be compared
Cost-utility	Therapies for which mortality and quality of life are important outcomes	Cost/QALY	Different therapies with different efficacies can be compared; includes patient-centered outcomes; difficult to comprehend

ABBREVIATION: QALY, quality-adjusted life year.

TABLE 68-3 Cost Effectiveness of Selected Mechanical Ventilation-Related Interventions

Intervention	Cost per QALY
Mechanical ventilation for respiratory failure related to pneumonia or ARDS[10,11]	$29,000 (estimated 2-month survival >70%)
	$44,000 (estimated 2-month survival 51–70%)
	$110,000 (estimated 2-month survival ≤ 50%)
	$32,000 (age <65 years)
	$46,000 (age >75 years)
ICU care for patients with acute respiratory failure without chronic lung disease[5]	$11,970[a]
ICU care for patients with acute respiratory failure *with* chronic lung disease[5]	$14,365[a]
ICU care for patients with acute renal failure[5]	$30,625[a]
Tissue plasminogen activator for acute myocardial infarction compared to streptokinase[12]	$30,300
Activated protein C for severe sepsis[13]	$27,400 (APACHE II ≥ 25)
	>$100,000 (APACHE II <25)
Ultrasound screening for deep vein thrombosis in ventilated patients with femoral vein catheters[14]	$12,793
Lung transplantation compared to standard care[15]	$44,000 (assuming 10-year survival)
	$204,000 (assuming 5-year survival)
In-hospital cardiopulmonary resuscitation[16]	$215,000

[a] Analysis did not include costs after hospital discharge.
ABBREVIATION: APACHE, Acute Physiology, Age, and Chronic Health Evaluation score; ARDS, acute respiratory distress syndrome; QALY, quality-adjusted life year.

analyses related to mechanical ventilation and ICU care are listed in Table 68-3.

The advantages of cost-utility analyses are that costs and benefits of different therapies involving different types of patients can be compared, and outcomes beyond survival are factored in. The disadvantage is that many clinicians have difficulty understanding the complexity of the studies, and the models can involve numerous assumptions that vary across patient populations. Therefore, strict guidelines[17] must be followed in conducting the studies to ensure transparency in how utilities are assigned, and rigorous testing in the form of sensitivity analyses should be performed to determine how variability in clinical factors could affect results of the models.

Cost-effectiveness analyses and cost-utility analyses are often referred to together as cost-effectiveness analyses. They can aid decision making by providing data on how much therapies cost relative to the outcomes that are achieved, particularly if one therapy has greater benefits than the alternative, but the costs are greater as well. When good cost-effectiveness data are provided, however, health systems and clinicians can still be challenged by difficult decisions. If a therapy costs more than the alternative, but provides better outcomes, how much is a health system willing to pay for the incremental benefit? In most Western health systems, an incremental cost per QALY of less than $20,000 is strong evidence for adoption of a therapy. Incremental costs per QALY of $50,000–$100,000 provide moderate evidence for adoption. If the incremental cost per QALY is >$100,000, the therapy is not considered cost effective. Ultimate decision making must take into account other factors such as seriousness of the health condition, availability of alternatives, and number of patients who would receive the therapy (total budgetary impact). If a therapy has slightly lower effectiveness than an alternative, but the cost savings associated with it are substantial, a society may consider it to be the preferred option.[2]

Costs of Mechanical Ventilation in the ICU

Recent economic analyses of Medicare data[1,7] indicate that average costs of care in an ICU range between $2462 and $2674 per day per patient. Average costs are only slightly less in ICUs in Europe and Canada.[4,5,18] ICU costs for Medicare patients have increased by 126% since 1985. The average total cost of hospitalization for a critically ill patient is $14,135, which is nearly three times the cost of a hospitalized patient managed on the medical or surgical floor ($5571).[7] Two-thirds of the costs associated with critically ill patients are accrued during their stay in the ICU. For those whose length of stay in the ICU is more than 5 days, as much as 80% of their hospital costs are accrued in the ICU.

Maintaining a mechanical ventilator accounts for only 15–20% of direct ICU costs. A ventilator includes a one-time cost of $20,000 to $38,000 for the hospital plus nominal maintenance charges, and it is used for a number of years. A respiratory therapist's time (when utilized) ranges from $70–$120 per day depending on local salary and staffing levels, and administrative costs are a smaller factor. Rather than the mechanical ventilator itself, the major contributor to ICU costs for a ventilated patient is the nursing time assigned to the patient[4,5] (see Table 68-1). Nursing requirements for ventilated patients can be substantial, especially if the patient is hemodynamically unstable and requires frequent suctioning of an endotracheal tube or sedation. The nurse/patient ratio for acutely ill mechanically ventilated patients is usually 1:1 or 1:2.

IS MECHANICAL VENTILATION COST EFFECTIVE?

Thorough economic analyses of mechanical ventilation have been limited because of difficulties in applying adequate study methods in this complex patient population. One high-quality study, however, addressed the question of cost effectiveness of mechanical ventilation in severely ill patients who required mechanical ventilation for pneumonia or acute respiratory distress syndrome (ARDS).[10] Patients with pneumonia or ARDS who were enrolled in the SUPPORT trial (Study to Understand Prognoses and Preferences for Outcomes and Risks of Treatments) and who received mechanical ventilation were compared to similar patients for whom mechanical ventilation was withheld when imminent death was likely. Utilities were estimated during patient interviews at baseline and 6 months later. Costs were determined from hospital fiscal data and Medicare data. In the analysis, patients were stratified based upon likelihood of 2-month survival (Table 68-4). The incremental cost per QALY of providing mechanical ventilation to these patients was $29,000 for low-risk patients (>70% estimated survival), $44,000 for medium-risk patients (51–70% estimated survival), and $110,000 for high-risk patients (≤50% estimated survival). Sensitivity analyses that increased mortality and costs to twice the baseline estimates resulted in incremental costs per QALY that were still less than $80,000 for low- and medium-risk patients. In another cost-utility analysis from France,[5] cost-utility ratios for ICU care of patients with acute respiratory failure were estimated to be $11,970 for patients without chronic lung disease and $14,365 for patients with chronic lung disease (see Table 68-3). This analysis did not include costs of care following discharge, so it is relevant only from the hospital's perspective.

These data suggest that mechanical ventilation for patients with acute respiratory failure caused by pneumonia or ARDS meets standard criteria for cost effectiveness for all but the highest-risk patients. It may be reasonable to assume that mechanical ventilation for patients with conditions that afford better prognoses, such as asthma, chronic obstructive pulmonary disease (COPD), or routine postoperative patients will be similarly cost effective, and mechanical ventilation for patients with worse prognoses, such as pulmonary or hematologic malignancies, may be less cost effective. Of course, it is rather difficult to apply these principles in bedside practice. The illness-severity measure used for the SUPPORT study applies to the study population as a whole, and application to patients outside of the study is not possible. A given patient's acute physiologic derangements will usually have more of an impact on outcome than their specific diagnosis. Physicians must discuss prognosis with their patient or their surrogate using the information at hand and their clinical judgment. Mechanical ventilation should then be utilized according to how the expected benefit matches with the patient's wishes for invasive care.

COSTS OF PROLONGED MECHANICAL VENTILATION

Patients who require more than 7 days of mechanical ventilation represent only 10% of ICU patients, but they consume up to 40% of ICU resources. Over 20% of those resources are consumed after the seventh day of ventilation.[19] When these patients were recognized as significant cost outliers in 1992, clinicians and hospitals were able to convince the Health Care Financing Administration for Medicare to create DRG 483 (tracheostomy except for face, mouth, and neck disease) as a way to fairly reimburse hospitals for their care. DRG 483 has maintained one of the highest severity weights in Medicare, and it reimburses at a high rate. The cost/payment ratio for DRG 483 has been 103%.[7] In July 2004, DRG 483 was replaced with DRG 541 (tracheostomy with mechanical ventilation 96+ hours or principal diagnosis except face, mouth, and neck diagnoses with major operating room [OR] procedure) and DRG 542 (tracheostomy with mechanical ventilation 96+ hours or principal diagnosis except face, mouth, and neck diagnoses without major OR procedure).[20] As a result, the amount of reimbursement for nonsurgical patients with prolonged ventilation will decrease significantly.

In the state of North Carolina, average Medicare reimbursements for patients discharged with DRG 483 ranged from $117,203 in 1992 to $102,776 in 2003, and payments

TABLE 68-4   Costs of Mechanical Ventilation for Patients with Acute Respiratory Failure Secondary to Pneumonia or Acute Respiratory Distress Syndrome

	>70% Estimated 2-Month Survival	51–70% Estimated 2-Month Survival	≤ 50% Estimated 2-Month Survival
Hospital costs	$59,096 ± $64,336	$70,130 ± $85,300	$59,310 ± $54,590
Physician costs	$5034 ± $6705	$6162 ± $5264	$6474 ± $7426
Costs through the year after discharge	$22,037 ± $44,847	$18,772 ± $42,253	$11,994 ± $34,475
Annual costs after the first year	$18,265 ± $48,078	$13,053 ± $26,519	$28,102 ± $86,998
1-Year survival	0.62	0.39	0.21
Costs per QALY	$29,000	$44,000	$110,000

Patients were enrolled in the SUPPORT trial. Index hospital costs were derived from hospital charges using Medicare cost/charge ratios. Physician costs and costs of hospitalization after the index hospital discharge were estimated from Medicare financial data. Two-month survival estimates were determined at the time of diagnosis of acute respiratory failure.

ABBREVIATION: QALY, quality-adjusted life year.

SOURCE: Modified, with permission, from Hamel et al.[10]

totaled $1.27 billion during the 10-year period.[21] The total number of patients discharged with DRG 483 increased dramatically during this period (owing in part to more frequent and earlier placement of tracheostomies in ventilated patients), resulting in an increase in yearly total hospital charges of 166%. Health care costs associated with prolonged ventilation remain high even after patients are liberated from mechanical ventilation and discharged from the hospital. Readmissions occur in up to 40% of patients within a year, and total health care costs that accrue for patients during the year after discharge are almost as high as their index hospital costs.[22]

One-year survival of patients requiring prolonged mechanical ventilation ranges from 23–40%.[23] Considering their poor long-term outcomes and very high costs, the question inevitably arises as to whether or not prolonged care for these patients is cost effective. One study at a single hospital in Canada attempted to address this question.[24] Costs for patients who required ICU care for more than 14 days were compared to those for patients who had life-sustaining therapies withdrawn. The incremental cost-effectiveness ratio was $65,219 Canadian per life saved, or $4350 Canadian per life-year saved. Although these data did not include costs associated with care for survivors after discharge, the study still suggests that prolonged ICU care is cost effective. Larger studies including longer follow-up and measures of quality of life should be conducted in the future.

Controlling Costs of Mechanical Ventilation

For acutely ill patients, the requirement for mechanical ventilation is a nearly universal indication for ICU admission. In the current DRG system for Medicare, more than half of the patients managed in the ICU generate costs that are greater than the average payment, leading to financial losses for the hospital.[7] This is less of a factor for some DRGs that are associated with mechanical ventilation (DRG 475: respiratory system diagnosis with ventilatory support; and DRG 483: tracheostomy except for face, mouth, and neck disease), which have payment/cost ratios of 99% and 103%, respectively. Other conditions, however, requiring ICU care and mechanical ventilation lead to significant losses. For example, DRG 014: specific cerebrovascular disorders except transient ischemia attack, has a payment/cost ratio of 68%, and DRG 127: heart failure and shock, has a payment/cost ratio of 73%. To control costs associated with mechanical ventilation, a patient's time on the ventilator and in the ICU must be limited as much as possible. Strategies to reduce duration of mechanical ventilation include prevention of intubation, efficient management of the ventilated patient, withholding or withdrawal of mechanical ventilation in terminally ill patients, and transfer of the ventilated patient to lower-intensity sites of care (Table 68-5).

PREVENTION OF INTUBATION

The two most effective means of preventing mechanical ventilation is to intervene with appropriate resuscitative

TABLE 68-5 Cost-Containment Strategies for Mechanical Ventilation

Proven strategies
Prevention of intubation
  Rapid response teams
  Noninvasive mechanical ventilation
Efficient management practices
  Daily screening and performance of spontaneous breathing trials
  Daily interruption of sedative infusions
  Prevention of ventilator-associated pneumonia
  Prevention of intravenous catheter–related infections
ICU organization
  Critical care–trained medical director
  Closed ICU format with full-time intensivist coverage
  Nurse-driven sedation protocols
  Nurse- or therapist-driven weaning protocols
  Flexible nurse staffing
  Continuous medical education
  Continuous quality improvement
Transfer to lower-intensity sites of care
  In-house respiratory care units
  Long-term acute care hospitals or regional weaning centers
  Acute rehabilitation hospitals with mechanical ventilation capabilities
  Skilled nursing facilities with mechanical ventilation capabilities
  Home mechanical ventilation
Unproven strategies
Withholding or withdrawing mechanical ventilation from terminally ill patients
  Advanced directives are uncommon and do not influence practice
  Very poor prognoses are often not evident until well into the ICU course
  Cost savings are reduced if patients require continued hospitalization for palliative care

efforts before respiratory failure occurs, and using noninvasive mechanical ventilation when appropriate. Early recognition and intervention for conditions that will predispose patients to respiratory failure, such as sepsis, cardiogenic pulmonary edema, or acute bronchospasm, may reverse processes enough to avoid intubation. Many hospitals are forming *rapid response teams* that consist of critical care–trained nurses and physicians who remain on call in the hospital to respond to floor patients who have acute changes in their hemodynamic, respiratory, or neurologic status. Enhancement of emergency department staffing to achieve more timely resuscitation of patients in shock is also being explored. Because these services will add to personnel costs, studies of patient outcomes and cost effectiveness are warranted.

NONINVASIVE MECHANICAL VENTILATION

Noninvasive ventilation for acute respiratory failure secondary to severe COPD exacerbations decreases the likelihood that a patient will need intubation. This is associated with significantly lower hospital mortality and decreased ICU and hospital length of stay. Noninvasive ventilation has also been shown to decrease the likelihood of intubation in patients with congestive heart failure without shock or ischemia, patients with community-acquired pneumonia if they have underlying COPD, patients with acute-on-chronic respiratory failure associated with obstructive sleep apnea, and in immunocompromised patients who have early ARDS.

Avoiding intubation does not eliminate all of the costs associated with mechanical ventilation. Noninvasive ventilation in the setting of acute respiratory failure still requires a significant investment in respiratory therapist time in addition to equipment and administrative costs. More importantly, if the patient requires monitoring in an ICU, the actual cost savings will be reduced.[25] Many hospitals manage patients with acute respiratory failure requiring noninvasive ventilation on a stepdown unit or hospital floor with lower nurse/patient ratios than in an ICU. While achieving cost savings, this approach should be considered only if well-trained staff and sufficient monitoring are available to be able to respond to patients who fail noninvasive ventilation. Utilization of noninvasive ventilation in patients with less severe COPD exacerbations would result in financial losses because it requires a higher level of monitoring than standard therapy and does not improve outcomes.

EFFICIENT MANAGEMENT PRACTICES

Because decreasing time on the ventilator and time in the ICU is the mainstay of cost reduction for mechanical ventilation, recent clinical trials have focused on these issues as important outcomes. Daily screening for readiness to wean and initiation of spontaneous breathing trials has been shown to reduce ventilator days by 1.5 days compared to usual care.[26] Similarly, daily awakening of patients receiving continuous infusions of sedatives can decrease ventilator days by 2.4 days compared to usual care.[27] Use of normal tidal volumes (6 ml/kg predicted body weight) in patients with acute lung injury or ARDS rather than tidal volumes of 12 ml/kg of predicted body weight results in fewer ventilator days in addition to lower mortality.[28] Because some of these practices have not been standard care at many medical centers, clinicians have been slow to adopt them into their daily routine. Practice guidelines and nurse- or therapist-driven protocols have been very useful in these settings. When evidence-based practices are applied systematically, the benefits are most likely to be translated into cost reductions in real clinical settings. Nurse-directed sedation protocols and therapist-driven weaning protocols have been successfully implemented in numerous settings.

Ventilator-associated pneumonia (VAP) occurs in up to 40% of ventilated patients. It is associated with longer time on the ventilator and increases ICU stays by approximately 4 days. VAP may result in higher patient mortality. Prevention of VAP is essential to minimizing costs. Practices that have been shown to decrease the incidence of VAP include semirecumbent positioning of the patient, use of a formal infection control program and adequate hand washing, avoidance of unnecessary antibiotics, maintenance of adequate pressure in endotracheal tube cuffs, scheduled drainage of condensate from ventilator circuits, and removal of nasogastric and endotracheal tubes as soon as possible.[29] Treatment of VAP can be limited to 8 days of intravenous antibiotics except in cases in which *Pseudomonas* species

have been cultured from respiratory specimens. Courses of antibiotics can be limited even further when a clinical scale is used to help confirm the presence of VAP or when more aggressive approaches to diagnosis are utilized using bronchoscopy. Bronchoscopic diagnosis of VAP helps to limit antibiotic therapy, but its cost-effectiveness relative to empiric antibiotic therapy is unknown.

An analysis of a large patient database has indicated that earlier tracheostomy for patients requiring more than 96 hours of mechanical ventilation is associated with lower hospital mortality.[21] In a recent randomized trial in a single hospital, early tracheostomy for patients with high illness severity resulted in lower hospital mortality and significantly fewer ventilator days and ICU days compared to tracheostomy after 14 days.[30] If these findings are duplicated in other settings, early tracheostomy may be another intervention that can improve outcomes and reduce hospital costs for ventilated patients. Direct and indirect costs associated with tracheostomy need to be adequately measured, however, especially if the patient is discharged with the tracheostomy in place.

ICU ORGANIZATION

A dedicated critical care–trained medical director is essential to maintaining an efficient ICU, and a closed ICU organization with intensivists managing all aspects of patient care is the ideal. The development, testing, and maintenance of clinical protocols require an individual who will remain current with rapidly changing literature and technology advances. Successful implementation of a clinical protocol requires a champion to maintain momentum and adherence. A clinician trained in critical care will be more likely to recognize the benefit of clinical innovations and understand approaches to implement them. If a medical director is able to work with a staff of full-time intensivists, education and buy-in for the protocol may require less effort. Even with the help of evidence-based protocols, management of the ventilated patient still requires a significant degree of clinical intuition, which is best developed through experience. Dedicated intensivists have a better opportunity to accrue this experience than clinicians with multiple competing clinical interests.

The rationale for maintaining high-intensity ICU staffing (mandatory intensivist consultation or a closed ICU setting) is supported by multiple studies in the literature, although none of them are randomized trials. A systematic review of studies comparing high-intensity staffing to settings with no intensivists or only elective intensivist consultation revealed a pooled estimate of relative risk for hospital mortality of 0.71 (95% confidence interval, 0.62–0.82).[31] While some studies noted greater use of ICU interventions such as mechanical ventilation or pulmonary artery catheters in the closed ICUs, high-intensity staffing reduced ICU length of stay in 14 of 18 studies including the two studies with case-mix adjustment. Importantly, the degree of illness severity increased for many of the ICUs when they adopted high-intensity staffing, suggesting that dedicated intensivists achieve more efficient use of ICU resources. While the closed ICU model is the norm in

Europe and Australia, only 30% of ICUs in the United States have adopted such forms of organization. This proportion may increase as quality initiatives by various health consortiums and industry groups have identified 24-hour intensivist coverage for ICU patients as an important priority.

WITHHOLDING OR WITHDRAWING MECHANICAL VENTILATION IN TERMINALLY ILL PATIENTS

Up to 12% of health care expenditures and 27% of Medicare expenditures are spent on patients during the last year of their life. For Medicare patients who die, 40% of their Medicare expenses are generated during the last month of their life. Seventy percent of their total expenses are spent on inpatient care. Dying patients often endure a period of critical illness before their death. Limiting ICU care for patients at the end of their life might seem like an obvious target for reducing ICU resource consumption and limiting health care costs. Although certain theoretical models have supported this assumption, realizing true cost savings in practice has been very difficult to accomplish for a number of reasons.[32]

Advance directives are relatively uncommon and often countermanded in the setting of acute respiratory failure if palliative measures are not already in place. The SUPPORT trial and other studies have demonstrated that interventions to make physicians more aware of patient prognoses and preferences for end-of-life care do not alter outcomes or result in reductions in resource use. Once patients have been intubated, early withdrawal of support for those with the worst prognoses could potentially result in cost savings, but only if it resulted in death in a much shorter period of time than would have occurred with continued care. Prolonged palliative care in an inpatient setting would significantly reduce any incremental cost savings. Unfortunately, 68% of the patients in the SUPPORT trial who received the most costly amounts of care had survival probabilities of 40–80% estimated on the day of ICU admission. Extremely poor prognoses did not become evident until after days or weeks of mechanical ventilation. The number of patients for whom dismal prognoses were evident on ICU admission were relatively few. Finally, since most costs of an ICU bed are fixed, aggressive efforts to limit mechanical ventilation in patients with extremely poor prognoses would result in significant cost savings only if consistent practice would lead to closing of ICU beds and layoff of employees.[32]

Cost effectiveness is not a reason to withhold or withdraw life-sustaining therapies such as mechanical ventilation from patients with acute respiratory failure when resources are available. Such decisions are best guided by considerations of whether the interventions are in the best interest of the patient in the context of his or her own wishes for life-sustaining care. This is true even for very old patients. Most studies have shown that advanced age is a minor risk factor for death in mechanically ventilated patients compared to acute illness severity and comorbidities. Despite these findings, critically ill elderly patients receive fewer resource-intensive interventions than younger patients. Because this is not associated with worse severity-adjusted mortality, overuse of resources in younger patients may be the relevant factor.[33]

TRANSFER TO LOWER-INTENSITY SITES OF CARE

For critically ill patients, the highest intensity of care usually occurs within the first few days of mechanical ventilation. As gas exchange and hemodynamics improve, the level of nursing required to manage patients decreases. As long as they remain in an ICU, however, the associated nursing commitment and costs remain substantial. When the lengths of stay for patients with DRG 483 (now DRG 541 and 542) extend beyond approximately 28 days, hospitals begin to assume considerable financial losses. Therefore, hospitals are quite motivated to find less-intensive sites of care for these patients. Prolonged occupancy of an acute hospital bed interferes with more efficient and well-reimbursed uses of that bed. The ICU bed occupied by a patient requiring 21 days of mechanical ventilation after coronary artery bypass grafting could have accommodated at least 8 other patients under the same DRG. If the ICU remained full and 8 elective cases were cancelled, the motivation to find alternative sites of care for the patient requiring prolonged ventilation would become extreme.

Options for lower-intensity sites of care for patients requiring prolonged mechanical ventilation include (1) stepdown units or dedicated respiratory care units within the acute hospital, (2) transfer to separate acute care hospitals dedicated to weaning patients from mechanical ventilation such as regional weaning centers, long-term acute care hospitals (LTACs) or specialized rehabilitation hospitals, (3) transfer to skilled nursing facilities that offer ventilator care, or (4) discharge to home with home ventilation. The number of free-standing facilities able to manage patients requiring prolonged mechanical ventilation has grown at a rate of 12% per year since 1992,[20] owing in part to the exemption from DRG-limited reimbursement for these facilities before 1998. Even after DRGs were established for long-term care facilities, they continued to proliferate because of the demand from acute hospitals for alternative sites of care and their relative profitability. Hospitals have been discharging patients to these facilities more frequently and earlier in their acute hospital course. Unfortunately, this trend has been associated with a significant increase in the proportion of chronically critically ill patients who are readmitted to acute care hospitals because of recurrence of severe acute illness.

Costs of Mechanical Ventilation in Post-ICU Settings

When mechanically ventilated patients are transferred from the acute ICU to lower-intensity settings, marginal cost savings are achieved primarily because of lower nurse/patient ratios. While 1:1 or 1:2 nurse/patient ratios are typical of most acute ICUs, ratios of 1:3 or 1:4 are standard for acute hospital stepdown units or respiratory care units, and ratios of 1:6 or 1:8 are often utilized in LTAC hospitals. Savings in nursing costs are balanced by additional expenses for respiratory therapists and physical and occupational therapists. Prolonged weaning of weak patients demands a high degree of therapist monitoring, and aggressive physical rehabilitation during weaning is felt to be important for good outcomes. Custodial care of ventilated patients in skilled nursing facilities that does not include active weaning or rehabilitation is less expensive on a daily basis, but complete failure to wean patients results in higher costs ultimately.

The timely transfer of a patient requiring prolonged mechanical ventilation to a long-term care hospital will help control costs for the referring acute hospital, but it is not completely clear whether such transfers are cost effective for payors. The Medicare Payment Advisory Commission (MedPAC) attempted to address this issue by comparing outcomes and costs for patients with DRG 483 who were treated in regions with LTAC hospitals versus regions without LTAC hospitals.[20] Using least-squares regression to control for illness severity, they found no difference in mortality between patients managed entirely in acute care hospitals and patients transferred to LTAC hospitals. When they used an instrumental variable approach to better adjust for selection bias, however, they found a higher mortality associated with LTAC transfer. Adjusted spending for the total episode of hospitalization (acute hospital and LTAC days) was lower for patients who used LTACs compared to those who did not. From this analysis, it appears that transferring a patient requiring prolonged mechanical ventilation to an LTAC results in equal or worse outcomes at lower costs. Clearly, prospective cost effectiveness analyses using validated measures of illness severity are necessary to adequately answer this important question. A randomized referral process would be ideal for such a study, but this would be difficult to implement considering the financial implications for the referring hospitals.

CONTROLLING COSTS IN POST-ICU SETTINGS

Cost containment in the post-ICU setting depends upon staffing and efficient patient management principles. As stated previously, the greatest cost savings are realized by limiting nursing coverage. Respiratory care units and LTAC hospitals should only accept patients that are hemodynamically stable and have stable airways via tracheostomy. The need for close bedside monitoring by nurses is greatly reduced in stable ventilated patients, and nurse/patient ratios can be maintained at levels from 1:6 to 1:8. Active weaning that includes prolonged spontaneous breathing trials creates periods of instability, but this can be monitored with the help of respiratory therapists.

Many of the efficient management practices in the acute ICU are relevant to the post-ICU setting. Prevention of ventilator-associated pneumonia and line infections are especially important because of the prolonged periods of risk. Therapist-driven weaning protocols have been shown to enhance the efficiency and safety of weaning in LTAC hospitals. Such protocols should be tailored to each facility's staffing patterns, and they should be frequently updated based on outcomes and new safety issues. The on-site presence of qualified physician staff around the clock might also enhance weaning efficiency. On-site physicians can address complications quickly, and communication with patients and families regarding goals of care occurs more regularly.

The Future

Continued advances in technology will increase the gap between what critical care medicine can do and what is economically feasible to do. The formal application of health economics to guide decision making in the delivery or organization of critical care is in its early stages. Economic analysis will become more influential as providers become more familiar with its benefits and its limitations. Increasing sophistication of clinical information systems and inclusion of economic components in the design of clinical trials will provide higher-quality data.[9] Investigators are continuing to refine quality-of-life assessments, and better understanding of long-term outcomes of critically ill patients is an area of growing research interest.[34] More research into the behavioral aspects of medicine including social and professional expectations for distribution of resources will provide guidance to societies and health plans on how to utilize the data from economic analyses.[35]

Economic pressures and financial constraints will continue to have a beneficial effect on efficiency of care in the ICU by minimizing waste and redundant services. ICU directors, however, need to exercise caution in the persistent drive for efficiency. Overly aggressive measures to discharge patients from the ICU and maintain high occupancy of only severely ill patients can worsen outcomes. For example, discharges from the ICU at night and ICU admissions during periods of peak occupancy and high nursing workload are associated with higher hospital mortality. From the perspective of society and health care systems, savings generated from reductions or restrictions in critical care services are justified only if those savings are invested in more effective services elsewhere in the system.[2]

Summary and Conclusions

The high costs of critical care services will always make this area of medicine a target for cost containment. Patients requiring mechanical ventilation consume a disproportionate share of hospital resources, especially those requiring prolonged ventilation. Despite the costs, mechanical ventilation for patients with acute respiratory failure meets current standards for cost effectiveness except for patients with the highest likelihood of short-term mortality. Strategies to reduce hospital costs are directed toward decreasing the duration of mechanical ventilation. These strategies include prevention of intubation by rapid response to illness and noninvasive ventilation when indicated, efficient evidence-based management practices, optimal ICU organization, and transfer to low-intensity sites of care when it is safe for the patient. Economic analyses will assume a greater role in decision making related to mechanical ventilation as investigators include cost and quality-of-life components in the design of clinical trials and as providers gain a better understanding of how to utilize the data.

References

1. Halpern NA, Pastores SM, Greenstein RJ. Critical care medicine in the United States 1985–2000: An analysis of bed numbers, use, and costs. Crit Care Med 2004; 32:1254–9.

2. Rubenfeld GD. Cost-effectiveness considerations in critical care. New Horiz 1998; 6:33–40.

3. Schramm W, Szucs TD. State-of-the-art principles and practices of medical economics. Haemophilia 1998; 4:491–7.

4. Noseworthy TW, Konopad E, Shustack A, et al. Cost accounting of adult intensive care: Methods and human and capital inputs. Crit Care Med 1998; 24:1168–72.

5. Sznajder M, Aegerter P, Launois R, et al. A cost-effectiveness analysis of stays in intensive care units. Intensive Care Med 2001; 27:146–153.

6. Rapoport J, Teres D, Lemeshow S, et al. A method for assessing the clinical performance and cost-effectiveness of intensive care units: A multicenter inception cohort study. Crit Care Med 1994; 22:1385–91.

7. Cooper LM, Linde-Zwirble WT. Medicare intensive care unit use: Analysis of incidence, cost, and payment. Crit Care Med 2004; 32:2247–53.

8. Keene AR, Cullen DJ. Therapeutic Intervention Scoring System: Update 1983. Crit Care Med 1983; 11:1–3.

9. Coughlin MT, Angus DC. Economic evaluation of new therapies in critical illness. Crit Care Med 2003; 31(Suppl.):S7–S16.

10. Hamel MB, Phillips RS, Davis RB, et al. Outcomes and cost-effectiveness of ventilator support and aggressive care for patients with acute respiratory failure due to pneumonia or acute respiratory distress syndrome. Am J Med 2000; 109:614–20.

11. Hamel MB, Phillips RS, Davis RB, et al. Are aggressive treatment strategies less cost-effective for older patients? The case of ventilator support and aggressive care for patients with acute respiratory failure. J Am Geriatr Soc 2001; 49:382–90.

12. Kalish SC, Gurwitz J, Krumholz HM, et al. A cost-effectiveness model of thrombolytic therapy for acute myocardial infarction. J Gen Intern Med 1995; 10:321–30.

13. Angus DC, Linde-Zwirble WT, Clermont G, et al. Cost-effectiveness of drotrecogin alfa (activated) in the treatment of severe sepsis. Crit Care Med 2003; 31:1–11.

14. Cox CE, Carson SS, Biddle AK. Cost-effectiveness of ultrasound in preventing femoral venous catheter-associated pulmonary embolism. Am J Respir Crit Care Med 2003; 168:1481–7.

15. Ramsey SD, Patrick DL, Albert RK, et al. The cost-effectiveness of lung transplantation. Chest 1995; 108:1594–601.

16. Lee KH, Angus DC, Abramson NS. Cardiopulmonary resuscitation: What cost to cheat death? Crit Care Med 1996; 14:2046–52.

17. Weinstein MD, Siegel JE, Gold MR, et al. Recommendations of the Panel on Cost-Effectiveness in Health and Medicine. JAMA 1996; 276:1253–8.

18. McCarthy TP, Yaculak G, Ringler B. A review of 2,487 mechanically ventilated patients: Ventilator length of stay (VLOS), base costs, ICU distribution, and mortality. Respir Care 1998; 43: 114–8.

19. Wagner DP. Economics of prolonged mechanical ventilation. Am Rev Respir Dis 1989; 140:S14–S18.

20. Medicare Payment Advisory Commission. Defining long-term care hospitals (Chapter 5, June 2004 report). Available at: www.medpac.gov/publications. Accessed November, 2004.

21. Cox CE, Carson SS, Holmes GM, et al. Increase in tracheostomy for prolonged mechanical ventilation in North Carolina, 1993–2002. Crit Care Med 2004; 32:2219–26.

22. Douglas SL, Daly BJ, Brennan PF, et al. Hospital readmission among long-term ventilator patients. Chest 2001; 120: 1278–86.

23. Carson SS, Bach PB. The epidemiology and costs of chronically critically ill patients. Crit Care Clin 2002; 18:461–76.

24. Heyland DK, Konopad E, Noseworthy TW, et al. Clinical investigations in critical care. Is it "worthwhile" to continue treating patients with a prolonged stay (>14 days) in the ICU? An economic evaluation. Chest 1998; 114:192–8.

25. Keenan SP, Gregor J, Sibbald WJ, et al. Noninvasive positive pressure ventilation in the setting of severe, acute exacerbations of chronic obstructive pulmonary disease: More effective and less expensive. Crit Care Med 2000; 28:2094–102.

26. Ely EW, Baker AM, Dunagan DP, et al. Effect on the duration of mechanical ventilation of identifying patients capable of breathing spontaneously. N Engl J Med 1996; 335:1864–9.

27. Kress JP, Pohlman AS, O'Connor MF, Hall JB. Daily interruption of sedative infusions in critically ill patients undergoing mechanical ventilation. N Engl J Med 2000; 342:1471–7.

28. The Acute Respiratory Distress Syndrome Network. Ventilation with lower tidal volumes as compared with traditional tidal volumes for acute lung injury and the acute respiratory distress syndrome. N Engl J Med 2000; 342:1301–8.

29. Kollef MH. The prevention of ventilator-associated pneumonia. N Engl J Med 1999; 340:627–34.

30. Rumbak MJ, Newton M, Truncale T, et al. A prospective, randomized, study comparing early percutaneous dilational tracheotomy to prolonged translaryngeal intubation (delayed tracheotomy) in critically ill medical patients. Crit Care Med 2004; 32:1689–94.

31. Pronovost PJ, Angus DC, Dorman T, et al. Physician staffing patterns and clinical outcomes in critically ill patients. A systematic review. JAMA 2002; 288:2151–62.

32. Luce JM, Rubenfeld GD. Critical Care Perspective. Can health care costs be reduced by limiting intensive care at the end of life? Am J Respir Crit Care Med 2002; 165:750–4.

33. Hamel MB, Davis RB, Teno JM, Knaus WA, et al. Older age, aggressiveness of care, and survival for seriously ill, hospitalized adults. Ann Intern Med 1999; 131:721–8.

34. Pronovost P, Angus DC. Economics of end-of-life care in the intensive care unit. Crit Care Med 2001; 29:N46–N51.

35. Fuchs VR. The future of health economics. J Health Econ 2000; 19:141–57.

PURCHASING
A VENTILATOR

JAMES B. FINK

Ventilators come in a broad range of configurations, modes, and monitoring capabilities, many without evidence to support clinical efficacy.[1] Developing and maintaining a fleet of ventilators is a complex administrative process, requiring a strategic plan, comprehensive analysis, and extensive evaluation.[2] Purchasing a ventilator should be based on a selection process with a compelling rationale.[3] Purchasing one or more ventilators is a strategic decision requiring involvement and support of numerous stakeholders. Ventilators are expensive capital equipment, costing as much as $50,000 per unit, with 20 ventilators costing> $1,000,000, competing for capital dollars with institutional priorities, such as monitoring and diagnostic imaging systems.

The assessment of need becomes the primary impetus for the design of the selection and evaluation process. From the needs assessment, the evaluation can be planned and organized according to time constraints, and resource limitations.[4] Critical items in the selection process must be identified and given higher value in the decision-making process.[5]

The Economic Argument for Proper Ventilator Evaluation

Well designed products may not work well in your clinical setting, and a poorly designed ventilator can be a disaster. Ventilators with similar specifications may function quite differently. Too many departments are populated with one or more very expensive and rarely used ventilators collecting dust. The goal is to select the ventilator with the best performance at the lowest relative cost.

Why Replace Ventilators?

Reasons to replace or add ventilators can range from aging devices that fail with increasing frequency to a perceived need for more advanced technology to support clinical practice. Chatburn et al[5] describe five generations of ventilators that evolved over the past 50 years, suggesting substantial advances in clinical capabilities. The purchasing decision should be based on an assessment of needs.[5] The assessment starts with an audit of existing resources and utilization, including a comprehensive list of each existing ventilator with the manufacturer, model, date of model release, date of purchase, primary areas of use, number of days per year in use, repair record, maintenance contracts, and costs. Overall estimates of ventilator utilization for the facility and each clinical area should reflect mean, as well as peak or maximum utilization. Ventilator rental patterns and costs should be tracked on an annual and month-by-month basis.

DEFINING NEEDS FOR NEW VENTILATORS

Once the needs assessment has identified resources and use patterns, the data should be analyzed to quantify needs and used to support a rationale for purchase. This rationale may include one or more of the following components:

1. A new service area is opening, with no existing ventilators available to support it. This is restricted to new facilities or expansion of capabilities in facilities with no capacity to share resources with other units.
2. Current ventilators are aging. Ventilators as capital equipment are typically depreciated over a 10-year cycle. Administrators tend to support scheduled replacement of capital devices on a relatively consistent schedule.
3. Increased device failure or maintenance costs. As ventilators age they become less reliable, with greater per annum costs for maintenance contracts or repair costs, with increased risk of device failure during use. These costs often escalate during the first 5 years of ventilator ownership.
4. Insufficient ventilators to meet current or anticipated demand. When ventilators are not available, both patient and institution are at considerable risk. Some institutions borrow or rent ventilators during peak periods. Using a machine without ensuring that is has received appropriate maintenance should not be done without review and approval by the hospital risk-management department. Monthly rental charges can represent 5–10% of the purchase price of a ventilator. Institutions renting ventilators 4 months a year will save money by purchasing by the end of year three.
5. Existing ventilators do not meet current clinical needs. This can range from units with limited flow rates, slow response times, and high work of breathing to ventilators that do not support desired clinical practices, such as pressure-controlled, pressure-release, heliox, noninvasive, high-frequency, or jet ventilation.[4]

6. Existing ventilators do not have the capability to manage the range of patients seen at the institution. Previous generations of technology have required separate ventilators capable of treating infants and adults. Acquisition of newer generation ventilators can reduce the number of different ventilators for staff to learn to use and maintain, and possibly the total number of ventilators required.[5]

7. Existing ventilators do not meet the environmental requirements for the facility. In areas where mains power is frequently interrupted and electrical back-up is inconsistent, ventilators with internal battery back-up may be essential. This category could also relate to size, mobility, noise level, or even power requirements.

DEFINING CHARACTERISTICS OF THE NEW VENTILATOR

Specific characteristics for the ventilator need to be identified based on patient populations, current practice preferences, and perceived needs to support current and future practices.[5–7]

Patients have distinct needs, and not all ventilators can support diverse populations. Few ventilators can effectively provide for the needs of both infants and adults. The type and severity of patients treated will dictate the range of ventilatory parameters, monitoring, and alarms best suited for a specific setting.

INTERFACE
Active video screens, liquid crystal displays (LCDs), and touch-screen technology provide the opportunity to improve accuracy of settings and scales while decreasing the number of analog controls. The profusion of ventilator modes, settings, and monitoring represents more options than can fit on a single panel or screen. This can result in poorly designed, nonintuitive interfaces that are difficult to navigate, and almost impossible to remember. Nonintuitive interfaces increase the potential that hard-to-access capabilities of the ventilator will be underutilized. Clinicians do not have time to repeatedly refer to instruction manuals to interpret poorly labeled controls, or to navigate multiple levels of software.

Considerations include whether a competent clinician can intuitively work through the layers of software after less than 5 minutes of initial orientation to the new interface. Can every feature be reached with three actions and activated by two actions?

MONITORING
The team should determine which monitoring capabilities will be used on a regular basis in the ICU. Avoid paying for monitoring capabilities that will seldom be used. For valuable measurements that are infrequently utilized, freestanding monitors constitute a better economic option. Other practical considerations include whether the display can be seen easily. It is important to get feedback from the staff as to whether the display can be read from across the room, under both high and low lighting conditions, and if it can easily be modified to reflect clinician preferences.

ACCESSORIES
Few ventilators come ready to be placed at the bedside without an array of accessories, often best purchased with the ventilator. They may include one or more of the following.

Carts, Brackets, and Carriers
Carts may be a simple base with wheels, or complex storage facilities with space to carry parts and supplies. Brackets may be used to mount the ventilator at the bedside. Carriers may be configured to attach to batteries and gas cylinders, which facilitate transport.

High-Pressure Gas Hoses and Connecting Hardware
Specify the quick connect required to interface with the piped gas outlets or tank regulators in the specific units. Assure sufficient hose length to reach the wall outlets.

External Blender
For ventilators without an internal blender, determine the type of blender, bracket, hoses, and attachment hardware required.

Internal Compressors versus Piped AIR
If the ventilator is to be used in areas where oxygen alone is piped in or is only available in cylinders, a compressor may be essential. Compressors add costs, both as for initial acquisition and regular maintenance, that often exceed the cost of maintaining the ventilator.

Heated Humidifiers
Active heated humidification is essential in treating infants and patients with thick secretions. Heated humidifiers range from a simple hot pot, to a microprocessor-driven, servo-controlled device, which can be used alone or with heated-wire circuits. Evaluate for initial acquisition as well as cost of use. Heated humidifiers require mounting brackets and an electricity source that will not compromise operation of the ventilator.

Ventilator Circuits
Circuits, probes, sensors, and adapters comprising the ventilator circuit may be disposable or reusable, with or without heated wires. Disposable, single-patient use circuits provide an element of convenience offset by cumulative operating costs, need for storage, and mounting requirements for proper disposal of contaminated medical waste, which burdens the environment with large amounts of plastic.[8] Reusable circuits require cleaning and sterilization or high-level disinfection between patients, requiring a substantial long-term commitment and operating costs. In addition to processing, circuits and individual parts may wear out or mistakenly be thrown out, requiring costly replacement. Institutional practices, such as extended use of ventilator circuits to 7 days or the length of the patient's ventilation, reduces circuit costs, and should be calculated into utilization/cost estimates.[9]

Filters
Inspiratory filters protect the patient from particulates in the piped or compressed gas supply. Expiratory filters eliminate

secondhand exposure to aerosols and protect the downstream sensors and components. Reusable filters tend to be expensive and require periodic testing to determine resistance to flow, and occasional visual aerosol challenge to assure that the filter element is still intact. Disposable filters are less expensive on a per unit basis and require no upkeep, but may have a greater impact on operating costs.

AEROSOL SYSTEMS

Over the past 50 years, it has been common for manufacturers to provide an internal gas source to drive a pneumatic jet nebulizer synchronized with the patient's inspiratory pattern. The pressure and flow delivered by the ventilator varies with ventilator model, and may be insufficient to efficiently drive the nebulizers.[10] Operating nebulizers at lower pressure and flow rates can increase particle size, reducing efficiency during mechanical ventilation. Gas sources to drive nebulizers should be evaluated to determine whether the pressure (>35 psi) and flow through the nebulizer meet the recommendations of the nebulizer manufacturer.

An alternative to the internal compressor is use of an external continuous gas source, typically at 50 psi, to provide the recommended flow to the nebulizer. This strategy provides consistent nebulizer performance, but changes the delivered flow rates and volumes secondary to the addition of the gas into the circuit, and adversely affects monitors and alarms. Because research has demonstrated the inefficiency of jet nebulizers as compared with pressurized metered dose inhalers (pMDIs), many manufacturers have eliminated gas output to drive nebulizers.[11] Ultrasonic nebulizers and electronic micropumps are severalfold more efficient than jet nebulizers,[12] but are relatively expensive to acquire, and are best ordered at the time of purchase of the ventilator.

SPECIAL NEEDS

Heliox

Use of helium-oxygen (heliox) mixtures requires ventilators and monitors capable of operation with this low-density gas.[13–18] While few ventilators are designed to work with heliox, some can work with calculations to compensate for gas density and flow rates, although other ventilators cannot work with heliox at all.[15–18] Bench evaluation with a volumetric test lung, or a monitor that can be adjusted for heliox concentrations provide valuable insight on the feasibility of using heliox.[18–19]

Anesthesia

Relatively few critical care ventilators have the capability for use with anesthetic agents. This capability can be of great value for supporting the difficult-to-ventilate patient during surgery, and should be a specific selection criterion in institutions in which the capability is desired.

Closed-Loop Ventilation and Lung-Recruitment Protocols

As clinical interest in closed-loop ventilation and lung-recruitment protocols increases,[20–24] manufacturers are introducing lung-recruitment, weaning and closed-loop ventilation protocols. If the premises of the algorithm does not agree with the premise of the clinician and cannot be adjusted by the user, these features may increase cost without being used.

COST ANALYSES

ESTIMATED PURCHASE AND OPERATING COSTS

Capital requests should include the number and general type of devices, purchase costs for the ventilator and accessories, and costs of contracts or routine maintenance.[2] The estimate should be sufficient to purchase your ideal ventilator, based on initial evaluation of device options and specifications. Specify how many units are being requested, and how many of those would be essential for the budget period. Cost-analysis considerations include the initial costs, ongoing costs, and added costs (Table 69-1).

It is not uncommon to be asked for a 5- or 10-year capital projection to help the institution plan for capital investment needs. Projecting future needs provides context for administration to better understand the context for the current request, and may improve chances of approval.

PREPARING A TENDER

Once it appears that funds will be available to make a purchase during the upcoming year, a document should be developed to communicate the essentials to the purchasing department. Often, the purchasing group issues a tender or request for quotation to solicit device options and costs from a variety of manufacturers, to purchase the least expensive device that meets the most basic of requirements. It is crucial

TABLE 69-1   Key Considerations for Cost Analysis

Initial acquisition costs
  Basic ventilator
  Accessories
    Monitor
    Compressor
    Cart
    Humidifier
    Nebulizer
    Blender
    Hoses and quick connects
Shipping
Taxes

Recurring operating costs
  Required sensors
    Disposable or reusable
  Filters
  Circuit requirements
    Disposable or reusable
  Scheduled maintenance contracts
  Repairs
  Upgrades

Administrative and staff costs
  Development of procedures
  Clinical staff training and support
  Biotech training and periodic testing and in-house maintenance
  Set-up and maintenance of parts/components inventory
  Parts and device processing between patients

TABLE 69-2 When to Evaluate Ventilators

To assess new technology
  How does it perform against its specifications?
  Identify advantages
  Identify disadvantages
  Evaluate the interface
  Evaluate safety
To understand existing technology
  How does it perform?
  Differentiate performance between device types
  Device failure analysis
When making purchasing decisions
  Establish suitability for use in clinical practice
  Establish cost/benefit relationships
  Comparative analysis across ventilator options

to establish the expectation that all candidate devices will meet all specifications and reserve the right to make final selection based on in-house evaluation of performance.

COMPARISON OF NEW VENTILATORS

TECHNICAL EVALUATION

Ventilators are evaluated to determine if they will be useful and serviceable in a specific environment. A ventilator should be evaluated as much to learn what it cannot do as to learn what it can. Marketing data, such as label specifications, emphasize what a product can do (from a narrow perspective), and is silent on what it cannot do. Only if device limitations are identified before adoption can one assure that patients will not be placed at risk by mistakenly extending the ventilator beyond those unspoken limitations (Table 69-2). More than just guiding purchasing decisions, these evaluations can help determine how best to apply the technology, and identify device limitations so that associated risks to the patient can be reduced or eliminated.

Ventilator evaluation is best performed in collaboration with a broad range of health care practitioners, in either the home or hospital setting.[3,4] Stakeholders with a direct interest should be involved in ventilator evaluation and the purchasing decision (Table 69-3).

TABLE 69-3 Key Participants in Ventilator Evaluation

Managers and supervisors
Clinical staff
Care providers
  Team members
    Nursing staff
    Physicians
    Primary users of the device
    Respiratory therapists
  Support services
    Biomed
    Central supply
    Central processing
Patients
Students
Educators

IDENTIFY CANDIDATE VENTILATORS

Candidate ventilators should be identified based on the characteristics, specifications, and options from the needs assessment. This process may require some translation of market branding of modes, accessories, and characteristics into common terms that can be related across devices. Two to four ventilators that best meet the initial wish list should be selected for additional evaluation.

TESTING TO SPECIFICATIONS

It is difficult to evaluate a ventilator based solely on its specifications. Few manufacturers provide sufficient detail on how they test their devices against label specification claims to permit the clinician to reproduce or even interpret their findings. This is in part a consequence of how specifications are created in the product-development process.[25] In-house methods to test or check a specification may be considerably different from those used by the manufacturer, and more clinically relevant.

TECHNICAL ANALYSIS

STEPS IN VENTILATOR EVALUATION

Background
Background information should be gathered and reviewed before initiating more extensive evaluation. A literature search can help you identify previous reviews, product alerts, and any published research.

Safety alerts and recalls can be found on the web at http://www.fda.gov/cdrh. ECRI publishes monthly publications such as Health Devices, Health Devices Alerts, and the searchable Health Device Index can be accessed on the web at www.ecri.org.[26]

Let the instruction manual be your guide. Manufacturer specifications and directions for use are essential reading before designing a device evaluation. Ask the manufacturer for contact information and references from current customers to help identify key performance parameters.

Bench Testing
Bench testing is easier, cheaper, and faster than clinical evaluations. Patients are complex and fragile, with many variables affecting how they react and how they interface with a device, making meaningful measurement and observation difficult. Bench testing allows you to better understand how the device works, when it works, and when it does not work. Once a model is shown to correlate with clinical experience, the in vitro-to-in vivo correlation becomes more meaningful and the bench model a reliable predictor of in vivo results.[27]

Limitations to in vitro Testing
While patient interfaces may be too complex to isolate individual performance issues, in vitro tests may be too simple (Table 69-4). Bench testing can seldom simulate the complexity of interactions in vivo.

Assessment of the Company
Beyond the characteristics and performance of a specific ventilator, consumers need to evaluate the company to

TABLE 69-4   Common Problems with Bench Evaluations

- Too many variables in a single experiment
- In vitro set-up does not sufficiently model some aspects of in vivo situations
- Inaccurate measurements
- Devices improperly or inconsistently used
- Data are not consistently or accurately recorded
- Too few repetitions
- Incorrect statistical methods are applied
- Methods are poorly described and not reproducible between ventilators
- Records are poorly maintained or scattered so experiments are not reproducible
- Results are not reported to full impact

TABLE 69-5   Preparing for a Bedside Evaluation

Select ventilators to be evaluated
  Bring units in for initial evaluation by stakeholders
  Formal presentation of devices
  Solicit feedback from stakeholders to reduce primary choices to three or fewer
Administrative components
  Arrange for extended evaluation for finalist ventilators
  Review instruction manuals
  Develop procedures for use for each ventilator
    Validate procedures
    Create a competency check-off sheet for use with each trained staff member
    Develop tools for collecting feedback
    Train all staff who will use the device
    Allow time for staff to play with the ventilator (simulated use before actual clinical use)
    Assure staff competency with device (use the check-off sheet)
  Acquire enough units for sufficient duration to gain experience (≥ 2 devices evaluated for up to 4 weeks)
Biomed safety evaluation and electrical check for each unit before use
Solicit feedback
Collect the feedback
Collate the feedback
Report findings to stakeholders

understand the quality systems in place, their ability to supply products as promised, and the ability to support products in the field. Any device can have problems in the field. The key is how the company responds to those problems in protecting patients and customers.

The ability of a company to supply a product in a timely manner is an important factor. Any delay can be a result of demand exceeding supply, or regulatory issues that embargo importation and delivery of the ventilator to a specific market.

Does the company provide good product support? Support varies between companies, based on dedicated resources and their distribution across service areas. These resources include clinical staff educator support, availability and promptness of in-house service and maintenance, and availability of replacement parts.

Introduction of new high-technology devices requires training of all staff that will operate and interface with the device, during both initial evaluation and installation of purchased units, and often requires extensive training on multiple shifts. Training of clinicians is best done by well-trained educators who understand both the technology and the clinical environment in which it will be used.

Repair services need to be available immediately, or within 24 hours when a device failure is identified. When this is not routinely available, the manufacturer should train in-house biomedical service personnel to do routine maintenance, troubleshooting, repair, and upgrades. A stock of common parts can be kept in the hospital, with the hospital paying as they are used.

Clinical Trials

Clinical experience with feedback from staff and stakeholders is valuable but expensive, costing up to $10,000 for each device. The steps for a well-planned evaluation are shown in Table 69-5. Evaluate sufficient numbers of each ventilator so staff can get meaningful experience in a short time. If necessary, rent or lease units for a month of evaluation. Ventilators should be inspected by the biomedical department. Designate a device champion who will be available to support first interactions with the ventilator and patients. Make feedback instruments available and encourage staff to fill them out and submit them on a daily basis. This feedback instrument provides the primary quantifiable evidence of how the device performed, and how the staff liked it.

Interaction with Hospital Administration

Hospital administrators seldom have the background to understand the resources necessary to support a critical care environment. Ongoing efforts to orient the responsible administrator, and to a more limited extent, the administrative hierarchy, can pay great dividends in developing an advocacy base within the system.

Developing and maintaining a fleet of ventilators is not dependent on a single purchase. It is a perpetual process. The strategy to justify and procure ventilators should be long-term, and negotiations for resources are an iterative process, with projected needs represented in capital budget forecasts on an annual basis. While it may be desirable to replace an entire fleet of ventilators in one purchase, limited capital resources may require negotiating a staged process over several capital cycles.

Project ventilator needs over a 3- to 5-year period so that the capital-budget committee is aware of the window in which allocations will be required. Negotiate whether the new ventilators should be purchased or leased.

The Future

Future options may include a profusion of new options with precious little evidence to guide the clinician as to which of these attributes add value and not just cost. It will remain incumbent on the buyer to identify which features make a positive difference for their unique patient population.

Summary and Conclusion

Starting, supplementing, and maintaining a fleet of ventilators that meets the diverse clinical needs within an institution is a strategic and political process within the organization. Planning, data gathering, assessment, evaluation, communication, and training are key components that support the process. Disciplined efforts can reap the rewards of always having sufficient ventilator resources to support patient needs.

References

1. Branson RD, Johannigman JA. What is the evidence base for the newer ventilator modes? Respir Care 2004; 49:742–60.
2. Fink JB, Fink AK. Respiratory therapist as manager: Tools for transition. Chicago: Year Book Medical Publishers, 1986.
3. Greenberg D, Pliskin JS, Peterburg Y. Decision making in acquiring medical technologies in Israeli medical centers: a preliminary study. Int J Technol Assess Health Care 2003; 19:194–201.
4. Grace K. The ventilator: selection of mechanical ventilators. Crit Care Clin 1998; 14:563–80.
5. Chatburn RL, Primiano FP. Decision analysis for large capital purchases: How to buy a ventilator. Respir Care 2001; 46: 1038–53.
6. Kacmarek RM. Introducing new mechanical ventilation technology: the hospital perspective. Respir Care 1995; 40:947–51.
7. Branson R. Understanding and implementing advances in ventilator capabilities. Curr Opin Crit Care 2004; 10:23–32.
8. Fink JB, Montague P. Ventilator circuits: disposables vs reusables. Respir Ther 1993; 6:540–42.
9. Fink JB. A rationale for change: reducing the frequency of ventilator circuit changes to seven days can cut costs without compromising patient care. Respir Ther 1993; 6:535–38.
10. McPeck, I'Riordan TG, Smaldone GC. Choice of mechanical ventilator: influence on nebulizer performance. Respir Care 1993; 38:887–95.
11. Fink JB, Tobin MJ, Dhand R. Bronchodilator therapy in mechanically ventilated patients. Respir Care 1999; 44:53–69.
12. Dhand R. Nebulizers that use a vibrating mesh or plate with multiple apertures to generate aerosol. Respir Care 2002; 47:1406–16.
13. Curtis J, Mahlmeister M, Stulbarg MS, et al. Use and availability of helium-oxygen gas therapy for the emergency treatment of inoperable airway obstruction. Chest 1986; 90:455–7.
14. Jaber S, Carlucci A, Boussarsar M, et al. Helium oxygen in the post extubation period decreases inspiratory effort. Am J Respir Crit Care Med 2001; 164:1–5.
15. Goode ML, Fink JB, Dhand R, Tobin MJ. Improvement in aerosol delivery with helium-oxygen mixtures during mechanical ventilation. Am J Respir Crit Care Med 2001; 163:109–14.
16. Oppenheim-Eden A, Cohen Y, Weissman C, Pizov R. The effect of helium on ventilator performance: study of five ventilators and a bedside Pitot tube spirometer. Chest 2001; 120:582–8.
17. Jaber S, Fodil R, Carlucci A, et al. Noninvasive ventilation with helium-oxygen in acute exacerbations of chronic obstructive pulmonary disease. Am J Respir Crit Care Med 2000; 161:1191–1200.
18. Tassaux D, Jolliet P, Roeseler J, Chevrolet JC. Effects of helium-oxygen on intrinsic positive end-expiratory pressure in intubated and mechanically ventilated patients with severe chronic obstructive pulmonary disease. Crit Care Med 2000; 28:2721–8.
19. Tassaux D, Jolliet P, Thouret JM, et al. Calibration of seven ICU ventilators for mechanical ventilation with helium-oxygen mixtures. Am J Respir Crit Care Med 1999; 160:22–32.
20. Ely EW, Bennett PA, Bowton DL, et al. Large scale implementation of a respiratory therapist-driven protocol for ventilator weaning. Am J Respir Crit Care Med 1999; 159:439–46.
21. Mancebo J, Albaladejo P, Touchard D, et al. Airway occlusion pressure to titrate positive end-expiratory pressure in patients with dynamic hyperinflation. Anesthesiology 2000; 93:81–90.
22. Dojat M, Brochard L. Knowledge-based systems for automatic ventilatory management. Respir Care Clin North Am 2001; 7:379–96.
23. Brunner JX. Principles and history of closed-loop controlled ventilation. Respir Care Clin North Am 2001; 7:341–62.
24. Lellouche F, Mancebo J, Roesler J, et al. Computer-driven ventilation reduces duration of weaning: a multicenter randomized controlled study. Intensive Care Med 2004; 30, supp 1:254–69.
25. Fink JB. Device and equipment evaluations. Respir Care 2004; 49:1157–64.
26. Intensive care ventilators. Health Devices 2002; 31:441–54.
27. Fink JB, Dhand R, Grychowski J, Fahey PJ, Tobin M. Reconciling in vitro and in vivo measurements of aerosol delivery from a metered-dose inhaler during mechanical ventilation and defining efficiency-enhancing factors. Am J Respir Crit Care Med 1999; 159:63–67.

Chapter 70

LONG-TERM OUTCOMES AFTER MECHANICAL VENTILATION

CATHERINE LEE HOUGH
J. RANDALL CURTIS

The use of mechanical ventilation in the intensive care unit (ICU) setting provides a potentially life-saving treatment for respiratory failure. In the past, research concerning the outcomes of mechanical ventilation focused on the short-term, with reports of physiologic endpoints such as oxygenation and ventilation, and clinical endpoints such as extubation rates, ICU survival, and hospital survival. Such outcomes are appropriate for many critical care studies concerning mechanical ventilation because of the high short-term mortality and life-threatening physiologic abnormalities in these patients. In recent years, increasing numbers of studies have examined longer-term outcomes in patients with acute respiratory failure requiring mechanical ventilation. These outcomes have included long-term morbidity and mortality, pulmonary function, quality of life, health status, neuropsychological and cognitive functioning, economic outcomes, and the effects on informal caregivers.

Why is it important that we know the long-term outcomes after mechanical ventilation for acute respiratory failure?

The answers vary depending on the category of the outcomes being considered. Long-term survival is important in order to know the prognosis that could play a role in decision making for the patient, his or her family, and the health care providers during the ICU admission, and in considering the utility of future ICU admissions. Knowledge of long-term survival may also be important in resource development and utilization planning.[1] Objectively measured physiologic outcomes such as pulmonary function can help connect events and therapy during the acute illness with other more patient-centered outcomes. These measurements may provide information about physiologic mechanisms of the acute illness and recovery and also may have predictive value. Patient-centered outcomes such as quality of life, health status, and symptoms are important to patients. Also, by understanding the prevalence and severity of decrements in these outcomes, we can begin to link them with possible etiologic factors during the critical illness that are potentially modifiable. In this way we can begin to develop strategies for patient management both during the critical illness and in follow-up, which may be able to prevent or minimize adverse long-term outcomes. Finally, we will also address emerging data of the effect of critical illness on the family and informal caregivers of critically ill patients.

This chapter will review what is known about long-term outcomes after mechanical ventilation for acute respiratory failure. For the most part, we will not be able to differentiate which outcomes are related to the use of mechanical ventilation and which are secondary either to the underlying condition for which mechanical ventilation was instituted or a variety of other factors, including the comorbidities that put patients at risk for acute respiratory failure and the effects of critical care therapies. The literature is most complete in the long-term outcomes after the acute respiratory distress syndrome (ARDS); therefore, follow-up studies of survivors of ARDS dominate this chapter.

We begin with a discussion of studies of long-term survival and mortality. Next, we discuss the use of physiologic outcomes as surrogates for long-term, patient-centered outcomes. We then focus on patient-centered outcomes, including quality of life, health status, neuropsychological and cognitive functioning, and symptoms. We also cover the long-term complications documented in survivors of mechanical ventilation. Mechanical ventilation may allow the occurrence or development of complications by allowing patients to survive acute respiratory failure, but may or may not be directly responsible for them. After a description of outcomes, we will briefly discuss possible etiologic factors where data exist to allow this, including whether mechanical ventilation may be implicated. Most of the data will be reported separately for the differing underlying conditions or types of acute respiratory failure, because the original studies most frequently report outcomes for a particular disease, but also because the underlying condition is likely an important determinant of outcome.

Long-Term Survival

There are no studies describing the impact of the therapy of mechanical ventilation on the long-term survival of patients who survive to hospital discharge. This will be a difficult topic to study because it is difficult to separate the effect of the respiratory failure from the effect of the therapy of mechanical ventilation. There are, however, two groups of studies addressing similar questions that are enlightening. One group looks at the association between ICU admission and long-term survival, either without a comparison group[2] or compared to other hospital[3] or population controls.[4,5] The reports from these studies do not specifically evaluate the independent effect of mechanical ventilation within the ICU patients, but do allow us to draw three conclusions. First, ICU admission is associated with increased short-term mortality (in-hospital), compared with hospitalized patients that are not in the ICU, and compared with population controls.[3] This undoubtedly relates largely to the severity of the illness resulting in the ICU admission. Second, ICU survivors continue to have a higher mortality than age- and gender-matched population controls for at least 1–2 years after hospital discharge.[4,5] Third, compared with patients admitted to the hospital but not to the ICU, the impact of ICU admission on long-term survival is "minimal."[3] That is, ICU admission is an independent risk factor for long-term mortality (odds ratio 1.21), but its impact is less than that of age, comorbidity, clinical diagnosis, and gender (Fig. 70-1).

FIGURE 70-1 Survival curves and 95% confidence intervals for intensive care unit (*ICU*) patients and hospital controls (*Controls*). For comparison, actuarial survival at 1, 2, and 3 years for the general population in British Columbia is shown. (*Reproduced, with permission, from Keenan et al.[3]*)

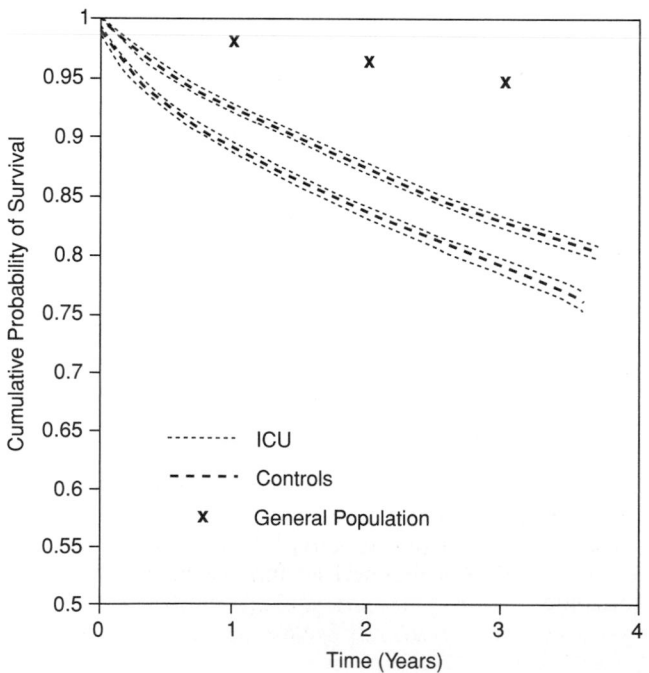

The second group of studies attempts to understand the impact of mechanical ventilation on long-term outcomes within the specific disease processes that cause respiratory failure. We will review studies that investigate the following causes of respiratory failure: chronic obstructive pulmonary disease (COPD), ARDS, and sepsis. For many common causes of acute respiratory failure, such as acute cardiogenic pulmonary edema, there are no studies of the impact of mechanical ventilation on long-term survival.[6,7]

LONG-TERM SURVIVAL IN PATIENTS WITH CHRONIC OBSTRUCTIVE PULMONARY DISEASE AND ACUTE RESPIRATORY FAILURE

Studies from the 1970s and 1980s suggested that once patients with COPD survive an episode of acute respiratory failure, their subsequent survival is similar to patients with the same degree of pulmonary dysfunction without an acute exacerbation of COPD.[8,9] In other words, the prognosis of a patient with COPD was dependent on their severity of COPD and was unaffected by a previous history of an episode of acute respiratory failure. Most patients in these studies, however, were not treated with mechanical ventilation.

Studies of patients with COPD and acute respiratory failure by Connors et al[10] and by Seneff et al[11] reported mortality at 6 months and 1 year (and 2 years for the Connors study). For the cohort of 1016 patients reported by Connors et al, mortality rates increased from the 11% hospital mortality to 33%, 43%, and 49%, respectively, for 6 months, 1 year, and 2 years of follow-up. Approximately one-third of patients received mechanical ventilation (348/1016). Increased mortality was observed in patients who required mechanical ventilation, 43% mortality at 6 months compared to 28% in patients who were not ventilated.

In the study by Seneff et al, specific long-term survival data after acute respiratory failure from COPD are limited to those patients aged 65 years or older. There were 216 who met this age criterion and complete data were available for 167. Overall mortality was 30% at hospital discharge, 47% at 6 months, and 59% at 1 year. Mortality figures for those receiving mechanical ventilation compared to those who did not were 37% versus 23% at hospital discharge, 54% versus 42% at 6 months, and 62% versus 56% at 1 year. Thus, hospital mortality, but not long-term survival, was higher in patients receiving mechanical ventilation (Fig. 70-2). When a multivariate analysis was performed to assess factors associated with mortality, however, mortality was explained by the physiologic abnormalities captured in the Acute Physiology and Chronic Health Evaluation (APACHE) III score and by pre-ICU hospital length of stay and mechanical ventilation was not independently significant.

In summary, although hospital survival for patients with COPD and acute respiratory failure is relatively good, there is a high cumulative mortality over the next 1–2 years. Ventilated patients have approximately twice the hospital mortality as nonventilated patients but mechanical ventilation did not influence subsequent long-term survival. The multivariate analysis finding that respiratory physiology and

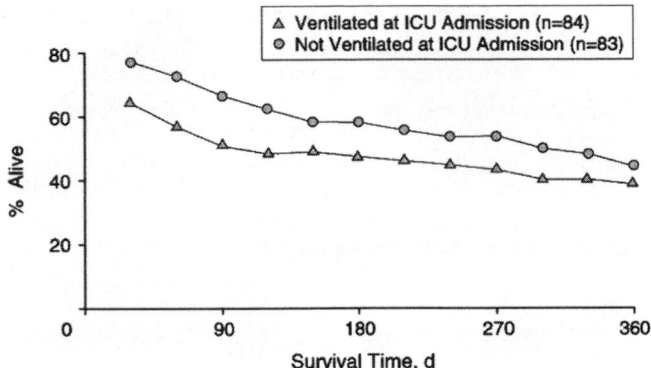

FIGURE 70-2 One-year survival curves for 167 patients aged 65 years or older admitted to an intensive care unit (ICU) for acute exacerbation of chronic obstructive pulmonary disease according to need for mechanical ventilation at ICU admission. (*Reproduced, with permission, from Seneff et al.[11]*)

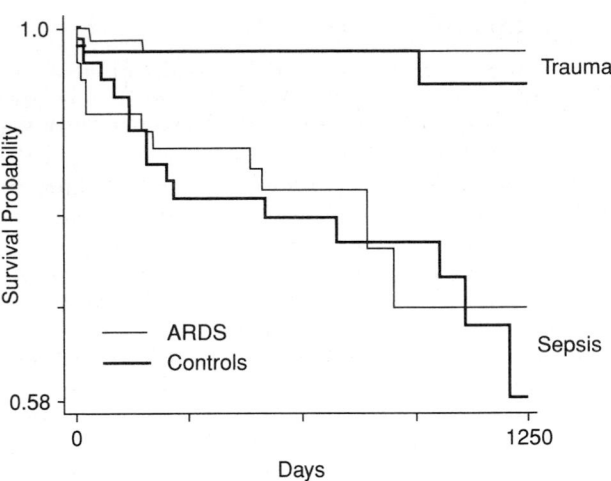

FIGURE 70-3 Survival plot of hospital survivors of ARDS and risk factor matched controls. (*Reproduced, with permission, from Davidson et al.[12]*)

severity of baseline COPD predicts mortality is relatively more important for long-term than short-term outcome.

LONG-TERM SURVIVAL IN THE ACUTE RESPIRATORY DISTRESS SYNDROME AND SEPSIS

Although many have reported the hospital mortality associated with ARDS, there has only been one study that specifically investigated the effects of ARDS on long-term survival compared with a control group. Davidson et al[12] conducted a prospective, matched parallel cohort study following 127 survivors of ARDS related to trauma or sepsis, and 127 control survivors with sepsis or trauma without ARDS. The control group was matched for severity of illness, using the Injury Severity Score for trauma patients and the APACHE III score for those with sepsis. The median follow-up period for both subjects and controls was approximately 2 years. This study found no difference in long-term mortality between the ARDS survivors and their matched controls (Fig. 70-3). Survival in both groups was correlated most significantly with risk factor, with a 3% late mortality in the trauma group compared to 22% in sepsis. Increased age and serious comorbidities in the sepsis patients were also associated with increased late mortality.

Many of the early sepsis studies focused on short-term mortality at 14 or 30 days from the onset of illness.[13] Two longer-term studies, however, suggest that there may be ongoing mortality for substantially longer than 30 days, which is directly related to the critical illness of sepsis and its complications.[14,15] These authors attempted to control for underlying comorbidities and their data suggests that the survival curve for patients with sepsis continues to separate from hospitalized controls without sepsis for over 1 year after hospital discharge. As recommended by the authors of these studies, interventional trials in sepsis are beginning to collect long-term outcomes for a more complete assessment of the effects of the intervention. The recent randomized controlled trial of recombinant human activated protein C (rhAPC; drotrecogin alfa) used 28-day mortality as a primary outcome measure, but also collected survival data

of subjects to 1 year and beyond.[16] While randomization to treatment with rhAPC was associated with increases in survival at 28 days and at hospital discharge, there was no statistically significant difference in survival at 3, 6, or 12 months after study enrollment.

LONG-TERM SURVIVAL OF CRITICALLY ILL ELDERLY PATIENTS

While there are many studies of the relation between age and survival to ICU and hospital discharge,[17–21] studies of differential long-term survival based on age are uncommon. Chelluri et al[22] reported long-term outcomes in critically ill patients aged 65 years and older, comparing those aged 75 years and older to those aged 65–74 years: 97 patients were studied, 54 aged 75 years or older and 43 aged 65–74 years. Hospital mortality and mortality at 1 year did not differ between the two groups (39 versus 40% and 63 versus 58%, respectively). Length of stay, hospital charges, and follow-up quality-of-life assessments were also the same between these groups. These authors concluded that age alone is not an adequate predictor of long-term survival and quality of life in critically ill elderly patients. Other studies have described poor long-term survival for elderly ICU survivors but did not include a comparison group of younger survivors to provide insight into the independent effect of age.[23]

Long-Term Follow-Up of Physiology and Pathology

Serial physiologic or radiologic studies in the months after acute respiratory failure may provide insight into the process and timing of lung repair. There is limited information available about serial pulmonary function studies, diagnostic imaging, and morphologic studies during recovery from acute respiratory failure treated with mechanical ventilation.

PULMONARY FUNCTION TESTING

Several studies have looked at the results of serial pulmonary function testing (PFT) after survival from acute respiratory failure associated with ARDS or COPD. Several studies of COPD patients have the advantage of having baseline PFTs before onset of respiratory failure, and show that, although recovery from mechanical ventilation is associated with an acute decrement of the forced expiratory volume in 1 second (FEV_1), most patients who survive the acute episode will return to their baseline pulmonary function.[8,9]

There have been two prospective studies of PFTs at multiple uniform time points after recovery from ARDS.[24,25] Unlike the studies in COPD, baseline PFTs were not available for survivors of ARDS, because most patients had no premorbid indication for testing. McHugh et al[24] enrolled 52 of 82 survivors of ARDS (63%), aiming to measure PFTs and self-perceived health scores at 2 weeks after extubation, and then again at 3, 6, and 12 months. The study showed that at extubation, forced vital capacity (FVC), total lung capacity (TLC), and diffusing capacity (D_LCO) were all markedly reduced. There was significant improvement in PFTs between extubation and 3 months. Function improved by a small additional amount by 6 months, at which point the FVC was still reduced in 55% of patients studied, the TLC was reduced in 45%, and the D_LCO was reduced in 79%. The degree of persisting impairment was mild in most patients. There was no additional improvement between 6 and 12 months. In a more recent study, Herridge et al[25] enrolled 109 ARDS survivors in a 12-month follow-up study that included PFTs. Of the 97 survivors at 12 months, 83 were evaluated (86% follow-up). Results were similar to those found by McHugh et al: patients had a mild restrictive defect and a moderate reduction in diffusion capacity at 3 months, with return of spirometry to the normal range in most patients by 6 months (median values were within 80% of predicted values) and continued improvement in D_LCO at between 6 and 12 months.

PATHOLOGY

The only studies providing information about the long-term effects of mechanical ventilation on lung histology in survivors of ARDS are case reports of four ARDS survivors. The scope and number of these investigations are quite limited, likely reflecting the invasive nature of obtaining tissue for evaluation. If these reports are generalizable, it appears that increased cellularity, organization, and fibroblast proliferation with fibrosis may be present early in the post-ARDS period and it normalizes over the first year of recovery.[26–28]

THORACIC IMAGING

There are few studies of the resolution of the radiographic changes coincident with acute respiratory failure in survivors of mechanical ventilation. These reports are limited to case series and prospective studies of patients recovering from ARDS. A review of 85 cases found that 19% of patients had persistent abnormalities on chest radiography at 3 or

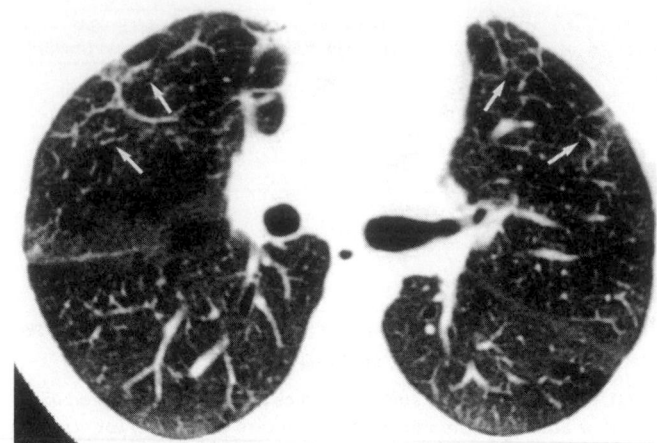

FIGURE 70-4 CT scan obtained in an 18-year-old survivor of ARDS. The image shows a limited extent of a reticular pattern, with associated distortion (*arrows*) of the anterior lung parenchyma. (*Reproduced, with permission, from Desai et al.[33]*)

more months after extubation; the most common findings were bibasilar interstitial infiltrates and reticular changes.[29] In a follow-up study by Herridge et al of over 100 ARDS survivors, 20% of patients had radiographic abnormalities at 1 year, with findings of linear fibrosis, small bullous cysts, and isolated areas of pleural thickening.[25,30]

There are a few small studies of the evolution of CT abnormalities in survivors of ARDS.[31–33] The largest study, by Desai et al, enrolled 27 patients with ARDS who had chest CTs in the acute phase.[33] Follow-up CTs were performed at nonuniform time points, ranging from 110 to 267 days after intubation.[33] Investigators looked for four types of parenchymal changes, and visually quantified involvement to determine extent. Ground-glass opacities were identified in all patients in the acute phase of ARDS, with a median extent of 68%. Intense parenchymal opacification was also seen in all 27 patients in the acute phase, largely in dependent regions with a median extent of 13%. On follow-up CTs, ground-glass opacities were seen in 17 of 27 patients but were not extensive (median extent of less than 1%). Of follow-up CTs, 23 of 27 demonstrated a coarse reticular pattern that distorted the underlying parenchyma, mainly in small anterior regions of the lung (Fig. 70-4). The other two studies had similar findings, noting that persistent radiographic abnormalities tended to be in the ventral distribution.[32]

SUMMARY

What have we learned from studies of diagnostic tests after recovery from acute respiratory failure and mechanical ventilation? Most patients with COPD who survive an episode of acute respiratory failure return to their baseline pulmonary function. For the most part, the abnormalities found in acute ARDS by PFTs and radiology improve over time and stabilize by 6 to 12 months. It is possible that the method of mechanical ventilation may have an impact on the timing and degree of lung repair, although no data are currently available to support this hypothesis. CT imaging may provide a sensitive and noninvasive surrogate for lung histology and may become a useful tool in the future studies of lung recovery after acute respiratory failure.

Patient-Centered Outcomes after Mechanical Ventilation

SYMPTOMS

Symptoms can be viewed as a patient-assessed outcome of import to patients and their families. There have been a few studies documenting significant symptom burden for critically ill patients while in the ICU,[34–36] but relatively few studies that explicitly examine the symptoms of survivors of critical illness. Studies of health status among survivors of critical illness incorporate the effect that these symptoms have on individual's lives. It may, however, also be important for investigators to explicitly examine the specific symptoms that are troubling to patients after a critical illness requiring mechanical ventilation as one way to understand the potential ways to decrease the symptom burden and the effect these symptoms have on patients' quality of life. For example, Angus et al[37] used the Quality of Well Being (QWB) questionnaire to assess the quality of life of 132 ARDS survivors. They found significant reductions in health status in the ARDS survivors and showed that the symptom domain of the QWB accounted for a larger decrement in quality of life than other domains including physical activity, social activity, and mobility. Symptoms accounted for about 70% of the reduction in health status seen in this study. The types of symptoms that were most bothersome included lower respiratory tract symptoms, but also depression and anxiety, constitutional symptoms, and cognitive symptoms (Table 70-1). In the follow-up study of 109 ARDS survivors, Herridge et al[25] also collected information on symptoms during standardized history and physical examinations. All subjects reported loss of muscle bulk, proximal weakness, and fatigue. Most had hair loss, with im-

TABLE 70-1 Proportion of ARDS Survivors with Persistent Symptoms at 6 and 12 Months

Symptom Groups	Symptoms at 6 Months (%)	Symptoms at 12 Months(%)
Musculoskeletal	69	71
Depression, anxiety, or insomnia	57	46
Constitutional	44	38
Neurologic	44	32
Lower respiratory	43	40
Cognitive	32	21
Upper respiratory	28	19
Auditory and dental	24	16
Gastrointestinal	21	23
Hoarseness/dysphonia	20	5
Dermatologic	15	25

Results from a follow-up study of 132 hospital survivors of ARDS.
SOURCE: Reproduced, with permission, from Angus et al.[37]

TABLE 70-2 Health-Related Quality of Life among ARDS Survivors and among Critically Ill Patients with Similar Severity of Illness but without ARDS

	ARDS Cases (n = 73) Mean (SD)	Matched Controls (n = 73) Mean (SD)	p Value
Physical functioning	62 (25)	84 (17)	<0.001
Role-physical	34 (34)	58 (32)	<0.001
Bodily pain	54 (25)	68 (20)	<0.001
General health	50 (20)	65 (19)	<0.001
Vitality	50 (19)	64 (14)	<0.001
Social functioning	61(27)	78 (18)	<0.001
Role-emotional	66 (40)	72 (36)	0.30
Mental health	64 (18)	75 (15)	<0.001

Results of Short Form 36 testing. Higher score indicates a better health-related quality of life.
SOURCE: Reproduced, with permission, from Davidson et al.[38]

provement by 6 months. Additionally, 10 subjects described persistent pain at chest tube insertion sites. These data provide some direction for investigators interested in decreasing the diverse symptom burden experienced by survivors of ARDS.

HEALTH-RELATED QUALITY OF LIFE AND HEALTH STATUS

There are an increasing number of studies that have examined the long-term effect of ARDS or other critical illnesses requiring mechanical ventilation on the quality of life and health status of survivors. McHugh et al, using the Sickness Impact Profile, demonstrated a significant decrement in health status among survivors of ARDS and showed that health status improved during the first 3 months after discharge from the hospital but remained relatively stable thereafter.[24] Davidson et al,[38] using the Medical Outcomes Study Short Form-36 (SF-36) and the St. George's Respiratory Questionnaire, showed that there were significant decrements in most domains of health status among survivors of ARDS and that these decrements were significantly worse for patients with ARDS compared to patients with a comparable severity of illness from sepsis or trauma, but who did not meet criteria for ARDS (Table 70-2). This study suggested decrements in physical function might be the most severe.

Similarly, in the largest and most complete follow-up study of ARDS survivors, Herridge et al found severe impairment in health status using the SF-36 at 3 months, with marked improvement at 6 months that continued to 1 year. Despite this improvement, at 1 year the median scores in all but one domain remained significantly reduced compared with age- and gender-matched controls.[25] Weinert et al studied 24 survivors of acute lung injury with the SF-36, also showing reductions in many domains of health status and particularly severe reductions in social functioning and mental health domains.[39] Finally, Angus et al used the Quality of Well Being to assess health status in a cohort of 200 previously healthy patients who developed ARDS and showed marked decrements in many domains of health status at 6 months and no significant change from 6 to 12 months.[37]

In addition to ARDS, studies have demonstrated reductions in health status for patients with other critical illnesses requiring prolonged mechanical ventilation, including sepsis,[40] multiple organ dysfunction,[41] and general ICU patients.[22,23,42] Although results vary, these studies also suggest decrements in a wide range of the domains of health status. Conversely, if intensive care and mechanical ventilation result from an elective surgical procedure, such as coronary artery bypass grafting,[43] spinal fusion,[44] or lung-volume reduction surgery,[45] survivors may experience significant long-term improvements in health-related quality of life.

PREDICTORS OF IMPAIRED QUALITY OF LIFE AND HEALTH STATUS

A number of studies have attempted to define the predictors of decreased health status among survivors of ARDS or other critical illness. Several studies suggest that the health status before admission to the ICU is a strong predictor of the health status after discharge.[46,47] A study by Wehler et al showed that patients with the best health status before critical illness were more likely to have reductions in their health status while those patients with the lowest health status prior to admission to an ICU were actually more likely to improve from their baseline health status.[46] Similarly, Konopad et al showed that among the very elderly, health status may actually increase from baseline after an ICU admission.[48] Severity of illness is also a significant predictor of health status after discharge from the ICU.[24,46,47] Increasing age predicts decreased health status after critical illness in some studies.[46,47] Other studies, however, did not find age to be an important independent predictor of health status[22] and suggest that even those over the age of 70, who receive more than 30 days of intensive care, are often satisfied with their health status and would choose to receive ICU care again if needed.[23] Schelling et al showed that pulmonary function impairment predicted worse health status, suggesting that treatment strategies designed to minimize lung injury may also improve health status in ARDS survivors.[49]

NEUROPSYCHOLOGICAL OUTCOMES

There has been increasing interest in examining the effect of critical illness, and especially ARDS, on the cognitive, emotional, and psychological functioning of survivors. There is mounting evidence suggesting that patients who survive critical illness may be left with decreased functioning in these realms.

COGNITIVE FUNCTION

In the landmark study published in 1999, Hopkins et al examined the cognitive function of 55 ARDS survivors.[50] At the time of hospital discharge, all 55 patients had significant impairment in cognitive and affective functioning. Patients improved over the first year of recovery, but 1 year after discharge from the hospital, 30% of patients still had generalized cognitive dysfunction and 78% had decrements in one or more of the following areas: attention, memory, concentration, and mental processing speed.[50] The authors attempted to identify predictors of cognitive impairment. They were limited, however, by their small sample size and by the collinearity of many of the important potential predictors, such as duration of mechanical ventilation, severity and duration of hypoxemia in the ICU, and duration and total dose of sedative medications used. Nonetheless, their analysis did show an association between the continuous oxygen saturation measurements and the severity of cognitive deficits.[50]

In a recently completed follow-up study,[51] Hopkins et al recruited 74 patients with ARDS who were enrolled in a randomized, controlled clinical trial of higher- versus lower-tidal-volume ventilator management.[52] Subjects were followed for 2 years with testing at uniform time points: hospital discharge, 1 year, and 2 years. As detected by a battery of tests chosen to interrogate multiple domains of cognitive function, 70% of subjects had neurocognitive impairment at hospital discharge. One year later, 45% of subjects still had impairment; there was no interval improvement between 1 and 2 years. The authors report that these subjects "found activities that require executive function, memory, attention or quick mental processing speed to be very difficult or impossible." This study again found a relationship between the duration of hypoxemia and cognitive impairment at hospital discharge, but this relationship was not significant at 1 or 2 years.

Another study assessed cognitive function in 46 survivors sometime between 1 and 12 years after ARDS (with a median of 6 years) and showed that 24% had mild or moderate cognitive impairment. This study suggested significant impact of this impairment on patients' lives by showing that 0 of 11 patients with cognitive impairment had returned to work, while 27 of 35 patients without cognitive impairment had returned to work.[53]

These three studies investigated only subjects with ARDS and therefore could not distinguish between the effects of ARDS on subsequent cognitive impairment and the effects of other aspects of critical illness and critical care therapies. A study of 6-month cognitive outcomes of medical ICU survivors found a similar degree of impairment as has been reported for ARDS patients.[54] One study compared neuropsychological outcomes in ARDS survivors with matched survivors of critical illness without ARDS and found that ARDS was independently associated with impaired cognitive function.[55] Although these studies are not definitive, they suggest that critical illness and mechanical ventilation may result in neurocognitive dysfunction in some patients and that ARDS is likely associated with increased risk for such dysfunction.

POSTTRAUMATIC STRESS DISORDER

Recognizing that critical illness can be a traumatic event, Schelling et al determined whether survivors of ARDS have an increased rate of symptoms of posttraumatic stress disorder (PTSD).[56] Using the previously validated PTSS-10 (Post Traumatic Stress Syndrome 10-Questions Inventory), they found that 28% of ARDS survivors had evidence of PTSD, significantly more than either hospital controls or United

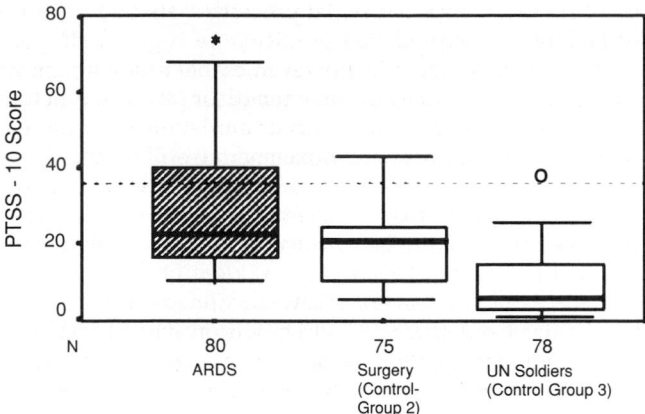

FIGURE 70-5 Comparison of scores of the German version of the Post Traumatic Stress Syndrome 10-Questions Inventory (PTSS-10) between patients with the acute respiratory distress syndrome (ARDS) and control groups 2 and 3. Hatched boxes indicate patients after the acute respiratory distress syndrome and open boxes indicate surgical patients and United Nations soldiers. The "whiskers" at the top and bottom of each box indicate the minimal and maximal values of the distribution, respectively. The top and bottom of each box indicate the 75th and 25th percentiles; the line through the box indicates the median (the 50th percentile). The dashed line indicates the PTSS-10 threshold for diagnosis of posttraumatic stress disorder (36 points). 0 indicates outliers. There was a significant difference of PTSS-10 scores in ARDS patients compared with all other groups (*p* <.001). (*Reproduced, with permission, from Schelling et al.[56]*)

Nations soldiers (Fig. 70-5). PTSD was associated with impaired health-related quality of life, and was highly correlated with the subjects' recollection of traumatic events from the ICU. The authors concluded "impairments in psychosocial function, including PTSD, occur in a subgroup of patients reporting adverse experiences during intensive care." The finding of high levels of PTSD in ARDS and general ICU survivors has been corroborated by subsequent investigations,[57–59] using the PTSS-10, the Impact of Events Scale, the *Diagnostic and Statistical Manual of Mental Disorders* (DSM-IV) diagnosis, and a novel measure, "The Experience after Treatment in Intensive Care 7 Item Scale."[59]

The results of the study by Schelling et al could lead one to hypothesize that memories of the ICU are detrimental, and critically ill patients would benefit from amnesia. This hypothesis is refuted by the study by Jones et al, which found that while delusional memories of intensive care were associated with symptoms of PTSD, factual memories appeared to be protective.[60] This study suggests that factual memories may allow ICU survivors to reject delusional memories and thereby decrease the symptoms of posttraumatic stress. It remains unclear, however, how to reduce delusional memories and increase recollection of factual experiences; additionally, it is unproven that interventions would translate into improved patient-centered outcomes.

We are not aware of any studies that investigated the effect of specific sedation protocols on memories after ICU discharge. In a small retrospective study, Nelson et al looked at the relationship between days and intensity of sedation use in patients with acute lung injury (ALI) and subsequent

PTSD and depression.[61] They found that duration of sedation was associated with an increase in the PTSD symptom score and an increase in depressive symptoms. These results are interesting but not conclusive, because the study design could not account for potential confounding by severity of illness. A randomized controlled trial of sedation protocols with patient follow-up and assessment of memories, PTSD, and health-related quality of life would be a more robust design with which to address this question.

In a follow-up study of subjects enrolled in the randomized controlled trial of daily sedative interruption,[62] Kress et al looked at the influence of sedation protocol on the long-term psychological outcomes of study survivors. While this is the optimal study design, they were limited by small numbers of subjects (18 subjects from the original study, and 14 additional "contemporaneous" patients who were not enrolled in the study).[63] Although memories from the ICU were not assessed, the investigators found that no subject managed with daily sedation interruption developed PTSD, compared with 32% of subjects managed without sedation interruption (*p* = 0.06). There was no difference in health-related quality of life, as assessed by the SF-36, between study groups. Again, these results are not conclusive, but suggest that using a protocol to limit sedation may reduce symptoms of PTSD.

EMOTIONAL OUTCOMES (ANXIETY AND DEPRESSION)

There are many reports of anxiety and depression in survivors of critical illness and mechanical ventilation.[25,37,39,50,51,64] These reports differ in the patient populations studied, the instruments used to assess emotional outcomes, and the timing of patient assessment. Using the CES-D (a self-report depression scale), Weinert et al found in a cross-sectional study that depression is very common in ARDS survivors in the first 15 months of recovery: 73% of patients had scores consistent with depression.[39] After 15 months, 25% of patients scored in the depressive range. In two studies that used the Beck Depression Inventory and the Beck Anxiety Index at 1 year after ARDS, Hopkins et al found that while patients reported some depressive symptoms, most did not report clinical levels of anxiety or depression.[50,51] Two years after ARDS, however, 23% of patients still had evidence of moderate-to-severe anxiety or depression. Investigators have also used the Hospital Anxiety and Depression (HAD) scale. One investigation using the HAD to study survivors of general ICU care reported significant depression in 43% of the 80 respondents, and significant anxiety in 30%.[57] These studies suggest that both anxiety and depression are common, but no study has yet definitively shown risk factors or demonstrated improved emotional outcomes after intervention.

IMPROVING NEUROPSYCHOLOGICAL OUTCOMES

Interventional studies designed to improve neuropsychological outcomes after mechanical ventilation are uncommon. In an interesting preliminary study, Schelling et al performed a small retrospective case-control study comparing patients who received corticosteroids for treatment of septic shock to similar patients who did not receive corticosteroids.[65] These authors found that the patients who received corticosteroids had a lower incidence of PTSD (5 of 27 compared to 16 of 27; $p = 0.002$) and higher scores on the mental health index of the SF-36. Although most of these studies are limited by small numbers and observational designs, they provide intriguing preliminary data to suggest that the way patients are managed in the ICU may have important effects on their long-term mental health and cognitive function. There is one published randomized controlled trial designed to evaluate the effectiveness of a self-help rehabilitation manual in improving physical and emotional outcomes in survivors of critical illness.[66] Remarkably, this simple intervention significantly improved subjects' physical function scores and tended to cause a decrease in depression (12% in the intervention group compared with 25% of controls). Further studies are needed to attempt to identify the components of long-term mechanical ventilation or critical illness that predispose patients to neuropsychological deficits. Efforts are needed to tease apart the potential causes, which include desaturation or decreased cerebral perfusion pressure during critical illness, inflammation and bio-trauma of sepsis and ARDS, duration and amount of sedation, and traumatic experiences during ICU stay. Because increasing severity of illness will portend increases in many of these variables, differentiating between the collinear potential causes will be challenging. Furthermore, randomized controlled trials of different mechanical ventilation and sedation strategies should also examine the potential effects on these neuropsychological outcomes.

NEUROMUSCULAR FUNCTION AFTER CRITICAL ILLNESS

Although pulmonary function normalizes in most survivors of ARDS, health-related quality of life remains markedly abnormal for years after recovery from critical illness.[24,25,64] These patients are more likely to describe symptoms of weakness and fatigue[25,37] than any other, and the most affected domains of general quality of life measures are those of strength and physical function. To measure overall physical function in ARDS survivors, Herridge et al had all subjects perform the six-minute walk test (a validated measure of physical function that measures distance walked in 6 minutes[25]) at 3, 6, and 12 months. Most patients demonstrated impairment that was severe at 3 months and improved over time. Even at 12 months, however, the majority of subjects remained impaired, with a median distance walked of 66% of predicted.

There are no other published studies that report results of long-term follow-up testing of strength or physical function of general survivors of mechanical ventilation. The etiology of this post-ICU functional impairment is still unknown, as is the role of ARDS as a specific risk factor. Insight, however, can be gained from a recent prospective study of consecutive patients who underwent mechanical ventilation for seven or more days. De Jonghe et al identified 25% of these patients as having severe muscle weakness, as measured by standardized clinical examination on day 7.[68] Electrophysiologic and pathologic testing of a subset with ICU-acquired paresis revealed both neuropathy and myopathy. A recent report identified clinical weakness in over one-third of COPD patients who required mechanical ventilation for exacerbations.[69] Using combinations of clinical, electrophysiologic, and pathologic assessment of all subjects, other studies have shown critical illness–related polyneuropathy or myopathy to be present in 33–100% of ICU patients receiving mechanical ventilation for 1 week or more.[70–77]

There have been no prospective, systematic follow-up studies in patients with critical illness–related polyneuropathy or myopathy; the timing of recovery and the prevalence of long-term sequelae remain unknown. It is likely that ICU-acquired damage to muscles and nerves is a significant contributor to impairments in function and quality of life. Interventions that decrease muscle and nerve damage, such as tight serum glucose control with intensive insulin therapy,[77] will likely improve long-term physical function, although this has not yet been shown (Table 70-3). Ongoing and future studies are needed to describe this epidemiology and test interventions to improve physical function after critical illness.

RETURN TO WORK

For young survivors of critical illness, the ability to return to work is an important outcome. This is particularly salient for survivors of ARDS, who tend to be under age 50 (median age 39 in the study of Davidson et al, and 45 years of age in the study of Herridge et al[25]), compared with a median age over 65 years among COPD survivors (mean age 66 in the study of Seneff et al,[11] and median age of 70 in the study of Connors et al[10]). Few follow-up studies have investigated return to work in ARDS survivors. At 1 year after hospital discharge,

---

TABLE 70-3 Effect of Intensive Insulin Therapy in Critically Ill Patients on Critical Illness Neuropathy and Myopathy: Electromyographic (EMG) Evidence in Subjects Requiring Seven or More Days of Intensive Care

	Conventional Treatment (n = 206)[a]	Intensive Treatment (n = 157)[a]	p Value
EMG-positive at least once[b]	51.9%	28.7%	<0.001
EMG-positive at least thrice[b]	18.9%	7.0%	<0.001

[a]Intensive insulin therapy was associated with reduced duration of mechanical ventilation.
[b]Electromyography performed once weekly for all patients remaining in the ICU, starting on ICU day 7.
SOURCE: Reproduced, with permission, from van den Berghe et al.[78]

McHugh et al found that only 44% of subjects had returned to work.[24] The results of Herridge et al were similar: at 1 year, 49% of survivors had returned to work, most to their original positions.[25] The reasons that were reported for not returning to previous employment included weakness and fatigue, and difficulty walking secondary to large joint immobility (heterotopic ossification) and foot-drop. Rothenhausler et al showed that decreased cognitive function was an important predictor of inability to return to work after recovery from acute respiratory failure.[53]

Long-Term Outcomes of Informal Caregivers

The effects of surviving critical illness do not end with ICU or hospital discharge, nor do the effects end with the patient. There is a growing body of literature that describes the short- and long-term effects of surviving critical illness on patients' families and informal caregivers. Most patients who receive mechanical ventilation in the ICU will continue to need informal caregiving (care provided by those who are not health care providers, usually family or spouse) for months after hospital or post–hospital institution discharge.[78] Caregivers may have deterioration of their own general health, particularly those with pre-existing health problems. Many caregivers must reduce work hours or quit jobs in response to the burden of caregiving, often leading to economic difficulties.[78,79]

The emotional and psychological toll of caring for ICU survivors is considerable. Significant levels of anxiety have been reported in 49–62% of caregivers of medical and surgical ICU survivors, persisting at least to 6 months after hospital discharge.[78,80–82] Depression is seen in 20–34% of these caregivers. Posttraumatic stress symptoms are also common among caregivers. A recent multi-center study evaluated 284 caregivers 90 days after their family member's death or ICU discharge.[80] Symptoms consistent with PTSD were found in 33% of caregivers; significantly more caregivers were at risk for PTSD if they participated in end-of-life decision making and if their family member died. Of caregivers who participated in end-of-life decision making, over 80% had symptoms of PTSD. Written information providing education concerning recovery from the ICU has been effective in reducing caregiver anxiety for patients with simple myocardial infarctions.[83] There has been one randomized controlled trial of similar written educational information for caregivers of ICU patients; this intervention had no effect on rates of anxiety, depression, or posttraumatic stress symptoms of the caregivers at 6 months after hospital discharge.[82]

Conclusions

Most of the available data of long-term outcomes after mechanical ventilation deal with the survivors of ALI/ARDS. Long-term survival for these patients appears to be related more to the underlying risk condition (sepsis versus trauma)

than to occurrence of acute lung injury. Similarly, the long-term survival in patients with COPD and cardiogenic pulmonary edema, once they have survived to hospital discharge, is more related to the severity of the underlying condition than to the episode of acute respiratory failure itself.

In the last 10 years, there has been an increasing amount of research regarding long-term patient-centered outcomes. Studies have shown that a significant proportion of survivors of ARDS survive with an impairment in their quality of life and health status. Lung function shows substantial return toward normal in most patients; impairment, when present, is typically mild to moderate and does not to appear to explain the reduced quality of life. Recent studies point to neuromuscular, neurocognitive, and psychological abnormalities, which persist at 1 year, as being the sequelae that are most troublesome to survivors.

It is difficult to identify the causative agent for the long-term sequelae in survivors of critical illness who have received mechanical ventilation. It is likely that many long-term complications after hospital discharge are caused by either the underlying disease process that led to respiratory failure or by the severity of illness and multiple organ dysfunction syndrome present in many critically ill patients. There are also many ways in which ICU management, including the method of ventilation and the sedatives and analgesics used, may affect long-term outcomes. For example, in addition to increasing hospital mortality, failure to use low tidal volumes may affect lung injury and the degree of successful repair. It is also conceivable that the sustained systemic inflammation from injurious ventilation may affect end-organ function in the long-term as well as short-term, including central nervous system and neuromuscular function.

Studies are needed to link the acute events occurring during the period of critical illness with the longer-term sequelae in order to identify modifiable factors and allow strategies that will prevent or minimize these burdensome residua of critical illness. In the meantime, critical care clinicians should look for ways to minimize complications and interventions in mechanically ventilated patients that may be associated with long-term effects on neuromuscular and neurocognitive, as well as pulmonary, functioning of these patients.

References

1. Angus DC, Black N. Improving care of the critically ill: institutional and health-care system approaches. Lancet 2004; 363:1314–20.
2. Jacobs CJ, van der Vliet JA, van Roozendaal MT, van der Linden CJ. Mortality and quality of life after intensive care for critical illness. Intensive Care Med 1988; 14:217–20.
3. Keenan SP, Dodek P, Chan K, et al. Intensive care unit admission has minimal impact on long-term mortality. Crit Care Med 2002; 30:501–7.
4. Niskanen M, Kari A, Halonen P. Five-year survival after intensive care—comparison of 12,180 patients with the general population. Finnish ICU Study Group. Crit Care Med 1996; 24:1962–7.

5. Ridley S, Plenderleith L. Survival after intensive care. Comparison with a matched normal population as an indicator of effectiveness. Anaesthesia 1994; 49:933–5.

6. Wiener RS, Moses HW, Richeson JF, Gatewood RP Jr. Hospital and long-term survival of patients with acute pulmonary edema associated with coronary artery disease. Am J Cardiol 1987; 60:33–5.

7. Adnet F, Le Toumelin P, Leberre A, et al. In-hospital and long-term prognosis of elderly patients requiring endotracheal intubation for life-threatening presentation of cardiogenic pulmonary edema. Crit Care Med 2001; 29:891–5.

8. Gottlieb LS, Balchum OJ. Course of chronic obstructive pulmonary disease following first onset of respiratory failure. Chest 1973; 63:5–8.

9. Martin TR, Lewis SW, Albert RK. The prognosis of patients with chronic obstructive pulmonary disease after hospitalization for acute respiratory failure. Chest 1982; 82:310–4.

10. Connors AF Jr, Dawson NV, Thomas C, et al. Outcomes following acute exacerbation of severe chronic obstructive lung disease. The SUPPORT investigators (Study to Understand Prognoses and Preferences for Outcomes and Risks of Treatments). Am J Respir Crit Care Med 1996; 154(4 Pt 1):959–67.

11. Seneff MG, Wagner DP, Wagner RP, Zimmerman JE, Knaus WA. Hospital and 1-year survival of patients admitted to intensive care units with acute exacerbation of chronic obstructive pulmonary disease. JAMA 1995; 274:1852–7.

12. Davidson TA, Rubenfeld GD, Caldwell ES, Hudson LD, Steinberg KP. The effect of acute respiratory distress syndrome on long-term survival. Am J Respir Crit Care Med 1999; 160:1838–42.

13. Bone RC, Fisher CJ Jr, Clemmer TP, et al. A controlled clinical trial of high-dose methylprednisolone in the treatment of severe sepsis and septic shock. N Engl J Med 1987; 317:653–8.

14. Sasse KC, Nauenberg E, Long A, et al. Long-term survival after intensive care unit admission with sepsis. Crit Care Med 1995; 23:1040–7.

15. Quartin AA, Schein RM, Kett DH, Peduzzi PN. Magnitude and duration of the effect of sepsis on survival. Department of Veterans Affairs Systemic Sepsis Cooperative Studies Group. JAMA 1997; 277:1058–63.

16. Angus DC, Laterre PF, Helterbrand J, et al. The effect of drotrecogin alfa (activated) on long-term survival after severe sepsis. Crit Care Med 2004; 32:2199–206.

17. Ely EW, Wheeler AP, Thompson BT, et al. Recovery rate and prognosis in older persons who develop acute lung injury and the acute respiratory distress syndrome. Ann Intern Med 2002; 136:25–36.

18. Angus DC, Linde-Zwirble WT, Lidicker J, et al. Epidemiology of severe sepsis in the United States: analysis of incidence, outcome, and associated costs of care. Crit Care Med 2001; 29:1303–10.

19. Ely EW, Angus DC, Williams MD, et al. Drotrecogin alfa (activated) treatment of older patients with severe sepsis. Clin Infect Dis 2003; 37:187–95.

20. Esteban A, Anzueto A, Frutos F, et al. Characteristics and outcomes in adult patients receiving mechanical ventilation: a 28-day international study. JAMA 2002; 287:345–55.

21. Chelluri L, Pinsky MR, Grenvik AN. Outcome of intensive care of the "oldest-old" critically ill patients. Crit Care Med 1992; 20:757–61.

22. Chelluri L, Grenvik A, Silverman M. Intensive care for critically ill elderly: mortality, costs, and quality of life. Review of the literature. Arch Intern Med 1995; 155:1013–22.

23. Montuclard L, Garrouste-Orgeas M, Timsit JF, et al. Outcome, functional autonomy, and quality of life of elderly patients with a long-term intensive care unit stay. Crit Care Med 2000; 28:3389–95.

24. McHugh LG, Milberg JA, Whitcomb ME, et al. Recovery of function in survivors of the acute respiratory distress syndrome. Am J Respir Crit Care Med 1994; 150:90–4.

25. Herridge MS, Cheung AM, Tansey CM, et al. One-year outcomes in survivors of the acute respiratory distress syndrome. N Engl J Med 2003; 348:683–93.

26. Alberts WM, Priest GR, Moser KM. The outlook for survivors of ARDS. Chest 1983; 84:272–4.

27. Lakshminarayan S, Stanford RE, Petty TL. Prognosis after recovery from adult respiratory distress syndrome. Am Rev Respir Dis 1976; 113:7–16.

28. Mittermayer C, Hassenstein J, Riede UN. Is shock-induced lung fibrosis reversible? A report on recovery from "shock-lung". Pathol Res Pract 1978; 162:73–87.

29. Lee CM, Hudson LD. Long-term outcomes after ARDS. Semin Respir Crit Care Med 2001; 22:327–36.

30. Herridge MS, Cheung AM, Tansey CM, et al. One year outcomes in survivors of the acute respiratory distress syndrome. N Engl J Med 2003; 348:683–93.

31. Owens CM, Evans TW, Keogh BF, Hansell DM. Computed tomography in established adult respiratory distress syndrome. Correlation with lung injury score. Chest 1994; 106:1815–21.

32. Nobauer-Huhmann IM, Eibenberger K, Schaefer-Prokop C, et al. Changes in lung parenchyma after acute respiratory distress syndrome (ARDS): assessment with high-resolution computed tomography. Eur Radiol 2001; 11:2436–43.

33. Desai SR, Wells AU, Rubens MB, Evans TW, Hansell DM. Acute respiratory distress syndrome: CT abnormalities at long-term follow-up. Radiology 1999; 210:29–35.

34. Nelson JE, Meier DE, Oei EJ, et al. Self-reported symptom experience of critically ill cancer patients receiving intensive care. Crit Care Med 2001; 29:277–82.

35. Puntillo KA. Pain experience of intensive care unit patients. Heart Lung 1990; 19:525–33.

36. A controlled trial to improve care for seriously ill hospitalized patients. The study to understand prognoses and preferences for outcomes and risks of treatments (SUPPORT). The SUPPORT Principal Investigators. JAMA 1995; 274:1591–8.

37. Angus DC, Musthafa AA, Clermont G, et al. Quality-adjusted survival in the first year after the acute respiratory distress syndrome. Am J Respir Crit Care Med 2001; 163:1389–94.

38. Davidson TA, Caldwell ES, Curtis JR, Hudson LD, Steinberg KP. Reduced quality of life in survivors of acute respiratory distress syndrome compared with critically ill control patients. JAMA 1999; 281:354–60.

39. Weinert CR, Gross CR, Kangas JR, Bury CL, Marinelli WA. Health-related quality of life after acute lung injury. Am J Respir Crit Care Med 1997; 156(4 Pt 1):1120–8.

40. Heyland DK, Hopman W, Coo H, Tranmer J, McColl MA. Long-term health-related quality of life in survivors of sepsis. Short Form 36: a valid and reliable measure of health-related quality of life. Crit Care Med 2000; 28:3599–605.

41. Pettila V, Kaarlola A, Makelainen A. Health-related quality of life of multiple organ dysfunction patients one year after intensive care. Intensive Care Med 2000; 26:1473–9.

42. Roche VM, Kramer A, Hester E, Welsh CH. Long-term functional outcome after intensive care. J Am Geriatr Soc 1999; 47:18–24.

43. Rumsfeld JS, Magid DJ, O'Brien M, et al. Changes in health-related quality of life following coronary artery bypass graft surgery. Ann Thorac Surg 2001; 72:2026–32.

44. Sasso RC, Kitchel SH, Dawson EG. A prospective, randomized controlled clinical trial of anterior lumbar interbody fusion using a titanium cylindrical threaded fusion device. Spine 2004; 29:113–22; discussion 21–2.

45. Fishman A, Martinez F, Naunheim K, et al. A randomized trial comparing lung-volume-reduction surgery with medical therapy for severe emphysema. N Engl J Med 2003; 348:2059–73.

46. Wehler M, Martus P, Geise A, et al. Changes in quality of life after medical intensive care. Intensive Care Med 2001; 27:154–9.

47. Mata GV, Fernandez RR, Carmona AG. Factors related to quality of life 12 months after discharge from an intensive care unit. Crit Care Med 1992; 20:1257–62.

48. Konopad E, Noseworthy TW, Johnston R, Shustack A, Grace M. Quality of life measures before and one year after admission to an intensive care unit. Crit Care Med 1995; 23:1653–9.

49. Schelling G, Stoll C, Vogelmeier C, et al. Pulmonary function and health-related quality of life in a sample of long-term survivors of the acute respiratory distress syndrome. Intensive Care Med 2000; 26:1304–11.

50. Hopkins RO, Weaver LK, Pope D, et al. Neuropsychological sequelae and impaired health status in survivors of severe acute respiratory distress syndrome. Am J Respir Crit Care Med 1999; 160:50–6.

51. Hopkins RO, Weaver LK, Collingridge D, et al. Two year cognitive, emotional and quality of life outcomes in acute respiratory distress syndrome. Am J Respir Crit Care Med 2005; 171: 340–7.

52. Ventilation with lower tidal volumes as compared with traditional tidal volumes for acute lung injury and the acute respiratory distress syndrome. The Acute Respiratory Distress Syndrome Network. N Engl J Med 2000; 342:1301–8.

53. Rothenhausler HB, Ehrentraut S, Stoll C, Schelling G, Kapfhammer HP. The relationship between cognitive performance and employment and health status in long-term survivors of the acute respiratory distress syndrome: results of an exploratory study. Gen Hosp Psychiatry 2001; 23:90–6.

54. Jackson JC, Hart RP, Gordon SM, et al. Six-month neuropsychological outcome of medical intensive care unit patients. Crit Care Med 2003; 31:1226–34.

55. Marquis KA, Curtis JR, Caldwell E, et al. Neuropsychological sequelae in survivors of ARDS compared with critically ill control patients. Am J Respir Crit Care Med 2000; 161:A383.

56. Schelling G, Stoll C, Haller M, et al. Health-related quality of life and posttraumatic stress disorder in survivors of the acute respiratory distress syndrome. Crit Care Med 1998; 26:651–9.

57. Scragg P, Jones A, Fauvel N. Psychological problems following ICU treatment. Anaesthesia 2001; 56:9–14.

58. Cuthbertson BH, Hull A, Strachan M, Scott J. Post-traumatic stress disorder after critical illness requiring general intensive care. Intensive Care Med 2004; 30:450–5.

59. Kapfhammer HP, Rothenhausler HB, Krauseneck T, Stoll C, Schelling G. Posttraumatic stress disorder and health-related quality of life in long-term survivors of acute respiratory distress syndrome. Am J Psychiatry 2004; 161:45–52.

60. Jones C, Griffiths RD, Humphris G, Skirrow PM. Memory, delusions, and the development of acute posttraumatic stress disorder-related symptoms after intensive care. Crit Care Med 2001; 29:573–80.

61. Nelson BJ, Weinert CR, Bury CL, Marinelli WA, Gross CR. Intensive care unit drug use and subsequent quality of life in acute lung injury patients. Crit Care Med 2000; 28:3626–30.

62. Kress JP, Pohlman AS, O'Connor MF, Hall JB. Daily interruption of sedative infusions in critically ill patients undergoing mechanical ventilation. N Engl J Med 2000; 342:1471–7.

63. Kress JP, Gehlbach B, Lacy M, et al. The long-term psychological effects of daily sedative interruption on critically ill patients. Am J Respir Crit Care Med 2003; 168:1457–61.

64. Orme J Jr, Romney JS, Hopkins RO, et al. Pulmonary function and health-related quality of life in survivors of acute respiratory distress syndrome. Am J Respir Crit Care Med 2003; 167:690–4.

65. Schelling G, Stoll C, Kapfhammer HP, et al. The effect of stress doses of hydrocortisone during septic shock on posttraumatic stress disorder and health-related quality of life in survivors. Crit Care Med 1999; 27:2678–83.

66. Jones C, Skirrow P, Griffiths RD, et al. Rehabilitation after critical illness: a randomized, controlled trial. Crit Care Med 2003; 31:2456–61.

67. Weisman IM, Zeballos RJ. Clinical exercise testing. Clin Chest Med 2001; 22:679–701, viii.

68. De Jonghe B, Sharshar T, Lefaucheur JP, et al. Paresis acquired in the intensive care unit: a prospective multicenter study. JAMA 2002; 288:2859–67.

69. Amaya-Villar R, Garnacho-Montero J, Garcia-Garmendia JL, et al. Steroid-induced myopathy in patients intubated due to exacerbation of chronic obstructive pulmonary disease. Intensive Care Med 2005; 31:157–61.

70. Deem S, Lee CM, Curtis JR. Acquired neuromuscular disorders in the intensive care unit. Am J Respir Crit Care Med 2003; 168: 735–9.

71. Coakley JH, Nagendran K, Honavar M, Hinds CJ. Preliminary observations on the neuromuscular abnormalities in patients with organ failure and sepsis. Intensive Care Med 1993; 19:323–8.

72. de Letter MA, Schmitz PI, Visser LH, et al. Risk factors for the development of polyneuropathy and myopathy in critically ill patients. Crit Care Med 2001; 29:2281–6.

73. Witt NJ, Zochodne DW, Bolton CF, et al. Peripheral nerve function in sepsis and multiple organ failure. Chest 1991; 99:176–84.

74. Helliwell TR, Coakley JH, Wagenmakers AJ, et al. Necrotizing myopathy in critically-ill patients. J Pathol 1991; 164:307–14.

75. Douglass JA, Tuxen DV, Horne M, et al. Myopathy in severe asthma. Am Rev Respir Dis 1992; 146:517–9.

76. Tennila A, Salmi T, Pettila V, et al. Early signs of critical illness polyneuropathy in ICU patients with systemic inflammatory response syndrome or sepsis. Intensive Care Med 2000; 26:1360–3.

77. van den Berghe G, Wouters P, Weekers F, et al. Intensive insulin therapy in the critically ill patients. N Engl J Med 2001; 345: 1359–67.

78. Im K, Belle SH, Schulz R, Mendelsohn AB, Chelluri L. Prevalence and outcomes of caregiving after prolonged (≥48 hours) mechanical ventilation in the ICU. Chest 2004; 125:597–606.

79. Covinsky KE, Goldman L, Cook EF, et al. The impact of serious illness on patients' families. SUPPORT Investigators. Study to Understand Prognoses and Preferences for Outcomes and Risks of Treatment. JAMA 1994; 272:1839–44.

80. Azoulay E, Pochard F, Kentish-Barnes N, et al. Risk of post-traumatic stress symptoms in family members of intensive care unit patients. Am J Respir Crit Care Med 2005; 171:987–94.

81. Young E, Eddleston J, Ingleby S, et al. Returning home after intensive care: A comparison of symptoms of anxiety and depression in ICU and elective cardiac surgery patients and their relatives. Intensive Care Med 2005; 31:86–91.

82. Jones C, Skirrow P, Griffiths RD, et al. Post-traumatic stress disorder-related symptoms in relatives of patients following intensive care. Intensive Care Med 2004; 30:456–60.

83. Hentinen M. Need for instruction and support of the wives of patients with myocardial infarction. J Adv Nurs 1983;8:519–24.

INDEX

The letter *f* or *t* following a page number indicates that either a figure or a table is being referenced.